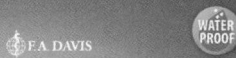
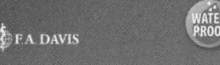

DAVIS'S
DRUG GUIDE AT A GLANCE

BEERS **REMS**

Ⓧ **cloZAPine** (kloe-za-peen)
Clozaril, ~~FazaClo~~, Versacloz
Classification
Therapeutic: antipsychotics

Risk Evaluation and Mitigation Systems (REMS) Icon

Tab for the AGS Beers Criteria for Potentially Inappropriate Medication Use in Older Adults

---

RED tab for High Alert medications

BEERS HIGH ALERT

Ⓧ **warfarin** (war-fa-rin)
~~Coumadin~~, Jantoven
Classification
Therapeutic: anticoagulants
Pharmacologic: coumarins

Icon for pharmacogenomic content

Indications
Prophylaxis and treatment of: Venous thrombosis, Pulmonary embolism, Atrial fibrillation with embolization. Management of MI. Prevention of thrombus formation and embolization after prosthetic valve placement.

Action
Interferes with hepatic synthesis of vitamin K-dependent clotting factors (II, VII, IX, and X). **Therapeutic Effects:** Prevention of thromboembolic events.

Life-threatening side effects in RED, CAPITALIZED letters

Pharmacokinetics
Absorption: Well absorbed from the GI tract after oral administration.
Distribution: Minimally distributed to tissues.
Protein Binding: 99%.
Metabolism and Excretion: Primarily metabolized by the liver via the CYP2C9 isoenzyme, with some metabolism via the CYP3A4 isoenzyme; Ⓧ the CYP2C9 isoenzyme exhibits genetic polymorphism (intermediate or poor metabolizers may have significantly ↑ (S)-warfarin concentrations and an ↑ risk of adverse reactions).
Half-life: 42 hr.

Drug-drug, drug-food, and drug-natural product interactions

TIME/ACTION PROFILE (effects on coagulation tests)

ROUTE	ONSET	PEAK	DURATION
PO	36–72 hr	5–7 days†	2–5 days‡

†At a constant dose
‡After discontinuation

Headings highlighting considerations for patient populations
- Geri—concerns for older adults
- OB and Lact—information for pregnant and breastfeeding patients
- Pedi—concerns for children
- Rep—considerations for patients of reproductive age

Contraindications/Precautions
Contraindicated in: Uncontrolled bleeding; Open wounds; Active ulcer disease; Recent brain, eye, or spinal cord injury or surgery; Severe hepatic impairment; Uncontrolled hypertension; OB: Pregnancy.
Use Cautiously in: Malignancy; History of ulcer, liver disease, or acute kidney injury; History of poor compliance; Ⓧ Asian patients or those who carry the CYP2C9*2 allele and/or CYP2C9*3 allele, or with the VKORC1 AA genotype (↑ risk of bleeding with standard dosing; lower initial doses should be considered); Rep: Women of reproductive potential; Pedi: Has been used safely in children, but may require more frequent PT/INR assessments; Geri: Appears on Beers list. ↑ risk of major bleeding when compared with direct acting oral anticoagulants (DOACs) in older adults. Avoid starting as initial therapy for treatment of nonvalvular atrial fibrillation or venous thromboembolism unless alternative

options (DOACs) are contraindicated or there are significant barriers to their use. If already using warfarin, it may be reasonable to continue treatment, especially if INR is well controlled (i.e., >70% time in therapeutic range) and no adverse effects.

Adverse Reactions/Side Effects
Derm: dermal necrosis. **GI:** cramps, nausea. **GU:** CALCIPHYLAXIS. **Hemat:** BLEEDING. **Misc:** fever.

Interactions
Drug-Drug: Androgens, capecitabine, cefotetan, chloramphenicol, clopidogrel, disulfiram, fluconazole, fluoroquinolones, itraconazole, metronidazole (including vaginal use), thrombolytics, eptifibatide, tirofiban, sulfonamides, quinidine, quinine, NSAIDs, valproates, and aspirin may ↑ the response to warfarin and ↑ the risk of bleeding. Chronic use of acetaminophen may ↑ the risk of bleeding. Chronic alcohol ingestion may ↓ action of warfarin; if chronic alcohol abuse results in significant liver damage, action of warfarin may be ↑ due to ↓ production of clotting factor. Acute alcohol ingestion may ↑ action of warfarin. Barbiturates, carbamazepine, rifampin, and hormonal contraceptives containing estrogen may ↓ the anticoagulant response to warfarin. Many other drugs may affect the activity of warfarin.
Drug-Natural Products: St. John's wort ↓ effect. ↑ bleeding risk with anise, arnica, chamomile, clove, dong quai, fenugreek, feverfew, garlic, ginger, ginkgo, Panax ginseng, licorice, and others.
Drug-Food: Ingestion of large quantities of foods high in vitamin K content (see list in Appendix J) may antagonize the anticoagulant effect of warfarin.

Route/Dosage
Ⓧ **PO (Adults):** 2–5 mg/day for 2–4 days; then adjust daily dose by results of INR. Initiate therapy with lower doses in older adults or in Asian patients or those with CYP2C9*2 and/or CYP2C9*3 alleles or VKORC1 AA genotype.
PO (Children >1 mo): *Initial loading dose:* 0.2 mg/kg (maximum dose: 10 mg) for 2–4 days then adjust daily dose by results of INR, use 0.1 mg/kg if hepatic impairment is present. *Maintenance dose range:* 0.05–0.34 mg/kg/day.

Availability (generic available)
Tablets: 1 mg, 2 mg, 2.5 mg, 3 mg, 4 mg, 5 mg, 6 mg, 7.5 mg, 10 mg.

NURSING IMPLICATIONS
Assessment
- Assess for signs of bleeding and hemorrhage (bleeding gums; nosebleed; unusual bruising; tarry, black stools; hematuria; fall in hematocrit or BP; guaiac-positive stools, urine, or nasogastric aspirate).

🍁 = Canadian drug name. Ⓧ = Genetic implication. ~~Strikethrough~~ = Discontinued. CAPITALS = life-threatening. <u>Underline</u> = most frequent.

NURSING IMPLICATIONS
Assessment
- Assess for signs of bleeding and hemorrhage (bleeding gums; nosebleed; unusual bruising; tarry, black stools; hematuria; fall in hematocrit or BP; guaiac-positive stools, urine, or nasogastric aspirate).

Clearly defined nursing responsibilities and priorities

1290   warfarin

- Assess for evidence of additional or increased thrombosis. Symptoms depend on area of involvement.

Lab Test Considerations
- Monitor PT, INR, and other clotting factors frequently during therapy; monitor more frequently in patients with renal impairment. Therapeutic PT ranges 1.3–1.5 times greater than control; however, the INR, a standardized system that provides a common basis for communicating and interpreting PT results, is usually referenced. Normal INR (not on anticoagulants) is 0.8–1.2. An INR of 2.5–3.5 is recommended for patients at very high risk of embolization (for example, patients with mitral valve replacement and ventricular hypertrophy). Lower levels are acceptable when risk is lower. Heparin may affect the PT/INR; draw blood for PT/INR in patients receiving both heparin and warfarin at least 5 hr after the IV bolus dose, 4 hr after cessation of IV infusion, or 24 hr after SUBQ heparin injection. ⌘ Asian patients and those who carry the CYP2C9*2 allele and/or the CYP2C9*3 allele, or those with VKORC1 AA genotype may require more frequent monitoring and lower doses.
- Geri: Patients over 60 yr exhibit greater than expected PT/INR response. Monitor for side effects at lower therapeutic ranges.
- Pedi: Achieving and maintaining therapeutic PT/INR ranges may be more difficult in pediatric patients. Assess PT/INR levels more frequently.
- Monitor hepatic function and CBC before and periodically throughout therapy.
- Monitor stool and urine for occult blood before and periodically during therapy.

Toxicity and Overdose
- Withholding 1 or more doses of warfarin is usually sufficient if INR is excessively elevated or if minor bleeding occurs. If overdose occurs or anticoagulation needs to be immediately reversed, the antidote is vitamin K (phytonadione). Administration of whole blood or plasma also may be required in severe bleeding because of the delayed onset of vitamin K.

Implementation
- **High Alert:** Do not confuse Jantoven with Janumet or Januvia.
- Because of the large number of medications capable of significantly altering warfarin's effects, careful monitoring is recommended when new agents are started or other agents are discontinued. Interactive potential should be evaluated for all new medications (Rx, OTC, and herbal products).
- **PO:** Administer medication at same time each day. Medication requires 3–5 days to reach effective levels; usually begun while patient is still on heparin.

- Do not interchange brands; potencies may not be equivalent.

Patient/Family Teaching

In-depth guidance for patient and family education

- Instruct patient to take medication as directed. Take missed doses as soon as remembered that day; do not double doses. Inform health care professional of missed doses at time of checkup or lab tests. Inform patients that anticoagulant effect may persist for 2–5 days following discontinuation. Advise patient to read *Medication Guide* before starting therapy and with each Rx refill in case of changes.
- Review foods high in vitamin K (see Appendix J). Patient should have consistent limited intake of these foods, as vitamin K is the antidote for warfarin, and alternating intake of these foods will cause PT levels to fluctuate. Advise patient to avoid cranberry juice or products during therapy.
- Caution patient to avoid IM injections and activities leading to injury. Instruct patient to use a soft toothbrush, not to floss, and to shave with an electric razor during warfarin therapy. Advise patient that venipunctures and injection sites require application of pressure to prevent bleeding or hematoma formation.
- Advise patient to report any symptoms of unusual bleeding or bruising (bleeding gums; nosebleed; black, tarry stools; hematuria; excessive menstrual flow) and pain, color, or temperature change to any area of your body to health care professional immediately. ⌘ Patients with a deficiency in protein C and/or S mediated anticoagulant response may be at greater risk for tissue necrosis.
- Instruct patient not to drink alcohol or take other Rx, OTC, or herbal products, especially those containing aspirin or NSAIDs, or to start or stop any new medications during warfarin therapy without advice of health care professional.
- Rep: May cause fetal harm. Advise females of reproductive potential to use effective contraception during and for 1 month after last dose. Advise patient to notify health care professional if pregnancy is planned or suspected or if breastfeeding.
- Instruct patient to carry identification describing medication regimen at all times and to inform all health care personnel caring for patient on anticoagulant therapy before lab tests, treatment, or surgery.
- Emphasize the importance of frequent lab tests to monitor coagulation factors.

More patient safety information than any other drug guide

Evaluation/Desired Outcomes
- Prolonged PT (1.3–2.0 times the control; may vary with indication) or INR of 2–4.5 without signs of hemorrhage.

Find enhanced Canadian content throughout—in the monographs, appendices, and index.

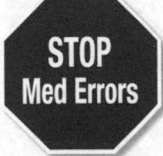

STOP
Med Errors

DAVIS'S DRUG GUIDE for NURSES®

NINETEENTH EDITION

April Hazard Vallerand, PhD, RN, FAAN

Director, PhD Program
Distinguished Professor
College of Nursing Alumni Endowed Professor
Wayne State University
College of Nursing
Detroit, Michigan

Cynthia A. Sanoski, BS, PharmD, BCPS, FCCP

Department Chair and Associate Professor
Thomas Jefferson University
Jefferson College of Pharmacy
Philadelphia, Pennsylvania

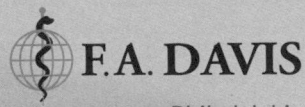

F.A. DAVIS

Philadelphia

F. A. Davis Company
1915 Arch Street
Philadelphia, PA 19103
www.fadavis.com

Printed in China

Last digit indicates print number 10 9 8 7 6 5 4 3 2 1
Editor-in-Chief, Nursing: Jean Rodenberger
Publisher, Nursing: Suzanne Toppy
Senior Content Project Manager: Amanda Minutola
Senior Project Editor, Content Solutions: Megan Schindele
Manager, Content Architecture: Robert Allen

NOTE: As new scientific information becomes available through basic and clinical research, recommended treatments and drug therapies undergo changes. The authors and publisher have done everything possible to make this book accurate, up to date, and in accord with accepted standards at the time of publication. However, the reader is advised always to check product information (package inserts) for changes and new information regarding dose and contraindications before administering any drug. Caution is especially urged when using new or infrequently ordered drugs.

Library of Congress Control Number: 2023950820

DEDICATION

To my son, Ben, whose sensitivity and sense of humor make even the toughest day easier.
To my daughter, Katharine, whose dedication and passion in seeking her goals is inspiring.
To my daughter-in-law, Amy, whose enthusiasm and commitment show great determination.
To my granddaughter, Claire, who brings joy and sunshine. Watching you grow into a strong and kind young lady fills me with love.
I am so proud of our wonderful family! Your support of my work inspires me. Thank you for sharing so much of your lives with me. I love you.

AHV

In loving memory of my mother, Geraldine, who provided me with 91 years of continual love, support, and wisdom as I pursued all of my personal and professional goals. My memories of her will always be a huge blessing in my life. I love you, Momma!

CAS

ACKNOWLEDGMENTS

We offer our thanks to the students and nurses who have used our book for more than 35 years. We hope our book provides you with the current knowledge of pharmacotherapeutics you need to continue to give quality care in our rapidly changing health care environment.

April and Cindy

Contributors

Wanda Edwards, PMHCNS-BC, NP
Instructor (Clinical)
Wayne State University
College of Nursing
Detroit, MI

Althea DuBose-Hayes, RDN
Consulting Renal Dietitian
Nephrology Associates of Michigan
Ann Arbor, MI

Kimberly Ferguson, DNP, APRN, FNP, PMHNP
Assistant Professor
East Tennessee State University
Johnson City, Tennessee

Margaret F. Galuardi, DNP, FNP-BC
Assistant Professor (Clinical)
Wayne State University College of Nursing
Detroit, Michigan

Margaret Mary Gingrich, RN, MSN, CRNP
Senior Professor/Adjunct Faculty
Harrisburg Area Community College
Harrisburg, Pennsylvania

Jason Micheal Kiernan, PhD, RN, ACNP
Assistant Professor
Michigan State University, College of Nursing
East Lansing, Michigan

Gladdi Tomlinson, RN, MSN
Professor of Nursing
Harrisburg Area Community College
Harrisburg, PA

Sally Villasenor, DNP, RN, ACNP-BC
Assistant Professor (Clinical)
Wayne State University College of Nursing
Detroit, Michigan

Erin Ziegler, PhD, NP-PHC
Assistant Professor
Daphne Cockwell School of Nursing, Ryerson University
Toronto, Ontario

CONTENTS

How To Use *Davis's Drug Guide for Nurses*

Davis's Drug Guide for Nurses provides comprehensive, current drug information in well-organized, nursing-focused monographs. It also includes extensive supplemental material in 14 appendices, addresses the issue of safe medication administration, and educates the reader about 45 different therapeutic classes of drugs. In this 19th edition, we continue to focus on safe medication administration by including **Medication Safety Tools** and even more information about health care's most vulnerable patients: children, the elderly, pregnant women, and breast feeding mothers. Look for more Pedi, Geri, OB, Lactation, and Rep headings in the monographs. A BEERS label appears at the top of applicable drug monographs for those medications listed in the most recent Beers Criteria developed by the American Geriatrics Society. These medications are potentially inappropriate for use in older adults because they are associated with more risk than benefit in this patient population. For Canadian students and nurses, we include an appendix comparing Canadian and U.S. pharmaceutical practices, more Canada-only combination drugs in the Combination Drugs appendix, and additional Canadian brand names in the drug monographs. To help you find this information quickly, a maple leaf icon (✤) appears in the index next to each Canadian entry. We have added pharmacogenomic information, marked with a double helix icon (⚕), in many monographs to help the nurse select and monitor various drug therapies. The following sections describe the organization of *Davis's Drug Guide for Nurses*.

Safe Medication Use Articles

This book includes several articles that describe the medication safety issues that confront clinicians and patients. "Medication Errors: Improving Practices and Patient Safety" familiarizes you with the systems issues and clinical situations repeatedly implicated in medication errors and suggests means to avoid them. It also teaches you about *high alert* medications, which have a greater potential to cause patient harm than other medications. "Detecting and Managing Adverse Drug Reactions" explains and provides guidance on identifying and managing adverse reactions. "Risk Evaluation and Mitigation Strategies (REMS)" explains strategies developed by the pharmaceutical industry and required by the Food and Drug Administration (FDA) to minimize adverse drug reactions from potentially dangerous drugs. We highlight the drugs that currently have approved REMS programs associated with their use by adding a REMS label at the top of applicable drug monographs. "Special Dosing Considerations" identifies the patient populations, such as neonates and patients with renal impairment, who require careful dose adjustments to ensure optimal therapeutic outcomes. "Educating Patients About Medication Use" reviews the most important teaching points for nurses to discuss with their patients and their families. Other critical information is highlighted in red in each drug monograph. In addition to these articles, please refer to the Medication Safety Tools in the back of the book for the BEERS criteria drug list, proper dosing for pediatric intravenous medications, confused drug names, FDA-approved Tall Man letters, and more.

Classifications

Medications in the same therapeutic class often share similar mechanisms of action, assessment guidelines, precautions, and interactions. The Classifications section provides summaries of the major therapeutic classifications we cover. It also provides patient teaching information common to all agents within the class. A list of drugs within each class can be found in the Comprehensive Index.

Drug Monographs

Drug monographs are organized in the following manner:

High Alert Status: Some medications, such as chemotherapeutic agents, anticoagulants, and insulins, have a greater potential for harm than others. These medications are identified by the *Institute for Safe Medication Practices* as **high alert drugs**. *Davis's Drug Guide for Nurses* includes a High Alert tab in the upper right corner of the monograph header in appropriate medications to alert the nurse to the medication's risk. The term "high alert" is used in other parts of the monograph to help the nurse administer these medications safely. See the article "Medication Errors: Improving Practices and Patient Safety" for a complete list of high alert medications in *Davis's Drug Guide for Nurses*.

Generic/Brand Name: The generic name appears first, with a pronunciation key, followed by an alphabetical list of trade names. Canadian trade names are preceded by a maple leaf (✢). Many brand names have been discontinued by the manufacturer, requiring nurses to know the generic names of drugs. Brand names that have been discontinued have a slash through them (Decadron).

Classification: The therapeutic classification, which categorizes drugs by the disease state they are used to treat, appears first, followed by the pharmacologic classification, which is based on the drug's mechanism of action.

Controlled Substance Schedule: All drugs regulated by federal law are placed into one of five schedules, based on the drug's medicinal value, harmfulness, and potential for abuse or addiction. Schedule I drugs, the most dangerous and having no medicinal value, are not included in *Davis's Drug Guide for Nurses*. (See Appendix H for Controlled Substances Schedules.)

Pregnancy Category: The FDA discontinued the Pregnancy Category system (A, B, C, D, and X) because this categorization may not appropriately communicate the risk that a drug may have during pregnancy or breast feeding. Therefore, Pregnancy Categories have been removed from all drug monographs and replaced with a *Rep* tag in drug prescribing information and Patient/Family Teaching sections. Here you will find information on the potential risk of using the drug during pregnancy and breast feeding, contraception suggestions, and potential impairment of fertility in women and men of reproductive potential.

Indications: Medications are approved by the FDA for specific disease states. This section identifies the diseases or conditions for which the drug is approved and includes significant unlabeled uses as well.

Action: This section contains a concise description of how the drug produces the desired therapeutic effect.

Pharmacokinetics: This section provides information on how the body processes a medication by absorption, distribution, metabolism, and excretion and includes information on the drug's half-life.

Absorption: Absorption is the process that follows drug administration and its subsequent delivery to systemic circulation. If only a small fraction is absorbed following oral administration (diminished bioavailability), then the oral dose must be much greater than the parenteral dose. Absorption into systemic circulation also follows other routes of administration such as topical, transdermal, intramuscular, subcutaneous, rectal, and ophthalmic routes. Drugs administered intravenously are 100% bioavailable.

Distribution: This section comments on the drug's distribution in body tissues and fluids. Distribution becomes important in choosing one drug over another, as in selecting an antibiotic that will penetrate the central nervous system to treat meningitis or in avoiding drugs that cross the placenta or concentrate in breast milk. Information on protein binding is included for drugs that are >95% bound to plasma proteins, which has implications for drug-drug interactions.

Metabolism and Excretion: Drugs are primarily eliminated from the body either by hepatic conversion to active or inactive compounds (metabolism or biotransformation) and subsequent excretion by the kidneys, or by renal elimination of unchanged drug. Therefore, drug metabolism and excretion information is important in determining dose regimens and intervals for patients with impaired renal or hepatic function. The creatinine clearance (CCr) helps quantify renal function and guides dose adjustments. Formulas to estimate CCr are included in Appendix E.

Half-Life: The half-life of a drug is the amount of time it takes for the drug concentration to decrease by 50% and roughly correlates with the drug's duration of action. Half-lives are given for drugs assuming the patient has normal renal or hepatic function. Conditions that alter the half-life are noted.

Time/Action Profile: The time/action profile table provides the drug's onset of action, peak effect, and duration of activity for each route. This information can aid in planning administration schedules and allows the reader to appreciate differences in choosing one route over another.

Contraindications and Precautions: Situations in which drug use should be avoided are listed as contraindications. In general, most drugs are contraindicated in pregnancy or lactation, unless the potential benefits outweigh the possible risks to the mother or baby (e.g., anticonvulsants, antihypertensives, and antiretrovirals). Contraindications may be absolute (i.e., the drug in question should be avoided completely) or relative, in which certain clinical situations may allow cautious use of the drug. The precautions portion includes disease states or clinical situations in which drug use involves risks or in which dose modification may be necessary. Extreme cautions are noted separately to draw attention to conditions under which use of the drug results in serious, potentially life-threatening consequences.

Adverse Reactions/Side Effects: It is not possible to list all reported reactions, but major side effects for all drugs are included. Life-threatening adverse reactions or side effects are **CAPITALIZED**, and the most frequent side effects are underlined. Those underlined generally have an incidence of >10%. Those not underlined occur in <10% but >1% of patients. Although life-threatening reactions may be rare (<1%), they are included because of their significance. For each body system, the most frequent adverse reactions are listed first alphabetically (including life-threatening); then all other reactions are subsequently listed alphabetically (including life-threatening). The following abbreviations are used for body systems:

CV: cardiovascular	**Hemat:** hematologic
Derm: dermatologic	**Local:** local
EENT: eye, ear, nose, and throat	**Metab:** metabolic
Endo: endocrinologic	**MS:** musculoskeletal
F and E: fluid and electrolyte	**Neuro:** neurologic
GI: gastrointestinal	**Resp:** respiratory
GU: genitourinary	**Misc:** miscellaneous

Interactions: Drug interactions are a significant risk for patients. As the number of medications a patient receives increases, so does the likelihood of drug-drug interactions. This section provides the most important drug-drug interactions and their physiological effects. Significant drug-food and drug-natural product interactions are also noted as are recommendations for avoiding or minimizing these interactions.

Route/Dosage: This section includes recommended doses for adults, children, and other more specific age groups by route. Dose units are expressed in the terms in which they are usually prescribed. For example, the penicillin G dose is given in units rather than in milligrams. Dosing intervals are also provided in the way they are frequently ordered. If a specific clinical situation (indication) requires a different dose or interval, this is listed separately for clarity. Specific dosing regimens for hepatic or renal impairment are also included.

Availability: This section lists the strengths and concentrations of available dose forms, which is useful in planning more convenient regimens (fewer tablets/capsules, less injection volume) and in determining whether certain dose forms are available (suppositories, oral concentrates, sustained- or extended-release forms). Flavors of oral liquids and chewable tablets have been included to improve compliance and adherence in pediatric patients.

Nursing Implications: This section helps the nurse apply the nursing process to pharmacotherapeutics. The subsections provide a guide to clinical assessment, implementation (drug administration), and evaluation of the outcomes of pharmacologic therapy.

Assessment: This section includes guidelines for assessing patient history and physical data before, during, and following drug therapy. Assessments specific to the drug's various indications are also included. **Lab Test Considerations** provide information regarding which laboratory tests to monitor and how the results may be affected by the medication. This section also includes dose modifications required for changes in lab values. **Toxicity and Overdose** identifies therapeutic serum drug concentrations that must be monitored, as well as signs and symptoms of toxicity. The antidote and treatment for toxicity or overdose are also included.

Implementation: Provides guidelines for administering medication. **High Alert** information relates to preventing medication errors with inherently dangerous drugs. Sound-alike look-alike name confusion alerts are also included here. Other headings in this section provide data regarding routes of administration. Dose modifications for side effects are included for drugs that provide this information. **PO** describes when and how to administer an oral drug, whether tablets may be crushed or capsules opened, and when to administer the medication in relation to food. The Do Not Crush (DNC) tag identifies drugs that should be swallowed whole. We have also identified which opioids have *abuse deterrent* properties and describe the mechanism of these properties. In the **IV Administration** section, bold, red headings are included to highlight the recommended **reconstitution**, **dilution**, and **concentration**. These headings complement the **rate** heading and make this critical information easy to find. **IV Push**, which refers to administering medications from a syringe directly into a saline lock, Y-site of IV tubing, or a 3-way stopcock, provides details for reconstitution, concentration, dilution, and rate. **Rate** is also included for other methods of IV administration. **Intermittent** and **Continuous Infusion** specify standard dilution solutions and amounts, stability information, and rates. In addition, a quick reference for information about dilution amounts in neonates and infants, who are extremely sensitive to excess fluids, is contained in the new **Medication Safety Tools** section. **Y-Site Compatibility/Incompatibility** identifies medications compatible or incompatible with each drug when administered via Y-site injection or 3-way stopcock in IV tubing. Information for drugs not included in these lists is conflicting or unavailable. Compatibility information is compiled from *Micromedex* and the manufacturer's package insert.

Patient/Family Teaching: This section includes information that should be taught to patients and/or families of patients. Side effects that should be reported, information on minimizing and managing side effects, details on administration, and follow-up requirements are presented. The nurse also should refer to the **Implementation** section for specific information to teach to the patient and family about taking the medication. The **Rep** tag identifies information on contraception, breast feeding, monitoring parameters for infants exposed to the drug, and fertility data. **Home Care Issues** discusses aspects to be considered for medications taken in the home setting.

Evaluation: Outcome criteria for determination of the effectiveness of the medication are provided.

Evidence-Based Practice and Pharmacotherapeutics

The purpose of evidence-based practice (EBP) is to use the best available evidence to make informed patient-care decisions that ultimately improve the treatment outcomes and safety of treatment for patients. How pharmacologic agents affect patients is often the subject of research; such research is required by the Food and Drug Administration (FDA) before and after drug approval. Any medication can be the subject of an evidence-based clinical review. But what does "evidence-based" mean, and how does it relate to nursing?

Evidence-based nursing practice can be viewed as a foundation of professional practice. It is an approach to making decisions, providing nursing care, and improving clinical practice based upon clinical expertise in combination with the most current and relevant research evidence. Still subject to debate are questions about the sufficiency and quality of evidence. For example, what kind of evidence is needed? How much evidence is necessary to support, modify, or change clinical practice? And were the studies reviewed of "good" quality and are their results valid?

Clinicians use a **hierarchy of evidence** to rank types of research reports from the most valuable and scientifically rigorous to the least useful. The hierarchy makes clear that some level of evidence about the effect of a particular treatment or condition exists, even if the evidence is considered weak. Figure 1 illustrates a hierarchy of evidence pyramid with widely accepted rankings: the most scientifically rigorous at the top, the least scientifically rigorous at the bottom. Clinicians should look for the highest level of available evidence to answer their clinical questions. It is important that clinicians also apply the second fundamental principle of EBP, which is that evidence alone is not sufficient to make clinical decisions. Decision makers must always trade off the benefits and risks, as well as the costs associated with alternative treatment options, and consider the patient's values and preferences.

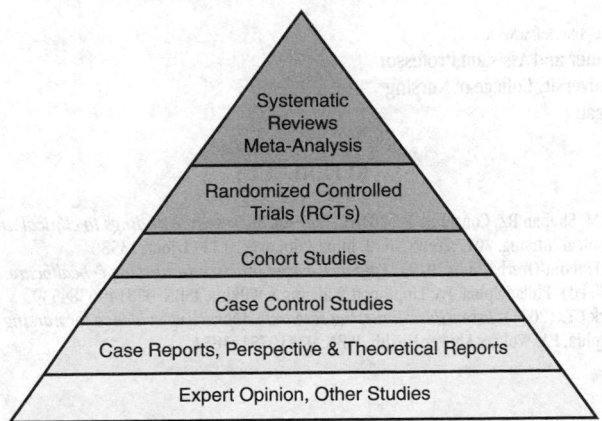

Figure 1: Hierarchy of Scientific Evidence Pyramid

Evidence-Based Practice and Its Importance in Pharmacology

Evidence-based practices in pharmacology generally are derived from well-designed randomized controlled trials (RCTs) or other experimental designs that investigate a drug's therapeutic and nontherapeutic effects. FDA-approved pharmacologic agents have undergone rigorous testing through RCTs, but nurses have the responsibility to evaluate the findings for the best scientific evidence available and to recognize the most appropriate, safest, and efficacious drugs for their patients.

One valuable and quickly accessible resource for evaluating the current highest level of pharmacologic evidence is the Cochrane Database of Systematic Reviews. The Cochrane library and databases provide full text of high-quality, regularly updated systematic reviews, protocols, and clinical trials.

AHRQ's Evidence-Based Practice Centers (EPCs) provide evidence reports and technology assessments that can assist nurses in their efforts to provide the highest quality and safest pharmacologic health care available. The EPCs systematically review the relevant scientific literature, conduct additional analyses (when appropriate) prior to developing their reports and assessments, and provide guideline comparisons.

Evidence-based systematic guidelines provide nurses with access to the most current knowledge, enabling them to critically appraise the scientific evidence and its appropriateness to their patient population. This is especially important given the need for nurses to keep abreast of the rapidly changing pharmacologic agents in use. New drugs are approved each month, compelling nurses to know these drugs' intended uses, therapeutic effects, interactions, and adverse effects.

Evidence-based practice requires a shift from the traditional paradigm of clinical practice—grounded in intuition, clinical experience, and pathophysiologic rationale—to a paradigm in which nurses must combine clinical expertise, patient values and preferences, and clinical circumstances with the integration of the best scientific evidence to make conscientious, well-informed, research-based decisions that affect nursing patient care.

***

Sally Villasenor, DNP, RN, ACNP-BC
Nurse Practitioner and Assistant Professor
Wayne State University College of Nursing
Detroit, Michigan

REFERENCES

1. Curtis K, Fry M, Shaban RZ, Considine J. (2016). *Translating research findings to clinical nursing practice.* Journal of Clinical Nursing. 2017;26:862-872. https://doi.org/10.1111/jocn.13586
2. Melnyk BM, Fineout-Overholt E. (2019). *Evidence-based practice in nursing & healthcare: A guide to best practice.* (4th ed). Philadelphia, PA: Lippincott Williams & Wilkins. ISBN: 9781496384539
3. Polit DF, Beck CT. (2021). *Essentials of nursing research: Appraising evidence for nursing practice.* (10th ed). Philadelphia, PA: Wolters Kluwer Health. ISBN: 9781975141851

Pharmacogenomics

Introduction

Multiple variables influence the selection and optimization of drug therapy for each individual patient. Pharmacogenomics, the study of the influence of individual genetic variations on drug response in patients, may yield additional information to further enhance safe and effective medication use. Originally the field focused on the effects of specific variants within individual genes on drug response (i.e., pharmaco *genetics*), however more recent research has focused on the role of multiple variants across the genome (i.e., pharmaco *genomics*) and their combined potential to modify and alter drug therapy outcomes.

The understanding of pharmacogenomics has increased considerably. Most emerging research has fallen into one of three domains:

- Gene variants that influence the function of drug transporter proteins (how efficiently drugs are delivered to their site(s) of activity)
- Gene variants that cause differences in the function of drug metabolizing enzymes (how quickly or slowly drugs are utilized and broken down in the body)
- Gene variants that alter a drugs' "target" proteins (variations in the genes coding for a target protein may alter the protein's three-dimensional shape, changing the binding affinity for drugs to that protein)

As the biological relevance of specific genetic variants has increased, it is understood that multiple variations across the genome can contribute to significant, yet *relatively predictable* treatment outcomes. Virtually every therapeutic area involving medication use includes a drug for which documented genetic variability has the potential to affect drug response. Some of this information is included in the FDA-approved package insert prescribing information. For some agents, the suitability of a specific drug or the determination of an appropriate initial dose for an individual patient based on pharmacogenetic information has been incorporated into dosing algorithms and patient care. As such, it is essential that health care professionals can interpret and utilize this information to facilitate safer and more effective use of medications for individual patients.

Genetic Variation Within the Human Genome

The human genome is comprised of approximately 3 billion nucleotide base pair sequences that encode for molecular DNA with each individual having his/her own unique human genome sequence (except for identical twins). Four nucleotide bases (adenine, guanine, cytosine, and thymine) for the sequence of each single strand of DNA. Variations in nucleotide sequences can occur and contribute to alterations in the expression and activities of certain genes as well as their protein products. The location of these variations within a DNA sequence on a particular chromosome can have a profound impact on the biological activity of that gene, however it should also be understood that some gene variants may lead to little or no discernable change to biologic activity at all. As new gene variants are discovered, the process of understanding the *degree of impact* becomes a focus for investigators.

Proteins are involved in most enzymatic, structural, and biologic functions associated with drug disposition and effects. The processes involved in DNA replication, RNA transcription, and translation to synthesized proteins are complex. Each of these processes is potentially susceptible to consequences of DNA sequence variations.

Genetic variations can take many forms, but most fall into three general categories:

- single nucleotide base substitutions (e.g., a cytosine substituted for an adenine)
- insertions or deletions of a nucleotide base within a sequence
- deletions or extra copies of entire DNA sequences (e.g., trisomy 21, in which an extra copy of *all* genes on the 21st chromosome are present)

Variations in DNA that occur at a frequency of greater than 1% in the population are called

7

polymorphisms. The most common gene varients in humans are single nucleotide polymorphisms (SNPs, pronounced as the word "snips" in dialogue). SNPs result from the substitution of one nucleotide base for another. The location of a SNP within a gene is important, as the location may or may not elicit a downstream effect on protein made from the gene. It is helpful to recall the importance of introns and exons for mRNA manufacturing when considering how SNPs can impact protein function. An important point to keep in mind is that *any* gene variant may have a spectrum-like impact on protein manufacture ranging from zero clinical consequences (no discernible effect on proteins) to complete lack of functional proteins associated with significant alterations in drug response. Also, pharmacogenomic clinical effects must always be considered within the larger sphere of environmental influences on drugs and drug responses. Finally, due to the commonality of polymorphisms, multiple gene variants may be present within one patient, making prediction of drug response particularly challenging.

Clinical Significance of Genetic Polymorphisms

SNPs and other genetic variations influence drug response at different levels through alterations in the activities of enzymes or proteins involved in drug absorption, transport, metabolism, elimination, or at the drug target receptor (site of drug action). Clinically relevant polymorphisms have been identified for genes that encode for most of the common enzymes involved in drug metabolism. Most enzymes are localized intracellularly throughout a wide variety of tissues in the body, including the enterocytes that line the intestine and within hepatocytes. Variants that cause diminished or absent enzyme activity decrease drug metabolism processes. In this case, if the drug is metabolized to an inactive product, then the prolonged persistence of the parent drug in the body could result in excessive pharmacologic effects and potential toxicities may occur. If the drug requires enzymatic conversion to a pharmacologically active metabolite, drug response may be reduced or absent. In contrast, if the variation is due to extra copies of a gene that results in increased enzymatic activity, opposite effects on drug metabolism and response can occur.

Similar outcomes can be associated with polymorphisms in genes that encode for membrane transporter proteins that are responsible for drug transport into cells (influx), as well as proteins that participate in energy-dependent processes that export drugs out of cells (efflux transporters). Polymorphisms in drug transport proteins can influence drug response by altering drug gastrointestinal absorption, uptake and distribution in tissues, exposure to intracellular drug metabolizing enzymes, and elimination via the bile or urine. Finally, some genes that encode for certain drug receptors are highly polymorphic, resulting in attenuated or exaggerated drug responses. The number of polymorphic genes responsible for variations in drug response at drug receptors is relatively small compared to those associated with drug metabolizing enzymes or transport proteins; however, this area has undergone the least amount of study to date.

Incorporating Pharmacogenomic Information into Clinical Practice

Most drugs are initiated in individual patients based on knowledge about their safety and effectiveness within the general population. Information regarding patient characteristics (e.g., age, ethnicity, renal/hepatic function, concomitant disease, etc.) known to contribute to variability in drug response, when available, is considered at this time. It is becoming more and more common, however, to consider gene variants as well when initiating drugs, as interindividual gene factors are thought to contribute to drug response variability in 15-30% of patients. Currently, there are more than 122 with pharmacogenomic information included in the package insert. For selected agents, dosing recommendations based on an individual's genetic information (i.e., genotype) for specific drugs and drug classes are also considered. Genomic biomarkers can play an important role in identifying responders and non-responders, avoiding drug toxicity, and adjusting the dose of drugs to optimize their efficacy and safety. However, the typical strategy for most drug therapy is to monitor the patient's response to treatment and modify regimens as necessary. Patients who develop exaggerated pharmacologic responses or elicit no pharmacologic effect may be expressing a phenotype suggestive of altered drug disposition or target receptor effect that could be associated with an underlying genetic polymorphism. As we continue to learn more about these associations and can incorporate pharmacogenomic information into decisions regarding drug therapy for individual patients, the ultimate goal is to improve therapeutic outcomes by limiting drug exposure to patients that are most likely to derive no therapeutic benefit and/or experience toxic drug effects.

For example, some genetic variants are associated with hypersensitivity reactions to a specific drug. A prescriber who is contemplating initiating that drug for a patient may need to determine whether the patient possesses that variant in their DNA. If that specific variant is present, the prescriber might select an alternate agent, thereby avoiding a potentially life-threatening hypersensitivity reaction. In another example, patients who are determined to have a genetic variant that results in an inactive metabolizing enzyme would not be appropriate candidates for an analgesic drug that requires that enzyme to convert the drug to the active analgesia-producing form. On the other hand, if that metabolizing enzyme is responsible for conversion of an active parent drug to an inactive metabolite, the starting dose of the drug may be reduced or perhaps an alternate drug might be selected.

Several Clinical Laboratory Improvement Amendment (CLIA)-approved laboratories offer pharmacogenetic testing to identify relevant genetic polymorphisms that predict drug response and can be used to initiate appropriate drugs and dosing regimens for individual patients. Some of these tests, while recommended in drug prescribing information, are costly and may not be covered by insurance. Patients may not fully understand the utility of undergoing genetic testing and providing a specimen for DNA analysis, which is typically performed on a blood, saliva, buccal swab, or other tissue collection. On the other hand, patients who are engaged in their medical care may be familiar with the concept of "personalized medicine" and seek information about available tests to "individualize" their own drug therapy. Many drugs are now required to have pharmacogenetic testing performed before they are prescribed. Other drugs have labeling that includes "test recommended" or "for information only." Health care professionals will need to be familiar with pharmacogenetic tests that are recommended for specific drug therapies, how to interpret the results of those tests, and how to incorporate pharmacogenetic data with other clinical information to optimize patient drug therapy and health care outcomes.

Pertinent Resources:

Benjeddou, M, Peiró, AM. (2021). Pharmacogenomics and prescription opioid use. *Pharmacogenomics,* 22(4), 235–245. https://doi.org/10.2217/pgs-2020-0032.

Carr, DF, Turner, RM. Pirmohamed. M. (2021). Pharmacogenomics of anticancer drugs: Personalising the choice and dose to manage drug response. *British journal of clinical pharmacology,* 87(2), 237–255. https://doi.org/10.1111/bcp.14407.

Cheek DJ, Bashore L, Brazeau DA. Pharmacogenomics and implications for nursing practice. *J Nurs Scolarsh* 2015;47:496–504.

NCBI Genetics Primer: http://www.ncbi.nlm.nih.gov/pmc/articles/PMC3860415/pdf/arcr-34-3-270.pdf

Nicholson, WT, Formea, CM, Matey, ET, et al. (2021). Considerations When Applying Pharmacogenomics to Your Practice. *Mayo Clinic proceedings,* 96(1), 218–230. https://doi.org/10.1016/j.mayocp.2020.03.011.

Roden, DM, McLeod, HL, Relling, MV, et al. (2019). Pharmacogenomics. *Lancet,* 394(10197), 521–532. https://doi.org/10.1016/S0140-6736(19)31276-0.

Rollinson, V, Turner, R, Pirmohamed, M. (2020). Pharmacogenomics for Primary Care: An Overview. *Genes,* 11(11), 1337. https://doi.org/10.3390/genes11111337.

van der Lee, M, Kriek, M, Guchelaar, HJ, Swen, JJ. (2020). Technologies for Pharmacogenomics: A Review. *Genes,* 11(12), 1456. https://doi.org/10.3390/genes11121456.

Wake, DT, Ilbawi, N, Dunnenberger, HM, Hulick, PJ. (2019). Pharmacogenomics: prescribing precisely. *The Medical Clinics of North America,* 103(6), 977–990. https://doi.org/10.1016/j.mcna.2019.07.002.

Medication Errors: Improving Practices and Patient Safety

It is widely acknowledged that medication errors result in thousands of adverse drug events, preventable reactions, and deaths per year. Nurses, physicians, pharmacists, patient safety organizations, the Food and Drug Administration, the pharmaceutical industry, Health Canada, and other parties share in the responsibility for determining how medication errors occur and designing strategies to reduce error.

One impediment to understanding the scope and nature of the problem has been the reactive "blaming, shaming, training" culture that singled out one individual as the cause of the error. Also historically, medication errors that did not result in patient harm—near-miss situations in which an error could have but didn't happen—or errors that did not result in serious harm were not reported. In contrast, serious errors often instigated a powerful punitive response in which one or a few persons were deemed to be at fault and, as a result, lost their jobs and sometimes their licenses.

In 1999, the Institute of Medicine (IOM) published *To Err Is Human: Building a Safer Health System*, which drew attention to the problem of medication errors. It pointed out that excellent health care providers do make medication errors, that many of the traditional processes involved in the medication-use system were error-prone, and that other factors, notably drug labeling and packaging, contributed to error. Furthermore, the IOM report, in conjunction with other groups such as the United States Pharmacopeia (USP) and the Institute for Safe Medication Practices (ISMP), called for the redesign of error-prone systems to include processes that anticipated the fallibility of humans working within the system. This initiative is helping shift the way the health care industry addresses medication errors from a single person/bad apple cause to a systems issue.

The National Coordinating Council for Medication Error Reporting and Prevention (NCC-MERP) developed the definition of a medication error that reflects this shift and captures the scope and breadth of the issue:

"A medication error is any preventable event that may cause or lead to inappropriate medication use or patient harm while the medication is in the control of the health care professional, patient, or consumer. Such events may be related to professional practice, health care products, procedures, and systems, including prescribing; order communication; product labeling, packaging, and nomenclature; compounding; dispensing; distribution; administration; education; monitoring; and use."

Inherent in this definition's mention of related factors are the human factors that are part of the medication use system. For example, a nurse or pharmacist may automatically reach into the bin where dobutamine is usually kept, see "do" and "amine" but select dopamine instead of dobutamine. Working amidst distractions, working long hours or shorthanded, and working in a culture where perfection is expected and questioning is discouraged are other examples of the human factors and environmental conditions that contribute to error.

The goal for the design of any individual or hospital-wide medication use system is to determine where systems are likely to fail and to build in safeguards that minimize the potential for error. One way to begin that process is to become familiar with medications or practices that have historically been shown to be involved in serious errors.

High Alert Medications

Some medications, because of a narrow therapeutic range or inherent toxic nature, have a high risk of causing devastating injury or death if improperly ordered, prepared, stocked, dispensed, administered, or monitored. Although these medications may not be involved in more errors, they require special attention due to the potential for serious, possibly fatal consequences. These have been termed **high-alert medications**, to communicate the need for extra care and safeguards. Many of these drugs are used commonly in the general population or are used frequently in urgent clinical situations. The Joint Commission (TJC) monitors the use of frequently prescribed high-alert medications, which include insulin, opioids, injectable potassium chloride (or phosphate) concentrate, intravenous anticoagulants (such as heparin), sodium chloride solutions with a concentration greater than 0.9%, and others. Visit the Institute for Safe Medication Practices at www.ismp.org for a complete list of High Alert Drugs.

Causes of Medication Errors

Many contributing factors and discrete causes of error have been identified, including failed communication, poor pharmaceutical supply chain distribution practices, dose miscalculations, drug packaging and drug-device related problems, incorrect drug administration, and lack of patient education.

Failed Communication: Failed communication covers many of the errors made in the ordering phase, and although ordering is performed by the prescriber, the nurse, the clerk, and the pharmacist who interpret that order are also involved in the communication process.

- *Poorly handwritten or verbal orders.* Handwriting is a major source of error and has led to inaccurate interpretations of the drug intended, the route of administration, the frequency, and dose. Telephone and verbal orders are likewise prone to misinterpretation. The current use of electronic drug order entry within hospitals and electronic prescribing to pharmacies contributes to increased legibility and consistency of medication orders and prescriptions.

- *Drugs with similar-sounding or similar-looking names.* Similar sounding names, or names that look similar when handwritten, are frequently confused. Doxorubicin hydrochloride and doxorubicin liposomal, or Lunesta® and Neulasta® are two examples. Mix-ups are more likely when each drug has similar dose ranges and frequencies.

Several of the sound-alike/look-alike drugs were targeted for labeling intervention by the FDA, which requested manufacturers with look-alike names to voluntarily revise the appearance of the established names. The revision visually differentiates the drug names by using "tall man" letters (capitals) to highlight distinguishing syllables (ex.: buPROPrion versus busPIRone or ceFAZolin versus cefTAZidime. See the TALL MAN Lettering table in the **Medication Safety Tools** section for the list of the pairs of drugs that are commonly confused, often with serious consequences.

- *Misuse of zeroes in decimal numbers.* Massive, ten-fold overdoses are traceable to not using a leading zero (.2 mg instead of 0.2 mg) or adding an unnecessary trailing zero (2.0 mg instead of 2 mg) in decimal expressions of dose. Similar overdoses are found in decimal expressions in which the decimal point is obscured by poor handwriting, stray marks, or lined orders sheets (e.g., reading 3.1 grams as 31 grams). Underdosing also may occur by the same mechanism and prevent a desired, perhaps life-saving effect.

- *Misinterpreted abbreviations.* Abbreviations can be misinterpreted or, when used in the dose part of the order, can result in incorrect dose of the correct medication. For example, lower or uppercase "U" for units has been read as a zero, making 10 u of insulin look like 100 units when handwritten. The Latin abbreviation "QOD" for every other day has been misinterpreted as QID (4 times per day). Current widespread use of electronic drug ordering and prescriptions increases legibility; frequency choices are often in plain language such as "every other day" instead of "QOD". See Table 1 for a list of confusing abbreviations and safer alternatives.

- *Ambiguous or incomplete orders.* Orders that do not clearly specify dose, route, frequency, or indication do not communicate complete information and are open to misinterpretation.

Poor Distribution Practices: Poor distribution includes error-prone storing practices such as keeping similar-looking products next to each other. Dispensing multidose floor stock vials of potentially dangerous drugs instead of unit (single) dose vials is also associated with error, as is allowing non-pharmacists to dispense medications in the absence of the pharmacist.

Dose Miscalculations: Dose miscalculations are a prime source of medication error. Also, many medications need to be dose-adjusted for renal or hepatic impairment, age, height and weight, and body composition (i.e., correct for obesity). Complicated dosing formulas provide many opportunities to introduce error. Often vulnerable populations, such as premature infants, children, older adults, and those with serious underlying illnesses, are at greatest risk.

Drug Packaging: Similar packaging or poorly designed packaging encourages error. Drug companies may use the same design for different formulations, or fail to highlight information about concentration or strength. Lettering, type size, color, and packaging methods can either help or hinder drug identification.

Drug Delivery Systems: Drug delivery systems include infusion pumps and drip rate controllers. Some models do not prevent free flow of medication, leading to sudden high dose infusion of potent and dangerous medications. The lack of safeguards preventing free flow and programming errors are among the problems encountered with infusion control devices. Newer models, which are integrated with the medication administration record (MAR) via scanned barcodes to match the patient with drug, dose, and timing, contribute to increased dosing safety; however, it is a nursing responsibility to verify the dose and determine that the infusion pump is delivering properly at the point of drug administration.

Incorrect Drug Administration: Incorrect drug administration covers many problems. Misidentification of a patient, incorrect route of administration, missed doses, or improper drug preparation are types of errors that occur during the administration phase. Barcode scanning to identify the patient and correlate with the correct MAR decreases the likelihood of incorrect drug administration.

Lack of Patient Education: Safe medication use is enhanced in the hospital and the home when the patient is well informed. The knowledgeable patient can recognize when something has changed in his or her medication regimen and can question the health care professional. At the same time, many issues related to medication errors, such as ambiguous directions, unfamiliarity with a drug, and confusing packaging, affect the patient as well as the health care professional, underscoring the need for careful education. Patient education also enhances adherence, which is a factor in proper medication use.

Prevention Strategies

Since medication use systems are complex and involve many steps and people, they are error-prone. On an individual basis, nurses can help reduce the incidence of error by implementing the following strategies:

- Clarify any order that is not obviously and clearly legible. Ask the prescriber to print orders using block style letters if handwritten.
- Do not accept orders with the abbreviation "u" or "IU" for units. Clarify the dosage and ask the prescriber to write out the word units.
- Clarify any abbreviated drug name or the abbreviated dosing frequencies q.d., QD, q.o.d., QOD, and q.i.d or QID. Suggest abandoning Latin abbreviations in favor of spelling out dosing frequency.
- Decimal point errors can be hard to see. Suspect a missed decimal point and clarify any order if the dose requires more than 3 dosing units.
- If dose ordered requires use of multiple dosage units or very small fractions of a dose unit, review the dose, have another health care provider check the original order and recalculate formulas, and confirm the dose with the prescriber.
- If taking a verbal order, ask prescriber to spell out the drug name and dosage to avoid sound-alike confusion (e.g., hearing Cerebyx for Celebrex, or fifty for fifteen). Read back the order to the prescriber after you have written it in the chart. Confirm and document the indication to further enhance accurate communication.
- Clarify any order that does not include metric weight, dosing frequency, or route of administration.
- Do not start a patient on new medication by borrowing medications from another patient. This action bypasses the double check provided by the pharmacist's review of the order.
- Always check the patient's name band before administering medications. Verbally addressing a

patient by name does not provide sufficient identification. If available, use of barcode scanning per institutional policy recommended.

- Use the facility's standard drug administration times to reduce the chance of an omission error.
- Be sure to fully understand any drug administration device before using it. This includes infusion pumps, inhalers, and transdermal patches.
- Have a second practitioner independently check original order, dose calculations, and infusion pump settings for high alert medications.
- Realize that the printing on packaging boxes, vials, ampules, prefilled syringes, or any container in which a medication is stored can be misleading. Be sure to differentiate clearly the medication and the number of milligrams per milliliter versus the total number of milligrams contained within. Massive overdoses have been administered by assuming that the number of milligrams per ml is all that is contained within the vial or ampule. Read the label when obtaining the medication, before preparing or pouring the medication, and after preparing or pouring the medication.
- Educate patients about the medications they take. Provide verbal and written instructions and ask the patient to restate important points.

REFERENCES

1. Billstein-Leber M, Carrillo C, Cassano AT, et al. ASHP guidelines on preventing medication errors in hospitals. *Am J Health Syst Pharm.* 2018;75: 1493−517.
2. Wang H, Tao D, Yan M. Effects of text enhancement on reduction of look-alike drug name confusion: A systematic review and meta-analysis. *Qual Manag Health Care* 2021;30:233−43.
3. ISMP. Targeted Medication Safety Best Practices for Hospitals *ISMP Guidelines.* February 9, 2022.https://www.ismp.org/guidelines/best-practices-hospitals
4. Koeck JA, Young NJ, Kontny U, et al. Interventions to reduce medication dispensing, administration, and monitoring errors in pediatric professional healthcare settings: A systematic review. *Front Pediatr.* 2021;9:633064.
5. Kohn LT, Corrigan JM, Donaldson MS (eds). *To Err Is Human: Building a Safer Health System.* National Academy Press, Washington, DC (1999).
6. Manias E, Snezana K, Wu A. Interventions to reduce medication errors in adult medical and surgical settings: a systematic review. *Ther Adv Drug Saf.* 2020;11:2042098620968309. http://dx.doi.org/10.1177/2042098620968309
7. National Coordinating Council for Medication Error Reporting and Prevention. (2023). *About Medication Errors: What is a Medication Error?* http://www.nccmerp.org/about-medication-errors
8. Strudwick G. Factors associated with barcode medication administration technology that contribute to patient safety: An integrative review. *J Nurs Care Qual.* 2018;33:79−85.

Table 1: Abbreviations and Symbols Associated with Medication Errors

Abbreviation/Symbol	Intended Meaning	Mistaken For	Recommendation
APAP	Acetaminophen	Not recognized as acetaminophen	Use full drug name
AT II	Angiotensin II	Antithrombin III	Use full drug name
AT III	Antithrombin III	Angiotensin II	Use full drug name
AZT	Zidovudine	Azithromycin, azathioprine, aztreonam	Use full drug name
CPZ	Compazine (prochlorperazine)	Chlorpromazine	Use full drug name
DOR	Doravirine	Dovato (dolutegravir/lamivudine)	Use full drug name
HCT	Hydrocortisone	Hydrochlorothiazide	Use full drug name
HCTZ	Hydrochlorothiazide	Hydrocortisone	Use full drug name
IV vanc	Intravenous vancomycin	Invanz (ertapenem)	Use full drug name
"Levo"	Levofloxacin	Levophed (norepinephrine)	Use full drug name
$MgSO_4$*	Magnesium sulfate	Morphine sulfate	Use full drug name
MS or MSO_4*	Morphine sulfate	Magnesium sulfate	Use full drug name
MTX	Methotrexate	Mitoxantrone	Use full drug name
Na at the beginning of a drug name (e.g., Na bicarbonate)	Sodium bicarbonate	No bicarbonate	Use full drug name
"Nitro" drip	Nitroglycerin infusion	Nitroprusside infusion	Use full drug name
NoAC	Novel/new oral anticoagulant	No anticoagulant	Use full drug name
OXY	Oxytocin	Oxycodone, Oxycontin	Use full drug name
PCA	Procainamide	Patient controlled analgesia	Use full drug name
PIT	Pitocin (oxytocin)	Pitressin (vasopressin)	Use full drug name
PNV	Prenatal vitamins	Penicillin VK	Use full drug name
PTU	Propylthiouracil	Mercaptopurine	Use full drug name
T3	Tylenol with codeine no. 3	Liothyronine	Use full drug name
TAC or tac	Triamcinolone or tacrolimus	Tetracaine, Adrenalin, cocaine, Taxotere, Adriamycin, cyclophosphamide	Use full drug name
TAF	Tenofovir alafenamide	Tenofovir disoproxil fumarate	Use full drug name
TDF	Tenofovir disoproxil fumarate	Tenofovir alafenamide	Use full drug name
TNK	TNKase	tPA	Use full drug name
TPA or tPA	Tissue plasminogen activator (alteplase)	TNKase (tenecteplase), TXA (tranexamic acid), Retevase (reteplase)	Use full drug name
TXA	Tranexamic acid	tPA	Use full drug name
$ZnSO_4$	Zinc sulfate	Morphine sulfate	Use full drug name
μg	Microgram	mg (milligram)	Use "mcg"
AD, AS, or AU	Right ear, left ear, both ears	Right eye, left eye, both eyes	Spell out "right ear," "left ear," or "both ears"
BIW or biw	2 times a week	2 times a day	Spell out "2 times weekly"
cc	cubic centimeters	u (units)	Use "ml"
D/C	Discharge or discontinue	One mistaken for the other	Spell out "discharge" or "discontinue"
HS or hs	Half strength or hours of sleep (at bedtime)	One mistaken for the other	Spell out "half strength" or use "HS" for at bedtime
IN	Intranasal	IM or IV	Spell out "intranasal" or use "NAS"
IT	Intrathecal	Intratracheal, intratumor, intratympanic, inhalation therapy	Spell out "intrathecal"

Abbreviation	Intended Meaning	Misinterpretation	Correction
IU*	International Units	IV or 10	Spell out "units"
l	Liter	1 (one)	Use uppercase "L"
M or K	Thousand	Million	Spell out "thousand"
ml	Milliliter	1 (one)	Use "mL" (with lowercase "m" and uppercase "L")
MM or M	Million	Thousand	Spell out "million"
Ng or ng	Nanogram	mg (milligram) or nasogastric	Spell out "nanogram"
OD, OS, or OU	Right eye, left eye, both eyes	Right ear, left ear, both ears	Spell out "right eye," "left eye," or "both eyes"
o.d. or OD	Once daily	Right eye	Spell out "daily"
OJ	Orange juice	OD (right eye), OS (left eye)	Spell out "orange juice"
q.d., qd, Q.D., or QD*	Every day	qid (4 times per day)	Spell out "daily"
q1d	Daily	qid (4 times per day)	Spell out "daily"
Qhs	Nightly at bedtime	qhr (every hour)	Spell out "nightly" or use "HS" for bedtime
q.o.d., qod, Q.O.D., or QOD*	Every other day	qid (4 times per day) or qd (daily)	Spell out "every other day"
SC, SQ, sq, or sub q	Subcutaneously	SC mistaken as SL (sublingual); SQ mistaken as "5 every"; q in sub q mistaken as "every"	Use "SUBQ" or write out "subcutaneously"
SSRI	Sliding scale regular insulin	Selective serotonin reuptake inhibitor	Spell out "sliding scale insulin"
TIW or tiw	3 times a week	3 times a day or twice a week	Spell out "3 times weekly"
u or U*	units	0 (zero), 4 (four) or cc	Spell out "units"
UD	As directed	Unit dose	Spell out "as directed"
/ (slash mark)	Per"	1 (one)	Spell out "per"
+	Plus sign	4 (four)	Spell out "and"
Zero **after** a decimal point (e.g., 1.0 mg)*	1 mg	10 mg	DO NOT USE zero after a decimal point
No zero **before** a decimal point (e.g., .1 mg)*	.1 mg	1 mg	ALWAYS USE zero before a decimal point
@	At	2 (two)	Use "at"
>	Greater than	<	Spell out "greater than"
<	Less than	4 or >	Spell out "less than"
&	And	2 (two)	Use "and"
°	Hour	Zero	Use "hr," "h," or "hour"
Drug name and dose run together. Example: Inderal 40 mg	Inderal 40 mg	Inderal 140 mg	Leave space between drug name, dose, and unit of measure
Numerical dose and unit of measure run together. Example: 10 mg	10 mg	100 mg	Leave space between drug dose and unit of measure

*Appears on The Joint Commission's "Do Not Use" list of abbreviations.
Modified from ISMP's List of Error-Prone Abbreviations, Symbols, and Dose Designations, 2021.

Detecting and Managing Adverse Drug Reactions

An *adverse drug reaction* (ADR) is any unexpected, undesired, or excessive response to a medication that results in:

- temporary or permanent serious harm or disability
- admission to a hospital, transfer to a higher level of care, or prolonged stay
- death.

Adverse drug reactions are distinguished from adverse drug events, in which causality is uncertain, and side effects, which may be bothersome to the patient and necessitate a change in therapy but are not considered serious. Although some ADRs are the result of medication errors, many are not.

Types of ADRs

The Food and Drug Administration (FDA) classifies ADRs into 2 broad categories: Type A and Type B. Type A reactions are predictable reactions based on the primary or secondary pharmacologic effect of the drug. Dose-related reactions and drug-drug interactions are examples of Type A reactions. Type B reactions are unpredictable, are not related to dose, and are not the result of the drug's primary or secondary pharmacologic effect. Idiosyncratic and hypersensitivity reactions are examples of Type B reactions.

Dose-Related Reactions (Toxic Reactions): In dose related reactions, the dose prescribed for the patient is excessive. Although a variety of mechanisms may interact, reasons for this type of reaction include:

- renal or hepatic impairment
- extremes in age (neonates and frail elderly)
- drug-drug or drug-food interactions
- underlying illness.

Dose-related reactions are often the result of preventable errors in prescribing in which physiologic factors such as age, renal impairment, and weight were not considered sufficiently, or in inadequate therapeutic monitoring. Medications with narrow therapeutic ranges (digoxin, aminoglycosides, antiepileptic drugs) and those that require careful monitoring or laboratory testing (anticoagulants, nephrotoxic drugs) are most frequently implicated in dose-related reactions. Dose-related reactions usually are managed successfully by temporarily discontinuing the drug and then reducing the dose or increasing the dosing interval. In some instances, the toxic effects need to be treated with another agent (e.g., Digibind for digoxin toxicity or protamine for heparin toxicity). Appropriately timed therapeutic drug level monitoring, review of new drugs added to an existing regimen that may affect the drug level, and frequent assessment of relevant laboratory values are critical to safe medical management and prevention of dose-related reactions.

Drug-Drug Interactions: Drug-drug interactions occur when the pharmacokinetic or pharmacodynamic properties of an individual drug affect another drug. Pharmacokinetics refers to the way the body processes a medication (absorption, distribution, metabolism, and elimination). In a drug-drug interaction, the pharmacokinetic properties of one drug can cause a change in drug concentration of another drug and an altered response. For example, one drug may block enzymes that metabolize a second drug. The concentration of the second drug is then increased and may become toxic or cause adverse reactions. Pharmacodynamic drug-drug interactions involve the known effects and side effects of the drugs. For example, two drugs with similar therapeutic effects may act together in a synergistic way. The increased antithrombotic effects that occur when warfarin and aspirin are taken together, or the increased central nervous system (CNS) depression that results when two drugs with CNS depressant effects potentiate each other, are examples of pharmacodynamic drug-drug interactions. Certain classes of drugs are more likely to result in serious drug-drug interactions, and patients receiving these agents should be monitored carefully. These medication classes include anticoagulants, oral hypoglycemic agents, nonsteroidal anti-inflammatory drugs, antihypertensives, antibiotics, antiepileptics, antiretrovirals, antidepressants, and antipsychotic agents.

Idiosyncratic Reactions: Idiosyncratic reactions occur without relation to dose and are unpredictable and sporadic. Reactions of this type may manifest in many different ways, including fever, blood dyscrasias, cardiovascular effects, or mental status changes. The time frame between the occurrence of a problem and initiation of therapy is sometimes the only clue linking drug to symptom. Some idiosyncratic reactions may be explained by genetic differences in drug-metabolizing enzymes.

Hypersensitivity Reactions: Hypersensitivity reactions are usually allergic responses. Manifestations of hypersensitivity reactions range from mild rashes, to nephritis, pneumonitis, hemolytic anemia, and anaphylaxis. Protein drugs (vaccines, enzymes) are frequently associated with hypersensitivity reactions. In most instances, antibody formation is involved in the process and therefore cross-sensitivity may occur. An example of this is hypersensitivity to penicillin and cross-sensitivity with other penicillins and/or cephalosporins. Documenting drugs to which the patient is allergic and the specific hypersensitivity reaction is very important. If the reaction to an agent is anaphylaxis, the nurse should monitor the patient during administration of a cross-hypersensitive agent, especially during the initial dose, and ensure ready access to emergency resuscitative equipment.

Recognizing an ADR

Adverse drug reactions should be suspected whenever there is a negative change in a patient's condition, particularly when a new drug has been introduced. Strategies that can enhance recognition include knowing the side effect/adverse reaction profile of medications. Nurses should be familiar with a drug's most commonly encountered side effects and adverse reactions before administering it. In *Davis's Drug Guide for Nurses*, most frequent ADRs are underlined, and life-threatening ADRs are CAPITALIZED and appear in second color in the **Adverse Reactions and Side Effects** section. Within each organ system in this section, ADRs occurring at a frequency of ≥10% are underlined and are listed first (in alphabetical order). Adverse drug reactions occurring at a frequency of <10% will not be underlined and will be listed (in alphabetical order) after the underlined ADRs. As always, monitoring the patient's response to a medication and ongoing assessment are key nursing actions. Learn to recognize patient findings that suggest an ADR has occurred. These include:

- rash
- change in respiratory rate, heart rate, blood pressure, or mental state
- seizure
- anaphylaxis
- diarrhea
- fever

Any of these findings can suggest an ADR and should be reported and documented promptly so that appropriate interventions, including discontinuation of suspect medications, can occur. Prompt intervention can prevent a mild adverse reaction from escalating into a serious health problem. Other steps taken by the health care team when identifying and treating an ADR include:

1. Determining that the drug ordered was the drug given and intended.
2. Determining that the drug was given in the correct dosage by the correct route.
3. Establishing the chronology of events: time drug was taken and onset of symptoms.
4. Stopping the drug and monitoring patient status for improvement (dechallenge).
5. Restarting the drug, if appropriate, and monitoring closely for adverse reactions (rechallenge).

Prevention

Health care organizations have responded to consumer, regulator, and insurer pressures by developing programs that aim to eliminate preventable ADRs. In the inpatient setting, computer systems can display the patient's age, height, weight, and creatinine clearance (or estimated glomerular filtratration rate) and send an alert to the clinician if a prescribed dose is out of range for any of the displayed parameters. Allergy alerts and drug-drug interaction alerts can be presented to the clinician at the time an order is entered.

In the outpatient setting, strategies that increase the patient's knowledge base and access to pharmacists and nurses may help prevent adverse reactions. Outpatient pharmacy computer systems that are linked within a chain of pharmacies may allow the pharmacist to view the patient's profile if the patient is filling a prescription in a pharmacy other than the usual one. Many pharmacy computers have dose limits and drug-drug interaction verification to assist pharmacists filling orders.

Such strategies are a valuable auxiliary to, but cannot replace, conscientious history taking, careful patient assessment, and ongoing monitoring. A thorough medication history including all prescription and nonprescription drugs, all side effects and adverse reactions encountered, allergies, and all pertinent physical data should be available to the prescriber. The prescriber is responsible for reviewing this data, along with current medications, laboratory values, and any other variable that affects drug response.

It is not expected that practitioners will remember all relevant information when prescribing. In fact, reliance on memory is error-fraught, and clinicians need to use available resources to verify drug interactions whenever adding a new drug to the regimen. Setting expectations that clinicians use evidence-based information rather than their memories when prescribing, dispensing, administering, or monitoring patients has the potential to reduce the incidence of preventable ADRs.

Reporting ADRs in the U.S.:

Food and Drug Administration MedWatch Program: To monitor and assess the incidence of adverse reactions, the FDA sponsors MedWatch, a program that allows health care practitioners and consumers the opportunity to report serious adverse reactions or product defects encountered from medications, medical devices, special nutritional products, or other FDA-regulated items. The FDA considers serious those reactions that result in death, life-threatening illness or injury, hospitalization, disability, congenital anomaly, or those that require medical/surgical intervention.

In addition to reporting serious ADRs, health care providers should also report problems related to suspected contamination, questionable stability, defective components, or poor packaging/labeling. Reports should be submitted even if there is some uncertainty about the cause/effect relationship or if some details are missing. This reporting form may be accessed at https://www.fda.gov/safety/medwatch-fda-safety-information-and-adverse-event-reporting-program. Reactions to vaccines should be reported to the Vaccine Adverse Event Reporting System (VAERS; https://vaers.hhs.gov/). Nurses share with other health care providers an obligation to report adverse reactions to the MedWatch program so that all significant data can be analyzed for opportunities to improve patient care.

Reporting ADRs in Canada:

The Marketed Health Products Directorate of Health Canada coordinates ADR reporting activities, and analyzes reports submitted from regional centers in each province. MedEffect Canada encourages health professionals, patients and regulatory authorities to report adverse reactions as they occur, either by email, mail, or the Health Canada website. Health care professionals reporting ADRs are required to supply information regarding patient characteristics, details about the reaction(s), current treatment, and outcomes. Information identifying the patient or health care provider remains confidential.

Adverse drug reaction reports are analyzed to investigate any associations with the health product. Based on the outcome, regulatory bodies decide on a course of action, which may include performing additional post-marketing studies, reassessment of the risk versus benefit of the product, packaging modification, addition of warnings in patient information leaflets, or issuing public alerts or market withdrawals. Updates regarding adverse reactions are published in the Health Product InfoWatch every month.

Access the following link for the Side Effect Reporting Form for consumers and health professionals: https://www.canada.ca/en/health-canada/services/drugs-health-products/medeffect-canada/adverse-reaction-reporting.html.

REFERENCES

1. Zazzara MB, Palmer K, Vetrano DL, et al. Adverse drug reactions in older adults: a narrative review of the literature. *Eur Geriatr Med*. 2021;12:463–73.
2. Schiavo G, Forgerini M, Lucchetta RC, et al. Cost of adverse drug events related to potentially inappropriate medication use: A systematic review. *J Am Pharm Assoc*. 2022;62:1463–76.
3. Ouellett GM, Ouellett JA, Tinetti ME. Principle of rational prescribing and deprescribing in older adults with multiple chronic conditions. *Ther Adv Drug Saf*. 2018;9:639–52.
4. Petrovic M, van der Cammen T, Onder G. Adverse drug reactions in older people: detection and prevention. *Drugs Aging*. 2012;29:453–62.
5. "Adverse Reaction Information." *MedEffect Canada*. October 2012. http://www.hc-sc.gc.ca/dhp-mps/medeff/advers-react-neg/index-eng.php#a5 (accessed November 7, 2023).

Overview of Risk Evaluation and Mitigation Systems (REMS)

Over the past several decades, the Food and Drug Administration (FDA) has employed a number of "risk management" programs designed to detect, evaluate, prevent, and mitigate drug adverse events for drugs with the potential for serious adverse drug reactions. Some of the risk management plans used by the FDA over the years have included the use of patient package inserts, medication guides, restricted access programs, and classification of drugs as controlled substances. These programs were acknowledged by the FDA as Risk Minimization Action Plans (RiskMAPS) in 2005. With these programs, the FDA only had the authority to mandate postmarketing commitments from drug manufacturers before the drug was approved; however, these requirements could not be enforced after the drug was approved.

The Food and Drug Administration Amendments Act of 2007 gave the FDA the authority to subject drugs to new risk identification and communication strategies in the postmarketing period. These new strategies, called Risk Evaluation and Mitigation Strategies (REMS), can be required for any drug or drug class that is associated with serious risks. The FDA can require a REMS if it believes that this program is necessary to ensure that the benefits outweigh the potential risks of the drug. The FDA can require a REMS either as part of the drug approval process or during the postmarketing period if new information becomes available regarding potentially harmful effects that are associated with the use of the drug.

Components of the REMS may include a medication guide, a patient package insert, and/or a communication plan. A REMS for New Drug Applications or Biologics License Applications requires a timetable for submission of assessment of the REMS. A variety of elements to ensure safe use of drugs can be required as part of the REMS if it is believed that a medication guide, patient package insert, or communication plan are not adequate to mitigate the serious risks associated with a particular drug. These elements may include the following:

- Health care providers who prescribe the drug are specifically trained and/or certified.
- Pharmacies, practitioners, or health care settings that dispense the drug are specifically trained and/or certified.
- The drug is dispensed to patients only in certain health care settings, such as hospitals.
- The drug is dispensed only to patients with evidence or other documentation of safe-use conditions, such as laboratory test results.
- Patients using the drug are subject to certain monitoring.
- Patients using the drug are enrolled in a registry.

The FDA maintains an updated list of these REMS programs at https://www.accessdata.fda.gov/scripts/cder/rems/index.cfm. A REMS tag has been added at the top of and within the monographs of drugs associated with these programs.

Special Dosing Considerations

For many patients the average dose range for a given drug can be toxic. The purpose of this section is to describe vulnerable patient populations for which special dosing considerations must be made to protect the patient and improve clinical outcomes.

The Pediatric Patient

Most drugs prescribed to children are not approved by the Food and Drug Administration (FDA) for use in pediatric populations. This does not mean it's wrong to prescribe these drugs to children, rather it means that the medications were not tested in children. The lack of pediatric drug information can result in patient harm or death, such as what occurred with the drug chloramphenicol. When given to very young children, chloramphenicol caused toxicity and multiple deaths. Referred to as "gray baby syndrome," this toxic reaction was eventually found to be dose dependent. The FDA now requires that new drugs that may be used in children include information for safe pediatric use.

The main reason for adjusting doses in pediatric patients is body size, which is measured by body weight or body surface area (BSA). Weight-based pediatric drug doses are expressed in number of milligrams per kilogram of body weight (mg/kg) while doses calculated on BSA are expressed in number of milligrams per meter squared (mg/m^2). BSA is determined using a BSA nomogram or calculated by using formulas (Appendix E).

The neonate and the premature infant require additional adjustments secondary to immature function of body systems. For example, absorption may be incomplete or altered due to differences in gastric pH or motility. Distribution may be altered because of varying amounts of total body water, and metabolism and excretion can be delayed due to immature liver and kidney function. Furthermore, rapid weight changes and progressive maturation of hepatic and renal function require frequent monitoring and careful dose adjustments. Gestational age, as well as weight, may be needed to properly dose some drugs in the neonate.

The Older Adult Patient

Absorption, distribution, metabolism, and excretion are altered in adults over 65 years of age, putting the older patient at risk for toxic reactions. Pharmacokinetic properties in older adults are affected by (1) diminished gastrointestinal (GI) motility and blood flow, which delays absorption; (2) changes in ratios of percentage of body fat, lean muscle mass, and total body water, which alter distribution; (3) decreased plasma proteins, especially in the malnourished patient, which alters distribution by allowing a larger proportion of free or unbound drug to circulate and exert effects; (4) diminished hepatic function, which slows metabolism; and (5) diminished renal function, which delays excretion.

Older adults should be prescribed the lowest effective dose at the initiation of therapy, followed by careful titration of doses. Monitor carefully for signs and symptoms of adverse drug reactions.

Another concern is that many older adult patients are prescribed multiple drugs and are at risk for polypharmacy. As the number of medications a patient takes increases, so does the risk for an adverse drug reaction. One drug may negate or potentiate the effects of another drug (drug-drug interaction). This situation is compounded by concurrent use of nonprescription or over-the-counter (OTC) drugs, herbal supplements, and vitamins. In general, doses of most medications (especially digoxin, sedative/hypnotics, anticoagulants, nonsteroidal anti-inflammatory agents, antibiotics, and antihypertensives) should be decreased in the older adult population. The Beers List/Criteria, which appears in the *Medication Safety Tools* section, is a list of drugs to be used with caution in older adults.

Females of Reproductive Potential

Generally, pregnant women should avoid medications, except when necessary. Both the mother and the fetus must be considered. The placenta is a membrane which allows rapid and complete diffusion of lipid soluble drugs and protects the fetus only from extremely large molecules. The fetus is particularly vulnerable during the first and the last trimesters of pregnancy. During the first trimester, vital organs are forming, and ingestion of teratogenic drugs may lead to fetal malformation or miscarriage. Unfortunately, this is the time when a woman is least likely to know that she is pregnant. In the third trimester, drugs administered to the mother and transferred to the fetus may not be safely metabolized and excreted by the fetus. This is especially true of drugs administered near term. After the infant is delivered, he or she no longer has the placenta to help with drug excretion, and drugs administered before delivery may result in toxicity.

Of course, many conditions, such as asthma, diabetes, gastrointestinal disorders, and mental illness affect pregnant women and require long-term medication use. When the medications are used, whether over-the-counter or prescription, prescribing the lowest effective dose for the shortest period of time necessary is the rule. The Centers for Disease Control and Prevention (CDC) has a variety of resources and treatment guidelines called Treating for Two: Medicine and Pregnancy. The Web address is https://www.cdc.gov/pregnancy/meds/treatingfortwo/.

The possibility of a medication altering sperm quality and quantity in a potential father is also an area of concern. Male patients should be informed of this risk when taking any medications known to have this potential.

Renal Impairment

The kidneys are the major organ of drug elimination. Failure to account for decreased renal function is a preventable source of adverse drug reactions. Renal function is measured by the creatinine clearance (CCr), which can be approximated in the absence of a 24-hour urine collection (Appendix E). In addition, doses in patients with renal impairment can be optimized by measuring blood levels of certain drugs (e.g., digoxin, aminoglycosides).

Patients with underlying renal impairment, premature infants with immature renal function, and older adults with an age-related decrease in renal function require careful dose adjustments. Renal function may fluctuate over time and should be reassessed periodically.

Hepatic Impairment

The liver is the major organ of drug metabolism. The cytochrome P-450 (CYP450) system changes a drug from a relatively fat-soluble compound to a more water-soluble substance, which means that the drug can then be excreted by the kidneys. Liver function is not as easily quantified as renal function, and it therefore is difficult to predict the correct dose for a patient with hepatic impairment based on laboratory tests.

A patient who is severely jaundiced or who has very low serum proteins (particularly albumin) can be expected to have some problems metabolizing drugs. In advanced liver disease, portal vascular congestion also impairs drug absorption. Examples of drugs that should be carefully dosed in patients with hepatic impairment include theophylline, diuretics, phenytoin, and sedatives. Some drugs (e.g., enalapril, carisoprodol) must be activated in the liver to exert their effect and are known as prodrugs. In patients with hepatic impairment, these drugs may not be converted to the active component, thereby resulting in decreased efficacy.

Heart Failure

Heart failure results in passive congestion of blood vessels in the gastrointestinal tract, which impairs drug absorption. Heart failure also slows drug delivery to the liver, delaying metabolism. Renal function is frequently compromised, adding to delayed elimination and prolonged drug action. Doses of drugs metabolized mainly by the liver or excreted mainly by the kidneys should be decreased in patients with chronic heart failure.

Body Size

Drug dosing is often based on total body weight. However, some drugs selectively penetrate fatty tissues. If the drug does not penetrate fatty tissues (e.g., digoxin, gentamicin), doses for the obese patient should be determined by ideal body weight or estimated lean body mass. Ideal body weight may be determined from tables of optimal weights or may be estimated using formulas for lean body mass when the patient's height and weight are known (Appendix E). If such adjustments are not made, considerable toxicity can result.

Body size is also a factor in patients who are grossly underweight. Older adults, chronic alcoholics, patients with acquired immune deficiency, and patients who are terminally ill from cancer or other debilitating illnesses need careful attention to dosing. Patients who have had a limb amputated also need to have this change in body size considered.

Drug Interactions

Use of multiple drugs, especially those known to interact with other drugs, may necessitate dose adjustments. Drugs highly bound to plasma proteins, such as warfarin and phenytoin, may be displaced by other highly protein-bound drugs. When this phenomenon occurs, the drug that has been displaced exhibits an increase in its activity because the free or unbound drug is thus available to be active.

Some drugs decrease the liver's ability to metabolize other drugs by inhibiting the CYP450 system. Drugs capable of doing this include cimetidine and ketoconazole. Co-administered drugs that are also highly metabolized by the liver may need to be administered in decreased doses. Other agents such as phenobarbital, other barbiturates, and rifampin can stimulate the liver to metabolize drugs more rapidly by inducing the CYP450 system, requiring larger doses to be administered. Co-administered drugs that are also highly metabolized by the liver may need to be administered in higher doses.

Drugs that significantly alter urine pH can affect excretion of drugs for which the excretory process is pH dependent. Alkalinizing the urine will hasten the excretion of acidic drugs. An example of this is administering sodium bicarbonate in cases of aspirin overdose to promote the renal excretion of aspirin. Alkalinizing the urine will increase reabsorption of alkaline drugs, which prolongs and enhances drug action. Acidification of the urine will hasten the excretion of alkaline drugs. Acidification of the urine will also enhance reabsorption of acidic drugs, prolonging and enhancing drug action.

Some drugs compete for enzyme systems with other drugs. Allopurinol inhibits the enzyme involved in uric acid production, but it also inhibits metabolism (inactivation) of 6-mercaptopurine, greatly increasing its toxicity. The dose of mercaptopurine needs to be significantly reduced when co-administered with allopurinol.

The same potential for interactions exists for some foods. Dietary calcium, found in high concentrations in dairy products, combines with tetracycline or fluoroquinolones and prevents their absorption. Foods high in pyridoxine (vitamin B_6) can negate the anti-Parkinsonian effect of levodopa. Grapefruit juice inhibits the enzyme that breaks down some drugs, and concurrent ingestion may significantly increase drug levels and the risk for toxicity.

Many commonly taken natural products interact with pharmaceutical drugs. St. John's wort, garlic, ephedra, and other natural products can interact with medications and cause known or unpredictable reactions.

Nurses and prescribers should consult drug references and remember that the average dosing range for drugs is intended for an average patient. Every patient is an individual with specific drug-handling capabilities. Taking these special dosing considerations into account allows for an individualized drug regimen that promotes the desired therapeutic outcome and minimizes the risk of toxicity.

REFERENCES

1. Burchum, J, Rosenthal, L. (2021). Lehne's Pharmacology for Nursing Care (11th ed.). St. Louis, Missouri: Elsevier.
2. Ziend, CS, Carvalho, MD. (2023). Applied Therapeutics: The clinical use of drugs. (12th ed.). Philadelphia, PA: Lippincott Williams & Wilkins.

The Cytochrome P450 System: What Is It and Why Should I Care?

Looking beyond the obvious takes time, energy, insight, and fortitude; yet this is what we are called to do. We are nurses—tireless care providers. Yet, when the subject of the liver's enzyme system, also called the cytochrome P450 system, is discussed, we feel the urge to run the other way . . . or better yet, to just ignore the conversation. Yet, can we do this as the tireless care provider? The answer to this question is clear and simple: no, we cannot. This is because numerous medications, nutrients, and herbal therapies are metabolized through the cytochrome P450 (CYP450) enzyme system. This system can be inhibited or induced by drugs, and once altered can be clinically significant in the development of drug-drug interactions that may cause unanticipated adverse reactions or therapeutic failures. This article will review the basic concepts of the CYP450 system and relate these concepts to clinically significant altered responses.

The CYP450 enzymes are essential for the production of numerous agents including cholesterol and steroids. Additionally, these enzymes are necessary for the detoxification of foreign chemicals and the metabolism of drugs. CYP450 enzymes are so named because they are bound to membranes within a cell (cyto) and contain a heme pigment (chrome and P) that absorbs light at a wavelength of 450 nm when exposed to carbon monoxide. There are more than 50 CYP450 enzymes, but the CYP1A2, CYP2C19, CYP2D6, CYP1A2, CYP3A4, and CYP3A5 enzymes are responsible for metabolizing 45% of drug metabolism. The CYP2D6 (20–30%), the CYP2C9 (10%), and the CYP2E1 and CYP1A2 (5%) complete this enzyme system.

Drugs that cause CYP450 drug interactions are referred to as either inhibitors or inducers. An inducing agent can increase the rate of another drug's metabolism by as much as two- to threefold that develops over a period of a week. When an inducing agent is prescribed with another medication, the dose of the other medication may need to be adjusted since the rate of metabolism is increased and the effect of the medication reduced. This can lead to a therapeutic failure of the medication. Conversely, if a medication is taken with an agent that inhibits its metabolism, then the drug level can rise and possibly result in a harmful or adverse effect. Information regarding a drug's CYP450 metabolism and its potential for inhibition or induction can be found on the drug label and accessed through the U.S. Food and Drug Administration (FDA) or manufacturer's websites.

When we assess our patients and provide management modalities, these are implemented within a framework of the patient's heritage, race, and culture. This is also true in pharmacology as well (i.e., "pharmacogenetics"). This concept is important to examine since we know that there exists genetic variability, which may influence a patient's response to commonly prescribed drug classes. This genetic variability can be defined as polymorphism. Seven percent of Caucasians and 2–7% of African Americans are poor metabolizers of drugs dependent on CYP2D6, which metabolizes many beta blockers, antidepressants, and opioids. This is because the drug's metabolism via CYP450 enzymes exhibits genetic variability.

Recently, researchers have studied the genetic variability in metabolism among women who were prescribed tamoxifen and medications that inhibit the CYP2D6 enzyme. To review, tamoxifen is biotransformed to the potent antiestrogen, endoxifen, by this enzyme. CYP2D6 genetic variation (individuals considered extensive metabolizers versus poor metabolizers) and inhibitors of the enzyme markedly reduce endoxifen plasma concentrations in tamoxifen-treated patients.

The researchers concluded that CYP2D6 metabolism is an "independent predictor of breast cancer outcome in post-menopausal women receiving tamoxifen for early breast cancer. Determination of CYP2D6 genotype may be of value in selecting adjuvant hormonal therapy and it appears CYP2D6 inhibitors should be avoided in tamoxifen-treated women." Do oncology patients come to us with only their cancer and its treatment? No, they come with multifaceted dimensions and co-morbid conditions such as hypertension, dyslipidemia, depression, seizure disorders, etc. For example, several antidepressants (paroxetine [Paxil] and fluoxetine [Prozac]) are inhibitors of metabolism when given with drugs metabolized through the CYP2D6 enzyme, such as haloperidol

(Haldol), metoprolol (Lopressor), and hydrocodone. Thus, the therapeutic response can be accentuated. Medications that inhibit the CYP3A4 enzyme, such as amiodarone and antifungals, can affect the therapeutic response of fentanyl, alprazolam (Xanax), and numerous statins; as a result, the effect of these drugs can be enhanced leading to potential toxic levels.

At times, these CYP450 inducers and inhibitors are commonly ingested items such as grapefruit juice and tobacco. In the case of grapefruit juice, there are numerous medications known to interact with grapefruit juice including statins, antiarrhythmic agents, immunosuppressive agents, and calcium channel blockers. Furthermore, the inhibition of the enzyme system seems to be dose dependent; thus, the more a patient drinks, the more the inhibition that occurs. Additionally, the effects can last for several days if grapefruit juice is consumed on a regular basis. Luckily, the effect of this is not seen with other citrus juices.

Hopefully, this brief review has opened the door to your inquisitive nature on how the liver's enzyme system is affected by numerous medications and why some patients experience clinically significant unanticipated adverse reactions or therapeutic failures.

CYP1A2		
Substrates	**Inhibitors**	**Inducers**
alosetron, amitriptyline, clozapine, cyclobenzaprine, desipramine, diazepam, duloxetine, fluvoxamine, imipramine, mexiletine, mirtazapine, olanzapine, propranolol, ropinirole, theophylline, warfarin	cimetidine, ciprofloxacin, fluvoxamine, ketoconazole, lidocaine, mexiletine	carbamazepine, cigarette smoke, phenobarbital, rifampin

CYP2C9		
Substrates	**Inhibitors**	**Inducers**
celecoxib, glimepiride, glipizide, losartan, montelukast, nateglinide, phenytoin, voriconazole, (S)-warfarin	amiodarone, efavirenz, fluconazole, fluvastatin, ketoconazole, zafirlukast	carbamazepine, phenobarbital, phenytoin, rifampin

CYP2C19		
Substrates	**Inhibitors**	**Inducers**
citalopram, diazepam, escitalopram, esomeprazole, imipramine, lansoprazole, nelfinavir, omeprazole, pantoprazole, phenytoin, rabeprazole, voriconazole	efavirenz, esomeprazole, fluoxetine, fluvoxamine, lansoprazole, omeprazole, rabeprazole, sertraline,	carbamazepine, phenytoin, rifampin

CYP2D6		
Substrates	**Inhibitors**	**Inducers**
amitriptyline, aripiprazole, atomoxetine, codeine, desipramine, dextromethorphan, duloxetine, flecainide, fluoxetine, haloperidol, imipramine, lidocaine, metoprolol, mexiletine, mirtazapine, nefazodone, nortriptyline, oxycodone, paroxetine, propafenone, propranolol, risperidone, ritonavir, tramadol, venlafaxine	amiodarone, cimetidine, clozapine, desipramine, duloxetine, fluoxetine, haloperidol, lidocaine, methadone, paroxetine, pimozide, quinidine, ritonavir, sertraline, ticlopidine	None

CYP3A

Substrates	Inhibitors	Inducers
alprazolam, amiodarone, aprepitant, aripiprazole, atorvastatin, buspirone, calcium channel blockers, carbamazepine, cilostazol, citalopram, clarithromycin, clonazepam, cyclosporine, dapsone, diazepam, disopyramide, efavirenz, ergot derivatives, erlotinib, erythromycin, escitalopram, estrogens, fentanyl, gefitinib, glucocorticoids, imatinib, indinavir, irinotecan, itraconazole, ketoconazole, lansoprazole, lidocaine, losartan, lovastatin, methadone, midazolam, mirtazapine, montelukast, nateglinide, nefazodone, nelfinavir, nevirapine, ondansetronoxycodone, paclitaxel, pimozide, protease inhibitors, quetiapine, quinidine, repaglinide, rifabutin, sildenafil, simvastatin, sirolimus, sorafenib, sunitinib, tacrolimus, tadalafil, tamoxifen, theophylline, tiagabine, vardenafil, (R)-warfarin, zolpidem, zonisamide	amiodarone, aprepitant, cimetidine, clarithromycin, cyclosporine, diltiazem, efavirenz, erythromycin, fluconazole, grapefruit juice, imatinib, indinavir, itraconazole, ketoconazole, metronidazole, nefazodone, nelfinavir, quinidine, ritonavir, saquinavir, sertraline, verapamil, voriconazole	carbamazepine, efavirenz, nevirapine, phenobarbital, phenytoin, rifabutin, rifampin, St. John's wort

REFERENCES

1. Arcangelo VP, Peterson AM, Wilbur V, Reinhold JA. (2021). *Pharmacotherapeutics for Advanced Practice: A Practical Approach* (5th ed). Philadelphia: Wolters Kluwer.
2. Krau SD. Cytochrome p450, part 1: what nurses really need to know. *Nurs Clin North Am* 2013;48:671–80.
3. Krau SD. Cytochrome p450, part 2: what nurses need to know about the cytochrome p450 family systems. *Nurs Clin North Am* 2013;48:681–96.
4. Krau SD. Cytochrome p450, part 3: drug interactions: essential concepts and considerations. *Nurs Clin North Am* 2013;48:697–706.

Educating Patients About Safe Medication Use

Research has shown that patients need information about several medication-related topics, no matter what the medication. A well-informed patient and/or family can help prevent medication errors by hospital staff and is less likely to make medication errors at home. Adherence to the medication regimen is another goal achieved through patient education.

Before beginning any teaching, however, always assess the patient's current knowledge by asking if he or she is familiar with the medication, how it is taken at home, what precautions or follow-up care is required, and other questions specific to each drug. Based on the patient's current knowledge level and taking into consideration factors such as readiness to learn, environmental and social barriers to learning or adherence, and cultural factors, discuss the following:

1. **Generic and brand names of the medication.** Patients should know both the brand and generic names of each medication for two reasons. It helps them identify their medications when a generic equivalent is substituted for a brand name version, and it prevents patients or health care providers from making sound-alike confusion errors when giving or documenting a medication history. An example of this is saying Celebrex but meaning or hearing Cerebyx.
2. **Purpose of the medication.** Patients have a right to know what the therapeutic benefit of the medication will be but also should be told the consequences of not taking the prescribed medication. This may enhance adherence. For example, a patient may be more likely to take blood pressure medication if told lowering high blood pressure will prevent heart attack, kidney disease, or stroke, rather than saying only that it will lower blood pressure.
3. **Dose and how to take the medication.** To derive benefit and avoid adverse reactions or other poor outcomes, the patient must know how much of the medication to take and when to take it. Refer to doses in metric weight (i.e., milligram, gram) rather than dosage unit (tablet) or volume (1 teaspoon). The patient must also be informed of the best time to take the medication, for example, on an empty or a full stomach, before bedtime, or with or without other medications. If possible, help the patient fit the medication schedule into his or her own schedule, so that taking the medication is not difficult or forgotten.
4. **What to do if a dose is missed.** Always explain to patients what to do if a dose is missed. Patients have reported taking a double dose of medication when a missed dose occurs, putting themselves at risk for side effects and adverse reactions.
5. **Duration of therapy.** It is not uncommon for patients to stop taking a medication when they feel better or to discontinue a medication when they cannot perceive a benefit. For very long term, even lifelong therapy, the patient may need to be reminded that the medication helps maintain the current level of wellness. Patients may need to be reminded to finish short-term courses of medications even though they frequently will feel much better before the prescription runs out. Some medications cannot be discontinued abruptly, and patients should be warned to consult a health care professional before discontinuing such agents. Patients will need to know to refill prescriptions several days before running out or to take extra medication if traveling.
6. **Minor side effects and what to do if they occur.** Inform the patient that all medications have potential side effects. Explain the most common side effects associated with the medication and how to avoid or manage them if they occur. An informed patient is less likely to stop taking a medication because of a minor and potentially avoidable side effect.
7. **Serious side effects and what to do if they occur.** Inform the patient of the possibility of serious side effects. Describe signs and symptoms associated with serious side effects, and tell the patient to immediately inform a health care professional should they occur. Tell the patient to call before the next dose of the medication is scheduled and to not assume that the medication is the source of the symptom and prematurely discontinue it.
8. **Medications to avoid.** Drug-drug interactions can dampen drug effects, enhance drug effects, or cause life-threatening adverse events such as cardiac dysrhythmias, hepatitis, renal failure, or

internal bleeding. The patient and family need to know which other medications, including which over-the-counter medications, to avoid.

9. **Foods to avoid and other precautions.** Food-drug interactions are not uncommon and can have effects similar to drug-drug interactions. Excessive sun exposure resulting in severe dermal reactions is not uncommon and represents an environmental-drug interaction. Likewise, the patient should be informed of what activities to avoid, in case the medication affects alertness or coordination, for example.

10. **How to store the medication:** Medications must be stored properly to maintain potency. Most medications should not be stored in the bathroom medicine cabinet because of excess heat and humidity. In addition, thoughtful storage practices, such as separating two family members' medications, can prevent mix-ups and inadvertent accessibility by children (or pets). Some medications, such as those with potential for abuse, must be kept in a safe/locked container away from children or others. Review storage with patients and ask about current methods for storing medications.

11. **Follow-up care.** Anyone taking medication requires ongoing care to assess effectiveness and appropriateness of medications. Many medications require invasive and noninvasive testing to monitor blood levels; hematopoietic, hepatic, or renal function; or other effects on other body systems. Ongoing medical evaluation may result in dosage adjustments, change in medication, or discontinuation of medication.

12. **What not to take.** Inform patients not to take expired medications or someone else's medication. Warn them not to self-medicate with older, no-longer-used prescriptions even if the remaining supply is not expired. Tell patients to keep a current record of all medications taken and to ask health care providers if new medications are meant to replace a current medication.

As you teach, encourage the patient and the family to ask questions. Providing feedback about medication questions will increase their understanding and help you identify areas that need reinforcement. Also, ask patients to repeat what you have said and return to demonstrate application or administration techniques.

Stress the importance of concurrent therapies. Medications often are only a part of a recommended therapy. Review with the patient and family other measures that will enhance or maintain health. Always consider the cultural context in which health information is provided and plan accordingly. This might include obtaining a same-gender translator or adjusting dosing times to avoid conflict with traditional rituals.

Finally, provide written instructions in a simple and easy-to-read format. Keep in mind that most health care information is written at a 10th grade reading level, while many patients read at a 5th grade level. Tell patients to keep the written instructions, so that they can be reviewed at home, when stress levels are lower and practical difficulties in maintaining the medication plan are known.

Classifications

• ANTI-ALZHEIMER'S AGENTS

Pharmacologic Profile

General Use
Management of Alzheimer's dementia.

General Action and Information
All agents act by ↑ the amount of acetylcholine in the CNS by inhibiting cholinesterase. No agents to date can slow the progression of Alzheimer's dementia. Current agents may temporarily improve cognitive function and therefore improve quality of life.

Contraindications
Hypersensitivity.

Precautions
Use cautiously in patients with a history of "sick sinus syndrome" or other supraventricular cardiac conduction abnormalities (may cause bradycardia). Cholinergic effects may result in adverse GI effects (nausea, vomiting, diarrhea, weight loss) and may also ↑ gastric acid secretion resulting in GI bleeding, especially during concurrent NSAID therapy. Other cholinergic effects may include urinary tract obstruction, seizures, or bronchospasm.

Interactions
Additive effects with other drugs having cholinergic properties. May exaggerate the effects of succinylcholine-type muscle relaxation during anesthesia. May ↓ therapeutic effects of anticholinergics.

Nursing Implications

Assessment
- Assess cognitive function (memory, attention, reasoning, language, ability to perform simple tasks) throughout therapy.
- Monitor heart rate periodically during therapy. May cause bradycardia.

Implementation

Patient/Family Teaching
- Instruct patient and caregiver that medication should be taken as directed.
- Advise patient and caregiver to notify health care professional if nausea, vomiting, diarrhea, or changes in color of stool occur or if new symptoms occur or previously noted symptoms increase in severity.

Evaluation/Desired Outcomes
- Improvement in cognitive function (memory, attention, reasoning, language, ability to perform simple tasks) in patients with Alzheimer's disease.

• ANTIANEMICS

Pharmacologic Profile

General Use
Prevention and treatment of anemias.

General Action and Information
Iron (ferric carboxymaltose, ferric citrate, ferric derisomaltose, ferric maltol, ferric pyrophosphate citrate, ferrous fumarate, ferrous gluconate, ferrous sulfate, ferumoxytol, iron dextran, iron

sucrose, polysaccharide-iron complex, sodium ferric gluconate complex) is required for production of hemoglobin, which is necessary for oxygen transport to cells. Cyanocobalamin and hydroxocobalamin (vitamin B_{12}) and folic acid are water-soluble vitamins that are required for red blood cell production. Darbepoetin, epoetin, and methoxy polyethylene glycol-epoetin beta stimulate production of red blood cells.

Contraindications
Undiagnosed anemias. Hemochromatosis, hemosiderosis, hemolytic anemia (Iron). Uncontrolled hypertension (darbepoetin, epoetin, and methoxy polyethylene glycol-epoetin beta).

Precautions
Use parenteral iron (ferric carboxymaltose, ferric derisomaltose, ferric pyrophosphate citrate, ferumoxytol, iron dextran, iron sucrose, sodium ferric gluconate complex) cautiously in patients with a history of allergy or hypersensitivity reactions.

Interactions
Oral iron can ↓ the absorption of tetracyclines, fluoroquinolones, bisphosphonates, mycophenolate mofetil, levothyroxine, or penicillamine. Concurrent use of proton pump inhibitors, H_2 antagonists, or antacids may ↓ absorption of oral iron. Phenytoin and other anticonvulsants may ↓ the absorption of folic acid.

Nursing Implications
Assessment
- Assess patient's nutritional status and dietary history to determine possible causes for anemia and need for patient teaching.

Implementation
- Iron salts are available in combination with many vitamins and minerals (see Appendix N).
- When administering parenteral iron, assess for hypersensitivity reactions and anaphylaxis (rash, dyspnea, loss of consciousness, hypotension, collapse, convulsions) for at least 30 min following injection. Equipment for resuscitation should be readily available.
- Monitor hemoglobin, hematocrit, serum ferritin, and transferrin saturation prior to and periodically during therapy.

Patient/Family Teaching
- Encourage patients to comply with diet recommendations of health care professional. Explain that the best source of vitamins and minerals is a well-balanced diet with foods from the four basic food groups.
- Patients self-medicating with vitamin and mineral supplements should be cautioned not to exceed RDA. The effectiveness of megadoses for treatment of various medical conditions is unproven and may cause side effects.

Evaluation/Desired Outcomes
- Resolution of anemia.

• ANTIANGINALS

Pharmacologic Profile
General Use
Nitrates are used to treat and prevent attacks of angina. Only nitrates (sublingual, translingual spray, transdermal ointment, or intravenous) may be used in the acute treatment of attacks of angina pectoris. Calcium channel blockers (CCBs), beta blockers, and ranolazine are used prophylactically in long-term management of angina.

General Action and Information
Several different groups of medications are used in the treatment of angina pectoris. The nitrates (isosorbide dinitrate, isosorbide mononitrate, and nitroglycerin) are available as a translingual

spray, sublingual tablets, intravenous solution, transdermal patch, transdermal ointment, and sustained-release oral dosage forms. Nitrates dilate coronary arteries and cause systemic vasodilation (↑ myocardial oxygen supply); they also ↓ myocardial wall tension (↓ myocardial oxygen demand). Dihydropyridine CCBs (e.g., amlodipine, nifedipine) dilate coronary arteries (↑ myocardial oxygen supply) and ↓ contractility and wall tension (↓ myocardial oxygen demand). Nondihydropyridine CCBs (e.g., diltiazem, verapamil) work similar to the dihydropyridine CCBs but also reduce heart rate (↑ myocardial oxygen supply and ↓ myocardial oxygen demand). Beta blockers ↓ heart rate, contractility and wall tension (↓ myocardial oxygen demand). Ranolazine ↓ wall tension and myocardial oxygen consumption (↓ myocardial oxygen demand).

Contraindications
Hypersensitivity. Avoid use of beta blockers and nondihydropyridine CCBs in sick sinus syndrome or 2nd/3rd degree heart block, cardiogenic shock, or decompensated HF. Avoid nitroglycerin in ↑ intracranial pressure and during concurrent use of phosphodiesterase (PDE)-5 inhibitors (avanafil, sildenafil, tadalafil, vardenafil), or riociguat.

Precautions
Beta blockers should be used cautiously in patients with diabetes mellitus or pulmonary disease.

Interactions
Nitrates, CCBs, and beta blockers may cause hypotension with other antihypertensives or acute ingestion of alcohol. Nitrates may also cause significant hypotension with PDE-5 inhibitors or riociguat. Verapamil, diltiazem, and beta blockers may ↑ risk of bradycardia when used with digoxin, ivabradine, or clonidine. Verapamil, diltiazem, and ranolazine have a number of other significant drug-drug interactions.

Nursing Implications

Assessment
- Assess location, duration, intensity, and precipitating factors of patient's anginal pain.
- Monitor BP and heart rate periodically throughout therapy.

Implementation
- Available in various dose forms. See specific drugs for information on administration.

Patient/Family Teaching
- Instruct patient on concurrent nitrate therapy and prophylactic antianginals to continue taking both medications as ordered and to use sublingual/translingual nitroglycerin as needed for anginal attacks.
- Advise patient to contact health care professional immediately if chest pain does not improve; worsens after therapy; is accompanied by diaphoresis or shortness of breath; or if severe, persistent headache occurs.
- Inform patient that headache is a common side effect of nitrates that should decrease with continuing therapy. Aspirin or acetaminophen may be ordered to treat headache.
- Caution patient to make position changes slowly to minimize orthostatic hypotension.
- Advise patient to avoid concurrent use of alcohol with these medications.

Evaluation/Desired Outcomes
- Decrease in frequency and severity of anginal attacks.
- Increase in activity tolerance.

● ANTIANXIETY AGENTS

Pharmacologic Profile

General Use
Antianxiety agents are used in the management of various forms of anxiety, including generalized anxiety disorder. Some agents are more suitable for intermittent or short-term use (benzodiaze-

pines) while others are more useful long-term (buspirone, fluoxetine, paroxetine, sertraline, venlafaxine).

General Action and Information

Most agents cause generalized CNS depression. Benzodiazepines may produce tolerance with long-term use and have potential for psychological or physical dependence. These agents have NO analgesic properties.

Contraindications

Hypersensitivity. Should not be used in comatose patients or in those with pre-existing CNS depression. Should not be used in patients with uncontrolled severe pain. Avoid use during pregnancy or lactation.

Precautions

Use cautiously in patients with hepatic impairment, severe renal impairment, or severe underlying pulmonary disease (benzodiazepines only). Use with caution in patients who may be suicidal or who may have had previous drug addictions. Patients may be more sensitive to CNS depressant effects; dosage ↓ may be required.

Interactions

Mainly for benzodiazepines; additive CNS depression with alcohol, antihistamines, some antidepressants, opioid analgesics, or phenothiazines may occur. Most agents should not be used with MAO inhibitors.

Nursing Implications

Assessment

- Monitor BP, heart rate, and respiratory status frequently throughout IV administration.
- Prolonged high-dose therapy may lead to psychological or physical dependence. Restrict the amount of drug available to patient, especially if patient is depressed, suicidal, or has a history of addiction.
- Assess degree of anxiety and level of sedation (ataxia, dizziness, slurred speech) before and periodically throughout therapy.

Implementation

- Patients changing to buspirone from other antianxiety agents should receive gradually ↓ doses. Buspirone will not prevent withdrawal symptoms.

Patient/Family Teaching

- May cause daytime drowsiness. Caution patient to avoid driving and other activities requiring alertness until response to medication is known.
- Advise patient to avoid the use of alcohol and other CNS depressants concurrently with these medications.
- Advise patient to inform health care professional if pregnancy is planned or suspected.

Evaluation/Desired Outcomes

- Decrease in anxiety level.

• ANTIARRHYTHMICS

Pharmacologic Profile

General Use

Suppression of cardiac arrhythmias.

General Action and Information

Correct cardiac arrhythmias by a variety of mechanisms, depending on the group used. The therapeutic goal is ↓ symptomatology and ↑ hemodynamic performance. Choice of agent depends on etiology of arrhythmia and individual patient characteristics. Treatable causes of arrhythmias should be corrected before therapy is initiated (e.g., electrolyte disturbances, other drugs). Anti-arrhythmics are generally classified by their effects on cardiac conduction tissue (see the following table). Adenosine, atropine, and digoxin are also used as antiarrhythmics.

MECHANISM OF ACTION OF MAJOR ANTIARRHYTHMIC DRUGS

CLASS	DRUGS	MECHANISM
IA	quinidine, procainamide, disopyramide	Na channel blockers, ↑ APD and ERP, ↓ membrane responsiveness
IB	lidocaine, phenytoin, mexiletine	Na channel blockers, ↓ APD and ERP
IC	flecainide, propafenone	Profound slowing of conduction by blocking Na channels; propafenone also has beta-blocking properties
II	esmolol, propranolol, metoprolol	Beta-blockers; ↓ AV nodal conduction, ↓ automaticity
III	amiodarone, dofetilide, dronedarone, ibutilide, sotalol	K channel blockers; amiodarone and dronedarone also have Na channel, beta-receptor, and Ca-channel blocking properties; sotalol also has beta-blocking properties
IV	diltiazem, verapamil	Non-dihydropyridine Ca channel blockers; ↓ AV nodal conduction

APD = action-potential duration; AV = atrioventricular; Ca = calcium; ERP = effective refractory period; K = potassium; Na = sodium.

Contraindications
Differ greatly among various agents. See individual drugs.

Precautions
Differ greatly among agents used. Appropriate dosage adjustments should be made in elderly patients and those with renal or hepatic impairment, depending on agent chosen. Correctable causes (electrolyte abnormalities, drug toxicity) should be evaluated. See individual drugs.

Interactions
Differ greatly among agents used. See individual drugs.

Nursing Implications

Assessment
- Monitor ECG, heart rate, and BP continuously throughout IV administration and periodically throughout oral administration.

Implementation
- Take heart rate before administration of oral doses. Withhold dose and notify physician or other health care professional if heart rate is <50 bpm.

Patient/Family Teaching
- Instruct patient to take oral doses around the clock, as directed, even if feeling better.
- Instruct patient or family member on how to take pulse. Advise patient to report changes in pulse rate or rhythm to health care professional.
- Caution patient to avoid taking OTC medications without consulting health care professional.
- Advise patient to carry identification describing disease process and medication regimen at all times.
- Emphasize the importance of follow-up exams to monitor progress.

Evaluation/Desired Outcomes
- Resolution of cardiac arrhythmias without detrimental side effects.

● ANTIASTHMATICS

Pharmacologic Profile

General Use
Management of acute and chronic episodes of reversible bronchoconstriction. Goal of therapy is to treat acute attacks (short-term control) and to ↓ incidence and intensity of future attacks

(long-term control). The choice of modalities depends on the continued requirement for short term control agents.

General Action and Information

Adrenergic bronchodilators and phosphodiesterase inhibitors both work by ↑ intracellular levels of cyclic-3', 5'-adenosine monophosphate (cAMP), which produces bronchodilation; adrenergics by ↑ production and phosphodiesterase inhibitors by ↓ breakdown of cAMP. Corticosteroids act by ↓ airway inflammation. Anticholinergics (ipratropium) produce bronchodilation by ↓ intracellular levels of cyclic guanosine monophosphate (cGMP). Leukotriene receptor antagonists and mast cell stabilizers ↓ the release of substances that can contribute to bronchospasm.

Contraindications

Inhaled corticosteroids, long-acting adrenergic agents, and mast cell stabilizers should not be used during acute attacks of asthma.

Precautions

Adrenergic bronchodilators and anticholinergics should be used cautiously in patients with cardiovascular disease. Chronic use of systemic corticosteroids should be avoided in children or during pregnancy or lactation. Patients with diabetes may experience loss of glycemic control during corticosteroid therapy. Corticosteroids should never be abruptly discontinued.

Interactions

Adrenergic bronchodilators and phosphodiesterase inhibitors may have additive CNS and cardiovascular effects with other adrenergic agents. Corticosteroids may ↓ the effectiveness of antidiabetics. Corticosteroids may cause hypokalemia, which may be additive with potassium-losing diuretics and may also ↑ the risk of digoxin toxicity.

Nursing Implications

Assessment

- Assess lung sounds and respiratory function prior to and periodically throughout therapy.
- Assess cardiovascular status of patients taking adrenergic bronchodilators or anticholinergics. Monitor for ECG changes and chest pain.

Implementation

- **Inhaln:** Shake inhaler well, and allow at least 1 min between inhalations of aerosol medication. Prime the inhaler before first use. Use of spacer recommended for children.

Patient/Family Teaching

- Instruct patient to take antiasthmatics as directed. Do not take more than prescribed or discontinue without discussing with health care professional.
- Advise patient to avoid smoking and other respiratory irritants.
- Instruct patient in correct use of metered-dose inhaler or other administration devices (see Appendix C).
- Advise patient to contact health care professional promptly if the usual dose of medication fails to produce the desired results, if symptoms worsen after treatment, or if toxic effects occur.
- Patients using inhalation medications and bronchodilators should be advised to use the bronchodilator first and allow 5 min to elapse before administering other medications, unless otherwise directed by health care professional.

Evaluation/Desired Outcomes

- Prevention of and reduction in symptoms of asthma.

• ANTICHOLINERGICS

Pharmacologic Profile

General Use

Atropine: Bradyarrhythmias; also used as ophthalmic mydriatic. **Ipratropium:** bronchospasm (inhalation) and rhinorrhea (intranasal). **Scopolamine:** Nausea and vomiting related to motion sickness and vertigo. **Glycopyrrolate:** Inhibits salivation and excessive respiratory secretions. **Benztropine and trihexyphenidyl:** Parkinson's disease; also used to manage drug-induced extrapyramidal effects. **Darifenacin, fesoterodine, oxybutynin, solifenacin, and tolterodine:** Overactive bladder.

General Action and Information

Competitively inhibit the action of acetylcholine. In addition, atropine, glycopyrrolate, and scopolamine are antimuscarinic in that they inhibit the action of acetylcholine at sites innervated by postganglionic cholinergic nerves.

Contraindications

Hypersensitivity, narrow-angle glaucoma, severe hemorrhage, tachycardia (due to thyrotoxicosis or cardiac insufficiency), or myasthenia gravis.

Precautions

Older adults and pediatric patients are more susceptible to adverse effects. Use cautiously in patients with urinary tract pathology; those at risk for GI obstruction; and those with chronic renal, hepatic, pulmonary, or cardiac disease.

Interactions

Additive anticholinergic effects (dry mouth, dry eyes, blurred vision, constipation) with other agents possessing anticholinergic activity, including antihistamines, antidepressants, quinidine, and disopyramide. May alter GI absorption of other drugs by inhibiting GI motility and ↑ transit time. Antacids may ↓ absorption of orally administered anticholinergics.

Nursing Implications

Assessment

- Assess vital signs and ECG frequently during IV drug therapy. Report any significant changes in heart rate or BP promptly.
- Monitor intake and output ratios in older adults or surgical patients; may cause urinary retention.
- Assess patient regularly for abdominal distention and auscultate for bowel sounds. Constipation may become a problem. Increasing fluids and adding bulk to the diet may help alleviate constipation.

Implementation

- **PO:** Administer oral doses of glycopyrrolate or scopolamine 30 min before meals.
- Scopolamine transdermal patch should be applied at least 4 hr before travel.

Patient/Family Teaching

- Instruct patient that frequent rinses, sugarless gum or candy, and good oral hygiene may help relieve dry mouth.
- May cause drowsiness. Caution patient to avoid driving or other activities requiring alertness until response to medication is known.
- **Ophth:** Advise patients that ophthalmic preparations may temporarily blur vision and impair ability to judge distances. Dark glasses may be needed to protect eyes from bright light.

Evaluation/Desired Outcomes

- Increase in heart rate.
- Decrease in nausea and vomiting related to motion sickness or vertigo.

C
L
A
S
S
I
F
I
C
A
T
I
O
N
S

- Dryness of mouth.
- Dilation of pupils.
- Decrease in GI motility.
- Resolution of signs and symptoms of Parkinson's disease.
- Decreased urinary frequency, urgency, and urge incontinence.

• ANTICOAGULANTS

Pharmacologic Profile

General Use

Prevention and treatment of thromboembolic disorders including deep vein thrombosis (DVT), pulmonary embolism (PE), and atrial fibrillation (AF)-induced stroke and systemic thromboembolism. Also used in the management of myocardial infarction (MI) sequentially or in combination with thrombolytics and/or antiplatelet agents.

General Action and Information

Anticoagulants are used to prevent clot extension and formation. They do not dissolve clots. The main types of anticoagulants in common use are parenteral heparins, oral warfarin, oral/parenteral direct thrombin inhibitors, and oral/parenteral factor Xa inhibitors. When initiating warfarin, unfractionated heparin or a low-molecular weight heparin is usually administered concomitantly initially since warfarin takes several days to produce therapeutic anticoagulation. Once a therapeutic anticoagulant effect is achieved with warfarin, the unfractionated heparin or low-molecular weight heparin will be discontinued. Unfractionated heparin (at lower doses), a low-molecular weight heparin (at lower doses), or fondaparinux are mostly used to prevent DVT after certain surgical procedures or situations in which prolonged bedrest increases the risk of thromboembolism. Argatroban is used to provide anticoagulation in patients who have developed thrombocytopenia during heparin therapy. Apixaban, dabigatran, edoxaban, and rivaroxaban are used to reduce the risk of stroke/systemic embolism associated with nonvalvular atrial fibrillation and to treat/prevent the recurrent of DVT and PE.

Contraindications

Underlying coagulation disorders, ulcer disease, malignancy, recent surgery, or active bleeding.

Precautions

Anticoagulation should be undertaken cautiously in any patient with a potential site for bleeding. Pregnant or lactating patients should not receive warfarin. Heparin does not cross the placenta. All anticoagulants should be used cautiously in patients receiving epidural analgesia.

Interactions

Warfarin is highly protein bound and may displace or be displaced by other highly protein-bound drugs. The resultant interactions depend on which drug is displaced. Bleeding may be potentiated by aspirin or large doses of penicillins or penicillin-like drugs, cefotetan, cefoperazone, valproic acid, or NSAIDs. Apixaban, dabigatran, edoxaban, and rivaroxaban have a number of other significant drug-drug interactions. See individual drugs.

Nursing Implications

Assessment

- Assess patient taking anticoagulants for signs of bleeding and hemorrhage (bleeding gums; nosebleed; unusual bruising; tarry, black stools; hematuria; fall in hematocrit or BP; guaiac-positive stools; urine; or nasogastric aspirate).
- Assess patient for evidence of additional or increased thrombosis. Symptoms will depend on area of involvement.
- **Lab Test Considerations:** Monitor prothrombin time (PT) or international normalized ratio (INR) with warfarin therapy, activated partial thromboplastin time (aPTT) with full-dose heparin therapy and hematocrit frequently during therapy.

- **Toxicity and Overdose:** If overdose occurs or anticoagulation needs to be immediately reversed, the antidote for heparins is protamine sulfate; for warfarin, the antidote is vitamin K (phytonadione); for dabigatran, the antidote is idarucizumab; for rivaroxaban and apixaban, the antidote is andexanet alfa. Administration of fresh frozen plasma or prothrombin complex concentrate may also be required in severe bleeding due to warfarin, the oral direct thrombin inhibitors, or the oral factor Xa inhibitors.

Implementation
- Inform all health care professionals caring for patient of anticoagulant therapy. Venipunctures and injection sites require application of pressure to prevent bleeding or hematoma formation.
- Use an infusion pump with continuous infusions to ensure accurate dosage.

Patient/Family Teaching
- Caution patient to avoid activities leading to injury, to use a soft toothbrush and electric razor, and to report any symptoms of unusual bleeding or bruising to health care professional immediately.
- Instruct patient not to take OTC medications, especially those containing aspirin, NSAIDs, or alcohol, without advice of health care professional.
- Review foods high in vitamin K (see Appendix J) with patients on warfarin. Patient should have consistent limited intake of these foods, as vitamin K is the antidote for warfarin and greatly alternating intake of these foods will cause the INR to fluctuate.
- Emphasize the importance of frequent lab tests to monitor the degree of anticoagulation with unfractionated heparin or warfarin.
- Instruct patient to carry identification describing medication regimen at all times and to inform all health care professionals caring for patient of anticoagulant therapy before laboratory tests, treatment, or surgery.

Evaluation/Desired Outcomes
- Prevention of undesired clotting and its sequelae without signs of hemorrhage. Prevention of stroke, MI, and death in patients at risk.

• ANTICONVULSANTS
Pharmacologic Profile
General Use
Anticonvulsants are used to ↓ the incidence and severity of seizures due to various etiologies. Some anticonvulsants are used parenterally in the immediate treatment of seizures. It is not uncommon for patients to require more than one anticonvulsant to control seizures on a long-term basis. Several anticonvulsants are evaluated with serum level monitoring. Several anticonvulsants also are used to treat neuropathic pain.

General Action and Information
Anticonvulsants include a variety of agents, all capable of depressing abnormal neuronal discharges in the CNS that may result in seizures. They may work by preventing the spread of seizure activity, depressing the motor cortex, raising seizure threshold, or altering levels of neurotransmitters, depending on the group. See individual drugs.

Contraindications
Previous hypersensitivity.

Precautions
Use cautiously in patients with severe hepatic or renal impairment; dose adjustment may be required. Choose agents carefully in pregnant and lactating women. Fetal hydantoin syndrome may occur in offspring of patients who receive phenytoin during pregnancy.

Interactions

Barbiturates stimulate the metabolism of other drugs that are metabolized by the liver, ↓ their effectiveness. Phenytoin is highly protein-bound and may displace or be displaced by other highly protein-bound drugs. Lamotrigine, tiagabine, and topiramate are capable of interacting with several other anticonvulsants. Many drugs are capable of lowering seizure threshold and may ↓ the effectiveness of anticonvulsants, including tricyclic antidepressants and phenothiazines. For more specific interactions, see individual drugs.

Nursing Implications

Assessment

- Assess location, duration, and characteristics of seizure activity.
- **Toxicity and Overdose:** Monitor serum drug levels routinely throughout anticonvulsant therapy, especially when adding or discontinuing other medications.

Implementation

- Administer anticonvulsants around the clock. Abrupt discontinuation may precipitate status epilepticus.
- Implement seizure precautions.

Patient/Family Teaching

- Instruct patient to take medication every day, exactly as directed.
- May cause drowsiness. Caution patient to avoid driving or other activities requiring alertness until response to medication is known. Do not resume driving until physician gives clearance based on control of seizures.
- Advise patient to avoid taking alcohol or other CNS depressants concurrently with these medications.
- Advise patient to carry identification describing disease process and medication regimen at all times.

Evaluation/Desired Outcomes

- Decrease or cessation of seizures without excessive sedation.
- Decreased neuropathic pain.

• ANTIDEPRESSANTS

Pharmacologic Profile

General Use

Used in the treatment of various forms of endogenous depression, often in conjunction with psychotherapy. Other uses include: Treatment of anxiety (duloxetine, fluoxetine, paroxetine, sertraline, venlafaxine); Enuresis (imipramine); Neuropathic pain (amitriptyline, duloxetine, imipramine, nortriptyline); Smoking cessation (bupropion); Bulimia (fluoxetine); Obsessive-compulsive disorder (fluoxetine, fluvoxamine, paroxetine, sertraline); Social anxiety disorder (paroxetine, sertraline, venlafaxine).

General Action and Information

Antidepressant activity is most likely due to preventing the reuptake of dopamine, norepinephrine, and serotonin by presynaptic neurons, resulting in accumulation of these neurotransmitters. The major classes of antidepressants are the tricyclic antidepressants (TCAs), the selective serotonin reuptake inhibitors (SSRIs), and the serotonin/norepinephrine reuptake inhibitors (SNRIs). Most TCAs (amitriptyline, amoxapine, desipramine, doxepin, imipramine, nortriptyline, trimipramine) possess significant anticholinergic and sedative properties, which explains many of their side effects. The SSRIs (citalopram, escitalopram, fluoxetine, paroxetine, sertraline, vortioxetine, vilazodone) are more likely to cause insomnia. The SNRIs include desvenlafaxine, duloxetine, levomilnacipran, milnacipran, and venlafaxine. Bupropion works by inhibiting the uptake of norepinephrine and dopamine.

Contraindications

Hypersensitivity. Should not be used in narrow-angle glaucoma, pregnancy/lactation, or immediately after MI.

Precautions

Use cautiously in older adults and those with pre-existing cardiovascular disease. Men with prostatic enlargement may be more susceptible to urinary retention. Anticholinergic side effects of TCAs (dry eyes, dry mouth, blurred vision, and constipation) may require dosage modification or drug discontinuation. Dosage requires slow titration; onset of therapeutic response may be 2−4 wk. May ↓ seizure threshold, especially bupropion.

Interactions

TCAs: May cause hypertension, tachycardia, and seizures when used with MAO inhibitors or MAO-inhibitor-like drugs. May prevent therapeutic response to some antihypertensives. Additive CNS depression with other CNS depressants. Sympathomimetic activity may be enhanced when used with other sympathomimetics. Additive anticholinergic effects with other drugs possessing anticholinergic properties. **SSRIs/SNRIs:** May cause hypertension, tachycardia, and seizures when used with MAO inhibitors or MAO-inhibitor-like drugs. May ↑ risk of serotonin syndrome when used with other drugs with serotonergic properties. These drugs have a number of other significant drug-drug interactions. See individual drugs.

Nursing Implications

Assessment

- Monitor mental status and affect. Assess for suicidal tendencies, especially during early therapy. Restrict amount of drug available to patient.

Implementation

- Administer drugs that are sedating at bedtime to avoid excessive drowsiness during waking hours, and administer drugs that cause insomnia in the morning.

Patient/Family Teaching

- Caution patient to avoid alcohol and other CNS depressants.
- Inform patient that dizziness or drowsiness may occur. Caution patient to avoid driving and other activities requiring alertness until response to the drug is known.
- Caution patient to make position changes slowly to minimize orthostatic hypotension.
- Advise patient to notify health care professional if dry mouth, urinary retention, or constipation occurs. Frequent rinses, good oral hygiene, and sugarless candy or gum may diminish dry mouth. An increase in fluid intake, fiber, and exercise may prevent constipation.
- Advise patient to notify health care professional of medication regimen and any herbal alternative therapies before treatment or surgery.
- Emphasize the importance of participation in psychotherapy and follow-up exams to evaluate progress.

Evaluation/Desired Outcomes

- Resolution of depression.
- Decrease in anxiety.
- Control of bedwetting in children over 6 yr of age.
- Management of chronic neuropathic pain.

● ANTIDIABETICS

Pharmacologic Profile

General Use

Insulin is used in the management of type 1 diabetes mellitus (DM). It may also be used in type 2 DM when diet and/or oral medications fail to adequately control blood sugar. The choice of insulin preparation (rapid-acting, intermediate-acting, long-acting) depends on the degree of control desired, daily blood glucose fluctuations, and history of previous reactions. Oral agents and non-insulin injectable agents are used primarily in type 2 DM. Oral agents are used when diet therapy alone fails to control blood glucose or symptoms or when patients are not amenable to using insulin or another injectable agent. Some oral agents may be used with insulin.

General Action and Information

Insulin, a hormone produced by the pancreas, lowers blood glucose by ↑ transport of glucose into cells and promotes the conversion of glucose to glycogen. It also promotes the conversion of amino acids to proteins in muscle, stimulates triglyceride formation, and inhibits the release of free fatty acids. Sulfonylureas, nateglinide, repaglinide, the dipeptidyl peptidase 4 (DPP-4) inhibitors (e.g., sitagliptin), and the glucagon-like peptide-1 (GLP-1) receptor agonists (e.g., semaglutide) ↓ blood glucose by stimulating endogenous insulin secretion by beta cells of the pancreas and by ↑ sensitivity to insulin at intracellular receptor sites. Intact pancreatic function is required. Acarbose and miglitol delay digestion of ingested carbohydrates, thus ↓ blood glucose, especially after meals. The thiazolidinediones (e.g., pioglitazone) and metformin ↑ insulin sensitivity. The sodium-glucose transporter 2 (SGLT2) inhibitors (e.g., empagliflozin) inhibit the reabsorption of glucose in the proximal renal tubule, thereby ↑ the excretion of glucose in the urine.

Contraindications

Insulin: Hypoglycemia. **Oral hypoglycemic agents:** Hypersensitivity (cross-sensitivity with other sulfonylureas and sulfonamides may exist). Hypoglycemia. Type 1 DM. Avoid use in patients with severe kidney, liver, thyroid, and other endocrine dysfunction. Should not be used in pregnancy or lactation. **DPP-4 inhibitors:** Type 1 DM. **GLP-1 agonists:** Personal or family history of medullary thyroid carcinoma. Multiple Endocrine Neoplasia syndrome type 2. Type 1 DM. **SGLT2 inhibitors:** Severe renal impairment. Type 1 DM.

Precautions

Insulin: Infection, stress, or changes in diet may alter requirements. **Oral hypoglycemic agents:** Use cautiously in older adults; dose ↓ may be necessary. Infection, stress, or changes in diet may alter requirements. Use sulfonylureas with caution in patients with a history of cardiovascular disease. Metformin may cause lactic acidosis. **DPP-4 inhibitors:** Use cautiously in patients with renal impairment, history of pancreatitis, or history of angioedema to another DPP-4 inhibitor. **GLP-1 agonists:** Use cautiously in patients with a history of pancreatitis, diabetic retinopathy, or history of angioedema to another GLP-1 agonist. **SGLT2 inhibitors:** Moderate renal impairment or use of loop diuretics may ↑ risk of hypotension and hypovolemia. History of pancreatitis, pancreatic surgery, reduced caloric intake due to illness or surgery, surgical procedures, or alcohol abuse may ↑ risk of ketoacidosis.

Interactions

Insulin: Additive hypoglycemic effects with oral hypoglycemic agents. **Oral hypoglycemic agents:** Ingestion of alcohol with sulfonylureas may result in disulfiram-like reaction with some agents. Alcohol, corticosteroids, rifampin, glucagon, and thiazide and loop diuretics may ↓ effectiveness. Anabolic steroids, chloramphenicol, MAO inhibitors, most NSAIDs, salicylates, sulfonamides, and warfarin may ↑ hypoglycemic effect. Beta blockers may produce hypoglycemia and mask signs and symptoms of hypoglycemia. **DPP-4 inhibitors:** Use with insulin or sulfonylureas may ↑ hypoglycemic effect. **GLP-1 agonists:** Use with insulin or sulfonylureas may ↑ hypoglycemic effect. **SGLT2 inhibitors:** Use with insulin or sulfonylureas may ↑ hypoglycemic effect. NSAIDs, diuretics, ACE inhibitors, or ARBs may ↑ risk of acute kidney injury.

Nursing Implications

Assessment

- Observe patient for signs and symptoms of hypoglycemic reactions.
- Metformin, acarbose, miglitol, and pioglitazone do not cause hypoglycemia when taken alone but may ↑ the hypoglycemic effect of other hypoglycemic agents.

- Patients who have been well controlled on metformin but develop illness or laboratory abnormalities should be assessed for ketoacidosis or lactic acidosis. Assess serum electrolytes, renal function, ketones, glucose, and, if indicated, blood pH and lactate and pyruvate levels. If either form of acidosis is present, discontinue metformin immediately and treat acidosis.
- **Lab Test Considerations:** Serum glucose and A1c should be monitored periodically throughout therapy to evaluate effectiveness of treatment.

Implementation

- Patients stabilized on a treatment regimen who are exposed to stress, fever, trauma, infection, or surgery may require sliding scale insulin. Withhold oral hypoglycemic agents and reinstitute after resolution of acute illness..
- **Insulin:** Available in different types and strengths and from different species. Check type, species, source, dose, and expiration date with another licensed nurse. Do not interchange insulins without physician's order. Use only insulin syringes to draw up dose. Use only U100 syringes to draw up insulin lispro dose.

Patient/Family Teaching

- Explain to patient that medication controls hyperglycemia but does not cure diabetes. Therapy is long-term.
- Review signs of hypoglycemia and hyperglycemia with patient. If hypoglycemia occurs, advise patient to take a glass of orange juice or 2–3 tsp of sugar, honey, or corn syrup dissolved in water (glucose, not table sugar, if taking miglitol), and notify health care professional.
- Encourage patient to follow prescribed diet, medication, and exercise regimen to prevent hypoglycemic or hyperglycemic episodes.
- Instruct patient in proper testing of serum glucose and ketones.
- Advise patient to notify health care professional if nausea, vomiting, or fever develops; if unable to eat usual diet; or if blood glucose levels are not controlled.
- Advise patient to carry sugar or a form of glucose and identification describing medication regimen at all times.
- Insulin is the recommended method of controlling blood glucose during pregnancy.
- **Insulin:** Instruct patient on proper technique for administration; include type of insulin, equipment (syringe and cartridge pens), storage, and syringe disposal. Discuss the importance of not changing brands of insulin or syringes, selection and rotation of injection sites, and compliance with therapeutic regimen.
- **Sulfonylureas:** Advise patient that concurrent use of alcohol may cause a disulfiram-like reaction (abdominal cramps, nausea, flushing, headache, and hypoglycemia).
- **Metformin:** Explain to patient the risk of lactic acidosis and the potential need for discontinuation of metformin therapy if a severe infection, dehydration, or severe or continuing diarrhea occurs or if medical tests or surgery is required.

Evaluation/Desired Outcomes

- Control of blood glucose levels without the appearance of hypoglycemic or hyperglycemic episodes.

• ANTIDIARRHEALS

Pharmacologic Profile

General Use

For the control and symptomatic relief of acute and chronic nonspecific diarrhea.

General Action and Information

Diphenoxylate/atropine, difenoxin/atropine, and loperamide slow intestinal motility and propulsion. Bismuth subsalicylate affects fluid content of the stool. Bismuth subsalicylate is also used as part of the management of peptic ulcer disease due to *Helicobacter pylori*. Polycarbophil acts as an antidiarrheal by taking on water within the bowel lumen to create a formed stool. Polycarbophil may also be used to treat constipation. Octreotide is used specifically for diarrhea associated with GI endocrine tumors.

Contraindications
Previous hypersensitivity. Severe abdominal pain of unknown cause, especially when associated with fever.

Precautions
Use cautiously in patients with severe liver disease or inflammatory bowel disease. Safety in pregnancy and lactation not established (diphenoxylate/atropine and loperamide). Octreotide may aggravate gallbladder disease.

Interactions
Polycarbophil ↓ the absorption of tetracycline. Octreotide may alter the response to insulin or oral hypoglycemic agents.

Nursing Implications
Assessment
- Assess the frequency and consistency of stools and bowel sounds before and throughout therapy.
- Assess patient's fluid and electrolyte status and skin turgor for dehydration.

Implementation
- Shake liquid preparations before administration.

Patient/Family Teaching
- Instruct patient to notify health care professional if diarrhea persists; or if fever, abdominal pain, or palpitations occur.

Evaluation/Desired Outcomes
- Decrease in diarrhea.

• ANTIEMETICS

Pharmacologic Profile
General Use
Phenothiazines, dolasetron, granisetron, metoclopramide, ondansetron, and palonosetron are used to manage nausea and vomiting of many causes, including surgery, anesthesia, and antineoplastic and radiation therapy. Aprepitant, fosaprepitant, netupitant, and rolapitant are used specifically with emetogenic chemotherapy. Dimenhydrinate, scopolamine, and meclizine are used almost exclusively to prevent motion sickness. Doxylamine/pyridoxine is used exclusively for the treatment of nausea and vomiting during pregnancy that has not responded to conservative management.

General Action and Information
Phenothiazines and doxylamine act on the chemoreceptor trigger zone to inhibit nausea and vomiting. Dimenhydrinate, scopolamine, and meclizine act as antiemetics mainly by diminishing motion sickness. Metoclopramide ↓ nausea and vomiting by its effects on gastric emptying. Dolasetron, granisetron, palonosetron, and ondansetron block the effects of serotonin at 5-HT$_3$ receptor sites. Aprepitant, fosaprepitant, netupitant, and rolapitant act as selective antagonists at substance P/neurokinin 1 receptors in the brain.

Contraindications
Previous hypersensitivity.

Precautions
Use phenothiazines cautiously in children who may have viral illnesses. Use dolasetron, granisetron, palonosetron, and ondansetron with caution in patients with QT interval prolongation.

Interactions

Additive CNS depression with other CNS depressants including antidepressants, antihistamines, opioid analgesics, and sedative/hypnotics. Phenothiazines may produce hypotension when used with antihypertensives, nitrates, or acute ingestion of alcohol. Dolasetron, granisetron, palonosetron, and ondansetron may ↑ the risk of serotonin syndrome when used with other serotonergic agents. Aprepitant, fosaprepitant, netupitant, and rolapitant have numerous drug interactions with CYP450 agents. See individual drugs.

Nursing Implications

Assessment

- Assess nausea, vomiting, bowel sounds, and abdominal pain before and following administration.
- Monitor hydration status and intake and output. Patients with severe nausea and vomiting may require IV fluids in addition to antiemetics.

Implementation

- For prophylactic administration, follow directions for specific drugs so that peak effect corresponds to time of anticipated nausea.

Patient/Family Teaching

- Advise patient and family to use general measures to decrease nausea (begin with sips of liquids and small, nongreasy meals; provide oral hygiene; and remove noxious stimuli from environment).
- May cause drowsiness. Advise patient to call for assistance when ambulating and to avoid driving or other activities requiring alertness until response to medication is known.
- Advise patient to make position changes slowly to minimize orthostatic hypotension.

Evaluation/Desired Outcomes

- Prevention of, or reduction in, nausea and vomiting.

● ANTIFUNGALS

Pharmacologic Profile

General Use

Treatment of fungal infections. Infections of skin or mucous membranes may be treated with topical or vaginal preparations. Deep-seated or systemic infections require oral or parenteral therapy. Lipid-based formulations of amphotericin employ lipid encapsulation technology designed to ↓ nephrotoxicity.

General Action and Information

Kill (fungicidal) or stop growth of (fungistatic) susceptible fungi by affecting the permeability of the fungal cell membrane or protein synthesis within the fungal cell itself.

Contraindications

Previous hypersensitivity.

Precautions

Because most systemic antifungals may have adverse effects on bone marrow function, use cautiously in patients with depressed bone marrow reserve. Amphotericin B commonly causes renal impairment. Fluconazole requires dosage adjustment in the presence of renal impairment. Adverse reactions to fluconazole may be more severe in HIV-positive patients. The IV formulation of voriconazole should be avoided in patients with renal impairment.

Interactions

Differ greatly among various agents. See individual drugs.

Nursing Implications
Assessment
- Assess patient for signs of infection and assess involved areas of skin and mucous membranes before and throughout therapy. Increased skin irritation may indicate need to discontinue medication.

Implementation
- Available in various dosage forms. Refer to specific drugs for directions for administration..
- **Topical:** Consult physician or other health care professional for cleansing technique before applying medication. Wear gloves during application. Do not use occlusive dressings unless specified by physician or other health care professional.

Patient/Family Teaching
- Instruct patient on proper use of medication form.
- Instruct patient to continue medication as directed for full course of therapy, even if feeling better.
- Advise patient to report increased skin irritation or lack of therapeutic response to health care professional.

Evaluation/Desired Outcomes
- Resolution of signs and symptoms of infection. Length of time for complete resolution depends on organism and site of infection. Deep-seated fungal infections may require prolonged therapy (weeks–months). Recurrent fungal infections may be a sign of serious systemic illness.

• ANTIHISTAMINES
Pharmacologic Profile
General Use
Relief of symptoms associated with allergies, including rhinitis, urticaria, and angioedema, and as adjunctive therapy in anaphylactic reactions. Some antihistamines are used to treat motion sickness (dimenhydrinate and meclizine), insomnia (diphenhydramine), and other nonallergic conditions.

General Action and Information
Antihistamines block the effects of histamine at the H_1 receptor. They do not block histamine release, antibody production, or antigen-antibody reactions. Most antihistamines have anticholinergic properties and may cause constipation, dry eyes, dry mouth, and blurred vision. In addition, many antihistamines cause sedation.

Contraindications
Hypersensitivity and angle-closure glaucoma. Should not be used in premature or newborn infants.

Precautions
Older adults may be more susceptible to adverse anticholinergic effects of antihistamines. Use cautiously in patients with pyloric obstruction, prostatic hypertrophy, hyperthyroidism, cardiovascular disease, or severe liver disease. Use cautiously in pregnancy and lactation.

Interactions
Additive sedation when used with other CNS depressants, including alcohol, antidepressants, opioid analgesics, and sedative/hypnotics. MAO inhibitors prolong and intensify the anticholinergic properties of antihistamines.

Nursing Implications
Assessment
- Assess allergy symptoms (rhinitis, conjunctivitis, hives) before and periodically throughout therapy.

- Monitor BP and heart rate before initiating and throughout IV therapy.
- Assess lung sounds and character of bronchial secretions. Maintain fluid intake of 1500–2000 mL/day to decrease viscosity of secretions.
- **Nausea and Vomiting:** Assess degree of nausea and frequency and amount of emesis when administering for nausea and vomiting.
- **Pruritus:** Observe the character, location, and size of affected area when administering for pruritic skin conditions.

Implementation

- When used for prophylaxis of motion sickness, administer at least 30 min and preferably 1–2 hr before exposure to conditions that may precipitate motion sickness.

Patient/Family Teaching

- Inform patient that drowsiness may occur. Avoid driving or other activities requiring alertness until response to drug is known.
- Caution patient to avoid using concurrent alcohol or CNS depressants.
- Advise patient that good oral hygiene, frequent rinsing of mouth with water, and sugarless gum or candy may help relieve dryness of mouth.
- Instruct patient to contact health care professional if symptoms persist.

Evaluation/Desired Outcomes

- Decrease in allergic symptoms.
- Prevention or decreased severity of nausea and vomiting.
- Relief of pruritus.
- Sedation when used as a hypnotic.

• ANTIHYPERTENSIVES

Pharmacologic Profile

General Use

Treatment of hypertension of many causes, most commonly essential hypertension. Parenteral products are used in the treatment of hypertensive emergencies. Oral treatment should be initiated as soon as possible and individualized to ensure adherence and compliance for long-term therapy.

General Action and Information

As a group, the antihypertensives are used to lower BP to a normal level (<130–140 systolic and <80–90 mm Hg diastolic) or to the lowest level tolerated. The goal of antihypertensive therapy is prevention of end-organ damage. Antihypertensives are classified into groups according to their site of action. These include alpha-1 receptor antagonists, centrally-acting alpha-adrenergic agonists; beta blockers; vasodilators; ACE inhibitors; angiotensin II receptor blockers (ARBs); calcium channel blockers; renin inhibitors; and diuretics. Hypertensive emergencies may be managed with parenteral agents, such as nitroglycerin, nitroprusside, nicardipine, or beta blockers (e.g., esmolol, labetalol).

Contraindications

Hypersensitivity to individual agents. Avoid aliskiren in patients with diabetes or moderate to severe renal impairment who are also taking an ACE inhibitor or ARB.

Precautions

Choose agents carefully in pregnancy and during lactation. ACE inhibitors, ARBs, and aliskiren should be avoided during pregnancy. Centrally acting alpha-adrenergic agonists and beta blockers should be used only in patients who are compliant with their medications because abrupt discontinuation of these agents may result in rapid and excessive ↑ in BP (rebound phenomenon). Thiazide and loop diuretics may ↑ the risk of hyperglycemia. Vasodilators may cause tachycardia if used alone and are commonly used in combination with beta blockers. Some antihypertensives (c.g., hydralazine, minoxidil) cause sodium and water retention and are usually combined with a diuretic.

Interactions
Many drugs can negate the therapeutic effectiveness of antihypertensives, including NSAIDs, sympathomimetics, decongestants, appetite suppressants, SNRIs, and MAO inhibitors. Hypokalemia from diuretics may ↑ the risk of digoxin toxicity. Potassium supplements and potassium-sparing diuretics may cause hyperkalemia when used with ACE inhibitors, ARBs, or aliskiren. ACE inhibitors, ARBs, and diuretics may ↑ the risk of lithium toxicity.

Nursing Implications
Assessment
- Monitor BP and heart rate frequently during dosage adjustment and periodically throughout therapy.
- Monitor intake and output ratios and daily weight with use of diuretics.
- Monitor frequency of prescription refills to determine compliance.

Implementation
- Many antihypertensives are available as combination products to enhance compliance (see Appendix N).

Patient/Family Teaching
- Instruct patient to continue taking medication, even if feeling well. Abrupt withdrawal may cause rebound hypertension. Medication controls, but does not cure, hypertension.
- Encourage patient to comply with additional interventions for hypertension (weight reduction, low-sodium diet, regular exercise, discontinuation of smoking, moderation of alcohol consumption, and stress management).
- Instruct patient and family on proper technique for monitoring BP. Advise them to check BP weekly and report significant changes.
- Caution patient to make position changes slowly to minimize orthostatic hypotension. Advise patient that exercise or hot weather may enhance hypotensive effects.
- Advise patient to consult health care professional before taking any OTC medications, especially cold remedies.
- Advise patient to inform health care professional of medication regimen before treatment or surgery.
- Patients taking ACE inhibitors, ARBs, or aliskiren should notify health care professional if pregnancy is planned or suspected.
- Emphasize the importance of follow-up exams to monitor progress.

Evaluation/Desired Outcomes
- Decrease in BP.

• ANTI-INFECTIVES

Pharmacologic Profile
General Use
Treatment and prophylaxis of various bacterial infections. See specific drugs for spectrum and indications. Some infections may require additional surgical intervention and supportive therapy.

General Action and Information
Kill (bactericidal) or inhibit the growth of (bacteriostatic) susceptible pathogenic bacteria. Not active against viruses or fungi. Anti-infectives are subdivided into categories depending on chemical similarities and antimicrobial spectrum.

Contraindications
Known hypersensitivity to individual agents. Cross-sensitivity among related agents may occur.

Precautions
Culture and susceptibility testing are desirable to optimize therapy. Dosage modification may be required in patients with hepatic or renal impairment. Use cautiously in pregnant and lactating women. Prolonged inappropriate use of broad spectrum anti-infective agents may lead to superinfection with fungi or resistant bacteria.

Interactions
Penicillins and aminoglycosides chemically inactivate each other and should not be physically admixed. Erythromycin and clarithromycin may ↓ hepatic metabolism of other drugs. Probenecid ↑ serum levels of penicillins and related compounds. Highly protein-bound anti-infectives such as sulfonamides may displace or be displaced by other highly bound drugs. Fluoroquinolone and tetracycline absorption may be ↓ by antacids, bismuth subsalicylate, calcium, iron salts, sucralfate, and zinc salts.

Nursing Implications

Assessment
- Assess patient for signs and symptoms of infection prior to and throughout therapy.
- Determine previous hypersensitivities in patients receiving penicillins or cephalosporins.
- Obtain specimens for culture and sensitivity prior to initiating therapy. First dose may be given before receiving results.
- Monitor bowel function. Diarrhea, abdominal cramping, fever, and bloody stools should be reported to health care professional promptly as a sign of *Clostridioides difficile*-associated diarrhea.

Implementation
- Most anti-infectives should be administered around the clock to maintain therapeutic serum drug levels.

Patient/Family Teaching
- Instruct patient to continue taking medication around the clock until finished completely, even if feeling better.
- Advise patient to report the signs of superinfection (black, furry overgrowth on the tongue; vaginal itching or discharge; loose or foul-smelling stools) and allergy to health care professional.
- Instruct patient to notify health care professional if fever and diarrhea develop, especially if stool contains pus, blood, or mucus. Advise patient not to treat diarrhea without consulting health care professional.
- Instruct patient to notify health care professional if symptoms do not improve.

Evaluation/Desired Outcomes
- Resolution of the signs and symptoms of infection. Length of time for complete resolution depends on organism and site of infection.

● ANTINEOPLASTICS

Pharmacologic Profile

General Use
Used in the treatment of various solid tumors, lymphomas, and leukemias. Also used in some autoimmune disorders such as rheumatoid arthritis (methotrexate). Often used in combinations to minimize individual toxicities and ↑ response. Chemotherapy may be combined with other treatment modalities such as surgery and radiation therapy. Dosages vary greatly, depending on extent of disease, other agents used, and patient's condition. Some agents (doxorubicin, irinotecan) are available in lipid-based formulations that have less toxicity with greater efficacy.

C
L
A
S
S
I
F
I
C
A
T
I
O
N
S

General Action and Information

Act by many different mechanisms (see the following table). Many affect DNA synthesis or function; others alter immune function or affect hormonal status of sensitive tumors. Action may not be limited to neoplastic cells.

MECHANISM OF ACTION OF SELECTED ANTINEOPLASTICS

MECHANISM OF ACTION	AGENT	EFFECTS ON CELL CYCLE
ALKYLATING AGENTS Cause cross-linking of DNA	busulfan carboplatin chlorambucil cisplatin cyclophosphamide ifosfamide melphalan procarbazine temozolamide	Cell cycle–nonspecific
ANTHRACYCLINES Interfere with DNA and RNA synthesis	daunorubicin doxorubicin epirubicin idarubicin	Cell cycle–nonspecific
ANTITUMOR ANTIBIOTIC Interfere with DNA and RNA synthesis	bleomycin mitomycin mitoxantrone	Cell cycle–nonspecific (except bleomycin)
ANTIMETABOLITES Take the place of normal proteins	cytarabine fluorouracil hydroxyurea methotrexate	Cell cycle–specific, work mostly in S phase (DNA synthesis)
ENZYMES Deplete asparagine	asparaginase pegaspargase	Cell cycle phase–specific
ENZYME INHIBITORS Inhibits topoisomerase	irinotecan topotecan	Cell cycle phase–specific
Inhibits kinase	imatinib	Unknown
HORMONAL AGENTS Alter hormonal status in tumors that are sensitive	bicalutamide flutamide leuprolide megestrol nilutamide tamoxifen testosterone (androgens) triptorelin	Unknown
HORMONAL AGENTS—AROMATASE INHIBITORS Inhibit enzyme responsible for activating estrogen	anastrozole letrozole	Unknown
IMMUNE MODULATORS	aldesleukin alemtuzumab gemtuzumab toremifene trastuzumab	Unknown
PODOPHYLLOTOXIN DERIVATIVES Damages DNA before mitosis	etoposide	Cell cycle phase–specific
TAXOIDS Interrupt interphase and mitosis	docetaxel paclitaxel	Cell cycle phase–specific
VINCA ALKALOIDS Interfere with mitosis	vinblastine vincristine vinorelbine	Cell cycle–specific, work during M phase (mitosis)

Contraindications
Previous bone marrow depression or hypersensitivity. Contraindicated in pregnancy and lactation.

Precautions
Use cautiously in patients with active infections, ↓ bone marrow reserve, radiation therapy, or other debilitating illnesses. Use cautiously in women of reproductive potential.

Interactions
Allopurinol ↓ metabolism of mercaptopurine. Toxicity from methotrexate may be ↑ by other nephrotoxic drugs or larger doses of aspirin or NSAIDs. Bone marrow depression is additive. See individual drugs.

Nursing Implications

Assessment
- Monitor for bone marrow depression. Assess for bleeding (bleeding gums, bruising, petechiae, guaiac stools, urine, and emesis) and avoid IM injections and rectal temperatures if platelet count is low. Apply pressure to venipuncture sites for 10 min. Assess for signs of infection during neutropenia. Anemia may occur. Monitor for ↑ fatigue, dyspnea, and orthostatic hypotension.
- Monitor intake and output ratios, appetite, and nutritional intake. Prophylactic antiemetics may be used. Adjusting diet as tolerated may help maintain fluid and electrolyte balance and nutritional status.
- Monitor IV site carefully and ensure patency. Discontinue infusion immediately if discomfort, erythema along vein, or infiltration occurs. Tissue ulceration and necrosis may result from infiltration.
- Monitor for symptoms of gout (↑ uric acid, joint pain, and edema). Encourage patient to drink at least 2 L of fluid each day. Allopurinol may be given to ↓ uric acid levels. Alkalinization of urine may be ordered to ↑ excretion of uric acid.

Implementation
- Solutions for injection should be prepared in a biologic cabinet. Wear gloves, gown, and mask while handling medication. Discard equipment in designated containers.
- Check dose carefully. Fatalities have resulted from dosing errors.

Patient/Family Teaching
- Caution patient to avoid crowds and persons with known infections. Health care professional should be informed immediately if symptoms of infection occur.
- Instruct patient to report unusual bleeding. Advise patient of thrombocytopenia precautions.
- These drugs may cause gonadal suppression; however, patient should still use birth control, as most antineoplastics are teratogenic. Advise patient to inform health care professional immediately if pregnancy is suspected.
- Discuss with patient the possibility of hair loss. Explore methods of coping.
- Instruct patient to inspect oral mucosa for erythema and ulceration. If ulceration occurs, advise patient to use sponge brush and to rinse mouth with water after eating and drinking. Topical agents may be used if mouth pain interferes with eating. Stomatitis pain may require treatment with opioid analgesics.
- Instruct patient not to receive any vaccinations without advice of health care professional. Antineoplastics may ↓ antibody response and ↑ risk of adverse reactions.
- Advise patient of need for medical follow-up and frequent lab tests.

Evaluation/Desired Outcomes
- Decrease in size and spread of tumor.
- Improvement in hematologic status in patients with leukemia.

**C
L
A
S
S
I
F
I
C
A
T
I
O
N
S**

• ANTIPARKINSON AGENTS

Pharmacologic Profile

General Use
Treatment of Parkinson's disease.

General Action and Information
Drugs used in the treatment of Parkinson's disease and other dyskinesias are aimed at restoring the natural balance of two major neurotransmitters in the CNS: acetylcholine and dopamine. The imbalance is a deficiency in dopamine that results in excessive cholinergic activity. Many of the drugs used are either anticholinergics (benztropine and trihexyphenidyl) or dopaminergic agonists (apomorphine, bromocriptine, levodopa/carbidopa, pramipexole, ropinirole, rotigotine). Entacapone and tolcapone inhibit the enzyme that breaks down levodopa, thereby enhancing its effects. Rasagiline and selegiline are MAO-B inhibitors that lead to ↑ concentrations of dopamine in the CNS.

Contraindications
Anticholinergics should be avoided in patients with angle-closure glaucoma.

Precautions
Use cautiously in patients with severe cardiac disease, pyloric obstruction, or prostatic enlargement.

Interactions
Pyridoxine, MAO inhibitors, benzodiazepines, phenytoin, phenothiazines, and haloperidol may antagonize the effects of levodopa. Agents that antagonize dopamine (phenothiazines, metoclopramide) may ↓ effectiveness of dopamine agonists.

Nursing Implications

Assessment
- Assess parkinsonian and extrapyramidal symptoms (akinesia, rigidity, tremors, pill rolling, mask facies, shuffling gait, muscle spasms, twisting motions, and drooling) before and throughout course of therapy. On-off phenomenon may cause symptoms to appear or improve suddenly.
- Monitor BP frequently during therapy. Instruct patient to remain supine during and for several hr after first dose of bromocriptine, as severe hypotension may occur.

Implementation
- In the carbidopa/levodopa combination, the number following the drug name represents the milligram of each respective drug.

Patient/Family Teaching
- May cause drowsiness or dizziness. Advise patient to avoid driving or other activities that require alertness until response to medication is known.
- Caution patient to make position changes slowly to minimize orthostatic hypotension.
- Instruct patient that frequent rinsing of mouth, good oral hygiene, and sugarless gum or candy may decrease dry mouth. Patient should notify health care professional if dryness persists (saliva substitutes may be used). Also notify the dentist if dryness interferes with use of dentures.
- Advise patient to confer with health care professional before taking OTC medications, especially cold remedies, or drinking alcoholic beverages. Patients receiving levodopa should avoid multivitamins because vitamin B_6 (pyridoxine) may interfere with levodopa's action.
- Caution patient that decreased perspiration may occur. Overheating may occur during hot weather. Patients should remain indoors in an air-conditioned environment during hot weather.
- Advise patient to increase activity, bulk, and fluid in diet to minimize constipating effects of medication.

- Advise patient to notify health care professional if confusion, rash, urinary retention, severe constipation, visual changes, or worsening of parkinsonian symptoms occur.

Evaluation/Desired Outcomes
- Resolution of parkinsonian signs and symptoms
- Resolution of drug-induced extrapyramidal symptoms.

● ANTIPLATELET AGENTS

Pharmacologic Profile

General Use
To treat and prevent thromboembolic events such as stroke and MI.

General Action and Information
Inhibit platelet aggregation and prevent MI or stroke (aspirin, clopidogrel, dipyridamole, ticlopidine, prasugrel, ticagrelor). The glycoprotein IIb/IIIa inhibitors (e.g., eptifibatide, tirofiban) are used in the management of acute coronary syndromes. These agents are often used concurrently/sequentially with anticoagulants and thrombolytics. Cangrelor is used as an adjunct to percutaneous coronary intervention in patients not currently receiving a $P2Y_{12}$ platelet inhibitor (e.g., clopidogrel, ticagrelor, prasugrel) and are not receiving a glycoprotein IIb/IIIa inhibitor.

Contraindications
Hypersensitivity, ulcer disease, active bleeding, and recent surgery.

Precautions
Use cautiously in patients at risk for bleeding (trauma, surgery) or a history of GI bleeding or ulcer disease.

Interactions
Concurrent use with NSAIDs, heparin, thrombolytics, warfarin, dabigatran, rivaroxaban, apixaban, or edoxaban may ↑ the risk of bleeding. All proton pump inhibitors, except pantoprazole, may ↓ the antiplatelet effects of clopidogrel.

Nursing Implications

Assessment
- Assess patient taking antiplatelet agents for symptoms of stroke, peripheral arterial disease, or MI periodically throughout therapy.

Implementation
- Use an infusion pump with continuous infusions to ensure accurate dosage.

Patient/Family Teaching
- Instruct patient to notify health care professional immediately if any bleeding is noted.

Evaluation/Desired Outcomes
- Prevention of stroke, MI, and vascular death in patients at risk.

● ANTIPSYCHOTICS

Pharmacologic Profile

General Use
Treatment of schizophrenia. Use of clozapine is limited to schizophrenia unresponsive to conventional therapy. Selected agents are also used for acute treatment of manic and mixed episodes associated with bipolar I disorder, maintenance treatment of bipolar I disorder, and as adjunctive treatment of depression.

C
L
A
S
S
I
F
I
C
A
T
I
O
N
S

General Action and Information

Block dopamine receptors in the brain; also alter dopamine release and turnover. Peripheral effects include anticholinergic properties and alpha-adrenergic blockade. Typical antipsychotics include the phenothiazines and haloperidol. Atypical antipsychotics may have fewer adverse reactions compared to the typical antipsychotics and include aripiprazole, asenapine, brexpiprazole, cariprazine, clozapine, iloperidone, lumateperone, lurasidone, olanzapine, paliperidone, pimavanserin, quetiapine, risperidone, and ziprasidone. Phenothiazines differ in their ability to produce sedation (greatest with chlorpromazine and thioridazine), extrapyramidal reactions (greatest with prochlorperazine and trifluoperazine), and anticholinergic effects (greatest with chlorpromazine).

Contraindications

Hypersensitivity. Cross-sensitivity may exist among phenothiazines. Should not be used in angle-closure glaucoma. Should not be used in patients who have CNS depression.

Precautions

Use cautiously in patients with symptomatic cardiac disease. Avoid exposure to extremes in temperature. Use cautiously in severely ill or debilitated patients and patients with respiratory insufficiency, diabetes, prostatic hypertrophy, or intestinal obstruction. May ↓ seizure threshold. Clozapine may cause agranulocytosis. Most agents are capable of causing neuroleptic malignant syndrome. Should not be used routinely for anxiety or agitation not related to psychoses.

Interactions

Additive hypotension with acute ingestion of alcohol, antihypertensives, or nitrates. Phenobarbital may ↑ metabolism and ↓ effectiveness. Additive CNS depression with other CNS depressants, including alcohol, antihistamines, antidepressants, opioid analgesics, or sedative/hypnotics. Lithium may ↓ blood levels and effectiveness of phenothiazines. May ↓ the therapeutic response to levodopa. May ↑ the risk of agranulocytosis with antithyroid agents. Many of the atypical antipsychotics have CYP450 interactions. See individual agents.

Nursing Implications

Assessment

- Assess patient's mental status (orientation, mood, behavior) before and periodically throughout therapy.
- Monitor BP (sitting, standing, lying), heart rate, and respiratory rate before and frequently during the period of dosage adjustment.
- Observe patient carefully when administering medication to ensure medication is actually taken and not hoarded.
- Monitor patient for onset of *akathisia*—restlessness or desire to keep moving—and extrapyramidal side effects; *parkinsonian effects*—difficulty speaking or swallowing, loss of balance control, pill rolling, mask-like face, shuffling gait, rigidity, tremors; and *dystonia*—muscle spasms, twisting motions, twitching, inability to move eyes, weakness of arms or legs—every 2 mo during therapy and 8–12 wk after therapy has been discontinued. Parkinsonian effects are more common in older adults and dystonias are more common in younger patients. Notify health care professional if these symptoms occur, as ↓ in dosage or discontinuation of medication may be necessary. Trihexyphenidyl or benztropine may be used to control these symptoms.
- Monitor for *tardive dyskinesia*—uncontrolled rhythmic movement of mouth, face, and extremities; lip smacking or puckering; puffing of cheeks; uncontrolled chewing; rapid or worm-like movements of tongue. Notify health care professional immediately if these symptoms occur; these side effects may be irreversible.
- Monitor for development of *neuroleptic malignant syndrome*—fever, respiratory distress, tachycardia, convulsions, diaphoresis, hypertension or hypotension, pallor, tiredness, severe muscle stiffness, loss of bladder control. Notify health care professional immediately if these symptoms occur.

Implementation

- Keep patient recumbent for at least 30 min following parenteral administration to minimize hypotensive effects.
- **PO:** Administer with **food, milk**, or a full glass of **water** to minimize gastric irritation.

Patient/Family Teaching

- Advise patient to take medication exactly as directed and not to skip doses or double up on missed doses. Abrupt withdrawal may lead to gastritis, nausea, vomiting, dizziness, headache, tachycardia, and insomnia.
- Advise patient to make position changes slowly to minimize orthostatic hypotension.
- Medication may cause drowsiness. Caution patient to avoid driving or other activities requiring alertness until response to the medication is known.
- Caution patient to avoid taking alcohol or other CNS depressants concurrently with this medication.
- Advise patient to use sunscreen and protective clothing when exposed to the sun to prevent photosensitivity reactions. Extremes of temperature should also be avoided, as these drugs impair body temperature regulation.
- Advise patient that ↑ activity, bulk, and fluids in the diet helps minimize the constipating effects of this medication.
- Instruct patient to use frequent mouth rinses, good oral hygiene, and sugarless gum or candy to minimize dry mouth.
- Advise patient to notify health care professional of medication regimen before treatment or surgery.
- Emphasize the importance of routine follow-up exams and continued participation in psychotherapy as indicated.

Evaluation/Desired Outcomes

- Decrease in excitable, paranoic, or withdrawn behavior. Decrease in incidence of mood swings in patients with bipolar disorders. Increase in sense of well-being in patients with depression.

● ANTIRETROVIRALS

Pharmacologic Profile

General Use

The goal of antiretroviral therapy in the management of HIV infection is to improve CD4 cell counts and ↓ viral load. If accomplished, this generally results in slowed progression of the disease, improved quality of life, and ↓ opportunistic infections. Perinatal use of agents also prevents transmission of the virus to the fetus. Postexposure and pre-exposure prophylaxis with certain antiretrovirals is also recommended.

General Action and Information

Because of the rapid emergence of resistance and toxicities of individual agents, HIV infection is almost always managed by a combination of agents. Selections and doses are based on individual toxicities, underlying organ system disease, concurrent drug therapy, and severity of illness.

Contraindications

Hypersensitivity. Because of highly varying toxicities among agents, see individual monographs for more specific information.

Precautions

Many agents require modification for renal impairment. Protease inhibitors may cause hyperglycemia and hyperlipidemia and should be used cautiously in patients with diabetes and patients at increased risk for cardiovascular disease. Hemophiliacs may also be at risk of bleeding when taking protease inhibitors. See individual monographs for specific information.

Interactions

There are many significant and potentially serious drug-drug interactions among the antiretrovirals. Many of these interactions involve the cytochrome P450 system. See individual agents.

Nursing Implications

Assessment

- Assess patient for change in severity of symptoms of HIV and for symptoms of opportunistic infections throughout therapy.
- **Lab Test Considerations:** Monitor viral load and CD4 counts prior to and periodically during therapy.

Implementation

- Administer doses around the clock.

Patient/Family Teaching

- Instruct patient to take medication exactly as directed. Emphasize the importance of complying with therapy, not taking more than prescribed amount, and not discontinuing without consulting health care professional. Missed doses should be taken as soon as remembered unless almost time for next dose; patient should not double doses.
- Inform patient that antiretroviral therapy does not cure HIV and does not ↓ the risk of transmission of HIV to others through sexual contact or blood contamination. Caution patient to use a condom during sexual contact and to avoid sharing needles or donating blood to prevent spreading the HIV virus to others.
- Advise patient to avoid taking any Rx, OTC, or herbal products without consulting health care professional.
- Emphasize the importance of regular follow-up exams and blood counts to determine progress and to monitor for side effects.

Evaluation/Desired Outcomes

- Decrease in viral load and increase in CD4 counts in patients with HIV.

• ANTIRHEUMATICS

Pharmacologic Profile

General Use

Antirheumatics are used to manage symptoms of rheumatoid arthritis (pain, swelling) and in more severe cases to slow down joint destruction and preserve joint function. NSAIDs, aspirin, and other salicylates are used to manage symptoms such as pain and swelling, allowing continued motility and improved quality of life. Corticosteroids are reserved for more advanced swelling and discomfort, primarily because of their ↑ side effects, especially with chronic use. They can be used to control acute flares of disease. Neither NSAIDs nor corticosteroids prevent disease progression or joint destruction. Disease-modifying antirheumatics drugs (DMARDs) slow the progression of rheumatoid arthritis and delay joint destruction. Several months of therapy may be required before benefit is noted and maintained.

General Action and Information

Both NSAIDs and corticosteroids have potent anti-inflammatory properties. DMARDs work by a variety of mechanisms. See individual agents, but most work by suppressing the autoimmune response thought to be responsible for joint destruction.

Contraindications

Hypersensitivity. Patients who are allergic to aspirin should not receive other NSAIDs. Corticosteroids should not be used in patients with active untreated infections. Many DMARDs have immunosuppressive properties and should be avoided in patients for whom immunosuppression poses a serious risk, including patients with active infections, underlying malignancy, and transplant recipients.

Precautions
NSAIDs and corticosteroids should be used cautiously in patients with a history of GI bleeding. Corticosteroids should be used with caution in patients with diabetes.

Interactions
NSAIDs may diminish the response to diuretics and other antihypertensives. Corticosteroids may augment hypokalemia from other medications and ↑ the risk of digoxin toxicity. DMARDs ↑ the risk of serious immunosuppression with other immunosuppressants. Live vaccines should not be given concurrently with DMARDs.

Nursing Implications
Assessment
- Assess patient monthly for pain, swelling, and range of motion.

Implementation
- Most agents require regular administration to obtain maximum effects.

Patient/Family Teaching
- Instruct patient to contact health care professional if no improvement is noticed within a few days.
- Instruct patient to contact health care professional promptly if signs or symptoms of infection develop.

Evaluation/Desired Outcomes
- Improvement in signs and symptoms of rheumatoid arthritis.

• ANTITUBERCULARS

Pharmacologic Profile
General Use
To treat and prevent tuberculosis. Combinations are used in the treatment of active tuberculosis to rapidly ↓ the infectious state and delay or prevent the emergence of resistant strains. In selected situations, intermittent (twice weekly) regimens may be employed. Rifampin is also used in the prevention of meningococcal meningitis and *Haemophilus influenzae* type B and in treatment of *S. aureus* infections (in combination with other antimicrobial agents).

General Action and Information
Kill (tuberculocidal) or inhibit the growth of (tuberculostatic) mycobacteria responsible for causing tuberculosis. Combination therapy with two or more agents is required, unless used as prophylaxis (isoniazid alone).

Contraindications
Hypersensitivity. Severe liver disease.

Precautions
Use cautiously in patients with a history of liver disease or in older adults. Ethambutol requires ophthalmologic follow-up. Compliance is required for optimal response.

Interactions
Isoniazid inhibits the metabolism of phenytoin. Rifampin significantly ↓ levels of many drugs.

Nursing Implications
Assessment
- Mycobacterial studies and susceptibility tests should be performed prior to and periodically throughout therapy to detect possible resistance.
- Assess lung sounds and character and amount of sputum periodically throughout therapy.

Implementation
- Most medications can be administered with food if GI irritation occurs.

C
L
A
S
S
I
F
I
C
A
T
I
O
N
S

Patient/Family Teaching

- Advise patient of the importance of continuing therapy even after symptoms have subsided.
- Emphasize the importance of regular follow-up exams to monitor progress and check for side effects.
- Inform patients taking rifampin that saliva, sputum, sweat, tears, urine, and feces may become red-orange to red-brown and that soft contact lenses may become permanently discolored.

Evaluation/Desired Outcomes
- Resolution of the signs and symptoms of tuberculosis. Negative sputum cultures.

• ANTIULCER AGENTS

Pharmacologic Profile

General Use
Treatment and prophylaxis of peptic ulcer and gastric hypersecretory conditions such as Zollinger-Ellison syndrome. H_2-receptor antagonists and proton pump inhibitors (PPIs) are also used in the management of gastroesophageal reflux disease.

General Action and Information
Because a great majority of peptic ulcer disease may be traced to GI infection with the organism *Helicobacter pylori*, eradication of the organism ↓ symptomatology and recurrence. Anti-infectives with significant activity against the organism include amoxicillin, clarithromycin, metronidazole, and tetracycline. Bismuth also has anti-infective activity against *H. pylori*. *H. pylori* treatment regimens usually include: a PPI, and 2 anti-infectives with or without bismuth subsalicylate for 10–14 days.. Other medications used in the management of gastric/duodenal ulcer disease are aimed at neutralizing gastric acid (antacids), ↓ acid secretion (H_2 antagonists, PPIs, misoprostol), or protecting the ulcer surface from further damage (misoprostol, sucralfate). H_2-receptor antagonists competitively inhibit the action of histamine at the H_2 receptor, located primarily in gastric parietal cells, resulting in inhibition of gastric acid secretion. Misoprostol ↓ gastric acid secretion and ↑ production of protective mucus. PPIs prevent the transport of hydrogen ions into the gastric lumen. Sucralfate forms a forms a protective coating that acts locally to protect the gastric lumen.

Contraindications
Hypersensitivity.

Precautions
Most H_2 antagonists require dose reduction in renal impairment and in older adults. Magnesium-containing antacids should be used cautiously in patients with renal impairment. Misoprostol should be used cautiously in women of reproductive potential. Long-term therapy (>1 yr) with PPIs may be associated with an ↑ risk of hip, wrist, or spine fractures; fundic gland polyps; and vitamin B_{12} deficiency.

Interactions
Calcium- and magnesium-containing antacids ↓ the absorption of tetracycline and fluoroquinolones. Omeprazole ↓ metabolism of phenytoin, diazepam, and warfarin. All agents that ↑ gastric pH will ↓ the absorption of itraconazole, ketoconazole, iron salts, erlotinib, nilotinib, atazanavir, nelfinavir, rilpivirine, and mycophenolate mofetil. All PPIs, except pantoprazole, may ↓ the antiplatelet effects of clopidogrel.

Nursing Implications

Assessment
- Assess patient routinely for epigastric or abdominal pain and frank or occult blood in the stool, emesis, or gastric aspirate.

- **Antacids:** Assess for heartburn and indigestion as well as the location, duration, character, and precipitating factors of gastric pain.
- **H$_2$ Receptor Antagonists:** Assess older adults and severely ill patients for confusion routinely. Notify health care professional promptly should this occur.
- **Misoprostol:** Assess women of reproductive potential for pregnancy. Medication is usually begun on 2nd or 3rd day of menstrual period following a negative serum pregnancy test within 2 wk of beginning therapy.

Implementation

- **Antacids:** Antacids cause premature dissolution and absorption of enteric-coated tablets and may interfere with absorption of other oral medications. Separate administration of antacids and other oral medications by at least 1 hr.
- Shake liquid preparations well before pouring. Follow administration with water to ensure passage to stomach. Liquid and powder dosage forms are considered to be more effective than chewable tablets.
- Chewable tablets must be chewed thoroughly before swallowing. Follow with half a glass of water.
- Administer 1 and 3 hr after meals and at bedtime for maximum antacid effect.
- **Misoprostol:** Administer with meals and at bedtime to reduce the severity of diarrhea.
- **PPIs:** Administer before meals, preferably in the morning. Capsules should be swallowed whole; do not open, crush, or chew.
- May be administered concurrently with antacids.
- **Sucralfate:** Administer on an empty stomach 1 hr before meals and at bedtime. Do not crush or chew tablets. Shake suspension well prior to administration. If nasogastric administration is required, consult pharmacist, as protein-binding properties of sucralfate have resulted in formation of a bezoar when administered with enteral feedings and other medications.

Patient/Family Teaching

- Instruct patient to take medication as directed for the full course of therapy, even if feeling better. If a dose is missed, it should be taken as soon as remembered but not if almost time for next dose. Do not double doses.
- Advise patient to avoid alcohol, products containing aspirin, NSAIDs, and foods that may cause an ↑ in GI irritation.
- Advise patient to report onset of black, tarry stools to health care professional promptly.
- Inform patient that cessation of smoking may help prevent the recurrence of duodenal ulcers.
- **Antacids:** Caution patient to consult health care professional before taking antacids for >2 wk or if problem is recurring. Advise patient to consult health care professional if relief is not obtained or if symptoms of gastric bleeding (black, tarry stools; coffee-ground emesis) occur.
- **Misoprostol:** Inform patient that misoprostol may cause spontaneous abortion. Women of reproductive potential must be informed of this effect through verbal and written information and must use contraception throughout therapy. If pregnancy is suspected, the woman should stop taking misoprostol and immediately notify her health care professional.
- **Sucralfate:** Advise patient that an ↑ in fluid intake, dietary bulk, and exercise may prevent drug-induced constipation.

Evaluation/Desired Outcomes

- Decrease in GI pain and irritation.
- Prevention of gastric irritation and bleeding.
- Decreased symptoms of GERD.
- Prevention of gastric ulcers in patients receiving chronic NSAID therapy (misoprostol only).

C L A S S I F I C A T I O N S

• ANTIVIRALS

Pharmacologic Profile

General Use

Acyclovir, docosanol, famciclovir, penciclovir, and valacyclovir are used in the management of herpes virus infections. Acyclovir and valacyclovir are also used in the management of chickenpox. Baloxavir, oseltamivir, peramivir, and zanamivir are used primarily in the prevention and/or treatment of influenza infection. Cidofovir, foscarnet, ganciclovir, letermovir, maribavir, and valganciclovir are used in the prevention and/or treatment of cytomegalovirus (CMV) infection. Molnupiravir, nirmatrelvir/ritonavir, and remdesivir are used in the treatment of COVID-19 infection.

General Action and Information

Most agents inhibit viral replication.

Contraindications

Previous hypersensitivity.

Precautions

Many antiviral agents require dose adjustment in renal impairment. Acyclovir may cause renal impairment. Acyclovir may cause CNS toxicity. Foscarnet ↑ risk of seizures.

Interactions

Acyclovir may have additive CNS and nephrotoxicity with drugs causing similar adverse reactions. Nirmatrelvir/ritonavir has numerous drug interactions involving the cytochrome P450 system.

Nursing Implications

Assessment

- Assess patient for signs and symptoms of infection before and throughout therapy.
- **Ophth:** Assess eye lesions before and daily during therapy.
- **Topical:** Assess lesions before and daily during therapy.

Implementation

- Most systemic antiviral agents should be administered around the clock to maintain therapeutic serum drug levels.

Patient/Family Teaching

- Instruct patient to continue taking medication around the clock for full course of therapy, even if feeling better.
- Advise patient that antivirals do not prevent transmission to others. Precautions should be taken to prevent spread of virus.
- Instruct patient in correct technique for topical or ophthalmic preparations.
- Instruct patient to notify health care professional if symptoms do not improve.

Evaluation/Desired Outcomes

- Prevention or resolution of the signs and symptoms of viral infection. Length of time for complete resolution depends on organism and site of infection.

• BETA BLOCKERS

Pharmacologic Profile

General Use

Management of hypertension, angina pectoris, tachyarrhythmias, migraine headache (prophylaxis), MI, glaucoma (ophthalmic use), HF (bisoprolol, carvedilol, and metoprolol succinate only) and hyperthyroidism (management of symptoms only).

General Action and Information

Beta blockers compete with adrenergic (sympathetic) neurotransmitters (epinephrine and norepinephrine) for adrenergic receptor sites. Beta$_1$-adrenergic receptor sites are located chiefly in the heart where stimulation results in increased heart rate and myocardial contractility. Beta$_2$-adrenergic receptors are found mainly in bronchial and vascular smooth muscle and the uterus. Stimulation of beta$_2$-adrenergic receptors produces vasodilation, bronchodilation, and uterine relaxation. Beta blockers may be relatively selective for beta$_1$-adrenergic receptors (acebutolol, atenolol, betaxolol, bisoprolol, esmolol, and metoprolol) or nonselective (carvedilol, labetalol, nadolol, pindolol, propranolol, and timolol) blocking both beta$_1$- and beta$_2$-adrenergic receptors. Carvedilol and labetalol have additional alpha-adrenergic blocking properties. Ophthalmic beta blockers ↓ production of aqueous humor.

Contraindications
Decompensated HF, acute bronchospasm, some forms of valvular heart disease, bradycardia, and 2nd/3rd degree heart block.

Precautions
Use cautiously in pregnant and lactating women (may cause fetal bradycardia and hypoglycemia), lung disease, diabetes, or severe liver disease.

Interactions
May cause additive bradycardia when used with other agents having these effects (digoxin, diltiazem, verapamil, clonidine, and ivabradine). May antagonize the therapeutic effects of bronchodilators. May alter the requirements for insulin or hypoglycemic agents in patients with diabetes.

Nursing Implications
Assessment
- Monitor BP and heart rate frequently during dosage adjustment and periodically throughout therapy.
- Monitor intake and output ratios and daily weight. Assess patient routinely for signs and symptoms of HF (dyspnea, rales/crackles, weight gain, peripheral edema, jugular venous distention).
- **Angina:** Assess frequency and severity of episodes of chest pain periodically throughout therapy.
- **Migraine Prophylaxis:** Assess frequency and severity of migraine headaches periodically throughout therapy.

Implementation
- Take apical pulse prior to administering. If heart rate is <50 bpm or if arrhythmias occur, hold medication and notify health care professional.

Patient/Family Teaching
- Instruct patient to continue taking medication, even if feeling well. Abrupt withdrawal may cause life-threatening arrhythmias, hypertension, or myocardial ischemia. Medication controls, but does not cure, hypertension.
- Encourage patient to comply with additional interventions for hypertension (weight reduction, low-sodium diet, regular exercise, smoking cessation, moderation of alcohol consumption, and stress management).
- Instruct patient and family on proper technique for monitoring BP and pulse. Advise them to check BP and pulse weekly and report significant changes to health care professional.
- Caution patient to make position changes slowly to minimize orthostatic hypotension. Advise patient that exercising or hot weather may enhance hypotensive effects.
- Advise patient to consult health care professional before taking any OTC medications or herbal/alternative therapies, especially cold remedies.
- Patients with diabetes should monitor blood glucose closely, especially if weakness, malaise, irritability, or fatigue occurs.
- Advise patient to advise health care professional of medication regimen prior to treatment or surgery.
- **Ophth:** Instruct patient in correct technique for administration of ophthalmic preparations.

Evaluation/Desired Outcomes

- Decrease in BP.
- Decrease in frequency and severity of anginal attacks.
- Control of arrhythmias.
- Prevention of myocardial reinfarction.
- Prevention of migraine headaches.
- Decrease in tremors.
- Lowering of intraocular pressure.

● BONE RESORPTION INHIBITORS

Pharmacologic Profile

General Use

Bone resorption inhibitors are primarily used to treat and prevent osteoporosis in postmenopausal women. Other uses include treatment of osteoporosis due to other causes, including corticosteroid therapy, treatment of Paget's disease of the bone, and management of hypercalcemia.

General Action and Information

Bisphosphonates (alendronate, ibandronate, pamidronate, risedronate, and zoledronic acid) inhibit resorption of bone by inhibiting hydroxyapatite crystal dissolution and osteoclast activity. Raloxifene binds to estrogen receptors, producing estrogen-like effects on bone including ↓ bone resorption and ↓ bone turnover. Denosumab is a monoclonal antibody that binds specifically to the human receptor activator of nuclear factor kappa-B-ligand (RANKL), which is inhibits osteoclast activity. Teriparatide and abaloparatide are analogs of parathyroid hormone and stimulate osteoblastic activity by increasing GI absorption and renal tubular reabsorption of calcium.

Contraindications

Hypersensitivity. Bisphosphonates and denosumab should not be used in patients with hypocalcemia. Bisphosphonates should not be used in patients with abnormalities of the esophagus that delay esophageal emptying. Raloxifene should not be used in women of reproductive potential or a history of thromboembolic disease. Teriparatide and abaloparatide should not be used in Paget's disease of the bone, elevated alkaline phosphatase, bone metastases or skeletal malignancies, prior external beam or implant radiation therapy involving the skeleton, hereditary disorders predisposing to osteosarcoma, hypercalcemia, or primary hyperparathyroidism.

Precautions

Use bisphosphonates cautiously in patients with renal impairment; some agents should be avoided in moderate to severe renal impairment. Invasive dental procedures, cancer, chemotherapy, corticosteroids, angiogenesis inhibitors, poor oral hygiene, diabetes, gingival infections, periodontal disease, dental disease, anemia, coagulopathy, infection, or poorly fitting dentures may ↑ risk of jaw osteonecrosis in patients receiving bisphosphonates or denosumab. Use teriparatide cautiously in patients with autoimmune disease or renal failure because of ↑ risk of calciphylaxis.

Interactions

Calcium supplements ↓ absorption of bisphosphonates. Aspirin and NSAIDs may ↑ GI adverse reactions with bisphosphonates. Corticosteroids and warfarin may ↑ risk of calciphylaxis with teriparatide.

Nursing Implications

Assessment

- Assess patients for low bone density before and periodically during therapy.
- Assess for symptoms of Paget's disease (bone pain, headache, decreased visual and auditory acuity, ↑ skull size).

- For patients receiving denosumab, monitor for signs and symptoms of hypersensitivity reactions (hypotension, dyspnea, upper airway edema, lip swelling, rash, pruritus, urticaria) after administration. Treat symptomatically and discontinue medication if symptoms occur.
- **Lab Test Considerations:** Monitor serum calcium in patients with osteoporosis. Monitor alkaline phosphatase in patients with Paget's disease.

Implementation
- Denosumab, teriparatide, and abaloparatide are administered SUBQ.

Patient/Family Teaching
- Instruct patient to take medication exactly as directed.
- Emphasize the importance of follow-up tests for bone mineral density.
- Discuss the importance of other treatments for osteoporosis (supplemental calcium and/or vitamin D, weight-bearing exercise, modification of behavioral factors such as smoking and/or alcohol consumption).
- Advise patient to take good care of teeth and gums (brush and floss regularly) and to inform health care professional of therapy prior to dental surgery.
- Inform patient of increased risk of fractures upon discontinuation of denosumab. If denosumab is discontinued, consider another bone resorption inhibitor.
- Teriparatide and abaloparatide may cause orthostatic hypotension during first several doses. Caution patient to administer medication in a lying or sitting position. If light-headedness or palpitations occur, lie down until symptoms resolve. Notify health care professional if symptoms persist or worsen.

Evaluation/Desired Outcomes
- Prevention of, or decrease in, the progression of osteoporosis with a reduction in fractures.
- Decrease in the progression of Paget's disease.

• BRONCHODILATORS

Pharmacologic Profile

General Use
Used in the treatment of reversible airway obstruction due to asthma or chronic obstructive pulmonary disease. Rapid-acting inhaled beta-agonist bronchodilators (not salmeterol, formoterol, arformoterol, olodaterol, or vilanterol) should be reserved as acute relievers of bronchospasm; repeated or chronic use indicates the need for additional long-term control agents, including inhaled corticosteroids, mast cell stabilizers, long-acting bronchodilators (oral theophylline, beta$_2$-agonists, or anticholinergics), and leukotriene modifiers (montelukast, zafirlukast).

General Action and Information
Beta$_2$-adrenergic agonists (albuterol, arformoterol, epinephrine, formoterol, levalbuterol, olodaterol, salmeterol, terbutaline, and vilanterol) produce bronchodilation by stimulating the production of cyclic adenosine monophosphate (cAMP). Onset of action allows use in management of acute attacks except for arformoterol, formoterol, olodaterol, salmeterol, and vilanterol, which have delayed onset. Phosphodiesterase inhibitors (aminophylline and theophylline) inhibit the breakdown of cAMP. Aclidinium, glycopyrrolate, ipratropium, revefenacin, tiotropium, and umeclidinium are anticholinergic compounds that produce bronchodilation by blocking the action of acetylcholine in the respiratory tract.

Contraindications
Hypersensitivity to agents or preservatives (bisulfites) used in their formulation. Avoid use in uncontrolled cardiac arrhythmias.

C
L
A
S
S
I
F
I
C
A
T
I
O
N
S

Precautions

Use beta$_2$ agonists cautiously in patients with diabetes, cardiovascular disease, or hyperthyroidism. Use anticholinergic agents cautiously in narrow-angle glaucoma, prostatic hyperplasia, or bladder neck obstruction.

Interactions

Therapeutic effectiveness of beta$_2$ agonists may be antagonized by concurrent use of beta blockers. Beta$_2$ agonists may have additive sympathomimetic effects with other adrenergic drugs, including vasopressors and decongestants. Use of anticholinergic agents with other agents with anticholinergic activity may result in additive anticholinergic effects (dry mouth, dry eyes, blurred vision, constipation).

Nursing Implications

Assessment

- Assess BP, heart rate, respiration, lung sounds, and character of secretions before and throughout therapy.
- Patients with a history of cardiovascular problems should be monitored for ECG changes and chest pain with use of beta$_2$ agonists.

Implementation

- Administer around the clock to maintain therapeutic plasma levels.

Patient/Family Teaching

- Emphasize the importance of taking only the prescribed dose at the prescribed time intervals.
- Encourage the patient to drink adequate liquids (2000 mL/day minimum) to ↓ the viscosity of the airway secretions.
- Advise patient to avoid OTC cough, cold, or breathing preparations without consulting health care professional and to minimize intake of xanthine-containing foods or beverages (colas, coffee, and chocolate), as these may ↑ side effects of theophylline.
- Caution patient to avoid smoking and other respiratory irritants.
- Instruct patient on proper use of metered-dose inhaler (see Appendix C).
- Advise patient to contact health care professional promptly if the usual dose of medication fails to produce the desired results, symptoms worsen after treatment, or toxic effects occur.
- Patients using other inhalation medications and bronchodilators should be advised to use bronchodilator first and allow 5 min to elapse before administering the other medication, unless otherwise directed by health care professional.

Evaluation/Desired Outcomes

- Decreased bronchospasm.
- Increased ease of breathing.

● CALCIUM CHANNEL BLOCKERS

Pharmacologic Profile

General Use

Used in the treatment of hypertension (amlodipine, diltiazem, felodipine, isradipine, nicardipine, nifedipine, nisoldipine, verapamil) or in the treatment and prophylaxis of angina pectoris or coronary artery spasm (amlodipine, diltiazem, felodipine, nicardipine, verapamil). Verapamil and diltiazem are also used as antiarrhythmics. Nimodipine is used to prevent neurologic damage due to certain types of cerebral vasospasm.

General Action and Information

Block calcium entry into cells of vascular smooth muscle and myocardium. Dilate coronary arteries in both normal and ischemic myocardium and inhibit coronary artery spasm. Diltiazem and verapamil also ↓ AV nodal conduction. Nimodipine has a relatively selective effect on cerebral blood vessels.

Contraindications

Hypersensitivity. Contraindicated in bradycardia, 2nd- or 3rd-degree heart block, or decompensated HF (all except for amlodipine and felodipine).

Precautions

Use cautiously in patients with liver disease or uncontrolled arrhythmias.

Interactions

May cause additive bradycardia when used with other agents having these effects (beta blockers, digoxin, clonidine, and ivabradine). Effectiveness may be ↓ by phenobarbital or phenytoin and ↑ by propranolol. Verapamil and diltiazem may ↑ serum digoxin levels and cause toxicity.

Nursing Implications

Assessment

- Monitor BP and heart rate frequently during dosage adjustment and periodically throughout therapy.
- Monitor intake and output ratios and daily weight. Assess patient routinely for signs and symptoms of HF (dyspnea, rales/crackles, weight gain, peripheral edema, jugular venous distention).
- **Angina:** Assess frequency and severity of episodes of chest pain periodically throughout therapy.
- **Arrhythmias:** ECG should be monitored continuously during IV therapy and periodically during long-term therapy with verapamil or diltiazem.
- **Cerebral Vasospasm:** Assess patient's neurological status (level of consciousness, movement) before and periodically during therapy with nimodipine.

Implementation

- May be administered without regard to meals.

Patient/Family Teaching

- Instruct patient to continue taking medication, even if feeling well.
- Caution patient to make position changes slowly to minimize orthostatic hypotension. Advise patient that exercising or hot weather may enhance hypotensive effects.
- Instruct patient on the importance of maintaining good dental hygiene and seeing dentist frequently for teeth cleaning to prevent tenderness, bleeding, and gingival hyperplasia (gum enlargement).
- Advise patient to consult health care professional before taking any OTC medications or herbal/alternative therapies, especially cold remedies.
- Advise patient to advise health care professional of medication regimen prior to treatment or surgery.
- **Angina:** Instruct patients on concurrent nitrate therapy to continue taking both medications as directed and using SL nitroglycerin as needed for anginal attacks. Advise patient to contact health care professional if chest pain worsens or does not improve after therapy, or is accompanied by diaphoresis or shortness of breath, or if severe, persistent headache occurs. Caution patient to discuss exercise precautions with health care professional prior to exertion.
- **Hypertension:** Encourage patient to comply with additional interventions for hypertension (weight reduction, low-sodium diet, regular exercise, smoking cessation, moderation of alcohol consumption, and stress management). Medication controls, but does not cure, hypertension.
- Instruct patient and family on proper technique for monitoring BP and pulse. Advise them to check BP and pulse weekly and report significant changes to health care professional.

Evaluation/Desired Outcomes
- Decrease in BP.
- Decrease in frequency and severity of anginal attacks.
- Decrease in need for nitrate therapy.
- Increase in activity tolerance and sense of well-being.
- Suppression and prevention of supraventricular tachyarrhythmias.
- Improvement in neurological deficits due to vasospasm following subarachnoid hemorrhage.

• CENTRAL NERVOUS SYSTEM STIMULANTS

Pharmacologic Profile

General Use
Used in the treatment of narcolepsy and as adjunctive treatment in the management of attention deficit hyperactivity disorder (ADHD).

General Action and Information
Produce CNS stimulation by ↑ levels of neurotransmitters in the CNS. Produce CNS and respiratory stimulation, dilated pupils, ↑ motor activity and mental alertness, and a diminished sense of fatigue. In patients with ADHD, these agents ↓ restlessness and ↑ attention span.

Contraindications
Hypersensitivity. Should not be used in pregnant or lactating women. Should not be used in hyperexcitable states, patients with psychotic personalities or suicidal/homicidal tendencies, glaucoma and severe cardiovascular disease.

Precautions
Use cautiously in patients with a history of cardiovascular disease, hypertension, diabetes mellitus, or in older adults.

Interactions
Additive sympathomimetic (adrenergic) effects. Use with MAO inhibitors can result in hypertensive crises. Alkalinizing the urine (sodium bicarbonate, acetazolamide) ↓ excretion and enhances effects of amphetamines. Acidification of the urine (ammonium chloride, large doses of ascorbic acid) ↓ effect of amphetamines.

Nursing Implications

Assessment
- Monitor BP, heart rate, and respiration before administering and periodically during therapy.
- Monitor weight biweekly and inform health care professional of significant weight loss.
- Monitor height periodically in children; inform health care professional if growth inhibition occurs.
- May produce false sense of euphoria and well-being. Provide frequent rest periods and observe patient for rebound depression after the effects of the medication have worn off.
- **ADHD:** Assess attention span, impulse control, and interactions with others. Therapy may be interrupted at intervals to determine if symptoms are sufficient to warrant continued therapy.
- **Narcolepsy:** Observe and document frequency of episodes.

Implementation
- Follow administration directions associated with individual formulations.

Patient/Family Teaching
- Instruct patient not to alter dose without consulting health care professional. Abrupt cessation with high doses may cause extreme fatigue and mental depression.
- Advise patient to avoid intake of large amounts of caffeine.
- Advise patient that many of these medications have known abuse potential. Caution patient to protect the medications from theft, and never give them to anyone other than the individual for

whom it was prescribed. Store the medications out of sight and reach of children, and in a location not accessible by others.

- Advise patient to notify health care professional if nervousness, insomnia, palpitations, vomiting, skin rash, fever, painful and prolonged erections, or circulation problems (fingers or toes feel numb, cool, painful; fingers or toes change color from pale, to blue, to red) occur.
- Medication may impair judgment. Caution patient to avoid driving or other activities requiring judgment until response to medication is known.
- Inform patient that periodic holidays from the drug may be used to assess progress and decrease dependence.

Evaluation/Desired Outcomes
- Decreased frequency of narcoleptic episodes.
- Improved attention span and social interactions.

● CORTICOSTEROIDS

Pharmacologic Profile

General Use
Used in replacement doses (20 mg of hydrocortisone or equivalent) systemically to treat adrenocortical insufficiency. Larger doses are usually used for their anti-inflammatory, immunosuppressive, or antineoplastic activity. Used adjunctively in many other situations, including autoimmune diseases. Topical corticosteroids are used in a variety of inflammatory and allergic conditions. Inhaled corticosteroids are used in the chronic management of asthma or chronic obstructive pulmonary disease; intranasal and ophthalmic corticosteroids are used in the management of chronic allergic and inflammatory conditions.

General Action and Information
Produce profound and varied metabolic effects, in addition to modifying the normal immune response and suppressing inflammation. Available in a variety of dosage forms, including oral, injectable, topical, ophthalmic, intranasal, and inhalation. Prolonged used of large amounts of topical, ophthalmic, intranasal, or inhaled agent may result in systemic absorption and/or adrenal suppression.

Contraindications
Serious infections (except for certain forms of meningitis). Do not administer live vaccines to patients on larger doses.

Precautions
Prolonged treatment will result in adrenal suppression. Use lowest dose possible for shortest time possible. Alternate-day therapy is preferable during long-term treatment. Do not discontinue abruptly. Additional doses may be needed during stress (surgery and infection). Long-term use in children will result in ↓ growth. May mask signs of infection.

Interactions
Additive hypokalemia with amphotericin B and potassium-losing diuretics. Hypokalemia may ↑ the risk of digoxin toxicity. May ↑ requirements for oral or injectable hypoglycemic agents. Phenytoin, phenobarbital, and rifampin stimulate metabolism and may ↓ effectiveness. Oral contraceptives may block metabolism of corticosteroids.

Nursing Implications

Assessment
- These drugs are indicated for many conditions. Assess involved systems prior to and periodically throughout course of therapy.
- Assess patient for signs of adrenal insufficiency (hypotension, weight loss, weakness, nausea, vomiting, anorexia, lethargy, confusion, restlessness) prior to and periodically throughout course of therapy.

C L A S S I F I C A T I O N S

- Children should have periodic evaluations of growth during chronic therapy.

Implementation

- If dose is ordered daily or every other day, administer in the morning to coincide with the body's normal secretion of cortisol..
- **PO:** Administer with meals to minimize gastric irritation.

Patient/Family Teaching

- Emphasize need to take medication exactly as directed. Review symptoms of adrenal insufficiency that may occur when stopping the medication and that may be life-threatening.
- These drugs cause immunosuppression and may mask symptoms of infection. Instruct patient to avoid people with known contagious illnesses and to report possible infections. Advise patient to consult health care professional before receiving any vaccinations.
- Advise patient to carry identification in the event of an emergency in which patient cannot relate medical history.

Evaluation/Desired Outcomes

- Suppression of the inflammatory and immune responses in autoimmune disorders, allergic reactions, and organ transplants.
- Replacement therapy in adrenal insufficiency.
- Resolution of skin inflammation, pruritus, or other dermatologic conditions.

● DIURETICS

Pharmacologic Profile

General Use
Thiazide diuretics and loop diuretics are used alone or in combination with other antihypertensives in the treatment of hypertension; they are also used for the treatment of edema due to HF or other causes. Potassium-sparing diuretics have weak diuretic and antihypertensive properties and are used mainly to conserve potassium in patients receiving thiazide or loop diuretics.

General Action and Information
Enhance the selective excretion of various electrolytes and water by affecting renal mechanisms for tubular secretion and reabsorption. Classes commonly used are thiazide diuretics and thiazide-like diuretics (chlorothiazide, chlorthalidone, hydrochlorothiazide, indapamide, and metolazone), loop diuretics (bumetanide, furosemide, and torsemide), and potassium-sparing diuretics (amiloride, spironolactone, and triamterene). Mechanisms vary, depending on agent.

Contraindications
Hypersensitivity. Thiazide and loop diuretics may exhibit cross-sensitivity with other sulfonamides. Potassium-sparing diuretics should be avoided in hyperkalemia or severe renal impairment.

Precautions
Use with caution in patients with renal or hepatic disease.

Interactions
Thiazide and loop diuretics may have additive hypokalemia with corticosteroids, amphotericin B, and piperacillin/tazobactam. Hypokalemia may ↑ the risk of digoxin toxicity. Thiazide and loop diuretics may ↑ the risk of lithium toxicity. Additive hypotension with other antihypertensives or nitrates. Potassium-sparing diuretics may cause hyperkalemia when used with potassium supplements, ACE inhibitors, angiotensin II receptor antagonists, and aliskiren.

Nursing Implications

Assessment
- Assess fluid status throughout therapy. Monitor daily weight, intake and output ratios, amount and location of edema, lung sounds, skin turgor, and mucous membranes.

- Assess patient for anorexia, muscle weakness, numbness, tingling, paresthesia, confusion, and excessive thirst. Notify health care professional promptly if these signs of electrolyte imbalance occur.
- **Hypertension:** Monitor BP before and during administration. Monitor frequency of prescription refills to determine compliance in patients treated for hypertension.
- **Lab Test Considerations:** Monitor electrolytes (especially potassium), blood glucose, BUN, serum creatinine, and serum uric acid levels before and periodically throughout course of therapy.

Implementation
- If administering once daily, give in the morning to prevent disruption of sleep cycle. If administering twice daily, give last dose no later than 5 PM to minimize disruption of sleep cycle.
- Many diuretics are available in combination with other antihypertensives or potassium-sparing diuretics (see Appendix N).

Patient/Family Teaching
- Instruct patient to take medication exactly as directed. Advise patients on antihypertensive regimen to continue taking medication, even if feeling better. Medication controls, but does not cure, hypertension.
- Caution patient to make position changes slowly to minimize orthostatic hypotension. Caution patient that the use of alcohol, exercise during hot weather, or standing for long periods during therapy may enhance orthostatic hypotension.
- Instruct patient to consult health care professional regarding dietary potassium guidelines.
- Instruct patient to monitor weight weekly and report significant changes.
- Caution patient to use sunscreen and protective clothing to prevent photosensitivity reactions with thiazide and loop diuretics.
- Advise patient to consult health care professional before taking OTC medication concurrently with this therapy.
- Instruct patient to notify health care professional of medication regimen before treatment or surgery.
- Advise patient to contact health care professional immediately if muscle weakness, cramps, nausea, dizziness, or numbness or tingling of extremities occurs.
- Reinforce the need to continue additional therapies for hypertension (weight loss, regular exercise, restricted sodium intake, stress reduction, moderation of alcohol consumption, and cessation of smoking).
- Instruct patients with hypertension in the correct technique for monitoring weekly BP.

Evaluation/Desired Outcomes
- Decreased BP.
- Increased urine output.
- Decreased edema.
- Prevention of hypokalemia in patients taking diuretics.

• HORMONES

Pharmacologic Profile
General Use
Used in the treatment of deficiency states including diabetes mellitus (insulin), diabetes insipidus (desmopressin), hypothyroidism (thyroid hormones), and menopause (estrogens or estrogens/progestins). Estrogenic and progestational hormones are used as contraceptive agents in various combinations and sequences. Hormones may be used to treat hormonally sensitive tumors (androgens, estrogens) and in other selected situations. See individual drugs.

General Action and Information
Natural or synthetic substances that have a specific effect on target tissue. Differ greatly in their effects, depending on individual agent and function of target tissue.

Contraindications
Differ greatly among individual agents; see individual entries.

Precautions
Differ greatly among individual agents; see individual entries.

Interactions
Differ greatly among individual agents; see individual entries.

Nursing Implications

Assessment
- Monitor patient for symptoms of hormonal excess or insufficiency.
- **Sex Hormones:** BP and hepatic function tests should be monitored periodically throughout therapy.

Implementation
- **Sex Hormones:** During hospitalization, continue to administer according to schedule followed prior to hospitalization.

Patient/Family Teaching
- Explain dose schedule (and withdrawal bleeding with female sex hormones).
- Emphasize the importance of follow-up exams to monitor effectiveness of therapy and to ensure proper development of children and early detection of possible side effects.
- **Female Sex Hormones:** Advise patient to report signs and symptoms of fluid retention, thromboembolic disorders, mental depression, or hepatic dysfunction to health care professional.

Evaluation/Desired Outcomes
- Resolution of clinical symptoms of hormone imbalance including menopause symptoms and contraception.
- Correction of fluid and electrolyte imbalances.
- Control of the spread of advanced metastatic breast or prostate cancer.
- Slowed progression of postmenopausal osteoporosis.

• IMMUNOSUPPRESSANTS

Pharmacologic Profile

General Use
Azathioprine, basiliximab, cyclosporine, everolimus, mycophenolate, sirolimus, and tacrolimus are used with corticosteroids in the prevention of transplantation rejection reactions. Muromonab-CD3 is used to manage rejection reactions not controlled by other agents. Azathioprine, cyclosporine, cyclophosphamide, and methotrexate are used in the management of selected autoimmune diseases (nephrotic syndrome of childhood and severe rheumatoid arthritis).

General Action and Information
Inhibit cell-mediated immune responses by different mechanisms. In addition to azathioprine and cyclosporine, which are used primarily for their immunomodulating properties, cyclophosphamide and methotrexate are used to suppress the immune responses in certain disease states (nephrotic syndrome of childhood and severe rheumatoid arthritis). Muromonab-CD3 is a recombinant immunoglobulin antibody that alters T-cell function. Basiliximab is a monoclonal antibody.

Contraindications
Hypersensitivity to drug or vehicle.

Precautions
Use cautiously in patients with infections.

Interactions
Allopurinol inhibits the metabolism of azathioprine. Drugs that alter liver-metabolizing processes may change the effect of cyclosporine, tacrolimus, or sirolimus. The risk of toxicity with methotrexate may be ↑ by other nephrotoxic drugs, large doses of aspirin, or NSAIDs. Muromonab-CD3 has additive immunosuppressive properties; concurrent immunosuppressive doses should be ↓ or eliminated.

Nursing Implications

Assessment
- Monitor for infection (vital signs, sputum, urine, stool, WBC). Notify physician or other health care professional immediately if symptoms occur.
- Assess for symptoms of organ rejection throughout therapy.
- **Lab Test Consideration:** Monitor CBC and differential throughout therapy.

Implementation
- Protect transplant patients from staff and visitors who may carry infection.
- Maintain protective isolation as indicated.

Patient/Family Teaching
- Reinforce the need for lifelong therapy to prevent transplant rejection. Review symptoms of rejection for transplanted organ and stress the need for patient to notify health care professional immediately if they occur.
- Advise patient to avoid contact with contagious persons. Patients should not receive vaccinations without first consulting with health care professional.
- Emphasize the importance of follow-up exams and lab tests.

Evaluation/Desired Outcomes
- Prevention or reversal of rejection of organ transplants.
- Decrease in symptoms of autoimmune disorders.

● LAXATIVES

Pharmacologic Profile

General Use
To treat or prevent constipation or to prepare the bowel for radiologic or endoscopic procedures.

General Action and Information
Induce one or more bowel movements per day. Groups include stimulants (bisacodyl, sennosides), saline laxatives (magnesium salts and phosphates), stool softeners (docusate), bulk-forming agents (polycarbophil and psyllium), and osmotic cathartics (lactulose, polyethylene glycol/electrolyte). ↑ fluid intake, exercising, and adding more dietary fiber are also useful in the management of chronic constipation.

Contraindications
Hypersensitivity. Contraindicated in persistent abdominal pain, nausea, or vomiting of unknown cause, especially if accompanied by fever or other signs of an acute abdomen.

Precautions
Excessive or prolonged use may lead to dependence. Should not be used in children unless advised by a physician or other health care professional.

Interactions
Theoretically may ↓ the absorption of other orally administered drugs by ↓ transit time.

Nursing Implications

Assessment

- Assess patient for abdominal distention, presence of bowel sounds, and usual pattern of bowel function.
- Assess color, consistency, and amount of stool produced.

Implementation

- May be administered at bedtime for morning results.
- Taking oral doses on an empty stomach will usually produce more rapid results.
- Do not crush or chew enteric-coated tablets. Take with a full glass of water or juice.
- Stool softeners and bulk laxatives may take several days for results.

Patient/Family Teaching

- Advise patients, other than those with spinal cord injuries, that laxatives should be used only for short-term therapy. Long-term therapy may cause electrolyte imbalance and dependence.
- Encourage patients to use other forms of bowel regulation: ↑ bulk in the diet, ↑ fluid intake, and ↑ mobility. Normal bowel habits are individualized and may vary from 3 times/day to 3 times/wk.
- Instruct patients with cardiac disease to avoid straining during bowel movements (Valsalva maneuver).
- Advise patient that laxatives should not be used when constipation is accompanied by abdominal pain, fever, nausea, or vomiting.

Evaluation/Desired Outcomes

- A soft, formed bowel movement.
- Evacuation of the colon.

● LIPID-LOWERING AGENTS

Pharmacologic Profile

General Use

Used as a part of a total plan including diet and exercise to ↓ blood lipids in an effort to ↓ the morbidity and mortality of atherosclerotic cardiovascular disease and its sequelae.

General Action and Information

HMG-CoA reductase inhibitors (atorvastatin, fluvastatin, lovastatin, pitavastatin, pravastatin, rosuvastatin, simvastatin) inhibit an enzyme involved in cholesterol synthesis. The PCSK9 inhibitors (alirocumab, evolocumab) facilitate clearing of LDL from the blood. Bile acid sequestrants (cholestyramine, colestipol, colesevelam) bind cholesterol in the GI tract. Ezetimibe inhibits the absorption of cholesterol in the small intestine. Bempedoic acid inhibits adenosine triphosphate-citrate lyase, which inhibits cholesterol synthesis in the liver and subsequently lowers LDL. Inclisiran acts as a small interfering ribonucleic acid that is taken up by hepatocytes, where it causes breakdown of mRNA for PCSK9, which ultimately lowers LDL. Fenofibrate, gemfibrozil, and niacin act by other mechanisms (see individual monographs).

Contraindications

Hypersensitivity. HMG-CoA reductase inhibitors, bempedoic acid, and inclisiran are contraindicated in pregnancy.

Precautions

Differ greatly among individual agents; see individual entries.

Interactions

Bile acid sequestrants (cholestyramine and colestipol) may bind lipid-soluble vitamins (A, D, E, and K) and other concurrently administered drugs in the GI tract. HMG-CoA reductase inhibitors have numerous drug interactions involving cytochrome P450 system. Bempedoic acid may ↑ risk of tendon rupture/injury with fluoroquinolones or corticosteroids.

Nursing Implications

Assessment

- Obtain a diet history, especially in regard to **fat** and alcohol consumption.
- Monitor for signs and symptoms of hyperuricemia or gout in patients taking bempedoic acid. Also monitor these patients for signs and symptoms of tendon rupture (joint pain, swelling, inflammation) periodically during therapy.
- **Lab Test Considerations:** Serum cholesterol, LDL, HDL, and triglyceride levels should be evaluated before initiating and periodically throughout therapy.
- Liver function tests should be assessed before and periodically throughout therapy with HMG Co-A reductase inhibitors, niacin, and fibric acid derivatives.

Implementation

- See specific medications to determine timing of doses in relation to meals.
- PCSK9 inhibitors and inclisiran are administered SUBQ.

Patient/Family Teaching

- Advise patient that these medications should be used in conjunction with diet restrictions (**fat**, **cholesterol**, **carbohydrates**, and alcohol), exercise, and cessation of smoking.
- Advise patients taking bempedoic acid to notify health care professional if signs and symptoms of hyperuricemia (severe foot pain, especially in the toe joint; tender joints; warm joints; joint redness; swelling), tendinitis (pain; swelling; tears; inflammation of tendons, including arm, shoulder, back of the ankle) or tendon rupture (hear or feel a snap or pop in a tendon area, bruising right after an injury in a tendon area, unable to move affected area or put weight on affected area) occur.

Evaluation/Desired Outcomes

- Decreased serum cholesterol, triglyceride, and LDL levels and improved HDL levels.

● NONOPIOID ANALGESICS

Pharmacologic Profile

General Use

Used to control mild to moderate pain and/or fever. Phenazopyridine is used only to treat urinary tract pain, and capsaicin is used topically for a variety of painful syndromes.

General Action and Information

Most nonopioid analgesics inhibit prostaglandin synthesis peripherally for analgesic effect and centrally for antipyretic effect.

Contraindications

Hypersensitivity and cross-sensitivity among NSAIDs may occur.

Precautions

Use cautiously in patients with severe hepatic or renal disease, chronic alcohol use/abuse, or malnutrition.

Interactions

Long-term use of acetaminophen with NSAIDs may ↑ the risk of adverse renal effects. Prolonged high-dose acetaminophen may ↑ the risk of bleeding with warfarin. Hepatotoxicity may be additive with other hepatotoxic agents, including alcohol. NSAIDs ↑ the risk of bleeding with warfarin, thrombolytic agents, antiplatelet agents, some cephalosporins, and valproate (effect is greatest with aspirin). NSAIDs may also ↓ the effectiveness of diuretics and antihypertensives.

C
L
A
S
S
I
F
I
C
A
T
I
O
N
S

Nursing Implications

Assessment

- Patients who have asthma, allergies, and nasal polyps or who are allergic to tartrazine are at an ↑ risk for developing hypersensitivity reactions.
- **Pain:** Assess pain and limitation of movement; note type, location, and intensity prior to and at the peak (see Time/Action Profile) following administration.
- **Fever:** Assess fever and note associated signs (diaphoresis, tachycardia, malaise, chills).
- **Lab Test Considerations:** Hepatic, hematologic, and renal function should be evaluated periodically throughout prolonged high-dose therapy. Aspirin and most NSAIDs prolong bleeding time due to suppressed platelet aggregation and, in large doses, may cause prolonged prothrombin time. Monitor hematocrit periodically in prolonged high-dose therapy to assess for GI blood loss.

Implementation

- **PO:** Administer salicylates and NSAIDs after meals or with food to minimize gastric irritation.

Patient/Family Teaching

- Instruct patient to take salicylates and NSAIDs with a full glass of water and to remain in an upright position for 15–30 min after administration.
- Acetaminophen should not be taken for longer than 10 days in adults and 5 days in children unless directed by health care professional. Short-term doses of acetaminophen with salicylates or NSAIDs should not exceed the recommended daily dose of either drug alone.
- Caution patient to avoid concurrent use of alcohol with this medication to minimize possible gastric irritation; three or more glasses of alcohol per day may ↑ the risk of GI bleeding with salicylates or NSAIDs. Caution patient to avoid taking acetaminophen, salicylates, or NSAIDs concurrently for more than a few days, unless directed by health care professional to prevent analgesic nephropathy.
- Advise patients on long-term therapy to inform health care professional of medication regimen prior to surgery. Salicylates and NSAIDs may need to be withheld prior to surgery.

Evaluation/Desired Outcomes

- Relief of mild to moderate discomfort.
- Reduction of fever.

• NONSTEROIDAL ANTI-INFLAMMATORY DRUGS (NSAIDS)

Pharmacologic Profile

General Use

NSAIDs are used to control mild to moderate pain, fever, and various inflammatory conditions, such as rheumatoid arthritis and osteoarthritis. Ophthalmic NSAIDs are used to ↓ postoperative ocular inflammation, to inhibit perioperative miosis, and to ↓ inflammation due to allergies.

General Action and Information

NSAIDs have analgesic, antipyretic, and anti-inflammatory properties. Analgesic and anti-inflammatory effects are due to inhibition of prostaglandin synthesis. Antipyretic action is due to vasodilation and inhibition of prostaglandin synthesis in the CNS. COX-2 inhibitors (celecoxib) may cause less GI bleeding.

Contraindications

Hypersensitivity to aspirin is a contraindication for the whole group of NSAIDs; cross-sensitivity may occur. Avoid use after 30 wk of gestation.

Precautions

Use cautiously in patients with a history of bleeding disorders, GI bleeding, and severe hepatic, renal, or cardiovascular disease. Use at or after 20 wk gestation may cause fetal or neonatal renal impairment; if treatment is necessary between 20 wk and 30 wk gestation, limit use to the lowest effective dose and shortest duration.

Interactions

NSAIDs prolong bleeding time and potentiate the effect of warfarin, thrombolytic agents, some cephalosporins, antiplatelet agents, and valproates. Prolonged use with aspirin may result in ↑ GI side effects and ↓ effectiveness. NSAIDs may also ↓ response to diuretics or antihypertensive therapy. COX-2 inhibitors do not negate the cardioprotective effect of low-dose aspirin.

Nursing Implications

Assessment

- Patients who have asthma, allergies, and nasal polyps or who are allergic to tartrazine are at an ↑ risk for developing hypersensitivity reactions.
- **Pain:** Assess pain and limitation of movement; note type, location, and intensity prior to and at the peak (see Time/Action Profile) following administration.
- **Fever:** Assess fever and note associated signs (diaphoresis, tachycardia, malaise, chills).
- **Lab Test Considerations:** Renal function, CBC, and liver function tests should be evaluated periodically in patients receiving prolonged therapy.

Implementation

- Administer oral NSAIDs after meals or with food to minimize gastric irritation.

Patient/Family Teaching

- Instruct patient to take NSAIDs with a full glass of water and to remain in an upright position for 15–30 min after administration.
- Caution patient to avoid concurrent use of alcohol with this medication to minimize possible gastric irritation; three or more glasses of alcohol per day may ↑ the risk of GI bleeding with salicylates or NSAIDs. Caution patient to avoid taking NSAIDs with acetaminophen or for more than a few days, unless directed by health care professional to prevent analgesic nephropathy.
- Advise patient on long-term therapy to inform health care professional of medication regimen prior to surgery. NSAIDs may need to be withheld prior to surgery.

Evaluation/Desired Outcomes

- Relief of mild to moderate discomfort
- Reduction of fever.

• OPIOID ANALGESICS

Pharmacologic Profile

General Use

Management of moderate to severe pain. Fentanyl is also used as a general anesthetic adjunct.

General Action and Information

Opioids bind to opiate receptors in the CNS, where they act as agonists of endogenously occurring opioid peptides (eukephalins and endorphins). The result is alteration to the perception of and response to pain.

Contraindications

Hypersensitivity to individual agents.

Precautions

Use cautiously in patients with undiagnosed abdominal pain, head trauma or pathology, liver disease, or history of addiction to opioids. Use smaller doses initially in older adults and those with respiratory diseases. Prolonged use may result in tolerance and the need for larger doses to relieve pain. Psychological or physical dependence may occur.

CLASSIFICATIONS

Interactions

↑ the CNS depressant properties of other drugs, including alcohol, antihistamines, antidepressants, sedative/hypnotics, phenothiazines, and MAO inhibitors. Use of partial-antagonist opioid analgesics (buprenorphine, butorphanol, and nalbuphine) may precipitate opioid withdrawal in physically dependent patients. Use with MAO inhibitors or procarbazine may result in severe paradoxical reactions (especially with meperidine). Methadone may ↑ the risk of QT interval prolongation when use with other QT interval prolonging medications.

Nursing Implications

Assessment

- Assess type, location, and intensity of pain prior to and at peak following administration. When titrating opioid doses, ↑ of 25–50% should be administered until there is either a 50% ↓ in the patient's pain rating on a numerical or visual analogue scale or the patient reports satisfactory pain relief. A repeat dose can be safely administered at the time of the peak if previous dose is ineffective and side effects are minimal.
- Opioid agonist-antagonists are not recommended for prolonged use or as first-line therapy for acute or cancer pain.
- An equianalgesic chart (see Appendix I) should be used when changing routes or when changing from one opioid to another.
- Assess BP, heart rate, and respirations before and periodically during administration. If respiratory rate is <10/min, assess level of sedation. Physical stimulation may be sufficient to prevent significant hypoventilation. Dose may need to be ↓ by 25–50%. Initial drowsiness will diminish with continued use.
- Assess prior analgesic history. Antagonistic properties of agonist-antagonists may induce withdrawal symptoms (vomiting, restlessness, abdominal cramps, and ↑ BP and temperature) in patients physically dependent on opioids.
- Prolonged use may lead to physical and psychological dependence and tolerance. This should not prevent patient from receiving adequate analgesia. Most patients who receive opioid analgesics for pain do not develop psychological dependence. Progressively higher doses may be required to relieve pain with chronic therapy.
- Assess bowel function routinely. Prevention of constipation should be instituted with ↑ intake of fluids and bulk, stool softeners, and laxatives to minimize constipating effects. Stimulant laxatives should be administered routinely if opioid use exceeds 2–3 days, unless contraindicated.
- Monitor intake and output ratios. If significant discrepancies occur, assess for urinary retention and inform physician or other health care professional.
- **Toxicity and Overdose:** If an opioid antagonist is required to reverse respiratory depression or coma, naloxone is the antidote. Dilute the 0.4-mg ampule of naloxone in 10 mL of 0.9% NaCl and administer 0.5 mL (0.02 mg) by IV push every 2 min. For children and patients weighing <40 kg, dilute 0.1 mg of naloxone in 10 mL of 0.9% NaCl for a concentration of 10 mcg/mL and administer 0.5 mcg/kg every 1–2 min. Naloxone may also be administered intranasally to reverse opioid-induced respiratory depression or coma. Administer 1 spray (2 mg or 4 mg) in one nostril; may repeat dose every 2–3 min (with each subsequent dose being administered in alternate nostril). Titrate dose to avoid withdrawal, seizures, and severe pain.

Implementation

- Explain therapeutic value of medication before administration to enhance the analgesic effect.
- Regularly administered doses may be more effective than prn ("as needed") administration. Analgesic is more effective if given before pain becomes severe.
- Coadministration with nonopioid analgesics may have additive analgesic effects and may permit lower doses.
- Medication should be discontinued gradually after long-term use to prevent withdrawal symptoms.

Patient/Family Teaching

- Instruct patient on how and when to ask for pain medication.
- Advise patient that opioid analgesics have known abuse potential. Advise the patient to protect these medications from theft, and never give them to anyone other than the individual for whom it was prescribed. Store out of sight and reach of children, and in a location not accessible by others.
- Medication may cause drowsiness or dizziness. Caution patient to call for assistance when ambulating or smoking and to avoid driving or other activities requiring alertness until response to medication is known.
- Advise patient to make position changes slowly to minimize orthostatic hypotension.
- Caution patient to avoid concurrent use of alcohol or other CNS depressants with this medication.
- Encourage patient to turn, cough, and breathe deeply every 2 hr to prevent atelectasis.

Evaluation/Desired Outcomes

- Decreased severity of pain without a significant alteration in level of consciousness or respiratory status.

● SEDATIVE/HYPNOTICS

Pharmacologic Profile

General Use

Sedatives are used to provide sedation, usually prior to procedures. Hypnotics are used to manage insomnia. Selected agents are useful as anticonvulsants (clorazepate, diazepam, phenobarbital), skeletal muscle relaxants (diazepam), adjuncts in the management of alcohol withdrawal syndrome (chlordiazepoxide, diazepam, oxazepam), adjuncts in general anesthesia (droperidol), or as amnestics (midazolam, diazepam).

General Action and Information

Cause generalized CNS depression. May produce tolerance with chronic use and have potential for psychological or physical dependence. These agents have NO analgesic properties.

Contraindications

Hypersensitivity. Should not be used in comatose patients or in those with pre-existing CNS depression. Should not be used in patients with uncontrolled severe pain. Avoid use during pregnancy or lactation.

Precautions

Use cautiously in patients with hepatic impairment, severe renal impairment, or severe underlying pulmonary disease. Use with caution in patients who may be suicidal or who may have had previous drug addictions. Hypnotic use should be short-term. Older adults may be more sensitive to CNS depressant effects; dosage ↓ may be required.

Interactions

Additive CNS depression with alcohol, antihistamines, some antidepressants, opioid analgesics, or phenothiazines. Should not be used with MAO inhibitors.

Nursing Implications

Assessment

- Monitor BP, heart rate, and respiratory status frequently throughout IV administration. Prolonged high-dose therapy may lead to psychological or physical dependence. Restrict the amount of drug available to patient, especially if patient is depressed, suicidal, or has a history of addiction.
- **Insomnia:** Assess sleep patterns before and periodically throughout course of therapy.

- **Seizures:** Observe and record intensity, duration, and characteristics of seizure activity. Institute seizure precautions.
- **Muscle Spasms:** Assess muscle spasms, associated pain, and limitation of movement before and throughout therapy.
- **Alcohol Withdrawal:** Assess patient experiencing alcohol withdrawal for tremors, agitation, delirium, and hallucinations. Protect patient from injury.

Implementation

- Supervise ambulation and transfer of patients following administration of hypnotic doses. Side rails should be raised and call bell within reach at all times. Keep bed in low position.

Patient/Family Teaching

- Discuss the importance of preparing the environment for sleep (dark room, quiet, avoidance of nicotine and caffeine). If less effective after a few weeks, consult health care professional; do not ↑ dose. Gradual withdrawal may be required to prevent reactions following prolonged therapy.
- May cause daytime drowsiness. Caution patient to avoid driving and other activities requiring alertness until response to medication is known.
- Advise patient to avoid the use of alcohol and other CNS depressants concurrently with these medications.
- Advise patient to inform health care professional if pregnancy is planned or suspected.

Evaluation/Desired Outcomes

- Improvement in sleep patterns.
- Control of seizures.
- Decrease in muscle spasms.
- More rational ideation when used for alcohol withdrawal.

• SKELETAL MUSCLE RELAXANTS

Pharmacologic Profile

General Use

Two major uses are spasticity associated with spinal cord diseases or lesions (baclofen and dantrolene) or adjunctive therapy in the symptomatic relief of acute painful musculoskeletal conditions (carisoprodol, chlorzoxazone, cyclobenzaprine, diazepam, metaxolone, and methocarbamol). IV dantrolene is also used to treat and prevent malignant hyperthermia.

General Action and Information

Act either centrally (baclofen, carisoprodol, chlorzoxazone, cyclobenzaprine, diazepam, metaxolone, and methocarbamol) or directly (dantrolene).

Contraindications

Baclofen and oral dantrolene should not be used in patients in whom spasticity is used to maintain posture and balance.

Precautions

Use cautiously in patients with a history of liver disease.

Interactions

Additive CNS depression with other CNS depressants, including alcohol, antihistamines, antidepressants, opioid analgesics, and sedative/hypnotics.

Nursing Implications

Assessment

- Assess patient for pain, muscle stiffness, and range of motion before and periodically throughout therapy.

Implementation
- Provide safety measures as indicated. Supervise ambulation and transfer of patients.

Patient/Family Teaching
- Encourage patient to comply with additional therapies prescribed for muscle spasm (rest, physical therapy, heat).
- Medication may cause drowsiness. Caution patient to avoid driving or other activities requiring alertness until response to drug is known.
- Advise patient to avoid concurrent use of alcohol or other CNS depressants with these medications.

Evaluation/Desired Outcomes
- Decreased musculoskeletal pain
- Decreased muscle spasticity
- Increased range of motion
- Prevention or decrease in temperature and skeletal rigidity in malignant hyperthermia.

• THROMBOLYTICS

Pharmacologic Profile

General Use
Acute management of ST-segment-elevation MI. Alteplase is also used in the management of acute pulmonary embolism and acute ischemic stroke.

General Action and Information
Directly convert plasminogen to plasmin, which then degrades fibrin in clots, resulting in lysis of the clot.

Contraindications
Hypersensitivity. Active internal bleeding, history of cerebrovascular accident, recent CNS trauma or surgery, neoplasm, or arteriovenous malformation, severe uncontrolled hypertension, and known bleeding tendencies.

Precautions
Recent (within 10 days) major surgery, trauma, GI or GU bleeding. Severe hepatic or renal disease. Subacute bacterial endocarditis or acute pericarditis. Use cautiously in older adults.

Interactions
Concurrent use with antiplatelet agents, NSAIDs, warfarin, dabigatran, rivaroxaban, apixaban, edoxaban, or heparins may ↑ the risk of bleeding, although these agents are frequently used together or in sequence. Risk of bleeding may also be ↑ by concurrent use with cefotetan and valproic acid.

Nursing Implications

Assessment
- Begin therapy as soon as possible after the onset of symptoms.
- Monitor vital signs continuously for coronary thrombosis and at least every 4 hr during therapy for other indications. Do not use lower extremities to monitor BP.
- Assess patient carefully for bleeding every 15 min during the 1st hr of therapy, every 15–30 min during the next 8 hr, and at least every 4 hr for the duration of therapy. Frank bleeding may occur from sites of invasive procedures or from body orifices. Internal bleeding may also occur (↓ neurologic status; abdominal pain with coffee-ground emesis or black, tarry stools; hematuria; joint pain). If uncontrolled bleeding occurs, stop medication and notify physician immediately.
- Assess neurologic status throughout therapy.

CLASSIFICATIONS

- Altered sensorium or neurologic changes may be indicative of intracranial bleeding.
- **Coronary Thrombosis:** Monitor BP, heart rate, and ECG continuously. Notify physician if significant arrhythmias occur. Cardiac enzymes should be monitored. Coronary angiography may be ordered following therapy.
- Monitor heart sounds and breath sounds frequently. Inform physician if signs of HF occur (rales/crackles, dyspnea, S3 heart sound, jugular venous distention).
- **Pulmonary Embolism:** Monitor BP, heart rate, hemodynamics, and respiratory status (rate, degree of dyspnea, arterial blood gases).
- **Cannula/Catheter Occlusion:** Monitor ability to aspirate blood as indicator of patency. Ensure that patient exhales and holds breath when connecting and disconnecting IV syringe to prevent air embolism.
- **Acute Ischemic Stroke:** Assess neurologic status. Determine time of onset of stroke symptoms. Alteplase must be administered within 3–4.5 hr of onset (within 3 hr in patients >80 yr, those taking oral anticoagulants, those with a baseline National Institutes of Health Stroke Scale score >25, or those with both a history of stroke and diabetes).
- **Lab Test Considerations:** Hematocrit, hemoglobin, platelet count, fibrin/fibrin degradation product titer, fibrinogen concentration, prothrombin time, thrombin time, and activated partial thromboplastin time may be evaluated prior to and frequently throughout therapy. Bleeding time may be assessed prior to therapy if patient has received platelet aggregation inhibitors. Obtain type and cross match and have blood available at all times in case of hemorrhage. Stools should be tested for occult blood loss and urine for hematuria periodically during therapy.
- **Toxicity and Overdose:** If local bleeding occurs, apply pressure to site. If severe or internal bleeding occurs, discontinue infusion. Clotting factors and/or blood volume may be restored through infusions of whole blood, packed RBCs, fresh frozen plasma, or cryoprecipitate. Do not administer dextran, as it has antiplatelet activity. Aminocaproic acid may be used as an antidote.

Implementation

- Starting two IV lines prior to therapy is recommended: one for the thrombolytic agent, the other for any additional infusions.
- Avoid invasive procedures, such as IM injections or arterial punctures, with this therapy. If such procedures must be performed, apply pressure to all arterial and venous puncture sites for at least 30 min. Avoid venipunctures at noncompressible sites (jugular vein, subclavian site).
- Systemic anticoagulation with heparin is usually begun several hr after the completion of thrombolytic therapy.

Patient/Family Teaching

- Explain purpose of medication and the need for close monitoring to patient and family. Instruct patient to report hypersensitivity reactions (rash, dyspnea) and bleeding or bruising.
- Explain need for bedrest and minimal handling during therapy to avoid injury. Avoid all unnecessary procedures such as shaving and vigorous tooth brushing.

Evaluation/Desired Outcomes

- Lysis of thrombi and restoration of blood flow
- Prevention of neurologic sequelae in acute ischemic stroke
- Cannula or catheter patency.

• VASCULAR HEADACHE SUPPRESSANTS

Pharmacologic Profile

General Use

Used for acute treatment of vascular headaches (migraine, cluster headaches, migraine variants). Other agents such as some beta blockers and some calcium channel blockers are used for suppression of frequently occurring vascular headaches.

General Action and Information
Ergot derivatives (ergotamine, dihydroergotamine) directly stimulate alpha-adrenergic and serotonergic receptors, producing vascular smooth muscle vasoconstriction. Almotriptan, eletriptan, frovatriptan, naratriptan, rizatriptan, sumatriptan, and zolmitriptan produce vasoconstriction by acting as serotonin ($5-HT_1$) agonists. Atogepant, erenumab, rimegepant, ubrogepant, and zavegepant bind to and inhibit the calcitonin gene-related peptide (CGRP) receptor, which reduces the neuroinflammatory and vasodilatory effects of CGRP (rimegepant, ubrogepant, and zavegepant are used for acute treatment of migraine headaches; atogepant, erenumab, and rimegepant are used for migraine prevention).

Contraindications
Use of ergot derivatives and the $5-HT_1$ agonists should be avoided in patients with ischemic cardiovascular disease.

Precautions
Use ergot derivatives and $5-HT_1$ agonists cautiously in patients who are at risk for cardiovascular disease. ↑ risk of serotonin syndrome with $5-HT_1$ agonists when used with serotonergic agents.

Interactions
Avoid concurrent use of ergot derivative agents with serotonin agonist agents; see also individual agents. Many of the CGRP antagonists have interactions involving the cytochrome P450 system.

Nursing Implications

Assessment
- Assess pain location, intensity, duration, and associated symptoms (photophobia, phonophobia, nausea, vomiting) during migraine attack and frequency of attacks.

Implementation
- Medications used for acute treatment of headache should be administered at the first sign of a headache.

Patient/Family Teaching
- Advise patient that lying down in a darkened room following medication administration may further help relieve headache.
- May cause dizziness or drowsiness. Caution patient to avoid driving or other activities requiring alertness until response to medication is known.
- Advise patient to avoid alcohol, which aggravates headaches.

Evaluation/Desired Outcomes
- Relief of migraine attack.

• WEIGHT CONTROL AGENTS

Pharmacologic Profile

General Use
These agents are used in the management of exogenous obesity as part of a regimen including a reduced-calorie diet. They are especially useful in the presence of other risk factors including hypertension, diabetes, or dyslipidemias.

General Action and Information
Phentermine is an anorexiant designed to ↓ appetite via its action in the CNS. Orlistat is a lipase inhibitor that ↓ absorption of dietary fat.

Contraindications
None of these agents should be used during pregnancy or lactation. Phentermine should not be used in patients with severe hepatic or renal disease, uncontrolled hypertension, known HF, or cardiovascular disease. Orlistat should not be used in patients with chronic malabsorption.

C
L
A
S
S
I
F
I
C
A
T
I
O
N
S

Precautions

Phentermine should be used cautiously in patients with a history of seizures, or angle-closure glaucoma and in geriatric patients.

Interactions

Phentermine may have additive, adverse effects with CNS stimulants, some vascular headache suppressants, MAO inhibitors, and some opioids (concurrent use should be avoided). Orlistat ↓ absorption of some fat-soluble vitamins and beta-carotene.

Nursing Implications

Assessment

- Monitor weight and dietary intake prior to and periodically during therapy. Adjust concurrent medications (antihypertensives, antidiabetics, lipid-lowering agents) as needed.

Implementation

Patient/Family Teaching

- Advise patient that regular physical activity, approved by health care professional, should be used in conjunction with medication and diet.

Evaluation/Desired Outcomes

- Slow, consistent weight loss when combined with a reduced-calorie diet.

A

⅏ abacavir/dolutegravir/ lamivudine

(ah-**back**-ah-veer/doe-loo-**teg**-ra-vir/la-**mi**-vyoo-deen)

Triumeq, Triumeq PD

Classification

Therapeutic: antiretrovirals (combination)
Pharmacologic: integrase strand transfer inhibitors (INSTI) (dolutegravir), nucleoside reverse transcriptase inhibitors (abacavir, lamivudine)

Indications

HIV-1 infection.

Action

Abacavir: Converted inside cells to carbovir triphosphate, its active metabolite. Carbovir triphosphate inhibits the activity of HIV-1 reverse transcriptase, which in turn terminates viral DNA growth. *Dolutegravir:* Inhibits HIV-1 integrase, which is required for viral replication. *Lamivudine:* After intracellular conversion to its active form (lamivudine-5-triphosphate), inhibits viral DNA synthesis by inhibiting the enzyme reverse transcriptase. **Therapeutic Effects:** Evidence of decreased viral replication and reduced viral load with slowed progression of HIV and its sequelae.

Pharmacokinetics

Abacavir

Absorption: Rapidly and extensively (83%) absorbed.

Distribution: Distributes into extravascular space and readily distributes into erythrocytes.

Metabolism and Excretion: Mostly metabolized by the liver; 1.2% excreted unchanged in urine.

Half-life: 1.5 hr.

Dolutegravir

Absorption: Absorption follows oral administration; bioavailability is unknown.

Distribution: Enters CSF.

Protein Binding: >98.9%.

Metabolism and Excretion: Metabolized primarily by the UGT1A1 enzyme system with some metabolism by CYP3A4. 53% excreted unchanged in feces. Metabolites are renally excreted, minimal renal elimination of unchanged drug. ⅏ Poor metabolizers of dolutegravir have ↑ levels and ↓ clearance.

Half-life: 14 hr.

Lamivudine

Absorption: Well absorbed after oral administration (86% in adults, 66% in infants and children).

Distribution: Distributes into the extravascular space. Some penetration into CSF; remainder of distribution unknown.

Metabolism and Excretion: Mostly excreted unchanged in urine; <5% metabolized by the liver.

Half-life: 13–19 hr.

TIME/ACTION PROFILE (plasma concentrations)

ROUTE	ONSET	PEAK	DURATION
PO	unknown	unknown	24 hr

Contraindications/Precautions

Contraindicated in: Hypersensitivity to any component (especially abacavir, rechallenge may be fatal); Resistance to any component; ⅏ Presence of HLA-B*5701 allele; Concurrent use of dofetilide; Concurrent administration of lamivudine or abacavir alone or in other combination antiretroviral dose forms; Hepatic impairment; CCr <30 mL/min; OB: Avoid use through first trimester of pregnancy (may ↑ risk of neural tube defects); Lactation: Breastfeeding not recommended for patients with HIV.

Use Cautiously in: Underlying hepatitis B or C (may worsen liver function); Women and obesity (↑ risk of lactic acidosis and severe hepatomegaly with steatosis); Underlying cardiovascular disease, including history of hypertension, hyperlipidemia, smoking history, or diabetes mellitus; OB: Can consider use during second or third trimester if potential maternal benefit justifies potential fetal risk; Pedi: Children <6 kg (safety and effectiveness not established).

Adverse Reactions/Side Effects

CV: MI. **F and E:** LACTIC ACIDOSIS. **GI:** exacerbation of hepatitis B, HEPATOMEGALY (WITH STEATOSIS), HEPATOTOXICITY (↑ WITH HEPATITIS B OR C). **Neuro:** fatigue, headache, insomnia. **Misc:** HYPERSENSITIVITY REACTIONS, immune reconstitution syndrome.

Interactions

Drug-Drug: Abacavir: Alcohol ↑ blood levels. May ↑ **methadone** metabolism in some patients; slight ↑ in **methadone** dosing may be needed. May ↑ levels and toxicity of **riociguat**; may need to ↓ riociguat dose. Combination therapy with **tenofovir** and **abacavir** may lead to virologic nonresponse; avoid use. **Dolutegravir:** May ↑ levels and toxicity from **dofetilide**; concurrent use contraindicated. Levels and effectiveness are ↓ by **etravirine** (should not be used concurrently without atazanavir/ritonavir, darunavir/ritonavir or lopinavir/ritonavir). Levels and effectiveness are ↓ by **efavirenz, fosamprenavir/ritonavir, tipranavir/ritonavir, carbamazepine,** and **rifampin**; ↑ dosage of dolutegravir recommended. Levels and effectiveness may be ↓ by **nevirapine**; avoid concurrent use. May ↑ levels and toxicity from **metformin**. Levels and effectiveness may be ↓ by other **metabolic inducers** including **oxcarbazepine, phenobarbital,** and **phenytoin**; avoid concurrent use. Absorption and effectiveness may be ↓ by cation-containing **antacids**

☀ = Canadian drug name. ⅏ = Genetic implication. S̶t̶r̶i̶k̶e̶t̶h̶r̶o̶u̶g̶h̶ = Discontinued. CAPITALS = life-threatening. <u>Underline</u> = most frequent.

or **laxatives**, as well as **buffered medications**, or **sucralfate**; should be taken 2 hr before or 6 hr after these medications. Absorption and effectiveness may be ↓ by **calcium supplements** (oral) or **iron supplements** (oral); under fasting conditions, abacavir/dolutegravir/lamivudine should be taken 2 hr before or 6 hr after these medications; when taken with food, abacavir/dolutegravir/lamivudine and calcium or iron supplements may be taken at the same time. May ↑ **dalfampridine** levels and risk of seizures. **Lamivudine: Trimethoprim/sulfamethoxazole** ↑ levels (dose alteration may be necessary in renal impairment). ↑ risk of pancreatitis with concurrent use of other **drugs causing pancreatitis**. ↑ risk of neuropathy with concurrent use of other **drugs causing neuropathy**. **Sorbitol** may ↓ levels; avoid concurrent use.

Drug-Natural Products: Levels and effectiveness may be ↓ **St. John's wort**; avoid concurrent use.

Route/Dosage

Tablets and tablets for oral suspension are NOT interchangeable on a milligram-per-milligram basis.

PO (Adults and Children ≥25 kg): *Triumeq:* One tablet (abacavir 600 mg/dolutegravir 50 mg/lamivudine 300 mg) once daily; *Concurrent efavirenz, fosamprenavir/ritonavir, tipranavir/ritonavir, carbamazepine, or rifampin:* additional 50–mg dose of dolutegravir (Tivicay) is required separated from Triumeq by 12 hr.

PO (Children 20–<25 kg): *Triumeq PD:* Six tablets once daily (total dose = abacavir 360 mg/dolutegravir 30 mg/lamivudine 180 mg). *Concurrent efavirenz, fosamprenavir/ritonavir, tipranavir/ritonavir, carbamazepine, or rifampin:* additional 30–mg dose of dolutegravir (Tivicay PD) is required separated from Triumeq PD by 12 hr.

PO (Children 14–<20 kg): *Triumeq PD:* Five tablets once daily (total dose = abacavir 300 mg/dolutegravir 25 mg/lamivudine 150 mg). *Concurrent efavirenz, fosamprenavir/ritonavir, tipranavir/ritonavir, carbamazepine, or rifampin:* additional 25–mg dose of dolutegravir (Tivicay PD) is required separated from Triumeq PD by 12 hr.

PO (Children 10–<14 kg): *Triumeq PD:* Four tablets once daily (total dose = abacavir 240 mg/dolutegravir 20 mg/lamivudine 120 mg). *Concurrent efavirenz, fosamprenavir/ritonavir, tipranavir/ritonavir, carbamazepine, or rifampin:* additional 20–mg dose of dolutegravir (Tivicay PD) is required separated from Triumeq PD by 12 hr.

PO (Children 6–<10 kg): *Triumeq PD:* Three tablets once daily (total dose = abacavir 180 mg/dolutegravir 15 mg/lamivudine 90 mg). *Concurrent efavirenz, fosamprenavir/ritonavir, tipranavir/ritonavir, carbamazepine, or rifampin:* additional 15-mg dose of dolutegravir (Tivicay PD) is required separated from Triumeq PD by 12 hr.

Availability (generic available)

Tablets: abacavir 600 mg/dolutegravir 50 mg/lamivudine 300 mg. **Tablets for oral suspension:** abacavir 60 mg/dolutegravir 5 mg/lamivudine 30 mg.

NURSING IMPLICATIONS

Assessment

● Assess patient for change in severity of HIV symptoms and for symptoms of opportunistic infections during therapy.

● Assess for signs of hypersensitivity reactions (fever; rash; GI—nausea, vomiting, diarrhea, abdominal pain; constitutional—malaise, fatigue, achiness; respiratory—dyspnea, cough, pharyngitis). May also cause elevated liver function tests, increased CK or serum creatinine, and lymphopenia. ⚠ Patients who carry the HLA-B*5701 allele are at high risk for hypersensitivity reaction. Discontinue promptly if hypersensitivity reaction is suspected. Regardless of HLA-B*5701 status, permanently discontinue if hypersensitivity cannot be ruled out, even when other diagnoses are possible. Following a hypersensitivity reaction, never restart abacavir-containing products. More severe symptoms may occur within hr and may include life-threatening hypotension and death. Symptoms usually resolve upon discontinuation.

● May cause lactic acidosis and severe hepatomegaly with steatosis. Monitor patient for signs (↑ serum lactate levels, ↑ liver enzymes, liver enlargement on palpation). Therapy should be suspended if clinical or laboratory signs occur.

● Monitor patient for signs and symptoms of peripheral neuropathy (tingling, burning, numbness, or pain in hands or feet); may be difficult to differentiate from peripheral neuropathy of severe HIV disease. May require discontinuation of therapy.

Lab Test Considerations

● Verify negative pregnancy test in adolescent and adult females of reproductive potential prior to starting therapy.

● Monitor viral load and CD4 cell count regularly during therapy.

● ⚠ Screen for HLA-B*5701 allele prior to initiation of therapy to decrease risk of hypersensitivity reaction. Screening is also recommended prior to reinitiation of abacavir in patients of unknown HLA-B*5701 status who have previously tolerated abacavir.

● Test for presence of hepatitis B virus (HBV) prior to or when starting therapy. Emergence of lamivudine-resistant HBV variants associated with lamivudine-containing antiretroviral regimens have been reported. Consider additional treatment for chronic HBV if used in patients co-infected with HIV-1 and HBV; or consider an alternative regimen.

● Monitor liver function periodically. May cause ↑ levels of AST, ALT, and alkaline phosphatase, which usually resolve after interruption of therapy. Patients with concurrent hepatitis B or C should be followed for at least several mo after stopping therapy. Lactic

acidosis may occur with hepatic toxicity, causing hepatic steatosis; may be fatal, especially in women.
- May cause ↑ serum glucose, lipase, and triglyceride levels.

Implementation
- *Triumeq* and *Triumeq PD* are not bioequivalent and are not interchangeable on a milligram-per-milligram basis. Dose adjustment is required when switching dose forms.
- **PO:** Administer without regard to food.
- **DNC: Pediatric patients**: Fully disperse *Triumeq PD* tablets for oral suspension in 20 mL of drinking water (if using 4, 5, or 6 tablets for oral suspension) or 15 mL (if using 3 tablets for oral suspension) in the supplied cup; swirl the suspension so that no lumps remain. After full dispersion, administer oral suspension within 30 min of mixing. Do not chew, cut, or crush the tablets. Administer *Triumeq* 2 hr before or 6 hr after antacids, laxatives, other medications containing aluminum, magnesium, sucralfate, or buffering agents, calcium, or iron. Supplements containing calcium or iron can be taken with *Triumeq* if taken with food.

Patient/Family Teaching
- Emphasize the importance of taking *Triumeq* as directed. Must always be used in combination with other antiretroviral drugs. Do not take more than prescribed amount, and do not stop taking without consulting health care professional. Take missed doses as soon as remembered unless almost time for next dose; do not double doses. Advise patient to read the *Medication Guide* prior to starting therapy and with each Rx refill in case of changes.
- Instruct patient or caregiver in how to disperse *Triumeq PD* tablets.
- Instruct patient not to share medication with others.
- Inform patient that medication does not cure HIV or prevent associated or opportunistic infections. Medication may reduce the risk of transmission of HIV to others through sexual contact or blood contamination. Caution patient to use a condom, and avoid sharing needles or donating blood to prevent spreading HIV to others. Advise patient that the long-term effects of medication are unknown at this time.
- Advise patient of potential for hypersensitivity reactions that may result in death. Instruct patient to discontinue medication and notify health care professional immediately if symptoms of hypersensitivity or signs of Immune Reconstitution Syndrome (signs and symptoms of inflammation from previous infections) occur. A warning card summarizing symptoms of hypersensitivity is provided with each prescription; instruct patient to carry card at all times.
- Instruct patient to notify health care professional immediately if symptoms of lactic acidosis (tiredness or weakness, unusual muscle pain, trouble breathing, stomach pain with nausea and vomiting, cold especially in arms or legs, dizziness, fast or irregular heartbeat) or if signs of hepatotoxicity (yellow skin or whites of eyes, dark urine, light-colored stools, lack of appetite for several days or longer, nausea, abdominal pain) occur. These symptoms may occur more frequently in patients that are female, obese, or have been taking medications for a long time.
- Instruct patient to notify health care professional promptly if signs of peripheral neuropathy or pancreatitis occur.
- Advise patient to avoid sugarless gum or candy due to sorbitol content; may ↓ medication effectiveness.
- Advise patient to notify health care professional of all Rx or OTC medications, vitamins, or herbal products being taken and to consult with health care professional before taking other medications, especially methadone, St. John's wort, and other antiretrovirals.
- Rep: May cause fetal harm and increase risk of neural tube defects. Advise adolescent and adult females of reproductive potential to use effective contraception and to avoid breastfeeding during therapy. Notify care professional if pregnancy is planned or suspected. Switch to another antiviral regimen during 1st trimester; may increase risk of neural tube defects. May consider *Triumeq* during 2nd and 3rd trimesters of pregnancy if expected benefit justifies potential risk to pregnant woman and fetus. Pregnant patients should be encouraged to enroll in the Antiretroviral Pregnancy Registry by calling 1-800-258-4263.
- Advise patient to carry hypersensitivity warning card with them at all times.
- Emphasize the importance of regular follow-up exams and blood counts to determine progress and monitor for side effects.

Evaluation/Desired Outcomes
- Delayed progression of AIDS, and decreased opportunistic infections in patients with HIV.
- Decrease in viral load and increase in CD4 cell counts.

⚕ abemaciclib
(a-bem-a-**sye**-klib)
Verzenio
Classification
Therapeutic: antineoplastics
Pharmacologic: kinase inhibitors

Indications
⚕ Adjuvant treatment of hormone receptor (HR)-positive, human epidermal growth factor 2 (HER2)-negative, node-positive, early breast cancer at high risk of recurrence (in combination with tamoxifen or an aro-

matase inhibitor). ☒ Advanced or metastatic HR-positive, HER2-negative breast cancer in patients with disease progression following endocrine therapy (in combination with fulvestrant). ☒ HR-positive, HER2-negative advanced or metastatic breast cancer in patients with disease progression following endocrine therapy and prior chemotherapy in the metastatic setting (as monotherapy). ☒ HR-positive, HER2-negative advanced or metastatic breast cancer (as initial endocrine-based therapy in combination with an aromatase inhibitor).

Action
Inhibits kinases (cyclin-dependent kinases 4 and 6) that are part of the signaling pathway for cell proliferation. **Therapeutic Effects:** Improved survival and decreased spread of breast cancer.

Pharmacokinetics
Absorption: 45% absorbed following oral administration.
Distribution: Extensively distributed to tissues.
Protein Binding: 96%.
Metabolism and Excretion: Primarily metabolized in the liver by CYP3A4 to several active metabolites; 81% excreted in feces, 3% in urine.
Half-life: 18.3 hr.

TIME/ACTION PROFILE (blood levels)

ROUTE	ONSET	PEAK	DURATION
PO	unknown	8 hr	24 hr

Contraindications/Precautions
Contraindicated in: OB: Pregnancy; Lactation: Lactation.
Use Cautiously in: Severe renal impairment (CCr <30 mL/min); Severe hepatic impairment (↓ dose); History of venous thromboembolism; Rep: Women of reproductive potential; Pedi: Safety and effectiveness not established in children.

Adverse Reactions/Side Effects
CV: peripheral edema, VENOUS THROMBOEMBOLISM. **Derm:** alopecia, pruritus, rash. **GI:** ↓ appetite, ↑ liver enzymes, abdominal pain, constipation, diarrhea, dry mouth, nausea, stomatitis, vomiting, HEPATOTOXICITY. **GU:** ↑ serum creatinine, ↓ fertility (males). **Hemat:** ANEMIA, LEUKOPENIA, NEUTROPENIA, THROMBOCYTOPENIA. **Metab:** ↓ weight. **MS:** arthralgia. **Neuro:** dizziness, dysgeusia, fatigue, headache. **Resp:** cough, INTERSTITIAL LUNG DISEASE/PNEUMONITIS. **Misc:** fever, INFECTION.

Interactions
Drug-Drug: Strong CYP3A inhibitors, including **itraconazole** or **ketoconazole** may ↑ abemaciclib levels and risk of toxicity; avoid concurrent use with ketoconazole; ↓ abemaciclib dose when using other strong CYP3A4 inhibitors (resume original dose after 3–5 half-lives of offending drug have passed following discontinuation). **Strong CYP3A inducers,** including

rifampin may ↓ abemaciclib levels and its effectiveness; avoid concurrent use.

Route/Dosage
PO (Adults): *With fulvestrant, tamoxifen, or an aromatase inhibitor:* 150 mg twice daily; for early breast cancer, continue for 2 years or until disease progression or unacceptable toxicity; for advanced or metastatic breast cancer, continue until disease progression or unacceptable toxicity. *As monotherapy:* 200 mg twice daily; continue until disease progression or unacceptable toxicity. *Concurrent use of strong CYP3A inhibitor (other then ketoconazole):* 100 mg twice daily (with fulvestrant, tamoxifen, an aromatase inhibitor, or as monotherapy); if dose already at 100 mg twice daily due to adverse reactions, ↓ dose to 50 mg twice daily; for early breast cancer, continue for 2 years or until disease progression or unacceptable toxicity; for advanced or metastatic breast cancer, continue until disease progression or unacceptable toxicity.

Hepatic Impairment
PO (Adults): *Severe hepatic impairment (Child-Pugh C):* With fulvestrant, tamoxifen or an aromatase inhibitor: 150 mg once daily; for early breast cancer, continue for 2 years or until disease progression or unacceptable toxicity; for advanced or metastatic breast cancer, continue until disease progression or unacceptable toxicity. As monotherapy: 200 mg once daily; continue until disease progression or unacceptable toxicity. Concurrent use of strong CYP3A inhibitor (other than ketoconazole): 100 mg once daily (with fulvestrant, tamoxifen, an aromatase inhibitor, or as monotherapy); if dose already at 100 mg once daily due to adverse reactions, ↓ dose to 50 mg once daily; for early breast cancer, continue for 2 years or until disease progression or unacceptable toxicity; for advanced or metastatic breast cancer, continue until disease progression or unacceptable toxicity.

Availability
Tablets: 50 mg, 100 mg, 150 mg, 200 mg.

NURSING IMPLICATIONS
Assessment
● Monitor for diarrhea, may result in dehydration and infection. *Grade 1:* no dose modification required. *Grade 2:* If diarrhea resolves in 24 hrs to ≤Grade 1, suspend therapy until resolution. No dose reduction required. *Grade 2 that persists or recurs after resuming same dose despite maximum supportive measures:* Hold dose until diarrhea resolves to ≤Grade 1. Resume at next lower dose. *Grade 3 or 4 diarrhea or diarrhea that requires hospitalization,* hold abemaciclib until diarrhea resolves to ≤Grade 1, then resume at next lower dose.
● Monitor for signs and symptoms of venous thrombosis and pulmonary embolism and treat as needed.

Lab Test Considerations
● Verify negative pregnancy test before starting therapy.

- Monitor CBC before starting, every 2 wk for first 2 mo, monthly for next 2 mo, and as clinically indicated. *Grade 1 or 2 neutropenia:* No dose reduction required. *Grade 3:* Hold dose until resolves to ≤Grade 2. *Grade 3 recurrent or Grade 4:* Hold therapy until resolved to ≤ Grade 2. Resume at next lower dose.
- Monitor ALT, AST, and serum bilirubin prior to starting therapy, every 2 wk for first 2 mo, monthly for next 2 mo, and as clinically indicated. *If Grade 1 (>ULN to 3 times ULN), Grade 2 (>3.0 to 5.0 times ULN, without ↑ in total bilirubin >2 times ULN):* no dose reduction required. *If persistent or recurrent Grade 2, or Grade 3 (>5.0–20.0 × ULN), without ↑ in total bilirubin above 2 × ULN:* Hold therapy until toxicity resolves to baseline or Grade 1. Resume at next lower dose. *If elevation in AST and/or ALT >3 × ULN with total bilirubin >2 × ULN, in the absence of cholestasis or Grade 4 (>20.0 × ULN):* discontinue therapy.
- May cause ↑ serum creatinine without glomerular function being affected. Monitor BUN, cystatin C, or calculated glomerular filtration rate to determine impaired renal function.

Implementation
- Dose Reduction Recommendations: *Starting dose,* 150 mg twice daily for therapy in combination with fulvestrant or an aromatase inhibitor OR 200 mg twice daily for monotherapy. *1st dose reduction,* 100 twice daily for combination therapy OR 150 mg twice daily for monotherapy. *2nd dose reduction,* 50 mg twice daily for combination therapy OR 100 mg twice daily for monotherapy. *3rd dose reduction,* discontinue combination therapy OR 50 mg twice daily for monotherapy.
- **PO:** Administer twice daily, at the same times each day, without regard to food. *DNC:* Swallow tablets whole; do not crush, break, or chew.

Patient/Family Teaching
- Instruct patient to take abemaciclib at the same times each day as directed. If patient vomits or misses a dose, omit dose and take next dose as scheduled. Do not ingest tablets that are broken, cracked, or not intact. Advise patient to read *Patient Information* before starting therapy and with each Rx refill in case of changes.
- Advise patient that at first sign of diarrhea, start antidiarrheal therapy (loperamide), increase oral fluids, and notify health care professional.
- Advise patient to notify health care professional if signs and symptoms of infection (fever, chills), liver problems (feeling very tired, pain on upper right side of abdomen, loss of appetite, unusual bleeding or bruising), or venous thromboembolism (pain or swelling in arms or legs, shortness of breath, chest pain, rapid breathing, rapid heart rate) occur.

- Instruct patient to notify health care professional of all Rx or OTC medications, vitamins, or herbal products being taken and to consult with health care professional before taking other medications.
- Rep: May cause fetal harm. Advise females of reproductive potential to use effective contraception and avoid breastfeeding during and for at least 3 wk after last dose of therapy. Inform male patient may impair fertility.

Evaluation/Desired Outcomes
- Decrease in the spread of breast cancer.

abiraterone (a-bi-ra-te-rone)
Yonsa, Zytiga
Classification
Therapeutic: antineoplastics
Pharmacologic: enzyme inhibitors

Indications
Zytiga: Treatment of metastatic castration-resistant prostate cancer (in combination with prednisone). **Zytiga:** Treatment of metastatic high-risk castration-sensitive prostate cancer (in combination with prednisone). **Yonsa:** Treatment of metastatic castration-resistant prostate cancer (in combination with methylprednisolone).

Action
Inhibits the enzyme 17α-hydroxylase/C17,20−lyase (CYP17), which is required for androgen production. May also result in increased mineralocortocoid production. **Therapeutic Effects:** Decreased androgen production with decreased spread of androgen-sensitive prostate cancer.

Pharmacokinetics
Absorption: Hydrolyzed to its active compound following oral administration.
Distribution: Widely distributed to tissues.
Protein Binding: >99%.
Metabolism and Excretion: Metabolized by esterases to inactive compounds; eliminated primarily in feces as unchanged drug and metabolites; 5% excreted in urine.
Half-life: 12 hr.

TIME/ACTION PROFILE (plasma concentrations)

ROUTE	ONSET	PEAK	DURATION
PO	unknown	2 hr	12 hr

Contraindications/Precautions
Contraindicated in: Severe hepatic impairment; Concurrent use of radium Ra 223 dichloride (↑ risk of fractures and mortality).
Use Cautiously in: HF, recent MI, other cardiovascular disease, ventricular arrhythmias; Electrolyte ab-

normalities or hypertension (correct/treat prior to initiation); Moderate hepatic impairment; Stress, infection, trauma, acute disease process (may result in adrenocortical insufficiency requiring additional corticosteroids); Rep: Men with female partners of reproductive potential.

Adverse Reactions/Side Effects

CV: hypertension, arrhythmia, edema, QT interval prolongation (in presence of hypokalemia), TORSADES DE POINTES (in presence of hypokalemia). **Derm:** hot flush. **Endo:** adrenocortical insufficiency (due to concurrent corticosteroid), hypoglycemia. **F and E:** hypokalemia. **GI:** diarrhea, dyspepsia, HEPATOTOXICITY. **GU:** ↓ fertility, nocturia, urinary frequency. **MS:** fracture, joint pain/discomfort. **Resp:** cough.

Interactions

Drug-Drug: May ↑ levels of and risk of toxicity from **CYP2D6 substrates**, including **thioridazine** and **dextromethorphan**; if concurrent use necessary, ↓ dose of CYP2D6 substrate. may be required. May ↑ levels of and risk of toxicity from **CYP2C8 substrates**, including **pioglitazone**; if concurrent use necessary, ↓ dose of CYP2C8 substrate may be required. **Strong CYP3A4 inducers**, including **carbamazepine**, **phenobarbital**, **phenytoin**, **rifabutin**, **rifapentine**, or **rifampin** may ↓ levels and effectiveness; avoid concurrent use. May ↑ risk of hypoglycemia when used with **pioglitazone** or **repaglinide**.

Route/Dosage

Zytiga and Yonsa are not interchangeable.

Zytiga

PO (Adults): 1000 mg once daily; *Concurrent use with strong CYP3A4 inducer:* 1000 mg twice daily.

Hepatic Impairment

PO (Adults): *Moderate hepatic impairment:* 250 mg once daily.

Yonsa

PO (Adults): 500 mg once daily; *Concurrent use with strong CYP3A4 inducer:* 500 mg twice daily.

Hepatic Impairment

PO (Adults): *Moderate hepatic impairment:* 125 mg once daily.

Availability (generic available)

Tablets (Zytiga): 250 mg, 500 mg. **Tablets (Yonsa):** 125 mg.

NURSING IMPLICATIONS

Assessment

- Monitor BP and assess for fluid retention at least monthly. Control hypertension during therapy.
- Monitor for signs and symptoms of adrenocortical insufficiency (hypotension, weight loss, weakness, nausea, vomiting, anorexia, lethargy, confusion, restlessness), especially in patients under stress or

who are withdrawn from or have decreased prednisone dose. Symptoms may be masked by abiraterone.

Lab Test Considerations

- Monitor AST, ALT, and bilirubin prior to starting therapy, every 2 wk for 3 mo, and monthly thereafter. Administer reduced dose to patients with baseline moderate hepatic impairment and monitor AST, ALT, and bilirubin prior to starting therapy, every wk for first mo, every 2 wk for 2 mo, and monthly thereafter. If clinical signs of hepatic toxicity occur, measure serum bilirubin, AST, and ALT promptly; monitor frequently if ↑ levels. If AST and/or ALT ↑ >5 times upper limit of normal (ULN) or bilirubin ↑ >3 times ULN in patients with baseline moderate hepatic impairment, interrupt abiraterone. Following return of liver function to baseline or AST and ALT ↑ >2.5 times ULN or bilirubin ↑ >1.5 times ULN may restart at a reduced dose of 750 mg once daily. Monitor serum transaminases and bilirubin every 2 wk for 3 mo and monthly thereafter. If hepatotoxicity recurs, may restart at 500 mg once daily following return to baseline or AST and ALT ↑ >2.5 times ULN or bilirubin ↑ >1.5 times ULN. If hepatotoxicity recurs at 500 mg dose, discontinue therapy. If concurrent ↑ ALT >3 times ULN and total bilirubin ↑ >2 times ULN without biliary obstruction or other causes, permanently discontinue therapy.
- Monitor serum potassium and sodium at least monthly during therapy. May cause hypokalemia; control during therapy.
- May cause ↑ triglycerides and ↓ phosphorous.

Implementation

- Control hypertension and correct hypokalemia prior to starting therapy.
- Patients should also receive a gonadotropin-releasing hormone analog concurrently or should have had bilateral orchiectomy.
- **Zytiga:** *For castration-resistant prostate cancer:* Administer once daily with twice daily prednisone 5 mg on an empty stomach at least 1 hr before or 2 hr after meals; food increases absorption and adverse reactions. Swallow tablets whole with water; do not crush, break, or chew. *For castration-sensitive prostate cancer:* Administer once daily with once daily prednisone 5 mg on an empty stomach at least 1 hr before or 2 hr after meals; food increases absorption. Swallow tablets whole with water; do not crush, break, or chew.
- **Yonsa:** Administer orally once daily in combination with methylprednisolone 4 mg administered orally twice daily. Administer without regard to meals. *DNC:* Swallow tablets whole; do not crush, break, or chew.

Patient/Family Teaching

- Instruct patient to take medications as directed and not to stop abiraterone, prednisone or methylprednisolone, or gonadotropin-releasing hormone ana-

log without consulting health care professional. If a dose is missed, take the following day. If more than 1 dose is missed, consult health care professional. Do not share medication with others, even if they have the same symptoms; may be dangerous. Advise patient to read *Patient Information* before starting therapy and with each Rx refill in case of changes.
- Advise patient to notify health care professional if signs and symptoms of high blood pressure, low potassium, and fluid retention (dizziness, fast heartbeats, feel faint or lightheaded, headache, confusion, muscle weakness, pain in legs, swelling in legs or feet), adrenal insufficiency, or hepatotoxicity (yellowing of skin and eyes, dark urine, pain in upper right quadrant, severe nausea or vomiting, difficulty concentrating, disorientation, confusion) occur or of side effects that are bothersome or persistent.
- Advise parents to notify health care professional of all Rx or OTC medications, vitamins, or herbal products being taken and to consult with health care professional before taking other medications.
- Rep: Male patients should use a condom and another form of contraception during sex with a women of reproductive potential during and for 3 wk after therapy. Pregnant women and women of reproductive potential should not touch tablets without wearing gloves. May impair reproductive function and fertility in males of reproductive potential.
- Explain need for continued follow-up exams and lab tests to assess possible side effects.

Evaluation/Desired Outcomes
- Decreased androgen production with decreased spread of androgen-sensitive prostate cancer.

✂ abrocitinib (a-broe-**sye**-ti-nib)
Cibinqo
Classification
Therapeutic: anti-inflammatories
Pharmacologic: kinase inhibitors

Indications
Refractory, moderate to severe atopic dermatitis in patients whose disease is not adequately controlled with other systemic drug products, including biologics, or when use of those therapies are not recommended (not to be used with other JAK inhibitors, biologic immunomodulators, or other immunosuppressants).

Action
Inhibits JAK enzymes which prevents the signaling of interleukin-4, interleukin-13, and other cytokines involved in the pathogenesis of atopic dermatitis. **Therapeutic Effects:** Improvement in clinical and symptomatic parameters of atopic dermatitis.

Pharmacokinetics
Absorption: Well absorbed following oral administration.
Distribution: Extensively distributed to tissues.
Metabolism and Excretion: Primarily metabolized by the liver via the CYP2C19, CYP2C9, CYP3A4, and CYP2B6 isoenzymes into two active metabolites (M1 and M2). ✂ 2% of Whites, 4% of Blacks, and 14% of Asians have CYP2C19 genotype that results in reduced metabolism of abrocitinib. Primarily excreted in urine (<1% as unchanged drug).
Half-life: 3–5 hr.

TIME/ACTION PROFILE (plasma concentrations)

ROUTE	ONSET	PEAK	DURATION
PO	rapid	<1 hr	unknown

Contraindications/Precautions
Contraindicated in: Concurrent use of antiplatelet therapies (excluding low-dose aspirin [≤81 mg/day]) for the first 3 mo of treatment; Active infection; Platelet count <150,000/mm^3, lymphocyte count <500 cells/mm^3, absolute neutrophil count <1000 cells/mm^3, or hemoglobin level <8 g/dL; Increased risk for thrombosis; Severe renal impairment or end-stage renal disease; Severe hepatic impairment; Lactation: Lactation.
Use Cautiously in: Patients who are >50 yr old and have ≥1 cardiovascular risk factor (↑ risk of all-cause mortality, cardiovascular death, MI, stroke, and thrombosis); Chronic or recurrent infection; Previously exposed to tuberculosis; History of serious or opportunistic infection; Resided or traveled in areas of endemic tuberculosis or endemic mycoses; Underlying conditions that predispose to infection; Malignancy (other than successfully treated non-melanoma skin cancer); ✂ Known or suspected CYP2C19 poor metabolizers (↓ dose); Moderate renal impairment (↓ dose); OB: Other agents for atopic dermatitis preferred in pregnancy; Pedi: Children <12 yr (safety and effectiveness not established); Geri: Older adults may have ↑ risk of lymphopenia, thrombocytopenia, and herpes infection.

Adverse Reactions/Side Effects
CV: CARDIOVASCULAR DEATH, DEEP VEIN THROMBOSIS (DVT), hypertension, MI. **Derm:** acne, contact dermatitis, impetigo. **EENT:** <u>nasopharyngitis</u>, retinal detachment. **GI:** nausea, abdominal pain, oropharyngeal pain, vomiting. **Hemat:** lymphopenia, thrombocytopenia. **Metab:** hyperlipidemia. **MS:** ↑ creatine kinase. **Neuro:** dizziness, fatigue, headache. **Resp:** PULMONARY EMBOLISM (PE). **Misc:** INFECTION (including tuberculosis, bacterial, invasive fungal, viral, or opportunistic infections), MALIGNANCY (including non-melanoma skin cancer).

✂ = Canadian drug name. ✂ = Genetic implication. ~~Strikethrough~~ = Discontinued. CAPITALS = life-threatening. <u>Underline</u> = most frequent.

Interactions

Drug-Drug: May ↑ risk of bleeding and thrombocytopenia when used with **antiplatelet drugs**, excluding low-dose **aspirin** (≤81 mg/day); concurrent use during first 3 mo of abrocitinib contraindicated. **Moderate-to-strong inhibitors of both CYP2C9 and CYP2C19**, including **fluconazole**, significantly ↑ levels and risk of toxicity; avoid concurrent use. **Strong CYP2C9 inducers** and **strong CYP2C19 inducers**, including **rifampin**, ↓ levels and effectiveness; avoid concurrent use. **Strong CYP2C19 inhibitors**, including **fluvoxamine**, may ↑ levels and risk of toxicity; ↓ abrocitinib dose. May ↑ levels and risk of toxicity of **P-glycoprotein substrates**, including **dabigatran**; closely monitor. May ↑ risk of adverse reactions and ↓ antibody response to **live vaccines**; avoid concurrent use.

Route/Dosage

PO (Adults and Children ≥12 yr): 100 mg once daily initially; if adequate response not achieved after 12 wk, may ↑ to 200 mg once daily. Discontinue therapy if inadequate response after dose ↑ to 200 mg once daily. *CYP2C19 poor metabolizers or concurrent use of strong CYP2C19 inhibitors:* 50 mg once daily initially; if adequate response not achieved after 12 wk, may ↑ to 100 mg once daily. Discontinue therapy if inadequate response after dose ↑ to 100 mg once daily.

Renal Impairment

PO (Adults and Children ≥12 yr): *Moderate renal impairment (CCr 30–59 mL/min):* 50 mg once daily initially; if adequate response not achieved after 12 wk, may ↑ to 100 mg once daily. Discontinue therapy if inadequate response after dose ↑ to 100 mg once daily.

Availability

Tablets: 50 mg, 100 mg, 200 mg.

NURSING IMPLICATIONS

Assessment

- Assess involved area of skin before starting and periodically during therapy.
- Determine tuberculosis (TB) infection status. Use of abrocitinib is not recommended in patients with active TB. For patients with latent TB or those with a negative latent TB test who are at high risk for TB, start preventive therapy for latent TB before starting abrocitinib.
- Conduct viral hepatitis screening in accordance with clinical guidelines. Starting abrocitinib is not recommended in patients with active hepatitis B or hepatitis C.
- Monitor for development of signs and symptoms of infection, including TB, during and after therapy with abrocitinib. If a serious or opportunistic infection, discontinue therapy. Begin diagnostic testing and antimicrobial therapy. Considered risks and benefits of therapy before reinitiating therapy.
- Monitor for signs and symptoms of major adverse cardiac events. Patients who are current or past smokers and patients with other cardiovascular risk factors are at greatest risk.
- Monitor for thrombosis, including DVT, PE, and arterial thrombosis. Avoid abrocitinib in patients that may be at increased risk of thrombosis. If symptoms of thrombosis occur, discontinue therapy and evaluate and treat patients.

Lab Test Considerations

- Monitor CBC at baseline, 4 wk after starting therapy and 4 wk after dose increase. Abrocitinib is not recommended in patients with a platelet count <150,000/mm³, an absolute lymphocyte count (ALC) <500/mm³, an absolute neutrophil count (ANC) <1,000/mm³, or a hemoglobin value <8 g/dL. *If platelet count <50,000/mm³,* discontinue therapy and follow with CBC until >100,000/mm³. *If ALC <500/mm³,* temporarily discontinue abrocitinib; may be restarted once ALC return above this value. *If ANC <1,000/mm³,* temporarily discontinue therapy; may be restarted once ANC return above this value. *If Hgb value <8 g/dL,* temporarily discontinue abrocitinib; may be restarted once Hgb returns above this value.
- May cause increased serum lipids. Monitor lipid levels after 4 wk of therapy and periodically thereafter.

Implementation

- Complete any necessary immunizations, including herpes zoster vaccinations, in agreement with current immunization guidelines prior to starting therapy.
- Abrocitinib can be used with or without topical corticosteroids.
- **PO:** Administer 100 mg daily without regard to food, at the same time each day. *DNC:* Swallow tablets whole with water; do not crush, split, or chew. If an adequate response is not achieved with 100 mg orally daily after 12 wk, may increase dose to 200 mg orally once daily. Discontinue therapy if inadequate response is seen after dose of 200 mg once daily.

Patient/Family Teaching

- Instruct patient to take abrocitinib as directed. Take missed dose as soon as possible unless <12 hrs before next dose. If <12 hrs before next dose, omit dose and resume dosing at the regular scheduled time.
- Advise patient to notify health care professional if signs and symptoms of infection (fever, sweating, or chills, blood in phlegm, diarrhea or stomach pain, muscle aches, weight loss, burning during urination or urinating more often than usual, cough or shortness of breath, warm, red, or painful skin or sores on body, feeling very tired).
- Caution patient with signs and symptoms of a heart attack or stroke (discomfort in the center of chest that lasts for more than a few minutes, or that goes away and comes back; severe tightness, pain, pressure, or heaviness in chest, throat, neck, or jaw; pain or discomfort in arms, back, neck, jaw, or

stomach; weakness in one part or on one side of your body; slurred speech; shortness of breath with or without chest discomfort; breaking out in a cold sweat; nausea or vomiting; feeling lightheaded) to notify health care professional immediately.

- Inform patient of increased risk of DVT and pulmonary embolism. If signs and symptoms (swelling, pain or tenderness in one or both legs; sudden, unexplained chest or upper back pain; shortness of breath or difficulty breathing) occur, stop therapy and get immediate medical care. Notify health care professional if you have had blood clots in the veins of your legs or lungs in the past.

- May increase risk of cancer. Advise patient to have skin checked for skin cancer during therapy. Limit amount of time spent in sunlight. Avoid using tanning beds or sunlamps. Wear protective clothing and use sunscreen with a high protection factor (SPF 30 and above). Especially important for patients with very fair skin or with a family history of skin cancer. Instruct patient to notify health care professional if you have ever had any type of cancer.

- Instruct patient to notify health care professional of all Rx or OTC medications, vitamins, or herbal products being taken and to consult with health care professional before taking other medications.

- Rep: Advise women of reproductive potential to notify health care professional if pregnancy is planned or suspected. Advise to avoid breastfeeding during and for 1 day after last dose. May impair female fertility; may be reversible. There is a pregnancy exposure registry that monitors pregnancy outcomes in women exposed to abrocitinib during pregnancy. Pregnant women exposed to abrocitinib and health care providers are encouraged to call 1-877-311-3770 or www.cibinqopregnancyregistry.com.

Evaluation/Desired Outcomes

- Improvement in clinical and symptomatic parameters of atopic dermatitis.

acetaminophen (oral, rectal)
(a-seet-a-**min**-oh-fen)
　　❋ Abenol, Acephen, ❋ Acet,
　　❋ Children Feverhalt, ❋ Fortolin, Infant's Feverall, ❋ Pediaphen,
　　❋ Pediatrix, ❋ Taminol, ❋ Tempra,
　　Tylenol

acetaminophen (intravenous)
~~Ofirmev~~
Classification
Therapeutic: antipyretics, nonopioid analgesics

Indications
PO, Rect: Treatment of: Mild pain, Fever. **IV:** Treatment of: Mild to moderate pain, Moderate to severe pain with opioid analgesics, Fever.

Action
Inhibits synthesis of prostaglandins that may serve as mediators of pain and fever, primarily in the CNS. Has no significant anti-inflammatory properties or GI toxicity. **Therapeutic Effects:** Analgesia. Antipyresis.

Pharmacokinetics
Absorption: Well absorbed following oral administration. Rectal absorption is variable. Intravenous administration results in complete bioavailability.
Distribution: Widely distributed. Crosses the placenta; enters breast milk in low concentrations.
Metabolism and Excretion: 85–95% metabolized by the liver (CYP2E1 enzyme system). Metabolites may be toxic in overdose situation. Metabolites excreted by the kidneys.
Half-life: Neonates: 7 hr; Infants and Children: 3–4 hr; Adults: 1–3 hr.

TIME/ACTION PROFILE (analgesia and antipyresis)

ROUTE	ONSET	PEAK	DURATION
PO	0.5–1 hr	1–3 hr	3–8 hr†
Rect	0.5–1 hr	1–3 hr	3–4 hr
IV‡	within 30 min	30 min	4–6 hr

†Depends on dose.
‡Antipyretic effects.

Contraindications/Precautions
Contraindicated in: Previous hypersensitivity; Products containing alcohol, aspartame, saccharin, sugar, or tartrazine (FDC yellow dye #5) should be avoided in patients who have hypersensitivity or intolerance to these compounds; Severe hepatic impairment/active liver disease.
Use Cautiously in: Hepatic disease/renal disease (lower chronic doses recommended); Alcoholism, chronic malnutrition, severe hypovolemia or severe renal impairment (CCr <30 mL/min, ↑ dosing interval and ↓ daily dose may be necessary); Chronic alcohol use/abuse; Malnutrition; OB: Use in pregnancy only if clearly needed (for IV); Lactation: Use cautiously (for IV).

Adverse Reactions/Side Effects
CV: hypertension (IV), hypotension (IV). **Derm:** ACUTE GENERALIZED EXANTHEMATOUS PUSTULOSIS, rash, STEVENS-JOHNSON SYNDROME, TOXIC EPIDERMAL NECROLYSIS, urticaria. **F and E:** hypokalemia (IV). **GI:** ↑ liver enzymes, constipation (↑ in children) (IV), HEPATOTOXICITY (↑ DOSES), nausea (IV), vomiting (IV). **GU:** renal failure (high doses/chronic use). **Hemat:** neutropenia, pancytopenia. **MS:** muscle spasms (IV), trismus (IV).
Neuro:

agitation (↑ in children) (IV), anxiety (IV), fatigue (IV), headache (IV), insomnia (IV). **Resp:** atelectasis (↑ in children) (IV), dyspnea (IV).

Interactions

Drug-Drug: Chronic high-dose acetaminophen (>2 g/day) may ↑ risk of bleeding with **warfarin** (INR should not exceed 4). Hepatotoxicity is additive with other **hepatotoxic substances,** including **alcohol.** Concurrent use of **isoniazid, rifampin, rifabutin, phenytoin, barbiturates,** and **carbamazepine** may ↑ the risk of acetaminophen-induced liver damage (limit self-medication); these agents will also ↓ therapeutic effects of acetaminophen. Concurrent use of **NSAIDs** may ↑ the risk of adverse renal effects (avoid chronic concurrent use). **Propranolol** ↓ metabolism and may ↑ effects. May ↓ effects of **lamotrigine** and **zidovudine.**

Route/Dosage

Children ≤12 yr should not receive >5 PO or rectal doses/24 hr without notifying physician or other health care professional. No dose adjustment needed when converting between IV and PO acetaminophen in adults and children ≥50 kg.

PO (Adults and Children >12 yr): 325–650 mg every 6 hr or 1 g 3–4 times daily or 1300 mg every 8 hr (not to exceed 3 g or 2 g/24 hr in patients with hepatic/renal impairment).

PO (Children 1–12 yr): 10–15 mg/kg/dose every 6 hr as needed (not to exceed 5 doses/24 hr).

PO (Infants): 10–15 mg/kg/dose every 6 hr as needed (not to exceed 5 doses/24 hr).

PO (Neonates): 10–15 mg/kg/dose every 6–8 hr as needed.

IV (Adults and Children ≥13 yr and ≥50 kg): 1000 mg every 6 hr or 650 mg every 4 hr (not to exceed 1000 mg/dose, 4 g/day [by all routes], and less than 4 hr dosing interval).

IV (Adults and Children ≥13 yr and <50 kg): 15 mg/kg every 6 hr or 12.5 mg/kg every 4 hr (not to exceed 15 mg/kg/dose [up to 750 mg/dose], 75 mg/kg/day [up to 3750 mg/day] [by all routes], and less than 4 hr dosing interval).

IV (Children 2–12 yr): 15 mg/kg every 6 hr or 12.5 mg/kg every 4 hr (not to exceed 15 mg/kg/dose [up to 750 mg/dose], 75 mg/kg/day [up to 3750 mg/day] [by all routes], and less than 4 hr dosing interval).

IV (Infants 29 days-2 yr): 15 mg/kg every 6 hr (not to exceed 60 mg/kg/day [by all routes]).

IV (Neonates Birth–28 days): 12.5 mg/kg every 6 hr (not to exceed 50 mg/kg [by all routes]).

Rect (Adults and Children >12 yr): 325–650 mg every 4–6 hr as needed or 1 g 3–4 times/day (not to exceed 4 g/24 hr).

Rect (Children 1–12 yr): 10–20 mg/kg/dose every 4–6 hr as needed.

Rect (Infants): 10–20 mg/kg/dose every 4–6 hr as needed.

Rect (Neonates): 10–15 mg/kg/dose every 6–8 hr as needed.

Availability (generic available)

Chewable tablets (fruit, bubblegum, or grape flavor): 80 mg^{OTC}, 160 mg^{OTC}. **Tablets:** 160 mg^{OTC}, 325 mg^{OTC}. **Caplets:** 325 mg^{OTC}. **Solution (berry, fruit, and grape flavor):** 100 mg/mL^{OTC}. **Liquid (mint):** 160 mg/5 mL^{OTC}. **Elixir (grape and cherry flavor):** 160 mg/5 mL^{OTC}. **Drops:** 160 mg/ 5 mL ^{OTC}. **Suspension:** ✱ 100 mg/mL^{OTC}, ✱ 160 mg/5 mL^{OTC}. **Syrup:** 160 mg/5 mL^{OTC}. **Suppositories:** 80 mg^{OTC}, 120 mg^{OTC}, 325 mg^{OTC}. **Solution for injection:** 10 mg/mL. *In combination with:* many other medications. See Appendix N.

NURSING IMPLICATIONS

Assessment

- Assess overall health status and alcohol usage before administering acetaminophen. Patients who are malnourished or chronically abuse alcohol are at higher risk of developing hepatotoxicity with chronic use of usual doses of this drug.
- Assess amount, frequency, and type of drugs taken in patients self-medicating, especially with OTC drugs. Prolonged use of acetaminophen increases risk of adverse hepatic and renal effects. For short-term use, combined doses of acetaminophen and salicylates should not exceed the recommended dose of either drug given alone. Do not exceed maximum daily dose of acetaminophen when considering all routes of administration and all combination products containing acetaminophen.
- Assess for rash periodically during therapy. May cause Stevens-Johnson syndrome. Discontinue therapy if rash (reddening of skin, blisters, and detachment of upper surface of skin peeling) or if accompanied with fever, general malaise, fatigue, muscle or joint aches, blisters, oral lesions, conjunctivitis, hepatitis, and/or eosinophilia.
- **Pain:** Assess type, location, and intensity prior to and 30–60 min following administration.
- **Fever:** Assess fever; note presence of associated signs (diaphoresis, tachycardia, and malaise).

Lab Test Considerations

- Evaluate hepatic, hematologic, and renal function periodically during prolonged, high-dose therapy.
- May alter results of blood glucose monitoring. May cause falsely ↓ values when measured with glucose oxidase/peroxidase method, but probably not with hexokinase/G6PD method. May also cause falsely ↑ values with certain instruments; see manufacturer's instruction manual.
- Increased serum bilirubin, LDH, AST, ALT, and prothrombin time may indicate hepatotoxicity.

Toxicity and Overdose

- If overdose occurs, **N-acetylcysteine** (Acetadote) is the antidote.

Implementation

- Do not confuse Tylenol with Tylenol PM. Do not confuse acetaminophen with acetazolamide.

- To prevent fatal medication errors ensure dose in milligrams (mg) and milliliters (mL) is not confused; dosing is based on weight for patients under 50 kg; program infusion pump for accuracy; and total daily dose of acetaminophen from all sources does not exceed maximum daily limits.
- When combined with opioids do not exceed the maximum recommended daily dose of acetaminophen.
- **PO:** Administer with a full glass of water.
- May be taken with food or on an empty stomach.

IV Administration
- **Intermittent Infusion:** *For 1000 mg dose,* insert vented IV set through septum of 100 mL vial; may be administered without further dilution. *For doses <1000 mg,* withdraw appropriate dose from vial and place in a separate empty, sterile container for IV infusion. Place small volume pediatric doses up to 60 mL in a syringe and administer via syringe pump. Solution is clear and colorless; do not administer solutions that are discolored or contain particulate matter. Administer within 6 hrs of breaking vial seal. *Rate:* Infuse over 15 min. Monitor end of infusion in order to prevent air embolism, especially if acetaminophen is primary infusion.
- **Y-Site Compatibility:** buprenorphine, butorphanol, cefazolin, ceftriaxone, clindamycin, D5W, defibrotide, dexamethasone, dexmedetomidine, D10W, D5/LR, D5/0.9% NaCl, diphenhydramine, droperidol, esmolol, gentamicin, granisetron, heparin, hydrocortisone, hydromorphone, ketamine, LR, labetalol, lidocaine, lorazepam, magnesium sulfate, mannitol, meperidine, methylprednisolone, metoclopramide, metoprolol, midazolam, morphine, nalbuphine, 0.9% NaCl, ondansetron, oxytocin, piperacillin/tazobactam, potassium chloride, prochlorperazine, protamine, sufentanil, vancomycin.
- **Y-Site Incompatibility:** acyclovir, atropine, blinatumomab, chlorpromazine, diazepam, metronidazole, phenobarbital, phenytoin, propofol.
- **Additive Incompatibility:** Do not mix with other medications.

Patient/Family Teaching
- Advise patient to take medication exactly as directed and not to take more than the recommended amount. Chronic excessive use of >4 g/day (2 g in chronic alcoholics) may lead to hepatotoxicity, renal, or cardiac damage. Adults should not take acetaminophen longer than 10 days and children not longer than 5 days unless directed by health care professional. Short-term doses of acetaminophen with salicylates or NSAIDs should not exceed recommended daily dose of either drug alone.
- Advise patient to avoid alcohol (3 or more glasses per day increase the risk of liver damage) if taking

more than an occasional 1–2 doses and to avoid taking concurrently with salicylates or NSAIDs for more than a few days, unless directed by health care professional.
- Advise patient to discontinue acetaminophen and notify health care professional if rash occurs.
- Inform patients with diabetes that acetaminophen may alter results of blood glucose monitoring. Advise patient to notify health care professional if changes are noted.
- Caution patient to check labels on all OTC products. Advise patients to avoid taking more than one product containing acetaminophen at a time to prevent toxicity.
- Advise patient to consult health care professional if discomfort or fever is not relieved by routine doses of this drug or if fever is greater than 39.5°C (103°F) or lasts longer than 3 days.
- Pedi: Advise parents or caregivers to check concentrations of liquid preparations. All OTC single ingredient acetaminophen liquid products now come in a single concentration of 160 mg/5 mL. Errors have resulted in serious liver damage. Have parents or caregivers determine the correct formulation and dose for their child (based on the child's age/weight), and demonstrate how to measure it using an appropriate measuring device.

Evaluation/Desired Outcomes
- Relief of mild to moderate pain.
- Reduction of fever.

acetylcysteine
(a-se-teel-**sis**-teen)
Acetadote, ~~Mucomyst~~
Classification
Therapeutic: antidotes (for acetaminophen toxicity), mucolytic

Indications
PO, IV: Antidote for the management of potentially hepatotoxic overdose of acetaminophen. **Inhaln:** Mucolytic in the management of conditions associated with thick viscid mucous secretions. **Unlabeled Use: PO:** Prevention of radiocontrast-induced renal impairment.

Action
PO, IV: Decreases the buildup of a hepatotoxic metabolite in acetaminophen overdosage. **Inhaln:** Degrades mucus, allowing easier mobilization and expectoration. **Therapeutic Effects: PO:** Prevention or lessening of liver damage following acetaminophen overdose. **Inhaln:** Lowers the viscosity of mucus.

Pharmacokinetics
Absorption: Absorbed from the GI tract following oral administration. Action is local following inhalation;

remainder may be absorbed from pulmonary epithelium. IV administration results in complete bioavailability.

Distribution: Well distributed to tissues.

Metabolism and Excretion: Partially metabolized by the liver, 22% excreted renally.

Half-life: *Adults:* 5.6 hr (↑ in hepatic impairment) *newborns:* 11 hr.

TIME/ACTION PROFILE

ROUTE	ONSET	PEAK	DURATION
PO (antidote)	unknown	30–60 min	4 hr
IV (antidote)	unknown	unknown	unknown
Inhaln (mucolytic)	1 min	5–10 min	short

Contraindications/Precautions

Contraindicated in: Hypersensitivity.

Use Cautiously in: Severe respiratory insufficiency, asthma, or history of bronchospasm; History of GI bleeding (oral only); OB: Use during pregnancy only if potential maternal benefit justifies potential fetal risk; Lactation: Safety not established in breastfeeding.

Adverse Reactions/Side Effects

CV: hypotension, tachycardia. **Derm:** rash, clamminess, pruritus, urticaria. **EENT:** rhinorrhea. **F and E:** fluid overload. **GI:** nausea, vomiting, stomatitis. **Neuro:** drowsiness. **Resp:** bronchospasm, ↑ secretions, bronchial/tracheal irritation, chest tightness. **Misc:** chills, fever, HYPERSENSITIVITY REACTIONS (including anaphylaxis and angioedema) (primarily with IV).

Interactions

Drug-Drug: **Activated charcoal** may adsorb orally administered acetylcysteine and ↓ its effectiveness as an antidote.

Route/Dosage

Acetaminophen Overdose

PO (Adults and Children): 140 mg/kg initially, followed by 70 mg/kg every 4 hr for 17 additional doses.

IV (Adults and Children): *Loading dose:* 150 mg/kg (maximum: 15 g) over 60 min initially followed by *First maintenance dose:* 50 mg/kg (maximum: 5 g) over 4 hr, then *second maintenance dose:* 100 mg/kg (maximum: 10 g) over 16 hr.

Mucolytic

Inhaln (Adults and Children 1–12 yr): *Nebulization via face mask:* 3–5 mL of 20% solution or 6–10 mL of the 10% solution 3–4 times daily; *nebulization via tent or croupette:* volume of 10–20% solution required to maintain heavy mist; *direct instillation:* 1–2 mL of 10–20% solution every 1–4 hr; *intratracheal instillation via tracheostomy:* 1–2 mL of 10–20% solution every 1–4 hr (up to 2–5 mL of 20% solution via tracheal catheter into particular segments of the bronchopulmonary tree).

Inhaln (Infants): *Nebulization:* 1–2 mL of 20% solution or 2–4 mL of 10% solution 3–4 times daily.

Prevention of Radiocontrast-Induced Renal Impairment

PO (Adults): 600 mg twice daily for 2 days, beginning the day before the procedure.

Availability (generic available)

Solution for inhalation: 10% (100 mg/mL), 20% (200 mg/mL). **Solution for injection:** 200 mg/mL.

NURSING IMPLICATIONS

Assessment

● **Antidote in Acetaminophen Overdose:** Assess type, amount, and time of acetaminophen ingestion. Assess plasma acetaminophen levels. Initial levels are drawn at least 4 hr after ingestion of acetaminophen. Plasma level determinations may be difficult to interpret following ingestion of extended-release preparations. Do not wait for results to administer dose.

● *IV:* Assess for anaphylaxis. Erythema and flushing are common, usually occurring 30–60 min after initiating infusion, and may resolve with continued administration. If rash, hypotension, wheezing, or dyspnea occur, initiate treatment for anaphylaxis (antihistamine and epinephrine). Interrupt acetylcysteine infusion until symptoms resolve and restart carefully. If anaphylaxis recurs, discontinue acetylcysteine and use alternative form of treatment.

● Assess patient for nausea, vomiting, and urticaria. Notify health care professional if these occur.

● Monitor for signs and symptoms of fluid overload (dyspnea, edema, increased BP) during therapy. Adjust volume of diluent as needed. May result in hyponatremia, seizures, and death.

● **Mucolytic:** Assess respiratory function (lung sounds, dyspnea) and color, amount, and consistency of secretions before and immediately following treatment to determine effectiveness of therapy.

Lab Test Considerations

● Monitor AST, ALT, and bilirubin levels along with INR every 24 hr for 96 hr in patients with plasma acetaminophen levels indicating potential hepatotoxicity.

● Monitor cardiac and renal function (serum creatinine, BUN), serum glucose, and electrolytes. Maintain fluid and electrolyte balance; correct hypoglycemia.

Implementation

● After opening, solution for inhalation may turn light purple; does not alter potency. Refrigerate open vials and discard after 96 hr.

● Drug reacts with rubber and metals (iron, nickel, copper); avoid contact.

● **PO:** Prepare oral solution by diluting 20% acetylcysteine solution with diet cola or other diet soft drink to a final concentration of 5% (add 3 mL of diluent for each 1 mL of 20% acetylcysteine solution; do not decrease the proportion of diluent). Water may be used as diluent if administered via gastric tube or Miller-Abbott tube. Dilution should be freshly prepared and administered within 1 hr. Undiluted solutions are stable for 96 hr if refrigerated.

- **Acetaminophen Overdose**—Empty stomach contents by inducing emesis or lavage prior to administration.

IV Administration
- **Intermittent Infusion:** Most effective if administered within 8 hr of acetaminophen ingestion. *Dilution:* Dilute in Sterile Water for Injection, D5W/ 0.45% NaCl, or D5W. Solution is colorless to slight pink or purple; do not administer solutions that are cloudy, discolored or contain particulate matter. Stable for 24 hr at room temperature. *Concentration:* **For loading dose:** *For patients 5–20 kg:* Dilute 150 mg in 3 mL/kg of diluent. *For patients 21–40 kg:* Dilute 150 mg/kg in 100 mL. *For patients 41–100 kg:* Dilute 150 mg/kg in 200 mL. **For Second Dose:** *For patients 5–20 kg:* Dilute 50 mg/kg in 7 mL/kg of diluent. *For patients 21–40 kg:* Dilute 50 mg/kg in 250 mL of diluent. *For patients 41–100 kg:* Dilute 50 mg/kg in 500 mL. **For Third Dose:** *For patients 5–20 kg:* Dilute 100 mg/kg in 14 mL/kg of diluent. *For patients 21–40 kg:* 100 mg/kg diluted in 500 mL of diluent. *For patients 41–100 kg:* Dilute 100 mg/kg in 1000 mL. Adjust fluid volume for patients requiring fluid restriction. Vials are single-use. Discard after using. Reconstituted solution is stable for 24 hr at room temperature. *Rate:* Administer **Loading Dose** over 1 hr.
- Administer **For Second Dose:** over 4 hr.
- Administer **For Third Dose:** over 16 hr.
- **Y-Site Compatibility:** heparin, naloxone, tigecycline, vancomycin.
- **Y-Site Incompatibility:** cefepime, ceftazidime.
- **Inhaln: Mucolytic**—Encourage adequate fluid intake (2000–3000 mL/day) to decrease viscosity of secretions.
- For nebulization, 20% solution may be diluted with 0.9% NaCl for injection or inhalation or sterile water for injection or inhalation. May use 10% solution undiluted. May be administered by nebulization, or 1–2 mL may be instilled directly into airway. During administration, when 25% of medication remains in nebulizer, dilute with equal amount of 0.9% NaCl or sterile water.
- An increased volume of liquefied bronchial secretions may occur following administration. Have suction equipment available for patients unable to effectively clear airways.
- If bronchospasm occurs during treatment, discontinue and consult health care professional regarding possible addition of bronchodilator to therapy. Patients with asthma or hyperactive airway disease should be given a bronchodilator prior to acetylcysteine to prevent bronchospasm.

- Rinse patient's mouth and wash face following treatment, as drug leaves a sticky residue.

Patient/Family Teaching
- Advise patient to notify health care professional if symptoms of hypersensitivity reaction or fluid overload occur.
- Rep: Advise females of reproductive potential to notify health care professional if pregnancy is planned or suspected and to avoid breastfeeding for 30 hr after administration.
- **Acetaminophen Overdose:** Explain purpose of medication to patient.
- **Inhaln:** Instruct patient to clear airway by coughing deeply before taking aerosol treatment.
- Inform patient that unpleasant odor of this drug becomes less noticeable as treatment progresses and medicine dissipates.

Evaluation/Desired Outcomes
- Decreased acetaminophen levels.
- No further increase in hepatic damage during acetaminophen overdose therapy.
- Decreased dyspnea and clearing of lung sounds when used as a mucolytic.
- Prevention of radiocontrast-induced renal dysfunction.

aclidinium/formoterol
(a-kli-**din**-ee-um/for-**moh**-te-rol)
❋ Duaklir Genuair, Duaklir Pressair
Classification
Therapeutic: bronchodilators
Pharmacologic: anticholinergics, adrenergics

Indications
Maintenance treatment of COPD.

Action
Aclidinium: Acts as an anticholinergic by inhibiting the M_3 receptor in bronchial smooth muscle. *Formoterol:* Beta$_2$-adrenergic agonist that stimulates adenyl cyclase, resulting in accumulation of cyclic adenosine monophosphate and subsequent bronchodilation. **Therapeutic Effects:** Improved airflow and ↓ exacerbations in COPD.

Pharmacokinetics
Absorption: *Aclidinium:* 6% systemically absorbed following inhalation; *Formoterol:* majority of inhaled drug is swallowed and absorbed.
Distribution: Unknown.
Metabolism and Excretion: *Aclidinium:* Rapidly hydrolyzed; metabolites are not pharmacologically active. Metabolites are eliminated in urine (54–65%) and feces (20–33%); <1% excreted unchanged in urine. *Formoterol:* Mostly metabolized by the liver; 10–18% excreted unchanged in urine.

Half-life: *Aclidinium:* 12 hr. *Formoterol:* 10 hr.

TIME/ACTION PROFILE (bronchodilation)

ROUTE	ONSET	PEAK	DURATION
Inhalation	1 hr	2–4 hr	12 hr

Contraindications/Precautions

Contraindicated in: Hypersensitivity; Severe hypersensitivity to milk proteins; Asthma; Acutely deteriorating COPD or acute respiratory symptoms.

Use Cautiously in: Narrow-angle glaucoma; Prostatic hyperplasia or bladder neck obstruction; Severe hypersensitivity to milk proteins; History of hypersensitivity to atropine (cross-sensitivity may occur); Cardiovascular disease (including angina, hypertension, and arrhythmias); Diabetes; Seizure disorders; Glaucoma; Hyperthyroidism; Pheochromocytoma; Excessive use (may lead to tolerance and paradoxical bronchospasm); OB: Use during pregnancy only if potential maternal benefit justifies potential fetal risk; may inhibit contractions during labor; Lactation: Use while breastfeeding only if potential maternal benefit justifies potential risk to infant; Pedi: Safety and effectiveness not established in children.

Adverse Reactions/Side Effects

CV: angina, arrhythmias, hypertension, hypotension, palpitations, tachycardia. **EENT:** worsening of narrow-angle glaucoma. **F and E:** hypokalemia. **GI:** dry mouth, nausea. **GU:** urinary retention. **Metab:** hyperglycemia. **MS:** arthralgia, muscle cramps. **Neuro:** dizziness, headache, insomnia, nervousness, tremor. **Resp:** cough, PARADOXICAL BRONCHOSPASM. **Misc:** HYPERSENSITIVITY REACTIONS (including anaphylaxis and angioedema).

Interactions

Drug-Drug: Concurrent use with **MAO inhibitors**, **tricyclic antidepressants**, or other **QT interval prolonging agents** may results in serious arrhythmias; use concurrently only with extreme caution. ↑ risk of hypokalemia with **theophylline, corticosteroids, loop diuretics**, and **thiazide diuretics. Beta blockers** may ↓ therapeutic effects. ↑ adrenergic effects may occur with concurrent use of **adrenergics**. May ↑ risk of anticholinergic effects with other **anticholingerics**.

Route/Dosage

Inhaln (Adults): One inhalation (aclidinium 400 mcg/formoterol 12 mcg) twice daily.

Availability

Powder for inhalation (contains lactose): aclidinium 400 mcg/formoterol 12 mcg/actuation.

NURSING IMPLICATIONS

Assessment

● Assess lung sounds, pulse, and BP before administration and during peak of medication. Note amount, color, and character of sputum produced. Closely monitor patients on higher dose for adverse effects.

● Monitor pulmonary function tests before initiating and periodically during therapy to determine effectiveness.

● Observe for paradoxical bronchospasm (wheezing, dyspnea, tightness in chest) and hypersensitivity reaction (rash; urticaria; swelling of the face, lips, or eyelids). If condition occurs, withhold medication and notify health care professional immediately.

● Monitor ECG periodically during therapy. May cause prolonged QTc interval.

● Monitor patient for signs of hypersensitivity reactions (difficulties in breathing or swallowing, swelling of tongue, lips and face), urticaria, or skin rash during therapy. Discontinue therapy and consider alternative if reaction occurs.

Lab Test Considerations

● May cause ↑ serum glucose and decreased serum potassium.

Implementation

● **Inhaln:** Administer as 1 inhalation twice daily, morning and evening. Inhaler is breath-activated.

Patient/Family Teaching

● Instruct patient to use medication as directed. Do not discontinue therapy without discussing with health care professional, even if feeling better. If a dose is missed skip dose and take next dose at regularly scheduled time. Do not double doses. Use a rapid-acting bronchodilator if symptoms occur before next dose is due. Caution patient not to use more than 1 time a day; may cause adverse effects, paradoxical bronchospasm, or loss of effectiveness of medication. Instruct patient to review *Patient Information* before starting therapy and with each Rx refill in case of changes.

● Caution patient not to use medication to treat acute symptoms. A rapid-acting inhaled beta-adrenergic bronchodilator should be used for relief of acute asthma attacks. Notify health care professional immediately if symptoms get worse or more inhalations than usual are needed from rescue inhaler.

● Instruct patient to contact health care professional immediately if shortness of breath is not relieved by medication or nausea, vomiting, shakiness, headache, fast or irregular heartbeat, sleeplessness, or signs and symptoms of narrow angle glaucoma (eye pain or discomfort, blurred vision, visual halos or colored images, red eyes) or urinary retention (difficulty passing urine, painful urination) occur.

● Advise patient to consult health care professional before taking any Rx, OTC, or herbal products or alcohol concurrently with this therapy. Caution patient also to avoid smoking and other respiratory irritants.

● Rep: Advise patient to notify health care professional if pregnancy is planned or suspected, or if breastfeeding.

Evaluation/Desired Outcomes
- Bronchodilation with decreased airflow obstruction.

acyclovir (ay-sye-kloe-veer)
Sitavig, Zovirax
Classification
Therapeutic: antivirals
Pharmacologic: purine analogues

Indications
PO: Treatment of: Recurrent genital herpes infections, Localized cutaneous herpes zoster infections (shingles) and chickenpox (varicella). **Buccal:** Recurrent herpes labialis (cold sores) in nonimmunosuppressed patients. **IV:** Treatment of: Severe initial episodes of genital herpes in nonimmunosuppressed patients, Mucosal or cutaneous herpes simplex infections or herpes zoster infections (shingles) in immunosuppressed patients, Herpes simplex encephalitis, Neonatal herpes simplex infections. **Topical:** *Cream:* Recurrent herpes labialis (cold sores). *Ointment:* Treatment of limited non–life-threatening herpes simplex infections in immunocompromised patients (systemic treatment is preferred).

Action
Interferes with viral DNA synthesis. **Therapeutic Effects:** Inhibition of viral replication, decreased viral shedding, and reduced time for healing of lesions.

Pharmacokinetics
Absorption: Despite poor absorption (15–30%), therapeutic plasma concentrations are achieved.
Distribution: Widely distributed. CSF concentrations are 50% of plasma.
Metabolism and Excretion: >90% eliminated unchanged by kidneys; remainder metabolized by liver.
Half-life: *Neonates:* 4 hr; *Children (1–12 yr):* 2–3 hr; *Adults:* 2–3.5 hr (↑ in renal failure).

TIME/ACTION PROFILE (plasma concentrations)

ROUTE	ONSET	PEAK	DURATION
PO	unknown	1.5–2.5 hr	4 hr
IV	prompt	end of infusion	8 hr
Buccal	unknown	12 hr (7 hr†)	unknown

† Salivary concentrations

Contraindications/Precautions
Contraindicated in: Hypersensitivity to acyclovir or valacyclovir; Hypersensitivity to milk protein concentrate (buccal only).
Use Cautiously in: Pre-existing serious neurologic, hepatic, pulmonary, or fluid and electrolyte abnormalities; Renal impairment (dose alteration recommended if CCr <50 mL/min); Obese patients (dose should be based on ideal body weight); Patients with hypoxia; OB: Use during pregnancy only if potential maternal benefit justifies potential fetal risk; systemic exposure minimal following buccal or topical administration; Lactation: Use while breastfeeding only if potential maternal benefit justifies potential risk to infant; systemic exposure minimal following buccal or topical administration; Pedi: Safety and effectiveness of buccal formulation not established in children; Geri: May need to ↓ dose in older adults due to age-related ↓ in renal function.

Adverse Reactions/Side Effects
Derm: acne, hives, rash, STEVENS-JOHNSON SYNDROME, unusual sweating. **Endo:** changes in menstrual cycle. **F and E:** polydipsia. **GI:** diarrhea, nausea, vomiting, ↑ liver enzymes, abdominal pain, anorexia, hyperbilirubinemia. **GU:** crystalluria, hematuria, RENAL FAILURE, renal pain. **Hemat:** THROMBOTIC THROMBOCYTOPENIC PURPURA/HEMOLYTIC UREMIC SYNDROME (high doses in immunosuppressed patients). **Local:** pain, phlebitis, local irritation. **MS:** joint pain. **Neuro:** dizziness, headache, hallucinations, SEIZURES, trembling.

Interactions
Drug-Drug: Probenecid and theophylline may ↑ levels and risk of toxicity. Valproic acid or phenytoin may ↓ levels and effectiveness. Concurrent use of other nephrotoxic drugs may ↑ risk nephrotoxicity. Zidovudine and intrathecal methotrexate may ↑ risk of CNS side effects.

Route/Dosage

Initial Genital Herpes
PO (Adults and Children): 200 mg every 4 hr while awake (5 times/day) for 7–10 days or 400 mg every 8 hr for 7–10 days; maximum dose in children: 80 mg/kg/day in 3–5 divided doses.
IV (Adults and Children ≥12 yr): 5 mg/kg every 8 hr for 5 days.

Chronic Suppressive Therapy for Recurrent Genital Herpes
PO (Adults and Children): 400 mg twice daily or 200 mg 3–5 times/day for up to 12 mo. Maximum dose in children: 80 mg/kg/day in 2–5 divided doses.

Intermittent Therapy for Recurrent Genital Herpes
PO (Adults and Children): 200 mg every 4 hr while awake (5 times/day) or 400 mg every 8 hr or 800 mg every 12 hr for 5 days, start at first sign of symptoms. Maximum dose in children: 80 mg/kg/day in 2–5 divided doses.

Acute Treatment of Herpes Zoster in Immunosuppressed Patients
PO (Adults): 800 mg every 4 hr while awake (5 times/day) for 7–10 days. *Prophylaxis:* 400 mg 5 times/day.
PO (Children): 250–600 mg/m²/dose 4–5 times/day.

Herpes Zoster in Immunocompetent Patients

PO (Adults and Children): 4000 mg/day in 5 divided doses for 5–7 days, maximum dose in children: 80 mg/kg/day in 5 divided doses.

Chickenpox

PO (Adults and Children): 20 mg/kg (not to exceed 800 mg/dose) 4 times daily for 5 days. Start within 24 hr of rash onset.

Mucosal and Cutaneous Herpes Simplex Infections in Immunosuppressed Patients

IV (Adults and Children >12 yr): 5 mg/kg every 8 hr for 7 days.
IV (Children 3 mo–12 yr): 10 mg/kg every 8 hr for 7 days.
Topical (Adults): 0.5 in. ribbon of 5% *ointment* for every 4-square-in. area every 3 hr (6 times/day) for 7 days.

Herpes Simplex Encephalitis

IV (Adults and Children ≥12 yr): 10 mg/kg every 8 hr for 10 days.
IV (Children 3 mo–12 yr): 20 mg/kg every 8 hr for 10 days.
IV (Children birth–3 mo): 20 mg/kg every 8 hr for 14–21 days.
IV (Neonates, premature): 10 mg/kg every 12 hr for 14–21 days.

Neonatal Herpes Simplex Infections

IV (Children post-menstrual age of ≥34 wk): 20 mg/kg every 8 hr for 21 days.
IV (Children post-menstrual age of <34 wk): 20 mg/kg every 12 hr for 21 days.

Varicella Zoster Infections in Immunosuppressed Patients

IV (Adults and Children ≥12 yr): 10 mg/kg every 8 hr for 7 days.
IV (Children <12 yr): 20 mg/kg every 8 hr for 7 days.

Renal Impairment

PO, IV (Adults and Children >3 mo): *CCr 25.1–50 mL/min/1.73 m²:* Normal dose every 12 hr; *CCr 10.1–25 mL/min/1.73 m²:* Normal dose every 24 hr; *CCr ≤10 mL/min/1.73 m²:* 50% of dose every 24 hr.

Herpes Labialis

Topical (Adults and Children >12 yr): Apply 5 times/day for 4 days; start at first symptoms.
Buccal (Adults): Apply one 50–mg buccal tablet to the upper gum region within 1 hr of onset of prodromal symptoms (but before appearance of any lesions).

Availability (generic available)

Tablets: ❀ 200 mg, 400 mg, 800 mg. **Capsules:** 200 mg. **Oral suspension (banana flavor):** 200 mg/5 mL. **Solution for injection:** ❀ 25 mg/mL, 50 mg/mL. **Buccal tablets:** 50 mg. **Cream:** 5%. **Ointment:** 5%. *In combination with:* hydrocortisone (Xerese). See Appendix N.

NURSING IMPLICATIONS

Assessment

- Assess lesions before and daily during therapy.
- Monitor frequency of recurrences.
- Monitor neurologic status in patients with herpes encephalitis.

Lab Test Considerations

- Monitor BUN, serum creatinine, and CCr before and during therapy. ↑ BUN and serum creatinine levels or ↓ CCr may indicate renal failure.

Implementation

- Do not confuse Zovirax with Zyvox.
- Start acyclovir treatment as soon as possible after herpes simplex symptoms appear and within 24 hr of a herpes zoster outbreak.
- **PO:** Acyclovir may be administered with food or on an empty stomach, with a full glass of water.
- Shake oral suspension well before administration.
- **Buccal:** Apply tablet with a dry finger to upper gum just above canine tooth immediately after taking out of blister. Hold in place with pressure on lip for 30 sec to ensure adhesion. May be more comfortable to apply rounded side of tablet to gum surface. Apply on same side as herpes labialis symptoms within 1 hr of onset of symptoms, before appearance of herpes labialis lesions. Once applied, stays in position and dissolves slowly during day; do not crush, suck, chew, or swallow. May eat and drink while tablet is in place; avoid interfering with adhesion of tablet (chewing gum, touching, or pressing tablet after placement, wearing upper denture, brushing teeth). If the teeth need to be cleaned while tablet is in place, rinse mouth gently. Drink plenty of liquids to prevent dry mouth.

IV Administration

- **IV:** Maintain adequate hydration (2000–3000 mL/day), especially during first 2 hr after IV infusion, to prevent crystalluria.
- Observe infusion site for phlebitis. Rotate infusion site to prevent phlebitis.
- Do not administer acyclovir injectable topically, IM, SUBQ, PO, or in the eye.
- **Intermittent Infusion:** Reconstitute 500-mg or 1-g vial with 10 mL or 20 mL, respectively, of sterile water for injection. Do not reconstitute with bacteriostatic water with benzyl alcohol or parabens. Shake well to dissolve completely. *Dilution:* Dilute in at least 100 mL of D5W, 0.9% NaCl, dextrose/saline combinations or LR. *Concentration:* 7 mg/mL. Patients requiring fluid restriction: 10 mg/mL. Acyclovir is an irritant at concentrations >7 mg/mL. Use reconstituted solution within 12 hr. Once diluted for infusion, use solution within 24 hr. Refrigeration results in precipitation, which dissolves at room temperature. *Rate:* Administer via infusion pump over 1 hr to minimize renal tubular damage.
- **Y-Site Compatibility:** alemtuzumab, allopurinol, amikacin, aminophylline, amphotericin deoxycho-

late, amphotericin B lipid complex, amphotericin B liposome, ampicillin, anidulafungin, argatroban, arsenic trioxide, atracurium, azithromycin, bivalirudin, bleomycin, bumetanide, buprenorphine, busulfan, butorphanol, calcium chloride, calcium gluconate, carboplatin, carmustine, cefazolin, cefotaxime, cefotetan, cefoxitin, ceftaroline, ceftazidime, ceftriaxone, cefuroxime, chloramphenicol, cisplatin, clindamycin, cyclophosphamide, cytarabine, dactinomycin, dantrolene, dexamethasone, dexmedetomidine, digoxin, dimenhydrinate, docetaxel, doxorubicin liposome, doxycycline, enalaprilat, ephedrine, ertapenem, erythromycin lactobionate, etoposide, etoposide phosphate, famotidine, fentanyl, filgrastim, fluconazole, fluorouracil, fosphenytoin, furosemide, glycopyrrolate, heparin, hetastarch, hydrocortisone, hydromorphone, ifosfamide, imipenem/cilastatin, insulin, regular, isoproterenol, LR, leucovorin calcium, linezolid, lorazepam, magnesium sulfate, mannitol, melphalan, methohexital, methotrexate, methylprednisolone, metoprolol, metronidazole, milrinone, mitoxantrone, multivitamins, nafcillin, nitroglycerin, octreotide, oxacillin, oxytocin, paclitaxel, pamidronate, pemetrexed, penicillin G potassium, pentobarbital, phenobarbital, potassium acetate, potassium chloride, propofol, propranolol, remifentanil, rituximab, rocuronium, sodium acetate, sodium bicarbonate, succinylcholine, sufentanil, theophylline, thiopental, thiotepa, tigecycline, tirofiban, tobramycin, trastuzumab, trimethoprim/sulfamethoxazole, vancomycin, vasopressin, vinblastine, vincristine, voriconazole, zidovudine, zoledronic acid.

- **Y-Site Incompatibility:** acetaminophen, amifostine, aminocaproic acid, amiodarone, ampicillin/sulbactam, aztreonam, cefepime, chlorpromazine, ciprofloxacin, dacarbazine, daptomycin, daunorubicin hydrochloride, dexrazoxane, diazepam, dobutamine, dopamine, doxorubicin hydrochloride, epinephrine, epirubicin, eptifibatide, esmolol, fludarabine, foscarnet, gemcitabine, gemtuzumab ozogamicin, haloperidol, hydralazine, hydroxyzine, idarubicin, irinotecan, ketamine, ketorolac, labetalol, levofloxacin, lidocaine, mesna, methadone, midazolam, mitomycin, mycophenolate, nicardipine, nitroprusside, ondansetron, palonosetron, pentamidine, phenylephrine, phenytoin, piperacillin/tazobactam, potassium phosphate, procainamide, prochlorperazine, promethazine, sargramostim, sodium phosphates, tacrolimus, topotecan, vecuronium, verapamil, vinorelbine.
- **Topical:** Apply to skin lesions only; do not use in the eye.

Patient/Family Teaching

- Instruct patient to take medication as directed for the full course of therapy. Take missed doses as soon as possible but not just before next dose is due; do not double doses. Acyclovir should not be used more frequently or longer than prescribed.
- Advise patients that the additional use of OTC creams, lotions, and ointments may delay healing and may cause spreading of lesions.
- Inform patient that acyclovir is not a cure; the virus lies dormant in the ganglia. Acyclovir will not prevent the spread of infection to others.
- Advise patient that condoms should be used during sexual contact and to avoid sexual contact while lesions are present.
- Instruct patient to consult health care professional if symptoms are not relieved after 7 days of topical therapy or if oral acyclovir does not decrease the frequency and severity of recurrences. Immunocompromised patients may require a longer time, usually 2 wk, for crusting over of lesions.
- Instruct women with genital herpes to have yearly Papanicolaou smears because they may be more likely to develop cervical cancer.
- Rep: Advise females of reproductive potential to notify health care professional if pregnancy is planned or suspected or if breastfeeding.
- **Topical:** Instruct patient to apply ointment in sufficient quantity to cover all lesions every 3 hr, 6 times/day for 7 days. 0.5-in. ribbon of ointment covers approximately 4 square in. Use a finger cot or glove when applying to prevent inoculation of other areas or spread to other people. Keep affected areas clean and dry. Loose-fitting clothing should be worn to prevent irritation.
- Avoid drug contact in or around eyes. Report any unexplained eye symptoms to health care professional immediately; ocular herpetic infection can lead to blindness.
- **Buccal:** Instruct patient on correct application and use of buccal tablet. If buccal tablet does not adhere or falls off within first 6 hrs, reposition immediately with same tablet. If tablet cannot be repositioned, apply new tablet. If swallowed within first 6 hrs, advise patient to drink a glass of water and apply a new tablet. Do not reapply if tablet falls out after 6 hrs.

Evaluation/Desired Outcomes

- Crusting over and healing of skin lesions.
- Decrease in frequency and severity of recurrences.
- Acceleration of complete healing and cessation of pain in herpes zoster.
- Decrease in intensity of chickenpox.

✱ = Canadian drug name. ▩ = Genetic implication. ~~Strikethrough~~ = Discontinued. CAPITALS = life-threatening. Underline = most frequent.

adalimumab (a-da-li-**mu**-mab)
Abrilada, ✿ Amgevita, Amjevita, Cyl-
tezo, Hadlima, Hulio, Humira, Hyri-
moz, Idacio, ✿ Simlandi, Yuflyma,
Yusimry
Classification
Therapeutic: antirheumatics
Pharmacologic: DMARDs, monoclonal anti-
bodies

Indications
**Abrilada, Amjevita, Cyltezo, Hadlima, Hulio, Hu-
mira, Idacio, Hyrimoz, Yuflyma, and Yusimry:**
Treatment of the following conditions: Moderately to
severely active rheumatoid arthritis (may be used alone
or with methotrexate or other non-biologic disease-
modifying antirheumatic drugs [DMARDs]), Psoriatic
arthritis (may be used alone or with other non-biologic
DMARDs), Active ankylosing spondylitis, Moderately to
severely active Crohn's disease in patients who have responded inadequately to conventional therapy, Moderately to severely active ulcerative colitis in patients who
have responded inadequately to immunosuppressants
such as corticosteroids, azathioprine, or 6-mercapto-
purine, Moderate to severely active polyarticular juvenile idiopathic arthritis (as monotherapy or with methotrexate), Moderate to severe chronic plaque psoriasis
in patients who are candidates for systemic therapy or
phototherapy and when other systemic therapies are
deemed inappropriate. **Abrilada, Amjevita, Cyltezo,
Hadlima, Humira, Hyrimoz, Yuflyma, and Yusimry only:** Treatment of the following condition:
Moderate to severe hidradenitis suppurativa, **Abrilada,
Amjevita, Cyltezo, Hulio, and Humira
only:** Treatment of the following condition: Non-infec-
tious intermediate, posterior and panuveitis.

Action
Neutralizes and prevents the action of tumor necrosis
factor (TNF), resulting in anti-inflammatory and antiproliferative activity. **Therapeutic Effects:** Decreased
pain and swelling with decreased rate of joint destruction in patients with rheumatoid arthritis, psoriatic arthritis, juvenile idiopathic arthritis, and ankylosing
spondylitis. Reduced signs and symptoms and maintenance of clinical remission of Crohn's disease. Induction and maintenance of clinical remission of ulcerative
colitis. Reduced severity of plaques. Reduced number
of abscesses and inflammatory nodules. Decreased
progression of uveitis.

Pharmacokinetics
Absorption: 64% absorbed after SUBQ administra-
tion.
Distribution: Synovial fluid concentrations are 31-
96% of serum.
Metabolism and Excretion: Unknown.
Half-life: 14 days (range 10-20 days).

TIME/ACTION PROFILE (improvement)
ROUTE	ONSET	PEAK	DURATION
SUBQ	8-26 wk	131 hr*	2 wk†

*Plasma concentration.
†Following discontinuation.

Contraindications/Precautions
Contraindicated in: Hypersensitivity; Concurrent
use of anakinra or abatacept; Active infection (including localized).
Use Cautiously in: History of chronic or recurrent
infection or underlying illness/treatment predisposing
to infection; History of exposure to tuberculosis; History of opportunistic infection; Patients residing, or
who have resided, where tuberculosis, histoplasmosis,
coccidioidomycoses, or blastomycosis is endemic; Pre-
existing or recent-onset CNS demyelinating disorders;
History of lymphoma; OB: Use during pregnancy only if
potential maternal benefit justifies potential fetal risk;
Lactation: Use while breastfeeding only if potential maternal benefit justifies potential risk to infant; Pedi: Children <2 yr (safety not established); ↑ risk of lymphoma
(including hepatosplenic T-cell lymphoma [HSTCL] in
patients with Crohn's disease or ulcerative colitis), leukemia, and other malignancies in children; Geri: ↑ risk
of infection/malignancy in older adults.

Adverse Reactions/Side Effects
CV: hypertension. **Derm:** rash, psoriasis. **EENT:** optic
neuritis. **GI:** abdominal pain, nausea. **GU:** hematuria.
Hemat: neutropenia, thrombocytopenia. **Local:** injection site reactions. **Metab:** hyperlipidemia. **MS:** back
pain. **Neuro:** headache, Guillain-Barré syndrome, multiple sclerosis. **Misc:** fever, HYPERSENSITIVITY REACTIONS
(including anaphylaxis and angioedema), INFECTION
(including reactivation tuberculosis [TB] and other opportunistic infections due to bacterial, invasive fungal,
viral, mycobacterial, and parasitic pathogens), MALIG-
NANCY (including lymphoma, HSTCL, leukemia, and
skin cancer).

Interactions
Drug-Drug: Concurrent use with **anakinra**, **abatacept**, or other **TNF-blocking agents** ↑ risk of serious
infections; concurrent use contraindicated. Concurrent
use with **azathioprine** and/or **methotrexate** may ↑
risk of HSTCL. **Live vaccinations** should not be given
concurrently. Risks and benefits should be considered
before using live vaccinations in an infant exposed to
adalimumab therapy *in utero*.

Route/Dosage
Rheumatoid Arthritis, Ankylosing Spondyli-
tis, and Psoriatic Arthritis
SUBQ (Adults): 40 mg every other wk. Methotrexate,
non-biologic DMARDs, corticosteroids, and/or analgesics may be continued during therapy. Patients not receiving concurrent methotrexate may receive additional
benefit by ↑ dose to 40 mg once weekly *or* 80 mg every
other wk.

Crohn's Disease

SUBQ (Adults): 160 mg initially on Day 1 (given in one day or over two consecutive days), followed by 80 mg 2 wk later on Day 15. Two wk later (Day 29), begin maintenance dose of 40 mg every other wk. Aminosalicylates, corticosteroids, and/or immunomodulatory agents (e.g. azathioprine, 6–mercaptopurine, methotrexate) may be continued during therapy.

SUBQ (Children ≥6 yr and ≥40 kg): *Abrilada, Amjevita, Hadlima, Hulio, Humira, Idacio, and Hyrimoz only:* 160 mg initially on Day 1 (given in one day or over two consecutive days), followed by 80 mg 2 wk later on Day 15. Two wk later (Day 29), begin maintenance dose of 40 mg every other wk. Aminosalicylates, corticosteroids, and/or immunomodulatory agents (e.g. azathioprine, 6–mercaptopurine, methotrexate) may be continued during therapy.

SUBQ (Children ≥6 yr and 17–<40 kg): *Abrilada, Amjevita, Hadlima, Hulio, and Humira only:* 80 mg initially on Day 1, followed by 40 mg 2 wk later on Day 15. Two wk later (Day 29), begin maintenance dose of 20 mg every other wk. Aminosalicylates, corticosteroids, and/or immunomodulatory agents (e.g. azathioprine, 6–mercaptopurine, methotrexate) may be continued during therapy.

Ulcerative Colitis

SUBQ (Adults): 160 mg initially on Day 1 (given in one day or over two consecutive days), followed by 80 mg 2 wk later on Day 15. Two wk later (Day 29), begin maintenance dose of 40 mg every other wk. Aminosalicylates, corticosteroids, and/or immunomodulatory agents (e.g. azathioprine, 6–mercaptopurine, methotrexate) may be continued during therapy. Should be continued only if patients have evidence of clinical remission by wk 8 of therapy.

SUBQ (Children ≥5 yr and ≥40 kg): *Humira only:* 160 mg initially on Day 1 (given in one day or over two consecutive days), followed by 80 mg 1 wk later on Day 8, and then followed by 80 mg 1 wk later on Day 15. Two wk later (Day 29), begin maintenance dose of either 80 mg every other wk *or* 40 mg every wk. Aminosalicylates, corticosteroids, and/or immunomodulatory agents (e.g. azathioprine, 6–mercaptopurine, methotrexate) may be continued during therapy.

SUBQ (Children ≥5 yr and 20–<40 kg): *Humira only:* 80 mg initially on Day 1, followed by 40 mg 1 wk later on Day 8, and then followed by 40 mg 1 wk later on Day 15. Two wk later (Day 29), begin maintenance dose of either 40 mg every other wk *or* 20 mg every wk. Aminosalicylates, corticosteroids, and/or immunomodulatory agents (e.g. azathioprine, 6–mercaptopurine, methotrexate) may be continued during therapy.

Juvenile Idiopathic Arthritis

SUBQ (Children 2–17 yr (Abrilada, Amjevita, Hadlima, Hulio, Humira, Idacio, and Hyrimoz); 4–17 yr (Cyltezo): *10–<15 kg (Abrilada, Hadlima,*

Humira, and Hyrimoz only): 10 mg every other wk; *15–<30 kg (Abrilada, Amjeveta, Hadlima, Hulio, and Humira only):* 20 mg every other wk; *≥30 kg:* 40 mg every other wk.

Plaque Psoriasis

SUBQ (Adults): 80 mg initially, then in 1 wk, begin regimen of 40 mg every other wk.

Uveitis

SUBQ (Adults): *Abrilada, Amjevita, Cyltezo, Hadlima, Hulio, or Humira only:* 80 mg initially, then in 1 wk, begin regimen of 40 mg every other wk.

SUBQ (Children ≥2 yr and ≥30 kg): *Humira only:* 40 mg every other wk.

SUBQ (Children ≥2 yr and 15–<30 kg): *Humira only:* 20 mg every other wk.

SUBQ (Children ≥2 yr and 10–<15 kg): *Humira only:* 10 mg every other wk.

Hidradenitis Suppurativa

SUBQ (Adults): *Abrilada, Amjevita, Cyltezo, Hadlima, Humira, or Yusimry:* 160 mg initially (given in one day or over two consecutive days), followed by 80 mg 2 wk later on Day 15. Two wk later (Day 29), begin maintenance dose of 40 mg every wk *or* 80 mg every other wk.

SUBQ (Children ≥12 yr and ≥60 kg): *Humira only:* 160 mg initially (given in one day or over two consecutive days), followed by 80 mg 2 wk later on Day 15. Two wk later (Day 29), begin maintenance dose of 40 mg every wk *or* 80 mg every other wk.

SUBQ (Children ≥12 yr and 30–59 kg): *Humira only:* 80 mg initially on Day 1, followed by 40 mg 1 wk later on Day 8. Two wk later (Day 22), begin maintenance dose of 40 mg every other wk.

Availability

Solution for injection (prefilled syringes): 10 mg/0.1 mL, 10 mg/0.2 mL, 20 mg/0.2 mL, 20 mg/0.4 mL, 40 mg/0.4 mL, 40 mg/0.8 mL, 80 mg/0.8 mL. **Solution for injection (vials):** 40 mg/0.8 mL. **Solution for injection (prefilled pens):** 40 mg/0.4 mL, 40 mg/0.8 mL, 80 mg/0.8 mL.

NURSING IMPLICATIONS

Assessment

- Assess for signs of infection (fever, dyspnea, flu-like symptoms, frequent or painful urination, redness or swelling at the site of a wound), including tuberculosis and hepatitis B virus (HBV), prior to and periodically during therapy. Adalimumab is contraindicated in patients with active infection. Monitor new infections closely; most common are upper respiratory tract infections, bronchitis, and urinary tract infections. Infections may be fatal, especially in patients taking immunosuppressive therapy.
- Assess patient for latent tuberculosis with a tuberculin skin test prior to initiation of therapy. Start treat-

ment of latent tuberculosis before therapy with adalimumab.

- Monitor for injection site reactions (redness and/or itching, rash, hemorrhage, bruising, pain, or swelling). Rash will usually disappear within a few days. Application of a towel soaked in cold water may relieve pain or swelling.

- Assess patient for latex allergy. Needle cover of syringe contains latex and should not be handled by persons sensitive to latex.

- Monitor patient for signs of anaphylaxis (urticaria, dyspnea, facial edema) following injection. Medications (antihistamines, corticosteroids, epinephrine) and equipment should be readily available in the event of a severe reaction. Discontinue adalimumab immediately if anaphylaxis or other severe allergic reaction occurs.

- Assess for signs and symptoms of systemic fungal infections (fever, malaise, weight loss, sweats, cough, dyspnea, pulmonary infiltrates, serious systemic illness with or without concomitant shock). Determine if patient lives in or has traveled to areas of endemic mycoses. Consider empiric antifungal treatment for patients at risk of histoplasmosis and other invasive fungal infections until pathogens are identified. Consult with an infectious diseases specialist. Consider stopping adalimumab until infection has been diagnosed and adequately treated.

- **Arthritis:** Assess pain and range of motion before and periodically during therapy.

- **Crohn's Disease or Ulcerative Colitis:** Monitor frequency and consistency of bowel movements periodically during therapy.

- **Plaque Psoriasis:** Assess skin lesions periodically during therapy.

- **Hidradenitis Suppurativa:** Monitor skin lesions (abscesses, inflammatory nodules, draining fistulas) during therapy.

- **Uveitis:** Monitor signs and symptoms of uveitis (red eye with or without pain, photosensitivity, blurry vision, seeing "floaters" all of a sudden) during therapy.

Lab Test Considerations

- Monitor CBC with differential periodically during therapy. May cause leukopenia, neutropenia, thrombocytopenia, and pancytopenia. Discontinue adalimumab if symptoms of blood dyscrasias (persistent fever) occur.

- Monitor for HBV blood tests before starting during, and for several mo after therapy is completed.

Implementation

- Administer a tuberculin skin test prior to administration of adalimumab. Patients with active latent TB should be treated for TB prior to therapy.

- Immunizations should be current prior to initiating therapy. Patients on adalimumab may receive concurrent vaccinations, except for live vaccines.

- Administer initial injection under supervision of a health care professional.

- Vial is for institutional use only. With training, patient may use pen and prefilled syringes at home.

- Do not administer solutions that are discolored or contain particulate matter. Discard unused solution.

- **SUBQ:** Solution may be left at room temperature for 15–30 min before injecting. Administer at a 45° angle in upper thighs or abdomen, avoiding the 2 inches around the navel. Put pressure on injection site for 10 sec, do not rub. Rotate injection sites; avoid areas that are tender, bruised, hard, or red. If multiple injections required per dose, administer in separate sites. Solution is clear to slightly opalescent, colorless to pale brownish-yellow; do not administer solutions that are cloudy, discolored, or contain particulate matter. Refrigerate prefilled syringes and pens.

Patient/Family Teaching

- Instruct patient on the correct technique for administering adalimumab. Review *Medication Guide*, preparation of dose, administration sites and technique, and disposal of equipment into a puncture-resistant container.

- If a dose is missed, instruct patient to administer as soon as possible, then take next dose according to regular schedule.

- Caution patient to notify health care professional immediately if signs of infection, HBV (muscle aches, clay-colored bowel movements, feeling very tired, fever, dark urine, chills, skin or eyes look yellow, stomach discomfort, little or no appetite, skin rash, vomiting), severe rash, swollen face, or difficulty breathing occurs or if nervous system problems (numbness or tingling, problems vision, weakness in arms or legs, dizziness) occur while taking adalimumab.

- Inform patient that an increase risk of cancer occurs when taking adalimumab.

- Advise patient to notify health care professional of all Rx or OTC medications, vitamins, or herbal products being taken and to consult with health care professional before taking other medications.

- Instruct patient to notify health care professional of medication regimen prior to treatment or surgery.

- Advise patient to avoid live vaccines during therapy.

- **Rep:** Advise females of reproductive potential to notify health care professional if pregnancy is planned or suspected or if breastfeeding.

- **Pen:** Clean area for injection with alcohol swab. Hold pen with gray cap pointing up. Check solution through window; if discolored, cloudy, or contains flakes, discard solution. Turn pen over and point cap down to make sure solution reaches fill line; if not, do not use and contact pharmacist. Remove gray cap exposing the needle and the plum cap exposing the button; removing the plum cap activates the pen. Pinch skin and place pen, with window visible, against skin at a 90° angle and press button until a click is heard. Hold pen in place until all solution is injected (10 sec) and yellow marker is visible in window and has stopped moving. Continue to pinch skin throughout injection. Remove needle and press with a gauze pad or cotton ball for 10 sec. Do not rub injection site. Dispose of pen into a puncture-resistant container.

Evaluation/Desired Outcomes
● Decreased pain and swelling with decreased rate of joint destruction in patients with rheumatoid arthritis.
● Decreased signs and symptoms, slowed progression of joint destruction, and improved physical function in patients with psoriatic arthritis.
● Reduced signs and symptoms of ankylosing spondylitis.
● Decreased signs and symptoms, and maintenance of remission, in patients with Crohn's disease or ulcerative colitis.
● Reduced pain and swelling in patients moderate to severe polyarticular juvenile idiopathic arthritis in children 2 yr of age and older.
● Reduced severity of plaques in patients with severe chronic plaque psoriasis.
● Improvement in skin lesions in patients with hidradenitis suppurativa.
● Decreased progression of uveitis.

---

adenosine (a-**den**-oh-seen)
~~Adenocard, Adenoscan~~
Classification
Therapeutic: antiarrhythmics

Indications
Conversion of paroxysmal supraventricular tachycardia to normal sinus rhythm when vagal maneuvers are unsuccessful. As a diagnostic agent (with noninvasive techniques) to assess myocardial perfusion defects occurring as a consequence of coronary artery disease.

Action
Restores normal sinus rhythm by interrupting re-entrant pathways in the AV node. Slows conduction time through the AV node. Also produces coronary artery vasodilation. **Therapeutic Effects:** Restoration of normal sinus rhythm.

Pharmacokinetics
Absorption: IV administration results in complete bioavailability.
Distribution: Taken up by erythrocytes and vascular endothelium.
Metabolism and Excretion: Rapidly converted to inosine and adenosine monophosphate.
Half-life: <10 sec.

TIME/ACTION PROFILE (antiarrhythmic effect)

ROUTE	ONSET	PEAK	DURATION
IV	immediate	unknown	1–2 min

Contraindications/Precautions
Contraindicated in: Hypersensitivity; 2nd- or 3rd-degree AV block or sick sinus syndrome, unless a functional artificial pacemaker is present; Myocardial ischemia/infarction (only when used as diagnostic agent); Lactation: Lactation.
Use Cautiously in: Asthma (may induce bronchospasm); Unstable angina; OB: Safety not established in pregnancy.

Adverse Reactions/Side Effects
CV: arrhythmias, chest pain, hypotension, MI, palpitations, VENTRICULAR TACHYCARDIA. **Derm:** facial flushing, burning sensation, sweating. **EENT:** blurred vision, throat tightness. **GI:** metallic taste, nausea. **MS:** neck and back pain. **Neuro:** apprehension, dizziness, head pressure, headache, lightheadedness., numbness, SEIZURES (only when used for diagnostic use), STROKE (only when used for diagnostic use), tingling. **Resp:** shortness of breath, chest pressure, hyperventilation. **Misc:** heaviness in arms, HYPERSENSITIVITY REACTIONS, pressure sensation in groin.

Interactions
Drug-Drug: Carbamazepine may ↑ risk of progressive heart block. **Dipyridamole** ↑ effects of adenosine; ↓ adenosine. Effects of adenosine ↓ by **theophylline** or **caffeine**; may need to ↑ adenosine dose. Concurrent use with **digoxin** may ↑ risk of ventricular fibrillation.

Route/Dosage
IV (Adults and Children >50 kg): *Antiarrhythmic:* 6 mg by rapid IV bolus; if no results, repeat 1–2 min later as 12-mg rapid bolus. This dose may be repeated (single dose not to exceed 12 mg). *Diagnostic use:* 140 mcg/kg/min for 6 min (0.84 mg/kg total).
IV (Children <50 kg): *Antiarrhythmic:* 0.05–0.1 mg/kg as a rapid bolus, may repeat in 1–2 min; if response is inadequate, may ↑ by 0.05–0.1 mg/kg until sinus rhythm is established or maximum dose of 0.3 mg/kg is used.

Availability (generic available)
Solution for injection: 3 mg/mL.

NURSING IMPLICATIONS
Assessment
● Monitor heart rate frequently (every 15–30 sec) and ECG continuously during therapy. A short, transient period of 1st-, 2nd-, or 3rd-degree heart block or asystole may occur following injection; usually resolves quickly due to short duration of adenosine. Once conversion to normal sinus rhythm is achieved, transient arrhythmias (premature ventricular contractions, atrial premature contractions, sinus tachycardia, sinus bradycardia, skipped beats,

AV nodal block) may occur, but generally last a few sec.
- Monitor BP during therapy.
- Assess respiratory status (breath sounds, rate) following administration. Patients with history of asthma may experience bronchospasm.

Implementation

IV Administration
- **IV:** Crystals may occur if adenosine is refrigerated. Warm to room temperature to dissolve crystals. Solution must be clear before use. Do not administer solutions that are discolored or contain particulate matter. Discard unused portions.
- **IV Push:** *Dilution:* Administer undiluted. *Concentration:* 3 mg/mL. *Rate:* Administer over 1–2 sec via peripheral IV as proximal as possible to trunk. Slow administration may cause increased heart rate in response to vasodilation. Follow each dose with 20 mL rapid saline flush to ensure injection reaches systemic circulation.
- **Intermittent Infusion (for use in diagnostic testing):** *Dilution:* Administer 30-mL vial undiluted. *Concentration:* 3 mg/mL. *Rate:* Administer at a rate of 140 mcg/kg/min over 6 min for a total dose of 0.84 mg/kg. Thallium-201 should be injected as close to the venous access as possible at the midpoint (after 3 min) of the infusion.

Patient/Family Teaching
- Caution patient to change positions slowly to minimize orthostatic hypotension. Doses >12 mg decrease BP by decreasing peripheral vascular resistance.
- Instruct patient to report facial flushing, shortness of breath, or dizziness.
- Advise patient to avoid products containing methylxanthines (caffeinated coffee, tea, carbonated drinks or drugs such as aminophylline or theophylline) prior to myocardial perfusion imaging study.

Evaluation/Desired Outcomes
- Conversion of supraventricular tachycardia to normal sinus rhythm.
- Diagnosis of myocardial perfusion defects.

⚠ ado-trastuzumab
(ado tras-**too**-zoo-mab)
Kadcyla
Classification
Therapeutic: antineoplastics
Pharmacologic: drug-antibody conjugates

Indications
⚠ HER2-positive metastatic breast cancer in patients previously treated with trastuzumab and a taxane who have either received prior therapy for metastatic disease or developed disease recurrence during or within 6 mo of completing adjuvant therapy. ⚠ Adjuvant treatment of HER2–positive early breast cancer in patients who have residual invasive disease after neoadjuvant taxane and trastuzumab-based therapy.

Action
A HER2-targeted antibody and microtubule inhibitor conjugate. Trastuzumab, the antibody, attaches to receptors and is taken into the cell, where the microtubule inhibitor, DM1, causes cell cycle arrest and death. **Therapeutic Effects:** Decreased spread of metastatic breast cancer, with improved progression-free survival.

Pharmacokinetics
Absorption: IV administration results in complete bioavailability.
Distribution: Unknown.
Metabolism and Excretion: DM1 is metabolized by CYP3A4/5.
Half-life: 4 days.

TIME/ACTION PROFILE (comparative improvement in progression-free survival)

ROUTE	ONSET	PEAK	DURATION
IV	4–6 mo	10–12 mo	2 yr

Contraindications/Precautions
Contraindicated in: Interstitial lung disease or pneumonitis; OB: Pregnancy; Lactation: Lactation.
Use Cautiously in: Underlying cardiovascular or pulmonary disease, including dyspnea at rest; Rep: Women of reproductive potential and men with female partners of reproductive potential should use effective contraception; Pedi: Safety and effectiveness not established in children.

Adverse Reactions/Side Effects
CV: HF, hypertension, peripheral edema. **Derm:** pruritus, rash. **EENT:** ↑ lacrimation, blurred vision, conjunctivitis, dry eyes. **F and E:** hypokalemia. **GI:** ↑ liver enzymes, constipation, nausea, altered taste, diarrhea, dry mouth, dyspepsia, HEPATOTOXICITY, stomatitis, vomiting. **GU:** ↓ fertility. **Hemat:** anemia, HEMORRHAGE, neutropenia, THROMBOCYTOPENIA. **MS:** musculoskeletal pain, arthralgia, myalgia. **Neuro:** fatigue, headache, peripheral neuropathy, dizziness, insomnia, weakness. **Resp:** cough, INTERSTITIAL LUNG DISEASE. **Misc:** chills, fever, HYPERSENSITIVITY REACTIONS, infusion-related reactions.

Interactions
Drug-Drug: **Strong CYP3A4 inhibitors,** including **atazanavir, clarithromycin, itraconazole, ketoconazole, nefazodone, nelfinavir, ritonavir,** and **voriconazole** may ↑ levels and risk of toxicity; avoid concurrent use. Concurrent use of **anticoagulants,** or **antiplatelet agents,** especially during the first cycle, may ↑ risk of bleeding.

Route/Dosage
Should not be used interchangeably with trastuzumab.

Metastatic Breast Cancer
IV (Adults): 3.6 mg/kg every 3 wk until disease progression or unacceptable toxicity.

Early Breast Cancer
IV (Adults): 3.6 mg/kg every 3 wk (21–day cycle) for a total of 14 cycles unless there is disease progression or unacceptable toxicity.

Availability
Lyophilized powder for injection: 100 mg/vial, 160 mg/vial.

NURSING IMPLICATIONS
Assessment
- Evaluate left ventricular function in all patients prior to and every 3 mo during therapy. **For patients with metastatic disease:** *If symptomatic HF:* discontinue ado-trastuzumab. *If left ventricular ejection fraction (LVEF) <40%:* Hold dose. Repeat LVEF assessment within 3 wk. If LVEF <40% is confirmed, discontinue therapy. *If LVEF 40% to ≤45% and decrease is ≥10% points from baseline:* Hold dose. Repeat LVEF within 3 wk. If LVEF has not recovered to within 10% points from baseline, discontinue therapy. *If LVEF 40% to ≤45% and decrease is <10% points from baseline:* Continue therapy with ado-trastuzumab. Repeat LVEF within 3 wk. *If LVEF >45%:* Continue therapy. Discontinue therapy if symptomatic heart failure occurs. **For patients with early breast cancer:** *If LVEF <45%:* Hold dose. Repeat LVEF within 3 wk. If LVEF < 45% confirmed, discontinue therapy. *If LVEF 45% to < 50% and decrease is ≥ 10% points from baseline:* Hold dose. Repeat LVEF within 3 wk. *If the LVEF < 50% and not recovered to < 10% points from baseline, discontinue therapy. If LVEF 45% to < 50% and decrease is < 10% points from baseline:* Continue therapy. Repeat LVEF within 3 wk. *If LVEF ≥ 50%:* Continue therapy. *If symptomatic heart failure, Grade 3-4 left ventricular systolic dysfunction or Grade 3-4 heart failure, or Grade 2 heart failure accompanied by LVEF < 45%:* Discontinue therapy.
- Monitor infusion site closely for infiltration and extravasation closely. Within 24 hrs erythema, tenderness, skin irritation, pain, or swelling at infusion site is seen if extravasation occurs.
- Assess for signs and symptoms of infusion reactions (fever, chills, flushing, dyspnea, hypotension, wheezing, bronchospasm, tachycardia). Slow or interrupt therapy if symptoms are severe. Observe closely during first infusion. Permanently discontinue for life-threatening reactions.
- Monitor neurologic status before and during treatment. Assess for paresthesia (numbness, tingling, pain, burning sensation), loss of deep tendon reflexes (Achilles reflex is usually first involved),

weakness (wrist drop or footdrop, gait disturbances), cranial nerve palsies (jaw pain, hoarseness, ptosis, visual changes), arthralgia, myalgia, muscle spasm, autonomic dysfunction (ileus, difficulty voiding, orthostatic hypotension, impaired sweating), and CNS dysfunction (decreased level of consciousness, agitation, hallucinations). Temporarily discontinue therapy in patients with Grade 3 or 4 peripheral neuropathy (severe symptoms; limiting self-care activities of daily living [ADL]) until resolution to ≤ Grade 2 (moderate symptoms; limiting instrumental ADL) neuropathy.
- Monitor for signs and symptoms of pulmonary toxicity (dyspnea, cough, fatigue, pulmonary infiltrates). Permanently discontinue therapy if interstitial lung disease or pneumonitis develops.
- Monitor for hemorrhage (central nervous system, respiratory, gastrointestinal hemorrhage) during therapy, especially in patients receiving anticoagulants, antiplatelet therapy, or who have thrombocytopenia.

Lab Test Considerations
- ⚕ HER2 protein overexpression is used to determine whether treatment with ado-trastuzumab is indicated. HER2 protein overexpression should be determined by labs with proficiency in specific technology used. Information on approved tests is available at http://www.fda.gov/CompanionDiagnostics.
- Verify negative pregnancy status before starting therapy.
- Monitor serum transaminases and bilirubin prior to starting therapy and before each dose. **For patients with metastatic disease:** *If AST/ALT is Grade 2 (>2.5 to ≤5× upper limit of normal [ULN]):* Treat at same dose. *If AST/ALT is Grade 3 (>5 to ≤20× ULN):* Do not administer ado-trastuzumab until AST/ALT recovers to Grade ≤2, and then reduce 1 dose level. *If AST/ALT is Grade 4 (>20× ULN):* Permanently discontinue ado-trastuzumab. *If serum bilirubin is Grade 2 (>1.5 to ≤3× ULN):* Hold dose until bilirubin recovers to Grade ≤1, then treat at same dose level. *If bilirubin is Grade 3 (>3 to ≤10× ULN):* Hold dose until bilirubin recovers to Grade ≤1, then reduce 1 dose level. *If bilirubin is Grade 4 (>10× ULN):* Permanently discontinue ado-trastuzumab. Permanently discontinue ado-trastuzumab in patients with AST/ALT >3× ULN and concomitant total bilirubin >2× ULN. **For patients with early breast cancer:** *If ALT Grade 2-3 (>3.0 to ≤ 20 × ULN on day of scheduled treatment):* Hold dose until ALT recovers to Grade ≤1, then reduce one dose level. *If ALT Grade 4 (> 20 × ULN at any time):* Permanently discontinue therapy. *If AST Grade 2 (> 3.0 to ≤ 5 × ULN on day of scheduled treatment):* Hold dose until AST recovers to Grade ≤1, then treat with same dose. *If AST Grade 3 (> 5*

to ≤ 20 × ULN on day of scheduled treatment):
Hold dose until AST recovers to Grade ≤1, then reduce one dose level. *If AST Grade 4 (>20 × ULN at
any time):* Permanently discontinue therapy. *If total bilirubin >1.0 to ≤ 2.0 × ULN on day of scheduled treatment:* Hold dose until total bilirubin ≤
1.0× ULN, then reduce one dose level. *If total bilirubin >2 × ULN at any time:* Permanently discontinue therapy.
- Monitor platelet count prior to starting therapy and
before each dose. Nadir of thrombocytopenia occurs
by Day 8 and generally improves to Grade 0 or 1 by
next scheduled dose. **For patients with metastatic
disease:** *If thrombocytopenia is Grade 3 (platelets 25,000/mm³ to <50,000/mm³:* Hold dose until
platelet count recovers to ≤Grade 1 (≥75,000/
mm³), then treat at same dose level. *If thrombocytopenia is Grade 4 (platelets <25,000/mm₃):* Hold
dose until platelet count recovers to ≤Grade 1, then
reduce 1 dose level. **For patients with early
breast cancer:** If Grade 2-3 on day of scheduled
treatment (25,000 to < 75,000/mm³): Hold dose
until platelet count recovers to Grade ≤1 (≥
75,000/mm³), then treat at the same dose level. If 2
delays required due to thrombocytopenia, reduce
dose by one level. *If Grade 4 at any time < 25,000/
mm³:* Hold dose until platelet count recovers to
Grade ≤1 (≥ 75,000/mm³), then reduce one dose
level.
- May cause ↓ hemoglobin, neutrophils, and serum
potassium.

Implementation
- *High Alert:* Do not confuse ado-trastuzumab with
trastuzumab. Double-check names. Trade name of
administered product should be clearly recorded in
patient file to improve traceability.
- *High Alert:* Fatalities have occurred with chemotherapeutic agents. Before administering, clarify all
ambiguous orders; double check single, daily, and
course-of-therapy dose limits; have second practitioner independently double check original order,
dose calculations and infusion pump settings.
- Dose reduction schedule is: *Starting dose:* 3.6 mg/
kg; *First dose reduction:* 3 mg/kg; *Second dose reduction:* 2.4 mg/kg; *Requirement for further dose
reduction:* discontinue therapy.
- Solution should be prepared in a biologic cabinet.
Wear gloves, gown, and mask while handling medication. Discard IV equipment in specially designated
containers.

IV Administration
- **Intermittent Infusion:** *Reconstitution:* Reconstitute by slowly injecting 5 or 8 mL of sterile water
for injection into 100 or 160 mg vial of ado-trastuzumab respectively, for a solution of 20 mg/mL.
Swirl gently until dissolved; do not shake. Solution is
clear, colorless to pale brown, and slightly opalescent; do not administer solutions that are discolored

or contain particulate matter. Use reconstituted vials
immediately or store in refrigerator up to 4 hr; then
discard. Do not freeze. Calculate amount of solution
needed. *Dilution:* Withdraw from vial and add to
infusion bag containing 250 mL of 0.9% NaCl; do not
use dextrose solutions. Gently invert bag to mix without foaming. Use diluted solution immediately; may
be stored in refrigerator up to 24 hrs prior to use,
then discard; do not freeze or shake. Administer
every 3 wk (21-day cycle); if cycle is delayed, administer as soon as possible. Do not wait until next
planned cycle; maintain 3-wk interval between
doses. *Rate:* Infuse through a 0.2 or 0.22 micron
in-line non-protein adsorptive polyethersulfone filter. Do not administer as IV push or bolus. *First infusion:* Infuse over 90 min; observe for infusion related reaction. *Subsequent infusions:* Infuse over
30 min if prior infusions were well tolerated. Observe patient during infusion and for at least 90 min
after infusion.
- Management of increased serum transaminases, hyperbilirubinemia, left ventricular dysfunction,
thrombocytopenia, pulmonary toxicity, or peripheral neuropathy may require temporary interruption, dose reduction, or discontinuation.
- **Y-Site Incompatibility:** Do not mix or administer
with other medications.

Patient/Family Teaching
- Explain purpose of medication to patient. If a dose is
missed administer as soon as possible; do not wait
until next scheduled dose. Adjust schedule to maintain 3 wk interval between doses.
- Inform patient of potential liver injury and HF. Advise patient to notify health care professional immediately if signs and symptoms of liver injury (nausea,
vomiting, abdominal pain, jaundice, dark urine,
pruritus, anorexia) or HF (new onset or worsening
shortness of breath, cough, swelling of ankles/legs,
palpitations, weight gain of >5 lbs in 24 hr, dizziness, loss of consciousness) occur.
- Advise patient to notify health care professional if
signs of peripheral neuropathy (burning, numbness,
pain in hands and feet/legs) occur.
- Rep: May cause fetal harm. Advise females of reproductive potential to use a highly effective method
(IUD, hormonal contraceptive, tubal ligation, partner's vasectomy) of contraception during and for at
least 7 mo after last dose. Advise males with a female
partner of reproductive potential to use highly effective contraception during and for at least 4 mo after
last dose. Instruct patient to notify health care professional promptly if pregnancy is suspected and to
avoid breastfeeding for at least 7 mo after last dose.
Encourage women who have been exposed to ado-
trastuzumab either directly or through seminal fluid,
to immediately report exposure to Genentech Adverse Event Line at 1-888-835-2555. May impair fertility in male and female patients.

Evaluation/Desired Outcomes

● Decreased spread of metastatic breast cancer.

⚛ aducanumab
(a-due-**kan**-ue-mab)
Aduhelm
Classification
Therapeutic: anti-Alzheimer's agents
Pharmacologic: monoclonal antibodies, anti-amyloid monoclonal antibodies

Indications
Alzheimer's disease in patients with mild cognitive impairment or mild dementia stage of disease.

Action
Acts as a monoclonal antibody directed against aggregated soluble and insoluble forms of amyloid beta.
Therapeutic Effects: Reduction in clinical decline. Reduction in beta amyloid plaques in the brain.

Pharmacokinetics
Absorption: IV administration results in complete bioavailability.
Distribution: Not widely distributed to extravascular tissues.
Metabolism and Excretion: Degraded into small peptides and amino acids via catabolic pathways.
Half-life: 24.8 days.

TIME/ACTION PROFILE (plasma concentrations)

ROUTE	ONSET	PEAK	DURATION
IV	rapid	unknown	4 wk

Contraindications/Precautions
Contraindicated in: None.
Use Cautiously in: ⚛ Apolipoprotein E ∈4 homozygotes (15% of patients with Alzheimer's disease) (↑ risk of amyloid-related imaging abnormalities); Previous localized superficial siderosis, ≥10 brain microhemorrhages, and/or brain hemorrhage; OB: Safety not established in pregnancy; Lactation: Safety not established in breastfeeding; Pedi: Safety and effectiveness not established in children.

Adverse Reactions/Side Effects
CNS: amyloid-related imaging abnormalities (ARIA) (including edema and hemosiderin deposition), SEIZURES. **Misc:** HYPERSENSITIVITY REACTIONS (including angioedema).

Interactions
Drug-Drug: None reported.

Route/Dosage
IV (Adults): 1 mg/kg every 4 wk for Infusions 1 and 2, then 3 mg/kg every 4 wk for Infusions 3 and 4, then 6 mg/kg every 4 wk for Infusions 5 and 6, then 10 mg/kg every 4 wk thereafter.

Availability
Solution for injection: 100 mg/mL.

NURSING IMPLICATIONS
Assessment
● Confirm the presence of amyloid beta pathology prior to starting therapy.
● Obtain recent (within 1 yr) brain magnetic resonance imaging (MRI) prior to starting therapy. Obtain MRIs prior to 5th infusion (first dose of 6 mg/kg), 7th infusion (first dose of 10 mg/kg), 9th infusion (third dose of 10 mg/kg), and 12th infusion (sixth dose of 10 mg/kg).
● May cause amyloid related imaging abnormalities-edema (ARIA-E), seen on MRI as brain edema or sulcal effusions, and amyloid related imaging abnormalities hemosiderin deposition (ARIA-H), includes microhemorrhage and superficial siderosis. Safety of aducanumab in patients with ≥10 brain microhemorrhages, any pretreatment localized superficial siderosis, and/or with a brain hemorrhage >1 cm within one year of start of therapy has not been established. Clinically, ARIA may cause headache, confusion, dizziness, visual disturbance, nausea, and seizures. *If mild ARIA-E changes occur on MRI but patient is asymptomatic or has mild symptoms,* continue dosing at current dose and schedule. *If symptoms are moderate or severe,* hold aducanumab until MRI demonstrates radiographic resolution and symptoms, if present, resolve. *If ARIA-H changes occur on MRI but patient is asymptomatic,* continue dosing at current dose and schedule. *If MRI changes are moderate and patient is symptomatic,* hold doses until MRI demonstrates radiographic resolution and symptoms, if present, resolve. *If MRI changes or symptoms are severe,* hold doses until MRI demonstrates radiographic stabilization and symptoms, if present, resolve; may consider continuing or discontinuing therapy.
● Monitor for signs and symptoms of hypersensitivity reaction (hives, urticaria, swelling of the face, lips, mouth, or tongue) during infusion. Discontinue infusion if symptoms occur.
● ⚛ Testing for ApoE ∈4 status should be performed prior to initiation of treatment to inform the risk of developing ARIA.

Implementation
● *Dilution:* Withdraw required volume of aducanumab from vial(s) and add to an infusion bag of 100 mL of 0.9% NaCl. Do not use other intravenous diluents. Gently invert infusion bag to mix completely; do not shake. After dilution, infuse immediately. If not administered immediately, store diluted solution in refrigerator for up to 3 days, or at room temperature

for up to 12 hr. Prior to infusion, allow diluted solution to warm to room temperature. Solution is clear to opalescent and colorless to yellow solution. Do not use if opaque particles, discoloration, or other foreign particles are present. Allow solutions to warm to room temperature before infusing. *Rate:* Infuse over 1 hr through a sterile, low-protein binding, 0.2 or 0.22 micron in-line filter. Promptly discontinue infusion on first sign of a hypersensitivity-type reaction.

Patient/Family Teaching

● Explain purpose of infusion to patient and family.
● Instruct patient to notify health care professional of signs and symptoms of ARIA or hypersensitivity reactions occur.
● Instruct patient to notify health care professional of all Rx or OTC medications, vitamins, or herbal products being taken and consult health care professional before taking any new medications.
● Rep: Advise females of reproductive potential to notify health care professional if pregnancy is planned or suspected or if breastfeeding.

Evaluation/Desired Outcomes

● Reduction in beta amyloid plaques in the brain.

▩ afatinib (a-fa-ti-nib)
Gilotrif, ◆ Giotrif
Classification
Therapeutic: antineoplastics
Pharmacologic: kinase inhibitors

Indications

▩ First-line treatment of metastatic non-small cell lung cancer (NSCLC) where the tumor has non-resistant epidermal growth factor receptor (EGFR) mutations. Treatment of metastatic squamous NSCLC progressing after platinum chemotherapy.

Action

Inhibits tyrosine kinases which results in slowed proliferation of specific tumor cell lines. **Therapeutic Effects:** Decreased spread of NSCLC.

Pharmacokinetics

Absorption: Well absorbed (92%) following oral administration; absorption is ↓ by high-fat meal.
Distribution: Unknown.
Metabolism and Excretion: Metabolites occur partly as protein-bound products. Excretion is primarily fecal (85%) as parent drug; 4% excreted in urine.
Half-life: 37 hr.

TIME/ACTION PROFILE (improved progression-free survival)

ROUTE	ONSET	PEAK	DURATION
PO	3 mo	12 mo	20 mo

Contraindications/Precautions

Contraindicated in: ▩ Tumors with resistant EGFR mutations; OB: Pregnancy; Lactation: Lactation.
Use Cautiously in: Concurrent use of corticosteroids, NSAIDs, or antiangiogenic drugs, history of GI ulceration, history of diverticular disease, or history of bowel metastases (↑ risk of GI perforation); Severe renal impairment (↓ dose); Severe hepatic impairment (dose adjustment may be necessary); ▩ Asian ethnicity (may be ↑ susceptible to interstitial lung disease); Rep: Women of reproductive potential; Pedi: Safety and effectiveness not established in children; Geri: ↑ risk of GI perforation in older adults.

Adverse Reactions/Side Effects

Derm: cutaneous reactions (including bullous/blistering/exfoliating reactions, acneiform eruptions and palmar-plantar erythrodysesthesia), dry skin, paronychia, pruritus, rash, STEVENS-JOHNSON SYNDROME, TOXIC EPIDERMAL NECROLYSIS. **EENT:** conjunctivitis, epistaxis, keratitis, rhinorrhea. **F and E:** hypokalemia. **GI:** ↓ appetite, ↓ weight, diarrhea, nausea, stomatitis, vomiting, GI PERFORATION, HEPATOTOXICITY, PANCREATITIS. **Resp:** INTERSTITIAL LUNG DISEASE (ILD). **Misc:** fever.

Interactions

Drug-Drug: P-glycoprotein (P-gp) inhibitors, including **amiodarone, cyclosporine, erythromycin, itraconazole, ketoconazole, quinidine ritonavir, tacrolimus,** or **verapamil,** may ↑ levels and risk of toxicity; dosage adjustment may be necessary (ritonavir may be given concurrently or 6 hr after). **P-gp inducers,** including **carbamazepine, phenobarbital, phenytoin,** or **rifampin** may ↓ levels and effectiveness; dosage adjustment may be necessary.

Route/Dosage

PO (Adults): 40 mg once daily until disease progression or unacceptable toxicity. *Concurrent use of P-gp inhibitors:* ↓ dose by 10 mg/day if necessary. *Concurrent use of P-gp inducers:* ↑ dose by 10 mg/day if necessary.

Renal Impairment

PO (Adults): *eGFR 15–29 mL/min:* 30 mg once daily until disease progression or unacceptable toxicity.

Availability

Tablets: 20 mg, 30 mg, 40 mg.

NURSING IMPLICATIONS

Assessment

● Monitor for diarrhea; occurs frequently. Provide patient with an antidiarrheal agent (loperamide) at the onset of diarrhea and until diarrhea ceases for 12 hr. If diarrhea is severe and lasts more than 48 hr despite use of antidiarrheal agent (Grade 2 or higher), withhold afatinib until diarrhea resolves to Grade 1 or less, then resume with reduced dose of 10 mg/day.
● Assess for cutaneous reactions (bullous, blistering, exfoliative lesions; rash, erythema, acneiform rash)

periodically during therapy. Discontinue afatinib if life-threatening lesions or prolonged Grade 2 cutaneous lesions lasting ≥7 days, intolerable Grade 2, or Grade 3 cutaneous reactions occur. Withhold afatinib until reaction resolves to Grade 1 or less and resume at 10 mg/day.

- Monitor for signs and symptoms of ILD (lung infiltration, pneumonitis, acute respiratory distress syndrome, allergic alveolitis); ░ may occur more commonly in patients of Asian ethnicity. Withhold afatinib if symptoms occur; discontinue if ILD is confirmed.
- Monitor for signs and symptoms of GI perforation (severe abdominal pain) during therapy. Permanently discontinue afatinib if perforation occurs.
- Monitor for signs and symptoms of keratitis (acute or worsening eye inflammation, lacrimation, light sensitivity, blurred vision, eye pain, red eye) during therapy. May require interruption or discontinuation of afatinib.

Lab Test Considerations
- Monitor liver function tests periodically during therapy. If severe decline in liver function occurs, discontinue afatinib. May cause ↑ AST and ALT.
- May cause hypokalemia.

Implementation
- **PO:** Administer once daily on an empty stomach, at least 1 hr before or 2 hr after meals.

Patient/Family Teaching
- Instruct patient to take afatinib as directed. Take missed dose as soon as remembered unless within 12 hr of next dose, then omit and take next dose at scheduled time; do not double doses. Advise patient to read *Patient Information* before starting therapy and with each Rx refill in case of changes.
- Caution patient to notify health care professional if signs and symptoms of keratitis (acute or worsening eye inflammation, lacrimation, light sensitivity, blurred vision, eye pain, and/or red eye) occur. Withhold if symptoms occur; if ulcerative keratitis is confirmed, discontinue afatinib. Advise patient that use of contact lenses is also a risk factor.
- Advise patient to wear sunscreen and protective clothing during therapy to minimize risk of skin disorders.
- Inform patient that diarrhea occurs in most patients and may cause dehydration and renal impairment. Notify health care professional if diarrhea is severe or persistent, if new or worsening lung symptoms (difficulty breathing, shortness of breath, cough, fever), symptoms of liver problems (yellow skin or whites of eyes, dark brown urine, pain on right side of abdomen, unusual bleeding or bruising, lethargy), severe abdominal pain, or if symptoms of left ventricular dysfunction (shortness of breath, exercise intolerance, cough, fatigue, swelling or ankles or feet, palpitations, sudden weight gain) occur.

- Advise patient to notify health care professional of all Rx or OTC medications, vitamins, or herbal products being taken and to consult with health care professional before taking other medications.
- Rep: May be teratogenic. Advise females of reproductive potential to use highly effective contraception and to avoid breastfeeding during and for at least 2 wk after last dose. If pregnancy occurs, instruct patient to notify health care professional immediately. May impair fertility in males and females.

Evaluation/Desired Outcomes
- Decreased spread of NSCLC.

---

albuterol (al-byoo-ter-ole)
~~Accuneb~~, ✦Airomir, Proair Digihaler, Proair HFA, Proair Respiclick, Proventil HFA, ✦Salbutamol, Ventolin HFA, ✦Ventolin Diskus, ✦Ventolin Nebules, ~~VoSpire ER~~

Classification
Therapeutic: bronchodilators
Pharmacologic: adrenergics

Indications
Treatment or prevention of bronchospasm in asthma or chronic obstructive pulmonary disease (COPD). **Inhaln:** Prevention of exercise-induced bronchospasm. **PO:** Treatment of bronchospasm in asthma or COPD.

Action
Binds to beta$_2$-adrenergic receptors in airway smooth muscle, leading to activation of adenyl cyclase and increased levels of cyclic-3', 5'-adenosine monophosphate (cAMP). Increases in cAMP activate kinases, which inhibit the phosphorylation of myosin and decrease intracellular calcium. Decreased intracellular calcium relaxes smooth muscle airways. Relaxation of airway smooth muscle with subsequent bronchodilation. Relatively selective for beta$_2$ (pulmonary) receptors. **Therapeutic Effects:** Bronchodilation.

Pharmacokinetics
Absorption: Well absorbed after oral administration but rapidly undergoes extensive metabolism.
Distribution: Small amounts appear in breast milk.
Metabolism and Excretion: Extensively metabolized by the liver and other tissues.
Half-life: Oral 2.7–5 hr; Inhalation: 3.8 hr.

TIME/ACTION PROFILE (bronchodilation)

ROUTE	ONSET	PEAK	DURATION
PO	15–30 min	2–3 hr	4–6 hr or more
Inhaln	5–15 min	60–90 min	3–6 hr

Contraindications/Precautions

Contraindicated in: Hypersensitivity to adrenergic amines.

Use Cautiously in: Cardiac disease; Hypertension; Hyperthyroidism; Diabetes; Glaucoma; Seizure disorders; Excess inhaler use may lead to tolerance and paradoxical bronchospasm; OB: Use during pregnancy only if potential maternal benefit justifies potential fetal risk; Lactation: Use while breastfeeding only if potential maternal benefit justifies potential risk to infant; Pedi: Children <2 yr (safety and effectiveness not established); Geri: ↑ risk of adverse reactions in older adults; may require dose ↓.

Adverse Reactions/Side Effects

CV: <u>chest pain</u>, <u>palpitations</u>, angina, arrhythmias, hypertension. **Endo:** hyperglycemia. **F and E:** hypokalemia. **GI:** nausea, vomiting. **Neuro:** <u>nervousness</u>, <u>restlessness</u>, <u>tremor</u>, headache, hyperactivity (children), insomnia. **Resp:** PARADOXICAL BRONCHOSPASM (excessive use of inhalers).

Interactions

Drug-Drug: Concurrent use with other **adrenergic agents** will have ↑ adrenergic side effects. Use with **MAO inhibitors** may lead to hypertensive crisis. **Beta blockers** may negate therapeutic effect. May ↓ serum **digoxin** levels. Cardiovascular effects are potentiated in patients receiving **tricyclic antidepressants**. Risk of hypokalemia ↑ concurrent use of **potassium-losing diuretics**. Hypokalemia ↑ the risk of **digoxin** toxicity.

Drug-Natural Products: Use with caffeine-containing herbs (**cola nut**, **guarana**, **tea**, **coffee**) ↑ stimulant effect.

Route/Dosage

PO (Adults and Children ≥12 yr): 2–4 mg 3–4 times daily (not to exceed 32 mg/day).

PO (Geriatric Patients): Initial dose should not exceed 2 mg 3–4 times daily, may be ↑ carefully (up to 32 mg/day).

PO (Children 6–12 yr): 2 mg 3–4 times daily; may be carefully ↑ as needed (not to exceed 8 mg/day).

PO (Children 2–6 yr): 0.1 mg/kg 3 times daily (not to exceed 2 mg 3 times daily initially); may be carefully ↑ to 0.2 mg/kg 3 times daily (not to exceed 4 mg 3 times daily).

Inhaln (Adults and Children ≥4 yr): *Via metered-dose inhaler or dry powder inhaler:* 2 inhalations every 4–6 hr (some patients may respond to 1 inhalation) or 2 inhalations 15 min before exercise; *NIH Guidelines for acute asthma exacerbation: Children:* 4–8 puffs every 20 min for 3 doses then every 1–4 hr; *Adults:* 4–8 puffs every 20 min for up to 4 hr then every 1–4 hr as needed.

Inhaln (Adults and Children >12 yr): *NIH Guidelines for acute asthma exacerbation via nebulization or IPPB:* 2.5–5 mg every 20 min for 3 doses then 2.5–10 mg every 1–4 hr as needed; *Continuous nebulization:* 10–15 mg/hr.

Inhaln (Children 2–12 yr): *NIH Guidelines for acute asthma exacerbation via nebulization or IPPB:* 0.15 mg/kg/dose (minimum dose 2.5 mg) every 20 min for 3 doses then 0.15–0.3 mg/kg (not to exceed 10 mg) every 1–4 hr as needed or 1.25 mg 3–4 times daily for children 10–15 kg or 2.5 mg 3–4 times daily for children >15 kg; *Continuous nebulization:* 0.5–3 mg/kg/hr.

Inhaln (Neonates): 1.25 mg/dose every 8 hr via nebulization or 1–2 puffs via MDI into the ventilator circuit every 6 hrs.

Availability (generic available)

Immediate-release tablets: 2 mg, 4 mg. **Oral syrup (strawberry-flavored):** 2 mg/5 mL. **Inhalation solution:** 0.63 mg/3 mL (0.021%), 1.25 mg/3 mL (0.042%), 2.5 mg/3 mL (0.083%), ✿ 1 mg/mL, ✿ 2 mg/mL, 5 mg/mL (0.5%). **Metered-dose aerosol:** 90 mcg/inhalation in 6.7-g, 8-g, 8.5-g, and 18-g canisters (200 metered inhalations), ✿ 100 mcg/spray. **Powder for inhalation (Proair Digihaler and Proair Respiclick):** 90 mcg/inhalation (200 metered inhalations). **Powder for inhalation (Ventolin Diskus):** ✿ 200 mcg. *In combination with:* budesonide (Airsupra); ipratropium (Combivent). See Appendix N.

NURSING IMPLICATIONS

Assessment

- Assess lung sounds, pulse, and BP before administration and during peak of medication. Note amount, color, and character of sputum produced.
- Monitor pulmonary function tests before initiating therapy and periodically during therapy.
- Observe for paradoxical bronchospasm (wheezing). If condition occurs, withhold medication and notify health care professional immediately.

Lab Test Considerations

- May cause transient ↓ in serum potassium concentrations with nebulization or higher-than-recommended doses.

Implementation

- **PO:** Administer oral medication with meals to minimize gastric irritation.
- **Inhaln:** Shake inhaler well, and allow at least 1 min between inhalations of aerosol medication. Prime the inhaler before first use by releasing 4 test sprays into the air away from the face. *Proair Respiclick* does not require priming. Pedi: Use spacer for children <8 yr of age.
- For nebulization or IPPB, the 0.5-, 0.83-, 1-, and 2-mg/mL solutions do not require dilution before administration. The 5 mg/mL (0.5%) solution must be diluted with 1–2.5 mL of 0.9% NaCl for inhalation. Diluted solutions are stable for 24 hr at room temperature or 48 hr if refrigerated.
- For nebulizer, compressed air or oxygen flow should be 6–10 L/min; a single treatment of 3 mL lasts about 10 min.
- IPPB usually lasts 5–20 min.

Patient/Family Teaching

- Instruct patient to take albuterol as directed. If on a scheduled dosing regimen, take missed dose as soon as remembered, spacing remaining doses at regular intervals. Do not double doses or increase the dose or frequency of doses. Caution patient not to exceed recommended dose; may cause adverse effects, paradoxical bronchospasm (more likely with first dose from new canister), or loss of effectiveness of medication.
- Instruct patient to contact health care professional immediately if shortness of breath is not relieved by medication or is accompanied by diaphoresis, dizziness, palpitations, or chest pain.
- Instruct patient to prime unit with 4 sprays before using and to discard canister after 200 sprays. Actuators should not be changed among products.
- Inform patient that these products contain hydrofluoroalkane (HFA) and the propellant and are described as non-CFC or CFC-free (contain no chlorofluorocarbons).
- Instruct patient to notify health care professional of all Rx or OTC medications, vitamins, or herbal products being taken and to consult health care professional before taking any OTC medications or alcoholic beverages concurrently with this therapy. Caution patient also to avoid smoking and other respiratory irritants.
- Inform patient that albuterol may cause an unusual or bad taste.
- Rep: Advise females of reproductive potential to notify health care professional if pregnancy is planned or suspected or if breastfeeding. Encourage patients who become pregnant during therapy to enroll in the pregnancy registry that monitors pregnancy outcomes in women exposed to asthma medications during pregnancy. For more information, contact the MothersToBaby Pregnancy Studies conducted by the Organization of Teratology Information Specialists at 1-877-311-8972 or visit http://mothertobaby.org/pregnancy-studies/.
- Inhaln: Instruct patient in the proper use of the metered-dose inhaler or nebulizer (see Appendix C).
- Advise patients to use albuterol first if using other inhalation medications and allow 5 min to elapse before administering other inhalant medications unless otherwise directed.
- Advise patient to rinse mouth with water after each inhalation dose to minimize dry mouth and clean the mouthpiece with water at least once a wk.
- Instruct patient to notify health care professional if there is no response to the usual dose or if contents of one canister are used in less than 2 wk. Asthma and treatment regimen should be re-evaluated and corticosteroids should be considered. Need for increased use to treat symptoms indicates decrease in asthma control and need to re-evaluate patient's therapy.

Evaluation/Desired Outcomes

- Prevention or relief of bronchospasm.

alclometasone, See CORTICOSTEROIDS (TOPICAL/LOCAL).

⚕ alectinib (al-ekti-nib)
Alecensa, ✲ Alecensaro
Classification
Therapeutic: antineoplastics
Pharmacologic: kinase inhibitors

Indications
⚕ Patients with metastatic non-small cell lung cancer (NSCLC) that is positive for anaplastic lymphoma kinase (ALK).

Action
Inhibits tyrosine kinase receptors targeting ALK and RET. **Therapeutic Effects:** Decreased spread of NSCLC.

Pharmacokinetics
Absorption: 37% absorbed following oral administration; high-fat, high-calorie meals ↑ absorption.
Distribution: Extensively distributed to tissues.
Protein Binding: 99%.
Metabolism and Excretion: Primarily metabolized by the liver via the CYP3A4 isoenzyme to its active metabolite, M4 (also metabolized by CYP3A4). 84% excreted in feces unchanged; minimal excretion in urine.
Half-life: *Alectinib:* 33 hr; *M4 active metabolite:* 31 hr.

TIME/ACTION PROFILE (plasma concentrations)

ROUTE	ONSET	PEAK	DURATION
PO	unknown	4 hr	unknown

Contraindications/Precautions
Contraindicated in: OB: Pregnancy; Lactation: Lactation.
Use Cautiously in: Severe renal impairment or end-stage renal disease; Severe hepatic impairment (↓ dose); Rep: Women of reproductive potential; Pedi: Safety and effectiveness not established in children.

Adverse Reactions/Side Effects
CV: bradycardia, edema. **Derm:** photosensitivity, rash. **EENT:** blurred vision, diplopia. **Endo:** hyperglycemia. **F and E:** hypocalcemia, hypokalemia, hyponatremia, hypophosphatemia. **GI:** constipation, diarrhea, hyperbilirubinemia, nausea, vomiting, HEPATOTOXICITY. **GU:** ↑ serum creatinine. **Hemat:** anemia, lymphopenia, BLEEDING, hemolytic anemia. **Metab:** ↑ weight. **MS:** ↑

✲= Canadian drug name. ⚕ = Genetic implication. ~~Strikethrough~~ = Discontinued. CAPITALS = life-threatening. Underline = most frequent.

creatine kinase, back pain, myalgia. **Neuro:** fatigue, headache. **Resp:** cough, dyspnea, INTERSTITIAL LUNG DISEASE (ILD), PULMONARY EMBOLISM.

Interactions
Drug-Drug: None reported.

Route/Dosage
PO (Adults): 600 mg twice daily.

Hepatic Impairment
PO (Adults): *Severe hepatic impairment:* 450 mg twice daily.

Availability
Capsules: 150 mg.

NURSING IMPLICATIONS
Assessment
- Monitor for signs and symptoms of ILD/pneumonitis (worsening of respiratory symptoms, dyspnea, cough, fever). Withhold therapy if symptoms occur and permanently discontinue if no other potential causes are identified.
- Monitor heart rate and BP regularly during therapy. *If symptomatic bradycardia occurs,* withhold therapy until asymptomatic or heart rate ≥60 bpm. If concomitant medication identified as contributing and is discontinued, or its dose adjusted, resume alectinib at previous dose upon recovery to asymptomatic bradycardia or to heart rate ≥60 bpm. If no contributing medication identified, or if contributing medications are not discontinued or dose modified, resume alectinib at reduced dose upon recovery to asymptomatic bradycardia or to heart rate of ≥60 bpm. *If life-threatening bradycardia occurs,* permanently discontinue alectinib if no contributing medication is identified. If contributing medication is identified and discontinued, or its dose is adjusted, resume alectinib at reduced dose upon recovery to asymptomatic bradycardia or to heart rate of ≥60 bpm, with frequent monitoring as clinically indicated. Permanently discontinue alectinib in case of recurrence.
- Assess for myalgia periodically during therapy.

Lab Test Considerations
- ⚡ For patient selection, determine presence of ALK positivity in tumor tissue or plasma specimens using FDA approved test. Information on FDA-approved tests for the detection of ALK rearrangements in NSCLC is available at http://www.fda.gov/CompanionDiagnostics.
- Dose reduction schedule: 1st dose reduction— 450 mg twice daily, 2nd dose reduction 300 mg twice daily. Discontinue if unable to tolerate 300 mg twice daily.
- Monitor liver function tests every 2 wk during first 3 mo of therapy, and then monthly and as clinically indicated during treatment. *If ALT or AST ↑ >5 times upper limit of normal (ULN) with total bilirubin ≤2 times ULN,* temporarily withhold until recovery to baseline or ≤3 times ULN, then resume at reduced dose. *If ALT or AST ↑ >3 times ULN with total bilirubin ↑ >2 times ULN in absence of cholestasis or hemolysis,* permanently discontinue alectinib. *If total bilirubin ↑ >3 times ULN,* temporarily withhold until recovery to baseline or to ≤1.5 times ULN, then resume at reduced dose.
- Assess CK every 2 wk during 1st mo of therapy and in patients reporting unexplained muscle pain, tenderness, or weakness. *If ↑ CK >5 times ULN,* temporarily withhold until recovery to baseline or ≤2.5 times ULN, then resume at same dose. *If ↑ CK >10 times ULN or 2nd occurrence of ↑ CK >5 times ULN,* temporarily withhold until recovery to baseline or ≤2.5 times ULN, then resume at reduced dose.
- Monitor serum creatinine periodically during therapy. *If Grade 3 renal impairment occurs,* hold doses until serum creatinine ≤ 1.5 times ULN, then resume at reduced dose. *If Grade 4 renal impairment occurs,* discontinue alectinib permanently.
- May cause hyperglycemia, hypocalcemia, hypokalemia, hypophosphatemia, and hyponatremia.
- May cause anemia and lymphopenia.

Implementation
- **PO:** Administer twice daily with food. *DNC:* Swallow capsules whole, do not open or dissolve capsule contents.

Patient/Family Teaching
- Instruct patient to take alectinib as directed. If a dose is missed or vomiting occurs after taking, omit dose and take next dose at scheduled time. Advise patient to read *Patient Information* before starting therapy and with each Rx refill in case of changes.
- Advise patient to use sunscreen and lip balm (SPF ≥50) and to wear protective clothing to prevent photosensitivity reaction.
- Advise patient to notify health care professional if signs and symptoms of liver problems (feeling tired, itchy skin, feeling less hungry than usual, nausea or vomiting, yellowing of skin or whites of eyes, pain on right side of stomach, dark urine, bleeding or bruising more easily than normal), respiratory problems (trouble breathing, shortness of breath, cough, fever), bradycardia (dizziness, lightheadedness, syncope), or myalgia (unexplained muscle pain, tenderness, or weakness) occur.
- Instruct patient to notify health care professional of all Rx or OTC medications, vitamins, or herbal products being taken and consult health care professional before taking any new medications.
- Rep: May cause fetal harm. Advise females of reproductive potential to use effective contraception and avoid breastfeeding during and for at least 1 wk following therapy. Advise males with female partners of reproductive potential to use effective contraception during and for 3 mo after last dose.

Evaluation/Desired Outcomes
- Decreased spread of NSCLC.

alendronate (a-len-drone-ate)
Binosto, Fosamax
Classification
Therapeutic: bone resorption inhibitors
Pharmacologic: bisphosphonates

Indications
Treatment and prevention of postmenopausal osteoporosis. Treatment of osteoporosis in men. Treatment of Paget's disease of the bone. Treatment of corticosteroid-induced osteoporosis in patients (men and women) who are receiving ≥7.5 mg of prednisone/day (or equivalent) with evidence of decreased bone mineral density.

Action
Inhibits resorption of bone by inhibiting osteoclast activity. **Therapeutic Effects:** Reversal of the progression of osteoporosis with decreased fractures. Decreased progression of Paget's disease.

Pharmacokinetics
Absorption: Poorly absorbed (0.6–0.8%) after oral administration.
Distribution: Transiently distributes to soft tissue, then distributes to bone.
Metabolism and Excretion: Excreted in urine.
Half-life: 10 yr (reflects release of drug from skeleton).

TIME/ACTION PROFILE (inhibition of bone resorption)

ROUTE	ONSET	PEAK	DURATION
PO	1 mo	3–6 mo	3 wk–7 mo†

†After discontinuation of alendronate.

Contraindications/Precautions
Contraindicated in: Abnormalities of the esophagus that delay esophageal emptying (e.g., strictures, achalasia); Inability to stand/sit upright for at least 30 min; Renal impairment (CCr <35 mL/min); OB: Pregnancy.
Use Cautiously in: History of upper GI disorders; Pre-existing hypocalcemia or vitamin D deficiency; Invasive dental procedures; cancer; receiving chemotherapy, corticosteroids, or angiogenesis inhibitors; poor oral hygiene; periodontal disease; dental disease; anemia; coagulopathy; infection; or poorly fitting dentures (may ↑ risk of jaw osteonecrosis); HF or hypertension (effervescent tablet only); Lactation: Safety not established in breastfeeding; Pedi: Safety and effectiveness not established in children.

Adverse Reactions/Side Effects
CV: atrial fibrillation. **Derm:** erythema, photosensitivity, rash. **EENT:** blurred vision, conjunctivitis, eye pain/inflammation. **GI:** abdominal distention, abdominal pain, acid regurgitation, constipation, diarrhea, dyspepsia, dysphagia, esophageal cancer, esophageal ulcer, esophagitis, flatulence, gastritis, nausea, taste perversion, vomiting. **MS:** musculoskeletal pain, femur fractures, osteonecrosis (primarily of jaw). **Neuro:** headache. **Resp:** asthma exacerbation.

Interactions
Drug-Drug: Calcium supplements, antacids, and **levothyroxine** may ↓ the absorption of alendronate. Doses >10 mg/day ↑ risk of adverse GI events when used with **NSAIDs**.
Drug-Food: Food significantly ↓ absorption. **Caffeine (coffee, tea, cola), mineral water,** and **orange juice** also ↓ absorption.

Route/Dosage
Treatment of Osteoporosis
PO (Adults): 10 mg once daily or 70 mg once weekly.
Prevention of Osteoporosis
PO (Adults): 5 mg once daily or 35 mg once weekly.
Paget's Disease
PO (Adults): 40 mg once daily for 6 mo. Retreatment may be considered for patients who relapse.
Treatment of Corticosteroid-Induced Osteoporosis in Men and Women
PO (Adults): *Men and premenopausal women:* 5 mg once daily. *Postmenopausal women not receiving estrogen:* 10 mg once daily.

Availability (generic available)
Tablets: 5 mg, 10 mg, 35 mg, 40 mg, 70 mg. **Effervescent tablets (strawberry flavor) (contains 603 mg of sodium/tablet) (Binosto):** 70 mg. **Oral solution (raspberry flavor):** 70 mg/75 mL. *In combination with:* cholecalciferol (Fosamax plus D). See Appendix N.

NURSING IMPLICATIONS
Assessment
- **Osteoporosis:** Assess patients for low bone mass before and periodically during therapy.
- **Paget's Disease:** Assess for symptoms of Paget's disease (bone pain, headache, decreased visual and auditory acuity, increased skull size).

Lab Test Considerations
- *Osteoporosis:* Assess serum calcium before and periodically during therapy. Correct hypocalcemia and vitamin D deficiency before initiating alendronate therapy. May cause mild, transient ↑ of calcium and phosphate.
- **Paget's Disease:** Monitor alkaline phosphatase before and periodically during therapy. Alendronate is indicated for patients with alkaline phosphatase twice the upper limit of normal.

Implementation

- **PO:** Administer first thing in the morning with 6–8 oz plain water 30 min before other medications, beverages, or food. Oral solution should be followed by at least 2 oz of water. *DNC:* Swallow tablets whole; do not crush, break, or chew.
- For *effervescent tablets* dissolve 1 tablet in half a glass (4 oz) of plain room temperature water (not mineral water or flavored water). Wait at least 5 min after the effervescence stops, stir the solution for approximately 10 sec and drink contents.

Patient/Family Teaching

- Instruct patient on the importance of taking exactly as directed, first thing in the morning, 30 min before other medications, beverages, or food. Waiting longer than 30 min will improve absorption. Take alendronate with 6–8 oz plain water (mineral water, orange juice, coffee, and other beverages decrease absorption). If a dose is missed, skip dose and resume the next morning; do not double doses or take later in the day. If a weekly dose is missed, take the morning after remembered and resume the following wk on the chosen day. Do not take 2 tablets on the same day. Do not discontinue without consulting health care professional. Advise patient to read *Medication Guide* before starting therapy and with each Rx refill in case of changes.
- Caution patient to remain upright for 30 min following dose to facilitate passage to stomach and minimize risk of esophageal irritation. Advise patient to discontinue alendronate and notify health care provider if pain or difficulty swallowing, retrosternal pain, or new/worsening heartburn occur.
- Caution patient not to swallow, chew, or allow undissolved effervescent tablet to dissolve in their mouth; may cause oropharyngeal irritation.
- Advise patient to eat a balanced diet and consult health care professional about the need for supplemental calcium and vitamin D.
- Encourage patient to participate in regular exercise and to modify behaviors that increase the risk of osteoporosis (stop smoking, reduce alcohol consumption).
- Advise parents to notify health care professional of all Rx or OTC medications, vitamins, or herbal products being taken and to consult with health care professional before taking other medications.
- Advise patient to inform health care professional of alendronate therapy prior to dental surgery.
- Caution patient to use sunscreen and protective clothing to prevent photosensitivity reactions.
- Advise patient to notify health care professional if blurred vision, eye pain, or inflammation occur.
- OB: Advise female patient to notify health care professional if pregnancy is planned or suspected or if breastfeeding.

Evaluation/Desired Outcomes

- Prevention of or decrease in the progression of osteoporosis in postmenopausal women. Reassess need for medication periodically. Consider discontinuation of alendronate after 3–5 yr in patients with low risk of fractures. If discontinued, reassess fracture risk periodically.
- Treatment of osteoporosis in men.
- Decrease in the progression of Paget's disease.
- Treatment of corticosteroid-induced osteoporosis.

alfuzosin (al-fyoo-zo-sin)
Uroxatral, ✤Xatral
Classification
Therapeutic: urinary tract antispasmodics
Pharmacologic: peripherally acting antiadrenergics

Indications
Management of symptomatic benign prostatic hyperplasia (BPH).

Action
Selectively blocks alpha$_1$-adrenergic receptors in the lower urinary tract to relax smooth muscle in the bladder neck and prostate. **Therapeutic Effects:** Increased urine flow and decreased symptoms of BPH.

Pharmacokinetics
Absorption: 49% absorbed following oral administration; food enhances absorption.
Distribution: Unknown.
Metabolism and Excretion: Mostly metabolized by the liver via the CYP3A4 isoenzyme system; 11% excreted unchanged in urine.
Half-life: 10 hr.

TIME/ACTION PROFILE

ROUTE	ONSET	PEAK	DURATION
PO-ER	within hr	8 hr	24 hr

Contraindications/Precautions
Contraindicated in: Hypersensitivity; Moderate to severe hepatic impairment; Concurrent use of strong CYP3A4 inhibitors; Concurrent use of other alpha-adrenergic blocking agents; Severe renal impairment.
Use Cautiously in: Congenital or acquired QTc prolongation or concurrent use of other drugs known to prolong QTc; Mild hepatic impairment; Symptomatic hypotension; Concurrent use of antihypertensive agents, phosphodiesterase type 5 inhibitors, or nitrates (↑ risk of postural hypotension); Previous hypotensive episode with other medications; Geri: Consider age-related changes in body mass and cardiac, renal, and hepatic function when prescribing in older adults.

Adverse Reactions/Side Effects
CV: postural hypotension. **Derm:** TOXIC EPIDERMAL NECROLYSIS. **EENT:** intraoperative floppy iris syndrome. **GI:** abdominal pain, constipation, dyspepsia, nausea. **GU:** erectile dysfunction, priapism. **Hemat:** thrombocytopenia. **Neuro:** dizziness, fatigue, headache. **Resp:** bronchitis, pharyngitis, sinusitis.

Interactions

Drug-Drug: **Strong CYP3A4 inhibitors,** including **ketoconazole, itraconazole,** and **ritonavir,** may significantly ↑ levels and risk of toxicity; concurrent use contraindicated. **Cimetidine, atenolol,** and **diltiazem** may ↑ levels and risk of toxicity. May ↑ levels and risk of toxicity of **atenolol** and **diltiazem;** monitor BP and heart rate. ↑ risk of hypotension with **antihypertensives, nitrates, phosphodiesterase type 5 inhibitors** (including **sildenafil, tadalafil,** and **vardenafil**) and acute ingestion of **alcohol.**

Route/Dosage
PO (Adults): 10 mg once daily.

Availability (generic available)
Extended-release tablets: 10 mg.

NURSING IMPLICATIONS

Assessment
● Assess for symptoms of BPH (urinary hesitancy, feeling of incomplete bladder emptying, interruption of urinary stream, impairment of size and force of urinary stream, terminal urinary dribbling, straining to start flow, dysuria, urgency) before and periodically during therapy.
● Assess for orthostatic reaction and syncope. Monitor BP (lying and standing) and pulse frequently during initial dose adjustment and periodically thereafter. May occur within a few hr after initial doses and occasionally thereafter.
● Rule out prostatic carcinoma before therapy; symptoms are similar.

Implementation
● **PO:** Administer with food at the same meal each day. Tablets must be swallowed whole; *DNC:* do not crush, break, or chew.

Patient/Family Teaching
● Instruct patient to take medication with the same meal each day. Take missed doses as soon as remembered. If not remembered until next day, omit; do not double doses.
● May cause dizziness or drowsiness. Advise patient to avoid driving or other activities requiring alertness until response to the medication is known.
● Caution patient to avoid sudden changes in position to decrease orthostatic hypotension.
● Advise patient to consult health care professional before taking any cough, cold, or allergy remedies.
● Instruct patient to notify health care professional of medication regimen before any surgery, especially cataract surgery.
● Advise patient to notify health care professional if priapism, angina, frequent dizziness, rash, or fainting occurs.
● Emphasize the importance of follow-up exams to evaluate effectiveness of medication.

● Geri: Assess risk for falls; implement fall prevention program and instruct patient and family in preventing falls at home.

Evaluation/Desired Outcomes
● Decreased symptoms of BPH.

alirocumab (a-li-**roe**-kyoo-mab)
Praluent
Classification
Therapeutic: lipid-lowering agents
Pharmacologic: proprotein convertase subtilisin kexin type 9 (PCSK9) inhibitors, monoclonal antibodies

Indications
Primary hyperlipidemia, including heterozygous familial hypercholesterolemia (HeFH) (as adjunct to diet, as monotherapy or in combination with other low-density lipoprotein cholesterol (LDL-C)-lowering therapies [e.g. statin, ezetimibe]). Reduction in risk of MI, stroke, and unstable angina requiring hospitalization in patients with established cardiovascular disease. Homozygous familial hypercholesterolemia (HoFH) (as adjunct to other LDL-C lowering therapies).

Action
A human monoclonal immunoglobulin (IgG1) produced in genetically engineered Chinese hamster ovary cells that binds to PCSK9, inhibiting its binding to the low density lipoprotein receptor (LDLR) resulting in ↑ number of LDLRs available to clear LDL from blood. **Therapeutic Effects:** Reduction in LDL-C in primary hyperlipidemia and HoFH. Reduction in risk of MI, stroke, and unstable angina requiring hospitalization.

Pharmacokinetics
Absorption: Well absorbed (85%) following SUBQ administration.
Distribution: Mostly distributed in the circulatory system.
Metabolism and Excretion: Eliminated by binding to PCSK9 and by proteolytic degradation.
Half-life: 17–20 days.

TIME/ACTION PROFILE (effect on circulating unbound PCSK9)

ROUTE	ONSET	PEAK	DURATION
SUBQ	rapid	4–8 hr	2 wk

Contraindications/Precautions
Contraindicated in: Serious hypersensitivity.
Use Cautiously in: Severe renal impairment; Severe hepatic impairment; OB: Safety not established in pregnancy; Lactation: Safety not established in breastfeeding; Pedi: Safety and effectiveness not established in children; Geri: Older adults may be more sensitive to drug effects.

Adverse Reactions/Side Effects
Local: injection site reactions. **Neuro:** confusion.
Misc: HYPERSENSITIVITY REACTIONS (including angioedema, vasculitis).

Interactions
Drug-Drug: None reported.

Route/Dosage

Primary Hyperlipidemia (including Heterozygous Familial Hypercholesterolemia) or Established Cardiovascular Disease
SUBQ (Adults): 75 mg every 2 wk *or* 300 mg every 4 wk; if desired LDL-C has not been achieved, may ↑ dose to 150 mg every 2 wk. *Patients with HeFH undergoing apheresis:* 150 mg every 2 wk.

Homozygous Familial Hypercholesterolemia
SUBQ (Adults): 150 mg every 2 wk.

Availability
Solution for injection (prefilled pens): 75 mg/mL, 150 mg/mL.

NURSING IMPLICATIONS

Assessment
- Obtain a diet history, especially with regard to fat consumption.
- Monitor for signs and symptoms of hypersensitivity reactions (pruritus, rash, urticaria, hypersensitivity vasculitis and hypersensitivity reactions requiring hospitalization) during therapy. If severe symptoms occur, discontinue alirocumab.

Lab Test Considerations
- Assess LDL-C levels within 4–8 wk of initiating or titrating alirocumab for patients taking every 2 wk or just before next dose for patients taking every 4 wk, to assess response and adjust dose, if needed.

Implementation
- **SUBQ:** Allow solution to warm to room temperature for 30–40 min before injecting. May be kept at room temperature for up to 30 days. Solution is clear and colorless to pale yellow; do not administer solutions that are cloudy or contain particulate matter. Do not shake. Inject into thigh, abdomen, or upper arm into areas not tender, bruised, red, or indurated. Rotate sites with each injection. Do not inject into areas with skin disease or injury (sunburns, rashes, inflammation, skin infections). Do not reuse prefilled pen or syringe. Do not administer other injectable drugs at same site. Store in refrigerator; keep in original container, protect from light. Do not freeze.
- Administer 300 mg dose as two 150 mg injections in 2 different sites.

Patient/Family Teaching
- Instruct patient in correct technique for self-injection, care and disposal of equipment. Administer

missed doses within 7 days, then resume original schedule. If not administered within 7 days, wait until next dose on original schedule. Advise patient to read *Patient Information* before starting therapy and with each Rx refill in case of changes.
- Advise patient that this medication should be used in conjunction with diet restrictions (fat, cholesterol, carbohydrates, alcohol), exercise, and cessation of smoking.
- Advise patient to notify health care professional immediately if signs and symptoms of hypersensitivity reactions occur.
- Instruct patient to notify health care professional of all Rx or OTC medications, vitamins, or herbal products being taken and to consult health care professional before taking any other Rx, OTC, or herbal products.
- Advise patient to notify health care professional of medication regimen prior to treatment or surgery.
- Rep: Advise patient to notify health care professional if pregnancy is planned or suspected or if breastfeeding. There is a pregnancy safety study for alirocumab. If alirocumab is administered during pregnancy, report alirocumab exposure by contacting Regeneron at 1-844-734-6643.

Evaluation/Desired Outcomes
- ↓ LDL-C levels.
- Reduction in risk of MI, stroke, and unstable angina requiring hospitalization.

✖ **allopurinol** (al-oh-**pure**-i-nole)
Aloprim, Zyloprim
Classification
Therapeutic: antigout agents, antihyperuricemics
Pharmacologic: xanthine oxidase inhibitors

Indications
PO: Prevention of attack of gouty arthritis and nephropathy. **PO, IV:** Treatment of secondary hyperuricemia, which may occur during treatment of tumors or leukemias.

Action
Inhibits the production of uric acid by inhibiting the action of xanthine oxidase. **Therapeutic Effects:** Lowering of serum uric acid levels.

Pharmacokinetics
Absorption: Well absorbed (80%) following oral administration.
Distribution: Widely distributed in tissue and breast milk.
Protein Binding: <1%.
Metabolism and Excretion: Metabolized to oxypurinol, an active compound with a long half-life. 12% excreted unchanged, 76% excreted as oxypurinol.
Half-life: 1–3 hr (oxypurinol 18–30 hr).

TIME/ACTION PROFILE (hypouricemic effect)

ROUTE	ONSET	PEAK	DURATION
PO, IV	1–2 days	1–2 wk	1–3 wk†

†Duration after discontinuation of allopurinol.

Contraindications/Precautions

Contraindicated in: Hypersensitivity; ≋ Presence of HLA-B*58:01 allele (↑ risk of hypersensitivity reactions); Lactation: Lactation.

Use Cautiously in: Acute attacks of gout; Renal impairment (dose ↓ required if CCr <20 mL/min); Dehydration (adequate hydration necessary); OB: Safety not established in pregnancy; Geri: Begin at lower end of dosage range in older adults.

Adverse Reactions/Side Effects

CV: bradycardia, flushing, heart failure (reported with IV administration), hypertension, hypotension. **Derm:** rash (discontinue drug at first sign of rash), DRUG REACTION WITH EOSINOPHILIA AND SYSTEMIC SYMPTOMS (DRESS), STEVENS-JOHNSON SYNDROME, TOXIC EPIDERMAL NECROLYSIS, urticaria. **GI:** diarrhea, hepatitis, nausea, vomiting. **GU:** hematuria, renal failure. **Hemat:** bone marrow depression. **Neuro:** drowsiness. **Misc:** HYPERSENSITIVITY REACTIONS.

Interactions

Drug-Drug: Use with **mercaptopurine** and **azathioprine** ↑ bone marrow depressant properties—doses of these drugs should be ↓. Use with **ampicillin** or **amoxicillin** ↑ risk of rash. Use with **oral hypoglycemic agents** and **warfarin** ↑ effects of these drugs. Use with **thiazide diuretics** or **ACE inhibitors** ↑ risk of hypersensitivity reactions. Large doses of allopurinol may ↑ risk of **theophylline** toxicity. May ↑ **cyclosporine** levels.

Route/Dosage

Gout

PO (Adults and Children >10 yr): *Initially:* 100 mg/day; ↑ at weekly intervals based on serum uric acid (not to exceed 800 mg/day). Doses >300 mg/day should be given in divided doses; *Maintenance dose:* 100–200 mg 2–3 times daily. Doses of ≤300 mg may be given as a single daily dose.

Renal Impairment

(Adults and Children): *CCr 10–50 mL/min:* ↓ dose to 50% of recommended; *CCr <10 mL/min:* ↓ dosage to 30% of recommended.

Secondary Hyperuricemia

PO (Adults and Children >10 yr): 600–800 mg/day in 2–3 divided doses starting 1–2 days before chemotherapy or radiation.

PO (Children 6–10 yr): 10 mg/kg/day in 2–3 divided doses (maximum 800 mg/day) or 300 mg daily in 2–3 divided doses.

PO (Children <6 yr): 10 mg/kg/day in 2–3 divided doses (maximum 800 mg/day) or 150 mg daily in 3 divided doses.

IV (Adults and Children >10 yr): 200–400 mg/m²/day (up to 600 mg/day) as a single daily dose or in divided doses every 8–24 hr.

IV (Children <10 yr): 200 mg/m²/day initially as a single daily dose or in divided doses every 8–24 hr (maximum dose 600 mg/day).

Renal Impairment

(Adults and Children): *CCr 10–50 mL/min:* ↓ dose to 50% of recommended; *CCr <10 mL/min:* ↓ dosage to 30% of recommended.

Availability (generic available)

Tablets: 100 mg, 200 mg, 300 mg. **Powder for injection:** 500 mg/vial.

NURSING IMPLICATIONS

Assessment

- Monitor intake and output ratios. Decreased kidney function can cause drug accumulation and toxic effects. Ensure that patient maintains adequate fluid intake (minimum 2500–3000 mL/day) to minimize risk of kidney stone formation.

- ≋ Consider testing for the HLA-B*58:01 allele in patients of African, Asian, and Native Hawaiian/Pacific Islander ancestry prior to using allopurinol; use not recommended if allele present.

- Assess patient for rash or more severe hypersensitivity reactions. Discontinue allopurinol immediately if rash occurs. Therapy should be discontinued permanently if reaction is severe. Therapy may be reinstated after a mild reaction has subsided, at a lower dose (50 mg/day with very gradual titration). If skin rash recurs, discontinue permanently.

- Monitor for signs and symptoms of DRESS (fever, rash, lymphadenopathy, and/or facial swelling, associated with involvement of other organ systems (hepatitis, nephritis, hematologic abnormalities, myocarditis, myositis) during therapy. May resemble an acute viral infection. Eosinophilia is often present. Discontinue therapy if signs occur.

- **Gout:** Monitor for joint pain and swelling. Addition of colchicine or NSAIDs may be necessary for acute attacks. Prophylactic doses of colchicine or an NSAID should be administered concurrently during first 3–6 mo of therapy because of an increased frequency of acute attacks of gouty arthritis during early therapy.

Lab Test Considerations

- Serum and urine uric acid levels usually begin to ↓ 2–3 days after initiation of oral therapy.

- Monitor blood glucose in patients receiving oral hypoglycemic agents. May cause hypoglycemia.

- Monitor hematologic, renal, and liver function tests before and periodically during therapy, especially during the first few mo. May cause ↑ serum alkaline phosphatase, bilirubin, AST, and ALT levels. ↓ CBC and platelets may indicate bone marrow depression. ↑ BUN, serum creatinine may indicate nephrotoxicity. These are usually reversed with discontinuation of therapy.

Implementation

- Do not confuse Zyloprim with zolpidem.
- **PO:** May be administered after milk or meals to minimize gastric irritation; give with plenty of fluid. May be crushed and given with fluid or mixed with food for patients who have difficulty swallowing.

IV Administration

- **Intermittent Infusion:** *Reconstitution:* Reconstitute each 500 mg vial with 25 mL of sterile water for injection. Solution is clear and almost colorless with only slight opalescence; do not administer solutions that are cloudy, discolored, or contain particulate matter. *Dilution:* Dilute to desired concentration with 0.9% NaCl or D5W. Administer within 10 hr of reconstitution; do not refrigerate. Do not administer solutions that are discolored or contain particulate matter. *Concentration:* Not >6 m g/mL. *Rate:* Infusion should be initiated 24–48 hr before start of chemotherapy known to cause tumor cell lysis. Rate of infusion depends on volume of infusate (100–300 mg doses may be infused over 30 min). May be administered as a single infusion or equally divided infusions at 6-, 8-, or 12-hr intervals.
- **Y-Site Compatibility:** acyclovir, aminophylline, amphotericin B lipid complex, anidulafungin, argatroban, arsenic trioxide, aztreonam, bivalirudin, bleomycin, bumetanide, buprenorphine, butorphanol, calcium gluconate, carboplatin, caspofungin, cefazolin, cefotetan, ceftazidime, ceftriaxone, cefuroxime, cisplatin, cyclophosphamide, dactinomycin, dexamethasone sodium phosphate, dexmedetomidine, docetaxel, doxorubicin liposome, enalaprilat, etoposide, famotidine, filgrastim, fluconazole, fludarabine, fluorouracil, fosphenytoin, furosemide, ganciclovir, gemcitabine, gemtuzumab ozogamicin, granisetron, heparin, hetastarch, hydrocortisone, hydromorphone, ifosfamide, leucovorin calcium, linezolid, lorazepam, mannitol, mesna, methotrexate, metronidazole, milrinone, mitoxantrone, morphine, octreotide, oxaliplatin, oxytocin, paclitaxel, pamidronate, pantoprazole, pemetrexed, piperacillin/tazobactam, potassium chloride, sodium acetate, thiotepa, tigecycline, tirofiban, trimethoprim/sulfamethoxazole, vancomycin, vasopressin, vinblastine, vincristine, voriconazole, zidovudine, zoledronic acid.
- **Y-Site Incompatibility:** alemtuzumab, amikacin, amiodarone, carmustine, cefotaxime, chlorpromazine, clindamycin, cytarabine, dacarbazine, daptomycin, daunorubicin hydrochloride, dexrazoxane, diltiazem, diphenhydramine, doxorubicin hydrochloride, doxycycline, droperidol, epirubicin, erta-

penem, etoposide phosphate, floxuridine, foscarnet, gentamicin, haloperidol, hydroxyzine, idarubicin, imipenem/cilastatin, irinotecan, meperidine, methadone, methylprednisolone, metoprolol, minocycline, mitomycin, moxifloxacin, mycophenolate, nalbuphine, ondansetron, palonosetron, potassium acetate, prochlorperazine, promethazine, sodium bicarbonate, tacrolimus, tobramycin, topotecan, vecuronium, vinorelbine.

Patient/Family Teaching

- Instruct patient to take allopurinol as directed. Take missed doses as soon as remembered. If dosing schedule is once daily, do not take if remembered the next day. If dosing schedule is more than once a day, take up to 300 mg for next dose.
- Instruct patient to continue taking allopurinol along with an NSAID or colchicine during an acute attack of gout. Allopurinol helps prevent, but does not relieve, acute gout attacks.
- Alkaline diet may be ordered. Urinary acidification with large doses of vitamin C or other acids may increase kidney stone formation (see Appendix J). Advise patient of need for increased fluid intake.
- May occasionally cause drowsiness. Caution patient to avoid driving or other activities requiring alertness until response to drug is known.
- Instruct patient to report skin rash, blood in urine, influenza symptoms (chills, fever, muscle aches and pains, nausea, or vomiting) or symptoms of DRESS to health care professional immediately; skin rash may indicate hypersensitivity.
- Advise patient that large amounts of alcohol increase uric acid concentrations and may decrease the effectiveness of allopurinol.
- Advise females of reproductive potential to notify health care professional if pregnancy is planned or suspected and to avoid breastfeeding during therapy and for 1 wk after last dose.
- Emphasize the importance of follow-up exams to monitor effectiveness and side effects.

Evaluation/Desired Outcomes

- Decreased serum and urinary uric acid levels. May take 2–6 wk to observe clinical improvement in patients treated for gout.

almotriptan (al-moe-**trip**-tan)
Axert
Classification
Therapeutic: vascular headache suppressants
Pharmacologic: 5-HT$_1$ agonists

Indications

Acute treatment of migraine headache (for adolescents, migraines should be ≥4 hr in duration).

Action

Acts as an agonist at specific 5-HT$_1$ receptor sites in intracranial blood vessels and sensory trigeminal nerves.

Therapeutic Effects: Cranial vessel vasoconstriction with associated decrease in release of neuropeptides and resultant decrease in migraine headache.

Pharmacokinetics
Absorption: Well absorbed following oral administration (70%).
Distribution: Widely distributed to tissues.
Metabolism and Excretion: 27% metabolized by monoamine oxidase-A (MAO-A); 12% metabolized by the CYP3A4 and CYP2D6 isoenzymes; 40% excreted unchanged in urine; 13% excreted in feces as unchanged and metabolized drug.
Half-life: 3–4 hr.

TIME/ACTION PROFILE (plasma concentrations)

ROUTE	ONSET	PEAK	DURATION
PO	unknown	1–3 hr	unknown

Contraindications/Precautions
Contraindicated in: Hypersensitivity; Ischemic cardiovascular, cerebrovascular, or peripheral vascular syndromes (including ischemic bowel disease); History of significant cardiovascular disease; Uncontrolled hypertension; Should not be used within 24 hr of other 5-HT$_1$ agonists or ergot-type compounds (dihydroergotamine); Basilar or hemiplegic migraine; Concurrent MAO-A inhibitor therapy or within 2 wk of discontinuing MAO-A inhibitor therapy.
Use Cautiously in: Cardiovascular risk factors (hypertension, hypercholesterolemia, cigarette smoking, obesity, diabetes, strong family history, menopausal women, or men >40 yr); use only if cardiovascular status has been evaluated and determined to be safe and first dose is administered under supervision; Renal impairment; Hepatic impairment; Hypersensitivity to sulfonamides (cross-sensitivity may occur); OB: Safety not established in pregnancy; Lactation: Safety not established in breastfeeding; Pedi: Children <12 yr (safety and effectiveness not established).

Adverse Reactions/Side Effects
CV: CORONARY ARTERY VASOSPASM, MI, myocardial ischemia, VENTRICULAR ARRHYTHMIAS. **GI:** dry mouth, nausea. **Neuro:** drowsiness, headache, paresthesia.

Interactions
Drug-Drug: Concurrent use with **MAO-A inhibitors** ↑ levels and the risk of toxicity; concurrent use or use within 2 wk or MAO inhibitor contraindicated. Concurrent use with other **5-HT$_1$ agonists** or **ergot-type compounds (dihydroergotamine)** may result in additive vasoactive properties; avoid use within 24 hr of each other. ↑ serotonin levels and serotonin syndrome may occur when used concurrently with **SSRIs** or **SNRIs. CYP3A4 inhibitors,** including **ketoconazole, itraconazole, ritonavir,** and **erythromycin,** may ↑ levels and risk of toxicity.

Route/Dosage
PO (Adults and Children ≥12 yr): 6.25–12.5 mg initially, may repeat in 2 hr; not to exceed 2 doses per 24-hr period.

Hepatic/Renal Impairment
PO (Adults): 6.25 mg initially, may repeat in 2 hr; not to exceed 2 doses per 24-hr period.

Availability (generic available)
Tablets: 6.25 mg, 12.5 mg.

NURSING IMPLICATIONS
Assessment
- Assess pain location, character, intensity, and duration and associated symptoms (photophobia, phonophobia, nausea, vomiting) during migraine attack.
- Assess for serotonin syndrome (mental changes [agitation, hallucinations, coma], autonomic instability [tachycardia, labile BP, hyperthermia], neuromuscular aberrations [hyperreflexia, incoordination], and/or GI symptoms [nausea, vomiting, diarrhea]), especially in patients taking other serotonergic drugs (SSRIs, SNRIs).

Implementation
- **PO:** Tablets should be swallowed whole with liquid.

Patient/Family Teaching
- Inform patient that almotriptan should only be used during a migraine attack. It is meant to be used for relief of migraine attacks but not to prevent or reduce the number of attacks.
- Instruct patient to administer almotriptan as soon as symptoms of a migraine attack appear, but it may be administered any time during an attack. If migraine symptoms return, a 2nd dose may be used. Allow at least 2 hr between doses, and do not use more than 2 doses in any 24-hr period.
- If first dose does not relieve headache, additional almotriptan doses are not likely to be effective; notify health care professional.
- Caution patient not to take almotriptan within 24 hr of another vascular headache suppressant.
- Advise patient that lying down in a darkened room following almotriptan administration may further help relieve headache.
- Advise patient that overuse (use more than 10 days/month) may lead to exacerbation of headache (migraine-like daily headaches, or as a marked increase in frequency of migraine attacks). May require gradual withdrawal of almotriptan and treatment of symptoms (transient worsening of headache).
- Advise patient to notify health care professional prior to next dose of almotriptan if pain or tightness in the chest occurs during use. If pain is severe or does not subside, notify health care professional immediately. If feelings of tingling, heat, flushing, heaviness, pressure,

drowsiness, dizziness, tiredness, or sickness develop discuss with health care professional at next visit.
- May cause dizziness or drowsiness. Caution patient to avoid driving or other activities requiring alertness until response to medication is known.
- Advise patient to avoid alcohol, which aggravates headaches, during almotriptan use.
- Advise patient to notify health care professional of all Rx or OTC medications, vitamins, or herbal products being taken and to consult with health care professional before taking other medications.
- Advise patient to notify health care professional immediately if signs or symptoms of serotonin syndrome occur.
- Rep: Advise females of reproductive potential to notify health care professional if pregnancy is planned or suspected, or if breastfeeding.

Evaluation/Desired Outcomes
- Relief of migraine attack.

alogliptin (al-oh-**glip**-tin)
Nesina
Classification
Therapeutic: antidiabetics
Pharmacologic: dipeptidyl peptidase-4 (DPP-4) inhibitors

Indications
Adjunct to diet and exercise to improve glycemic control in type 2 diabetes mellitus.

Action
Acts as a competitive inhibitor of dipeptidyl peptidase-4 (DPP-4) which slows the inactivation of incretin hormones, thereby increasing their concentrations and reducing fasting and postprandial glucose concentrations. **Therapeutic Effects:** Improved control of blood glucose.

Pharmacokinetics
Absorption: Completely absorbed following oral administration (100%).
Distribution: Well distributed to tissues.
Metabolism and Excretion: Not extensively metabolized, 76% excreted unchanged in urine.
Half-life: 21 hr.

TIME/ACTION PROFILE (inhibition of DPP-4)

ROUTE	ONSET	PEAK†	DURATION
PO	unknown	1–2 hr	24 hr

†Multiple dosing.

Contraindications/Precautions
Contraindicated in: Type 1 diabetes; Diabetic ketoacidosis; Previous severe hypersensitivity reactions.
Use Cautiously in: Hepatic impairment; Renal impairment (dose ↓ required if CCr <60 mL/min); HF or renal impairment (↑ risk for worsening HF); OB: Use

during pregnancy only if potential maternal benefit justifies potential fetal risk; Lactation: Use while breastfeeding only if potential maternal benefit justifies potential risk to infant; Pedi: Safety and effectiveness not established in children; Geri: Older adults may have ↑ sensitivity to effects.

Adverse Reactions/Side Effects
CV: HF. **Derm:** bullous pemphigoid, STEVENS-JOHNSON SYNDROME (SJS). **GI:** ↑ liver enzymes, HEPATOTOXICITY, PANCREATITIS. **MS:** arthralgia, RHABDOMYOLYSIS. **Neuro:** headache. **Misc:** HYPERSENSITIVITY REACTIONS (including anaphylaxis or angioedema).

Interactions
Drug-Drug: ↑ risk of hypoglycemia with **sulfonylureas** and **insulin**; dose adjustments may be necessary.

Route/Dosage
PO (Adults): 25 mg once daily.

Renal Impairment
PO (Adults): *CCr 30–59 mL/min:* 12.5 mg once daily; *CCr 15–29 mL/min:* 6.25 mg once daily; *CCr <15 mL/min or requiring hemodialysis:* 6.25 mg once daily.

Availability
Tablets: 6.25 mg, 12.5 mg, 25 mg. *In combination with:* metformin (Kazano), pioglitazone (Oseni).

NURSING IMPLICATIONS
Assessment
- Observe for signs and symptoms of hypoglycemic reactions (abdominal pain, sweating, hunger, weakness, dizziness, headache, tremor, tachycardia, anxiety).
- Monitor for signs of pancreatitis (nausea, vomiting, anorexia, persistent severe abdominal pain, sometimes radiating to the back) during therapy. If pancreatitis occurs, discontinue alogliptin and monitor serum and urine amylase, amylase/CCr ratio, electrolytes, serum calcium, glucose, and lipase.
- Assess for signs and symptoms of HF (increasing shortness of breath, rapid increase in weight, swelling of feet) periodically during therapy.
- Assess for rash periodically during therapy. May cause SJS. Discontinue therapy if severe or if accompanied with fever, general malaise, fatigue, muscle or joint aches, blisters, oral lesions, conjunctivitis, hepatitis, and/or eosinophilia.

Lab Test Considerations
- Monitor hemoglobin A1C prior to and periodically during therapy.
- Monitor liver function tests prior to starting and periodically during therapy. Interrupt therapy and determine cause if significant ↑ in enzymes or abnormal tests persist or worsen. Do not restart therapy without explanation for abnormalities.
- Monitor renal function prior to and periodically during therapy.

Implementation
- Patients stabilized on a diabetic regimen who are exposed to stress, fever, trauma, infection, or surgery may require administration of insulin.
- **PO:** May be administered without regard to food.

Patient/Family Teaching
- Instruct patient to take alogliptin as directed. Take missed doses as soon as remembered, unless it is almost time for next dose; do not double dose. Advise patient to read *Medication Guide* before starting and with each Rx refill in case of changes.
- Explain to patient that alogliptin helps control hyperglycemia but does not cure diabetes. Therapy is usually long term.
- Instruct patient not to share this medication with others, even if they have the same symptoms; it may harm them.
- Encourage patient to follow prescribed diet, medication, and exercise regimen to prevent hyperglycemic or hypoglycemic episodes.
- Review signs of hypoglycemia and hyperglycemia with patient. If hypoglycemia occurs, advise patient to take a glass of orange juice or 2–3 tsp of sugar, honey, or corn syrup dissolved in water, and notify health care professional.
- Instruct patient in proper testing of blood glucose and urine ketones. These tests should be monitored closely during periods of stress or illness and health care professional notified if significant changes occur.
- Advise patient to stop taking alogliptin and notify health care professional promptly if symptoms of hypersensitivity reactions (rash; hives; swelling of face, lips, tongue, and throat; difficulty in breathing or swallowing), liver dysfunction (fatigue, nausea, vomiting, anorexia, right upper abdominal discomfort, dark urine, yellowing of skin or whites of eyes), HF, or pancreatitis occur.
- Advise patient to notify health care professional of all Rx or OTC medications, vitamins, or herbal products being taken and to consult with health care professional before taking other medications.
- Instruct patient to notify health care professional if severe joint pain occurs.
- OB: Advise patient to notify health care professional if pregnancy is planned or suspected or if breastfeeding.

Evaluation/Desired Outcomes
- Improved hemoglobin A1C, fasting plasma glucose and 2-hr postprandial glucose levels.

⚕ alpelisib (al-pe-lisib)
Piqray, Vijoice
Classification
Therapeutic: antineoplastics
Pharmacologic: kinase inhibitors

Indications
Piqray ⚕ Treatment of postmenopausal women and men with hormone receptor-positive, human epidermal growth factor receptor 2-negative, PIK3CA-mutated, advanced or metastatic breast cancer (in combination with fulvestrant). **Vijoice** ⚕ Severe manifestations of PIK3CA-related overgrowth spectrum in patients who require systemic therapy.

Action
⚕ Acts as an inhibitor of phosphatidylinositol 3–kinase (PI3K). Mutations in the gene encoding the catalytic α-subunit of PI3K (PIK3CA) lead to activation of PI3Kα and Akt-signaling, cellular transformation, and tumor generation. Alpelisib inhibits phosphorylation of PI3K downstream targets (including Akt) and demonstrated activity in cell lines harboring a PIK3CA mutation. Activating mutations in PIK3CA may induce overgrowths and malformations in PROS. **Therapeutic Effects:** Decreased progression of breast cancer. Reduction in lesion volume in PIK3CA-related overgrowth spectrum.

Pharmacokinetics
Absorption: Well absorbed following oral administration.
Distribution: Widely distributed to tissues.
Metabolism and Excretion: Primarily metabolized via hydrolysis; also metabolized to a lesser extent by CYP3A4. Excreted in feces (36% as unchanged drug; 32% as metabolites) and urine (2% as unchanged drug; 7% as metabolites).
Half-life: 8–9 hr.

TIME/ACTION PROFILE (plasma concentrations)

ROUTE	ONSET	PEAK	DURATION
PO	unknown	2–4 hr	24 hr

Contraindications/Precautions
Contraindicated in: History of serious hypersensitivity reactions including anaphylaxis, Stevens-Johnson syndrome, erythema multiforme, or toxic epidermal necrolysis; Concurrent use of strong CYP3A inducers; OB: Pregnancy; Lactation: Lactation.
Use Cautiously in: Diabetes or risk factors for hyperglycemia (obesity, elevated fasting plasma glucose, elevated HbA1c, concurrent use of systemic corticosteroids or age ≥75 yr); Severe renal impairment (CCr ≤30 mL/min) (Piqray only); Rep: Women of reproductive potential and men with female partners of reproductive potential; Pedi: Safety and effectiveness not established in children <18 yr (breast cancer) or <2 yr (PIK3CA-related overgrowth spectrum); Geri: Older adults may be more sensitive to drug effects.

Adverse Reactions/Side Effects
CV: peripheral edema. **Derm:** alopecia, DRUG REACTION WITH EOSINOPHILIA AND SYSTEMIC SYMPTOMS (DRESS),

---

dry skin, ERYTHEMA MULTIFORM (EM), pruritus, rash, STEVENS-JOHNSON SYNDROME (SJS), TOXIC EPIDERMAL NECROLYSIS (TEN), cellulitis, eczema. **Endo:** hyperglycemia, hypoglycemia, hyperglycemic hyperosmolar nonketotic syndrome, KETOACIDOSIS. **F and E:** hyperkalemia, hypocalcemia, hypokalemia, hypomagnesemia, hyponatremia, hypophosphatemia. **GI:** ↓ appetite, ↑ lipase, ↑ liver enzymes, abdominal pain, DIARRHEA, hyperbilirubinemia, metallic taste, nausea, stomatitis, vomiting, colitis. **GU:** ↑ serum creatinine, ↓ fertility, acute kidney injury. **Hemat:** anemia, lymphocytopenia, thrombocytopenia. **Metab:** ↓ weight, hypercholesterolemia, hypertriglyceridemia, hypoalbuminemia. **Neuro:** fatigue, headache, insomnia. **Resp:** cough, PNEUMONITIS. **Misc:** fever, INFECTION, HYPERSENSITIVITY REACTIONS (including anaphylaxis and angioedema).

Interactions

Drug–Drug: Strong CYP3A4 inducers may ↓ levels and effectiveness; avoid concurrent use. **Breast cancer resistance protein inhibitors** may ↑ levels and risk of toxicity; avoid concurrent use. May ↓ levels of **CYP2C9 substrates**, including **warfarin**.

Route/Dosage

Breast Cancer

PO (Adults): 300 mg once daily until disease progression or unacceptable toxicity.

PIK3CA-Related Overgrowth Spectrum

PO (Adults): 250 mg once daily until disease progression or unacceptable toxicity.
PO (Children 6–<18 yr): 50 mg once daily until disease progression or unacceptable toxicity. After 24 wk, may ↑ to 125 mg once daily to optimize clinical/radiological response; continue until disease progression or unacceptable toxicity. Once patient becomes 18 yr old, gradually ↑ to 250 mg once daily.
PO (Children 2–<6 yr): 50 mg once daily until disease progression or unacceptable toxicity.

Availability

Tablets (Piqray): 50 mg, 150 mg, 200 mg. **Tablets (Vijoice):** 50 mg, 125 mg, 200 mg.

NURSING IMPLICATIONS

Assessment

- Monitor for signs and symptoms of hypersensitivity reactions (dyspnea, flushing, rash, fever, tachycardia) during therapy. If symptoms occur, permanently discontinue alpelisib.
- Assess for severe cutaneous adverse reactions including SJS, EM, TEN, and DRESS (prodrome of fever, flu-like symptoms, mucosal lesions, progressive skin rash) during therapy. *If rash is Grade 1 (< 10% body surface area [BSA] with active skin toxicity);* No dose adjustment needed. Initiate topical corticosteroid treatment. Consider adding oral antihistamine to manage symptoms. If rash is not im-

proved within 28 days of treatment, add a low dose systemic corticosteroid. If the cause is SJS, EM, TEN, or DRESS, permanently discontinue alpelisib. *If Grade 2 (10-30% BSA with active skin toxicity);* No dose adjustment necessary. Initiate or intensify topical corticosteroid and oral antihistamines. Consider low dose systemic corticosteroid treatment. If rash improves to Grade ≤ 1 within 10 days, systemic corticosteroid may be discontinued. If the cause is SJS, EM, TEN, or DRESS, permanently discontinue alpelisib. *If Grade 3 (severe rash not responsive to medical management and >30% BSA with active skin toxicity):* Hold alpelisib. Initiate or intensify topical/systemic corticosteroid and oral antihistamines. If the cause is SJS, EM, TEN, or DRESS, permanently discontinue alpelisib. If the etiology is not SJS, EM, TEN, or DRESS, hold dose until improvement to Grade ≤ 1, then resume alpelisib at next lower dose. *If Grade 4 (severe bullous, blistering or exfoliating skin conditions and any % BSA associated with extensive superinfection, with IV antibiotics indicated; life-threatening):* Permanently discontinue alpelisib.
- Monitor for signs and symptoms of pneumonitis (hypoxia, cough, dyspnea, interstitial infiltrates) during therapy. If pneumonitis is confirmed, discontinue alpelisib permanently.
- Monitor for signs and symptoms of diarrhea and colitis (abdominal pain, mucus or blood in stool) during therapy. *If Grade 1 diarrhea occurs,* do not adjust alpelisib dose. Start antidiarrheal therapy and monitor symptoms. *If Grade 2 diarrhea occurs,* start or intensify antidiarrheal therapy and monitor symptoms. May add enteric-acting and/or systemic steroids to therapy for Grade 2 or Grade 3 colitis. Hold alpelisib until recovery to Grade ≤1, then resume at same dose. *If Grade 3 diarrhea occurs,* start or intensify antidiarrheal therapy and monitor symptoms. Hold alpelisib until recovery to Grade ≤1, then resume at the next lower dose. *If Grade 4 diarrhea occurs,* permanently discontinue alpelisib.

Lab Test Considerations

- Verify negative pregnancy test before starting therapy. ⊠ Information on FDA approved tests for the detection of PIK3CA mutations in breast cancer is available at: http://www.fda.gov/CompanionDiagnostics.
- May cause hyperglycemia. Before starting alpelisib therapy, test fasting blood glucose (FBG) and HbA1c; optimize blood glucose. After starting therapy, monitor blood glucose at least weekly for first 2 wk, then at least once every 4 wk, and as indicated. Monitor HbA1c every 3 mo and as indicated. If hyperglycemia develops, monitor FBG at least twice weekly until FBG decreases to normal. During treatment with anti-diabetic agents, continue monitoring FBG at least weekly for 8 wk, then once every 2 wk and as needed clinically. *If Grade 1 FBG >ULN-160 mg/dL,* No dose adjustment needed. Begin or intensify anti-diabetic treatment. *If Grade 2 FBG >160-*

250 mg/dL: No dose adjustment needed. Begin or further intensify anti-diabetic therapy. If FBG does not decrease to ≤ 160 mg/dL within 21 days, reduce alpelisib dose by 1 dose level and follow FBG value recommendations. *If Grade 3 >250-500 mg/dL,* Hold alpelisib. Begin or intensify oral anti-diabetic therapy and consider additional anti-diabetic agents for 1-2 days until hyperglycemia improves. Administer intravenous hydration and consider added intervention for electrolyte/ketoacidosis/hyperosmolar disturbances). If FBG decreases to ≤160 mg/dL within 3 to 5 days under appropriate anti-diabetic therapy, resume alpelisib at 1 lower dose level. If FBG does not decrease to ≤160 mg/dL within 3 to 5 days under appropriate anti-diabetic therapy, consult with a specialist in the treatment of hyperglycemia. If FBG does not decrease to ≤160 mg/dL within 21 days following appropriate anti-diabetic therapy, permanently discontinue alpelisib. *If Grade 4 >500 m g/dL:* Hold alpelisib. Begin or intensify appropriate anti-diabetic therapy (administer intravenous hydration and consider appropriate intervention for electrolyte/ketoacidosis/hyperosmolar disturbances), recheck FBG within 24 hr and as indicated. If FBG decreases to ≤500 mg/dL, follow FBG recommendations for Grade 3. If FBG is confirmed at >500 m g/dL, discontinue alpelisib permanently.

Implementation

- When starting at *Piqray* at 300 mg once daily, two 150 mg tablets, dose adjustments for adverse reactions include *First-dose reduction:* 250 mg once daily, one 200 mg tablet and one 50 mg tablet. *Second-dose reduction:* 200 mg tablet once daily.
- Dose reductions for *Vijoice* include *First dose reduction:* 125 mg once daily. *Second dose reduction:* 50 mg once daily. If adult or pediatric patients cannot tolerate 50 mg, discontinue alpelisib.
- **PO:** Administer with food once daily at same time of day. *DNC:* Swallow tablets whole, do not crush, break, or chew. For patients with difficulty swallowing, administer *Vijoice* as an oral suspension with food. Place *Vijoice* tablets 2–4 ounces of water and let stand for 5 min. Make suspension with water only. Crush tablets with a spoon and stir until an oral suspension is obtained. Administer immediately after preparation. Discard oral suspension if not administered within 60 min after preparation. After administration, add 2–3 tbsp of water to same glass. Stir with same spoon to resuspend any remaining particles and administer entire contents. Repeat if particles remain.
- When administered with fulvestrant, fulvestrant 500 mg is usually given on Days 1, 15, and 29, and once monthly thereafter.

Patient/Family Teaching

- Instruct patient to take alpelisib as directed. Take missed doses with food within 9 hr of time usually

taken. If >9 hr, omit dose and take next dose next day at usual time. If patient vomits after dose, skip dose and take next dose next day. Advise patient to read *Patient Information* before starting and with each Rx refill in case of changes.
- Advise patients to notify health care professional of the signs and symptoms of hypersensitivity reactions, skin reactions, hyperglycemia (e.g., excessive thirst, urinating more often than usual or higher amount of urine than usual, or increased appetite with weight loss), and lung problems occur. Advise patients to immediately report new or worsening respiratory symptoms.
- If diarrhea occurs, advise patient to start antidiarrheal treatment, increase oral fluids, and notify health care professional.
- Advise patient to notify health care professional of all Rx or OTC medications, vitamins, or herbal products being taken and to consult health care professional before taking any new medications.
- Rep: May cause fetal harm. Advise females of reproductive potential and males with female partners of reproductive potential to use effective contraception during and for 1 wk after last dose. Advise patient to avoid breastfeeding during and for 1 wk after last dose. May impair fertility in male and female patients.

Evaluation/Desired Outcomes

- Decreased progression of breast cancer.
- Reduction in lesion volume in PIK3CA-related overgrowth spectrum.

BEERS

ALPRAZolam (al-pray-zoe-lam)
Xanax, Xanax XR
Classification
Therapeutic: antianxiety agents
Pharmacologic: benzodiazepines

Schedule IV

Indications
Generalized anxiety disorder. Panic disorder. Anxiety associated with depression.

Action
Acts at many levels in the CNS to produce anxiolytic effect. May produce CNS depression. Effects may be mediated by GABA, an inhibitory neurotransmitter. **Therapeutic Effects:** Relief of anxiety.

Pharmacokinetics
Absorption: Well absorbed (90%) from the GI tract; absorption is slower with extended-release tablets.
Distribution: Widely distributed, crosses blood-brain barrier. Probably crosses the placenta and enters breast milk. Accumulation is minimal.

Metabolism and Excretion: Metabolized by the liver by the CYP3A4 isoenzyme to an active compound that is subsequently rapidly metabolized.
Half-life: 12–15 hr.

TIME/ACTION PROFILE (sedation)

ROUTE	ONSET	PEAK	DURATION
PO	1–2 hr	1–2 hr	up to 24 hr

Contraindications/Precautions

Contraindicated in: Hypersensitivity; Cross-sensitivity with other benzodiazepines may exist; Pre-existing CNS depression; Severe uncontrolled pain; Angle-closure glaucoma; Obstructive sleep apnea or pulmonary disease; Concurrent use with itraconazole or ketoconazole; Lactation: Lactation.
Use Cautiously in: Renal impairment (↓ dose required); Hepatic impairment (↓ dose required); History of suicide attempt or alcohol/drug dependence, debilitated patients (↓ dose required); OB: Use late in pregnancy can result in sedation (respiratory depression, lethargy, hypotonia) and/or withdrawal symptoms (hyperreflexia, irritability, restlessness, tremors, inconsolable crying, and feeding difficulties) in neonates; Pedi: Safety and effectiveness not established in children; Geri: Appears on Beers list. ↑ risk of cognitive impairment, delirium, falls, fractures, and motor vehicle accidents in older adults. If possible, avoid use in older adults.

Adverse Reactions/Side Effects

Derm: rash. **EENT:** blurred vision. **GI:** constipation, diarrhea, nausea, vomiting, weight gain. **Neuro:** dizziness, drowsiness, lethargy, confusion, depression, hangover, headache, paradoxical excitation. **Misc:** physical dependence, psychological dependence, tolerance.

Interactions

Drug-Drug: Use with **opioids** or other **CNS depressants**, including other **benzodiazepines**, **non-benzodiazepine sedative/hypnotics**, **anxiolytics**, **general anesthetics**, **muscle relaxants**, **antipsychotics**, and **alcohol** may cause profound sedation, respiratory depression, coma, and death; reserve concurrent use for when alternative treatment options are inadequate. **Hormonal contraceptives, disulfiram, fluoxetine, isoniazid, metoprolol, propranolol, valproic acid, CYP3A4 inhibitors (erythromycin, ketoconazole, itraconazole, fluvoxamine, cimetidine, nefazodone)** ↑ levels and effects; dose adjustments may be necessary; concurrent use with ketoconazole and itraconazole contraindicated. May ↓ efficacy of **levodopa. CYP3A4 inducers (rifampin, carbamazepine, or barbiturates)** ↓ levels and effects. Sedative effects may be ↓ by **theophylline. Cigarette smoking** ↑ levels and effects.
Drug-Natural Products: **Kava-kava, valerian,** or **chamomile** can ↑ CNS depression.
Drug-Food: Concurrent ingestion of **grapefruit juice** ↑ levels and effects.

Route/Dosage

Anxiety
PO (Adults): 0.25–0.5 mg 2–3 times daily (not to exceed 4 mg/day).
PO (Geriatric Patients): Begin with 0.25 mg 2–3 times daily.

Panic Attacks
PO (Adults): 0.5 mg 3 times daily; may be ↑ by 1 mg or less every 3–4 days as needed (not to exceed 10 mg/day). *Extended-release tablets:* 0.5–1 mg once daily in the morning, may be ↑ every 3–4 days by not more than 1 mg/day; up to 10 mg/day (usual range 3–6 mg/day).

Availability (generic available)

Tablets: 0.25 mg, 0.5 mg, 1 mg, 2 mg. **Extended-release tablets:** 0.5 mg, 1 mg, 2 mg, 3 mg. **Orally disintegrating tablets (orange-flavor):** 0.25 mg, 0.5 mg, 1 mg, 2 mg. **Oral solution (concentrate):** 1 mg/mL.

NURSING IMPLICATIONS

Assessment

- Assess degree and manifestations of anxiety and mental status (orientation, mood, behavior) prior to and periodically during therapy.
- Assess patient for drowsiness, light-headedness, and dizziness. These symptoms usually disappear as therapy progresses. Dose should be reduced if these symptoms persist.
- Geri: Assess CNS effects and risk of falls. Institute falls prevention strategies.
- Assess risk for addiction, abuse, or misuse prior to administration and periodically during therapy.
- Prolonged high-dose therapy may lead to psychological or physical dependence. Risk is greater in patients taking >4 mg/day. Restrict the amount of drug available to patient. Assess regularly for continued need for treatment.

Lab Test Considerations
- Monitor CBC and liver and renal function periodically during long-term therapy. May cause ↓ hematocrit and neutropenia.

Toxicity and Overdose
- Flumazenil is the antidote for alprazolam toxicity or overdose. (Flumazenil may induce seizures in patients with a history of seizures disorder or who are taking tricyclic antidepressants).

Implementation
- Do not confuse Xanax with Fanapt.
- Do not confuse alprazolam with clonazepam or lorazepam.
- If early morning anxiety or anxiety between doses occurs, same total daily dose should be divided into more frequent intervals.
- **PO:** May be administered with food if GI upset occurs. Administer greatest dose at bedtime to avoid daytime sedation.

- Tablets may be crushed and taken with food or fluids if patient has difficulty swallowing. *DNC:* Do not crush, break, or chew extended-release tablets.
- Taper by 0.5 mg every 3 days to prevent withdrawal; may require even more gradual taper if withdrawal symptoms (heightened sensory perception, impaired concentration, dysosmia, clouded sensorium, paresthesias, muscle cramps, muscle twitch, diarrhea, blurred vision, appetite decrease, weight loss) occur. Some patients may require longer tapering period (weeks to >12 mo).
- For *orally disintegrating tablets:* Remove tablet from bottle with dry hands just prior to taking medication. Place tablet on tongue. Tablet will dissolve with saliva; may also be taken with water. Remove cotton from bottle and reseal tightly to prevent moisture from entering bottle. If only ½ tablet taken, discard unused portion immediately; may not remain stable.

Patient/Family Teaching

- Instruct patient to take medication as directed; do not skip or double up on missed doses. If a dose is missed, take within 1 hr; otherwise, skip the dose and return to regular schedule. If medication is less effective after a few wk, check with health care professional; do not increase dose. Caution patient not to stop taking alprazolam without consulting health care professional. Abrupt withdrawal may cause sweating, vomiting, muscle cramps, tremors, and seizures; may be life-threatening.
- Advise patient to avoid drinking grapefruit juice during therapy.
- Advise patient to not take more than prescribed or share medication with anyone.
- Advise patient that alprazolam is a drug with known abuse potential. Protect it from theft, and never give to anyone other than the individual for whom it was prescribed. Store out of sight and reach of children, and in a location not accessible by others.
- May cause drowsiness or dizziness. Caution patient to avoid driving and other activities requiring alertness until response to the medication is known. Geri: Instruct patient and family how to reduce falls risk at home.
- Advise patient to avoid the use of alcohol or other CNS depressants, including opioids, concurrently with alprazolam, may cause respiratory depression and overdose. Instruct patient to consult health care professional before taking Rx, OTC, or herbal products concurrently with this medication.
- Inform patient that benzodiazepines are usually prescribed for short-term use and do not cure underlying problems.
- Rep: May cause fetal harm. Advise patient to notify health care professional if pregnancy is planned or suspected or if breastfeeding. Monitor neonates ex-

posed to benzodiazepines during pregnancy (especially during 3rd trimester) and labor for signs of sedation (respiratory depression, lethargy, hypotonia) and/or withdrawal symptoms (hyperreflexia, irritability, restlessness, tremors, inconsolable crying, and feeding difficulties) in the neonate. Monitor neonates and infants exposed to alprazolam during breastfeeding for sedation and withdrawal symptoms. Inform women who take alprazolam during pregnancy about the National Pregnancy Registry for Other Psychiatric Medications to monitor pregnancy outcomes in women exposed to alprazolam during pregnancy. Enroll patient by calling 1-866-961-2388 or visiting online at https://womensmentalhealth.org/research/pregnancyregistry/.

Evaluation/Desired Outcomes

- Decreased sense of anxiety without CNS side effects.
- Decreased frequency and severity of panic attacks.
- Decreased symptoms of premenstrual syndrome.

alteplase, See THROMBOLYTIC AGENTS.

amcinonide, See CORTICOSTEROIDS (TOPICAL/LOCAL).

amifostine (a-mi-**fos**-teen)
Ethyol
Classification
Therapeutic: cytoprotective agents

Indications
Reduces renal toxicity from cisplatin. Reduces the incidence of moderate to severe xerostomia from postoperative radiation for head and neck cancer in which the radiation port includes a large portion of the parotid glands.

Action
Converted by alkaline phosphatase in tissue to a free thiol compound that binds and detoxifies damaging metabolites of cisplatin and reactive oxygen species generated by radiation. **Therapeutic Effects:** Decreased renal damage from cisplatin. Decreased severity of xerostomia following radiation for head and neck cancer.

Pharmacokinetics
Absorption: IV administration results in complete bioavailability.
Distribution: Unknown.
Metabolism and Excretion: Rapidly cleared from plasma; converted to cytoprotective compounds by alkaline phosphatase in tissues.

Half-life: 8 min.

TIME/ACTION PROFILE

ROUTE	ONSET	PEAK	DURATION
IV	unknown	unknown	unknown

Contraindications/Precautions

Contraindicated in: Hypersensitivity to aminothiol compounds; Hypotension or dehydration; Concurrent antineoplastic therapy for other tumors (especially malignancies of germ cell origin); OB: Pregnancy; Lactation: Lactation.

Use Cautiously in: Cardiovascular disease (↑ risk of adverse reactions); Pedi: Safety and effectiveness not established in children; Geri: ↑ risk of adverse reactions in older adults.

Adverse Reactions/Side Effects

CV: hypotension. **Derm:** DRUG REACTION WITH EOSINOPHILIA AND SYSTEMIC SYMPTOMS (DRESS), ERYTHEMA MULTIFORME, EXFOLIATIVE DERMATITIS, flushing, STEVENS-JOHNSON SYNDROME, TOXIC EPIDERMAL NECROLYSIS, TOXODERMA. **EENT:** blurred vision, diplopia, sneezing. **F and E:** hypocalcemia. **GI:** nausea, vomiting, hiccups. **Neuro:** dizziness, somnolence. **Misc:** ANAPHYLAXIS, chills, injection site reactions.

Interactions

Drug-Drug: Concurrent use of **antihypertensives** ↑ risk of hypotension.

Route/Dosage

Reduction of Renal Damage with Cisplatin

IV (Adults): 910 mg/m² once daily, within 30 min before chemotherapy; if full dose is poorly tolerated, subsequent doses should be ↓ to 740 mg/m².

Reduction of Xerostomia from Radiation

IV (Adults): 200 mg/m² once daily starting 15–30 min before standard fraction radiation therapy.

Availability (generic available)

Powder for injection: 500 mg/vial.

NURSING IMPLICATIONS

Assessment

- Monitor BP before and every 5 min during infusion. Discontinue antihypertensives 24 hr prior to treatment. If significant hypotension requiring interruption of therapy occurs, place patient in Trendelenburg position and administer an infusion of 0.9% NaCl using a separate IV line. If BP returns to normal in 5 min and patient is asymptomatic, infusion may be resumed so that full dose may be given.
- Assess fluid status before administration. Correct dehydration before instituting therapy. Nausea and vomiting are frequent and may be severe. Administer prophylactic antiemetics including dexamethasone 20 mg IV and a serotonin-antagonist antiemetic

(granisetron, ondansetron, palonosetron) before and during infusion. Monitor fluid status closely.
- Observe patient for signs and symptoms of anaphylaxis (rash, pruritus, laryngeal edema, wheezing). Discontinue the drug and notify physician or other health care professional immediately if these problems occur. Keep epinephrine, an antihistamine, and resuscitation equipment close by in case of an anaphylactic reaction.
- Monitor patient for skin reactions before, during, and after amifostine administration; reactions may be delayed by several wk after initiation of therapy. Permanently discontinue amifostine in patients who experience serious or severe cutaneous reactions or cutaneous reactions associated with fever or other symptoms of unknown cause. Withhold therapy and obtain dermatologic consultation and biopsy for cutaneous reactions or mucosal lesions of unknown cause appearing outside of injection site or radiation port, and for erythematous, edematous, or bullous lesions on the palms of the hand or soles of the feet.
- Monitor for signs and symptoms of DRESS (fever, rash, lymphadenopathy, and/or facial swelling), associated with involvement of other organ systems (hepatitis, nephritis, hematologic abnormalities, myocarditis, myositis) during therapy. May resemble an acute viral infection. Eosinophilia is often present. Discontinue therapy if signs occur.
- **Xerostomia:** Assess patient for dry mouth and mouth sores periodically during therapy.

Lab Test Considerations
- Monitor serum calcium concentrations before and periodically during therapy. May cause hypocalcemia. Calcium supplements may be necessary.

Implementation

IV Administration
- **Intermittent Infusion:** *Dilution:* Reconstitute with 9.7 mL of sterile 0.9% NaCl. Dilute further with 0.9% NaCl. Do not administer solutions that are discolored or contain particulate matter. Solution is stable for 5 hr at room temperature or 24 hr if refrigerated. *Concentration:* Adults: dilute dose to a final volume of 50 mL; Children: 5–40 mg/mL. *Rate: For renal toxicity:* Administer over 15 min within 30 min before chemotherapy administration. Longer infusion times are not as well tolerated. *For xerostomia:* Administer over 3 min starting 15–30 min prior to radiation therapy.
- **Y-Site Compatibility:** alemtuzumab, amikacin, aminophylline, amphotericin B liposomal, ampicillin, ampicillin/sulbactam, anidulafungin, argatroban, aztreonam, bivalirudin, bleomycin, bumetanide, buprenorphine, butorphanol, calcium gluconate, carboplatin, carmustine, caspofungin, cefazolin, cefotaxime, cefotetan, cefoxitin, ceftazidime, ceftriaxone, cefuroxime, ciprofloxacin, clindamycin, cyclophosphamide, cytarabine, dacarbazine, dactinomycin, daptomycin, daunorubicin, dexametha-

sone, dexmedetomidine, dexrazoxane, diltiazem, diphenhydramine, dobutamine, docetaxel, docetaxel, dopamine, doxorubicin hydrochloride, doxycycline, droperidol, enalaprilat, epirubicin, ertapenem, etoposide, etoposide phosphate, famotidine, floxuridine, fluconazole, fludarabine, fluorouracil, foscarnet, fosphenytoin, furosemide, gemcitabine, gentamicin, granisetron, haloperidol, heparin, hetastarch, hydrocortisone, hydromorphone, idarubicin, ifosfamide, imipenem/cilastatin, irinotecan, leucovorin, levofloxacin, linezolid, lorazepam, magnesium sulfate, mannitol, meperidine, mesna, methotrexate, methylprednisolone, metoclopramide, metronidazole, milrinone, mitomycin, morphine, moxifloxacin, nalbuphine, octreotide, ondansetron, oxaliplatin, paclitaxel, palonosetron, pamidronate, pantoprazole, pemetrexed, piperacillin/tazobactam, potassium acetate, potassium chloride, promethazine, rituximab, sodium acetate, sodium bicarbonate, tacrolimus, thiotepa, tigecycline, tirofiban, tobramycin, trastuzumab, trimethoprim/sulfamethoxazole, vancomycin, vasopressin, vecuronium, vinblastine, vincristine, vinorelbine, voriconazole, zidovudine, zoledronic acid.

- **Y-Site Incompatibility:** acyclovir, amiodarone, amphotericin B deoxycholate, amphotericin B lipid complex, chlorpromazine, cisplatin, ganciclovir, hydroxyzine, minocycline, mycophenolate, prochlorperazine, topotecan.

Patient/Family Teaching

- Explain the purpose of amifostine infusion to patient.
- Inform patient that amifostine may cause hypotension, nausea, vomiting, flushing, chills, dizziness, somnolence, hiccups, and sneezing.
- Advise patient to notify health care professional if skin reactions, or signs and symptoms of anaphylaxis or DRESS occur.
- OB: Advise patient to notify health care professional if pregnancy is suspected or if breastfeeding.

Evaluation/Desired Outcomes

- Prevention of renal toxicity associated with repeated administration of cisplatin in patients with ovarian cancer.
- Decreased severity of xerostomia from radiation treatment of head and neck cancer.

amikacin, See AMINOGLYCOSIDES.

aMILoride, See DIURETICS (POTASSIUM-SPARING).

aminocaproic acid
(a-mee-noe-ka-**pro**-ik **a**-sid)
Amicar
Classification
Therapeutic: hemostatic agents
Pharmacologic: fibrinolysis inhibitors

Indications

Treatment of acute, life-threatening hemorrhage due to systemic hyperfibrinolysis or urinary fibrinolysis. **Unlabeled Use:** Prevention of recurrent subarachnoid hemorrhage. Prevention of bleeding following oral surgery in hemophiliacs. Management of severe hemorrhage caused by thrombolytic agents.

Action

Inhibits activation of plasminogen. **Therapeutic Effects:** Inhibition of fibrinolysis. Stabilization of clot formation.

Pharmacokinetics

Absorption: Rapidly absorbed following oral administration.
Distribution: Widely distributed.
Metabolism and Excretion: Mostly eliminated unchanged by the kidneys.
Half-life: Unknown.

TIME/ACTION PROFILE (plasma concentrations)

ROUTE	ONSET	PEAK	DURATION
PO	unknown	2 hr	N/A
IV	unknown	2 hr	N/A

Contraindications/Precautions

Contraindicated in: Active intravascular clotting.
Use Cautiously in: Upper urinary tract bleeding; Cardiac, renal, or liver disease (dose ↓ may be required); Disseminated intravascular coagulation (should be used concurrently with heparin); OB: Safety not established in pregnancy; Lactation: Safety not established in breastfeeding; Pedi: Do not use products containing benzyl alcohol with neonates.

Adverse Reactions/Side Effects

CV: arrhythmias, hypotension (IV only). **EENT:** nasal stuffiness, tinnitus. **GI:** anorexia, bloating, cramping, diarrhea, nausea. **GU:** diuresis, renal failure. **MS:** myopathy. **Neuro:** dizziness, malaise.

Interactions

Drug-Drug: Concurrent use with **estrogens, conjugated** may result in a hypercoagulable state. Concurrent use with **clotting factors** may ↑ risk of thromboses.

Route/Dosage

Acute Bleeding Syndromes due to Elevated Fibrinolytic Activity

PO (Adults): 5 g during the 1st hr, followed by 1–1.25 g every hr for 8 hr or until hemorrhage is controlled; or 6 g over 24 hr after prostate surgery (not >30 g/day).

IV (Adults): 4–5 g over 1st hr, followed by 1 g/hr for 8 hr or until hemorrhage is controlled; or 6 g over 24 hr after prostate surgery (not >30 g/day).

PO, IV (Children): 100 mg/kg or 3 g/m² over 1st hr, followed by continuous infusion of 33.3 mg/kg/hr; or 1 g/m²/hr (total dose not >18 g/m²/24 hr).

Subarachnoid Hemorrhage

PO (Adults): *To follow IV:* 3 g every 2 hr (36 g/day). If no surgery is performed, continue for 21 days after bleeding stops, then ↓ to 2 g every 2 hr (24 g/day) for 3 days, then 1 g every 2 hr (12 g/day) for 3 days.

IV (Adults): 36 g/day for 10 days followed by PO.

Prevention of Bleeding Following Oral Surgery in Hemophiliacs

PO (Adults): 75 mg/kg (up to 6 g) immediately after procedure, then every 6 hr for 7–10 days; syrup may also be used as an oral rinse of 1.25 g (5 mL) 4 times a day for 7–10 days.

IV, PO (Children): *Also for epistaxis:* 50–100 mg/kg/dose administered IV every 6 hr for 2–3 days starting 4 hr before the procedure. After completion of IV therapy, aminocaproic acid should be given as 50–100 mg/kg/dose orally every 6 hr for 5–7 days.

Availability (generic available)

Tablets: 500 mg, 1000 mg. **Oral syrup (raspberry flavor):** 1.25 g/5 mL. **Solution for injection:** 250 mg/mL.

NURSING IMPLICATIONS

Assessment

- Monitor BP, pulse, and respiratory status as indicated by severity of bleeding.
- Monitor for overt bleeding every 15–30 min during acute bleed and periodically during therapy.
- Monitor neurologic status (pupils, level of consciousness, motor activity) in patients with subarachnoid hemorrhage.
- Monitor intake and output ratios frequently; notify health care professional if significant discrepancies occur.
- Assess for thromboembolic complications (especially in patients with history). Notify health care professional of positive Homans' sign, leg pain and edema, hemoptysis, dyspnea, or chest pain.

Lab Test Considerations

- Monitor platelet count and clotting factors prior to and periodically throughout therapy in patients with systemic fibrinolysis.
- ↑ CK may indicate myopathy.
- May ↑ serum potassium.

Implementation

- **PO:** Syrup may be used as an oral rinse, swished for 30 sec 4 times/day for 7–10 days for the control of bleeding during dental and oral surgery in hemophilic patients. Small amounts may be swallowed, except during 1st and 2nd trimesters of pregnancy. Syrup may be applied with an applicator in children or unconscious patients.

IV Administration

- **IV:** Stabilize IV catheter to minimize thrombophlebitis. Monitor site closely.
- **Intermittent Infusion:** *Dilution:* Do not administer undiluted. Dilute initial 4–5 g dose in 250 mL of sterile water for injection, 0.9% NaCl, D5W, or LR. Do not dilute with sterile water in patients with subarachnoid hemorrhage. *Concentration:* 20 mg/mL. *Rate:* Single doses: Administer over 1 hr. Rapid infusion rate may cause hypotension, bradycardia, or other arrhythmias.
- **Continuous Infusion:** Administer IV solution using infusion pump to ensure accurate dose. Administer via slow IV infusion.
- *Rate:* Initial dose may be followed by a continuous infusion of 1–1.25 g/hr in adults or 33.3 mg/kg/hr in children.
- **Y-Site Compatibility:** alemtuzumab, amikacin, aminophylline, amphotericin B deoxycholate, amphotericin B lipid complex, amphotericin B liposomal, ampicillin, ampicillin/sulbactam, anidulafungin, argatroban, arsenic trioxide, atracurium, azithromycin, aztreonam, bivalirudin, bleomycin, bumetanide, buprenorphine, butorphanol, calcium chloride, calcium gluconate, carboplatin, carmustine, cefazolin, cefepime, cefotaxime, cefotetan, cefoxitin, ceftazidime, ceftriaxone, cefuroxime, cisatracurium, clindamycin, cyclophosphamide, cyclosporine, cytarabine, dacarbazine, daptomycin, dexamethasone, dexmedetomidine, digoxin, diltiazem, diphenhydramine, dobutamine, docetaxel, dopamine, droperidol, enalaprilat, ephedrine, epinephrine, epirubicin, ertapenem, erythromycin, esmolol, etoposide, etoposide phosphate, famotidine, fentanyl, fluconazole, fludarabine, foscarnet, fosphenytoin, furosemide, gemcitabine, gentamicin, granisetron, haloperidol, heparin, hetastarch, hydrocortisone, hydromorphone, idarubicin, ifosfamide, imipenem/cilastatin, irinotecan, isoproterenol, ketorolac, labetalol, leucovorin calcium, levofloxacin, lidocaine, linezolid, lorazepam, magnesium sulfate, mannitol, meperidine, meropenem, mesna, methohexital, methylprednisolone, metoclopramide, metoprolol, metronidazole, milrinone, mitoxantrone, morphine, nalbuphine, naloxone, nitroglycerin, nitroprusside, octreotide, ondansetron, oxaliplatin, oxytocin, palonosetron, pamidronate, pantoprazole, pemetrexed, pentamidine, pentobarbital, phenobarbital, phenylephrine, piperacillin/tazobactam, potassium acetate, potassium chloride, potassium phosphate, procainamide, promethazine,

propranolol, remifentanil, rocuronium, sargramostim, sodium bicarbonate, sodium phosphate, succinylcholine, sufentanil, tacrolimus, theophylline, thiotepa, tigecycline, tirofiban, tobramycin, trimethoprim/sulfamethoxazole, vancomycin, vasopressin, vecuronium, verapamil, vincristine, voriconazole, zidovudine, zoledronic acid.

- **Y-Site Incompatibility:** acyclovir, amiodarone, caspofungin, chlorpromazine, ciprofloxacin, diazepam, doxycycline, filgrastim, ganciclovir, midazolam, mycophenolate, nicardipine, phenytoin, prochlorperazine, thiopental.

Patient/Family Teaching

- Instruct patient to notify the nurse immediately if bleeding recurs or if thromboembolic symptoms develop.
- **IV:** Caution patient to make position changes slowly to avoid orthostatic hypotension.
- OB: Advise patient to notify health care professional if pregnancy is planned or suspected or if breastfeeding.

Evaluation/Desired Outcomes

- Cessation of bleeding.
- Prevention of rebleeding in subarachnoid hemorrhage without occurrence of undesired clotting.

☒ AMINOGLYCOSIDES

amikacin (am-i-**kay**-sin)
~~Amikin~~, Arikayce
gentamicin† (jen-ta-**mye**-sin)
~~Garamycin~~
neomycin (neo-oh-**mye**-sin)
streptomycin (strep-toe-**mye**-sin)
tobramycin† (toe-bra-**mye**-sin)
Bethkis, Kitabis Pak, TOBI, TOBI Podhaler
Classification
Therapeutic: anti-infectives
Pharmacologic: aminoglycosides

†See Appendix B for ophthalmic use

Indications

Amikacin, gentamicin, and tobramycin: Treatment of serious gram-negative bacterial infections and infections caused by staphylococci when penicillins or other less toxic drugs are contraindicated. **Streptomycin:** In combination with other agents in the management of active tuberculosis. **Neomycin:** Used orally to prepare the GI tract for surgery, to decrease the number of ammonia-producing bacteria in the gut as part of the management of hepatic encephalopathy, and to treat diarrhea caused by *Escherichia coli.* **Amikacin by inhalation:** Treatment of *Mycobacterium avium* complex (MAC) lung disease in patients who have lim-

ited or no other treatment options and who do not achieve negative sputum cultures after ≥6 consecutive mo of a multidrug treatment regimen (in combination with other antibacterial drugs). **Tobramycin by inhalation:** Management of *Pseudomonas aeruginosa* in cystic fibrosis patients. **Gentamicin, streptomycin:** In combination with other agents in the management of serious enterococcal infections. **Gentamicin IV:** Prevention of infective endocarditis. **Gentamicin (topical):** Treatment of localized infections caused by susceptible organisms. **Unlabeled Use: Amikacin:** In combination with other agents in the management of *Mycobacterium avium* complex infections.

Action

Inhibits protein synthesis in bacteria at level of 30S ribosome. **Therapeutic Effects:** Bactericidal action. **Spectrum:** Most aminoglycosides notable for activity against: *P. aeruginosa, Klebsiella pneumoniae, E.coli, Proteus, Serratia, Acinetobacter, Staphylococcus aureus.* In treatment of enterococcal infections, synergy with a penicillin is required. Streptomycin and amikacin also active against *Mycobacterium.*

Pharmacokinetics

Absorption: Well absorbed after IM administration. IV administration results in complete bioavailability. Some absorption follows administration by other routes. Minimal systemic absorption with neomycin (may accumulate in patients with renal failure).

Distribution: Widely distributed throughout extracellular fluid; cross the placenta; small amounts enter breast milk. Poor penetration into CSF (↑ when meninges are inflamed).

Metabolism and Excretion: Excretion is >90% renal.

Half-life: 2–4 hr (↑ in renal impairment).

TIME/ACTION PROFILE (plasma concentrations*)

ROUTE	ONSET	PEAK	DURATION
PO (neomycin)	rapid	1–4 hr	N/A
IM	rapid	30–90 min	6–24 hr
IV	rapid	15–30 min†	6–24 hr

*All parenterally administered aminoglycosides.
†Postdistribution peak occurs 30 min after the end of a 30-min infusion and 15 min after the end of a 1-hr infusion.

Contraindications/Precautions

Contraindicated in: Hypersensitivity to aminoglycosides; Most parenteral products contain bisulfites and should be avoided in patients with known intolerance; Intestinal obstruction (neomycin only); OB: Avoid use of tobramycin (IV/IM), streptomycin, and inhaled amikacin during pregnancy; Pedi: Products containing benzyl alcohol should be avoided in neonates.

Use Cautiously in: Renal impairment (dose adjustments necessary; blood level monitoring useful in preventing ototoxicity and nephrotoxicity); Hearing impairment; ⌘ Mitochondrial DNA variants in the 12S rRNA gene (*MTRNR1*) or maternal history of ototoxicity (↑ risk of ototoxicity); Neuromuscular diseases such as myasthenia gravis; Obese patients (dose should be based on ideal body weight); COPD or asthma (amikacin inhalation may worsen condition); OB: Minimal systemic absorption anticipated (inhalation formulations); Lactation: Safety not established in breastfeeding; Pedi: Neonates have ↑ risk of neuromuscular blockade; difficulty in assessing auditory and vestibular function and immature renal function; safety and effectiveness of amikacin inhalation not established in children; Geri: Difficulty in assessing auditory and vestibular function and age-related renal impairment in older adults.

Adverse Reactions/Side Effects

Derm: rash (amikacin inhalation only). **EENT:** ototoxicity (vestibular and cochlear), voice alteration (amikacin inhalation only), epistaxis (amikacin inhalation only), oral candidiasis (amikacin inhalation only). **F and E:** hypomagnesemia. **GI:** diarrhea (amikacin inhalation only), nausea (amikacin inhalation only), diarrhea (neomycin only), dry mouth (amikacin inhalation only), metallic taste (amikacin inhalation only), nausea (neomycin only), vomiting (amikacin inhalation and neomycin only). **GU:** nephrotoxicity. **Metab:** ↓ weight (amikacin inhalation only). **MS:** muscle paralysis (high parenteral doses). **Neuro:** ataxia, headache (amikacin inhalation only), ↑ neuromuscular blockade, anxiety (amikacin inhalation only), vertigo. **Resp:** bronchospasm (amikacin inhalation only), cough (amikacin inhalation only), hemoptysis (amikacin inhalation only), apnea, bronchospasm (tobramycin inhalation only), hypersensitivity pneumonitis (amikacin inhalation only), wheezing (tobramycin inhalation only). **Misc:** hypersensitivity reactions.

Interactions

Drug-Drug: Inactivated by **penicillins** and **cephalosporins** when coadministered to patients with renal insufficiency. Possible respiratory paralysis after **inhalation anesthetics** or **neuromuscular blocking agents**. ↑ incidence of ototoxicity with **loop diuretics** or **mannitol (IV)**. ↑ incidence of nephrotoxicity with other **nephrotoxic drugs**. Neomycin may ↑ anticoagulant effects of **warfarin**. Neomycin may ↓ absorption of **digoxin** and **methotrexate**.

Route/Dosage

Amikacin

IM, IV (Adults and Children): 5 mg/kg every 8 hr or 7.5 mg/kg every 12 hr (not to exceed 1.5 g/day). *Mycobacterium avium complex:* 7.5–15 mg/kg/day divided every 12–24 hr.

IM, IV (Neonates): *Loading dose:* 10 mg/kg; *Maintenance dose:* 7.5 mg/kg every 12 hr.

Inhaln (Adults): 590 mg once daily.

Renal Impairment

IM, IV (Adults): *Loading dose:* 7.5 mg/kg, further dosing based on blood level monitoring and renal function assessment.

Gentamicin

Many regimens are used; most involve dosing adjusted on the basis of blood level monitoring and assessment of renal function.

IM, IV (Adults): 1–2 mg/kg every 8 hr (up to 6 mg/kg/day in 3 divided doses). *Once-daily dosing (unlabeled):* 4–7 mg/kg every 24 hr.

IM, IV (Children >5 yr): 2–2.5 mg/kg/dose every 8 hr; *Once daily:* 5–7.5 mg/kg/dose every 24 hr; *Cystic fibrosis:* 2.5–3.3 mg/kg/dose every 6–8 hr; *Hemodialysis:* 1.25–1.75 mg/kg/dose postdialysis.

IM, IV (Children 1 mo–5 yr): 2.5 mg/kg/dose every 8 hr; *Once daily:* 5–7.5 mg/kg/dose every 24 hr; *Cystic fibrosis:* 2.5–3.3 mg/kg/dose every 6–8 hr; *Hemodialysis:* 1.25–1.75 mg/kg/dose postdialysis.

IM, IV (Neonates full term and/or >1 wk): *Weight <1200 g:* 2.5 mg/kg/dose every 18–24 hr; *Weight 1200–2000 g:* 2.5 mg/kg/dose every 8–12 hr; *Weight >2000 g:* 2.5 mg/kg/dose every 8 hr; *ECMO:* 2.5 mg/kg/dose every 18 hr, subsequent doses based on serum concentrations; *Once daily:* 3.5–5 mg/kg/dose every 24 hr.

IM, IV (Neonates premature and/or ≤1 wk): *Weight <1000 g:* 3.5 mg/kg/dose every 24 hr; *Weight 1000–1200 g:* 2.5 mg/kg/dose every 18–24 hr; *Weight >1200 g:* 2.5 mg/kg/dose every 12 hr; *Once daily:* 3.5–4 mg/kg/dose every 24 hr.

IT (Adults): 4–8 mg/day.

IT (Infants >3 mo and Children): 1–2 mg/day.

IT (Neonates): 1 mg/day.

Topical (Adults and Children >1 mo): Apply cream or ointment 3–4 times daily.

Renal Impairment

IM, IV (Adults): Initial dose of 2 mg/kg. Subsequent doses/intervals based on blood level monitoring and renal function assessment.

Neomycin

PO (Adults): *Preoperative intestinal antisepsis:* 1 g every hr for 4 doses, then 1 g every 4 hr for 5 doses *or* 1 g at 1 PM, 2 PM, and 11 PM on day before surgery; *Hepatic encephalopathy:* 1–3 g every 6 hr for 5–6 days; may be followed by 4 g/day chronically.

PO (Children): *Preoperative intestinal antisepsis:* 15 mg/kg every 4 hr for 2 days *or* 25 mg/kg at 1 PM, 2 PM, and 11 PM on day before surgery; *Hepatic encephalopathy:* 12.5–25 mg/kg every 6 hr for 5–6 days (maximum dose = 12 g/day).

Streptomycin

IM (Adults): *Tuberculosis:* 1 g/day initially, ↓ to 1 g 2–3 times weekly; *Other infections:* 250 mg–1 g every 6 hr *or* 500 mg–2 g every 12 hr.

IM (Children): *Tuberculosis:* 20 mg/kg/day (not to exceed 1 g/day); *Other infections:* 5–10 mg/kg every 6 hr *or* 10–20 mg/kg every 12 hr.

Renal Impairment
IM (Adults): 1 g initially, further dosing determined by blood level monitoring and assessment of renal function.

Tobramycin
IM, IV (Adults): 1–2 mg/kg every 8 hr *or* 4–6.6 mg/kg/day every 24 hr.

IM, IV (Adults): 3–6 mg/kg/day in 3 divided doses, or 4–6.6 mg/kg once daily.

IM, IV (Children >5 yr): 6–7.5 mg/kg/day divided every 8 hr, up to 13 mg/kg/day divided every 6–8 hr in cystic fibrosis patients (dosing interval may vary from every 6 hr–every 24 hr, depending on clinical situation).

IM, IV (Children 1 mo–5 yr): 7.5 mg/kg/day divided every 8 hr, up to 13 mg/kg/day divided every 6–8 hr in cystic fibrosis.

IM, IV (Neonates): *Preterm <1000 g:* 3.5 mg/kg/dose every 24 hr; *0–4 weeks, <1200 g:* 2.5 mg/kg/dose every 18 hr; *Postnatal age <7 days:* 2.5 mg/kg/dose every 12 hr; *Postnatal age ≥8 days, 1200–2000 g:* 2.5 mg/kg/dose every 8–12 hr; *Postnatal age ≥8 days, >2000 g:* 2.5 mg/kg/dose every 8 hr.

Inhaln (Adults and Children ≥6 yr): *Nebulizer solution:* 300 mg twice daily for 28 days, then off for 28 days, then repeat cycle; *Powder for inhalation:* Inhale contents of four 28-mg capsules twice daily for 28 days, then off for 28 days, then repeat cycle.

Renal Impairment
IM, IV (Adults): 1 mg/kg initially, further dosing determined by blood level monitoring and assessment of renal function.

Availability

Amikacin (generic available)
Solution for injection: 250 mg/mL. **Suspension for oral inhalation:** 590 mg/8.4 mL.

Gentamicin (generic available)
Premixed infusion: 60 mg/50 mL, 80 mg/50 mL, 80 mg/100 mL, 100 mg/50 mL, 100 mg/100 mL, 120 mg/100 mL. **Solution for injection:** 10 mg/mL, 40 mg/mL. **Topical cream:** 0.1%. **Topical ointment:** 0.1%.

Neomycin (generic available)
Tablets: 500 mg. *In combination with:* other topical antibiotics or anti-inflammatory agents for skin, ear, and eye infections. See Appendix N.

Streptomycin (generic available)
Lyophilized powder for injection: 1 g/vial.

Tobramycin (generic available)
Lyophilized powder for injection: 1200 mg/vial. **Nebulizer solution (Bethkis):** 300 mg/4 mL. **Nebulizer solution (TOBI, Kitabis Pak):** 300 mg/5 mL. **Powder for inhalation (TOBI Podhaler):** 28 mg/capsule. **Solution for injection:** 10 mg/mL, 40 mg/mL.

NURSING IMPLICATIONS

Assessment
- Assess for infection (vital signs, wound appearance, sputum, urine, stool, WBC) at beginning of and throughout therapy.
- Obtain specimens for culture and sensitivity before initiating therapy. First dose may be given before receiving results.
- Evaluate eighth cranial nerve function by audiometry before and throughout therapy. Hearing loss is usually in high-frequency range. Prompt recognition and intervention are essential in preventing permanent damage. Monitor for vestibular dysfunction (vertigo, ataxia, nausea, vomiting). Eighth cranial nerve dysfunction is associated with persistently elevated peak aminoglycoside levels. Discontinue aminoglycosides if tinnitus or subjective hearing loss occurs.
- Monitor intake and output and daily weight to assess hydration status and renal function.
- Assess for signs of superinfection (fever, upper respiratory infection, vaginal itching or discharge, increasing malaise, diarrhea).
- **Hepatic Encephalopathy:** Monitor neurologic status. Before administering oral medication, assess patient's ability to swallow.

Lab Test Considerations
- Monitor renal function by urinalysis, specific gravity, BUN, serum creatinine, and CCr before and during therapy.
- May cause ↑ BUN, AST, ALT, serum alkaline phosphatase, bilirubin, creatinine, and LDH concentrations.
- May cause ↓ serum calcium, magnesium, potassium, and sodium concentrations (streptomycin and tobramycin).

Toxicity and Overdose
- Monitor blood levels periodically during oral, IM, and IV therapy; not needed for inhalation therapy. Timing of blood levels is important in interpreting results. Draw blood for peak levels 1 hr after IM injection and 30 min after a 30-min IV infusion is completed. Draw trough levels just before next dose. Peak level for **amikacin** is 20–30 mcg/mL; trough level should be <10 mcg/mL. Peak level for **gentamicin** and **tobramycin** should not exceed 10 mcg/mL; trough level should not exceed 2 mcg/mL. Peak level for **streptomycin** should not exceed 25 mcg/mL.

Implementation
- Do not confuse gentamicin with gentian violet.
- Keep patient well hydrated (1500–2000 mL/day) during therapy.
- **Preoperative Bowel Prep:** Neomycin is usually used in conjunction with erythromycin, a low-residue diet, and a cathartic or enema.

- **PO:** Neomycin may be administered without regard to meals.
- **IM:** IM administration should be deep into a well-developed muscle. Alternate injection sites.
- **IV:** If aminoglycosides and penicillins or cephalosporins must be administered concurrently, administer in separate sites, at least 1 hr apart.

Amikacin

IV Administration

- **Intermittent Infusion:** *Dilution:* Dilute with D5W, D10W, 0.9% NaCl, dextrose/saline combinations, or LR. Solution may be pale yellow without decreased potency. Stable for 24 hr at room temperature. *Concentration:* 10 mg/mL. *Rate:* Infuse over 30–60 min for adults and children and over 1–2 hr in infants.
- **Y-Site Compatibility:** acyclovir, aldesleukin, alemtuzumab, amifostine, aminophylline, amiodarone, anidulafungin, arsenic trioxide, ascorbic acid, atracurium, atropine, aztreonam, benztropine, bivalirudin, bleomycin, bumetanide, buprenorphine, butorphanol, calcium chloride, calcium gluconate, cangrelor, carboplatin, carmustine, caspofungin, cefazolin, cefepime, cefotaxime, cefotetan, cefoxitin, ceftaroline, ceftazidime, ceftriaxone, cefuroxime, chloramphenicol, chlorpromazine, cisatracurium, cisplatin, clindamycin, cyanocobalamin, cyclophosphamide, cyclosporine, cytarabine, dactinomycin, daptomycin, daunorubicin hydrochloride, dexamethasone, dexmedetomidine, digoxin, diltiazem, diphenhydramine, dobutamine, docetaxel, dopamine, doxorubicin hydrochloride, doxycycline, enalaprilat, ephedrine, epinephrine, epirubicin, epoetin alfa, eptifibatide, ertapenem, erythromycin, esmolol, etoposide, etoposide phosphate, famotidine, fentanyl, filgrastim, fluconazole, fludarabine, fluorouracil, foscarnet, fosphenytoin, furosemide, gemcitabine, gentamicin, glycopyrrolate, granisetron, hydrocortisone, hydromorphone, idarubicin, ifosfamide, imipenem/cilastatin, irinotecan, isoproterenol, ketamine, ketorolac, labetalol, leucovorin calcium, levofloxacin, lidocaine, linezolid, lorazepam, magnesium sulfate, mannitol, melphalan, meperidine, mesna, methotrexate, methylprednisolone, metoclopramide, metoprolol, midazolam, milrinone, mitoxantrone, morphine, multivitamins, mycophenolate, nafcillin, nalbuphine, naloxone, nicardipine, nitroglycerin, nitroprusside, norepinephrine, octreotide, ondansetron, oxaliplatin, oxytocin, paclitaxel, palonosetron, pamidronate, pemetrexed, papaverine, penicillin G, phenobarbital, phentolamine, phenylephrine, phytonadione, piperacillin/tazobactam, posaconazole, potassium acetate, potassium chloride, procainamide, prochlorperazine, promethazine, propranolol, protamine, pyridoxine, remifentanil, rituximab, rocuronium, sargramostim, sodium acetate, sodium bicarbonate, succinylcholine, sufentanil, tacrolimus, theophylline, thiamine, thiotepa, tigecycline, tirofiban, tobramycin, topotecan, vancomycin, vasopressin, vecuronium, verapamil, vinblastine, vincristine, vinorelbine , voriconazole, warfarin, zidovudine, zoledronic acid.
- **Y-Site Incompatibility:** allopurinol, amphotericin B colloidal, amphotericin B lipid complex, amphotericin B liposomal, azathioprine, dacarbazine, dantrolene, diazepam, diazoxide, folic acid, ganciclovir, heparin, hetastarch, indomethacin, mitomycin, pentamidine, pentobarbital, phenytoin, propofol, trastuzumab, trimethoprim/sulfamethoxazole.
- **Inhaln:** If using a bronchodilator or with known hyperreactive airway disease, chronic obstructive pulmonary disease, asthma, or bronchospasm, pretreat with short-acting selective beta-2 agonists.
- Allow to come to room temperature before administering with *Lamira™ Nebulizer System* only. Shake vial well for 10–15 sec. until contents appear uniform and well mixed. Flip up plastic top of vial and pull down on metal ring to open. Remove metal ring and rubber stopper carefully. Pour contents of vial into medication reservoir of the nebulizer handset.

Gentamicin

IV Administration

- **Intermittent Infusion:** *Dilution:* Dilute each dose with D5W, 0.9% NaCl, or LR. Do not use solutions that are discolored or that contain a precipitate. *Concentration:* 10 mg/mL. *Rate:* Infuse slowly over 30 min–2 hr.
- **Y-Site Compatibility:** aldesleukin, alemtuzumab, alprostadil, amifostine, amikacin, aminophylline, amiodarone, anidulafungin, argatroban, ascorbic acid, atropine, aztreonam, benztropine, bivalirudin, bleomycin, bumetanide, buprenorphine, butorphanol, calcium chloride, calcium gluconate, carboplatin, carmustine, caspofungin, chlorpromazine, ciprofloxacin, cisatracurium, cisplatin, clindamycin, cyanocobalamin, cyclophosphamide, cyclosporine, cytarabine, dactinomycin, daptomycin, dexmedetomidine, dexrazoxane, digoxin, diltiazem, dimenhydrinate, diphenhydramine, dobutamine, docetaxel, dopamine, doxapram, doxorubicin, doxorubicin liposomal, doxycycline, enalaprilat, ephedrine, epinephrine, epirubicin, epoetin alfa, eptifibatide, ertapenem, erythromycin, esmolol, etoposide, etoposide phosphate, famotidine, fentanyl, fluconazole, fludarabine, fluorouracil, foscarnet, fosphenytoin, gemcitabine, glycopyrrolate, granisetron, hydromorphone, ifosfamide, imipenem/cilastatin, irinotecan, isoproterenol, ketamine, ketorolac, labetalol, leucovorin calcium, levofloxacin, lidocaine, linezolid, lorazepam, magnesium sulfate, mannitol, melphalan, meperidine, meropenem, mesna, methylprednisolone, metoclopramide, metoprolol, metronidazole, midazolam, milrinone, mitoxantrone, morphine, multivitamins, mycophenolate, nalbuphine, naloxone, nicardipine, nitroglycerin, nitroprusside, -

norepinephrine, octreotide, ondansetron, oxaliplatin, oxytocin, paclitaxel, palonosetron, pamidronate, papaverine, phenobarbital, phentolamine, phenylephrine, phytonadione, posaconazole, potassium acetate, potassium chloride, procainamide, prochlorperazine, promethazine, propranolol, protamine, pyridoxine, remifentanil, rituximab, rocuronium, sargramostim, sodium acetate, sodium bicarbonate, succinylcholine, sufentanil, tacrolimus, telavancin, theophylline, thiamine, thiotepa, tigecycline, tirofiban, tobramycin, topotecan, trastuzumab, vancomycin, vasopressin, vecuronium, verapamil, vinblastine, vincristine, vinorelbine, voriconazole, zidovudine, zoledronic acid.

- **Y-Site Incompatibility:** allopurinol, amphotericin B colloidal, amphotericin B lipid complex, amphotericin B liposomal, azathioprine, cangrelor, cefotetan, dacarbazine, dantrolene, diazepam, diazoxide, folic acid, ganciclovir, idarubicin, indomethacin, methotrexate, pemetrexed, pentamidine, pentobarbital, phenytoin, propofol, trimethoprim/sulfamethoxazole.

Tobramycin

IV Administration
- **Intermittent Infusion:** *Dilution:* Dilute each dose of tobramycin in 50–100 mL of D5W, D10W, D5/0.9% NaCl, 0.9% NaCl, Ringer's or lactated Ringer's solution. *Concentration:* not >10 m g/mL. Pediatric doses may be diluted in proportionately smaller amounts. Stable for 24 hr at room temperature, 96 hr if refrigerated. *Rate:* Infuse slowly over 30–60 min in both adult and pediatric patients.
- **Y-Site Compatibility:** acyclovir, aldesleukin, alemtuzumab, alprostadil, alteplase, amifostine, aminophylline, amiodarone, anidulafungin, argatroban, ascorbic acid, atropine, aztreonam, benztropine, bivalirudin, bleomycin, bumetanide, buprenorphine, butorphanol, calcium chloride, calcium gluconate, carboplatin, carmustine, caspofungin, chloramphenicol, chlorpromazine, ciprofloxacin, cisatracurium, cisplatin, clindamycin, cyanocobalamin, cyclophosphamide, cyclosporine, cytarabine, dactinomycin, daptomycin, daunorubicin hydrochloride, dexmedetomidine, dexrazoxane, digoxin, diltiazem, dimenhydrinate, diphenhydramine, dobutamine, docetaxel, dopamine, doxorubicin hydrochloride, doxorubicin liposomal, doxycycline, enalaprilat, ephedrine, epinephrine, epirubicin, epoetin alfa, ertapenem, esmolol, etoposide, etoposide phosphate, famotidine, fentanyl, filgrastim, fluconazole, fludarabine, fluorouracil, foscarnet, furosemide, gemcitabine, gentamicin, glycopyrrolate, granisetron, hydromorphone, idarubicin, ifosfamide, imipenem/cilastatin, irinotecan, isoproterenol, ketamine, ketorolac, labetalol, leucovorin calcium, lev-

ofloxacin, lidocaine, linezolid, lorazepam, magnesium sulfate, mannitol, melphalan, meperidine, mesna, methotrexate, methylprednisolone, metoclopramide, metoprolol, metronidazole, midazolam, milrinone, mitomycin, mitoxantrone, morphine, multivitamins, mycophenolate, nalbuphine, naloxone, nicardipine, nitroglycerin, nitroprusside, norepinephrine, octreotide, ondansetron, oxaliplatin, oxytocin, paclitaxel, palonosetron, pamidronate, papaverine, phenobarbital, phentolamine, phenylephrine, phytonadione, potassium acetate, potassium chloride, procainamide, prochlorperazine, promethazine, propranolol, protamine, pyridoxine, remifentanil, rituximab, rocuronium, sodium acetate, sodium bicarbonate, succinylcholine, sufentanil, tacrolimus, telavancin, theophylline, thiamine, thiotepa, tigecycline, tirofiban, topotecan, trastuzumab, vancomycin, vasopressin, vecuronium, verapamil, vinblastine, vincristine, vinorelbine, voriconazole, zidovudine, zoledronic acid.

- **Y-Site Incompatibility:** allopurinol, amphotericin B colloidal, amphotericin B lipid complex, amphotericin B liposomal, azathioprine, cangrelor, cefazolin, cefotetan, ceftriaxone, dacarbazine, dantrolene, dexamethasone, diazepam, diazoxide, folic acid, ganciclovir, hetastarch, indomethacin, oxacillin, pemetrexed, pentamidine, pentobarbital, phenytoin, piperacillin/tazobactam, propofol, sargramostim, trimethoprim/sulfamethoxazole.
- **Topical:** Cleanse skin before application. Wear gloves during application.
- **Inhaln:** Do not mix *TOBI* with dornase alpha in nebulizer.
- *TOBI Podhaler* capsules are not for oral use. Store capsules in blister until immediately before use. Use new Podhaler device provided with each weekly packet. Check to see capsule is empty after inhaling. If powder remains in capsule, repeat inhalation until capsule is empty.

Patient/Family Teaching
- Instruct patient to report signs of hypersensitivity, tinnitus, vertigo, hearing loss, rash, dizziness, or difficulty urinating.
- Advise patient of the importance of drinking plenty of liquids.
- Teach patients with a history of rheumatic heart disease or valve replacement the importance of using antimicrobial prophylaxis before invasive medical or dental procedures.
- Rep: Advise females of reproductive potential to notify health care professional if pregnancy is planned or suspected or if breastfeeding. Avoid tobramycin (IV/IM), streptomycin, and inhaled amikacin during pregnancy; may cause fetal harm. May cause irreversible deafness in babies.
- PO: Instruct patient to take neomycin as directed for full course of therapy. Take missed doses as soon as

possible if not almost time for next dose; do not take double doses.

- Caution patient that neomycin may cause nausea, vomiting, or diarrhea.
- **Topical:** Instruct patient to wash affected skin gently and pat dry. Apply a thin film of ointment. Apply occlusive dressing only if directed by health care professional. Patient should assess skin and inform health care professional if skin irritation develops or infection worsens.
- **Inhaln: Amikacin:** Advise patient to omit missed doses and administer next dose next day; do not double doses. Instruct patient to read *Medication Guide* before starting and with each Rx refill in case of changes.
- Advise patient to notify health care professional if signs and symptoms of allergic inflammation of lungs (fever, wheezing, coughing, shortness of breath, fast breathing), hemoptysis (coughing up blood), bronchospasm (shortness of breath, difficult or labored breathing, wheezing, coughing, chest tightness) or worsening of COPD occur. **Tobramycin:** Instruct patient to take inhalation twice daily as close to 12 hr apart as possible; not <6 hr apart. Solution is colorless to pale yellow and may darken with age without effecting quality. Administer over 15-min period using a handheld PARI LC PLUS reusable nebulizer with a *PARI VIOS (for Bethkis) or DeVibiss Pulmo Aide (for TOBI)* compressor. Instruct patient on multiple therapies to take others first and use *tobramycin* last. Tobramycin-induced bronchospasm may be reduced if tobramycin is administered after bronchodilators. Instruct patient to sit or stand upright during inhalation and breathe normally through mouthpiece of nebulizer. Nose clips may help patient breath through mouth. Store at room temperature for up to 28 days. Advise patient to disinfect the nebulizer parts (except tubing) by boiling them in water for a full 10 min every other treatment day.
- Instruct patient in correct technique for use of *TOBI Podhaler*. Wipe mouthpiece with clean, dry cloth after use; do not wash with water.

Evaluation/Desired Outcomes

- Resolution of the signs and symptoms of infection. If no response is seen within 3–5 days, new cultures should be taken.
- Prevention of infection in intestinal surgery (neomycin).
- Improved neurologic status in hepatic encephalopathy (neomycin).
- Endocarditis prophylaxis (gentamicin).

BEERS HIGH ALERT

amiodarone (am-ee-oh-da-rone)
Nexterone, Pacerone
Classification
Therapeutic: antiarrhythmics (class III)

Indications
Life-threatening ventricular arrhythmias unresponsive to less toxic agents. **Unlabeled Use: PO:** Supraventricular tachyarrhythmias. **IV:** As part of the Advanced Cardiac Life Support (ACLS) and Pediatric Advanced Life Support (PALS) guidelines for the management of ventricular fibrillation (VF)/pulseless ventricular tachycardia (VT) after cardiopulmonary resuscitation and defibrillation have failed; also for other life-threatening tachyarrhythmias.

Action
Prolongs action potential and refractory period. Inhibits adrenergic stimulation. Slows the sinus rate, increases PR and QT intervals, and decreases peripheral vascular resistance (vasodilation). **Therapeutic Effects:** Suppression of arrhythmias.

Pharmacokinetics
Absorption: Slowly and variably absorbed from the GI tract (35–65%). IV administration results in complete bioavailability.
Distribution: Distributed to and accumulates slowly in body tissues. Reaches high levels in fat, muscle, liver, lungs, and spleen. Crosses the placenta and enters breast milk.
Protein Binding: 96% bound to plasma proteins.
Metabolism and Excretion: Metabolized by the liver, excreted into bile. Minimal renal excretion. One metabolite has antiarrhythmic activity.
Half-life: 13–107 days.

TIME/ACTION PROFILE (suppression of ventricular arrhythmias)

ROUTE	ONSET	PEAK	DURATION
PO	2–3 days (up to 2–3 mo)	3–7 hr	wk–mos
IV	2 hr	3–7 hr	unknown

Contraindications/Precautions
Contraindicated in: Cardiogenic shock; Severe sinus node dysfunction; 2nd- and 3rd-degree AV block; Bradycardia (unless a pacemaker is in place); Hypersensitivity to amiodarone or iodine; Lactation: Lactation.

Use Cautiously in: Thyroid disorders; Corneal refractive laser surgery; Severe pulmonary or liver disease; OB: Should only be used during pregnancy when arrhythmias are refractory to other treatments or when other treatments are contraindicated; Pedi: Safety and effectiveness not established in children; Geri: Appears on Beers list. Avoid use as first-line therapy for rhythm control in atrial fibrillation in older adults unless HF or significant left ventricular hypertrophy present.

Adverse Reactions/Side Effects
CV: bradycardia, hypotension, HF, QT interval prolongation, WORSENING OF ARRHYTHMIAS. **Derm:** photosensitivity, blue discoloration, TOXIC EPIDERMAL NECROLYSIS (rare). **EENT:** corneal microdeposits, abnormal sense

of smell, dry eyes, optic neuritis, optic neuropathy, photophobia. **Endo:** <u>hypothyroidism</u>, hyperthyroidism. **GI:** <u>anorexia</u>, <u>constipation</u>, <u>nausea</u>, <u>vomiting</u>, ↑ liver enzymes, abdominal pain, abnormal sense of taste. **GU:** ↓ libido, epididymitis. **Neuro:** <u>ataxia</u>, <u>dizziness</u>, <u>fatigue</u>, <u>involuntary movement</u>, <u>malaise</u>, <u>paresthesia</u>, <u>peripheral neuropathy</u>, <u>poor coordination</u>, <u>tremor</u>, confusional states, disorientation, hallucinations, headache, insomnia. **Resp:** ACUTE RESPIRATORY DISTRESS SYNDROME, PULMONARY FIBROSIS.

Interactions

Drug-Drug: ↑ risk of QT interval prolongation with **fluoroquinolones**, **macrolides**, and **azole antifungals** (undertake concurrent use with caution). ↑ levels of **digoxin** (↓ dose of digoxin by 50%). ↑ levels of **class I antiarrhythmics (quinidine, mexiletine, lidocaine,** or **flecainide**— ↓ doses of other drugs by 30–50%). ↑ levels of **cyclosporine, dextromethorphan, methotrexate, phenytoin, carvedilol,** and **theophylline. Phenytoin** ↓ amiodarone levels. ↑ activity of **warfarin** (↓ dose of warfarin by 33–50%). ↑ risk of bradyarrhythmias, sinus arrest, or AV heart block with **beta blockers, verapamil, diltiazem, digoxin, ivabradine,** or **clonidine.** ↑ risk of bradycardia when used with **sofosbuvir, ledipasvir/sofosbuvir, sofosbuvir/velpatasvir,** or **sofosbuvir/velpatasvir/voxilaprevir**; concurrent use not recommended. **Cholestyramine** may ↓ amiodarone levels. **Cimetidine** and **ritonavir** ↑ amiodarone levels. Risk of myocardial depression is ↑ by **volatile anesthetics.** ↑ risk of myopathy with **lovastatin** and **simvastatin** (do not exceed 40 mg/day of lovastatin or 20 mg/day of simvastatin).

Drug-Natural Products: St. John's wort induces enzymes that metabolize amiodarone; may ↓ levels and effectiveness. Avoid concurrent use.

Drug-Food: Grapefruit juice inhibits enzymes in the GI tract that metabolize amiodarone resulting in ↑ levels and risk of toxicity; avoid concurrent use.

Route/Dosage

Ventricular Arrhythmias

PO (Adults): 800–1600 mg/day in 1–2 doses for 1–3 wk, then 600–800 mg/day in 1–2 doses for 1 mo, then 400 mg/day maintenance dose.
PO (Children): 10 mg/kg/day (800 mg/1.72 m^2/day) for 10 days or until response or adverse reaction occurs, then 5 mg/kg/day (400 mg/1.72 m^2/day) for several wk, then ↓ to 2.5 mg/kg/day (200 mg/1.72 m^2/day) or lowest effective maintenance dose.
IV (Adults): 150 mg over 10 min, followed by 360 mg over the next 6 hr and then 540 mg over the next 18 hr. Continue infusion at 0.5 mg/min until oral therapy is initiated. If arrhythmia recurs, a small loading infusion of 150 mg over 10 min should be given; in addition, the rate of the maintenance infusion may be ↑. *Conversion*

to initial oral therapy: If duration of IV infusion was <1 wk, oral dose should be 800–1600 mg/day; if IV infusion was 1–3 wk, oral dose should be 600–800 mg/day; if IV infusion was >3 wk, oral dose should be 400 mg/day. *ACLS guidelines for pulseless VF/VT:* 300 mg IV push, may repeat once after 3–5 min with 150 mg IV push (maximum cumulative dose 2.2 g/24 hr; unlabeled).

IV: Intraosseous (Children and infants): *PALS guidelines for pulseless VF/VT:* 5 mg/kg as a bolus; *Perfusion tachycardia:* 5 mg/kg loading dose over 20–60 min (maximum of 15 mg/kg/day; unlabeled).

Supraventricular Tachycardia

PO (Adults): 600–800 mg/day for 1 wk or until desired response occurs or side effects develop, then ↓ to 400 mg/day for 3 wk, then maintenance dose of 200–400 mg/day.
PO (Children): 10 mg/kg/day (800 mg/1.72 m^2/day) for 10 days or until response or side effects occur, then 5 mg/kg/day (400 mg/1.72 m^2/day) for several wk, then ↓ to 2.5 mg/kg/day (200 mg/1.72 m^2/day) or lowest effective maintenance dose.

Availability (generic available)

Premixed infusion (Nexterone): 150 mg/100 mL D5W (does not contain polysorbate 80 or benzyl alcohol), 360 mg/200 mL D5W (does not contain polysorbate 80 or benzyl alcohol). **Solution for injection:** 50 mg/mL. **Tablets:** 100 mg, 200 mg, 400 mg.

NURSING IMPLICATIONS

Assessment

- Monitor ECG continuously during IV therapy or initiation of oral therapy. Monitor heart rate and rhythm throughout therapy; PR prolongation, slight QRS widening, and T-wave amplitude reduction with T-wave widening and bifurcation may occur. QT prolongation may be associated with worsening of arrhythmias; monitor closely during IV therapy. Report bradycardia or increase in arrhythmias promptly; patients receiving IV therapy may require slowing rate, discontinuing infusion, or inserting a temporary pacemaker.
- Assess pacing and defibrillation threshold in patients with pacemakers and implanted defibrillators at beginning and periodically during therapy.
- Assess for signs of pulmonary toxicity (rales/crackles, decreased breath sounds, pleuritic friction rub, fatigue, dyspnea, cough, wheezing, pleuritic pain, fever, hemoptysis, hypoxia). Chest x-ray and pulmonary function tests are recommended before therapy. Monitor chest x-ray every 3–6 mo during therapy to detect diffuse interstitial changes or alveolar infiltrates. Bronchoscopy or gallium radionuclide scan may also be used for diagnosis. Usually reversible after withdrawal, but fatalities have occurred.

✦ = Canadian drug name. ▓ = Genetic implication. ~~Strikethrough~~ = Discontinued. CAPITALS = life-threatening. <u>Underline</u> = most frequent.

- **IV:** Assess for signs and symptoms of ARDS during therapy. Report dyspnea, tachypnea, or rales/crackles promptly. Bilateral, diffuse pulmonary infiltrates are seen on chest x-ray.
- **Monitor BP** frequently. Hypotension usually occurs during first several hrs of therapy and is related to rate of infusion. If hypotension occurs, slow rate.
- **PO:** Assess for neurotoxicity (ataxia, proximal muscle weakness, tingling or numbness in fingers or toes, uncontrolled movements, tremors); common during initial therapy, but may occur within 1 wk to several mo of initiation of therapy and may persist for more than 1 yr after withdrawal. Dose reduction is recommended. Assist patient during ambulation to prevent falls.
- Ophthalmic exams should be performed before and regularly during therapy and whenever visual changes (photophobia, halos around lights, decreased acuity) occur. May cause permanent loss of vision.
- Assess for signs of thyroid dysfunction, especially during initial therapy. Lethargy; weight gain; edema of the hands, feet, and periorbital region; and cool, pale skin suggest hypothyroidism and may require decrease in dose or discontinuation of therapy and thyroid supplementation. Tachycardia; weight loss; nervousness; sensitivity to heat; insomnia; and warm, flushed, moist skin suggest hyperthyroidism and may require discontinuation of therapy and treatment with antithyroid agents.

Lab Test Considerations
- Monitor liver and thyroid functions before and every 6 mo during therapy. Drug effects persist long after discontinuation. Thyroid function abnormalities are common, but clinical thyroid dysfunction is uncommon.
- Monitor AST, ALT, and alkaline phosphatase at regular intervals during therapy, especially in patients receiving high maintenance dose. If liver function studies are 3 times normal or double in patients with elevated baseline levels or if hepatomegaly occurs, dose should be reduced.
- May cause asymptomatic ↑ in ANA titer concentrations.
- Monitor serum potassium, calcium, and magnesium prior to starting and periodically during therapy. Hypokalemia, hypocalcemia, and/or hypomagnesemia may ↓ effectiveness or cause additional arrhythmias; correct levels before beginning therapy. Monitor closely when converting from IV to oral therapy, especially in geriatric patients.

Implementation
- **High Alert:** IV vasoactive medications are inherently dangerous; fatalities have occurred from medication errors involving amiodarone. Before administering, have second practitioner check original order, dose calculations, and infusion pump settings. Patients should be hospitalized and monitored

closely during IV therapy and initiation of oral therapy. IV therapy should be administered only by clinicians experienced in treating life-threatening arrhythmias.
- Do not confuse amiodarone with amantadine.
- **PO:** May be administered with meals and in divided doses if GI intolerance occurs or if daily dose exceeds 1000 mg.

IV Administration
- **IV:** Administer via volumetric pump; drop size may be reduced, causing altered dosing with drop counter infusion sets.
- Administer through an in-line filter.
- Infusions exceeding 2 hr must be administered in glass or polyolefin bottles to prevent adsorption. However, polyvinyl chloride (PVC) tubing must be used during administration because concentrations and infusion rate recommendations have been based on PVC tubing.
- **IV Push:** *Dilution:* Administer undiluted. May also be diluted in 20–30 mL of D5W or 0.9% NaCl. *Concentration:* 50 mg/mL. *Rate:* Administer IV push.
- **Intermittent Infusion:** *Dilution:* Dilute 150 mg of amiodarone in 100 mL of D5W. Infusion stable for 2 hr in PVC bag, or use pre-mixed bags. *Concentration:* 1.5 mg/mL. *Rate:* Infuse over 10 min. Do not administer IV push.
- **Continuous Infusion:** *Dilution:* Dilute 900 mg (18 mL) of amiodarone in 500 mL of D5W. Infusion stable for 24 hr in glass or polyolefin bottle. *Concentration:* 1.8 mg/mL. Concentration may range from 1–6 mg/mL (concentrations >2 mg/mL must be administered via central venous catheter). *Rate:* Infuse at a rate of 1 mg/min for the first 6 hr, then decrease infusion rate to 0.5 mg/min and continue until oral therapy initiated.
- **Y-Site Compatibility:** alemtuzumab, amikacin, amphotericin B lipid complex, anidulafungin, arsenic trioxide, atracurium, atropine, bleomycin, buprenorphine, busulfan, butorphanol, calcium chloride, cangrelor, carboplatin, carmustine, caspofungin, cefepime, ceftaroline, ceftolozane/tazobactam, chlorpromazine, ciprofloxacin, cisatracurium, cisplatin, clindamycin, cyclophosphamide, cyclosporine, dacarbazine, dactinomycin, daptomycin, daunorubicin hydrochloride, dexmedetomidine, dexrazoxane, diltiazem, diphenhydramine, docetaxel, dopamine, doxycycline, droperidol, enalaprilat, ephedrine, epinephrine, erythromycin lactobionate, esmolol, etoposide, etoposide phosphate, famotidine, fluconazole, gemcitabine, gentamicin, glycopyrrolate, granisetron, hetastarch, hydralazine, hydromorphone, idarubicin, ifosfamide, irinotecan, isavuconazonium, isoproterenol, ketamine, labetalol, lidocaine, linezolid, lorazepam, mannitol, meperidine, mesna, methadone, metoclopramide, metoprolol, metronidazole, midazolam, milrinone, mitoxantrone, morphine, moxifloxacin, mycophenolate, nafcillin, nalbuphine, naloxone, nicardipine, ni-

troglycerin, octreotide, ondansetron, oxaliplatin, palonosetron, pemetrexed, penicillin G potassium, pentamidine, phentolamine, phenylephrine, procainamide, prochlorperazine, promethazine, propranolol, remifentanil, rifampin, rocuronium, succinylcholine, sufentanil, tacrolimus, tedizolid, theophylline, tirofiban, tobramycin, topotecan, vancomycin, vasopressin, vecuronium, vinblastine, vincristine, vinorelbine, voriconazole, zidovudine, zoledronic acid.

- **Y-Site Incompatibility:** acyclovir, allopurinol, amifostine, aminocaproic acid, aminophylline, ampicillin, ampicillin/sulbactam, azithromycin, bivalirudin, cefotaxime, cefotetan, ceftazidime, chloramphenicol, cytarabine, dantrolene, dexamethasone, diazepam, digoxin, doxorubicin hydrochloride, doxorubicin liposomal, eravacycline, ertapenem, fludarabine, fluorouracil, foscarnet, fosphenytoin, ganciclovir, gemtuzumab ozogamicin, heparin, hydrocortisone, imipenem-cilastatin, ketorolac, LR, leucovorin calcium, levofloxacin, melphalan, meropenem, meropenem/vaborbactam, methotrexate, micafungin, mitomycin, paclitaxel, pentobarbital, phenobarbital, phenytoin, piperacillin/tazobactam, plazomicin, potassium acetate, potassium phosphate, sodium acetate, sodium bicarbonate, sodium phosphate, thiopental, thiotepa, tigecycline, trimethoprim/sulfamethoxazole, verapamil.

Patient/Family Teaching

- Instruct patient to take amiodarone as directed. If a dose is missed, do not take at all. Consult health care professional if more than two doses are missed. Advise patient to read the *Medication Guide* prior to first dose and with each Rx refill in case of changes.
- Advise patient to avoid drinking grapefruit juice during therapy.
- Inform patient that side effects may not appear until several days, weeks, or yr after initiation of therapy and may persist for several mo after withdrawal.
- Teach patients to monitor pulse daily and report abnormalities.
- Advise patients that photosensitivity reactions may occur through window glass, thin clothing, and sunscreens. Protective clothing and sunblock are recommended during and for 4 mo after therapy. If photosensitivity occurs, dose reduction may be useful.
- Inform patients that bluish discoloration of the face, neck, and arms is a possible side effect of this drug after prolonged use. This is usually reversible and will fade over several mo. Notify health care professional if this occurs.
- Instruct male patients to notify health care professional if signs and symptoms of epididymitis (pain and swelling in scrotum) occur. May require reduction in dose.

- Advise patient to notify health care professional of all Rx or OTC medications, vitamins, or herbal products being taken and to consult with health care professional before taking other medications, especially St. John's wort.
- Instruct patient to notify health care professional of medication regimen before treatment or surgery.
- Advise patient to notify health care professional if signs and symptoms of thyroid dysfunction occur.
- Rep: May cause fetal harm. Advise females of reproductive potential to use effective contraception and to avoid breastfeeding during therapy. May cause neonatal bradycardia, QT prolongation, periodic ventricular extrasystoles; neonatal hypothyroidism (with or without goiter) detected antenatally or in the newborn and reported even after a few days of exposure; neonatal hyperthyroxinemia; neurodevelopmental abnormalities independent of thyroid function, including speech delay and difficulties with written language and arithmetic, delayed motor development, and ataxia; jerk nystagmus with synchronous head titubation; fetal growth retardation; and premature birth. Advise patient to notify health care professional if pregnancy is planned or suspected.
- Emphasize the importance of follow-up exams, including chest x-ray and pulmonary function tests every 3–6 mo and ophthalmic exams after 6 mo of therapy, and then annually.

Evaluation/Desired Outcomes

- Cessation of life-threatening ventricular arrhythmias. Adverse effects may take up to 4 mo to resolve.

BEERS

⚹ amitriptyline
(a-mee-**trip**-ti-leen)
✤Elavil
Classification
Therapeutic: antidepressants
Pharmacologic: tricyclic antidepressants

Indications

Depression. **Unlabeled Use:** Anxiety, insomnia, treatment-resistant depression. Chronic pain syndromes (i.e., fibromyalgia, neuropathic pain/chronic pain, headache, low back pain).

Action

Potentiates the effect of serotonin and norepinephrine in the CNS. Has significant anticholinergic properties. **Therapeutic Effects:** Antidepressant action.

Pharmacokinetics

Absorption: Well absorbed from the GI tract.
Distribution: Widely distributed.
Protein Binding: 95% bound to plasma proteins.
Metabolism and Excretion: Extensively metabolized by the liver, primarily by the CYP2D6 isoenzyme;

the CYP2D6 enzyme system exhibits genetic polymorphism (~7% of population may be poor metabolizers and may have significantly ↑ amitriptyline concentrations and an ↑ risk of adverse effects). Some metabolites have antidepressant activity. Undergoes enterohepatic recirculation and secretion into gastric juices. Probably crosses the placenta and enters breast milk. **Half-life:** 10–50 hr.

TIME/ACTION PROFILE (antidepressant effect)

ROUTE	ONSET	PEAK	DURATION
PO	2–3 wk (up to 30 days)	2–6 wk	days–wk

Contraindications/Precautions

Contraindicated in: Angle-closure glaucoma; Known history of QTc interval prolongation, recent MI, or HF; Lactation: Lactation.

Use Cautiously in: May ↑ risk of suicide attempt/ideation especially during dose early treatment or dose adjustment; risk may be greater in children or adolescents; Patients with pre-existing cardiovascular disease; Prostatic hyperplasia (↑ risk of urinary retention); History of seizures (threshold may be ↓); OB: Use during pregnancy only if potential maternal benefit justifies potential fetal risk; Pedi: Children <12 yr (safety and effectiveness not established); Geri: Appears on Beers list. ↑ risk of adverse reactions in older adults, including falls secondary to sedative and anticholinergic effects and orthostatic hypotension. Avoid use in older adults.

Adverse Reactions/Side Effects

CV: hypotension, ARRHYTHMIAS, QT interval prolongation, TORSADES DE POINTES. **Derm:** photosensitivity. **EENT:** blurred vision, dry eyes, dry mouth. **Endo:** changes in blood glucose, gynecomastia. **GI:** constipation, hepatitis, paralytic ileus. **GU:** ↓ libido, urinary retention. **Hemat:** blood dyscrasias. **Metab:** ↑ appetite, weight gain. **Neuro:** lethargy, sedation, SUICIDAL THOUGHTS.

Interactions

Drug-Drug: Amitriptyline is metabolized in the liver by the cytochrome P450 2D6 enzyme, and its action may be affected by drugs that compete for metabolism by this enzyme, including other **antidepressants**, **phenothiazines**, **carbamazepine**, **class 1C antiarrhythmics** including **propafenone**, and **flecainide**; when these drugs are used concurrently with amitriptyline, may need to ↓ dose of one or the other or both. Concurrent use of other drugs that inhibit the activity of the enzyme, including **cimetidine**, **quinidine**, **amiodarone**, and **ritonavir**, may result in ↑ effects of amitriptyline. May cause hypotension, tachycardia, and potentially fatal reactions when used with **MAO inhibitors** (avoid concurrent use—discontinue 2 wk before starting amitriptyline). Concurrent use with **SSRIs** may result in ↑ toxicity and should be avoided (**fluoxetine** should be stopped 5 wk before starting amitriptyline). Concurrent use with **clonidine** may result in hypertensive crisis and should be avoided. Concurrent use with **levodopa** may result in delayed or ↓ absorption of levodopa or hypertension. Blood levels and effects may be ↓ by **rifampin**, **rifapentine**, and **rifabutin**. Concurrent use with **moxifloxacin** ↑ risk of adverse cardiovascular reactions. ↑ CNS depression with other **CNS depressants** including **alcohol**, **antihistamines**, **clonidine**, **opioids**, and **sedative/hypnotics**. **Barbiturates** may alter blood levels and effects. **Adrenergic** and **anticholinergic** side effects may be ↑ with other agents having **anticholinergic** properties. **Phenothiazines** or **oral contraceptives** ↑ levels and may cause toxicity. **Nicotine** may ↑ metabolism and alter effects.

Drug-Natural Products: St. John's wort may ↓ serum concentrations and efficacy. Concomitant use of **kava-kava**, **valerian**, or **chamomile** can ↑ CNS depression. ↑ anticholinergic effects with **jimson weed** and **scopolia**.

Route/Dosage

PO (Adults): 75 mg/day in divided doses; may be ↑ up to 150 mg/day *or* 50–100 mg at bedtime, may ↑ by 25–50 mg up to 150 mg (in hospitalized patients, may initiate with 100 mg/day, and ↑ total daily dose up to 300 mg).

PO (Geriatric Patients): 10–25 mg at bedtime; may ↑ by 10–25 mg weekly if tolerated (usual dose range = 25–150 mg/day).

Availability (generic available)

Tablets: 10 mg, 25 mg, 50 mg, 75 mg, 100 mg, 150 mg.

NURSING IMPLICATIONS

Assessment

- Obtain weight and BMI initially and periodically during treatment.
- Assess fasting glucose and cholesterol levels in overweight/obese individuals.
- Monitor BP and pulse before and during initial therapy. Notify health care professional of decreases in BP (10–20 mm Hg) or sudden increase in pulse rate. Monitor ECG before and periodically during therapy in patients taking high doses or with a history of cardiovascular disease.
- **Depression:** Monitor mental status (orientation, mood behavior) frequently. Assess for suicidal tendencies, especially during early therapy. Restrict amount of drug available to patient.
- Assess for suicidal tendencies, especially during early therapy. Restrict amount of drug available to patient. Risk may be increased in children, adolescents, and adults ≤24 yrs. After starting therapy, children, adolescents, and young adults should be seen by health care professional at least weekly for 4 wk, every 3 wk for next 4 wk, and on advice of health care professional thereafter.

- **Pain:** Assess intensity, quality, and location of pain periodically during therapy. May require several wk for effects to be seen. Use pain scale to monitor effectiveness of medication. Assess for sexual dysfunction (decreased libido; erectile dysfunction). Geri: Geriatric patients started on amitriptyline may be at an increased risk for falls; start with low dose and monitor closely. Assess for anticholinergic effects (weakness and sedation).

Lab Test Considerations

- Assess leukocyte and differential blood counts, liver function, and serum glucose before and periodically during therapy. May cause an ↑ serum bilirubin and alkaline phosphatase. May cause bone marrow depression. Serum glucose may be ↑ or ↓.

Implementation

- Dose increases should be made at bedtime due to sedation. Dose titration is a slow process; may take wks to mos. May give entire dose at bedtime. Sedative effect may be apparent before antidepressant effect is noted. May require tapering to avoid withdrawal effects.
- **PO:** Administer medication with or immediately after a meal to minimize gastric upset. Tablet may be crushed and given with food or fluids.

Patient/Family Teaching

- Instruct patient to take medication as directed. If a dose is missed, take as soon as possible unless almost time for next dose; if regimen is a single dose at bedtime, do not take in the morning because of side effects. Advise patient that drug effects may not be noticed for at least 2 wk. Abrupt discontinuation may cause nausea, vomiting, diarrhea, headache, trouble sleeping with vivid dreams, and irritability.
- May cause drowsiness and blurred vision. Caution patient to avoid driving and other activities requiring alertness until response to drug is known.
- Orthostatic hypotension, sedation, and confusion are common during early therapy, especially in geriatric patients. Protect patient from falls and advise patient to make position changes slowly. Institute fall precautions. Advise patient to make position changes slowly. Refer as appropriate for nutrition/weight management and medical management.
- Advise patient to avoid alcohol or other CNS depressant drugs during and for 3–7 days after therapy has been discontinued.
- Advise patient, family and caregivers to look for suicidality, especially during early therapy or dose changes. Notify health care professional immediately if thoughts about suicide or dying, attempts to commit suicide, new or worse depression or anxiety, agitation or restlessness, panic attacks, insomnia, new or worse irritability, aggressiveness, acting on dangerous impulses, mania, or other changes in mood or behavior occur.

- Instruct patient to notify health care professional if urinary retention, dry mouth, or constipation persists. Sugarless candy or gum may diminish dry mouth, and an increase in fluid intake or bulk may prevent constipation. If symptoms persist, dose reduction or discontinuation may be necessary. Consult health care professional if dry mouth persists for >2 wk.
- Caution patient to use sunscreen and protective clothing to prevent photosensitivity reactions. Alert patient that medication may turn urine blue-green in color.
- Inform patient of need to monitor dietary intake. Increase in appetite may lead to undesired weight gain.
- Advise patient to notify health care professional of medication regimen before treatment or surgery. Medication should be discontinued as long as possible before surgery.
- Rep: May cause fetal harm. Advise patient to notify health care professional if pregnancy is planned or suspected and to avoid breastfeeding. Assess neonates of women taking amitriptyline during pregnancy for irritability, jitteriness, increased crying, constipation, problems with urinating, respiratory distress, nausea and convulsions. Patients exposed to antidepressants during pregnancy are encouraged to enroll in the National Pregnancy Registry for Antidepressants. Patients 18 to 45 years of age or their health care providers may contact the registry by calling 844-405-6185. Enrollment should be done as early in pregnancy as possible.

Evaluation/Desired Outcomes

- Increased sense of well-being.
- Renewed interest in surroundings.
- Increased appetite.
- Improved energy level.
- Improved sleep.
- Decrease in chronic pain symptoms.
- Full therapeutic effects may be seen 2–6 wk after initiating therapy.

---

amLODIPine (am-loe-di-peen)
Katerzia, Norliqva, Norvasc
Classification
Therapeutic: antianginals, antihypertensives
Pharmacologic: calcium channel blockers

Indications

Hypertension (as monotherapy or in combination with other antihypertensive agents). Chronic stable angina (as monotherapy or in combination with other antianginal agents). Vasospastic (Prinzmetal's) angina (as monotherapy or in combination with other antianginal agents). Recently documented coronary artery disease by angiography and without HF or an ejection fraction <40%.

Action
Inhibits the transport of calcium into myocardial and vascular smooth muscle cells, resulting in inhibition of excitation-contraction coupling and subsequent contraction. **Therapeutic Effects:** Reduction in BP. Decreased frequency and severity of attacks of angina. Reduction in risk of hospitalization for angina or coronary revascularization in patients with recently documented coronary artery disease.

Pharmacokinetics
Absorption: Well absorbed after oral administration (64–90%).
Distribution: Probably crosses the placenta.
Protein Binding: 95–98%.
Metabolism and Excretion: Mostly metabolized by the liver by the CYP3A4 isoenzyme.
Half-life: 30–50 hr (↑ in geriatric patients and patients with hepatic impairment).

TIME/ACTION PROFILE (cardiovascular effects)

ROUTE	ONSET	PEAK	DURATION
PO	unknown	6–9 hr	24 hr

Contraindications/Precautions
Contraindicated in: Hypersensitivity; Systolic BP <90 mm Hg.
Use Cautiously in: Severe hepatic impairment (dose ↓ recommended); Aortic stenosis; History of HF; OB: Use during pregnancy only if potential maternal benefit justifies potential fetal risk; other calcium channel blockers preferred in pregnancy; Lactation: Use while breastfeeding only if potential maternal benefit justifies potential risk to infant; Pedi: Children <6 yr (safety and effectiveness not established); Geri: ↑ risk of hypotension in older adults (dose ↓ recommended).

Adverse Reactions/Side Effects
CV: peripheral edema, angina, bradycardia, hypotension, palpitations. **Derm:** flushing. **GI:** gingival hyperplasia, nausea. **Neuro:** dizziness, fatigue.

Interactions
Drug-Drug: Strong CYP3A4 inhibitors, including **ketoconazole**, **itraconazole**, **clarithromycin**, and **ritonavir** may ↑ levels. Additive hypotension may occur when used concurrently with **fentanyl**, other **antihypertensives**, **nitrates**, acute ingestion of **alcohol**, or **quinidine**. Antihypertensive effects may be ↓ by concurrent use of **NSAIDs**. May ↑ risk of neurotoxicity with **lithium**. ↑ risk of myopathy with **simvastatin** (do not exceed 20 mg/day of simvastatin). May ↑ **cyclosporine** and **tacrolimus** levels.

Route/Dosage
PO (Adults): 5–10 mg once daily.
PO (Geriatric Patients): *Antihypertensive:* Initiate therapy at 2.5 mg/day, ↑ as required/tolerated (up to 10 mg/day); *Antianginal:* initiate therapy at 5 mg/day, ↑ as required/tolerated (up to 10 mg/day).

PO (Children >6 yr): 2.5–5 mg once daily.

Hepatic Impairment
PO (Adults): *Antihypertensive:* Initiate therapy at 2.5 mg/day, ↑ as required/tolerated (up to 10 mg/day); *Antianginal:* initiate therapy at 5 mg/day, ↑ as required/tolerated (up to 10 mg/day).

Availability (generic available)
Tablets: 2.5 mg, 5 mg, 10 mg. **Oral solution (Norliqva) (peppermint flavor):** 1 mg/mL. **Oral suspension (Katerzia):** 1 mg/mL. *In combination with:* atorvastatin (Caduet), benazepril (Lotrel), olmesartan (Azor), olmesartan/hydrochlorothiazide (Tribenzor), telmisartan, valsartan (Exforge), and valsartan/hydrochlorothiazide (Exforge HCT). See Appendix N.

NURSING IMPLICATIONS

Assessment
- Monitor BP and pulse before therapy, during dose titration, and periodically during therapy. Monitor ECG periodically during prolonged therapy.
- Monitor intake and output ratios and daily weight. Assess for signs of HF (peripheral edema, rales/crackles, dyspnea, weight gain, jugular venous distention).
- Monitor frequency of prescription refills to determine adherence.
- **Angina:** Assess location, duration, intensity, and precipitating factors of patient's anginal pain.

Lab Test Considerations
- Total serum calcium concentrations are not affected by calcium channel blockers.

Implementation
- Do not confuse amlodipine with amiloride.
- **PO:** May be administered without regard to meals.
- *Norliqva* is a pale straw colored solution. *Katerzia* is a white to off-white liquid suspension. Shake before using.

Patient/Family Teaching
- Advise patient to take medication as directed, even if feeling well. Take missed doses as soon as possible within 12 hrs of missed dose. If >12 hrs since missed dose, skip dose and take next dose at scheduled time; do not double doses. May need to be discontinued gradually.
- Caution patient to change positions slowly to minimize orthostatic hypotension.
- May cause drowsiness or dizziness. Advise patient to avoid driving or other activities requiring alertness until response to the medication is known.
- Instruct patient on importance of maintaining good dental hygiene and seeing dentist frequently for teeth cleaning to prevent tenderness, bleeding, and gingival hyperplasia (gum enlargement).
- Instruct patient to notify health care professional of all Rx or OTC medications, vitamins, or herbal products being taken, to avoid alcohol, and to consult

health care professional before taking any new medications, especially cold preparations.

- Advise patient to notify health care professional if irregular heartbeats, dyspnea, swelling of hands and feet, pronounced dizziness, nausea, constipation, or hypotension occurs or if headache is severe or persistent.
- Advise patient to inform health care professional of medication regimen before treatment or surgery.
- Rep: Advise females of reproductive potential to notify health care professional if pregnancy is planned or suspected or if breastfeeding.
- Angina: Instruct patient on concurrent nitrate or beta-blocker therapy to continue taking both medications as directed and to use SL nitroglycerin as needed for anginal attacks.
- Advise patient to contact health care professional if chest pain does not improve or worsens after therapy, if it occurs with diaphoresis, if shortness of breath occurs, or if severe, persistent headache occurs.
- Caution patient to discuss exercise restrictions with health care professional before exertion.
- Hypertension: Encourage patient to comply with other interventions for hypertension (weight reduction, low-sodium diet, smoking cessation, moderation of alcohol consumption, regular exercise, and stress management). Medication controls but does not cure hypertension.
- Instruct patient and family in proper technique for monitoring BP. Advise patient to take BP weekly and to report significant changes to health care professional.

Evaluation/Desired Outcomes

- Decrease in BP.
- Decrease in frequency and severity of anginal attacks.
- Decrease in need for nitrate therapy.
- Increase in activity tolerance and sense of well-being.
- Reduction in risk of hospitalization for angina or coronary revascularization in patients with recently documented coronary artery disease.

amoxicillin (a-mox-i-sill-in)
Amoxil, ✸ Novamoxin, Trimox
Classification
Therapeutic: anti-infectives, antiulcer agents
Pharmacologic: aminopenicillins

Indications

Treatment of: Skin and skin structure infections, Otitis media, Sinusitis, Respiratory infections, Genitourinary infections. Endocarditis prophylaxis. Postexposure inhalational anthrax prophylaxis. Management of ulcer disease due to *Helicobacter pylori*. **Unlabeled Use:** Lyme disease.

Action

Binds to bacterial cell wall, causing cell death. **Therapeutic Effects:** Bactericidal action; spectrum is broader than penicillins. **Spectrum:** Active against: Streptococci, Pneumococci, Enterococci, *Haemophilus influenzae*, *Escherichia coli*, *Proteus mirabilis*, *Neisseria meningitidis*, *N. gonorrhoeae*, *Shigella*, *Chlamydia trachomatis*, *Salmonella*, *Borrelia burgdorferi*, *H. pylori*.

Pharmacokinetics

Absorption: Well absorbed from duodenum (75–90%). More resistant to acid inactivation than other penicillins.

Distribution: Diffuses readily into most body tissues and fluids. CSF penetration increased when meninges are inflamed. Crosses placenta; enters breast milk in small amounts.

Metabolism and Excretion: 70% excreted unchanged in the urine; 30% metabolized by the liver.

Half-life: Neonates: 3.7 hr; Infants and Children: 1–2 hr; Adults: 0.7–1.4 hr.

TIME/ACTION PROFILE (plasma concentrations)

ROUTE	ONSET	PEAK	DURATION
PO	30 min	1–2 hr	8–12 hr

Contraindications/Precautions

Contraindicated in: Hypersensitivity to penicillins (cross-sensitivity exists to cephalosporins and other beta-lactams).

Use Cautiously in: Severe renal impairment (↓ dose if CCr <30 mL/min); Infectious mononucleosis, acute lymphocytic leukemia, or cytomegalovirus infection (↑ risk of rash).

Adverse Reactions/Side Effects

Derm: <u>rash</u>, ACUTE GENERALIZED EXANTHEMATOUS PUSTULOSIS, DRUG REACTION WITH EOSINOPHILIA AND SYSTEMIC SYMPTOMS, STEVENS-JOHNSON SYNDROME, TOXIC EPIDERMAL NECROLYSIS, urticaria. **GI:** <u>diarrhea</u>, ↑ liver enzymes, CLOSTRIDIOIDES DIFFICILE-ASSOCIATED DIARRHEA (CDAD), nausea, vomiting. **Hemat:** blood dyscrasias. **Neuro:** SEIZURES (high doses). **Misc:** HYPERSENSITIVITY REACTIONS (including anaphylaxis), SERUM SICKNESS, superinfection.

Interactions

Drug-Drug: Probenecid ↓ renal excretion and ↑ blood levels of amoxicillin—therapy may be combined for this purpose. May ↑ effect of **warfarin**. May ↓ effectiveness of **oral contraceptives**. **Allopurinol** may ↑ frequency of rash.

Route/Dosage

Most Infections

PO (Adults): 250–500 mg every 8 hr *or* 500–875 mg every 12 hr (not to exceed 2–3 g/day).

PO (Children >3 mo): 25–50 mg/kg/day in divided doses every 8 hr *or* 25–50 mg/kg/day in divided doses every 12 hr; *Acute otitis media due to highly resistant strains of S. pneumoniae:* 80–90 mg/kg/day in divided doses every 12 hr; *Postexposure inhalational anthrax prophylaxis:* <40 kg: 45 mg/kg/day in divided doses every 8 hr; >40 kg: 500 mg every 8 hr.

PO (Infants ≤3 mo and neonates): 20–30 mg/kg/day in divided doses every 12 hr.

Renal Impairment

PO (Adults): *CCr 10–30 mL/min:* 250–500 mg every 12 hr; *CCr <10 mL/min:* 250–500 mg every 24 hr.

Helicobacter pylori

PO (Adults): *Triple therapy:* 1000 mg amoxicillin twice daily with lansoprazole 30 mg twice daily and clarithromycin 500 mg twice daily for 14 days *or* 1000 mg amoxicillin twice daily with omeprazole 20 mg twice daily and clarithromycin 500 mg twice daily for 14 days *or* amoxicillin 1000 mg twice daily with esomeprazole 40 mg daily and clarithromycin 500 mg twice daily for 10 days. *Dual therapy:* 1000 mg amoxicillin three times daily with lansoprazole 30 mg three times daily for 14 days.

Endocarditis Prophylaxis

PO (Adults): 2 g 1 hr prior to procedure.
PO (Children): 50 mg/kg 1 hr prior to procedure (not to exceed adult dose).

Gonorrhea

PO (Adults and Children ≥40 kg): 3 g as a single dose.
PO (Children >2 yr and <40 kg): 50 mg/kg with probenecid 25 mg/kg as a single dose.

Availability (generic available)

Capsules: 250 mg, 500 mg. **Tablets:** 500 mg, 875 mg. **Chewable tablets (cherry, banana, peppermint flavors):** 125 mg, 250 mg. **Powder for oral suspension (strawberry [125 mg/5 mL] and bubblegum [200 mg/5 mL, 250 mg/5 mL, 400 mg/5 mL] flavors):** 125 mg/5 mL, 200 mg/5 mL, 250 mg/5 mL, 400 mg/5 mL. *In combination with:* clarithromycin and lansoprazole in a compliance package; omeprazole and clarithromycin (Omeclamox-Pak); omeprazole and rifabutin (Talicia); clarithromycin and vonoprazan in a compliance package (Voquenza Triple Pak); vonoprazan in a compliance package (Voquenza Dual Pak). See Appendix N.

NURSING IMPLICATIONS

Assessment

- Assess for infection (vital signs; appearance of wound, sputum, urine, and stool; WBC) at beginning of and throughout therapy.

- Obtain a history before initiating therapy to determine previous use of and reactions to penicillins or cephalosporins. Persons with a negative history of penicillin sensitivity may still have an allergic response.
- Monitor for signs and symptoms of anaphylaxis (rash, pruritus, laryngeal edema, wheezing). Notify health care professional immediately if these occur.
- Obtain specimens for culture and sensitivity prior to therapy. First dose may be given before receiving results.
- Monitor bowel function. Diarrhea, abdominal cramping, fever, and bloody stools should be reported to health care professional promptly as a sign of CDAD. May begin up to several wk following cessation of therapy.

Lab Test Considerations
- May cause ↑ serum alkaline phosphatase, LDH, AST, and ALT concentrations.
- May cause false-positive direct Coombs' test result.

Implementation

- **PO:** Administer around the clock. May be given without regard to meals or with meals to decrease GI side effects. Capsule contents may be emptied and swallowed with liquids.
- Shake oral suspension before administering. Suspension may be given straight or mixed in formula, milk, fruit juice, water, or ginger ale. Administer immediately after mixing. Discard refrigerated reconstituted suspension after 10 days.

Patient/Family Teaching

- Instruct patients to take medication around the clock and to finish the drug completely as directed, even if feeling better. Advise patients that sharing of this medication may be dangerous.
- Pedi: Teach parents or caregivers to calculate and measure doses accurately. Reinforce importance of using measuring device supplied by pharmacy or with product, not household items.
- Advise patient to report the signs of superinfection (furry overgrowth on the tongue, vaginal itching or discharge, loose or foul-smelling stools) and allergy.
- Instruct patient to notify health care professional immediately if diarrhea, abdominal cramping, fever, or bloody stools occur and not to treat with antidiarrheals without consulting health care professional.
- Instruct the patient to notify health care professional if symptoms do not improve.
- Teach patients with a history of rheumatic heart disease or valve replacement the importance of using antimicrobial prophylaxis before invasive medical or dental procedures.
- Rep: Caution female patients taking oral contraceptives to use an alternate or additional nonhormonal method of contraception during therapy with amoxicillin and until next menstrual period.

Evaluation/Desired Outcomes

- Resolution of the signs and symptoms of infection. Length of time for complete resolution depends on the organism and site of infection.
- Endocarditis prophylaxis.
- Eradication of *H. pylori* with resolution of ulcer symptoms.
- Prevention of inhalational anthrax (postexposure).

amoxicillin/clavulanate
(a-mox-i-**sill**-in/klav-yoo-**lan**-ate)
Augmentin, Augmentin ES,
✤ Clavulin
Classification
Therapeutic: anti-infectives
Pharmacologic: aminopenicillins/beta-lactamase inhibitors

Indications

Treatment of a variety of infections including: Skin and skin structure infections, Otitis media, Sinusitis, Respiratory tract infections, Genitourinary tract infections.

Action

Binds to bacterial cell wall, causing cell death; spectrum of amoxicillin is broader than penicillin. Clavulanate resists action of beta-lactamase, an enzyme produced by bacteria that is capable of inactivating some penicillins. **Therapeutic Effects:** Bactericidal action against susceptible bacteria. **Spectrum:** Active against: Streptococci, Pneumococci, Enterococci, *Haemophilus influenzae*, *Escherichia coli*, *Proteus mirabilis*, *Neisseria meningitidis*, *N. gonorrhoeae*, *Staphylococcus aureus*, *Klebsiella pneumoniae*, *Shigella*, *Salmonella*, *Moraxella catarrhalis*.

Pharmacokinetics

Absorption: Well absorbed from the duodenum (75–90%). More resistant to acid inactivation than other penicillins.
Distribution: Diffuses readily into most body tissues and fluids. Does not readily enter brain/CSF; CSF penetration is ↑ in the presence of inflamed meninges. Crosses the placenta and enters breast milk in small amounts.
Metabolism and Excretion: 70% excreted unchanged in the urine; 30% metabolized by the liver.
Half-life: 1–1.3 hr.

TIME/ACTION PROFILE (peak blood levels)

ROUTE	ONSET	PEAK	DURATION
PO	30 min	1–2 hr	8–12 hr

Contraindications/Precautions

Contraindicated in: Hypersensitivity to penicillins or clavulanate; Suspension and chewable tablets contain aspartame and should be avoided in phenylketonurics; History of amoxicillin/clavulanate-associated cholestatic jaundice.
Use Cautiously in: Severe renal impairment (dose ↓ necessary); Infectious mononucleosis (↑ risk of rash); Hepatic impairment (dose cautiously, monitor liver function).

Adverse Reactions/Side Effects

Derm: rash, ACUTE GENERALIZED EXANTHEMATOUS PUSTULOSIS, DRUG REACTION WITH EOSINOPHILIA AND SYSTEMIC SYMPTOMS, STEVENS-JOHNSON SYNDROME, TOXIC EPIDERMAL NECROLYSIS, urticaria. **GI:** diarrhea, CLOSTRIDIOIDES DIFFICILE-ASSOCIATED DIARRHEA (CDAD), hepatic impairment, nausea, vomiting. **GU:** vaginal candidiasis. **Hemat:** blood dyscrasias. **Neuro:** SEIZURES (high doses). **Misc:** ALLERGIC REACTIONS (including anaphylaxis and serum sickness), superinfection.

Interactions

Drug-Drug: Probenecid ↓ renal excretion and ↑ blood levels of amoxicillin—therapy may be combined for this purpose. May ↑ the effect of **warfarin**. Concurrent **allopurinol** therapy ↑ risk of rash. May ↓ the effectiveness of **hormonal contraceptives**.
Drug-Food: Clavulanate absorption is ↓ by a **high fat meal**.

Route/Dosage

Most Infections (Dosing based on amoxicillin component)
PO (Adults and Children >40 kg): 250 mg every 8 hr or 500 mg every 12 hr.

Serious Infections and Respiratory Tract Infections
PO (Adults and Children >40 kg): 875 mg every 12 hr *or* 500 mg every 8 hr; *Acute bacterial sinusitis:* 2000 mg every 12 hr for 10 days as extended release product; *Community-acquired pneumonia:* 2000 mg every 12 hr for 7–10 days as extended release product.

Recurrent/persistent acute otitis media due to Multidrug-resistant *Streptococcus pneumoniae*, *H. influenzae*, or *M. catarrhalis*
PO (Children <40 kg): 80–90 mg/kg/day in divided doses every 12 hr for 10 days (as ES formulation only).

Renal Impairment
PO (Adults): *CCr 10–30 mL/min:* 250–500 mg every 12 hr (do not use 875 mg tablet); *CCr <10 mL/ min:* 250–500 mg every 24 hr.

Otitis Media, Sinusitis, Lower Respiratory Tract Infections, Serious Infections
PO (Children ≥3 mo): *200 mg/5 mL or 400 mg/5 mL suspension:* 45 mg/kg/day divided every 12 hr; *125 mg/5 mL or 250 mg/5 mL suspension:* 40 mg/kg/day divided every 8 hr.

✤ = Canadian drug name. ⚄ = Genetic implication. ~~Strikethrough~~ = Discontinued. CAPITALS = life-threatening. <u>Underline</u> = most frequent.

Less Serious Infections

PO (Children ≥3 mo): *200 mg/5 mL or 400 mg/5 mL suspension:* 25 mg/kg/day divided every 12 hr *or* 20 mg/kg/day divided every 8 hr (as 125 mg/5 mL or 250 mg/5 mL suspension).
PO (Children <3 mo): 15 mg/kg every 12 hr (125 mg/mL suspension recommended).

Availability (generic available)

Immediate-release tablets: 250 mg amoxicillin with 125 mg clavulanate, 500 mg amoxicillin with 125 mg clavulanate, 875 mg amoxicillin with 125 mg clavulanate. **Chewable tablets (cherry-banana flavor):** 200 mg amoxicillin with 28.5 mg clavulanate, 400 mg amoxicillin with 57 mg clavulanate. **Extended-release tablets (scored):** 1000 mg amoxicillin with 62.5 mg clavulanate. **Powder for oral suspension (200 mg/5 mL is fruit flavor; 250 mg/5 mL is orange flavor; 400 mg/5 mL is fruit flavor; 600 mg/5 mL is orange or strawberry-creme flavor):** 200 mg amoxicillin with 28.5 mg clavulanate/5 mL, 250 mg amoxicillin with 62.5 mg clavulanate/5 mL, 400 mg amoxicillin with 57 mg clavulanate/5 mL, 600 mg amoxicillin with 42.9 mg clavulanate/5 mL (ES formulation).

NURSING IMPLICATIONS

Assessment

- Assess for infection (vital signs; appearance of wound, sputum, urine, and stool; WBC) at beginning of and during therapy.
- Obtain a history before initiating therapy to determine previous use of and reactions to penicillins or cephalosporins. Persons with a negative history of penicillin sensitivity may still have an allergic response.
- Observe for signs and symptoms of anaphylaxis (rash, pruritus, laryngeal edema, wheezing). Notify health care professional immediately if these occur.
- Obtain specimens for culture and sensitivity prior to therapy. First dose may be given before receiving results.
- Monitor bowel function. Diarrhea, abdominal cramping, fever, and bloody stools should be reported to health care professional promptly as a sign of CDAD. May begin up to several wk following cessation of therapy.

Lab Test Considerations

- May cause ↑ serum alkaline phosphatase, LDH, AST, and ALT concentrations. Elderly men and patients receiving prolonged treatment are at ↑ risk for hepatic impairment.
- May cause false-positive direct Coombs' test result.

Implementation

- **PO:** Administer around the clock. Administer at the start of a meal to enhance absorption and to de-

crease GI side effects. Do not administer with high fat meals; clavulanate absorption is decreased. Extended-release tablet is scored and can be broken for ease of administration. Capsule contents may be emptied and swallowed with liquids. Chewable tablets should be crushed or chewed before swallowing with liquids. Shake oral suspension before administering. Refrigerated reconstituted suspension should be discarded after 10 days.

- Two 250-mg tablets are not bioequivalent to one 500-mg tablet; 250-mg tablets and 250-mg chewable tablets are also not interchangeable. Two 500-mg tablets are not interchangeable with one 1000-mg extended release tablet; amounts of clavulanic acid and durations of action are different. Augmentin ES 600 (600 mg/5 mL) does not contain the same amount of clavulanic acid as any of the other Augmentin suspensions. Suspensions are not interchangeable.
- **Pedi:** Do not administer 250-mg chewable tablets to children <40 kg due to clavulanate content. Children <3 mo should receive the 125-mg/5 mL oral solution.

Patient/Family Teaching

- Instruct patients to take medication around the clock and to finish the drug completely as directed, even if feeling better. Advise patients that sharing of this medication may be dangerous.
- **Pedi:** Teach parents or caregivers to calculate and measure doses accurately. Reinforce importance of using measuring device supplied by pharmacy or with product, not household items.
- Advise patient to report the signs of superinfection (furry overgrowth on the tongue, vaginal itching or discharge, loose or foul-smelling stools) and allergy.
- Instruct patient to notify health care professional immediately if diarrhea, abdominal cramping, fever, or bloody stools occur and not to treat with antidiarrheals without consulting health care professionals.
- Instruct the patient to notify health care professional if symptoms do not improve or if nausea or diarrhea persists when drug is administered with food.
- **Rep:** Instruct females of reproductive potential taking oral contraceptives to use an alternate or additional method of contraception during therapy and until next menstrual period; may decrease effectiveness of hormonal contraceptives. Advise patient to notify health care professional if pregnancy is planned or suspected or if breastfeeding.

Evaluation/Desired Outcomes

- Resolution of the signs and symptoms of infection. Length of time for complete resolution depends on the organism and site of infection.

amphetamine mixtures
(am-**fet**-a-meen)
Adderall, Adderall XR, Mydayis
Classification
Therapeutic: central nervous system stimulants

Schedule II

Indications
Attention-deficit/hyperactivity disorder (ADHD). Narcolepsy.

Action
Causes release of norepinephrine from nerve endings. Pharmacologic effects are: CNS and respiratory stimulation, Vasoconstriction, Mydriasis (pupillary dilation). **Therapeutic Effects:** Increased motor activity, mental alertness, and decreased fatigue in narcoleptic patients. Increased attention span in ADHD.

Pharmacokinetics
Absorption: Well absorbed after oral administration.
Distribution: Widely distributed in body tissues, with high concentrations in the brain and CSF.
Metabolism and Excretion: Some metabolism by the liver. Urinary excretion is pH-dependent. Alkaline urine promotes reabsorption and prolongs action.
Half-life: *Children 6–12 yrs:* 9–11 hr; *Adults:* 10–13 hr (depends on urine pH).

TIME/ACTION PROFILE (CNS stimulation)

ROUTE	ONSET	PEAK	DURATION
PO	tablet: 0.5–1 hr	tablet: 3 hr capsule: 7 hr	4–6 hr

Contraindications/Precautions
Contraindicated in: Hypersensitivity; Hyperexcitable states including hyperthyroidism; Psychotic personalities; Concurrent use or use within 14 days of monoamine oxidase (MAO) inhibitors or MAO-like drugs (linezolid or methylene blue); Suicidal or homicidal tendencies; Chemical dependence; Glaucoma; Structural cardiac abnormalities (may ↑ the risk of sudden death); End-stage renal disease; Lactation: Lactation.
Use Cautiously in: Cardiovascular disease (sudden death has occurred in children with structural cardiac abnormalities or other serious heart problems); History of substance use disorder (misuse may result in serious cardiovascular events/sudden death); Hypertension; Diabetes mellitus; Tourette's syndrome (may exacerbate tics); Severe renal impairment (↓ dose); OB: Use during pregnancy only if potential maternal benefit justifies potential fetal risk; may lead to premature delivery and low birth weight infants; Geri: Older adults may be more susceptible to side effects.

Adverse Reactions/Side Effects
CV: <u>palpitations</u>, <u>tachycardia</u>, cardiomyopathy (↑ with prolonged use or high doses), hypertension, hypotension, peripheral vasculopathy, SUDDEN DEATH. **Derm:** alopecia, urticaria. **EENT:** blurred vision, mydriasis. **Endo:** growth inhibition (with long term use in children). **GI:** <u>anorexia</u>, constipation, cramps, diarrhea, dry mouth, intestinal ischemia, nausea, vomiting. **GU:** libido changes, erectile dysfunction, priapism. **MS:** RHABDOMYOLYSIS. **Neuro:** <u>hyperactivity</u>, insomnia, restlessness, tremor, aggression, anger, behavioral disturbances, dizziness, dysgeusia, hallucinations, headache, irritability, mania, paresthesia, skin picking, talkativeness, thought disorder, tics. **Misc:** HYPERSENSITIVITY REACTIONS (including anaphylaxis and angioedema), psychological dependence.

Interactions
Drug-Drug: Concurrent use with **MAO inhibitors** or **MAO-inhibitor-like drugs**, such as **linezolid** or **methylene blue** may result in serious, potentially fatal reactions; wait at least 14 days following discontinuation of MAO inhibitor before initiation of amphetamine mixtures. Drugs that affect serotonergic neurotransmitter systems, including **MAO inhibitors**, **tricyclic antidepressants**, **selective serotonin reuptake inhibitors**, **serotonin/norepinephrine reuptake inhibitors**, **fentanyl**, **buspirone**, **tramadol**, **lithium**, and **triptans** ↑ risk of serotonin syndrome. ↑ adrenergic effects with other **adrenergics** or **thyroid preparations**. Drugs that alkalinize urine (**sodium bicarbonate**, **acetazolamide**) ↓ excretion, ↑ effects. Drugs that acidify urine (large doses of **ascorbic acid**) ↑ excretion, ↓ effects. ↑ risk of hypertension and bradycardia with **beta blockers**. ↑ risk of arrhythmias with **digoxin**. Tricyclic antidepressants may ↑ effect of amphetamine but may ↑ risk of arrhythmias, hypertension, or hyperpyrexia. **Proton pump inhibitors** may ↑ effects.
Drug-Natural Products: Use with **St. John's wort** may ↑ risk of serotonin syndrome.
Drug-Food: Foods that alkalinize the urine (fruit juices) can ↑ effect of amphetamine.

Route/Dosage
Dose is expressed in total amphetamine content (amphetamine + dextroamphetamine).

Attention-Deficit/Hyperactivity Disorder
PO (Adults): *Immediate-release tablets:* 5 mg 1–2 times daily; may ↑ daily dose in 5–mg increments at weekly intervals; usual dose range = 5–40 mg/day in 1–3 divided doses. *Extended-release capsules (Adderall XR):* 20 mg once daily; *Extended-release capsules (Mydayis):* 12.5–25 mg once daily in the morning upon awakening; may ↑ daily dose in 12.5–mg increments at weekly intervals. (maximum dose = 50 mg/day).

PO (Children ≥13 yr): *Immediate-release tablets:* 5 mg 1–2 times daily; may ↑ daily dose in 5–mg increments at weekly intervals; usual dose range = 5–40 mg/day in 1–3 divided doses. *Extended-release capsules (Adderall XR):* 10 mg once daily in the morning; may ↑ to 20 mg once daily in the morning after 1 wk; *Extended-release capsules (Mydayis):* 12.5 mg once daily in the morning upon awakening; may ↑ daily dose in 12.5–mg increments at weekly intervals (maximum dose = 25 mg/day).

PO (Children 6–12 yr): *Immediate-release tablets:* 5 mg 1–2 times daily; may ↑ daily dose in 5–mg increments at weekly intervals; usual dose range = 5–40 mg/day in 1–3 divided doses. *Extended-release capsules (Adderall XR):* 5–10 mg once daily in the morning; may ↑ daily dose in 5–10–mg increments at weekly intervals (maximum dose = 30 mg/day).

PO (Children 3–5 yr): *Immediate-release tablets:* 2.5 mg once daily in the morning; may ↑ daily dose in 2.5–mg increments at weekly intervals; usual dose range = 2.5–40 mg/day in 1–3 divided doses.

Renal Impairment

PO (Adults): *GFR 15–29 mL/min/1.73 m²:* Extended-release capsules (Adderall XR) — 15 mg once daily in the morning; Extended–release capsules (Mydayis) — 12.5 mg once daily in the morning upon awakening; may ↑ daily dose in 12.5–mg increments at weekly intervals (maximum dose = 25 mg/day).

Renal Impairment

(Children ≥13 yr): *GFR 15–29 mL/min/1.73 m²:* Extended–release capsules (Mydayis) — 12.5 mg once daily in the morning upon awakening (maximum dose = 12.5 mg/day).

Renal Impairment

(Children ≥6 yr): *GFR 15–29 mL/min/1.73 m²:* Extended–release capsules (Adderall XR) — 5 mg once daily in the morning (maximum dose = 20 mg/day in children 6–12 yrs).

Narcolepsy

PO (Adults and Children ≥13 yr): *Immediate-release tablets:* 10 mg once daily in the morning; may ↑ daily dose in 10–mg increments at weekly intervals; usual dosage range = 5–60 mg/day in 1–3 divided doses.

PO (Children 6–12 yr): *Immediate-release tablets:* 5 mg once daily; may ↑ daily dose in 5–mg increments at weekly intervals; usual dose range = 5–60 mg/day in 1–3 divided doses.

Availability (generic available)

Amount is expressed in total amphetamine content (amphetamine + dextroamphetamine).
Immediate-release tablets: 5 mg, 7.5 mg, 10 mg, 12.5 mg, 15 mg, 20 mg, 30 mg. **Extended-release capsules (Adderall XR):** 5 mg, 10 mg, 15 mg, 20 mg, 25 mg, 30 mg. **Extended-release capsules (Mydayis):** 12.5 mg, 25 mg, 37.5 mg, 50 mg.

NURSING IMPLICATIONS

Assessment

- Monitor BP, pulse, and respiration before and periodically during therapy. Obtain a history (including assessment of family history of sudden death or ventricular arrhythmia), physical exam to assess for cardiac disease, and further evaluation (ECG and echocardiogram), if indicated. If exertional chest pain, unexplained syncope, or other cardiac symptoms occur, evaluate promptly.
- May produce a false sense of euphoria and well-being. Provide frequent rest periods and observe patient for rebound depression after the effects of the medication have worn off.
- Monitor closely for behavior change during therapy.
- Assess for risk of abuse before starting therapy. Monitor for signs and symptoms of abuse (increased heart rate, respiratory rate, blood pressure, sweating, dilated pupils, hyperactivity, restlessness, insomnia, decreased appetite, loss of coordination, tremors, flushed skin, vomiting, abdominal pain, anxiety, psychosis, hostility, aggression, suicidal or homicidal ideation) during therapy. Has high dependence and abuse potential. Tolerance to medication occurs rapidly; do not increase dose.
- Assess infants born to mothers taking amphetamines for symptoms of withdrawal (feeding difficulties, irritability, agitation, excessive drowsiness).
- **ADHD:** Monitor weight biweekly and height periodically and inform health care professional of significant loss.
- Assess child's attention span, impulse control, and interactions with others. Therapy may be interrupted at intervals to determine whether symptoms are sufficient to continue therapy.
- **Narcolepsy:** Observe and document frequency of narcoleptic episodes.

Lab Test Considerations

- May interfere with urinary steroid determinations.
- May cause ↑ plasma corticosteroid concentrations; greatest in evening.

Implementation

- *High Alert:* Do not confuse Adderall with Adderall XR.
- **PO:** Administer in the morning to prevent insomnia. May be taken without regard to food. Individualize dose to therapeutic needs and response of patient. Use the lowest effective dose.
- Administer short acting doses 4–6 hr apart.
- *DNC:* Extended-release capsules may be swallowed whole or opened and sprinkled on applesauce; swallow contents without chewing. Applesauce should be swallowed immediately; do not store. Do not divide contents of capsule; entire contents of capsule should be taken.
- **ADHD:** Pedi: When symptoms are controlled, dose reduction or interruption of therapy may be possible during summer months or may be given on each of

the 5 school days, with medication-free weekends and holidays.

Patient/Family Teaching

● Instruct patient to take medication once in the early morning as directed. With extended release capsule, avoid afternoon doses to prevent insomnia. Omit missed doses and resume schedule next day. Do not double doses. Discuss safe use, risks, and proper storage and disposal of amphetamines with patients and caregivers with each Rx. Advise patient and parents to read the *Medication Guide* prior to starting therapy and with each Rx refill in case of changes. Instruct patient not to alter dose without consulting health care professional. Abrupt cessation of high doses may cause extreme fatigue and mental depression.

● Advise patient that amphetamine mixtures are drugs with known abuse potential. Protect them from theft, and never give to anyone other than the individual for whom they were prescribed. Store out of sight and reach of children, and in a location not accessible by others. Amphetamine mixtures are a federally controlled substance (CII) because it can be abused or lead to dependence. Keep this medication in a safe place to prevent misuse and abuse. Selling or giving away amphetamines may harm others, and is against the law.

● Caution patients to inform health care professional if they have ever abused or been dependent on alcohol or drugs, or if they are now abusing or dependent on alcohol or drugs.

● Inform patient that the effects of drug-induced dry mouth can be minimized by rinsing frequently with water or chewing sugarless gum or candies.

● Advise patient to limit intake of foods that alkalinize the urine (fruit juices).

● May impair judgment. Advise patient to use caution when driving or during other activities requiring alertness until response to medication is known.

● Advise patient to notify health care professional of all Rx or OTC medications, vitamins, or herbal products being taken and to consult with health care professional before taking other medications, especially St. John's wort.

● Inform patient that periodic holidays from the drug may be used to assess progress and decrease dependence. Pedi: Children should be given a drug-free holiday each yr to reassess symptoms and treatment. Doses will change as children age due to pharmacokinetic changes such as slower hepatic metabolism. If reduced appetite and weight loss occur, advise parents to provide high calorie meals when drug levels are low (at breakfast and or bedtime).

● Advise patient and/or parents to notify health care professional of behavioral changes (new or worse behavior and thought problems, bipolar illness, or aggressive behavior or hostility; new psychotic symptoms such as hearing voices, believing things that are not true, are suspicious, or new manic symptoms).

● Advise patient to notify health care professional if symptoms of heart problems (chest pain, shortness of breath, fainting), nervousness, restlessness, insomnia, dizziness, anorexia, or dry mouth becomes severe.

● Inform patients of risk of peripheral vasculopathy. Instruct patients to notify health care professional of any new numbness; pain; skin color change from pale, to blue, to red; or coolness or sensitivity to temperature in fingers or toes, and call if unexplained wounds appear on fingers or toes.

● Rep: Advise patient to notify health care professional if pregnancy is planned or suspected, and to avoid breastfeeding. May cause birth complications. Amphetamines cause vasoconstriction and may decrease placental perfusion and can stimulate uterine contractions, increasing risk of premature delivery and low birth weight. Monitor infants born to mothers taking amphetamines for symptoms of withdrawal (feeding difficulties, irritability, agitation, excessive drowsiness). Enroll women exposed to amphetamine mixtures during pregnancy by calling the National Pregnancy Registry for Psychiatric Medications at 1-866-961-2388 or online at https://womensmentalhealth.org/clinical-and-research-programs/pregnancyregistry/othermedications/.

● Emphasize the importance of routine follow-up exams to monitor progress.

● **Home Care Issues:** Advise parents to notify school nurse of medication regimen.

Evaluation/Desired Outcomes

● Improved attention span in patients with ADHD.

● Increased motor activity, mental alertness, and decreased fatigue in patients with narcolepsy.

ampicillin/sulbactam
(am-pi-**sil**-in/sul-**bak**-tam)
   Unasyn
Classification
Therapeutic: anti-infectives
Pharmacologic: aminopenicillins/beta-lactamase inhibitors

Indications

Treatment of the following infections: Skin and skin structure infections, soft-tissue infections, Otitis media, Intra-abdominal infections, Sinusitis, Respiratory infections, Genitourinary infections, Meningitis, Septicemia.

Action

Binds to bacterial cell wall, resulting in cell death; spectrum is broader than that of penicillin. Addition of sulbactam increases resistance to beta-lactamases, enzymes produced by bacteria that may inactivate ampicillin. **Therapeutic Effects:** Bactericidal action. **Spectrum:** Active against: Streptococci, Pneumococci, Enterococci, *Haemophilus influenzae, Escherichia coli, Proteus mirabilis, Neisseria meningitidis, N. gonorrhoeae, Shigella, Salmonella, Bacteroides fragilis, Moraxella catarrhalis.* Use should be reserved for infections caused by beta-lactamase–producing strains.

Pharmacokinetics
Absorption: Well absorbed from IM sites.
Distribution: Ampicillin diffuses readily into bile, blister and tissue fluids. Poor CSF penetration unless meninges are inflamed.
Metabolism and Excretion: Ampicillin is variably metabolized by the liver (12–50%). Renal excretion is also variable. Sulbactam is eliminated unchanged in urine.
Protein Binding: *Ampicillin:* 28%; *sulbactam:* 38%.
Half-life: *Ampicillin:* 1–1.8 hr; *sulbactam:* 1–1.3 hr.

TIME/ACTION PROFILE (plasma concentrations)

ROUTE	ONSET	PEAK	DURATION
IM	rapid	1 hr	6–8 hr
IV	immediate	end of infusion	6–8 hr

Contraindications/Precautions
Contraindicated in: Hypersensitivity to penicillins or sulbactam; History of cholestatic jaundice or hepatic impairment with ampicillin/sulbactam.
Use Cautiously in: Severe renal impairment (↓ dosage if CCr <30 mL/min); Epstein-Barr virus infection, acute lymphocytic leukemia, or cytomegalovirus infection (↑ risk of rash); OB: Safety not established in pregnancy; Lactation: Use while breastfeeding only if potential maternal benefit justifies potential risk to infant.

Adverse Reactions/Side Effects
Derm: rash, ACUTE GENERALIZED EXANTHEMATOUS PUSTULOSIS, ERYTHEMA MULTIFORME, STEVENS-JOHNSON SYNDROME, TOXIC EPIDERMAL NECROLYSIS, urticaria. **GI:** diarrhea, cholestasis, CLOSTRIDIOIDES DIFFICILE-ASSOCIATED DIARRHEA (CDAD), HEPATOTOXICITY, nausea, vomiting. **Hemat:** blood dyscrasias. **Local:** pain at injection site, phlebitis. **Neuro:** SEIZURES (high doses). **Misc:** HYPERSENSITIVITY REACTIONS (including anaphylaxis and myocardial ischemia [with or without mi]), superinfection.

Interactions
Drug-Drug: Probenecid ↓ renal excretion and ↑ levels of ampicillin—therapy may be combined for this purpose. May potentiate the effect of **warfarin**. Concurrent **allopurinol** therapy (↑ risk of rash). May ↓ levels and effectiveness of **hormonal contraceptives**.

Route/Dosage
Dosage based on ampicillin component.
IM, IV (Adults and Children ≥40 kg): 1–2 g ampicillin every 6–8 hr (not to exceed 12 g ampicillin/day).
IM, IV (Children ≥1 yr): 100–200 mg ampicillin/kg/day divided every 6 hr; *Meningitis:* 200–400 mg ampicillin/kg/day divided every 6 hr; maximum dose: 8 g ampicillin/day.
IM, IV (Infants >1 mo): 100–150 mg ampicillin/kg/day divided every 6 hr.

Renal Impairment
IM, IV (Adults , Children, and Infants): *CCr 15–29 mL/min:* Administer every 12 hr; *CCr 5–14:* Administer every 24 hr.

Availability (generic available)
Powder for injection: 1.5 g/vial (1 g ampicillin with 500 mg sulbactam), 3 g/vial (2 g ampicillin with 1 g sulbactam), 15 g/vial (10 g ampicillin with 5 g sulbactam).

NURSING IMPLICATIONS
Assessment
- Assess patient for infection (vital signs, wound appearance, sputum, urine, stool, and WBCs) at beginning and throughout therapy.
- Obtain a history before initiating therapy to determine previous use of, and reactions to, penicillins or cephalosporins. Persons with a negative history of penicillin sensitivity may still have an allergic response.
- Obtain specimens for culture and sensitivity before therapy. First dose may be given before receiving results.
- Monitor for signs and symptoms of anaphylaxis (rash, pruritus, laryngeal edema, wheezing). Discontinue drug and notify health care professional immediately if these occur. Keep epinephrine, an antihistamine, and resuscitation equipment close by in the event of an anaphylactic reaction.
- Monitor bowel function. Diarrhea, abdominal cramping, fever, and bloody stools should be reported to health care professional promptly as a sign of CDAD. May begin up to several mo following cessation of therapy.
- Monitor for rash, may lead to severe skin reactions.

Lab Test Considerations
- Monitor hepatic function periodically during therapy. May cause ↑ AST, ALT, LDH, bilirubin, alkaline phosphatase, BUN, and serum creatinine.
- May cause ↓ hemoglobin, hematocrit, RBC, WBC, neutrophils, and lymphocytes.
- May cause transient ↓ estradiol, total conjugated estriol, estriol-glucuronide, or conjugated estrone in pregnant women.
- May cause a false-positive Coombs' test result.

Implementation
- **IM:** Reconstitute for IM use by adding 3.2 mL of sterile water or 0.5% or 2% lidocaine HCl to the 1.5-g vial or 6.4 mL to the 3-g vial. Administer within 1

hr of preparation, deep IM into well-developed muscle.

IV Administration

- **IV Push:** *Reconstitution:* Reconstitute 1.5-g vial with 3.2 mL of sterile water for injection and the 3-g vial with 6.4 mL. *Concentration:* 375 mg ampicillin/sulbactam per mL. *Rate:* Administer over at least 10–15 min within 1 hr of reconstitution. More rapid administration may cause seizures.
- **Intermittent Infusion:** *Reconstitution:* Reconstitute vials as per directions above. *Dilution:* Further dilute in 50–100 mL of 0.9% NaCl, D5W, D5/0.45% NaCl, or LR. Stability of solution varies from 2–8 hr at room temperature or 3–72 hr if refrigerated, depending on concentration and diluent. *Concentration:* Final concentration of infusion should be 3–45 mg of ampicillin/sulbactam per mL. *Rate:* Infuse over 15–30 min.
- **Y-Site Compatibility:** alemtuzumab, amifostine, aminocaproic acid, anidulafungin, argatroban, azithromycin, bivalirudin, bleomycin, cangrelor, carboplatin, carmustine, cefepime, cisplatin, cyclophosphamide, cytarabine, dactinomycin, daptomycin, dexmedetomidine, dexrazoxane, docetaxel, doxorubicin liposomal, eptifibatide, etoposide, etoposide phosphate, filgrastim, fludarabine, fluorouracil, foscarnet, fosphenytoin, gemcitabine, granisetron, hydromorphone, ifosfamide, irinotecan, leucovorin calcium, levofloxacin, linezolid, mesna, methotrexate, metronidazole, milrinone, mitomycin, octreotide, oxaliplatin, paclitaxel, palonosetron, pamidronate, pantoprazole, pemetrexed, potassium acetate, remifentanil, rituximab, rocuronium, sodium acetate, telavancin, thiotepa, tigecycline, tirofiban, trastuzumab, vecuronium, vinblastine, vincristine, voriconazole, zoledronic acid.
- **Y-Site Incompatibility:** acyclovir, amiodarone, amphotericin B deoxycholate, amphotericin B lipid complex, amphotericin B liposomal, azathioprine, caspofungin, chlorpromazine, ciprofloxacin, dacarbazine, dantrolene, daunorubicin hydrochloride, diazepam, diazoxide, dobutamine, doxorubicin hydrochloride, doxycycline, epirubicin, ganciclovir, haloperidol, hydralazine, hydrocortisone, hydroxyzine, idarubicin, lansoprazole, lorazepam, methylprednisolone, midazolam, mitoxantrone, mycophenolate, nicardipine, ondansetron, papaverine, pentamidine, phenytoin, prochlorperazine, promethazine, protamine, sargramostim, topotecan, tranexamic acid, trimethoprim/sulfamethoxazole, verapamil, vinorelbine, If aminoglycosides and penicillins must be given concurrently, administer in separate sites at least 1 hr apart.

Patient/Family Teaching

- Advise patient to report rash, signs of superinfection (furry overgrowth on the tongue, vaginal itching or discharge, loose or foul-smelling stools) and allergy.

- Caution patient to notify health care professional if fever and diarrhea occur, especially if stool contains blood, pus, or mucus. Advise patient not to treat diarrhea without consulting health care professional. May occur up to several wk after discontinuation of medication.
- Rep: Caution patients taking oral contraceptives to use an alternative or additional nonhormonal method of contraception while taking ampicillin/sulbactam and until next menstrual period. Advise patient to notify health care professional if pregnancy is planned or suspected or if breastfeeding.
- Instruct the patient to notify health care professional if symptoms do not improve.

Evaluation/Desired Outcomes

- Resolution of signs and symptoms of infection. Length of time for complete resolution depends on the organism and site of infection.

anastrozole (a-nass-troe-zole)
Arimidex
Classification
Therapeutic: antineoplastics
Pharmacologic: aromatase inhibitors

Indications

Adjuvant treatment of postmenopausal hormone receptor-positive early breast cancer. Initial therapy in women with postmenopausal hormone receptor-positive or hormone receptor unknown, locally advanced, or metastatic breast cancer. Advanced postmenopausal breast cancer in women with disease progression despite tamoxifen therapy.

Action

Inhibits the enzyme aromatase, which is partially responsible for conversion of precursors to estrogen. **Therapeutic Effects:** Lowers levels of circulating estrogen, which may halt progression of estrogen-sensitive breast cancer.

Pharmacokinetics

Absorption: 83–85% absorbed following oral administration.
Distribution: Unknown.
Metabolism and Excretion: 85% metabolized by the liver; 11% excreted renally.
Half-life: 50 hr.

TIME/ACTION PROFILE (lowering of serum estradiol)

ROUTE	ONSET	PEAK	DURATION
PO	within 24 hr	14 days	6 days†

†Following cessation of therapy.

Contraindications/Precautions

Contraindicated in: OB: Pregnancy; Lactation: Lactation.

Use Cautiously in: Ischemic heart disease; Rep: Women of reproductive potential; Pedi: Safety and effectiveness not established in children.

Adverse Reactions/Side Effects

CV: angina, MI, peripheral edema. **Derm:** hot flashes, rash, sweating. **EENT:** pharyngitis. **F and E:** hypercalcemia. **GI:** nausea, abdominal pain, anorexia, constipation, diarrhea, dry mouth, vomiting. **GU:** ↓ fertility (females), pelvic pain, vaginal bleeding, vaginal dryness. **Metab:** ↑ weight, hypercholesterolemia. **MS:** back pain, arthritis, bone pain, carpal tunnel syndrome, fracture, myalgia. **Neuro:** headache, weakness, dizziness., paresthesia. **Resp:** cough, dyspnea. **Misc:** pain, HYPERSENSITIVITY REACTIONS (including anaphylaxis and angiooedema).

Interactions

Drug-Drug: None reported.

Route/Dosage

PO (Adults): 1 mg once daily.

Availability (generic available)

Tablets: 1 mg.

NURSING IMPLICATIONS

Assessment

* Assess patient for pain and other side effects periodically during therapy.

Lab Test Considerations

* Obtain a negative pregnancy test before starting therapy. May cause ↑ GGT, AST, ALT, alkaline phosphatase, total cholesterol, and LDL cholesterol levels.

Implementation

* **PO:** Take medication consistently with regard to food.

Patient/Family Teaching

* Instruct patient to take medication as directed. Take missed doses as soon as remembered unless it is almost time for next dose. Do not double doses. Advise patient to read the *Patient Information* leaflet before starting and with each Rx refill; changes may occur.
* Inform patient of potential for adverse reactions, and advise patient to notify health care professional immediately if allergic reactions (swelling of the face, lips, tongue, and/or throat, difficulty in swallowing and/or breathing), liver problems (general feeling of not being well, yellowing of skin or whites of eyes, pain on the right side of abdomen), skin reactions (lesions, ulcers, or blisters), or chest pain occurs.
* Advise patient that vaginal bleeding may occur during first few wk after changing over from other hormonal therapy. Continued bleeding should be evaluated.

* Teach patient to report increase in pain so treatment can be initiated.
* Rep: May cause fetal harm. Advise female patients of reproductive potential to use effective contraception during and for at least 3 wk after last dose of therapy, to avoid breastfeeding for at least 2 wk after last dose, and to notify health care professional immediately if pregnancy is planned or suspected. May impair female fertility.

Evaluation/Desired Outcomes

* Slowing of disease progression in women with advanced breast cancer.

⚙ ANGIOTENSIN-CONVERTING ENZYME (ACE) INHIBITORS

benazepril (ben-**aye**-ze-pril)
  Lotensin
captopril (**kap**-toe-pril)
  ~~Capoten~~
enalapril/enalaprilat
  (e-**nal**-a-pril/e-**nal**-a-pril-at)
  Epaned, Vasotec, ✷ Vasotec IV
fosinopril (foe-**sin**-oh-pril)
  ~~Monopril~~
lisinopril (lyse-**in**-oh-pril)
  ~~Prinivil~~, Qbrelis, Zestril
moexipril (moe-**eks**-i-pril)
  ~~Univasc~~
perindopril (pe-**rin**-do-pril)
  ~~Aceon~~, ✷ Coversyl
quinapril (**kwin**-a-pril)
  Accupril
ramipril (ra-**mi**-pril)
  Altace
trandolapril (tran-**doe**-la-pril)
  ✷ Mavik

Classification
Therapeutic: antihypertensives
Pharmacologic: ACE inhibitors

Indications

Hypertension (as monotherapy or in combination with other antihypertensives). **Captopril, enalapril, fosinopril, lisinopril, quinapril, ramipril, trandolapril:** HF. **Captopril, lisinopril, ramipril, trandolapril:** Reduction of risk of death or development of HF following MI. **Enalapril:** Slowed progression of left ventricular dysfunction into overt HF. **Ramipril:** Reduction of the risk of MI, stroke, and death from cardiovascular disease in patients at risk (>55 yr old with a history of CAD, stroke, peripheral vascular disease, or diabetes with another cardiovascular risk factor). **Captopril:** ↓ progression of diabetic nephropathy. **Perindopril:** Reduction of risk of death from cardiovascular causes or nonfatal MI in patients with stable CAD.

A

Action

ACE inhibitors block the conversion of angiotensin I to the vasoconstrictor angiotensin II. ACE inhibitors also prevent the degradation of bradykinin and other vasodilatory prostaglandins. ACE inhibitors also ↑ plasma renin levels and ↓ aldosterone levels. Net result is systemic vasodilation. **Therapeutic Effects:** Lowering of BP in hypertensive patients. Improved symptoms in patients with HF (selected agents only). ↓ development of overt heart failure (enalapril only). Improved survival and ↓ development of overt HF after MI (selected agents only). ↓ risk of death from cardiovascular causes or MI in patients with stable CAD (perindopril only). ↓ risk of MI, stroke or death from cardiovascular causes in high-risk patients (ramipril only). ↓ progression of diabetic nephropathy (captopril only).

Pharmacokinetics

Absorption: *Benazepril:* 37% absorbed after oral administration. *Captopril:* 60–75% absorbed after oral administration (↓ by food). *Enalapril:* 55–75% absorbed after oral administration. *Enalaprilat:* IV administration results in complete bioavailability. *Fosinopril:* 36% absorbed after oral administration. *Lisinopril:* 25% absorbed after oral administration (much variability). *Moexipril:* 13% bioavailability as moexiprilat after oral administration (↓ by food). *Perindopril:* 25% bioavailability as perindoprilat after oral administration. *Quinapril:* 60% absorbed after oral administration (high-fat meal may ↓ absorption). *Ramipril:* 50–60% absorbed after oral administration. *Trandolapril:* 70% bioavailability as trandolapril at after oral administration.

Distribution: All ACE inhibitors cross the placenta. *Benazepril, captopril, enalapril, fosinopril, quinapril,* and *trandolapril:* Enter breast milk. *Lisinopril:* Minimal penetration of CNS. *Ramipril:* Probably does not enter breast milk. *Trandolapril:* Enters breast milk.

Protein Binding: *Benazepril:* 95%, *Fosinopril:* 99.4%, *Moexipril:* 90%, *Quinapril:* 97%.

Metabolism and Excretion: *Benazepril:* Converted by the liver to benazeprilat, the active metabolite. 20% excreted by kidneys; 11–12% nonrenal (biliary elimination). *Captopril:* 50% metabolized by the liver to inactive compounds, 50% excreted unchanged by the kidneys. *Enalapril, enalaprilat:* Enalapril is converted by the liver to enalaprilat, the active metabolite; primarily eliminated by the kidneys. *Fosinopril:* Converted by the liver and GI mucosa to fosinoprilat, the active metabolite— 50% excreted in urine, 50% in feces. *Lisinopril:* 100% eliminated by the kidneys. *Moexipril:* Converted by liver and GI mucosa to moexiprilat, the active metabolite; 13% excreted in urine, 53% in feces. *Perindopril:* Converted by the liver to perindoprilat, the active metabolite; primarily excreted in urine. *Quinapril:* Converted by the liver, GI mucosa, and tissue to quinaprilat, the active metabolite: 96% eliminated by the kid-

neys. *Ramipril:* Converted by the liver to ramiprilat, the active metabolite; 60% excreted in urine, 40% in feces. *Trandolapril:* Converted by the liver to trandolaprilat, the active metabolite; 33% excreted in urine, 66% in feces.

Half-life: *Benazeprilat:* 10–11 hr. *Captopril:* 2 hr (↑ in renal impairment). *Enalapril:* 2 hr (↑ in renal impairment). *Enalaprilat:* 35–38 hr (↑ in renal impairment). *Fosinoprilat:* 12 hr. *Lisinopril:* 12 hr (↑ in renal impairment). *Moexiprilat:* 2–9 hr (↑ in renal impairment). *Perindoprilat:* 3–10 hr (↑ in renal impairment). *Quinaprilat:* 3 hr (↑ in renal impairment). *Ramiprilat:* 13–17 hr (↑ in renal impairment). *Trandolaprilat:* 22.5 hr (↑ in renal impairment).

TIME/ACTION PROFILE (effect on BP— single dose†)

ROUTE	ONSET	PEAK	DURATION
Benazepril	within 1 hr	2–4 hr	24 hr
Captopril	15–60 min	60–90 min	6–12 hr
Enalapril PO	1 hr	4–8 hr	12–24 hr
Enalapril IV	15 min	1–4 hr	4–6 hr
Fosinopril	within 1 hr	2–6 hr	24 hr
Lisinopril	1 hr	6 hr	24 hr
Moexipril	within 1 hr	3–6 hr	up to 24 hr
Perindoprilat	within 1–2 hr	3–7 hr	up to 24 hr
Quinapril	within 1 hr	2–4 hr	up to 24 hr
Ramipril	within 1–2 hr	3–6 hr	24 hr
Trandolapril	within 1–2 hr	4–10 hr	up to 24 hr

†Full effects may not be noted for several wks.

Contraindications/Precautions

Contraindicated in: Hypersensitivity; History of angioedema with previous use of ACE inhibitors (also in absence of previous use of ACE inhibitors for benazepril); Concurrent use with aliskiren in patients with diabetes or moderate to severe renal impairment (CCr <60 mL/min); Concurrent use with sacubitril/valsartan; must be a 36-hr washout period after switching to/from sacubitril/valsartan; OB: Pregnancy; Lactation: Lactation.

Use Cautiously in: Renal impairment, hepatic impairment, hypovolemia, hyponatremia, concurrent diuretic therapy; ⚎ Black patients with hypertension (monotherapy less effective, may require additional therapy; ↑ risk of angioedema); Rep: Women of reproductive potential; Surgery/anesthesia (hypotension may be exaggerated); Pedi: Safety and effectiveness not established in children <18 yr (moexipril, perindopril, quinapril ramipril, trandolapril) or <6 yr (benazepril, fosinopril, lisinopril); Geri: Initial dose ↓ recommended for most agents in older adults due to age-related ↓ in renal function.

Exercise Extreme Caution in: Family history of angioedema.

Adverse Reactions/Side Effects

CV: <u>hypotension</u>, chest pain, edema, tachycardia. **Derm:** flushing, pruritus, rashes. **Endo:** hyperuricemia. **F and E:** hyperkalemia. **GI:** taste disturbances, abdominal pain, anorexia, constipation, diarrhea, nausea, vomiting. **GU:** erectile dysfunction, proteinuria, renal dysfunction, renal failure. **Hemat:** AGRANULOCYTOSIS, neutropenia (captopril only). **MS:** back pain, muscle cramps, myalgia. **Neuro:** dizziness, drowsiness, fatigue, headache, insomnia, vertigo, weakness. **Resp:** cough, dyspnea. **Misc:** ANGIOEDEMA, fever.

Interactions

Drug-Drug: Concurrent use with **sacubitril** ↑ risk of angioedema; concurrent use contraindicated; do not administer within 36 hr of switching to/from **sacubitril/valsartan**. Excessive hypotension may occur with concurrent use of **diuretics** and other **antihypertensives**. ↑ risk of hyperkalemia with concurrent use of **potassium supplements**, **potassium-sparing diuretics**, or **potassium-containing salt substitutes**. ↑ risk of hyperkalemia, renal dysfunction, hypotension, and syncope with concurrent use of **angiotensin II receptor blockers** or **aliskiren**; avoid concurrent use with aliskiren in patients with diabetes or CCr <60 mL/min; avoid concurrent use with angiotensin II receptor blockers. **NSAIDs** and selective **COX-2 inhibitors** may blunt the antihypertensive effect and ↑ the risk of renal dysfunction. Absorption of fosinopril may be ↓ by **antacids** (separate administration by 1–2 hr). ↑ levels and may ↑ risk of **lithium** toxicity. Quinapril may ↓ absorption of **tetracycline**, **doxycycline**, and **fluoroquinolones** (because of magnesium in tablets). ↑ risk of angioedema with **temsirolimus**, **sirolimus**, or **everolimus**.

Drug-Food: Food significantly ↓ absorption of captopril and moexipril (administer drugs 1 hr before meals).

Route/Dosage

Benazepril

ℨ **PO (Adults):** 10 mg once daily, ↑ gradually to maintenance dose of 20–40 mg/day in 1–2 divided doses (begin with 5 mg/day in patients receiving diuretics).
PO (Children ≥6 yr): 0.2 mg/kg once daily; may be titrated up to 0.6 mg/kg/day (or 40 mg/day).

Renal Impairment
PO (Adults): *CCr <30 mL/min:* Initiate therapy with 5 mg once daily.

Renal Impairment
PO (Children ≥6 yr): *CCr <30 mL/min:* Contraindicated.

Captopril

PO (Adults): *Hypertension:* 12.5–25 mg 2–3 times daily, may be ↑ at 1–2 wk intervals up to 150 mg 3 times daily (begin with 6.25–12.5 mg 2–3 times daily in patients receiving diuretics) (maximum dose = 450 mg/day); *HF:* 25 mg 3 times daily (6.25–12.5 mg 3 times daily in patients who have been vigorously diuresed); titrated up to target dose of 50 mg 3 times daily; *Post-MI:* 6.25-mg test dose, followed by 12.5 mg

3 times daily, may be ↑ up to 50 mg 3 times daily; *Diabetic nephropathy:* 25 mg 3 times daily.
PO (Children): *HF:* 0.3–0.5 mg/kg/dose 3 times daily, titrate up to a maximum of 6 mg/kg/day in 2–4 divided doses; *Older Children:* 6.25–12.5 mg/dose every 12–24 hr, titrate up to a maximum of 6 mg/kg/day in 2–4 divided doses.
PO (Infants): *HF:* 0.15–0.3 mg/kg/dose, titrate up to a maximum of 6 mg/kg/day in 1–4 divided doses.
PO (Neonates): *HF:* 0.05–0.1 mg/kg/dose every 8–24 hr, may ↑ as needed up to 0.5 mg/kg every 6–24 hr; *Premature neonates:* 0.01 mg/kg/dose every 8–12 hr.

Renal Impairment
PO (Adults): *CCr 10–50 mL/min:* Administer 75% of dose; *CCr <10 mL/min:* Administer 50% of dose.

Enalapril/Enalaprilat

PO (Adults): *Hypertension:* 2.5–5 mg once daily, ↑ as required up to 40 mg/day in 1–2 divided doses (initiate therapy at 2.5 mg once daily in patients receiving diuretics); *HF:* 2.5 mg 1–2 times daily, titrated up to target dose of 10 mg twice daily; begin with 2.5 mg once daily in patients with hyponatremia (serum sodium <130 mEq/L); *Asymptomatic left ventricular dysfunction:* 2.5 mg twice daily, titrated up to a target dose of 10 mg twice daily.
PO (Children >1 mo): *Hypertension:* 0.08 mg/kg once daily; may be slowly titrated up to a maximum of 0.58 mg/kg/day.
IV (Adults): *Hypertension:* 0.625–1.25 mg (0.625 mg if receiving diuretics) every 6 hr; can be titrated up to 5 mg every 6 hr.
IV (Children >1 mo): *Hypertension:* 5–10 mcg/kg/dose given every 8–24 hr.

Renal Impairment
PO, IV (Adults): *Hypertension CCr 10–50 mL/min:* Administer 75% of dose; *CCr <10 mL/min:* Administer 50% of dose.

Renal Impairment
PO, IV (Children >1 mo): *CCr <30 mL/min:* Contraindicated.

Fosinopril

PO (Adults): *Hypertension:* 10 mg once daily, may be ↑ as required up to 80 mg/day. *HF:* 10 mg once daily (5 mg once daily in patients who have been vigorously diuresed), may be ↑ over several wk up to 40 mg/day.
PO (Children ≥6 yr and >50 kg): *Hypertension:* 5–10 mg once daily.

Lisinopril

PO (Adults): *Hypertension:* 10 mg once daily, can be ↑ up to 20–40 mg/day (initiate therapy at 5 mg/day in patients receiving diuretics); *HF:* 5 mg once daily; may be titrated every 2 wk up to 40 mg/day; begin with 2.5 mg once daily in patients with hyponatremia (serum sodium <130 mEq/L); *Post-MI:* 5 mg once daily for 2 days, then 10 mg daily.

PO (Children ≥6 yr): *Hypertension:* 0.07 mg/kg once daily (up to 5 mg/day), may be titrated every 1–2 wk up to 0.6 mg/kg/day (or 40 mg/day).

Renal Impairment
PO (Adults): *CCr 10–30 mL/min:* Begin with 5 mg once daily; may be slowly titrated up to 40 mg/day; *CCr <10 mL/min:* Begin with 2.5 mg once daily; may be slowly titrated up to 40 mg/day.

Renal Impairment
(Children ≥6 yr): *CCr <30 mL/min:* Contraindicated.

Moexipril
PO (Adults): 7.5 mg once daily, may be ↑ up to 30 mg/day in 1–2 divided doses (begin with 3.75 mg/day in patients receiving diuretics).

Renal Impairment
PO (Adults): *CCr ≤40 mL/min:* Initiate therapy at 3.75 mg once daily, may be titrated upward carefully to 15 mg/day.

Perindopril
PO (Adults): *Hypertension:* 4 mg once daily, may be slowly titrated up to 16 mg/day in 1–2 divided doses (should not exceed 8 mg/day in elderly patients) (begin with 2–4 mg/day in 1–2 divided doses in patients receiving diuretics); *Stable CAD:* 4 mg once daily for 2 wk, may be ↑, if tolerated, to 8 mg once daily; for elderly patients, begin with 2 mg once daily for 1 wk (may be ↑, if tolerated, to 4 mg once daily for 1 wk, then, ↑ as tolerated to 8 mg once daily).

Renal Impairment
PO (Adults): *CCr 30–60 mL/min:* 2 mg/day initially, may be slowly titrated up to 8 mg/day in 1–2 divided doses.

Quinapril
PO (Adults): *Hypertension:* 10–20 mg once daily initially, may be titrated every 2 wk up to 80 mg/day in 1–2 divided doses (initiate therapy at 5 mg/day in patients receiving diuretics); *HF:* 5 mg twice daily initially, may be titrated at weekly intervals up to 20 mg twice daily.

Renal Impairment
PO (Adults): *CCr >60 mL/min:* Initiate therapy at 10 mg/day; *CCr 30–60 mL/min:* Initiate therapy at 5 mg/day; *CCr 10–30 mL/min:* Initiate therapy at 2.5 mg/day.

Ramipril
PO (Adults): *Hypertension:* 2.5 mg once daily, may be ↑ slowly up to 20 mg/day in 1–2 divided doses (initiate therapy at 1.25 mg/day in patients receiving diuretics). *HF post-MI:* 1.25–2.5 mg twice daily initially, may be ↑ slowly up to 5 mg twice daily. *Reduction in risk of MI, stroke, and death from cardiovascular causes:* 2.5 mg once daily for 1 wk, then 5 mg once daily for 3 wk, then ↑ as tolerated to 10 mg once daily (can also be given in 2 divided doses).

Renal Impairment
PO (Adults): *CCr <40 mL/min:* Initiate therapy at 1.25 mg once daily, may be slowly titrated up to 5 mg/day in 1–2 divided doses.

Trandolapril
💰 PO (Adults): *Hypertension:* 1 mg once daily (2 mg once daily in black patients); *HF post-MI:* Initiate therapy at 1 mg once daily, titrate up to 4 mg once daily if possible.

Renal Impairment
PO (Adults): *CCr <30 mL/min:* Initiate therapy at 0.5 mg once daily, may be slowly titrated upward (maximum dose = 4 mg/day).

Hepatic Impairment
PO (Adults): Initiate therapy at 0.5 mg once daily, may be slowly titrated upward (maximum dose = 4 mg/day).

Availability

Benazepril (generic available)
Tablets: 5 mg, 10 mg, 20 mg, 40 mg. *In combination with:* amlodipine (Lotrel) and hydrochlorothiazide (Lotensin HCT). See Appendix N.

Captopril (generic available)
Tablets: 12.5 mg, 25 mg, 50 mg, 100 mg. *In combination with:* hydrochlorothiazide.

Enalapril (generic available)
Tablets: 2.5 mg, 5 mg, 10 mg, 20 mg. **Oral solution (mixed berry flavor):** 1 mg/mL. *In combination with:* hydrochlorothiazide (Vaseretic). See Appendix N.

Enalaprilat (generic available)
Solution for injection: 1.25 mg/mL.

Fosinopril (generic available)
Tablets: 10 mg, 20 mg, 40 mg. *In combination with:* hydrochlorothiazide.

Lisinopril (generic available)
Tablets: 2.5 mg, 5 mg, 10 mg, 20 mg, 30 mg, 40 mg. **Oral solution:** 1 mg/mL. *In combination with:* hydrochlorothiazide (Zestoretic). See Appendix N.

Moexipril (generic available)
Tablets: 7.5 mg, 15 mg.

Perindopril (generic available)
Tablets: 2 mg, 4 mg, 8 mg.

Quinapril (generic available)
Tablets: 5 mg, 10 mg, 20 mg, 40 mg. *In combination with:* hydrochlorothiazide.

Ramipril (generic available)
Capsules: 1.25 mg, 2.5 mg, 5 mg, 10 mg, ❁ 15 mg.

Trandolapril (generic available)
Tablets: ❁ 0.5 mg, 1 mg, 2 mg, 4 mg. *In combination with:* verapamil.

NURSING IMPLICATIONS

Assessment

- **Hypertension:** Monitor BP and pulse frequently during initial dose adjustment and periodically during therapy. Notify health care professional of significant changes.
- Monitor frequency of prescription refills to determine adherence.
- Assess patient for signs of angioedema (swelling of face, extremities, eyes, lips, tongue, difficulty in swallowing or breathing); may occur at any time during therapy. Discontinue medication and provide supportive care.
- **HF:** Monitor weight and assess patient routinely for resolution of fluid overload (peripheral edema, rales/crackles, dyspnea, weight gain, jugular venous distention).

Lab Test Considerations

- Monitor BUN, serum creatinine, and electrolyte levels periodically. Serum potassium, BUN and creatinine may be ↑, whereas sodium levels may be ↓. If ↑ BUN or serum creatinine concentrations occur, dose reduction or withdrawal may be required.
- Monitor CBC periodically during therapy. Certain drugs may rarely cause slight ↓ in hemoglobin and hematocrit, leukopenia, and eosinophilia.
- May cause ↑ AST, ALT, alkaline phosphatase, serum bilirubin, uric acid, and glucose.
- Assess urine protein prior to and periodically during therapy for up to 1 yr in patients with renal impairment or those receiving >150 mg/day of captopril. If excessive or ↑ proteinuria occurs, re-evaluate ACE inhibitor therapy.
- *Captopril:* May cause positive ANA titer.
- *Captopril:* May cause false-positive test results for urine acetone.
- *Captopril:* Monitor CBC with differential prior to initiation of therapy, every 2 wk for first 3 mo, and periodically for up to 1 yr in patients at risk for neutropenia (patients with renal impairment or collagen-vascular disease) or at first sign of infection. Discontinue therapy if neutrophil count is <1000/mm^3.

Implementation

- Do not confuse Accupril with Aciphex. Do not confuse benazepril with Benadryl. Do not confuse captopril with carvedilol. Do not confuse Zestril with Zegerid, Zetia, or Zyprexa.
- Correct volume depletion, if possible, before initiation of therapy.
- **PO:** Precipitous drop in BP during first 1–3 hr after first dose may require volume expansion with normal saline but is not usually considered an indication for stopping therapy. Discontinuing diuretic therapy or cautiously increasing salt intake 2–3 days before initiation may ↓ risk of hypotension. Monitor closely for at least 1 hr after BP has stabilized. Resume diuretics if BP is not controlled.

Benazepril

- **PO:** For patients with difficulty swallowing tablets, pharmacist may compound oral suspension; stable for 30 days if refrigerated. Shake suspension before each use.

Captopril

- **PO:** Administer 1 hr before or 2 hr after meals. May be crushed if patient has difficulty swallowing. Tablets may have a sulfurous odor.
- An oral solution may be prepared by crushing a 25-mg tablet and dissolving it in 25–100 mL of water. Shake for at least 5 min and administer within 30 min.

Enalapril

- **PO:** For patients with difficulty swallowing tablets, oral solution is available ready to use. Shake solution before each use. Solution is stable at controlled room temperature for 60 days.

Enalaprilat

IV Administration

- **IV Push:** *Dilution:* May be administered undiluted. *Concentration:* 1.25 mg/mL. *Rate:* Administer over at least 5 min.
- **Intermittent Infusion:** *Dilution:* Dilute in up to 50 mL of D5W, 0.9% NaCl, D5/0.9% NaCl, or D5/LR. Diluted solution is stable for 24 hr. *Rate:* Administer as a slow infusion over at least 5 min.
- **Y-Site Compatibility:** acyclovir, alemtuzumab, allopurinol, amifostine, amikacin, aminocaproic acid, aminophylline, amiodarone, amphotericin B lipid complex, amphotericin B liposomal, anidulafungin, argatroban, arsenic trioxide, ascorbic acid, atropine, azathioprine, azithromycin, aztreonam, benztropine, bivalirudin, bleomycin, bumetanide, buprenorphine, butorphanol, calcium chloride, calcium gluconate, cangrelor, carboplatin, carmustine, cefazolin, cefotaxime, cefotetan, cefoxitin, ceftaroline, ceftazidime, ceftriaxone, cefuroxime, chloramphenicol, chlorpromazine, cisatracurium, cisplatin, cladribine, clindamycin, cyanocobalamin, cyclophosphamide, cyclosporine, cytarabine, dacarbazine, dactinomycin, daptomycin, daunorubicin hydrochloride, dexamethasone, dexmedetomidine, dexrazoxane, digoxin, diltiazem, diphenhydramine, dobutamine, docetaxel, dopamine, doxorubicin hydrochloride, doxorubicin liposomal, doxycycline, ephedrine, epinephrine, epirubicin, epoetin alfa, eptifibatide, ertapenem, erythromycin, esmolol, etoposide, etoposide phosphate, famotidine, fentanyl, filgrastim, fluconazole, fludarabine, fluorouracil, folic acid, foscarnet, fosphenytoin, furosemide, ganciclovir, gemcitabine, gentamicin, glycopyrrolate, granisetron, heparin, hetastarch, hydrocortisone, hydromorphone, idarubicin, ifosfamide, imipenem/cilastatin, indomethacin, insulin, regular, irinotecan, isoproterenol, ketorolac, labetalol, lactated Ringer's, leucovorin calcium, levofloxacin, lidocaine, linezo-

lid, lorazepam, magnesium sulfate, mannitol, melphalan, meperidine, meropenem, mesna, methadone, methotrexate, methylprednisolone, metoclopramide, metoprolol, metronidazole, midazolam, milrinone, mitomycin, mitoxantrone, morphine, moxifloxacin, multivitamins, mycophenolate, nafcillin, nalbuphine, naloxone, nicardipine, nitroglycerin, nitroprusside, norepinephrine, octreotide, ondansetron, oxacillin, oxaliplatin, oxytocin, paclitaxel, palonosetron, pamidronate, papaverine, pemetrexed, penicillin G, pentamidine, pentobarbital, phenobarbital, phentolamine, phenylephrine, phytonadione, piperacillin/tazobactam, potassium acetate, potassium chloride, potassium phosphate, procainamide, prochlorperazine, promethazine, propofol, propranolol, protamine, pyridoxine, remifentanil, rituximab, rocuronium, sodium acetate, sodium bicarbonate, succinylcholine, sufentanil, tacrolimus, tetracycline, theophylline, thiamine, thiotepa, tigecycline, tirofiban, tobramycin, topotecan, trastuzumab, vancomycin, vasopressin, vecuronium, verapamil, vinblastine, vincristine, vinorelbine, voriconazole, zoledronic acid.

- **Y-Site Incompatibility:** amphotericin B deoxycholate, caspofungin, cefepime, dantrolene, diazepam, diazoxide, gemtuzumab ozogamicin, phenytoin.

Lisinopril
- **PO:** Oral solution is clear to slightly opalescent. Administer without dilution.

Moexipril
- **PO:** Administer moexipril on an empty stomach, 1 hr before a meal.

Ramipril
- **PO:** Capsules may be opened and sprinkled on applesauce, or dissolved in 4 oz water or apple juice for patients with difficulty swallowing. Effectiveness is same as capsule. Prepared mixtures can be stored for up to 24 hr at room temperature or up to 48 hr if refrigerated.

Trandolapril
- **PO:** May be taken with or without food.

Patient/Family Teaching
- Instruct patient to take medication as directed at the same time each day, even if feeling well. Take missed doses as soon as possible but not if almost time for next dose. Do not double doses. Warn patient not to discontinue ACE inhibitor therapy unless directed by health care professional.
- Caution patient to avoid salt substitutes or foods containing high levels of potassium or sodium unless directed by health care professional (see Appendix J).
- Caution patient to change positions slowly to minimize hypotension. Use of alcohol, standing for long periods, exercising, and hot weather may ↑ orthostatic hypotension. Instruct patient to notify health care professional of all Rx or OTC medications, vitamins, or herbal products being taken and consult health care professional before taking any new medications, especially cough, cold, or allergy remedies.
- May cause dizziness. Caution patient to avoid driving and other activities requiring alertness until response to medication is known.
- Advise patient to inform health care professional of medication regimen prior to treatment or surgery.
- Advise patient that medication may cause impairment of taste that generally resolves within 8–12 wk, even with continued therapy.
- Instruct patient to notify health care professional immediately if rash; mouth sores; sore throat; fever; swelling of hands or feet; irregular heart beat; chest pain; dry cough; hoarseness; swelling of face, eyes, lips, or tongue; difficulty swallowing or breathing occur; or if taste impairment or skin rash persists. Persistent dry cough may occur and may not subside until medication is discontinued. Consult health care professional if cough becomes bothersome. Also notify health care professional if nausea, vomiting, or diarrhea occurs and continues.
- Advise diabetic patients to monitor blood glucose closely, especially during first mo of therapy; may cause hypoglycemia.
- Rep: May cause fetal harm. Advise females of reproductive potential to use effective contraception during therapy and notify health care professional if pregnancy is planned or suspected. If pregnancy is detected, discontinue medication as soon as possible. Closely observe infants with histories of in utero exposure to ACE inhibitors for hypotension, oliguria, and hyperkalemia. If oliguria or hypotension occur, support blood pressure and renal perfusion. Exchange transfusions or dialysis may be required as a means of reversing hypotension and substituting for disordered renal function. Advise patient to avoid breastfeeding during therapy.
- Emphasize the importance of follow-up examinations to monitor progress.
- **Hypertension:** Encourage patient to comply with additional interventions for hypertension (weight reduction, low sodium diet, discontinuation of smoking, moderation of alcohol consumption, regular exercise, and stress management). Medication controls but does not cure hypertension.
- Instruct patient and family on correct technique for monitoring BP. Advise them to check BP at least weekly and to report significant changes to health care professional.

Evaluation/Desired Outcomes
- Decrease in BP without appearance of excessive side effects.
- Decrease in signs and symptoms of HF (some drugs may also improve survival).

🍁 = Canadian drug name. 🜨 = Genetic implication. ~~Strikethrough~~ = Discontinued. CAPITALS = life-threatening. <u>Underline</u> = most frequent.

- Decrease in development of overt HF (enalapril).
- Reduction of risk of death or development of HF following MI.
- Reduction of risk of death from cardiovascular causes and MI in patients with stable CAD (perindopril).
- Reduction of risk of MI, stroke, or death from cardiovascular causes in patients at high-risk for these events (ramipril).
- Decrease in progression of diabetic nephropathy (captopril).

⚡ ANGIOTENSIN II RECEPTOR ANTAGONISTS

azilsartan (a-zill-**sar**-tan)
  Edarbi
candesartan (can-de-**sar**-tan)
  Atacand
irbesartan (ir-be-**sar**-tan)
  Avapro
losartan (loe-**sar**-tan)
  Cozaar
olmesartan (ole-me-**sar**-tan)
  Benicar, ✿ Olmetec
telmisartan (tel-mi-**sar**-tan)
  Micardis
valsartan (val-**sar**-tan)
  Diovan
Classification
Therapeutic: antihypertensives
Pharmacologic: angiotensin II receptor antagonists

Indications

Hypertension (as monotherapy or in combination with other antihypertensives). Diabetic nephropathy in patients with type 2 diabetes and hypertension (irbesartan and losartan only). HF (New York Heart Association class II-IV) in patients who cannot tolerate ACE inhibitors (candesartan and valsartan only) or in combination with an ACE inhibitor and beta-blocker (candesartan only). Prevention of stroke in patients with hypertension and left ventricular hypertrophy (losartan only). Reduction of risk of death from cardiovascular causes in patients with left ventricular systolic dysfunction after MI (valsartan only). Reduction of risk of myocardial infarction, stroke, or cardiovascular death in patients ≥55 yr who are at high risk for cardiovascular events and are unable to take ACE inhibitors (telmisartan only).

Action

Blocks vasoconstrictor and aldosterone-producing effects of angiotensin II at receptor sites, including vascular smooth muscle and the adrenal glands. **Therapeutic Effects:** Lowering of BP. Slowed progression of diabetic nephropathy (irbesartan and losartan only). Reduced cardiovascular death and hospitalizations due to HF in patients with HF (candesartan and valsartan only). Decreased risk of cardiovascular death in patients with left ventricular systolic dysfunction who are post-MI (valsartan only). Decreased risk of stroke in patients with hypertension and left ventricular hypertrophy (effect may be less in black patients) (losartan only).

Pharmacokinetics

Absorption: *Azilsartan:* Azilsartan medoxomil is converted to azilsartan, the active component. 60% absorbed; *Candesartan:* Candesartan cilexetil is converted to candesartan, the active component; 15% bioavailability of candesartan; *Irbesartan:* 60–80% absorbed after oral administration; *Losartan:* well absorbed, with extensive first-pass hepatic metabolism, resulting in 33% bioavailability; *Olmesartan:* Olmesartan medoxomil is converted to olmesartan, the active component; 26% bioavailability of olmesartan; *Telmisartan:* 42–58% absorbed following oral administration (bioavailability ↑ in patients with hepatic impairment); *Valsartan:* 10–35% absorbed following oral administration; systemic exposure 60% higher with the oral solution compared to tablets.

Distribution: All angiotensin receptor blockers (ARBs) cross the placenta; *Candesartan:* enters breast milk.

Protein Binding: All ARBs are >90% protein-bound.

Metabolism and Excretion: *Azilsartan:* 50% metabolized by the liver, primarily by the CYP2C9 enzyme system. 55% eliminated in feces, 42% in urine (15% as unchanged drug); *Candesartan:* Minor metabolism by the liver; 33% excreted in urine, 67% in feces (via bile); *Irbesartan:* Some hepatic metabolism; 20% excreted in urine, 80% in feces; *Losartan:* Undergoes extensive first-pass hepatic metabolism; 14% is converted to an active metabolite. 4% excreted unchanged in urine; 6% excreted in urine as active metabolite; some biliary elimination; *Olmesartan:* 30–50% excreted unchanged in urine, remainder eliminated in feces via bile; *Telmisartan:* Excreted mostly unchanged in feces via biliary excretion; *Valsartan:* Minor metabolism by the liver; 13% excreted in urine, 83% in feces.

Half-life: *Azilsartan:* 11 hr; *Candesartan:* 9 hr; *Irbesartan:* 11–15 hr; *Losartan:* 2 hr (6–9 hr for metabolite); *Olmesartan:* 13 hr; *Telmisartan:* 24 hr; *Valsartan:* 6 hr.

TIME/ACTION PROFILE (antihypertensive effect with chronic dosing)

DRUG	ONSET	PEAK	DURATION
Azilsartan	within 2 hr	18 hr	24 hr
Candesartan	2–4 hr	4 wk	24 hr
Irbesartan	within 2 hr	2 wk	24 hr
Losartan	6 hr	3–6 wk	24 hr
Olmesartan	within 1 wk	2 wk	24 hr
Telmisartan	within 3 hr	4 wk	24 hr
Valsartan	within 2 hr	4 wk	24 hr

Contraindications/Precautions

Contraindicated in: Hypersensitivity; Concurrent use with aliskiren in patients with diabetes or moderate to severe renal impairment (CCr <60 mL/min); Severe hepatic impairment (candesartan); OB: Pregnancy; Lactation: Lactation.

Use Cautiously in: HF (may result in azotemia, oliguria, acute renal failure, and/or death); Volume- or salt-depleted patients or patients receiving high doses of diuretics (correct deficits before initiating therapy and initiate at lower doses); ☒ Black patients (may not be effective); Impaired renal function due to primary renal disease or HF (may worsen renal function); Obstructive biliary disorders (telmisartan) or hepatic impairment (losartan, telmisartan); Severe renal impairment (CCr <30 mL/min) (valsartan); Rep: Women of reproductive potential; Pedi: Safety and effectiveness not established in children <18 yr (azilsartan, candesartan, irbesartan, telmisartan), <6 yr (losartan, olmesartan), and <1 yr (valsartan).

Adverse Reactions/Side Effects

CV: <u>hypotension</u>, chest pain, edema, tachycardia. **Derm:** rash. **EENT:** nasal congestion, pharyngitis, rhinitis, sinusitis. **F and E:** hyperkalemia. **GI:** abdominal pain, diarrhea, drug-induced hepatitis, dyspepsia, nausea, vomiting. **GU:** impaired renal function. **MS:** arthralgia, back pain, myalgia. **Neuro:** dizziness, anxiety, depression, fatigue, headache, insomnia, weakness. **Misc:** ANGIOEDEMA.

Interactions

Drug-Drug: NSAIDs and selective **COX-2 inhibitors** may blunt the antihypertensive effect and ↑ the risk of renal dysfunction. ↑ antihypertensive effects with other **antihypertensives** and **diuretics**. Telmisartan may ↑ serum **digoxin** levels. Concurrent use of **potassium-sparing diuretics**, **potassium-containing salt substitutes**, or **potassium supplements** may ↑ risk of hyperkalemia. ↑ risk of hyperkalemia, renal dysfunction, hypotension, and syncope with concurrent use of **ACE inhibitors** or **aliskiren**; avoid concurrent use with aliskiren in patients with diabetes or CCr <60 mL/min; avoid concurrent use with ACE inhibitors. Candesartan, valsartan, and irbesartan may ↑ **lithium** levels. Irbesartan and losartan may ↑ effects of **amiodarone**, **fluoxetine**, **glimepiride**, **glipizide**, **phenytoin**, and **warfarin**. **Rifampin** may ↓ effects of losartan. ↑ risk of renal dysfunction when telmisartan used with **ramipril** (concurrent use not recommended). **Colesevelam** may ↓ olmesartan levels; administer olmesartan ≥4 hr before colesevelam.

Route/Dosage

Azilsartan

PO (Adults): 80 mg once daily, initial dose may be ↓ to 40 mg once daily if high doses of diuretics are used concurrently.

Candesartan

PO (Adults): *Hypertension:* 16 mg once daily; may ↑ up to 32 mg/day in 1–2 divided doses (begin therapy at a lower dose in patients who are receiving diuretics or are volume depleted). *HF:* 4 mg once daily initially, dose may be doubled at 2 wk intervals up to target dose of 32 mg once daily.

PO (Children 6–16 yr and >50 kg): 8–16 mg/day (in 1–2 divided doses); may ↑ up to 32 mg/day (in 1–2 divided doses).

PO (Children 6–16 yr and <50 kg): 4–8 mg/day (in 1–2 divided doses); may ↑ up to 16 mg/day (in 1–2 divided doses).

PO (Children 1–5 yr): 0.20 mg/kg/day (in 1–2 divided doses); may ↑ up to 0.4 mg/kg/day (in 1–2 divided doses).

Hepatic Impairment

PO (Adults): *Moderate hepatic impairment:* Initiate at 8 mg once daily.

Irbesartan

PO (Adults): *Hypertension:* 150 mg once daily; may ↑ to 300 mg once daily. Initiate therapy at 75 mg once daily in patients who are receiving diuretics or are volume depleted. *Type 2 diabetic nephropathy:* 300 mg once daily.

Losartan

PO (Adults): *Hypertension:* 50 mg once daily initially (range 25–100 mg/day as a single daily dose or 2 divided doses) (initiate therapy at 25 mg once daily in patients who are receiving diuretics or are volume depleted). *Prevention of stroke in patients with hypertension and left ventricular hypertrophy:* 50 mg once daily initially; hydrochlorothiazide 12.5 mg once daily should be added and/or dose of losartan ↑ to 100 mg once daily followed by an ↑ in hydrochlorothiazide to 25 mg once daily based on BP response. *Type 2 diabetic nephropathy:* 50 mg once daily, may ↑ to 100 mg once daily depending on BP response.

Hepatic Impairment

PO (Adults): 25 mg once daily initially; may ↑ as tolerated.

PO (Children >6 yr): *Hypertension:* 0.7 mg/kg once daily (up to 50 mg/day), may titrate up to 1.4 mg/kg/day (or 100 mg/day).

Renal Impairment

PO (Children >6 yr): *CCr <30 mL/min:* Contraindicated.

Olmesartan

PO (Adults): 20 mg once daily; may ↑ up to 40 mg once daily (patients who are receiving diuretics or are volume-depleted should be started on lower doses).

PO (Children 6–16 yr): ≥*35 kg:* 20 mg once daily; may ↑ after 2 wk up to 40 mg once daily; *20–34.9 kg:* 10 mg once daily; may ↑ after 2 wk up to 20 mg once daily.

Telmisartan

PO (Adults): *Hypertension:* 40 mg once daily (volume-depleted patients should start with 20 mg once daily); may be titrated up to 80 mg/day; *Cardiovascular risk reduction:* 80 mg once daily.

Valsartan

Oral tablets and solution are NOT interchangeable on a mg-per-mg basis. These dosage forms should not be combined to arrive at a particular dose.

PO (Adults): *Hypertension:* 80 mg or 160 mg once daily initially in patients who are not volume-depleted; may ↑ to 320 mg once daily; *HF:* 40 mg twice daily, may be titrated up to target dose of 160 mg twice daily as tolerated; *Post-MI:* 20 mg twice daily (may be initiated ≥ 12 hr after MI); dose may be titrated up to target dose of 160 mg twice daily, as tolerated.

PO (Children 1–16 yr): *Hypertension:* 1 mg/kg once daily (maximum dose = 40 mg/day) (may consider using starting dose of 2 mg/kg once daily if greater BP reduction needed); may ↑ up to 4 mg/kg once daily (maximum dose = 160 mg/day).

Availability

Azilsartan (generic available)
Tablets: 40 mg, 80 mg. *In combination with:* chlorthalidone (Edarbyclor); see Appendix N.

Candesartan (generic available)
Tablets: 4 mg, 8 mg, 16 mg, 32 mg. *In combination with:* hydrochlorothiazide (Atacand HCT); see Appendix N.

Irbesartan (generic available)
Tablets: 75 mg, 150 mg, 300 mg. *In combination with:* hydrochlorothiazide (Avalide); see Appendix N.

Losartan (generic available)
Tablets: 25 mg, 50 mg, 100 mg. *In combination with:* hydrochlorothiazide (Hyzaar); see Appendix N.

Olmesartan (generic available)
Tablets: 5 mg, 20 mg, 40 mg. *In combination with:* hydrochlorothiazide (Benicar HCT); amlodipine (Azor); amlodipine and hydrochlorothiazide (Tribenzor); see Appendix N.

Telmisartan (generic available)
Tablets: 20 mg, 40 mg, 80 mg. *In combination with:* hydrochlorothiazide (Micardis HCT); amlodipine; see Appendix N.

Valsartan (generic available)
Tablets: 40 mg, 80 mg, 160 mg, 320 mg. **Oral solution (grape flavor):** 4 mg/mL. *In combination with:* amlodipine (Exforge); hydrochlorothiazide (Diovan HCT); amlodipine and hydrochlorothiazide (Exforge HCT); see Appendix N.

NURSING IMPLICATIONS

Assessment
- Assess BP (lying, sitting, standing) and pulse periodically during therapy. Notify health care professional of significant changes.
- Monitor frequency of prescription refills to determine adherence.
- Assess patient for signs of angioedema (dyspnea, facial swelling). May rarely cause angioedema.
- **HF:** Monitor daily weight and assess patient routinely for resolution of fluid overload (peripheral edema, rales/crackles, dyspnea, weight gain, jugular venous distention).

Lab Test Considerations
- Monitor renal function and electrolyte levels periodically. Serum potassium, BUN, and serum creatinine may be ↑.
- May cause ↑ AST, ALT, and serum bilirubin (candesartan and olmesartan only).
- May cause ↑ uric acid, slight ↓ in hemoglobin and hematocrit, neutropenia, and thrombocytopenia.

Implementation
- Do not confuse Atacand with antacid. Do not confuse Cozaar with Colace or Zocor.
- Correct volume depletion, if possible, prior to initiation of therapy.
- **PO:** May be administered without regard to meals.

Losartan
- **PO:** For patients with difficulty swallowing tablets, pharmacist can compound oral suspension; stable for 4 wk if refrigerated. Shake suspension before each use.

Valsartan
- For pediatric patients unable to swallow tablets, solution can be prepared by pharmacist. Tablets and suspension are not interchangeable. Do not combine tablets and suspension. Solution should be used for pediatric patients aged 1 to 5 yr, for patients >5 yr of age who cannot swallow tablets and for pediatric patients for whom the calculated dose (mg/kg) does not correspond to the available tablet strengths of valsartan.

Patient/Family Teaching
- Instruct patient to take as medication directed, even if feeling well. Take missed doses as soon as remembered if not almost time for next dose; do not double doses. Instruct patient to take medication at the same time each day. Warn patient not to discontinue therapy unless directed by health care professional.
- Caution patient to avoid salt substitutes containing potassium or food containing high levels of potassium or sodium unless directed by health care professional. See Appendix J.
- Caution patient to avoid sudden changes in position to decrease orthostatic hypotension. Use of alcohol, standing for long periods, exercising, and hot weather may increase orthostatic hypotension.
- May cause dizziness. Caution patient to avoid driving or other activities requiring alertness until response to medication is known.
- Instruct patient to notify health care professional of all Rx or OTC medications, vitamins, or herbal prod-

ucts being taken and consult health care professional before taking any new medications, especially NSAIDs and cough, cold, or allergy remedies.

- Instruct patient to notify health care professional of medication regimen prior to treatment or surgery.
- Instruct patient to notify health care professional immediately if swelling of face, eyes, lips, or tongue occurs, or if difficulty swallowing or breathing occurs.
- Rep: May cause fetal harm. Advise females of reproductive potential to use contraception and notify health care professional if pregnancy is planned or suspected, or if breastfeeding. If pregnancy is detected, discontinue medication as soon as possible. In patients taking during pregnancy, perform serial ultrasound examinations to assess the intra-amniotic environment. Fetal testing may be appropriate, based on the week of gestation. Patients should be aware, however, that oligohydramnios may not appear until after the fetus has sustained irreversible injury. If oligohydramnios is observed, consider alternative drug treatment. Closely observe neonates with histories of in utero exposure to valsartan for hypotension, oliguria, and hyperkalemia. In neonates with a history of in utero exposure to valsartan, if oliguria or hypotension occurs, support blood pressure and renal perfusion. Exchange transfusions or dialysis may be required as a means of reversing hypotension and replacing renal function.
- Emphasize the importance of follow-up exams to evaluate effectiveness of medication.
- **Hypertension:** Encourage patient to comply with additional interventions for hypertension (weight reduction, low-sodium diet, discontinuation of smoking, moderation of alcohol consumption, regular exercise, stress management). Medication controls but dose not cure hypertension.
- Instruct patient and family on proper technique for monitoring BP. Advise them to check BP at least weekly and to report significant changes.

Evaluation/Desired Outcomes
- Decrease in BP without appearance of excessive side effects.
- Slowed progression of diabetic nephropathy (irbesartan, losartan).
- Decreased cardiovascular death and HF-related hospitalizations in patients with HF (candesartan).
- Decreased hospitalizations in patients with HF (valsartan).
- Decreased risk of cardiovascular death in patients with left ventricular systolic dysfunction after MI (valsartan).
- Reduced risk of stroke in patients with hypertension and left ventricular hypertrophy (losartan).
- Reduction of risk of MI, stroke, or cardiovascular death (telmisartan).

anidulafungin
(a-**ni**-du-la-fun-gin)
    Eraxis
Classification
Therapeutic: antifungals
Pharmacologic: echinocandins

Indications
Candidemia and other serious candidal infections including intra-abdominal abscess, peritonitis. Esophageal candidiasis.

Action
Inhibits the synthesis of fungal cell wall. **Therapeutic Effects:** Death of susceptible fungi. **Spectrum:** Active against *Candida albicans*, *C. glabrata*, *C. parapsilosis*, and *C. tropicalis*.

Pharmacokinetics
Absorption: IV administration results in complete bioavailability.
Distribution: Widely distributed to tissues.
Metabolism and Excretion: Undergoes chemical degradation without hepatic metabolism; <1% excreted in urine.
Half-life: 40–50 hr.

TIME/ACTION PROFILE (plasma concentrations)

ROUTE	ONSET	PEAK	DURATION
IV	rapid	end of infusion	24 hr

Contraindications/Precautions
Contraindicated in: Hypersensitivity; Known or suspected hereditary fructose intolerance.
Use Cautiously in: Underlying liver disease (may worsen); OB: Safety not established in pregnancy; other antifungal agents preferred in pregnancy for infections caused by *Candida*; Lactation: Use while breastfeeding only if potential maternal benefit justifies potential risk to infant; Pedi: Safety and effectiveness not established in children <1 mo (candidemia and intra-abdominal abscess and peritonitis caused by *Candida* or <18 yr (esophageal candidiasis); may lead to polysorbate toxicity in low-birth weight infants.

Adverse Reactions/Side Effects
CV: hypotension. **Derm:** flushing, rash, urticaria. **F and E:** hypokalemia. **GI:** ↑ liver enzymes, diarrhea. **Resp:** bronchospasm, dyspnea. **Misc:** ANAPHYLAXIS, infusion reactions.

Interactions
Drug-Drug: None reported.

✸= Canadian drug name. ፠ = Genetic implication. S̶t̶r̶i̶k̶e̶t̶h̶r̶o̶u̶g̶h̶ = Discontinued. CAPITALS = life-threatening. <u>Underline</u> = most frequent.

Route/Dosage

Candidemia and Intra-abdominal Abscess or Peritonitis Caused by *Candida*

IV (Adults): 200 mg loading dose on Day 1, then 100 mg once daily. Continue therapy for ≥14 days after last positive culture.

IV (Children ≥1 mo): 3 mg/kg (max = 200 mg) loading dose on Day 1, then 1.5 mg/kg (max = 100 mg) once daily. Continue therapy for ≥14 days after last positive culture.

Esophageal Candidiasis

IV (Adults): 100 mg loading dose on Day 1, then 50 mg once daily. Continue therapy for a minimum of 14 days and for ≥7 days following resolution of symptoms.

Availability

Lyophilized powder for injection (contains fructose and polysorbate 80): 50 mg/vial, 100 mg/vial.

NURSING IMPLICATIONS

Assessment

- Assess infected area and monitor cultures before and periodically during therapy.
- Obtain specimens for culture before starting therapy. Therapy may be started before results are obtained.
- Monitor for signs and symptoms of anaphylaxis (rash, urticaria, flushing, pruritus, bronchospasm, dyspnea, hypotension); usually related to histamine release. To decrease risk, do not exceed a rate of infusion of 1.1 mg/min.

Lab Test Considerations

- May cause ↑ ALT, AST, alkaline phosphatase, and hepatic enzymes.
- May cause hypokalemia.
- May cause neutropenia and leukopenia.

Implementation

IV Administration

- **Adults: Intermittent Infusion:** *Reconstitution:* Reconstitute each 50 mg vial with 15 mL or the 100 mg vial with 30 mL of sterile water for injection. *Concentration:* 3.33 mg/mL. Stable at room temperature for up to 24 hr. *Adults: Dilution:* Further dilute within 24 hr by transferring contents of reconstituted vial into IV bag of D5W or 0.9% NaCl. For the 50 mg dose, dilute with 50 mL for an infusion volume of 65 mL. For the 100 mg dose, dilute with 100 mL for an infusion volume of 130 mL. For the 200 mg dose, dilute with 200 mL for a total infusion volume of 260 mL. *Concentration:* Final concentration is 0.77 mg/mL. Do not administer solutions that are discolored or contain particulate matter. Solution is stable for up to 48 hr at room temperature. *Rate:* Infuse over at least 45 min for the 50 mg dose, 90 min for the 100 mg dose, or 180 min for the 200 mg dose.

- **Pediatric Patients: Intermittent Infusion:** *Reconstitution:* Reconstitute each vial with sterile water for injection. *Concentration:* 3.33 mg/mL. *Dilution:* Dilute with 0.9% NaCl or D5W. *Concentration:* Final concentration is 0.77 mg/mL. Prepare in infusion syringe or IV infusion bag. *Rate:* Administer at a rate not to exceed 1.1 mg/min (1.4 mL/min or 84 mL/hr).

- **Y-Site Compatibility:** acyclovir, alemtuzumab, allopurinol, amifostine, amikacin, aminophylline, amiodarone, amphotericin B lipid complex, amphotericin B liposomal, ampicillin, ampicillin/sulbactam, argatroban, arsenic trioxide, atracurium, azithromycin, aztreonam, bivalirudin, bleomycin, bumetanide, buprenorphine, busulfan, butorphanol, calcium chloride, calcium gluconate, carboplatin, carmustine, caspofungin, cefazolin, cefepime, cefotaxime, cefotetan, cefoxitin, ceftazidime, ceftriaxone, cefuroxime, chloramphenicol, ciprofloxacin, cisatracurium, cisplatin, clindamycin, cyclophosphamide, cyclosporine, cytarabine, dacarbazine, dactinomycin, daunorubicin hydrochloride, dexamethasone, dexmedetomidine, digoxin, diltiazem, diphenhydramine, dobutamine, docetaxel, dopamine, doxorubicin hydrochloride, doxorubicin liposomal, doxycycline, droperidol, enalaprilat, ephedrine, epinephrine, epirubicin, eptifibatide, erythromycin, esmolol, etoposide, etoposide phosphate, famotidine, fentanyl, fluconazole, fludarabine, fluorouracil, foscarnet, fosphenytoin, furosemide, ganciclovir, gemcitabine, gentamicin, glycopyrrolate, granisetron, haloperidol, heparin, hydralazine, hydrocortisone, hydromorphone, idarubicin, ifosfamide, imipenem/cilastatin, insulin, irinotecan, isoproterenol, ketorolac, labetalol, leucovorin calcium, levofloxacin, linezolid, lorazepam, mannitol, melphalan, meperidine, meropenem, mesna, methotrexate, methylprednisolone, metoclopramide, metoprolol, metronidazole, midazolam, milrinone, mitomycin, mitoxantrone, morphine, mycophenolate, nafcillin, naloxone, nicardipine, nitroglycerin, nitroprusside, norepinephrine, octreotide, ondansetron, oxaliplatin, oxytocin, paclitaxel, palonosetron, pamidronate, pantoprazole, pentamidine, pentobarbital, phenobarbital, phentolamine, phenylephrine, piperacillin/tazobactam, potassium acetate, potassium chloride, procainamide, prochlorperazine, promethazine, propranolol, remifentanil, rocuronium, sodium acetate, succinylcholine, sufentanil, tacrolimus, theophylline, thiopental, thiotepa, tirofiban, tobramycin, topotecan, trimethoprim/sulfamethoxazole, vancomycin, vasopressin, vecuronium, verapamil, vinblastine, vincristine, vinorelbine, voriconazole, zidovudine, zoledronic acid.

- **Y-Site Incompatibility:** amphotericin B deoxycholate, dantrolene, diazepam, ertapenem, magnesium sulfate, nalbuphine, pemetrexed, phenytoin, potassium phosphate, sodium bicarbonate, sodium phosphate.

Patient/Family Teaching

- Explain purpose of medication to patient.
- Instruct patient to notify health care professional if signs and symptoms of anaphylaxis occur or if diarrhea becomes pronounced.
- Inform patient that anidulafungin contains fructose. May be life-threatening when administered to patients with hereditary fructose intolerance.
- Rep: Advise patient to notify health care professional if pregnancy is planned or suspected or if breastfeeding.

Evaluation/Desired Outcomes

- Resolution of clinical and laboratory indications of fungal infections. Duration of therapy should be based on the patients clinical response. Therapy should be continued for at least 14 days after the last positive culture. For esophageal candidiasis, treatment should continue for at least 7 days following resolution of symptoms.

---

anifrolumab (an-i-frol-ue-mab)
   Saphnelo
   Classification
   Therapeutic: none assigned
   Pharmacologic: monoclonal antibodies, interferon receptor antagonists

Indications

Moderate to severe systemic lupus erythematosus (SLE) in patients who are receiving standard therapy.

Action

Monoclonal antibody that binds to subunit 1 of the type I interferon receptor which inhibits type I interferon signaling and reduces inflammatory and immunological processes that occur in SLE. **Therapeutic Effects:** Reduction in SLE disease activity.

Pharmacokinetics

Absorption: IV administration results in complete bioavailability.
Distribution: Not widely distributed to extravascular tissues.
Metabolism and Excretion: Unknown.
Half-life: Unknown.

TIME/ACTION PROFILE (plasma concentrations)

ROUTE	ONSET	PEAK	DURATION
IV	unknown	unknown	unknown

Contraindications/Precautions

Contraindicated in: Hypersensitivity; Active infection; Concurrent use with other biologic therapies.
Use Cautiously in: Chronic infection, history of recurrent infections, or risk factors for infection; Risk

factors for malignancy; OB: Safety not established in pregnancy; Lactation: Safety not established in breastfeeding; Pedi: Safety and effectiveness not established in children.

Adverse Reactions/Side Effects

Resp: cough. **Misc:** INFECTION, HYPERSENSITIVITY REACTIONS (including anaphylaxis and angioedema), infusion-related reactions, MALIGNANCY.

Interactions

Drug-Drug: ↑ risk of adverse reactions and ↓ immune response to **live vaccines** or **live-attenuated vaccines**; avoid concurrent use.

Route/Dosage

IV (Adults): 300 mg every 4 wk.

Availability

Solution for injection: 150 mg/mL.

NURSING IMPLICATIONS

Assessment

- Assess patient for lupus symptoms before starting and periodically during therapy.
- Monitor for signs and symptoms of infections (fever, sore throat, shortness of breath, rash, urinary burning or frequency) during therapy. May require interruption of therapy.
- Monitor for signs and symptoms of hypersensitivity reactions (swelling of face, tongue, or mouth, breathing difficulties, and/or fainting, dizziness, feeling lightheaded) during therapy.

Implementation

- Update immunizations, according to current immunization guidelines, before starting therapy.
- **Intermittent Infusion: *Dilution:*** Solution is clear to opalescent, colorless to slightly yellow; do not administer solutions that are cloudy, discolored, or contain particulate matter. Withdraw and discard 2 mL of solution from a 100 mL 0.9% NaCl infusion bag. Withdraw 2 mL of solution from vial of anifrolumab and add it to infusion bag. Mix the solution by gentle inversion. Do not shake. Administer immediately after mixing. Diluted solution is stable for 4 hr at room temperature and up to 24 hr if refrigerated. Allow solution to reach room temperature before administering. *Rate:* Administer over 30 min through an infusion line containing a sterile, low-protein binding 0.2 or 0.22 micron in-line filter. Flush infusion set with 25 mL of 0.9% NaCl to ensure all solution has been administered.

Patient/Family Teaching

- Explain purpose of anifrolumab to patient. Advise patient to read *Patient Information* before starting anifrolumab and periodically during therapy in case of changes.

- Advise patient to notify health care professional if signs and symptoms of infection (fever or flu-like symptoms; muscle aches; cough; shortness of breath; burning on urination or urinating more often than usual; diarrhea or stomach pain; shingles [a red skin rash that can cause pain and burning]) or hypersensitivity reactions occur.
- Instruct patient to avoid live or live-attenuated vaccines during therapy.
- Instruct patient to notify health care professional of all Rx or OTC medications, vitamins, or herbal products being taken and consult health care professional before taking any new medications.
- Rep: Advise females of reproductive potential to notify health care professional if pregnancy is planned or suspected or if breastfeeding. Inform patient of pregnancy exposure registry monitors pregnancy outcomes in women exposed to anifrolumab during pregnancy. For more information about the registry or to report a pregnancy while on *Saphnelo*, contact AstraZeneca at 1-877-693-9268.

Evaluation/Desired Outcomes

- Decrease in disease activity of SLE.

ANTIFUNGALS (TOPICAL)
butenafine (byoo-**ten**-a-feen)
 Lotrimin Ultra
ciclopirox (sye-kloe-**peer**-ox)
 Ciclodan, Loprox, ~~Penlac~~, ✦Stieprox
clotrimazole (kloe-**trye**-ma-zole)
 Alevazol, ✦Canesten,
 ✦Clotrimaderm, Votriza-AL
econazole (ee-**kon**-a-zole)
 Ecoza
efinaconazole (eff-in-a-**kon**-a-zole)
 Jublia
ketoconazole (kee-toe-**koe**-na-zole)
 Ketodan, ✦Ketoderm
luliconazole (loo-li-**kon**-a-zole)
 Luzu
miconazole (mye-**kon**-a-zole)
 Fungoid, Lotrimin AF, Micatin,
 ✦Micozole, Zeasorb-AF
naftifine (**naff**-ti-feen)
 Naftin
nystatin (nye-**stat**-in)
 ~~Mycostatin~~, Nyamyc, ✦Nyaderm,
 Nystop
oxiconazole (ox-i-**kon**-a-zole)
 Oxistat
sertaconazole (ser-ta-**kon**-a-zole)
 Ertaczo
sulconazole (sul-**kon**-a-zole)
 Exelderm

tavaborole (ta-va-**bor**-ole)
 Kerydin
terbinafine (ter-**bin**-a-feen)
 ✦Lamisil, Lamisil AT
tolnaftate (tol-**naff**-tate)
 Tinactin
Classification
Therapeutic: antifungals (topical)

Indications
Treatment of a variety of cutaneous fungal infections, including cutaneous candidiasis, tinea pedis (athlete's foot), tinea cruris (jock itch), tinea corporis (ringworm), tinea versicolor, seborrheic dermatitis, dandruff, and onychomycosis of fingernails and toenails.

Action
Butenafine, nystatin, clotrimazole, econazole, efinaconazole, ketoconazole, luliconazole, miconazole, naftifine, oxiconazole, sertaconazole, sulconazole, and terbinafine affect the synthesis of the fungal cell wall, allowing leakage of cellular contents. Tolnaftate distorts the hyphae and stunts mycelial growth in fungi. Ciclopirox inhibits the transport of essential elements in the fungal cell, disrupting the synthesis of DNA, RNA, and protein. Tavaborole inhibits fungal protein synthesis via inhibition of aminoacyl-transfer ribonucleic acid (tRNA) synthetase. **Therapeutic Effects:** Decrease in symptoms of fungal infection.

Pharmacokinetics
Absorption: Absorption through intact skin is minimal.
Distribution: Distribution after topical administration is primarily local.
Metabolism and Excretion: Metabolism and excretion not known following local application.
Half-life: *Butenafine:* 35 hr; *Ciclopirox:* 5.5 hr (gel); *Efinaconazole:* 29.9 hr; *Terbinafine:* 21 hr.

TIME/ACTION PROFILE (resolution of symptoms/lesions†)

ROUTE	ONSET	PEAK	DURATION
Butenafine	unknown	up to 4 wk	unknown
Luliconazole	unknown	3–4 wk	unknown
Tolnaftate	24–72 hr	unknown	unknown

† Only the drugs with known information included in this table.

Contraindications/Precautions
Contraindicated in: Hypersensitivity to active ingredients, additives, preservatives, or bases; Some products contain alcohol or bisulfites and should be avoided in patients with known intolerance.
Use Cautiously in: Nail and scalp infections (may require additional systemic therapy); OB, Lactation: Safety not established.

Adverse Reactions/Side Effects
Local: burning, itching, local hypersensitivity reactions, redness, stinging.

Interactions
Drug-Drug: Econazole may ↑ levels of and risk of bleeding from **warfarin**.

Route/Dosage
Butenafine
Topical (Adults and Children >12 yr): Apply once daily for 2 wk for tinea corporis, tinea cruris, or tinea versicolor. Apply once daily for 4 wk or once daily for 7 days for tinea pedis.

Ciclopirox
Topical (Adults and Children >10 yr): *Cream/lotion:* Apply twice daily for 2–4 wk; *Topical solution (nail lacquer):* Apply to nails at bedtime or 8 hr prior to bathing for up to 48 wk. Each daily application should be made over the previous coat and then removed with alcohol every 7 days; *Gel:* Apply twice daily for 4 wk; *Shampoo:* 5–10 mL applied to scalp, lather and leave on for 3 min, rinse; repeat twice weekly for 4 wk (at least 3 days between applications).

Clotrimazole
Topical (Adults and Children >3 yr): Apply twice daily for 1–4 wk.

Econazole
Topical (Adults and Children): Apply once daily for tinea pedis (for 4 wk), tinea cruris (for 2 wk), tinea corporis (for 2 wk), or tinea versicolor (for 2 wk). Apply twice daily for cutaneous candidiasis (for 2 wk).

Efinaconazole
Topical (Adults and Children ≥6 yr): Apply to affected toenails once daily for 48 wk.

Ketoconazole
Topical (Adults): Apply cream once daily for cutaneous candidiasis (for 2 wk), tinea corporis (for 2 wk), tinea cruris (for 2 wk), tinea pedis (for 6 wk), or tinea versicolor (for 2 wk). Apply cream twice daily for seborrheic dermatitis (for 4 wk). For dandruff, use shampoo twice weekly (wait 3–4 days between treatments) for 4 wk, then intermittently.

Luliconazole
Topical (Adults and Children ≥12 yr): *Interdigital tinea pedis:* Apply to affected and surrounding areas once daily for 2 wk; *Tinea cruris:* Apply to affected and surrounding areas once daily for 1 wk.
Topical (Adults and Children ≥2 yr): *Tinea corporis:* Apply to affected and surrounding areas once daily for 1 wk.
Topical (Adults): *Interdigital tinea pedis:* Apply to affected and surrounding areas once daily for 2 wk; *Tinea cruris and tinea corporis:* Apply to affected and surrounding areas once daily for 1 wk.

Miconazole
Topical (Adults and Children >2 yr): Apply twice daily. Treat tinea cruris for 2 wk and tinea pedis or tinea corporis for 4 wk.

Naftifine
Topical (Adults): *Interdigital tinea pedis:* Apply cream or gel once daily for 2 wk; *Tinea cruris or tinea corporis:* apply cream once daily for 2 wk.
Topical (Children ≥12 yr): *Interdigital tinea pedis:* Apply cream or gel once daily for 2 wk.
Topical (Children ≥2 yr): *Tinea corporis:* Apply cream once daily for 2 wk.

Nystatin
Topical (Adults and Children): Apply 2–3 times daily until healing is complete.

Oxiconazole
Topical (Adults and Children): Apply cream or lotion 1–2 times daily for tinea pedis (for 4 wk), tinea corporis (for 2 wk), or tinea cruris (for 2 wk). Apply cream once daily for tinea versicolor (for 2 wk).

Sertaconazole
Topical (Adults and Children >12 yr): Apply twice daily for 4 wk.

Sulconazole
Topical (Adults): Apply 1–2 times daily (twice daily for tinea pedis). Treat tinea corporis, tinea cruris, or tinea versicolor for 3 wk, and tinea pedis for 4 wk.

Tavaborole
Topical (Adults and Children ≥6 yr): Apply to affected nail once daily for 48 wk.

Terbinafine
Topical (Adults): Apply twice daily for tinea pedis (for 1 wk) or daily for tinea cruris or tinea corporis for 1 wk.

Tolnaftate
Topical (Adults): Apply twice daily for tinea cruris (for 2 wk), tinea pedis (for 4 wk), or tinea corporis (for 4 wk).

Availability
Butenafine (generic available)
Cream: 1%^{Rx, OTC}.

Ciclopirox (generic available)
Cream: 0.77%. **Gel:** 0.77%. **Lotion:** ✲ 1%. **Nail lacquer:** 8%. **Shampoo:** 1%, ✲ 1.5%. **Suspension:** 0.77%.

Clotrimazole (generic available)
Cream: 1%^{OTC}. **Solution:** 1%^{OTC}. *In combination with:* betamethasone.

Econazole (generic available)
Cream: 1%. **Foam:** 1%.

Efinaconazole (generic available)
Solution: 10%.

Ketoconazole (generic available)
Cream: 2%. **Foam:** 2%. **Gel:** 2%. **Shampoo:** 2%.

Luliconazole (generic available)
Cream: 1%.

Miconazole (generic available)
Cream: 2%$^{Rx, OTC}$. Ointment: 2%^{OTC}. Powder: 2%^{OTC}. Solution: 2%^{OTC}. Spray powder: 2%^{OTC}. *In combination with:* zinc oxide (Vusion). See Appendix N.

Naftifine
Cream: 1%, 2%. Gel: 1%, 2%.

Nystatin (generic available)
Cream: 100,000 units/g$^{Rx, OTC}$. Ointment: 100,000 units/g$^{Rx, OTC}$. Powder: 100,000 units/g$^{Rx, OTC}$. *In combination with:* triamcinolone.

Oxiconazole (generic available)
Cream: 1%. Lotion: 1%.

Sertaconazole
Cream: 2%.

Sulconazole (generic available)
Cream: 1%. Solution: 1%.

Tavaborole (generic available)
Solution: 5%.

Terbinafine (generic available)
Cream: 1%^{OTC}. Spray liquid: 1%^{OTC}.

Tolnaftate (generic available)
Cream: 1%^{OTC}. Powder: 1%^{OTC}. Solution: 1%^{OTC}. Spray powder: 1%^{OTC}.

NURSING IMPLICATIONS
Assessment
- Inspect involved areas of skin and mucous membranes before and frequently during therapy. Increased skin irritation may indicate need to discontinue medication.

Implementation
- Consult health care professional for proper cleansing technique before applying medication.
- Choice of vehicle is based on use. Ointments, creams, and liquids are used as primary therapy. Lotion is usually preferred in intertriginous areas; if cream is used, apply sparingly to avoid maceration. Powders are usually used as adjunctive therapy but may be used as primary therapy for mild conditions (especially for moist lesions).
- **Topical:** Apply small amount to cover affected area completely. Avoid use of occlusive wrappings or dressings unless directed by health care professional.
- **Nail lacquer:** Avoid contact with skin other than skin immediately surrounding treated nail. Avoid contact with eyes or mucous membranes. Removal of unattached, infected nail, as frequently as monthly, by health care professional is needed with use of this medication. Up to 48 wk of daily application and professional removal may be required to achieve clear or almost clear nail. 6 mo of treatment may be required before results are noticed.

- **Ciclopirox or ketoconazole shampoo:** Moisten hair and scalp thoroughly with water. Apply sufficient shampoo to produce enough lather to wash scalp and hair and gently massage it over the entire scalp area for approximately 1 min. Rinse hair thoroughly with warm water. Repeat process, leaving shampoo on hair for an additional 3 min. After the 2nd shampoo, rinse and dry hair with towel or warm air flow. Shampoo twice a wk for 4 wk with at least 3 days between each shampooing and then intermittently as needed to maintain control.
- **Ketoconazole or econazole foam:** Hold container upright and dispense foam into cap of can or other smooth surface; dispensing directly on to hand is not recommended as the foam begins to melt immediately on contact with warm skin. Pick up small amounts with fingertips and gently massage into affected areas until absorbed. Move hair to allow direct application to skin.

Patient/Family Teaching
- Instruct patient to apply medication as directed for full course of therapy, even if feeling better. Emphasize the importance of avoiding the eyes.
- Caution patient that some products may stain fabric, skin, or hair. Check label information. Fabrics stained from cream or lotion can usually be cleaned by hand washing with soap and warm water; stains from ointments can usually be removed with standard cleaning fluids.
- Patients with athlete's foot should be taught to wear well-fitting, ventilated shoes, to wash affected areas thoroughly, and to change shoes and socks at least once a day.
- Advise patient to report increased skin irritation or lack of response to therapy to health care professional.
- **Nail lacquer:** File away loose nail and trim nails every 7 days after solution is removed with alcohol. Do not use nail polish on treated nails. Inform health care professional if patient has diabetes mellitus before using.

Evaluation/Desired Outcomes
- Decrease in skin irritation and resolution of infection. Early relief of symptoms may be seen in 2–3 days. For *Candida*, tinea cruris, and tinea corporis, 2 wk are needed, and for tinea pedis, therapeutic response may take 3–4 wk. Recurrent fungal infections may be a sign of systemic illness.

ANTIFUNGALS (VAGINAL)
butoconazole (byoo-toe-**kon**-a-zole)
  Gynezole-1
clotrimazole (kloe-**trye**-ma-zole)
  ♣ Canesten, ♣ Clotrimaderm
miconazole (mye-**kon**-a-zole)
terconazole (ter-**kon**-a-zole)

tioconazole (tye-oh-**kon**-a-zole)
Monistat-1Day
Classification
Therapeutic: antifungals (vaginal)

Indications
Treatment of vulvovaginal candidiasis.

Action
Affects the permeability of the fungal cell wall, allowing leakage of cellular contents. Not active against bacteria. **Therapeutic Effects:** Inhibited growth and death of susceptible *Candida*, with decrease in accompanying symptoms of vulvovaginitis (vaginal burning, itching, discharge).

Pharmacokinetics
Absorption: Absorption through intact skin is minimal.
Distribution: Unknown. Action is primarily local.
Metabolism and Excretion: Negligible with local application.
Half-life: Not applicable.

TIME/ACTION PROFILE

ROUTE	ONSET	PEAK	DURATION
All agents	rapid	unknown	24 hr

Contraindications/Precautions
Contraindicated in: Hypersensitivity to active ingredients, additives, or preservatives; OB: Safety not established in pregnancy; Lactation: Safety not established in breastfeeding.
Use Cautiously in: None noted.

Adverse Reactions/Side Effects
Derm: *terconazole:* TOXIC EPIDERMAL NECROLYSIS. **GU:** itching, pelvic pain, vulvovaginal burning. **Misc:** *terconazole:* ANAPHYLAXIS.

Interactions
Drug-Drug: Concurrent use of vaginal miconazole with **warfarin** ↑ risk of bleeding/bruising (appropriate monitoring recommended).

Route/Dosage

Butoconazole
Vag (Adults and Children ≥12 yr): one applicatorful single dose (Gynezole-1).

Clotrimazole
Vag (Adults and Children >12 yr): 1 applicatorful (5 g) of 1% cream at bedtime for 7 days *or* 1 applicatorful (5 g) of 2% cream at bedtime for 3 days.

Miconazole
Vag (Adults and Children ≥12 yr): *Vaginal suppositories:* one 100-mg suppository at bedtime for 7 days *or* one 200-mg suppository at bedtime for 3 days *or* one 1200-mg suppository as a single dose. *Vaginal cream:* 1 applicatorful of 2% cream at bedtime for 7 days *or* 1 applicatorful of 4% cream at bedtime for 3 days. *Combination packages:* contain a cream or suppositories as well as an external vaginal cream (may be used twice daily for up to 7 days, as needed, for symptomatic management of itching).

Terconazole
Vag (Adults): *Vaginal cream:* 1 applicatorful (5 g) of 0.4% cream at bedtime for 7 days *or* 1 applicatorful (5 g) of 0.8% cream at bedtime for 3 days. *Vaginal suppositories:* 1 suppository (80 mg) at bedtime for 3 days.

Tioconazole
Vag (Adults and Children ≥12 yr): 1 applicatorful (4.6 g) at bedtime as a single dose.

Availability

Butoconazole
Vaginal cream: 2%^{Rx, OTC}.

Clotrimazole (generic available)
Vaginal cream: 1%^{OTC}, 2%^{OTC}.

Miconazole (generic available)
Vaginal cream: 2%^{OTC}, 4%^{OTC}. **Vaginal suppositories:** 100 mg^{OTC}, 200 mg^{Rx, OTC}. *In combination with:* combination package of three 200-mg suppositories and 2% external cream^{OTC}; one 1200-mg suppository and 2% external cream^{OTC}; 4% vaginal cream and 2% external cream^{OTC}; seven 100-mg suppositories and 2% external cream^{OTC}; 2% vaginal cream and 2% external cream^{OTC}.

Terconazole (generic available)
Vaginal cream: 0.4%, 0.8%. **Vaginal suppositories:** 80 mg.

Tioconazole
Vaginal ointment: 6.5%^{OTC}.

NURSING IMPLICATIONS

Assessment
- Inspect involved areas of skin and mucous membranes before and frequently during therapy. Increased skin irritation may indicate need to discontinue medication.

Implementation
- Consult health care professional for proper cleansing technique before applying medication.
- **Vag:** Applicators are supplied for vaginal administration.

Patient/Family Teaching
- Instruct patient to apply medication as directed for full course of therapy, even if feeling better. Therapy should be continued during menstrual period.
- Instruct patient on proper use of vaginal applicator. Medication should be inserted high into the vagina at

bedtime. Instruct patient to remain recumbent for at least 30 min after insertion. Advise use of sanitary napkins to prevent staining of clothing or bedding.

- Advise patient to avoid using tampons while using this product.
- Advise patient to consult health care professional regarding intercourse during therapy. Vaginal medication may cause minor skin irritation in sexual partner. Advise patient to refrain from sexual contact during therapy or have male partner wear a condom. Some products may weaken latex contraceptive devices. Another method of contraception should be used during treatment.
- Advise patient to report to health care professional increased skin irritation or lack of response to therapy. A second course may be necessary if symptoms persist.
- Instruct patient to stop using medication and notify health care professional if rash or signs and symptoms of anaphylaxis (wheezing, rash, hives, shortness of breath) occur.
- Advise patient to dispose of applicator after each use (except for terconazole).
- OB: Advise patient to notify health care professional if pregnancy is suspected or if breastfeeding.

Evaluation/Desired Outcomes

- Decrease in skin irritation and vaginal discomfort. Therapeutic response is usually seen after 1 wk. Diagnosis should be reconfirmed with smears or cultures before a second course of therapy to rule out other pathogens associated with vulvovaginitis. Recurrent vaginal infections may be a sign of systemic illness.

---

apixaban (a-pix-a-ban)
Eliquis
Classification
Therapeutic: anticoagulants
Pharmacologic: factor Xa inhibitors

Indications
Reduction in risk of stroke/systemic embolism associated with nonvalvular atrial fibrillation. Prevention of deep vein thrombosis (DVT) that may lead to pulmonary embolism (PE) following knee or hip replacement surgery. Treatment of and reduction in risk of recurrence of DVT or PE.

Action
Acts as a selective, reversible site inhibitor of factor Xa, inhibiting both free and bound factor. Does not affect platelet aggregation directly, but does inhibit thrombin-induced platelet aggregation. Decreases thrombin generation and thrombus development. **Therapeutic Effects:** Treatment and prevention of thromboembolic events.

Pharmacokinetics
Absorption: 50% absorbed following oral administration.

Distribution: Unknown.
Metabolism and Excretion: Primarily metabolized by the liver by the CYP3A4 isoenzyme; excreted in urine and feces. Biliary and direct intestinal excretion account for fecal elimination.
Half-life: 6 hr (12 hr after repeated dosing due to prolonged absorption).

TIME/ACTION PROFILE (effect on hemostasis)

ROUTE	ONSET	PEAK	DURATION
PO	unknown	3–4 hr†	24 hr

†Blood levels.

Contraindications/Precautions
Contraindicated in: Previous severe hypersensitivity reactions; Active pathological bleeding; Severe hepatic impairment; Prosthetic heart valves; PE with hemodynamic instability or requiring thrombolysis or pulmonary embolectomy; Triple-positive antiphospholipid syndrome (↑ risk of thrombosis); Lactation: Lactation.
Use Cautiously in: Neuroaxial spinal anesthesia or spinal puncture, especially if concurrent with an indwelling epidural catheter, drugs affecting hemostasis, history of traumatic/repeated spinal puncture or spinal deformity (↑ risk of spinal hematoma); Surgery; Renal impairment (dose ↓ may be required); Moderate hepatic impairment (↑ risk of bleeding); Rep: Women of reproductive potential; OB: Use during pregnancy only if potential maternal benefit justifies potential fetal risk; Pedi: Safety and effectiveness not established in children.

Adverse Reactions/Side Effects
Hemat: BLEEDING. **Misc:** HYPERSENSITIVITY REACTIONS (including anaphylaxis) .

Interactions
Drug-Drug: ↑ risk of bleeding with other **anticoagulants, aspirin, clopidogrel, ticagrelor, prasugrel, fibrinolytics, NSAIDs, SNRIs,** or **SSRIs.** Concurrent use of strong inhibitors of both CYP3A4 and P-glycoprotein (P-gp), including **itraconazole, ketoconazole,** and **ritonavir,** ↑ levels and bleeding risk; may need to ↓ apixaban dose or avoid concurrent use. Inducers of CYP3A4 and P-gp system, including **carbamazepine, phenytoin, rifampin,** will ↓ levels and may ↑ risk of thromboses; avoid concomitant use.
Drug-Natural Products: Concurrent use **St. John's wort,** a strong dual inducer of the CYP3A4 and P-gp enzyme systems can ↓ levels and ↑ risk of thromboses and should be avoided.

Route/Dosage

Reduction in Risk of Stroke/Systemic Embolism in Nonvalvular Atrial Fibrillation
PO (Adults): 5 mg twice daily; *Any 2 of the following: age ≥80 yr, weight ≤60 kg, serum creatinine ≥1.5 mg/dL:* 2.5 mg twice daily; *Concurrent use of strong*

inhibitors of both CYP3A4 and P-gp: 2.5 mg twice daily; if patient already taking 2.5 mg twice daily, avoid concomitant use.

Renal Impairment
PO (Adults): *Hemodialysis:* 5 mg twice daily; *HD and either age ≥80 yr or weight ≤60 kg:* 2.5 mg twice daily.

Prevention of Deep Vein Thrombosis Following Knee or Hip Replacement Surgery
PO (Adults): 2.5 mg twice daily, initiated 12–24 hr postoperatively (when hemostasis is achieved) continued for 35 days after hip replacement or 12 days after knee replacement; *Concurrent use of strong inhibitors of both CYP3A4 and P-gp:* Avoid concomitant use.

Treatment of Deep Vein Thrombosis or Pulmonary Embolism
PO (Adults): 10 mg twice daily for 7 days, then 5 mg twice daily; *Concurrent use of strong inhibitors of both CYP3A4 and P-gp:* 2.5 mg twice daily.

Reduction in Risk of Recurrence of Deep Vein Thrombosis or Pulmonary Embolism
PO (Adults): 2.5 mg twice daily after ≥6 mo of treatment of DVT or PE; *Concurrent use of strong inhibitors of both CYP3A4 and P-gp:* Avoid concomitant use.

Availability (generic available)
Tablets: 2.5 mg, 5 mg.

NURSING IMPLICATIONS
Assessment
- Assess patient for symptoms of stroke, DVT, PE, bleeding, or peripheral vascular disease periodically during therapy.

Toxicity and Overdose
- Antidote is andexanet alfa. Effects persist for at least 24 hrs after last dose. Oral activated charcoal decreases apixaban absorption, lowering plasma concentrations. Other agents and hemodialysis do not have a significant effect.

Implementation
- **High Alert:** Do not confuse apixaban with axitinib.
- When *converting from warfarin*, discontinue warfarin and start apixaban when INR is <2.0.
- When *converting from apixaban to warfarin*, apixaban affects INR, so INR measurements may not be useful for determining appropriate dose of warfarin. If continuous anticoagulation is necessary, discontinue apixaban and begin both a parenteral anticoagulant and warfarin at time of next dose of apixaban, discontinue parenteral anticoagulant when INR reaches acceptable range.
- When *switching between apixaban and anticoagulants other than warfarin*, discontinue one being taken and begin the other at the next scheduled dose.

- *For surgery*, discontinue apixaban at least 48 hrs before invasive or surgical procedures with a moderate or high risk of unacceptable or clinically significant bleeding or at least 24 hrs prior to procedures with a low risk of bleeding or where the bleeding would be non-critical in location and easily controlled.
- **PO:** Administer twice daily without regard to food.
- For patients who cannot swallow tablet, 5 mg and 2.5 mg tablets can be crushed, suspended in water, D5W, or apple juice, or mixed with applesauce and administered immediately orally. May also be suspended in 60 mL of water or D5W and promptly administered through a nasogastric tube.

Patient/Family Teaching
- Instruct patient to take apixaban as directed. Take missed doses as soon as remembered on the same day and resume twice daily administration; do not double doses. Do not discontinue without consulting health care professional; may increase risk of having a stroke, DVT, or PE. If temporarily discontinued, restart as soon as possible. Store apixaban at room temperature. Advise patient to read *Medication Guide* before beginning therapy and with each Rx refill in case of changes.
- Inform patient that they may bruise and bleed more easily or longer than usual. Advise patient to notify health care professional immediately if signs of bleeding (unusual bruising, pink or brown urine, red or black, tarry stools, coughing up blood, vomiting blood, pain or swelling in a joint, headache, dizziness, weakness, recurring nose bleeds, unusual bleeding from gums, heavier than normal menstrual bleeding, dyspepsia, abdominal pain, epigastric pain) occurs or if injury occurs, especially head injury.
- Caution patient to notify health care professional if skin rash or signs of severe allergic reaction (chest pain or tightness, swelling of face or tongue, trouble breathing or wheezing, feeling dizzy or faint) occur.
- Advise patient to notify health care professional of medication regimen prior to treatment or surgery.
- Instruct patient to notify health care professional of all Rx or OTC medications, vitamins, or herbal products being taken and consult health care professional before taking any new medications, especially St. John's wort. Risk of bleeding is increased with aspirin, NSAIDs, warfarin, heparin, SSRIs or SNRIs.
- Inform patient having had neuraxial anesthesia or spinal puncture to watch for signs and symptoms of spinal or epidural hematomas (numbness or weakness of legs, bowel or bladder dysfunction). Notify health care professional immediately if symptoms occur.
- Rep: Advise females of reproductive potential to notify health care professional if pregnancy is planned or suspected and to avoid breastfeeding during therapy. May increase risk of uterine bleeding in preg-

nant women, fetus, and neonate; advise patient to notify health care professional if significant uterine bleeding occurs.

Evaluation/Desired Outcomes

- Reduction in the risk and treatment of stroke and systemic embolism.

---

apremilast (a-pre-mil-ast)
Otezla
Classification
Therapeutic: antirheumatics, antipsoriatics
Pharmacologic: phosphodiesterase type 4 inhibitors

Indications

Active psoriatic arthritis. Plaque psoriasis in patients who are candidates for phototherapy or systemic therapy. Oral ulcers associated with Behcet's Disease.

Action

Acts as an inhibitor of phosphodiesterase type 4 (PDE4). Inhibition of PDE4 results in ↑ intracellular levels of cyclic adenosine monophosphate. **Therapeutic Effects:** Reduction in severity of psoriatic arthritis with improved joint function. Reduction in severity of plaques. Reduction in number of and pain associated with oral ulcers.

Pharmacokinetics

Absorption: 73% absorbed following oral administration.
Distribution: Unknown.
Metabolism and Excretion: Extensively metabolized (mostly by CYP3A4); metabolites are not pharmacologically active. Excreted in urine (58%) and feces (39%) as inactive metabolites; 3% excreted unchanged in urine, 7% in feces.
Half-life: 6–9 hr.

TIME/ACTION PROFILE (blood levels†)

ROUTE	ONSET	PEAK	DURATION
PO	unknown	2.5 hr	12–24 hr

† Improvement in joint symptoms make take up to 4 mos.

Contraindications/Precautions

Contraindicated in: Hypersensitivity; Concurrent use of CYP450 enzyme inducers.
Use Cautiously in: History of depression or suicidal ideation; Severe renal impairment (dose ↓ required for CCr <30 mL/min); Taking diuretics or antihypertensive medications (may be at higher risk of complications from severe nausea, vomiting, and diarrhea); OB: Use during pregnancy only if potential maternal benefits justify potential fetal risks; Lactation: Use while breastfeeding only if potential maternal benefits justify potential risks to infant; Pedi: Safety and effectiveness not established in children; Geri: Older adults may be at ↑ risk of complications from severe nausea, vomiting, and diarrhea.

Adverse Reactions/Side Effects

GI: diarrhea, nausea, upper abdominal pain, vomiting. **Metab:** weight loss. **Neuro:** depression, headache. **Misc:** HYPERSENSITIVITY REACTIONS (including anaphylaxis and angioedema).

Interactions

Drug-Drug: Concurrent use of CYP450 inducers, including **carbamazepine**, **phenobarbital**, **phenytoin** and **rifampin** may ↓ blood levels and effectiveness; concurrent use should be avoided.

Route/Dosage

PO (Adults): *Day 1:* 10 mg in the morning; *Day 2:* 10 mg in the morning and 10 mg in the evening; *Day 3:* 10 mg in the morning and 20 mg in the evening; *Day 4:* 20 mg in the morning and 20 mg in the evening; *Day 5:* 20 mg in the morning and 30 mg in the evening; *Day 6 and thereafter:* 30 mg in the morning and 30 mg in the evening.

Renal Impairment

PO (Adults CCr <30 mL/min): *Days 1–3:* 10 in the morning; *days 4–5:* 20 mg in the morning; *day 6 and thereafter:* 30 mg in the morning.

Availability (generic available)

Tablets: 10 mg, 20 mg, 30 mg.

NURSING IMPLICATIONS

Assessment

- Assess pain and range of motion before and periodically during therapy.
- Monitor mental status for signs and symptoms of depression (orientation, mood behavior) frequently. Assess for suicidal tendencies, especially during early therapy.
- Obtain weight and BMI initially and periodically during treatment. If clinically significant weight loss occurs, evaluate weight loss and consider discontinuation of therapy.

Implementation

- Follow titration guidelines when beginning therapy to minimize GI side effects.
- PO: Administer without regard for meals. *DNC:* Swallow tablet whole; do not crush, break, or chew.

Patient/Family Teaching

- Instruct patient to take apremilast as directed.
- Advise patient, family and caregivers to look for suicidality, especially during early therapy or dose changes. Notify health care professional immediately if thoughts about suicide or dying, attempts to commit suicide, new or worse depression or anxiety, agitation or restlessness, panic attacks, insomnia, new or worse irritability, aggressiveness, acting on dangerous impulses, mania, or other changes in mood or behavior occur.
- Inform patient of risk of nausea, vomiting, and diarrhea. Instruct patient to notify health care professional if severe nausea, vomiting or diarrhea occur;

may need to consider dose reduction or interruption of therapy.

● Inform patient of need to monitor weight regularly. Notify health care professional if unexplained or clinically significant weight loss occurs: may need to discontinue therapy.

● Advise patient to notify health care professional of all Rx or OTC medications, vitamins, or herbal products being taken and to consult with health care professional before taking other medications.

● Rep: Advise patient to notify health care professional if pregnancy is planned or suspected or if breastfeeding. Encourage patients to enroll in pregnancy registry for women who have taken apremilast during pregnancy 1-877-311-8972 to enroll or visit https://mothertobaby.org/ongoing-study/otezla/ .

Evaluation/Desired Outcomes

● Improvement in pain and function in patients with psoriatic arthritis.

● Increased healing of lesions in plaque psoriasis.

● Improvement in oral ulcers associated with Behçet's Disease.

aprepitant (a-prep-i-tant)
Aponvie, Cinvanti, Emend
Classification
Therapeutic: antiemetics
Pharmacologic: neurokinin antagonists

Indications

IV, PO: Prevention of: Acute and delayed nausea and vomiting associated with initial and repeat courses of highly emetogenic chemotherapy (in combination with other antiemetic agents) (Cinvanti and Emend); Nausea and vomiting associated with initial and repeat courses of moderately emetogenic chemotherapy (in combination with other antiemetic agents) (Cinvanti and Emend). **IV:** Prevention of delayed nausea and vomiting associated with initial and repeat courses of moderately emetogenic chemotherapy (in combination with other antiemetic agents) (Cinvanti). **IV:** Prevention of postoperative nausea and vomiting (Aponvie).

Action

Acts as a selective antagonist at substance P/neurokinin 1 (NK_1) receptors in the brain. **Therapeutic Effects:** Decreased nausea and vomiting associated with chemotherapy or surgical procedures. Augments the antiemetic effects of dexamethasone and 5-HT$_3$ antagonists in patients receiving chemotherapy.

Pharmacokinetics

Absorption: 60–65% absorbed following oral administration. IV administration results in complete bioavailability.

Distribution: Crosses the blood brain barrier; remainder of distribution unknown.

Protein Binding: 95–99%.

Metabolism and Excretion: Mostly metabolized by the liver (CYP3A4 enzyme system); not renally excreted.

Half-life: 9–13 hr.

TIME/ACTION PROFILE (antiemetic effect)

ROUTE	ONSET	PEAK	DURATION
PO	1 hr	4 hr*	24 hr
IV	rapid	end of infusion*	24 hr

*Plasma concentration.

Contraindications/Precautions

Contraindicated in: Hypersensitivity; Concurrent use with pimozide; OB: Pregnancy (IV only; contains alcohol).

Use Cautiously in: OB: Safety not established in pregnancy (PO only); Rep: Women of reproductive potential; Lactation: Safety not established in breastfeeding; Pedi: Safety and effectiveness not established in children <18 yr (IV) or <6 mo (PO).

Adverse Reactions/Side Effects

CV: dizziness, fatigue, weakness. **Derm:** STEVENS-JOHNSON SYNDROME. **GI:** diarrhea. **Neuro:** headache. **Misc:** hiccups, HYPERSENSITIVITY REACTIONS (including anaphylaxis).

Interactions

Drug-Drug: May significantly ↑ levels of **pimozide**, which can ↑ risk of torsades de pointes; concurrent use contraindicated. May ↑ levels of **CYP3A4 substrates**, including **docetaxel, paclitaxel, etoposide, irinotecan, ifosfamide, imatinib, vinorelbine, vinblastine, vincristine, midazolam, triazolam**, and **alprazolam**; concurrent use should be undertaken with caution. **Moderate or strong CYP3A4 inhibitors**, including **ketoconazole, itraconazole, nefazodone, clarithromycin, ritonavir, nelfinavir**, and **diltiazem**) may ↑ levels and risk of adverse reactions. **Strong CYP3A4 inducers**, including **rifampin, carbamazepine**, and **phenytoin** may ↓ levels and effects. ↑ levels and effects of **dexamethasone** (regimen reflects a 50% dose ↓); a similar effect occurs with **methylprednisolone** (↓ IV dose by 25%, ↓ PO dose by 50% when used concurrently). May ↓ the effects of **warfarin** (carefully monitor INR for 2 wk), **oral contraceptives** (use alternate method), and **phenytoin**.

Route/Dosage

Prevention of Acute and Delayed Nausea and Vomiting Associated with Highly Emetogenic Chemotherapy

PO (Adults and Children ≥12 yr): *Capsules:* 125 mg given 1 hr prior to chemotherapy (Day 1), then 80 mg once daily for 2 days (Days 2 and 3). *Suspension (if unable to swallow capsules):* 3 mg/kg (max dose

= 125 mg) given 1 hr prior to chemotherapy (Day 1), then 2 mg/kg (max dose = 80 mg) once daily for 2 days (Days 2 and 3).

IV (Adults): *Cinvanti:* 130 mg given 30 min prior to chemotherapy on Day 1 only.

PO (Children 6 mo–<12 yr and >6 kg): *Suspension:* 3 mg/kg (max dose = 125 mg) given 1 hr prior to chemotherapy (Day 1), then 2 mg/kg (max dose = 80 mg) once daily for 2 days (Days 2 and 3).

Prevention of Nausea and Vomiting Associated with Moderately Emetogenic Chemotherapy

PO (Adults and Children ≥12 yr): *Capsules:* 125 mg given 1 hr prior to chemotherapy (Day 1), then 80 mg once daily for 2 days (Days 2 and 3). *Suspension (if unable to swallow capsules):* 3 mg/kg (max dose = 125 mg) given 1 hr prior to chemotherapy (Day 1), then 2 mg/kg (max dose = 80 mg) once daily for 2 days (Days 2 and 3).

IV (Adults): *Cinvanti (single–dose regimen for delayed nausea/vomiting):* 130 mg given 30 min prior to chemotherapy on Day 1 (with dexamethasone 12 mg PO given 30 min prior to chemotherapy and a 5-HT$_3$ antagonist prior to chemotherapy). *Cinvanti (3–day regimen):* 100 mg given 30 min prior to chemotherapy on Day 1 (with dexamethasone 12 mg PO given 30 min prior to chemotherapy and a 5-HT$_3$ antagonist prior to chemotherapy). Continue aprepitant 80 mg PO on Days 2 and 3.

PO (Children 6 mo–<12 yr and >6 kg): *Suspension:* 3 mg/kg (max dose = 125 mg) given 1 hr prior to chemotherapy (Day 1), then 2 mg/kg (max dose = 80 mg) once daily for 2 days (Days 2 and 3).

Prevention of Postoperative Nausea and Vomiting

IV (Adults): *Aponvie:* 32 mg as a single dose administered prior to induction of anesthesia.

Availability (generic available)

Capsules (Emend): 40 mg, 80 mg, 125 mg. **Powder for oral suspension (Emend):** 125 mg/pouch. **Emulsion for injection (Aponvie, Cinvanti) (contains alcohol):** 7.2 mg/mL.

NURSING IMPLICATIONS

Assessment

- Assess nausea, vomiting, appetite, bowel sounds, and abdominal pain prior to and following administration.
- Monitor hydration, nutritional status, and intake and output. Patients with severe nausea and vomiting may require IV fluids in addition to antiemetics.
- Assess for rash periodically during therapy. May cause Stevens-Johnson syndrome. Discontinue therapy if severe rash or if accompanied with fever, general malaise, fatigue, muscle or joint aches, blisters, skin peeling, sores, oral lesions, conjunctivitis, hepatitis, and/or eosinophilia.

- Monitor for signs and symptoms of infusion site reaction (erythema, edema, pain, thrombophlebitis). Treat symptomatically. Avoid infusion into small veins or through a butterfly catheter.
- Monitor for signs and symptoms of hypersensitivity reactions (flushing, erythema, dyspnea, hypotension, syncope) periodically during therapy. If symptoms occur, discontinue therapy and treat symptoms; do not reinitiate therapy if symptoms occur with first use.

Lab Test Considerations

- Monitor clotting status closely during the 2 wk period, especially at 7–10 days, following aprepitant therapy in patients on chronic warfarin therapy.
- May cause mild, transient ↑ in alkaline phosphatase, AST, ALT, and BUN.
- May cause proteinuria, erythrocyturia, leukocyturia, hyperglycemia, hyponatremia, and ↑ leukocytes.
- May cause ↓ hemoglobin and WBC.

Implementation

- For chemotherapy, aprepitant is given as part of a regimen that includes a corticosteroid and a 5-HT$_3$ antagonist (see Route/Dosage).
- **PO:** Administer daily for 3 days. *Day 1:* administer 1 hr prior to chemotherapy. *Days 2 and 3:* administer once in the morning. May be administered without regard to food. *DNC:* Swallow capsules whole; do not open, crush, or chew.
- Oral suspension may be used for pediatric patients or those with difficulty swallowing. Follow manufacture's instructions for preparing suspension. Refrigerate suspension; may be stored at room temperature for up to 3 hrs before use. To administer, take cap off, place dispenser in patient's mouth along inner cheek. Dispense slowly. Discard after 72 hrs.

IV Administration

Cinvanti

- Complete injection or infusion 30 min prior to chemotherapy.
- **IV Push:** Withdraw 18 mL for the 130 mg dose or 14 mL for the 100 mg dose from the vial. Do not dilute. *Rate:* Inject over 2 min. Flush line with 0.9% NaCl before and after injection.
- **Intermittent Infusion:** *Dilution:* 0.9% NaCl or D5W. *For Highly-Emetogenic Chemotherapy:* Using 130 mL of diluent, withdraw 18 mg aprepitant from vial and add to bag for 148 mL. *For Moderately-Emetogenic Chemotherapy:* Using 100 mL of diluent, withdraw 14 mL aprepitant from vial and add to bag for 114 mL. Mix by gently inverting bag 4–5 times. Solution is an opaque, off-white emulsion. Do not administer solutions that are discolored or contain particulate matter. May be stored at room temperature for 6 hrs if mixed with 0.9% NaCl or 12 hrs if mixed with D5W or in refrigerator for up to 72 hrs. *Rate:* Infuse over 30 min.

- **Y-Site Incompatibility:** Incompatible with solutions containing divalent cations (calcium, magnesium), including LR and Hartmann's Solution.

Emend
- Complete injection or infusion 30 min prior to chemotherapy.
- **Intermittent Infusion:** *Reconstitution:* Inject 5 mL of 0.9% NaCl into vial along the vial wall to prevent foaming. Swirl vial gently. Avoid shaking and jetting 0.9% NaCl into the vial. *Dilution:* Withdraw entire volume from vial and transfer to infusion bag containing 145 mL of 0.9% NaCl for a volume of 150 mL. *Concentration:* Final concentration of 1 mg/mL. Gently invert bag 2 to 3 times. Solution is stable for 24 hrs at room temperature. Discard unused portion. *Rate:* Infuse over 20–30 min for adults, over 30 min for children 12–17 yrs, or over 60 min for children 6 mos to <12 yrs. For children may also be given as a 3–day regimen via central venous catheter. *For children 12–17 yrs,* Day 1: infuse 115 mg over 30 min; Day 2 and 3: infuse 80 mg over 30 min. *For children 6 mos to <12 yrs,* Day 1: infuse 3 mg/kg up to 115 mg over 60 min; Day 2 and 3: infuse 2 mg/kg up to 80 mg over 60 min.
- **Y-Site Incompatibility:** Incompatible with solutions containing divalent cations (calcium, magnesium), including LR and Hartmann's Solution.

Aponvie
- **IV Push:** Withdraw 4.4 mL from vial. Solution is opaque and off-white to amber. Do not administer solutions that are discolored or contain particulate matter. Flush the infusion line with 0.9% NaCl before and after administration. *Rate:* Administer over 30 sec prior to induction of anesthesia.
- **Y-Site Incompatibility:** Incompatible with solutions containing divalent cations (calcium, magnesium), including LR and Hartmann's Solution.

Patient/Family Teaching
- Instruct patient to take aprepitant as directed. Direct patient to read the *Patient Package Insert* before starting therapy and each time Rx renewed in case of changes.
- Instruct patient to notify health care professional if nausea and vomiting occur prior to administration.
- Advise patient to notify health care professional immediately if symptoms of hypersensitivity reaction (hives, rash, itching, redness of the face/skin, difficulty in breathing or swallowing) occur.
- Instruct patient to notify health care professional of all Rx or OTC medications, vitamins, or herbal products being taken and consult health care professional before taking any new medications.
- Advise patient and family to use general measures to decrease nausea (begin with sips of liquids and small, non-greasy meals; provide oral hygiene; remove noxious stimuli from environment).

- Rep: Caution females of reproductive potential that aprepitant may decrease efficacy of oral contraceptives. Advise patient to use effective alternate nonhormonal methods of contraception during and for 1 mo following treatment. Advise females of reproductive potential that *Cinvanti* contains alcohol and may cause fetal harm including central nervous system abnormalities, behavioral disorders, and impaired intellectual development. Avoid use of *Cinvanti* during pregnancy. Advise patient to notify health care professional if pregnancy is planned or suspected or if breastfeeding.

Evaluation/Desired Outcomes
- Decreased nausea and vomiting associated with chemotherapy or surgery.
- Augmentation of antiemetic effects of dexamethasone and 5-HT$_3$ antagonists in patients receiving chemotherapy.

HIGH ALERT

argatroban (ar-**gat**-tro-ban)
Classification
Therapeutic: anticoagulants
Pharmacologic: thrombin inhibitors

Indications
Prophylaxis or treatment of thrombosis in patients with heparin-induced thrombocytopenia (HIT). As an anticoagulant in patients with or at risk for heparin-induced thrombocytopenia who are undergoing percutaneous coronary intervention (PCI).

Action
Inhibits thrombin by binding to its receptor sites. Inhibition of thrombin prevents activation of factors V, VIII, and XII; the conversion of fibrinogen to fibrin; platelet adhesion and aggregation. **Therapeutic Effects:** Decreased thrombus formation and extension with decreased sequelae of thrombosis (emboli, postphlebitic syndromes).

Pharmacokinetics
Absorption: IV administration results in complete bioavailability.
Distribution: Unknown.
Metabolism and Excretion: Mostly metabolized by the liver; excreted primarily in feces via biliary excretion. 16% excreted unchanged in urine, 14% excreted unchanged in feces.
Half-life: 39–51 min (↑ in hepatic impairment).

TIME/ACTION PROFILE (anticoagulant effect)

ROUTE	ONSET	PEAK	DURATION
IV	immediate	1–3 hr	2–4 hr

Contraindications/Precautions

Contraindicated in: Major bleeding; Hypersensitivity.

Use Cautiously in: Hepatic impairment (↓ initial infusion rate recommended); OB: Use during pregnancy only if potential maternal benefit justifies potential fetal risk; Lactation: Use while breastfeeding only if potential maternal benefit justifies potential risk to infant; Pedi: Safety and effectiveness not established in children.

Adverse Reactions/Side Effects

CV: hypotension. **GI:** diarrhea, nausea, vomiting. **Hemat:** BLEEDING. **Misc:** fever, HYPERSENSITIVITY REACTIONS (including anaphylaxis).

Interactions

Drug-Drug: Risk of bleeding may be ↑ by concurrent use of **antiplatelet agents**, **thrombolytic agents**, or **other anticoagulants**.
Drug-Natural Products: ↑ bleeding risk with **anise**, **arnica**, **chamomile**, **clove**, **feverfew**, **garlic**, **ginger**, **ginkgo**, **Panax ginseng**, and others.

Route/Dosage

IV (Adults): 2 mcg/kg/min as a continuous infusion; adjust infusion rate on the basis of activated partial thromboplastin time (aPTT). *Patients undergoing PCI:* 350 mcg/kg bolus followed by infusion at 25 mcg/kg/min, activated clotting time (ACT) should be assessed 5–10 min later. If ACT is 300–450 sec, procedure may be started. If ACT <300 sec, give additional bolus of 150 mcg/kg and ↑ infusion rate to 30 mcg/kg/min. If ACT is >450 sec infusion rate should be ↓ to 15 mcg/kg/min and ACT rechecked after 5–10 min. If thrombotic complications occur or ACT drops to <300 sec, an additional bolus of 150 mcg/kg may be given and the infusion rate ↑ to 40 mcg/kg/min followed by ACT monitoring. If anticoagulation is required after surgery, lower infusion rates should be used.

Hepatic Impairment

IV (Adults): 0.5 mcg/kg/min as a continuous infusion; adjust infusion rate on the basis of aPTT.

Availability (generic available)

Premixed infusion: 50 mg/50 mL. **Solution for injection:** 100 mg/mL.

NURSING IMPLICATIONS

Assessment

- Monitor vital signs periodically during therapy. Unexplained decreases in BP may indicate hemorrhage. Assess patient for bleeding. Minimize arterial and venous punctures, IM injections, and use of urinary catheters, nasotracheal intubation, and nasogastric tubes. Avoid noncompressible sites for IV access. Monitor for blood in urine, lower back pain, pain or burning on urination. If bleeding cannot be controlled with pressure, decrease dose or discontinue argatroban immediately.

- Monitor for signs of anaphylaxis (rash, coughing, dyspnea) during therapy.

Lab Test Considerations

- Monitor aPTT prior to initiation of continuous infusion, 2 hrs after initiation of therapy, and periodically during therapy to confirm aPTT is within desired therapeutic range.

- For patients undergoing PCI, monitor ACT as described in Route and Dose section.

- Assess hemoglobin, hematocrit, and platelet count prior to, and periodically during, argatroban therapy. May cause ↓ hemoglobin and hematocrit. Unexplained ↓ hematocrit may indicate hemorrhage.

- Use of argatroban concurrently with multiple doses of warfarin will result in more prolonged prothrombin time and international normalized ratio (INR) (although there is not an ↑ in vitamin K-dependent factor X_a activity) than when warfarin is used alone. Monitor INR daily during concomitant therapy. Repeat INR 4–6 hr after argatroban is discontinued. If repeat value is below desired therapeutic value for warfarin alone, restart argatroban therapy and continue until desired therapeutic range for warfarin alone is reached. To obtain the INR for warfarin alone when dose of argatroban is >2 mcg/kg/min, temporarily reduce argatroban dose to 2 mcg/kg/min; INR for combined therapy may then be obtained 4–6 hr after argatroban dose was reduced.

Toxicity and Overdose

- There is no specific antidote for argatroban. If overdose occurs, discontinue argatroban. Anticoagulation parameters usually return to baseline within 2–4 hr after discontinuation.

Implementation

- Do not confuse argatroban with Aggrastat.
- Discontinue all parenteral anticoagulants before argatroban therapy is started. Oral anticoagulation may be initiated with maintenance dose of warfarin; do not administer loading dose. Discontinue argatroban therapy when INR for combined therapy is >4.

IV Administration

- **IV:** Do not administer solutions that are cloudy or contain particulate matter. Discard unused portion.
- **IV Push:** *Dilution:* Bolus dose of 350 mcg/kg should be given prior to continuous infusion in patients undergoing PCI. For Diluent information, see Continuous Infusion section below. *Rate:* Administer bolus over 3–5 min.
- **Continuous Infusion:** *Dilution:* Dilute each 100 mg/mL in 250 mL of 0.9% NaCl, D5W, or LR. *Concentration:* 1 mg/mL. Mix by repeated inversion for 1 min. Diluted solution is slightly viscous, clear, and colorless to pale yellow; may show a slight haziness that disappears upon mixing; solution must be clear before use. Solution is stable at controlled room temperature and ambient light for 24 hrs, or for 96 hrs at controlled room temperature or refrig-

erated and protected from light; do not expose to direct sunlight. Pre-mixed solutions are clear and colorless. Store at room temperature, do not refrigerate or freeze. *Rate:* Based on patient's weight (See Route/Dosage section). Dose adjustment may be made 2 hr after starting infusion or changing dose until steady-state aPTT is 1.5–3 times the initial baseline value (not to exceed 100 sec).

● **Y-Site Compatibility:** acyclovir, alemtuzumab, allopurinol, amifostine, amikacin, aminocaproic acid, aminophylline, amiodarone, amphotericin B lipid complex, amphotericin B liposomal, ampicillin, ampicillin/sulbactam, anidulafungin, arsenic trioxide, atracurium, atropine, azithromycin, aztreonam, bivalirudin, bleomycin, bumetanide, buprenorphine, busulfan, butorphanol, calcium acetate, calcium chloride, calcium gluconate, carboplatin, carmustine, caspofungin, cefazolin, cefotaxime, cefotetan, cefoxitin, ceftazidime, ceftriaxone, cefuroxime, chloramphenicol, chlorpromazine, ciprofloxacin, cisatracurium, cisplatin, clindamycin, cyclophosphamide, cyclosporine, cytarabine, dacarbazine, dactinomycin, dantrolene, daptomycin, daptomycin, daunorubicin hydrochloride, dexamethasone, dexmedetomidine, dexrazoxane, digoxin, diltiazem, diphenhydramine, dobutamine, docetaxel, dopamine, doxorubicin hydrochloride, doxorubicin liposomal, doxycycline, droperidol, enalaprilat, ephedrine, epinephrine, epirubicin, eptifibatide, ertapenem, erythromycin, esmolol, etoposide, etoposide phosphate, famotidine, fentanyl, fluconazole, fludarabine, fluorouracil, foscarnet, fosphenytoin, furosemide, ganciclovir, gemcitabine, gemtuzumab ozogamicin, gentamicin, glycopyrrolate, granisetron, haloperidol, heparin, hydralazine, hydrocortisone, hydromorphone, ibutilide, idarubicin, ifosfamide, imipenem/cilastatin, insulin, regular, irinotecan, isoproterenol, ketorolac, labetalol, leucovorin, levofloxacin, lidocaine, linezolid, lorazepam, magnesium sulfate, mannitol, melphalan, meperidine, meropenem, mesna, methadone, methotrexate, methylprednisolone, metoclopramide, metoprolol, midazolam, milrinone, mitomycin, mitoxantrone, morphine, moxifloxacin, mycophenolate, nafcillin, nalbuphine, naloxone, nicardipine, nitroglycerin, nitroprusside, norepinephrine, octreotide, ondansetron, oxaliplatin, oxytocin, paclitaxel, palonosetron, pamidronate, pantoprazole, pentamidine, pentobarbital, phenobarbital, phentolamine, phenylephrine, phenytoin, piperacillin/tazobactam, potassium acetate, potassium chloride, potassium phosphate, procainamide, prochlorperazine, promethazine, propranolol, remifentanil, rocuronium, sodium acetate, sodium bicarbonate, sodium phosphate, succinylcholine, sufentanil, tacrolimus, theophylline, thiopental, thiotepa, tigecycline, tirofiban, tobramycin, topotecan, trimethoprim/sulfamethoxazole, vancomycin, vaso-

pressin, vecuronium, verapamil, vinblastine, vincristine, vinorelbine, voriconazole, zidovudine, zoledronic acid.

● **Y-Site Incompatibility:** cefepime, dantrolene, diazepam, phenytoin.

Patient/Family Teaching

● Explain the purpose of argatroban to patient.
● Advise patient to avoid other products known to affect bleeding.
● Instruct patient to notify health care professional immediately if any bleeding or signs and symptoms of allergic reaction is noted.
● Rep: Advise females or reproductive potential to notify health care professional if pregnancy is planned or suspected or if breastfeeding.

Evaluation/Desired Outcomes

● Decreased thrombus formation and extension.
● Decreased sequelae of thrombosis (emboli, postphlebitic syndromes).

BEERS

⚉ARIPiprazole (a-ri-**pip**-ra-zole)
Abilify, Abilify Asimtufii, Abilify Maintena, Abilify Mycite, Aristada, Aristada Initio
Classification
Therapeutic: antipsychotics, mood stabilizers
Pharmacologic: serotonin-dopamine activity modulators (SDAM)

Indications
Schizophrenia (Abilify, Abilify Asimtufii, Abilify Maintena, Abilify Mycite, and Aristada). Acute treatment of manic and mixed episodes associated with bipolar I disorder (as monotherapy or with lithium or valproate) (Abilify and Abilify Mycite). Maintenance treatment of bipolar I disorder (as monotherapy) (Abilify Asimtufii and Abilify Maintena). Maintenance treatment of bipolar I disorder (as monotherapy or with lithium or valproate) (Abilify Mycite). Adjunctive treatment of depression (Abilify and Abilify Mycite). Agitation associated with schizophrenia or bipolar disorder (Abilify only). Irritability associated with autistic disorder (Abilify only). Tourette's disorder (Abilify only).

Action
Psychotropic activity may be due to agonist activity at dopamine D_2 and serotonin 5-HT$_{1A}$ receptors and antagonist activity at the 5-HT$_{2A}$ receptor. Also has alpha$_1$ adrenergic blocking activity. **Therapeutic Effects:** Decreased manifestations of schizophrenia. Decreased mania in bipolar patients. Decreased symptoms of depression. Decreased agitation associated with schizophrenia or bipolar disorder. Decreased emotional and behavioral symptoms of irritability. Decreased incidence of tics.

Pharmacokinetics

Absorption: Well absorbed (87%) following oral administration; 100% following IM injection.
Distribution: Extensive extravascular distribution.
Protein Binding: >99%.
Metabolism and Excretion: Mostly metabolized by the liver by the CYP3A4 and CYP2D6 isoenzymes; ≋ the CYP2D6 enzyme system exhibits genetic polymorphism; ~7% of population may be poor metabolizers (PMs) and may have significantly ↑ aripiprazole concentrations and an ↑ risk of adverse effects (↓ dose by 50% in PMs); one metabolite (dehydro-aripiprazole) has antipsychotic activity. 18% excreted unchanged in feces; <1% excreted unchanged in urine.
Half-life: *Aripiprazole:* 75 hr; *dehydro-aripiprazole: 94 hr*; ER injectable suspension: 30–46 days (Abilify Maintena); 29–35 days (Aristada).

TIME/ACTION PROFILE (antipsychotic effect)

ROUTE	ONSET	PEAK	DURATION
PO	unknown	2 wk	unknown
ER-IM	unknown	unknown	unknown

Contraindications/Precautions

Contraindicated in: Hypersensitivity; CYP2D6 PMs or concurrent use of strong CYP3A4 inhibitors, strong CYP2D6 inhibitors, or strong CYP3A4 inducers (Aristada Initio only).
Use Cautiously in: Known cardiovascular or cerebrovascular disease; Conditions which cause hypotension (dehydration, treatment with antihypertensives or diuretics); Diabetes (may ↑ risk of hyperglycemia); Seizure disorders; Patients at risk for aspiration pneumonia or falls; OB: Use during pregnancy only if potential maternal benefit justifies potential fetal risk; neonates at ↑ risk for extrapyramidal symptoms and withdrawal after delivery when exposed during the 3rd trimester; Lactation: Use while breastfeeding only if potential maternal benefit justifies potential risk to infant; Pedi: May ↑ risk of suicide attempt/ideation especially during dose early treatment or dose adjustment; risk may be greater in children, adolescents, and young adults taking antidepressants (safety in children/adolescents not established); Geri: Appears on Beers list. ↑ risk of stroke, cognitive decline, and mortality in older adults with dementia. Avoid use in older adults, except for schizophrenia, bipolar disorder, or adjunctive treatment of major depressive disorder.

Adverse Reactions/Side Effects

CV: bradycardia, chest pain, edema, hypertension, orthostatic hypotension, tachycardia. **Derm:** DRUG REACTION WITH EOSINOPHILIA AND SYSTEMIC SYMPTOMS (DRESS), dry skin, ecchymosis, skin ulcer, sweating. **EENT:** blurred vision, conjunctivitis, ear pain. **Endo:** ↓ prolactin, hyperglycemia. **GI:** constipation, ↑ salivation, anorexia, nausea, vomiting. **GU:** urinary incontinence. **Hemat:** AGRANULOCYTOSIS, anemia, leukopenia, neutropenia. **Metab:** dyslipidemia, weight gain, weight loss. **MS:** muscle cramps, neck pain. **Neuro:** drowsiness, extrapyramidal reactions, tremor, abnormal gait, akathisia, confusion, depression, fatigue, hostility, impaired cognitive function, impulse control disorders (eating/binge eating, gambling, sexual, shopping), insomnia, lightheadedness, manic reactions, nervousness, restlessness, sedation, SEIZURES, SUICIDAL THOUGHTS, tardive dyskinesia. **Resp:** dyspnea. **Misc:** ↓ heat regulation, HYPERSENSITIVITY REACTIONS, injection site reactions, NEUROLEPTIC MALIGNANT SYNDROME.

Interactions

Drug-Drug: **Strong CYP3A4 inhibitors**, including **ketoconazole** and **clarithromycin** may ↑ levels and risk of toxicity; ↓ aripiprazole dose by 50%. **Strong CYP2D6 inhibitors**, including **quinidine, fluoxetine**, or **paroxetine** may ↑ levels and risk of toxicity; ↓ aripiprazole dose by at least 50%. **CYP3A4 inducers** may ↓ levels and effectiveness; double aripiprazole dose.

Route/Dosage

If used concurrently with combination of strong, moderate, or weak CYP3A4 and CYP2D6 inhibitors, ↓ oral aripiprazole dose by 75%. Aripiprazole dose should be ↓ by 75% in CYP2D6 PMs who are concomitantly receiving a strong CYP3A4 inhibitor. Do NOT substitute Aristada Initio for Aristada.

Schizophrenia

PO (Adults): 10 or 15 mg once daily; doses up to 30 mg/day have been used; increments in dosing should not be made before 2 wk at a given dose.
PO (Children 13–17 yr): 2 mg once daily; ↑ to 5 mg once daily after 2 days, and then to target dose of 10 mg once daily after another 2 days; may further ↑ dose in 5-mg increments if needed (max: 30 mg/day).
IM (Adults): *Abilify Maintena:* 400 mg every mo; after 1st injection, continue treatment with oral aripiprazole (10–20 mg/day) for 14 days; if no adverse reactions to 400 mg/mo dose, may ↓ dose to 300 mg every mo. *CYP2D6 PMs:* ↓ dose to 300 mg monthly; *CYP2D6 PMs concomitantly receiving strong CYP3A4 inhibitor:* ↓ dose to 200 mg monthly; *Concomitant therapy with strong CYP2D6 or CYP3A4 inhibitor:* ↓ dose to 300 mg monthly (if originally receiving 400 mg monthly) or 200 mg monthly (if originally receiving 300 mg monthly); *Concomitant therapy with strong CYP2D6 and CYP3A4 inhibitor:* ↓ dose to 200 mg monthly (if originally receiving 400 mg monthly) or 160 mg monthly (if originally receiving 300 mg monthly); *Concomitant therapy with CYP3A4 inducer:* Avoid use.
IM (Adults): *Abilify Asimtufii and receiving oral antipsychotics:* 960 mg every 2 mo (56 days after previous injection); after 1st injection, if previously receiving oral aripiprazole, continue treatment with oral aripiprazole (10–20 mg/day) for 14 days. If previously stable on another oral antipsychotic (but known to tolerate aripiprazole), after 1st injection, continue treatment

with oral antipsychotic for 14 days. *Abilify Asimtufii and previously receiving Abilify Maintena:* 960 mg every 2 mo in place of the next scheduled Abilify Maintena injection; the 1st injection may be administered in place of the 2nd or later injection of Abilify Maintena; *CYP2D6 PMs:* ↓ dose to 720 mg every 2 mo; *CYP2D6 PMs concomitantly receiving strong CYP3A4 inhibitor:* Avoid use; *Concomitant therapy with strong CYP2D6 or CYP3A4 inhibitor:* ↓ dose to 720 mg every 2 mo; *Concomitant therapy with strong CYP2D6 and CYP3A4 inhibitor:* Avoid use; *Concomitant therapy with CYP3A4 inducer:* Avoid use.

IM (Adults): *Aristada with Aristada Initio:* administer 675–mg injection of Aristada Initio with first injection of Aristada (dose is based on total daily dose of oral aripiprazole; if patient receiving 10 mg/day of oral aripiprazole, administer 441 mg every mo; if patient receiving 15 mg/day of oral aripiprazole, administer 662 mg every mo, 882 mg every 6 wk, or 1064 mg every 2 mo; if patient receiving ≥20 mg/day of oral aripiprazole, administer 882 mg every mo) (initial Aristada dose can be given on same day as or within 10 days of Aristada Initio) AND one dose of oral aripiprazole 30 mg; *Aristada without Aristada Initio:* Dose is based on total daily dose of oral aripiprazole; if patient receiving 10 mg/day of oral aripiprazole, administer 441 mg every mo; if patient receiving 15 mg/day of oral aripiprazole, administer 662 mg every mo, 882 mg every 6 wk, or 1064 mg every 2 mo; if patient receiving ≥20 mg/day of oral aripiprazole, administer 882 mg every mo; after 1st injection; continue treatment with oral aripiprazole for 21 days; *Concomitant therapy with strong CYP2D6 or CYP3A4 inhibitor for >2 wk:* ↓ dose of Aristada to 441 mg monthly (if originally receiving 662 mg monthly) or 662 mg monthly (if originally receiving 882 mg monthly); no dose adjustment necessary if originally receiving 441 mg monthly; avoid use of Aristada Initio; *CYP2D6 PMs concomitantly receiving strong CYP3A4 inhibitor for >2 wk:* ↓ dose of Aristada to 441 mg monthly (if originally receiving 662 mg or 882 mg monthly); no dose adjustment necessary if originally receiving 441 mg monthly; avoid use of Aristada Initio; *Concomitant therapy with strong CYP2D6 and CYP3A4 inhibitor:* avoid use of Aristada in patients requiring 662 mg or 882 mg monthly dose; no dose adjustment of Aristada necessary if originally receiving 441 mg monthly; avoid use of Aristada Initio; *Concomitant therapy with CYP3A4 inducer:* ↑ dose of Aristada to 662 mg monthly (if originally receiving 441 mg monthly); no dose adjustment if Aristada necessary if originally receiving 662 mg or 882 mg monthly; avoid use of Aristada Initio.

Acute Manic or Mixed Episodes Associated with Bipolar I Disorder

PO (Adults): 15 mg once daily as monotherapy or 10–15 mg once daily with lithium or valproate; target

dose is 15 mg once daily; may ↑ to 30 mg once daily, if needed.
PO (Children 10–17 yr): 2 mg once daily; ↑ to 5 mg once daily after 2 days, and then to target dose of 10 mg once daily after another 2 days; may further ↑ dose in 5-mg increments if needed (max: 30 mg/day).

Maintenance Treatment of Bipolar I Disorder

PO (Adults): *Abilify Mycite:* 15 mg once daily as monotherapy or 10–15 mg once daily with lithium or valproate; target dose is 15 mg once daily; may ↑ to 30 mg once daily, if needed.
IM (Adults): *Abilify Maintena:* 400 mg every mo; after 1st injection, continue treatment with oral aripiprazole (10–20 mg/day) for 14 days; if no adverse reactions to 400 mg/mo dose, may ↓ dose to 300 mg every mo. *CYP2D6 PMs:* ↓ dose to 300 mg monthly; *CYP2D6 PMs concomitantly receiving strong CYP3A4 inhibitor:* ↓ dose to 200 mg monthly; *Concomitant therapy with strong CYP2D6 or CYP3A4 inhibitor:* ↓ dose to 300 mg monthly (if originally receiving 400 mg monthly) or 200 mg monthly (if originally receiving 300 mg monthly); *Concomitant therapy with strong CYP2D6 and CYP3A4 inhibitor:* ↓ dose to 200 mg monthly (if originally receiving 400 mg monthly) or 160 mg monthly (if originally receiving 300 mg monthly); *Concomitant therapy with CYP3A4 inducer:* Avoid use.

IM (Adults): *Abilify Asimtufii and receiving oral antipsychotics:* 960 mg every 2 mo (56 days after previous injection); after 1st injection, if previously receiving oral aripiprazole, continue treatment with oral aripiprazole (10–20 mg/day) for 14 days. If previously stable on another oral antipsychotic (but known to tolerate aripiprazole), after 1st injection, continue treatment with oral antipsychotic for 14 days. *Abilify Asimtufii and previously receiving Abilify Maintena:* 960 mg every 2 mo in place of the next scheduled Abilify Maintena injection; the 1st injection may be administered in place of the 2nd or later injection of Abilify Maintena; *CYP2D6 PMs:* ↓ dose to 720 mg every 2 mo; *CYP2D6 PMs concomitantly receiving strong CYP3A4 inhibitor:* Avoid use; *Concomitant therapy with strong CYP2D6 or CYP3A4 inhibitor:* ↓ dose to 720 mg every 2 mo; *Concomitant therapy with strong CYP2D6 and CYP3A4 inhibitor:* Avoid use; *Concomitant therapy with CYP3A4 inducer:* Avoid use.

Depression
PO (Adults): 2–5 mg once daily, may titrate upward at 1-wk intervals to 5–10 mg once daily (max: 15 mg/day).

Irritability Associated with Autistic Disorder
PO (Children 6–17 yr): 2 mg once daily; ↑ to 5 mg once daily after at least 1 wk; may further ↑ dose in 5-mg increments if needed at ≥1-wk intervals (max: 15 mg/day).

Tourette's Disorder

PO (Children 6–18 yr and ≥50 kg): 2 mg once daily; ↑ to target dose of 5 mg once daily after 2 days; may further ↑ dose if needed at ≥1-wk intervals (max: 10 mg/day).

PO (Children 6–18 yr and <50 kg): 2 mg once daily; ↑ to 5 mg once daily after 2 days, and then to target dose of 10 mg once daily after 5 days; may further ↑ dose in 5-mg increments if needed at ≥1-wk intervals (max: 20 mg/day).

Availability (generic available)

Immediate-release tablets: 2 mg, 5 mg, 10 mg, 15 mg, 20 mg, 30 mg. **Immediate-release tablets with sensor (Abilify Mycite):** 2 mg, 5 mg, 10 mg, 15 mg, 20 mg, 30 mg. **Orally disintegrating tablets (vanilla flavor):** 10 mg, 15 mg. **Oral solution (orange cream):** 1 mg/mL. **Extended-release suspension for injection (Abilify Maintena) (prefilled syringes or vials):** 300 mg, 400 mg. **Extended-release suspension for injection (Aristada) (prefilled syringes):** 441 mg/1.6 mL, 662 mg/2.4 mL, 882 mg/3.2 mL, 1064 mg/3.9 mL. **Extended-release suspension for injection (Aristada Initio) (prefilled syringes):** 675 mg/2.4 mL. **Extended-release suspension for injection (Abilify Asimtufii) (prefilled syringes):** 720 mg/2.4 mL, 960 mg/3.2 mL.

NURSING IMPLICATIONS

Assessment

- Assess mental status (orientation, mood, behavior) before and periodically during therapy. Assess for suicidal tendencies, especially during early therapy for depression. Restrict amount of drug available to patient. Risk may be increased in children, adolescents, and adults ≤24 yrs.
- Assess weight and BMI initially and during therapy. Compare weight of children and adolescents with that expected during normal growth.
- Monitor BP (sitting, standing, lying), pulse, and respiratory rate before and periodically during therapy.
- Observe patient carefully when administering medication to ensure that medication is actually taken and not hoarded or cheeked.
- Monitor patient for onset of akathisia (restlessness or desire to keep moving) and extrapyramidal side effects (*parkinsonian:* difficulty speaking or swallowing, loss of balance control, pill rolling of hands, masklike face, shuffling gait, rigidity, tremors; and *dystonic:* muscle spasms, twisting motions, twitching, inability to move eyes, weakness of arms or legs) periodically during therapy. Report these symptoms.
- Monitor for tardive dyskinesia (uncontrolled rhythmic movement of mouth, face, and extremities; lip smacking or puckering; puffing of cheeks; uncontrolled chewing; rapid or worm-like movements of tongue). Notify health care professional immediately if these symptoms occur, as these side effects may be irreversible.

- Monitor for development of neuroleptic malignant syndrome (fever, muscle rigidity, altered mental status, respiratory distress, tachycardia, seizures, diaphoresis, hypertension or hypotension, pallor, tiredness, loss of bladder control). Notify health care professional immediately if these symptoms occur.
- Assess for falls risk. Drowsiness, orthostatic hypotension, and motor and sensory instability increase risk. Institute prevention as indicated.

Lab Test Considerations

- May cause ↑ CK.
- Monitor CBC frequently during initial mos of therapy in patients with pre-existing or history of low WBC. May cause leukopenia, neutropenia, or agranulocytosis. Discontinue therapy if this occurs.
- Monitor blood glucose and cholesterol levels prior to starting and periodically during therapy. Patients with diabetes or risk factors for diabetes mellitus (obesity, family history of diabetes), who are starting treatment with atypical antipsychotics should undergo fasting blood glucose testing at beginning and periodically during therapy.

Implementation

- Do not confuse aripiprazole with rabeprazole or proton pump inhibitors.
- *Aristada Initio* is only used as a one-time dose to initiate *Aristada* therapy or if doses of *Aristada* are missed. Administer missed doses as soon as possible, may supplement next *Aristada* injection with *Aristada Initio*. **If last Aristada injection 441 mg** *and time since last injection ≤6 wk,* do not supplement; *if >6 wk and ≤7 wk since last dose,* supplement with single dose of *Aristada Initio*; *if >7 wk since last dose,* re-initiate with a single dose of *Aristada Initio* and a single dose of oral aripiprazole 30 mg. **If last Aristada injection 662 mg or 882 mg** *and time since last injection ≤8 wk,* do not supplement; *if >8 wk and ≤12 wk since last dose,* supplement with single dose of *Aristada Initio*; *if ≥12 wk since last dose,* re-initiate with a single dose of *Aristada Initio* and a single dose of oral aripiprazole 30 mg. **If last Aristada injection 1064 mg** *and time since last injection ≤10 wk,* do not supplement; *if >8 wk and ≤12 wk since last dose,* supplement with single dose of *Aristada Initio*; *if ≥12 wk since last dose,* re-initiate with a single dose of *Aristada Initio* and a single dose of oral aripiprazole 30 mg.
- **PO:** Administer once daily without regard to meals.
- *Orally disintegrating tablets:* Do not open blister until ready to administer. For single tablet removal, open package and peel back foil on blister to expose tablet. Do not push tablet through foil; may damage tablet. Immediately upon opening blister, using dry hands, remove tablet and place entire oral disintegrating tablet on tongue. Tablet disintegration occurs rapidly in saliva. Take tablet without liquid; but if needed, it can be taken with liquid. Do not attempt to split tablet.

- **Abilify Mycite:** Comprised of aripiprazole tablets embedded with an ingestible event marker (IEM) sensor to track drug ingestion. Kit includes tablets, a wearable sensor (Mycite patch) that detects signal from IEM after ingestion and transmits to a smartphone, a smartphone app (Mycite app) to display information for patient, and a web-based portal for health care professionals and caregivers. Ensure patient is capable and willing before use. Download app, follow instructions, ensure app is compatible with smartphone and paired with patch. When instructed by app, apply patch to left side of body just above lower edge of rib cage for *1-component patch* or to right or left side for *2–component patch*. Avoid applying patch in areas where skin is scraped, cracked, inflamed, or irritated, or in a location that overlaps area of most recently removed patch; if skin irritation occurs remove patch. Change patch at least weekly; do not remove for showering, swimming, or exercising. Ingestion is usually detected within 30 min, but may take up to 2 hr. If ingestion is not detected, do not repeat dose. Administer tablet without regard to food. *DNC:* Swallow tablet whole; do not divide, crush, or chew.
- **Extended-Release IM:** *Abilify Maintena* is available in vials or dual chamber prefilled syringes. *For vials,* reconstitute 300 mg dose with 1.5 mL and 400 mg dose with 1.9 mL of sterile water for injection; discard extra sterile water. Withdraw air to equalize pressure in vial. Shake vial vigorously for 30 sec until suspension is uniform; suspension is opaque and milky white. If injection is not given immediately, shake vial vigorously to resuspend prior to injection. Do not store suspension in syringe. Determine volume needed for dose: from 400 mg vial: 400 mg = 2 mL, 300 mg = 1.5 mL, 200 mg = 1.0, and 160 mg = 0.8 mL. From 300 mg vial: 300 mg = 1.5 mL, 200 mg = 1 mL, and 160 mg = 0.8 mL. *For prefilled syringes,* push plunger rod slightly to engage threads. Rotate plunger rod until rod stops rotating to release diluent; middle stopper will be at indicator line. Vertically shake syringe vigorously for 20 sec until drug is uniformly milky-white. *For deltoid site,* use 23 gauge needle, 1 inch in length for nonobese patients and 22 gauge 1.5 inch for obese patients. *For gluteal site,* use 22 gauge needle, 1.5 inches in length for non-obese patients and 22 gauge, 2 inch for obese patients. Inject deep into deltoid or gluteal site; do not massage. Continue oral dosing of aripiprazole for 2 wk after first dose of *Abilify Maintena.*
- If 2nd or 3rd doses of *Abilify Maintena* are missed and >4 wk and <5 wk since last injection, administer injection as soon as possible. If >5 wk since last injection, restart concomitant oral aripiprazole for 14 days with next administered injection. If fourth or subsequent doses are missed and >4 wk and <6 wk since last injection, administer injection as soon as possible. If >6 wk since last injection, restart concomitant oral aripiprazole for 14 days with next administered injection.
- *Aristada* comes in a kit with several needle sizes. Tap syringe at least 10 times to dislodge settled material and shake syringe vigorously for at least 30 sec to ensure suspension is uniform. Shake again if syringe not used within 15 min. Select needle and injection site. Deltoid may be used for 441 mg dose only. May use gluteal site for all doses. Remove air from syringe. Inject entire contents rapidly and continuously over <10 sec.
- *Abilify Asimtufii* must be administered as an intramuscular gluteal injection by a health care professional. Do not administer by any other route. For patients who have never taken aripiprazole, establish tolerability with oral aripiprazole prior to initiating treatment with *Abilify Asimtufii.* Due to the half-life of oral aripiprazole, it may take up to 2 weeks to fully assess tolerability. The suspension should appear to be a uniform, homogeneous suspension that is opaque and milky-white in color. Do not use *Abilify Asimtufii* prefilled syringe if the suspension is discolored, or contains particulate matter. Tap syringe on your hand at least 10 times. After tapping, shake syringe vigorously for at least 10 sec, until medication is uniform. For non-obese patients use a 22-gauge, 1.5-inch needle; for obese patients use a 21-gauge, 2-inch needle. Slowly inject the entire contents of prefilled syringe IM into gluteal muscle of patient; do not massage injection site.

Patient/Family Teaching

- Advise patient to take medication as directed and not to skip doses or double up on missed doses. Take missed doses as soon as remembered unless almost time for the next dose. Emphasize importance of maintaining regular scheduled injections when taking *Abilify Maintena or Aristada. Abilify Asimtufii* If >8 wk and <14 wk have elapsed since last injection, administer next dose of *Abilify Asimitufii* as soon as possible. Resume the once every 2 mo schedule. If >14 wk elapsed since last injection, restart concomitant oral aripiprazole for 14 days with the next administered injection of *Abilify Asimtufii.*
- Inform patient of possibility of extrapyramidal symptoms and tardive dyskinesia. Instruct patient to report these symptoms immediately.
- Advise patient to make position changes slowly to minimize orthostatic hypotension.
- Medication may cause drowsiness and lightheadedness. Caution patient to avoid driving or other activities requiring alertness until response to medication is known.
- Advise patient and family to notify health care professional if thoughts about suicide or dying, attempts to

commit suicide; new or worse depression; new or worse anxiety; feeling very agitated or restless; panic attacks; trouble sleeping; new or worse irritability; acting aggressive; being angry or violent; acting on dangerous impulses; an extreme increase in activity and talking; other unusual changes in behavior or mood or if signs and symptoms of high blood sugar (feel very thirsty, urinating more than usual, feel very hungry, feel weak or tired, nausea, confusion, breath smells fruity) occur.

- Inform patient that aripiprazole may cause weight gain. Advise patient to monitor weight periodically. Notify health care professional of significant weight gain.
- Instruct patient to notify health care professional of all Rx or OTC medications, vitamins, or herbal products being taken and to consult health care professional before taking any new medications. Caution patient to avoid taking alcohol or other CNS depressants concurrently with this medication.
- Advise patient that extremes in temperature should be avoided, because this drug impairs body temperature regulation.
- Advise patient to notify health care professional if new or increased eating/binge eating, gambling, sexual, shopping, or other impulse control disorders occur.
- Advise patient to notify health care professional of medication regimen prior to treatment or surgery.
- Rep: Advise females of reproductive potential to notify health care professional if pregnancy is planned or suspected or if breastfeeding. Extrapyramidal and/or withdrawal symptoms, (agitation, hypertonia, hypotonia, tremor, somnolence, respiratory distress, feeding disorder) have been reported in neonates who were exposed to antipsychotic drugs, during the third trimester of pregnancy. Monitor neonates closely. Encourage pregnant patients to enroll in pregnancy exposure registry that monitors outcomes of women exposed to aripiprazole during pregnancy by contacting National Pregnancy Registry for Atypical Antipsychotics at 1-866-961-2388 or visit http://womensmentalhealth.org/clinical-and-research-programs/pregnancyregistry/.
- Emphasize the importance of routine follow-up exams and continued participation in psychotherapy as indicated.
- Abilify Mycite: Advise patient referred for MRI test to remove patch and replace with a new patch as soon as possible.

Evaluation/Desired Outcomes

- Decrease in excitable, paranoid, or withdrawn behavior.
- Decrease incidence of mood swings in patients with bipolar disorders.
- Increased sense of well-being in patients with depression.
- Decreased agitation associated with schizophrenia or bipolar disorder.

- Decreased emotional and behavioral symptoms of irritability.
- Decrease in tics.

BEERS

asenapine (a-sen-a-peen)
Saphris, Secuado
Classification
Therapeutic: antipsychotics, mood stabilizers
Pharmacologic: dibenzo-oxepino pyrroles

Indications
SL, Transdermal: Schizophrenia. **SL:** Acute treatment of manic/mixed episodes associated with bipolar I disorder (as monotherapy or with lithium or valproate). **SL:** Maintenance treatment of manic/mixed episodes associated with bipolar I disorder (as monotherapy).

Action
May act through combined antagonism of dopaminergic (D_2) and $5-HT_{2A}$ receptors. **Therapeutic Effects:** Decreased symptoms of acute schizophrenia and mania/mixed episodes of bipolar I disorder.

Pharmacokinetics
Absorption: 35% absorbed following SL administration; 60% released from transdermal system.
Distribution: Extensively distributed to extravascular tissues.
Protein Binding: 95%.
Metabolism and Excretion: Primarily metabolized by CYP1A2 and UGTA14 enzyme systems; 50% excreted in urine, 40% in feces, primarily as metabolites.
Half-life: 24 hr.

TIME/ACTION PROFILE (plasma concentrations)

ROUTE	ONSET	PEAK	DURATION
SL	unknown	0.5–1.5 hr	12 hr
TD	unknown	12–24 hr	24 hr

Contraindications/Precautions
Contraindicated in: Hypersensitivity; Dementia-related psychoses; Severe hepatic impairment.
Use Cautiously in: History of cardiac arrhythmias, congenital QT prolongation, electrolyte abnormalities (especially hypomagnesemia or hypokalemia; correct prior to use) or concurrent use of medications known to prolong the QTc interval (may ↑ risk of life-threatening arrhythmias); History of seizures or conditions/medications known to ↓ seizure threshold; History of leukopenia/neutropenia; Strenuous exercise, exposure to extreme heat, concurrent medications with anticholinergic activity, or risk of dehydration; History of suicide attempt; Dehydration, hypovolemia, concurrent use of antihypertensive medications, history of MI/ischemic heart disease/HF/conduction abnormalities/cerebrovascular disease (↑ risk of hypotension); Patients at risk for falls; OB: Neonates at ↑ risk for extra-

pyramidal symptoms and withdrawal after delivery when exposed during the 3rd trimester; use during pregnancy only if potential maternal benefit justifies potential fetal risk; Lactation: Safety not established in breastfeeding; Pedi: Children <10 yr (safety and effectiveness not established); Geri: Appears on Beers list. ↑ risk of stroke, cognitive decline, and mortality in older adults with dementia. Avoid use in older adults, except for schizophrenia or bipolar disorder.

Adverse Reactions/Side Effects
CV: bradycardia, orthostatic hypotension, QT interval prolongation, tachycardia. **Endo:** hyperglycemia, hyperprolactinemia. **GI:** oral hypoesthesia, dry mouth, dyspepsia, dysphagia, oral blisters, oral inflammation, oral peeling/sloughing, oral ulcers. **Hemat:** AGRANULOCYTOSIS, leukopenia, neutropenia. **Local:** application site reactions (↑ in African Americans). **Metab:** weight gain, ↑ appetite, dyslipidemia. **Neuro:** akathisia, dizziness, drowsiness, extrapyramidal symptoms, anxiety, fatigue, NEUROLEPTIC MALIGNANT SYNDROME, SEIZURES, SUICIDAL THOUGHTS, syncope, tardive dyskinesia. **Misc:** HYPERSENSITIVITY REACTIONS (including anaphylaxis and angioedema).

Interactions
Drug-Drug: Concurrent use of **QTc interval prolonging drugs** including **Class 1A antiarrhythmics** such as **quinidine** and **procainamide** or **Class 3 antiarrhythmics** including **amiodarone** and **sotalol** or other **antipsychotics** including **ziprasidone**, **chlorpromazine** or **thioridazine** or certain **antibiotics** such as **moxifloxacin**; may ↑ risk of torsades de pointes and/or sudden death; avoid concurrent use. **Strong CYP1A2 inhibitors**, including **fluvoxamine**, may ↑ levels and risk of toxicity. **CYP2D6 inhibitors**, including **paroxetine**, may ↑ levels and risk of toxicity. ↑ risk of CNS depression with other **CNS depressants** including **antihistamines**, some **antidepressants**, **sedative/hypnotics**, and **alcohol**.

Route/Dosage
Schizophrenia
SL (Adults): 5 mg twice daily; may ↑ to 10 mg twice daily after 1 wk.
Transdermal (Adults): Apply 3.8 mg/24 hours patch once daily; may ↑ to 5.7 mg/24 hours or 7.6 mg/24 hours patch once daily after 1 week.

Acute Manic/Mixed Episodes Associated with Bipolar I Disorder
SL (Adults): *Monotherapy:* 10 mg twice daily; may ↓ to 5 mg twice daily if tolerated poorly; continue on the dose that caused stabilization as maintenance therapy; *Adjunctive therapy with lithium or valproate:* 5 mg twice daily; may ↑ to 10 mg twice daily.
SL (Children 10–17 yr): *Monotherapy:* 2.5 mg twice daily; may ↑ to 5 mg twice daily after 3 days; may ↑ to 10 mg twice daily after another 3 days.

Availability (generic available)
Sublingual tablets (Saphris) (black cherry flavor): 2.5 mg, 5 mg, 10 mg. **Transdermal patch (Secuado):** 3.8 mg/24 hours, 5.7 mg/24 hours, 7.6 mg/24 hours.

NURSING IMPLICATIONS
Assessment
- Monitor for clinical worsening and emergence of suicidal thoughts and behaviors, especially during the first few months of drug therapy and at times of dose changes. Assess mental status (orientation, mood, behavior) before and periodically during therapy. Assess for suicidal tendencies. Restrict amount of drug available to patient. Risk may be increased in children, adolescents, and adults ≤24 yrs.
- Assess weight and BMI initially and during therapy.
- Monitor BP (sitting, standing, lying) and pulse before and periodically during therapy.
- Observe patient carefully when administering medication to ensure that medication is actually taken and not hoarded.
- Monitor patient for onset of akathisia (restlessness or desire to keep moving) and extrapyramidal side effects (*parkinsonian:* difficulty speaking or swallowing, loss of balance control, pill rolling of hands, masklike face, shuffling gait, rigidity, tremors; and *dystonic:* muscle spasms, twisting motions, twitching, inability to move eyes, weakness of arms or legs) periodically throughout therapy. Report these symptoms.
- Monitor for tardive dyskinesia (uncontrolled rhythmic movement of mouth, face, and extremities; lip smacking or puckering; puffing of cheeks; uncontrolled chewing; rapid or worm-like movements of tongue). Notify health care professional immediately if these symptoms occur, as these side effects may be irreversible.
- Monitor for development of neuroleptic malignant syndrome (fever, muscle rigidity, altered mental status, respiratory distress, tachycardia, seizures, diaphoresis, hypertension or hypotension, pallor, tiredness, loss of bladder control). Discontinue asenapine and notify health care professional immediately if these symptoms occur.
- Monitor for symptoms related to hyperprolactinemia (menstrual abnormalities, galactorrhea, sexual dysfunction).
- Assess for falls risk. Drowsiness, orthostatic hypotension, and motor and sensory instability increase risk. Institute prevention if indicated.
- Assess patient for signs and symptoms of hypersensitivity reactions, including anaphylaxis, angioedema, hypotension, tachycardia, swollen tongue, dyspnea, itching, wheezing, and rash.

- Monitor for symptoms related to hyperprolactinemia (menstrual abnormalities, galactorrhea, sexual dysfunction).

Lab Test Considerations
- Obtain fasting blood glucose, lipid profile, and cholesterol levels initially and periodically during therapy.
- Monitor CBC frequently during initial mo of therapy in patients with pre-existing or history of low WBC. May cause leukopenia, neutropenia, or agranulocytosis. Monitor patients with neutropenia for fever or other symptoms of infection and treat promptly. Discontinue therapy if ANC <1000/mm³ occurs.
- May cause transient ↑ in serum ALT.

Implementation

- **SL:** Open packet immediately before use by firmly pressing thumb button and pulling out tablet pack. Do not push tablet through or cut or tear tablet pack. Peel back colored tab and gently remove tablet. Place tablet under tongue and allow to dissolve completely; dissolves in saliva within sec. *DNC:* Do not split, crush, chew, or swallow tablets. Avoid eating or drinking for 10 min after administration. Slide tablet pack back into case until it clicks.
- **Transdermal patch:** Once each day, apply to clean, dry, and intact skin of upper arm, upper back, abdomen, or hip. Rotate site with each application. Do not cut open pouch until ready to apply and do not use if pouch seal is broken or appears to be damaged. Do not cut patch; apply whole patch. If patch lifts at edges, reattach by pressing firmly and smoothing down edges. If patch comes off completely, apply a new patch. Remove old patch; apply only 1 patch at a time. Discard by folding patch so that adhesive side sticks to itself and safely discard. If irritation or a burning sensation occurs while wearing patch, remove the system and apply a new patch to a new application site. May wear during shower, but use during swimming or taking a bath has not been evaluated. Do not apply external heat sources (heating pad) over patch; prolonged application of heat over patch increases plasma concentrations of asenapine.

Patient/Family Teaching

- Instruct patient to take medication as directed and not to skip doses or double up on missed doses. Take missed doses as soon as remembered unless almost time for the next dose. Advise patient to read *Instructions for Use* before starting asenapine.
- Inform patient of possibility of extrapyramidal symptoms and tardive dyskinesia. Instruct patient to report these symptoms immediately.
- Advise patient to make position changes slowly to minimize orthostatic hypotension. Protect from falls.
- Medication may cause drowsiness and dizziness. Caution patient to avoid driving or other activities requiring alertness until response to medication is known.

- Advise patient and family to notify health care professional if thoughts about suicide or dying, attempts to commit suicide; new or worse depression; new or worse anxiety; feeling very agitated or restless; panic attacks; trouble sleeping; new or worse irritability; acting aggressive; being angry or violent; acting on dangerous impulses; an extreme increase in activity and talking; other unusual changes in behavior or mood or if signs and symptoms of hypersensitivity reactions (difficulty breathing, itching, swelling of the face, tongue or throat, feeling lightheaded) occur.
- Instruct patient to notify health care professional of all Rx or OTC medications, vitamins, or herbal products being taken, to avoid alcohol, and to consult health care professional before taking any new medications and to avoid taking alcohol or other CNS depressants concurrently with this medication.
- Advise patient that extremes in temperature should be avoided, because this drug impairs body temperature regulation.
- Counsel patients on signs and symptoms of hyperprolactinemia and to contact their health care professional if these abnormalities occur.
- Advise patient to notify health care professional of medication regimen prior to treatment or surgery.
- Rep: May cause fetal harm. Advise females of reproductive potential to notify health care professional if pregnancy is planned or suspected and to avoid breastfeeding during therapy. If used during 3rd trimester may cause extrapyramidal and or withdrawal symptoms in infant (agitation, hypertonia, hypotonia, tremor, somnolence, respiratory distress, feeding disorder). Monitor neonates closely. Encourage pregnant patients to enroll in registry by contacting National Pregnancy Registry for Atypical Antipsychotics at 1-866-961-2388 or visit http://womensmentalhealth.org/clinical-and-research-programs/pregnancyregistry/.
- Emphasize the importance of routine follow-up exams and continued participation in psychotherapy as indicated.
- **SL:** Inform patient that oral ulcers, blisters, peeling/sloughing, and inflammation may occur at application site. Advise patient to notify health care professional if these occur, may require discontinuation. Inform patient that numbness or tingling of mouth or throat may occur shortly after administration of asenapine; usually resolves within 1 hr.
- **Transdermal patch:** Instruct patient in correct application of patch. May cause erythema, pruritus, papules, discomfort, pain, edema, or irritation at site of application during wear time or immediately after removal; occurs more frequently in African Americans. Risk increases if worn longer that 24 hr or if site is used repeatedly.

Evaluation/Desired Outcomes

- Decrease in excitable, paranoic, or withdrawn behavior.

- Decrease incidence of mood swings in patients with bipolar disorders.
- Decreased agitation associated with schizophrenia or bipolar disorder.

BEERS

aspirin (as-pir-in)

Acuprin, ✹Asaphen, Aspergum, Aspir-Low, Aspirtab, Bayer Aspirin, Bayer Timed-Release Arthritic Pain Formula, Easprin, Ecotrin, 8-Hour Bayer Timed-Release, Empirin, ✹Entrophen, Halfprin, Healthprin, ✹Lowprin, Norwich Aspirin, ✹Novasen, ✹Rivasa, Sloprin, St. Joseph Adult Chewable Aspirin, Therapy Bayer, Vazalore, ZORprin

Classification
Therapeutic: antiplatelet agents, antipyretics, nonopioid analgesics
Pharmacologic: salicylates, nonsteroidal antiinflammatory drugs (NSAIDs)

Indications

Inflammatory disorders including: Rheumatoid arthritis, Osteoarthritis. Mild to moderate pain. Fever. Prophylaxis of transient ischemic attacks and MI. **Unlabeled Use:** Adjunctive treatment of Kawasaki disease.

Action

Produce analgesia and reduce inflammation and fever by inhibiting the production of prostaglandins. Decreases platelet aggregation. **Therapeutic Effects:** Analgesia. Reduction of inflammation. Reduction of fever. Decreased incidence of transient ischemic attacks and MI.

Pharmacokinetics

Absorption: Well absorbed from the upper small intestine; absorption from enteric-coated preparations may be unreliable; rectal absorption is slow and variable.

Distribution: Rapidly and widely distributed; crosses the placenta and enters breast milk.

Metabolism and Excretion: Extensively metabolized by the liver; inactive metabolites excreted by the kidneys. Amount excreted unchanged by the kidneys depends on urine pH; as pH increases, amount excreted unchanged increases from 2–3% up to 80%.

Half-life: 2–3 hr for low doses; up to 15–30 hr with larger doses because of saturation of liver metabolism.

TIME/ACTION PROFILE (analgesia/fever reduction)

ROUTE	ONSET	PEAK	DURATION
PO	5–30 min	1–3 hr	3–6 hr

Contraindications/Precautions

Contraindicated in: Hypersensitivity to aspirin or other salicylates; Cross-sensitivity with other NSAIDs may exist (less with nonaspirin salicylates); Bleeding disorders or thrombocytopenia; OB: Avoid use after 30 wk gestation; Pedi: May ↑ risk of Reye's syndrome in children or adolescents with viral infections.

Use Cautiously in: History of GI bleeding or ulcer disease; Chronic alcohol use/abuse; Severe hepatic or renal disease; OB: Use at or after 20 wk gestation may cause fetal or neonatal renal impairment; if NSAID treatment is necessary between 20 wk and 30 wk gestation, limit use to the lowest effective dose and shortest duration possible; Lactation: Safety not established in breastfeeding; Geri: Appears on Beers list. ↑ risk of major bleeding in older adults. Avoid use for primary prevention of cardiovascular disease in older adults. Avoid chronic use for pain (at doses >325 mg/day) in older adults unless other alternatives are not effective and the patient can take a gastroprotective agent; avoid short-term use for pain (at doses >325 mg/day) in older adults in combination with oral or parenteral corticosteroids, anticoagulants, or antiplatelet agents unless other alternatives are not effective and the patient can take a gastroprotective agent.

Adverse Reactions/Side Effects

Derm: DRUG REACTION WITH EOSINOPHILIA AND SYSTEMIC SYMPTOMS (DRESS), rash, urticaria. **EENT:** tinnitus. **GI:** dyspepsia, epigastric distress, nausea, abdominal pain, anorexia, GI BLEEDING, hepatotoxicity, vomiting. **Hemat:** anemia, hemolysis. **Misc:** HYPERSENSITIVITY REACTIONS (including anaphylaxis and laryngeal edema).

Interactions

Drug-Drug: May ↑ the risk of bleeding with **warfarin**, **heparin**, **heparin-like agents**, **thrombolytic agents**, **dipyridamole**, **clopidogrel**, **tirofiban**, or **eptifibatide**, although these agents are frequently used safely in combination and in sequence. **Ibuprofen:** may negate the cardioprotective antiplatelet effects of low-dose aspirin. May ↑ risk of bleeding with **cefotetan** and **valproic acid**. May ↑ activity of **penicillins**, **phenytoin**, **methotrexate**, **valproic acid**, **oral hypoglycemic agents**, and **sulfonamides**. **Urinary acidification** ↑ reabsorption and may ↑ serum salicylate levels. **Alkalinization of the urine** or the ingestion of large amounts of **antacids** ↑ excretion and ↓ serum salicylate levels. May blunt the therapeutic response to **diuretics** and **ACE inhibitors**. ↑ risk of GI irritation with **NSAIDs**.

Drug-Natural Products: ↑ anticoagulant effect and bleeding risk with **arnica**, **chamomile**, **clove**, **feverfew**, **garlic**, **ginger**, **ginkgo**, **Panax ginseng**, and others.

Drug-Food: **Foods capable of acidifying the urine** (see Appendix J) may ↑ serum salicylate levels.

✹= Canadian drug name. ▩ = Genetic implication. S̶t̶r̶i̶k̶e̶t̶h̶r̶o̶u̶g̶h̶ = Discontinued. CAPITALS = life-threatening. Underline = most frequent.

Route/Dosage

Pain/Fever
PO, Rect (Adults): 325–1000 mg every 4–6 hr (not to exceed 4 g/day). *Extended-release tablets:* 650 mg every 8 hr or 800 mg every 12 hr.
PO, Rect (Children 2–11 yr): 10–15 mg/kg/dose every 4–6 hr; maximum dose: 4 g/day.

Inflammation
PO (Adults): 2.4 g/day initially; ↑ to maintenance dose of 3.6–5.4 g/day in divided doses (up to 7.8 g/day for acute rheumatic fever).
PO (Children): 60–100 mg/kg/day in divided doses (up to 130 mg/kg/day for acute rheumatic fever).

Prevention of Transient Ischemic Attacks
PO (Adults): 50–325 mg once daily.

Prevention of Myocardial Infarction/Antiplatelet Effects
PO (Adults): 80–325 mg once daily. *Suspected acute MI:* 160 mg as soon as MI is suspected.
PO (Children): 3–10 mg/kg/day given once daily (round dose to a convenient amount).

Kawasaki Disease
PO (Children): 80–100 mg/kg/day in 4 divided doses until fever resolves; may be followed by maintenance dose of 3–5 mg/kg/day as a single dose for up to 8 wk.

Availability (generic available)
Immediate-release tablets: 81 mg[OTC], 162.5 mg[OTC], 325 mg[OTC], 500 mg[OTC], 650 mg[OTC], ✲975 mg[OTC]. **Immediate-release capsules:** 325 mg[OTC]. **Extended-release tablets:** ✲325 mg[OTC], 650 mg[OTC], 800 mg. **Enteric-coated (delayed-release) tablets:** 80 mg[OTC], 165 mg[OTC], ✲300 mg[OTC], 325 mg[OTC], 500 mg[OTC], ✲600 mg[OTC], 650 mg[OTC], 975 mg[OTC]. **Delayed-release capsules:** ✲325 mg[OTC], ✲500 mg[OTC]. **Chewable tablets:** ✲80 mg[OTC], 81 mg[OTC]. **Dispersible tablets:** 325 mg[OTC], 500 mg[OTC]. **Suppositories:** 60 mg[OTC], 120 mg[OTC], 125 mg[OTC], 130 mg[OTC], ✲150 mg[OTC], ✲160 mg[OTC], 195 mg[OTC], 200 mg[OTC], 300 mg[OTC], ✲320 mg[OTC], 325 mg[OTC], 600 mg[OTC], ✲640 mg[OTC], 650 mg[OTC], 1.2 g[OTC]. *In combination with:* antihistamines, decongestants, cough suppressants[OTC], and opioids. See Appendix N.

NURSING IMPLICATIONS

Assessment
- Patients who have asthma, allergies, and nasal polyps or who are allergic to tartrazine are at an increased risk for developing hypersensitivity reactions.
- Monitor for signs and symptoms of DRESS (fever, rash, lymphadenopathy, facial swelling) periodically during therapy. Discontinue therapy if symptoms occur.
- **Pain:** Assess pain and limitation of movement; note type, location, and intensity before and 60 min after administration.
- **Fever:** Assess fever and note associated signs (diaphoresis, tachycardia, malaise, chills).

Lab Test Considerations
- Monitor hepatic function before antirheumatic therapy and if symptoms of hepatotoxicity occur; more likely in patients, especially children, with rheumatic fever, systemic lupus erythematosus, juvenile arthritis, or pre-existing hepatic disease. May cause ↑ serum AST, ALT, and alkaline phosphatase, especially when plasma concentrations exceed 25 mg/100 mL. May return to normal despite continued use or dose reduction. If severe abnormalities or active liver disease occurs, discontinue and use with caution in future.
- Monitor serum salicylate levels periodically with prolonged high-dose therapy to determine dose, safety, and efficacy, especially in children with Kawasaki disease.
- May alter results of serum uric acid, urine vanillylmandelic acid (VMA), protirelin-induced thyroid-stimulating hormone (TSH), urine hydroxyindoleacetic acid (5-HIAA) determinations, and radionuclide thyroid imaging.
- Prolongs bleeding time for 4–7 days and, in large doses, may cause prolonged prothrombin time. Monitor hematocrit periodically in prolonged high-dose therapy to assess for GI blood loss.

Toxicity and Overdose
- Monitor for the onset of tinnitus, headache, hyperventilation, agitation, mental confusion, lethargy, diarrhea, and sweating. If these symptoms appear, withhold medication and notify health care professional immediately.

Implementation
- Use lowest effective dose for shortest period of time.
- **PO:** Administer after meals or with food or an antacid to minimize gastric irritation. Food slows but does not alter the total amount absorbed.
- *DNC:* Do not crush or chew enteric-coated tablets. Do not take antacids within 1–2 hr of enteric-coated tablets. Chewable tablets may be chewed, dissolved in liquid, or swallowed whole. Some extended-release tablets may be broken or crumbled but must not be ground up before swallowing. See manufacturer's prescribing information for individual products.

Patient/Family Teaching
- Instruct patient to take aspirin with a full glass of water and to remain in an upright position for 15–30 min after administration.
- Advise patient to report tinnitus; unusual bleeding of gums; bruising; black, tarry stools; or fever lasting longer than 3 days.
- Caution patient to avoid concurrent use of alcohol with this medication to minimize possible gastric irritation; 3 or more glasses of alcohol per day may increase risk of GI bleeding. Caution patient to

avoid taking concurrently with acetaminophen or NSAIDs for more than a few days, unless directed by health care professional to prevent analgesic nephropathy.

- Instruct patients on a sodium-restricted diet to avoid effervescent tablets or buffered-aspirin preparations.
- Tablets with an acetic (vinegar-like) odor should be discarded.
- Advise patients on long-term therapy to inform health care professional of medication regimen before surgery. Aspirin may need to be withheld for 1 wk before surgery.
- Rep: May cause fetal harm. Advise females of reproductive potential to notify health care professional if pregnancy is planned or suspected or if breastfeeding. Advise women to avoid aspirin in the 3rd trimester of pregnancy (after 29 wk), may cause premature closure of the fetal ductus arteriosus. Use of aspirin after 20 wk may cause fetal renal dysfunction leading to oligohydramnios. May cause reversible infertility in women attempting to conceive; may consider discontinuing aspirin.
- Pedi: Centers for Disease Control and Prevention warns against giving aspirin to children or adolescents with varicella (chickenpox) or influenza-like or viral illnesses because of a possible association with Reye's syndrome.
- **Transient Ischemic Attacks or MI:** Advise patients receiving aspirin prophylactically to take only prescribed dose. Increasing dose has not been found to provide additional benefits.

Evaluation/Desired Outcomes
- Relief of mild to moderate discomfort.
- Increased ease of joint movement. May take 2–3 wk for maximum effectiveness.
- Reduction of fever.
- Prevention of transient ischemic attacks.
- Prevention of MI.

atenolol (a-ten-oh-lole)
Tenormin
Classification
Therapeutic: antianginals, antihypertensives
Pharmacologic: beta blockers

Indications
Hypertension. Angina pectoris. MI.

Action
Blocks stimulation of beta$_1$(myocardial)-adrenergic receptors. Does not usually affect beta$_2$(pulmonary, vascular, uterine)-receptor sites. **Therapeutic Effects:** Decreased BP and heart rate. Decreased frequency of attacks of angina pectoris. Reduction of cardiovascular mortality associated with MI.

Pharmacokinetics
Absorption: 50–60% absorbed after oral administration.
Distribution: Minimal penetration of CNS.
Metabolism and Excretion: 40–50% excreted unchanged by the kidneys; remainder excreted in feces as unabsorbed drug.
Half-life: 6–9 hr.

TIME/ACTION PROFILE (cardiovascular effects)

ROUTE	ONSET	PEAK	DURATION
PO	1 hr	2–4 hr	24 hr

Contraindications/Precautions
Contraindicated in: Uncompensated HF; Pulmonary edema; Cardiogenic shock; Bradycardia or heart block.

Use Cautiously in: Renal impairment (dosage ↓ recommended if CCr ≤35 mL/min); Hepatic impairment; Pulmonary disease (including asthma; beta selectivity may be lost at higher doses); Diabetes mellitus (may mask signs of hypoglycemia); Thyrotoxicosis (may mask symptoms); Patients with a history of severe allergic reactions (intensity of reactions may be ↑); OB: Crosses the placenta and may cause fetal/neonatal bradycardia, hypotension, hypoglycemia, or respiratory depression; Lactation: Use while breastfeeding only if potential maternal benefit justifies potential risk to infant; Pedi: Safety and effectiveness not established in children; Geri: Older adults may have ↑ sensitivity to beta blockers (initial dose ↓ recommended).

Adverse Reactions/Side Effects
CV: BRADYCARDIA, HF, hypotension, peripheral vasoconstriction. **Derm:** rash. **EENT:** blurred vision, stuffy nose. **Endo:** hyperglycemia, hypoglycemia. **GI:** ↑ liver enzymes, constipation, diarrhea, nausea, vomiting. **GU:** erectile dysfunction, ↓ libido, urinary frequency. **MS:** arthralgia, back pain, joint pain. **Neuro:** fatigue, weakness, anxiety, depression, dizziness, drowsiness, insomnia, memory loss, mental status changes, nervousness, nightmares. **Resp:** bronchospasm, PULMONARY EDEMA, wheezing. **Misc:** drug-induced lupus syndrome.

Interactions
Drug-Drug: General anesthesia, phenytoin, and **verapamil** may cause additive myocardial depression. Additive bradycardia may occur with **clonidine, digoxin, diltiazem, ivabradine,** and **verapamil**. Additive hypotension may occur with other **antihypertensives,** acute ingestion of **alcohol,** or **nitrates.** Concurrent use with **amphetamine, cocaine, ephedrine, epinephrine, norepinephrine, phenylephrine,** or **pseudoephedrine** may result in unopposed alpha-adrenergic stimulation (excessive hypertension, bradycardia). Concurrent **thyroid** admin-

istration may ↓ effectiveness. May alter the effectiveness of **insulins** or **oral hypoglycemic agents** (dosage adjustments may be necessary). May ↓ the effectiveness of **theophylline**. May ↓ the beneficial beta₁-cardiovascular effects of **dopamine** or **dobutamine**. Use cautiously within 14 days of **MAO inhibitor** therapy; may result in hypertension.

Route/Dosage
PO (Adults): *Antianginal:* 50 mg once daily; may be ↑ after 1 wk to 100 mg/day (up to 200 mg/day). *Antihypertensive:* 25–50 mg once daily; may be ↑ after 2 wk to 50–100 mg once daily. *MI:* 50 mg, then 50 mg 12 hr later, then 100 mg/day as a single dose or in 2 divided doses for 6–9 days or until hospital discharge.

Renal Impairment
PO (Adults): *CCr 15–35 mL/min:* dosage should not exceed 50 mg/day; *CCr <15 mL/min:* dosage should not exceed 50 mg every other day.

Availability (generic available)
Tablets: 25 mg, 50 mg, 100 mg. *In combination with:* chlorthalidone (Tenoretic). See Appendix N.

NURSING IMPLICATIONS
Assessment
- Monitor BP, ECG, and pulse frequently during dose adjustment period and periodically throughout therapy.
- Monitor intake and output ratios and daily weights. Assess routinely for HF (dyspnea, rales/crackles, weight gain, peripheral edema, jugular venous distention).
- Monitor frequency of prescription refills to determine adherence.
- **Angina:** Assess frequency and characteristics of angina periodically during therapy.

Lab Test Considerations
- May cause ↑ BUN, serum lipoprotein, potassium, triglyceride, and uric acid levels.
- May cause ↑ ANA titers.
- May cause ↑ in blood glucose levels.

Toxicity and Overdose
- Monitor patients receiving beta blockers for signs of overdose (bradycardia, severe dizziness or fainting, severe drowsiness, dyspnea, bluish fingernails or palms, seizures). Notify health care professional immediately if these signs occur.

Implementation
- **PO:** Take apical pulse before administering drug. If <50 bpm or if arrhythmia occurs, withhold medication and notify health care professional.

Patient/Family Teaching
- Instruct patient to take atenolol as directed at the same time each day, even if feeling well; do not skip or double up on missed doses. Take missed doses as soon as possible up to 8 hr before next dose. Abrupt

withdrawal may cause life-threatening arrhythmias, hypertension, or myocardial ischemia.
- Advise patient to make sure enough medication is available for weekends, holidays, and vacations. A written prescription may be kept in wallet in case of emergency.
- Teach patient and family how to check pulse and BP. Instruct them to check pulse daily and BP biweekly and to report significant changes.
- May cause drowsiness or dizziness. Caution patients to avoid driving or other activities that require alertness until response to the drug is known.
- Advise patients to change positions slowly to minimize orthostatic hypotension.
- Caution patient that atenolol may increase sensitivity to cold.
- Instruct patient to notify health care professional of all Rx or OTC medications, vitamins, or herbal products being taken, to avoid alcohol, and to consult health care professional before taking any new medications, especially cold preparations.
- Patients with diabetes should closely monitor blood glucose, especially if weakness, malaise, irritability, or fatigue occurs. Medication does not block sweating as a sign of hypoglycemia.
- Advise patient to notify health care professional if slow pulse, difficulty breathing, wheezing, cold hands and feet, dizziness, light-headedness, confusion, depression, rash, fever, sore throat, unusual bleeding, or bruising occurs.
- Instruct patient to inform health care professional of medication regimen before treatment or surgery.
- Rep: Advise females of reproductive potential to notify health care professional if pregnancy is planned or suspected or if breastfeeding.
- Advise patient to carry identification describing disease process and medication regimen at all times.
- **Hypertension:** Reinforce the need to continue additional therapies for hypertension (weight loss, sodium restriction, stress reduction, regular exercise, moderation of alcohol consumption, and smoking cessation). Medication controls but does not cure hypertension.

Evaluation/Desired Outcomes
- Decrease in BP.
- Reduction in frequency of angina.
- Increase in activity tolerance.
- Prevention of MI.

⚠ atezolizumab
(a-te-zoe-**liz**-ue-mab)
Tecentriq
Classification
Therapeutic: antineoplastics
Pharmacologic: monoclonal antibodies, programmed death ligand 1 (PD-L1) inhibitors

Indications

⚡ First-line treatment of metastatic non-small cell lung cancer (NSCLC) in patients whose tumors have high PD-L1 expression (PD-L1 stained ≥50% of tumor cells or PD-L1 stained tumor-infiltrating immune cells covering ≥ 10% of the tumor area) and have no epidermal growth factor receptor (EGFR) or anaplastic lymphoma kinase (ALK) genomic tumor aberrations (as monotherapy). ⚡ Metastatic NSCLC in patients who have disease progression during or following platinum-containing chemotherapy (as monotherapy). Patients with EGFR or ALK genomic tumor aberrations should have disease progression on FDA-approved therapy for these aberrations prior to receiving atezolizumab. Stage II to IIIA NSCLC as adjuvant treatment following resection and platinum-based chemotherapy in patients whose tumors have PD-L1 expression on ≥ 1% of tumor cells (as monotherapy). ⚡ Metastatic non-squamous, NSCLC as first-line therapy in patients whose tumors have no EGFR or ALK genomic tumor aberrations (in combination with bevacizumab, paclitaxel, and carboplatin). ⚡ Metastatic non-squamous NSCLC as first-line therapy in patients whose tumors have no EGFR or ALK genomic tumor aberrations (in combination with paclitaxel protein bound and carboplatin). Extensive-stage small cell lung cancer as first-line therapy (in combination with carboplatin and etoposide). Unresectable or metastatic hepatocellular carcinoma in patients who have not previously received systemic therapy (in combination with bevacizumab). ⚡ BRAF V600 mutation-positive unresectable or metastatic melanoma (in combination with cobimetinib and vemurafenib). Unresectable or metastatic alveolar soft part sarcoma (as monotherapy).

Action

Binds to (PD-L1 to prevent its interaction with the programmed cell death-1 (PD-1) and B7.1 (or CD80) receptors, which activates the anti-tumor immune response. **Therapeutic Effects:** Decreased spread of NSCLC, small cell lung cancer, hepatocellular carcinoma, and melanoma with increased survival. Decreased spread of alveolar soft part sarcoma.

Pharmacokinetics

Absorption: IV administration results in complete bioavailability.
Distribution: Minimally distributed to tissues.
Metabolism and Excretion: Unknown.
Half-life: 27 days.

TIME/ACTION PROFILE (plasma concentrations)

ROUTE	ONSET	PEAK	DURATION
IV	unknown	unknown	unknown

Contraindications/Precautions

Contraindicated in: OB: Pregnancy; Lactation: Lactation.

Use Cautiously in: Allogeneic hematopoietic stem cell transplant recipients (↑ risk of transplantation complications); Rep: Women of reproductive potential; Pedi: Children <2 yr (alveolar soft part sarcoma) or <18 yr (all other indications) (safety and effectiveness not established).

Adverse Reactions/Side Effects

CV: peripheral edema, myocarditis, pericarditis. **Derm:** pruritus, rash, DRUG REACTION WITH EOSINOPHILIA AND SYSTEMIC SYMPTOMS (DRESS), STEVENS-JOHNSON SYNDROME (SJS), TOXIC EPIDERMAL NECROLYSIS (TEN). **Endo:** hypothyroidism, ADRENAL INSUFFICIENCY, hyperglycemia, hyperthyroidism, hypophysitis, type 1 diabetes mellitus. **F and E:** hyponatremia, dehydration. **GI:** ↓ appetite, COLITIS/DIARRHEA, constipation, HEPATOTOXICITY, nausea, vomiting, ↑ liver enzymes, abdominal pain, PANCREATITIS. **GU:** hematuria, ↓ fertility (females), ↑ serum creatinine, acute kidney injury, nephritis, urinary obstruction. **Hemat:** lymphopenia, anemia. **Metab:** hypoalbuminemia. **MS:** arthralgia. **Neuro:** Guillain-Barre syndrome, ENCEPHALITIS, MENINGITIS, MYASTHENIA GRAVIS, myelitis, nerve paresis. **Resp:** cough, dyspnea, INTERSTITIAL LUNG DISEASE. **Misc:** fatigue, fever, INFECTIONS (including herpes encephalitis and tuberculosis), INFUSION-RELATED REACTIONS.

Interactions

Drug-Drug: None reported.

Route/Dosage

Non-Small Cell Lung Cancer

IV (Adults): *As monotherapy (metastatic NSCLC):* 840 mg every 2 wk until disease progression or unacceptable toxicity or 1200 mg every 3 wk until disease progression or unacceptable toxicity or 1680 mg every 4 wk until disease progression or unacceptable toxicity. *As monotherapy (adjuvant treatment):* 840 mg every 2 wk for up to 1 yr unless there is disease recurrence or unacceptable toxicity or 1200 mg every 3 wk for up to 1 yr unless there is disease recurrence or unacceptable toxicity or 1680 mg every 4 wk for up to 1 yr unless there is disease recurrence or unacceptable toxicity. *Combination therapy:* 840 mg every 2 wk until disease progression or unacceptable toxicity or 1200 mg every 3 wk until disease progression or unacceptable toxicity or 1680 mg every 4 wk until disease progression or unacceptable toxicity. Administer prior to bevacizumab and chemotherapy when given on same day.

Small Cell Lung Cancer

IV (Adults): 840 mg every 2 wk until disease progression or unacceptable toxicity or 1200 mg every 3 wk until disease progression or unacceptable toxicity or 1680 mg every 4 wk until disease progression or unacceptable toxicity. Administer prior to carboplatin and etoposide when given on same day.

Hepatocellular Carcinoma
IV (Adults): 840 mg every 2 wk until disease progression or unacceptable toxicity *or* 1200 mg every 3 wk until disease progression or unacceptable toxicity *or* 1680 mg every 4 wk until disease progression or unacceptable toxicity. Administer prior to bevacizumab when given on same day.

Melanoma
IV (Adults): 840 mg every 2 wk until disease progression or unacceptable toxicity *or* 1200 mg every 3 wk until disease progression or unacceptable toxicity *or* 1680 mg every 4 wk until disease progression or unacceptable toxicity. A 28-day treatment cycle of cobimetinib and vemurafenib should be administered prior to starting atezolizumab therapy.

Alveolar Soft Part Sarcoma
IV (Adults): 840 mg every 2 wk until disease progression or unacceptable toxicity *or* 1200 mg every 3 wk until disease progression or unacceptable toxicity *or* 1680 mg every 4 wk until disease progression or unacceptable toxicity.

IV (Children ≥2 yr): 15 mg/kg (max dose = 1200 mg) every 3 wk until disease progression or unacceptable toxicity.

Availability
Solution for injection: 60 mg/mL.

NURSING IMPLICATIONS
Assessment
● Monitor for signs and symptoms of pneumonitis (new or worsening cough, dyspnea, chest pain) during therapy. Monitor with x-rays as needed. *For ≥Grade 2 pneumonitis,* hold atezolizumab and administer corticosteroids at a dose of 1–2 mg/kg/day prednisolone equivalents followed by a taper. Resume after taper corticosteroid if Grade 0–1. If no complete or partial resolution within 12 wk of starting corticosteroids or inability to reduce prednisone to ≤10 mg per day within 12 wk of starting steroids, permanently discontinue atezolizumab. *For Grade 3 or 4 pneumonitis,* permanently discontinue atezolizumab.
● Monitor for signs and symptoms of hepatitis (jaundice, severe nausea or vomiting, pain on right side of abdomen, lethargy, dark urine, unusual bleeding or bruising, anorexia) periodically during therapy.
● Monitor for signs and symptoms of diarrhea or colitis (blood in stools, dark tarry stools, abdominal pain or tenderness) periodically during therapy. *For Grade 2 or 3,* hold atezolizumab until Grade 1 or resolved and corticosteroid dose ≤prednisone 10 mg per day (or equivalent). *For Grade 4,* permanently discontinue atezolizumab.
● Monitor for signs and symptoms of adrenal insufficiency (extreme tiredness, dizziness or fainting, frequent urination, nausea or vomiting, changes in mood or behavior, ↓ sex drive, irritability, forgetfulness), hypophysitis (unusual headaches, persistent headaches, vision problems), hyperthyroidism, and Type 1 diabetes periodically during therapy. *If Grades 2, 3, or 4 occur,* hold dose until Grade 1 or resolved and clinically stable on hormone replacement therapy.
● Monitor for signs and symptoms of immune-mediated skin reactions (rash, pruritus, blistering, painful sores in mouth, nose, throat, genital area) periodically during therapy. Topical emollients and/or topical corticosteroids may treat mild to moderate non-exfoliative rashes. May cause exfoliative dermatitis (SJS, TEN, DRESS). *If SJS, TEN, or DRESS is suspected,* hold atezolizumab. *If SJS, TEN, or DRESS are confirmed,* permanently discontinue atezolizumab.
● Monitor for signs and symptoms of meningitis or encephalitis (fever, confusion, changes in mood or behavior, extreme sensitivity to light, neck stiffness) during therapy. If symptoms occur, permanently discontinue atezolizumab. Administer 1–2 mg/kg/day methylprednisolone or equivalent. Convert to oral prednisone 60 mg/day or equivalent once improved. When symptoms improve to ≤ Grade 1, taper steroids over ≥1 mo.
● Monitor for signs and symptoms of motor or sensory neuropathy (severe muscle weakness, numbness or tingling in hands or feet) periodically during therapy. For Grade 2 neurological toxicities, hold atezolizumab and administer corticosteroids at a dose of 1–2 mg/kg/day prednisolone equivalents followed by a taper. Resume after taper corticosteroid if Grade 0–1. If no complete or partial resolution within 12 wk of starting corticosteroids or inability to reduce prednisone to ≤10 mg per day within 12 wk of starting steroids, permanently discontinue atezolizumab. *If Grades 3 or 4 or symptoms of myasthenic syndrome/myasthenia gravis or Guillain-Barre syndrome occur,* permanently discontinue atezolizumab. Institute treatment as needed.
● Monitor for signs and symptoms of pancreatitis (abdominal pain) during therapy. *If Grade 2 or 3 pancreatitis,* hold atezolizumab. Treat with methylprednisolone IV 1–2 mg/kg/day or equivalent. Once symptoms improve, follow with 1–2 mg/kg/day of oral prednisone or equivalent. Resume atezolizumab if symptoms of pancreatitis resolved and corticosteroid reduced to ≤10 mg/day oral prednisone or equivalent. *For Grade 4 or recurrent pancreatitis,* permanently discontinue atezolizumab.
● Monitor for signs and symptoms of infection (fever, cough, frequent urination, flu-like symptoms, painful urination) periodically during therapy. Treat suspected or confirmed infections with antibiotics. *For ≥Grade 3 or 4 infections,* withhold atezolizumab until Grade 1 or resolved.
● Monitor for signs and symptoms of infusion-related reactions (chills or shaking, itching or rash, flushing, dyspnea, wheezing, dizziness, fever, feeling faint, back or neck pain, facial swelling) during therapy. *For Grade 1 or 2,* interrupt or slow infusion. *For Grade 3 or 4 infusion reactions,* permanently discontinue atezolizumab.

• Monitor for signs and symptoms of myocarditis (chest pain, irregular heartbeat, shortness of breath, swelling of ankles) during therapy. *If Grade 2, 3, or 4 myocarditis occurs,* discontinue atezolizumab permanently.

Lab Test Considerations
• Verify a negative pregnancy test before starting therapy.
• ⅔ Confirm PD-L1 expression in melanoma via tests and BRAF V600 in unresectable or metastatic melanoma at http://www.fda.gov/CompanionDiagnostics. An FDA-approved test for the detection of other BRAF V600 mutations for this use is not currently available.
• For patients with hepatitis with no tumor involvement of the liver, monitor AST, ALT, and serum bilirubin prior to and periodically during therapy. *If AST or ALT >3 and ≤ 8× upper limit of normal (ULN) or total bilirubin >1.5 and ≤ 3× ULN* hold dose until Grade 1 or resolved and corticosteroid dose ≤prednisone 10 mg per day (or equivalent). *If AST or ALT >8× ULN or total bilirubin >3× ULN,* permanently discontinue atezolizumab. For patients with hepatitis with tumor involvement of the liver, *If baseline AST or ALT >1 and ≤3× ULN and increases to >5 and ≤10× ULN or baseline AST or ALT >3 and ≤5× ULN and increases to >8 and ≤10× ULN,* hold atezolizumab and administer corticosteroids at a dose of 1–2 mg/kg/day prednisolone equivalents followed by a taper. Resume after taper corticosteroid if Grade 0–1. If no complete or partial resolution within 12 wk of starting corticosteroids or inability to reduce prednisone to ≤10 mg per day within 12 wk of starting steroids, permanently discontinue atezolizumab. *If AST or ALT increases to >10× ULN or total bilirubin increases to >3× ULN,* permanently discontinue atezolizumab.
• Monitor thyroid function prior to and periodically during therapy. *If asymptomatic,* continue therapy. *For symptomatic hypothyroidism (extreme tiredness, weight gain, constipation, feeling cold, hair loss, deepening voice),* withhold atezolizumab and begin thyroid replacement therapy as needed without corticosteroids. *For symptomatic hyperthyroidism (hunger, irritability, mood swings, weight loss),* hold atezolizumab until Grade 1 or resolved and clinically stable on hormone replacement therapy. Resume therapy when symptoms of hyper- or hypothyroidism are controlled and thyroid function is improving.
• Monitor blood glucose periodically during therapy. For type 1 diabetes, begin treatment with insulin. For ≥Grade 2, 3, or 4 hyperglycemia (fasting glucose >250–500 mg/dL), hold atezolizumab until Grade 1 or resolved and control is achieved on insulin replacement therapy.

• Monitor serum amylase or lipase in patients with symptoms of pancreatitis. If serum amylase or lipase levels ≥Grade 3 (>2× upper limit of normal), withhold atezolizumab. Treat with methylprednisolone IV 1–2 mg/kg/day or equivalent. Once symptoms improve, follow with 1–2 mg/kg/day of oral prednisone or equivalent. Resume atezolizumab if symptoms of pancreatitis resolved and corticosteroid ↓ to ≤10 mg/day oral prednisone or equivalent.
• Monitor renal function prior to and periodically during therapy. *If serum creatinine increases to Grades 2 or 3,* hold atezolizumab and administer corticosteroids at a dose of 1–2 mg/kg/day prednisolone equivalents followed by a taper. Resume after taper corticosteroid if Grade 0–1. If no complete or partial resolution within 12 wk of starting corticosteroids or inability to reduce prednisone to ≤10 mg per day within 12 wk of starting steroids, permanently discontinue atezolizumab. *If serum creatinine increases to Grade 4,* permanently discontinue atezolizumab.
• May cause lymphopenia, hyponatremia, anemia, ↑ alkaline phosphatase, ↑ serum creatinine, and hypoalbuminemia.

Implementation

IV Administration
• **Intermittent Infusion:** *Dilution:* Dilute with 0.9% NaCl in a polyvinyl chloride, polyethylene, or polyolefin infusion bag. *Concentration:* 3.2 mg/mL to 16.8 mg/mL. Gently invert to dilute; do not shake. Solution is clear and colorless to slightly yellow. Do not administer solutions that are discolored or contain particulate matter. Administer immediately once prepared or store for ≤6 hrs at room temperature (including infusion time) or ≤24 hrs if refrigerated. Do not freeze.
• Administer atezolizumab before chemotherapy or other antineoplastic drugs when given on same day. *Rate:* Administer over 60 min with or without a sterile, non-pyrogenic, low-protein binding in-line filter (0.2–0.22 micron); do not administer via IV push or bolus. If first infusion is tolerated, subsequent infusions may be infused over 30 min.
• **Y-Site Incompatibility:** Do not administer other drugs through same IV line.

Patient/Family Teaching
• Explain purpose of atezolizumab to patient. Advise patient to read the *Medication Guide* before starting and periodically during therapy in case of changes.
• Advise patient to notify health care professional immediately if symptoms of pneumonitis, hepatitis, colitis, endocrine problems, meningitis, nervous system problems, ocular inflammatory toxicity (blurry or double vision, eye pain or redness), pancreatitis, infection, infusion-related reactions, or rash occur.

✱ = Canadian drug name. ⅔ = Genetic implication. ~~Strikethrough~~ = Discontinued. CAPITALS = life-threatening. <u>Underline</u> = most frequent.

- Advise patient to notify health care professional of all Rx or OTC medications, vitamins, or herbal products being taken and to consult with health care professional before taking other medications.
- Rep: May cause fetal harm. Advise females of reproductive potential to use effective contraception and to avoid breastfeeding during and for at least 5 mo after last dose. Inform females that atezolizumab may impair fertility during therapy.

Evaluation/Desired Outcomes

- Decreased spread of NSCLC, SCLC, HCC, and melanoma with increased survival.
- Decreased spread of alveolar soft part sarcoma.

atogepant (a-toe-je-pant)
Qulipta
Classification
Therapeutic: vascular headache suppressants
Pharmacologic: calcitonin gene-related peptide receptor antagonists

Indications
Preventive treatment of migraines.

Action
Binds to and inhibits the calcitonin gene-related peptide (CGRP) receptor, which reduces the neuroinflammatory and vasodilatory effects of CGRP. **Therapeutic Effects:** Reduction in number of monthly migraine days.

Pharmacokinetics
Absorption: Well absorbed following oral administration.
Distribution: Well distributed to tissues.
Metabolism and Excretion: Primarily metabolized in the liver via the CYP3A4 isoenzyme. Primarily excreted as unchanged drug in feces (42%) and urine (5%).
Half-life: 11 hr.

TIME/ACTION PROFILE (plasma concentrations)

ROUTE	ONSET	PEAK	DURATION
PO	rapid	1–2 hr	unknown

Contraindications/Precautions
Contraindicated in: Hypersensitivity; Severe renal impairment (CCr 15–29 mL/min) or end-stage renal disease (CCr <15 mL/min) (for chronic migraine prevention); Severe hepatic impairment.
Use Cautiously in: Severe renal impairment (CCr 15–29 mL/min) or end-stage renal disease (CCr <15 mL/min) (for episodic migraine prevention); OB: Oral CGRP antagonists not currently recommended for prevention of migraine during pregnancy; Lactation: Oral CGRP antagonists not currently recommended for prevention of migraine while breastfeeding; Pedi: Safety and effectiveness not established in children.

Adverse Reactions/Side Effects
GI: constipation, nausea. **Metab:** ↓ appetite, ↓ weight. **Neuro:** dizziness, fatigue, sedation. **Misc:** HYPERSENSITIVITY REACTIONS (including anaphylaxis).

Interactions
Drug-Drug: Strong CYP3A4 inhibitors, including **itraconazole**, may ↑ levels and risk of toxicity; ↓ dose for episodic migraine prevention and avoid concurrent use for chronic migraine prevention. **Strong CYP3A4 inducers**, including **rifampin**, **moderate CYP3A4 inducers**, or **weak CYP3A4 inducers**, including **topiramate** may ↓ levels and effectiveness; ↑ dose for episodic migraine prevention and avoid concurrent use for chronic migraine prevention. **OATP inhibitors**, including **rifampin** may ↑ levels and risk of toxicity; ↓ dose for episodic or chronic migraine prevention.

Route/Dosage
Episodic Migraine
PO (Adults): 10 mg, 30 mg, or 60 mg once daily. *Concurrent use of strong CYP3A4 inhibitors:* 10 mg once daily. *Concurrent use of strong, moderate, or weak CYP3A4 inducers:* 30 mg or 60 mg once daily. *Concurrent use of OATP inhibitors:* 10 mg or 30 mg once daily.

Renal Impairment
PO (Adults): *Severe renal impairment or end-stage renal disease:* 10 mg once daily.

Chronic Migraine
PO (Adults): 60 mg once daily. *Concurrent use of strong CYP3A4 inhibitors:* Avoid concurrent use. *Concurrent use of strong, moderate, or weak CYP3A4 inducers:* Avoid concurrent use. *Concurrent use of OATP inhibitors:* 30 mg once daily.

Renal Impairment
PO (Adults): *Severe renal impairment or end-stage renal disease:* Avoid use.

Availability
Tablets: 10 mg, 30 mg, 60 mg.

NURSING IMPLICATIONS
Assessment
- Assess pain location, character, intensity, duration, and associated symptoms (photophobia, phonophobia, nausea, vomiting) of migraine pain.
- Monitor frequency of migraine headaches.
- Monitor for signs and symptoms of hypersensitivity reactions (anaphylaxis, dyspnea, rash, pruritus, urticaria, facial edema). Hypersensitivity reactions can occur days after administration. If a hypersensitivity reaction occurs, discontinue atogepant and begin therapy as needed.

Implementation
- Doses for episodic and chronic migraines are different.
- PO: Administer without regard to food.

Patient/Family Teaching

- Instruct patient to take atogepant as directed. Advise patients taking triptans, ergotamine derivatives, NSAIDs, acetaminophen, and opioids for headache treatment, use while taking atogepant is acceptable. Advise patient to read *Patient Information* before starting and with each Rx refill in case of changes.
- Advise patient to avoid alcohol, which aggravates headaches, during atogepant use.
- Advise patient that lying down in a darkened room following atogepant administration may further help relieve headache.
- Inform patients of potential for hypersensitivity reaction and that these reactions can occur days after administration of atogepant. Advise patients to notify health care professional immediately if signs or symptoms of hypersensitivity reactions (shortness of breath, rash) occur. Atogepant should be discontinued if hypersensitivity reaction occurs.
- Advise patient to notify health care professional of all Rx or OTC medications, vitamins, or herbal products being taken and to consult with health care professional before taking other medications.
- Rep: Advise females of reproductive potential to notify health care professional if pregnancy is planned or suspected or if breastfeeding.

Evaluation/Desired Outcomes

- Decrease in number of migraines/month.

💥 atomoxetine (a-to-mox-e-teen)

Strattera

Classification

Therapeutic: agents for attention deficit disorder

Pharmacologic: selective norepinephrine reuptake inhibitors

Indications

Attention-deficit/hyperactivity disorder (ADHD).

Action

Selectively inhibits the presynaptic transporter of norepinephrine. **Therapeutic Effects:** Increased attention span.

Pharmacokinetics

Absorption: Well absorbed following oral administration.

Distribution: Unknown.

Protein Binding: 98%.

Metabolism and Excretion: Mostly metabolized by the liver (CYP2D6 enzyme pathway); 💥 the CYP2D6 enzyme system exhibits genetic polymorphism (~7% of population may be poor metabolizers and may have significantly ↑ atomoxetine concentrations and an ↑ risk of adverse effects).

Half-life: 5 hr.

TIME/ACTION PROFILE

ROUTE	ONSET	PEAK	DURATION
PO	unknown	1–2 hr	12–24 hr

Contraindications/Precautions

Contraindicated in: Hypersensitivity; Concurrent or within 2 wk therapy with monoamine oxidase (MAO) inhibitors; Angle-closure glaucoma; Pheochromocytoma; Hypertension, tachycardia, cardiovascular, or cerebrovascular disease.

Use Cautiously in: Personal or family history of bipolar disorder, mania, or hypomania; Concurrent albuterol or vasopressors (↑ risk of adverse cardiovascular reactions); CYP2D6 poor metabolizers (↓ dose); OB: Use during pregnancy only if potential maternal benefit justifies potential fetal risk; Lactation: Safety not established in breastfeeding; Pedi: May ↑ risk of suicide attempt/ideation especially during dose early treatment or dose adjustment; risk may be greater in children or adolescents; Pedi: Children <6 yr (safety and effectiveness not established).

Adverse Reactions/Side Effects

CV: hypertension, orthostatic hypotension, QT interval prolongation, syncope, tachycardia. **Derm:** ↑ sweating, rash, urticaria. **GI:** <u>nausea</u>, <u>vomiting</u>, dyspepsia, HEPATOTOXICITY; *Adults:* constipation, dry mouth. **GU:** *Adults:* dysmenorrhea, ejaculatory problems, erectile dysfunction, libido changes, priapism, urinary hesitation, urinary retention. **Metab:** ↓ appetite, weight/growth loss. **MS:** RHABDOMYOLYSIS. **Neuro:** <u>dizziness</u>, <u>fatigue</u>, <u>insomnia</u>, <u>mood swings</u>, aggression, behavioral disturbances, delusions, hallucinations, hostility, mania, paresthesia, SUICIDAL THOUGHTS, thought disorder. **Misc:** HYPERSENSITIVITY REACTIONS (including anaphylaxis and angioedema).

Interactions

Drug-Drug: Concurrent use with **MAO inhibitors** may result in serious, potentially fatal reactions (do not use within 2 wk of each other). ↑ risk of cardiovascular effects with **albuterol** or **vasopressors** (use cautiously). **CYP2D6 inhibitors,** including **quinidine, fluoxetine,** or **paroxetine,** may ↑ levels and risk of toxicity; dose ↓ recommended.

Route/Dosage

PO (Children and Adolescents ≥6 yr and <70 kg): 0.5 mg/kg/day initially; may ↑ every 3 days to a daily target dose of 1.2 mg/kg, given as a single dose in the morning or evenly divided doses in the morning and late afternoon/early evening (not to exceed 1.4 mg/kg/day or 100 mg/day whichever is less). *Concurrent use of CYP2D6 inhibitor (quinidine, fluoxetine, paroxetine) or CYP2D6 poor metabolizer:* 0.5 mg/kg/day initially, may ↑ if needed to 1.2 mg/kg/day after 4 wk.

PO (Adults , Adolescents, and Children ≥6 yr and >70 kg): 40 mg/day initially; may ↑ every 3 days to a daily target dose of 80 mg/day given as a single dose in the morning or evenly divided doses in the morning and late afternoon/early evening; may further ↑ after 2–4 wk up to 100 mg/day. *Concurrent use of CYP2D6 inhibitor (quinidine, fluoxetine, paroxetine):* 40 mg/day initially, may ↑ if needed to 80 mg/day after 4 wk.

Hepatic Impairment

PO (Adults and Children): *Moderate hepatic impairment (Child-Pugh Class B):* ↓ initial and target dose by 50%; *Severe hepatic impairment (Child-Pugh Class C):* ↓ initial and target dose to 25% of normal.

Availability (generic available)

Capsules: 10 mg, 18 mg, 25 mg, 40 mg, 60 mg, 80 mg, 100 mg.

NURSING IMPLICATIONS

Assessment

- Assess attention span, impulse control, and interactions with others.
- Assess for bipolar disorder (screen patients for a personal or family history of bipolar disorder, mania, or hypomania) before starting therapy with atomoxetine.
- Monitor BP and pulse periodically during therapy. Obtain a history (including assessment of family history of sudden death or ventricular arrhythmia), physical exam to assess for cardiac disease, and further evaluation (ECG and echocardiogram), if indicated. If exertional chest pain, unexplained syncope, or other cardiac symptoms occur, evaluate promptly.
- Monitor growth, body height, and weight in children.
- Assess for signs of liver injury (pruritus, dark urine, jaundice, right upper quadrant tenderness, unexplained "flu-like" symptoms) during therapy. Monitor liver function tests at first sign of liver injury. Discontinue and do not restart atomoxetine in patients with jaundice or laboratory evidence of liver injury.
- Monitor closely for notable changes in behavior that could indicate the emergence or worsening of suicidal thoughts or behavior or depression. Psychotic or manic symptoms (hallucinations, delusional thinking, mania) in patients without a history of psychotic illness or mania can be caused by atomoxetine at usual doses. If symptoms occur, consider discontinuing atomoxetine.

Implementation

- Do not confuse atomoxetine with atorvastatin.
- **PO:** *DNC:* Administer without regard to food. Swallow capsules whole; do not open, crush, or chew. Doses may be discontinued without tapering.

Patient/Family Teaching

- Instruct patient to take medication as directed. Take missed doses as soon as possible, but should not take more than the total daily amount in any 24-hr period. Advise patient and parents to read the *Medication Guide* prior to starting therapy and with each Rx refill in case of changes.
- Inform patient that sharing this medication may be dangerous.
- Advise patient and family to notify health care professional if thoughts about suicide or dying, attempts to commit suicide; new or worse depression; new or worse anxiety; feeling very agitated or restless; panic attacks; trouble sleeping; new or worse irritability; acting aggressive or hostile; being angry or violent; acting on dangerous impulses; an extreme increase in activity and talking; other unusual changes in behavior or mood occur or if signs and symptoms of severe liver injury (pruritus, dark urine, jaundice, right upper quadrant tenderness, or unexplained "flu-like" symptoms) occur.
- Instruct patient to notify health care professional of all Rx or OTC medications, vitamins, or herbal products being taken and consult health care professional before taking any new medications.
- May cause dizziness. Caution patient to avoid driving or other activities requiring alertness until response to medication is known.
- Rep: Advise female patients to notify health care professional if pregnancy is planned or suspected or if they are breastfeeding. Register patients who took atomoxetine during pregnancy in Pregnancy Exposure Registry to monitor pregnancy outcomes by calling the National Pregnancy Registry for ADHD Medications at 1-866-961-2388 or visiting https://womensmentalhealth.org/adhd-medications/.

Evaluation/Desired Outcomes

- Improved attention span and social interactions in ADHD.

---

atorvastatin, See HMG-CoA REDUCTASE INHIBITORS (statins).

---

atovaquone (a-toe-va-kwone)
Mepron
Classification
Therapeutic: anti-infectives

Indications

Treatment of mild to moderate *Pneumocystis jirovecii* pneumonia (PJP) in patients who are unable to tolerate trimethoprim/sulfamethoxazole. Prophylaxis of *PJP*.

Action

Inhibits the action of enzymes necessary to nucleic acid and ATP synthesis. **Therapeutic Effects:** Active against *P. jirovecii*.

Pharmacokinetics

Absorption: Absorption is poor but is increased by food, particularly fat.

Distribution: Enters CSF in very low concentrations (<1% of plasma levels).
Protein Binding: >99.9%.
Metabolism and Excretion: Undergoes enterohepatic recycling; elimination occurs in feces.
Half-life: 2.2–2.9 days.

TIME/ACTION PROFILE (plasma concentrations)

ROUTE	ONSET	PEAK	DURATION
PO	unknown	1–8 hr; 24–96 hr†	12 hr

†Two peaks are due to enterohepatic recycling.

Contraindications/Precautions

Contraindicated in: Hypersensitivity; Lactation: Breastfeeding not recommended for women with HIV.
Use Cautiously in: ↓ hepatic, renal, or cardiac function (dose modification may be necessary); GI disorders (absorption may be limited); OB: Use during pregnancy only if potential maternal benefit justifies potential fetal risk; Pedi: Children <13 yr (safety and effectiveness not established).

Adverse Reactions/Side Effects

Derm: <u>rash</u>. **GI:** <u>diarrhea</u>, <u>nausea</u>, <u>vomiting</u>. **Neuro:** <u>headache</u>, <u>insomnia</u>. **Resp:** <u>cough</u>. **Misc:** <u>fever</u>.

Interactions

Drug-Drug: **Rifampin** or **rifabutin** may ↓ levels and efficacy; concurrent use not recommended. **Tetracycline** may ↓ levels and efficacy; use caution when using concurrently. **Metoclopramide** may ↓ levels and efficacy; use only if no other alternative available.
Drug-Food: Food ↑ absorption.

Route/Dosage

Treatment of Mild to Moderate *Pneumocystis jirovecii* Pneumonia

PO (Adults and Children ≥13 yr): 750 mg twice daily for 21 days.

Prevention of *Pneumocystis jirovecii* Pneumonia

PO (Adults and Children ≥13 yr): 1500 mg once daily.

Availability (generic available)

Suspension (citrus flavor): 750 mg/5 mL. *In combination with:* proguanil (Malarone). See Appendix N.

NURSING IMPLICATIONS

Assessment

- Assess patient for signs of infection (vital signs, lung sounds, sputum, WBCs) at beginning of and throughout therapy.
- Obtain specimens prior to initiating therapy. First dose may be given before receiving results.

Lab Test Considerations
- Monitor hematologic and hepatic functions. May cause mild, transient anemia and neutropenia. May also cause ↑ serum amylase, AST, ALT, and alkaline phosphatase.
- Monitor electrolytes. May cause hyponatremia.

Implementation

- **PO:** Administer with food twice daily for 21 days for treatment and once daily for prevention.
- Shake suspension gently prior to administration.

Patient/Family Teaching

- Instruct patient to take atovaquone as directed around the clock for full course of therapy, even if feeling better. Emphasize the importance of taking atovaquone with food, especially foods high in fat; taking without food may decrease plasma concentrations and effectiveness.
- Advise patient to notify health care professional if rash occurs.
- Rep: Advise females of reproductive potential to notify health care professional if pregnancy is planned or suspected or if breastfeeding.

Evaluation/Desired Outcomes

- Resolution of the signs and symptoms of infection.

BEERS

atropine† (at-ro-peen)

Classification
Therapeutic: antiarrhythmics
Pharmacologic: anticholinergics, antimuscarinics

†See Appendix B for ophthalmic use

Indications

IV: Given preoperatively to decrease oral and respiratory secretions. **IV:** Sinus bradycardia and heart block. **IV:** Reversal of adverse muscarinic effects of anticholinesterase agents (neostigmine or pyridostigmine). **IV:** Anticholinesterase (organophosphate pesticide) poisoning. **Inhaln:** Exercise-induced bronchospasm.

Action

Inhibits the action of acetylcholine at postganglionic sites located in: Smooth muscle, Secretory glands, CNS (antimuscarinic activity). Low doses decrease: Sweating, Salivation, Respiratory secretions. Intermediate doses result in: Mydriasis (pupillary dilation), Cycloplegia (loss of visual accommodation), Increased heart rate. GI and GU tract motility are decreased at larger doses. **Therapeutic Effects:** Increased heart rate. Decreased GI and respiratory secretions. Reversal of muscarinic effects. May have a spasmolytic action on the biliary and genitourinary tracts.

Pharmacokinetics

Absorption: Well absorbed following SUBQ administration. IV administration results in complete bioavailability.

Distribution: Readily crosses the blood-brain barrier. Crosses the placenta and enters breast milk.

Metabolism and Excretion: Mostly metabolized by the liver; 30–50% excreted unchanged by the kidneys.

Half-life: Children <2 yr: 4–10 hr; Children >2 yr: 1.5–3.5 hr; Adults: 4–5 hr.

TIME/ACTION PROFILE (inhibition of salivation)

ROUTE	ONSET	PEAK	DURATION
SUBQ	rapid	15–50 min	4–6 hr
IV	immediate	2–4 min	4–6 hr

Contraindications/Precautions

Contraindicated in: Hypersensitivity; Angle-closure glaucoma; Acute hemorrhage; Tachycardia secondary to cardiac insufficiency or thyrotoxicosis; Obstructive disease of the GI tract.

Use Cautiously in: Intra-abdominal infections; Prostatic hyperplasia; Chronic renal, hepatic, pulmonary, or cardiac disease; OB: Safety not established in pregnancy; Lactation: Use while breastfeeding only if potential maternal benefit justifies potential risk to infant; Pedi: Infants with Down syndrome have ↑ sensitivity to cardiac effects and mydriasis. Children may have ↑ susceptibility to adverse reactions. Exercise care when prescribing in children with spastic paralysis or brain damage; Geri: Appears on Beers list. ↑ risk of adverse reactions in older adults due to anticholinergic effects. Avoid use of all formulations in older adults except for ophthalmic formulations.

Adverse Reactions/Side Effects

CV: tachycardia, arrhythmias, palpitations. **Derm:** ↓ sweating, flushing. **EENT:** blurred vision, cycloplegia, dry eyes, mydriasis, photophobia. **GI:** dry mouth, constipation, impaired GI motility. **GU:** urinary hesitancy, impotency, retention. **Neuro:** drowsiness, confusion. **Resp:** pulmonary edema, tachypnea.

Interactions

Drug-Drug: ↑ anticholinergic effects with other **anticholinergics,** including **antihistamines, tricyclic antidepressants, quinidine,** and **disopyramide.** Anticholinergics may alter the absorption of other **orally administered drugs** by slowing motility of the GI tract. **Antacids** ↓ absorption of **anticholinergics.** May ↑ GI mucosal lesions in patients taking oral **potassium chloride** tablets. May alter response to **beta-blockers.**

Route/Dosage

Preanesthesia (To Decrease Salivation/Secretions)

IV, SUBQ (Adults): 0.4–0.6 mg 30–60 min preop.

IV, SUBQ (Children >5 kg): 0.01–0.02 mg/kg/dose 30–60 min preop to a maximum of 0.4 mg/dose; minimum: 0.1 mg/dose.

IV, SUBQ (Children <5 kg): 0.02 mg/kg/dose 30–60 min preop then every 4–6 hr as needed.

Bradycardia

IV (Adults): 0.5–1 mg; may repeat as needed every 5 min, not to exceed a total of 2 mg (every 3–5 min in Advanced Cardiac Life Support guidelines) or 0.04 mg/kg (total vagolytic dose).

IV (Children): 0.02 mg/kg (maximum single dose is 0.5 mg in children and 1 mg in adolescents); may repeat every 5 min up to a total dose of 1 mg in children (2 mg in adolescents).

Endotracheal (Children): use the IV dose and dilute before administration.

Reversal of Adverse Muscarinic Effects of Anticholinesterases

IV (Adults): 0.6–12 mg for each 0.5–2.5 mg of neostigmine or 10–20 mg of pyridostigmine concurrently with anticholinesterase.

Organophosphate Poisoning

IV (Adults): 1–2 mg/dose every 10–20 min until atropinic effects observed then every 1–4 hr for 24 hr; up to 50 mg in first 24 hr and 2 g over several days may be given in severe intoxication.

IV (Children): 0.02–0.05 mg/kg every 10–20 min until atropinic effects observed then every 1–4 hr for 24 hr.

Bronchospasm

Inhaln (Adults): 0.025–0.05 mg/kg/dose every 4–6 hr as needed; maximum 2.5 mg/dose.

Inhaln (Children): 0.03–0.05 mg/kg/dose 3–4 times/day; maximum 2.5 mg/dose.

Availability (generic available)

Solution for injection: 0.05 mg/mL, 0.1 mg/mL, 0.4 mg/mL, 1 mg/mL.

NURSING IMPLICATIONS

Assessment

- Assess vital signs and ECG tracings frequently during IV drug therapy. Report any significant changes in heart rate or BP, or increased ventricular ectopy or angina to health care professional promptly.
- Monitor intake and output ratios in elderly or surgical patients because atropine may cause urinary retention.

- Assess patients routinely for abdominal distention and auscultate for bowel sounds. If constipation becomes a problem, increasing fluids and adding bulk to the diet may help alleviate constipation.

Implementation

IV Administration

- **IV Push:** *Dilution:* Administer undiluted. *Rate:* Administer over 1 min; more rapid administration may be used during cardiac resuscitation (follow with 20 mL saline flush). Slow administration (over >1 min) may cause a paradoxical bradycardia (usually resolved in approximately 2 min).
- **Y-Site Compatibility:** amikacin, aminophylline, amiodarone, argatroban, ascorbic acid, azathioprine, aztreonam, benztropine, bivalirudin, bumetanide, buprenorphine, butorphanol, calcium chloride, calcium gluconate, cangrelor, cefazolin, cefotaxime, cefotetan, cefoxitin, ceftazidime, ceftriaxone, cefuroxime, chloramphenicol, chlorpromazine, clindamycin, cyanocobalamin, cyclosporine, dexamethasone, dexmedetomidine, digoxin, diphenhydramine, dobutamine, dopamine, doxycycline, enalaprilat, ephedrine, epinephrine, epoetin alfa, eptifibatide, erythromycin, esmolol, etomidate, famotidine, fentanyl, fluconazole, folic acid, furosemide, ganciclovir, gentamicin, glycopyrrolate, heparin, hydrocortisone, hydromorphone, imipenem/cilastatin, indomethacin, insulin, regular, isoproterenol, ketamine, ketorolac, labetalol, LR, lidocaine, magnesium sulfate, mannitol, meperidine, meropenem, methadone, methylprednisolone, metoclopramide, metoprolol, midazolam, morphine, multivitamins, nafcillin, nalbuphine, naloxone, nitroglycerin, nitroprusside, norepinephrine, ondansetron, oxacillin, oxytocin, palonosetron, papaverine, penicillin G, pentamidine, pentobarbital, phenobarbital, phentolamine, phenylephrine, phytonadione, potassium chloride, procainamide, prochlorperazine, promethazine, propranolol, protamine, pyridoxine, sodium bicarbonate, succinylcholine, sufentanil, theophylline, thiamine, tirofiban, tobramycin, vancomycin, vasopressin, verapamil.
- **Y-Site Incompatibility:** acetaminophen, dantrolene, diazepam, pantoprazole, phenytoin, trimethoprim/sulfamethoxazole, thiopental.
- **Endotracheal:** Dilute with 5–10 mL of 0.9% NaCl.
- *Rate:* Inject directly into the endotracheal tube followed by several positive pressure ventilations.

Patient/Family Teaching

- Explain purpose of atropine to patient.
- May cause drowsiness. Caution patients to avoid driving or other activities requiring alertness until response to medication is known.
- Instruct patient that oral rinses, sugarless gum or candy, and frequent oral hygiene may help relieve dry mouth.

- Caution patients that atropine impairs heat regulation. Strenuous activity in a hot environment may cause heat stroke. Advise patient to notify health care professional of all Rx or OTC medications, vitamins, or herbal products being taken and to consult with health care professional before taking other medications.
- Rep: Advise patient to notify health care professional if pregnancy is planned or suspected or if breastfeeding.
- Pedi: Instruct parents or caregivers that medication may cause fever and to notify health care professional before administering to a febrile child.
- Geri: Inform male patients with benign prostatic hyperplasia that atropine may cause urinary hesitancy and retention. Changes in urinary stream should be reported to health care professional.

Evaluation/Desired Outcomes

- Increase in heart rate.
- Dryness of mouth.
- Reversal of muscarinic effects.

---

avanafil (av-an-a-fil)
Stendra
Classification
Therapeutic: erectile dysfunction agents
Pharmacologic: phosphodiesterase type 5 inhibitors

Indications
Treatment of erectile dysfunction.

Action
Enhances effects of nitric oxide released during sexual stimulation. Nitric oxide activates guanylate cyclase, which produces ↑ levels of cyclic guanosine monophosphate (cGMP). cGMP produces smooth muscle relaxation of the corpus cavernosum, which promotes ↑ blood flow and subsequent erection. Inhibits the enzyme phosphodiesterase type 5 (PDE5), PDE5 inactivates cGMP. **Therapeutic Effects:** Enhanced blood flow to the corpus cavernosum and erection sufficient to allow sexual intercourse. Requires sexual stimulation.

Pharmacokinetics
Absorption: Rapidly absorbed following oral administration.
Distribution: Minimal amounts enter semen.
Protein Binding: 99%.
Metabolism and Excretion: Mostly metabolized by the liver (primarily by the CYP3A4 enzyme system), metabolites excreted in feces (62%) and urine (21%). One metabolite had inhibitory activity on PDE5.
Half-life: 5 hr.

TIME/ACTION PROFILE (effect on BP)

ROUTE	ONSET	PEAK	DURATION
PO	within 1 hr	1–2 hr	unknown

Contraindications/Precautions

Contraindicated in: Hypersensitivity; Concurrent use of nitrates, riociguat, or vericiguat; Severe renal or hepatic impairment; Concurrent use of strong CYP3A4 inhibitors; Serious underlying cardiovascular disease (including history of MI, stroke, or serious arrhythmia within 6 mo), cardiac failure, or coronary artery disease with unstable angina, angina with sexual intercourse; History of HF, coronary artery disease, uncontrolled hypertension (BP >170/110 mm Hg) or hypotension (BP <90/50 mm Hg), dehydration, autonomic dysfunction, or severe left ventricular outflow obstruction; Hereditary degenerative retinal disorders; Women.

Use Cautiously in: Serious underlying cardiovascular disease or conditions in which sexual activity is not advised; History of sudden severe vision loss or non-arteritic ischemic optic neuropathy (NAION); may ↑ risk of recurrence; Low cup to disk ratio, age >50 yr, diabetes, hypertension, coronary artery disease, hyperlipidemia, or smoking (↑ risk of NAION); Alpha adrenergic blockers (patients should be on stable dose of alpha blockers before treatment, initiate with 50 mg dose); Anatomic penile deformity (angulation, cavernosal fibrosis, Peyronie disease); Conditions associated with priapism (sickle cell anemia, multiple myeloma, leukemia); Concurrent use of moderate CYP3A4 inhibitors (initiate with 50 mg dose); History of hearing loss; Bleeding disorders or peptic ulceration; Pedi: Safety not established in children; Geri: older adults may be more sensitive to drug effects.

Adverse Reactions/Side Effects

Derm: flushing. **EENT:** nasal congestion, nasopharyngitis, sudden hearing/vision loss. **GU:** priapism. **MS:** back pain. **Neuro:** headache, dizziness.

Interactions

Drug-Drug: Concurrent use of **nitrates** may cause serious, life-threatening hypotension and is contraindicated. Concurrent use of **riociguat** or **vericiguat** may result in severe hypotension; concurrent use contraindicated. Blood levels and effects may be ↑ by **CYP3A4 inhibitors**, concurrent use of **strong CYP3A4 inhibitors** including **atazanavir, clarithromycin, itraconazole, ketoconazole, nefazodone**, and **nelfinavir** is contraindicated. A similar but lesser effect is expected with **moderate CYP3A4 inhibitors** including **erythromycin, aprepitant, diltiazem, fluconazole, fosamprenavir, ritonavir**, and **verapamil**; initial dose should not exceed 50 mg/24 hr. ↑ risk of hypotension with **alpha-adrenergic blockers, antihypertensives**, and **alcohol** (more than 3 units); dosage adjustments may be necessary.

Route/Dosage

PO (Adults): 100 mg 15 min prior to sexual activity, not to exceed once daily (range 50–200 mg, use lowest effective dose); *Concurrent alpha-blockers or moderate CYP3A4 inhibitors:* 50 mg, not to exceed once daily.

Availability

Tablets: 50 mg, 100 mg, 200 mg.

NURSING IMPLICATIONS

Assessment

* Determine erectile dysfunction before administration. Avanafil has no effect in the absence of sexual stimulation.

Implementation

* **PO:** Administer dose as needed for erectile dysfunction at least 15 min prior to sexual activity.
* May be administered without regard to food.

Patient/Family Teaching

* Instruct patient to take avanafil as needed for ED at least 15 min before sexual activity and not more than once per day. Inform patient that sexual stimulation is required for an erection to occur after taking avanafil.
* Advise patient that avanafil is not indicated for use in women.
* Caution patient not to take avanafil concurrently with alpha adrenergic blockers (unless on a stable dose) or nitrates. If chest pain occurs after taking avanafil, instruct patient to seek immediate medical attention.
* Advise patient to avoid excess alcohol intake (≥3 units) in combination with avanafil; may increase risk of orthostatic hypotension, increased heart rate, decreased standing BP, dizziness, headache.
* Instruct patient to notify health care professional promptly if erection lasts longer than 4 hr, if they are not satisfied with their sexual performance, develop unwanted side effects or if they experience sudden or decreased vision loss in one or both eyes or loss or decrease in hearing, ringing in the ears, or dizziness.
* Advise patient to notify health care professional of all Rx or OTC medications, vitamins, or herbal products being taken and to consult with health care professional before taking other medications that may interact with avanafil.
* Inform patient that avanafil offers no protection against sexually transmitted diseases. Counsel patient that protection against sexually transmitted diseases and HIV infection should be considered.

Evaluation/Desired Outcomes

* Male erection sufficient to allow intercourse.

azaTHIOprine
(ay-za-**thye**-oh-preen)
Azasan, Imuran
Classification
Therapeutic: immunosuppressants
Pharmacologic: purine antagonists

Indications

Prevention of renal transplant rejection (with corticosteroids, local radiation, or other cytotoxic agents). Treatment of severe, active, erosive rheumatoid arthritis unresponsive to more conventional therapy. **Unlabeled Use:** Management of Crohn's disease or ulcerative colitis.

Action

Antagonizes purine metabolism with subsequent inhibition of DNA and RNA synthesis. **Therapeutic Effects:** Suppression of cell-mediated immunity and altered antibody formation.

Pharmacokinetics

Absorption: Readily absorbed after oral administration. IV administration results in complete bioavailability.

Distribution: Unknown.

Metabolism and Excretion: Metabolized to 6–mercaptopurine, which is further metabolized ※ (one route is by thiopurine methyltransferase [TPMT] to form an inactive metabolite; nucleotide diphosphatase [NUDT15] is also involved in inactivation process). Minimal renal excretion of unchanged drug.

Half-life: 3 hr.

TIME/ACTION PROFILE

ROUTE	ONSET	PEAK	DURATION
PO (anti-inflammatory)	6–8 wk	12 wk	unknown

Contraindications/Precautions

Contraindicated in: Hypersensitivity; Concurrent use of mycophenolate; OB: Pregnancy; Lactation: Lactation.

Use Cautiously in: Infection; Malignancies; ↓ bone marrow reserve; Previous or concurrent radiation therapy; Severe renal impairment/oliguria (↑ sensitivity); ※ TPMT or NUDT15 enzyme deficiency (alternative therapy or substantial dose ↓ are required to avoid hematologic adverse events); Rep: Women of reproductive potential; Pedi: ↑ risk of hepatosplenic T-cell lymphoma (HSTCL) in children with inflammatory bowel disease.

Adverse Reactions/Side Effects

CV: Raynaud's phenomenon. **Derm:** alopecia, rash. **EENT:** retinopathy. **GI:** anorexia, hepatotoxicity, nausea, vomiting, diarrhea, mucositis, pancreatitis. **Hemat:** anemia, leukopenia, pancytopenia, thrombocytopenia. **MS:** arthralgia. **Neuro:** PROGRESSIVE MULTIFOCAL LEUKOENCEPHALOPATHY. **Resp:** pulmonary edema. **Misc:** chills, fever, MALIGNANCY (including post-transplant lymphoma, HSTCL, and skin cancer), SERUM SICKNESS.

Interactions

Drug-Drug: Febuxostat may ↑ levels and risk of toxicity; concurrent use not recommended. Additive myelosuppression with **antineoplastics**, **cyclosporine**, and **myelosuppressive agents**. **Allopurinol** may ↑ levels and risk of toxicity. ↓ azathioprine dose to 25–33% of the usual dose. May ↓ antibody response to **live-virus vaccines** and ↑ the risk of adverse reactions.

Drug-Natural Products: Concomitant use with **echinacea** and **melatonin** may interfere with immunosuppression.

Route/Dosage

Renal Allograft Rejection Prevention

PO, IV (Adults and Children): 3–5 mg/kg/day initially; maintenance dose 1–3 mg/kg/day.

Rheumatoid Arthritis

PO, IV (Adults and Children): 1 mg/kg/day for 6–8 wk, ↑ by 0.5 mg/kg/day every 4 wk until response or up to 2.5 mg/kg/day, then ↓ by 0.5 mg/kg/day every 4–8 wk to minimal effective dose.

Inflammatory Bowel Disease (Crohn's Disease or Ulcerative Colitis) (unlabeled use)

PO (Adults and Children): 50 mg once daily; may ↑ by 25 mg/day every 1–2 wk as tolerated to target dose of 2–3 mg/kg/day.

Availability (generic available)

Tablets: 50 mg, 75 mg, 100 mg. **Powder for injection:** 100 mg/vial.

NURSING IMPLICATIONS

Assessment

- Assess for infection (vital signs, sputum, urine, stool, WBC) during therapy.
- Monitor intake and output and daily weight. Decreased urine output may lead to toxicity with this medication.
- **Rheumatoid Arthritis:** Assess range of motion; degree of swelling, pain, and strength in affected joints; and ability to perform activities of daily living before and periodically during therapy.

Lab Test Considerations

- Monitor renal, hepatic, and hematologic functions before beginning therapy, weekly during the 1st mo, bimonthly for the next 2–3 mo, and monthly thereafter.
- Leukocyte count of <3000/mm^3 or platelet count of <100,000/mm^3 may necessitate a reduction in dose or temporary discontinuation.

✦ = Canadian drug name. ※ = Genetic implication. S̶t̶r̶i̶k̶e̶t̶h̶r̶o̶u̶g̶h̶ = Discontinued. CAPITALS = life-threatening. Underline = most frequent.

- ↓ in hemoglobin may indicate bone marrow suppression.
- Hepatotoxicity may be manifested by ↑ alkaline phosphatase, bilirubin, AST, ALT, and amylase concentrations. Usually occurs within 6 mo of transplant, rarely with rheumatoid arthritis, and is reversible on discontinuation of azathioprine.
- May ↓ serum and urine uric acid and plasma albumin.

Implementation
- Do not confuse azathioprine with azacitidine.
- Protect transplant patients from staff members and visitors who may carry infection. Maintain protective isolation as indicated.
- **PO:** May be administered with or after meals or in divided doses to minimize nausea.
- **IV: *Reconstitution:*** Add 10 mL of sterile water for injection, and swirl until a clear solution results. Solution is equivalent to 100 mg of azathioprine; it is for IV use only, has a pH of approximately 9.6, and should be used within 24 hr. *Dilution:* Further dilute with 0.9% NaCl or D5W; final volume depends on time for the infusion, usually 30 to 60 min, but as short as 5 min and as long as 8 hr for the daily dose. Inspect solution for particulate matter and discoloration prior to administration. *Rate:* Infuse over 30–60 min; 5 min to 8 hr have been used.

Patient/Family Teaching
- Instruct patient to take azathioprine as directed. If a dose is missed on a once-daily regimen, omit dose; if on several-times-a-day dosing, take as soon as possible or double next dose. Consult health care professional if more than 1 dose is missed or if vomiting occurs shortly after dose is taken. Do not discontinue without consulting health care professional.
- Advise patient to report unusual tiredness or weakness; cough or hoarseness; fever or chills; lower back or side pain; painful or difficult urination; severe diarrhea; black, tarry stools; blood in urine; or transplant rejection to health care professional immediately.
- Reinforce the need for lifelong therapy to prevent transplant rejection.
- Inform patient of increased risk of malignancy. For patients with increased risk for skin cancer, exposure to sunlight and ultraviolet light should be limited by wearing protective clothing and using a sunscreen with a high protection factor.
- Instruct patient to notify health care professional of all Rx or OTC medications, vitamins, or herbal products being taken and consult health care professional before taking any new medications or receiving any vaccinations while taking this medication.
- Advise patient to avoid contact with persons with contagious diseases and persons who have recently taken oral poliovirus vaccine or other live viruses.
- Rep: May cause fetal harm. Advise patient to use contraception during and for at least 4 mo after therapy is completed and to avoid breastfeeding during therapy.
- Emphasize the importance of follow-up exams and lab tests.
- **Rheumatoid Arthritis:** Concurrent therapy with salicylates, NSAIDs, or corticosteroids may be necessary. Patient should continue physical therapy and adequate rest. Explain that joint damage will not be reversed; goal is to slow or stop disease process.

Evaluation/Desired Outcomes
- Prevention of transplant rejection.
- Decreased stiffness, pain, and swelling in affected joints in 6–8 wk in rheumatoid arthritis. Therapy is discontinued if no improvement in 12 wk.

---

azelastine† (a-zel-as-teen)
Astepro Allergy
Classification
Therapeutic: allergy, cold, and cough remedies, antihistamines

† See Appendix B for ophthalmic use

Indications
Temporary relief of nasal congestion, runny nose, sneezing, and itchy nose due to hay fever or other upper respiratory allergies.

Action
Locally antagonizes the effects of histamine at H_1-receptor sites; does not bind to or inactivate histamine.
Therapeutic Effects: Decreased sneezing, nasal rhinitis, pruritus and postnasal drip.

Pharmacokinetics
Absorption: 40% absorbed after intranasal administration.
Distribution: Widely distributed to tissues.
Metabolism and Excretion: Most of absorbed azelastine is metabolized by the liver (converted to an active metabolite.
Half-life: 22–25 hr.

TIME/ACTION PROFILE (relief of symptoms)

ROUTE	ONSET	PEAK	DURATION
Intranasal	rapid	2–3 hr†	12 hr

†Plasma concentration.

Contraindications/Precautions
Contraindicated in: Hypersensitivity.
Use Cautiously in: OB: Safety not established in pregnancy; Lactation: Safety not established in breastfeeding; Pedi: Safety not established in children <6 yr.

Adverse Reactions/Side Effects
EENT: epistaxis, nasal burning, pharyngitis, sinusitis, sneezing. **GI:** bitter taste, dry mouth, nausea. **Metab:** ↑ weight. **MS:** myalgia. **Neuro:** drowsiness, dizziness, dysesthesia, fatigue, headache.

Interactions

Drug-Drug: Additive CNS depression with **CNS depressants**, including **alcohol, sedative/hypnotics**, and **opioid analgesics**. Concurrent use of **cimetidine** ↑ blood levels.
Drug-Natural Products: Concomitant use of **kava, valerian, skullcap, chamomile**, or **hops** can ↑ CNS depression.

Route/Dosage

Intranasal (Adults and Children ≥12 yr): 2 sprays/nostril once daily *or* 1–2 sprays/nostril twice daily.
Intranasal (Children 6–11 yr): 1 spray/nostril twice daily.

Availability (generic available)

Nasal spray: 205.5 mcg/spray (60–200 sprays/bottle) ᴼᵀᶜ. *In combination with:* fluticasone (Dymista); see Appendix N.

NURSING IMPLICATIONS

Assessment

● Assess allergy symptoms (rhinitis, sneezing, conjunctivitis, hives) before and periodically during therapy.
● Assess lung sounds and character of bronchial secretions. Maintain fluid intake of 1500–2000 mL/day to decrease viscosity of secretions.

Lab Test Considerations

● May cause false-negative allergy skin testing. Discontinue antihistamines at least 72 hr before testing.

Implementation

● **Intranasal:** Before initial use, remove the safety clip on the bottle and prime the delivery system with 6 sprays or until a fine mist appears. When ≥3 days have elapsed since last use, reprime the unit with 2 sprays or until a fine mist appears.

Patient/Family Teaching

● Instruct patient in the proper technique for administration of azelastine. Keep head tilted downward toward toes during instillation of intranasal spray to decrease bitter taste.
● May cause drowsiness. Caution patient to avoid driving or other activities requiring alertness until effects of the medication are known.
● Advise patient to avoid taking alcohol or other CNS depressants concurrently with this drug.
● Advise patient that good oral hygiene, frequent rinsing of the mouth, and sugarless gum or candy may help relieve dry mouth. Patient should notify dentist if dry mouth persists >2 wk.
● Instruct patient to notify health care professional of all Rx or OTC medications, vitamins, or herbal products being taken and consult health care professional before taking any new medications.

● Rep: Advise females of reproductive potential to notify health care professional if pregnancy is planned or suspected or if breastfeeding.
● Instruct patient to contact health care professional if symptoms persist.

Evaluation/Desired Outcomes

● Decreased sneezing, nasal rhinitis, pruritus and postnasal drip.

---

azilsartan, See ANGIOTENSIN II RECEPTOR ANTAGONISTS.

---

azithromycin
(aye-**zith**-roe-mye-sin)
Zithromax, ~~Zmax~~
Classification
Therapeutic: agents for atypical mycobacterium, anti-infectives
Pharmacologic: macrolides

Indications

Treatment of the following infections due to susceptible organisms: Upper respiratory tract infections, including streptococcal pharyngitis, acute bacterial exacerbations of chronic bronchitis and tonsillitis, Lower respiratory tract infections, including bronchitis and pneumonia, Acute otitis media, Skin and skin structure infections, Nongonococcal urethritis, cervicitis, gonorrhea, and chancroid. Prevention of disseminated *Mycobacterium avium* complex (MAC) infection in patients with advanced HIV infection. **Unlabeled Use:** Prevention of bacterial endocarditis. Treatment of cystic fibrosis lung disease. Treatment and post-exposure prophylaxis of pertussis in infants.

Action

Inhibits protein synthesis at the level of the 50S bacterial ribosome. **Therapeutic Effects:** Bacteriostatic action against susceptible bacteria. **Spectrum:** Active against the following gram-positive aerobic bacteria: *Staphylococcus aureus, Streptococcus pneumoniae, S. pyogenes* (group A strep). Active against these gram-negative aerobic bacteria: *Haemophilus influenzae, Moraxella catarrhalis, Neisseria gonorrhoeae*. Also active against: *Bordetella pertussis, Mycoplasma, Legionella, Chlamydia pneumoniae, Ureaplasma urealyticum, Borrelia burgdorferi, M. avium*. Not active against methicillin-resistant *S. aureus*.

Pharmacokinetics

Absorption: Rapidly absorbed (40%) after oral administration. IV administration results in complete bioavailability.

Distribution: Widely distributed to body tissues and fluids. Intracellular and tissue levels exceed those in serum; low CSF levels.

Protein Binding: 7–51%.

Metabolism and Excretion: Mostly excreted unchanged in bile; 4.5% excreted unchanged in urine.

Half-life: 11–14 hr after single dose; 2–4 days after several doses.

TIME/ACTION PROFILE (serum)

ROUTE	ONSET	PEAK	DURATION
PO	rapid	2.5–3.2 hr	24 hr
IV	rapid	end of infusion	24 hr

Contraindications/Precautions

Contraindicated in: Hypersensitivity to azithromycin, erythromycin, or other macrolide anti-infectives; History of cholestatic jaundice or hepatic dysfunction with prior use of azithromycin; QT interval prolongation, hypokalemia, hypomagnesemia, or bradycardia; Concurrent use of quinidine, procainamide, dofetilide, amiodarone, or sotalol.

Use Cautiously in: Severe hepatic impairment (dose adjustment may be required); Severe renal impairment (CCr <10 mL/min); Myasthenia gravis (may worsen symptoms); OB: Use during pregnancy only if potential maternal benefit justifies potential fetal risk; Lactation: Use while breastfeeding only if potential maternal benefit justifies potential risk to infant; Pedi: Neonates (↑ risk of infantile hypertrophic pyloric stenosis at up to 42 days of life); Geri: Older adults may have ↑ risk of QT interval prolongation.

Adverse Reactions/Side Effects

CV: CARDIOVASCULAR DEATH, chest pain, hypotension, palpitations, QT interval prolongation, TORSADES DE POINTES. **Derm:** ACUTE GENERALIZED EXANTHEMATOUS PUSTULOSIS, DRUG REACTION WITH EOSINOPHILIA AND SYSTEMIC SYMPTOMS (DRESS), photosensitivity, rash, STEVENS-JOHNSON SYNDROME, TOXIC EPIDERMAL NECROLYSIS. **EENT:** ototoxicity. **F and E:** hyperkalemia. **GI:** abdominal pain, diarrhea, nausea, ↑ liver enzymes, cholestatic jaundice, CLOSTRIDIOIDES DIFFICILE-ASSOCIATED DIARRHEA (CDAD), dyspepsia, flatulence, HEPATOTOXICITY, melena, oral candidiasis, pyloric stenosis. **GU:** nephritis, vaginitis. **Hemat:** anemia, leukopenia, thrombocytopenia. **Neuro:** dizziness, drowsiness, fatigue, headache, seizures. **Misc:** HYPERSENSITIVITY REACTIONS (including anaphylaxis and angioedema).

Interactions

Drug-Drug: **Quinidine**, **procainamide**, **dofetilide**, **sotalol**, and **amiodarone** may ↑ risk of QT interval prolongation; concurrent use should be avoided. **Aluminum-** and **magnesium-containing antacids** ↓ peak levels. **Nelfinavir** ↑ levels (monitor carefully); azithromycin also ↓ nelfinavir levels. **Efavirenz** ↑ lev-

els. May ↑ the effects and risk of toxicity of **warfarin** and **zidovudine**. Other macrolide anti-infectives have been known to ↑ levels and effects of **digoxin**, **theophylline**, **ergotamine**, **dihydroergotamine**, **triazolam**, **carbamazepine**, **cyclosporine**, **tacrolimus**, and **phenytoin**; careful monitoring of concurrent use is recommended.

Route/Dosage

Most Respiratory and Skin Infections

PO (Adults): 500 mg on 1st day, then 250 mg/day for 4 more days (total dose of 1.5 g); *Acute bacterial sinusitis:* 500 mg once daily for 3 days.

PO (Children ≥ 6 mo): *Pneumonia/Pertussis:* 10 mg/kg (not to exceed 500 mg/dose) on 1st day, then 5 mg/kg once daily (not to exceed 250 mg/dose) for 4 more days. *Pharyngitis/tonsilitis:* 12 mg/kg once daily for 5 days (not to exceed 500 mg/dose); *Acute bacterial sinusitis:* 10 mg/kg once daily for 3 days.

PO (Neonates): *Pertussis, treatment and post-exposure prophylaxis:* 10 mg/kg once daily for 5 days.

Otitis Media

PO (Children ≥6 mo): 30 mg/kg single dose (not to exceed 1500 mg/dose) *or* 10 mg/kg once daily (not to exceed 500 mg/dose) for 3 days *or* 10 mg/kg (not to exceed 500 mg/dose) on 1st day, then 5 mg/kg once daily (not to exceed 250 mg/dose) for 4 more days.

Acute Bacterial Exacerbations of Chronic Bronchitis

PO (Adults): 500 mg on 1st day, then 250 mg once daily for 4 more days (total dose of 1.5 g) *or* 500 mg once daily for 3 days.

Community-Acquired Pneumonia

IV, PO (Adults): *More severe:* 500 mg IV every 24 hr for at least 2 doses, then 500 mg PO every 24 hr for a total of 7–10 days; *Less severe:* 500 mg PO, then 250 mg/day PO for 4 more days.

PO (Children >6 mo): 10 mg/kg on 1st day, then 5 mg/kg once daily for 4 more days.

Pelvic Inflammatory Disease

IV, PO (Adults): 500 mg IV every 24 hr for 1–2 days, then 250 mg PO every 24 hr for a total of 7 days.

Endocarditis Prophylaxis

PO (Adults): 500 mg 1 hr before procedure.

PO (Children): 15 mg/kg 1 hr before procedure.

Nongonococcal Urethritis, Cervicitis, Chancroid, Chlamydia

PO (Adults): Single 1-g dose.

PO (Children): *Chancroid:* Single 20-mg/kg dose (not to exceed 1000 mg/dose). *Urethritis or cervicitis:* Single 10-mg/kg dose (not >1000 mg/dose).

Gonorrhea

PO (Adults): Single 2-g dose.

Prevention of Disseminated MAC Infection

PO (Adults): 1.2 g once weekly (alone or with rifabutin).

PO (Children): 5 mg/kg once daily (not >250 mg/dose) or 20 mg/kg (not >1200 mg/dose) once weekly (alone or with rifabutin).

Cystic Fibrosis

PO (Children ≥6 yrs, ≥40 kg): 500 mg every Monday, Wednesday, and Friday.

PO (Children ≥6 yrs, 25 kg to <40 kg): 250 mg every Monday, Wednesday, and Friday.

Availability (generic available)

Tablets: 250 mg, 500 mg, 600 mg. Powder for oral suspension (cherry and banana flavor) : 1 g/pkt. Powder for oral suspension (cherry, creme de vanilla, and banana flavor) : 100 mg/5 mL, 200 mg/5 mL. Powder for injection : 500 mg/vial.

NURSING IMPLICATIONS

Assessment

- Assess patient for infection (vital signs; appearance of wound, sputum, urine, and stool; WBC) at beginning of and throughout therapy.
- Obtain specimens for culture and sensitivity before initiating therapy. First dose may be given before receiving results.
- Observe for signs and symptoms of anaphylaxis (rash, pruritus, laryngeal edema, wheezing). Notify health care professional immediately if these occur.
- Assess patient for skin rash frequently during therapy. Discontinue azithromycin at first sign of rash; may be life-threatening. Stevens-Johnson syndrome or toxic epidermal necrolysis may develop. Treat symptomatically; may recur once treatment is stopped.

Lab Test Considerations

- May cause ↑ serum bilirubin, AST, ALT, LDH, and alkaline phosphatase concentrations.
- May cause ↑ creatine phosphokinase, potassium, prothrombin time, BUN, serum creatinine, and blood glucose concentrations.
- May occasionally cause ↓ WBC and platelet count.

Implementation

- PO: Administer 1 hr before or 2 hr after meals.
- For administration of single 1-g packet, thoroughly mix entire contents of packet with 2 oz (60 mL) of water. Drink entire contents immediately; add an additional 2 oz of water, mix and drink to assure complete consumption of dose. Do not use the single packet to administer doses other than 1000 mg of azithromycin. Pedi: 1-g packet is not for pediatric use.

IV Administration

- Intermittent Infusion: *Reconstitution:* Reconstitute each 500-mg vial with 4.8 mL of sterile water for injection to achieve a concentration of 100 mg/mL. Reconstituted solution is stable for 24 hr at

room temperature. *Dilution:* Further dilute the 500-mg dose in 250 mL or 500 mL of 0.9% NaCl, 0.45% NaCl, D5W, LR, D5/0.45% NaCl, or D5/LR. Infusion is stable for 24 hr at room temperature or for 7 days if refrigerated. *Concentration:* Final concentration of infusion is 1 – 2 mg/mL. *Rate:* Administer the 1-mg/mL solution over 3 hr or the 2-mg/mL solution over 1 hr. Do not administer as a bolus.

- Y-Site Compatibility: acyclovir, alemtuzumab, aminocaproic acid, aminophylline, amphotericin B lipid complex, amphotericin B liposome, ampicillin, ampicillin/sulbactam, anidulafungin, argatroban, arsenic trioxide, atracurium, bivalirudin, bleomycin, bumetanide, buprenorphine, butorphanol, calcium chloride, calcium gluconate, cangrelor, carboplatin, carmustine, cefazolin, cefepime, cefotetan, cefoxitin, ceftaroline, ceftazidime, ceftolozane/tazobactam, cisatracurium, cisplatin, cyclophosphamide, cyclosporine, cytarabine, dacarbazine, daptomycin, dexamethasone, dexmedetomidine, dexrazoxane, digoxin, diltiazem, diphenhydramine, dobutamine, docetaxel, dopamine, doxorubicin liposome, doxycycline, droperidol, enalaprilat, ephedrine, epinephrine, eptifibatide, ertapenem, esmolol, etoposide, etoposide phosphate, fluconazole, fluorouracil, foscarnet, fosphenytoin, ganciclovir, gemcitabine, granisetron, haloperidol, heparin, hetastarch, hydrocortisone, hydromorphone, idarubicin, ifosfamide, irinotecan, isoproterenol, labetalol, LR, leucovorin, lidocaine, linezolid, lorazepam, magnesium sulfate, mannitol, meperidine, meropenem, meropenem/vaborbactam, mesna, methadone, methohexital, methotrexate, methylprednisolone, metoclopramide, milrinone, nalbuphine, naloxone, nitroglycerin, nitroprusside, octreotide, ondansetron, oxaliplatin, oxytocin, paclitaxel, palonosetron, pamidronate, pantoprazole, pemetrexed, pentobarbital, phenobarbital, phenylephrine, plazomicin, potassium acetate, potassium phosphate, procainamide, prochlorperazine, promethazine, propranolol, remifentanil, rocuronium, sodium acetate, sodium bicarbonate, sodium phosphate, succinylcholine, sufentanil, tacrolimus, telavancin, thiotepa, tigecycline, tirofiban, trimethoprim/sulfamethoxazole, vancomycin, vasopressin, vecuronium, verapamil, vincristine, voriconazole, zidovudine, zoledronic acid.
- Y-Site Incompatibility: amiodarone, amphotericin B deoxycholate, chlorpromazine, diazepam, doxorubicin hydrochloride, epirubicin, gemtuzumab ozogamicin, midazolam, mitoxantrone, mycophenolate, nicardipine, pentamidine, phenytoin, thiopental.

Patient/Family Teaching

- Instruct patients to take medication as directed and to finish the drug completely, even if they are feeling better. Take missed doses as soon as possible unless almost time for next dose; do not double doses. Advise patients that sharing of this medication may be dangerous.

- Instruct patient not to take azithromycin with food or antacids.
- May cause drowsiness and dizziness. Caution patient to avoid driving or other activities requiring alertness until response to medication is known.
- Advise patient to use sunscreen and protective clothing to prevent photosensitivity reactions.
- Advise patient to report symptoms of chest pain, palpitations, yellowing of skin or eyes, or signs of superinfection (black, furry overgrowth on the tongue; vaginal itching or discharge; loose or foul-smelling stools) or rash.
- Instruct patient to notify health care professional if fever and diarrhea develop, especially if stool contains blood, pus, or mucus. Advise patient not to treat diarrhea without advice of health care professional.
- Advise patients being treated for nongonococcal urethritis or cervicitis that sexual partners should also be treated.
- Instruct parents, caregivers, or patient to notify health care professional if symptoms do not improve.
- Rep: Advise females of reproductive potential to notify health care professional if pregnancy is planned or suspected or if breastfeeding. Advise women to monitor breastfed infant for diarrhea, vomiting, or rash.

Evaluation/Desired Outcomes

- Resolution of the signs and symptoms of infection. Length of time for complete resolution depends on the organism and site of infection.

aztreonam (az-tree-oh-nam)
Azactam, Cayston

Classification
Therapeutic: anti-infectives
Pharmacologic: monobactams

Indications

IM, IV: Treatment of serious gram-negative infections including: Septicemia, Skin and skin structure infections, Intra-abdominal infections, Gynecologic infections, Respiratory tract infections, Urinary tract infections. Useful for treatment of multiresistant strains of some bacteria including aerobic gram-negative pathogens. **Inhaln:** To improve respiratory symptoms in cystic fibrosis (CF) patients with *Pseudomonas aeruginosa*.

Action

Binds to the bacterial cell wall membrane, causing cell death. **Therapeutic Effects:** Bactericidal action against susceptible bacteria. **Spectrum:** Displays significant activity against gram-negative aerobic organisms

only: *Escherichia coli, Serratia, Klebsiella oxytoca or pneumoniae, Citrobacter, Proteus mirabilis, Pseudomonas aeruginosa, Enterobacter, Haemophilus influenzae.* Not active against: *Staphylococcus aureus, Enterococcus, Bacteroides fragilis, Streptococci.*

Pharmacokinetics

Absorption: Well absorbed following IM administration. IV administration results in complete bioavailability. Low absorption follows administration by oral inhalation.

Distribution: Widely distributed to tissues. High concentrations achieved in sputum with inhalation.

Metabolism and Excretion: 60–70% excreted unchanged by the kidneys. 10% of inhaled dose excreted unchanged in urine. Small amounts metabolized by the liver.

Half-life: *Adults:* 1.5–2 hr; *Children:* 1.7 hr; *Neonates:* 2.4–9 hr (↑ in renal impairment).

TIME/ACTION PROFILE (plasma concentrations)

ROUTE	ONSET	PEAK	DURATION
IM	rapid	60 min	6–8 hr
IV	rapid	end of infusion	6–8 hr
Inhaln	rapid	unknown	Several hr

Contraindications/Precautions

Contraindicated in: Hypersensitivity; Lactation: Lactation (IV/IM formulation).

Use Cautiously in: Renal impairment (dosage ↓ required if CCr 30 mL/min or less); Cross-sensitivity with penicillins or cephalosporins may occur rarely. Has been used safely in patients with a history of penicillin or cephalosporin allergy; Patients with FEV₁ <25% or >75% predicted, or patients colonized with *Burkholderia cepacia* (safety and effectiveness not established); OB: Safety of IV/IM formulation not established in pregnancy. Systemic absorption of oral inhalation expected to be minimal; Lactation: Systemic absorption of oral inhalation expected to be minimal; Pedi: Children <7 yr (oral inhalation) (safety and effectiveness not established); Geri: Consider age-related ↓ in renal function in older adults.

Adverse Reactions/Side Effects

CV: chest discomfort (oral inhalation). **Derm:** rash. **EENT:** nasal congestion (oral inhalation), nasopharyngeal pain (oral inhalation). **GI:** abdominal pain (oral inhalation), altered taste, CLOSTRIDIOIDES DIFFICILE-ASSOCIATED DIARRHEA (CDAD), diarrhea, nausea, vomiting. **Local:** pain at IM site, phlebitis at IV site. **Neuro:** SEIZURES. **Resp:** cough (oral inhalation), wheezing (oral inhalation), bronchospasm (oral inhalation). **Misc:** fever (inhalation), HYPERSENSITIVITY REACTIONS (including anaphylaxis), superinfection.

Interactions

Drug-Drug: Levels may be ↑ by **furosemide** or **probenecid**.

Route/Dosage

IM, IV (Adults): *Moderately severe infections:* 1–2 g every 8–12 hr; *severe or life-threatening infections (including those due to Pseudomonas aeruginosa):* 2 g every 6–8 hr; *urinary tract infections:* 0.5–1 g every 8–12 hr.

IV (Children 1 mo–16 yr): *Mild to moderate infections:* 30 mg/kg every 8 hr; *moderate to severe infections:* 30 mg/kg every 6–8 hr; *cystic fibrosis:* 50 mg/kg every 6–8 hr.

IV (Neonates >2 kg): 30 mg/kg every 6–8 hr.

IV (Neonates ≤2 kg): 30 mg/kg every 8–12 hr.

Inhaln (Adults and Children >7 yr): 75 mg three times daily for 28 days.

Renal Impairment

IV (Adults): *CCr 10–30 mL/min:* 1–2 g initially, then 50% of usual dosage at usual interval; *CCr <10 mL/min:* 500 mg–2 g initially, then 25% of usual dosage at usual interval (⅛ of initial dose should also be given after each hemodialysis session).

Availability (generic available)

Powder for injection: 1 g/vial, 2 g/vial. **Lyophilized powder for use with diluent provided in Altera Nebulizer System only (Cayston):** 75 mg/vial with 1 mL ampule of diluent (0.17% sodium chloride).

NURSING IMPLICATIONS

Assessment

- Assess for infection (vital signs; wound appearance, sputum, urine, and stool; WBC) at beginning of and throughout therapy.
- Obtain a history before initiating therapy to determine previous use of and reactions to penicillins and cephalosporins. Patients allergic to these drugs may exhibit hypersensitivity reactions to aztreonam. However, aztreonam can often be used in these patients.
- Obtain specimens for culture and sensitivity before initiating therapy. First dose may be given before receiving results.
- Assess respiratory status prior to and following inhalation therapy.
- Observe for signs and symptoms of anaphylaxis (rash, pruritus, laryngeal edema, wheezing). Notify the health care professional immediately if these occur.
- Monitor bowel function. Report diarrhea, abdominal cramping, fever, and bloody stools to health care professional promptly as a sign of CDAD. May begin up to several wk following cessation of therapy.

Lab Test Considerations

- May cause ↑ in AST, ALT, alkaline phosphatase, LDH, and serum creatinine. May cause ↑ prothrombin and partial thromboplastin times, and positive Coombs' test.

Implementation

- After adding diluent to vial, shake immediately and vigorously. Not for multidose use; discard unused solution. IV route is recommended if single dose >1 g or for severe or life-threatening infection.
- **IM:** Dilute each gram of aztreonam with at least 3 mL of 0.9% NaCl, or sterile or bacteriostatic water for injection. Stable at room temperature for 48 hr or 7 days if refrigerated.
- Administer into large, well-developed muscle.

IV Administration

- **IV Push:** Reconstitute each vial with 6–10 mL of sterile water for injection. *Rate:* Administer slowly over 3–5 min by direct injection or into tubing of a compatible solution.
- **Intermittent Infusion:** Reconstitute each vial with 3 mL of sterile water for injection. *Dilution:* Dilute further with 0.9% NaCl, Ringer's or LR, D5W, D10W, D5/0.9% NaCl, D5/0.45% NaCl, D5/0.2% NaCl, D5/ LR, or sodium lactate. *Concentration:* Do not exceed 50 mg/mL. Solution is stable for 48 hr at room temperature and 7 days if refrigerated. Solutions range from colorless to light, straw yellow or may develop a pink tint upon standing; this does not affect potency. *Rate:* Infuse over 20–60 min.
- **Y-Site Compatibility:** alemtuzumab, allopurinol, amifostine, amikacin, aminophylline, amphotericin B lipid complex, anidulafungin, argatroban, ascorbic acid, atracurium, atropine, benztropine, bivalirudin, bleomycin, bumetanide, buprenorphine, butorphanol, calcium chloride, calcium gluconate, carboplatin, carmustine, caspofungin, cefazolin, cefepime, cefotaxime, cefotetan, cefoxitin, ceftazidime, ceftriaxone, cefuroxime, chloramphenicol, ciprofloxacin, cisatracurium, cisplatin, clindamycin, cyanocobalamin, cyclophosphamide, cyclosporine, cytarabine, dacarbazine, dactinomycin, daptomycin, dexamethasone, dexmedetomidine, digoxin, diltiazem, dobutamine, docetaxel, dopamine, doxorubicin hydrochloride, doxorubicin liposomal, doxycycline, droperidol, enalaprilat, ephedrine, epinephrine, epirubicin, epoetin alfa, eptifibatide, ertapenem, esmolol, etoposide, etoposide phosphate, famotidine, fentanyl, filgrastim, floxuridine, fluconazole, fludarabine, fluorouracil, folic acid, foscarnet, furosemide, gemcitabine, gentamicin, glycopyrrolate, granisetron, heparin, hetastarch, hydrocortisone, hydromorphone, idarubicin, ifosfamide, insulin, regular, irinotecan, isoproterenol, ketorolac, labetalol, leucovorin calcium, levofloxacin, lidocaine, linezolid, magnesium sulfate, mannitol, melphalan, meperidine, mesna, methotrexate, methylprednisolone, metoclopramide, metoprolol, midazolam, milrinone, morphine, multivitamins, nafcillin, nalbuphine, naloxone, nicardipine, nitroglycerin, nitroprusside, norepinephrine, octreotide, ondansetron, oxacillin, oxaliplatin, oxytocin, pacli-

taxel, palonosetron, pamidronate, pemetrexed, penicillin G, phenobarbital, phentolamine, phenylephrine, phytonadione, piperacillin/tazobactam, potassium acetate, potassium chloride, procainamide, propofol, propranolol, protamine, pyridoxine, remifentanil, rituximab, rocuronium, sargramostim, sodium acetate, sodium bicarbonate, succinylcholine, sufentanil, tacrolimus, theophylline, thiamine, thiotepa, tigecycline, tirofiban, tobramycin, vasopressin, vecuronium, verapamil, vinblastine, vincristine, vinorelbine, voriconazole, zidovudine, zoledronic acid.

- **Y-Site Incompatibility:** acyclovir, amphotericin B deoxycholate, amphotericin B liposomal, azathioprine, azithromycin, chlorpromazine, dantrolene, daunorubicin hydrochloride, diazepam, diazoxide, erythromycin, ganciclovir, indomethacin, lorazepam, metronidazole, mitomycin, mitoxantrone, mycophenolate, pantoprazole, papaverine, pentamidine, pentobarbital, phenytoin, prochlorperazine, trastuzumab.

- **Inhaln:** Open glass aztreonam vial by removing metal ring and pulling tab, and removing gray rubber stopper. Twist tip of diluent ampule and squeeze contents into glass aztreonam vial. Replace rubber stopper and swirl gently until contents are completely dissolved. Administer immediately after reconstitution using *Altera Nebulizer System.* Pour reconstituted solution into handset of nebulizer. Turn unit on. Place mouthpiece into mouth and breathe normally only through mouth. Administration takes 2–3 min. Do not use other nebulizers or mix with other medications. Do not administer IV or IM. Refrigerate aztreonam and diluent; may be stored at room temperature for up to 28 days. Protect from light.

- Administer short-acting bronchodilator between 15 min and 4 hr or long-acting bronchodilator between 30 min and 12 hr prior to treatment. If taking multiple inhaled therapies, administer in the following order: bronchodilator, mucolytic, and lastly, aztreonam.

Patient/Family Teaching

- Advise patient to report the signs of superinfection (furry overgrowth on the tongue, vaginal itching or discharge, loose or foul-smelling stools) and allergy.
- Instruct patient to notify health care professional if fever and diarrhea develop, especially if stool contains blood, pus, or mucus. Advise patient not to treat diarrhea without consulting health care professional.
- Advise patient to notify health care professional if new or worsening symptoms occur or if signs or symptoms of anaphylaxis occur.
- Rep: Advise females of reproductive potential to notify health care professional if pregnancy is planned or suspected or if breastfeeding. Patients receiving IV aztreonam should consider temporarily discontinuing breastfeeding or using formula during therapy.
- **Inhaln:** Instruct patient to use aztreonam as directed for the full 28-day course, even if feeling better. If a dose is missed, take all 3 daily doses, as long as doses are at least 4 hr apart. Skipping doses or not completing full course of therapy may decrease effectiveness and increase likelihood of bacterial resistance not treatable in the future. Inform patient of the importance of using a bronchodilator prior to treatment and in use and cleaning of nebulizer. Advise patient to read *Patient Information* before starting therapy.

Evaluation/Desired Outcomes

- Resolution of signs and symptoms of infection. Length of time for complete resolution depends on the organism and site of infection.
- Improvement in respiratory symptoms in patients with CF.

baclofen (bak-loe-fen)

Fleqsuvy, Gablofen, Lioresal, Lyvispah, Ozobax

Classification

Therapeutic: antispasticity agents, skeletal muscle relaxants (centrally acting)

Indications

PO: Treatment of reversible spasticity due to multiple sclerosis or spinal cord lesions. **IT:** Treatment of severe spasticity of cerebral or spinal origin (should be reserved for patients who do not respond or are intolerant to oral baclofen) (should wait at least one yr in patients with traumatic brain injury before considering therapy). **Unlabeled Use:** Management of pain in trigeminal neuralgia.

Action

Inhibits reflexes at the spinal level. **Therapeutic Effects:** Decreased muscle spasticity; bowel and bladder function may also be improved.

Pharmacokinetics

Absorption: Well absorbed after oral administration. **Distribution:** Widely distributed; crosses the placenta. **Protein Binding:** 30%. **Metabolism and Excretion:** 70–80% eliminated unchanged by the kidneys. **Half-life:** 2.5–4 hr.

TIME/ACTION PROFILE (effects on spasticity)

ROUTE	ONSET	PEAK	DURATION
PO	hr–wk	unknown	unknown
IT	0.5–1 hr	4 hr	4–8 hr

Contraindications/Precautions

Contraindicated in: Hypersensitivity.

Use Cautiously in: Patients in whom spasticity maintains posture and balance; Patients with epilepsy (may ↓ seizure threshold); Renal impairment (↓ dose may be required); OB: Safety not established in pregnancy; Lactation: Use while breastfeeding only if potential maternal benefit justifies potential risk to infant; Pedi: Children <4 yr (intrathecal) (safety and effectivenessnot established); Geri: ↑ risk of CNS side effects in older adults.

Adverse Reactions/Side Effects

CV: edema, hypotension. **Derm:** pruritus, rash. **EENT:** nasal congestion, tinnitus. **GI:** <u>nausea</u>, constipation. **GU:** frequency. **Metab:** ↑ weight, hyperglycemia. **Neuro:** dizziness, <u>drowsiness</u>, fatigue, weakness, ataxia, confusion, depression, headache, insomnia, SEIZURES (IT). **Misc:** hypersensitivity reactions, sweating.

Interactions

Drug-Drug: ↑ CNS depression with other **CNS depressants** including **alcohol, antihistamines, opioid analgesics,** and **sedative/hypnotics.** Use with **MAO inhibitors** may lead to ↑ CNS depression or hypotension.

Drug-Natural Products: Concomitant use of **kava-kava, valerian,** or **chamomile** can ↑ CNS depression.

Route/Dosage

PO (Adults): 5 mg 3 times daily. May ↑ every 3 days by 5 mg/dose up to 80 mg/day (some patients may have a better response to 4 divided doses).

PO (Children ≥8 yr): 30–40 mg daily divided every 8 hr; titrate to a maximum of 120 mg/day.

PO (Children 2–7 yr): 20–30 mg daily divided every 8 hr; titrate to a maximum of 60 mg/day.

PO (Children <2 yr): 10–20 mg daily divided every 8 hr; titrate to a maximum of 40 mg/day.

IT (Adults): 100–800 mcg/day infusion; dose is determined by response during screening phase.

IT (Children ≥4 yr): 25–1200 mcg/day infusion (average 275 mcg/day); dose is determined by response during screening phase.

Availability (generic available)

Tablets: 5 mg, 10 mg, 20 mg. **Oral granules:** 5 mg/pkt, 10 mg/pkt, 20 mg/pkt. **Oral solution (grape flavor):** 1 mg/mL. **Oral suspension (grape flavor):** 5 mg/mL. **Solution for intrathecal injection:** 50 mcg/mL, 500 mcg/mL, 1000 mcg/mL, 2000 mcg/mL.

NURSING IMPLICATIONS

Assessment

- Assess muscle spasticity before and periodically during therapy.
- Observe patient for drowsiness, dizziness, or ataxia. May be alleviated by a change in dose.
- **IT:** Monitor patient closely during test dose and titration. Have resuscitative equipment immediately available for life-threatening or intolerable side effects.

Lab Test Considerations

- May cause ↑ in serum glucose, alkaline phosphatase, AST, and ALT levels.

Implementation

- **PO:** Administer with milk or food to minimize gastric irritation.
- **Oral suspension**: Shake oral suspension well before use. Use a calibrated measuring device to measure and deliver dose accurately; household teaspoon or tablespoon is not an adequate measuring device. Discard unused portion 2 mo after first opening. **Oral granules:** Empty entire contents of packet of oral granules *into mouth*. Granules will

dissolve in mouth or can be swallowed. May be taken *with up to 15 mL of liquids or soft foods (apple sauce, yogurt, pudding).*Administer no >2 hrs after mixing. If multiple packets are to be used, mix each packet separately. May also be administered via *enteral feeding tubes* (nasogastric (NG) at sizes 8 FR or higher, gastrostomy (G) at sizes 12 FR or higher, percutaneous endoscopic gastrostomy (PEG) at sizes 14 FR or higher, and gastrojejunostomy (GJ) tubes at sizes 16 FR or higher). Flush feeding tube with up to 15 mL of water using a catheter tip syringe. Open and empty full contents of one packet in 15 mL of liquid, such as apple juice or milk, in a clean container. Mix suspension to ensure all granules are wetted. Draw up suspension into a syringe immediately after mixing and administer dose via the feeding tube. Administer no longer than 2 hrs after mixing. If syringe is allowed to stand for 15 min before administration, invert syringe 3 times. Refill syringe with 15 mL of water and flush feeding tube. If multiple packets are to be administered, mix each packet with a separate volume of liquid.

- IT: For *screening phase, Dilution:* dilute for a concentration of 50 mcg/mL with sterile preservative-free NaCl for injection. Test dose should be administered over at least 1 min. Observe patient for a significant decrease in muscle tone or frequency or severity of spasm. If response is inadequate, 2 additional test doses, each 24 hr apart, 75 mcg/1.5 mL and 100 mcg/2 mL respectively, may be administered. Patients with an inadequate response should not receive chronic IT therapy. Avoid use of prefilled syringes for filling reservoir of pump; prefilled syringes are not sterile.
- Dose titration for implantable IT pumps is based on patient response. If no substantive response after dose increase, check pump function and catheter patency.

Patient/Family Teaching

- Instruct patient to take baclofen as directed. Take a missed dose within 1 hr; do not double doses. Caution patient to avoid abrupt withdrawal of this medication; may precipitate an acute withdrawal reaction (hallucinations, increased spasticity, seizures, mental changes, restlessness). Discontinue baclofen gradually over 2 wk or more.
- May cause dizziness and drowsiness. Advise patient to avoid driving or other activities requiring alertness until response to drug is known.
- Instruct patient to change positions slowly to minimize orthostatic hypotension.
- Advise patient to avoid concurrent use of alcohol or other CNS depressants while taking this medication.
- Instruct patient to notify health care professional if frequent urge to urinate or painful urination, constipation, nausea, headache, insomnia, tinnitus, depression, or confusion persists.
- Advise patient to report signs and symptoms of hypersensitivity (rash, itching) promptly.

- Rep: Advise females of reproductive potential to notify health care professional if pregnancy is planned or suspected or if breastfeeding. Inform patient that use during pregnancy or breastfeeding may cause withdrawal symptoms (increased muscle tone, tremor, jitteriness, seizures) in infants starting hrs to days after delivery.
- IT: Caution patient and caregiver not to discontinue IT therapy abruptly. May result in fever, mental status changes, exaggerated rebound spasticity, and muscle rigidity. Advise patient not to miss scheduled refill appointments and to notify health care professional promptly if signs of withdrawal occur.

Evaluation/Desired Outcomes

- Decrease in muscle spasticity and associated musculoskeletal pain with an increased ability to perform activities of daily living.
- Decreased pain in patients with trigeminal neuralgia. May take wk to obtain optimal effect.

baloxavir (ba-lox-a-veer)
Xofluza
Classification
Therapeutic: antivirals
Pharmacologic: endonuclease inhibitors

Indications

Treatment of acute uncomplicated influenza in patients who have been symptomatic for ≤48 hr and who are otherwise healthy or at high risk of developing influenza-related complications. Post-exposure prophylaxis of influenza following contact with an individual who has influenza.

Action

Inhibits the endonuclease activity of the polymerase acidic protein in the viral RNA polymerase complex that is required for viral gene transcription, thereby resulting in inhibition of influenza virus replication. **Therapeutic Effects:** Reduced duration of flu-related symptoms.

Pharmacokinetics

Absorption: Administered as a prodrug (baloxavir marboxil) which is rapidly absorbed from the GI tract and converted by the liver to the active form, baloxavir. **Distribution:** Extensively distributed to tissues. **Protein Binding:** 93–94%. **Metabolism and Excretion:** Rapidly metabolized by the liver by UGT1A3 to baloxavir, the active metabolite. Primarily excreted in feces (80%); 15% excreted in urine (3% as active metabolite). **Half-life:** 79 hr.

TIME/ACTION PROFILE (plasma concentrations)

ROUTE	ONSET	PEAK	DURATION
PO	unknown	4 hr	unknown

Contraindications/Precautions

Contraindicated in: Hypersensitivity.

Use Cautiously in: OB: Safety not established during pregnancy; Lactation: Safety not established in breastfeeding; Pedi: Children <5 yr (↑ risk of treatment-emergent resistance).

Adverse Reactions/Side Effects

EENT: nasopharyngitis. **GI:** diarrhea, nausea. **Neuro:** headache. **Misc:** HYPERSENSITIVITY REACTIONS (including anaphylaxis and angioedema).

Interactions

Drug-Drug: Medications containing divalent or trivalent cations, including **calcium**, **iron**, **magnesium**, **selenium**, or **zinc** may ↓ absorption of baloxavir; avoid concurrent use. May ↓ the therapeutic effect of the **live attenuated influenza vaccine**.

Drug-Food: **Calcium** in foods or **dairy products** may ↓ absorption of baloxavir; avoid concurrent administration.

Route/Dosage

PO (Adults and Children ≥5 yr and ≥80 kg): 80 mg as a single dose (as tablets or oral suspension).

PO (Adults and Children ≥5 yr and 20–<80 kg): 40 mg as a single dose (as tablets or oral suspension).

PO (Adults and Children ≥5 yr and <20 kg): 2 mg/kg as a single dose (as oral suspension).

Availability

Oral suspension (strawberry flavor): 2 mg/mL. **Tablets:** 40 mg, 80 mg.

NURSING IMPLICATIONS

Assessment

- Monitor influenza symptoms (sudden onset of fever, cough, headache, fatigue, muscular weakness, sore throat). Additional supportive treatment may be indicated to treat symptoms.
- Monitor for signs and symptoms of hypersensitivity reactions (anaphylaxis, angioedema, urticaria, erythema multiforme) following therapy.

Implementation

- Administer as soon as possible after influenza symptom onset or exposure to influenza.
- PO: Administer 2 tablets without regard to food within 48 hr of onset of symptoms. Avoid taking dairy products, calcium-fortified beverages, polyvalent cation-containing laxatives, antacids, or oral supplements (calcium, iron, magnesium, selenium, or zinc) at same time.
- Suspension may be used for patients with difficulty swallowing or who require enteral administration. Gently tap bottom of bottle to loosen granules (white to light yellow) and constitute with 20 mL of drinking water or sterile water. Swirl to mix granules evenly; do not shake. Solution is stable for 10 hr

since constitution at room temperature; write expiration time and date on label. Measure dose with oral syringe to ensure correct dose; may require more than 1 bottle. Patient must sit upright when taking baloxavir; do not give while patient is lying down. Do not mix suspension with soft food or another liquid.

- For administration via feeding tube, draw up suspension with an enteral syringe. Flush with 1 mL of water before and after administration.

Patient/Family Teaching

- Instruct patient to take baloxavir as directed. Advise patient to read *Patient Information* before taking baloxavir.
- Advise patient to notify health care professional immediately if signs and symptoms of hypersensitivity reactions (rash, hives, difficulty breathing, swelling of lips, face, and throat) occur.
- Advise patient to consult health care professional before receiving a live attenuated influenza vaccine after taking baloxavir.
- Advise patient that baloxavir is not a substitute for a flu shot. Patients should receive annual flu shot according to immunization guidelines.
- Advise patient to notify health care professional of all Rx or OTC medications, vitamins, or herbal products being taken and to consult health care professional before taking any new medications.
- Rep: Advise females of reproductive potential to notify health care professional if pregnancy is planned or suspected, or if breastfeeding. Pregnant women are at higher risk of severe complications from influenza, which may lead to adverse pregnancy and/or fetal outcomes, including maternal death, stillbirth, birth defects, preterm delivery, low birth weight, and small for gestational age.

Evaluation/Desired Outcomes

- Reduced duration or prevention of flu-related symptoms.

baricitinib (bar-i-**sye**-ti-nib)
Olumiant
Classification
Therapeutic: antirheumatics
Pharmacologic: kinase inhibitors

Indications

Moderately to severely active rheumatoid arthritis (RA) in patients who have had an inadequate response/intolerance to ≥1 tumor necrosis factor inhibitor therapies (as monotherapy or in combination with methotrexate or other nonbiologic disease-modifying antirheumatic drugs [DMARDs]) (not to be used with other Janus kinase [JAK] inhibitors, biologic DMARDs or potent immunosuppressants including azathioprine and cyclosporine). Coronavirus disease 2019 (COVID-19) in hospitalized patients requiring supplemental oxygen, noninvasive or invasive mechanical ventilation, or extracorporeal membrane oxygenation (ECMO). Severe alopecia areata (not to be used with other JAK inhibitors, biologic immunomodulates, or cyclosporine, or other potent immunosuppressants).

Action

Acts as a JAK inhibitor which prevents the activation of signal transducers and activators of transcription resulting in a reduction in immunoglobulins and C-reactive protein. **Therapeutic Effects:** Improvement in clinical and symptomatic parameters of RA. Shortened time to recovery and reduction in death from COVID-19. Improvement in scalp hair coverage in alopecia areata.

Pharmacokinetics

Absorption: Well absorbed following oral administration (80%).

Distribution: Widely distributed into tissues.

Metabolism and Excretion: Metabolized by the liver by CYP3A4; primarily excreted in the urine (69% as unchanged drug); 15% excreted in feces as unchanged drug.

Half-life: 12 hr.

TIME/ACTION PROFILE (clinical improvement)

ROUTE	ONSET	PEAK	DURATION
PO	1 wk	3 mo	unknown

Contraindications/Precautions

Contraindicated in: Active infection; Severe renal impairment (eGFR <30 mL/min/1.73 m²) (for treatment of RA); Patients with end-stage renal disease (ESRD) or acute kidney injury or undergoing dialysis (eGFR <15 mL/min/1.73 m²) (for treatment of COVID-19); Severe hepatic impairment (for treatment of RA or alopecia areata); Increased risk for thrombosis; History of MI or stroke; Absolute lymphocyte count <500 cells/mm³, absolute neutrophil count (ANC) <1000 cells/mm³, or hemoglobin levels <8 g/dL; Lactation: Lactation.

Use Cautiously in: Patients who are >50 yr old and have ≥1 cardiovascular risk factor (↑ risk of all-cause mortality, cardiovascular death, MI, stroke, and thrombosis); Current or past history of smoking (↑ risk of malignancy, cardiovascular death, MI, or stroke); Known malignancy; Severe hepatic impairment (use for treatment of COVID-19 only if potential benefit outweighs potential risk); Diverticulitis (↑ risk of GI perforation); OB: Use during pregnancy only if potential maternal benefit justifies potential fetal risk; Pedi: Safety and effectiveness not established in children; Geri: Infection risk may be ↑ in older adults.

Adverse Reactions/Side Effects

CV: ARTERIAL THROMBOSIS, CARDIOVASCULAR DEATH, DEEP VEIN THROMBOSIS, MI. **GI:** ↑ liver enzymes, GI PERFORA-

TION, nausea. **GU:** ↑ serum creatinine. **Hemat:** anemia, lymphopenia, neutropenia, thrombocytosis. **Metab:** ↑ lipids. **MS:** ↑ creatine kinase. **Neuro:** STROKE. **Resp:** PULMONARY EMBOLISM. **Misc:** DEATH, HYPERSENSITIVITY REACTIONS (including angioedema), INFECTION (including tuberculosis, bacterial, invasive fungal infections, viral, and other infections due to opportunistic pathogens), MALIGNANCY.

Interactions

Drug-Drug: Organic anion transporter 3 (OAT3) inhibitors, including **probenecid** may ↑ levels and risk of toxicity; avoid concurrent use.

Route/Dosage

Rheumatoid Arthritis

PO (Adults): 2 mg once daily. *Concurrent use of OAT3 inhibitors (if recommended baricitinib dose is 2 mg once daily):* 1 mg once daily. *Concurrent use of OAT3 inhibitors (if recommended baricitinib dose is 1 mg once daily):* Consider discontinuing OAT3 inhibitor. *Concurrent use of OAT3 inhibitors:* 1 mg once daily.

Renal Impairment

PO (Adults): *eGFR 30– <60 mL/min/m²:* 1 mg once daily. *eGFR <30 mL/min/m²:* Not recommended.

COVID-19

PO (Adults): 4 mg once daily for 14 days or until hospital discharge, whichever occurs first. *Concurrent use of OAT3 inhibitors (if recommended baricitinib dose is 4 mg once daily):* 2 mg once daily. *Concurrent use of OAT3 inhibitors (if recommended baricitinib dose is 2 mg once daily):* 1 mg once daily. *Concurrent use of OAT3 inhibitors (if recommended baricitinib dose is 1 mg once daily):* Consider discontinuing OAT3 inhibitor.

Renal Impairment

PO (Adults): *eGFR 30– <60 mL/min/m²:* 2 mg once daily. *eGFR 15– <30 mL/min/m²:* 1 mg once daily. *eGFR <15 mL/min/m²:* Not recommended.

Alopecia Areata

PO (Adults): 2 mg once daily; may ↑ to 4 mg once daily if response inadequate. For patients with nearly complete or complete scalp hair loss, with or without substantial eyelash or eyebrow hair loss, consider starting treatment with 4 mg once daily. In patients receiving 4 mg once daily (as initial therapy or after a dose ↑), ↓ to 2 mg once daily once adequate response achieved. *Concurrent use of OAT3 inhibitors (if recommended baricitinib dose is 4 mg once daily):* 2 mg once daily. *Concurrent use of OAT3 inhibitors (if recommended baricitinib dose is 2 mg once daily):* 1 mg once daily. *Concurrent use of OAT3 inhibitors (if recommended baricitinib dose is 1 mg once daily):* Consider discontinuing OAT3 inhibitor.

Renal Impairment

PO (Adults): *eGFR 30– <60 mL/min/m² (if recommended baricitinib dose is 4 mg once daily):* 2 mg once daily. *eGFR 30– <60 mL/min/m²* (*if recommended baricitinib dose is 2 mg once daily*): 1 mg once daily. *eGFR <30 mL/min/m²:* Not recommended.

Availability
Film-coated tablets: 1 mg, 2 mg, 4 mg.

NURSING IMPLICATIONS
Assessment
- Assess pain and range of motion before and periodically during therapy.
- Assess for signs of infection (fever, dyspnea, flu-like symptoms, frequent or painful urination, redness or swelling at the site of a wound), including tuberculosis and hepatitis B virus (HBV), prior to and periodically during therapy. Baricitinib is contraindicated in patients with active infection. New infections should be monitored closely; most common are upper respiratory tract infections, bronchitis, and urinary tract infections. Infections may be fatal, especially in patients taking immunosuppressive therapy.
- Assess patients, except those with COVID-19, for latent tuberculosis with a tuberculin skin test prior to initiation of therapy. Treatment of latent tuberculosis should be started before therapy with baricitinib.
- Monitor for signs and symptoms of hypersensitivity reactions (hives, rash, pruritus, swelling of lips, face, or tongue, dyspnea) during therapy. Discontinue baricitinib promptly if symptoms occur.

Lab Test Considerations
- May cause neutropenia. Monitor ANC at baseline and periodically during therapy. *Patients with RA or alopecia areata: If ANC ≥1000 cells/mm³*, maintain dose. *If ANC <1000 cells/mm³*, hold baricitinib until ANC ≥1000 cells/mm³. *Patients with COVID-19:* Do not start therapy if ANC <500 cells/mm³.
- May cause lymphopenia. *Patients with RA or alopecia areata:* Monitor absolute lymphocyte count (ALC) at baseline and periodically during therapy. *If ALC ≥500 cells/mm³*, maintain dose. *If ALC <500 cells/mm³*, hold baricitinib until ALC ≥500 cells/mm³. Do not start therapy if ALC <500 cells/mm³. *Patients with COVID-19:* Do not start therapy if ALC <200 cells/mm³.
- May cause anemia. *Patients with RA or alopecia areata:* Monitor hemoglobin at baseline and periodically during therapy. *If hemoglobin ≥8 g/dL*, maintain dose. *If hemoglobin <8 g/dL*, hold baricitinib until hemoglobin ≥8 g/dL. Do not start therapy if hemoglobin <8 g/dL.
- Monitor liver enzymes at baseline and periodically during therapy. If elevations in AST or ALT and liver injury is suspected, hold baricitinib until cause determined.
- May cause elevations in serum lipids. Monitor total cholesterol, low-density lipoprotein (LDL) choles-

terol, and high-density lipoprotein (HDL) cholesterol 12 wk after starting therapy.
- Monitor renal function at baseline and periodically during therapy.

Implementation
- Administer a tuberculin skin test prior to administration of baricitinib. Patients with active latent TB should be treated for TB prior to therapy.
- Immunizations for patients with RA and alopecia areata should be current prior to initiating therapy. Patients on baricitinib may receive concurrent vaccinations, except for live vaccines.
- **PO:** Administer once daily without regard to food.
- For patients unable to swallow tablets, tablets may be dispersed in water. Place tablets in a container with 10 mL (5 mL minimum) of room temperature water, disperse by gently swirling the tablet(s) and administer immediately orally. Rinse container with 10 mL (5 mL minimum) of water and swallow entire contents.
- *Administration via G tube:* Place tablet(s) in a container with approximately 15 mL (10 mL minimum) of room temperature water and disperse with gentle swirling. Ensure tablet(s) are sufficiently dispersed to allow free passage through tip of syringe. Withdraw entire contents into an appropriate syringe and immediately administer through gastric feeding tube. Rinse container with approximately 15 mL (10 mL minimum) of room temperature water, withdraw contents into syringe, and administer through the tube.
- *Administration via NG or OG tube:* Place tablet(s) into a container with approximately 30 mL of room temperature water and disperse with gentle swirling. Ensure tablet(s) are sufficiently dispersed to allow free passage through tip of syringe. Withdraw entire contents into an appropriate syringe and immediately administer through enteral feeding tube. To avoid clogging of small diameter tubes (smaller than 12 Fr), syringe can be held horizontally and shaken during administration. Rinse container with at least 15 mL of room temperature water, withdraw contents into syringe, and administer through the tube.

Patient/Family Teaching
- Instruct patient to take baricitinib as directed. Advise patient to read *Medication Guide* before starting therapy and with each Rx refill in case of changes.
- Advise patient to notify health care professional if signs and symptoms of infections (fever; sweating; chills; muscle aches; cough; shortness of breath; blood in your phlegm; weight loss; warm, red, or painful skin or sores on body; diarrhea or stomach pain; burning during urination or urinating more often than normal, feeling tired) blood clots in legs (swelling, pain, or tenderness in leg, sudden unexplained chest pain, shortness of breath), stomach

problems (fever, stomach-area pain that does not go away, change in bowel habits), or hypersensitivity reactions occur.

- Advise patient to notify health care professional of all Rx or OTC medications, vitamins, or herbal products being taken and to consult with health care professional before taking other medications.
- Inform patients that baricitinib may increase risk of certain cancers. Instruct patients to notify health care professional if they have ever had any type of cancer.
- Advise patient to avoid live vaccines during therapy.
- Rep: May cause fetal harm. Advise females of reproductive potential to notify health care professional if pregnancy is planned or suspected, and to avoid breastfeeding during and for 4 days after last dose of therapy.

Evaluation/Desired Outcomes

- Decreased pain and swelling with decreased rate of joint destruction in patients with rheumatoid arthritis.
- Shortened time to recovery and reduction in death from COVID-19.
- Improvement in scalp hair coverage in alopecia areata.

---

basiliximab (ba-sil-**ix**-i-mab)
Simulect
Classification
Therapeutic: immunosuppressants
Pharmacologic: monoclonal antibodies

Indications
Prevention of acute organ rejection in patients undergoing renal transplantation (in combination with corticosteroids and cyclosporine).

Action
Binds to and blocks specific interleukin-2 (IL-2) receptor sites on activated T lymphocytes. **Therapeutic Effects:** Prevention of acute organ rejection following renal transplantation.

Pharmacokinetics
Absorption: IV administration results in complete bioavailability.
Distribution: Moderately distributed to tissues.
Metabolism and Excretion: Unknown.
Half-life: 7.2 days.

TIME/ACTION PROFILE (effect on immune function)

ROUTE	ONSET	PEAK	DURATION
IV	2 hr	unknown	36 days

Contraindications/Precautions
Contraindicated in: Hypersensitivity; Lactation: Lactation.

Use Cautiously in: Rep: Women of reproductive potential; OB: Safety not established in pregnancy.

Adverse Reactions/Side Effects
Noted for patients receiving corticosteroids and cyclosporine in addition to basiliximab.
CV: edema, hypertension, angina, arrhythmias, HF, hypotension. **Derm:** acne, wound complications, hypertrichosis, pruritus. **EENT:** abnormal vision, cataracts. **Endo:** hyperglycemia, hypoglycemia. **F and E:** acidosis, hyperkalemia, hypocalcemia, hypokalemia, hypophosphatemia. **GI:** abdominal pain, constipation, diarrhea, dyspepsia, moniliasis, nausea, vomiting, gingival hyperplasia, stomatitis. **Hemat:** BLEEDING, coagulation abnormalities. **Metab:** ↑ weight, hypercholesterolemia, hyperuricemia. **MS:** pain. **Neuro:** dizziness, headache, insomnia, tremor, weakness, neuropathy, paresthesia. **Resp:** cough. **Misc:** infection, chills, HYPERSENSITIVITY REACTIONS (including anaphylaxis).

Interactions
Drug-Drug: Immunosuppression may be ↑ with other **immunosuppressants**.
Drug-Natural Products: Concurrent use with **echinacea** and **melatonin** may interfere with immunosuppression.

Route/Dosage
IV (Adults and Children ≥35 kg): 20 mg given 2 hr before transplantation; repeated 4 days after transplantation. Second dose should be withheld if complication or graft loss occurs.
IV (Children <35 kg): 10 mg given 2 hr before transplantation; repeated 4 days after transplantation. Second dose should be withheld if complication or graft loss occurs.

Availability
Powder for injection: 10 mg/vial, 20 mg/vial.

NURSING IMPLICATIONS
Assessment

- Monitor for signs of anaphylactic or hypersensitivity reactions (hypotension, tachycardia, cardiac failure, dyspnea, wheezing, bronchospasm, pulmonary edema, respiratory failure, urticaria, rash, pruritus, sneezing) at each dose. Onset of symptoms is usually within 24 hr. Resuscitation equipment and medications for treatment of severe hypersensitivity should be readily available. If a severe hypersensitivity reaction occurs, basiliximab therapy should be permanently discontinued. Patients who have previously received basiliximab should only receive subsequent therapy with extreme caution.
- Monitor for infection (fever, chills, rash, sore throat, purulent discharge, dysuria). Notify physician immediately if these symptoms occur; may necessitate discontinuation of therapy.

Lab Test Considerations
- May cause ↑ or ↓ hemoglobin, hematocrit, serum glucose, potassium, and calcium concentrations.

- May cause ↑ serum cholesterol levels.
- May cause ↑ BUN, serum creatinine, and uric acid concentrations.
- May cause ↓ serum magnesium, phosphate, and platelet levels.

Implementation
IV Administration
- Basiliximab is usually administered concurrently with cyclosporine and corticosteroids.
- Reconstitute with 2.5 mL or 5 mL of sterile water for injection for the 10 mg or 20 mg vial, respectively. Shake gently to dissolve powder.
- **IV Push:** *Dilution:* May be administered undiluted. Bolus administration may be associated with nausea, vomiting, and local reactions (pain). *Concentration:* 4 mg/mL. *Rate:* Administer over 20–30 min via peripheral or central line.
- **Intermittent Infusion:** *Dilution:* Dilute further with 25–50 mL of 0.9% NaCl or D5W. Gently invert bag to mix; do not shake, to avoid foaming. Solution is clear to opalescent and colorless; do not administer solutions that are discolored or contain particulate matter. Discard unused portion. Administer within 4 hr or may be refrigerated for up to 24 hr. Discard after 24 hr. *Concentration:* 0.08–0.16 mg/mL. *Rate:* Administer over 20–30 min via peripheral or central line.
- **Additive Incompatibility:** Do not admix; do not administer in IV line containing other medications.

Patient/Family Teaching
- Explain purpose of medication to patient. Explain that patient will need to resume lifelong therapy with other immunosuppressive drugs after completion of basiliximab course.
- May cause dizziness. Caution patient to avoid driving or other activities requiring alertness until response is known.
- Instruct patient to continue to avoid crowds and persons with known infections, because basiliximab also suppresses the immune system.
- Rep: Advise females of reproductive potential to notify health care professional if pregnancy is planned or suspected or if breastfeeding.

Evaluation/Desired Outcomes
- Prevention of acute organ rejection in patients receiving renal transplantation.

becaplermin (be-kap-lerm-in)
Regranex
Classification
Therapeutic: wound/ulcer/decubiti healing agent
Pharmacologic: platelet-derived growth factors

Indications
Lower extremity diabetic neuropathic ulcers extending to SUBQ tissue or beyond and having adequate blood supply.

Action
Promotes chemotaxis of cells involved in wound repair and enhances formation of granulation tissue. **Therapeutic Effects:** Improved healing.

Pharmacokinetics
Absorption: Minimal absorption (<3%).
Distribution: Action is primarily local.
Metabolism and Excretion: Unknown.
Half-life: Unknown.

TIME/ACTION PROFILE (improvement in ulcer healing)

ROUTE	ONSET	PEAK	DURATION
Topical	within 10 wk	unknown	unknown

Contraindications/Precautions
Contraindicated in: Known hypersensitivity to becaplermin or parabens; Known neoplasm at site of application; Wounds that close by primary intention.
Use Cautiously in: Known malignancy; OB: Safety not established in pregnancy; Lactation: Safety not established in breastfeeding; Pedi: Children <16 yr (safety and effectiveness not established).

Adverse Reactions/Side Effects
Derm: erythematous rash at application site. **Misc:** MALIGNANCY.

Interactions
Drug-Drug: None reported.

Route/Dosage
Topical (Adults and Children ≥16 yr): Length of gel *in inches* from 15- or 7.5-g tube = length × width of ulcer area × 0.6; from the 2-g tube = length × width of ulcer area × 1.3. Length of gel *in centimeters* from 15- or 7.5-g tube = length × width of ulcer area ÷ 4; from the 2-g tube = length × width of ulcer area ÷ 2; for 12 hr each day.

Availability
Gel: 0.01%.

NURSING IMPLICATIONS
Assessment
- Assess size, color, drainage, and skin surrounding wound at weekly or biweekly intervals. Amount of gel to be applied is recalculated based on wound size.

Implementation
- **Topical:** Calculated amount is applied as a thin layer (1/16 in. thick) and covered with a moist saline dressing for 12 hr; dressing is removed, ulcer rinsed and

redressed with moist dressing without becaplermin for rest of day. Process is repeated daily.

- Store gel in refrigerator; do not freeze. Do not use beyond expiration date on crimped end of tube.

Patient/Family Teaching

- Instruct patient on proper technique for application. Wash hands before applying gel and use cotton swab or tongue depressor to aid in application. Tip of tube should not come in contact with ulcer or any other surface; recap tightly after each use. Squeeze calculated amount of gel onto a clean, firm, nonabsorbable surface (wax paper). Spread gel with swab or tongue depressor over the ulcer surface in an even layer to the thickness of a dime. Cover with a saline-moistened gauze dressing.
- Do not apply more than calculated amount; has not been shown to be beneficial. If a dose is missed, apply as soon as remembered. If not remembered until next day, skip dose and return to regular dosing schedule. Do not double doses.
- After 12 hr, rinse ulcer gently with saline or water to remove residual gel and cover with saline-moistened gauze.
- Emphasize the importance of strict wound care and non–weight-bearing program.
- Rep: Advise females of reproductive potential to notify health care professional if pregnancy is planned or suspected or if breastfeeding.

Evaluation/Desired Outcomes

- Improved healing of ulcers. If the ulcer does not decrease in size by 30% within 10 wk or if complete healing has not occurred within 20 wk, continuation of therapy should be reassessed.

---

beclomethasone, See CORTICOSTEROIDS (INHALATION).

---

beclomethasone, See CORTICOSTEROIDS (NASAL).

---

belatacept (be-lat-a-sept)
Nulojix
Classification
Therapeutic: immunosuppressants
Pharmacologic: fusion proteins

Indications

Prevention of organ rejection following kidney transplant in adult patients (in combination with basiliximab induction, mycophenolate, and corticosteroids).

Action

Binds to CD80 and CD86 sites, thereby blocking T-cell costimulation; result is inhibition of T-lymphocyte proliferation and cytokine production. **Therapeutic Effects:** Prolonged graft survival with decreased production of antidonor antibodies following kidney transplantation.

Pharmacokinetics

Absorption: IV administration results in complete bioavailability.
Distribution: Not widely distributed to tissues.
Metabolism and Excretion: Unknown.
Half-life: 9.8 days.

TIME/ACTION PROFILE

ROUTE	ONSET	PEAK	DURATION
IV	unknown	end of infusion	up to 4 wk

Contraindications/Precautions

Contraindicated in: Epstein-Barr virus (EBV) seronegativity or unknown EBV serostatus; Liver transplantation; Lactation: Lactation.

Use Cautiously in: Cytomegalovirus (CMV) infection/T-cell depleting therapy (↑ risk of post-transplant lymphoproliferative disorder [PTLD]), CMV prophylaxis recommended for 3 mo following transplant; Change in body weight >10% (dose adjustment recommended); Unknown tuberculosis status (latent infection should be treated prior to use); Evidence of polyoma virus-associated nephropathy, ↓ immunosuppression may be necessary; Patients being converted from a calcineurin inhibitor based maintenance regimen (↑ risk of rejection) (conversion is only recommended if patient is intolerant to calcineurin inhibitor); OB: Use during pregnancy only if potential maternal benefit justifies potential fetal risk; Pedi: Safety and effectiveness not established in children.

Adverse Reactions/Side Effects

CV: hypertension, peripheral edema. **Endo:** diabetes mellitus. **F and E:** hyperkalemia, hypokalemia. **GI:** constipation, diarrhea, nausea, vomiting. **GU:** proteinuria. **Hemat:** anemia, leukopenia. **Neuro:** headache, PROGRESSIVE MULTIFOCAL LEUKOENCEPHALOPATHY (PML). **Resp:** cough. **Misc:** fever, graft dysfunction, INFECTION, infusion reactions, MALIGNANCY, PTLD.

Interactions

Drug-Drug: May ↓ antibody response to and ↑ risk of adverse reactions from **live virus vaccines**; avoid use during treatment. May ↑ levels and risk of toxicity of **mycophenolate mofetil**; ↓ dose of mycophenolate mofetil. Concurrent use with **antithymocyte globulin** may ↑ risk of venous thrombosis of renal allograft; separate administration by 12 hr.

Route/Dosage

Prescribed dose must be evenly divisible by 12.5 to ensure accurate preparation.
IV (Adults): *Initial phase:* 10 mg/kg on day of transplant/prior to implantation, day 5 (96 hr after day 1 dose), and at end of wk 2, 4, 8, and 12 following transplantation; *Maintenance phase:* 10 mg/kg at end of wk 16 and then every 4 wk (±3 days).

Availability

Lyophilized powder for injection: 250 mg/vial.

NURSING IMPLICATIONS

Assessment

- Assess for symptoms of organ rejection throughout therapy.
- Assess for signs of PML (hemiparesis, apathy, confusion, cognitive deficiencies, and ataxia) periodically during therapy.
- Monitor for signs and symptoms of infection (fever, dyspnea) periodically during therapy.
- Assess for signs and symptoms of PTLD (changes in mood or usual behavior, confusion, problems thinking, loss of memory, changes in walking or talking, decreased strength or weakness on one side of the body, changes in vision) during and for at least 36 mo post-transplant.
- Monitor for infusion reactions (hypotension, hypertension) during therapy.

Lab Test Considerations

- Determine EBV status before starting therapy. Only administer to patients who are EBV seropositive. May cause hyperkalemia, hypokalemia, hypophosphatemia, hyperglycemia, hypocalcemia, hypercholesterolemia, hypomagnesemia, and hyperuricemia.

Implementation

- Premedication is not required.
- Cortisone doses should be consistent with clinical trials experience. Cortisone doses were tapered to between 10–20 mg/day by first 6 wk after transplant, then remained at 10 mg (5–10 mg) per day for first 6 mo after transplant.
- Treat patient for latent tuberculosis prior to therapy.
- Prophylaxis for *Pneumocystis jiroveci* infection is recommended after transplant.

IV Administration

- **Intermittent Infusion:** Calculate number of vials required for total infusion dose. *Reconstitution:* Reconstitute contents of each vial with 10.5 mL of sterile water for injection, 0.9% NaCl or D5W using the silicone-free disposable syringe provided and an 18–21 gauge needle for a concentration of 25 mg/mL. Direct stream of diluent to wall of vial. Rotate and invert vial gently; do not shake to avoid foaming. Solution is clear to slightly opalescent and colorless to pale yellow; do not use if opaque particles, discoloration, or other particles are present. Calculate total volume needed for infusion dose. *Dilution:* Dilute further with 0.9% NaCl or D5W if reconstituted with sterile water for injection, 0.9% NaCl if reconstituted with 0.9% NaCl, or with D5W if reconstituted with D5W. *Concentration:* 2 mg/mL. Withdraw amount of diluent from infusion container equal to volume of infusion dose. Using same *silicone-free disposable syringe* used for

reconstitution, withdraw required amount of belatacept solution from vial, inject into infusion container, and rotate gently to mix. Typical infusion volume is 100 mL, but may range from 50–250 mL. Transfer from vial to infusion container immediately; infusion must be completed within 24 hr of reconstitution. May be refrigerated and protected from light for 24 hr. Do not administer solutions that are discolored or contain particulate matter. Discard unused solution in vials. *Rate:* Infuse over 30 min using a nonpyrogenic, low-protein-binding filter with 0.2–1.2 micron pore size.

- **Y-Site Incompatibility:** Do not mix or infuse in same line with other agents.

Patient/Family Teaching

- Explain purpose of belatacept to patient.
- Reinforce the need for lifelong therapy to prevent transplant rejection. Review symptoms of rejection for the transplanted organ, and stress need to notify health care professional immediately if signs of rejection or infection occur.
- Advise patient to avoid contact with persons with contagious diseases.
- Inform patient of the increased risk of skin cancer and other malignancies. Advise patient to use sunscreen with a high protection factor and wear protective clothing to decrease risk of skin cancer.
- Advise patient to notify health care professional of all Rx or OTC medications, vitamins, or herbal products being taken and to consult with health care professional before taking other medications.
- Advise patient to notify health care professional immediately if signs or symptoms of infection, PTLD, or PML occur.
- Advise patients to avoid live vaccines during therapy.
- Rep: Advise female patients to notify health care professional if pregnancy is planned or suspected or if breastfeeding. Encourage patients who become pregnant or whose partners have received belatacept to register with the Transplant Pregnancy Registry International by calling 1-877-955-6877.
- Emphasize the importance of routine follow-up laboratory tests.

Evaluation/Desired Outcomes

- Prevention of rejection of transplanted kidneys.

belimumab (be-li-moo-mab)
Benlysta
Classification
Therapeutic: immunosuppressants
Pharmacologic: monoclonal antibodies

Indications

Active autoantibody-positive systemic lupus erythematosus in patients currently receiving standard therapy. Active lupus nephritis in patients currently receiving standard therapy.

Action

A monoclonal antibody produced by recombinant DNA technique that specifically binds to B-lymphocyte stimulator protein (BLyS), thereby inactivating it. **Therapeutic Effects:** ↓ survival of B cells, including autoreactive ones and ↓ differentiation into immunoglobulin-producing plasma cells. Result is ↓ disease activity with lessened damage/improvement in mucocutaneous, musculoskeletal, and immunologic manifestations of SLE. Improvement in or stabilization of renal function in lupus nephritis.

Pharmacokinetics

Absorption: 74% absorbed after SUBQ administration; IV administration results in complete bioavailability.
Distribution: Unknown.
Metabolism and Excretion: Unknown.
Half-life: 19.4 days.

TIME/ACTION PROFILE (reduction in activated B cells)

ROUTE	ONSET	PEAK	DURATION
IV or SUBQ	8 wk	unknown	52 wk†

†With continuous treatment.

Contraindications/Precautions

Contraindicated in: Hypersensitivity; Concurrent use of live vaccines; Receiving therapy for chronic infection.
Use Cautiously in: Concurrent use of other biologicals or rituximab; Infections (consider temporary withdrawal for acute infections, treat aggressively); Previous history of depression or suicidal ideation (may worsen); OB: Use during pregnancy only if potential maternal benefit justifies potential fetal risk; Lactation: Safety not established in breastfeeding; Rep: Women of reproductive potential; Pedi: Children <5 yr (safety and effectiveness not established); Geri: Older adults may be more sensitive to drug effects.

Adverse Reactions/Side Effects

Derm: rash. **GI:** diarrhea, nausea. **GU:** cystitis. **Hemat:** leukopenia. **MS:** extremity pain, myalgia. **Neuro:** depression, insomnia, migraine, anxiety, fatigue, PROGRESSIVE MULTIFOCAL LEUKOENCEPHALOPATHY (PML), SUICIDAL IDEATION/BEHAVIOR. **Misc:** fever, infusion reactions, ANAPHYLAXIS, facial edema, INFECTION.

Interactions

Drug-Drug: ↑ risk of adverse reactions and ↓ immune response to **live vaccines**; should not be given concurrently. ↑ risk of serious infections and post-injection systemic reactions when used with **rituximab**.

Route/Dosage

Systemic Lupus Erythematosus

IV (Adults and Children ≥5 yr): 10 mg/kg every 2 wk for 3 doses, then 10 mg/kg every 4 wk.

SUBQ (Adults): 200 mg once weekly; if transitioning from IV therapy, give first SUBQ dose 1–4 wk after last IV dose.

Lupus Nephritis

IV (Adults and Children ≥5 yr): 10 mg/kg every 2 wk for 3 doses, then 10 mg/kg every 4 wk.
SUBQ (Adults): 400 mg (given as two, 200–mg injections) once weekly for 4 wk, then 200 mg once weekly. May transition from IV therapy after completing first two IV doses, give first SUBQ dose 1–2 wk after last IV dose.

Availability

Lyophilized powder for injection: 120 mg/vial, 400 mg/vial. **Solution for injection (prefilled syringes and autoinjectors):** 200 mg/mL.

NURSING IMPLICATIONS

Assessment

- Monitor patient for signs of anaphylaxis (hypotension, angioedema, urticaria, rash, pruritus, wheezing, dyspnea, facial edema) during and following injection. Medications (antihistamines, corticosteroids, epinephrine) and equipment should be readily available in the event of a severe reaction. Discontinue belimumab immediately if anaphylaxis or other severe allergic reaction occurs.
- Monitor for infusion reactions (headache, nausea, skin reactions, bradycardia, myalgia, rash, urticaria, hypotension). Infusion rate may be slowed or interrupted if an infusion reaction occurs.
- Assess for signs of infection (fever, dyspnea, flu-like symptoms, frequent or painful urination, redness or swelling at the site of a wound), including tuberculosis, prior to injection. Belimumab is contraindicated in patients with active infection. New infections should be monitored closely; most common are upper respiratory tract infections, bronchitis, and urinary tract infections. Signs and symptoms of inflammation may be lessened due to suppression from belimumab. Infections may be fatal, especially in patients taking immunosuppressive therapy. If patient develops a serious infection, consider discontinuing belimumab until infection is controlled.
- Assess mental status and mood changes. Inform health care professional if patient demonstrates significant ↑ in depressed mood, anxiety, nervousness, or insomnia.
- Assess for signs of progressive multifocal leukoencephalopathy (hemiparesis, apathy, confusion, cognitive deficiencies, and ataxia) periodically during therapy.

Implementation

- Consider premedication for prophylaxis against infusion reactions and hypersensitivity reactions.
- **SUBQ:** Allow autoinjector or prefilled syringe to sit at room temperature for 30 min prior to injection; do not use other methods of warming. Solution is

clear to opalescent and colorless to pale yellow. Do not inject solutions that are discolored or contain particulate matter. Administer first injection under supervision of health care professional into abdomen or thigh. Rotate injection sites each wk. Avoid areas of tenderness, bruising, redness, or hardness. Refrigerate autoinjectors and prefilled syringes prior to use; do not freeze or shake. Avoid exposure to heat. May be stored at room temperature if protected from sunlight for up to 12 hrs.

IV Administration

- **Intermittent Infusion:** Remove belimumab from refrigerator and allow to stand 10–15 min to reach room temperature. *Reconstitution:* Using a 21–25 gauge needle, reconstitute 120 mg vial with 1.5 mL and 400 mg vial with 4.8 mL of sterile water for injection by directing stream toward side of vial to minimize foaming. Swirl gently for 60 sec. Allow vial to sit at room temperature during reconstitution, swirling gently for 60 sec every 5 min until powder is dissolved. Do not shake. Reconstitution usually takes 10–15 min, but may take up to 30 min. Protect from sunlight. Solution is opalescent and colorless to pale yellow and without particles. Small bubbles are expected and acceptable. *Concentration:* 80 mg/mL. *Dilution:* 0.9% NaCl, 0.45% NaCl or LR. Remove volume of patient's dose from a 250 mL infusion bag and discard. Replace with required amount of reconstituted solution. Gently invert bag to mix. Do not administer solutions that are discolored or contain particulate matter. Discard unused solution in vial. If not used immediately, refrigerate or store at room temperature and protect from light. Total time from reconstitution to completion of infusion should not exceed 8 hrs. *Rate:* Infuse over 1 hr; may slow or interrupt rate if patient develops an infusion reaction.
- **Y-Site Incompatibility:** Do not administer with dextrose solutions or other solutions or medications.

Patient/Family Teaching

- Instruct patient in correct technique for SUBQ injection, care, and disposal of equipment. Inject on the same day each wk. Inject missed doses as soon as remembered, then resume on usual day or start a new weekly schedule from the day missed dose was administered. Do not inject 2 doses on same day. Advise patient to read *Medication Guide* prior to each treatment session in case of changes.
- Caution patient to notify health care professional immediately if signs of infection (fever, sweating, chills, muscle aches, cough, shortness of breath, blood in phlegm, weight loss, warm, red or painful skin or sores, diarrhea or stomach pain, burning on urination, urinary frequency, feeling tired), progressive multifocal leukoencephalopathy, severe rash, swollen face, or difficulty breathing occurs while taking.

- Advise patient, family, and caregivers to look for depression and suicidality, especially during early therapy or dose changes. Notify health care professional immediately if thoughts about suicide or dying, attempts to commit suicide; new or worse depression or anxiety; agitation or restlessness; panic attacks; insomnia; new or worse irritability; aggressiveness; acting on dangerous impulses, mania, or other changes in mood or behavior, or if symptoms of serotonin syndrome occur.
- Caution patient to avoid receiving live vaccines for 30 days before and during belimumab therapy.
- Instruct patient to notify health care professional of all Rx or OTC medications, vitamins, or herbal products being taken and consult health care professional before taking any new medications.
- Rep: Advise females of reproductive potential to use effective contraception during and for at least 4 mo after final treatment and to notify health care professional if breastfeeding. Encourage pregnant patients to enroll in pregnancy registry by calling 1-877-311-8972 or visiting https://mothertobaby.org/ongoing-study/benlysta-belimumab/.

Evaluation/Desired Outcomes

- Improvement in mucocutaneous, musculoskeletal, and immunologic disease activity in patients with SLE.
- Improvement in or stabilization of renal function in lupus nephritis.

---

bempedoic acid
(bem-pe-doe-ik as-id)
Nexletol
Classification
Therapeutic: lipid-lowering agents
Pharmacologic: adenosine triphosphate citrate lyase inhibitors

Indications

Heterozygous familial hypercholesterolemia or established atherosclerotic cardiovascular disease in patients who require additional lowering of low-density lipoprotein cholesterol (LDL-C) levels (as adjunct to diet and maximally tolerated statin therapy).

Action

Inhibits adenosine triphosphate-citrate lyase, which inhibits cholesterol synthesis in the liver and subsequently lowers LDL-C. **Therapeutic Effects:** Reduction in LDL-C levels.

Pharmacokinetics

Absorption: Unknown.
Distribution: Some distribution to extravascular tissues.
Metabolism and Excretion: Metabolized in liver to active metabolite (ESP15228); both parent drug and

ESP15228 are also metabolized via glucuronidation to inactive metabolites. 70% excreted in urine and 30% excreted in feces primarily as metabolites (<5% excreted as unchanged drug in urine and feces).
Half-life: 21 hr.

TIME/ACTION PROFILE (plasma concentrations)

ROUTE	ONSET	PEAK	DURATION
PO	unknown	3.5 hr	24 hr

Contraindications/Precautions

Contraindicated in: OB: Pregnancy (may cause fetal harm); Lactation: Lactation.
Use Cautiously in: History of gout; Concurrent use of corticosteroids or fluoroquinolones, renal failure, or previous tendon disorders (↑ risk of tendon rupture/injury); Severe renal impairment or end-stage renal disease; Severe hepatic impairment; Pedi: Safety and effectiveness in children not established; Geri: ↑ risk of tendon rupture/injury in patients >60 yr.

Adverse Reactions/Side Effects

CV: atrial fibrillation. **GI:** ↑ liver enzymes, abdominal pain. **GU:** ↑ blood urea nitrogen, ↑ serum creatinine, benign prostatic hyperplasia. **Hemat:** anemia. **Metab:** hyperuricemia, gout. **MS:** ↑ creatine kinase, back pain, muscle spasm, tendon rupture/injury. **Resp:** upper respiratory tract infection.

Interactions

Drug-Drug: Concurrent therapy with **corticosteroids** or **fluoroquinolones** may ↑ the risk of tendon rupture/injury. May ↑ levels of and risk of myopathy with **pravastatin** and **simvastatin**; do not exceed 40 mg/day of pravastatin or 20 mg/day of simvastatin.

Route/Dosage

PO (Adults): 180 mg once daily.

Availability

Tablets: 180 mg.

NURSING IMPLICATIONS

Assessment

- Obtain a diet history, especially with regard to fat consumption.
- Monitor for signs and symptoms of hyperuricemia (gout) periodically during therapy. May occur within 4 wk of therapy. Initiate treatment with urate-lowering drugs as appropriate.
- Monitor for signs and symptoms of tendon rupture (joint pain, swelling, inflammation) periodically during therapy. May occur within days to months of starting therapy and more frequently in patients >60 years of age, taking corticosteroid or fluoroquinolones, with renal failure, and with previous tendon disorders. Consider discontinuing therapy if symptoms occur and discontinue therapy if tendon rupture occurs.

Lab Test Considerations

- Evaluate serum cholesterol levels before initiating, after 8–12 wk of therapy, and periodically thereafter.
- Monitor serum uric acid levels periodically if symptoms of hyperuricemia occur.
- May cause ↑ BUN and serum creatinine.
- May cause ↓ hemoglobin and leukocytes and ↑ platelet count.
- May cause ↑ AST, ALT, and creatine kinase.

Implementation

- **PO:** Administer once daily without regard to food.

Patient/Family Teaching

- Instruct patient to take medication as directed. Advise patient to read Patient Information before starting and with each Rx refill in case of changes.
- Advise patient that this medication should be used in conjunction with diet restrictions (fat, cholesterol, carbohydrates, alcohol), exercise, and cessation of smoking.
- Advise patient to notify health care professional if signs and symptoms of hyperuricemia (severe foot pain especially in the toe joint, tender joints, warm joints, joint redness, swelling) occur.
- Advise patient to rest at the first sign of tendinitis (pain, swelling, tears, inflammation of tendons including arm, shoulder, back of the ankle) or tendon rupture (hear or feel a snap or pop in a tendon area, bruising right after an injury in a tendon area, unable to move affected area or put weight on affected area) and stop medication and contact health care professional if tendinitis or tendon rupture symptoms occur.
- Instruct patient to notify health care professional of all Rx or OTC medications, vitamins, or herbal products being taken and consult health care professional before taking any new medications.
- Rep: Advise females of reproductive potential to notify health care professional if pregnancy is planned or suspected or if breastfeeding. Bempedoic acid should be discontinued during pregnancy and lactation.

Evaluation/Desired Outcomes

- Reduction in LDL-C levels. Evaluate in 8–12 wk.

---

benazepril, See ANGIOTENSIN-CONVERTING ENZYME (ACE) INHIBITORS.

---

benralizumab
(ben-ra-**liz**-ue-mab)
Fasenra
Classification
Therapeutic: anti-asthmatics
Pharmacologic: monoclonal antibodies, interleukin antagonists

Indications

Add-on maintenance treatment of severe asthma that is of an eosinophilic phenotype.

Action

Interleukin-5 (IL-5) antagonist that inhibits binding of IL-5 to the surface of the eosinophil, which reduces the production and survival of eosinophils. **Therapeutic Effects:** Decreased incidence of asthma exacerbations. Reduction in use of maintenance oral corticosteroid therapy.

Pharmacokinetics

Absorption: 58% absorbed following SUBQ administration.

Distribution: Minimally distributed to tissues.

Metabolism and Excretion: Degraded by proteolytic enzymes located throughout the body.

Half-life: 15 days.

TIME/ACTION PROFILE (plasma concentrations)

ROUTE	ONSET	PEAK	DURATION
SUBQ	unknown	unknown	unknown

Contraindications/Precautions

Contraindicated in: Hypersensitivity; Acute bronchospasm or status asthmaticus.

Use Cautiously in: Pre-existing helminth infections; OB: Use during pregnancy only if potential maternal benefit outweighs potential fetal risk; Lactation: Safety not established in breastfeeding; Pedi: Children <12 yr (safety and effectiveness not established).

Adverse Reactions/Side Effects

EENT: pharyngitis. **Neuro:** headache. **Misc:** fever, HYPERSENSITIVITY REACTIONS (including anaphylaxis, angioedema, urticaria, and rash), injection site reactions.

Interactions

Drug-Drug: None reported.

Route/Dosage

SUBQ (Adults and Children ≥12 yr): 30 mg every 4 wk for first three doses, then 30 mg every 8 wk thereafter.

Availability

Solution for injection (prefilled syringes or autoinjectors): 30 mg/mL.

NURSING IMPLICATIONS

Assessment

- Assess lung sounds, pulse, and BP periodically during therapy. Note amount, color, and character of sputum produced.
- Monitor for signs and symptoms of hypersensitivity reactions (rash, pruritus, hives, swelling of face and neck, dyspnea, fainting, dizziness, feeling light-headed) periodically during therapy; usually occur within hrs, but may occur days after injection. Discontinue medication if reaction occurs.

Implementation

- Treat pre-existing helminth infections before starting therapy.
- Prefilled syringe is for administration by a health care professional. Autoinjector can be administered by patient or caregiver with training.
- **SUBQ:** Administer every 4 wk for the 1st three doses and every 8 wk thereafter in upper arm, thigh or abdomen. Store in refrigerator; protect from light. Do not freeze or shake. Leave carton at room temperature for 30 min before administration. Solution is clear to opalescent, colorless to slightly yellow; may contain a few translucent or white to off-white particles. Do not administer if liquid is cloudy, discolored, or contains large particles or foreign particulate matter. Do not expel the air bubble prior to administration. Pinch skin to inject medication.

Patient/Family Teaching

- Instruct patient to have medication administered by health care professional as scheduled. Instruct patient in correct technique for injection, care, and disposal of equipment. Advise patient to read *Patient Information* before starting therapy and with each Rx refill in case of changes.
- Advise patient that benralizumab should not be used to treat an acute asthma attack. Patient should continue asthma medications, including corticosteroids, unless otherwise instructed by health care professional.
- Advise patient to stop using medication and notify health care professional immediately if signs and symptoms of hypersensitivity reactions occur.
- Instruct patient to notify health care professional of all Rx or OTC medications, vitamins, or herbal products being taken and to consult health care professional before taking any OTC medications or alcoholic beverages concurrently with this therapy. Caution patient also to avoid smoking and other respiratory irritants.
- Instruct patient whose systemic corticosteroids have been recently reduced or withdrawn to carry a warning card indicating the need for supplemental systemic corticosteroids in the event of stress or severe asthma attack unresponsive to bronchodilators.
- Advise patient to have helminth infections treated before starting benralizumab therapy.
- Rep: Advise females of reproductive potential to notify health care professional if pregnancy is planned or suspected or if breastfeeding. Encourage health care professional or pregnant patients to enroll in pregnancy registry to monitor outcomes of women exposed to benralizumab during pregnancy by calling 1-877-311-8972 or visiting mothertobaby.org/Fasenra.

Evaluation/Desired Outcomes
● Decreased incidence of asthma exacerbations. Reduction in use of maintenance oral corticosteroid therapy.

BEERS

benztropine (benz-troe-peen)
~~Cogentin~~
Classification
Therapeutic: antiparkinson agents
Pharmacologic: anticholinergics

Indications
Adjunctive treatment of all forms of Parkinson's disease, including drug-induced extrapyramidal effects and acute dystonic reactions.

Action
Blocks cholinergic activity in the CNS, which is partially responsible for the symptoms of Parkinson's disease. Restores the natural balance of neurotransmitters in the CNS. **Therapeutic Effects:** Reduction of rigidity and tremors.

Pharmacokinetics
Absorption: Well absorbed following PO and IM administration. IV administration results in complete bioavailability.
Distribution: Unknown.
Metabolism and Excretion: Unknown.
Half-life: Unknown.

TIME/ACTION PROFILE (antidyskinetic activity)

ROUTE	ONSET	PEAK	DURATION
PO	1–2 hr	several days	24 hr
IM, IV	within min	unknown	24 hr

Contraindications/Precautions
Contraindicated in: Hypersensitivity; Angle-closure glaucoma; Tardive dyskinesia; Pedi: Children <3 yr.
Use Cautiously in: Prostatic hyperplasia; Seizure disorders; Cardiac arrhythmias; OB, Lactation: Safety not established; Geri: Appears on Beers list. Not recommended for prevention or treatment of extrapyramidal symptoms due to antipsychotics in older adults; more effective agents available for treatment of Parkinson's disease. Avoid use of oral formulation in older adults.

Adverse Reactions/Side Effects
CV: arrhythmias, hypotension, palpitations, tachycardia. **Derm:** ↓ sweating. **EENT:** blurred vision, dry eyes, mydriasis. **GI:** constipation, dry mouth, ileus, nausea. **GU:** hesitancy, urinary retention. **Neuro:** confusion, depression, dizziness, hallucinations, headache, sedation, weakness.

Interactions
Drug-Drug: Additive anticholinergic effects with **drugs sharing anticholinergic properties**, such as **antihistamines, phenothiazines, quinidine, disopyramide**, and **tricyclic antidepressants**. Counteracts the cholinergic effects of **bethanechol**. Antacids and **antidiarrheals** may ↓ absorption.
Drug-Natural Products: ↑ anticholinergic effect with **angel's trumpet, jimson weed**, and **scopolia**.

Route/Dosage
Parkinsonism
PO (Adults): 1–2 mg/day in 1–2 divided doses (range 0.5–6 mg/day).

Acute Dystonic Reactions
IM, IV (Adults): 1–2 mg, then 1–2 mg PO twice daily.

Drug-Induced Extrapyramidal Reactions
PO, IM, IV (Adults): 1–4 mg given once or twice daily (1–2 mg 2–3 times daily may also be used PO).

Availability (generic available)
Tablets: 0.5 mg, 1 mg, 2 mg. Solution for injection: 1 mg/mL.

NURSING IMPLICATIONS
Assessment
● Assess parkinsonian and extrapyramidal symptoms (restlessness or desire to keep moving, rigidity, tremors, pill rolling, masklike face, shuffling gait, muscle spasms, twisting motions, difficulty speaking or swallowing, loss of balance control) before and during therapy.
● Assess bowel function daily. Monitor for constipation, abdominal pain, distention, or absence of bowel sounds.
● Monitor intake and output ratios and assess patient for urinary retention (dysuria, distended abdomen, infrequent voiding of small amounts, overflow incontinence).
● Patients with mental illness are at risk of developing exaggerated symptoms of their disorder during early therapy with benztropine. Hold benztropine and notify health care professional if significant behavioral changes occur.
● **IM/IV:** Monitor pulse and BP closely and maintain bedrest for 1 hr after administration. Advise patients to change positions slowly to minimize orthostatic hypotension.

Implementation
● **PO:** Administer with food or immediately after meals to minimize gastric irritation. May be crushed and administered with food if patient has difficulty swallowing.
● **IM:** Parenteral route is used only for dystonic reactions.

IV Administration
● **IV Push:** IV route is rarely used because onset is same as with IM route. *Rate:* Administer at a rate of 1 mg over 1 min.

- **Y-Site Compatibility:** amikacin, aminophylline, ascorbic acid, atracurium, atropine, azathioprine, aztreonam, bumetanide, buprenorphine, butorphanol, calcium chloride, calcium gluconate, cefazolin, cefotaxime, cefotetan, cefoxitin, ceftazidime, ceftriaxone, cefuroxime, chlorpromazine, clindamycin, cyanocobalamin, cyclosporine, dexamethasone, digoxin, diphenhydramine, dobutamine, dopamine, doxycycline, enalaprilat, ephedrine, epinephrine, epoetin alfa, erythromycin, esmolol, famotidine, fentanyl, fluconazole, folic acid, gentamicin, glycopyrrolate, heparin, hydrocortisone, imipenem/cilastatin, insulin, regular, isoproterenol, ketorolac, labetalol, LR, lidocaine, magnesium sulfate, mannitol, meperidine, meropenem, methylprednisolone, metoclopramide, metoprolol, midazolam, morphine, multivitamins, nafcillin, nalbuphine, naloxone, nitroglycerin, nitroprusside, norepinephrine, ondansetron, oxacillin, oxytocin, papaverine, penicillin G, pentamidine, phenobarbital, phentolamine, phenylephrine, phytonadione, potassium chloride, procainamide, prochlorperazine, promethazine, propranolol, protamine, pyridoxine, sodium bicarbonate, succinylcholine, sufentanil, tacrolimus, theophylline, thiamine, tobramycin, vancomycin, vasopressin, verapamil.
- **Y-Site Incompatibility:** chloramphenicol, dantrolene, diazepam, furosemide, ganciclovir, indomethacin, pentobarbital, phenytoin, sulfamethoxazole/trimethoprim.

Patient/Family Teaching

- Encourage patient to take benztropine as directed. Take missed doses as soon as possible, up to 2 hr before the next dose. Taper gradually when discontinuing or a withdrawal reaction may occur (anxiety, tachycardia, insomnia, return of parkinsonian or extrapyramidal symptoms).
- May cause drowsiness or dizziness. Advise patient to avoid driving or other activities that require alertness until response to the drug is known.
- Instruct patient that frequent rinsing of mouth, good oral hygiene, and sugarless gum or candy may decrease dry mouth. Patient should notify health care professional if dryness persists (saliva substitutes may be used). Also, notify the dentist if dryness interferes with use of dentures.
- Caution patient to change positions slowly to minimize orthostatic hypotension.
- Instruct patient to notify health care professional if difficulty with urination, constipation, abdominal discomfort, rapid or pounding heartbeat, confusion, eye pain, or rash occurs.
- Advise patient to confer with health care professional before taking OTC medications, especially cold remedies, or drinking alcoholic beverages.
- Caution patient that this medication decreases perspiration. Overheating may occur during hot

weather. Patient should notify health care professional if unable to remain indoors in an air-conditioned environment during hot weather.
- Advise patient to avoid taking antacids or antidiarrheals within 1–2 hr of this medication.
- Emphasize the importance of routine follow-up exams.
- Rep: Advise females of reproductive potential to notify health care professional if pregnancy is planned or suspected or if breastfeeding.

Evaluation/Desired Outcomes

- Decrease in tremors and rigidity and an improvement in gait and balance. Therapeutic effects are usually seen 2–3 days after the initiation of therapy.

betamethasone, See CORTICOSTEROIDS (SYSTEMIC).

betamethasone, See CORTICOSTEROIDS (TOPICAL/LOCAL).

bevacizumab
(be-va-**siz**-uh-mab)
✤ Abevmy, Alymsys, Avastin,
✤ Aybintio, ✤ Bambevi, Mvasi, Vegzelma, Zirabev
Classification
Therapeutic: antineoplastics
Pharmacologic: monoclonal antibodies

Indications
Alymsys, Avastin, Mvasi, Vegzelma, and Zirabev: Treatment of the following conditions: First- or second-line treatment of metastatic colorectal cancer (in combination with IV 5–fluorouracil-based chemotherapy), Second-line treatment of metastatic colorectal cancer in patients who have progressed on a first-line regimen containing bevacizumab (in combination with fluoropyrimidine-irinotecan- or fluoropyrimidine-oxaliplatin-based chemotherapy), First-line treatment of patients with unresectable, locally advanced, recurrent or metastatic non-squamous, non-small cell lung cancer (in combination with carboplatin and paclitaxel), Recurrent glioblastoma (as monotherapy), Metastatic renal cell carcinoma (in combination with interferon alfa), Persistent, recurrent, or metastatic cervical cancer (in combination with paclitaxel and cisplatin or paclitaxel and topotecan), Platinum-resistant recurrent epithelial ovarian, fallopian tube, or primary peritoneal cancer in patients who have received ≤2 previous chemotherapy regimens (in combination with paclitaxel, pegylated liposomal doxorubicin, or topotecan). **Avastin, Mvasi, Vegzelma, and Zirabev:** Treatment of the following

conditions: Platinum-sensitive recurrent epithelial ovarian, fallopian tube, or primary peritoneal cancer (in combination with carboplatin and paclitaxel or with carboplatin and gemcitabine), Stage III or IV epithelial ovarian, fallopian tube, or primary peritoneal cancer following initial surgical resection (in combination with carboplatin and paclitaxel followed by bevacizumab as a single agent). **Avastin only:** Unresectable or metastatic hepatocellular carcinoma (HCC) in patients who have not previously received systemic therapy (in combination with atezolizumab).

Action
A monoclonal antibody that binds to vascular endothelial growth factor (VEGF), preventing its attachment to binding sites on vascular endothelium, thereby inhibiting growth of new blood vessels (angiogenesis). **Therapeutic Effects:** Decreased metastatic disease progression and microvascular growth.

Pharmacokinetics
Absorption: IV administration results in complete bioavailability.
Distribution: Unknown.
Metabolism and Excretion: Unknown.
Half-life: 20 days (range 11–50 days).

TIME/ACTION PROFILE

ROUTE	ONSET	PEAK	DURATION
IV	rapid	end of infusion	14 days

Contraindications/Precautions
Contraindicated in: Hypersensitivity; Recent hemoptysis or other serious recent bleeding episode; First 28 days after major surgery; OB: Pregnancy; Lactation: Lactation.
Use Cautiously in: Cardiovascular disease; Diabetes (↑ risk of arterial thromboembolic events); Previous use of anthracyclines (↑ risk of HF); Esophageal varices (in patients with HCC); Rep: Women of reproductive potential; Pedi: Safety and effectiveness not established in children; cases of non-mandibular osteonecrosis reported; Geri: ↑ risk of serious adverse reactions including arterial thromboembolic events in older adults.

Adverse Reactions/Side Effects
CV: HF, hypertension, hypotension. **Derm:** NECROTIZING FASCIITIS. **GI:** GI PERFORATION. **GU:** ↑ serum creatinine, nephrotic syndrome, ovarian failure, proteinuria. **Hemat:** BLEEDING, THROMBOEMBOLIC EVENTS. **Neuro:** POSTERIOR REVERSIBLE ENCEPHALOPATHY SYNDROME (PRES). **Resp:** HEMOPTYSIS, nasal septum perforation, non-gastrointestinal fistulas. **Misc:** impaired wound healing, INFUSION REACTIONS, WOUND DEHISCENCE.

Interactions
Drug-Drug: ↑ blood levels of SN 38 (the active metabolite of **irinotecan**); significance is not known. ↑ risk of microangiopathic hemolytic anemia when used with **sunitinib**; concurrent use should be avoided.

Route/Dosage
Colorectal Cancer
IV (Adults): 5 mg/kg every 14 days when given with bolus-IFL chemotherapy regimen *or* 10 mg/kg every 14 days when given with FOLFOX4 chemotherapy regimen *or* 5 mg/kg every 14 days or 7.5 mg/kg every 21 days when given with a fluoropyrimidine-irinotecan or fluoropyrimidine-oxaliplatin based chemotherapy regimen.

Lung Cancer or Cervical Cancer
IV (Adults): 15 mg/kg every 3 wk.

Glioblastoma or Renal Cell Carcinoma
IV (Adults): 10 mg/kg every 2 wk.

Platinum-Resistant Epithelial Ovarian, Fallopian Tube, or Primary Peritoneal Cancer
IV (Adults): 10 mg/kg every 2 wk when given with paclitaxel, pegylated liposomal doxorubicin, or topotecan (weekly) *or* 15 mg/kg every 3 wk when given with topotecan (every 3 wk).

Platinum-Sensitive Epithelial Ovarian, Fallopian Tube, or Primary Peritoneal Cancer
IV (Adults): 15 mg/kg every 3 wk when given with carboplatin and paclitaxel for 6–8 cycles, followed by 15 mg/kg every 3 wk as a single agent *or* 15 mg/kg every 3 wk when given with carboplatin and gemcitabine for 6–10 cycles, followed by 15 mg/kg every 3 wk as a single agent.

Stage III or IV Epithelial Ovarian, Fallopian Tube, or Primary Peritoneal Cancer Following Surgical Resection
IV (Adults): 15 mg/kg every 3 wk when given with carboplatin and paclitaxel for up to 6 cycles, followed by 15 mg/kg every 3 wk as a single agent for a total up to 22 cycles or until disease progression, whichever occurs earlier.

Hepatocellular Carcinoma
IV (Adults): 15 mg/kg every 3 wk (administer after atezolizumab on same day) until disease progression or unacceptable toxicity.

Availability
Solution for injection: 25 mg/mL.

NURSING IMPLICATIONS
Assessment
- Assess for signs of GI perforation (abdominal pain associated with constipation, fever, nausea, and vomiting), fistula formation, and wound dehiscence during therapy; discontinue therapy if this occurs.
- Assess for signs of hemorrhage (epistaxis, hemoptysis, bleeding) and thromboembolic events (stroke, MI, deep vein thrombosis, pulmonary embolus) during therapy. If Grade 3 or 4 hemorrhage, severe arterial thromboembolism, or Grade 4 venous thromboembolism occurs, discontinue therapy. Hold bevacizumab for patients with recent history of hemoptysis of ≥1/2 teaspoon (2.5 mL) of red blood.

- Monitor BP every 2–3 wk during therapy. Temporarily suspend therapy during severe hypertension not controlled with medical management; permanently discontinue if hypertensive crisis or encephalopathy occurs.
- Assess for infusion reactions (stridor, wheezing, hypertension, oxygen desaturation, chest pain, headache, rigors, diaphoresis) during therapy. May require epinephrine, corticosteroids, IV antihistamines, bronchodilators and/or oxygen. If clinically significant reaction occurs, hold therapy until resolved and resume at decreased rate. Stop therapy if severe reaction occurs.
- Assess for signs of HF (dyspnea, peripheral edema, rales/crackles, jugular venous distension) during therapy. Discontinue therapy if symptoms occur.
- Monitor for signs of PRES (headache, seizure, lethargy, confusion, blindness). Hypertension may or may not be present. May occur within 16 hr to 1 yr of initiation of therapy. Treat hypertension if present and discontinue bevacizumab therapy. Symptoms usually resolve within days.
- Monitor wound healing. *If wound healing complications occur,* hold bevacizumab until adequate wound healing. *If necrotizing fasciitis occurs,* discontinue therapy.

Lab Test Considerations
- Monitor serial urinalysis for proteinuria during therapy. Patients with a 2+ or greater urine dipstick require further testing with a 24-hr urine collection. Hold therapy for ≥2 grams of proteinuria/24 hr and resume when proteinuria is <2 g/24 hr. Discontinue therapy in patients with nephrotic syndrome.
- May cause leukopenia, thrombocytopenia, hypokalemia, and hyperbilirubinemia.
- May cause ↑ serum creatinine.

Implementation
- Avoid administration for at least 28 days before elective surgery and at least 28 days following major surgery; surgical incision should be fully healed due to potential for impaired wound healing.

IV Administration
- **Intermittent Infusion: *Dilution:*** Dilute prescribed dose in 100 mL of 0.9% NaCl. Do not shake. Discard unused portions. Solution is colorless to pale yellow; do not administer solution that is discolored or contains particulate matter. Stable if refrigerated for up to 4 hr (*Alymsys*), 8 hr (*Avastin, Mvasi, Zirabev*), 24 hr (*Vegzelma*) or at room temperature up to 4 hr (*Vegzelma*). *Rate:* Administer initial dose over 90 min. If well tolerated, second infusion may be administered over 60 min. If well tolerated, all subsequent infusions may be administered over 30 min. **Do not administer as an IV push or bolus.**
- **Additive Incompatibility:** Do not mix or administer with dextrose solutions.

Patient/Family Teaching
- Inform patient of purpose of medication.
- Advise patient of the need for monitoring BP periodically during therapy; notify health care professional if BP is elevated.
- Advise patient to report any signs of bleeding, unusual bleeding, high fever, rigors, sudden onset of worsening neurological function, or persistent or severe abdominal pain, severe constipation, or vomiting immediately to health care professional.
- Inform patient of increased risk of wound healing complications and arterial thromboembolic events.
- Rep: Bevacizumab may cause fetal harm. Advise females of reproductive potential to use effective contraception and avoid breastfeeding during and for 6 mo after last dose. Inform female patient of reproductive potential of risk of ovarian failure that may lead to sterility following therapy.

Evaluation/Desired Outcomes
- Decreased metastatic disease progression and microvascular growth.

bezlotoxumab
(bez-loe-**tox**-ue-mab)
Zinplava
Classification
Therapeutic: antidiarrheals
Pharmacologic: monoclonal antibodies

Indications
Reduction in recurrence of *Clostridioides difficile* infection (CDI) in patients who are receiving antibacterial drug treatment of CDI and are at a high risk for CDI recurrence.

Action
Binds to *Clostridioides difficile* toxin B and neutralizes its effects. **Therapeutic Effects:** Reduced CDI recurrence.

Pharmacokinetics
Absorption: IV administration results in complete bioavailability.
Distribution: Minimally distributed to tissues.
Metabolism and Excretion: Eliminated primarily through catabolism.
Half-life: 19 days.

TIME/ACTION PROFILE (plasma concentrations)

ROUTE	ONSET	PEAK	DURATION
IV	unknown	unknown	unknown

Contraindications/Precautions
Contraindicated in: None.
Use Cautiously in: HF; OB: Safety not established in pregnancy; Lactation: Safety not established in breast-

feeding; Pedi: Children <1 yr (safety and effectiveness not established).

Adverse Reactions/Side Effects
CV: HF. GI: nausea. Neuro: headache. Misc: infusion reactions, fever.

Interactions
Drug-Drug: None reported.

Route/Dosage
IV (Adults and Children ≥1 yr): 10 mg/kg as a single dose.

Availability
Solution for injection: 25 mg/mL.

NURSING IMPLICATIONS

Assessment
● Assess for signs and symptoms of CDI prior to and following therapy.

Implementation
● Not for treatment of CDI; must be used with antibacterial agents.

IV Administration
● Intermittent Infusion: *Dilution:* Withdraw volume from bezlotoxumab vial based on patient weight and transfer to IV bag of 0.9% NaCl or D5W. Invert gently to mix; do not shake. Solution is clear to moderately opalescent, colorless to pale yellow; do not administer solutions that are discolored or contain particulate matter. *Concentration:* 1 mg/mL to 10 mg/mL. Store in refrigerator for up to 24 hrs or at room temperature protected from light for up to 16 hrs prior to preparation; do not freeze. *Rate:* Infuse over 60 min using a sterile, non-pyrogenic, low-protein binding 0.205 micron in-line or add-on filter. Do not administer as IV push or bolus. May be infused via central line or peripheral catheter.
● Y-Site Incompatibility: Do not administer other drugs simultaneously through same infusion line.

Patient/Family Teaching
● Inform patient that bezlotoxumab does not replace antibacterial treatment for their CDI infection. Antibacterial medications must be continued as directed.
● Rep: Advise females of reproductive potential to notify health care professional if pregnancy is planned or suspected or if breastfeeding.

Evaluation/Desired Outcomes
● Decrease in recurrence of CDI.

---

bicalutamide
(bye-ka-**loot**-a-mide)
Casodex
Classification
Therapeutic: antineoplastics
Pharmacologic: antiandrogens

Indications
Metastatic prostate cancer (in combination with a luteinizing hormone-releasing hormone (LHRH) analog).

Action
Antagonizes the effects of androgen at the cellular level.
Therapeutic Effects: Decreased spread of prostate cancer.

Pharmacokinetics
Absorption: Well absorbed following oral administration.
Distribution: Unknown.
Protein Binding: 96%.
Metabolism and Excretion: Mostly metabolized by the liver. Excreted in the urine and feces.
Half-life: 5.8 days.

TIME/ACTION PROFILE (plasma concentrations)

ROUTE	ONSET	PEAK	DURATION
PO	unknown	31.3 hr	unknown

Contraindications/Precautions
Contraindicated in: Hypersensitivity.
Use Cautiously in: Moderate to severe liver impairment; Rep: Men with female partners of reproductive potential.

Adverse Reactions/Side Effects
CV: chest pain, hypertension, peripheral edema. Derm: hot flashes, alopecia, photosensitivity, rash, sweating. Endo: breast pain, gynecomastia, hyperglycemia. GI: constipation, diarrhea, nausea, ↑ liver enzymes, abdominal pain, HEPATOTOXICITY, vomiting. GU: ↓ fertility, erectile dysfunction, hematuria, incontinence, nocturia, urinary tract infections. Hemat: anemia. Metab: ↓ weight. MS: pain. Neuro: weakness, dizziness, headache, insomnia, paresthesia. Resp: dyspnea. Misc: flu-like syndrome, infection.

Interactions
Drug-Drug: May ↑ the effect of warfarin.

Route/Dosage
PO (Adults): 50 mg once daily.

Availability (generic available)
Tablets: 50 mg.

NURSING IMPLICATIONS

Assessment
● Assess patient for adverse GI effects. Diarrhea is the most common cause of discontinuation of therapy.

Lab Test Considerations
● Monitor serum prostate-specific antigen periodically to determine response to therapy. If levels rise, assess patient for disease progression. May require periodic LHRH analog administration without bicalutamide.
● Monitor serum transaminases before, regularly during first 4 mo of therapy, and periodically during

therapy. May cause ↑ serum alkaline phosphatase, AST, ALT, and bilirubin concentrations. If patient is jaundiced or if transaminases ↑>2 times upper limit of normal, discontinue bicalutamide; levels usually return to normal after discontinuation.
- May cause ↑ BUN and serum creatinine, and ↓ hemoglobin and WBCs.
- May cause ↓ glucose tolerance in males taking LHRH agonists concurrently; monitor blood glucose in patients receiving bicalutamide in combination with LHRH analog.
- Monitor PT/INR closely in patients taking warfarin. May lead to severe bleeding.

Implementation
- Start treatment with bicalutamide at the same time as LHRH analog.
- **PO:** May be administered in the morning or evening, without regard to food.

Patient/Family Teaching
- Instruct patient to take bicalutamide along with the LHRH analog as directed at the same time each day. If a dose is missed, omit and take the next dose at regular time; do not double doses. Do not discontinue without consulting health care professional. Advise patient to read *Patient Information* prior to starting and with each Rx refill in case of changes.
- May cause dizziness. Caution patient to avoid driving or other activities requiring alertness until response to medication is known.
- Advise patient to stop taking bicalutamide and notify health care professional immediately of symptoms of liver dysfunction (nausea, vomiting, abdominal pain, fatigue, anorexia, "flu-like" symptoms, dark urine, jaundice, or right upper quadrant tenderness) or interstitial lung disease (trouble breathing with or without a cough or fever).
- Advise patient to notify health care professional of all Rx or OTC medications, vitamins, or herbal products being taken and to consult health care professional before taking any new medications.
- Instruct patient to report severe or persistent diarrhea.
- Discuss with patient the possibility of hair loss, breast enlargement and breast pain. Explore methods of coping.
- Advise patient to use sunscreen, avoid sunlight or sunlamps and tanning beds, and wear protective clothing to prevent photosensitivity reactions.
- Rep: Advise male patients with female partners of reproductive potential to use effective contraception during and for 130 days after last dose of therapy. Advise male patients that bicalutamide may impair fertility.
- Emphasize the importance of regular follow-up exams and blood tests to determine progress; monitor for side effects.

Evaluation/Desired Outcomes
- Decreased spread of prostate cancer.

bictegravir/emtricitabine/tenofovir alafenamide
(bik-**teg**-ra-vir/em-trye-**sye**-ta-been/ten-**of**-oh-veer al-a-**fen**-a-mide)
Biktarvy
Classification
Therapeutic: antiretrovirals
Pharmacologic: nucleoside reverse transcriptase inhibitors, integrase strand transfer inhibitors (INSTI)

Indications
Management of HIV infection in patients who have no antiretroviral treatment history or in those on a stable antiretroviral regimen who are virologically suppressed (with HIV-1 RNA <50 copies/mL) and no history of treatment failure or no known substitutions associated with resistance to the individual components of the medication (to replace their current antiretroviral regimen).

Action
Bictegravir: Inhibits HIV-1 integrase, which is required for viral replication; *Emtricitabine:* Phosphorylated intracellularly where it inhibits HIV reverse transcriptase, resulting in viral DNA chain termination; *Tenofovir:* Phosphorylated intracellularly where it inhibits HIV reverse transcriptase resulting in disruption of DNA synthesis. **Therapeutic Effects:** Slowed progression of HIV infection and decreased occurrence of sequelae.

Pharmacokinetics
Absorption: *Bictegravir:* Extent of absorption following oral administration unknown; *Emtricitabine:* Well absorbed (93%) following oral administration; *Tenofovir:* Tenofovir alafenamide is a prodrug, which is hydrolyzed into tenofovir, the active component; absorption enhanced by high-fat meals.

Distribution: *Bictegravir, emtricitabine, and tenofovir:* Unknown.

Protein Binding: *Bictegravir:* >99%.

Metabolism and Excretion: *Bictegravir:* Primarily metabolized by the CYP3A4 isoenzyme and UGT1A1 in the liver; 60% excreted in feces, 35% excreted in urine; *Emtricitabine:* Undergoes some metabolism, 70% excreted in urine, 14% excreted in feces; *Tenofovir:* Tenofovir is phosphorylated to tenofovir diphosphate (active metabolite); 32% excreted in feces, <1% excreted in urine.

Half-life: *Bictegravir:* 17.3 hr; *Emtricitabine:* 10.4 hr; *Tenofovir alafenamide:* 0.51 hr; *Tenofovir diphosphate:* 150–180 hr.

✱= Canadian drug name. ℨℨ = Genetic implication. ~~Strikethrough~~ = Discontinued. CAPITALS = life-threatening. <u>Underline</u> = most frequent.

TIME/ACTION PROFILE (plasma concentrations)

ROUTE	ONSET	PEAK	DURATION
bictegravir PO	unknown	2–4 hr	24 hr
emtricitabine PO	unknown	1.5–2 hr	24 hr
tenofovir PO	unknown	0.5–2 hr	24 hr

Contraindications/Precautions

Contraindicated in: Concurrent use of dofetilide or rifampin; Severe renal impairment (CCr 15–30 mL/min) or end-stage renal disease (CCr <15 mL/min) not receiving hemodialysis; Patients with no antiretroviral treatment history and end-stage renal disease (CCr <15 mL/min) who are receiving chronic hemodialysis; Severe hepatic impairment; Lactation: Breastfeeding not recommended in patients with HIV.

Use Cautiously in: Hepatitis B co-infection; History of suicidal ideation or depression (↑ risk of suicidal thoughts); Renal impairment or receiving nephrotoxic medications (↑ risk of renal impairment); OB: Use during pregnancy only if potential benefit justifies potential fetal risk; Pedi: Children weighing <14 kg (safety and effectiveness not established).

Adverse Reactions/Side Effects

GI: ↑ amylase, ↑ liver enzymes, diarrhea, LACTIC ACIDOSIS/HEPATOMEGALY WITH STEATOSIS, nausea. **GU:** ACUTE RENAL FAILURE/FANCONI SYNDROME. **Hemat:** neutropenia. **Metab:** hyperlipidemia. **MS:** ↑ creatine kinase. **Neuro:** abnormal dreams, dizziness, fatigue, headache, insomnia. **Misc:** ACUTE EXACERBATION OF HEPATITIS B, immune reconstitution syndrome.

Interactions

Drug-Drug: Bictegravir may ↑ **dofetilide** levels and the risk of torsades de pointes; concurrent use contraindicated. **Rifampin** may ↓ bictegravir levels and its effectiveness; concurrent use contraindicated. Medications that compete for active tubular secretion, including **acyclovir, cidofovir, ganciclovir, valacyclovir, valganciclovir,** or **aminoglycosides** may ↑ emtricitabine and tenofovir levels and toxicity. Nephrotoxic agents, including **NSAIDs** ↑ risk of nephrotoxicity with tenofovir; avoid concurrent use. **Carbamazepine, oxcarbazepine, phenobarbital, phenytoin, rifabutin,** and **rifapentine** may ↓ bictegravir and tenofovir levels and their effectiveness; avoid concurrent use. Administration with **antacids**, containing **magnesium** or **aluminum** ↓ absorption of bictegravir; take ≥2 hr before or ≥6 hr after magnesium- or aluminum-containing antacids. Administration with supplements or antacids containing **calcium** or **iron**↓ absorption of bictegravir; take at the same time as calcium or iron supplements with food (and not on an empty stomach). May ↑ **metformin** levels.

Drug-Natural Products: St. John's wort may ↓ bictegravir and tenofovir levels and their effectiveness; avoid concurrent use.

Route/Dosage

PO (Adults and Children ≥25 kg): 1 tablet (bictegravir 50 mg/emtricitabine 200 mg/tenofovir alafenamide 25 mg) once daily.

PO (Children 14–24 kg): 1 tablet (bictegravir 30 mg/emtricitabine 120 mg/tenofovir alafenamide 15 mg) once daily.

Renal Impairment

PO (Adults): *Virologically suppressed with CCr <15 mL/min and receiving chronic hemodialysis:* 1 tablet (bictegravir 50 mg/emtricitabine 200 mg/tenofovir alafenamide 25 mg) once daily (on days of hemodialysis, give dose after hemodialysis session).

Availability

Tablets: bictegravir 30 mg/emtricitabine 120 mg/tenofovir alafenamide 15 mg, bictegravir 50 mg/emtricitabine 200 mg/tenofovir alafenamide 25 mg.

NURSING IMPLICATIONS

Assessment

- Assess patient for change in severity of HIV symptoms and for symptoms of opportunistic infections during therapy.
- May cause lactic acidosis and severe hepatomegaly with steatosis. Monitor patient for signs (increased serum lactate levels, elevated liver enzymes, liver enlargement on palpation). Suspended therapy if clinical or laboratory signs occur.

Lab Test Considerations

- Monitor viral load and CD4 cell count regularly during therapy.
- Test patients for chronic hepatitis B virus (HBV) before initiating therapy. Medication is not indicated for treatment of HBV. Exacerbations of HBV have occurred upon discontinuation of therapy.
- Assess serum creatinine, estimated CCr, urine glucose and urine protein prior to and periodically during therapy. Also monitor serum phosphorous in patients with chronic kidney disease. Discontinue therapy in patients who develop clinically significant ↓ renal function or evidence of Fanconi syndrome.
- Monitor liver function tests in patients co-infected with HIV and HBV who discontinue *Biktarvy*. May cause an exacerbation of hepatitis B. May cause ↑ AST, ALT, bilirubin, creatine kinase, serum amylase, serum lipase, and triglycerides.
- May cause ↓ neutrophil count.
- May cause ↑ LDL cholesterol.

Implementation

- **PO:** Administer once daily without regard for food.
- Administer medication at least 2 hr before or 6 hr after antacids containing aluminum or magnesium. Medication may be taken with food at same time as supplements or antacids containing iron or calcium.
- *For virologically-suppressed adults with estimated creatinine clearance <15 mL per min who are receiving chronic hemodialysis:* On days of he-

modialysis, administer daily dose after completion of hemodialysis treatment.

Patient/Family Teaching

● Emphasize the importance of taking medication as directed. Do not take more than prescribed amount and do not stop taking without consulting health care professional. Take missed doses as soon as remembered, but not if almost time for next dose; do not double doses. Advise patient to read *Patient Information* before starting therapy and with each Rx refill in case of changes.

● Instruct patient that medication should not be shared with others.

● Inform patient that medication does not cure AIDS or prevent associated or opportunistic infections. Therapy may reduce the risk of transmission of HIV to others through sexual contact or blood contamination. Caution patient to use a condom and to avoid sharing needles or donating blood to prevent spreading the AIDS virus to others.

● Instruct patient to notify health care professional immediately if symptoms of lactic acidosis (tiredness or weakness, unusual muscle pain, trouble breathing, stomach pain with nausea and vomiting, cold especially in arms or legs, dizziness, fast or irregular heartbeat) or if signs of hepatotoxicity (yellow skin or whites of eyes, dark urine, light colored stools, lack of appetite for several days or longer, nausea, abdominal pain) occur.

● Instruct patient to notify health care professional of all Rx or OTC medications, vitamins, or herbal products being taken and consult health care professional before taking any new medications, especially St. John's wort.

● Advise patient to notify health care professional if signs and symptoms of immune reconstitution syndrome (signs and symptoms of an infection) occur.

● Rep: May cause fetal harm. Advise patient taking oral contraceptives to use a nonhormonal method of birth control during therapy. If pregnancy is suspected notify health care professional promptly. Inform pregnant women about the Antiretroviral Pregnancy Registry. Enroll patient by calling 1-800-258-4263. Advise female patient to avoid breastfeeding.

● Emphasize the importance of regular follow-up exams and blood counts to determine progress and monitor for side effects.

Evaluation/Desired Outcomes

● Delayed progression of AIDS and decreased opportunistic infections in patients with HIV.

● Decrease in viral load and increase in CD4 cell counts.

⌘ **binimetinib** (bin-i-me-ti-nib)
Mektovi
Classification
Therapeutic: antineoplastics
Pharmacologic: kinase inhibitors

Indications
⌘ Treatment of metastatic/unresectable melanoma with the BRAF V600E or V600K mutation (in combination with encorafenib).

Action
Inhibits the activity of mitogen-activated extracellular kinase (MEK) 1 and 2, which are enzymes that normally promote cellular proliferation. **Therapeutic Effects:** Decreased progression of melanoma and improved survival.

Pharmacokinetics
Absorption: At least 50% absorbed following oral administration.
Distribution: Extensively distributed to tissues.
Protein Binding: 97%.
Metabolism and Excretion: Mostly metabolized by the liver via glucuronidation. 62% excreted in feces (32% as unchanged drug); 31% excreted in urine (6.5% as unchanged drug).
Half-life: 3.5 hr.

TIME/ACTION PROFILE (plasma concentrations)

ROUTE	ONSET	PEAK	DURATION
PO	unknown	1.6 hr	unknown

Contraindications/Precautions
Contraindicated in: OB: Pregnancy; Lactation: Lactation.
Use Cautiously in: Left ventricular ejection fraction <50%; History of retinal vein occlusion; Uncontrolled glaucoma or history of hypercoagulability (↑ risk of retinal vein occlusion); Moderate or severe hepatic impairment (↓ dose); Rep: Women of reproductive potential; Pedi: Safety and effectiveness not established in children.

Adverse Reactions/Side Effects
CV: <u>hypertension</u>, peripheral edema, CARDIOMYOPATHY, DEEP VENOUS THROMBOSIS (DVT). **Derm:** <u>rash</u>. **EENT:** retinopathy, visual impairment, macular edema, retinal detachment, retinal vein occlusion (RVO), uveitis. **F and E:** hyponatremia. **GI:** ↑ <u>liver enzymes</u>, <u>abdominal pain</u>, <u>constipation</u>, <u>diarrhea</u>, <u>nausea</u>, <u>vomiting</u>, colitis, HEPATOTOXICITY. **GU:** ↑ serum creatinine. **Hemat:** <u>anemia</u>, HEMORRHAGE, leukopenia, lymphopenia, neutropenia. **MS:** ↑ creatine kinase, RHABDOMYOLYSIS. **Neuro:** <u>dizziness</u>, <u>fatigue</u>. **Resp:** INTERSTITIAL LUNG DISEASE (ILD), PULMONARY EMBOLISM (PE). **Misc:** <u>fever</u>.

Interactions
Drug-Drug: None reported.

Route/Dosage
PO (Adults): 45 mg twice daily; continue until disease progression or unacceptable toxicity.

Hepatic Impairment
PO (Adults): *Moderate or severe hepatic impairment:* 30 mg twice daily; continue until disease progression or unacceptable toxicity.

Availability
Tablets: 15 mg.

NURSING IMPLICATIONS
Assessment
- Monitor cardiac function (LVEF) by ECG or multigated acquisition (MUGA) scan before starting therapy with binimetinib, one mo after initiation of therapy, and then at 2- to 3-mo intervals during therapy. *If asymptomatic, absolute decrease in LVEF >10% from baseline that is also below lower limit of normal (LLN) occurs,* hold binimetinib for up to 4 wk and evaluate LVEF every 2 wk. Resume binimetinib at reduced dose if present: LVEF ≥ LLN and absolute decrease from baseline is ≤10% and patient is asymptomatic. If LVEF does not recover within 4 wk, permanently discontinue binimetinib. *If symptomatic HF occurs with absolute decrease in LVEF >20% from baseline that is also below LLN,* discontinue binimetinib permanently.
- Monitor for signs and symptoms of venous thromboembolism (shortness of breath, chest pain, arm or leg swelling, cool or pale arm or leg) during therapy. *If uncomplicated DVT or PE occurs,* hold binimetinib. If improves to Grade 0-1, resume at reduced dose. If not improved, permanently discontinue. *If life-threatening PE occurs,* permanently discontinue binimetinib.
- Assess for visual symptoms at each visit. Perform regular ophthalmologic exams. Monitor for signs and symptoms of ocular toxicities (blurred vision, loss of vision, other vision changes, see color dots, halo around objects), swelling, redness, photophobia, eye pain). *If symptomatic retinopathy/retinal pigment epithelial detachments occur,* hold binimetinib for up to 10 days. If improves and becomes asymptomatic, resume at same dose. If not improved, resume at a lower dose or permanently discontinue. *If any grade RVO occurs,* permanently discontinue binimetinib. *If Grade 1–3 uveitis occurs,* if Grade 1 or 2 does not respond to specific ocular therapy, or for Grade 3 uveitis, withhold binimetinib for up to 6 wk. If improved, resume at same or reduced dose. If not improved, permanently discontinue binimetinib. *If Grade 4 uveitis occurs,* permanently discontinue therapy.
- Monitor for signs and symptoms of ILD or pneumonitis (cough, dyspnea, hypoxia, pleural effusion, infiltrates) during therapy. *If Grade 2 occurs,* hold binimetinib for up to 4 wk. If improved to Grade 0–1, resume at reduced dose. If not resolved within 4 wk, permanently discontinue binimetinib. *If Grade 3 or 4 occurs,* discontinue binimetinib permanently.
- Assess for bleeding (headaches, dizziness, feeling weak, coughing up blood or blood clots, vomiting blood or vomit looks like "coffee grounds", red or black stools that look like tar) during therapy. *If recurrent Grade 2 or first occurrence of Grade 3 occurs,* hold binimetinib for up to 4 wk. If improves to Grade 0–1 or to pretreatment/baseline levels, resume at reduced dose. If no improvement, permanently discontinue binimetinib. *If first occurrence of Grade 4 hemorrhagic event occurs,* permanently discontinue binimetinib, or hold for up to 4 wk. If improves to Grade 0–1 or to pretreatment/baseline levels, resume at reduced dose. If no improvement, permanently discontinue. *If recurrent Grade 3 hemorrhagic event occurs,* consider discontinuing binimetinib permanently. *If recurrent Grade 4 hemorrhagic event occurs,* permanently discontinue therapy.

Lab Test Considerations
- Verify negative pregnancy test prior to starting therapy.
- ⚎ Confirm presence of BRAF V600E or V600K mutation in tumor specimens before starting therapy. Information on FDA-approved tests for the detection of BRAF V600 mutations in melanoma is available at: http://www.fda.gov/CompanionDiagnostics.
- Monitor liver function tests before starting therapy, monthly during therapy, and as indicated. *If Grade 2 AST or ALT increased,* continue dose. If no improvement within 2 wk, hold binimetinib until improved to Grade 0–1 or to pretreatment/baseline levels and resume at same dose. *If Grade 3 or 4 AST or increased ALT occurs,* consider permanently discontinuing binimetinib.
- May cause rhabdomyolysis. Monitor CK and serum creatinine levels prior to starting therapy, periodically during therapy, and as indicated. *If Grade 4 asymptomatic CK elevation or any Grade CK elevation with symptoms or with renal impairment occurs,* hold dose for up to 4 wk. If improved to Grade 0–1 resume at reduced dose. If not resolved within 4 wk, permanently discontinue binimetinib.

Implementation
- Dose adjustments for adverse reactions include: *First dose reduction,* 30 mg twice daily. *If patient unable to tolerate 30 mg twice daily,* discontinue binimetinib.
- **PO:** Administer twice daily, about 12 hr apart, without regard to food. Usually taken with encorafenib.

Patient/Family Teaching
- Instruct patient to take medication as directed. Take missed doses as soon as remembered, but not closer

than 6 hr to next dose. If patient vomits after dose, omit and take next dose when scheduled.

- Advise patient to notify health care professional promptly if signs and symptoms of HF, venous thromboembolism (sudden onset of difficulty breathing, leg pain, swelling), changes in vision, ILD (new or worsening cough or dyspnea), hepatotoxicity (jaundice, dark urine, nausea, vomiting, loss of appetite, fatigue, bruising, bleeding), rhabdomyolysis (unusual or new onset weakness, myalgia, darkened urine), or hemorrhage occur.
- Rep: May cause fetal harm. Advise females of reproductive potential to use effective contraception during and for at least 30 days after last dose and to avoid breastfeeding for 3 days after last dose. Advise patient to notify health care professional if pregnancy is planned or suspected.

Evaluation/Desired Outcomes

- Decreased progression of melanoma and improved survival.

---

bisacodyl (bis-a-**koe**-dill)
Dulcolax, Ex-Lax Ultra
Classification
Therapeutic: laxatives
Pharmacologic: stimulant laxatives

Indications
Constipation. Evacuation of the bowel before radiologic studies or surgery. Part of a bowel regimen in spinal cord injury patients.

Action
Stimulates peristalsis. Alters fluid and electrolyte transport, producing fluid accumulation in the colon. **Therapeutic Effects:** Evacuation of the colon.

Pharmacokinetics
Absorption: Variable absorption follows oral administration; rectal absorption is minimal; action is local in the colon.
Distribution: Small amounts of metabolites excreted in breast milk.
Metabolism and Excretion: Small amounts absorbed are metabolized by the liver.
Half-life: Unknown.

TIME/ACTION PROFILE (evacuation of bowel)

ROUTE	ONSET	PEAK	DURATION
PO	6–12 hr	unknown	unknown
Rectal	15–60 min	unknown	unknown

Contraindications/Precautions
Contraindicated in: Hypersensitivity; Abdominal pain; Obstruction; Nausea or vomiting (especially with fever or other signs of an acute abdomen).

Use Cautiously in: Severe cardiovascular disease; Anal or rectal fissures; Excess or prolonged use (may result in dependence).

Adverse Reactions/Side Effects
F and E: hypokalemia (with chronic use). **GI:** <u>abdominal cramps</u>, <u>nausea</u>, diarrhea, rectal burning. **MS:** muscle weakness (with chronic use). **Misc:** protein-losing enteropathy, tetany (with chronic use).

Interactions
Drug-Drug: **Antacids**, **histamine H$_2$-receptor antagonists**, and **proton pump inhibitors** may remove enteric coating of tablets resulting in gastric irritation/dyspepsia. May ↓ the absorption of other **orally administered drugs** because of ↑ motility and ↓ transit time.
Drug-Food: **Milk** may remove enteric coating of tablets, resulting in gastric irritation/dyspepsia.

Route/Dosage
PO (Adults and Children ≥12 yr): 5–15 mg/day (up to 30 mg/day) as a single dose.
PO (Children 3–11 yr): 5–10 mg/day (0.3 mg/kg) as a single dose.
Rect (Adults and Children ≥12 yr): 10 mg/day single dose.
Rect (Children 2–11 yr): 5–10 mg/day single dose.
Rect (Children <2 yr): 5 mg/day single dose.

Availability (generic available)
Enteric-coated tablets: 5 mg^{OTC}. **Rectal suppositories:** 10 mg^{OTC}. **Rectal enema:** 10 mg/30 mL^{OTC}.

NURSING IMPLICATIONS

Assessment
- Assess patient for abdominal distention, presence of bowel sounds, and usual pattern of bowel function.
- Assess color, consistency, and amount of stool produced.

Implementation
- Do not confuse Dulcolax (bisacodyl) with Dulcolax (docusate sodium).
- May be administered at bedtime for morning results.
- PO: Taking on an empty stomach will produce more rapid results.
- *DNC:* Do not crush or chew enteric-coated tablets. Take with a full glass of water or juice.
- Do not administer oral doses within 1 hr of milk or antacids; this may lead to premature dissolution of tablet and gastric or duodenal irritation.
- **Rect:** Rectal suppository or enema can be given at the time a bowel movement is desired. Lubricate suppositories with water or water-soluble lubricant before insertion. Encourage patient to retain the suppository or enema 15–30 min before expelling.

✦ = Canadian drug name. ▩ = Genetic implication. ~~Strikethrough~~ = Discontinued. CAPITALS = life-threatening. <u>Underline</u> = most frequent.

Patient/Family Teaching

- Advise patients, other than those with spinal cord injuries, that laxatives should be used only for short-term therapy. Prolonged therapy may cause electrolyte imbalance and dependence.
- Advise patient to increase fluid intake to at least 1500–2000 mL/day during therapy to prevent dehydration.
- Encourage patients to use other forms of bowel regulation (increasing bulk in the diet, increasing fluid intake, or increasing mobility). Normal bowel habits may vary from 3 times/day to 3 times/wk.
- Instruct patients with cardiac disease to avoid straining during bowel movements (Valsalva maneuver).
- Advise patient that bisacodyl should not be used when constipation is accompanied by abdominal pain, fever, nausea, or vomiting.

Evaluation/Desired Outcomes

- Soft, formed bowel movement when used for constipation.
- Evacuation of colon before surgery or radiologic studies, or for patients with spinal cord injuries.

---

bisoprolol (bis-oh-proe-lol)
~~Zebeta~~
Classification
Therapeutic: antihypertensives
Pharmacologic: beta blockers

Indications
Hypertension.

Action
Blocks stimulation of beta$_1$(myocardial)-adrenergic receptors. Does not usually affect beta$_2$(pulmonary, vascular, uterine)-receptor sites. **Therapeutic Effects:** Decreased BP and heart rate.

Pharmacokinetics
Absorption: Well absorbed after oral administration, but 20% undergoes first-pass hepatic metabolism.
Distribution: Widely distributed to tissues.
Metabolism and Excretion: 50% excreted unchanged by the kidneys; remainder renally excreted as metabolites; 2% excreted in feces.
Half-life: 9–12 hr.

TIME/ACTION PROFILE (antihypertensive effect)

ROUTE	ONSET	PEAK	DURATION
PO	unknown	1–4 hr	24 hr

Contraindications/Precautions
Contraindicated in: Uncompensated HF; Pulmonary edema; Cardiogenic shock; Bradycardia or heart block.

Use Cautiously in: Renal impairment (dosage ↓ recommended); Hepatic impairment (dosage ↓ recommended); Pulmonary disease (including asthma; beta$_1$ selectivity may be lost at higher doses); avoid use if possible; Diabetes mellitus (may mask signs of hypoglycemia); Thyrotoxicosis (may mask symptoms); History of severe allergic reactions (intensity of reactions may be ↑); OB: Safety not established in pregnancy; Lactation: Safety not established in breastfeeding; Pedi: Safety and effectiveness not established in children; Geri: Older adults may have ↑ sensitivity to beta blockers (initial dosage ↓ recommended).

Adverse Reactions/Side Effects
CV: BRADYCARDIA, HF, hypotension, peripheral vasoconstriction. **Derm:** rash. **EENT:** blurred vision, stuffy nose. **Endo:** hyperglycemia, hypoglycemia. **GI:** ↑ liver enzymes, constipation, diarrhea, nausea, vomiting. **GU:** erectile dysfunction, ↓ libido, urinary frequency. **MS:** arthralgia, back pain, joint pain. **Neuro:** fatigue, weakness, anxiety, depression, dizziness, drowsiness, insomnia, memory loss, mental status changes, nervousness, nightmares. **Resp:** bronchospasm, PULMONARY EDEMA, wheezing. **Misc:** drug-induced lupus syndrome.

Interactions
Drug-Drug: General anesthetics, phenytoin, and verapamil may cause additive myocardial depression. Additive bradycardia may occur with clonidine, digoxin, diltiazem, ivabradine, or verapamil. Additive hypotension may occur with other antihypertensives, acute ingestion of alcohol, or nitrates. Concurrent use with amphetamine, cocaine, ephedrine, epinephrine, norepinephrine, phenylephrine, or pseudoephedrine may result in unopposed alpha-adrenergic stimulation (excessive hypertension, bradycardia). Concurrent thyroid preparation administration may ↓ effectiveness. May alter the effectiveness of insulins or oral hypoglycemic agents (dose adjustments may be necessary). May ↓ the effectiveness of theophylline. May ↓ the beta$_1$-cardiovascular effects of dopamine or dobutamine. Use cautiously within 14 days of MAO inhibitor therapy (may result in hypertension).

Route/Dosage
PO (Adults): 5 mg once daily, may be ↑ to 10 mg once daily (range 2.5–20 mg/day).

Renal Impairment
PO (Adults): *CCr <40 mL/min:* Initiate therapy with 2.5 mg/day, titrate cautiously.

Hepatic Impairment
PO (Adults): *Hepatitis/Cirrhosis:* Initiate therapy with 2.5 mg/day, titrate cautiously.

Availability (generic available)
Tablets: 5 mg, 10 mg. *In combination with:* hydrochlorothiazide (Ziac). See Appendix N.

NURSING IMPLICATIONS
Assessment
- Monitor BP, ECG, and pulse frequently during dosage adjustment period and periodically throughout therapy.
- Monitor intake and output ratios and daily weights. Assess routinely for signs and symptoms of HF (dyspnea, rales/crackles, weight gain, peripheral edema, jugular venous distention).
- Monitor frequency of prescription refills to determine adherence.

Lab Test Considerations
- May cause ↑ BUN, serum triglyceride, and uric acid levels.
- May cause ↑ in ANA titers.
- May cause ↑ in blood glucose levels.

Implementation
- **PO:** Take apical pulse before administering. If <50 bpm or if arrhythmia occurs, withhold medication and notify physician or other health care professional.
- May be administered without regard to meals.

Patient/Family Teaching
- Instruct patient to take medication exactly as directed, at the same time each day, even if feeling well; do not skip or double up on missed doses. If a dose is missed, it should be taken as soon as possible up to 4 hr before next dose. Abrupt withdrawal may precipitate life-threatening arrhythmias, hypertension, or myocardial ischemia.
- Teach patient and family how to check pulse and BP. Instruct them to check pulse daily and BP biweekly and to report significant changes to health care professional.
- May cause drowsiness. Caution patients to avoid driving or other activities that require alertness until response to the drug is known.
- Advise patients to change positions slowly to minimize orthostatic hypotension.
- Caution patient that this medication may increase sensitivity to cold.
- Instruct patient to notify health care professional of all Rx or OTC medications, vitamins, or herbal products being taken and to consult health care professional before taking any Rx, OTC, or herbal products, especially cold preparations, concurrently with this medication. Patients on antihypertensive therapy should also avoid excessive amounts of coffee, tea, and cola.
- Diabetics should closely monitor blood glucose, especially if weakness, malaise, irritability, or fatigue occurs. Medication does not block dizziness or sweating as signs of hypoglycemia.
- Advise patient to notify health care professional if slow pulse, difficulty breathing, wheezing, cold hands and feet, dizziness, light-headedness, confusion, depression, rash, fever, sore throat, unusual bleeding, or bruising occurs.
- Instruct patient to inform health care professional of medication regimen before treatment or surgery.
- Advise patient to carry identification describing disease process and medication regimen at all times.
- Rep: Advise females of reproductive potential to notify health care professional if pregnancy is planned or suspected or if breastfeeding.
- **Hypertension:** Reinforce the need to continue additional therapies for hypertension (weight loss, sodium restriction, stress reduction, regular exercise, moderation of alcohol consumption, and smoking cessation). Medication controls but does not cure hypertension.

Evaluation/Desired Outcomes
- Decrease in BP.

HIGH ALERT

bivalirudin (bi-val-i-**roo**-din)
Angiomax
Classification
Therapeutic: anticoagulants
Pharmacologic: thrombin inhibitors

Indications
Patients undergoing percutaneous coronary intervention (PCI), including those with heparin-induced thrombocytopenia (HIT) or heparin-induced thrombocytopenia and thrombosis syndrome (HITTS).

Action
Specifically and reversibly inhibits thrombin by binding to its receptor sites. Inhibition of thrombin prevents activation of factors V, VIII, and XII; the conversion of fibrinogen to fibrin; platelet adhesion and aggregation. **Therapeutic Effects:** Decreased acute ischemic complications in patients with unstable angina (death, MI, or the urgent need for revascularization procedures).

Pharmacokinetics
Absorption: IV administration results in complete bioavailability.
Distribution: Unknown.
Metabolism and Excretion: Cleared from plasma by a combination of renal mechanisms and proteolytic breakdown.
Half-life: 25 min (↑ in renal impairment).

TIME/ACTION PROFILE (anticoagulant effect)

ROUTE	ONSET	PEAK	DURATION
IV	immediate	unknown	1–2 hr

Contraindications/Precautions
Contraindicated in: Active major bleeding; Hypersensitivity.

Use Cautiously in: Any disease state associated with an ↑ risk of bleeding; Heparin-induced thrombocytopenia or heparin-induced thrombocytopenia-thrombosis syndrome; Patients with unstable angina not undergoing PCI; Patients with other acute coronary syndromes; Concurrent use with other platelet aggregation inhibitors (safety not established); Renal impairment (↓ infusion rate if CCr <30 mL/min); OB: Safety not established in pregnancy; Lactation: Use while breastfeeding only if potential maternal benefit justifies potential risk to infant; Pedi: Safety and effectiveness not established in children.

Adverse Reactions/Side Effects
CV: hypotension, ACUTE STENT THROMBOSIS (especially in patients with ST-segment elevation MI undergoing PCI), bradycardia, hypertension. **GI:** nausea, abdominal pain, dyspepsia, vomiting. **Hemat:** BLEEDING. **Local:** injection site pain. **MS:** pain. **Neuro:** headache, anxiety, insomnia, nervousness. **Misc:** fever.

Interactions
Drug-Drug: Risk of bleeding may be ↑ by concurrent use of **heparin, low molecular weight heparins, clopidogrel, thrombolytics,** or any other **drugs that inhibit coagulation.**
Drug-Natural Products: ↑ risk of bleeding with **arnica, chamomile, clove, dong quai, feverfew, garlic, ginger, gingko, Panax ginseng,** and others.

Route/Dosage
IV (Adults): 0.75 mg/kg as a bolus injection, followed by an infusion at a rate of 1.75 mg/kg/hr for the duration of the PCI procedure. An activated clotting time (ACT) should be performed 5 min after bolus dose and an additional bolus dose of 0.3 mg/kg may be administered if needed. Continuation of the infusion (at a rate of 1.75 mg/kg/hr) for up to 4 hr post-procedure is optional (should be considered in patients with ST-segment elevation MI). Therapy should be initiated prior to the procedure and given in conjunction with aspirin.

Renal Impairment
IV (Adults): No ↓ in the bolus dose is needed in any patient with renal impairment. *CCr <30 mL/min:* ↓ infusion rate to 1 mg/kg/hr; *Hemodialysis:* ↓ infusion rate to 0.25 mg/kg/hr.

Availability (generic available)
Lyophilized powder for injection: 250 mg/vial.
Premixed infusion: 250 mg/50 mL (as ready-to-use vial).

NURSING IMPLICATIONS
Assessment
● Assess for bleeding. Most common is oozing from the arterial access site for cardiac catheterization. Minimize use of arterial and venous punctures, IM injections, and use of urinary catheters, nasotracheal intubation, and nasogastric tubes. Avoid noncompressible sites for IV access. If bleeding cannot be controlled with pressure, discontinue bivalirudin immediately.
● Monitor vital signs. May cause bradycardia, hypertension, or hypotension. An unexplained decrease in BP may indicate hemorrhage.
● Monitor patients with STEMI undergoing primary PCI with bivalirudin for acute stent thrombosis for at least 24 hrs in a facility capable of managing ischemic complications.

Lab Test Considerations
● Assess hemoglobin, hematocrit, and platelet count prior to bivalirudin therapy and periodically during therapy. May cause ↓ hemoglobin and hematocrit. An unexplained ↓ in hematocrit may indicate hemorrhage.
● Bivalirudin interferes with INR measurements; INR may not be useful in determining appropriate dose of warfarin.
● Monitor ACT periodically in patients with renal dysfunction.

Implementation
● Administer IV just prior to PCI, in conjunction with aspirin 300 mg to 325 mg/day. Do not administer IM.

IV Administration
● **IV Push:** (for bolus dose) *Reconstitution:* Reconstitute each 250-mg vial with 5 mL of sterile water for injection. Reconstituted vials are stable for 24 hr if refrigerated. *Dilution:* Further dilute in 50 mL of D5W or 0.9% NaCl. Withdraw bolus dose out of bag. Infusion is stable for 24 hr at room temperature. *Concentration:* Final concentration of infusion is 5 mg/mL. *Rate:* Administer as a bolus injection.
● **Intermittent Infusion:** *Reconstitution:* Reconstitute each 250-mg vial as per the above directions. *Dilution:* Further dilute in 50 mL of D5W or 0.9% NaCl. If infusion is to be continued after 4 hr (at a rate of 0.2 mg/kg/hr), reconstituted vial should be diluted in 500 mL of D5W or 0.9% NaCl. Infusion is stable for 24 hr at room temperature. Premixed infusion is stable for 24 hr at room temperature or 14 days if refrigerated. *Concentration:* 5 mg/mL (for infusion rate of 1.75 mg/kg/hr); 0.5 mg/mL (for infusion rate of 0.2 mg/kg/hr). *Rate:* Based on patient's weight (see Route/Dosage section).
● **Y-Site Compatibility:** acyclovir, allopurinol, amifostine, amikacin, aminocaproic acid, aminophylline, amphotericin B liposome, ampicillin, ampicillin/sulbactam, anidulafungin, argatroban, arsenic trioxide, atropine, azithromycin, aztreonam, bivacin, bumetanide, buprenorphine, busulfan, butorphanol, calcium chloride, calcium gluconate, cangrelor, carboplatin, carmustine, cefazolin, cefepime, cefotaxime, cefotetan, cefoxitin, ceftazidime, cef-

triaxone, cefuroxime, chloramphenicol, ciprofloxacin, cisatracurium, cisplatin, clindamycin, cyclophosphamide, cyclosporine, cytarabine, dacarbazine, dactinomycin, daptomycin, daunorubicin hydrochloride, dexamethasone, dexmedetomidine, dexrazoxane, digoxin, diltiazem, diphenhydramine, docetaxel, dopamine, doxorubicin hydrochloride, doxorubicin liposomal, doxycycline, droperidol, enalaprilat, ephedrine, epinephrine, epirubicin, epoprostenol, eptifibatide, ertapenem, erythromycin, esmolol, etoposide, etoposide phosphate, fentanyl, fluconazole, fludarabine, fluorouracil, foscarnet, fosphenytoin, furosemide, ganciclovir, gemcitabine, gentamicin, glycopyrrolate, granisetron, heparin, hydralazine, hydrocortisone, hydromorphone, idarubicin, ifosfamide, imipenem/cilastatin, insulin, regular, irinotecan, isoproterenol, ketorolac, leucovorin calcium, levofloxacin, lidocaine, linezolid, magnesium sulfate, mannitol, melphalan, meperidine, meropenem, mesna, methotrexate, methylprednisolone, metoclopramide, metoprolol, metronidazole, midazolam, milrinone, mitomycin, mitoxantrone, morphine, moxifloxacin, mycophenolate, nafcillin, nalbuphine, naloxone, nicardipine, nitroglycerin, nitroprusside, norepinephrine, octreotide, ondansetron, oxaliplatin, oxytocin, paclitaxel, palonosetron, pamidronate, pemetrexed, pentobarbital, phenobarbital, phenylephrine, piperacillin/tazobactam, potassium acetate, potassium chloride, potassium phosphate, procainamide, propranolol, remifentanil, rocuronium, sodium acetate, sodium bicarbonate, sodium phosphate, succinylcholine, sufentanil, tacrolimus, theophylline, thiopental, thiotepa, tigecycline, tirofiban, tobramycin, topotecan, trimethoprim/sulfamethoxazole, vasopressin, vecuronium, verapamil, vinblastine, vincristine, vinorelbine, voriconazole, warfarin, zidovudine, zoledronic acid.

- **Y-Site Incompatibility:** alteplase, amiodarone, amphotericin B lipid complex, caspofungin, chlorpromazine, dantrolene, diazepam, dobutamine, pentamidine, phenytoin, prochlorperazine, reteplase, vancomycin.

Patient/Family Teaching

- Inform patient of the purpose of bivalirudin.
- Instruct patient to notify health care professional immediately if any bleeding or bruising is noted.
- Instruct patient to notify health care professional of all Rx or OTC medications, vitamins, or herbal products being taken and consult health care professional before taking any new medications.
- Rep: May cause fetal harm. Advise females of reproductive potential to notify health care professional if pregnancy is planned or suspected or if breastfeeding.

Evaluation/Desired Outcomes

- Decreased acute ischemic complications in patients with unstable angina (death, MI, or the urgent need for revascularization procedures).

HIGH ALERT

bleomycin (blee-oh-**mye**-sin)

Classification
Therapeutic: antineoplastics
Pharmacologic: antitumor antibiotics

Indications
Treatment of: Lymphomas, Squamous cell carcinoma, Testicular embryonal cell carcinoma, Choriocarcinoma, Teratocarcinoma. Intrapleural administration to prevent the reaccumulation of malignant effusions.

Action
Inhibits DNA and RNA synthesis. **Therapeutic Effects:** Death of rapidly replicating cells, particularly malignant ones.

Pharmacokinetics
Absorption: IV administration results in complete bioavailability. Well absorbed from IM and SUBQ sites. Absorption follows intrapleural and intraperitoneal administration.

Distribution: Widely distributed; concentrates in skin, lungs, peritoneum, kidneys, and lymphatics.

Metabolism and Excretion: 60–70% excreted unchanged by the kidneys.

Half-life: 2 hr (↑ in renal impairment).

TIME/ACTION PROFILE (tumor response)

ROUTE	ONSET	PEAK	DURATION
IV, IM, SUBQ	2–3 wk	unknown	unknown

Contraindications/Precautions
Contraindicated in: Hypersensitivity; OB: Pregnancy; Lactation: Lactation.

Use Cautiously in: Renal impairment (dose ↓ required if CCr <35 mL/min); Pulmonary disease; Rep: Women of reproductive potential; Geri: ↑ risk of pulmonary toxicity and renal impairment in older adults.

Adverse Reactions/Side Effects
CV: hypotension, peripheral vasoconstriction. **Derm:** hyperpigmentation, mucocutaneous toxicity, alopecia, erythema, rash, urticaria, vesiculation. **GI:** ↓ weight, anorexia, nausea, stomatitis, vomiting. **Hemat:** anemia, leukopenia, thrombocytopenia. **Local:** pain at tumor site, phlebitis at IV site. **Neuro:** aggressive behavior, disorientation, weakness. **Resp:** pneumonitis, PULMONARY FIBROSIS. **Misc:** chills, fever, ANAPHYLACTOID REACTIONS.

Interactions
Drug-Drug: Hematologic toxicity ↑ with concurrent use of **radiation therapy** and other **antineoplastics**.

✱ = Canadian drug name. ⚏ = Genetic implication. ~~Strikethrough~~ = Discontinued. CAPITALS = life-threatening. <u>Underline</u> = most frequent.

Concurrent use with **cisplatin** ↓ elimination of bleomycin and may ↑ toxicity. ↑ risk of pulmonary toxicity with other **antineoplastics** or thoracic **radiation therapy**. **General anesthesia** ↑ the risk of pulmonary toxicity. ↑ risk of Raynaud's phenomenon when used with **vinblastine**.

Route/Dosage

Patients with lymphoma should receive initial test doses of 2 units or less for the first 2 doses.

IV, IM, SUBQ (Adults and Children): 0.25–0.5 unit/kg (10–20 units/m²) weekly or twice weekly initially. If favorable response, lower maintenance doses given (1 unit/day or 5 units/wk IM or IV). May also be given as continuous IV infusion at 0.25 unit/kg or 15 units/m²/day for 4–5 days.

Intrapleural (Adults): 15–20 units instilled for 4 hr, then removed.

Availability (generic available)

Powder for injection: 15 units/vial, 30 units/vial.

NURSING IMPLICATIONS

Assessment

- Monitor vital signs before and frequently during therapy.
- Assess for fever and chills. May occur 3–6 hr after administration and last 4–12 hr.
- Monitor for anaphylactic (fever, chills, hypotension, wheezing) and idiosyncratic (confusion, hypotension, fever, chills, wheezing) reactions. Keep resuscitation equipment and medications on hand. Patients with lymphoma are at particular risk for idiosyncratic reactions that may occur immediately or several hr after therapy, usually after the 1st or 2nd dose.
- Assess respiratory status for dyspnea and rales/crackles. Monitor chest x-ray before and periodically during therapy. Pulmonary toxicity occurs primarily in geriatric patients (age 70 or older) who have received 400 or more units or at lower doses in patients who received other antineoplastics or thoracic radiation. May occur 4–10 wk after therapy. Discontinue and do not resume bleomycin if pulmonary toxicity occurs.
- Assess nausea, vomiting, and appetite. Weigh weekly. Modify diet as tolerated. Antiemetics may be given before administration.

Lab Test Considerations

- Monitor CBC before and periodically during therapy. May cause thrombocytopenia and leukopenia (nadir occurs in 12 days and usually returns to pretreatment levels by day 17).
- Monitor baseline and periodic renal and hepatic function.

Implementation

- *High Alert:* Fatalities have occurred with chemotherapeutic agents. Before administering, clarify all ambiguous orders; double-check single, daily, and course-of-therapy dose limits; have second practitioner independently double-check original order and dose calculations.
- Prepare solution in a biologic cabinet. Wear gloves, gown, and mask while handling medication. Discard equipment in specially designated containers.
- Patients with lymphoma should receive a 1- or 2-unit test dose 2–4 hr before initiation of therapy. Monitor closely for anaphylactic reaction. May not detect reactors.
- Premedication with acetaminophen, corticosteroids, and diphenhydramine may reduce drug fever and risk of anaphylaxis.
- Reconstituted solution is stable for 24 hr at room temperature and for 14 days if refrigerated.
- **IM SUBQ:** Reconstitute vial with 1–5 mL of sterile water for injection, 0.9% NaCl, or bacteriostatic water for injection. Do not reconstitute with diluents containing benzyl alcohol when used for neonates.

IV Administration

- **Intermittent Infusion:** Prepare IV doses by diluting 15-unit vial with at least 5 mL of 0.9% NaCl. *Dilution:* Further dilute dose in 50 to 1000 mL of D5W or 0.9% NaCl. *Rate:* Administer slowly over 10 min.
- **Y-Site Compatibility:** allopurinol, amifostine, aminocaproic acid, aminophylline, amiodarone, anidulafungin, atracurium, aztreonam, bivalirudin, bumetanide, busulfan, calcium chloride, calcium gluconate, carboplatin, carmustine, caspofungin, cefepime, chlorpromazine, cimetidine, cisatracurium, cisplatin, cyclophosphamide, cyclosporine, cytarabine, dacarbazine, dactinomycin, daptomycin, daunorubicin hydrochloride, dexamethasone, dexmedetomidine, dexrazoxane, digoxin, diltiazem, diphenhydramine, dobutamine, docetaxel, dopamine, doxorubicin hydrochloride, doxorubicin liposomal, droperidol, enalaprilat, epinephrine, epirubicin, ertapenem, esmolol, etoposide, etoposide phosphate, famotidine, filgrastim, fludarabine, fluorouracil, fosphenytoin, furosemide, gemcitabine, glycopyrrolate, granisetron, haloperidol, heparin, hetastarch, hydralazine, hydrocortisone, idarubicin, ifosfamide, insulin, regular, isoproterenol, ketorolac, labetalol, leucovorin calcium, levofloxacin, lidocaine, magnesium sulfate, mannitol, melphalan, meperidine, mesna, methotrexate, methylprednisolone, metoclopramide, metoprolol, milrinone, mitomycin, mitoxantrone, naloxone, nicardipine, nitroglycerin, norepinephrine, octreotide, ondansetron, oxaliplatin, paclitaxel, palonosetron, pantoprazole, pemetrexed, phentolamine, phenylephrine, piperacillin/tazobactam, potassium chloride, potassium phosphate, procainamide, rituximab, sargramostim, sodium acetate, thiotepa, tirofiban, trastuzumab, vinblastine, vincristine, vinorelbine, voriconazole.
- **Y-Site Incompatibility:** amphotericin B liposomal, dantrolene, phenytoin, tigecycline.

- **Intrapleural:** Dissolve 60 units in 50–100 mL of 0.9% NaCl.
- May be administered through thoracotomy tube. Position patient as directed.

Patient/Family Teaching

- Instruct patient to notify health care professional if fever, chills, wheezing, faintness, diaphoresis, shortness of breath, prolonged nausea and vomiting, or mouth sores occur.
- Encourage patient not to smoke because this may worsen pulmonary toxicity.
- Explain to the patient that skin toxicity may manifest itself as skin sensitivity, hyperpigmentation (especially at skin folds and points of skin irritation), and skin rashes and thickening.
- Instruct patient to inspect oral mucosa for erythema and ulceration. If ulceration occurs, advise patient to use sponge brush and rinse mouth with water after eating and drinking. Opioid analgesics may be required if pain interferes with eating.
- Discuss with patient the possibility of hair loss. Explore coping strategies.
- Instruct patient not to receive any vaccinations without advice of health care professional.
- Rep: May cause fetal harm. Advise patient of the need for contraception during therapy. Advise females of reproductive potential to notify health care professional if pregnancy is planned or suspected or if breastfeeding.
- Emphasize need for periodic lab tests to monitor for side effects.

Evaluation/Desired Outcomes

- Decrease in tumor size without evidence of hypersensitivity or pulmonary toxicity.

---

bortezomib (bor-tez-o-mib)
Velcade
Classification
Therapeutic: antineoplastics
Pharmacologic: proteasome inhibitors

Indications
Multiple myeloma (as initial therapy or after progression) (in combination with melphalan and prednisone). Mantle cell lymphoma.

Action
Inhibits proteasome, a regulator of intracellular protein catabolism, resulting in disruption of various intracellular processes. Cytotoxic to a variety of cancerous cells. **Therapeutic Effects:** Decreased progression and improved survival in multiple myeloma and mantle cell lymphoma.

Pharmacokinetics
Absorption: IV administration results in complete bioavailability.

Distribution: Widely distributed to tissues.
Metabolism and Excretion: Mostly metabolized by the liver via the CYP2C19, CYP3A4, and CYP1A2 isoenzymes, and to a lesser extent by the CYP2D6 and CYP2C9 isoenzymes; excretion pathway unknown.
Half-life: 9–15 hr.

TIME/ACTION PROFILE

ROUTE	ONSET	PEAK	DURATION
IV	unknown	38 days*	unknown

*Median time to response based on clinical parameters.

Contraindications/Precautions
Contraindicated in: Hypersensitivity to bortezomib, boron, or mannitol; Intrathecal administration (may cause death); OB: Pregnancy; Lactation: Lactation.
Use Cautiously in: Moderate to severe hepatic impairment; History of or risk factors for HF; Rep: Women of reproductive potential and men with female partners of reproductive potential; Pedi: Safety and effectiveness not established in children.

Adverse Reactions/Side Effects
CV: <u>hypotension</u>, HF. **Derm:** STEVENS-JOHNSON SYNDROME, TOXIC EPIDERMAL NECROLYSIS. **EENT:** blurred vision, diplopia. **GI:** <u>anorexia</u>, <u>constipation</u>, <u>diarrhea</u>, <u>nausea</u>, <u>vomiting</u>, LIVER FAILURE. **Hemat:** <u>anemia</u>, <u>neutropenia</u>, <u>thrombocytopenia</u>, BLEEDING, THROMBOTIC THROMBOCYTOPENIC PURPURA/HEMOLYTIC UREMIC SYNDROME. **Neuro:** <u>fatigue</u>, <u>malaise</u>, <u>peripheral neuropathy</u>, <u>weakness</u>, dizziness, POSTERIOR REVERSIBLE ENCEPHALOPATHY SYNDROME (PRES), syncope. **Resp:** pneumonia. **Misc:** <u>fever</u>, tumor lysis syndrome.

Interactions
Drug-Drug: Concurrent neurotoxic medications including **amiodarone**, some **antivirals**, **nitrofurantoin**, **isoniazid**, or **HMG-CoA reductase inhibitors** may ↑ risk of peripheral neuropathy.

Route/Dosage

Previously Untreated Multiple Myeloma
IV, SUBQ (Adults): 1.3 mg/m² twice weekly for Cycles 1–4 (days 1, 4, 8, 11, 22, 25, 29, and 32; no treatment during cycle 3), then once weekly for Cycles 5–9 (days 1, 8, 22, and 29; no treatment during Cycle 7); further cycles/doses depend on response and toxicity.

Hepatic Impairment
IV (Adults): *Moderate or severe hepatic impairment:* 0.7 mg/m² per injection for the first cycle, then may ↑ to 1 mg/m² per injection or ↓ further to 0.5 mg/m² per injection, based on tolerability.

Previously Untreated Mantle Cell Lymphoma
IV, SUBQ (Adults): 1.3 mg/m² twice weekly on days 1, 4, 8, and 11, followed by a 10-day rest (days 12–21);

repeat for 5 additional cycles; further cycles/doses depend on response and toxicity.

Hepatic Impairment
IV (Adults): *Moderate or severe hepatic impairment:* 0.7 mg/m² per injection for the first cycle, then may ↑ to 1 mg/m² per injection or ↓ further to 0.5 mg/m² per injection, based on tolerability.

Relapsed Multiple Myeloma and Mantle Cell Lymphoma
IV, SUBQ (Adults): 1.3 mg/m² twice weekly for 2 wk (days 1, 4, 8, and 11), followed by a 10-day rest; further cycles/doses depend on response and toxicity. Patients with multiple myeloma who have previously responded to bortezomib therapy and who have relapsed ≥6 mo after prior bortezomib therapy can be started on their last tolerated dose; dose should be given twice weekly (days 1, 4, 8, and 11) every 3 wk for a maximum of 8 cycles.

Hepatic Impairment
IV (Adults): *Moderate or severe hepatic impairment:* 0.7 mg/m² per injection for the first cycle, then may ↑ to 1 mg/m² per injection or ↓ further to 0.5 mg/m² per injection, based on tolerability.

Availability (generic available)
Lyophilized powder for injection: 3.5 mg/vial. **Solution for injection:** 1 mg/mL, 2.5 mg/mL.

NURSING IMPLICATIONS
Assessment
- Monitor vital signs frequently during therapy. May cause fever and orthostatic hypotension requiring adjustment of antihypertensives, hydration, or administration of mineralocorticoids.
- Monitor for GI adverse effects. May require antidiarrheals, antiemetics, and fluid and electrolyte replacement to prevent dehydration. Weigh weekly; modify diet as tolerated.
- Monitor for signs and symptoms of peripheral neuropathy (burning sensation, hyperesthesia, hypoesthesia, paresthesia, discomfort, neuropathic pain, weakness) during therapy. *If peripheral neuropathy is Grade 1 (paresthesia or loss of reflexes without pain or loss of function)* continue prescribed dose. *If paresthesia is Grade 1 with pain or Grade 2 (interfering with function but not with daily activities)* reduce dose to 1.0 mg/m². *If peripheral neuropathy is Grade 2 with pain or Grade 3 (interfering with activities of daily living)* withhold dose until toxicity resolves, then reinitiate with a reduced dose of 0.7 mg/m² and decrease frequency to once/wk. *If peripheral neuropathy is Grade 4 (permanent sensory loss that interferes with daily function)* discontinue bortezomib.
- Monitor for signs and symptoms of tumor lysis syndrome (tachypnea, tachycardia, hypotension, pulmonary edema). Patients with high tumor burden prior to treatment are at increased risk.

- Monitor for signs of PRES (headache, seizure, lethargy, confusion, blindness). Hypertension may or may not be present. May occur within 16 hr to 1 yr of initiation of therapy. Treat hypertension if present and discontinue bortezomib therapy. Symptoms usually resolve within days.
- Monitor for signs and symptoms of thrombotic angiopathy (thrombocytopenia, microangiopathic hemolytic anemia, thrombotic thrombocytopenic purpura/hemolytic uremic syndrome, acute kidney injury). Discontinue therapy immediately if clinical or lab symptoms occur.

Lab Test Considerations
- Verify negative pregnancy test before starting therapy. Monitor CBC frequently during therapy. Assess platelet count before each dose. Dose modifications for hematologic toxicity are made based on indication and concurrent drug therapy; see manufacturer's recommendations. The nadir of thrombocytopenia is day 11 and recovery is usually by next cycle. Occurs more commonly in cycles 1 and 2, but may occur throughout therapy. May require discontinuation of therapy.
- Monitor blood glucose levels closely in patients taking oral hypoglycemic agents; may require adjustment of antidiabetic agent dose.

Implementation
- Should be administered under the supervision of a physician experienced in the use of antineoplastic therapy.
- Solution should be prepared in a biologic cabinet. Wear gloves, gown, and mask while handling medication. Discard IV equipment in specially designated containers.

IV Administration
- **SUBQ:** *Reconstitution:* Reconstitute each vial with 1.4 mL of 0.9% NaCl. *Concentration:* 2.5 mg/mL. Solution should be clear and colorless; do not administer solutions that are discolored or contain particulate matter. May inject into thigh or abdomen; rotate injection sites. Inject into sites at least 1 inch from other sites and avoid tender, bruised, erythematous, or indurated sites. If local injection site reactions occur, may inject a less concentrated (1 mg/mL) solution.
- **IV Push:** *Reconstitution:* Reconstitute each vial with 3.5 mL of 0.9% NaCl. Solution should be clear and colorless; do not administer solutions that are discolored or contain particulate matter. *Concentration:* 1 mg/mL. Administer reconstituted solution within 8 hr at room temperature; 3 of the 8 hr may be stored in a syringe. *Rate:* Administer as a 3–5 sec bolus injection twice weekly for 2 wk followed by a 10-day rest period. At least 72 hr should elapse between consecutive doses.

Patient/Family Teaching
- Caution the patient that dehydration may occur with vomiting or diarrhea. Advise patient to maintain fluid

intake and to notify health care professional if dizziness or fainting occurs.
- Instruct patient to contact health care professional if they experience new or worsening signs of peripheral neuropathy (tingling, numbness, pain, burning feeling in the feet or hands, weakness in the arms or legs), PML (progressive weakness on one side of the body or clumsiness of limbs; disturbance of vision; changes in thinking, memory, and orientation leading to confusion and personality changes), or if symptoms of dehydration (dizziness, fainting) due to vomiting or diarrhea; rash; shortness of breath; cough; swelling of feet, ankles, or legs; bleeding, infection, convulsions; persistent headache; reduced eyesight; increase in BP or blurred vision occur.
- May cause dizziness and blurred vision. Caution patient to avoid driving or other activities requiring alertness until response to medication is known.
- Advise patient to notify health care professional of all Rx or OTC medications, vitamins, or herbal products being taken and consult health care professional before taking Rx, OTC, or herbal products, especially St. John's wort.
- Advise diabetic patients taking oral hypoglycemic agents to monitor blood glucose frequently and notify health care professional of changes in blood sugar.
- Rep: Advise females of reproductive potential to use effective contraception during and for 7 mo after last dose and to avoid breastfeeding during therapy and for 2 mo after therapy. Advise males with female partner of reproductive potential to use effective contraception for 4 mo after last dose of bortezomib. Patient should notify health care professional immediately if pregnancy is suspected. May impair fertility for male and female patients.

Evaluation/Desired Outcomes
- Decrease in serum and urine myeloma protein.
- Decrease in size and spread of malignancy.

bremelanotide
(bre-me-**lan**-oh-tide)
Vyleesi
Classification
Therapeutic: sexual dysfunction agents
Pharmacologic: melanocortin receptor agonists

Indications
Treatment of premenopausal women with acquired, generalized hypoactive sexual desire disorder (HSDD) that is characterized by low sexual desire that causes marked distress or interpersonal difficulty and is NOT due to a concomitant medical or psychiatric condition, relationship problems, or the effects of a medication or drug substance.

Action
Stimulates various melanocortin receptors, with the most notable being MC4R (present in the CNS) and MC4l (present on melanocytes). The precise mechanism by which this receptor activation improves HSDD is unknown. **Therapeutic Effects:** Improved sexual desire.

Pharmacokinetics
Absorption: Completely absorbed following SUBQ administration.
Distribution: Not distributed to the tissues.
Metabolism and Excretion: Primarily undergoes hydrolysis; 65% excreted in urine, 23% in feces.
Half-life: 2.7 hr.

TIME/ACTION PROFILE (plasma concentrations)

ROUTE	ONSET	PEAK	DURATION
SUBQ	unknown	1 hr	unknown

Contraindications/Precautions
Contraindicated in: Uncontrolled hypertension; Cardiovascular disease; OB: Pregnancy.
Use Cautiously in: Patients at high risk for cardiovascular disease; Patients with dark skin (↑ risk for focal hyperpigmentation); Severe hepatic impairment; Severe renal impairment (CCr <30 mL/min); Lactation: Use while breastfeeding only if potential maternal benefit justifies potential risk to infant; Rep: Women of reproductive potential; Pedi: Safety and effectiveness not established in children.

Adverse Reactions/Side Effects
CV: ↓ heart rate, ↑ blood pressure. **Derm:** flushing, focal hyperpigmentation. **EENT:** nasal congestion, rhinorrhea. **GI:** nausea, abdominal pain, diarrhea, vomiting. **Local:** injection site reactions. **MS:** ↑ creatine kinase, arthralgia, myalgia, pain. **Neuro:** headache, dizziness, fatigue, paresthesia, restless leg syndrome. **Resp:** cough.

Interactions
Drug-Drug: May ↓ absorption of concomitantly administered medications; avoid using bremelanotide when using antibiotics or analgesics. May ↓ **naltrexone** levels; avoid using bremelanotide in patients using naltrexone for substance use disorders.

Route/Dosage
PO (Adults): 1.75 mg given on an as needed basis ≥45 min before anticipated sexual activity (not to exceed one dose/24 hr or 8 doses/mo). Discontinue after 8 wk if no improvement in symptoms.

Availability
Solution for injection (auto-injectors): 1.75 mg/0.3 mL.

NURSING IMPLICATIONS
Assessment
- Assess sexual desire prior to and periodically during therapy.
- Assess cardiovascular risk and control of BP periodically during therapy. Systolic BP ↑ 6 mmHg, diastolic BP ↑ 3 mmHg and HR ↓ up to 5 bpm transiently after dose; usually return to normal within 12 hr of dose.
- Assess for focal hyperpigmentation of face, gingiva, and breasts periodically during therapy. More common in patients with dark skin or with >8 doses/month. Consider discontinuation of therapy if hyperpigmentation occurs; may not resolve with discontinuation.
- Assess for nausea during therapy; may require antiemetics. Usually improves with 2nd dose; may require discontinuation.

Implementation
- **SUBQ:** Using auto-injector, inject into abdomen or thigh 45 min before anticipated sexual activity. Do not administer more than 1 dose/24 hr or more than 8 doses/month.

Patient/Family Teaching
- Instruct patient to take medication as directed with no more than 1 dose/24 hr or no more than 8 doses/month. Advise patient to read *Patient Information* before starting and with each Rx refill in case of changes.
- Inform patient that increases in BP and decreases in HR may occur after each dose; usually resolve within 12 hr.
- Inform patient that darkening of the skin of the face, gums, and breasts may occur, especially in patients with darker skin. Risks increase with daily use. Advise patient that changes may not resolve after stopping the medication. Contact health care professional for concerns about skin changes.
- Inform patient that nausea may occur, especially after first dose, lasting 2 or more hr. May require antiemetics. Advise patient to notify health care professional if nausea is problematic.
- Instruct patient to notify health care professional of all Rx or OTC medications, vitamins, or herbal products being taken and consult health care professional before taking any new medications.
- Rep: Advise women of reproductive potential to use effective contraception during therapy and to notify health care professional if pregnancy is planned or expected or if breastfeeding. Discontinue bremelanotide if pregnancy is suspected. Encourage pregnant women exposed to bremelanotide to call the VYLEESI Pregnancy Exposure Registry at (877) 411-2510.

Evaluation/Desired Outcomes
- Improved sexual desire in premenopausal women. If no improvement in 8 wk, discontinue medication.

⚕ brentuximab vedotin
(bren-**tux**-i-mab)
Adcetris
Classification
Therapeutic: antineoplastics
Pharmacologic: drug-antibody conjugates

Indications
Classical Hodgkin lymphoma (cHL) in patients who have failed autologous hematopoietic stem cell transplant (auto-HSCT) or who have failed ≥2 prior multiagent chemotherapies and are not candidates for auto-HSCT. Previously untreated, high-risk cHL (in combination with doxorubicin, vincristine, etoposide, prednisone, and cyclophosphamide). cHL in patients who are at high risk of relapse or progression as post-auto-HSCT consolidation. Previously untreated stage III or IV cHL (in combination with doxorubicin, vinblastine, and dacarbazine). Systemic anaplastic large cell lymphoma after failure of ≥1 multi-agent chemotherapy regimen. ⚕ Primary cutaneous anaplastic large cell lymphoma or CD30-expressing mycosis fungoides in patients who have received prior systemic therapy. ⚕ Previously untreated systemic anaplastic large cell lymphoma or other CD30-expressing peripheral T-cell lymphoma (in combination with cyclophosphamide, doxorubicin, and prednisone).

Action
⚕ An antibody-drug conjugate made up of three parts: an antibody specific for human CD30 (cAC10, a cell membrane protein of the tumor necrosis factor receptor), a microtubule disrupting agent monomethyl auristatin (MMAE), and a protease-cleavable linker that attaches MMAE covalently to cAC10. The combination disrupts the intracellular microtubule network causing cell-cycle arrest and apoptotic cellular death. **Therapeutic Effects:** Decreased spread of lymphoma.

Pharmacokinetics
Absorption: IV administration results in complete bioavailability.
Distribution: Unknown.
Metabolism and Excretion: Small amounts of MMAE that are released are metabolized by the liver and eliminated mostly by the kidneys.
Half-life: *ADC:* 4–6 days.

TIME/ACTION PROFILE (plasma concentrations)

ROUTE	ONSET	PEAK	DURATION
IV (ADC)	unknown	end of infusion	3 wk
IV (MMAE)	unknown	1–3 days	3 wk

Contraindications/Precautions
Contraindicated in: Concurrent use of bleomycin (↑ risk of pulmonary toxicity); Severe renal impairment (CCr <30 mL/min); Moderate or severe hepatic impairment; OB: Pregnancy; Lactation: Lactation.

Use Cautiously in: Preexisting GI involvement (↑ risk of GI perforation); High BMI or diabetes (↑ risk of hyperglycemia); Rep: Women of reproductive potential and males with female partners of reproductive potential; Pedi: Children <2 yr (safety and effectiveness not established).

Adverse Reactions/Side Effects

CV: peripheral edema. **Derm:** alopecia, night sweats, pruritus, rash, STEVENS-JOHNSON SYNDROME, TOXIC EPIDERMAL NECROLYSIS, dry skin. **Endo:** hyperglycemia. **F and E:** KETOACIDOSIS. **GI:** ↓ appetite, abdominal pain, BOWEL OBSTRUCTION, constipation, diarrhea, GI HEMORRHAGE, GI PERFORATION, GI ULCER, HEPATOTOXICITY, ILEUS, nausea, PANCREATITIS, vomiting, ENTEROCOLITIS, NEUTROPENIC COLITIS, ulcer. **GU:** ↓ fertility. **Hemat:** anemia, NEUTROPENIA, THROMBOCYTOPENIA. **Metab:** weight loss. **MS:** arthralgia, back pain, extremity pain, myalgia, muscle spasm. **Neuro:** anxiety, dizziness, fatigue, headache, insomnia, peripheral neuropathy, PROGRESSIVE MULTIFOCAL LEUKOENCEPHALOPATHY (PML). **Resp:** ACUTE RESPIRATORY DISTRESS SYNDROME, cough, dyspnea, INTERSTITIAL LUNG DISEASE, oropharyngeal pain. **Misc:** fever, lymphadenopathy, chills, INFUSION REACTIONS (including anaphylaxis), TUMOR LYSIS SYNDROME.

Interactions

Drug-Drug: MMAE is both a substrate and inhibitor of the CYP3A4/5 enzyme system. **Bleomycin** may ↑ risk of pulmonary toxicity; concurrent use contraindicated. **Strong CYP3A4 inhibitors**, including **ketoconazole** may ↑ levels and risk of adverse reactions. **Strong CYP3A4 inducers**, including **rifampin**, may ↓ levels and effectiveness.

Route/Dosage

Relapsed Classical Hodgkin Lymphoma or Relapsed Systemic Anaplastic Large Cell Lymphoma

IV (Adults): 1.8 mg/kg (max dose = 180 mg) every 3 wk until disease progression or unacceptable toxicity.

Renal Impairment
IV (Adults): *CCr <30 mL/min:* Avoid use.

Hepatic Impairment
IV (Adults): *Mild (Child-Pugh A):* 1.2 mg/kg (max dose = 120 mg) every 3 wk until disease progression or unacceptable toxicity; *Moderate (Child-Pugh B) or severe (Child-Pugh C):* Avoid use.

Previously Untreated, High-Risk Classical Hodgkin Lymphoma

IV (Children ≥2 yr): 1.8 mg/kg (max dose = 180 mg) every 3 wk until a maximum of 5 doses completed.

Renal Impairment
IV (Children ≥2 yr): *CCr <30 mL/min:* Avoid use.

Hepatic Impairment
IV (Children ≥2 yr): *Mild (Child-Pugh A):* 1.2 mg/kg (max dose = 120 mg) every 3 wk until a maximum of 5 doses completed; *Moderate (Child-Pugh B) or severe (Child-Pugh C):* Avoid use.

Classical Hodgkin Lymphoma Consolidation

IV (Adults): 1.8 mg/kg (max dose = 180 mg) every 3 wk until a maximum of 16 cycles completed, disease progression, or unacceptable toxicity. Initiate therapy within 4–6 wk post-auto-HSCT or upon recovery of auto-HSCT.

Renal Impairment
IV (Adults): *CCr <30 mL/min:* Avoid use.

Hepatic Impairment
IV (Adults): *Mild (Child-Pugh A):* 1.2 mg/kg (max dose = 120 mg) every 3 wk until a maximum of 16 cycles completed, disease progression, or unacceptable toxicity; *Moderate (Child-Pugh B) or severe (Child-Pugh C):* Avoid use.

Previously Untreated Stage III or IV Classical Hodgkin Lymphoma

IV (Adults): 1.2 mg/kg (max dose = 120 mg) every 2 wk until a maximum of 12 doses completed, disease progression, or unacceptable toxicity.

Renal Impairment
IV (Adults): *CCr <30 mL/min:* Avoid use.

Hepatic Impairment
IV (Adults): *Mild (Child-Pugh A):* 0.9 mg/kg (max dose = 90 mg) every 2 wk until a maximum of 12 doses completed, disease progression, or unacceptable toxicity; *Moderate (Child-Pugh B) or severe (Child-Pugh C):* Avoid use.

Relapsed Primary Cutaneous Anaplastic Large Cell Lymphoma or CD-30 Expressing Mycosis Fungoides

IV (Adults): 1.8 mg/kg (max dose = 180 mg) every 3 wk until a maximum of 16 cycles completed, disease progression, or unacceptable toxicity.

Renal Impairment
IV (Adults): *CCr <30 mL/min:* Avoid use.

Hepatic Impairment
IV (Adults): *Mild (Child-Pugh A):* 1.2 mg/kg (max dose = 120 mg) every 3 wk until a maximum of 16 cycles completed, disease progression, or unacceptable toxicity; *Moderate (Child-Pugh B) or severe (Child-Pugh C):* Avoid use.

Previously Untreated Systemic Anaplastic Large Cell Lymphoma or Other CD-30 Expressing Peripheral T-Cell Lymphomas

IV (Adults): 1.8 mg/kg (max dose = 180 mg) every 3 wk with each cycle of chemotherapy for 6–8 doses.

Renal Impairment
IV (Adults): *CCr <30 mL/min:* Avoid use.

Hepatic Impairment

IV (Adults): *Mild (Child-Pugh A):* 1.2 mg/kg (max dose = 120 mg) every 3 wk with each cycle of chemotherapy for 6–8 doses; *Moderate (Child-Pugh B) or severe (Child-Pugh C):* Avoid use.

Availability

Lyophilized powder for injection: 50 mg/vial.

NURSING IMPLICATIONS

Assessment

● Monitor for signs and symptoms of peripheral neuropathy (hypoesthesia, hyperesthesia, paresthesia, discomfort, burning, neuropathic pain, weakness). *For new or worsening neuropathy Grade 2:* Reduce dose of vincristine per prescribing information. Continue dosing with brentuximab. If neuropathy improves to Grade ≤1 by day 8 of next cycle, then resume vincristine at full dose. *For Grade 3,* Discontinue vincristine. For first occurrence, delay next dose until neuropathy improves to ≤ Grade 1, then restart at brentuximab at 1.2 mg/kg up to 120 mg. For second occurrence, hold therapy until improvement to ≤ Grade 2 then restart at 0.8 mg/kg up to a maximum of 80 mg. *For third occurrence,* discontinue brentuximab. *If Grade 4 peripheral neuropathy occurs,* discontinue brentuximab and vincristine.

● Monitor temperature periodically during therapy, especially if neutropenic.

● Assess for signs and symptoms of infusion-related reaction, including anaphylaxis (rash, pruritus, dyspnea, swelling of face and neck). If anaphylaxis occurs, discontinue infusion immediately; do not restart. Treat other infusion-related reactions by stopping and treating symptoms. Premedicate patient prior to subsequent infusions with acetaminophen, an antihistamine, and a corticosteroid.

● Monitor for tumor lysis syndrome due to rapid reduction in tumor volume (acute renal failure, hyperkalemia, hypocalcemia, hyperuricemia, or hypophosphatemia). Risks are higher in patients with greater tumor burden and rapidly proliferating tumors; may be fatal. Correct electrolyte abnormalities, monitor renal function and fluid balance, and administer supportive care, including dialysis, as indicated.

● Assess for skin rash frequently during therapy. Discontinue at first sign of rash; may be life-threatening. Stevens-Johnson syndrome may develop. Treat symptomatically; may recur once treatment is stopped.

● Assess for any new signs or symptoms that may be suggestive of PML, an opportunistic infection of the brain caused by the JC virus, that leads to death or severe disability; withhold dose and notify health care professional promptly. PML symptoms may begin gradually but usually worsen rapidly. Symptoms vary depending on which part of brain is infected (mental function declines rapidly and progressively, causing dementia; speaking becomes increasingly difficult; partial blindness; difficulty walking; rarely, headaches and seizures occur). Diagnosis is usually made via gadolinium-enhanced MRI and CSF analysis. Risk of PML increases with the number of infusions. Withhold brentuximab at first sign of PML.

● Monitor for signs and symptoms of pulmonary toxicity (cough, dyspnea) during therapy. If new or worsening pulmonary symptoms occur, hold brentuximab during assessment and until symptoms improve.

● Monitor for severe abdominal pain during therapy; may cause pancreatitis.

Lab Test Considerations

● Verify negative pregnancy status prior to starting therapy.

● Monitor CBC prior to each dose and more frequently in patients with Grade 3 or 4 neutropenia. Prolonged (≥1 wk) severe neutropenia may occur. Hold dose of brentuximab for Grade 3 or 4 neutropenia until resolution to baseline or ≤Grade 2. Consider growth factor support for subsequent cycles for patients who developed Grade 3 or 4 neutropenia. Discontinue brentuximab or reduce dose to 1.2 mg/kg (up to 120 mg) in patients with recurrent Grade 4 neutropenia despite use of growth factors.

● Monitor liver enzymes and bilirubin periodically during therapy. Signs of new, worsening, or recurrent hepatotoxicity may require decrease in dose, or interruption or discontinuation of therapy.

● Monitor blood glucose frequently during therapy. May occur more frequently in patients with high body mass index or diabetes. If hyperglycemia develops, administer antihyperglycemic agents as clinically indicated.

Implementation

IV Administration

● Premedicate patients with previously untreated Stage III, IV cHL and PTCL who are treated with brentuximab in combination with chemotherapy with G-CSF beginning with Cycle 1.

● **Intermittent Infusion:** Calculate dose and number of brentuximab vials needed. Calculate for 100 kg for patients weighing >100 kg. *Reconstitution:* Reconstitute each 50 mg vial with 10.5 mL of Sterile Water for Injection. Direct stream to side of vial. Swirl gently; do not shake. *Concentration:* 5 mg/mL. Solution should be clear to slightly opalescent, and colorless. Do not administer solutions that are discolored or contain a precipitate. Withdraw volume of brentuximab dose from infusion bag of at least 100 mL. *Dilution:* 0.9% NaCl, D5W, or LR. *Concentration:* 0.4–1.8 mg/mL. Invert bag gently to mix. Dilute immediately into infusion bag or store solution in refrigerator; use within 24 hr of reconstitution. Do not freeze. *Rate:* Infuse over 30 min. Do not administer as IV push or bolus.

- **Y-Site Incompatibility:** Do not administer with other mediations or solutions.

Patient/Family Teaching

- Instruct patient to notify health care professional of any numbness or tingling of hands or feet or any muscle weakness.
- Advise patient to notify health care professional immediately if signs and symptoms of infection (fever of ≥100.5°F, chills, cough, pain on urination), hepatotoxicity (fatigue, anorexia, right upper abdominal discomfort, dark urine, jaundice), PML (changes in mood or usual behavior, confusion, thinking problems, loss of memory, changes in vision, speech, or walking, decreased strength or weakness on one side of body), pulmonary toxicity, GI complications or pancreatitis (abdominal pain, nausea, vomiting, diarrhea, rash), or infusion reactions (fever, chills, rash, breathing problems within 24 hr of infusion) occur.
- Educate patient about signs and symptoms of hyperglycemia (blurred vision; drowsiness; dry mouth; flushed, dry skin; fruit-like breath odor; increased urination; ketones in urine; loss of appetite; stomachache; nausea or vomiting; tiredness; rapid, deep breathing; unusual thirst; unconsciousness). Advise patient to notify health care professional if symptoms occur.
- Advise patient to notify health care professional of all Rx or OTC medications, vitamins, or herbal products being taken and to consult with health care professional before taking other medications.
- Rep: May cause fetal harm. Advise females of reproductive potential and males with a partner of reproductive potential to use effective contraception during therapy and for at least 6 mo after last dose and to avoid breastfeeding during therapy. If pregnancy is suspected, notify health care professional promptly. Inform male patients therapy may impair fertility.

Evaluation/Desired Outcomes

- Decreased spread of lymphoma.

REMS

brexanolone (brex-an-oh-lone)
Zulresso

Classification
Therapeutic: antidepressants
Pharmacologic: corticosteroids, gamma aminobutyric acid (GABA) enhancers

Schedule IV

Indications
Postpartum depression.

Action
Although not fully understood, thought to be related to positive allosteric modulation of GABA-A receptors. **Therapeutic Effects:** Reduction in depressive symptoms.

Pharmacokinetics
Absorption: IV administration results in complete absorption.
Distribution: Extensively distributed to tissues.
Metabolism and Excretion: Extensively metabolized via keto-reduction, glucuronidation, and sulfation to inactive metabolites. Primarily excreted in feces (47%) and urine (42%) as metabolites.
Half-life: 9 hr.

TIME/ACTION PROFILE (reduction in depressive symptoms)

ROUTE	ONSET	PEAK	DURATION
IV	1–2 hr	60–72 hr	At least 30 days

Contraindications/Precautions
Contraindicated in: End-stage renal disease (CCr <15 mL/min) (↑ accumulation of solubilizing agent).
Use Cautiously in: OB: Safety not established; Lactation: Enters breast milk; use while breastfeeding only if potential maternal benefit justifies potential risk to infant; Pedi: May ↑ risk of suicidal thoughts/behaviors; Pedi: Children <15 yr (safety and effectiveness not established).

Adverse Reactions/Side Effects
CV: tachycardia. **Derm:** flushing. **GI:** dry mouth, diarrhea, dyspepsia, oropharyngeal pain. **Neuro:** dizziness, presyncope, sedation, vertigo, altered consciousness, loss of consciousness, SUICIDAL THOUGHTS/BEHAVIORS.

Interactions
Drug-Drug: Use with **benzodiazepines** or other **CNS depressants**, including **opioids, non-benzodiazepine sedative/hypnotics, anxiolytics, muscle relaxants,** and **alcohol** may cause profound sedation, loss of consciousness, and/or respiratory depression; avoid concurrent use, if possible.

Route/Dosage
IV (Adults and Children ≥15 yr): 30 mcg/kg/hr for 4 hr, then ↑ to 60 mcg/kg/hr for 20 hr, then ↑ to 90 mcg/kg/hr for 28 hr, then ↓ to 60 mcg/kg/hr for 4 hr, then ↓ to 30 mcg/kg/hr for 4 hr, then discontinue. Total duration of infusion = 60 hr.

Availability
Solution for injection: 5 mg/mL.

NURSING IMPLICATIONS
Assessment
- Monitor for hypoxia using continuous pulse oximetry equipped with alarm. Assess for excessive seda-

tion every 2 hr during planned, non-sleep periods. Stop infusion immediately if signs or symptoms of excessive sedation occur. Time to full recovery from loss or altered state of consciousness ranges from 15–60 min after infusion is stopped. Infusion may be resumed at same or lower dose after symptoms resolve. If hypoxia occurs, immediately stop infusion and do not resume.

● Assess for suicidal tendencies, especially during early therapy. Risk may be increased in adults ≤24 yr. Consider changing therapeutic regimen, including discontinuing brexanolone, in patients whose depression becomes worse or who experience emergent suicidal thoughts and behaviors.

Implementation

● Start brexanolone therapy early enough during the day to allow for recognition of excessive sedation.

● *REMS:* Brexanolone is only available through a restricted Risk Evaluation and Mitigation Strategy (REMS) called the Zulresso REMS due to potential harm from excessive sedation or sudden loss of consciousness. Healthcare facilities must enroll to ensure medication is only given to patients enrolled in program. Pharmacies must be certified with the program. Patients must be enrolled before receiving brexanolone.

● **Continuous Infusion:** Prepare 5 infusion bags for 60 hr period, more if patient weighs ≥90 kg. For each bag, prepare and store in polyolefin, non-DEHP, nonlatex bag, only. Dilute in infusion bag immediately after initial puncture of vial. Withdraw 20 mL of brexanolone from vial and place in infusion bag. *Dilution:* Dilute with 40 mL of sterile water for injection, and further dilute with 40 mL of 0.9% NaCl 100 mL volume. *Concentration:* 1 mg/mL. Immediately place infusion bag in refrigerator until use. Solution is clear and colorless; do not administer solutions that are discolored or contain particulate matter. Solution is stable for up to 96 hr if refrigerated. Diluted solution is stable for 12 hr at room temperature. Each 60 hr infusion requires at least 5 bags. Discard bag after 12 hr of infusion. *Rate:* Use a programmable peristaltic infusion pump to ensure accurate delivery. See Route and Dosage for rate. Use a dedicated line; do not mix with other medications in bag or line. Prime infusion line with admixture before inserting into pump and connecting to venous catheter. Use a PVC, non-DEHP, nonlatex infusion set. Do not use in-line filter infusion sets.

Patient/Family Teaching

● *REMS:* Explain purpose of medication to patient and family and requirements of Zulresso REMS program. Advise patient to read *Medication Guide* before starting brexanolone.

● Advise patient to notify health care professional if excessive sedation occurs during infusion. Patients must not be the primary caregiver of dependents and must be accompanied during interactions with their child(ren).

● Caution patient to avoid driving and activities requiring alertness until response from medication is known.

● Instruct patient to notify health care professional of all Rx or OTC medications, vitamins, or herbal products being taken and consult health care professional before taking any new medications. Advise patient to avoid taking other CNS depressants or alcohol.

● Rep: Advise females of reproductive potential to notify health care professional if they could possibly be pregnant prior to therapy. Advise pregnant women and females of reproductive potential of the potential risk to a fetus. Encourage patient to enroll in the registry that monitors pregnancy outcomes in women exposed to antidepressants during pregnancy. To register patients, healthcare professionals should call the National Pregnancy Registry for Antidepressants at 1-844-405-6185 or online at https://womensmentalhealth.org/clinical-and-researchprograms/pregnancyregistry/antidepressants/.

Evaluation/Desired Outcomes

● Decreased symptoms of postpartum depression.

BEERS

✄ brexpiprazole
(brex-**pip**-ra-zole)
Rexulti
Classification
Therapeutic: antipsychotics, antidepressants
Pharmacologic: serotonin-dopamine activity modulators (SDAM)

Indications
Schizophrenia. Adjunctive treatment of major depressive disorder. Agitation associated with dementia due to Alzheimer's disease.

Action
Psychotropic activity may be due to partial agonist activity at dopamine D_2 and serotonin 5-HT$_{1A}$ receptors and antagonist activity at the 5-HT$_{2A}$ receptor. **Therapeutic Effects:** Decreased manifestations of schizophrenia including excitable, paranoic, or withdrawn behavior. Improvement in symptoms of depression with increased sense of wellbeing. Decreased agitation associated with dementia due to Alzheimer's disease.

Pharmacokinetics
Absorption: Well absorbed (95%) following oral administration.
Distribution: Displays extravascular distribution.
Protein Binding: >99%.
Metabolism and Excretion: Primarily metabolized by the liver via the CYP3A4 and CYP2D6 isoenzymes; ✄ the CYP2D6 enzyme system exhibits genetic

B

polymorphism (~7% of population may be poor metabolizers and may have significantly ↑ brexpiprazole concentrations and an ↑ risk of adverse effects). 25% excreted in urine (<1% unchanged), 46% in feces (14% unchanged).
Half-life: 91 hr.

TIME/ACTION PROFILE (improvement in symptoms)

ROUTE	ONSET	PEAK	DURATION
PO (schizophrenia)	within 1–2 wk	4–6 wk	unknown
PO (depression)	within 1 wk	5 wk	unknown

Contraindications/Precautions

Contraindicated in: Hypersensitivity.
Use Cautiously in: History of seizures or concurrent use of medications that may ↓ seizure threshold; Pre-existing cardiovascular disease, dehydration, hypotension, concurrent antihypertensives, diuretics, electrolyte imbalance (↑ risk of orthostatic hypotension, correct deficits before treatment); Pre-existing low WBC (may ↑ risk of leukopenia/neutropenia); History of diabetes, metabolic syndrome or dyslipidemia (may exacerbate); Patients <24 yr (may ↑ suicidal ideation/behaviors, monitor carefully); Patients at risk for falls; ⚥ Poor CYP2D6 metabolizers (PM), dose ↓ required; OB: Use during third trimester may result in extrapyramidal/withdrawal symptoms in infant; use during pregnancy only if potential maternal benefit justifies potential fetal risk; Lactation: Safety not established during breastfeeding; Pedi: Antidepressants may ↑ risk of suicidal ideation/behaviors in children; safety and effectiveness not established in children <18 yr (major depressive disorder) or <13 yr (schizophrenia); Geri: Appears on Beers list. ↑ risk of stroke, cognitive decline, and mortality in older adults with dementia. Avoid use in older adults, except for schizophrenia, adjunctive treatment of major depressive disorder, or agitation associated with dementia due to Alzheimer's disease.

Adverse Reactions/Side Effects

CV: cerebrovascular adverse reactions (↑ in elderly patients with dementia-related psychoses), orthostatic hypotension/syncope. **EENT:** blurred vision. **Endo:** hyperglycemia/diabetes. **GI:** abdominal pain, constipation, diarrhea, dry mouth, dysphagia, excess salivation, flatulence. **Hemat:** agranulocytosis, leukopenia, neutropenia. **Metab:** ↑ weight, ↑ appetite, dyslipidemia. **Neuro:** akathisia, abnormal dreams, dizziness, drowsiness, dystonia, extrapyramidal symptoms, headache, NEUROLEPTIC MALIGNANT SYNDROME, restlessness, SEIZURES, tardive dyskinesia, tremor, urges (eating, gambling, sexual, shopping). **Misc:** body temperature dysregulation, HYPERSENSITIVITY REACTIONS (including anaphylaxis).

Interactions

Drug-Drug: Strong CYP3A4 inhibitors, including **clarithromycin**, **itraconazole** or **ketoconazole**, may ↑ levels and risk of toxicity; ↓ brexpiprazole dose. **Strong CYP2D6 inhibitors**, including **fluoxetine**, **paroxetine**, or **quinidine** may ↑ levels and risk of toxicity; ↓ brexpiprazole dose. Combined use of **strong or moderate CYP3A4 inhibitors with strong or moderate CYP2D6 inhibitors** in addition to brexpiprazole including the following combinations: **itraconazole + quinidine, fluconazole + paroxetine, itraconazole + duloxetine** or **fluconazole + duloxetine** may ↑ levels and risk of toxicity; ↓ brexpiprazole dose. **Strong CYP3A4 inducers**, including **rifampin**, may ↓ levels and effectiveness; ↑ brexpiprazole dose. Concurrent use of **antihypertensives** or **diuretics** may ↑ the risk of hypotension. Concurrent use of **medications that may ↓ seizure threshold** may ↑ the risk of seizures.
Drug-Natural Products: St. John's wort may ↓ levels and effectiveness; ↑ brexpiprazole dose.

Route/Dosage

Schizophrenia

PO (Adults): 1 mg once daily on Days 1–4, then ↑ to 2 mg once daily on Days 5–7, then ↑ to 4 mg once daily on Day 8 (not to exceed 4 mg once daily). *Known CYP2D6 poor metabolizers:* use 50% of the usual dose. *Concurrent use of strong CYP2D6 inhibitors (schizophrenia only) or CYP3A4 inhibitors:* use 50% of the usual dose; *Concurrent use of strong/moderate CYP2D6 inhibitors AND strong/moderate CYP3A4 inhibitors:* use 25% of the usual dose; *Known CYP2D6 poor metabolizer taking concurrent strong/moderate CYP3A4 inhibitors:* use 25% of the usual dose; *Concurrent use of strong CYP3A4 inducers:* double usual dose over 1–2 wk; titrate by clinical response.
PO (Children 13–17 yr): 0.5 mg once daily on Days 1–4, then ↑ to 1 mg once daily on Days 5–7, then ↑ to 2 mg once daily on Day 8. May ↑ dose by 1 mg/day on weekly basis (not to exceed 4 mg once daily). *Known CYP2D6 poor metabolizers:* use 50% of the usual dose. *Concurrent use of strong CYP2D6 inhibitors (schizophrenia only) or CYP3A4 inhibitors:* use 50% of the usual dose; *Concurrent use of strong/moderate CYP2D6 inhibitors AND strong/moderate CYP3A4 inhibitors:* use 25% of the usual dose; *Known CYP2D6 poor metabolizer taking concurrent strong/moderate CYP3A4 inhibitors:* use 25% of the usual dose; *Concurrent use of strong CYP3A4 inducers:* double usual dose over 1–2 wk; titrate by clinical response.

Renal Impairment

PO (Adults and Children 13–17 yr): *Moderate/severe/end-stage renal impairment [CCr <60 mL/min]:* maximum daily dose should not exceed 3 mg.

✳ = Canadian drug name. ⚥ = Genetic implication. ~~Strikethrough~~ = Discontinued. CAPITALS = life-threatening. <u>Underline</u> = most frequent.

Hepatic Impairment

(Adults and Children 13 – 17 yr): *Moderate to severe hepatic impairment [Child-Pugh score ≥7]:* maximum daily dose should not exceed 3 mg.

Major Depressive Disorder

PO (Adults): 0.5 or 1 mg once daily initially, may be ↑ to 2 mg once daily (not to exceed 3 mg once daily); *Known CYP2D6 poor metabolizers:* use 50% of the usual dose. *Concurrent use of strong CYP2D6 inhibitors (schizophrenia only) or CYP3A4 inhibitors:* use 50% of the usual dose; *Concurrent use of strong/ moderate CYP2D6 inhibitors AND strong/moderate CYP3A4 inhibitors:* use 25% of the usual dose; *Known CYP2D6 poor metabolizer taking concurrent strong/ moderate CYP3A4 inhibitors:* use 25% of the usual dose; *Concurrent use of strong CYP3A4 inducers:* double usual dose over 1 – 2 wk; titrate by clinical response.

Renal Impairment

PO (Adults): *Moderate/severe/end-stage renal impairment [CCr <60 mL/min]:* maximum daily dose should not exceed 2 mg.

Hepatic Impairment

PO (Adults): *Moderate to severe hepatic impairment [Child-Pugh score ≥7]:* maximum daily dose should not exceed 2 mg.

Agitation Associated with Dementia Due to Alzheimer's Disease

PO (Adults): 0.5 mg once daily on Days 1 – 7, then ↑ to 1 mg once daily on Days 8 – 14, then ↑ to 2 mg once daily on Day 15. May ↑ to 3 mg once daily after ≥14 days based on clinical response and tolerability. *Known CYP2D6 poor metabolizers:* use 50% of the usual dose. *Concurrent use of strong CYP2D6 inhibitors (schizophrenia only) or CYP3A4 inhibitors:* use 50% of the usual dose; *Concurrent use of strong/moderate CYP2D6 inhibitors AND strong/moderate CYP3A4 inhibitors:* use 25% of the usual dose; *Known CYP2D6 poor metabolizer taking concurrent strong/moderate CYP3A4 inhibitors:* use 25% of the usual dose; *Concurrent use of strong CYP3A4 inducers:* double usual dose over 1 – 2 wk; titrate by clinical response.

Renal Impairment

PO (Adults): *Moderate/severe/end-stage renal impairment [CCr <60 mL/min]:* maximum daily dose should not exceed 2 mg.

Hepatic Impairment

PO (Adults): *Moderate to severe hepatic impairment [Child-Pugh score ≥7]:* maximum daily dose should not exceed 2 mg.

Availability (generic available)

Tablets: 0.25 mg, 0.5 mg, 1 mg, 2 mg, 3 mg, 4 mg.

NURSING IMPLICATIONS
Assessment

- Assess mental status (orientation, mood, behavior) before and periodically during therapy. Assess for

suicidal tendencies, especially during early therapy for depression. Restrict amount of drug available to patient. Risk may be increased in children, adolescents, and adults ≤24 yrs.
- Assess weight and BMI initially and throughout therapy.
- Obtain fasting blood glucose and cholesterol levels initially and periodically during therapy.
- Monitor BP (sitting, standing, lying), pulse, and respiratory rate before and periodically during therapy.
- Observe patient carefully when administering medication to ensure that medication is actually taken and not hoarded or cheeked.
- Monitor patient for onset of akathisia (restlessness or desire to keep moving) and extrapyramidal side effects (*parkinsonian:* difficulty speaking or swallowing, loss of balance control, pill rolling of hands, masklike face, shuffling gait, rigidity, tremors; and *dystonic:* muscle spasms, twisting motions, twitching, inability to move eyes, weakness of arms or legs) periodically during therapy. Report these symptoms.
- Monitor for tardive dyskinesia (uncontrolled rhythmic movement of mouth, face, and extremities; lip smacking or puckering; puffing of cheeks; uncontrolled chewing; rapid or worm-like movements of tongue). Notify health care professional immediately if these symptoms occur; symptoms may partially or completely resolve, but may be irreversible.
- Monitor for development of neuroleptic malignant syndrome (fever, muscle rigidity, altered mental status, respiratory distress, tachycardia, seizures, diaphoresis, hypertension or hypotension, pallor, tiredness, loss of bladder control, elevated CK, myoglobinuria/rhabdomyolysis, acute renal failure). Notify health care professional immediately if these symptoms occur.
- Assess for falls risk. Drowsiness, orthostatic hypotension, and motor and sensory instability increase risk. Institute prevention if indicated.

Lab Test Considerations

- Monitor CBC frequently during initial mo of therapy in patients with pre-existing or history of low WBC. May cause leukopenia, neutropenia, or agranulocytosis. Discontinue therapy if severe neutropenia (ANC <1000 mm^3 occurs).
- Monitor blood glucose and cholesterol levels initially and periodically during therapy.

Implementation

- Brexpiprazole is not indicated as an as needed ("prn") treatment for agitation associated with dementia due to Alzheimer's disease.
- **PO:** Administer once daily without regard to meals.

Patient/Family Teaching

- Advise patient to take medication as directed and not to skip doses or double up on missed doses. Take missed doses as soon as remembered unless almost time for the next dose. Do not stop taking brexiprazole without consulting health care professional. Advise patient to read *Medication Guide* before starting and with each Rx refill in case of changes.

- Inform patient of possibility of extrapyramidal symptoms and tardive dyskinesia. Instruct patient to report these symptoms immediately.
- Advise patient to make position changes slowly to minimize orthostatic hypotension. Protect from falls.
- Medication may cause drowsiness and lightheadedness. Caution patient to avoid driving or other activities requiring alertness until response to medication is known.
- Advise patient and family to notify health care professional if thoughts about suicide or dying, attempts to commit suicide; new or worse depression; new or worse anxiety; feeling very agitated or restless; panic attacks; trouble sleeping; new or worse irritability; acting aggressive; being angry or violent; acting on dangerous impulses; an extreme increase in activity and talking; other unusual changes in behavior or mood occur or if signs and symptoms of high blood sugar (feel very thirsty, urinating more than usual, feel very hungry, feel weak or tired, nausea, confusion, breath smells fruity) occur.
- Inform patient that brexipiprazole may cause weight gain. Advise patient to monitor weight periodically. Notify health care professional of significant weight gain.
- Instruct patient to notify health care professional of all Rx or OTC medications, vitamins, or herbal products being taken and to consult health care professional before taking any new medications. Caution patient to avoid taking alcohol or other CNS depressants concurrently with this medication.
- Advise patient that extremes in temperature should be avoided, because this drug impairs body temperature regulation.
- Advise patient to notify health care professional if new or increased eating/binge eating, gambling, sexual, shopping, or other impulse control disorders occur.
- Advise patient to notify health care professional of medication regimen prior to treatment or surgery.
- Rep: May cause fetal harm. Advise females of reproductive potential to notify health care professional if pregnancy is planned or suspected and to avoid breastfeeding during therapy. May cause extrapyramidal and/or withdrawal symptoms (agitation, hypertonia, hypotonia, tremor, somnolence, respiratory distress, feeding disorder) in neonates whose mothers were exposed to antipsychotic drugs during third trimester of pregnancy. Symptoms vary in severity. Some neonates recover within hr or days without specific treatment; others require prolonged hospitalization. Monitor neonates for extrapyramidal and/or withdrawal symptoms and manage symptoms appropriately. Encourage pregnant patients to enroll in registry by contacting National Pregnancy Registry for Atypical Antipsychotics at 1-866-961-2388 or visit http://womensmentalhealth.org/clinical-and-research-programs/pregnancyregistry/.
- Emphasize the importance of routine follow-up exams and continued participation in psychotherapy as indicated.

Evaluation/Desired Outcomes

- Decrease in excitable, paranoic, or withdrawn behavior.
- Increased sense of wellbeing in patients with depression.
- Decreased agitation associated with dementia due to Alzheimer's disease.

XXX **brigatinib** (bri-ga-ti-nib)
Alunbrig
Classification
Therapeutic: antineoplastics
Pharmacologic: kinase inhibitors

Indications
XXX Metastatic non-small cell lung cancer (NSCLC) that is positive for anaplastic lymphoma kinase (ALK).

Action
Inhibits receptor tyrosine kinases including anaplastic lymphoma kinase (ALK), insulin-like growth factor-1 receptor (IGF-1R), ROS1, and FMS-like tyrosine kinase-3 (FLT-3). **Therapeutic Effects:** Improved progression free survival in NSCLC.

Pharmacokinetics
Absorption: Well absorbed following oral administration. Bioavailability reduced by high fat meals.
Distribution: Extensively distributed to tissues.
Metabolism and Excretion: Mostly metabolized by the liver (CYP2C8 and CYP3A4 isoenzymes); also induces CYP3A. 27% excreted in feces unchanged, 22% eliminated unchanged in urine.
Half-life: 25 hr.

TIME/ACTION PROFILE (blood levels)

ROUTE	ONSET	PEAK	DURATION
PO	unknown	1–4 hr	unknown

Contraindications/Precautions
Contraindicated in: Concurrent use of moderate or strong inhibitors/inducers of the CYP3A enzyme system; OB: Pregnancy (may cause fetal harm); Lactation: Lactation.
Use Cautiously in: Diabetes; Severe renal or hepatic impairment; Rep: Women of reproductive potential and men with female sexual partners of reproductive potential; Pedi: Safety and effectiveness not established in children.

Adverse Reactions/Side Effects

CV: hypertension, bradycardia. **Derm:** rash, photosensitivity. **EENT:** ↓ visual acuity, blurred vision, diplopia, cataracts, macular edema, photophobia. **Endo:** hyperglycemia. **F and E:** hypophosphatemia. **GI:** ↓ appetite, ↑ amylase, ↑ lipase, ↑ liver enzymes, abdominal pain, constipation, diarrhea, nausea, vomiting. **Hemat:** ↑ activated partial thromboplastin time, anemia, lymphopenia. **MS:** ↑ creatine kinase, arthralgia, back pain, muscle spasms, myalgia. **Neuro:** headache, insomnia, peripheral neuropathy. **Resp:** cough, dyspnea, hypoxia, INTERSTITIAL LUNG DISEASE/PNEUMONITIS, pneumonia. **Misc:** fatigue, fever.

Interactions

Drug-Drug: Strong or moderate CYP3A inhibitors, including, **clarithromycin, cobicistat, conivaptan, itraconazole, ketoconazole, lopinavir, nefazodone, nelfinavir, posaconazole, ritonavir,** and **voriconazole** may ↑ levels; concurrent use should be avoided; if concurrent therapy must be used, ↓ brigatinib dose. **Strong CYP3A inducers,** including **carbamazepine, phenytoin,** and **rifampin** may ↓ levels and effectiveness; concurrent use should be avoided; if concurrent therapy with moderate CYP3A inducer must be used, ↓ brigatinib dose. **Beta-blockers, verapamil, diltiazem, digoxin,** and **clonidine** may ↑ risk of bradycardia; avoid concurrent use, if possible.

Drug-Natural Products: Concurrent use of **St. John's wort** may ↓ levels and effectiveness and should be avoided.

Drug-Food: Grapefruit or **grapefruit juice** may ↑ levels and should be avoided.

Route/Dosage

PO (Adults): 90 mg once daily for 7 days, then 180 mg once daily. Continue until disease progression or unacceptable toxicity. *Concurrent use of strong CYP3A inhibitor:* If previously taking 180 mg once daily, ↓ dose to 90 mg once daily; if previously taking 90 mg once daily, ↓ dose to 60 mg once daily; *Concurrent use of moderate CYP3A inhibitor:* If previously taking 180 mg once daily, ↓ dose to 120 mg once daily; if previously taking 120 mg once daily, ↓ dose to 90 mg once daily; if previously taking 90 mg once daily, ↓ dose to 60 mg once daily; *Concurrent use of moderate CYP3A inducer:* ↑ daily dose in 30-mg increments after 7 days of treatment with the dose used prior to initiation of moderate CYP3A inducer; dose may be ↑ up to a maximum of twice the dose that was tolerated prior to initiating the moderate CYP3A inducer.

Renal Impairment

PO (Adults): *Severe renal impairment (CCr 15–29 mL/min):* If previously taking 180 mg once daily, ↓ dose to 90 mg once daily; if previously taking 90 mg once daily, ↓ dose to 60 mg once daily.

Hepatic Impairment

PO (Adults): *Severe hepatic impairment (Child–Pugh C):* If previously taking 180 mg once daily, ↓ dose to 120 mg once daily; if previously taking 120 mg once daily, ↓ dose to 90 mg once daily; if previously taking 90 mg once daily, ↓ dose to 60 mg once daily.

Availability

Film-coated tablets: 30 mg, 90 mg, 180 mg.

NURSING IMPLICATIONS

Assessment

- Assess respiratory function (lung sounds, dyspnea, oxygen saturation) periodically during therapy.
- Monitor for signs and symptoms of interstitial lung disease (ILD) or pneumonitis (difficulty breathing, shortness or breath, cough with or without mucus, fever) periodically during therapy. **Grade 1:** *If new pulmonary symptoms occur during first 7 days of therapy,* hold brigatinib until recovery to baseline, then resume at same dose; do not escalate to 180 mg if ILD/pneumonitis is suspected. *If new pulmonary symptoms occur after first 7 days of therapy,* hold brigatinib until recovery to baseline, then resume at same dose. *If ILD/pneumonitis recurs,* permanently discontinue brigatinib. **Grade 2:** *If new pulmonary symptoms occur during first 7 days of therapy,* hold brigatinib until recovery to baseline, then resume at same dose; do not escalate to 180 mg if ILD/pneumonitis is suspected. *If new pulmonary symptoms occur after first 7 days of therapy,* hold brigatinib until recovery to baseline. If ILD/pneumonitis is suspected, resume at next lower dose; if not, resume at same dose. *If ILD/pneumonitis recurs,* permanently discontinue brigatinib. **Grade 3 or 4:** Permanently discontinue brigatinib for ILD/pneumonitis.
- Monitor BP prior to therapy, after 2 wk, and monthly during therapy. Control BP prior to therapy. Monitor blood pressure after 2 wk and at least monthly during therapy. *If Grade 3 hypertension (SBP ≥160 mm Hg or DBP ≥100 mm Hg) occurs,* hold brigatinib until hypertension ≤Grade 1 (SBP <140 mm Hg and DBP <90 mm Hg), then resume brigatinib at next lower dose. *If recurrence of Grade 3:* withhold therapy until recovery to ≤Grade 1, and resume at next lower dose or permanently discontinue treatment. *If Grade 4 hypertension (life-threatening consequences, urgent intervention indicated) occurs,* hold brigatinib until ≤Grade 1, and resume at next lower dose or permanently discontinue. *Grade 4 recurrence:* permanently discontinue brigatinib.
- Monitor for bradycardia (HR <60 bpm) periodically during therapy, especially if concurrent medications decrease HR. *If symptomatic bradycardia (dizziness, lightheadedness, fainting) occurs,* hold brigatinib until asymptomatic bradycardia or resting heart rate of ≥60 bpm. *If concomitant medication known to cause bradycardia is identified and discontinued or dose reduced,* resume at same dose once asymptomatic or resting heart rate of ≥60 bpm. *If no concomitant medication known to cause bradycardia, or if contributing concomi-*

B

tant medications are not discontinued or dose re-duced, resume brigatinib at next lower dose upon recovery to asymptomatic bradycardia or to resting heart rate of ≥60 bpm. *If bradycardia with life-threatening consequences or urgent intervention needed,* permanently discontinue brigatinib if no contributing concomitant medication is identified. *If contributing concomitant medication is identi-fied and discontinued or dose reduced,* resume therapy at next lower dose when recovered to asymptomatic bradycardia or to a resting heart rate of ≥60 bpm, with frequent monitoring. *Grade 4 re-currence:* permanently discontinue therapy.

- Treat hypertension before starting therapy. Monitor BP after 2 wks and at least monthly during therapy. *If Grade 3 hypertension (SBP ≥160 mmHg or DBP ≥100 mmHg) occurs,* hold brigatinib until hyper-tension ≤Grade 1 (SBP <140 mmHg and DBP <90 mmHg), then resume therapy at same dose. If hyper-tension recurs, hold brigatinib until ≤Grade 1; re-sume at next lower dose or permanently discontinue therapy. *If Grade 4 hypertension (life-threaten-ing) occurs,* hold brigatinib until ≤Grade 1; resume at next lower dose or permanently discontinue ther-apy. If Grade 4 hypertension recurs, permanently discontinue brigatinib.

- Monitor for visual changes (blurred vision, diplopia, reduced visual acuity) periodically during therapy. *If Grade 2 or 3 visual disturbance occurs,* hold doses until recovery to Grade 1 or baseline, then resume at next lower dose. *If Grade 4 visual disturbance oc-curs,* discontinue brigatinib permanently.

Lab Test Considerations

- Verify negative pregnancy before starting therapy.▓ Information on FDA-approved tests for the detection of ALK rearrangements in NSCLC is available at http://www.fda.gov/CompanionDiagnostics.Monitor CK levels periodically during therapy. *If Grade 3 CK ↑ (>5× upper limit of normal [ULN]) occurs,* hold therapy until ≤Grade 1 (≤2.5× ULN) or to baseline, then resume at same dose. *If Grade 4 CK ↑ (>10× ULN) or recurrence of Grade 3 ↑ occurs,* hold bri-gatinib until ≤Grade 1 (≤2.5× ULN) or to baseline, then resume therapy at next lower dose.

- Monitor serum lipase and amylase periodically dur-ing therapy. *If Grade 3 lipase or amylase ↑ (>2× ULN) occurs,* hold brigatinib until ≤Grade 1 (≤1.5× ULN) or baseline, then resume brigatinib at same dose. *If Grade 4 lipase or amylase ↑ (>5× ULN) or recurrence of Grade 3 ↑ occurs,* hold bri-gatinib until ≤Grade 1 (≤ 1.5× ULN) or baseline, then resume therapy at next lower dose.

- Monitor fasting serum glucose prior to starting and periodically during therapy. May cause new or wors-ening hyperglycemia. Use antihyperglycemic medi-cations as needed. If Grade 3 (>250 mg/dL) or Grade 4 hyperglycemia occurs, hold brigatinib until adequate hyperglycemic control is achieved and re-sume at next lower dose or discontinue brigatinib.

- Monitor AST, ALT, and total bilirubin during therapy, especially during first 3 mo. *If Grade 3 or 4 eleva-tion (>5× ULN) of either ALT or AST with biliru-bin ≤2× ULN,* hold brigatinib until recovery to ≤ Grade 1 (≤ 3x ULN) or to baseline, then resume at next lower dose. *If Grade 2 to 4 elevation (>3× ULN) of ALT or AST with concurrent total bilirubin elevation >2× ULN in the absence of cholestasis or hemolysis,* permanently discontinue brigatinib.

Implementation

- Dose reductions for adverse reactions. **Patients taking 90 mg once daily:** *First reduction:* 60 mg once daily. *Second reduction:* permanently discon-tinue brigatinib. **Patients taking 180 mg once daily:** *First reduction:* 120 mg once daily. *Second reduction:* 90 mg once daily. *Third reduction:* 60 mg once daily.

- **PO:** Administer daily without regard to food. *DNC:* Swallow tablets whole; do not crush, break, or chew.If therapy is interrupted for 14 days or longer, other than adverse reactions, resume therapy at 90 mg once daily for 7 days before increasing to previ-ously tolerated dose.

Patient/Family Teaching

- Instruct patient to take brigatinib as directed. If pa-tient vomits or misses a dose, omit dose and take next dose as scheduled. Do not double doses. Advise patient to read *Patient Information* before starting therapy and with each Rx refill in case of changes.

- Advise patient to avoid eating grapefruit or drinking grapefruit juice during therapy.

- Advise patient to notify health care professional if signs and symptoms of lung problems (cough, chest pain, fever), hypertension (headaches, dizziness, blurred vision, chest pain, shortness of breath), bradycardia (dizziness, lightheadedness, feeling faint), visual changes (double vision, seeing flashes of light, blurry vision, light hurting eyes, new or in-creased floaters), symptoms of pancreatitis (upper abdominal pain, weight loss, nausea), new or wors-ening symptoms of myalgia (unexplained muscle pain, tenderness, or weakness), or hyperglycemia (feeling very thirsty, needing to urinate more than usual, feeling very hungry, nausea, feeling weak or tired, feeling confused) occur, may require dose re-duction or discontinuation.

- Advise patients to limit sun exposure while taking brigatinib, and for at least 5 days after stopping ther-apy. Wear a hat and protective clothing, and use a broad-spectrum Ultraviolet A (UVA)/ Ultraviolet B (UVB) sunscreen and lip balm (SPF ≥30) to help protect against sunburn. Sunburn may require inter-rupting or discontinuing therapy based on severity.

✸= Canadian drug name. ▓ = Genetic implication. ~~Strikethrough~~ = Discontinued. CAPITALS = life-threatening. Underline = most frequent.

- Instruct patient to notify health care professional of all Rx or OTC medications, vitamins, or herbal products being taken and consult health care professional before taking any new medications, especially St. John's wort.
- Rep: May cause fetal harm. Advise females of reproductive potential to use effective non-hormonal contraception during and for at least 4 mo after final dose. Advise males with female partners of reproductive potential to use effective contraception during and for at least 3 mo after last dose of brigatinib. Advise patient to avoid breastfeeding during and for 1 wk after last dose. Inform male patient that brigatinib may impair fertility.

Evaluation/Desired Outcomes
- Decreased spread in lung cancer.

▧ brivaracetam
(briv-a-**ra**-se-tam)
Briviact, ✦ Brivlera
Classification
Therapeutic: anticonvulsants

Schedule V

Indications
Partial-onset seizures.

Action
Displays a high and selective affinity for synaptic vesicle protein 2A (SV2A) in the brain, which may contribute to its anticonvulsant effect. **Therapeutic Effects:** Decreased incidence of seizures.

Pharmacokinetics
Absorption: Rapidly and completely absorbed following oral administration. IV administration results in complete bioavailability.

Distribution: Widely distributed to tissues.

Metabolism and Excretion: Hepatic and extrahepatic amidase-mediated hydrolysis of the amide moiety to form carboxylic acid metabolite (primary route) and hydroxylation primarily by the CYP2C19 isoenzyme to form the hydroxy metabolite (secondary route) (all metabolites inactive). ▧ The CYP2C19 isoenzyme exhibits genetic polymorphism (2% of Whites, 4% of Blacks, and 14% of Asians may be poor metabolizers and may have significantly ↑ brivaracetam concentrations and an ↑ risk of adverse effects). >95% excreted by the kidneys (<10% excreted unchanged).

Half-life: 9 hr.

TIME/ACTION PROFILE (plasma concentrations)

ROUTE	ONSET	PEAK	DURATION
PO	unknown	1–4hr†	unknown
IV	unknown	end of infusion	unknown

† 1 hr in fasting state; 4 hr with high-fat meal.

Contraindications/Precautions
Contraindicated in: Hypersensitivity; End-stage renal disease.

Use Cautiously in: All patients (may ↑ risk of suicidal thoughts/behaviors); ▧ Patients who are known or suspected to be poor CYP2C19 metabolizers (may require dose ↓); Hepatic impairment (dose ↓ recommended); OB: Safety not established in pregnancy; Lactation: Safety not established in breastfeeding; Pedi: Children <1 mo (safety and effectiveness not established); Geri: Dose adjustment may be needed because of ↓ renal and hepatic function in older adults.

Adverse Reactions/Side Effects
EENT: nystagmus. **GI:** constipation, nausea, vomiting. **Hemat:** leukopenia. **Local:** infusion site pain. **Neuro:** aggression, agitation, anger, anxiety, apathy, belligerence, depression, dizziness, drowsiness, hallucinations, irritability, mood swings, paranoia, psychosis, restlessness, SUICIDAL THOUGHTS/BEHAVIOR, tearfulness, vertigo, ataxia, balance disorder, coordination difficulties, dysgeusia, euphoria, fatigue. **Misc:** HYPERSENSITIVITY REACTIONS (including bronchospasm and angioedema).

Interactions
Drug-Drug: CYP2C19 inducers including **rifampin** may ↓ levels and effectiveness; ↑ brivaracetam dose by up to 100%. Concurrent use with **carbamazepine** may ↑ levels of carbamazepine-epoxide (active metabolite); consider ↓ dose of carbamazepine if tolerability issues occur. May ↑ levels of **phenytoin**.

Route/Dosage
IV route should only be used when oral therapy is not feasible.

PO, IV (Adults and Children ≥16 yr): 50 mg twice daily; may titrate down to 25 mg twice daily or up to 100 mg twice daily based on tolerability and effectiveness.

PO, IV (Children ≥1 mo and ≥50 kg): 25–50 mg twice daily; may titrate up to 100 mg twice daily based on tolerability and effectiveness.

PO, IV (Children ≥1 mo and 20–<50 kg): 0.5-1 mg/kg twice daily; may titrate up to 2 mg/kg twice daily based on tolerability and effectiveness.

PO, IV (Children ≥1 mo and 11–<20 kg): 0.5-1.25 mg/kg twice daily; may titrate up to 2.5 mg/kg twice daily based on tolerability and effectiveness.

PO, IV (Children ≥1 mo and <11 kg): 0.75-1.5 mg/kg twice daily; may titrate up to 3 mg/kg twice daily based on tolerability and effectiveness.

Hepatic Impairment
PO, IV (Adults and Children ≥16 yr): 25 mg twice daily; may titrate up to 75 mg twice daily based on tolerability and effectiveness.

Hepatic Impairment
PO, IV (Children ≥1 mo and ≥50 kg): 25 mg twice daily; may titrate up to 75 mg twice daily based on tolerability and effectiveness.

Hepatic Impairment
PO, IV (Children ≥1 mo and 20–<50 kg): 0.5 mg/kg twice daily; may titrate up to 1.5 mg/kg twice daily based on tolerability and effectiveness.

Hepatic Impairment
PO, IV (Children ≥1 mo and 11–<20 kg): 0.5 mg/kg twice daily; may titrate up to 2 mg/kg twice daily based on tolerability and effectiveness.

Hepatic Impairment
PO, IV (Children ≥1 mo and <11 kg): 0.75 mg/kg twice daily; may titrate up to 2.25 mg/kg twice daily based on tolerability and effectiveness.

Availability (generic available)
Tablets: 10 mg, 25 mg, 50 mg, 75 mg, 100 mg. **Oral solution (raspberry-flavored):** 10 mg/mL. **Solution for injection:** 10 mg/mL.

NURSING IMPLICATIONS
Assessment
● Assess mental status (orientation, mood, behavior) before and periodically during therapy. Monitor closely for notable changes in behavior that could indicate the emergence or worsening of suicidal thoughts or behavior or depression.
● Monitor for signs and symptoms of bronchospasm (wheezing, dyspnea) and angioedema (rash, pruritus, perioral swelling) during therapy. If signs of hypersensitivity occur discontinue brivaracetam.

Lab Test Considerations
● May cause ↓ WBC and neutrophil counts.

Implementation
● *High Alert:* Do not confuse Briviact with Brilinta.
● Initiate therapy with oral or IV administration. IV administration may be used when oral dose is not feasible; administer at same dose and frequency as oral doses.
● **PO:** Administer twice daily without regard to food. *DNC:* Swallow tablets whole with liquid; do not crush or chew.
● Use a calibrated measuring device for accuracy with oral solution. Dilution is not necessary, May be administered via nasogastric or gastrostomy tube. Oral solution is stable for 5 mo after opening.

IV Administration
● **Intermittent Infusion:** *Dilution:* May be administered undiluted or diluted with 0.9% NaCl, LR, or D5W. Solution is clear and colorless; do not administer solutions that are discolored or contain particulate matter. Solution is stable for up to 4 hr at room temperature; may be stored in polyvinyl chloride bags. *Rate:* Administer over 2–15 min.

Patient/Family Teaching
● Instruct patient to take brivaracetam as directed. Decrease dose gradually; do not stop abruptly to minimize risk of increased seizure frequency and status epilepticus. Advise patient to read *Medication Guide* prior to therapy and with each Rx refill in case of changes.
● May cause drowsiness, fatigue, dizziness, and balance problems. Caution patient to avoid driving or other activities requiring alertness until response to medication is known. Do not resume driving until physician gives clearance based on control of seizure disorder.
● Advise patient and family to notify health care professional if behavioral changes, thoughts about suicide or dying, attempts to commit suicide; new or worse depression; new or worse anxiety; feeling very agitated or restless; panic attacks; trouble sleeping; new or worse irritability; acting aggressive; being angry or violent; acting on dangerous impulses; an extreme increase in activity and talking; other unusual changes in behavior or mood occur.
● Advise patient to notify health care professional of all Rx or OTC medications, vitamins, or herbal products being taken and to consult with health care professional before taking other medications.
● Rep: Advise females of reproductive potential to notify health care professional if pregnancy is planned or suspected or if breastfeeding. Encourage patients who become pregnant to enroll in the North American Antiepileptic Drug (NAAED) Pregnancy Registry by calling 1-888-233-2334 or on the web at www.aedpregnancyregistry.org. Enrollment must be done by patients themselves.

Evaluation/Desired Outcomes
● Decreased incidence of partial-onset seizures.

REMS

brodalumab (broe-dal-ue-mab)
Siliq
Classification
Therapeutic: antipsoriatics
Pharmacologic: interleukin antagonists

Indications
Moderate to severe plaque psoriasis in patients who are candidates for systemic therapy or phototherapy and have failed to respond or have lost response to other systemic therapies.

Action
A monoclonal antibody that acts as an antagonist of interleukin (IL)–17RA by selectively binding to it and preventing its interaction with numerous IL cytokines. Antagonism prevents production of inflammatory cytokines and chemokines. **Therapeutic Effects:** Decreased plaque formation and spread.

Pharmacokinetics
Absorption: 55% absorbed following SUBQ administration.
Distribution: Minimally distributed to tissues.
Metabolism and Excretion: Primarily eliminated by being catabolized into small peptides and amino acids.
Half-life: Unknown.

TIME/ACTION PROFILE (plasma concentrations)

ROUTE	ONSET	PEAK	DURATION
SUBQ	unknown	3 days	unknown

Contraindications/Precautions
Contraindicated in: Crohn's disease (may worsen disease); Active tuberculosis (TB).
Use Cautiously in: History of suicidality or depression; Chronic infection or history of recurrent infection; OB: Safety not established in pregnancy; Lactation: Safety not established in breastfeeding; Pedi: Safety and effectiveness not established in children.

Adverse Reactions/Side Effects
EENT: oropharyngeal pain. **GI:** Crohn's disease, diarrhea, nausea. **Hemat:** neutropenia. **Local:** injection site reactions. **MS:** arthralgia, myalgia. **Neuro:** headache, SUICIDAL THOUGHTS/BEHAVIORS. **Misc:** fatigue, INFECTION (including reactivation TB).

Interactions
Drug-Drug: May ↓ antibody response to **live-virus vaccine** and ↑ risk of adverse reactions (do not administer concurrently). May affect activity of CYP450 enzymes and may alter the effectiveness/toxicity of drugs that are substrates of CYP450 (including **warfarin** and **cyclosporine**); close monitoring is recommended and necessary dose modifications undertaken.

Route/Dosage
SUBQ (Adults): 210 mg at Wk 0, 1, and 2 then 210 mg every 2 wk; consider discontinuing therapy if adequate response not achieved after 12–16 wk of therapy.

Availability
Solution for SUBQ injection (prefilled syringes): 210 mg/1.5 mL.

NURSING IMPLICATIONS

Assessment
- Assess skin lesions prior to and periodically during therapy.
- Assess for TB infection prior to starting therapy. Begin treatment for latent TB prior to brodalumab administration; do not administer to patients with active TB infection.
- Assess for new or worsening symptoms of depression, anxiety, other mood disorders, or suicidality. Refer to mental health professional as appropriate. Re-evaluate risks and benefits of brodalumab if depression occurs.

- Monitor for signs and symptoms of infection (fever, sweats, chills, muscle aches, cough, dyspnea, sore throat or difficulty swallowing, warm, red, or painful skin or sores, diarrhea or stomach pain, burning or frequency of urination) during therapy. If serious infection develops or is not responding to therapy, monitor patient closely and discontinue brodalumab until infection resolves.

Implementation
- Available only through restricted program called Siliq REMS due to suicide risks. Providers must be certified, patients must sign a Patient-Provider Agreement form, and pharmacies must be certified and only dispense to patients authorized to receive brodalumab. Further information and a list of qualified pharmacies can be found at www.SILIQREMS.com or by calling 855-511-6135.
- **SUBQ:** Allow prefilled syringe to reach room temperature for approximately 30 min before injecting. Do not warm any other way. Solution is clear to slightly opalescent, colorless to slightly yellow. A few translucent to white, amorphous proteinaceous particles may be present; do not administer if solution is cloudy or discolored. Inject full dose (1.5 mL) into thigh, abdomen, or upper arm. Pinch skin and inject at a 45° or 90° angle. Do not rub injection site. Do not inject in skin areas that are tender, bruised, red, hard, thick, scaly, or affected by psoriasis. Store in refrigerator or at room temperature for up to 14 days; do not return to refrigerator after room temperature. Protect from light. Do not freeze.

Patient/Family Teaching
- Advise patient to administer injection as directed, according to schedule. Health care professional should supervise first self-injection. Instruct patient to inject full dose, and to use proper technique for syringe and needle disposal. Inform patient that they must enroll in SILIQ REMS program and to carry SILIQ Patient Wallet Card at all times and share with other health care professionals. Card describes symptoms that, if experienced, should prompt patient to seek immediate medical evaluation. Provide patient with telephone number and website for pharmacies participating in SILIQ REMS program.
- Caution patient to avoid live vaccines during therapy.
- May cause depression or suicide. Instruct patients and caregivers to monitor for emergence of suicidal thoughts and behaviors. Notify health care professional immediately if suicidal thoughts, new or worsening depression, anxiety, changes in behavior or mood, thoughts of suicide, dying, or hurting self, or acting on dangerous impulses occur. Instruct patient to carry wallet card and to call the national Suicide Prevention Lifeline at 1-800-273-8255 if they experience suicidal thoughts.
- Instruct patient to notify health care professional if signs and symptoms of infection occur.
- Instruct patient to notify health care professional of all Rx or OTC medications, vitamins, or herbal prod-

ucts being taken and consult health care professional before taking any new medications.

- Rep: Advise female patient to notify health care professional if pregnancy is planned or suspected or if breastfeeding.

Evaluation/Desired Outcomes

- Decrease in plaque formation and spread of plaque psoriasis. Consider discontinuing if adequate response not achieved after 12–16 wk. Treatment beyond 16 wk in patients without an adequate response is not likely to result in greater success.

budesonide/formoterol/ glycopyrrolate

(byoo-**des**-oh-nide/for-**moe**-te-rol/ glye-koe-**pye**-roe-late)
Breztri Aerosphere
Classification
Therapeutic: anti-inflammatories (steroidal), bronchodilators
Pharmacologic: corticosteroids, long-acting beta₂-adrenergic agonists (LABAs), anticholinergics

Indications

Maintenance treatment of COPD.

Action

Budesonide: Potent, locally acting anti-inflammatory; *formoterol:* a beta₂-adrenergic agonist that stimulates adenyl cyclase, resulting in accumulation of cyclic adenosine monophosphate at beta₂–adrenergic receptors resulting in bronchodilation; *glycopyrrolate:* acts as an anticholinergic by inhibiting M3 muscarinic receptors in bronchial smooth muscle resulting in bronchodilation. **Therapeutic Effects:** Bronchodilation with decreased airflow obstruction.

Pharmacokinetics

Budesonide
Absorption: Unknown.
Distribution: Extensively distributed to extravascular tissues.
Metabolism and Excretion: Primarily metabolized by the liver by the CYP3A4 isoenzyme into inactive metabolites; primarily excreted in urine and feces as metabolites.
Half-life: 5 hr.
Formoterol
Absorption: Unknown.
Distribution: Extensively distributed to extravascular tissues.
Metabolism and Excretion: Primarily metabolized by the liver by glucuronidation and O-demethylation to inactive metabolites; 62% of drug excreted in urine, 24% excreted in feces.

Half-life: 10 hr.
Glycopyrrolate
Absorption: Unknown.
Distribution: Extensively distributed to extravascular tissues.
Metabolism and Excretion: Primarily metabolized by the liver, with the CYP2D6 isoenzyme playing a minor role in elimination; 85% excreted in urine.
Half-life: 15 hr.

TIME/ACTION PROFILE (improvement in FEV₁)

ROUTE	ONSET	PEAK	DURATION
Inhalation	within 5 min	4 wk	unknown

Contraindications/Precautions

Contraindicated in: Hypersensitivity; Asthma; Acutely deteriorating COPD or acute respiratory symptoms.

Use Cautiously in: Systemic corticosteroid therapy (should not be abruptly discontinued when inhaled therapy is started; additional corticosteroids needed during stress or trauma); Prolonged immobilization, family history of osteoporosis, postmenopausal status, cigarette smoking, advanced age, or poor nutrition (↑ risk of osteoporosis); Narrow-angle glaucoma; Seizure disorders; Thyrotoxicosis; Urinary retention, prostatic hyperplasia, bladder-neck obstruction; Diabetes; Severe hepatic impairment; Severe renal impairment (CCr <30 mL/min) or end-stage renal disease requiring dialysis (use only if expected benefit exceeds potential risk); OB: Safety not established in pregnancy; Lactation: Use while breastfeeding only if potential maternal benefit justifies potential risk to infant; Pedi: Safety and effectiveness not established in children.

Exercise Extreme Caution in: Concurrent use of MAO inhibitors, tricyclic antidepressants, or drugs that prolong the QTc interval.

Adverse Reactions/Side Effects

CV: arrhythmias, hypertension, tachycardia. **EENT:** cataracts, glaucoma, sinusitis. **Endo:** adrenal suppression (high dose, long-term therapy only), hyperglycemia. **F and E:** hypokalemia. **GI:** diarrhea, oropharyngeal candidiasis. **MS:** ↓ bone density, muscle spasms. **Resp:** bronchospasm, cough, pneumonia. **Misc:** HYPERSENSITIVITY REACTIONS (including angioedema, urticaria, or rash).

Interactions

Drug-Drug: Strong **CYP3A4 inhibitors**, including **atazanavir, clarithromycin, itraconazole, ketoconazole, nefazodone, nelfinavir,** and **ritonavir** may ↑ levels and risk of toxicity. **Anticonvulsants, oral corticosteroids,** and **proton pump inhibitors** may ↑ risk of osteoporosis. Concurrent use with other **adrenergics** may ↑ adrenergic adverse reactions of formoterol (↑ heart rate, ↑ BP, jitteriness). **Xanthine derivatives**, **corticosteroids**, **diuretics** may ↑ risk of hypokalemia or ECG changes with formoterol. ↑ risk of serious adverse cardiovascular effects with **MAO inhibitors**, **tricyclic antidepressants**, **QT-interval prolonging drugs**; use with extreme caution. Effectiveness of formoterol may be ↓ by **beta-blockers**; use cautiously and only when necessary. ↑ risk of anticholinergic adverse reactions with glycopyrrolate when used concurrently with other **anticholinergics**; avoid concurrent use.

Route/Dosage
Inhaln (Adults): 2 inhalations twice daily.

Availability
Inhalation aerosol: budesonide 160 mcg/glycopyrrolate 9 mcg/formoterol 4.8 mcg per inhalation in 10.7-g canister (120 inhalations).

NURSING IMPLICATIONS
Assessment
- Assess lung sounds, pulse, and BP before administration and during peak of medication. Note amount, color, and character of sputum produced.
- Observe for paradoxical bronchospasm (wheezing, dyspnea, tightness in chest) and hypersensitivity reaction (rash; urticaria; swelling of the face, lips, or eyelids). If condition occurs, withhold medication and notify health care professional immediately.
- Monitor patient for signs of hypersensitivity reactions (difficulties in breathing or swallowing; swelling of tongue, lips, and face; urticaria; skin rash) during therapy. Discontinue therapy and consider alternative if reaction occurs.

Lab Test Considerations
- May ↑ serum glucose and ↓ serum potassium.

Implementation
- **Inhaln:** Administer as 2 inhalations twice daily, morning and evening. Shake well prior to use. Prime by releasing 4 sprays into air away from face before 1st use and by releasing 2 sprays if unused for more than 7 days. After inhalation, rinse mouth with water without swallowing. See Appendix C for use of metered-dose inhalers.

Patient/Family Teaching
- Instruct patient to use medication as directed. Do not discontinue therapy without discussing with health care professional, even if feeling better. If a dose is missed, skip dose and take next dose at regularly scheduled time. Do not double doses. Use a rapid-acting bronchodilator if symptoms occur before next dose is due. Caution patient not to use more than 2 times a day; may cause adverse effects, paradoxical bronchospasm, or loss of effectiveness of medication. Instruct patient to review *Medication Guide* before starting therapy and with each Rx refill in case of changes.

- Advise patient that inhaler should be discarded when display window indicates zero or 3 mo (120-inhalation canister) or 3 wk (28-inhalation canister) after removal of canister from pouch, whichever comes first. Never immerse the canister into water to determine the amount remaining in the canister ("float test").
- Caution patient not to use medication to treat acute symptoms. A rapid-acting inhaled beta-adrenergic bronchodilator should be used for relief of acute asthma attacks. Notify health care professional immediately if symptoms get worse or more inhalations than usual are needed from rescue inhaler.
- Advise patient to rinse the mouth with water without swallowing after inhalation to help reduce the risk of getting a fungus infection (thrush) in the mouth and throat.
- Instruct patient to contact health care professional immediately if shortness of breath is not relieved by medication or nausea, vomiting, shakiness, headache, fast or irregular heartbeat, sleeplessness, or signs and symptoms of narrow angle glaucoma (eye pain or discomfort, blurred vision, visual halos or colored images, red eyes), urinary retention (difficulty passing urine, painful urination) or pneumonia (increase in mucus (sputum) production, change in mucus color, fever, chills, increased cough, increased breathing problems) occur.
- Advise patient to consult health care professional before taking any Rx, OTC, or herbal products or alcohol concurrently with this therapy. Caution patient also to avoid smoking and other respiratory irritants.
- Rep: Advise females of reproductive potential to notify health care professional if pregnancy is planned or suspected or if breastfeeding.

Evaluation/Desired Outcomes
- Bronchodilation with decreased airflow obstruction.

budesonide, See CORTICOSTEROIDS (INHALATION).

budesonide, See CORTICOSTEROIDS (NASAL).

budesonide, See CORTICOSTEROIDS (SYSTEMIC).

BEERS

bumetanide (byoo-met-a-nide)
~~Bumex~~, ✦Burinex

Classification
Therapeutic: diuretics
Pharmacologic: loop diuretics

Indications

Edema due to heart failure, hepatic disease, or renal impairment. **Unlabeled Use:** Reversal of oliguria in preterm neonates.

Action

Inhibits the reabsorption of sodium and chloride from the loop of Henle and distal renal tubule. Increases renal excretion of water, sodium chloride, magnesium, potassium, and calcium. Effectiveness persists in impaired renal function. **Therapeutic Effects:** Diuresis and subsequent mobilization of excess fluid (edema, pleural effusions).

Pharmacokinetics

Absorption: Well absorbed after oral or IM administration. IV administration results in complete bioavailability.

Distribution: Widely distributed.
Protein Binding: 72–96%.
Metabolism and Excretion: Partially metabolized by liver; 50% eliminated unchanged by kidneys and 20% excreted in feces.
Half-life: 60–90 min (6 hr in neonates).

TIME/ACTION PROFILE (diuretic effect)

ROUTE	ONSET	PEAK	DURATION
PO	30–60 min	1–2 hr	4–6 hr
IM	30–60 min	1–2 hr	4–6 hr
IV	2–3 min	15–45 min	2–3 hr

Contraindications/Precautions

Contraindicated in: Hypersensitivity; Cross-sensitivity with thiazides and sulfonamides may occur; Hepatic coma or anuria; Lactation: Lactation.

Use Cautiously in: Severe liver disease (may precipitate hepatic coma; concurrent use with potassium-sparing diuretics may be necessary); Electrolyte depletion; Diabetes mellitus; Increasing azotemia; Pedi: Potent displacer of bilirubin and should be used cautiously in critically ill or jaundiced neonates because of risk of kernicterus. Injection contains benzyl alcohol, which may cause gasping syndrome in neonates. Safety and effectiveness not established in children; Geri: Appears on Beers list. May worsen or cause hyponatremia in older adults. Use with caution in older adults and monitor sodium concentrations closely when initiating therapy or ↑ the dose.

Adverse Reactions/Side Effects

CV: hypotension. **Derm:** photosensitivity, pruritus, rash, STEVENS-JOHNSON SYNDROME, TOXIC EPIDERMAL NECROLYSIS. **EENT:** hearing loss, tinnitus. **Endo:** hyperglycemia, hyperuricemia. **F and E:** <u>dehydration</u>, <u>hypochloremia</u>, <u>hypokalemia</u>, <u>hypomagnesemia</u>, <u>hyponatremia</u>, <u>hypovolemia</u>, <u>metabolic alkalosis</u>, hypocalcemia. **GI:** diarrhea, dry mouth, nausea, vomiting. **GU:** ↑ BUN. **MS:** arthralgia, muscle cramps, myalgia. **Neuro:** dizziness, encephalopathy, headache.

Interactions

Drug-Drug: ↑ risk of hypotension with **antihypertensives**, **nitrates**, or acute ingestion of **alcohol**. ↑ risk of hypokalemia with other **diuretics**, **amphotericin B**, **stimulant laxatives**, and **corticosteroids**. Hypokalemia may ↑ risk of **digoxin** toxicity. ↓ **lithium** excretion, may cause **lithium** toxicity. ↑ risk of ototoxicity with **aminoglycosides**. **NSAIDs** ↓ effects of bumetanide.

Route/Dosage

PO (Adults): 0.5–2 mg/day given in 1–2 doses; titrate to desired response (maximum daily dose = 10 mg/day).
PO (Infants and Children): 0.015–0.1 mg/kg/dose every 6–24 hrs (maximum: 10 mg/day).
PO (Neonates): 0.01–0.05 mg/kg/dose every 12–24 hr in term neonates or every 24–48 hr in preterm neonates.
IM, IV (Adults): 0.5–1 mg/dose, may repeat every 2–3 hr as needed (up to 10 mg/day).
IM, IV (Infants and Children): 0.015–0.1 mg/kg/dose every 6–24 hr (maximum: 10 mg/day).
IM, IV (Neonates): 0.01–0.05 mg/kg/dose every 12–24 hr in term neonates or every 24–48 hr in preterm neonates.

Availability (generic available)

Tablets: 0.5 mg, 1 mg, 2 mg, ✿ 5 mg. **Solution for injection:** 0.25 mg/mL.

NURSING IMPLICATIONS

Assessment

- Assess fluid status during therapy. Monitor daily weight, intake and output ratios, amount and location of edema, lung sounds, skin turgor, and mucous membranes. Notify health care professional if thirst, dry mouth, lethargy, weakness, hypotension, or oliguria occurs.
- Monitor BP and pulse before and during administration. Monitor frequency of prescription refills to determine compliance.
- Assess patients receiving digoxin for anorexia, nausea, vomiting, muscle cramps, paresthesia, and confusion; ↑ risk of digoxin toxicity due to potassium-depleting effect of diuretic. Potassium supplements or potassium-sparing diuretics may be used concurrently to prevent hypokalemia.
- Assess patient for tinnitus and hearing loss. Audiometry is recommended for patients receiving prolonged high-dose IV therapy. Hearing loss is most common after rapid or high-dose IV administration in patients with decreased renal function or those taking other ototoxic drugs.
- Assess for allergy to sulfonamides.
- Assess patient for skin rash frequently during therapy. Discontinue bumetanide at first sign of rash;

may be life-threatening. Stevens-Johnson syndrome or toxic epidermal necrolysis may develop. Treat symptomatically; may recur once treatment is stopped.

● Geri: Diuretic use is associated with increased risk for falls in older adults. Assess falls risk and implement fall prevention strategies.

Lab Test Considerations

● Monitor electrolytes, renal and hepatic function, serum glucose, and uric acid levels before and periodically during therapy. May cause ↓ serum sodium, potassium, calcium, and magnesium concentrations. May also cause ↑ BUN, serum glucose, creatinine, and uric acid levels.

Implementation

● If administering twice daily, give last dose no later than 5 PM to minimize disruption of sleep cycle.

● IV is preferred over IM for parenteral administration.

● PO: May be taken with food to minimize gastric irritation.

IV Administration

● **IV Push:** *Dilution:* Administer undiluted. *Concentration:* 0.25 mg/mL. *Rate:* Administer slowly over 1–2 min.

● **Continuous Infusion:** *Dilution:* May dilute in D5W or 0.9% NaCl. May also administer as undiluted drug. Protect from light. *Concentration:* Not to exceed 0.25 mg/mL. *Rate:* Infuse over 5 min. May be administered over 12 hr for patients with renal impairment.

● **Y-Site Compatibility:** acyclovir, allopurinol, amifostine, amikacin, aminocaproic acid, aminophylline, amiodarone, amphotericin B lipid complex, amphotericin B liposome, anidulafungin, argatroban, ascorbic acid, atropine, azithromycin, aztreonam, benztropine, bivalirudin, bleomycin, buprenorphine, butorphanol, calcium chloride, calcium gluconate, carboplatin, carmustine, caspofungin, cefazolin, cefepime, cefotaxime, cefoxitin, ceftaroline, ceftazidime, ceftriaxone, cefuroxime, chloramphenicol, cisatracurium, cisplatin, cladribine, clindamycin, cyanocobalamin, cyclophosphamide, cyclosporine, cytarabine, dactinomycin, daptomycin, dexamethasone, dexmedetomidine, dexrazoxane, digoxin, diltiazem, diphenhydramine, dobutamine, docetaxel, dopamine, doxorubicin hydrochloride, doxorubicin liposomal, doxycycline, enalaprilat, ephedrine, epinephrine, epirubicin, epoetin alfa, eptifibatide, ertapenem, erythromycin, esmolol, etoposide, etoposide phosphate, famotidine, fentanyl, filgrastim, fluconazole, fludarabine, fluorouracil, folic acid, furosemide, gemcitabine, gentamicin, glycopyrrolate, granisetron, heparin, hetastarch, hydrocortisone sodium succinate, hydromorphone, idarubicin, ifosfamide, imipenem/cilastatin, indomethacin, insulin, irinotecan, isoproterenol, ketorolac, labetalol, leucovorin calcium, levofloxacin, lidocaine, linezolid, lorazepam, magnesium sulfate, mannitol, melphalan, meperidine, methotrexate, methylprednisolone sodium succinate, metoclopramide, metoprolol, metronidazole, micafungin, milrinone, mitoxantrone, morphine, moxifloxacin, multivitamins, mycophenolate, nafcillin, nalbuphine, naloxone, nitroglycerin, nitroprusside, norepinephrine, octreotide, ondansetron, oxacillin, oxaliplatin, oxytocin, paclitaxcel, palonosetron, pamidronate, pantoprazole, pemetrexed, penicillin G, pentobarbital, phenobarbital, phentolamine, phenylephrine, phytonadione, piperacillin/tazobactam, potassium acetate, potassium chloride, procainamide, promethazine, propofol, propranolol, protamine, pyridoxine, remifentanil, rifampin, rituximab, rocuronium, sodium acetate, sodium bicarbonate, succinylcholine, sufentanil, tacrolimus, theophylline, thiamine, thiotepa, tigecycline, tirofiban, tobramycin, trastuzumab, vancomycin, vasopressin, vecuronium, verapamil, vinblastine, vincristine, vinorelbine, voriconazole, zoledronic acid.

● **Y-Site Incompatibility:** alemtuzumab, amphotericin B deoxycholate, azathioprine, chlorpromazine, dantrolene, diazepam, diazoxide, ganciclovir, haloperidol, papaverine, pentamidine, phenytoin, trimethoprim/sulfamethoxazole.

Patient/Family Teaching

● Instruct patient to take bumetanide as directed. Take missed doses as soon as possible; do not double doses.

● Caution patient to change positions slowly to minimize orthostatic hypotension. Caution patient that drinking alcohol, exercising during hot weather, or standing for long periods may enhance orthostatic hypotension.

● Instruct patient to consult health care professional regarding a diet high in potassium. See Appendix J.

● Advise patient to contact health care professional of gain more than 3 lbs in one day.

● Instruct patient to notify health care professional of all Rx or OTC medications, vitamins, or herbal products being taken and to consult health care professional before taking any OTC medications concurrently with this therapy.

● Instruct patient to notify health care professional of medication regimen before treatment or surgery.

● Caution patient to use sunscreen and protective clothing to prevent photosensitivity reactions.

● Advise patient to contact health care professional immediately if rash, muscle weakness, cramps, nausea, dizziness, numbness, or tingling of extremities occurs.

● Advise patients with diabetes to monitor blood glucose closely; may cause increased levels.

● Rep: Advise females of reproductive potential to notify health care professional if pregnancy is planned or suspected and to avoid breastfeeding. Diuretics

have the potential to decrease milk volume and suppress lactation.
● Emphasize the importance of routine follow-up examinations.
● Geri: Caution older patients or their caregivers about increased risk for falls. Suggest strategies for fall prevention.

Evaluation/Desired Outcomes

● Decrease in edema.
● Decrease in abdominal girth and weight.
● Increase in urinary output.

REMS HIGH ALERT

buprenorphine
(byoo-pre-**nor**-feen)
Belbuca, Brixadi, Buprenex, Butrans, Sublocade, ~~Subutex~~

Classification
Therapeutic: opioid analgesics
Pharmacologic: opioid agonists/antagonists

Schedule III

Indications

IM, IV: Management of moderate to severe acute pain. **Buccal, Transdermal:** Pain that is severe enough to require daily, around-the-clock long-term opioid treatment and for which alternative treatment options (e.g. non-opioid analgesics or immediate-release opioids) are inadequate. **SL:** Treatment of opioid use disorder (preferred for induction only); suppresses withdrawal symptoms in opioid detoxification. **SUBQ:** Treatment of moderate to severe opioid use disorder in patients who have initiated treatment with a buprenorphine-containing product for ≥7 days (Sublocade). **SUBQ:** Treatment of moderate to severe opioid use disorder in patients who have initiated treatment with a single dose of a transmucosal buprenorphine product or who are already being treated with buprenorphine (Brixadi).

Action

Binds to opiate receptors in the CNS. Alters the perception of and response to painful stimuli while producing generalized CNS depression. Has partial antagonist properties that may result in opioid withdrawal in physically dependent patients when used as an analgesic. **Therapeutic Effects: IM, IV, Transdermal:** Decreased severity of pain. **SL:** Suppression of withdrawal symptoms during detoxification and maintenance from heroin or other opioids. Produces a relatively mild withdrawal compared to other agents. **SUBQ:** Continued cessation of opioid use.

Pharmacokinetics

Absorption: Well absorbed after IM and SL use; 46–65% absorbed with buccal use; 15% of transdermal dose absorbed through skin; IV administration results in complete bioavailability.
Distribution: Crosses the placenta; enters breast milk. CNS concentration is 15–25% of plasma.
Protein Binding: 96%.
Metabolism and Excretion: Mostly metabolized by the liver mostly via the CYP3A4 isoenzyme; one metabolite is active; 70% excreted in feces; 27% excreted in urine.
Half-life: 2–3 hr (IV); 27 hr (buccal); 26 hr (transdermal); 37 hr (SL); 24–48 hr (subdermal); 43–60 days (SUBQ).

TIME/ACTION PROFILE (analgesia)

ROUTE	ONSET	PEAK	DURATION
IM	15 min	60 min	6 hr†
IV	rapid	less than 60 min	6 hr†
SL	unknown	unknown	unknown
Transdermal	unknown	unknown	7 days
Buccal	unknown	unknown	unknown
SUBQ	unknown	unknown	unknown

†4–5 hr in children.

Contraindications/Precautions

Contraindicated in: Hypersensitivity; Significant respiratory depression (transdermal, buccal); Acute or severe bronchial asthma (transdermal, buccal); Paralytic ileus (transdermal, buccal); Acute, mild, intermittent, or postoperative pain (transdermal); Long QT syndrome; Concurrent use of class I or III antiarrhythmics; Lactation: Lactation.

Use Cautiously in: ↑ intracranial pressure; Compromised respiratory function including COPD, cor pulmonale, diminished respiratory reserve, hypoxia, hypercapnia, or respiratory depression of other causes; Severe renal impairment; Moderate or severe hepatic impairment (dose ↓ needed for severe impairment); Hypothyroidism; Seizure disorders; Adrenal insufficiency; Alcoholism; Biliary tract disease; Acute pancreatitis; Debilitated patients (dose ↓ required); Oral mucositis (dose ↓ required) (buccal); Undiagnosed abdominal pain; Hypokalemia, hypomagnesemia, unstable atrial fibrillation, symptomatic bradycardia, unstable HF, QT interval prolongation, or myocardial ischemia; Prostatic hyperplasia; OB: Safety not established in pregnancy; prolonged use of buccal, transdermal, or SL buprenorphine during pregnancy can result in neonatal opioid withdrawal syndrome; Pedi: Safety and effectiveness not established in children <18 yr (SL and transdermal) or <2 yr (parenteral); Geri: ↑ risk of respiratory depression in older adults (dose ↓ required).

Adverse Reactions/Side Effects

CV: hypertension, hypotension, palpitations, QT interval prolongation. **Derm:** <u>sweating</u>, clammy feeling, erythema, pruritus, rash. **EENT:** blurred vision, diplopia, miosis (high doses). **Endo:** adrenal insufficiency. **GI:** nausea, constipation, dry mouth, HEPATOTOXICITY, ileus, vomiting. **GU:** urinary retention. **Neuro:** confusion, dysphoria, hallucinations, sedation, dizziness, euphoria, floating feeling, headache, unusual dreams. **Resp:** RESPIRATORY DEPRESSION (including central sleep apnea and sleep-related hypoxemia). **Misc:** HYPERSENSITIVITY REACTIONS (including anaphylaxis, angioedema, and bronchospasm), injection site reactions, physical dependence, psychological dependence, tolerance.

Interactions

Drug-Drug: Concurrent use with **class Ia antiarrhythmics, class III antiarrhythmics,** or other **QT interval prolonging medications** may ↑ risk of QT interval prolongation; avoid concurrent use. Use with **benzodiazepines** or other **CNS depressants** including other **opioids, non-benzodiazepine sedative/ hypnotics, anxiolytics, general anesthetics, muscle relaxants, antipsychotics,** and **alcohol** may cause profound sedation, respiratory depression, coma, and death; reserve concurrent use for when alternative treatment options are inadequate. Use with extreme caution in patients receiving **MAO inhibitors** (↑ CNS and respiratory depression and hypotension— ↓ buprenorphine dose by 50%; may need to ↓ **MAO inhibitor** dose; do not use transdermal formulation within 14 days of **MAO inhibitor**). May ↓ effectiveness of other **opioid analgesics. CYP3A4 inhibitors,** including **itraconazole, ketoconazole, erythromycin, ritonavir, atazanavir,** or **fosamprenavir** may ↑ levels and risk of toxicity; may need to ↓ buprenorphine dose. **CYP3A4 inducers,** including **carbamazepine, rifampin,** or **phenytoin** may ↓ levels and effectiveness; buprenorphine dose modification may be necessary during concurrent use. Concurrent abuse of buprenorphine and **benzodiazepines** may result in coma and death. Drugs that affect serotonergic neurotransmitter systems, including **tricyclic antidepressants, SSRIs, SNRIs, MAO inhibitors, TCAs, tramadol, trazodone, mirtazapine, 5–HT₃ receptor antagonists, linezolid, methylene blue,** and **triptans** ↑ risk of serotonin syndrome.

Drug-Natural Products: Concomitant use of **kava-kava, valerian, chamomile,** or **hops** can ↑ CNS depression.

Route/Dosage

Analgesia

IM, IV (Adults): 0.3 mg every 4–6 hr as needed. May repeat initial dose after 30 min (up to 0.3 mg every 4 hr or 0.6 mg every 6 hr); 0.6-mg doses should be given only IM.

IM, IV (Children 2–12 yr): 2–6 mcg (0.002–0.006 mg)/kg every 4–6 hr.

Transdermal (Adults): *Opioid-naïve:* Transdermal system delivering 5–20 mcg/hr applied every 7 days. Initiate with 5 mcg/hr system; each dose titration may occur after 72 hr; do not exceed dose of 20 mcg/hr (due to ↑ risk of QT interval prolongation); *Previously*

taking <30 mg/day of morphine or equivalent: Initiate with 5 mcg/hr system; each dose titration may occur after 72 hr; do not exceed dose of 20 mcg/hr (due to ↑ risk of QT interval prolongation); apply patch every 7 days; *Previously taking 30–80 mg/day of morphine or equivalent:* Initiate with 10 mcg/hr system; each dose titration may occur after 72 hr; do not exceed dose of 20 mcg/hr (due to ↑ risk of QT interval prolongation); apply patch every 7 days; *Previously taking >80 mg/day of morphine or equivalent:* Consider use of alternate analgesic.

Buccal (Adults): *Opioid-naïve:* Initiate therapy with 75 mcg once daily or every 12 hr for ≥4 days, then ↑ dose to 150 mcg every 12 hr; may then titrate dose in increments of 150 mcg every 12 hr no more frequently than every 4 days; do not exceed dose of 450 mcg every 12 hr (based on clinical studies); *Previously taking <30 mg/day of morphine or equivalent:* Initiate therapy with 75 mcg once daily or every 12 hr for ≥4 days, then ↑ dose to 150 mcg every 12 hr; may then titrate dose in increments of 150 mcg every 12 hr no more frequently than every 4 days; do not exceed dose of 900 mcg every 12 hr (due to ↑ risk of QT interval prolongation); *Previously taking 30–89 mg/day of morphine or equivalent:* Initiate therapy with 150 mcg every 12 hr for ≥4 days; may titrate dose in increments of 150 mcg every 12 hr no more frequently than every 4 days; do not exceed dose of 900 mcg every 12 hr (due to ↑ risk of QT interval prolongation); *Previously taking 90–160 mg/day of morphine or equivalent:* Initiate therapy with 300 mcg every 12 hr for ≥4 days; may then titrate dose in increments of 150 mcg every 12 hr no more frequently than every 4 days; do not exceed dose of 900 mcg every 12 hr (due to ↑ risk of QT interval prolongation); *Previously taking >160 mg/day of morphine or equivalent:* Consider use of alternate analgesic; *Patients with oral mucositis:* ↓ initial dose by 50% then titrate dose in increments of 75 mcg every 12 hr no more frequently than every 4 days.

Hepatic Impairment

Transdermal (Adults): *Mild to moderate hepatic impairment:* Initiate with 5 mcg/hr system.

Hepatic Impairment

Buccal (Adults): *Severe hepatic impairment:* ↓ initial dose by 50% then titrate dose in increments of 75 mcg every 12 hr no more frequently than every 4 days.

Treatment of Opioid Use Disorder

SL (Adults): *Induction:* 8 mg once daily on Day 1, then 16 mg once daily on Day 2–4; *Maintenance:* Patients should preferably be transitioned to buprenorphine/naloxone; if patient cannot tolerate naloxone, then can use buprenorphine (usual dosage range = 4–24 mg/day); recommended target dose = 16 mg/day; dose can be ↑ or ↓ by 2–4 mg, as needed to prevent signs/symptoms of opioid withdrawal.

SUBQ (Adults): *Sublocade:* 300 mg once monthly for 2 mo, then 100 mg once monthly; may ↑ maintenance dose to 300 mg once monthly if patient reports illicit opioid use or has positive urine drug screen for illicit opioid use.

SUBQ (Adults): *Patients not currently receiving buprenorphine treatment (Brixadi [weekly formulation] only):* To avoid precipitating an opioid withdrawal syndrome, a single 4-mg test dose of transmucosal buprenorphine-containing product should be administered prior to administration of Brixadi weekly injection. If the test dose is tolerated without precipitating withdrawal, administer 16 mg (weekly formulation) initially, followed by an additional 8 mg (weekly formulation) within 3 days of the initial dose for a total recommended weekly dose of 24 mg. If needed, during the 1st wk of treatment, may administer an additional 8 mg (weekly formulation) after ≥24 hr after the previous dose, for a total weekly dose of 32 mg. Administer subsequent injections (weekly formulation) once weekly based on the total weekly dose that was established during Wk 1 (16–32 mg). Dose adjustments can be made at weekly intervals (max dose = 32 mg once weekly). *Patients currently receiving buprenorphine treatment (Brixadi [weekly formulation]):* If daily dose of SL buprenorphine ≤6 mg, administer 8 mg once weekly (weekly formulation). If daily dose of SL buprenorphine 8–10 mg, administer 16 mg once weekly (weekly formulation). If daily dose of SL buprenorphine 12–16 mg, administer 24 mg once weekly (weekly formulation). If daily dose of SL buprenorphine 18–24 mg, administer 32 mg once weekly (weekly formulation). *Patients currently receiving buprenorphine treatment (Brixadi [monthly formulation]):* If daily dose of SL buprenorphine 8–10 mg, administer 64 mg once monthly (monthly formulation). If daily dose of SL buprenorphine 12–16 mg, administer 96 mg once monthly (monthly formulation). If daily dose of SL buprenorphine 18–24 mg, administer 128 mg once monthly (monthly formulation). *Transitioning between Brixadi (monthly formulation) and Brixadi (monthly formulation):* If dose of weekly formulation 16 mg once weekly, convert to 64 mg once monthly (monthly formulation). If dose of weekly formulation 24 mg once weekly, convert to 96 mg once monthly (monthly formulation). If dose of weekly formulation 32 mg once weekly, convert to 128 mg once monthly (monthly formulation).

Hepatic Impairment
SL (Adults): *Severe hepatic impairment:* ↓ initial dose and adjustment dose by 50%.

Availability (generic available)
Buccal film (Belbuca): 75 mcg, 150 mcg, 300 mcg, 450 mcg, 600 mcg, 750 mcg, 900 mcg. **Extended-release solution for SUBQ injection (prefilled syringes) (Sublocade):** 100 mg/0.5 mL, 300 mg/1.5 mL. **Extended-release solution for SUBQ injection (prefilled syringes) (Brixadi [weekly]):** 8 mg/0.16 mL, 16 mg/0.32 mL, 24 mg/0.48 mL, 32 mg/0.64 mL.

Extended-release solution for SUBQ injection (prefilled syringes) (Brixadi [monthly]): 64 mg/0.18 mL, 96 mg/0.27 mL, 128 mg/0.36 mL. **Solution for injection (Buprenex):** 300 mcg (0.3 mg)/mL. **Sublingual tablets:** 2 mg, 8 mg. **Transdermal systems (Butrans):** 5 mcg/hr, 7.5 mcg/hr, 10 mcg/hr, 15 mcg/hr, 20 mcg/hr. *In combination with:* naloxone (Suboxone, Zubsolv). See Appendix N.

NURSING IMPLICATIONS
Assessment
- Monitor for signs and symptoms of adrenal insufficiency (nausea, vomiting, anorexia, fatigue, weakness, dizziness, and low blood pressure) during therapy. If adrenal insufficiency is suspected, confirm with diagnostic testing. If confirmed, treat with physiologic doses of replacement corticosteroids. Wean patient off opioid to allow adrenal recovery and continue corticosteroids until adrenal function recovers. Other opioids may be tried.
- **Pain:** Assess type, location, and intensity of pain before and 1 hr after IM and 5 min (peak) after IV administration. When titrating opioid doses, increases of 25–50% should be administered until there is either a 50% reduction in the patient's pain rating on a numerical or visual analogue scale or the patient reports satisfactory pain relief. A repeat dose can be safely administered at the time of the peak if previous dose is ineffective and side effects are minimal. Single doses of 600 mcg (0.6 mg) should be administered IM. Patients requiring doses higher than 600 mcg (0.6 mg) should be converted to an opioid agonist. Buprenorphine is not recommended for prolonged use (except buccal or transdermal) or as first-line therapy for acute or cancer pain. SL formulations should not be used to relieve pain.
- An equianalgesic chart (see Appendix I) should be used when changing routes or when changing from one opioid to another.
- Assess level of consciousness, BP, pulse, and respirations before and periodically during administration, especially within first 24–72 hrs of buccal therapy. If respiratory rate is <10/min, assess level of sedation. Dose may need to be decreased by 25–50%. Buprenorphine 0.3–0.4 mg has approximately equal analgesic and respiratory depressant effects to morphine 10 mg. Monitor for respiratory depression, especially during initiation or following dose increase; serious, life-threatening, or fatal respiratory depression may occur. May cause sleep-related breathing disorders (central sleep apnea, sleep-related hypoxemia).
- Assess previous analgesic history. Antagonistic properties may induce withdrawal symptoms (vomiting, restlessness, abdominal cramps, increased BP and temperature) in patients who are physically dependent on opioid agonists. Symptoms may occur up to

15 days after discontinuation and persist for 1–2 wk.

- Buprenorphine has a lower potential for dependence than other opioids; however, prolonged use may lead to physical and psychological dependence and tolerance. This should not prevent patient from receiving adequate analgesia. Most patients receiving buprenorphine for pain rarely develop psychological dependence. If tolerance develops, changing to an opioid agonist may be required to relieve pain.
- Assess bowel function routinely. Prevent constipation with increased intake of fluids and bulk, and laxatives to minimize constipating effects. Administer stimulant laxatives routinely if opioid use exceeds 2–3 days, unless contraindicated. Consider drugs for opioid-induced constipation.
- **Transdermal:** Assess risk for opioid addiction, abuse, or misuse prior to administration. Monitor for respiratory depression, especially during initiation or following dose increase; serious, life-threatening, or fatal respiratory depression may occur. Misuse or abuse of *Butrans* by chewing, swallowing, snorting or injecting buprenorphine extracted from transdermal system will result in the uncontrolled delivery of buprenorphine and risk of overdose and death.
- Maintain frequent contact during periods of changing analgesic requirements, including initial titration, between the prescriber, other members of the health care team, the patient, and the caregiver/family.
- **Treatment of Opioid Dependence:** Assess patient for signs and symptoms of opioid withdrawal before and during therapy.

Lab Test Considerations
- May cause ↑ serum amylase and lipase levels.
- Monitor liver function tests prior to and periodically during opioid dependence therapy.

Toxicity and Overdose
- If an opioid antagonist is required to reverse respiratory depression or coma, naloxone is the antidote. Dilute the 0.4-mg ampule of naloxone in 10 mL of 0.9% NaCl and administer 0.5 mL (0.02 mg) by IV push every 2 min. For children and patients weighing <40 kg, dilute 0.1 mg of naloxone in 10 mL of 0.9% NaCl for a concentration of 10 mcg/mL and administer 0.5 mcg/kg every 1–2 min. Titrate dose to avoid withdrawal, seizures, and severe pain. Naloxone may not completely reverse respiratory depressant effects of buprenorphine; may require mechanical ventilation, oxygen, IV fluids, and vasopressors.

Implementation
- Do not confuse buprenorphine with hydromorphone.
- **Pain:** Explain therapeutic value of medication before administration to enhance the analgesic effect.
- Regularly administered doses may be more effective than prn administration. Analgesic is more effective if given before pain becomes severe.

- Coadministration with non-opioid analgesics has additive effects and may permit lower opioid doses.
- For patients taking forms of long-acting buprenorphine, if acute pain management or anesthesia is needed, treat with a non-opioid analgesic, if possible. Patients requiring opioid therapy for analgesia may be treated with a high-affinity full opioid analgesic under the supervision of a physician, with particular attention to respiratory function. Higher doses may be required for analgesic effect. Monitor patient closely.
- **REMS:** FDA strongly encourages health care professionals to complete a REMS-compliant education program that includes all the elements of the FDA Education *Blueprint for Health Care Providers Involved in the Management or Support of Patients with Pain,* available at www.fda.gov/Opioid-AnalgesicREMSBlueprint. Information on programs can be found at 1-800-503-0784 or www.opioidanalgesicrems.com.
- Discuss availability of naloxone for emergency treatment of opioid overdose with the patient and caregiver and assess the potential need for access to naloxone, both when initiating and renewing therapy, especially if patient has household members (including children) or other close contacts at risk for accidental exposure or overdose. Consider prescribing naloxone, based on the patient's risk factors for overdose, such as concomitant use of CNS depressants, a history of opioid use disorder, or prior opioid overdose. However, the presence of risk factors for overdose should not prevent the proper management of pain in any patient.
- **Buccal:** Have patient wet inside of cheek with tongue or rinse mouth with water. Apply film immediately after removal from package. Place yellow side of film against inside of cheek. Hold film in place with dry fingers for 5 sec, then leave in place on inside of cheek until fully dissolved. If chewed or swallowed, may result in lower peak concentrations and lower bioavailability. Do not administer if package seal is broken or film is cut, damaged, or changed. Avoid applying to areas of mouth with sores or lesions. To dispose of unused film, remove from foil package, drop into toilet, and flush.
- **IM:** Administer IM injections deep into well-developed muscle. Rotate sites of injections.

IV Administration
- **IV Push:** May give IV undiluted. *High Alert:* Administer slowly. Rapid administration may cause respiratory depression, hypotension, and cardiac arrest. *Rate:* Give over at least 2 min.
- **Y-Site Compatibility:** acetaminophen, acyclovir, allopurinol, amifostine, amikacin, aminocaproic acid, amiodarone, amphotericin B lipid complex, amphotericin B liposomal, anidulafungin, argatroban, arsenic trioxide, ascorbic acid, atracurium, atropine, azithromycin, aztreonam, benztropine, bivalirudin, bleomycin, bumetanide, butorphanol,

calcium chloride, calcium gluconate, carboplatin, carmustine, cefazolin, cefepime, cefotaxime, cefotetan, cefoxitin, ceftazidime, ceftriaxone, cefuroxime, chloramphenicol, chlorpromazine, cisatracurium, cisplatin, cladribine, clindamycin, cyanocobalamin, cyclophosphamide, cyclosporine, cytarabine, dacarbazine, dactinomycin, daptomycin, daunorubicin hydrochloride, dexamethasone, dexmedetomidine, dexrazoxane, digoxin, diltiazem, diphenhydramine, dobutamine, docetaxel, dopamine, doxorubicin hydrochloride, doxycycline, enalaprilat, ephedrine, epinephrine, epirubicin, epoetin alfa, eptifibatide, ertapenem, erythromycin, esmolol, etoposide, etoposide phosphate, famotidine, fentanyl, filgrastim, fluconazole, fludarabine, foscarnet, fosphenytoin, gemcitabine, gentamicin, glycopyrrolate, granisetron, heparin, hetastarch, hydrocortisone, idarubicin, ifosfamide, imipenem/cilastatin, insulin, regular, irinotecan, isoproterenol, ketorolac, labetalol, leucovorin calcium, levofloxacin, lidocaine, linezolid, lorazepam, magnesium sulfate, mannitol, melphalan, meperidine, mesna, methotrexate, methylprednisolone, metoclopramide, metoprolol, metronidazole, midazolam, milrinone, mitomycin, mitoxantrone, morphine, multivitamins, mycophenolate, nafcillin, nalbuphine, naloxone, nicardipine, nitroglycerin, nitroprusside, norepinephrine, octreotide, ondansetron, oxacillin, oxaliplatin, oxytocin, paclitaxel, palonosetron, pamidronate, papaverine, pemetrexed, penicillin G, pentamidine, phentolamine, phenylephrine, phytonadione, piperacillin/tazobactam, potassium acetate, potassium chloride, procainamide, prochlorperazine, promethazine, propofol, propranolol, protamine, pyridoxine, remifentanil, rituximab, rocuronium, sodium acetate, succinylcholine, sufentanil, tacrolimus, theophylline, thiamine, thiotepa, tigecycline, tirofiban, tobramycin, topotecan, trastuzumab, vancomycin, vasopressin, vecuronium, verapamil, vinblastine, vincristine, vinorelbine, voriconazole, zoledronic acid.

- **Y-Site Incompatibility:** alemtuzumab, aminophylline, ampicillin, azathioprine, dantrolene, diazepam, diazoxide, doxorubicin liposomal, fluorouracil, gemtuzumab ozogamicin, indomethacin, pantoprazole, pentobarbital, phenobarbital, phenytoin, sodium bicarbonate, trimethoprim/sulfamethoxazole.
- **Transdermal:** Buprenorphine may cause withdrawal in patients who are already taking opioids. For conversion from other opioids to buprenorphine transdermal, taper current around-the-clock opioids for up to 7 days to no more than 30 mg of morphine or equivalent per day before beginning treatment with buprenorphine transdermal. May use short-acting analgesics as needed until analgesic efficacy with buprenorphine transdermal is attained. Buprenorphine transdermal may not provide ade-

quate analgesia for patients requiring greater than 80 mg/day oral morphine equivalents.
- Apply system to flat, hairless, nonirritated, and nonirradiated site on the upper outer arm, upper chest, upper back or the side of the chest. If skin preparation is necessary, use clear water and clip, do not shave, hair. Allow skin to dry completely before application. Apply immediately after removing from package. Do not alter the system (i.e., cut) in any way before application. Remove liner from adhesive layer and press firmly in place with palm of hand for 30 sec, especially around the edges, to make sure contact is complete. Remove used system and fold so that adhesive edges are together. Flush system down toilet immediately on removal or follow the institutional policy. Apply new system to a different site. After removal, wait a minimum of 3 wk before applying to the same site. If patch falls off during 7-day dosing interval, dispose of patch and place a new patch on at a different site.
- May be titrated no less than every 72 hrs. Dose adjustments in 5 mcg/hr, 7.5 mcg/hr, or 10 mcg/hr increments may be used by using no more than two patches.
- To discontinue, taper dose gradually to prevent signs and symptoms of withdrawal; consider introduction of immediate-release opioid medication. For patients taking buprenorphine regularly for a week or more, initiate taper by a small enough increment (no more than 10% to 25% of the total daily dose) to avoid withdrawal symptoms, and proceed with dose-lowering at an interval of every 2 to 4 wk or longer. Provision of lower dose strengths may be necessary for a successful taper. Monitor for withdrawal symptoms (restlessness, lacrimation, rhinorrhea, yawning, perspiration, chills, myalgia, mydriasis, irritability, anxiety, backache, joint pain, weakness, abdominal cramps, insomnia, nausea, anorexia, vomiting, diarrhea, increased blood pressure, respiratory rate, or heart rate) during taper. If withdrawal symptoms occur, it may be necessary to pause the taper for a period of time or raise the dose of the opioid analgesic to the previous dose, and then proceed with a slower taper. Monitor for changes in mood, emergence of suicidal thoughts, or use of other substances.
- **Treatment of Opioid Use Disorder:** Must be prescribed by health care professional with special training.
- **SL:** Induction is usually started with buprenorphine SL over 3–4 days. Initial dose should be administered at least 4 hr after last opioid dose and preferably when early signs of opioid withdrawal appear. Once patient is on a stable dose, maintenance therapy with buprenorphine/naloxone (Suboxone) is preferred for continued, unsupervised treatment.

- Administer sublingually. Usually takes 2–10 min for tablets to dissolve. If more than one tablet is prescribed, place multiple tablets under the tongue or 2 at a time until all tablets are dissolved. Do not chew or swallow; decreases amount of medication absorbed. Not used for analgesia; may cause death in opioid naïve patients.
- **SUBQ:** *Sublocade* is for patients who have initiated treatment with a transmucosal buprenorphine product followed by dose adjustment for at least 7 days. Prepare and administer only by health care professional monthly with a minimum of 26 days between doses. Use syringe and needle provided by manufacturer. Remove from refrigerator at least 15 min before injection to allow to reach room temperature. Do not open foil pouch until patient has arrived. Discard if left at room temperature for >7 days. Do not administer solutions that are discolored or contain particulate matter. Pinch injection site and administer into abdomen; do not rub. May cause a lump that will decrease over several wk. Do not administer IV or IM. If discontinued, withdrawal effects will be delayed (2–5 mo) due to long half-life. Monitor patients discontinuing for withdrawal signs and symptoms. May use transmucosal buprenorphine to treat withdrawal. In patients taking *Sublocade* for 4–6 months or more, plasma and urine levels of buprenorphine may be detectable for 12 months or longer following discontinuation. Administer missed doses as soon as possible with following dose given at least 26 days later. For patients with regular therapy of 100 mg monthly, a two-month dosing interval may be used on occasion (e.g., extended travel); a single 300 mg dose may be given to cover a two-month period, then resume 100 mg monthly regimen. Caution patient that 300 mg dose may cause sedation.
- **REMS:** *Brixandi* is only available through a restricted program called the *Brixandi REMS*. Health care settings and pharmacies that order and dispense *Brixandi* must be certified in this program and comply with REMS requirements.
- **Treatment of Opioid Use Disorder**: There are two formulations of *Brixandi*; one lasting 7 days and one lasting 1 month. Doses of *Brixandi* (weekly) cannot be combined to yield a monthly dose.
- Only health care providers should prepare and administer *Brixandi*. Administer *Brixandi* as a single injection. Do not divide.
- For patients not currently receiving buprenorphine, begin with a test dose of 4 mg transmucosal buprenorphine to establish that buprenorphine is tolerated without precipitated withdrawal, and then transition to *Brixandi* (weekly).
- *Brixandi* is only for SUBQ injection; do not administer IV, IM, or intradermally.
- **SUBQ:** Inject slowly at a 90° angle into SUBQ tissue of the buttock, thigh, abdomen, or upper arm. Hold safety syringe in place for an additional 2 seconds keeping plunger pressed down fully. Rotate injection

sites. In patients not currently receiving buprenorphine, for *Brixandi* (weekly), use the upper arm site only after steady-state has been achieved (4 consecutive doses). Injection in the arm site was associated with approximately 10% lower plasma levels than other sites.
- Needle cap is synthetically derived from natural rubber latex; may cause allergic reactions in latex-sensitive individuals.
- If a dose of *Brixandi* (weekly) is missed, administer next dose as soon as possible. *Brixandi* (weekly) should be administered in 7-day intervals and *Brixandi* monthly should be administered every 28 days.

Patient/Family Teaching

- **REMS:** Instruct patient on risk of addiction, abuse, and misuse, which could lead to death. Discuss safe use, risks, and proper storage and disposal of opioid analgesics with patients and caregivers with each Rx. *The Patient Counseling Guide* is available at www.fda.gov/OpioidAnalgesicREMSPCG. Advise patient not to share buprenorphine with others and to protect from theft or misuse. Advise patient to avoid abrupt discontinuation; may lead to withdrawal symptoms.
- Educate patients and caregivers on how to recognize respiratory depression and emphasize the importance of calling 911 or getting emergency medical help right away in the event of a known or suspected overdose. Inform patients and caregivers about various ways to obtain naloxone as permitted by individual state naloxone dispensing and prescribing requirements or guidelines (by prescription, directly from a pharmacist, or as part of a community-based program).
- Medication may cause drowsiness or dizziness. Advise patient to call for assistance when ambulating and to avoid driving or other activities requiring alertness until response to medication is known, especially within 24–48 hrs after subdermal implant insertion.
- Advise patient to avoid concurrent use of alcohol or other CNS depressants.
- Instruct patient to notify health care professional of all Rx or OTC medications, vitamins, or herbal products being taken and to consult health care professional before taking any Rx, OTC, or herbal products, especially CNS depressants.
- Advise patient and family members to inform health care professionals of physical dependence on an opioid and of buprenorphine therapy.
- Rep: Advise patient to notify health care professional if pregnancy is planned or suspected, and to avoid breastfeeding during therapy. Inform patient of potential for neonatal opioid withdrawal syndrome with prolonged use during pregnancy. Chronic use of buprenorphine may impair male and female fertility. Monitor infant for signs and symptoms of neonatal opioid withdrawal syndrome (irritability, hyperactivity and abnormal sleep pattern, high pitched

cry, tremor, vomiting, diarrhea, and/or failure to gain weight); usually occur in the first days after birth.
- **Pain:** Instruct patient on how and when to ask for pain medication.
- Encourage patients on bedrest to turn, cough, and deep-breathe every 2 hr to prevent atelectasis.
- Instruct patient to change positions slowly to minimize orthostatic hypotension.
- Advise patient that good oral hygiene, frequent mouth rinses, and sugarless gum or candy may decrease dry mouth.
- **Buccal:** Instruct patient on proper technique of buccal film and to avoid eating or drinking until film dissolves. Apply at same time each day. Avoid touching or moving buccal film with tongue or fingers. After product has completely dissolved, take a sip of water, swish gently around teeth and gums, and swallow. Wait for at least 1 hr after taking *Belbuca* before brushing teeth. Do not stop using buprenorphine without consulting health care professional. Advise patient to read *Instructions for Use* prior to starting therapy and with each Rx refill in case of changes.
- Advise patient to notify health care professional if the dose does not control pain.
- **Transdermal:** Instruct patient in correct method for application, removal, storage, and disposal of transdermal system. Wear patches for 7 days. May be worn while bathing, showering, or swimming. Do not discontinue or change dose without consulting health care professional. Instruct patient to read the *Medication Guide* prior to starting and with each Rx refill.
- Advise patients and caregivers/family members of the potential side effects. Instruct patient to notify health care professional if pain is not controlled or if bothersome side effects occur. Contact immediately if difficulty or changes in breathing, unusual deep "sighing" breathing, slow or shallow breathing, new or unusual snoring, slow heartbeat, severe sleepiness, cold, clammy skin, feeling faint, dizzy, confused, or cannot think, walk, or talk normally, or if swelling or blistering around patch occurs.
- Advise patient that fever, electric blankets, heating pads, saunas, hot tubs, and heated water beds increase release of buprenorphine from patch.
- Advise patient referred for MRI test to discuss patch with referring health care professional and MRI facility to determine if removal of patch is necessary prior to test and for directions for replacing patch.
- **Opioid Use Disorder:** Explain techniques for use to patient.
- Caution patient that buprenorphine may be a target for people who abuse drugs; store medications in a safe place to protect them from theft. Selling or giving this medication to others is against the law.

- Caution patient that injection of *Suboxone* can lead to severe withdrawal symptoms.
- Advise patient if admitted to the emergency department to inform treating health care professional and emergency room staff of physical dependence on opioids and of treatment regimen.
- Advise patient to notify health care professional promptly if faintness, dizziness, confusion, slowed breathing, skin or whites of eyes turn yellow, urine turns dark, light-colored stools, decreased appetite, nausea, or abdominal pain occur.
- **SL:** Instruct patient in correct use of medication; directions for use must be followed exactly. Medication must be used regularly, not occasionally. Take missed doses as soon as remembered; if almost time for next dose, skip missed dose and return to regular dosing schedule. Do not take 2 doses at once unless directed by health care professional. Do not discontinue use without consulting health care professional; abrupt discontinuation may cause withdrawal symptoms. If medication is discontinued, flush unused tablets down the toilet if a drug takeback option is not readily available. **SUBQ *REMS*:** Inform patient *Sublocade* and *Brixandi* are only available through a restricted program, *Sublocade* or *Brixandi* REMS program. *Sublocade* can only be dispensed to directly to a health care provider. *Brixandi* can only be administered by a health care provider.

Evaluation/Desired Outcomes
- Decrease in severity of pain without a significant alteration in level of consciousness or respiratory status.
- Suppression of withdrawal symptoms during detoxification and maintenance from heroin or other opioids.
- Continued cessation of opioid use.

---

buPROPion (byoo-**proe**-pee-on)
Aplenzin, Forfivo XL, ~~Wellbutrin~~, Wellbutrin SR, Wellbutrin XL, ❋Zyban

Classification
Therapeutic: antidepressants, smoking deterrents
Pharmacologic: aminoketones

Indications
Major depressive disorder. Depression with seasonal affective disorder. Smoking cessation.

Action
Decreases neuronal reuptake of dopamine in the CNS. Diminished neuronal uptake of serotonin and norepinephrine (less than tricyclic antidepressants). **Therapeutic Effects:** Diminished depression. Decreased craving for cigarettes.

Pharmacokinetics

Absorption: Although well absorbed, rapidly and extensively metabolized by the liver.

Distribution: Unknown.

Metabolism and Excretion: Extensively metabolized by the liver into 3 active metabolites (CYP2B6 isoenzyme involved in formation of one of the active metabolites).

Half-life: 14 hr (active metabolites may have longer half-lives).

TIME/ACTION PROFILE (antidepressant effect)

ROUTE	ONSET	PEAK	DURATION
PO	1–3 wk	unknown	unknown

Contraindications/Precautions

Contraindicated in: Hypersensitivity; Concurrent use of MAO inhibitors or MAO-like drugs (linezolid or methylene blue); Concurrent use of ritonavir; Seizure disorders; Arteriovenous malformation, severe head injury, CNS tumor, CNS infection, severe stroke, anorexia nervosa, bulimia, or abrupt discontinuation of alcohol, benzodiazepines, barbiturates, or antiepileptic drugs (↑ risk of seizures).

Use Cautiously in: Renal/hepatic impairment (↓ dose recommended) (Forfivo XL not recommended in patients with renal or hepatic impairment); Recent history of MI; History of suicide attempt; Unstable cardiovascular status; May ↑ risk of suicide attempt/ideation especially during early treatment or dose adjustment; this risk appears to be greater in adolescents or children; Psychiatric illness; Angle-closure glaucoma; OB: Use during pregnancy only if potential maternal benefit justifies potential fetal risk; Lactation: Use while breastfeeding only if potential maternal benefit justifies potential risk to infant; Pedi: May ↑ risk of suicide attempt/ideation especially during early treatment or dose adjustment in children/adolescents; safety and effectiveness not established in children; Geri: ↑ risk of drug accumulation and ↑ sensitivity to effects in older adults.

Adverse Reactions/Side Effects

CV: hypertension. **Derm:** photosensitivity. **Endo:** hyperglycemia, hypoglycemia, syndrome of inappropriate antidiuretic hormone secretion. **GI:** dry mouth, nausea, vomiting, change in appetite, weight gain, weight loss. **Neuro:** agitation, headache, tremor, aggression, anxiety, delusions, depression, hallucinations, HOMICIDAL THOUGHTS/BEHAVIOR, hostility, insomnia, mania, panic, paranoia, psychoses, SEIZURES, SUICIDAL THOUGHTS/BEHAVIOR.

Interactions

Drug-Drug: Concurrent use with **MAO-inhibitors** may ↑ risk of hypertensive reactions; concurrent use contraindicated; at least 14 days should elapse between discontinuation of MAO inhibitor and initiation of bupropion (or visa versa). Concurrent use with **MAO-inhibitor like drugs**, such as **linezolid** or **methylene**

blue may ↑ risk of hypertensive reactions; concurrent use contraindicated; do not start therapy in patients receiving **linezolid** or **methylene blue**; if **linezolid** or **methylene blue** need to be started in a patient receiving bupropion, immediately discontinue bupropion and monitor for 2 wk or until 24 hr after last dose of linezolid or methylene blue, whichever comes first (may resume bupropion therapy 24 hr after last dose of linezolid or methylene blue). ↑ risk of adverse reactions when used with **amantadine** or **levodopa**. ↑ risk of seizures with **phenothiazines**, **antidepressants**, **theophylline**, **corticosteroids**, **OTC stimulants/anorectics**, or cessation of **alcohol** or **benzodiazepines** (avoid or minimize alcohol use). **Ritonavir**, **lopinavir/ritonavir**, and **efavirenz** may ↓ levels; may need to ↑ bupropion dose. May ↑ **citalopram** levels. **Carbamazepine** may ↓ blood levels and effectiveness. Concurrent use with **nicotine** replacement may cause hypertension. ↑ risk of bleeding with **warfarin**. Bupropion and one of its metabolites inhibit the CYP2D6 isoenzyme and may ↑ levels and risk of toxicity of **antidepressants** (SSRIs and tricyclic), **haloperidol**, **risperidone**, **thioridazine**, **beta blockers**, **flecainide**, and **propafenone**. May ↓ levels and efficacy of **tamoxifen**. May ↓ the efficacy of **tamoxifen**. May ↓ **digoxin** levels.

Route/Dosage

Depression

PO (Adults): *Immediate-release:* 100 mg twice daily initially; after 3 days may ↑ to 100 mg 3 times daily; after at least 4 wk of therapy, may ↑ up to 450 mg/day in divided doses (not to exceed 150 mg/dose; wait at least 6 hr between doses at the 300 mg/day dose or at least 4 hr between doses at the 450-mg/day dose). *12–hr sustained-release:* 150 mg once daily in the morning; after 3 days, may ↑ to 150 mg twice daily with at least 8 hr between doses; after at least 4 wk of therapy, may ↑ to a maximum daily dose of 400 mg given as 200 mg twice daily. *24–hr extended-release (Wellbutrin XL):* 150 mg once daily in the morning, may be ↑ after 4 days to 300 mg once daily; some patients may require up to 450 mg/day as a single daily dose. *24–hr extended-release (Aplenzin):* 174 mg once daily in the morning, may be ↑ after 4 days to 348 mg once daily; some patients may require up to 522 mg/day as a single daily dose. *24–hr extended-release (Forfivo XL):* 450 mg once daily (should NOT be used as initial therapy; it should only be used in patients who have been receiving 300 mg/day of another bupropion formulation for at least 2 wk and require titration up to 450 mg/day or in those patients receiving 450 mg/day of another bupropion formulation).

Hepatic Impairment

PO (Adults): *Moderate-to-severe hepatic impairment (Aplenzin):* Max dose: 174 mg every other day.

Seasonal Affective Disorder

PO (Adults): *24–hr extended-release (Wellbutrin XL):* 150 mg/day in the morning; if dose is well tolerated, ↑ to 300 mg/day in one wk. Doses should be tapered to 150 mg/day for 2 wk before discontinuing; *24-hr extended-release (Aplenzin):* 174 mg once daily in the morning, may be ↑ after 7 days to 348 mg once daily.

Hepatic Impairment
PO (Adults): *Moderate-to-severe hepatic impairment (Aplenzin):* Max dose: 174 mg every other day.

Smoking cessation
PO (Adults): *12-hr sustained release:* 150 mg once daily for 3 days, then 150 mg twice daily for 7-12 wk (doses should be at least 8 hr apart).

Availability (generic available)
Immediate-release tablets: 75 mg, 100 mg. **12-hour sustained-release tablets:** 100 mg, 150 mg, 200 mg. **24-hour extended-release tablets (Wellbutrin XL):** 150 mg, 300 mg. **24-hour extended-release tablets (Aplenzin):** 174 mg, 348 mg, 522 mg. **24-hour extended-release tablets (Forfivo XL):** 450 mg. *In combination with:* dexamethasone (Auvelity); naltrexone (Contrave). See Appendix N.

NURSING IMPLICATIONS

Assessment
- Assess mental status and mood changes in all patients, especially during initial few mo of therapy and during dose changes. Risk may be increased in children, adolescents, and adults ≤24 yrs. Inform health care professional if patient demonstrates significant increase in signs of depression (depressed mood, loss of interest in usual activities, significant change in weight and/or appetite, insomnia or hypersomnia, psychomotor agitation or retardation, increased fatigue, feelings of guilt or worthlessness, slowed thinking or impaired concentration, suicide attempt or suicidal/homicidal ideation). If so, restrict amount of drug available to patient.

Lab Test Considerations
- Monitor hepatic and renal function closely in patients with kidney or liver impairment to prevent ↑ serum and tissue bupropion concentrations.
- May cause false-positive urine test for amphetamines.

Implementation
- Do not confuse bupropion with buspirone. Do not confuse Wellbutrin SR with Wellbutrin XL.
- Administer doses in equally spaced time increments during the day to minimize the risk of seizures. Risk of seizures increases fourfold in doses >450 mg per day.
- May be initially administered concurrently with sedatives to minimize agitation. This is not usually required after the 1st wk of therapy.

- Insomnia may be decreased by avoiding bedtime doses. May require treatment during 1st wk of therapy.
- Nicotine patches, gum, inhalers, and spray may be used concurrently with bupropion.
- When converting from other brands of bupropion to *Aplenzin* 522 mg/day *Aplenzin* is equivalent to 450 mg/day bupropion hydrochloride, 348 mg/day *Aplenzin* is equivalent to 300 mg/day bupropion hydrochloride, and 174 mg/day *Aplenzin* is equivalent to 150 mg/day bupropion hydrochloride.
- **PO:** *DNC:* Swallow sustained-release or extended-release tablets whole; do not break, crush, or chew.
- May be administered with food to lessen GI irritation.
- **Seasonal Affective Disorder:** Begin administration in autumn prior to the onset of depressive symptoms. Continue therapy through winter and begin to taper and discontinue in early spring.

Patient/Family Teaching
- Instruct patient to take bupropion as directed at the same time each day. Missed doses should be omitted. Do not double doses or take more than prescribed. May require 4 wk or longer for full effects. Do not discontinue without consulting health care professional. May require gradual reduction before discontinuation. Advise patient to read *Medication Guide* before starting and with each Rx refill in case of changes.
- May impair judgment or motor and cognitive skills. Caution patient to avoid driving and other activities requiring alertness until response to medication is known.
- Advise patient, family, and caregivers to look for suicidality, especially during early therapy or dose changes. Notify health care professional immediately if thoughts about suicide or dying, attempts to commit suicide, new or worse depression or anxiety, agitation or restlessness, panic attacks, insomnia, new or worse irritability, aggressiveness, acting on dangerous impulses, mania, or other changes in mood or behavior occur.
- Instruct patient to notify health care professional of all Rx or OTC medications, vitamins, or herbal products being taken, to avoid alcohol during therapy and to consult with health care professional before taking other medications with bupropion.
- Inform patient that frequent mouth rinses, good oral hygiene, and sugarless gum or candy may minimize dry mouth. If dry mouth persists for more than 2 wk, consult health care professional regarding use of saliva substitute.
- Advise patient to notify health care professional if rash or other troublesome side effects occur.
- Inform patient that unused shell of XL tablets may appear in stool; this is normal.

✤ = Canadian drug name. ⬚ = Genetic implication. ~~Strikethrough~~ = Discontinued. CAPITALS = life-threatening. <u>Underline</u> = most frequent.

- Advise patient to use sunscreen and protective clothing to prevent photosensitivity reactions.
- Advise patient to notify health care professional of medication regimen before treatment or surgery.
- Rep: Instruct females of reproductive potential to inform health care professional if pregnancy is planned or suspected or if breastfeeding. Inform patient about pregnancy exposure registry to monitor pregnancy outcomes in women exposed to antidepressants during pregnancy. Register patients by calling the National Pregnancy Registry for Antidepressants at 1-844-405-6185 or visiting online at https://womensmentalhealth.org/clinical-and-researchprograms/pregnancyregistry/antidepressants/.
- Emphasize the importance of follow-up exams to monitor progress.
- **Smoking Cessation:** Smoking should be stopped during the 2nd wk of therapy to allow for the onset of bupropion and to maximize the chances of quitting.
- Advise patient to stop taking bupropion and contact a health care professional immediately if agitation, depressed mood, and any changes in behavior that are not typical of nicotine withdrawal, or if suicidal thoughts or behavior occur.

Evaluation/Desired Outcomes

- Increased sense of well-being.
- Renewed interest in surroundings. Acute episodes of depression may require several mo of treatment.
- Cessation of smoking.

---

bupropion/naltrexone
(byoo-**proe**-pee-on nal-**trex**-one)
Contrave
Classification
Therapeutic: weight control agents
Pharmacologic: aminoketones, opioid antagonists

Indications
Adjunct to calorie-reduced diet and increased physical activity for chronic weight management in obese patients (BMI ≥30 kg/m^2) or overweight patients (BMI ≥27 kg/m^2) with at least one other comorbidity (hypertension, type 2 diabetes, or dyslipidemia).

Action
Bupropion: antidepressant that acts as a weak inhibitor of neuronal reuptake of dopamine and norepinephrine. *Naltrexone:* acts as an opioid antagonist. In combination they affect two different brain areas involved in food intake: the hypothalamic appetite regulatory center and mesolimbic dopamine circuit reward system.
Therapeutic Effects: Decreased appetite with associated weight loss.

Pharmacokinetics
Bupropion
Absorption: Well absorbed but rapidly metabolized by the liver. Absorption is enhanced by a high-fat meal.
Distribution: Parent drug and metabolites enter breast milk.
Metabolism and Excretion: Extensively metabolized; three metabolites are pharmacologically active. Excretion is mostly renal as metabolites, minimal renal excretion of unchanged drug.
Half-life: 21 hr (longer for some metabolites).
Naltrexone
Absorption: Well absorbed orally, undergoes extensive first pass hepatic metabolism resulting in 5–40% bioavailability. Absorption is enhanced by a high-fat meal.
Distribution: Parent drug and metabolites enter breast milk.
Metabolism and Excretion: Metabolized to 6–beta-naltrexol. Both parent drug and metabolite are pharmacologically active. Excretion is mostly renal as metabolite, less than 2% as unchanged drug.
Half-life: *naltrexone:* 5 hr; 6–beta-naltrexol: 13 hr.

TIME/ACTION PROFILE (weight loss)

ROUTE	ONSET	PEAK	DURATION
PO	within 4 wk	6 mo	unknown

Contraindications/Precautions
Contraindicated in: Known hypersensitivity to bupropion or naltrexone; Uncontrolled hypertension; End-stage renal disease; Severe hepatic impairment; Seizure disorders; Anorexia or bulimia; During withdrawal from or discontinuation of alcohol, benzodiazepines, barbiturates, or antiepileptics; Chronic opioid/opiate agonist or partial agonist use or acute opiate withdrawal; During/within 14 days of MAO inhibitors; Concurrent use of CYP2B6 inducers; Concurrent use of other bupropion-containing medications; OB: Pregnancy; Pedi: Not recommended for use in children.
Use Cautiously in: History of suicidal behavior/ideation; History of seizure risk (avoid administration with a high-fat meal, adhere to recommended dose); Cardiac/cerebrovascular disease; Angle-closure glaucoma; Diabetes mellitus (weight loss may result in hypoglycemia if treatment is not adjusted); Moderate or severe renal impairment (use lower dose); Moderate hepatic impairment (use lower dose); Lactation: Use while breastfeeding only if potential maternal benefit justifies potential risk to infant; Geri: Older adults may have ↑ sensitivity to adverse CNS reactions.

Adverse Reactions/Side Effects
CV: hypertension, tachycardia. **Derm:** hot flush, sweating. **EENT:** angle-closure glaucoma (bupropion), tinnitus. **GI:** constipation, nausea, vomiting, abdominal pain, diarrhea, dry mouth, hepatotoxicity (naltrexone). **Neuro:** headache, aggression, agitation, anxiety, delu-

sions, depression, dizziness, dysgeusia, hallucinations, HOMICIDAL THOUGHTS/BEHAVIOR, hostility, insomnia, mania, panic, paranoia, psychosis, SEIZURES, SUICIDAL THOUGHTS/BEHAVIOR, tremor. **Misc:** HYPERSENSITIVITY REACTIONS (including anaphylaxis and anaphylactoid reactions).

Interactions
Drug-Drug: Concurrent or use within 14 days with **MAO inhibitors** ↑ risk of hypertensive reactions. May ↑ levels and risk of toxicity of **CYP2D6 substrates**, including **SSRIs, tricyclic antidepressants, haloperidol, risperidone, thioridazine, metoprolol, flecainide,** and **propafenone. CYP2B6 inducers** including **carbamazepine, efavirenz, ritonavir, lopinavir, phenobarbital,** and **phenytoin** may ↓ levels and effectiveness; avoid concurrent use. **CYP2B6 inhibitors,** including **clopidogrel,** may ↑ levels and risk of toxicity; not to exceed one tablet twice daily. Concurrent use of **drugs that ↓ seizure threshold** may ↑ risk of seizures. **Dopaminergic drugs** including **amantadine** and **levodopa** may ↑ risk of CNS toxicity. Concurrent ingestion of **alcohol** may ↑ risk of neuropsychiatric reactions (reduce consumption or avoid). May ↓ renal excretion of and ↑ levels/risk of toxicity from **amantadine, amiloride, cimetidine, dopamine, famotidine, memantine, metformin, pindolol, procainamide, varenicline,** and **oxaliplatin**. May ↓ analgesic effects of **opioids**.

Route/Dosage
PO (Adults): *Week 1:* one tablet in the morning; *Week 2:* one tablet in the morning and one tablet in the evening; *Week 3:* two tablets in the morning and one tablet in the evening; *Week 4 and onward:* two tablets in the morning and two tablets in the evening. *Concurrent use of CYP2B6 inhibitors:* dose should not exceed one tablet twice daily.

Renal Impairment
PO (Adults): *Moderate or severe renal impairment:* Dose should not exceed one tablet in the morning and one tablet in the evening.

Hepatic Impairment
PO (Adults): *Moderate hepatic impairment:* Dose should not exceed one tablet in the morning and one tablet in the evening.

Availability
Extended-release tablets: 90 mg bupropion/8 mg naltrexone.

NURSING IMPLICATIONS
Assessment
- Monitor for weight loss and adjust concurrent medications (antihypertensives, antidiabetics, lipid-lowering agents) as needed.
- Assess mental status and mood changes, especially during initial few mo of therapy. Risk may be in-

creased in children, adolescents, and adults ≤24 yr. Inform health care professional if patient demonstrates significant increase in signs of depression (depressed mood, loss of interest in usual activities, insomnia or hypersomnia, psychomotor agitation or retardation, increased fatigue, feelings of guilt or worthlessness, slowed thinking or impaired concentration, irritability, hostility, suicide or homicide attempt or suicidal ideation). Restrict amount of drug available to patient.
- Monitor BP and heart rate periodically during therapy, especially in patient with hypertension.
- Monitor for signs and symptoms of anaphylactic reactions (pruritus, urticaria, hives, angioedema, dyspnea). Discontinue therapy and treat symptomatically.

Lab Test Considerations
- Monitor blood glucose prior to and during therapy in patients with type 2 diabetes; may cause hypoglycemia.
- May cause false-positive urine test for amphetamines.

Implementation
- **PO:** Administer in the morning and evening according to dose escalation schedule. *DNC:* Swallow tablets whole; do not break, crush, or chew.
- Do not administer with a high-fat meal; may ↑ risk of seizures.

Patient/Family Teaching
- Instruct patient to take medication as directed, following the dose escalation schedule. If a dose is missed, omit and wait until next scheduled dose; do not double doses. Advise patient to read *Medication Guide* before starting therapy and with each Rx refill in case of changes.
- Instruct patient to adhere to a reduced-calorie diet and increased physical activity.
- Advise patient, family, and caregivers to look for suicidality, especially during early therapy. Notify health care professional immediately if thoughts about suicide, homicide, or dying, attempts to commit suicide, new or worse depression or anxiety, agitation or restlessness, panic attacks, insomnia, new or worse irritability, aggressiveness, hostility, acting on dangerous impulses, mania, or other changes in mood or behavior occur.
- Advise patient to notify health care professional if signs and symptoms of liver damage (stomach pain lasting more than a few days, dark urine, yellowing of skin and whites of eyes, tiredness) occurs.
- Advise patients they may be less sensitive to opioids during therapy. Advise patients to notify health care professional of bupropion/naltrexone therapy.
- Advise patient to notify health care professional of all Rx or OTC medications, vitamins, or herbal products

being taken and to consult with health care professional before taking other medications and to minimize or avoid alcohol during therapy.

● Rep: Instruct females of reproductive potential to notify health care professional if pregnancy is planned or suspected and to avoid breastfeeding during therapy. Advise pregnant patients to discontinue medication as appropriate weight gain based on pre-pregnancy weight is recommended for all pregnant patients, including those who are overweight or obese, due to the weight gain that occurs in maternal tissues during pregnancy.

Evaluation/Desired Outcomes

● Decreased appetite with associated weight loss. Evaluate therapy after 12 wk at maintenance dose. If patient has not lost 5% of baseline body weight discontinue medication; clinically meaningful weight loss is unlikely.

---

busPIRone (byoo-**spye**-rone)
~~BuSpar~~
Classification
Therapeutic: antianxiety agents

Indications
Anxiety.

Action
Binds to serotonin and dopamine receptors in the brain. Increases norepinephrine metabolism in the brain. **Therapeutic Effects:** Relief of anxiety.

Pharmacokinetics
Absorption: Rapidly absorbed.
Distribution: Widely distributed to tissues.
Protein Binding: 95%.
Metabolism and Excretion: Extensively metabolized by the liver via the CYP3A4 isoenzyme; 20–40% excreted in feces.
Half-life: 2–3 hr.

TIME/ACTION PROFILE (relief of anxiety)

ROUTE	ONSET	PEAK	DURATION
PO	7–10 days	3–4 wk	unknown

Contraindications/Precautions
Contraindicated in: Hypersensitivity; Severe renal impairment; Severe hepatic impairment; Concurrent use of MAO inhibitors; Lactation: Lactation.
Use Cautiously in: Patients receiving other antianxiety agents (other agents should be slowly withdrawn to prevent withdrawal or rebound phenomenon); Patients receiving other psychotropics; OB: Safety not established in pregnancy; Pedi: Children <6 yr (safety and effectiveness not established).

Adverse Reactions/Side Effects
CV: chest pain, palpitations, tachycardia, hypertension, hypotension, syncope. **Derm:** rash, sweating, alopecia,

blisters, bruising, dry skin, edema, flushing, pruritus. **EENT:** blurred vision, nasal congestion, sore throat, tinnitus, altered taste or smell, conjunctivitis. **Endo:** irregular menses. **GI:** nausea, abdominal pain, constipation, diarrhea, dry mouth, vomiting. **GU:** changes in libido, dysuria, urinary frequency, urinary hesitancy. **MS:** myalgia. **Neuro:** dizziness, drowsiness, excitement, fatigue, headache, incoordination, insomnia, nervousness, numbness, paresthesia, weakness, personality changes, tremor. **Resp:** chest congestion, hyperventilation, shortness of breath. **Misc:** clamminess, fever.

Interactions
Drug-Drug: Concurrent use with **MAO inhibitors** may ↑ risk of hypertensive reactions; concurrent use contraindicated; at least 14 days should elapse between discontinuation of MAO inhibitor and initiation of buspirone (or vice versa). **CYP3A4 inhibitors**, including **erythromycin, nefazodone, ketoconazole, itraconazole**, and **ritonavir**, may ↑ levels and risk of toxicity; ↓ dose to 2.5 mg twice daily with erythromycin; ↓ dose to 2.5 mg once daily with nefazodone. **CYP3A4 inducers**, including **rifampin, dexamethasone, phenytoin, phenobarbital**, and **carbamazepine**, may ↓ levels and effectiveness. Avoid concurrent use with **alcohol**.
Drug-Natural Products: Concomitant use of **kava-kava, valerian**, or **chamomile** can ↑ CNS depression.
Drug-Food: Grapefruit juice ↑ levels and risk of toxicity; ingestion of large amounts of grapefruit juice is not recommended.

Route/Dosage
PO (Adults): 7.5 mg twice daily; may ↑ by 5 mg/day every 2–4 days as needed (not to exceed 60 mg/day). Usual dose is 10–15 mg twice daily.
PO (Children ≥6 yr): 5 mg once daily; may ↑ by 5 mg/day every 2–7 days as needed. Usual dose is 7.5–30 mg twice daily.

Availability (generic available)
Tablets: 5 mg, 7.5 mg, 10 mg, 15 mg, 30 mg.

NURSING IMPLICATIONS
Assessment
● Assess degree and manifestations of anxiety before and periodically during therapy.
● Buspirone does not appear to cause physical or psychological dependence or tolerance. However, patients with a history of substance use disorder should be assessed for tolerance or impaired control. Restrict amount of drug available to these patients.

Implementation
● Do not confuse buspirone with bupropion.
● Patients changing from other antianxiety agents should receive gradually decreasing doses. Buspirone will not prevent withdrawal symptoms.

- **PO:** May be administered with food to minimize gastric irritation. Food slows but does not alter extent of absorption.

Patient/Family Teaching

- Instruct patient to take buspirone exactly as directed. Take missed doses as soon as possible if not just before next dose; do not double doses. Do not take more than amount prescribed.
- May cause dizziness or drowsiness. Caution patient to avoid driving or other activities requiring alertness until response to the medication is known.
- Advise patient to avoid concurrent use of alcohol or other CNS depressants.
- Instruct patient to notify health care professional of all Rx or OTC medications, vitamins, or herbal products being taken and to consult health care professional before taking any Rx, OTC, or herbal products.
- Instruct patient to notify health care professional if any chronic abnormal movements occur (dystonia, motor restlessness, involuntary movements of facial or cervical muscles).
- Emphasize the importance of follow-up exams to determine effectiveness of medication.
- Rep: Advise females of reproductive potential to notify health care professional if pregnancy is planned or suspected or if breastfeeding.

Evaluation/Desired Outcomes

- Increase in sense of well-being.
- Decrease in subjective feelings of anxiety. Some improvement may be seen in 7–10 days. Optimal results take 3–4 wk of therapy. Buspirone is usually used for short-term therapy (3–4 wk). If prescribed for long-term therapy, efficacy should be periodically assessed.

HIGH ALERT

busulfan (byoo-sul-fan)
Busulfex, Myleran
Classification
Therapeutic: antineoplastics
Pharmacologic: alkylating agents

Indications

PO: Chronic myelogenous leukemia (CML) and bone marrow disorders. **IV:** Conditioning regimen before allogenic hematopoietic progenitor cell transplantation for CML (in combination with cyclophosphamide).

Action

Disrupts nucleic acid function and protein synthesis (cell-cycle phase–nonspecific). **Therapeutic Effects:** Death of rapidly growing cells, especially malignant ones.

Pharmacokinetics

Absorption: Rapidly absorbed from the GI tract following oral administration. IV administration results in complete bioavailability.
Distribution: Unknown.
Metabolism and Excretion: Extensively metabolized by the liver.
Half-life: 2.5 hr.

TIME/ACTION PROFILE (effect on blood counts)

ROUTE	ONSET	PEAK	DURATION
PO	1–2 wk	weeks	up to 1 mo†
IV	unknown	unknown	13 days‡

†Complete recovery may take up to 20 mo.
‡After administration of last dose.

Contraindications/Precautions

Contraindicated in: Hypersensitivity; Failure to respond to previous courses; OB: Pregnancy; Lactation: Lactation.
Use Cautiously in: Active infection; ↓ bone marrow reserve; Obese patients (base dose on ideal body weight); Other chronic debilitating diseases; Rep: Women of reproductive potential and men with female partners of reproductive potential; Geri: Begin therapy at lower end of dose range in older adults due to ↑ frequency of impaired cardiac, hepatic, or renal function.

Adverse Reactions/Side Effects

Incidence and severity of adverse reactions and side effects are increased with IV use.
CV: *PO:* CARDIAC TAMPONADE (WITH HIGH-DOSE CYCLO-PHOSPHAMIDE); *IV:* chest pain, hypotension, tachycardia, thrombosis, arrhythmias, atrial fibrillation, cardiomegaly, ECG changes, edema, heart block, HF, hypertension, pericardial effusion, ventricular extrasystoles. **Derm:** *PO:* itching, rash, acne, alopecia, erythema nodosum, exfoliative dermatitis, hyperpigmentation. **EENT:** *PO:* cataracts; *IV:* epistaxis, pharyngitis, ear disorders. **Endo:** *PO and IV:* hyperuricemia; *IV:* hyperglycemia; *PO:* sterility, gynecomastia. **F and E:** hypokalemia, hypomagnesemia, hypophosphatemia. **GI:** *PO:* drug-induced hepatitis, nausea, vomiting; *IV:* abdominal enlargement, anorexia, constipation, diarrhea, dry mouth, hematemesis, nausea, rectal discomfort, vomiting, abdominal pain, dyspepsia, hepatic veno-occlusive disease (↑ in allogenic transplantation), hepatomegaly, pancreatitis, stomatitis. **GU:** oliguria, dysuria, hematuria, ↓ fertility. **Hemat:** BONE MARROW DEPRESSION. **Local:** inflammation/pain at injection site. **MS:** arthralgia, myalgia, back pain. **Neuro:** *IV:* anxiety, confusion, depression, dizziness, headache, weakness., CEREBRAL HEMORRHAGE/COMA, encephalopathy, mental status changes, SEIZURES. **Resp:** *PO:* PULMONARY FIBROSIS; *IV:* alveolar hemorrhage, asthma, atelectasis, cough, hemoptysis, hypoxia, pleural effusion, pneumonia, rhini-

tis, sinusitis. **Misc:** allergic reactions, chills, fever, infection.

Interactions

Drug-Drug: Concurrent or previous (within 72 hr) use of **acetaminophen** may ↓ elimination and ↑ toxicity. Concurrent use with high-dose **cyclophosphamide** in patients with thalassemia may result in cardiac tamponade. **Itraconazole**, **metronidazole**, or **deferasirox** may ↑ levels and risk of toxicity. **Phenytoin** may ↓ levels and effectiveness. Long-term continuous therapy with **thioguanine** may ↑ risk of hepatic toxicity. ↑ bone marrow suppression with other **antineoplastics** or **radiation therapy.** May ↓ the antibody response to and ↑ risk of adverse reactions from **live-virus vaccines**.

Route/Dosage

PO (Adults): *Induction:* 1.8 mg/m²/day or 0.06 mg/kg/day until WBCs <15,000/mm³. Usual dose is 4–8 mg/day (range 1–12 mg/day). *Maintenance:* 1–3 mg/day.
PO (Children): 0.06–0.12 mg/kg/day or 1.8–4.6 mg/m²/day initially. Titrate dose to maintain WBC of approximately 20,000/mm³.
IV (Adults): 0.8 mg/kg every 6 hr (dose based on ideal body weight or actual weight, whichever is less; in obese patients, dosage should be based on adjusted ideal body weight) for 4 days (total of 16 doses); given in combination with cyclophosphamide.

Availability (generic available)

Tablets: 2 mg. **Solution for injection:** 6 mg/mL.

NURSING IMPLICATIONS

Assessment

● **High Alert:** Monitor for bone marrow depression. Assess for bleeding (bleeding gums, bruising, petechiae, guaiac stools, urine, emesis) and avoid IM injections and taking rectal temperatures. Apply pressure to venipuncture sites for at least 10 min. Assess for signs of infection (fever, chills, sore throat, cough, hoarseness, lower back or side pain, difficult or painful urination) during neutropenia. Anemia may occur. Monitor for increased fatigue, dyspnea, and orthostatic hypotension. Notify health care professional if these symptoms occur.
● Monitor intake and output ratios and daily weights. Report significant changes in totals.
● Monitor for symptoms of gout (increased uric acid, joint pain, lower back or side pain, swelling of feet or lower legs). Encourage patient to drink at least 2 L of fluid each day. Allopurinol may be given to decrease uric acid levels. Alkalinization of urine may be ordered to increase excretion of uric acid.
● Assess for pulmonary fibrosis (fever, cough, shortness of breath) periodically during and after therapy. Discontinue therapy at the first sign of pulmonary fibrosis. Usually occurs 8 mo– 10 yr (average 4 yr) after initiation of therapy.

Lab Test Considerations

● Monitor CBC with differential and platelet count before and weekly during therapy. The nadir of leukopenia occurs within 10–15 days and the nadir of WBC at 11–30 days. Recovery usually occurs within 12–20 wk. Notify health care professional if WBC is <15,000/mm³ or if a precipitous drop occurs. Institute thrombocytopenia precautions if platelet count is <150,000/mm³. Bone marrow depression may be severe and progressive, with recovery taking 1 mo–2 yr after discontinuation of therapy.
● Monitor serum ALT, bilirubin, alkaline phosphatase, and uric acid before and periodically during therapy. May cause ↑ uric acid levels.
● May cause false-positive cytology results of breast, bladder, cervix, and lung tissues.

Implementation

● **High Alert:** Fatalities have occurred with chemotherapeutic agents. Before administering, clarify all ambiguous orders; double check single, daily, and course-of-therapy dose limits; have second practitioner independently double check original order, calculations, and infusion pump settings.
● **High Alert:** Do not confuse Myleran with Leukeran.
● **IV:** Premedicate patient with phenytoin before IV administration to minimize the risk of seizures.
● Administer antiemetics before IV administration and on a fixed schedule during IV administration.
● **PO:** Administer at the same time each day. Administer on an empty stomach to decrease nausea and vomiting.

IV Administration

● **IV:** Prepare solution in a biologic cabinet. Wear gloves, gown, and mask while handling IV medication. Discard IV equipment in specially designated containers.
● **Intermittent Infusion:** *Dilution:* Dilute with 10 times the volume of busulfan using 0.9% NaCl or D5W. *Concentration:* ≥0.5 mg/mL. When drawing busulfan from vial, use needle with 5-micron nylon filter provided, remove calculated volume from vial, remove needle and filter, replace needle and inject busulfan into diluent. Do not use polycarbonate syringes with busulfan. Only use filters provided with busulfan. Always add busulfan to diluent, not diluent to busulfan. Add 9.3 mL busulfan to 93 mL of 0.9 NaCl or D5W for final solution. Mix by inverting several times. Before and after infusion, flush catheter with 5 mL of 0.9% NaCl or D5W. Solution diluted with 0.9% NaCl or D5W is stable for 8 hr at room temperature and solution diluted with 0.9% NaCl is stable for 12 hr if refrigerated. Administration must be completed during this time. Solution is clear and colorless; do not administer solutions that are discolored or contain a precipitate. *Rate:* Administer via central venous catheter over 2 hr every 6 hr for 4 days for a total of 16 doses. Use infusion pump to administer entire dose over 2 hr.

- **Y-Site Compatibility:** acyclovir, amiodarone, amphotericin B lipid complex, amphotericin B liposomal, anidulafungin, argatroban, arsenic trioxide, bivalirudin, bleomycin, caspofungin, dacarbazine, daptomycin, dexmedetomidine, dexrazoxane, diltiazem, docetaxel, ertapenem, foscarnet, fosphenytoin, granisetron, hetastarch, hydromorphone, leucovorin calcium, levofloxacin, linezolid, lorazepam, meperidine, mesna, metronidazole, milrinone, moxifloxacin, octreotide, ondansetron, paclitaxel, palonosetron, piperacillin/tazobactam, potassium acetate, rituximab, sodium acetate, tacrolimus, tigecycline, tirofiban, trastuzumab, vasopressin, vinblastine, zoledronic acid.
- **Y-Site Incompatibility:** idarubicin, thiotepa, vecuronium, voriconazole.

Patient/Family Teaching

- Instruct patient to take medication as directed, at the same time each day, even if nausea and vomiting are a problem. Consult health care professional if vomiting occurs shortly after dose is taken. If a dose is missed, do not take at all; do not double doses.
- Advise patient to notify health care professional if fever; sore throat; signs of infection; lower back or side pain; difficult or painful urination; sores in the mouth or on the lips; chills; dyspnea; persistent cough; bleeding gums; bruising; petechiae; or blood in urine, stool, or emesis occurs. Instruct patient to use soft toothbrush and electric razor. Caution patient not to drink alcoholic beverages or take products containing aspirin or NSAIDs.
- Caution patient to avoid crowds and persons with known infections. Health care professional should be informed immediately if symptoms of infection occur.
- Discuss with patient the possibility of hair loss. Explore methods of coping.

- Instruct patient not to receive any vaccinations without advice of health care professional.
- Advise patient to notify health care professional if unusual bleeding; bruising; or flank, stomach, or joint pain occurs. Advise patients on long-term therapy to notify health care professional immediately if cough, shortness of breath, and fever occur or if darkening of skin, diarrhea, dizziness, fatigue, anorexia, confusion, or nausea and vomiting become pronounced.
- Inform patient of increased risk of a second malignancy with busulfan.
- Rep: May cause fetal harm. Advise female patients of reproductive potential to use effective contraception during and for 6 mo after last dose and to avoid breastfeeding during therapy. Advise men with female partners of reproductive potential to use effective contraception during and for 3 mo after last dose of therapy. Women need to use contraception even if amenorrhea occurs. May impair fertility in male and female patients.
- Advise patient of the importance of periodic blood counts.

Evaluation/Desired Outcomes

- Decrease in leukocyte count to within normal limits.
- Decreased night sweats.
- Increase in appetite.
- Increased sense of well-being. Therapy is resumed when leukocyte count reaches 50,000/mm³.

---

butenafine, See ANTIFUNGALS (TOPICAL).

---

butoconazole, See ANTIFUNGALS (VAGINAL).

---

cabazitaxel (ka-ba-zi-**tax**-el)
Jevtana
Classification
Therapeutic: antineoplastics
Pharmacologic: taxoids

Indications
Hormone-refractory metastatic prostate cancer previously treated with a regimen including docetaxel (in combination with prednisone).

Action
Binds to intracellular tubulin and promotes its assembly into microtubules while inhibiting disassembly. Result is inhibition of mitosis and interphase. **Therapeutic Effects:** Death of rapidly replicating cells, particularly malignant ones, with ↓ spread of metastatic prostate cancer.

Pharmacokinetics
Absorption: IV administration results in complete bioavailability.
Distribution: Equally distributed between blood and plasma.
Metabolism and Excretion: Extensively (>95%) metabolized by the liver, 80–90% by the CYP3A4/5 isoenzymes. Metabolites are excreted in urine and feces. Minimal renal excretion.
Half-life: 95 hr.

TIME/ACTION PROFILE (plasma concentrations)

ROUTE	ONSET	PEAK	DURATION
IV	rapid	end of infusion	unknown

Contraindications/Precautions
Contraindicated in: Severe hypersensitivity to cabazitaxel or polysorbate 80; Neutrophil count ≤1,500/mm³; Hepatic impairment (total bilirubin ≥3× upper limit of normal [ULN]); Concurrent use of strong CYP3A4 inhibitors or inducers.
Use Cautiously in: Patients with neutropenia or a history of pelvic radiation, adhesions, ulceration, or GI bleeding (↑ risk of GI and urinary adverse reactions); Concomitant use of steroids, NSAIDs, or antithrombotics (↑ risk of GI adverse reactions); Severe renal impairment (CCr <30 mL/min) or end-stage renal disease; Hemoglobin <10 g/dL; Lung disease (↑ risk of pulmonary toxicity); Mild or moderate hepatic impairment (dose ↓ required); Poor performance status, previous episodes of febrile neutropenia, extensive prior radiation ports, or poor nutritional status (↑ risk of complications from prolonged neutropenia); Rep: Men with female partners of reproductive potential; Pedi: Safety and effectiveness not established in children; Geri: ↑ risk of adverse reactions

in older adults (especially prolonged neutropenia and febrile neutropenia).

Adverse Reactions/Side Effects
CV: arrhythmias, hypotension. **Derm:** alopecia. **F and E:** electrolyte imbalance. **GI:** abdominal pain, abnormal taste, anorexia, constipation, DIARRHEA, GI BLEED, GI PERFORATION, nausea, vomiting, dyspepsia, ENTEROCOLITIS, ILEUS. **GU:** hematuria, cystitis, RENAL FAILURE. **Hemat:** anemia, leukopenia, NEUTROPENIA, THROMBOCYTOPENIA. **MS:** arthralgia, back pain, muscle spasms. **Neuro:** peripheral neuropathy, weakness, fatigue. **Resp:** dyspnea, ACUTE RESPIRATORY DISTRESS SYNDROME, INTERSTITIAL LUNG DISEASE. **Misc:** fever, HYPERSENSITIVITY REACTIONS (including anaphylaxis).

Interactions
Drug-Drug: **Strong CYP3A inhibitors** including **ketoconazole, itraconazole, clarithromycin, atazanavir, nefazodone, nelfinavir, ritonavir,** and **voriconazole** ↑ levels and risk of toxicity; concurrent use contraindicated. **Strong CYP3A inducers** including **phenytoin, carbamazepine, rifampin, rifabutin, rifapentin,** and **phenobarbital** may ↓ levels and effectiveness; concurrent use contraindicated.
Drug-Natural Products: **St. John's wort** may ↓ levels and effectiveness; concomitant use contraindicated.

Route/Dosage
IV (Adults): 20 mg/m² every 3 wk (with prednisone 10 mg PO daily). A dose of 25 mg/m² may be considered in select patients.

Hepatic Impairment
IV (Adults): *Mild hepatic impairment (total bilirubin >1× to ≤1.5× ULN or AST >1.5× ULN):* 20 mg/m² every 3 wk (with prednisone 10 mg PO daily); *Moderate hepatic impairment (total bilirubin >1.5× to ≤3× ULN):* 15 mg/m² every 3 wk (with prednisone 10 mg PO daily); *Severe hepatic impairment (total bilirubin >3× ULN):* Contraindicated.

Availability (generic available)
Viscous solution for injection: 40 mg/mL (contains polysorbate 80); comes with diluent (5.7 mL of 13% [w/w] ethanol in water for injection). **Solution for injection:** 10 mg/mL.

NURSING IMPLICATIONS
Assessment
- Assess for hypersensitivity reactions (generalized rash/erythema, hypotension, bronchospasm, swelling of face). May occur within min following initiation of infusion. If severe reactions occur, discontinue infusion immediately and provide supportive therapy.
- Assess for signs and symptoms of GI toxicity (abdominal pain and tenderness, fever, persistent constipation, nausea, vomiting, severe diarrhea); may result in death due to electrolyte imbalance. Pre-

medication is recommended. Treat with rehydration, antidiarrheal, or antiemetic therapy as needed. If Grade ≥3 diarrhea or persisting diarrhea occurs despite appropriate medication, fluid and electrolyte replacement, delay treatment until improvement or resolution, then reduce dose to 20 mg/mL.

- Assess for signs and symptoms of peripheral neuropathy (pain, burning, numbness in hands, feet, or legs) during therapy. *If Grade 2 occurs,* withhold until improvement or resolution, then reduce dose to 20 mg/mL. *If ≥Grade 3 occurs,* discontinue therapy.
- Monitor for signs and symptoms of respiratory compromise (trouble breathing, dyspnea, chest pain, cough, fever) during therapy. Interrupt therapy if new or worsening symptoms occur. Consider discontinuation.

Lab Test Considerations

- Monitor CBC weekly during cycle 1 and before each treatment cycle thereafter. Do not administer if neutrophils ≤1500/mm^3. If prolonged grade 3 neutropenia (>1 wk) despite appropriate medication including filgrastim, delay treatment until neutrophil count is >1500 mm^3, then reduce dose to 20 mg/m^2. Use filgrastim for secondary prophylaxis. Risk is ↑ in elderly patients.
- If febrile neutropenia occurs, delay therapy until improvement or resolution and neutrophil count is >1500/mm^3, then reduce dose to 20 mg/m^2. Use filgrastim for primary or secondary prophylaxis.
- Discontinue cabazitaxel if prolonged Grade 3 neutropenia, febrile neutropenia, or Grade 3 diarrhea occur at the 20 mg/m^2 dose.
- May cause hematuria.
- May cause Grade 3–4 ↑ AST, ↑ ALT, and ↑ bilirubin.

Implementation

- **High Alert:** Fatalities have occurred with chemotherapeutic agents. Before administering, clarify all ambiguous orders; double-check single, daily, and course-of-therapy dose limits; have second practitioner independently double-check original order and dose calculations.
- Prepare solution in a biologic cabinet. Wear gloves, gown, and mask while handling medication. Discard equipment in specially designated containers. If solution comes in contact with skin or mucosa, wash with soap and water immediately.
- Premedicate at least 30 min before each dose with antihistamine (diphenhydramine 25 mg or equivalent), corticosteroid (dexamethasone 8 mg or equivalent), and H$_2$ antagonist (famotidine 20 mg or equivalent). Antiemetic prophylaxis, PO or IV, is recommended.
- Begin prophylaxis with G-CSF (filgrastim) in all patients receiving a dose of 25 mg/m^2 to minimize complications due to prolonged neutropenia.

IV Administration

- Two dilutions are required. Do not use PVC infusion containers or polyurethane infusion sets for preparation or infusion.
- **First Dilution:** *Reconstitution:* Mix vial with entire contents of supplied diluent. Direct needle to inside wall of vial and inject slowly to avoid foaming. Mix gently by repeated inversions for at least 45 sec; do not shake. Let stand for a few min to allow foam to dissipate. *Concentration:* 10 mg/mL. **Second Dilution:** *Dilution:* Withdraw recommended dose from cabazitaxel solution and dilute further into a sterile 250 mL PVC-free container of 0.9% NaCl or D5W. If dose >65 mg is required, use a larger volume of infusion vehicle so concentration does not exceed 0.26 mg/mL. Gently invert container to mix. *Concentration:* 0.10–0.26 mg/mL. Stable for 8 hr (including 1 hr infusion) at room temperature or 24 hr if refrigerated. May crystallize over time. Do not use if crystallized, discolored, or contains particulate matter; discard. *Rate:* Infuse over 1 hr at room temperature through a 0.22 micrometer nominal pore size filter.
- **Y-Site Incompatibility:** Do not mix with other medication.

Patient/Family Teaching

- Instruct patient to take oral prednisone as prescribed and to notify health care professional if a dose is missed or not taken in time.
- Advise patient to notify health care professional immediately if signs or symptoms of hypersensitivity reactions; fever; sore throat; signs of infection; lower back or side pain; difficult or painful urination; sores on the mouth or on the lips; bleeding gums; bruising; petechiae; blood in urine, stool, or emesis; unusual swelling, shortness of breath, trouble breathing, chest pain, cough, or fever occur. Caution patient to avoid crowds and persons with known infections. Instruct patient to use soft toothbrush and electric razor and to avoid falls. Patient should also be cautioned not to drink alcoholic beverages or to take products containing aspirin or NSAIDs; may precipitate GI hemorrhage.
- May cause dizziness. Caution patient to avoid driving or other activities requiring alertness until response to medication is known.
- Instruct patient to notify health care professional of all Rx or OTC medications, vitamins, or herbal products being taken and consult health care professional before taking any new medications, especially St. John's wort.
- Instruct patient not to receive any vaccinations without advice of health care professional.
- Rep: Advise male patients with female partners of reproductive potential to use effective contraception during and for at least 4 mo after last dose of cabazitaxel. May impair fertility in males.

- Emphasize need for periodic lab tests to monitor for side effects. Advise patient to monitor temperature frequently.

Evaluation/Desired Outcomes

- ↓ in size and spread of metastatic prostate cancer.

---

cabotegravir (ka-boe-teg-ra-vir)
Apretude, Vocabria
Classification
Therapeutic: antiretrovirals
Pharmacologic: integrase strand transfer inhibitors (INSTIs)

Indications

PO: Short-term treatment of HIV-1 infection in patients who are virologically suppressed (HIV-1 RNA <50 copies/mL) on a stable antiretroviral regimen with no history of treatment failure and with no known or suspected resistance to either cabotegravir or rilpivirine (in combination with rilpivirine). To be used in one of the following situations: 1) As an oral lead-in therapy to assess the tolerability of cabotegravir prior to administration of cabotegravir/rilpivirine extended-release injection (Cabenuva); or 2) As oral therapy for patients who will miss planned dosing with the cabotegravir/rilpivirine extended-release injection (Cabenuva). **PO, IM:** Pre-exposure prophylaxis (PrEP) to reduce the risk of sexually acquired HIV-1 infection in at-risk individuals. To be used in one of the following situations: 1) As an oral lead-in therapy to assess the tolerability of cabotegravir prior to administration of cabotegravir extended-release injection (Apretude); or 2) As oral PrEP for patients who will miss planned dosing with the cabotegravir extended-release injection (Apretude).

Action

Inhibits HIV-1 integrase, which is required for viral replication. **Therapeutic Effects:** Evidence of decreased viral replication and reduced viral load with slowed progression of HIV and its sequelae. Reduction in risk of sexually acquired HIV infection in at-risk individuals.

Pharmacokinetics

Absorption: Increased with high-fat meals after oral administration.
Distribution: Widely distributed to extravascular tissues.
Protein Binding: >99%.
Metabolism and Excretion: Primarily metabolized by the uridine diphosphate glucuronosyltransferase (UGT) 1A1 enzyme system, with some involvement of UGT1A9. Primarily excreted in feces as unchanged drug (47%), with 27% excreted in urine as metabolites.
Half-life: *PO:* 41 hr; *IM:* 5.6–11.5 wk.

TIME/ACTION PROFILE (plasma concentrations)

ROUTE	ONSET	PEAK	DURATION
PO	unknown	3 hr	24 hr
IM	unknown	7 days	2 mo

Contraindications/Precautions

Contraindicated in: Hypersensitivity; Concurrent use of carbamazepine, oxcarbazepine, phenobarbital, phenytoin, rifampin, or rifapentine; Unknown or positive HIV-1 status (for HIV-1 PrEP only); Lactation: Breastfeeding not recommended in patients with HIV.
Use Cautiously in: Severe hepatic impairment; End-stage renal disease (CCr <15 mL/min); Severe renal impairment (CCr 15–<30 mL/min) (injection only); OB: Safety not established in pregnancy; Pedi: Safety and effectiveness not established in children <12 yr; Geri: Use with caution in older adults, considering concurrent disease states, drug therapy, and age-related ↓ in hepatic and renal function.

Adverse Reactions/Side Effects

GI: diarrhea, HEPATOTOXICITY, nausea. **Local:** injection site reactions. **MS:** ↑ creatine kinase (injection). **Neuro:** abnormal dreams, anxiety, depression, dizziness, fatigue, headache, insomnia, mood disturbances. **Misc:** fever, HYPERSENSITIVITY REACTIONS (including angioedema).

Interactions

Drug-Drug: **Strong UGT1A1 inducers,** including **carbamazepine, oxcarbazepine, phenobarbital, phenytoin, rifampin, rifapentine,** may significantly ↓ levels and effectiveness; concurrent use contraindicated. **Antacids** containing polyvalent cations, including **aluminum hydroxide, calcium carbonate,** or **magnesium hydroxide,** may ↓ absorption and effectiveness of cabotegravir; administer antacids ≥2 hr before or ≥4 hr after cabotegravir. May ↓ **methadone** levels and effectiveness.

Route/Dosage

HIV-1 Treatment

Oral Lead-in Dosing to Assess Tolerability of Cabotegravir

PO (Adults and Children ≥12 yr and ≥35 kg): 30 mg once daily (taken with rilpivirine 25 mg once daily). Continue for ≥28 days to assess tolerability prior to initiating cabotegravir/rilpivirine extended-release injection (Cabenuva) therapy. The last dose of oral cabotegravir should be taken on the same day that cabotegravir/rilpivirine extended-release injection (Cabenuva) therapy is initiated.

Oral Dosing to Replace Planned Missed Doses of Cabotegravir/Rilpivirine Extended-Release Injection (Cabenuva)

PO (Adults and Children ≥12 yr and ≥35 kg): *To replace planned missed cabotegravir/rilpivirine extended-release injections (Cabenuva) for patients*

C

on monthly dosing schedule (if patient plans to miss scheduled monthly injection by >7 days): 30 mg once daily (with rilpivirine 25 mg once daily) initiated at the same time as missed injection of cabotegravir/rilpivirine and then continued until day the cabotegravir/rilpivirine extended-release injection (Cabenuva) is restarted (oral replacement therapy can be continued for up to 2 mo). *To replace planned missed cabotegravir/rilpivirine extended-release injections (Cabenuva) for patients on every 2-month dosing schedule (if patient plans to miss scheduled every 2-month injection by >7 days):* 30 mg once daily (with rilpivirine 25 mg once daily) initiated the same time as missed injection of cabotegravir/rilpivirine and then continued until day the cabotegravir/rilpivirine extended-release injection (Cabenuva) is restarted (oral replacement therapy can be continued for up to 2 mo).

HIV-1 Pre-exposure Prophylaxis
May initiate with cabotegravir oral lead-in therapy (to assess tolerability of cabotegravir) prior to cabotegravir IM injections or may precede directly to cabotegravir IM injections without oral lead-in.

Oral Lead-in Therapy
PO (Adults and Children ≥12 yr and ≥35 kg): 30 mg once daily. Continue for ≥28 days to assess tolerability prior to initiating IM therapy (see Initiation Injections section below).

Initiation Injections
IM (Adults and Children ≥12 yr and ≥35 kg):
With oral lead-in therapy: 600 mg once monthly for 2 consecutive mo (second initiation injection may be administered up to 7 days before or after the date the individual is scheduled to receive the injection), then proceed with Continuation Injections. First initiation injection should be given on the last day of oral cabotegravir lead-in therapy or within 3 days of the last dose of oral cabotegravir lead-in therapy (see Oral Lead-in Therapy section above to assess tolerability of cabotegravir). *Without oral lead-in therapy:* 600 mg once monthly for 2 consecutive mo (second initiation injection may be administered up to 7 days before or after the date the individual is scheduled to receive the injection), then proceed with Continuation Injections.

Continuation Injections
IM (Adults and Children ≥12 yr and ≥35 kg): 600 mg every 2 mo starting 2 mo after the last initiation injection (injection may be administered up to 7 days before or after the date the individual is scheduled to receive the injection).

Missed Doses of Injection
PO (Adults and Children ≥12 yr and ≥35 kg):
Planned missed injections: If a patient plans to miss a scheduled every 2-mo dose of cabotegravir extended-release injection (Apretude) by >7 days, use cabotegravir 30 mg once daily to replace one every 2-mo injection. The first dose of oral therapy should be taken approximately 2 mo after the last dose of cabotegravir extended-release injection (Apretude) and continued until the day that injection dosing is restarted or within 3 days of injection dosing being restarted. For oral PrEP durations >2 months, use an alternative oral regimen for PrEP. *Unplanned missed injections:* If a scheduled injection visit is missed or delayed by >7 days and oral dosing has not been taken in the interim, clinically reassess to determine if injection therapy remains appropriate.

Availability
Tablets (Vocabria): 30 mg. **Extended-release suspension for injection (Apretude):** 200 mg/mL.

NURSING IMPLICATIONS
Assessment
- Assess patient for change in severity of HIV symptoms and for symptoms of opportunistic infections during therapy.
- Monitor for anxiety, depression (especially in patients with a history of psychiatric illness), suicidal ideation, and paranoia during therapy.
- Monitor for signs and symptoms of hypersensitivity reactions (severe rash, or rash accompanied by fever, general malaise, fatigue, muscle or joint aches, blisters, oral blisters or lesions, conjunctivitis, facial edema, hepatitis, eosinophilia, angioedema, difficulty breathing) during therapy. Discontinue cabotegravir immediately if reactions occur.

Lab Test Considerations
- Monitor liver functions tests periodically during therapy.

Implementation
- Oral lead-in is used for at least 28 days concurrently with rilpivirine to assess the tolerability of cabotegravir prior to the initiation of cabotegravir/rilpivirine. Administer last oral dose on same day injections with cabotegravir/rilpivirine are started.
- If taking to replace a missed scheduled injection of cabotegravir/rilpivirine, take first dose of oral therapy approximately 1 mo after last injection dose and continue until the day injection dosing is restarted.
- **PO:** Administer once daily with a meal at the same time each day.
- **IM:** *Apretude*: Before starting *Apretude* for HIV-1 PrEP, ask seronegative individuals about recent (in past month) potential exposure events (condomless sex or condom breaking during sex with a partner of unknown HIV-1 status or unknown viremic status, a recent sexually transmitted infection [STI]), and evaluate for current or recent signs or symptoms consistent with acute HIV-1 infection (fever, fatigue, myalgia, skin rash). If recent (<1 mo) exposures to

HIV-1 are suspected or symptoms consistent with acute HIV-1 infection are present, use an FDA-approved test as an aid in diagnosis of acute or primary HIV-1 infection. When using *Apretude* for HIV-1 PrEP, test for HIV-1 before each injection and upon diagnosis of any other STIs. If an individual has confirmed HIV-1 infection, then individual must be transitioned to a complete HIV-1 treatment regimen. *Apretude* may be initiated with oral cabotegravir prior to intramuscular injections, or patient may proceed directly to injection of *Apretude* without an oral lead-in.

• Prior to starting *Apretude*, carefully select individuals who agree to the required injection dosing and testing schedule and counsel individuals about the importance of adherence to scheduled dosing visits to help reduce the risk of acquiring HIV-1 infection and development of resistance.

• Bring to room temperature prior to administration. Administer undiluted in the ventrogluteal or dorsogluteal site; do not administer by any other route or anatomical site. Consider the body mass index (BMI) of the individual to ensure that the needle length is sufficient to reach the gluteus muscle. Longer needle lengths may be required for individuals with higher BMI (>30 kg/m²) to ensure injection is administered IM and not SUBQ. Solution is white to light pink; do not administer solutions that are discolored or contain particulate matter. Do not freeze. Do not mix with any other product or diluent. Administer dose as soon as possible; may remain in the syringe for up to 2 hr.

Patient/Family Teaching

• Instruct patient to take cabotegravir as directed. Take missed doses as soon as remembered. Do not stop taking cabotegravir without consulting health care professional. Instruct patient to read *Patient Information* before starting cabotegravir and with each Rx refill in case of changes.

• Advise patient to notify health care professional if signs and symptoms of allergic reaction (fever, generally ill feeling, tiredness, muscle or joint aches, trouble breathing, blisters or sores in mouth, blisters, redness or swelling of eyes, swelling of mouth, face, lips, or tongue), liver problems (yellow skin or white part of eyes, dark or "tea-colored" urine, light-colored stools, nausea or vomiting, loss of appetite, pain, aching, or tenderness on the right side of stomach area, itching) or depression (feeling sad or hopeless, feeling anxious or restless, have thoughts of hurting yourself [suicide] or have tried to hurt yourself) occur.

• Apretude is not always effective in preventing HIV-1. Encourage consistent and correct condom use; knowledge of partner(s)' HIV-1 status, including viral suppression status; regular testing for STIs that can facilitate HIV-1 transmission.

• Instruct patient to notify health care professional of all Rx or OTC medications, vitamins, or herbal products being taken and consult health care professional before taking any new medications.

• Rep: May cause fetal harm. Advise females of reproductive potential to use effective contraception during therapy and avoid breastfeeding. Cabotegravir is detected in systemic circulation for ≥12 mo after discontinuing *Apretude*. Inform patient of pregnancy exposure registry that monitors pregnancy outcomes in women exposed to cabotegravir during pregnancy. Register patients by calling the Antiretroviral Pregnancy Registry at 1-800-258-4263.

Evaluation/Desired Outcomes

• Decrease in viral load and improvement in CD4 cell counts.

• Delayed progression of AIDS and decreased opportunistic infections in patients with HIV.

cabotegravir/rilpivirine
(ka-boe-**teg**-ra-vir/**ril**-pi-vir-een)
Cabenuva
Classification
Therapeutic: antiretrovirals
Pharmacologic: integrase strand transfer inhibitors (INSTIs), non-nucleoside reverse transcriptase inhibitors

Indications

Management of HIV-1 infection to replace the current antiretroviral regimen in patients who are virologically suppressed (HIV-1 RNA <50 copies/mL) on a stable antiretroviral regimen with no history of treatment failure and with no known or suspected resistance to either cabotegravir or rilpivirine.

Action

Cabotegravir: Inhibits HIV-1 integrase, which is required for viral replication; *Rilpivirine:* Inhibits HIV-replication by noncompetitively inhibiting HIV reverse transcriptase. **Therapeutic Effects:** Evidence of decreased viral replication and reduced viral load with slowed progression of HIV and its sequelae.

Pharmacokinetics
Cabotegravir
Absorption: Increased with high-fat meals.
Distribution: Distributed to extravascular tissues.
Protein Binding: >99%.
Metabolism and Excretion: Primarily metabolized by the uridine diphosphate glucuronosyltransferase (UGT) 1A1 enzyme system, with some involvement of UGT1A9. Primarily excreted in feces as unchanged drug (47%), with 27% excreted in urine as metabolites.
Half-life: 41 hr.
Rilpivirine
Absorption: Well absorbed following oral administration.
Distribution: Unknown.

Protein Binding: 99.7%.
Metabolism and Excretion: Primarily metabolized by the liver via the CYP3A isoenzyme; 25% excreted in feces unchanged, <1% excreted unchanged in urine.
Half-life: 50 hr.

TIME/ACTION PROFILE (plasma concentrations)

ROUTE	ONSET	PEAK	DURATION
cabotegravir IM	unknown	7 days	unknown
rilpivirine IM	unknown	3–4 days	unknown

Contraindications/Precautions

Contraindicated in: Hypersensitivity to cabotegravir or rilpivirine; Concurrent use of carbamazepine, dexamethasone (more than a single dose), oxcarbazepine, phenobarbital, phenytoin, rifabutin, rifampin, rifapentine, or St. John's wort; OB: Pregnancy; Lactation: Breastfeeding not recommended in patients with HIV.
Use Cautiously in: History of depression or suicide attempt; Hepatic impairment; Severe renal impairment (CCr 15–30 mL/min) or end-stage renal disease (CCr <15 mL/min); Pedi: Children <12 yr (safety and effectiveness not established); Geri: Use with caution in older adults, considering concurrent disease states, drug therapy, and age-related ↓ in hepatic and renal function.

Adverse Reactions/Side Effects

CV: QT interval prolongation. **Derm:** DRUG REACTION WITH EOSINOPHILIA AND SYSTEMIC SYMPTOMS (DRESS), rash. **GI:** ↑ lipase, HEPATOTOXICITY, nausea. **Local:** injection site reactions. **Metab:** ↑ weight. **MS:** ↑ creatine kinase, pain. **Neuro:** depression, dizziness, fatigue, headache, insomnia, mood disturbances, negative thoughts, somnolence, SUICIDAL THOUGHTS/BEHAVIORS. **Misc:** fever, HYPERSENSITIVITY REACTIONS (including angioedema).

Interactions

Drug-Drug: Strong UGT1A1 inducers or CYP3A inducers, including **carbamazepine, oxcarbazepine, phenobarbital, phenytoin, rifabutin, rifampin**, or **rifapentine** may significantly ↓ cabotegravir and rilpivirine levels and effectiveness; concurrent use contraindicated. Use of more than a single dose of **dexamethasone** may significantly ↓ rilpivirine levels and effectiveness; concurrent use contraindicated. **Macrolide antibiotics,** including **azithromycin, clarithromycin,** and **erythromycin** may ↑ rilpivirine levels and risk of toxicity, including QT interval prolongation; use alternative antibiotic therapy. **QT interval prolonging drugs** may ↑ risk of QT interval prolongation and torsades de pointes. May ↓ levels and effects of **methadone**.

Drug-Natural Products: St. John's wort may significantly ↓ rilpivirine levels and effectiveness; concurrent use contraindicated.

Route/Dosage

Lead-in therapy with oral cabotegravir and oral rilpivirine must be used for at least 28 days to assess tolerability to both cabotegravir and rilpivirine prior to initiating cabotegravir/rilpivirine extended-release injection therapy.

Monthly Dosing

IM (Adults and Children ≥12 yr and ≥35 kg): *Initiation injections:* Cabotegravir 600 mg as single injection and rilpivirine 900 mg as single injection, both administered on the final day of lead-in therapy with oral cabotegravir and oral rilpivirine. *Continuation injections:* Cabotegravir 400-mg injection and rilpivirine 600-mg injection once monthly (administer both injections during same visit). Start continuation injections 1 mo following initiation injections. Monthly injections may be given within 7 days of originally scheduled date of injection. *Switching to every 2-mo injection dosing:* Administer cabotegravir 600-mg injection and rilpivirine 900-mg injection 1 mo after the last monthly continuation injection and then every 2 mo thereafter. *Planned missed injections:* If patient plans to miss a scheduled injection visit by >7 days, give oral cabotegravir 30 mg once daily and oral rilpivirine 25 mg once daily initiated at the same time as missed injection of cabotegravir/rilpivirine and then continued until day the cabotegravir/rilpivirine extended-release injection is restarted (oral replacement therapy can be continued for up to 2 mo). If time since last injection ≤2 mo, resume injection with cabotegravir 400-mg injection and rilpivirine 600-mg injection once monthly. If time since last injection >2 mo, resume injection with initiation injection of cabotegravir 600-mg single injection and rilpivirine 900-mg single injection followed in 1 mo by continuation injections of cabotegravir 400-mg injection and rilpivirine 600-mg injection once monthly (start continuation injections 1 mo following initiation injections). *Unplanned missed injections:* If monthly injections are missed or delayed by >7 days and oral cabotegravir and oral rilpivirine therapy have not been taken in the interim, reassess patient to determine if resumption of injection dosing remains appropriate.

Every 2-Month Dosing

IM (Adults and Children ≥12 yr and ≥35 kg): *Initiation injections:* Cabotegravir 600-mg injection and rilpivirine 900-mg injection once monthly for 2 consecutive mo, with the first set of injections being administered on the final day of lead-in therapy with oral cabotegravir and oral rilpivirine. Second initiation injection may be given within 7 days of originally scheduled date of injection. *Continuation injections:* Cabotegravir

600-mg injection and rilpivirine 900-mg injection every 2 mo (administer both injections during same visit). Start continuation injections 2 mo following second initiation injection. Every 2-mo injections may be given within 7 days of originally scheduled date of injection. *Switching to monthly injection dosing:* Administer cabotegravir 400-mg injection and rilpivirine 600-mg injection 2 mo after the last monthly continuation injection and then once monthly thereafter. *Planned missed injections:* If patient plans to miss a scheduled injection visit by >7 days, give oral cabotegravir 30 mg once daily and oral rilpivirine 25 mg once daily initiated at the same time as missed injection of cabotegravir/rilpivirine and then continued until day the cabotegravir/rilpivirine extended-release injection is restarted (oral replacement therapy can be continued for up to 2 mo). If time since second initiation injection ≤2 mo, resume initiation injection with cabotegravir 600-mg injection and rilpivirine 900-mg injection, followed by continuation injections every 2 mo (starting 2 mo following second initiation injection). If time since second initiation injection >2 mo, restart the two initiation injections (see above) given once monthly for 2 consecutive months, followed by the continuation injections (see above) given every 2 mo. If patient misses a continuation injection by ≤3 mo, resume injection with cabotegravir 600-mg injection and rilpivirine 900-mg injection every 2 mo. If time since last injection >3 mo, restart the two initiation injections (see above) given once monthly for 2 consecutive mo followed by the continuation injections (see above) given every 2 mo. *Unplanned missed injections:* If monthly injections are missed or delayed by >7 days and oral cabotegravir and oral rilpivirine therapy have not been taken in the interim, reassess patient to determine if resumption of injection dosing remains appropriate.

Availability

Extended-release suspension for injection: 400-mg/600-mg kit (200 mg/mL vial of cabotegravir and 300 mg/mL vial of rilpivirine), 600-mg/900-mg kit (200 mg/mL vial of cabotegravir and 300 mg/mL vial of rilpivirine).

NURSING IMPLICATIONS

Assessment

- Assess patient for change in severity of HIV symptoms and for symptoms of opportunistic infections during therapy.
- Monitor for anxiety, depression (especially in patients with a history of psychiatric illness), suicidal ideation, and paranoia during therapy.
- Monitor for signs and symptoms of hypersensitivity reactions (severe rash, or rash accompanied by fever, general malaise, fatigue, muscle or joint aches, blisters, oral blisters or lesions, conjunctivitis, facial edema, hepatitis, eosinophilia, angioedema, difficulty breathing) during therapy. Discontinue cabotegravir immediately if reactions occur.

- Observe patient for 10 min following injections for post-injection reactions (dyspnea, agitation, abdominal cramping, flushing, sweating, oral numbness, changes in blood pressure).

Lab Test Considerations

- Monitor liver function tests periodically during therapy. Discontinue therapy if hepatotoxicity is suspected.

Implementation

- Lead-in therapy with oral cabotegravir and oral rilpivirine must be used for at least 28 days to assess tolerability to both cabotegravir and rilpivirine prior to initiating cabotegravir/rilpivirine extended-release injection therapy. Start injections of cabotegravir/rilpivirine on last day of PO lead-in therapy.
- Injection must be administered by health care provider.
- **IM:** Administer cabotegravir and rilpivirine at separate gluteal (preferably ventrogluteal) injection sites (on opposite sides or 2 cm apart) during the same visit. Use needles long enough for IM injection. Allow suspensions to come to room temperature for 15 min before administration. Stable at room temperature for up to 6 hr. Shake suspensions vigorously to mix. Do not administer solutions that contain particulate matter. Administer within 2 hr of drawing into syringe; if >2 hr, discard injection. Do not refrigerate syringes. Start continuation injections a month after the initiation injections. Injections may be given 7 days before or after the date to receive the injection.

Patient/Family Teaching

- Instruct patient in the importance of adhering to monthly schedule of injections. *Planned Missed Injections:* If a scheduled injection visit by >7 days, take daily PO therapy to replace up to 2 consecutive monthly injection visits. Take first dose of PO therapy approximately 1 mo after the last injection dose and continued until the day injection dosing is restarted. *Unplanned Missed Injections:* If monthly injections are missed or delayed by >7 days and PO therapy has not been taken in the interim, health care professional will reassess patient to determine if resumption of injection dosing remains appropriate. Instruct patient to read *Patient Information* before starting cabotegravir/rilpivirine therapy and with each injection in case of changes.
- Advise patient to notify health care professional if signs and symptoms of allergic reaction (fever, generally ill feeling, tiredness, muscle or joint aches, trouble breathing, blisters or sores in mouth, blisters, redness or swelling of eyes, swelling of mouth, face, lips, or tongue), post-injection reactions (trouble breathing, stomach cramps, sweating, numbness of mouth, feeling anxious, feeling warm, feeling lightheaded or faint, blood pressure changes), liver problems (yellow skin or white part of eyes, dark or "tea-colored" urine, light-colored stools, nausea or

vomiting, loss of appetite, pain, aching, or tenderness on the right side of stomach area, itching), or depression (feeling sad or hopeless, feeling anxious or restless, have thoughts of hurting yourself [suicide] or have tried to hurt yourself) occur.

- Instruct patient to notify health care professional of all Rx or OTC medications, vitamins, or herbal products being taken and consult health care professional before taking any new medications, especially St. John's wort.
- Rep: May cause fetal harm. Advise females of reproductive potential to use effective contraception during therapy and to avoid breastfeeding. Cabotegravir is detected in systemic circulation for ≥12 mo after discontinuing cabotegravir/rilpivirine. Inform patient of pregnancy exposure registry that monitors pregnancy outcomes in women exposed to cabotegravir during pregnancy. Register patients by calling the Antiretroviral Pregnancy Registry at 1-800-258-4263.

Evaluation/Desired Outcomes
- Decrease in viral load and improvement in CD4 cell counts.
- Delayed progression of AIDS and decreased opportunistic infections in patients with HIV.

---

calcifediol, See VITAMIN D COMPOUNDS.

---

calcitriol, See VITAMIN D COMPOUNDS.

HIGH ALERT

CALCIUM SALTS
calcium acetate (25% Ca or 12.6 mEq/g) (kal-see-um ass-e-tate)
~~PhosLo~~
calcium carbonate (40% Ca or 20 mEq/g)
(kal-see-um kar-bo-nate)
~~Caltrate~~, Maalox , Titralac, Tums, Tums E-X
calcium chloride (27% Ca or 13.6 mEq/g) (kal-see-um kloh-ride)
❦ Calciject
calcium citrate (21% Ca or 12 mEq/g) (kal-see-um si-trate)
Cal-Citrate
calcium gluconate (9% Ca or 4.5 mEq/g)
(kal-see-um gloo-koh-nate)

calcium lactate (13% Ca or 6.5 mEq/g) (kal-see-um lak-tate)
Classification
Therapeutic: mineral and electrolyte replacements/supplements
Pharmacologic: antacids

Indications
PO, IV: Treatment and prevention of hypocalcemia. **PO:** Adjunct in the prevention of postmenopausal osteoporosis. **IV:** Emergency treatment of hyperkalemia and hypermagnesemia and adjunct in cardiac arrest or calcium channel blocking agent toxicity (calcium chloride, calcium gluconate). **Calcium carbonate:** May be used as an antacid. **Calcium acetate:** Control of hyperphosphatemia in end-stage renal disease.

Action
Essential for nervous, muscular, and skeletal systems. Maintain cell membrane and capillary permeability. Act as an activator in the transmission of nerve impulses and contraction of cardiac, skeletal, and smooth muscle. Essential for bone formation and blood coagulation. Binds to dietary phosphate to form an insoluble calcium phosphate complex, which is excreted in the feces, resulting in decreased serum phosphorus concentrations (calcium acetate). **Therapeutic Effects:** Replacement of calcium in deficiency states. Control of hyperphosphatemia in end-stage renal disease without promoting aluminum absorption (calcium acetate).

Pharmacokinetics
Absorption: Absorption from the GI tract requires vitamin D. IV administration results in complete bioavailability.
Distribution: Readily enters extracellular fluid. Crosses the placenta and enters breast milk.
Metabolism and Excretion: Excreted mostly in the feces; 20% eliminated by the kidneys.
Half-life: Unknown.

TIME/ACTION PROFILE (effects on serum calcium)

ROUTE	ONSET	PEAK	DURATION
PO	unknown	unknown	unknown
IV	immediate	immediate	0.5–2 hr

Contraindications/Precautions
Contraindicated in: Hypercalcemia; Renal calculi; Ventricular fibrillation; Concurrent use of calcium supplements (calcium acetate).
Use Cautiously in: Patients receiving digoxin; Severe respiratory insufficiency; Renal impairment; Cardiac disease; OB: Hypercalcemia may ↑ risk of maternal and fetal complications; Lactation: Breastfeeding not expected to harm infant provided that serum calcium levels monitored.

❦ = Canadian drug name. ▩ = Genetic implication. ~~Strikethrough~~ = Discontinued. CAPITALS = life-threatening. <u>Underline</u> = most frequent.

Adverse Reactions/Side Effects

CV: <u>arrhythmias</u>, bradycardia, CARDIAC ARREST (IV only). **F and E:** <u>hypercalcemia</u>. **GI:** <u>constipation</u>, diarrhea (oral solution only), nausea, vomiting. **GU:** calculi, hypercalciuria. **Local:** <u>phlebitis</u> (IV only). **Neuro:** syncope (IV only), tingling.

Interactions

Drug-Drug: Hypercalcemia ↑ the risk of **digoxin** toxicity. Chronic use with **antacids** in renal insufficiency may lead to milk-alkali syndrome. **Calcium supplements**, including calcium-containing antacids, may ↑ risk of hypercalcemia; avoid concurrent use. Ingestion by mouth ↓ the absorption of orally administered **phenytoin** and **iron salts**; take 1 hr before or 3 hr after oral calcium supplements. Excessive amounts may ↓ the effects of **calcium channel blockers**. Calcium acetate may ↓ absorption of orally administered **tetracyclines**; take ≥1 hr before calcium acetate. Calcium acetate may ↓ absorption of orally administered **fluoroquinolones**; take ≥2 hr before or 6 hr after calcium acetate. Calcium acetate may ↓ absorption of orally administered **levothyroxine**; take ≥4 hr before or 4 hr after calcium acetate. ↓ absorption of **risedronate** (do not take within 2 hr of calcium supplements). Concurrent use with **diuretics (thiazide)** may result in hypercalcemia. May ↓ the ability of **sodium polystyrene sulfonate** to decrease serum potassium.

Drug-Food: **Cereals**, **spinach**, or **rhubarb** may ↓ the absorption of calcium supplements.

Route/Dosage

Doses are expressed in mg, g, or mEq of calcium.

PO (Adults): *Prevention of hypocalcemia, treatment of depletion, osteoporosis:* 1–2 g/day. *Antacid:* 0.5–1.5 g as needed (calcium carbonate only). *Hyperphosphatemia in end-stage renal disease (calcium acetate only):* 1334 mg with each meal, may ↑ gradually (in absence of hypercalcemia) to achieve target serum phosphate levels (usual dose = 2001–2668 mg with each meal).

PO (Children): *Supplementation:* 45–65 mg/kg/day.

PO (Infants): *Neonatal hypocalcemia:* 50–150 mg/kg (not to exceed 1 g).

IV (Adults): *Emergency treatment of hypocalcemia, cardiac standstill:* 7–14 mEq. *Hypocalcemic tetany:* 4.5–16 mEq; repeat until symptoms are controlled. *Hyperkalemia with cardiac toxicity:* 2.25–14 mEq; may repeat in 1–2 min. *Hypermagnesemia:* 7 mEq.

IV (Children): *Emergency treatment of hypocalcemia:* 1–7 mEq. *Hypocalcemic tetany:* 0.5–0.7 mEq/kg 3–4 times daily.

IV (Infants): *Emergency treatment of hypocalcemia:* <1 mEq. *Hypocalcemic tetany:* 2.4 mEq/kg/day in divided doses.

Availability (generic available)

Calcium Acetate
Tablets: 667 mg (169 mg elemental Ca). **Gelcaps:** 667 mg (169 mg elemental Ca).

Calcium Carbonate
Tablets: 600 mg (240 mg Ca)^OTC, 650 mg (260 mg Ca)^OTC, 1.25 g (500 mg Ca)^OTC, 1.5 g (600 mg Ca)^OTC. **Chewable tablets:** 420 mg (168 mg Ca)^OTC, 500 mg (200 mg Ca)^OTC, 750 mg (300 mg Ca)^OTC, 1 g (400 mg Ca)^OTC, 1.25 g (500 mg Ca)^OTC. **Oral suspension:** 1.25 g (500 mg Ca)/5 mL^OTC. **Powder:** 6.5 g (2400 mg Ca)/packet^OTC.

Calcium Chloride
Solution for injection: 10% (1.36 mEq/mL).

Calcium Citrate
Tablets: 200 mg^OTC, 250 mg^OTC. **Capsules:** 150 mg.

Calcium Gluconate
Tablets: 500 mg (45 mg Ca)^OTC. **Premixed infusion (in sodium chloride):** 1 g/50 mL (4.65 mEq/50 mL), 2 g/100 mL (9.3 mEq/100 mL). **Solution for injection:** 10% (0.45 mEq/mL).

Calcium Lactate
Tablets: 100 mg ^OTC.

NURSING IMPLICATIONS

Assessment

- **Calcium Supplement/Replacement:** Observe patient closely for symptoms of hypocalcemia (paresthesia, muscle twitching, laryngospasm, colic, cardiac arrhythmias, Chvostek's or Trousseau's sign). Notify health care professional if these occur. Protect symptomatic patients by elevating and padding siderails and keeping bed in low position.
- Monitor BP, pulse, and ECG frequently during parenteral therapy. May cause vasodilation with resulting hypotension, bradycardia, arrhythmias, and cardiac arrest. Transient increases in BP may occur during IV administration, especially in geriatric patients or in patients with hypertension.
- Assess IV site for patency. Extravasation may cause cellulitis, necrosis, and sloughing.
- Monitor patient on digoxin for signs of toxicity.
- **Antacid:** When used as an antacid, assess for heartburn, indigestion, and abdominal pain. Inspect abdomen; auscultate bowel sounds.

Lab Test Considerations

- Monitor serum calcium or ionized calcium, chloride, sodium, potassium, magnesium, albumin, and parathyroid hormone (PTH) concentrations before and periodically during therapy for treatment of hypocalcemia.
- *For patients with hyperphosphatemia:* Monitor serum calcium twice weekly during adjustment phase. If serum calcium level is >12 mg/dL, discontinue therapy and start hemodialysis as needed; lower dose or temporarily stop therapy for calcium level between 10.5 and 11.9 mg/dL.

C

• May cause ↓ serum phosphate concentrations with excessive and prolonged use. When used to treat hyperphosphatemia in renal failure patients, monitor phosphate levels.

Toxicity and Overdose
• Assess patient for nausea, vomiting, anorexia, thirst, severe constipation, paralytic ileus, and bradycardia. Contact health care professional immediately if these signs of hypercalcemia occur.

Implementation
• *High Alert:* Errors with IV calcium gluconate and chloride have occurred secondary to confusion over which salt is ordered. Clarify incomplete orders. Confusion has occurred with milligram doses of calcium chloride and calcium gluconate, which are not equal. Chloride and gluconate forms are routinely available on most hospital crash carts; specify form of calcium desired.
• Do not confuse Os-Cal with Asacol.
• In arrest situations, the use of calcium chloride is now limited to patients with hyperkalemia, hypocalcemia, and calcium channel blocker toxicity.
• **PO:** Administer calcium carbonate or phosphate 1–1.5 hr after meals and at bedtime. Chewable tablets should be well chewed before swallowing. Follow oral doses with a full glass of water, except when using calcium carbonate as a phosphate binder in renal dialysis. Administer on an empty stomach before meals to optimize effectiveness in patients with hyperphosphatemia.
• **IM:** IM administration of calcium salts can cause severe necrosis and tissue sloughing. Do not administer IM.

IV Administration
• **IV:** IV solution should be warmed to body temperature and given through a small-bore needle in a large vein to minimize phlebitis. Do not administer through a scalp vein. May cause cutaneous burning sensation, peripheral vasodilation, and drop in BP. Patient should remain recumbent for 30–60 min after IV administration.
• If infiltration occurs, discontinue IV. May be treated with application of heat, elevation, and local infiltration of normal saline, 1% procaine, or hyaluronidase.
• *High Alert:* Administer slowly. High concentrations may cause cardiac arrest. Rapid administration may cause tingling, sensation of warmth, and a metallic taste. Halt infusion if these symptoms occur, and resume infusion at a slower rate when they subside.
• Do not administer solutions that are not clear or that contain a precipitate.

Calcium Chloride
IV Administration
• **IV Push:** May be administered undiluted by IV push.
• **Intermittent/Continuous Infusion:** May be diluted with D5W, D10W, 0.9% NaCl, D5/0.25% NaCl, D5/0.45% NaCl, D5/0.9% NaCl, or D5/LR.
• *Rate:* Maximum rate for adults is 0.7–1.4 mEq/min (0.5–1 mL of 10% solution); for children, 0.5 mL/min.
• **Y-Site Compatibility:** acyclovir, alemtuzumab, amikacin, aminocaproic acid, aminophylline, amiodarone, anidulafungin, argatroban, arsenic trioxide, ascorbic acid, atropine, azithromycin, aztreonam, benztropine, bivalirudin, bleomycin, buprenorphine, butorphanol, calcium gluconate, carboplatin, carmustine, caspofungin, cefotaxime, cefotetan, cefoxitin, ceftaroline, ceftolozane/tazobactam, chloramphenicol, chlorpromazine, cisplatin, clindamycin, cyanocobalamin, cyclophosphamide, cyclosporine, cytarabine, dacarbazine, dactinomycin, daptomycin, daunorubicin hydrochloride, dexmedetomidine, dexrazoxane, digoxin, diltiazem, diphenhydramine, dobutamine, docetaxel, dopamine, doxorubicin hydrochloride, doxycycline, enalaprilat, ephedrine, epinephrine, epirubicin, epoetin alfa, eptifibatide, eravacycline, ertapenem, erythromycin, esmolol, etoposide, etoposide phosphate, famotidine, fentanyl, fluconazole, fludarabine, furosemide, ganciclovir, gemcitabine, gentamicin, glycopyrrolate, granisetron, heparin, hetastarch, hydromorphone, idarubicin, ifosfamide, insulin, regular, irinotecan, isavuconazonium, isoproterenol, labetalol, LR, leucovorin calcium, lidocaine, linezolid, lorazepam, mannitol, meperidine, meropenem, mesna, methadone, methotrexate, metoclopramide, metoprolol, metronidazole, micafungin, midazolam, milrinone, mitomycin, mitoxantrone, morphine, moxifloxacin, multivitamin, mycophenolate, nafcillin, nalbuphine, naloxone, nicardipine, nitroglycerin, nitroprusside, norepinephrine, octreotide, ondansetron, oxytocin, paclitaxel, palonosetron, papaverine, penicillin G, pentobarbital, phenobarbital, phentolamine, phenylephrine, phytonadione, piperacillin/tazobactam, potassium acetate, potassium chloride, procainamide, promethazine, propranolol, protamine, pyridoxine, rocuronium, succinylcholine, sufentanil, tacrolimus, theophylline, thiamine, thiotepa, tigecycline, tirofiban, tobramycin, topotecan, vancomycin, vasopressin, vecuronium, verapamil, vinblastine, vincristine, vinorelbine, voriconazole.
• **Y-Site Incompatibility:** amphotericin B deoxycholate, amphotericin B lipid complex, amphotericin B liposomal, azathioprine, cefazolin, ceftazidime, ceftriaxone, cefuroxime, dantrolene, diazepam, doxorubicin liposomal, fluorouracil, folic acid, foscarnet, fosphenytoin, gemtuzumab ozogamicin, haloperidol, indomethacin, ketorolac, magnesium sulfate, mero-

penem/vaborbactam, methylprednisolone, minocycline, oxacillin, oxaliplatin, pantoprazole, pemetrexed, phenytoin, plazomicin, potassium phosphate, prochlorperazine, propofol, sodium bicarbonate, sodium phosphate, trimethoprim/sulfamethoxazole.

Calcium Gluconate

IV Administration

- **IV Push:** Administer slowly by IV push. *Rate:* Maximum administration rate for adults is 1.5–2 mL/min.
- **Continuous Infusion:** May be further diluted in 1000 mL of D5W, D10W, D20W, D5/0.9% NaCl, 0.9% NaCl, D5/LR, or LR.
- *Rate:* Administer at a rate not to exceed 200 mg/min over 12–24 hr.
- **Y-Site Compatibility:** acyclovir, aldesleukin, alemtuzumab, allopurinol, amifostine, amikacin, aminocaproic acid, aminophylline, anidulafungin, argatroban, arsenic trioxide, ascorbic acid, azathioprine, azithromycin, aztreonam, benztropine, bivalirudin, bleomycin, bumetanide, buprenorphine, butorphanol, calcium chloride, carboplatin, carmustine, caspofungin, cefazolin, cefepime, cefotaxime, cefotetan, ceftaroline, ceftazidime, ceftolozane/tazobactam, cefuroxime, chloramphenicol, chlorpromazine, ciprofloxacin, cisatracurium, cisplatin, cladribine, clindamycin, cyanocobalamin, cyclophosphamide, cyclosporine, cytarabine, dacarbazine, dactinomycin, daptomycin, daunorubicin hydrochloride, dexmedetomidine, dexrazoxane, digoxin, diltiazem, diphenhydramine, dobutamine, docetaxel, dopamine, doxapram, doxorubicin hydrochloride, doxorubicin liposomal, doxycycline, enalaprilat, epinephrine, epirubicin, epoetin alfa, eptifibatide, eravacycline, ertapenem, erythromycin, esmolol, etoposide, etoposide phosphate, famotidine, fentanyl, filgrastim, fludarabine, fluorouracil, folic acid, furosemide, ganciclovir, gemcitabine, gentamicin, glycopyrrolate, granisetron, heparin, hetastarch, hydromorphone, idarubicin, ifosfamide, insulin regular, irinotecan, isavuconazonium, isoproterenol, ketamine, labetalol, LR, leucovorin calcium, levofloxacin, lidocaine, linezolid, lorazepam, magnesium sulfate, mannitol, melphalan, meperidine, meropenem/vaborbactam, mesna, methadone, methohexital, methotrexate, metoclopramide, metoprolol, metronidazole, micafungin, midazolam, milrinone, mitomycin, mitoxantrone, morphine, moxifloxacin, multivitamins, nafcillin, nalbuphine, naloxone, nicardipine, nitroglycerin, nitroprusside, norepinephrine, octreotide, ondansetron, oritavancin, oxaliplatin, oxytocin, paclitaxel, palonosetron, papaverine, penicillin G, pentamidine, pentobarbital, phenobarbital, phentolamine, phenylephrine, phytonadione, piperacillin/tazobactam, plazomicin, potassium acetate, potassium chloride, procainamide, prochlorperazine, promethazine, propofol, propranolol, prot-

amine, pyridoxine, remifentanil, rituximab, rocuronium, sargramostim, sodium acetate, succinylcholine, sufentanil, tacrolimus, telavancin, theophylline, thiamine, thiotepa, tigecycline, tirofiban, tobramycin, trastuzumab, vancomycin, vasopressin, vecuronium, verapamil, vinblastine, vincristine, vinorelbine, voriconazole.

- **Y-Site Incompatibility:** amphotericin B deoxycholate, amphotericin B lipid complex, amphotericin B liposomal, cangrelor, ceftriaxone, dantrolene, diazepam, foscarnet, fosphenytoin, gemtuzumab ozogamicin, indomethacin, methylprednisolone, minocycline, mycophenolate, oxacillin, pemetrexed, phenytoin, potassium phosphate, sodium bicarbonate, sodium phosphate, tedizolid, topotecan, trimethoprim/sulfamethoxazole.

Patient/Family Teaching

- Instruct patient to take medication as directed. Instruct patients on a regular schedule to take missed doses as soon as possible, then go back to regular schedule.
- Instruct patient not to take enteric-coated tablets within 1 hr of calcium carbonate; this will result in premature dissolution of the tablets.
- Do not administer concurrently with foods containing large amounts of oxalic acid (spinach, rhubarb), phytic acid (brans, cereals), or phosphorus (milk or dairy products). Administration with milk products may lead to milk-alkali syndrome (nausea, vomiting, confusion, headache). Do not take within 1–2 hr of other medications if possible.
- Advise patient that calcium carbonate may cause constipation. Review methods of preventing constipation (increasing bulk in diet, increasing fluid intake, increasing mobility) and using laxatives. Severe constipation may indicate toxicity.
- Advise patient to avoid excessive use of tobacco or beverages containing alcohol or caffeine.
- Rep: Advise females with reproductive potential to notify health care professional if pregnancy is planned or suspected, or if breastfeeding. Monitor infants born to mothers with hypocalcemia for signs of hypocalcemia or hypercalcemia (neuromuscular irritability, apnea, cyanosis, and cardiac rhythm disorders).
- **Calcium Supplement:** Encourage patients to maintain a diet adequate in vitamin D (see Appendix J).
- **Osteoporosis:** Advise patients that exercise has been found to arrest and reverse bone loss. Patient should discuss any exercise limitations with health care professional before beginning program.
- **Hyperphosphatemia:** Advise patient to notify health care professional promptly if signs and symptoms of hypercalcemia (constipation, anorexia, nausea, vomiting, confusion, stupor) occur.
- Advise patient to avoid taking calcium-containing supplements, including calcium-based antacids, during therapy.

Evaluation/Desired Outcomes
- Increase in serum calcium levels.
- Decrease in the signs and symptoms of hypocalcemia.
- Resolution of indigestion.
- Control of hyperphosphatemia in patients with renal failure (calcium acetate only).

BEERS

canagliflozin (kan-a-gli-**floe**-zin)
Invokana
Classification
Therapeutic: antidiabetics
Pharmacologic: sodium-glucose co-transporter 2 (SGLT2) inhibitors

Indications
Adjunct to diet and exercise in the management of type 2 diabetes mellitus. To reduce the risk of major adverse cardiovascular events in patients with type 2 diabetes mellitus and established cardiovascular disease. To reduce the risk of end-stage kidney disease (ESKD), doubling of serum creatinine, cardiovascular death, and hospitalization for HF in patients with type 2 diabetes mellitus and diabetic nephropathy with albuminuria >300 m g/day.

Action
Inhibits proximal renal tubular sodium-glucose cotransporter 2 (SGLT2), which determines reabsorption of glucose from the tubular lumen. Inhibits reabsorption of glucose, lowers renal threshold for glucose, and increases excretion of glucose in urine. **Therapeutic Effects:** Improved glycemic control. Reduction in risk of cardiovascular death, nonfatal MI, and nonfatal stroke. Reduction in risk of ESKD, doubling of serum creatinine, cardiovascular death, and HF hospitalizations.

Pharmacokinetics
Absorption: Well absorbed (65%) following oral administration.
Distribution: Extensive tissue distribution.
Protein Binding: 99%.
Metabolism and Excretion: Mostly metabolized by UDP-glucuronyl transferases (UGT) to inactive metabolites, minimal metabolism by CYP3A4 (7%). 50% excreted in feces as parent drug and metabolites, 33% as metabolites in urine, <1% excreted in urine as unchanged drug.
Half-life: 10.6 hr.

TIME/ACTION PROFILE (effects on A1C)

ROUTE	ONSET	PEAK	DURATION
PO	unknown	unknown	24 hr

Contraindications/Precautions
Contraindicated in: Hypersensitivity; Type 1 diabetes; Severe hepatic impairment; Lactation: Lactation.
Use Cautiously in: History of pancreatitis, pancreatic surgery, reduced caloric intake due to illness or surgery, surgical procedures or alcohol abuse (↑ risk of ketoacidosis); Hypovolemia, chronic kidney disease (eGFR <60 mL/min/1.73 m²), or concurrent use of loop diuretics (↑ risk of volume depletion or hypotension); Previous amputation, peripheral vascular disease, neuropathy, or diabetic foot infection (↑ risk of lower limb amputation); Hypotension (correct prior to treatment, especially if eGFR 30–60 mL/min, age >75 yr, or concurrent use of loop diuretics, ACE inhibitors, or ARBs); OB: Use during pregnancy only if potential maternal benefit justifies potential fetal risk; Pedi: Safety and effectiveness not established in children; Geri: Appears on Beers list. Older adults may have ↑ risk of urogenital infections (especially women in the 1st mo of treatment) and euglycemic diabetic ketoacidosis. Use with caution in older adults.

Adverse Reactions/Side Effects
CV: hypotension. **Endo:** hypoglycemia (↑ with other medications). **F and E:** hypermagnesemia, hyperphosphatemia, KETOACIDOSIS, thirst. **GI:** abdominal pain, constipation, nausea. **GU:** female mycotic infections, ↓ renal function, ↑ urination, acute kidney injury, glucosuria, male mycotic infections, NECROTIZING FASCIITIS OF PERINEUM (FOURNIER'S GANGRENE), urinary tract infection (including pyelonephritis), UROSEPSIS, vulvovaginal pruritus. **Metab:** hyperlipidemia. **MS:** bone fractures, lower limb amputation. **Misc:** HYPERSENSITIVITY REACTIONS (including anaphylaxis or angioedema).

Interactions
Drug-Drug: Blood levels are ↓ by **UGT inducers** including **phenobarbital**, **phenytoin**, **rifampin**, and **ritonavir**; ↑ dose may be required. ↑ risk of hypoglycemia with **insulin** or **insulin secretagogues**; dose adjustments may be required. May ↑ blood levels and effects of **digoxin**; levels should be monitored. ↑ risk of hyperkalemia with **potassium-sparing diuretics** or **medications that interfere with the renin-angiotensin-aldosterone system**. Concurrent use with **loop diuretics**, may ↑ risk of hypovolemia and hypotension. May ↓ **lithium** levels and effectiveness.

Route/Dosage
PO (Adults): 100 mg once daily initially, may ↑ to 300 mg once daily; *Concurrent use of UGT inducers (phenobarbital, phenytoin, rifampin, ritonavir):* If patient tolerating canagliflozin 100 mg once daily, ↑ to 200 mg once daily; if patient tolerating canagliflozin 200 mg once daily and requires addition glycemic control, ↑ to 300 mg once daily.

✹= Canadian drug name. ⚏ = Genetic implication. ~~Strikethrough~~ = Discontinued. CAPITALS = life-threatening. Underline = most frequent.

Renal Impairment
PO (Adults): *eGFR 30– <60 mL/min/1.73 m²:* 100 mg once daily. *eGFR <30 mL/min/1.73 m²:* Initiation of therapy not recommended; patients with albuminuria >300 m g/day who are already receiving therapy may continue with 100 mg once daily to reduce the risk of ESKD, doubling of serum creatinine, cardiovascular death, and hospitalization for HF. *Concurrent use of UGT inducers (phenobarbital, phenytoin, rifampin, ritonavir) and eGFR <60 mL/min/1.73 m²:* If patient tolerating canagliflozin 100 mg once daily, ↑ to 200 mg once daily; if patient requires additional glycemic control, consider adding another antihyperglycemic agent.

Availability
Tablets: 100 mg, 300 mg. *In combination with:* metformin (Invokamet); metformin XR (Invokamet XR). See Appendix N.

NURSING IMPLICATIONS
Assessment
- Observe patient for signs and symptoms of hypoglycemic reactions (abdominal pain, sweating, hunger, weakness, dizziness, headache, tremor, tachycardia, anxiety).
- Monitor for signs and symptoms of volume depletion (dizziness, feeling faint, weakness, orthostatic hypotension) after initiating therapy.
- Monitor for infection, new pain, tenderness, erythema, swelling, sores, or ulcers involving lower limbs, with fever or malaise; discontinue canagliflozin if these occur.

Lab Test Considerations
- Monitor hemoglobin A1C prior to and periodically during therapy.
- May cause ↑ uric acid levels.
- Monitor renal function prior to and periodically during therapy, especially in patients with eGFR <60 mL/min/1.73 m². May ↑ serum creatinine and ↓ eGFR.
- May cause ↑ serum potassium, magnesium, and phosphate levels. Monitor electrolytes periodically during therapy.
- May cause ↑ LDL-C. Monitor serum lipid levels periodically during therapy.
- Causes positive test for urine glucose.
- Monitor for ketoacidosis, especially during prolonged fasting for illness or surgery. May require temporary discontinuation of therapy.

Implementation
- Patients stabilized on a diabetic regimen who are exposed to stress, fever, trauma, infection, or surgery may require administration of insulin.
- Correct volume depletion prior to beginning therapy with canagliflozin.
- **PO:** Administer before the first meal of the day.

Patient/Family Teaching
- Instruct patient to take canagliflozin as directed. Take missed doses as soon as remembered, unless it is almost time for next dose; do not double doses. Advise patient to read the *Medication Guide* before starting and with each Rx refill in case of changes.
- Explain to patient that canagliflozin helps control hyperglycemia but does not cure diabetes. Therapy is usually long term.
- Instruct patient not to share this medication with others, even if they have the same symptoms; it may harm them.
- Encourage patient to follow prescribed diet, medication, preventative foot care, and exercise regimen to prevent hyperglycemic or hypoglycemic episodes.
- Review signs of hypoglycemia and hyperglycemia with patient. If hypoglycemia occurs, advise patient to take a glass of orange juice or 2–3 tsp of sugar, honey, or corn syrup dissolved in water and notify health care professional.
- Instruct patient in proper testing of blood glucose and urine ketones, especially during periods of stress or illness. Inform patient that canagliflozin will cause a positive test result when testing for urine glucose. Notify health care professional if significant changes occur.
- Advise patient to notify health care professional if new pain or tenderness, sores or ulcers, or infections involving the leg or foot occur and to immediately seek care if pain or tenderness, redness, or swelling of the genitals or area from the genitals back to the rectum, along with a fever above 100.4°F or malaise occur.
- Inform patient that canagliflozin may cause yeast infections. Women may have signs and symptoms of a vaginal yeast infection (vaginal odor, white or yellow vaginal discharge [may be lumpy or look like cottage cheese], vaginal itching). Men may have signs and symptoms of a yeast infection of the penis (redness, itching, or swelling of penis; rash on penis; foul smelling discharge from penis; pain in skin around penis). Advise patient to notify health care professional if yeast infection occurs.
- Advise patient to notify health care professional promptly if rash; hives; or swelling of face, lips, or throat occurs.
- Advise patient to notify health care professional of medication regimen before treatment or surgery. Holding doses for at least 3 days before surgery may be required.
- Inform patient of increased risk for urinary tract infections, hypotension, and bone fractures and discuss factors that may increase risk.
- Advise patient to notify health care professional of all Rx or OTC medications, vitamins, or herbal products being taken and to consult with health care professional before taking other medications, especially other oral hypoglycemic medications.
- Rep: May cause fetal harm. Advise females of reproductive potential to use effective contraception and avoid breastfeeding during therapy; especially avoid canagliflozin during the 2nd and 3rd trimesters. Ad-

vise patient to notify health care professional if pregnancy is planned or suspected.

Evaluation/Desired Outcomes

- Improved hemoglobin A1C and glycemic control in adults with Type II diabetes.
- Reduction in risk of cardiovascular death, nonfatal MI, and nonfatal stroke.
- Reduction in risk of ESKD, doubling of serum creatinine, cardiovascular death, and HF hospitalizations.

---

candesartan, See ANGIOTENSIN II RECEPTOR ANTAGONISTS.

---

cangrelor (kan-grel-or)
Kengreal
Classification
Therapeutic: antiplatelet agents
Pharmacologic: platelet aggregation inhibitors

Indications

Adjunct to percutaneous coronary intervention (PCI) in patients not currently receiving a $P2Y_{12}$ platelet inhibitor and are not receiving a glycoprotein IIb/IIIa inhibitor.

Action

Inhibits platelet aggregation by reversibly interacting with platelet $P2Y_{12}$ADP-receptors, preventing signal transduction and platelet activation. **Therapeutic Effects:** ↓ risk of periprocedural MI, repeat coronary revascularization or stent thrombosis associated with PCI.

Pharmacokinetics

Absorption: IV administration results in complete bioavailability.
Distribution: Minimally distributed to tissues.
Protein Binding: 97–98%.
Metabolism and Excretion: Metabolized rapidly in the bloodstream; metabolites do not have antiplatelet activity. 58% excreted by kidneys, 35% in feces.
Half-life: 3–6 min.

TIME/ACTION PROFILE (antiplatelet effect)

ROUTE	ONSET	PEAK	DURATION
IV	rapid	2 min	1 hr†

† following discontinuation.

Contraindications/Precautions

Contraindicated in: Hypersensitivity; Significant severe bleeding.
Use Cautiously in: OB: Use during pregnancy only if potential maternal benefit justifies potential fetal risk;

Lactation: Safety not established in breastfeeding; Pedi: Safety and effectiveness not established in children.

Adverse Reactions/Side Effects

Hemat: bleeding. **Resp:** dyspnea. **Misc:** HYPERSENSITIVITY REACTIONS (including anaphylaxis).

Interactions

Drug-Drug: Concurrent use of other $P2Y_{12}$ inhibitors, including **clopidogrel**, **prasugrel**, or **ticagrelor**, ↑ risk of bleeding. Blocks antiplatelet effects of concurrently administered **clopidogrel** or **prasugrel**; administer clopidogrel or prasugrel after cangrelor infusion is discontinued.

Route/Dosage

IV (Adults): 30 mcg/kg bolus prior to PCI, then 4 mcg/kg/min infusion for 2 hr or duration of procedure, whichever is longer; should be followed by initiation of an oral $P2Y_{12}$ platelet inhibitor.

Availability

Lyophilized powder for injection: 50 mg/vial.

NURSING IMPLICATIONS

Assessment

- Monitor for signs and symptoms of bleeding during and following infusion.
- Monitor for signs and symptoms of hypersensitivity reaction (bronchospasm, angioedema, stridor) during therapy. Discontinue therapy and treat symptomatically.

Implementation

- **IV Push:** *Reconstitution:* Reconstitute each 50 mg vial with 5 mL of sterile water for injection. Swirl gently until dissolved; avoid vigorous mixing. Allow foam to settle. Solution is clear and colorless to pale yellow; do not administer solutions that are discolored or contain particulate matter. *Dilution:* Withdraw reconstituted solution and add to 250 mL of 0.9% NaCl or D5W. Dilute immediately. Stable for 12 hr if diluted with D5W or 24 hr if diluted with 0.9% NaCl at room temperature. Discard unused portion. *Concentration:* 200 mcg/mL. Patients >100 kg will require at least 2 bags. *Rate:* Administer rapidly over <1 min from diluted bag via IV push or pump. Ensure bolus completely administered before beginning infusion.
- **Intermittent Infusion:** Start infusion immediately after administration of bolus. *Rate:* 4 mcg/kg/min for at least 2 hr or duration of PCI, whichever is longer.
- **Y-Site Incompatibility:** Infusion requires a dedicated line.
- To maintain platelet inhibition, administer either ticagrelor 180 mg PO at any time during or immediately after discontinuation, or prasugrel 60 mg PO or clopidogrel 600 mg PO immediately after discontin-

---

✦ = Canadian drug name. ⚇ = Genetic implication. ~~Strikethrough~~ = Discontinued. CAPITALS = life-threatening. <u>Underline</u> = most frequent.

uation of infusion; do not administer prasugrel or clopidogrel prior to discontinuation of infusion.

Patient/Family Teaching

● Caution patient to notify health care professional if bleeding occurs.

● Rep: Advise females of reproductive potential to notify health care professional if pregnancy is suspected or if breastfeeding. Avoid neuraxial blockade procedures and, when possible, discontinue cangrelor 1 hr prior to labor, delivery, or neuraxial blockade.

Evaluation/Desired Outcomes

● ↓ risk of periprocedural MI, repeat coronary revascularization or stent thrombosis associated with PCI.

cannabidiol (kan-a-bi-**dye**-ol)
Epidiolex
Classification
Therapeutic: anticonvulsants
Pharmacologic: cannabinoids

Schedule V

Indications

Seizures associated with Lennox-Gastaut syndrome, Dravet syndrome, or tuberous sclerosis complex.

Action

Cannabidiol is a cannabinoid that naturally occurs in the *Cannabis sativa* plant. Mechanism of anticonvulsant effect unknown; does not work by interacting with cannabinoid receptors. **Therapeutic Effects:** Reduction in frequency of atonic, tonic, clonic, and tonic-clonic seizures.

Pharmacokinetics

Absorption: Extent of absorption unknown. High fat/high calorie meals increase extent of absorption.
Distribution: Extensively distributed to tissues.
Protein Binding: >94%.
Metabolism and Excretion: Primarily metabolized in the liver by the CYP2C9 and CYP3A4 isoenzymes to an active metabolite (7-OH-CBD). Primarily excreted in feces.
Half-life: 56–61 hr.

TIME/ACTION PROFILE (plasma concentrations)

ROUTE	ONSET	PEAK	DURATION
PO	unknown	2.5–5 hr	unknown

Contraindications/Precautions

Contraindicated in: Hypersensitivity to cannabidiol or sesame oil.
Use Cautiously in: Concurrent use of valproic acid or clobazam; Concurrent use of sedatives, hypnotics, or other psychoactive drugs (↑ risk of adverse effects); Elevated liver enzymes (at baseline); Moderate to severe

hepatic impairment; OB: Use during pregnancy only if the potential maternal benefit justifies the potential fetal risk; Lactation: Use while breastfeeding only if the potential maternal benefit justifies the potential risk to the infant; Pedi: Children <2 yr (safety and effectiveness not established); Geri: Choose dose carefully in older adults, considering concurrent disease states, drug therapy, and age-related ↓ in hepatic and renal function.

Adverse Reactions/Side Effects

Derm: rash. **EENT:** dry mouth. **GI:** ↓ appetite, ↑ liver enzymes, diarrhea, ↓ weight, abdominal pain, hepatotoxicity. **GU:** ↑ serum creatinine. **Hemat:** anemia. **Neuro:** fatigue, insomnia, sedation, aggressive behavior, agitation, ataxia, SUICIDAL THOUGHTS/BEHAVIORS. **Misc:** HYPERSENSITIVITY REACTIONS (including angioedema), infection, physical dependence, psychological dependence (high doses or prolonged therapy).

Interactions

Drug-Drug: Concurrent use of **valproic acid** may ↑ risk of hepatotoxicity. **Moderate or strong CYP2C9 inhibitors** and **moderate or strong CYP3A4 inhibitors** may ↑ levels and risk of toxicity; consider ↓ cannabidiol dose. **Strong CYP2C9 inducers** or **strong CYP3A4 inducers** may ↓ levels and effectiveness; consider ↑ cannabidiol dose. May ↑ levels of **CYP1A2 substrates**, including **theophylline** and **tizanidine**; consider ↓ dose of CYP1A2 substrate. May ↑ levels of **CYP2B6 substrates**, including **bupropion** and **efavirenz**; consider ↓ dose of CYP2B6 substrate. May ↑ levels and risk of toxicity of **CYP2C8 substrates** and **CYP2C9 substrates**; consider ↓ dose of CYP2C8 or CYP2C9 substrate. May ↑ levels of **CYP2C19 substrates**, including **diazepam**; consider ↓ dose of CYP2C19 substrate. May ↑ levels of active metabolite of **clobazam** which may ↑ risk of toxicity associated with clobazam. May ↑ levels and risk of toxicity of **stiripentol** and **everolimus**. Additive CNS depression with **alcohol, antihistamines, barbiturates, benzodiazepines, muscle relaxants, opioid analgesics,** and **sedative/hypnotics**.

Route/Dosage

Seizures Associated with Lennox-Gastaut Syndrome or Dravet Syndrome

PO (Adults and Children ≥1 yr): 2.5 mg/kg twice daily; can ↑ dose to 5 mg/kg twice daily in 1 wk. If further reduction in seizure frequency needed, may continue to ↑ dose on weekly basis (every other day if more rapid titration warranted) in increments of 2.5 mg/kg twice daily (max dose = 10 mg/kg twice daily).

Hepatic Impairment

PO (Adults and Children ≥1 yr): *Moderate hepatic impairment (Child–Pugh B):* 1.25 mg/kg twice daily; can ↑ dose to 2.5 mg/kg twice daily in 1 wk. If further reduction in seizure frequency needed, may continue to ↑ dose on weekly basis (every other day if more rapid titration warranted) in increments of 1.25 mg/kg twice daily (max dose = 5 mg/kg twice daily); *Severe hepatic impairment (Child–Pugh C):* 0.5 mg/kg twice daily; can ↑ dose to 1 mg/kg twice daily in 1 wk. If further reduction in seizure frequency needed, may continue to ↑ dose on weekly basis (every other day if more rapid titration warranted) in increments of 0.5 mg/kg twice daily (max dose = 2 mg/kg twice daily).

Seizures Associated with Tuberous Sclerosis Complex

PO (Adults and Children ≥1 yr): 2.5 mg/kg twice daily; can ↑ dose on weekly basis (every other day if more rapid titration warranted) in increments of 2.5 mg/kg twice daily to recommended maintenance dosage of 12.5 mg/kg twice daily.

Hepatic Impairment

PO (Adults and Children ≥1 yr): *Moderate hepatic impairment (Child–Pugh B):* 1.25 mg/kg twice daily; can ↑ dose on weekly basis (every other day if more rapid titration warranted) in increments of 1.25 mg/kg twice daily to recommended maintenance dosage of 6.25 mg/kg twice daily; *Severe hepatic impairment (Child–Pugh C):* 0.5 mg/kg twice daily; can ↑ dose on weekly basis (every other day if more rapid titration warranted) in increments of 0.5 mg/kg twice daily to recommended maintenance dosage of 2.5 mg/kg twice daily.

Availability

Oral solution (strawberry flavor): 100 mg/mL.

NURSING IMPLICATIONS

Assessment

- Assess location, duration, and characteristics of seizure activity. Institute seizure precautions.
- Monitor closely for notable changes in behavior that could indicate the emergence or worsening of suicidal thoughts, behavior, or depression.
- Monitor for signs and symptoms of hepatotoxicity (unexplained nausea, vomiting, right upper quadrant abdominal pain, fatigue, anorexia, jaundice and/or dark urine). If signs and symptoms occur, promptly measure serum transaminases and total bilirubin and interrupt or discontinue treatment with cannabidiol.
- Monitor for signs and symptoms of hypersensitivity reactions (pruritus, erythema, and angioedema) during therapy. Discontinue cannabidiol if symptoms occur.

Lab Test Considerations

- Obtain serum transaminases (ALT, AST) and total bilirubin levels before starting therapy. Elevations usually respond to decreased dose or discontinuation of therapy. Monitor levels at 1, 3, and 6 mo after starting therapy, within 1 mo following dose changes, and as needed thereafter. Discontinue cannabidiol if transaminase levels >3 times upper limit

of normal (ULN) and bilirubin levels >2 times ULN. Also discontinue therapy if transaminase persistently >5 times ULN.

Implementation

- **PO:** Administer orally twice daily with consistency in regard to food; food may effect cannabidiol levels. Use calibrated measuring device included with cannabidiol to ensure accurate dosing. Solution is strawberry flavored clear, colorless to yellow. Store at room temperature; do not refrigerate or freeze. Discard 12 wk after bottle is first opened.
- May be administered enterally via silicone feeding (nasogastric, gastrostomy) tubes. Flush with approximately 5 times the priming volume of the tube with room-temperature drinking water after each dose. Volume may need to be modified in patients with fluid restrictions. Do not use with tubes made of polyvinyl chloride (PVC) or polyurethane and avoid use of silicone nasogastric tubes with short lengths and narrow diameters (e.g., less than 50 cm and less than 5 FR).

Patient/Family Teaching

- Instruct patient to take cannabidiol as directed. Advise patient not to stop cannabidiol without consulting health care professional; must be gradually discontinued to prevent seizures. Advise patient to read the *Medication Guide* before starting therapy and with each Rx refill in case of changes.
- May cause drowsiness. Caution patient to avoid driving or other activities requiring alertness until response to medication is known. Tell patient not to resume driving until health care professional gives clearance based on control of seizure disorder and response to medication is known.
- Advise patient to notify health care professional promptly if signs and symptoms of hepatotoxicity occur.
- Instruct patient to notify health care professional of all Rx or OTC medications, vitamins, or herbal products being taken and consult health care professional before taking any new medications and to avoid alcohol during therapy.
- Inform patients and families of risk of suicidal thoughts and behavior and advise that behavioral changes, emergency or worsening signs and symptoms of depression, unusual changes in mood, or emergence of suicidal thoughts, behavior, or thoughts of self-harm should be reported to health care professional immediately.
- Inform patients of potential for positive cannabis drug screens.
- Rep: Advise females of reproductive potential to notify health care professional if pregnancy is planned or suspected or if breastfeeding. Encourage patients who become pregnant to enroll in the North American Antiepileptic Drug (NAAED) Pregnancy Registry

by calling 1-888-233-2334 or on the web at www.aedpregnancyregistry.org to collect information about the safety of antiepileptic medicines during pregnancy. Enrollment must be done by patients themselves.

Evaluation/Desired Outcomes
* Decreased frequency and intensity of seizure activity.

capsaicin (kap-**say**-sin)
Capzasin-HP, Capzasin-P, DiabetAid Pain and Tingling Relief, Qutenza, ~~Zostrix~~, Zostrix-HP
Classification
Therapeutic: nonopioid analgesics (topical)

Indications
Temporary management of pain due to rheumatoid arthritis and osteoarthritis. Pain associated with postherpetic neuralgia (topical and transdermal) or diabetic neuropathy. **Unlabeled Use:** Postmastectomy pain syndrome. Complex regional pain syndrome.

Action
Topical: May deplete and prevent the reaccumulation of a chemical (substance P) responsible for transmitting painful impulses from peripheral sites to the CNS. **Transdermal**: Initially stimulates the transient receptor potential vanilloid 1 (TRPV1) receptors on nociceptive nerve fibers in the skin; this is followed by pain relief thought to be due to a reduction in TRPV1– expressing nociceptive nerve endings. **Therapeutic Effects:** Relief of discomfort associated with painful peripheral syndromes.

Pharmacokinetics
Absorption: Unknown.
Distribution: Unknown.
Metabolism and Excretion: Unknown.
Half-life: Unknown.

TIME/ACTION PROFILE

ROUTE	ONSET	PEAK	DURATION
topical	1–2 wk	2–4 wk†	unknown
transdermal	unknown	unknown	unknown

†May take up to 6 wk for head and neck neuralgias.

Contraindications/Precautions
Contraindicated in: Hypersensitivity to capsaicin or hot peppers; Not for use near eyes or on open or broken skin.
Use Cautiously in: OB: Safety not established in pregnancy; Lactation: Safety not established in breastfeeding; Pedi: Safety not established in children <18 yr (transdermal) or <2 yr (topical).

Adverse Reactions/Side Effects
CV: *Patch:* ↑ BP. **Derm:** pain (after application of patch), transient burning. **Neuro:** ↓ sensory function. **Resp:** cough.

Interactions
Drug-Drug: None reported.

Route/Dosage
Topical (Adults and Children ≥2 yr): Apply to affected areas 3–4 times daily.
Transdermal (Adults): *Postherpetic neuralgia:* Apply up to 4 patches for 60 min (single use); may be repeated every 3 mo, as needed based on pain (should not be used more frequently than every 3 mo); *Diabetic neuropathy of feet:* Apply up to 4 patches for 30 min (single use); may be repeated every 3 mo, as needed based on pain (should not be used more frequently than every 3 mo).

Availability (generic available)
Cream: 0.025%^{OTC}, 0.035%^{OTC}, 0.075%^{OTC}, 0.1%^{OTC}.
Gel: 0.025%^{OTC}. **Lotion:** 0.025%^{OTC}. **Topical liquid:** 0.15%^{OTC}. **Transdermal patch:** 0.0225%, 0.025%, 0.03%, 0.0375%, 0.05%, 8%. *In combination with:* methylsalicylate (Ziks^{OTC}). See Appendix N.

NURSING IMPLICATIONS

Assessment
* Assess pain intensity and location before and periodically during therapy.
* May cause temporary, minor reductions in sensory function. Assess patients with pre-existing sensory deficits, signs of sensory deterioration or loss, prior to each application. If sensory deterioration or loss is detected or pre-existing sensory deficit worsens, reconsider continued use of capsaicin.
* **Transdermal:** Monitor BP periodically during application.

Implementation
* **Topical:** Apply to affected area not more than 3–4 times daily. Avoid getting medication into eyes or on broken or irritated skin. Do not bandage tightly.
* Topical lidocaine may be applied during the first 1–2 wk of treatment to reduce initial discomfort.
* **Transdermal:** Examine area for lesions before application. Identify treatment area (painful area including areas of hypersensitivity and allodynia) and mark on the skin. If needed, clip hair (do not shave) in and around treatment area to promote patch adherence. Cut patch to size and shape of treatment area. Gently wash area with mild soap and water and dry thoroughly. Topical anesthetic may be applied to the entire treatment area and surrounding 1–2 cm and keep the local anesthetic in place until skin is anesthetized prior to the application of patch. Remove the topical anesthetic with a dry wipe. Gently wash treatment area with mild soap and water and dry. Administer in a well-ventilated area. Use a face mask and protective glasses during administration. Use only nitrile gloves when handling capsaicin and cleaning capsaicin residue from skin; latex gloves do not provide adequate protection. Apply patch to dry, intact skin. Apply patch within 2 hr of opening

C

pouch. Tear pouch open along the three dashed lines and remove patch. Inspect patch and identify the outer surface backing layer with the printing on one side and the capsaicin-containing adhesive on the other side. Adhesive side of the patch is covered by a clear, unprinted, diagonally cut release liner. Cut patch before removing protective release liner. Peel a small section of the release liner back and place adhesive side of patch on treatment area. While slowly peeling back release liner from under patch with one hand, use other hand to smooth the patch down on to skin. Once patch is applied, leave in place for 60 min for postherpetic neuralgia and for 30 min for diabetic peripheral neuropathy. To ensure patch maintains contact with treatment area, a dressing, such as rolled gauze, may be used. Instruct the patient not to touch the patch or treatment area.

- Even following use of a local anesthetic prior to administration of capsaicin, patients may experience substantial procedural pain. Treat acute pain during and following application with local cooling (ice pack) and/or appropriate analgesic medication.
- May apply up to 4 patches at the same time. Do not apply more frequently than every 3 mo.
- Remove patches by gently and slowly rolling inward. After removal, generously apply *Cleansing Gel* to treatment area and leave on for at least 1 min. Remove *Cleansing Gel* with a dry wipe and gently wash area with mild soap and water and dry thoroughly. Aerosolization of capsaicin can occur upon rapid removal of patches. Remove patches gently and slowly by rolling adhesive side inward. If irritation of eyes or airways occurs, remove affected individual from the vicinity. Flush eyes and mucous membranes with cool water. Inhalation of airborne capsaicin can result in coughing or sneezing. Provide supportive care if shortness of breath develops. If skin not intended to be treated comes in contact with capsaicin, apply *Cleansing Gel* for 1 min and wipe off with dry gauze. After *Cleansing Gel* has been wiped off, wash area with soap and water.

Patient/Family Teaching

- **Topical:** Instruct patient on the correct method for application of capsaicin. Rub cream into affected area well so that little or no cream is left on the surface. Gloves should be worn during application or hands should be washed immediately after application. If application is to hands for arthritis, do not wash hands for at least 30 min after application.
- Advise patient to apply missed doses as soon as possible unless almost time for next dose. Pain relief lasts only as long as capsaicin is used regularly.
- Advise patient that transient burning may occur with application, especially if applied fewer than 3–4

times daily. Burning usually disappears after the first few days but may continue for 2–4 wk or longer. Burning is increased by heat, sweating, bathing in warm water, humidity, and clothing. Burning usually decreases in frequency and intensity the longer capsaicin is used. Decreasing number of daily doses will not lessen burning but may decrease amount of pain relief and may prolong period of burning.

- Caution patient to flush area with water if capsaicin gets into eyes and to wash with warm, but not hot, soapy water if capsaicin gets on other sensitive areas of the body.
- Instruct patient with herpes zoster (shingles) not to apply capsaicin cream until lesions have healed completely.
- Advise patient to discontinue use and notify health care professional if pain persists longer than 1 mo, worsens, or if signs of infection are present.
- **Transdermal:** Inform patient that treated area may be sensitive for a few days to heat (e.g., hot showers or baths, direct sunlight, vigorous exercise).
- Advise patient that exposure of skin to capsaicin may result in transient erythema and burning sensation. Instruct patients not to touch patch and if they accidentally touch patch it may burn and/or sting.
- Instruct patient to notify health care professional immediately if irritation of eyes or airways occurs, or if any of the side effects become severe.
- If opioids are used to treat pain from patch, caution patient that opioids may cause drowsiness and to avoid driving or other activities requiring alertness until response to medication is known.
- May cause transient increases in BP. Instruct patients to inform health care professional if they have experienced any recent cardiovascular event.
- Rep: Advise females of reproductive potential to notify health care professional if pregnancy is planned or suspected or if breastfeeding. Advise breastfeeding patient to avoid application to nipple and areola. Capsaicin is negligibly absorbed systemically following topical administration, and fetal exposure is not expected following maternal use.

Evaluation/Desired Outcomes

- Decrease in discomfort associated with:
- Postherpetic neuropathy.
- Diabetic peripheral neuropathy.
- Rheumatoid arthritis.
- Osteoarthritis. Pain relief usually begins within 1–2 wk with arthritis, 2–4 wk with neuralgias, and 4–6 wk with neuralgias of the head and neck.

---

captopril, See ANGIOTENSIN-CONVERTING ENZYME (ACE) INHIBITORS.

℞ carBAMazepine
(kar-ba-**maz**-e-peen)
Carbatrol, Epitol, Equetro, TEGretol,
✤ TEGretol CR, TEGretol XR
Classification
Therapeutic: anticonvulsants, mood stabilizers

Indications
Tonic-clonic, mixed, and complex-partial seizures. Pain in trigeminal neuralgia. **Equetro only:** Acute manic or mixed episodes associated with bipolar I disorder.

Action
Decreases synaptic transmission in the CNS by affecting sodium channels in neurons. **Therapeutic Effects:** Prevention of seizures. Relief of pain in trigeminal neuralgia. Decreased mania.

Pharmacokinetics
Absorption: Absorption is slow but complete. Suspension produces earlier, higher peak, and lower trough levels.

Distribution: Widely distributed. Crosses the blood-brain barrier. Crosses the placenta rapidly and enters breast milk in high concentrations.

Protein Binding: *Carbamazepine:* 75–90%; *epoxide:* 50%.

Metabolism and Excretion: Extensively metabolized in the liver by the CYP3A4 isoenzyme to active epoxide metabolite; epoxide metabolite has anticonvulsant and antineuralgic activity.

Half-life: *Carbamazepine:* single dose—25–65 hr, chronic dosing—*Children:* 8–14 hr; *Adults:* 12–17 hr; *epoxide:* 34±9 hr.

TIME/ACTION PROFILE (anticonvulsant activity)

ROUTE	ONSET	PEAK	DURATION
PO	up to 1 mo†	4–5 hr‡	6–12 hr
PO-ER	up to 1 mo†	2–3–12 hr‡	12 hr

†Onset of antineuralgic activity is 8–72 hr.
‡Listed for tablets; peak level occurs 1.5 hr after a chronic dose of suspension.

Contraindications/Precautions
Contraindicated in: Hypersensitivity to carbamazepine or tricyclic antidepressants; Bone marrow suppression; Concomitant use or use within 14 days of MAO inhibitors; Concurrent use of nefazodone or NNRTIs that are CYP3A4 substrates; Lactation: Lactation.

Use Cautiously in: All patients (may ↑ risk of suicidal thoughts/behaviors); Cardiac or hepatic disease; Renal failure (dosing adjustment required for CCr <10 mL/min); ↑ intraocular pressure; OB: Use during pregnancy only if potential maternal benefits outweigh potential fetal risks; additional vitamin K during last wk of pregnancy has been recommended; Geri: Appears on Beers list. May worsen or cause syndrome of inappropriate antidiuretic hormone (SIADH) secretion in older adults. Use with caution in older adults and closely monitor sodium concentrations when starting therapy or ↑ dose.

Exercise Extreme Caution in: ℞ Patients positive for HLA-B*1502 or HLA-A*3101 alleles (unless benefits clearly outweigh the risks) (↑ risk of serious skin reactions).

Adverse Reactions/Side Effects
CV: HF, edema, heart block, hypertension, hypotension, syncope. **Derm:** DRUG REACTION WITH EOSINOPHILIA AND SYSTEMIC SYMPTOMS (DRESS), nail shedding, photosensitivity, rash, STEVENS-JOHNSON SYNDROME, TOXIC EPIDERMAL NECROLYSIS, urticaria. **EENT:** blurred vision, corneal opacities, nystagmus. **Endo:** SIADH. **F and E:** hyponatremia. **GI:** ↑ liver enzymes, HEPATOTOXICITY, PANCREATITIS. **GU:** hesitancy, urinary retention. **Hemat:** AGRANULOCYTOSIS, APLASTIC ANEMIA, eosinophilia, leukopenia, lymphadenopathy, THROMBOCYTOPENIA. **Metab:** weight gain. **Neuro:** ataxia, drowsiness, fatigue, psychosis, sedation, SUICIDAL THOUGHTS, vertigo. **Resp:** pneumonitis. **Misc:** chills, fever.

Interactions
Drug-Drug: May significantly ↓ levels of **nefazodone** or **NNRTIs** that are CYP3A4 substrates; concurrent use contraindicated. Concurrent or recent (within 2 wk) use of **MAO inhibitors** may result in hyperpyrexia, hypertension, seizures, and death; use contraindicated. May ↓ levels/effectiveness of **acetaminophen, alprazolam, aprepitant, buprenorphine, bupropion, calcium channel blockers, citalopram, clonazepam, corticosteroids, cyclosporine, doxycycline, estrogen-containing contraceptives, everolimus, haloperidol, imatinib, itraconazole, lamotrigine, levothyroxine, methadone. midazolam, olanzapine, paliperidone, phenytoin, protease inhibitors, risperidone, sertraline, sirolimus, tacrolimus, tadalafil, theophylline, tiagabine, topiramate, tramadol, trazodone, tricyclic antidepressants, valproic acid, warfarin, ziprasidone,** and **zonisamide.** May ↓ **aripiprazole** levels; double the aripiprazole dose. May ↓ **temsirolimus** and **lapatinib** levels; avoid concurrent use. May ↓ levels and effectiveness of **apixaban, dabigatran, edoxaban,** and **rivaroxaban**; avoid concurrent use. **Aprepitant, cimetidine, ciprofloxacin, clarithromycin, danazol, dantrolene, diltiazem, erythromycin, fluconazole, fluoxetine, fluvoxamine, isoniazid, itraconazole, ketoconazole, loratadine, olanzapine, omeprazole, oxybutynin, protease inhibitors, trazodone, voriconazole,** and **verapamil** may ↑ carbamazepine levels; may ↑ risk of toxicity. Enzyme inducers such as **rifampin, phenobarbital,** and **phenytoin** may ↓ levels. May ↑ risk of hepatotoxicity from

isoniazid. May ↑ risk of CNS toxicity from lithium. May ↓ effects of nondepolarizing neuromuscular blocking agents. May ↑ risk of toxicity from cyclophosphamide.

Drug-Food: Grapefruit juice ↑ serum levels and oral bioavailability by 40% and therefore may ↑ effects.

Route/Dosage

When converting from immediate-release to extended-release formulation, administer same total daily dose (in 2 divided doses).

Seizures

PO (Adults and Children >12 yr): 200 mg twice daily (immediate-release [IR] tablets and extended-release [ER] tablets/capsules) or 100 mg 4 times daily (suspension); ↑ by up to 200 mg/day in divided doses (every 12 hr for ER tablets; every 6–8 hr for IR tablets and suspension) every 7 days until therapeutic levels are achieved (usual range = 600–1200 mg/day); not to exceed 1000 mg/day in children 12–15 yrs old or 1200 mg/day in children 15–18 yrs old or 1600 mg/day in adults.

PO (Children 6–12 yr): 100 mg twice daily (IR tablets or ER tablets/capsules) or 50 mg 4 times daily (suspension). ↑ by up to 100 mg/day in divided doses (every 12 hr for ER tablets; every 6–8 hr for IR tablets and suspension) every 7 days until therapeutic levels are achieved (usual range = 400–800 mg/day); not to exceed 1000 mg/day.

PO (Children <6 yr): 10–20 mg/kg/day in 2–3 divided doses (IR tablets) or in 4 divided doses (suspension); may be ↑ at weekly intervals until optimal response and therapeutic levels are achieved; not to exceed 35 mg/kg/day.

Trigeminal Neuralgia

PO (Adults): 100 mg twice daily (IR or ER tablets), 200 mg once daily (ER capsules), or 50 mg 4 times daily (suspension); ↑ by up to 200 mg/day in divided doses (every 12 hr for IR tablets or ER tablets/capsules; every 6 hr for suspension) as needed until pain is relieved (usual range = 400–800 mg/day); not to exceed 1200 mg/day.

Acute Manic or Mixed Episodes Associated with Bipolar I Disorder

PO (Adults): *Equetro:* 200 mg twice daily; ↑ by 200 mg/day until optimal response is achieved; not to exceed 1600 mg/day.

Availability (generic available)

Immediate-release tablets: 200 mg. **Chewable tablets:** 100 mg, ✽ 200 mg. **Extended-release capsules (Carbatrol, Equetro):** 100 mg, 200 mg, 300 mg. **Extended-release tablets (Tegretol XR):** 100 mg, 200 mg, 400 mg. **Oral suspension (citrus-vanilla flavor):** 100 mg/5 mL.

NURSING IMPLICATIONS

Assessment

- Monitor closely for changes in behavior that could indicate the emergence or worsening of suicidal thoughts or behavior or depression.
- ▩ Monitor for changes in skin condition in early therapy. Stevens-Johnson syndrome and toxic epidermal necrolysis are significantly more common in patients with a particular human leukocyte antigen (HLA) allele, HLA-B*1502 (occurs almost exclusively in patients with Asian ancestry, including South Asian Indians). Screen patients of Asian ancestry for the HLA-B*1502 allele before starting treatment with carbamazepine. If positive, carbamazepine should not be started unless the expected benefit outweighs increased risk of serious skin reactions. Patients who have been taking carbamazepine for more than a few mo without developing skin reactions are at low risk of these events ever developing.
- Monitor for signs and symptoms of DRESS syndrome (fever, rash, and/or lymphadenopathy with organ system involvement [hepatitis, nephritis, hematologic abnormalities, myocarditis, myositis]) resembling an acute viral infection with eosinophilia. Discontinue carbamazepine if other cause not determined.
- **Seizures:** Assess frequency, location, duration, and characteristics of seizure activity.
- **Trigeminal Neuralgia:** Assess for facial pain (location, intensity, duration). Ask patient to identify stimuli that may precipitate facial pain (hot or cold foods, bedclothes, touching face).
- **Bipolar Disorder:** Assess mental status (mood, orientation, behavior) and cognitive abilities before and periodically during therapy.

Lab Test Considerations

- Monitor CBC, including platelet count, reticulocyte count, and serum iron, at baseline, weekly during the first 2 mo, and yearly thereafter for evidence of potentially fatal blood cell abnormalities. Discontinue therapy if bone marrow depression occurs.
- ▩ Perform genetic testing for the HLA-B*1502 allele in patients of Asian ancestry prior to beginning therapy.
- Perform liver function tests, urinalysis, electrolytes, serum creatinine, and BUN at baseline and routinely performed. May cause ↑ AST, ALT, serum alkaline phosphatase, bilirubin, BUN, urine protein, and urine glucose levels.
- Monitor serum-ionized calcium levels every 6 mo or if seizure frequency increases. Thyroid function tests and ionized serum calcium concentrations may be ↓ hypocalcemia ↓ seizure threshold.
- Monitor ECG and serum electrolytes before and periodically during therapy. May cause hyponatremia.
- May occasionally cause ↑ serum cholesterol, high-density lipoprotein, and triglyceride concentrations.

✽= Canadian drug name. ▩ = Genetic implication. ~~Strikethrough~~ = Discontinued. CAPITALS = life-threatening. <u>Underline</u> = most frequent.

- May cause false-negative pregnancy test results with tests that determine human chorionic gonadotropin.

Toxicity and Overdose
- Serum blood levels should be routinely monitored during therapy. Therapeutic levels range from 4 to 12 mcg/mL.

Implementation
- Do not confuse carbamazepine with oxcarbazepine. Do not confuse Tegretol with Tegretol XR.
- Implement seizure precautions as indicated.
- **PO:** Administer medication with food to minimize gastric irritation. May take at bedtime to reduce daytime sedation. *DNC:* Do not crush or chew extended-release tablets. Extended-release capsules may be opened and the contents sprinkled on applesauce or other similar foods.
- Do not administer suspension simultaneously with other liquid medications or diluents; mixture produces an orange rubbery mass.

Patient/Family Teaching
- Instruct patient to take carbamazepine around the clock, as directed. Take missed doses as soon as possible but not just before next dose; do not double doses. Notify health care professional if more than one dose is missed. Discontinue gradually to prevent seizures. Instruct patient to read the *Medication Guide* before starting and with each Rx refill in case of changes.
- Advise patient to avoid grapefruit and grapefruit juice during therapy.
- May cause dizziness or drowsiness. Advise patients to avoid driving or other activities requiring alertness until response to medication is known.
- Advise patient to notify health care professional of all Rx or OTC medications, vitamins, or herbal products being taken and to consult with health care professional before taking other medications.
- Instruct patient to report behavioral changes, skin rash, fever, sore throat, mouth ulcers, easy bruising, petechiae, unusual bleeding, abdominal pain, chills, rash, pale stools, dark urine, or jaundice to health care professional immediately. Advise patient and family to notify health care professional if thoughts about suicide or dying, attempts to commit suicide; new or worse depression; new or worse anxiety; feeling very agitated or restless; panic attacks; trouble sleeping; new or worse irritability; acting aggressive; being angry or violent; acting on dangerous impulses; an extreme increase in activity and talking, other unusual changes in behavior or mood occur.
- Inform patient that coating of *Tegretol XR* is not absorbed but is excreted in feces and may be visible in stool.
- Advise patient not to take alcohol or other CNS depressants concurrently with this medication.
- Caution patients to use sunscreen and protective clothing to prevent photosensitivity reactions.

- Inform patient that frequent mouth rinses, good oral hygiene, and sugarless gum or candy may help reduce dry mouth. Saliva substitute may be used. Consult dentist if dry mouth persists >2 wk.
- Instruct patient to notify health care professional of medication regimen before treatment or surgery.
- Rep: May cause fetal harm. Advise females of reproductive potential to use a nonhormonal form of contraception while taking carbamazepine, to avoid breastfeeding during therapy, and to notify health care professional if pregnancy is planned or suspected or if breastfeeding. May reduce effects of estrogen-containing contraceptives. Encourage patients who become pregnant to enroll in the North American Antiepileptic Drug Pregnancy Registry by calling 1-888-233-2334 or on the web at www.aedpregnancyregistry.org. Enrollment must be done by patients themselves.
- Emphasize the importance of follow-up lab tests and eye exams to monitor for side effects.
- **Seizures:** Advise patients to carry identification describing disease and medication regimen at all times.

Evaluation/Desired Outcomes
- Absence or reduction of seizure activity.
- Decrease in trigeminal neuralgia pain. Patients with trigeminal neuralgia who are pain-free should be reevaluated every 3 mo to determine minimum effective dose.
- Decreased mania and depressive symptoms in bipolar I disorder.

carbidopa/levodopa
(kar-bi-doe-pa/**lee**-voe-doe-pa)
Dhivy, Duopa, ❋Duodopa, Rytary, Sinemet, ~~Sinemet CR~~
Classification
Therapeutic: antiparkinson agents
Pharmacologic: dopamine agonists

Indications
Parkinson's disease, postencephalitic parkinsonism, and symptomatic parkinsonism that may follow carbon monoxide intoxication or manganese intoxication.

Action
Levodopa is converted to dopamine in the CNS, where it serves as a neurotransmitter. Carbidopa, a decarboxylase inhibitor, prevents peripheral destruction of levodopa. **Therapeutic Effects:** Relief of tremor and rigidity in Parkinson's syndrome.

Pharmacokinetics
Absorption: Well absorbed following oral administration.
Distribution: Widely distributed. *Levodopa:* enters the CNS in small concentrations. *Carbidopa:* does not cross the blood-brain barrier but does cross the placenta.

Metabolism and Excretion: *Levodopa:* mostly metabolized by the GI tract and liver. *Carbidopa:* 30% excreted unchanged by the kidneys.

Half-life: *Levodopa:* 1 hr; *carbidopa:* 1–2 hr.

TIME/ACTION PROFILE (antiparkinson effects)

ROUTE	ONSET	PEAK	DURATION
Carbidopa	unknown	unknown	5–24 hr
Levodopa	10–15 min	unknown	5–24 hr or more
Carbidopa/levodopa sustained release	unknown	2 hr	12 hr

Contraindications/Precautions

Contraindicated in: Hypersensitivity; Angle-closure glaucoma; Nonselective MAO inhibitor therapy; Malignant melanoma; Undiagnosed skin lesions; Some products contain tartrazine, phenylalanine, or aspartame and should be avoided in patients with known hypersensitivity.

Use Cautiously in: History of cardiac, psychiatric, or ulcer disease; OB: Safety not established in pregnancy; Lactation: May ↓ serum prolactin; levodopa enters breast milk; use while breastfeeding only if potential maternal benefit justifies potential risk to infant; Pedi: Safety and effectiveness not established in children.

Adverse Reactions/Side Effects

CV: orthostatic hypotension. **Derm:** melanoma. **EENT:** blurred vision, mydriasis. **GI:** constipation, nausea, vomiting, anorexia, bezoar (enteral suspension), dry mouth, GI HEMORRHAGE (enteral suspension), GI ISCHEMIA (enteral suspension), GI OBSTRUCTION (enteral suspension), GI PERFORATION (enteral suspension), HEPATOTOXICITY, INTUSSUSCEPTION (enteral suspension), PANCREATITIS (enteral suspension), PERITONITIS (enteral suspension). **Hemat:** hemolytic anemia, leukopenia. **MS:** dyskinesias. **Neuro:** depression, involuntary movements, anxiety, confusion, dizziness, drowsiness, hallucinations, memory loss, neuropathy, psychiatric problems, sudden sleep onset, urges (gambling, sexual). **Resp:** aspiration pneumonia (enteral suspension). **Misc:** darkening of urine or sweat, MELANOMA, SEPSIS (enteral suspension).

Interactions

Drug-Drug: Use with **nonselective MAO inhibitors** may result in hypertensive reactions; concurrent use contraindicated (MAO inhibitor must be discontinued ≥2 wk before initiating carbidopa/levodopa). ↑ risk of arrhythmias with **inhalation hydrocarbon anesthetics** (especially **halothane**; if possible discontinue 6–8 hr before anesthesia). **Phenothiazines**, **haloperidol**, **papaverine**, and **phenytoin** may ↓ ef-

fect of levodopa. Large doses of **pyridoxine** may ↓ beneficial effects of levodopa. ↑ hypotension may result with concurrent **antihypertensives**. **Anticholinergics** may ↓ absorption of levodopa. ↑ risk of adverse reactions with **selegiline** or **cocaine**.

Drug-Natural Products: Kava-kava may ↓ levodopa effectiveness.

Drug-Food: Ingestion of foods containing large amounts of **pyridoxine** may ↓ effect of levodopa.

Route/Dosage

Carbidopa/Levodopa

PO (Adults): 25 mg carbidopa/100 mg levodopa 3 times daily; may be ↑ every 1–2 days until desired effect is achieved (max = 8 tablets of 25 mg carbidopa/100 mg levodopa/day).

Enteral (Adults): Patients must be converted to and be on stable dose of PO immediate-release carbidopa/levodopa tablets before initiation of enteral suspension therapy. *Morning dose for Day 1 (mL) (to be administered over 10–30 min)* = (Amount of levodopa [in mg] in first dose of immediate-release carbidopa/levodopa taken by patient on previous day * 0.8); *Continuous dose for Day 1 (mL) (to be administered over 16 hr)* = Determine amount of levodopa (in mg) patient received from immediate-release carbidopa/levodopa doses throughout 16 waking hr of previous day (do not include doses of immediate-release carbidopa/levodopa taken at night when calculating the levodopa amount). Then, subtract amount of first levodopa dose (in mg) taken by patient on previous day. Divide result by 20 to obtain the # of mL to be administered over 16 hr. Do not exceed dose of 2000 mg. At end of daily 16-hr infusion, patients will disconnect the pump from feeding tube and take their nighttime dose of oral immediate-release carbidopa/levodopa tablets. Total daily dose can be titrated after Day 1 based on patient response and tolerability.

Carbidopa/Levodopa Extended-Release (doses of all other dosage forms of carbidopa/levodopa and Rytary are not interchangeable)

PO (Adults): *Patients not currently receiving levodopa (Sinemet CR):* 50 mg carbidopa/200 mg levodopa twice daily (minimum of 6 hr apart) initially. *Patients not currently receiving levodopa (Rytary):* 23.75 mg carbidopa/95 mg levodopa 3 times daily for 3 days, then 36.25 mg carbidopa/145 mg levodopa 3 times daily. May continue to ↑ dose as needed (max dose = 97.5 mg carbidopa/390 mg levodopa 3 times daily). May also ↑ frequency of administration up to 5 times daily (max dose = 612.5 mg carbidopa/2450 mg levodopa/day). *Conversion from immediate-release (IR) carbidopa/levodopa to Sinemet CR:* initiate therapy with at least 10% more levodopa content/day (may

✦= Canadian drug name. ▓ = Genetic implication. S̶t̶r̶i̶k̶e̶t̶h̶r̶o̶u̶g̶h̶ = Discontinued. CAPITALS = life-threatening. Underline = most frequent.

need up to 30% more) given at 4–8 hr intervals while awake. Allow 3 days between dosage changes; some patients may require larger doses and shorter dosing intervals. *Conversion from IR carbidopa/levodopa to Rytary:* If taking 400–549 mg/day of IR levodopa, give 3 capsules of Rytary 23.75 mg carbidopa/95 mg levodopa 3 times daily. If taking 550–749 mg/day of IR levodopa, give 4 capsules of Rytary 23.75 mg carbidopa/95 mg levodopa 3 times daily. If taking 750–949 mg/day of IR levodopa, give 3 capsules of Rytary 36.25 mg carbidopa/145 mg levodopa 3 times daily. If taking 950–1249 mg/day of IR levodopa, give 3 capsules of Rytary 48.75 mg carbidopa/195 mg levodopa 3 times daily. If taking ≥1250 mg/day of IR levodopa, give 4 capsules of Rytary 48.75 mg carbidopa/195 mg levodopa 3 times daily or 3 capsules of Rytary 61.25 mg carbidopa/245 mg levodopa 3 times daily; may then titrate as needed (max daily dose = 612.5 mg carbidopa/2450 mg levodopa).

Availability (generic available)

Immediate-release tablets: carbidopa 10 mg/levodopa 100 mg, carbidopa 25 mg/levodopa 100 mg, carbidopa 25 mg/levodopa 250 mg. **Extended-release capsules (Rytary):** carbidopa 23.75 mg/levodopa 95 mg, carbidopa 36.25 mg/levodopa 145 mg, carbidopa 48.75 mg/levodopa 195 mg, carbidopa 61.25 mg/levodopa 245 mg. **Extended-release tablets:** carbidopa 25 mg/levodopa 100 mg, carbidopa 50 mg/levodopa 200 mg. **Enteral suspension (Duopa):** carbidopa 4.63 mg/levodopa 20 mg/mL, ✿ carbidopa 5 mg/levodopa 20 mg/mL. *In combination with:* entacapone (Stalevo); see Appendix N.

NURSING IMPLICATIONS

Assessment

- Assess parkinsonian symptoms (akinesia, rigidity, tremors, pill rolling, shuffling gait, mask-like face, twisting motions, and drooling) during therapy. "On-off phenomenon" may cause symptoms to appear or improve suddenly.
- Assess BP and pulse frequently during period of dose adjustment.
- **Duopa:** Monitor for signs and symptoms of GI complications (abdominal pain, prolonged constipation, nausea, vomiting, fever, melanotic stool) during therapy.

Lab Test Considerations

- May cause false-positive test results in Coombs' test.
- May cause ↑ serum glucose. Dipstick for urine ketones may reveal false-positive results.
- Monitor hepatic and renal function and CBC periodically in patients on long-term therapy. May cause ↑ AST, ALT, bilirubin, alkaline phosphatase, LDH, and serum protein-bound iodine concentrations.
- May cause ↓ hemoglobin, ↓ hematocrit, agranulocytosis, hemolytic and nonhemolytic anemia, thrombocytopenia, leukopenia, and ↑ WBC.

Toxicity and Overdose

- Assess for signs of toxicity (involuntary muscle twitching, facial grimacing, spasmodic eye winking, exaggerated protrusion of tongue, behavioral changes). Consult health care professional if symptoms occur.

Implementation

- Do not confuse Sinemet with Janumet.
- In the carbidopa/levodopa combination, the number following the drug name represents the milligrams of each respective drug.
- In preoperative patients or patients who are NPO, confer with health care professional about continuing medication administration using oral disintegrating tablets.
- **PO:** Administer on a regular schedule. Hospitalized patients should be continued on same schedule as at home. Administer while awake, not around the clock to improve sleep and prevent side effects.
- *DNC:* Controlled-release tablets may be administered as whole or half tablets, but they should not be crushed or chewed.
- Each *Dhivy* tablet is scored in three segments with each segment containing 6.25 mg of carbidopa and 25 mg of levodopa to help with titration.
- *For enteral administration,* administer *Duopa* into the jejunum through a percutaneous endoscopic gastrostomy with jejunal tube (PEG-J) with CADD-Legacy 1400 portable infusion pump. Take suspension out of refrigerator 20 min prior to use; must be at room temperature for use. Administer over 16 hr. If extra dose is needed, set function at 1 mL (20 mg of levodopa) when starting; may be adjusted in 0.2 mL increments. Limit to 1 extra dose every 2 hr. Frequent extra doses may cause or worsen dyskinesias. Discontinue gradually; do not stop abruptly.
- *For extended-release capsules,* administer without regard to food. *DNC:* Swallow capsules whole; do not chew, divide, or crush. For patients with difficulty swallowing, open capsule and sprinkle entire contents on 1–2 tablespoons of applesauce; consume immediately. Do not store mixture for future use. Inform patients that first dose of day may be taken 1–2 hr before eating, as a high-fat, high-calorie meal may delay the absorption of levodopa and onset of action by 2–3 hr. Discontinue gradually; do not stop abruptly. When adjusting dose of extended-release capsules, keep dose of other Parkinson's medications stable; dose may need to be increased in patients taking COMT inhibitor. Extended-release capsules may be administered 3–5 times daily if more frequent dosing is needed and tolerated.

Patient/Family Teaching

- Instruct patient to take medication at regular intervals as directed. Do not change dose regimen or take additional antiparkinson drugs, including more carbidopa/levodopa, without consulting health care professional. Take missed doses as soon as remembered, unless next scheduled dose is within 2 hr; do not double doses.

- Explain that gastric irritation may be decreased by eating food shortly after taking medications but that high-protein meals may impair levodopa's effects. Dividing daily protein intake among all the meals may help ensure adequate protein intake and drug effectiveness. Do not drastically alter diet during carbidopa/levodopa therapy without consulting health care professional.
- May cause sudden onset of sleep, drowsiness, or dizziness. Advise patient to avoid driving and other activities that require alertness until response to drug is known.
- Caution patient to change positions slowly to minimize orthostatic hypotension. Notify health care professional if orthostatic hypotension occurs.
- Instruct patient that frequent rinsing of mouth, good oral hygiene, and sugarless gum or candy may decrease dry mouth.
- Caution patient to monitor skin lesions for any changes. Notify health care professional promptly because carbidopa/levodopa may activate malignant melanoma.
- Advise patient to notify health care professional of all Rx or OTC medications, vitamins, or herbal products being taken and to consult with health care professional before taking other medications, especially cold remedies. Large amounts of vitamin B_6 (pyridoxine) and iron may interfere with the action of levodopa.
- Inform patient that harmless darkening of saliva, urine, or sweat may occur.
- Advise patient to notify health care professional if signs and symptoms of GI complications, palpitations, urinary retention, involuntary movements, behavioral changes, severe nausea and vomiting, new skin lesions, or new or increased gambling, sexual, binge or compulsive eating, or other intense urges occur. Dose reduction may be required.
- Inform patient that sometimes a "wearing-off" effect may occur at end of dosing interval. Notify health care professional if this poses a problem to lifestyle.
- Rep: Advise female patients to notify health care professional if pregnancy is planned or suspected or if breastfeeding. May inhibit lactation.

Evaluation/Desired Outcomes

- Resolution of parkinsonian signs and symptoms. Therapeutic effects usually become evident after 2–3 wk of therapy but may require up to 6 mo. Patients who take this medication for several yr may experience a decrease in the effectiveness of this drug.

HIGH ALERT

CARBOplatin (kar-boe-pla-tin)
Paraplatin
Classification
Therapeutic: antineoplastics
Pharmacologic: alkylating agents

C

Indications
Advanced ovarian carcinoma (in combination with other agents). Palliative treatment of ovarian carcinoma unresponsive to other modalities.

Action
Inhibits DNA synthesis by producing cross-linking of parent DNA strands (cell-cycle phase–nonspecific). **Therapeutic Effects:** Death of rapidly replicating cells, particularly malignant ones.

Pharmacokinetics
Absorption: IV administration results in complete bioavailability.
Distribution: Well distributed to tissues.
Protein Binding: Platinum is irreversibly bound to plasma proteins.
Metabolism and Excretion: Excreted mostly by the kidneys.
Half-life: *Carboplatin:* 2.6–5.9 hr (↑ in renal impairment); *platinum:* 5 days.

TIME/ACTION PROFILE (effects on blood counts)

ROUTE	ONSET	PEAK	DURATION
IV	unknown	21 days	28 days

Contraindications/Precautions
Contraindicated in: Hypersensitivity to carboplatin, cisplatin, or mannitol; OB: Pregnancy; Lactation: Lactation.
Use Cautiously in: Hearing loss; Electrolyte abnormalities; Renal impairment (dose ↓ recommended if CCr <60 mL/min); Active infection; Diminished bone marrow reserve (dose ↓ recommended); Rep: Women of reproductive potential; Pedi: Safety and effectiveness not established in children; Geri: ↑ risk of thrombocytopenia in older adults; consider renal function in dose determination.

Adverse Reactions/Side Effects
Derm: alopecia, rash. **EENT:** ototoxicity. **F and E:** hypocalcemia, hypokalemia, hypomagnesemia, hyponatremia. **GI:** abdominal pain, nausea, vomiting, constipation, diarrhea, hepatitis, stomatitis. **GU:** gonadal suppression, nephrotoxicity. **Hemat:** ANEMIA, LEUKOPENIA, THROMBOCYTOPENIA. **Metab:** hyperuricemia. **Neuro:** peripheral neuropathy, weakness. **Misc:** HYPERSENSITIVITY REACTIONS (including anaphylaxis).

Interactions

Drug-Drug: ↑ nephrotoxicity and ototoxicity with other **aminoglycosides** and **loop diuretics**. ↑ bone marrow depression with other **bone marrow–depressing drugs** or **radiation therapy**. May ↓ antibody response to **live-virus vaccines** and ↑ risk of adverse reactions.

Route/Dosage

IV (Adults): *Initial treatment:* 300 mg/m² with cyclophosphamide at 4-wk intervals. *Treatment of refractory tumors:* 360 mg/m² as a single dose; may be repeated at 4-wk intervals, depending on response.

Renal Impairment

IV (Adults): *CCr 41–59 mL/min:* initial dose 250 mg/m²; *CCr 16–40 mL/min:* initial dose 200 mg/m².

Availability (generic available)

Solution for injection: 10 mg/mL.

NURSING IMPLICATIONS

Assessment

● Assess for nausea and vomiting; often occur 6–12 hr after therapy (1–4 hr for aqueous solution) and may persist for 24 hr. Prophylactic antiemetics may be used. Adjust diet as tolerated to maintain fluid and electrolyte balance and ensure adequate nutritional intake. May require discontinuation of therapy.

● Monitor for bone marrow depression. Assess for bleeding (bleeding gums, bruising, petechiae, guaiac stools, urine, and emesis) and avoid IM injections and rectal temperatures if platelet count is low. Apply pressure to venipuncture sites for 10 min. Assess for signs of infection during neutropenia. Anemia may occur and may be cumulative; transfusions are frequently required. Monitor for increased fatigue, dyspnea, and orthostatic hypotension.

● Monitor for signs of anaphylaxis (rash, urticaria, pruritus, facial swelling, wheezing, tachycardia, hypotension). Discontinue medication immediately and notify physician if these occur. Epinephrine and resuscitation equipment should be readily available.

● Audiometry is recommended before initiation of therapy and subsequent doses. Ototoxicity manifests as tinnitus and unilateral or bilateral hearing loss in high frequencies and becomes more frequent and severe with repeated doses. Ototoxicity is more pronounced in children.

Lab Test Considerations

● Monitor CBC, differential, and clotting studies before and weekly during therapy. The nadirs of thrombocytopenia and leukopenia occur after 21 days and recover by 30 days after a dose. Nadir of granulocyte counts usually occurs after 21–28 days and recovers by day 35. Withhold subsequent doses until neutrophil count is >2000/mm³ and platelet count is >100,000/mm³.

● Monitor renal function and serum electrolytes before initiation of therapy and before each course of carboplatin.

● Monitor hepatic function before and periodically during therapy. May cause ↑ serum bilirubin, alkaline phosphatase, and AST concentrations.

Implementation

● **High Alert:** Fatalities have occurred with chemotherapeutic agents. Before administering, clarify all ambiguous orders; double-check single, daily, and course-of-therapy dose limits; have second practitioner independently double-check original order, calculations, and infusion pump settings.

● **High Alert:** Do not confuse carboplatin with cisplatin.

● **High Alert:** Carboplatin should be administered in a monitored setting under the supervision of a physician experienced in cancer chemotherapy.

IV Administration

● Solution should be prepared in a biologic cabinet. Wear gloves, gown, and mask while handling medication. Discard equipment in specially designated containers.

● Do not use aluminum needles or equipment during preparation or administration; aluminum reacts with the drug.

● **Intermittent Infusion:** *Concentration:* 0.5 mg/mL. Stable for 8 hr at room temperature. *Rate:* Infuse over 15–60 min.

● **Y-Site Compatibility:** acyclovir, alemtuzumab, allopurinol, amifostine, amikacin, aminocaproic acid, aminophylline, amiodarone, amphotericin B lipid complex, amphotericin B liposomal, ampicillin, ampicillin/sulbactam, anidulafungin, argatroban, atracurium, azithromycin, aztreonam, bivalirudin, bleomycin, bumetanide, buprenorphine, butorphanol, calcium chloride, calcium gluconate, caspofungin, cefazolin, cefepime, cefotaxime, cefotetan, cefoxitin, ceftazidime, ceftriaxone, cefuroxime, ciprofloxacin, cisatracurium, cisplatin, cladribine, clindamycin, cyclophosphamide, cyclosporine, cytarabine, dacarbazine, daptomycin, dexamethasone, dexmedetomidine, dexrazoxane, digoxin, diltiazem, diphenhydramine, docetaxel, dopamine, doxorubicin hydrochloride, doxycycline, droperidol, enalaprilat, ephedrine, ertapenem, erythromycin, esmolol, etoposide, etoposide phosphate, famotidine, fentanyl, filgrastim, fluconazole, fludarabine, fluorouracil, foscarnet, fosphenytoin, furosemide, ganciclovir, gemcitabine, gentamicin, glycopyrrolate, granisetron, haloperidol, heparin, hetastarch, hydrocortisone, hydromorphone, idarubicin, ifosfamide, imipenem/cilastatin, insulin, regular, isoproterenol, ketorolac, labetalol, levofloxacin, lidocaine, linezolid, lorazepam, magnesium sulfate, mannitol, melphalan, meperidine, meropenem, mesna, methotrexate, methylprednisolone, metoclopramide, metoprolol, metronidazole, micafungin, midazolam, milrinone, mitomycin, mitoxantrone, morphine, moxifloxacin, nafcillin, nalbuphine, naloxone, nicardipine, nitroglycerin, nitroprusside, norepinephrine, octreotide, ondansetron, oxaliplatin, paclitaxel, palonosetron, pamidronate, pantoprazole, pemetrexed, pentamidine, pentobarbital, phenobarbital, phenylephrine, piperacillin/tazobactam, potassium acetate, potassium chloride, potassium phosphate, prochlorperazine, promethazine, propofol, propranolol, remifentanil, rituximab, rocuronium, sargramostim, sodium acetate, sodium bicarbonate, sodium phosphate, succinylcholine, sufentanil, tacrolimus, theophylline, thiotepa, tigecycline, tirofiban, tobramycin, trastuzumab, trimethoprim/sulfamethoxazole, vancomycin, vecuronium, verapamil, vinblastine, vincristine, vinorelbine, voriconazole, zidovudine, zoledronic acid.

- **Y-Site Incompatibility:** amphotericin B deoxycholate, chlorpromazine, diazepam, leucovorin calcium, phenytoin, procainamide, thiopental.

Patient/Family Teaching

- Instruct patient to notify health care professional promptly if fever; chills; sore throat; signs of infection; lower back or side pain; difficult or painful urination; bleeding gums; bruising; pinpoint red spots on skin; blood in stools, urine, or emesis; increased fatigue, dyspnea, or orthostatic hypotension occurs.
- Caution patient to avoid crowds and persons with known infections. Instruct patient to use soft toothbrush and electric razor and to avoid falls. Caution patients not to drink alcoholic beverages or take medication containing aspirin or NSAIDs because they may precipitate gastric bleeding.
- Instruct patient to promptly report any numbness or tingling in extremities or face, decreased coordination, difficulty with hearing or ringing in the ears, unusual swelling, or weight gain to health care professional.
- Instruct patient not to receive any vaccinations without advice of health care professional and to avoid contact with persons who have received oral polio vaccine within the past several mo.
- Advise patient of the need for contraception (if patient is not infertile as a result of surgical or radiation therapy).
- Instruct patient to inspect oral mucosa for erythema and ulceration. If ulceration occurs, advise patient to notify health care professional, rinse mouth with water after eating, and use sponge brush. Mouth pain may require treatment with opioids.
- Discuss with patient the possibility of hair loss. Explore methods of coping.
- Emphasize the need for periodic lab tests to monitor for side effects.
- Rep: Advise females of reproductive potential to notify health care professional if pregnancy is planned

or suspected or if breastfeeding. Advise patient of the need for contraception during therapy.

Evaluation/Desired Outcomes

- Decrease in size or spread of ovarian carcinoma.

BEERS

cariprazine (kar-ip-ra-zeen)
Vraylar
Classification
Therapeutic: antipsychotics

Indications
Schizophrenia. Acute treatment of mania/mixed episodes associated with bipolar I disorder. Depressive episodes associated with bipolar I disorder. Adjunctive treatment of major depressive disorder (in combination with antidepressants).

Action
Acts as a partial agonist at dopamine D_2 receptors in the CNS and serotonin $5-HT_{1A}$; also acts an antagonist at $5-HT_{2A}$ receptors. **Therapeutic Effects:** Decreased incidence and severity of symptoms of schizophrenia. Decreased occurrence and severity of mania associated with bipolar 1 disorder. Antidepressant action.

Pharmacokinetics
Absorption: Well absorbed following oral administration.
Distribution: Unknown.
Protein Binding: 91–97%.
Metabolism and Excretion: Two metabolites, desmethyl cariprazine (DCAR) and didesmethyl cariprazine (DDCAR), have antipsychotic activity. Metabolism occurs mostly via the CYP3A4 enzyme system, with further metabolism resulting in inactive metabolites; 21% excreted urine, 1.2% as unchanged drug.
Half-life: Cariprazine—2–4 days; *DDCAR*: 1–3 wk.

TIME/ACTION PROFILE (improvement in symptoms)

ROUTE	ONSET	PEAK	DURATION
PO (schizophrenia)	within 1–2 wk	4–6 wk	2 wk†
PO (mania due to bipolar 1 disorder)	within 5–7 days	2–3 wk	2 wk†

†Plasma concentrations of drug and active metabolites following discontinuation.

Contraindications/Precautions
Contraindicated in: Hypersensitivity.
Use Cautiously in: Known cerebrovascular/cardiovascular disease, dehydration, concurrent use of diuretics/antihypertensives or syncope (↑ risk of orthostatic hypotension); Pre-existing ↓ WBC or ANC or

✹ = Canadian drug name. ⅺ = Genetic implication. ~~Strikethrough~~ = Discontinued. CAPITALS = life-threatening. <u>Underline</u> = most frequent.

history of drug-induced leukopenia/neutropenia; At risk of aspiration or falls; OB: Neonates exposed in the third trimester may experience extrapyramidal symptoms/withdrawal; Lactation: Use while breastfeeding only if potential maternal benefit justifies potential risk to infant; Pedi: Safety and effectiveness not established; may ↑ risk of suicide attempt/ideation in children or adolescents; Geri: Appears on Beers list. ↑ risk of stroke, cognitive decline, and mortality in older adults with dementia. Avoid use in older adults, except for schizophrenia, bipolar disorder, or adjunctive treatment of major depressive disorder.

Adverse Reactions/Side Effects

CV: hypertension, orthostatic hypotension, tachycardia. **Derm:** rash, STEVENS-JOHNSON SYNDROME. **EENT:** blurred vision. **Endo:** hyperglycemia/diabetes mellitus. **GI:** dyspepsia, nausea, ↑ liver enzymes, constipation, diarrhea, dry mouth, dysphagia (↑ aspiration risk), vomiting. **Hemat:** AGRANULOCYTOSIS, leukopenia, neutropenia. **Metab:** ↓ appetite, dyslipidemia, weight gain. **MS:** arthralgia, back pain, extremity pain. **Neuro:** akathisia, drowsiness, extrapyramidal symptoms, headache, agitation, dizziness, fatigue, insomnia, NEUROLEPTIC MALIGNANT SYNDROME, restlessness, SUICIDAL THOUGHTS/BEHAVIORS, tardive dyskinesia. **Resp:** cough. **Misc:** body temperature dysregulation.

Interactions

Drug-Drug: Levels, effects, and risk of toxicity ↑ by concurrent use of **strong CYP3A4 inhibitors** including **itraconazole** and **ketoconazole**; concurrent use not recommended. Levels and effectiveness may be ↓ by concurrent use of **strong CYP3A4 inducers** including **carbamazepine** and **rifampin**; concurrent use not recommended. Concurrent use of **diuretics** or **antihypertensives** may ↑ risk of orthostatic hypotension/syncope.

Route/Dosage

Schizophrenia or Acute Treatment of Mania/Mixed Episodes Associated with Bipolar I Disorder

PO (Adults): 1.5 mg once daily; may ↑ to 3 mg once daily on Day 2; further dosage adjustments can be made in increments of 1.5 mg or 3 mg depending on response/tolerability (max dose = 6 mg once daily). *Initiation of strong CYP3A4 inhibitor while on stable dose of cariprazine:* ↓ dose by 50%; *Initiation of cariprazine while on stable dose of strong CYP3A4 inhibitor:* 1.5 mg once daily on Days 1 and 3 (no dose on Day 2), then 1.5 mg once daily starting on Day 4; may titrate depending on response/tolerance up to max dose of 3 mg once daily.

Depressive Episodes Associated with Bipolar I Disorder or Adjunctive Treatment of Major Depressive Disorder

PO (Adults): 1.5 mg once daily; may ↑ to 3 mg once daily on Day 15 depending on response/tolerability (max dose = 3 mg once daily); *Initiation of strong CYP3A4 inhibitor while on stable dose of cariprazine:* ↓ dose by 50%; *Initiation of cariprazine while on stable dose of strong CYP3A4 inhibitor:* 1.5 mg once daily on Days 1 and 3 (no dose on Day 2), then 1.5 mg once daily starting on Day 4; may titrate depending on response/tolerance up to max dose of 3 mg once daily.

Availability

Capsules: 1.5 mg, 3 mg, 4.5 mg, 6 mg.

NURSING IMPLICATIONS

Assessment

- Assess mental status (orientation, mood, behavior) before and periodically during therapy. Monitor for worsening depression and emergence of suicidal thoughts and behaviors.
- Assess weight and BMI at baseline and frequently during therapy.
- Monitor BP (sitting, standing, lying), pulse, and respiratory rate before and periodically during therapy.
- Observe patient carefully when administering medication to ensure that medication is actually taken and not hoarded or cheeked.
- Monitor for adverse reactions and patient response for several wk after starting therapy and after each dose increase. Due to long action, may not occur for several wk. Consider reducing dose or discontinuing drug if severe adverse reactions occur.
- Monitor patient for onset of akathisia (restlessness or desire to keep moving) and extrapyramidal side effects (*parkinsonian:* difficulty speaking or swallowing, loss of balance control, pill rolling of hands, masklike face, shuffling gait, rigidity, tremors; and *dystonic:* muscle spasms, twisting motions, twitching, inability to move eyes, weakness of arms or legs) periodically throughout therapy. Report these symptoms.
- Monitor for tardive dyskinesia (uncontrolled rhythmic movement of mouth, face, and extremities; lip smacking or puckering; puffing of cheeks; uncontrolled chewing; rapid or worm-like movements of tongue). Notify health care professional immediately if these symptoms occur, as these side effects may be irreversible.
- Monitor for development of neuroleptic malignant syndrome (fever, muscle rigidity, altered mental status, respiratory distress, tachycardia, seizures, diaphoresis, hypertension or hypotension, pallor, tiredness, loss of bladder control). Notify health care professional immediately if these symptoms occur.
- Assess for skin reactions (rash, toxic skin reactions, bullous exanthema).
- Assess for falls risk. Drowsiness, orthostatic hypotension, and motor and sensory instability increase risk. Institute prevention if indicated.

Lab Test Considerations

- Monitor CBC frequently during therapy in patients with pre-existing or history of low WBC. May cause

leukopenia, neutropenia, or agranulocytosis. Discontinue therapy if severe neutropenia (ANC <1000 mm³) occurs.
● Monitor fasting blood glucose and lipid profile before, soon after starting, and periodically during therapy.

Implementation
● **PO:** Administer once daily without regard to food.

Patient/Family Teaching
● Advise patient to take medication as directed and not to skip doses or double up on missed doses. Take missed doses as soon as remembered unless almost time for the next dose. Do not stop taking cariprazine without consulting health care professional.
● Inform patient of possibility of extrapyramidal symptoms and tardive dyskinesia. Instruct patient to report these symptoms immediately.
● Advise patient to make position changes slowly to minimize orthostatic hypotension. Protect from falls.
● Medication may cause drowsiness. Caution patient to avoid driving or other activities requiring alertness until response to medication is known.
● Advise patient and family to notify health care professional of new or worse depression; new or worse anxiety; feeling very agitated or restless; panic attacks; trouble sleeping; new or worse irritability; acting aggressive; being angry or violent; acting on dangerous impulses; an extreme increase in activity and talking; other unusual changes in behavior or mood; or rash occur.
● Inform patient that cariprazine may cause weight gain. Advise patient to monitor weight periodically. Notify health care professional of significant weight gain.
● Instruct patient to notify health care professional of all Rx or OTC medications, vitamins, or herbal products being taken and to consult health care professional before taking any new medications. Caution patient to avoid taking alcohol or other CNS depressants concurrently with this medication.
● Advise patient that extremes in temperature should be avoided, because this drug impairs body temperature regulation.
● Advise patient to notify health care professional of medication regimen prior to treatment or surgery.
● Rep: May cause fetal harm. Advise female patients to notify health care professional if pregnancy is planned or suspected during therapy. Encourage pregnant patients to enroll in registry by contacting National Pregnancy Registry for Atypical Antipsychotics at 1-866-961-2388 or visit http://womensmentalhealth.org/clinical-and-research-programs/pregnancyregistry/. May cause extrapyramidal and/or withdrawal symptoms (agitation, hypertonia, hypotonia, tremor, somnolence, respiratory distress feeding disorder) in neonates whose mothers were exposed to antipsychotic drugs during third trimester of pregnancy. Symptoms vary in severity. Some neonates recover within hrs or days without specific treatment; others required prolonged hospitalization. Monitor neonates of women pregnant while taking cariprazine for extrapyramidal and/or withdrawal symptoms and manage symptoms appropriately.

Evaluation/Desired Outcomes
● Decrease in excitable, paranoid, or withdrawn behavior.
● Decreased occurrence and severity of mania associated with bipolar 1 disorder.
● Increased sense of well-being.
● Renewed interest in surroundings.

⌾ **carvedilol** (kar-ve-di-lole)
Coreg, Coreg CR
Classification
Therapeutic: antihypertensives
Pharmacologic: beta blockers

Indications
Hypertension. HF (ischemic or cardiomyopathic) with digoxin, diuretics, and ACE inhibitors. Left ventricular dysfunction after MI.

Action
Blocks stimulation of beta₁ (myocardial) and beta₂ (pulmonary, vascular, and uterine)-adrenergic receptor sites. Also has alpha₁ blocking activity, which may result in orthostatic hypotension. **Therapeutic Effects:** Decreased heart rate and BP. Improved cardiac output, slowing of the progression of HF and decreased risk of death.

Pharmacokinetics
Absorption: Well absorbed but rapidly undergoes extensive first-pass hepatic metabolism, resulting in 25–35% bioavailability. Food slows absorption.
Distribution: Widely distributed to tissues.
Protein Binding: 98%.
Metabolism and Excretion: Extensively metabolized by the liver via the CYP2D6 and CYP2C9 isoenzymes; ⌾ the CYP2D6 enzyme system exhibits genetic polymorphism; ~7% of population may be poor metabolizers and may have significantly ↑ carvedilol concentrations and an ↑ risk of adverse effects. Excreted in feces via bile, <2% excreted unchanged in urine.
Half-life: 7–10 hr.

TIME/ACTION PROFILE (cardiovascular effects)

ROUTE	ONSET	PEAK	DURATION
PO	within 1 hr	1–2 hr	12 hr
PO-CR	unknown	5 hr	24 hr

Contraindications/Precautions

Contraindicated in: Hypersensitivity; Pulmonary edema; Cardiogenic shock; Bradycardia, heart block, or sick sinus syndrome (unless a pacemaker is in place); Decompensated HF requiring IV inotropic agents (wean before starting carvedilol); Severe hepatic impairment; Asthma or other bronchospastic disorders.

Use Cautiously in: Diabetes mellitus (may mask signs of hypoglycemia); Thyrotoxicosis (may mask symptoms); Peripheral vascular disease; History of severe allergic reactions (intensity of reactions may be ↑); Patients undergoing cataract surgery (↑ risk of intraoperative floppy iris syndrome); OB: Crosses placenta and may cause fetal/neonatal bradycardia, hypotension, hypoglycemia, or respiratory depression; Lactation: Use while breastfeeding only if potential maternal benefit justifies potential risk to infant; Pedi: Safety and effectiveness not established in children; Geri: Older adults may have ↑ sensitivity to beta blockers; initial dose ↓ recommended.

Adverse Reactions/Side Effects

CV: BRADYCARDIA, HF. **Derm:** itching, rash, STEVENS-JOHNSON SYNDROME, TOXIC EPIDERMAL NECROLYSIS, urticaria. **EENT:** blurred vision, dry eyes, intraoperative floppy iris syndrome, nasal stuffiness. **Endo:** hyperglycemia, hypoglycemia. **GI:** diarrhea, constipation, nausea. **GU:** erectile dysfunction, ↓ libido. **MS:** arthralgia, back pain, muscle cramps. **Neuro:** dizziness, fatigue, weakness, anxiety, depression, drowsiness, insomnia, memory loss, mental status changes, nervousness, nightmares, paresthesia. **Resp:** bronchospasm, PULMONARY EDEMA, wheezing. **Misc:** drug-induced lupus syndrome, HYPERSENSITIVITY REACTIONS (including anaphylaxis and angioedema).

Interactions

Drug-Drug: General **anesthetics, phenytoin, diltiazem,** and **verapamil** may cause ↑ myocardial depression. ↑ risk of bradycardia with **clonidine, digoxin, diltiazem, ivabradine,** and **verapamil.** **Amiodarone, cimetidine,** and **fluconazole** may ↑ levels and risk of toxicity. ↑ hypotension may occur with other **antihypertensives,** acute ingestion of **alcohol,** or **nitrates.** May ↑ withdrawal phenomenon from **clonidine;** discontinue carvedilol first. Concurrent administration of **thyroid preparations** may ↓ effectiveness. May alter the effectiveness of **insulins** or **oral hypoglycemic agents;** dose adjustments may be necessary. May ↓ effectiveness of **theophylline.** May ↓ beneficial beta₁-cardiovascular effects of **dopamine** or **dobutamine.** Use cautiously within 14 days of **MAO inhibitor** therapy; may result in hypotension/bradycardia. **NSAIDs** may ↓ antihypertensive effects. **Rifampin** may ↓ levels and effectiveness. May ↑ levels and risk of toxicity of **digoxin** and **cyclosporine;** closely monitor levels.

Route/Dosage

Hypertension

PO (Adults): *Immediate release:* 6.25 mg twice daily; may be ↑ every 7–14 days up to 25 mg twice daily; *Extended release:* 20 mg once daily; dose may be doubled every 7–14 days up to 80 mg once daily.

Heart Failure

PO (Adults): *Immediate release:* 3.125 mg twice daily; dose may be doubled every 2 wk as tolerated (not to exceed 25 mg twice daily in patients <85 kg or 50 mg twice daily in patients >85 kg); *Extended release:* 10 mg once daily; dose may be doubled every 2 wk as tolerated up to 80 mg once daily.

Left Ventricular Dysfunction After Myocardial Infarction

PO (Adults): *Immediate release:* 6.25 mg twice daily; ↑ after 3–10 days to 12.5 twice daily, then to target dose of 25 mg twice daily; some patients may require lower initial doses and slower titration; *Extended release:* 20 mg once daily; dose may be doubled every 3–10 days up to 80 mg once daily.

Availability (generic available)

Extended-release capsules: 10 mg, 20 mg, 40 mg, 80 mg. **Tablets:** 3.125 mg, 6.25 mg, 12.5 mg, 25 mg.

NURSING IMPLICATIONS

Assessment

- Monitor BP and pulse frequently during dose adjustment period and periodically during therapy. Assess for orthostatic hypotension when assisting patient up from supine position. If heart rate decreases below 55 beats/min, decrease dose.
- Monitor intake and output ratios and daily weight. Assess patient routinely for evidence of fluid overload (peripheral edema, dyspnea, rales/crackles, fatigue, weight gain, jugular venous distention). Patients may experience worsening of symptoms during initiation of therapy for HF.
- **Hypertension:** Check frequency of refills to determine adherence.

Lab Test Considerations
- May cause ↑ BUN, triglycerides, and uric acid levels.
- May cause ↑ in ANA titers.
- May cause ↑ in blood glucose levels.

Toxicity and Overdose
- Monitor patients receiving beta blockers for signs of overdose (bradycardia, severe dizziness or fainting, severe drowsiness, dyspnea, bluish fingernails or palms, seizures). Notify health care professional immediately if these signs occur.

Implementation

- Do not confuse carvedilol with captopril.
- Discontinuation of concurrent clonidine should be gradual, with carvedilol discontinued first over 1–2 wk with limitation of physical activity; then, after several days, discontinue clonidine.

- **PO:** Take apical pulse before administering. If <50 bpm or if arrhythmia occurs, withhold medication and notify health care professional.
- Administer with food to minimize orthostatic hypotension.
- Administer extended-release capsules in the morning. *DNC:* Swallow whole; do not crush or chew. Extended-release capsules may be opened and sprinkled on cold applesauce and taken immediately; do not store mixture.
- To convert from immediate-release to extended-release product, doses of 3.125 mg twice daily can be converted to 10 mg daily; doses of 6.25 mg twice daily can be converted to 20 mg daily; doses of 12.5 mg twice daily can be converted to 40 mg daily; and doses of 25 mg twice daily can be converted to 80 mg daily.

Patient/Family Teaching

- Instruct patient to take medication as directed, at the same time each day, even if feeling well. Do not skip or double up on missed doses. Take missed doses as soon as possible up to 4 hr before next dose. Abrupt withdrawal may precipitate life-threatening arrhythmias, hypertension, or myocardial ischemia. Discontinue carvedilol slowly over 1–2 wk. Advise patient to read *Patient Information* before starting therapy and with each Rx refill in case of changes.
- Advise patient to make sure enough medication is available for weekends, holidays, and vacations. A written prescription may be kept in wallet in case of emergency.
- Teach patient and family how to check pulse and BP. Instruct them to check pulse daily and BP biweekly. Advise patient to hold dose and contact health care professional if pulse is <50 bpm or BP changes significantly.
- May cause drowsiness or dizziness. Caution patients to avoid driving or other activities that require alertness until response to the drug is known.
- Advise patient to change positions slowly to minimize orthostatic hypotension, especially during initiation of therapy or when dose is increased.
- Caution patient that this medication may increase sensitivity to cold.
- Instruct patient to notify health care professional of all Rx or OTC medications, vitamins, or herbal products being taken and to consult health care professional before taking other Rx, OTC, or herbal products, especially cold preparations, concurrently with this medication.
- Advise patients with diabetes to closely monitor blood glucose, especially if weakness, malaise, irritability, or fatigue occurs. Medication may mask some signs of hypoglycemia, but dizziness and sweating may still occur.
- Advise patient to notify health care professional if slow pulse, difficulty breathing, wheezing, cold hands and feet, dizziness, confusion, depression, rash, fever, sore throat, unusual bleeding, or bruising occurs.
- Instruct patient to inform health care professional of medication regimen before treatment or surgery.
- Advise patient to carry identification describing disease process and medication regimen at all times.
- Rep: Advise females of reproductive potential to notify health care professional if pregnancy is planned or suspected, or if breastfeeding. If carvedilol is taken during third trimester, monitor newborn for symptoms of hypotension, bradycardia, hypoglycemia, and respiratory depression and manage accordingly.
- **Hypertension:** Reinforce the need to continue additional therapies for hypertension (weight loss, sodium restriction, stress reduction, regular exercise, moderation of alcohol consumption, and smoking cessation). Medication controls but does not cure hypertension.

Evaluation/Desired Outcomes

- Decrease in BP without appearance of detrimental side effects.
- Decrease in severity of HF.

---

caspofungin (kas-po-**fun**-gin)
Cancidas
Classification
Therapeutic: antifungals
Pharmacologic: echinocandins

Indications

Invasive aspergillosis refractory to, or intolerant of, other therapies. Candidemia and associated serious infections (intra-abdominal abscesses, peritonitis, pleural space infections). Esophageal candidiasis. Suspected fungal infections in febrile neutropenic patients.

Action

Inhibits the synthesis of β (1, 3)-D-glucan, a necessary component of the fungal cell wall. **Therapeutic Effects:** Death of susceptible fungi.

Pharmacokinetics

Absorption: IV administration results in complete bioavailability.
Distribution: Widely distributed to tissues.
Protein Binding: 97%.
Metabolism and Excretion: Slowly and extensively metabolized; <1.5% excreted unchanged in urine.
Half-life: Polyphasic: β *phase:* 9–11 hr; γ *phase:* 40–50 hr.

TIME/ACTION PROFILE

ROUTE	ONSET	PEAK	DURATION
IV	unknown	end of infusion	24 hr

Contraindications/Precautions

Contraindicated in: Hypersensitivity; OB: Pregnancy.

Use Cautiously in: Moderate hepatic impairment (↓ maintenance dose recommended); Lactation: Use while breastfeeding only if potential maternal benefit justifies potential risk to infant.

Adverse Reactions/Side Effects

Derm: flushing, pruritus, rash, STEVENS-JOHNSON SYNDROME (SJS), TOXIC EPIDERMAL NECROLYSIS. **GI:** ↑ liver enzymes, diarrhea, nausea, vomiting. **GU:** ↑ serum creatinine. **Local:** venous irritation at injection site. **Neuro:** headache. **Resp:** bronchospasm. **Misc:** chills, fever, HYPERSENSITIVITY REACTIONS (including anaphylaxis and angioedema).

Interactions

Drug-Drug: ↑ risk of hepatotoxicity with **Cyclosporine**; closely monitor liver enzymes during concurrent therapy. May ↓ levels and effectiveness of **tacrolimus**. **Rifampin** may ↓ levels and effectiveness; maintenance dose should be ↑ to 70 mg/day (in patients with normal hepatic function). **Efavirenz, nelfinavir, nevirapine, phenytoin, dexamethasone,** or **carbamazepine** may ↓ levels and effectiveness; an ↑ in the maintenance dose to 70 mg/day should be considered in patients who are not clinically responding.

Route/Dosage

IV (Adults): 70 mg initially followed by 50 mg once daily; duration determined by clinical situation and response; *Esophageal candidiasis:* 50 mg once daily; duration determined by clinical situation and response.

IV (Children ≥3 mo): 70 mg/m² (max = 70 mg) initially followed by 50 mg/m² once daily (max = 70 mg/day); duration determined by clinical situation and response.

IV (Infants 1 to <3 mo and Neonates): 25 mg/m² once daily.

Hepatic Impairment

IV (Adults): *Moderate hepatic impairment:* 70 mg initially followed by 35 mg once daily; duration determined by clinical situation and response.

Availability (generic available)

Powder for injection: 50 mg/vial, 70 mg/vial.

NURSING IMPLICATIONS

Assessment

- Assess patient for signs and symptoms of fungal infections prior to and periodically during therapy.
- Assess for skin rash frequently during therapy. Discontinue at first sign of rash; may be life-threatening. SJS may develop. Treat symptomatically; may recur once treatment is stopped.

- Monitor patient for signs of anaphylaxis (rash, dyspnea, stridor, facial swelling, angioedema, pruritus, sensation of warmth, bronchospasm) during therapy.

Lab Test Considerations

- May cause ↑ serum alkaline phosphatase, serum creatinine, AST, ALT, eosinophils, and urine protein and RBCs. May also cause ↓ serum potassium, hemoglobin, hematocrit, and WBCs.

Implementation

IV Administration

- **Intermittent Infusion:** Allow refrigerated vial to reach room temperature. *For 70-mg or 50-mg dose:* Reconstitute vials with 10.8 mL of 0.9% NaCl, sterile water for injection, bacteriostatic water for injection with methylparaben and propylparaben, or bacteriostatic water for injection with 0.9% benzyl alcohol. Use preservative-free diluents for neonates. Do not dilute with dextrose solutions. Reconstituted solution is stable for 1 hr at room temperature. *Dilution:* Withdraw 10 mL from vial and add to 250 mL of 0.9% NaCl, 0.45% NaCl, 0.225% NaCl, or LR. The 50-mg dose also can be diluted in 100 mL when volume restriction is necessary. Infusion is stable for 24 hr at room temperature or 48 hr if refrigerated. *For 35-mg dose:* Reconstitute a 50-mg or 70-mg vial as per the directions above. Remove the volume of drug equal to the calculated loading dose or calculated maintenance dose based on a concentration of 7 mg/mL (if reconstituted from the 70-mg vial) or a concentration of 5 mg/mL (if reconstituted from the 50-mg vial). White cake should dissolve completely. Mix gently until a clear solution is obtained. Do not use a solution that is cloudy, discolored, or contains precipitates. *Concentration:* 0.14–0.47 mg/mL. *Rate:* Infuse over 1 hr.
- **Y-Site Compatibility:** alemtuzumab, allopurinol, amifostine, amikacin, aminophylline, amiodarone, anidulafungin, argatroban, arsenic trioxide, atracurium, aztreonam, bleomycin, bumetanide, busulfan, butorphanol, calcium acetate, calcium chloride, calcium gluconate, carboplatin, carmustine, chlorpromazine, ciprofloxacin, cisatracurium, cisplatin, cyclophosphamide, cyclosporine, dacarbazine, dactinomycin, daptomycin, daunorubicin hydrochloride, dexmedetomidine, dexrazoxane, diltiazem, diphenhydramine, dobutamine, docetaxel, dopamine, doxorubicin hydrochloride, doxorubicin liposomal, doxycycline, droperidol, epinephrine, epirubicin, erythromycin, esmolol, etoposide, etoposide phosphate, famotidine, fentanyl, fluconazole, fludarabine, ganciclovir, gemcitabine, gentamicin, glycopyrrolate, granisetron, haloperidol, hydrocortisone, hydromorphone, idarubicin, ifosfamide, imipenem/cilastatin, insulin, regular, irinotecan, isoproterenol, labetalol, leucovorin, levofloxacin, linezolid, magnesium sulfate, mannitol, melphalan, meperidine, meropenem, mesna, metoclopramide, metoprolol, mid-

azolam, milrinone, mitomycin, mitoxantrone, morphine, moxifloxacin, mycophenolate, nalbuphine, naloxone, nicardipine, nitroglycerin, norepinephrine, octreotide, ondansetron, oxaliplatin, oxytocin, paclitaxel, palonosetron, pentamidine, phentolamine, phenylephrine, posaconazole, potassium acetate, potassium chloride, procainamide, prochlorperazine, promethazine, propranolol, remifentanil, rocuronium, succinylcholine, sufentanil, tacrolimus, telavancin, theophylline, thiopental, thiotepa, tigecycline, tirofiban, tobramycin, topotecan, vancomycin, vasopressin, vecuronium, verapamil, vinblastine, vincristine, vinorelbine, voriconazole, zidovudine, zoledronic acid.

- **Y-Site Incompatibility:** aminocaproic acid, amphotericin B lipid complex, amphotericin B liposomal, ampicillin, ampicillin/sulbactam, bivalirudin, blinatumomab, cefazolin, cefepime, cefotaxime, cefotetan, cefoxitin, ceftaroline, ceftazidime, ceftriaxone, cefuroxime, chloramphenicol, clindamycin, dantrolene, dexamethasone, diazepam, digoxin, enalaprilat, ephedrine, ertapenem, fluorouracil, foscarnet, fosphenytoin, furosemide, heparin, ketorolac, lidocaine, methotrexate, methylprednisolone, nafcillin, nitroprusside, pamidronate, pemetrexed, pentobarbital, phenobarbital, phenytoin, piperacillin/tazobactam, potassium phosphate, sodium acetate, sodium bicarbonate, sodium phosphate, trimethoprim/sulfamethoxazole.
- **Solution Incompatibility:** Solutions containing dextrose.

Patient/Family Teaching
- Explain the purpose of caspofungin to patient and family.
- Advise patient to notify health care professional immediately if symptoms of allergic reactions (rash, facial swelling, pruritus, sensation of warmth, difficulty breathing) occur.
- Rep: Advise females of reproductive potential to notify health care professional if pregnancy is planned or suspected or if breastfeeding.

Evaluation/Desired Outcomes
- Decrease in signs and symptoms of fungal infections. Duration of therapy is determined based on severity of underlying disease, recovery from immunosuppression, and clinical response.

cefaclor, See CEPHALOSPORINS— SECOND GENERATION.

cefadroxil, See CEPHALOSPORINS— FIRST GENERATION.

ceFAZolin, See CEPHALOSPORINS— FIRST GENERATION.

cefdinir, See CEPHALOSPORINS— THIRD GENERATION.

cefepime (seff-e-peem)
~~Maxipime~~
Classification
Therapeutic: anti-infectives
Pharmacologic: fourth-generation cephalosporins

Indications
Treatment of the following infections caused by susceptible organisms: Uncomplicated skin and skin structure infections, Bone and joint infections, Uncomplicated and complicated urinary tract infections, Respiratory tract infections, Complicated intra-abdominal infections (with metronidazole), Septicemia. Empiric treatment of febrile neutropenic patients.

Action
Binds to the bacterial cell wall membrane, causing cell death. **Therapeutic Effects:** Bactericidal action against susceptible bacteria. **Spectrum:** Similar to that of second- and third-generation cephalosporins, but activity against staphylococci is less, whereas activity against gram-negative pathogens is greater, even for organisms resistant to first-, second-, and third-generation agents. Notable is increased action against: *Enterobacter*, *Haemophilus influenzae* (including β-lactamase-producing strains), *Escherichia coli*, *Klebsiella pneumoniae*, *Neisseria*, *Proteus*, *Providencia*, *Pseudomonas aeruginosa*, *Serratia*, *Moraxella catarrhalis* (including β-lactamase-producing strains). Not active against methicillin-resistant staphylococci or enterococci.

Pharmacokinetics
Absorption: Well absorbed after IM administration; IV administration results in complete bioavailability.
Distribution: Widely distributed. Some CSF penetration.
Metabolism and Excretion: 85% excreted unchanged in urine.
Half-life: *Adults:* 2 hr (↑ in renal impairment); *Children 2 mo–6 yr:* 1.7–1.9 hr.

TIME/ACTION PROFILE (plasma concentrations)

ROUTE	ONSET	PEAK	DURATION
IM	rapid	1–2 hr	12 hr
IV	rapid	end of infusion	12 hr

Contraindications/Precautions

Contraindicated in: Hypersensitivity to cephalosporins; Serious hypersensitivity to penicillins.
Use Cautiously in: Renal impairment (↓ dosing/↑ dosing interval recommended if CCr ≤60 mL/min); History of GI disease, especially colitis; Hepatic impairment or poor nutritional status (may be at ↑ risk of bleeding); OB: Safety not established in pregnancy; Lactation: Safety not established in breastfeeding; Geri: Dose adjustment due to age-related ↓ in renal function may be necessary in older adults.

Adverse Reactions/Side Effects

Derm: rash, pruritus, urticaria. **GI:** CLOSTRIDIOIDES DIFFICILE-ASSOCIATED DIARRHEA (CDAD), diarrhea, nausea, vomiting. **Hemat:** bleeding, eosinophilia, hemolytic anemia, neutropenia, thrombocytopenia. **Local:** pain at IM site, phlebitis at IV site. **Neuro:** aphasia, ENCEPHALOPATHY, headache, SEIZURES (↑ risk in renal impairment). **Misc:** fever, HYPERSENSITIVITY REACTIONS (including anaphylaxis), superinfection.

Interactions

Drug-Drug: Probenecid ↓ excretion and ↑ levels. Concurrent use of **loop diuretics** or **aminoglycosides** may ↑ risk of nephrotoxicity.

Route/Dosage

IM (Adults): *Mild to moderate uncomplicated or complicated urinary tract infections due to Escherichia coli:* 0.5–1 g every 12 hr.
IV (Adults): *Moderate to severe pneumonia:* 1–2 g every 12 hr. *Mild to moderate uncomplicated or complicated urinary tract infections:* 0.5–1 g every 12 hr. *Severe uncomplicated or complicated urinary tract infections, moderate to severe uncomplicated skin and skin structure infections, complicated intra-abdominal infections:* 2 g every 12 hr. *Empiric treatment of febrile neutropenia:* 2 g every 8 hr.
IV (Children 1 mo–16 yr): *Uncomplicated and complicated urinary tract infections, uncomplicated skin and skin structure infections, pneumonia:* 50 mg/kg every 12 hr (not to exceed 2 g/dose). *Febrile neutropenia:* 50 mg/kg every 8 hr (not to exceed 2 g/dose).
IV (Neonates postnatal age ≥14 days): 50 mg/kg every 12 hr.
IV (Neonates postnatal age <14 days): 30 mg/kg every 12 hr; consider 50 mg/kg every 12 hr for *Pseudomonas* infections.

Renal Impairment

IM, IV (Adults): (See Manufacturer's specific recommendations) *CCr 30–60 mL/min:* 0.5–1 g every 24 hr or 2 g every 12–24 hr; *CCr 11–29 mL/min:* 0.5–2 g every 24 hr; *CCr <11 mL/min:* 250 mg–1 g every 24 hr.

Availability (generic available)

Powder for injection: 1 g, 2 g. **Premixed infusion:** 1 g/50 mL D5W, 2 g/100 mL D5W.

NURSING IMPLICATIONS

Assessment

- Assess patient for infection (vital signs; appearance of wound, sputum, urine, and stool; WBC) at beginning of and throughout therapy.
- Before initiating therapy, obtain a history to determine previous use of and reactions to penicillins or cephalosporins. Persons with a negative history of penicillin sensitivity may still have an allergic response.
- Obtain specimens for culture and sensitivity before initiating therapy. First dose may be given before receiving results.
- Observe patient for signs and symptoms of anaphylaxis (rash, pruritus, laryngeal edema, wheezing). Discontinue the drug and notify health care professional immediately if these symptoms occur. Keep epinephrine, an antihistamine, and resuscitation equipment close by in the event of an anaphylactic reaction.
- Monitor bowel function. Diarrhea, abdominal cramping, fever, and bloody stools should be reported to health care professional promptly as a sign of CDAD. May begin up to several wk following cessation of therapy.

Lab Test Considerations

- May cause positive results for Coombs' test in patients receiving high doses or in neonates whose mothers were given cephalosporins before delivery.
- May cause ↑ AST, ALT, bilirubin, BUN, and serum creatinine.
- May rarely cause leukopenia, neutropenia, thrombocytopenia, and eosinophilia.

Implementation

- **IM:** *Reconstitution:* Reconstitute IM doses with sterile or bacteriostatic water for injection, 0.9% NaCl, or D5W. May be diluted with lidocaine to minimize injection discomfort.
- Inject deep into a well-developed muscle mass; massage well.
- IM route should only be used for treatment of mild to moderate uncomplicated or complicated urinary tract infections due to *Escherichia coli*.

IV Administration

- **IV:** Monitor injection site frequently for phlebitis (pain, redness, swelling). Change sites every 48–72 hr to prevent phlebitis.
- If aminoglycosides are administered concurrently, administer in separate sites, if possible, at least 1 hr apart. If second site is unavailable, flush lines between medications.
- **Intermittent Infusion:** *Reconstitution:* Reconstitute with 10 mL sterile water, 0.9% NaCl, or D5W for the 1-g or 2-g vials. *Dilution:* Dilute further in 50–100 mL of D5W, 0.9% NaCl, D10W, D5/0.9% NaCl, or D5/LR. *Concentration:* Maximum 40 mg/mL.

C

- Solution is stable for 24 hr at room temperature and 7 days if refrigerated. *Rate:* Administer over 20–30 min.
- **Y-Site Compatibility:** amikacin, aminocaproic acid, amiodarone, amphotericin B lipid complex, ampicillin/sulbactam, anidulafungin, arsenic trioxide, azithromycin, aztreonam, bivalirudin, bleomycin, bumetanide, buprenorphine, butorphanol, calcium gluconate, carboplatin, carmustine, ceftolozane/tazobactam, cyclophosphamide, cytarabine, dactinomycin, daptomycin, dexamethasone, dexmedetomidine, docetaxel, doxorubicin liposomal, eptifibatide, eravacycline, esmolol, fluconazole, fludarabine, fluorouracil, foscarnet, fosphenytoin, furosemide, gentamicin, granisetron, hetastarch, hydrocortisone, hydromorphone, imipenem/cilastatin, insulin, regular, ketamine, LR, leucovorin calcium, levofloxacin, linezolid, lorazepam, melphalan, meropenem/vaborbactam, mesna, methadone, methotrexate, methylprednisolone, metoprolol, metronidazole, milrinone, octreotide, oxytocin, paclitaxel, palonosetron, pamidronate, piperacillin/tazobactam, potassium acetate, remifentanil, rocuronium, sargramostim, sodium acetate, sodium bicarbonate, sufentanil, tedizolid, telavancin, thiotepa, tigecycline, tirofiban, tobramycin, trimethoprim/sulfamethoxazole, valproate sodium, vasopressin, zidovudine, zoledronic acid.
- **Y-Site Incompatibility:** acetylcysteine, acyclovir, alemtuzumab, amphotericin B deoxycholate, amphotericin B liposomal, argatroban, caspofungin, chlorpromazine, ciprofloxacin, cisplatin, dacarbazine, daunorubicin hydrochloride, dexrazoxane, diazepam, diltiazem, diphenhydramine, doxorubicin hydrochloride, droperidol, enalaprilat, epirubicin, erythromycin, etoposide, etoposide phosphate, famotidine, filgrastim, floxuridine, ganciclovir, gemcitabine, gemtuzumab ozogamicin, haloperidol, hydroxyzine, idarubicin, ifosfamide, irinotecan, isavuconazonium, labetalol, magnesium sulfate, mannitol, meperidine, metoclopramide, midazolam, mitomycin, mitoxantrone, nalbuphine, ondansetron, oxaliplatin, pantoprazole, pemetrexed, phenytoin, prochlorperazine, promethazine, tacrolimus, theophylline, vecuronium, vinblastine, vincristine, vinorelbine, voriconazole.

Patient/Family Teaching

- Advise patient to report signs of superinfection (furry overgrowth on the tongue, vaginal itching or discharge, loose or foul-smelling stools) and allergy.
- Instruct patient to notify health care professional if fever and diarrhea develop, especially if stool contains blood, pus, or mucus. Advise patient not to treat diarrhea without consulting health care professional.

- Rep: Advise females of reproductive potential to notify health care professional if pregnancy is planned or suspected or if breastfeeding.

Evaluation/Desired Outcomes

- Resolution of the signs and symptoms of infection. Length of time for complete resolution depends on the organism and site of infection.

cefiderocol (sef-i-der-oh-kol)
Fetroja
Classification
Therapeutic: anti-infectives
Pharmacologic: cephalosporin derivatives

Indications
Complicated urinary tract infections, including pyelonephritis, in patients who have limited or no alternative treatment options. Hospital-acquired bacterial pneumonia and ventilator-associated bacterial pneumonia.

Action
Functions as a siderophore and binds to extracellular free ferric iron. Iron transport systems then deliver cefiderocol across the outer membrane of gram-negative bacilli where it binds to the bacterial cell wall membrane, causing cell death. **Therapeutic Effects:** Bactericidal action against susceptible bacteria. **Spectrum:** Active against the following gram-negative bacilli: *Acinetobacter baumannii*, *Enterobacter cloacae*, *Escherichia coli*, *Klebsiella pneumoniae*, *Proteus mirabilis*, *Pseudomonas aeruginosa*, and *Serratia marcescens*.

Pharmacokinetics
Absorption: IV administration results in complete bioavailability.
Distribution: Some distribution to tissues.
Metabolism and Excretion: Undergoes minimal metabolism by liver; primarily excreted in urine (99%; 91% as unchanged drug).
Half-life: 2–3 hr.

TIME/ACTION PROFILE (plasma concentrations)

ROUTE	ONSET	PEAK	DURATION
IV	rapid	end of infusion	8 hr

Contraindications/Precautions
Contraindicated in: Known serious hypersensitivity to cefiderocol or other beta-lactams.
Use Cautiously in: Carbapenem-resistant gram-negative bacterial infections, including nosocomial pneumonia, bloodstream infections, and sepsis (↑ risk of mortality); Seizure disorders; Renal impairment (dosage ↓ required for CCr <60 mL/min); OB: Use

during pregnancy only if potential maternal benefit justifies potential fetal risk; Lactation: Use while breastfeeding only if potential maternal benefit justifies potential risk to infant; Pedi: Safety and effectiveness not established in children; Geri: Dose adjustment may be necessary in older adults for age-related ↓ in renal function.

Adverse Reactions/Side Effects

Derm: rash. **EENT:** thrush. **F and E:** hypokalemia. **GI:** ↑ liver enzymes, CLOSTRIDIOIDES DIFFICILE-ASSOCIATED DIARRHEA (CDAD), constipation, diarrhea, nausea, vomiting. **GU:** candiduria, vaginal candidiasis. **Local:** infusion site reactions. **Neuro:** headache, SEIZURES. **Resp:** cough. **Misc:** HYPERSENSITIVITY REACTIONS (including anaphylaxis).

Interactions

Drug-Drug: None reported.

Route/Dosage

IV (Adults): *CCr ≥120 mL/min:* 2 g every 6 hr for 7–14 days; *CCr 60–119 mL/min:* 2 g every 8 hr for 7–14 days.

Renal Impairment

IV (Adults): *CCr 30–59 mL/min:* 1.5 g every 8 hr for 7–14 days; *CCr 15–29 mL/min:* 1 g every 8 hr for 7–14 days; *CCr <15 mL/min (with or without hemodialysis):* 0.75 g every 12 hr for 7–14 days (in patients receiving hemodialysis, administer dose immediately following hemodialysis session); *Continuous renal replacement therapy:* Effluent flow rate ≥4.1 L/hr: 2 g every 8 hr for 7–14 days; effluent flow rate 3.1–4 L/hr: 1.5 g every 8 hr for 7–14 days; Effluent flow rate 2.1–3 L/hr: 2 g every 12 hr for 7–14 days; Effluent flow rate ≤2 L/hr: 1.5 g every 12 hr for 7–14 days.

Availability

Lyophilized powder for injection: 1 g/vial.

NURSING IMPLICATIONS

Assessment

- Assess for infection (vital signs, appearance of urine, WBC) at beginning of and during therapy. Monitor clinical response to therapy closely.
- Obtain a history before initiating therapy to determine previous use of and reactions to penicillins or cephalosporins. Persons with a negative history of penicillin sensitivity may still have an allergic response.
- Observe for signs and symptoms of anaphylaxis (rash, pruritus, laryngeal edema, wheezing). Notify health care professional immediately if these occur.
- Obtain specimens for culture and sensitivity prior to therapy. First dose may be given before receiving results.
- Monitor bowel function. Diarrhea, abdominal cramping, fever, and bloody stools should be reported to health care professional promptly as a sign of CDAD. May begin up to several wk following cessation of therapy.

Lab Test Considerations

- May cause false-positive results in dipstick tests (urine protein, ketones, occult blood). Use alternate clinical laboratory methods of testing to confirm positive tests.

Implementation

- **Intermittent Infusion:** *Reconstitution:* Reconstitute with 10 mL 0.9% NaCl or D5W; gently shake to dissolve. Allow vial to stand until foaming has disappeared; usually 2 min. *Concentration:* 0.089 gram/mL. *Dilution:* Withdraw appropriate volume from vial and dilute in 100 mL 0.9% NaCl or D5W immediately after reconstitution. Solution is clear and colorless; do not administer solutions that are discolored, cloudy, or contain particulate matter. Reconstituted solution is stable for 1 hr at room temperature. Solution diluted in IV bag is stable for up to 6 hr at room temperature and 24 hr if refrigerated and protected from light. *Rate:* Infusion must be completed within 6 hr.

Patient/Family Teaching

- Explain purpose of cefiderocol and the importance of completing full course of therapy to patient. Skipping doses or not completing full course of therapy may decrease effectiveness of the immediate treatment and increase the likelihood that bacteria will develop resistance and will not be treatable by cefiderocol or other antibacterial drugs in the future.
- Advise patient to report the signs of superinfection (furry overgrowth on the tongue, vaginal itching or discharge, loose or foul-smelling stools) and allergy.
- Instruct patient to notify health care professional immediately if diarrhea, abdominal cramping, fever, or bloody stools or signs and symptoms of anaphylaxis occur and not to treat with antidiarrheals without consulting health care professional.
- Inform patient of risk of seizures, especially in patient with a seizure disorder. Advise patient to notify health care professional immediately if seizure occurs.
- Rep: Advise females of reproductive potential to notify health care professional if pregnancy is planned or suspected or if breastfeeding.

Evaluation/Desired Outcomes

- Resolution of the signs and symptoms of infection.

---

cefixime, See CEPHALOSPORINS—THIRD GENERATION.

---

cefotaxime, See CEPHALOSPORINS—THIRD GENERATION.

---

cefoTEtan, See CEPHALOSPORINS—SECOND GENERATION.

cefOXitin, See CEPHALOSPORINS—SECOND GENERATION.

cefpodoxime, See CEPHALOSPORINS—THIRD GENERATION.

cefprozil, See CEPHALOSPORINS—SECOND GENERATION.

ceftaroline (sef-tar-oh-leen)
Teflaro
Classification
Therapeutic: anti-infectives
Pharmacologic: cephalosporin derivatives

Indications
Acute bacterial skin/skin structure infections. Community-acquired pneumonia.

Action
Binds to bacterial cell wall membrane, causing cell death. **Therapeutic Effects:** Bactericidal action against susceptible bacteria. **Spectrum:** Active against *Staphylococcus aureus* (including methicillin-susceptible and -resistant strains), *Streptococcus pneumoniae*, *Streptococcus pyogenes*, *Streptococcus agalactiae*, *Escherichia coli*, *Haemophilus influenzae*,*Haemophilus influenzae Klebsiella pneumoniae*, and *Klebsiella oxytoca*.

Pharmacokinetics
Absorption: IV administration results in complete bioavailability of parent drug.
Distribution: Well distributed to tissues.
Metabolism and Excretion: Ceftaroline fosamil is rapidly converted by plasma phosphatases to ceftaroline, the active metabolite; 88% excreted in urine, 6% in feces.
Half-life: 2.6 hr (after multiple doses).

TIME/ACTION PROFILE (plasma concentrations)

ROUTE	ONSET	PEAK	DURATION
IV	rapid	end of infusion	12 hr

Contraindications/Precautions
Contraindicated in: Known serious hypersensitivity to cephalosporins.
Use Cautiously in: Known hypersensitivity to other beta-lactams; Renal impairment (dosage ↓ required for CCr ≤50 mL/min in adults); OB: Safety not established

in pregnancy; Lactation: Use while breastfeeding only if potential maternal benefit justifies potential risk to infant; Pedi: Neonates <34 wk (gestational age) or <12 days (postnatal age) (acute bacterial skin/skin structure infections) and infants <2 mo (community-acquired pneumonia) (safety and effectiveness not established); Geri: Dose adjustment may be necessary in older adults for age-related ↓ in renal function.

Adverse Reactions/Side Effects
Derm: rash. **GI:** CLOSTRIDIOIDES DIFFICILE-ASSOCIATED DIARRHEA (CDAD), diarrhea, nausea. **Hemat:** hemolytic anemia. **Local:** phlebitis at injection site. **Neuro:** ENCEPHALOPATHY, SEIZURES. **Misc:** HYPERSENSITIVITY REACTIONS (including anaphylaxis).

Interactions
Drug-Drug: None reported.

Route/Dosage
Acute Bacterial Skin/Skin Structure Infections
IV (Adults): 600 mg every 12 hr for 5–14 days.
IV (Children 2–17 yr and >33 kg): 400 mg every 8 hr for 5–14 days *or* 600 mg every 12 hr for 5–14 days.
IV (Children 2–17 yr and ≤33 kg): 12 mg/kg every 8 hr for 5–14 days.
IV (Children 2 mo–<2 yr): 8 mg/kg every 8 hr for 5–14 days.
IV (Neonates 0–<2 mo): 6 mg/kg every 8 hr for 5–14 days.

Renal Impairment
IV (Adults): *CCr >30 to ≤50 mL/min:* 400 mg every 12 hr; *CCr ≥15 to ≤30 mL/min:* 300 mg every 12 hr; *CCr <15 mL/min including hemodialysis:* 200 mg every 12 hr.

Community-Acquired Pneumonia
IV (Adults): 600 mg every 12 hr for 5–7 days.
IV (Children 2–17 yr and >33 kg): 400 mg every 8 hr for 5–14 days *or* 600 mg every 12 hr for 5–14 days.
IV (Children 2–17 yr and ≤33 kg): 12 mg/kg every 8 hr for 5–14 days.
IV (Children 2 mo–<2 yr): 8 mg/kg every 8 hr for 5–14 days.

Renal Impairment
IV (Adults): *CCr >30 to ≤50 mL/min:* 400 mg every 12 hr; *CCr ≥15 to ≤30 mL/min:* 300 mg every 12 hr; *CCr <15 mL/min including hemodialysis:* 200 mg every 12 hr.

Availability (generic available)
Powder for injection: 400 mg/vial, 600 mg/vial.

NURSING IMPLICATIONS
Assessment
● Assess for infection (vital signs; appearance of wound, sputum, urine, and stool; WBC) at beginning of and throughout therapy.

- Before initiating therapy, obtain a history to determine previous use of and reactions to penicillins, cephalosporins, or carbapenems. Persons with a negative history of sensitivity may still have an allergic response.
- Obtain specimens for culture and sensitivity before initiating therapy. First dose may be given before receiving results.
- Observe patient for signs and symptoms of anaphylaxis (rash, pruritus, laryngeal edema, wheezing). Discontinue the drug and notify health care professional immediately if these symptoms occur. Keep epinephrine, an antihistamine, and resuscitation equipment close by in the event of an anaphylactic reaction.
- Monitor bowel function. Diarrhea, abdominal cramping, fever, and bloody stools should be reported to health care professional promptly as a sign of CDAD. May begin up to several mo following cessation of therapy.

Lab Test Considerations
- May cause seroconversion from a negative to a positive direct Coombs' test. If anemia develops during or after therapy, perform a direct Coombs' test. If drug-induced hemolytic anemia is suspected, discontinue ceftaroline and provide supportive care.

Implementation

IV Administration
- **Intermittent Infusion:** *Reconstitution:* Reconstitute with 20 mL of sterile water for injection, 0.9% NaCl, D5W, or LR. *Dilution:* Dilute further with 50–250 mL of same diluent unless reconstituted with sterile water for injection, then use 0.9% NaCl, D5W, D2.5W, 0.45% NaCl, or LR. Mix gently to dissolve. Solution is clear to light or dark yellow; do not administer solutions that are discolored or contain particulate matter. Solution is stable for 6 hr at room temperature or 24 hr if refrigerated. *Rate:* Infuse over 5–60 min.
- **Y-Site Compatibility:** acyclovir, amikacin, aminophylline, amiodarone, azithromycin, bumetanide, calcium chloride, calcium gluconate, ceftolozane/tazobactam, ciprofloxacin, cisatracurium, clindamycin, cyclosporine, dexamethasone, digoxin, diltiazem, diphenhydramine, dopamine, enalaprilat, esomeprazole, famotidine, fentanyl, fluconazole, furosemide, gentamicin, granisetron, haloperidol, heparin, hydrocortisone, hydromorphone, insulin, regular, insulin lispro, levofloxacin, lidocaine, lorazepam, mannitol, meperidine, methylprednisolone, metoclopramide, metoprolol, midazolam, milrinone, morphine, moxifloxacin, multivitamins, norepinephrine, ondansetron, pantoprazole, plazomicin, potassium chloride, promethazine, propofol, remifentanil, sodium bicarbonate, tobramycin, trimethoprim/sulfamethoxazole, vasopressin, voriconazole.

- **Y-Site Incompatibility:** caspofungin, diazepam, eravacycline, filgrastim, isavuconazonium, labetalol, meropenem/vaborbactam, potassium phosphate, sodium phosphate, tedizolid.

Patient/Family Teaching
- Explain the purpose of ceftaroline to patient. Emphasize the importance of completing therapy, even if feeling better.
- Instruct patient to notify health care professional if fever and diarrhea develop, especially if stool contains blood, pus, or mucus. Advise patient not to treat diarrhea without consulting health care professional.
- Rep: Advise females of reproductive potential to notify health care professional if pregnancy is planned or suspected or if breastfeeding.

Evaluation/Desired Outcomes
- Resolution of the signs and symptoms of infection. Length of time for complete resolution depends on the organism and site of infection.

---

cefTAZidime, See CEPHALOSPORINS—THIRD GENERATION.

---

ceftazidime/avibactam
(sef-**tay**-zi-deem/a-vi-**bak**-tam)
  Avycaz
Classification
Therapeutic: anti-infectives
Pharmacologic: third-generation cephalosporins, beta-lactamase inhibitors

Indications
Complicated intra-abdominal infections (in combination with metronidazole). Complicated urinary tract infections (including pyelonephritis). Hospital-acquired and ventilator-associated bacterial pneumonia.

Action
Ceftazidime: Binds to the bacterial cell wall membrane, causing cell death. *Avibactam:* Inhibits beta-lactamase, an enzyme that destroys penicillins and cephalosporins. **Therapeutic Effects:** Death of susceptible bacteria with resolution of infection. **Spectrum:** Active against *Escherichia coli, Klebsiella pneumoniae, Proteus mirabilis, Haemophilus influenzae, Enterobacter cloacae, Klebsiella oxytoca, Pseudomonas aeruginosa, Citrobacter freundii,* and *Serratia marcescens.*

Pharmacokinetics
Absorption: IV administration results in complete bioavailability.
Distribution: *Ceftazidime:* Widely distributed, enters breast milk in low concentrations; *avibactam:* widely distributed.

Metabolism and Excretion: *ceftazidime:* minimally metabolized, 80–90% excreted unchanged in urine; *avibactam:* minimally metabolized, mainly excreted unchanged in urine.

Half-life: *Ceftazidime:* 2.8–3.3 hr (↑ in renal impairment); *avibactam:* 2.2–2.7 hr.

TIME/ACTION PROFILE (blood levels)

ROUTE	ONSET	PEAK	DURATION
IV	rapid	end of infusion	8 hr (↑ in renal impairment)

Contraindications/Precautions

Contraindicated in: Known hypersensitivity to ceftazidime, other cephalosporins or avibactam-containing products; cross-sensitivity with other penicillins, carbapenems, and cephalosporins may occur.
Use Cautiously in: CCr 30–50 mL/min (efficacy may be ↓, monitor renal function frequently and adjust dose if necessary); OB: Use during pregnancy only if potential material benefit justifies potential fetal risk; Lactation: Use while breastfeeding only if potential maternal benefit justifies potential risk to infant; Pedi: Children <3 mo (safety and effectiveness not established); Geri: Consider age-related impairment of renal function.

Adverse Reactions/Side Effects

F and E: hypokalemia. **GI:** CLOSTRIDIOIDES DIFFICILE-ASSOCIATED DIARRHEA (CDAD), diarrhea, nausea, vomiting. **Hemat:** eosinophilia, thrombocytopenia. **Neuro:** anxiety, dizziness, headache, SEIZURES (↑ in renal impairment). **Misc:** HYPERSENSITIVITY REACTIONS (including anaphylaxis and serious skin reactions).

Interactions

Drug-Drug: Probenecid may ↓ renal excretion of avibactam; concurrent administration is not recommended.

Route/Dosage

IV (Adults): 2.5 g (2 g ceftazidime/0.5 g avibactam) every 8 hr. Duration of therapy = 5–14 days (complicated intra-abdominal infections); 7–14 days (complicated urinary tract infections or hospital-/ventilator-acquired bacterial pneumonia).
IV (Children ≥2 yr): 62.5 mg/kg (50 mg/kg ceftazidime/12.5 mg/kg avibactam) (max dose = 2.5 g [2 g ceftazidime/0.5 g avibactam]) every 8 hr. Duration of therapy = 5–14 days (complicated intra-abdominal infections); 7–14 days (complicated urinary tract infections or hospital-/ventilator-acquired bacterial pneumonia).
IV (Children 6 mo–<2 yr): 62.5 mg/kg (50 mg/kg ceftazidime/12.5 mg/kg avibactam) every 8 hr. Duration of therapy = 5–14 days (complicated intra-abdominal infections); 7–14 days (complicated urinary

tract infections or hospital-/ventilator-acquired bacterial pneumonia).
IV (Children 3 mo–<6 mo): 50 mg/kg (40 mg/kg ceftazidime/10 mg/kg avibactam) every 8 hr. Duration of therapy = 5–14 days (complicated intra-abdominal infections); 7–14 days (complicated urinary tract infections or hospital-/ventilator-acquired bacterial pneumonia).

Renal Impairment

IV (Adults): *CCr 31–50 mL/min:* 1.25 g (1 g ceftazidime/0.25 g avibactam) every 8 hr; *CCr 16–30 mL/min:* 0.94 g (0.75 g ceftazidime/0.19 g avibactam) every 12 hr; *CCr 6–15 mL/min:* 0.94 g (0.75 g ceftazidime/0.19 g avibactam) every 24 hr; *CCr ≤5 mL/min:* 0.94 g (0.75 g ceftazidime/0.19 g avibactam) every 48 hr: *Hemodialysis:* Administer dose after hemodialysis on hemodialysis days.

Renal Impairment

IV (Children ≥2 yr): *CCr 31–50 mL/min:* 31.25 mg/kg (25 mg/kg ceftazidime/6.25 mg/kg avibactam) (max dose = 1.25 g [1 g ceftazidime/0.25 g avibactam]) every 8 hr; *CCr 16–30 mL/min:* 23.75 mg/kg (19 mg/kg ceftazidime/4.75 mg/kg avibactam) (max dose = 0.94 g [0.75 g ceftazidime/0.19 g avibactam]) every 12 hr; *CCr 6–15 mL/min:* 23.75 mg/kg (19 mg/kg ceftazidime/4.75 mg/kg avibactam) (max dose = 0.94 g [0.75 g ceftazidime/0.19 g avibactam]) every 24 hr; *CCr ≤5 mL/min:* 23.75 mg/kg (19 mg/kg ceftazidime/4.75 mg/kg avibactam) (max dose = 0.94 g [0.75 g ceftazidime/0.19 g avibactam]) every 48 hr; *Hemodialysis:* Administer dose after hemodialysis or on hemodialysis days.

Availability

Powder for injection: ceftazidime 2 g/avibactam 0.5 g/vial.

NURSING IMPLICATIONS

Assessment

- Assess for infection (vital signs; appearance of wound, sputum, urine, and stool; WBC) at beginning of and during therapy.
- Before initiating therapy, obtain a history to determine previous use of and reactions to penicillins, cephalosporins, or carbapenems. Persons with a negative history of sensitivity may still have an allergic response.
- Obtain specimens for culture and sensitivity before initiating therapy. First dose may be given before receiving results.
- Observe patient for signs and symptoms of anaphylaxis (rash, pruritus, laryngeal edema, wheezing). Discontinue the drug and notify health care professional immediately if these symptoms occur. Keep epinephrine, an antihistamine, and resuscitation equipment close by in the event of an anaphylactic reaction.

- Monitor bowel function. Diarrhea, abdominal cramping, fever, and bloody stools should be reported to health care professional promptly as a sign of CDAD. May begin up to several mo following cessation of therapy.
- Monitor for signs and symptoms of encephalopathy (disturbance of consciousness including confusion, hallucinations, stupor, coma), myoclonus, and seizures during and following therapy. May require immediate treatment, dose adjustment, or discontinuation of therapy.

Lab Test Considerations
- May cause seroconversion from a negative to a positive direct Coombs' test. If anemia develops during or after therapy, perform a direct Coombs' test.
- May cause a false-positive reaction for glucose in urine with certain methods; use enzymatic glucose oxidase reactions.

Implementation

IV Administration
- **Intermittent Infusion:** *Reconstitution:* Reconstitute with 10 mL of sterile water for injection. 0.9% NaCl, D5W, D5/0.9% NaCl, D5/0.45% NaCl, D2.5/0.9% NaCl, D2.5/0.45% NaCl, or LR. Mix gently. *Dilution:* Use same diluent used for reconstitution for a volume between 50 mL and 250 mL. *Concentration:* 40 and 10 mg/mL of ceftazidime and avibactam, respectively to 8 and 2 mg/mL of ceftazidime and avibactam, respectively. Solution ranges from clear to light yellow; do not administer solutions that are discolored or contain particulate matter. Solution is stable for 12 hr at room temperature or 24 hr if refrigerated. *Rate:* Infuse over 2 hr.
- **Y-Site Compatibility:** aztreonam, amikacin, azithromycin, ceftaroline, daptomycin, dexmedetomidine, dopamine, eravacycline, ertapenem, furosemide, gentamicin, heparin, imipenem/cilastatin, levofloxacin, linezolid, magnesium sulfate, meropenem, meropenem/vaborbactam, metronidazole, norepinephrine, phenylephrine, plazomicin, potassium chloride, potassium phosphates, sodium bicarbonate, tedizolid, tobramycin, vasopressin, vecuronium.

Patient/Family Teaching
- Explain the purpose of ceftazidime/avibactam to patient.
- Instruct patient to notify health care professional if fever and diarrhea develop, especially if stool contains blood, pus, or mucus. Advise patient not to treat diarrhea without consulting health care professional.
- Advise patient to notify health care professional immediately if signs and symptoms of allergic reactions or nervous system reactions occur.
- Advise females of reproductive potential to notify health care professional if pregnancy is planned or suspected or if breastfeeding.

Evaluation/Desired Outcomes
- Resolution of the signs and symptoms of infection. Length of time for complete resolution depends on the organism and site of infection.

ceftolozane/tazobactam
(sef-**tol**-o-zane/taz-oh-**bak**-tam)
Zerbaxa
Classification
Therapeutic: anti-infectives
Pharmacologic: cephalosporin derivatives, beta-lactamase inhibitors

Indications
Complicated intra-abdominal infections (in combination with metronidazole). Complicated urinary tract infections (including pyelonephritis). Hospital-acquired bacterial pneumonia and ventilator-associated bacterial pneumonia.

Action
Ceftolozane: binds to bacterial cell wall membrane, causing cell death. Spectrum is extended compared with other penicillins. Tazobactam: Inhibits beta-lactamase, an enzyme that can destroy penicillins. **Therapeutic Effects:** Death of susceptible bacteria. **Spectrum:** Active against *Bacteroides fragilis*, *Enterobacter cloacae*, *Escherichia coli*, *Haemophilus influenzae*, *Klebsiella oxytoca*, *Klebsiella pneumoniae*, *Proteus mirabilis*, *Pseudomonas aeruginosa*, *Serratia marcesens*, *Streptococcus anginosus*, *Streptococcus constellatus*, and *Streptococcus salivarius*.

Pharmacokinetics
Absorption: IV administration results in complete bioavailability.
Distribution: Unknown.
Metabolism and Excretion: *Ceftolozane:* minimal metabolism, excreted almost entirely (>95%) unchanged in urine; *tazobactam:* 80% excreted unchanged in urine, some metabolized to an inactive M1 metabolite which is excreted unchanged in urine.
Half-life: *Ceftolozane:* 2.8 hr; *tazobactam:* 0.9 hr.

TIME/ACTION PROFILE

ROUTE	ONSET	PEAK	DURATION
IV	rapid	end of infusion	8 hr

Contraindications/Precautions
Contraindicated in: Known serious hypersensitivity to ceftolozane/tazobactam, piperacillin/tazobactam or other beta-lactams; Pedi: eGFR ≤50 mL/min/1.73 m². **Use Cautiously in:** CCr 30–<50 mL/min (effectiveness may be ↓ in adults); CCr <50 mL/min (dose adjustment recommended in adults); OB: Use during pregnancy only if potential benefit outweighs potential risks; Lactation: Use cautiously if breastfeeding.

Adverse Reactions/Side Effects

CV: atrial fibrillation, hypotension. **Derm:** rash. **F and E:** hypokalemia. **GI:** diarrhea, abdominal pain, CLOS-TRIDIOIDES DIFFICILE-ASSOCIATED DIARRHEA (CDAD), constipation, nausea, vomiting. **Hemat:** anemia, thrombocytosis. **Neuro:** anxiety, dizziness, headache, insomnia. **Misc:** HYPERSENSITIVITY REACTIONS (including anaphylaxis).

Interactions

Drug-Drug: None reported.

Route/Dosage

Complicated Intra-abdominal Infections or Complication Urinary Tract Infections

IV (Adults): 1.5 g (1 g ceftolozane/0.5 g tazobactam) every 8 hr for 4–14 days for complicated intra-abdominal infection or 7 days for complicated urinary tract infection.

IV (Children <18 yr and eGFR >50 mL/min/1.73 m²): 30 mg/kg (max dose = 1.5 g) every 8 hr for 5–14 days for complicated intra-abdominal infection or 7–14 days for complicated urinary tract infection.

Renal Impairment

(Adults): *CCr 30–50 mL/min:* 750 mg (500 mg ceftolozane/250 mg tazobactam) every 8 hr; *CCr 15–29 mL/min:* 375 mg (250 mg ceftolozane/125 mg tazobactam) every 8 hr; *End-stage renal disease on hemodialysis:* Single loading dose of 750 mg (500 mg ceftolozane/250 mg tazobactam), then 150 mg (100 mg ceftolozane/50 mg tazobactam) every 8 hr (on dialysis days administer as soon as possible after dialysis).

Hospital-Acquired Bacterial Pneumonia or Ventilator-Associated Bacterial Pneumonia

IV (Adults): 3 g (2 g ceftolozane/1 g tazobactam) every 8 hr for 8–14 days.

Renal Impairment

(Adults): *CCr 30–50 mL/min:* 1.5 g (1 g ceftolozane/0.5 g tazobactam) every 8 hr; *CCr 15–29 mL/min:* 750 mg (500 mg ceftolozane/250 mg tazobactam) every 8 hr; *End-stage renal disease on hemodialysis:* Single loading dose of 2.25 g (1.5 g ceftolozane/0.75 g tazobactam), then 450 mg (300 mg ceftolozane/150 mg tazobactam) every 8 hr (on dialysis days administer as soon as possible after dialysis).

Availability

Powder for injection: 1 g ceftolozane/0.5 g tazobactam/vial.

NURSING IMPLICATIONS

Assessment

- Assess for infection (vital signs; appearance of wound, sputum, urine, and stool; WBC) at beginning of and throughout therapy.
- Before initiating therapy, obtain a history to determine previous use of and reactions to penicillins, cephalosporins, or other beta-lactams. Persons with a negative history of sensitivity may still have an allergic response.
- Obtain specimens for culture and sensitivity before initiating therapy. First dose may be given before receiving results.
- Observe patient for signs and symptoms of anaphylaxis (rash, pruritus, laryngeal edema, wheezing). Discontinue the drug and notify health care professional immediately if these symptoms occur. Keep epinephrine, an antihistamine, and resuscitation equipment close by in the event of an anaphylactic reaction.
- Monitor bowel function. Diarrhea, abdominal cramping, fever, and bloody stools should be reported to health care professional promptly as a sign of CDAD. May begin up to several mo following cessation of therapy.

Lab Test Considerations

- Monitor CCr at least daily in patients with changing renal function and adjust dose accordingly.

Implementation

IV Administration

- **Intermittent Infusion:** *Reconstitution:* Reconstitute with 10 mL of sterile water for injection or 0.9% NaCl for injection; shake gently to dissolve for final volume of 11.4 mL. *Dilution:* Withdraw 11.4 mL for 1.5 g (1.0 g/0.5 g dose, 5.7 mL for 750 mg (500 mg/250 mg) dose, 2.9 mL for 375 mg (250 mg/125 mg) dose, or 1.2 mL for 150 mg (100 mg/50 mg) dose and add to 100 mL of 0.9% NaCl or D5W. Solution is clear, colorless to slightly yellow; do not administer solutions that are discolored or contain particulate matter. Solution is stable for 24 hr at room temperature or 7 days if refrigerated; do not freeze. *Rate:* Infuse over 1 hr.
- **Y-Site Compatibility:** amikacin, ampicillin/sulbactam, anidulafungin, azithromycin, aztreonam, bumetanide, calcium chloride, calcium gluconate, cefazolin, cefepime, ceftaroline, ceftazidime, ceftriaxone, cefuroxime, ciprofloxacin, cisatracurium, daptomycin, dexamethasone, dexmedetomidine, digoxin, diltiazem, diphenhydramine, dobutamine, dopamine, doxycycline, ephedrine, epinephrine, eptifibatide, eravacycline, ertapenem, esmolol, esomeprazole, famotidine, fentanyl, filgrastim, fosphenytoin, furosemide, gentamicin, heparin, hydrocortisone, hydromorphone, insulin, regular, isavuconazonium, labetalol, levofloxacin, lidocaine, linezolid, lorazepam, magnesium sulfate, mannitol, meperidine, meropenem, meropenem/vaborbactam, mesna, metoclopramide, micafungin, midazolam, milrinone, morphine, mycophenolate, naloxone, nicardipine, nitroglycerin, nitroprusside, norepinephrine, octreotide, ondansetron, pantoprazole, penicillin G, phenylephrine, piperacillin/tazobactam, plazomicin,

potassium chloride, potassium phosphate, rocuronium, sodium bicarbonate, sodium phosphate, tacrolimus, tedizolid, tigecycline, tobramycin, vancomycin, vasopressin, vecuronium.
- **Y-Site Incompatibility:** albumin human, amphotericin B lipid complex, amphotericin B liposome, caspofungin, cyclosporine, phenytoin, propofol.

Patient/Family Teaching
- Explain the purpose of ceftolozane/tazobactam to patient.
- Instruct patient to notify health care professional if fever and diarrhea develop, especially if stool contains blood, pus, or mucus. Advise patient not to treat diarrhea without consulting health care professional.
- Advise female patient to notify health care professional if pregnancy is planned or suspected or if breastfeeding.

Evaluation/Desired Outcomes
- Resolution of the signs and symptoms of infection. Length of time for complete resolution depends on the organism and site of infection.

---

cefTRIAXone, See CEPHALOSPORINS—THIRD GENERATION.

---

cefuroxime, See CEPHALOSPORINS—SECOND GENERATION.

℥ celecoxib (sel-e-kox-ib)
CeleBREX, Elyxyb
Classification
Therapeutic: antirheumatics
Pharmacologic: COX-2 inhibitors

Indications
Osteoarthritis. Rheumatoid arthritis. Ankylosing spondylitis. Juvenile rheumatoid arthritis. Acute pain. Primary dysmenorrhea. Acute treatment of migraine (with or without aura) (oral solution only).

Action
Inhibits the enzyme COX-2. This enzyme is required for the synthesis of prostaglandins. Has analgesic, anti-inflammatory, and antipyretic properties. **Therapeutic Effects:** Decreased pain and inflammation caused by osteoarthritis, rheumatoid arthritis, ankylosing spondylitis, or juvenile rheumatoid arthritis. Decreased acute pain.

Pharmacokinetics
Absorption: Bioavailability unknown.
Distribution: Extensively distributed to tissues.
Protein Binding: 97%.

Metabolism and Excretion: Mostly metabolized by the liver via the CYP2C9 isoenzyme; ℥ the CYP2C9 isoenzyme exhibits genetic polymorphism; poor metabolizers may have significantly ↑ celecoxib concentrations and an ↑ risk of adverse effects; <3% excreted unchanged in urine and feces.
Half-life: 11 hr.

TIME/ACTION PROFILE (pain reduction)

ROUTE	ONSET	PEAK	DURATION
PO	24–48 hr	unknown	12–24 hr†

†After discontinuation.

Contraindications/Precautions
Contraindicated in: Hypersensitivity; Cross-sensitivity may exist with other NSAIDs, including aspirin; History of allergic-type reactions to sulfonamides; History of allergic-type reactions to aspirin or other NSAIDs, including the aspirin triad (asthma, nasal polyps, and severe hypersensitivity reactions to aspirin); Advanced renal disease; Severe hepatic impairment; Coronary artery bypass graft (CABG) surgery; HF; OB: Avoid use after 30 wk gestation.

Use Cautiously in: Cardiovascular disease or risk factors for cardiovascular disease (may ↑ risk of serious cardiovascular thrombotic events, myocardial infarction, and stroke, especially with prolonged use or use of higher doses); avoid use in patients with recent MI or HF; Renal impairment, hepatic impairment, dehydration, or concurrent diuretic, ACE inhibitor, or angiotensin receptor blocker therapy (↑ risk of renal impairment); History of long duration of NSAID use, smoking, alcohol use, advanced liver disease, coagulopathy, and poor general health (↑ risk of GI bleeding); Hypertension or fluid retention; Asthma; ℥ Patients who are known or suspected to be poor CYP2C9 metabolizers (↓ initial dose by 50%; in patients with juvenile rheumatoid arthritis, use alternative treatment); Asthma; OB: Use at or after 20 wk gestation may cause fetal or neonatal renal impairment; if treatment is necessary between 20 wk and 30 wk gestation, limit use to the lowest effective dose and shortest duration possible; Pedi: Safety not established in children <2 yr or for longer than 6 mo; Geri: ↑ risk of GI bleeding and renal impairment in older adults.

Exercise Extreme Caution in: History of peptic ulcer disease or GI bleeding.

Adverse Reactions/Side Effects
CV: edema, HF, hypertension, MI, THROMBOSIS. **Derm:** ACUTE GENERALIZED EXANTHEMATOUS PUSTULOSIS, DRUG REACTION WITH EOSINOPHILIA AND SYSTEMIC SYMPTOMS (DRESS), EXFOLIATIVE DERMATITIS, rash, STEVENS-JOHNSON SYNDROME (SJS), TOXIC EPIDERMAL NECROLYSIS. **F and E:** hyperkalemia. **GI:** abdominal pain, diarrhea, dyspepsia, flatulence, GI BLEEDING, nausea. **GU:** renal impairment. **Hemat:** anemia. **Neuro:** dizziness, headache, insomnia, STROKE.

Interactions

Drug-Drug: CYP2C9 inhibitors may ↑ levels and risk of toxicity. May ↓ effectiveness of **ACE inhibitors**, **thiazide diuretics**, and **furosemide**. **Fluconazole** ↑ levels (use lowest recommended dosage). ↑ risk of GI bleeding with **anticoagulants, aspirin, clopidogrel, ticagrelor, prasugrel, corticosteroids, fibrinolytics, SNRIs**, or **SSRIs**. May ↑ levels and risk of toxicity of **lithium** and **methotrexate**. May ↑ risk of nephrotoxicity associated with **cyclosporine**. May ↑ risk of myelosuppression, and renal and GI toxicity associated with **pemetrexed**.

Route/Dosage

Osteoarthritis

PO (Adults): 200 mg once daily *or* 100 mg twice daily. *CYP2C9 poor metabolizers:* ↓ dose by 50%.

Hepatic Impairment

PO (Adults): *Moderate hepatic impairment:* ↓ dose by 50%.

Rheumatoid Arthritis

PO (Adults): 100–200 mg twice daily (capsules). *CYP2C9 poor metabolizers:* ↓ dose by 50%.

Hepatic Impairment

PO (Adults): *Moderate hepatic impairment:* ↓ dose by 50%.

Ankylosing Spondylitis

PO (Adults): 200 mg once daily (capsules) *or* 100 mg twice daily (capsules); may ↑ dose after 6 wk to 400 mg/day. *CYP2C9 poor metabolizers:* ↓ dose by 50%.

Hepatic Impairment

PO (Adults): *Moderate hepatic impairment:* ↓ dose by 50%.

Juvenile Rheumatoid Arthritis

PO (Children ≥2 yr, 10–25 kg): 50 mg twice daily (capsules).
PO (Children ≥2 yr, ≥25 kg): 100 mg twice daily (capsules).

Hepatic Impairment

PO (Children ≥2 yr): *Moderate hepatic impairment:* ↓ dose by 50%.

Acute Pain or Primary Dysmenorrhea

PO (Adults): 400 mg initially, then a 200-mg dose if needed on the first day; then 200 mg twice daily as needed (capsules). *CYP2C9 poor metabolizers:* ↓ dose by 50%.

Hepatic Impairment

PO (Adults): *Moderate hepatic impairment:* ↓ dose by 50%.

Acute Treatment of Migraine

PO (Adults): 120 mg as a single dose (not to exceed 120 mg/24 hr). *CYP2C9 poor metabolizers:* 60 mg as a single dose (not to exceed 60 mg/24 hr).

Hepatic Impairment

PO (Adults): *Moderate hepatic impairment:* 60 mg as a single dose (not to exceed 60 mg/24 hr).

Availability (generic available)

Capsules: 50 mg, 100 mg, 200 mg, 400 mg. **Oral solution:** 25 mg/mL.

NURSING IMPLICATIONS

Assessment

- Assess range of motion, degree of swelling, and pain in affected joints before and periodically during therapy.
- Assess patient for allergy to sulfonamides, aspirin, or NSAIDs. Patients with these allergies should not receive celecoxib.
- Assess patient for skin rash frequently during therapy. Discontinue at first sign of rash; may be life-threatening. SJS may develop. Treat symptomatically; may recur once treatment is stopped.
- Monitor for signs and symptoms of DRESS (fever, rash, lymphadenopathy, facial swelling) periodically during therapy. Discontinue therapy if symptoms occur.
- **Migraines:** Assess intensity and frequency of migraine pain.

Lab Test Considerations

- May cause ↑ AST and ALT levels.
- May cause hypophosphatemia, hyperkalemia, and ↑ BUN.

Implementation

- Do not confuse Celebrex with Celexa or Cerebyx.
- Use lowest effective dose for shortest period of time.
- **PO:** May be administered without regard to meals. Capsules may be opened and sprinkled on applesauce and ingested immediately with water. Mixture may be stored in the refrigerator for up to 6 hr.
- Solution is clear and colorless.
- Limit *Elyxyb* use to ≤10 days per month to avoid medication-overuse headache.

Patient/Family Teaching

- Instruct patient to take celecoxib as directed. Do not take more than prescribed dose. Increasing doses does not appear to increase effectiveness. Advise patient to read *Medication Guide* before starting therapy and with each Rx refill in case of changes.
- Caution patient to avoid use of more than one NSAID or aspirin at a time; increases risk of GI toxicity. Increasing dose or adding an NSAID or aspirin does not provide increased pain relief but may increase incidence of side effects.
- Advise patient to notify health care professional promptly if signs or symptoms of GI toxicity (abdominal pain, black stools), skin rash, unexplained weight gain, or edema occurs. Patients should discontinue celecoxib and notify health care profes-

sional if signs and symptoms of hepatotoxicity (nausea, fatigue, lethargy, pruritus, jaundice, upper right quadrant tenderness, flu-like symptoms) occur.
- May cause hypertension. Instruct patient in correct technique for monitoring BP and to notify health care professional if significant changes occur.
- Inform patient of increased risk of MI and stroke. Use lowest effective dose for shortest time. Advise patient to notify health care professional immediately if signs and symptoms (shortness of breath or trouble breathing, chest pain, weakness in one part or side of body, slurred speech, swelling of the face or throat) occur.
- Rep: May cause fetal harm. Advise females of reproductive potential to notify health care professional if pregnancy is planned or suspected or if breastfeeding. Advise women to avoid celecoxib in the 3rd trimester of pregnancy (after 29 wk), may cause premature closure of the fetal ductus arteriosus. Use of celecoxib after 20 wk may cause fetal renal dysfunction leading to oligohydramnios. May cause reversible infertility in women attempting to conceive; may consider discontinuing celecoxib.

Evaluation/Desired Outcomes
- Reduction in joint pain in patients with osteoarthritis.
- Reduction in joint tenderness, pain, and joint swelling in patients with rheumatoid arthritis, juvenile rheumatoid arthritis, and ankylosing spondylitis.
- Decreased pain.
- Decreased pain with dysmenorrhea.
- Decrease in acute migraine pain.

---

cephalexin, See CEPHALOSPORINS—FIRST GENERATION.

CEPHALOSPORINS—FIRST GENERATION
cefadroxil (sef-a-**drox**-ill)
~~Duricef~~
ceFAZolin (sef-**a**-zoe-lin)
~~Ancef~~
cephalexin (sef-a-**lex**-in)
~~Keflex~~
Classification
Therapeutic: anti-infectives
Pharmacologic: first-generation cephalosporins

Indications
Treatment of the following infections caused by susceptible organisms: Skin and skin structure infections (including burn wounds), Pneumonia, Urinary tract infections, Bone and joint infections, Septicemia. Not suitable for the treatment of meningitis. **Cefadroxil:** Pharyngitis and/or tonsillitis. **Cefazolin:** Perioperative prophylaxis, biliary tract infections, genital infections, bacterial endocarditis prophylaxis for dental and upper respiratory tract procedures. **Cephalexin:** Otitis media.

Action
Bind to bacterial cell wall membrane, causing cell death. **Therapeutic Effects:** Bactericidal action against susceptible bacteria. **Spectrum:** Active against many gram-positive cocci including: *Streptococcus pneumoniae*, Group A beta-hemolytic streptococci, Penicillinase-producing staphylococci. Not active against: Methicillin-resistant staphylococci, *Bacteroides fragilis*, *Enterococcus*. Active against some gram-negative rods including: *Klebsiella pneumoniae*, *Proteus mirabilis*, *Escherichia coli*.

Pharmacokinetics
Absorption: *Cefadroxil* and *cephalexin* are well absorbed following oral administration. *Cefazolin* is well absorbed following IM administration.

Distribution: Widely distributed. Cefazolin penetrates bone and synovial fluid well. Minimal CSF penetration.

Metabolism and Excretion: Excreted almost entirely unchanged by the kidneys.

Half-life: *Cefadroxil:* 60–120 min; *cefazolin:* 90–150 min; *cephalexin:* 50–80 min (all are ↑ in renal impairment).

TIME/ACTION PROFILE (blood levels)

ROUTE	ONSET	PEAK	DURATION
Cefadroxil PO	rapid	1.5–2 hr	12–24 hr
Cefazolin IM	rapid	0.5–2 hr	6–12 hr
Cefazolin IV	rapid	5 min	6–12 hr
Cephalexin PO	rapid	1 hr	6–12 hr

Contraindications/Precautions
Contraindicated in: Hypersensitivity to cephalosporins; Serious hypersensitivity to penicillins.

Use Cautiously in: Renal impairment (dosage ↓ and/or ↑ dosing interval recommended for: *cefadroxil* and *cephalexin*, if CCr ≤50 mL/min, and *cefazolin*, if CCr <50 mL/min (adults) or <70 mL/min (children); History of GI disease, especially colitis; OB, Lactation: Half-life is shorter and blood levels lower during pregnancy; have been used safely; Geri: Dose adjustment due to age-related ↓ in renal function may be necessary.

Adverse Reactions/Side Effects
Derm: rash, pruritus, STEVENS-JOHNSON SYNDROME (SJS), urticaria. **GI:** diarrhea, nausea, vomiting, CLOSTRIDIOIDES DIFFICILE-ASSOCIATED DIARRHEA (CDAD), cramps. **Hemat:** agranulocytosis, eosinophilia, hemolytic anemia, neutropenia, thrombocytopenia. **Local:** pain at IM site, phlebitis at IV site. **Neuro:** SEIZURES (high doses). **Misc:** HYPERSENSITIVITY REACTIONS (including anaphylaxis and serum sickness), superinfection.

Interactions

Drug-Drug: Probenecid ↓ excretion and ↑ blood levels of renally excreted cephalosporins. Concurrent use of **loop diuretics** or **aminoglycosides** may ↑ risk of renal toxicity.

Route/Dosage

Cefadroxil

PO (Adults): *Pharyngitis and tonsillitis:* 500 mg every 12 hr or 1 g every 24 hr for 10 days. *Skin and soft-tissue infections:* 500 mg every 12 hr or 1 g every 24 hr. *Urinary tract infections:* 500 mg– 1 g every 12 hr or 1– 2 g every 24 hr.

PO (Children): *Pharyngitis, tonsillitis, or impetigo:* 15 mg/kg every 12 hr or 30 mg/kg every 24 hr for 10 days. *Skin and soft-tissue infections:* 15 mg/kg every 12 hr. *Urinary tract infections:* 15 mg/kg every 12 hr.

Renal Impairment

PO (Adults): *CCr 25– 50 mL/min:* 500 mg every 12 hr; *CCr 10– 25 mL/min:* 500 mg every 24 hr; *CCr <10 mL/min:* 500 mg every 36 hr.

Cefazolin

IM, IV (Adults): *Moderate-to-severe infections:* 500 mg– 1 g every 6– 8 hr. *Mild infections with gram-positive cocci:* 250– 500 mg every 8 hr. *Uncomplicated urinary tract infection:* 1 g every 12 hr. *Pneumococcal pneumonia:* 500 mg every 12 hr. *Severe, life-threatening infections (e.g., infective endocarditis or septicemia):* 1– 1.5 g every 6 hr. *Perioperative prophylaxis:* 1– 2 g within 30– 60 min prior to incision (an additional 500 mg– 1 g should be given for surgeries ≥2 hr). 500 mg– 1 g should then be given for all surgeries every 6– 8 hr for 24 hr following the surgery.

IV (Children ≥10 yr and ≥50 kg): *Perioperative prophylaxis:* 2 g within 30– 60 min prior to incision (an additional 500 mg– 1 g should be given for surgeries ≥2 hr). 500 mg– 1 g should then be given for all surgeries every 6– 8 hr for 24 hr following the surgery.

IV (Children ≥10 yr and <50 kg): *Perioperative prophylaxis:* 1 g within 30– 60 min prior to incision (an additional 500 mg– 1 g should be given for surgeries ≥2 hr). 500 mg– 1 g should then be given for all surgeries every 6– 8 hr for 24 hr following the surgery.

IV (Children): *Mild to moderate infections:* 25– 50 mg/kg/day divided into 3 or 4 equal doses. *Severe infections:* 100 mg/kg/day divided into 3 or 4 equal doses.

Renal Impairment

IV (Adults): *CCr 30– 49 mL/min:* 1– 2 g every 8– 12 hr; *CCr 10– 29 mL/min:* 1 g every 12 hr; *CCr ≤10 mL/min:* 500 mg– 1 g every 24 hr. *Hemodialysis:* 500 mg– 1 g every 24 hr (on hemodialysis days, give dose after dialysis). *Peritoneal dialysis:* 500 mg every 12 hr *or* 1 g every 24 hr.

Renal Impairment

(Children): *CCr 40– 70 mL/min:* Give 60% of normal daily dose in 2 divided doses (every 12 hr). *CCr 20– 40 mL/min:* Give 25% of normal daily dose in 2 divided doses (every 12 hr). *CCr 5– 20 mL/min:* Give 10% of normal daily dose every 24 hr.

Cephalexin

PO (Adults): *Most infections:* 250– 500 mg every 6 hr. *Uncomplicated cystitis, skin and soft-tissue infections, streptococcal pharyngitis:* 500 mg every 12 hr.

PO (Children): *Most infections:* 25– 50 mg/kg/day divided every 6– 8 hr (can be administered every 12 hr in skin/skin structure infections or streptococcal pharyngitis). *Otitis media:* 18.75– 25 mg/kg every 6 hr (maximum = 4 g/day).

Renal Impairment

PO (Adults): *CCr 10– 50 mL/min:* 500 mg every 8– 12 hr; *CCr <10 mL/min:* 250– 500 mg every 12– 24 hr.

Availability

Cefadroxil (generic available)

Capsules: 500 mg. **Tablets:** 1 g. **Oral suspension (orange-pineapple flavor):** 250 mg/5 mL, 500 mg/5 mL.

Cefazolin (generic available)

Powder for injection: 500 mg/vial, 1 g/vial, 2 g/vial, 3 g/vial, 10 g/vial, 20 g/vial, 100 g/vial, 300 g/vial. **Premixed containers:** 1 g/50 mL D5W, 2 g/50 mL D5W.

Cephalexin (generic available)

Capsules: 250 mg, 500 mg, 750 mg. **Tablets:** 250 mg, 500 mg. **Oral suspension:** 125 mg/5 mL, 250 mg/5 mL.

NURSING IMPLICATIONS

Assessment

- Assess for infection (vital signs; appearance of wound, sputum, urine, and stool; WBC) at beginning and during therapy.
- Before initiating therapy, obtain a history to determine previous use of and reactions to penicillins or cephalosporins. Persons with a negative history of penicillin sensitivity may still have an allergic response.
- Obtain specimens for culture and sensitivity before initiating therapy. First dose may be given before receiving results.
- Observe patient for signs and symptoms of anaphylaxis (rash, pruritus, laryngeal edema, wheezing). Discontinue drug and notify health care professional immediately if these problems occur. Keep epinephrine, an antihistamine, and resuscitation equipment close by in case of an anaphylactic reaction.
- Monitor bowel function. Diarrhea, abdominal cramping, fever, and bloody stools should be reported to

health care professional promptly as a sign of CDAD. May begin up to several wk following cessation of therapy.

● Assess patient for skin rash frequently during therapy. Discontinue cephalosporins at first sign of rash; may be life-threatening. SJS may develop. Treat symptomatically; may recur once treatment is stopped.

Lab Test Considerations

● May cause positive results for Coombs' test in patients receiving high doses or in neonates whose mothers were given cephalosporins before delivery.

● May cause ↑ AST, ALT, alkaline phosphatase, bilirubin, LDH, BUN, and serum creatinine.

● May rarely cause leukopenia, neutropenia, agranulocytosis, thrombocytopenia, or eosinophilia.

Implementation

● Do not confuse cefazolin with cefotetan, cefoxitin, ceftazidime, or ceftriaxone.

● **PO:** Administer around the clock. May be administered on full or empty stomach. Administration with food may minimize GI irritation. Shake oral suspension well before administering. Use calibrated measuring device with liquid preparations. Refrigerate oral suspensions.

Cefazolin

● *Reconstitution:* For IM, IV push, and IV intermittent infusion, reconstitute 500-mg vial and 1-g vial with 2 mL and 2.5 mL, respectively, of sterile water for injection to achieve a final concentration of 225 mg/mL or 330 mg/mL, respectively.

● **IM:** Inject deep into a well-developed muscle mass; massage well.

IV Administration

● **IV:** Monitor site frequently for thrombophlebitis (pain, redness, swelling). Change sites every 48–72 hr to prevent phlebitis.

● Do not use solutions that are cloudy or contain a precipitate.

● If aminoglycosides are administered concurrently, administer in separate sites, if possible, at least 1 hr apart. If second site is unavailable, flush line between medications.

● **IV Push:** *Dilution:* 0.9% NaCl, D5W, D10W, dextrose/saline combinations, D5/LR. *Concentration:* 100 mg/mL. May use up to 138 mg/mL in fluid-restricted patients. *Rate:* May administer over 3–5 min.

● **Intermittent Infusion:** *Dilution:* Reconstituted 500-mg or 1-g solution may be diluted in 50–100 mL of 0.9% NaCl, D5W, D10W, dextrose/saline combinations, D5/LR. Solution is stable for 24 hr at room temperature and 10 days if refrigerated. *Concentration:* 20 mg/mL. *Rate:* Administer over 10–60 min.

● **Y-Site Compatibility:** acetaminophen, acyclovir, allopurinol, alprostadil, amifostine, aminocaproic acid, aminophylline, amphotericin B lipid complex, amphotericin B liposomal, anidulafungin, argatroban, arsenic trioxide, ascorbic acid, atracurium, atropine, azithromycin, aztreonam, benztropine, bivalirudin, bleomycin, bumetanide, buprenorphine, butorphanol, calcium gluconate, cangrelor, carboplatin, carmustine, cefotetan, cefoxitin, ceftazidime, ceftolozane/tazobactam, ceftriaxone, cefuroxime, chloramphenicol, cisplatin, clindamycin, cyanocobalamin, cyclophosphamide, cyclosporine, cytarabine, dactinomycin, daptomycin, dexamethasone, dexmedetomidine, digoxin, diltiazem, docetaxel, doxapram, doxorubicin liposomal, enalaprilat, ephedrine, epinephrine, epirubicin, epoetin alfa, eptifibatide, esmolol, etoposide, etoposide phosphate, fentanyl, filgrastim, fluconazole, fludarabine, fluorouracil, folic acid, foscarnet, furosemide, gemcitabine, glycopyrrolate, granisetron, heparin, hydrocortisone, ifosfamide, imipenem/cilastatin, indomethacin, insulin, regular, irinotecan, isoproterenol, ketamine, ketorolac, LR, leucovorin calcium, lidocaine, linezolid, lorazepam, mannitol, melphalan, meperidine, meropenem, meropenem/vaborbactam, mesna, methadone, methotrexate, methylprednisolone, metoclopramide, metoprolol, metronidazole, midazolam, milrinone, morphine, multivitamins, nafcillin, nalbuphine, nicardipine, nitroglycerin, nitroprusside, norepinephrine, octreotide, ondansetron, oxacillin, oxaliplatin, oxytocin, paclitaxel, palonosetron, pamidronate, penicillin G, phenobarbital, phenylephrine, plazomicin, phytonadione, potassium acetate, potassium chloride, procainamide, propofol, propranolol, remifentanil, rituximab, sargramostim, sodium acetate, sodium bicarbonate, succinylcholine, sufentanil, tacrolimus, tedizolid, theophylline, thiamine, thiotepa, tigecycline, tirofiban, topotecan, trastuzumab, vasopressin, vecuronium, verapamil, vinblastine, vincristine, voriconazole, zoledronic acid.

● **Y-Site Incompatibility:** alemtuzumab, amphotericin B deoxycholate, azathioprine, calcium chloride, caspofungin, cefotaxime, chlorpromazine, dacarbazine, dantrolene, daunorubicin hydrochloride, diazepam, diphenhydramine, dobutamine, dopamine, doxorubicin hydrochloride, doxycycline, erythromycin, ganciclovir, gemtuzumab ozogamicin, haloperidol, hydralazine, hydroxyzine, idarubicin, isavuconazonium, levofloxacin, minocycline, mitomycin, mitoxantrone, mycophenolate, papaverine, pemetrexed, pentamidine, pentobarbital, phentolamine, phenytoin, prochlorperazine, promethazine, protamine, pyridoxine, tobramycin, trimethoprim/sulfamethoxazole, vinorelbine.

Patient/Family Teaching

● Instruct patient to take medication around the clock at evenly spaced times and to finish the medication completely as directed, even if feeling better. Take missed doses as soon as possible unless almost time for next dose; do not double doses. Instruct parents or caregivers to use calibrated measuring device with liquid preparations. Advise patient that sharing this medication may be dangerous.

● Advise patient to report signs of superinfection (furry overgrowth on the tongue, vaginal itching or discharge, loose or foul-smelling stools) and allergy.

● Instruct patient to notify health care professional if rash or fever and diarrhea develop, especially if diarrhea contains blood, mucus, or pus. Advise patient not to treat diarrhea without consulting health care professional.

● Rep: Advise females of reproductive potential to notify health care professional if pregnancy is planned or suspected or if breastfeeding.

Evaluation/Desired Outcomes

● Resolution of signs and symptoms of infection. Length of time for complete resolution depends on the organism and site of infection.

● Decreased incidence of infection when used for prophylaxis.

CEPHALOSPORINS — SECOND GENERATION
cefaclor (sef-a-klor)
cefoTEtan (sef-oh-**tee**-tan)
~~Cefotan~~
cefOXitin (se-**fox**-i-tin)
~~Mefoxin~~
cefprozil (sef-**proe**-zil)
cefuroxime (se-fyoor-**ox**-eem)
~~Ceftin, Zinacef~~

Classification
Therapeutic: anti-infectives
Pharmacologic: second-generation cephalosporins

Indications
Treatment of the following infections caused by susceptible organisms: Respiratory tract infections, Skin and skin structure infections, Bone and joint infections (not cefaclor or cefprozil), Urinary tract infections (not cefprozil). **Cefotetan and cefoxitin:** Intra-abdominal and gynecologic infections. **Cefuroxime:** Meningitis, gynecologic infections, and Lyme disease. **Cefaclor, cefprozil, cefuroxime:** Otitis media. **Cefoxitin and cefuroxime:** Septicemia. **Cefotetan, cefoxitin, cefuroxime:** Perioperative prophylaxis.

Action
Bind to bacterial cell wall membrane, causing cell death. **Therapeutic Effects:** Bactericidal action against susceptible bacteria. **Spectrum:** Similar to that of first-generation cephalosporins but have ↑ activity against several other gram-negative pathogens including: *Haemophilus influenzae, Escherichia coli, Klebsiella pneumoniae, Morganella morganii, Neisseria*

gonorrhoeae (including penicillinase-producing strains), *Proteus, Providencia, Serratia marcescens, Moraxella catarrhalis*. Not active against methicillin-resistant staphylococci or enterococci. **Cefuroxime:** Active against *Borrelia burgdorferi*. **Cefotetan and cefoxitin:** Active against *Bacteroides fragilis*.

Pharmacokinetics
Absorption: *Cefotetan, cefoxitin,* and *cefuroxime:* well absorbed following IM administration. *Cefaclor, cefprozil,* and *cefuroxime:* well absorbed following oral administration.

Distribution: Widely distributed. Penetration into CSF is poor, but adequate for cefuroxime (IV) to be used in treating meningitis.

Metabolism and Excretion: Excreted primarily unchanged by the kidneys.

Half-life: *Cefaclor:* 30–60 min; *cefotetan:* 3–4.6 hr; *cefoxitin:* 40–60 min; *cefprozil:* 90 min; *cefuroxime:* 60–120 min (all are ↑ in renal impairment).

TIME/ACTION PROFILE

ROUTE	ONSET	PEAK	DURATION
Cefaclor PO	rapid	30–60 min	6–12 hr
Cefaclor PO-CD	unknown	unknown	12 hr
Cefotetan IM	rapid	1–3 hr	12 hr
Cefotetan IV	rapid	end of infusion	12 hr
Cefoxitin IM	rapid	30 min	4–8 hr
Cefoxitin IV	rapid	end of infusion	4–8 hr
Cefprozil PO	unknown	1–2 hr	12–24 hr
Cefuroxime PO	unknown	2–3 hr	8–12 hr
Cefuroxime IM	rapid	15–60 min	6–12 hr
Cefuroxime IV	rapid	end of infusion	6–12 hr

Contraindications/Precautions
Contraindicated in: Hypersensitivity to cephalosporins; Serious hypersensitivity to penicillins.

Use Cautiously in: Renal impairment (↓ dose/↑ dosing interval recommended for: *cefotetan* if CCr ≤30 mL/min, *cefoxitin* if CCr ≤50 mL/min, *cefprozil* if CCr <30 mL/min, *cefuroxime* if CCr <30 mL/min); Patients with hepatic dysfunction, poor nutritional state, or cancer may be at ↑ risk for bleeding; History of GI disease, especially colitis; *Cefprozil (oral suspension)* contains aspartame and should be avoided in patients with phenylketonuria; Geri: Dose adjustment due to age-related ↓ in renal function may be necessary; may also be at ↑ risk for bleeding with *cefotetan* or *cefoxitin*; OB, Lactation: Have been used safely.

Adverse Reactions/Side Effects
Derm: <u>rash</u>, urticaria. **GI:** <u>diarrhea</u>, CLOSTRIDIOIDES DIFFICILE-ASSOCIATED DIARRHEA (CDAD), cramps, nau-

---

sea, vomiting. **Hemat:** agranulocytosis, bleeding (↑ with cefotetan and cefoxitin), eosinophilia, hemolytic anemia, neutropenia, thrombocytopenia. **Local:** <u>pain</u> at IM site, <u>phlebitis</u> at IV site. **Neuro:** SEIZURES (high doses). **Misc:** HYPERSENSITIVITY REACTIONS (including anaphylaxis and serum sickness), superinfection.

Interactions

Drug-Drug: **Probenecid** ↓ excretion and ↑ blood levels. If **alcohol** is ingested within 48–72 hr of cefotetan, a disulfiram-like reaction may occur. Cefotetan may ↑ risk of bleeding with **anticoagulants, antiplatelet agents, thrombolytics,** and **NSAIDs. Antacids** ↓ absorption of cefaclor. Concurrent use of **aminoglycosides** or **loop diuretics** may ↑ risk of nephrotoxicity.

Route/Dosage

Cefaclor

PO (Adults): 250–500 mg every 8 hr or 500 mg every 12 hr as extended-release tablets.
PO (Children >1 mo): 6.7–13.4 mg/kg every 8 hr or 10–20 mg/kg every 12 hr (up to 1 g/day).

Cefotetan

IM, IV (Adults): *Most infections:* 1–2 g every 12 hr. *Severe/life-threatening infections:* 2–3 g every 12 hr. *Urinary tract infections:* 500 mg–2 g every 12 hr *or* 1–2 g every 24 hr. *Perioperative prophylaxis:* 1–2 g 30–60 min before initial incision (one-time dose).

Renal Impairment

IM, IV (Adults): *CCr 10–30 mL/min:* Usual adult dose every 24 hr *or* ½ usual adult dose every 12 hr; *CCr <10 mL/min:* Usual adult dose every 48 hr *or* ¼ usual adult dose every 12 hr.

Cefoxitin

IM, IV (Adults): *Most infections:* 1 g every 6–8 hr. *Severe infections:* 1 g every 4 hr *or* 2 g every 6–8 hr. *Life-threatening infections:* 2 g every 4 hr *or* 3 g every 6 hr. *Perioperative prophylaxis:* 2 g 30–60 min before initial incision, then 2 g every 6 hr for up to 24 hr.
IM, IV (Children and Infants >3 mo): *Most infections:* 13.3–26.7 mg/kg every 4 hr *or* 20–40 mg/kg every 6 hr. *Perioperative prophylaxis:* 30–40 mg/kg within 60 min of initial incision, then 30–40 mg/kg every 6 hr for up to 24 hr.

Renal Impairment

IM, IV (Adults): *CCr 30–50 mL/min:* 1–2 g every 8–12 hr; *CCr 10–29 mL/min:* 1–2 g every 12–24 hr; *CCr 5–9 mL/min:* 0.5–1 g every 12–24 hr; *CCr <5 mL/min:* 0.5–1 g every 24–48 hr.

Cefprozil

PO (Adults): *Most infections:* 250–500 mg every 12 hr *or* 500 mg every 24 hr.
PO (Children 6 mo–12 yr): *Otitis media:* 15 mg/kg every 12 hr. *Acute sinusitis:* 7.5–15 mg/kg every 12 hr (higher dose should be used for moderate-to-severe infections).

PO (Children 2–12 yr): *Pharyngitis/tonsillitis:* 7.5 mg/kg every 12 hr. *Skin/skin structure infections:* 20 mg/kg every 24 hr.

Renal Impairment

PO (Adults and Children ≥6 mo): *CCr <30 mL/min:* ½ of usual dose at normal dosing interval.

Cefuroxime

PO (Adults and Children >12 yr): *Pharyngitis/tonsillitis, maxillary sinusitis, uncomplicated UTIs:* 250 mg every 12 hr. *Bronchitis, uncomplicated skin/skin structure infections:* 250–500 mg every 12 hr. *Gonorrhea:* 1 g (single dose). *Lyme disease:* 500 mg every 12 hr for 20 days.
PO (Children 3 mo–12 yr): *Otitis media, acute bacterial maxillary sinusitis, impetigo:* 250 mg every 12 hr.
IM, IV (Adults): *Uncomplicated urinary tract infections, skin/skin structure infections, disseminated gonococcal infections, uncomplicated pneumonia:* 750 mg every 8 hr. *Bone/joint infections, severe or complicated infections:* 1.5 g every 8 hr. *Life-threatening infections:* 1.5 g every 6 hr. *Meningitis:* 3 g every 8 hr. *Perioperative prophylaxis:* 1.5 g IV 30–60 min before initial incision; 750 mg IM/IV every 8 hr can be given when procedure prolonged. *Prophylaxis during open-heart surgery:* 1.5 g IV at induction of anesthesia and then every 12 hr for 3 additional doses. *Gonorrhea:* 1.5 g IM (750 mg in two sites) with 1 g probenecid PO.
IM, IV (Children and Infants >3 mo): *Most infections:* 12.5–25 mg/kg every 6 hr *or* 16.7–33.3 mg/kg every 8 hr (max dose = 6 g/day). *Bone and joint infections:* 50 mg/kg every 8 hr (max dose = 6 g/day). *Bacterial meningitis:* 50–60 mg/kg every 6 hr *or* 66.7–80 mg/kg every 8 hr.

Renal Impairment

IM, IV (Adults): *CCr 10–29 mL/min:* Give standard dose every 24 hr; *CCr <10 mL/min (no hemodialysis):* Give standard dose every 48 hr; *Hemodialysis:* Give an additional dose at end of each dialysis session.

Availability

Cefaclor (generic available)

Capsules: 250 mg, 500 mg. **Extended-release tablets:** 500 mg. **Oral suspension (strawberry):** 125 mg/5 mL, 250 mg/5 mL, 375 mg/5 mL.

Cefotetan (generic available)

Powder for injection: 1 g/vial, 2 g/vial.

Cefoxitin (generic available)

Powder for injection: 1 g/vial, 2 g/vial, 10 g/vial.

Cefprozil (generic available)

Oral suspension (bubblegum flavor): 125 mg/5 mL, 250 mg/5 mL. **Tablets:** 250 mg, 500 mg.

Cefuroxime (generic available)

Tablets: 250 mg, 500 mg. **Powder for oral suspension (tutti frutti flavor):** ✳125 mg/5 mL. **Powder for injection :** 750 mg/vial, 1.5 g/vial.

NURSING IMPLICATIONS

Assessment

- Assess for infection (vital signs; appearance of wound, sputum, urine, and stool; WBC) at beginning and during therapy.
- Before initiating therapy, obtain a history to determine previous use of and reactions to penicillins or cephalosporins. Persons with a negative history of penicillin sensitivity may still have an allergic response.
- Obtain specimens for culture and sensitivity before initiating therapy. First dose may be given before receiving results.
- Observe patient for signs and symptoms of anaphylaxis (rash, pruritus, laryngeal edema, wheezing). Discontinue the drug immediately if these symptoms occur. Keep epinephrine, an antihistamine, and resuscitation equipment close by in the event of an anaphylactic reaction.
- Monitor bowel function. Diarrhea, abdominal cramping, fever, and bloody stools should be reported to health care professional promptly as a sign of CDAD. May begin up to several wk following cessation of therapy.

Lab Test Considerations

- May cause positive results for Coombs' test in patients receiving high doses or in neonates whose mothers were given cephalosporins before delivery.
- *Cefotetan:* monitor prothrombin time and assess patient for bleeding (guaiac stools; check for hematuria, bleeding gums, ecchymosis) daily in high-risk patients; may cause hypoprothrombinemia.
- May cause ↑ AST, ALT, alkaline phosphatase, bilirubin, LDH, BUN, and serum creatinine.
- *Cefoxitin* may cause falsely ↑ test results for serum and urine creatinine; do not obtain serum samples within 2 hr of administration.
- May rarely cause leukopenia, neutropenia, agranulocytosis, thrombocytopenia, and eosinophilia.

Implementation

- Do not confuse cefotetan with cefazolin, cefoxitin, ceftazidime, or ceftriaxone. Do not confuse cefoxitin with cefazolin, cefotetan, ceftazidime, or cetriaxone. Do not confuse cefuroxime with sulfasalazine.
- **PO:** Administer around the clock. May be administered on full or empty stomach. Administration with food may minimize GI irritation. Shake oral suspension well before administering.
- Administer cefaclor extended-release tablets with food; *DNC:* Do not crush, break, or chew.
- Do not administer *cefaclor* within 1 hr of antacids.
- *Cefuroxime.DNC:* tablets should be swallowed whole, not crushed; crushed tablets have a strong, persistent bitter taste. Tablets may be taken without regard to meals.
- **IM:** *Reconstitution:* Reconstitute IM doses with sterile or bacteriostatic water for injection or 0.9%

NaCl for injection. May be diluted with lidocaine to minimize injection discomfort.
- Inject deep into a well-developed muscle mass; massage well.

IV Administration

- **IV:** Change sites every 48–72 hr to prevent phlebitis. Monitor site frequently for thrombophlebitis (pain, redness, swelling).
- If aminoglycosides are administered concurrently, administer in separate sites if possible, at least 1 hr apart. If second site is unavailable, flush line between medications.

Cefotetan

- **IV Push:** *Reconstitution:* Reconstitute each gram with at least 10 mL of sterile or bacteriostatic water for injection, 0.9% NaCl, or D5W. Do not use preparations containing benzyl alcohol for neonates. *Concentration:* 95 mg/mL. *Rate:* Administer slowly over 3–5 min.
- **Intermittent Infusion:** *Dilution:* Reconstituted solution may be further diluted in 50–100 mL of D5W or 0.9% NaCl. Solution may be colorless or yellow. Solution is stable for 24 hr at room temperature or 96 hr if refrigerated. *Concentration:* 10–40 mg/mL. *Rate:* Administer over 20–30 min.
- **Y-Site Compatibility:** acyclovir, allopurinol, amifostine, aminocaproic acid, aminophylline, amphotericin B lipid complex, anidulafungin, argatroban, arsenic trioxide, ascorbic acid, atropine, azithromycin, aztreonam, benztropine, bivalirudin, bleomycin, bumetanide, buprenorphine, butorphanol, calcium chloride, calcium gluconate, carboplatin, carmustine, cefazolin, cefotaxime, cefoxitin, ceftazidime, ceftriaxone, cefuroxime, chloramphenicol, cisplatin, clindamycin, cyanocobalamin, cyclophosphamide, cyclosporine, cytarabine, dacarbazine, dactinomycin, daptomycin, dexamethasone, dexmedetomidine, dexrazoxane, digoxin, diltiazem, docetaxel, dopamine, doxorubicin liposomal, enalaprilat, ephedrine, epinephrine, epoetin alfa, eptifibatide, etoposide, etoposide phosphate, fentanyl, filgrastim, fluconazole, fludarabine, fluorouracil, folic acid, foscarnet, fosphenytoin, furosemide, gemcitabine, glycopyrrolate, granisetron, heparin, hetastarch, hydrocortisone, hydromorphone, ifosfamide, imipenem/cilastatin, irinotecan, isoproterenol, ketorolac, LR, leucovorin calcium, levofloxacin, lidocaine, linezolid, lorazepam, magnesium sulfate, mannitol, melphalan, mesna, methadone, methotrexate, methylprednisolone, metoclopramide, metoprolol, metronidazole, milrinone, mitoxantrone, morphine, multivitamins, nafcillin, nalbuphine, naloxone, nicardipine, nitroglycerin, nitroprusside, norepinephrine, octreotide, oxacillin, oxaliplatin, oxytocin, paclitaxel, palonosetron, pamidronate, penicillin G, phenylephrine, phytonadione, potassium acetate, potassium chloride, procainamide, propofol, pro-

pranolol, pyridoxine, remifentanil, rituximab, rocuronium, sargramostim, sodium acetate, succinylcholine, sufentanil, tacrolimus, theophylline, thiamine, thiotepa, tigecycline, tirofiban, topotecan, vasopressin, vecuronium, verapamil, vinblastine, vincristine, voriconazole, zoledronic acid.

- **Y-Site Incompatibility:** alemtuzumab, amiodarone, amphotericin B liposomal, azathioprine, caspofungin, chlorpromazine, dantrolene, daunorubicin hydrochloride, diazepam, diphenhydramine, dobutamine, doxorubicin hydrochloride, doxycycline, epirubicin, erythromycin, esmolol, ganciclovir, gemtuzumab ozogamicin, gentamicin, haloperidol, hydralazine, hydroxyzine, idarubicin, indomethacin, labetalol, minocycline, mitomycin, mycophenolate, pantoprazole, papaverine, pemetrexed, pentamidine, pentobarbital, phenobarbital, phentolamine, phenytoin, prochlorperazine, promethazine, protamine, sodium bicarbonate, tobramycin, trastuzumab, trimethoprim/sulfamethoxazole, vinorelbine.

Cefoxitin

- **IV Push: *Reconstitution:*** Reconstitute each gram with at least 10 mL of sterile or bacteriostatic water for injection, 0.9% NaCl, or D5W. Do not use preparations containing benzyl alcohol for neonates. ***Concentration:*** 200 mg/mL. ***Rate:*** Administer slowly over 3–5 min.
- **Intermittent Infusion: *Dilution:*** Reconstituted solution may be further diluted in 50–100 mL of D5W, D10W, 0.9% NaCl, dextrose/saline combinations, D5/LR, Ringer's or LR. Stable for 24 hr at room temperature and 1 wk if refrigerated. Darkening of powder does not alter potency. ***Concentration:*** 40 mg/mL. ***Rate:*** Administer over 30–60 min.
- **Continuous Infusion:** May be diluted in 500–1000 mL for continuous infusion.
- **Y-Site Compatibility:** acetaminophen, acyclovir, amifostine, aminocaproic acid, aminophylline, amphotericin B deoxycholate, amphotericin B lipid complex, amphotericin B liposomal, anidulafungin, argatroban, arsenic trioxide, ascorbic acid, atropine, azithromycin, aztreonam, benztropine, bivalirudin, bleomycin, bumetanide, buprenorphine, butorphanol, calcium chloride, calcium gluconate, cangrelor, carboplatin, carmustine, cefazolin, cefotaxime, cefotetan, ceftazidime, ceftriaxone, cefuroxime, chloramphenicol, cisplatin, clindamycin, cyanocobalamin, cyclophosphamide, cyclosporine, cytarabine, dacarbazine, dactinomycin, daptomycin, dexamethasone, dexmedetomidine, dexrazoxane, digoxin, diltiazem, docetaxel, dopamine, doxorubicin liposomal, enalaprilat, ephedrine, epinephrine, epoetin alfa, eptifibatide, esmolol, etoposide, etoposide phosphate, fentanyl, fluconazole, fludarabine, fluorouracil, folic acid, foscarnet, fosphenytoin, furosemide, gemcitabine, glycopyrrolate, granisetron, heparin, hetastarch, hydrocortisone, hydromorphone, ifosfamide, imipenem/cilastatin, indomethacin, irinotecan, isoproterenol, ketorolac, LR, leucovorin calcium, lidocaine, linezolid, lorazepam, magnesium sulfate, mannitol, meperidine, meropenem, mesna, methotrexate, metoclopramide, metoprolol, metronidazole, midazolam, milrinone, mitomycin, morphine, multivitamins, nafcillin, nalbuphine, naloxone, nicardipine, nitroglycerin, nitroprusside, norepinephrine, octreotide, ondansetron, oxacillin, oxaliplatin, oxytocin, paclitaxel, palonosetron, pamidronate, penicillin G, phenylephrine, phytonadione, potassium acetate, potassium chloride, procainamide, propofol, propranolol, pyridoxine, remifentanil, rituximab, rocuronium, sodium acetate, succinylcholine, sufentanil, tacrolimus, theophylline, thiamine, thiotepa, tigecycline, tirofiban, topotecan, vasopressin, vecuronium, verapamil, vinblastine, vincristine, voriconazole, zoledronic acid.

- **Y-Site Incompatibility:** alemtuzumab, azathioprine, caspofungin, chlorpromazine, dantrolene, daunorubicin hydrochloride, diazepam, diphenhydramine, dobutamine, doxorubicin hydrochloride, doxycycline, epirubicin, erythromycin, filgrastim, ganciclovir, gemtuzumab ozogamicin, haloperidol, hetastarch, hydralazine, hydroxyzine, idarubicin, insulin, regular, labetalol, levofloxacin, methylprednisolone, minocycline, mitoxantrone, mycophenolate, papaverine, pemetrexed, pentamidine, pentobarbital, phenobarbital, phentolamine, phenytoin, prochlorperazine, promethazine, protamine, sodium bicarbonate, trastuzumab, trimethoprim/sulfamethoxazole, vinorelbine.

Cefuroxime

- **IV Push: *Reconstitution:*** Reconstitute 750 mg vial with 8.3 mL and 1.5 g vial with 16 mL of sterile water for injection, respectively. Do not use preparations containing benzyl alcohol for neonates. ***Rate:*** Administer slowly over 3–5 min.
- **Intermittent Infusion: *Dilution:*** Dilute further in 50–100 mL of 0.9% NaCl, D5W, or 0.45% NaCl. Stable for 24 hr at room temperature and 7 days if refrigerated. . ***Concentration:*** 10–40 mg/mL. ***Rate:*** Administer over 15–60 min.
- **Continuous Infusion:** May also be diluted in 500–1000 mL 0.9% NaCl, D5W, D10W, D5/0.9% NaCl, D5/.45 NaCl, or 1/6 M sodium lactate injection for continuous infusion.
- **Y-Site Compatibility:** acetaminophen, acyclovir, allopurinol, amifostine, aminocaproic acid, aminophylline, amphotericin B lipid complex, amphotericin B liposomal, anidulafungin, argatroban, arsenic trioxide, ascorbic acid, atracurium, atropine, aztreonam, benztropine, bivalirudin, bleomycin, bumetanide, buprenorphine, butorphanol, calcium gluconate, cangrelor, carboplatin, carmustine, cefazolin, cefotaxime, cefotetan, cefoxitin, ceftazidime, ceftolozane/tazobactam, ceftriaxone, chloramphenicol, cisplatin, clindamycin, cyclophosphamide, cyanocobalamin, cyclophosphamide, cyclosporine, cytarabine, dacarbazine, dactinomycin, daptomycin,

dexmedetomidine, dexrazoxane, digoxin, diltiazem, docetaxel, dopamine, doxorubicin liposomal, enalaprilat, ephedrine, epinephrine, epoetin alfa, eptifibatide, erythromycin, esmolol, etoposide, etoposide phosphate, famotidine, fentanyl, fludarabine, fluorouracil, folic acid, foscarnet, fosphenytoin, furosemide, gemcitabine, gemtuzumab ozogamicin, glycopyrrolate, granisetron, heparin, hetastarch, hydrocortisone, hydromorphone, ifosfamide, imipenem/cilastatin, indomethacin, insulin, regular, irinotecan, isoproterenol, ketamine, ketorolac, LR, leucovorin calcium, levofloxacin, lidocaine, linezolid, lorazepam, mannitol, melphalan, meperidine, meropenem, meropenem/vaborbactam, mesna, methadone, methotrexate, methylprednisolone, metoclopramide, metoprolol, milrinone, morphine, multivitamins, nafcillin, nalbuphine, naloxone, nitroglycerin, nitroprusside, norepinephrine, octreotide, ondansetron, oxacillin, oxaliplatin, oxytocin, paclitaxel, palonosetron, pamidronate, pemetrexed, penicillin G, phenylephrine, phytonadione, plazomicin, potassium acetate, potassium chloride, procainamide, propofol, propranolol, pyridoxine, remifentanil, rituximab, rocuronium, sargramostim, sodium acetate, succinylcholine, sufentanil, tacrolimus, tedizolid, theophylline, thiamine, thiotepa, tigecycline, tirofiban, topotecan, trastuzumab, vasopressin, vecuronium, verapamil, vinblastine, vincristine, voriconazole, zoledronic acid.

- **Y-Site Incompatibility:** alemtuzumab, azathioprine, calcium chloride, caspofungin, chlorpromazine, dantrolene, daunorubicin hydrochloride, dexamethasone, diazepam, diphenhydramine, dobutamine, doxorubicin hydrochloride, doxycycline, epirubicin, filgrastim, ganciclovir, haloperidol, hydralazine, hydroxyzine, idarubicin, isavuconazonium, labetalol, magnesium sulfate, midazolam, minocycline, mitomycin, mitoxantrone, mycophenolate, nicardipine, papaverine, pentamidine, pentobarbital, phenobarbital, phentolamine, phenytoin, prochlorperazine, promethazine, protamine, sodium bicarbonate, trimethoprim/sulfamethoxazole, vinorelbine.

Patient/Family Teaching

- Instruct patient to take medication around the clock at evenly spaced times and to finish the medication completely, even if feeling better. Take missed doses as soon as possible unless almost time for next dose; do not double doses. Use calibrated measuring device with liquid preparations. Advise patient that sharing of this medication may be dangerous.
- Advise patient to report signs of superinfection (furry overgrowth on the tongue, vaginal itching or discharge, loose or foul-smelling stools) and allergy.
- Caution patients that concurrent use of alcohol with *cefotetan* may cause a disulfiram-like reaction (ab-

dominal cramps, nausea, vomiting, headache, hypotension, palpitations, dyspnea, tachycardia, sweating, flushing). Alcohol and alcohol-containing medications should be avoided during and for several days after therapy.

- Instruct patient to notify health care professional if fever and diarrhea develop, especially if stool contains blood, pus, or mucus. Advise patient not to treat diarrhea without consulting health care professional.
- Rep: Advise females of reproductive potential to notify health care professional if pregnancy is planned or suspected, or if breastfeeding.

Evaluation/Desired Outcomes

- Resolution of signs and symptoms of infection. Length of time for complete resolution depends on the organism and site of infection.
- Decreased incidence of infection when used for prophylaxis.

CEPHALOSPORINS—THIRD GENERATION

cefdinir (**sef**-di-nir)
~~Omnicef~~
cefixime (sef-**ik**-seem)
Suprax
cefotaxime (sef-oh-**taks**-eem)
~~Claforan~~
cefpodoxime (sef-poe-**dox**-eem)
~~Vantin~~
cefTAZidime (sef-**tay**-zi-deem)
~~Fortaz~~, Tazicef
cefTRIAXone (sef-try-**ax**-one)
~~Rocephin~~
Classification
Therapeutic: anti-infectives
Pharmacologic: third-generation cephalosporins

Indications

Treatment of the following infections caused by susceptible organisms: Skin and skin structure infections (not cefixime), Urinary and gynecologic infections (not cefdinir), Respiratory tract infections (not cefdinir). **Cefotaxime, ceftazidime, ceftriaxone:** Meningitis and bone/joint infections. **Cefotaxime, ceftazidime, ceftriaxone:** Intra-abdominal infections and septicemia. **Cefdinir, cefixime, cefpodoxime, ceftriaxone:** Otitis media. **Cefotaxime, ceftriaxone:** Perioperative prophylaxis. **Ceftazidime:** Febrile neutropenia. **Cefotaxime, ceftriaxone:** Lyme disease.

Action

Bind to the bacterial cell wall membrane, causing cell death. **Therapeutic Effects:** Bactericidal action against susceptible bacteria. **Spectrum:** Similar to that of second-generation cephalosporins, but activity against staphylococci is less, whereas activity against gram-negative pathogens is greater, even for organisms resistant to first- and second-generation agents. Notable is increased action against: *Enterobacter, Haemophilus influenzae, Escherichia coli, Klebsiella pneumoniae, Neisseria gonorrhoeae, Citrobacter, Morganella, Proteus, Providencia, Serratia, Moraxella catarrhalis, Borrelia burgdorferi*. Some agents have activity against *N. meningitidis* (cefotaxime, ceftazidime, ceftriaxone). Some agents have enhanced activity against *Pseudomonas aeruginosa* (ceftazidime). Not active against methicillin-resistant staphylococci or enterococci. Some agents have activity against anaerobes, including *Bacteroides fragilis* (cefotaxime, ceftriaxone).

Pharmacokinetics

Absorption: *Cefotaxime, ceftazidime,* and *ceftriaxone* are well absorbed after IM administration. *Cefixime* 40–50% absorbed after oral administration (oral suspension); *cefdinir* 16–25% absorbed after oral administration. *Cefpodoxime proxetil* is a prodrug that is converted to its active component in GI tract during absorption (50% absorbed).
Distribution: Widely distributed. CSF penetration better than with first- and second-generation agents.
Protein Binding: *Ceftriaxone* ≥90%.
Metabolism and Excretion: *Cefdinir* and *ceftazidime*>85% excreted in urine. *Cefpodoxime:* 30% excreted in urine. *Ceftriaxone* and *cefotaxime:* partly metabolized and partly excreted in the urine. *Cefixime:* 50% excreted unchanged in urine, ≥10% in bile.
Half-life: *Cefdinir:* 1.7 hr; *cefixime:* 3–4 hr; *cefotaxime:* 1–1.5 hr; *cefpodoxime:* 2–3 hr; *ceftazidime:* 2 hr; *ceftriaxone:* 6–9 hr (all except *ceftriaxone* are ↑ in renal impairment).

TIME/ACTION PROFILE

ROUTE	ONSET	PEAK	DURATION
Cefdinir PO	rapid	2–4 hr	12–24 hr
Cefixime PO	rapid	2–6 hr	24 hr
Cefotaxime IM	rapid	0.5 hr	4–12 hr
Cefotaxime IV	rapid	end of infusion	4–12 hr
Cefpodoxime PO	unknown	2–3 hr	12 hr
Ceftazidime IM	rapid	1 hr	6–12 hr
Ceftazidime IV	rapid	end of infusion	6–12 hr
Ceftriaxone IM	rapid	1–2 hr	12–24 hr
Ceftriaxone IV	rapid	end of infusion	12–24 hr

Contraindications/Precautions

Contraindicated in: Hypersensitivity to cephalosporins; Serious hypersensitivity to penicillins; Pedi: Premature neonates up to a postmenstrual age of 41 wk (ceftriaxone only); Pedi: Hyperbilirubinemic neonates (may lead to bilirubin encephalopathy); Pedi: Neonates ≤28 days requiring calcium-containing IV solutions (↑ risk of precipitation formation).

Use Cautiously in: Renal impairment (↓ dosing/↑ dosing interval recommended for: *cefdinir* if CCr <30 mL/min, *cefixime* if CCr ≤60 mL/min, *cefotaxime* if CCr <20 mL/min, *cefpodoxime* if CCr <30 mL/min, *ceftazidime* if CCr ≤50 mL/min); Combined severe hepatic and renal impairment (↑ risk of neurological adverse reactions with *ceftriaxone*; dose ↓/↑ dosing interval recommended); Diabetes (*cefdinir* suspension contain sucrose); Phenylketonuria (*cefixime* chewable tablets contain aspartame); History of GI disease, especially colitis; Pedi: ↑ risk of urolithiasis and acute renal failure (ceftriaxone only); Geri: Dose adjustment due to age-related ↓ in renal function may be necessary.

Adverse Reactions/Side Effects

Derm: rash, STEVENS-JOHNSON SYNDROME (SJS), urticaria. **GI:** diarrhea, nausea, vomiting, cholelithiasis (ceftriaxone), CLOSTRIDIOIDES DIFFICILE ASSOCIATED DIARRHEA (CDAD), cramps, pancreatitis (ceftriaxone). **GU:** acute renal failure (ceftriaxone), hematuria, urolithiasis (ceftriaxone), vaginal moniliasis. **Hemat:** agranulocytosis, bleeding, eosinophilia, hemolytic anemia, lymphocytosis, neutropenia, thrombocytopenia, thrombocytosis. **Local:** pain at IM site, phlebitis at IV site. **Neuro:** encephalopathy, headache, SEIZURES (high doses). **Misc:** HYPERSENSITIVITY REACTIONS (including anaphylaxis and serum sickness), superinfection.

Interactions

Drug-Drug: **Probenecid** ↓ excretion and ↑ serum levels (cefdinir, cefixime, cefotaxime, cefpodoxime, ceftriaxone). Concurrent use of **loop diuretics**, **aminoglycosides**, or **NSAIDs** may ↑ risk of nephrotoxicity. **Antacids** ↓ absorption of cefdinir and cefpodoxime. **Iron supplements** ↓ absorption of cefdinir. **H₂-receptor antagonists** ↓ absorption of cefpodoxime. Cefixime may ↑ **carbamazepine** levels. Ceftriaxone should not be administered concomitantly with any calcium-containing solutions. Ceftriaxone may ↑ risk of bleeding with **warfarin**.

Route/Dosage

Cefdinir

PO (Adults ≥13 yr): 300 mg every 12 hr *or* 600 mg every 24 hr (use every 12 hr dosing only for community-acquired pneumonia or skin and skin structure infections).
PO (Children 6 mo–12 yr): 7 mg/kg every 12 hr (use only for skin/skin structure infections) *or* 14 mg/kg every 24 hr; dose should not exceed 600 mg/day.

Renal Impairment

PO (Adults and Children ≥13 yr): *CCr <30 mL/min:* 300 mg every 24 hr.

Renal Impairment

PO (Children 6 mo–12 yr): *CCr <30 mL/min:* 7 mg/kg every 24 hr.

Cefixime

PO (Adults and Children >12 yr or >45 kg): *Most infections:* 400 mg once daily; *Gonorrhea:* 400 mg single dose.

C

PO (Children 6 mo–12 yr): 8 mg/kg once daily *or* 4 mg/kg every 12 h.

Renal Impairment
PO (Adults): *CCr 21–60 mL/min:* 75% of standard dose once daily; *CCr ≤20 mL/min:* 50% of standard dose once daily.

Cefotaxime
IM, IV (Adults and Children >12 yr): *Most uncomplicated infections:* 1 g every 12 hr. *Moderate or severe infections:* 1–2 g every 6–8 hr. *Life-threatening infections:* 2 g every 4 hr (maximum dose = 12 g/day). *Gonococcal urethritis/cervicitis or rectal gonorrhea in females:* 500 mg IM (single dose). *Rectal gonorrhea in males:* 1 g IM (single dose). *Perioperative prophylaxis:* 1 g 30–90 min before initial incision (one-time dose).

IM, IV (Children 1 mo–12 yr): *<50 kg :* 100–200 mg/kg/day divided every 6–8 hr. *Meningitis:* 200 mg/kg/day divided every 6 hr. *Invasive pneumococcal meningitis:* 225–300 mg/kg/day divided every 6–8 hr. *≥50 kg:* see adult dosing.

IV (Neonates 1–4 wk): 50 mg/kg every 6–8 hr.

IV (Neonates ≤1 wk): 50 mg/kg every 8–12 hr.

Renal Impairment
(Adults): *CCr <20 mL/min:* ↓ dose by 50%.

Cefpodoxime
PO (Adults): *Most infections:* 200 mg every 12 hr. *Skin and skin structure infections:* 400 mg every 12 hr. *Urinary tract infections/pharyngitis:* 100 mg every 12 hr. *Gonorrhea:* 200 mg single dose.

PO (Children 2 mo–12 yr): *Pharyngitis/tonsillitis/otitis media/acute maxillary sinusitis:* 5 mg/kg every 12 hr (not to exceed 200 mg/dose).

Renal Impairment
PO (Adults): *CCr <30 mL/min:* ↑ dosing interval to every 24 hr.

Ceftazidime
IM, IV (Adults and Children ≥12 yr): *Pneumonia and skin/skin structure infections:* 500 mg–1 g every 8 hr. *Bone and joint infections:* 2 g every 12 hr. *Severe and life-threatening infections:* 2 g every 8 hr. *Complicated urinary tract infections:* 500 mg every 8–12 hr. *Uncomplicated urinary tract infections:* 250 mg every 12 hr. *Cystic fibrosis lung infection caused by* P. acruginosa— 30–50 mg/kg every 8 hr (maximum dose = 6 g/day).

IM, IV (Children 1 mo–12 yr): 33.3–50 mg/kg every 8 hr (maximum dose = 6 g/day).

IM, IV (Neonates ≤4 wk): 50 mg/kg every 8–12 hr.

Renal Impairment
IM, IV (Adults): *CCr 31–50 mL/min:* 1 g every 12 hr; *CCr 16–30 mL/min:* 1 g every 24 hr; *CCr 6–15 mL/min:* 500 mg every 24 hr; *CCr <5 mL/min:* 500 mg every 48 hr.

Ceftriaxone
IM, IV (Adults): *Most infections:* 1–2 g every 12–24 hr. *Gonorrhea:* 250 mg IM (single dose). *Meningitis:* 2 g every 12 hr. *Perioperative prophylaxis:* 1 g 30–120 min before initial incision (single dose).

IM, IV (Children): *Most infections:* 25–37.5 mg/kg every 12 hr *or* 50–75 mg/kg every 24 hr; dose should not exceed 2 g/day. *Meningitis:* 100 mg/kg every 24 hr *or* 50 mg/kg every 12 hr; dose should not exceed 4 g/day. *Acute otitis media:* 50 mg/kg IM single dose; dose should not exceed 1 g. *Uncomplicated gonorrhea:* 125 mg IM (single dose).

Hepatic/Renal Impairment
IM, IV (Adults): *Hepatic impairment with significant renal impairment:* Not to exceed 2 g/day.

Availability

Cefdinir (generic available)
Capsules: 300 mg. Oral suspension (strawberry): 125 mg/5 mL, 250 mg/5 mL.

Cefixime (generic available)
Capsules: 400 mg. Chewable tablets (contain aspartame): 100 mg, 150 mg, 200 mg. Oral suspension (strawberry): 100 mg/5 mL, 200 mg/5 mL, 500 mg/5 mL. Tablets: 400 mg.

Cefotaxime (generic available)
Powder for injection: 500 mg/vial, 1 g/vial, 2 g/vial, 10 g/vial.

Cefpodoxime (generic available)
Oral suspension (lemon creme): 50 mg/5 mL, 100 mg/5 mL. Tablets: 100 mg, 200 mg.

Ceftazidime (generic available)
Powder for injection: 1 g/vial, 2 g/vial, 6 g/vial. Premixed infusion: 1 g/50 mL, 2 g/50 mL.

Ceftriaxone (generic available)
Powder for injection: 250 mg/vial, 500 mg/vial, 1 g/vial, 2 g/vial, 10 g/vial, 100 g/vial. Premixed infusion: 1 g/50 mL, 2 g/50 mL.

NURSING IMPLICATIONS
Assessment
- Assess for infection (vital signs; appearance of wound, sputum, urine, and stool; WBC) at beginning of and throughout therapy.
- Before initiating therapy, obtain a history to determine previous use of and reactions to penicillins or cephalosporins. Persons with a negative history of penicillin sensitivity may still have an allergic response.
- Obtain specimens for culture and sensitivity before initiating therapy. First dose may be given before receiving results.
- Observe for signs and symptoms of anaphylaxis (rash, pruritus, laryngeal edema, wheezing). Dis-

✦ = Canadian drug name. ⅏ = Genetic implication. S̶t̶r̶i̶k̶e̶t̶h̶r̶o̶u̶g̶h̶ = Discontinued. CAPITALS = life-threatening. <u>Underline</u> = most frequent.

continue drug and notify health care professional immediately if these symptoms occur. Keep epinephrine, an antihistamine, and resuscitation equipment close by in the event of an anaphylactic reaction.
- Monitor bowel function. Diarrhea, abdominal cramping, fever, and bloody stools should be reported to health care professional promptly as a sign of CDAD. May begin up to several wk following cessation of therapy.
- Assess patient for skin rash frequently during therapy. Discontinue at first sign of rash; may be life-threatening. SJS may develop. Treat symptomatically; may recur once treatment is stopped.
- Pedi: Assess newborns for jaundice and hyperbilirubinemia before making decision to use ceftriaxone (should not be used in jaundiced or hyperbilirubinemic neonates).

Lab Test Considerations
- May cause positive results for Coombs' test in patients receiving high doses or in neonates whose mothers were given cephalosporins before delivery.
- May cause ↑ AST, ALT, alkaline phosphatase, bilirubin, LDH, BUN, and serum creatinine.
- May rarely cause leukopenia, neutropenia, agranulocytosis, thrombocytopenia, eosinophilia, lymphocytosis, and thrombocytosis.

Implementation
- Do not confuse ceftazidime with cefazolin, cefoxitin, cefotetan, or ceftriaxone. Do not confuse ceftriaxone with cefazolin, cefotetan, cefoxitin, or ceftazidime.
- PO: Administer around the clock. May be administered on full or empty stomach. Administration with food may minimize GI irritation. Shake oral suspension well before administering. Administer *cefpodoxime tablets* with meals to enhance absorption (suspension may be administered without regard to meals.
- *Cefixime oral suspension* should be used to treat otitis media (results in higher peak concentrations than tablets).
- Do not administer *cefdinir* or *cefpodoxime* within 2 hr before or after an antacid. Do not administer *cefpodoxime* within 2 hr before or after an H₂ receptor antagonist. Do not administer *cefdinir* within 2 hr before or after iron supplements.
- IM: *Reconstitution:* Reconstitute IM doses with sterile or bacteriostatic water for injection or 0.9% NaCl for injection. May be diluted with lidocaine to minimize injection discomfort. Do not administer lidocaine-containing ceftriaxone IV.
- Inject deep into a well-developed muscle mass; massage well.

IV Administration
- IV: Monitor injection site frequently for phlebitis (pain, redness, swelling). Change sites every 48–72 hr to prevent phlebitis.
- If aminoglycosides are administered concurrently, administer in separate sites, if possible, at least 1 hr

apart. If second site is unavailable, flush lines between medications.

Cefotaxime
- IV Push: *Reconstitution:* Reconstitute 500-mg, 1-g and 2-g vials in at least 10 mL of sterile water for injection. *Concentration:* 50 mg/mL (500 mg), 95 mg/mL (1 g), and 180 mg/mL (2 g). Do not use preparations containing benzyl alcohol for neonates. *Rate:* Administer slowly over 3–5 min.
- Intermittent Infusion: *Dilution:* Reconstituted solution may be further diluted in D5W, D10W, lactated Ringer's solution, D5/0.25% NaCl, D5/0.45% NaCl, D5/0.9% NaCl, or 0.9% NaCl. *Concentration:* 20–60 mg/mL. Solution may appear light yellow to amber. Solution is stable for 24 hr at room temperature and 5 days if refrigerated. *Rate:* Administer over 20–30 min.
- Y-Site Compatibility: acetaminophen, acyclovir, alprostadil, amifostine, amikacin, aminocaproic acid, aminophylline, amphotericin B lipid complex, anidulafungin, argatroban, arsenic trioxide, ascorbic acid, atracurium, atropine, aztreonam, benztropine, bivalirudin, bleomycin, bumetanide, buprenorphine, butorphanol, calcium chloride, calcium gluconate, cangrelor, carboplatin, carmustine, cefotetan, cefoxitin, ceftriaxone, cefuroxime, cisplatin, clindamycin, cyanocobalamin, cyclophosphamide, cyclosporine, cytarabine, dactinomycin, daptomycin, dexamethasone, dexmedetomidine, dexrazoxane, digoxin, diltiazem, dimenhydrinate, docetaxel, dopamine, doxorubicin liposomal, doxycycline, enalaprilat, ephedrine, epinephrine, epirubicin, epoetin alfa, eptifibatide, erythromycin, esmolol, etoposide, etoposide phosphate, famotidine, fentanyl, fludarabine, fluorouracil, folic acid, foscarnet, fosphenytoin, furosemide, glycopyrrolate, granisetron, heparin, hetastarch, hydrocortisone, ifosfamide, imipenem/cilastatin, indomethacin, insulin, regular, isoproterenol, ketamine, ketorolac, LR, leucovorin calcium, lidocaine, linezolid, lorazepam, magnesium sulfate, mannitol, melphalan, meperidine, meropenem, mesna, methadone, methotrexate, metoclopramide, metoprolol, midazolam, milrinone, morphine, multivitamins, nafcillin, nalbuphine, naloxone, nicardipine, nitroglycerin, nitroprusside, norepinephrine, octreotide, ondansetron, oxacillin, oxaliplatin, oxytocin, paclitaxel, palonosetron, pamidronate, penicillin G, phenylephrine, phytonadione, potassium acetate, potassium chloride, procainamide, propofol, propranolol, pyridoxine, remifentanil, rituximab, rocuronium, sargramostim, sodium acetate, succinylcholine, sufentanil, tacrolimus, theophylline, thiamine, thiotepa, tigecycline, tirofiban, tobramycin, topotecan, vasopressin, verapamil, vinblastine, vinorelbine, voriconazole, zoledronic acid.
- Y-Site Incompatibility: alemtuzumab, allopurinol, amiodarone, amphotericin B liposomal, azathioprine, caspofungin, cefazolin, ceftazidime, chloramphenicol, chlorpromazine, dacarbazine, dantrolene,

daunorubicin hydrochloride, diazepam, diphenhydramine, dobutamine, doxorubicin hydrochloride, filgrastim, ganciclovir, gemcitabine, gemtuzumab ozogamicin, haloperidol, hetastarch, hydralazine, hydroxyzine, idarubicin, irinotecan, labetalol, methylprednisolone, minocycline, mitomycin, mitoxantrone, mycophenolate, pantoprazole, papaverine, pemetrexed, pentamidine, pentobarbital, phenobarbital, phenytoin, prochlorperazine, promethazine, protamine, sodium bicarbonate, trastuzumab, trimethoprim/sulfamethoxazole, vecuronium.

Ceftazidime

- **IV Push:** *Reconstitution:* Reconstitute 500-mg, 1-g and 2-g vials with 5.3 mL, 10 mL or 10 mL, respectively, of sterile water for injection. *Concentration:* 100 mg/mL (500 mg), 100 mg/mL (1 g), and 170 mg/mL (2 g). Do not use preparations containing benzyl alcohol for neonates. *Rate:* Administer slowly over 3–5 min.
- **Intermittent Infusion:** *Dilution:* Reconstituted solution may be further diluted in at least 1 g/10 mL of 0.9% NaCl, D5W, D10W, dextrose/saline combinations, or LR. Dilution causes CO_2 to form inside vial, resulting in positive pressure; vial may require venting after dissolution to preserve sterility of vial. Solution may appear yellow to amber; darkening does not alter potency. Solution is stable for 18 hr at room temperature and 7 days if refrigerated. *Concentration:* 40 mg/mL. *Rate:* Administer over 15–30 min.
- **Y-Site Compatibility:** acetaminophen, acyclovir, allopurinol, amifostine, aminocaproic acid, aminophylline, amphotericin B lipid complex, anakinra, anidulafungin, argatroban, arsenic trioxide, atropine, aztreonam, benztropine, bivalirudin, bleomycin, bumetanide, buprenorphine, butorphanol, calcium gluconate, cangrelor, carboplatin, carmustine, cefazolin, cefotetan, cefoxitin, ceftolozane/tazobactam, ceftriaxone, cefuroxime, ciprofloxacin, cisplatin, clindamycin, cyanocobalamin, cyclophosphamide, cyclosporine, cytarabine, dacarbazine, dactinomycin, daptomycin, dexamethasone, dexmedetomidine, dexrazoxane, digoxin, diltiazem, dimenhydrinate, docetaxel, dopamine, enalaprilat, ephedrine, epinephrine, epoetin alfa, eptifibatide, eravacycline, esmolol, etoposide, etoposide phosphate, famotidine, fentanyl, filgrastim, fludarabine, fluorouracil, folic acid, foscarnet, fosphenytoin, furosemide, gemcitabine, glycopyrrolate, granisetron, heparin, hetastarch, hydrocortisone, hydromorphone, ibuprofen lysine, ifosfamide, imipenem/cilastatin, indomethacin, insulin, regular, irinotecan, isoproterenol, ketamine, ketorolac, labetalol, LR, leucovorin calcium, levofloxacin, lidocaine, linezolid, lorazepam, magnesium sulfate, mannitol, melphalan, meperidine, meropenem, meropenem/vaborbactam, mesna, methadone, methotrexate, methylprednisolone, metoclopramide, metoprolol, metronidazole, milrinone, mitomycin, morphine, multivitamins, nafcillin, nalbuphine, naloxone, nitroglycerin, norepinephrine, octreotide, oxacillin, oxaliplatin, oxytocin, paclitaxel, palonosetron, pamidronate, penicillin G, phenobarbital, phentolamine, phenylephrine, phytonadione, plazomicin, potassium acetate, potassium chloride, procainamide, propranolol, pyridoxine, remifentanil, rituximab, rocuronium, sodium acetate, sodium bicarbonate, succinylcholine, sufentanil, tacrolimus, tedizolid, telavancin, thiotepa, tigecycline, tirofiban, trastuzumab, vasopressin, vecuronium, vinblastine, vincristine, vinorelbine, voriconazole, zidovudine, zoledronic acid.

- **Y-Site Incompatibility:** acetylcysteine, alemtuzumab, amiodarone, amphotericin B deoxycholate, amphotericin B liposomal, ascorbic acid, azathioprine, blinatumomab, calcium chloride, caspofungin, cefotaxime, chloramphenicol, chlorpromazine, dantrolene, daunorubicin hydrochloride, diazepam, diphenhydramine, doxorubicin hydrochloride, doxorubicin liposomal, doxycycline, epirubicin, ganciclovir, gemtuzumab ozogamicin, haloperidol, hydralazine, hydroxyzine, idarubicin, isavuconazonium, midazolam, minocycline, mitoxantrone, mycophenolate, nitroprusside, papaverine, pemetrexed, pentamidine, phenytoin, prochlorperazine, promethazine, protamine, thiamine, topotecan, trimethoprim/sulfamethoxazole, verapamil.

Ceftriaxone

- **Intermittent Infusion:** *Reconstitution:* Reconstitute each 250-mg vial with 2.4 mL, each 500-mg vial with 4.8 mL, each 1-g vial with 9.6 mL, and each 2-g vial with 19.2 mL of sterile water for injection, 0.9% NaCl, or D5W for a concentration of 100 mg/mL. *Dilution:* Solution should be further diluted in 50–100 mL of 0.9% NaCl, D5W, D10W, D5/0.45% NaCl, or D5/0.9% NaCl. Solution may appear light yellow to amber. Solution is stable for 3 days at room temperature. *Concentration:* 40 mg/mL. *Rate:* Infuse over 30 min.
- **Y-Site Compatibility:** acetaminophen, acyclovir, allopurinol, amifostine, aminocaproic acid, aminophylline, amphotericin B lipid complex, amphotericin B liposomal, anidulafungin, argatroban, arsenic trioxide, atropine, aztreonam, benztropine, bivalirudin, bleomycin, bumetanide, buprenorphine, butorphanol, cangrelor, carboplatin, carmustine, cefazolin, cefotaxime, cefotetan, cefoxitin, ceftazidime, ceftolozane/tazobactam, cefuroxime, cisatracurium, cisplatin, cyanocobalamin, cyclophosphamide, cyclosporine, cytarabine, dactinomycin, daptomycin, dexamethasone, dexmedetomidine, dexrazoxane, digoxin, diltiazem, docetaxel, dopamine, doxorubicin liposomal, doxycycline, enalaprilat, ephedrine, epi-

nephrine, epoetin alfa, eptifibatide, erythromycin, esmolol, etoposide, etoposide phosphate, fentanyl, fludarabine, fluorouracil, folic acid, foscarnet, fosphenytoin, furosemide, gemcitabine, glycopyrrolate, granisetron, heparin, hydrocortisone, hydromorphone, ifosfamide, indomethacin, insulin, regular, isoproterenol, ketorolac, levofloxacin, lidocaine, linezolid, lorazepam, mannitol, melphalan, meperidine, meropenem, meropenem/vaborbactam, mesna, methadone, methotrexate, methylprednisolone, metoclopramide, metoprolol, metronidazole, midazolam, milrinone, mitomycin, morphine, multivitamins, nafcillin, nalbuphine, naloxone, nicardipine, nitroglycerin, nitroprusside, norepinephrine, octreotide, oxacillin, oxaliplatin, oxytocin, paclitaxel, palonosetron, pamidronate, pantoprazole, pemetrexed, penicillin G, phenobarbital, phentolamine, phenylephrine, phytonadione, plazomicin, potassium acetate, potassium chloride, procainamide, propranolol, pyridoxine, remifentanil, rituximab, rocuronium, sargramostim, sodium acetate, sodium bicarbonate, succinylcholine, sufentanil, tacrolimus, tedizolid, telavancin, theophylline, thiamine, thiotepa, tigecycline, tirofiban, topotecan, trastuzumab, vasopressin, vecuronium, verapamil, vinblastine, vincristine, voriconazole, zidovudine, zoledronic acid.

- **Y-Site Incompatibility:** alemtuzumab, amphotericin B deoxycholate, ascorbic acid, azathioprine, blinatumomab, calcium chloride, calcium gluconate, caspofungin, chloramphenicol, chlorpromazine, clindamycin, dacarbazine, dantrolene, daunorubicin hydrochloride, diazepam, diphenhydramine, dobutamine, doxorubicin hydrochloride, epirubicin, filgrastim, ganciclovir, gemtuzumab ozogamicin, haloperidol, hetastarch, hydralazine, hydroxyzine, idarubicin, imipenem/cilastatin, irinotecan, isavuconazonium, labetalol, leucovorin calcium, minocycline, mitoxantrone, mycophenolate, papaverine, pentamidine, pentobarbital, phenytoin, prochlorperazine, promethazine, protamine, tobramycin, trimethoprim/sulfamethoxazole, vinorelbine., Calcium-containing solutions, including parenteral nutrition, should not be mixed or co-administered, even via different infusion lines at different sites in patients <28 days old. In older patients, flush line thoroughly between infusions

Patient/Family Teaching

- Instruct patient to take medication around the clock and to finish the medication completely, even if feeling better. Take missed doses as soon as possible unless almost time for next dose; do not double doses. Advise patient that sharing of this medication may be dangerous.
- Pedi: Instruct parents or caregivers to use calibrated measuring device with liquid preparations.
- Advise patient to report signs of superinfection (furry overgrowth on the tongue, vaginal itching or discharge, loose or foul-smelling stools) and allergy.

- Instruct patient to notify health care professional if rash, fever, and diarrhea develop, especially if stool contains blood, pus, or mucus. Advise patient not to treat diarrhea without consulting health care professional.
- Rep: Advise females of reproductive potential to notify health care professional if pregnancy is planned or suspected, or if breastfeeding.

Evaluation/Desired Outcomes

- Resolution of the signs and symptoms of infection. Length of time for complete resolution depends on the organism and site of infection.
- Decreased incidence of infection when used for prophylaxis.

⚠ **ceritinib** (se-ri-ti-nib)
Zykadia
Classification
Therapeutic: antineoplastics
Pharmacologic: kinase inhibitors

Indications
⚠ Anaplastic lymphoma kinase (ALK)-positive, metastatic non-small cell lung cancer (NSCLC).

Action
Acts as a tyrosine kinase inhibitor, inhibiting anaplastic lymphoma kinase as well as other kinases, resulting in decreased growth of certain malignant cell lines. **Therapeutic Effects:** Slowed progression of metastatic NSCLC.

Pharmacokinetics
Absorption: Absorption follows oral administration; food significantly ↑ absorption and may ↑ risk of adverse reactions.
Distribution: Slight preference to distribute from plasma into red blood cells.
Metabolism and Excretion: Metabolized in the liver (mostly by CYP3A) and is a substrate of P-glycoprotein (P-gp); 68% eliminated unchanged in feces, 1.3% in urine.
Half-life: 41 hr.

TIME/ACTION PROFILE (clinical response)

ROUTE	ONSET	PEAK	DURATION
PO	unknown	4–6 hr (blood level)	7.1–7.4 mo

Contraindications/Precautions
Contraindicated in: Congenital long QT syndrome; OB: Pregnancy; Lactation: Lactation.
Use Cautiously in: Moderate to severe hepatic impairment/severe renal impairment (CCr <30 mL/min); HF, bradycardia, electrolyte abnormalities, or concurrent use of QT prolonging medications; Concurrent use of strong CYP3A4 inhibitors; Rep: Women of reproductive potential and men with female partners of repro-

ductive potential; Pedi: Safety and effectiveness not established in children.

Adverse Reactions/Side Effects

CV: BRADYCARDIA, QT interval prolongation, TORSADES DE POINTES. **Derm:** rash, photosensitivity. **Endo:** hyperglycemia. **F and E:** hypophosphatemia. **GI:** ↓ appetite, ↑ lipase, ↑ liver enzymes, abdominal pain, constipation, diarrhea, esophagitis/reflux/dysphagia, nausea, vomiting, HEPATOTOXICITY, PANCREATITIS. **GU:** ↑ serum creatinine. **Hemat:** anemia. **Neuro:** fatigue. **Resp:** INTERSTITIAL LUNG DISEASE/PNEUMONITIS.

Interactions

Drug-Drug: Concurrent use of strong **CYP3A inhibitors** including **ketoconazole, nefazodone,** and **ritonavir** ↑ levels and risk of toxicity; avoid concurrent use; if unavoidable, ↓ ceritinib dose. Strong **CYP3A inducers,** including **carbamazepine, phenytoin,** and **rifampin** may ↓ levels and effectiveness; avoid concurrent use. May ↑ levels and risk of toxicity of CYP3A substrates, including **midazolam;** avoid concurrent use; if unavoidable, ↓ dose of CYP3A substrate. May ↑ levels and risk of toxicity of CYP2C9 substrates, including **warfarin;** avoid concurrent use; if unavoidable, ↓ dose of CYP2C9 substrate. **Beta-blockers, diltiazem, verapamil, digoxin,** and **clonidine** may ↑ risk of bradycardia; avoid concurrent use, if possible. Concurrent use of **QT interval prolonging medications** may ↑ risk of QT interval prolongation and torsades de pointes.

Drug-Natural Products: St. John's wort ↓ levels and effectiveness; avoid concurrent use.

Drug-Food: Grapefruit/grapefruit juice ↑ levels and the risk of toxicity; avoid concurrent ingestion.

Route/Dosage

PO (Adults): 450 mg once daily; continue until disease progression or unacceptable toxicity; *Concurrent use of strong CYP3A inhibitors:* ↓ dose by ⅓, rounded to the nearest 150-mg strength.

Hepatic Impairment

PO (Adults): *Severe hepatic impairment:* ↓ dose by ⅓, rounded to the nearest 150-mg strength.

Availability

Tablets: 150 mg.

NURSING IMPLICATIONS

Assessment

● Assess for signs and symptoms of interstitial lung disease or pneumonitis (trouble breathing, shortness of breath, fever, cough with or without mucus, chest pain). If these symptoms occur, discontinue therapy permanently.

● Monitor ECG periodically during therapy. *If QTc interval is >500 msec on at least 2 separate ECGs,* hold ceritinib until QTc interval <481 msec or recovery to baseline if QTc ≥481 msec, then resume ceritinib with a 150-mg dose reduction. *If QTc interval prolongation occurs in combination with torsades de pointes or polymorphic ventricular tachycardia or signs and symptoms of serious arrhythmia,* discontinue ceritinib permanently.

● *If symptomatic bradycardia that is not life-threatening occurs,* hold ceritinib until recovery to asymptomatic bradycardia or a heart rate ≥60 bpm, evaluate concurrent medications causing bradycardia, and adjust dose of ceritinib. *If clinically significant bradycardia requiring intervention or life-threatening bradycardia in patients taking concurrent medication known to cause bradycardia or a medication known to cause hypotension occurs,* hold ceritinib until recovery to asymptomatic bradycardia or a heart rate ≥60 bpm. *If concurrent medication can be adjusted or discontinued,* resume ceritinib with a 150-mg dose reduction and frequent monitoring. *If life-threatening bradycardia occurs in patients not taking medications known to cause bradycardia or hypotension,* discontinue ceritinib permanently.

● Assess for nausea, vomiting, diarrhea. If severe or intolerable nausea, vomiting, or diarrhea continue despite optimal antiemetic or antidiarrheal therapy, hold ceritinib until improved; then resume with a 150-mg dose reduction.

Lab Test Considerations

● ⚗ Test patient for ALK positivity in tumor specimens through an FDA approved test prior to starting therapy.

● Monitor liver function tests at least monthly. *If ALT or AST >5 times the upper limit of normal (ULN) and total bilirubin is ≤2 times ULN,* hold ceritinib until recovery to baseline or ≤3 times ULN, then resume ceritinib with a 150-mg dose reduction. *If ALT or AST >3 times ULN and total bilirubin is >2 times ULN in the absence of cholestasis or hemolysis,* permanently discontinue ceritinib.

● Monitor fasting blood glucose prior to and periodically during therapy. *If persistent hyperglycemia >250 mg/dL despite anti-hyperglycemic therapy,* hold ceritinib until hyperglycemia is adequately controlled, then resume with a 150-mg dose reduction. *If adequate hyperglycemic control cannot be achieved,* discontinue therapy.

● May cause ↓ hemoglobin and serum phosphate; ↑ serum creatinine.

● Monitor serum lipase and amylase prior to and periodically during therapy. May cause ↑ serum lipase and amylase. *If ↑ lipase or amylase >2 times ULN,* hold ceritinib and monitor serum lipase and amylase. *When recovery to <1.5 times ULN,* resume with 150-mg dose reduction.

Implementation

- **PO:** Administer on an empty stomach, at least 1 hr before or 2 hr after meals.

Patient/Family Teaching

- Instruct patient to take ceritinib as directed. Take missed doses as soon as remembered unless within 12 hr of next dose. If vomiting occurs, do not administer additional dose, continue with next scheduled dose. Instruct patient to read *Patient Information* prior to starting therapy and with each Rx refill in case of changes.
- Inform patient to avoid consuming grapefruit and grapefruit juice during therapy.
- Advise patient to notify health care professional if nausea, vomiting, and diarrhea is severe or persistent; if signs and symptoms of hepatotoxicity (feeling tired, itchy skin, skin or whites of eyes turn yellow, nausea and vomiting, decreased appetite, pain on right side of stomach, dark or brown, tea-colored urine, bleed or bruise easily); pneumonitis; QTc interval prolongation or bradycardia (new chest pain, changes in heartbeat, palpitations, dizziness, fainting, or changes in or use of a new heart or BP medication); hyperglycemia (increased thirst, increased hunger, headaches, trouble thinking or concentration, urinating often, blurred vision, tiredness, breath smells like fruit), or pancreatitis (upper abdominal pain that may spread to the back and get worse with eating) occur.
- Instruct patient to notify health care professional of all Rx or OTC medications, vitamins, or herbal products being taken and to consult health care professional before taking other Rx, OTC, or herbal products, especially St. John's wort.
- Rep: May cause fetal harm. Advise females of reproductive potential to use effective contraceptives during and for 6 mo and to avoid breastfeeding during and for 2 wk following completion of therapy. Advise patient to notify health care provider if pregnancy is planned or suspected. Advise males with female partners of reproductive potential to use condoms during therapy and for 3 mo following completion of therapy.

Evaluation/Desired Outcomes

- Slowed progression of metastatic NSCLC.

---

certolizumab (ser-toe-liz-u-mab)
Cimzia
Classification
Therapeutic: gastrointestinal anti-inflammatories, antirheumatics
Pharmacologic: tumor necrosis factor blockers, DMARDs, monoclonal antibodies

Indications

Moderately to severely active Crohn's disease when response to conventional therapy has been inadequate. Moderately to severely active rheumatoid arthritis. Active psoriatic arthritis. Active ankylosing spondylitis. Moderate to severe plaque psoriasis in patients who are not candidates for systemic therapy or phototherapy. Active non-radiographic axial spondyloarthritis with objective signs of inflammation.

Action

Neutralizes tumor necrosis factor (TNF), a prime mediator of inflammation; pegylation provides a long duration of action. **Therapeutic Effects:** Decreased signs/symptoms of Crohn's disease. Decreased pain and swelling, decreased rate of joint destruction and improved physical function in rheumatoid arthritis. Decreased joint swelling and pain in psoriatic arthritis. Decreased spinal pain and inflammation in ankylosing spondylitis. Reduced severity of plaques. Decreased pain and swelling, reduced C-reactive protein levels, and improved physical function in axial spondyloarthritis.

Pharmacokinetics

Absorption: 80% absorbed following SUBQ administration.
Distribution: Minimally distributed to tissues.
Metabolism and Excretion: Unknown.
Half-life: 14 days.

TIME/ACTION PROFILE (plasma concentrations)

ROUTE	ONSET	PEAK	DURATION
SUBQ	unknown	50–120 hr	2–4 wk

Contraindications/Precautions

Contraindicated in: Hypersensitivity; Active infection (including localized); Concurrent use of anakinra.
Use Cautiously in: History of chronic or recurrent infection or underlying illness/treatment predisposing to infection; History of exposure to tuberculosis (TB); History of opportunistic infection; Patients residing, or who have resided, where TB, histoplasmosis, coccidioidomycoses, or blastomycosis is endemic; History of demyelinating disorders (may exacerbate); History of HF; OB: Use during pregnancy only if potential maternal benefits justify potential fetal risk; Lactation: Use while breastfeeding only if potential maternal benefits justify potential risk to infant; Pedi: Safety and effectiveness not established in children; Geri: May ↑ risk of infection in older adults.

Adverse Reactions/Side Effects

Derm: psoriasis, skin reactions (rarely severe). **Hemat:** hematologic reactions. **MS:** arthralgia. **Misc:** INFECTION (including reactivation TB, hepatitis B virus [HBV] reactivation, and other opportunistic infections due to bacterial, invasive fungal, viral, mycobacterial, and parasitic pathogens), HYPERSENSITIVITY REACTIONS (including anaphylaxis, angioedema, serum sickness, and urticaria), lupus-like syndrome, MALIGNANCY (including lymphoma, hepatosplenic T-cell lymphoma [HSTCL], leukemia, and skin cancer).

Interactions

Drug-Drug: Anakinra ↑ risk of serious infections; concurrent use contraindicated. Concurrent use with **azathioprine** and/or **methotrexate** may ↑ risk of HSTCL. May ↓ antibody response to or ↑ risk of adverse reactions to **live vaccines**; avoid concurrent use.

Route/Dosage

Crohn's Disease
SUBQ (Adults): 400 mg (given as two 200-mg injections) initially, repeat 2 and 4 wk later; may be followed by maintenance dose of 400 mg (given as two 200-mg injections) every 4 wk.

Rheumatoid Arthritis or Psoriatic Arthritis
SUBQ (Adults): 400 mg (given as two 200-mg injections) initially, repeat 2 and 4 wk later; then maintenance dose of 200 mg every 2 wk (400 mg [given as two 200-mg injections] every 4 wk may be used alternatively).

Ankylosing Spondylitis or Non-Radiographic Axial Spondyloarthritis
SUBQ (Adults): 400 mg (given as two 200-mg injections) initially, repeat 2 and 4 wk later; then maintenance dose of 200 mg every 2 wk or 400 mg (given as two 200-mg injections) every 4 wk.

Plaque Psoriasis
SUBQ (Adults): 400 mg (given as two 200-mg injections) every 2 wk; *Patients ≤90 kg:* may consider giving 400 mg (given as two 200-mg injections) initially, then repeat 2 and 4 wk later; then maintenance dose of 200 mg every 2 wk.

Availability
Lyophilized powder for injection: 200 mg/vial. **Solution for injection (prefilled syringes):** 200 mg/mL.

NURSING IMPLICATIONS
Assessment
- **Crohn's Disease:** Assess abdominal pain and frequency, quantity, and consistency of stools at beginning and during therapy.
- **Arthritis/Ankylosing Spondylitis:** Assess pain and range of motion before and periodically during therapy.
- Assess for signs of infection (fever, sore throat, dyspnea, WBC) prior to and during therapy. Monitor all patients for active TB (persistent cough, wasting, weight loss, low-grade fever) during therapy, even if initial test was negative. Do not begin certolizumab during an active infection, including chronic or localized infections. If infection develops, monitor closely and discontinue certolizumab if infection becomes serious.
- Evaluate patients at risk for HBV infection for prior evidence of HBV infection before initiating therapy. Monitor carriers of HBV closely for clinical and lab

signs of active HBV infection during and for several mo following discontinuation of therapy. If HBV reactivation occurs, discontinue certolizumab and initiate antiviral therapy.
- Monitor for signs of hypersensitivity reactions (angioedema, dyspnea, hypotension, rash, serum sickness, urticaria). If reactions occur, discontinue certolizumab and treat symptomatically.
- Assess for signs and symptoms of systemic fungal infections (fever, malaise, weight loss, sweats, cough, dyspnea, pulmonary infiltrates, serious systemic illness with or without concomitant shock). Ascertain if patient lives in or has traveled to areas of endemic mycoses. Consider empiric antifungal treatment for patients at risk of histoplasmosis and other invasive fungal infections until the pathogens are identified. Consult with an infectious diseases specialist. Consider stopping certolizumab until the infection has been diagnosed and adequately treated.

Lab Test Considerations
- May cause anemia, leukopenia, pancytopenia, and thrombocytopenia.
- Monitor CBC with differential periodically during therapy. May cause leukopenia, neutropenia, thrombocytopenia, and pancytopenia. Discontinue certolizumab if symptoms of blood dyscrasias (persistent fever) occur.
- May ↑ liver enzymes.
- May erroneously ↑ aPTT.

Implementation
- Perform test for latent TB. If positive for latent TB, active TB in whom an adequate course of treatment cannot be confirmed, and for patients with a negative test for TB who have risk factors for tuberculosis infection, begin treatment for TB prior to starting certolizumab therapy. Monitor for TB throughout therapy, even if latent TB test is negative.
- Allow vial to sit at room temperature for 30 min prior to reconstituting; do not use other warming methods. Reconstitute vial by adding 1 mL of sterile water for injection, using a 20-gauge needle, for a concentration of 200 mg/mL. Gently swirl so all powder comes into contact with sterile water; do not shake. Leave vial undisturbed for as long as 30 min to fully reconstitute. Solution is clear and colorless to pale yellow; do not administer solutions that are cloudy, discolored, or contain particulate matter. Do not leave reconstituted solution at room temperature for >2 hr prior to injection. May be refrigerated for up to 24 hr prior to injection; do not freeze.
- **SUBQ:** Allow solution to sit at room temperature for 30 min prior to injection; do not use other warming methods. Give 400-mg dose as two injections of 200 mg each. Using a new 20-gauge needle for each vial, withdraw reconstituted solution into 2 separate syringes each containing 1 mL (200 mg/mL) of certo-

lizumab. Switch each 20-gauge needle to a 23-gauge needle and inject the full contents of each syringe SUBQ into separate sides of the abdomen or thigh. Avoid areas of skin tenderness, bruising, redness or hardness, or scars or stretch marks.
- Assess for latex allergies. Needle shield inside the removable cap of prefilled syringes contains a derivative of natural rubber latex.

Patient/Family Teaching
- Advise patient of potential benefits and risks of certolizumab. Instruct patient in correct technique for injection, and care and disposal of equipment. Advise patient to read the *Medication Guide* prior to starting therapy.
- Inform patient of risk of infection. Advise patient to notify health care professional if symptoms of infection (fever, cough, flu-like symptoms, or open cuts or sores), including TB or reactivation of HBV infection, occur.
- Counsel patient about possible risk of lymphoma and other malignancies while receiving certolizumab.
- Advise patient to notify health care professional if signs of hypersensitivity reactions (rash, swollen face, difficulty breathing), or new or worsening medical conditions such as heart or neurological disease or autoimmune disorders occur and to report signs of bone marrow depression (bruising, bleeding, or persistent fever).
- Advise patient to notify health care professional of all Rx or OTC medications, vitamins, or herbal products being taken and to consult with health care professional before taking other medications.
- Rep: Advise patient to notify health care professional if pregnancy is planned or suspected or if breastfeeding. Encourage women who become pregnant to enroll in the MotherToBaby Pregnancy Studies conducted by the Organization of Teratology Information Specialists (OTIS). The OTIS AutoImmune Diseases Study at 1-877-311-8972 or visit http://mothertobaby.org/pregnancy-studies/.

Evaluation/Desired Outcomes
- Decrease in signs and symptoms of Crohn's disease.
- Decreased pain and swelling with decreased rate of joint destruction in patients with rheumatoid arthritis.
- Decreased joint swelling and pain in psoriatic arthritis.
- Decreased spinal pain and inflammation in ankylosing spondylitis.
- Reduced severity of plaques.
- Decreased pain and swelling, reduced C-reactive protein levels, and improved physical function in axial spondyloarthritis.

---

cetirizine (se-ti-ra-zeen)
Quzyttir, ✿ Reactine, ZyrTEC
Classification
Therapeutic: allergy, cold, and cough remedies, antihistamines
Pharmacologic: piperazines (peripherally selective)

Indications
PO: Relief of allergic symptoms caused by histamine release including: Seasonal and perennial allergic rhinitis, Chronic urticaria. **IV**: Acute urticaria.

Action
Antagonizes the effects of histamine at H_1-receptor sites; does not bind to or inactivate histamine. Anticholinergic effects are minimal, and sedation is dose related. **Therapeutic Effects:** Decreased symptoms of histamine excess (sneezing, rhinorrhea, ocular tearing and redness, pruritus).

Pharmacokinetics
Absorption: Well absorbed following oral administration. IV administration results in complete bioavailability.
Distribution: Unknown.
Protein Binding: 93%.
Metabolism and Excretion: Excreted primarily unchanged by the kidneys.
Half-life: 7.4–9 hr ($\downarrow$ in children to 6.2 hr, $\uparrow$ in renal impairment up to 19–21 hr).

TIME/ACTION PROFILE (antihistaminic effects)

ROUTE	ONSET	PEAK	DURATION
PO	30 min	4–8 hr	24 hr
IV	unknown	unknown	unknown

Contraindications/Precautions
Contraindicated in: Hypersensitivity to cetirizine, levocetirizine, hydroxyzine, or any component; Pedi: Children <6 yr with renal or hepatic impairment.
Use Cautiously in: Patients with hepatic or renal impairment (dose $\downarrow$ recommended if CCr ≤31 mL/min or hepatic function is impaired); OB: Use during pregnancy only if potential maternal benefit justifies potential fetal risk; Lactation: Use while breastfeeding only if potential maternal benefit justifies potential risk to infant; Pedi: Children <6 mo (safety and effectiveness not established); Geri: Initiate at lower doses in older adults.

Adverse Reactions/Side Effects
Derm: acute generalized exanthematous pustulosis. **EENT:** pharyngitis. **GI:** dry mouth. **Neuro:** dizziness, drowsiness (significant with oral doses >10 mg/day), fatigue.

Interactions
Drug-Drug: Additive CNS depression may occur with **alcohol**, **opioid analgesics**, or **sedative/hypnotics**. **Theophylline** may $\downarrow$ clearance and $\uparrow$ toxicity.

Route/Dosage
PO (Adults and Children ≥6 yr): 5–10 mg given once or divided twice daily.
PO (Children 2–5 yr): 2.5 mg once daily initially, may be $\uparrow$ to 5 mg once daily or 2.5 mg every 12 hr.
PO (Children 1–2 yr): 2.5 mg once daily initially; may be $\uparrow$ to 2.5 mg every 12 hr.

PO (Children 6–12 mo): 2.5 mg once daily.
IV (Adults and Children ≥12 yr): 10 mg every 24 hr as needed.
IV (Children 6–11 yr): 5–10 mg every 24 hr as needed.
IV (Children 6 mo–5 yr): 2.5 mg every 24 hr as needed.

Hepatic/Renal Impairment
PO (Adults and Children ≥12 yr): *CCr ≤31 mL/ min, hepatic impairment or hemodialysis:* 5 mg once daily.

Hepatic/Renal Impairment
PO (Children 6–11 yr): start therapy at <2.5 mg/ day.

Availability (generic available)
Capsules: 10 mg^OTC. Chewable tablets: 5 mg^OTC, 10 mg^OTC. Orally disintegrating tablets: 10 mg. Syrup (banana-grape and bubblegum flavors): 1 mg/ mL^OTC. Tablets: 5 mg^OTC, 10 mg^OTC, ✱ 20 mg. Solution for injection: 10 mg/mL. *In combination with:* pseudoephedrine (Zyrtec-D 12 hr) (See Appendix N).

NURSING IMPLICATIONS
Assessment
- Assess allergy symptoms (rhinitis, conjunctivitis, hives) before and periodically during therapy.
- Assess lung sounds and character of bronchial secretions. Maintain fluid intake of 1500–2000 mL/ day to decrease viscosity of secretions.
- Assess severity of urticaria before and periodically after injection.

Lab Test Considerations
- May cause false-negative result in allergy skin testing.

Implementation
- Do not confuse cetirizine with sertraline. Do not confuse Zyrtec with Lipitor, Zocor, Zyprexa, or Zyrtec-D.
- PO: Administer once daily without regard to food.

IV Administration
- IV Push: Administer undiluted. Solution is clear and colorless; do not administer solutions that are cloudy, discolored, or contain precipitate matter. *Rate:* Administer IV push over 1–2 min.

Patient/Family Teaching
- Instruct patient to take medication as directed.
- May cause dizziness and drowsiness. Caution patient to avoid driving or other activities requiring alertness until response to medication is known.
- Advise patient to avoid taking alcohol or other CNS depressants, including opioids, concurrently with this drug.

- Advise patient that good oral hygiene, frequent rinsing of mouth with water, and sugarless gum or candy may minimize dry mouth. Patient should notify dentist if dry mouth persists >2 wk.
- Instruct patient to contact health care professional if rash or dizziness occurs or if symptoms persist.
- Rep: Advise females of reproductive potential to notify health care professional if pregnancy is planned or suspected or if breastfeeding.

Evaluation/Desired Outcomes
- Decrease in allergic symptoms.

cetuximab (se-tux-i-mab)
Erbitux
Classification
Therapeutic: antineoplastics
Pharmacologic: monoclonal antibodies

Indications
Locally or regionally advanced squamous cell carcinoma of the head and neck (in combination with radiation therapy). Recurrent or metastatic squamous cell carcinoma of the head and neck progressing after platinum-based therapy. Recurrent or metastatic squamous cell carcinoma of the head and neck (in combination with platinum-based therapy with 5-fluorouracil). *K-ras* wild-type, epidermal growth factor receptor (EGFR)-expressing metastatic colorectal cancer in patients who have not responded to irinotecan and oxaliplatin or are intolerant to irinotecan. *K-ras* wild-type, EGFR-expressing metastatic colorectal cancer in patients who have not responded to irinotecan alone (in combination with irinotecan). First-line treatment of *K-ras* wild-type, EGFR-expressing metastatic colorectal cancer (in combination with irinotecan, 5-fluorouracil, and leucovorin [FOLFIRI]). Metastatic colorectal cancer with a BRAF V600E mutation (in combination with encorafenib).

Action
Binds specifically to EGFR, thereby preventing the binding of endogenous epidermal growth factor. This prevents cell growth and differentiation processes. **Therapeutic Effects:** Decreased tumor growth and spread.

Pharmacokinetics
Absorption: IV administration results in complete bioavailability.
Distribution: Minimally distributed to tissues.
Metabolism and Excretion: Unknown.
Half-life: 97–114 hr.

TIME/ACTION PROFILE

ROUTE	ONSET	PEAK	DURATION
IV	unknown	unknown	unknown

✱= Canadian drug name. = Genetic implication. ~~Strikethrough~~ = Discontinued. CAPITALS = life-threatening. <u>Underline</u> = most frequent.

Contraindications/Precautions

Contraindicated in: Hypersensitivity to cetuximab or murine (mouse) proteins; ▒ *RAS*-mutant metastatic colorectal cancer or unknown *RAS* mutation status (↑ mortality and tumor progression); OB: Pregnancy; Lactation: Lactation.

Use Cautiously in: Exposure to sunlight (may exacerbate dermatologic toxicity); History of tick bites, red meat allergy, or in presence of IgE antibodies directed against galactose-α-1,3-galactose (alpha-gal) (↑ risk of anaphylaxis); Rep: Women of reproductive potential; Pedi: Safety and effectiveness not established in children.

Adverse Reactions/Side Effects

Most adverse reactions reflect combination therapy with irinotecan.
CV: CARDIOPULMONARY ARREST, peripheral edema, SUDDEN CARDIAC DEATH. **Derm:** acneform dermatitis, hypertrichosis, nail disorder, pruritus, skin desquamation, skin infection, STEVENS-JOHNSON SYNDROME (SJS), TOXIC EPIDERMAL NECROLYSIS (TEN). **EENT:** conjunctivitis, ulcerative keratitis. **F and E:** dehydration, hypomagnesemia. **GI:** abdominal pain, constipation, diarrhea, nausea, vomiting, ↓ weight, anorexia, stomatitis. **GU:** ↓ fertility (females), renal failure. **Hemat:** anemia, leukopenia. **MS:** back pain. **Neuro:** malaise, depression, headache, insomnia. **Resp:** cough, dyspnea, INTERSTITIAL LUNG DISEASE, PULMONARY EMBOLISM. **Misc:** fever, INFUSION REACTIONS (including anaphylaxis).

Interactions

Drug-Drug: None reported.

Route/Dosage

Head and Neck Cancer with Radiation

IV (Adults): 400 mg/m² administered 1 wk prior to initiation of radiation therapy, followed by 250 mg/m² once weekly for the duration of radiation therapy or until disease progression or unacceptable toxicity (complete infusion 1 hr prior to radiation therapy).

Head and Neck Cancer Monotherapy or in Combination with Platinum-Based Therapy and 5-Fluorouracil

IV (Adults): *Monotherapy (weekly regimen):* 400 mg/m² initially, followed by 250 mg/m² once weekly until disease progression or unacceptable toxicity. *Monotherapy (biweekly regimen):* 500 mg/m² every 2 wk until disease progression or unacceptable toxicity. *Combination therapy with platinum-based therapy and 5-fluorouracil (weekly regimen):* 400 mg/m² initially, followed by 250 mg/m² once weekly until disease progression or unacceptable toxicity (complete infusion 1 hr to prior to administering platinum-based therapy with 5-fluorouracil). *Combination therapy with platinum-based therapy and 5-fluorouracil (biweekly regimen):* 500 mg/m² every 2 wk until disease progression or unacceptable toxicity (complete infusion 1 hr prior to administering platinum-based therapy with 5-fluorouracil).

Colorectal Cancer

IV (Adults): *Monotherapy (weekly regimen):* 400 mg/m² initially, followed by 250 mg/m² once weekly until disease progression or unacceptable toxicity. *Monotherapy (biweekly regimen):* 500 mg/m² every 2 wk until disease progression or unacceptable toxicity. *Combination therapy with irinotecan or FOLFIRI (weekly regimen):* 400 mg/m² initially, followed by 250 mg/m² once weekly until disease progression or unacceptable toxicity (complete infusion 1 hr prior to administering irinotecan or FOLFIRI). *Combination therapy with irinotecan or FOLFIRI (biweekly regimen):* 500 mg/m² every 2 wk until disease progression or unacceptable toxicity (complete infusion 1 hr prior to administering irinotecan or FOLFIRI). *Combination therapy with encorafenib:* 400 mg/m² initially, followed by 250 mg/m² once weekly until disease progression or unacceptable toxicity.

Availability

Solution for injection: 2 mg/mL.

NURSING IMPLICATIONS

Assessment

● Assess for infusion reaction (rapid onset of airway obstruction [bronchospasm, stridor, hoarseness], urticaria, hypotension, loss of consciousness, myocardial infarction, cardiopulmonary arrest) for at least 1 hr following infusion. Longer observation periods may be required for those who experience infusion reactions. Risk of anaphylactic reactions may be increased in patients with a history of tick bites, red meat allergy, or in the presence of IgE antibodies directed against galactose-α-1,3-galactose (alpha-gal). Most reactions occur during first dose, but may also occur in later doses. For severe reactions, immediately stop infusion and discontinue cetuximab permanently. Epinephrine, corticosteroids, IV antihistamines, bronchodilators, and oxygen should be available for reactions. Mild to moderate reactions (chills, fever, dyspnea) may be managed by slowing rate of infusion and administration of antihistamines. *If infusion reaction is Grade 1 or 2,* reduce infusion rate by 50%. *If infusion reaction is Grade 3 or 4,* discontinue immediately and permanently.

● Assess for acute onset or worsening of pulmonary symptoms. Delay infusion 1–2 wk; if condition improves, continue at dose that was being administered at the time of occurrence. If no improvement in 2 wk or interstitial lung disease is confirmed, discontinue cetuximab and treat appropriately.

● Assess for dermatologic toxicities (acneform rash, skin drying and fissuring, inflammatory and infectious sequelae [blepharitis, cheilitis, cellulitis, cyst]). Treat symptomatically. Acneform rash usually occurs within initial 2 wk of therapy and resolves following cessation, but may continue up to 28 days following therapy. *For 1st occurrence of dermato-*

logic toxicities; Grade 3 or 4, delay infusion 1–2 wk; if improvement, continue at 250 mg/m², if no improvement, discontinue cetuximab. *For 2nd occurrence; Grade 3 or 4,* delay infusion 1–2 wk; if improvement, reduce dose to 200 mg/m², if no improvement, discontinue cetuximab. *For 3rd occurrence; Grade 3 or 4,* delay infusion 1–2 wk; if improvement, reduce dose to 150 mg/m², if no improvement, discontinue cetuximab. *For 4th occurrence; Grade 3 or 4,* discontinue cetuximab.

Lab Test Considerations
- Verify negative pregnancy test before starting therapy. ⚷ Determine Ras mutation and EGFR-expression status using FDA-approved tests prior to initiating treatment. Only patients whose tumors are *K-ras* wild-type should receive cetuximab. Determine BRAF V600E mutation before use for metastatic colon cancer. Information on FDA-approved tests for the detection of *K-ras* or BRAF V600E mutations in patients with metastatic colorectal cancer is available at: http://www.fda.gov/CompanionDiagnostics.
- Consider testing patients for alpha-gal IgE antibodies using FDA-cleared methods before starting therapy. Negative results for alpha-gal antibodies do not rule out the risk of severe infusion reactions.
- May cause anemia and leukopenia.
- Monitor serum electrolytes, especially serum magnesium, potassium, and calcium, closely during and periodically for at least 8 wk following infusion. May cause hypomagnesemia, hypocalcemia, and hypokalemia; may occur from days to mo after initiation of therapy. May require electrolyte replacement. May lead to cardiopulmonary arrest and sudden death.

Implementation
- Premedicate with histamine₁ antagonist (diphenhydramine 50 mg) 30–60 min prior to first dose; base subsequent administration on presence and severity of infusion reactions.

IV Administration
- Administer through a low protein binding 0.22-micrometer in-line filter placed as proximal to patient as possible. Solution should be clear and colorless and may contain a small amount of white amorphous cetuximab particles. Do not shake or dilute.
- Can be administered via infusion pump or syringe pump. Cetuximab should be piggybacked to the patient's infusion line.
- Observe patient for 1 hr following infusion.
- **Intermittent Infusion:** *For administration via infusion pump:* Draw up volume of a vial using vented spike needle or other transfer device. Transfer to a sterile evacuated container or bag. Repeat with new needle for each vial until calculated volume is in container. Affix infusion line and prime with cetuximab before starting infusion.

- *For administration via syringe pump:* Draw up volume of a vial using sterile syringe attached to an appropriate vented spike needle. Place syringe into syringe driver of a syringe pump and set rate. Connect infusion line and prime with cetuximab. Use a new needle and filter for each vial. *Dilution:* Do not dilute. *Concentration:* 2 mg/mL. *Rate:* Administer over 2 hr at a rate not to exceed 10 mg/min. Use 0.9% NaCl to flush line at end of infusion.
- Cetuximab infusion must be completed 1 hr prior to FOLFIRI (irinotecan, 5-fluorouracil, leucovorin) regimen. May infuse subsequent weekly infusions over 1 hr.

Patient/Family Teaching
- Explain purpose of cetuximab and potential side effects to patient.
- Advise patient to notify health care professional promptly if dermatologic changes (itchy, dry, scaly, or cracking skin, and inflammation, infection or swelling at base of nails or loss of the nails), conjunctivitis, blepharitis, or decreased vision, and signs and symptoms of pulmonary toxicity (new or worsening cough, chest pain, shortness of breath), infusion reactions (fever, chills, or breathing problems) promptly. Risk for infusion reactions in patients who have had a tick bite or red meat allergy.
- Caution patient to wear sunscreen and hats and limit sun exposure during therapy and for 2 mo following last dose of cetuximab.
- Rep: May cause fetal harm. Advise females of reproductive potential to use effective contraception during and for 2 mo after last dose of therapy and to avoid breastfeeding during and for 2 mo following therapy. May impair female fertility.

Evaluation/Desired Outcomes
- Decreased tumor growth and spread.

---

chlorothiazide, See DIURETICS (THIAZIDE).

---

chlorthalidone (thiazide-like), See DIURETICS (THIAZIDE).

---

cholecalciferol, See VITAMIN D COMPOUNDS.

---

ciclesonide, See CORTICOSTEROIDS (NASAL).

---

ciclesonide (inhalation), See CORTICOSTEROIDS (INHALATION).

ciclopirox, See ANTIFUNGALS (TOPICAL).

cimetidine, See HISTAMINE H₂ ANTAGONISTS.

cinacalcet (sin-a-kal-set)
Sensipar
Classification
Therapeutic: hypocalcemics
Pharmacologic: calcimimetic agents

Indications
Secondary hyperparathyroidism in patients with chronic kidney disease on dialysis. Hypercalcemia caused by parathyroid carcinoma. Severe hypercalcemia in patients with primary hyperparathyroidism who are unable to undergo parathyroidectomy.

Action
Increases sensitivity of calcium-sensing receptors located on the surface of chief cells of parathyroid gland to levels of extracellular calcium. This decreases parathyroid hormone (PTH) production with resultant decrease in serum calcium. **Therapeutic Effects:** Decreased bone turnover and fibrosis. Decreased serum calcium.

Pharmacokinetics
Absorption: Well absorbed following oral administration; absorption is enhanced by food and further enhanced by a high-fat meal.
Distribution: Extensively distributed to tissues.
Protein Binding: 93–97%.
Metabolism and Excretion: Primarily metabolized by the liver via the CYP3A4, CYP2D6, and CYP1A2 isoenzymes; 80% excreted in urine as metabolites, 15% in feces.
Half-life: 30–40 hr.

TIME/ACTION PROFILE (effect on PTH levels)

ROUTE	ONSET	PEAK	DURATION
PO	rapid	2–6 hr	6–12 hr

Contraindications/Precautions
Contraindicated in: Hypersensitivity; Hypocalcemia.

Use Cautiously in: History of seizure disorder (↑ risk of seizures with hypocalcemia); Chronic kidney disease patients who are not being dialyzed (↑ risk of hypocalcemia); Intact parathyroid hormone (iPTH) level <150 pg/mL (dose ↓ or discontinuation may be warranted); Moderate or severe hepatic impairment; Congenital long QT syndrome, QT interval prolongation, family history of long QT syndrome or sudden cardiac death, or concurrent use of QT-interval-prolonging medications; OB: Safety not established in pregnancy; Lactation: Use while breastfeeding only if potential maternal benefit justifies potential risk to infant; Pedi: Safety and effectiveness not established in children.

Adverse Reactions/Side Effects
CV: ARRHYTHMIA, HF exacerbation, hypotension, QT interval prolongation, TORSADES DE POINTES. **F and E:** HYPOCALCEMIA. **GI:** nausea, vomiting. **Metab:** adynamic bone disease. **Neuro:** SEIZURES.

Interactions
Drug-Drug: Concurrent use of **QT interval prolonging medications** may ↑ risk of QT interval prolongation and/or torsade de pointes, especially in patients with hypocalcemia. May ↑ levels and risk of toxicity of **CYP2D6 substrates**, including **flecainide**, **vinblastine, thioridazine, metoprolol, carvedilol**, and most **tricyclic antidepressants**; dose adjustments may be necessary. **Strong CYP3A4 inhibitors**, including **ketoconazole, itraconazole**, and **erythromycin**, may ↑ levels and risk of toxicity; monitoring and dose adjustment may be necessary.

Route/Dosage

Secondary Hyperparathyroidism in Patients with Chronic Kidney Disease on Dialysis
PO (Adults): 30 mg once daily; may ↑ dose every 2–4 wk (dose range 30–180 mg once daily) based on iPTH levels. *Switching from etecalcetide:* Discontinue etecalcetide for ≥4 wk and ensure corrected serum calcium is at or above lower limit of normal prior to starting cinacalcet.

Parathyroid Carcinoma or Primary Hyperparathyroidism
PO (Adults): 30 mg twice daily; may ↑ every 2–4 wk up to 90 mg 3–4 times daily based on serum calcium levels.

Availability (generic available)
Tablets: 30 mg, 60 mg, 90 mg.

NURSING IMPLICATIONS
Assessment
- Monitor for signs and symptoms of hypocalcemia (paresthesias, myalgias, cramping, tetany, convulsions) during therapy. If calcium levels decrease to below normal, serum calcium may be increased by adjusting dose (see Lab Test Considerations) and providing supplemental serum calcium, initiating or increasing dose of calcium-based phosphate binder or vitamin D.
- Monitor ECG for prolonged QT interval periodically during therapy.

Lab Test Considerations
- Monitor serum calcium and phosphorus levels within 1 wk after initiation of therapy or dose adjust-

ment and monthly for patients with hyperparathyroidism or every 2 mo for patients with parathyroid carcinoma once maintenance dose has been established, especially in patients with a history of seizure disorder. Therapy should not be initiated in patients with serum calcium less than the lower limit of normal (8.4 mg/dL).

- If serum calcium ↓ below 8.4 mg/dL but remains above 7.5 mg/dL, or if symptoms of hypocalcemia occur, use calcium-containing phosphate binders and/or vitamin D sterols to ↑ serum calcium. If serum calcium ↓ below 7.5 mg/dL, or if symptoms of hypocalcemia persist and the dose of vitamin D cannot be ↑, withhold administration of cinacalcet until serum calcium levels reach 8.0 mg/dL and/or symptoms of hypocalcemia resolve. Reinitiate therapy using next lowest dose of cinacalcet.
- Monitor serum iPTH levels 1 to 4 wk after initiation of therapy or dose adjustment, and every 1 to 3 mo after maintenance dose has been established. If iPTH levels ↓ below 150–300 pg/mL, reduce dose or discontinue cinacalcet. Assess iPTH levels no earlier than 12 hr after dose.
- Monitor liver function tests in patients with moderate to severe hepatic impairment during therapy.

Implementation
- Cinacalcet may be used alone or in combination with vitamin D and/or phosphate binders.
- **PO:** Administer with food or shortly after a meal. Take tablets whole; *DNC:* do not crush, break, or chew.

Patient/Family Teaching
- Instruct patient to take cinacalcet as directed.
- Advise patient to report signs and symptoms of hypocalcemia, GI bleeding (black tarry stools, abdominal pain), nausea, and vomiting to health care professional promptly.
- Rep: Advise females of reproductive potential to notify health care professional if pregnancy is planned or suspected, or if breastfeeding.
- Emphasize the importance of follow-up lab tests to monitor safely and efficacy.

Evaluation/Desired Outcomes
- Decreased serum calcium levels.

---

ciprofloxacin, See FLUOROQUINOLONES.

HIGH ALERT

CISplatin (sis-pla-tin)
~~Platinol~~
Classification
Therapeutic: antineoplastics
Pharmacologic: alkylating agents

Indications
Metastatic testicular and ovarian carcinoma. Advanced bladder cancer. Head and neck cancer. Cervical cancer. Lung cancer.

Action
Inhibits DNA synthesis by producing cross-linking of parent DNA strands (cell-cycle phase–nonspecific). **Therapeutic Effects:** Death of rapidly replicating cells, particularly malignant ones.

Pharmacokinetics
Absorption: IV administration results in complete bioavailability.
Distribution: Widely distributed; accumulates for months.
Metabolism and Excretion: Excreted mainly by the kidneys.
Half-life: 30–100 hr.

TIME/ACTION PROFILE (effects on blood counts)

ROUTE	ONSET	PEAK	DURATION
IV	unknown	18–23 days	39 days

Contraindications/Precautions
Contraindicated in: Hypersensitivity; OB: Pregnancy; Lactation: Lactation.
Use Cautiously in: Hearing loss; Renal impairment (dosage ↓ recommended); HF; Electrolyte abnormalities; Active infections; Bone marrow depression; Rep: Women of reproductive potential; Geri: ↑ risk of nephrotoxicity and peripheral neuropathy in older adults.

Adverse Reactions/Side Effects
Derm: alopecia. **EENT:** ototoxicity, tinnitus. **F and E:** hypocalcemia, hypokalemia, hypomagnesemia. **GI:** nausea, vomiting, diarrhea, HEPATOTOXICITY. **GU:** nephrotoxicity, sterility. **Hemat:** anemia, LEUKOPENIA, THROMBOCYTOPENIA. **Local:** phlebitis at IV site. **Metab:** hyperuricemia. **Neuro:** malaise, peripheral neuropathy, REVERSIBLE POSTERIOR LEUKOENCEPHALOPATHY SYNDROME (RPLS), SEIZURES, weakness. **Misc:** anaphylactoid reactions.

Interactions
Drug-Drug: ↑ risk of nephrotoxicity and ototoxicity with other **aminoglycosides** and **loop diuretics**. ↑ risk of hypokalemia and hypomagnesemia with **loop diuretics** and **amphotericin B**. May ↓ **phenytoin** levels and effectiveness. ↑ bone marrow depression with other **antineoplastics** or **radiation therapy**. May ↓ antibody response to **live-virus vaccines** and ↑ adverse reactions.

Route/Dosage
IV (Adults): *Metastatic testicular tumors:* 20 mg/m² daily for 5 days repeated every 3–4 wk. *Metastatic ovarian cancer:* 75–100 mg/m², repeat every 4 wk in

combination with cyclophosphamide *or* 100 mg/m^2 every 3 wk if used as a single agent. *Advanced bladder cancer:* 50–70 mg/m^2 every 3–4 wk as a single agent.

Availability (generic available)
Solution for injection: 1 mg/mL.

NURSING IMPLICATIONS
Assessment
* Monitor vital signs frequently during administration. Report significant changes.
* Monitor intake and output and specific gravity frequently during therapy. To reduce risk of nephrotoxicity, maintain urinary output of at least 100 mL/hr for 4 hr before initiating and for at least 24 hr after administration.
* Encourage patient to drink 2000–3000 mL/day of water to promote excretion of uric acid. Allopurinol and alkalinization of urine may be used to help prevent uric acid nephropathy.
* Assess patency of IV site frequently during therapy. Cisplatin may cause severe irritation and necrosis of tissue if extravasation occurs. If a large amount of highly concentrated cisplatin solution extravasates, mix 4 mL of 10% sodium thiosulfate with 6 mL of sterile water or 1.6 mL of 25% sodium thiosulfate with 8.4 mL of sterile water and inject 1–4 mL (1 mL for each mL extravasated) through existing line or cannula. Inject SUBQ if needle has been removed. Sodium thiosulfate inactivates cisplatin.
* Severe and protracted nausea and vomiting usually occur 1–4 hr after a dose; vomiting may last for 24 hr. Administer parenteral antiemetic agents 30–45 min before therapy and routinely around the clock for the next 24 hr. Monitor amount of emesis and notify health care professional if emesis exceeds guidelines to prevent dehydration. Nausea and anorexia may persist for up to 1 wk.
* Monitor for bone marrow depression. Assess for bleeding (bleeding gums, bruising, petechiae, stools, urine, and emesis) and avoid IM injections and taking rectal temperatures if platelet count is low. Apply pressure to venipuncture sites for 10 min. Assess for signs of infection during neutropenia. Anemia may occur. Monitor for increased fatigue, dyspnea, and orthostatic hypotension.
* Monitor for signs of anaphylaxis (facial edema, wheezing, dizziness, fainting, tachycardia, hypotension). Discontinue medication immediately and report symptoms. Epinephrine and resuscitation equipment should be readily available.
* Medication may cause ototoxicity and neurotoxicity. Assess patient frequently for dizziness, tinnitus, hearing loss, loss of coordination, loss of taste, or numbness and tingling of extremities; may be irreversible. Notify health care professional promptly if these occur. Audiometry should be performed before initiation of therapy and before subsequent doses. Hearing loss is more frequent with children and usually

occurs first with high frequencies and may be unilateral or bilateral.
* Monitor for inadvertent cisplatin overdose. Doses >100 m g/m^2/cycle once every 3–4 wk are rarely used. Differentiate daily doses from total dose/cycle. Symptoms of high cumulative doses include muscle cramps (localized, painful involuntary skeletal muscle contractions of sudden onset and short duration) and are usually associated with advanced stages of peripheral neuropathy.
* Monitor for signs of RPLS (headache, seizure, lethargy, confusion, blindness). Hypertension may or may not be present. May occur within 16 hr to 1 yr of initiation of therapy. Treat hypertension if present and discontinue cisplatin therapy. Symptoms usually resolve within days.

Lab Test Considerations
* Monitor CBC with differential and platelet count before and routinely throughout therapy. The nadir of leukopenia, thrombocytopenia, and anemia occurs within 18–23 days and recovery 39 days after a dose. Withhold further doses until WBC is >4000/mm^3 and platelet count is >100,000/mm^3.
* Monitor BUN, serum creatinine, and CCr before initiation of therapy and before each course of cisplatin to detect nephrotoxicity. May cause ↑ BUN and creatinine and ↓ calcium, magnesium, phosphate, sodium, and potassium levels that usually occur 2nd wk after a dose. Do not administer additional doses until BUN is <25 mg/dL and serum creatinine is <1.5 mg/dL. May cause ↑ uric acid level, which usually peaks 3–5 days after a dose.
* May cause transiently ↑ serum bilirubin and AST concentrations.
* May cause positive Coombs' test result.

Implementation
* *High Alert:* Fatalities have occurred with chemotherapeutic agents. Before administering, clarify all ambiguous orders; double-check single, daily, and course-of-therapy dose limits; have second practitioner independently double-check original order, calculations, and infusion pump settings.
* Do not confuse cisplatin with carboplatin. To prevent confusion, orders should include generic and brand names. Administer under supervision of a physician experienced in use of cancer chemotherapeutic agents.
* Solution should be prepared in a biologic cabinet. Wear gloves, gown, and mask while handling medication. If powder or solution comes in contact with skin or mucosa, wash thoroughly with soap and water. Discard equipment in specially designated containers.
* Hydrate patient with at least 1–2 L of IV fluid 8–12 hr before initiating therapy with cisplatin. Amifostine may be administered to minimize nephrotoxicity.
* Do not use aluminum needles or equipment during preparation or administration. Aluminum reacts

with this drug, forms a black or brown precipitate, and renders the drug ineffective.

- Unopened vials of powder and constituted solution must not be refrigerated.

IV Administration
- **Intermittent Infusion:** Solution should be clear and colorless; discard if turbid or if it contains precipitates.
- *Dilution:* Dilution in 2 L of 5% dextrose in 0.3% or 0.45% NaCl containing 37.5 g of mannitol is recommended. *Concentration:* Keep under 0.5 mg/mL to prevent tissue necrosis. *Rate:* Variable. Administer over 6–8 hr. Maximum rate 1 mg/min.
- **Continuous Infusion:** Has been administered as continuous infusion over 24 hr to 5 days with resultant decrease in nausea and vomiting. *High Alert:* Clarify dose to ensure cumulative dose is not confused with daily dose; errors may be fatal.
- **Y-Site Compatibility:** acyclovir, allopurinol, amikacin, aminophylline, amiodarone, ampicillin, ampicillin/sulbactam, anidulafungin, argatroban, azithromycin, aztreonam, bivalirudin, bleomycin, bumetanide, buprenorphine, butorphanol, calcium chloride, calcium gluconate, carmustine, caspofungin, cefazolin, cefotaxime, cefotetan, ceftazidime, ceftriaxone, cefuroxime, chlorpromazine, ciprofloxacin, cisatracurium, cladribine, clindamycin, cyclophosphamide, cyclosporine, cytarabine, dactinomycin, daptomycin, daunorubicin hydrochloride, dexamethasone, dexmedetomidine, dexrazoxane, digoxin, diltiazem, diphenhydramine, dobutamine, docetaxel, dopamine, doxorubicin, doxorubicin liposomal, doxycycline, droperidol, enalaprilat, ephedrine, epinephrine, epirubicin, ertapenem, erythromycin, esmolol, etoposide, etoposide phosphate, famotidine, fentanyl, filgrastim, fluconazole, fludarabine, fluorouracil, foscarnet, fosphenytoin, furosemide, ganciclovir, gemcitabine, gentamicin, glycopyrrolate, granisetron, haloperidol, heparin, hetastarch, hydrocortisone, hydromorphone, idarubicin, ifosfamide, imipenem/cilastatin, indomethacin, irinotecan, isoproterenol, ketorolac, labetalol, leucovorin calcium, levofloxacin, lidocaine, linezolid, lorazepam, magnesium sulfate, mannitol, melphalan, meperidine, meropenem, methotrexate, methylprednisolone, metoclopramide, metoprolol, metronidazole, midazolam, milrinone, mitomycin, mitoxantrone, moxifloxacin, nafcillin, naloxone, nicardipine, nitroglycerin, nitroprusside, norepinephrine, octreotide, ondansetron, oxaliplatin, paclitaxel, palonosetron, pamidronate, pemetrexed, pentamidine, pentobarbital, phenobarbital, phenylephrine, phenytoin, potassium acetate, potassium chloride, potassium phosphate, procainamide, prochlorperazine, promethazine, propofol, propranolol, remifentanil, rituximab, sargramostim, sodium acetate, sodium bicarbonate, sodium phosphate, succinylcholine, sufentanil, tacrolimus, theophylline, thiopental, tigecycline, tirofiban, tobramycin, topotecan, trastuzumab, vancomycin, vasopressin, vecuronium, verapamil, vinblastine, vincristine, vinorelbine, voriconazole, zidovudine, zoledronic acid.

- **Y-Site Incompatibility:** amifostine, amphotericin B deoxycholate, amphotericin B lipid complex, amphotericin B liposomal, cefepime, dantrolene, diazepam, insulin, regular, pantoprazole, piperacillin/tazobactam, thiotepa.

Patient/Family Teaching
- Instruct patient to report pain at injection site immediately.
- Instruct patient to notify health care professional promptly if fever; chills; cough; hoarseness; sore throat; signs of infection; lower back or side pain; painful or difficult urination; bleeding gums; bruising; petechiae; blood in stools, urine, or emesis; increased fatigue; dyspnea; or orthostatic hypotension occurs. Caution patient to avoid crowds and persons with known infections. Instruct patient to use soft toothbrush and electric razor and to avoid falls. Caution patient not to drink alcoholic beverages or take medication containing aspirin or NSAIDs; may precipitate gastric bleeding.
- Instruct patient to report promptly any numbness or tingling in extremities or face, difficulty with hearing or tinnitus, unusual swelling, or joint pain.
- Instruct patient not to receive any vaccinations without advice of health care professional.
- Emphasize the need for periodic lab tests to monitor for side effects.
- Rep: Advise females of reproductive potential to notify health care professional if pregnancy is planned or suspected or if breastfeeding. Advise patient of the need for contraception, although cisplatin may cause infertility.

Evaluation/Desired Outcomes
- Decrease in size or spread of malignancies. Therapy should not be administered more frequently than every 3–4 wk, and only if lab values are within acceptable parameters and patient is not exhibiting signs of ototoxicity or other serious adverse effects.

BEERS

⁂ **citalopram** (si-tal-oh-pram)
CeleXA
Classification
Therapeutic: antidepressants
Pharmacologic: selective serotonin reuptake inhibitors (SSRIs)

Indications
Depression. **Unlabeled Use:** Premenstrual dysphoric disorder. Obsessive-compulsive disorder. Panic disor-

der. Generalized anxiety disorder. Post-traumatic stress disorder. Social anxiety disorder (social phobia).

Action
Selectively inhibits the reuptake of serotonin in the CNS. **Therapeutic Effects:** Antidepressant action.

Pharmacokinetics
Absorption: 80% absorbed after oral administration.
Distribution: Enters breast milk.
Metabolism and Excretion: Mostly metabolized by the liver (10% by the CYP3A4 and CYP2C19 isoenzymes); ♀ the CYP2C19 isoenzyme exhibits genetic polymorphism (2% of Whites, 4% of Blacks, and 14% of Asians may be poor metabolizers and may have significantly ↑ citalopram concentrations and an ↑ risk of adverse effects). Excreted unchanged in the urine.
Half-life: 35 hr.

TIME/ACTION PROFILE (antidepressant effect)

ROUTE	ONSET	PEAK	DURATION
PO	1–4 wk	unknown	unknown

Contraindications/Precautions
Contraindicated in: Hypersensitivity; Concurrent use of MAO inhibitors or MAO-like drugs (linezolid or methylene blue); Concurrent use of pimozide; Congenital long QT syndrome, bradycardia, hypokalemia, hypomagnesemia, recent myocardial infarction, decompensated heart failure (↑ risk of QT interval prolongation); Concurrent use of QT interval prolonging drugs.
Use Cautiously in: History of mania; History of suicide attempt/ideation (↑ risk during early therapy and during dose adjustment); History of seizure disorder; Illnesses or conditions that are likely to result in altered metabolism or hemodynamic responses; Severe renal or hepatic impairment (maximum dose of 20 mg/day in patients with hepatic impairment); ♀ Poor CYP2C19 metabolizers (↑ risk of QT interval prolongation) (maximum dose of 20 mg/day); Concurrent use of CYP2C19 inhibitors (↑ risk of QT interval prolongation) (maximum dose of 20 mg/day); Angle-closure glaucoma; **OB:** Use during pregnancy only if potential maternal benefit justifies potential fetal risk; Lactation: Use while breastfeeding only if potential maternal benefit justifies potential risk to infant; Pedi: May ↑ risk of suicide attempt/ideation especially during early treatment or dose adjustment in children/adolescents; safety and effectiveness not established in children; Geri: Appears on Beers list. May worsen or cause syndrome of inappropriate antidiuretic hormone (SIADH) secretion and/or hyponatremia in older adults. Use with caution in older adults and closely monitor sodium concentrations when starting therapy or ↑ dose. Maximum dose of 20 mg/day in patients >60 yr.

Adverse Reactions/Side Effects
CV: QT interval prolongation, postural hypotension, tachycardia, TORSADES DE POINTES. **Derm:** sweating,

photosensitivity, pruritus, rash. **EENT:** abnormal accommodation. **Endo:** SIADH. **F and E:** hyponatremia. **GI:** ↑ salivation, abdominal pain, anorexia, diarrhea, dry mouth, dyspepsia, flatulence, nausea, altered taste, vomiting. **GU:** ↓ libido, amenorrhea, delayed/absent orgasm, dysmenorrhea, ejaculatory delay/failure, erectile dysfunction, polyuria. **Hemat:** BLEEDING. **Metab:** ↑ appetite, weight gain, weight loss. **MS:** arthralgia, myalgia. **Neuro:** apathy, confusion, drowsiness, insomnia, tremor, weakness, ↓ libido, ↑ depression, agitation, amnesia, anxiety, dizziness, fatigue, impaired concentration, migraine headache, NEUROLEPTIC MALIGNANT SYNDROME, paresthesia, SUICIDAL THOUGHTS. **Resp:** cough. **Misc:** fever, SEROTONIN SYNDROME, yawning.

Interactions
Drug-Drug: May cause serious, potentially fatal reactions when used with **MAO inhibitors**; concurrent use contraindicated; allow at least 14 days between citalopram and **MAO inhibitors**. Concurrent use with **MAO-inhibitor like drugs**, such as **linezolid** or **methylene blue**, may ↑ risk of serotonin syndrome; concurrent use contraindicated; do not start therapy in patients receiving **linezolid** or **methylene blue**; if linezolid or methylene blue need to be started in a patient receiving citalopram, immediately discontinue citalopram and monitor for signs/symptoms of serotonin syndrome for 2 wk or until 24 hr after last dose of linezolid or methylene blue, whichever comes first (may resume citalopram therapy 24 hr after last dose of linezolid or methylene blue). Concurrent use with **pimozide** may result in prolongation of the QT interval and is contraindicated. **QT interval prolonging drugs** may ↑ the risk of QT interval prolongation and torsades de pointes (concurrent use should be avoided). **CYP2C19 inhibitors,** including **cimetidine** may ↑ levels and the risk of toxicity (maximum dose = 20 mg/day). Drugs that affect serotonergic neurotransmitter systems, including **tricyclic antidepressants, SNRIs, fentanyl, lithium, buspirone, tramadol, meperidine, methadone, amphetamines,** and **triptans** (↑ risk of serotonin syndrome). Use cautiously with other **centrally acting drugs** (including **alcohol, antihistamines, opioid analgesics,** and **sedative/hypnotics;** concurrent use with **alcohol** is not recommended). Serotonergic effects may be ↑ by **lithium** (concurrent use should be carefully monitored). **Ketoconazole, itraconazole, erythromycin,** and **omeprazole** may ↑ levels. **Carbamazepine** may ↓ blood levels. May ↑ levels of **metoprolol.** Use cautiously with **tricyclic antidepressants** due to unpredictable effects on serotonin and norepinephrine reuptake. ↑ risk of bleeding with **NSAIDs, aspirin, clopidogrel, prasugrel, ticagrelor, dabigatran, apixaban, edoxaban, rivaroxaban,** or **warfarin.**
Drug-Natural Products: ↑ risk of serotonergic side effects including serotonin syndrome with **St. John's wort** and **SAMe.**

Route/Dosage

PO (Adults): 20 mg once daily initially, may be ↑ in 1 wk to 40 mg/day (maximum dose); *CYP2C19 poor metabolizers or concurrent use of CYP2C19 inhibitor:* Not to exceed 20 mg/day.

PO (Geriatric Patients): 20 mg once daily initially (not to exceed 20 mg/day in patients >60 yr).

Hepatic Impairment

PO (Adults): 20 mg once daily (not to exceed 20 mg/day).

Availability (generic available)

Capsules: 30 mg. **Tablets:** 10 mg, 20 mg, ✿ 30 mg, 40 mg. **Oral solution (peppermint flavor):** 10 mg/5 mL.

NURSING IMPLICATIONS

Assessment

● Screen patient for a personal or family history of bipolar disorder, mania, or hypomania before starting therapy; may precipitate a mixed/manic episode.
● Monitor mood changes during therapy.
● Assess for suicidal tendencies, especially during early therapy and dose changes. Restrict amount of drug available to patient. Risk may be increased in children, adolescents, and adults ≤24 yr. After starting therapy, children, adolescents, and young adults should be seen by health care professional at least weekly for 4 wk, every 3 wk for the next 4 wk, and on advice of health care professional thereafter.
● Assess sexual function before starting citalopram. Assess for changes in sexual function during treatment, including timing of onset; patient may not report.
● Assess for serotonin syndrome (mental changes [agitation, hallucinations, coma], autonomic instability [tachycardia, labile BP, hyperthermia], neuromuscular aberrations [hyperreflexia, incoordination], and/or GI symptoms [nausea, vomiting, diarrhea]), especially in patients taking other serotonergic drugs (SSRIs, SNRIs, triptans).

Lab Test Considerations

● Monitor electrolytes (potassium and magnesium) in patients at risk for electrolyte imbalances prior to and periodically during therapy.

Implementation

● Do not confuse with Celexa with Celebrex, Cerebyx, or Zyprexa. Do not confuse citalopram with escitalopram.
● **PO:** Administer as a single dose in the morning or evening without regard to food.

Patient/Family Teaching

● Instruct patient to take citalopram as directed. Take missed doses as soon as remembered unless almost time for next dose; do not double doses. Do not stop abruptly; may cause anxiety, irritability, high or low mood, feeling restless or changes in sleep habits, headache, sweating, nausea, dizziness, electric shock-like sensations, shaking, and confusion. Advise patient to read the *Medication Guide* prior to starting therapy and with each refill in case of changes.
● May cause drowsiness, dizziness, impaired concentration, and blurred vision. Caution patient to avoid driving and other activities requiring alertness until response to the drug is known.
● Instruct patient to notify health care professional of all Rx or OTC medications, vitamins, or herbal products being taken and to consult health care professional before taking any other Rx, OTC, or herbal products, especially alcohol or other CNS depressants, including opioids, and St. John's wort.
● Caution patient to change positions slowly to minimize dizziness.
● Advise patient, family, and caregivers to look for suicidality, especially during early therapy or dose changes. Notify health care professional immediately if thoughts about suicide or dying, attempts to commit suicide, new or worse depression or anxiety, agitation or restlessness, panic attacks, insomnia, new or worse irritability, aggressiveness, acting on dangerous impulses, mania, or other changes in mood or behavior or if symptoms of serotonin syndrome occur.
● Advise patient to use sunscreen and wear protective clothing to prevent photosensitivity reactions.
● Inform patient that frequent mouth rinses, good oral hygiene, and sugarless gum or candy may minimize dry mouth. If dry mouth persists for more than 2 wk, consult health care professional regarding use of saliva substitute.
● Inform patient that citalopram may cause symptoms of sexual dysfunction. In males, ejaculatory delay or failure, decreased libido, and erectile dysfunction may occur. In female patients, may result in decreased libido and delayed or absent orgasm. Advise patient to notify health care professional if symptoms occur.
● Rep: Instruct females of reproductive potential to notify health care professional if pregnancy is planned or suspected or if breastfeeding. If used during pregnancy, should be tapered during 3rd trimester to avoid neonatal serotonin syndrome and increased risk of maternal postpartum hemorrhage. Monitor infants exposed to citalopram for excess sedation, restlessness, agitation, poor feeding, poor weight gain, respiratory distress; may ↑ risk of persistent pulmonary hypertension of the newborn. Inform patient of pregnancy exposure registry that monitors pregnancy outcomes in women exposed to

✿= Canadian drug name. ⬚ = Genetic implication. S̶t̶r̶i̶k̶e̶t̶h̶r̶o̶u̶g̶h̶ = Discontinued. CAPITALS = life-threatening. <u>Underline</u> = most frequent.

antidepressants during pregnancy. Register patients by calling the National Pregnancy Registry for Antidepressants at 1-866-961-2388 or visiting online at https://womensmentalhealth.org/research/pregnancyregistry/antidepressants/.

- Emphasize the importance of follow-up exams to monitor progress.

Evaluation/Desired Outcomes

- Increased sense of well-being.
- Renewed interest in surroundings. May require 1–4 wk of therapy to obtain antidepressant effects.

---

clindamycin (klin-da-**mye**-sin)
Cleocin, Cleocin T, Clinda-Derm, ✣ Clinda-T, Clindagel, Clindesse, ~~Clindets~~, ✣ Dalacin C, ✣ Dalacin Vaginal, Xaciato
Classification
Therapeutic: anti-infectives

Indications
PO, IM, IV: Treatment of: Skin and skin structure infections, Respiratory tract infections, Septicemia, Intra-abdominal infections, Gynecologic infections, Osteomyelitis, Endocarditis prophylaxis. **Topical:** Severe acne. **Vag:** Bacterial vaginosis. **Unlabeled Use: PO, IM, IV:** Treatment of *Pneumocystis jiroveci* pneumonia, CNS toxoplasmosis, and babesiosis.

Action
Inhibits protein synthesis in susceptible bacteria at the level of the 50S ribosome. **Therapeutic Effects:** Bactericidal or bacteriostatic, depending on susceptibility and concentration. **Spectrum:** Active against most gram-positive aerobic cocci, including: Staphylococci, *Streptococcus pneumoniae*, other streptococci, but not enterococci. Has good activity against those anaerobic bacteria that cause bacterial vaginosis, including *Bacteroides fragilis*, *Gardnerella vaginalis*, *Mobiluncus* spp., *Mycoplasma hominis*, and *Corynebacterium*. Also active against *Pneumocystis jirovecii*, *Propionibacterium acnes*, and *Toxoplasma gondii*.

Pharmacokinetics
Absorption: Well absorbed following PO/IM administration. Minimal absorption following topical/vaginal use.
Distribution: Widely distributed. Does not significantly cross blood-brain barrier. Crosses the placenta; enters breast milk.
Protein Binding: 94%.
Metabolism and Excretion: Mostly metabolized by the liver by the CYP3A4 isoenzyme.
Half-life: *Neonates:* 3.6–8.7 hr; *Infants up to 1 yr:* 3 hr; *Children and adults:* 2–3 hr.

TIME/ACTION PROFILE (plasma concentrations)

ROUTE	ONSET	PEAK	DURATION
PO	rapid	60 min	6–8 hr
IM	rapid	1–3 hr	6–8 hr
IV	rapid	end of infusion	6–8 hr

Contraindications/Precautions
Contraindicated in: Hypersensitivity; Regional enteritis or ulcerative colitis (topical foam); Previous *Clostridioides difficile*-associated diarrhea (CDAD); Severe hepatic impairment; Diarrhea; Known alcohol intolerance (topical solution, suspension).
Use Cautiously in: OB: Safety not established in pregnancy for topical administration; systemic administration during 2nd and 3rd trimesters not associated with ↑ risk of congenital abnormalities; approved for vaginal use in 3rd trimester of pregnancy; injection contains benzyl alcohol which can cross placenta; Lactation: Use while breastfeeding only if potential maternal benefit justifies potential risk to infant; Pedi: Injection contains benzyl alcohol which can cause gasping syndrome in infants and neonates.

Adverse Reactions/Side Effects
CV: arrhythmias, hypotension. **Derm:** DRUG REACTION WITH EOSINOPHILIA AND SYSTEMIC SYMPTOMS (DRESS), ERYTHEMA MULTIFORME, rash, STEVENS-JOHNSON SYNDROME, TOXIC EPIDERMAL NECROLYSIS, urticaria. **GI:** diarrhea, CDAD, bitter or metallic taste, nausea, vomiting. **Local:** local irritation (topical products), phlebitis at IV site. **Neuro:** dizziness, headache, vertigo. **Misc:** HYPERSENSITIVITY REACTIONS (including anaphylaxis).

Interactions
Drug-Drug: May enhance the neuromuscular blocking action of other **neuromuscular blocking agents**. **CYP3A4 inhibitors** may ↑ levels. **CYP3A4 inducers**, including **rifampin**, may ↓ levels and lead to therapeutic failure. **Topical:** Concurrent use with **irritants, abrasives**, or **desquamating agents** may result in additive irritation.

Route/Dosage
PO (Adults): *Most infections:* 150–450 mg every 6 hr. *Pneumocystis jiroveci pneumonia:* 1200–1800 mg/day in divided doses with 15–30 mg primaquine/day (unlabeled). *CNS toxoplasmosis:* 1200–2400 mg/day in divided doses with pyrimethamine 50–100 mg/day (unlabeled); *Bacterial endocarditis prophylaxis:* 600 mg 1 hr before procedure.
PO (Children >1 mo): 10–30 mg/kg/day divided every 6–8 hr; maximum dose 1.8 g/day. *Bacterial endocarditis prophylaxis:* 20 mg/kg 1 hr before procedure.
IM, IV (Adults): *Most infections:* 300–600 mg every 6–8 hr *or* 900 mg every 8 hr (up to 4.8 g/day IV has been used; single IM doses of >600 mg are not recommended). *Pneumocystis jiroveci pneumonia:* 2400–

2700 mg/day in divided doses with primaquine (unlabeled). *Toxoplasmosis:* 1200–4800 mg/day in divided doses with pyrimethamine. *Bacterial endocarditis prophylaxis:* 600 mg 30 min before procedure.
IM, IV (Children >1 mo): 20–40 mg/kg/day (based on total body weight) divided every 6–8 hr; maximum dose: 4.8 g/day. *Bacterial endocarditis prophylaxis:* 20 mg/kg 30 min before procedure; maximum dose: 600 mg.
Vag (Adults and Adolescents): *Cleocin, Clindamax:* 1 applicatorful (5 g) at bedtime for 3 or 7 days (7 days in pregnant patients); *Clindesse:* one applicatorful (5 g) single dose; *or* 1 suppository (100 mg) at bedtime for 3 nights. *Xaciato:* one applicatorful (5 g) single dose.
Topical (Adults and Adolescents): *Solution:* 1% solution/suspension applied twice daily (range 1–4 times daily). *Foam, gel:* 1% foam or gel applied once daily.

Availability (generic available)
Capsules: 75 mg, 150 mg, 300 mg. **Oral solution:** 75 mg/5 mL. **Solution for injection:** 150 mg/mL. **Premixed infusion:** 300 mg/50 mL 0.9% NaCl, 600 mg/50 mL 0.9% NaCl, 900 mg/50 mL 0.9% NaCl. **Topical:** 1% lotion, gel, foam, solution, suspension, single-use applicators. **Vaginal cream:** 2%. **Vaginal gel:** 2%. **Vaginal suppositories (ovules):** 100 mg. *In combination with:* benzoyl peroxide (Acanya, Onexton), tretinoin (Veltin, Ziana); (see Appendix N).

NURSING IMPLICATIONS
Assessment
● Assess for infection (vital signs; appearance of wound, sputum, urine, and stool; WBC) at beginning of and during therapy.
● Obtain specimens for culture and sensitivity prior to initiating therapy. First dose may be given before receiving results.
● Monitor bowel elimination. Report diarrhea, abdominal cramping, fever, and bloody stools to health care professional promptly as a sign of CDAD). May begin up to several wk following the cessation of therapy.
● Assess patient for hypersensitivity (skin rash, urticaria).

Lab Test Considerations
● Monitor CBC; may cause transient ↓ in leukocytes, eosinophils, and platelets.
● May cause ↑ alkaline phosphatase, bilirubin, CK, AST, and ALT concentrations.

Implementation
● **PO:** Administer with a full glass of water. May be given with or without meals. Shake liquid preparations well. Do not refrigerate. Stable for 14 days at room temperature.

● **IM:** Inject undiluted. Do not administer >600 mg in a single IM injection.

IV Administration
● **Intermittent Infusion:** *Dilution:* Vials must be diluted before use. Dilute a dose of 300 mg or 600 mg in 50 mL and a dose of 900 mg or 1200 mg in 100 mL. Compatible diluents include D5W, 0.9% NaCl, D5/0.9% NaCl, D5/0.45% NaCl, or LR. Admixed solution stable for 16 days at room temperature. Premixed infusion is already diluted and ready to use. *Concentration:* Not to exceed 18 mg/mL. *Rate:* Infuse over 10–60 min. Not to exceed 30 mg/min. Hypotension and cardiopulmonary arrest have been reported following rapid IV administration.
● **Y-Site Compatibility:** acetaminophen, acyclovir, alemtuzumab, amifostine, amikacin, aminocaproic acid, aminophylline, amiodarone, amphotericin B lipid complex, amphotericin B liposomal, anakinra, anidulafungin, argatroban, arsenic trioxide, ascorbic acid, atropine, aztreonam, benztropine, bivalirudin, bleomycin, bumetanide, buprenorphine, butorphanol, calcium chloride, calcium gluconate, cangrelor, carboplatin, carmustine, cefazolin, cefotaxime, cefotetan, cefoxitin, ceftaroline, ceftazidime, cefuroxime, chloramphenicol, cisatracurium, cisplatin, cyanocobalamin, cyclophosphamide, cyclosporine, cytarabine, dacarbazine, dactinomycin, daptomycin, dexamethasone, dexmedetomidine, dexrazoxane, digoxin, diltiazem, diphenhydramine, dobutamine, docetaxel, dopamine, doxorubicin hydrochloride, doxorubicin liposomal, doxycycline, enalaprilat, ephedrine, epinephrine, epirubicin, epoetin alfa, eptifibatide, esmolol, etoposide, etoposide phosphate, famotidine, fentanyl, fludarabine, fluorouracil, folic acid, foscarnet, fosphenytoin, furosemide, gemcitabine, gemtuzumab ozogamicin, gentamicin, glycopyrrolate, granisetron, heparin, hetastarch, hydrocortisone, hydromorphone, ifosfamide, imipenem/cilastatin, indomethacin, insulin, regular, irinotecan, isoproterenol, ketamine, ketorolac, LR, leucovorin calcium, levofloxacin, lidocaine, linezolid, lorazepam, magnesium sulfate, mannitol, melphalan, meperidine, meropenem, mesna, methadone, methotrexate, methylprednisolone, metoclopramide, metoprolol, milrinone, morphine, multivitamins, nafcillin, nalbuphine, naloxone, nitroglycerin, nitroprusside, norepinephrine, octreotide, ondansetron, oxacillin, oxaliplatin, oxytocin, paclitaxel, palonosetron, pamidronate, pemetrexed, penicillin G, phenobarbital, phenylephrine, phytonadione, piperacillin/tazobactam, potassium acetate, potassium chloride, procainamide, propofol, propranolol, protamine, pyridoxine, remifentanil, rituximab, rocuronium, sargramostim, sodium acetate, sodium bicarbonate, succinylcholine, sufentanil, tacrolimus, theophylline, thiamine, thiotepa, tigecycline, tirofiban, tobramycin, vancomycin, vaso-

pressin, vecuronium, verapamil, vinblastine, vincristine, vinorelbine, voriconazole, zidovudine, zoledronic acid.
- **Y-Site Incompatibility:** allopurinol, azathioprine, caspofungin, ceftriaxone, chlorpromazine, dantrolene, daunorubicin hydrochloride, diazepam, filgrastim, ganciclovir, haloperidol, hydroxyzine, idarubicin, minocycline, mitomycin, mitoxantrone, mycophenolate, oritavancin, papaverine, pentamidine, pentobarbital, phentolamine, phenytoin, prochlorperazine, promethazine, topotecan, trastuzumab, trimethoprim/sulfamethoxazole.
- **Vag:** Applicators are supplied for vaginal administration. When treating bacterial vaginosis, concurrent treatment of male partner is not usually necessary.
- **Topical:** Contact with eyes, mucous membranes, and open cuts should be avoided during topical application. If accidental contact occurs, rinse with copious amounts of cool water.
- Wash affected areas with warm water and soap, rinse, and pat dry prior to application. Apply to entire affected area.

Patient/Family Teaching
- Instruct patient to take medication around the clock at evenly spaced times and to finish completely as directed, even if feeling better. Take missed doses as soon as possible unless almost time for next dose. Do not double doses. Advise patient that sharing of this medication may be dangerous.
- Instruct patient to notify health care professional immediately if diarrhea, abdominal cramping, fever, or bloody stools occur and not to treat with antidiarrheals without consulting health care professional.
- Advise patient to report signs of superinfection (furry overgrowth on the tongue, vaginal or anal itching or discharge).
- Notify health care professional if no improvement within a few days.
- Patients with a history of rheumatic heart disease or valve replacement need to be taught the importance of antimicrobial prophylaxis before invasive medical or dental procedures.
- Rep: Advise females of reproductive potential to notify health care professional if pregnancy is planned or suspected or if breastfeeding. Use with caution during 1st trimester. If breastfeeding, alternate drugs are preferred. If breastfeeding continued, monitor infant for diarrhea, thrush, and diaper rash.
- **IV:** Inform patient that bitter or metallic taste occurring with IV administration is not clinically significant.
- **Vag:** Instruct patient on proper use of vaginal applicator. Insert high into vagina at bedtime. Instruct patient to remain recumbent for at least 30 min following insertion. Advise patient to use sanitary napkin to prevent staining of clothing or bedding. Continue therapy during menstrual period.

- Advise patient to refrain from vaginal sexual intercourse during treatment.
- Caution patient that mineral oil in clindamycin cream may weaken latex or rubber contraceptive devices. Such products should not be used within 72 hr of vaginal cream.
- **Topical:** Caution patient applying topical clindamycin that solution is flammable (vehicle is isopropyl alcohol). Avoid application while smoking or near heat or flame.
- Advise patient to notify health care professional if excessive drying of skin occurs.
- Advise patient to wait 30 min after washing or shaving area before applying.

Evaluation/Desired Outcomes
- Resolution of the signs and symptoms of infection. Length of time for complete resolution depends on the organism and site of infection.
- Endocarditis prophylaxis.
- Improvement in acne vulgaris lesions. Improvement should be seen in 6 wk but may take 8–12 wk for maximum benefit.

clobetasol, See CORTICOSTEROIDS (TOPICAL/LOCAL).

clocortolone, See CORTICOSTEROIDS (TOPICAL/LOCAL).

BEERS

clonazePAM (kloe-na-ze-pam)
KlonoPIN, ✿Rivotril
Classification
Therapeutic: anticonvulsants
Pharmacologic: benzodiazepines

Schedule IV

Indications
Lennox-Gastaut, akinetic, or myoclonic seizures. Panic disorder with or without agoraphobia. **Unlabeled Use:** Uncontrolled leg movements during sleep. Neuralgias. Infantile spasms. Sedation. Adjunct management of acute mania, acute psychosis, or insomnia.

Action
Anticonvulsant effects may be due to presynaptic inhibition. Produces sedative effects in the CNS, probably by stimulating inhibitory GABA receptors. **Therapeutic Effects:** Prevention of seizures. Decreased manifestations of panic disorder.

Pharmacokinetics
Absorption: Well absorbed from the GI tract.
Distribution: Probably crosses the blood-brain barrier.

Protein Binding: 85%.
Metabolism and Excretion: Mostly metabolized by the liver.
Half-life: 18–50 hr.

TIME/ACTION PROFILE (anticonvulsant activity)

ROUTE	ONSET	PEAK	DURATION
PO	20–60 min	1–2 hr	6–12 hr

Contraindications/Precautions

Contraindicated in: Hypersensitivity to clonazepam or other benzodiazepines; Severe hepatic impairment.

Use Cautiously in: All patients (may ↑ risk of suicidal thoughts/behaviors); Angle-closure glaucoma; Obstructive sleep apnea; Chronic respiratory disease; History of porphyria; OB: Use late in pregnancy can result in sedation (respiratory depression, lethargy, hypotonia) and/or withdrawal symptoms (hyperreflexia, irritability, restlessness, tremors, inconsolable crying, and feeding difficulties) in neonates; Lactation: Use while breastfeeding only if potential maternal benefit justifies potential risk to infant; Pedi: Safety and effectiveness not established in children for panic disorder; Geri: Appears on Beers list. ↑ risk of cognitive impairment, delirium, falls, fractures, and motor vehicle accidents. If possible, avoid use in older adults.

Adverse Reactions/Side Effects

CV: palpitations. **Derm:** rash. **EENT:** diplopia, nystagmus. **GI:** constipation, diarrhea, hepatitis. **GU:** dysuria, nocturia, urinary retention. **Hemat:** anemia, eosinophilia, leukopenia, thrombocytopenia. **Metab:** weight gain. **Neuro:** ataxia, behavioral changes, drowsiness, fatigue, hypotonia, sedation, slurred speech, SUICIDAL THOUGHTS. **Resp:** ↑ secretions. **Misc:** fever, physical dependence, psychological dependence, tolerance.

Interactions

Drug-Drug: Use with **opioids** or other **CNS depressants**, including other **benzodiazepines, nonbenzodiazepine sedative/hypnotics, anxiolytics, general anesthetics, muscle relaxants, antipsychotics,** and **alcohol** may cause profound sedation, respiratory depression, coma, and death; reserve concurrent use for when alternative treatment options are inadequate. **Cimetidine, hormonal contraceptives, disulfiram, fluoxetine, isoniazid, ketoconazole, metoprolol, propranolol,** or **valproic acid** may ↓ metabolism and ↑ toxicity of clonazepam. May ↓ efficacy of **levodopa. Rifampin** or **barbiturates** may ↑ metabolism and ↓ effectiveness. Sedative effects may be ↓ by **theophylline.** May ↑ **phenytoin** levels. **Phenytoin** may ↓ levels.

Drug-Natural Products: Concomitant use of **kava-kava, valerian,** or **chamomile** can ↑ CNS depression.

Route/Dosage

PO (Adults): 0.5 mg 3 times daily; may ↑ by 0.5–1 mg every 3 days. Total daily maintenance dose not to exceed 20 mg. *Panic disorder:* 0.125 mg twice daily; ↑ after 3 days toward target dose of 1 mg/day (some patients may require up to 4 mg/day).
PO (Children ≤10 yr or ≤30 kg): Initial daily dose 0.01–0.03 mg/kg/day (not to exceed 0.05 mg/kg/day) given in 2–3 equally divided doses; ↑ by no more than 0.25–0.5 mg every 3 days until therapeutic blood levels are reached (not to exceed 0.2 mg/kg/day).

Availability (generic available)

Tablets: ✿ 0.25 mg, 0.5 mg, 1 mg, 2 mg. **Orally disintegrating tablets:** 0.125 mg, 0.25 mg, 0.5 mg, 1 mg, 2 mg.

NURSING IMPLICATIONS

Assessment

- Observe and record intensity, duration, and location of seizure activity.
- Assess degree and manifestations of anxiety and mental status (orientation, mood, behavior) prior to and periodically during therapy.
- Assess need for continued treatment regularly.
- Assess patient for drowsiness, unsteadiness, and clumsiness. These symptoms are dose related and most severe during initial therapy; may decrease in severity or disappear with continued or long-term therapy.
- Monitor closely for notable changes in behavior that could indicate the emergence or worsening of suicidal thoughts or behavior or depression.
- Assess risk for addiction, abuse, or misuse prior to administration and periodically during therapy.

Lab Test Considerations
- Patients on prolonged therapy should have CBC and liver function test results evaluated periodically. May cause an ↑ in serum bilirubin, AST, and ALT.
- May cause ↓ thyroidal uptake of ^{123}I, and ^{131}I.

Toxicity and Overdose
- Therapeutic serum concentrations are 20–80 mg/mL. Flumazenil antagonizes clonazepam toxicity or overdose (may induce seizures in patients with history of seizure disorder or who are on tricyclic antidepressants).

Implementation

- Do not confuse clonazepam with alprazolam, clonidine, clozapine, clobazam, or lorazepam. Do not confuse Klonopin with clonidine.
- Institute seizure precautions for patients on initial therapy or undergoing dose manipulations.
- **PO:** Administer with food to minimize gastric irritation. Tablets may be crushed if patient has difficulty swallowing. Administer largest dose at bedtime to avoid daytime sedation. Taper by 0.25 mg every 3

✿ = Canadian drug name. ⚇ = Genetic implication. ~~Strikethrough~~ = Discontinued. CAPITALS = life-threatening. <u>Underline</u> = most frequent.

days to decrease signs and symptoms of withdrawal. Some patients may require longer taper period (months).

- Orally disintegrating tablets should be left in the package until use. Remove from the blister pouch. Do not push tablet through the blister; peel open the blister pack with dry hands and place tablet on tongue. Tablet will dissolve rapidly and be swallowed with saliva. No liquid is needed to take the orally disintegrating tablet.
- Gradually taper to discontinue or reduce the dose to reduce risk of withdrawal reactions, increased seizure frequency, and status epilepticus. Taper by decreasing total daily dose on a weekly basis until discontinued. If patient develops withdrawal symptoms, pause taper or increase dose to previous tapered dose level; decrease dose more slowly. Some patients may require longer tapering period (weeks to >12 mo).

Patient/Family Teaching

- Instruct patient to take medication exactly as directed. Take missed doses within 1 hr or omit; do not double doses. Abrupt withdrawal of clonazepam may cause status epilepticus, tremors, nausea, vomiting, and abdominal and muscle cramps. Instruct patient to read the *Medication Guide* before starting and with each Rx refill; changes may occur.
- Advise patient that clonazepam is usually prescribed for short-term use and does not cure underlying problems.
- Advise patient that clonazepam is a drug with known abuse potential. Protect it from theft, and never give to anyone other than the individual for whom it was prescribed. Store out of sight and reach of children, and in a location not accessible by others.
- Advise patient to not share medication with others.
- May cause drowsiness or dizziness. Advise patient to avoid driving or other activities requiring alertness until response to drug is known.
- Instruct patient to notify health care professional of all Rx or OTC medications, vitamins, or herbal products being taken and to consult health care professional before taking any other Rx, OTC, or herbal products. Caution patient to avoid taking alcohol or other CNS depressants, including opioids, concurrently with this medication, may cause respiratory depression and overdose.
- Advise patient to notify health care professional of medication regimen prior to treatment or surgery.
- Instruct patient and family to notify health care professional of unusual tiredness, bleeding, sore throat, fever, clay-colored stools, yellowing of skin, or behavioral changes. Advise patient and family to notify health care professional if thoughts about suicide or dying, attempts to commit suicide; new or worse depression; new or worse anxiety; feeling very agitated or restless; panic attacks; trouble sleeping; new or worse irritability; acting aggressive; being angry or violent; acting on dangerous impulses; an extreme

increase in activity and talking; other unusual changes in behavior or mood occur.

- Rep: Advise females of reproductive potential to notify health care professional if pregnancy is planned or suspected or if breastfeeding. Monitor infants exposed to clonazepam during 2nd and 3rd trimester or immediately prior to or during childbirth for decreased fetal movement and/or fetal heart rate variability, "floppy infant syndrome," dependence, sedation (respiratory depression, lethargy, hypotonia) and symptoms of withdrawal (hypertonia, hyperreflexia, hypoventilation, irritability, tremors, diarrhea, vomiting, restlessness, inconsolable crying, and feeding difficulties); may occur shortly after delivery up to 3 wk after birth. Monitor breastfed infants for sedation, poor sucking, poor feeding and poor weight gain. Encourage pregnant patients to enroll in North American Antiepileptic Drug Pregnancy Registry to collect information about safety of antiepileptic drugs during pregnancy. To enroll, patients can call 1-888-233-2334 or visit http://www.aedpregnancyregistry.org/.
- Patient on anticonvulsant therapy should carry identification at all times describing disease process and medication regimen.
- Emphasize the importance of follow-up exams to determine effectiveness of the medication.

Evaluation/Desired Outcomes

- Decrease or cessation of seizure activity without undue sedation. Dose adjustments may be required after several mo of therapy.
- Decrease in frequency and severity of panic attacks.
- Relief of leg movements during sleep.
- Decrease in pain from neuralgia.

BEERS

cloNIDine (klon-i-deen)
~~Catapres~~, Catapres-TTS, Duraclon, Kapvay, Nexiclon XR

Classification
Therapeutic: antihypertensives
Pharmacologic: adrenergics (centrally acting)

Indications
PO, Transdermal: Hypertension. **PO:** Attention-deficit hyperactivity disorder (ADHD) (as monotherapy or as adjunctive to stimulants) (Kapvay only). **Epidural:** Cancer pain unresponsive to opioids alone. **Unlabeled Use:** Opioid withdrawal. Neuropathic pain (as adjunctive treatment).

Action
Stimulates alpha-adrenergic receptors in the CNS, which results in decreased sympathetic outflow inhibiting cardioacceleration and vasoconstriction centers. Prevents pain signal transmission to the CNS by stimulating alpha-adrenergic receptors in the spinal cord. **Therapeutic Effects:** Decreased BP. Decreased pain. Improved ADHD symptoms.

C

Pharmacokinetics

Absorption: Well absorbed from the GI tract and skin. Enters systemic circulation following epidural use.

Distribution: Widely distributed; enters CNS. Crosses the placenta readily; enters breast milk in high concentrations.

Metabolism and Excretion: Mostly metabolized by the liver; 40–60% eliminated unchanged in urine.

Half-life: *Neonates:* 44–72 hr; *Children:* 8–12 hr; *Adults: Plasma:* 12–16 hr (↑ in renal impairment); *CNS:* 1.3 hr.

TIME/ACTION PROFILE (PO, TD = antihypertensive effect; epidural = analgesia)

ROUTE	ONSET	PEAK	DURATION
PO	30–60 min	1–3 hr	8–12 hr
Transdermal	2–3 days	unknown	7 days†
Epidural	unknown	unknown	unknown

†8 hr following removal of patch.

Contraindications/Precautions

Contraindicated in: Hypersensitivity; *Epidural:* injection site infection, anticoagulant therapy, or bleeding problems.

Use Cautiously in: Serious cardiac or cerebrovascular disease; Renal impairment; OB: Use during pregnancy only if potential maternal benefit justifies potential fetal risk; Lactation: Use while breastfeeding only if potential maternal benefit justifies potential risk to infant; Pedi: Safety and efficacy not established in children <6 yr (ADHD); evaluation for cardiac disease should precede initiation of therapy for ADHD in children; Geri: Appears on Beers list. ↑ risk of CNS effects, orthostatic hypotension, and bradycardia in older adults. Avoid use as first-line treatment of hypertension in older adults.

Adverse Reactions/Side Effects

CV: bradycardia, heart block, hypotension (↑ with epidural), palpitations. **Derm:** rash, sweating. **EENT:** dry eyes. **F and E:** sodium retention. **GI:** dry mouth, constipation, nausea, vomiting. **GU:** ↓ fertility, erectile dysfunction. **Metab:** weight gain. **Neuro:** drowsiness, depression, dizziness, hallucinations, nervousness, nightmares, paresthesia.

Interactions

Drug-Drug: Additive sedation with **CNS depressants,** including **alcohol, antihistamines, opioid analgesics,** and **sedative/hypnotics.** Additive hypotension with other **antihypertensives** and **nitrates.** Additive bradycardia with **beta blockers, diltiazem, verapamil,** or **digoxin. MAO inhibitors, amphetamines,** or **tricyclic antidepressants** may ↓ antihypertensive effect. Withdrawal phenomenon may be ↑ by discontinuation of **beta blockers.** Epidural cloni-

dine prolongs the effects of epidurally administered **local anesthetics.** May ↓ effectiveness of **levodopa.**

Route/Dosage

PO (Adults and Children ≥12 yr): *Hypertension (immediate-release):* 0.1 mg twice daily, ↑ by 0.1–0.2 mg/day every 2–4 days until BP is controlled; usual maintenance dose is 0.2–0.6 mg/day in 2–3 divided doses (up to 2.4 mg/day). *Hypertension (extended-release):* 0.17 mg once daily, ↑ by 0.09 mg/day at weekly intervals until BP is controlled; usual maintenance dose is 0.17–0.52 mg/day. *Urgent treatment of hypertension (immediate-release):* 0.2 mg loading dose, then 0.1 mg every hr until BP is controlled or 0.8 mg total has been administered; follow with maintenance dosing; *Opioid withdrawal (immediate-release):* 0.3 mg–1.2 mg/day, may be ↓ by 50%/day for 3 days, then discontinued or ↓ by 0.1–0.2 mg/day.

PO (Geriatric Patients): *Hypertension (immediate-release):* 0.1 mg at bedtime initially, ↑ as needed.

PO (Children): *Hypertension (immediate-release):* Initial 5–10 mcg/kg/day divided into 2 or 3 doses, then ↑ gradually to 5–25 mcg/kg/day in divided doses every 6 hr; maximum dose: 0.9 mg/day. *ADHD (Kapvay-extended release) (children >6 yr):* 0.1 mg once daily at bedtime; after 1 wk, ↑ dose to 0.1 mg in AM and at bedtime; after 1 wk, ↑ dose to 0.1 mg in AM and 0.2 mg at bedtime; after 1 wk, ↑ dose to 0.2 mg in AM and at bedtime (max dose = 0.4 mg/day). *ADHD (Immediate-release) (children >6 yr, <45 kg):* 0.05 mg once daily at bedtime; then ↑ every 3–7 days to 0.05 mg twice daily; then 0.05 mg 3 times daily; then 0.05 mg 4 times daily. *Neuropathic pain (immediate-release):* 2 mcg/kg/dose every 4–6 hr then ↑ gradually over days up to 4 mcg/kg/dose every 4–6 hr.

PO (Neonates): *Neonatal abstinence syndrome:* 0.5–1 mcg/kg/dose every 4–6 hr. Once stabilized taper by 0.25 mcg/kg/dose every 6 hr.

Transdermal (Adults): *Hypertension:* Transdermal system delivering 0.1–0.3 mg/24 hr applied every 7 days. Initiate with 0.1 mg/24 hr system; dosage increments may be made every 1–2 wk when system is changed.

Transdermal (Children): Once stable oral dose is reached, children may be switched to a transdermal system equivalent closest to the total daily oral dose.

Epidural (Adults): 30 mcg/hr initially; titrated according to need.

Epidural (Children): 0.5 mcg/kg/hr initially; titrated according to need up to 2 mcg/kg/hr.

Availability (generic available)

Immediate-release tablets: ✤ 0.025 mg, 0.1 mg, 0.2 mg, 0.3 mg. **Extended-release tablets (Kapvay):** 0.1 mg. **Extended-release tablets (Nexiclon XR):** 0.17 mg, 0.26 mg. **Solution for epidural injection (Duraclon):** 100 mcg/mL, 500 mcg/mL. **Trans-**

✤ = Canadian drug name. ▓ = Genetic implication. ~~Strikethrough~~ = Discontinued. CAPITALS = life-threatening. <u>Underline</u> = most frequent.

dermal systems: 0.1 mg/24 hr, 0.2 mg/24 hr, 0.3 mg/24 hr.

NURSING IMPLICATIONS

Assessment

- **Hypertension:** Monitor intake and output ratios and daily weight, and assess for edema daily, especially at beginning of therapy.
- Monitor BP and pulse prior to starting, frequently during initial dose adjustment and dose increases and periodically during therapy. Titrate slowly in patients with cardiac conditions or those taking other sympatholytic drugs. Report significant changes.
- **Pain:** Assess location, character, and intensity of pain prior to, frequently during first few days, and routinely during administration.
- Monitor for fever as potential sign of catheter infection.
- **Opioid Withdrawal:** Monitor patient for signs and symptoms of opioid withdrawal (tachycardia, fever, runny nose, diarrhea, sweating, nausea, vomiting, irritability, stomach cramps, shivering, unusually large pupils, weakness, difficulty sleeping, gooseflesh).
- **ADHD:** Assess attention span, impulse control, and interactions with others.

Lab Test Considerations

- May cause transient ↑ in blood glucose levels.
- May cause ↓ urinary catecholamine and vanillylmandelic acid (VMA) concentrations; these may ↑ on abrupt withdrawal.
- May cause weakly positive Coombs' test result.

Implementation

- Do not confuse clonidine with clonazepam (Klonopin) or clozapine.
- Do not substitute between clonidine products on a mg-per-mg basis, because of differing pharmacokinetic profiles.
- In the perioperative setting, continue clonidine up to 4 hr prior to surgery and resume as soon as possible thereafter. Do not interrupt *transdermal clonidine* during surgery. Monitor BP carefully.
- **PO:** Administer last dose of the day at bedtime. May be taken without regard for food.
- *DNC:* Swallow extended-release tablets whole; do not crush, break, or chew.
- **Transdermal:** Transdermal system should be applied once every 7 days. May be applied to any hairless site; avoid cuts or calluses. Absorption is greater when placed on chest or upper arm and decreased when placed on thigh. Rotate sites. Wash area with soap and water; dry thoroughly before application. Apply firm pressure over patch to ensure contact with skin, especially around edges. Remove old system and discard. System includes a protective adhesive overlay to be applied over medication patch to ensure adhesion, should medication patch loosen.
- **Epidural:** Dilute 500 mcg/mL with 0.9% NaCl for a concentration of 100 mcg/mL. Do not administer solutions that are discolored or contain a precipitate. Discard unused portion.

Patient/Family Teaching

- Instruct patient to take clonidine at the same time each day, even if feeling well. Take missed dose as soon as remembered. If dose of extended-release product is missed, omit dose and take next dose as scheduled. Do not take more than the prescribed daily dose in any 24 hr. If more than 1 oral dose in a row is missed or if transdermal system is late in being changed by 3 or more days, consult health care professional. All routes of clonidine should be gradually discontinued over 2–4 days to prevent rebound hypertension. Advise patients taking oral and transdermal forms to read *Patient Information* before starting and with each Rx refill in case of changes.
- Advise patient to make sure enough medication is available for weekends, holidays, and vacations. A written prescription may be kept in wallet in case of emergency.
- May cause drowsiness, which usually diminishes with continued use. Advise patient to avoid driving or other activities requiring alertness until response to medication is known.
- Caution patient to avoid sudden changes in position to decrease orthostatic hypotension. Use of alcohol, standing for long periods, exercising, and hot weather may increase orthostatic hypotension.
- If dry mouth occurs, frequent mouth rinses, good oral hygiene, and sugarless gum or candy may decrease effect. If dry mouth continues for more than 2 wk, consult health care professional.
- Caution patients with contact lenses that clonidine may cause dryness of eyes.
- Caution patient to avoid concurrent use of alcohol or other CNS depressants, including opioids, with this medication.
- Instruct patient to notify health care professional of all Rx or OTC medications, vitamins, or herbal products being taken and to consult health care professional before taking any other Rx, OTC, or herbal products, especially cough, cold, or allergy remedies.
- Advise patient to notify health care professional of medication regimen prior to treatment or surgery.
- Advise patient to notify health care professional if itching or redness of skin (with transdermal patch), mental depression, swelling of feet and lower legs, paleness or cold feeling in fingertips or toes, or vivid dreams or nightmares occur. May require discontinuation of therapy, especially with depression.
- **Hypertension:** Encourage patient to comply with additional interventions for hypertension (weight reduction, low-sodium diet, discontinuation of smoking, moderation of alcohol consumption, regular exercise, and stress management). Medication helps control but does not cure hypertension.

- Instruct patient and family on proper technique for BP monitoring. Advise them to check BP at least weekly and report significant changes.
- **Transdermal:** Instruct patient on proper application of transdermal system. Do not cut or trim unit. Transdermal system can remain in place during bathing or swimming.
- Advise patient referred for MRI test to discuss patch with referring health care professional and MRI facility to determine if removal of patch is necessary prior to test and for directions for replacing patch.
- Pedi: Advise parents to notify school nurse of medication regimen.
- Rep: Advise females of reproductive potential to notify health care professional if pregnancy is planned or suspected or if breastfeeding. Monitor breastfeeding infants exposed to *Kapvay* through breast milk for symptoms of hypotension and/or bradycardia such as sedation, lethargy, tachypnea, and poor feeding. May impair female and male fertility. There is a pregnancy exposure registry that monitors pregnancy outcomes in women exposed to ADHD medications during pregnancy. Register patients by calling the National Pregnancy Registry for ADHD Medications at 1-866-961-2388 or visiting https://womensmentalhealth.org/adhd-medications/.

Evaluation/Desired Outcomes

- Decrease in BP.
- Decrease in severity of pain.
- Decrease in the signs and symptoms of opioid withdrawal.
- Improved attention span and social interactions in ADHD.

※ clopidogrel (kloh-pid-oh-grel)
Plavix
Classification
Therapeutic: antiplatelet agents
Pharmacologic: platelet aggregation inhibitors

Indications
Acute coronary syndrome (ST-segment elevation MI, non-ST-segment elevation MI, or unstable angina). Patients with established peripheral arterial disease, recent MI, or recent stroke.

Action
Inhibits platelet aggregation by irreversibly inhibiting the binding of ATP to platelet receptors. **Therapeutic Effects:** Reduction in risk of MI and stroke.

Pharmacokinetics
Absorption: Well absorbed following oral administration; rapidly metabolized to an active antiplatelet compound. Parent drug has no antiplatelet activity.
Distribution: Unknown.

Protein Binding: *Clopidogrel:* 98%; *active metabolite:* 94%.
Metabolism and Excretion: Rapidly and extensively converted by the liver via the CYP2C19 isoenzyme to its active metabolite, which is then eliminated 50% in urine and 45% in feces; ※ 2% of Whites, 4% of Blacks, and 14% of Asians have CYP2C19 genotype that results in reduced metabolism of clopidogrel (poor metabolizers) into its active metabolite (may result in ↓ antiplatelet effects).
Half-life: 6 hr (active metabolite 30 min).

TIME/ACTION PROFILE (effects on platelet function)

ROUTE	ONSET	PEAK	DURATION
PO	within 24 hr	3–7 days	5 days†

†Following discontinuation.

Contraindications/Precautions
Contraindicated in: Hypersensitivity to clopidogrel or prasugrel; Pathologic bleeding (peptic ulcer, intracranial hemorrhage); Concurrent use of omeprazole or esomeprazole; ※ CYP2C19 poor metabolizers.
Use Cautiously in: Patients at risk for bleeding (trauma, surgery, or other pathologic conditions); History of GI bleeding/ulcer disease; Severe hepatic impairment; Hypersensitivity to another thienopyridine (prasugrel); OB: Use should not be withheld, if needed for emergent treatment of stroke or MI during pregnancy. Discontinue use 5 to 7 days prior to labor, delivery, or neuraxial blockade, if possible, due to ↑ risk of maternal bleeding and hemorrhage; Lactation: Use while breastfeeding only if potential maternal benefit justifies potential risk to infant; Pedi: Safety and effectiveness not established in children.

Adverse Reactions/Side Effects
CV: chest pain, edema, hypertension. **Derm:** ACUTE GENERALIZED EXANTHEMATOUS PUSTULOSIS, DRUG RASH WITH EOSINOPHILIA AND SYSTEMIC SYMPTOMS, pruritus, purpura, rash, STEVENS-JOHNSON SYNDROME, TOXIC EPIDERMAL NECROLYSIS. **EENT:** epistaxis. **GI:** abdominal pain, diarrhea, dyspepsia, gastritis, GI BLEEDING. **Hemat:** BLEEDING, NEUTROPENIA, THROMBOTIC THROMBOCYTOPENIC PURPURA. **Metab:** hypercholesterolemia. **MS:** arthralgia, back pain. **Neuro:** depression, dizziness, fatigue, headache. **Resp:** cough, dyspnea, eosinophilic pneumonia. **Misc:** fever, HYPERSENSITIVITY REACTIONS (including anaphylaxis).

Interactions
Drug-Drug: Concurrent **eptifibatide, tirofiban, aspirin, dipyridamole, NSAIDs, heparin, LMWHs, thrombolytic agents, SSRIs, SNRIs,** or **warfarin** may ↑ risk of bleeding. **Strong CYP2C19 inducers,** including **rifampin,** may ↑ risk of bleeding; avoid concurrent use. May ↓ metabolism and ↑ effects of **phenytoin, repaglinide, tamoxifen, torsemide, fluvas-**

tatin, and many **NSAIDs**; avoid concurrent use with **repaglinide**. Concurrent use with the CYP2C19 inhibitors, **omeprazole**, or **esomeprazole** may ↓ antiplatelet effects; avoid concurrent use; may consider using **H₂ antagonist** or **pantoprazole**. **Opioids** may ↓ absorption of clopidogrel and its active metabolite and ↓ antiplatelet effects; consider using parenteral antiplatelet in patients with acute coronary syndrome if concurrent use of opioids needed.

Drug-Natural Products: ↑ bleeding risk with **anise**, **arnica**, **chamomile**, **clove**, **fenugreek**, **feverfew**, **garlic**, **ginger**, **ginkgo**, **Panax ginseng**, and others.

Route/Dosage

Recent MI, Stroke, or Peripheral Arterial Disease
PO (Adults): 75 mg once daily.

Acute Coronary Syndrome
PO (Adults): 300 mg initially, then 75 mg once daily; aspirin 75–325 mg once daily should be given concurrently.

Availability (generic available)
Tablets: 75 mg, 300 mg.

NURSING IMPLICATIONS

Assessment
- Assess patient for symptoms of stroke, peripheral vascular disease, or MI periodically during therapy.
- Monitor patient for signs of thrombotic thrombocytopenic purpura (thrombocytopenia, microangiopathic hemolytic anemia, neurologic findings, renal dysfunction, fever). May rarely occur, even after short exposure (<2 wk). Requires prompt treatment.

Lab Test Considerations
- Monitor bleeding time during therapy. Prolonged bleeding time, which is time- and dose-dependent, is expected.
- Monitor CBC with differential and platelet count periodically during therapy. Neutropenia and thrombocytopenia may rarely occur.
- May cause ↑ serum bilirubin, hepatic enzymes, total cholesterol, nonprotein nitrogen, and uric acid concentrations.

Implementation
- Do not confuse Plavix with Paxil or Pradaxa.
- Discontinue clopidogrel 5–7 days before planned surgical procedures. If clopidogrel must be temporarily discontinued, restart as soon as possible. Premature discontinuation of therapy may increase risk of cardiovascular events.
- **PO:** Administer once daily without regard to food.

Patient/Family Teaching
- Instruct patient to take medication exactly as directed. Take missed doses as soon as possible unless almost time for next dose; do not double doses.

Do not discontinue clopidogrel without consulting health care professional; may increase risk of cardiovascular events. Advise patient to read the *Medication Guide* before starting clopidogrel and with each Rx refill in case of changes.
- Advise patient to notify health care professional promptly if signs and symptoms of bleeding (unexpected bleeding or bleeding that lasts a long time; blood in urine [pink, red, or brown urine], red or black stools [looks like tar], bruises without known cause or get larger; cough up blood or blood clots; vomit blood or vomit looks like coffee grounds); fever, weakness, chills, sore throat, rash, unusual bleeding or bruising, extreme skin paleness, purple skin patches, yellowing of skin or eyes, or neurological changes occur.
- Advise patient to notify health care professional of medication regimen prior to treatment or surgery.
- Caution patient to avoid taking omeprazole or esomeprazole during therapy. Consult health care professional for other options.
- Instruct patient to notify health care professional of all Rx or OTC medications, vitamins, or herbal products being taken and to consult health care professional before taking any other Rx, OTC, or herbal products, especially those containing aspirin or NSAIDs or proton pump inhibitors.
- Rep: Advise females of reproductive potential to notify health care professional if pregnancy is planned or suspected, or if breastfeeding. Therapy should not be withheld because of potential concerns regarding effects of clopidogrel on the fetus. Use during labor or delivery increases risk of maternal bleeding and hemorrhage. Avoid neuraxial blockade during clopidogrel use due to risk of spinal hematoma. When possible, discontinue clopidogrel 5 to 7 days prior to labor, delivery, or neuraxial blockade.

Evaluation/Desired Outcomes
- Prevention of stroke, MI, and vascular death in patients at risk.

---

clotrimazole, See ANTIFUNGALS (TOPICAL).

---

clotrimazole, See ANTIFUNGALS (VAGINAL).

| BEERS REMS |

℞℞℞ cloZAPine (kloe-za-peen)
Clozaril, ~~FazaClo~~, Versacloz
Classification
Therapeutic: antipsychotics

Indications
Schizophrenia unresponsive to or intolerant of standard therapy with other antipsychotics (treatment re-

C

fractory). To reduce recurrent suicidal behavior in
schizophrenic patients.

Action

Binds to dopamine receptors in the CNS. Also has anticholinergic and alpha-adrenergic blocking activity.
Produces fewer extrapyramidal reactions and less tardive dyskinesia than standard antipsychotics but carries
high risk of hematologic abnormalities. **Therapeutic
Effects:** Diminished schizophrenic behavior. Diminished suicidal behavior.

Pharmacokinetics

Absorption: Well absorbed after oral administration.
Distribution: Rapid and extensive distribution;
crosses blood-brain barrier.
Protein Binding: 95%.
Metabolism and Excretion: Mostly metabolized
through the liver by the CYP1A2, CYP2D6, and CYP3A4
isoenzymes; ⚯ (the CYP2D6 enzyme system exhibits genetic polymorphism; ~7% of population may be poor
metabolizers and may have significantly ↑ clozapine
concentrations and an ↑ risk of adverse effects).
Half-life: 8–12 hr.

TIME/ACTION PROFILE (antipsychotic effect)

ROUTE	ONSET	PEAK	DURATION
PO	unknown	wk	4–12 hr

Contraindications/Precautions

Contraindicated in: Hypersensitivity; Bone marrow
depression; Severe CNS depression/coma; Uncontrolled
epilepsy; Clozapine-induced agranulocytosis or severe
granulocytopenia; Lactation: Lactation.
Use Cautiously in: Long QT syndrome; Risk factors
for QT interval prolongation or ventricular arrhythmias
(i.e., recent myocardial infarction, heart failure, arrhythmias); Concurrent use of CYP1A2, CYP2D6, or
CYP3A4 inhibitors or QT-interval prolonging drugs; Hypokalemia or hypomagnesemia; Presence/history of
constipation, urinary retention, or prostatic hypertrophy; Angle-closure glaucoma; Malnourished or dehydrated patients and patients with cardiovascular, cerebrovascular, hepatic, or renal disease, or patients on
antihypertensives (use lower initial dose, titrate more
slowly); Risk factors for stroke (↑ risk of stroke in patients with dementia); Diabetes; Seizure disorder; Patients at risk for falls; OB: Use during pregnancy only if
potential maternal benefit justifies potential fetal risk;
neonates at ↑ risk for extrapyramidal symptoms and
withdrawal after delivery when exposed during the 3rd
trimester; Pedi: Children <16 yr (safety and effectiveness not established); Geri: Appears on Beers list. ↑
risk of stroke, cognitive decline, and mortality in older
adults with dementia. Avoid use in older adults, except
for schizophrenia, bipolar disorder, or psychosis in
Parkinson's disease.

Adverse Reactions/Side Effects

CV: hypotension, tachycardia, bradycardia, CARDIAC AR-
REST, DEEP VEIN THROMBOSIS, HF, hypertension, MITRAL
VALVE INCOMPETENCE, MYOCARDITIS, QT interval prolon-
gation, syncope, TORSADES DE POINTES, VENTRICULAR AR-
RHYTHMIAS. **Derm:** rash, sweating. **EENT:** visual distur-
bances. **Endo:** hyperglycemia. **GI:** constipation, ↑
salivation, abdominal discomfort, dry mouth, GI ISCHE-
MIA/INFARCTION/NECROSIS, GI OBSTRUCTION, GI PERFORA-
TION, HEPATOTOXICITY, nausea, ulceration, vomiting.
GU: nocturnal enuresis. **Hemat:** AGRANULOCYTOSIS, LEU-
KOPENIA. **Metab:** hyperlipidemia, weight gain. **Neuro:**
dizziness, sedation, extrapyramidal reactions, NEURO-
LEPTIC MALIGNANT SYNDROME, SEIZURES. **Resp:** PULMO-
NARY EMBOLISM. **Misc:** fever.

Interactions

Drug-Drug: ↑ anticholinergic effects with other **anticholinergic drugs**, including **antihistamines**,
quinidine, disopyramide, and **antidepressants**;
avoid concurrent use. Concurrent use with strong
CYP1A2 inhibitors, including **fluvoxamine** or **ciprofloxacin** may ↑ levels; ↓ clozapine dose to ⅓ of the
original dose during concurrent use. Concurrent use
with moderate or weak **CYP1A2 inhibitors**, including
oral contraceptives or **caffeine** may ↑ levels; consider ↓ clozapine dose. Concurrent use with **CYP2D6
inhibitors** or **CYP3A4 inhibitors**, including **cimetidine, escitalopram, erythromycin, paroxetine,
bupropion, fluoxetine, quinidine, duloxetine,
terbinafine,** or **sertraline** may ↑ levels; consider ↓
clozapine dose. Concurrent use with **CYP1A2 inducers** or **CYP3A4 inducers**, including **nicotine, carbamazepine, phenytoin,** or **rifampin** may ↓ levels;
concurrent use with strong CYP3A4 inducers not recommended. ↑ CNS depression with **alcohol, antidepressants, antihistamines, opioid analgesics,** or
sedative/hypnotics. ↑ hypotension with **nitrates,**
acute ingestion of **alcohol,** or **antihypertensives.** ↑
risk of bone marrow suppression with **antineoplastics** or **radiation therapy.** Use with **lithium** ↑ risk of
adverse CNS reactions, including seizures. ↑ risk of QT
interval prolongation with other **QT interval prolonging agents.**
Drug-Natural Products: Caffeine-containing
herbs (**cola nut, tea, coffee**) may ↑ levels and side effects. **St. John's wort** may ↓ blood levels and efficacy.

Route/Dosage

PO (Adults): 12.5 mg 1–2 times daily initially; ↑ by
25–50 mg/day over a period of 2 wk to target dose
of 300–450 mg/day. May then be ↑ by up to 100 mg/
day once or twice weekly (not to exceed 900 mg/day).
Treatment should be continued for at least 2 yr in patients with suicidal behavior.

Availability (generic available)

Tablets (Clozaril): 25 mg, 50 mg, 100 mg, 200 mg.
Orally disintegrating tablets (mint): 12.5 mg, 25

mg, 100 mg, 150 mg, 200 mg. **Oral suspension (Versacloz):** 50 mg/mL.

NURSING IMPLICATIONS

Assessment

- Monitor patient's mental status (orientation, mood, behavior) before and periodically during therapy. Titrate slowly and monitor closely; may cause orthostatic hypotension, bradycardia, syncope, and cardiac arrest.
- Monitor BP (sitting, standing, lying) and pulse rate before and frequently during initial dose titration.
- Assess weight and BMI initially and periodically during therapy. Refer as appropriate for nutritional/weight management and medical management.
- Observe patient carefully when administering medication to ensure that medication is actually taken and not hoarded or cheeked.
- Monitor for signs of myocarditis (unexplained fatigue, dyspnea, tachypnea, fever, chest pain, palpitations, other signs and symptoms of heart failure, ECG changes, such as ST-T wave abnormalities, arrhythmias, or tachycardia during first mo of therapy). If these occur, clozapine should be discontinued and not restarted.
- Monitor patient for onset of akathisia (restlessness or desire to keep moving) and extrapyramidal side effects (*parkinsonian:* difficulty speaking or swallowing, loss of balance control, pill-rolling motion of hands, mask-like face, shuffling gait, rigidity, tremors and dystonic muscle spasms, twisting motions, twitching, inability to move eyes, weakness of arms or legs) every 2 mo during therapy and 8–12 wk after therapy has been discontinued. Notify health care professional if these symptoms occur; reduction in dose or discontinuation of medication may be necessary. Trihexyphenidyl or benzotropine may be used to control these symptoms.
- Monitor for possible tardive dyskinesia (uncontrolled rhythmic movement of mouth, face, and extremities; lip smacking or puckering; puffing of cheeks; uncontrolled chewing; rapid or worm-like movements of tongue). Report these symptoms immediately; may be irreversible.
- Monitor frequency and consistency of bowel movements and assess for symptoms of hypomotility (nausea, vomiting, abdominal distension, abdominal pain). Symptoms range from constipation to paralytic ileus; risk increased with use of other anticholinergic medications. Increasing bulk and fluids in the diet, and laxatives may help to minimize constipation. Prophylactic laxatives may be used for high-risk patients.
- Clozapine lowers the seizure threshold. Institute seizure precautions for patients with history of seizure disorder.
- Transient fevers may occur, especially during first 3 wk of therapy. Fever is usually self-limiting but may require discontinuation of medication. Also, monitor for development of neuroleptic malignant syndrome (fever, respiratory distress, tachycardia, seizures, diaphoresis, hypertension or hypotension, pallor, tiredness). Notify health care professional immediately if these symptoms occur.
- Assess respiratory status during therapy. If deep-vein thrombosis, acute dyspnea, chest pain, or other respiratory signs and symptoms occur, consider pulmonary embolism.
- Assess for falls risk. Drowsiness, orthostatic hypotension, and motor and sensory instability increase risk. Institute prevention if indicated.
- Monitor for signs and symptoms of hepatotoxicity (fatigue, malaise, anorexia, nausea, jaundice, hyperbilirubinemia, coagulopathy, hepatic encephalopathy). May require permanent discontinuation if combined with elevated transaminases.

Lab Test Considerations

- Monitor WBC, absolute neutrophil count (ANC), and differential count before starting therapy. ANC must be $\geq 1500/mm^3$ for the general population and $\geq 1000/mm^3$ for patients with documented Benign Ethnic Neutropenia (BEN) for patient to begin therapy. Monitor ANC weekly for the first 6 mo, then biweekly for the second 6 mo, then, if maintained within acceptable parameters, monthly after 12 mo. *If mild neutropenia (ANC 1000–1499/mm³) occurs,* continue therapy and monitor ANC 3 times/wk until ANC $\geq 1500/mm^3$. Once ANC $\geq 1500/mm^3$, return to patient's last ANC monitoring interval. *If moderate neutropenia (ANC 500–999/mm³) occurs,* recommend hematology consultation. Interrupt therapy for suspected clozapine-induced neutropenia. Resume therapy once ANC $\geq 1000/mm^3$. Monitor ANC daily until ANC $\geq 1000/mm^3$ then 3 times/wk until ANC $\geq 1500/mm^3$. Once ANC $\geq 1500/mm^3$, check ANC weekly for 4 wk, then return to patient's last ANC monitoring interval. *If severe neutropenia (<500/mm³) occurs,* recommend hematology consultation. Interrupt therapy for suspected clozapine-induced neutropenia. Do not rechallenge unless benefit outweighs risk. Monitor ANC daily until ANC $\geq 1000/mm^3$, then 3 times/wk until ANC $\geq 1500/mm^3$. If patient rechallenged, resume therapy as a new patient using normal monitoring once ANC $\geq 1500/mm^3$. For patients with **Benign Ethnic Neutropenia (BEN)**, obtain at least 2 baseline ANC levels before starting therapy. Monitor ANC weekly for the first 6 mo, then biweekly for the second 6 mo, then, if maintained within acceptable parameters, monthly after 12 mo. *If neutropenia (ANC 500–999/mm³) occurs,* recommend hematology consultation and continue therapy. Monitor ANC 3 times/wk until ANC $\geq 1000/mm^3$ or at patient's known baseline. Once ANC $\geq 1000/mm^3$, check ANC weekly for 4 wk, then return to patient's last ANC monitoring interval. *If severe neutropenia (<500/mm³) occurs,* recommend hematology consultation. Interrupt therapy for suspected clozapine-induced neutropenia. Do not rechallenge. Monitor ANC daily until ANC $\geq$500/mm³, then 3 times/wk until ANC $\geq$ patient's baseline. If patient rechallenged, resume therapy as a new patient using normal monitoring once ANC $\geq$1000/mm³ or at patient's baseline.

- Assess fasting blood glucose and cholesterol levels initially and throughout therapy.
- Monitor liver function tests periodically during therapy or if clinical signs of hepatotoxicity occur.

Toxicity and Overdose

- Overdose is treated with activated charcoal and supportive therapy. Monitor patient for several days because of risk of delayed effects.
- Avoid use of epinephrine and its derivatives when treating hypotension, and avoid quinidine and procainamide when treating arrhythmias.

Implementation

- Do not confuse clozapine with clonazepam or clonidine. Do not confuse Clozaril with Colazal.
- *REMS:* Because of the risk of severe neutropenia, clozapine is only available through a restricted program called *Clozapine REMS Program*. Health care professionals must be trained and certified to prescribe clozapine. Patients must be enrolled in the program and comply with ANC testing and monitoring requirements. Pharmacies dispensing clozapine must be trained and certified with program and must dispense only to patients eligible to receive clozapine.
- Discontinue therapy over 1–2 wk. For abrupt discontinuation unrelated to neutropenia, continue ANC monitoring for general population patients until ANC $\geq$1500/mm³ and for BEN patients until their ANC is $\geq$1000/mm³ or above their baseline. Monitor for recurrence of psychotic symptoms and symptoms related to cholinergic rebound (profuse sweating, headache, nausea, vomiting, diarrhea).
- When restarting clozapine in patients after even a brief interruption in therapy, dose must be reduced to minimize risk of hypotension, bradycardia, and syncope. If one day's dosing has been missed, resume treatment at 40% to 50% of the established dose. If two days dosing has been missed, resume dose at approximately 25% of established dosage. For longer interruptions, re-initiate with a dose of 12.5 mg once daily or twice daily. If these doses are well tolerated, the dose may be increased to previous dose more quickly than recommended for initial treatment.
- **PO:** Administer capsules with food or milk to decrease gastric irritation.
- Leave oral disintegrating tablet in blister until time of use. Do not push tablet through foil. Just before use, peel foil and gently remove disintegrating tablet. Immediately place tablet in mouth and allow to disintegrate and swallow with saliva. If ½ tablet dose used, destroy other half of tablet.
- Oral solution may be taken without regard to food. Shake bottle for suspension for 10 sec prior to withdrawing. Use oral syringes and oral adaptor provided for accurate dosing. Do not store dose in syringe; wash between doses.

Patient/Family Teaching

- Instruct patient to take medication as directed. If clozapine is stopped for >2 days, do not restart medication, notify health care professional for new dosing instructions. Patients on long-term therapy may need to discontinue gradually over 1–2 wk.
- *REMS:* Explain purpose and procedures of *Clozapine REMS Program* to patient.
- Inform patient of possibility of extrapyramidal symptoms. Instruct patient to report these symptoms immediately.
- Inform patient that cigarette smoking can decrease clozapine levels. Risk for relapse increases if patient begins or increases smoking.
- Advise patient to change positions slowly to minimize orthostatic hypotension. Protect from falls.
- May cause seizures and drowsiness. Caution patient to avoid driving or other activities requiring alertness while taking clozapine.
- Instruct patient to notify health care professional of all Rx or OTC medications, vitamins, or herbal products being taken and to consult health care professional before taking any other medications. Caution patient to avoid concurrent use of alcohol and other CNS depressants.
- Instruct patient to use frequent mouth rinses, good oral hygiene, and sugarless gum or candy to minimize dry mouth.
- Advise patient to notify health care professional of medication regimen before treatment or surgery.
- Instruct patient to notify health care professional promptly if unexplained fatigue, dyspnea, tachypnea, chest pain, palpitations, sore throat, fever, lethargy, weakness, malaise, constipation, or flu-like symptoms occur.
- Rep: May cause fetal harm. Advise females of reproductive potential to notify health care professional if pregnancy is planned or suspected, or if breastfeeding. Consider early screening for gestational diabetes if used during pregnancy. Neonates exposed to antipsychotic drugs during third trimester are at risk for extrapyramidal and/or withdrawal symptoms following delivery. Monitor neonates for symptoms of agitation, hypertonia, hypotonia, tremor, somnolence, respiratory distress, excessive sedation, and feeding difficulties. Monitor infants exposed to clozapine through breast milk for excessive sedation.
- Advise patient of need for continued medical follow-up for psychotherapy, eye exams, and laboratory tests.

Evaluation/Desired Outcomes

- Decreased positive symptoms (delusions, hallucinations) of schizophrenia.
- Decrease in negative symptoms (social withdrawal; flat, blunt affect) of schizophrenia.

⚠ **cobimetinib** (koe-bi-**me**-ti-nib)
Cotellic

Classification

Therapeutic: antineoplastics
Pharmacologic: kinase inhibitors

Indications

⚠ Metastatic/unresectable melanoma with the BRAF V600E or V600K mutation (in combination with vemurafenib). Histiocytic neoplasms.

Action

Inhibits the activity of mitogen-activated extracellular kinase (MEK) 1 and 2, which are enzymes that normally promote cellular proliferation. **Therapeutic Effects:** Decreased progression of melanoma and histiocytic neoplasms.

Pharmacokinetics

Absorption: 46% absorbed following oral administration.

Distribution: Extensively distributed to tissues.

Protein Binding: 95%.

Metabolism and Excretion: Mostly metabolized by the liver (via CYP3A4 enzyme system and glucuronidation). 6.6% excreted in feces unchanged; 20% excreted in urine (mostly as metabolites).

Half-life: 44 hr.

TIME/ACTION PROFILE (blood levels)

ROUTE	ONSET	PEAK	DURATION
PO	unknown	2.4 hr	unknown

Contraindications/Precautions

Contraindicated in: Concurrent use of strong or moderate CYP3A4 inhibitors or inducers; OB: Pregnancy; Lactation: Lactation.

Use Cautiously in: Left ventricular ejection fraction <50%; Severe renal impairment (CCr <30 mL/min); Rep: Women of reproductive potential; Pedi: Safety and effectiveness not established in children.

Adverse Reactions/Side Effects

CV: CARDIOMYOPATHY, hypertension. **Derm:** alopecia, erythema, photosensitivity, rash. **EENT:** retinopathy. **F and E:** hyperkalemia, hypocalcemia, hypokalemia, hyponatremia, hypophosphatemia. **GI:** diarrhea, hypoalbuminemia, nausea, stomatitis, vomiting, HEPATOTOXICITY. **GU:** ↑ serum creatinine, ↓ fertility. **Hemat:** anemia, HEMORRHAGE, lymphopenia, thrombocytopenia. **MS:** ↑ creatine kinase, RHABDOMYOLYSIS. **Misc:** fever, MALIGNANCY.

Interactions

Drug-Drug: Strong or moderate CYP3A4 inhibitors, including **itraconazole**, may ↑ levels; avoid concurrent use. Strong or moderate CYP3A4 inducers, including **carbamazepine**, **efavirenz**, **phenytoin**, and **rifampin**, may ↓ levels; avoid concurrent use.

Drug-Natural Products: St. John's wort may ↓ levels; avoid concurrent use.

Route/Dosage

PO (Adults): 60 mg once daily for days 1–21 of each 28-day cycle; continue until disease progression or unacceptable toxicity; *Concurrent short-term use of moderate CYP3A4 inhibitor:* 20 mg once daily; resume 60 mg once daily once 3A4 inhibitor discontinued (avoid use of strong or moderate CYP3A4 inhibitor if patient already taking reduced dose of 20–40 mg once daily).

Availability

Tablets: 20 mg.

NURSING IMPLICATIONS

Assessment

- Assess skin prior to starting therapy and every 2 mo during and for 6 mo following therapy for new lesions. If new lesions appear, evaluate and remove as needed. If Grade 2 (intolerable), Grade 3, or Grade 4 rash or other skin reactions occur, withhold or reduce dose.
- Monitor for bleeding and hemorrhage periodically during therapy. *If Grade 3 hemorrhage occurs,* hold therapy for up to 4 wk. If improved to Grade 0 or 1, resume at next lower dose. If not improved within 4 wk, permanently discontinue. *If Grade 4 hemorrhage occurs,* permanently discontinue therapy.
- Monitor left ventricular ejection fraction (LVEF) prior to initiation, 1 mo after initiation, and every 3 mo until discontinuation. *If asymptomatic, absolute ↓ LVEF from baseline of >10% and <institutional lower limit of normal (LLN),* hold therapy for 2 wk; repeat LVEF. *Resume at next lower dose if all of following are present:* LVEF is ≥LLN and absolute ↓ from baseline LVEF ≤10%. *Discontinue permanently if any of following are present:* LVEF is <LLN or absolute ↓ from baseline LVEF >10%. *If symptomatic LVEF ↓ from baseline,* hold therapy for up to 4 wk, repeat LVEF. *Resume at next lower dose if all of following are present:* symptoms resolve and LVEF is ≥LLN and absolute ↓ from baseline LVEF is ≤10%. *Discontinue permanently if any of following are present:* symptoms persist, or LVEF <LLN, or absolute ↓ from baseline LVEF >10%. If restarting cobimetinib after a dose reduction or interruption, evaluate LVEF at approximately 2 wk, 4 wk, 10 wk, and 16 wk, and as clinically indicated.
- Perform ophthalmological evaluations periodically during therapy and if patient reports new or worsen-

ing visual disturbances. *If serious retinopathy occurs,* hold therapy for up to 4 wk. If signs and symptoms improve, resume at next lower dose. If not improved or symptoms recur at lower dose within 4 wk, permanently discontinue. *If retinal vein occlusion occurs,* permanently discontinue therapy.

- Assess for photosensitivity during therapy. *If Grade 2 (intolerable), Grade 3, or Grade 4 photosensitivity occurs,* withhold therapy up to 4 wk. If improved to Grade 0 or 1, resume at next lower dose. If not improved within 4 wk, permanently discontinue.

Lab Test Considerations
- ⅜ Confirm presence of BRAF V600E or V600K mutation in tumor specimens starting therapy with cobimetinib with vemurafenib. Information on FDA-approved tests for the detection of BRAF V600 mutations in melanoma is available at: http://www.fda.gov/CompanionDiagnostics. May cause ↑ AST, ALT, alkaline phosphatase, and GGT. Monitor liver function tests before starting and monthly during therapy, and as clinically indicated. *For 1st occurrence of Grade 4 hepatotoxicity,* hold therapy up to 4 wk. If improved to Grade 0 or 1, resume at next lower dose. If not improved to Grade 0 or 1 within 4 wk, permanently discontinue. *If Grade 4 hepatotoxicity recurs,* discontinue therapy permanently.

- Obtain CK and serum creatinine levels at baseline and periodically during therapy. If Grade 4 CK ↑ or any CK ↑ and myalgia occur, hold therapy up to 4 wk. If improved to Grade 3 or lower, resume at next lower dose level. If not improved within 4 wk, permanently discontinue.

- May cause hypophosphatemia, hyponatremia, hypoalbuminemia, hypokalemia, hyperkalemia, and hypocalcemia.

- May cause anemia, lymphopenia, and thrombocytopenia.

Implementation
- Dose reduction guidelines: *1st dose reduction,* 40 mg once daily. *2nd dose reduction,* 20 mg once daily. *Subsequent modification,* discontinue therapy permanently if unable to tolerate 20 mg once daily.
- PO: Administer three 20-mg tablets once daily without regard to food.

Patient/Family Teaching
- Instruct patient to take cobimetinib as directed. If dose is missed or vomiting occurs after dose, do not repeat, take next dose as scheduled.
- Advise patient to notify health care professional immediately if skin changes (new wart, skin sore that bleeds or does not heal, change in size or color of mole), signs and symptoms of bleeding (blood in urine, red or black stools, unusual or excessive vagi-

nal bleeding, bleeding of gums, abdominal pain, headache, dizziness, feeling weak), cardiomyopathy (persistent coughing or wheezing, tiredness, shortness of breath, increased heart rate, swelling of ankles and feet), eye problems (blurred vision, halos, distorted vision, other vision changes, partly missing vision), liver injury (yellowing of skin or white of eyes, feeling tired or weak, dark or brown [tea color] urine, loss of appetite, nausea or vomiting), rhabdomyolysis (muscle aches, dark, reddish urine, muscle spasms, weakness), or rash occur.
- Advise patient to avoid sun exposure, wear protective clothing and use a broad-spectrum UVA/UVB sunscreen and lip balm (SPF ≥30) when outdoors. May require dose reduction or discontinuation.
- Advise patient to notify health care professional of all Rx or OTC medications, vitamins, or herbal products being taken and to consult with health care professional before taking other medications, especially St. John's wort.
- Rep: May cause fetal harm. Advise patient use effective contraception and avoid breastfeeding during and for at least 2 wk following therapy. May reduce fertility in females and males of reproductive potential.

Evaluation/Desired Outcomes
- Decrease in progression of melanoma and histiocytic neoplasms.

```
                              REMS   HIGH ALERT
```

⅜ codeine (koe-deen)
Classification
Therapeutic: allergy, cold, and cough remedies, antitussives, opioid analgesics
Pharmacologic: opioid agonists

Schedule II, III, IV, V (depends on content)

Indications
Mild to moderate pain. Antitussive (in smaller doses).

Action
Binds to opiate receptors in the CNS. Alters the perception of and response to painful stimuli while producing generalized CNS depression. Decreases cough reflex. Decreases GI motility. **Therapeutic Effects:** Decreased severity of pain. Suppression of the cough reflex.

Pharmacokinetics
Absorption: 50% absorbed from the GI tract.
Distribution: Widely distributed to tissues.
Metabolism and Excretion: Mostly metabolized by the liver via the CYP2D6 isoenzyme); 10% converted to morphine; ⅜ the CYP2D6 enzyme system exhibits genetic polymorphism (some patients [1–10% Whites,

---

✦ = Canadian drug name. ⅜ = Genetic implication. ~~Strikethrough~~ = Discontinued. CAPITALS = life-threatening. <u>Underline</u> = most frequent.

3% African Americans, 16–28% North Africans/Ethiopians/Arabs] may be ultra-rapid metabolizers and may have ↑ morphine concentrations and an ↑ risk of adverse effects); 5–15% excreted unchanged in urine. **Half-life:** 2.5–4 hr.

TIME/ACTION PROFILE (analgesia)

ROUTE	ONSET	PEAK	DURATION
PO	30–45 min	60–120 min	4 hr

Contraindications/Precautions

Contraindicated in: Hypersensitivity; Significant respiratory depression; Acute or severe bronchial asthma (in unmonitored setting or in absence of resuscitative equipment); Known or suspected GI obstruction (including paralytic ileus); Concurrent use of MAO inhibitors (or use within the past 14 days); ⚕ Ultra-rapid CYP2D6 metabolizers of codeine; Lactation: Lactation; Pedi: Children <12 yr, children <18 yr following tonsillectomy and/or adenoidectomy, and children 12–18 yr who are postoperative; have obstructive sleep apnea, obesity, or severe pulmonary disease, neuromuscular disease; or are taking other medications that cause respiratory depression (↑ risk of respiratory depression and death).

Use Cautiously in: Head trauma; ↑ intracranial pressure; Severe renal impairment; Severe hepatic impairment; Severe pulmonary disease; Hypothyroidism; Adrenal insufficiency; Alcoholism; Prostatic hyperplasia; Undiagnosed abdominal pain; OB: Has been used during labor; respiratory depression may occur in the newborn; Geri: Older adults may be more susceptible to CNS depression and constipation (dose ↓ required).

Adverse Reactions/Side Effects

CV: hypotension, bradycardia. **Derm:** flushing, sweating. **EENT:** blurred vision, diplopia, miosis. **GI:** constipation, nausea, vomiting. **GU:** urinary retention. **Neuro:** confusion, sedation, dysphoria, euphoria, floating feeling, hallucinations, headache, unusual dreams. **Resp:** RESPIRATORY DEPRESSION (including central sleep apnea [CSA] and sleep-related hypoxemia). **Misc:** physical dependence, psychological dependence, tolerance.

Interactions

Drug-Drug: MAO inhibitors ↑ risk of adverse reactions; concurrent use or use within previous 14 days contraindicated. Additive CNS depression with **alcohol**, **antidepressants**, **antihistamines**, **benzodiazepines**, and **sedative/hypnotics**. CYP3A4 inhibitors, including **erythromycin**, **clarithromycin**, **ketoconazole**, **itraconazole**, and **protease inhibitors** may ↑ levels and risk of respiratory depression. **CYP3A4 inducers** may ↓ levels and effectiveness. **CYP2D6 inhibitors**, including **amiodarone** and **quinidine** may ↓ analgesic effects. **Mixed agonist/antagonist analgesics**, including **nalbuphine** or **butorphanol** and **partial agonist analgesics**, including **buprenorphine**, may ↓ meperidine's analgesic effects and/or

precipitate opioid withdrawal in physically dependent patients. Drugs that affect serotonergic neurotransmitter systems, including **tricyclic antidepressants**, **SSRIs**, **SNRIs**, **MAO inhibitors**, **TCAs**, **tramadol**, **trazodone**, **mirtazapine**, **5–HT₃ receptor antagonists**, **linezolid**, **methylene blue**, and **triptans** ↑ risk of serotonin syndrome.

Drug-Natural Products: Concomitant use of **kava-kava**, **valerian**, **skullcap**, **chamomile**, or **hops** can ↑ CNS depression.

Route/Dosage

PO (Adults): *Analgesic:* 15–60 mg every 4 hr as needed (not to exceed 360 mg/day). *Antitussive:* 10–20 mg every 4–6 hr as needed (not to exceed 120 mg/day). *Antidiarrheal:* 30 mg up to 4 times daily.

Renal Impairment

(Adults): *CCr 10–50 mL/min:* Administer 75% of the dose; *CCr <10 mL/min:* Administer 50% of the dose.

Availability (generic available)

Tablets: 15 mg, 30 mg, 60 mg. **Oral solution:** ✦ 25 mg/5 mL.

NURSING IMPLICATIONS

Assessment

- Assess BP, pulse, and respirations before and periodically during administration. If respiratory rate is <10/min, assess level of sedation. Physical stimulation may be sufficient to prevent significant hypoventilation. Dose may need to be decreased by 25–50%. Initial drowsiness will diminish with continued use. Monitor for respiratory depression, especially during initiation or following dose increase; serious, life-threatening, or fatal respiratory depression may occur. May cause sleep-related breathing disorders (CSA, sleep-related hypoxemia).
- Assess bowel function routinely. Prevention of constipation should be instituted with increased intake of fluids, bulk, and laxatives to minimize constipating effects. Stimulant laxatives should be administered routinely if opioid use exceeds 2–3 days, unless contraindicated. Consider drugs for opioid induced constipation.
- Assess risk for opioid addiction, abuse, or misuse prior to administration.
- **Pain:** Assess type, location, and intensity of pain before and 1 hr (peak) after administration. When titrating opioid doses, increases of 25–50% should be administered until there is either a 50% reduction in the patient's pain rating on a numerical or visual analogue scale or the patient reports satisfactory pain relief. A repeat dose can be safely administered at the time of the peak if previous dose is ineffective and side effects are minimal.
- An equianalgesic chart (see Appendix I) should be used when changing routes or when changing from one opioid to another.
- Prolonged use may lead to physical and psychological dependence and tolerance. This should not pre-

vent patient from receiving adequate analgesia. Most patients who receive codeine for pain do not develop psychological dependence. If progressively higher doses are required, consider conversion to a stronger opioid.

- **Cough:** Assess cough and lung sounds during antitussive use.

Lab Test Considerations

- May cause ↑ plasma amylase and lipase concentrations.

Toxicity and Overdose

- If an opioid antagonist is required to reverse respiratory depression or coma, naloxone is the antidote. Dilute the 0.4-mg ampule of naloxone in 10 mL of 0.9% NaCl and administer 0.5 mL (0.02 mg) by IV push every 2 min. For children and patients weighing <40 kg, dilute 0.1 mg of naloxone in 10 mL of 0.9% NaCl for a concentration of 10 mcg/mL and administer 0.5 mcg/kg every 2 min. Titrate dose to avoid withdrawal, seizures, and severe pain.

Implementation

- ***High Alert:*** Accidental overdosage of opioid analgesics has resulted in fatalities. Before administering, clarify all ambiguous orders.
- Explain therapeutic value of medication before administration to enhance the analgesic effect.
- Regularly administered doses may be more effective than prn administration. Analgesic is more effective if given before pain becomes severe.
- Coadministration with nonopioid analgesics may have additive analgesic effects and permit lower doses.
- ***REMS:*** FDA strongly encourages health care professionals to complete a REMS-compliant education program that includes all the elements of the FDA Education *Blueprint for Health Care Providers Involved in the Management or Support of Patients with Pain,* available at www.fda.gov/OpioidAnalgesicREMSBlueprint. Information on programs can be found at 1-800-503-0784 or www.opioidanalgesicrems.com. Discuss availability of naloxone for emergency treatment of opioid overdose with the patient and caregiver and assess the potential need for access to naloxone, both when initiating and renewing therapy, especially if patient has household members (including children) or other close contacts at risk for accidental exposure or overdose. Consider prescribing naloxone, based on the patient's risk factors for overdose, such as concomitant use of CNS depressants, a history of opioid use disorder, or prior opioid overdose. However, the presence of risk factors for overdose should not prevent the proper management of pain in any patient. When combined with nonopioid analgesics (aspirin, acetaminophen) #2 = 15 mg, #3 = 30 mg, #4 = 60 mg codeine. Codeine as an individ-

ual drug is a Schedule II substance. In combination with other drugs, tablet form is Schedule III, and elixir or cough suppressant is Schedule V (see Appendix H).

- **PO:** Oral doses may be administered with food or milk to minimize GI irritation.
- If administered regularly for ≥1 wk, discontinue by tapering dose gradually by a small enough increment (no >10% to 25% of total daily dose) to avoid withdrawal symptoms, and proceed with dose-lowering at an interval of every 2 to 4 wk or longer. Monitor for withdrawal symptoms (restlessness, lacrimation, rhinorrhea, yawning, perspiration, chills, myalgia, mydriasis, irritability, anxiety, backache, joint pain, weakness, abdominal cramps, insomnia, nausea, anorexia, vomiting, diarrhea, increased blood pressure, respiratory rate, or heart rate) during taper. If withdrawal symptoms occur, it may be necessary to pause the taper for a period of time or raise the dose of the opioid analgesic to the previous dose, and then proceed with a slower taper. Monitor for changes in mood, emergence of suicidal thoughts, or use of other substances.

Patient/Family Teaching

- Instruct patient on how and when to ask for and take pain medication. Do not stop abruptly without consulting health care professional.
- Advise patient that codeine is a drug with known abuse potential. Protect it from theft, and never give to anyone other than the individual for whom it was prescribed.
- ***REMS:*** Instruct patient on risk of addiction, abuse, and misuse, which could lead to death. Discuss safe use, risks, and proper storage and disposal of opioid analgesics with patients and caregivers with each Rx. The Patient Counseling Guide is available at www.fda.gov/OpioidAnalgesicREMSPCG. Advise patient not to share codeine with others and to protect from theft or misuse.
- Advise patient that codeine is a drug with known abuse potential. Protect it from theft, and never give to anyone other than the individual for whom it was prescribed. Store out of sight and reach of children, and in a location not accessible by others.
- Educate patients and caregivers on how to recognize respiratory depression and emphasize the importance of calling 911 or getting emergency medical help right away in the event of a known or suspected overdose. Inform patients and caregivers about various ways to obtain naloxone as permitted by individual state naloxone dispensing and prescribing requirements or guidelines (by prescription, directly from a pharmacist, or as part of a community-based program).
- May cause drowsiness or dizziness. Advise patient to call for assistance when ambulating or smoking.

Caution ambulatory patient to avoid driving or other activities requiring alertness until response to medication is known.

- Advise patient to change positions slowly to minimize orthostatic hypotension.
- Caution patient to avoid concurrent use of alcohol or other CNS depressants with this medication.
- Encourage patient to turn, cough, and breathe deeply every 2 hr to prevent atelectasis.
- Advise patient that good oral hygiene, frequent mouth rinses, and sugarless gum or candy may decrease dry mouth.
- Rep: Advise patient to notify health care professional if pregnancy is planned or suspected, or if breastfeeding. Inform patient of potential for neonatal opioid withdrawal syndrome with prolonged use during pregnancy. Monitor neonate for signs and symptoms of withdrawal symptoms (irritability, hyperactivity and abnormal sleep pattern, high pitched cry, tremor, vomiting, diarrhea, and/or failure to gain weight); usually occur the first days after birth. Monitor infants exposed to codeine through breast milk for excess sedation and respiratory depression.

Evaluation/Desired Outcomes

- Decrease in severity of pain without a significant alteration in level of consciousness or respiratory status.
- Suppression of cough.
- Control of diarrhea.

HIGH ALERT

colchicine (kol-chi-seen)
Colcrys, Gloperba, Lodoco, Mitigare
Classification
Therapeutic: antigout agents

Indications

Treatment of gout flares (Colcrys and generic tablets only). Prophylaxis of gout flares (Gloperba, Mitigare, and generic capsules only). Familial Mediterranean fever (Colcrys and generic tablets only). To reduce the risk of MI, stroke, coronary revascularization, and cardiovascular death in patients with established atherosclerotic disease or with multiple risk factors for cardiovascular disease (Lodoco only).

Action

Interferes with the functions of WBCs in initiating and perpetuating the inflammatory response to monosodium urate crystals. **Therapeutic Effects:** Decreased pain and inflammation in acute attacks of gout. Reduced number of attacks of gout and familial Mediterranean fever. Reduction in risk of MI, stroke, coronary revascularization, and cardiovascular death in patients with established atherosclerotic disease or with multiple risk factors for cardiovascular disease.

Pharmacokinetics

Absorption: 45% absorbed from the GI tract, then re-enters GI tract from biliary secretions, when more absorption may occur.

Distribution: Extensively distributed to tissues.

Metabolism and Excretion: Partially metabolized by the liver by the CYP3A4 isoenzyme; also a substrate for P-glycoprotein. Secreted in bile back into GI tract; eliminated in the feces. 40–65% excreted in the urine as unchanged drug.

Half-life: 19–31 hr.

TIME/ACTION PROFILE (anti-inflammatory activity)

ROUTE	ONSET	PEAK	DURATION
PO	12 hr	24–72 hr	unknown

Contraindications/Precautions

Contraindicated in: Hypersensitivity; Concurrent use of P-glycoprotein (P-gp) inhibitors or strong CYP3A4 inhibitors in patients with renal or hepatic impairment (generic tablets or Colcrys only); Concurrent use of drugs that inhibit both P-gp and CYP3A4 in patients with renal or hepatic impairment (Gloperba or Mitigare only); Concurrent use of strong P-glycoprotein inhibitors or strong CYP3A4 inhibitors (Lodoco only); Presence of both renal and hepatic impairment (Gloperba and Mitigare only); Renal failure (CCr <15 mL/min) (Lodoco only); Severe hepatic impairment (Lodoco only); Pre-existing blood dyscrasias (Lodoco only).

Use Cautiously in: Renal impairment (dose ↓ suggested if CCr <80 mL/min); OB: Use during pregnancy only if potential maternal benefit justifies potential fetal risk; Lactation: Use while breastfeeding only if potential maternal benefit justifies potential risk to infant; Pedi: Safety and effectiveness not established in children (for gout or cardiovascular risk reduction); Geri: ↑ risk of toxicity in older adults with renal impairment.

Adverse Reactions/Side Effects

Derm: alopecia. **GI:** diarrhea, nausea, vomiting, abdominal pain. **Hemat:** AGRANULOCYTOSIS, APLASTIC ANEMIA, leukopenia, thrombocytopenia. **MS:** myalgia, RHABDOMYOLYSIS. **Neuro:** peripheral neuritis.

Interactions

Drug-Drug: Concurrent use of strong **CYP3A4 inhibitors**, including **atazanavir, clarithromycin, darunavir/ritonavir, itraconazole, ketoconazole, lopinavir/ritonavir, nefazodone, nelfinavir, ritonavir,** or **tipranavir/ritonavir,** may ↑ levels and risk of toxicity; ↓ colchicine dose in patients with normal renal or hepatic function; concurrent use in patients with renal or hepatic impairment is contraindicated; concurrent use with Lodoco is contraindicated. Concurrent use of strong **P-gp inhibitors,** including **cyclosporine** or **ranolazine** may ↑ levels and risk of toxicity; ↓ colchicine dose in patients with normal renal or hepatic function; concurrent use in patients with renal or hepatic impairment is contraindicated; concurrent use with Lodoco is contraindicated. Moderate **CYP3A4 inhibitors**, including **aprepitant, diltiazem, erythromycin, fluconazole, fosamprenavir,** or **verapamil** may ↑ levels and risk of toxicity; ↓ colchicine dose in patients with normal renal or hepatic function; avoid concurrent use of Lodoco in patients with renal or hepatic impairment. Additive bone marrow depression may occur with **bone marrow depressants** or **radiation therapy**. ↑ risk of rhabdomyolysis with **HMG-CoA reductase inhibitors, gemfibrozil, fenofibrate, digoxin,** or **cyclosporine**. Additive adverse GI effects with **NSAIDs**. May cause reversible malabsorption of **vitamin B$_{12}$**.

Drug-Food: **Grapefruit juice** may ↑ levels and risk of toxicity; ↓ colchicine dose (for all formulations, except Lodoco); avoid concurrent use with Lodoco.

Route/Dosage

Treatment of Gout Flares (Colcrys and Generic Tablets Only)
PO (Adults): 1.2 mg initially, then 0.6 mg 1 hr later (maximum dose of 1.8 mg in 1 hr); *Concomitant use of strong CYP3A4 inhibitors in patients with normal renal and hepatic function (atazanavir, clarithromycin, darunavir/ritonavir, itraconazole, ketoconazole, lopinavir/ritonavir, nefazodone, nelfinavir, ritonavir, tipranavir/ritonavir):* 0.6 mg initially, then 0.3 mg 1 hr later (do not repeat treatment course for ≥3 days); *Concomitant use of moderate CYP3A4 inhibitors (aprepitant, diltiazem, erythromycin, fluconazole, fosamprenavir, grapefruit juice, verapamil):* 1.2 mg as single dose (do not repeat for ≥3 days); *Concomitant use of strong P-gp inhibitors (cyclosporine, ranolazine) in patients with normal renal and hepatic function:* 0.6 mg as single dose (do not repeat for ≥3 days).

Renal Impairment
PO (Adults): *CCr <30 mL/min:* 1.2 mg initially, then 0.6 mg 1 hr later; do not repeat treatment course for ≥2 wk; *Dialysis:* 0.6 mg as single dose; do not repeat treatment course for ≥2 wk.

Prevention of Gout Flares (Gloperba, Mitigare, and Generic Capsules Only)
PO (Adults): 0.6 mg once or twice daily; *Concomitant use of strong CYP3A4 inhibitors (atazanavir, clarithromycin, darunavir/ritonavir, itraconazole, ketoconazole, lopinavir/ritonavir, nefazodone, nelfinavir, ritonavir, tipranavir/ritonavir) or strong P-gp inhibitors (cyclosporine, ranolazine) in patients with normal renal and hepatic function:* if original dose was 0.6 mg twice daily, ↓ to 0.3 mg once daily; if original dose was 0.6 mg once daily, ↓ to 0.3 mg every other day; *Concomitant use of moderate CYP3A4 inhibitors (aprepitant, diltiazem, erythromycin, flu-*

conazole, fosamprenavir, grapefruit juice, verapamil):* if original dose was 0.6 mg twice daily, ↓ to 0.3 mg twice daily or 0.6 mg once daily; if original dose was 0.6 mg once daily, ↓ to 0.3 mg once daily.

Renal Impairment
PO (Adults): *CCr <30 mL/min:* 0.3 mg once daily; *Dialysis:* 0.3 mg twice weekly.

Familial Mediterranean Fever (Colcrys and Generic Tablets Only)
PO (Adults and Children >12 yr): 1.2–2.4 mg/day (in 1–2 divided doses); may ↑ or ↓ dose in 0.3-mg/day increments based on safety and efficacy; *Concomitant use of strong CYP3A4 inhibitors (atazanavir, clarithromycin, darunavir/ritonavir, itraconazole, ketoconazole, lopinavir/ritonavir, nefazodone, nelfinavir, ritonavir, tipranavir/ritonavir) or strong P-gp inhibitors (cyclosporine, ranolazine) in patients with normal renal and hepatic function:* Do not exceed 0.6 mg/day (may be given as 0.3 mg twice daily); *Concomitant use of moderate CYP3A4 inhibitors (aprepitant, diltiazem, erythromycin, fluconazole, fosamprenavir, grapefruit juice, verapamil):* Do not exceed 1.2 mg/day (may be given as 0.6 mg twice daily).
PO (Children 6–12 yr): 0.9–1.8 mg/day (in 1–2 divided doses).
PO (Children 4–6 yr): 0.3–1.8 mg/day (in 1–2 divided doses).

Renal Impairment
PO (Adults): *CCr 30–50 mL/min:* dose ↓ may be necessary; *CCr <30 mL/min or dialysis:* 0.3 mg/day.

Reduction in Risk of MI, Stroke, Coronary Revascularization, and Cardiovascular Death
PO (Adults): 0.5 mg once daily.

Availability (generic available)
Tablets (Colcrys): 0.6 mg. **Tablets (Lodoco):** 0.5 mg. **Capsules (Mitigare):** 0.6 mg. **Oral solution (cherry flavor) (Gloperba):** 0.6 mg/5 mL. *In combination with:* probenecid.

NURSING IMPLICATIONS
Assessment
- Monitor intake and output ratios. Fluids should be encouraged to promote a urinary output of at least 2000 mL/day.
- **Gout:** Assess involved joints for pain, mobility, and edema throughout therapy. During initiation of therapy, monitor for drug response every 1–2 hr.
- **Familial Mediterranean fever:** Assess for signs and symptoms of familial Mediterranean fever (abdominal pain, chest pain, fever, chills, recurrent joint pain, red and swollen skin lesions) periodically during therapy.

✱= Canadian drug name. ▧ = Genetic implication. ~~Strikethrough~~ = Discontinued. CAPITALS = life-threatening. <u>Underline</u> = most frequent.

Lab Test Considerations

● In patients receiving prolonged therapy, monitor baseline and periodic CBC; report significant ↓ in values. May cause ↓ platelet count, leukopenia, aplastic anemia, and agranulocytosis.

● May cause ↑ in AST and alkaline phosphatase.

● May cause false-positive results for urine hemoglobin.

● May interfere with results of urinary 17-hydroxycorticosteroid concentrations.

Toxicity and Overdose

● *High Alert:* Assess patient for toxicity (muscle pain or weakness, tingling or numbness in fingers or toes; pale or gray color to lips, tongue, or palms of hands; severe diarrhea or vomiting; unusual bleeding, bruising, sore throat, fatigue, malaise, or weakness or tiredness). If these symptoms occur, discontinue colchicine and treat symptomatically.

Implementation

● Do not confuse colchicine with Cortrosyn.

● Intermittent therapy with 3 days between courses may be used to decrease risk of toxicity.

● **PO:** Administer without regard to meals.

● Use an accurate measuring device for solution; a teaspoon is not accurate. Solution is slightly hazy, red liquid with a cherry odor.

Patient/Family Teaching

● Instruct patient to take colchicine as directed. Review medication administration schedule. Take missed doses as soon as remembered unless almost time for next dose. Do not double doses.

● Instruct patients taking prophylactic doses not to increase to therapeutic doses during an acute attack to prevent toxicity. An NSAID or corticosteroid, preferably via intrasynovial injection, should be used to treat acute attacks.

● Advise patient to avoid grapefruit and grapefruit juice during therapy; may increase risk of toxicity.

● Advise patient to follow recommendations of health care professional regarding weight loss, diet, and alcohol consumption.

● Instruct patient to report muscle pain or weakness, tingling or numbness in fingers or toes; pale or gray color to lips, tongue, or palms of hands; severe diarrhea or vomiting; unusual bleeding, bruising, sore throat, fatigue, malaise, or weakness or tiredness promptly. Hold colchicine if symptoms of toxicity occur.

● Instruct patient to notify health care professional of all Rx or OTC medications, vitamins, or herbal products being taken and to notify health care professional before taking any other Rx, OTC, or herbal products.

● Surgery may precipitate an acute attack of gout. Advise patient to confer with health care professional regarding dose 3 days before surgical or dental procedures.

● Rep: Advise females of reproductive potential to notify health care professional if pregnancy is planned or suspected or if breastfeeding. Monitor breastfed infants for diarrhea. Inform males that colchicine may cause infertility that reverses when colchicine is stopped.

Evaluation/Desired Outcomes

● Decrease in pain and swelling in affected joints within 12 hr.

● Relief of symptoms within 24–48 hr.

● Prevention of acute gout attacks.

● Reduced number of attacks of familial Mediterranean fever.

● Reduction in risk of MI, stroke, coronary revascularization, and cardiovascular death in patients with established atherosclerotic disease or with multiple risk factors for cardiovascular disease.

colesevelam (koe-le-sev-e-lam)
✦Lodalis, Welchol
Classification
Therapeutic: lipid-lowering agents
Pharmacologic: bile acid sequestrants

Indications

Adjunctive therapy to diet and exercise for the reduction of LDL cholesterol in patients with primary hypercholesterolemia; may be used alone or in combination with statins. Adjunctive therapy to diet and exercise for the reduction of LDL cholesterol in children 10–17 yr with heterozygous familial hypercholesterolemia if diet therapy fails (LDL cholesterol remains ≥190 mg/dL or remains ≥160 mg/dL [with family history of premature cardiovascular disease or ≥2 risk factors for cardiovascular disease]); may be used alone or in combination with statin. Adjunctive therapy to diet and exercise to improve glycemic control in patients with type 2 diabetes.

Action

Binds bile acids in the GI tract. Results in increased clearance of cholesterol. Mechanism for lowering blood glucose unknown. **Therapeutic Effects:** Decreased cholesterol and blood glucose.

Pharmacokinetics

Absorption: Not absorbed; action is primarily local in the GI tract.
Distribution: Unknown.
Metabolism and Excretion: Unknown.
Half-life: Unknown.

TIME/ACTION PROFILE (cholesterol-lowering effect)

ROUTE	ONSET	PEAK	DURATION
PO	24–48 hr	2 wk	unknown

Contraindications/Precautions

Contraindicated in: Hypersensitivity; Bowel obstruction; Triglycerides >500 mg/dL; History of pancreatitis due to hypertriglyceridemia.

Use Cautiously in: Triglycerides >300 mg/dL; Dysphagia, swallowing disorders, severe GI motility disorders, or major GI tract surgery; Phenylketonuria (oral suspension packets contain phenylalanine); OB: Use during pregnancy not expected to result in fetal exposure (not systemically absorbed); Lactation: Not expected to be present in breast milk (not systemically absorbed); Pedi: Safety and effectiveness not established in children <10 yr (hyperlipidemia) or <18 yr (type 2 diabetes).

Adverse Reactions/Side Effects

GI: constipation, dyspepsia.

Interactions

Drug-Drug: May ↓ absorption of **glyburide, glimepiride, glipizide, levothyroxine, olmesartan, phenytoin, cyclosporine, warfarin,** and **estrogen-containing oral contraceptives** (give ≥4 hr before colesevelam). May ↑ levels of **metformin extended-release**.

Route/Dosage

Hyperlipidemia

PO (Adults and Children 10–17 yr): 6 tablets once daily *or* 3 tablets twice daily *or* one 3.75-g packet once daily.

Type 2 Diabetes

PO (Adults): 6 tablets once daily *or* 3 tablets twice daily *or* one 3.75-g packet once daily.

Availability (generic available)

Granules for oral suspension: 3.75 g/packet (contains 27 mg phenylalanine). **Tablets:** 625 mg.

NURSING IMPLICATIONS

Assessment

- **Hypercholesterolemia:** Obtain a diet history, especially in regard to fat consumption.
- **Type 2 Diabetes:** Observe patient for signs and symptoms of hypoglycemic reactions (sweating, hunger, weakness, dizziness, tremor, tachycardia, anxiety).

Lab Test Considerations

- Monitor serum total cholesterol, LDL, and triglyceride levels before initiating, 4–6 wk after starting, and periodically during therapy. May cause hypertriglyceridemia.
- Monitor serum glucose and glycosylated hemoglobin periodically during therapy in patients with diabetes.

Implementation

- Patients stabilized on a diabetic regimen who are exposed to stress, fever, trauma, infection, or surgery may require administration of insulin.
- **PO:** Administer once or twice daily with meals. Colesevelam should be taken with a liquid. For oral suspension, empty the entire contents of one packet into a glass or cup. Add 1 cup (8 oz) of water, fruit juice, or a diet soft drink; do not take in dry form to avoid esophageal distress.

Patient/Family Teaching

- Instruct patient to take medication as directed; do not skip doses or double up on missed doses.
- Advise patients taking oral vitamin supplementation or oral contraceptives to take their vitamins at least 4 hr prior to colesevelam, especially those taking warfarin. Colesevelam may decrease absorption of fat-soluble vitamins A, D, E, and K.
- Instruct patient to consume a diet that promotes bowel regularity. Patients should be instructed to promptly discontinue colesevelam and notify health care professional if severe abdominal pain or severe constipation or symptoms of acute pancreatitis (severe abdominal pain with or without nausea and vomiting) occur.
- Instruct patient to notify health care professional of all Rx or OTC medications, vitamins, or herbal products being taken and consult health care professional before taking other Rx, OTC, or herbal products.
- Rep: Insulin is the recommended method of controlling blood sugar during pregnancy. Counsel females of reproductive potential that colesevelam may reduce efficacy of oral contraceptives; advise patients to take oral contraceptives at least 4 hr prior to taking colesevelam or use a form of contraception other than oral contraceptives and to notify health care professional promptly if pregnancy is planned or suspected.
- **Hypercholesterolemia:** Advise patient that this medication should be used in conjunction with diet restrictions (fat, cholesterol, carbohydrates, alcohol), exercise, and cessation of smoking.
- **Diabetes:** Explain to patient that this medication controls hyperglycemia but does not cure diabetes. Therapy is long term.
- Review signs of hypoglycemia and hyperglycemia with patient. If hypoglycemia occurs, advise patient to drink a glass of orange juice or ingest 2–3 tsp of sugar, honey, or corn syrup dissolved in water or an appropriate number of glucose tablets and notify health care professional.
- Encourage patient to follow prescribed diet, medication, and exercise regimen to prevent hypoglycemic or hyperglycemic episodes.
- Instruct patient in proper testing of serum glucose and ketones. These tests should be closely moni-

tored during periods of stress or illness and health care professional notified if significant changes occur.

- Advise patient to carry a form of sugar (sugar packets, candy) and identification describing disease process and medication regimen at all times.

Evaluation/Desired Outcomes

- Decrease in serum total cholesterol, LDL cholesterol, apolipoprotein, and blood glucose levels.
- Control of blood glucose levels without the appearance of hypoglycemic or hyperglycemic episodes.

conivaptan (con-i-vap-tan)
Vaprisol
Classification
Therapeutic: electrolyte modifiers
Pharmacologic: vasopressin antagonists

Indications
Hospitalized patients with euvolemic or hypervolemic hyponatremia.

Action
Antagonizes vasopressin at V_2 receptor sites in renal collecting ducts, resulting in excretion of free water. **Therapeutic Effects:** Increased serum sodium concentrations. Improved fluid status.

Pharmacokinetics
Absorption: IV administration results in complete bioavailability.
Distribution: Unknown.
Protein Binding: 99%.
Metabolism and Excretion: Primarily metabolized by the liver via the CYP3A4 isoenzyme. 83% excreted in feces as metabolites, 12% in urine (as metabolites).
Half-life: 5 hr.

TIME/ACTION PROFILE (plasma concentrations)

ROUTE	ONSET	PEAK	DURATION
IV	unknown	12 hr	end of infusion

Contraindications/Precautions
Contraindicated in: Hypersensitivity; Hypovolemic hyponatremia; Concurrent use of ketonconazole, itraconazole, clarithromycin, or ritonavir; Lactation: Lactation.
Use Cautiously in: Moderate or severe hepatic impairment (↓ dose recommended); Severe renal impairment (not recommended if CCr <30 mL/min); OB: Safety not established in pregnancy; Pedi: Safety and effectiveness not established in children.

Adverse Reactions/Side Effects
CV: hypertension, hypotension. **F and E:** dehydration, hypokalemia, hypomagnesemia, hyponatremia, thirst. **GI:** diarrhea. **GU:** ↓ fertility (females), polyuria.

Neuro: headache, confusion, insomnia. **Misc:** infusion reactions, fever.

Interactions
Drug-Drug: CYP3A4 inhibitors, including ketoconazole, itraconazole, clarithromycin, and ritonavir, may ↑ levels and risk of toxicity; concurrent use contraindicated. May ↑ levels and risk of toxicity of CYP3A4 substrates, including midazolam, simvastatin, lovastatin, and amlodipine; careful monitoring recommended. May ↑ digoxin levels and risk of toxicity.

Route/Dosage
IV (Adults): 20 mg loading dose initially, followed by 20 mg/day as a continuous infusion for 2–4 days. May titrate conivaptan up to 40 mg/day as a continuous infusion if serum sodium is not rising at desired rate. Total duration of therapy should not exceed 4 days.

Hepatic Impairment
(Adults): *Moderate or severe hepatic impairment:* 10-mg loading dose initially, followed by 10 mg/day as a continuous infusion for 2–4 days; may titrate up to 20 mg/day as a continuous infusion if serum sodium is not rising at desired rate.

Availability
Premixed infusion: 20 mg/100 mL D5W.

NURSING IMPLICATIONS
Assessment
- Monitor injection site during administration. Frequently causes erythema, pain, swelling, and phlebitis. May require discontinuation of therapy.
- Monitor vital signs frequently during therapy. Discontinue therapy if patient becomes hypovolemic and hypotensive. Therapy may be resumed at a reduced dose once patient is euvolemic and no longer hypotensive, if patient remains hyponatremic.
- Assess neurologic status during administration. Overly rapid rise in serum sodium may cause neurologic sequelae.

Lab Test Considerations
- Monitor serum sodium concentration frequently during therapy. If serum sodium rises at an undesirably rapid rate (>12 mEq/L/24 hr), discontinue administration of conivaptan. If serum sodium continues to rise, do not resume therapy. If hyponatremia persists or recurs (after discontinuation for rapid rise of serum sodium) and patient has no evidence of neurologic sequelae from rapid increase, conivaptan may be resumed at a reduced dose.
- May cause hyperglycemia, hypoglycemia, hypokalemia, hypomagnesemia, and hyponatremia.

Implementation
IV Administration
- Administer IV through large veins and rotate infusion site every 24 hr to minimize risk of vascular irritation.

Loading Dose
- **Intermittent Infusion:** *Dilution:* Premixed containers require no further dilution. *Concentration:* 0.2 mg/mL. *Rate:* Administer over 30 min.

Continuous Infusion
- **Continuous Infusion:** *Dilution:* Premixed containers require no further dilution. *Concentration:* 0.2 mg/mL. *Rate:* Administer continuous infusion at a rate of 20 mg/24 hr. If patient requires 40 mg/24 hr continuous infusion, infuse 20 mg over 12 hr, followed by 20 mg over 12 hr.
- **Additive Incompatibility:** Do not admix with LR, furosemide, or combine with any other product in the same IV line or bag.

Patient/Family Teaching
- Explain purpose of medication to patient.
- Instruct patient to notify health care professional if pain or redness occurs at infusion site.
- Rep: Advise females of reproductive potential to notify health care professional if pregnancy is planned or suspected or if breastfeeding.

Evaluation/Desired Outcomes
- Restoration of normal fluid and electrolyte balance.

CONTRACEPTIVES, HORMONAL
MONOPHASIC ORAL CONTRACEPTIVES

estetrol/drospirenone
(**es**-te-trol/droe-**spy**-re-nown)
Nextstellis

ethinyl estradiol/desogestrel
(**eth**-in-il es-tra-**dye**-ole/dess-oh-**jess**-trel)
Apri-28, Cyred EQ, Enskyce, Isibloom, Juleber, Kalliga, Reclipsen

ethinyl estradiol/drospirenone
(**eth**-in-il es-tra-**dye**-ole/droe-**spy**-re-nown)
Beyaz, Jasmiel, Lo-Zumandimine, Loryna, Nikki, Ocella, Safyral, Syeda, Tydemy, Vestura, Yasmin, Yaz, Zumandimine

ethinyl estradiol/ethynodiol
(**eth**-in-il es-tra-**dye**-ole/e-thye-noe-**dye**-ole)
Kelnor 1/35, Kelnor 1/50, Zovia 1/35

ethinyl estradiol/levonorgestrel
(**eth**-in-il es-tra-**dye**-ole/lee-voe-nor-**jess**-trel)
Afirmelle, Altavera, Aubra EQ, Aviane, Ayuna, Balcoltra, Chateal EQ, Falmina, Joyeaux, Kurvelo, Lessina, Levora-28, Lutera, Marlissa, Portia-28, Sronyx, Tyblume, Vienva

ethinyl estradiol/norethindrone
(**eth**-in-il es-tra-**dye**-ole/nor-eth-in-drone)
Alyacen 1/35, Aurovela 1/20, Aurovela 1.5/30, Aurovela 24 Fe, Aurovela Fe 1/20, Aurovela Fe 1.5/30, Balziva, Blisovi 24 Fe, Blisovi Fe 1/20, Blisovi Fe 1.5/30, Briellyn, Charlotte 24 Fe, Cyonanz, Dasetta 1/35, Finzala, Fyavolv, Gemmily, Generess Fe, Hailey 1.5/30, Hailey 24 Fe, Hailey Fe 1/20, Hailey Fe 1.5/30, Jinteli, Junel 1/20, Junel 1.5/30, Junel Fe 1/20, Junel Fe 1.5/30, Junel Fe 24, Kaitlib Fe, Larin 1/20, Larin 1.5/30, Larin 24 Fe, Larin Fe 1/20, Larin Fe 1.5/30, Layolis Fe, Loestrin 1/20, Loestrin 1.5/30, Loestrin Fe 1/20, Loestrin Fe 1.5/30, Merzee, Mibelas 24 Fe, Microgestin 1/20, Microgestin 1.5/30, Microgestin 24 Fe, Microgestin Fe 1/20, Microgestin Fe 1.5/30, Minastrin 24 Fe, Necon 0.5/35, Nexesta Fe, Nortrel 0.5/35, Nortrel 1/35, Nylia 1/35, Philith, Tarina 24 Fe, Tarina Fe 1/20 EQ, Taysofy, Taytulla, Tilia Fe, Vyfemla, Wera, Wymzya Fe, Zenchent Fe

ethinyl estradiol/norgestimate
(**eth**-in-il es-tra-**dye**-ole/nor-**jes**-ti-mate)
Estarylla, Mili, Mono-Linyah, Nymyo, Previfem, Sprintec-28, VyLibra

ethinyl estradiol/norgestrel
(**eth**-in-il es-tra-**dye**-ole/nor-**jess**-trel)
Cryselle-28, Elinest, Low-Ogestrel

C

BIPHASIC ORAL CONTRACEPTIVES

ethinyl estradiol/desogestrel
(eth-in-il es-tra-**dye**-ole/dess-oh-**jess**-trel)
Azurette, Bekyree, Kariva, Mircette, Pimtrea, Simliya, Viorele, Volnea

ethinyl estradiol/norethindrone
(eth-in-il es-tra-**dye**-ole/nor-eth-**in**-drone)
Lo Loestrin Fe

TRIPHASIC ORAL CONTRACEPTIVES

ethinyl estradiol/desogestrel
(eth-in-il es-tra-**dye**-ole/dess-oh-**jess**-trel)
Velivet

ethinyl estradiol/levonorgestrel
(eth-in-il ess-tra-**dye**-ole/lee-voe-nor-**jess**-trel)
Enpresse-28, Levonest, Trivora-28

ethinyl estradiol/norethindrone
(eth-in-il es-tra-**dye**-ole/nor-eth-**in**-drone)
Alyacen 7/7/7, Aranelle, Dasetta 7/7/7, Leena, Nortrel 7/7/7, Nylia 7/7/7, Tri-Legest Fe

ethinyl estradiol/norgestimate
(eth-in-il es-tra-**dye**-ole/nor-**jess**-ti-mate)
Tri-Estarylla, Tri-Linyah, Tri-Lo-Estarylla, Tri-Lo-Marzia, Tri-Lo-Mili, Tri-Lo-Sprintec, Tri-Mili, Tri-Nymyo, Tri-Sprintec, Tri-VyLibra, Tri-VyLibra Lo

FOURPHASIC ORAL CONTRACEPTIVES

estradiol valerate/dienogest
(es-tra-**dye**-ole **val**-er-ate/dye-**en**-oh-jest)
Natazia

EXTENDED-CYCLE ORAL CONTRACEPTIVE

ethinyl estradiol/levonorgestrel
(eth-in-il ess-tra-**dye**-ole/lee-voe-nor-**jess**-trel)
Amethia, Amethyst, Ashlyna, Camrese, Camrese Lo, Daysee, Dolishale, Iclevia, Introvale, Jaimiess, Jolessa, LoJaimiess, LoSeasonique, Quartette, Rivelsa, Seasonique, Setlakin, Simpesse

PROGESTIN-ONLY ORAL CONTRACEPTIVES

norethindrone (nor-eth-**in**-drone)
Aygestin, Camila, Deblitane, Emzahh, Errin, Heather, Incassia, Jencycla, Lyleq, Nora-BE, Sharobel

drospirenone
Slynd

CONTRACEPTIVE IMPLANT

etonogestrel (e-toe-no-**jess**-trel)
Nexplanon

EMERGENCY CONTRACEPTIVE

levonorgestrel
(lee-voe-nor-**jess**-trel)
Aftera, Athentia Next, Curae, EContra One-Step, Her Style, My Choice, My Way, New Day, Opcicon One-Step, Plan B One-Step, Take Action

ulipristal (u-li-**priss**-tal)
Ella

INJECTABLE CONTRACEPTIVE

medroxyprogesterone
(me-**drox**-ee-proe-**jess**-te-rone)
Depo-Provera, Depo-subQ Provera 104

INTRAUTERINE CONTRACEPTIVE

levonorgestrel
(lee-voe-nor-**jess**-trel)
Kyleena, Liletta, Mirena, Skyla

VAGINAL RING CONTRACEPTIVE

ethinyl estradiol/etonogestrel
(eth-in-il ess-tra-**dye**-ole/e-toe-noe-**jess**-trel)
EluRyng, Enilloring, Haloette, NuvaRing

TRANSDERMAL CONTRACEPTIVE

ethinyl estradiol/levonorgestrel
(eth-in-il ess-tra-**dye**-ole/**lee**-voe-nor-**jess**-trel)
Twirla

ethinyl estradiol/norelgestromin
(eth-in-il ess-tra-**dye**-ole/nor-el-**jess**-troe-min)
Xulane, Zafemy

Classification
Therapeutic: contraceptive hormones

Indications

Prevention of pregnancy. Regulation of menstrual cycle. Emergency contraception (some products). Treatment

C

of heavy menstrual bleeding in women who choose to use intrauterine contraception as their method of contraception. Treatment of heavy menstrual bleeding in women who choose to use an oral contraceptive as their method of contraception. Treatment of premenstrual dysphoric disorder. Management of acne in women >14 yr who desire contraception, have no health problems, and have failed topical treatment. Increase folate levels in women who desire oral contraception to reduce the risk of neural tube defects in a pregnancy that occurs while taking or shortly after discontinuing the product.

Action
Monophasic Oral Contraceptives: Provide a fixed dosage of estrogen/progestin over a 21-day cycle. Ovulation is inhibited by suppression of follicle-stimulating hormone (FSH) and luteinizing hormone (LH). May alter cervical mucus and the endometrial environment, preventing penetration by sperm and implantation of the egg. **Biphasic Oral Contraceptives:** Ovulation is inhibited by suppression of FSH and LH. May alter cervical mucus and the endometrial environment, preventing penetration by sperm and implantation of the egg. In addition, smaller dose of progestin in phase 1 allows for proliferation of endometrium. Larger amount in phase 2 allows for adequate secretory development. **Triphasic Oral Contraceptives:** Ovulation is inhibited by suppression of FSH and LH. May alter cervical mucus and the endometrial environment, preventing penetration by sperm and implantation of the egg. Varying doses of estrogen/progestin may more closely mimic natural hormonal fluctuations. **Fourphasic Oral Contraceptives:** Ovulation is inhibited by suppression of FSH and LH. May alter cervical mucus and the endometrial environment, preventing penetration by sperm and implantation of the egg. Doses of estrogen decrease while doses of progestin increase over the 28-day cycle. **Extended-cycle:** Provides continuous estrogen/progestin for 84 days, then off for 7 days (low-dose estrogen-only tablet taken during these 7 days with LoSeasonique and Seasonique), resulting in 4 menstrual periods/yr. **Progressive Estrogen:** Contains constant amount of progestin with 3 progressive doses of estrogen. **Progestin-Only Contraceptives/Contraceptive Implant/Intrauterine Levonorgestrel/Medroxyprogesterone Injection:** Mechanism not clearly known. May alter cervical mucus and the endometrial environment, preventing penetration by sperm and implantation of the egg. Ovulation may also be suppressed. **Emergency Contraceptive Pills:** Inhibit ovulation/fertilization; may also alter tubal transport of sperm/egg and prevent implantation. **Vaginal Ring, Transdermal Patch:** Inhibits ovulation, decreases sperm entry into uterus, decreases likelihood of implantation. **Anti-acne effect:** Combination of estrogen/progestin may increase sex hormone binding

globulin resulting in decreased unbound testosterone, which may be a cause of acne. **Therapeutic Effects:** Prevention of pregnancy. Decreased severity of acne. Decrease in menstrual blood loss. Decrease in premenstrual dysphoric disorder. Decrease in vasomotor symptoms or symptoms of vulvar and vaginal atrophy due to menopause. Increase in folate levels and prevention of neural tube defects.

Pharmacokinetics
Absorption: *Ethinyl estradiol:* rapidly absorbed; *Norethindrone:* 65% absorbed; *Desogestrel and levonorgestrel:* 100% absorbed; *Dienogest:* 91% absorbed. Others are well absorbed after oral administration. Slowly absorbed from implant, SUBQ or IM injection. Some absorption follows intrauterine implantation.

Distribution: Unknown.

Protein Binding: *Ethinyl estradiol:* 97–98%; *Drospirenone:* 97%; *Dienogest:* 90%; *Ulipristal:* >94%.

Metabolism and Excretion: *Ethinyl estradiol and norethindrone:* undergo extensive first-pass hepatic metabolism. *Desogestrel:* is rapidly metabolized to 3-keto-desogestrel, the active metabolite. Most agents are metabolized by the liver.

Half-life: *Ethinyl estradiol:* 6–20 hr; *Levonorgestrel:* 45 hr; *Norethindrone:* 5–14 hr; *Desogestrel (metabolite):* 38 ± 20 hr; *Drospirenone:* 30 hr; *Norgestimate (metabolite):* 12–20 hr; *Dienogest:* 11 hr; *others:* unknown; *Ulipristal:* 32 hr.

TIME/ACTION PROFILE (prevention of pregnancy)

ROUTE	ONSET	PEAK	DURATION
PO	1 mo	1 mo	1 mo†
Implant	1 mo	1 mo	5 yr
Intrauterine system	1 mo	1 mo	5 yr
IM	1 mo	1 mo	3 mo
SUBQ	unknown	1 wk	3 mo

†Only during mo of taking contraceptive.

Contraindications/Precautions
Contraindicated in: Hypersensitivity; History of cigarette smoking and age >35 yr (↑ risk of cardiovascular or thromboembolic phenomenon); History of deep vein thrombosis or pulmonary embolism; Inherited or acquired coagulopathies; Cerebrovascular disease; Coronary artery disease; Thrombogenic valvular heart disease or thrombogenic heart rhythms; Major surgery with extended periods of immobility; Diabetes and >35 yr old; diabetes with hypertension, vascular disease, or end-organ damage; or diabetes for >20 yr; Headache with focal neurologic symptoms or migraine headaches with aura; Women >35 yr old with migraine headaches; Uncontrolled hypertension or hypertension with vascular disease; Breast cancer, endo-

metrial cancer, or any other estrogen- or progestin-sensitive cancer (current or history of); Abnormal genital bleeding; Cholestatic jaundice of pregnancy or jaundice with prior contraceptive use; Hepatic adenoma or carcinoma; Hypersensitivity to and parabens (injectable only); *Drosperinone-containing products only:* Renal impairment, liver disease, or adrenal insufficiency (↑ risk of hyperkalemia); *Intrauterine levonorgestrel only:* Intrauterine anomaly, postpartum endometriosis, multiple sexual partners, pelvic inflammatory disease, liver disease, genital actinomycosis, immunosuppression, IV drug abuse, untreated genitourinary infection, history of ectopic pregnancy; *Ethinyl estradiol/levonorgestrel and ethinyl estradiol/norelgestromin transdermal patches only:* Body mass index ≥30 kg/m² (↑ risk of venous thromboembolism); OB: Pregnancy; Lactation: Avoid use; ↑ risk of uterine rupture/perforation with intrauterine levonorgestrel.

Use Cautiously in: Presence of other cardiovascular risk factors (obesity, hyperglycemia, hypertension); History or family history of hypertriglyceridemia (↑ risk of pancreatitis); Diabetes mellitus, bleeding disorders, concurrent anticoagulant therapy or headaches; Hereditary angioedema; Chloasma; *Estetrol/drospirenone:* BMI >30 k g/m² (↓ effectiveness); *Ethinyl estradiol/norelgestromin transdermal patch only:* Weight >90 kg (↓ effectiveness); *Ethinyl estradiol/levonorgestrel transdermal patch only:* Body mass index 25−<30 kg/m (↓ effectiveness); Pedi: Avoid use before menarche.

Adverse Reactions/Side Effects

CV: edema, hypertension, Raynaud's phenomenon, THROMBOEMBOLISM, thrombophlebitis. **Derm:** melasma, rash. **EENT:** contact lens intolerance, optic neuritis, retinal thrombosis. **Endo:** hyperglycemia. **F and E:** *Drosperinone-containing products only:* hyperkalemia. **GI:** abdominal cramps, bloating, cholestatic jaundice, gallbladder disease, liver tumors, nausea, PANCREATITIS, vomiting. **GU:** *Intrauterine levonorgestrel only:* amenorrhea, breakthrough bleeding, dysmenorrhea, spotting, uterine imbedment/uterine rupture. **MS:** *Injectable medroxyprogesterone only:* bone loss. **Neuro:** depression, headache. **Misc:** BREAST CANCER (especially with prolonged use), HYPERSENSITIVITY REACTIONS (including anaphylaxis and angioedema), weight change.

Interactions

Drug-Drug: Oral contraceptive efficacy may be ↓ by **penicillins, chloramphenicol, barbiturates**, chronic **alcohol** use, **carbamazepine, oxcarbazepine, bosentan, felbamate,** systemic **corticosteroids, phenytoin, topiramate, primidone, modafinil, rifampin, rifabutin, nelfinavir, ritonavir, darunavir/ritonavir, fosamprenavir/ritonavir, lopinavir/ritonavir, tipranavir/ritonavir, nevirapine, efavirenz, colesevelam,** or **tetracyclines. CYP3A4 inducers,** including **barbiturates, bosen-**

tan, **carbamazepine, oxcarbazepine, phenytoin, topiramate, felbamate, rifampin** may ↓ effectiveness of ulipristal; avoid concomitant use. May ↑ effects/risk of toxicity of some **benzodiazepines, beta blockers, corticosteroids, cyclosporine, tizanidine, theophylline,** and **voriconazole.** ↑ risk of hepatotoxicity with **dantrolene** (estrogen only). **Atazanavir/ritonavir, etravirine, itraconazole, ketoconazole, fluconazole, voriconazole, rosuvastatin,** and **atorvastatin** may ↑ effects/risk of toxicity. **Smoking** ↑ risk of thromboembolic phenomena (estrogen only). May ↓ levels of **acetaminophen, temazepam, lamotrigine, lorazepam, oxazepam,** or **morphine.** Concurrent use of combinations containing **ombitasvir/paritaprevir/ritonavir** or **glecaprevir/pibrentasvir** with ethinyl estradiol-containing products may ↑ risk of elevated liver enzymes; avoid concurrent use. *Drosperinone-containing products only:* concurrent use with **NSAIDs, potassium-sparing diuretics, potassium supplements, ACE inhibitors, aldosterone receptor antagonists,** or **angiotensin II receptor antagonists** may result in hyperkalemia. *Drosperinone-containing products only:* concurrent use with strong **CYP3A4 inhibitors,** including **ketoconazole, itraconazole, voriconazole, protease inhibitors,** or **clarithromycin** may ↑ risk of hyperkalemia; consider monitoring K+ concentrations. Ulipristal may ↑ levels of **P-glycoprotein substrates,** including **dabigatran** and **digoxin.**

Drug-Natural Products: Concomitant use with **St. John's wort** may ↓ contraceptive efficacy and cause breakthrough bleeding and irregular menses.

Drug-Food: **Grapefruit juice** may ↑ effects/risk of toxicity.

Route/Dosage

Monophasic Oral Contraceptives

PO (Adults): On 21-day regimen, take first tablet on first Sunday after menses begins (take on Sunday if menses begins on Sunday) for 21 days, then skip 7 days and begin again. Regimen may also be started on first day of menses, continue for 21 days, then skip 7 days and begin again. Some regimens contain 7 placebo tablets, so that 1 tablet is taken every day for 28 days.

Biphasic Oral Contraceptives

PO (Adults): Given in 2 phases. First phase is 10 days of smaller amount of progestin. Second phase is larger amount of progestin. Amount of estrogen remains constant for same length of time (total of 21 days), then skip 7 days and begin again. Some regimens contain 7 placebo tablets for 28-day regimen.

Triphasic Oral Contraceptives

PO (Adults): Progestin amount varies throughout 21-day cycle. Estrogen component stays the same or may vary. Some regimens contain 7 placebo tablets for 28-day regimen.

Fourphasic Oral Contraceptives
PO (Adults): Given in 4 phases. First phase contains higher amount of estrogen and no progestin. Second and third phases contain lower amount of estrogen, and increasing amounts of progestin. Fourth phase contains low dose of estrogen only. Also contains 2 placebo tablets to complete 28-day regimen.

Extended-Cycle Contraceptive
PO (Adults): *Daysee, LoSeasonique, Quartette,* and *Seasonique.* Start taking first active pill on first Sunday after menses begins (if first day is Sunday, begin then), continue for 84 days of active pill, followed by 7 days of placebo tablets (low-dose estrogen tablets for Daysee, LoSeasonique, Quartette, and Seasonique), then resume 84/7 cycle again.

Progestin-Only Oral Contraceptives
PO (Adults): Start on first day of menses. Taken daily and continuously.

Progressive Estrogen Oral Contraceptives
PO (Adults): Estrogen amount increases every 7 days throughout 21-day cycle. Progestin component stays the same. Some regimens contain 7 placebo tablets for 28-day regimen.

Emergency Contraceptive
PO (Adults and Adolescents): *Levonorgestrel:* 1 tablet within 72 hr of unprotected intercourse; *Lo/Ovral:* 4 white tablets within 72 hr of unprotected intercourse followed by 4 more white tablets 12 hr later; *Ulipristal:* 1 tablet as soon as possible within 120 hr (5 days) after unprotected intercourse or known/suspected contraceptive failure.

Injectable Contraceptive
Medroxyprogesterone (Depo-Provera)
IM (Adults): 150 mg within first 5 days of menses or within 5 days postpartum, if not breastfeeding. If breastfeeding, give 6 wk postpartum; repeat every 3 mo.

Medroxyprogesterone (Depo-Sub Q Provera 104)
SUBQ (Adults): 104 mg within first 5 days of menses or within 5 days postpartum, if not breastfeeding. If breastfeeding, give 6 wk postpartum; repeat every 12–14 wk.

Intrauterine Contraceptive
Intrauterine (Adults): Insert one device into uterine cavity within 7 days of menses or immediately after 1st trimester abortion. Skyla should be removed or replaced after 3 yr. Kyleena, should be removed or replaced after 5 yr. Mirena and Liletta should be removed or replaced after 5 yr (for treatment of heavy menstrual bleeding) or 8 yr (contraception).

Vaginal Ring Contraceptive
Vag (Adults): One ring inserted on or prior to day 5 of menstrual cycle. Ring is left in place for 3 wk, then removed for 1 wk, then a new ring is inserted.

Transdermal Patch
Transdermal (Adults): *Ethinyl estradiol/norelgestromin transdermal patch:* Patch is applied on day 1 of menstrual cycle (or convenient day in first wk), changed weekly thereafter for 3 wk. Wk 4 is patch-free. Cycle is then repeated. *Ethinyl estradiol/levonorgestrel transdermal patch:* Patch is applied during first 24 hr of menstruation and then changed weekly thereafter for 3 wk. Wk 4 is patch-free. Cycle is then repeated.

Acne
PO (Adults): Take daily for 21 days, off for 7 days.

Availability
Combination Estrogen/Progestin Oral Contraceptives (generic available)
Oral contraceptive tablets: Usually in monthly packs with enough (21) active tablets to complete a 28-day cycle. Some contain 7 inert tablets to complete the cycle with or without supplemental iron, Beyaz and Safyral —contain 0.451 mg of levomefolate calcium/tablet.

Extended-Cycle Contraceptive
Tablets: *LoSeasonique:* active tablets containing 0.02 mg ethinyl estradiol, 0.1 mg levonorgestrel, and 7 tablets containing 0.01 mg ethinyl estradiol; *Quartette:* 42 tablets containing 0.02 mg ethinyl estradiol and 0.15 mg levonorgestrel, 21 tablets containing 0.025 mg ethinyl estradiol and 0.15 mg levonorgestrel, 21 tablets containing 0.03 mg ethinyl estradiol and 0.15 mg levonorgestrel, and 7 tablets containing 0.01 mg ethinyl estradiol; *Daysee* and *Seasonique:* active tablets containing 0.03 mg ethinyl estradiol, 0.15 mg levonorgestrel, and 7 tablets containing 0.01 mg ethinyl estradiol.

Levonorgestrel (generic available)
Emergency contraceptive: 1.5 mg OTC. **Intrauterine system (Kyleena):** contains 19.5 mg levonorgestrel (releases 9 mcg/day). **Intrauterine system (Liletta):** contains 52 mg levonorgestrel (releases 14.7 mcg/day). **Intrauterine system (Mirena):** contains 52 mg levonorgestrel (releases 20 mcg/day). **Intrauterine system (Skyla):** contains 13.5 mg levonorgestrel (releases 14 mcg/day).

Etonorgestrel
Implant: Rod contains 68 mg etonogestrel.

Ulipristal
Tablets: 30 mg.

Medroxyprogesterone (generic available)
Injectable IM: 150 mg/mL. **Injectable SUBQ:** 104 mg/0.65 mL (in prefilled syringes).

Vaginal Ring Contraceptive
Ring: delivers 0.015 mg ethinyl estradiol and 0.120 mg etonogestrel/day.

Transdermal Patch
Patch (Xulane or Onsura): contains 0.53 mg ethinyl estradiol and 4.86 mg of norelgestromin; releases 35

mcg ethinyl estradiol/150 mcg norelgestromin per 24 hr. **Patch (Twirla):** contains 2.3 mg ethinyl estradiol and 2.6 mg of levonorgestrel; releases 30 mcg ethinyl estradiol/120 mcg levonorgestrel per 24 hr.

NURSING IMPLICATIONS
Assessment
- Assess BP before and periodically during therapy.
- Exclude the possibility of pregnancy on the basis or history and/or physical exam or a pregnancy test before administering emergency contraceptives.
- **Acne:** Assess skin lesions before and periodically during therapy.
- **Menopausal Symptoms:** Assess vasomotor symptoms or symptoms of vulvar and vaginal atrophy due to menopause prior to and periodically during therapy.

Lab Test Considerations
- Monitor hepatic function periodically during therapy.
- *Estrogens only:* May cause ↑ serum glucose, sodium, triglyceride, HDL, total cholesterol, prothrombin, and factors VII, VIII, IX, and X levels. May cause ↓ LDL and antithrombin III levels.
- May cause false interpretations of thyroid function tests.
- *Progestins only:* May cause ↑ LDL concentrations. May cause ↓ serum alkaline phosphatase and HDL concentrations.
- *Drosperinone-containing contraceptives:* monitor serum potassium during first treatment cycle in women on long-term treatment with strong CYP3A4 inhibitors; may ↑ serum potassium concentration.

Implementation
- Do not confuse Slynd with Syeda. Do not confuse Yasmin with Yaz.
- **PO:** Oral doses may be administered with or immediately after food to reduce nausea. Chewable tablets may be swallowed whole or chewed; if chewed follow with 8 oz of liquid.
- For extended-cycle tablets,*Jolessa, Quartette, Seasonique*, or *LoSeasonique:* take active tablets for 84 days followed by the placebo tablets for 7 days.
- For *Emergency Contraception:* Tablets are taken as soon as possible and within 72 hr after unprotected intercourse. Two doses are taken 12 hr apart. Emergency contraception products are available without a prescription to all women of reproductive potential.
- *Ulipristal:* Administer 1 tablet as soon as possible within 120 hr (5 days) after unprotected intercourse or a known or suspected contraceptive failure. May be taken without regard to food. If vomiting occurs within 3 hr of dose, may repeat. May be taken at any time during the menstrual cycle. Ulipristal may be less effective in women with a body mass index >30 kg/m².
- **SUBQ:** Shake vigorously before use to form a uniform suspension. Inject slowly (over 5–7 sec) at a 45° angle into fatty area of anterior thigh or abdomen every 12 to 14 wk. If more than 14 wk elapse

between injections, rule out pregnancy prior to administration. Do not rub area after injection.
- When switching from other hormonal contraceptives, administer within dosing period (7 days after taking last active pill, removing patch or ring, or within the dosing period for IM injection).
- **IM:** Shake vial vigorously just before use to ensure uniform suspension. Administer deep IM into gluteal or deltoid muscle. If period between injections is >14 wk, determine that patient is not pregnant before administering the drug.
- Injectable medroxyprogesterone may lead to bone loss, especially in women younger than 21 yr. Injectable medroxyprogesterone should be used for >2 yr only if other methods of contraception are inadequate. If used long term, women should use supplemental calcium and vitamin D, and monitor bone mineral density.
- **Intrauterine system:** Health care providers are advised to become thoroughly familiar with the insertion instructions before attempting insertion. Following insertion, counsel patient on what to expect. Give patient *Follow-up Reminder Card* provided with product. Discuss expected bleeding patterns during the first mo of use. Prescribe analgesics, if indicated. Patients should be reexamined and evaluated 4 to 12 wk after insertion and once a yr thereafter, or more frequently if clinically indicated.

Patient/Family Teaching
- Instruct patient to take oral medication as directed at the same time each day. Pills should be taken in proper sequence and kept in the original container. Advise patient not to skip pills even if not having sex very often. Advise patient to read *Patient Guide* before starting and with each Rx refill in case of changes.
- *If single daily dose is missed:* Take as soon as remembered; if not until next day, take 2 tablets and continue on regular dosing schedule. *If 2 days in a row are missed:* Take 2 tablets a day for the next 2 days and continue on regular dosing schedule, using a 2nd method of birth control for the remaining cycle. *If 3 days in a row are missed:* Discontinue medication and use another form of birth control until period begins or pregnancy is ruled out; then begin a new cycle of tablets. *For 28-day dosing schedule:* If schedule is followed for first 21 days and 1 dose is missed of the last 7 tablets, it is important to take the 1st tablet of next month's cycle on the regularly scheduled day. Advise patient taking *Natazia* to follow *Patient Guide* for what to do if a pill is missed.
- Advise patient taking *Jolessa, Quartette, Seasonique*, or *LoSeasonique* that withdrawal bleeding should occur during the 7 days following discontinuation of the active tablets. If withdrawal bleeding does not occur, notify health care professional. Advise patient taking *Lybrel* that no withdrawal bleeding should occur.

- For initial use of *Jolessa, Quartette, Seasonique,* or *LoSeasonique,* caution patient to use a nonhormonal method of contraception until she has taken the first 7 days of active tablets. Each 91-day cycle should start on the same day of the wk. If started later than the proper day or 2 or more days are missed, a 2nd nonhormonal method of contraception should be used until she has taken the pink tablet for 7 days. Transient spotting or bleeding may occur. If bleeding is persistent or prolonged, notify health care professional.
- Advise patient taking extended cycle tablets that spotting or light bleeding may occur, especially during first 3 mo. Continue medication; notify health care professional if bleeding lasts >70 days.
- Advise patient of the need to use another form of contraception for the first 3 wk when beginning to use *oral contraceptives.*
- Instruct patient to notify health care professional of all Rx or OTC medications, vitamins, or herbal products being taken and consult health care professional before taking any new medications.
- Advise patient that a 2nd method of birth control should also be used during each cycle in which any of the following are used: *Oral contraceptives:* ampicillin, corticosteroids, antiretroviral protease inhibitors, barbiturates, carbamazepine, chloramphenicol, dihydroergotamine, corticosteroids (systemic), mineral oil, oral neomycin, oxcarbazepine, penicillin VK, primidone, rifampin, sulfonamides, tetracyclines, topiramate, bosentan, or valproic acid.
- Explain dose schedule and maintenance routine. Discontinuing medication suddenly may cause withdrawal bleeding.
- If nausea becomes a problem, advise patient that eating solid food often provides relief. If nausea persists or vomiting or diarrhea occurs, use a nonhormonal method of contraception and notify health care professional.
- Advise patient to report signs and symptoms of fluid retention (swelling of ankles and feet, weight gain), thromboembolic disorders (pain, swelling, tenderness in extremities, headache, chest pain, blurred vision), mental depression, hepatic dysfunction (yellowed skin or eyes, pruritus, dark urine, light-colored stools), or abnormal vaginal bleeding. Women with a strong family history of breast cancer, fibrocystic breast disease, abnormal mammograms, or cervical dysplasia should be monitored for breast cancer at least yearly. Risk of thromboembolism is highest in 1st yr of use and increased when a combination hormonal contraceptive is restarted after a break in use of at least 4 wk.
- Caution patient that cigarette smoking during estrogen therapy may increase risk of serious side effects, especially for women over age 35.

- Caution patients to use sunscreen and protective clothing to prevent increased pigmentation.
- Caution patient that hormonal contraceptives do not protect against HIV or other sexually transmitted diseases.
- Advise patient to notify health care professional of medication regimen before treatment or surgery.
- Rep: Instruct patient to stop taking medication and notify health care professional if pregnancy is suspected.
- Emphasize the importance of routine follow-up physical exams including BP; breast, abdomen, and pelvic examinations; and Papanicolaou smears every 6–12 mo.
- **Emergency Contraception:** Instruct patient to take emergency contraceptive as directed. Advise patient that they should not take emergency contraceptives if they know or suspect they are pregnant; emergency contraceptives are not for use to end an existing pregnancy. Advise patient to contact health care professional if they vomit within 3 hr after taking *ulipristal.*
- Inform patient that *ulipristal* may reduce the effectiveness of hormonal contraceptives. Advise patient to use a nonhormonal contraceptive during that menstrual cycle. Advise patient to wait at least 5 days after taking *ulipristal* to resume taking hormonal contraceptives.
- Advise patient to notify health care professional and consider the possibility of pregnancy if their period is delayed by more than 1 wk beyond the expected date after taking *ulipristal.*
- Inform patient that emergency contraceptives are not to be used as a routine form of contraception or to be used repeatedly within the same menstrual cycle.
- Advise patient to notify health care professional if severe lower abdominal pain occurs 3–5 wk after taking *ulipristal* to be evaluated for an ectopic pregnancy.
- Advise female patients to avoid breastfeeding if taking *ulipristal.*
- **IM SUBQ:** Advise patient to maintain adequate amounts of dietary calcium and vitamin D to help prevent bone loss.
- **Transdermal:** Instruct patient on application of patch. First patch should be applied within 24 hr of menstrual period. If applied after Day 1 of menstrual period, a nonhormonal method of contraception should be used for the next 7 days. Day of application becomes *Patch Change Day.* Patches are worn for 1 wk and changed on the same day of each wk for 3 wk. Wk 4 is patch-free. Withdrawal bleeding is expected during this time.
- Apply patch to clean, dry, intact, healthy skin on buttock, abdomen, upper outer arm, or upper torso in a place where it won't be rubbed by tight clothing. Do not place on skin that is red, irritated, or cut, and

do not place on breasts. Do not apply make-up, creams, lotions, powders, or other topical products to area of patch application.

- To apply patch, open foil pouch by tearing along edge using fingers. Peel pouch apart and open flat. Grasp a corner of the patch firmly and remove gently from foil pouch. Use fingernail to lift one corner of the patch and peel patch **and** the plastic liner off the foil liner. Do not remove clear liner as patch is removed. Peel away half of the clear liner without touching sticky surface. Apply the sticky surface and remove the rest of the liner. Press down firmly with palm of hand for 10 sec; make sure the edges stick well.

- On *Patch Change Day* remove patch and apply new one immediately. Used patch still contains some active hormones; fold in half so it sticks to itself and throw away. Apply new patches to a new spot to prevent skin irritation; may be applied in same anatomic area.

- Following patch-free wk, apply a new patch on *Patch Change Day*, the day after Day 28, no matter when the menstrual cycle begins.

- If patch becomes partially or completely detached for less than 1 day, reapply patch or apply new patch. If patch is detached for more than 1 day, apply a new patch immediately and use a nonhormonal form of contraception for the next 7 days. Cycle will now start over with a new *Patch Change Day*. If patch is no longer sticky, apply a new patch; do not use tape or wraps to keep patch in place.

- If patch is not changed on *Patch Change Day* in the first wk of the cycle, apply new patch immediately upon remembering and use a nonhormonal method of contraception for next 7 days. If patch change is missed for 1 or 2 days during Wk 2 or 3, apply new patch immediately and apply next patch on usual *Patch Change Day*. No backup contraception is needed. If patch change is missed for more than 2 days during Wk 2 or 3, stop the cycle and start a new 4-wk contraceptive cycle by applying new patch immediately and using a nonhormonal method of contraception for the next 7 days. If patch is not removed on *Patch Change Day* in Wk 4, remove as soon as remembered and start next cycle on usual *Patch Change Day*. No additional contraception is needed.

- Advise patient referred for MRI test to discuss patch with referring health care professional and MRI facility to determine if removal of patch is necessary prior to test and for directions for replacing patch.

- **NuvaRing:** *If a hormonal contraceptive was not used in the past mo*, insert *NuvaRing* between Days 1 and 5 of the menstrual cycle (Day 1 = first day of menstrual period), even if bleeding has not finished. Use a nonhormonal method of birth control other than a diaphragm during the first 7 days of ring use. *If switching from a combination estrogen/progesterone oral contraceptive*, insert *NuvaRing* any time during first 7 days after last tablet and no later

than the day a new pill cycle would have started. No extra birth control is needed. *If switching from a mini-pill*, start using *NuvaRing* on any day of the mo; do not skip days between last pill and first day of *NuvaRing* use. *If switching from an implant*, start using *NuvaRing* on same day implant is removed. *If switching from an injectable contraceptive*, start using *NuvaRing* on the day when next injection is due. *If switching from a progestin-containing IUD*, start using *NuvaRing* on the same day as IUD is removed. A nonhormonal method of contraception, other than the diaphragm, should be used for the first 7 days of *NuvaRing* use when switching from the mini-pill, implant, injectable contraceptive, or IUD.

- *NuvaRing* comes in a reclosable foil pouch. Instruct patient to wash hands, then remove *NuvaRing* from pouch; keep pouch for ring disposal. Using a position of comfort (lying down, squatting, or standing with one leg up), hold *NuvaRing* between thumb and index finger and press opposite sides of the ring together. Gently push folded ring into vagina. Exact position is not important for function of *NuvaRing*. Most women do not feel *NuvaRing* once it is in place. If discomfort is felt, *NuvaRing* may not be inserted far enough into vagina; use finger to push further into vagina. *There is no danger of NuvaRing being pushed in too far or getting lost*. Once inserted, leave *NuvaRing* in place for 3 wk.

- Remove ring 3 wk after insertion on same day and time of insertion. Remove by hooking finger under forward rim or by holding ring between index and middle finger and pulling out. Place ring in foil pouch and dispose; do not throw in toilet. Menstrual period will usually start 2–3 days after ring is removed and may not have finished before next ring is inserted. To continue contraceptive protection, new ring must be inserted 1 wk after last one was removed, even if menstrual period has not stopped.

- If *NuvaRing* slips out of vagina and has been out less than 3 hr, contraceptive protection is still in place. *NuvaRing* can be rinsed in cool to tepid water and should be reinserted as soon as possible. If ring is lost, insert a new ring and continue same schedule as lost ring. If *NuvaRing* has been out of vagina for more than 3 hr, a nonhormonal method of contraception, other than a diaphragm, should be used for the next 7 days.

- *If NuvaRing has been left in for an extra wk or less (4 wk total or less)*, remove and insert a new ring after a 1-wk ring-free break. If *NuvaRing* has been left in place for more than 4 wk, woman should check to be sure she is not pregnant. A nonhormonal method of contraception, other than a diaphragm, must be used for the next 7 days.

- Advise patient to avoid using other female barrier contraceptives (diaphragm, cervical cap, female condom) with *NuvaRing*.

- **Intrauterine system:** Advise patient to notify health care professional if pelvic pain or pain during sex, unusual vaginal discharge or genital sores, unexplained fever, exposure to sexually transmitted infections, very severe or migraine headaches, yellowing of skin or whites of the eyes, very severe vaginal bleeding or bleeding that lasts a long time occurs, if a menstrual period is missed, or if *Mirena*'s threads cannot be felt.

Evaluation/Desired Outcomes
- Prevention of pregnancy.
- Regulation of the menstrual cycle.
- Decrease in menstrual blood loss.
- Decrease in acne.
- Decrease in symptoms of premenstrual dysphoric disorder.
- Decrease in vasomotor symptoms or symptoms of vulvar and vaginal atrophy due to menopause.

CORTICOSTEROIDS (INHALATION)
beclomethasone
(be-kloe-**meth**-a-sone)
✹ QVAR, QVAR Redihaler
budesonide (byoo-**dess**-oh-nide)
Pulmicort Flexhaler,
✹ Pulmicort Nebuamp, Pulmicort Respules, ✹ Pulmicort Turbuhaler
ciclesonide (inhalation)
(si-**kless**-o-nide)
Alvesco
fluticasone (floo-**ti**-ka-sone)
✹ Aermony Respiclick, Armonair Digihaler, Arnuity Ellipta, ~~Flovent Diskus~~, ~~Flovent HFA~~
mometasone (mo-**met**-a-sone)
Asmanex HFA, Asmanex Twisthaler
Classification
Therapeutic: anti-asthmatics, anti-inflammatories (steroidal)
Pharmacologic: corticosteroids (inhalation)

Indications
Maintenance treatment of asthma as prophylactic therapy. May decrease the need for or eliminate use of systemic corticosteroids in patients with asthma.

Action
Potent, locally acting anti-inflammatory and immune modifier. **Therapeutic Effects:** Decreased frequency and severity of asthma attacks. Improves asthma symptoms.

Pharmacokinetics
Absorption: *Beclomethasone:* 20%; *budesonide:* 6–13% (Flexhaler), 6% (Respules); *ciclesonide:* negligible; *fluticasone:* <7% (aerosol), 8–14% (pow-

der); *mometasone:* <1%. Action is primarily local after inhalation.

Distribution: All cross the placenta and enter breast milk in small amounts.

Metabolism and Excretion: *Beclomethasone:* after inhalation, beclomethasone dipropionate is converted to beclomethasone monopropionate, an active metabolite that adds to its potency, primarily excreted in feces (<10% excreted in urine; *Budesonide, fluticasone, mometasone:* metabolized by the liver (primarily by CYP3A4) after absorption from lungs; *Budesonide:* 60% excreted in urine, 40% in feces; *ciclesonide:* converted by esterases to des-ciclesonide, the active drug, which is subsequently metabolized by the liver. Some further metabolites may be pharmacologically active. Mostly eliminated in feces via biliary excretion; <20% of des-ciclesonide is excreted in urine; *fluticasone:* primarily excreted in feces (<5% excreted in urine); *mometasone:* 75% excreted in feces.

Half-life: *Beclomethasone:* 2.8 hr; *budesonide:* 2–3.6 hr; *ciclesonide:* 0.7 hr (ciclesonide); 6–7 hr (des-ciclesonide); *fluticasone:* 7.8 hr (propionate); 24 hr (furoate); *mometasone:* 5 hr.

TIME/ACTION PROFILE (improvement in symptoms)

ROUTE	ONSET	PEAK	DURATION
Inhalation	within 24 hr‡	1–4 wk†	unknown

†Improvement in pulmonary function; ↓ airway responsiveness may take longer.
‡2–8 days for budesonide respule.

Contraindications/Precautions
Contraindicated in: Some products contain alcohol or lactose and should be avoided in patients with known hypersensitivity or intolerance; Acute attack of asthma/status asthmaticus.

Use Cautiously in: Active untreated infections; Diabetes or glaucoma; Underlying immunosuppression (due to disease or concurrent therapy); Systemic corticosteroid therapy (should not be abruptly discontinued when inhalation therapy is started; additional corticosteroids needed in stress or trauma); Hepatic impairment (fluticasone); OB, Lactation: Safety not established; Pedi: Prolonged or high-dose therapy may lead to complications.

Adverse Reactions/Side Effects
EENT: <u>dysphonia</u>, <u>hoarseness</u>, cataracts, glaucoma, nasal congestion, pharyngitis, sinusitis. **Endo:** ↓ bone mineral density, adrenal suppression (↑ dose, long-term therapy only), ↓ growth (children). **GI:** diarrhea, dry mouth, dyspepsia, esophageal candidiasis, nausea, taste disturbances. **MS:** back pain. **Neuro:** headache, agitation, depression, dizziness, fatigue, insomnia, restlessness. **Resp:** bronchospasm, cough, wheezing. **Misc:** CHURG-STRAUSS SYNDROME, HYPERSENSITIVITY RE-

ACTIONS (including anaphylaxis, laryngeal edema, urticaria, and bronchospasm).

Interactions
Drug-Drug: Strong **CYP3A4 inhibitors**, including **ritonavir, atazanavir, clarithromycin, conivaptan, itraconazole, ketoconazole, lopinavir, nefazodone, nelfinavir,** and **voriconazole** ↓ metabolism and ↑ levels of budesonide, mometasone, and fluticasone; concurrent use with fluticasone not recommended.

Route/Dosage
Beclomethasone
Inhaln (Adults and Children ≥12 yr): *No prior treatment with inhaled corticosteroid:* 40–80 mcg twice daily (max dose = 320 mcg twice daily); *Prior treatment with inhaled corticosteroid:* 40–320 mcg twice daily (starting dose should be based on dose of previous inhaled corticosteroid and disease severity) (max dose = 320 mcg twice daily).
Inhaln (Children 4–11 yr): *No prior treatment with inhaled corticosteroid:* 40 mcg twice daily (max = 80 mcg twice daily); *Prior treatment with inhaled corticosteroid:* 40 mcg twice daily (max = 80 mcg twice daily).

Budesonide (Pulmicort Flexhaler)
Inhaln (Adults): 180–360 mcg twice daily (not to exceed 720 mcg twice daily).
Inhaln (Children ≥6 yr): 180–360 mcg twice daily (not to exceed 360 mcg twice daily).

Budesonide (Pulmicort Respules)
Inhaln (Children 1–8 yr): *Previously on bronchodilators alone:* 0.5 mg once daily or 0.25 mg twice daily (not to exceed 0.5 mg/day); *Previously on other inhaled corticosteroids:* 0.5 mg once daily or 0.25 mg twice daily (not to exceed 1 mg/day); *Previously on oral corticosteroids:* 1 mg once daily or 0.5 mg twice daily (not to exceed 1 mg/day).

Ciclesonide
Inhaln (Adults and Children ≥12 yr): *Previous therapy with bronchodilators alone:* 80 mcg twice daily, may be ↑ to 160 mcg twice daily; *Previous therapy with inhaled corticosteroids:* 80 mcg twice daily, may be ↑ to 320 mcg twice daily; *Previous therapy with oral corticosteroids:* 320 mcg twice daily.

Fluticasone (Aerosol Inhaler)
Inhaln (Adults and Children ≥12 yr): *Previously on bronchodilators alone:* 88 mcg twice daily initially, may be ↑ up to 440 mcg twice daily; *Previously on other inhaled corticosteroids:* 88–220 mcg twice daily initially, may be ↑ up to 440 mcg twice daily; *Previously on oral corticosteroids:* 440 mcg twice daily initially, may be ↑ up to 880 mcg twice daily.
Inhaln (Children 4–11 yr): 88 mcg twice daily (not to exceed 88 mcg twice daily).

Fluticasone (Dry Powder Inhaler)
Inhaln (Adults and Children ≥12 yr): *No prior treatment with inhaled corticosteroid:* Propionate (Flovent Diskus generic): 100 mcg twice daily initially, may ↑ dose in 2 wk if not adequately responding (max dose = 1,000 mcg twice daily); Propionate (Armonair Digihaler): 55 mcg twice daily initially, may ↑ dose in 2 wk if not adequately responding (max dose = 232 mcg twice daily); Furoate: 100 mcg once daily, may ↑ dose in 2 wk to 200 mcg once daily if not adequately responding (max dose = 200 mcg once daily); *Prior treatment with inhaled corticosteroid:* Propionate (Armonair Digihaler): 55–232 mcg twice daily (starting dose should be based on dose of previous inhaled corticosteroid and disease severity) (max dose = 232 mcg twice daily); Furoate: 100–200 mcg once daily (max dose = 200 mcg once daily).
Inhaln (Children 5–11 yr): Furoate: 50 mcg once daily.
Inhaln (Children 4–11 yr): *No prior treatment with inhaled corticosteroid:* Propionate (Flovent Diskus generic): 50 mcg twice daily initially, may ↑ dose in 2 wk to 100 mcg twice daily if not adequately responding (max dose = 100 mcg twice daily).

Mometasone (Aerosol Inhaler)
Inhaln (Adults and Children ≥12 yr): *Previously on medium-dose inhaled corticosteroids:* Two 100-mcg inhalations twice daily; *Previously on high-dose inhaled corticosteroids or oral corticosteroids:* Two 200-mcg inhalations twice daily (not to exceed 800 mcg/day).

Mometasone (Dry Powder Inhaler)
Inhaln (Adults and Children ≥12 yr): *Previously on bronchodilators or other inhaled corticosteroids:* 220 mcg once daily in evening, up to 440 mcg/day as a single dose or 2 divided doses; *Previously on oral corticosteroids:* 440 mcg twice daily (not to exceed 880 mcg/day).
Inhaln (Children 4–11 yr): 110 mcg once daily in evening (not to exceed 110 mcg/day).

Availability
Beclomethasone
Inhalation aerosol: 40 mcg/metered inhalation in 10.6-g canister (delivers 120 metered inhalations), ❋ 50 mcg/metered inhalation in 6.5-g canister (delivers 100 metered inhalations) and 12.4-g canister (delivers 200 metered inhalations), 80 mcg/metered inhalation in 10.6-g canister (delivers 120 metered inhalations), ❋ 100 mcg/metered inhalation in 6.5-g canister (delivers 100 metered inhalations) and 12.4-g canister (delivers 200 metered inhalations).

Budesonide (generic available)
Inhalation powder (Flexhaler): 90 mcg/metered inhalation (delivers 60 metered inhalations), 180 mcg/metered inhalation (delivers 120 metered inhalations).
Inhalation powder (Turbuhaler): ❋ 100 mcg/metered inhalation (delivers 200 metered inhalations), ❋

200 mcg/metered inhalation (delivers 200 metered inhalations), ✹ 400 mcg/metered inhalation (delivers 200 metered inhalations). **Inhalation suspension (Respules):** 0.25 mg/2 mL in single-dose ampules (5 ampules/envelope), 0.5 mg/2 mL in single-dose ampules (5 ampules/envelope), 1 mg/2 mL in single-dose ampules (5 ampules/envelope). *In combination with:* albuterol (Airsupra); formoterol (Breyna, Symbicort); formoterol and glycopyrrolate (Breztri Aerosphere). See Appendix N.

Ciclesonide
Inhalation aerosol (contains HFA-134A as a propellant): 80 mcg/actuation in 6.1-g canisters of 60 actuations, 160 mcg/actuation in 6.1-g canisters of 60 actuations.

Fluticasone
Inhalation aerosol (propionate) (Flovent-HFA generic): 44 mcg/metered inhalation in 10.6-g canisters (delivers 120 metered inhalations), ✹ 50 mcg/metered inhalation in 13-g canisters (delivers 120 metered inhalations), 110 mcg/metered inhalation in 12-g canisters (delivers 120 metered inhalations), ✹ 125 mcg/metered inhalation in 7.5-g canisters (delivers 60 metered inhalations) and 13-g canisters (delivers 120 metered inhalations), 220 mcg/metered inhalation in 12-g canisters (delivers 120 metered inhalations), ✹ 250 mcg/metered inhalation in 7.5-g canisters (delivers 60 metered inhalations) and 13-g canisters (delivers 120 metered inhalations). **Powder for inhalation (propionate) (Flovent Diskus generic):** 50 mcg/blister, 100 mcg/blister, 250 mcg/blister, ✹ 500 mcg/blister. **Powder for inhalation (propionate) (Armonair Digihaler):** 55 mcg/metered inhalation (delivers 60 metered inhalations), 113 mcg/metered inhalation (delivers 60 metered inhalations), 232 mcg/metered inhalation (delivers 60 metered inhalations). **Powder for inhalation (furoate) (Arnuity Ellipta):** 50 mcg/blister, 100 mcg/blister, 200 mcg/blister. *In combination with:* salmeterol (Advair Diskus, Advair HFA, AirDuo Digihaler, AirDuo RespiClick, Wixhela Inhub); vilanterol (Breo Ellipta); umeclidinium and vilanterol (Trelegy Ellipta). See Appendix N.

Mometasone
Inhalation aerosol (Asmanex HFA): 50 mcg/metered inhalation in 13-g canisters (120 metered inhalations), 100 mcg/metered inhalation in 13-g canisters (120 metered inhalations), 200 mcg/metered inhalation in 13-g canisters (120 metered inhalations). **Powder for inhalation (Asmanex Twisthaler):** ✹ 100 mcg/metered inhalation (30 metered inhalations), 110 mcg (delivers 100 mcg/metered inhalation; in packages of 7 and 30 inhalation units), ✹ 200 mcg/metered inhalation (60 metered inhalations), 220 mcg (delivers 200 mcg/metered inhalation; in packages of 14, 30, 60, and 120 inhalation units), ✹ 400 mcg/metered inhala-

tion (30 and 60 metered inhalations). *In combination with:* formoterol (Dulera). See Appendix N.

NURSING IMPLICATIONS
Assessment
- Monitor respiratory status and lung sounds. Assess pulmonary function tests periodically during and for several mo after a transfer from systemic to inhalation corticosteroids.
- Assess patients changing from systemic corticosteroids to inhalation corticosteroids for signs of adrenal insufficiency (anorexia, nausea, weakness, fatigue, hypotension, hypoglycemia) during initial therapy and periods of stress. If these signs appear, notify health care professional immediately; condition may be life-threatening.
- Monitor for withdrawal symptoms (joint or muscular pain, lassitude, depression) during withdrawal from oral corticosteroids.
- Monitor growth rate in children receiving chronic therapy; use lowest possible dose.
- May cause decreased bone mineral density during prolonged therapy. Monitor patients with increased risk (prolonged immobilization, family history of osteoporosis, postmenopausal status, tobacco use, advanced age, poor nutrition, chronic use of drugs that can reduce bone mass [anticonvulsants, oral corticosteroids]) for fractures.
- Monitor for signs and symptoms of hypersensitivity reactions (rash, pruritus, swelling of face and neck, dyspnea) periodically during therapy.

Lab Test Considerations
- Periodic adrenal function tests may be ordered to assess degree of hypothalamic-pituitary-adrenal (HPA) axis suppression in chronic therapy. Children and patients using higher than recommended doses are at highest risk for HPA suppression.
- May cause ↑ serum and urine glucose concentrations if significant absorption occurs.

Implementation
- Do not confuse Flovent with Flonase.
- After desired clinical effect has been obtained, attempts should be made to decrease dose to lowest amount required to control symptoms. Gradually decrease dose every 2–4 wk as long as desired effect is maintained. If symptoms return, dose may briefly return to starting dose.
- **Inhaln:** Allow at least 1 min between inhalations.

Patient/Family Teaching
- Advise patient to take medication as directed. Take missed doses as soon as remembered unless almost time for next dose. Instruct patient to read the *Patient Information and Instructions for Use* before using and with each Rx refill, in case of changes. Advise patient not to discontinue medication without

consulting health care professional; gradual decrease is required.

- Advise patients using inhalation corticosteroids and bronchodilator to use bronchodilator first and to allow 5 min to elapse before administering the corticosteroid, unless otherwise directed by health care professional.
- Advise patient that inhalation corticosteroids should not be used to treat an acute asthma attack but should be continued even if other inhalation agents are used.
- Patients using inhalation corticosteroids to control asthma may require systemic corticosteroids for acute attacks. Advise patient to use regular peak flow monitoring to determine respiratory status.
- Caution patient to avoid smoking, known allergens, and other respiratory irritants.
- Advise patient to notify health care professional if sore throat or sore mouth occurs.
- Advise patient to stop using medication and notify health care professional immediately if signs and symptoms of hypersensitivity reactions occur.
- Instruct patient whose systemic corticosteroids have been recently reduced or withdrawn to carry a warning card indicating the need for supplemental systemic corticosteroids in the event of stress or severe asthma attack unresponsive to bronchodilators.
- Advise patient to have regular eye exams. May increase risk for eye problems (glaucoma, cataracts, blurred vision).
- Rep: Advise females of reproductive potential to notify health care professional if pregnancy is planned or suspected or if breastfeeding.
- **Metered-Dose Inhaler:** Instruct patient in proper use of metered-dose inhaler. Most inhalers require priming before first use. Shake inhaler well. Exhale completely, and then close lips firmly around mouthpiece. While breathing in deeply and slowly, press down on canister. Hold breath for as long as possible to ensure deep instillation of medication. Remove inhaler from mouth and breathe out gently. Allow 1–2 min between inhalations. Rinse mouth with water or mouthwash after each use to minimize fungal infections, dry mouth, and hoarseness. Clean mouthpiece weekly with clean, dry tissue or cloth. Do not place in water (see Appendix C).
- **Pulmicort Flexhaler:** Advise patient to follow instructions supplied. Before first-time use, prime unit by turning cover and lifting off; hold upright with mouthpiece up and twist brown grip fully to right, then fully to left until it clicks. To administer dose, hold upright, twist brown grip fully to right, then fully to left until it clicks. Turn head away from inhaler and exhale (do not blow into inhaler). Do not shake inhaler. Place mouthpiece between lips and inhale deeply and forcefully. Remove inhaler from mouth and exhale (do not exhale into mouthpiece). Repeat procedure if 2nd dose required. Replace cover; rinse mouth with water (do not swallow).

- **Pulmicort Respules:** Administer with a jet nebulizer connected to adequate air flow, equipped with a mouthpiece or face mask. Adjust face mask to avoid exposing eyes to nebulized medication. Wash face after use of face mask. Ultrasonic nebulizers are not adequate for administration and not recommended. Store respules upright, away from heat and protected from light. Do not refrigerate or freeze. Respules are stable for 2 wk at room temperature after opening aluminum foil envelope. Open respules must be used promptly. Unused respules should be returned to aluminum foil envelope.
- **Arnuity Ellipta:** Do not use with a spacer. Exhale completely and then close lips firmly around mouthpiece. While breathing in deeply and slowly, press down on canister. Hold breath for as long as possible to ensure deep instillation of medication. Remove inhaler from mouth and breathe out gently. Allow 1–2 min between inhalations. After inhalation, rinse mouth with water and spit out (see Appendix C). Never wash the mouthpiece or any part of the Diskus inhaler. Discard Diskus inhaler device (Flovent Diskus) 6 wk (50-mcg strength) or 2 mo (100-mcg and 250-mcg strengths) or blister tray (Arnuity Ellipta) 6 wk after removal from protective foil overwrap pouch or after all blisters have been used (whichever comes first).
- **Asmanex Twisthaler:** Advise patient to remove cap while device is in upright position. To administer dose, exhale fully, then place mouthpiece between lips and inhale deeply and forcefully. Remove device from mouth and hold breath for 10 sec before exhaling (do not exhale into mouthpiece). Wipe the mouthpiece dry, if necessary, and replace the cap on the device. Rinse mouth with water. Advise patient to discard twisthaler 45 days from opening or when dose counter reads "00," whichever comes first.

Evaluation/Desired Outcomes
- Decreased frequency and severity of asthma attacks.
- Improvement in symptoms of asthma.

CORTICOSTEROIDS (NASAL)
beclomethasone
(be-kloe-**meth**-a-sone)
~~Beconase AQ~~, QNASL, ✳ ~~Rivanase AQ~~
budesonide (byoo-**dess**-oh-nide)
Rhinocort Allergy, ✳ Rhinocort Aqua
ciclesonide (sye-**kles**-oh-nide)
Omnaris, Zetonna
fluticasone (floo-**ti**-ka-sone)
✳ Avamys, Flonase Allergy Relief,
Flonase Sensimist Allergy Relief,
Xhance
mometasone (moe-**met**-a-sone)
~~Nasonex~~

triamcinolone
(trye-am-**sin**-oh-lone)
Nasacort Allergy 24 HR, ✦ Nasacort AQ
Classification
Therapeutic: anti-inflammatories (steroidal)
Pharmacologic: corticosteroids (nasal)

Indications

Seasonal or perennial allergic rhinitis. Nonallergic rhinitis (fluticasone). Chronic rhinosinusitis with nasal polyps.

Action

Potent, locally acting anti-inflammatory and immune modifier. **Therapeutic Effects:** ↓ in symptoms of allergic or nonallergic rhinitis. ↓ in symptoms of nasal polyps.

Pharmacokinetics

Absorption: *Beclomethasone:* 27–44% absorbed; *budesonide:* 34% absorbed; *ciclesonide, fluticasone, mometasone:* negligible absorption. Action of all agents is primarily local following nasal use.
Distribution: All agents cross the placenta and enter breast milk in small amounts.
Metabolism and Excretion: Following absorption from nasal mucosa, corticosteroids are rapidly and extensively metabolized by the liver.
Half-life: *Beclomethasone:* 2.7 hr; *budesonide:* 2–3 hr; *ciclesonide:* unknown; *fluticasone:* 7.8 hr; *mometasone:* 5.8 hr; *triamcinolone:* 3–5.4 hr.

TIME/ACTION PROFILE (improvement in symptoms)

ROUTE	ONSET	PEAK	DURATION
Beclomethasone	1–3 days	up to 2 wk	unknown
Budesonide	1–2 days	2 wk	unknown
Ciclesonide	1–2 days	2–5 wk	unknown
Flunisolide	few days	up to 3 wk	unknown
Fluticasone	few days	unknown	unknown
Mometasone	within 2 days	1–2 wk	unknown
Triamcinolone	few days	3–4 days	unknown

Contraindications/Precautions

Contraindicated in: Some products contain alcohol, propylene, or polyethylene glycol and should be avoided in patients with known hypersensitivity or intolerance.
Use Cautiously in: Active untreated infections; Diabetes or glaucoma; Underlying immunosuppression (due to disease or concurrent therapy); Systemic corticosteroid therapy (should not be abruptly discontinued when intranasal therapy is started); History of ↑ intraocular pressure, glaucoma, or cataracts; Recent nasal trauma, septal ulcers, or surgery (wound healing may be impaired by nasal corticosteroids); OB, Lactation, Pedi: Pregnancy; lactation; or children <12 yr (beclomethasone]), <6 yr (budesonide, ciclesonide), <4 yr

(fluticasone [Flonase Allergy Relief]), or <2 yr (fluticasone [Flonase Sensimist], mometasone, triamcinolone) (safety not established; prolonged or high-dose therapy may lead to complications).

Adverse Reactions/Side Effects

Derm: rash (fluticasone), urticaria (fluticasone). **EENT:** ↑ intraocular pressure, blurred vision, cataracts, epistaxis, glaucoma, nasal burning, nasal congestion, nasal irritation, nasal perforation, nasal ulceration, pharyngitis, rhinorrhea, sneezing, tearing eyes. **Endo:** adrenal suppression (high-dose, long-term therapy only), growth suppression (children). **GI:** dry mouth, esophageal candidiasis, nausea, vomiting. **Neuro:** dizziness, headache. **Resp:** bronchospasm, cough. **Misc:** HYPERSENSITIVITY REACTIONS (including anaphylaxis and angioedema).

Interactions

Drug-Drug: **Strong CYP3A4 inhibitors**, including **atazanavir, clarithromycin, cobicistat, itraconazole, ketoconazole, nefazodone, nelfinavir,** and **ritonavir** may ↑ levels of budesonide, ciclesonide, fluticasone, and mometasone and ↑ the risk of adverse reactions.

Route/Dosage

Beclomethasone

Intranasal (Adults and Children ≥12 yr): 2 sprays in each nostril once daily.
Intranasal (Children 4–11 yr): 1 spray in each nostril once daily.

Budesonide

Intranasal (Adults and Children ≥12 yr): 1 spray in each nostril once daily (not to exceed 4 sprays in each nostril once daily). For OTC use, administer 2 sprays in each nostril once daily; once symptoms improve, ↓ to 1 spray in each nostril once daily.
Intranasal (Children 6–11 yr): 1 spray in each nostril once daily (not to exceed 2 sprays in each nostril once daily).

Ciclesonide

Intranasal (Adults and Children ≥12 yr): *Omnaris (for perennial allergic rhinitis only):* 2 sprays in each nostril once daily (not to exceed 2 sprays in each nostril/day); *Zetonna:* 1 spray in each nostril once daily (not to exceed 1 spray in each nostril/day).
Intranasal (Adults and Children ≥6 yr): *Omnaris (for seasonal allergic rhinitis only):* 2 sprays in each nostril once daily (not to exceed 2 sprays in each nostril/day).

Flunisolide

Intranasal (Adults and Children >14 yr): 2 sprays in each nostril twice daily, may be ↑ to 2 sprays in each nostril 3 times daily if greater effect needed after 4–7 days (not to exceed 8 sprays in each nostril/day).

Intranasal (Children 6–14 yr): 1 spray in each nostril 3 times daily or 2 sprays in each nostril twice daily (not to exceed 4 sprays in each nostril/day).

Fluticasone

Intranasal (Adults): *Fluticasone Rx:* 2 sprays in each nostril once daily or 1 spray in each nostril twice daily (not to exceed 2 sprays in each nostril/day); after several days, attempt to ↓ dose to 1 spray in each nostril once daily. *Xbance:* 1 spray in each nostril twice daily; may adjust to 2 sprays in each nostril twice daily.

Intranasal (Adults and Children ≥12 yr): *Flonase Sensimist Allergy Relief (OTC) and Flonase Allergy Relief (OTC):* 2 sprays in each nostril once daily; after 1 wk, may adjust to 1–2 sprays in each nostril once daily; discuss with health care professional if need to continue longer than 6 mo.

Intranasal (Children 4–11 yr): *Flonase Allergy Relief (OTC):* 1 spray in each nostril once daily; discuss with health care professional if need to continue longer than 2 mo.

Intranasal (Children ≥4 yr): *Fluticasone Rx:* 1 spray in each nostril once daily; may ↑ to 2 sprays in each nostril once daily if no response; once symptoms controlled, attempt to ↓ dose to 1 spray in each nostril once daily.

Intranasal (Children 2–11 yr): *Flonase Sensimist Allergy Relief (OTC):* 1 spray in each nostril once daily; discuss with health care professional if need to continue longer than 2 mo.

Mometasone

Intranasal (Adults and Children >12 yr): *Treatment of seasonal and perennial allergic rhinitis:* 2 sprays in each nostril once daily (not to exceed 2 sprays in each nostril once daily).

Intranasal (Adults): *Nasal polyps:* 2 sprays in each nostril twice daily (not to exceed 2 sprays in each nostril twice daily).

Intranasal (Children 2–11 yr): *Treatment of seasonal and perennial allergic rhinitis:* 1 spray in each nostril once daily.

Triamcinolone

Intranasal (Adults and Children ≥12 yr): 2 sprays in each nostril once daily; not to be used in children for longer than 2 mo.

Intranasal (Children 6–11 yr): 1 spray in each nostril once daily (not to exceed 2 sprays in each nostril/day); not to be used for longer than 2 mo.

Intranasal (Children 2–5 yr): 1 spray in each nostril once daily not to be used for longer than 2 mo.

Availability

Beclomethasone

Nasal spray: 40 mcg/metered spray in 4.9-g bottles (delivers 60 metered sprays), 80 mcg/metered spray in 8.7-g bottles (delivers 120 metered sprays).

Budesonide (generic available)

Nasal spray (Rhinocort Allergy): 32 mcg/metered spray in 5-mL bottle (delivers 60 metered sprays)[OTC],

and 8.43-mL bottle (delivers 120 metered sprays)[OTC].
Nasal spray (Rhinocort Aqua): ✸ 64 mcg/metered spray (delivers 120 metered sprays).

Ciclesonide

Nasal spray (Zetonna): 37 mcg/actuation in 6.1-g bottle (delivers 60 metered sprays). Nasal suspension (Omnaris): 50 mcg/metered spray in 12.5-g bottle (delivers 120 metered sprays).

Flunisolide (generic available)

Nasal solution: 25 mcg/actuation in 25-mL bottle (delivers 200 metered sprays).

Fluticasone (generic available)

Nasal spray: 50 mcg/metered spray in 16-g bottle (delivers 120 metered sprays). Nasal spray (Flonase Allergy Relief): 50 mcg/metered spray in 9.9-mL bottle (delivers 60 metered sprays)[OTC]. Nasal spray (Flonase Sensimist Allergy Relief): 27.5 mcg/spray in 9.9-mL bottle (delivers 60 metered sprays)[OTC]. Nasal spray (Avamys): ✸ 27.5 mcg/spray in 4.5-g bottle (delivers 30 metered sprays) and 10-g bottle (delivers 120 metered sprays). Nasal spray (Xhance): 93 mcg/spray in 16-mL bottle (delivers 120 metered sprays). *In combination with:* azelastine (Dymista); see Appendix N.

Mometasone (generic available)

Nasal spray (scent-free): 50 mcg/metered spray in 17-g bottle (delivers 120 metered sprays). *In combination with:* olopatadine (Ryaltris). See Appendix N.

Triamcinolone (generic available)

Nasal spray: 55 mcg/metered spray in 6.7-mL bottle (delivers 30 metered sprays)[OTC], 10.8-mL bottle (delivers 60 metered sprays)[OTC], and 16.9-mL bottle (delivers 120 metered sprays)[OTC].

NURSING IMPLICATIONS

Assessment

- Monitor degree of nasal stuffiness, amount and color of nasal discharge, and frequency of sneezing.
- Monitor for signs of adverse effects on nasal mucosa (nasal discomfort, epistaxis, nasal ulceration, *Candida albicans* infection, nasal septal perforation, impaired wound healing) periodically during therapy. Avoid use in patients with recent nasal ulcers, nasal surgery, or nasal trauma.
- Patients on long-term therapy should have periodic otolaryngologic examinations to monitor nasal mucosa and passages for infection or ulceration.
- Monitor growth rate in children receiving chronic therapy; use lowest possible dose.

Lab Test Considerations

- Periodic adrenal function tests may be ordered to assess degree of hypothalamic-pituitary-adrenal (HPA) axis suppression in chronic therapy. Children and patients using higher than recommended doses are at highest risk for HPA suppression.

Implementation
- Do not confuse Flonase with Flovent.
- After desired clinical effect is obtained, decrease dose to lowest effective amount. Gradually decrease dose every 2–4 wk as long as desired effect is maintained. If symptoms return, dose may briefly return to starting dose.
- **Intranasal:** Patients also using a nasal decongestant should be given decongestant 5–15 min before corticosteroid nasal spray. If patient is unable to breathe freely through nasal passages, instruct patient to blow nose gently in advance of medication administration.

Patient/Family Teaching
- Advise patient to take medication as directed. Take missed doses as soon as remembered unless almost time for next dose.
- Caution patient not to exceed maximal daily dose of nasal spray.
- Instruct patient in correct technique for administering nasal spray (see Appendix C). Most nasal sprays include directions with pictures. Instruct patient to read patient information sheet prior to use. Most nasal sprays require priming prior to first use or use after 7 days. Shake well before use. Warn patient that temporary nasal stinging may occur.
- Instruct patient to gently blow nose to clear nostrils prior to administering dose.
- Instruct patient to stop medication and notify health care professional immediately if signs of anaphylaxis (rash, hives, difficulty breathing, swollen lips or throat) or if changes in vision occur.
- Instruct patient to notify health care professional of all Rx or OTC medications, vitamins, or herbal products being taken and consult health care professional before taking other Rx, OTC, or herbal products.
- Rep: Advise females of reproductive potential to notify health care professional if pregnancy is planned or suspected or if breastfeeding.
- Instruct patient to notify health care professional if symptoms do not improve within 1 mo, if symptoms worsen, or if sneezing or nasal irritation occurs.

Evaluation/Desired Outcomes
- Resolution of nasal stuffiness, discharge, and sneezing in seasonal or perennial allergic rhinitis or nonallergic rhinitis.
- Reduction in symptoms of nasal polyps.

CORTICOSTEROIDS (SYSTEMIC)
short-acting corticosteroids
hydrocortisone
(hye-droe-**kor**-ti-sone)
Alkindi Sprinkle, Cortef, Cortenema, Solu-CORTEF

intermediate-acting corticosteroids
methylPREDNISolone
(meth-ill-pred-**niss**-oh-lone)
Depo-Medrol, Medrol, Solu-MEDROL
prednisoLONE (pred-**niss**-oh-lone)
~~Orapred~~, Millipred, Orapred ODT, Pediapred
predniSONE (pred-ni-sone)
Rayos, ✹ Winipred
triamcinolone
(trye-am-**sin**-oh-lone)
Hexatrione, Kenalog, ✹ Trispan, Zilretta

long-acting corticosteroids
betamethasone
(bay-ta-**meth**-a-sone)
✹ ~~Betaject~~, Celestone Soluspan, ~~Celestone~~
budesonide (byoo-**dess**-oh-nide)
✹ Cortiment, ✹ Entocort, ✹ Jorveza, ~~Entocort EC~~, Ortikos, Tarpeyo, Uceris
dexAMETHasone
(dex-a-**meth**-a-sone)
~~Decadron~~, Hemady
Classification
Therapeutic: anti-asthmatics, corticosteroids
Pharmacologic: corticosteroids (systemic)

Indications
Hydrocortisone: Management of adrenocortical insufficiency. **Betamethasone, dexamethasone, hydrocortisone, prednisolone, prednisone, methylprednisolone, triamcinolone:** Used systemically and locally in a wide variety of chronic diseases including: Inflammatory, Allergic, Hematologic, Neoplastic, Autoimmune disorders. **Methylprednisolone, prednisone:** With other immunosuppressants in the prevention of organ rejection in transplantation surgery. Asthma. **Dexamethasone:** Cerebral edema: Diagnostic agent in adrenal disorders., Multiple myeloma (in combination with other anti-myeloma agents). **Budesonide (3-mg Delayed-Release Capsules and Ortikos):** Treatment of mild to moderate Crohn's disease involving ileum and/or ascending colon. **Budesonide (3-mg Delayed-Release Capsules and Ortikos):** Maintenance of clinical remission for up to 3 mo of mild to moderate Crohn's disease involving ileum and/or ascending colon. **Budesonide (Uceris):** Induction of remission of active, mild to moderate ulcerative colitis. **Budesonide (Tarpeyo):** Reduction of proteinuria in patients with primary immunoglobulin A nephropathy who are at risk of rapid disease progression (i.e., a urine protein-to-creatinine ratio [UPCR] ≥ 1.5 g/g).

✹ = Canadian drug name. ⚇ = Genetic implication. ~~Strikethrough~~ = Discontinued. CAPITALS = life-threatening. <u>Underline</u> = most frequent.

Unlabeled Use: Short-term administration to high-risk mothers before delivery to prevent respiratory distress syndrome in the newborn (betamethasone, dexamethasone). Adjunctive therapy of hypercalcemia (prednisone, prednisolone, methylprednisolone). Management of acute spinal cord injury (methylprednisolone). Adjunctive management of nausea and vomiting from chemotherapy (dexamethasone, prednisone, prednisolone, methylprednisolone). Management of croup (dexamethasone). Treatment of airway edema prior to extubation (dexamethasone). Facilitation of ventilator weaning in neonates with bronchopulmonary dysplasia (dexamethasone).

Action

In pharmacologic doses, all agents suppress inflammation and the normal immune response. All agents have numerous intense metabolic effects (see Adverse Reactions/Side Effects). Suppress adrenal function at chronic doses of *betamethasone:* 0.6 mg/day; *hydrocortisone:* 20 mg/day; *dexamethasone:* 0.75 mg/day; *methylprednisolone, triamcinolone:* 4 mg/day; *prednisone/prednisolone:* 5 mg/day. **Hydrocortisone:** Replace endogenous cortisol in deficiency states. **Hydrocortisone:** Have potent mineralocorticoid (sodium-retaining) activity. **Prednisolone, prednisone:** Have minimal mineralocorticoid activity. **Betamethasone, dexamethasone, methylprednisolone, triamcinolone:** Have negligible mineralocorticoid activity. **Budesonide:** Local anti-inflammatory activity in the lumen of the GI tract in Crohn's disease and ulcerative colitis; modulates activity of B-cells in ileum to decrease production of galactose-deficient IgA1 antibodies, which cause IgA nephropathy. **Therapeutic Effects:** Suppression of inflammation and modification of the normal immune response. Replacement therapy in adrenal insufficiency. **Budesonide:** Improvement in symptoms/sequelae of Crohn's disease, induction of remission of ulcerative colitis, and reduction in UPCR.

Pharmacokinetics

Absorption: Well absorbed after oral administration (except budesonide). Sodium phosphate and sodium succinate salts are rapidly absorbed after IM administration. Acetate and acetonide salts are slowly but completely absorbed after IM administration. Absorption from local sites (intra-articular, intralesional) is slow but complete. Bioavailability of budesonide is 9–21%.
Distribution: All are widely distributed.
Metabolism and Excretion: All are metabolized mostly by the liver to inactive metabolites. *Prednisone* is converted by the liver to prednisolone, which is then metabolized by the liver.
Half-life: *Betamethasone:* 3–5 hr (plasma), 36–54 hr (tissue). *Budesonide:* 2.0–3.6 hr (3-mg delayed-release capsules, Ortikos, Uceris); 5–6.8 hr (Tarpeyo). *Dexamethasone:* 3–4.5 hr (plasma), 36–54 hr (tissue). *Hydrocortisone:* 1.5–2 hr (plasma), 8–12 hr (tissue). *Methylprednisolone:* >3.5 hr (plasma), 18–36 hr (tissue). *Prednisolone:* 2.1–3.5 hr (plasma), 18–36 hr (tissue). *Prednisone:* 3.4–3.8 hr (plasma), 18–36 hr (tissue). *Triamcinolone:* 2–5 hr (plasma), 18–36 hr (tissue).

TIME/ACTION PROFILE (anti-inflammatory activity)

ROUTE	ONSET	PEAK	DURATION
Betamethasone IM (acetate/sodium phosphate)	1–3 hr	unknown	1 wk
Budesonide PO	unknown	unknown	unknown
Dexamethasone PO	unknown	1–3 hr	2.75 days
Dexamethasone IM, IV (sodium phosphate)	rapid	unknown	2.75 days
Hydrocortisone PO	unknown	1–2 hr	1.25–1.5 days
Hydrocortisone IM (sodium succinate)	rapid	1 hr	variable
Hydrocortisone IV (sodium succinate)	rapid	unknown	unknown
Methylprednisolone PO	unknown	1–2 hr	1.25–1.5 days
Methylprednisolone IM (acetate)	6–48 hr	4–8 days	1–4 wk
Methylprednisolone IM, IV (sodium succinate)	rapid	unknown	unknown
Prednisolone PO	unknown	1–2 hr	1.25–1.5 days
Prednisone PO	unknown	1–2 hr	1.25–1.5 days
Triamcinolone IM (acetonide)	24–48 hr	unknown	1–6 wk
Triamcinolone Intralesional (hexacetonide)	slow	unknown	4 days–4 wk

Contraindications/Precautions

Contraindicated in: Active untreated infections (may be used in patients being treated for some forms of meningitis); Lactation: Avoid chronic use; Known alcohol, bisulfite, cow's milk, or tartrazine hypersensitivity or intolerance (some products contain these and should be avoided in susceptible patients); Administration of live virus vaccines.

Use Cautiously in: Chronic treatment (will lead to adrenal suppression; use lowest possible dose for shortest period of time); Hypothyroidism; Immunosuppression; Cirrhosis; Stress (surgery, infections); supplemental doses may be needed; Potential infections may mask signs (fever, inflammation); Traumatic brain injury (high doses may be associated with ↑ mortality); OB: Safety not established; Pedi: Children (chronic use will result in ↓ growth; use lowest possible dose for shortest period of time); Pedi: Neonates (avoid use of benzyl alcohol containing injectable preparations; use preservative-free formulations).

Adverse Reactions/Side Effects

Adverse reactions/side effects are much more common with high-dose/long-term therapy.

C

CV: hypertension. **Derm:** ↓ wound healing, acne, ecchymoses, fragility, hirsutism, petechiae. **EENT:** ↑ intraocular pressure, cataracts. **Endo:** adrenal suppression, cushingoid appearance (moon face, buffalo hump), hyperglycemia, PHEOCHROMOCYTOMA. **F and E:** fluid retention (long-term high doses), hypokalemia, hypokalemic alkalosis. **GI:** anorexia, nausea, PEPTIC ULCERATION, vomiting. **Hemat:** leukocytosis, THROMBOEMBOLISM, thrombophlebitis. **Metab:** weight gain. **MS:** muscle wasting, osteoporosis, avascular necrosis of joints, muscle pain. **Neuro:** depression, euphoria, ↑ intracranial pressure (children only), headache, personality changes, psychoses, restlessness. **Misc:** ↑ susceptibility to infection.

Interactions

Drug-Drug: ↑ risk of hypokalemia with **thiazide** and **loop diuretics**, or **amphotericin B**. Hypokalemia may ↑ risk of **digoxin** toxicity. May increase requirement for **insulin** or **oral hypoglycemic agents**. **Phenytoin, phenobarbital,** and **rifampin** ↑ metabolism; may ↓ effectiveness. **Hormonal contraceptives** may ↓ metabolism. ↑ risk of adverse GI effects with **NSAIDs** (including aspirin). At chronic doses that suppress adrenal function, may ↓ antibody response to and ↑ risk of adverse reactions from **live-virus vaccines**. May ↑ serum concentrations of **cyclosporine** and **tacrolimus**. May ↑ risk of tendon rupture from **fluoroquinolones. Antacids** ↓ absorption of prednisone and dexamethasone. **CYP3A4 inhibitors**, including **clarithromycin, cobicistat, itraconazole, ketoconazole,** or **ritonavir** may ↑ levels and the risk of toxicity. May ↓ **isoniazid** levels and effectiveness. May antagonize the effects of **anticholinergic agents** in myasthenia gravis.
Drug-Food: Grapefruit juice ↑ serum levels and effects of budesonide (avoid concurrent use).

Route/Dosage

Betamethasone

IM (Adults): 0.5–9 mg as betamethasone sodium phosphate/acetate suspension. *Prevention of respiratory distress syndrome in newborn:* 12 mg daily for 2–3 days before delivery (unlabeled).
IM (Children): *Adrenocortical insufficiency:* 17.5 mcg/kg/day (500 mcg/m²/day) in 3 divided doses every 3rd day or 5.8–8.75 mcg/kg (166–250 mcg/m²)/day as a single dose.

Budesonide

PO (Adults): *Active Crohn's disease:* 9 mg once daily in the morning for ≤8 wk; may repeat 8-wk course for recurring episodes. *Maintenance of remission of Crohn's disease:* 6 mg once daily for up to 3 mo; once symptoms are controlled, taper to complete cessation; *Induction of remission of ulcerative colitis:* 9 mg once daily for up to 8 wk; once symptoms are controlled, taper to complete cessation; *Reduction in pro-*

teinuria associated with primary immunoglobulin A nephropathy: 16 mg once daily in the morning for 9 mo, then 8 mg once daily in the morning for 2 wk.
PO (Children 8–17 yr and >25 kg): *Active Crohn's disease:* 9 mg once daily in the morning for up to 8 wk, then 6 mg once daily in the morning for 2 wk.

Hepatic Impairment

(Adults): *Moderate hepatic impairment (Child-Pugh Class B):* 3 mg once daily in the morning.

Dexamethasone

PO, IM, IV (Adults): *Anti-inflammatory:* 0.75–9 mg daily in divided doses every 6–12 hr. *Airway edema or extubation:* 0.5–2 mg/kg/day divided every 6 hr; begin 24 hr prior to extubation and continue for 24 hr post-extubation. *Cerebral edema:* 10 mg IV, then 4 mg IM or IV every 6 hr until maximal response achieved, then switch to PO regimen and taper over 5–7 days.
PO, IM, IV (Children): *Airway edema or extubation:* 0.5–2 mg/kg/day divided every 6 hr; begin 24 hr prior to extubation and continue for 24 hr post-extubation. *Anti-inflammatory:* 0.08–0.3 mg/kg/day or 2.5–10 mg/m²/day divided every 6–12 hr. *Physiologic replacement:* 0.03–0.15 mg/kg/day or 0.6–0.75 mg/m²/day divided every 6–12 hr.
PO (Adults): *Suppression test:* 1 mg at 11 PM or 0.5 mg every 6 hr for 48 hr. *Multiple myeloma:* 20–40 mg once daily on specific days (based on protocol being used).
IV (Children): *Chemotherapy-induced emesis:* 5–20 mg given 15–30 min before treatment; *Cerebral edema:* Loading dose 1–2 mg/kg followed by 1–1.5 mg/kg/day divided every 4–6 hr for 5 days (not to exceed 16 mg/day); then taper over 1–6 wk; *Bacterial meningitis:* 0.6 mg/kg/day divided every 6 hr for 4 days (start at time of first antibiotic dose).
IV, PO (Adults): *Chemotherapy-induced emesis:* 10–20 mg given 15–30 min before each treatment or 10 mg every 12 hr on each treatment day; *Delayed nausea/vomiting:* 4–10 mg PO 1–2 times/day for 2–4 days or 8 mg PO every 12 hr for 2 days, then 4 mg PO every 12 hr for 2 days or 20 mg PO 1 hr before chemotherapy, then 10 mg PO every 12 hr after chemotherapy, then 8 mg PO every 12 hr for 2 days, then 4 mg PO every 12 hr for 2 days.
IS (Adults): 0.4–6 mg/day.

Hydrocortisone

PO (Adults): 20–240 mg/day in 1–4 divided doses.
PO (Children): *Adrenocortical insufficiency/replacement therapy:* 8–10 mg/m²/day in 2–3 divided doses; *Anti-inflammatory or immunosuppressive:* 2.5–10 mg/kg/day or 75–300 mg/m²/day in 3–4 divided doses.
IM, IV (Adults): 100–500 mg every 2–6 hr (range 100–8000 mg/day).
IM, IV (Children): *Adrenocortical insufficiency:* 0.186–0.28 mg/kg/day (10–12 mg/m²/day) in 3 di-

vided doses. *Other uses:* 0.666–4 mg/kg (20–120 mg/m^2) every 12–24 hr.
Rect (Adults): *Retention enema:* 100 mg nightly for 21 days or until remission occurs.

Methylprednisolone

PO (Adults): *Multiple sclerosis:* 160 mg/day for 7 days, then 64 mg every other day for 1 mo. *Other uses:* 2–60 mg/day as a single dose or in 2–4 divided doses. *Asthma exacerbations:* 120–180 mg/day in divided doses 3–4 times/day for 48 hr, then 60–80 mg/day in 2 divided doses.
PO (Children): *Anti-inflammatory/Immunosuppressive:* 0.5–1.7 mg/kg/day (5–25 mg/m^2/day) in divided doses every 6–12 hr. *Asthma exacerbations:* 1 mg/kg every 6 hr for 48 hr, then 1–2 mg/kg/day (maximum: 60 mg/day) divided twice daily.
IM, IV (Adults): *Most uses: methylprednisolone sodium succinate:* 40–250 mg every 4–6 hr. *High-dose "pulse" therapy: methylprednisolone sodium succinate:* 30 mg/kg IV every 4–6 hr for up to 72 hr. *Status asthmaticus: methylprednisolone sodium succinate:* 2 mg/kg IV, then 0.5–1 mg/kg IV every 6 hr for up to 5 days. *Multiple sclerosis: methylprednisolone sodium succinate:* 160 mg/day for 7 days, then 64 mg every other day for 1 mo. *Adjunctive therapy of* P. jiroveci *pneumonia in AIDS patients: methylprednisolone sodium succinate:* 30 mg twice daily for 5 days, then 30 mg once daily for 5 days, then 15 mg once daily for 10 days. *Acute spinal cord injury: methylprednisolone sodium succinate:* 30 mg/kg IV over 15 min initially, followed in 45 min with a continuous infusion of 5.4 mg/kg/hr for 23 hr (unlabeled).
IM, IV (Children): *Anti-inflammatory/Immunosuppressive:* 0.5–1.7 mg/kg/day (5–25 mg/m^2/day) in divided doses every 6–12 hr. *Acute spinal cord injury: methylprednisolone sodium succinate:* 30 mg/kg IV over 15 min initially, followed in 45 min with a continuous infusion of 5.4 mg/kg/hr for 23 hr (unlabeled). *Status asthmaticus:* 2 mg/kg IV, then 0.5–1 mg/kg IV every 6 hr. *Lupus nephritis:* 30 mg/kg IV every other day for 6 doses.
IM (Adults): *Methylprednisolone acetate:* 40–120 mg daily, weekly, or every 2 wk.

Prednisolone

PO (Adults): *Most uses:* 5–60 mg/day as a single dose or in divided doses. *Multiple sclerosis:* 200 mg/day for 7 days, then 80 mg every other day for 1 mo. *Asthma exacerbations:* 120–180 mg/day in divided doses 3–4 times/day for 48 hr, then 60–80 mg/day in 2 divided doses.
PO (Children): *Anti-inflammatory/Immunosuppressive:* 0.1–2 mg/kg/day in 1–4 divided doses; *Nephrotic syndrome:* 2 mg/kg/day (60 mg/m^2/day) in 1–3 divided doses daily (maximum dose: 80 mg/day) until urine is protein-free for 4–6 wk, followed by 2 mg/kg/day (40 mg/m^2/dose) every other day in the morning; gradually taper off over 4–6 wk; *Asthma exacerbations:* 1 mg/kg every 6 hr for 48 hr, then 1–2 mg/kg/day (maximum: 60 mg/day) divided twice daily.

Prednisone

PO (Adults): *Most uses:* 5–60 mg/day as a single dose or in divided doses. *Multiple sclerosis:* 200 mg/day for 1 wk, then 80 mg every other day for 1 mo. *Adjunctive therapy of* P. jiroveci *pneumonia in AIDS patients:* 40 mg twice daily for 5 days, then 40 mg once daily for 5 days, then 20 mg once daily for 10 days.
PO (Children): *Nephrotic syndrome:* 2 mg/kg/day initially given in 1–3 divided doses (maximum 80 mg/day) until urine is protein-free for 4–6 wk. Maintenance dose of 2 mg/kg/day every other day in the morning, gradually taper off after 4–6 wk. *Asthma exacerbation:* 1 mg/kg every 6 hr for 48 hr, then 1–2 mg/kg/day (maximum 60 mg/day) in divided doses twice daily.

Triamcinolone

IM (Adults): *Triamcinolone acetonide:* 40–80 mg every 4 wk.
Intra-articular (Adults): *Triamcinolone hexacetonide:* 2–20 mg every 3–4 wk (dose depends on size of joint to be injected, amount of inflammation, and amount of fluid present); *Triamcinolone acetonide:* 32 mg as a single dose into the knee joint.
IM (Children): *Triamcinolone acetonide:* 40 mg every 4 wk or 30–200 mcg/kg (1–6.25 mg/m^2) every 1–7 days.

Availability

Betamethasone (generic available)
Suspension for injection (sodium phosphate and acetate): 6 mg (total)/mL.

Budesonide (generic available)
Delayed-release capsules: 3 mg. **Delayed-release capsules (Tarpeyo):** 4 mg. **Extended-release capsules (Ortikos):** 6 mg, 9 mg. **Extended-release tablets (Uceris):** 9 mg. **Orally disintegrating tablets (Jorveza):** ✸ 1 mg.

Dexamethasone (generic available)
Tablets: 0.5 mg, 0.75 mg, 1 mg, 1.5 mg, 2 mg, 4 mg, 6 mg, 20 mg. **Elixir (raspberry flavor):** 0.5 mg/5 mL. **Oral solution (cherry flavor):** 0.5 mg/5 mL, 1 mg/mL. **Solution for injection (sodium phosphate):** 4 mg/mL, 10 mg/mL.

Hydrocortisone (generic available)
Tablets: 5 mg, 10 mg, 20 mg. **Oral granules (Alkindi Sprinkle):** 0.5 mg, 1 mg, 2 mg, 5 mg. **Enema:** 100 mg/60 mL. **Lyophilized powder for injection (sodium succinate):** 100 mg/vial, 250 mg/vial, 500 mg/vial, 1 g.

Methylprednisolone (generic available)
Tablets: 2 mg, 4 mg, 8 mg, 16 mg, 32 mg. **Powder for injection (sodium succinate):** 40 mg/vial, 125 mg/vial, 500 mg/vial, 1 g/vial, 2 g/vial. **Suspension for injection (acetate):** 20 mg/mL, 40 mg/mL, 80 mg/mL.

Prednisolone (generic available)
Tablets: 5 mg. **Orally disintegrating tablets (grape flavor):** 10 mg, 15 mg, 30 mg. **Oral solution:** 5 mg/5 mL, 10 mg/5 mL, 15 mg/5 mL, 20 mg/5 mL, 25 mg/5 mL.

Prednisone (generic available)
Tablets: 1 mg, 2.5 mg, 5 mg, 10 mg, 20 mg, 50 mg. **Delayed-release tablets:** 1 mg, 2 mg, 5 mg. **Oral solution:** 5 mg/5 mL, 5 mg/mL.

Triamcinolone (generic available)
Extended-release suspension for intra-articular injection (acetonide) (requires reconstitution) (Zilretta): 32 mg/vial. **Suspension for intra-articular injection (hexacetonide):** 20 mg/mL. **Suspension for intramuscular injection (acetonide):** 10 mg/mL, 40 mg/mL, 80 mg/mL.

NURSING IMPLICATIONS
Assessment
● These drugs are indicated for many conditions. Assess involved systems before and periodically during therapy.
● Assess for signs of adrenal insufficiency (hypotension, weight loss, weakness, nausea, vomiting, anorexia, lethargy, confusion, restlessness) before and periodically during therapy. When switching other oral hydrocortisone formulations to *Alkindi Sprinkle*, use the same total daily hydrocortisone dose. Closely monitor patients after switching to *Alkindi Sprinkle* for symptoms of adrenocortical insufficiency. If symptoms of adrenal insufficiency occur after switching, increase total daily dose of *Alkindi Sprinkle*.
● Monitor intake and output ratios and daily weights. Observe patient for peripheral edema, steady weight gain, rales/crackles, or dyspnea. Notify health care professional if these occur.
● Children should have periodic evaluations of growth; may slow growth.
● **Cerebral Edema:** Assess for changes in level of consciousness and headache during therapy.
● **Budesonide:** Assess signs of Crohn's disease and ulcerative colitis (diarrhea, crampy abdominal pain, fever, bleeding from rectum) during therapy. Monitor frequency and consistency of bowel movements periodically during therapy.
● **Rect:** Assess symptoms of ulcerative colitis (diarrhea, bleeding, weight loss, anorexia, fever, leukocytosis) periodically during therapy.

Lab Test Considerations
● Verify negative pregnancy test before starting therapy with *Hemady*. Monitor serum electrolytes and glucose. May cause hyperglycemia, especially in persons with diabetes. May cause hypokalemia. Patients on prolonged therapy should routinely have CBC, serum electrolytes, and serum and urine glucose evaluated. May ↓ WBCs. May ↓ serum potassium and calcium and ↑ serum sodium concentrations.
● Guaiac-test stools. Promptly report presence of guaiac-positive stools.
● May ↑ serum cholesterol and lipid values. May ↓ uptake of thyroid ¹²³I or ¹³¹I.
● Suppress reactions to allergy skin tests.
● Periodic adrenal function tests may be ordered to assess degree of hypothalamic-pituitary-adrenal axis suppression in systemic and chronic topical therapy.
● **Dexamethasone Suppression Test:** To diagnose Cushing's syndrome: Obtain baseline cortisol level; administer dexamethasone at 11 PM and obtain cortisol levels at 8 AM the next day. Normal response is a ↓ cortisol level.
● Alternative method: Obtain baseline 24-hr urine for 17-hydroxycorticosteroid concentrations, then begin 48-hr administration of dexamethasone. Second 24-hr urine for 17-hydroxycorticosteroid is obtained after 24 hr of dexamethasone.

Implementation
● Do not confuse prednisone with prednisolone. Do not confuse dexamethasone with dexmedetomidine. Do not confuse methylprednisolone with medroxyprogesterone or methyltestosterone. Do not confuse Solu-Cortef with Solu-Medrol. Do not confuse Depo-Medrol with Solu-Medrol.
● If dose is ordered daily or every other day, administer in the morning to coincide with the body's normal secretion of cortisol.
● Periods of stress, such as surgery, may require supplemental systemic corticosteroids.
● Patients with mild to moderate Crohn's disease may be switched from oral prednisolone without adrenal insufficiency by gradually decreasing prednisolone doses and adding budesonide.
● **PO:** Administer with meals to minimize GI irritation.
● **DNC:** Swallow *Ortikos* (budesonide) tablets whole; do not crush or chew. Other tablets may be crushed and administered with food or fluids for patients with difficulty swallowing. *DNC:* Capsules and extended-release tablets should be swallowed whole; do not open, crush, break, or chew.
● *Entocort EC* (budesonide) capsules can be opened and contents sprinkled onto 1 tbsp of applesauce for patients unable to swallow capsule. Applesauce must not be hot and must be soft enough to swallow without chewing. Mix granules with applesauce and consume entire contents within 30 min of mixing. Do not chew or crush the granules. Do not save the applesauce and granules for future use. Follow with a glass (8 oz) of cool water to ensure complete swallowing of granules.
● *Alkindi Sprinkle* (hydrocortisone) are granules in capsules. Do not swallow capsules; do not crush or

chew granules. Do not use with nasogastric or gastric tubes; may cause blockage of tube. To open capsule, hold capsule so that printed strength is at the top and tap to ensure all granules are in the lower half of the capsule. Squeeze bottom of capsule gently and twist off top of capsule. Granules may be poured directly onto patient's tongue, poured onto a spoon and placed in patient's mouth, or sprinkled onto a spoonful of cold or room temperature soft food (yogurt or fruit puree). Swallow granules within 5 min to avoid bitter taste as the outer taste masking cover can dissolve. Tap capsule to ensure all granules are removed. Avoid wetting capsule on the tongue or soft food; may result in granules remaining in capsule. Immediately follow administration with fluids (water, milk, breast milk, formula) to ensure all granules are swallowed. Do not add granules to liquid; may result in reductions of dose administered and may result in a bitter taste.

- Use calibrated measuring device to ensure accurate dose of liquid forms.
- For orally disintegrating tablets, remove tablet from blister just prior to dosing. Peel blister pack open, and place tablet on tongue; may be swallowed whole or allowed to dissolve in mouth, with or without water. Tablets are friable; do not cut, split, or break.
- Avoid consumption of grapefruit juice during therapy with budesonide or methylprednisolone.
- **IM SUBQ:** Shake suspension well before drawing up. IM doses should not be administered when rapid effect is desirable. Do not dilute with other solution or admix. Do not administer suspensions IV.

Dexamethasone

IV Administration

- **IV Push:** *Dilution:* May be given undiluted. *Concentration:* 4–10 mg/mL. *Rate:* Administer over 1–4 min if dose is <10 mg.
- **Intermittent Infusion:** *Dilution:* High-dose therapy should be added to D5W or 0.9% NaCl solution. Solution is clear and colorless to light yellow; use diluted solution within 24 hr. *Concentration:* Up to 10 mg/mL. *Rate:* Administer infusions over 15–30 min.
- **Y-Site Compatibility:** acetaminophen, acyclovir, allopurinol, amifostine, amikacin, aminocaproic acid, aminophylline, amphotericin B deoxycholate, amphotericin B lipid complex, amphotericin B liposomal, anidulafungin, argatroban, arsenic trioxide, ascorbic acid, atracurium, atropine, azithromycin, aztreonam, benztropine, bivalirudin, bleomycin, bumetanide, buprenorphine, butorphanol, cangrelor, carboplatin, carmustine, cefazolin, cefepime, cefotaxime, cefotetan, cefoxitin, ceftaroline, ceftazidime, ceftolozane/tazobactam, ceftriaxone, chloramphenicol, cisatracurium, cisplatin, cladribine, clindamycin, cyanocobalamin, cyclophosphamide, cyclosporine, cytarabine, dacarbazine, dactinomy-

cin, daptomycin, dexmedetomidine, digoxin, diltiazem, dimenhydrinate, docetaxel, dopamine, doxorubicin hydrochloride, doxorubicin liposomal, enalaprilat, ephedrine, epinephrine, epoetin alfa, eptifibatide, ertapenem, etoposide, etoposide phosphate, famotidine, fentanyl, filgrastim, fluconazole, fludarabine, fluorouracil, folic acid, fosaprepitant, foscarnet, fosphenytoin, furosemide, ganciclovir, gemcitabine, glycopyrrolate, granisetron, heparin, hetastarch, hydrocortisone, hydromorphone, ifosfamide, imipenem/cilastatin, indomethacin, insulin, regular, irinotecan, isavuconazonium, isoproterenol, ketorolac, leucovorin calcium, levofloxacin, lidocaine, linezolid, lorazepam, mannitol, melphalan, meropenem, meropenem/vaborbactam, mesna, methohexital, methylprednisolone, metoclopramide, metoprolol, metronidazole, milrinone, mitomycin, morphine, moxifloxacin, multivitamin, nafcillin, nalbuphine, naloxone, nitroglycerin, nitroprusside, norepinephrine, octreotide, ondansetron, oxaliplatin, oxytocin, paclitaxel, palonosetron, pamidronate, pemetrexed, penicillin G, pentobarbital, phenobarbital, phenylephrine, phytonadione, piperacillin/tazobactam, plazomicin, potassium acetate, potassium chloride, procainamide, prochlorperazine, propofol, propranolol, pyridoxine, remifentanil, rituximab, sargramostim, sodium acetate, sodium bicarbonate, succinylcholine, sufentanil, tacrolimus, tedizolid, telavancin, theophylline, thiamine, thiotepa, tigecycline, tirofiban, trastuzumab, vancomycin, vasopressin, vecuronium, verapamil, vinblastine, vincristine, vinorelbine, voriconazole, zidovudine, zoledronic acid.

- **Y-Site Incompatibility:** alemtuzumab, amiodarone, blinatumomab, caspofungin, cefuroxime, ciprofloxacin, dacarbazine, dantrolene, daunorubicin hydrochloride, diazepam, diphenhydramine, dobutamine, doxycycline, epirubicin, esmolol, gemtuzumab ozogamicin, haloperidol, hydroxyzine, idarubicin, labetalol, magnesium sulfate, midazolam, minocycline, mitoxantrone, mycophenolate, nicardipine, pantoprazole, papaverine, pentamidine, phenytoin, prochlorperazine, protamine, tobramycin, topotecan, trimethoprim/sulfamethoxazole.

Hydrocortisone Sodium Succinate

IV Administration

- **IV Push:** *Reconstitution:* Reconstitute with provided solution (i.e., Act-O-Vials) or 2 mL of bacteriostatic water or saline for injection. *Concentration:* 50 mg/mL. *Rate:* Administer each 100 mg over at least 30 sec. Doses 500 mg and larger should be infused over at least 10 min.
- **Intermittent/Continuous Infusion:** *Dilution:* May be added to 50–1000 mL of D5W, 0.9% NaCl, or D5/0.9% NaCl. Diluted solutions should be used within 24 hr. *Concentration:* 1–5 mg/mL.

Concentrations of up to 60 mg/mL have been used in fluid restricted adults. *Rate:* Administer over 20–30 min or at prescribed rate.

- **Y-Site Compatibility:** acetaminophen, acyclovir, alemtuzumab, allopurinol, amifostine, amikacin, aminophylline, amphotericin B deoxycholate, amphotericin B lipid complex, amphotericin B liposomal, anidulafungin, argatroban, ascorbic acid, atracurium, atropine, azithromycin, aztreonam, benztropine, bivalirudin, bleomycin, bumetanide, buprenorphine, butorphanol, cangrelor, carboplatin, carmustine, caspofungin, cefazolin, cefepime, cefotaxime, cefotetan, cefoxitin, ceftaroline, ceftazidime, ceftriaxone, cefuroxime, chloramphenicol, chlorpromazine, cisatracurium, cisplatin, cladribine, clindamycin, cyanocobalamin, cyclophosphamide, cyclosporine, cytarabine, dactinomycin, daptomycin, daunorubicin hydrochloride, defibrotide, dexamethasone, dexmedetomidine, dexrazoxane, digoxin, docetaxel, dopamine, doxorubicin hydrochloride, doxorubicin liposomal, droperidol, enalaprilat, ephedrine, epinephrine, epirubicin, epoetin alfa, eptifibatide, ertapenem, erythromycin, estrogens, conjugated, etoposide, famotidine, fentanyl, filgrastim, fluconazole, fludarabine, fluorouracil, folic acid, foscarnet, fosphenytoin, furosemide, gemcitabine, glycopyrrolate, granisetron, heparin, hetastarch, hydromorphone, ifosfamide, imipenem/cilastatin, indomethacin, insulin, regular, irinotecan, isoproterenol, ketamine, ketorolac, leucovorin calcium, levofloxacin, lidocaine, linezolid, lorazepam, mannitol, melphalan, meropenem/vaborbactam, mesna, methotrexate, methylergonovine, metoclopramide, metoprolol, metronidazole, milrinone, mitoxantrone, morphine, moxifloxacin, multivitamins, nafcillin, naloxone, neostigmine, nitroglycerin, nitroprusside, norepinephrine, octreotide, ondansetron, oxacillin, oxaliplatin, oxytocin, paclitaxel, palonosetron, pamidronate, pantoprazole, pemetrexed, penicillin G, pentobarbital, phenobarbital, phentolamine, phenylephrine, phytonadione, piperacillin/tazobactam, plazomicin, potassium acetate, potassium chloride, procainamide, prochlorperazine, propofol, propranolol, pyridostigmine, remifentanil, rituximab, scopolamine, sodium acetate, sodium bicarbonate, succinylcholine, sufentanil, tacrolimus, tedizolid, telavancin, theophylline, thiotepa, tigecycline, tirofiban, topotecan, trastuzumab, vasopressin, vecuronium, verapamil, vinblastine, vincristine, vinorelbine, voriconazole, zoledronic acid.
- **Y-Site Incompatibility:** amiodarone, ampicillin/sulbactam, azathioprine, ciprofloxacin, dantrolene, diazepam, diazoxide, dobutamine, doxycycline, ganciclovir, gemtuzumab ozogamicin, haloperidol, idarubicin, labetalol, midazolam,

mycophenolate, nalbuphine, pentamidine, phenytoin, protamine, pyridoxine, rocuronium, sargramostim, thiamine, trimethoprim/sulfamethoxazole.

Methylprednisolone Sodium Succinate

IV Administration

- **IV Push:** *Reconstitution:* Reconstitute with provided solution (Act-O-Vials, Univials) or 2 mL of bacteriostatic water (with benzyl alcohol) for injection. Use preservative-free diluent for use in neonates. Acetate injection is not for IV use. *Concentration:* Maximum concentration 125 mg/mL. *Rate:* Low dose (<1.8 mg/kg or <125 mg/dose): May be administered IV push over 1 to several min. Moderate dose (2 mg/kg or 250 mg/dose): give over 15–30 min. High dose (15 mg/kg or 500 mg/dose): give over 30 min. Doses 15 mg/kg or 1 g give over 1 hr.
- **Intermittent/Continuous Infusion:** *Dilution:* May be diluted further in D5W, 0.9% NaCl, or D5/0.9% NaCl and administered as intermittent or continuous infusion at the prescribed rate. *Concentration:* Maximum 2.5 mg/mL. Solution may form a haze upon dilution.
- **Y-Site Compatibility:** acetaminophen, acyclovir, alprostadil, amifostine, amikacin, aminophylline, amphotericin B deoxycholate, amphotericin B lipid complex, amphotericin B liposomal, anidulafungin, argatroban, arsenic trioxide, ascorbic acid, atracurium, atropine, azithromycin, aztreonam, benztropine, bivalirudin, bleomycin, bumetanide, buprenorphine, butorphanol, cangrelor, carboplatin, carmustine, cefazolin, cefepime, cefotetan, ceftaroline, ceftazidime, ceftriaxone, cefuroxime, chloramphenicol, chlorpromazine, cisplatin, cladribine, clindamycin, cyanocobalamin, cyclophosphamide, cyclosporine, cytarabine, dactinomycin, daptomycin, dexamethasone, dexmedetomidine, digoxin, dobutamine, dopamine, doxorubicin liposomal, enalaprilat, ephedrine, epinephrine, epoetin alfa, eptifibatide, ertapenem, erythromycin, etoposide, fentanyl, fluconazole, fludarabine, fluorouracil, folic acid, fosaprepitant, furosemide, gentamicin, glycopyrrolate, granisetron, hetastarch, hydromorphone, ifosfamide, imipenem/cilastatin, insulin, regular, isoproterenol, ketorolac, labetalol, levofloxacin, linezolid, lorazepam, mannitol, melphalan, meropenem/vaborbactam, mesna, methotrexate, metoclopramide, metoprolol, metronidazole, milrinone, morphine, moxifloxacin, multivitamin, nafcillin, naloxone, nitroglycerin, nitroprusside, norepinephrine, octreotide, oxaliplatin, oxytocin, pamidronate, pemetrexed, penicillin G, pentobarbital, phenobarbital, phenylephrine, piperacillin/tazobactam, potassium acetate, procainamide, prochlorperazine, propranolol, remifentanil, rituximab, sodium acetate, sodium

bicarbonate, succinylcholine, sufentanil, tacrolimus, tedizolid, theophylline, thiotepa, tirofiban, tobramycin, topotecan, trastuzumab, vasopressin, verapamil, vincristine, voriconazole, zoledronic acid.

- **Y-Site Incompatibility:** alemtuzumab, allopurinol, ampicillin/sulbactam, blinatumomab, calcium chloride, calcium gluconate, caspofungin, cefotaxime, cefoxitin, ciprofloxacin, dacarbazine, dantrolene, daunorubicin hydrochloride, dexrazoxane, diazepam, diazoxide, diphenhydramine, docetaxel, doxycycline, epirubicin, etoposide phosphate, filgrastim, foscarnet, ganciclovir, gemcitabine, gemtuzumab ozogamicin, haloperidol, hydralazine, idarubicin, irinotecan, isavuconazonium, magnesium sulfate, mitoxantrone, mycophenolate, nalbuphine, paclitaxel, palonosetron, pantoprazole, papaverine, pentamidine, phenytoin, promethazine, propofol, protamine, pyridoxine, rocuronium, sargramostim, thiamine, trimethoprim/sulfamethoxazole, vancomycin, vecuronium, vinorelbine.

Patient/Family Teaching

- Instruct patient on correct technique of medication administration. Advise patient to take medication as directed. Take missed doses as soon as remembered unless almost time for next dose. Do not double doses. If full dose is not administered due to regurgitating or vomiting of granules, instruct patients and/or caregivers to contact their health care professional. A repeat dose may be required to avoid adrenal insufficiency. Stopping the medication suddenly may result in adrenal insufficiency (anorexia, nausea, weakness, fatigue, dyspnea, hypotension, hypoglycemia). If these signs appear, notify health care professional immediately. This can be life threatening. Advise patient to read *Patient Information* before starting and with each Rx refill in case of changes.
- Advise patient to avoid consumption of grapefruit juice during therapy with *budesonide* or *methylprednisolone*; may increase blood levels.
- Corticosteroids cause immunosuppression and may mask symptoms of infection. Instruct patient to avoid people with known contagious illnesses and to report possible infections immediately.
- *Pediapred* solution may be refrigerated.
- Caution patient to avoid vaccinations without first consulting health care professional.
- Review side effects with patient. Instruct patient to inform health care professional promptly if severe abdominal pain or tarry stools occur. Patient should also report unusual swelling, weight gain, tiredness, bone pain, bruising, nonhealing sores, visual disturbances, or behavior changes. Advise patient to notify health care professional if signs and symptoms of hypercorticism (acne, thicker or more hair on body and face; bruise easily; fatty pad or hump between shoulders [buffalo hump], rounding of face [moon face], pink or purple stretch marks on skin of abdomen, thighs, breasts and arms; ankle swelling), ad-

renal suppression (tiredness, weakness, nausea and vomiting, low blood pressure), worsening of allergies (eczema, rhinitis), and infection (fever, chills, pain, feeling tired, aches, nausea, and vomiting). May worsen existing tuberculosis, fungal, bacterial, viral, or parasitic infections, or ocular herpes simplex.

- Instruct patient to notify health care professional of all Rx or OTC medications, vitamins, or herbal products being taken and to consult health care professional before taking any Rx, OTC, or herbal products.
- Instruct patient to notify health care professional immediately if exposed to chicken pox or measles.
- Advise patient to notify health care professional of medication regimen before treatment or surgery.
- Discuss possible effects on body image. Explore coping mechanisms.
- Instruct patient to inform health care professional if symptoms of underlying disease return or worsen.
- Rep: Advise females of reproductive potential to notify health care professional if pregnancy is planned or suspected or if breastfeeding. *Hemady* may cause fetal harm. Advise females taking *Hemady* to use effective contraception during and for at least one month after last dose. Monitor infants born to mothers who have received substantial doses of corticosteroids during pregnancy for signs of hypoglycemia and hypoadrenalism. Advise women not to breastfeed during and for 2 wks after last dose. May impair male fertility.
- Advise patient to carry identification describing disease process and medication regimen in the event of emergency in which patient cannot relate medical history.
- Explain need for continued medical follow-up to assess effectiveness and possible side effects of medication. Periodic lab tests and eye exams may be needed.
- **Long-term Therapy:** Encourage patient to eat a diet high in protein, calcium, and potassium, and low in sodium and carbohydrates (see Appendix J). Alcohol should be avoided during therapy; may ↑ risk of GI irritation.
- If rectal dose used 21 days, decrease to every other night for 2–3 wk to decrease gradually.

Evaluation/Desired Outcomes

- Decrease in presenting symptoms with minimal systemic side effects.
- Suppression of the inflammatory and immune responses in autoimmune disorders, allergic reactions, and neoplasms.
- Management of symptoms in adrenal insufficiency.
- Improvement of symptoms/sequelae of Crohn's disease and ulcerative colitis (decreased frequency of liquid stools, decreased abdominal complaints, improved sense of well-being).

- Improvement in symptoms of ulcerative colitis. Clinical symptoms usually improve in 3–5 days. Mucosal appearance may require 2–3 mo to improve.
- Induction of remission of ulcerative colitis.
- Treatment of adults with multiple myeloma.

C

CORTICOSTEROIDS (TOPICAL/LOCAL)

alclometasone (al-kloe-**met**-a-sone)
~~Aclovate~~

amcinonide (am-**sin**-oh-nide)

betamethasone (bay-ta-**meth**-a-sone)
♣ Betaderm, ♣ Beteflam, ♣ Celestoderm V, ♣ Celestoderm V/2, Diprolene, ~~Diprolene AF~~, ♣ Diprosone, Sernivo

clobetasol (kloe-**bay**-ta-sol)
Clobex, Clodan, ♣ Dermovate, Impoyz, Olux-E, ~~Temovate~~, ~~Temovate E~~, Tovet

clocortolone (kloe-**kore**-toe-lone)
Cloderm

desonide (**des**-oh-nide)
~~Desonate~~, DesOwen, Tridesilon, Verdeso

desoximetasone (dess-ox-i-**met**-a-sone)
Topicort

diflorasone (dye-**flor**-a-sone)
Apexicon E

fluocinolone (floo-oh-**sin**-oh-lone)
Capex, Derma-Smoothe/FS, Synalar

fluocinonide (floo-oh-**sin**-oh-nide)
♣ Lidemol, ♣ Lyderm, ♣ Tiamol, Vanos

flurandrenolide (flure-an-**dren**-oh-lide)
Cordran, ~~Cordran SP~~

fluticasone (floo-**ti**-ka-sone)
~~Cutivate~~

halcinonide (hal-**sin**-oh-nide)
Halog

halobetasol (hal-oh-**bay**-ta-sol)
Bryhali, Lexette, Ultravate

hydrocortisone (hye-droe-**kor**-ti-sone)
Ala-Cort, Ala-Scalp, Anusol HC, ♣ Barriere-HC, Cortaid, Cortifoam, ♣ Cortoderm, ♣ Hyderm, ♣ Hydroval, Locoid, Pandel, ♣ Sarna HC, Texacort

mometasone (moe-**met**-a-sone)
♣ Elocom, ~~Elocon~~

triamcinolone (trye-am-**sin**-oh-lone)
♣ Aristocort C, ♣ Aristocort R, Kenalog, ♣ Triaderm, Triderm, Tritocin

Classification
Therapeutic: anti-inflammatories (steroidal)
Pharmacologic: corticosteroids (topical)

Indications
Moderate to severe plaque psoriasis. Inflammation and pruritus associated with corticosteroid-responsive dermatoses.

Action
Suppress normal immune response and inflammation. **Therapeutic Effects:** Suppression of dermatologic inflammation and immune processes. Clearing of plaques.

Pharmacokinetics
Absorption: Minimal. Prolonged use on large surface areas, application of large amounts, or use of occlusive dressings may ↑ systemic absorption.
Distribution: Remain primarily at site of action.
Metabolism and Excretion: Usually metabolized in skin; some have been modified to resist local metabolism and have a prolonged local effect.
Half-life: *Betamethasone:* 3–5 hr (plasma), 36–54 hr (tissue). *Dexamethasone:* 3–4.5 hr (plasma), 36–54 hr (tissue). *Hydrocortisone:* 1.5–2 hr (plasma), 8–12 hr (tissue). *Triamcinolone:* 2–>5 hr (plasma), 18–36 hr (tissue).

TIME/ACTION PROFILE (response depends on condition being treated)

ROUTE	ONSET	PEAK	DURATION
Topical	min–hr	hr–days	hr–days

Contraindications/Precautions
Contraindicated in: Hypersensitivity or known intolerance to corticosteroids or components of vehicles (ointment or cream base, preservative, alcohol); Untreated bacterial or viral infections.
Use Cautiously in: Hepatic impairment; Diabetes mellitus, cataracts, glaucoma, or tuberculosis (use of large amounts of high-potency agents may worsen condition); Patients with pre-existing skin atrophy; OB, Lactation: Chronic use at high dosages may result in adrenal suppression in mother and growth suppression in children; Pedi: Children may be more susceptible to adrenal and growth suppression. Clobetasol not recommended for children <18 yr (cream, lotion, shampoo, spray) or <12 yr (foam, gel, ointment, solution); desoximetasone not recommended for children <10 yr (cream, ointment, gel) or <18 yr (spray); halobetasol not recommended for children <12 yr.

♣= Canadian drug name. ⬚ = Genetic implication. ~~Strikethrough~~ = Discontinued. CAPITALS = life-threatening. <u>Underline</u> = most frequent.

Adverse Reactions/Side Effects

Derm: allergic contact dermatitis, atrophy, burning, dryness, edema, folliculitis, hypersensitivity reactions, hypertrichosis, hypopigmentation, irritation, maceration, miliaria, perioral dermatitis, secondary infection, striae. **EENT:** cataracts, glaucoma. **Misc:** adrenal suppression (↑ dose, long-term therapy).

Interactions

Drug-Drug: None significant.

Route/Dosage

Topical (Adults and Children): 1–4 times daily (depends on product, preparation, and condition being treated).
Rect (Adults): hydrocortisone *Aerosol foam:* 90 mg 1–2 times/day for 2–3 wk; then adjusted.

Availability

Alclometasone (generic available)
Cream: 0.05%. **Ointment:** 0.05%.

Amcinonide (generic available)
Cream: 0.1%. **Lotion:** 0.1%. **Ointment:** 0.1%.

Betamethasone (generic available)
Aerosol foam: 0.12%. **Cream:** 0.05%, 0.1%. **Gel:** 0.05%. **Lotion:** 0.05%, 0.1%. **Ointment:** 0.05%, 0.1%. **Spray:** 0.05%. *In combination with:* calcipotriene (Enstilar, Taclonex, Wynzora), clotrimazole (Lotrisone); see Appendix N.

Clobetasol (generic available)
Cream: 0.025%, 0.05%. **Foam:** 0.05%. **Gel:** 0.05%. **Lotion:** 0.05%. **Ointment:** 0.05%. **Scalp solution:** 0.05%. **Shampoo:** 0.05%. **Spray:** 0.05%.

Clocortolone (generic available)
Cream: 0.1%.

Desonide (generic available)
Cream: 0.05%. **Foam:** 0.05%. **Gel:** 0.05%. **Lotion:** 0.05%. **Ointment:** 0.05%.

Desoximetasone (generic available)
Cream: 0.05%, 0.25%. **Gel:** 0.05%. **Ointment:** 0.05%, 0.25%. **Spray:** 0.25%.

Diflorasone (generic available)
Cream: 0.05%. **Ointment:** 0.05%.

Fluocinolone (generic available)
Cream: 0.01%, 0.025%. **Oil:** 0.01%. **Ointment:** 0.025%. **Shampoo:** 0.01%. **Solution:** 0.01%. *In combination with:* hydroquinone and tretinoin (Tri-Luma); neomycin (Neo-Synalar). See Appendix N.

Fluocinonide (generic available)
Cream: 0.05%, 0.1%. **Gel:** 0.05%. **Ointment:** 0.05%. **Solution:** 0.05%.

Flurandrenolide (generic available)
Lotion: 0.05%. **Ointment:** 0.05%. **Tape:** 4 mcg/cm².

Fluticasone (generic available)
Cream: 0.05%. **Lotion:** 0.05%. **Ointment:** 0.005%.

Halcinonide (generic available)
Cream: 0.1%. **Ointment:** 0.1%. **Solution:** 0.1%.

Halobetasol (generic available)
Cream: 0.05%. **Foam:** 0.05%. **Lotion:** 0.01%, 0.05%. **Ointment:** 0.05%. *In combination with:* tazarotene (Duobrii). See Appendix N.

Hydrocortisone (generic available)
Cream: 0.1%, 0.2%, 0.5%$^{Rx, OTC}$, 1%$^{Rx, OTC}$, 2.5%. **Gel:** 2%$^{Rx, OTC}$. **Lotion:** 0.1%, 1%$^{Rx, OTC}$, 2%. **Ointment:** 0.1%, 0.2%, 0.5%$^{Rx, OTC}$, 1%$^{Rx, OTC}$, 2.5%. **Rectal cream:** 1%, 2.5%. **Solution:** 0.1%, 1%, 2.5%. *In combination with:* acetic acid, antifungals, anti-infectives, antihistamines, urea, and benzoyl peroxide in various otic and topical preparations. See Appendix N.

Mometasone (generic available)
Cream: 0.1%. **Ointment:** 0.1%. **Lotion:** ✿ 0.1%. **Solution:** 0.1%.

Triamcinolone (generic available)
Cream: 0.025%, 0.1%, 0.5%. **Lotion:** 0.025%, 0.1%. **Ointment:** 0.025%, 0.05%, 0.1%, 0.5%. **Spray:** 0.147 mg/g. *In combination with:* acetic acid, antifungals, anti-infectives, antihistamines, urea, and benzoyl peroxide in various otic and topical preparations. See Appendix N.

NURSING IMPLICATIONS

Assessment

- Assess affected skin before and daily during therapy. Note degree of inflammation, pruritus, and/or plaques. Notify health care professional if symptoms of infection (increased pain, erythema, purulent exudate) develop.

Lab Test Considerations

- Adrenal function tests may be ordered to assess degree of hypothalamic-pituitary-adrenal (HPA) axis suppression in long-term topical therapy. Children and patients with dose applied to a large area, using an occlusive dressing, or using high-potency products are at highest risk for HPA suppression.
- May cause ↑ serum and urine glucose concentrations if significant absorption occurs.

Implementation

- Choice of vehicle depends on site and type of lesion. Ointments are more occlusive and preferred for dry, scaly lesions. Creams should be used on oozing or intertriginous areas, where the occlusive action of ointments might cause folliculitis or maceration. Creams may be preferred for esthetic reasons even though they may dry skin more than ointments. Gels, aerosols, lotions, and solutions are useful in hairy areas.
- **Topical:** Apply *ointments, creams,* or *gels* sparingly as a thin film to clean, slightly moist skin. Wear gloves. Apply occlusive dressing only if specified by health care professional.
- Apply *lotion, solution,* or *gel* to hair by parting hair and applying a small amount to affected area.

Rub in gently. Protect area from washing, clothing, or rubbing until medication has dried. Hair may be washed as usual but not right after applying medication.

- Use *aerosols* by shaking well and spraying on affected area, holding container 3–6 in. away. Spray for about 2 sec to cover an area the size of a hand. Do not inhale. If spraying near face, cover eyes.
- Shake *Sernivo spray* before using. Spray affected area and rub in gently. Discontinue if control not achieved or after 4 wk of use.

Patient/Family Teaching

- Instruct patient on correct technique of medication administration. Emphasize importance of avoiding the eyes. Apply missed doses as soon as remembered unless almost time for the next dose.
- Caution patient to use only as directed. Avoid using cosmetics, bandages, dressings, or other skin products over the treated area unless directed by health care professional.
- Advise parents of pediatric patients not to apply tight-fitting diapers or plastic pants on a child treated in the diaper area; these garments work as an occlusive dressing and may cause more of the drug to be absorbed.
- Advise patient to consult health care professional before using medicine for condition other than indicated.
- Rep: Caution females of reproductive potential that medication should not be used extensively, in large amounts, or for protracted periods if they are pregnant or planning to become pregnant. Advise female patients of reproductive potential to notify health care professional if pregnancy is planned or suspected, or if breastfeeding.
- Instruct patient to inform health care professional if symptoms of underlying disease return or worsen or if symptoms of infection develop.
- **Fluticasone:** Advise patient to avoid excessive natural or artificial exposure (tanning booth, sun lamp) to areas where lotion is applied.

Evaluation/Desired Outcomes

- Resolution of skin inflammation, pruritus, or other dermatologic conditions.
- Clearing of plaques in plaque psoriasis.

---

crisaborole (kris-a-**bor**-ole)
Eucrisa
Classification
Therapeutic: anti-inflammatories
Pharmacologic: phosphodiesterase type 4 inhibitors

Indications

Mild to moderate atopic dermatitis.

Action

Inhibits phosphodiesterase 4 (PDE-4) resulting in ↑ intracellular cyclic adenosine monophosphate levels. **Therapeutic Effects:** Decreased severity of atopic dermatitis.

Pharmacokinetics

Absorption: Minimal systemic absorption through intact skin.
Distribution: Local distribution after topical administration.
Protein Binding: 97%.
Metabolism and Excretion: Metabolized through liver into inactive metabolites; metabolites excreted in urine.
Half-life: Unknown.

TIME/ACTION PROFILE (improvement in symptoms)

ROUTE	ONSET	PEAK	DURATION
Topical	8 days	unknown	unknown

Contraindications/Precautions

Contraindicated in: Hypersensitivity.
Use Cautiously in: OB: Safety not established in pregnancy; Lactation: Safety not established in breastfeeding; Pedi: Children <3 mo (safety and effectiveness not established).

Adverse Reactions/Side Effects

Derm: burning, stinging. **Misc:** hypersensitivity reactions.

Interactions

Drug-Drug: None reported.

Route/Dosage

Topical (Adults and Children ≥3 mo): Apply a thin layer to affected areas twice daily. Once clinical effect achieved, may ↓ frequency of application to once daily.

Availability

Ointment: 2%.

NURSING IMPLICATIONS

Assessment

- Assess skin lesions periodically during therapy.

Implementation

- **Topical:** Apply a thin layer to affected areas twice daily. Do not apply to ophthalmic, oral, or vaginal areas. Wash hands after applying ointment.

Patient/Family Teaching

- Instruct patient or parent to apply as directed. For topical use only.
- Advise patient or parent to discontinue therapy and notify health care professional if signs and symptoms of hypersensitivity (pruritus, swelling, erythema) at application site or a distant site occur.

✱= Canadian drug name. ⚏ = Genetic implication. ~~Strikethrough~~ = Discontinued. CAPITALS= life-threatening. <u>Underline</u> = most frequent.

- Instruct patient to notify health care professional of all Rx or OTC medications, vitamins, or herbal products being taken and consult health care professional before taking any new medications.
- Rep: Advise females of reproductive potential to notify health care professional if pregnancy is planned or suspected or if breastfeeding.

Evaluation/Desired Outcomes
- Decreased severity of atopic dermatitis.

---

crizanlizumab
(kriz-an-liz-ue-mab)
Adakveo
Classification
Therapeutic: none assigned
Pharmacologic: monoclonal antibodies, selectin inhibitors

Indications
Vaso-occlusive crises in patients with sickle cell disease.

Action
Binds to P-selectin on the surface of the activated endothelium and platelets to prevent their interaction with endothelial cells, platelets, red blood cells, and white blood cells. **Therapeutic Effects:** Reduction in frequency of vaso-occlusive crises.

Pharmacokinetics
Absorption: IV administration results in complete bioavailability.
Distribution: Minimally distributed to extravascular tissues.
Metabolism and Excretion: Metabolized by catabolic pathways into smaller peptides; excretion pathway unknown.
Half-life: 10.6 days.

TIME/ACTION PROFILE (plasma concentrations)

ROUTE	ONSET	PEAK	DURATION
IV	unknown	unknown	unknown

Contraindications/Precautions
Contraindicated in: None reported.
Use Cautiously in: OB: Use during pregnancy only if potential maternal benefit justifies potential fetal risk; Lactation: Use while breastfeeding only if potential maternal benefit justifies potential risk to infant; Pedi: Children <16 yr (safety and effectiveness not established).

Adverse Reactions/Side Effects
Derm: pruritus. **GI:** abdominal pain, nausea, diarrhea, vomiting. **Local:** infusion-site reaction. **MS:** arthralgia, back pain, myalgia. **Misc:** fever, infusion-related reactions.

Interactions
Drug-Drug: None reported.

Route/Dosage
IV (Adults and Children ≥16 yr): 5 mg/kg initially, then in 2 wk, and then every 4 wk thereafter.

Availability
Solution for injection: 10 mg/mL.

NURSING IMPLICATIONS
Assessment
- Monitor frequency of vaso-occlusive crises during therapy.
- Monitor for signs and symptoms of infusion-related reactions (severe pain, fever, chills, nausea, vomiting, fatigue, dizziness, pruritus, urticaria, sweating, shortness of breath, wheezing) during and within 24 hr of infusion. For mild to moderate reactions, interrupt infusion or slow rate of infusion. Begin symptomatic therapy (acetaminophen, NSAIDs, opioids, antihistamines, intravenous fluids, and/or oxygen therapy). Consider premedication and/or reduce infusion rate of subsequent infusions. Discontinue therapy for severe reactions.

Lab Test Considerations
- May interfere with automated platelet counts (platelet clumping), in particular when blood samples are collected in tubes containing ethylenediaminetetraacetic acid. Run blood samples within 4 hr of blood collection or collect blood samples in tubes containing citrate. When needed, estimate platelet count via peripheral blood smear.

Implementation
- **Intermittent Infusion:** Obtain number of vials needed; one vial for every 10 mL crizanlizumab. Allow vials to reach room temperature for up to 4 hr before preparing. Solution is clear to opalescent, colorless, or may have a slightly brownish-yellow tint; do not use solutions with particulate matter. *Dilution:* Dilute in 0.9% NaCl or D5W to a total volume of 100 mL in an infusion bag of either polyvinyl chloride, polyethylene, or polypropylene by withdrawing the volume to be added. Gently invert to mix; do not shake. Solution is stable for up to 4.5 hr at room temperature, including infusion time and up to 24 hr if refrigerated and protected from light. *Rate:* Infuse over 30 min through a sterile, nonpyrogenic 0.2 micron inline filter. Flush the line with at least 25 mL of 0.9% NaCl or D5W following infusion.
- **Y-Site Incompatibility:** Do not mix or coadminister with other drugs through the same IV line.

Patient/Family Teaching
- Explain the purpose of crizanlizumab to patient. Do not stop receiving crizanlizumab without consulting health care professional. If an appointment is missed, contact health care professional as soon as possible to reschedule. Advise patient to read *Medication Guide* before starting and periodically during therapy in case of changes.
- Advise patient to notify health care professional if signs and symptoms of infusion reactions (fever,

chills or shivering, nausea, vomiting, tiredness, dizziness, sweating, hives, itching, shortness of breath, wheezing) occur.

- Instruct patient to inform health care professional of crizanlizumab therapy before blood tests due to potential interference with laboratory tests used to measure platelet counts.
- Advise patient to notify health care professional of all Rx or OTC medications, vitamins, or herbal products being taken and to consult with health care professional before taking other medications.
- Rep: May cause fetal harm. Advise patient to notify health care professional if pregnancy is planned or suspected or if breastfeeding.

Evaluation/Desired Outcomes

- Decreased frequency of vaso-occlusive crises in patients with sickle cell disease.

cyanocobalamin, See VITAMIN B₁₂ PREPARATIONS.

BEERS

cyclobenzaprine
(sye-kloe-**ben**-za-preen)
Amrix, Fexmid, Flexeril
Classification
Therapeutic: skeletal muscle relaxants (centrally acting)

Indications
Acute painful musculoskeletal conditions associated with muscle spasm. **Unlabeled Use:** Fibromyalgia.

Action
Reduces tonic somatic muscle activity at the level of the brain stem. Structurally similar to tricyclic antidepressants. **Therapeutic Effects:** Reduction in muscle spasm and hyperactivity without loss of function.

Pharmacokinetics
Absorption: Well absorbed from the GI tract.
Distribution: Unknown.
Protein Binding: 93%.
Metabolism and Excretion: Mostly metabolized by the liver.
Half-life: 1–3 days.

TIME/ACTION PROFILE (skeletal muscle relaxation)

ROUTE	ONSET	PEAK†	DURATION
PO	within 1 hr	3–8 hr	12–24 hr
Extended release	unknown	unknown	24 hr

†Full effects may not occur for 1–2 wk.

Contraindications/Precautions
Contraindicated in: Hypersensitivity; Concurrent use of or use within 14 days of MAO inhibitor therapy; Immediate period after MI; Severe or symptomatic cardiovascular disease; Cardiac conduction disturbances; Hyperthyroidism.
Use Cautiously in: Cardiovascular disease; OB: Use during pregnancy only if potential maternal benefit justifies potential fetal risk; Lactation: Use while breastfeeding only if potential maternal benefit justifies potential risk to infant; Pedi: Children <15 yr (safety and effectiveness not established); Geri: Appears on Beers list. ↑ risk of anticholinergic adverse reactions, sedation, and fractures in older adults. Avoid use in older adults.

Adverse Reactions/Side Effects
CV: arrhythmias. **EENT:** dry mouth, blurred vision. **GI:** constipation, dyspepsia, nausea, unpleasant taste. **GU:** urinary retention. **Neuro:** dizziness, drowsiness, confusion, fatigue, headache, nervousness.

Interactions
Drug-Drug: Additive CNS depression with other **CNS depressants**, including **alcohol, antihistamines, opioid analgesics**, and **sedative/hypnotics**. Additive anticholinergic effects with **drugs possessing anticholinergic properties**, including **antihistamines, antidepressants, atropine, disopyramide, haloperidol**, and **phenothiazines**. Avoid use within 14 days of **MAO inhibitors** (hyperpyretic crisis, seizures, and death may occur). Drugs that affect serotonergic neurotransmitter systems, including **tricyclic antidepressants, SSRIs, SNRIs, fentanyl, buspirone, tramadol**, and **triptans** ↑ risk of serotonin syndrome.
Drug-Natural Products: Concomitant use of **kava-kava, valerian, chamomile**, or **hops** can ↑ CNS depression.

Route/Dosage
PO (Adults and Children ≥15 yo): *Acute painful musculoskeletal conditions:* Immediate-release: 10 mg 3 times daily (range 20–40 mg/day in 2–4 divided doses; not to exceed 60 mg/day); Extended-release: 15–30 mg once daily. *Fibromyalgia:* 5–40 mg at bedtime (unlabeled).

Availability (generic available)
Immediate-release tablets: 5 mg, 7.5 mg, 10 mg.
Extended-release capsules (Amrix): 15 mg, 30 mg.

NURSING IMPLICATIONS
Assessment
- Assess patient for pain, muscle stiffness, and range of motion before and periodically during therapy.
- Geri: Assess geriatric patients for anticholinergic effects (sedation and weakness).
- Assess for serotonin syndrome (mental changes [agitation, hallucinations, coma], autonomic instability

[tachycardia, labile BP, hyperthermia], neuromuscular aberrations [hyperreflexia, incoordination], and/or GI symptoms [nausea, vomiting, diarrhea]), especially in patients taking other serotonergic drugs (SSRIs, SNRIs, triptans).

Implementation
- **PO:** Administer doses at same time each day. May be administered with meals to minimize gastric irritation.
- **DNC:** Swallow extended-release capsules whole; do not open, crush, or chew. Capsules may be opened and contents sprinkled onto applesauce; swallow immediately without chewing. Rinse mouth to make sure contents have been swallowed.

Patient/Family Teaching
- Instruct patient to take medication as directed, at the same time each day; do not take more than the prescribed amount. Take missed doses within 1 hr of time ordered; otherwise, return to normal dose schedule. Do not double doses. Do not stop abruptly, may cause nausea, headache, and malaise; discontinue gradually.
- Medication may cause drowsiness, dizziness, and blurred vision. Caution patient to avoid driving or other activities requiring alertness until response to drug is known.
- Advise patient to avoid concurrent use of alcohol or other CNS depressants with this medication.
- If constipation becomes a problem, advise patient that increasing fluid intake and bulk in diet and stool softeners may alleviate this condition.
- Instruct patient to notify health care professional of all Rx or OTC medications, vitamins, or herbal products being taken and to consult health care professional before taking any other Rx, OTC, or herbal products.
- Advise patient to notify health care professional if symptoms of urinary retention (distended abdomen, feeling of fullness, overflow incontinence, voiding small amounts) occur.
- Instruct patient to notify health care professional immediately if signs and symptoms of serotonin syndrome, irregular or abnormal heartbeat, fast heartbeat, or allergic reaction (difficulty breathing, hives, swelling of face or tongue, itching) occur.
- Inform patient that good oral hygiene, frequent mouth rinses, and sugarless gum or candy may help relieve dry mouth.
- **Rep:** Advise females of reproductive potential to notify health care professional if pregnancy is planned or suspected or if breastfeeding.

Evaluation/Desired Outcomes
- Relief of muscular spasm in acute skeletal muscle conditions. Maximum effects may not be evident for 1–2 wk. Use is usually limited to 2–3 wk; however, has been effective for at least 12 wk in the management of fibromyalgia.

cycloPHOSphamide
(sye-kloe-**fos**-fa-mide)
~~Cytoxan~~, ✳ Procytox
Classification
Therapeutic: antineoplastics, immunosuppressants
Pharmacologic: alkylating agents

Indications
Alone or with other modalities in the management of: Hodgkin's disease, Malignant lymphomas, Multiple myeloma, Leukemias, Mycosis fungoides, Neuroblastoma, Ovarian carcinoma, Breast carcinoma, and a variety of other tumors. Minimal change nephrotic syndrome in children. **Unlabeled Use:** Severe active rheumatoid arthritis or granulomatosis with polyangiitis.

Action
Interferes with DNA replication and RNA transcription, ultimately disrupting protein synthesis (cell-cycle phase–nonspecific). **Therapeutic Effects:** Death of rapidly replicating cells, particularly malignant ones. Also has immunosuppressant action in smaller doses.

Pharmacokinetics
Absorption: Inactive parent drug is well absorbed from the GI tract. IV administration results in complete bioavailability.
Distribution: Widely distributed. Limited penetration of the blood-brain barrier.
Metabolism and Excretion: Converted to active drug by the liver; 30% eliminated unchanged by the kidneys.
Half-life: 4–6.5 hr.

TIME/ACTION PROFILE (effects on blood counts)

ROUTE	ONSET	PEAK	DURATION
PO, IV	7 days	7–15 days	21 days

Contraindications/Precautions
Contraindicated in: Hypersensitivity; OB: Pregnancy; Lactation: Lactation.
Use Cautiously in: Active infections; Bone marrow depression; Other chronic debilitating illnesses; Rep: Women of reproductive potential.

Adverse Reactions/Side Effects
CV: hypotension, MYOCARDIAL FIBROSIS. **Derm:** alopecia. **Endo:** gonadal suppression, syndrome of inappropriate antidiuretic hormone (SIADH). **GI:** anorexia, nausea, vomiting. **GU:** hematuria, ↓ fertility, HEMORRHAGIC CYSTITIS. **Hemat:** thrombocytopenia, anemia, LEUKOPENIA. **Metab:** hyperuricemia. **Resp:** PULMONARY FIBROSIS. **Misc:** SECONDARY MALIGNANCY.

Interactions
Drug-Drug: Phenobarbital or **rifampin** may ↑ toxicity of cyclophosphamide. Concurrent **allopurinol** or **thiazide diuretics** may exaggerate bone marrow depression. May prolong neuromuscular blockade from **succinylcholine.** Cardiotoxicity may be additive with other **cardiotoxic agents** (e.g., **cytarabine, daunorubicin, doxorubicin**). May ↓ **digoxin** levels and effectiveness. Additive bone marrow depression with other **antineoplastics** or **radiation therapy.** May potentiate the effects of **warfarin.** May ↓ antibody response to **live-virus vaccines** and ↑ risk of adverse reactions. Prolongs the effects of **cocaine.**

Route/Dosage
PO (Adults): 1–5 mg/kg/day.
PO (Children): *Induction:* 2–8 mg/kg/day (60–250 mg/m²/day) in divided doses for 6 days or longer. *Maintenance:* 2–5 mg/kg (50–150 mg/m²/day) twice weekly.
IV (Adults): 40–50 mg/kg in divided doses over 2–5 days *or* 10–15 mg/kg every 7–10 days *or* 3–5 mg/kg twice weekly *or* 1.5–3 mg/kg/day. Other regimens may use larger doses.
IV (Children): *Induction:* 2–8 mg/kg/day (60–250 mg/m²/day) in divided doses for 6 days or longer. Total dose for 7 days may be given as a single weekly dose. *Maintenance:* 10–15 mg/kg every 7–10 days or 30 mg/kg every 3–4 wk.

Availability (generic available)
Capsules: 25 mg, 50 mg. **Tablets:** 25 mg, 50 mg. **Lyophilized powder for injection:** ✿ 200 mg/vial, 500 mg/vial, 1 g/vial, 2 g/vial. **Solution for injection:** 200 mg/mL, 500 mg/mL.

NURSING IMPLICATIONS
Assessment
● Monitor BP, pulse, respiratory rate, and temperature frequently during administration. Report significant changes.
● Monitor urinary output frequently during therapy. To reduce the risk of hemorrhagic cystitis and to promote excretion of uric acid, fluid intake should be at least 3000 mL/day for adults and 1000–2000 mL/day for children. May be administered with mesna. Alkalinization of the urine may be used to help prevent uric acid nephropathy.
● Monitor for bone marrow depression. Assess for bleeding (bleeding gums, bruising, petechiae, guaiac stools, urine, and emesis) and avoid IM injections and taking rectal temperatures if platelet count is low. Apply pressure to venipuncture sites for 10 min. Assess for signs of infection during neutropenia. Anemia may occur. Monitor for increased fatigue, dyspnea, and orthostatic hypotension.
● Assess nausea, vomiting, and appetite. Weigh weekly. Antiemetics may be given 30 min before administra-

tion of medication to minimize GI effects. Anorexia and weight loss can be minimized by feeding frequent light meals.
● Assess cardiac and respiratory status for dyspnea, rales/crackles, cough, weight gain, edema. Pulmonary toxicity may occur after prolonged therapy. Cardiotoxicity may occur early in therapy and is characterized by symptoms of HF.

Lab Test Considerations
● Monitor CBC with differential and platelet count before and periodically during therapy. The nadir of leukopenia occurs in 7–12 days (recovery in 17–21 days). Leukocytes should be maintained at 2500–4000/mm³. May also cause thrombocytopenia (nadir 10–15 days), and rarely causes anemia.
● Monitor BUN, serum creatinine, and uric acid before and frequently during therapy to detect nephrotoxicity.
● Monitor ALT, AST, LDH, and serum bilirubin before and frequently during therapy to detect hepatotoxicity.
● Urinalysis should be evaluated before initiating therapy and frequently during therapy to detect hematuria or change in specific gravity indicative of SIADH.
● May suppress positive reactions to skin tests for *Candida*, mumps, *Trichophyton*, and tuberculin purified-protein derivative (PPD). May also produce false-positive results in Papanicolaou smears.

Implementation
● *High Alert:* Fatalities have occurred with chemotherapeutic agents. Before administering, clarify all ambiguous orders; double-check single, daily, and course-of-therapy dose limits; have second practitioner independently double-check original order, calculations, and infusion pump settings.
● Do not confuse cyclophosphamide with cyclosporine or cycloserine.
● Administer antiemetics before dosing with cyclophosphamide.
● **PO:** Administer in the morning. *DNC:* Swallow tablets whole; do not crush, break, or chew.

IV Administration
● Provide adequate fluids (PO or IV) during or immediately after IV administration, to force diuresis and reduce the risk of urinary tract toxicity.
● **IV:** Solution should be prepared in a biologic cabinet. Wear gloves, gown, and mask while handling medication. If powder or solution comes in contact with skin or mucosa, wash thoroughly with soap and water. Discard equipment in specially designated containers.
● **IV Push:** *Dilution:* Withdraw prescribed dose of cyclophosphamide from vial with a syringe and dilute with 0.9% NaCl. Do not dilute with sterile water for injection; results in a hypotonic solution not suitable for IV push. Solution is clear, colorless to slight

✿ = Canadian drug name. ░ = Genetic implication. ~~Strikethrough~~ = Discontinued. CAPITALS = life-threatening. <u>Underline</u> = most frequent.

yellow; do not administer solutions that are cloudy, discolored, or contain particulate matter. *Concentration:* 20 mg/mL. *Rate:* Inject very slowly. Monitor IV site; may be an irritant.

- **Intermittent Infusion: *Dilution:*** Withdraw prescribed dose of cyclophosphamide from vial and dilute to a concentration of 2 mg per mL with 0.9% NaCl, 0.45% NaCl, D5W, D5/0.45% NaCl. Swirl gently to dissolve. Solutions diluted with 0.9% NaCl or 0.45% NaCl may be stored at room temperature for 24 hr or if refrigerated for 6 days. Solutions diluted with D5W or D5/0.45% NaCl are stable up to 24 hr at room temperature or 36 hr if refrigerated. *Concentration:* minimum 2 mg/mL. *Rate:* Infuse very slowly. Monitor IV site; may be an irritant. May reduce rate-dependent adverse reactions (facial swelling, headache, nasal congestion, scalp burning).

- **Y-Site Compatibility:** acyclovir, alemtuzumab, allopurinol, amifostine, amikacin, aminocaproic acid, aminophylline, amiodarone, amphotericin B lipid complex, amphotericin B liposomal, ampicillin/sulbactam, anidulafungin, argatroban, arsenic trioxide, atropine, atracurium, azithromycin, aztreonam, bivalirudin, bleomycin, bumetanide, buprenorphine, butorphanol, calcium chloride, calcium gluconate, carboplatin, carmustine, caspofungin, cefazolin, cefepime, cefotaxime, cefotetan, cefoxitin, ceftazidime, ceftriaxone, cefuroxime, chloramphenicol, chlorpromazine, ciprofloxacin, cisatracurium, cisplatin, cladribine, clindamycin, cyclosporine, cytarabine, dacarbazine, dactinomycin, daptomycin, daunorubicin hydrochloride, dexamethasone, dexmedetomidine, dexrazoxane, digoxin, diltiazem, diphenhydramine, dobutamine, docetaxel, dopamine, doxorubicin hydrochloride, doxorubicin liposomal, doxycycline, droperidol, enalaprilat, ephedrine, epinephrine, epirubicin, ertapenem, erythromycin, esmolol, etoposide, etoposide phosphate, famotidine, fentanyl, filgrastim, fluconazole, fludarabine, fluorouracil, foscarnet, fosphenytoin, furosemide, ganciclovir, gemcitabine, gentamicin, granisetron, haloperidol, heparin, hetastarch, hydralazine, hydrocortisone, hydromorphone, idarubicin, imipenem/cilastatin, insulin, regular, irinotecan, isoproterenol, ketorolac, labetalol, leucovorin calcium, levofloxacin, lidocaine, linezolid, lorazepam, magnesium sulfate, mannitol, melphalan, meperidine, meropenem, mesna, methadone, methotrexate, methylprednisolone, metoclopramide, metoprolol, metronidazole, midazolam, milrinone, mitomycin, mitoxantrone, morphine, moxifloxacin, nafcillin, nalbuphine, naloxone, nicardipine, nitroglycerin, nitroprusside, norepinephrine, octreotide, ondansetron, oxacillin, oxaliplatin, oxytocin, paclitaxel, palonosetron, pamidronate, pantoprazole, pemetrexed, penicillin G, pentamidine, pentobarbital, phenobarbital, phentolamine, phenylephrine, piperacillin/tazobactam, potassium acetate, potassium chloride, potassium phosphate, procainamide, pro-

chlorperazine, promethazine, propofol, propranolol, remifentanil, rituximab, rocuronium, sargramostim, sodium acetate, sodium bicarbonate, sodium phosphate, succinylcholine, sufentanil, tacrolimus, theophylline, thiopental, thiotepa, tigecycline, tirofiban, tobramycin, topotecan, trastuzumab, trimethoprim/sulfamethoxazole, vancomycin, vasopressin, vecuronium, verapamil, vinblastine, vincristine, vinorelbine, voriconazole, zidovudine, zoledronic acid.

- **Y-Site Incompatibility:** amphotericin B deoxycholate, diazepam, gemtuzumab ozogamicin, phenytoin.

Patient/Family Teaching

- Instruct patient to take dose in early morning. Emphasize need for adequate fluid intake for 72 hr after therapy. Patient should void frequently to decrease bladder irritation from metabolites excreted by the kidneys. Report hematuria immediately. If a dose is missed, contact health care professional. Advise caregivers to use gloves when handling capsules. If capsule opens, wash hands thoroughly.

- Instruct patient to notify health care professional promptly if fever; sore throat; signs of infection; lower back or side pain; difficult or painful urination; sores in the mouth or on the lips; yellow discoloration of skin or eyes; bleeding gums; bruising; petechiae; blood in urine, stool, or emesis; unusual swelling of ankles or legs; joint pain; shortness of breath; cough; palpitations; weight gain of more than 5 lb in 24 hr; dizziness; loss of consciousness or confusion occurs. Caution patient to avoid crowds and persons with known infections. Instruct patient to use soft toothbrush and electric razor and to avoid falls. Patient should also be cautioned not to drink alcoholic beverages or to take products containing aspirin or NSAIDs; may precipitate GI hemorrhage.

- Discuss with patient the possibility of hair loss. Explore methods of coping. May also cause darkening of skin and fingernails.

- Instruct patient not to receive any vaccinations without advice of health care professional.

- Rep: May cause fetal harm. Advise females of reproductive potential use highly effective contraceptive measures for up to 1 yr after last dose and to avoid breastfeeding during and for 1–6 wk after last dose. Advise males with female partners of reproductive potential to wear condoms during and for at least 4 mo after last dose of therapy. Advise patient or notify health care professional if pregnancy is planned or suspected. Patients treated for rheumatic and musculoskeletal diseases should consider discontinuing cyclophosphamide 3 to 6 mo prior to conception to allow for disease monitoring and potential change to another immunosuppressant. Discontinue cyclophosphamide 12 wk before attempting conception in patients with rheumatic and musculoskeletal diseases who are planning to father a child. Inform patient that this medication may cause sterility and menstrual irregularities or cessation of menses.

Evaluation/Desired Outcomes

- Decrease in size or spread of malignant tumors.
- Improvement of hematologic status in patients with leukemia. Maintenance therapy is instituted if leukocyte count remains between 2500 and 4000/mm³ and if patient does not demonstrate serious side effects.
- Management of minimal change nephrotic syndrome in children.

cycloSPORINE†
(sye-kloe-spor-een)
Gengraf, Neoral, SandIMMUNE
Classification
Therapeutic: immunosuppressants, antirheumatics (DMARD)
Pharmacologic: polypeptides (cyclic)
†See Appendix B for ophthalmic use

Indications

PO, IV: Prevention and treatment of rejection in renal, cardiac, and hepatic transplantation (with corticosteroids). **PO:** Treatment of severe active rheumatoid arthritis (Neoral only). Treatment of severe recalcitrant psoriasis in adult nonimmunocompromised patients (Neoral only). **Unlabeled Use:** Management of recalcitrant ulcerative colitis. Treatment of steroid-resistant nephrotic syndrome. Treatment of severe steroid-resistant autoimmune disease. Prevention and treatment of graft vs. host disease in bone marrow transplant patients.

Action

Inhibits normal immune responses (cellular and humoral) by inhibiting interleukin-2, a factor necessary for initiation of T-cell activity. **Therapeutic Effects:** Prevention of rejection reactions. Slowed progression of rheumatoid arthritis or psoriasis.

Pharmacokinetics

Absorption: Erratically absorbed (range 10–60%) after oral administration, with significant first-pass metabolism by the liver. Microemulsion (Neoral) has better bioavailability. IV administration results in complete bioavailability.
Distribution: Widely distributed, mainly into extracellular fluid and blood cells.
Protein Binding: 90–98%.
Metabolism and Excretion: Extensively metabolized by the liver by the CYP3A4 isoenzyme (first pass); excreted in bile, small amounts excreted unchanged in urine.
Half-life: *Children:* 7 hr; *Adults:* 19 hr.

TIME/ACTION PROFILE (plasma concentrations)

ROUTE	ONSET	PEAK	DURATION
PO	unknown†	2–6 hr	unknown
IV	unknown	end of infusion	unknown

†Onset of action in rheumatoid arthritis is 4–8 wk and may last 4 wk after discontinuation; for psoriasis, onset is 2–6 wk and lasts 6 wk following discontinuation.

Contraindications/Precautions

Contraindicated in: Hypersensitivity to cyclosporine or polyoxyethylated castor oil (vehicle for IV form); Disulfiram therapy or known alcohol intolerance (IV and oral liquid dose forms contain alcohol); Patients with psoriasis receiving immunosuppressants or radiation; Renal impairment (in rheumatoid arthritis or psoriasis); Uncontrolled hypertension; Lactation: Lactation.
Use Cautiously in: Severe hepatic impairment (dose ↓ recommended); Renal impairment (frequent dose changes may be necessary); Active infection; OB: An acceptable immunosuppressant when used following a kidney, heart, or liver transplant; not a preferred agent for other indications; Pedi: Larger or more frequent doses may be required in children.

Adverse Reactions/Side Effects

CV: hypertension. **Derm:** hirsutism, acne, psoriasis. **F and E:** hyperkalemia, hypomagnesemia. **GI:** diarrhea, nausea, vomiting, abdominal discomfort, anorexia, HEPATOTOXICITY, PANCREATITIS. **GU:** nephrotoxicity. **Hemat:** anemia, leukopenia, thrombocytopenia. **Metab:** hyperlipidemia, hyperuricemia. **MS:** lower extremity pain. **Neuro:** tremor, confusion, flushing, headache, hyperesthesia, paresthesia, POSTERIOR REVERSIBLE ENCEPHALOPATHY SYNDROME (PRES), PROGRESSIVE MULTIFOCAL LEUKOENCEPHALOPATHY (PML), psychiatric problems, SEIZURES. **Misc:** gingival hyperplasia, hypersensitivity reactions, infection (including activation of latent viral infections such as BK virus-associated nephropathy), MALIGNANCY.

Interactions

Drug-Drug: Azithromycin, clarithromycin, allopurinol, amiodarone, bromocriptine, colchicine, danazol, digoxin, diltiazem, erythromycin, fluconazole, fluoroquinolones, imatinib, itraconazole, ketoconazole, voriconazole, metoclopramide, methylprednisolone, nefazodone, nicardipine, protease inhibitors, verapamil, or hormonal contraceptives may ↑ levels and risk of toxicity. ↑ immunosuppression with other **immunosuppressants** (cyclophosphamide, azathioprine, corticosteroids). **Carbamazepine, nafcillin, octreotide, orlistat, oxcarbazepine, phenobarbital, phenytoin, rifampin, rifabutin,** or **terbinafine** may

↓ levels and effect. **Bosentan** may significantly ↓ levels; avoid concurrent use. ↑ risk of hyperkalemia with **potassium-sparing diuretics, potassium supplements**, or **ACE inhibitors**. May ↑ levels and risk of toxicity of **aliskiren, bosentan, colchicine, digoxin, etoposide, HMG-CoA reductase inhibitors, methotrexate, nifedipine, repaglinide**, and **sirolimus**. May ↑ levels and risk of toxicity of **ambrisentan**; do not titrate dose of ambrisentan up to maximum daily dose. May ↑ levels of and risk of bleeding with **dabigatran**; avoid concurrent use. May ↓ antibody response to **live-virus vaccines** and ↑ risk of adverse reactions; avoid concurrent use. Concurrent use with **tacrolimus** should be avoided. ↑ risk of renal impairment with **ciprofloxacin, aminoglycosides, vancomycin, trimethoprim/sulfamethoxazole, melphalan, amphotericin B, ketoconazole, colchicine, NSAIDs, cimetidine**, or **fibric acid derivatives**.

Drug-Natural Products: Concomitant use with **echinacea** and **melatonin** may interfere with immunosuppression. Use with **St. John's wort** may cause ↓ serum levels and organ rejection for transplant patients.

Drug-Food: Concurrent ingestion of **grapefruit or grapefruit juice** may ↑ serum levels and should be avoided. **Food** ↓ absorption of microemulsion products (Neoral).

Route/Dosage
Doses are adjusted on the basis of serum level monitoring.

Prevention of Transplant Rejection (Sandimmune)
PO (Adults and Children): 14–18 mg/kg/dose 4–12 hr before transplant then 5–15 mg/kg/day divided every 12–24 hr postoperatively, taper by 5% weekly to maintenance dose of 3–10 mg/kg/day.
IV (Adults and Children): 5–6 mg/kg/dose 4–12 hr before transplant, then 2–10 mg/kg/day in divided doses every 8–24 hr; change to PO as soon as possible.

Prevention of Transplant Rejection (Neoral)
PO (Adults and Children): 4–12 mg/kg/day divided every 12 hr (dose varies depending on organ transplanted).

Rheumatoid Arthritis (Neoral only)
PO (Adults and Children): 2.5 mg/kg/day given in 2 divided doses; may ↑ by 0.5–0.75 mg/kg/day after 8 and 12 wk, up to 4 mg/kg/day. ↓ dose by 25–50% if adverse reactions occur.

Severe Psoriasis (Neoral only)
PO (Adults): 2.5 mg/kg/day given in 2 divided doses, for at least 4 wk; then may ↑ by 0.5 mg/kg/day every 2 wk, up to 4 mg/kg/day. ↓ dose by 25–50% if adverse reactions occur.

Autoimmune Diseases (Neoral only)
PO (Adults and Children): 1–3 mg/kg/day.

Availability (generic available)
Microemulsion soft gelatin capsules (Gengraf, Neoral): 25 mg, 50 mg, 100 mg. **Microemulsion oral solution (Gengraf, Neoral):** 100 mg/mL. **Soft gelatin capsules (Sandimmune):** 25 mg, 100 mg. **Oral solution (Sandimmune):** 100 mg/mL. **Solution for injection (Sandimmune):** 50 mg/mL.

NURSING IMPLICATIONS
Assessment
- Monitor serum creatinine level, intake and output ratios, daily weight, and BP during therapy. Report significant changes.
- Assess for any new signs or symptoms that may be suggestive of PML, an opportunistic infection of the brain caused by the Jakob Cruzfeldt (JC) virus, that may be fatal; withhold dose and notify health care professional promptly. PML symptoms may begin gradually (hemiparesis, apathy, confusion, cognitive deficiencies, and ataxia) and may include deteriorating renal function and renal graft loss.
- Monitor for signs and symptoms of PRES (impaired consciousness, convulsions, visual disturbances including blindness, loss of motor function, movement disorders and psychiatric disturbances, papilledema, visual impairment). Usually reversible with discontinuation of cyclosporine. Occurs more often in patients with liver transplant than kidney transplant.
- **Prevention of Transplant Rejection:** Assess for symptoms of organ rejection during therapy.
- **IV:** Monitor patient for signs and symptoms of hypersensitivity (wheezing, dyspnea, flushing of face or neck) continuously during at least the first 30 min of each treatment and frequently thereafter. Oxygen, epinephrine, and equipment for treatment of anaphylaxis should be available with each IV dose.
- **Arthritis:** Assess pain and limitation of movement prior to and during administration.
- Prior to initiating therapy, perform a physical exam including BP on 2 occasions to determine baseline. Monitor BP every 2 wk during initial 3 mo, then monthly if stable. If hypertension occurs, dose should be reduced.
- **Psoriasis:** Assess skin lesions prior to and during therapy.

Lab Test Considerations
- Measure serum creatinine, BUN, CBC, magnesium, potassium, uric acid, and lipids at baseline, every 2 wk during initial therapy, and then monthly if stable. Nephrotoxicity may occur; report significant increases.
- May cause hepatotoxicity; monitor for ↑ AST, ALT, alkaline phosphatase, amylase, and bilirubin.
- May cause ↑ serum potassium and uric acid levels and ↓ serum magnesium levels.
- Serum lipid levels may be ↑.

Toxicity and Overdose

- Evaluate serum cyclosporine levels periodically during therapy. Dose may be adjusted daily, in response to levels, during initiation of therapy. Guidelines for desired serum levels will vary among institutions.

Implementation

- Do not confuse cyclosporine with cyclophosphamide or cycloserine. Do not confuse Sandimmune with Sandostatin.
- Administer initial dose 4–12 hrs before transplantation.
- Given with adrenal corticosteroids; avoid other immunosuppressive agents. Protect transplant patients from staff and visitors who may carry infection. Maintain protective isolation as indicated.
- Microemulsion products (Neoral) and other products (Sandimmune) are not interchangeable.
- **PO:** Draw up oral solution in the syringe provided; do not rinse syringe either before or after use. Introduction of water into the product by any means will cause variation in dose. Mix oral solution with milk, chocolate milk, apple juice, or orange juice, preferably at room temperature. Stir well and drink at once. Use a glass container and rinse with more diluent to ensure that total dose is taken. Administer oral doses with meals.

IV Administration

- Due to risk of anaphylaxis, IV dose should be reserved for patients who are unable to take the soft gelatin capsules or oral solution.
- **Intermittent Infusion:** *Dilution:* Dilute each 1 mL (50 mg) of IV concentrate immediately before use with 20–100 mL of D5W or 0.9% NaCl for injection. Solution is stable for 24 hr in D5W. In 0.9% NaCl, it is stable for 6 hr in a polyvinylchloride container and 12 hr in a glass container at room temperature. *Concentration:* 2.5 mg/mL. *Rate:* Infuse slowly over 2–6 hr via infusion pump.
- **Continuous Infusion:** May be administered over 24 hr.
- **Y-Site Compatibility:** alemtuzumab, amikacin, aminocaproic acid, aminophylline, amiodarone, amphotericin B lipid complex, anidulafungin, argatroban, arsenic trioxide, ascorbic acid, atropine, azithromycin, aztreonam, benztropine, bivalirudin, bleomycin, bumetanide, buprenorphine, butorphanol, calcium chloride, calcium gluconate, carboplatin, carmustine, caspofungin, cefazolin, cefotaxime, cefotetan, cefoxitin, ceftaroline, ceftazidime, ceftriaxone, cefuroxime, chloramphenicol, chlorpromazine, cisplatin, clindamycin, cyclophosphamide, cytarabine, dacarbazine, dactinomycin, daptomycin, daunorubicin hydrochloride, dexamethasone, dexmedetomidine, dexrazoxane, digoxin, diltiazem, diphenhydramine, dobutamine, docetaxel, dopamine, doxorubicin hydrochloride, dox-

orubicin liposomal, doxycycline, enalaprilat, ephedrine, epinephrine, epirubicin, epoetin alfa, ertapenem, erythromycin, esmolol, etoposide, etoposide phosphate, famotidine, fentanyl, fluconazole, fludarabine, fluorouracil, folic acid, foscarnet, fosphenytoin, furosemide, ganciclovir, gemcitabine, gentamicin, glycopyrrolate, granisetron, heparin, hetastarch, hydrocortisone, hydromorphone, ifosfamide, imipenem/cilastatin, indomethacin, irinotecan, isoproterenol, ketorolac, labetalol, leucovorin calcium, levofloxacin, lidocaine, linezolid, lorazepam, mannitol, meperidine, meropenem, methotrexate, methylprednisolone, metoclopramide, metoprolol, metronidazole, micafungin, midazolam, milrinone, mitoxantrone, morphine, moxifloxacin, multivitamins, nafcillin, nicardipine, nitroglycerin, nitroprusside, norepinephrine, octreotide, ondansetron, oxacillin, oxaliplatin, oxytocin, paclitaxel, palonosetron, pamidronate, papaverine, pemetrexed, penicillin G, pentamidine, phentolamine, phenylephrine, phytonadione, piperacillin/tazobactam, potassium acetate, potassium chloride, procainamide, prochlorperazine, promethazine, propofol, propranolol, protamine, pyridoxine, sargramostim, sodium acetate, sodium bicarbonate, succinylcholine, sufentanil, tacrolimus, theophylline, thiamine, thiotepa, tigecycline, tirofiban, tobramycin, topotecan, vancomycin, vasopressin, vecuronium, verapamil, vinblastine, vincristine, vinorelbine, zoledronic acid.

- **Y-Site Incompatibility:** amphotericin B liposomal, ceftolozane/tazobactam, cyanocobalamin, dantrolene, diazepam, gemtuzumab ozogamicin, idarubicin, isavuconazonium, nalbuphine, pentobarbital, phenobarbital, phenytoin, rituximab, trastuzumab, trimethoprim/sulfamethoxazole, voriconazole.

Patient/Family Teaching

- Instruct patient to take medication at the same time each day with meals, as directed. Take missed doses as soon as remembered within 12 hr. Do not skip doses or double up on missed doses. Do not discontinue medication without advice of health care professional.
- Reinforce the need for lifelong therapy to prevent transplant rejection. Review symptoms of rejection for transplanted organ, and stress need to notify health care professional immediately if they occur.
- Instruct patients and/or parents to notify health care professional if diarrhea develops; decreases absorption of cyclosporine and can result in rejection.
- Instruct patient to avoid grapefruit and grapefruit juice to prevent interaction with cyclosporine.
- Advise patient of common side effects (nephrotoxicity, ↑ BP, hand tremors, increased facial and body hair, gingival hyperplasia). Advise patients that if hair growth is excessive, depilatories or waxing can be used.

🍁 = Canadian drug name. ▨ = Genetic implication. S̶t̶r̶i̶k̶e̶t̶h̶r̶o̶u̶g̶h̶ = Discontinued. CAPITALS = life-threatening. Underline = most frequent.

- Teach patient the correct method for monitoring BP. Instruct patient to notify health care professional of significant changes in BP or if hematuria, increased frequency, cloudy urine, decreased urine output, fever, sore throat, tiredness, or unusual bruising occurs.
- Instruct patient on proper oral hygiene. Meticulous oral hygiene and dental examinations for teeth cleaning and plaque control every 3 mo will help decrease gingival inflammation and hyperplasia.
- Instruct patient to notify health care professional of all Rx or OTC medications, vitamins, or herbal products being taken and consult health care professional before taking other Rx, OTC, or herbal products or receiving any vaccinations while taking this medication.
- Rep: Advise patient to notify health care professional if pregnancy is planned or suspected, and to avoid breastfeeding.
- Emphasize the importance of follow-up exams and lab tests.

Evaluation/Desired Outcomes

- Prevention of rejection of transplanted tissues.
- Decrease in severity of pain in patients with rheumatoid arthritis.
- Increased ease of joint movement in patients with rheumatoid arthritis.
- Decrease in progression of psoriasis.

HIGH ALERT

cytarabine (sye-tare-a-been)
Cytosar-U
Classification
Therapeutic: antineoplastics
Pharmacologic: antimetabolites

Indications

IV: Treatment of leukemias and non-Hodgkin's lymphomas (in combination with other agents). **IT:** Prophylaxis and treatment of meningeal leukemia.

Action

Inhibits DNA synthesis by inhibiting DNA polymerase (cell-cycle S-phase–specific). **Therapeutic Effects:** Death of rapidly replicating cells, particularly malignant ones.

Pharmacokinetics

Absorption: Absorption occurs from SUBQ sites, but blood levels are lower than with IV administration; IT administration results in negligible systemic exposure.

Distribution: Widely distributed; IV- and SUBQ-administered cytarabine crosses the blood-brain barrier but not in sufficient quantities.

Metabolism and Excretion: Metabolized mostly by the liver; <10% excreted unchanged by the kidneys. Metabolism to inactive drug in the CSF is negligible because the enzyme that metabolizes it is present in very low concentrations in the CSF.

Half-life: *IV, SUBQ:* 1–3 hr; *IT:* 100–236 hr.

TIME/ACTION PROFILE (IV, SUBQ— effects on WBCs; IT—levels in CSF)

ROUTE	ONSET	PEAK	DURATION
SUBQ, IV (1st phase)	24 hr	7–9 days	12 days
SUBQ, IV (2nd phase)	15–24 days	15–24 days	25–34 days
IT	rapid	5 hr	14–28 days

Contraindications/Precautions

Contraindicated in: Hypersensitivity; Active meningeal infection (IT only); OB: Pregnancy; Lactation: Lactation.

Use Cautiously in: Active infection; ↓ bone marrow reserve; Renal impairment; Hepatic impairment; Rep: Women of reproductive potential.

Adverse Reactions/Side Effects

CV: edema. **Derm:** alopecia, rash. **EENT:** corneal toxicity (high dose), hemorrhagic conjunctivitis (high dose), visual disturbances (including blindness). **GI:** nausea, vomiting, GI ulceration (high dose), HEPATOTOXICITY, stomatitis. **GU:** sterility, urinary incontinence. **Hemat:** *(less with IT use):* anemia, leukopenia, thrombocytopenia. **Metab:** hyperuricemia. **Neuro:** *IT:* abnormal gait, CHEMICAL ARACHNOIDITIS, CNS dysfunction (high dose), confusion, drowsiness, headache. **Resp:** PULMONARY EDEMA (high dose). **Misc:** cytarabine syndrome, fever.

Interactions

Drug-Drug: ↑ bone marrow depression with other **antineoplastics** or **radiation therapy**. ↑ risk of cardiomyopathy when used in high-dose regimens with **cyclophosphamide**. May ↓ antibody response to **live-virus vaccines** and ↑ risk of adverse reactions. May ↓ absorption of **digoxin** tablets. May ↓ the efficacy of **gentamicin** when used to treat *Klebsiella pneumoniae* infections. Recent treatment with **asparaginase** may ↑ risk of pancreatitis. ↑ risk of neurotoxicity with concurrently administered **IT antineoplastics** (IT only).

Route/Dosage

Dose regimens vary widely.

IV (Adults): *Induction dose:* 200 mg/m^2/day for 5 days every 2 wk as a single agent *or* 2–6 mg/kg/day (100–200 mg/m^2/day) as a single daily dose *or* in 2–3 divided doses for 5–10 days or until remission occurs as part of combination chemotherapy. *Maintenance:* 70–200 mg/m^2/day for 2–5 days monthly. *Refractory leukemias/lymphomas:* 3 g/m^2 every 12 hr for up to 12 doses.

SUBQ (Adults): *Maintenance:* 1–1.5 mg/kg every 1–4 wk.

IT (Adults): Usual dose = 30 mg/m^2 every 4 days; range = 5–75 mg/m^2 once daily for 4 days or every 4 days until CNS findings normalize, followed by one additional treatment.

Availability (generic available)

Solution for injection: 20 mg/mL, 100 mg/mL. *In combination with:* daunorubicin (Vyxeos). See Appendix N.

NURSING IMPLICATIONS

Assessment

* Monitor for bone marrow depression. Assess for bleeding (bleeding gums, bruising, petechiae, guaiac stools, urine, and emesis) and avoid IM injections and taking rectal temperatures if platelet count is low. Apply pressure to venipuncture sites for 10 min. Assess for signs of infection during neutropenia. Anemia may occur. Monitor for increased fatigue, dyspnea, and orthostatic hypotension.
* Monitor intake and output ratios and daily weights. Report significant changes in totals.
* Monitor for symptoms of gout (increased uric acid, joint pain, edema). Encourage patient to drink at least 2 L of fluid each day. Allopurinol may decrease uric acid levels. Alkalinization of urine may increase excretion of uric acid.
* Assess nutritional status. Nausea and vomiting may occur within 1 hr of administration, especially if IV dose is administered rapidly, less severe if medication is infused slowly. Administering an antiemetic prior to and periodically throughout therapy and adjusting diet as tolerated may help maintain fluid and electrolyte balance and nutritional status.
* Monitor patient for development of *cytarabine* (fever, myalgia, bone pain, chest pain, maculopapular rash, conjunctivitis, malaise), which usually occurs 6–12 hr following administration. Corticosteroids may be used for treatment or prevention. If patient responds to corticosteroids, continue cytarabine and corticosteroids.
* Assess patient for respiratory distress and pulmonary edema. Occurs with high doses rarely; may be fatal.
* Monitor patient for signs of anaphylaxis (rash, dyspnea, swelling). Epinephrine, corticosteroids, and resuscitation equipment should be readily available.
* **IT:** CSF flow should be evaluated prior to IT therapy. Administer directly into CSF via an intraventricular reservoir or by direct injection into the lumbar sac slowly over 1–5 min. Following administration by lumbar puncture, patient should lie flat for 1 hr. Chemical arachnoiditis (nausea, vomiting, headache, fever, back pain, CSF pleocytosis and neck rigidity, neck pain, or meningism) is an expected side effect of IT cytarabine. Incidence and severity of symptoms may be decreased with coadministration of dexamethasone. 4 mg bid, PO or IV, for 5 days beginning on day of injection.
* Monitor patients receiving IT therapy continuously for the development of neurotoxicity (myelopathy, personality changes, dysarthria, ataxia, confusion,

somnolence, coma). If neurotoxicity develops, decrease amount of subsequent doses and discontinue if neurotoxicity persists. Risk may be increased if cytarabine is administered intrathecally and IV within a few days.

Lab Test Considerations

* Monitor CBC with differential and platelet count prior to and frequently during therapy. Leukocyte counts begin to drop within 24 hr of administration. The initial nadir occurs in 7–9 days. After a small ↑ in the count, the second, deeper nadir occurs 15–24 days after administration. Platelet counts begin to ↓ 5 days after a dose, with a nadir at 12–15 days. Leukocyte and platelet counts usually begin to ↑ 10 days after the nadirs. Therapy is usually withdrawn if leukocyte count is <1000/mm³ or platelet count is <50,000/mm³. Bone marrow aspirations are recommended every 2 wk until remission occurs.
* Monitor renal (BUN and serum creatinine) and hepatic function (AST, ALT, bilirubin, alkaline phosphatase, and LDH) prior to and routinely during therapy.
* May cause ↑ uric acid concentrations.

Implementation

* *High Alert:* Fatalities have occurred with chemotherapeutic agents. Before administering, clarify all ambiguous orders; double-check single, daily, and course-of-therapy dose limits; have second practitioner independently double-check original order, calculations, and infusion pump settings.
* *High Alert:* Do not confuse high-dose and regular therapy. Fatalities have occurred with high-dose therapy.
* Solution should be prepared in a biologic cabinet. Wear gloves, gown, and mask while handling IV medication. Discard IV equipment in specially designated containers.
* May be given SUBQ, direct IV, intermittent IV, continuous IV, or IT.

IV Administration

* **IV Push:** *Dilution:* Administer undiluted. *Concentration:* 100 mg/mL. *Rate:* Administer each 100 mg over 1–3 min.
* **Intermittent Infusion:** *Dilution:* May be further diluted in 0.9% NaCl, D5W, D10W, D5/0.9% NaCl, Ringer's solution, LR, or D5/LR. *Concentration:* Dilute doses in 100 mL of diluent. *Rate:* Infuse over 15–30 min.
* **Continuous Infusion:** Rate and concentration for IV infusion are ordered individually.
* **Y-Site Compatibility:** acyclovir, alemtuzumab, amifostine, amikacin, aminocaproic acid, aminophylline, amphotericin B lipid complex, amphotericin B liposomal, ampicillin, ampicillin/sulbactam, anidulafungin, argatroban, azithromycin, aztreonam, bivalirudin, bleomycin, bumetanide, buprenorphine,

butorphanol, calcium chloride, calcium gluconate, carboplatin, carmustine, cefazolin, cefepime, cefotaxime, cefotetan, cefoxitin, ceftazidime, ceftriaxone, cefuroxime, chlorpromazine, ciprofloxacin, cisatracurium, cisplatin, cladribine, clindamycin, cyclophosphamide, cyclosporine, dacarbazine, daunorubicin hydrochloride, dexamethasone, dexmedetomidine, dexrazoxane, digoxin, diltiazem, diphenhydramine, dobutamine, docetaxel, dopamine, doxorubicin hydrochloride, doxorubicin liposomal, doxycycline, droperidol, enalaprilat, ephedrine, epinephrine, ertapenem, erythromycin, esmolol, etoposide, etoposide phosphate, famotidine, fentanyl, filgrastim, fluconazole, fludarabine, foscarnet, fosphenytoin, furosemide, gemcitabine, gentamicin, granisetron, haloperidol, heparin, hydrocortisone, hydromorphone, idarubicin, ifosfamide, imipenem/cilastatin, insulin, regular, irinotecan, isoproterenol, ketorolac, labetalol, leucovorin, levofloxacin, lidocaine, linezolid, lorazepam, magnesium sulfate, mannitol, melphalan, meperidine, meropenem, mesna, methohexital, methotrexate, methylprednisolone, metoclopramide, metoprolol, metronidazole, midazolam, milrinone, mitoxantrone, morphine, moxifloxacin, nalbuphine, naloxone, nicardipine, nitroglycerin, nitroprusside, norepinephrine, octreotide, ondansetron, oxaliplatin, paclitaxel, palonosetron, pamidronate, pantoprazole, pemetrexed, pentamidine, pentobarbital, phenobarbital, phenylephrine, piperacillin/tazobactam, potassium acetate, potassium chloride, potassium phosphate, procainamide, prochlorperazine, promethazine, propofol, propranolol, remifentanil, rituximab, rocuronium, sargramostim, sodium acetate, sodium bicarbonate, sodium phosphate, succinylcholine, sufentanil, tacrolimus, theophylline, thiopental, thiotepa, tigecycline, tirofiban, tobramycin, trastuzumab, trimethoprim/sulfamethoxazole, vancomycin, vasopressin, vecuronium, verapamil, vincristine, vinorelbine, voriconazole, zidovudine, zoledronic acid.

- **Y-Site Incompatibility:** allopurinol, amiodarone, amphotericin B deoxycholate, daptomycin, diazepam, ganciclovir, phenytoin.

- **IT:** Reconstitute IT doses with preservative-free 0.9% NaCl or autologous spinal fluid. Use immediately to prevent bacterial contamination. Instruct patient to lie flat for 1 hr following IT injection. Monitor for immediate toxic reactions.

Patient/Family Teaching

- Caution patient to avoid crowds and persons with known infections. Report symptoms of infection (fever, chills, cough, hoarseness, sore throat, lower back or side pain, painful or difficult urination) immediately.
- Instruct patient to report unusual bleeding. Advise patient of thrombocytopenia precautions (use soft toothbrush and electric razor, avoid falls, do not drink alcoholic beverages or take medication containing aspirin or NSAIDs; may precipitate gastric bleeding).
- Instruct patient to inspect oral mucosa for redness and ulceration. If mouth sores occur, advise patient to use sponge brush and rinse mouth with water after eating and drinking. Stomatitis may require treatment with opioid analgesics.
- Instruct patient not to receive any vaccinations without advice of health care professional.
- Rep: Advise patient that this medication may have teratogenic effects. Contraception should be used during therapy and for at least 4 mo after therapy is concluded.
- Emphasize the need for periodic lab tests to monitor for side effects.
- **IT:** Inform patient about the expected side effects (headache, nausea, vomiting, fever) and about early signs of neurotoxicity. Instruct patient to notify health care professional if these signs occur.

Evaluation/Desired Outcomes

- Improvement of hematopoietic values in leukemias.
- Decrease in size and spread of the tumor in non-Hodgkin's lymphomas. Therapy is continued every 2 wk until patient is in complete remission or platelet count or leukocyte count falls below acceptable levels.
- Treatment of lymphomatous meningitis.

dabigatran (da-bi-**gat**-ran)
Pradaxa
Classification
Therapeutic: anticoagulants
Pharmacologic: thrombin inhibitors

Indications
Reduction in the risk of stroke/systemic embolization associated with nonvalvular atrial fibrillation (AF). Treatment of venous thromboembolic events (VTE) (including deep vein thrombosis [DVT] or pulmonary embolism [PE]) in patients who have been treated with a parenteral anticoagulant for ≥5 days. Reduction in the risk of recurrence of VTE in patients who have been previously treated. Prevention of DVT and PE following hip replacement surgery.

Action
Acts as a direct inhibitor of thrombin. **Therapeutic Effects:** Reduced risk of thrombotic sequelae (stroke and systemic embolism) in nonvalvular AF. Reduced risk of recurrent PE and DVT. Resolution of DVT and PE.

Pharmacokinetics
Absorption: 3–7% absorbed following oral administration. Bioavailability of oral pellets higher than that of capsules in adults.
Distribution: Unknown.
Metabolism and Excretion: Of the amount absorbed, mostly excreted by kidneys (80%); 86% of ingested dose is eliminated in feces due to poor bioavailability.
Half-life: 12–17 hr.

TIME/ACTION PROFILE (effects on coagulation)

ROUTE	ONSET	PEAK	DURATION
PO	within hrs	unknown	2 days†

†Following discontinuation, 3–5 days in renal impairment.

Contraindications/Precautions
Contraindicated in: Hypersensitivity; Active pathologic bleeding; Concurrent use of P-glycoprotein (P-gp) inducers; Prosthetic heart valves (mechanical or bioprosthetic); Triple-positive antiphospholipid syndrome (↑ risk of thrombosis); OB: Pregnancy; Lactation: Lactation.
Use Cautiously in: Neuroaxial spinal anesthesia or spinal puncture, especially if concurrent with an indwelling epidural catheter, drugs affecting hemostasis, history of traumatic/repeated spinal puncture or spinal deformity (↑ risk of spinal hematoma); Concurrent medications/pre-existing conditions that ↑ bleeding risk (other anticoagulants, antiplatelet agents, fibrinolytics, heparins, chronic NSAID use, labor and delivery); Renal impairment; Surgical procedures (discontinue

1–2 days prior if CCr ≥50 mL/min or 3–4 days prior if CCr <50 mL/min; Rep: Women of reproductive potential; Pedi: Safety and effectiveness in children <3 mo (treatment and reduction in risk of VTE) and <18 yr (all other indications) not established; Geri: Appears on Beers list. ↑ risk of bleeding in older adults. Use caution in selecting dabigatran over apixaban for long-term treatment of nonvalvular AF or VTE.

Adverse Reactions/Side Effects
GI: abdominal pain, diarrhea, dyspepsia, gastritis, esophageal ulceration, nausea. **Hemat:** BLEEDING, thrombocytopenia. **Misc:** HYPERSENSITIVITY REACTIONS (including anaphylaxis and angioedema).

Interactions
Drug-Drug: Concurrent use of other **anticoagulants, antiplatelet agents, fibrinolytics, heparins, prasugrel, clopidogrel,** or chronic use of **NSAIDs** ↑ risk of bleeding. Concurrent use of **P-gp inducers** including **rifampin** ↓ levels and effectiveness; avoid concurrent use. **P-gp inhibitors,** including **dronedarone, ketoconazole (systemic), verapamil, quinidine,** and **ticagrelor** may ↑ levels and the risk of bleeding; concomitant use should be avoided in patients with CCr 15–30 mL/min.

Route/Dosage
Do not interchange capsules and oral pellets on a milligram-to-milligram basis and do not combine these dose forms to achieve the total dose.

Reduction in Risk of Stroke/Systemic Embolism in Nonvalvular Atrial Fibrillation
PO (Adults): *Capsules:* 150 mg twice daily.

Renal Impairment
PO (Adults): *CCr 30–50 mL/min and taking dronedarone or systemic ketoconazole:* Capsules: 75 mg twice daily; *CCr <30 mL/min and taking P-gp inhibitor:* Avoid concomitant use; *CCr 15–30 mL/min:* Capsules: 75 mg twice daily; *CCr <15 mL/min or on dialysis:* Not recommended.

Treatment of and Reduction in Risk of Recurrence of Deep Vein Thrombosis or Pulmonary Embolism
Capsules
PO (Adults): 150 mg twice daily.
PO (Children 8–<18 yr and ≥81 kg actual body weight): 260 mg (one 150-mg capsule + one 110-mg capsule *or* one 110-mg capsule + two 75-mg capsules) twice daily.
PO (Children 8–<18 yr and 61–<81 kg actual body weight): 220 mg (two 110-mg capsules) twice daily.
PO (Children 8–<18 yr and 41–<61 kg actual body weight): 185 mg (one 110-mg capsule + one 75-mg capsule) twice daily.

✤ = Canadian drug name. ☒ = Genetic implication. ~~Strikethrough~~ = Discontinued. CAPITALS = life-threatening. Underline = most frequent.

PO (Children 8–<18 yr and 26–<41 kg actual body weight): 150 mg (one 150-mg capsule *or* two 75-mg capsules) twice daily.

PO (Children 8–<18 yr and 16–<26 kg actual body weight): 110 mg (one 110-mg capsule) twice daily.

PO (Children 8–<18 yr and 11–<16 kg actual body weight): 75 mg (one 75-mg capsule) twice daily.

Oral Pellets

PO (Children 2–<12 yr and ≥41 kg actual body weight): 260 mg (one 110-mg pkt + one 150-mg pkt) twice daily.

PO (Children 2–<12 yr and 21–<41 kg actual body weight): 220 mg (two 110-mg pkts) twice daily.

PO (Children 2–<12 yr and 16–<21 kg actual body weight): 170 mg (one 20-mg pkt + one 150-mg pkt) twice daily.

PO (Children 2–<12 yr and 13–<16 kg actual body weight): 140 mg (one 30-mg pkt + one 110-mg pkt) twice daily.

PO (Children 2–<12 yr and 11–<13 kg actual body weight): 110 mg (one 110-mg pkt) twice daily.

PO (Children 2–<12 yr and 9–<11 kg actual body weight): 90 mg (one 40-mg pkt + one 50-mg pkt) twice daily.

PO (Children 2–<12 yr and 7–<9 kg actual body weight): 70 mg (one 30-mg pkt + one 40-mg pkt) twice daily.

PO (Children 18 mo–<2 yr and 21–<26 kg actual body weight): 180 mg (one 30-mg pkt + one 150-mg pkt) twice daily.

PO (Children 12 mo–<2 yr and 16–<21 kg actual body weight): 140 mg (one 30-mg pkt + one 110-mg pkt) twice daily.

PO (Children 11 mo–<2 yr and 13–<16 kg actual body weight): 140 mg (one 30-mg pkt + one 110-mg pkt) twice daily.

PO (Children 10 mo–<11 mo and 13–<16 kg actual body weight): 100 mg (two 50-mg pkts) twice daily.

PO (Children 18 mo–<2 yr and 11–<13 kg actual body weight): 110 mg (one 110-mg pkt) twice daily.

PO (Children 8 mo–<18 mo and 11–<13 kg actual body weight): 100 mg (two 50-mg pkts) twice daily.

PO (Children 11 mo–<2 yr and 9–<11 kg actual body weight): 90 mg (one 40-mg pkt + one 50-mg pkt) twice daily.

PO (Children 6–<11 mo and 9–<11 kg actual body weight): 80 mg (two 40-mg pkts) twice daily.

PO (Children 5–<6 mo and 9–<11 kg actual body weight): 60 mg (two 30-mg pkts) twice daily.

PO (Children 9 mo–<2 yr and 7–<9 kg actual body weight): 70 mg (one 30-mg pkt + one 40-mg pkt) twice daily.

PO (Children 4–<9 mo and 7–<9 kg actual body weight): 60 mg (two 30-mg pkts) twice daily.

PO (Children 3–<4 mo and 7–<9 kg actual body weight): 50 mg (one 50-mg pkt) twice daily.

PO (Children 5 mo–<2 yr and 5–<7 kg actual body weight): 50 mg (one 50-mg pkt) twice daily.

PO (Children 3–<5 mo and 5–<7 kg actual body weight): 40 mg (one 40-mg pkt) twice daily.

PO (Children 3–<10 mo and 4–<5 kg actual body weight): 40 mg (one 40-mg pkt) twice daily.

PO (Children 3–<6 mo and 3–<4 kg actual body weight): 30 mg (one 30-mg pkt) twice daily.

Renal Impairment

PO (Adults): *CCr <50 mL/min and taking P-gp inhibitor:* Avoid concomitant use; *CCr <30 mL/min or on dialysis:* Not recommended.

Renal Impairment

(Children 8–<18 yr and ≥11 kg): *eGFR <50 mL/min/1.73 m²:* Not recommended.

Prevention of Deep Vein Thrombosis and Pulmonary Embolism Following Hip Replacement Surgery

PO (Adults): *Capsules:* 110 mg taken 1–4 hr after surgery and once hemostasis achieved, then 220 mg once daily for 28–35 days; if unable to start on day of surgery, once hemostasis achieved, start with 220 mg once daily.

Renal Impairment

PO (Adults): *CCr <50 mL/min and taking P-gp inhibitor:* Avoid concomitant use; *CCr ≤30 mL/min or on dialysis:* Not recommended.

Availability (generic available)

Capsules: 75 mg, 110 mg, 150 mg. **Oral pellets:** 20 mg/pkt, 30 mg/pkt, 40 mg/pkt, 50 mg/pkt, 110 mg/pkt, 150 mg/pkt.

NURSING IMPLICATIONS

Assessment

- Assess for symptoms of stroke or peripheral vascular disease periodically during therapy.
- Assess for symptoms of bleeding and blood loss; may be fatal. If reversal of anticoagulant effect is required, may use idarucizumab.

Lab Test Considerations

- Use aPTT or ecarin clotting time (ECT), not INR, to assess anticoagulant activity, if needed.
- Monitor renal function prior to and periodically during therapy. Patients with renal impairment may require dose reduction or discontinuation.

Toxicity and Overdose

- Should dabigatran need to be reversed, the reversal agent is idarucizumab; has not been tested in pediatric patients.

Implementation

- Do not confuse dabigatran with vigabatrin. Do not confuse Pradaxa with Plavix.
- Do not exchange capsule for oral pellets. Doses are not equal.

D

- When *converting from warfarin*, discontinue warfarin and start dabigatran when INR is <2.0.
- When *converting from dabigatran to warfarin*, adjust starting time based on CCr. For *CCr >50 mL/min*, start warfarin 3 days before discontinuing dabigatran. For *CCr 31–50 mL/min*, start warfarin 2 days before discontinuing dabigatran. For *CCr 15–30 mL/min*, start warfarin 1 day before discontinuing dabigatran. For *CCr <15 mL/min*, no recommendations can be made. INR will better reflect warfarin's effect after dabigatran has been stopped for at least 2 days.
- When *converting from parenteral anticoagulants*, start PO dabigatran up to 2 hr before next dose of parenteral drug is due or at time of discontinuation of parenteral therapy.
- When *converting from dabigatran to parenteral anticoagulants*, wait 12 hrs (CCr ≥30 mL/min) or 24 hr (CCr <30 mL/min) after last dose of dabigatran before initiating parenteral anticoagulant therapy.
- *For surgery*, discontinue dabigatran 1–2 days (CCr ≥50 mL/min) or 3–5 days (CCr <50 mL/min) before invasive or surgical procedures; consider longer times for major surgery, spinal puncture, or placement of a spinal or epidural catheter. If surgery cannot be delayed, bleeding risk is ↑. Assess bleeding risk with ECT or aPTT, if ECT is not available.
- **PO:** Administer twice daily, at the same time each day, about 12 hr apart with a full glass of water without regard to food. Give with food to decrease GI distress. *DNC:* Swallow capsule whole; do not open, crush, or chew; may result in increased exposure.
- Administer pellets immediately after mixing or within 30 min after mixing. If not administered within 30 min of mixing, discard dose, and prepare a new dose. Mix pellets with 2 teaspoons of soft food (mashed carrots, apple sauce, mashed banana) at room temperature or spoon pellets directly into mouth and swallowed apple juice or added to 1–2 oz of apple juice for drinking. Do not administer pellets via syringes or feeding tubes, or with milk, milk products, or soft foods containing milk products.
- If dabigatran is discontinued, consider starting another anticoagulant; discontinuation of dabigatran increases risk of thromboembolic events.

Patient/Family Teaching
- Instruct patient to take dabigatran as directed. Take missed doses as soon as remembered within 6 hr. If <6 hr until next dose, skip dose and take next dose when scheduled; do not double doses. Do not discontinue without consulting health care professional. If temporarily discontinued, restart as soon as possible. Store dabigatran at room temperature. After opening bottle, use within 4 mo; discard unused dabigatran after 4 mo. Advise patient to read *Medication Guide* before starting therapy and with each Rx refill in case of changes.

- Inform patient that they may bleed more easily or longer than usual. Advise patient to notify health care professional immediately if signs of bleeding (unusual bruising; pink or brown urine; red or black, tarry stools; coughing up blood; vomiting blood; pain or swelling in a joint; headache; dizziness; weakness; recurring nose bleeds; unusual bleeding from gums; heavier than normal menstrual bleeding; dyspepsia; abdominal pain; epigastric pain) occur.
- Advise patient to notify health care professional of medication regimen prior to treatment or surgery.
- Instruct patient to notify health care professional of all Rx or OTC medications, vitamins, or herbal products being taken and consult health care professional before taking any new medications.
- Rep: May cause fetal harm. Advise females of reproductive potential to notify health care professional if pregnancy is planned or suspected and to avoid breastfeeding during therapy. May increase risk of bleeding in the fetus and neonate. Monitor neonates for bleeding. May increase risk of uterine bleeding; advise patient to notify health care professional if significant uterine bleeding occurs.

Evaluation/Desired Outcomes
- Reduction in the risk of stroke and systemic embolism associated with nonvalvular AF.
- Reduced risk of recurrent PE and DVT.
- Resolution of DVT and PE.

⚇ **dabrafenib** (da-**braf**-e-nib)
Tafinlar
Classification
Therapeutic: antineoplastics
Pharmacologic: kinase inhibitors

Indications
⚇ Metastatic or unresectable melanoma in patients with the BRAF V600E mutation (as monotherapy). ⚇ Metastatic or unresectable melanoma in patients with the BRAF V600E or V600K mutation (in combination with trametinib). ⚇ Adjuvant treatment of melanoma in patients with the BRAF V600E or V600K mutation and lymph node involvement following complete resection (in combination with trametinib). ⚇ Metastatic non-small cell lung cancer (NSCLC) in patients with the BRAF V600E mutation (in combination with trametinib). ⚇ Locally advanced or metastatic anaplastic thyroid cancer in patients with the BRAF V600E mutation and no satisfactory locoregional treatment options (in combination with trametinib). ⚇ Unresectable or metastatic solid tumors with the BRAF V600E mutation in patients who have progressed following prior treatment and have no satisfactory alternative treatment options (in combination with trametinib). ⚇ Low-grade glioma with a BRAF V600E mutation in patients who require systemic therapy (in combination with trametinib).

Action

Inhibits kinase, an enzyme that promotes cell proliferation. **Therapeutic Effects:** Decreased spread/progression of melanoma, NSCLC, anaplastic thyroid cancer, low-grade gliomas, and other solid tumors.

Pharmacokinetics

Absorption: Well absorbed (95%) following oral administration.

Distribution: Unknown.

Protein Binding: 99.7%.

Metabolism and Excretion: Mostly metabolized by the CYP2C8 and CYP3A4 isoenzymes; two metabolites (hydroxy-dabrafenib and desmethyl-1–dabrafenib) have antineoplastic activity. Excreted as metabolites in feces (72%) and urine (23%).

Half-life: *Dabrafenib:* 8 hr; *hydroxy-dabrafenib:* 10 hr, *desmethyl-1–dabrafenib:* 21–22 hr.

TIME/ACTION PROFILE (progression-free survival)

ROUTE	ONSET	PEAK	DURATION
PO	within 1 mo	1–2 mo	8 mo

Contraindications/Precautions

Contraindicated in: BRAF wild-type solid tumors (may ↑ proliferation); OB: Pregnancy; Lactation: Lactation.

Use Cautiously in: ⚥ History of glucose-6–phosphate dehydrogenase (G6PD) deficiency (may cause hemolytic anemia); Diabetes; Moderate or severe hepatic impairment; Moderate or severe renal impairment; Rep: Women of reproductive potential and men with female partners of reproductive potential; Pedi: Safety and effectiveness not established in children <18 yr (as monotherapy) or <1 yr (in combination with trametinib for unresectable or metastatic solid tumors or low-grade gliomas with BRAF V600E mutation).

Adverse Reactions/Side Effects

CV: HF, THROMBOEMBOLISM. **Derm:** alopecia, hyperkeratosis, palmar-plantar erythrodysesthesia, papilloma, cutaneous squamous cell carcinoma, DRUG REACTION WITH EOSINOPHILIA AND SYSTEMIC SYMPTOMS (DRESS), STEVENS-JOHNSON SYNDROME. **EENT:** iritis, retinal detachment, uveitis. **Endo:** hyperglycemia. **F and E:** hypophosphatemia, hyponatremia. **GI:** constipation, PANCREATITIS. **Hemat:** BLEEDING, hemophagocytic lymphohistiocytosis. **MS:** arthralgia, back pain, myalgia. **Neuro:** headache, fatigue. **Resp:** cough, nasopharyngitis. **Misc:** fever (including serious febrile reactions), chills, MALIGNANCY.

Interactions

Drug-Drug: Concurrent use of **strong CYP3A4 inhibitors** or **strong CYP2C8 inhibitors**, including **ketoconazole, nefazodone, clarithromycin,** and **gemfibrozil** may ↑ levels and ↑ the risk of toxicity and should be avoided. Concurrent use of **strong CYP3A4 inducers** or **strong CYP2C8 inducers**, including **carbamazepine, phenobarbital, phenytoin,** and **rifampin** may ↓ levels and ↓ effectiveness. **Drugs that** ↑ **gastric pH** including **antacids, H₂–receptor antagonists** and **proton pump inhibitors** may ↓ levels and effectiveness. May ↓ effectiveness of other **CYP3A4 substrates** and **CYP2C9 substrates**, including **midazolam, warfarin, dexamethasone,** and **hormonal contraceptives**.

Drug-Natural Products: St. John's wort ↓ levels and may ↓ effectiveness; concurrent use should be avoided.

Route/Dosage

Treatment of Unresectable/Metastatic Melanoma, Metastatic Non-Small Cell Lung Cancer, or Locally Advanced/Metastatic Anaplastic Thyroid Cancer

Capsules

PO (Adults): 150 mg twice daily until disease progression or unacceptable toxicity.

Tablets for Oral Suspension

PO (Adults ≥51 kg): 150 mg twice daily until disease progression or unacceptable toxicity.

PO (Adults 46–50 kg): 130 mg twice daily until disease progression or unacceptable toxicity.

PO (Adults 42–45 kg): 110 mg twice daily until disease progression or unacceptable toxicity.

PO (Adults 38–41 kg): 100 mg twice daily until disease progression or unacceptable toxicity.

PO (Adults 34–37 kg): 90 mg twice daily until disease progression or unacceptable toxicity.

PO (Adults 30–33 kg): 80 mg twice daily until disease progression or unacceptable toxicity.

PO (Adults 26–29 kg): 70 mg twice daily until disease progression or unacceptable toxicity.

PO (Adults 22–25 kg): 60 mg twice daily until disease progression or unacceptable toxicity.

PO (Adults 18–21 kg): 50 mg twice daily until disease progression or unacceptable toxicity.

PO (Adults 14–17 kg): 40 mg twice daily until disease progression or unacceptable toxicity.

PO (Adults 10–13 kg): 30 mg twice daily until disease progression or unacceptable toxicity.

PO (Adults 8–9 kg): 20 mg twice daily until disease progression or unacceptable toxicity.

Adjuvant Treatment of Unresectable/Metastatic Melanoma

Capsules

PO (Adults): 150 mg twice daily; continue until disease recurrence or unacceptable toxicity for up to 1 yr.

Tablets for Oral Suspension

PO (Adults ≥51 kg): 150 mg twice daily until disease progression or unacceptable toxicity for up to 1 yr.

PO (Adults 46–50 kg): 130 mg twice daily until disease progression or unacceptable toxicity for up to 1 yr.

PO (Adults 42–45 kg): 110 mg twice daily until disease progression or unacceptable toxicity for up to 1 yr.

PO (Adults 38–41 kg): 100 mg twice daily until disease progression or unacceptable toxicity for up to 1 yr.
PO (Adults 34–37 kg): 90 mg twice daily until disease progression or unacceptable toxicity for up to 1 yr.
PO (Adults 30–33 kg): 80 mg twice daily until disease progression or unacceptable toxicity for up to 1 yr.
PO (Adults 26–29 kg): 70 mg twice daily until disease progression or unacceptable toxicity for up to 1 yr.
PO (Adults 22–25 kg): 60 mg twice daily until disease progression or unacceptable toxicity for up to 1 yr.
PO (Adults 18–21 kg): 50 mg twice daily until disease progression or unacceptable toxicity for up to 1 yr.
PO (Adults 14–17 kg): 40 mg twice daily until disease progression or unacceptable toxicity for up to 1 yr.
PO (Adults 10–13 kg): 30 mg twice daily until disease progression or unacceptable toxicity for up to 1 yr.
PO (Adults 8–9 kg): 20 mg twice daily until disease progression or unacceptable toxicity for up to 1 yr.

Treatment of Unresectable/Metastatic Solid Tumors
Capsules
PO (Adults): 150 mg twice daily until disease progression or unacceptable toxicity.
PO (Children ≥1 yr and ≥51 kg): 150 mg twice daily until disease progression or unacceptable toxicity.
PO (Children ≥1 yr and 38–50 kg): 100 mg twice daily until disease progression or unacceptable toxicity.
PO (Children ≥1 yr and 26–37 kg): 75 mg twice daily until disease progression or unacceptable toxicity.

Tablets for Oral Suspension
PO (Adults and Children ≥1 yr and ≥51 kg): 150 mg twice daily until disease progression or unacceptable toxicity.
PO (Adults and Children ≥1 yr and 46–50 kg): 130 mg twice daily until disease progression or unacceptable toxicity.
PO (Adults and Children ≥1 yr and 42–45 kg): 110 mg twice daily until disease progression or unacceptable toxicity.
PO (Adults and Children ≥1 yr and 38–41 kg): 100 mg twice daily until disease progression or unacceptable toxicity.
PO (Adults and Children ≥1 yr and 34–37 kg): 90 mg twice daily until disease progression or unacceptable toxicity.
PO (Adults and Children ≥1 yr and 30–33 kg): 80 mg twice daily until disease progression or unacceptable toxicity.
PO (Adults and Children ≥1 yr and 26–29 kg): 70 mg twice daily until disease progression or unacceptable toxicity.
PO (Adults and Children ≥1 yr and 22–25 kg): 60 mg twice daily until disease progression or unacceptable toxicity.

PO (Adults and Children ≥1 yr and 18–21 kg): 50 mg twice daily until disease progression or unacceptable toxicity.
PO (Adults and Children ≥1 yr and 14–17 kg): 40 mg twice daily until disease progression or unacceptable toxicity.
PO (Adults and Children ≥1 yr and 10–13 kg): 30 mg twice daily until disease progression or unacceptable toxicity.
PO (Adults and Children ≥1 yr and 8–9 kg): 20 mg twice daily until disease progression or unacceptable toxicity.

Treatment of Low-Grade Glioma
Capsules
PO (Children ≥1 yr and ≥51 kg): 150 mg twice daily until disease progression or unacceptable toxicity.
PO (Children ≥1 yr and 38–50 kg): 100 mg twice daily until disease progression or unacceptable toxicity.
PO (Children ≥1 yr and 26–37 kg): 75 mg twice daily until disease progression or unacceptable toxicity.

Tablets for Oral Suspension
PO (Children ≥1 yr and ≥51 kg): 150 mg twice daily until disease progression or unacceptable toxicity.
PO (Children ≥1 yr and 46–50 kg): 130 mg twice daily until disease progression or unacceptable toxicity.
PO (Children ≥1 yr and 42–45 kg): 110 mg twice daily until disease progression or unacceptable toxicity.
PO (Children ≥1 yr and 38–41 kg): 100 mg twice daily until disease progression or unacceptable toxicity.
PO (Children ≥1 yr and 34–37 kg): 90 mg twice daily until disease progression or unacceptable toxicity.
PO (Children ≥1 yr and 30–33 kg): 80 mg twice daily until disease progression or unacceptable toxicity.
PO (Children ≥1 yr and 26–29 kg): 70 mg twice daily until disease progression or unacceptable toxicity.
PO (Children ≥1 yr and 22–25 kg): 60 mg twice daily until disease progression or unacceptable toxicity.
PO (Children ≥1 yr and 18–21 kg): 50 mg twice daily until disease progression or unacceptable toxicity.
PO (Children ≥1 yr and 14–17 kg): 40 mg twice daily until disease progression or unacceptable toxicity.
PO (Children ≥1 yr and 10–13 kg): 30 mg twice daily until disease progression or unacceptable toxicity.
PO (Children ≥1 yr and 8–9 kg): 20 mg twice daily until disease progression or unacceptable toxicity.

Availability
Capsules: 50 mg, 75 mg. **Tablets for oral suspension:** 10 mg.

NURSING IMPLICATIONS
Assessment
- Perform skin examinations before starting therapy and every 2 mo during and for 6 mo after completion of therapy. *If intolerable Grade 2 skin toxicity, Grade 3, or Grade 4 occurs,* hold dabrafenib for up

to 3 wk. If improved, resume at a lower dose. If not improved, permanently discontinue.

- Monitor temperature. *If temperature is >100.3°F,* hold dabrafenib or dabrafenib and trametinib. Fever may include hypotension, rigors or chills, dehydration, or renal failure. Evaluate for signs and symptoms of infection and monitor serum creatinine and other evidence of renal function during and following severe pyrexia. Dabrafenib and trametinib may be restarted if the patient has recovered from febrile reaction for ≥ 24 hours, either at the same or lower dose. Administer antipyretics as secondary prophylaxis when resuming dabrafenib. Administer corticosteroids (prednisone 10 mg daily) for ≥ 5 days for second or subsequent pyrexia if temperature does not return to baseline within 3 days of onset of pyrexia, or for pyrexia associated with complications (dehydration, hypotension, renal failure, severe chills/rigors) and there is no evidence of active infection.

- Monitor for signs and symptoms of ocular toxicities (blurred vision, loss of vision, other vision changes, see color dots, halo around objects, swelling, redness, photophobia, eye pain). May require steroid and mydriatic ophthalmic drops. *If iritis occurs,* do not modify dabrafenib dose. If severe uveitis or mild to moderate uveitis that does not respond to ocular therapy, hold dabrafenib for up to 6 wk. If improved to Grade 0–1, resume at same or lower dose. If not improved, permanently discontinue therapy.

- Monitor cardiac function (LVEF) by ECG or multigated acquisition (MUGA) scan before starting therapy with dabrafenib with trametinib, 1 mo after initiation of therapy, and then at 2- to 3-mo intervals during therapy. *If symptomatic HF occurs with absolute decrease in LVEF >20% from baseline that is below lower limit of normal (LLN),* hold dabrafenib until improved to institutional LLN and absolute decrease to ≤10% compared to baseline, then resume at same dose.

- Monitor for signs and symptoms of venous thromboembolism (shortness of breath, chest pain, arm or leg swelling, cool or pale arm or leg) during therapy. *If uncomplicated deep vein thrombosis or pulmonary embolus (PE) occurs,* do not modify dabrafenib dose. Withhold trametinib for up to 3 wk. If improved to Grade 0–1, resume at lower dose. If not improved, permanently discontinue. *If life-threatening PE occurs,* permanently discontinue dabrafenib and trametinib.

- Monitor for signs and symptoms of interstitial lung disease or pneumonitis (cough, dyspnea, hypoxia, pleural effusion, infiltrates) during therapy. If signs and symptoms occur, do not modify dabrafenib dose; permanently discontinue trametinib.

- Assess for bleeding (headaches, dizziness, feeling weak, coughing up blood or blood clots, vomiting blood or vomit looks like "coffee grounds," red or black stools that look like tar) during therapy. *If*

Grade 3 hemorrhagic event occurs, hold dabrafenib and trametinib for up to 3 wk, if improved resume at lower level. *If Grade 4 hemorrhagic event occurs,* permanently discontinue dabrafenib and trametinib.

Lab Test Considerations

- Verify negative pregnancy test prior to starting therapy. Confirm presence of BRAF V600E mutation in tumor specimens prior to therapy with dabrafenib and confirm the presence of BRAF V600E or V600K mutation in tumor specimens prior to therapy with dabrafenib and trametinib. Confirm presence of BRAF V600E mutation in tumor specimens before starting treatment for solid tumors or low-grade gliomas with dabrafenib and trametinib. Information on FDA-approved tests for the detection of BRAF V600 mutations in melanoma and NSCLC is available at http://www.fda.gov/CompanionDiagnostics. No FDA-approved test for detection of BRAF V600E mutation in anaplastic thyroid cancer is available.May cause hyperglycemia requiring increase in dose of or initiation of insulin or oral hypoglycemic agents. Monitor serum glucose levels in patients with pre-existing diabetes or hyperglycemia.

- May cause hypophosphatemia, ↑ alkaline phosphatase, and hyponatremia.

- Monitor for hemolytic anemia in patients with G6PD deficiency.

Implementation

- Dose reduction recommendations: **Adults:** *If taking 75 mg twice daily,* 1st dose reduction, 50 mg PO twice daily. Permanently discontinue if unable to tolerate 50 mg twice daily. *If taking 100 mg twice daily,* 1st dose reduction, 75 mg PO twice daily, 2nd dose reduction, 50 mg PO twice daily. Permanently discontinue if unable to tolerate 50 mg twice daily. *If taking 150 mg twice daily,* 1st dose reduction, 100 mg PO twice daily, 2nd dose reduction, 75 mg PO twice daily, 3rd dose reduction, 50 mg PO twice daily. If patient is unable to tolerate 50 mg twice daily, permanently discontinue dabrafenib. **Pediatric Patients:** *If 8–9 kg, taking 20 mg twice daily,* discontinue dabrafenib if unable to tolerate 10 mg PO twice daily. *If 10–13 kg, taking 30 mg twice daily,* 1st dose reduction, 20 mg PO twice daily, 2nd dose reduction, 10 mg PO twice daily. *If 14–17 kg, taking 40 mg twice daily,* 1st dose reduction, 30 mg PO twice daily, 2nd dose reduction, 20 mg PO twice daily, 3rd dose reduction, 10 mg PO twice daily. *If 18–21 kg, taking 50 mg twice daily,* 1st dose reduction, 30 mg PO twice daily, 2nd dose reduction, 20 mg PO twice daily, 3rd dose reduction, 10 mg PO twice daily. *If 22–25 kg, taking 60 mg twice daily,* 1st dose reduction, 40 mg PO twice daily, 2nd dose reduction, 30 mg PO twice daily, 3rd dose reduction, 20 mg PO twice daily. *If 26–29 kg, taking 70 mg twice daily,* 1st dose reduction, 50 mg PO twice daily, 2nd dose reduction, 40 mg PO twice daily, 3rd dose reduction, 20 mg PO twice daily. *If 30–33 kg, taking 80 mg twice daily,* 1st dose reduction, 50 mg PO twice daily, 2nd dose reduction, 40 mg PO twice daily, 3rd dose reduction, 30 mg PO twice daily. *If 34–37 kg, taking 90 mg twice daily,* 1st dose reduction, 60 mg PO twice daily, 2nd dose reduction, 50 mg PO twice daily, 3rd dose reduction, 30 mg PO twice daily. *If 38–41 kg, taking 100 mg twice daily,* 1st dose reduction, 70 mg PO twice daily, 2nd dose reduction, 50 mg PO twice daily, 3rd dose reduction, 30 mg PO twice daily. *If 42–45 kg, taking 110 mg twice daily,* 1st dose reduction, 70 mg PO twice daily, 2nd dose reduction, 60 mg PO twice daily, 3rd dose reduction, 40 mg PO twice daily. *If 46–50 kg, taking 130 mg twice daily,* 1st dose reduction, 90 mg PO twice daily, 2nd dose reduction, 70 mg PO twice daily, 3rd dose reduction, 40 mg PO twice daily. *If ≥ 51 kg, taking 150 mg twice daily,* 1st dose reduction, 100 mg PO twice daily, 2nd dose reduction, 80 mg PO twice daily, 3rd dose reduction, 50 mg PO twice daily.

● **PO:** Administer capsules twice daily about 12 hr apart. Administer on an empty stomach at least 1 hr before or 2 hr after a meal. *DNC:* Swallow capsules whole; do not open, crush, break, or chew.

● When administered with trametinib, administer once-daily dose of trametinib at same time each day with either morning or evening dose of dabrafenib.

● For tablets for oral suspension, use only dosing cups provided. Add cool drinking water to markings on cup, if dose is 1–4 tablets use 5 mL of water, if dose is 5–15 tablets use 10 mL of water. Put tablets in cup with water and gently stir with the handle of a teaspoon until tablets break apart, may take up to 3 min. Suspension is cloudy white and may contain small pieces. Administer suspension within 30 min of preparing; if outside 30 min, dispose of suspension and begin the process again. To access medicine residue in cup, add 5 mL of drinking water, stir and drink the water and residual mixture. If 1–4 tablets were used, rinse and drink once; if 5–15 tablets used, repeat rinse procedure twice.

● For tablets for oral suspension for use with oral syringe or feeding tube, use directions for oral suspension above. If dose is 1–3 tablets, the minimum size feeding tube that may be used is 10 French. If dose is 4 to 15 tablets, the minimum size feeding tube that may be used is 12 French. Flush feeding tube before administering suspension. Draw up all oral suspension from dosing cup into a syringe. If giving the dose through a feeding tube, give oral suspension into the feeding tube according to feeding tube manufacturer's instructions. If giving dose of oral suspension using an oral syringe, place the open end of the oral syringe inside the mouth with the tip pointing toward the inside of either cheek. If giving dose

of oral suspension to a child, make sure they are sitting upright. Slowly push the plunger all the way down on the plunger to give the full dose. Add 5 mL of water to empty dosing cup. Stir to loosen medicine residue inside the cup. Draw up water and medicine residue mixture. Give water and medicine residue mixture into the feeding tube or into the inside of the cheek. Repeat procedure 3 times.

Patient/Family Teaching

● Instruct patient to take dabrafenib as directed at least 1 hr before or 2 hr after meals. Take missed doses as soon as remembered unless within 6 hr of next dose, then skip missed dose and take regularly scheduled dose. If vomiting occurs after administration, do not take an additional dose. Take next dose at the scheduled time. Advise patient to read *Medication Guide* before starting therapy and with each Rx refill in case of changes.

● Inform patient that dabrafenib increases risk of developing new cutaneous malignancies. Notify health care professional immediately if new lesions (wart, skin sore, or reddish bump that bleeds or does not heal) or changes in size or color of existing moles or lesions occur.

● Advise patient to notify health care professional of all Rx or OTC medications, vitamins, or herbal products being taken and to consult with health care professional before taking other medications, especially St. John's wort.

● Inform patient of potential side effects. Advise patient to notify health care professional if fever, signs and symptoms of hyperglycemia (increased thirst, urinating more often than normal, breath smells like fruit), or eye problems (blurred vision, loss of vision, vision changes, see color dots, halo [see blurred outline around objects], eye pain, swelling, redness), bleeding (headaches, dizziness, or feeling weak, cough up blood or blood clots, vomit blood or vomit looks like "coffee grounds," red or black stool that looks like tar), skin reactions (blisters or peeling of skin, blisters on lips, or around mouth or eyes, mouth sores, high fever or flu-like symptoms, enlarged lymph nodes), thromboembolism, HF (heart pounding or racing, shortness of breath, swelling of ankles and feet, feeling lightheaded) occur.

● Rep: Advise females of reproductive potential and males (including those who have had vasectomies) with female partner of reproductive potential to use a highly effective form of contraception during and for at least 2 wk after last dose of dabrafenib. Use a nonhormonal form of contraception; dabrafenib may decrease effectiveness of hormonal contraceptives. Advise patient to notify health care professional if pregnancy is suspected and to avoid breastfeeding during and for 2 wk after last dose. Advise patients to seek counseling on fertility and family planning before beginning therapy; may permanently impair fertility in females and males.

Evaluation/Desired Outcomes

● Decrease in progression of malignant melanoma, NSCLC, anaplastic thyroid cancer, low-grade gliomas, and other solid tumors.

HIGH ALERT

dacarbazine (da-kar-ba-zeen)
Classification
Therapeutic: antineoplastics
Pharmacologic: alkylating agents

Indications

Metastatic malignant melanoma. Hodgkin's disease as second-line therapy (in combination with other agents).

Action

Disrupts DNA and RNA synthesis (cell-cycle phase–nonspecific). **Therapeutic Effects:** Death of rapidly growing tissue cells, especially malignant ones.

Pharmacokinetics

Absorption: IV administration results in complete bioavailability.
Distribution: Widely distributed to tissues; probably concentrates in liver; some CNS penetration.
Metabolism and Excretion: 50% metabolized by the liver, 50% excreted unchanged by the kidneys.
Half-life: 5 hr ($\uparrow$ in renal and hepatic impairment).

TIME/ACTION PROFILE (effects on blood counts)

ROUTE	ONSET	PEAK	DURATION
IV (WBCs)	16–20 days	21–25 days	3–5 days
IV (platelets)	unknown	16 days	3–5 days

Contraindications/Precautions

Contraindicated in: Hypersensitivity; OB: Pregnancy; Lactation: Lactation.
Use Cautiously in: Active infection; Bone marrow depression; Renal impairment; Hepatic impairment; Pedi: Safety and effectiveness not established in children.

Adverse Reactions/Side Effects

Derm: alopecia, facial flushing, photosensitivity, rash. **Endo:** gonadal suppression. **GI:** anorexia, nausea, vomiting, diarrhea, HEPATIC NECROSIS, hepatic vein thrombosis. **Hemat:** anemia, leukopenia, thrombocytopenia. **Local:** pain at IV site, phlebitis at IV site, tissue necrosis. **MS:** myalgia. **Neuro:** facial paresthesia, malaise. **Misc:** ANAPHYLAXIS, fever, flu-like syndrome.

Interactions

Drug-Drug: Additive bone marrow depression with other **antineoplastics**. **Carbamazepine**, **phenobarbital**, and **rifampin** may $\downarrow$ levels and effectiveness.

Amiodarone, **ciprofloxacin**, **fluvoxamine**, **ketoconazole**, **ofloxacin**, **isoniazid**, or **miconazole** may $\uparrow$ levels and risk of toxicity. May $\downarrow$ antibody response to **live-virus vaccines** and $\uparrow$ risk of adverse reactions.

Route/Dosage

Malignant Melanoma
IV (Adults): 2–4.5 mg/kg/day for 10 days administered every 4 wk *or* 250 mg/m²/day for 5 days administered every 3 wk.

Hodgkin's Disease
IV (Adults): 150 mg/m²/day for 5 days (in combination with other agents) administered every 4 wk *or* 375 mg/m² (in combination with other agents) administered every 15 days.

Availability

Powder for injection: 100 mg/vial, 200 mg/vial.

NURSING IMPLICATIONS

Assessment

● Monitor vital signs prior to and frequently during therapy.
● Monitor for bone marrow depression. Assess for bleeding (bleeding gums, bruising, petechiae, guaiac stools, urine, and emesis) and avoid IM injections and rectal temperatures if platelet count is low. Apply pressure to venipuncture sites for 10 min. Assess for signs of infection during neutropenia. Anemia may occur. Monitor for increased fatigue, dyspnea, and orthostatic hypotension.
● Monitor IV site closely. Dacarbazine is an irritant. Instruct patient to notify health care professional immediately if discomfort at IV site occurs. Discontinue IV immediately if infiltration occurs. Applications of hot packs may relieve pain, burning sensation, and irritation at injection site.
● Monitor intake and output, appetite, and nutritional intake. Assess for nausea and vomiting, which may be severe and last 1–12 hr. Administration of an antiemetic prior to and periodically during therapy, restricting oral intake for 4–6 hr prior to administration, and adjusting diet as tolerated may help maintain fluid and electrolyte balance and nutritional status. Nausea usually decreases on subsequent doses.

Lab Test Considerations
● Monitor CBC and differential prior to and periodically throughout therapy. The nadir of thrombocytopenia occurs in 16 days. The nadir of leukopenia occurs in 3–4 wk. Recovery begins in 5 days. Withhold dose and notify physician if platelet count is <100,000/mm³ or leukocyte count is <4000/mm³.
● Monitor for increased AST, ALT, BUN, and serum creatinine. May cause hepatic necrosis.

Implementation

● *High Alert:* Fatalities have occurred with chemotherapeutic agents. Before administering, clarify all ambiguous orders; double-check single, daily, and course-of-therapy dose limits; have second practitioner independently double-check original order, calculations, and infusion pump settings.

IV Administration
● Prepare solution in a biologic cabinet. Wear gloves, gown, and mask while handling medication. Discard equipment in designated containers.
● Reconstitute each 100-mg and 200-mg vial with 9.9 mL and 19.7 mL, respectively, of sterile water for injection. Solution is colorless or clear yellow. Do not use solution that has turned pink. *Concentration:* 10 mg/mL. Solution is stable for 8 hr at room temperature and for 72 hr if refrigerated.
● **Intermittent Infusion:** *Dilution:* Further dilute with up to 250 mL of D5W or 0.9% NaCl. Stable for 24 hr if refrigerated or 8 hr at room temperature. *Rate:* Administer over 30–60 min.
● **Y-Site Compatibility:** amifostine, aztreonam, bivalirudin, caspofungin, daptomycin, dexmedetomidine, docetaxel, doxorubicin liposomal, ertapenem, etoposide phosphate, filgrastim, fludarabine, granisetron, hetastarch, levofloxacin, melphalan, octreotide, ondansetron, oxaliplatin, paclitaxel, palonosetron, sargramostim, thiotepa, tigecycline, tirofiban, vinorelbine, voriconazole.
● **Y-Site Incompatibility:** allopurinol, amphotericin B liposomal, cefepime, pantoprazole, pemetrexed, piperacillin/tazobactam.

Patient/Family Teaching
● Instruct patient to notify health care professional if fever; chills; sore throat; signs of infection; bleeding gums; bruising; petechiae; abdominal pain; yellowing of eyes; or blood in urine, stool, or emesis occur. Caution patient to avoid crowds and persons with known infections. Instruct patient to use soft toothbrush and electric razor. Patients should be cautioned not to drink alcoholic beverages or take products containing aspirin or NSAIDs; may increase GI irritation.
● May cause photosensitivity. Instruct patient to avoid sunlight or wear protective clothing and use sunscreen for 2 days after therapy.
● Instruct patient to inform health care professional if flu-like syndrome occurs. Symptoms include fever, myalgia, and general malaise. May occur after several courses of therapy. Usually occurs 1 wk after administration. May persist for 1–3 wk. Acetaminophen may be used for relief of symptoms.
● Discuss with patient the possibility of hair loss. Explore coping strategies.
● Rep: Advise females of reproductive potential to notify health care professional if pregnancy is planned or suspected or if breastfeeding. Advise patient of the need for a nonhormonal method of contraception.
● Instruct patient not to receive any vaccinations without advice of health care professional.

Evaluation/Desired Outcomes
● Decrease in size and spread of malignant melanoma or Hodgkin's lymphoma.

---

dalbavancin (dal-ba-van-sin)
Dalvance, ✦Xydalba
Classification
Therapeutic: anti-infectives
Pharmacologic: lipoglycopeptides

Indications
Acute bacterial skin/skin structure infections due to susceptible bacteria.

Action
Binds to bacterial cell wall resulting in cell death.
Therapeutic Effects: Bactericidal action against susceptible bacteria with resolution of infection. **Spectrum:** Active against *Staphylococcus aureus* (including methicillin-susceptible and methicillin-resistant strains), *Streptococcus agalactiae, Streptococcus dysgalactiae, Streptococcus anginosus* (including *S. anginosus, S. intermedius,* and *S. constellatus*), *Streptococcus pyogenes,* and *Enterococcus faecalis* (only isolates susceptible to vancomycin).

Pharmacokinetics
Absorption: IV administration results in complete bioavailability.
Distribution: Penetrates tissues and fluids.
Metabolism and Excretion: 33% eliminated unchanged in urine, 12% eliminated as inactive metabolite, 20% excreted in feces.
Half-life: 346 hr.

TIME/ACTION PROFILE (plasma concentrations)

ROUTE	ONSET	PEAK	DURATION
IV	unknown	end of infusion	1 wk

Contraindications/Precautions
Contraindicated in: Hypersensitivity.
Use Cautiously in: Renal impairment (dose adjustment required for adults with CCr <30 mL/min and not receiving hemodialysis); Moderate to severe hepatic impairment; OB: Safety not established in pregnancy; Lactation: Safety not established in breastfeeding; Geri: Consider age-related ↓ in renal function in older adults.

Adverse Reactions/Side Effects
Derm: pruritus, rash. **GI:** ↑ liver enzymes, CLOSTRIDIOIDES DIFFICILE-ASSOCIATED DIARRHEA (CDAD), nausea.
Neuro: headache. **Misc:** HYPERSENSITIVITY REACTIONS (including anaphylaxis), infusion reactions (including infusion-related reaction resembling vancomycin flushing syndrome).

Interactions
Drug-Drug: None reported.

Route/Dosage
IV (Adults): 1500 mg as a single dose *or* 1000 mg followed 1 wk later by 500 mg.
IV (Children 6–<18 yr): *CCr ≥30 mL/min/1.73 m²:* 18 mg/kg (max dose = 1500 mg) as a single dose.
IV (Children Birth–<6 yr): *CCr ≥30 mL/min/1.73 m²:* 22.5 mg/kg (max dose = 1500 mg) as a single dose.

Renal Impairment
IV (Adults): *CCr <30 mL/min (with no hemodialysis):* 1125 mg as a single dose *or* 750 mg followed 1 wk later by 375 mg.

Availability
Lyophilized powder for injection: 500 mg/vial.

NURSING IMPLICATIONS
Assessment
● Assess for infection (vital signs; appearance of wound, sputum, urine, and stool; WBC) at beginning of and during therapy.
● Obtain specimens for culture and sensitivity prior to therapy. First dose may be given before receiving results.
● Monitor bowel function. Diarrhea, abdominal cramping, fever, and bloody stools should be reported to health care professional promptly as a sign of CDAD. May begin up to 2 mo following cessation of therapy.
● Monitor for infusion reactions (infusion-related reaction resembling vancomycin flushing syndrome—flushing of upper body, urticaria, pruritus, rash, back pain). May resolve with stopping or slowing infusion.

Lab Test Considerations
● Monitor hepatic function tests. May cause ↑ ALT, AST, and bilirubin.

Implementation
IV Administration
● **Intermittent Infusion:** *Reconstitution:* Reconstitute with 25 mL of sterile water or D5W in each 500-mg vial. Alternate gentle swirling and inverting to avoid foaming, until completely dissolved. Do not shake. Reconstituted vial contains a clear colorless to yellow solution. Do not administer solutions that are discolored or contain particulate matter. Transfer reconstituted solution into D5W. *Concentration:* 1 mg/mL to 5 mg/mL. Discard unused solution. May be refrigerated or kept at room temperature; do not freeze. Infuse within 48 hr of reconstitution. Do not administer solutions containing particulate matter. *Rate:* Infuse over 30 min.
● **Y-Site Incompatibility:** Do not infuse with other medications or electrolytes. Saline solutions may cause precipitation. Flush line before and after infusion with D5W.

Patient/Family Teaching
● Explain purpose of dalbavancin to patient.
● Instruct patient to notify health care professional if signs and symptoms of hypersensitivity reactions (rash, hives, dyspnea, facial swelling) occur.
● Instruct patient to notify health care professional immediately if diarrhea, abdominal cramping, fever, or bloody stools occur and not to treat with antidiarrheals without consulting health care professionals.
● Advise patient to notify health care professional of all Rx or OTC medications, vitamins, or herbal products being taken and to consult with health care professional before taking other medications.
● Rep: Advise females of reproductive potential to notify health care professional if pregnancy is planned or suspected or if breastfeeding.
● Instruct the patient to notify health care professional if symptoms do not improve.

Evaluation/Desired Outcomes
● Resolution of the signs and symptoms of infection. Length of time for complete resolution depends on the organism and site of infection.

---

dalfampridine
(dal-**fam**-pri-deen)
Ampyra, ✤Fampyra
Classification
Therapeutic: anti-multiple sclerosis agents
Pharmacologic: potassium channel blockers

Indications
To improve walking speed in patients with multiple sclerosis.

Action
Acts as a potassium channel blocker, which may increase conduction of action potentials. **Therapeutic Effects:** Increased walking speed in patients with multiple sclerosis.

Pharmacokinetics
Absorption: Rapidly and completely absorbed (96%).
Distribution: Unknown.
Metabolism and Excretion: 96% eliminated in urine, 0.5% in feces.
Half-life: 5.2–6.5 hr.

TIME/ACTION PROFILE (improvement in walking speed)

ROUTE	ONSET	PEAK	DURATION
PO	unknown	3–4 hr	24 hr

Contraindications/Precautions
Contraindicated in: Hypersensitivity; History of seizures; Moderate/severe renal impairment (CCr ≤50 mL/min) (↑ risk of seizures).

Use Cautiously in: Mild renal impairment (CCr 51–80 mL/min) (↑ risk of seizures); OB: Safety not established in pregnancy; Lactation: Safety not established in breastfeeding; Pedi: Safety and effectiveness not established in children; Geri: Consider age-related ↓ in renal function in older adults.

Adverse Reactions/Side Effects
EENT: nasopharyngitis, pharyngolaryngeal pain. **GI:** constipation, dyspepsia, nausea. **GU:** urinary tract infection. **MS:** back pain. **Neuro:** dizziness, headache, insomnia, multiple sclerosis relapse, paresthesia, SEIZURES, vertigo, weakness. **Misc:** ANAPHYLAXIS.

Interactions
Drug-Drug: Cimetidine may ↑ levels and ↑ risk of seizures.

Route/Dosage
PO (Adults): 10 mg twice daily.

Availability (generic available)
Extended-release tablets: 10 mg.

NURSING IMPLICATIONS
Assessment
- Assess walking speed in patients with multiple sclerosis prior to and periodically during therapy.
- Monitor for seizures during therapy, risk increases with increased dose. If seizure occurs, discontinue therapy.
- Monitor for signs and symptoms of anaphylaxis (dyspnea, wheezing, urticaria, angioedema of the throat or tongue) during therapy.

Lab Test Considerations
- Monitor CCr prior to and at least yearly during therapy; renal impairment may require dose reduction or discontinuation.

Implementation
- Administer tablets twice daily approximately 12 hr apart without regard to food. *DNC:* Swallow tablets whole; do not break, crush, chew, or dissolve.

Patient/Family Teaching
- Instruct patient to take dalfampridine as directed, with approximately 12 hr between tablets. If a dose is missed, omit and take next scheduled dose on time; do not double doses. May increase risk of seizures. Advise patient to read *Medication Guide* prior to beginning therapy and with each Rx refill in case of changes.
- May cause vertigo, dizziness, and seizures. Caution patient to avoid driving and other activities requiring alertness until response to the drug is known.
- Instruct patient to notify health care professional of all Rx or OTC medications, vitamins, or herbal products being taken and consult health care professional before taking any new medications.

- If a seizure or signs or symptoms of anaphylaxis occur, advise patient to notify health care professional immediately, to discontinue dalfampridine, and to not restart medication.
- Advise females of reproductive potential to notify health care professional if pregnancy is planned or suspected or if breastfeeding.

Evaluation/Desired Outcomes
- Improved walking and increased walking speed in patients with multiple sclerosis.

---

dalteparin, See HEPARINS (LOW MOLECULAR WEIGHT).

---

dantrolene (dan-troe-leen)
Dantrium, Revonto, Ryanodex
Classification
Therapeutic: skeletal muscle relaxants (direct acting)

Indications
PO: Treatment of spasticity associated with: Spinal cord injury, Stroke, Cerebral palsy, Multiple sclerosis. Prevention of malignant hyperthermia in patients at high risk. **IV:** Emergency treatment of malignant hyperthermia. Prevention of malignant hyperthermia in patients at high risk. **Unlabeled Use:** Management of moderate to severe neuroleptic malignant syndrome.

Action
Acts directly on skeletal muscle, causing relaxation by decreasing calcium release from sarcoplasmic reticulum in muscle cells. Prevents intense catabolic process associated with malignant hyperthermia. **Therapeutic Effects:** Reduction of muscle spasticity. Treatment and prevention of malignant hyperthermia.

Pharmacokinetics
Absorption: 35% absorbed after oral administration. IV administration results in complete bioavailability.
Distribution: Widely distributed to tissues.
Metabolism and Excretion: Almost entirely metabolized by the liver.
Half-life: 8.7–11.4 hr.

TIME/ACTION PROFILE (effects on spasticity)

ROUTE	ONSET	PEAK	DURATION
PO	1 wk	unknown	6–12 hr
IV	rapid	rapid	unknown

🍁 = Canadian drug name. ⚎ = Genetic implication. ~~Strikethrough~~ = Discontinued. CAPITALS = life-threatening. <u>Underline</u> = most frequent.

Contraindications/Precautions

Contraindicated in: Situations in which spasticity is used to maintain posture or balance (PO only); Lactation: Lactation.

Use Cautiously in: Cardiac, pulmonary, or previous liver disease; Women and patients >35 yr (↑ risk of hepatotoxicity); OB: Use during pregnancy only if potential maternal benefit justifies potential fetal risk; Geri: Use lowest possible dose in older adults (may have ↑ risk of hepatotoxicity).

Adverse Reactions/Side Effects

CV: changes in BP, HF, tachycardia. **Derm:** flushing, pruritus, sweating, urticaria. **EENT:** excessive lacrimation, visual disturbances. **GI:** diarrhea, anorexia, cramps, dysphagia, GI bleeding, HEPATOTOXICITY, nausea, vomiting. **GU:** crystalluria, dysuria, erectile dysfunction, frequency, incontinence, nocturia. **Hemat:** anemia, aplastic anemia, eosinophilia, leukopenia, thrombocytopenia. **Local:** irritation at IV site, phlebitis. **MS:** myalgia. **Neuro:** drowsiness, muscle weakness, confusion, dizziness, headache, insomnia, malaise, nervousness. **Resp:** dyspnea, pleural effusion, respiratory depression. **Misc:** ANAPHYLAXIS, chills, drooling, fever.

Interactions

Drug-Drug: Calcium channel blockers may ↑ risk of cardiovascular collapse; avoid concomitant use. Additive CNS depression with **CNS depressants**, including **alcohol**, **antihistamines**, **opioid analgesics**, **sedative/hypnotics**, and parenteral **magnesium sulfate**. ↑ risk of hepatotoxicity with other **hepatotoxic agents** or **estrogens**. ↑ risk of arrhythmias with **verapamil**. ↑ neuromuscular blocking effects of **vecuronium**.

Drug-Natural Products: Concomitant use of **kava-kava**, **valerian**, **chamomile**, or **hops** can ↑ CNS depression.

Route/Dosage

Spasticity

PO (Adults): 25 mg once daily for 7 days, then 25 mg 2 times daily for 7 days, then 50 mg 3 times daily for 7 days, then 100 mg 3 times daily; may ↑ to 100 mg 4 times daily, if needed.

PO (Children ≥5 yr): 0.5 mg/kg once daily for 7 days, then 0.5 mg/kg 3 times daily for 7 days, then 1 mg/kg 3 times daily for 7 days, then 2 mg/kg 3 times daily (not to exceed 400 mg/day).

Prevention of Malignant Hyperthermia

PO (Adults and Children ≥5 yr): 4–8 mg/kg/day in 3–4 divided doses for 1–2 days before procedure, with last dose 3–4 hr preoperatively.

IV (Adults and Children): 2.5 mg/kg given 75 min before surgery.

Treatment of Malignant Hyperthermia

IV (Adults and Children): At least 1 mg/kg, continued until symptoms ↓ or a cumulative dose of 10 mg/kg has been given. If symptoms reappear, dose may be repeated.

Neuroleptic Malignant Syndrome (unlabeled)

IV (Adults): 1–2.5 mg/kg initially; if rapid resolution of hyperthermia and rigidity is observed, may follow with 1 mg/kg every 6 hours (max dose = 10 mg/kg/day). After the patient is stabilized and symptoms have resolved, consider taper over days to weeks (do not abruptly discontinue).

Availability (generic available)

Capsules: 25 mg, 50 mg, 100 mg. **Powder for injection:** 20 mg/vial, 250 mg/vial.

NURSING IMPLICATIONS

Assessment

- Assess bowel function periodically. Persistent diarrhea may warrant discontinuation of therapy.
- **Muscle Spasticity:** Assess neuromuscular status and muscle spasticity prior to and periodically during therapy to determine response.
- **Malignant Hyperthermia:** Assess previous anesthesia history of all surgical patients. Also assess for family history of reactions to anesthesia (malignant hyperthermia or perioperative death).
- Monitor ECG, vital signs, electrolytes, and urine output continuously when administering IV for malignant hyperthermia.
- Monitor patient for difficulty swallowing and choking during meals on the day of administration.

Lab Test Considerations

- Monitor liver function frequently during therapy. Liver function abnormalities (↑ AST, ALT, alkaline phosphatase, bilirubin, GGT) may require discontinuation of therapy.
- Evaluate renal function and CBC before and periodically during therapy in patients receiving prolonged therapy.

Implementation

- **PO:** If gastric irritation becomes a problem, may be administered with food. Oral suspensions may be made by opening capsules and adding them to fruit juices or other liquids. Drink immediately after mixing.

IV Administration

- *Reconstitution:* Reconstitute each 20 mg of **Dantrium** with 60 mL of sterile water for injection (without a bacteriostatic agent). Shake until solution is clear. Solution must be used within 6 hr. Protect diluted solution from direct light.
- *Reconstitution:* Reconstitute **Ryanodex** by adding 5 mL of sterile water for injection; do not reconstitute with other solutions. Shake vial to ensure uniform orange suspension. Do not administer solutions that are discolored or contain particulate matter. Solution is stable for 6 hr at room temperature.

Treatment of Malignant Hyperthermia

- **IV Push:** Administer reconstituted solution without further dilution. *Rate:* Administer each single dose by rapid continuous IV push through Y-site. Follow immediately with subsequent doses as indicated. Medication is very irritating to tissues; observe infusion site frequently to avoid extravasation.

Prevention of Malignant Hyperthermia

- **IV Push:** Rates of products for prevention differ. *Rate:* Inject **Ryanodex** over at least 1 min starting 75 min before surgery into catheter with free-flowing 0.9% NaCl or D5W or into a patent indwelling catheter; flush before and after injection.
- **Intermittent Infusion:** Reconstitute required number of **Dantrium** vials as above and transfer to a larger volume sterile plastic bag (do not use glass bottles). *Rate:* Administer over 1 hr beginning 75 min before anesthesia.
- **Y-Site Compatibility:** acyclovir, paclitaxel, palonosetron.
- **Y-Site Incompatibility:** alemtuzumab, amikacin, aminophylline, amphotericin B deoxycholate, amphotericin B lipid complex, ampicillin, ampicillin/sulbactam, anidulafungin, argatroban, arsenic trioxide, ascorbic acid, atropine, azathioprine, aztreonam, benztropine, bivalirudin, bleomycin, bumetanide, buprenorphine, butorphanol, calcium chloride, calcium gluconate, carmustine, caspofungin, cefotaxime, cefotetan, cefoxitin, ceftazidime, ceftriaxone, cefuroxime, chloramphenicol, chlorpromazine, cisplatin, clindamycin, cyanocobalamin, cyclosporine, dactinomycin, daptomycin, daunorubicin hydrochloride, dexamethasone, dexrazoxane, diazepam, diazoxide, digoxin, diltiazem, diphenhydramine, dobutamine, docetaxel, dopamine, doxorubicin liposomal, doxycycline, enalaprilat, ephedrine, epinephrine, epoetin alfa, ertapenem, erythromycin, esmolol, etoposide, etoposide phosphate, famotidine, fentanyl, fluconazole, fludarabine, folic acid, foscarnet, fosphenytoin, furosemide, ganciclovir, gemcitabine, gemtuzumab ozogamicin, gentamicin, glycopyrrolate, granisetron, haloperidol, heparin, hetastarch, hydralazine, hydrocortisone, hydromorphone, hydroxyzine, idarubicin, imipenem/cilastatin, indomethacin, insulin, regular, irinotecan, isoproterenol, ketorolac, labetalol, leucovorin calcium, lidocaine, linezolid, lorazepam, magnesium sulfate, mannitol, meperidine, mesna, methylprednisolone, metoclopramide, metoprolol, metronidazole, midazolam, milrinone, mitoxantrone, morphine, moxifloxacin, multivitamins, mycophenolate, nafcillin, nalbuphine, naloxone, nitroglycerin, nitroprusside, norepinephrine, octreotide, ondansetron, oxacillin, oxaliplatin, oxytocin, pamidronate, pantoprazole, papaverine, pemetrexed, penicillin G, pentamidine, pentobarbital, phenobarbital, phentolamine, phenylephrine, phenytoin, phytonadione, piperacillin/tazobactam, potassium acetate, potassium chloride, procainamide, prochlorperazine, promethazine, propranolol, protamine, pyridoxine, sodium acetate, sodium bicarbonate, succinylcholine, sufentanil, tacrolimus, theophylline, thiamine, thiotepa, tigecycline, tirofiban, tobramycin, topotecan, trimethoprim/sulfamethoxazole, vancomycin, vasopressin, vecuronium, verapamil, vinblastine, vinorelbine, voriconazole, zoledronic acid.

Patient/Family Teaching

- Advise patient not to take more medication than the amount prescribed, to minimize risk of hepatotoxicity and other side effects. If a dose is missed, do not take unless remembered within 1 hr. Do not double doses.
- May cause dizziness, drowsiness, visual disturbances, and muscle weakness. Advise patient to avoid driving and other activities requiring alertness until response to drug is known. After IV dose for surgery, patients may experience decreased grip strength, leg weakness, light-headedness, and difficulty swallowing for up to 48 hr. Caution patients to avoid activities requiring alertness and to use caution when walking down stairs and eating during this period.
- Advise patient to avoid taking alcohol or other CNS depressants concurrently with this medication.
- Instruct patient to notify health care professional if rash; itching; yellow eyes or skin; dark urine; or clay-colored, bloody, or black, tarry stools occur or if nausea, weakness, malaise, fatigue, or diarrhea persists. May require discontinuation of therapy.
- Advise patient to wear sunscreen and protective clothing to prevent photosensitivity reactions.
- Rep: Advise females of reproductive potential to notify health care professional if pregnancy is planned or suspected and to avoid breastfeeding during and for 3 days after last dose. Monitor infants breastfed during therapy for respiratory depression and muscle weakness.
- Emphasize the importance of follow-up exams to check progress in long-term therapy and blood tests to monitor for side effects.
- **Malignant Hyperthermia:** Patients with malignant hyperthemia should carry identification describing disease process at all times.

Evaluation/Desired Outcomes

- Relief of muscle spasm in musculoskeletal conditions. One wk or more may be required to see improvement; if there is no observed improvement in 45 days, the medication is usually discontinued.
- Prevention of or decrease in temperature and skeletal rigidity in malignant hyperthermia.

✹ = Canadian drug name. ▓ = Genetic implication. ~~Strikethrough~~ = Discontinued. CAPITALS = life-threatening. <u>Underline</u> = most frequent.

dapagliflozin (dap-a-gli-**floe**-zin)
Farxiga, ✳ Forxiga
Classification
Therapeutic: antidiabetics
Pharmacologic: sodium-glucose co-transporter 2 (SGLT2) inhibitors

Indications
Type 2 diabetes mellitus (as adjunct to diet and exercise). To reduce the risk of hospitalization for HF in patients with type 2 diabetes mellitus and established cardiovascular disease or multiple cardiovascular risk factors. To reduce the risk of cardiovascular death, hospitalization for HF, and urgent visits for HF in patients with HF. To reduce the risk of sustained eGFR decline, end-stage kidney disease, cardiovascular death, and hospitalization for HF in patients with chronic kidney disease at risk of progression.

Action
Inhibits proximal renal tubular sodium-glucose cotransporter 2 (SGLT2), which determines reabsorption of glucose from the tubular lumen. Inhibits reabsorption of glucose, lowers renal threshold for glucose and increases excretion of glucose in urine. **Therapeutic Effects:** Improved glycemic control. Reduction in risk of HF hospitalizations in patients with type 2 diabetes mellitus. Reduction in risk of cardiovascular death, HF hospitalizations, and urgent visits for HF in patients with HF. Reduction in risk of sustained eGFR decline, end-stage kidney disease, cardiovascular death, and HF hospitalizations in patients with chronic kidney disease at risk of progression.

Pharmacokinetics
Absorption: 78% absorbed following oral administration.
Distribution: Unknown.
Metabolism and Excretion: Extensively metabolized by UGT1A9 to inactive metabolites which are primarily excreted in urine. 15% excreted in feces as unchanged drug.
Half-life: 12.9 hr.

TIME/ACTION PROFILE (decrease in HbA1c)

ROUTE	ONSET	PEAK	DURATION
PO	within 4 wk	12 wk	unknown

Contraindications/Precautions
Contraindicated in: Hypersensitivity; Moderate renal impairment (eGFR <45 mL/min/1.73 m²) (use not recommended to improve glycemic control in patients with type 2 diabetes mellitus); Dialysis; Type 1 diabetes; Diabetic ketoacidosis; Active bladder cancer; OB: Not recommended for use during 2nd and 3rd trimesters of pregnancy (may cause adverse renal effects in infant); Lactation: Lactation.

Use Cautiously in: History of pancreatitis, pancreatic surgery, reduced caloric intake due to illness or surgery, or alcohol abuse (↑ risk of ketoacidosis); Renal impairment (eGFR <60 mL/min/1.73 m²), age >65 yr, or concurrent use of loop diuretics (↑ risk of hypovolemia and hypotension); History of bladder cancer; Polycystic kidney disease or recent history of immunosuppressive therapy for kidney disease (use not recommended for treatment of chronic kidney disease); OB: Use during 1st trimester of pregnancy only if potential maternal benefit justifies potential fetal risk (other agents recommended in pregnancy); Pedi: Safety and effectiveness not established in children; Geri: Appears on Beers list. Older adults may have ↑ risk of urogenital infections (especially women in the 1st mo of treatment) and euglycemic diabetic ketoacidosis. Use with caution in older adults.

Adverse Reactions/Side Effects
Endo: hypoglycemia (↑ with other medications). **F and E:** hyperphosphatemia, hypovolemia, KETOACIDOSIS. **GU:** ↑ urination, acute kidney injury, genital mycotic infections, NECROTIZING FASCIITIS OF PERINEUM (FOURNIER'S GANGRENE), renal impairment, urinary tract infection (including pyelonephritis), UROSEPSIS. **Misc:** HYPERSENSITIVITY REACTIONS (including anaphylaxis or angioedema).

Interactions
Drug-Drug: ↑ risk of hypoglycemia with **insulin** or **insulin secretagogues**; dose adjustments may be required. Concurrent use with **loop diuretics**, may ↑ risk of hypovolemia and associated complications. May ↓ **lithium** levels and effectiveness.

Route/Dosage

Type 2 Diabetes Mellitus (for Glycemic Control)
PO (Adults): *eGFR ≥45 mL/min/1.73 m²:* 5 mg once daily, may ↑ to 10 mg once daily, if needed.

Renal Impairment
PO (Adults): *eGFR <45 mL/min/1.73 m²:* Use not recommended.

Type 2 Diabetes (for Reduction in Risk of HF Hospitalizations), HF, or Chronic Kidney Disease
PO (Adults): *eGFR ≥25 mL/min/1.73 m²:* 10 mg once daily.

Renal Impairment
PO (Adults): *eGFR <25 mL/min/1.73 m²:* Initiation of therapy not recommended; however, patients currently taking dapagliflozin may continue with 10 mg once daily.

Availability (generic available)
Tablets: 5 mg, 10 mg. *In combination with:* metformin XR (Xigduo XR); saxagliptin (Qtern). See Appendix N.

NURSING IMPLICATIONS

Assessment

- Observe for signs and symptoms of hypoglycemic reactions (sweating, hunger, weakness, dizziness, tremor, tachycardia, anxiety), especially in patients taking insulin or other hypoglycemic agents.
- Assess cardiovascular status (BP, edema, dyspnea) before starting and periodically during therapy.
- Assess volume status and correct before starting dapagliflozin. Patients with impaired renal function (eGFR less than 60 mL/min/1.73 m^2), older adults, or patients on loop diuretics may be at increased risk for volume depletion or hypotension. Monitor BP after initiating and periodically during therapy; may cause hypotension.
- Monitor for signs and symptoms of urinary tract infection (burning during urination, frequent urination, urgency, pain in pelvis, blood in urine, fever, back pain, nausea, vomiting) during therapy. Treat promptly.
- Monitor for infection, new pain, tenderness, erythema, swelling, sores, or ulcers involving genital or perianal area, with fever or malaise; assess for necrotizing fasciitis. If suspected, start treatment immediately with broad-spectrum antibiotics and, if necessary, surgical debridement. Discontinue dapagliflozin if these occur.

Lab Test Considerations

- Monitor serum glucose and HbA1c periodically during therapy to evaluate effectiveness of treatment. May cause ketoacidosis.
- Evaluate renal function prior to starting and periodically during therapy; may cause ↑ serum creatinine and ↓ eGFR.
- May cause an ↑ hematocrit and serum phosphorous.
- Will cause urine to test positive for glucose.
- Monitor for ketoacidosis, especially during prolonged fasting for illness or surgery. Consider temporarily discontinuing therapy for at least 3 days prior to surgery.

Toxicity and Overdose

- Overdose is manifested by symptoms of hypoglycemia. Mild hypoglycemia may be treated with administration of oral glucose. Treat severe hypoglycemia with IV D50W followed by continuous IV infusion of more dilute dextrose solution at a rate sufficient to keep serum glucose at approximately 100 mg/dL.

Implementation

- Do not confuse Farxiga with Fetzima.
- Patients stabilized on a diabetic regimen who are exposed to stress, fever, trauma, infection, or surgery may require administration of insulin.
- **PO:** Administer once daily in the morning without regard to food.

Patient/Family Teaching

- Instruct patient to take medication at same time each day. Take missed doses as soon as remembered unless almost time for next dose; do not double doses. Advise patient to read *Medication Guide* before starting and with each Rx refill in case of changes.
- Explain to patient that this medication controls hyperglycemia but does not cure diabetes. Therapy is long term.
- Inform patient dapagliflozin may cause dehydration and hypotension. Maintain adequate hydration and notify health care professional if dizziness, fainting, weakness, or orthostatic hypotension occur.
- Advise patient to notify health care professional if signs and symptoms of urinary tract infections or genital mycotic infections; females (vaginal odor, white or yellowish vaginal discharge, vaginal itching), males (rash or redness of glans or foreskin of penis, foul-smelling discharge from penis, pain in skin around penis) occur. Instruct patient on treatment options and when to notify health care professional.
- Review signs of hypoglycemia and hyperglycemia with patient. If hypoglycemia occurs, advise patient to drink a glass of orange juice or ingest 2–3 tsp of sugar, honey, or corn syrup dissolved in water or an appropriate number of glucose tablets and notify health care professional.
- Encourage patient to follow prescribed diet, medication, and exercise regimen to prevent hypoglycemic or hyperglycemic episodes.
- Instruct patient in proper testing of serum glucose and ketones, especially during periods of stress or illness. Inform patient that dapagliflozin will cause a positive test result when testing for urine glucose. Notify health care professional if significant changes occur.
- Advise patient to notify health care professional immediately if new pain or tenderness, sores or ulcers, or infections involving the leg or foot occur and to immediately seek care if pain or tenderness, redness, or swelling of the genitals or area from the genitals back to the rectum, along with a fever above 100.4°F or malaise occur.
- Advise patient to notify health care professional of all Rx or OTC medications, vitamins, or herbal products being taken and to consult with health care professional before taking other medications.
- Advise patient to inform health care professional of medication regimen prior to treatment or surgery.
- Advise patient to notify health care professional promptly if signs and symptoms of hypersensitivity reactions (rash; raised red patches on skin; swelling of face, lips, tongue, throat; difficulty breathing or swallowing) or bladder cancer (blood or red color in urine, painful urination) occur.
- Advise patient to carry a form of sugar (sugar packets, candy) and identification describing disease process and medication regimen at all times.

- Rep: Insulin is the recommended method of controlling blood sugar during pregnancy. Advise patient to notify health care professional if pregnancy is planned or suspected and to avoid breastfeeding during therapy. Effective contraception should be used especially during the 2nd and 3rd trimesters of pregnancy.
- Emphasize the importance of routine follow-up exams.

Evaluation/Desired Outcomes

- Control of blood glucose levels without the appearance of hypoglycemic or hyperglycemic episodes.
- Reduction in risk of HF hospitalizations.
- Reduction in risk of sustained eGFR decline, end-stage kidney disease, cardiovascular death, and HF hospitalizations in patients with chronic kidney disease at risk of progression.

DAPTOmycin (dap-to-mye-sin)
~~Cubicin, Cubicin RF~~

Classification
Therapeutic: anti-infectives
Pharmacologic: cyclic lipopeptide antibacterial agents

Indications
Complicated skin and skin structure infections caused by gram-positive bacteria. *Staphylococcus aureus* bacteremia, including right-sided infective endocarditis caused by methicillin-susceptible and methicillin-resistant strains (in adults). *Staphylococcus aureus* bacteremia (in pediatric patients).

Action
Causes rapid depolarization of membrane potential following binding to bacterial membrane; this results in inhibition of protein, DNA, and RNA synthesis. **Therapeutic Effects:** Death of bacteria with resolution of infection. **Spectrum:** Active against *Staphylococcus aureus* (including methicillin-resistant strains), *Streptococcus pyogenes*, *Streptococcus agalactiae*, some *Streptococcus dysgalactiae*, and *Enterococcus faecalis* (vancomycin-susceptible strains).

Pharmacokinetics
Absorption: IV administration results in complete bioavailability.
Distribution: Unknown.
Protein Binding: 92%.
Metabolism and Excretion: Metabolism not known; mostly excreted by kidneys.
Half-life: 8.1 hr.

TIME/ACTION PROFILE

ROUTE	ONSET	PEAK	DURATION
IV	rapid	end of infusion	24 hr

Contraindications/Precautions
Contraindicated in: Hypersensitivity.
Use Cautiously in: CCr <30 mL/min (dose ↓ required); Moderate-to-severe renal impairment (may have ↓ clinical response); OB: Safety not established in pregnancy; Lactation: Safety not established in breastfeeding; Pedi: Children <1 yr (↑ risk of muscular, neuromuscular, and CNS effects; avoid use); Geri: Older adults may have ↓ clinical response with ↑ risk of adverse reactions.

Adverse Reactions/Side Effects
CV: hypertension, hypotension. **Derm:** DRUG RASH WITH EOSINOPHILIA AND SYSTEMIC SYMPTOMS (DRESS), pruritus, rash. **GI:** ↑ liver enzymes, CLOSTRIDIOIDES DIFFICILE-ASSOCIATED DIARRHEA (CDAD), constipation, diarrhea, nausea, vomiting. **GU:** renal impairment. **Hemat:** anemia. **Local:** injection site reactions. **MS:** ↑ creatine kinase. **Neuro:** dizziness. **Resp:** dyspnea, EOSINOPHILIC PNEUMONIA. **Misc:** ANGIOEDEMA, fever.

Interactions
Drug-Drug: Tobramycin ↑ blood levels. Concurrent **HMG-CoA reductase inhibitors** may ↑ the risk of myopathy.

Route/Dosage

Complicated Skin/Skin Structure Infections
IV (Adults): 4 mg/kg every 24 hr for 7–14 days.
IV (Children 12–17 yr): 5 mg/kg every 24 hr for up to 14 days.
IV (Children 7–11 yr): 7 mg/kg every 24 hr for up to 14 days.
IV (Children 2–6 yr): 9 mg/kg every 24 hr for up to 14 days.
IV (Children 1–<2 yr): 10 mg/kg every 24 hr for up to 14 days.

Renal Impairment
IV (Adults): *CCr <30 mL/min:* 4 mg/kg every 48 hr for 7–14 days; *Hemodialysis and CAPD:* 4 mg/kg every 48 hr for 7–14 days with dose administered after hemodialysis on hemodialysis days.

Staphylococcus aureus Bacteremia/Right-Sided Infective Endocarditis
IV (Adults): 6 mg/kg every 24 hr for 2–6 wk.

Renal Impairment
IV (Adults): *CCr <30 mL/min:* 6 mg/kg every 48 hr for 2–6 wk; *Hemodialysis and CAPD:* 6 mg/kg every 48 hr for 2–6 wk with dose administered after hemodialysis on hemodialysis days.

Staphylococcus aureus Bacteremia
IV (Children 12–17 yr): 7 mg/kg every 24 hr for up to 42 days.
IV (Children 7–11 yr): 9 mg/kg every 24 hr for up to 42 days.
IV (Children 1–6 yr): 12 mg/kg every 24 hr for up to 42 days.

Availability (generic available)

Lyophilized powder for injection: 350 mg/vial, 500 mg/vial.

NURSING IMPLICATIONS

Assessment

- Assess for infection (vital signs; appearance of wound, sputum, urine, and stool; WBC) at beginning of and during therapy.
- Monitor bowel function. Diarrhea, abdominal cramping, fever, and bloody stools should be reported to health care professional promptly as a sign of CDAD. May begin up to several wk following cessation of therapy.
- Monitor for signs and symptoms of eosinophilic pneumonia (new onset or worsening fever, dyspnea, difficulty breathing, new infiltrates on chest imaging studies). Discontinue daptomycin if symptoms occur.
- Monitor for signs and symptoms of DRESS (fever, rash, lymphadenopathy, and/or facial swelling), associated with involvement of other organ systems (hepatitis, nephritis, hematologic abnormalities, myocarditis, myositis) during therapy. May resemble an acute viral infection. Eosinophilia is often present. Discontinue therapy if signs occur.
- Monitor for development of muscle pain or weakness, particularly of distal extremities. Discontinue daptomycin in patients with unexplained signs and symptoms of myopathy in conjunction with CK elevation >1000 units/L, or in patients without reported symptoms who have marked elevations in CK >2000 units/L. Consider temporarily suspending agents associated with rhabdomyolysis (HMG-CoA reductase inhibitors) in patients receiving daptomycin.

Lab Test Considerations

- Monitor CK weekly, more frequently in patients with unexplained ↑. Discontinue daptomycin if CK >1000 units/L and signs and symptoms of myopathy occur. In patients with renal insufficiency, monitor both renal function and CK more frequently.
- May cause false prolongation of PT and ↑ INR.
- Monitor renal function prior to and periodically during therapy. If new or worsening renal impairment occurs, evaluate renal function. If tubulointerstitial nephritis is suspected, discontinue daptomycin and begin treatment.

Implementation

- Do not confuse daptomycin with dactinomycin.

IV Administration

- **IV Push:** *Reconstitution:* Reconstitute 500-mg vial with 10 mL of 0.9% NaCl inserted toward wall of vial. Rotate vial gently to wet powder. Allow to stand for 10 min undisturbed. Swirl vial gently to completely reconstitute solution. Reconstituted vials are stable for 12 hr at room temperature or 48 hr if refrigerated. *Concentration:* 50 mg/mL. *Rate:* Administer over 2 min (for adults only).
- **Intermittent Infusion:** *Adults: Dilution:* Dilute further in 50 mL of 0.9% NaCl for adults, adolescents and children ≥7 yrs. Solution is stable for 12 hr at room temperature or 48 hr if refrigerated. Do not administer solutions that are cloudy or contain a precipitate. *Rate:* Infuse over 30 min.
- **Intermittent Infusion:** *Children 1–6 yrs: Dilution:* Dilute further into a 25 mL IV infusion bag of 0.9% NaCl. *Rate:* Infuse over 60 min at a rate of 0.42 mL/min.
- **Intermittent Infusion:** *Children 7–17 yrs: Dilution:* Dilute further into a 50 mL IV infusion bag of 0.9% NaCl. *Rate:* Infuse over 30 min at a rate of 1.67 mL/min.
- **Y-Site Compatibility:** amifostine, amikacin, aminocaproic acid, aminophylline, amiodarone, amphotericin B liposomal, ampicillin, ampicillin/sulbactam, argatroban, azithromycin, aztreonam, bivalirudin, bleomycin, bumetanide, buprenorphine, busulfan, butorphanol, calcium chloride, calcium gluconate, cangrelor, carboplatin, carmustine, caspofungin, cefazolin, cefepime, cefotaxime, cefotetan, cefoxitin, ceftazidime, ceftazidime/avibactam, ceftolozane/tazobactam, ceftriaxone, cefuroxime, chloramphenicol, chlorpromazine, ciprofloxacin, cisatracurium, cisplatin, clindamycin, cyclophosphamide, cyclosporine, dacarbazine, dactinomycin, daunorubicin hydrochloride, dexamethasone, dexmedetomidine, dexrazoxane, digoxin, diltiazem, diphenhydramine, dobutamine, docetaxel, dopamine, doxorubicin hydrochloride, doxorubicin liposomal, doxycycline, droperidol, enalaprilat, ephedrine, epinephrine, epirubicin, eptifibatide, ertapenem, erythromycin, esmolol, etoposide, etoposide phosphate, famotidine, fentanyl, fluconazole, fludarabine, fluorouracil, foscarnet, fosphenytoin, furosemide, ganciclovir, gentamicin, glycopyrrolate, granisetron, haloperidol, heparin, hydralazine, hydrocortisone, hydromorphone, idarubicin, ifosfamide, insulin, regular, irinotecan, isavuconazonium, isoproterenol, ketorolac, labetalol, leucovorin calcium, levofloxacin, lidocaine, linezolid, lorazepam, magnesium sulfate, mannitol, melphalan, meperidine, meropenem, mesna, methadone, methylprednisolone, metoclopramide, metoprolol, midazolam, milrinone, mitoxantrone, morphine, moxifloxacin, mycophenolate, nafcillin, nalbuphine, naloxone, nicardipine, nitroprusside, norepinephrine, octreotide, ondansetron, oxaliplatin, oxytocin, paclitaxel, palonosetron, pamidronate, pemetrexed, pentamidine, phenobarbital, phentolamine, phenylephrine, piperacillin/tazobactam, posaconazole, potassium acetate, potassium chloride, potassium phosphate, procainamide, prochlorperazine, promethazine, propranolol, rocu-

---

♣= Canadian drug name. ⚏ = Genetic implication. ~~Strikethrough~~ = Discontinued. CAPITALS = life-threatening. <u>Underline</u> = most frequent.

ronium, sodium acetate, sodium bicarbonate, sodium phosphate, succinylcholine, tacrolimus, tedizolid, theophylline, thiotepa, tigecycline, tirofiban, tobramycin, topotecan, trimethoprim/sulfamethoxazole, vasopressin, vecuronium, verapamil, vinblastine, vincristine, vinorelbine, voriconazole, zidovudine, zoledronic acid.

- **Y-Site Incompatibility:** acyclovir, alemtuzumab, allopurinol, amphotericin B lipid complex, blinatumomab, cytarabine, D5W, dantrolene, gemcitabine, gemtuzumab ozogamicin, imipenem/cilastatin, meropenem/vaborbactam, methotrexate, metronidazole, minocycline, mitomycin, nitroglycerin, pantoprazole, pentobarbital, phenytoin, plazomicin, remifentanil, sufentanil, thiopental, vancomycin.

Patient/Family Teaching
- Inform patient of purpose of daptomycin.
- Instruct patient to notify health care professional if fever and diarrhea develop, especially if stool contains blood, pus, or mucus. Advise patient not to treat diarrhea without consulting health care professional.
- May cause dizziness. Caution patient to avoid driving or other activities requiring alertness until response to medication is known.
- Advise patient to notify health care professional immediately if weakness, numbness, or tingling in forearms and lower legs, or signs and symptoms of eosinophilic pneumonia or DRESS occur.
- Advise patient to notify health care professional of all Rx or OTC medications, vitamins, or herbal products being taken and to consult with health care professional before taking other medications.
- Rep: Advise females of reproductive potential to notify health care professional if pregnancy is planned or suspected, or if breastfeeding. Monitor infants exposed to daptomycin through breast milk for GI disturbances.

Evaluation/Desired Outcomes
- Resolution of the signs and symptoms of infection. Length of time for complete resolution depends on the organism and site of infection.

---

darbepoetin (dar-be-**poh**-e-tin)
Aranesp
Classification
Therapeutic: antianemics
Pharmacologic: erythropoiesis stimulating agents (ESA)

Indications
Anemia associated with chronic kidney disease (CKD). Chemotherapy-induced anemia in patients with nonmyeloid malignancies when there is ≥2 additional mo of planned chemotherapy.

Action
Stimulates erythropoiesis (production of RBCs). **Therapeutic Effects:** Maintains and may elevate RBC counts, decreasing the need for transfusions.

Pharmacokinetics
Absorption: 30–50% following SUBQ administration; IV administration results in complete bioavailability.
Distribution: Confined to the intravascular space.
Metabolism and Excretion: Unknown.
Half-life: *SUBQ:* 49 hr; *IV:* 21 hr.

TIME/ACTION PROFILE (↑ in RBCs)

ROUTE	ONSET	PEAK	DURATION
IV, SUBQ	2–6 wk	unknown	unknown

Contraindications/Precautions
Contraindicated in: Hypersensitivity; Uncontrolled hypertension; Patients with cancer receiving hormonal agents, biologic products, or radiotherapy, unless also receiving concomitant myelosuppressive chemotherapy; Patients receiving chemotherapy when anticipated outcome is cure; Patients with cancer receiving myelosuppressive chemotherapy in whom the anemia can be managed by transfusion; Patients who require immediate correction of anemia when RBC transfusions can be used instead.
Use Cautiously in: Cardiovascular disease or stroke; Underlying hematologic diseases, including hemolytic anemia, sickle-cell anemia, thalassemia, and porphyria (safety not established); OB: Use during pregnancy only if potential maternal benefit justifies potential fetal risk; Lactation: Safety not established in breastfeeding.

Adverse Reactions/Side Effects
CV: hypertension, hypotension, chest pain, DEEP VEIN THROMBOSIS (especially with Hgb >11 g/dL), edema, HF, MI. **Derm:** ERYTHEMA MULTIFORME, pruritus, STEVENS-JOHNSON SYNDROME (SJS), TOXIC EPIDERMAL NECROLYSIS (TEN). **GI:** abdominal pain, diarrhea, nausea, vomiting, constipation. **Hemat:** pure red cell aplasia. **MS:** myalgia, arthralgia, back pain, limb pain. **Neuro:** dizziness, fatigue, headache, SEIZURES, STROKE, weakness. **Resp:** cough, dyspnea, bronchitis, PULMONARY EMBOLISM (especially with Hgb >11 g/dL). **Misc:** fever, ↑ MORTALITY AND ↑ TUMOR GROWTH (especially with Hgb >11 g/dL), HYPERSENSITIVITY REACTIONS (including anaphylaxis and angioedema), sepsis.

Interactions
Drug-Drug: None reported.

Route/Dosage

Anemia Due to Chronic Kidney Disease
(Do not initiate if Hgb ≥10 g/dL; should only consider initiating therapy in patients not on dialysis if rate of hemoglobin decline indicates likelihood of requiring a RBC transfusion and a goal is to reduce the risk of alloimmunization and/or RBC transfusion risks.)

IV, SUBQ (Adults): *Starting treatment with darbepoetin (no previous epoetin):* 0.45 mcg/kg once weekly or 0.75 mcg/kg every 2 wk (for patients on dialysis); 0.45 mcg/kg every 4 wk (for patients not on dialysis); use lowest dose sufficient to ↓ the need for RBC transfusions (do not exceed Hgb of 10 g/dL [patients not on dialysis] or 11 g/dL [patients on dialysis]); if Hgb ↑ by >1 g/dL in 2 wk, ↓ dose by 25%; if Hgb ↑ by <1 g/dL after 4 wk of therapy (with adequate iron stores), ↑ dose by 25%; do not ↑ dose more frequently than every 4 wk. *Conversion from epoetin to darbepoetin:* weekly epoetin dose <2500 units = 6.25 mcg/wk darbepoetin; weekly epoetin dose 2500–4999 units = 12.5 mcg/wk darbepoetin; weekly epoetin dose 5000–10,999 units = 25 mcg/wk darbepoetin; weekly epoetin dose 11,000–17,999 units = 40 mcg/wk darbepoetin; weekly epoetin dose 18,000–33,999 units = 60 mcg/wk darbepoetin; weekly epoetin dose 34,000–89,999 units = 100 mcg/wk darbepoetin; weekly epoetin dose >90,000 units = 200 mcg/wk darbepoetin.

IV, SUBQ (Children): *Starting treatment with darbepoetin (no previous epoetin):* 0.45 mcg/kg once weekly (may also start with 0.75 mcg/kg every 2 wk in patients not on dialysis); use lowest dose sufficient to ↓ the need for RBC transfusions (do not exceed Hgb of 12 g/dL; if Hgb ↑ by >1.0 g/dL in 2 wk, ↓ dose by 25%; if Hgb ↑ by <1 g/dL after 4 wk of therapy (with adequate iron stores), ↑ dose by 25%; do not ↑ dose more frequently than every 4 wk.

Anemia Due to Chemotherapy
(Use only for chemotherapy-related anemia and discontinue when chemotherapy course is completed; do not initiate if Hgb ≥10 g/dL).
SUBQ (Adults): 2.25 mcg/kg weekly or 500 mcg every 3 wk; target Hgb should not exceed 12 g/dL. If Hgb ↑ by >1 g/dL in 2 wk or reaches a level needed to avoid RBC transfusions, ↓ dose by 40%; if Hgb ↑ by <1 g/dL after 6 wk of therapy, ↑ dose to 4.5 mcg/kg weekly.

Availability
Solution for injection (single-dose vials): 25 mcg/mL, 40 mcg/mL, 60 mcg/mL, 100 mcg/mL, 200 mcg/mL, 300 mcg/mL. **Solution for injection (prefilled syringes):** 10 mcg/0.4 mL, 25 mcg/0.42 mL, 40 mcg/0.4 mL, 60 mcg/0.3 mL, 100 mcg/0.5 mL, 150 mcg/0.3 mL, 200 mcg/0.4 mL, 300 mcg/0.6 mL, 500 mcg/1 mL.

NURSING IMPLICATIONS
Assessment
- Monitor BP before and during therapy. Inform health care professional if severe hypertension is present or if BP begins to increase. Additional antihypertensive therapy may be required during initiation of therapy.
- Monitor response for symptoms of anemia (fatigue, dyspnea, pallor).

- Monitor dialysis shunts (thrill and bruit) and status of artificial kidney during hemodialysis. May need to increase heparin dose to prevent clotting. Monitor patients with underlying vascular disease for impaired circulation.
- Monitor for allergic reactions (rash, urticaria). Discontinue darbepoetin if signs of anaphylaxis (dyspnea, laryngeal swelling) occur.
- Assess patient for skin rash frequently during therapy. Discontinue darbepoetin at first sign of rash; may be life-threatening. SJS or TEN may develop. Treat symptomatically; may recur once treatment is stopped.
- **Lab Test Considerations:** May cause ↑ in WBCs and platelets. May ↓ bleeding times.
- Monitor serum ferritin, transferrin, and iron levels prior to and during therapy to assess need for concurrent iron therapy. Administer supplemental iron therapy if transferrin saturation <20% or serum ferritin is <100 mcg/mL.
- Monitor Hgb weekly until the Hgb level is stable and sufficient to minimize the need for RBC transfusion after starting therapy and after each dose adjustment.
- **Anemia due to Chemotherapy:** Monitor Hgb before and weekly during initial therapy, for 4 wk after a change in dose, and regularly after target range has been reached and maintenance dose is determined. Monitor other hematopoietic parameters (CBC with differential and platelet count) before and periodically during therapy. *If Hgb ↑ by more than 1 g/dL in any 2-wk period or Hgb reaches a level needed to avoid RBC transfusion,* ↓ dose by 40%. *If Hgb exceeds a level needed to avoid RBC transfusion,* withhold dose until Hgb approaches level where RBC transfusions may be required and reinitiate at a dose 40% below the previous dose. *If Hgb ↑ by less than 1 g/dL and remains below 10 g/dL after 6 wk of therapy,* ↑ dose to 4.5 mcg/kg/wk (if on weekly therapy) or do not adjust dose (if on every 3-wk schedule). *If there is no response as measured by Hgb or if RBC transfusions are still required after 8 wk of therapy,* following completion of a chemotherapy course, discontinue darbepoetin. Hgb >11 g/dL increases the likelihood of life-threatening cardiovascular complications, cardiac arrest, neurologic events (seizures, stroke), hypertensive reactions, HF, vascular thrombosis/ischemia/infarction, MI, and fluid overload/edema.
- **Anemia of CKD:** Monitor Hgb at least weekly until stable, then at least monthly. Do not ↑ dose more frequently than once every 4 wk. Decreases in dose can be made more frequently. Avoid frequent dose adjustments. *If Hgb ↑ by >1 g/dL in a 2-wk period,* ↓ dose by 25% or more. *If Hgb ↑ by <1 g/dL over 4 wk (and iron stores are adequate),* ↑ dose by 25%. *If no response after 12 wk of escalation,* fur-

ther dose ↑ is unlikely to improve response and may increase risks. Use lowest dose that will maintain Hgb level sufficient to reduce need for RBC transfusions.

- **Adults with Anemia of CKD on Dialysis**: Start darbepoetin when Hgb >10 g/dL. If Hgb ≥11 g/dL, reduce or hold dose. **Adults with Anemia of CKD not on Dialysis**: Start darbepoetin only when Hgb <10 g/dL AND rate of Hgb decline indicates likelihood of requiring a RBC transfusion AND reducing risk of alloimmunization and/or other RBC transfusion-related risks is a goal. If Hgb level >10 g/dL, reduce or hold dose, and use lowest darbepoetin dose sufficient to reduce need for RBC transfusions. **Children with Anemia of CKD**: Start epoetin only when Hgb <10 g/dL. If Hgb level >12 g/dL, reduce or hold dose. Monitor renal function studies and electrolytes closely; resulting increased sense of well-being may lead to decreased compliance with other therapies for renal failure. Increases in BUN, serum creatinine, uric acid, phosphorus, and potassium may occur.

Implementation

- Transfusions are still required for severe symptomatic anemia. Supplemental iron should be initiated with darbepoetin and continued during therapy. Correct deficiencies of folic acid or vitamin B_{12} prior to therapy.
- Institute seizure precautions in patients who experience greater than a 1 g/dL ↑ in Hgb in a 2-wk period or exhibit any change in neurologic status.
- *For conversion from epoetin alfa to darbepoetin,* if epoetin was administered 2–3 times/wk, administer darbepoetin once a wk. If patient was receiving epoetin once/wk, darbepoetin may be administered once every 2 wk. Route of administration should remain consistent.
- Dose adjustments should not be more frequent than once/mo.
- Do not shake vial; inactivation of medication may occur. Do not administer vials containing solution that is discolored or contains particulate matter. Discard vial immediately after withdrawing dose. Do not pool unused portions.
- **SUBQ:** This route is often used for patients not requiring dialysis.

IV Administration
- **IV Push:** Administer undiluted. *Rate:* May be administered as direct injection or bolus over 1–3 min into IV tubing or via venous line at end of dialysis session.
- **Y-Site Incompatibility:** Do not administer in conjunction with other drugs or solutions.

Patient/Family Teaching

- Instruct patient to read the *Medication Guide* prior to beginning therapy and with each Rx refill in case of changes. Inform patients of risks and benefits of darbepoetin.

- Discuss ways of preventing self-injury in patients at risk for seizures. Driving and activities requiring continuous alertness should be avoided.
- Advise patient to stop darbepoetin and notify health care professional immediately if severe skin reactions (skin rash with itching, blisters, skin sores, peeling, areas of skin coming off) or signs and symptoms of serious allergic reactions (rash, itching, shortness of breath, wheezing, dizziness and fainting due to drop in blood pressure, swelling around mouth or eyes, fast pulse, sweating) occur.
- Inform patient that use of darbepoetin may result in shortened overall survival and/or ↓ time to tumor progression. May also cause MI or stroke. Advise patient to notify health care professional immediately if chest pain; trouble breathing or shortness of breath; pain in legs, with or without swelling; a cool or pale arm or leg; sudden confusion, trouble speaking, or trouble understanding others' speech; sudden numbness or weakness in face, arm, or leg, especially on one side of body; sudden trouble seeing; sudden trouble walking, dizziness, loss of balance or coordination; loss of consciousness (fainting); or hemodialysis vascular access stops working.
- Advise patient to notify health care professional of darbepoetin prior to surgery.
- Rep: Advise females of reproductive potential to notify health care professional if pregnancy is planned or suspected or if breastfeeding.
- **Anemia of CKD**: Stress importance of compliance with dietary restrictions, medications, and dialysis. Foods high in iron and low in potassium include liver, pork, veal, beef, mustard and turnip greens, peas, eggs, broccoli, kale, blackberries, strawberries, apple juice, watermelon, oatmeal, and enriched bread. Darbepoetin will result in increased sense of well-being, but it does not cure underlying disease.
- **Home Care Issues:** Home dialysis patients determined to be able to safely and effectively administer darbepoetin should be taught proper dose, administration technique with syringe, auto-injector or IV use, and disposal of equipment. *Information for Patients and Caregivers* should be provided to patient along with medication.

Evaluation/Desired Outcomes

- Increase in Hgb not to exceed 11 g/dL with improvement in symptoms of anemia in patients with CKD or with chemotherapy-induced anemia.

---

daridorexant (dar-i-doe-**rex**-ant)
Quviviq
Classification
Therapeutic: sedative/hypnotics
Pharmacologic: orexin receptor antagonists

Schedule IV

Indications
Insomnia associated with difficulty in sleep onset and/or maintenance.

Action
Antagonizes the effects of orexins A and B, naturally occurring neuropeptides that promote wakefulness, by binding to their receptors. **Therapeutic Effects:** Improved sleep.

Pharmacokinetics
Absorption: 62% absorbed following oral administration; a high-fat meal will delay absorption and sleep onset.
Distribution: Well distributed to tissues.
Protein Binding: 99.7%.
Metabolism and Excretion: Primarily metabolized in the liver via the CYP3A4 isoenzyme. Primarily excreted as metabolites in the feces (57%), with some excretion in the urine (28%).
Half-life: 8 hr.

TIME/ACTION PROFILE (sleep)

ROUTE	ONSET	PEAK	DURATION
PO	30 min	unknown	6 hr†

†Excess sedation may persist for several days after discontinuation.

Contraindications/Precautions
Contraindicated in: Narcolepsy; Severe hepatic impairment.
Use Cautiously in: History of substance abuse or drug dependence; Depression; Underlying pulmonary disease; Moderate hepatic impairment (↓ dose); OB: Safety not established in pregnancy; Lactation: Use while breastfeeding only if potential maternal benefit justifies potential risk to infant; Pedi: Safety and effectiveness not established in children; Geri: ↑ risk of falls in older adults.

Adverse Reactions/Side Effects
GI: nausea, vomiting. **Neuro:** drowsiness, cataplexy, complex sleep behaviors (including sleep driving, sleep walking, or engaging in other activities while sleeping), dizziness, hallucinations (during sleep), headache, sleep paralysis, SUICIDAL IDEATION, worsening of depression.

Interactions
Drug-Drug: Strong CYP3A4 inhibitors, including **itraconazole**, ↑ levels and risk of toxicity; concurrent use not recommended. **Moderate CYP3A4 inhibitors**, including **diltiazem**, may ↑ levels and risk of toxicity; ↓ daridorexant dose. **Strong CYP3A4 inducers**, including **rifampin**, and **moderate CYP3A4 inducers**, including **efavirenz**, ↓ levels and effectiveness; concurrent use not recommended. Risk of CNS depression, next-day impairment, "sleep-driving" and other

complex behaviors while not fully awake ↑ with other **CNS depressants** including **alcohol**, some **antihistamines**, **opioids**, other **sedative/hypnotics** (including **benzodiazepines**) and **tricyclic antidepressants**; concurrent alcohol use should be avoided; for patients receiving other CNS depressants, dose adjustments of daridorexant and/or CNS depressants may be necessary.

Route/Dosage
PO (Adults): 25–50 mg within 30 min of going to bed; dose may not be repeated on a single night and should be taken when ≥7 hr of sleep time is anticipated before planned awakening. *Concurrent use of moderate CYP3A4 inhibitors:* 25 mg within 30 min of going to bed; dose may not be repeated on a single night and should be taken when ≥7 hr of sleep time is anticipated before planned awakening.

Hepatic Impairment
PO (Adults): *Moderate hepatic impairment:* 25 mg within 30 min of going to bed; dose may not be repeated on a single night and should be taken when ≥7 hr of sleep time is anticipated before planned awakening.

Availability
Tablets: 25 mg, 50 mg.

NURSING IMPLICATIONS
Assessment
- Assess sleep patterns prior to and during administration. Continued insomnia after 7–10 days of therapy may indicate primary psychiatric or mental illness.
- Assess mental status and potential for abuse prior to administration. Prolonged use of >7–10 days may lead to physical and psychological dependence. Limit amount of drug available to the patient.

Implementation
- **PO:** Administer within 30 min of going to bed with ≥7 hrs remaining prior to planned awakening. Time to sleep onset may be delayed if taken with or soon after a meal.

Patient/Family Teaching
- Instruct patient to take daridorexant within 30 min of going to bed, as directed. Do not take daridorexant if alcohol was consumed that evening. Do not increase dose or discontinue without notifying health care professional. CNS-depressant effects may persist in some patients for up to several days after discontinuing. Advise patient to read *Medication Guide* before starting therapy and with each Rx refill in case of changes.
- May cause daytime and next-day drowsiness. Caution patient to avoid driving or other activities requiring alertness until response to medication is known.

- Caution patient that daridorexant may cause complex sleep behaviors (sleep walking, sleep driving, making and eating food, talking on the phone, having sex) while unaware. Patient may not remember anything done during the night; increased risk with alcohol or other CNS depressants. Discontinue daridorexant immediately and notify health care professional if complex sleep behaviors occur.
- Inform patients and their families that daridorexant may cause sleep paralysis, an inability to move or speak for several min during sleep-wake transitions and hypnagogic/hypnopompic hallucinations, including vivid and disturbing perceptions.
- Advise patient that daridorexant is a drug with known abuse potential. Protect it from theft, and never give to anyone other than the individual for whom it was prescribed. Store out of sight and reach of children, and in a location not accessible by others.
- Instruct patient to notify health care professional of all Rx or OTC medications, vitamins, or herbal products being taken and to consult health care professional before taking any other Rx, OTC, or herbal products.
- Caution patient to avoid concurrent use of alcohol or other CNS depressants, including opioids.
- Advise patient to notify health care professional if signs and symptoms of allergic reaction (swelling of tongue or throat, trouble breathing, nausea and vomiting) occur.
- Rep: Advise females of reproductive potential to notify health care professional if pregnancy is planned or suspected, or if breastfeeding. Infants exposed to daridorexant through breast milk should be monitored for excessive sedation. Inform females there is a Pregnancy Exposure Registry that monitors pregnancy outcomes in females exposed to daridorexant during pregnancy. Pregnant women exposed to daridorexant and health care professionals are encouraged to call Idorsia Pharmaceuticals Ltd at 1-833-400-9611.

Evaluation/Desired Outcomes
- Improved sleep.

𝕏 darifenacin (dar-i-fen-a-sin)
✤Enablex
Classification
Therapeutic: urinary tract antispasmodics
Pharmacologic: anticholinergics

Indications
Overactive bladder with symptoms (urge incontinence, urgency, frequency).

Action
Acts as a muscarinic (cholinergic) receptor antagonist; antagonizes bladder smooth muscle contraction. **Therapeutic Effects:** Decreased symptoms of overactive bladder.

Pharmacokinetics
Absorption: 15–19% absorbed.
Distribution: Unknown.
Protein Binding: 98%.
Metabolism and Excretion: Extensively metabolized in the liver by the CYP2D6 isoenzyme, with some metabolism by the CYP3A4 isoenzyme; 𝕏 the CYP2D6 isoenzyme exhibits genetic polymorphism (~7% of population may be poor metabolizers and may have significantly ↑ darifenacin concentrations and an ↑ risk of adverse effects). 60% excreted by the kidneys as metabolites, 40% in feces as metabolites.
Half-life: 13–19 hr.

TIME/ACTION PROFILE

ROUTE	ONSET	PEAK	DURATION
PO	unknown	7 hr	24 hr

Contraindications/Precautions
Contraindicated in: Hypersensitivity; Urinary retention; Gastric retention; Uncontrolled angle-closure glaucoma; Severe hepatic impairment.
Use Cautiously in: Moderate hepatic impairment (lower dose recommended); Bladder outflow obstruction; GI obstructive disorders, ↓ GI motility, severe constipation or ulcerative colitis; Myasthenia gravis; Angle-closure glaucoma; OB: Safety not established in pregnancy; Lactation: Safety not established in breastfeeding; Pedi: Safety and effectiveness not established in children.

Adverse Reactions/Side Effects
EENT: blurred vision. **GI:** constipation, dry mouth, dyspepsia, nausea. **Metab:** heat intolerance. **Neuro:** confusion, dizziness, drowsiness, hallucinations, headache. **Misc:** ANGIOEDEMA.

Interactions
Drug-Drug: **Strong CYP3A4 inhibitors**, including **ketoconazole**, **itraconazole**, **ritonavir**, **nelfinavir**, **clarithromycin**, and **nefazodone** may ↑ levels and risk of toxicity; daily dose should not exceed 7.5 mg. Concurrent use of **moderate CYP3A4 inhibitors**, especially those with narrow therapeutic indices, including **flecainide**, **thioridazine**, and **tricyclic antidepressants**, should be undertaken with caution.

Route/Dosage
PO (Adults): 7.5 mg once daily, may ↑ after 2 wk to 15 mg once daily.

Availability (generic available)
Extended-release tablets: 7.5 mg, 15 mg.

NURSING IMPLICATIONS
Assessment
- Monitor voiding pattern and assess symptoms of overactive bladder (urinary urgency, urinary incontinence, urinary frequency) to and periodically during therapy.

Implementation
- **PO:** Administer once daily without regard to food. **DNC:** Swallow extended-release tablets whole; do not break, crush, or chew.

Patient/Family Teaching
- Instruct patient to take darifenacin as directed. If a dose is missed, skip dose and take next day; do not take 2 doses in same day. Advise patient to read *Patient Information* before starting therapy and with each Rx refill in case of changes.
- Do not share darifenacin with others; may be dangerous.
- Inform patient of potential anticholinergic side effects (constipation, urinary retention, blurred vision, heat prostration in a hot environment).
- May cause dizziness, drowsiness, confusion, and blurred vision. Caution patient to avoid driving and other activities that require alertness until response to medication is known.
- Instruct patient to notify health care professional of all Rx or OTC medications, vitamins, or herbal products being taken and consult health care professional before taking any new medications.
- Advise females of reproductive potential to notify health care professional if pregnancy is planned or suspected or if breastfeeding.

Evaluation/Desired Outcomes
- Decrease in symptoms of overactive bladder (urge urinary incontinence, urgency, frequency).

℞ darunavir/cobicistat/emtricitabine/tenofovir alafenamide
(da-**roo**-na-veer/koe-**bik**-i-stat/em-tri-**si**-ti-been/te-**noe**-fo-veer al-a-**fen**-a-mide)
Symtuza
Classification
Therapeutic: antiretrovirals, pharmacoenhancers
Pharmacologic: protease inhibitors, enzyme inhibitors, nucleoside reverse transcriptase inhibitors

Indications
HIV-1 infection in patients who have no prior antiretroviral treatment history or who are virologically suppressed (HIV-1 RNA <50 copies/mL) on a stable antiretroviral regimen for ≥6 mo and have no known substitutions associated with resistance to darunavir or tenofovir.

Action
Darunavir: Inhibits HIV-1 protease, selectively inhibiting the cleavage of HIV-encoded specific polyproteins in infected cells. This prevents the formation of mature virus particles. *Cobicistat:* Strongly inhibits CYP3A enzymes, enhancing systemic exposure to darunavir. *Emtricitabine:* Phosphorylated intracellularly where it inhibits HIV reverse transcriptase, resulting in viral DNA chain termination. *Tenofovir alafenamide:* Phosphorylated intracellularly where it inhibits HIV reverse transcriptase resulting in disruption of DNA synthesis.
Therapeutic Effects: Increased CD4 cell counts and decreased viral load with subsequent slowed progression of HIV infection and its sequelae.

Pharmacokinetics
Darunavir
Absorption: Food enhances oral absorption.
Distribution: Unknown.
Protein Binding: 95%.
Metabolism and Excretion: Extensively metabolized by the liver via the CYP3A isoenzyme; 41% excreted unchanged in feces, 8% in urine.
Half-life: 9.4 hr.
Cobicistat
Absorption: Absorption follows oral administration.
Distribution: Unknown.
Protein Binding: 97–98%.
Metabolism and Excretion: Metabolized by the liver primarily by the CYP3A isoenzyme and to a lesser extent by the CYP2D6 isoenzyme; 86.2% excreted in feces, 8.2% in urine.
Half-life: 3.2 hr.
Emtricitabine
Absorption: 93% absorbed following oral administration.
Distribution: Unknown.
Metabolism and Excretion: Not significantly metabolized; 86% excreted in urine, 14% in feces.
Half-life: 7.5 hr.
Tenofovir Alafenamide
Absorption: Tenofovir alafenamide is a prodrug, which is hydrolyzed into tenofovir, the active component; absorption enhanced by high-fat meals.
Distribution: Unknown.
Metabolism and Excretion: Tenofovir is phosphorylated to tenofovir diphosphate (active metabolite); 32% excreted in feces, <1% in urine.
Half-life: 0.5 hr.

TIME/ACTION PROFILE (plasma concentrations)

ROUTE	ONSET	PEAK	DURATION
Darunavir (PO)	unknown	3 hr	24 hr
Cobicistat (PO)	unknown	3 hr	24 hr
Emtricitabine (PO)	rapid	1.5 hr	24 hr
Tenofovir (PO)	unknown	0.5 hr	24 hr

Contraindications/Precautions

Contraindicated in: Concurrent use of alfuzosin, carbamazepine, dronedarone, colchicine (in renal/hepatic impairment), elbasvir/grazoprevir, ergot derivatives, ivabradine, lomitapide, lovastatin, lurasidone, midazolam (PO), naloxegol, phenobarbital, phenytoin, pimozide, ranolazine, rifampin, sildenafil (Revatio), simvastatin, triazolam, or St. John's wort; Severe renal impairment; Severe hepatic impairment; OB: Pregnancy (significantly lower concentrations of darunavir and cobicistat during 2nd and 3rd trimesters); Lactation: Breastfeeding not recommended in women with HIV.
Use Cautiously in: Hepatitis B virus (HBV) or hepatitis C virus infection; Sulfonamide allergy; Hemophilia (↑ risk of bleeding); Pedi: Children <40 kg (safety and effectiveness not established); Geri: Consider age-related impairment in hepatic function, concurrent chronic disease states and drug therapy in older adults.

Adverse Reactions/Side Effects

Derm: rash, ACUTE GENERALIZED EXANTHEMATOUS PUSTULOSIS, DRUG REACTION WITH EOSINOPHILIA AND SYSTEMIC SYMPTOMS (DRESS), STEVENS-JOHNSON SYNDROME (SJS), TOXIC EPIDERMAL NECROLYSIS (TEN). **Endo:** Graves' disease, hyperglycemia. **GI:** abdominal pain, ACUTE EXACERBATION OF HBV, autoimmune hepatitis, diarrhea, flatulence, HEPATOTOXICITY, LACTIC ACIDOSIS/HEPATOMEGALY WITH STEATOSIS, nausea. **GU:** acute renal failure, Fanconi syndrome, proximal renal tubulopathy. **Metab:** body fat redistribution, hyperlipidemia. **MS:** polymyositis. **Neuro:** Guillain-Barré syndrome, fatigue, headache. **Misc:** immune reconstitution syndrome.

Interactions

Drug-Drug: ↑ levels and risk of toxicity from **alfuzosin**, **dronedarone**, **elbasvir/grazoprevir**, **ergot derivatives** (**dihydroergotamine, ergotamine, methylergonovine**), **ivabradine, lomitapide, lovastatin, lurasidone, midazolam (oral), pimozide, ranolazine, sildenafil (Revatio), simvastatin,** and **triazolam**; concurrent use contraindicated. May ↑ **naloxegol** levels, which can precipitate opioid withdrawal symptoms; concurrent use contraindicated. **Strong CYP3A4 inducers,** including **carbamazepine, phenobarbital, phenytoin,** and **rifampin** may ↓ cobicistat, darunavir, and tenofovir levels and their effectiveness; concurrent use contraindicated. ↑ levels/ risk of adverse reactions with **colchicine**; concurrent use in patients with renal/hepatic impairment contraindicated; for others ↓ dose (*for gout flare:* 0.6 mg followed by 0.3 mg 1 hr later, may repeat no sooner than 3 days, *for prophylaxis of gout flare:* if dose was originally 0.6 mg twice daily, ↓ to 0.3 mg once daily, if original regimen was 0.6 mg once daily, ↓ to 0.3 mg every other day, *for treatment of familial Mediterranean fever:* dose should not exceed 0.6 mg once daily or 0.3 mg twice daily). **Clarithromycin** and **erythromycin** may ↑ levels of darunavir and cobicistat; consider alter-

native anti-infectives. ↑ levels/risk of toxicity with **dasatinib, nilotinib, vinblastine,** and **vincristine**; careful monitoring for toxicity and dose adjustments recommended. May ↑ bleeding risk with **apixaban** and **rivaroxaban**; may need to adjust apixaban dose; avoid concurrent use with rivaroxaban. Effect on **warfarin** is not known; monitor INR. **Oxcarbazepine** and **eslicarbazepine** may ↓ cobicistat and tenofovir levels and their effectiveness; consider alternative anticonvulsant or antiretroviral therapy. May ↑ levels of **clonazepam**; careful anticonvulsant monitoring recommended. May ↑ levels/effects of **tricyclic antidepressants** and **trazodone**; careful dosing of antidepressants recommended (effect on **SSRIs** is unknown). May ↑ levels of **ketoconazole, isavuconazonium,** and **itraconazole**; effect on **voriconazole** unknown; concurrent use with voriconazole not recommended. Effects are unknown with **artemether/lumefantrine**; monitor for ↓ antimalarial activity or QT prolongation. ↑ levels/ effects/risk of adverse reaction including neutropenia and uveitis with **rifabutin**; lower rifabutin dose to 150 mg every other day. **Rifapentine**↓ darunavir and tenofovir levels; concurrent use not recommended. May ↑ levels/effects of **neuroleptics that are metabolized by CYP3A or CYP2D6**, including **perphenazine, risperidone,** and **thioridazine**; ↓ dose of neuroleptic may be necessary. May ↑ levels of **quetiapine**; if taking quetiapine when initiating therapy, consider alternative antiretroviral therapy or ↓ quetiapine dose to ⅙ of the original dose and monitor for adverse effects. ↑ levels/ effects of **beta blockers metabolized by CYP2D6**, including **metoprolol, carvedilol,** and **timolol**; clinical monitoring recommended. ↑ levels/effects of **calcium channel blockers metabolized by CYP3A**, including **amlodipine, diltiazem, felodipine, nifedipine,** or **verapamil**; careful monitoring recommended. ↑ level and risk of toxicity with **antiarrhythmics** including **amiodarone, disopyramide, flecainide, mexiletine, propafenone,** and **quinidine**; careful monitoring and titration is recommended. May ↑ levels and risk of toxicity with **digoxin**; closely monitor digoxin levels and adjust dose as needed. **Dexamethasone** may ↓ levels of cobicistat and darunavir; consider use of alternative corticosteroid, such as prednisone or prednisolone. May ↑ levels of **corticosteroids** (all routes of administration) primarily metabolized by the CYP3A isoenzyme (e.g., **betamethasone, budesonide, ciclesonide, fluticasone, methylprednisolone, mometasone,** or **triamcinolone**, which may ↑ the risk of Cushing's disease and adrenal suppression; consider alternative corticosteroid such as beclomethasone, prednisone, or prednisolone. Concurrent use with **bosentan** may result in ↑ levels/toxicity of bosentan and ↓ levels darunavir and cobicistat; dose alteration is required (*initiating bosentan in patients already receiving darunavir/cobicistat/emtricitabine/tenofovir alafenamide for ≥10 days:* bosentan 62.5 mg daily or every other day, depending on tolerance; *initiating darunavir/cobicistat/emtricitabine/tenofovir alafenamide in patient already receiving bosentan:* discontinue bosentan for 10 days, resume bosentan at 62.5 mg daily or every other day, depending on tolerance). May ↑ levels of **glecaprevir/pibrentasvir**; concurrent use not recommended. Nephrotoxic agents, including **NSAIDs**, ↑ risk of nephrotoxicity; avoid concurrent use. May ↓ levels and contraceptive efficacy of some combined **hormonal contraceptives**; additional or alternative methods of nonhormonal contraception recommended. May ↑ risk of hyperkalemia when used with **drospirenone**. ↑ levels and risk of toxicity from **immunosuppressants metabolized by CYP3A**, including **cyclosporine, everolimus, sirolimus**, and **tacrolimus**; therapeutic monitoring recommended. May ↑ levels of **irinotecan**; discontinue darunavir/cobicistat/emtricitabine/tenofovir alafenamide ≥1 wk before starting irinotecan therapy. ↑ levels of **salmeterol** and may ↑ risk of serious adverse cardiovascular events; concurrent use is not recommended. ↑ levels and risk of myopathy from **atorvastatin, fluvastatin, pitavastatin, pravastatin**, or **rosuvastatin**; use lowest dose of these agents; do not exceed atorvastatin or rosuvastatin dose of 20 mg/day. May ↑ levels/risk of respiratory depression with opioids, including **buprenorphine, buprenorphine/naloxone, fentanyl, oxycodone**, and **tramadol**; carefully monitor for **opioid** effects, dose adjustment of opioid may be necessary. May ↑ levels and risk of adverse cardiovascular, ophthalmic, and genitourinary effects of **PDE-5 inhibitors**, including **avanafil, sildenafil, tadalafil**, and **vardenafil**; **avanafil** use is not recommended, *sildenafil:* use for pulmonary hypertension is contraindicated, when used for erectile dysfunction single dose should not exceed 25 mg/48 hr; *tadalafil:* for pulmonary hypertension-initiating tadalafil in patients receiving darunavir/cobicistat/emtricitabine/tenofovir alafenamide for ≥7 days—20 mg once daily initially, may be titrated to 40 mg once daily, initiating darunavir/cobicistat/emtricitabine/tenofovir alafenamide in patients receiving tadalafil—discontinue tadalafil 24 hr prior to initiating therapy, after 7 days reinstitute tadalafil at 20 mg once daily, may be ↑ to 40 mg once daily; for erectile dysfunction single dose should not exceed 10 mg/72 hr; *vardenafil:* for erectile dysfunction single dose should not exceed 2.5 mg/72 hr. May ↑ levels and risk of bleeding with **ticagrelor**; concurrent use not recommended. May ↓ antiplatelet effects of **clopidogrel**; concurrent use not recommended. ↑ levels/ effects and risk of excess sedation/respiratory depression from some **sedative/hypnotics metabolized by CYP3A** including **buspirone, diazepam**, and **parenteral midazolam**; concurrent with **other sedative/hypnotics metabolized by CYP3A** should be undertaken with caution; dose ↓ may be necessary. May ↑ **fesoterodine** and **solifenacin** levels; should not exceed fesoterodine dose of 4 mg once daily or solifenacin dose of 5 mg once daily.

Drug-Natural Products: St. John's wort may ↓ cobicistat, darunavir, and tenofovir levels and their effectiveness; concurrent use contraindicated.

Route/Dosage
PO (Adults and Children ≥40 kg): One tablet (darunavir 800 mg/cobicistat 150 mg/emtricitabine 200 mg/tenofovir alafenamide 10 mg) once daily.

Availability
Tablets: darunavir 800 mg/cobicistat 150 mg/emtricitabine 200 mg/tenofovir alafenamide 10 mg.

NURSING IMPLICATIONS
Assessment
- Assess patient for change in severity of HIV symptoms and for symptoms of opportunistic infections during therapy.
- Assess for allergy to sulfonamides.
- Monitor for development of rash. May cause SJS or TEN. Discontinue therapy if severe or if accompanied with fever, general malaise, fatigue, muscle or joint aches, blisters, oral lesions, conjunctivitis, hepatitis, and/or eosinophilia.

Lab Test Considerations
- Monitor viral load and CD4 count before and routinely during therapy to determine response.
- Assess for HBV. *Symtuza* is not approved for administration in patients with HIV and HBV. If therapy is discontinued, may cause severe exacerbation of HBV. Monitor liver function in coinfected patients for several mo after stopping therapy.
- Monitor liver function tests prior to, during, and following therapy. May cause ↑ LDL cholesterol, total cholesterol, and triglyceride concentrations. Lactic acidosis may occur with hepatic toxicity causing hepatic steatosis; may be fatal, especially in women. Discontinue therapy if symptoms occur.
- Monitor serum creatinine, CCr, urine glucose, and urine protein prior to and periodically during therapy and when clinically indicated. In patients with chronic kidney disease, assess serum creatinine, creatinine clearance, serum phosphorus, urine glucose, and urine protein prior to and periodically during therapy. May cause hypophosphatemia in patients with renal impairment.
- May cause hyperglycemia and glycosuria.

Implementation
- **PO:** Administer once daily with food. For patients who are unable to swallow the whole tablet, may be split into two pieces using a tablet cutter, and consume entire dose immediately after splitting.

Patient/Family Teaching
- Instruct patient on the importance of taking medication as directed, even if feeling better. Do not take

more than prescribed amount and do not stop taking without consulting health care professional. Discontinuing therapy may lead to severe exacerbations. Take missed doses as soon as remembered unless almost time for next dose; do not double doses. Advise patient to read *Patient Information* prior to starting therapy and with each Rx refill in case of changes. Caution patient not to share or trade *Symtuza* with others.

- Inform patient of importance of HBV testing before starting antiretroviral therapy.
- Inform patient that *Symtuza* does not cure AIDS and may reduce the risk of transmission of HIV to others through sexual contact or blood contamination. Caution patient to use a condom and avoid sharing needles or donating blood to prevent spreading HIV to others.
- Advise patient to notify health care professional immediately if symptoms of lactic acidosis (nausea, vomiting, unusual or unexpected stomach discomfort, unusual muscle pain, difficulty breathing, feeling cold, especially in arms and legs, dizziness, fast or irregular heartbeat, and weakness or tiredness), liver problems (yellow skin or whites of eyes, dark urine, light colored stools, loss of appetite, nausea, stomach pain), or signs of immune reconstitution syndrome (signs and symptoms of an infection or inflammation) occur.
- Instruct patient to notify health care professional of all Rx or OTC medications, vitamins, or herbal products being taken and consult health care professional before taking any new medications, especially St. John's wort.
- Inform patient that redistribution and accumulation of body fat may occur, causing central obesity, dorsocervical fat enlargement (buffalo hump), peripheral wasting, breast enlargement, and cushingoid appearance. The cause and long-term effects are not known.
- Rep: Advise females of reproductive potential to notify health care professional if pregnancy is planned or suspected. Encourage pregnant women to enroll in the Antiretroviral Pregnancy Registry by calling 1-800-258-4263 to monitor pregnancy outcomes. Advise female patient that pregnancy is not recommended during *Symtuza* and avoid breastfeeding during therapy.
- Emphasize the importance of regular follow-up exams and blood counts to determine progress and monitor for side effects.

Evaluation/Desired Outcomes

- Delayed progression of AIDS and decreased opportunistic infections in patients with HIV.
- Decrease in viral load and improvement in CD4 cell counts.

HIGH ALERT

DAUNOrubicin hydrochloride
(daw-noe-**roo**-bi-sin **hye**-dro-**klor**-ide)
✤Cerubidine

Classification
Therapeutic: antineoplastics
Pharmacologic: anthracyclines

Indications
Remission induction of various leukemias.

Action
Forms a complex with DNA, which subsequently inhibits DNA and RNA synthesis (cell-cycle phase-nonspecific). **Therapeutic Effects:** Death of rapidly replicating cells, particularly malignant ones. Also has immunosuppressive properties.

Pharmacokinetics
Absorption: IV administration results in complete bioavailability.
Distribution: Widely distributed to tissues.
Metabolism and Excretion: Extensively metabolized by the liver. Converted partially to a compound that also has antineoplastic activity (daunorubicinol); 40% eliminated by biliary excretion.
Half-life: *Daunorubicin:* 18.5 hr. *Daunorubicinol:* 26.7 hr.

TIME/ACTION PROFILE (effects on blood counts)

ROUTE	ONSET	PEAK	DURATION
IV	7–10 days	10–14 days	21 days

Contraindications/Precautions
Contraindicated in: Hypersensitivity to daunorubicin or any other components in the formulation; Symptomatic HF or arrhythmias; OB: Pregnancy; Lactation: Lactation.
Use Cautiously in: Active infections or decreased bone marrow reserve; Previous radiation therapy (may reactivate skin lesions); Renal impairment (↓ dose recommended if serum creatinine >3 mg/dL); Hepatic impairment (↓ dose recommended if serum bilirubin >1.2 mg/dL); Previous anthracycline therapy or underlying cardiovascular disease (↑ risk of cardiotoxicity); Rep: Women of reproductive potential; Geri: ↓ dose recommended for patients ≥60 yr.

Adverse Reactions/Side Effects
CV: arrhythmias, CARDIOTOXICITY. **Derm:** alopecia. **EENT:** rhinitis, abnormal vision, sinusitis. **GI:** nausea, vomiting, esophagitis, hepatoxicity, stomatitis. **GU:** red urine, gonadal suppression. **Hemat:** anemia, leukopenia, thrombocytopenia. **Local:** phlebitis at IV site. **Metab:** hyperuricemia. **Misc:** chills, fever.

Interactions

Drug-Drug: Additive myelosuppression with other **antineoplastics.** May ↓ antibody response to **live-virus vaccines** and ↑ risk of adverse reactions. **Cyclophosphamide** and **trastuzumab** ↑ risk of cardiotoxicity; avoid use of daunorubicin for up to 7 mo after discontinuing trastuzumab. May ↑ risk of hepatotoxicity with other **hepatotoxic agents**.

Route/Dosage

In adults, cumulative dose should not exceed 550 mg/m² (450 mg/m² if previous chest radiation).

IV (Adults <60 yr): 45 mg/m²/day for 3 days in first course, then for 2 days of second course (as part of combination regimen).

IV (Adults ≥60 yr): 30 mg/m²/day for 3 days in first course, then for 2 days of second course (as part of combination regimen).

IV (Children >2 yr): 25 mg/m² once weekly (as part of combination regimen). In children <2 yr or BSA <0.5 m², dose should be determined on a mg/kg basis.

Availability (generic available)

Powder for injection: ✹ 20 mg/vial. **Solution for injection:** 5 mg/mL.

NURSING IMPLICATIONS
Assessment

- Monitor vital signs before and frequently during therapy.
- Monitor for bone marrow depression. Assess for bleeding (bleeding gums; bruising; petechiae; guaiac stools, urine, and emesis) and avoid IM injections and taking rectal temperatures if platelet count is low. Apply pressure to venipuncture sites for 10 min. Assess for signs of infection during neutropenia. Anemia may occur. Monitor for increased fatigue, dyspnea, and orthostatic hypotension.
- Assess IV site frequently for inflammation or infiltration. Instruct patient to notify nurse immediately if pain or irritation at injection site occurs. If extravasation occurs, infusion must be stopped and restarted in another vein to avoid damage to SUBQ tissue. Notify health care professional immediately. Daunorubicin is a vesicant. If extravasation occurs, stop infusion immediately and disconnect (leave cannula/needle in place); gently aspirate extravasated solution (do NOT flush line); remove needle/cannula; elevate extremity. Initiate antidote (dexrazoxane [adult] or dimethyl sulfate [DMSO]). Apply dry cold compresses for 20 min 4 times daily for 1 to 2 days; hold cooling beginning 15 min before dexrazoxane infusion; continue holding cooling until 15 min after infusion is completed. Do not administer topical DMSO in combination with dexrazoxane; may lessen dexrazoxane efficacy.
- Monitor intake and output, appetite, and nutritional intake. Assess for nausea and vomiting, which, although mild, may persist for 24–48 hr. Administration of an antiemetic before and periodically during therapy and adjusting diet as tolerated may help maintain fluid and electrolyte balance and nutritional status. Encourage fluid intake of 2000–3000 mL/day. Allopurinol and alkalinization of the urine may be used to help prevent urate stone formation.
- Assess for evidence of cardiotoxicity which manifests as HF (peripheral edema, dyspnea, rales/crackles, weight gain, jugular venous distention) and usually occurs 1–6 mo after initiation of therapy. Obtain chest x ray, echocardiography, ECGs, and radionuclide angiography determination of ejection fraction before each course of therapy and periodically during therapy. A 30% decrease in QRS voltage and decrease in systolic ejection fraction are early signs of cardiotoxicity. Patients who receive total cumulative doses >550/mm², who have a history of cardiac disease, or who have received mediastinal radiation are at greater risk of developing cardiotoxicity. Cardiotoxicity may develop if cumulative dose exceeds 400 to 550 mg/m² in adults, 300 mg/m² in children older than 2 yr, or 10 mg/kg in children younger than 2 yr. May be irreversible and fatal, but usually responds to early treatment.

Lab Test Considerations
- Monitor uric acid levels periodically during therapy.
- Monitor CBC and differential before and frequently during therapy. The leukocyte count nadir occurs 10–14 days after administration. Recovery usually occurs within 21 days after administration of daunorubicin.
- Monitor AST, ALT, LDH, and serum bilirubin prior to each course of therapy. May cause transiently ↑ serum alkaline phosphatase, bilirubin, and AST concentrations.
- Monitor renal function before each course of therapy.

Implementation
- **High Alert:** Fatalities have occurred with chemotherapeutic agents. Before administering, clarify all ambiguous orders; double-check single, daily, and course-of-therapy dose limits; have second practitioner independently double-check original order, calculations, and infusion pump settings.
- Do not confuse daunorubicin hydrochloride with doxorubicin or idarubicin. To prevent confusion, orders should include generic and brand name.
- Provide antiemetics before each infusion.

IV Administration
- Solution should be prepared in a biologic cabinet. Wear gloves, gown, and mask while handling IV medication. Discard IV equipment in specially designated containers.
- **IV: *Reconstitution:*** Reconstitute each 20 mg with 4 mL of sterile water for injection for a concentra-

tion of 5 mg/mL. Shake gently to dissolve. Reconstituted medication is stable for 24 hr if refrigerated. Protect from sunlight.

- Do not use aluminum needles when reconstituting or injecting daunorubicin, as aluminum darkens the solution.
- **IV Push:** *Dilution:* Dilute further in 10–15 mL of 0.9% NaCl. Administer IV push through Y-site into free-flowing infusion of 0.9% NaCl or D5W. *Rate:* Administer over at least 2–3 min. Rapid administration rate may cause facial flushing or erythema along the vein.
- **Intermittent Infusion:** *Dilution:* May also be diluted in 50–100 mL of 0.9% NaCl. *Rate:* Administer 50 mL over 10–15 min or 100 mL over 30–45 min.
- **Y-Site Compatibility:** alemtuzumab, amifostine, amikacin, amiodarone, anidulafungin, argatroban, arsenic trioxide, atracurium, bivalirudin, bleomycin, bumetanide, buprenorphine, butorphanol, calcium chloride, calcium gluconate, carboplatin, carmustine, caspofungin, chlorpromazine, ciprofloxacin, cisatracurium, cisplatin, cyclophosphamide, cyclosporine, cytarabine, dacarbazine, dactinomycin, daptomycin, dexmedetomidine, dexrazoxane, digoxin, diltiazem, diphenhydramine, dobutamine, docetaxel, dopamine, doxycycline, droperidol, enalaprilat, ephedrine, epinephrine, erythromycin, esmolol, etoposide, etoposide phosphate, famotidine, fentanyl, filgrastim, fluconazole, gemcitabine, gemtuzumab ozogamicin, gentamicin, glycopyrrolate, granisetron, haloperidol, hetastarch, hydralazine, hydrocortisone, hydromorphone, idarubicin, imipenem/cilastatin, insulin regular, irinotecan, isoproterenol, labetalol, leucovorin calcium, lidocaine, linezolid, lorazepam, magnesium sulfate, mannitol, melphalan, meperidine, meropenem, methotrexate, metoclopramide, metoprolol, metronidazole, midazolam, milrinone, mitomycin, morphine, moxifloxacin, nalbuphine, naloxone, nitroglycerin, norepinephrine, octreotide, ondansetron, oxaliplatin, paclitaxel, palonosetron, pentamidine, phentolamine, phenylephrine, potassium acetate, potassium chloride, potassium phosphate, procainamide, prochlorperazine, promethazine, propranolol, remifentanil, rituximab, sodium acetate, sodium bicarbonate, sodium phosphate, succinylcholine, sufentanil, tacrolimus, theophylline, thiotepa, tigecycline, tobramycin, topotecan, trastuzumab, vancomycin, vecuronium, verapamil, vinblastine, vincristine, vinorelbine, voriconazole, zidovudine, zoledronic acid.
- **Y-Site Incompatibility:** acyclovir, allopurinol, aminophylline, amphotericin B lipid complex, amphotericin B liposomal, ampicillin, ampicillin/sulbactam, aztreonam, cefazolin, cefepime, cefotaxime, cefotetan, cefoxitin, ceftazidime, ceftriaxone, cefuroxime, chloramphenicol, clindamycin, dantrolene, dexamethasone, diazepam, ertapenem, fludarabine, foscarnet, fosphenytoin, furosemide, ganciclovir, heparin, indomethacin, ketorolac, levofloxacin, methohexital, methylprednisolone, mitoxantrone, nafcillin, nitroprusside, pantoprazole, pemetrexed, pentobarbital, phenobarbital, phenytoin, piperacillin/tazobactam, thiopental, trimethoprim/sulfamethoxazole.
- **Additive Incompatibility:** Manufacturer does not recommend admixing daunorubicin hydrochloride.

Patient/Family Teaching
- Instruct patient to notify health care professional if fever; chills; sore throat; signs of infection; bleeding gums; bruising; petechiae; or blood in urine, stool, or emesis occurs. Caution patient to avoid crowds and persons with known infections. Instruct patient to use soft toothbrush and electric razor. Patient should be cautioned not to drink alcoholic beverages or take products containing aspirin or NSAIDs.
- Instruct patient to inspect oral mucosa for erythema and ulceration. If ulceration occurs, advise patient to use sponge brush and rinse mouth with water after eating and drinking. Stomatitis pain may require management with opioid analgesics. Period of highest risk is 3–7 days after administration of dose.
- Instruct patient to notify health care professional immediately if irregular heartbeat, shortness of breath, or swelling of lower extremities occurs.
- Discuss with patient possibility of hair loss. Explore methods of coping. Regrowth of hair usually begins within 5 wk after discontinuing therapy.
- Inform patient that medication may turn urine reddish color for 1–2 days after administration.
- Instruct patient not to receive any vaccinations without advice of health care professional.
- Rep: May cause fetal harm. Advise females of reproductive potential and males with a partner of reproductive potential to use effective contraception during therapy and for at least 4 mo after last dose and to avoid breastfeeding during therapy. Inform patient that daunorubicin may cause irreversible gonadal suppression.
- Emphasize the need for periodic lab tests to monitor for side effects.

Evaluation/Desired Outcomes
- Improvement of hematologic status in patients with leukemia.

deferoxamine
(de-fer-**ox**-a-meen)
Desferal
Classification
Therapeutic: antidotes
Pharmacologic: heavy metal antagonists

Indications
Acute toxic iron ingestion. Secondary iron overload syndromes associated with multiple transfusion therapy.

Action
Chelates unbound iron, forming a water-soluble complex (ferrioxamine) in plasma that is easily excreted by the kidneys. **Therapeutic Effects:** Removal of excess iron. Also chelates aluminum.

Pharmacokinetics
Absorption: Poorly absorbed after oral administration. Well absorbed after IM administration and SUBQ administration. IV administration results in complete bioavailability.
Distribution: Appears to be widely distributed.
Metabolism and Excretion: Metabolized by tissues and plasma enzymes. Unchanged drug and chelated form excreted by the kidneys; 33% of iron removed is eliminated in the feces via biliary excretion.
Half-life: 1 hr.

TIME/ACTION PROFILE (effects on hematologic parameters)

ROUTE	ONSET	PEAK	DURATION
IV	rapid	unknown	unknown
IM	unknown	unknown	unknown
SUBQ	unknown	unknown	unknown

Contraindications/Precautions
Contraindicated in: Severe renal impairment; Anuria; Lactation: Lactation.
Use Cautiously in: OB: Safety not established in pregnancy. Treatment should not be withheld in pregnant women with acute iron toxicity; Pedi: Children <3 yr (safety and effectiveness not established).

Adverse Reactions/Side Effects
CV: hypotension, tachycardia. **Derm:** erythema, flushing, urticaria. **EENT:** blurred vision, cataracts, ototoxicity. **GI:** abdominal pain, diarrhea. **GU:** red urine. **Local:** induration at injection site, pain at injection site. **MS:** leg cramps. **Misc:** fever, HYPERSENSITIVITY REACTIONS (including anaphylaxis), shock (after rapid IV administration).

Interactions
Drug-Drug: **Ascorbic acid** may ↑ effectiveness of deferoxamine but may also ↑ cardiac iron toxicity.

Route/Dosage
Acute Iron Ingestion
IM, IV (Adults and Children ≥3 yr): 1 g, then 500 mg every 4 hr for 2 doses. Additional doses of 500 mg every 4–12 hr may be needed (not to exceed 6 g/24 hr).

Chronic Iron Overload
IM, IV (Adults and Children ≥3 yr): 500 mg–1 g daily IM; additional doses of 2 g should be given IV for each unit of blood transfused (not to exceed 1 g/day in absence of transfusions; 6 g/day if patient receives transfusions).

SUBQ (Adults and Children ≥3 yr): 1–2 g/day (20–40 mg/kg/day) infused over 8–24 hr.

Availability (generic available)
Powder for injection: 500 mg/vial, 2 g/vial.

NURSING IMPLICATIONS
Assessment
- In acute poisoning, assess time, amount, and type of iron preparation ingested.
- Monitor signs of iron toxicity: early acute (abdominal pain, bloody diarrhea, emesis), late acute (decreased level of consciousness, shock, metabolic acidosis).
- Monitor vital signs closely, especially during IV administration. Report hypotension, erythema, urticaria, or signs of allergic reaction. Keep epinephrine, an antihistamine, and resuscitation equipment close by in the event of an anaphylactic reaction.
- May cause oculotoxicity or ototoxicity. Report decreased visual acuity or hearing loss. Audiovisual exams should be performed every 3 mo in patients with chronic iron overload.
- Monitor intake and output and urine color. Inform health care professional if patient is anuric. Chelated iron is excreted primarily by the kidneys; urine may turn red.

Lab Test Considerations
- Monitor serum iron, total iron binding capacity (TIBC), ferritin levels, and urinary iron excretion before and periodically during therapy.
- Monitor liver function studies to assess damage from iron poisoning.

Implementation
- IM route is preferred in acute iron intoxication unless patient is in shock.
- **Reconstitution:** Reconstitute 500-mg vial with 2 mL and 2-g vial with 8 mL of sterile water for injection. Dissolve powder completely before administration. Solution is yellow and is stable for 1 wk after reconstitution if protected from light. Discard unused portion. **Concentration:** 213 mg/mL. Used in conjunction with induction of emesis or gastric aspiration and lavage with sodium bicarbonate, and supportive measures for shock and metabolic acidosis in acute poisoning.
- **IM:** Administer deep IM and massage well. Rotate sites. IM administration may cause transient severe pain.
- **SUBQ:** Reconstitute 500-mg vial with 5 mL and 2-g vial with 20 mL of sterile water for injection. **Concentration:** 95 mg/mL. SUBQ route used to treat chronically elevated iron therapy is administered into abdominal SUBQ tissue via infusion pump for 8–24 hr per treatment.

IV Administration

- **IV:** *Reconstitution:* Reconstitute 500-mg vial with 5 mL and 2-g vial with 20 mL of sterile water for injection. *Concentration:* 95 mg/mL. *Dilution:* D5W, 0.9% NaCl, 0.45% NaCl, or LR. Dissolve powder completely before administration. Solution is clear and colorless to slightly yellow. Administer within 3 hr of reconstitution; 24 hr if prepared under laminar flow hood. Discard unused portion. *Rate:* Maximum infusion rate is 15 mg/kg/hr for first 1000 mg. May be followed by 500 mg infused over 4 hr at a slower rate not to exceed 125 mg/hr. Rapid infusion rate may cause hypotension, erythema, urticaria, wheezing, convulsions, tachycardia, or shock.
- May be administered at the same time as blood transfusion in persons with chronically elevated serum iron levels. Use separate site for administration.

Patient/Family Teaching

- Reinforce need to keep iron preparations, all medications, and hazardous substances out of the reach of children.
- Reassure patient that red coloration of urine is expected and reflects excretion of excess iron.
- May cause dizziness or impairment of vision or hearing. Caution patient to avoid driving or other activities requiring alertness until response from medication is known.
- Advise patient not to take vitamin C preparations without consulting health care professional, because tissue toxicity may increase.
- Encourage patients requiring chronic therapy to keep follow-up appointments for lab tests. Eye and hearing exams may be monitored every 3 mo.
- Rep: Advise females of reproductive potential to notify health care professional if pregnancy is planned. Breastfeeding should be avoided during therapy and for 1 wk after the last dose.

Evaluation/Desired Outcomes

- Return of serum iron concentrations to a normal level (50–150 mcg/100 mL).

---

delafloxacin, See FLUOROQUINOLONES.

REMS

denosumab (de-no-su-mab)
Prolia, Xgeva
Classification
Therapeutic: bone resorption inhibitors
Pharmacologic: monoclonal antibodies

Indications

Prolia. Treatment of osteoporosis in postmenopausal women who are at high risk for fracture or those who have failed/are intolerant of conventional osteoporosis therapy. To increase bone mass in men with osteoporosis who are at high risk for fracture or those who have failed/are intolerant of conventional osteoporosis therapy. Treatment of glucocorticoid-induced osteoporosis in men and women at high risk for fracture who are initiating or continuing systemic glucocorticoids at a daily dosage of ≥7.5 mg of prednisone and are expected to remain on glucocorticoids for ≥6 mo. To increase bone mass in men receiving androgen deprivation therapy for nonmetastatic prostate cancer who are at high risk for fracture. To increase bone mass in women receiving adjuvant aromatase inhibitor therapy for breast cancer who are at high risk for fracture. **Xgeva.** Prevention of skeletal-related events in patients with multiple myeloma and in patients with bone metastases from solid tumors. Giant cell tumor of bone that is unresectable or where surgical resection is likely to result in severe morbidity. Hypercalcemia of malignancy that is refractory to bisphosphonate therapy.

Action

A monoclonal antibody that binds specifically to the human receptor activator of nuclear factor kappa-B-ligand (RANKL), which is required for formation, function, and survival of osteoclasts. Binding inhibits osteoclast formation, function, and survival. **Therapeutic Effects:** ↓ bone resorption with ↓ occurrence of fractures (vertebral, nonvertebral, hip) or other skeletal-related events (e.g., radiation therapy to bone, surgery to bone, spinal cord compression). ↑ bone mass.

Pharmacokinetics

Absorption: Well absorbed following SUBQ administration.
Distribution: Unknown.
Metabolism and Excretion: Unknown.
Half-life: 25.4 days.

TIME/ACTION PROFILE (effects on bone resorption)

ROUTE	ONSET	PEAK	DURATION
SUBQ	1 mo	unknown†	12 mo‡

†Maximum ↓ in serum calcium occurs at 10 days.
‡Following discontinuation.

Contraindications/Precautions

Contraindicated in: Hypersensitivity; Hypocalcemia (correct before administration); adequate supplemental calcium and vitamin D required; OB: Pregnancy; Lactation: Lactation.

Use Cautiously in: Conditions associated with hypocalcemia including hypoparathyroidism, previous thyroid/parathyroid surgery, malabsorption syndromes, history of small intestinal excision, inadequate/no calcium supplementation, renal impairment/hemodialysis (CCr <30 mL/min and/or on dialysis); monitoring of calcium levels and calcium and vitamin D intake recommended; Invasive dental procedures, cancer, receiving chemotherapy, corticosteroids, or angiogenesis inhibitors, poor oral hygiene, diabetes, gingival infections, periodontal disease, dental disease, anemia, coagulopathy, infection, or poorly-fitting dentures (may ↑ risk of jaw osteonecrosis); History of osteoporosis or prior fractures (↑ risk of multiple vertebral fractures upon drug discontinuation); Concurrent use of immunosuppressants or diseases resulting in immunosuppression (↑ risk of infection); Rep: Women of reproductive potential; Pedi: Safety and effectiveness not established in children; Geri: Older adults may be more sensitive to drug effects.

Adverse Reactions/Side Effects

Derm: dermatitis, eczema, rashes. **F and E:** <u>hypocalcemia</u>, <u>hypophosphatemia</u>, hypercalcemia. **GI:** <u>diarrhea</u>, nausea, PANCREATITIS. **GU:** <u>cystitis</u>. **Metab:** hypercholesterolemia. **MS:** <u>back pain</u>, <u>extremity pain</u>, <u>musculoskeletal pain</u>, atypical femoral fracture, osteonecrosis of the jaw, suppression of bone turnover. **Neuro:** headache. **Resp:** <u>dyspnea</u>, cough. **Misc:** HYPERSENSITIVITY REACTIONS (including anaphylaxis), infection.

Interactions

Drug-Drug: Concurrent use of **immunosuppressants** ↑ risk of infection. Concurrent use of **calcimimetic drugs** may ↑ risk of hypocalcemia.

Route/Dosage

Prolia

SUBQ (Adults): 60 mg every 6 mo.

Xgeva

SUBQ (Adults): *Multiple myeloma or bone metastasis from solid tumors:* 120 mg every 4 wk; *Giant cell tumor of bone:* 120 mg every 4 wk, with additional doses of 120 mg given on Days 8 and 15 of first mo of therapy; *Hypercalcemia of malignancy:* 120 mg every 4 wk, with additional doses of 120 mg given on Days 8 and 15 of first mo of therapy.

Availability

Solution for injection (Prolia) (prefilled syringe): 60 mg/mL. **Solution for injection (Xgeva):** 120 mg/1.7 mL.

NURSING IMPLICATIONS

Assessment

● Assess patients via bone density study for low bone mass before and periodically during therapy.
● Perform a routine oral exam prior to initiation of therapy. Dental exam with appropriate preventative dentistry should be considered prior to therapy. Patients with history of tooth extraction, poor oral hygiene, gingival infections, diabetes, or use of a dental appliance or those taking immunosuppressive therapy, angiogenesis inhibitors, or systemic corticosteroids are at greater risk for osteonecrosis of the jaw.

● Monitor for signs and symptoms of hypersensitivity reactions (hypotension, dyspnea, upper airway edema, lip swelling, rash, pruritus, urticaria). Treat symptomatically and discontinue medication if symptoms occur.

Lab Test Considerations

● Verify negative pregnancy status of patient before starting therapy.
● Assess serum calcium, phosphorous, and magnesium levels before and periodically during therapy, especially during first wk of therapy. Correct hypocalcemia and vitamin D deficiency before starting therapy. May cause mild, transient ↑ of calcium and phosphate. Supplement with calcium, magnesium, and vitamin D as needed.
● May cause hypercalcemia within the yr following discontinuation. Monitor for signs and symptoms of hypercalcemia, assess serum calcium periodically, re-evaluate the patient's calcium and vitamin D supplementation requirements and manage as clinically.
● May cause anemia.
● May cause hypercholesterolemia.

Implementation

● **SUBQ:** Remove from refrigerator and bring to room temperature by standing in original container for 15–30 min prior to administration; do not warm in any other way. Do not shake. Administer using a 27-gauge needle in the upper arm, upper thigh, or abdomen. Solution is clear and colorless to pale yellow, and may contain trace amounts of translucent to white proteinaceous particles. Do not use if solution is discolored or contains many particles. Manually activate the green safety guard *after* the injection is given, not before.
● Patients should receive calcium 1000 mg and vitamin D 400 IU daily.

Patient/Family Teaching

● Explain the purpose of denosumab to patient. If a dose is missed, administer injection as soon as possible.
● Advise patient once treatment is stopped there may be an increased risk of having broken bones in the spine, especially in patients who have had a fracture or who have had osteoporosis. Advise patients not to interrupt therapy without their health care professional advice.
● Advise patient to eat a balanced diet and consult health care professional about the need for supplemental calcium and vitamin D (see Appendix J).
● Advise patient to notify health care professional immediately if signs of hypersensitivity, hypocalcemia (spasms, twitches, or cramps in muscles; numbness or tingling in fingers, toes, or around mouth), infection (fever, chills, skin that is red, swollen, hot, or

tender to touch; severe abdominal pain, frequent or urgent need to urinate or burning during urination), or skin reactions (redness, itching, rash, dry or leathery feeling, blisters that ooze or become crusty, peeling), or osteonecrosis of the jaw (pain, numbness, swelling of or drainage from the jaw, mouth, or teeth) occur.

● Encourage patient to participate in regular exercise and to modify behaviors that ↑ the risk of osteoporosis (stop smoking, reduce alcohol consumption).

● Advise patient to take good care of teeth and gums (brush and floss regularly) and to inform health care professional of therapy prior to dental surgery.

● Inform patient of increased risk of fractures upon discontinuation. If denosumab is discontinued, consider another bone resorption inhibitor.

● Rep: Instruct female of reproductive potential to use highly effective contraception during and for at least 5 mo after therapy is completed. Advise patient to notify health care professional if pregnancy is planned or suspected or if breastfeeding.

Evaluation/Desired Outcomes

● Reversal of the progression of osteoporosis with ↓ fractures and other sequelae.

● ↑ bone mass.

● Decreased growth of giant cell tumors.

● Reduction in hypercalcemia of malignancy that is refractory to bisphosphonate therapy.

BEERS

※ desipramine
(dess-**ip**-ra-meen)
~~Norpramin~~

Classification
Therapeutic: antidepressants
Pharmacologic: tricyclic antidepressants

Indications
Depression. **Unlabeled Use:** Chronic pain syndromes. Anxiety. Insomnia.

Action
Potentiates the effect of serotonin and norepinephrine in the CNS. Has significant anticholinergic properties. **Therapeutic Effects:** Antidepressant action (may develop only over several wk).

Pharmacokinetics
Absorption: Well absorbed from the GI tract.
Distribution: Widely distributed.
Protein Binding: 90–92%.
Metabolism and Excretion: Mostly metabolized by the liver by the CYP2D6 isoenzyme; one metabolite is pharmacologically active (2-hydroxydesipramine); ※ the CYP2D6 enzyme system exhibits genetic polymorphism; ~7% of population may be poor metabolizers (PMs) and may have significantly ↑ desipramine concentrations and an ↑ risk of adverse effects. Small amounts enter breast milk.

Half-life: 12–27 hr.

TIME/ACTION PROFILE (antidepressant effect)

ROUTE	ONSET	PEAK	DURATION
PO	2–3 wk	2–6 wk	days–wk

Contraindications/Precautions
Contraindicated in: Angle-closure glaucoma; Recent MI, HF, known history of QTc interval prolongation.

Use Cautiously in: Pre-existing cardiovascular disease; Family history of sudden death, cardiac arrhythmias, or conduction disturbances; Prostatic hyperplasia (↑ susceptibility to urinary retention); History of seizures (threshold may be ↓ seizures may precede the development of cardiac arrhythmias or death); May ↑ risk of suicide attempt/ideation especially during early treatment or dose adjustment; risk may be greater in children or adolescents; OB: Use during pregnancy only if potential maternal benefit outweighs risk to fetus; Lactation: Use while breastfeeding only if potential maternal benefit outweighs risk to infant; Pedi: Children <12 yr (safety not established); Geri: Appears on Beers list. ↑ risk of adverse reactions in older adults, including falls secondary to sedative and anticholinergic effects and orthostatic hypotension. Avoid use in older adults.

Adverse Reactions/Side Effects
CV: hypotension, ARRHYTHMIAS, ECG changes. **Derm:** photosensitivity. **EENT:** blurred vision, dry eyes. **Endo:** changes in blood glucose, gynecomastia. **GI:** constipation, dry mouth, hepatitis, paralytic ileus. **GU:** ↓ libido, urinary retention. **Hemat:** blood dyscrasias. **Metab:** ↑ appetite, weight gain. **Neuro:** drowsiness, fatigue.

Interactions
Drug-Drug: Desipramine is metabolized in the liver by the CYP2D6 isoenzyme and its action may be affected by drugs that compete for metabolism or alter the activity of this enzyme including other **antidepressants**, **phenothiazines**, **carbamazepine**, **class 1C antiarrhythmics** (**propafenone** or **flecainide**); when used concurrently dose ↓ of one or the other or both may be necessary. Concurrent use of other drugs that inhibit the activity of the enzyme, including **cimetidine**, **quinidine**, **amiodarone**, and **ritonavir**, may result in ↑ effects. May cause hypotension, tachycardia, and potentially fatal reactions when used with **MAO inhibitors** (avoid concurrent use—discontinue 2 wk prior to). Concurrent use with **SSRIs** may result in ↑ toxicity and should be avoided (fluoxetine should be stopped 5 wk before). Concurrent use with **clonidine** may result in hypertensive crisis and should be avoided. **Phenytoin** may ↓ levels and effectiveness; ↑ doses of desipramine may be required to treat depression. Concurrent use with **levodopa** may result in delayed/↓ absorption of levodopa or hypertension. Blood levels and effects may be ↓ by **rifampin**, **carbamazepine**, and **barbi-**

turates. Concurrent use with **moxifloxacin** ↑ risk of adverse cardiovascular reactions. ↑ CNS depression with other **CNS depressants** including **alcohol, antihistamines, clonidine, opioid analgesics,** and **sedative/hypnotics. Barbiturates** may alter blood levels and effects. **Adrenergic** and **anticholinergic** side effects may be ↑ with other **agents having these properties. Hormonal contraceptives** ↑ levels and may cause toxicity. **Cigarette smoking** may ↑ metabolism and alter effects.

Drug-Natural Products: Concomitant use of **kava-kava, valerian,** or **chamomile** can ↑ CNS depression. ↑ anticholinergic effects with **jimson weed** and **scopolia.**

Route/Dosage
PO (Adults): 100–200 mg/day as a single dose or in divided doses (up to 300 mg/day).
PO (Geriatric Patients): 25–50 mg/day in divided doses (up to 150 mg/day).
PO (Children >12 yr): 25–50 mg/day in divided doses, may ↑ as needed up to 100 mg/day.
PO (Children 6–12 yr): 10–30 mg/day (1–5 mg/kg/day) in divided doses.

Availability (generic available)
Tablets: 10 mg, 25 mg, 50 mg, 75 mg, 100 mg, 150 mg.

NURSING IMPLICATIONS
Assessment
● Monitor for weight gain. Obtain weight and BMI initially and periodically during therapy.
● Refer as appropriate for nutrition/weight management and medical management.
● Monitor BP and pulse prior to and during initial therapy. Notify health care professional of decreases in BP (10–20 mm Hg) or sudden increase in pulse rate. Monitor ECG prior to and periodically during therapy in patients taking high doses or with a history of cardiovascular disease.
● **Depression:** Monitor mental status (orientation, mood, behavior) frequently. Assess for suicidal tendencies, especially during early therapy. Restrict amount of drug available to patient.
● Assess mental status and mood changes, especially during initial few mo of therapy and during dose changes. Risk may be increased in children, adolescents, and adults ≤24 yrs. Inform health care professional if patient demonstrates significant increase in signs of depression (depressed mood, loss of interest in usual activities, significant change in weight and/or appetite, insomnia or hypersomnia, psychomotor agitation or retardation, increased fatigue, feelings of guilt or worthlessness, slowed thinking or impaired concentration, suicide attempt or suicidal ideation). Restrict amount of drug available to patient.

● **Pain:** Assess intensity, quality, and location of pain periodically during therapy.

Lab Test Considerations
● Assess leukocyte and differential blood counts, liver function, and serum glucose periodically. May cause an ↑ serum bilirubin and alkaline phosphatase. May cause bone marrow depression. Serum glucose may be ↑ or ↓.
● Serum levels may be monitored in patients who fail to respond to usual therapeutic dose.
● Assess fasting blood glucose and cholesterol levels for overweight/obese individuals.

Implementation
● Do not confuse despiramine with disopyramide.
● Begin dose increases at bedtime due to sedation. Dose titration is a slow process; may take wks to mos. May give entire dose at bedtime.
● When discontinuing, taper to avoid withdrawal effects. Reduce dose by half for 3 days then reduce again by half for 3 days, then discontinue; may require 2–4 wk to discontinue.
● **PO:** Administer medication with or immediately after a meal to minimize gastric upset. Tablet may be crushed and given with food or fluids.

Patient/Family Teaching
● Instruct patient to take desipramine as directed. Take missed doses as soon as possible unless almost time for next dose; if regimen is a single dose at bedtime, do not take in the morning because of side effects. Advise patient that drug effects may not be noticed for at least 2 wk. Abrupt discontinuation may cause nausea; vomiting; diarrhea; headache; trouble sleeping, with vivid dreams; and irritability; decrease dose gradually. Instruct patient to read the *Medication Guide* prior to starting and with each Rx refill in case of changes.
● May cause drowsiness and blurred vision. Caution patient to avoid driving and other activities requiring alertness until response to drug is known.
● Orthostatic hypotension, sedation, and confusion are common during early therapy, especially in the elderly. Protect patient from falls. Institute fall precautions. Advise patient to make position changes slowly.
● Advise patient to avoid alcohol or other CNS depressant drugs, including opioids, during and for 3–7 days after therapy has been discontinued.
● Advise patient, family, and caregivers to look for suicidality, especially during early therapy or dose changes. Notify health care professional immediately if thoughts about suicide or dying, attempts to commit suicide, new or worse depression or anxiety, agitation or restlessness, panic attacks, insomnia, new or worse irritability, aggressiveness, acting on dangerous impulses, mania, or other changes in mood or behavior occur.

- Instruct patient to notify health care professional if urinary retention, dry mouth, or constipation persists. Sugarless candy or gum may diminish dry mouth, and an increase in fluids or bulk may prevent constipation. If symptoms persist, dose reduction or discontinuation may be necessary. Consult health care professional if dry mouth persists for more than 2 wk.
- Caution patient to use sunscreen and protective clothing to prevent photosensitivity reactions.
- Inform patient of need to monitor dietary intake. Increase in appetite may lead to undesired weight gain.
- Alert patient that medication may turn urine blue-green in color.
- Advise patient to notify health care professional of medication regimen prior to treatment or surgery.
- Rep: Advise females of reproductive potential to notify health care professional if pregnancy is planned or suspected or if breastfeeding. Enroll pregnant patients in National Pregnancy Registry for Antidepressants at 1-844-405-6185 or http://womensmentalhealth.org/clinical-and-researchprograms/pregnancyregistry/antidepressants to monitor pregnancy outcomes in women exposed to antidepressants; enroll as early as possible.
- Therapy for depression is usually prolonged. Emphasize the importance of follow-up exams to monitor effectiveness and side effects and to improve coping skills.

Evaluation/Desired Outcomes
- Increased sense of well-being.
- Renewed interest in surroundings.
- Increased appetite.
- Improved energy level.
- Improved sleep.
- Decrease in chronic pain symptoms.
- Full therapeutic effects may be seen 2–6 wk after initiating therapy.

BEERS

desmopressin
(des-moe-**press**-in)
❋Bipazen, DDAVP, ❋DDAVP Melt, Nocdurna, ❋Octostim
Classification
Therapeutic: hormones
Pharmacologic: antidiuretic hormones

Indications
PO, SL, SUBQ, IV, Intranasal: Central diabetes insipidus caused by a deficiency of vasopressin. **IV:** Bleeding in certain types of hemophilia and von Willebrand's disease. **Intranasal, SL:** Nocturia due to nocturnal polyuria in patients who awaken ≥2 times per night to void (Nocdurna only). **PO, SL:** Primary nocturnal enuresis.

Action
An analogue of naturally occurring vasopressin (antidiuretic hormone). Primary action is enhanced reabsorption of water in the kidneys. **Therapeutic Effects:** Prevention of nocturnal enuresis. Reduction in number of episodes of nocturia. Maintenance of appropriate body water content in diabetes insipidus. Control of bleeding in certain types of hemophilia or von Willebrand's disease.

Pharmacokinetics
Absorption: <1% absorbed following oral or SL administration; nasal solution 10–20% absorbed; nasal spray 3–4% absorbed.
Distribution: Distribution not fully known.
Metabolism and Excretion: Primarily excreted in urine.
Half-life: *PO:* 1.5–2.5 hr; *SL:* 2.8 hr; *IV:* 75 min (↑ in renal impairment); *Intranasal:* 1.8–3.5 hr.

TIME/ACTION PROFILE (PO, intranasal = antidiuretic effect; IV = effect on factor VIII activity)

ROUTE	ONSET	PEAK	DURATION
PO	1 hr	4–7 hr	unknown
SL	unknown	unknown	unknown
Intranasal	1 hr	1–5 hr	8–20 hr
IV	within min	15–30 min	3 hr†

†4–24 hr in mild hemophilia A.

Contraindications/Precautions
Contraindicated in: Hypersensitivity; Hypersensitivity to chlorobutanol; Patients with severe type I, type IIB, or platelet-type (pseudo) von Willebrand's disease, hemophilia A with factor VIII levels <5%, or hemophilia B; Renal impairment (CCr <50 mL/min); Current or a history of hyponatremia; Polydipsia (Nocdurna only); Concurrent use with loop diuretics or systemic/inhaled glucocorticoids (Nocdurna only); Known or suspected syndrome of inappropriate antidiuretic hormone secretion (Nocdurna only); Conditions that can lead to electrolyte or fluid imbalances, including gastroenteritis, salt-wasting nephropathies, or infection (Nocdurna only); HF (New York Heart Association class II-IV) (Nocdurna only); Uncontrolled hypertension (Nocdurna only); OB: Nocdurna not recommended for treatment of nocturia in pregnancy.
Use Cautiously in: Angina pectoris; Hypertension; Patients at risk for hyponatremia; Patients at risk for ↑ intracranial hypertension (Nocdurna only); Urinary retention (Nocdurna only); Women (↑ risk of hyponatremia; require ↓ dose) (Nocdurna only); Patients who require use of other intranasal medications; Pedi: Safety and effectiveness not established in children (Nocdurna only); Geri: Appears on Beers list. ↑ risk of hyponatremia in older adults. Avoid use for treatment of nocturia or nocturnal polyuria in older adults.

Adverse Reactions/Side Effects
CV: edema, hypertension, hypotension, tachycardia (large IV doses only). **Derm:** flushing. **EENT:** *intrana-*

sal: epistaxis, nasal congestion, nasal discomfort, rhinitis, sneezing. **F and E:** HYPONATREMIA. **GI:** dry mouth, mild abdominal cramps, nausea. **GU:** vulval pain. **Local:** phlebitis at IV site. **MS:** back pain. **Neuro:** dizziness, drowsiness, headache, listlessness, SEIZURES. **Resp:** dyspnea.

Interactions

Drug-Drug: Loop diuretics, systemic glucocorticoids, or inhaled glucocorticoids ↑ risk of severe hyponatremia; concurrent use with Nocdurna contraindicated. Carbamazepine, chlorpromazine, lamotrigine, NSAIDs, opioids, SSRIs, sulfonylureas, TCAs, or thiazide diuretics may ↑ risk of fluid retention and hyponatremia. Demeclocycline, lithium, or norepinephrine may diminish the antidiuretic response to desmopressin. Large doses may enhance the effects of vasopressors.

Route/Dosage

Primary Nocturnal Enuresis
PO (Adults and Children ≥6 yr): 0.2 mg at bedtime; may be titrated up to 0.6 mg at bedtime to achieve desired response.
SL (Adults and Children): 120 mcg 1 hr before bedtime; may be titrated up to 360 mcg at bedtime to achieve desired response.

Diabetes Insipidus
PO (Adults and Children): 0.05 mg twice daily; adjusted as needed (usual range: 0.1–1.2 mg/day for adults or 0.1–0.8 mg/day for children in 2–3 divided doses).
SL (Adults and Children): 60 mcg 3 times daily; adjusted as needed (usual range: 120–720 mcg/day in 2–3 divided doses).
Intranasal (Adults and Children ≥12 yr): *DDAVP:* 5–40 mcg (0.05–0.4 mL) in 1–3 divided doses.
Intranasal (Children 3 mo–12 yr): *DDAVP:* 5–30 mcg (0.05–0.3 mL) in 1–2 divided doses.
SUBQ, IV (Adults and Children ≥12 yr): 2–4 mcg/day in 2 divided doses.
SUBQ, IV (Children <12 yr): 0.1–1 mcg/day in 1–2 divided doses.

Hemophilia A/von Willebrand's Disease
IV (Adults and Children >3 mo): 0.3 mcg/kg, repeated as needed.

Nocturia
SL (Adults): *Women:* 27.7 mcg 1 hr before bedtime; *Men:* 55.3 mcg 1 hr before bedtime.

Availability (generic available)
Tablets: 0.1 mg, 0.2 mg. **Sublingual tablet (Nocdurna):** 27.7 mcg, 55.3 mcg, ✹ 60 mcg, ✹ 120 mcg. **Nasal spray:** 10 mcg/spray in 5-mL bottle (contains 50 sprays). **Solution for injection:** 4 mcg/mL, ✹ 15 mcg/mL.

NURSING IMPLICATIONS

Assessment
- Restrict free water intake and monitor for hyponatremia.
- **Nocturnal Enuresis:** Monitor frequency of enuresis during therapy. Use cautiously in patients at risk for water intoxication with hyponatremia.
- Do not use intranasal form for nocturnal enuresis.
- **Nocturia:** Assess for possible causes of nocturia (adults who awaken at least 2 times per night to void), including excessive fluid intake before bedtime, and address other treatable causes of nocturia.
- **Diabetes Insipidus:** Monitor serum sodium, urine and plasma osmolality and urine volume frequently. Assess patient for symptoms of dehydration (excessive thirst, dry skin and mucous membranes, tachycardia, poor skin turgor). Weigh patient daily and assess for edema.
- **Hemophilia:** Monitor plasma factor VIII coagulant, factor VIII antigen, and ristocetin cofactor. May also assess activated partial thromboplastin time (aPTT) for hemophilia A and skin bleeding time for von Willebrand's disease. Assess patient for signs of bleeding.
- Monitor BP and pulse during IV infusion.
- Monitor intake and output and adjust fluid intake (especially in children and elderly) to avoid overhydration in patients receiving desmopressin for hemophilia.

Lab Test Considerations
- Begin *Nocdurna* with a normal serum sodium level. Determine that serum sodium concentration is normal before starting or resuming *Nocdurna*, within 1 wk, 1 mo after starting, and periodically during therapy. Patients ≥65 yrs and older and patients at ↑ risk of hyponatremia may require more frequent monitoring. May need to hold or discontinue therapy if hyponatremia occurs.
- *Nocdurna:* Obtain a 24-hr urine collection to confirm diagnosis of nocturnal polyuria before starting therapy.

Toxicity and Overdose
- Signs and symptoms of water intoxication include confusion, drowsiness, headache, weight gain, difficulty urinating, seizures, and coma.
- Treatment of overdose includes decreasing dose and, if symptoms are severe, administration of furosemide.

Implementation
- Do not confuse desmopressin with vasopressin.
- IV desmopressin has 10 times the antidiuretic effect of intranasal desmopressin.
- **PO:** Begin oral doses 12 hr after last intranasal dose. Monitor response closely.
- **SL:** Administer 1 hr before bedtime. Place tablet under tongue until dissolved completely. *Nocdurna:*

✹ = Canadian drug name. ⌘ = Genetic implication. ~~Strikethrough~~ = Discontinued. CAPITALS = life-threatening. <u>Underline</u> = most frequent.

Limit fluid intake for at least 1 hr before until 8 hrs after administration. Use without fluid reduction may lead to fluid retention and hyponatremia.
- **Diabetes Insipidus:** Parenteral dose for antidiuretic effect is administered IV push or SUBQ.
- **Hemophilia:** Parenteral dose for control of bleeding is administered via IV infusion. If used preoperatively, administer 30 min prior to procedure.

IV Administration
- **IV Push:** (for diabetes insipidus). *Dilution:* Administer undiluted. *Concentration:* 4 mcg/mL. *Rate:* Administer over 1 min.
- **Intermittent Infusion (for hemophilia and von Willebrand's disease):** *Dilution:* Dilute each dose in 50 mL of 0.9% NaCl for adults and children >10 kg and in 10 mL in children weighing <10 kg. Inspect solution; do not administer solutions that are cloudy, discolored, or contain particulate matter. *Concentration:* Maximum 0.5 mcg/mL. *Rate:* Infuse slowly over 15–30 min.
- **Y-Site Compatibility:** naloxone.
- **Intranasal** If intranasal dose is used preoperatively, administer 2 hr before procedure.

Patient/Family Teaching
- Explain purpose of desmopressin to patient.
- Advise patient to notify health care professional if bleeding is not controlled or if headache, dyspnea, heartburn, nausea, abdominal cramps, vulval pain, or severe nasal congestion or irritation occurs.
- Caution patient to avoid concurrent use of alcohol with this medication.
- Instruct patient to notify health care professional of all Rx or OTC medications, vitamins, or herbal products being taken and to consult with health care professional before taking other medications.
- Rep: Advise females of reproductive potential to notify health care professional if pregnancy is planned or suspected or if breastfeeding.
- **Diabetes Insipidus:** If nasal spray is used, prime pump prior to first use by pressing down 4 times. Caution patient that nasal spray should not be used beyond the labeled number of sprays; subsequent sprays may not deliver accurate dose. Do not attempt to transfer remaining solution to another bottle. Instruct patient to take missed doses as soon as remembered but not if it is almost time for the next dose. Do not double doses. Advise patient that rhinitis or upper respiratory infection may decrease effectiveness of this therapy. If increased urine output occurs, patient should contact health care professional for dose adjustment. Patients with diabetes insipidus should carry identification at all times describing disease process and medication regimen.
- **Nocturia:** Instruct patient to place tablet under tongue 1 hr before bedtime and empty bladder immediately before bedtime.
- Advise patient to limit fluid intake before bedtime and to avoid caffeine and alcohol before bedtime.

- Advise patient to notify health care professional immediately if signs and symptoms of hyponatremia (headache, feeling restless, drowsiness, muscle cramps, nausea or vomiting, fatigue, dizziness, change in mental condition [hallucinations, confusion, decreased awareness or alertness]) occur.
- Instruct patient to notify health care professional if fever, infection, or diarrhea occurs. May need to hold medication.

Evaluation/Desired Outcomes
- Decreased frequency of nocturnal enuresis.
- Decrease in urine volume.
- Relief of polydipsia.
- Increased urine osmolality.
- Control of bleeding in hemophilia and von Willebrand's disease.
- Reduced frequency of episodes of nocturia.

desonide, See CORTICOSTEROIDS (TOPICAL/LOCAL).

desoximetasone, See CORTICOSTEROIDS (TOPICAL/LOCAL).

BEERS

desvenlafaxine
(**des**-ven-la-**fax**-een)
~~Khedezla, Pristiq~~
Classification
Therapeutic: antidepressants
Pharmacologic: selective serotonin/norepinephrine reuptake inhibitors

Indications
Major depressive disorder.

Action
Inhibits serotonin and norepinephrine reuptake in the CNS. **Therapeutic Effects:** Decrease in depressive symptomatology, with fewer relapses/recurrences.

Pharmacokinetics
Absorption: 80% absorbed following oral administration.
Distribution: Widely distributed to tissues.
Metabolism and Excretion: 55% metabolized by the liver, 45% excreted unchanged in urine.
Half-life: 10 hr.

TIME/ACTION PROFILE (plasma concentrations)

ROUTE	ONSET	PEAK	DURATION
PO	unknown	7.5 hr	24 hr

Contraindications/Precautions
Contraindicated in: Hypersensitivity to venlafaxine or desvenlafaxine; Concurrent use of MAO inhibitors or

MAO-like drugs (linezolid or methylene blue); Should not be used concurrently with venlafaxine.

Use Cautiously in: Untreated cerebrovascular or cardiovascular disease, including untreated hypertension (control BP before initiating therapy); Bipolar disorder (may activate mania/hypomania); Moderate or severe renal impairment; History of seizures or neurologic impairment; Moderate or severe hepatic impairment; Angle-closure glaucoma; OB: Safety not established in pregnancy; Lactation: Use while breastfeeding only if potential maternal benefit justifies potential risk to infant; Pedi: ↑ risk of suicidal thinking and behavior (suicidality) in children and adolescents with major depressive disorder and other psychiatric disorders; Geri: Appears on Beers list. May worsen or cause syndrome of inappropriate antidiuretic hormone (SIADH) secretion and/or hyponatremia in older adults. Use with caution in older adults and closely monitor sodium concentrations when starting therapy or ↑ dose .

Adverse Reactions/Side Effects

CV: hypertension. **Derm:** sweating, ERYTHEMA MULTIFORME, STEVENS-JOHNSON SYNDROME (SJS), TOXIC EPIDERMAL NECROLYSIS. **EENT:** ↑ intraocular pressure, mydriasis. **Endo:** SIADH. **F and E:** hyponatremia. **GI:** ↓ appetite, constipation, nausea, PANCREATITIS. **GU:** ↓ libido, delayed/absent orgasm, ejaculatory delay/failure, erectile dysfunction. **Hemat:** BLEEDING. **Metab:** hyperlipidemia. **Neuro:** anxiety, dizziness, drowsiness, insomnia, headache, NEUROLEPTIC MALIGNANT SYNDROME, SEIZURES, SUICIDAL THOUGHTS, teeth grinding, vertigo. **Resp:** eosinophilic pneumonia, interstitial lung disease. **Misc:** discontinuation syndrome, SEROTONIN SYNDROME.

Interactions

Drug-Drug: Concurrent use with **MAO inhibitors** may result in serious, potentially fatal reactions (wait at least 2 wk after stopping MAO inhibitor before initiating desvenlafaxine; wait at least 1 wk after stopping desvenlafaxine before starting an MAO inhibitor). Concurrent use with **MAO-inhibitor like drugs**, such as **linezolid** or **methylene blue** may ↑ risk of serotonin syndrome; concurrent use contraindicated; do not start therapy in patients receiving **linezolid** or **methylene blue**; if **linezolid** or **methylene blue** need to be started in a patient receiving desvenlafaxine, immediately discontinue desvenlafaxine and monitor for signs/symptoms of serotonin syndrome for 2 wk or until 24 hr after last dose of linezolid or methylene blue, whichever comes first (may resume desvenlafaxine therapy 24 hr after last dose of linezolid or methylene blue). ↑ risk of bleeding with **NSAIDs, aspirin, clopidogrel, prasugrel, ticagrelor, dabigatran, apixaban, edoxaban, rivaroxaban,** or **warfarin**. Use cautiously with other **CNS-active drugs,** including **alcohol** or **sedative/hypnotics;** effects of combination are unknown. Drugs that affect serotonergic neurotransmitter

systems, including **tricyclic antidepressants, SNRIs, fentanyl, lithium, buspirone, tramadol, meperidine, methadone, amphetamines,** and **triptans** ↑ risk of serotonin syndrome. **Ketoconazole** may ↑ the effects of desvenlafaxine. May ↑ levels of CYP2D6 substrates, including **desipramine, atomoxetine, dextromethorphan, metoprolol, nebivolol, perphenazine,** and **tolterodine;** if using desvenlafaxine at dose of 400 mg/day, ↓ dose of CYP2D6 substrate by 50%.

Route/Dosage

PO (Adults): 50 mg once daily (range = 50–400 mg/day).

Renal Impairment
PO (Adults): *CCr 30–50 mL/min:* 50 mg once daily; *CCr <30 mL/min:* 50 mg every other day or 25 mg once daily.

Hepatic Impairment
PO (Adults): *Moderate-to-severe hepatic impairment:* 50 mg once daily (not to exceed 100 mg/day).

Availability (generic available)
Extended-release tablets: 25 mg, 50 mg, 100 mg.

NURSING IMPLICATIONS

Assessment

- Assess mental status and mood changes, especially during initial few mo of therapy and during dose changes. Inform health care professional if patient demonstrates significant increase in signs of depression (depressed mood, loss of interest in usual activities, significant change in weight and/or appetite, insomnia or hypersomnia, psychomotor agitation or retardation, increased fatigue, feelings of guilt or worthlessness, slowed thinking or impaired concentration, suicide attempt or suicidal ideation).
- Assess suicidal tendencies, especially in early therapy. Restrict amount of drug available to patient. Risk may be increased in children, adolescents, and adults ≤24 yr.
- Monitor BP before and periodically during therapy. Sustained hypertension may be dose related; decrease dose or discontinue therapy if this occurs.
- Monitor appetite and nutritional intake; weigh weekly. Report continued weight loss. Adjust diet as tolerated to support nutritional status.
- Assess for serotonin syndrome (mental changes [agitation, hallucinations, coma], autonomic instability [tachycardia, labile BP, hyperthermia], neuromuscular aberrations [hyperreflexia, incoordination], and/or GI symptoms [nausea, vomiting, diarrhea]), especially in patients taking other serotonergic drugs (SSRIs, SNRIs, triptans).
- Assess patient for skin rash frequently during therapy. Discontinue at first sign of rash; may be life-

threatening. SJS may develop. Treat symptomatically; may recur once treatment is stopped.

• Assess sexual function before starting desvenlafaxine. Assess for changes in sexual function during treatment, including timing of onset; patient may not report.

Lab Test Considerations

• May cause ↑ fasting serum total cholesterol, LDL cholesterol, and triglycerides.

• May cause transient proteinuria, not usually associated with ↑ BUN or serum creatinine.

• May cause hyponatremia.

• May cause false-positive immunoassay screening tests for phencyclidine and amphetamine.

Implementation

• **PO:** Administer at the same time each day, with or without food. *DNC:* Swallow tablets whole; do not crush, break, chew, or dissolve.

Patient/Family Teaching

• Instruct patient to take medication exactly as directed at the same time each day. Take missed doses as soon as possible unless almost time for next dose. Do not double doses or discontinue abruptly; gradually decrease before discontinuation to prevent dizziness, nausea, headache, irritability, insomnia, diarrhea, anxiety, fatigue, abnormal dreams, and hyperhidrosis; discontinuation may take several mo.

• Advise patient, family, and caregivers to look for suicidality, especially during early therapy or dose changes. Notify health care professional immediately if thoughts about suicide or dying, attempts to commit suicide, new or worse depression or anxiety, agitation or restlessness, panic attacks, insomnia, new or worse irritability, aggressiveness, acting on dangerous impulses, mania, or other changes in mood or behavior or if symptoms of serotonin syndrome occur.

• May cause drowsiness or dizziness. Caution patient to avoid driving or other activities requiring alertness until response to the drug is known.

• Caution patient to avoid taking alcohol or other CNS-depressant drugs, including opioids during therapy and of increased risk of bleeding with concomitant use of NSAIDs, aspirin, or other drugs that affect coagulation. Instruct patient to notify health care professional of all Rx or OTC medications, vitamins, or herbal products being taken, especially St. John's wort, and to consult health care professional before taking other Rx, OTC, or herbal products.

• Instruct patient to notify health care professional if signs of allergy (rash, hives, swelling, difficulty breathing) occur.

• Inform patient that desvenlafaxine may cause symptoms of sexual dysfunction. In males, ejaculatory delay or failure, decreased libido, and erectile dysfunction may occur. In female patients, may result in decreased libido and delayed or absent orgasm. Advise patient to notify health care professional if symptoms occur.

• Inform patient that remains of tablet may pass into stool, but medication has already been absorbed.

• Rep: May cause fetal harm. Advise females of reproductive potential to notify health care professional if pregnancy is planned or suspected or if breastfeeding. Exposure to desvenlafaxine in mid- to late pregnancy may increase risk for preeclampsia and exposure near delivery may increase risk of postpartum hemorrhage. Fetal exposure late in pregnancy may lead to increased risk for neonatal complications requiring prolonged hospitalization, respiratory support, and tube feeding. Monitor neonates exposed to desvenlafaxine in the third trimester for drug discontinuation syndrome. Inform patient of pregnancy exposure registry to monitor pregnancy outcomes in women exposed to antidepressants during pregnancy. Register patients by calling the National Pregnancy Registry for Antidepressants at 1-866-961-2388.

• Emphasize the importance of follow-up exams to monitor progress.

Evaluation/Desired Outcomes

• Increased sense of well-being.

• Renewed interest in surroundings. Need for therapy should be periodically reassessed. Therapy is usually continued for several mo.

deucravacitinib
(doo-krav-a-**sye**-ti-nib)
   Sotyktu
Classification
Therapeutic: antipsoriatics
Pharmacologic: kinase inhibitors

Indications

Moderate-to-severe plaque psoriasis in patients who are candidates for systemic therapy or phototherapy.

Action

Acts as a inhibitor of tyrosine kinase 2. Its exact mechanism for effect in plaque psoriasis is unknown. **Therapeutic Effects:** Decreased formation and spread of plaques.

Pharmacokinetics

Absorption: Well absorbed (99%) following oral administration.

Distribution: Extensively distributed to tissues.

Protein Binding: 82–90%.

Metabolism and Excretion: Primarily metabolized by the liver via the CYP1A2 isoenzyme to form an active metabolite (BMT-153261). Also metabolized by CYP2B6, CYP2D6, carboxylesterase 2, and UGT1A9. 26% and 13% excreted in feces and urine, respectively, as unchanged drug.

Half-life: 10 hr.

TIME/ACTION PROFILE (plasma concentrations)

ROUTE	ONSET	PEAK	DURATION
PO	unknown	2–3 hr	24 hr

Contraindications/Precautions

Contraindicated in: Hypersensitivity; Active or serious infection (including tuberculosis [TB] and hepatitis B/C); Severe hepatic impairment.

Use Cautiously in: Chronic or recurrent infection, exposure to tuberculosis, history of opportunistic infection, underlying conditions that predispose to infection; Malignancy (other than successfully treated non-melanoma skin cancer); OB: Safety not established in pregnancy; Lactation: Use while breastfeeding only if potential maternal benefit justifies potential risk to infant; Pedi: Safety and effectiveness not established in children.

Adverse Reactions/Side Effects

Derm: acne. **GI:** ↑ liver enzymes, mouth ulcers. **Metab:** hypertriglyceridemia. **MS:** ↑ creatine kinase, RHABDOMYOLYSIS. **Misc:** INFECTION, HYPERSENSITIVITY REACTIONS (including angioedema), MALIGNANCY (including lymphoma).

Interactions

Drug-Drug: Avoid concurrent use with **live vaccines**.

Route/Dosage

PO (Adults): 6 mg once daily.

Availability

Tablets: 6 mg.

NURSING IMPLICATIONS

Assessment

- Assess skin lesions and concurrent symptoms (absence of itch, pain, burning, stinging, and skin tightness) before and periodically during therapy.
- Monitor for signs and symptoms of hypersensitivity (feeling faint; swelling of face, eyelids, lips, mouth, tongue, or throat; trouble breathing or throat tightness; chest tightness; skin rash; hives). If symptoms occur, discontinue therapy.
- Assess for signs and symptoms of infection (fever, sweats, chills, muscle aches, weight loss, cough, shortness of breath, blood in phlegm [mucus], warm, red, or painful skin or sores on body different from psoriasis, diarrhea or stomach pain, burning during urination or urinating more often than normal, feeling very tired) during and after treatment. Administer diagnostic tests and begin antimicrobial therapy promptly. If serious infection occurs, discontinue therapy until infection resolved. May cause reactivation of herpes virus infection.

Lab Test Considerations

- May cause rhabdomyolysis and asymptomatic CK elevation. Discontinue deucravacitinib if markedly elevated CK levels occur or myopathy is diagnosed or suspected.
- Periodically evaluate serum triglycerides. May cause hyperlipidemia.
- Assess liver enzymes at baseline and periodically thereafter in patients with known or suspected liver disease. If increases in liver enzymes occur and drug-induced liver injury is suspected, interrupt therapy until a diagnosis of liver injury is excluded.

Implementation

- Evaluate for acute and latent TB before starting therapy. If positive, begin therapy for TB before starting deucravacitinib.
- Update age-appropriate immunizations before starting therapy, including prophylactic herpes zoster vaccination. Avoid use of live vaccines during therapy.
- **PO:** Administer tablet once daily without regard to food. *DNC:* Swallow tablets whole, do not break, crush, or chew.

Patient/Family Teaching

- Instruct patient to take deucravacitinib as directed. Advise patient to read *Medication Guide* before starting therapy and with each Rx refill in case of changes.
- Instruct patients to promptly report any unexplained muscle pain, tenderness or weakness, particularly if accompanied by malaise or fever.
- Advise patient to avoid live vaccines during therapy.
- Advise patient to notify health care professional of all Rx or OTC medications, vitamins, or herbal products being taken and to consult with health care professional before taking other medications.
- Inform patients that medication may increase their risk of developing malignancies, including lymphomas.
- Rep: Advise females of reproductive potential to notify health care professional if pregnancy is planned or suspected or if breastfeeding. If pregnancy occurs, report pregnancies to the Bristol-Myers Squibb Company's Adverse Event reporting line at 1-800-721-5072.
- Encourage patient to maintain follow-up lab tests to monitor blood levels.

Evaluation/Desired Outcomes

- Absence or decrease in psoriatic symptoms (absence of itch, pain, burning, stinging, and skin tightness).

dexAMETHasone, See CORTICOSTEROIDS (SYSTEMIC).

℥ **dexlansoprazole**
(dex-lan-**soe**-pra-zole)
Dexilant
Classification
Therapeutic: antiulcer agents
Pharmacologic: proton-pump inhibitors

Indications
Erosive esophagitis. Maintenance of healed erosive esophagitis and relief of heartburn. Treatment of heartburn from nonerosive gastroesophageal reflux disease (GERD).

Action
Binds to an enzyme in the presence of acidic gastric pH, preventing the final transport of hydrogen ions into the gastric lumen. **Therapeutic Effects:** Diminished accumulation of acid in the gastric lumen, with lessened acid reflux.

Pharmacokinetics
Absorption: Well absorbed following oral administration.
Distribution: Unknown.
Protein Binding: 96–99%.
Metabolism and Excretion: Extensively metabolized by the liver, primarily by the CYP2C19 and CYP3A4 isoenzymes; ℥ the CYP2C19 isoenzyme exhibits genetic polymorphism (15–20% of Asian patients and 3–5% of Caucasian and Black patients may be poor metabolizers and may have significantly ↑ dexlansoprazole concentrations and an ↑ risk of adverse effects); no active metabolites. No renal elimination.
Half-life: 1–2 hr.

TIME/ACTION PROFILE (plasma concentrations)

ROUTE	ONSET	PEAK*	DURATION
PO	unknown	1–2 hr (1st); 4–5 hr (2nd)	24 hr

*Reflects effects of delayed release capsule.

Contraindications/Precautions
Contraindicated in: Hypersensitivity to dexlansoprazole or related drugs (benzimidazoles); Severe hepatic impairment; Concurrent use of rilpivirine.
Use Cautiously in: Moderate hepatic impairment; Patients using high doses for >1 yr (↑ risk of hip, wrist, or spine fractures and fundic gland polyps); Patients using therapy for >3 yr (↑ risk of vitamin B$_{12}$ deficiency); Pre-existing risk of hypocalcemia; OB: Safety not established in pregnancy; Lactation: Safety not established in breastfeeding; Pedi: Children <12 yr (safety and effectiveness not established); ↑ risk of heart valve thickening in children <2 yr; Geri: Appears on Beers list. ↑ risk of *Clostridioides difficile* infection, pneumonia, GI malignancies, bone loss, and frac-

tures in older adults. Avoid scheduled use for >8 wk in older adults unless for high-risk patients (e.g., oral corticosteroid or chronic NSAID use) or patients with erosive esophagitis, Barrett's esophagitis, pathological hypersecretory condition, or demonstrated need for maintenance therapy (e.g., failure of H$_2$ antagonist).

Adverse Reactions/Side Effects
Derm: ACUTE GENERALIZED EXANTHEMATOUS PUSTULOSIS, cutaneous lupus erythematosus, DRUG REACTION WITH EOSINOPHILIA AND SYSTEMIC SYMPTOMS (DRESS), STEVENS-JOHNSON SYNDROME (SJS), TOXIC EPIDERMAL NECROLYSIS (TEN). **F and E:** hypocalcemia (especially if treatment duration ≥3 mo), hypokalemia (especially if treatment duration ≥3 mo), hypomagnesemia (especially if treatment duration ≥3 mo). **GI:** abdominal pain, diarrhea, CLOSTRIDIOIDES DIFFICILE-ASSOCIATED DIARRHEA (CDAD), flatulence, fundic gland polyps, nausea, vomiting. **GU:** acute tubulointerstitial nephritis. **Hemat:** vitamin B$_{12}$ deficiency. **MS:** bone fracture. **Misc:** HYPERSENSITIVITY REACTIONS (including anaphylaxis, angioedema, or acute tubulointerstitial nephritis), systemic lupus erythematosus.

Interactions
Drug-Drug: May ↓ absorption of drugs requiring acid pH, including **ketoconazole, itraconazole, atazanavir, nelfinavir, rilpivirine, ampicillin esters, iron salts, erlotinib,** and **mycophenolate mofetil;** concurrent use with rilpivirine contraindicated; avoid concurrent use with atazanavir and nelfinavir. May ↑ levels of **digoxin, methotrexate,** and **tacrolimus.** May ↑ effect of **warfarin.** Hypomagnesemia and hypokalemia ↑ risk of **digoxin** toxicity.

Route/Dosage
PO (Adults and Children ≥12 yr): *Healing of erosive esophagitis:* 60 mg once daily for up to 8 wk; *Maintenance of healed erosive esophagitis:* 30 mg once daily for up to 6 mo (adults) and up to 16 wk (12–17 yr old); *GERD:* 30 mg once daily for 4 wk.

Hepatic Impairment
PO (Adults): *Moderate hepatic impairment:* Not to exceed 30 mg/day.

Availability (generic available)
Delayed-release capsules: 30 mg, 60 mg.

NURSING IMPLICATIONS
Assessment
- Assess patient routinely for epigastric or abdominal pain and for frank or occult blood in stool, emesis, or gastric aspirate.
- Monitor bowel elimination. Diarrhea, abdominal cramping, fever, and bloody stools should be reported to health care professional promptly as a sign of CDAD.
- Monitor for signs and symptoms of decreased renal function (malaise, nausea, anorexia) periodically during therapy. If symptoms occur, discontinue dexlansoprazole and evaluate patient for acute tubulointerstitial nephritis.

- Monitor for severe cutaneous adverse reactions (SJS, TEN, DRESS). Discontinue dexlansoprazole at first signs or symptoms of severe skin reactions and consider further evaluation.

Lab Test Considerations
- May cause abnormal liver function tests, including ↑ AST, ALT, and ↑ or ↓ serum bilirubin.
- May cause ↑ serum creatinine and BUN, ↑ blood glucose, and ↑ serum potassium, and ↓ serum magnesium levels. Consider monitoring magnesium and calcium levels prior to starting and periodically during therapy in patients with a pre-existing risk of hypocalcemia (hypoparathyroidism). Supplement with magnesium and/or calcium as necessary. If hypocalcemia is refractory to treatment, consider discontinuing therapy.
- May cause ↓ platelet levels.
- May also cause ↑ gastrin and total protein levels.
- Monitor INR and prothrombin time in patients taking warfarin.

Implementation
- Do not confuse Dexilant with duloxetine.
- **PO:** May be administered without regard to food. *DNC:* Swallow capsules whole or may be opened and sprinkled on 1 tbsp of applesauce and swallowed immediately, without crushing or chewing, for patients with difficulty swallowing.
- Capsules may be opened and granules emptied into 20 mL water. Withdraw entire mixture into syringe; swirl gently to mix. Administer mixture into mouth or nasogastric tube immediately; do not save for later. Rinse syringe with 10 mL of water twice to ensure all medication administered.
- Administer for shortest time possible to minimize risk of osteoporosis-related fractures and cutaneous or systemic lupus erythematosus.

Patient/Family Teaching
- Instruct patient to take medication as directed for the full course of therapy, even if feeling better. Take missed doses as soon as remembered but not if just before next scheduled dose; do not double doses.
- Advise patient to avoid alcohol, products containing aspirin or NSAIDs, and foods that may cause an increase in GI irritation.
- Advise patient to report onset of black, tarry stools; diarrhea; or abdominal pain to health care professional promptly, especially if accompanied by fever or bloody stools. Do not treat with antidiarrheals without consulting health care professional.
- Advise patient to notify health care professional if signs and symptoms of hypomagnesemia (seizures, dizziness, abnormal or fast heartbeat, jitteriness, jerking movements or shaking [tremors], muscle weakness, spasms of the hands and feet, cramps or muscle aches, spasm of the voice box) occur.

- Instruct patient to notify health care professional of all Rx or OTC medications, vitamins, or herbal products being taken and to consult with health care professional before taking other medications.
- Rep: Advise females of reproductive potential to notify health care professional if pregnancy is planned or suspected or if breastfeeding.

Evaluation/Desired Outcomes
- Decrease in abdominal pain, heartburn, gastric irritation, and bleeding in patients with GERD; may require up to 4 wk of therapy.
- Healing in patients with erosive esophagitis; may require up to 8 wk of therapy for healing and 6 mo of therapy for maintenance.

---

dexmedeTOMIDine
(dex-me-de-**to**-mi-deen)
Igalmi, Precedex
Classification
Therapeutic: sedative/hypnotics
Pharmacologic: alpha adrenergic agonists

Indications
IV: Sedation of initially intubated and mechanically ventilated patients during treatment in an intensive care setting; should not be used for >24 hr. **IV:** Sedation of nonintubated patients before and/or during surgical and other procedures. **Buccal, SL:** Acute treatment of agitation associated with schizophrenia or bipolar I or II disorder.

Action
Acts as a relatively selective alpha-2 adrenergic agonist with sedative properties. **Therapeutic Effects:** Sedation. Decreased agitation.

Pharmacokinetics
Absorption: IV administration results in complete bioavailability. 72% absorbed following SL administration; 82% absorbed following buccal administration.
Distribution: Widely distributed to extravascular tissues.
Protein Binding: 94%.
Metabolism and Excretion: Mostly metabolized by the liver, some metabolism by P450 enzyme system. Metabolites are mostly excreted in urine.
Half-life: *IV:* 2 hr; *SL/buccal:* 2.8 hr.

TIME/ACTION PROFILE (sedation)

ROUTE	ONSET	PEAK	DURATION
IV	rapid	unknown	unknown
SL/buccal	20–30 min	60–90 min	2 hr

Contraindications/Precautions
Contraindicated in: Hypersensitivity; Hypotension; Advanced heart block; Severe left ventricular dysfunc-

tion; History of syncope; QT interval prolongation, arrhythmias, symptomatic bradycardia, hypokalemia, hypomagnesemia, or concurrent use of QT interval prolonging medications.

Use Cautiously in: Hepatic impairment (lower doses may be required); Hypovolemia, diabetes, and/or chronic hypertension (↑ risk of hypotension and bradycardia); OB: Safety not established in pregnancy; Lactation: Use while breastfeeding only if potential maternal benefit justifies potential risk to infant; Pedi: Children <1 mo (safety and effectiveness not established); Geri: ↑ risk of bradycardia and hypotension in older adults (consider dose ↓).

Adverse Reactions/Side Effects

CV: <u>hypotension</u>, BRADYCARDIA, QT interval prolongation, SINUS ARREST, transient hypertension. **GI:** dry mouth, nausea, oral numbness, vomiting. **Hemat:** anemia. **Neuro:** somnolence, dizziness. **Resp:** hypoxia. **Misc:** fever, hyperthermia.

Interactions

Drug-Drug: Sedation is enhanced by **anesthetics**, other **sedative/hypnotics**, and **opioid analgesics**. **QT interval prolonging medications** may ↑ the risk of QT interval prolongation and torsades de pointes; avoid concurrent use.

Drug-Natural Products: Concomitant use of **kava-kava, valerian, skullcap, chamomile,** or **hops** can ↑ CNS depression.

Route/Dosage

ICU Sedation

IV (Adults): *Loading infusion:* 1 mcg/kg over 10 min followed by *Maintenance infusion:* 0.2–0.7 mcg/kg/hr for maximum of 24 hr; rate is adjusted to achieve desired level of sedation.

Procedural Sedation

IV (Adults): *Loading infusion:* 1 mcg/kg (0.5 mcg/kg for ophthalmic surgery or patients >65 yr) over 10 min followed by *maintenance infusion* of 0.6 mcg/kg/hr; rate is adjusted to achieve desired level of sedation (usual range 0.2–1 mcg/kg/hr) (maintenance infusion of 0.7 mcg/kg/hr recommended for fiberoptic intubation until endotracheal tube secured).

IV (Children ≥2 yr): *Loading infusion:* 2 mcg/kg over 10 min followed by *maintenance infusion* of 1.5 mcg/kg/hr; rate is adjusted to achieve desired level of sedation (usual range 0.5–1.5 mcg/kg/hr).

IV (Children 1 mo–<2 yr): *Loading infusion:* 1.5 mcg/kg over 10 min followed by *maintenance infusion* of 1.5 mcg/kg/hr; rate is adjusted to achieve desired level of sedation (usual range 0.5–1.5 mcg/kg/hr).

Acute Treatment of Agitation Associated with Schizophrenia or Bipolar I or II Disorder.

Buccal, SL (Adults <65 yr): *Mild or moderate agitation:* 120 mcg initially; if agitation continues, up to two

additional doses of 60 mcg may be administered ≥2 hours apart (max total dose = 240 mcg/day). *Severe agitation:* 180 mcg initially; if agitation continues, up to two additional doses of 90 mcg may be administered ≥2 hours apart (max total dose = 360 mcg/day).

Buccal, SL (Geriatric Patients ≥65 yr): *Mild, moderate, or severe agitation:* 120 mcg initially; if agitation continues, up to two additional doses of 60 mcg may be administered ≥2 hours apart (max total dose = 240 mcg/day).

Hepatic Impairment

Buccal, SL (Adults): *Mild or moderate hepatic impairment:* Mild or moderate agitation: 90 mcg initially; if agitation continues, up to two additional doses of 60 mcg may be administered ≥2 hours apart (max total dose = 210 mcg/day). Severe agitation: 120 mcg initially; if agitation continues, up to two additional doses of 60 mcg may be administered ≥2 hours apart (max total dose = 240 mcg/day). *Severe hepatic impairment:* Mild or moderate agitation: 60 mcg initially; if agitation continues, up to two additional doses of 60 mcg may be administered ≥2 hours apart (max total dose = 180 mcg/day). Severe agitation: 120 mcg initially; if agitation continues, up to two additional doses of 60 mcg may be administered ≥2 hours apart (max total dose = 240 mcg/day).

Availability (generic available)

Sublingual/buccal film (Igalmi): 120 mcg, 180 mcg. **Premixed infusion (in 0.9% NaCl):** 80 mcg/20 mL, 200 mcg/50 mL, 400 mcg/100 mL, 1000 mcg/250 mL. **Solution for injection:** ✿ 4 mcg/mL, 100 mcg/mL.

NURSING IMPLICATIONS

Assessment

- Assess level of sedation during therapy. Dose is adjusted based on level of sedation.
- Monitor ECG and BP continuously during therapy. May cause hypotension, bradycardia, and sinus arrest.
- Monitor for hypotension, orthostatic hypotension, and bradycardia. Ensure patient is adequately hydrated and keep in sitting or lying position until vital signs are stable. If unable to sit or lie down, take precautions to prevent falls.
- Monitor for signs and symptoms of withdrawal (nausea, vomiting, agitation); may lead to tachycardia and hypertension. Usually occur within 24-48 hr of discontinuing dexmedetomidine. Treat symptomatically.

Toxicity and Overdose
- Atropine IV may be used to modify the vagal tone.

Implementation

- Do not confuse dexmedetomidine with dexamethasone.
- Dexmedetomidine should be administered only in intensive care settings with continuous monitoring.
- A loading dose may not be required when converting patient from another sedative.
- **Buccal, SL:** Administer under the supervision of a health care professional. Monitor vital signs and

alertness after administration to prevent falls and syncope. Open pouch and give to patients. Instruct patient to remove the from pouch with clean dry hands. *For SL dose,* instruct patient to place film under tongue; film will stick in place. Advise patient not to eat or drink for 15 min after SL administration. *For buccal dose,* instruct patient to place film behind lower lip; film will stick in place. Advise patient not to eat or drink for 1 hr after administration. Instruct patient to close their mouth; allow film to dissolve. Do not chew or swallow film.

IV Administration

- **Continuous Infusion:** *Dilution:* To prepare infusion, withdraw 2 mL of dexmedetomidine and add to 48 mL of 0.9% NaCl for a total of 50 mL. *Concentration:* 4 mcg/mL. Shake gently. Solution should be clear; do not administer solutions that are discolored or contain particulate matter. Ampules and vials are for single use only. *Rate:* Administer *loading infusion* over 10 min, followed by *maintenance infusion* of 0.2–0.7 mcg/kg/hr for ICU sedation and 0.2–1.0 mcg/kg/hr for procedural sedation. Adjust dose to achieve desired level of sedation. Administer via infusion pump to ensure accurate rate.

- **Y-Site Compatibility:** acetaminophen, acyclovir, alemtuzumab, allopurinol, amifostine, amikacin, aminophylline, amiodarone, amphotericin B liposome, ampicillin, ampicillin/sulbactam, anidulafungin, argatroban, arsenic trioxide, atropine, azithromycin, aztreonam, bivalirudin, bleomycin, bumetanide, buprenorphine, busulfan, butorphanol, calcium chloride, calcium gluconate, carboplatin, carmustine, caspofungin, cefazolin, cefepime, cefotaxime, cefotetan, cefoxitin, ceftazidime, ceftazidime/avibactam, ceftozolane/tazobactam, ceftriaxone, cefuroxime, chlorpromazine, ciprofloxacin, cisatracurium, cisplatin, clindamycin, cyclophosphamide, cyclosporine, cytarabine, D5W, dacarbazine, dactinomycin, daptomycin, daunorubicin hydrochloride, dexamethasone, dexrazoxane, digoxin, diltiazem, diphenhydramine, dobutamine, docetaxel, dopamine, doxorubicin hydrochloride, doxorubicin liposome, doxycycline, droperidol, enalaprilat, ephedrine, epinephrine, eravacycline, ertapenem, erythromycin, esmolol, etomidate, etoposide, etoposide phosphate, famotidine, fentanyl, fluconazole, fludarabine, fluorouracil, foscarnet, fosphenytoin, furosemide, ganciclovir, gemcitabine, gentamicin, glycopyrrolate, granisetron, haloperidol, heparin, hetastarch, hydrocortisone, hydromorphone, idarubicin, ifosfamide, imipenem/cilastatin, imipenem/cilastatin/relebactam, insulin, regular, isavuconazonium, isoproterenol, ketorolac, labetalol, LR, leucovorin calcium, levofloxacin, lidocaine, linezolid, lorazepam, magnesium sulfate, mannitol, meperidine, meropenem, meropenem/vaborbactam, mesna, methadone, methohexital, methotrexate, methylprednisolone, metoclopramide, metoprolol, metronidazole, midazolam, milrinone, mitomycin, mitoxantrone, morphine, moxifloxacin, mycophenolate, nalbuphine, naloxone, nicardipine, nitroglycerin, nitroprusside, norepinephrine, 0.9% NaCl, octreotide, ondansetron, oritavancin, oxaliplatin, oxytocin, paclitaxel, palonosetron, pamidronate, pemetrexed, pentamidine, pentobarbital, phenobarbital, phenylephrine, piperacillin/tazobactam, plazomicin, potassium acetate, potassium chloride, potassium phosphate, prochlorperazine, promethazine, propofol, propranolol, remifentanil, rocuronium, sodium acetate, sodium bicarbonate, sodium phosphate, succinylcholine, sufentanil, tacrolimus, tedizolid, theophylline, thiopental, thiotepa, tigecycline, tirofiban, tobramycin, topotecan, trimethoprim/sulfamethoxazole, vancomycin, vasopressin, vecuronium, verapamil, vinblastine, vincristine, vinorelbine, voriconazole, zidovudine, zoledronic acid.

- **Y-Site Incompatibility:** amphotericin B deoxycholate, amphotericin B lipid complex, diazepam, gemtuzumab ozogamicin, irinotecan, pantoprazole, phenytoin.

Patient/Family Teaching

- Explain to patient and family the purpose of the medication.
- May cause drowsiness. Caution patient to avoid driving and other activities requiring alertness until response to drug is known.
- Rep: May cause fetal harm. Advise patient to notify health care professional if pregnancy is suspected or if breastfeeding. Advise women to monitor breastfed infants for irritability.

Evaluation/Desired Outcomes

- Sedation for up to 24 hr.
- Decreased agitation.

---

dexrazoxane (dex-ra-**zox**-ane)

~~Totect~~, ✹ Zinecard

Classification
Therapeutic: cardioprotective agents

Indications

Reducing incidence and severity of cardiomyopathy from doxorubicin in women with metastatic breast cancer who have already received a cumulative dose of doxorubicin >300 mg/m^2 and who will continue to receive doxorubicin therapy to maintain tumor control. Treatment of extravasation resulting from IV anthracycline chemotherapy.

Action

Acts as an intracellular chelating agent. **Therapeutic Effects:** Diminishes the cardiotoxic effects of doxorubicin. Decreased damage from extravasation of anthracyclines.

Pharmacokinetics

Absorption: IV administration results in complete bioavailability.
Distribution: Well distributed to tissues.
Metabolism and Excretion: Some metabolism occurs; 42% eliminated in urine.
Half-life: 2.1–2.5 hr.

TIME/ACTION PROFILE (cardioprotective effect)

ROUTE	ONSET	PEAK	DURATION
IV	rapid	unknown	unknown

Contraindications/Precautions

Contraindicated in: Any other type of chemotherapy except other anthracyclines (doxorubicin-like agents); Hepatic impairment (for treatment of extravasation only); OB: Pregnancy; Lactation: Lactation.
Use Cautiously in: Renal impairment (CCr <40 mL/min) (↓ dose); Rep: Women of reproductive potential and men with female partners of reproductive potential; Pedi: Safety and effectiveness not established in children.

Adverse Reactions/Side Effects

GU: ↓ fertility (males). **Hemat:** leukopenia, NEUTROPENIA, thrombocytopenia. **Local:** pain at injection site. **Misc:** HYPERSENSITIVITY REACTIONS (including anaphylaxis and angioedema), MALIGNANCY.

Interactions

Drug-Drug: Myelosuppression may be ↑ by **antineoplastics** or **radiation therapy**. Antitumor effects of concurrent combination chemotherapy with **fluorouracil** and **cyclophosphamide** may be ↓ by dexrazoxane.

Route/Dosage

Cardioprotective
IV (Adults): 10 mg of dexrazoxane/1 mg doxorubicin.
Renal Impairment
IV (Adults): *CCr <40 mL/min:* ↓ dose by 50%.

Extravasation Treatment
IV (Adults): 1000 mg/m² (maximum 2000 mg) given on days 1 and 2, and followed by a dose of 500 mg/m² (maximum 1000 mg) on day 3.
Renal Impairment
IV (Adults): *CCr <40 mL/min:* ↓ dose by 50%.

Availability (generic available)

Lyophilized powder for injection: 250 mg/vial, 500 mg/vial.

NURSING IMPLICATIONS

Assessment

● **Cardioprotective:** Assess extent of cardiomyopathy (cardiomegaly on x ray, basilar rales, S_3 gallop, dyspnea, decline in left ventricular ejection fraction) prior to and periodically during therapy.

● **Extravasation protection:** Assess site of extravasation for pain, burning, swelling, and redness. Assess site during and after therapy until resolution. Dexrazoxane is not effective against the effects of vesicants other than anthracyclines.

Lab Test Considerations
● Verify negative pregnancy test before starting therapy. Monitor CBC and platelet count before each course of therapy and frequently during therapy. Thrombocytopenia, leukopenia, neutropenia, and granulocytopenia from chemotherapy may be more severe at nadir with dexrazoxane therapy.

● Monitor liver function tests periodically during therapy. May cause reversible ↑ of liver enzymes.

Implementation

IV Administration
● Solution should be prepared in a biologic cabinet. Wear gloves, gown, and mask while handling IV medication. Discard IV equipment in specially designated containers.

● Solution is slightly yellow. Do not administer solutions that are discolored or contain particulate matter. Reconstituted solution and diluted solution are stable in an IV bag for 6 hr at room temperature or if refrigerated. Discard unused solutions.

● **Extravasation Protection:** Administer as soon as possible within 6 hr of extravasation in a large caliber vein in an extremity/area other than the one affected by the extravasation. Remove cooling procedures, such as ice packs, at least 15 min before administration to allow sufficient blood flow to area of extravasation. Start treatment on Day 2 and Day 3 at same hr (+/- 3 hr) as on first day.

● **Intermittent Infusion:** *Reconstitution:* Reconstitute with 50 mL sterile water for injection. *Concentration:* 10 mg/mL. *Dilution:* Withdraw dose volume within 30 min of reconstitution and inject into 1000 mL bag of LR. Solution is stable for 4 hr at room temperature or 12 hr if refrigerated. *Rate:* Infuse over 1–2 hr in a large caliber vein.

● **Cardioprotective:** Doxorubicin should be administered within 30 min following dexrazoxane administration.

● **Intermittent Infusion:** *Reconstitution:* Reconstitute with 25 mL sterile water for injection for 250-mg vial or 50 mL for 500-mg vial. *Concentration:* 10 mg/mL. *Dilution:* Dilute reconstituted solution further in LR. *Concentration:* 1.3–5 mg/mL. Solution is stable for 1 hr at room temperature or 4 hr if refrigerated. *Rate:* Infuse over 15 min. Administer doxorubicin within 30 min of completion of infusion. Do not administer via IV push.

● **Additive Incompatibility:** Do not mix with other medications.

● **Y-Site Compatibility:** alemtuzumab, amifostine, amikacin, amiodarone, ampicillin, ampicillin/sulbactam, anidulafungin, argatroban, arsenic trioxide, atracurium, azithromycin, aztreonam, bivalirudin,

bleomycin, bumetanide, buprenorphine, busulfan, butorphanol, calcium chloride, calcium gluconate, carboplatin, carmustine, caspofungin, cefazolin, cefotaxime, cefotetan, cefoxitin, ceftazidime, ceftriaxone, cefuroxime, chloramphenicol, chlorpromazine, ciprofloxacin, cisatracurium, cisplatin, clindamycin, cyclophosphamide, cyclosporine, cytarabine, dactinomycin, daptomycin, daunorubicin hydrochloride, dexmedetomidine, digoxin, diltiazem, diphenhydramine, docetaxel, dopamine, doxorubicin hydrochloride, doxorubicin liposomal, doxycycline, droperidol, enalaprilat, ephedrine, epinephrine, epirubicin, eptifibatide, ertapenem, erythromycin, esmolol, etoposide, etoposide phosphate, famotidine, fentanyl, fluconazole, fludarabine, fluorouracil, foscarnet, fosphenytoin, gemcitabine, gentamicin, glycopyrrolate, granisetron, haloperidol, heparin, hetastarch, hydralazine, hydrocortisone, hydromorphone, idarubicin, ifosfamide, imipenem/cilastatin, insulin, regular, irinotecan, isoproterenol, ketorolac, leucovorin calcium, levofloxacin, lidocaine, linezolid, lorazepam, magnesium sulfate, mannitol, melphalan, meperidine, meropenem, mesna, metoclopramide, metoprolol, midazolam, milrinone, mitoxantrone, morphine, moxifloxacin, mycophenolate, nalbuphine, naloxone, nicardipine, nitroglycerin, nitroprusside, norepinephrine, octreotide, ondansetron, oxaliplatin, paclitaxel, palonosetron, pamidronate, pemetrexed, pentamidine, phenobarbital, phentolamine, phenylephrine, piperacillin/tazobactam, polmyxin B, potassium acetate, potassium chloride, potassium phosphate, procainamide, prochlorperazine, promethazine, propranolol, remifentanil, rituximab, rocuronium, sodium acetate, sodium bicarbonate, succinylcholine, sufentanil, tacrolimus, theophylline, thiotepa, tigecycline, tirofiban, tobramycin, topotecan, vancomycin, vasopressin, vecuronium, verapamil, vinblastine, vincristine, vinorelbine, voriconazole, zoledronic acid.
- **Y-Site Incompatibility:** acyclovir, allopurinol, aminophylline, amphotericin B lipid complex, amphotericin B liposomal, cefepime, dantrolene, diazepam, dobutamine, furosemide, ganciclovir, gemtuzumab ozogamicin, methotrexate, methylprednisolone, mitomycin, nafcillin, pantoprazole, pentobarbital, phenytoin, sodium phosphate, thiopental, trimethoprim/sulfamethoxazole, zidovudine.

Patient/Family Teaching
- Explain the purpose of the medication to the patient.
- Emphasize the need for continued monitoring of cardiac function.
- Rep: Dexrazoxane may cause fetal harm. Advise females of reproductive potential to use highly effective contraception during and for 6 mo after last dose of dexrazoxane and to avoid breastfeeding dur-

ing and for 2 wk after last dose. Advise males with female partners of reproductive potential to use highly effective contraception during and for 3 mo after last dose. Advise patient to notify health care professional immediately if pregnancy is suspected. May impair fertility in males.

Evaluation/Desired Outcomes
- Reduction of incidence and severity of cardiomyopathy associated with doxorubicin administration in women with metastatic breast cancer.
- Decrease in late sequelae (site pain, fibrosis, atrophy, and local sensory disturbance) following extravasation of anthracycline chemotherapeutic agents.

dextromethorphan
(dex-troe-meth-**or**-fan)
✤Balminil DM, ✤Benylin DM, ✤Bronchophan Forte DM, ✤Buckley's DM, ✤Cough Syrup DM, Creo-Terpin, Creomulsion Adult Formula, Creomulsion for Children, Delsym, ✤Delsym DM, ✤DM Children's Cough Syrup, ✤DM Cough Syrup, ✤Dry Cough Syrup, Father John's, Hold DM, ✤Koffex DM, ✤Neocitran Thin Strips Cough, Pediacare Children's Long-Acting Cough, Robafin Cough, Robitussin Children's Cough Long-Acting, Robitussin Cough Long-Acting, Robitussin CoughGels Long-Acting, Robitussin Lingering Cold Long-Acting Cough-Gels, Scot-Tussin Diabetes, ✤Sedatuss DM, ✤Sucrets Cough Control, ✤Sucrets DM, ✤Triaminic DM, ✤Triaminic Long-Acting Cough, Triaminic Thin Strips Children's Long-Acting Cough, Triaminic Children's Cough Long-Acting, Vicks 44 Cough Relief, ✤Vicks Custom Care Dry Cough, Vicks DayQuil Cough, Vicks Nature Fusion Cough
Classification
Therapeutic: allergy, cold, and cough remedies, antitussives

Indications
Symptomatic relief of coughs caused by minor viral upper respiratory tract infections or inhaled irritants.

Most effective for chronic nonproductive cough. A common ingredient in nonprescription cough and cold preparations.

Action
Suppresses the cough reflex by a direct effect on the cough center in the medulla. Related to opioids structurally but has no analgesic properties. **Therapeutic Effects:** Relief of irritating nonproductive cough.

Pharmacokinetics
Absorption: Rapidly absorbed from the GI tract. Extended-release product is slowly absorbed.
Distribution: Unknown. Probably crosses the placenta and enters breast milk.
Metabolism and Excretion: Metabolized to dextrorphan, an active metabolite. Dextromethorphan and dextrorphan are renally excreted.
Half-life: Unknown.

TIME/ACTION PROFILE (cough suppression)

ROUTE	ONSET	PEAK	DURATION
PO	15–30 min	unknown	3–6 hr†
PO-ER	unknown	unknown	9–12 hr

†Up to 8 hr for gelcaps.

Contraindications/Precautions
Contraindicated in: Hypersensitivity; Patients taking MAO inhibitors or SSRIs; Should not be used for chronic productive coughs; Some products contain alcohol and should be avoided in patients with known intolerance.
Use Cautiously in: Cough that lasts more than 1 wk or is accompanied by fever, rash, or headache— health care professional should be consulted; History of drug abuse or drug-seeking behavior (capsules have been abused resulting in deaths); Diabetes (some products contain sucrose); Lactation: Lactation; Pedi: Children <4 yr (OTC cough and cold products containing this medication should be avoided).

Adverse Reactions/Side Effects
GI: nausea. **Neuro:** *high dose:* dizziness, sedation.

Interactions
Drug-Drug: Use with **MAO inhibitors** may result in serotonin syndrome (nausea, confusion, changes in BP); concurrent use should be avoided. ↑ CNS depression with **antihistamines, alcohol, antidepressants, sedative/hypnotics**, or **opioids. Amiodarone, fluoxetine**, or **quinidine** may ↑ blood levels and adverse reactions from dextromethorphan.

Route/Dosage
PO (Adults and Children >12 yr): 10–20 mg every 4 hr *or* 30 mg every 6–8 hr *or* 60 mg of extended-release preparation bid (not to exceed 120 mg/day).

PO (Children 6–12 yr): 5–10 mg every 4 hr *or* 15 mg every 6–8 hr *or* 30 mg of extended-release preparation every 12 hr (not to exceed 60 mg/day).
PO (Children 4–6 yr): 2.5–5 mg every 4 hr *or* 7.5 mg every 6–8 hr *or* 15 mg of extended-release preparation every 12 hr (not to exceed 30 mg/day).

Availability (generic available)
Gelcaps: 30 mg^{OTC}. **Lozenges (cherry):** 2.5 mg^{OTC}, 5 mg^{OTC}. **Liquid (cherry, grape):** 3.5 mg/5 mL^{OTC}, 5 mg/5 mL, 7.5 mg/5 mL^{OTC}, 15 mg/5 mL^{OTC}, 30 mg/5 mL^{OTC}. **Syrup (cherry, cherry bubblegum):** 7.5 mg/ 5 mL^{OTC}, 15 mg/15 mL^{OTC}, 10 mg/5 mL^{OTC}. **Extended-release suspension (orange):** 30 mg/5 mL^{OTC}. **Drops (Grape):** 7.5 mg/0.8 mL^{OTC}, 7.5 mg/1 mL^{OTC}. **Orally-disintegrating strips (cherry, grape):** 7.5 mg^{OTC}, 15 mg^{OTC}. *In combination with:* antihistamines, decongestants, and expectorants in cough and cold preparations^{OTC}; bupropion (Auvelity); quinidine sulfate (Nuedexta). See Appendix N.

NURSING IMPLICATIONS
Assessment
- Assess frequency and nature of cough, lung sounds, and amount and type of sputum produced. Unless contraindicated, maintain fluid intake of 1500–2000 mL to decrease viscosity of bronchial secretions.

Implementation
- **PO:** Do not give fluids immediately after administering to prevent dilution of vehicle. Shake oral suspension well before administration.

Patient/Family Teaching
- Instruct patient to cough effectively: Sit upright and take several deep breaths before attempting to cough.
- Advise patient to minimize cough by avoiding irritants, such as cigarette smoke, fumes, and dust. Humidification of environmental air, frequent sips of water, and sugarless hard candy may also decrease the frequency of dry, irritating cough.
- Caution patient to avoid taking more than the recommended dose or taking alcohol or other CNS depressants concurrently with this medication; fatalities have occurred. Caution parents to avoid OTC cough and cold products while breastfeeding or to children <4 yrs.
- May occasionally cause dizziness. Caution patient to avoid driving or other activities requiring alertness until response to the medication is known.
- Advise patient that any cough lasting over 1 wk or accompanied by fever, chest pain, persistent headache, or skin rash warrants medical attention.

Evaluation/Desired Outcomes
- Decrease in frequency and intensity of cough without eliminating patient's cough reflex.

✗✗ diazePAM (dye-az-e-pam)
Diastat, Valium, Valtoco

Classification
Therapeutic: antianxiety agents, anticonvulsants, sedative/hypnotics, skeletal muscle relaxants (centrally acting)
Pharmacologic: benzodiazepines

Schedule IV

Indications
Anxiety disorders. Preoperative sedation. Conscious sedation (provides light anesthesia and anterograde amnesia). Status epilepticus/uncontrolled seizures. Acute treatment of intermittent, stereotypic episodes of frequent seizure activity that are distinct from a patient's usual seizure pattern (not status epilepticus) (nasal spray). Skeletal muscle spasms. Alcohol withdrawal.

Action
Depresses the CNS, probably by potentiating GABA, an inhibitory neurotransmitter. Produces skeletal muscle relaxation by inhibiting spinal polysynaptic afferent pathways. Has anticonvulsant properties due to enhanced presynaptic inhibition. **Therapeutic Effects:** Relief of anxiety. Sedation. Amnesia. Skeletal muscle relaxation. Decreased seizure activity.

Pharmacokinetics
Absorption: Rapidly absorbed from the GI tract. Absorption from IM sites may be slow and unpredictable. Well absorbed from rectal mucosa (90%) and nasal mucosa (97%). IV administration results in complete bioavailability.

Distribution: Widely distributed. Crosses the blood-brain barrier.

Metabolism and Excretion: Primarily metabolized in the liver via the CYP2C19 and CYP3A4 isoenzymes; ✗✗ the CYP2C19 isoenzyme exhibits genetic polymorphism; 5–20% of Asian patients and 3–5% of Caucasian and Black patients may be poor metabolizers and may have significantly ↑ diazepam concentrations and an ↑ risk of adverse effects. Some products of metabolism are active as CNS depressants.

Half-life: *Neonates:* 50–95 hr; *Infants (1 mo–2 yr):* 40–50 hr; *Children 2–12 yr:* 15–21 hr; *Children 12–16 yr:* 18–20 hr; *Adults:* 20–50 hr (up to 100 hr for metabolites).

TIME/ACTION PROFILE (sedation)

ROUTE	ONSET	PEAK	DURATION
PO	30–60 min	1–2 hr	up to 24 hr
IM	within 20 min	0.5–1.5 hr	unknown
IV	1–5 min	15–30 min	15–60 min†
Rectal	2–10 min	1–2 hr	4–12 hr

†In status epilepticus, anticonvulsant duration is 15–20 min.

Contraindications/Precautions
Contraindicated in: Hypersensitivity; Cross-sensitivity with other benzodiazepines may occur; Comatose patients; Myasthenia gravis; Severe pulmonary impairment; Sleep apnea; Severe hepatic impairment; Pre-existing CNS depression; Uncontrolled severe pain; Angle-closure glaucoma; Some products contain alcohol, propylene glycol, or tartrazine and should be avoided in patients with known hypersensitivity or intolerance; Lactation: Lactation; Pedi: Children <6 mo (for oral; safety not established).

Use Cautiously in: Severe renal impairment; History of suicide attempt or drug dependence; Debilitated patients (dose ↓ required); Patients with low albumin; OB: Use late in pregnancy can result in sedation (respiratory depression, lethargy, hypotonia) and/or withdrawal symptoms (hyperreflexia, irritability, restlessness, tremors, inconsolable crying, and feeding difficulties) in neonates; Pedi: Metabolites can accumulate in neonates. Injection contains benzyl alcohol, which can cause potentially fatal gasping syndrome in neonates; Geri: Appears on Beers list. ↑ risk of cognitive impairment, delirium, falls, fractures, and motor vehicle accidents. If possible, avoid use in older adults.

Adverse Reactions/Side Effects
CV: hypotension (IV only). **Derm:** rash. **EENT:** ↑ intra-ocular pressure, blurred vision, epistaxis (nasal spray only), nasal congestion (nasal spray only), nasal discomfort (nasal spray only). **GI:** constipation, diarrhea (may be caused by propylene glycol content in oral solution), nausea, vomiting. **Local:** pain (IM), phlebitis (IV). **Metab:** weight gain. **Neuro:** dizziness, drowsiness, lethargy, ataxia, depression, dysgeusia (nasal spray only), hangover, headache, paradoxical excitation, slurred speech. **Resp:** RESPIRATORY DEPRESSION. **Misc:** physical dependence, psychological dependence, tolerance.

Interactions
Drug-Drug: Use with **opioids** or other **CNS depressants**, including other **benzodiazepines**, **non-benzodiazepine sedative/hypnotics**, **anxiolytics**, **general anesthetics**, **muscle relaxants**, **antipsychotics**, and **alcohol** may cause profound respiratory depression, coma, and death; reserve concurrent use for when alternative treatment options are inadequate. **Cimetidine**, **hormonal contraceptives**, **disulfiram**, **fluoxetine**, **isoniazid**, **ketoconazole**, **metoprolol**, **propranolol**, or **valproic acid** may ↓ the metabolism of diazepam, enhancing its actions. May ↓ the efficacy of **levodopa**. **Rifampin** or **barbiturates** may ↑ the metabolism and ↓ effectiveness of diazepam. Sedative effects may be ↓ by **theophylline**. Concurrent use of **ritonavir** is not recommended.

Drug-Natural Products: Concomitant use of **kava-kava**, **valerian**, or **chamomile** can ↑ CNS depression.

✦= Canadian drug name. ✗✗ = Genetic implication. ~~Strikethrough~~ = Discontinued. CAPITALS= life-threatening. <u>Underline</u> = most frequent.

Route/Dosage
Anxiety
PO (Adults): 2–10 mg 2–4 times daily.
IM, IV (Adults): 2–10 mg, may repeat in 3–4 hr as needed.
PO (Children >6 mo): 1–2.5 mg 3–4 times daily.
IM, IV (Children >1 mo): 0.04–0.3 mg/kg/dose every 2–4 hr to a maximum of 0.6 mg/kg within an 8-hr period if necessary.

Pre-Endoscopy
IV (Adults): 2.5–20 mg.
IM (Adults): 5–10 mg 30 min pre-endoscopy.

Pediatric Conscious Sedation for Procedures
PO (Children >6 mo): 0.2–0.3 mg/kg (not to exceed 10 mg/dose) 45–60 min prior to procedure.

Status Epilepticus/Acute Seizure Activity
IV (Adults): 5–10 mg, may repeat every 10–15 min to a total of 30 mg, may repeat regimen again in 2–4 hr (IM route may be used if IV route unavailable); larger doses may be required.
IM, IV (Children ≥5 yr): 0.05–0.3 mg/kg/dose given over 3–5 min every 15–30 min to a total dose of 10 mg, repeat every 2–4 hr.
IM, IV (Children 1 mo–5 yr): 0.05–0.3 mg/kg/dose given over 3–5 min every 15–30 min to maximum dose of 5 mg, repeat in 2–4 hr if needed.
IV (Neonates): 0.1–0.3 mg/kg/dose given over 3–5 min every 15–30 min to maximum dose of 2 mg.
Intranasal (Adults and Children ≥12 yr and ≥76 kg): 0.2 mg/kg as single dose (total dose = 20 mg; administered using one 10-mg spray devices, with one spray [10 mg] from each device administered into each nostril). May administer another dose, if needed, ≥4 hr after initial dose (max = 2 doses/seizure episode).
Intranasal (Adults and Children ≥12 yr and 51–75 kg): 0.2 mg/kg as single dose (total dose = 15 mg; administered using two 7.5–mg spray devices, with one spray [7.5 mg] from each device administered into each nostril). May administer another dose, if needed, ≥4 hr after initial dose (max = 2 doses/seizure episode).
Intranasal (Adults and Children ≥12 yr and 28–50 kg): 0.2 mg/kg as single dose (total dose = 10 mg; administered using one 10-mg spray device, with one spray [10 mg] from device administered into one nostril). May administer another dose, if needed, ≥4 hr after initial dose (max = 2 doses/seizure episode).
Intranasal (Adults and Children ≥12 yr and 14–27 kg): 0.2 mg/kg as single dose (total dose = 5 mg; administered using one 5-mg spray device, with one spray [5 mg] from device administered into one nostril). May administer another dose, if needed, ≥4 hr after initial dose (max = 2 doses/seizure episode).
Intranasal (Children 6–11 yr and 56–74 kg): 0.3 mg/kg as single dose (total dose = 20 mg; administered using two 10-mg spray devices, with one spray [10 mg] from each device administered into each nostril). May administer another dose, if needed, ≥4 hr after initial dose (max = 2 doses/seizure episode).
Intranasal (Children 6–11 yr and 38–55 kg): 0.3 mg/kg as single dose (total dose = 15 mg; administered using two 7.5-mg spray devices, with one spray [7.5 mg] from each device administered into each nostril). May administer another dose, if needed, ≥4 hr after initial dose (max = 2 doses/seizure episode).
Intranasal (Children 6–11 yr and 19–37 kg): 0.3 mg/kg as single dose (total dose = 10 mg; administered using one 10-mg spray device, with one spray [10 mg] from device administered into one nostril). May administer another dose, if needed, ≥4 hr after initial dose (max = 2 doses/seizure episode).
Intranasal (Children 6–11 yr and 10–18 kg): 0.3 mg/kg as single dose (total dose = 5 mg; administered using one 5-mg spray device, with one spray [5 mg] from device administered into one nostril). May administer another dose, if needed, ≥4 hr after initial dose (max = 2 doses/seizure episode).
Rect (Adults and Children >12 yr): 0.2 mg/kg; may repeat 4–12 hr later.
Rect (Children 6–11 yr): 0.3 mg/kg; may repeat 4–12 hr later.
Rect (Children 2–5 yr): 0.5 mg/kg; may repeat 4–12 hr later.

Febrile Seizure Prophylaxis
PO (Children >1 mo): 1 mg/kg/day divided every 8 hr at first sign of fever and continue for 24 hr after fever is gone.

Skeletal Muscle Relaxation
PO (Adults): 2–10 mg 3–4 times daily.
PO (Geriatric Patients or Debilitated Patients): 2–2.5 mg 1–2 times daily initially.
PO (Children >6 mo): 1–2.5 mg 3–4 times daily.
IM, IV (Adults): 5–10 mg; may repeat in 2–4 hr (larger doses may be required for tetanus).
IM, IV (Geriatric Patients or Debilitated Patients): 2–5 mg; may repeat in 2–4 hr (larger doses may be required for tetanus).
IM, IV (Children ≥5 yr): *Tetanus:* 5–10 mg every 3–4 hr.
IM, IV (Children >1 mo): *Tetanus:* 1–2 mg every 3–4 hr.

Alcohol Withdrawal
PO (Adults): 10 mg 3–4 times in first 24 hr, ↓ to 5 mg 3–4 times daily.
IM, IV (Adults): 10 mg initially, then 5–10 mg in 3–4 hr as needed; larger or more frequent doses have been used.

Availability (generic available)
Tablets: 2 mg, 5 mg, 10 mg. **Oral solution:** 1 mg/mL, 5 mg/mL (Intensol). **Rectal gel delivery system:** 2.5 mg, 10 mg, 20 mg. **Nasal spray:** 5 mg/device, 7.5 mg/device, 10 mg/device. **Solution for injection:** 5 mg/mL (contains 10% alcohol and 40% propylene glycol).

NURSING IMPLICATIONS
Assessment
- Monitor BP, pulse, and respiratory rate prior to and periodically during therapy and frequently during IV therapy.
- Assess IV site frequently during administration; diazepam may cause phlebitis and venous thrombosis.
- Prolonged high-dose therapy may lead to psychological or physical dependence. Restrict amount of drug available to patient. Observe depressed patients closely for suicidal tendencies.
- Assess risk for addiction, abuse, or misuse prior to administration.
- Conduct regular assessment of continued need for treatment.
- Geri: Assess risk of falls and institute fall prevention strategies.
- **Anxiety:** Assess mental status (orientation, mood, behavior) and degree of anxiety.
- Assess level of sedation (ataxia, dizziness, slurred speech) prior to and periodically throughout therapy.
- **Seizures:** Observe and record intensity, duration, and location of seizure activity. The initial dose of diazepam offers seizure control for 15–20 min after administration. Institute seizure precautions.
- **Muscle Spasms:** Assess muscle spasm, associated pain, and limitation of movement prior to and during therapy.
- **Alcohol Withdrawal:** Assess patient experiencing alcohol withdrawal for tremors, agitation, delirium, and hallucinations. Protect patient from injury.

Lab Test Considerations
- Evaluate hepatic and renal function and CBC periodically during prolonged therapy. May cause ↑ AST, ALT, and alkaline phosphatase.

Toxicity and Overdose
- Flumazenil is an adjunct in the management of toxicity or overdose. Flumazenil may induce seizures in patients with a history of seizures disorder or who are on tricyclic antidepressants.

Implementation
- Do not confuse diazepam with diltiazem.
- Patient should be kept on bed rest and observed for at least 3 hr following parenteral administration.
- If opioid analgesics are used concurrently with parenteral diazepam, decrease opioid dose by ⅓ and titrate dose to effect.
- Use lowest effective dose. Taper by 2 mg every 3 days to decrease withdrawal symptoms. Some patients may require longer taper periods (mo).
- **PO:** Tablets may be crushed and taken with food or water if patient has difficulty swallowing.
- **IM:** IM injections are painful and erratically absorbed. If IM route is used, inject deeply into deltoid muscle for maximum absorption.

IV Administration
- **IV:** Resuscitation equipment should be available when diazepam is administered IV.
- **IV Push:** *Dilution:* For IV administration do not dilute or mix with any other drug. If IV push is not feasible, administer IV push into tubing as close to insertion site as possible. Continuous infusion is not recommended due to precipitation in IV fluids and absorption of diazepam into infusion bags and tubing. Injection may cause burning and venous irritation; avoid small veins. *Concentration:* 5 mg/mL. *Rate:* Administer slowly at a rate of 5 mg/min in adults. Infants and children should receive 1–2 mg/min. Rapid injection may cause apnea, hypotension, bradycardia, or cardiac arrest.
- **Y-Site Compatibility:** docetaxel, piperacillin/tazobactam.
- **Y-Site Incompatibility:** acetaminophen, acyclovir, alemtuzumab, amikacin, aminocaproic acid, aminophylline, amphotericin B deoxycholate, amphotericin B lipid complex, amphotericin B liposomal, ampicillin, ampicillin/sulbactam, anidulafungin, arsenic trioxide, argatroban, ascorbic acid, atracurium, atropine, azathioprine, azithromycin, aztreonam, benztropine, bivalirudin, bleomycin, bumetanide, buprenorphine, butorphanol, calcium chloride, calcium gluconate, carboplatin, carmustine, caspofungin, cefazolin, cefepime, cefotaxime, cefotetan, cefoxitin, ceftaroline, ceftazidime, ceftriaxone, cefuroxime, chloramphenicol, chlorpromazine, cisplatin, clindamycin, cyanocobalamin, cyclophosphamide, cyclosporine, cytarabine, dactinomycin, dantrolene, daunorubicin hydrochloride, dexamethasone, dexmedetomidine, dexrazoxane, diazoxide, digoxin, diltiazem, diphenhydramine, dopamine, doxorubicin hydrochloride, doxorubicin liposomal, doxycycline, enalaprilat, ephedrine, epinephrine, epirubicin, epoetin alfa, eptifibatide, ertapenem, erythromycin, esmolol, etoposide, etoposide phosphate, famotidine, fluconazole, fludarabine, fluorouracil, folic acid, foscarnet, furosemide, ganciclovir, gemcitabine, gemtuzumab ozogamicin, gentamicin, glycopyrrolate, granisetron, haloperidol, heparin, hetastarch, hydralazine, hydrocortisone, hydroxocobalamin, hydroxyzine, idarubicin, ifosfamide, imipenem/cilastatin, indomethacin, insulin, regular, irinotecan, isoproterenol, ketorolac, labetalol, leucovorin calcium, levofloxacin, lidocaine, linezolid, magnesium chloride, mannitol, meperidine, meropenem, methotrexate, methylprednisolone, metoclopramide, metoprolol, metronidazole, midazolam, milrinone, mitoxantrone, multivitamin, mycophenolate, nalbuphine, naloxone, nitroglycerin, nitroprusside, norepinephrine, octreotide, oxacillin, oxaliplatin, oxytocin, paclitaxel, palonosetron, pantoprazole, papaverine, pemetrexed, penicillin G, pentamidine, pentobarbi-

tal, phenobarbital, phentolamine, phenylephrine, phenytoin, phytonadione, potassium acetate, potassium chloride, procainamide, prochlorperazine, promethazine, propofol, propranolol, protamine, pyridoxine, rocuronium, sodium acetate, sodium bicarbonate, succinylcholine, tacrolimus, theophylline, thiamine, thiotepa, tigecycline, tirofiban, tobramycin, trimethoprim/sulfamethoxazole, vancomycin, vasopressin, vecuronium, verapamil, vinblastine, vincristine, vinorelbine, vitamin B complex with C, voriconazole, zoledronic acid.

- **Intranasal:** Do not prime before use. Only used for seizure clusters. Ensure caregiver is able to distinguish cluster seizures from patient's usual seizure activity. A 2nd dose, when required, may be administered >4 hrs after initial dose; use a new blister pack. Do not use >2 doses to treat a single episode and no more than one episode every 5 days and no more than 5 episodes per mo.
- **Rect:** Only used for seizure clusters. Ensure caregiver is able to distinguish cluster seizures from patient's usual seizure activity; have been instructed to administer rectal dose; understands explicitly which seizure manifestations may or may not be treated with diazepam rectal gel; and are able to monitor the clinical response and recognize when that response is such that immediate professional medical evaluation is required.

Patient/Family Teaching
- Instruct patient to take medication as directed and not to take more than prescribed or increase dose if less effective after a few wk without checking with health care professional. Review *Medication Guide* for *Valtoco* and *Diastat* rectal gel with patient/caregiver prior to administration. Abrupt withdrawal of diazepam may cause insomnia, unusual irritability or nervousness, and seizures. Advise patient that sharing of this medication may be dangerous.
- Advise patient that diazepam is a drug with known abuse potential. Protect it from theft, and never give to anyone other than the individual for whom it was prescribed. Store out of sight and reach of children, and in a location not accessible by others.
- Medication may cause drowsiness, clumsiness, or unsteadiness. Advise patient to avoid driving or other activities requiring alertness until response to medication is known. Geri: Advise geriatric patients of increased risk for CNS effects and potential for falls.
- Caution patient to avoid taking alcohol or other CNS depressants, including opioids, concurrently with this medication, may cause an overdose.
- Instruct patient to notify health care professional of all Rx or OTC medications, vitamins, or herbal products being taken and consult health care professional before taking any new medications.
- Rep: May cause fetal harm. Advise patient to notify health care professional if pregnancy is planned or suspected or if breastfeeding. Use in late pregnancy can result in sedation (respiratory depression, leth-

argy, hypotonia) and/or withdrawal symptoms (hyperreflexia, irritability, restlessness, tremors, inconsolable crying, and feeding difficulties) in the neonate. Monitor neonates exposed to diazepam during pregnancy or labor for signs of sedation and monitor neonates exposed to diazepam during pregnancy for signs of withdrawal. Monitor infants exposed to diazepam through breast milk for sedation, poor feeding, and poor weight gain. Encourage women who take diazepam during pregnancy to enroll in the North American Antiepileptic Drug Pregnancy Registry by calling 1-888-233-2334 or visiting http://www.aedpregnancyregistry.org to monitor pregnancy outcomes in women exposed to antiepileptic drugs.
- Emphasize the importance of follow-up examinations to determine effectiveness of the medication.
- **Intranasal:** Instruct caregiver in correct technique for administration and how to monitor patient after dose.
- **Rect:** Instruct caregiver in correct technique for administration and monitoring. Turn patient on side and administer rectal gel. Stay with patient and monitor for changes in resting breathing rate, changes in color, and side effects. A second dose, if prescribed, may be given 4–12 hours after the first dose, when required.
- **Seizures:** Patients on anticonvulsant therapy should carry identification describing disease process and medication regimen at all times.

Evaluation/Desired Outcomes
- Decrease in anxiety level. Full therapeutic antianxiety effects occur after 1–2 wk of therapy.
- Decreased recall of surgical or diagnostic procedures.
- Control of seizures.
- Decrease in muscle spasms.
- Decreased tremulousness and more rational ideation when used for alcohol withdrawal.

BEERS

DICLOFENAC† (dye-kloe-fen-ak)
diclofenac (oral)
   Zorvolex
diclofenac potassium (oral)
   Cambia, ~~Cataflam~~, Lofena, Zipsor
diclofenac sodium (oral)
   ✦Voltaren, ✦Voltaren SR, ~~Voltaren XR~~
diclofenac sodium (rectal suppository)
   ✦Voltaren
diclofenac sodium (topical gel)
   ~~Solaraze~~, Voltaren
diclofenac sodium (topical solution)
   Pennsaid

diclofenac epolamine (topical patch)
Flector, Licart

Classification
Therapeutic: antirheumatics, nonopioid analgesics
Pharmacologic: nonsteroidal anti-inflammatory drugs (NSAIDs)

†For ophthalmic use see Appendix B

Indications

PO: Management of inflammatory disorders including: Rheumatoid arthritis, Osteoarthritis, Ankylosing spondylitis. Primary dysmenorrhea. Relief of mild to moderate pain. Acute treatment of migraines (powder for oral solution). **Topical:** Management of: Actinic keratosis (3% gel), Osteoarthritis (Voltaren Gel, Pennsaid [for knees]). Acute pain due to minor strains, sprains, and contusions (patch).

Action

Inhibits prostaglandin synthesis. **Therapeutic Effects:** Suppression of pain and inflammation. Relief of acute migraine attacks. **Topical (3% gel):** Clearance of actinic keratosis lesions.

Pharmacokinetics

Absorption: Undergoes first-pass metabolism by liver which results in 50% bioavailability. Oral diclofenac sodium is a delayed-release dose form. Diclofenac potassium is an immediate-release dose form. 6–10% of topical gel is systemically absorbed.
Distribution: Crosses the placenta.
Protein Binding: >99%.
Metabolism and Excretion: Primarily metabolized by the liver via the CYP2C9 isoenzyme to several metabolites; 65% excreted in urine, 35% in bile.
Half-life: 2 hr.

TIME/ACTION PROFILE

ROUTE	ONSET	PEAK	DURATION
PO (inflammation)	few days–1 wk	≥2 wk	unknown
PO (pain)	30 min	unknown	up to 8 hr
Top (gel and patch)	unknown	10–20 hr	unknown
Top (solution)	unknown	unknown	unknown

Contraindications/Precautions

Contraindicated in: Hypersensitivity to diclofenac or other components of formulation; Cross-sensitivity may occur with other NSAIDs, including aspirin; Active GI bleeding/ulcer disease; Coronary artery bypass graft surgery; Exudative dermatitis, eczema, infectious lesions, burns, or wounds; OB: Avoid use after 30 wk gestation.

Use Cautiously in: Severe renal/hepatic impairment; Cardiovascular disease or risk factors for cardiovascular disease (may ↑ risk of serious cardiovascular thrombotic events, myocardial infarction, and stroke, especially with prolonged use or use of higher doses); avoid use in patients with recent MI or HF; HF or edema; History of porphyria; History of peptic ulcer disease and/or GI bleeding; Bleeding tendency or concurrent anticoagulant therapy; OB: Use at or after 20 wk gestation may cause fetal or neonatal renal impairment; if treatment is necessary between 20 wk and 30 wk gestation, limit use to the lowest effective dose and shortest duration possible; Pedi: Safety and effectiveness only established for patch in children ≥6 yr and diclofenac potassium (Zipsor) in children ≥12 yr; Geri: Appears on Beers list. ↑ risk GI bleeding or peptic ulcer disease in older adults. Avoid chronic use unless other alternatives are not effective and the patient can take a gastroprotective agent; avoid short-term use in combination with oral or parenteral corticosteroids, anticoagulants, or antiplatelet agents unless other alternatives are not effective and the patient can take a gastroprotective agent.

Adverse Reactions/Side Effects

CV: edema, HF, hypertension, MI. **Derm:** pruritus, rash, DRUG REACTION WITH EOSINOPHILIA AND SYSTEMIC SYMPTOMS (DRESS), eczema, EXFOLIATIVE DERMATITIS, photosensitivity, STEVENS-JOHNSON SYNDROME (SJS), TOXIC EPIDERMAL NECROLYSIS (TEN). **EENT:** tinnitus. **F and E:** hyperkalemia. **GI:** abdominal pain, constipation, diarrhea, dyspepsia, flatulence, GI BLEEDING, heartburn, HEPATOTOXICITY, nausea, vomiting. **GU:** acute renal failure, hematuria. **Hemat:** anemia, prolonged bleeding time. **Local:** Topical only: contact dermatitis, dry skin, exfoliation. **Neuro:** dizziness, headache, STROKE. **Misc:** HYPERSENSITIVITY REACTIONS (including anaphylaxis).

Interactions

Primarily noted for oral administration.

Drug-Drug: ↑ adverse GI effects with **aspirin**, other **NSAIDs**, or **corticosteroids**. May ↓ effectiveness of **diuretics** or **antihypertensives**. May ↑ levels/risk of toxicity from **cyclosporine**, **lithium**, or **methotrexate**. ↑ risk of bleeding with **anticoagulants**, **aspirin**, **clopidogrel**, **ticagrelor**, **prasugrel**, **corticosteroids**, **fibrinolytics**, **SNRIs**, or **SSRIs**. **CYP2C9** inhibitors, including **voriconazole** may ↑ levels/risk of toxicity. **CYP2C9 inducers**, including **rifampin**, may ↓ levels/effectiveness. Concurrent use of oral **NSAIDs** during topical diclofenac therapy should be minimized.

Drug-Natural Products: ↑ bleeding risk with **arnica**, **chamomile**, **clove**, **dong quai**, **feverfew**, **garlic**, **ginger**, **ginkgo**, **Panax ginseng**, and others.

Route/Dosage

Different formulations of oral diclofenac (diclofenac capsules, diclofenac sodium enteric-coated tablets, diclofenac sodium extended-release tablets, and diclofenac potassium immediate-release tablets) are not bioequivalent and should not be substituted on a mg-to-mg basis.

Diclofenac
PO (Adults): *Acute pain:* 18–35 mg 3 times daily; *Osteoarthritis:* 35 mg 3 times daily.

Hepatic Impairment
PO (Adults): Do not exceed dose of 18 mg 3 times daily.

Diclofenac Potassium
PO (Adults): *Analgesic/antidysmenorrheal (Cataflam):* 100 mg initially, then 50 mg 3 times daily as needed; *Mild-to-moderate acute pain (Zipsor):* 25 mg 4 times daily; *Rheumatoid arthritis (Cataflam):* 50 mg 3–4 times daily; *Osteoarthritis (Cataflam):* 50 mg 2–3 times daily; *Osteoarthritis (Cambia):* one packet (50 mg) given as a single dose.
PO (Children ≥12 yr): *Mild-to-moderate acute pain (Zipsor):* 25 mg 4 times daily.

Diclofenac Sodium
PO (Adults): *Rheumatoid arthritis (delayed-release [enteric-coated] tablets):* 50 mg 3–4 times daily *or* 75 mg twice daily (usual maintenance dose 25 mg 3 times daily). *Rheumatoid arthritis (extended-release tablets):* 100 mg once daily; if unsatisfactory response, dose may be ↑ to 100 mg twice daily. *Osteoarthritis (delayed-release [enteric-coated] tablets):* 50 mg 2–3 times daily *or* 75 mg twice daily. *Osteoarthritis (extended-release tablets):* 100 mg once daily. *Ankylosing spondylitis (delayed-release [enteric-coated] tablets):* 25 mg 4 times daily, with an additional 25 mg given at bedtime, if necessary.
Topical (Adults): *3% topical gel:* Apply to lesions twice daily for 60–90 days; *Voltaren gel:* Lower extremities (knees, ankles, feet): Apply 4 g to affected area 4 times daily (maximum of 16 g per joint/day); Upper extremities (elbows, wrists, hands): Apply 2 g to affected area 4 times daily (maximum of 8 g per joint/day). Maximum total body dose should not exceed 32 g/day; *Pennsaid:* Apply 40 drops to affected knee(s) 4 times daily.
Rect (Adults): Insert 50 mg or 100 mg as single dose to substitute for final oral daily dose (max combined dose [rectal and oral]: 100 mg/day).

Diclofenac Epolamine
Topical (Adults and Children ≥6 yr): *Flector:* Apply 1 patch to most painful area twice daily. *Licart:* Apply 1 patch to most painful area once daily.

Availability (generic available)
Diclofenac potassium immediate-release tablets (Cataflam): 50 mg. **Diclofenac potassium liquid-filled capsules (Zipsor):** 25 mg. **Diclofenac potassium powder for oral solution (Cambia):** 50 mg/packet. **Diclofenac capsules (Zorvolex):** 18 mg, 35 mg. **Diclofenac sodium delayed-release (enteric-coated) tablets:** 25 mg, 50 mg, 75 mg. **Diclofenac sodium extended-release tablets:** ✱ 75 mg, 100 mg. **Diclofenac sodium topical gel:** 1% (Voltaren gel)^OTC, 3%. **Diclofenac sodium topical solution:** 1.5%, 2%. **Diclofenac epolamine transdermal patch:** 1.3%. **Diclofenac sodium rectal suppository:** ✱ 50 mg. *In combination with:* misoprostol (Arthrotec). See Appendix N.

NURSING IMPLICATIONS

Assessment
- Patients who have asthma, aspirin-induced allergy, and nasal polyps are at ↑ risk for developing hypersensitivity reactions.
- Monitor BP closely during initiation of treatment and periodically during therapy in patients with hypertension.
- Assess patient for skin rash frequently during therapy. Discontinue at first sign of rash; may be life-threatening. SJS may develop. Treat symptomatically; may recur once treatment is stopped.
- Monitor for signs and symptoms of DRESS (fever, rash, lymphadenopathy, facial swelling) periodically during therapy. Discontinue therapy if symptoms occur.
- **Pain:** Assess pain and limitation of movement; note type, location, and intensity before and 30–60 min after administration.
- **Migraine:** Assess pain location, character, intensity, and duration and associated symptoms (photophobia, phonophobia, nausea, vomiting) during migraine attack.
- **Arthritis:** Assess arthritic pain (note type, location, intensity) and limitation of movement before and periodically during therapy.
- **Actinic Keratosis:** Assess lesions prior to and periodically during therapy.

Lab Test Considerations
- Diclofenac has minimal effect on bleeding time and platelet aggregation.
- May cause ↓ in hemoglobin and hematocrit.
- Monitor CBC and liver function tests within 4–8 wk of initiating diclofenac and periodically during therapy. May cause ↑ serum alkaline phosphatase, LDH, AST, and ALT concentrations.
- Monitor BUN and serum creatinine periodically during therapy. May cause ↑ BUN and serum creatinine.

Implementation
- Various brands and dose forms are not interchangeable.
- Administration in higher than recommended doses does not provide increased effectiveness but may cause increased side effects. Use lowest effective dose for shortest period of time.
- **PO:** Take with food or milk to minimize gastric irritation. May take first 1–2 doses on an empty stomach for more rapid onset. *DNC:* Do not crush or chew enteric-coated or extended-release tablets. Administer *Zorvolex* capsules on an empty stomach; food may reduce effectiveness.

D

- **Dysmenorrhea:** Administer as soon as possible after the onset of menses. Prophylactic treatment has not been shown to be effective.
- **Migraine:** Empty contents of one packet into a cup containing 1–2 oz or 2–4 tablespoons (30–60 mL) of water, mix well and drink immediately. Do not use liquids other than water. Take on empty stomach; food may reduce effectiveness. Use only for acute migraine pain; not indicated for prophylaxis.
- **Topical: Gel** should be applied to intact skin; do not use on open wounds. An adequate amount of gel should be applied to cover the entire lesion.
- **Topical:** Dispense **solution** 10 drops at a time either directly onto knee or first into the hand and then onto knee. Spread solution evenly around front, back, and sides of the knee. Repeat until 40 drops have been applied and knee is completely covered with solution.
- **Transdermal:** Apply patch to the most painful area once (*Licart*) or twice (*Flector*) a day. Do not apply to nonintact or damaged skin resulting from any etiology (exudative dermatitis, eczema, infected lesion, burns, wounds). Avoid contact with eyes; wash hands after applying, handling, or removing patch.

Patient/Family Teaching

- Instruct patient to take diclofenac as directed and not take more than recommended. Advise patient to read *Medication Guide* before starting diclofenac and with each Rx refill in case of changes.
- *Migraine:* Advise patient that overuse (use more than 10 days/mo) may lead to exacerbation of headache (migraine-like daily headaches, or as a marked increase in frequency of migraine attacks). May require gradual withdrawal of diclofenac and treatment of symptoms (transient worsening of headache).
- Instruct patient to notify health care professional of medication regimen before treatment or surgery.
- Caution patient to avoid concurrent use of alcohol, aspirin, acetaminophen, other NSAIDs, or other OTC medications without consulting health care professional.
- May cause serious side effects: cardiovascular (MI or stroke), GI (ulcers, bleeding), skin (exfoliative dermatitis, SJS, TEN), and hypersensitivity (anaphylaxis). May occur without warning symptoms. Advise patient to stop medication and notify health care professional immediately if symptoms of cardiovascular side effects (chest pain, shortness of breath, weakness, slurring of speech), GI side effects (epigastric pain, dyspepsia, melena, hematemesis), skin side effects (skin rash, blisters, fever, itching), or hypersensitivity reactions (difficulty breathing or swelling of face or throat) occur. Inform patient that risk for heart attack or stroke that can lead to death increases with longer use of NSAIDs and in people

who have heart disease and that risk of ulcer increases with concurrent use of corticosteroids and anticoagulants, longer use, smoking, drinking alcohol, older age, and having poor health.
- Advise patient to notify health care professional promptly if unexplained weight gain, swelling of arms and legs or hands and feet, nausea, fatigue, lethargy, rash, pruritus, yellowing of skin or eyes, itching, stomach pain, vomiting blood, bloody or tarry stools, or flu-like symptoms occur.
- Instruct patient to notify health care professional of all Rx or OTC medications, vitamins, or herbal products being taken and to consult with health care professional before taking other medications, especially other NSAIDs or aspirin.
- Rep: May cause fetal harm. Advise females of reproductive potential to notify health care professional if pregnancy is planned or suspected or if breastfeeding. Advise women to avoid diclofenac in the 3rd trimester of pregnancy (after 29 wk); may cause premature closure of the fetal ductus arteriosus. Use of diclofenac after 20 wk may cause fetal renal dysfunction leading to oligohydramnios. May cause reversible infertility in women attempting to conceive; may consider discontinuing diclofenac.
- **PO:** Instruct patient to take diclofenac with a full glass of water and to remain in an upright position for 15–30 min after administration. Take missed doses as soon as possible within 1–2 hr if taking once or twice a day or unless almost time for next dose if taking more than twice a day. Do not double doses.
- May cause drowsiness or dizziness. Caution patient to avoid driving or other activities requiring alertness until response to medication is known.
- Caution patient to wear sunscreen and protective clothing to prevent photosensitivity reactions.
- **Topical:** Advise patient to minimize use of concurrent NSAIDs during topical therapy. Instruct patient to read *Medication Guide* before starting therapy and with each Rx refill in case changes have been made.
- *Pennsaid:* Instruct patient to avoid touching treated knee and allowing another person to touch knee until completely dry. Cover knee with clothing until completely dry. Avoid covering lesion with occlusive dressing or tight clothing, and avoid applying sunscreen, insect repellent, lotion, moisturizer, or cosmetics to the affected area. Do not use heating pads, sunlamps, and tanning beds. Protect treated knee from sunlight; wear protective clothes when in sunlight. Avoid showers or baths for at least 30 min after application.
- *Voltaren:* Measure dose using the dosing card supplied in the drug product carton. Dosing card is clear polypropylene; use for each application. Apply gel within the rectangular area of the dosing card up to the 2-g or 4-g line (2 g for each elbow, wrist, or hand, and 4 g for each knee, ankle, or foot). Apply gel using dosing card. Use hands to gently rub gel

into skin. After using dosing card, hold with fingertips, rinse, and dry. If treatment site is the hands, patient should wait at least 1 hr to wash hands.

- **3% gel:** Advise patient that it may take 60–90 days for complete healing of the lesion to occur.
- **Transdermal:** Instruct patient on correct application procedure for patch. Apply patch to most painful area. Change patch every 24 hr (*Licart*) or 12 hr (*Flector*). Remove patch if irritation occurs. Fold used patches so adhesive sticks to itself and discard where children and pets cannot get them. Encourage patient to read the *NSAID Medication Guide* that accompanies the prescription.
- Do not wear patch during bathing or showering. Bathing should take place between scheduled patch removal and application.
- Instruct patients if patch begins to peel off to tape the edges. Patient may overlay the topical system with a mesh netting sleeve to secure topical systems applied to ankles, knees, or elbows. Mesh netting sleeve (Curad® Hold Tite™, Surgilast® Tubular Elastic Dressing) must allow air to pass through and not be occlusive.
- Advise patient referred for MRI test to discuss patch with referring health care professional and MRI facility to determine if removal of patch is necessary prior to test and for directions for replacing patch.

Evaluation/Desired Outcomes

- Decrease in severity of mild-to-moderate pain.
- Increased ease of joint movement. Patients who do not respond to one NSAID may respond to another. May require 2 wk or more for maximum effects.
- Decrease in severity of acute migraine pain.
- Decrease in or healing of lesions in actinic keratosis. Lesions that do not heal should be re-evaluated.

---

dicloxacillin, See PENICILLINS, PENICILLINASE RESISTANT.

---

diflorasone, See CORTICOSTEROIDS (TOPICAL/LOCAL).

BEERS HIGH ALERT

digoxin (di-jox-in)
Lanoxin
Classification
Therapeutic: antiarrhythmics, inotropics
Pharmacologic: digitalis glycosides

Indications

HF. Atrial fibrillation and atrial flutter (slows ventricular rate). Paroxysmal atrial tachycardia.

Action

Increases the force of myocardial contraction. Prolongs refractory period of the AV node. Decreases conduction through the SA and AV nodes. **Therapeutic Effects:** Increased cardiac output (positive inotropic effect) and slowing of the heart rate (negative chronotropic effect).

Pharmacokinetics

Absorption: 60–80% absorbed after oral administration of tablets; 70–85% absorbed after administration of elixir; 80% absorbed from IM sites (IM route not recommended due to pain/irritation). IV administration results in complete bioavailability.

Distribution: Widely distributed to tissues.

Metabolism and Excretion: Excreted almost entirely unchanged by the kidneys.

Half-life: 36–48 hr (↑ in renal impairment).

TIME/ACTION PROFILE (antiarrhythmic or inotropic effects, provided that a loading dose has been given)

ROUTE	ONSET	PEAK	DURATION
PO	30–120 min	2–8 hr	2–4 days†
IM	30 min	4–6 hr	2–4 days†
IV	5–30 min	1–4 hr	2–4 days†

†Duration listed is that for normal renal function; in impaired renal function, duration will be longer.

Contraindications/Precautions

Contraindicated in: Hypersensitivity; Uncontrolled ventricular arrhythmias; Heart block (in absence of pacemaker); Idiopathic hypertrophic subaortic stenosis; Constrictive pericarditis; Known alcohol intolerance (elixir only).

Use Cautiously in: Hypokalemia (↑ risk of digoxin toxicity); Hypercalcemia (↑ risk of toxicity, especially with mild hypokalemia); Hypomagnesemia (↑ risk of digoxin toxicity); Diuretic use (may cause electrolyte abnormalities including hypokalemia and hypomagnesemia); Hypothyroidism; MI; Renal impairment (↓ dose); Obesity (base dose on ideal body weight); OB: Monitor neonates for signs/symptoms of digoxin toxicity; monitor levels in mother during pregnancy as levels may fluctuate during pregnancy and postpartum periods; may lead to ↑ risk of arrhythmias during labor and delivery; Lactation: Use with caution while breastfeeding; Geri: Appears on Beers list. Avoid use as first-line therapy for rate control in atrial fibrillation or for HF in older adults; if used, avoid using dose >0.125 mg/day.

Adverse Reactions/Side Effects

CV: bradycardia, ARRHYTHMIAS, ECG changes, heart block. **EENT:** blurred vision, yellow or green vision. **GI:** anorexia, nausea, vomiting, diarrhea. **Hemat:** thrombocytopenia. **Neuro:** fatigue, headache, weakness.

Interactions

Drug-Drug: **Thiazide** and **loop diuretics**, **piperacillin/tazobactam**, **amphotericin B**, **corticosteroids**, and excessive use of **laxatives** may cause hypokalemia which may ↑ risk of toxicity. **Quinidine** and **ritonavir** may ↑ levels and lead to toxicity; ↓ digoxin dose by 30–50%. **Amiodarone** and **dronedarone** may ↑ levels and lead to toxicity; ↓ digoxin dose by 50%. **Cyclosporine, itraconazole, mirabegron, propafenone, quinine, spironolactone,** and **verapamil** may ↑ levels and lead to toxicity; serum level monitoring/dose ↓ may be required. Levels may be ↓ by some **antineoplastics (bleomycin, carmustine, cyclophosphamide, cytarabine, doxorubicin, methotrexate, procarbazine, vincristine),** activated charcoal, cholestyramine, colestipol, metoclopramide, penicillamine, rifampin,** or **sulfasalazine**. In a small percentage (10%) of patients gut bacteria metabolize digoxin to inactive compounds; **macrolide anti-infectives (erythromycin, azithromycin, clarithromycin)** and **tetracyclines,** by killing these bacteria, will cause ↑ levels and toxicity; dose may need to be ↓ for up to 9 wk. Additive bradycardia may occur with **beta blockers, diltiazem, verapamil, clonidine, ivabradine,** and other **antiarrhythmics (quinidine, disopyramide)**. Concurrent use of **sympathomimetics** may ↑ risk of arrhythmias. **Thyroid hormones** may ↓ therapeutic effects.

Drug-Natural Products: Licorice and stimulant natural products (**aloe**) may ↑ risk of potassium depletion. **St. John's wort** may ↓ levels and effect.

Drug-Food: Concurrent ingestion of a **high-fiber meal** may ↓ absorption. Administer digoxin 1 hr before or 2 hrs after such a meal.

Route/Dosage

For rapid effect, a larger initial loading dose should be given in several divided doses over 12–24 hr. Maintenance doses are determined for digoxin by renal function. All dosing must be evaluated by individual response. In general, doses required for atrial arrhythmias are higher than those for inotropic effect.

IV, IM (Adults): *Loading dose:* 0.5–1 mg given as 50% of the dose initially and one quarter of the initial dose in each of 2 subsequent doses at 6–12 hr intervals.

IV, IM (Children >10 yr): *Loading dose:* 8–12 mcg/kg given as 50% of the dose initially and one quarter of the initial dose in each of 2 subsequent doses at 6–12 hr intervals.

IV, IM (Children 5–10 yr): *Loading dose:* 15–30 mcg/kg given as 50% of the dose initially and one quarter of the initial dose in each of 2 subsequent doses at 6–12 hr intervals.

IV, IM (Children 2–5 yr): *Loading dose:* 25–35 mcg/kg given as 50% of the dose initially and one quarter of the initial dose in each of 2 subsequent doses at 6–12 hr intervals.

IV, IM (Children 1–24 mo): *Loading dose:* 30–50 mcg/kg given as 50% of the dose initially and one quarter of the initial dose in each of 2 subsequent doses at 6–12 hr intervals.

IV, IM (Infants –full term): *Loading dose:* 20–30 mcg/kg given as 50% of the dose initially and one quar-

ter of the initial dose in each of 2 subsequent doses at 6–12 hr intervals.

IV, IM (Infants –premature): *Loading dose:* 15–25 mcg/kg given as 50% of the dose initially and one quarter of the initial dose in each of 2 subsequent doses at 6–12 hr intervals.

PO (Adults): *Loading dose:* 0.75–1.5 mg given as 50% of the dose initially and one quarter of the initial dose in each of 2 subsequent doses at 6–12 hr intervals. *Maintenance dose:* 0.125–0.5 mg/day depending on patient's lean body weight, renal function, and serum level.

PO (Geriatric Patients): Initial daily dose should not exceed 0.125 mg.

PO (Children >10 yr): *Loading dose:* 10–15 mcg/kg given as 50% of the dose initially and one quarter of the initial dose in each of 2 subsequent doses at 6–12 hr intervals. *Maintenance dose:* 2.5–5 mcg/kg given daily as a single dose.

PO (Children 5–10 yr): *Loading dose:* 20–35 mcg/kg given as 50% of the dose initially and one quarter of the initial dose in each of 2 subsequent doses at 6–12 hr intervals. *Maintenance dose:* 5–10 mcg/kg given daily in 2 divided doses.

PO (Children 2–5 yr): *Loading dose:* 30–40 mcg/kg given as 50% of the dose initially and one quarter of the initial dose in each of 2 subsequent doses at 6–12 hr intervals. *Maintenance dose:* 7.5–10 mcg/kg given daily in 2 divided doses.

PO (Children 1–24 mo): *Loading dose:* 35–60 mcg/kg given as 50% of the dose initially and one quarter of the initial dose in each of 2 subsequent doses at 6–12 hr intervals. *Maintenance dose:* 10–15 mcg/kg given daily in 2 divided doses.

PO (Infants –full term): *Loading dose:* 25–35 mcg/kg given as 50% of the dose initially and one quarter of the initial dose in each of 2 subsequent doses at 6–12 hr intervals. *Maintenance dose:* 6–10 mcg/kg given daily in 2 divided doses.

PO (Infants –premature): *Loading dose:* 20–30 mcg/kg given as 50% of the dose initially and one quarter of the initial dose in each of 2 subsequent doses at 6–12 hr intervals. *Maintenance dose:* 5–7.5 mcg/kg given daily in 2 divided doses.

Availability (generic available)

Tablets: 0.0625 mg, 0.125 mg, 0.25 mg. **Oral solution (lime flavor):** 0.05 mg/mL. **Solution for injection:** 0.25 mg/mL. **Solution for injection (pediatric):** 0.1 mg/mL.

NURSING IMPLICATIONS
Assessment

- Monitor apical pulse for 1 full min before administering. Hold dose and notify health care professional if pulse rate is <60 bpm in an adult, <70 bpm in a child, or <90 bpm in an infant. Notify health care professional promptly of any significant changes in rate, rhythm, or quality of pulse.

- Pedi: Heart rate varies in children depending on age; ask health care professional to specify at what heart rates digoxin should be withheld.
- Monitor BP periodically in patients receiving IV digoxin.
- Monitor ECG during IV administration and 6 hr after each dose. Notify health care professional if bradycardia or new arrhythmias occur.
- Observe IV site for redness or infiltration; extravasation can lead to tissue irritation and sloughing.
- Monitor intake and output ratios and daily weights. Assess for peripheral edema, and auscultate lungs for rales/crackles during therapy.
- Before administering initial loading dose, determine whether patient has taken any digoxin in the preceding 2–3 wk.

Lab Test Considerations
- Evaluate serum electrolyte levels (especially potassium, magnesium, and calcium) and renal and hepatic function periodically during therapy. Notify health care professional before giving dose if patient is hypokalemic. Hypokalemia, hypomagnesemia, or hypercalcemia may make the patient more susceptible to digitalis toxicity. Pedi: Neonates may have falsely elevated serum digoxin concentrations due to a naturally occurring substance chemically similar to digoxin.

Toxicity and Overdose
- Therapeutic serum digoxin concentrations range from 0.5–2 ng/mL. Serum levels may be drawn 6–8 hr after a dose is administered; usually drawn immediately before the next dose. Geri: Older adults are at increased risk for toxic effects of digoxin (on Beers list) due to age-related decreased renal clearance; may exist even when serum creatinine is normal. Digoxin requirements in older adult may change and a formerly therapeutic dose can become toxic.
- Observe for signs and symptoms of toxicity. *In adults and older children,* first symptoms of toxicity usually include abdominal pain, anorexia, nausea, vomiting, visual disturbances, bradycardia, and other arrhythmias. *In infants and small children,* first signs of overdose are usually cardiac arrhythmias. If these appear, withhold drug and notify health care professional immediately.
- If signs of toxicity occur and are not severe, discontinuation of digoxin may be all that is required.
- Correct electrolyte abnormalities, thyroid dysfunction, and concomitant medications. Administer potassium to maintain serum potassium between 4.0 and 5.5 mEq/L. Monitor ECG for evidence of potassium toxicity (peaked T waves).
- Treatment of life-threatening arrhythmias may include administration of digoxin immune Fab *(Digibind)*, which binds to the digitalis glycoside molecule in the blood and is excreted by the kidneys.

Implementation
- Do not confuse Lanoxin with levothyroxine or naloxone.
- *High Alert:* Digoxin has a narrow therapeutic range. Medication errors associated with digoxin include miscalculation of pediatric doses and insufficient monitoring of digoxin levels.
- For rapid digitalization, initial dose is higher than maintenance dose; 50% of total digitalizing dose is given initially. Administer remainder of dose in 25% increments at 4–8 hr intervals.
- When changing from parenteral to oral dose forms, dose adjustments may be necessary because of pharmacokinetic variations in percentage of digoxin absorbed: 100 mcg (0.1 mg) digoxin injection = 125 mcg (0.125 mg) tablet or 125 mcg (0.125 mg) of elixir.
- PO: Administer oral preparations consistently with regard to meals. Tablets can be crushed and administered with food or fluids if patient has difficulty swallowing. Use calibrated measuring device for elixir; calibrated dropper is not accurate for doses of less than 0.2 mL or 10 mcg.
- IM: Administer deep into gluteal muscle and massage well to reduce painful local reactions. Do not administer more than 2 mL of digoxin in each IM site. IM administration is not generally recommended.

IV Administration
- IV Push: *Dilution:* May be administered undiluted. May also dilute 1 mL of digoxin in 4 mL of sterile water for injection, D5W, or 0.9% NaCl. Less diluent will cause precipitation. Use diluted solution immediately. *Rate:* Administer over at least 5 min.
- Y-Site Compatibility: acyclovir, alemtuzumab, amikacin, aminocaproic acid, aminophylline, amphotericin B lipid complex, anidulafungin, argatroban, ascorbic acid, atracurium, atropine, azathioprine, azithromycin, aztreonam, benztropine, bivalirudin, bleomycin, bumetanide, buprenorphine, butorphanol, calcium chloride, calcium gluconate, cangrelor, carboplatin, carmustine, cefazolin, cefotaxime, cefotetan, cefoxitin, ceftaroline, ceftazidime, ceftolozane/tazobactam, ceftriaxone, cefuroxime, chloramphenicol, chlorpromazine, ciprofloxacin, cisatracurium, cisplatin, clindamycin, cyanocobalamin, cyclophosphamide, cyclosporine, cytarabine, dacarbazine, dactinomycin, daptomycin, daunorubicin hydrochloride, dexamethasone, dexmedetomidine, dexrazoxane, diltiazem, dimenhydrinate, diphenhydramine, dobutamine, docetaxel, dopamine, doxorubicin liposomal, doxycycline, enalaprilat, ephedrine, epinephrine, epirubicin, epoetin alfa, eptifibatide, ertapenem, erythromycin, esmolol, etoposide, etoposide phosphate, famotidine, fentanyl, fludarabine, fluorouracil, folic acid, fosphenytoin, furosemide, ganciclovir, gemcitabine, gentamicin, glycopyrrolate, granisetron, heparin, hetastarch, hydrocortisone, hydromorphone, ifosfamide, imipenem/cilastatin, indomethacin, irinotecan, isavuconazonium, isoproterenol, ketamine, ketorolac,

labetalol, LR, leucovorin calcium, levofloxacin, lidocaine, linezolid, lorazepam, magnesium sulfate,
mannitol, meperidine, meropenem, meropenem/va-
borbactam, mesna, methadone, methohexital, methotrexate, methylprednisolone, metoclopramide, metoprolol, metronidazole, midazolam, milrinone,
mitomycin, morphine, moxifloxacin, multivitamins,
mycophenolate, nafcillin, nalbuphine, naloxone, nicardipine, nitroglycerin, nitroprusside, norepinephrine, octreotide, ondansetron, oxacillin, oxaliplatin,
oxytocin, palonosetron, pamidronate, pantoprazole,
papaverine, pemetrexed, penicillin G, pentobarbital,
phenobarbital, phentolamine, phenylephrine, phytonadione, piperacillin/tazobactam, plazomicin, potassium acetate, potassium chloride, procainamide,
prochlorperazine, promethazine, propranolol, protamine, pyridoxine, remifentanil, rituximab, rocuronium, sodium acetate, sodium bicarbonate, streptomycin, succinylcholine, sufentanil, tacrolimus,
theophylline, thiamine, thiotepa, tigecycline, tirofiban, tobramycin, trastuzumab, vancomycin, vasopressin, vecuronium, verapamil, vinblastine, vincristine, vinorelbine, voriconazole, zoledronic acid.
- **Y-Site Incompatibility:** amiodarone, amphotericin B deoxycholate, amphotericin B liposomal, caspofungin, dantrolene, diazepam, doxorubicin hydrochloride, foscarnet, gemtuzumab ozogamicin,
idarubicin, minocycline, mitoxantrone, paclitaxel,
pentamidine, phenytoin, propofol, telavancin, topotecan, trimethoprim/sulfamethoxazole.

Patient/Family Teaching
- Instruct patient to take medication as directed, at
same time each day. Teach parents or caregivers of
infants and children how to accurately measure
medication. Take missed doses within 12 hr of
scheduled dose or omit. Do not double doses. Consult health care professional if doses for 2 or more
days are missed. Do not discontinue medication
without consulting health care professional.
- Teach patient to take pulse and to contact health
care professional before taking medication if pulse
rate is <60 or >100.
- Pedi: Teach parents or caregivers that changes in
heart rate, especially bradycardia, are among the
first signs of digoxin toxicity in infants and children.
Instruct parents or caregivers in apical heart rate assessment and ask them to notify health care professional if heart rate is outside of range set by health
care professional before administering the next
scheduled dose.
- Review signs and symptoms of digitalis toxicity with
patient and family. Advise patient to notify health
care professional immediately if these or symptoms
of HF occur. Inform patient that these symptoms may
be mistaken for those of colds or flu.
- Instruct patient to keep digoxin tablets in their original container and not to mix in pill boxes with other

medications; may look similar to and may be mistaken for other medications.
- Advise patient that sharing of this medication can be
dangerous.
- Instruct patient to notify health care professional of
all Rx or OTC medications, vitamins, or herbal products being taken and to consult health care professional before taking other Rx, OTC, or herbal products, especially St. John's wort. Advise patient to
avoid taking antacids or antidiarrheals within 2 hr of
digoxin.
- Advise patient to notify health care professional of
this medication regimen before treatment.
- Patients taking digoxin should carry identification
describing disease process and medication regimen
at all times.
- Geri: Review fall prevention strategies with older
adults and their families.
- Rep: Advise females of reproductive potential to notify health care professional if pregnancy is planned
or suspected, may increase risk for low birth weight
or preterm birth. Digoxin is recommended as a first-
line agent for chronic treatment of highly symptomatic supraventricular tachycardia in pregnancy.
Monitor for maternal arrhythmias during labor and
delivery. Monitor maternal serum digoxin concentrations; may require dose adjustments during pregnancy and postpartum; may lead to ↑ risk of arrhythmias during labor and delivery. Monitor neonates
for signs and symptoms of digoxin toxicity (vomiting,
cardiac arrhythmias). Monitor neonates for signs/
symptoms of digoxin toxicity.
- Emphasize the importance of routine follow-up exams to determine effectiveness and to monitor for
toxicity.

Evaluation/Desired Outcomes
- Decrease in severity of HF.
- Increase in cardiac output.
- Decrease in ventricular response in atrial fibrillation
or atrial flutter.
- Termination of paroxysmal atrial tachycardia.

---

dilTIAZem (dil-tye-a-zem)
Cardizem, Cardizem CD, Cardizem
LA, Cartia XT, Matzim LA, Taztia XT,
Tiadylt ER, Tiazac, ✦Tiazac XC
Classification
Therapeutic: antianginals, antiarrhythmics
(class IV), antihypertensives
Pharmacologic: calcium channel blockers

Indications
Hypertension. Angina pectoris and vasospastic (Prinzmetal's) angina. Supraventricular tachyarrhythmias and
rapid ventricular rates in atrial flutter or fibrillation.

Action

Inhibits transport of calcium into myocardial and vascular smooth muscle cells, resulting in inhibition of excitation-contraction coupling and subsequent contraction. **Therapeutic Effects:** Systemic vasodilation resulting in decreased BP. Coronary vasodilation resulting in decreased frequency and severity of attacks of angina. Reduction of ventricular rate in atrial fibrillation or flutter.

Pharmacokinetics

Absorption: Well absorbed, but rapidly metabolized after oral administration.
Distribution: Unknown.
Protein Binding: 70–80%.
Metabolism and Excretion: Primarily metabolized by the liver via the CYP3A4 isoenzyme. Excreted in the urine and feces.
Half-life: 3.5–9 hr.

TIME/ACTION PROFILE

ROUTE	ONSET	PEAK	DURATION
PO	30 min	2–3 hr	6–8 hr
PO–CD, LA, XT	unknown	14 days†	up to 24 hr
IV	2–5 min	2–4 hr	unknown

†Maximum antihypertensive effect with chronic therapy.

Contraindications/Precautions

Contraindicated in: Hypersensitivity; Sick sinus syndrome; 2nd- or 3rd-degree AV block (unless an artificial pacemaker is in place); Systolic BP <90 mm Hg; Recent MI or pulmonary congestion; Concurrent use of rifampin; Lactation: Lactation.
Use Cautiously in: Severe hepatic impairment (↓ dose recommended); Severe renal impairment; Serious ventricular arrhythmias or HF; OB: Use during pregnancy only if potential maternal benefit justifies potential fetal risk ; Pedi: Safety and effectiveness not established in children ; Geri: ↓ dose and slower IV infusion rate recommended in older adults; ↑ risk of hypotension; consider age-related decrease in body mass, ↓ hepatic/renal/cardiac function, concurrent drug therapy, and other disease states.

Adverse Reactions/Side Effects

CV: peripheral edema, ARRHYTHMIA, bradycardia, chest pain, HF, hypotension, palpitations, syncope, tachycardia. **Derm:** dermatitis, erythema multiforme, flushing, photosensitivity, pruritus/urticaria, rash, STEVENS-JOHNSON SYNDROME (SJS), sweating. **EENT:** blurred vision, disturbed equilibrium, epistaxis, tinnitus. **Endo:** gynecomastia, hyperglycemia. **GI:** ↑ liver enzymes, anorexia, constipation, diarrhea, dry mouth, dyspepsia, nausea, vomiting. **GU:** dysuria, nocturia, polyuria, sexual dysfunction, urinary frequency. **Hemat:** anemia, leukopenia, thrombocytopenia. **Metab:** weight gain. **MS:** joint stiffness, muscle cramps. **Neuro:** abnormal dreams, anxiety, confusion, dizziness, drowsiness, dysgeusia, headache, nervousness, paresthesia, psychiatric disturbances, tremor, weakness. **Resp:** cough, dyspnea. **Misc:** gingival hyperplasia.

Interactions

Drug-Drug: ↑ hypotension may occur when used with **fentanyl**, other **antihypertensives, nitrates,** acute ingestion of **alcohol,** or **quinidine.** Antihypertensive effects may be ↓ by **NSAIDs.** May ↑ **digoxin** levels. May ↑ levels of and risk of myopathy from **simvastatin** and **lovastatin.** Concurrent use with **beta blockers, clonidine, digoxin, disopyramide, ivabradine,** or **phenytoin** may result in bradycardia, conduction defects, or HF; avoid concurrent use with ivabradine. **Phenobarbital** and **phenytoin** may ↑ metabolism and ↓ effectiveness. May ↓ metabolism of and ↑ risk of toxicity from **cyclosporine, quinidine,** or **carbamazepine. Cimetidine** ↑ levels and effects. May ↑ or ↓ the effects of **lithium** or **theophylline.**
Drug-Food: Grapefruit juice ↑ levels and effect.

Route/Dosage

PO (Adults): 30–120 mg 3–4 times daily or 180–240 mg once daily as CD or XR capsules or LA tablets (up to 360 mg/day); *Concurrent simvastatin therapy:* Diltiazem dose should not exceed 240 mg/day and simvastatin dose should not exceed 10 mg/day.
IV (Adults): 0.25 mg/kg; may repeat in 15 min with a dose of 0.35 mg/kg. May follow with continuous infusion at 10 mg/hr (range 5–15 mg/hr) for up to 24 hr.

Availability (generic available)

Tablets: 30 mg, 60 mg, 90 mg, 120 mg. **Extended-release capsules (Cardizem CD, Tiazac, Tiadylt ER, Cartia XT, Taztia XT):** 120 mg, 180 mg, 240 mg, 300 mg, 360 mg, 420 mg. **Extended-release tablets (Cardizem LA, Matzim LA):** 120 mg, 180 mg, 240 mg, 300 mg, 360 mg, 420 mg. **Premixed infusion:** 125 mg/125 mL D5W, 250 mg/250 mL D5W. **Solution for injection:** 5 mg/mL.

NURSING IMPLICATIONS

Assessment

● Monitor BP and pulse prior to therapy, during dose titration, and periodically during therapy. Monitor ECG periodically during prolonged therapy. May cause prolonged PR interval.
● Monitor intake and output ratios and daily weight. Assess for signs of HF (peripheral edema, rales/crackles, dyspnea, weight gain, jugular venous distention).
● Monitor frequency of prescription refills to determine adherence.
● Patients receiving digoxin concurrently with calcium channel blockers should have routine serum digoxin levels checked and be monitored for signs and symptoms of digoxin toxicity.
● Assess for rash periodically during therapy. May cause SJS. Discontinue therapy if severe or if accompanied with fever, general malaise, fatigue, muscle or joint aches, blisters, oral lesions, conjunctivitis, hepatitis and/or eosinophilia.

- **Angina:** Assess location, duration, intensity, and precipitating factors of patient's anginal pain.
- **Arrhythmias:** Monitor ECG continuously during administration. Report bradycardia or prolonged hypotension promptly. Emergency equipment and medication should be available. Monitor BP and pulse before and frequently during administration.

Lab Test Considerations
- Total serum calcium concentrations are not affected by calcium channel blockers.
- Monitor serum potassium periodically. Hypokalemia ↑ the risk of arrhythmias and should be corrected.
- Monitor renal and hepatic functions periodically during long-term therapy. May cause ↑ in hepatic enzymes after several days of therapy, which return to normal on discontinuation of therapy.

Implementation
- Do not confuse Cardizem with Cardene. Do not confuse Tiazac with Ziac. Do not confuse diltiazem with diazepam.
- **PO:** May be administered without regard to meals. May be administered with meals if GI irritation becomes a problem.
- *DNC:* Do not open, crush, break, or chew extended-release tablets. Empty tablets that appear in stool are not significant.

IV Administration
- **IV Push:** *Dilution:* Administer bolus dose undiluted. *Concentration:* 5 mg/mL. *Rate:* Administer over 2 min.
- **Continuous Infusion:** *Dilution:* Dilute 125 mg in 100 mL, 250 mg in 250 mL, or 250 mg in 500 mL of 0.9% NaCl, D5W, or D5/0.45% NaCl. Infusion is stable for 24 hr at room temperature or if refrigerated. *Concentration:* 125 mg/125 mL (1 mg/mL), 250 mg/300 mL (0.83 mg/mL), 250 mg/550 mL (0.45 mg/mL). *Rate:* See Route/Dosage section. Titrate to patient's heart rate and BP response.
- **Y-Site Compatibility:** albumin, alemtuzumab, amifostine, amikacin, aminocaproic acid, amiodarone, amphotericin B deoxycholate, anidulafungin, argatroban, arsenic trioxide, atracurium, azithromycin, aztreonam, bivalirudin, bleomycin, bumetanide, buprenorphine, busulfan, butorphanol, calcium chloride, calcium gluconate, cangrelor, carboplatin, carmustine, caspofungin, cefazolin, cefotaxime, cefotetan, cefoxitin, ceftaroline, ceftazidime, ceftolozane/tazobactam, ceftriaxone, cefuroxime, chlorpromazine, ciprofloxacin, cisatracurium, cisplatin, clindamycin, cyclophosphamide, cyclosporine, cytarabine, dacarbazine, dactinomycin, daptomycin, daunorubicin hydrochloride, dexamethasone, dexmedetomidine, dexrazoxane, digoxin, diphenhydramine, dobutamine, docetaxel, dopamine, doxorubicin hydrochloride, doxycycline, droperidol, enalaprilat, ephedrine, epinephrine, epirubicin, ep-

tifibatide, eravacycline, ertapenem, erythromycin, esmolol, etoposide, etoposide phosphate, famotidine, fentanyl, fluconazole, fludarabine, foscarnet, fosphenytoin, gemcitabine, gentamicin, glycopyrrolate, granisetron, haloperidol, hetastarch, hydralazine, hydromorphone, idarubicin, ifosfamide, imipenem/cilastatin, irinotecan, isoproterenol, isavuconazonium, labetalol, leucovorin calcium, levofloxacin, lidocaine, linezolid, lorazepam, magnesium sulfate, mannitol, melphalan, meperidine, meropenem, meropenem/vaborbactam, mesna, methadone, metoclopramide, metoprolol, metronidazole, midazolam, milrinone, mitoxantrone, morphine, moxifloxacin, multivitamins, mycophenolate, nalbuphine, naloxone, nicardipine, nitroglycerin, nitroprusside, norepinephrine, octreotide, ondansetron, oxacillin, oxaliplatin, oxytocin, paclitaxel, palonosetron, pamidronate, pemetrexed, penicillin G potassium, pentamidine, phentolamine, phenylephrine, plazomicin, potassium acetate, potassium chloride, potassium phosphate, prochlorperazine, promethazine, propranolol, remifentanil, rocuronium, sodium acetate, succinylcholine, sufentanil, tacrolimus, telavancin, theophylline, thiotepa, tigecycline, tirofiban, tobramycin, topotecan, trimethoprim/sulfamethoxazole, vancomycin, vasopressin, vecuronium, verapamil, vinblastine, vincristine, vinorelbine, voriconazole, zidovudine, zoledronic acid.
- **Y-Site Incompatibility:** allopurinol, amphotericin B lipid complex, amphotericin B liposomal, cefepime, chloramphenicol, dantrolene, diazepam, doxorubicin liposomal, fluorouracil, furosemide, ganciclovir, gemtuzumab ozogamicin, ketorolac, methotrexate, micafungin, mitomycin, pantoprazole, pentobarbital, phenobarbital, phenytoin, piperacillin/tazobactam, rifampin, thiopental.

Patient/Family Teaching
- Advise patient to take medication as directed at the same time each day, even if feeling well. Take missed doses as soon as possible unless almost time for next dose; do not double doses. May need to be discontinued gradually.
- Advise patient to avoid large amounts of grapefruit juice (6–8 glasses/day) during therapy.
- Instruct patient on correct technique for monitoring pulse. Instruct patient to contact health care professional if heart rate is <50 bpm.
- Caution patient to change positions slowly to minimize orthostatic hypotension.
- May cause drowsiness or dizziness. Advise patient to avoid driving or other activities requiring alertness until response to the medication is known.
- Instruct patient on importance of maintaining good dental hygiene and seeing dentist frequently for teeth cleaning to prevent tenderness, bleeding, and gingival hyperplasia (gum enlargement).

- Instruct patient to notify health care professional of all Rx or OTC medications, vitamins, or herbal products being taken and to avoid concurrent use of alcohol or OTC medications and herbal products, especially NSAIDs and cold preparations, without consulting health care professional.
- Advise patient to notify health care professional if rash, irregular heartbeat, dyspnea, swelling of hands and feet, pronounced dizziness, nausea, constipation, or hypotension occurs or if headache is severe or persistent.
- Caution patient to wear protective clothing and use sunscreen to prevent photosensitivity reactions.
- Rep: Advise females of reproductive potential to notify health care professional if pregnancy is planned or suspected or if breastfeeding.
- **Angina:** Instruct patient on concurrent nitrate or beta-blocker therapy to continue taking both medications as directed and to use SL nitroglycerin as needed for anginal attacks.
- Advise patient to contact health care professional if chest pain does not improve, worsens after therapy, or occurs with diaphoresis; if shortness of breath occurs; or if severe, persistent headache occurs.
- Caution patient to discuss exercise restrictions with health care professional before exertion.
- **Hypertension:** Encourage patient to comply with other interventions for hypertension (weight reduction, low-sodium diet, smoking cessation, moderation of alcohol consumption, regular exercise, and stress management). Medication controls but does not cure hypertension.
- Instruct patient and family in proper technique for monitoring BP. Advise patient to take BP weekly and to report significant changes to health care professional.

Evaluation/Desired Outcomes

- Decrease in BP.
- Decrease in frequency and severity of anginal attacks.
- Decrease in need for nitrate therapy.
- Increase in activity tolerance and sense of well-being.
- Suppression and prevention of supraventricular tachyarrhythmias.

---

dimethyl fumarate
(dye-**meth**-il **fue**-ma-rate)
Tecfidera
Classification
Therapeutic: anti-multiple sclerosis agents

Indications

Relapsing forms of multiple sclerosis (MS), including clinically isolated syndrome, relapsing-remitting disease, and active secondary progressive disease.

Action

Activates nuclear factor (Nrf2) pathway involved in cellular response to oxidative stress. **Therapeutic Effects:** Decreased incidence/severity of relapse with decreased progression of lesions and disability.

Pharmacokinetics

Absorption: Following oral administration rapidly converted to active metabolite monomethyl fumarate (MMF) by enzymes in GI tract, blood, and tissue.
Distribution: Unknown.
Metabolism and Excretion: MMF is metabolized by the tricarboxylic acid cycle. 60% eliminated via exhalation of CO_2. Minor amounts eliminated by renal (16%) and fecal (1%) routes, trace amounts in urine.
Half-life: *MMF:* 1 hr.

TIME/ACTION PROFILE (effects on disability)

ROUTE	ONSET	PEAK	DURATION
PO	24 wk	60 wk	Unknown

Contraindications/Precautions

Contraindicated in: Hypersensitivity.
Use Cautiously in: Serious infections (treatment may be withheld); Persistent lymphopenia (>6 mo) (↑ risk of progressive multifocal leukoencephalopathy [PML]); OB: Use during pregnancy only if potential maternal benefit justifies potential fetal risk; Lactation: Safety not established in breastfeeding; Pedi: Safety and effectiveness not established in children.

Adverse Reactions/Side Effects

Derm: flushing, erythema, pruritus, rash. **GI:** abdominal pain, diarrhea, nausea, ↑ liver enzymes, dyspepsia, HEPATOTOXICITY, vomiting. **Hemat:** lymphopenia. **Neuro:** PML. **Misc:** HYPERSENSITIVITY REACTIONS (including anaphylaxis and angioedema), INFECTION (bacterial, viral [especially herpes zoster], and fungal).

Interactions

Drug-Drug: None reported.

Route/Dosage

PO (Adults): 120 mg twice daily for one wk, then 240 mg twice daily.

Availability (generic available)

Extended-release capsules: 120 mg, 240 mg.

NURSING IMPLICATIONS

Assessment

- Monitor for signs and symptoms of infections (fever, sore throat, herpes zoster, fungal and bacterial infections). Consider withholding medication until serious infections are resolved.
- Monitor for signs and symptoms of PML (progressive weakness on one side of body or clumsiness of limbs, disturbance of vision, changes in thinking, memory, and orientation causing confusion and personality changes). Symptoms are diverse, progress

over days to weeks. Withhold medication and obtain diagnostic evaluation.
- Monitor for signs and symptoms of hypersensitivity reactions (difficulty breathing, urticaria, swelling of throat and tongue) during therapy.

Lab Test Considerations
- Monitor CBC with lymphocyte count before initiating therapy, after 6 mo, and every 6–12 mo thereafter. If lymphocyte count is <0.5 × 10⁹/L for >6 mo, may interrupt therapy. Consider withholding therapy for patients with serious infections.
- Assess AST, ALT, alkaline phosphatase, and total bilirubin levels prior to starting therapy and as clinically indicated. May cause ↑ AST and ALT. Discontinue therapy if clinically significant liver injury is suspected.
- May cause transient ↑ mean eosinophil count during first 2 mo of therapy.

Implementation
- **PO:** Administer 120 mg twice daily for 7 days then increase to maintenance dose of 240 mg twice daily without regard to food. For patients with difficulty tolerating maintenance dose, may temporarily decrease to 120 mg twice daily; resume maintenance dose within 4 wk. **DNC:** Swallow capsules whole; do not open, crush, chew, or sprinkle on food. Discard any unused capsules 90 days after opening.

Patient/Family Teaching
- Instruct patient to take dimethyl fumarate as directed. Advise patient to read *Patient Information* before starting therapy and with each Rx refill in case of changes.
- Caution patient not to share medication with others, even if they have the same symptoms; may be dangerous.
- May cause flushing (warmth, redness, itching, and/or burning sensation). Usually begins after starting and resolves over time. Administration of dimethyl fumarate with food or administration of nonenteric coated aspirin (up to a dose of 325 mg) 30 min prior to dimethyl fumarate dosing may decrease incidence or severity of flushing.
- Advise patient to notify health care professional if signs or symptoms of infections or liver injury (fatigue, anorexia, right upper abdominal discomfort, dark urine, jaundice) occur.
- Advise patient to notify health care professional promptly if signs and symptoms of PML (new or worsening weakness; trouble using their arms or legs; or changes to thinking, eyesight, strength or balance) or hypersensitivity reactions (difficulty breathing, urticaria, swelling of throat and tongue) occur.
- Advise patient to notify health care professional of all Rx or OTC medications, vitamins, or herbal products

being taken and to consult with health care professional before taking other medications.
- Rep: Advise female patient to notify health care professional if pregnancy is planned or suspected, or if breastfeeding. Encourage patients who become pregnant to join the pregnancy registry by calling 1-866-810-1462 or visiting www.tecfiderapregnancyregistry.com.

Evaluation/Desired Outcomes
- Decreased incidence/severity of relapse of MS.

dinoprostone
(dye-noe-**prost**-one)
Cervidil, Prepidil
Classification
Therapeutic: cervical ripening agent
Pharmacologic: oxytocics, prostaglandins

Indications
Used to "ripen" the cervix in pregnancy at or near term when induction of labor is indicated.

Action
Produces contractions similar to those occurring during labor at term by stimulating the myometrium (oxytocic effect). Initiates softening, effacement, and dilation of the cervix ("ripening"). Also stimulates GI smooth muscle. **Therapeutic Effects:** Initiation of labor.

Pharmacokinetics
Absorption: Rapidly absorbed.
Distribution: Unknown. Action is mostly local.
Metabolism and Excretion: Metabolized by enzymes in lung, kidneys, spleen, and liver tissue.
Half-life: 2.5–5 min.

TIME/ACTION PROFILE

ROUTE	ONSET	PEAK	DURATION
Cervical ripening (gel)	rapid	30–45 min	unknown
Cervical ripening (insert)	rapid	unknown	12 hr

Contraindications/Precautions
Contraindicated in: Hypersensitivity to prostaglandins or additives in the gel or suppository; Should be avoided in situations in which prolonged uterine contractions should be avoided, including: Previous cesarean section or uterine surgery; Cephalopelvic disproportion; Traumatic delivery or difficult labor; Multiparity (≥6 term pregnancies); Hyperactive or hypertonic uterus; Fetal distress (if delivery is not imminent); Unexplained vaginal bleeding; Placenta previa; Vasa previa; Active herpes genitalis; Obstetric emergency requiring surgical intervention; Situations in

which vaginal delivery is contraindicated; Presence of acute pelvic inflammatory disease or ruptured membranes; Concurrent oxytocic therapy (wait for 30 min after removing insert before using oxytocin).

Use Cautiously in: Uterine scarring; Asthma; Hypotension; Cardiac disease; Adrenal disorders; Anemia; Jaundice; Diabetes mellitus; Seizure disorders; Glaucoma; Renal impairment; Hepatic impairment; Pulmonary disease; Multiparity (up to five previous term pregnancies); Women >30 yr, those with complications during pregnancy, and those with a gestational age >40 wk (↑ risk of disseminated intravascular coagulation).

Adverse Reactions/Side Effects

GU: uterine contractile abnormalities, warm feeling in vagina. **MS:** back pain. **Misc:** AMNIOTIC FLUID EMBOLISM, fever.

Interactions

Drug-Drug: Augments the effects of other **oxytocics**.

Route/Dosage

Vag (Adults, Cervical): *Endocervical gel:* 0.5 mg; if response is unfavorable, may repeat in 6 hr (not to exceed 1.5 mg/24 hr). *Vaginal insert:* one 10-mg insert.

Availability

Endocervical gel (Prepidil): 0.5 mg dinoprostone in 3 g of gel vehicle in a prefilled syringe with catheters. **Vaginal insert (Cervidil):** 10 mg.

NURSING IMPLICATIONS

Assessment

● Monitor uterine activity, fetal status, and dilation and effacement of cervix continuously throughout therapy. Assess for hypertonus, sustained uterine contractility, and fetal distress. Insert should be removed at the onset of active labor.

Implementation

● **Vaginal Insert:** Place vaginal insert transversely in the posterior vaginal fornix immediately after removing from foil package. Warming of insert and sterile conditions are not required. Use vaginal insert only with a retrieval system. Use minimal amount of water-soluble lubricant during insertion; avoid excess because it may hamper release of dinoprostone from insert. Patient should remain supine for 2 hr after insertion, then may ambulate. Store vaginal inserts in freezer.
● Vaginal insert delivers dinoprostone 0.3 mg/hr over 12 hr. Remove insert at the onset of active labor, before amniotomy, or after 12 hr.
● Oxytocin should not be used during or <30 min after removal of insert.
● **Endocervical Gel:** Determine degree of effacement before insertion of the endocervical catheter. Do not administer above the level of the internal os. Use a 20-mm endocervical catheter if no effacement is present and a 10-mm catheter if the cervix is 50% effaced.

● Use caution to prevent contact of dinoprostone gel with skin. Wash hands thoroughly with soap and water after administration.
● Bring gel to room temperature just before administration. Do not force warming with external sources (water bath, microwave). Remove peel-off seal from end of syringe; then remove the protective end cap and insert end cap into plunger stopper assembly in barrel of syringe. Aseptically remove catheter from package. Firmly attach catheter hub to syringe tip; click is evidence of attachment. Fill catheter with sterile gel by pushing plunger to expel air from catheter before administration to patient. Gel is stable for 24 mo if refrigerated.
● Patient should be in dorsal position with cervix visualized using a speculum. Introduce gel with catheter into cervical canal using sterile technique. Administer gel by gentle expulsion from syringe and then remove catheter. Do not attempt to administer small amount of gel remaining in syringe. Use syringe for only 1 patient; discard syringe, catheter, and unused package contents after using.
● Patient should remain supine for 15–30 min after administration to minimize leakage from cervical canal.
● Oxytocin may be administered 6–12 hr after desired response from dinoprostone gel. If no cervical/uterine response to initial dose of dinoprostone is obtained, repeat dose may be administered in 6 hr.

Patient/Family Teaching

● Explain purpose of medication and vaginal exams.
● **Cervical Ripening:** Inform patient that she may experience a warm feeling in her vagina during administration.
● Advise patient to notify health care professional if contractions become prolonged.

Evaluation/Desired Outcomes

● Cervical ripening and induction of labor.

BEERS

diphenhydrAMINE (oral, parenteral)

(dye-fen-**hye**-dra-meen)

✦Aller-Aide, ✦Allerdryl, ✦Allergy Formula, AllerMax, ✦Allernix, Banophen, Benadryl Dye-Free Allergy, Benadryl Allergy, Benadryl, ✦Benylin, ✦Calmex, Compoz, Compoz Nighttime Sleep Aid, ✦Dimetane Allergy, Diphen AF, Diphen Cough, ✦Diphenhist, ✦Dormex, ✦Dormiphen, Genahist, 40 Winks, Hyrexin-50, ✦Insomnal, Maximum Strength Nytol, Maximum Strength Sleepinal, Midol PM, Miles Nervine, ✦Nadryl, Nighttime Sleep

Aid, Nytol, Scot-Tussin Allergy DM, Siladril, Silphen, Sleep-Eze 3, Sleep-well 2-night, Sominex, Snooze Fast, Sominex, Tusstat, Twilite, Unisom Nighttime Sleep-Aid

D

Classification
Therapeutic: allergy, cold, and cough remedies, antihistamines, antitussives

Indications
Relief of allergic symptoms caused by histamine release including: Anaphylaxis, Seasonal and perennial allergic rhinitis, Allergic dermatoses. Parkinson's disease and dystonic reactions from medications. Mild nighttime sedation. Prevention of motion sickness. Antitussive (syrup only).

Action
Antagonizes the effects of histamine at H_1-receptor sites; does not bind to or inactivate histamine. Significant CNS depressant and anticholinergic properties. **Therapeutic Effects:** Decreased symptoms of histamine excess (sneezing, rhinorrhea, nasal and ocular pruritus, ocular tearing and redness, urticaria). Relief of acute dystonic reactions. Prevention of motion sickness. Suppression of cough.

Pharmacokinetics
Absorption: Well absorbed after oral or IM administration but 40–60% of an oral dose reaches systemic circulation due to first-pass metabolism.
Distribution: Widely distributed. Crosses the placenta; enters breast milk.
Metabolism and Excretion: 95% metabolized by the liver.
Half-life: 2.4–7 hr.

TIME/ACTION PROFILE (antihistaminic effects)

ROUTE	ONSET	PEAK	DURATION
PO	15–60 min	2–4 hr	4–8 hr
IM	20–30 min	2–4 hr	4–8 hr
IV	rapid	unknown	4–8 hr

Contraindications/Precautions
Contraindicated in: Hypersensitivity; Acute attacks of asthma; Known alcohol intolerance (some liquid products); Lactation: Lactation.
Use Cautiously in: Severe liver disease; Angle-closure glaucoma; Seizure disorders; Prostatic hyperplasia; Peptic ulcer; May cause paradoxical excitation in young children; Hyperthyroidism; OB: Safety not established in pregnancy; Geri: Appears on Beers list. ↑ risk of anticholinergic adverse reactions in older adults, including falls, delirium, and dementia. Avoid use of oral formulations in older adults.

Adverse Reactions/Side Effects
CV: hypotension, palpitations. **Derm:** photosensitivity.
EENT: blurred vision, tinnitus. **GI:** anorexia, dry mouth, constipation, nausea. **GU:** dysuria, urinary frequency, urinary retention. **Local:** pain at IM site.
Neuro: drowsiness, dizziness, headache, paradoxical excitation (↑ in children). **Resp:** chest tightness, thickened bronchial secretions, wheezing.

Interactions
Drug-Drug: ↑ risk of CNS depression with other **antihistamines**, **alcohol**, **opioid analgesics**, and **sedative/hypnotics**. ↑ anticholinergic effects with **tricyclic antidepressants**, **quinidine**, or **disopyramide**. **MAO inhibitors** intensify and prolong the anticholinergic effects of antihistamines.
Drug-Natural Products: Concomitant use of **kava-kava**, **valerian**, or **chamomile** can ↑ CNS depression.

Route/Dosage
PO (Adults and Children >12 yr): *Antihistaminic/antiemetic/antivertiginic:* 25–50 mg every 4–6 hr, not to exceed 300 mg/day. *Antitussive:* 25 mg every 4 hr as needed, not to exceed 150 mg/day. *Antidyskinetic:* 25–50 mg every 4 hr (not to exceed 400 mg/day). *Sedative/hypnotic:* 50 mg 20–30 min before bedtime.
PO (Children 6–12 yr): *Antihistaminic/antiemetic/antivertiginic:* 12.5–25 mg every 4–6 hr (not to exceed 150 mg/day). *Antidyskinetic:* 1–1.5 mg/kg every 6–8 hr as needed (not to exceed 300 mg/day). *Antitussive:* 12.5 mg every 4 hr (not to exceed 75 mg/day). *Sedative/hypnotic:* 1 mg/kg/dose 20–30 min before bedtime (not to exceed 50 mg).
PO (Children 2–6 yr): *Antihistaminic/antiemetic/antivertiginic:* 6.25–12.5 mg every 4–6 hr (not to exceed 37.5 mg/day). *Antidyskinetic:* 1–1.5 mg/kg every 4–6 hr as needed (not to exceed 300 mg/day). *Antitussive:* 6.25 mg every 4 hr (not to exceed 37.5 mg/24 hr). *Sedative/hypnotic:* 1 mg/kg/dose 20–30 min before bedtime (not to exceed 50 mg).
IM, IV (Adults): 25–50 mg every 4 hr as needed (may need up to 100-mg dose, not to exceed 400 mg/day).
IM, IV (Children): 1.25 mg/kg (37.5 mg/m²) 4 times daily (not to exceed 300 mg/day).
Topical (Adults and Children ≥2 yr): Apply to affected area up to 3–4 times daily.

Availability (generic available)
Capsules: 25 mg$^{Rx, OTC}$, 50 mg$^{Rx, OTC}$. **Tablets:** ✸ 12.5 mg$^{Rx, OTC}$, 25 mg$^{Rx, OTC}$, 50 mg$^{Rx, OTC}$. **Chewable tablets (grape flavor):** 25 mg$^{Rx, OTC}$. **Orally disintegrating strips (cherry and grape flavor):** 12.5 mg$^{Rx, OTC}$, 25 mg^{OTC}. **Orally disintegrating tablets:** 12.5 mg^{OTC}, 25 mg^{OTC}, 50 mg$^{Rx, OTC}$. **Elixir (cherry and other flavors):** 12.5 mg/5 mL$^{Rx, OTC}$. **Syrup (cherry and rasp-**

berry flavor): ✸ 6.25 mg/5 mL^Rx, OTC, 12.5 mg/5 mL^Rx, OTC. **Cream:** 1%^Rx, OTC, 2%^Rx, OTC. **Topical gel:** 2%^OTC. **Topical spray:** 2%^OTC. **Topical stick:** 2%^OTC. **Solution for injection:** 50 mg/mL. *In combination with:* analgesics, decongestants, and expectorants, in OTC pain, sleep, cough, and cold preparations. See Appendix N.

NURSING IMPLICATIONS
Assessment
* Diphenhydramine has multiple uses. Determine why the medication was ordered and assess symptoms that apply to the individual patient. Geri: Appears in the *Beers list.* May cause sedation and confusion due to increased sensitivity to anticholinergic effects. Monitor carefully, assess for confusion, delirium, other anticholinergic side effects and fall risk. Institute measures to prevent falls.
* **Prevention and Treatment of Anaphylaxis:** Assess for urticaria and for patency of airway.
* **Allergic Rhinitis:** Assess degree of nasal stuffiness, rhinorrhea, and sneezing.
* **Parkinsonism and Extrapyramidal Reactions:** Assess movement disorder before and after administration.
* **Insomnia:** Assess sleep patterns.
* **Motion Sickness:** Assess nausea, vomiting, bowel sounds, and abdominal pain.
* **Cough Suppressant:** Assess frequency and nature of cough, lung sounds, and amount and type of sputum produced. Unless contraindicated, maintain fluid intake of 1500–2000 mL daily to decrease viscosity of bronchial secretions.
* **Pruritus:** Assess degree of itching, skin rash, and inflammation.

Lab Test Considerations
* May ↓ skin response to allergy tests. Discontinue 4 days before skin testing.

Implementation
* Do not confuse Benadryl with benazepril. Do not confuse diphenhydramine with dimenhydrinate.
* When used for insomnia, administer 20–30 min before bedtime and schedule activities to minimize interruption of sleep.
* When used for prophylaxis of motion sickness, administer at least 30 min and preferably 1–2 hr before exposure to conditions that may precipitate motion sickness.
* **PO:** Administer with meals or milk to minimize GI irritation. Capsule may be emptied and contents taken with water or food.
* Orally disintegrating tablets and strips should be left in the package until use. Remove from the blister pouch. Do not push tablet through the blister; peel open the blister pack with dry hands and place tablet on tongue. Tablet will dissolve rapidly and be swallowed with saliva. No liquid is needed to take the orally disintegrating tablet.

* **IM:** Administer 50 mg/mL into well-developed muscle. Avoid SUBQ injections.

IV Administration
* **IV Push: *Dilution:*** May be further diluted in 0.9% NaCl, 0.45% NaCl, D5W, D10W, dextrose/saline combinations, Ringer's solution, LR, and dextrose/Ringer's combinations. ***Concentration:*** 25 mg/mL. ***Rate:*** Infuse at a rate not to exceed 25 mg/min. For pediatric patients, may further dilute as an intermittent infusion over 10 to 15 min.
* **Y-Site Compatibility:** acetaminophen, aldesleukin, alemtuzumab, amifostine, amikacin, aminocaproic acid, amiodarone, amphotericin B lipid complex, amphotericin B liposome, anidulafungin, argatroban, ascorbic acid, atracurium, atropine, azithromycin, benztropine, bivalirudin, bleomycin, bumetanide, buprenorphine, butorphanol, calcium chloride, calcium gluconate, carboplatin, carmustine, caspofungin, ceftaroline, ceftolozane/tazobactam, chlorpromazine, ciprofloxacin, cisatracurium, cisplatin, cladribine, clindamycin, cyanocobalamin, cyclophosphamide, cyclosporine, cytarabine, dacarbazine, dactinomycin, daptomycin, daunorubicin hydrochloride, dexmedetomidine, dexrazoxane, digoxin, diltiazem, dobutamine, docetaxel, dopamine, doxorubicin hydrochloride, doxorubicin liposomal, doxycycline, enalaprilat, ephedrine, epinephrine, epirubicin, epoetin alfa, eptifibatide, ertapenem, erythromycin, esmolol, etoposide, etoposide phosphate, famotidine, fentanyl, filgrastim, fluconazole, fludarabine, folic acid, fosphenytoin, gemcitabine, gemtuzumab ozogamicin, gentamicin, glycopyrrolate, granisetron, hetastarch, hydromorphone, idarubicin, ifosfamide, imipenem/cilastatin, irinotecan, isoproterenol, ketamine, labetalol, LR, leucovorin calcium, levofloxacin, lidocaine, linezolid, lorazepam, magnesium sulfate, mannitol, melphalan, meperidine, meropenem, mesna, methotrexate, methadone, metoclopramide, metoprolol, metronidazole, midazolam, mitomycin, mitoxantrone, morphine, moxifloxacin, multiple vitamins, mycophenolate, nalbuphine, naloxone, nicardipine, nitroglycerin, norepinephrine, octreotide, ondansetron, oxaliplatin, oxytocin, paclitaxel, palonosetron, pamidronate, papaverine, pemetrexed, penicillin G, pentamidine, phentolamine, phenylephrine, phytonadione, piperacillin/tazobactam, plazomicin, potassium acetate, potassium chloride, procainamide, prochlorperazine, promethazine, propofol, propranolol, protamine, pyridoxine, remifentanil, rituximab, rocuronium, sargramostim, sodium acetate, succinylcholine, sufentanil, tacrolimus, theophylline, thiamine, thiotepa, tigecycline, tirofiban, tobramycin, topotecan, trastuzumab, vancomycin, vasopressin, vecuronium, verapamil, vinblastine, vincristine, vinorelbine, voriconazole, zoledronic acid.
* **Y-Site Incompatibility:** allopurinol, aminophylline, amphotericin B deoxycholate, ampicillin, azathioprine, cefazolin, cefepime, cefotaxime, cefotetan,

cefoxitin, ceftazidime, ceftriaxone, cefuroxime, chloramphenicol, dantrolene, dexamethasone, diazepam, fluorouracil, foscarnet, furosemide, ganciclovir, heparin, indomethacin, insulin, regular, ketorolac, meropenem/vaborbactam, methylprednisolone, milrinone, nitroprusside, oxacillin, pantoprazole, pentobarbital, phenobarbital, phenytoin, sodium bicarbonate, trimethoprim/sulfamethoxazole.

- **Topical:** Apply a thin coat and rub gently until absorbed. Only for topical use; avoid ingestion.

Patient/Family Teaching

- Instruct patient to take medication as directed; do not exceed recommended amount. Caution patient not to use oral OTC diphenhydramine products with any other product containing diphenhydramine, including products used topically.
- May cause drowsiness. Caution patient to avoid driving or other activities requiring alertness until response to drug is known.
- May cause dry mouth. Inform patient that frequent oral rinses, good oral hygiene, and sugarless gum or candy may minimize this effect. Notify health care professional if dry mouth persists for more than 2 wk.
- Teach sleep hygiene techniques (dark room, quiet, bedtime ritual, limit daytime napping, avoidance of nicotine and caffeine) to patients taking diphenhydramine to aid sleep.
- Advise patient to use sunscreen and protective clothing to prevent photosensitivity reactions.
- Caution patient to avoid use of alcohol and other CNS depressants, including opioids, concurrently with this medication.
- Rep: Advise females of reproductive potential to notify health care professional if pregnancy is planned or suspected and to avoid breastfeeding during therapy. Monitor infants exposed to diphenhydramine through breast milk for irritability and drowsiness.
- Pedi: Can cause excitation in children. Caution parents or caregivers about proper dose calculation; overdose, especially in infants and children, can cause hallucinations, seizures, or death. Caution parents to avoid OTC cough and cold products while breastfeeding or to children <4 yr.
- Geri: Instruct older adults to avoid OTC products that contain diphenhydramine due to increased sensitivity to anticholinergic effects and potential for adverse reactions related to these effects.
- Advise patients taking diphenhydramine in OTC preparations to notify health care professional if symptoms worsen or persist for more than 7 days.

Evaluation/Desired Outcomes

- Prevention of, or decreased urticaria in, anaphylaxis or other allergic reactions.
- Decreased dyskinesia in parkinsonism and extrapyramidal reactions.

- Sedation when used as a sedative/hypnotic.
- Prevention of or decrease in nausea and vomiting caused by motion sickness.
- Decrease in frequency and intensity of cough without eliminating cough reflex.

DIURETICS (POTASSIUM-SPARING)
aMILoride (a-**mill**-oh-ride)
☘ Midamor
spironolactone (speer-oh-no-**lak**-tone)
Aldactone, Carospir
triamterene (trye-**am**-ter-een)
Dyrenium
Classification
Therapeutic: diuretics
Pharmacologic: potassium-sparing diuretics

Indications
Counteract potassium loss caused by other diuretics. Used with other agents (thiazides) to treat edema or hypertension. Primary hyperaldosteronism (spironolactone only). New York Heart Association (NYHA) class III-IV HF (spironolactone only). **Unlabeled Use:** Acne (spironolactone only). Hormone therapy for transgender females (male-to-female) (spironolactone only).

Action
Inhibition of sodium reabsorption in the kidney while saving potassium and hydrogen ions (spironolactone achieves this effect by antagonizing aldosterone receptors). **Therapeutic Effects:** Weak diuretic and antihypertensive response when compared with other diuretics. Conservation of potassium. Improved survival in patients with NYHA class II-IV HF.

Pharmacokinetics
Absorption: *Amiloride:* 30–90% absorbed; *spironolactone:* >90% absorbed; oral suspension results in 15–37% higher serum concentrations compared to tablets; *triamterene:* 30–70% absorbed.
Distribution: *Amiloride* and *triamterene:* widely distributed; all cross the placenta and enter breast milk.
Protein Binding: *Spironolactone* >90%.
Metabolism and Excretion: *Amiloride:* 50% eliminated unchanged in urine, 40% excreted in the feces; *spironolactone:* converted by the liver to its active diuretic compound (canrenone); *triamterene:* 80% metabolized by the liver, some excretion of unchanged drug.
Half-life: *Amiloride:* 6–9 hr; *spironolactone:* 78–84 min (spironolactone); 13–24 hr (canrenone); *triamterene:* 1.7–2.5 hr.

TIME/ACTION PROFILE (diuretic effect)

ROUTE	ONSET	PEAK	DURATION
Amiloride	2 hr†	6–10 hr†	24 hr†
Spironolactone	unknown	2–3 days‡	2–3 days‡
Triamterene	2–4 hr†	1–several days‡	7–9 hr†

†Single dose.
‡Multiple doses.

Contraindications/Precautions

Contraindicated in: Hypersensitivity; Hyperkalemia; Anuria; Acute renal insufficiency; Significant renal impairment (CCr ≤30 mL/min or serum creatinine >2.5 mg/dL).

Use Cautiously in: Hepatic impairment; Diabetes (↑ risk of hyperkalemia); History of gout or kidney stones (triamterene only); Concurrent use of potassium supplements or potassium-containing salt substitutes; OB, Lactation, Pedi: Safety not established; Geri: Presence of age-related renal impairment may lead to ↑ risk of hyperkalemia.

Adverse Reactions/Side Effects

CV: arrhythmias. **GI:** *amiloride:* constipation, nausea, vomiting. **GU:** *spironolactone:* erectile dysfunction; *triamterene:* nephrolithiasis. **Derm:** STEVENS-JOHNSON SYNDROME (SJS), TOXIC EPIDERMAL NECROLYSIS (TEN); *triamterene:* photosensitivity. **Endo:** *spironolactone:* breast tenderness, gynecomastia, irregular menses, voice deepening. **F and E:** hyperkalemia, hyponatremia. **Hemat:** *spironolactone:* agranulocytosis; *triamterene:* hemolytic anemia, thrombocytopenia. **MS:** muscle cramps. **Neuro:** dizziness; *spironolactone only:* clumsiness, headache. **Misc:** allergic reactions.

Interactions

Drug-Drug: ↑ hypotension with acute ingestion of **alcohol**, other **antihypertensives**, or **nitrates**. Use with **ACE inhibitors**, **angiotensin II receptor antagonists**, **NSAIDs**, **potassium supplements**, **cyclosporine**, or **tacrolimus** ↑ risk of hyperkalemia. May ↑ levels/risk of toxicity from **lithium**. Effectiveness may be ↓ by **NSAIDs**. Spironolactone may ↑ levels and risk of toxicity of **digoxin**; monitor levels closely. Spironolactone may ↑ levels and risk of toxicity of **CYP2C8 substrates**, including **repaglinide**. Spironolactone may ↑ levels and risk of toxicity of **CYP3A4/5 substrates**, including **midazolam**, **sirolimus**, or **tacrolimus**.

Route/Dosage

Amiloride

PO (Adults): *Hypertension:* 5–10 mg/day (up to 20 mg).

PO (Children 1–17 yr): 0.4–0.625 mg/kg/day (maximum = 20 mg/day) (unlabeled use).

Spironolactone

Oral suspension is not therapeutically equivalent to tablets. If patient requires a dose >100 mg, use tablets, NOT suspension. Suspension doses >100 mg may result in higher than expected spironolactone concentrations.

PO (Adults): *Edema:* Tablets: 25–200 mg/day as a single dose or 2 divided doses. Suspension: 75 mg/day as a single dose or 2 divided doses. *Hypertension:* Tablets: 25–100 mg/day as a single dose or 2 divided doses; may titrate dose every 2 wk (max dose = 100 mg/day). Suspension: 20–75 mg/day as a single dose or 2 divided doses; may titrate dose every 2 wk (max dose = 75 mg/day). *Diuretic-induced hypokalemia:* 25–100 mg/day in 1–2 divided doses. *Diagnosis of primary hyperaldosteronism:* 100–400 mg/day in 1–2 divided doses. *HF with serum potassium ≤5 mEq/L and eGFR >50 mL/min/1.73 m²:* Tablet: 25 mg once daily; may then ↑ to 50 mg once daily; if develop hyperkalemia with 25 mg once daily, ↓ dose to 25 mg every other day. Suspension: 20 mg once daily; may then ↑ to 37.5 mg once daily; if develop hyperkalemia with 20 mg once daily, ↓ dose to 20 mg every other day. *HF with serum potassium ≤5 mEq/L and eGFR 30–50 mL/min/1.73 m²:* Tablets: 25 mg every other day. Suspension: 10 mg once daily. *Acne (off-label use):* 50–200 mg once daily. *Hormone therapy for transgender females (off-label use):* 25 mg once or twice daily in combination with other appropriate agents. Increase at 1-wk intervals based on serum testosterone levels and tolerability to a usual dose of 50–150 mg twice daily (max dose = 200 mg twice daily).

PO (Children 1–17 yr): *Diuretic, Hypertension:* 1 mg/kg/day in 1–2 divided doses (should not exceed 3.3 mg/kg/day or 100 mg/day) (unlabeled use). *Diagnosis of primary hyperaldosteronism:* 125–375 mg/m²/day in 1–2 divided doses (unlabeled use).

PO (Neonates): 1–3 mg/kg/day in 1–2 divided doses.

Triamterene

PO (Adults): *Hypertension:* 100 mg twice daily (not to exceed 300 mg/day; lower doses in combination products).

PO (Children): *Hypertension:* 1–2 mg/kg/day in 2 divided doses; should not exceed 4 mg/kg/day or 300 mg/day.

Availability

Amiloride (generic available)

Tablets: 5 mg. *In combination with:* hydrochlorothiazide.

Spironolactone (generic available)

Tablets: 25 mg, 50 mg, 100 mg. **Oral suspension (banana-flavor):** 25 mg/5 mL. *In combination with:* hydrochlorothiazide.

Triamterene

Capsules: 50 mg, 100 mg. *In combination with:* hydrochlorothiazide (Maxzide). See Appendix N.

NURSING IMPLICATIONS

Assessment

- Monitor intake and output ratios and daily weight during therapy.
- If medication is given as an adjunct to antihypertensive therapy, monitor BP before administering.
- Assess patient frequently for development of hyperkalemia (fatigue, muscle weakness, paresthesia, confusion, dyspnea, ECG changes, cardiac arrhythmias). Patients who have diabetes mellitus or kidney disease and geriatric patients are at increased risk of developing these symptoms.
- Periodic ECGs are recommended in patients receiving prolonged therapy.
- Assess patient for skin rash frequently during therapy. Discontinue diuretic at first sign of rash; may be life-threatening. SJS or TEN may develop. Treat symptomatically; may recur once treatment is stopped.

Lab Test Considerations

- Evaluate serum potassium levels before and routinely during therapy. Hold drug and notify health care professional if patient becomes hyperkalemic.
- Monitor BUN, serum creatinine, and electrolytes before and periodically during therapy. May cause ↑ serum magnesium, BUN, creatinine, potassium, and urinary calcium excretion levels. May also cause ↓ sodium levels.
- Discontinue potassium-sparing diuretics 3 days before a glucose tolerance test because of risk of severe hyperkalemia.
- *Spironolactone* may cause false ↑ of plasma cortisol concentrations. Spironolactone should be withdrawn 4–7 days before test.
- Monitor platelet count and total and differential leukocyte count periodically during therapy in patients taking *triamterene*.

Implementation

- Do not confuse amiloride with amlodipine.
- *Carospir* is not therapeutically equivalent to *Aldactone*; do not interchange.
- **PO:** Administer in AM to avoid interrupting sleep pattern.
- Administer with food or milk to minimize gastric irritation and to increase bioavailability. Administer with or without food, but take consistently with respect to food.
- *Triamterene* capsules may be opened and contents mixed with food or fluids for patients with difficulty swallowing.

Patient/Family Teaching

- Emphasize the importance of continuing to take this medication, even if feeling well. Instruct patient to take medication at the same time each day. Take missed doses as soon as remembered unless almost time for next dose. Do not double doses.
- Caution patient to avoid salt substitutes and foods that contain high levels of potassium or sodium unless prescribed by health care professional.
- May cause dizziness. Caution patient to avoid driving or other activities requiring alertness until response to medication is known.
- Instruct patient to notify health care professional of all Rx or OTC medications, vitamins, or herbal products being taken and to consult health care professional before taking any OTC medications concurrently with this therapy, especially OTC decongestants, cough or cold preparations, or appetite suppressants due to potential for increased BP.
- Advise patients taking *triamterene* to use sunscreen and protective clothing to prevent photosensitivity reactions.
- Instruct patient to notify health care professional of medication regimen before treatment or surgery.
- Advise patient to notify health care professional if rash, muscle weakness or cramps; fatigue; or severe nausea, vomiting, or diarrhea occurs.
- Inform male patients that spironolactone may cause gynecomastia; may require dose decrease. Usually reversible.
- Rep: Advise females of reproductive potential to notify health care professional if pregnancy is planned or suspected or if breastfeeding.
- Emphasize the need for follow-up exams to monitor progress.
- **Hypertension:** Reinforce need to continue additional therapies for hypertension (weight loss, restricted sodium intake, stress reduction, moderation of alcohol intake, regular exercise, and cessation of smoking). Medication helps control but does not cure hypertension.
- Teach patient and family the correct technique for checking BP weekly.

Evaluation/Desired Outcomes

- Increase in diuresis and decrease in edema while maintaining serum potassium level in an acceptable range.
- Decrease in BP.
- Prevention of hypokalemia in patients taking diuretics.
- Treatment of hyperaldosteronism.
- Improved survival in patients with NYHA class II-IV HF.
- Reduced male characteristics in male-to-female transgender patients.

DIURETICS (THIAZIDE)
chlorothiazide (klor-oh-**thye**-a-zide)
  Diuril
chlorthalidone (**thiazide-like**)
(klor-**thal**-i-doan)
  Thalitone
hydroCHLOROthiazide
(hye-droe-klor-oh-**thye**-a-zide)
  ~~Microzide~~

Classification
Therapeutic: antihypertensives, diuretics
Pharmacologic: thiazide diuretics

Indications
Management of mild to moderate hypertension. Treatment of edema associated with: HF, Renal impairment, Cirrhosis, Glucocorticoid therapy, Estrogen therapy.

Action
Increases excretion of sodium and water by inhibiting sodium reabsorption in the distal tubule. Promotes excretion of chloride, potassium, magnesium, and bicarbonate. May produce arteriolar dilation. **Therapeutic Effects:** Lowering of BP in hypertensive patients and diuresis with mobilization of edema.

Pharmacokinetics
Absorption: All are rapidly absorbed after oral administration.
Distribution: All cross the placenta and enter breast milk.
Metabolism and Excretion: All are excreted mainly unchanged by the kidneys.
Half-life: *Chlorothiazide:* 1–2 hr; *chlorthalidone:* 35–50 hr; *hydrochlorothiazide:* 6–15 hr.

TIME/ACTION PROFILE (diuretic effect)

ROUTE	ONSET	PEAK	DURATION
Chlorothia-zide PO	2 hr	4 hr	6–12 hr
Chlorothia-zide IV	15 min	30 min	2 hr
Chlorthali-done	2 hr	2 hr	48–72 hr
Hydro-chlorothia-zide†	2 hr	3–6 hr	6–12 hr

†Onset of antihypertensive effect is 3–4 days and does not become maximal for 7–14 days of dosing.

Contraindications/Precautions
Contraindicated in: Hypersensitivity (cross-sensitivity with other thiazides or sulfonamides may exist); Some products contain tartrazine and should be avoided in patients with known intolerance; Anuria; Lactation: Lactation.
Use Cautiously in: Renal or hepatic impairment; OB: Pregnancy (jaundice or thrombocytopenia may be seen in the newborn).

Adverse Reactions/Side Effects
CV: hypotension. **Derm:** photosensitivity, rash, SKIN CANCER (non-melanoma), STEVENS-JOHNSON SYNDROME (SJS). **EENT:** acute angle-closure glaucoma (hydrochlorothiazide), acute myopia (hydrochlorothiazide). **Endo:** hyperglycemia. **F and E:** hypokalemia, dehydration, hypercalcemia, hypochloremic alkalosis, hypomagnesemia, hyponatremia, hypophosphatemia, hypovolemia. **GI:** anorexia, cramping, hepatitis, nausea, pancreatitis, vomiting. **Hemat:** thrombocytopenia. **Metab:** hypercholesterolemia, hyperuricemia. **MS:** muscle cramps. **Neuro:** dizziness, drowsiness, lethargy, weakness.

Interactions
Drug-Drug: Additive hypotension with other **antihypertensives**, acute ingestion of **alcohol**, or **nitrates**. Additive hypokalemia with **corticosteroids**, **amphotericin B**, or **piperacillin/tazobactam**. May ↑ **lithium** levels. **Cholestyramine** or **colestipol** ↓ absorption. Hypokalemia ↑ risk of **digoxin** toxicity. **NSAIDs** may ↓ effectiveness.

Route/Dosage
When used as a diuretic in adults, generally given daily, but may be given every other day or 2–3 days/wk.

Chlorothiazide
PO (Adults): 125 mg–2 g/day in 1–2 divided doses.
PO (Children >6 mo): 20 mg/kg/day in 1–2 divided doses (maximum dose = 1 g/day).
PO (Neonates ≤6 mo): 10–20 mg/kg every 12 hr (maximum dose = 375 mg/day).
IV (Adults): 500 mg–1 g/day in 1–2 divided doses.
IV (Children >6 mo): 4 mg/kg/day in 1–2 divided doses (maximum dose = 20 mg/kg/day) (unlabeled use).
IV (Neonates ≤6 mo): 1–4 mg/kg every 12 hr (maximum dose = 20 mg/kg/day) (unlabeled use).

Chlorthalidone
PO (Adults): 12.5–100 mg once daily (daily doses above 25 mg are associated with greater likelihood of electrolyte abnormalities).

Hydrochlorothiazide
PO (Adults): 12.5–100 mg/day in 1–2 divided doses (up to 200 mg/day); not to exceed 50 mg/day for hypertension; daily doses above 25 mg are associated with greater likelihood of electrolyte abnormalities.
PO (Children >6 mo): 1–3 mg/kg/day in 2 divided doses (not to exceed 37.5 mg/day).
PO (Children <6 mo): 1–3 mg/kg/day in 2 divided doses.

Availability

Chlorothiazide (generic available)
Oral suspension: 250 mg/5 mL. **Powder for injection:** 500 mg/vial.

Chlorthalidone (generic available)
Tablets: ❀ 12.5 mg, 15 mg, 25 mg, 50 mg. *In combination with:* atenolol (Tenoretic); azilsartan (Edarbyclor). See Appendix N.

Hydrochlorothiazide (generic available)

Tablets: 12.5 mg, 25 mg, 50 mg, ✿ 100 mg. **Capsules:** 12.5 mg. *In combination with:* numerous antihypertensive agents. See Appendix N.

NURSING IMPLICATIONS

Assessment

- Monitor BP, intake, output, and daily weight and assess feet, legs, and sacral area for edema daily.
- Assess patient, especially if taking digoxin, for anorexia, nausea, vomiting, muscle cramps, paresthesia, and confusion. Notify health care professional if these signs of electrolyte imbalance occur. Patients taking digoxin are at risk of digoxin toxicity because of the potassium-depleting effect of the diuretic.
- If hypokalemia occurs, consideration may be given to potassium supplements or ↓ dose of diuretic.
- Assess patient for allergy to sulfonamides. Assess patient for skin rash frequently during therapy. Discontinue diuretic at first sign of rash; may be life-threatening. SJS may develop. Treat symptomatically; may recur once treatment is stopped.
- **Hypertension:** Monitor BP before and periodically during therapy.
- Monitor frequency of prescription refills to determine compliance.

Lab Test Considerations

- Monitor electrolytes (especially potassium), blood glucose, BUN, serum creatinine, and uric acid levels before and periodically during therapy.
- May cause ↑ in serum and urine glucose in diabetic patients.
- May cause ↑ in serum bilirubin, calcium, creatinine, and uric acid, and ↓ in serum magnesium, potassium, sodium, and urinary calcium concentrations.
- May cause ↑ serum cholesterol, low-density lipoprotein, and triglyceride concentrations.

Implementation

- Do not confuse hydrochlorothiazide with hydroxyzine, hydralazine, or hydroxychloroquine.
- Administer in the morning to prevent disruption of sleep cycle.
- Intermittent dose schedule may be used for continued control of edema.
- PO: May give with food or milk to minimize GI irritation. Tablets may be crushed and mixed with fluid to facilitate swallowing.

IV Administration

- **Intermittent Infusion:** *Reconstitution:* Reconstitute chlorothiazide with at least 18 mL of sterile water for injection. Shake to dissolve. Stable for 24 hr at room temperature. *Dilution:* May be given undiluted or may be diluted further with D5W or 0.9% NaCl. *Concentration:* Up to 28 mg/mL. *Rate:* If administered undiluted may give by IV push over 3–5 min. If diluted, may infuse over 30 min.

- **Y-Site Compatibility:** alprostadil, aminophylline, atropine, calcium chloride, calcium gluconate, chloramphenicol, cyclophosphamide, dexamethasone, digoxin, epinephrine, erythromycin, furosemide, gentamicin, heparin, hydrocortisone, isoproterenol, lidocaine, methohexital, norepinephrine, oxytocin, penicillin G, phenobarbital, phentolamine, potassium chloride, procainamide, propranolol, succinylcholine.
- **Y-Site Incompatibility:** chlorpromazine, hydralazine, prochlorperazine, promethazine.

Patient/Family Teaching

- Instruct patient to take this medication at the same time each day. Take missed dose as soon as remembered but not just before next dose is due. Do not double doses.
- Instruct patient to monitor weight biweekly and notify health care professional of significant changes.
- Caution patient to change positions slowly to minimize orthostatic hypotension. This may be potentiated by alcohol.
- Advise patient to use sunscreen and protective clothing to prevent photosensitivity reactions. Advise patient of importance of regular skin cancer screenings.
- Instruct patient to discuss dietary potassium requirements with health care professional (see Appendix J).
- Instruct patient to notify health care professional of medication regimen before treatment or surgery.
- Advise patient to report rash, muscle weakness, cramps, nausea, vomiting, diarrhea, or dizziness to health care professional.
- Rep: Advise patient to notify health care professional if pregnancy is planned or suspected or if breastfeeding.
- Emphasize the importance of routine follow-up exams.
- **Hypertension:** Advise patient to continue taking the medication even if feeling better. Medication controls but does not cure hypertension.
- Encourage patient to comply with additional interventions for hypertension (weight reduction, low-sodium diet, regular exercise, smoking cessation, moderation of alcohol consumption, and stress management).
- Instruct patient and family in correct technique for monitoring weekly BP.
- Instruct patient to notify health care professional of all Rx or OTC medications, vitamins, or herbal products being taken and to consult health care professional before taking other Rx, OTC, or herbal products, especially cough or cold preparations.

Evaluation/Desired Outcomes

- Decrease in BP.
- Increase in urine output.
- Decrease in edema.

✿ = Canadian drug name. ▓ = Genetic implication. ~~Strikethrough~~ = Discontinued. CAPITALS = life-threatening. <u>Underline</u> = most frequent.

divalproex sodium, See VALPROATES.

DOBUTamine
(doe-**byoo**-ta-meen)
~~Dobutrex~~
Classification
Therapeutic: inotropics
Pharmacologic: adrenergics

Indications
Short-term management of HF caused by depressed contractility from organic heart disease or surgical procedures.

Action
Stimulates beta$_1$(myocardial)-adrenergic receptors with relatively minor effect on heart rate or peripheral blood vessels. **Therapeutic Effects:** Increased cardiac output without significantly increased heart rate.

Pharmacokinetics
Absorption: IV administration results in complete bioavailability.
Distribution: Unknown.
Metabolism and Excretion: Metabolized by the liver and other tissues.
Half-life: 2 min.

TIME/ACTION PROFILE (inotropic effects)

ROUTE	ONSET	PEAK	DURATION
IV	1–2 min	10 min	brief (min)

Contraindications/Precautions
Contraindicated in: Hypersensitivity to dobutamine or bisulfites; Idiopathic hypertrophic subaortic stenosis.
Use Cautiously in: Hypertension (↑ risk of exaggerated pressor response); MI; Atrial fibrillation; History of ventricular atopic activity (may be exacerbated); Hypovolemia (correct before administration); OB: Safety not established in pregnancy; Lactation: Safety not established in breastfeeding.

Adverse Reactions/Side Effects
CV: hypertension, premature ventricular contractions, tachycardia, angina, arrhythmias, hypotension, palpitations. **GI:** nausea, vomiting. **Local:** phlebitis. **Neuro:** headache. **Resp:** shortness of breath. **Misc:** hypersensitivity reactions, nonanginal chest pain.

Interactions
Drug-Drug: **Beta blockers** may negate the effect of dobutamine. ↑ risk of arrhythmias or hypertension with some **anesthetics** (**cyclopropane**, **halothane**), **MAO inhibitors**, **oxytocics**, or **tricyclic antidepressants**.

Route/Dosage
IV (Adults and Children): 2.5–15 mcg/kg/min; titrate to response (max dose = 40 mcg/kg/min).
IV (Neonates): 2–15 mcg/kg/min.

Availability (generic available)
Solution for injection (requires dilution): 12.5 mg/mL. **Premixed infusion:** 250 mg/250 mL, 500 mg/250 mL, 1000 mg/250 mL.

NURSING IMPLICATIONS
Assessment
- Monitor BP, heart rate, ECG, pulmonary capillary wedge pressure (PCWP), cardiac output, central venous pressure (CVP), and urinary output continuously during the administration. Report significant changes in vital signs or arrhythmias. Consult physician for parameters for pulse, BP, or ECG changes for adjusting dose or discontinuing medication.
- Palpate peripheral pulses and assess appearance of extremities routinely during dobutamine administration. Notify health care professional if quality of pulse deteriorates or if extremities become cold or mottled.

Lab Test Considerations
- Monitor potassium concentrations during therapy; may cause hypokalemia.
- Monitor electrolytes, BUN, creatinine, and prothrombin time weekly during prolonged therapy.

Toxicity and Overdose
- If overdose occurs, reduction or discontinuation of therapy is the only treatment necessary because of the short duration of dobutamine.

Implementation
- *High Alert:* IV vasoactive medications are potentially dangerous. Have second practitioner independently check original order, dose calculations, and infusion pump settings. Do not confuse dobutamine with dopamine. If available as floor stock, store in separate areas.
- Correct hypovolemia with volume expanders before initiating dobutamine therapy.
- Administer into a large vein and assess administration site frequently. Extravasation may cause pain and inflammation.

IV Administration
- **Continuous Infusion:** *Dilution:* Vials must be diluted before use. Dilute 250–1000 mg in 250–500 mL of D5W, 0.9% NaCl, 0.45% NaCl, D5/0.45% NaCl, D5/0.9% NaCl, or LR. Admixed infusions stable for 48 hr at room temperature and 7 days if refrigerated. Premixed infusions are already diluted and ready to use. *Concentration:* 0.25–5 mg/mL. *Rate:* Based on patient's weight (see Route/Dosage section). Administer via infusion pump to ensure precise amount delivered. Titrate to patient response (heart rate, presence of ectopic activity, BP, urine output, CVP, PCWP, cardiac index). Dose should be

titrated so heart rate does not increase by >10% of baseline.

- **Y-Site Compatibility:** alemtuzumab, alprostadil, amifostine, amikacin, aminocaproic acid, anidulafungin, argatroban, arsenic trioxide, ascorbic acid, atracurium, atropine, azithromycin, aztreonam, benztropine, bleomycin, bumetanide, buprenorphine, butorphanol, calcium chloride, calcium gluconate, cangrelor, carboplatin, caspofungin, chlorpromazine, ciprofloxacin, cisatracurium, cisplatin, cladribine, clindamycin, cyanocoblamin, cyclophosphamide, cyclosporine, cytarabine, dactinomycin, daptomycin, daunorubicin hydrochloride, dexmedetomidine, digoxin, diltiazem, diphenhydramine, docetaxel, dopamine, doxorubicin hydrochloride, doxorubicin liposomal, doxycycline, enalaprilat, ephedrine, epinephrine, epirubicin, epoetin alfa, eptifibatide, erythromycin, esmolol, etoposide phosphate, famotidine, fentanyl, fluconazole, fludarabine, gemcitabine, gentamicin, glycopyrrolate, granisetron, hetastarch, hydromorphone, idarubicin, ifosfamide, irinotecan, isoproterenol, ketamine, labetalol, leucovorin calcium, levofloxacin, lidocaine, linezolid, lorazepam, magnesium sulfate, mannitol, meperidine, mesna, methylprednisolone, metoclopramide, metoprolol, milrinone, mitoxantrone, morphine, moxifloxacin, multivitamins, mycophenolate, nafcillin, nalbuphine, naloxone, nicardipine, nitroglycerin, norepinephrine, octreotide, ondansetron, oxaliplatin, oxytocin, paclitaxel, palonosetron, pamidronate, papaverine, pentamidine, phentolamine, phenylephrine, posaconazole, potassium acetate, potassium chloride, procainamide, prochlorperazine, promethazine, propranolol, protamine, pyridoxine, remifentanil, rituximab, rocuronium, sodium acetate, succinylcholine, sufentanil, tacrolimus, televancin, theophylline, thiamine, thiotepa, tigecycline, tirofiban, tobramycin, topotecan, trastuzumab, vancomycin, vasopressin, vecuronium, verapamil, voriconazole, zidovudine, zoledronic acid.
- **Y-Site Incompatibility:** acyclovir, alteplase, aminophylline, amphotericin B deoxycholate, amphotericin B lipid complex, amphotericin B liposomal, ampicillin, ampicillin/sulbactam, azathioprine, bivalirudin, carmustine, cefazolin, cefotaxime, cefotetan, cefoxitin, ceftriaxone, cefuroxime, chloramphenicol, dacarbazine, dantrolene, dexamethasone, dexrazoxane, diazoxide, ertapenem, fluorouracil, folic acid, foscarnet, fosphenytoin, ganciclovir, hydrocortisone, ibuprofen, indomethacin, ketorolac, methotrexate, micafungin, mitomycin, oxacillin, pantoprazole, pemetrexed, penicillin G, pentobarbital, phenobarbital, phenytoin, piperacillin/tazobactam, sodium bicarbonate, thiopental, trimethoprim/sulfamethoxazole.

Patient/Family Teaching
- Explain to patient the dobutamine and the need for frequent monitoring.
- Advise patient to inform nurse immediately if chest pain; dyspnea; or numbness, tingling, or burning of extremities occurs.
- Instruct patient to notify nurse immediately of pain or discomfort at the site of administration.
- Rep: Advise females of reproductive potential to notify health care professional if pregnancy is planned or suspected or if breastfeeding.
- **Home Care Issues:** Instruct caregiver on proper care of IV equipment.
- Instruct caregiver to report signs of worsening HF (shortness of breath, orthopnea, decreased exercise tolerance), abdominal pain, and nausea or vomiting to health care professional promptly.

Evaluation/Desired Outcomes
- Increase in cardiac output.
- Improved hemodynamic parameters.
- Increased urine output.

HIGH ALERT

DOCEtaxel (doe-se-tax-el)
~~Taxotere~~
Classification
Therapeutic: antineoplastics
Pharmacologic: taxoids

Indications
Locally advanced or metastatic breast cancer after failure of prior chemotherapy. Adjuvant treatment of operable node-positive breast cancer (in combination with doxorubicin and cyclophosphamide). Locally advanced or metastatic non-small cell lung cancer (NSCLC) after failure of prior platinum-based regimen. Unresectable, locally advanced or metastatic NSCLC in patients who have not previously received chemotherapy for this condition (in combination with cisplatin). Metastatic castration-resistant prostate cancer (in combination with prednisone). Locally advanced squamous cell carcinoma of the head and neck (in combination with cisplatin and fluorouracil). Advanced gastric adenocarcinoma (including adenocarcinoma of the gastroesophageal junction) in patients who have not received prior chemotherapy for advanced disease (in combination with cisplatin and fluorouracil).

Action
Interferes with normal cellular microtubule function required for interphase and mitosis. **Therapeutic Effects:** Death of rapidly replicating cells, particularly malignant ones.

Pharmacokinetics
Absorption: IV administration results in complete bioavailability.

Distribution: Widely distributed to tissues.
Metabolism and Excretion: Extensively metabolized by the liver via the CYP3A isoenzyme; metabolites undergo fecal elimination.
Half-life: 116 hr.

TIME/ACTION PROFILE (effect on blood counts)

ROUTE	ONSET	PEAK	DURATION
IV	rapid	5–9 days	7 days

Contraindications/Precautions

Contraindicated in: Hypersensitivity to docetaxel, paclitaxel, or medications formulated with polysorbate 80; Known alcohol intolerance; Neutrophil count <1500/mm^3; Liver impairment (serum bilirubin > upper limit of normal [ULN], ALT and/or AST >1.5x ULN, with alkaline phosphatase >2.5x ULN); OB: Pregnancy; Lactation: Lactation.
Use Cautiously in: Rep: Women of reproductive potential and men with female partners of reproductive potential; Pedi: Safety and effectiveness not established in children.

Adverse Reactions/Side Effects

CV: peripheral edema, CARDIAC TAMPONADE, PERICARDIAL EFFUSION. **Derm:** alopecia, edema, rash, ACUTE GENERALIZED EXANTHEMATOUS PUSTULOSIS (AGEP), dermatitis, desquamation, erythema, nail disorders, STEVENS-JOHNSON SYNDROME (SJS), TOXIC EPIDERMAL NECROLYSIS (TEN). **EENT:** cystoid macular edema. **GI:** diarrhea, nausea, stomatitis, vomiting, ASCITES, ENTEROCOLITIS, NEUTROPENIC COLITIS. **GU:** ↓ fertility (males), amenorrhea. **Hemat:** anemia, leukopenia, thrombocytopenia. **Local:** injection site reactions. **MS:** myalgia, arthralgia. **Neuro:** fatigue, weakness, alcohol intoxication, neurosensory deficits, peripheral neuropathy. **Resp:** ACUTE RESPIRATORY DISTRESS SYNDROME, bronchospasm, dyspnea, INTERSTITIAL LUNG DISEASE, PULMONARY EDEMA, PULMONARY FIBROSIS. **Misc:** HYPERSENSITIVITY REACTIONS (including anaphylaxis), MALIGNANCY (including leukemias, myelodysplastic syndrome, non-Hodgkin's lymphoma, and renal cancer), tumor lysis syndrome.

Interactions

Drug-Drug: ↑ bone marrow depression may occur with other **antineoplastics** or **radiation therapy**. Strong inhibitors of CYP3A4, including **atazanavir, clarithromycin, itraconazole, ketoconazole, nefazodone, nelfinavir, ritonavir,** or **voriconazole** ↑ levels and the risk of toxicity; avoid concomitant use (if need to use, ↓ docetaxel dose by 50%).

Route/Dosage

IV (Adults): *Breast cancer:* 60–100 mg/m^2 every 3 wk; *Breast cancer adjuvant therapy:* 75 mg/m^2 every 3 wk for 6 cycles (with doxorubicin and cyclophosphamide); *Non-small cell lung cancer:* 75 mg/m^2 every 3 wk (alone or with platinum); *Prostate cancer:* 75 mg/ m^2 every 3 wk (with oral prednisone); *Squamous cell head and neck cancer:* 75 mg/m^2 every 3 wk for 3–4 cycles (with cisplatin and fluorouracil); *Gastric adenocarcinoma:* 75 mg/m^2 every 3 wk (with cisplatin and fluorouracil).

Availability (generic available)

Solution for injection (concentrate): 10 mg/mL (dose of 100 mg/m^2 contains 0.15 g/m^2 of ethanol), 20 mg/mL (dose of 100 mg/m^2 contains 1.975 g/m^2 of ethanol).

NURSING IMPLICATIONS

Assessment

- Monitor vital signs before and after administration.
- Assess infusion site for patency. Docetaxel is not a vesicant. If extravasation occurs, discontinue docetaxel immediately and aspirate the IV needle. Apply cold compresses to the site for 24 hr.
- Monitor for signs and symptoms of hypersensitivity reactions (bronchospasm, hypotension, erythema) continuously during infusion; most common after first and second doses of docetaxel. Treat mild to moderate reactions symptomatically and slow or stop infusion until reaction subsides. Discontinue therapy if severe reactions occur. Do not readminister docetaxel to patients with previous severe reactions. Severe edema may also occur. Weigh patients before each treatment. Fluid accumulation may result in edema, ascites, and pleural or pericardial effusions. Pretreatment with corticosteroids is recommended to minimize edema and hypersensitivity reactions. PO furosemide may be used to treat edema. For hormone-refractory metastatic prostate cancer (given with prednisone), premedicate with dexamethasone.
- Monitor for bone marrow depression. Assess for bleeding (bleeding gums, bruising, petechiae; guaiac stools, urine, and emesis) and avoid IM injections and taking rectal temperatures if platelet count is low. Apply pressure to venipuncture sites for 10 min. Assess for signs of infection during neutropenia. Anemia may occur. Monitor for increased fatigue, dyspnea, and orthostatic hypotension.
- Assess for rash. May occur on feet or hands but may also occur on arms, face, or thorax, usually with pruritus. Rash usually occurs within 1 wk after infusion and resolves before next infusion. May cause SJS, TEN, and AGEP; permanently discontinue docetaxel if severe cutaneous reactions occur.
- Assess for development of neurosensory deficit (paresthesia, dysesthesia, pain, burning). May also cause weakness. Pyridoxine may be used to minimize symptoms. Severe symptoms may require dose reduction or discontinuation.
- Assess for arthralgia and myalgia, which are usually relieved by nonopioid analgesics but may be severe enough to require treatment with opioid analgesics.
- Assess for diarrhea and stomatitis especially in patients receiving docetaxel with cisplatin and fluoro-

uracil *If Grade 3 diarrhea occurs,* 1st episode: reduce fluorouracil dose by 20%. 2nd episode: reduce docetaxel dose by 20%. *If Grade 4 diarrhea occurs,* 1st episode: reduce docetaxel and fluorouracil doses by 20%. 2nd episode: discontinue treatment. *If Grade 3 stomatitis/mucositis occurs,* 1st episode: reduce fluorouracil dose by 20%. 2nd episode: stop fluorouracil only, at all subsequent cycles. 3rd episode: reduce docetaxel dose by 20%. *If Grade 4 stomatitis/mucositis occurs,* 1st episode: stop fluorouracil only, at all subsequent cycles. 2nd episode: reduce docetaxel dose by 20%.

- Monitor for tumor lysis syndrome due to rapid reduction in tumor volume (acute renal failure, hyperkalemia, hypocalcemia, hyperuricemia, or hypophosphatemia). Risks are higher in patients with greater tumor burden and rapidly proliferating tumors; may be fatal. Correct electrolyte abnormalities, monitor renal function and fluid balance, and administer supportive care, including dialysis, as indicated.
- Monitor for signs and symptoms of fluid retention (edema, weight gain), usually begins with peripheral edema in lower extremities. May be treated with sodium restriction and diuretics.
- Monitor patients for second primary malignancies.

Lab Test Considerations

- Verify negative pregnancy test before starting therapy. Monitor CBC and differential before each treatment. Frequently causes neutropenia (<2000 neutrophils/mm³); may require dose adjustment. *If neutrophil count <1500/mm³,* hold dose. Neutropenia is reversible and not cumulative. The nadir is 8 days, with a duration of 7 days. May also cause thrombocytopenia and anemia.
- Monitor liver function studies (AST, ALT, alkaline phosphatase, bilirubin) before each cycle. *If AST/ ALT >2.5 to ≤5 times ULN and alkaline phosphatase ≤2.5 times ULN, or AST/ALT >1.5 to ≤5 × ULN, and alkaline phosphatase >2.5 to ≤5 × ULN,* reduce dose by 20%. *If AST/ALT >5 × upper limit of normal and/or alkaline phosphatase >5 times ULN,* discontinue therapy.

Implementation

- **High Alert:** Fatalities have occurred with chemotherapeutic agents. Before administering, clarify all ambiguous orders; double-check single, daily, and course-of-therapy dose limits; have second practitioner independently double-check original order, calculations, and infusion pump settings.
- Do not confuse docetaxel with paclitaxel.
- Premedicate with dexamethasone 8 mg twice daily for 3 days starting 1 day before docetaxel infusion to reduce incidence and severity of fluid retention and hypersensitivity reactions. Premedicate patients with hormone-refractory metastatic prostate cancer with

PO dexamethasone 8 mg, at 12 hr, 3 hr, and 1 hr before docetaxel infusion.

IV Administration

- Solution should be prepared in a biologic cabinet. Wear gloves, gown, and mask while handling medication. If powder or solution comes in contact with skin or mucosa, wash thoroughly with soap and water. Discard equipment in specially designated containers.
- **Intermittent Infusion:** *One-vial formulation:* Do not dilute one-vial formulation. Solution is ready to add to infusion solution. *For injection concentrate:* Before dilution, allow vials to stand at room temperature for 5 min. Solution is pale yellow to brownish yellow. Use a 21-gauge needle to withdraw docetaxel from vial; larger bore needles may result in stopper coring and rubber particles. *Dilution:* Withdraw required amount and inject into 250-mL bag of 0.9% NaCl or D5W. If a dose >200 mg is required, use a larger volume diluent so that concentration of 0.74 mg/mL is not exceeded. Rotate gently to mix. Do not administer solutions that are cloudy or contain a precipitate. Diluted solution must be infused within 6 hr. *Concentration:* 0.3 mg/mL to 0.74 mg/mL. Solution is supersaturated and may crystallize over time. If crystals appear, solution must be discarded. *Rate:* Administer over 1 hr.
- **Y-Site Compatibility:** acyclovir, allopurinol, amifostine, amikacin, aminocaproic acid, aminophylline, amiodarone, amphotericin B lipid complex, ampicillin, ampicillin/sulbactam, anidulafungin, argatroban, atracurium, azithromycin, aztreonam, bivalirudin, bleomycin, bumetanide, buprenorphine, busulfan, butorphanol, calcium chloride, calcium gluconate, carboplatin, carmustine, caspofungin, cefazolin, cefepime, cefotaxime, cefotetan, cefoxitin, ceftazidime, ceftriaxone, cefuroxime, chlorpromazine, ciprofloxacin, cisatracurium, cisplatin, clindamycin, cyclophosphamide, cyclosporine, cytarabine, dacarbazine, dactinomycin, daptomycin, daunorubicin hydrochloride, dexamethasone, dexmedetomidine, dexrazoxane, diazepam, digoxin, diltiazem, diphenhydramine, dobutamine, dopamine, doxorubicin hydrochloride, doxycycline, droperidol, enalaprilat, ephedrine, epinephrine, epirubicin, ertapenem, erythromycin, esmolol, etoposide, etoposide phosphate, famotidine, fentanyl, fluconazole, fludarabine, fluorouracil, foscarnet, fosphenytoin, furosemide, ganciclovir, gemcitabine, gentamicin, glycopyrrolate, granisetron, haloperidol, heparin, hetastarch, hydralazine, hydrocortisone, hydromorphone, ifosfamide, imipenem/cilastatin, insulin regular, irinotecan, isoproterenol, ketorolac, labetalol, leucovorin calcium, levofloxacin, lidocaine, linezolid, lorazepam, magnesium sulfate, mannitol, meperidine, meropenem, mesna, methadone, methotrexate, metoclopramide, metoprolol,

metronidazole, midazolam, milrinone, mitoxantrone, morphine, moxifloxacin, nafcillin, naloxone, nicardipine, nitroglycerin, nitroprusside, norepinephrine, octreotide, ondansetron, oxaliplatin, palonosetron, pamidronate, pantoprazole, pemetrexed, pentamidine, pentobarbital, phenobarbital, phentolamine, phenylephrine, piperacillin/tazobactam, potassium acetate, potassium chloride, potassium phosphate, procainamide, prochlorperazine, promethazine, propranolol, remifentanil, rituximab, rocuronium, sodium acetate, sodium bicarbonate, sodium phosphate, succinylcholine, sufentanil, tacrolimus, theophylline, thiotepa, tigecycline, tirofiban, tobramycin, trastuzumab, trimethoprim/sulfamethoxazole, vancomycin, vasopressin, vecuronium, verapamil, vinblastine, vincristine, vinorelbine, voriconazole, zidovudine, zoledronic acid.

- **Y-Site Incompatibility:** amphotericin B liposomal, dantrolene, doxorubicin liposomal, idarubicin, methylprednisolone, mitomycin, nalbuphine, phenytoin.

Patient/Family Teaching

- Explain purpose of docetaxel to patient.
- Instruct patient to report symptoms of hypersensitivity reactions (trouble breathing; sudden swelling of face, lips, tongue, throat; trouble swallowing; hives; rash; redness all over body) to health care professional immediately.
- Advise patient to notify health care professional if fever >101°F; chills; sore throat; signs of infection; bleeding gums; bruising; petechiae; or blood in urine, stool, or emesis occur. Caution patient to avoid crowds and persons with known infections. Instruct patient to use soft toothbrush and electric razor.
- Patient should be cautioned to avoid alcohol and products containing aspirin or NSAIDs.
- Fatigue is a frequent side effect of docetaxel. Advise patient that frequent rest periods and pacing of activities may minimize fatigue.
- Instruct patient to notify health care professional if signs of fluid retention (peripheral edema in the lower extremities, weight gain, dyspnea), colitis (abdominal pain or tenderness, diarrhea, with or without fever), yellow skin, weakness, paresthesia, gait disturbances, swelling of the feet, or joint or muscle aches occur.
- Alcohol content of docetaxel may impair CNS. Caution patient to avoid driving or other activities requiring alertness until response to medication is known.
- Instruct patient to inspect oral mucosa for redness and ulceration. If mouth sores occur, advise patient to use sponge brush and rinse mouth with water after eating and drinking.
- Instruct patient to notify health care professional of all Rx or OTC medications, vitamins, or herbal products being taken and consult health care professional before taking any new medications.
- Advise patient to notify health care professional if changes in vision occur. Obtain a prompt and comprehensive ophthalmologic examination. May require discontinuation of docetaxel and use of a nontaxane cancer therapy.
- Discuss with patient the possibility of hair loss. Complete hair loss usually begins after 1 or 2 treatments and is reversible after discontinuation of therapy. Explore coping strategies.
- Instruct patient not to receive any vaccinations without advice of health care professional.
- Rep: Advise females of reproductive potential to use effective contraception during and for 2 mo after last dose of therapy and to avoid breastfeeding during and for 1 wk after last dose. Advise men with female partners of reproductive potential to use effective contraception during and for 4 mo after last dose of therapy. May impair fertility in male patients.
- Emphasize the need for periodic lab tests to monitor for side effects.

Evaluation/Desired Outcomes

- Decrease in size or spread of malignancy in women with advanced breast cancer.
- Decrease in size or spread of malignancy in locally advanced or metastatic non-small cell lung cancer, squamous cell carcinoma of the head and neck, and gastric adenocarcinoma.
- Decreased size or spread of advanced metastatic hormone-refractory prostate cancer.

DOCUSATE (dok-yoo-sate)
docusate calcium
docusate sodium

Colace, DOK, Dulcolax Stool Softener, Enemeez Mini, ✹Selax, Silace, ✹Soflax

Classification
Therapeutic: laxatives
Pharmacologic: stool softeners

Indications
PO: Prevention of constipation (in patients who should avoid straining, such as after MI or rectal surgery). **Rect:** Used as enema to soften fecal impaction.

Action
Promotes incorporation of water into stool, resulting in softer fecal mass. May also promote electrolyte and water secretion into the colon. **Therapeutic Effects:** Softening and passage of stool.

Pharmacokinetics
Absorption: Small amounts may be absorbed from the small intestine after oral administration. Absorption from the rectum is not known.
Distribution: Unknown.
Metabolism and Excretion: Amounts absorbed after oral administration are eliminated in bile.

Half-life: Unknown.

TIME/ACTION PROFILE (softening of stool)

ROUTE	ONSET	PEAK	DURATION
PO	12–72 hr	unknown	unknown
Rectal	2–15 min	unknown	unknown

Contraindications/Precautions

Contraindicated in: Hypersensitivity; Abdominal pain, nausea, or vomiting, especially when associated with fever or other signs of an acute abdomen.
Use Cautiously in: Excessive or prolonged use may lead to dependence; Should not be used if prompt results are desired; OB, Lactation: Has been used safely.

Adverse Reactions/Side Effects

Derm: rash. **EENT:** throat irritation. **GI:** diarrhea, mild cramps.

Interactions

Drug-Drug: None significant.

Route/Dosage

Docusate Calcium
PO (Adults): 240 mg once daily.

Docusate Sodium
PO (Adults and Children >12 yr): 50–400 mg in 1–4 divided doses.
PO (Children 6–12 yr): 40–150 mg in 1–4 divided doses.
PO (Children 3–6 yr): 20–60 mg in 1–4 divided doses.
PO (Children <3 yr): 10–40 mg in 1–4 divided doses.
PO (Infants): 5 mg/kg/day in 1–4 divided doses.
Rect (Adults): 50–100 mg or 1 unit containing 283 mg docusate sodium, soft soap, and glycerin.

Availability (generic available)

Docusate Calcium
Capsules: 240 mg^OTC.

Docusate Sodium (generic available)
Tablets: 100 mg^OTC. **Capsules:** 100 mg^OTC, 250 mg^OTC. **Syrup:** 60 mg/15 mL^OTC. **Liquid:** 50 mg/5 mL^OTC, 100 mg/10 mL^OTC. **Enema:** 283 mg/5 mL^OTC. *In combination with:* stimulant laxatives^OTC. See Appendix N.

NURSING IMPLICATIONS

Assessment
- Assess for abdominal distention, presence of bowel sounds, and usual pattern of bowel function.
- Assess color, consistency, and amount of stool produced.

Implementation
- Do not confuse Colace with Cozaar. Do not confuse Dulcolax (docusate sodium) with Dulcolax (bisacodyl).
- This medication does not stimulate intestinal peristalsis; stimulant laxative may be required for constipation.
- **PO:** Administer with a full glass of water or juice. May be administered on an empty stomach for more rapid results.
- Oral solution may be diluted in milk, infant formula, or fruit juice to decrease bitter taste.
- Do not administer within 2 hr of other laxatives, especially mineral oil. May cause increased absorption.
- **Rect:** Administer as a retention or flushing enema.

Patient/Family Teaching
- Advise patients that laxatives should be used only for short-term therapy. Long-term therapy may cause electrolyte imbalance and dependence.
- Encourage patients to use other forms of bowel regulation, such as increasing bulk in the diet, increasing fluid intake (6–8 full glasses/day), and increasing mobility. Normal bowel habits are variable and may vary from 3 times/day to 3 times/wk.
- Instruct patients with cardiac disease to avoid straining during bowel movements (Valsalva maneuver).
- Advise patient not to use laxatives when abdominal pain, nausea, vomiting, or fever is present.
- Advise patient not to take docusate within 2 hr of other laxatives.
- Rep: Advise females of reproductive potential to notify health care professional is pregnancy is planned or suspected or if breastfeeding.

Evaluation/Desired Outcomes
- A soft, formed bowel movement, usually within 24–48 hr. Therapy may take 3–5 days for results. Rectal dose forms produce results within 2–15 min.

dofetilide (doe-fet-il-ide)
Tikosyn
Classification
Therapeutic: antiarrhythmics (class III)

Indications
Maintenance of normal sinus rhythm (delay in time to recurrence of atrial fibrillation/atrial flutter [AF/AFl]) in patients with AF/AFl lasting more than 1 wk, and who have been converted to normal sinus rhythm. Conversion of AF and AFl to normal sinus rhythm.

Action
Blocks cardiac ion channels responsible for transport of potassium. Increases monophasic action potential duration. Increases effective refractory period. **Thera-**

peutic Effects: Prevention of recurrent AF/AFl. Conversion of AF/AFl to normal sinus rhythm.

Pharmacokinetics

Absorption: Well absorbed (>90%) following oral administration.
Distribution: Widely distributed to tissues.
Metabolism and Excretion: Primarily metabolized in the liver via the CYP3A4 isoenzyme; 80% excreted by kidneys via cationic renal secretion, mostly as unchanged drug; 20% excreted as inactive metabolites.
Half-life: 10 hr.

TIME/ACTION PROFILE (plasma concentrations)

ROUTE	ONSET	PEAK	DURATION
PO	within hrs	2–3 hr†	12–24 hr

†Steady state levels are achieved after 2–3 days.

Contraindications/Precautions

Contraindicated in: Hypersensitivity; Congenital or acquired prolonged QT syndromes; Baseline QTc interval >440 msec (500 msec in patients with ventricular conduction abnormalities); CCr <20 mL/min; Concurrent use of verapamil, cimetidine, dolutegravir, ketoconazole, itraconazole, trimethoprim, megestrol, prochlorperazine, hydrochlorothiazide, or other QT-interval prolonging drugs; Lactation: Lactation.
Use Cautiously in: Underlying electrolyte abnormalities (↑ risk of serious arrhythmias; correct prior to administration); CCr 20–60 mL/min (dose ↓ recommended); Severe hepatic impairment; OB: Use during pregnancy only if potential maternal benefit justifies potential fetal risk; Pedi: Safety and effectiveness not established in children.

Adverse Reactions/Side Effects

CV: chest pain, QT interval prolongation, TORSADES DE POINTES. **Neuro:** dizziness, headache.

Interactions

Drug-Drug: **Hydrochlorothiazide, verapamil, cimetidine, ketoconazole, itraconazole, trimethoprim, megestrol, dolutegravir,** and **prochlorperazine** ↑ levels and the risk of QT interval prolongation with arrhythmias; concurrent use contraindicated. **QT interval prolonging drugs** may ↑ the risk of QT interval prolongation with arrhythmias; concurrent use contraindicated. **Amiloride, metformin,** and **triamterene** may ↑ levels; use with caution. **CYP3A4 inhibitors,** including **macrolides, azole antifungals, protease inhibitors, amiodarone, diltiazem,** and **nefazodone,** may ↑ levels and the risk of arrhythmias; concurrent use should be undertaken with caution. Should not be used concurrently with other **class I or III antiarrhythmics** due to ↑ risk of arrhythmias. Hypokalemia or hypomagnesemia from **potassium-depleting diuretics** ↑ the risk of arrhythmias; correct abnormalities prior to administration. Concurrent use of **digoxin** may ↑ the risk of arrhythmias.

Drug-Food: Grapefruit juice may ↑ levels; avoid concurrent use.

Route/Dosage

Dosing should be adjusted according to renal function and assessment of QT interval.
PO (Adults): *Starting dose:* 500 mcg twice daily; *maintenance dose:* 250 mcg twice daily (not to exceed 500 mcg twice daily).

Renal Impairment

PO (Adults): *CCr 40–60 mL/min Starting dose:* 250 mcg twice daily; *maintenance dose:* 125 mcg twice daily; *CCr 20–40 mL/min Starting dose:* 125 mcg twice daily; *maintenance dose:* 125 mcg once daily.

Availability (generic available)

Capsules: 125 mcg, 250 mcg, 500 mcg.

NURSING IMPLICATIONS

Assessment

- Monitor ECG, pulse, and BP continuously during initiation of therapy and for at least 3 days or a minimum of 12 hr after electrical or pharmacological conversion to normal sinus rhythm, whichever is greater, then periodically during therapy. Evaluate QTc interval (or QT interval if heart rate <60 bpm) before starting therapy and every 3 mo during therapy. If QTc interval exceeds 440 msec (500 msec in patients with ventricular conduction abnormalities), discontinue dofetilide and monitor patient until QTc interval returns to baseline.
- Within 2–3 hr after first dose, evaluate QTc interval (or QT interval if heart rate <60 bpm). If QTc or QT interval ↑ by >15% compared to baseline or if QTc or QT interval >500 msec (550 msec in patients with ventricular conduction abnormalities), adjust doses as follows: *if initial dose was 500 mcg twice daily,* change to 250 mcg twice daily; *if initial dose was 250 mcg twice daily,* change to 125 mcg twice daily; *if initial dose was 125 mcg twice daily,* change to 125 mcg once a day. Determine QTc or QT interval within 2–3 hr after each subsequent dose for hospital doses 2–5. No further down titration of dose is recommended. Discontinue dofetilide if at any time after second dose is given QTc or QT interval >500 msec (550 msec in patients with ventricular conduction abnormalities).
- Assess the patient's medication history including OTC, Rx, and natural/herbal products, with emphasis on those that interact with dofetilide (see Interactions).

Lab Test Considerations

- Calculate CCr prior to administration to determine dose and every 3 mo during therapy.
- Correct hypokalemia before starting therapy. Maintain serum potassium in normal range during dofetilide therapy.

Implementation

- Dofetilide must be initiated or reinitiated and monitored for at least 3 days in a setting that provides continuous ECG monitoring and has personnel trained in the management of serious ventricular arrhythmias. Due to the potential for life-threatening ventricular arrhythmias, dofetilide is usually used for patients with highly symptomatic AF/AFl.
- Patients with AF should be anticoagulated according to usual protocol prior to electrical or pharmacological cardioversion.
- Make sure patient has an adequate supply of dofetilide prior to discharge to prevent interruption of therapy.
- Patients should not be discharged from the hospital within 12 hr of electrical or pharmacological conversion to normal sinus rhythm.
- **PO:** Administer at the same time each day without regard to food.

Patient/Family Teaching

- Instruct patient to take medication as directed, even if feeling well. If a dose is missed, skip dose; do not double next dose. Take next dose at usual time.
- Advise patient to avoid grapefruit juice during therapy; may increase drug levels.
- Advise patient to read *Medication Guide* prior to starting therapy and each Rx refill in case of changes. Emphasize need for adherence with therapy, potential for drug interactions, and need for periodic monitoring to minimize the risk of serious arrhythmias.
- Instruct patient or family member on how to take pulse. Advise patient to report changes in pulse rate or rhythm to health care professional.
- May cause dizziness. Caution patient to avoid driving or other activities requiring alertness until response to medication is known.
- Advise patient to inform health care professional of medication regimen prior to treatment or surgery.
- Instruct patient to notify health care professional of all Rx or OTC medications, vitamins, or herbal products being taken and to consult health care professional before taking other Rx, OTC, or herbal products.
- Advise patient to consult health care professional immediately if they faint, become dizzy, or have fast heartbeat. If health care professional is unavailable, instruct patient to go to nearest hospital emergency department, take remaining dofetilide capsules to hospital, and show them to health care professional. If symptoms associated with altered electrolyte balance such as excessive or prolonged diarrhea, sweating, or vomiting or loss of appetite or thirst occur, notify health care professional immediately.
- Rep: Advise females of reproductive potential to notify health care professional if pregnancy is planned or suspected or if breastfeeding.

- Emphasize the importance of routine follow-up exams to monitor progress.

Evaluation/Desired Outcomes

- Prevention of recurrent AF/AFl.
- Conversion of AF/AFl to normal sinus rhythm.
- If patients do not convert to normal sinus rhythm within 24 hr of initiation of therapy, electrical conversion should be considered.

⚙ dolutegravir/lamivudine
(doe-loo-**teg**-ra-vir/la-**mi**-vyoo-deen)
Dovato
Classification
Therapeutic: antiretrovirals
Pharmacologic: integrase strand transfer inhibitors (INSTI), nucleoside reverse transcriptase inhibitors

Indications

HIV-1 infection in patients with no antiretroviral treatment history and with no known substitutions associated with resistance to dolutegravir or lamivudine. HIV-1 infection as a replacement for the current antiretroviral regimen in patients who are virologically suppressed (HIV-1 RNA <50 copies/mL), taking a stable antiretroviral regimen, have no history of treatment failure, and have no known substitutions associated with resistance to dolutegravir or lamivudine.

Action

Dolutegravir: Inhibits HIV-1 integrase, which is required for viral replication. *Lamivudine:* After intracellular conversion to its active form (lamivudine-5-triphosphate), inhibits viral DNA synthesis by inhibiting the enzyme reverse transcriptase. **Therapeutic Effects:** Evidence of decreased viral replication and reduced viral load with slowed progression of HIV and its sequelae.

Pharmacokinetics

Dolutegravir
Absorption: Bioavailability unknown.
Distribution: Unknown.
Protein Binding: >98.9%.
Metabolism and Excretion: Metabolized primarily by the UGT1A1 enzyme system with some metabolism by the CYP3A4 isoenzyme. ⚙ Poor UGT1A1 metabolizers have ↑ dolutegravir concentrations and an ↑ risk of adverse effects. 64% excreted in feces (53% as unchanged drug), 31% excreted in urine (<1% as unchanged drug).
Half-life: 14 hr.

Lamivudine
Absorption: Well absorbed after oral administration.
Distribution: Unknown.

Metabolism and Excretion: Mostly excreted unchanged in urine (70% as unchanged drug).
Half-life: 13–19 hr.

TIME/ACTION PROFILE (plasma concentrations)

ROUTE	ONSET	PEAK	DURATION
Dolutegravir (PO)	unknown	2.5 hr	24 hr
Lamivudine (PO)	unknown	1 hr	24 hr

Contraindications/Precautions

Contraindicated in: Prior hypersensitivity reaction to dolutegravir; Concurrent use of dofetilide; Severe renal impairment; Severe hepatic impairment; OB: Avoid use through first trimester of pregnancy (may ↑ risk of neural tube defects); Lactation: Breastfeeding not recommended in women with HIV.

Use Cautiously in: Coinfection with hepatitis B virus (HBV) (hepatitis may recur after discontinuation of lamivudine and ↑ risk of lamivudine-resistant HBV); Underlying hepatic disease, including HBV or hepatitis C (↑ risk of hepatotoxicity); Women and obesity (↑ risk of lactic acidosis and severe hepatomegaly with steatosis); OB: Can consider use during second or third trimester if potential maternal benefit justifies potential fetal risk; Rep: Women of reproductive potential; Pedi: Safety and effectiveness not established in children; Geri: Consider age-related ↓ in cardiac, renal and hepatic function, chronic disease states and concurrent medications in older adults.

Adverse Reactions/Side Effects

Endo: hyperglycemia. **F and E:** hypophosphatemia, LACTIC ACIDOSIS. **GI:** ↑ lipase, ↑ liver enzymes, diarrhea, HEPATOMEGALY WITH STEATOSIS, HEPATOTOXICITY (↑ with HBV or hepatitis C), nausea. **Metab:** hyperlipidemia. **MS:** ↑ creatine kinase. **Neuro:** dizziness, fatigue, headache, insomnia. **Misc:** hypersensitivity reactions (including rash, constitutional symptoms, and liver injury), immune reconstitution syndrome.

Interactions

Drug-Drug: May ↑ levels and risk of toxicity from **dofetilide**; concurrent use contraindicated. May ↑ levels and risk of toxicity of **metformin**. **Carbamazepine** and **rifampin** may ↓ levels and effectiveness of dolutegravir; additional 50-mg dose of dolutegravir should be given 12 hr after dose of dolutegravir/lamivudine. **Oxcarbazepine, phenobarbital,** and **phenytoin** may ↓ levels and effectiveness of dolutegravir; avoid concurrent use. Absorption and effectiveness may be ↓ by cation-containing **antacids** or **laxatives**, as well as **buffered medications,** or **sucralfate**; dolutegravir should be taken 2 hr before or 6 hr after these medications. Absorption and effectiveness may be ↓ by **calcium supplements** (oral) or **iron supplements** (oral); under fasting conditions, dolutegravir should be taken 2 hr before or 6 hr after these medications; when

taken with food, dolutegravir and calcium or iron supplements may be taken at the same time. May ↑ **dalfampridine** levels and risk of seizures. **Sorbitol** may ↓ levels of lamivudine; avoid concurrent use. May ↑ **dalfampridine** levels and risk of seizures.

Drug-Natural Products: St. John's wort may ↓ levels and effectiveness of dolutegravir; avoid concurrent use.

Route/Dosage

PO (Adults): One tablet (dolutegravir 50 mg/lamivudine 300 mg) once daily.

Availability

Tablets: dolutegravir 50 mg/lamivudine 300 mg.

NURSING IMPLICATIONS

Assessment

- Assess for change in severity of HIV symptoms and for symptoms of opportunistic infections during therapy.
- Monitor for signs and symptoms of hypersensitivity reactions (rash, fever, malaise, fatigue, muscle or joint aches, blisters or peeling of skin, oral blisters or lesions, conjunctivitis, facial edema, hepatitis, eosinophilia, angioedema, difficulty breathing). Discontinue therapy and do not restart.

Lab Test Considerations

- Verify negative pregnancy test before starting therapy. Monitor viral load and CD4 counts regularly during therapy.
- Assess for HBV. *Dovato* is not approved for administration in patients with HIV and HBV. If therapy is discontinued, may cause severe exacerbation of HBV. Monitor liver function in coinfected patients for several months after stopping therapy.
- Monitor liver function tests prior to, during and following therapy. May cause ↑ LDL cholesterol, total cholesterol, and triglyceride concentrations. Lactic acidosis may occur with hepatic toxicity causing hepatic steatosis; may be fatal, especially in women. Discontinue therapy if symptoms occur.

Implementation

- **PO:** Administer once daily without regard to food.
- Iron and calcium supplements may be taken with dolutegravir/lamivudine and food. If taken separately, administer dolutegravir/lamivudine ≥2 hr before or ≥6 hr after iron and calcium supplements.

Patient/Family Teaching

- Instruct patient on the importance of taking medication as directed, even if feeling better. Take missed dose as soon as remembered; do not double doses. Do not take more than prescribed amount and do not stop taking without consulting health care professional. Discontinuing therapy may lead to severe exacerbations. Take missed doses as soon as remembered unless almost time for next dose; do not double doses. Advise patient to read *Patient Infor-*

mation prior to starting therapy and with each Rx refill in case of changes. Caution patient not to share or trade *Dovato* with others.

- Inform patient of importance of HBV testing before starting antiretroviral therapy.
- Inform patient that *Dovato* does not cure AIDS and may reduce the risk of transmission of HIV to others through sexual contact or blood contamination. Caution patient to use a condom and avoid sharing needles or donating blood to prevent spreading HIV to others.
- Advise patient to notify health care professional immediately if symptoms of hypersensitivity reactions, lactic acidosis (nausea, vomiting, unusual or unexpected stomach discomfort, unusual muscle pain, difficulty breathing, feeling cold, especially in arms and legs, dizziness, fast or irregular heartbeat, and weakness or tiredness), liver problems (yellow skin or whites of eyes, dark urine, light colored stools, loss of appetite, nausea, stomach pain), or signs of Immune Reconstitution Syndrome (signs and symptoms of an infection or inflammation) occur.
- Instruct patient to notify health care professional of all Rx or OTC medications, vitamins, or herbal products being taken and consult health care professional before taking any new medications, especially St. John's wort.
- Rep: Advise females of reproductive potential to use effective contraception during *Dovato* therapy and to avoid breastfeeding during therapy. Advise patient to notify health care professional if pregnancy is planned or suspected. Enroll pregnant women in the Antiretroviral Pregnancy Registry by calling 1-800-258-4263.
- Emphasize the importance of regular follow-up exams and blood counts to determine progress and monitor for side effects.

Evaluation/Desired Outcomes
- Slowed progression of HIV infection and decreased occurrence of sequelae.

donepezil (doe-**nep**-i-zill)
Adlarity, Aricept, ~~Aricept ODT~~
Classification
Therapeutic: anti-Alzheimer's agents
Pharmacologic: cholinergics (cholinesterase inhibitors)

Indications
Mild, moderate, or severe dementia/neurocognitive disorder associated with Alzheimer's disease.

Action
Inhibits acetylcholinesterase thus improving cholinergic function by making more acetylcholine available.
Therapeutic Effects: May temporarily lessen some of the dementia associated with Alzheimer's disease. Enhances cognition. Does not cure the disease.

Pharmacokinetics
Absorption: Well absorbed after oral administration. Bioavailability of transdermal formulation comparable to that of oral tablets.
Distribution: Widely distributed to extravascular tissues.
Protein Binding: 96%.
Metabolism and Excretion: Partially metabolized by the liver (CYP2D6 and CYP3A4 isoenzymes) and partially excreted by kidneys (17% unchanged). Two metabolites are pharmacologically active. 🐾 The CYP2D6 enzyme system exhibits genetic polymorphism (~7% of population may be poor metabolizers and may have significantly ↑ donepezil concentrations and an ↑ risk of adverse effects).
Half-life: *Oral:* 70 hr. *Transdermal:* 91 hr.

TIME/ACTION PROFILE (improvement in symptoms)

ROUTE	ONSET	PEAK	DURATION
PO	unknown	several wk	6 wk†
Transdermal	unknown	several wk	6 wk†

†Return to baseline after discontinuation.

Contraindications/Precautions
Contraindicated in: Hypersensitivity to donepezil or piperidine derivatives; History of allergic contact dermatitis with transdermal donepezil.
Use Cautiously in: Underlying cardiac disease, especially sick sinus syndrome or supraventricular conduction defects; History of ulcer disease or currently taking NSAIDs; History of seizures; History of asthma or obstructive pulmonary disease; OB: Safety not established in pregnancy; Lactation: Use while breastfeeding only if potential maternal benefit justifies potential risk to infant; Pedi: Safety and effectiveness not established in children.

Adverse Reactions/Side Effects
CV: atrial fibrillation, hypertension, hypotension, vasodilation. **Derm:** allergic contact dermatitis (transdermal), ecchymoses. **Endo:** hot flashes. **GI:** diarrhea, nausea, anorexia, vomiting. **GU:** frequent urination. **Metab:** weight loss. **MS:** arthritis, muscle cramps. **Neuro:** headache, abnormal dreams, depression, dizziness, drowsiness, fatigue, insomnia, syncope.

Interactions
Drug-Drug: Exaggerates muscle relaxation from **succinylcholine**. Interferes with the action of **anticholinergics**. ↑ cholinergic effects of **bethanechol**. May ↑ risk of GI bleeding from **NSAIDs**. **Quinidine** and **ketoconazole** ↓ metabolism of donepezil. **Rifampin, carbamazepine, dexamethasone, phenobarbital,** and **phenytoin** induce the enzymes that metabolize donepezil and may ↓ its effects.

❋= Canadian drug name. 🐾 = Genetic implication. ~~Strikethrough~~ = Discontinued. CAPITALS = life-threatening. <u>Underline</u> = most frequent.

Drug-Natural Products: Jimson weed and **scopolia** may antagonize cholinergic effects.

Route/Dosage

Mild to Moderate Alzheimer's Disease

PO (Adults): 5 mg once daily; may ↑ to 10 mg once daily after 4–6 wk (dose should not exceed 5 mg/day in frail, elderly females).

Transdermal (Adults): Apply one 5 mg/day transdermal system once weekly; may ↑ to one 10 mg/day transdermal system once weekly after 4–6 wk. *Switching from oral to transdermal donepezil:* If patient taking 5 mg/day of oral donepezil, switch to one 5 mg/day transdermal system applied once weekly; if receiving 5 mg/day of oral donepezil for ≥4–6 wk, can switch to one 10 mg/day transdermal system applied once weekly. If patient taking 10 mg/day of oral donepezil, switch to one 10 mg/day transdermal system applied once weekly.

Severe Alzheimer's Disease

PO (Adults): 5 mg once daily; may ↑ to 10 mg once daily after 4–6 wk; after 3 mo, may then ↑ to 23 mg once daily.

Transdermal (Adults): Apply one 5 mg/day transdermal system once weekly; may ↑ to one 10 mg/day transdermal system once weekly after 4–6 wk. *Switching from oral to transdermal donepezil:* If patient taking 5 mg/day of oral donepezil, switch to one 5 mg/day transdermal system applied once weekly; if receiving 5 mg/day of oral donepezil for ≥4–6 wk, can switch to one 10 mg/day transdermal system applied once weekly. If patient taking 10 mg/day of oral donepezil, switch to one 10 mg/day transdermal system applied once weekly.

Availability (generic available)

Tablets: 5 mg, 10 mg, 23 mg. **Orally disintegrating tablets:** 5 mg, 10 mg. **Transdermal patch (Adlarity):** 5 mg/day, 10 mg/day. *In combination with:* memantine (Namzaric). See Appendix N.

NURSING IMPLICATIONS

Assessment

- Assess cognitive function (memory, attention, reasoning, language, ability to perform simple tasks) periodically during therapy.
- Monitor heart rate periodically during therapy. May cause bradycardia.

Implementation

- Do not confuse Aricept with Aciphex or Azilect.
- **PO:** Administer in the evening just before going to bed. May be taken without regard to food.
- *Oral disintegrating tablets* should be allowed to dissolve on tongue; follow with water.
- Swallow *23-mg tablet* whole. *DNC:* Do not split, crush, or chew; may increase rate of absorption.
- **Transdermal:** Take patch from refrigerator and allow to reach room temperature; do not use external

heat sources to warm. Do not apply a cold transdermal system. Recommended application site is the back, avoiding the spine or a site that would be rubbed by tight clothing. May use the upper buttocks or the upper outer thigh. Do not use same location for application site for at least 2 weeks (14 days). Do not apply to an area where medication, cream, lotion, or powder has recently been applied. Do not apply to red, irritated, or cut skin. Do not shave site. Press down firmly for 30 sec to ensure good contact with skin at edges of transdermal system. May be worn while bathing or in hot weather. Avoid long exposure to external heat sources (excessive sunlight, saunas, solariums, heating pads). If patch falls off or a dose is missed, apply a new transdermal system immediately and then replace this transdermal system 7 days later to start a new 1-week cycle.

Patient/Family Teaching

- Emphasize the importance of taking donepezil daily, as directed. Missed doses should be skipped and regular schedule returned to the following day. Do not take more than prescribed; higher doses do not increase effects but may increase side effects.
- Inform patient/family that it may take weeks before improvement in baseline behavior is observed.
- Caution patient and caregiver that donepezil may cause dizziness. Advise patient to avoid driving and other activities requiring alertness until response to medication is known.
- Advise patient and caregiver to notify health care professional if nausea, vomiting, diarrhea, or changes in color of stool occur or if new symptoms occur or previously noted symptoms increase in severity.
- Instruct patient to notify health care professional of all Rx or OTC medications, vitamins, or herbal products being taken and to consult health care professional before taking other Rx, OTC, or herbal products.
- Advise patient and caregiver to notify health care professional of medication regimen before treatment or surgery.
- Advise females of reproductive potential to notify health care professional if pregnancy is planned or suspected or if breastfeeding.
- Emphasize the importance of follow-up exams to monitor progress.
- **Transdermal:** Instruct patients or caregivers to fold the transdermal system in half after use and discard it in the trash, out of the reach and sight of children and pets. Inform patients or caregivers that drug still remains in the transdermal system after 7-day usage and that used transdermal systems should not be flushed down the toilet.

Evaluation/Desired Outcomes

- Improvement in cognitive function (memory, attention, reasoning, language, ability to perform simple tasks) in patients with Alzheimer's disease.

DOPamine (dope-a-meen)
Classification
Therapeutic: inotropics, vasopressors
Pharmacologic: adrenergics

Indications
Adjunct to standard measures to improve: BP, Cardiac output, Urine output in treatment of shock unresponsive to fluid replacement. Increase renal perfusion (low doses).

Action
Small doses (0.5–3 mcg/kg/min) stimulate dopaminergic receptors, producing renal vasodilation. Larger doses (2–10 mcg/kg/min) stimulate dopaminergic and beta₁-adrenergic receptors, producing cardiac stimulation and renal vasodilation. Doses greater than 10 mcg/kg/min stimulate alpha-adrenergic receptors and may cause renal vasoconstriction. **Therapeutic Effects:** Increased cardiac output, increased BP, and improved renal blood flow.

Pharmacokinetics
Absorption: IV administration results in complete bioavailability.
Distribution: Widely distributed but does not cross the blood-brain barrier.
Metabolism and Excretion: Metabolized in liver, kidneys, and plasma.
Half-life: 2 min.

TIME/ACTION PROFILE (hemodynamic effects)

ROUTE	ONSET	PEAK	DURATION
IV	1–2 min	up to 10 min	<10 min

Contraindications/Precautions
Contraindicated in: Tachyarrhythmias; Pheochromocytoma; Hypersensitivity to bisulfites (some products).
Use Cautiously in: Hypovolemia; MI; Occlusive vascular diseases; OB: Safety not established in pregnancy; Lactation: Safety not established in breastfeeding; Geri: Older adults may be more susceptible to adverse effects.

Adverse Reactions/Side Effects
CV: arrhythmias, hypotension, angina, palpitations, vasoconstriction. **Derm:** piloerection. **EENT:** mydriasis (high dose). **GI:** nausea, vomiting. **Local:** irritation at IV site. **Neuro:** headache. **Resp:** dyspnea.

Interactions
Drug-Drug: Use with **MAO inhibitors**, **ergot alkaloids (ergotamine)**, **doxapram**, or some **antidepressants** results in severe hypertension. Use with IV **phenytoin** may cause hypotension and bradycardia.

Use with **general anesthetics** may result in arrhythmias. **Beta blockers** may antagonize cardiac effects.

Route/Dosage
IV (Adults): *Dopaminergic (renal vasodilation) effects:* 1–5 mcg/kg/min continuous infusion. *Beta-adrenergic (cardiac stimulation) effects:* 5–15 mcg/kg/min continuous infusion. *Alpha-adrenergic (increased peripheral vascular resistance) effects:* >15 mcg/kg/min continuous infusion; infusion rate may be ↑ as needed.
IV (Children and Infants): 1–20 mcg/kg/min continuous infusion, depending on desired response (1–5 mcg/kg/min has been used to improve renal blood flow).
IV (Neonates): 1–20 mcg/kg/min continuous infusion.

Availability (generic available)
Solution for injection: 40 mg/mL. **Premixed infusion:** 200 mg/250 mL, 400 mg/250 mL, 400 mg/500 mL, 800 mg/250 mL, 800 mg/500 mL.

NURSING IMPLICATIONS
Assessment
- Monitor BP, heart rate, pulse pressure, ECG, pulmonary capillary wedge pressure (PCWP), cardiac output, central venous pressure (CVP), and urinary output continuously during administration. Report significant changes in vital signs or arrhythmias. Consult physician for parameters for pulse, BP, or ECG changes for adjusting dose or discontinuing medication.
- Monitor urine output frequently throughout administration. Report decreases in urine output promptly.
- Palpate peripheral pulses and assess appearance of extremities routinely during dopamine administration. Notify physician if quality of pulse deteriorates or if extremities become cold or mottled.
- If hypotension occurs, administration rate should be increased. If hypotension continues, more potent vasoconstrictors (norepinephrine) may be administered.

Toxicity and Overdose
- If excessive hypertension occurs, rate of infusion should be decreased or temporarily discontinued until BP is decreased.

Implementation
- *High Alert:* IV vasoactive medications are potentially dangerous. Have second practitioner independently check original order, dose calculations, and infusion pump settings. Do not confuse dopamine with dobutamine. If both are available as floor stock, store in separate areas.
- Correct hypovolemia with volume expanders before initiating dopamine therapy.

- Extravasation may cause severe irritation, necrosis, and sloughing of tissue. Administer into a large vein and assess administration site frequently. If extravasation occurs, affected area should be infiltrated liberally with 10–15 mL of 0.9% NaCl containing 5–10 mg of phentolamine. For pediatric patients, use 1 mL of phentolamine dilution to infiltrate (do not exceed 5 mg total). Infiltration within 12 hr of extravasation produces immediate hyperemic changes.

IV Administration
- **Continuous Infusion:** *Dilution:* Dopamine vials must be diluted before use. Dilute 200–800 mg of dopamine in 250–500 mL of 0.9% NaCl, D5W, D5/LR, D5/0.45% NaCl, D5/0.9% NaCl, or LR. Admixed solution is stable for 24 hr. Discard solutions that are cloudy, discolored, or contain a precipitate. Premixed infusions are already diluted and ready to use. *Concentration:* 0.8–3.2 mg/mL. *Rate:* Based on patient's weight (see Route/Dosage section). Infusion must be administered via infusion pump to ensure precise amount delivered. Titrate to response (BP, heart rate, urine output, peripheral perfusion, presence of ectopic activity, PCWP, CVP, cardiac index). Decrease rate gradually when discontinuing to prevent marked decreases in BP.
- **Y-Site Compatibility:** alemtuzumab, alprostadil, amifostine, amikacin, aminocaproic acid, aminophylline, amiodarone, anidulafungin, argatroban, arsenic trioxide, ascorbic acid, atracurium, atropine, azithromycin, aztreonam, benztropine, bivalirudin, bleomycin, bumetanide, buprenorphine, butorphanol, calcium chloride, calcium gluconate, cangrelor, carboplatin, carmustine, caspofungin, cefotaxime, cefotetan, cefoxitin, ceftaroline, ceftazidime, ceftazidime/avibactam, ceftolozane/tazobactam, ceftriaxone, cefuroxime, chlorpromazine, ciprofloxacin, cisatracurium, cisplatin, cladribine, clindamycin, cyanocobalamin, cyclophosphamide, cyclosporine, cytarabine, dactinomycin, daptomycin, daunorubicin hydrochloride, dexamethasone, dexmedetomidine, dexrazoxane, digoxin, diltiazem, diphenhydramine, dobutamine, docetaxel, doxorubicin hydrochloride, doxorubicin liposomal, doxycycline, droperidol, enalaprilat, ephedrine, epinephrine, epirubicin, epoetin alpha, eptifibatide, eravacycline, ertapenem, erythromycin, esmolol, etoposide, etoposide phosphate, famotidine, fentanyl, fluconazole, fludarabine, fluorouracil, folic acid, foscarnet, gemcitabine, gemtuzumab ozogamicin, gentamicin, glycopyrrolate, granisetron, heparin, hetastarch, hydrocortisone, hydromorphone, idarubicin, ifosfamide, imipenem/cilastatin/relebactam, imipenem/cilastatin, irinotecan, isavuconazonium, isoproterenol, ketamine, ketorolac, labetalol, LR, leucovorin calcium, levofloxacin, lidocaine, linezolid, lorazepam, magnesium sulfate, mannitol, meperidine, meropenem/vaborbactam, mesna, methylprednisolone, metoclopramide, metoprolol, metronidazole, micafungin, midazolam, milrinone, mitoxantrone, morphine, moxifloxacin, multivitamins, mycophenolate, nafcillin, nalbuphine, naloxone, nicardipine, nitroglycerin, nitroprusside, norepinephrine, octreotide, ondansetron, oritavancin, oxaliplatin, oxytocin, paclitaxel, palonosetron, pamidronate, papaverine, pemetrexed, penicillin G, pentamidine, pentobarbital, phenobarbital, phenylephrine, phytonadione, piperacillin/tazobactam, plazomicin, potassium acetate, potassium chloride, procainamide, prochlorperazine, promethazine, propranolol, protamine, pyridoxine, remifentanil, sargramostim, sodium acetate, succinylcholine, sufentanil, tacrolimus, tedizolid, telavancin, theophylline, thiamine, thiotepa, tigecycline, tirofiban, tobramycin, topotecan, trastuzumab, vancomycin, vasopressin, vecuronium, verapamil, vinblastine, vincristine, vinorelbine, voriconazole, warfarin, zidovudine, zoledronic acid.
- **Y-Site Incompatibility:** acyclovir, alteplase, amphotericin B deoxycholate, amphotericin B lipid complex, amphotericin B liposomal, azathioprine, cefazolin, chloramphenicol, dacarbazine, dantrolene, diazepam, esomeprazole, ganciclovir, ibuprofen lysine, indomethacin, methotrexate, mitomycin, phenytoin, sodium bicarbonate, thiopental, trimethoprim/sulfamethoxazole.

Patient/Family Teaching
- Explain purpose of dopamine to patient and the need for frequent monitoring.
- Advise patient to inform nurse immediately if chest pain; dyspnea; numbness, tingling, or burning of extremities occurs.
- Instruct patient to inform nurse immediately of pain or discomfort at the site of administration.
- Rep: Advise females of reproductive potential to notify health care professional if pregnancy is planned or suspected or if breastfeeding.

Evaluation/Desired Outcomes
- Increase in BP.
- Increase in peripheral circulation.
- Increase in urine output.

---

doravirine/lamivudine/tenofovir disoproxil fumarate
(**dor**-a-**vir**-een/la-**mi**-vyoo-deen/te-**noe**-fo-veer dye-soe-**prox**-il **fue**-ma-rate)
   Delstrigo

Classification
Therapeutic: antiretrovirals
Pharmacologic: non-nucleoside reverse transcriptase inhibitors, nucleoside reverse transcriptase inhibitors

---

Indications
HIV-1 infection in patients with no prior antiretroviral treatment history. To replace the current antiretroviral

regimen in patients with HIV-1 infection who are virologically suppressed (HIV-1 RNA <50 copies/mL), receiving a stable antiretroviral regimen with no history of treatment failure, and have no known substitutions associated with resistance to doravirine, lamivudine, or tenofovir disoproxil fumarate.

Action

Doravirine: Binds to the enzyme reverse transcriptase, which results in disrupted viral DNA synthesis. *Lamivudine:* After intracellular conversion to its active form (lamivudine-5-triphosphate), inhibits viral DNA synthesis by inhibiting the enzyme HIV reverse transcriptase. *Tenofovir disoproxil fumarate:* Phosphorylated intracellularly where it inhibits HIV reverse transcriptase resulting in disruption of DNA synthesis. **Therapeutic Effects:** Evidence of decreased viral replication and reduced viral load with slowed progression of HIV and its sequelae.

Pharmacokinetics

Doravirine
Absorption: 64% absorbed following oral administration.
Distribution: Extensively distributed to tissues.
Metabolism and Excretion: Primarily metabolized in the liver by CYP3A enzymes. Primarily excreted in feces (as metabolites), 6% unchanged in urine.
Half-life: 15 hr.

Lamivudine
Absorption: 86% absorbed after oral administration.
Distribution: Extensively distributed to tissues.
Metabolism and Excretion: 71% excreted unchanged in urine by glomerular filtration and active tubular secretion.
Half-life: 5–7 hr.

Tenofovir Disoproxil Fumarate
Absorption: 25% absorbed after oral administration.
Distribution: Extensively distributed to tissues.
Metabolism and Excretion: 70–80% excreted unchanged in urine by glomerular filtration and active tubular secretion.
Half-life: 17 hr.

TIME/ACTION PROFILE (plasma concentrations)

ROUTE	ONSET	PEAK	DURATION
Doravirine (PO)	unknown	2 hr	24 hr
Lamivudine (PO)	unknown	unknown	24 hr
Tenofovir (PO)	unknown	1 hr	24 hr

Contraindications/Precautions

Contraindicated in: Previous hypersensitivity reaction to lamivudine; Concurrent use of carbamazepine, enzalutamide, mitotane, oxcarbazepine, phenobarbital, phenytoin, rifampin, rifapentine, and St. John's wort; Concurrent or recent use of nephrotoxic medications; CCr <50 mL/min; Lactation: Breastfeeding not recommended in women with HIV.

Use Cautiously in: Coinfection with hepatitis B virus (HBV) (hepatitis may recur after discontinuation of lamivudine and ↑ risk of lamivudine-resistant HBV); Severe hepatic impairment; OB: Safety of doravirine not established in pregnancy; Pedi: Children <35 kg (safety and effectiveness not established); Geri: Consider age-related ↓ in organ function and body mass, concurrent disease states and medications in older adults.

Adverse Reactions/Side Effects

Derm: rash. **Endo:** Graves' disease. **GI:** ↑ lipase, ↑ liver enzymes, autoimmune hepatitis, diarrhea, HEPATOTOXICITY (↑ with HBV or hepatitis C), hyperbilirubinemia, nausea. **GU:** ↑ serum creatinine, ACUTE RENAL FAILURE/FANCONI SYNDROME. **MS:** ↓ bone mineral density, ↑ creatine kinase, arthralgia, muscle weakness, myalgia, osteomalacia, polymyositis. **Neuro:** abnormal dreams, dizziness, Guillan-Barré syndrome, insomnia, sedation. **Misc:** immune reconstitution syndrome.

Interactions

Drug-Drug: Strong CYP3A inducers, including **carbamazepine, enzalutamide, mitotane, oxcarbazepine, phenobarbital, phenytoin, rifampin,** and **rifapentine** may significantly ↓ levels and effectiveness of doravirine; concurrent use contraindicated; should discontinue these medications for ≥4 wk before initiating doravirine/lamivudine/tenofovir disoproxil fumarate therapy. **Rifabutin** may ↓ levels and effectiveness of doravirine; take one doravirine 100-mg tablet 12 hr after doravirine/lamivudine/tenofovir disoproxil fumarate dose. Nephrotoxic drugs, including **acyclovir, aminoglycosides, cidofovir, ganciclovir, NSAIDs, valacyclovir,** or **valganciclovir** may ↑ risk of nephrotoxicity; avoid recent or concurrent use. **Ledipasvir/sofosbuvir** and **sofosbuvir/velpatasvir** may ↑ tenofovir levels and risk of toxicity; closely monitor. Medications containing **sorbitol** may ↓ lamivudine levels; avoid concurrent use.

Drug-Natural Products: **St. John's wort** may significantly ↓ levels and effectiveness of doravirine; concurrent use contraindicated; should discontinue this medication for ≥4 wk before initiating doravirine therapy.

Route/Dosage

PO (Adults and Children ≥35 kg): One tablet (doravirine 100 mg/lamivudine 300 mg/tenofovir disoproxil fumarate 300 mg) once daily.

✹ = Canadian drug name. ▨ = Genetic implication. ~~Strikethrough~~ = Discontinued. CAPITALS = life-threatening. <u>Underline</u> = most frequent.

Availability
Tablets: doravirine 100 mg/lamivudine 300 mg/tenofovir disoproxil fumarate 300 mg.

NURSING IMPLICATIONS
Assessment
- Assess for change in severity of HIV symptoms and for symptoms of opportunistic infections during therapy.
- Assess bone mineral density in patients with HIV who have a history of pathologic bone fracture or other risk factors for osteoporosis or bone loss. Consider supplementation with calcium and vitamin D.

Lab Test Considerations
- Monitor viral load and CD4 cell count regularly during therapy.
- Assess for HBV. Not approved for administration in patients with HIV and HBV. If therapy is discontinued, may cause severe exacerbation of hepatitis B. Monitor liver function in coinfected patients for several mo after stopping therapy.
- Monitor liver function tests before and periodically during therapy, especially in patients with underlying liver disease or marked ↑ transaminases. May cause ↑ serum creatinine, AST, ALT, total bilirubin, total cholesterol, LDL, and triglycerides. May cause lactic acidosis and severe hepatomegaly with steatosis. These events are more likely to occur if patients are female, obese, or receiving nucleoside analogue medications for extended periods of time. Monitor patient for signs (increased serum lactate levels, elevated liver enzymes, liver enlargement on palpation). Therapy should be suspended if clinical or laboratory signs occur.
- Assess serum creatinine, CCr, urine glucose, and urine protein before starting and periodically during therapy. Also assess serum phosphorous in patients with chronic kidney disease. Patients taking nephrotoxic agents, including NSAIDs, are at increased risk for renal impairment.

Implementation
- Administer once daily without regard to meals.

Patient/Family Teaching
- Instruct patient on the importance of taking medication as directed, even if feeling better. Do not take more than prescribed amount and do not stop taking without consulting health care professional. Discontinuing therapy may lead to severe exacerbations. Take missed doses as soon as remembered unless almost time for next dose; do not double doses. Advise patient to read *Patient Information* prior to starting therapy and with each Rx refill in case of changes. Caution patient not to share or trade *Delstrigo*™ with others.
- Inform patient of importance of hepatitis B testing before starting antiretroviral therapy.
- Inform patient that *Delstrigo*™ does not cure HIV and may reduce the risk of transmission of HIV to others through sexual contact or blood contamination. Caution patient to use a condom and avoid sharing needles or donating blood to prevent spreading HIV to others.
- Advise patient to notify health care professional if bone pain (bone pain that does not go away or worsening bone pain; pain in arms, legs, hands or feet; broken bones, muscle pain or weakness). May be symptoms of a bone or kidney problem.
- Advise patient to notify health care professional if signs and symptoms of immune reconstitution syndrome (signs and symptoms of an infection) occur.
- Instruct patient to notify health care professional of all Rx or OTC medications, vitamins, or herbal products being taken and consult health care professional before taking any new medications, especially St. John's wort.
- Rep: Advise patient to notify health care professional if pregnancy is planned or suspected. Encourage pregnant women to enroll in the Antiretroviral Pregnancy Registry by calling 1-800-258-4263. Advise female patient that pregnancy is not recommended and to avoid breastfeeding during therapy.
- Emphasize the importance of regular follow-up exams and blood counts to determine progress and monitor for side effects.

Evaluation/Desired Outcomes
- Delayed progression of AIDS and decreased opportunistic infections in patients with HIV.
- Decrease in viral load and increase in CD4 cell counts.

BEERS

doxazosin (dox-ay-zoe-sin)
Cardura, Cardura XL
Classification
Therapeutic: antihypertensives
Pharmacologic: peripherally acting antiadrenergics

Indications
Hypertension (as monotherapy or in combination with other antihypertensive agents) (immediate-release only). Symptomatic benign prostatic hyperplasia (BPH).

Action
Dilates both arteries and veins by blocking postsynaptic alpha$_1$-adrenergic receptors. **Therapeutic Effects:** Lowering of BP. Increased urine flow and decreased symptoms of BPH.

Pharmacokinetics
Absorption: Well absorbed following oral administration.
Distribution: Unknown.
Protein Binding: 98–99%.
Metabolism and Excretion: Extensively metabolized by the liver.
Half-life: 22 hr.

TIME/ACTION PROFILE

ROUTE	ONSET	PEAK	DURATION
PO†	1–2 hr	2–6 hr	24 hr
PO-XL‡	5 wk	unknown	unknown

†Antihypertensive effect.
‡Improved urinary flow and BPH symptoms.

Contraindications/Precautions
Contraindicated in: Hypersensitivity.
Use Cautiously in: Hepatic impairment; GI narrowing (XL only); Patients undergoing cataract surgery (↑ risk of intraoperative floppy iris syndrome); OB: Not a preferred antihypertensive during pregnancy ; Pedi: Safety and effectiveness not established in children; Geri: Appears on Beers list. ↑ risk of orthostatic hypotension in older adults. Avoid use for treatment of hypertension in older adults.

Adverse Reactions/Side Effects
CV: first-dose orthostatic hypotension, arrhythmias, chest pain, edema, palpitations. **Derm:** flushing, rash, urticaria. **EENT:** blurred vision, conjunctivitis, epistaxis, intraoperative floppy iris syndrome. **GI:** abdominal discomfort, constipation, diarrhea, dry mouth, flatulence, nausea, vomiting. **GU:** ↓ libido, priapism, sexual dysfunction. **MS:** arthralgia, myalgia. **Neuro:** dizziness, headache, depression, drowsiness, fatigue, nervousness, weakness.. **Resp:** dyspnea.

Interactions
Drug-Drug: ↑ risk of hypotension with **sildenafil, tadalafil, vardenafil,** other **antihypertensives, nitrates,** or acute ingestion of **alcohol. NSAIDs, sympathomimetics,** or **estrogens** may ↓ effects of antihypertensive therapy.

Route/Dosage
Hypertension
PO (Adults): 1 mg once daily, may be gradually ↑ at 2-wk intervals to 2–16 mg/day; incidence of postural hypotension greatly ↑ at doses >4 mg/day.

Benign Prostatic Hyperplasia
PO (Adults): *Immediate release:* 1 mg once daily, may be ↑ every 1–2 wk up to 8 mg/day; *Extended release:* 4 mg once daily (with breakfast), may be ↑ in 3–4 wk to 8 mg/day.

Availability (generic available)
Tablets: 1 mg, 2 mg, 4 mg, 8 mg. **Extended-release tablets:** 4 mg, 8 mg.

NURSING IMPLICATIONS
Assessment
- Monitor BP and pulse 2–6 hr after first dose, with each increase in dose, and periodically during therapy. Report significant changes.
- Assess for first-dose orthostatic hypotension and syncope. Incidence may be dose related. Observe patient closely during this period and take precautions to prevent injury.
- Monitor intake and output ratios and daily weight, and assess for edema daily, especially at beginning of therapy. Report weight gain or edema.
- **BPH:** Assess patient for symptoms of prostatic hyperplasia (urinary hesitancy, feeling of incomplete bladder emptying, interruption of urinary stream, impairment of size and force of urinary stream, terminal urinary dribbling, straining to start flow, dysuria, urgency) prior to and periodically during therapy.

Implementation
- **PO:** Administer daily dose at bedtime.
- **DNC:** XL tablets should be swallowed whole; do not break, crush, or chew.
- **Hypertension:** May be administered concurrently with a diuretic or other antihypertensive.

Patient/Family Teaching
- Emphasize the importance of continuing to take this medication, even if feeling well. Instruct patient to take doxazosin at the same time each day. Take missed doses as soon as remembered unless almost time for next dose. Do not double doses.
- May cause drowsiness or dizziness. Advise patient to avoid driving or other activities requiring alertness until response to medication is known.
- Caution patient to change positions slowly to decrease orthostatic hypotension. May cause syncopal episodes, especially within first 24 hr of therapy, with dose increase, and with resumption of therapy after interruption.
- Instruct patient to notify health care professional of all Rx or OTC medications, vitamins, or herbal products being taken and to avoid concurrent use of alcohol or OTC medications and herbal products, especially cold preparations, without consulting health care professional, especially cough, cold, or allergy remedies.
- Advise patient to notify other physicians of drug therapy.
- Advise male patient to notify health care professional if priapism or erection of longer than 4 hr occurs; may lead to permanent impotence if not treated.
- Rep: Advise females of reproductive potential to notify health care professional if pregnancy is planned or suspected or if breastfeeding.
- Emphasize the importance of follow-up visits to determine effectiveness of therapy.
- **Hypertension:** Instruct patient and family on proper technique for BP monitoring. Advise them to check BP at least weekly and report significant changes.
- Encourage patient to comply with additional interventions for hypertension (weight reduction, low-sodium diet, smoking cessation, moderation of alco-

hol consumption, regular exercise, and stress management).

Evaluation/Desired Outcomes

- Decrease in BP without appearance of side effects.
- Decrease in urinary symptoms of BPH.

---

doxercalciferol, See VITAMIN D COMPOUNDS.

HIGH ALERT

DOXOrubicin hydrochloride
(dox-oh-**roo**-bi-sin)
Adriamycin, ✳Caelyx
Classification
Therapeutic: antineoplastics
Pharmacologic: anthracyclines

Indications

Breast cancer. Acute lymphoblastic leukemia. Acute myeloblastic leukemia. Hodgkin's lymphoma. Non-Hodgkin's lymphoma. Metastatic Wilms' tumor. Metastatic neuroblastoma. Metastatic soft tissue sarcoma. Metastatic bone sarcoma. Metastatic ovarian carcinoma.

Action

Inhibits DNA and RNA synthesis by forming a complex with DNA; action is cell-cycle S-phase specific. Also has immunosuppressive properties. **Therapeutic Effects:** Death of rapidly replicating cells, particularly malignant ones.

Pharmacokinetics

Absorption: IV administration results in complete bioavailability.

Distribution: Widely distributed to tissues; does not cross the blood-brain barrier.

Metabolism and Excretion: Primarily metabolized by the liver via the CYP2D6 and CYP3A4 isoenzymes to an active metabolite. Excreted predominantly in the bile, 50% as unchanged drug. Less than 5% eliminated unchanged in the urine.

Half-life: 16.7 hr.

TIME/ACTION PROFILE (effect on blood counts)

ROUTE	ONSET	PEAK	DURATION
IV	10 days	14 days	21–24 days

Contraindications/Precautions

Contraindicated in: Hypersensitivity; OB: Pregnancy; Lactation: Lactation.

Use Cautiously in: History of cardiac disease or high cumulative doses of anthracyclines; Depressed bone marrow reserve; Hepatic impairment (↓ dose if serum bilirubin >1.2 mg/dL); Rep: Women of reproductive potential and men with female partners of re-

productive potential; Pedi, Geri: Children, older adults, mediastinal radiation, concurrent cyclophosphamide (↑ risk of cardiotoxicity).

Adverse Reactions/Side Effects

CV: CARDIOMYOPATHY, ECG changes. **Derm:** alopecia, photosensitivity. **Endo:** prepubertal growth failure with temporary gonadal impairment (children only). **GI:** diarrhea, esophagitis, nausea, stomatitis, vomiting. **GU:** red urine, sterility. **Hemat:** anemia, leukopenia, thrombocytopenia. **Local:** phlebitis at IV site, tissue necrosis. **Metab:** hyperuricemia. **Resp:** recall pneumonitis. **Misc:** hypersensitivity reactions.

Interactions

Drug-Drug: **CYP2D6 inhibitors**, **CYP3A4 inhibitors**, and **P-glycoprotein inhibitors** may ↑ risk of toxicity; avoid concurrent use. **CYP2D6 inducers**, **CYP3A4 inducers**, and **P-glycoprotein inducers** may ↓ effectiveness; avoid concurrent use. ↑ bone marrow depression with other **antineoplastics** or **radiation therapy**. Pediatric patients who have received concurrent doxorubicin and **dactinomycin** have an ↑ risk of recall pneumonitis at variable times following local radiation therapy. May ↑ skin reactions at previous **radiation therapy** sites. If **paclitaxel** is administered first, clearance of doxorubicin is ↓ and the incidence and severity of neutropenia and stomatitis are ↑ (problem is diminished if doxorubicin is administered first). Hematologic toxicity is ↑ and prolonged by concurrent use of **cyclosporine**; risk of coma and seizures is also ↑. Incidence and severity of neutropenia and thrombocytopenia are ↑ by concurrent **progesterone**. **Phenobarbital** may ↑ clearance and ↓ effects of doxorubicin. Doxorubicin may ↓ metabolism and ↑ effects of **phenytoin**. **Streptozocin** may ↑ the half-life of doxorubicin (dosage ↓ of doxorubicin recommended). May ↑ risk of hemorrhagic cystitis from **cyclophosphamide**. May ↑ risk of hepatotoxicity from **mercaptopurine**. Cardiac toxicity may be ↑ by **radiation therapy** or **cyclophosphamide**. ↑ risk of cardiac toxicity with **trastuzumab**; avoid use of doxorubicin for up to 7 mo after discontinuing trastuzumab. If **dexrazoxane** is administered at initiation of doxorubicin-containing regimens, may ↑ risk of therapeutic failure and tumor progression. May ↓ antibody response to **live-virus vaccines** and ↑ risk of adverse reactions.

Route/Dosage

IV (Adults): 60–75 mg/m² daily, repeat every 21 days; or 25–30 mg/m² daily for 2–3 days, repeat every 3–4 wk or 20 mg/m²/wk. Total cumulative dose should not exceed 550 mg/m² without monitoring of cardiac function or 400 mg/m² in patients with previous chest radiation or other cardiotoxic chemotherapy.

IV (Children): 30 mg/m²/day for 3 days every 4 wk.

Hepatic Impairment

IV (Adults): *Serum bilirubin 1.2–3 mg/dL:* ↓ dose by 50%; *Serum bilirubin 3.1–5 mg/dL:* ↓ dose by 75%.

Availability (generic available)
Powder for injection: 10 mg/vial, 50 mg/vial, ✸ 150 mg/vial. **Solution for injection:** 2 mg/mL.

NURSING IMPLICATIONS
Assessment
- Monitor BP, pulse, respiratory rate, and temperature frequently during administration. Report significant changes.
- Monitor for bone marrow depression. Assess for bleeding (bleeding gums, bruising, petechiae, guaiac stools, urine, and emesis) and avoid IM injections and taking rectal temperatures if platelet count is low. Apply pressure to venipuncture sites for 10 min. Assess for signs of infection during neutropenia. Anemia may occur. Monitor for increased fatigue, dyspnea, and orthostatic hypotension.
- Monitor intake and output ratios, and report occurrence of significant discrepancies. Encourage fluid intake of 2000–3000 mL/day. Allopurinol and alkalinization of the urine may be used to decrease serum uric acid levels and to help prevent urate stone formation.
- Severe and protracted nausea and vomiting may occur as early as 1 hr after therapy and may last 24 hr. Administer parenteral antiemetics 30–45 min prior to therapy and routinely around the clock for the next 24 hr as indicated. Monitor amount of emesis and notify health care professional if emesis exceeds guidelines to prevent dehydration.
- Monitor for development of signs of cardiac toxicity, which may be either acute and transient (ST segment depression, flattened T wave, sinus tachycardia, and extrasystoles) or late onset (usually occurs 1–6 mo after initiation of therapy) and characterized by intractable HF (peripheral edema, dyspnea, rales/crackles, weight gain). Chest x ray, echocardiography, ECGs, and radionuclide angiography may be ordered prior to and periodically during therapy. Cardiotoxicity is more prevalent in children younger than 2 yr and geriatric patients. Dexrazoxane may be used to prevent cardiotoxicity in patients receiving cumulative doses of >300 mg/m².
- Assess injection site frequently for redness, irritation, or inflammation during and for up to 2 hr after completion of infusion. Doxorubicin is a vesicant but may infiltrate painlessly even if blood returns on aspiration of infusion needle. Severe tissue damage may occur if doxorubicin extravasates. If extravasation occurs, stop infusion immediately, restart, and complete dose in another vein. Local infiltration of antidote is not recommended. If extravasation is suspected, intermittent application of ice to site for 15 min, 4 times daily for 3 days may be useful. Because of the progressive nature of extravasation reactions, close observation and plastic surgery consultation are recommended. Blistering, ulceration, and/or persistent pain are indications for wide excision surgery, followed by split-thickness skin grafting. May use dexrazoxane to treat extravasation. Administer first infusion of dexrazoxane as soon as possible within 6 hr of extravasation. Remove ice packs for at least 15 min prior to and during dexrazoxane administration. Recommended dose of dexrazoxane for day 1 is 1000 mg/m² (up to 2000 mg); the dose for day 2 is 1000 mg/m² (up to 2000 mg); the dose for day 3 is 500 mg/m² (up to 1000 mg). Dexrazoxane is administered as an IV infusion over 1–2 hr. If swelling, redness, and/or pain persists beyond 48 hr, immediate consultation for possible debridement is indicated.
- Assess oral mucosa frequently for development of stomatitis. Increased dosing interval and/or decreasing dose is recommended if lesions are painful or interfere with nutrition.

Lab Test Considerations
- Verify negative pregnancy test before starting therapy. Monitor CBC and differential prior to and periodically during therapy. WBC nadir occurs 10–14 days after administration, and recovery usually occurs by the 21st day. Thrombocytopenia and anemia may also occur. Increased dosing interval and/or decreased dose is recommended if ANC is <1000 cells/mm³ and/or platelet count is <50,000 cells/mm³.
- Monitor renal (BUN and serum creatinine) and hepatic (AST, ALT, LDH, and serum bilirubin) function prior to and periodically during therapy. Dose reduction is required for bilirubin >1.2 mg/dL or serum creatinine >3 mg/dL.
- May cause ↑ serum and urine uric acid concentrations.

Implementation
- **High Alert:** Fatalities have occurred with incorrect administration of chemotherapeutic agents. Before administering, clarify all ambiguous orders; double-check single, daily, and course-of-therapy dose limits; have second practitioner independently double-check original order, calculations, and infusion pump settings.
- **High Alert:** Do not confuse doxorubicin hydrochloride with doxorubicin liposomal, daunorubicin hydrochloride, or idarubicin. Clarify orders that do not include both generic and brand names.
- Monitor cumulative dose of doxorubicin and other anthracyclines received; risk for cardiomyopathy increases as the cumulative dose increases (>250 mg/m² in pediatric patients <18 years of age and 550 mg/m² in patients >18 years of age).
- Solution should be prepared in a biologic cabinet. Wear gloves, gown, and mask while handling medication. Discard IV equipment in specially designated containers.
- Aluminum needles may be used to administer doxorubicin but should not be used during storage, be-

cause prolonged contact results in discoloration of solution and formation of a dark precipitate. Solution is red.

IV Administration

● **IV Push:** *Reconstitution:* Dilute each 10 mg with 5 mL of 0.9% NaCl (nonbacteriostatic) for injection. Shake to dissolve completely. Do not add to IV solution. Reconstituted medication is stable for 24 hr at room temperature and 48 hr if refrigerated. Protect from sunlight. *Concentration:* 2 mg/mL. *Rate:* Administer each dose over 3–10 min through Y-site of a free-flowing infusion of 0.9% NaCl or D5W. Facial flushing and erythema along involved vein frequently occur when administration is too rapid.

● **Intermittent Infusion:** May be further diluted in 50–1000 mL of D5W or 0.9% NaCl. *Rate:* Infuse over 30–60 min.

● **Y-Site Compatibility:** alemtuzumab, amifostine, amikacin, anidulafungin, argatroban, arsenic trioxide, aztreonam, bivalirudin, bleomycin, bumetanide, buprenorphine, butorphanol, calcium chloride, calcium gluconate, carboplatin, carmustine, caspofungin, chlorpromazine, ciprofloxacin, cisplatin, cladribine, clindamycin, cyclophosphamide, cyclosporine, cytarabine, D5W, dacarbazine, dactinomycin, daptomycin, dexamethasone, dexmedetomidine, dexrazoxane, diltiazem, diphenhydramine, dobutamine, docetaxel, dopamine, doxycycline, droperidol, enalaprilat, ephedrine, epinephrine, erythromycin, esmolol, etoposide, etoposide phosphate, famotidine, fentanyl, filgrastim, fluconazole, fludarabine, gemcitabine, gentamicin, granisetron, haloperidol, hetastarch, hydrocortisone, hydromorphone, ifosfamide, imipenem/cilastatin, irinotecan, isoproterenol, ketorolac, labetalol, leucovorin calcium, lidocaine, linezolid, lorazepam, mannitol, melphalan, meperidine, mesna, methadone, methotrexate, metoclopramide, metoprolol, midazolam, milrinone, mitomycin, morphine, moxifloxacin, nalbuphine, naloxone, nicardipine, nitroglycerin, nitroprusside, 0.9% NaCl, octreotide, ondansetron, oxaliplatin, paclitaxel, palonosetron, pamidronate, phenylephrine, potassium acetate, potassium chloride, procainamide, prochlorperazine, promethazine, propranolol, sargramostim, sodium acetate, sufentanil, tacrolimus, theophylline, thiotepa, tigecycline, tirofiban, tobramycin, topotecan, trastuzumab, vancomycin, vasopressin, vecuronium, verapamil, vinblastine, vincristine, vinorelbine, zidovudine, zoledronic acid.

● **Y-Site Incompatibility:** acyclovir, allopurinol, aminophylline, amiodarone, amphotericin B deoxycholate, amphotericin B lipid complex, amphotericin B liposomal, ampicillin, ampicillin/sulbactam, azithromycin, cefazolin, cefepime, cefotaxime, cefotetan, cefoxitin, ceftazidime, ceftriaxone, cefuroxime, diazepam, digoxin, ertapenem, foscarnet, fosphenytoin, ganciclovir, gemtuzumab ozogamicin, magnesium sulfate, meropenem, methohexital, minocycline, pantoprazole, pemetrexed, pentamidine,

pentobarbital, phenobarbital, phenytoin, piperacillin/tazobactam, potassium phosphate, propofol, rituximab, sodium phosphate, thiopental, trimethoprim/sulfamethoxazole, voriconazole.

Patient/Family Teaching

● Explain purpose of doxorubicin to patient.

● Instruct patient to notify health care professional promptly if fever; sore throat; signs of infection; bleeding gums; bruising; petechiae; blood in stools, urine, or emesis; increased fatigue; dyspnea; or orthostatic hypotension occurs. Caution patient to avoid crowds and persons with known infections. Instruct patient to use soft toothbrush and electric razor and to avoid falls. Caution patient not to drink alcoholic beverages or take medication containing aspirin or NSAIDs, because these may precipitate gastric bleeding.

● Instruct patient to report pain at injection site immediately.

● Instruct patient to inspect oral mucosa for erythema and ulceration. If ulceration occurs, advise patient to use sponge brush, rinse mouth with water after eating and drinking, and confer with health care professional if mouth pain interferes with eating. Pain may require treatment with opioid analgesics. The risk of developing stomatitis is greatest 5–10 days after a dose; usual duration is 3–7 days.

● Instruct patient to notify health care professional immediately if irregular heartbeat, shortness of breath, swelling of lower extremities, or skin irritation (swelling, pain, or redness of feet or hands) occurs.

● Discuss the possibility of hair loss with patient. Explore methods of coping. Regrowth usually occurs 2–3 mo after discontinuation of therapy.

● Instruct patient not to receive any vaccinations without advice of health care professional.

● Inform patient that medication may cause urine to appear red for 1–2 days.

● Instruct patient to notify health care professional if skin irritation occurs at site of previous radiation therapy.

● Advise family and/or caregivers to take precautions (i.e., latex gloves) in handling body fluids for at least 5 days post-treatment.

● Instruct patient to notify health care professional of all Rx or OTC medications, vitamins, or herbal products being taken and to consult health care professional before taking other Rx, OTC, or herbal products.

● Inform patient that doxorubicin may increase risk of developing secondary cancers.

● Rep: May cause fetal harm. Advise females of reproductive potential to use effective contraception during and for 6 mo after last dose and to avoid breastfeeding during and for 10 days to 6 wk after last dose. Advise males with female partners of reproductive potential to use effective contraception during and for 3–6 mo after last dose of doxorubicin. A pregnancy registry is available for all cancers diagnosed during pregnancy at Cooper Health (877-635-4499). Inform patient before initiating therapy that this medication may cause irreversible gonadal suppression, or irreversible amenorrhea or early menopause.

- Emphasize the need for periodic lab tests to monitor for side effects.

Evaluation/Desired Outcomes

- Decrease in size or spread of malignancies in solid tumors.
- Improvement of hematologic status in leukemias.

doxycycline, See TETRACYCLINES.

doxylamine/pyridoxine
(dox-**il**-a-meen peer-ih-**dox**-een)
Bonjesta, Diclegis, ✤Diclectin
Classification
Therapeutic: antiemetics
Pharmacologic: antihistamines, vitamin B6 analogues

Indications
Treatment of nausea and vomiting during pregnancy that has not responded to conservative management.

Action
Combination of an antihistamine and a vitamin B_6 analog. Mechanism not known. **Therapeutic Effects:** Decreased nausea and vomiting associated with pregnancy.

Pharmacokinetics
Absorption: Well absorbed following oral administration. Food delays/↓ absorption.
Distribution: Doxylamine probably enters breast milk.
Metabolism and Excretion: Doxylamine is mostly metabolized by the liver, inactive metabolites are renally excreted. Pyridoxine is a pro-drug, converted to its active metabolite by the liver.
Half-life: *Doxylamine:* 12.5 hr; *pyridoxine:* 0.4–0.5 hr.

TIME/ACTION PROFILE (anti-emetic effect)

ROUTE	ONSET	PEAK	DURATION
PO	unknown	unknown	8–24 hr

Contraindications/Precautions
Contraindicated in: Hypersensitivity to doxylamine or pyridoxine; Concurrent use of monoamine oxidase (MAO) inhibitors; Lactation: Doxylamine probably enters breast milk and may cause irritability, excitement, or sedation in infants; breastfeeding should be avoided.

Use Cautiously in: ↑ intraocular pressure or narrow angle glaucoma; Stenosing peptic ulcer or pyloroduodenal obstruction; Urinary bladder-neck obstruction; Pedi: Safety and effectiveness not established in children.

Adverse Reactions/Side Effects
Neuro: drowsiness.

Interactions
Drug-Drug: MAO inhibitors ↑ intensity/duration of adverse CNS (anticholinergic) reactions; concurrent use contraindicated. ↑ risk of CNS depression with other **CNS depressants** including **alcohol**, other **antihistamines**, **opioid analgesics**, and **sedative/hypnotics**.

Route/Dosage
Delayed-Release Tablets
PO (Adults): *Day 1:* 2 tablets (doxylamine 10 mg/pyridoxine 10 mg) at bedtime; if symptoms are controlled continue this regimen; *Day 2, if symptoms persist into afternoon on day 2:* 2 tablets at bedtime on day 2 and then 1 tablet in the morning on day 3 and 2 tablets in the evening; if symptoms are controlled, continue this regimen; *Day 4, if symptoms persist:* 1 tablet in the morning, 1 tablet mid-afternoon and 2 tablets at bedtime (not to exceed 4 tablets daily).

Extended-Release Tablets
PO (Adults): *Day 1:* 1 tablet (doxylamine 20 mg/pyridoxine 20 mg) at bedtime; if symptoms are controlled, continue this regimen; *Day 2, if symptoms persist on day 2:* 1 tablet in AM and 1 tablet at bedtime on day 2; if symptoms are controlled, continue this regimen (not to exceed two tablets daily).

Availability (generic available)
Delayed-release tablets (Diclegis): doxylamine 10 mg/pyridoxine 10 mg. **Extended-release tablets (Bonjesta):** doxylamine 20 mg/pyridoxine 20 mg.

NURSING IMPLICATIONS
Assessment
- Assess for frequency and amount of emesis daily during therapy. Reassess need for medication as pregnancy progresses.
- Monitor hydration status to prevent dehydration.

Lab Test Considerations
- May cause false positive urine screening tests for methadone, opiates, and PCP.

Implementation
- **PO:** Administer on an empty stomach with a full glass of water; food delays onset of medication. *DNC:* Swallow tablets whole; do not crush, break, or chew.

Patient/Family Teaching

- Instruct patient to take as directed. Do not take more than prescribed amount.
- May cause drowsiness. Caution patient to avoid driving and other activities requiring alertness until response to medication is known.
- Advise patient to avoid alcohol and CNS depressants, including sedatives, tranquilizers, antihistamines, opioids, and some cough and cold medications with doxylamine pyridoxine.
- Instruct patient to notify health care professional of all Rx or OTC medications, vitamins, or herbal products being taken and consult health care professional before taking any new medications.
- Rep: Advise female patient to avoid breastfeeding during therapy.

Evaluation/Desired Outcomes

- Decrease in frequency of nausea and vomiting during pregnancy.

---

drospirenone, See CONTRACEPTIVES, HORMONAL.

---

dulaglutide (doo-la-**gloo**-tide)
Trulicity
Classification
Therapeutic: antidiabetics
Pharmacologic: glucagon-like peptide-1 (GLP-1) receptor agonists

Indications

Type 2 diabetes (as adjunct to diet and exercise). To reduce the risk of major cardiovascular events in patients with type 2 diabetes who have established cardiovascular disease or multiple risk factors for cardiovascular disease.

Action

Acts as an acylated human glucagon-like peptide-1 (GLP-1, an incretin) receptor agonist; increases intracellular cyclic AMP (cAMP) leading to insulin release when glucose is elevated, which then subsides as blood glucose decreases toward euglycemia. Also decreases glucagon secretion and delays gastric emptying. **Therapeutic Effects:** Improved glycemic control. Reduction in risk of cardiovascular death, nonfatal MI, or nonfatal stroke.

Pharmacokinetics

Absorption: *0.75 mg dose:* 65% absorbed following SUBQ administration; *1.5 mg dose:* 47% absorbed following SUBQ administration.
Distribution: Unknown.
Metabolism and Excretion: Degraded by protein catabolic processes.
Half-life: 5 days.

TIME/ACTION PROFILE ($\downarrow$ in A$_{1c}$)

ROUTE	ONSET	PEAK	DURATION
SUBQ	within 4 wk	13 wk	unknown

Contraindications/Precautions

Contraindicated in: Hypersensitivity; Personal or family history of medullary thyroid carcinoma; Multiple Endocrine Neoplasia syndrome type 2; History of pancreatitis; Type 1 diabetes; Diabetic ketoacidosis; Severe gastrointestinal disease (including severe gastroparesis).
Use Cautiously in: History of angioedema or anaphylaxis to another GLP-1 receptor agonist; Hepatic/renal impairment; Diabetic retinopathy (may $\uparrow$ risk of complications); OB: Use during pregnancy only if potential maternal benefit justifies potential fetal risk; Lactation: Use while breastfeeding only if potential maternal benefit justifies potential risk to infant; Pedi: Children <10 yr (safety and effectiveness not established).

Adverse Reactions/Side Effects

Derm: pruritus, rash. **Endo:** THYROID C-CELL TUMORS. **GI:** abdominal pain, nausea, vomiting, $\downarrow$ appetite, cholecystitis, cholelithiasis, constipation, diarrhea, dyspepsia, PANCREATITIS. **GU:** acute renal failure. **Local:** injection site reactions. **Neuro:** fatigue. **Misc:** HYPERSENSITIVITY REACTIONS (including anaphylaxis and angioedema).

Interactions

Drug-Drug: Concurrent use with **insulin** or **agents that increase insulin secretion** including **sulfonylureas** may $\uparrow$ the risk of serious hypoglycemia; use cautiously and consider dose $\downarrow$ of insulin or agents increasing insulin secretion. May alter absorption of concomitantly administered **oral medications** due to delayed gastric emptying.

Route/Dosage

Type 2 Diabetes

SUBQ (Adults): 0.75 mg once weekly; after $\geq$4 wk, may $\uparrow$ to 1.5 mg once weekly to obtain glycemic control; if additional glycemic control still needed, may then $\uparrow$ to 3 mg once weekly after $\geq$4 wk; if additional glycemic control still needed, may then $\uparrow$ to 4.5 mg once weekly after $\geq$4 wk.
SUBQ (Children $\geq$10 yr): 0.75 mg once weekly; after $\geq$4 wk, may $\uparrow$ to 1.5 mg once weekly to obtain glycemic control.

Risk Reduction of Major Cardiovascular Events

SUBQ (Adults): 0.75 mg once weekly; after $\geq$4 wk, may $\uparrow$ to 1.5 mg once weekly to obtain glycemic control; if additional glycemic control still needed, may then $\uparrow$ to 3 mg once weekly after $\geq$4 wk; if additional glycemic control still needed, may then $\uparrow$ to 4.5 mg once weekly after $\geq$4 wk.

Availability
Solution for injection (single-dose, prefilled pens): 0.75 mg/0.5 mL, 1.5 mg/0.5 mL, 3 mg/0.5 mL, 4.5 mg/0.5 mL.

NURSING IMPLICATIONS
Assessment
- Observe patient taking concurrent insulin for signs and symptoms of hypoglycemic reactions (sweating, hunger, weakness, dizziness, tremor, tachycardia, anxiety, headache, blurred vision, slurred speech, irritability).
- If thyroid nodules or elevated serum calcitonin are noted, patient should be referred to an endocrinologist.
- Monitor for pancreatitis (persistent severe abdominal pain, sometimes radiating to the back, with or without vomiting). If pancreatitis is suspected, discontinue dulaglutide; if confirmed, do not restart dulaglutide.

Lab Test Considerations
- Monitor serum A_{1c} periodically during therapy to evaluate effectiveness.
- May ↑ lipase and pancreatic amylase.

Implementation
- Do not confuse Trulicity with Toujeo, Tradjenta, or Tresiba.
- Patients stabilized on a diabetic regimen who are exposed to stress, fever, trauma, infection, or surgery may require administration of insulin.
- **SUBQ:** Administer once weekly at any time of the day, without regard to food. Day of wk may be changed as long as at least 72 hr before next dose. Inject into abdomen, thigh, or upper arm. Solution should be clear and colorless; do not administer solutions that are discolored or contain particulate matter.

Patient/Family Teaching
- Instruct patient on use of pen and to take dulaglutide as directed. Follow manufacturer's instructions for pen use. Pen should never be shared between patients, even if needle is changed. Store pen in refrigerator; do not freeze. After initial use, pen may be stored at room temperature up to 14 days. Advise patient to read the *Medication Guide* before starting dulaglutide and with each Rx refill in case of changes.
- Take missed dose as soon as remembered as long as 3 days (72 hr) until next scheduled dose. If less than 3 days until next scheduled dose, skip and take next scheduled dose.
- Inform patient that nausea is the most common side effect, but usually decreases over time.
- Advise patient taking insulin and dulaglutide to never mix insulin and dulaglutide together. Give as 2 separate injections. Both injections may be given in the same body area, but should not be given right next to each other.
- Explain to patient that this medication controls hyperglycemia but does not cure diabetes. Therapy is long-term.
- Review signs of hypoglycemia and hyperglycemia with patient. If hypoglycemia occurs, advise patient to take a glass of orange juice or 2–3 tsp of sugar, honey, or corn syrup dissolved in water and notify health care professional.
- Encourage patient to follow prescribed diet, medication, and exercise regimen to prevent hypoglycemic or hyperglycemic episodes.
- Instruct patient in proper testing of serum glucose and ketones. These tests should be closely monitored during periods of stress or illness, and health care professional should be notified if significant changes occur.
- Advise patient to notify health care professional if changes in vision occur during therapy.
- Advise patient to notify health care professional of all Rx or OTC medications, vitamins, or herbal products being taken and consult health care professional before taking any new medications.
- Advise patient to notify health care professional immediately if signs of pancreatitis (nausea, vomiting, abdominal pain) or hypersensitivity (swelling of face, lips, tongue or throat, problems breathing or swallowing, severe rash or itching, fainting or feeling dizzy, very rapid heartbeat) occur.
- Inform patient of risk of benign and malignant thyroid C-cell tumors. Advise patient to notify health care professional if symptoms of thyroid tumors (lump in neck, hoarseness, trouble swallowing, shortness of breath) or if signs of allergic reaction (swelling of face, lips, tongue, or throat; fainting or feeling dizzy; very rapid heartbeat; problems breathing or swallowing; severe rash or itching) occur.
- Advise patient to inform health care professional of medication regimen before treatment or surgery.
- Advise patient to carry a form of sugar (sugar packets, candy) and identification describing disease process and medication regimen at all times.
- Rep: Insulin is the preferred method of controlling blood glucose during pregnancy. Counsel female patients to notify health care professional if pregnancy is planned or suspected or if breastfeeding.
- Emphasize the importance of routine follow-up exams.

Evaluation/Desired Outcomes
- Improved glycemic control.
- Reduction in risk of cardiovascular death, nonfatal MI, or nonfatal stroke.

☒ DULoxetine (do-lox-e-teen)
Cymbalta
Classification
Therapeutic: antidepressants
Pharmacologic: selective serotonin/norepi-
nephrine reuptake inhibitors

Indications
Major depressive disorder. Diabetic peripheral neuropathic pain. Generalized anxiety disorder. Chronic
musculoskeletal pain (including chronic lower back
pain and chronic pain from osteoarthritis). Fibromyalgia.

Action
Inhibits serotonin and norepinephrine reuptake in the
CNS. Both antidepressant and pain inhibition are cen-
trally mediated. **Therapeutic Effects:** Decreased de-
pressive symptomatology. Decreased neuropathic pain.
Decreased symptoms of anxiety. Decreased pain.

Pharmacokinetics
Absorption: Well absorbed following oral administration.
Distribution: Unknown.
Protein Binding: >90%.
Metabolism and Excretion: Primarily metabolized in the liver via the CYP2D6 and CYP1A2 isoenzymes; ☒ the CYP2D6 isoenzyme exhibits genetic polymorphism; ~7% of population may be poor
metabolizers and may have significantly ↑ duloxetine
concentrations and an ↑ risk of adverse effects.
Half-life: 12 hr.

TIME/ACTION PROFILE (plasma concentrations)

ROUTE	ONSET	PEAK	DURATION
PO	unknown	6 hr	12 hr

Contraindications/Precautions
Contraindicated in: Hypersensitivity; Concurrent
use of MAO inhibitors or MAO-like drugs (linezolid or
methylene blue); Severe renal impairment (CCr <30
mL/min); Hepatic impairment or substantial alcohol
use (↑ risk of hepatitis).
Use Cautiously in: History of suicide attempt or
ideation; History of mania (may activate mania/hypo-
mania); History of seizure disorder; Diabetes (may
worsen glycemic control); Angle-closure glaucoma;
OB: Use during 3rd trimester may result in neonatal serotonin syndrome requiring prolonged hospitalization,
respiratory and nutritional support; may ↑ risk of postpartum hemorrhage in mother when used in the month
before delivery; Lactation: Use while breastfeeding only
if potential maternal benefit justifies potential risk to infant; Pedi: May ↑ risk of suicide attempt/ideation especially during dose early treatment or dose adjustment;
risk may be greater in children or adolescents. Safety

and effectiveness not established in children <7 yr
(generalized anxiety disorder) or <13 yr (fibromyalgia); Geri: Appears on Beers list. May worsen or cause
syndrome of inappropriate antidiuretic hormone
(SIADH) secretion and/or hyponatremia in older
adults. Use with caution in older adults and closely
monitor sodium concentrations when starting therapy
or ↑ dose.

Adverse Reactions/Side Effects
CV: hypertension, orthostatic hypotension. **Derm:** ↑
sweating, ERYTHEMA MULTIFORME, pruritus, rash, STEV-
ENS-JOHNSON SYNDROME (SJS). **EENT:** ↑ intraocular
pressure, blurred vision. **Endo:** SIADH. **F and E:** hyponatremia. **GI:** ↓ appetite, constipation, dry mouth, nausea, ↑ liver enzymes, diarrhea, gastritis, HEPATOTOXIC-
ITY, PANCREATITIS, vomiting. **GU:** dysuria, ↓ libido,
delayed/absent orgasm, ejaculatory delay/failure, erectile dysfunction, urinary retention. **Hemat:** BLEEDING.
Neuro: drowsiness, fatigue, insomnia, activation of mania, dizziness, fainting, falls, NEUROLEPTIC MALIGNANT
SYNDROME, nightmares, SEIZURES, SUICIDAL THOUGHTS,
tremor. **Misc:** SEROTONIN SYNDROME.

Interactions
Drug-Drug: Concurrent use with **MAO inhibitors**
may result in serious potentially fatal reactions (Do not
use within 14 days of discontinuing MAO inhibitor. Wait
at least 5 days after stopping duloxetine to start MAO inhibitor). Concurrent use with **MAO-inhibitor-like
drugs**, such as **linezolid** or **methylene blue** may ↑
risk of serotonin syndrome; concurrent use contraindicated; do not start therapy in patients receiving **linezolid** or **methylene blue**; if **linezolid** or **methylene
blue** need to be started in a patient receiving duloxetine, immediately discontinue duloxetine and monitor
for signs/symptoms of serotonin syndrome for 5 days
or until 24 hr after last dose of linezolid or methylene
blue, whichever comes first (may resume duloxetine
therapy 24 hr after last dose of linezolid or methylene
blue). ↑ risk of hepatotoxicity with alcohol use disor-
der/**alcohol** abuse. Drugs that affect serotonergic neurotransmitter systems, including **tricyclic antidepressants, SNRIs, fentanyl, lithium, buspirone,
tramadol, meperidine, methadone, amphetam-
mines**, and **triptans** ↑ risk of serotonin syndrome.
Strong CYP1A2 inhibitors, including **cimetidine,
ciprofloxacin**, and **fluvoxamine**, may ↑ levels; avoid
concurrent use. **CYP2D6 inhibitors**, including **paroxetine, fluoxetine**, and **quinidine** ↑ levels of duloxetine and may increase the risk of adverse reactions.
May ↑ levels and risk of toxicity of **CYP2D6 substrates**, including **TCAs, phenothiazines**, and **class
Ic antiarrhythmics** (**propafenone** and **flecainide**);
concurrent use should be undertaken with caution. ↑
risk of serious arrhythmias with **thioridazine**; avoid
concurrent use. ↑ risk of bleeding with **NSAIDs, aspirin, clopidogrel, prasugrel, ticagrelor, dabigatran, apixaban, edoxaban, rivaroxaban**, or **warfarin**.

Drug-Natural Products: Use with **St. John's wort** ↑ serotonin syndrome.

Route/Dosage

Major Depressive Disorder
PO (Adults): 40–60 mg/day (as 20 mg or 30 mg twice daily or as 60 mg once daily) as initial therapy, then 60 mg once daily as maintenance therapy.

Generalized Anxiety Disorder
PO (Adults ≥65 yr): 30 mg once daily for 2 wk; may then consider ↑ to 60 mg once daily, then may ↑ by 30 mg once daily to maintenance dose of 60–120 mg once daily.
PO (Adults <65 yr): 30–60 mg once daily as initial therapy (if initiated on 30 mg once daily, should titrate to 60 mg once daily after 1 wk), then may ↑ by 30 mg once daily to maintenance dose of 60–120 mg once daily.
PO (Children ≥7 yr): 30 mg once daily for 2 wk; may then consider ↑ to 60 mg once daily; recommended maintenance dose = 30–60 mg once daily (not to exceed 120 mg once daily).

Diabetic Peripheral Neuropathic Pain
PO (Adults): 60 mg once daily.

Fibromyalgia
PO (Adults): 30 mg once daily for 1 wk, then ↑ to 60 mg once daily.
PO (Children ≥13 yr): *Cymbalta only:* 30 mg once daily; may ↑ to 60 mg once daily based on response and tolerability.

Chronic Musculoskeletal Pain
PO (Adults): 30 mg once daily for 1 wk, then ↑ to 60 mg once daily.

Availability (generic available)
Delayed-release capsules: 20 mg, 30 mg, 40 mg, 60 mg.

NURSING IMPLICATIONS

Assessment
- Monitor BP before and periodically during therapy. Sustained hypertension may be dose related; decrease dose or discontinue therapy if this occurs.
- Monitor appetite and nutritional intake. Weigh weekly. Report continued weight loss. Adjust diet as tolerated to support nutritional status.
- Assess sexual function before starting duloxetine. Assess for changes in sexual function during treatment, including timing of onset; patient may not report.
- Monitor closely for notable changes in behavior that could indicate the emergence or worsening of suicidal thoughts or behavior or depression, especially in early therapy or during dose changes. Risk may be increased in children, adolescents, and adults ≤24 yr. Restrict amount of drug available to patient.

- Assess for serotonin syndrome (mental changes [agitation, hallucinations, coma], autonomic instability [tachycardia, labile BP, hyperthermia], neuromuscular aberrations [hyperreflexia, incoordination], and/or GI symptoms [nausea, vomiting, diarrhea]), especially in patients taking other serotonergic drugs (SSRIs, SNRIs, triptans).
- Assess for rash periodically during therapy. May cause SJS. Discontinue therapy if severe or if accompanied with fever, general malaise, fatigue, muscle or joint aches, blisters, oral lesions, conjunctivitis, hepatitis and/or eosinophilia.
- **Depression or Anxiety:** Assess mental status (orientation, mood, and behavior). Inform health care professional if patient demonstrates significant increase in anxiety, nervousness, or insomnia.
- **Pain or Fibromyalgia:** Assess intensity, quality, and location of pain periodically during therapy. May require several wk for effects to be seen.

Lab Test Considerations
- May cause ↑ ALT, AST, bilirubin, CK, and alkaline phosphatase.
- May cause hyponatremia.
- Monitor blood sugar and A1c. May cause slight ↑ in blood glucose.

Implementation
- Do not confuse duloxetine with fluoxetine, paroxetine, or Dexilant. Do not confuse Cymbalta with Symbyax.
- **PO:** May be administered without regard to meals. *DNC:* Swallow capsules whole; do not crush, chew, or open and sprinkle contents on food or liquids; may affect enteric coating.

Patient/Family Teaching
- Instruct patient to take duloxetine as directed at the same time each day. Take missed doses as soon as possible unless time for next dose. Do not stop abruptly; may cause dizziness, headache, nausea, diarrhea, paresthesia, irritability, vomiting, insomnia, anxiety, hyperhidrosis, and fatigue; must be decreased gradually. Advise patient to read *Medication Guide* before starting therapy and with each Rx refill in case of changes.
- Encourage patient and family to be alert for emergence of anxiety, agitation, panic attacks, insomnia, irritability, hostility, impulsivity, akathisia, hypomania, mania, worsening of depression and suicidal ideation, especially during early antidepressant therapy. If these symptoms occur, notify health care professional.
- May cause drowsiness. Caution patient to avoid driving or other activities requiring alertness until response to medication is known.
- Advise patient to make position changes slowly to minimize orthostatic hypotension and falls, especially in elderly patients and those taking antihypertensive medications.

- Instruct patient to notify health care professional of all Rx or OTC medications, vitamins, or herbal products being taken and to consult with health care professional before taking other medications, especially NSAIDs or aspirin.
- Instruct patient to notify health care professional if signs of serotonin syndrome (mental status changes: agitation, hallucinations, coma); autonomic instability (tachycardia, labile BP, hyperthermia); neuromuscular aberrations (hyperreflexia, incoordination); and/or gastrointestinal symptoms (nausea, vomiting, diarrhea); liver damage (pruritus, dark urine, jaundice, right upper quadrant tenderness, unexplained "flu-like" symptoms), bleeding (ecchymoses, hematomas, epistaxis, petechiae, hemorrhage), or rash occur.
- Advise patient to avoid taking alcohol during duloxetine therapy.
- Inform patient that duloxetine may cause symptoms of sexual dysfunction. In males, ejaculatory delay or failure, decreased libido, and erectile dysfunction may occur. In female patients, may result in decreased libido and delayed or absent orgasm. Advise patient to notify health care professional if symptoms occur.
- Rep: May cause fetal harm. Advise females of reproductive potential to notify health care professional if pregnancy is planned or suspected or if breastfeeding. Use late in 3rd trimester may result in neonatal serotonin syndrome requiring prolonged hospitalization, respiratory support, and tube feeding; may occur immediately upon delivery. Symptoms include respiratory distress, cyanosis, apnea, seizures, temperature instability, feeding difficulty, vomiting, hypoglycemia, hypotonia, hypertonia, hyperreflexia, tremor, jitteriness, irritability, and constant crying. Use of duloxetine in last month of pregnancy may increase risk of postpartum hemorrhage. There is a pregnancy exposure registry that monitors pregnancy outcomes in women exposed to antidepressants during pregnancy. Encourage health care professionals to register patients by contacting the National Pregnancy Registry for Antidepressants at 1-866-961-2388 or online at https://womensmentalhealth.org/research/pregnancyregistry/. Monitor infants exposed to duloxetine via breastfeeding for sedation, poor feeding, and poor weight gain.

Evaluation/Desired Outcomes

- Increased sense of well-being.
- Renewed interest in surroundings. Need for therapy should be periodically reassessed. Patients may notice improvement within 1–4 wk, but should be advised to continue therapy as directed. Therapy is usually continued for several mo.
- Decrease in neuropathic pain associated with diabetic peripheral neuropathy.
- Decrease in chronic musculoskeletal pain and pain and soreness associated with fibromyalgia.
- Decrease in anxiety.

dupilumab (doo-pil-ue-mab)
Dupixent

Classification
Therapeutic: anti-inflammatories, anti-asthmatics
Pharmacologic: interleukin antagonists

Indications
Moderate-to-severe atopic dermatitis not controlled by other prescription therapies or when these therapies cannot be used (with or without topical corticosteroids). Add-on maintenance treatment of moderate-to-severe asthma that is of an eosinophilic phenotype or that is dependent on oral corticosteroids. Add-on maintenance treatment of inadequately controlled chronic rhinosinusitis with nasal polyposis. Eosinophilic esophagitis. Prurigo nodularis.

Action
Monoclonal antibody that inhibits interleukin-4 (IL-4) and IL-13, which inhibits cytokine-induced inflammatory responses. Mechanism in asthma not fully established. **Therapeutic Effects:** Decreased severity of atopic dermatitis. Decreased incidence of asthma exacerbations. Reduction in nasal polyps and nasal congestion. Achievement of remission and reduction in dysphagia in eosinophilic esophagitis. Reduction in itching associated with prurigo nodularis.

Pharmacokinetics
Absorption: 61–64% absorbed following SUBQ administration.
Distribution: Minimally distributed to tissues.
Metabolism and Excretion: Degraded by proteolytic enzymes located throughout the body.
Half-life: Unknown.

TIME/ACTION PROFILE (plasma concentrations)

ROUTE	ONSET	PEAK	DURATION
SUBQ	unknown	1 wk	unknown

Contraindications/Precautions
Contraindicated in: Hypersensitivity; Acute bronchospasm or status asthmaticus.
Use Cautiously in: Pre-existing helminth infections; OB: Use during pregnancy only if potential maternal benefit justifies potential fetal risk; Lactation: Use while breastfeeding only if potential maternal benefit justifies potential risk to infant; Pedi: Safety and effectiveness not established in children <6 mo (atopic dermatitis); <6 yr (asthma); <12 yr (eosinophilic esophagitis); or <18 yr (chronic rhinosinusitis with nasal polyposis).

Adverse Reactions/Side Effects
CV: vasculitis. EENT: conjunctivitis, keratitis. Hemat: eosinophilia. MS: arthralgia. Resp: eosinophilic pneumonia. Misc: HYPERSENSITIVITY REACTIONS (including anaphylaxis), injection site reactions.

Interactions

Drug-Drug: Avoid use of **live vaccines**.

Route/Dosage

Atopic Dermatitis

SUBQ (Adults and Children ≥6 yr and ≥60 kg):
600 mg (given as two 300-mg injections) initially, then
300 mg in 2 wk, then 300 mg every 2 wk.
SUBQ (Children ≥6 yr and 30–<60 kg): 400 mg
(given as two 200-mg injections) initially, then 200 mg
in 2 wk, then 200 mg every 2 wk.
SUBQ (Children ≥6 yr and 15–<30 kg): 600 mg
(given as two 300-mg injections) initially, then 300 mg
in 4 wk, then 300 mg every 4 wk.
SUBQ (Children 6 mo-5 yr and 15–<30 kg): 300
mg every 4 wk.
SUBQ (Children 6 mo-5 yr and 5–<15 kg): 200
mg every 4 wk.

Asthma

SUBQ (Adults): 400 mg (given as two 200-mg injections) initially, then 200 mg in 2 wk, then 200 mg every
2 wk *or* 600 mg (given as two 300-mg injections) initially, then 300 mg in 2 wk, then 300 mg every 2 wk.
*Patients with oral corticosteroid-dependent asthma,
concomitant moderate-to-severe atopic dermatitis,
or concomitant chronic rhinosinusitis with nasal
polyposis:* 600 mg (given as two 300-mg injections)
initially, then 300 mg in 2 wk, then 300 mg every 2 wk.
SUBQ (Children ≥12 yr): 400 mg (given as two 200-
mg injections) initially, then 200 mg in 2 wk, then 200
mg every 2 wk *or* 600 mg (given as two 300-mg injections) initially, then 300 mg in 2 wk, then 300 mg every
2 wk. *Patients with oral corticosteroid-dependent
asthma or concomitant moderate-to-severe atopic
dermatitis:* 600 mg (given as two 300-mg injections)
initially, then 300 mg in 2 wk, then 300 mg every 2 wk.
SUBQ (Children 6–11 yr and ≥30 kg): 200 mg
every 2 wk. *Patients with concomitant moderate-to-
severe atopic dermatitis:* 400 mg (given as two 200-
mg injections) initially, then 200 mg in 2 wk, then 200
mg every 2 wk.
SUBQ (Children 6–11 yr and 15–<30 kg): 100
mg every 2 wk *or* 300 mg every 4 wk. *Patients with
concomitant moderate-to-severe atopic dermatitis:*
600 mg (given as two 300-mg injections) initially, then
300 mg in 4 wk, then 300 mg every 4 wk.

Chronic Rhinosinusitis with Nasal Polyposis

SUBQ (Adults): 300 mg every 2 wk.

Eosinophilic Esophagitis

SUBQ (Adults and Children ≥12 yr and ≥40 kg):
300 mg every week.

Prurigo Nodularis

SUBQ (Adults): 600 mg (given as two 300-mg injections) initially, then 300 mg in 2 wk, then 300 mg every
2 wk.

Availability

Solution for injection (prefilled syringes): 100
mg/0.67 mL, 200 mg/1.14 mL, 300 mg/2 mL. **Solution
for injection (prefilled pens):** 200 mg/1.14 mL, 300
mg/2 mL.

NURSING IMPLICATIONS

Assessment

- Monitor for signs and symptoms of hypersensitivity
  reactions (rash, urticaria, erythema nodosum, serum sickness) during therapy. If severe reaction occurs, treat symptomatically and discontinue dupilumab.
- Monitor for signs and symptoms of conjunctivitis
  and keratitis (eye redness or irritation) periodically
  during therapy.
- Monitor lung sounds periodically during therapy.
- Monitor for signs and symptoms of rhinosinusitis periodically during therapy.
- **Atopic Dermatitis:** Monitor skin lesions before
  starting and periodically during therapy.
- **Asthma:** Assess lung sounds, pulse, and BP before
  administration and during peak of medication. Note
  amount, color, and character of sputum produced.

Implementation

- Complete all age-appropriate vaccinations as recommended by current immunization guidelines before
  starting therapy.
- Prefilled pen is for adults and children ≥2 yr; prefilled syringe is for adults and children ≥6 mo.
- Before injection, remove dupilumab from the refrigerator and allow to reach room temperature (45
  min for the 300 mg/2 mL prefilled syringe or prefilled pen, 30 min for the 200 mg/1.14 mL prefilled syringe or prefilled pen, and 100 mg/0.67 mL prefilled
  syringe) without removing the needle cap. After removal from the refrigerator, must be used within 14
  days or discarded.
- **SUBQ:** Dose must be divided into two injections for
  400 mg and 600 mg doses. Administer at different
  sites. Thigh and abdomen may be used if patient ad-
  ministers dose. May also use upper arm if administered by caregiver. Rotate site with each injection; do
  not inject in skin that is tender, damaged, bruised,
  or scarred. Allow solution to reach room temperature (45 min for 300 mg dose, 30 min for 200 mg
  dose) before injecting. Solution is clear to slightly
  opalescent, colorless to pale yellow; do not administer solutions that are cloudy, discolored, or contain
  particulate matter.

Patient/Family Teaching

- Instruct patient and caregiver in correct injection
  technique and disposal of equipment. If a weekly
  dose is missed, administer dose as soon as possible,
  and start a new weekly schedule from the date of the
  last administered dose. If every other week missed

dose as soon as remembered if within 7 days, then resume original schedule. If longer than 7 days, skip dose and resume with next scheduled dose. If every 4 wk dose is missed, administer injection within 7 days from missed dose and resume original schedule. If missed dose is not administered within 7 days, administer dose and start a new schedule based on this date. Advise patient to read *Instructions for Use* before starting therapy and with each Rx refill in case of changes.

- Inform patient that dupilumab is not used for acute asthma symptoms or exacerbations. Instruct patient to notify health care professional if asthma symptoms remain uncontrolled or worsen after starting dupilumab therapy.
- Advise patient to notify health care professional if new onset or worsening eye symptoms occur.
- Instruct patient to notify health care professional of all Rx or OTC medications, vitamins, or herbal products being taken and to consult health care professional before taking other Rx, OTC, or herbal products.
- Advise patient to avoid live vaccines during therapy.
- Advise patient to have helminth infections treated before starting dupilumab therapy. If patient becomes infected while receiving treatment with dupilumab and does not respond to antihelminth treatment, discontinue treatment with dupilumab until infection resolves.
- Rep: Advise females of reproductive potential to notify health care professional if pregnancy is planned or suspected or if breastfeeding. Inform patient of pregnancy exposure registry that monitors pregnancy outcomes in women exposed to dupilumab during pregnancy. Health care professionals and patients may call 1-877-311-8972 or go to https://mothertobaby.org/ongoing-study/dupixent/ to enroll in or to obtain information about the registry.

Evaluation/Desired Outcomes

- Decreased severity of atopic dermatitis.
- Decreased incidence of asthma exacerbations.
- Reduction in symptoms of chronic rhinosinusitis with nasal polyposis.
- Achievement of remission and reduction in dysphagia in eosinophilic esophagitis.
- Reduction in itching associated with prurigo nodularis.

---

dutasteride (doo-tas-te-ride)
Avodart
Classification
Therapeutic: benign prostatic hyperplasia (BPH) agents
Pharmacologic: androgen inhibitors

Indications

Management of the symptoms of benign prostatic hyperplasia (BPH) in men with an enlarged prostate gland (as monotherapy or in combination with tamsulosin).

Action

Inhibits the enzyme 5-alpha-reductase, which is responsible for converting testosterone to its potent metabolite 5-alpha-dihydrotestosterone in the prostate gland and other tissues. 5-Alpha-dihydrotestosterone is partly responsible for prostatic hyperplasia. **Therapeutic Effects:** Reduced prostate size with associated decrease in urinary symptoms.

Pharmacokinetics

Absorption: Well absorbed (60%) following oral administration; also absorbed through skin.
Distribution: 11.5% of serum concentration partitions into semen.
Protein Binding: 99% bound to albumin; 96.6% bound to alpha-1 glycoprotein.
Metabolism and Excretion: Mostly metabolized by the liver via the CYP3A4 isoenzyme; metabolites are excreted in feces.
Half-life: 5 wk.

TIME/ACTION PROFILE (↓ in dihydrotestosterone levels†)

ROUTE	ONSET	PEAK	DURATION
PO	unknown	1–2 wk	unknown

†Symptoms may only improve over 3–12 mo.

Contraindications/Precautions

Contraindicated in: Hypersensitivity; Cross-sensitivity with other 5-alpha-reductase inhibitors may occur.
Use Cautiously in: Hepatic impairment.

Adverse Reactions/Side Effects

Derm: rash, urticaria. **Endo:** gynecomastia. **GU:** ↓ libido, ejaculation disorders, erectile dysfunction, PROSTATE CANCER (high-grade), testicular pain, testicular swelling. **Neuro:** depression. **Misc:** HYPERSENSITIVITY REACTIONS (including angioedema).

Interactions

Drug-Drug: **CYP3A4 inhibitors**, including **ritonavir, ketoconazole, verapamil, diltiazem, cimetidine**, and **ciprofloxacin** may ↑ levels and risk of toxicity.

Route/Dosage

PO (Adults): 0.5 mg once daily.

Availability (generic available)

Soft gelatin capsules: 0.5 mg. *In combination with:* tamsulosin (Jalyn); see Appendix N.

NURSING IMPLICATIONS
Assessment

- Assess patient for symptoms of BPH (urinary hesitancy, feeling of incomplete bladder emptying, interruption of urinary stream, impairment of size and force of urinary stream, terminal urinary dribbling, straining to start flow, dysuria, urgency) before and periodically during therapy.

D

- Digital rectal examinations should be performed before and periodically during therapy for BPH.

Lab Test Considerations
- Serum prostate-specific antigen (PSA) concentrations, used to screen for prostate cancer, ↓ by about 20% within the 1st mo of therapy and stabilize at about 50% of the pretreatment level within 6 mo. New baseline PSA concentrations should be established at 3 and 6 mo of therapy and evaluated periodically during therapy. Any ↑ in PSA during dutasteride therapy may be a sign of prostate cancer and should be evaluated, even those within normal limits. Isolated PSA values from men taking dutasteride for 3 mo or more should be doubled for comparison in untreated men.

Implementation
- **PO:** Administer once daily with or without meals. *DNC:* Do not break, crush, or chew capsule.

Patient/Family Teaching
- Instruct patient to take dutasteride at the same time each day as directed, even if symptoms improve or are unchanged. Take missed doses as soon as re-

membered later in the day or omit dose. Do not make up by taking double doses the next day.
- Caution patient that sharing of dutasteride may be dangerous.
- Inform patient that the volume of ejaculate may be decreased during therapy but that this will not interfere with normal sexual function.
- Advise patient to avoid donating blood for at least 6 mo after last dose of dutasteride to prevent a pregnant female from receiving dutasteride through a blood transfusion.
- Inform patient of potential increase risk in high-grade prostate cancer.
- Emphasize the importance of periodic follow-up exams to determine whether a clinical response has occurred.
- Rep: Caution patient that dutasteride poses a potential risk to a male fetus. Women who are pregnant or may become pregnant should avoid exposure to semen of a partner taking dutasteride and should not handle dutasteride because of the potential for absorption.

Evaluation/Desired Outcomes
- Decrease in urinary symptoms of BPH.

econazole, See ANTIFUNGALS (TOPICAL).

edaravone (e-dar-a-vone)
Radicava, Radicava ORS
Classification
Therapeutic: agents for amyotrophic lateral sclerosis

Indications
Amyotrophic lateral sclerosis (ALS).

Action
Unknown. **Therapeutic Effects:** Improved functional ability.

Pharmacokinetics
Absorption: IV administration results in complete bioavailability. 57% bioavailability of oral suspension (absorption significantly ↓ when taken with food).
Distribution: Well distributed to tissues.
Protein Binding: 92%.
Metabolism and Excretion: Metabolized via sulfation and glucuronidation into inactive metabolites. Primarily eliminated in urine (1% as unchanged drug).
Half-life: *IV*: 4.5–6 hr. *Oral suspension*: 4.5–9 hr.

TIME/ACTION PROFILE (blood levels)

ROUTE	ONSET	PEAK	DURATION
IV	unknown	1 hr	unknown
PO	unknown	30 min	24 hr

Contraindications/Precautions
Contraindicated in: Hypersensitivity; Sulfite allergy.
Use Cautiously in: Severe renal impairment; OB: Safety not established in pregnancy; Lactation: Safety not established in breastfeeding; Pedi: Safety and effectiveness not established in children.

Adverse Reactions/Side Effects
Derm: contusion, dermatitis, eczema, fungal infection (tinea). **GU:** glycosuria. **Neuro:** gait abnormality, headache. **Misc:** HYPERSENSITIVITY REACTIONS (including anaphylaxis).

Interactions
Drug-Drug: None known.

Route/Dosage
PO (Adults): 105 mg once daily in the morning on an empty stomach (after overnight fasting) for 14 days, followed by a drug-free period of 14 days. Each subsequent cycle should consist of 105 mg once daily in the morning on an empty stomach (after overnight fasting) for 10 days out of 14 days, followed by a drug-free period of 14 days.
IV (Adults): 60 mg once daily for 14 days, followed by a drug-free period of 14 days. Each subsequent cycle should consist of 60 mg once daily for 10 days out of 14 days, followed by a drug-free period of 14 days.

Availability
Oral suspension: 105 mg/5 mL. **Premixed infusion:** 30 mg/100 mL.

NURSING IMPLICATIONS

Assessment
- Assess respiratory and functional status prior to and periodically during therapy.
- Monitor for signs and symptoms of hypersensitivity reactions or sulfite allergic reactions (redness, wheals, erythema multiforme, urticaria, decreased blood pressure, dyspnea) with each infusion. If reaction occurs, discontinue therapy and treat with standard care.

Implementation
- Patients treated with 60 mg of *Radicava* IV may be switched to 105 mg (5 mL) *Radicava ORS* using the same dosing frequency.
- PO: Administer orally or via feeding tube in the morning after overnight fasting. *If patient consumed a high-fat meal (800–1,000 calories, 50% fat)*, must be fasting 8 hrs before administration and 1 hr after administration. *If patient consumed a low-fat meal (400–500 calories, 25% fat)*, must be fasting 4 hrs before administration and 1 hr after administration. *If patient is taking a caloric supplement (250 calories, e.g., protein drink)*, must be fasting 2 hrs before administration and 1 hr after administration. Invert bottle and shake vigorously for 30 sec. Administer using syringe provided; household teaspoon is not an adequate measuring device. Dispose of medication not used within 15 days after opening bottle.
- If administering via nasogastric (NG) tubes or percutaneous endoscopic gastrostomy (PEG) tubes made of silicone, polyvinyl chloride, or polyurethane can be used. Before and after administration, use a catheter-tip syringe to flush the tube with ≥1 ounce (30 mL) of water.

IV Administration
- **Intermittent Infusion:** Do not use if oxygen indicator has turned blue or purple before opening package. Use within 24 hrs of opening overwrap. Solution is clear and colorless; do not administer solutions that are discolored or contain particulate matter. *Rate:* Infuse over 60 min at 1 mg/min.
- **Y-Site Incompatibility:** Do not mix with other medications.

Patient/Family Teaching
- Explain purpose of medication to patient. Advise patient to read *Patient Information* before starting therapy.
- Instruct patient to notify health care professional immediately if signs and symptoms of hypersensitivity or allergic reactions (hives; swelling of lips, tongue, face; fainting; breathing problems; dizziness; itching; wheezing) occur.

- Rep: **Advise patient to notify health care professional if pregnancy is planned or suspected or if breastfeeding.**

Evaluation/Desired Outcomes
- Improved functional ability.

edoxaban (e-**dox**-a-ban)
❦Lixiana, Savaysa
Classification
Therapeutic: anticoagulants
Pharmacologic: factor Xa inhibitors

Indications
Reduction of stroke/systemic embolization risk associated with nonvalvular atrial fibrillation (AF). Treatment of deep vein thrombosis (DVT) and pulmonary embolism (PE) following 5–10 days of initial therapy with a parenteral anticoagulant.

Action
Selective inhibitor of factor Xa. Does not inhibit platelet aggregation directly, but does inhibit thrombin-induced platelet aggregation. Decreases thrombin generation and thrombus development. **Therapeutic Effects:** Decreased thrombotic events associated with AF, including stroke and systemic embolization. Resolution of DVT and PE.

Pharmacokinetics
Absorption: 62% absorbed following oral administration.
Distribution: Widely distributed to tissues.
Metabolism and Excretion: Minimal metabolism; one metabolite is pharmacologically active. Excreted mostly unchanged in urine.
Half-life: 10–14 hr.

TIME/ACTION PROFILE (anticoagulant effect)

ROUTE	ONSET	PEAK	DURATION
PO	unknown	1–2 hr	24 hr

Contraindications/Precautions
Contraindicated in: Active bleeding; CCr >95 mL/min (↓ effectiveness); Concurrent use of other anticoagulants or rifampin; Presence of mechanical heart valves or severe mitral stenosis; Moderate to severe hepatic impairment; Triple-positive antiphospholipid syndrome (↑ risk of thrombosis); Lactation: Lactation.
Use Cautiously in: Elective/planned invasive/surgical procedures (discontinue at least 24 hr prior to ↓ risk of bleeding); Premature discontinuation (↑ risk of ischemic events); Neuroaxial anesthesia/spinal puncture (↑ risk of spinal/epidural hematoma and potential paralysis); Renal impairment (↓ dose for CCr 15–50 mL/min); Deteriorating or improving renal function (may require dose change); Body weight ≤60 kg (requires

lower dose); Rep: **Women of reproductive potential;** OB: Use during pregnancy only if potential maternal benefit justifies potential fetal risk; Pedi: **Safety and effectiveness not established in children.**

Adverse Reactions/Side Effects
GI: ↑ liver enzymes. **Hemat:** anemia, BLEEDING.

Interactions
Drug-Drug: Rifampin may ↓ levels and effectiveness; concurrent use contraindicated. ↑ risk of bleeding with other **anticoagulants, aspirin, clopidogrel, ticagrelor, prasugrel, fibrinolytics, NSAIDs, SNRIs,** or **SSRIs.** P-glycoprotein (P-gp) inhibitors, including **azithromycin, clarithromycin, erythromycin, itraconazole** (oral), **ketoconazole** (oral), **quinidine,** or **verapamil,** ↑ levels and the risk of bleeding; lower dose required.

Route/Dosage
Treatment of Nonvalvular Atrial Fibrillation
PO (Adults): 60 mg once daily.

Renal Impairment
PO (Adults): *CCr 15–50 mL/min:* 30 mg once daily.

Treatment of Deep Vein Thrombosis/Pulmonary Embolism
PO (Adults >60 kg): 60 mg once daily. *Concurrent use of P-gp inhibitors (verapamil, quinidine, azithromycin, clarithromycin, erythromycin, itraconazole [PO], or ketoconazole [PO]):* 30 mg once daily.
PO (Adults ≤60 kg): 30 mg once daily.

Renal Impairment
PO (Adults): *CCr 15–50 mL/min:* 30 mg once daily.

Availability
Tablets: 15 mg, 30 mg, 60 mg.

NURSING IMPLICATIONS
Assessment
- Monitor for bleeding. Discontinue edoxaban if active bleeding occurs. Concomitant drugs (aspirin, other antiplatelet agents, other antithrombotic agents, fibrinolytic therapy, chronic use of NSAIDs) may ↑ risk of bleeding. Anticoagulant effects of edoxaban persist for about 24 hr after last dose. Anticoagulant effects cannot be reliably monitored with standard laboratory tests. No reversal agent is available; protamine sulfate, vitamin K, and tranexamic acid do not reverse anticoagulant activity. May consider prothrombin complex concentrate (PCC), or other procoagulant reversal agents such as activated prothrombin complex concentrate or recombinant factor VIIa. If PCC is used, monitoring anticoagulation effect of edoxaban using clotting test (PT, INR, or aPTT) or anti-FXa activity is not useful. Hemodialysis does not significantly contribute to edoxaban clearance.
- Monitor frequently for signs and symptoms of neurological impairment (numbness or weakness of legs,

bowel, or bladder dysfunction, back pain, tingling, muscle weakness); if noted, urgent treatment is required. Intrathecal or epidural catheters should not be removed earlier than 12 hr after last dose of edoxaban. Next dose of edoxaban should not be given less than 2 hr after removal of catheter.

Lab Test Considerations
● Assess CCr using Cockcroft-Gault equation CCr = (140 – age) × (weight in kg) × (0.85 if female)/(72 × serum creatinine in mg/dL) before starting therapy.

Implementation
● Discontinue edoxaban at least 24 hr prior to invasive or surgical procedures; may ↑ risk of bleeding. Edoxaban may be restarted as soon as adequate hemostasis is established; time to onset of pharmacodynamic effect is 1–2 hr.
● **PO:** Tablets may be crushed and mixed with 2–3 oz of water and immediately administered by mouth or through a gastric tube. May also mix with applesauce and administered immediately.
● *If transitioning from warfarin or other vitamin K antagonists to edoxaban,* discontinue warfarin and start edoxaban when INR ≤2.5. *If transitioning from oral anticoagulants other than warfarin or other vitamin K antagonists to edoxaban,* discontinue current oral anticoagulant and start edoxaban at time of next scheduled dose of other oral anticoagulant. *If transitioning from low molecular weight heparin (LMWH) to edoxaban,* discontinue LMWH and start edoxaban at time of next scheduled administration of LMWH. *If transitioning from unfractionated heparin to edoxaban,* discontinue infusion and start edoxaban 4 hr later.
● *If transitioning from edoxaban to warfarin,* Oral Option: For patients taking 60 mg of edoxaban, ↓ dose to 30 mg and begin warfarin concomitantly. For patients taking 30 mg of edoxaban, ↓ dose to 15 mg and begin warfarin concomitantly. Measure INR at least weekly and just prior to daily dose of edoxaban to minimize influence of edoxaban on INR measurements. Once stable INR ≥2.0 achieved, discontinue edoxaban and continue warfarin. Parenteral Option: Discontinue edoxaban and administer a parenteral anticoagulant and warfarin at time of next scheduled edoxaban dose. Once stable INR ≥2.0 achieved, discontinue parenteral anticoagulant and continue warfarin. *If transitioning from edoxaban to non-vitamin-K dependant oral anticoagulant,* discontinue edoxaban and start other oral anticoagulant at time of next dose of edoxaban. *If transitioning from edoxaban to parenteral anticoagulant,* discontinue edoxaban and start parenteral anticoagulant at time of next dose of edoxaban.

Patient/Family Teaching
● Instruct patient to take edoxaban as directed. Take missed doses as soon as remembered on same day. Return to regular schedule next day. Do not double

doses in one day. Do not discontinue without consulting health care professional; stopping may increase risk of stroke. Advise patient to read *Medication Guide* before starting therapy and with each Rx refill in case of changes.
● Caution patient that they may bleed more easily, longer, or bruise more easily during therapy. Advise patient to notify health care professional immediately if bleeding or a fall, especially with head injury, occurs.
● Advise patient to notify health care professional of all Rx or OTC medications, vitamins, or herbal products being taken and to consult with health care professional before taking other medications, especially other aspirin or NSAIDs.
● Advise patient to notify health care professional of therapy before surgery, medical, or dental procedures are scheduled.
● Rep: Advise female patient to notify health care professional if pregnancy is planned or suspected and to avoid breastfeeding during therapy. May ↑ risk of uterine bleeding in females of reproductive potential and those with abnormal uterine bleeding. Monitor neonates for bleeding.

Evaluation/Desired Outcomes
● Decreased thrombotic events (stroke and systemic embolization) associated with nonvalvular AF.
● Treatment of deep vein thrombosis DVT and pulmonary embolism PE.

efavirenz/lamivudine/tenofovir disoproxil fumarate
(e-**fav**-e-renz/la-**mi**-vyoo-deen/te-**noe**-fo-veer dye-soe-**prox**-il fue-ma-rate)
Symfi, Symfi Lo
Classification
Therapeutic: antiretrovirals
Pharmacologic: non-nucleoside reverse transcriptase inhibitors, nucleoside reverse transcriptase inhibitors

Indications
HIV-1 infection.

Action
Efavirenz: Inhibits HIV reverse transcriptase, which results in disruption of DNA synthesis. *Lamivudine:* After intracellular conversion to its active form (lamivudine-5-triphosphate), inhibits viral DNA synthesis by inhibiting the enzyme HIV reverse transcriptase. *Tenofovir:* Phosphorylated intracellularly where it inhibits HIV reverse transcriptase resulting in disruption of DNA synthesis. **Therapeutic Effects:** Slowed progression of HIV infection and decreased occurrence of sequelae.

Pharmacokinetics
Efavirenz
Absorption: 50% absorbed when ingested following a high-fat meal.

Distribution: Unknown.
Protein Binding: >99%.
Metabolism and Excretion: Mostly metabolized by the liver by the CYP3A and CYP2B6 isoenzymes. 16–61% excreted in feces as unchanged drug, 14–34% excreted in urine (primarily as metabolites).
Half-life: *Following single dose:* 52–76 hr. *Following multiple doses:* 40–55 hr.

Lamivudine
Absorption: 86% absorbed after oral administration.
Distribution: Unknown.
Metabolism and Excretion: Mostly excreted unchanged in urine; <5% metabolized by the liver.
Half-life: 5–7 hr.

Tenofovir Disoproxil Fumarate
Absorption: Tenofovir disoproxil fumarate is a prodrug, which is split into tenofovir, the active component; absorption enhanced by food.
Distribution: Unknown.
Metabolism and Excretion: 70–80% excreted unchanged in urine by glomerular filtration and active tubular secretion.
Half-life: 17 hr.

TIME/ACTION PROFILE (plasma concentrations)

ROUTE	ONSET	PEAK	DURATION
Efavirenz (PO)	rapid	3–5 hr	24 hr
Lamivudine (PO)	unknown	0.9 hr	24 hr
Tenofovir (PO)	unknown	2 hr	24 hr

Contraindications/Precautions

Contraindicated in: Hypersensitivity; Concurrent use of elbasvir and grazoprevir; Coinfection with hepatitis B virus (HBV) (hepatitis may recur after discontinuation of lamivudine or tenofovir) (lamivudine dose not appropriate for patients coinfected with HBV); Concurrent or recent use of nephrotoxic medications; Concurrent use with ribavirin and/or interferon alfa (↑ risk of hepatic decompensation); Moderate or severe hepatic impairment; CCr <50 mL/min; OB: May cause fetal harm during 1st trimester of pregnancy; Lactation: Breastfeeding not recommended for women with HIV.
Use Cautiously in: Mental illness, substance abuse, or use of psychiatric medications (↑ risk of psychiatric symptoms); Seizures disorders (↑ risk of seizures); Rep: Women of reproductive potential; Pedi: Children with a prior history of antiretroviral exposure or history of pancreatitis (↑ risk of pancreatitis); Pedi: Children <40 kg (Symfi) or <35 kg (Symfi Lo) (safety and effectiveness not established); Geri: Cautious initial dosing in older adults due to ↑ incidence of renal, hepatic, or cardiac dysfunction.

Adverse Reactions/Side Effects

CV: QT interval prolongation. **Derm:** rash, ERYTHEMA MULTIFORME, STEVENS-JOHNSON SYNDROME (SJS). **Endo:** Graves' disease. **F and E:** diarrhea. **GI:** ↑ amylase, ↑ liver enzymes, abdominal pain, autoimmune hepatitis, dyspepsia, HEPATOMEGALY WITH STEATOSIS, HEPATOTOXICITY, LACTIC ACIDOSIS, nausea, PANCREATITIS, vomiting. **GU:** ACUTE RENAL FAILURE/FANCONI SYNDROME, hematuria. **Hemat:** neutropenia. **Metab:** fat redistribution, hyperlipidemia. **MS:** ↑ creatine kinase, pain, ↓ bone mineral density, arthralgia, muscle weakness, myalgia, osteomalacia, polymyositis. **Neuro:** depression, headache, abnormal dreams, aggressive behavior, anxiety, ataxia, catatonia, delusions, dizziness, drowsiness, encephalopathy, fatigue, Guillain-Barré syndrome, hallucinations, impaired concentration, insomnia, manic episodes, nervousness, paranoia, peripheral neuropathy, psychoses, sedation, SEIZURES, SUICIDAL THOUGHTS/BEHAVIORS. **Misc:** fever, immune reconstitution syndrome.

Interactions

Drug-Drug: May lead to loss of virologic response to **elbasvir/grazoprevir**; concurrent use contraindicated. Nephrotoxic drugs, including **acyclovir, aminoglycosides, cidofovir, ganciclovir, NSAIDs, valacyclovir,** or **valganciclovir,** may ↑ risk of nephrotoxicity; avoid recent or concurrent use. May ↑ risk of hepatic decompensation with **ribavirin** or **interferon alfa**; avoid concurrent use. Concurrent use with other **QT interval prolonging medications** may ↑ risk of QT interval prolongation or torsades de pointes. May alter the effects of **warfarin**. Concurrent use with **carbamazepine** may ↓ levels of carbamazepine and efavirenz; use alternative anticonvulsant agent. Concurrent use with **phenytoin** or **phenobarbital** may ↓ levels of phenytoin, carbamazepine, and efavirenz. May ↓ levels of **bupropion** and **sertraline**; may need to ↑ antidepressant dose. May ↓ **posaconazole** levels; avoid concurrent use. May ↓ **itraconazole** or **ketoconazole** levels; use alternative antifungal agent. May ↓ **clarithromycin** levels; consider using alternative antibiotic that does not cause QT interval prolongation. May ↓ **rifabutin** levels; ↑ daily dose of rifabutin by 50%. **Rifampin** may ↓ levels; ↑ dose of efavirenz. May ↓ **artemether/lumefantrine** levels; consider alternative antimalarial that does not cause QT interval prolongation. May ↓ **atovaquone/proguanil** levels; concurrent use not recommended. May ↓ levels of **calcium channel blockers**; may need to ↑ calcium channel blocker dose. May ↓ levels of **atorvastatin, pravastatin,** and **simvastatin**. May ↓ therapeutic effects of **pibrentasvir/glecaprevir, velpatasvir/sofosbuvir,** and **velpatasvir/sofosbuvir/voxilaprevir**; concurrent use not recommended. **Ledipasvir/sofosbuvir** may ↑ tenofovir levels. May ↓ the effectiveness of **progestin-containing hormonal contraceptives** (e.g., etonogestrel, norelgestromin, levonorgestrel); additional barrier contraceptive should be used. May ↓ levels of **cyclosporine, tacrolimus,**

E

and **sirolimus**; may need to adjust dose of immunosuppressant. May ↓ **methadone** levels. Medications containing **sorbitol** may ↓ lamivudine levels.

Route/Dosage

PO (Adults and Children ≥40 kg): *Symfi:* 1 tablet (efavirenz 600 mg/lamivudine 300 mg/tenofovir disoproxil fumarate 300 mg) once daily.
PO (Adults and Children ≥35 kg): *Symfi Lo:* 1 tablet (efavirenz 400 mg/lamivudine 300 mg/tenofovir disoproxil fumarate 300 mg) once daily.

Availability (generic available)

Tablets (Symfi): efavirenz 600 mg/lamivudine 300 mg/tenofovir disoproxil fumarate 300 mg. **Tablets (Symfi Lo):** efavirenz 400 mg/lamivudine 300 mg/tenofovir disoproxil fumarate 300 mg.

NURSING IMPLICATIONS

Assessment

* Assess patient for change in severity of HIV symptoms and for symptoms of opportunistic infections during therapy.
* Assess patient for CNS and psychiatric symptoms (dizziness, impaired concentration, somnolence, abnormal dreams, insomnia, suicidal thoughts and behaviors) during therapy. Symptoms usually begin during 1st or 2nd day of therapy and resolve after 2–4 wk. Administration at bedtime may minimize symptoms. Concurrent use with alcohol or psychoactive agents may cause additive CNS symptoms.
* Assess for rash, especially during 1st mo of therapy. Onset is usually within 2 wk and resolves with continued therapy within 1 mo. May range from mild maculopapular with erythema and pruritus to exfoliative dermatitis and SJS. Occurs more often and may be more severe in children. If rash is severe or accompanied by blistering, desquamation, mucosal involvement, or fever, therapy must be discontinued immediately. *Symfi* may be reinstated concurrently with antihistamines or corticosteroids in patients discontinuing due to rash.
* Monitor for signs and symptoms of pancreatitis (abdominal pain with or without nausea and vomiting) during therapy. Discontinue therapy immediately if symptoms occur.
* Monitor for seizures during therapy. Institute seizure precautions.
* Assess bone mineral density in adult and pediatric patients with a history of pathologic bone fracture or other risk factors for osteoporosis or bone loss. May supplement with calcium and vitamin D.

Lab Test Considerations

* Verify negative pregnancy test before starting therapy.
* Monitor viral load and CD4 count before and routinely during therapy to determine response.
* Assess for HBV. *Symfi* and *Symfi Lo* are not approved for administration in patients with HIV and HBV. If therapy is discontinued, may cause severe exacerbation of HBV. Monitor liver function in coinfected patients for several months after stopping therapy.

* Monitor liver function prior to, during and following therapy. May cause ↑ LDL cholesterol, total cholesterol, and triglyceride concentrations. Lactic acidosis may occur with hepatic toxicity causing hepatic steatosis; may be fatal, especially in women. Discontinue therapy if symptoms occur.
* Calculate serum creatinine, CCr, urine glucose, and urine protein prior to and periodically during therapy and when clinically indicated. In patients with chronic kidney disease, assess serum creatinine, CCr, serum phosphorus, urine glucose, and urine protein prior to and periodically during therapy. May cause hypophosphatemia in patients with renal impairment.
* May cause ↑ lipids. Monitor total cholesterol and triglycerides before starting and periodically during therapy.
* May cause hyperglycemia and glycosuria.

Implementation

* **PO:** Administer once daily on an empty stomach, preferably at bedtime to minimize drowsiness.

Patient/Family Teaching

* Instruct patient on the importance of taking medication as directed, even if feeling better. Do not take more than prescribed amount and do not stop taking without consulting health care professional. Discontinuing therapy may lead to severe exacerbations. Take missed doses as soon as remembered unless almost time for next dose; do not double doses. Advise patient to read *Patient Information* prior to starting therapy and with each Rx refill in case of changes. Caution patient not to share or trade *Symfi* or *Symfi Lo* with others.
* Inform patient of importance of HBV testing before starting antiretroviral therapy.
* Inform patient that *Symfi* and *Symfi Lo* do not cure AIDS and may reduce the risk of transmission of HIV to others through sexual contact or blood contamination. Caution patient to use a condom and avoid sharing needles or donating blood to prevent spreading HIV to others.
* May cause dizziness, impaired concentration, or drowsiness. Caution patient to avoid driving or other activities requiring alertness until response to medication is known.
* Instruct patient to notify health care professional immediately if rash or suicidal thoughts or behaviors occur.
* Advise patient to notify health care professional immediately if symptoms of lactic acidosis (nausea, vomiting, unusual or unexpected stomach discomfort; unusual muscle pain; difficulty breathing; feeling cold, especially in arms and legs; dizziness; fast or irregular heartbeat; and weakness or tiredness) liver problems (yellow skin or whites of eyes, dark urine, light-colored stools, loss of appetite, nausea, stomach pain) or signs of immune reconstitution syndrome (signs and symptoms of an infection or inflammation) occur.

- Advise patient to notify health care professional if bone pain (bone pain that does not go away or worsening bone pain; pain in arms, legs, hands, or feet; broken bones; muscle pain or weakness). May be symptoms of a bone or kidney problem.
- Instruct patient to notify health care professional of all Rx or OTC medications, vitamins, or herbal products being taken and consult health care professional before taking any new medications, especially St. John's wort.
- Inform patient of risk of developing late-onset neurotoxicity (ataxia, encephalopathy); may occur months to years after starting therapy.
- Rep: May cause fetal harm; may cause neural tube defects if administered during 1st trimester. Advise females of reproductive potential taking oral contraceptives to use a nonhormonal method of birth control during therapy and for at least 12 wk following discontinuation and to avoid breastfeeding. Advise patient to notify health care professional if they become pregnant while taking *Symfi* or *Symfi Lo*. Encourage patients who become pregnant during therapy to join Antiretroviral Pregnancy Registry that monitors pregnancy outcomes in women exposed to efavirenz during pregnancy. Enroll patient by calling 1-800-258-4263.
- Emphasize the importance of regular follow-up exams and blood counts to determine progress and monitor for side effects.

Evaluation/Desired Outcomes
- Delayed progression of AIDS and decreased opportunistic infections in patients with HIV.
- Decrease in viral load and increase in CD4 cell counts.

---

efinaconazole, See ANTIFUNGALS (TOPICAL).

---

elagolix (el-a-goe-lix)
Orilissa
Classification
Therapeutic: analgesics
Pharmacologic: GnRH antagonist

Indications
Moderate to severe pain associated with endometriosis.

Action
Competitively binds to and inhibits gonadotropin-releasing hormone receptors in the pituitary gland, causing a decrease in the release of estradiol and progesterone by the ovaries. **Therapeutic Effects:** Reduction in dysmenorrhea and nonmenstrual pelvic pain.

Pharmacokinetics
Absorption: Rapidly absorbed.
Distribution: Unknown.
Metabolism and Excretion: Primarily metabolized in the liver via the CYP3A isoenzyme with some metabolism by the CYP2D6 and CYP2C8 isoenzymes as well as UGT. 90% of dose excreted in feces, <3% in urine.
Half-life: 4–6 hr.

TIME/ACTION PROFILE (plasma concentrations)

ROUTE	ONSET	PEAK	DURATION
PO	unknown	1 hr	24 hr

Contraindications/Precautions
Contraindicated in: Hypersensitivity; Osteoporosis (may ↑ risk of bone loss); Severe hepatic impairment; Concurrent use of strong organic anion transporting polypeptide (OATP) 1B1 inhibitors; OB: Pregnancy (may ↑ risk of early pregnancy loss).
Use Cautiously in: History of low-trauma fracture or other risk factors for osteoporosis; History of suicidal thoughts/behaviors or depression; Moderate hepatic impairment (use lower dose); Lactation: Use while breastfeeding only if potential maternal benefit justifies potential risk to infant; Rep: Women of reproductive potential; Pedi: Safety and effectiveness not established in children.

Adverse Reactions/Side Effects
Derm: rash. **Endo:** hot flush, night sweats. **GI:** nausea, ↑ liver enzymes, abdominal pain, constipation, diarrhea. **GU:** ↓ libido, menstrual irregularities. **Metab:** ↑ weight, dyslipidemia. **MS:** ↓ bone density, arthralgia. **Neuro:** headache, anxiety, depression, dizziness, insomnia, mood swings, SUICIDAL THOUGHTS/BEHAVIOR. **Misc:** HYPERSENSITIVITY REACTIONS (including anaphylaxis and angioedema).

Interactions
Drug-Drug: Strong OATP1B1 inhibitors, including **cyclosporine** and **gemfibrozil** may significantly ↑ levels; concurrent use contraindicated. **Estrogen-containing oral contraceptives** may ↓ effectiveness; impact of **progestin-containing oral contraceptives** on effectiveness unknown; recommended to use nonhormonal contraceptives. May ↑ estrogen exposure when used with **estrogen-containing contraceptives**, which may ↑ risk of thromboembolic events. May ↓ levels of **levonorgestrel-containing oral contraceptives**, which may ↓ effectiveness. May ↓ levels of **CYP3A substrates**, including **midazolam**. May ↑ levels of **CYP2C19 substrates**, including **omeprazole**; consider ↓ omeprazole dose when using higher doses (>40 mg/day). May ↑ levels of **P-glycoprotein substrates**, including **digoxin**; closely monitor digoxin levels. **Strong CYP3A inhibitors** may ↑ levels; limit concurrent use with elagolix 200 mg twice daily to ≤1 mo; limit concurrent use with elagolix 150 mg once daily to ≤6

✳ = Canadian drug name. ▓ = Genetic implication. S̶t̶r̶i̶k̶e̶t̶h̶r̶o̶u̶g̶h̶ = Discontinued. CAPITALS = life-threatening. <u>Underline</u> = most frequent.

mo. **CYP3A inducers**, including **rifampin** may ↓ levels; concurrent use with elagolix 200 mg twice daily not recommended; limit concurrent use with elagolix 150 mg once daily to ≤6 mo. May ↓ **rosuvastatin** levels; consider ↑ rosuvastatin dose.

Route/Dosage
PO (Adults): *No dyspareunia:* 150 mg once daily for max duration of 24 mo; *Coexisting dyspareunia:* 200 mg twice daily for max duration of 6 mo.

Hepatic Impairment
PO (Adults): *Moderate hepatic impairment:* 150 mg once daily for max duration of 6 mo.

Availability
Tablets: 150 mg, 200 mg. *In combination with:* estradiol/norethindrone (Oriahnn). See Appendix N.

NURSING IMPLICATIONS
Assessment
- Assess bone mineral density in patients with a history of a low-trauma fracture or other risk factors for osteoporosis or bone loss. Vitamin D and calcium supplements may be considered.
- Assess for depression and mood changes during therapy. Refer patients with new or worsening depression, anxiety or other mood changes, suicidal ideation and behavior to a mental health professional. Consider benefits and risks of continuing elagolix.

Lab Test Considerations
- Verify negative pregnancy test before starting therapy. Use lowest effective dose for limited duration to minimize bone loss.
- Monitor liver function tests periodically during therapy. May cause ↑ AST and ALT.
- May cause ↑ lipid levels during first 2 mo of therapy, then usually remains stable.

Implementation
- **PO:** Administer at the same time each day without regard to food.

Patient/Family Teaching
- Instruct patient to take elagolix as directed. Take missed doses as soon as remembered if same day as missed dose, then return to regular dosing schedule; do not double doses. Advise patient to read *Medication Guide* before starting and with each Rx refill in case of changes.
- Inform patient that elagolix may change menstrual periods (irregular bleeding or spotting, a decrease in menstrual bleeding, no bleeding at all), and make it hard to know if you are pregnant. Watch for other signs of pregnancy (breast tenderness, weight gain, nausea).
- Advise patient and family to notify health care professional if signs and symptoms of mood or behavior changes (thoughts about suicide or dying, try to commit suicide, new or worse depression, new or worse anxiety, other unusual changes in behavior or mood)

or liver problems (yellowing of skin or whites of eyes, dark amber-colored urine, feeling tired, nausea and vomiting, generalized swelling, right upper abdomen pain, bruising easily) occur.
- Advise patient to notify health care professional of all Rx or OTC medications, vitamins, or herbal products being taken and to consult with health care professional before taking other medications, especially birth control pills.
- Rep: May result in pregnancy loss if used in early pregnancy. Advise females of reproductive potential to use effective nonhormonal contraception during and for 28 days after last dose. Hormonal contraceptives may decrease effectiveness of elagolix and may increase risk of thromboembolic and vascular disorders. Advise patient to notify health care professional if pregnancy is planned or suspected, or if breastfeeding. Encourage patient to enroll in pregnancy registry to monitor outcomes of women who become pregnant while taking elagolix by calling 1-833-782-7241. Discontinue elagolix if pregnancy occurs.

Evaluation/Desired Outcomes
- Reduction in dysmenorrhea and nonmenstrual pelvic pain.

elagolix/estradiol/ norethindrone
(**el**-a-**goe**-lix/es-tra-**dye**-ole/nor-eth-**in**-drone)
   Oriahnn
Classification
Therapeutic: hemostatic agents, hormones
Pharmacologic: GnRH antagonist, estrogens, progestins

Indications
Heavy menstrual bleeding associated with uterine fibroids in premenopausal women.

Action
Elagolix: competitively binds to and inhibits gonadotropin-releasing hormone receptors in the pituitary gland, causing a decrease in the release of estradiol and progesterone by the ovaries, reducing bleeding associated with uterine fibroids. *Estradiol:* binds to estrogen receptors and reduces the increase in bone resorption and potential bone loss associated with elagolix. *Norethindrone:* protects uterus from potential adverse endometrial effects caused by unopposed estrogen use. **Therapeutic Effects:** Reduced menstrual blood loss.

Pharmacokinetics
Elagolix
Absorption: Rapidly absorbed following oral administration.
Distribution: Unknown.
Metabolism and Excretion: Primarily metabolized in the liver via the CYP3A isoenzyme with some metabolism by the CYP2D6 and CYP2C8 isoenzymes as well as UGT. 90% of dose excreted in feces, <3% in urine.

Half-life: 4–6 hr.

Estradiol

Absorption: Well absorbed following oral administration.

Distribution: Widely distributed.

Protein Binding: 98%.

Metabolism and Excretion: Metabolized by the liver via the CYP3A isoenzyme; also undergoes sulfation and glucuronidation. Enterohepatic recirculation occurs, and more absorption may occur from the GI tract.

Half-life: 8–20 hr.

Norethindrone

Absorption: Rapidly absorbed following oral administration.

Distribution: Unknown.

Protein Binding: 97%.

Metabolism and Excretion: Metabolized by the liver via the CYP3A isoenzyme.

Half-life: 5–13 hr.

TIME/ACTION PROFILE (plasma concentrations)

ROUTE	ONSET	PEAK	DURATION
PO	rapid	1–2 hr	unknown

Contraindications/Precautions

Contraindicated in: Hypersensitivity to elagolix, estradiol, or norethindrone; History of cigarette smoking and age >35 yr (↑ risk of cardiovascular or thromboembolic phenomenon); Thromboembolic disease (e.g., deep vein thrombosis [DVT], pulmonary embolism [PE], MI, stroke); Cerebrovascular disease, coronary artery disease, or peripheral vascular disease; Valvular heart disease or thrombogenic heart rhythms; Protein C, protein S, or antithrombin deficiency or other thrombophilic disorder; Headache with focal neurological symptoms or migraine headaches with aura in women >35 yr; Uncontrolled hypertension; Major surgery with extended periods of immobility; Osteoporosis (may ↑ risk of bone loss); Breast cancer or other hormone-sensitive malignancy; ↑ risk for hormone sensitive malignancy; Hepatic impairment; Undiagnosed abnormal uterine bleeding; Concurrent use of strong organic anion transporting polypeptide (OATP) 1B1 inhibitors; OB: Pregnancy.

Use Cautiously in: Aspirin hypersensitivity (contains tartrazine, which may cause allergic reaction); History of low-trauma fracture or other risk factors for osteoporosis; History of suicidal thoughts/behaviors or depression; Controlled hypertension; Diabetes; Hypertriglyceridemia (↑ risk of pancreatitis); Lactation: Use while breastfeeding only if potential maternal benefit justifies potential risk to infant; Rep: Women of reproductive potential; Pedi: Safety and effectiveness not established in children.

Adverse Reactions/Side Effects

CV: ↑ BP, DVT, MI. **Derm:** alopecia. **Endo:** hot flush, hyperglycemia. **GI:** ↑ liver enzymes, cholelithiasis, vomiting. **GU:** ↓ libido, metrorrhagia. **Metab:** ↑ weight, hyperlipidemia. **MS:** ↓ bone density, arthralgia. **Neuro:** depression, headache, mood swings, STROKE, SUICIDAL THOUGHTS/BEHAVIOR. **Resp:** PE. **Misc:** fatigue, MALIGNANCY (BREAST, ENDOMETRIAL, OVARIAN).

Interactions

Drug-Drug: Strong OATP1B1 inhibitors, including **rifampin** may significantly ↑ elagolix levels and risk of toxicity; concurrent use contraindicated. **Corticosteroids, anticonvulsants,** and **proton pump inhibitors** may ↑ risk for bone loss. Elagolix may ↓ levels of **CYP3A substrates,** including **midazolam**; consider ↑ midazolam dose. Elagolix may ↑ levels of **CYP2C19 substrates,** including **omeprazole**; consider ↓ omeprazole dose when using higher doses (>40 mg/day). Elagolix may ↑ levels of **P-glycoprotein substrates,** including **digoxin**; closely monitor digoxin levels. May ↓ **rosuvastatin** levels; consider ↑ rosuvastatin dose. **Strong CYP3A inhibitors** may ↑ elagolix, estradiol, and norethindrone levels and risk of toxicity; concurrent use not recommended. **Strong CYP3A inducers** may ↓ elagolix, estradiol, and norethindrone levels and effectiveness.

Route/Dosage

PO (Adults): One capsule (elagolix 300 mg/estradiol 1 mg/norethindrone 0.5 mg) every AM and elagolix 300 mg every PM. Continue for no longer than 24 mo.

Availability

Capsules: elagolix 300 mg/estradiol 1 mg/norethindrone 0.5 mg (AM); elagolix 300 mg (PM).

NURSING IMPLICATIONS

Assessment

- Monitor amount of menstrual bleeding during therapy.
- Monitor for signs and symptoms of thromboembolic disorders and vascular events (pain, swelling, tenderness in extremities; headache; chest pain; blurred vision; sudden unexplained partial or complete loss of vision; proptosis; diplopia; papilledema retinal vascular lesions) during therapy. Discontinue therapy if symptoms occur or are suspected. Evaluate for retinal vein thrombosis if visual changes occur.
- Assess bone mineral density by dual-energy x-ray absorptiometry (DXA) at baseline and periodically during therapy. Consider discontinuing therapy if risk associated with bone loss exceeds potential benefit of treatment. Consider calcium and vitamin D supplementation for patients with inadequate dietary intake.
- Assess for new or worsening depression, anxiety, or other mood changes periodically during therapy. Consider referral to mental health professional. Re-

evaluate benefits and risks of therapy if such events occur.

● Monitor BP prior to and periodically during therapy. Hold therapy for significant increases in BP.

Lab Test Considerations

● Verify negative pregnancy test within 7 days from onset of menses.

● May cause ↑ AST and ALT.

● May decrease glucose tolerance and ↑ blood glucose levels. Monitor blood glucose more frequently in women with prediabetes and diabetes.

● Monitor lipid levels periodically during therapy. May cause ↑ total cholesterol, low-density lipoprotein cholesterol, high-density lipoprotein cholesterol, and serum triglycerides.

Implementation

● **PO:** Administer morning and evening doses at same times each day without regard to food.

Patient/Family Teaching

● Instruct patient to take medication as directed at the same times each day. Take missed doses within 4 hr of time it was supposed to be taken and take next dose at usual time. If more than 4 hr since capsule is usually taken, omit dose and take next dose at usual time. Take only one morning and one evening capsule each day. Advise patient to read *Medication Guide* before starting therapy and with each Rx refill in case of changes.

● Advise patient to stop taking medication and notify health care professional immediately if signs and symptoms of cardiovascular conditions (leg pain or swelling that will not go away; sudden shortness of breath; double vision; bulging of the eyes; sudden blindness, partial or complete; pain or pressure in chest, arm, or jaw; sudden, severe headache unlike usual headaches; weakness or numbness in an arm or leg; trouble speaking) occur.

● Inform patient of risk of bone loss. Advise patient to take supplementary calcium and vitamin D and to avoid taking iron supplements at same time.

● Instruct patient to pay attention to changes in mood, behaviors, thoughts, or feelings. Advise patients to notify health care professional immediately if signs and symptoms of suicidal ideation and behavior (thoughts about suicide or dying, attempts to commit suicide, new or worse depression, new or worse anxiety, other unusual changes in behavior or mood) occur.

● Advise patient to notify health care professional if signs and symptoms of liver injury (jaundice, dark amber-colored urine, feeling tired, nausea and vomiting, generalized swelling, right upper stomach area pain, bruising easily) occur.

● Advise patient that alopecia, hair loss, and hair thinning in no specific pattern, may occur and may not completely resolve after discontinuing therapy. Advise patient to consult health care professional with concerns about changes to hair.

● Instruct patient to notify health care professional of all Rx or OTC medications, vitamins, or herbal products being taken and to avoid concurrent use of Rx, OTC, and herbal products without consulting health care professional.

● Dispose unused medication via a take-back option if available. Otherwise, follow FDA instructions for disposing medication in the household trash: www.fda.gov/drugdisposal. Do NOT flush down the toilet.

● Rep: Inform patient that *Oriahnn* may decrease menstrual bleeding or result in no menstrual bleeding, making it hard to know if you are pregnant; watch for other signs of pregnancy (breast tenderness, weight gain, nausea). May result in pregnancy loss if used in early pregnancy. Advise females of reproductive potential to use effective nonhormonal contraception during and for 1 wk after last dose. Hormonal contraceptives may decrease effectiveness of elagolix and may increase risk of thromboembolic and vascular disorders. Advise patient to notify health care professional if pregnancy is planned or suspected, or if breastfeeding. Encourage patients who become pregnant during therapy to enroll in pregnancy exposure registry to monitor pregnancy outcomes by calling 1-833-782-7241.

Evaluation/Desired Outcomes

● Reduced menstrual blood loss.

⚕ elexacaftor/tezacaftor/ivacaftor
(e-lex-a-**kaf**-tor/tez-a-**kaf**-tor/**eye**-va-**kaf**-tor)
Trikafta
Classification
Therapeutic: cystic fibrosis therapy adjuncts
Pharmacologic: transmembrane conductance regulator potentiators

Indications

⚕ Cystic fibrosis (CF) in patients who have ≥1 *F508del* mutation in the cystic fibrosis transmembrane conductance regulator *(CFTR)* gene or a mutation in the *CFTR* gene that is responsive based on *in vitro* data.

Action

Elexacaftor and tezacaftor: facilitate the cellular processing and trafficking of *F508del*-CFTR to increase the amount of mature CFTR protein delivered to the cell surface. *Ivacaftor:* acts as a potentiator of the CFTR protein (a chloride channel on the surface of endothelial cells) facilitating chloride transport by increasing the channel-open probability (gating). **Therapeutic Effects:** Improved lung function.

Pharmacokinetics
Elexacaftor

Absorption: Well absorbed (88%) following oral administration; absorption is enhanced 2-fold by moderate-fat-containing foods.

Distribution: Well distributed to tissues.
Protein Binding: >99%.
Metabolism and Excretion: Primarily metabolized in liver via the CYP3A4 and CYP3A5 isoenzymes; one metabolite (M23) is pharmacologically active; 87% excreted in feces (primarily as metabolite); <1% excreted in urine.
Half-life: 30 hr.

Tezacaftor
Absorption: Some absorption following oral administration.
Distribution: Widely distributed to tissues.
Protein Binding: >99%.
Metabolism and Excretion: Primarily metabolized in liver via the CYP3A4 and CYP3A5 isoenzymes; one metabolite (M1) is pharmacologically active; 72% excreted in feces as unchanged drug or metabolite; 14% excreted in urine (primarily as metabolite).
Half-life: 15 hr.

Ivacaftor
Absorption: Some absorption following oral administration; absorption is enhanced 3-fold by fat-containing foods.
Distribution: Widely distributed to tissues.
Protein Binding: >99%.
Metabolism and Excretion: Primarily metabolized in liver via the CYP3A4 and CYP3A5 isoenzymes; one metabolite (M1) is pharmacologically active; 87.8% eliminated in feces; negligible urinary elimination.
Half-life: 14 hr.

TIME/ACTION PROFILE (plasma concentrations)

ROUTE	ONSET	PEAK	DURATION
Elexacaftor (PO)	unknown	6 hr	24 hr
Tezacaftor (PO)	unknown	4 hr	12 hr
Ivacaftor (PO)	unknown	6 hr	12 hr

Contraindications/Precautions
Contraindicated in: Concurrent use of strong CYP3A inducers; Severe hepatic impairment.
Use Cautiously in: Moderate hepatic impairment (not recommended; if necessary, use only if benefit outweighs risk; dose ↓ recommended); Severe renal impairment (CCr <30 mL/min) or end-stage renal disease; OB: Safety not established in pregnancy; Lactation: Safety not established in breastfeeding; Pedi: Children <6 yr (safety and effectiveness not established).

Adverse Reactions/Side Effects
Derm: rash. **EENT:** nasal congestion, cataracts, rhinitis, rhinorrhea, sinusitis. **GI:** ↑ liver enzymes, abdominal pain, diarrhea, HEPATOTOXICITY, hyperbilirubinemia. **MS:** ↑ creatine kinase. **Neuro:** headache. **Resp:** upper respiratory tract infection. **Misc:** HYPERSENSITIVITY REACTIONS (including anaphylaxis), influenza.

Interactions
Drug-Drug: Strong CYP3A inducers, including **carbamazepine, phenobarbital, phenytoin, rifabutin,** and **rifampin,** may ↓ elexacaftor, tezacaftor, and ivacaftor levels and effectiveness; avoid concurrent use. Strong CYP3A inhibitors, including **clarithromycin, itraconazole, ketoconazole, posaconazole,** and **voriconazole** as well as **moderate CYP3A inhibitors,** including **erythromycin** and **fluconazole** may ↑ elexacaftor, tezacaftor, and ivacaftor levels and risk of toxicity; dose adjustment recommended. May ↑ levels and risk of bleeding with **warfarin**; monitor INR closely. May ↑ levels and risk of hypoglycemia with **glimepiride** or **glipizide**. May ↑ levels of **P-glycoprotein substrates,** including **cyclosporine, digoxin, everolimus, sirolimus,** and **tacrolimus**. May ↑ levels of **glyburide, nateglinide, repaglinide,** and **statins**. Hormonal contraceptives may ↑ risk of rash.
Drug-Natural Products: St. John's wort may ↓ elexacaftor, tezacaftor, and ivacaftor levels and effectiveness; avoid concurrent use.
Drug-Food: Grapefruit juice may ↑ elexacaftor, tezacaftor, and ivacaftor levels; avoid concurrent use.

Route/Dosage
PO (Adults and Children ≥12 yr): Two elexacaftor 100-mg/tezacaftor 50-mg/ivacaftor 75-mg tablets in AM and one ivacaftor 150-mg tablet in PM (approximately 12 hr apart) with fat-containing food. *Concurrent use of strong CYP3A inhibitor:* Two elexacaftor 100-mg/tezacaftor 50-mg/ivacaftor 75-mg tablets given twice weekly (3–4 days apart) in AM. Do not give PM ivacaftor dose on any of the days. *Concurrent use of moderate CYP3A inhibitor:* Two elexacaftor 100-mg/tezacaftor 50-mg/ivacaftor 75-mg tablets in AM on Day 1, then one ivacaftor 150-mg tablet in AM on Day 2; continue this regimen on alternate days in AM. Do not give PM ivacaftor dose on any of the days.
PO (Children 6–11 yr and ≥30 kg): Two elexacaftor 100-mg/tezacaftor 50-mg/ivacaftor 75-mg tablets in AM and one ivacaftor 150-mg tablet in PM (approximately 12 hr apart) with fat-containing food. *Concurrent use of strong CYP3A inhibitor:* Two elexacaftor 100-mg/tezacaftor 50-mg/ivacaftor 75-mg tablets given twice weekly (3–4 days apart) in AM. Do not give PM ivacaftor dose on any of the days. *Concurrent use of moderate CYP3A inhibitor:* Two elexacaftor 100-mg/tezacaftor 50-mg/ivacaftor 75-mg tablets in AM on Day 1, then one ivacaftor 150-mg tablet in AM on Day 2; continue this regimen on alternate days in AM. Do not give PM ivacaftor dose on any of the days.
PO (Children 6–11 yr and <30 kg): Two elexacaftor 50-mg/tezacaftor 25-mg/ivacaftor 37.5-mg tablets in AM and one ivacaftor 75-mg tablet in PM (approximately 12 hr apart) with fat-containing food. *Concurrent use of*

strong CYP3A inhibitor: Two elexacaftor 50-mg/teza-caftor 25-mg/ivacaftor 37.5-mg tablets given twice weekly (3–4 days apart) in AM. Do not give PM ivacaftor dose on any of the days. *Concurrent use of moderate CYP3A inhibitor:* Two elexacaftor 50-mg/tezacaftor 25-mg/ivacaftor 37.5-mg tablets in AM on Day 1, then one ivacaftor 75-mg tablet in AM on Day 2; continue this regimen on alternate days in AM. Do not give PM ivacaftor dose on any of the days.

PO (Children 2–5 yr and ≥14 kg): One packet (containing elexacaftor 100 mg/tezacaftor 50 mg/ivacaftor 75 mg oral granules) in AM and one packet (containing ivacaftor 75-mg oral granules) in PM (approximately 12 hr apart) with fat-containing food. *Concurrent use of strong CYP3A inhibitor:* One packet (containing elexacaftor 100 mg/tezacaftor 50 mg/ivacaftor 75 mg oral granules) twice weekly (given 3–4 days apart). Do not give PM ivacaftor dose on any of the days. *Concurrent use of moderate CYP3A inhibitor:* One packet (containing elexacaftor 100 mg/tezacaftor 50 mg/ivacaftor 75 mg oral granules) in AM on Day 1, then one packet (containing ivacaftor 75-mg oral granules) in AM on Day 2; continue this regimen on alternate days in AM. Do not give PM ivacaftor dose on any of the days.

PO (Children 2–5 yr and <14 kg): One packet (containing elexacaftor 80 mg/tezacaftor 40 mg/ivacaftor 60 mg oral granules) in AM and one packet (containing ivacaftor 59.5-mg oral granules) in PM (approximately 12 hr apart) with fat-containing food. *Concurrent use of strong CYP3A inhibitor:* One packet (containing elexacaftor 80 mg/tezacaftor 40 mg/ivacaftor 60 mg oral granules) twice weekly (given 3–4 days apart). Do not give PM ivacaftor dose on any of the days. *Concurrent use of moderate CYP3A inhibitor:* One packet (containing elexacaftor 80 mg/tezacaftor 40 mg/ivacaftor 60 mg oral granules) in AM on Day 1, then one packet (containing ivacaftor 59.5-mg oral granules) in AM on Day 2; continue this regimen on alternate days in AM. Do not give PM ivacaftor dose on any of the days.

Hepatic Impairment
(Adults and Children ≥12 yr): *Moderate hepatic impairment:* Two elexacaftor 100-mg/tezacaftor 50-mg/ivacaftor 75-mg tablets in AM on Day 1, then one elexacaftor 100-mg/tezacaftor 50-mg/ivacaftor 75-mg tablet in AM on Day 2. Continue this regimen on alternate days in AM. Do not give ivacaftor 150-mg tablet in PM on any day.

Hepatic Impairment
(Adults and Children 6–11 yr and ≥30 kg): *Moderate hepatic impairment:* Two elexacaftor 100-mg/tezacaftor 50-mg/ivacaftor 75-mg tablets in AM on Day 1, then one elexacaftor 100-mg/tezacaftor 50-mg/ivacaftor 75-mg tablet in AM on Day 2. Continue this regimen on alternate days in AM. Do not give ivacaftor 150-mg tablet in PM on any day.

Hepatic Impairment
(Adults and Children 6–11 yr and <30 kg): *Moderate hepatic impairment:* Two elexacaftor 50-mg/tezacaftor 25-mg/ivacaftor 37.5-mg tablets in AM on Day 1,

then one elexacaftor 50-mg/tezacaftor 25-mg/ivacaftor 37.5-mg tablet in AM on Day 2. Continue this regimen on alternate days in AM. Do not give ivacaftor 75-mg tablet in PM on any day.

Hepatic Impairment
(Adults and Children 2–5 yr and ≥14 kg): *Moderate hepatic impairment:* One packet (containing elexacaftor 100 mg/tezacaftor 50 mg/ivacaftor 75 mg oral granules) in AM on Days 1–3. No dose on Day 4. One packet (containing elexacaftor 100 mg/tezacaftor 50 mg/ivacaftor 75 mg oral granules) in AM on Days 5 and 6. No dose on Day 7. Continue this weekly dosing schedule in AM. Do not give PM ivacaftor dose on any day of weekly dosing schedule.

Hepatic Impairment
(Adults and Children 2–5 yr and <14 kg): *Moderate hepatic impairment:* One packet (containing elexacaftor 80 mg/tezacaftor 40 mg/ivacaftor 60 mg oral granules) in AM on Days 1–3. No dose on Day 4. One packet (containing elexacaftor 80 mg/tezacaftor 40 mg/ivacaftor 60 mg oral granules) in AM on Days 5 and 6. No dose on Day 7. Continue this weekly dosing schedule in AM. Do not give PM ivacaftor dose on any day of weekly dosing schedule.

Availability
Tablets: elexacaftor 50 mg/tezacaftor 25 mg/ivacaftor 37.5 mg (combo) + ivacaftor 75 mg (separate tablets), elexacaftor 100 mg/tezacaftor 50 mg/ivacaftor 75 mg (combo) + ivacaftor 150 mg (separate tablets). **Oral granules:** elexacaftor 80 mg/tezacaftor 40 mg/ivacaftor 60 mg (combo) + ivacaftor 59.5 mg (separate oral granules), elexacaftor 100 mg/tezacaftor 50 mg/ivacaftor 75 mg (combo) + ivacaftor 75 mg (separate oral granules).

NURSING IMPLICATIONS
Assessment
- Monitor lung function (FEV, lung sounds) before and periodically during therapy.
- Assess eyes for cataracts/opacities prior to and periodically during therapy.
- Monitor for signs of hypersensitivity reactions (angioedema, anaphylaxis) during therapy. Discontinue therapy if signs occur.

Lab Test Considerations
- ▓ Determine patient's genotype prior to starting therapy. If genotype is unknown, use an FDA-cleared CF mutation test to detect the presence of a CFTR mutation followed by verification with bidirectional sequencing when recommended by the mutation test instructions for use.
- Monitor liver function (AST, ALT, bilirubin) prior to starting therapy, every 3 mo during 1st year, and yearly thereafter. May cause ↑ serum transaminases and bilirubin. Monitor AST and ALT before, every 3 mo for the first year, and annually thereafter. If AST

or ALT >3 × upper limit of normal (ULN) with bilirubin >2 × ULN, interrupt therapy. Once AST or ALT have returned to normal, consider benefits and risks before resuming therapy.

Implementation

● **PO:** Administer tablets twice daily, 12 hr apart, with fat-containing food (meals or snacks that contain fat are those prepared with butter or oils or those containing eggs, cheeses, nuts, whole milk, or meats). *DNC:* Swallow tablets whole; do not crush, break or chew.

● Administer oral granules immediately before or after ingestion of fat-containing food. Mix entire contents of each packet of oral granules with one teaspoon (5 mL) of age-appropriate soft food or liquid (pureed fruits or vegetables, yogurt, applesauce, water, milk, juice) that is at or below room temperature. Once mixed, consume product completely within one hour.

Patient/Family Teaching

● Instruct patient to take as directed with a fat-containing meal to increase absorption. Fat-containing foods include eggs, butter, peanut better, cheese pizza. Take missed doses within 6 hr of missed dose. If >6 hr since missed morning dose, take missed dose as soon as possible and omit the evening dose. Take next scheduled morning dose at usual time. If missed evening dose, omit the missed dose. Take next scheduled morning dose at usual time. Do not take morning and evening doses at same time. Advise patient to read *Patient Information* before starting therapy and with each Rx refill in case of changes.

● Advise patient to avoid eating grapefruit or drinking grapefruit juice during therapy.

● May cause dizziness. Advise patient to avoid driving and other activities requiring alertness until response to medication is known.

● Advise patient to notify health care professional immediately if symptoms of liver problems (pain or discomfort in right abdominal area, yellowing of skin or whites of eyes, loss of appetite, nausea, vomiting, dark amber-colored urine) occur.

● Instruct patient to notify health care professional of all Rx or OTC medications, vitamins, or herbal products being taken and to consult with health care professional before taking other medications, especially St. John's wort.

● Rep: Advise females of reproductive potential to notify health care professional if pregnancy is planned or suspected or if breastfeeding.

● Emphasize the importance of blood tests to monitor liver function and eye examinations.

Evaluation/Desired Outcomes

● Improved lung function.

elvitegravir/cobicistat/ emtricitabine/tenofovir alafenamide

(el-vi-**teg**-ra-vir/koe-**bik**-i-stat/em-trye-**sye**-ta-been/ten-**of**-oh-vir al-a-**fen**-a-mide)

Genvoya

Classification

Therapeutic: antiretrovirals

Pharmacologic: integrase strand transfer inhibitors (INSTI), enzyme inhibitors, nucleoside reverse transcriptase inhibitors

Indications

HIV infection in treatment-naive adults. HIV infection in patients with HIV-1 RNA <50 copies/mL (to replace their current antiretroviral regimen) who are on a stable antiretroviral regimen for ≥6 mo, have no history of treatment failure, and have no known substitutions associated with resistance to the individual medications in the combination product.

Action

Elvitegravir: An integrase strand transfer inhibitor that inhibits an enzyme necessary for viral replication. *Cobicistat:* A pharmacokinetic enhancer (inhibits the CYP3A and CYP2D6 isoenzymes) that increases systemic exposure to elvitegravir. *Emtricitabine:* Phosphorylated intracellularly where it inhibits HIV reverse transcriptase, resulting in viral DNA chain termination. *Tenofovir alafenamide:* Phosphorylated intracellularly where it inhibits HIV reverse transcriptase resulting in disruption of DNA synthesis. When compared to tenofovir disoproxil fumarate, tenofovir alafenamide is associated with fewer episodes of renal impairment and reductions in bone mineral density. **Therapeutic Effects:** Slowed progression of HIV infection and decreased occurrence of sequelae.

Pharmacokinetics

Elvitegravir

Absorption: Absorption follows oral administration.

Distribution: Unknown.

Protein Binding: 98–99%.

Metabolism and Excretion: Metabolized by the liver via the CYP3A isoenzyme; 94.5% eliminated in feces, 6.7% in urine.

Half-life: 12.9 hr.

Cobicistat

Absorption: Absorption follows oral administration.

Distribution: Unknown.

Protein Binding: 97–98%.

Metabolism and Excretion: Metabolized by the liver via the CYP3A isoenzyme and to a lesser extent by the CYP2D6 isoenzyme; 86.2% eliminated in feces, 8.2% in urine.

Half-life: 3.5 hr.
Emtricitabine
Absorption: Rapidly and extensively absorbed; 93% bioavailable.
Distribution: Unknown.
Metabolism and Excretion: Some metabolism; 86% eliminated in urine, 14% in feces.
Half-life: 10 hr.
Tenofovir Alafenamide
Absorption: Tenofovir alafenamide is a prodrug, which is hydrolyzed into tenofovir, the active component; absorption enhanced by high-fat meals.
Distribution: Unknown.
Metabolism and Excretion: Tenofovir is phosphorylated to tenofovir diphosphate (active metabolite); 32% excreted in feces, <1% in urine.
Half-life: 0.51 hr.

TIME/ACTION PROFILE (plasma concentrations)

ROUTE	ONSET	PEAK	DURATION
Elvitegravir PO	unknown	4 hr	24 hr
Cobicistat PO	unknown	3 hr	24 hr
Emtricitabine PO	rapid	1–2 hr	24 hr
Tenofovir alafenamide PO	unknown	0.5 hr	24 hr

Contraindications/Precautions

Contraindicated in: Severe hepatic impairment; Concurrent use of alfuzosin, carbamazepine, ergot derivatives, lomitapide, lovastatin, lurasidone, phenobarbital, phenytoin, pimozide, rifampin, sildenafil (Revatio), simvastatin, triazolam, or St. John's wort; Severe renal impairment or end-stage renal disease not receiving hemodialysis; Severe hepatic impairment; OB: Not recommended in pregnancy (significantly lower concentrations of elvitegravir and cobicistat); Lactation: Breastfeeding not recommended in women with HIV.
Use Cautiously in: Female patients or obese patients (may be at ↑ risk for lactic acidosis/hepatic steatosis); Chronic hepatitis B virus (HBV) infection (may exacerbate following discontinuation); Concurrent use of nephrotoxic drugs (↑ risk of renal impairment); Pedi: Children <25 kg (safety and effectiveness not established); Geri: Older adults may be more sensitive to drug effects; consider age-related ↓ in renal, hepatic, and cardiovascular function, as well as concurrent disease states and medications.
Exercise Extreme Caution in: HBV (may cause severe acute exacerbation).

Adverse Reactions/Side Effects

Endo: Graves' disease. **F and E:** hypophosphatemia. **GI:** nausea, autoimmune hepatitis, diarrhea, LACTIC ACIDOSIS/HEPATOMEGALY WITH STEATOSIS, POST-TREATMENT ACUTE EXACERBATION OF HBV. **GU:** proteinuria, ACUTE RENAL FAILURE/FANCONI SYNDROME. **Metab:** hyperlipidemia.

MS: polymyositis. **Neuro:** Guillain-Barré syndrome, headache. **Misc:** fatigue, immune reconstitution syndrome.

Interactions

Drug-Drug: May significantly ↑ levels and risk of toxicity of **alfuzosin, dihydroergotamine, ergotamine, lomitapide, lovastatin, lurasidone, methylergonovine, pimozide, sildenafil** (when used for pulmonary hypertension), **simvastatin,** and **triazolam**; concurrent use contraindicated. **Carbamazepine, phenobarbital, phenytoin,** or **rifampin** may significantly ↓ levels/effectiveness of cobicistat and elvitegravir and ↑ risk of resistance; concurrent use contraindicated. Nephrotoxic agents, including **NSAIDs** and **aminoglycosides,** may ↑ risk of nephrotoxicity; avoid concurrent use. **Acyclovir, cidofovir, ganciclovir, valacyclovir,** and **valganciclovir** may ↓ renal elimination and ↑ levels/toxicity of emtricitabine and tenofovir alafenamide. May ↑ levels/toxicity of **amiodarone, digoxin, disopyramide, flecainide, lidocaine, mexiletine, propafenone** and **quinidine;** careful monitoring recommended. May alter effects of **warfarin;** careful monitoring of INR recommended. Concurrent use with **clarithromycin** may ↑ levels/toxicity of clarithromycin and/or cobicistat (for patients with CCr 50–60 mL/min, ↓ dose of clarithromycin by 50%). May ↑ levels/toxicity of **ethosuximide;** clinical monitoring recommended. **Oxcarbazepine** may ↓ levels/effectiveness of cobicistat, elvitegravir, and tenofovir alafenamide; consider using alternative anticonvulsant. May ↑ levels/toxicity of **SSRIs** (except sertraline), **tricyclic antidepressants,** and **trazodone;** careful titration and monitoring recommended. Concurrent use with **itraconazole, ketoconazole,** or **voriconazole** may ↑ levels/toxicity of itraconazole, ketoconazole, voriconazole, elvitegravir, and cobicistat (max dose of ketoconazole or itraconazole = 300 mg/day; assess risk vs. benefit before using voriconazole). May ↑ levels/toxicity of **colchicine;** concurrent use contraindicated in renal or hepatic impairment; *Dosing adjustment for gout flares:* 0.6 mg, then 0.3 mg 1 hr later, do not repeat for ≥3 days; *Dosing adjustment for gout flare prophylaxis:* 0.3 mg once daily if original regimen was 0.6 mg twice daily, 0.3 mg every other day if original regimen was 0.6 mg once daily; *Dosing adjustment for treatment of familial Mediterranean fever:* not to exceed 0.6 mg daily, may be given as 0.3 mg twice daily. **Rifabutin** or **rifapentine** may ↓ levels/effectiveness of cobicistat, elvitegravir, and tenofovir alafenamide and may foster resistance; concurrent use not recommended. May ↑ levels/toxicity of **beta blockers;** careful monitoring recommended; ↓ dose of beta blocker if necessary. May ↑ levels/toxicity of **calcium channel blockers** including **amlodipine, diltiazem, felodipine, nicardipine, nifedipine,** and **verapamil;** careful monitoring recommended. Concurrent use of corticosteroids that are CYP3A inducers, including **betamethasone, budesonide, ciclesonide, dexamethasone, fluticasone, methylprednisolone, mometasone, prednisone,** and **triamcinolone,** may

↓ levels/effectiveness and ↑ risk of resistance to elvitegravir; consider use of other corticosteroids, such as beclomethasone or prednisolone. Concurrent use of corticosteroids that are CYP3A substrates, including **betamethasone, budesonide, ciclesonide, dexamethasone, fluticasone, methylprednisolone, mometasone, prednisone,** and **triamcinolone,** may ↑ risk of Cushing's disease and adrenal suppression; consider use of other corticosteroids, such as beclomethasone or prednisolone. May ↑ levels/toxicity of **bosentan**; initiate bosentan at 62.5 mg once daily or every other day if already receiving elvitegravir/cobicistat/emtricitabine/tenofovir alafenamide for ≥10 days; if already receiving bosentan, discontinue bosentan ≥36 hr prior to starting elvitegravir/cobicistat/emtricitabine/tenofovir alafenamide; after 10 days, bosentan may be restarted at 62.5 mg once daily or every other day. May ↑ levels/toxicity of **atorvastatin**; initiate atorvastatin at lowest dose titrate cautiously; do not exceed dose of 20 mg/day. May ↑ levels/toxicity of **norgestimate** and ↓ levels of **ethinyl estradiol**; due to unpredictable effects, nonhormonal contraceptive methods should be considered. ↑ risk of hyperkalemia with contraceptives containing **drospirenone**; closely monitor serum potassium concentrations. May ↑ levels/toxicity of **immunosuppressants**, including **cyclosporine, sirolimus,** and **tacrolimus**; careful monitoring recommended. **Cyclosporine** may ↑ levels/toxicity of cobicistat and elvitegravir; careful monitoring recommended. May ↑ levels/toxicity of **buprenorphine** and ↓ levels of **naloxone**; carefully monitor for sedation and altered cognitive effects. May ↑ levels of **fentanyl**, and **tramadol**; monitor for respiratory depression; consider ↓ tramadol dose. May ↑ levels of and risk of adverse cardiovascular effects with **salmeterol**, concurrent use not recommended. ↑ levels/toxicity of **neuroleptics**, including **perphenazine, risperidone,** and **thioridazine**; may need to ↓ dose of neuroleptic. May ↑ levels of **quetiapine**; if taking quetiapine when initiating therapy, consider alternative antiretroviral therapy or ↓ quetiapine dose to ⅙ of the original dose and monitor for adverse effects. May ↑ levels/toxicity of **PDE5 inhibitors**, including **sildenafil, tadalafil,** and **vardenafil**; *Dosing adjustment for pulmonary hypertension:* sildenafil is contraindicated; in patients who have received elvitegravir/cobicistat/emtricitabine/tenofovir alafenamide for ≥7 days, start tadalafil at 20 mg once daily and carefully titrate if tolerating to 40 mg once daily; in patients already receiving tadalafil, discontinue tadalafil for ≥24 hr before initiating elvitegravir/cobicistat/emtricitabine/tenofovir alafenamide; after ≥1 wk, resume tadalafil at 20 mg once daily and titrate if tolerating to 40 mg once daily; *Dosing adjustment for erectile dysfunction:* sildenafil dose should not exceed 25 mg in 48 hr, vardenafil dose should not exceed 2.5 mg in 72 hr, and tadalafil dose should not exceed 10 mg in 72 hr. ↑ levels/toxicity of **sedative/hypnotics**, including **midazolam** (parenteral), **diazepam, buspirone,** and **zolpidem**; con-

sider dose ↓ of parenteral midazolam; clinical monitoring and dose ↓, if necessary, is recommended for other sedative/hypnotics. May ↑ bleeding risk with **rivaroxaban**; avoid concurrent use. May ↑ bleeding risk with **apixaban**; if taking apixaban 5–10 mg twice daily, ↓ apixaban dose by 50%; if taking apixaban 2.5 mg twice daily, avoid concurrent use. May ↑ bleeding risk with **dabigatran**; may need to avoid concurrent use if patient has moderate or severe renal impairment (depends on dabigatran indication). May ↑ bleeding risk with **edoxaban**; ↓ edoxaban dose by 50% when used for treatment of venous thromboembolism in patients with moderate or severe renal impairment. May ↑ bleeding risk with **ticagrelor**; concurrent use not recommended. May ↓ antiplatelet effects of **clopidogrel** and ↑ risk of thromboembolic events; concurrent use not recommended. Medications containing polyvalent cations, including **calcium, magnesium, aluminum, iron,** or **zinc,** may ↓ levels and effectiveness of elvitegravir; separate administration by ≥2 hr.

Drug-Natural Products: St. John's wort may significantly ↓ levels and effectiveness of cobicistat and elvitegravir and ↑ risk of resistance; concurrent use contraindicated.

Route/Dosage
PO (Adults and Children ≥25 kg): One tablet once daily.

Renal Impairment
PO (Adults): *CCr <15 mL/min AND receiving chronic hemodialysis:* One tablet once daily (give after dialysis on dialysis days).

Availability
Tablets: elvitegravir 150 mg/cobicistat 150 mg/emtricitabine 200 mg/tenofovir alafenamide 10 mg.

NURSING IMPLICATIONS
Assessment
● Assess patient for change in severity of HIV symptoms and for symptoms of opportunistic infections during therapy.

Lab Test Considerations
● Monitor viral load and CD4 count before and routinely during therapy to determine response.
● Assess for HBV. *Genvoya* is not approved for administration in patients with HIV and HBV. If therapy is discontinued, may cause severe exacerbation of hepatitis B. Monitor liver function in coinfected patients for several mo after stopping therapy.
● Monitor liver function tests prior to, during and following therapy. May cause ↑ LDL cholesterol, total cholesterol, and triglyceride concentrations. Lactic acidosis may occur with hepatic toxicity causing hepatic steatosis; may be fatal, especially in women. Discontinue therapy if symptoms occur.
● Calculate serum creatinine, CCr, urine glucose, and urine protein prior to and periodically during ther-

apy and when clinically indicated. In patients with chronic kidney disease, assess serum creatinine, CCr, serum phosphorus, urine glucose, and urine protein prior to and periodically during therapy. May cause hypophosphatemia in patients with renal impairment.
● May cause hyperglycemia and glycosuria.

Implementation
● Do not confuse elvitegravir, cobicistat, emtricitabine, and tenofovir alafenamide with elvitegravir, cobicistat, emtricitabine, and tenofovir disoproxil fumarate.
● PO: Administer once daily with food.
● Administer antacids at least 2 hr before or after medication.

Patient/Family Teaching
● Instruct patient on the importance of taking medication as directed, even if feeling better. Do not take more than prescribed amount and do not stop taking without consulting health care professional. Discontinuing therapy may lead to severe exacerbations. Take missed doses as soon as remembered unless almost time for next dose; do not double doses. Advise patient to read *Patient Information* prior to starting therapy and with each Rx refill in case of changes. Caution patient not to share or trade *Genvoya* with others.
● Inform patient of importance of HBV testing before starting antiretroviral therapy.
● Advise patient if antacids containing aluminum, magnesium hydroxide, or calcium carbonate, take at least 2 hr before or after *Genvoya*.
● Instruct patient to notify health care professional of all Rx or OTC medications, vitamins, or herbal products being taken and consult health care professional before taking any new medications, especially St. John's wort.
● Advise patient to notify health care professional immediately if symptoms of lactic acidosis (nausea, vomiting, unusual or unexpected stomach discomfort; unusual muscle pain; difficulty breathing; feeling cold, especially in arms and legs; dizziness; fast or irregular heartbeat; and weakness or tiredness) liver problems (yellow skin or whites of eyes, dark urine, light-colored stools, loss of appetite, nausea, stomach pain) or signs of immune reconstitution syndrome (signs and symptoms of an infection or inflammation, can occur many months after start of therapy) occur.
● Inform patient that *Genvoya* does not cure AIDS and may reduce the risk of transmission of HIV to others through sexual contact or blood contamination. Caution patient to use a condom and avoid sharing needles or donating blood to prevent spreading HIV to others.
● Rep: Advise patient to notify health care professional if pregnancy is planned or suspected. Monitor viral load closely during pregnancy. Encourage patients who become pregnant during therapy to join the Antiretroviral Pregnancy Registry that monitors pregnancy outcomes in women exposed to *Genvoya* during pregnancy. Enroll patient by calling

1-800-258-4263. Advise female patient to avoid breastfeeding during therapy.
● Emphasize the importance of regular follow-up exams and blood counts to determine progress and monitor for side effects.

Evaluation/Desired Outcomes
● Delayed progression of AIDS and decreased opportunistic infections in patients with HIV.
● Decrease in viral load and increase in CD4 cell counts.

BEERS

empagliflozin
(em-pa-gli-**floe**-zin)
Jardiance
Classification
Therapeutic: antidiabetics
Pharmacologic: sodium-glucose co-transporter 2 (SGLT2) inhibitors

Indications
Type 2 diabetes (as adjunct to diet and exercise). To reduce risk of cardiovascular death in patients with type 2 diabetes and established cardiovascular disease. To reduce the risk of cardiovascular death and hospitalization for HF in patients with HF.

Action
Inhibits proximal renal tubular sodium-glucose cotransporter 2 (SGLT2), which determines reabsorption of glucose from the tubular lumen. Inhibits reabsorption of glucose, lowers renal threshold for glucose, and increases excretion of glucose in urine. **Therapeutic Effects:** Improved glycemic control. Reduced death due to cardiovascular causes in patients with type 2 diabetes and cardiovascular disease. Reduced death due to cardiovascular causes and hospitalizations due to HF in patients with HF.

Pharmacokinetics
Absorption: Well absorbed following oral administration.
Distribution: Enters red blood cells, remainder of distribution unknown.
Metabolism and Excretion: Minimally metabolized; excreted in feces (41.2% mostly as unchanged drug) and urine (54.4% half as unchanged drug, half as metabolites).
Half-life: 12.4 hr.

TIME/ACTION PROFILE (↓ in A1c)

ROUTE	ONSET	PEAK	DURATION
PO	within 6 wk	12 wk	unknown

Contraindications/Precautions
Contraindicated in: Hypersensitivity; Severe renal impairment (eGFR <30 mL/min/1.73 m² [patients with type 2 diabetes] or eGFR <20 mL/min/1.73 m² [patients with heart failure]) or receiving dialysis; Type 1 diabetes; Diabetic ketoacidosis; Lactation: Lactation.

Use Cautiously in: eGFR <60 mL/min/1.73 m² or concurrent use of loop diuretics (↑ risk of volume depletion or hypotension); History of pancreatitis, pancreatic surgery, reduced caloric intake due to illness or surgery, surgical procedures, or alcohol abuse (↑ risk of ketoacidosis); OB: Use during pregnancy only if potential maternal benefit justifies potential fetal risk; Pedi: Children <10 yr (safety and effectiveness not established); Geri: Appears on Beers list. Older adults may have ↑ risk of urogenital infections (especially women in the 1st mo of treatment) and euglycemic diabetic ketoacidosis. Use with caution in older adults.

Adverse Reactions/Side Effects
CV: hypotension, volume depletion. **Endo:** hypoglycemia (↑ with other medications). **F and E:** hyperphosphatemia, KETOACIDOSIS. **GU:** ↑ urination, acute kidney injury, genital mycotic infections, NECROTIZING FASCIITIS OF PERINEUM (FOURNIER'S GANGRENE), renal impairment, urinary tract infection (including pyelonephritis), UROSEPSIS. **Metab:** hyperlipidemia. **Misc:** HYPERSENSITIVITY REACTIONS (including angioedema).

Interactions
Drug-Drug: ↑ risk of hypotension with **antihypertensives** or **diuretics**. ↑ risk of hypoglycemia with other **antidiabetics** (dose adjustments may be required). ↑ risk of acute kidney injury with **diuretics**, **ACE inhibitors**, **angiotensin receptor blockers**, or **NSAIDs**. May ↓ **lithium** levels and effectiveness.

Route/Dosage
Type 2 Diabetes
PO (Adults and Children ≥10 yr): 10 mg once daily, may ↑ to 25 mg once daily for additional glycemic control.

Type 2 Diabetes in Patients with Established Cardiovascular Disease
PO (Adults): 10 mg once daily, may ↑ to 25 mg once daily for additional glycemic control.

Heart Failure
PO (Adults): 10 mg once daily.

Availability (generic available)
Tablets: 10 mg, 25 mg. *In combination with:* linagliptin (Glyxambi); linagliptin and metformin XR (Trijardy XR); metformin (Synjardy); metformin XR (Synjardy XR). See Appendix N.

NURSING IMPLICATIONS
Assessment
- Observe patient for signs and symptoms of hypoglycemic reactions (sweating, hunger, weakness, dizziness, confusion, headache, tremor, tachycardia, irritability, drowsiness).
- Monitor for signs and symptoms of volume depletion (dizziness, feeling faint, weakness, orthostatic hypotension) after initiating therapy, especially in elderly

patients and patients with renal impairment, low systolic BP, or on diuretics.
- Monitor for signs and symptoms of urinary tract infection during therapy. Treat promptly.
- Monitor for infection (pain or burning on urination, frequency, new pain, tenderness, erythema, swelling, sores, or ulcers involving genital or perianal area, with fever or malaise; assess for necrotizing fasciitis. If suspected, start treatment immediately with broad-spectrum antibiotics and, if necessary, surgical debridement. Discontinue empagliflozin if these occur.
- Assess for ketoacidosis in patients presenting with signs and symptoms of dehydration and metabolic acidosis (nausea, vomiting, abdominal pain, malaise, shortness of breath), regardless of blood glucose level. Discontinue empagliflozin and treat promptly (insulin, fluid and caloric replacement) if suspected. Consider risk factors for ketoacidosis (pancreatic insulin deficiency, caloric restriction, alcohol abuse) before starting empagliflozin.

Lab Test Considerations
- Monitor A1C prior to and periodically during therapy.
- May ↑ serum creatinine and ↓ eGFR. Monitor renal function prior to starting and periodically during therapy. Do not begin therapy if eGFR <30 mL/min/1.73 m². Discontinue therapy if eGFR is persistently <30 mL/min/1.73 m².
- May cause ↑ serum phosphate levels. Monitor electrolytes periodically during therapy.
- May cause ↑ LDL-C. Monitor serum lipid levels periodically during therapy.
- May cause ↑ hematocrit.
- Monitor for ketoacidosis, especially during prolonged fasting for illness or surgery. May require temporary discontinuation of therapy.

Implementation
- Patients stabilized on a diabetic regimen who are exposed to stress, fever, trauma, infection, or surgery may require administration of insulin.
- Correct volume depletion before starting therapy with empagliflozin.
- **PO:** Administer once daily in the morning with or without food.

Patient/Family Teaching
- Instruct patient to take empagliflozin as directed. Take missed doses as soon as remembered, unless it is almost time for next dose; do not double doses. Advise patient to read the *Medication Guide* before starting and with each Rx refill in case of changes.
- Explain to patient that empagliflozin helps control hyperglycemia but does not cure diabetes. Therapy is usually long term.
- Instruct patient not to share this medication with others, even if they have the same symptoms; it may harm them.

- Encourage patient to follow prescribed diet, medication, and exercise regimen to prevent hyperglycemic or hypoglycemic episodes.
- Review signs of hypoglycemia and hyperglycemia with patient. If hypoglycemia occurs, advise patient to take a glass of orange juice or 2–3 tsp of sugar, honey, or corn syrup dissolved in water, and notify health care professional.
- Instruct patient in proper testing of serum glucose and ketones, especially during periods of stress or illness. Inform patient that empagliflozin will cause a positive test result when testing for urine glucose. Notify health care professional if significant changes occur.
- Advise patient to inform health care professional of therapy before surgery. Consider temporarily discontinuing empagliflozin for at least 3 days before surgery. Monitor for ketoacidosis during and after surgery. Advise patient discontinue empagliflozin and to notify health care professional immediately if signs and symptoms of ketoacidosis occur.
- Advise patient to notify health care professional immediately if new pain or tenderness, sores or ulcers, or infections involving the leg or foot occur and to immediately seek care if pain or tenderness, redness, or swelling of the genitals or area from the genitals back to the rectum, along with a fever above 100.4°F or malaise occur.
- Advise patient to notify health care professional if signs and symptoms of hypotension occur and to maintain adequate hydration as dehydration may increase risk of hypotension.
- Inform patient that empagliflozin may cause mycotic (yeast) infections. Women may have signs and symptoms of a vaginal yeast infection (vaginal odor, white or yellow vaginal discharge [may be lumpy or look like cottage cheese], vaginal itching). Men may have signs and symptoms of a yeast infection of the penis (redness, itching or swelling of penis; rash on penis; foul-smelling discharge from penis; pain in skin around penis). Advise patient to notify health care professional if yeast infection occurs.
- Advise patient to notify health care professional if signs and symptoms of urinary tract infection (burning feeling when passing urine, cloudy urine, pain in pelvis or back) occur.
- Advise patient to notify health care professional of all Rx or OTC medications, vitamins, or herbal products being taken and to consult with health care professional before taking other medications, especially other oral hypoglycemic medications.
- Advise patient to notify health care professional promptly if signs and symptoms of hypersensitivity reactions (rash; raised red patches on skin; swelling of face, lips, tongue, throat; difficulty breathing or swallowing) occur.
- Rep: Insulin is the recommended method of controlling blood sugar during pregnancy. Advise females of reproductive potential to notify health care profes-

sional if pregnancy is planned or suspected and to avoid breastfeeding during therapy.
- Emphasize importance of routine follow up with routine lab tests for blood glucose and renal function.

Evaluation/Desired Outcomes
- Improved A1C and glycemic control in adults and children >10 yrs with type 2 diabetes.
- Reduced risk of cardiovascular death in patients with type 2 diabetes and established cardiovascular disease.
- Reduced death due to cardiovascular causes and hospitalizations due to HF in patients with HF.

emtricitabine/rilpivirine/tenofovir alafenamide
(em-tri-**sye**-ti-been/**ril**-pi-vir-een/te-**noe**-fo-veer al-a-**fen**-a-mide)
Odefsey
Classification
Therapeutic: antiretrovirals
Pharmacologic: nucleoside reverse transcriptase inhibitors, non-nucleoside reverse transcriptase inhibitors

Indications
Management of HIV infection in treatment-naive patients with HIV-1 RNA <100,000 copies/mL at the start of therapy (for use as a complete regimen). Management of HIV infection in patients on a stable antiretroviral regimen with HIV-1 RNA <50 copies/mL for ≥6 mo and have no history of treatment failure or no known substitutions associated with resistance to the individual components of the medication (to replace their current antiretroviral regimen).

Action
Emtricitabine: Phosphorylated intracellularly where it inhibits HIV reverse transcriptase, resulting in viral DNA chain termination. *Rilpivirine:* Inhibits HIV-replication by noncompetitively inhibiting HIV reverse transcriptase. *Tenofovir:* Phosphorylated intracellularly where it inhibits HIV reverse transcriptase resulting in disruption of DNA synthesis. **Therapeutic Effects:** Slowed progression of HIV infection and decreased occurrence of sequelae.

Pharmacokinetics
Emtricitabine
Absorption: Rapidly and extensively absorbed; 93% bioavailable.
Distribution: Unknown.
Metabolism and Excretion: Some metabolism, 86% renally excreted, 14% fecal excretion.
Half-life: 10 hr.
Rilpivirine
Absorption: Well absorbed following oral administration.
Distribution: Unknown.

Protein Binding: 99.7%.
Metabolism and Excretion: Primarily metabolized by the liver via the CYP3A isoenzyme; 25% excreted in feces unchanged, <1% excreted unchanged in urine.
Half-life: 50 hr.

Tenofovir Alafenamide
Absorption: Tenofovir alafenamide is a prodrug, which is hydrolyzed into tenofovir, the active component; absorption enhanced by high-fat meals.
Distribution: Unknown.
Metabolism and Excretion: Tenofovir is phosphorylated to tenofovir diphosphate (active metabolite); 32% excreted in feces, <1% in urine.
Half-life: 0.51 hr.

TIME/ACTION PROFILE (plasma concentrations)

ROUTE	ONSET	PEAK	DURATION
Emtricitabine PO	rapid	1–2 hr	24 hr
Rilpivirine PO	unknown	4–5 hr	24 hr
Tenofovir PO	unknown	1 hr	24 hr

Contraindications/Precautions
Contraindicated in: Concurrent use of carbamazepine, oxcarbazepine, phenobarbital, phenytoin, rifampin, rifapentine, proton pump inhibitors, dexamethasone (>1 dose), or St. John's wort; Severe renal impairment or end-stage renal disease not receiving hemodialysis; Lactation: Breastfeeding is not recommended in women with HIV.
Use Cautiously in: History of suicidal ideation or depression; HIV-1 RNA >100,000 copies/mL (↑ risk of virologic failure); Hepatitis B virus (HBV) or hepatitis C infection or hepatic impairment; Renal impairment or receiving nephrotoxic medications (↑ risk of renal impairment); Severe hepatic impairment; OB: Monitor viral load closely when used during pregnancy; Pedi: Children <12 yr or <35 kg (safety and effectiveness not established).

Adverse Reactions/Side Effects
CV: QT interval prolongation. **Derm:** DRUG REACTION WITH EOSINOPHILIA AND SYSTEMIC SYMPTOMS (DRESS). **Endo:** Graves' disease. **GI:** ACUTE EXACERBATION OF HBV, autoimmune hepatitis, HEPATOTOXICITY, LACTIC ACIDOSIS/HEPATOMEGALY WITH STEATOSIS. **GU:** ACUTE RENAL FAILURE/FANCONI SYNDROME. **Metab:** hyperlipidemia. **MS:** polymyositis. **Neuro:** depression, Guillain-Barré syndrome, headache, sleep disturbances, SUICIDAL ATTEMPTS/THOUGHTS. **Misc:** immune reconstitution syndrome.

Interactions
Drug-Drug: Strong CYP3A4 inducers, including carbamazepine, oxcarbazepine, phenobarbital, phenytoin, dexamethasone (more than a single dose), rifampin, and rifapentine may ↓ rilpivirine levels and its effectiveness; concurrent use contraindicated. Proton pump inhibitors including esomeprazole, lansoprazole, omeprazole, pantoprazole, and rabeprazole ↑ gastric pH and may ↓ rilpivirine levels and its effectiveness; concurrent use contraindicated. Concurrent use of QT interval prolonging medications may ↑ risk of torsades de pointes. Medications that compete for active tubular secretion, including acyclovir, cidofovir, ganciclovir, valacyclovir, valganciclovir, or aminoglycosides may ↑ emtricitabine and tenofovir levels and toxicity; avoid if possible. Antacids including aluminum hydroxide, magnesium hydroxide, and calcium carbonate ↑ gastric pH and may ↓ rilpivirine levels; administer antacid ≥2 hr before or ≥4 hr after. H₂-antagonists, including cimetidine, famotidine, and nizatidine, ↑ gastric pH and may ↓ rilpivirine levels; administer H₂-antagonist ≥12 hr before or ≥4 hr after rilpivirine. Nephrotoxic agents, including NSAIDs, ↑ risk of nephrotoxicity; avoid concurrent use. Rifabutin may ↓ rilpivirine and tenofovir alafenamide levels and their effectiveness; concurrent use not recommended. Fluconazole, itraconazole, ketoconazole, posaconazole, and voriconazole may ↑ rilpivirine and tenofovir alafenamide levels and risk of toxicity. May ↓ ketoconazole levels. May alter requirements for methadone maintenance. Clarithromycin or erythromycin may ↑ rilpivirine levels and risk of toxicity; consider azithromycin as an alternative. Ledipasvir/sofosbuvir, sofosbuvir/velpatasvir, and sofosbuvir/velpatasvir/voxilaprevir may ↑ tenofovir levels and risk of toxicity.
Drug-Natural Products: St. John's wort may ↓ rilpivirine levels and its effectiveness; concurrent use contraindicated.

Route/Dosage
PO (Adults and Children ≥12 yr and ≥35 kg): 1 tablet once daily.

Renal Impairment
PO (Adults and Children ≥12 yr and ≥35 kg): *End-stage renal disease (CCr <15 mL/min) AND receiving hemodialysis:* 1 tablet once daily (to be given after hemodialysis).

Availability
Tablets: emtricitabine 200 mg/rilpivirine 25 mg/tenofovir alafenamide 25 mg.

NURSING IMPLICATIONS
Assessment
- Assess for change in severity of HIV symptoms and for symptoms of opportunistic infections during therapy.
- Monitor for signs and symptoms of DRESS (fever; rash with fever, blisters, mucosal involvement, eye inflammation [conjunctivitis]); lymphadenopathy, and/or facial swelling, associated with involvement of other organ systems (hepatitis, nephritis, hematologic abnormalities, myocarditis, myositis) during

therapy. May resemble an acute viral infection. Eosinophilia is often present. Discontinue therapy if signs occur.

- Assess mental status (orientation, mood, behavior) before and periodically during therapy. Monitor closely for notable changes in behavior that could indicate the emergence or worsening of suicidal thoughts or behavior or depression.

Lab Test Considerations
- Monitor viral load and CD4 cell count regularly during therapy.
- Assess for HBV. *Odefsey* is not approved for administration in patients with HIV and HBV. If therapy is discontinued, may cause severe exacerbation of hepatitis B. Monitor liver function in coinfected patients for several mo after stopping therapy.
- Monitor liver function tests before and periodically during therapy, especially in patients with underlying liver disease or marked ↑ transaminase. May cause ↑ serum creatinine, AST, ALT, total bilirubin, total cholesterol, low-density lipoprotein cholesterol, and triglycerides. May cause lactic acidosis and severe hepatomegaly with steatosis. These events are more likely to occur if patients are female, obese, or receiving nucleoside analogue medications for extended periods of time. Monitor patient for signs (increased serum lactate levels, elevated liver enzymes, liver enlargement on palpation). Therapy should be suspended if clinical or laboratory signs occur.
- Assess serum creatinine, creatinine clearance, urine glucose, and urine protein before starting and periodically during therapy. Also assess serum phosphorous in patients with chronic kidney disease. Patients taking nephrotoxic agents, including NSAIDs, are at increased risk for renal impairment.

Implementation
- **PO:** Administer once daily with a meal.

Patient/Family Teaching
- Instruct patient to take medication as directed. Avoid missing doses, may result in development of resistance. Do not stop taking *Odefsey* without consulting health care professional. Advise patient to read *Patient Information* before starting and with each Rx refill in case of changes.
- Instruct patient that *Odefsey* should not be shared with others.
- Inform patient that *Odefsey* does not cure AIDS and may reduce the risk of transmission of HIV to others through sexual contact or blood contamination. Caution patient to use a condom and avoid sharing needles or donating blood to prevent spreading HIV to others.
- Advise patient to notify health care professional immediately if symptoms of lactic acidosis (nausea, vomiting, unusual or unexpected stomach discomfort, and weakness), hypersensitivity (swelling of face, eyes, lips, mouth, tongue or throat; difficulty swallowing; shortness of breath), severe liver prob-

lems (yellow skin or white part of eyes, dark "tea-colored" urine, light-colored stools, loss of appetite, nausea, stomach-area pain), or DRESS occur.
- Inform patients and families of risk of suicidal thoughts and behavior and advise that behavioral changes, emergency or worsening signs and symptoms of depression, unusual changes in mood, or emergence of suicidal thoughts, behavior, or thoughts of self-harm should be reported to health care professional immediately.
- Immune reconstitution syndrome may trigger opportunistic infections or autoimmune disorders. Notify health care professional if symptoms (signs and symptoms of an infection or inflammation) occur.
- Advise patient to notify health care professional of all Rx or OTC medications, vitamins, or herbal products being taken and to consult with health care professional before taking other medications, especially St. John's wort.
- Rep: Advise patient to notify health care professional if pregnancy is planned or suspected. Advise patient to avoid breastfeeding during *Odefsey* therapy. Monitor viral load closely during pregnancy. Encourage women who become pregnant during *Odefsey* therapy to join the Antiviral Pregnancy Registry that monitors pregnancy outcomes in women exposed to *Odefsey* during pregnancy. Enroll patient by calling 1-800-258-4263.

Evaluation/Desired Outcomes
- Delayed progression of AIDS and decreased opportunistic infections in patients with HIV.
- Decrease in viral load and increase in CD4 cell counts.

emtricitabine/tenofovir disoproxil fumarate
(em-tri-**sye**-ti-been/te-**noe**-fo-veer dye-soe-**prox**-il **fue**-ma-rate)
  Truvada
Classification
Therapeutic: antiretrovirals
Pharmacologic: nucleoside reverse transcriptase inhibitors

Indications
HIV infection (in combination with other antiretroviral agents). Pre-exposure prophylaxis (PrEP) to reduce the risk of sexually acquired HIV-1 infection in at-risk individuals.

Action
Emtricitabine and tenofovir disoproxil fumarate: Phosphorylated intracellularly where it inhibits HIV reverse transcriptase, resulting in inhibition of viral replication. **Therapeutic Effects:** Slowed progression of HIV infection and decreased occurrence of sequelae. Reduction in risk of sexually acquired HIV infection in at-risk individuals.

Pharmacokinetics

Emtricitabine

Absorption: Rapidly and extensively absorbed (93% bioavailable).

Distribution: Unknown.

Metabolism and Excretion: Undergoes some metabolism with 86% renally excreted and 14% excreted in feces as metabolites.

Half-life: 10 hr.

Tenofovir Disoproxil Fumarate

Absorption: Tenofovir disoproxil fumarate is a prodrug and undergoes hydrolysis to be converted to tenofovir, the active component.

Distribution: Unknown.

Metabolism and Excretion: 70–80% excreted unchanged in urine by glomerular filtration and active tubular secretion.

Half-life: 17 hr.

TIME/ACTION PROFILE (plasma concentrations)

ROUTE	ONSET	PEAK	DURATION
Emtricitabine PO	rapid	1–2 hr	24 hr
Tenofovir PO	rapid	1–2 hr	24 hr

Contraindications/Precautions

Contraindicated in: Unknown or positive HIV status (for PrEP); Severe renal impairment (HIV treatment) (CCr <30 mL/min); Moderate or severe renal impairment (PrEP) (CCr <60 mL/min); Lactation: Breastfeeding should be avoided in mothers infected with HIV.

Use Cautiously in: Hepatitis B virus (HBV) (may lead to acute exacerbation of HBV upon discontinuation); Moderate renal impairment (CCr 30–49 mL/min) (adjust dosing interval); History of pathologic fractures/osteoporosis/bone loss; OB: Use during pregnancy only if potential maternal benefit justifies potential fetal risk (in women with HIV, monitor viral load closely); Pedi: Safety and effectiveness not established in children who weigh <17 kg (HIV treatment) or <35 kg (PrEP).

Adverse Reactions/Side Effects

Endo: Graves' disease. **F and E:** hypophosphatemia. **GI:** ↑ liver enzymes, abdominal pain, autoimmune hepatitis, LACTIC ACIDOSIS/HEPATOMEGALY WITH STEATOSIS, POST-TREATMENT ACUTE EXACERBATION OF HEPATITIS B. **GU:** ACUTE RENAL FAILURE/FANCONI SYNDROME, renal impairment. **Metab:** ↓ weight. **MS:** ↓ bone mineral density, bone pain, muscle pain, osteomalacia, polymyositis. **Neuro:** Guillain-Barré syndrome, headache. **Misc:** immune reconstitution syndrome.

Interactions

Drug-Drug: Nephrotoxic agents, including **NSAIDs**, ↑ risk of nephrotoxicity; avoid concurrent use. Other drugs eliminated by active tubular secretion, including **acyclovir, adefovir, aminoglycosides, cidofovir, ganciclovir, valacyclovir,** and **valganciclovir,** may ↑ levels. May ↓ **atazanavir** levels and effectiveness; administer atazanavir with ritonavir when used with emtricitabine/tenofovir disoproxil fumarate. **Lopinavir/ritonavir, atazanavir/ritonavir,** or **darunavir/ritonavir** may ↑ tenofovir levels and risk of toxicity; closely monitor. **Sofosbuvir/velpatasvir, sofosbuvir/velpatasvir/voxilaprevir,** or **ledipasvir/sofosbuvir** may ↑ tenofovir levels and risk of toxicity; closely monitor.

Route/Dosage

HIV-1 Infection

PO (Adults and Children ≥35 kg): One tablet (emtricitabine 200 mg/tenofovir disoproxil fumarate 300 mg) once daily.

PO (Children 28–<35 kg): One tablet (emtricitabine 167 mg/tenofovir disoproxil fumarate 250 mg) once daily.

PO (Children 22–<28 kg): One tablet (emtricitabine 133 mg/tenofovir disoproxil fumarate 200 mg) once daily.

PO (Children 17–<22 kg): One tablet (emtricitabine 100 mg/tenofovir disoproxil fumarate 150 mg) once daily.

Renal Impairment

PO (Adults ≥35 kg): *CCr 30–49 mL/min:* One tablet (emtricitabine 200 mg/tenofovir disoproxil fumarate 300 mg) every 48 hr. *CCr <30 mL/min (including hemodialysis):* Not recommended.

HIV-1 PrEP

PO (Adults and Children ≥35 kg): One tablet (emtricitabine 200 mg/tenofovir disoproxil fumarate 300 mg) once daily.

Availability (generic available)

Tablets: emtricitabine 100 mg/tenofovir disoproxil fumarate 150 mg, emtricitabine 133 mg/tenofovir disoproxil fumarate 200 mg, emtricitabine 167 mg/tenofovir disoproxil fumarate 250 mg, emtricitabine 200 mg/tenofovir disoproxil fumarate 300 mg.

NURSING IMPLICATIONS

Assessment

- Assess for change in severity of HIV symptoms and for symptoms of opportunistic infections during therapy.
- Monitor weight periodically during therapy; may require dose modification.
- Monitor bone mineral density in patients who have a history of pathologic bone fracture or are at risk for osteoporosis or bone loss. Calcium and vitamin D supplementation may be beneficial for all patients.

Lab Test Considerations

- Screen patients for HIV-1 infection immediately before starting therapy for *HIV-1 PrEP* and at least every 3 mo during therapy, and upon diagnosis of any sexually transmitted infections. If recent (<1 mo) exposures to HIV-1 are suspected (condomless sex or condom breaking during sex with a partner of unknown HIV-1 status, unknown viremic status, or a recent sexually transmitted infection) or clinical symptoms consistent with acute HIV-1 infection occur, use a test approved by the FDA as an aid in the diagnosis of acute or primary HIV-1 infection. If HIV-1 test indicates possible HIV-1 infection, or symptoms consistent with acute HIV-1 infection develop following a potential exposure event, convert *HIV-1 PrEP* regimen to HIV treatment regimen until negative infection status is confirmed. Monitor viral load and CD4 cell count regularly during therapy.

- Assess for HBV. *Truvada* is not approved for administration in patients with HIV and HBV. If therapy is discontinued, may cause severe exacerbation of hepatitis B. Monitor liver function in coinfected patients for several months after stopping therapy. May use anti-hepatitis therapy. Offer vaccination to patients uninfected with HIV.
- Monitor liver function tests before and periodically during therapy, especially in patients with underlying liver disease or marked ↑ transaminase. May cause ↑ serum creatinine, AST, ALT, total bilirubin, total cholesterol, low-density lipoprotein cholesterol, and triglycerides. May cause lactic acidosis and severe hepatomegaly with steatosis. These events are more likely to occur if patients are female, obese, or receiving nucleoside analogue medications for extended periods of time. Monitor patient for signs (increased serum lactate levels, elevated liver enzymes, liver enlargement on palpation). Therapy should be suspended if clinical or laboratory signs occur.
- Monitor CCr, serum creatinine, urine glucose, and urine protein prior to therapy. CCr should be >70 mL/min before starting therapy. Monitor CCr, urine glucose, and urine protein in all patients periodically during therapy and serum phosphorous in patients with chronic kidney disease. Assess patients with persistent or worsening bone pain, pain in extremities, fractures and/or muscular pain, or weakness for proximal renal tubulopathy; evaluate renal function promptly.

Implementation
- **PO:** Administer once daily without regard to food.

Patient/Family Teaching
- Emphasize the importance of taking *Truvada* as directed. Do not take more than prescribed amount and do not stop taking without consulting health care professional. Uninfected individuals who miss doses are at greater risk of acquiring HIV-1. Advise patient to read *Medication Guide* prior to starting therapy and with each Rx refill in case of changes.
- Advise patients taking *Truvada* for *HIV-1 PrEP* to only take *Truvada* if confirmed HIV-1 negative. Some HIV-1 tests can miss HIV-1 infection in patients recently infected. Notify health care professional if flu-like symptoms (tiredness, fever, joint or muscle aches, headache, sore throat, vomiting or diarrhea,

rash, night sweats, enlarged lymph nodes in the neck or groin) occur. Advise patient to use condoms consistently and correctly to lower chances of sexual contact with any body fluids (semen, vaginal secretions, blood), the importance of knowing their HIV-1 status and the HIV-1 status of their partner(s), the need to get tested at least every 3 mo or more frequently for HIV-1 and other sexually transmitted infections (syphilis, chlamydia, gonorrhea), and to ask their partner to get tested. Advise patient if they become HIV-1 positive, more antiretroviral medication than *Truvada* is needed to treat HIV-1.

- Advise patients taking *Truvada* to *treat HIV-1 infection* that *Truvada* alone is not a complete treatment for HIV-1; other antiretroviral medications are required.
- Instruct patient that *Truvada* should not be shared with others.
- Inform patient that *Truvada* does not cure AIDS or prevent other sexually transmitted infections, associated or opportunistic infections. *Truvada* may reduce the risk of transmission of HIV to others through sexual contact or blood contamination. Caution patient to use a condom and to avoid sharing needles or donating blood to prevent spreading HIV to others.
- Advise patient to notify health care professional immediately if signs and symptoms of lactic acidosis (nausea, vomiting, unusual or unexpected stomach discomfort, and weakness) or severe liver problems (yellow skin or white part of eyes, dark "tea-colored" urine, light-colored stools, loss of appetite, nausea, stomach-area pain) occur.
- Immune reconstitution syndrome may trigger opportunistic infections or autoimmune disorders (Graves' disease, polymyositis, Guillain-Barré syndrome, autoimmune hepatitis). Notify health care professional if symptoms (signs and symptoms of an infection or inflammation) occur.
- Advise patient to notify health care professional of all Rx or OTC medications, vitamins, or herbal products being taken and to consult with health care professional before taking other medications.
- Rep: Advise patient to notify health care professional if pregnancy is planned or suspected. Advise patient to avoid breastfeeding during *Truvada* therapy. Encourage women who become pregnant during *Truvada* therapy to join the Antiretroviral Pregnancy Registry that monitors pregnancy outcomes in women exposed to *Truvada* during pregnancy. Enroll patient by calling 1-800-258-4263.
- Emphasize the importance of regular follow-up exams and blood counts to determine progress and monitor for side effects.

Evaluation/Desired Outcomes
- Delayed progression of AIDS and decreased opportunistic infections in patients with HIV.
- Decrease in viral load and increase in CD4 cell counts.

- Reduced risk of sexually acquired HIV-1 infection in at-risk individuals.

enalapril/enalaprilat, See ANGIOTENSIN-CONVERTING ENZYME (ACE) INHIBITORS.

Ⅹ encorafenib (en-koe-raf-e-nib)
Braftovi
Classification
Therapeutic: antineoplastics
Pharmacologic: kinase inhibitors

Indications
Ⅹ Metastatic or unresectable melanoma in patients with a BRAF V600E or V600K mutation (in combination with binimetinib). Ⅹ Metastatic colorectal cancer (CRC) in patients with a BRAF V600E mutation (in combination with cetuximab).

Action
Kinase inhibitor that targets BRAF V600E, a mutated enzyme that promotes tumor cell proliferation. **Therapeutic Effects:** Improvement in progression-free survival and overall survival in patients with melanoma and CRC.

Pharmacokinetics
Absorption: Well absorbed (86%) following oral administration.
Distribution: Extensively distributed to tissues.
Metabolism and Excretion: Primarily metabolized by the liver via the CYP3A4 and CYP2C19 isoenzymes. Primarily excreted as metabolites in feces (42%) and urine (45%).
Half-life: 3.5 hr.

TIME/ACTION PROFILE (plasma concentrations)

ROUTE	ONSET	PEAK	DURATION
PO	unknown	2 hr	24 hr

Contraindications/Precautions
Contraindicated in: Ⅹ Wild-type BRAF melanoma (may ↑ proliferation); Long QT syndrome, bradyarrhythmias, severe or decompensated HF, hypokalemia, or hypomagnesemia (↑ risk of QT interval prolongation); Concurrent use of QT-interval prolonging medications; Baseline QTc interval >500 msec; OB: Pregnancy; Lactation: Lactation.
Use Cautiously in: Moderate or severe hepatic impairment; Severe renal impairment; Rep: Women of reproductive potential; Pedi: Safety and effectiveness not established in children.

Adverse Reactions/Side Effects
CV: QT interval prolongation. **Derm:** alopecia, dry skin, hyperkeratosis, pruritus, rash, BASAL CELL CARCINOMA, CUTANEOUS SQUAMOUS CELL CARCINOMA, nodule formation. **EENT:** uveitis. **Endo:** hyperglycemia. **F and E:** hypermagnesemia, hyponatremia. **GI:** ↑ liver enzymes, abdominal pain, constipation, nausea, vomiting, GI HEMORRHAGE, PANCREATITIS. **GU:** ↑ serum creatinine, ↓ fertility (males). **Hemat:** anemia, BLEEDING, leukopenia, lymphopenia, neutropenia. **MS:** arthralgia, myalgia. **Neuro:** dizziness, fatigue, headache, peripheral neuropathy, facial paralysis, INTRACRANIAL HEMORRHAGE. **Misc:** fever, HYPERSENSITIVITY REACTIONS, MALIGNANCY.

Interactions
Drug-Drug: QT interval prolonging drugs may ↑ the risk of QT interval prolongation and torsades de pointes; avoid concurrent use. **Strong or moderate CYP3A4 inhibitors,** including **diltiazem** and **posaconazole** may ↑ levels and risk of toxicity; avoid concurrent use, if possible (if must use concurrently, ↓ encorafenib dose). **Strong or moderate CYP3A4 inducers** may ↓ levels and effectiveness; avoid concurrent use. May ↓ effectiveness of **hormonal contraceptives**; avoid concurrent use. May ↑ levels and risk of toxicity of **OATP1B1 substrates, OATP1B3 substrates,** or **BRCP substrates.**
Drug-Natural Products: St. John's wort may ↓ levels and effectiveness; avoid concurrent use.
Drug-Food: Grapefruit juice may ↑ levels and risk of toxicity; avoid concurrent use.

Route/Dosage

BRAF V600E or V600K Mutation-Positive Unresectable or Metastatic Melanoma
PO (Adults): 450 mg once daily until disease progression or unacceptable toxicity. *Concurrent use of moderate CYP3A4 inhibitor:* 225 mg once daily (if planned dose 450 mg once daily); 150 mg once daily (if planned dose 300 mg once daily); 75 mg once daily (if planned dose 225 mg once daily); *Concurrent use of strong CYP3A4 inhibitor:* 150 mg once daily (if planned dose 450 mg once daily); 75 mg once daily (if planned dose 300 mg once daily or 225 mg once daily).

BRAF V600E Mutation-Positive Metastatic CRC
PO (Adults): 300 mg once daily until disease progression or unacceptable toxicity. *Concurrent use of moderate CYP3A4 inhibitor:* 150 mg once daily (if planned dose 300 mg once daily); 75 mg once daily (if planned dose 225 mg once daily or 150 mg once daily); *Concurrent use of strong CYP3A4 inhibitor:* 75 mg once daily (if planned dose 300 mg once daily, 225 mg once daily, or 150 mg once daily).

Availability
Capsules: 75 mg.

✦ = Canadian drug name. Ⅹ = Genetic implication. ~~Strikethrough~~ = Discontinued. CAPITALS = life-threatening. <u>Underline</u> = most frequent.

NURSING IMPLICATIONS
Assessment

- Assess skin for lesions prior to starting, every 2 months during, and for up to 6 months following discontinuation of therapy. Manage suspicious skin lesions with excision and dermatopathologic evaluation. *For Grade 2 reaction,* if no improvement in 2 wk, hold encorafenib until Grade 0-1. Resume at same dose. *For Grade 3,* hold encorafenib until Grade 0-1. Resume at same dose if first occurrence or reduce dose if recurrent. *For Grade 4,* discontinue encorafenib permanently.
- Monitor for noncutaneous RAS mutation-positive malignancies. Permanently discontinue encorafenib if these malignancies occur.
- Monitor for signs and symptoms of hemorrhage (bleeding GI, rectal, anal, hemorrhoidal) periodically during therapy. *If Grade 2 or 1st occurrence of Grade 3:* Withhold encorafenib up to 4 wk. If improves to Grade 0-1 or to pretreatment level, resume at reduced dose. If no improvement, permanently discontinue encorafenib. *If 1st occurrence of Grade 4:* Discontinue encorafenib permanently or withhold up to 4 wk. If improves to Grade 0-1 or to pretreatment level, resume at reduced dose. If no improvement, permanently discontinue encorafenib. *If recurrent Grade 3:* Consider permanently discontinuing encorafenib. *If recurrent Grade 4:* permanently discontinue encorafenib.
- Monitor ECG in patients who already have or are at risk of QTc prolongation, including patients with known long QT syndromes, clinically significant bradyarrhythmias, severe or uncontrolled heart failure, and those taking other medications leading to QT prolongation. *If QTcF >500 ms and ≤60 ms increase from baseline,* hold encorafenib until QTcF ≤500 ms. Resume at reduced dose. If occurs more than once, permanently discontinue encorafenib. *If QTcF >500 ms and >60 ms increase from baseline,* discontinue encorafenib permanently.
- Assess for signs and symptoms of uveitis (visual changes, eye pain) during therapy. Perform ophthalmologic exam regularly and for new or worsening visual disturbances; follow new or persistent ophthalmologic findings. *If Grade 1 or 2 does not respond to ocular therapy, or for Grade 3 uveitis,* hold encorafenib for up to 6 wk. If improved, resume at same or reduced dose. If not improved, permanently discontinue encorafenib. *If Grade 4 uveitis occurs,* permanently discontinue encorafenib.

Lab Test Considerations

- Verify negative pregnancy status of females of reproductive potential prior to starting therapy.
- ✖ Confirm presence of a BRAF V600E or V600K mutation in tumor specimens before starting therapy for melanoma and of BRAF V600E mutation before starting therapy for CRC. Information on FDA-approved tests for the detection of BRAF V600E and V600K mutations is available at: http://www.fda.gov/CompanionDiagnostics.

- Monitor serum electrolytes periodically during therapy. Correct hypokalemia and hypomagnesemia prior to and during therapy. May also cause hyponatremia and hyperglycemia.
- May cause anemia, leukopenia, lymphopenia, and neutropenia.
- Monitor liver function periodically during therapy. May cause ↑ serum creatinine, GGT, AST, ALT, and alkaline phosphatase. *If Grade 2 AST or ALT ↑:* Continue encorafenib dose. If no improvement within 4 wk, hold encorafenib until Grade 0-1 or to baseline levels, then resume at same dose. If no improvement, permanently discontinue encorafenib. *If Grade 3 AST or ALT ↑:* Consider permanently discontinuing encorafenib. *If Grade 4 AST or ALT ↑:* Permanently discontinue encorafenib.

Implementation

- **Melanoma reduced dose recommendations**: If binimetinib is held, reduce encorafenib to maximum dose of 300 mg once daily until binimetinib is resumed. *First dose reduction:* 300 mg (four 75-mg capsules) orally once daily. *Second dose reduction:* 225 mg (three 75-mg capsules) orally once daily. *Subsequent modification:* Permanently discontinue if unable to tolerate encorafenib 225 mg (three 75-mg capsules) once daily. **CRC reduced dose recommendations**: If cetuximab is discontinued, discontinue encorafenib. *First dose reduction:* 225 mg (three 75-mg capsules) orally once daily. *Second dose reduction:* 150 mg (two 75-mg capsules) orally once daily. *Subsequent modification:* Permanently discontinue if unable to tolerate encorafenib 150 mg (two 75-mg capsules) once daily.
- **PO:** Administer once daily without regard to food. Store in original, tightly capped bottle at room temperature; do not remove desiccant, protect from moisture.

Patient/Family Teaching

- Instruct patient to take encorafenib as directed. Take missed dose within 12 hr of missed dose; do not take dose within 12 hr of next dose. If vomiting occurs, skip dose; continue with next scheduled dose. Advise patient to read *Medication Guide* before starting therapy and with each Rx refill in case of changes.
- Inform patient that grapefruit products may increase amount of encorafenib in the body. Avoid grapefruit and grapefruit juice during therapy.
- Inform patient that encorafenib increases risk of developing new cutaneous malignancies. Notify health care professional immediately if new lesions (wart, skin sore or reddish bump that bleeds or does not heal) or changes in size or color of existing moles or lesions occur.
- Advise patient to notify health care professional immediately if signs and symptoms of bleeding (headaches, dizziness, weakness, coughing up blood or blood clots, vomiting blood or vomit looks like "coffee grounds," red or black stools that look like tar); liver dysfunction (yellow skin or whites of eyes, feel-

ing tired, urine turns dark or brown, nausea or vomiting, loss of appetite, pain on right side of stomach), changes in heart rhythm (feeling faint, lightheaded, dizzy, heart beating irregularly or fast); or eye problems (blurred vision, loss of vision, other vision changes, seeing colored dots, seeing halos or blurred outline around objects, eye pain, swelling, redness) occur.

- Advise patient to notify health care professional of all Rx or OTC medications, vitamins, or herbal products being taken and to consult with health care professional before taking other medications, especially St. John's wort.
- Rep: May cause fetal harm. Encorafenib may decrease effectiveness of hormonal contraceptives. Advise female patient to use a highly effective nonhormonal form of contraception during and for 2 wk after last dose. Advise patient to notify health care professional if pregnancy is suspected and to avoid breastfeeding during and for at least 2 wk after last dose. May impair fertility in males.
- Inform patient that regular assessments of skin and assessments for signs and symptoms of other malignancies must be done every 2 mo during and for up to 6 mo after therapy. Advise patient to notify health care professional immediately if any changes in skin occur.

Evaluation/Desired Outcomes
- Decreased spread of melanoma and CRC.

enoxaparin, See HEPARINS (LOW MOLECULAR WEIGHT).

entacapone (en-tak-a-pone)
Comtan
Classification
Therapeutic: antiparkinson agents
Pharmacologic: catechol-*O*-methyltransferase (COMT) inhibitors

Indications
Parkinson's disease when signs and symptoms of end-of-dose "wearing-off" (so-called fluctuating patients) occur (in combination with levodopa/carbidopa).

Action
Acts as a selective and reversible inhibitor of the enzyme catechol *O*-methyltransferase (COMT). Inhibition of COMT prevents the breakdown of levodopa, increasing availability to the CNS. **Therapeutic Effects:** Prolongs duration of response to levodopa with end-of-dose motor fluctuations. Decreased signs and symptoms of Parkinson's disease.

Pharmacokinetics
Absorption: 35% absorbed following oral administration; absorption is rapid.

Distribution: Widely distributed to tissues.
Protein Binding: 98%.
Metabolism and Excretion: Minimal amounts excreted unchanged; highly metabolized followed by biliary excretion.
Half-life: *Initial phase:* 0.4–0.7 hr; *second phase:* 2.4 hr.

TIME/ACTION PROFILE (inhibition of COMT)

ROUTE	ONSET	PEAK	DURATION
PO	unknown	unknown	up to 8 hr

Contraindications/Precautions
Contraindicated in: Hypersensitivity; Psychotic disorder.
Use Cautiously in: Hepatic impairment; Concurrent use of drugs that are metabolized by COMT; OB: Safety not established in pregnancy; Lactation: Safety not established in breastfeeding; Pedi: Safety and effectiveness not established in children.

Adverse Reactions/Side Effects
CV: hypotension. **Derm:** MELANOMA. **GI:** abdominal pain, colitis, diarrhea, nausea (during initiation), retroperitoneal fibrosis. **GU:** brownish-orange discoloration of urine. **MS:** dyskinesia, RHABDOMYOLYSIS. **Neuro:** aggressive behavior, agitation, confusion, delirium, disorientation, dizziness, hallucinations, NEUROLEPTIC MALIGNANT SYNDROME, paranoid ideation, syncope, urges (gambling, sexual). **Resp:** pleural effusion, pleural thickening, pulmonary infiltrates.

Interactions
Drug-Drug: Concurrent use with selective **MAO inhibitors** is not recommended; both agents inhibit the metabolic pathways of catecholamines. Concurrent use of drugs that are metabolized by COMT, including **isoproterenol**, **epinephrine**, **norepinephrine**, **dopamine**, and **dobutamine**, may ↑ risk of tachycardia, ↑ BP, and arrhythmias. **Probenecid**, **cholestyramine**, **erythromycin**, **rifampin**, **ampicillin**, and **chloramphenicol** may interfere with biliary elimination of entacapone; use concurrently with caution.

Route/Dosage
PO (Adults): 200 mg with each dose of levodopa/carbidopa up to a maximum of 8 times daily.

Availability (generic available)
Tablets: 200 mg. *In combination with:* levodopa/carbidopa (Stalevo), see Appendix N.

NURSING IMPLICATIONS
Assessment
- Assess parkinsonian and extrapyramidal symptoms (restlessness or desire to keep moving, rigidity, tremors, pill rolling, mask-like face, shuffling gait, muscle spasms, twisting motions, difficulty speaking or swal-

lowing, loss of balance control) prior to and during therapy. Dyskinesia may increase with therapy.
- Monitor patient for development of diarrhea. Usually occurs within 4 to 12 wk of start of therapy, but may occur as early as the first wk and as late as mo after initiation of therapy.
- Monitor patient for signs and symptoms of neuroleptic malignant syndrome (elevated temperature, muscular rigidity, altered consciousness, elevated CK). Symptoms have been associated with rapid dose reduction or withdrawal of other dopaminergic drugs. Withdrawal should be gradual.

Implementation
- **PO:** Always administer entacapone with levodopa/carbidopa. Entacapone has no antiparkinsonism effects of its own.

Patient/Family Teaching
- Encourage patient to take entacapone as directed. Take missed doses as soon as possible, up to 2 hr before the next dose. Taper gradually when discontinuing or a withdrawal reaction may occur.
- May cause dizziness or hallucinations. Advise patient to avoid driving or other activities that require alertness until response to the drug is known.
- Inform patient that nausea may occur, especially at initiation of therapy, and diarrhea. Advise patient with diarrhea to drink fluids to maintain adequate hydration and monitor for weight loss. If diarrhea is prolonged, may resolve with discontinuation. Therapy may cause change in urine color to brownish orange.
- Caution patient to change positions slowly to minimize orthostatic hypotension.
- Advise patient to notify health care professional if suspicious or unusual skin changes, agitation, aggression, delirium, hallucinations, or new or increased gambling, sexual, or other intense urges occur.
- Rep: Advise females of reproductive potential to notify health care professional if pregnancy is planned or suspected or if breastfeeding.
- Emphasize the importance of routine follow-up exams.

Evaluation/Desired Outcomes
- Decreased signs and symptoms of Parkinson's disease.

entecavir (en-tek-aveer)
Baraclude
Classification
Therapeutic: antivirals
Pharmacologic: nucleoside analogues

Indications
Chronic hepatitis B virus (HBV) infection with evidence of active viral replication and either persistent elevations in AST or ALT or histologically active disease.

Action
Phosphorylated intracellularly to active form, which acts as an analogue of guanosine, interfering with viral DNA synthesis. **Therapeutic Effects:** Decreased hepatic damage due to chronic HBV infection.

Pharmacokinetics
Absorption: Well absorbed following oral administration.
Distribution: Extensive tissue distribution.
Metabolism and Excretion: 62–73% excreted unchanged by kidneys.
Half-life: Plasma: 128–149 hr; intracellular: 15 hr.

TIME/ACTION PROFILE (plasma concentrations)

ROUTE	ONSET	PEAK	DURATION
PO	rapid	0.5–1 hr	24 hr

Contraindications/Precautions
Contraindicated in: Hypersensitivity.
Use Cautiously in: Renal impairment (dose ↓ recommended if CCr <50 mL/min; Liver transplant recipients (careful monitoring of renal function recommended); Patients coinfected with HIV (unless receiving highly active antiretroviral therapy; at ↑ risk for resistance); OB: Other agents preferred for treatment of HBV during pregnancy; Lactation: Use during breastfeeding only if benefit to patient outweighs potential risk to infant; Pedi: Children <2 yr (safety and effectiveness not established); Geri: ↑ risk of toxicity in older adults due to age-related ↓ in renal function.

Adverse Reactions/Side Effects
Derm: alopecia, rash. **F and E:** LACTIC ACIDOSIS. **GI:** HEPATOMEGALY (WITH STEATOSIS), dyspepsia, nausea. **Neuro:** dizziness, fatigue, headache.

Interactions
Drug-Drug: Concurrent use of drugs that may impair renal function may ↑ levels and risk of toxicity.

Route/Dosage
PO (Adults): *Compensated liver disease:* 0.5 mg once daily; *Decompensated liver disease or history of lamivudine resistance:* 1 mg once daily.
PO (Children ≥2 yr and >30 kg): 0.5 mg once daily (1 mg once daily if history of lamivudine resistance).
PO (Children ≥2 yr and >26–30 kg): 0.45 mg once daily (0.9 mg once daily if history of lamivudine resistance).
PO (Children ≥2 yr and >23–26 kg): 0.4 mg once daily (0.8 mg once daily if history of lamivudine resistance).
PO (Children ≥2 yr and >20–23 kg): 0.35 mg once daily (0.7 mg once daily if history of lamivudine resistance).
PO (Children ≥2 yr and >17–20 kg): 0.3 mg once daily (0.6 mg once daily if history of lamivudine resistance).
PO (Children ≥2 yr and >14–17 kg): 0.25 mg once daily (0.5 mg once daily if history of lamivudine resistance).

PO (Children ≥2 yr and >11–14 kg): 0.2 mg once daily (0.4 mg once daily if history of lamivudine resistance).
PO (Children ≥2 yr and 10–11 kg): 0.15 mg once daily (0.3 mg once daily if history of lamivudine resistance).

Renal Impairment
PO (Adults): *CCr 30– <50 mL/min:* 0.25 mg once daily or 0.5 mg every 48 hr (0.5 mg once daily or 1 mg every 48 hr if lamivudine-resistant or decompensated liver disease). *CCr 10– <30 mL/min:* 0.15 mg once daily or 0.5 mg every 72 hr (0.3 mg once daily or 1 mg every 72 hr if lamivudine-resistant or decompensated liver disease). *CCr <10 mL/min, hemodialysis, or CAPD:* 0.05 mg once daily or 0.5 mg every 7 days (0.1 mg once daily or 1 mg every 7 days if lamivudine-resistant or decompensated liver disease).

Availability (generic available)
Oral solution (orange flavor): 0.05 mg/mL. **Tablets:** 0.5 mg, 1 mg.

NURSING IMPLICATIONS
Assessment
- Monitor signs of HBV (jaundice, fatigue, anorexia, pruritus) during and for several mo following discontinuation of therapy. Exacerbations may occur when therapy is discontinued.
- May cause lactic acidosis and severe hepatomegaly with steatosis. Monitor patient for signs (↑ serum lactate levels, elevated liver enzymes, liver enlargement on palpation). Suspend therapy if clinical or laboratory signs occur.

Lab Test Considerations
- Monitor liver function closely during and for several mo following discontinuation of therapy. May cause ↑ serum AST, ALT, bilirubin, amylase, lipase, creatinine, and glucose. May cause ↓ serum albumin.

Implementation
- **PO:** Administer on an empty stomach at least 2 hr before or after a meal. Use oral solution for dose <0.5 mg and children up to 30 kg. Children >30 kg can use oral solution or tablet. Oral solution is ready to use; do not dilute or mix with water or any other liquid. Hold spoon in a vertical position and fill gradually to mark corresponding to prescribed dose. Rinse dosing spoon with water after each daily dose. Store in outer carton at room temperature. After opening, solution can be used until expiration date on bottle.

Patient/Family Teaching
- Instruct patient to take entecavir as directed. Advise patient to read the *Patient Information* with each refill and to take entecavir as directed. Take missed doses as soon as possible unless almost time for next dose. Do not run out of entecavir; get more when supply runs low. Do not double doses. Emphasize the importance of compliance with full course of therapy, not taking more than the prescribed amount, and not discontinuing without consulting health care professional. Inform patient that hepatitis exacerbation may occur upon discontinuation of therapy. Caution patient not to share medication with others.
- Inform patient that entecavir does not cure HBV disease, but may lower the amount of HBV in the body, lower the ability of HBV to multiply and infect new liver cells, and may improve the condition of the liver. Entecavir does not reduce the risk of transmission of HBV to others through sexual contact or blood contamination. Caution patient to use a condom during sexual contact and avoid sharing needles or donating blood to prevent spreading HBV to others.
- Advise patient to notify health care professional promptly if signs of lactic acidosis (weakness or tiredness; unusual muscle pain; trouble breathing; stomach pain with nausea and vomiting; feeling cold, especially in arms or legs; dizziness; fast or irregular heartbeat) or hepatotoxicity (jaundice, dark urine, light-colored bowel movements, anorexia, nausea, lower stomach pain) occur.
- May cause dizziness. Caution patient to avoid driving or other activities requiring alertness until response to medication is known.
- Instruct patient to notify health care professional of all Rx or OTC medications, vitamins, or herbal products being taken and to consult with health care professional before taking other medications.
- Discuss the possibility of hair loss with patient. Explore methods of coping.
- Rep: Advise patient to notify health care professional if pregnancy is planned or suspected. Encourage pregnant women to enroll in the Antiretroviral Pregnancy Registry by calling 1-800-258-4263. Advise female patient to avoid breastfeeding during therapy.
- Emphasize the importance of regular follow-up exams and blood tests to determine progress and monitor for side effects.

Evaluation/Desired Outcomes
- Decreased hepatic damage due to chronic HBV infection.

enzalutamide
(en-za-**loo**-ta-mide)
Xtandi
Classification
Therapeutic: antineoplastics
Pharmacologic: androgen receptor inhibitors

Indications
Castration-resistant prostate cancer. Metastatic, castration-sensitive prostate cancer.

Action

Acts as an androgen receptor inhibitor, preventing the binding of androgen; also inhibits androgen nuclear translocation and DNA interaction. Decreases proliferation and induces cell death of prostate cancer cells.
Therapeutic Effects: Decreased growth and spread of prostate cancer.

Pharmacokinetics

Absorption: Well absorbed following oral administration.
Distribution: Widely distributed to tissues.
Protein Binding: *Enzalutamide:* 97–98%; *N-desmethylenzalutamide:* 95%.
Metabolism and Excretion: Extensively metabolized by the liver via the CYP2C8 and CYP3A4 isoenzymes; one metabolite (N-desmethylenzalutamide) has antineoplastic activity. Metabolites are primarily renally excreted, only minimal amounts as unchanged drug.
Half-life: *Enzalutamide:* 5.8 days; *N-desmethylenzalutamide:* 7.8–8.6 days.

TIME/ACTION PROFILE (improved survival)

ROUTE	ONSET	PEAK	DURATION
PO	3 mo	unknown	unknown

Contraindications/Precautions

Contraindicated in: None reported.
Use Cautiously in: History of seizures, underlying brain pathology, cerebrovascular accident, transient ischemic attack (within 12 mo), brain metastases, or brain arteriovenous malformation (may ↑ risk of seizures); Rep: Men with female partners of reproductive potential; Geri: Older adults may be more sensitive to drug effects.

Adverse Reactions/Side Effects

CV: peripheral edema, hypertension, ISCHEMIC HEART DISEASE. **Derm:** hot flush, dry skin, pruritus. **EENT:** epistaxis. **GI:** diarrhea. **GU:** hematuria, urinary frequency. **MS:** arthralgia, musculoskeletal pain, fracture, muscular stiffness, muscular weakness. **Neuro:** headache, weakness, anxiety, dizziness, hallucinations, hypoesthesia, insomnia, paresthesia, POSTERIOR REVERSIBLE ENCEPHALOPATHY SYNDROME (PRES), SEIZURES, SPINAL CORD COMPRESSION/CAUDA EQUINA SYNDROME. **Misc:** falls, HYPERSENSITIVITY REACTIONS (including angioedema).

Interactions

Drug-Drug: **Strong CYP2C8 inhibitors,** including **gemfibrozil,** may ↑ levels and risk of toxicity; avoid concurrent use (if concurrent administration necessary, ↓ enzalutamide dose). **Strong CYP3A4 inducers,** including **carbamazepine, phenobarbital, phenytoin, rifabutin, rifampin,** and **rifapentine** may ↓ levels and response; avoid concurrent use (if concurrent administration necessary, ↑ enzalutamide dose). May ↓ levels of **CYP3A4, CYP2C9, and CYP2C19 substrates** that have narrow therapeutic indexes including **cyclospor-**ine, **fentanyl, phenytoin, sirolimus, tacrolimus,** and **warfarin;** avoid concurrent use. **Drugs that ↓ seizure threshold** may ↑ risk of seizures.
Drug-Natural Products: St. John's wort may ↓ levels and response; avoid concurrent use (if concurrent administration necessary, ↑ enzalutamide dose).

Route/Dosage

Patients taking enzalutamide should also receive gonadotropin-releasing hormone analog concurrently or should have had bilateral orchiectomy.
PO (Adults): 160 mg once daily. *Concurrent use of strong CYP2C8 inhibitors:* 80 mg once daily; *Concurrent use of strong CYP3A4 inducers:* 240 mg once daily.

Availability (generic available)

Capsules: 40 mg. **Film-coated tablets:** 40 mg, 80 mg.

NURSING IMPLICATIONS

Assessment

- Monitor for seizures. Implement seizure precautions. If a seizure occurs during therapy, permanently discontinue enzalutamide therapy.
- Monitor for signs and symptoms of PRES (seizure, headache, lethargy, confusion, blindness, other visual and neurological disturbances, hypertension) during therapy. Diagnosis is made with MRI. Discontinue enzalutamide in patients who develop PRES.
- Monitor for signs and symptoms of hypersensitivity reactions (swelling of face, tongue, lips or throat; dyspnea). Discontinue enzalutamide if serious hypersensitivity reactions occur.
- Monitor for signs and symptoms of ischemic heart disease (chest pain, fainting, dyspnea). Permanently discontinue enzalutamide if Grade 3 or 4 ischemic heart disease symptoms occur.
- Assess risk of falls and fractures periodically during therapy. May consider bone-targeted agents.

Lab Test Considerations
- May cause hematuria.

Implementation

- **PO:** Administer (two 80-mg tablets or four 40-mg tablets or four 40-mg capsules) once daily without regard to food. *DNC:* Swallow capsules whole; do not open, dissolve, or chew.
- If ≥Grade 3 toxicity or intolerable side effects occur, hold dose for 1 wk or until symptoms improve to <Grade 2, then resume at same or reduced dose (120 mg or 80 mg).

Patient/Family Teaching

- Instruct patient to take enzalutamide as directed at the same time each day. Take missed doses as soon as remembered within the same day. If a whole day is missed, omit dose and take next day's scheduled dose; do not double dose. Advise patient not to interrupt, modify dose, or stop taking enzalutamide without consulting health care professional. Advise patient to read *Patient Information* before starting therapy and with each Rx refill in case of changes.

- May cause seizures, dizziness, mental impairment, paresthesia, hypoesthesia, falls, and hallucinations. Caution patient to avoid driving and other activities requiring alertness until response to medication is known. Notify health care professional immediately if loss of consciousness, seizure, chest pain, or signs and symptoms of PRES or hypersensitivity reactions occur.
- Inform patient of common side effects associated with enzalutamide: asthenia/fatigue, back pain, diarrhea, arthralgia, hot flush, peripheral edema, musculoskeletal pain, headache, upper and lower respiratory infection, muscular weakness, dizziness, insomnia, spinal cord compression, cauda equina syndrome, hematuria, paresthesia, anxiety, and hypertension. Notify health care professional if falls or problems thinking clearly, or if side effects are bothersome.
- Instruct patient to notify health care professional of all Rx or OTC medications, vitamins, or herbal products being taken and to consult health care professional before taking other Rx, OTC, or herbal products, especially St. John's wort.
- Rep: May cause fetal harm and loss of pregnancy. Instruct females of reproductive potential to avoid handling enzalutamide tablets. Advise males with female partners of reproductive potential to use a condom and effective contraception during and for 3 mo after last dose. May impair fertility in males.

Evaluation/Desired Outcomes
- Decreased growth and spread of prostate cancer.

HIGH ALERT

EPINEPHrine (ep-i-nef-rin)
Adrenaclick, Adrenalin, ✹ Allerject, ✹ Anapen, ✹ Anapen Junior, ~~AsthmaNefrin~~, Auvi-Q, EpiPen, Primatene Mist, ✹ S-2 (racepinephrine), Symjepi, ~~Twin-Ject~~

Classification
Therapeutic: anti-asthmatics, bronchodilators, vasopressors
Pharmacologic: adrenergics

See Appendix B for ophthalmic use

Indications
SUBQ, IM, IV: Severe allergic reactions. **IV:** Hypotension associated with septic shock. **Inhaln:** Upper airway obstruction and croup (racemic epinephrine). Temporary relief of mild symptoms of intermittent asthma (over-the-counter). **Local/Spinal:** Adjunct in the localization/prolongation of anesthesia. **Unlabeled Use:** IV, Intracardiac, Intratracheal, Intraosseous (part of advanced cardiac life support [ACLS] and pediatric advanced life support [PALS] guidelines): Cardiac arrest.

SUBQ, IM: Reversible airway disease due to asthma or COPD.

Action
Results in the accumulation of cyclic adenosine monophosphate (cAMP) at beta-adrenergic receptors. Affects both beta$_1$ (cardiac)-adrenergic receptors and beta$_2$ (pulmonary)-adrenergic receptor sites. Produces bronchodilation. Also has alpha-adrenergic agonist properties, which result in vasoconstriction. Inhibits the release of mediators of immediate hypersensitivity reactions from mast cells. **Therapeutic Effects:** Bronchodilation. Maintenance of heart rate and BP. Localization/prolongation of local/spinal anesthetic.

Pharmacokinetics
Absorption: IV administration results in complete bioavailability; well absorbed following SUBQ administration; some absorption may occur following repeated inhalation of large doses.
Distribution: Does not cross the blood-brain barrier; crosses the placenta and enters breast milk.
Metabolism and Excretion: Action is rapidly terminated by metabolism and uptake by nerve endings.
Half-life: Unknown.

TIME/ACTION PROFILE (bronchodilation)

ROUTE	ONSET	PEAK	DURATION
Inhaln	1 min	unknown	1–3 hr
SUBQ	5–10 min	20 min	<1–4 hr
IM	6–12 min	unknown	<1–4 hr
IV	rapid	20 min	20–30 min

Contraindications/Precautions
Contraindicated in: Hypersensitivity to adrenergic amines; Some products may contain bisulfites and should be avoided in patients with known hypersensitivity or intolerance.
Use Cautiously in: Cardiac disease (angina, tachycardia, MI); Hypertension; Hyperthyroidism; Parkinson's disease; Pheochromocytoma; Diabetes; Cerebral arteriosclerosis; Glaucoma (except for ophthalmic use); Excessive use may lead to tolerance and paradoxical bronchospasm (inhaler); OB: Use during pregnancy only if potential maternal benefit justifies potential fetal risk; Lactation: High IV doses of epinephrine might ↓ milk production or letdown. Low-dose epidural, topical, inhaled, or ophthalmic epinephrine are unlikely to interfere with breastfeeding; Pedi: Children <12 yr (over-the-counter product only); Geri: Older adults more susceptible to adverse reactions; may require ↓ dose.

Adverse Reactions/Side Effects
CV: angina, arrhythmias, hypertension, tachycardia. **Derm:** skin and soft tissue infections (including necrotizing fasciitis and myonecrosis). **Endo:** hyperglycemia. **GI:** nausea, vomiting. **GU:** renal impairment. **Neuro:** nervousness, restlessness, tremor, headache, insomnia. **Resp:** PARADOXICAL BRONCHOSPASM (with excessive use of inhalers), pulmonary edema.

Interactions

Drug-Drug: Concurrent use with other **adrenergic agents** will have additive adrenergic side effects. Use with **MAO inhibitors** may lead to hypertensive crisis. **Beta blockers** may negate therapeutic effect. **Tricyclic antidepressants** enhance pressor response to epinephrine.

Drug-Natural Products: Use with caffeine-containing herbs (**cola nut, guarana, mate, tea, coffee**) ↑ stimulant effect.

Route/Dosage

SUBQ, IM (Adults and Children ≥30 kg): *Severe anaphylaxis:* 0.3–0.5 mg (single dose not to exceed 0.5 mg); may repeat every 10–15 min as needed.

SUBQ (Children <30 kg): *Severe anaphylaxis:* 0.01 mg/kg (not to exceed 0.3 mg/dose); may repeat every 10–15 min as needed; *Auvi-Q or Symjepi (15–30 kg):* 0.15 mg; may repeat if anaphylactic symptoms persist; *Auvi-Q (7.5–15 kg):* 0.1 mg; may repeat if anaphylactic symptoms persist.

IV (Adults): *Severe anaphylaxis:* 0.1–0.25 mg every 5–15 min; may be followed by 1–4 mcg/min continuous infusion; *Cardiopulmonary resuscitation (ACLS guidelines):* 1 mg every 3–5 min; *Bradycardia (ACLS guidelines):* 2–10 mcg/min continuous infusion; *Hypotension associated with septic shock:* 0.05–2 mcg/kg/min continuous infusion; titrate every 10–15 min by 0.05–0.2 mcg/kg/min to achieve desired mean arterial pressure.

IV (Children): *Severe anaphylaxis:* 0.1 mg (less in younger children); may be followed by 0.1 mcg/kg/min continuous infusion (may be ↑ up to 1.5 mcg/kg/min); *Symptomatic bradycardia/pulseless arrest (PALS guidelines):* 0.01 mg/kg, may be repeated every 3–5 min, higher doses (up to 0.1–0.2 mg/kg) may be considered; may also be given by the intraosseous route. May also be given by the endotracheal route in doses of 0.1–0.2 mg/kg diluted to a volume of 3–5 mL with normal saline followed by several positive pressure ventilations.

Inhaln (Adults): *Inhalation solution:* 1 inhalation of 1% solution; may be repeated after 1–2 min; additional doses may be given every 3 hr; *Racepinephrine:* Via hand nebulizer, 2–3 inhalations of 2.25% solution; may repeat in 5 min with 2–3 more inhalations, up to 4–6 times daily.

Inhaln (Children >1 mo): 0.25–0.5 mL of 2.25% racemic epinephrine solution diluted in 3 mL normal saline.

Inhaln (Adults and Children ≥12 yr): *Over-the-counter inhaler:* 1–2 inhalations every 4 hr as needed (max = 8 inhalations/day).

IV, Intratracheal (Neonates): 0.01–0.03 mg/kg every 3–5 min as needed.

Intracardiac (Adults): 0.3–0.5 mg.

Endotracheal (Adults): *Cardiopulmonary resuscitation (ACLS guidelines):* 2–2.5 mg.

Topical (Adults and Children ≥6 yr): *Nasal decongestant:* Apply 1% solution as drops, spray, or with a swab.

Intraspinal (Adults and Children): 0.2–0.4 mL of 1:1000 solution.

With Local Anesthetics (Adults and Children): Use 1:200,000 solution with local anesthetic.

Availability (generic available)

Inhalation aerosol: 0.125 mg/inhalation (160 metered inhalations)^OTC. **Inhalation solution (racepinephrine):** ✿ 2.25%. **Intranasal solution:** 1 mg/mL (1:1000). **Premixed infusion:** 2 mg/250 mL 0.9% NaCl, 4 mg/250 mL 0.9% NaCl, 5 mg/250 mL 0.9% NaCl, 8 mg/250 mL 0.9% NaCl, 10 mg/250 mL 0.9% NaCl. **Solution for injection:** 1 mg/mL (1:1000). **Solution for injection (autoinjectors) (Adrenaclick, Auvi-Q, EpiPen):** 0.1 mg/0.1 mL (1:1000), 0.15 mg/0.15 mL (1:1000), 0.15 mg/0.3 mL (1:2000), 0.3 mg/0.3 mL (1:1000). **Solution for injection (prefilled syringes):** 0.1 mg/mL (1:10,000), 0.15 mg/0.3 mL (1:2000), 0.3 mg/0.3 mL (1:1000).

NURSING IMPLICATIONS

Assessment

- Monitor IV infusion site for extravasation (cold, hard, pallid appearance). If blanching occurs, may change infusion site to allow effects of local vasoconstriction to subside. If extravasation occurs, infiltrate area liberally with 10 mL to 15 mL of 0.9% NaCl with 5 mg–10 mg of phentolamine using a syringe with a fine needle within 12 hr of extravasation. Local hyperemic changes are immediate.

- **Bronchodilator:** Assess lung sounds, respiratory pattern, pulse, and BP before administration and during peak of medication. Note amount, color, and character of sputum produced, and notify health care professional of abnormal findings.

- Monitor pulmonary function tests before and periodically during therapy.

- Observe for paradoxical bronchospasm (wheezing). If condition occurs, withhold medication and notify health care professional immediately.

- Observe patient for drug tolerance and rebound bronchospasm. Patients requiring more than 3 inhalation treatments in 24 hr should be under close supervision. If minimal or no relief is seen after 3–5 inhalation treatments within 6–12 hr, further treatment with aerosol alone is not recommended.

- Assess for hypersensitivity reaction (rash; urticaria; swelling of the face, lips, or eyelids). If condition occurs, withhold medication and notify health care professional immediately.

- **Vasopressor:** Monitor BP, pulse, ECG, and respiratory rate frequently during IV administration. Continuous ECG, hemodynamic parameters, and urine output should be monitored continuously during IV administration.

- Monitor for chest pain, arrhythmias, heart rate >110 bpm, and hypertension. Consult health care professional for parameters of pulse, BP, and ECG changes for adjusting dose or discontinuing medication.

- **Shock:** Assess volume status. Correct hypovolemia prior to administering epinephrine IV.

- **Nasal Decongestant:** Assess for nasal and sinus congestion prior to and periodically during therapy.

Lab Test Considerations
- May cause transient ↓ in serum potassium concentrations with nebulization or at higher than recommended doses.
- May cause an ↑ in blood glucose and serum lactic acid concentrations.

Toxicity and Overdose
- Symptoms of overdose include persistent agitation, chest pain or discomfort, decreased BP, dizziness, hyperglycemia, hypokalemia, seizures, tachyarrhythmias, persistent trembling, and vomiting.
- Treatment includes discontinuing adrenergic bronchodilator and other beta-adrenergic agonists and symptomatic, supportive therapy. Cardioselective beta blockers are used cautiously because they may induce bronchospasm.

Implementation

- Do not confuse epinephrine with ephedrine.
- *High Alert:* Patient harm or fatalities have occurred from medication errors with epinephrine. Epinephrine is available in various concentrations, strengths, and percentages and used for different purposes. Packaging labels may be confused or products incorrectly diluted. Dilutions should be prepared by a pharmacist. IV doses should be expressed in milligrams not ampules, concentration, or volume. Prior to administration, have second practitioner independently check original order, dose calculations, concentration, route of administration, and infusion pump settings.
- Medication should be administered promptly at the onset of bronchospasm.
- Use a tuberculin syringe with a 26-gauge ½-in. needle for SUBQ injection to ensure that correct amount of medication is administered.
- Tolerance may develop with prolonged or excessive use. Effectiveness may be restored by discontinuing for a few days and then readministering.
- Do not use solutions that are pinkish or brownish or that contain a precipitate.
- For anaphylactic shock, volume replacement should be administered concurrently with epinephrine. Antihistamines and corticosteroids may be used in conjunction with epinephrine.
- **IM, SUBQ:** Administer into anterolateral thigh, through clothing if necessary for anaphylaxis. Hold child's leg firmly to limit movement during injection to prevent lacerations, bent needles, and broken/embedded needles. Avoid injecting into gluteal muscle; may not be effective for anaphylaxis and may cause infection. Medication can cause irritation of tissue. Rotate injection sites to prevent tissue necrosis. Massage injection sites well after administration to enhance absorption and to decrease local vasoconstriction. Avoid IM administration in gluteal muscle.

IV Administration
- **IV Push:** *Dilution:* The 1:10,000 solution can be administered undiluted. Dilute 1 mg (1 mL) of a 1:1000 solution in 9 mL of 0.9% NaCl to prepare a 1:10,000 solution. *Concentration:* 0.1 mg/mL (1:10,000). *Rate:* Administer each 1 mg (10 mL) of a 1:10,000 solution over at least 1 min; more rapid administration may be used during cardiac resuscitation. Follow each dose with 20 mL IV saline flush.
- **Continuous Infusion:** *Dilution:* Dilute 1 mg (1 mL) of a 1:1000 solution in 250 mL of D5W or 0.9% NaCl. Protect from light. Infusion stable for 24 hr. *Concentration:* 4 mcg/mL. *Rate:* See Route/Dosage section. Titrate to response (BP, heart rate, respiratory rate).
- **Y-Site Compatibility:** alprostadil, eravacycline, hydrocortisone, imipenem/cilastatin, meropenem/vaborbactam, milrinone, plazomicin.
- **Inhaln:** When using epinephrine inhalation solution, 10 drops of 1% base solution should be placed in the reservoir of the nebulizer.
- The 2.25% inhalation solution of racepinephrine must be diluted for use in the combination nebulizer/respirator.
- Allow 1–2 min to elapse between inhalations of epinephrine inhalation solution to make certain the second inhalation is necessary.
- When epinephrine is used concurrently with corticosteroid or ipratropium inhalations, administer bronchodilator first and other medications 5 min apart to prevent toxicity from inhaled fluorocarbon propellants.
- **Endotracheal:** Epinephrine can be injected directly into the bronchial tree via the endotracheal tube if the patient has been intubated. Perform 5 rapid insufflations; forcefully administer 10 mL containing 2–2.5 mg epinephrine (1 mg/mL) directly into tube; follow with 5 quick insufflations.

Patient/Family Teaching

- Instruct patient to take medication exactly as directed. If on a scheduled dosing regimen, take a missed dose as soon as possible; space remaining doses at regular intervals. Do not double doses. Caution patient not to exceed recommended dose; may cause adverse effects, paradoxical bronchospasm, or loss of effectiveness of medication.
- Instruct patient to contact health care professional immediately if shortness of breath is not relieved by medication or is accompanied by diaphoresis, dizziness, palpitations, or chest pain.
- Advise patient to consult health care professional before taking any OTC medications or alcoholic beverages concurrently with this therapy. Caution patient also to avoid smoking and other respiratory irritants.
- Rep: Advise females of reproductive potential to notify health care professional if pregnancy is planned or suspected or if breastfeeding.

- **Inhaln:** Review correct administration technique (aerosolization, IPPB) with patient.
- Do not spray inhaler near eyes.
- Advise patient to use bronchodilator first if using other inhalation medications, and allow 5 min to elapse before administering other inhalant medications, unless otherwise directed.
- Advise patient to rinse mouth with water after each inhalation dose to minimize dry mouth.
- Advise patient to maintain adequate fluid intake (2000–3000 mL/day) to help liquefy tenacious secretions.
- Advise patient to consult health care professional if respiratory symptoms are not relieved or worsen after treatment or if chest pain, headache, severe dizziness, palpitations, nervousness, or weakness occurs.
- **Autoinjector:** Instruct patients using auto-injector for anaphylactic reactions to remove gray safety cap, placing black tip on thigh at right angle to leg. Press hard into thigh until auto-injector functions, hold in place for 10 sec, remove, and discard properly. Massage injected area for 10 sec. Pedi: Teach parents or caregivers signs and symptoms of anaphylaxis, how to use auto-injector safely, and to get the child to a hospital as soon as possible. Instruct parents or caregivers to teach child how to manage his or her allergy, how to self-inject, and what to do in an emergency. For children too young to self-inject and who will be separated from parent, tell parents to always discuss allergy and use of auto-injector with responsible adult.

Evaluation/Desired Outcomes

- Prevention or relief of bronchospasm.
- Increase in ease of breathing.
- Prevention of bronchospasm or reduction of frequency of acute asthma attacks in patients with chronic asthma.
- Prevention of exercise-induced asthma.
- Reversal of signs and symptoms of anaphylaxis.
- Increase in cardiac rate and output, when used in cardiac resuscitation.
- Increase in BP, when used as a vasopressor.
- Localization of local anesthetic.
- Decrease in sinus and nasal congestion.

---

eplerenone (e-ple-re-none)
Inspra
Classification
Therapeutic: antihypertensives
Pharmacologic: aldosterone antagonists

Indications

Hypertension (HTN) (as monotherapy or in combination with other antihypertensive agents). Symptomatic HF with reduced ejection fraction (≤40%) after an acute MI.

Action

Blocks the effects of aldosterone by attaching to mineralocorticoid receptors. **Therapeutic Effects:** Lowering of BP. Improved survival in patients with evidence of HF post-MI.

Pharmacokinetics

Absorption: Well absorbed following oral administration.
Distribution: Unknown.
Metabolism and Excretion: Primarily metabolized by the liver via the CYP3A isoenzyme; <5% excreted unchanged by the kidneys.
Half-life: 4–6 hr.

TIME/ACTION PROFILE (antihypertensive effect)

ROUTE	ONSET	PEAK	DURATION
PO	unknown	4 wk	unknown

Contraindications/Precautions

Contraindicated in: Serum potassium >5.5 mEq/L; Type 2 diabetes with microalbuminuria (for patients with HTN; ↑ risk of hyperkalemia); Serum creatinine >2 mg/dL in males or >1.8 mg/dL in females (for patients with HTN); CCr ≤30 mL/min (for all patients); CCr <50 mL/min (for patients with HTN); Concurrent use of potassium supplements or potassium-sparing diuretics (for patients with HTN); Concurrent use of strong inhibitors of the CYP3A4 enzyme system; Lactation: Lactation.
Use Cautiously in: Moderate hepatic impairment; OB: Use during pregnancy only if potential maternal benefit justifies potential fetal risk; Pedi: Safety and effectiveness not established in children; Geri: ↑ risk of hyperkalemia in older adults due to age-related ↓ in renal function.

Adverse Reactions/Side Effects

Endo: gynecomastia. **F and E:** HYPERKALEMIA. **GI:** ↑ liver enzymes, abdominal pain, diarrhea. **GU:** abnormal vaginal bleeding, albuminuria. **Metab:** hypercholesterolemia, hypertriglyceridemia. **Neuro:** dizziness, fatigue. **Misc:** flu-like symptoms.

Interactions

Drug-Drug: Concurrent use of strong CYP3A inhibitors, including **ketoconazole, itraconazole, nefazodone, clarithromycin, ritonavir,** or **nelfinavir** may ↑ levels and risk of toxicity; concurrent use contraindicated. Concurrent use of moderate CYP3A inhibitors, including **erythromycin, fluconazole,** or **verapamil,** may ↑ levels and risk of toxicity; ↓ eplerenone dose. **NSAIDs** may ↓ antihypertensive effects. Concurrent use of **ACE inhibitors** or **angiotensin II receptor blockers** may ↑ risk of hyperkalemia.

Route/Dosage

Hypertension

PO (Adults): 50 mg once daily initially; may ↑ to 50 mg twice daily; *Concurrent use of moderate CYP3A4 inhibitors (erythromycin, verapamil, or fluconazole):* 25 mg once daily initially; may ↑ to 25 mg twice daily.

Heart Failure with Reduced Ejection Fraction Post-Myocardial Infarction

PO (Adults): 25 mg daily once initially; ↑ in 4 wk to 50 mg once daily; *Concurrent use of moderate CYP3A4 inhibitors (erythromycin, verapamil, or fluconazole):* Do not exceed 25 mg once daily.

Availability (generic available)
Tablets: 25 mg, 50 mg.

NURSING IMPLICATIONS
Assessment
• Monitor BP periodically during therapy.
• Monitor prescription refills to determine adherence.

Lab Test Considerations
• May cause hyperkalemia. Monitor serum potassium levels prior to starting therapy, within the first wk, at 1 mo following start of therapy or dose adjustment, and periodically thereafter. Monitor serum potassium and serum creatinine in 3–7 days in patients who start taking a moderate CYP3A4 inhibitor.
• May cause ↓ serum sodium and ↑ serum triglyceride, cholesterol, ALT, GGT, creatinine, and uric acid levels.

Implementation
• Do not confuse Inspra with Spiriva.
• **PO:** Administer once daily. May be increased to twice daily if response is inadequate.

Patient/Family Teaching
• Instruct patient to take medication as directed at the same time each day, even if feeling well.
• Encourage patient to comply with additional interventions for HTN (weight reduction, discontinuation of smoking, moderation of alcohol consumption, regular exercise, stress management). Medication controls but does not cure HTN.
• Instruct patient and family on correct technique for monitoring BP. Advise them to monitor BP at least weekly, and notify health care professional of significant changes.
• Inform patient not to use potassium supplements, salt substitutes containing potassium, or other Rx, OTC, or herbal products without consulting health care professional.
• May cause dizziness. Caution patient to avoid driving or other activities requiring alertness until response to medication is known.
• Advise patient to notify health care professional if dizziness, diarrhea, vomiting, rapid or irregular heartbeat, lower extremity edema, or difficulty breathing occur.
• Advise patient to inform health care professional of treatment regimen prior to treatment or surgery.
• Rep: Advise females of reproductive potential to notify health care professional if pregnancy is planned or suspected. Advise patient to avoid breastfeeding during therapy. May impair male fertility.

• Emphasize the importance of follow-up exams to check serum potassium.

Evaluation/Desired Outcomes
• Decrease in BP without appearance of side effects.
• Improvement in survival in patients with evidence of HF post-MI.

epoetin (e-poe-e-tin)
Epogen, ✤Eprex, Procrit, Retacrit
Classification
Therapeutic: antianemics
Pharmacologic: hormones, erythropoiesis stimulating agents (ESA)

Indications
Anemia associated with chronic kidney disease (CKD). Anemia secondary to zidovudine therapy in patients infected with HIV. Anemia from chemotherapy in patients with nonmyeloid malignancies when there is ≥2 additional mo of planned chemotherapy. Reduction of need for allogeneic RBC transfusions in patients undergoing elective, noncardiac, nonvascular surgery.

Action
Stimulates erythropoiesis (production of RBCs). **Therapeutic Effects:** Maintains and may elevate RBCs, decreasing the need for transfusions.

Pharmacokinetics
Absorption: Well absorbed after SUBQ administration.
Distribution: Concentrated in kidneys, liver, and bone marrow.
Metabolism and Excretion: Unknown.
Half-life: *Children and Adults:* 4–13 hr; *Neonates:* 11–17 hr.

TIME/ACTION PROFILE (increase in RBCs)

ROUTE	ONSET†	PEAK	DURATION
IV, SUBQ	7–10 days	within 2 mo	2 wk‡

†Increase in reticulocytes.
‡After discontinuation.

Contraindications/Precautions
Contraindicated in: Hypersensitivity to albumin or mammalian cell-derived products; Uncontrolled hypertension; Erythropoietin levels >200 mUnits/mL; Patients with cancer receiving hormonal agents, biologic products, or radiotherapy, unless also receiving concomitant myelosuppressive chemotherapy; Patients receiving chemotherapy when anticipated outcome is cure; Patients with cancer receiving myelosuppressive chemotherapy in whom the anemia can be managed by transfusion; Patients who require immediate correction of anemia when RBC transfusions can be used instead; Patients scheduled for surgery who are willing to donate

autologous blood; Patients undergoing cardiac or vascular surgery; OB, Lactation: Multidose vials should not be used as they contain benzyl alcohol and may cause fatal gasping syndrome in fetus in utero and breastfed infants; Pedi: Neutropenia in newborns; multidose vials should not be used in neonates and infants, as they contain benzyl alcohol, which can cause potentially fatal gasping syndrome.

Use Cautiously in: History of seizures or stroke; Cardiovascular disease; History of porphyria; Lactation: Use while breastfeeding only if potential maternal benefit justifies potential risk to infant.

Adverse Reactions/Side Effects

CV: hypertension, HF, MI, THROMBOEMBOLIC EVENTS (especially with Hgb >11 g/dL). **Derm:** ERYTHEMA MULTIFORME, STEVENS-JOHNSON SYNDROME, TOXIC EPIDERMAL NECROLYSIS, transient rash. **Endo:** restored fertility, resumption of menses. **Neuro:** headache, SEIZURES, STROKE. **Misc:** ↑ MORTALITY AND ↑ TUMOR GROWTH (especially with Hgb >12 g/dL).

Interactions

Drug-Drug: May ↑ requirement for **heparin** anticoagulation during hemodialysis.

Route/Dosage

Anemia of Chronic Kidney Disease

(Do not initiate if Hgb ≥10 g/dL).
SUBQ, IV (Adults): 50–100 units/kg 3 times weekly initially; use lowest dose sufficient to ↓ the need for RBC transfusions (do not exceed Hgb of 11 g/dL [patients on dialysis] or 10 g/dL [patients not on dialysis]); if Hgb ↑ by >1.0 g/dL in 2 wk, ↓ dose by 25%; if Hgb ↑ by <1.0 g/dL after 4 wk of therapy (with adequate iron stores), ↑ dose by 25%; do not ↑ dose more frequently than every 4 wk.
SUBQ, IV (Children 1 mo–16 yr): 50 units/kg 3 times weekly initially; use lowest dose sufficient to ↓ the need for RBC transfusions (do not exceed Hgb of 12 g/dL; if Hgb ↑ by >1.0 g/dL in 2 wk, ↓ dose by 25%; if Hgb ↑ by <1.0 g/dL after 4 wk of therapy (with adequate iron stores), ↑ dose by 25%; do not ↑ dose more frequently than every 4 wk.

Anemia Secondary to Zidovudine Therapy

SUBQ, IV (Adults): 100 units/kg 3 times weekly for 8 wk; if inadequate response, may ↑ by 50–100 units/kg every 4–8 wk (max: 300 units/kg 3 times weekly).
SUBQ, IV (Children 8 mo–17 yr): 50–400 units/kg 2–3 times weekly.

Anemia From Chemotherapy

(Use only for chemotherapy-related anemia and discontinue when chemotherapy course is completed; do not initiate if Hgb ≥10 g/dL).
SUBQ (Adults): 150 units/kg 3 times weekly or 40,000 units weekly; adjust dose to maintain lowest Hgb level sufficient to avoid RBC transfusions (do not exceed Hgb of 12 g/dL; if Hgb ↑ by >1.0 g/dL in 2 wk or reaches a level needed to avoid RBC transfusions, ↓ dose by 25%; if Hgb ↑ by <1.0 g/dL (and remains <10 g/dL) after ini-

tial 4 wk of therapy (with adequate iron stores), ↑ dose to 300 units/kg 3 times weekly or 60,000 units weekly.
IV (Children 5–18 yr): 600 units/kg weekly; adjust dose to maintain lowest hemoglobin level sufficient to avoid RBC transfusions (do not exceed Hgb of 12 g/dL); if Hgb ↑ by >1.0 g/dL in 2 wk or reaches a level needed to avoid RBC transfusions, ↓ dose by 25%; if Hgb ↑ by <1.0 g/dL (and remains <10 g/dL) after initial 4 wk of therapy (with adequate iron stores), ↑ dose to 900 units/kg (maximum = 60,000 units) weekly.

Surgery

SUBQ (Adults): 300 units/kg/day for 10 days before surgery, day of surgery, and 4 days after or 600 units/kg 21, 14, and 7 days before surgery and on day of surgery.

Availability

Solution for injection: 2,000 units/mL, 3,000 units/mL, 4,000 units/mL, 10,000 units/mL, 20,000 units/mL, 40,000 units/mL. **Solution for injection (prefilled syringes):** ✸ 1,000 units/0.5 mL, ✸ 2,000 units/0.5 mL, ✸ 3,000 units/0.3 mL, ✸ 4,000 units/0.4 mL, ✸ 5,000 units/0.5 mL, ✸ 6000 units/0.6 mL, ✸ 8,000 units/0.8 mL, ✸ 10,000 units/1 mL, ✸ 20,000 units/0.5 mL, ✸ 30,000 units/0.75 mL, ✸ 40,000 units/1 mL.

NURSING IMPLICATIONS

Assessment

● Monitor BP before and during therapy. Inform health care professional if severe hypertension is present or if BP begins to increase. Additional antihypertensive therapy may be required during initiation of therapy.
● Monitor for symptoms of anemia (fatigue, dyspnea, pallor).
● Monitor dialysis shunts (thrill and bruit) and status of artificial kidney during hemodialysis. Heparin dose may need to be increased to prevent clotting. Monitor patients with underlying vascular disease for impaired circulation.

Lab Test Considerations

● May cause ↑ in WBCs and platelets. May ↓ bleeding times.
● Monitor serum ferritin, transferrin, and iron levels to assess need for concurrent iron therapy. Administer supplemental iron therapy when serum ferritin <100 mcg/L or when serum transferrin saturation <20%.
● Monitor Hgb weekly until the Hgb level is stable and sufficient to minimize the need for RBC transfusion after starting therapy and after each dose adjustment.
● **Anemia of CKD:** Monitor Hgb at least weekly until stable, then at least monthly. Do not ↑ dose more frequently than once every 4 wk. A ↓ in dose can be made more frequently. Avoid frequent dose adjustments. *If Hgb ↑ >12 g/dL in a 2-wk period*, ↓ dose by 25% or more. *If Hgb ↑ by <1 g/dL over 4 wk (and iron stores are adequate)*, ↑ dose by 25%. If no response after 12 wk of escalation, further dose ↑ is unlikely to improve response and may ↑ risks. Use lowest dose that will maintain Hgb level sufficient to reduce need for RBC transfusions.

- **Adults With Anemia of CKD on Dialysis:** Start epoetin when Hgb >10 g/dL. If Hgb ≥11 g/dL, reduce or hold dose.
- **Adults With Anemia of CKD not on Dialysis:** Start epoetin only when Hgb <10 g/dL AND rate of Hgb decline indicates likelihood of requiring a RBC transfusion AND reducing risk of alloimmunization and/or other RBC transfusion-related risks is a goal. If Hgb level >10 g/dL, reduce or hold dose, and use lowest epoetin dose sufficient to reduce need for RBC transfusions.
- **Children With Anemia of CKD:** Start epoetin only when Hgb <10 g/dL. If Hgb level >12 g/dL, reduce or hold dose.
- Monitor renal function studies and electrolytes closely; resulting increased sense of well-being may lead to decreased compliance with other therapies for renal failure. Increases in BUN, serum creatinine, uric acid, phosphorus, and potassium may occur.
- **Anemia Secondary to Zidovudine Therapy:** Before initiating therapy, determine serum erythropoietin level before transfusion. Patients receiving zidovudine with endogenous serum erythropoietin levels >500 mUnits/mL may not respond to therapy. *If Hgb does not ↑ after 8 wk of therapy,* ↑ dose by 50–100 units/kg at 4–8 wk intervals until Hgb reaches level needed to avoid RBC transfusions or 300 units/kg. *If Hgb ≥12 g/dL,* hold dose until Hgb drops to <11 g/dL, then ↓ dose by 25%. *If ↑ in Hgb is not achieved at a dose of 300 Units/kg for 8 wk,* discontinue therapy.
- **Anemia From Chemotherapy:** Start epoetin only if Hgb ≥10 g/dL and there is an additional 2 mo of planned chemotherapy. Patients with lower baseline serum erythropoietin levels may respond more rapidly; not recommended if levels >200 mUnits/mL. *If Hgb ↑ by >1 g/dL in any 2-wk period or Hgb reaches level needed to avoid RBC transfusion,* ↓ dose by 25%. *If Hgb ↑ by <1 g/dL after 4 wk in absence of RBC transfusion and remains <10 g/dL,* ↑ dose to 300 units/kg three times per wk in adults or 60,000 units weekly (adults) or 900 units/kg (max: 60,000 units) in children. *If no response in Hgb levels or if RBC transfusions are still required after 8 wk of therapy,* discontinue epoetin.
- **Surgery:** Implement prophylaxis of deep venous thrombosis during therapy.

Implementation

IV Administration
- Transfusions are still required for severe symptomatic anemia. Supplemental iron should be initiated with epoetin and continued throughout therapy.
- Institute seizure precautions in patients who experience greater than a 4-point increase in hematocrit in a 2-wk period or exhibit any change in neurologic status. Risk of seizures is greatest during the first 90 days of therapy.
- Do not shake vial; inactivation of medication may occur. Solution is clear and colorless; do not adminis-

ter solutions that are discolored, cloudy, or contain a precipitate. Discard vial immediately after withdrawing dose from single-use 1-mL vial. Refrigerate multidose vials; stable for 21 days after initial entry.
- **SUBQ:** This route is often used for patients not requiring dialysis.
- May be admixed in syringe immediately before administration with 0.9% NaCl with benzyl alcohol 0.9% in a 1:1 ratio to prevent injection site discomfort.
- **IV Push:** *Dilution:* Administer undiluted or dilute with an equal amount of 0.9% NaCl. *Concentration:* 1000–40,000 units/mL. *Rate:* May be administered as direct injection or bolus over 1–3 min into IV tubing or via venous line at end of dialysis session.
- **Y-Site Compatibility:** amikacin, aminophylline, ascorbic acid, atracurium, atropine, azathioprine, aztreonam, benztropine, bumetanide, buprenorphine, butorphanol, calcium chloride, calcium gluconate, cefazolin, cefotaxime, cefotetan, cefoxitin, ceftazidime, ceftriaxone, cefuroxime, chloramphenicol, clindamycin, cyanocobalamin, cyclosporine, dexamethasone, digoxin, diphenhydramine, dobutamine, dopamine, doxycycline, enalaprilat, ephedrine, epinephrine, erythromycin, esmolol, famotidine, fentanyl, fluconazole, folic acid, furosemide, ganciclovir, gentamicin, glycopyrrolate, heparin, hydrocortisone, imipenem/cilastatin, indomethacin, insulin, regular, isoproterenol, ketorolac, labetalol, LR, lidocaine, magnesium sulfate, mannitol, meperidine, methylprednisolone, metoclopramide, metoprolol, morphine, multivitamins, nafcillin, nalbuphine, naloxone, nitroglycerin, nitroprusside, norepinephrine, ondansetron, oxacillin, oxytocin, penicillin G, pentobarbital, phenobarbital, phentolamine, phenylephrine, phytonadione, potassium chloride, procainamide, promethazine, propranolol, protamine, pyridoxine, sodium bicarbonate, succinylcholine, sufentanil, theophylline, tobramycin, vasopressin, verapamil.
- **Y-Site Incompatibility:** amphotericin B deoxycholate, chlorpromazine, dantrolene, diazepam, haloperidol, midazolam, minocycline, pentamidine, phenytoin, prochlorperazine, trimethoprim/sulfamethoxazole, vancomycin.

Patient/Family Teaching
- Advise patient to read the *Medication Guide* prior to initiating therapy and with each Rx refill in case of changes. Patient must sign the patient–health care provider acknowledgment form before each course of therapy.
- Explain rationale for concurrent iron therapy (increased RBC production requires iron).
- Discuss ways of preventing self-injury in patients at risk for seizures. Driving and activities requiring continuous alertness should be avoided.
- Inform patient that use of epoetin may result in shortened overall survival and/or ↓ time to tumor progression.

- Advise patient to notify health care professional immediately if signs and symptoms of blood clots (chest pain, trouble breathing or shortness of breath; pain in the legs, with or without swelling; a cool or pale arm or leg; sudden confusion; trouble speaking or trouble understanding others' speech; sudden numbness or weakness in the face, arm, or leg, especially on one side of the body; sudden trouble seeing; sudden trouble walking, dizziness, loss of balance or coordination; loss of consciousness or fainting; hemodialysis vascular access stops working), allergic reactions (rash, itching, shortness of breath, wheezing, dizziness and fainting, swelling around mouth or eyes, fast pulse, sweating), skin reactions (blisters, skin sores, peeling, or areas of skin coming off) occur.
- Advise patient to inform health care professional of medication prior to treatment or surgery.
- Rep: Discuss possible return of menses and fertility with health care professional. Advise female patients of reproductive potential to notify health care professional if pregnancy is planned or suspected or if breastfeeding.
- **Anemia of CKD:** Stress importance of compliance with dietary restrictions, medications, and dialysis. Foods high in iron and low in potassium include liver, pork, veal, beef, mustard and turnip greens, peas, eggs, broccoli, kale, blackberries, strawberries, apple juice, watermelon, oatmeal, and enriched bread. Epoetin will result in increased sense of well-being, but it does not cure underlying disease.
- **Home Care Issues:** Home dialysis patients determined to be able to safely and effectively administer epoetin should be taught proper dosage, administration technique, and disposal of equipment. *Information for Home Dialysis Patients* should be provided to patient along with medication.

Evaluation/Desired Outcomes

- Increase in hematocrit to 30–36% with improvement in symptoms of anemia in patients with chronic renal failure.
- Increase in hematocrit in anemia secondary to zidovudine therapy.
- Increase in hematocrit in patients with anemia resulting from chemotherapy.
- Reduction of need for RBC transfusions after surgery.

HIGH ALERT

eptifibatide (ep-ti-fib-a-tide)
Integrilin
Classification
Therapeutic: antiplatelet agents
Pharmacologic: glycoprotein IIb/IIIa inhibitors

Indications
Acute coronary syndrome (unstable angina/non-ST-elevation MI), including patients who will be managed medically and those who will undergo percutaneous coronary intervention (PCI). Patients undergoing PCI, including intracoronary stenting.

Action
Decreases platelet aggregation by reversibly antagonizing the binding of fibrinogen to the glycoprotein IIb/IIIa binding site on platelet surfaces. **Therapeutic Effects:** Reduction in risk of death or new MI in patients with acute coronary syndrome. Reduction in risk of death, new MI, or need for urgent intervention in patients undergoing PCI.

Pharmacokinetics
Absorption: IV administration results in complete bioavailability.
Distribution: Unknown.
Metabolism and Excretion: 50% excreted by the kidneys.
Half-life: 2.5 hr.

TIME/ACTION PROFILE (effects on platelet function)

ROUTE	ONSET	PEAK	DURATION
IV	immediate	following bolus	brief†

†Inhibition is reversible following cessation of infusion.

Contraindications/Precautions
Contraindicated in: Hypersensitivity; Active internal bleeding or history of bleeding within previous 30 days; Severe uncontrolled hypertension (systolic BP >200 mm Hg and/or diastolic BP >110 mm Hg); Major surgical procedure within 6 wk; History of hemorrhagic stroke or other stroke within 30 days; Concurrent use of other glycoprotein IIb/IIIa receptor antagonists; Platelet count <100,000/mm³; Severe renal impairment (serum creatinine ≥4 mg/dL) or dependency on renal dialysis.

Use Cautiously in: Renal impairment (↓ infusion rate if CCr <50 mL/min); OB: Safety not established in pregnancy; Lactation: Safety not established in breastfeeding; Pedi: Safety and effectiveness not established in children; Geri: ↑ risk of bleeding in older adults.

Adverse Reactions/Side Effects
Noted for patients receiving heparin and aspirin in addition to eptifibatide.
CV: hypotension. **Hemat:** BLEEDING (including GI and intracranial bleeding, hematuria, and hematomas), thrombocytopenia.

Interactions
Drug-Drug: ↑ risk of bleeding with other drugs that affect hemostasis (**heparins, warfarin, NSAIDs, thrombolytic agents, dipyridamole, clopidogrel,** some **cephalosporins, valproates**).
Drug-Natural Products: ↑ bleeding risk with **arnica, chamomile, clove, dong quai, feverfew, garlic, ginger, ginkgo,** and ***Panax ginseng***.

Route/Dosage

Acute Coronary Syndrome

IV (Adults): 180 mcg/kg (max = 22.6 mg) as a bolus dose, followed by 2 mcg/kg/min (max = 15 mg/hr) infusion until hospital discharge or initiation of coronary artery bypass graft surgery (up to 72 hr). If a patient is to undergo PCI, the infusion should be continued until hospital discharge or for up to 18–24 hr after the PCI, whichever comes first, allowing for up to 96 hr of therapy.

Renal Impairment

IV (Adults): *CrCl <50 mL/min:* 180 mcg/kg (max = 22.6 mg) as a bolus dose, followed by 1 mcg/kg/min (max = 7.4 mg/hr) infusion until hospital discharge or initiation of coronary artery bypass graft surgery (up to 72 hr). If a patient is to undergo PCI, the infusion should be continued until hospital discharge or for up to 18–24 hr after the PCI, whichever comes first, allowing for up to 96 hr of therapy.

Percutaneous Coronary Intervention

IV (Adults): 180 mcg/kg (max = 22.6 mg) as a bolus dose, immediately before PCI, followed by 2 mcg/kg/min (max = 15 mg/hr) infusion; a 2nd bolus of 180 mcg/kg (max = 22.6 mg) is given 10 min after 1st bolus. Infusion should be continued until hospital discharge, or for up to 18 to 24 hr, whichever comes first (minimum of 12 hr).

Renal Impairment

(Adults): *CrCl <50 mL/min:* 180 mcg/kg (max = 22.6 mg) bolus followed by 1 mcg/kg/min (max = 7.4 mg/hr) infusion; a 2nd bolus of 180 mcg/kg (max = 22.6 mg) is given 10 min after 1st bolus.

Availability (generic available)

Solution for injection: 20 mg/10 mL, 75 mg/100 mL, 200 mg/100 mL.

NURSING IMPLICATIONS

Assessment

- Assess for bleeding. Most common sites are arterial access site for cardiac catheterization or GI or GU tract. Minimize arterial and venous punctures, IM injections, and use of urinary catheters, nasotracheal intubation, and nasogastric tubes. Avoid noncompressible sites for IV access. If bleeding cannot be controlled with pressure, discontinue eptifibatide and heparin immediately.

Lab Test Considerations

- Prior to eptifibatide therapy, assess hemoglobin or hematocrit, platelet count, serum creatinine, and PT/aPTT. Activated clotting time (ACT) should also be measured in patients undergoing PCI.
- Maintain the aPTT between 50 and 70 sec unless PCI is to be performed. Maintain ACT between 300 and 350 sec during PCI.

- Arterial sheath should not be removed unless aPTT <45 sec.
- If platelet count decreases to <100,000 and is confirmed, discontinue eptifibatide and heparin and monitor and treat condition.

Implementation

- *High Alert:* Accidental overdose of antiplatelet medications has resulted in patient harm or death from internal hemorrhage or intracranial bleeding. Have second practitioner independently check original order, dose calculations, and infusion pump settings.
- Most patients receive heparin and aspirin concurrently with eptifibatide.
- After PCI, femoral artery sheath may be removed during eptifibatide treatment only after heparin has been discontinued and its effects mostly reversed.
- Do not administer solutions that are discolored or contain particulate matter. Discard unused portion.

IV Administration

- **IV Push:** *High Alert: Dilution:* Withdraw appropriate loading dose from bolus vial (20 mg/10-mL vial) into a syringe. Administer undiluted. *Concentration:* 2 mg/mL. *Rate:* Administer over 1–2 min.
- **Continuous Infusion:** *Dilution:* Administer undiluted directly from the 100-mL vial via an infusion pump. *Concentration:* 0.75 mg/mL or 2 mg/mL (depends on vial used). *Rate:* Based on patient's weight (see Route/Dosage section).
- **Y-Site Compatibility:** alemtuzumab, alteplase, amikacin, amiodarone, amphotericin B lipid complex, amphotericin B liposomal, ampicillin, ampicillin/sulbactam, anidulafungin, argatroban, arsenic trioxide, atracurium, atropine, azithromycin, aztreonam, bivalirudin, bumetanide, buprenorphine, butorphanol, calcium chloride, calcium gluconate, cangrelor, cefepime, cefotaxime, cefotetan, ceftazidime, ceftolozane/tazobactam, ceftriaxone, cefuroxime, ciprofloxacin, cisatracurium, clindamycin, cyclosporine, daptomycin, dexamethasone, dexrazoxane, D5/0.9% NaCl, digoxin, diltiazem, diphenhydramine, dobutamine, dopamine, doxorubicin liposomal, doxycycline, droperidol, enalaprilat, ephedrine, epinephrine, ertapenem, erythromycin, esmolol, famotidine, fentanyl, fluconazole, foscarnet, fosphenytoin, ganciclovir, gentamicin, granisetron, haloperidol, heparin, hydrocortisone, hydromorphone, imipenem/cilastatin, isavuconazonium, isoproterenol, ketorolac, labetalol, leucovorin calcium, levofloxacin, lidocaine, linezolid, lorazepam, magnesium sulfate, mannitol, meperidine, meropenem, meropenem/vaborbactam, methylprednisolone, metoclopramide, metoprolol, micafungin, midazolam, milrinone, morphine, nalbuphine, naloxone, nicardipine, nitroglycerin, nitroprusside, octreotide, ondansetron, oxytocin, palonosetron, pemetrexed, pentobarbital, phenobarbital, phenylephrine, piperacillin/tazobactam, plazomicin, potassium acetate, potassium chloride, potassium

phosphate, procainamide, prochlorperazine, promethazine, propranolol, remifentanil, rocuronium, sodium bicarbonate, sodium phosphate, succinylcholine, sufentanil, tedizolid, theophylline, tigecycline, tirofiban, tobramycin, vancomycin, vecuronium, verapamil, zidovudine, zoledronic acid.

- **Y-Site Incompatibility:** acyclovir, amphotericin B deoxycholate, chlorpromazine, diazepam, furosemide, gemtuzumab ozogamicin, methohexital, mycophenolate, pentamidine, phenytoin, thiopental.

Patient/Family Teaching

- Inform patient of the purpose of eptifibatide.
- Instruct patient to notify health care professional immediately if any bleeding is noted.
- Advise patient to notify health care professional of all Rx or OTC medications, vitamins, or herbal products being taken and to consult with health care professional before taking other medications.
- Advise females of reproductive potential to notify health care professional if pregnancy is planned or suspected or if breastfeeding.

Evaluation/Desired Outcomes

- Reduction in risk of death or new MI in patients with acute coronary syndrome.
- Reduction in risk of death, new MI, or need for urgent intervention in patients undergoing PCI.

---

erenumab (e-ren-ue-mab)
Aimovig
Classification
Therapeutic: vascular headache suppressants
Pharmacologic: monoclonal antibodies, calcitonin gene-related peptide receptor antagonists

Indications
Migraine prevention.

Action
Monoclonal antibody that binds to the calcitonin gene-related peptide (CGRP) receptor, which reduces the neuroinflammatory and vasodilatory effects of CGRP.
Therapeutic Effects: Reduction in frequency of migraines.

Pharmacokinetics
Absorption: Well absorbed (82%) following SUBQ administration.
Distribution: Some tissue distribution.
Metabolism and Excretion: *Low concentrations:* Eliminated through saturable binding to CGRP receptor; *High concentrations:* Eliminated through nonspecific, nonsaturable proteolytic pathway.
Half-life: 28 days.

TIME/ACTION PROFILE (plasma concentrations)

ROUTE	ONSET	PEAK	DURATION
SUBQ	unknown	6 days	1 mo

Contraindications/Precautions
Contraindicated in: Hypersensitivity.
Use Cautiously in: Hypertension; OB: Safety not established in pregnancy; Lactation: Safety not established in breastfeeding; Pedi: Safety and effectiveness not established in children; Geri: Choose dose carefully in older adults, considering concurrent disease states, drug therapy, and age-related ↓ in hepatic and renal function.

Adverse Reactions/Side Effects
CV: hypertension. **GI:** constipation. **Local:** injection site reactions. **MS:** muscle spasm. **Misc:** HYPERSENSITIVITY REACTIONS (including anaphylaxis and angioedema).

Interactions
Drug-Drug: Medications that ↓ GI motility may ↑ risk of more severe constipation.

Route/Dosage
SUBQ (Adults): 70 mg once monthly; may ↑ dose, if needed, to 140 mg once monthly.

Availability
Solution for injection (prefilled syringes and autoinjectors): 70 mg/mL, 140 mg/mL.

NURSING IMPLICATIONS
Assessment

- Assess frequency and intensity of migraines.
- Assess for latex allergy. Needle shield within white or orange cap of prefilled autoinjector and gray needle cap of prefilled syringe contain dry natural rubber (a derivative of latex), may cause allergic reactions in individuals sensitive to latex.
- Monitor for new-onset hypertension, or worsening of pre-existing hypertension. May require discontinuation.
- Monitor for signs and symptoms of hypersensitivity reactions (rash, angioedema, anaphylaxis); usually occur within hr of injection but >1 wk after injection. If reaction is severe, discontinue erenumab and treat as needed.

Implementation

- **SUBQ:** Prior to use allow vial to sit at room temperature for at least 30 min, protect from direct sunlight. Do not use other methods to warm solution (hot water or microwave). Do not shake. Solution is clear to opalescent, colorless to light yellow; do not administer solutions that are discolored, cloudy, or contain particulate matter. Store in refrigerator in original carton to protect from light; do not freeze. May be stored up to 7 days at room temperature.
- Inject entire contents into abdomen, thigh, or upper arm. Do not inject into areas where the skin is tender, bruised, red, or hard.

Patient/Family Teaching

- Instruct patient to take as directed. Administer missed doses as soon as possible and schedule next dose 1 mo from last dose administered. Educate patient and/or caregiver on correct technique for injection and disposal of equipment. Advise patient to read *Patient Information* before starting therapy and with each Rx refill in case of changes.

- Instruct patient to notify health care professional immediately if signs and symptoms of hypersensitivity reaction (swelling of face, mouth, tongue or throat, trouble breathing, rash) occur.
- Advise patient to notify health care professional if severe constipation occurs; may cause serious complications.
- Advise patient to notify health care professional of all Rx or OTC medications, vitamins, or herbal products being taken and to consult with health care professional before taking other medications.
- Rep: Advise females of reproductive potential to notify health care professional if pregnancy is planned or suspected or if breastfeeding.

Evaluation/Desired Outcomes

- Decrease in frequency and intensity of migraines.

---

ergocalciferol, See VITAMIN D COMPOUNDS.

⚹ erlotinib (er-lo-ti-nib)

Tarceva

Classification

Therapeutic: antineoplastics

Pharmacologic: enzyme inhibitors

Indications

⚹ Treatment of metastatic non–small-cell lung cancer (NSCLC) that has epidermal growth factor exon 19 deletions or exon 21 substitution mutations in patients who are receiving first-line, maintenance, or second or greater line treatment after progression following ≥1 previous chemotherapy regimen. First-line therapy for locally advanced, surgically unresectable, or metastatic pancreatic cancer (in combination with gemcitabine).

Action

⚹ Inhibits the enzyme tyrosine kinase, which is associated with human epidermal growth factor receptor (EGFR); blocks growth stimulation signals in cancer cells. **Therapeutic Effects:** Decreased spread of lung or pancreatic cancer with increased survival.

Pharmacokinetics

Absorption: 60% absorbed; bioavailability ↑ to 100% with food.

Distribution: Unknown.

Protein Binding: 93% protein bound.

Metabolism and Excretion: Mostly metabolized by the liver, primarily by the CYP3A4 isoenzyme. 83% excreted in feces (<1% as unchanged drug) and 8% excreted in urine (<1% as unchanged drug).

Half-life: 36 hr.

TIME/ACTION PROFILE (plasma concentrations)

ROUTE	ONSET	PEAK	DURATION
PO	unknown	4 hr	24 hr

Contraindications/Precautions

Contraindicated in: OB: Pregnancy; Lactation: Lactation.

Use Cautiously in: Hepatic impairment; Previous chemotherapy/radiation, pre-existing lung disease, metastatic lung disease (may ↑ risk of interstitial lung disease); Rep: Women of reproductive potential; Pedi: Safety and effectiveness not established in children.

Adverse Reactions/Side Effects

CV: MYOCARDIAL INFARCTION/ISCHEMIA (pancreatic cancer patients). **Derm:** rash, BULLOUS AND EXFOLIATIVE SKIN DISORDERS, dry skin, pruritus. **EENT:** ↓ tear production, abnormal eyelash growth, conjunctivitis, corneal perforation, corneal ulceration, keratitis. **GI:** diarrhea, HEPATOTOXICITY, ↑ liver enzymes, abdominal pain, anorexia, GI PERFORATION, nausea, stomatitis, vomiting. **GU:** RENAL FAILURE. **Hemat:** microangiopathic hemolytic anemia with thrombocytopenia (pancreatic cancer patients). **Neuro:** CEREBROVASCULAR ACCIDENT (pancreatic cancer patients), fatigue. **Resp:** dyspnea, cough, INTERSTITIAL LUNG DISEASE.

Interactions

Drug-Drug: Strong CYP3A4 inhibitors, including **atazanavir, clarithromycin, itraconazole, ketoconazole, nefazodone, nelfinavir, ritonavir,** or **voriconazole** ↑ levels and the risk of toxicity; consider alternative therapy or ↓ erlotinib dose. **Strong CYP3A4 inducers,** including **rifampin, rifabutin, rifapentine, phenytoin, carbamazepine,** or **phenobarbital,** ↓ levels and may ↓ response; consider alternative therapy or ↑ erlotinib dose. **CYP1A2 inhibitors,** including **ciprofloxacin,** may ↑ levels and the risk of toxicity; consider ↓ erlotinib dose if used with CYP3A4 inhibitor. **Smoking** may ↓ levels and may ↓ response; avoid smoking during therapy or consider ↑ erlotinib dose if smoking continues. **Moderate CYP1A2 inducers,** including **teriflunomide, rifampin,** or **phenytoin;** avoid concurrent use or ↑ erlotinib dose. May ↓ **midazolam** levels. May ↑ risk of bleeding with **warfarin.** ↓ levels with **proton pump inhibitors, H₂ blockers,** and **antacids;** avoid concurrent use with **proton pump inhibitors;** take 10 hr after **H₂ antagonist** and ≥2 hr before next dose of **H₂ antagonist;** separate from **antacid** by several hr.

Drug-Natural Products: St. John's wort may ↓ levels and may ↓ response; alternative therapy or ↑ dose should be considered.

Drug-Food: Grapefruit juice or grapefruit, a strong CYP3A4 inhibitor, ↑ levels and the risk of toxicity; consider dose ↓.

⚹ = Canadian drug name. ⚹ = Genetic implication. ~~Strikethrough~~ = Discontinued. CAPITALS = life-threatening. <u>Underline</u> = most frequent.

Route/Dosage

Non–Small-Cell Lung Cancer

PO (Adults): 150 mg once daily; *Concurrent use of strong CYP3A4 inhibitor or concurrent use of CYP3A4 and CYP1A2 inhibitor (e.g., ciprofloxacin):* Consider ↓ dose in 50-mg increments (avoid concomitant use, if possible); *Concurrent use of strong CYP3A4 inducer:* consider ↑ dose by 50 mg every 2 wk (max dose = 450 mg/day) (avoid concomitant use, if possible); *Concurrent cigarette smoking or concurrent use of moderate CYP1A2 inducer:* ↑ dose by 50 mg every 2 wk (max dose = 300 mg/day); immediately ↓ dose to recommended initial dose for indication upon smoking cessation.

Pancreatic Cancer

PO (Adults): 100 mg once daily. *Concurrent use of strong CYP3A4 inhibitor or concurrent use of CYP3A4 and CYP1A2 inhibitor (e.g., ciprofloxacin):* Consider ↓ dose in 50-mg increments (avoid concomitant use, if possible); *Concurrent use of strong CYP3A4 inducer:* consider ↑ dose by 50 mg every 2 wk (max dose = 450 mg/day) (avoid concomitant use, if possible); *Concurrent cigarette smoking or concurrent use of moderate CYP1A2 inducer:* ↑ dose by 50 mg every 2 wk (max dose = 300 mg/day); immediately ↓ dose to recommended initial dose for indication upon smoking cessation.

Availability (generic available)

Tablets: 25 mg, 100 mg, 150 mg.

NURSING IMPLICATIONS

Assessment

- Assess respiratory status prior to and periodically during therapy. If dyspnea, cough, or fever occur, discontinue erlotinib, assess for interstitial lung disease, and institute treatment as needed.
- Assess for diarrhea. Usually responds to loperamide but may require dose reduction or discontinuation of therapy if unresponsive to therapy or patient becomes dehydrated.
- Assess skin during therapy. If bullous, blistering, and exfoliative skin conditions, including Stevens-Johnson syndrome/toxic epidermal necrolysis, occur, interrupt or discontinue treatment. Skin rash may require treatment with corticosteroids or anti-infectives with anti-inflammatory properties; acne treatments may aggravate dry skin and erythema.
- Assess eyes periodically during therapy. Discontinue erlotinib if corneal ulceration occurs. Hold erlotinib if Grade 3 or 4 keratitis, or Grade 2 lasting >2 wk, or if acute or worsening eye pain or disorders occur.
- Assess for GI pain. Patients receiving concomitant antiangiogenic agents, corticosteroids, NSAIDs, and/or taxane-based chemotherapy, or who have prior history of peptic ulceration or diverticular disease, are at increased risk for GI perforation. Permanently discontinue erlotinib in patients who develop gastrointestinal perforation.

Lab Test Considerations

- ⚗ Test patients for EGFR exon 19 deletions or exon 21 (L858R) substitution mutations in plasma or tumor specimens prior to starting therapy; presence is required for therapy. Information on FDA-approved tests for the detection of EGFR mutations in NSCLC is available at: http://www.fda.gov/CompanionDiagnostics.
- Monitor liver function tests (AST, ALT, bilirubin, alkaline phosphatase) periodically during therapy. Consider dose reduction or discontinuation of therapy if severe changes in liver function (doubling or tripling of transaminase levels in *patients with pre-existing hepatic impairment* or total bilirubin ≥3 times upper limit of normal and/or transaminases ≥5 times upper limit of normal in *patients without pre-existing hepatic impairment*) occur.
- Monitor renal function and electrolytes in patients at risk for dehydration. Withhold therapy if dehydration or Grade 3 or 4 renal toxicity occurs.
- Monitor INR regularly in patients taking warfarin. May cause ↑ INR.

Implementation

- Do not confuse Tarceva with Tresiba.
- **PO:** Administer at least 1 hr before or 2 hr after food.

Patient/Family Teaching

- Instruct patient to take erlotinib as directed.
- Advise patient to notify health care professional if severe or persistent diarrhea, nausea, anorexia, vomiting, onset or worsening of skin rash, unexplained dyspnea or cough, eye irritation, or signs and symptoms of a cerebrovascular accident (sudden weakness; paralysis [an inability to move] or numbness of the face, arms, or legs, especially on one side of the body; confusion; trouble speaking or understanding speech; trouble seeing in one or both eyes; problems breathing; dizziness, trouble walking, loss of balance or coordination, unexplained falls; loss of consciousness; sudden and severe headache) occur.
- Instruct patient to avoid proton pump inhibitors and if antacids are necessary, separate antacids and erlotinib dose by several hr. If therapy with H₂ antagonists is required, take erlotinib 10 hr after H₂ antagonist and at least 2 hr before next dose of H₂ antagonist.
- Advise patient to notify health care professional of all Rx or OTC medications, vitamins, or herbal products being taken and consult health care professional before taking any new medications.
- Advise patient to wear sunscreen and protective clothing to decrease skin reactions.
- Instruct patient to discontinue smoking during therapy; smoking decreases blood levels of erlotinib.
- Rep: May cause fetal harm. Caution females of reproductive potential to use highly effective contraceptive during and for at least 1 mo after completion of therapy and to avoid breastfeeding during and for at least 2 wk following last dose. Advise female patients to notify health care professional if pregnancy is planned or suspected.

Evaluation/Desired Outcomes

- Decrease in spread of non–small-cell lung or pancreatic cancer with increased survival.

ertapenem (er-ta-**pen**-em)
~~INVanz~~
Classification
Therapeutic: anti-infectives
Pharmacologic: carbapenems

Indications

Complicated intra-abdominal infections. Complicated skin and skin structure infections (including diabetic foot infections with osteomyelitis). Community acquired pneumonia. Complicated urinary tract infections (including pyelonephritis). Acute pelvic infections (including postpartum endomyometritis, septic abortion, and postsurgical gynecologic infections). Prophylaxis of surgical site infection following elective colorectal surgery.

Action

Binds to bacterial cell wall, resulting in cell death. Ertapenem resists the actions of many enzymes that degrade most other penicillins and penicillin-like anti-infectives. **Therapeutic Effects:** Bactericidal action against susceptible bacteria. **Spectrum:** Active against the following aerobic gram-positive organisms: *Staphylococcus aureus* (methicillin-susceptible strains only), *Staphylococcus epidermidis*, *Streptococcus agalactiae*, *S. pneumoniae* (penicillin-susceptible strains only), and *S. pyogenes.* Also active against the following gram-negative aerobic organisms: *Escherichia coli, Haemophilus influenzae* (beta-lactamase negative strains), *Klebsiella pneumonia, Moraxella catarrhalis,* and *Providencia rettgeri.* Additional anaerobic spectrum includes *Bacteroides fragilis, B. distasonis, B. ovatus, B. thetaiotamicron, B. uniformis, B. vulgatis, Clostridioides clostrioforme, Eubacterium lentum, Peptostreptococcus, Porphyromonas asaccharolytica,* and *Prevotella bivia.*

Pharmacokinetics

Absorption: 90% after IM administration; IV administration results in complete bioavailability.
Distribution: Enters breast milk.
Metabolism and Excretion: Mostly excreted by the kidneys.
Half-life: 1.8 hr (↑ in renal impairment).

TIME/ACTION PROFILE (blood levels)

ROUTE	ONSET	PEAK	DURATION
IM	rapid	2 hr	24 hr
IV	rapid	end of infusion	24 hr

Contraindications/Precautions

Contraindicated in: Hypersensitivity; Cross-sensitivity may occur with penicillins, cephalosporins, and other carbapenems; Hypersensitivity to lidocaine (may be used as a diluent for IM administration).
Use Cautiously in: History of multiple hypersensitivity reactions; Seizure disorders; Renal impairment; OB: Safety not established in pregnancy; Lactation: Use during breastfeeding only if potential maternal benefit to patient justifies potential risk to infant; Pedi: Safety and effectiveness not established in children; Geri: ↑ sensitivity due to age-related ↓ in renal function in older adults.

Adverse Reactions/Side Effects

Derm: ACUTE GENERALIZED EXANTHEMATOUS PUSTULOSIS. **GI:** CLOSTRIDIOIDES DIFFICILE-ASSOCIATED DIARRHEA (CDAD), diarrhea, nausea, vomiting. **GU:** vaginitis. **Local:** pain at IM site, phlebitis at IV site. **Neuro:** headache, SEIZURES. **Misc:** HYPERSENSITIVITY REACTIONS (including anaphylaxis).

Interactions

Drug-Drug: Probenecid ↓ excretion and ↑ levels. May ↓ serum **valproate** levels (↑ risk of seizures).

Route/Dosage

IV, IM (Adults and Children ≥13 yrs): 1 g once daily for up to 14 days (IV) or 7 days (IM).
IV, IM (Children 3 mo–12 yrs): 15 mg/kg twice daily (not to exceed 1 g/day) for up to 14 days (IV) or 7 days (IM).

Renal Impairment

IM, IV (Adults): $CCr \leq 30 \ mL/min/1.73 \ m^2$: 500 mg once daily.

Availability (generic available)

Powder for injection: 1 g/vial.

NURSING IMPLICATIONS

Assessment

- Assess for infection (vital signs; appearance of wound, sputum, urine, and stool; WBC) at beginning of and during therapy.
- Obtain a history before initiating therapy to determine previous use of and reactions to penicillins, cephalosporins, or carbapenems. Persons with a negative history of penicillin sensitivity may still have an allergic response.
- Obtain specimens for culture and sensitivity before initiating therapy. First dose may be given before receiving results.
- Observe patient for signs and symptoms of anaphylaxis (rash, pruritus, laryngeal edema, wheezing). Discontinue the drug and notify healthcare professional immediately if these occur. Have epinephrine, an antihistamine, and resuscitative equipment close by in the event of an anaphylactic reaction.
- Monitor bowel function. Diarrhea, abdominal cramping, fever, and bloody stools should be reported to health care professional promptly as a sign of *Clostridioides difficile*-associated diarrhea

E

(CDAD). May begin up to several wk following cessation of therapy.

Lab Test Considerations
- May cause ↑ AST, ALT, serum alkaline phosphatase levels.
- May cause ↑ platelet and eosinophil counts.

Implementation
- **IM:** Reconstitute 1-g vial with 3.2 mL of 1% lidocaine without epinephrine. Shake well to form solution. Immediately withdraw contents and inject deep into large muscle mass. Use reconstituted solution within 1 hr.

IV Administration
- **Intermittent Infusion:** *Reconstitution:* Reconstitute 1-g vial with 10 mL of sterile water for injection or 0.9% NaCl using a 21-gauge or smaller diameter needle and shake well. *Dilution: For adults and pediatric patients 13 yrs and older:* further dilute in 50 mL of 0.9% NaCl. *For pediatric patients 3 mo to 12 yr:* immediately withdraw a volume equal to 15 mg/kg (not to exceed 1 g/day) and dilute in 0.9% NaCl to a final concentration of 20 mg/mL or less. Administer within 6 hr of reconstitution. *Rate:* Infuse over 30 min.
- **Y-Site Compatibility:** acyclovir, amifostine, amikacin, aminocaproic acid, aminophylline, amphotericin B lipid complex, amphotericin B liposomal, argatroban, arsenic trioxide, atracurium, azithromycin, aztreonam, bivalirudin, bleomycin, bumetanide, buprenorphine, busulfan, butorphanol, calcium chloride, calcium gluconate, cangrelor, carboplatin, carmustine, ceftazidime/avibactam, chloramphenicol, cisatracurium, cisplatin, cyclophosphamide, cyclosporine, cytarabine, dacarbazine, dactinomycin, daptomycin, dexamethasone, dexmedetomidine, dexrazoxane, digoxin, diltiazem, diphenhydramine, docetaxel, dopamine, doxorubicin liposomal, doxycycline, enalaprilat, ephedrine, epinephrine, eptifibatide, erythromycin, esmolol, etoposide, etoposide phosphate, famotidine, fluconazole, fludarabine, fluorouracil, foscarnet, fosphenytoin, furosemide, ganciclovir, gemcitabine, gemtuzumab ozogamicin, gentamicin, glycopyrrolate, granisetron, haloperidol, heparin, hetastarch, hydrocortisone, hydromorphone, ifosfamide, insulin, regular, irinotecan, isoproterenol, ketorolac, labetalol, leucovorin calcium, levofloxacin, lidocaine, linezolid, lorazepam, magnesium sulfate, mannitol, melphalan, meperidine, meropenem/vaborbactam, mesna, methadone, methotrexate, methylprednisolone, metoclopramide, metronidazole, milrinone, mitomycin, morphine, moxifloxacin, nalbuphine, naloxone, nitroglycerin, nitroprusside, norepinephrine, octreotide, oxaliplatin, oxytocin, paclitaxel, pamidronate, pantoprazole, pemetrexed, pentobarbital, phenobarbital, phentolamine, phenylephrine, plazomicin, potassium acetate, potassium chloride, potassium phosphate, procainamide, propranolol, remifentanil, rocuronium, sodium acetate, sodium bicarbonate, sodium phosphate, succinylcholine, sufentanil, tacrolimus, telavancin, theophylline, thiotepa, tigecycline, tirofiban, tobramycin, trimethoprim/sulfamethoxazole, vancomycin, vasopressin, vecuronium, vinblastine, vincristine, vinorelbine, voriconazole, zidovudine, zoledronic acid.
- **Y-Site Incompatibility:** alemtuzumab, allopurinol, amiodarone, anidulafungin, caspofungin, chlorpromazine, dantrolene, daunorubicin hydrochloride, diazepam, dobutamine, doxorubicin hydrochloride, droperidol, epirubicin, hydralazine, hydroxyzine, idarubicin, isavuconazonium, midazolam, minocycline, mitoxantrone, nicardipine, ondansetron, pentamidine, phenytoin, prochlorperazine, promethazine, thiopental, topotecan, verapamil.

Patient/Family Teaching
- Advise patient to report the signs of superinfection (black, furry overgrowth on the tongue; vaginal itching or discharge; loose or foul-smelling stools) and allergy.
- Caution patient to notify health care professional if fever and diarrhea occur, especially if stool contains blood, pus, or mucus. Advise patient not to treat diarrhea without consulting health care professional. May occur up to several wk after discontinuation of medication. Consult health care professional before treating with antidiarrheals.
- Instruct patient to notify health care professional of all Rx or OTC medications, vitamins, or herbal products being taken and to consult health care professional before taking any new medications.
- Rep: Advise females of reproductive potential to notify health care professional if pregnancy is planned or suspected or if breastfeeding.

Evaluation/Desired Outcomes
- Resolution of the signs and symptoms of infection. Length of time for complete resolution depends on the organism and site of infection.

BEERS

escitalopram (ess-sit-al-o-pram)
❦ Cipralex, Lexapro

Classification
Therapeutic: antidepressants
Pharmacologic: selective serotonin reuptake inhibitors (SSRIs)

Indications
Major depressive disorder. Generalized anxiety disorder. **Unlabeled Use:** Panic disorder. Obsessive-compulsive disorder. Post-traumatic stress disorder. Social anxiety disorder (social phobia). Premenstrual dysphoric disorder.

Action
Selectively inhibits the reuptake of serotonin in the CNS. **Therapeutic Effects:** Antidepressant action.

Pharmacokinetics

Absorption: 80% absorbed following oral administration.

Distribution: Enters breast milk.

Metabolism and Excretion: Mostly metabolized by the liver, primarily by the CYP3A4 and CYP2C19 isoenzymes; 7% excreted unchanged by kidneys.

Half-life: 27–32 hr (↑ in elderly and hepatic impairment).

TIME/ACTION PROFILE (antidepressant effect)

ROUTE	ONSET	PEAK	DURATION
PO	within 1–4 wk	unknown	unknown

Contraindications/Precautions

Contraindicated in: Hypersensitivity; Concurrent use of pimozide; Concurrent use of MAO inhibitors or MAO-like drugs (linezolid or methylene blue); Concurrent use of citalopram; Angle-closure glaucoma.

Use Cautiously in: Personal or family history of bipolar disorder, mania, or hypomania (may activate mania/hypomania); History of seizures; Patients at risk for suicide; Hepatic impairment (↓ dose); Severe renal impairment; OB: Use during pregnancy only if potential maternal benefit justifies potential fetal risk; Lactation: Use while breastfeeding only if potential maternal benefit justifies potential risk to infant; Pedi: May ↑ risk of suicide attempt/ideation especially during early treatment or dose adjustment; safety not established in children <12 yr (major depressive disorder) or <7 yr (generalized anxiety disorder); Geri: Appears on Beers list. May worsen or cause syndrome of inappropriate antidiuretic hormone (SIADH) secretion and/or hyponatremia in older adults. Use with caution in older adults and closely monitor sodium concentrations when starting therapy or ↑ dose.

Adverse Reactions/Side Effects

Derm: sweating. **Endo:** SIADH. **F and E:** hyponatremia. **GI:** diarrhea, <u>nausea</u>, abdominal pain, constipation, dry mouth, indigestion. **GU:** ↓ libido, delayed/absent orgasm, ejaculatory delay/failure, erectile dysfunction. **Hemat:** BLEEDING. **Metab:** ↑ appetite. **Neuro:** <u>insomnia</u>, dizziness, drowsiness, fatigue, NEUROLEPTIC MALIGNANT SYNDROME, SUICIDAL THOUGHTS. **Misc:** SEROTONIN SYNDROME.

Interactions

Drug-Drug: May cause serious, potentially fatal reactions when used with **MAO inhibitors**; allow at least 14 days between escitalopram and **MAO inhibitors**. Concurrent use with **MAO-inhibitor-like drugs**, such as **linezolid** or **methylene blue** may ↑ risk of serotonin syndrome; concurrent use contraindicated; do not start therapy in patients receiving **linezolid** or **methylene blue**; if **linezolid** or **methylene blue** need to be started in a patient receiving escitalopram, immediately discontinue escitalopram and monitor for signs/symptoms of serotonin syndrome for 2 wk or until 24 hr after last dose of linezolid or methylene blue, whichever comes first (may resume escitalopram therapy 24 hr after last dose of linezolid or methylene blue). Concurrent use with **pimozide** may result in prolongation of the QT interval and is contraindicated. Use cautiously with other **centrally acting drugs** (including **alcohol, antihistamines, opioid analgesics**, and **sedative/hypnotics**; concurrent use with **alcohol** is not recommended). Drugs that affect serotonergic neurotransmitter systems, including **tricyclic antidepressants, SNRIs, fentanyl, lithium, buspirone, tramadol, meperidine, methadone, amphetamines**, and **triptans** ↑ risk of serotonin syndrome. **Cimetidine** may ↑ levels. Serotonergic effects may be ↑ by **lithium** (concurrent use should be carefully monitored). **Carbamazepine** may ↓ levels. May ↑ levels of **metoprolol**. Use cautiously with **tricyclic antidepressants** due to unpredictable effects on serotonin and norepinephrine reuptake. ↑ risk of bleeding with **NSAIDs, aspirin, clopidogrel, prasugrel, ticagrelor, dabigatran, apixaban, edoxaban, rivaroxaban**, or **warfarin**.

Drug-Natural Products: ↑ risk of serotonin syndrome with **St. John's wort** and **SAMe**.

Route/Dosage

Major Depressive Disorder

PO (Adults): 10 mg once daily, may ↑ to 20 mg once daily after 1 wk.

PO (Geriatric Patients): 10 mg once daily.

PO (Children ≥12 yr): 10 mg once daily, may ↑ to 20 mg once daily after 3 wk.

Hepatic Impairment
PO (Adults): 10 mg once daily.

Generalized Anxiety Disorder

PO (Adults): 10 mg once daily, may ↑ to 20 mg once daily after 1 wk.

PO (Geriatric Patients): 10 mg once daily.

PO (Children ≥7 yr): 10 mg once daily, may ↑ to 20 mg once daily after 2 wk.

Hepatic Impairment
PO (Adults): 10 mg once daily.

Availability (generic available)

Tablets: 5 mg, 10 mg, 20 mg. **Orally disintegrating tablets:** ✹ 10 mg, ✹ 20 mg. **Oral solution (peppermint flavor):** 1 mg/mL.

NURSING IMPLICATIONS

Assessment

- Screen patient for a personal or family history of bipolar disorder, mania, or hypomania before starting therapy; may precipitate a mixed/manic episode.
- Monitor mood changes and level of anxiety during therapy.

- Assess for suicidal tendencies, especially during early therapy. Restrict amount of drug available to patient. Risk may be increased in children, adolescents, and adults ≤24 yr. After starting therapy, children, adolescents, and young adults should be seen by health care professional face-to-face at least weekly for 4 wk, then every other wk for next 4 wk, then at 12 wk, and then on advice of health care professional thereafter.
- Assess sexual function before starting escitalopram. Assess for changes in sexual function during treatment, including timing of onset; patient may not report.
- Assess for serotonin syndrome (mental changes [agitation, hallucinations, coma], autonomic instability [tachycardia, labile BP, hyperthermia], neuromuscular aberrations [hyperreflexia, incoordination], and/or GI symptoms [nausea, vomiting, diarrhea]), especially in patients taking other serotonergic drugs (SSRIs, SNRIs, triptans).

Implementation
- Do not confuse escitalopram with citalopram.
- Do not administer escitalopram and citalopram concomitantly. Taper to avoid potential withdrawal reactions. Reduce dose by 50% for 3 days, then again by 50% for 3 days, then discontinue.
- **PO:** Administer as a single dose in the morning or evening without regard to meals.

Patient/Family Teaching
- Instruct patient to take escitalopram as directed. Take missed doses on the same day as soon as remembered and consult health care professional. Resume regular dosing schedule next day. Do not double doses. Do not stop abruptly; should be discontinued gradually. Instruct patient to read *Medication Guide* before starting and with each Rx refill in case of changes.
- May cause dizziness. Caution patient to avoid driving or other activities requiring alertness until response to medication is known.
- Advise patient, family, and caregivers to watch for suicidality, especially during early therapy or dose changes. Notify health care professional immediately if thoughts about suicide or dying, attempts to commit suicide, new or worse depression or anxiety, agitation or restlessness, panic attacks, insomnia, new or worse irritability, aggressiveness, acting on dangerous impulses, mania, or other changes in mood or behavior or if rash or symptoms of serotonin syndrome occur.
- Instruct patient to notify health care professional of all Rx or OTC medications, vitamins, or herbal products being taken and to consult health care professional before taking any other Rx, OTC, or herbal products, especially St. John's wort, alcohol or other CNS depressants.
- Inform patient that escitalopram may cause symptoms of sexual dysfunction. In males, ejaculatory delay or failure, decreased libido, and erectile dysfunc-

tion may occur. In female patients, may result in decreased libido and delayed or absent orgasm. Advise patient to notify health care professional if symptoms occur.
- Rep: Advise females of reproductive potential to notify health care professional if pregnancy is planned or suspected or if breastfeeding. Use late in 3rd trimester may result in neonatal serotonin syndrome requiring prolonged hospitalization, respiratory support, and tube feeding; may occur immediately upon delivery. Symptoms include respiratory distress, cyanosis, apnea, seizures, temperature instability, feeding difficulty, vomiting, hypoglycemia, hypotonia, hypertonia, hyperreflexia, tremor, jitteriness, irritability, and constant crying. Use of escitalopram in last month of pregnancy may increase risk of postpartum hemorrhage. Inform patient of pregnancy exposure registry that monitors pregnancy outcomes in women exposed to antidepressants during pregnancy. Register patients by calling the National Pregnancy Registry for Antidepressants at 1-866-961-2388 or visiting online at https://womensmentalhealth.org/clinical-and-researchprograms/pregnancyregistry/antidepressants/. Monitor infants exposed to escitalopram via breastfeeding for sedation, poor feeding, and poor weight gain.
- Emphasize importance of follow-up exams to monitor progress.

Evaluation/Desired Outcomes
- Increased sense of well-being.
- Renewed interest in surroundings. May require 1–4 wk of therapy to obtain antidepressant effects. Full antidepressant effects occur in 4–6 wk.
- Decrease in anxiety.

REMS

esketamine (es-ket-a-meen)
Spravato
Classification
Therapeutic: antidepressants
Pharmacologic: N-methyl-D-aspartate antagonist

Schedule III

Indications
Treatment-resistant depression (in combination with an oral antidepressant). Depressive symptoms in patients with major depressive disorder with acute suicidal ideation or behavior (in combination with an oral antidepressant).

Action
Acts as a non-competitive N-methyl-D-aspartate receptor antagonist; the exact mechanism by which it exerts its antidepressant effect is unknown. **Therapeutic Effects:** Decreased severity of depressive symptoms and prolonged time to relapse.

Pharmacokinetics

Absorption: 48% absorbed following nasal administration.

Distribution: Extensively distributed to tissues.

Metabolism and Excretion: Primarily metabolized to noresketamine (active metabolite) in liver by CYP2B6 and CYP3A4 isoenzymes, and to lesser extent by CYP2C9 and CYP2C19 isoenzymes. Primarily excreted in urine (≥78%; <1% as unchanged drug); ≤2% excreted in feces.

Half-life: 7–12 hr.

TIME/ACTION PROFILE (plasma concentrations)

ROUTE	ONSET	PEAK	DURATION
Intranasal	unknown	20–40 min	unknown

Contraindications/Precautions

Contraindicated in: Hypersensitivity to esketamine or ketamine; Aneurysmal vascular disease (including thoracic and abdominal aorta, intracranial and peripheral arterial vessels) or arteriovenous malformation; History of intracerebral hemorrhage; Severe hepatic impairment; OB: Pregnancy; Lactation: Lactation.

Use Cautiously in: History of hypertensive encephalopathy; Psychosis; Moderate hepatic impairment; Rep: Women of reproductive potential; Pedi: Safety and effectiveness not established in children; may ↑ risk of suicide attempt/ideation especially during early treatment or dose adjustment.

Adverse Reactions/Side Effects

CV: ↑ BP, tachycardia. **Derm:** ↑ sweating. **EENT:** nasal irritation, throat irritation. **GI:** <u>nausea</u>, <u>vomiting</u>, constipation, diarrhea, dry mouth. **GU:** urinary tract infection. **Neuro:** <u>anxiety</u>, <u>depersonalization</u>, <u>derealization</u>, <u>dissociative changes</u>, <u>dizziness</u>, <u>dysgeusia</u>, <u>fatigue</u>, <u>headache</u>, <u>hypoesthesia</u>, <u>sedation</u>, <u>vertigo</u>, cognitive impairment, insomnia, loss of consciousness, slurred/slow speech, SUICIDAL THOUGHTS/BEHAVIORS, tremor. **Misc:** physical dependence, psychological dependence, tolerance.

Interactions

Drug-Drug: Concurrent use with **psychostimulants**, including **amphetamines**, **methylphenidate**, or **modafinil**, or **armodafinil**, as well as **MAO inhibitors** may ↑ BP. Use with **opioids** or other **CNS depressants**, including **benzodiazepines**, **non-benzodiazepine sedative/hypnotics**, **anxiolytics**, **general anesthetics**, **muscle relaxants**, **antipsychotics**, and **alcohol** may cause profound sedation.

Route/Dosage

Treatment-Resistant Depression

Intranasal (Adults): *Induction phase (Wk 1–4):* 56 mg (2 sprays in each nostril) twice weekly; may ↑ dose (after first dose) based on response and tolerability up to 84 mg (3 sprays in each nostril) twice weekly. *Main-* *tenance phase (Wk 5–8):* 56 mg (2 sprays in each nostril) or 84 mg (3 sprays in each nostril) once weekly. *Maintenance phase (Wk 9 and beyond):* 56 mg (2 sprays in each nostril) or 84 mg (3 sprays in each nostril) once weekly or every other wk (use least frequent dosing to maintain remission/response).

Depressive Symptoms in Patients With Major Depressive Disorder With Acute Suicidal Ideation or Behavior

Intranasal (Adults): 84 mg (3 sprays in each nostril) twice weekly for 4 wk; may ↓ dosage to 56 mg (2 sprays in each nostril) twice weekly based on tolerability. Reevaluate patient for continued need for treatment after 4 wk.

Availability

Nasal spray: 28 mg/device (14 mg/spray).

NURSING IMPLICATIONS

Assessment

- Monitor patient for sedation for at least 2 hr after each dose.
- Monitor BP before and 40 min after administration and periodically during 2 hr after administration. If BP elevated before administration, may hold dose. If elevated following dose, continue to monitor patient.
- Assess for history of psychosis. May cause dissociative or perceptual changes (distortion of time, space, and illusions), derealization and depersonalization. Monitor for 2 hr after each dose.
- Monitor for worsening and emergence of suicidal thoughts and behaviors, especially during initial few mo of drug therapy and at times of dose changes.
- Monitor for urinary tract and bladder symptoms during therapy and refer to an appropriate health care professional as clinically warranted.

Implementation

- Do not confuse Spravato with Steglatro.
- Must be administered under the supervision of a health care professional.
- ***REMS:*** Due to risks of serious adverse outcomes from sedation, dissociation, and abuse and misuse, available only through a restricted program under *Spravato REMS*. Health care settings and pharmacies must be certified and patients must be enrolled in REMS program. Esketamine is only administered in health care settings under direct observation of health care professional and patients must be monitored for at least 2 hr after administration.
- Advise patient to avoid food for at least 2 hr and liquids for 30 min prior to administration.
- If nasal corticosteroid or nasal decongestant is administered on a dosing day, administer at least 1 hr before esketamine administration.
- Esketamine is given in conjunction with an oral antidepressant.

- May cause dissociative or perceptual changes (including distortion of time, space, and illusions), derealization, and depersonalization; carefully assess patients with psychosis before administering esketamine.
- **Intranasal:** Use 2 devices (for a 56-mg dose) or 3 devices (for an 84-mg dose), with a 5-min rest between use of each device. Do not prime device. Advise patient to gently blow nose before first dose. Check that indicator shows 2 or 3 green dots. Instruct patient to recline head back 45°. Have patient insert device into nostril until nose rest is between nostrils. Close opposite nostril. Sniff gently after administering dose. Take device from patient; confirm no green dots. Instruct patient to recline and rest for 5 min between doses; do not blow nose. Repeat for each dose. Discard according to institution guidelines for Schedule III drugs.

Patient/Family Teaching

- **REMS:** Explain purpose of esketamine, administration procedure, and *Spravato REMS* program to patient. Advise patient to read *Medication Guide* before starting therapy. If a treatment session is missed and no worsening of depressive symptoms occurs, continue current dosing schedule. If depressive symptoms worsen, may return to previous dosing schedule.
- May cause sedation, dissociative symptoms, perception disturbances, dizziness, vertigo, and anxiety. Caution patient to avoid driving or activities requiring alertness until next day after a restful sleep.
- Advise patient, family, and caregivers to look for changes in behavior and suicidality, especially during early therapy or dose changes. Notify health care professional immediately if thoughts about suicide or dying, attempts to commit suicide; new or worse depression or anxiety; agitation or restlessness; panic attacks; insomnia; new or worse irritability; aggressiveness; acting on dangerous impulses, mania, or other changes in mood or behavior.
- Instruct patient to notify health care professional of all Rx or OTC medications, vitamins, or herbal products being taken and to avoid concurrent use of Rx, OTC, and herbal products without consulting health care professional.
- Rep: May cause fetal harm. Advise females of reproductive potential to use effective contraception during therapy and to avoid breastfeeding. Notify health care professional promptly if pregnancy is planned or suspected, or if breastfeeding. Inform patients who become pregnant during therapy of pregnancy registry that monitors pregnancy outcomes in women exposed to antidepressants. Enroll patients by contacting the National Pregnancy Registry for Antidepressants at 1-866-961-2388 or online at https://womensmentalhealth.org/clinical-and-researchprograms/pregnancyregistry/antidepressants/.

Evaluation/Desired Outcomes

- Decreased severity of depressive symptoms and prolonged time to relapse.

HIGH ALERT

esmolol (es-moe-lol)
Brevibloc
Classification
Therapeutic: antiarrhythmics (class II)
Pharmacologic: beta blockers

Indications
Sinus tachycardia. Supraventricular arrhythmias.

Action
Blocks stimulation of beta$_1$(myocardial)-adrenergic receptors. Does not usually affect beta$_2$(pulmonary, vascular, or uterine)-receptor sites. **Therapeutic Effects:** Decreased heart rate. Decreased AV conduction.

Pharmacokinetics
Absorption: IV administration results in complete bioavailability.
Distribution: Rapidly and widely distributed.
Metabolism and Excretion: Metabolized by enzymes in RBCs and liver.
Half-life: 9 min.

TIME/ACTION PROFILE (antiarrhythmic effect)

ROUTE	ONSET	PEAK	DURATION
IV	within min	unknown	1–20 min

Contraindications/Precautions
Contraindicated in: Uncompensated HF; Pulmonary edema; Cardiogenic shock; Bradycardia or heart block; Known alcohol intolerance; Lactation: Lactation.
Use Cautiously in: Thyrotoxicosis (may mask symptoms); Diabetes mellitus (may mask symptoms of hypoglycemia); Patients with a history of severe allergic reactions (intensity of reactions may be ↑); OB: Use during pregnancy only if potential maternal benefit justifies potential fetal risk; Pedi: Safety and effectiveness not established in children; Geri: ↑ sensitivity to the effects of beta blockers.

Adverse Reactions/Side Effects
CV: hypotension, peripheral ischemia. **Derm:** sweating. **Endo:** hypoglycemia. **GI:** nausea, vomiting. **Local:** injection site reactions. **Neuro:** fatigue, agitation, confusion, dizziness, drowsiness, weakness.

Interactions
Drug-Drug: **General anesthesia**, IV **phenytoin**, and **verapamil** may cause additive myocardial depression. Additive bradycardia may occur with **digoxin**. Additive hypotension may occur with other **antihypertensives**, acute ingestion of **alcohol**, or **nitrates**. Concurrent use with **amphetamine**, **cocaine**, **ephedrine**, **epinephrine**, **norepinephrine**,

phenylephrine, or **pseudoephedrine** may result in unopposed alpha-adrenergic stimulation (excessive hypertension, bradycardia). Concurrent **thyroid hormone** administration may ↓ effectiveness. May alter the effectiveness of **insulins** or **oral hypoglycemic agents** (dose adjustments may be necessary). May ↓ effectiveness of **theophylline**. May ↓ beneficial beta cardiovascular effects of **dopamine** or **dobutamine**. Use cautiously within 14 days of **MAO inhibitor** therapy (may result in hypertension).

Route/Dosage

IV (Adults): *Antiarrhythmic:* 500-mcg/kg loading dose over 1 min initially, followed by 50-mcg/kg/min infusion for 4 min; if no response within 5 min, give 2nd loading dose of 500 mcg/kg over 1 min, then ↑ infusion to 100 mcg/kg/min for 4 min. If no response, repeat loading dose of 500 mcg/kg over 1 min and ↑ infusion rate by 50-mcg/kg/min increments (not to exceed 200 mcg/kg/min for 48 hr). As therapeutic end point is achieved, eliminate loading doses and decrease dose increments to 25 mcg/kg/min. *Intraoperative antihypertensive/antiarrhythmic:* 250–500-mcg/kg loading dose over 1 min initially, followed by 50-mcg/kg/min infusion for 4 min; if no response within 5 min, give 2nd loading dose of 250–500 mcg/kg over 1 min, then ↑ infusion to 100 mcg/kg/min for 4 min. If no response, repeat loading dose of 250–500 mcg/kg over 1 min and ↑ infusion rate by 50-mcg/kg/min increments (not to exceed 200 mcg/kg/min for 48 hr).

IV (Children): *Antiarrhythmic:* 50 mcg/kg/min, may be ↑ every 10 min up to 300 mcg/kg/min.

Availability (generic available)

Solution for injection (for use as loading dose): 10 mg/mL. **Premixed infusion:** 2000 mg/100 mL, 2500 mg/250 mL.

NURSING IMPLICATIONS

Assessment

- Monitor BP, ECG, and pulse frequently during dose adjustment period and periodically during therapy. The risk of hypotension is greatest within the first 30 min of starting esmolol infusion.
- Monitor intake and output ratios and daily weights. Assess routinely for signs and symptoms of HF (dyspnea, rales/crackles, weight gain, peripheral edema, jugular venous distention).
- Assess infusion site frequently during therapy. Concentrations >10 mg/mL may cause redness, swelling, skin discoloration, and burning at the injection site. Do not use butterfly needles for administration. If venous irritation occurs, stop the infusion and resume at another site.
- Monitor for signs and symptoms of hypoglycemia (tachycardia). Symptoms may be prevented by esmolol. If hypoglycemia occurs, seek emergency treatment.

Toxicity and Overdose
- Monitor patients receiving esmolol for signs of overdose (bradycardia, severe dizziness or fainting, severe drowsiness, dyspnea, bluish fingernails or palms, seizures).
- IV glucagon and symptomatic care are used in the treatment of esmolol overdose. Because of the short action of esmolol, discontinuation of therapy may relieve acute toxicity.

Implementation

- ***High Alert:*** IV vasoactive medications are inherently dangerous. Esmolol is available in different concentrations; fatalities have occurred when loading dose vial is confused with concentrated solution for injection, which contains 2500 mg in 10 mL (250 mg/mL) and must be diluted. Before administering, have second practitioner independently check original order, dose calculations, and infusion pump settings.
- ***High Alert:*** Do not confuse Brevibloc with Brevital. If both are available as floor stock, store in separate areas.
- To convert to other antiarrhythmics following esmolol administration, administer the 1st dose of the antiarrhythmic agent and decrease the esmolol dose by 50% after 30 min. If an adequate response is maintained for 1 hr following the 2nd dose of the antiarrhythmic agent, discontinue esmolol.

IV Administration
- **IV Push:** *Dilution:* The 10-mg/mL and 20-mg/mL vials should be used for the loading dose. These vials are already diluted. No further dilution is needed. *Rate:* Administer 1 mg/kg over 30 sec or 500 mcg/kg over 1 min.
- **Continuous Infusion:** *Dilution:* Premixed infusions are already diluted and ready to use. Solution is clear, colorless to light yellow; do not administer solutions that are discolored or contain particulate matter. *Concentration:* 10 mg/mL. *Rate:* Based on patient's weight (see Route/Dosage section). Titration of dose is based on desired heart rate or undesired decrease in BP. Esmolol infusions should not be abruptly discontinued; the infusion rate should be tapered.
- **Y-Site Compatibility:** acetaminophen, albumin, human, alemtuzumab, amikacin, aminophylline, amiodarone, amphotericin B liposomal, anidulafungin, argatroban, ascorbic acid, atracurium, atropine, aztreonam, benztropine, bivalirudin, bleomycin, bumetanide, buprenorphine, butorphanol, calcium chloride, calcium gluconate, cangrelor, carboplatin, carmustine, caspofungin, cefazolin, cefepime, cefotaxime, cefoxitin, ceftazidime, ceftolozane/tazobactam, ceftriaxone, cefuroxime, chlorpromazine, cisatracurium, cisplatin, clindamycin, cyanocobalamin, cyclophosphamide, cyclosporine, cytarabine, D5W, D5/LR, D5/Ringer's, D5/0.45% NaCl, D5/0.9% NaCl, 0.45% NaCl, 0.9% NaCl, dacarbazine, dactinomycin, daptomycin, daunorubicin hydrochloride, dexmede-

---

✱ = Canadian drug name. ░ = Genetic implication. ~~Strikethrough~~ = Discontinued. CAPITALS = life-threatening. <u>Underline</u> = most frequent.

tomidine, dexrazoxane, digoxin, diltiazem, diphenhydramine, dobutamine, docetaxel, dopamine, doxorubicin hydrochloride, doxorubicin liposomal, doxycycline, enalaprilat, ephedrine, epinephrine, epoetin alfa, eptifibatide, eravacycline, ertapenem, erythromycin, etoposide, etoposide phosphate, famotidine, fentanyl, fluconazole, fludarabine, fluorouracil, folic acid, foscarnet, fosphenytoin, gemcitabine, gentamicin, glycopyrrolate, granisetron, heparin, hetastarch, hydrocortisone, hydromorphone, idarubicin, ifosfamide, imipenem/cilastatin, insulin (regular), irinotecan, isavuconazonium, isoproterenol, labetalol, LR, leucovorin calcium, levofloxacin, levothyroxine, lidocaine, linezolid, lorazepam, magnesium sulfate, mannitol, meperidine, meropenem, meropenem/vaborbactam, mesna, methadone, methotrexate, metoclopramide, metoprolol, metronidazole, micafungin, midazolam, mitoxantrone, morphine, moxifloxacin, multivitamins, mycophenolate, nalbuphine, naloxone, nicardipine, nitroglycerin, nitroprusside, norepinephrine, octreotide, ondansetron, oxaliplatin, oxytocin, paclitaxel, palonosetron, papaverine, pemetrexed, penicillin G, pentamidine, phentolamine, phenylephrine, phytonadione, piperacillin/tazobactam, plazomicin, potassium acetate, potassium chloride, potassium phosphates, procainamide, prochlorperazine, promethazine, propofol, propranolol, protamine, pyridoxine, remifentanil, rocuronium, sodium acetate, succinylcholine, sufentanil, tacrolimus, theophylline, thiamine, thiotepa, tigecycline, tirofiban, tobramycin, topotecan, vancomycin, vasopressin, vecuronium, verapamil, vinblastine, vincristine, voriconazole, zoledronic acid.

- **Y-Site Incompatibility:** acyclovir, amphotericin B deoxycholate, amphotericin B lipid complex, azathioprine, cefotetan, dantrolene, dexamethasone, diazepam, furosemide, ganciclovir, gemtuzumab ozogamicin, ibuprofen, indomethacin, ketorolac, milrinone, mitomycin, oxacillin, pantoprazole, pentobarbital, phenobarbital, sodium bicarbonate, tedizolid, warfarin.

Patient/Family Teaching

- Explain purpose of esmolol to patient.
- May cause drowsiness. Caution patients receiving esmolol to call for assistance during ambulation or transfer.
- Advise patients to change positions slowly to minimize orthostatic hypotension.
- Patients with diabetes should closely monitor blood glucose, especially if weakness, malaise, irritability, or fatigue occurs. Medication does not block dizziness or sweating as signs of hypoglycemia.
- Rep: May cause fetal harm. Advise females of reproductive potential to notify health care professional if pregnant. Avoid breastfeeding during therapy. May cause fetal bradycardia.

Evaluation/Desired Outcomes

- Control of arrhythmias without appearance of detrimental side effects.

✗✗✗ esomeprazole
(es-oh-**mep**-ra-zole)
NexIUM, NexIUM 24hr
Classification
Therapeutic: antiulcer agents
Pharmacologic: proton-pump inhibitors

Indications

PO, IV: GERD/erosive esophagitis (IV therapy should only be used if PO therapy is not possible/appropriate). **IV:** Reduction in risk of rebleeding following therapeutic endoscopy for acute bleeding gastric or duodenal ulcers. **PO:** Hypersecretory conditions, including Zollinger-Ellison syndrome. **PO:** Eradication of *Helicobacter pylori* in duodenal ulcer disease or history of duodenal ulcer disease (in combination with amoxicillin and clarithromycin). **PO:** Reduction in risk of gastric ulcer during continuous NSAID therapy. **OTC:** Heartburn occurring at least twice/wk.

Action

Binds to an enzyme on gastric parietal cells in the presence of acidic gastric pH, preventing the final transport of hydrogen ions into the gastric lumen. **Therapeutic Effects:** Diminished accumulation of acid in the gastric lumen with lessened gastroesophageal reflux. Healing of duodenal ulcers. Decreased incidence of gastric ulcer during continuous NSAID therapy.

Pharmacokinetics

Absorption: 90% absorbed following oral administration; food ↓ absorption.
Distribution: Unknown.
Protein Binding: 97%.
Metabolism and Excretion: Primarily metabolized by the liver via the CYP2C19 isoenzyme, with some metabolism by the CYP3A4 isoenzyme; ✗ (the CYP2C19 enzyme system exhibits genetic polymorphism; 15–20% of Asian patients and 3–5% of Caucasian and Black patients may be poor metabolizers and may have significantly ↑ esomeprazole concentrations and an ↑ risk of adverse effects); <1% excreted unchanged in urine.
Half-life: *Children 1–11 yr:* 0.42–0.88 hr; *Adults:* 1.0–1.5 hr.

TIME/ACTION PROFILE (plasma concentrations*)

ROUTE	ONSET	PEAK	DURATION
PO	rapid	1.6 hr	24 hr
IV	rapid	end of infusion	24 hr

*Resolution of symptoms takes 5–8 days.

Contraindications/Precautions

Contraindicated in: Hypersensitivity to esomeprazole or related drugs (benzimidazoles); Hypersensitivity; Concurrent use of rilpivirine.

Use Cautiously in: Severe hepatic impairment; Patients using high-doses for >1 yr (↑ risk of hip, wrist, or spine fractures and fundic gland polyps); Patients using therapy for >3 yr ($\uparrow$ risk of vitamin B$_{12}$ deficiency); Pre-existing risk of hypocalcemia; OB: Safety not established in pregnancy; Lactation: Safety not established in breast-feeding; Geri: Appears on Beers list. $\uparrow$ risk of *Clostridioides difficile* infection, pneumonia, GI malignancies, bone loss, and fractures in older adults. Avoid scheduled use for >8 wk in older adults unless for high-risk patients (e.g. oral corticosteroid or chronic NSAID use) or patients with erosive esophagitis, Barrett's esophagitis, pathological hypersecretory condition, or demonstrated need for maintenance therapy (e.g. failure of H$_2$ antagonist).

Adverse Reactions/Side Effects

Derm: ACUTE GENERALIZED EXANTHEMATOUS PUSTULOSIS, cutaneous lupus erythematosus, DRUG REACTION WITH EOSINOPHILIA AND SYSTEMIC SYMPTOMS (DRESS), STEVENS-JOHNSON SYNDROME, TOXIC EPIDERMAL NECROLYSIS. **F and E:** hypocalcemia (especially if treatment duration ≥3 mo), hypokalemia (especially if treatment duration ≥3 mo), hypomagnesemia (especially if treatment duration ≥3 mo). **GI:** abdominal pain, CLOSTRIDIOIDES DIFFICILE-ASSOCIATED DIARRHEA (CDAD), constipation, diarrhea, dry mouth, flatulence, fundic gland polyps, nausea. **GU:** acute tubulointerstitial nephritis. **Hemat:** vitamin B$_{12}$ deficiency. **MS:** bone fracture. **Neuro:** headache. **Misc:** HYPERSENSITIVITY REACTIONS (including anaphylaxis, angioedema, or tubulointerstitial nephritis), systemic lupus erythematosus.

Interactions

Drug-Drug: May significantly ↓ levels of **rilpivirine**; concurrent use contraindicated. May ↓ levels of **atazanavir** and **nelfinavir**; avoid concurrent use with either of these antiretrovirals. May ↓ absorption of drugs requiring acid pH, including **ketoconazole**, **itraconazole**, **ampicillin esters**, **iron salts**, **erlotinib**, and **mycophenolate mofetil**. May ↑ levels of **digoxin** and **methotrexate**. May ↑ risk of bleeding with **warfarin** (monitor INR and PT). **Voriconazole** may ↑ levels. May ↓ the antiplatelet effects of **clopidogrel**; avoid concurrent use. May ↑ levels of **cilostazol**; consider ↓ dose of cilostazol from 100 mg twice daily to 50 mg twice daily. **Rifampin** may ↓ levels and may ↓ response (avoid concurrent use). Hypomagnesemia and hypokalemia ↑ risk of **digoxin** toxicity. May ↑ levels of **tacrolimus** and **methotrexate**.

Drug-Natural Products: **St. John's wort** may ↓ levels and may ↓ response (avoid concurrent use).

Route/Dosage

Gastroesophageal Reflux Disease

PO (Adults): *Healing of erosive esophagitis:* 20 mg or 40 mg once daily for 4–8 wk; *Maintenance of healing of erosive esophagitis:* 20 mg once daily; *Symptomatic GERD:* 20 mg once daily for 4 wk (additional 4 wk may be considered for nonresponders); *Heartburn:* 20 mg once daily for 2 wk.

PO (Children 12–17 yr): *Short-term treatment of GERD:* 20–40 mg once daily for up to 8 wk.
PO (Children 1–11 yr): *Short-term treatment of GERD:* 10 mg once daily for up to 8 wk; *Healing of erosive esophagitis:* <20 kg: 10 mg once daily for 8 wk; ≥20 kg: 10–20 mg once daily for 8 wk.
PO (Infants and Children 1 mo–<1 yr): *>7.5–12 kg:* 10 mg once daily for up to 6 wk; *>5–7.5 kg:* 5 mg once daily for up to 6 wk; *3–5 kg:* 2.5 mg once daily for up to 6 wk.
IV (Adults): 20 or 40 mg once daily.
IV (Children 1–17 yr): *<55 kg:* 10 mg once daily; *≥55 kg:* 20 mg once daily.
IV (Children 1 mo–<1 yr): 0.5 mg/kg once daily.

Hepatic Impairment
PO, IV (Adults): *Severe hepatic impairment:* Dose should not exceed 20 mg/day.

Reduction of Risk of Rebleeding of Gastric or Duodenal Ulcers After Therapeutic Endoscopy
IV (Adults): 80 mg over 30 min, then 8 mg/hr continuous infusion for 71.5 hr.

Hepatic Impairment
IV (Adults): *Mild to moderate hepatic impairment:* Do not exceed continuous infusion rate of 6 mg/hr; *Severe hepatic impairment:* Do not exceed continuous infusion rate of 4 mg/hr.

H. pylori Eradication to Reduce the Risk of Duodenal Ulcer Recurrence (Triple Therapy)
PO (Adults): 40 mg once daily for 10 days with amoxicillin 1000 mg twice daily for 10 days and clarithromycin 500 mg twice daily for 10 days.

Hepatic Impairment
PO (Adults): *Severe hepatic impairment:* Dose should not exceed 20 mg/day.

Reduction in Risk of Gastric Ulcer During Continuous NSAID Therapy
PO (Adults): 20 or 40 mg once daily for up to 6 mo.

Hepatic Impairment
PO (Adults): *Severe hepatic impairment:* Dose should not exceed 20 mg/day.

Pathological Hypersecretory Conditions Including Zollinger-Ellison Syndrome
PO (Adults): 40 mg twice daily.

Hepatic Impairment
PO (Adults): *Severe hepatic impairment:* Dose should not exceed 20 mg/day.

Availability (generic available)
Delayed-release tablets: 20 mg^{OTC}. **Delayed-release capsules:** 20 mg$^{Rx, OTC}$, 40 mg. **Delayed-release oral suspension packets:** 2.5 mg/pkt, 5 mg/pkt, 10 mg/pkt, 20 mg/pkt, 40 mg/pkt. **Powder for injection:** 40 mg/vial. *In combination with:* naproxen (generic only).

NURSING IMPLICATIONS

Assessment

- Assess routinely for epigastric or abdominal pain and frank or occult blood in the stool, emesis, or gastric aspirate.
- Monitor bowel function. Diarrhea, abdominal cramping, fever, and bloody stools should be reported to health care professional promptly as a sign of CDAD).

Lab Test Considerations

- May cause ↑ serum creatinine, uric acid, total bilirubin, alkaline phosphatase, AST, and ALT.
- May alter hemoglobin, WBC, platelets, serum sodium, potassium, and thyroxine levels.
- May cause hypomagnesemia. Monitor serum magnesium prior to and periodically during therapy.
- May cause false positive results in diagnostic investigations for neuroendocrine tumors due to ↑ serum chromogranin A (CgA) levels secondary to drug-induced ↓ gastric acidity. Temporarily stop esomeprazole at least 14 days before assessing CgA levels and consider repeating test if initial CgA levels are high.

Implementation

- *High Alert:* Do not confuse Nexium with Nexavar.
- Antacids may be used while taking esomeprazole.
- **PO:** Administer at least 1 hr before meals. *DNC:* Swallow tablets and capsules whole.
- *Delayed-release capsules:* For patients with difficulty swallowing, place 1 tbsp of applesauce in an empty bowl. Open capsule and empty the pellets inside onto applesauce. Mix pellets with applesauce and swallow immediately. Applesauce should not be hot and should be soft enough to swallow without chewing. Do not store applesauce mixture for future use. Tap water, orange juice, apple juice, and yogurt have also been used. Do not crush or chew pellets.
- *For patients with an NG tube,* delayed-release capsules can be opened and intact granules emptied into a 60-mL syringe and mixed with 50 mL of water. Replace plunger and shake syringe vigorously for 15 sec. Hold syringe with tip up and check for granules in tip. Attach syringe to NG tube and administer solution. After administering, flush syringe with additional water. Do not administer if granules have dissolved or disintegrated. Administer immediately after mixing.
- For *Delayed-release oral suspension:* Mix contents of packet with 1 tbsp (15 mL) of water, leave 2–3 min to thicken, stir and drink within 30 min.
- For *delayed-release oral suspension NG or gastric tube:* Add 15 mL of water to a syringe and then add contents of packet. Shake syringe, leave 2–3 min to thicken. Shake syringe and inject through NG or gastric tube within 30 min.

IV Administration

- **IV Push:** *Reconstitution:* Reconstitute each vial with 5 mL of 0.9% NaCl. Do not administer solutions that are discolored or contain a precipitate. Stable at room temperature for up to 12 hr. Do not administer with other medication or solutions. Flush line with 0.9% NaCl before and after administration. *Rate:* Administer over at least 3 min.
- **Intermittent Infusion:** *Dilution:* Dilute reconstituted solution to a volume of 45 mL with *D5W, 0.9% NaCl, or LR for adults* and *with 0.9% NaCl for pediatric patients. Concentration:* 0.8 mg/mL (40-mg vial) or 0.4 mg/mL (20-mg vial). Solutions diluted with 0.9% NaCl or LR are stable for 12 hr and those diluted with D5W are stable for 6 hr at room temperature. *Rate:* Administer over 10–30 min.
- **Continuous Infusion:** *For 80-mg loading dose,* reconstitute two 40-mg vials with 5 mL of 0.9% NaCl. *Dilution:* Further diluted in 100 mL 0.9% NaCl. *Rate:* Administer *loading dose* over 30 min. Follow with infusion at a rate of 8 mg/hr for 71.5 hrs.
- **Continuous Infusion:** *For 80 mg dose, Reconstitution:* reconstitute two 40 mg vials with 5 mL of 0.9% NaCl. *Dilution:* Further diluted in 100 mL 0.9% NaCl. *Rate:* Follow loading dose with infusion at a rate of 8 mg/hr for 71.5 hrs.
- **Y-Site Compatibility:** ceftaroline, ceftolozane/tazobactam, D5W, fentanyl, furosemide, hydrocortisone, insulin, regular, LR, meropenem/vaborbactam, methadone, metoprolol, nitroglycerin, tedizolid.
- **Y-Site Incompatibility:** dobutamine, dopamine, esmolol, isavuconazonium, labetalol, midazolam, morphine, plazomicin, tacrolimus, telavancin, tigecycline.

Patient/Family Teaching

- Instruct patient to take medication as directed for the full course of therapy, even if feeling better. Take missed doses as soon as remembered but not if almost time for next dose. Do not double doses. Advise patient to read the *Patient Information* sheet before starting therapy and with each Rx refill in case of changes.
- Advise patient to avoid alcohol, products containing aspirin or NSAIDs, and foods that may cause an increase in GI irritation.
- Advise patient to report onset of black, tarry stools; diarrhea; abdominal pain; or persistent headache to health care professional promptly.
- Instruct patient to notify health care professional of all Rx or OTC medications, vitamins, or herbal products being taken and consult health care professional before taking any new medications, especially St. John's wort.
- Advise patient to notify health care professional if signs of hypomagnesemia (seizures, dizziness, abnormal or fast heartbeat, jitteriness, jerking movements or shaking, muscle weakness, spasms of the hands and feet, cramps or muscle aches, spasm of the voice box) occur.
- Caution patient to notify health care professional if fever and diarrhea occur, especially if stool contains blood, pus, or mucus. Advise patient not to treat diarrhea without consulting health care professional.

- Rep: Advise females of reproductive potential to notify health care professional if pregnancy is planned or suspected or if breastfeeding.

Evaluation/Desired Outcomes
- Decrease in abdominal pain or prevention of gastric irritation and bleeding. Healing of duodenal ulcers can be seen on x-ray examination or endoscopy.
- Decrease in symptoms of GERD and erosive esophagitis. Sustained resolution of symptoms usually occurs in 5–8 days. Therapy is continued for 4–8 wk after initial episode.
- Decreased incidence of gastric ulcer during continuous NSAID therapy.
- Eradication of *H. pylori* in duodenal ulcer disease.
- Decrease in symptoms of hypersecretory conditions, including Zollinger-Ellison.

---

estetrol/drospirenone, See CONTRACEPTIVES, HORMONAL.

ESTRADIOL (es-tra-**dye**-ole)
estradiol cypionate
  Depo-Estradiol
estradiol tablets
  Estrace
estradiol transdermal gel
  Divigel, Elestrin, EstroGel
estradiol transdermal spray
  EvaMist
estradiol transdermal system
  Alora, Climara, Dotti, Estraderm, ♣ Estradot, Lyllana, Menostar, Minivelle, ♣ Oesclim, Vivelle-Dot
estradiol vaginal cream
  Estrace
estradiol vaginal insert
  Imvexxy
estradiol vaginal ring
  Estring, Femring
estradiol vaginal tablet
  Vagifem, Yuvafem
estradiol valerate
  Delestrogen
Classification
Therapeutic: hormones
Pharmacologic: estrogens

Indications
PO, IM, Transdermal: Replacement of estrogen to diminish moderate to severe vasomotor symptoms of menopause and of various estrogen deficiency states including: Female hypogonadism, Ovariectomy, Primary

ovarian failure. Treatment and prevention of postmenopausal osteoporosis (not vaginal dose forms). **PO:** Inoperable metastatic postmenopausal breast or prostate carcinoma. **Vag:** Management of: Atrophic vaginitis due to menopause, Moderate to severe dyspareunia due to menopause.

Action
Estrogens promote growth and development of female sex organs and the maintenance of secondary sex characteristics in women. Metabolic effects include reduced blood cholesterol, protein synthesis, and sodium and water retention. **Therapeutic Effects:** Restoration of hormonal balance in various deficiency states, including menopause. Treatment of hormone-sensitive tumors.

Pharmacokinetics
Absorption: Well absorbed after oral administration. Readily absorbed through skin and mucous membranes.
Distribution: Widely distributed to tissues.
Metabolism and Excretion: Mostly metabolized by the liver and other tissues. Enterohepatic recirculation occurs, and more absorption may occur from the GI tract.
Half-life: Gel: 36 hr.

TIME/ACTION PROFILE (estrogenic effects)

ROUTE	ONSET	PEAK	DURATION
PO	unknown	unknown	unknown
IM	unknown	unknown	unknown
Transdermal	unknown	unknown	3–4 days (Estraderm), 7 days (Climara)
Topical	unknown	unknown	unknown
Vaginal insert	unknown	unknown	3–4 days
Vaginal ring	unknown	unknown	90 days

Contraindications/Precautions
Contraindicated in: History of anaphylaxis or angioedema to estradiol; Thromboembolic disease (e.g., deep vein thrombosis, pulmonary embolism, MI, stroke); Protein C, protein S, or antithrombin deficiency or other thrombophilic disorder; History of breast cancer; History of estrogen-dependent cancer; Hepatic impairment; Undiagnosed vaginal bleeding; OB: Pregnancy.
Use Cautiously in: Underlying cardiovascular disease; Severe renal impairment; History of porphyria; History of hereditary angioedema; Lactation: Use while breastfeeding only if potential maternal benefit justifies potential risk to infant.

Adverse Reactions/Side Effects
CV: edema, hypertension, MI, THROMBOEMBOLISM.
Derm: oily skin, acne, pigmentation, urticaria. **EENT:** intolerance to contact lenses, worsening of myopia or

astigmatism. **Endo:** gynecomastia (men), hyperglycemia. **F and E:** hypercalcemia, sodium and water retention. **GI:** nausea, weight changes, anorexia, jaundice, vomiting. **GU:** *women:* amenorrhea, dysmenorrhea, breakthrough bleeding, cervical erosions, loss of libido, vaginal candidiasis; *men:* erectile dysfunction, testicular atrophy. **Metab:** ↑ appetite. **MS:** leg cramps. **Neuro:** headache, dementia, dizziness, lethargy, STROKE. **Misc:** breast tenderness, MALIGNANCY (BREAST, ENDOMETRIAL, OVARIAN).

Interactions
Drug-Drug: May alter requirement for **warfarin**, **oral hypoglycemic agents**, or **insulins**. **Barbiturates** or **rifampin** may ↓ effectiveness. **Smoking** ↑ risk of adverse CV reactions.

Route/Dosage
Estrogens should be used in the lowest doses for the shortest period of time consistent with desired therapeutic outcome. Concurrent use of progestin is recommended during cyclical therapy to decrease the risk of endometrial carcinoma in patients with an intact uterus.

Symptoms of Menopause, Atrophic Vaginitis, Moderate to Severe Dyspareunia, Female Hypogonadism, Ovarian Failure/Osteoporosis
PO (Adults): 0.45–2 mg once daily or in a cycle.
IM (Adults): 1–5 mg monthly (estradiol cypionate) *or* 10–20 mg (estradiol valerate) monthly.
Topical Gel (Adults): Apply contents of one packet *(Divigel)* or one actuation from pump *(EstroGel, Elestrin)* once daily.
Topical Spray *EvaMist* **(Adults):** 1 spray once daily, may be ↑ to 2–3 sprays once daily.
Transdermal (Adults): *Climara:* 25 mcg/24-hr transdermal patch applied weekly. *Vivelle-Dot:* 25–50 mcg/24-hr transdermal patch applied twice weekly. *Menostar:* 14 mcg/24-hr transdermal patch applied every 7 days. Progestin may be administered for 10–14 days of each mo. *Dotti, Lyllana, or Minivelle:* 37.5 mcg/24-hr transdermal patch applied twice weekly (for treatment of vasomotor symptoms); 25 mcg/24-hr transdermal patch applied twice weekly (for prevention of postmenopausal osteoporosis).
Vag (Adults): *Cream:* 2–4 g (0.2–0.4 mg estradiol) once daily for 1–2 wk, then ↓ to 1–2 g/day for 1–2 wk; then maintenance dose of 1 g 1–3 times weekly for 3 wk, then off for 1 wk; then repeat cycle once vaginal mucosa has been restored; *Vaginal ring (Estring):* 2-mg (releases 7.5 mcg estradiol/24 hr) every 3 mo; *Vaginal ring (Femring):* 12.4 mg (releases 50 mcg estradiol/24 hr) every 3 mo or 24.8 mg (releases 100 mcg estradiol/24 hr) every 3 mo (*Femring* requires concurrent progesterone); *Vaginal insert (Vagifem, Yuvafem, or Imvexxy):* 1 insert once daily for 2 wk, then 1 insert twice weekly.

Postmenopausal Breast Cancer
PO (Adults): 10 mg 3 times daily.

Prostate Cancer
PO (Adults): 1–2 mg 3 times daily.
IM (Adults): 30 mg every 1–2 wk (estradiol valerate).

Availability (generic available)
Estradiol
Tablets: 0.5 mg, 1 mg, 2 mg. *In combination with:* dienogest (Natazia); drospirenone (Angeliq); elagolix/norethindrone (Oriahnn); norethindrone (Activella, Amabelz, Mimvey); norgestimate (Prefest); progesterone (Bijuva); relugolix/norethindrone (Myfembree). See Appendix N.

Estradiol Cypionate
Injection (in oil): 5 mg/mL.

Estradiol Transdermal Preparations
Gel packet (Divigel): 0.25 mg/pkt, 0.5 mg/pkt, 0.75 mg/pkt, 1 mg/pkt, 1.25 mg/pkt. **Gel pump (Elestrin):** 0.52 mg/actuation. **Gel pump (Estrogel):** 0.75 mg/actuation. **Transdermal patch:** 14 mcg/24-hr release rate, 25 mcg/24-hr release rate, 37.5 mcg/24-hr release rate, 50 mcg/24-hr release rate, 60 mcg/24-hr release rate, 75 mcg/24-hr release rate, 100 mcg/24-hr release rate. **Spray:** 1.53 mg/spray. *In combination with:* levonorgestrel (Climara Pro); norethindrone (Combipatch). See Appendix N.

Estradiol Vaginal Preparations
Vaginal cream: 0.01%. **Vaginal tablet (Vagifem or Yuvafem):** 10 mcg. **Vaginal insert (Imvexxy):** 4 mcg, 10 mcg. **Vaginal ring (Estring):** 2 mg (releases 7.5 mcg/day over 90 days). **Vaginal ring (Femring):** 12.4 mg (releases 50 mcg/day over 90 days), 24.8 mg (releases 100 mcg/day over 90 days).

Estradiol Valerate
Injection (in oil): 10 mg/mL, 20 mg/mL, 40 mg/mL.

NURSING IMPLICATIONS
Assessment
● Assess BP before and periodically during therapy.
● Monitor intake and output ratios and weekly weight. Report significant discrepancies or steady weight gain.
● **Menopause:** Assess frequency and severity of vasomotor symptoms.

Lab Test Considerations
● May cause ↑ HDL and triglycerides and ↓ serum LDL and total cholesterol concentrations.
● May cause ↑ serum glucose, sodium, cortisol, prolactin, prothrombin, and factor VII, VIII, IX, and X levels. May ↓ serum folate, pyridoxine, antithrombin III, and urine pregnanediol concentrations.
● Monitor hepatic function before and periodically during therapy.
● May cause false interpretations of thyroid function tests, false ↑ in norepinephrine platelet-induced aggregability, and false ↓ in metyrapone tests.
● May cause hypercalcemia in patients with metastatic bone lesions.

Implementation

- **PO:** Administer with or immediately after food to reduce nausea.
- **Vag:** Manufacturer provides applicator with cream. Dose is marked on the applicator. Wash applicator with mild soap and warm water after each use.
- **Transdermal:** When switching from PO form, begin transdermal therapy 1 wk after the last dose or when symptoms reappear.
- **Topical:** Apply *Divigel* individual-use once-daily packets of quick drying gel to an area measuring 5 inches by 7 inches (size of 2 palm prints) on the thigh. Do not wash area for at least 1 hr after gel has dried.
- Start with 1 pump daily and apply *Elestrin* to skin of upper arm to shoulder in a thin layer.
- Before first use of *Estrogel*, remove large canister cover and fully depress pump 5 times. Discard unused gel by rinsing down the sink or placing it in the household trash. After priming, pump is ready to use. Apply a thin layer over the entire arm on the inside and outside from wrist to shoulder.
- Spray *EvaMist* on inside of forearm at the same time each day. Do not massage or rub the spray into the skin. Allow to dry for 2 min before dressing and at least 1 hr before washing. Never spray *EvaMist* around breast or vagina. Do not use more than 56 doses, even if fluid remains in pump.
- **IM:** Injection has oil base. Roll syringe to ensure even dispersion. Administer deep IM. Avoid IV administration.

Patient/Family Teaching

- Instruct patient on correct method of administration. Instruct patient to take medication as directed. Take missed doses as soon as remembered as long as it is not just before next dose. If a dose of *EvaMist* is missed, apply if more than 12 hr before next dose; if less than 12 hr, omit dose and return to regular schedule. Do not double doses.
- Explain dose schedule and maintenance routine. Discontinuing medication suddenly may cause withdrawal bleeding.
- If nausea becomes a problem, advise patient that eating solid food often provides relief.
- Advise patient to report signs and symptoms of fluid retention (swelling of ankles and feet, weight gain), thromboembolic disorders (pain, swelling, tenderness in extremities, headache, chest pain, blurred vision), mental depression, or hepatic dysfunction (yellowed skin or eyes, pruritus, dark urine, light-colored stools) to health care professional.
- Advise patient to notify health care professional of medication regimen before treatment or surgery.
- Caution patient that cigarette smoking during estrogen therapy may cause increased risk of serious side effects, especially for women over age 35.

- Caution patient to use sunscreen and protective clothing to prevent increased pigmentation.
- Advise patient treated for osteoporosis that exercise has been found to arrest and reverse bone loss. Patient should discuss any exercise limitations with health care professional before beginning program.
- Inform patient that estrogens should not be used to decrease risk of cardiovascular disease. Estrogens may increase risk of cardiovascular disease (MI, stroke), dementia, and breast cancer.
- **Rep:** Instruct females of reproductive potential to stop taking medication and notify health care professional if pregnancy is planned or suspected, or if breastfeeding.
- Emphasize the importance of routine follow-up physical exams, including BP; breast, abdomen, and pelvic examinations; Papanicolaou smears every 6–12 mo; and mammogram every 12 mo or as directed. Health care professional will evaluate possibility of discontinuing medication every 3–6 mo. If on continuous (not cyclical) therapy or without concurrent progestins, endometrial biopsy may be recommended, if uterus is intact.
- **Vag:** Instruct patient in the correct use of applicator. Patient should remain recumbent for at least 30 min after administration. May use sanitary napkin to protect clothing, but do not use tampon. If a dose is missed, do not use the missed dose, but return to regular dosing schedule.
- Instruct patient to use applicator provided with vaginal tablet. Insert as high up in the vagina as comfortable, without using force.
- **Vaginal Ring:** Instruct patient to press ring into an oval and insert into the upper third of the vaginal vault. Exact position is not critical. Once ring is inserted, patient should not feel anything. If discomfort is felt, ring is probably not in far enough; gently push farther into vagina. Leave in place continuously for 90 days. Ring does not interfere with sexual intercourse. If straining at defecation makes ring move to lower vagina, push up with finger. If expelled totally, rinse ring with lukewarm water and reinsert. To remove, hook a finger through the ring and pull it out.
- **Transdermal:** Instruct patient to wash and dry hands first. Apply disc to intact skin on hairless portion of abdomen (do not apply to breasts or waistline). Apply patch to lower abdomen or buttocks. Press disc/patch for 10 sec to ensure contact with skin (especially around edges). Avoid areas where clothing may rub disc loose. Change site with each administration to prevent skin irritation. Do not reuse site for 1 wk; disc may be reapplied if it falls off.
- Advise patient referred for MRI test to discuss patch with referring health care professional and MRI facility to determine if removal of patch is necessary prior to test and for directions for replacing patch.
- *Evamist*: Caution patient to make sure children are not exposed to *Evamist* and do not come into contact

with any skin area where the drug was applied. Women who cannot avoid contact with children should wear a garment with long sleeves to cover the application site.

Evaluation/Desired Outcomes
● Resolution of menopausal vasomotor symptoms.
● Decreased vaginal and vulvar itching, inflammation, or dryness associated with menopause.
● Normalization of estrogen levels in patients with ovariectomy or hypogonadism.
● Control of the spread of advanced metastatic breast or prostate cancer.
● Prevention of osteoporosis.

---

estradiol valerate/dienogest, See CONTRACEPTIVES, HORMONAL.

BEERS

estrogens, conjugated
(ess-troe-jenz con-joo-gae-ted)
✦C.E.S, Premarin
Classification
Therapeutic: hormones
Pharmacologic: estrogens

Indications
PO: Moderate to severe vasomotor symptoms of menopause. Vulvar and vaginal atrophy associated with menopause. Estrogen deficiency states, including: Female hypogonadism, Ovariectomy, Primary ovarian failure. Prevention of postmenopausal osteoporosis. Advanced inoperable metastatic breast and prostatic carcinoma. **IM, IV:** Uterine bleeding resulting from hormonal imbalance. **Vag:** Atrophic vaginitis. Moderate to severe dyspareunia due to menopause. Concurrent use of progestin is recommended during cyclical therapy to decrease the risk of endometrial carcinoma in patients with an intact uterus.

Action
Estrogens promote the growth and development of female sex organs and the maintenance of secondary sex characteristics in women. **Therapeutic Effects:** Restoration of hormonal balance in various deficiency states and treatment of hormone-sensitive tumors.

Pharmacokinetics
Absorption: Well absorbed after oral administration. Readily absorbed through skin and mucous membranes. IV administration results in complete bioavailability.
Distribution: Widely distributed to tissues.
Metabolism and Excretion: Mostly metabolized by liver via the CYP3A4 isoenzyme. Enterohepatic recirculation occurs, with more absorption from GI tract.
Half-life: Unknown.

TIME/ACTION PROFILE (estrogenic effects†)

ROUTE	ONSET	PEAK	DURATION
PO	rapid	unknown	24 hr
IM	delayed	unknown	6–12 hr
IV	rapid	unknown	6–12 hr

†Tumor response may take several wk.

Contraindications/Precautions
Contraindicated in: History of anaphylaxis or angioedema to estrogen; Thromboembolic disease (e.g., DVT, PE, MI, stroke); Undiagnosed vaginal bleeding; History of breast cancer; History of estrogen-dependent cancer; Hepatic impairment; Protein C, protein S, or antithrombin deficiency or other thrombophilic disorder; OB: Pregnancy; Lactation: Lactation.
Use Cautiously in: Long-term use (more than 4–5 yr); may ↑ risk of myocardial infarction, stroke, invasive breast cancer, pulmonary emboli, deep vein thrombosis, and dementia in postmenopausal women; Underlying cardiovascular disease; Hypertriglyceridemia; History of hereditary angioedema; Geri: Appears on Beers list. ↑ risk of breast and endometrial cancer, heart disease, thromboembolic events, and dementia in older adults. Avoid use of systemic estrogens in older adults. Vaginal cream is acceptable to use for treatment of dyspareunia, recurrent lower urinary tract infections, and other vaginal symptoms in older adults.

Adverse Reactions/Side Effects
(Systemic use) **CV:** edema, hypertension, MI, THROMBOEMBOLISM. **Derm:** acne, oily skin, pigmentation, urticaria. **Endo:** gynecomastia (men), hyperglycemia. **F and E:** hypercalcemia. **GI:** nausea, weight changes, anorexia, jaundice, vomiting. **GU:** *women:* amenorrhea, breakthrough bleeding, breast tenderness, dysmenorrhea, cervical erosion, loss of libido, vaginal candidiasis; *men:* erectile dysfunction, testicular atrophy. **Metab:** ↑ appetite. **MS:** leg cramps. **Neuro:** headache, depression, dizziness, insomnia, lethargy. **Misc:** ANAPHYLAXIS, ANGIOEDEMA, MALIGNANCY (BREAST, ENDOMETRIAL, OVARIAN).

Interactions
Drug-Drug: May alter requirement for **warfarin, oral hypoglycemic agents,** or **insulins. Barbiturates, carbamazepine,** or **rifampin** may ↓ effectiveness. **Smoking** ↑ risk of adverse CV reactions. **Erythromycin, clarithromycin, itraconazole, ketoconazole,** and **ritonavir** may ↑ risk of adverse effects.
Drug-Food: Grapefruit juice may ↑ risk of adverse effects.

Route/Dosage
Estrogens should be used in the lowest doses for the shortest period of time consistent with desired therapeutic outcome.

Ovariectomy, Primary Ovarian Failure
PO (Adults): 1.25 mg once daily administered cyclically (3 wk on, 1 wk off).

Osteoporosis/Menopausal Symptoms
PO (Adults): 0.3–1.25 mg once daily or in a cycle.

Female Hypogonadism
PO (Adults): 0.3–0.625 mg once daily administered cyclically (3 wk on, 1 wk off).

Inoperable Breast Carcinoma—Men and Postmenopausal Women
PO (Adults): 10 mg 3 times daily.

Inoperable Prostate Carcinoma
PO (Adults): 1.25–2.5 mg 3 times daily.

Uterine Bleeding
IM, IV (Adults): 25 mg, may repeat in 6–12 hr if necessary.

Atrophic Vaginitis
PO (Adults): 0.3–1.25 mg once daily.
Vag (Adults): 0.5–2 g cream (0.3125 mg–1.25 g conjugated estrogens) once daily for 3 wk, off for 1 wk, then repeat.

Moderate to Severe Dyspareunia
Vag (Adults): 0.5 g cream (0.3125 mg conjugated estrogens) twice weekly continuously or daily for 3 wk, off for 1 wk, then repeat.

Availability
Tablets: 0.3 mg, 0.45 mg, 0.625 mg, 0.9 mg, 1.25 mg. **Powder for injection:** 25 mg/vial. **Vaginal cream:** 0.625 mg/g. *In combination with:* bazedoxifene (Duavee); medroxyprogesterone (Prempro and Premphase [compliance package]). See Appendix N.

NURSING IMPLICATIONS
Assessment
- Assess BP before and periodically during therapy.
- Monitor intake and output ratios and weekly weight. Report significant discrepancies or steady weight gain.
- **Menopause:** Assess frequency and severity of vasomotor symptoms.

Lab Test Considerations
- May cause ↑ HDL and triglycerides, and ↓ serum LDL and total cholesterol concentrations.
- May cause ↑ serum glucose, sodium, cortisol, prolactin, prothrombin, and factor VII, VIII, IX, and X levels. May ↓ serum folate, pyridoxine, antithrombin III, and urine pregnanediol concentrations.
- Monitor hepatic function before and periodically during therapy.
- May cause false interpretations of thyroid function tests.
- May cause hypercalcemia in patients with metastatic bone lesions.

Implementation
- Estrogens should be used in the lowest doses for the shortest period of time consistent with desired therapeutic outcome.
- **PO:** Administer with or immediately after food to reduce nausea.
- **Vag:** Manufacturer provides applicator with cream. Dose is marked on the applicator. Wash applicator with mild soap and warm water after each use.
- **IM:** To reconstitute, withdraw at least 5 mL of air from dry container and then slowly introduce the sterile diluent (bacteriostatic water for injection) against the container side. Gently agitate container to dissolve; do not shake vigorously. Solution is stable for 60 days if refrigerated. Do not use if precipitate is present or if solution is darkened.
- IV is preferred parenteral route because of rapid response.

IV Administration
- **IV Push:** *Reconstitution:* Reconstitute as for IM. Inject into distal port tubing of free-flowing IV of 0.9% NaCl, D5W, or lactated Ringer's solution. *Concentration:* 5 mg/mL. *Rate:* Administer slowly (no faster than 5 mg/min) to prevent flushing.
- **Y-Site Incompatibility:** pantoprazole.

Patient/Family Teaching
- Instruct patient to take oral medication as directed. Advise patient to avoid drinking grapefruit juice during therapy. Take missed doses as soon as remembered, but not just before next dose. Do not double doses.
- Explain dose schedule and maintenance routine. Discontinuing medication suddenly may cause withdrawal bleeding. Bleeding is anticipated during the wk when conjugated estrogens are withheld.
- If nausea becomes a problem, advise patient that eating solid food often provides relief. Inform patient that estrogens should not be used to decrease risk of cardiovascular disease. Estrogens may increase risk of cardiovascular disease and breast cancer.
- Advise patient to report signs and symptoms of fluid retention (swelling of ankles and feet, weight gain), thromboembolic disorders (pain, swelling, tenderness in extremities; headache; chest pain; blurred vision), depression, hepatic dysfunction (yellowed skin or eyes, pruritus, dark urine, light-colored stools), or abnormal vaginal bleeding to health care professional.
- Caution patient that cigarette smoking during estrogen therapy may increase risk of serious side effects, especially for women over age 35.
- Inform patient that *Premarin* tablet may appear in stool; this is not harmful.
- Caution patient to use sunscreen and protective clothing to prevent increased pigmentation.
- Instruct patient to notify health care professional of all Rx or OTC medications, vitamins, or herbal products being taken and to consult with health care professional before taking other medications.
- Advise patient to notify health care professional of medication regimen before treatment or surgery.

✳ = Canadian drug name. ▓ = Genetic implication. ~~Strikethrough~~ = Discontinued. CAPITALS = life-threatening. <u>Underline</u> = most frequent.

- Advise patient treated for osteoporosis that exercise has been found to arrest and reverse bone loss. The patient should discuss any exercise limitations with health care professional before beginning program.
- Rep: May cause fetal harm. Instruct patient to stop taking medication and notify health care professional if pregnancy is planned or suspected, and to avoid breastfeeding during therapy.
- Emphasize the importance of routine follow-up physical exams, including BP; breast, abdomen, and pelvic examinations; Papanicolaou (Pap) smears every 6–12 mo; and mammogram every 12 mo or as directed. Health care professional will evaluate possibility of discontinuing medication every 3–6 mo. If on continuous (not cyclical) therapy or without concurrent progestins, endometrial biopsy may be recommended if uterus is intact.
- Vag: Instruct patient in the correct use of applicator. Patient should remain recumbent for at least 30 min after administration. May use sanitary napkin to protect clothing, but do not use tampon. If a dose is missed, do not use the missed dose, but return to regular dosing schedule.

Evaluation/Desired Outcomes

- Resolution of menopausal vasomotor symptoms.
- Decreased vaginal and vulvar itching, inflammation, or dryness associated with menopause.
- Normalization of estrogen levels in patients with ovariectomy or hypogonadism.
- Control of the spread of advanced metastatic breast or prostate cancer.
- Prevention of osteoporosis.
- Relief of moderate to severe dyspareunia due to menopause.

BEERS

eszopiclone (es-zop-i-klone)
Lunesta
Classification
Therapeutic: sedative/hypnotics
Pharmacologic: cyclopyrrolones

Schedule IV

Indications
Insomnia.

Action
Interacts with GABA-receptor complexes; not a benzodiazepine. **Therapeutic Effects:** Improved sleep with decreased latency and increased maintenance of sleep.

Pharmacokinetics
Absorption: Rapidly absorbed after oral administration.
Distribution: Unknown.
Metabolism and Excretion: Extensively metabolized by the liver by the CYP3A4 and CYP2E1 isoenzymes; metabolites are renally excreted, <10% excreted unchanged in urine.

Half-life: 6 hr.

TIME/ACTION PROFILE (plasma concentrations)

ROUTE	ONSET	PEAK	DURATION
PO	rapid	1 hr	6 hr

Contraindications/Precautions
Contraindicated in: Hypersensitivity; History of experiencing complex sleep behaviors with zolpidem.
Use Cautiously in: Debilitated patients may have ↓ metabolism or increased sensitivity; use lower initial dose; Conditions that may alter metabolic or hemodynamic function; Severe hepatic impairment (↓ dose); OB: Safety not established in pregnancy; Lactation: Occasional use while breastfeeding an older infant should pose little risk; Pedi: Safety and effectiveness not established in children; Geri: Appears on Beers list. ↑ risk of cognitive impairment, delirium, falls, fractures, and motor vehicle accidents in older adults. Avoid use in older adults.

Adverse Reactions/Side Effects
CV: chest pain, peripheral edema. **Derm:** rash. **GI:** dry mouth, unpleasant taste. **Neuro:** abnormal thinking, behavior changes, COMPLEX SLEEP BEHAVIORS (including sleep driving, sleep walking, or engaging in other activities while sleeping), depression, hallucinations, headache, next day impairment.

Interactions
Drug-Drug: ↑ risk of CNS depression and next day impairment with other **CNS depressants** including **antihistamines, antidepressants, opioids, sedative/hypnotics,** and **antipsychotics.** ↑ levels and risk of CNS depression with **CYP3A4 inhibitors,** including **ketoconazole, itraconazole, clarithromycin, nefazodone, ritonavir,** and **nelfinavir.** Levels and effectiveness may be ↓ by **CYP3A4 inducers,** including **rifampin.**

Route/Dosage
PO (Adults): 1 mg immediately before bedtime; may be ↑ to 2–3 mg if needed; *Geriatric patients:* 1 mg immediately before bedtime; may be ↑ to 2 mg if needed; *Concurrent use of CYP3A4 inhibitors:* 1 mg immediately before bedtime; may be ↑ to 2 mg if needed.

Hepatic Impairment
PO (Adults): *Severe hepatic impairment:* 1 mg immediately before bedtime; may be ↑ to 2 mg if needed.

Availability (generic available)
Tablets: 1 mg, 2 mg, 3 mg.

NURSING IMPLICATIONS
Assessment
- Assess sleep patterns prior to and during administration. Continued insomnia after 7–10 days of therapy may indicate primary psychiatric or mental illness.
- Assess mental status and potential for abuse prior to administration. Prolonged use of >7–10 days may

lead to physical and psychological dependence. Limit amount of drug available to the patient.

Implementation

- Do not confuse Lunesta with Neulasta.
- **PO:** Onset is rapid. Administer immediately before going to bed or after patient has gone to bed and has experienced difficulty falling asleep, only on nights when patient is able to get 8 or more hr of sleep before being active again.
- *DNC:* Swallow tablet whole; do not break, crush, or chew.
- Eszopiclone is more effective if not taken with or before a high-fat, heavy meal.

Patient/Family Teaching

- Instruct patient to take eszopiclone immediately before going to bed, as directed. May result in short-term memory impairment, hallucinations, impaired coordination, and dizziness. Do not take eszopiclone if consumed alcohol that evening. Do not increase dose or discontinue without notifying health care professional. Dose may need to be decreased gradually to minimize withdrawal symptoms. Rebound insomnia and/or anxiety may occur upon discontinuation and usually resolves within 1–2 nights. Advise patient to read *Medication Guide* before starting therapy and with each Rx refill in case of changes.
- May cause daytime and next-day drowsiness. Caution patient to avoid driving or other activities requiring alertness until response to medication is known.
- Caution patient that eszopiclone may cause complex sleep behaviors (sleep walking, sleep driving, making and eating food, talking on the phone, having sex) while unaware. Patient may not remember anything done during the night; increased risk with alcohol or other CNS depressants. Discontinue eszopiclone immediately and notify health care professional if complex sleep behaviors occur.
- Instruct patient to notify health care professional of all Rx or OTC medications, vitamins, or herbal products being taken and to consult health care professional before taking any other Rx, OTC, or herbal products.
- Caution patient to avoid concurrent use of alcohol or other CNS depressants, including opioids.
- Advise patient to notify health care professional if signs and symptoms of allergic reaction (swelling of tongue or throat, trouble breathing, nausea and vomiting) occur.
- Rep: Advise females of reproductive potential to notify health care professional if pregnancy is planned or suspected, or if breastfeeding.

Evaluation/Desired Outcomes

- Decreased sleep latency and improved sleep maintenance.

etanercept (e-tan-er-sept)
✶Brenzys, Enbrel, ✶Erelzi

Classification
Therapeutic: antirheumatics (DMARDs)
Pharmacologic: anti-TNF agents

E

Indications
Moderately to severely active rheumatoid arthritis (as monotherapy or in combination with methotrexate). Moderate to severely active polyarticular juvenile idiopathic arthritis. Active ankylosing spondylitis. Psoriatic arthritis (as monotherapy or in combination with methotrexate). Moderate to severe chronic plaque psoriasis in patients who are candidates for systemic therapy or phototherapy.

Action
Binds to tumor necrosis factor (TNF), making it inactive. TNF is a mediator of inflammatory response. **Therapeutic Effects:** Decreased pain and swelling with decreased rate of joint destruction in patients with rheumatoid arthritis, psoriatic arthritis, juvenile idiopathic arthritis, and ankylosing spondylitis. Reduced severity of plaques.

Pharmacokinetics
Absorption: 60% absorbed after SUBQ administration.
Distribution: Unknown.
Metabolism and Excretion: Unknown.
Half-life: 115 hr (range 98–300 hr).

TIME/ACTION PROFILE (symptom reduction)

ROUTE	ONSET	PEAK	DURATION
SUBQ	2–4 wk	unknown	unknown

Contraindications/Precautions
Contraindicated in: Hypersensitivity; Active infection (including localized); Untreated infections; Granulomatosis with polyangiitis (receiving immunosuppressive agents); Concurrent cyclophosphamide or anakinra; Lactation: Lactation.
Use Cautiously in: History of chronic or recurrent infection or underlying illness/treatment predisposing to infection (including advanced or poorly controlled diabetes); History of exposure to tuberculosis; History of opportunistic infection; History of hepatitis B; Patients residing, or who have resided, where tuberculosis, histoplasmosis, coccidioidomycoses, or blastomycosis is endemic; Pre-existing or recent demyelinating disorders (multiple sclerosis, myelitis, optic neuritis); Latex allergy (needle cover of diluent syringe contains latex); OB: Use during pregnancy only if potential maternal benefit justifies potential fetal risk; Pedi: Children with significant exposure to varicella virus (temporarily discontinue etanercept; consider varicella zoster immune

globulin); ↑ risk of lymphoma (including hepatosplenic T-cell lymphoma [HSTCL]), leukemia, and other malignancies; Pedi: Safety and effectiveness not established in children <2 yr (juvenile idiopathic arthritis) or <4 yr (plaque psoriasis); Geri: Older adults may have ↑ risk of infection.

Adverse Reactions/Side Effects

Derm: psoriasis, rash. **EENT:** rhinitis, pharyngitis. **GI:** abdominal pain, dyspepsia. **Hemat:** pancytopenia. **Local:** injection site reactions. **Neuro:** headache, dizziness, weakness.. **Resp:** upper respiratory tract infection, cough, respiratory disorder. **Misc:** HYPERSENSITIVITY REACTIONS (including anaphylaxis), INFECTION (including reactivation tuberculosis and other opportunistic infections due to bacterial, invasive fungal, viral, mycobacterial, and parasitic pathogens), MALIGNANCY (including lymphoma, HSTCL, leukemia, and skin cancer), SARCOIDOSIS.

Interactions

Drug-Drug: Concurrent use with **anakinra** ↑ risk of serious infections (not recommended). Concurrent use of **cyclophosphamide** may ↑ risk of malignancies. Concurrent use with **azathioprine** and/or **methotrexate** may ↑ risk of HSTCL. May ↓ antibody response to **live-virus vaccine** and ↑ risk of adverse reactions (do not administer concurrently).

Route/Dosage

Rheumatoid Arthritis, Psoriatic Arthritis, and Ankylosing Spondylitis

SUBQ (Adults): 50 mg once weekly.

Plaque Psoriasis

SUBQ (Adults): 50 mg twice weekly for 3 mo, then 50 mg once weekly, may also be given as 25–50 mg once weekly as an initial dose.
SUBQ (Children ≥4 yr and ≥63 kg): 50 mg once weekly.
SUBQ (Children ≥4 yr and <63 kg): *Enbrel:* 0.8 mg/kg once weekly.

Juvenile Idiopathic Arthritis

SUBQ (Children ≥2 yr and ≥63 kg): 50 mg once weekly.
SUBQ (Children ≥2 yr and <63 kg): 0.8 mg/kg once weekly.

Availability

Powder for injection: 25 mg/vial. **Solution for injection:** 25 mg/0.5 mL (prefilled syringe and single-dose vial), 50 mg/mL (prefilled syringe and autoinjector).

NURSING IMPLICATIONS

Assessment

- Assess range of motion, degree of swelling, and pain in affected joints before and periodically during therapy.
- Assess for injection site reaction (erythema, pain, itching, swelling). Reactions are usually mild to moderate and last 3–5 days after injection.
- Monitor patients who develop a new infection while taking etanercept closely. Discontinue therapy in patients who develop a serious infection or sepsis. Do not start etanercept in patients with active infections.
- Assess for signs and symptoms of systemic fungal infections (fever, malaise, weight loss, sweats, cough, dyspnea, pulmonary infiltrates, serious systemic illness with or without concomitant shock). Ascertain if patient lives in or has traveled to areas of endemic mycoses. Consider empiric antifungal treatment for patients at risk of histoplasmosis and other invasive fungal infections until the pathogens are identified. Consult with an infectious diseases specialist. Consider stopping etanercept until the infection has been diagnosed and adequately treated.

Lab Test Considerations

- Monitor CBC with differential periodically during therapy. May cause leukopenia, neutropenia, thrombocytopenia, and pancytopenia. Discontinue etanercept if symptoms of blood dyscrasias (persistent fever) occur.

Implementation

- Do not confuse Enbrel with Levbid.
- Administer a tuberculin skin test prior to administration of etanercept. Patients with active latent TB should be treated for TB prior to therapy.
- **SUBQ:** Prepare injection with single dose prefilled syringe, single-dose vial or multidose vial for reconstitution.
- Allow solution in prefilled syringe to reach room temperature (15–30 min); do not remove needle cap during this time.
- For single-dose vial, allow solution to reach room temperature for at least 30 min before injecting. Solution may contain small white particles of protein; do not use if discolored, cloudy, or contains other particulate matter. Discard unused solution. Individual single-dose prefilled syringes, SureClick autoinjectors, single-dose vials, or Enbrel Mini cartridges can also be stored at room temp for up to 30 days.
- For multidose vial, *Reconstitution:* reconstitute with 1 mL of the bacteriostatic sterile water supplied by manufacturer for a concentration of 25 mg/mL. If the vial is used for multiple doses, use a 25-gauge needle for reconstituting and withdrawing solution and apply "Mixing Date" sticker with date of reconstitution entered. Inject diluent slowly into vial to avoid foaming. Some foaming will occur. Swirl gently for dissolution; do not shake or vigorously agitate to prevent excess foaming. Solution should be clear and colorless; do not administer solution that is discolored or contains particulate matter. Dissolution usually takes <10 min. Withdraw solution into syringe. Some foam may remain in vial. Amount in syringe should approximate 1 mL. Do not filter reconstituted solution during preparation or administration. Attach a 27-gauge needle to inject. Administer as soon as possible after reconstitution; stable up to 6 hr if refrigerated. Solution and prefilled syringes are stable if

refrigerated and used within 14 days. May be injected into abdomen, thigh, or upper arm. Rotate sites. Do not administer within 1 in. of an old site or into area that is tender, red, hard, or bruised.

- **Syringe Incompatibility:** Do not mix with other solutions or dilute with other diluents.

Patient/Family Teaching

- Instruct patient on self-administration technique, storage, and disposal of equipment. First injection should be administered under the supervision of health care professional. Provide patient with a puncture-proof container for used equipment. Advise patient to read *Medication Guide* before starting therapy and with each Rx refill in case of changes.
- Advise patient not to receive live vaccines during therapy. Parents should be advised that children should complete immunizations to date before starting etanercept. Patients with significant exposure to varicella virus (chickenpox) should temporarily discontinue therapy and varicella immune globulin should be considered.
- Instruct patient to notify health care professional of all Rx or OTC medications, vitamins, or herbal products being taken and to consult health care professional before taking any other Rx, OTC, or herbal products.
- Advise patient that methotrexate, analgesics, NSAIDs, corticosteroids, and salicylates may be continued during therapy.
- Instruct patient to notify health care professional if upper respiratory or other infections occur. Therapy may need to be discontinued if serious infection occurs.
- Advise patient of risk of malignancies such as hepatosplenic T-cell lymphoma. Instruct patient to report signs and symptoms (splenomegaly, hepatomegaly, abdominal pain, persistent fever, night sweats, weight loss) to health care professional promptly.
- Rep: Instruct females of reproductive potential to notify health care professional if pregnancy is planned or suspected and to avoid breastfeeding during therapy. Advise patients who become pregnant during therapy to notify health care professional. May limit administration of live vaccines to infant.

Evaluation/Desired Outcomes

- Reduction in symptoms of rheumatoid arthritis. Symptoms may return within 1 mo of discontinuation of therapy.
- Reduced severity of plaques in chronic plaque psoriasis.

---

ethambutol (e-tham-byoo-tole)
✦Etibi, Myambutol
Classification
Therapeutic: antituberculars

Indications
Active tuberculosis or other mycobacterial diseases (in combination with ≥1 other drug).

Action
Inhibits the growth of mycobacteria. **Therapeutic Effects:** Tuberculostatic effect against susceptible organisms.

Pharmacokinetics
Absorption: Rapidly and well absorbed (80%) from the GI tract.
Distribution: Widely distributed; crosses blood-brain barrier in small amounts.
Metabolism and Excretion: 50% metabolized by the liver, 50% eliminated unchanged by the kidneys.
Half-life: 3.3 hr (↑ in renal or hepatic impairment).

TIME/ACTION PROFILE (plasma concentrations)

ROUTE	ONSET	PEAK	DURATION
PO	rapid	2–4 hr	24 hr

Contraindications/Precautions
Contraindicated in: Hypersensitivity; Optic neuritis.
Use Cautiously in: Renal impairment (dose ↓ required); Severe hepatic impairment (dose ↓ required); OB: Although safety not established, ethambutol has been used with isoniazid in pregnant women without fetal adverse effects; Lactation: Use while breastfeeding only if potential maternal benefit justifies potential risk to infant.

Adverse Reactions/Side Effects
EENT: optic neuritis. **GI:** abdominal pain, anorexia, HEPATITIS, nausea, vomiting. **Metab:** hyperuricemia. **MS:** joint pain. **Neuro:** confusion, dizziness, hallucinations, headache, malaise, peripheral neuritis. **Resp:** pulmonary infiltrates. **Misc:** anaphylactoid reactions, fever.

Interactions
Drug-Drug: Neurotoxicity may be ↑ with other **neurotoxic agents**. **Aluminum hydroxide** may ↓ absorption (space doses 4 hr apart).

Route/Dosage
PO (Adults and Children >13 yr): 15–25 mg/kg/day (max = 2.5 g/day) *or* 50 mg/kg (up to 2.5 g) twice weekly *or* 25–30 mg/kg (up to 2.5 g) 3 times weekly.
PO (Children 1 mo–13 yr): *HIV negative:* 15–20 mg/kg/day once daily (max = 1 g/day) or 50 mg/kg/dose twice weekly (max = 2.5 g/dose); *HIV-exposed/-infected:* 15–25 mg/kg/day once daily (max = 2.5 g/day); *MAC, secondary prophylaxis, or treatment in HIV-exposed/-infected:* 15–25 mg/kg/day once daily (max = 2.5 g/day) with clarithromycin (or azithromycin) with or without rifabutin; *Nontuberculous mycobacterial infection:* 15–25 mg/kg/day once daily (max = 2.5 g/day).

Availability (generic available)
Tablets: 100 mg, 400 mg.

NURSING IMPLICATIONS
Assessment
- Mycobacterial studies and susceptibility tests should be performed before and periodically during therapy to detect possible resistance.
- Assess lung sounds and character and amount of sputum periodically during therapy.
- Assessments of visual function should be made frequently during therapy. Advise patient to report blurring of vision, constriction of visual fields, or changes in color perception immediately. Visual impairment, if not identified early, may lead to permanent sight impairment.

Lab Test Considerations
- Monitor renal and hepatic functions, CBC, and uric acid levels routinely. Frequently causes elevated uric acid concentrations, which may precipitate an attack of gout.

Implementation
- Ethambutol is given as a single daily dose and should be taken at the same time each day. Some regimens require dosing 2–3 times/wk. Usually administered concurrently with other antitubercular medications to prevent development of bacterial resistance.
- **PO:** Administer with food or milk to minimize GI irritation.
- **PO:** Tablets may be crushed and mixed with apple juice or apple sauce.

Patient/Family Teaching
- Instruct patient to take medication as directed. Take missed doses as soon as possible unless almost time for next dose; do not double up on missed doses. A full course of therapy may take mo to yr. Do not discontinue without consulting health care professional, even though symptoms may disappear.
- Instruct patient to notify health care professional if no improvement is seen in 2–3 wk. Health care professional should also be notified if unexpected weight gain or decreased urine output occurs.
- Emphasize the importance of routine exams to evaluate progress and ophthalmic examinations if signs of optic neuritis occur.
- Rep: Advise females of reproductive potential to notify health care professional if pregnancy is planned or suspected or if breastfeeding.

Evaluation/Desired Outcomes
- Resolution of clinical symptoms of tuberculosis.
- Decrease in acid-fast bacteria in sputum samples.
- Improvement seen in chest x rays. Therapy for tuberculosis is usually continued for at least 1–2 yr.

---

ethinyl estradiol/desogestrel, See CONTRACEPTIVES, HORMONAL.

---

ethinyl estradiol/drospirenone, See CONTRACEPTIVES, HORMONAL.

---

ethinyl estradiol/ethynodiol, See CONTRACEPTIVES, HORMONAL.

---

ethinyl estradiol/etonogestrel, See CONTRACEPTIVES, HORMONAL.

---

ethinyl estradiol/levonorgestrel, See CONTRACEPTIVES, HORMONAL.

---

ethinyl estradiol/norelgestromin, See CONTRACEPTIVES, HORMONAL.

---

ethinyl estradiol/norethindrone, See CONTRACEPTIVES, HORMONAL.

---

ethinyl estradiol/norgestimate, See CONTRACEPTIVES, HORMONAL.

---

ethinyl estradiol/norgestrel, See CONTRACEPTIVES, HORMONAL.

---

etonogestrel, See CONTRACEPTIVES, HORMONAL.

---

everolimus (e-ver-oh-li-mus)
Afinitor, Afinitor Disperz, Zortress
Classification
Therapeutic: antineoplastics, immunosuppressants
Pharmacologic: kinase inhibitors

Indications
Afinitor. Advanced renal cell carcinoma that has failed treatment with sunitinib or sorafenib. Subependymal giant cell astrocytoma associated with tuberous sclerosis complex in patients who are not candidates for curative surgical resection. Tuberous sclerosis complex–associated partial-onset seizures (adjunctive treatment). Progressive neuroendocrine tumors of pancreatic origin in patients with unresectable, locally advanced, or metastatic disease. Progressive, well-differentiated, nonfunctional neuroendocrine tumors of GI or lung origin in patients with unresectable, locally advanced, or metastatic disease. Renal angiomyoli-

poma with tuberous sclerosis complex in patients not requiring immediate surgery. 🎇 Treatment of postmenopausal women with advanced hormone receptor-positive, HER2-negative breast cancer after failure of treatment with letrozole or anastrozole (in combination with exemestane). **Zortress**. Prevention of organ rejection in patients who have received a kidney transplant and are at low to moderate immunologic risk. Prevention of organ rejection in patients who have received a liver transplant.

Action

Acts as a kinase inhibitor, decreasing cell proliferation. Inhibits activation and proliferation of T and B lymphocytes. **Therapeutic Effects:** Decreased spread of renal cell carcinoma and breast cancer. Improvement in progression-free survival in patients with progressive neuroendocrine tumors. Decreased volume of subependymal giant cell astrocytoma and angiomyolipoma lesions. Prevention of kidney and liver transplant rejection. Reduction in seizure frequency.

Pharmacokinetics

Absorption: Well absorbed following oral administration.

Distribution: 20% confined to plasma.

Metabolism and Excretion: Mostly metabolized by liver via the CYP3A4 isoenzyme; metabolites are mostly excreted in feces (80%) and urine (5%).

Half-life: 30 hr.

TIME/ACTION PROFILE (plasma concentrations)

ROUTE	ONSET	PEAK	DURATION
PO	unknown	1–2 hr	24 hr

Contraindications/Precautions

Contraindicated in: Hypersensitivity to everolimus or other rapamycins; Severe hepatic impairment; use only if benefit exceeds risk for renal cell carcinoma, progressive neuroendocrine tumors, breast cancer, and renal angiomyolipoma with tuberous sclerosis complex; Concurrent use with strong CYP3A4 inhibitors; Heart transplantation (Zortress) (↑ risk of mortality); Functional carcinoid tumors; OB: Pregnancy; Lactation: Lactation.

Use Cautiously in: Mild or moderate hepatic impairment (dose ↓ required); Exposure to sunlight/UV light (may ↑ risk of malignant skin changes); Patients undergoing radiation treatment before, during, or after therapy (↑ risk of radiation sensitization and radiation recall); Rep: Women of reproductive potential and men with female partners of reproductive potential; Pedi: Safety not established in children for indications other than SEGA and TSC-associated partial-onset seizures; Geri: Older adults may be more sensitive to drug effects; consider age-related ↓ in hepatic function, concurrent disease states, and drug therapy.

Adverse Reactions/Side Effects

CV: peripheral edema. **Derm:** delayed wound healing, dry skin, pruritus, rash. **GI:** anorexia, constipation, diarrhea, mouth ulcers, mucositis, nausea, stomatitis, vomiting, HEPATIC ARTERY THROMBOSIS. **GU:** ↓ fertility, acute renal failure, amenorrhea, kidney arterial/venous thrombosis (Zortress), menstrual irregularities, proteinuria. **Hemat:** anemia, leukopenia, thrombocytopenia, HEMOLYTIC UREMIC SYNDROME, THROMBOTIC MICROANGIOPATHY, THROMBOTIC THROMBOCYTOPENIC PURPURA. **Metab:** hyperglycemia, hyperlipidemia, hypertriglyceridemia. **MS:** extremity pain. **Neuro:** fatigue, weakness, dysgeusia, headache. **Resp:** cough, dyspnea, pulmonary embolism, INTERSTITIAL LUNG DISEASE, PULMONARY HYPERTENSION. **Misc:** fever, HYPERSENSITIVITY REACTIONS (including anaphylaxis and angioedema), INFECTION (including activation of latent viral infections such as BK virus-associated nephropathy), LYMPHOMA/SKIN CANCER (Zortress).

Interactions

Drug-Drug: **Strong CYP3A4 inhibitors**, including **atazanavir, clarithromycin, itraconazole, ketoconazole, nefazodone, nelfinavir, ritonavir,** or **voriconazole**, significantly ↑ levels and the risk of toxicity; avoid concurrent use. **Moderate CYP3A4 inhibitors**, including **aprepitant, diltiazem, erythromycin, fluconazole, fosamprenavir,** and **verapamil**, may ↑ levels and the risk of toxicity; ↓ dose of everolimus (Afinitor). **Strong CYP3A4 inducers**, including **carbamazepine, dexamethasone, phenobarbital, phenytoin, rifabutin,** and **rifampin**, may ↓ levels and effectiveness; avoid concurrent use, if possible. If concurrent use unavoidable, ↑ dose of everolimus may be required. ↑ risk of nephrotoxicity with **aminoglycosides, amphotericin B, cisplatin,** or **cyclosporine**. **ACE inhibitors** may ↑ risk of angioedema. May ↓ antibody formation and ↑ risk of adverse reactions from **live-virus vaccines**; avoid use of live-virus vaccines during treatment.

Drug-Natural Products: **St. John's wort** may ↓ levels and efficacy; avoid concurrent use.

Drug-Food: **Grapefruit juice** may ↑ levels and the risk of toxicity; avoid concurrent use.

Route/Dosage

Advanced Renal Cell Carcinoma, Advanced Progressive Neuroendocrine Tumors, Advanced Neuroendocrine Tumors, Advanced Hormone Receptor-Positive, HER2-Negative Breast Cancer, and Renal Angiomyolipoma with Tuberous Sclerosis Complex (Afinitor)

PO (Adults): 10 mg once daily until disease progression or unacceptable toxicity; *Concurrent use of P-glycoprotein (P-gp) inhibitor and moderate CYP3A4 inhibitor:* 2.5 mg once daily until disease progression or unacceptable toxicity; *Concurrent use of P-gp inducer and strong CYP3A4 inducer:* ↑ dose in 5 mg increments up to 20 mg once daily; continue until disease progression or unacceptable toxicity.

Hepatic Impairment

PO (Adults): *Mild hepatic impairment:* 7.5 mg once daily until disease progression or unacceptable toxicity; may ↓ to 5 mg once daily if not well tolerated; *Moderate hepatic impairment:* 5 mg once daily until disease progression or unacceptable toxicity; may ↓ to 2.5 mg once daily if not well tolerated; *Severe hepatic impairment:* 2.5 mg once daily until disease progression or unacceptable toxicity.

Subependymal Giant Cell Astrocytoma with Tuberous Sclerosis Complex (Afinitor)

PO (Adults and Children ≥1 yr): 4.5 mg/m² once daily. Titrate, as needed, at 2-wk intervals to achieve recommended whole blood trough concentration. Continue until disease progression or unacceptable toxicity; *Concurrent use of P-gp inhibitor and moderate CYP3A4 inhibitor:* 2.25 mg/m² once daily. Titrate, as needed, at 2-wk intervals to achieve recommended whole blood trough concentration. Continue until disease progression or unacceptable toxicity; *Concurrent use of P-gp inducer and strong CYP3A4 inducer:* 9 mg/m² once daily. Titrate, as needed, at 2-wk intervals to achieve recommended whole blood trough concentration. Continue until disease progression or unacceptable toxicity.

Hepatic Impairment

PO (Adults and Children ≥1 yr): *Severe hepatic impairment:* 2.5 mg/m² once daily. Titrate, as needed, at 2-wk intervals to achieve recommended whole blood trough concentration. Continue until disease progression or unacceptable toxicity.

Tuberous Sclerosis Complex-Associated Partial-Onset Seizures (Afinitor)

PO (Adults and Children ≥2 yr): 5 mg/m² once daily. Titrate, as needed, at 2-wk intervals to achieve recommended whole blood trough concentration. Continue until disease progression or unacceptable toxicity; *Concurrent use of P-gp inhibitor and moderate CYP3A4 inhibitor:* 2.5 mg/m² once daily. Titrate, as needed, at 2-wk intervals to achieve recommended whole blood trough concentration. Continue until disease progression or unacceptable toxicity; *Concurrent use of P-gp inducer and strong CYP3A4 inducer:* 10 mg/m² once daily. Titrate, as needed, at 2-wk intervals to achieve recommended whole blood trough concentration. Continue until disease progression or unacceptable toxicity.

Hepatic Impairment

PO (Adults and Children ≥2 yr): *Severe hepatic impairment:* 2.5 mg/m² once daily. Titrate, as needed, at 2-wk intervals to achieve recommended whole blood trough concentration. Continue until disease progression or unacceptable toxicity.

Kidney Transplantation (Zortress)

PO (Adults): 0.75 mg twice daily (with reduced-dose cyclosporine); titrate to achieve recommended whole blood trough concentration.

Hepatic Impairment

PO (Adults): *Mild hepatic impairment :* ↓ daily dose by 33%; *Moderate or severe hepatic impairment:* ↓ daily dose by 50%.

Liver Transplantation (Zortress)

PO (Adults): 1 mg twice daily (with reduced-dose tacrolimus) (start ≥30 days post-transplant); titrate to achieve recommended whole blood trough concentration.

Hepatic Impairment

PO (Adults): *Mild hepatic impairment :* ↓ daily dose by 33%; *Moderate or severe hepatic impairment:* ↓ daily dose by 50%.

Availability (generic available)

Tablets (Afinitor): 2.5 mg, 5 mg, 7.5 mg, 10 mg. **Tablets for oral suspension (Afinitor Disperz):** 2 mg, 3 mg, 5 mg. **Tablets (Zortress):** 0.25 mg, 0.5 mg, 0.75 mg, 1 mg.

NURSING IMPLICATIONS
Assessment

- Assess for symptoms of noninfectious pneumonitis (hypoxia, pleural effusion, cough, dyspnea) during therapy. If symptoms are mild, therapy may continue. *If Grade 2 pneumonitis occurs:* hold therapy until Grade 0–1; reinitiate everolimus at a 50% dose. Permanently discontinue if does not resolve or improve to Grade 1 within 4 wk. *If Grade 3 pneumonitis occurs:* hold therapy until Grade 0–1; resume at 50% of previous dose. Change to every other day if dose is lower than lowest available strength. Permanently discontinue if Grade 3 pneumonitis recurs. *If Grade 4 pneumonitis occurs:* permanently discontinue.
- Assess for mouth ulcers, stomatitis, or oral mucositis; usually occurs within first 8 wk of therapy. Begin dexamethasone alcohol-free oral solution as a swish and spit mouthwash when starting therapy to reduce incidence and severity of stomatitis. Topical treatments may be used; avoid peroxide-containing mouthwashes and antifungals unless fungal infection has been diagnosed. *If stomatitis Grade 2 occurs:* hold therapy until Grade 0–1; resume at previous dose. If Grade 2 recurs, withhold until Grade 0–1; resume at 50% dose. Change to every other day if dose is lower than lowest available strength. *If Grade 3 stomatitis occurs:* hold therapy until Grade 0–1; hold until Grade 0–1; resume at 50% of previous dose. Change to every other day if dose is lower than lowest available strength. *If Grade 4 stomatitis occurs:* discontinue permanently.
- Assess for signs and symptoms of systemic fungal infections (fever, malaise, weight loss, sweats, cough, dyspnea, pulmonary infiltrates, serious systemic illness with or without concomitant shock). Withhold

therapy until infection has been diagnosed and adequately treated.

● Monitor for signs and symptoms of hypersensitivity reactions (anaphylaxis, dyspnea, flushing, chest pain, angioedema) during therapy. Permanently discontinue therapy if severe reactions occur.

Lab Test Considerations

● Verify negative pregnancy test before starting therapy.

● Monitor renal function prior to and periodically during therapy. May cause ↑ BUN, serum creatinine, and proteinuria.

● Monitor fasting serum glucose and lipid profile prior to and periodically during therapy. May cause ↑ cholesterol, triglycerides, glucose. Attempt to achieve optimal glucose and lipid control prior to therapy. *If Grade 3 metabolic events (hyperglycemia, dyslipidemia) occur:* hold until improvement to Grade 0, 1, or 2. Resume at 50% of previous dose. Change to every other day if dose is lower than lowest available strength.

● Monitor CBC prior to and every 6 mo for 1st yr of therapy and annually thereafter; may cause ↓ hemoglobin, lymphocytes, neutrophils, and platelets. *If Grade 2 thrombocytopenia occurs:* hold dose until Grade 0–1; resume at same dose. *If Grade 3 or 4 thrombocytopenia occurs:* hold until improvement to Grade 0, 1, or 2. Resume at 50% of previous dose. Change to every other day if dose is lower than lowest available strength. *If Grade 3 neutropenia occurs:* hold dose until Grade 0–1; resume at same dose. *If Grade 4 neutropenia occurs:* hold until improvement to Grade 0, 1, or 2. Resume at 50% of previous dose. Change to every other day if dose is lower than lowest available strength. *If Grade 3 febrile neutropenia occurs:* hold until improvement to Grade 0, 1, or 2 and no fever. Resume at 50% of previous dose. Change to every other day if dose is lower than lowest available strength. *If Grade 4 febrile neutropenia occurs:* discontinue permanently.

● May cause ↑ AST, ALT, phosphate, and bilirubin.

● **Afinitor:** Monitor *Afinitor* trough levels 2 wk after initiation of therapy, a change in dose, a change in coadministration of CYP3A4 and/or P-gp inducers or inhibitors, change in hepatic function, or change in dose form between everolimus tablets and *Disperz*. Once at a stable dose, monitor trough concentrations every 3–6 mo in patients with changing body surface area or every 6–12 mo in patients with stable body surface area for duration of treatment. Therapeutic blood concentrations are 5–15 ng/mL (*Afinitor*). If trough concentration is <5 ng/mL, ↑ daily dose by 2.5 mg in patients taking tablets and 2 mg for *Disperz*. If trough concentration is >15 ng/mL, ↓ daily dose by 2.5 mg in patients taking tablets and 2 mg for *Disperz*. If dose ↓ is required with lowest dose, administer every other day. Do not combine dose forms to achieve dose. **Zortress:** Therapeutic blood concentrations are 3–8 ng/mL via the LCMSMS assay (*Zortress*). Base dose adjustments of *Zortress* on trough concentrations obtained 4 or 5 days after a previous dosing change. Adjust dose if trough concentration is <3 ng/mL by doubling dose using available tablet strengths (0.25 mg, 0.5 mg or 0.75 mg). If trough concentration is >8 ng/mL on 2 consecutive measures, ↓ dose of *Zortress* by 0.25 mg twice daily.

Implementation

● May impair wound healing. Hold everolimus for at least 1 wk before and at least 2 wk after elective surgery to ensure adequate wound healing.

● **PO:** Administer at the same time each day consistently with or without food, followed by a whole glass of water. *DNC:* Swallow tablets whole; do not break, crush, or chew.

● Do not combine the 2 dose forms (*Afinitor Tablets* and *Afinitor Disperz*) to achieve the desired total dose. Use one dose form or the other.

● Administer *Disperz*, dispersible tablet, as a suspension only. Wear gloves to avoid possible contact with everolimus when preparing suspensions for another person. Place dose in 10 mL syringe; do not exceed 10 mg/syringe. If higher dose required, use additional syringe. Do not break or crush tablets. Draw 5 mL water and 4 mL of air into syringe. Place filled syringe into container (tip up) for 3 min until tablets are in suspension. Invert syringe five times immediately prior to administration. Administer immediately after preparation; discard suspension if not administered within 60 min after preparation. After administration, draw 5 mL of water and 4 mL of air into same syringe, and swirl contents to suspend remaining particles. Administer entire contents of syringe. Can also be dispersed using same technique and 25 mL water in small glass.

Patient/Family Teaching

● Instruct patient to take everolimus at the same time each day as directed. Take missed doses as soon as remembered up to 6 hr after time of normal dose. If more than 6 hr after normal dose, omit dose for that day and take next dose next day; do not take two doses to make up missed dose. Do not eat grapefruit or drink grapefruit juice during therapy. Advise patient to read *Patient Information* prior to beginning therapy and with each Rx refill in case of new information.

● Advise patient to report worsening respiratory symptoms or signs of infection (new or worsening cough, shortness of breath, chest pain, difficulty breathing or wheezing, fever, chills, skin rash, joint pain and inflammation, tiredness, loss of appetite, nausea, pale stool or dark urine, yellowing of the skin, pain in upper right side) or severe allergic reaction (rash, itching, hives, flushing, trouble breathing or swallowing, chest pain, dizziness, trouble breathing, swelling of tongue, mouth, or throat) to health care professional promptly.

- Inform patient that mouth sores may occur. Consult health care professional for treatment if pain, discomfort, or open sores in mouth occur. May require special mouthwash or gel.
- Instruct patient to avoid use of live vaccines and close contact with those who have received live vaccines.
- Instruct patient to notify health care professional of all Rx or OTC medications, vitamins, or herbal products being taken and to consult with health care professional before taking other medications, especially St. John's wort.
- Notify health care professional of everolimus therapy before treatment or surgery. May require temporarily stopping everolimus.
- Rep: May cause fetal harm. Advise females of reproductive potential to use effective contraception during and for up to 8 wk after last dose, male patients with female partners of reproductive potential to use effective contraception during and for up to 4 wk after last dose, and to notify health care professional if pregnancy is planned or suspected. Advise female patients to avoid breastfeeding during and for 2 wk after last dose. May impair fertility in female and male patients.
- Emphasize the importance of routine blood tests to determine effectiveness and side effects.

Evaluation/Desired Outcomes

- Decreased spread of tumor. Continue treatment as long as clinical benefit is observed or until unacceptable toxicity occurs.
- Prevention of kidney or liver transplant rejection.
- Reduced seizure frequency.

---

evolocumab (e-vo-lo-kyoo-mab)
Repatha
Classification
Therapeutic: lipid-lowering agents
Pharmacologic: proprotein convertase subtilisin kexin type 9 (PCSK9) inhibitors, monoclonal antibodies

---

Indications
Primary hyperlipidemia (including heterozygous familial hypercholesterolemia [HeFH]) in adults (as an adjunct to diet as monotherapy or in combination with other low-density lipoprotein cholesterol [LDL-C]-lowering therapies). Homozygous familial hypercholesterolemia (in combination with other LDL-C lowering therapies). HeFH in pediatric patients ≥10 yr (as an adjunct to diet in combination with other LDL-C-lowering therapies). To reduce the risk of MI, stroke, and coronary revascularization in patients with cardiovascular disease.

Action
A human monoclonal immunoglobulin produced in genetically engineered Chinese hamster ovary cells that binds to PCSK9, inhibiting its binding to the low density lipoprotein receptor (LDLR) resulting in ↑ number of LDLRs available to clear LDL-C from blood. **Therapeutic Effects:** Reduction in LDL-C. Reduction in the risk of MI, stroke, and coronary revascularization.

Pharmacokinetics
Absorption: Well absorbed (72%) following SUBQ administration.
Distribution: Minimally distributed to tissues.
Metabolism and Excretion: Eliminated by binding to PCSK9 and by proteolytic degradation.
Half-life: 11–17 days.

TIME/ACTION PROFILE (effect on circulating unbound PCSK9)

ROUTE	ONSET	PEAK	DURATION
SUBQ	rapid	4 hr	2–4 wk

Contraindications/Precautions
Contraindicated in: Hypersensitivity.
Use Cautiously in: Severe renal impairment; Severe hepatic impairment; OB: Safety not established in pregnancy; Lactation: Safety not established in breastfeeding; Pedi: Children <10 yr (safety and effectiveness not established); Geri: Older adults may be more sensitive to drug effects.

Adverse Reactions/Side Effects
Local: injection site reactions. **MS:** back pain. **Misc:** HYPERSENSITIVITY REACTIONS (including angioedema).

Interactions
Drug-Drug: None reported.

Route/Dosage

Established Cardiovascular Disease or Primary Hyperlipidemia
SUBQ (Adults): 140 mg every 2 wk *or* 420 mg once monthly.

Heterozygous Familial Hypercholesterolemia
SUBQ (Children ≥10 yr): 140 mg every 2 wk *or* 420 mg once monthly.

Homozygous Familial Hypercholesterolemia
SUBQ (Adults and Children ≥10 yr): 420 mg once monthly; if inadequate response after 12 wk, may ↑ to 420 mg every 2 wk. *Patients on lipid apheresis:* 420 mg every 2 wk (administered after apheresis session completed).

Availability
Solution for injection (needle cover contains latex derivative): 420 mg/3.5 mL (Pushtronex system), 140 mg/mL (prefilled syringes and autoinjectors).

NURSING IMPLICATIONS
Assessment
- Obtain a diet history, especially with regard to fat consumption.

- Monitor for signs and symptoms of hypersensitivity reactions (rash, urticaria) during therapy. If symptoms occur, discontinue therapy.
- Assess for latex allergy. Needle cover of the glass prefilled syringe and the autoinjector contain dry natural rubber (a derivative of latex); may cause allergic reactions.

Lab Test Considerations
- Assess LDL-C levels within 4–8 wk of initiating; response to therapy depends on degree of LDLR function. For patients on a monthly regimen, measure LDL-C just prior to next scheduled dose.

Implementation
- Needle cover of glass single-dose prefilled syringe and single-dose prefilled autoinjector contain latex; avoid with latex allergies.
- **SUBQ:** To administer the 140-mg or 420-mg dose using *Single-Use Prefilled SureClick Autoinjector*, give 1 injection (140-mg dose) or give 3 injections (420-mg dose), using 3 separate pens/syringes in 3 separate sites, consecutively within 30 min. When switching dose regimens, administer first dose of new regimen on next scheduled date of prior regimen. If stored in refrigerator allow solution to warm to room temperature for at least 30 min before injecting. May also be stored at room temperature, but only stable for 30 days. Solution is clear to opalescent and colorless to pale yellow; do not administer solutions that are cloudy or contain particulate matter. Do not shake. Stretch or pinch skin. Inject into thigh, abdomen, or upper arm at a 90° angle. Injection may take 15 sec. Window turns from clear to yellow when the injection is done. Rotate sites with each injection. Do not inject into areas that are tender, bruised, red, or indurated. Do not reuse prefilled pen or syringe. Do not administer other injectable drugs at same site.
- To administer the 420-mg dose using *Pushtronex on-body infusor system:* Remove on-body infusor and prefilled cartridge from refrigerator 45 min prior to use to allow to reach room temperature; do not use other sources of warming. Prepare injection site with little hair (may trim) and firm and flat skin surface by cleaning with alcohol and allowing to dry. May use thigh, abdomen (except 2 inches from umbilicus) or outer area of upper arm if not self-administered. Avoid areas that are tender, bruised, red, or hard, or areas with wrinkles, skin folds, scars, stretch marks, moles, and excessive hair. Solution in cartridge should be clear and colorless to slightly yellow; do not administer solutions that are discolored or contain particular matter. Clean bottom of cartridge with alcohol and load into on-body infusor; press firmly on top of unit to secure. Administer injection within 5 min after loading the cartridge; >5 min may dry out medication. Swing door close until it snaps. Peel away both green pull tabs to show adhesive. When blue light flashes, infusor is on. If using abdo-

men, stretch skin prior to applying; do not stretch skin for thigh placement. Apply infusor to skin making sure blue light is visible and firmly press start button. Flashing green light and click indicates infusion has begun; may beep and patient may feel a pinch. Solution is injected over 5 min. When green light changes to solid, infusion is complete. Remove from skin and check medicine window for green light to be off. Dispose of on-body infusor in a sharps container.

Patient/Family Teaching
- Instruct patient in correct technique for self-injection or on-body infusor, care and disposal of equipment. Administer missed doses within 7 days, then resume original schedule. If not administered within 7 days, wait until next dose on original schedule. Advise patient to read *Patient Information* before starting therapy and with each Rx refill in case of changes.
- Advise patient that this medication should be used in conjunction with diet restrictions (fat, cholesterol, carbohydrates, alcohol), exercise, and cessation of smoking.
- Instruct patient to notify health care professional of all Rx or OTC medications, vitamins, or herbal products being taken and to consult health care professional before taking any other Rx, OTC, or herbal products.
- Advise patient to notify health care professional of medication regimen prior to treatment or surgery.
- Rep: Advise patient to notify health care professional if pregnancy is planned or suspected or if breastfeeding. Inform pregnant patients of pregnancy safety study that monitors pregnancy outcomes in women exposed to evolocumab during pregnancy. Enroll patient by contacting Amgen at 1-800-77-AMGEN (1-800-772-6436).

Evaluation/Desired Outcomes
- Decreased LDL-C levels.
- Reduction in the risk of MI, stroke, and coronary revascularization.

⚸ **exemestane** (ex-e-**mes**-tane)
Aromasin
Classification
Therapeutic: antineoplastics
Pharmacologic: aromatase inhibitors

Indications
⚸ Adjuvant treatment of breast cancer in postmenopausal women who have estrogen-receptor positive early disease and who have already received 2–3 yr of tamoxifen and are then switched to exemestane to complete a total of 5 yr of adjuvant therapy. Treatment of advanced postmenopausal breast cancer that has progressed despite tamoxifen therapy.

Action

Inhibits aromatase, an enzyme responsible for the conversion of androgen to estrogen. In postmenopausal women, the primary source of estrogen is androgen. Decreases circulating estrogen. **Therapeutic Effects:** Decreased spread of estrogen-sensitive breast cancer.

Pharmacokinetics

Absorption: 42% absorbed following oral administration.

Distribution: Extensively distributed to tissues.

Metabolism and Excretion: Mostly metabolized by the liver via the CYP3A4 isoenzyme; metabolites are excreted in urine (40%) and feces (40%); <1% excreted unchanged in urine.

Half-life: 24 hr.

TIME/ACTION PROFILE (suppression of circulating estrogen)

ROUTE	ONSET	PEAK	DURATION
PO	unknown	2–3 days	4–5 days

Contraindications/Precautions

Contraindicated in: Hypersensitivity; Premenopausal status; OB: Pregnancy; Lactation: Lactation.

Use Cautiously in: Rep: Women of reproductive potential;.

Adverse Reactions/Side Effects

CV: hypertension, THROMBOEMBOLISM. **Derm:** ↑ sweating, alopecia, hot flush, dermatitis. **EENT:** visual disturbances. **GI:** diarrhea, nausea. **GU:** endometrial hyperplasia, uterine polyps. **MS:** arthralgia, carpal tunnel syndrome, muscle cramps, osteoporosis, pain. **Neuro:** fatigue, depression, insomnia, neuropathy, paresthesia.

Interactions

Drug-Drug: Strong CYP3A4 inducers, including **rifampin** or **phenytoin**, may ↓ levels and effectiveness. **Estrogens** can interfere with action.

Route/Dosage

PO (Adults): 25 mg once daily; *Concurrent use with strong CYP3A4 inducers:* 50 mg once daily.

Availability (generic available)

Tablets: 25 mg.

NURSING IMPLICATIONS

Assessment

- Assess patient for pain and other side effects periodically during therapy.
- Monitor patients for bone mineral density loss and treat as appropriate.

Lab Test Considerations

- Verify negative pregnancy test within 7 days of starting exemestane.
- May cause ↑ GGT, AST, ALT, alkaline phosphatase, bilirubin, and serum creatinine levels.

- Assess 25-hydroxy vitamin D levels prior to starting therapy. Supplement vitamin D deficiency with vitamin D due to high prevalence of vitamin D deficiency in women with early breast cancer.

Implementation

- Take 1 tablet daily after a meal.

Patient/Family Teaching

- Instruct patient to take exemestane as directed at the same time each day. Take missed doses as soon as remembered unless it is almost time for next dose. Do not double doses. Advise patient to read the *Patient Information* leaflet before starting and with each Rx refill in case of changes.
- Advise patient not to take other estrogen-containing agents; may interfere with action of exemestane.
- Inform patient that lower level of estrogen may lead to decreased bone mineral density over time and increased risk of osteoporosis and fracture. Women with osteoporosis or at risk of osteoporosis should have their bone mineral density formally assessed by bone densitometry at end of treatment.
- Advise patient to notify health care professional immediately if chest pain or signs of heart failure or stroke occur.
- Advise patient to notify health care professional of all Rx or OTC medications, vitamins, or herbal products being taken and to consult with health care professional before taking other medications.
- Rep: May cause fetal harm. Advise females of reproductive potential to use effective contraception and avoid breastfeeding during therapy and for at least 1 mo after last dose. May impair female and male fertility.
- Explain need for follow-up blood tests to check liver and kidney function.

Evaluation/Desired Outcomes

- Slowing of disease progression in women with breast cancer.

---

exenatide (ex-en-a-tide)

Bydureon BCise, Byetta

Classification
Therapeutic: antidiabetics
Pharmacologic: incretin mimetic agents

Indications

Type 2 diabetes mellitus (as adjunct to diet and exercise).

Action

Mimics the action of incretin, which promotes endogenous insulin secretion and promotes other mechanisms of glucose lowering. **Therapeutic Effects:** Improved control of blood glucose.

Pharmacokinetics

Absorption: Well absorbed following SUBQ administration.

Distribution: Widely distributed to tissues.
Metabolism and Excretion: Excreted mostly by glomerular filtration followed by degradation.
Half-life: *Immediate-release:* 2.4 hr.

TIME/ACTION PROFILE (effects on postprandial blood glucose)

ROUTE	ONSET	PEAK	DURATION
SUBQ (immediate-release)	within 30 min	2.1 hr	8 hr
SUBQ (extended-release)	unknown	9 wk	unknown

Contraindications/Precautions

Contraindicated in: Hypersensitivity; History of drug-induced immune-mediated thrombocytopenia from exenatide; Type 1 diabetes or diabetic ketoacidosis; Severe renal impairment or end-stage renal disease (CCr <30 mL/min) (immediate-release only); CCr <45 mL/min (extended-release); Severe GI disease; Personal or family history of medullary thyroid carcinoma (extended-release only); Multiple Endocrine Neoplasia syndrome type 2 (extended-release only).
Use Cautiously in: History of pancreatitis; Concurrent use of ACE inhibitors, NSAIDs, or diuretics (↑ risk of renal impairment); OB: Use during pregnancy only if maternal benefit outweighs potential fetal risk; Lactation: Use during breastfeeding only if potential maternal benefit outweighs potential risk to infant; Pedi: Safety and effectiveness not established in children <18 yr (Byetta) or <10 yr (Bydureon BCise).

Adverse Reactions/Side Effects

Derm: ↑ sweating. **Endo:** hypoglycemia, THYROID C-CELL TUMORS (extended-release). **GI:** diarrhea, nausea, vomiting, ↓ appetite, ↓ weight, cholecystitis, cholelithiasis, dyspepsia, gastrointestinal reflux, PANCREATITIS. **GU:** acute renal failure, renal impairment. **Hemat:** THROMBOCYTOPENIA. **Local:** injection site reactions. **Neuro:** dizziness, headache, jitteriness, weakness. **Misc:** injection site reactions.

Interactions

Drug-Drug: Concurrent use with **sulfonylureas** or **insulin** may ↑ risk of hypoglycemia (↓ dose of sulfonylurea or insulin if hypoglycemia occurs). Concurrent use with **nateglinide** or **repaglinide** may ↑ risk of hypoglycemia. Due to slowed gastric emptying, may ↓ absorption of **orally administered medications**, especially those requiring rapid GI absorption or require a specific level for efficacy; take oral **anti-infectives** and **oral contraceptives** at least 1 hr before injecting exenatide). Concurrent use of **ACE inhibitors, NSAIDs,** or **diuretics** may ↑ risk of renal impairment.

Route/Dosage
Immediate Release (Byetta)

SUBQ (Adults): 5 mcg within 60 min before morning and evening meal; after 1 mo, dose may be ↑ to 10 mcg depending on response.

Renal Impairment
SUBQ (Adults): *CCr 30–50 mL/min:* Use caution when ↑ dose from 5 mcg to 10 mcg.

Extended Release (Bydureon BCise)
SUBQ (Adults and Children ≥10 yr): 2 mg every 7 days.

Availability
Solution for injection (Byetta) (prefilled pens): 300 mcg/1.2 mL (delivers 5 mcg/dose), 600 mcg/2.4 mL (delivers 10 mcg/dose). **Suspension for injection (Bydureon BCise) (prefilled autoinjectors):** 2 mg/0.85 mL.

NURSING IMPLICATIONS
Assessment

- Observe for signs and symptoms of hypoglycemic reactions (abdominal pain, sweating, hunger, weakness, dizziness, headache, drowsiness, tremor, tachycardia, anxiety, confusion, irritability, jitteriness), especially when combined with oral sulfonylureas.
- Assess for signs and symptoms of pancreatitis (persistent severe abdominal pain, sometimes radiating to the back, may or may not be accompanied by vomiting) at beginning of therapy and with dose increases. If suspected, promptly discontinue therapy and initiate appropriate management. If pancreatitis is confirmed, do not restart exenatide. Consider other antidiabetic therapies in patients with a history of pancreatitis.

Lab Test Considerations
- Monitor serum glucose and HbA1c periodically during therapy to evaluate effectiveness of therapy.
- Monitor renal function prior to and periodically during therapy. Renal dysfunction may be reversed with discontinuation of therapy.

Implementation

- Some medications (anti-infectives, oral contraceptives) may need to be taken 1 hr before exenatide.
- Patients stabilized on a diabetic regimen who are exposed to stress, fever, trauma, infection, or surgery may require administration of insulin.
- SUBQ: *Immediate release:* Follow directions for *New Pen Setup* in *Information for Patient* prior to use of each new pen. Inject exenatide in thigh, abdomen, or upper arm at any time within the 60-min period **before** the morning and evening meals. Do not administer after a meal. Do not mix with insulin. Solution should be clear and colorless; do not administer solutions that are discolored or contain particulate matter. Refrigerate; discard pen 30 days after 1st

use, even if some drug remains in pen. Do not freeze. Do not store pen with needle attached; medication may leak from pen or air bubbles may form in the cartridge.

- **SUBQ:** *Extended release:* Remove from refrigerator 15 min prior to mixing. Dilute with diluent and needles included in tray. Suspension should be white or off-white and cloudy. Mix by shaking vigorously for 15 sec. Do not inject solutions that are discolored or contain particulate matter. Administer without regard to meals. Inject into upper arm, abdomen, or thigh; change site each wk. Refrigerate; each tray can be kept at room temperature if not >77°F for up to 4 wk. Store *Bydureon BCise* flat. Do not use beyond expiration date.
- Do not mix insulin in the same syringe with exenatide. Injection of *Bydureon Bcise* and insulin may be administered in the same body area, but not right next to each other.
- If switching from immediate-release to extended-release, discontinue other forms of exenatide before starting *Bydureon BCise*. When switching from another extended-release product, may change with next scheduled dose. May cause transient ↑ in blood glucose for 2–4 wk.

Patient/Family Teaching

- Instruct patient to take exenatide *immediate release* as directed within 60 min before a meal. Do not take after a meal. If a dose is missed, skip the dose and take the next dose at the prescribed time. Do not take an extra dose or increase the amount of the next dose to make up for missed dose. If a dose of exenatide *extended release* is missed, administer as soon as remembered as long as the next dose is due at least 3 days later; if 1 or 2 days later skip dose and administer next dose as scheduled. The day of weekly administration can be changed as long as the last dose was administered 3 or more days before. Advise patient to read *Medication Guide* before starting therapy and with each Rx refill.
- Instruct patient in proper technique for administration, timing of dose, and concurrent oral medications, storage of medication, and disposal of used needles. Patients should read the *Information for Patient* insert prior to initiation of therapy and with each Rx refill. Advise patient that *New Pen Setup* should be done only with each new pen, not with each dose.
- Inform patient that pen needles are not included with pen and must be purchased separately. Advise patient which needle length and gauge should be used. Caution patient not to share pen and needles.
- Caution patient to never share pen with others, even if needle is changed. May cause transmission of bloodborne pathogens.
- Explain to patient that exenatide helps control hyperglycemia but does not cure diabetes. Therapy is usually long term.

- Encourage patient to follow prescribed diet, medication, and exercise regimen to prevent hyperglycemic or hypoglycemic episodes.
- Review signs of hypoglycemia and hyperglycemia with patient. If hypoglycemia occurs, advise patient to take a glass of orange juice or 2–3 tsp of sugar, honey, or corn syrup dissolved in water, and notify health care professional. Risk of hypoglycemia is increased if sulfonylureas are taken concurrently with exenatide.
- Advise patient to notify health care professional immediately if symptoms of pancreatitis (unexplained, persistent, severe abdominal pain that may or may not be accompanied by vomiting) occur.
- Inform patient that therapy may result in reduction of appetite, food intake, and/or body weight. Dose modification is not necessary. Nausea is more common at initiation of therapy and usually decreases over time.
- Instruct patient to notify health care professional of all Rx or OTC medications, vitamins, or herbal products being taken and to consult health care professional before taking any other Rx, OTC, or herbal products. Exenatide delays stomach emptying. Some medications (such as anti-infectives and oral contraceptives) may need to be taken 1 hr before exenatide injection.
- Instruct patient in proper testing of blood glucose and urine ketones. Monitor closely during periods of stress or illness; notify health care professional if significant changes occur.
- Advise patient to inform health care professional of medication regimen before treatment or surgery.
- Advise patient to carry a form of sugar (sugar packets, candy) and identification describing disease process and medication regimen at all times.
- Rep: Insulin is the recommended method of controlling blood sugar during pregnancy. Advise patient to notify health care professional if pregnancy is suspected or planned, or if breastfeeding.
- Emphasize the importance of routine follow-up exams and regular testing of blood glucose and HbA1c.

Evaluation/Desired Outcomes

- Control of blood glucose levels without the appearance of hypoglycemic or hyperglycemic episodes.

ezetimibe (e-zet-i-mibe)
⭐ Ezetrol, Zetia
Classification
Therapeutic: lipid-lowering agents
Pharmacologic: cholesterol absorption inhibitors

Indications

Primary hyperlipidemia, including heterozygous familial hypercholesterolemia (as monotherapy [in adults only] or in combination with a statin). Mixed hyperlipidemia (in combination with fenofibrate). Homozygous familial hypercholesterolemia (in combination with a statin and other low-density lipoprotein cholesterol [LDL-C] lowering therapies). Familial sitosterolemia.

Action
Inhibits absorption of cholesterol in the small intestine. **Therapeutic Effects:** Reduction of LDL-C concentrations. Reduction of sitosterol and campesterol concentrations.

Pharmacokinetics
Absorption: Following absorption, rapidly converted to ezetimibe-glucuronide, which is active. Bioavailability is variable.
Distribution: Unknown.
Metabolism and Excretion: Undergoes enterohepatic recycling, mostly eliminated in feces, minimal renal excretion.
Half-life: 22 hr.

TIME/ACTION PROFILE

ROUTE	ONSET	PEAK	DURATION
PO	unknown	unknown	unknown

Contraindications/Precautions
Contraindicated in: Hypersensitivity; When a statin, fenofibrate, or other LDL-C lowering therapy is contraindicated (when used in combination with statin, fenofibrate, or other LDL-C lowering therapy); Moderate or severe hepatic impairment.
Use Cautiously in: OB: Safety not established in pregnancy; Lactation: Safety not established in breastfeeding; Pedi: Children <10 yr (safety and effectiveness not established).

Adverse Reactions/Side Effects
Derm: rash. **GI:** ↑ liver enzymes, cholecystitis, cholelithiasis, nausea, pancreatitis. **MS:** myopathy, RHABDOMYOLYSIS. **Misc:** ANGIOEDEMA.

Interactions
Drug-Drug: Effects may be ↓ by **cholestyramine** or other **bile acid sequestrants**. Concurrent use of **fibrates** may ↑ levels and the risk of cholelithiasis. **Cyclosporine** may ↑ levels. May ↑ risk of rhabdomyolysis when used with **HMG CoA-reductase inhibitors**.

Route/Dosage
PO (Adults): 10 mg once daily.

Renal Impairment
PO (Adults): *CCr <60 mL/min and concurrent use with simvastatin:* Not to exceed simvastatin dose of 20 mg/day.

Availability (generic available)
Tablets: 10 mg. *In combination with:* rosuvastatin (Roszet); simvastatin (Vytorin); see Appendix N.

NURSING IMPLICATIONS
Assessment
- Obtain a diet history, especially with regard to fat consumption.

Lab Test Considerations
- Evaluate serum cholesterol and triglyceride levels before initiating, after 2–4 wk of therapy, and periodically thereafter.
- May cause ↑ liver transaminases when administered with HMG-CoA reductase inhibitors. Monitor liver enzymes prior to initiation and during therapy according to recommendations of HMG-CoA reductase inhibitor. Elevations are usually asymptomatic and return to baseline with continued therapy.

Implementation
- Do not confuse Zetia with Zestril.
- **PO:** Administer without regard to meals. May be taken at the same time as HMG-CoA reductase inhibitors or fenofibrate. Administer at least 2 hr before or at least 4 hr after bile acid sequestrants.

Patient/Family Teaching
- Instruct patient to take ezetimibe as directed, at the same time each day, even if feeling well. Take missed doses as soon as remembered, but do not take more than 1 dose/day. Medication helps control but does not cure elevated serum cholesterol levels. Advise patient to read *Patient Information* before starting therapy and with each Rx refill in case of change.
- Advise patient that this medication should be used in conjunction with diet restrictions (fat, cholesterol, carbohydrates, alcohol), exercise, and cessation of smoking. Ezetimibe does not assist with weight loss.
- Instruct patient to notify health care professional if unexplained muscle pain, tenderness, or weakness occur. Risk may increase when used with HMG-CoA reductase inhibitors.
- Instruct patient to notify health care professional of all Rx or OTC medications, vitamins, or herbal products being taken and to consult health care professional before taking any other Rx, OTC, or herbal products.
- Advise patient to notify health care professional of medication regimen prior to treatment or surgery.
- Rep: Advise females of reproductive potential to notify health care professional promptly if pregnancy is planned or suspected or if breastfeeding. If regimen includes HMG-CoA reductase inhibitors, they are contraindicated in pregnancy.
- Emphasize the importance of follow-up exams to determine effectiveness and to monitor for side effects.

Evaluation/Desired Outcomes
- Decrease in serum LDL-C and total cholesterol levels.

---

famciclovir (fam-sye-kloe-veer)
Famvir
Classification
Therapeutic: antivirals

Indications
Acute herpes zoster infections (shingles). Treatment/ suppression of recurrent herpes genitalis in immuno- competent patients. Treatment of recurrent herpes labi- alis (cold sores) in immunocompetent patients. Treat- ment of recurrent mucocutaneous herpes simplex virus (HSV) infection in patients with HIV.

Action
Inhibits viral DNA synthesis in herpes-infected cells only. **Therapeutic Effects:** Decreased duration of her- pes zoster infection with decreased duration of viral shedding. Decreased time to healing for cold sores. De- creased lesion formation and improved healing in re- current HSV infection.

Pharmacokinetics
Absorption: Following absorption, famciclovir is rapidly converted in the intestinal wall to penciclovir, the active compound.
Distribution: Unknown.
Metabolism and Excretion: Penciclovir is mostly excreted by the kidneys.
Half-life: *Penciclovir:* 2.1–3 hr (↑ in renal impair- ment).

TIME/ACTION PROFILE (penciclovir plasma concentrations)

ROUTE	ONSET	PEAK	DURATION
PO	rapid	0.9 hr	8–12 hr

Contraindications/Precautions
Contraindicated in: Hypersensitivity.
Use Cautiously in: Renal impairment (↑ dose in- terval/↓ dose if CCr <40–60 mL/min); OB: Use during pregnancy only if potential maternal benefit justifies po- tential fetal risk; Lactation: Use during breastfeeding only if potential maternal benefit justifies potential risk to infant; Pedi: Safety and effectiveness not established in children; Geri: Consider age-related ↓ in renal func- tion in older adults.

Adverse Reactions/Side Effects
CV: palpitations. **Derm:** hypersensitivity vasculitis. **GI:** diarrhea, nausea, vomiting. **GU:** ↓ fertility (males). **Neuro:** headache, dizziness, fatigue, SEIZURES. **Misc:** ANAPHYLAXIS.

Interactions
Drug-Drug: Probenecid ↑ levels of penciclovir.

Route/Dosage
Herpes Zoster
PO (Adults): 500 mg every 8 hr for 7 days.

Renal Impairment
PO (Adults): *CCr 40–59 mL/min:* 500 mg every 12 hr; *CCr 20–39 mL/min:* 500 mg every 24 hr; *CCr <20 mL/min:* 250 mg every 24 hr; *Hemodialysis:* 250 mg after each dialysis.

Recurrent Genital Herpes Simplex Infec- tions
PO (Adults): 1000 mg twice daily for one day.

Renal Impairment
PO (Adults): *CCr 40–59 mL/min:* 500 mg twice daily for 1 day; *CCr 20–39 mL/min:* 500 mg as a single dose; *CCr <20 mL/min:* 250 mg as a single dose; *He- modialysis:* 250 mg as a single dose after dialysis.

Suppression of Recurrent Herpes Simplex Infections
PO (Adults): 250 mg every 12 hr for up to 1 yr.

Renal Impairment
PO (Adults): *CCr 20–39 mL/min:* 125 mg every 12 hr for 5 days; *CCr <20 mL/min:* 125 mg every 24 hr for 5 days; *Hemodialysis:* 125 mg after each dialysis.

Recurrent Herpes Labialis Infections (Cold Sores)
PO (Adults): 1500 mg as a single dose.

Renal Impairment
PO (Adults): *CCr 40–59 mL/min:* 750 mg as a single dose; *CCr 20–39 mL/min:* 500 mg as a single dose; *CCr <20 mL/min:* 250 mg as a single dose; *Hemodial- ysis:* 250 mg as a single dose after dialysis.

Herpes Simplex in Patients with HIV
PO (Adults): 500 mg every 12 hr for 7 days.

Renal Impairment
PO (Adults): *CCr 20–39 mL/min:* 500 mg every 24 hr for 7 days; *CCr <20 mL/min:* 250 mg every 24 hr for 7 days; *Hemodialysis:* 250 mg after each dialysis.

Availability (generic available)
Tablets: 125 mg, 250 mg, 500 mg.

NURSING IMPLICATIONS
Assessment
- Assess lesions prior to and daily during therapy.
- Assess patient for postherpetic neuralgia periodically during and following therapy.

Implementation
- Famciclovir therapy should be started as soon as herpes zoster is diagnosed, at least within 72 hr, preferably within 48 hr.
- **PO:** Famciclovir may be administered without re- gard to meals.

Patient/Family Teaching
- Instruct patient to take famciclovir as directed for the full course of therapy. Take missed doses as soon as remembered, if not just before next dose.
- Inform patient that famciclovir does not prevent the spread of infection to others. Until all lesions have

crusted, precautions should be taken around others who have not had chickenpox or varicella vaccine or people who are immunosuppressed.

- Advise patient to use condoms during sexual contact and to avoid sexual contact while lesions are present.
- May cause dizziness. Caution patient to avoid driving and other activities requiring alertness until response to medication is known.
- Advise patient to notify health care professional immediately if seizures or signs and symptoms of anaphylaxis (rash, facial swelling, difficulty breathing) occur.
- Instruct women with genital herpes to have yearly Papanicolaou (Pap) smears because of increased risk of cervical cancer.
- Rep: Advise women of childbearing potential to notify health care professional if pregnancy is planned or suspected or if breastfeeding. Encourage women who become pregnant while taking famciclovir to enroll in the pregnancy reporting system to monitor maternal-fetal outcomes. Report pregnancies and pregnancy outcomes to the Novartis Adverse Event reporting line at 1-888-NOW-NOVA (669-6682). May cause decreased fertility in male patients.

Evaluation/Desired Outcomes

- Decrease in time to full crusting, loss of vesicles, loss of ulcers, and loss of crusts in patients with acute herpes zoster (shingles).
- Crusting over and healing of lesions in herpes labialis, genital herpes, and in recurrent mucocutaneous HSV infection in patients with HIV.
- Prevention of recurrence of herpes genitalis.
- Decreased time to healing for cold sores.

---

famotidine, See HISTAMINE H₂ ANTAGONISTS.

✂ fam-trastuzumab deruxtecan

(fam tras-**tu**-zoo-mab de-**rux**-te-can)

Enhertu

Classification

Therapeutic: antineoplastics
Pharmacologic: monoclonal antibodies, enzyme inhibitors

Indications

✂ Unresectable or metastatic human epidermal growth factor receptor 2 (HER2)-positive breast cancer in patients who have previously received ≥2 anti-HER2-based regimens either in the metastatic setting or in the neoadjuvant or adjuvant setting and have developed dis-

ease recurrence during or within 6 mo of completing therapy. ✂ Unresectable or metastatic HER2-low (IHC 1+ or IHC 2+/ISH-) breast cancer in patients who have previously received chemotherapy in the metastatic setting or developed disease recurrence during or within 6 mo of completing adjuvant chemotherapy. ✂ Locally advanced or metastatic HER2-positive gastric or gastroesophageal junction adenocarcinoma in patients who have previously received a trastuzumab-based regimen. ✂ Unresectable or metastatic non-small cell lung cancer (NSCLC) in patients whose tumors have activating HER2 (ERBB2) mutations and who have received a prior systemic therapy.

Action

Acts as a HER2-directed antibody-drug conjugate composed of a humanized IgG1 monoclonal antibody (which has the same amino acid sequence as trastuzumab [and targets HER2]), a cleavable linker, and a topoisomerase I inhibitor (DXd) (the cytotoxic component that causes DNA damage and apoptosis). **Therapeutic Effects:** Regression of breast cancer and metastases. Improved survival in gastric or gastroesophageal junction adenocarcinoma. Decreased spread of NSCLC.

Pharmacokinetics

Absorption: IV administration results in complete bioavailability.

Distribution: Minimally distributed to extravascular tissues.

Protein Binding: 97%.

Metabolism and Excretion: Monoclonal antibody component is degraded into smaller peptides via catabolism. DxD primarily metabolized by the liver via CYP3A4 isoenzyme. Excretion pathway unknown.

Half-life: *Fam-trastuzumab deruxtecan:* 5.7 days; *DXd:* 5.8 days.

TIME/ACTION PROFILE (plasma concentrations)

ROUTE	ONSET	PEAK	DURATION
IV	unknown	unknown	unknown

Contraindications/Precautions

Contraindicated in: OB: Pregnancy; Lactation: Lactation.

Use Cautiously in: Severe renal impairment (CCr <30 mL/min); Severe hepatic impairment (total bilirubin >3−10× upper limit of normal [ULN] or AST > ULN); Rep: Women of reproductive potential and men with female partners of reproductive potential; Pedi: Safety and effectiveness not established in children; Geri: Older adults may have ↑ risk of adverse reactions.

Exercise Extreme Caution in: Pre-existing cardiac dysfunction.

Adverse Reactions/Side Effects

CV: ↓ left ventricular ejection fraction (LVEF), HF. **Derm:** alopecia, rash. **EENT:** dry eye, epistaxis. **F and**

E: hypokalemia. **GI:** ↑ liver enzymes, abdominal pain, constipation, diarrhea, dyspepsia, nausea, stomatitis, vomiting. **GU:** ↓ fertility (males). **Hemat:** anemia, leukopenia, NEUTROPENIA, thrombocytopenia. **Metab:** ↓ appetite. **Neuro:** dizziness, fatigue, headache. **Resp:** cough, dyspnea, INTERSTITIAL LUNG DISEASE (ILD)/PNEUMONITIS, upper respiratory tract infection.

Interactions
Drug-Drug: None reported.

Route/Dosage
Do NOT substitute fam-trastuzumab deruxtecan with trastuzumab or ado-trastuzumab emtansine.

Metastatic Breast Cancer or Unresectable/Metastatic Non-Small Cell Lung Cancer
IV (Adults): 5.4 mg/kg every 3 wk. Continue until disease progression or unacceptable toxicity.

Locally Advanced or Metastatic Gastric or Gastroesophageal Junction Adenocarcinoma
IV (Adults): 6.4 mg/kg every 3 wk. Continue until disease progression or unacceptable toxicity.

Availability
Lyophilized powder for injection: 100 mg/vial.

NURSING IMPLICATIONS
Assessment
- Assess for signs and symptoms of ILD/pneumonitis (cough, dyspnea, fever, and/or any new or worsening respiratory symptoms) periodically during therapy. If asymptomatic (Grade 1), hold medication until resolved to Grade 0, then: if resolved in <28 days from date of onset, maintain dose. If resolved in >28 days from date of onset, reduce dose one level. Consider corticosteroid therapy as soon as ILD/pneumonitis is suspected. If symptomatic ILD/pneumonitis occurs (≥Grade 2), discontinue therapy permanently and start corticosteroid therapy.
- Assess for signs and symptoms of left ventricular dysfunction (LVEF) before starting and at regular intervals during therapy as clinically indicated. If LVEF >45% and absolute decrease from baseline is 10–20%, continue with therapy. If LVEF is 40–45% and absolute decrease from baseline is <10%, continue with therapy. Repeat LVEF assessment within 3 wk. If LVEF is 40–45% and absolute decrease from baseline is 10–20%, hold therapy and repeat LVEF assessment within 3 wk. If LVEF has not recovered to within 10% from baseline, permanently discontinue therapy. If LVEF recovers to within 10% from baseline, resume therapy at the same dose. If LVEF <40% or absolute decrease from baseline >20%, hold therapy and repeat LVEF assessment within 3 wk. If LVEF <40% or absolute decrease from baseline of >20% is confirmed, permanently discontinue therapy. If symptomatic HF occurs, discontinue therapy permanently.

Lab Test Considerations
- Verify negative pregnancy test before starting therapy.
- ▓ Patient selection for patients with locally advanced or metastatic gastric cancer is based on HER2 protein overexpression or HER2 gene amplification. Reassess HER2 status if it is feasible to obtain a new tumor specimen after prior trastuzumab-based therapy and before treatment with *Enhertu*. Select patients for treatment of unresectable or metastatic HER2-low breast cancer with *Enhertu* based on HER2 expression (IHC 1+ or IHC 2+/ISH–). Select patients for treatment of unresectable or metastatic HER2-mutant NSCLC with *Enhertu* based on the presence of activating HER2 (ERBB2) mutations in tumor or plasma specimens (see Clinical Studies [14.3]). If no mutation is detected in a plasma specimen, test tumor tissue. Information on FDA-approved tests available at: http://www.fda.gov/CompanionDiagnostics.
- Monitor CBC prior to start of therapy and before each dose, and as clinically indicated. *If neutropenia of Grade 3 (less than $1.0 - 0.5 \times 10^9/L$) occurs,* hold therapy until resolved to ≤Grade 2, then resume at same dose. *If Grade 4 neutropenia (less than $0.5 \times 10^9/L$) occurs,* hold therapy until resolved to ≤Grade 2, then reduce dose by 1 level. *If febrile neutropenia (absolute neutrophil count of $<1.0 \times 10^9/L$ and temperature $>38.3°C$ or a sustained temperature of $\geq 38°C$ for >1 hr),* hold therapy until resolved. Reduce dose by 1 level. *If Grade 3 (platelets <50 to $25 \times 10^9/L$) thrombocytopenia occurs,* interrupt *Enhertu* until resolved to ≤Grade 1, then maintain dose. *If Grade 4 (platelets $<25 \times 10^9/L$) occur,* hold *Enhertu* until resolved to $10^9/L$) ≤Grade 1. Reduce dose by one level.

Implementation
- Do not substitute fam-traztuzumab deruxtecan for or with trastuzumab or ado-trastuzumab.
- *Enhertu* is moderately emetogenic and may cause delayed nausea and/or vomiting. Administer prophylactic antiemetic medications per local institutional guidelines for prevention of chemotherapy-induced nausea and vomiting.
- **Dose reduction schedule:** *Breast cancer:* Starting dose 5.4 mg/kg. First dose reduction to 4.4 mg/kg. Second reduction to 3.2 mg/kg. If further dose reduction is needed, discontinue therapy. Do not re-escalate dose after dose reduction is made.
- *Gastric Cancer:* Starting dose 6.4 mg/kg. First dose reduction to 5.4 mg/kg. Second reduction to 4.4 mg/kg. If further dose reduction is needed, discontinue therapy. Do not re-escalate dose after dose reduction is made.

IV Administration
- **Intermittent Infusion:** *Reconstitution:* Reconstitute immediately before dilution with 5 mL sterile water for injection for each 100 mg vial. *Concentration:* 20 mg/mL. Swirl gently to dissolve; do not

shake. Solution is clear and colorless to light yellow; do not use if solution is cloudy, discolored, or contains particulate matter. Reconstituted solution is stable if refrigerated for 24 hr. *Dilution:* Dilute in 100 mL of D5W; do not dilute with 0.9% NaCl. Gently invert to mix; do not shake. Cover infusion bag to protect from light. Diluted solution is stable for 4 hr at room temperature and up to 24 hr if refrigerated; do not freeze. Allow refrigerated solution to reach room temperature before infusion. *Rate:* Infuse 1st infusion over 90 min via an infusion set of polyolefin or polybutadiene and a 0.20 or 0.22 micron in-line polyethersulfone or polysulfone filter. If tolerated, subsequent infusions can be infused over 30 min. Slow rate or interrupt infusion if patient develops infusion-related symptoms. If reaction is severe, discontinue medication. Do not administer IV push or bolus.

● **Y-Site Incompatibility:** Do not mix with other drugs or with other drugs in the same line.

Patient/Family Teaching
● Explain purpose of therapy to patient. Advise patient to read *Medication Guide* before starting therapy.
● Advise patient to notify health care professional immediately if signs and symptoms of lung problems (cough, trouble breathing or shortness of breath, fever, other new or worsening breathing symptoms [chest tightness, wheezing]), infection (fever, chills), or heart problems (new or worsening shortness of breath, coughing, feeling tired, swelling of ankles or legs, irregular heartbeat, sudden weight gain, dizziness or feeling lightheaded, loss of consciousness) occur.
● Instruct patient to notify health care professional of all Rx or OTC medications, vitamins, or herbal products being taken and to consult with health care professional before taking other medications.
● Rep: May cause fetal harm. Advise females of reproductive potential to use effective contraception and avoid breastfeeding during and for at least 7 mo after last dose. Advise males with female partners of reproductive potential to use effective contraception during and for at least 4 mo after last dose. May impair male fertility.

Evaluation/Desired Outcomes
● Regression of breast cancer and metastases.
● Improved survival in gastric or gastroesophageal junction adenocarcinoma.
● Decreased spread of NSCLC.

febuxostat (fe-**bux**-o-stat)
Uloric
Classification
Therapeutic: antigout agents
Pharmacologic: xanthine oxidase inhibitors

Indications
Chronic management of hyperuricemia in patients with gout who have an inadequate response to a maximally titrated dose of allopurinol, who are intolerant to allopurinol, or in whom allopurinol is not an appropriate treatment option.

Action
Decreases production of uric acid by inhibiting xanthine oxidase. **Therapeutic Effects:** Lowering of serum uric acid levels with resultant decrease in gouty attacks.

Pharmacokinetics
Absorption: Well absorbed (49%) following oral administration.
Distribution: Widely distributed to tissues.
Protein Binding: 99.2%.
Metabolism and Excretion: Extensively metabolized by the liver; minimal renal excretion of unchanged drug, 45% eliminated in feces as unchanged drug, remainder is eliminated in urine and feces as inactive metabolites.
Half-life: 5–8 hr.

TIME/ACTION PROFILE (plasma concentrations)

ROUTE	ONSET	PEAK	DURATION
PO	rapid	1–1.5 hr*	24 hr

*Maximum lowering of uric acid may take 2 wk.

Contraindications/Precautions
Contraindicated in: Concurrent use of azathioprine or mercaptopurine.
Use Cautiously in: Cardiovascular disease (↑ risk of cardiovascular death compared to allopurinol) (consider using low-dose aspirin when using febuxostat in these patients); Severe renal impairment (CCr <30 mL/min); Severe hepatic impairment; Previous skin reaction with allopurinol; OB: Use during pregnancy only when potential maternal benefit justifies potential fetal risk; Lactation: Safety not established in breastfeeding; Pedi: Safety and effectiveness not established in children.

Adverse Reactions/Side Effects
Derm: DRUG REACTION WITH EOSINOPHILIA AND SYSTEMIC SYMPTOMS (DRESS), rash, STEVENS-JOHNSON SYNDROME, TOXIC EPIDERMAL NECROLYSIS. **GI:** ↑ liver enzymes, nausea. **MS:** arthralgia, gout flare.

Interactions
Drug-Drug: Significantly ↑ levels of and risk of serious toxicity from **azathioprine** and **mercaptopurine**; concurrent use contraindicated. May ↑ levels of **theophylline**; use cautiously together.

Route/Dosage
PO (Adults): 40 mg once daily initially; if serum uric acid does not ↓ to <6 mg/dL, ↑ to 80 mg once daily.

Renal Impairment
PO (Adults): *CCr <30 mL/min:* Maximum dose = 40 mg/day.

Availability (generic available)
Tablets: 40 mg, 80 mg.

NURSING IMPLICATIONS
Assessment
- Assess for joint pain and swelling, especially during early therapy. Changing serum uric acid levels from mobilization of urate from tissue deposits may cause gout flares. Use prophylactic NSAID or colchicine therapy for up to 6 mo. If a gout flare occurs, continue febuxostat therapy and treat flare concurrently.
- Monitor for signs and symptoms of MI and stroke.
- Assess patient for skin reactions throughout therapy. Reactions may be severe and life threatening. Discontinue therapy if severe reactions or moderate rashes with systemic symptoms occur.

Lab Test Considerations
- Monitor serum uric acid levels prior to, 2 wk after initiating, and periodically thereafter. *If serum uric acid levels are ≥6 mg/dL after 2 wk of daily 40 mg therapy,* ↑ dose to 80 mg daily.
- Monitor liver function at 2 and 4 mo of therapy and periodically thereafter. May cause ↑ AST, ALT, CK, LDH, and alkaline phosphatase.
- May cause prolonged aPTT and PT, and ↓ hematocrit, hemoglobin, RBC, platelet count, and lymphocyte, neutrophil counts. May cause ↑ or ↓ WBC.
- May cause ↓ serum bicarbonate and ↑ serum sodium, glucose, potassium, and TSH levels.
- May cause ↑ serum cholesterol, triglycerides, amylase, and low-density lipoprotein cholesterol levels.
- May cause ↑ BUN and serum creatinine and proteinuria.

Implementation
- **PO:** May be taken with or without food and with antacids.

Patient/Family Teaching
- Instruct patient to take febuxostat as directed. If a gout flare occurs, continue febuxostat and consult health care professional; medications to manage gout flare may be added.
- Advise patient to notify health care professional if rash, chest pain, shortness of breath, dizziness, rapid or irregular heartbeat, or stroke symptoms (weakness, blurred vision, headache, confusion, slurred speech) occur or if side effects are persistent or bothersome.
- Instruct patient to notify health care professional of all Rx or OTC medications, vitamins, or herbal products being taken and to consult health care professional before taking any other Rx, OTC, or herbal products.
- Rep: Advise females of reproductive potential to notify health care professional if pregnancy is planned or suspected or if breastfeeding.

- Emphasize the importance of follow-up lab tests to monitor therapy.

Evaluation/Desired Outcomes
- Reduction in serum uric acid levels and resultant gout attacks.

---

fenofibrate (fen-o-fi-brate)
Antara, Fenoglide, ✦Lipidil EZ, ✦Lipidil Supra, Lipofen, Tricor, ~~Triglide~~
Classification
Therapeutic: lipid-lowering agents
Pharmacologic: fibric acid derivatives

Indications
With dietary therapy to decrease LDL cholesterol, total cholesterol, triglycerides, and apolipoprotein B in adult patients with hypercholesterolemia or mixed dyslipidemia. With dietary management in the treatment of severe hypertriglyceridemia (types IV and V hyperlipidemia) in patients who are at risk for pancreatitis and do not respond to nondrug therapy.

Action
Fenofibric acid primarily inhibits triglyceride synthesis. **Therapeutic Effects:** Lowering of cholesterol and triglycerides with subsequent decreased risk of pancreatitis.

Pharmacokinetics
Absorption: Well absorbed (60%) after oral administration; absorption ↑ by food.
Distribution: Unknown.
Protein Binding: 99%.
Metabolism and Excretion: Rapidly converted to fenofibric acid, which is the active metabolite; fenofibric acid is metabolized by the liver. Fenofibric acid and its metabolites are primarily excreted in urine (60%).
Half-life: 20 hr.

TIME/ACTION PROFILE (lowering of triglycerides)

ROUTE	ONSET	PEAK	DURATION
PO	unknown	2 wk	unknown

Contraindications/Precautions
Contraindicated in: Hypersensitivity; Hepatic impairment (including primary biliary cirrhosis); Pre-existing gallbladder disease; Severe renal impairment; Concurrent use of HMG-CoA reductase inhibitors; Lactation: Lactation.

Use Cautiously in: Concurrent warfarin or HMG-CoA reductase inhibitor therapy; OB: Safety not established in pregnancy; Pedi: Safety and effectiveness not established in children; Geri: Age-related ↓ in renal function may make older patients more susceptible to adverse reactions.

Adverse Reactions/Side Effects

CV: arrhythmia, DEEP VEIN THROMBOSIS. **Derm:** <u>rash</u>, DRUG REACTION WITH EOSINOPHILIA AND SYSTEMIC SYMPTOMS (DRESS), STEVENS-JOHNSON SYNDROME, TOXIC EPIDERMAL NECROLYSIS, urticaria. **GI:** ↑ liver enzymes, cholelithiasis, HEPATOTOXICITY, pancreatitis. **Metab:** ↓ HDL levels. **MS:** rhabdomyolysis. **Neuro:** <u>fatigue/weakness</u>, headache. **Resp:** INTERSTITIAL LUNG DISEASE, PULMONARY EMBOLISM. **Misc:** HYPERSENSITIVITY REACTIONS (including anaphylaxis and angioedema).

Interactions

Drug-Drug: ↑ anticoagulant effects of **warfarin**. **HMG-CoA reductase inhibitors** ↑ risk of rhabdomyolysis (concurrent use should be avoided). Absorption is ↓ by **bile acid sequestrants** (fenofibrate should be given 1 hr before or 4–6 hr after). ↑ risk of nephrotoxicity with **cyclosporine**. Concurrent use with **colchicine** may ↑ risk of rhabdomyolysis.

Route/Dosage

Primary Hypercholesterolemia/Mixed Dyslipidemia

PO (Adults): *Antara:* 130 mg once daily; *Fenoglide:* 120 mg once daily; *Tricor:* 145 mg once daily; *Lipofen:* 150 mg once daily.

Renal Impairment

PO (Adults): *CCr 30–89 mL/min: Antara:* 43 mg once daily initially; may titrate, if needed, up to 130 mg once daily. *Fenoglide:* 40 mg once daily initially; may titrate, if needed, up to 120 mg once daily. *Lipofen:* 50 mg once daily initially; may titrate, if needed, up to 150 mg once daily. *Tricor:* 48 mg once daily initially; may titrate, if needed, up to 145 mg once daily.

Hypertriglyceridemia

PO (Adults): *Antara:* 43–130 mg once daily; *Fenoglide:* 40–120 mg once daily; *Tricor:* 48–145 mg once daily; *Lipofen:* 50–150 mg once daily.

Renal Impairment

PO (Adults): *CCr 30–89 mL/min: Antara:* 43 mg once daily initially; may titrate, if needed, up to 130 mg once daily. *Fenoglide:* 40 mg once daily initially; may titrate, if needed, up to 120 mg once daily. *Lipofen:* 50 mg once daily initially; may titrate, if needed, up to 150 mg once daily. *Tricor:* 48 mg once daily initially; may titrate, if needed, up to 145 mg once daily.

Availability (generic available)

Capsules (Lipofen): 50 mg, 150 mg. **Micronized capsules (Antara):** 43 mg, 130 mg. **Tablets (Fenoglide):** 40 mg, 120 mg. **Tablets (Tricor):** 48 mg, 145 mg.

NURSING IMPLICATIONS

Assessment

- Obtain a diet history, especially with regard to fat consumption. Attempt to obtain normal serum triglyceride levels with diet, exercise, and weight loss in obese patients before fenofibrate therapy is instituted.
- Assess patient for cholelithiasis. If symptoms occur, gallbladder studies are indicated. Discontinue therapy if gallstones are found.
- Assess patient for skin reactions throughout therapy. Reactions may be severe and life threatening. Discontinue therapy if severe reactions or moderate rashes with systemic symptoms occur.

Lab Test Considerations

- Monitor serum lipids before therapy to determine consistent elevations, then monitor periodically during therapy.
- Monitor serum AST, ALT, and total bilirubin at baseline and periodically during therapy. May cause ↑ levels. Therapy should be discontinued if levels rise >3 times the normal limit. *If signs or symptoms of liver injury occur or if elevated enzyme levels persist (ALT or AST >3 × upper limit of normal, or if accompanied by elevation of bilirubin),* discontinue fenofibrate. Do not restart fenofibrate if there is no alternative explanation for the liver injury.
- If patient develops muscle tenderness during therapy, monitor CK levels. If CK levels are markedly ↑ or myopathy occurs, discontinue therapy.
- May cause mild to moderate ↓ in hemoglobin, hematocrit, and WBCs. Monitor periodically during first 12 mo of therapy. Levels usually stabilize during long-term therapy.
- Monitor prothrombin levels frequently until levels stabilize in patients taking anticoagulants concurrently.

Implementation

- Do not confuse Tricor with Tracleer.
- Place patients on a triglyceride-lowering diet before therapy and encourage them to remain on this diet during therapy.
- Dose may be increased after repeated serum triglyceride levels every 4–8 wk.
- Brands are not interchangeable.
- **PO:** Administer *Fenoglide, and Lipofen,* products with meals. *Antara* and *Tricor* can be administered without regard to meals. *DNC:* Swallow capsules whole; do not open, break, dissolve, or chew.

Patient/Family Teaching

- Instruct patient to take medication as directed, not to skip doses or double up on missed doses. Medication helps control but does not cure elevated serum triglyceride levels.
- Advise patient that this medication should be used in conjunction with diet restrictions (fat, cholesterol, carbohydrates, alcohol), exercise, and cessation of smoking.
- Instruct patient to notify health care professional if signs and symptoms of liver injury (jaundice, ab-

F

dominal pain, nausea, malaise, dark urine, abnormal stool, pruritus), unexplained muscle pain, tenderness, or weakness occurs, especially if accompanied by fever or malaise.

- Instruct patient to notify health care professional of all Rx or OTC medications, vitamins, or herbal products being taken and to consult health care professional before taking other Rx, OTC, or herbal products.
- Advise patient to notify health care professional of medication regimen before treatment or surgery.
- Rep: Advise females of reproductive potential to notify health care professional promptly if pregnancy is planned or suspected and to avoid breastfeeding during and for at least 5 days after last dose of therapy.
- Emphasize the importance of follow-up exams to determine effectiveness and to monitor for side effects.

Evaluation/Desired Outcomes

- Decrease in serum triglycerides and cholesterol to normal levels. Therapy should be discontinued in patients who do not have an adequate response in 2 mo of therapy.

HIGH ALERT

fentaNYL (parenteral)
(fen-ta-nil)
~~Sublimaze~~
Classification
Therapeutic: opioid analgesics
Pharmacologic: opioid agonists

Schedule II

Indications

Analgesic supplement to general anesthesia; usually with other agents (ultra–short-acting barbiturates, neuromuscular blocking agents, and inhalation anesthetics) to produce balanced anesthesia. Induction/maintenance of anesthesia (in combination with oxygen or oxygen/nitrous oxide and a neuromuscular blocking agent). Neuroleptanalgesia/neuroleptanesthesia (with or without nitrous oxide). Supplement to regional/local anesthesia. Preoperative and postoperative analgesia. **Unlabeled Use:** Continuous IV infusion as part of patient-controlled analgesia.

Action

Binds to opiate receptors in the CNS, altering the response to and perception of pain. Produces CNS depression. **Therapeutic Effects:** Supplement in anesthesia. Decreased pain.

Pharmacokinetics

Absorption: Well absorbed after IM administration. IV administration results in complete bioavailability.
Distribution: Extensively distributed to CNS and tissues.

Metabolism and Excretion: Primarily metabolized by the liver via the CYP3A4 isoenzyme; 10–25% excreted unchanged by the kidneys.
Half-life: *Children:* Bolus dose—2.4 hr, long-term continuous infusion—11–36 hr; *Adults:* 2–4 hr (↑ after cardiopulmonary bypass and in geriatric patients).

TIME/ACTION PROFILE (analgesia*)

ROUTE	ONSET	PEAK	DURATION
IM	7–15 min	20–30 min	1–2 hr
IV	1–2 min	3–5 min	0.5–1 hr

*Respiratory depression may last longer than analgesia.

Contraindications/Precautions

Contraindicated in: Hypersensitivity; cross-sensitivity among agents may occur; Known intolerance; Concurrent use of MAO inhibitors.

Use Cautiously in: Diabetes; Severe renal impairment; Severe hepatic impairment; Severe pulmonary disease; CNS tumors; ↑ intracranial pressure; Head trauma; Adrenal insufficiency; Undiagnosed abdominal pain; Hypothyroidism; Alcoholism; Cardiac disease (arrhythmias); OB: Use during pregnancy only if potential maternal benefit justifies potential fetal risk. Chronic maternal treatment with opioids during pregnancy may result in neonatal abstinence syndrome; Lactation: Use while breastfeeding only if potential maternal benefit justifies potential risk to infant (may cause infant sedation and/or respiratory depression); Geri: Older adults may be more sensitive to effects and may have an ↑ risk of adverse reactions; titrate dosage carefully.

Adverse Reactions/Side Effects

CV: arrhythmias, bradycardia, hypotension. **Derm:** facial itching. **EENT:** blurred/double vision. **Endo:** adrenal insufficiency. **GI:** biliary spasm, nausea, vomiting. **MS:** skeletal and thoracic muscle rigidity (with rapid IV infusion). **Neuro:** confusion, paradoxical excitation/delirium, postoperative drowsiness. **Resp:** allergic bronchospasm, APNEA, LARYNGOSPASM, RESPIRATORY DEPRESSION (including central sleep apnea and sleep-related hypoxemia).

Interactions

Drug-Drug: Concurrent use or within previous 14 days of **MAO inhibitors** may produce unpredictable, potentially fatal reactions and is contraindicated. **CYP3A4 inhibitors,** including **ritonavir, ketoconazole, itraconazole, clarithromycin, nelfinavir, nefazodone, diltiazem, aprepitant, fluconazole, fosamprenavir, verapamil,** and **erythromycin,** may ↑ levels and ↑ risk of CNS and respiratory depression. **CYP3A4 inducers,** including **barbiturates, carbamazepine, efavirenz, corticosteroids, modafinil, nevirapine, oxcarbazepine, phenobarbital, phenytoin, rifabutin,** or **rifampin,** may ↓ levels and analgesia; if inducers are discontinued or dosage ↓, patients should be monitored for signs of opioid toxicity and necessary dose adjustments should be made. Use with **benzodiazepines** or other **CNS depressants,**

including other **opioids, non-benzodiazepine sedative/hypnotics, anxiolytics, general anesthetics, muscle relaxants, antipsychotics,** and **alcohol,** may cause profound sedation, respiratory depression, coma, and death; reserve concurrent use for when alternative treatment options are inadequate. ↑ risk of hypotension with **benzodiazepines. Nalbuphine** or **buprenorphine** may ↓ analgesia. Drugs that affect serotonergic neurotransmitter systems, including **tricyclic antidepressants, SSRIs, SNRIs, MAO inhibitors, TCAs, tramadol, trazodone, mirtazapine, 5–HT$_3$ receptor antagonists, linezolid, methylene blue,** and **triptans,** ↑ risk of serotonin syndrome. **Drug-Food:** Grapefruit juice may ↑ levels and the risk of respiratory and CNS depression.

Route/Dosage

Preoperative Use
IM, IV (Adults and Children >12 yr): 50–100 mcg 30–60 min before surgery.

Adjunct to General Anesthesia
IM, IV (Adults and Children >12 yr): *Low dose–minor surgery:* 2 mcg/kg. *Moderate dose–major surgery:* 2–20 mcg/kg. *High dose–major surgery:* 20–50 mcg/kg.

Adjunct to Regional Anesthesia
IM, IV (Adults and Children >12 yr): 50–100 mcg.

Postoperative Use (Recovery Room)
IM, IV (Adults and Children >12 yr): 50–100 mcg; may repeat in 1–2 hr.

General Anesthesia
IV (Adults and Children >12 yr): 50–100 mcg/kg (up to 150 mcg/kg).
IV (Children 1–12 yr): 2–3 mcg/kg.

Sedation/Analgesia
IV (Adults and Children >12 yr): 0.5–1 mcg/kg/dose, may repeat after 30–60 min.
IV (Children 1–12 yr): *Bolus:* 1–2 mcg/kg/dose, may repeat at 30–60 min intervals. *Continuous infusion:* 1–5 mcg/kg/hr following bolus dose.
IV (Neonates): *Bolus:* 0.5–3 mcg/kg/dose. *Continuous infusion:* 0.5–2 mcg/kg/hr following bolus dose. *Continuous infusion during ECMO:* 5–10 mcg/kg bolus followed by 1–5 mcg/kg/hr; may require up to 20 mcg/kg/hr after 5 days of therapy.

Availability (generic available)
Solution for injection: 50 mcg/mL.

NURSING IMPLICATIONS

Assessment
- Assess type, location, and intensity of pain prior to and 30 min following IM and 5 min (peak) following IV administration. When titrating opioid doses, increases of 25–50% should be administered until there is either a 50% reduction in the patient's pain rating on a numerical or visual analogue scale or the patient reports satisfactory pain relief.
- Monitor respiratory rate and BP frequently during therapy, especially when starting therapy or when given with other drugs that depress respiration. May cause sleep-related breathing disorders (central sleep apnea, sleep-related hypoxemia). Report significant changes immediately. The respiratory depressant effects of fentanyl may last longer than the analgesic effects. Initial doses of other opioids should be reduced by 25–33% of the usually recommended dose. Monitor closely.
- Geri: Opioids have been associated with increased risk of falls in older adults. Assess risk and implement fall prevention strategies.
- Assess type, location, and intensity of pain before and 30 min after IM administration or 3–5 min after IV administration when fentanyl is used to treat pain.
- Assess risk for opioid addiction, abuse, or misuse prior to administration.

Lab Test Considerations
- May cause ↑ serum amylase and lipase concentrations.

Toxicity and Overdose
- Symptoms of toxicity include respiratory depression, hypotension, arrhythmias, bradycardia, and asystole. Atropine may be used to treat bradycardia. If respiratory depression persists after surgery, prolonged mechanical ventilation may be required. If an opioid antagonist is required to reverse respiratory depression or coma, naloxone is the antidote. Dilute the 0.4-mg ampule of naloxone in 10 mL of 0.9% NaCl and administer 0.5 mL (0.02 mg) by IV push every 2 min. Pedi: For children and patients weighing <40 kg, dilute 0.1 mg of naloxone in 10 mL of 0.9% NaCl for a concentration of 10 mcg/mL and administer 0.5 mcg/kg every 2 min. Titrate dose to avoid withdrawal, seizures, and severe pain. Administration of naloxone in these circumstances, especially in cardiac patients, has resulted in hypertension and tachycardia, occasionally causing left ventricular failure and pulmonary edema.

Implementation
- *High Alert:* Accidental overdosage of opioid analgesics has resulted in fatalities. Before administering, clarify all ambiguous orders; have second practitioner independently check original order, dose calculations, route of administration, and infusion pump programming.
- Do not confuse fentanyl with sufentanil.
- Benzodiazepines may be administered before or after administration of fentanyl to reduce the induction dose requirements, decrease the time to loss of consciousness, and produce amnesia. This combination

may also increase the risk of hypotension and respiratory depression.

- Explain therapeutic value of medication prior to administration to enhance the analgesic effect.
- Regularly administered doses may be more effective than prn administration. Analgesic is more effective if given before pain becomes severe.
- Coadministration with nonopioid analgesics may have additive analgesic effects and permit lower opioid doses.
- Medication should be discontinued gradually after long-term use to prevent withdrawal symptoms.
- May cause muscle rigidity, particularly involving muscles of respiration; effects are related to the dose and speed of injection. Effects can be reduced by: 1) administration of up to 1/4 of the full paralyzing dose of a non-depolarizing neuromuscular blocking agent just prior to administration of fentanyl; 2) administration of a full paralyzing dose of a neuromuscular blocking agent following loss of eyelash reflex when fentanyl is used in anesthetic doses titrated by slow intravenous infusion; or, 3) simultaneous administration of fentanyl and a full paralyzing dose of a neuromuscular blocking agent when fentanyl is used in rapidly administered anesthetic doses.

IV Administration

- **IV Push:** *Dilution:* Administer undiluted. *Concentration:* 50 mcg/mL. *Rate:* Inject slowly over 1–3 min. Administer doses >5 mcg/kg over 5–10 min. Slow IV administration may reduce the incidence and severity of muscle rigidity, bradycardia, or hypotension. Neuromuscular blocking agents may be administered concurrently to decrease chest wall muscle rigidity.
- **Intermittent Infusion:** *Dilution:* May be diluted in D5W or 0.9% NaCl. *Concentration:* Up to 50 mcg/mL. *Rate:* see IV Push.
- **Y-Site Compatibility:** acetaminophen, acyclovir, alemtuzumab, alprostadil, amikacin, aminocaproic acid, aminophylline, amiodarone, amphotericin B deoxycholate, amphotericin B lipid complex, amphotericin B liposomal, ampicillin/sulbactam, anidulafungin, argatroban, arsenic trioxide, ascorbic acid, atracurium, atropine, azathioprine, aztreonam, benztropine, bivalirudin, bleomycin, bumetanide, buprenorphine, butorphanol, calcium chloride, calcium gluconate, cangrelor, carboplatin, carmustine, caspofungin, cefazolin, cefotaxime, cefotetan, cefoxitin, ceftaroline, ceftazidime, ceftolozane/tazobactam, ceftriaxone, cefuroxime, chloramphenicol, chlorpromazine, cisatracurium, cisplatin, clindamycin, cyanocobalamin, cyclophosphamide, cyclosporine, cytarabine, dacarbazine, dactinomycin, daptomycin, daunorubicin hydrochloride, dexamethasone, dexmedetomidine, dexrazoxane, digoxin, diltiazem, diphenhydramine, dobutamine, docetaxel, dopamine, doxorubicin, doxorubicin liposomal, doxycycline, enalaprilat, ephedrine, epinephrine, epirubicin, epoetin alfa, eptifibatide, eravacycline, erythromycin,

esmolol, etomidate, etoposide, etoposide phosphate, famotidine, fluconazole, fludarabine, fluorouracil, folic acid, foscarnet, fosphenytoin, furosemide, ganciclovir, gemcitabine, gentamicin, glycopyrrolate, granisetron, haloperidol, heparin, hetastarch, hydrocortisone, hydromorphone, idarubicin, ifosfamide, imipenem/cilastatin, imipenem/cilastatin/relebactam, indomethacin, insulin, regular, irinotecan, isavuconazonium, isoproterenol, ketorolac, labetalol, leucovorin calcium, levofloxacin, lidocaine, linezolid, lorazepam, magnesium sulfate, mannitol, meperidine, meropenem/vaborbactam, mesna, methotrexate, methylprednisolone, metoclopramide, metoprolol, midazolam, milrinone, mitomycin, mitoxantrone, morphine, multivitamins, mycophenolate, nafcillin, nalbuphine, naloxone, nicardipine, nitroglycerin, nitroprusside, norepinephrine, octreotide, ondansetron, oritavancin, oxacillin, oxaliplatin, oxytocin, paclitaxel, palonosetron, pamidronate, papaverine, pemetrexed, penicillin G, pentamidine, pentobarbital, phenobarbital, phentolamine, phenylephrine, phytonadione, piperacillin/tazobactam, plazomicin, potassium acetate, potassium chloride, procainamide, prochlorperazine, promethazine, propofol, propranolol, protamine, pyridoxine, remifentanil, rituximab, rocuronium, sargramostim, scopolamine, sodium acetate, sodium bicarbonate, succinylcholine, sufentanil, tacrolimus, tedizolid, theophylline, thiamine, thiopental, thiotepa, tigecycline, tirofiban, tobramycin, topotecan, trastuzumab, vancomycin, vasopressin, vecuronium, verapamil, vinblastine, vincristine, vinorelbine, voriconazole, zoledronic acid.

- **Y-Site Incompatibility:** dantrolene, diazoxide, gemtuzumab ozogamicin, pantoprazole, phenytoin, trimethoprim/sulfamethoxazole.

Patient/Family Teaching

- Discuss the use of anesthetic agents and the sensations to expect with the patient before surgery.
- Instruct patient on how and when to ask for pain medication. Explain pain assessment scale to patient.
- Advise patient to notify health care professional if pain control is not adequate or if side effects occur.
- Caution patient to change positions slowly to minimize orthostatic hypotension. Geri: Older adults may be at a greater risk for orthostatic hypotension and, consequently, falls. Teach patient to take precautions until drug effects have completely resolved.
- Medication causes dizziness and drowsiness. Advise patient to call for assistance during ambulation and transfer, and to avoid driving or other activities requiring alertness for 24 hr after administration during outpatient surgery.
- Instruct patient to notify health care professional of all Rx or OTC medications, vitamins, or herbal products being taken and consult health care professional before taking any new medications.

- Encourage patient to turn, cough, and breathe deeply every 2 hr to prevent atelectasis.
- Instruct patient to avoid alcohol or other CNS depressants for 24 hr after administration for outpatient surgery.
- Rep: Advise females of reproductive potential to notify health care professional if pregnancy is planned or suspected, or if breastfeeding. Inform patient of potential for neonatal opioid withdrawal syndrome with prolonged use during pregnancy. Monitor neonate for signs and symptoms of withdrawal symptoms (irritability, hyperactivity and abnormal sleep pattern, high pitched cry, tremor, vomiting, diarrhea, and/or failure to gain weight); usually occur the first days after birth. Monitor infants exposed to fentanyl through breast milk for excess sedation and respiratory depression.

Evaluation/Desired Outcomes

- General quiescence.
- Reduced motor activity.
- Pronounced analgesia.

REMS HIGH ALERT

fentaNYL (transdermal)
(fen-ta-nil)
~~Duragesic~~
Classification
Therapeutic: opioid analgesics
Pharmacologic: opioid agonists

Schedule II

Indications
Moderate to severe chronic pain in opioid-tolerant patients requiring use of daily, around-the-clock long-term opioid treatment and for which alternative treatment options are inadequate (extended-release). Transdermal fentanyl is not recommended for the control of postoperative, mild, or intermittent pain, and it should not be used for short-term pain relief.

Action
Binds to opiate receptors in the CNS, altering the response to and perception of pain. **Therapeutic Effects:** Decrease in severity of chronic pain.

Pharmacokinetics
Absorption: Well absorbed (92% of dose) through skin surface under transdermal patch, creating a depot in the upper skin layers. Release from transdermal system into systemic circulation ↑ gradually to a constant rate, providing continuous delivery for 72 hr.
Distribution: Crosses the placenta; enters breast milk.
Metabolism and Excretion: Mostly metabolized by the liver via the CYP3A4 isoenzyme; 10–25% excreted unchanged by the kidneys.

Half-life: 17 hr after removal of a single application patch, ↑ to 21 hr after removal of multiple patches (because of continued release from deposition of drug in skin layers).

TIME/ACTION PROFILE (↓ pain)

ROUTE	ONSET	PEAK	DURATION
Transdermal	6 hr†	12–24 hr	72 hr‡

†Achievement of blood levels associated with analgesia. Maximal response and dose titration may take up to 6 days. ‡While patch is worn.

Contraindications/Precautions
Contraindicated in: Hypersensitivity to fentanyl or adhesives; Patients who are not opioid tolerant; Acute, mild, intermittent, or postoperative pain; Significant respiratory depression; Acute or severe bronchial asthma; Paralytic ileus; Severe hepatic or renal impairment; Alcohol intolerance (small amounts of alcohol released into skin); OB: Not recommended during labor and delivery; Lactation: Lactation.
Use Cautiously in: Diabetes; Patients with severe pulmonary disease; Mild or moderate hepatic or renal impairment; CNS tumors; ↑ intracranial pressure; Head trauma; Adrenal insufficiency; Undiagnosed abdominal pain; Hypothyroidism; Alcoholism; Cardiac disease (particularly bradyarrhythmias); Fever or situations that ↑ body temperature (↑ release of fentanyl from delivery system); Cachectic or debilitated patients (dose ↓ suggested because of altered drug disposition); OB: Use during pregnancy only if the potential maternal benefit justifies the potential fetal risk; Pedi: Children <2 yr (safety not established); pediatric patients initiating therapy at 25 mcg/hr should be opioid tolerant and receiving at least 60 mg oral morphine equivalents per day; Geri: ↑ risk of respiratory depression in older adults (dose ↓ suggested).

Adverse Reactions/Side Effects
CV: bradycardia, hypotension. **Derm:** <u>sweating</u>, erythema. **Endo:** adrenal insufficiency. **GI:** <u>anorexia</u>, <u>constipation</u>, <u>dry mouth</u>, nausea, vomiting. **Local:** application site reactions. **MS:** skeletal and thoracic muscle rigidity. **Neuro:** <u>confusion</u>, <u>sedation</u>, <u>weakness</u>, dizziness, restlessness. **Resp:** APNEA, bronchoconstriction, laryngospasm, RESPIRATORY DEPRESSION (including central sleep apnea and sleep-related hypoxemia). **Misc:** physical dependence, psychological dependence.

Interactions
Drug-Drug: Avoid use in patients who have received **MAO inhibitors** within the previous 14 days (may produce unpredictable, potentially fatal reactions). Concomitant use of **CYP3A4 inhibitors** including **ritonavir, ketoconazole, itraconazole, clarithromycin, nelfinavir, nefazodone, amiodarone, diltiazem, aprepitant, fluconazole, fosamprenavir, verapamil,** and **erythromycin** may result in ↑ plasma

levels and ↑ risk of CNS and respiratory depression. Levels and effectiveness may be ↓ by **CYP3A4 inducers** including **rifampin**, **carbamazepine**, and **phenytoin**. Use with **benzodiazepines** or other **CNS depressants** including other **opioids**, **non-benzodiazepine sedative/hypnotics**, **anxiolytics**, **general anesthetics**, **muscle relaxants**, **antipsychotics**, and **alcohol** may cause profound sedation, respiratory depression, coma, and death; reserve concurrent use for when alternative treatment options are inadequate. **Mixed agonist/antagonist analgesics**, including **nalbuphine** or **butorphanol** and **partial agonist analgesics**, including **buprenorphine**, may ↓ fentanyl's analgesic effects and/or precipitate opioid withdrawal in physically dependent patients. Drugs that affect serotonergic neurotransmitter systems, including **tricyclic antidepressants**, **SSRIs**, **SNRIs**, **MAO inhibitors**, **TCAs**, **tramadol**, **trazodone**, **mirtazapine**, **5–HT₃ receptor antagonists**, **linezolid**, **methylene blue**, and **triptans** ↑ risk of serotonin syndrome.

Drug-Natural Products: Concomitant use of **kava-kava**, **valerian**, or **chamomile** can ↑ CNS depression.

Drug-Food: **Grapefruit juice** is a moderate inhibitor of the CYP3A4 enzyme system; concurrent use may ↑ blood levels and the risk of respiratory and CNS depression. Careful monitoring and dose adjustment is recommended.

Route/Dosage
Transdermal (Adults): 25 mcg/hr is the initial dose; patients who have not been receiving opioids should receive not more than 25 mcg/hr. To calculate the dose of transdermal fentanyl required in patients who are already receiving opioid analgesics, assess the 24-hr requirement of currently used opioid. Using the equianalgesic table in Appendix I, convert this to an equivalent amount of morphine/24 hr. Conversion to fentanyl transdermal may be accomplished by using the fentanyl conversion table (Appendix I). During dose titration, additional short-acting opioids should be available for breakthrough pain. Morphine 10 mg IM or 60 mg PO every 4 hr (60 mg/24 hr IM or 360 mg/24 hr PO) is considered to be approximately equivalent to transdermal fentanyl 100 mcg/hr. Transdermal patch lasts 72 hr in most patients. Some patients require a new patch every 48 hr.

Transdermal (Adults >60 yr, Debilitated, or Cachectic Patients): Initial dose should be 25 mcg/hr unless previous opioid use was >135 mg morphine PO/day (or other opioid equivalent).

Hepatic Impairment
Transdermal (Adults): *Mild-to-moderate hepatic impairment:* 12 mcg/hr is the initial dose.

Renal Impairment
Transdermal (Adults): *Mild-to-moderate renal impairment:* 12 mcg/hr is the initial dose.

Availability (generic available)
Transdermal systems: 12.5 mcg/hr, 25 mcg/hr, 37.5 mcg/hr, 50 mcg/hr, 62.5 mcg/hr, 75 mcg/hr, 87.5 mcg/hr, 100 mcg/hr.

NURSING IMPLICATIONS
Assessment
- Assess type, location, and intensity of pain before and 24 hr after application and periodically during therapy. Monitor pain frequently during initiation of therapy and dose changes to assess need for supplementary analgesics for breakthrough pain.
- Assess BP, pulse, and respirations before and periodically during administration. If respiratory rate is <10/min, assess level of sedation. Physical stimulation may be sufficient to prevent significant hypoventilation. Dose may need to be decreased by 25–50%. Initial drowsiness will diminish with continued use. Monitor for respiratory depression, especially during initiation or following dose increase; serious, life-threatening, or fatal respiratory depression may occur. May cause sleep-related breathing disorders (central sleep apnea, sleep-related hypoxemia).
- Prolonged use may lead to physical and psychological dependence and tolerance. This should not prevent patient from receiving adequate analgesia. Most patients who receive opioid analgesics for pain rarely develop psychological dependence.
- Progressively higher doses may be required to relieve pain with long-term therapy. It may take up to 6 days after increasing doses to reach equilibrium, so patients should wear higher dose through 2 applications before increasing dose again. Increased doses and prolonged use may increase risk of overdose. Prolonged use of opioids should be reserved for patients whose pain remains severe enough to require them and alternative treatment options continue to be inadequate. Many acute pain conditions treated in the outpatient setting require no more than a few days of an opioid pain medicine.
- Assess bowel function routinely. Prevent constipation with increased intake of fluids and bulk, and laxatives to minimize constipating effects. Administer stimulant laxatives routinely if opioid use exceeds 2–3 days, unless contraindicated. Consider drugs for opioid induced constipation.
- Assess risk for opioid addiction, abuse, or misuse prior to administration. Misuse or abuse of *transdermal fentanyl* by chewing, swallowing, snorting or injecting fentanyl extracted from transdermal system will result in the uncontrolled delivery of fentanyl and risk of overdose and death.

Lab Test Considerations
- May ↑ plasma amylase and lipase levels.

Toxicity and Overdose
- If an opioid antagonist is required to reverse respiratory depression or coma, naloxone is the antidote. Dilute the 0.4-mg ampule of naloxone in 10 mL of

0.9% NaCl and administer 0.5 mL (0.02 mg) by IV push every 2 min. For patients weighing <40 kg, dilute 0.1 mg of naloxone in 10 mL of 0.9% NaCl for a concentration of 10 mcg/mL and administer 0.5 mcg/kg every 2 min. Titrate dose to avoid withdrawal, seizures, and severe pain. Monitor patient closely; dose may need to be repeated or may need to be administered as an infusion because of long duration of action despite removal of patch.

Implementation

- Do not confuse fentanyl with sufentanil.
- **High Alert:** Accidental overdose of opioid analgesics has resulted in fatalities. Before administering, confirm patient is opioid tolerant and clarify ambiguous orders.
- 12-mcg patch delivers 12.5 mcg/hr of fentanyl. Use supplemental doses of short-acting opioid analgesics to manage pain until relief is obtained with the transdermal system. Patients may continue to require supplemental opioids for breakthrough pain. If >100 mcg/hr is required, use multiple transdermal systems.
- Titrate dose based on patient's report of pain until adequate analgesia (50% reduction in patient's pain rating on numerical or visual analogue scale or patient reports satisfactory relief) is attained. Determine dose by calculating the previous 24-hr analgesic requirement and converting to the equianalgesic morphine dose using Appendix I. The conversion ratio from morphine to transdermal fentanyl is conservative; 50% of patients may require a dose increase after initial application. Increase after 3 days based on required daily doses of supplemental analgesics. Base increases on ratio of 45 mg/24 hr of oral morphine to 12.5 mcg/hr increase in transdermal fentanyl dose.
- Coadministration with nonopioid analgesics may have additive analgesic effects and permit lower opioid doses.
- To convert to another opioid analgesic, remove transdermal fentanyl system and begin treatment with half the equianalgesic dose of the new analgesic in 12–18 hr.
- Discontinue medication gradually after long-term use to prevent withdrawal symptoms. May be necessary to provide patient with a lower dose strength for a successful taper. Monitor frequently to manage pain and withdrawal symptoms (restlessness, lacrimation, rhinorrhea, yawning, perspiration, chills, myalgia, mydriasis, irritability, anxiety, backache, joint pain, weakness, abdominal cramps, insomnia, nausea, anorexia, vomiting, diarrhea, or increased blood pressure, respiratory rate, or heart rate). If withdrawal symptoms occur, pause the taper for a period of time or raise the dose of opioid analgesic to the previous dose, and then proceed with a slower taper. Also, monitor patients for changes in mood, emergence of suicidal thoughts, or use of other substances. A multimodal approach to pain management may optimize the treatment of chronic pain, as well as assist with the successful tapering of the opioid analgesic.
- **REMS:** FDA strongly encourages health care professionals to complete a REMS-compliant education program that includes all the elements of the FDA Education *Blueprint for Health Care Providers Involved in the Management or Support of Patients with Pain,* available at www.fda.gov/OpioidAnalgesicREMSBlueprint. Information on programs can be found at 1-800-503-0784 or www.opioidanalgesicrems.com.
- Discuss availability of naloxone for emergency treatment of opioid overdose with the patient and caregiver and assess the potential need for access to naloxone, both when initiating and renewing therapy, especially if patient has household members (including children) or other close contacts at risk for accidental exposure or overdose. Consider prescribing naloxone, based on the patient's risk factors for overdose, such as concomitant use of CNS depressants, a history of opioid use disorder, or prior opioid overdose. However, the presence of risk factors for overdose should not prevent the proper management of pain in any patient.
- **Transdermal:** Apply system to flat, nonirritated, and nonirradiated skin such as chest, back, flank, or upper arm. If skin preparation is necessary, use clear water and clip, do not shave, hair. Allow skin to dry completely before application. Apply immediately after removing from package. Do not alter the system (cut) in any way before application. Remove liner from adhesive layer and press firmly in place with palm of hand for 30 sec, especially around the edges, to make sure contact is complete. Remove used system and fold so that adhesive edges are together. Flush system down toilet immediately on removal or follow the institutional disposal policy. Apply new system to a different site.

Patient/Family Teaching

- **REMS:** Instruct patient in how and when to ask for and take pain medication. Do not increase doses without discussing with health care professional, may lead to overdose. Discuss safe use, risks, and proper storage and disposal of opioid analgesics with patients and caregivers with each Rx. The Patient Counseling Guide (PCG) is available at www.fda.gov/OpioidAnalgesicREMSPCG. Advise patient to read *Medication Guide* before starting therapy and with each Rx refill in case of changes.
- Instruct patient in correct method for application and disposal of transdermal system. Fatalities have occurred from children having access to improperly

discarded patches. May be worn while bathing, showering, or swimming.

- Advise patient to avoid grapefruit juice during therapy.
- Advise patient that fentanyl is a drug with known abuse potential. Protect it from theft, and never give to anyone other than the individual for whom it was prescribed. Store out of sight and reach of children, and in a location not accessible by others.
- Educate patients and caregivers on how to recognize respiratory depression and emphasize the importance of calling 911 or getting emergency medical help right away in the event of a known or suspected overdose. Inform patients and caregivers about various ways to obtain naloxone as permitted by individual state naloxone dispensing and prescribing requirements or guidelines (by prescription, directly from a pharmacist, or as part of a community-based program).
- May cause drowsiness or dizziness. Caution patient to call for assistance when ambulating or smoking and to avoid driving or other activities requiring alertness until response to medication is known.
- Advise patient to change positions slowly to minimize dizziness.
- Caution patient to avoid concurrent use of alcohol or other CNS depressants with this medication.
- Caution patient that fever, electric blankets, heating pads, saunas, hot tubs, and heated water beds increase the release of fentanyl from the patch.
- Advise patient that good oral hygiene, frequent mouth rinses, and sugarless gum or candy may decrease dry mouth.
- Advise patient to notify health care professional of all Rx or OTC medications, vitamins, or herbal products being taken and to consult with health care professional before taking other medications.
- Advise patient referred for MRI test to discuss patch with referring health care professional and MRI facility to determine if removal of patch is necessary prior to test and for directions for replacing patch.
- Rep: Instruct females of reproductive potential to notify health care professional if pregnancy is planned or suspected and to avoid breastfeeding during therapy. Inform patient of potential for neonatal opioid withdrawal syndrome with prolonged use during pregnancy. Monitor neonate for signs and symptoms of withdrawal symptoms (irritability, hyperactivity and abnormal sleep pattern, high pitched cry, tremor, vomiting, diarrhea, and/or failure to gain weight); usually occur the first days after birth. Monitor infants exposed to fentanyl through breast milk for excess sedation and respiratory depression. Chronic use may reduce fertility in females and males.

Evaluation/Desired Outcomes

- Decrease in severity of pain without a significant alteration in level of consciousness, respiratory status, or BP.

REMS HIGH ALERT

FENTANYL (transmucosal)
(fen-ta-nil)
fentaNYL (buccal tablet)
Fentora
fentaNYL (oral transmucosal lozenge)
Actiq
Classification
Therapeutic: opioid analgesics
Pharmacologic: opioid agonists

Schedule II

Indications
Management of breakthrough pain in patients with cancer who are already receiving opioids and are tolerant to around-the-clock opioids for persistent cancer pain (60 mg/day of oral morphine or equivalent).

Action
Binds to opioid receptors in the CNS, altering the response to and perception of pain. **Therapeutic Effects:** Decrease in severity of breakthrough pain.

Pharmacokinetics
Absorption: *Buccal tablet:* 65% absorbed from buccal mucosa; 50% is absorbed transmucosally, remainder is swallowed and is absorbed slowly from the GI tract. Buccal absorption is enhanced by an effervescent reaction in the dose form; *Transmucosal lozenge:* Initial rapid absorption (25%) from buccal mucosa is followed by more prolonged absorption (25%) from GI tract (combined bioavailability 50%).

Distribution: Readily crosses the placenta and enters breast milk.

Metabolism and Excretion: Mostly metabolized in the liver and intestinal mucosa via the CYP3A4 isoenzyme; inactive metabolites are excreted in urine; <7% excreted unchanged in urine.

Half-life: *Buccal tablet:* 2.6–11.7 hr (↑ with dose); *Transmucosal lozenge:* 7 hr.

TIME/ACTION PROFILE (↓ pain)

ROUTE	ONSET	PEAK	DURATION
Buccal tablet	15 min	40–60 min	60 min
Transmucosal lozenge	rapid	15–30 min	several hr

Contraindications/Precautions
Contraindicated in: Known intolerance or hypersensitivity; Acute/postoperative pain, including headache/migraine, dental pain, or emergency room use; Opioid-naive (nontolerant) patients; Concurrent use of MAO inhibitors; OB: Labor and delivery; Lactation: Lactation.

Use Cautiously in: Chronic obstructive pulmonary disease or pre-existing medical conditions predisposing to hypoventilation; Concurrent use of CNS active drugs; History of substance abuse; Severe renal/hepatic impairment (use lowest effective starting dose); Brady-arrhythmias; OB: Use during pregnancy only if the potential maternal benefit justifies the potential fetal risk; Pedi: Safety and effectiveness not established in children; Geri: Older adults may be more sensitive to effects and may have an ↑ risk of adverse reactions; titrate dosage carefully.

Exercise Extreme Caution in: Patients susceptible to intracranial effects of CO_2 retention, including those with ↑ intracranial pressure, head injuries, or impaired consciousness.

Adverse Reactions/Side Effects

CV: hypotension. **Endo:** adrenal insufficiency. **GI:** <u>constipation</u>, <u>nausea</u>, <u>vomiting</u>, abdominal pain, anorexia, dry mouth. **Neuro:** <u>dizziness</u>, <u>drowsiness</u>, <u>headache</u>, confusion, depression, fatigue, hallucinations, headache, insomnia, weakness. **Resp:** dyspnea, RESPIRATORY DEPRESSION (including central sleep apnea and sleep-related hypoxemia). **Misc:** HYPERSENSITIVITY REACTIONS (including anaphylaxis), physical dependence, psychological dependence.

Interactions

Drug-Drug: Should not be used within 14 days of **MAO inhibitors** because of possible severe and unpredictable reactions. **CYP3A4 inhibitors**, including **ritonavir, ketoconazole, itraconazole, fluconazole, clarithromycin, erythromycin, nefazodone, diltiazem, verapamil, nelfinavir,** and **fosamprenavir,** ↑ levels and risk of opioid toxicity; careful monitoring during initiation, dose changes, or discontinuation of the inhibitor is recommended. **CYP3A4 inducers,** including **barbiturates, carbamazepine, efavirenz, corticosteroids, modafinil, nevirapine, oxcarbazepine, phenobarbital, phenytoin, rifabutin,** or **rifampin,** may ↓ levels and analgesia; if inducers are discontinued or dosage ↓, patients should be monitored for signs of opioid toxicity and necessary dose adjustments should be made. Use with **benzodiazepines** or other **CNS depressants** including other **opioids, non-benzodiazepine sedative/hypnotics, anxiolytics, general anesthetics, muscle relaxants, antipsychotics,** and **alcohol** may cause profound sedation, respiratory depression, coma, and death; reserve concurrent use for when alternative treatment options are inadequate. Drugs that affect serotonergic neurotransmitter systems, including **tricyclic antidepressants, SSRIs, SNRIs, MAO inhibitors, TCAs, tramadol, trazodone, mirtazapine, 5−HT$_3$ receptor antagonists, linezolid, methylene blue,** and **triptans** ↑ risk of serotonin syndrome.

Drug-Natural Products: **St. John's wort** is an inducer of CYP3A4; concurrent use may ↓ levels and analgesia; if inducers are discontinued or dosage decreased, patients should be monitored for signs of opioid toxicity and necessary dosage adjustments made.

Drug-Food: **Grapefuit juice** is a moderate inhibitor of CYP3A4 enzyme system; concurrent use may ↑ levels and the risk of CNS and respiratory depression. Careful monitoring and dose adjustment may be necessary.

Route/Dosage

Transmucosal products are not equivalent on a mcg-to-mcg basis.

Buccal (Adults): *Tablets:* 100 mcg, then titrate to dose that provides adequate analgesia without undue side effects.

Oral transmucosal (Adults): One 200-mcg unit dissolved in mouth (see Implementation section) over 15 min; additional unit may be used 15 min after first unit is completed. If more than 1 unit is required per episode (as evaluated over several episodes), dose may be ↑ as required to control pain. Optimal usage/titration should result in using no more than 4 units/day.

Availability (generic available)

Buccal tablets: 100 mcg, 200 mcg, 400 mcg, 600 mcg, 800 mcg. **Oral transmucosal lozenge on a stick (berry flavor-sugar free):** 200 mcg, 400 mcg, 600 mcg, 800 mcg, 1200 mcg, 1600 mcg.

NURSING IMPLICATIONS

Assessment

- Monitor type, location, and intensity of pain before and 1 hr after administration of transmucosal fentanyl.
- Assess BP, pulse, and respirations before and periodically during administration, especially when starting therapy or when given with other drugs that depress respiration. May cause sleep-related breathing disorders (central sleep apnea, sleep-related hypoxemia). If respiratory rate is <10 min, assess level of sedation. Physical stimulation may be sufficient to prevent hypoventilation. Subsequent doses may need to be decreased. Patients tolerant to opioid analgesics are usually tolerant to the respiratory depressant effects also. Monitor for respiratory depression; serious, life-threatening, or fatal respiratory depression may occur.
- Monitor for application site reactions (paresthesia, ulceration, bleeding, pain, ulcer, irritation). Reactions are usually self-limited and rarely require discontinuation.
- Assess risk for opioid addiction, abuse, or misuse prior to administration.

Lab Test Considerations

- May cause anemia, neutropenia, thrombocytopenia, and leukopenia.
- May cause hypokalemia, hypoalbuminemia, hypercalcemia, hypomagnesemia, and hyponatremia.

Toxicity and Overdose

- If an opioid antagonist is required to reverse respiratory depression or coma, naloxone is the antidote.

Dilute the 0.4-mg ampule of naloxone in 10 mL of 0.9% NaCl and administer 0.5 mL (0.02 mg) by IV push every 2 min. For patients weighing <40 kg, dilute 0.1 mg of naloxone in 10 mL of 0.9% NaCl for a concentration of 10 mcg/mL and administer 0.5 mcg every 2 min. Use extreme caution when titrating dose in patients physically dependent on opioid analgesics to avoid withdrawal, seizures, and severe pain. Duration of respiratory depression may be longer than duration of opioid antagonist, requiring repeated doses.

Implementation

- **High Alert:** Accidental overdose of opioid analgesics has resulted in fatalities. Before administering, clarify all ambiguous orders.
- Do not confuse fentanyl with sufentanil.
- Patients considered opioid-tolerant are those who are taking ≥60 mg of oral morphine/day, at least 25 mcg transdermal fentanyl/hr, 30 mg of oxycodone/day, 8 mg of hydromorphone/day or an equianalgesic dose of another opioid for ≥1 wk.
- **High Alert:** Dose may be lethal to a child; keep out of reach of children.
- Do not substitute fentanyl products; doses are not equivalent.
- For patients no longer requiring opioid therapy, consider discontinuing, along with a gradual downward titration of other opioids to minimize possible withdrawal effects. In patients who continue to take their chronic opioid therapy for persistent pain, but no longer require treatment for breakthrough pain, therapy can usually be discontinued immediately.
- Discuss availability of naloxone for emergency treatment of opioid overdose with the patient and caregiver and assess the potential need for access to naloxone, both when initiating and renewing therapy, especially if patient has household members (including children) or other close contacts at risk for accidental exposure or overdose. Consider prescribing naloxone, based on the patient's risk factors for overdose, such as concomitant use of CNS depressants, a history of opioid use disorder, or prior opioid overdose. However, the presence of risk factors for overdose should not prevent the proper management of pain in any patient.
- **REMS:** Health care professionals who prescribe transmucosal immediate-release fentanyl (TIRF) medicines for outpatient use are required to enroll in the TIRF REMS Access program. Health care professionals already enrolled in an individual Risk Evaluation and Mitigation Strategy (REMS) program for at least one TIRF medicine, will be automatically transitioned to the shared TIRF REMS Access program, and do not need to re-enroll. Enrollment renewal in TIRF REMS program is required every 2 yr from the date of enrollment. Information can be found at www.TIRFREMSaccess.com. A TIRF REMS Access Patient-Prescriber Agreement Form must be signed with each new patient before writing the patient's first TIRF prescription and health care professionals must also provide patients with a copy of the *Medication Guide* during counseling about the proper use of their TIRF medicine. Pharmacists who dispense TIRF medicines are also required to enroll in the TIRF REMS program and re-enroll every 2 yr. Patients are enrolled in the TIRF REMS Access program by the pharmacy at the time their first prescription is filled. Patients can locate a participating pharmacy by consulting their prescriber or calling the TIRF REMS Access program at 1-866-822-1483.

- **Buccal:** *Fentora*: Do not attempt to push tablet through blister, may cause damage to tablet. Open by tearing along perforations to separate from blister card. Then bend blister unit on line where indicated. Blister backing should then be peeled to expose tablets. Use immediately; do not store, may damage integrity of tablet. Tablets are not to be sucked, chewed, or swallowed whole; this will reduce medication effectiveness. Place between cheek and gum above a molar or under tongue and allow medication to dissolve, usually 14–25 min. May cause bubbling sensation between teeth and gum while tablet dissolves. Do not attempt to split tablet. After 30 min, if remnants of tablet remain, swallow with glass of water.
- For patients not previously using transmucosal fentanyl, initial dose should be 100 mcg. Titrate to provide adequate relief while minimizing side effects. For patients switching from oral transmucosal fentanyl to fentanyl buccal, if transmucosal dose is 200–400 mcg, switch to 100 mcg buccal; if transmucosal dose is 600–800 mcg, switch to 200 mcg buccal; if transmucosal dose is 1200–1600 mcg, switch to 400 mcg buccal fentanyl.
- Dose may be repeated once during a single episode of breakthrough pain if not adequately relieved. Redose may occur 30 min after start of administration of fentanyl buccal and the same dose should be used.
- If more than 1 dose is required per breakthrough pain episode for several consecutive episodes, dose of maintenance opioid and fentanyl buccal tablets should be adjusted. To increase dose, use multiples of 100 mcg tablet, use two 100-mcg tablets (1 on each side of mouth in buccal cavity). If unsuccessful in controlling breakthrough pain episode, two 100-mcg tablets may be placed on each side of mouth in buccal cavity (four 100-mcg tablets). Titrate above 400 mcg by 200 mcg increments. To reduce risk of overdose, patients should have only one strength available at any one time.
- Once a successful dose has been established, instruct patient to use only one dose for each breakthrough episode; if pain is not relieved in 30 min after completion, only one additional use of the same strength can be used for that episode. Instruct patient to wait 4 hr before treating another episode of breakthrough pain. If more than 4 breakthrough

pain episodes/day occur, re-evaluate opioid dose for persistent pain.

- Inform patient if medication is no longer needed they should contact Teva Pharmaceuticals at 1-888-483-8279 or remove from blister pack and flush any remaining product down toilet.
- **Transmucosal:** *Actiq*: Open the foil package immediately before use. Instruct patient to place unit in the mouth between the cheek and lower gum, moving it from one side to the other using the handle. Patient should suck, not chew, the lozenge. If it is chewed and swallowed, lower peak concentrations and lower bioavailability may occur. Instruct patient to consume lozenge over 15-min period; longer or shorter periods may be less efficacious. If signs of excessive opioid effects occur, remove from patient's mouth immediately and decrease future doses.
- Initial dose for breakthrough pain should be 200 mcg. Six 200-mcg units should be prescribed and should be used before increasing to a higher dose. If one unit is ineffective, a 2nd unit may be started 15 min after the completion of the first unit. Do not use more than 2 units during a single episode of breakthrough pain during titration phase. With each new dose during titration, 6 units should be prescribed, allowing treatment of several episodes of breakthrough pain. Adequate dose is determined based on effective analgesia with acceptable side effects. Side effects during titration period are usually greater than after effective dose is determined.
- Once an effective dose is determined, instruct patient to use only one *Actiq* unit for each breakthrough episode; if pain is not relieved in 15 min after completion, only one additional use of the same strength can be used for that episode. Instruct patient to wait 4 hr before treating another episode of breakthrough pain.
- Discontinue with a gradual decrease in dose to prevent signs and symptoms of abrupt withdrawal.
- To dispose of remaining unit, using wire-cutting pliers cut off the drug matrix end so that it falls into the toilet. Flush remaining drug matrix down toilet. Drug remaining on handle may be removed by placing under running warm water until dissolved. Dispose of drug-free handle according to institutional protocol. *High Alert:* Partially consumed units are no longer protected by child-resistant pouch; dose may still be fatal. A temporary child-resistant storage bottle is provided for partially consumed units that cannot be disposed of properly.

Patient/Family Teaching

- Instruct patient to take fentanyl transmucosal as directed. Instruct patient in correct technique for use and disposal. Do not take more often than prescribed, keep out of reach of children, protect it

from being stolen, and do not share with others, even if they have the same symptoms. Open only when ready to administer. Advise patient to review *Medication Guide* before and with each Rx refill in case of changes. Advise patient to notify health care professional if breakthrough pain is not alleviated, worsens, if >4 units/day are required to control pain, or if excessive opioid effects occur.

- *REMS:* Explain TIRF REMS program to patient and caregiver. Patients must sign the Patient-Prescriber Agreement Form to confirm they understand the risks, appropriate use, and storage of fentanyl transmucosal.
- Educate patients and caregivers on how to recognize respiratory depression and emphasize the importance of calling 911 or getting emergency medical help right away in the event of a known or suspected overdose. Inform patients and caregivers about various ways to obtain naloxone as permitted by individual state naloxone dispensing and prescribing requirements or guidelines (by prescription, directly from a pharmacist, or as part of a community-based program).
- Advise patient to avoid grapefruit juice during therapy.
- Advise patient that transmucosal fentanyl is a drug with known abuse potential. Protect it from theft, and never give to anyone other than the individual for whom it was prescribed. Store out of sight and reach of children and in a location not accessible by others.
- Caution patient to make position changes slowly to minimize orthostatic hypotension.
- Medication causes dizziness and drowsiness. Advise patient to call for assistance during ambulation and transfer, and to avoid driving or other activities requiring alertness until response to medication is known.
- Instruct patient to avoid concurrent use of alcohol or other CNS depressants, such as sleep aids.
- Advise patient to notify health care professional if sores on gums or inside cheek become a problem.
- Advise patient to notify health care professional of all Rx or OTC medications, vitamins, or herbal products being taken and to consult with health care professional before taking other medications.
- Rep: Instruct females of reproductive potential to notify health care professional if pregnancy is planned or suspected and to avoid breastfeeding during therapy. Inform patient of potential for neonatal opioid withdrawal syndrome with prolonged use during pregnancy. Monitor neonate for signs and symptoms of withdrawal symptoms (irritability, hyperactivity and abnormal sleep pattern, high pitched cry, tremor, vomiting, diarrhea, and/or failure to gain weight); usually occur the first days after birth. Monitor infants exposed to fentanyl through

breast milk for excess sedation and respiratory depression. Chronic use may reduce fertility in females and males.

- *Actiq:* Inform patient that this drug may contain sugar and may cause dry mouth. Advise patient to maintain good oral hygiene and regular dental exams.

Evaluation/Desired Outcomes

- Decrease in severity of pain during episodes of breakthrough pain in patients receiving and tolerant to long-acting opioids.

ferrous sulfate (30% elemental iron) (fer-us sul-fate)
Classification
Therapeutic: antianemics
Pharmacologic: iron supplements

Indications
PO: Treatment and prevention of iron deficiency anemia.

Action
An essential mineral found in hemoglobin, myoglobin, and many enzymes. Enters the bloodstream and is transported to the organs of the reticuloendothelial system (liver, spleen, bone marrow) where it becomes part of iron stores. **Therapeutic Effects:** Resolution or prevention of iron deficiency anemia.

Pharmacokinetics
Absorption: Approximately 5–10% of dietary iron is absorbed (up to 30% in deficiency states). Therapeutically administered PO iron is up to 60% absorbed via active and passive transport processes.
Distribution: Remains in the body for many months.
Protein Binding: ≥90%.
Metabolism and Excretion: Mostly recycled; small daily losses occurring via desquamation, sweat, urine, and bile.
Half-life: Unknown.

TIME/ACTION PROFILE (effects on erythropoiesis)

ROUTE	ONSET	PEAK	DURATION
PO	4 days	7–10 days	2–4 mo

Contraindications/Precautions
Contraindicated in: Anemia not due to iron deficiency; Hemochromatosis; Hemosiderosis; Hypersensitivity to iron products.
Use Cautiously in: Peptic ulcer disease; Ulcerative colitis or regional enteritis (condition may be aggravated); Alcoholism; Severe hepatic impairment; Severe renal impairment.

Adverse Reactions/Side Effects
GI: constipation, dark stools, epigastric pain, nausea, GI bleeding, vomiting. **Neuro:** dizziness, headache,

syncope. **Misc:** temporary staining of teeth (liquid preparations).

Interactions
Drug-Drug: May ↓ absorption and effects of **tetracyclines, fluoroquinolones, bisphosphonates, levodopa, levothyroxine, mycophenolate mofetil,** and **penicillamine** (simultaneous administration should be avoided). Concurrent administration of **proton pump inhibitors, H₂ antagonists,** and **cholestyramine** may ↓ absorption of iron. Doses of **ascorbic acid** ≥200 mg may ↑ absorption of iron by up to 30%. **Chloramphenicol** and **vitamin E** may ↓ hematologic response to iron therapy.
Drug-Food: Iron absorption is ↓ 33–50% by concurrent administration of food.

Route/Dosage
Oral iron dosages are expressed as mg of elemental iron. Multiple salt forms exist—see approximate equivalent doses below or consider % elemental iron of each salt for dose conversions.

Approximate Equivalent Doses (mg of iron salt): *Ferrous fumarate:* 197; *Ferrous gluconate:* 560; *Ferrous sulfate:* 324; *Ferrous sulfate, exsiccated:* 217.
PO (Adults): *Deficiency:* 2–3 mg/kg/day in 2–4 divided doses or 60–100 mg elemental iron twice daily. *Prophylaxis:* 60–100 mg elemental iron daily.
PO (Infants and Children): *Severe deficiency:* 4–6 mg/kg/day in 3 divided doses. *Mild to moderate deficiency:* 3 mg/kg/day in 1–2 divided doses. *Prophylaxis:* 1–2 mg/kg/day in 1–2 divided dose (maximum: 15 mg/day).
PO (Neonates, premature): 2–4 mg/kg/day in 1–2 divided doses, maximum of 15 mg/day.

Availability
Tablets: 325 mg^OTC. **Delayed-release tablets:** 142 mg^OTC, 160 mg^OTC, 325 mg^OTC. **Solution:** 75 mg/mL^OTC, 300 mg/5 mL^OTC. **Elixir:** 220 mg/5 mL^OTC.

NURSING IMPLICATIONS
Assessment
- Assess nutritional status and dietary history to determine possible cause of anemia and need for patient teaching.
- Assess bowel function for constipation or diarrhea. Notify health care professional and use appropriate nursing measures should these occur.

Lab Test Considerations
- Monitor hemoglobin, hematocrit, and reticulocyte values prior to and every 3 wk during the first 2 mo of therapy and periodically thereafter. Serum ferritin and iron levels may also be monitored to assess effectiveness of therapy.
- Occult blood in stools may be obscured by black coloration of iron in stool. Guaiac test results may occasionally be false-positive. Benzidine test results are not affected by iron preparations.

Toxicity and Overdose
- Early symptoms of overdose include stomach pain, fever, nausea, vomiting (may contain blood), and diarrhea. Late symptoms include bluish lips, fingernails, and palms; drowsiness; weakness; tachycardia; seizures; metabolic acidosis; hepatic injury; and cardiovascular collapse. Patient may appear to recover prior to the onset of late symptoms. Therefore, hospitalization continues for 24 hr after patient becomes asymptomatic to monitor for delayed onset of shock or GI bleeding. Late complications of overdose include intestinal obstruction, pyloric stenosis, and gastric scarring.
- If patient is comatose or seizing, gastric lavage with sodium bicarbonate is performed. Deferoxamine is the antidote. Additional supportive treatments to maintain fluid and electrolyte balance and correction of metabolic acidosis are also indicated.

Implementation
- Discontinue oral iron preparations prior to parenteral administration.
- Oral preparations are most effectively absorbed if administered 1 hr before or 2 hr after meals. If gastric irritation occurs, administer with meals. Take tablets with a full glass of water or juice. *DNC:* Do not crush or chew enteric-coated tablets.
- Liquid preparations may stain teeth. Dilute in water or fruit juice, full glass (240 mL) for adults and ½ glass (120 mL) for children, and administer with a straw or place drops at back of throat.
- Avoid using antacids, coffee, tea, dairy products, eggs, or whole-grain breads with or within 1 hr after administration of ferrous salts. Iron absorption is decreased by 33% if iron is given with meals.

Patient/Family Teaching
- Explain purpose of iron therapy to patient.
- Encourage patient to comply with medication regimen. Take missed doses as soon as remembered within 12 hr; otherwise, return to regular dosing schedule. Do not double doses.
- Advise patient that stools may become dark green or black.
- Instruct patient to follow a diet high in iron (see Appendix J).
- Discuss with parents the risk of a child overdosing on iron. Medication should be stored in the original childproof container and kept out of reach of children. Do not refer to vitamins as candy. In the event of a suspected overdose, parents should contact poison control center (1-800-222-1222) or emergency medical services (911) immediately.
- Rep: Advise females of reproductive potential to notify health care professional if pregnancy is planned or suspected or if breastfeeding.

Evaluation/Desired Outcomes
- Increase in hemoglobin, which may reach normal parameters after 1–2 mo of therapy. May require 3–6 mo for normalization of body iron stores.
- Improvement in or prevention of iron deficiency anemia.

℀ fesoterodine
(fes-oh-**ter**-o-deen)
Toviaz
Classification
Therapeutic: urinary tract antispasmodics
Pharmacologic: anticholinergics

Indications
Overactive bladder with symptoms of urinary frequency, urgency, and urge incontinence. Neurogenic detrusor overactivity.

Action
Acts as a competitive muscarinic receptor antagonist resulting in inhibition of cholinergically mediated bladder contraction. **Therapeutic Effects:** Decreased urinary frequency, urgency, and urge incontinence in overactive bladder. Increase in maximum cystometric bladder capacity in neurogenic detrusor overactivity.

Pharmacokinetics
Absorption: Rapidly absorbed following oral administration, but is rapidly converted to its active metabolite (bioavailability of metabolite 52%).
Distribution: Unknown.
Metabolism and Excretion: Primarily metabolized in the liver via the CYP2D6 and CYP3A4 isoenzymes; ℀ the CYP2D6 enzyme system exhibits genetic polymorphism; ~7% of population may be poor metabolizers and may have significantly ↑ fesoterodine concentrations and an ↑ risk of adverse effects. 16% of active metabolite is excreted in urine, most of the remainder of inactive metabolites are renally excreted. 7% excreted in feces.
Half-life: 7 hr (following oral administration).

TIME/ACTION PROFILE (plasma concentrations of active metabolite)

ROUTE	ONSET	PEAK	DURATION
PO	rapid	5 hr	24 hr

Contraindications/Precautions
Contraindicated in: Hypersensitivity; Urinary retention; Significant bladder outlet obstruction (↑ risk of retention); Gastric retention; ↓ GI motility including severe constipation; Severe hepatic impairment; Uncontrolled narrow-angle glaucoma; Pedi: eGFR <15 mL/min/1.73 m² or requiring dialysis (children ≥6 yr and >35 kg); Pedi: eGFR <30 mL/min/1.73 m² or requiring dialysis (children ≥6 yr and 25–35 kg).

Use Cautiously in: CCr <30 mL/min (dose adjustment required in adults); Treated narrow-angle glaucoma (use only if benefits outweigh risks); Myasthenia gravis; OB: Safety not established in pregnancy; Lactation: Safety not established in breastfeeding; Pedi: Safety and effectiveness not established in children <18 yr (overactive bladder) or <6 yr or <25 kg (neurogenic detrusor overactivity); Geri: ↑ risk of anticholinergic side effects in patients >75 yr.

Adverse Reactions/Side Effects

CV: tachycardia (dose related). **GI:** dry mouth, constipation, nausea, upper abdominal pain. **GU:** dysuria, urinary retention. **MS:** back pain. **Neuro:** dizziness, drowsiness, headache. **Misc:** HYPERSENSITIVITY REACTIONS (including angioedema).

Interactions

Drug-Drug: **Strong CYP3A4 inhibitors,** including **ketoconazole, itraconazole,** and **clarithromycin,** ↑ levels and risk of toxicity; daily dose should not exceed 4 mg in adults and children ≥6 yr and >35 kg; avoid concurrent use in children ≥6 yr and 25–35 kg. Additive anticholinergic effects with other **anticholinergic drugs,** including **antihistamines, phenothiazines, quinidine, disopyramide,** and **tricyclic antidepressants.** May ↓ GI absorption of other drugs.

Route/Dosage

Overactive Bladder

PO (Adults): 4 mg once daily initially; may ↑ to 8 mg/daily, if needed based on response and tolerability; *Concurrent use of strong CYP3A4 inhibitors:* Do not exceed 4 mg/day.

Renal Impairment

PO (Adults): *CCr <30 mL/min:* Do not exceed 4 mg/day.

Neurogenic Detrusor Overactivity

PO (Children ≥6 yr and >35 kg): 4 mg once daily, then ↑ to 8 mg once daily after 1 wk; *Concurrent use of strong CYP3A4 inhibitors:* Do not exceed 4 mg/day. **PO (Children ≥6 yr and 25–35 kg):** 4 mg once daily; ↑ to 8 mg once daily, if needed; *Concurrent use of strong CYP3A4 inhibitors:* Use not recommended.

Renal Impairment

PO (Children ≥6 yr and >35 kg): *eGFR 15–29 mL/min/1.73 m²:* Do not exceed 4 mg/day; *eGFR <15 mL/min/1.73 m² or requiring dialysis:* Use not recommended.

Renal Impairment

PO (Children ≥6 yr and 25–35 kg): *eGFR 30–89 mL/min/1.73 m²:* Do not exceed 4 mg/day; *eGFR <30 mL/min/1.73 m² or requiring dialysis:* Use not recommended.

Availability (generic available)

Extended-release tablets: 4 mg, 8 mg.

NURSING IMPLICATIONS

Assessment

- Assess for urinary urgency, frequency, and urge incontinence periodically during therapy.
- Monitor for signs and symptoms of angioedema (swelling of face, lips, tongue, and/or larynx). May occur with first or subsequent doses. Discontinue therapy and prove supportive therapy. Have epinephrine, corticosteroids, and resuscitation equipment available.

Lab Test Considerations
- May cause ↑ ALT and GGT.

Implementation

- **PO:** Administer with liquid without regard to food.
- *DNC:* Swallow extended-release tablets whole; do not break, crush, or chew.

Patient/Family Teaching

- Instruct patient to take fesoterodine as directed. If a dose is missed, omit and begin taking again the next day; do not take 2 doses the same day. Advise patient to read the *Patient Information* sheet prior to initiation of therapy and with each Rx refill in case of changes.
- May cause drowsiness, dizziness, and blurred vision. Caution patient to avoid driving or other activities requiring alertness until response to medication is known.
- Advise patient to avoid alcohol; may increase drowsiness.
- Advise patient to use caution in hot environments; may cause decreased sweating and severe heat illness.
- Instruct patient to notify health care professional of all Rx or OTC medications, vitamins, or herbal products being taken and to consult with health care professional before taking other medications.
- Advise patient to stop medication and notify health care professional if signs and symptoms of angioedema occur.
- Rep: Advise females of reproductive potential to notify health care professional if pregnancy is planned or suspected or if breastfeeding.

Evaluation/Desired Outcomes

- Decreased urinary frequency, urgency, and urge incontinence.
- Increase in maximum cystometric bladder capacity in neurogenic detrusor overactivity.

fexofenadine
(fex-oh-**fen**-a-deen)
~~Allegra~~, Allegra Allergy, Children's Allegra Allergy, ~~Children's Allegra Hives~~, ~~Mucinex Allergy~~

Classification
Therapeutic: allergy, cold, and cough remedies
Pharmacologic: antihistamines

Indications
Relief of symptoms of seasonal allergic rhinitis. Management of chronic idiopathic urticaria.

Action
Antagonizes the effects of histamine at peripheral histamine−1 (H_1) receptors, including pruritus and urticaria. Also has a drying effect on the nasal mucosa. **Therapeutic Effects:** Decreased sneezing, rhinorrhea, itchy eyes, nose, and throat associated with seasonal allergies. Decreased urticaria.

Pharmacokinetics
Absorption: Rapidly absorbed after oral administration.
Distribution: Unknown.
Metabolism and Excretion: 80% excreted in urine, 11% excreted in feces.
Half-life: 14.4 hr (↑ in renal impairment).

TIME/ACTION PROFILE (antihistaminic effect)

ROUTE	ONSET	PEAK	DURATION
PO	within 1 hr	2–3 hr	12–24 hr

Contraindications/Precautions
Contraindicated in: Hypersensitivity.
Use Cautiously in: Renal impairment (↑ dosing interval recommended); OB: Use only if potential maternal benefit justifies potential fetal risk; Lactation: Safety not established in breastfeeding.

Adverse Reactions/Side Effects
GI: dyspepsia. **GU:** dysmenorrhea. **Neuro:** drowsiness, fatigue.

Interactions
Drug-Drug: **Magnesium and aluminum-containing antacids** ↓ absorption and may decrease effectiveness.
Drug-Food: **Apple**, **orange**, and **grapefruit juice** ↓ absorption and may decrease effectiveness.

Route/Dosage
PO (Adults and Children ≥12 yr): 60 mg twice daily, or 180 mg once daily.
PO (Children 2–11 yr): 30 mg twice daily.
PO (Children 6 mo–2 yr): 15 mg twice daily.

Renal Impairment
PO (Adults): 60 mg once daily as a starting dose.
PO (Children 6–11 yr): 30 mg once daily as a starting dose.

Availability (generic available)
Tablets: 60 mg^OTC, ✽ 120 mg^OTC, 180 mg^OTC. **Orally disintegrating tablets:** 30 mg^OTC. **Suspension (berry flavor):** 30 mg/5 mL^OTC. *In combination with:* pseudoephedrine (Allegra-D). See Appendix N.

NURSING IMPLICATIONS
Assessment
- Assess allergy symptoms (rhinitis, conjunctivitis, hives) before and periodically during therapy.
- Assess lung sounds and character of bronchial secretions. Maintain fluid intake of 1500–2000 mL/day to decrease viscosity of secretions.

Lab Test Considerations
- Will cause false-negative reactions on allergy skin tests; discontinue 3 days before testing.

Implementation
- Do not confuse Allegra with Viagra. Do not confuse Allegra (fexofenadine) with Allegra Anti-Itch Cream (diphenhydramine/allantoin).
- **PO:** Administer with food or milk to decrease GI irritation. Administer capsules and tablets with water or milk, not juice. Shake solution bottle well before use.

Patient/Family Teaching
- Instruct patient to take medication as directed. Take missed doses as soon as remembered unless almost time for next dose. Do not take more than recommended.
- Instruct patient or parents to avoid taking fexofenadine with fruit juices (apple, orange, grapefruit) or antacids containing aluminum or magnesium; may decrease effectiveness of fexofenadine.
- Inform patient that fexofenadine may cause drowsiness, although it is less likely to occur than with other antihistamines. Avoid driving or other activities requiring alertness until response to drug is known.
- Rep: Advise females of reproductive potential to notify health care professional if pregnancy is planned or suspected or if breastfeeding.
- Instruct patient to contact health care professional if symptoms persist.

Evaluation/Desired Outcomes
- Decrease in allergic symptoms.
- Decrease in urticaria.

fezolinetant (fez-oh-lin-e-tant)
Veozah
Classification
Therapeutic: menopausal agents
Pharmacologic: neurokinin 3 receptor antagonists

Indications
Moderate to severe vasomotor symptoms due to menopause.

Action
Acts as a neurokinin 3 receptor antagonist that blocks neurokinin B binding on the kisspeptin/neurokinin B/dynorphin neuron to regulate neuronal activity in the thermoregulatory center. **Therapeutic Effects:** Reduction in frequency and severity of vasomotor symptoms due to menopause.

Pharmacokinetics
Absorption: Extent of absorption unknown.
Distribution: Extensively distributed to tissues.
Metabolism and Excretion: Primarily metabolized by the liver via the CYP1A2 isoenzyme, with some metabolism by the CYP2C9 and CYP2C19 isoenzymes. Primarily excreted in the urine (77%; 1% as unchanged drug), with 15% excreted in the feces (<1% as unchanged drug).
Half-life: 9.6 hr.

TIME/ACTION PROFILE (plasma concentrations)

ROUTE	ONSET	PEAK	DURATION
PO	unknown	1–4 hr	24 hr

Contraindications/Precautions
Contraindicated in: Cirrhosis; Severe renal impairment or end-stage renal disease; Concurrent use with CYP1A2 inhibitors.
Use Cautiously in: None.

Adverse Reactions/Side Effects
Derm: hot flush. **GI:** ↑ liver enzymes, abdominal pain, diarrhea. **MS:** back pain. **Neuro:** insomnia.

Interactions
Drug-Drug: CYP1A2 inhibitors, including **fluvoxamine**, **mexiletine**, and **cimetidine** ↑ levels and risk of toxicity; concurrent use contraindicated.

Route/Dosage
PO (Adults): 45 mg once daily.

Availability
Tablets: 45 mg.

NURSING IMPLICATIONS

Assessment
● Assess vasomotor symptoms (feelings of warmth in the face, neck, and chest, or sudden intense feelings of heat and sweating (hot flashes or hot flushes) before starting and periodically during therapy.

Lab Test Considerations
● Monitor for hepatic function and injury with ALT, AST, and serum bilirubin (total and direct) before starting therapy and 3 mo, 6 mo, and 9 mo after starting therapy and when symptoms (nausea, vomiting, yellowing of the skin or eyes) occur suggesting

liver injury. Do not start therapy if concentration of ALT or AST ≥ two times the upper limit of normal (ULN) or if total bilirubin is elevated (≥2× ULN) for the evaluating laboratory.

Implementation
● **PO:** Administer once daily without regard to food, at the same time each day. *DNC:* Swallow tablets whole; do not break, crush, or chew.

Patient/Family Teaching
● Instruct patient to take fezolinetant as directed. Take missed doses as soon as remembered, unless there is <12 hr before next dose is due. Return to regular schedule next day. Advise patient to read *Patient Information* before starting and with each Rx refill in case of changes.
● Advise patient to notify health care professional promptly if signs and symptoms of liver problems (nausea, vomiting, yellowing of the eyes or skin, pain in the right upper abdomen) occur.
● Instruct patient to notify health care professional of all Rx or OTC medications, vitamins, or herbal products being taken and to consult with health care professional before taking other medications.
● Rep: Advise females of reproductive potential to notify health care professional if pregnancy is planned or suspected or if breastfeeding.

Evaluation/Desired Outcomes
● Decrease in frequency and severity of vasomotor symptoms due to menopause.

---

fidaxomicin (fi-dax-oh-**mye**-sin)
Dificid
Classification
Therapeutic: anti-infectives
Pharmacologic: macrolides

Indications
Treatment of diarrhea associated with *Clostridioides difficile*.

Action
Bactericidal action mostly against clostridia; inhibits RNA synthesis. Acts locally in the GI tract to eliminate *Clostridioides difficile*. **Therapeutic Effects:** Elimination of diarrhea caused by *Clostridioides difficile*.

Pharmacokinetics
Absorption: Minimal systemic absorption.
Distribution: Stays primarily in the GI tract.
Metabolism and Excretion: Mostly transformed via hydrolysis in the GI tract to OP-1118, its active metabolite. Eliminated mostly (>92%) in feces: <1% excreted in urine.
Half-life: *Fidaxomicin:* 11.7 hr; *OP-1118:* 11.2 hr.

TIME/ACTION PROFILE

ROUTE	ONSET	PEAK	DURATION
PO	unknown	unknown	unknown

Contraindications/Precautions

Contraindicated in: Hypersensitivity to fidaxomicin or macrolides (cross-sensitivity may occur).
Use Cautiously in: OB: Use during pregnancy only if potential maternal benefit justifies potential fetal risk; Lactation: Use while breastfeeding only if potential maternal benefit justifies potential risk to infant; Pedi: Children <6 mo (safety and effectiveness not established).

Adverse Reactions/Side Effects

GI: <u>nausea</u>, abdominal pain, GI HEMORRHAGE. **Hemat:** anemia, neutropenia. **Misc:** HYPERSENSITIVITY REACTIONS (including angioedema).

Interactions

Drug-Drug: None reported.

Route/Dosage

PO (Adults): 200 mg twice daily for 10 days.
PO (Children ≥6 mo and ≥12.5 kg): *Tablets:* 200 mg twice daily for 10 days (if unable to swallow tablets, use granules for oral suspension).
PO (Children ≥6 mo and 9–<12.5 kg): *Granules for oral suspension:* 160 mg twice daily for 10 days.
PO (Children ≥6 mo and 7–<9 kg): *Granules for oral suspension:* 120 mg twice daily for 10 days.
PO (Children ≥6 mo and 4–<7 kg): *Granules for oral suspension:* 80 mg twice daily for 10 days.

Availability

Granules for oral suspension (berry flavor): 40 mg/mL. **Tablets:** 200 mg.

NURSING IMPLICATIONS

Assessment

● Monitor bowel function for diarrhea, abdominal cramping, fever, and bloody stools. May begin up to several wk following cessation of antibiotic therapy.
● Monitor for signs and symptoms of hypersensitivity reactions (dyspnea, pruritus, rash, angioedema of mouth, throat, and face) periodically during therapy. Risk increases with a macrolide allergy.

Lab Test Considerations

● May cause ↑ serum alkaline phosphatase, and hepatic enzymes.
● May cause ↓ serum bicarbonate, ↓ platelet count, anemia, and neutropenia.
● May cause hyperglycemia and metabolic acidosis.

Implementation

● **PO:** Administer twice daily, about 12 hr apart, without regard to food.
● For oral suspension, shake the glass bottle to ensure the granules move around freely and no caking has occurred. Measure 130 mL of purified water, add to glass bottle, and cap tightly. Hold bottle in a horizontal position and shake bottle vigorously in that position for at least 2 minutes. Verify that suspension is

homogeneous; shake again. Once suspension is homogeneous, shake an additional 30 seconds. Let bottle stand for 1 min. Verify that suspension is still homogeneous. If not, repeat previous steps. Once reconstituted, oral suspension is white to yellowish white. Write discard date (current date plus 12 days) on the bottle. Stable in refrigerator for up to 12 days; discard after 12 days. Remove bottle from refrigerator 15 min before administration. Shake vigorously until suspension is homogenous. Administer orally with or without food using an oral dosing syringe to ensure accurate dose.

Patient/Family Teaching

● Instruct patient to take fidaxomicin twice daily, 12 hr apart, as directed for the full course of therapy, even if feeling better. Skipping doses or not completing full course of therapy may decrease effectiveness of therapy and increase risk that bacteria will develop resistance and not be treatable in the future.
● Advise patient to notify health care professional of all Rx or OTC medications, vitamins, or herbal products being taken and to consult with health care professional before taking other medications.
● Rep: Advise females of reproductive potential to notify health care professional if pregnancy is planned or suspected or if breastfeeding.

Evaluation/Desired Outcomes

● Decrease in diarrhea caused by *Clostridioides difficile*.

---

filgrastim (fil-gra-stim)
Granix, ✶Grastofil, Neupogen, Nivestym, Releuko, Zarxio
Classification
Therapeutic: colony-stimulating factors

Indications

Prevention of febrile neutropenia and associated infection in patients who have received bone marrow–depressing antineoplastics for the treatment of nonmyeloid malignancies. Reduction of time for neutrophil recovery and duration of fever in patients undergoing induction and consolidation chemotherapy for acute myelogenous leukemia. Reduction of time to neutrophil recovery and sequelae of neutropenia in patients with nonmyeloid malignancies undergoing myeloablative chemotherapy followed by bone marrow transplantation. Mobilization of hematopoietic progenitor cells into peripheral blood for collection by leukapheresis. Management of severe chronic neutropenia. Survival improvement in patients acutely exposed to myelosuppressive doses of radiation. **Unlabeled Use:** Neutropenia associated with HIV infection. Neonatal neutropenia.

✶ = Canadian drug name. ⚇ = Genetic implication. ~~Strikethrough~~ = Discontinued. CAPITALS = life-threatening. <u>Underline</u> = most frequent.

Action

A glycoprotein, filgrastim binds to and stimulates immature neutrophils to divide and differentiate. Also activates mature neutrophils. **Therapeutic Effects:** Decreased incidence of infection in patients who are neutropenic from chemotherapy or other causes. Improved harvest of progenitor cells for bone marrow transplantation. Improved survival in patients exposed to myelosuppressive doses of radiation.

Pharmacokinetics

Absorption: Well absorbed after SUBQ administration.
Distribution: Unknown.
Metabolism and Excretion: Unknown.
Half-life: *Adults:* 3.5 hr; *Neonates:* 4.4 hr.

TIME/ACTION PROFILE

ROUTE	ONSET	PEAK	DURATION
IV, SUBQ	unknown	unknown	4 days†

†Return of neutrophil count to baseline.

Contraindications/Precautions

Contraindicated in: Hypersensitivity to filgrastim or *Escherichia coli*-derived proteins.
Use Cautiously in: Congenital neutropenia (↑ risk of myelodysplastic syndrome or acute myeloid leukemia); Patients with breast or lung cancer receiving chemotherapy and/or radiotherapy (↑ risk of myelodysplastic syndrome or acute myeloid leukemia); Patients with sickle cell disease (↑ risk of sickle cell crisis); Malignancy with myeloid characteristics; Pre-existing cardiac disease; OB: Use only if potential maternal benefit justifies potential fetal risk; Lactation: Use while breastfeeding only if potential maternal benefit justifies potential risk to infant.

Adverse Reactions/Side Effects

CV: aortitis, vasculitis. **EENT:** hemoptysis. **GI:** SPLENIC RUPTURE, splenomegaly. **GU:** glomerulonephritis. **Hemat:** ACUTE MYELOID LEUKEMIA, excessive leukocytosis, MYELODYSPLASTIC SYNDROME, sickle cell crises, thrombocytopenia. **Local:** pain at injection site. **MS:** medullary bone pain. **Resp:** ACUTE RESPIRATORY DISTRESS SYNDROME, pulmonary infiltrates. **Misc:** HYPERSENSITIVITY REACTIONS (including anaphylaxis).

Interactions

Drug-Drug: Simultaneous use with **antineoplastics** may have adverse effects on rapidly proliferating neutrophils—avoid use for 24 hr before and 24 hr after chemotherapy. **Lithium** may potentiate the release of neutrophils; concurrent use should be undertaken cautiously.

Route/Dosage

After Myelosuppressive Chemotherapy

IV, SUBQ (Adults and Children): 5 mcg/kg/day as a single SUBQ injection, by short IV infusion, or via continuous IV infusion for up to 2 wk or until ANC reaches 10,000/mm³. Initiate at least 24 hr after chemotherapy. Dose may be ↑ by 5 mcg/kg during each cycle of chemotherapy, depending on blood counts.

After Bone Marrow Transplantation

IV (Adults): 10 mcg/kg/day as a continuous IV infusion for up to 24 hr; initiate at least 24 hr after chemotherapy and at least 24 hr after bone marrow transplantation. Subsequent dose is adjusted according to blood counts.

Peripheral Blood Progenitor Cell Collection and Therapy

SUBQ (Adults): 10 mcg/kg/day for at least 4 days before first leukapheresis and continued until last leukapheresis; Discontinue if WBC >100,000 cells/mm³.

Severe Chronic Neutropenia

SUBQ (Adults): *Congenital neutropenia:* 6 mcg/kg twice daily. *Idiopathic/cyclical neutropenia:* 5 mcg/kg daily (↓ if ANC remains >10,000/mm³).

After Myelosuppressive Radiation

SUBQ (Adults): 10 mcg/kg once daily; initiate as soon as possible after exposure to radiation doses greater than 2 gray (Gy); continue until ANC remains >1000/mm³ for 3 consecutive blood counts (performed every 3 days) or is >10,000/mm³ after a radiation-induced nadir.

Neonatal Neutropenia

IV, SUBQ (Neonates): 5–10 mcg/kg/day once daily for 3–5 days.

Availability

Solution for injection (prefilled syringes): 300 mcg/0.5 mL, 480 mcg/0.8 mL. **Solution for injection (vials):** 300 mcg/1 mL, 480 mcg/1.6 mL.

NURSING IMPLICATIONS

Assessment

- Monitor heart rate, BP, and respiratory status before and periodically during therapy.
- Assess bone pain during therapy. Pain is usually mild to moderate and controllable with nonopioid analgesics, but may require treatment with opioid analgesics, especially in patients receiving high-dose IV therapy. Loratadine 10 mg PO administered before filgrastim dose has been used to prevent bone pain.
- Monitor for signs and symptoms of allergic reactions (rash, urticaria, facial edema, wheezing, dyspnea, hypotension, tachycardia). Usually occur within 30 min of administration. Treatment includes antihistamines, steroids, bronchodilators, and/or epinephrine; may recur with rechallenge.
- Assess for signs and symptoms of acute respiratory distress syndrome (fever, lung infiltrates, or respiratory distress). If symptoms occur, withhold filgrastim until symptoms resolve or discontinue.
- Monitor for signs and symptoms of splenic enlargement or rupture (left upper abdominal or shoulder pain).
- May cause transient positive bone-imaging changes.

Lab Test Considerations

- *After chemotherapy,* obtain a CBC with differential, including examination for the presence of blast cells, and platelet count before chemotherapy and twice weekly during therapy to avoid leukocytosis. Monitor ANC. A transient rise is seen 1–2 days after initiation of therapy, but therapy should not be discontinued until ANC >10,000/mm³.
- *After bone marrow transplant,* the daily dose is titrated by the neutrophil response. When the ANC is >1000/mm³ for 3 consecutive days, reduce dose to 5 mcg/kg/day. If the ANC remains >1000/mm³ for 3 or more consecutive days, discontinue filgrastim. If the ANC decreases to <1000/mm³, resume filgrastim at 5 mcg/kg/day.
- *For chronic severe neutropenia,* monitor CBC with differential and platelet count twice weekly during initial 4 wk of therapy and during 2 wk after any dose adjustment.
- May cause ↓ platelet count and transient ↑ in uric acid, LDH, and alkaline phosphatase concentrations.
- May cause myelodysplastic syndrome and acute myeloid leukemia in patient with severe chronic neutropenia, breast, or lung cancer. Monitor for signs and symptoms (tiredness, fever, easy bruising or bleeding).

Implementation

- Administer no earlier than 24 hr after cytotoxic chemotherapy, at least 24 hr after bone marrow infusion, and not during the 24 hr before administration of chemotherapy.
- Refrigerate; do not freeze. Do not shake. Warm to room temperature for at least 30 min and up to 24 hr before injection. Discard if left at room temperature for >24 hr. Vial is for one-time use only.
- **SUBQ:** May be administered in outer area of upper arms, abdomen, thighs, or outer areas of buttock. If dose requires >1 mL of solution, may be divided into 2 injection sites.
- Cap of needle contains latex; avoid administration by persons with latex allergy.
- May also be administered as a continuous SUBQ infusion over 24 hr after bone marrow transplantation.

IV Administration

- Continuous Infusion: *Dilution:* Dilute in D5W; do not dilute with 0.9% NaCl, will precipitate. Refrigerate; do not freeze. Do not shake. May warm to room temperature for up to 4 hr (*Releuko*) or 24 hr (*Neupogen, Zarxio*) before injection. Vial is for one-time use only. *Concentration:* Dilute to a final concentration of at least 15 mcg/mL. If the final concentration is <15 mcg/mL, human albumin in a concentration of 2 mg/mL must be added to D5W before filgrastim to prevent adsorption of the components of the drug delivery system. May be stored

at room temperature for up to 4 hr (*Releuko*) or 24 hr (*Neupogen, Zarxio*). *Rate: After chemotherapy* dose is administered via infusion over 15–60 min.
- *After chemotherapy* dose may also be administered as a continuous infusion.
- *After bone marrow transplant,* administer dose as an infusion over 4 or 24 hr.
- **Y-Site Compatibility:** acyclovir, allopurinol, amikacin, aminophylline, ampicillin, ampicillin/sulbactam, aztreonam, bleomycin, bumetanide, buprenorphine, butorphanol, calcium gluconate, carboplatin, carmustine, cefazolin, cefotetan, ceftazidime, chlorpromazine, cisplatin, cyclophosphamide, cytarabine, dacarbazine, daunorubicin hydrochloride, dexamethasone, diphenhydramine, doxorubicin hydrochloride, doxycycline, droperidol, enalaprilat, famotidine, floxuridine, fluconazole, fludarabine, ganciclovir, granisetron, haloperidol, hydrocortisone, hydromorphone, idarubicin, ifosfamide, leucovorin calcium, levofloxacin, lorazepam, melphalan, meperidine, mesna, methotrexate, metoclopramide, mitoxantrone, morphine, nalbuphine, ondansetron, posaconazole, potassium chloride, promethazine, rituximab, sodium acetate, sodium bicarbonate, tobramycin, trastuzumab, trimethoprim/sulfamethoxazole, vancomycin, vinblastine, vincristine, vinorelbine, zidovudine.
- **Y-Site Incompatibility:** aminocaproic acid, cefepime, cefotaxime, cefoxitin, ceftaroline, ceftriaxone, cefuroxime, clindamycin, dactinomycin, etoposide, fluorouracil, furosemide, heparin, isavuconazonium, mannitol, methylprednisolone, metronidazole, mitomycin, prochlorperazine, thiotepa.

Patient/Family Teaching

- Explain purpose of filgrastim to patient. Instruct patient and caregiver on correct technique for injection, care and disposal of equipment. Advise patient to notify health care professional regarding when to give next dose if a dose is missed. Instruct patient and caregiver to read *Instructions for Patients and Caregivers* before starting therapy and with each Rx refill in case of changes.
- Instruct patient to notify health care professional immediately if signs and symptoms of spleen enlargement or rupture, allergic reaction, ARDS, glomerulonephritis (swelling of face or ankles, dark colored urine or blood in urine, decrease in urine production), MDS, AML, or vasculitis (skin redness, purple spots on skin) occur. Discuss risk of sickle cell crisis with patients with sickle cell disease before administering.
- Advise patient to notify health care professional of all Rx or OTC medications, vitamins, or herbal products being taken and to consult with health care professional before taking other medications.

- Rep: Advise females of reproductive potential to notify health care professional if pregnancy is planned or suspected or if breastfeeding.
- **Home Care Issues:** Instruct patient on correct technique and proper disposal for home administration. Caution patient not to reuse needle, vial, or syringe. Provide patient with a puncture-proof container for needle and syringe disposal.

Evaluation/Desired Outcomes

- Decreased incidence of infection in patients who receive bone marrow–depressing antineoplastics.
- Reduction of duration and sequelae of neutropenia after bone marrow transplantation.
- Reduction of the incidence and duration of sequelae of neutropenia in patients with severe chronic neutropenia.
- Improved harvest of progenitor cells for bone marrow transplantation.
- Improved survival in patients exposed to myelosuppressive doses of radiation.

finasteride (fi-nas-teer-ide)

Propecia, Proscar

Classification
Therapeutic: benign prostatic hyperplasia (BPH) agents, hair regrowth stimulants
Pharmacologic: androgen inhibitors

Indications

Benign prostatic hyperplasia (BPH); can be used with doxazosin. Androgenetic alopecia (male pattern baldness) in men only.

Action

Inhibits the enzyme 5-alpha-reductase, which is responsible for converting testosterone to its potent metabolite 5-alpha-dihydrotestosterone in prostate, liver, and skin; 5-alpha-dihydrotestosterone is partially responsible for prostatic hyperplasia and hair loss. **Therapeutic Effects:** Reduced prostate size with associated decrease in urinary symptoms. Decreases hair loss; promotes hair regrowth.

Pharmacokinetics

Absorption: Well absorbed after oral administration (63%).
Distribution: Enters prostatic tissue and crosses the blood-brain barrier. Remainder of distribution not known.
Protein Binding: 90%.
Metabolism and Excretion: Mostly metabolized; 39% excreted in urine as metabolites; 57% excreted in feces.
Half-life: 6 hr (range 6–15 hr; slightly ↑ in patients >70 yr).

TIME/ACTION PROFILE (↓ in dihydrotestosterone levels†)

ROUTE	ONSET	PEAK	DURATION
PO	rapid	8 hr	2 wk

†Clinical effects as noted by urinary tract symptoms and hair regrowth may not be evident for several mo and remain for 4 mo after discontinuation.

Contraindications/Precautions

Contraindicated in: Hypersensitivity.
Use Cautiously in: Hepatic impairment; Obstructive uropathy.

Adverse Reactions/Side Effects

Endo: gynecomastia. **GU:** ↓ libido, ↓ volume of ejaculate, erectile dysfunction, infertility, PROSTATE CANCER (HIGH-GRADE). **Misc:** ANGIOEDEMA, BREAST CANCER.

Interactions

Drug-Drug: None reported.

Route/Dosage

Benign Prostatic Hypertrophy
PO (Adults): *Proscar:* 5 mg once daily.

Androgenetic Alopecia
PO (Adults): *Propecia:* 1 mg once daily.

Availability (generic available)

Tablets (Proscar): 5 mg. **Tablets (Propecia):** 1 mg.
In combination with: tadalafil (Entadfi). See Appendix N.

NURSING IMPLICATIONS

Assessment

- Assess for symptoms of prostatic hyperplasia (urinary hesitancy, feeling of incomplete bladder emptying, interruption of urinary stream, impairment of size and force of urinary stream, terminal urinary dribbling, straining to start flow, dysuria, urgency) before and periodically during therapy.
- Digital rectal examinations should be performed before and periodically during therapy for BPH.

Lab Test Considerations
- Evaluate serum prostate-specific antigen (PSA) concentrations, which are used to screen for prostate cancer, before and periodically during therapy. Finasteride may cause a ↓ in serum PSA levels. Any confirmed increase from lowest PSA value while on *Propecia* may be a sign of prostate cancer and should be evaluated, even if PSA levels are within the normal range for men not taking a 5α-reductase inhibitor.

Implementation
- Do not confuse Proscar with Prograf or Provera.
- **PO:** Administer once daily with or without meals.

Patient/Family Teaching
- Instruct patient to take finasteride as directed, even if symptoms improve or are unchanged. At least 6–

12 mo of therapy may be necessary to determine whether or not an individual will respond to finasteride. If a dose is missed, omit and take next tablet at usual time. Advise patient to read the *Patient Package Insert* prior to starting therapy and with each Rx refill in case of changes.

- Inform patient that the volume of ejaculate may be decreased and erectile dysfunction and decreased libido may occur during therapy and after therapy is completed.
- Advise patient to notify health care professional promptly if changes in breasts (lumps, pain, nipple discharge) occur.
- Inform patient that there is an increased risk of high grade prostate cancer in men taking this drug.
- Rep: May cause fetal harm. Caution patient that finasteride poses a potential risk to a male fetus. Women who are pregnant or may become pregnant should avoid exposure to semen of a partner taking finasteride and should not handle crushed finasteride due to potential absorption.
- Emphasize the importance of periodic follow-up exams to determine whether a clinical response has occurred.

Evaluation/Desired Outcomes
- Decrease in urinary symptoms of benign prostatic hyperplasia.
- Hair regrowth in androgenetic alopecia. Evidence of hair growth usually requires 3 mo or longer. Continued use is recommended to sustain benefit. Withdrawal leads to reversal of effect within 12 mo.

---

finerenone (fin-er-e-none)
Kerendia
Classification
Therapeutic: none assigned
Pharmacologic: mineralocorticoid receptor antagonists (non-steroidal)

Indications
Chronic kidney disease (CKD) associated with type 2 diabetes.

Action
Acts as a nonsteroidal, selective antagonist of the mineralocorticoid receptor, which results in reduction in sodium reabsorption and a reduction in fibrosis and inflammation in the heart, blood vessels, and kidneys. **Therapeutic Effects:** Reduction in the risk of a sustained eGFR decline, end-stage kidney disease, cardiovascular death, nonfatal MI, and hospitalization for HF in CKD associated with type 2 diabetes.

Pharmacokinetics
Absorption: 44% absorbed following oral administration.

Distribution: Widely distributed to tissues.
Protein Binding: 92%.
Metabolism and Excretion: Primarily metabolized in the liver via the CYP3A4 isoenzyme, and to a lesser extent by the CYP2C8 isoenzyme to inactive metabolites. Primarily excreted in the urine (80%) as metabolites, with 20% being excreted in feces.
Half-life: 2–3 hr.

TIME/ACTION PROFILE (plasma concentrations)

ROUTE	ONSET	PEAK	DURATION
PO	rapid	30 min–1.25 hr	unknown

Contraindications/Precautions
Contraindicated in: Concurrent use of strong CYP3A4 inhibitors; Adrenal insufficiency; Hyperkalemia (serum potassium >5 mEq/L); eGFR <25 mL/min/m²; Severe hepatic impairment; Lactation: Lactation.
Use Cautiously in: Renal impairment (↑ risk of hyperkalemia) (adjust dose); Moderate hepatic impairment; OB: Safety not established in pregnancy; Pedi: Safety and effectiveness not established in children.

Adverse Reactions/Side Effects
CV: hypotension. **F and E:** <u>hyperkalemia</u>, hyponatremia.

Interactions
Drug-Drug: Strong CYP3A4 inhibitors may significantly ↑ levels and risk of hyperkalemia; concurrent use contraindicated. **Moderate CYP3A4 inhibitors**, including **erythromycin** or **weak CYP3A4 inhibitors**, including **amiodarone**, may ↑ levels and risk of hyperkalemia; closely monitor serum potassium levels after initiation of or after dosage adjustment of either the CYP3A4 inhibitor or finerenone. **Strong CYP3A4 inducers**, including **rifampin**, or **moderate CYP3A4 inducers**, including **efavirenz**, may ↓ levels and effectiveness; avoid concurrent use. Use with **ACE inhibitors, NSAIDs, potassium supplements, angiotensin II receptor antagonists, potassium-sparing diuretics, angiotensin converting enzyme inhibitors**, or **cyclosporine** ↑ risk of hyperkalemia.
Drug-Food: Grapefruit juice or **grapefruit** may ↑ levels and risk of hyperkalemia; avoid concomitant use.

Route/Dosage
PO (Adults): 20 mg once daily.

Renal Impairment
PO (Adults): *eGFR 25– <60 mL/min/m²:* 10 mg once daily; after 4 wk, may ↑ to 20 mg once daily if serum potassium ≤4.8 mEq/L.

Availability

Tablets: 10 mg, 20 mg.

NURSING IMPLICATIONS

Assessment

*   Monitor for signs and symptoms of hyperkalemia (fatigue, muscle weakness, paresthesia, confusion, dyspnea, cardiac arrhythmias) during therapy. If symptoms occur, confirm with serum potassium.

Lab Test Considerations

*   Measure serum potassium levels and eGFR before starting therapy. Do not start therapy if serum potassium is >5.0 mEq/L.
*   Measure serum potassium 4 wk after starting therapy and adjust dose. If serum potassium is ≤4.8 mEq/L, ↑ dose to 20 mg, if at 10 mg/day or maintain 20 mg/day dose. If serum potassium levels are >4.8 to 5.5 mEq/L, maintain current 10 mg/day or 20 mg/day dose. If serum potassium is >5.5 mEq/L, hold finerenone dose. If at 10 mg/day dose, consider restarting at 10 mg/day once serum potassium is ≤5.0 mEq/L. If at 20 mg/day dose, restart at 10 mg/day when serum potassium is ≤5.0 mEq/L. Monitor serum potassium 4 weeks after a dose adjustment and throughout treatment, and adjust the dose as needed.

Implementation

*   **PO:** For patients unable to swallow tablets whole, tablets may be crushed and mixed with water or soft foods (applesauce) immediately before use.

Patient/Family Teaching

*   Instruct patient to take finerenone as directed. Take missed dose as soon as remembered, but only on same day. Do not double doses.
*   Advise patients to consult with health care professional before using potassium supplements or salt substitutes containing potassium.
*   Caution patient to avoid grapefruit and grapefruit juice during therapy; may increase the plasma concentration of finerenone.
*   Advise patient to notify health care professional of all Rx or OTC medications, vitamins, or herbal products being taken and to consult with health care professional before taking other medications.
*   Rep: Advise females of reproductive potential to notify health care professional if pregnancy is planned or suspected and to avoid breastfeeding during and for 1 day after last dose.
*   Emphasize the importance of regular lab test to monitor potassium levels.

Evaluation/Desired Outcomes

*   Reduction of the risk of sustained eGFR decline, end-stage kidney disease, cardiovascular death, nonfatal MI, and hospitalization for HF in patients with CKD associated with type 2 diabetes.

fingolimod (fin-go-li-mod)

Gilenya, Tascenso ODT

Classification
Therapeutic: anti-multiple sclerosis agents
Pharmacologic: receptor modulators

Indications

Relapsing forms of multiple sclerosis (MS), including clinically isolated syndrome, relapsing-remitting disease, and active secondary progressive disease.

Action

Converted by sphingosine kinase to the active metabolite fingolimod-phosphate, which binds to sphingosine 1–phosphate receptors, resulting in ↓ migration of lymphocytes into peripheral blood. This may ↓ lymphocyte migration into the CNS. **Therapeutic Effects:** ↓ frequency of relapses/delayed accumulation of disability.

Pharmacokinetics

Absorption: Well absorbed (93%) following oral administration.

Distribution: Extensively distributed to body tissues; 86% of parent drug distributes into red blood cells; active metabolite uptake 17%.

Metabolism and Excretion: Converted to its active metabolite, then metabolized mostly by the CYP4F2 enzyme system, with further degradation by other enzymes). Most inactive metabolites excreted in urine (81%); <2.5% excreted as fingolimod and fingolimod-phosphate in feces.

Protein Binding: >99.7%.

Half-life: 6–9 days.

TIME/ACTION PROFILE

ROUTE	ONSET	PEAK	DURATION
PO	unknown	1–2 mo*	2 mo†

*Time to steady state plasma concentrations, peak plasma concentrations after a single dose at 12–16 hr.
†Time for complete elimination.

Contraindications/Precautions

Contraindicated in: Hypersensitivity; MI, unstable angina, stroke, transient ischemic attack, or class III or IV HF within previous 6 mo; 2nd- or 3rd-degree heart block or sick sinus syndrome (in the absence of a pacemaker); QT interval ≥500 msec; Cardiac arrhythmias requiring use of class Ia or III antiarrhythmics; Active acute/chronic untreated infections; OB: Pregnancy.

Use Cautiously in: Concurrent use of beta blockers, diltiazem, verapamil, or digoxin (↑ risk of bradycardia/heart block); History of ischemic heart disease, MI, HF, cerebrovascular disease, uncontrolled hypertension, AV or SA heart block, symptomatic bradycardia, recurrent syncope, cardiac arrest, or severe untreated sleep apnea (↑ risk of bradycardia/heart block); QT interval prolongation before doing or during observation period (>450 msec in adult and pediatric males, >470 msec in adult females, >460 msec in pediatric females), hypokalemia, hypomagnesemia, congenital long QT syndrome, or concurrent use of QT interval prolonging medications (↑ risk of QT interval prolongation); Severe hepatic impairment (↑ blood levels and risk of adverse reactions); Diabetes mellitus/history of uveitis (↑ risk of macular edema); Negative history for chickenpox or vaccination against varicella zoster virus (VZV) vaccination; Lactation: Use while breastfeeding only if potential maternal benefit justifies potential risk to infant; Rep: Women of reproductive potential; Pedi: Children <10 yr (safety and effectiveness not established); Geri: Risk of adverse reactions may be ↑ in older adults; consider age-related ↓ in cardiac/renal/hepatic function, chronic illnesses, and concurrent drug therapy.

Adverse Reactions/Side Effects

CV: ASYSTOLE, BRADYCARDIA, HEART BLOCK, QT interval prolongation, hypertension, syncope. **Derm:** BASAL/SQUAMOUS CELL CARCINOMA, MELANOMA. **EENT:** blurred vision, eye pain, macular edema. **GI:** ↑ liver enzymes, diarrhea, HEPATOTOXICITY. **Hemat:** leukopenia, lymphopenia. **MS:** back pain. **Neuro:** headache, POSTERIOR REVERSIBLE ENCEPHALOPATHY SYNDROME (PRES), PROGRESSIVE MULTIFOCAL LEUKOENCEPHALOPATHY (PML), tumefactive MS. **Resp:** cough, ↓ pulmonary function. **Misc:** HYPERSENSITIVITY REACTIONS (including angioedema), IMMUNE RECONSTITUTION INFLAMMATORY SYNDROME (IRIS), INFECTION (including bacterial, viral and fungal), LYMPHOMA.

Interactions

Drug-Drug: Class Ia or class III antiarrhythmics may ↑ risk of serious arrhythmias; concurrent use contraindicated. Concurrent use of **beta blockers, diltiazem, verapamil, ivabradine, clonidine,** or **digoxin** may ↑ risk of bradycardia; careful monitoring recommended. Concurrent use of **QT-interval prolonging medications** may ↑ risk of QT interval prolongation and torsades de pointes. Concurrent use of **ketoconazole** may ↑ blood levels and risk of adverse reactions. ↑ risk of immunosuppression with **antineoplastics, immunosuppressants,** or **immune modulating therapies. Live-attenuated vaccines** ↑ risk of infection.

Route/Dosage

PO (Adults and Children ≥10 yr and >40 kg): 0.5 mg once daily.
PO (Children ≥10 yr and ≤40 kg): 0.25 mg once daily.

Availability (generic available)

Capsules: 0.25 mg, 0.5 mg. **Orally disintegrating tablets:** 0.25 mg, 0.5 mg.

NURSING IMPLICATIONS

Assessment

● Perform *first-dose monitoring* in all patients when starting therapy, when restarting therapy after drug was discontinued for ≥ 14 days, when therapy is interrupted ≥1 day within first 2 wk of therapy; when therapy is interrupted for >7 days during wk 3 and 4 of therapy, and in pediatric patients when increasing dose.
● *First dose monitoring:* Monitor pulse and BP hourly for bradycardia for at least 6 hr following first dose and periodically during therapy. Obtain baseline ECG before first dose and at end of observation period. *If after 6 hr of therapy* patient develops heart rate <45 bpm in adults, <55 bpm in pediatric patients ≥12 yr, or <60 bpm in pediatric patients 10 or 11 yr of age; heart rate 6 hr postdose is at lowest value postdose, maximum pharmacodynamic effect on the heart may not have occurred; ECG 6 hr postdose shows new onset second degree or higher AV block, continue monitoring until resolves. If pharmacological treatment is required, continue monitoring overnight and repeat 6-hr monitoring after the second dose. Monitor ECG continuously overnight if pharmacologic intervention for symptomatic bradycardia required, patient has preexisting heart or cerebrovascular condition, patient has a prolonged QTc interval before dosing or during 6-hr observation, or at risk for QT prolongation, or on concurrent therapy with QT prolonging drugs.
● Monitor for signs of infection (fever, tiredness, body aches, chills, nausea, vomiting, headache, sore throat) during and for 2 mo after discontinuation of therapy. Consider suspending therapy if serious infection develops.
● Perform an ophthalmologic exam prior to starting fingolimod, at 3–4 mo after starting therapy, and if visual disturbances occur. Monitor visual acuity at baseline and during routine exams. Patients with diabetes or history of uveitis are at ↑ risk and should have regular ophthalmologic exams.
● Monitor pulmonary function tests for decline periodically during therapy. Obtain spirometry and diffusion lung capacity for carbon monoxide when indicated clinically.
● Assess for any new signs or symptoms that may be suggestive of PML, an opportunistic infection of the brain caused by the Jakob Cruzfeldt virus, that may be fatal; hold dose and notify health care professional promptly. PML symptoms may begin gradually (hemiparesis, apathy, confusion, cognitive deficiencies, and ataxia) and may include deteriorating renal function. Monitoring MRI every 6 mo may identify PML before clinical signs and symptoms occur. Discontinue therapy if PML is confirmed.
● Monitor for development of IRIS. Signs include clinical decline in patient's condition that may be rapid,

can lead to serious neurological complications or death, and is often associated with characteristic changes on MRI. The time to onset of IRIS in patients with PML was generally within a few months after receptor modulator discontinuation.

- May cause severe increase in disability upon discontinuation of therapy. Monitor patients for increase in disability 12–24 wk following discontinuation.

Lab Test Considerations
- Verify negative pregnancy test before starting therapy.
- Obtain baseline AST, ALT, and total bilirubin levels before starting, periodically during, and for 2 mo after therapy discontinued. If patient has symptoms of liver injury and ALT >3 × upper limit of normal (ULN) and total bilirubin >2 × ULN, hold therapy until cause is determined. If cause is fingolimod, permanently discontinue therapy. Monitor liver function tests if symptoms develop and discontinue therapy if liver injury is confirmed.
- Before initiating therapy, obtain a recent (within 6 mo) CBC. May cause ↓ lymphocyte counts.
- Test patients for antibodies to varicella zoster virus (VZV) before starting therapy.
- May cause decreased lymphocyte count for up to 2 mo following discontinuation.

Implementation
- Administer VZV vaccine to patients who are antibody negative before starting therapy. Complete all immunizations, including human papilloma virus, in accordance with current immunization guidelines for pediatric patients before starting therapy. Cancer screening, including Papanicolaou (Pap) test, is recommended before starting therapy.
- **PO:** Administer once daily without regard to food.
- For ODT tablet: open blister pack with dry hands. Peel back foil covering of one blister and gently remove orally disintegrating tablet (ODT). Do not push ODT through the foil. Remove the ODT and place on the tongue and allow it to dissolve before swallowing. The ODT may be taken with or without water. Take the ODT immediately after opening blister pack. Do not store the ODT outside the blister pack for future use.

Patient/Family Teaching
- Instruct patient to take fingolimod as directed. If a dose is missed, contact health care professional before taking next dose; may need to be observed by a health care professional for at least 6 hrs after taking next dose. Do not discontinue therapy without consulting health care professional, may cause severe increase in disability. Advise patient to read the *Medication Guide* prior to starting therapy and with each Rx refill in case of changes.
- Advise patient to notify health care professional if signs and symptoms of liver dysfunction (unexplained nausea, vomiting, abdominal pain, fatigue, anorexia, jaundice, dark urine), infection, PML, new

onset of dyspnea, PRES (sudden headache, confusion, seizures, loss of vision, weakness), hypersensitivity reactions (rash or itchy hives, swelling of lips, tongue, or face), skin nodules (shiny pearly nodules), patches or open sores that do not heal within weeks, or changes in vision develop.

- Instruct patient not to receive live-attenuated vaccines during and for 2 mo after treatment due to risk of infection. Patients who have not had a health care professional confirmed history of chickenpox or documentation of a full course vaccination should be tested for antibodies to VZV virus before starting therapy. Antibody-negative patients should receive vaccination prior to starting therapy, then postpone start of fingolimod for 1 mo to allow for full effect of vaccination.
- Advise patient to notify health care professional of all Rx or OTC medications, vitamins, or herbal products being taken and to consult with health care professional before taking other medications.
- May cause basal cell carcinoma, melanoma, and lymphoma. Caution patient to use sunscreen with a high protection factor, wear protective clothing, and limit exposure to sunlight and ultraviolet light.
- Rep: May cause fetal harm. Advise female patients to use contraception during and for at least 2 mo after discontinuation of therapy and to notify health care professional immediately if pregnancy is planned or suspected or if breastfeeding. Inform pregnant patients of pregnancy exposure registry that monitors pregnancy outcomes in women exposed to fingolimod during pregnancy. To enroll patient in the pregnancy registry, call 1-877-598-7237 or visit www.gilenyapregnancyregistry.com.

Evaluation/Desired Outcomes
- Reduction in frequency of clinical exacerbations and delay of accumulation of physical disability in patients with relapsing forms of MS.

REMS

✕ flibanserin (flib-an-ser-in)
Addyi
Classification
Therapeutic: sexual dysfunction agents

Indications
Treatment of premenopausal women with hypoactive sexual desire disorder unrelated to concurrent medical/psychiatric diagnoses, relationship issues, or substance abuse (does not enhance sexual performance).

Action
May be explained by agonist activity at $5-HT_{1A}$ receptors and antagonist activity at $5-HT_{2A}$ receptors; also has moderate antagonist activity at $5-HT_{2B}$, $5-HT_{2C}$, and dopamine D_4 receptors. **Therapeutic Effects:** ↑ sexual desire with ↓ distress and interpersonal dysfunction.

Pharmacokinetics

Absorption: Moderately absorbed (33%) following oral administration.

Distribution: Unknown.

Protein Binding: 98%.

Metabolism and Excretion: Primarily metabolized in the liver, via the CYP3A4 isoenzyme, and to a lesser extent by the CYP2C19 isoenzyme; ⊠ the CYP2C19 isoenzyme exhibits genetic polymorphism; poor metabolizers may have significantly ↑ flibanserin concentrations and an ↑ risk of adverse effects. 44% excreted in urine, 51% in feces almost entirely as metabolites, which do not appear to be pharmacologically active.

Half-life: 11 hr.

TIME/ACTION PROFILE (plasma concentrations)

ROUTE	ONSET	PEAK	DURATION
PO	within 1 hr	1 hr	24 hr

Contraindications/Precautions

Contraindicated in: Hypersensitivity; Concurrent use of strong/moderate CYP3A4 inhibitors; Hepatic impairment; Lactation: Lactation.

Use Cautiously in: Alcohol ingestion within 2 hr of flibanserin dose (excess risk of hypotension/syncope); ⊠ CYP2C19 poor metabolizers (↑ risk of adverse reactions including hypotension, syncope, and drowsiness); OB: Safety not established in pregnancy.

Adverse Reactions/Side Effects

CV: HYPOTENSION/SYNCOPE. **Derm:** rash. **GI:** nausea, constipation, dry mouth. **Neuro:** dizziness, drowsiness, anxiety, fatigue, insomnia, vertigo. **Misc:** HYPERSENSITIVITY REACTIONS (including anaphylaxis and angioedema).

Interactions

Drug-Drug: Concurrent use of **strong or moderate CYP3A4 inhibitors**, including **atazanavir**, **ciprofloxacin**, **clarithromycin**, **conivaptan**, **diltiazem**, **erythromycin**, **fluconazole**, **fosamprenavir**, **itraconazole**, **ketoconazole**, **nelfinavir**, **posaconazole**, **ritonavir**, and **verapamil**, significantly ↑ levels and the risk of toxicity; concurrent use contraindicated. Wait 2 wk after discontinuing inhibitor before initiating flibanserin. If initiating inhibitor, wait two days after last dose of flibanserin. Concurrent use with **alcohol** ↑ risk of hypotension/syncope and excess sedation; wait ≥2 hr after consuming 1–2 standard alcoholic drinks before taking dose at bedtime; skip bedtime dose if consumed ≥3 standard alcoholic drinks. Concurrent use of **oral hormonal contraceptives** and **weak CYP3A4 inhibitors** including **cimetidine** and **fluoxetine** may ↑ levels and the risk of toxicity; avoid concurrent use with multiple weak CYP3A4 inhibitors. **Strong**

CYP2C19 inhibitors, including **proton pump inhibitors**, **SSRIs**, **benzodiazepines**, and **antifungals**, ↑ levels and the risk of toxicity; concurrent use should be undertaken with caution. **CYP3A4 inducers**, including **carbamazepine**, **phenobarbital**, **phenytoin**, **rifabutin**, **rifampin**, and **rifapentine**, ↓ levels and effectiveness; concurrent use not recommended. ↑ **digoxin** and **sirolimus** levels and the risk of toxicity; careful monitoring recommended. ↑ risk of CNS depression with other **CNS depressants**, including **alcohol**, **antihistamines**, **opioids**, **sedative/hypnotics**, some **anti-anxiety agents**, **antidepressants**, and **antipsychotics**.

Natural-Natural: Concurrent use with **gingko** may ↑ levels and the risk of toxicity; avoid use with other weak CYP3A4 inhibitors. **St. John's wort** ↓ levels and effectiveness; concurrent use not recommended.

Drug-Food: Grapefruit juice ↑ levels and the risk of toxicity; concurrent ingestion contraindicated.

Route/Dosage

PO (Adults): 100 mg once daily at bedtime.

Availability

Tablets: 100 mg.

NURSING IMPLICATIONS

Assessment

- Assess sexual desire and related distress and interpersonal dysfunction before and periodically during therapy.
- Monitor for hypotension and syncope. Have patient lie supine if dizziness occurs.
- Assess likelihood of patient following alcohol restrictions, taking into account the patient's current and past drinking behavior, and other pertinent social and medical history. Counsel patients who are prescribed flibanserin about the importance of following guidelines for alcohol use; interaction with alcohol increases risk of hypotension and syncope.

Implementation

- Administer once daily at bedtime; administration during waking hr increases risks of hypotension, syncope, accidental injury, and CNS depression.

Patient/Family Teaching

- Instruct patient to take flibanserin only at bedtime as directed. If dose is missed, omit and take next dose at bedtime on next day. Advise patient to read *Medication Guide* before starting therapy and with each Rx refill in case of changes.
- Advise patient to avoid grapefruit juice during therapy.
- Caution patient to follow alcohol guidelines during therapy. Wait at least 2 hr after drinking 1 or 2 standard alcoholic drinks (one 12-oz regular beer; 5 oz of wine; 1.5 oz or a shot of brandy, gin, rum, tequila,

vodka, or whiskey) before taking flibanserin at bedtime. If you drink 3 or more standard alcoholic drinks in the evening, skip your flibanserin dose at bedtime. After you have taken your flibanserin at bedtime do not drink alcohol until the following day. Alcohol increases hypotensive effects. May cause dizziness and fainting.

- Advise patient if dizziness occurs, immediately lie supine and promptly seek medical help if symptoms do not resolve.
- May cause drowsiness. Caution patient to avoid driving and other activities requiring alertness until 6 hr after each dose or until response to medication is known.
- Advise patient to stop taking flibanserin and notify health care professional immediately if signs and symptoms of hypersensitivity reaction (swelling of the face, lips, and mouth; pruritus; urticaria) occur.
- Instruct patient to notify health care professional of all Rx or OTC medications, vitamins, or herbal products being taken and consult health care professional before taking any new medications, especially St. John's wort.
- Rep: Advise females of reproductive potential to notify health care professional if pregnancy is planned or suspected or if breastfeeding.

Evaluation/Desired Outcomes
- Increase in sexual desire in premenopausal women. If no improvement in 8 wk, discontinue flibanserin.

---

fluconazole (floo-kon-a-zole)
Diflucan
Classification
Therapeutic: antifungals (systemic)

Indications
PO, IV: Fungal infections caused by susceptible organisms, including: Oropharyngeal or esophageal candidiasis, Serious systemic candidal infections, Urinary tract infections, Peritonitis, Cryptococcal meningitis. Prevention of candidiasis in patients who have undergone bone marrow transplantation. **PO:** Single-dose oral treatment of vaginal candidiasis. **Unlabeled Use:** Prevention of recurrent vaginal yeast infections.

Action
Inhibits synthesis of fungal sterols, a necessary component of the cell membrane. **Therapeutic Effects:** Fungistatic action against susceptible organisms. May be fungicidal in higher concentrations. **Spectrum:** *Cryptococcus neoformans. Candida* spp.

Pharmacokinetics
Absorption: Well absorbed after oral administration.
Distribution: Widely distributed, good penetration into CSF, saliva, sputum, vaginal fluid, skin, eye, and peritoneum.
Metabolism and Excretion: >80% excreted unchanged by the kidneys; <10% metabolized by the liver.

Half-life: *Premature neonates:* 46–74 hr; *Children:* 19–25 hr (PO) and 15–17 hr (IV); *Adults:* 30 hr (↑ in renal impairment).

TIME/ACTION PROFILE (plasma concentrations)

ROUTE	ONSET	PEAK	DURATION
PO	unknown	2–4 hr	24 hr
IV	rapid	end of infusion	24 hr

Contraindications/Precautions
Contraindicated in: Hypersensitivity to fluconazole or other azole antifungals; Concurrent use with pimozide, erythromycin, or quinidine; OB: Pregnancy; may consider using for severe or life-threatening fungal infection if anticipated maternal benefit justifies potential fetal risk.

Use Cautiously in: Renal impairment (dose ↓ required if CCr <50 mL/min); Underlying liver disease; Structural heart disease, electrolyte abnormalities, or concurrent use of other QT interval-prolonging medications; Geri: ↑ risk of adverse reactions in older adults; consider age-related ↓ in renal function in determining dose.

Adverse Reactions/Side Effects
CV: QT interval prolongation, TORSADES DE POINTES. **Derm:** STEVENS-JOHNSON SYNDROME. **Endo:** adrenal insufficiency, hypertriglyceridemia, hypokalemia. **GI:** abdominal discomfort, diarrhea, HEPATOTOXICITY, nausea, vomiting. **Neuro:** dizziness, headache, seizures. **Misc:** HYPERSENSITIVITY REACTIONS (including anaphylaxis).

Interactions
Drug-Drug: May ↑ levels of **pimozide, erythromycin,** and **quinidine** which can prolong the QT interval and ↑ the risk of torsades de pointes; concurrent use contraindicated. May ↑ levels of **amiodarone** (especially with high-dose fluconazole [800 mg]), which can cause QT interval prolongation. May ↑ levels of and the risk of bleeding with **warfarin. Rifampin, rifabutin,** and **isoniazid** ↓ levels. ↑ hypoglycemic effects of **glyburide,** or **glipizide.** ↑ levels and risk of toxicity from **cyclosporine, carbamazepine, celecoxib, rifabutin, tacrolimus, sirolimus, theophylline, zidovudine,** and **phenytoin.** ↑ levels and effects of **benzodiazepines, amlodipine, felodipine, isradipine, nifedipine, nisoldipine, verapamil, atorvastatin, fluvastatin, lovastatin, simvastatin, methadone, flurbiprofen, prednisone, tricyclic antidepressants,** and **losartan.** ↑ levels of **tofacitinib;** ↓ tofacitinib dose to 5 mg once daily. May ↑ levels and risk of toxicity of **ivacaftor;** ↓ ivacaftor dose. May ↑ levels and risk of toxicity of **lurasidone;** ↓ lurasidone dose. May ↑ risk of bleeding with **warfarin.** May antagonize effects of **amphotericin B.** May ↑ levels and risk of toxicity of **abrocitinib, lemborexant,** and **voriconazole;** avoid concurrent use. May ↑ **olaparib** levels; concurrent use not recommended. May ↑ levels and

risk of toxicity of **ibrutinib**; ↓ ibrutinib dose. May ↑ levels and risk of toxicity of **tolvaptan**; ↓ tolvaptan dose. May ↑ levels and risk of toxicity of **ivacaftor**; ↓ ivacaftor dose. May ↑ levels and risk of toxicity of **lurasidone**; ↓ lurasidone dose.

Route/Dosage
Oropharyngeal Candidiasis
PO, IV (Adults): 200 mg initially, then 100 mg daily for at least 2 wk.
PO, IV (Children >14 days): 6 mg/kg initially, then 3 mg/kg/day for at least 2 wk.
PO, IV (Neonates <14 days, 30–36 wk gestation): same dose as older children except frequency is every 48 hr; Premature neonates <29 wk gestation: 5–6 mg/kg/dose every 48–72 hr.

Renal Impairment
PO, IV (Adults): *CCr ≤50 mL/min (no hemodialysis):* Give 50% of the usual dose; *Hemodialysis:* Give 100% of the usual dose after each dialysis session; give reduced dose based on CCr on non-dialysis days.

Esophageal Candidiasis
PO, IV (Adults): 200 mg initially, then 100 mg once daily for at least 3 wk (up to 400 mg/day).
PO, IV (Children >14 days): 6 mg/kg initially, then 3–12 mg/kg/day for at least 3 wk.
PO, IV (Neonates <14 days, 30–36 wk gestation): same dose as older children except frequency is every 48 hr; Premature neonates <29 wk gestation: 5–6 mg/kg/dose every 48–72 hr.

Renal Impairment
PO, IV (Adults): *CCr ≤50 mL/min (no hemodialysis):* Give 50% of the usual dose; *Hemodialysis:* Give 100% of the usual dose after each dialysis session; give reduced dose based on CCr on non-dialysis days.

Vaginal Candidiasis
PO (Adults): 150-mg single dose; prevention of recurrence (unlabeled)—150 mg daily for 3 days then weekly for 6 mo.

Systemic Candidiasis
PO, IV (Adults): 400 mg/day initially, then 200–800 mg/day for 28 days.
PO, IV (Children >14 days): 6–12 mg/kg/day for 28 days.
PO, IV (Neonates <14 days, 30–36 wk gestation): same dose as older children except frequency is every 48 hr; Premature neonates <29 wk gestation: 5–6 mg/kg/dose every 48–72 hr.

Renal Impairment
PO, IV (Adults): *CCr ≤50 mL/min (no hemodialysis):* Give 50% of the usual dose; *Hemodialysis:* Give 100% of the usual dose after each dialysis session; give reduced dose based on CCr on non-dialysis days.

Cryptococcal Meningitis
PO, IV (Adults): *Treatment:* 400 mg once daily until favorable clinical response, then 200–800 mg once daily for at least 10–12 wk after clearing of CSF; change to oral therapy as soon as possible. *Suppressive therapy:* 200 mg once daily.
PO, IV (Children >14 days): 12 mg/kg/day initially, then 6–12 mg/kg/day for at least 10–12 wk after clearing of CSF; change to oral therapy as soon as possible. *Suppressive therapy:* 6 mg/kg/day.
PO, IV (Neonates <14 days, 30–36 wk gestation): same dose as older children except frequency is every 48 hr; Premature neonates <29 wk gestation: 5–6 mg/kg/dose every 48–72 hr.

Renal Impairment
PO, IV (Adults): *CCr ≤50 mL/min (no hemodialysis):* Give 50% of the usual dose; *Hemodialysis:* Give 100% of the usual dose after each dialysis session; give reduced dose based on CCr on non-dialysis days.

Prevention of Candidiasis after Bone Marrow Transplant
PO, IV (Adults): 400 mg once daily; begin several days before procedure if severe neutropenia is expected, and continue for 7 days after ANC >1000 /mm³.
PO, IV (Children >14 days): 10–12 mg/kg/day, not to exceed 600 mg/day.

Renal Impairment
PO, IV (Adults): *CCr ≤50 mL/min (no hemodialysis):* Give 50% of the usual dose; *Hemodialysis:* Give 100% of the usual dose after each dialysis session; give reduced dose based on CCr on non-dialysis days.

Availability (generic available)
Tablets: 50 mg, 100 mg, 150 mg, 200 mg. **Powder for oral suspension (orange flavor):** 10 mg/mL, 40 mg/mL. **Premixed infusion:** 200 mg/100 mL 0.9% NaCl, 400 mg/200 mL 0.9% NaCl.

NURSING IMPLICATIONS
Assessment
- Assess infected area and monitor CSF cultures before and periodically during therapy.
- Obtain specimens for culture before instituting therapy. Therapy may be started before results are obtained.
- Assess patient for rash (mild to moderate rash usually occurs in the 2nd wk of therapy and resolves within 1–2 wk of continued therapy). If rash is severe (extensive erythematous or maculopapular rash with moist desquamation or angioedema), accompanied by systemic symptoms (serum sickness-like reaction, Stevens-Johnson syndrome, toxic epidermal necrolysis), or occurs during treatment for a su-

perficial fungal infection, therapy must be discontinued immediately.

Lab Test Considerations

● Monitor BUN and serum creatinine before and periodically during therapy; patients with renal dysfunction will require dose adjustment.

● Monitor liver function tests before and periodically during therapy. May cause ↑ AST, ALT, serum alkaline phosphate, and bilirubin concentrations.

Implementation

● Do not confuse Diflucan with Diprivan.

● **PO:** Administer at the same time each day. Shake oral suspension well before administration.

IV Administration

● **Intermittent Infusion: *Dilution:*** Premixed infusions are prediluted and ready to use. Do not unwrap until ready to use. Some opacity of the plastic is normal and does not affect the solution quality or safety; opacity will diminish gradually. Do not administer solution that is cloudy or has a precipitate. Check for leaks by squeezing inner bag. If leaks are found, discard container as unsterile. ***Concentration:*** 2 mg/mL. ***Rate:*** Infuse over 1–2 hr. Do not exceed a rate of 200 mg/hr. Pedi: For children receiving doses >6 mg/kg/day, give over 2 hr.

● **Y-Site Compatibility:** acyclovir, aldesleukin, alemtuzumab, allopurinol, amifostine, amikacin, aminocaproic acid, aminophylline, amiodarone, anidulafungin, argatroban, arsenic trioxide, ascorbic acid, atracurium, atropine, azathioprine, azithromycin, aztreonam, benztropine, bivalirudin, bleomycin, bumetanide, buprenorphine, butorphanol, calcium chloride, cangrelor, carboplatin, carmustine, caspofungin, cefazolin, cefepime, cefotetan, cefoxitin, ceftaroline, chlorpromazine, cisatracurium, cisplatin, cyanocobalamin, cyclophosphamide, cyclosporine, cytarabine, dacarbazine, dactinomycin, daptomycin, daunorubicin hydrochloride, defibrotide, dexamethasone, dexmedetomidine, dexrazoxane, diltiazem, diphenhydramine, dobutamine, docetaxel, dopamine, doxorubicin hydrochloride, doxorubicin liposomal, doxycycline, droperidol, enalaprilat, ephedrine, epinephrine, epirubicin, epoetin alfa, eptifibatide, eravacycline, ertapenem, erythromycin, esmolol, etoposide, etoposide phosphate, famotidine, fentanyl, filgrastim, fludarabine, fluorouracil, folic acid, foscarnet, fosphenytoin, ganciclovir, gemcitabine, gentamicin, glycopyrrolate, granisetron, heparin, hetastarch, hydrocortisone, hydromorphone, idarubicin, ifosfamide, immune globulin, indomethacin, insulin, regular, irinotecan, isoproterenol, ketorolac, labetalol, LR, leucovorin calcium, levofloxacin, lidocaine, linezolid, lorazepam, magnesium sulfate, mannitol, melphalan, meperidine, meropenem, mesna, methadone, methotrexate, methylprednisolone, metoclopramide, metoprolol, metronidazole, midazolam, milrinone, mitomycin, mitoxantrone, morphine, multivitamins, mycophenolate, nafcillin, nalbuphine, naloxone, nicardipine, nitroglycerin, nitroprusside, norepinephrine, octreotide, ondansetron, oritavancin, oxacillin, oxaliplatin, oxytocin, paclitaxel, palonosetron, pamidronate, papaverine, pemetrexed, penicillin G, pentobarbital, phenobarbital, phentolamine, phenylephrine, phytonadione, piperacillin/tazobactam, plazomicin, potassium acetate, potassium chloride, procainamide, prochlorperazine, promethazine, propofol, propranolol, protamine, pyridoxine, remifentanil, rituximab, rocuronium, sargramostim, sodium acetate, sodium bicarbonate, succinylcholine, sufentanil, tacrolimus, telavancin, theophylline, thiotepa, tigecycline, tirofiban, tobramycin, topotecan, trastuzumab, vancomycin, vasopressin, vecuronium, verapamil, vinblastine, vincristine, vinorelbine, voriconazole, zidovudine, zoledronic acid.

● **Y-Site Incompatibility:** amphotericin B deoxycholate, amphotericin B lipid complex, ampicillin, dantrolene, diazepam, gemtuzumab ozogamicin, pantoprazole, trimethoprim/sulfamethoxazole.

Patient/Family Teaching

● Instruct patient to take medication as directed, at the same time each day, even if feeling better. Take missed doses as soon as remembered, but not if almost time for next dose. Do not double doses.

● May cause dizziness or seizures. Caution patient to avoid driving and other activities requiring alertness until response to fluconazole is known.

● Instruct patient to notify health care professional if skin rash, abdominal pain, fever, or diarrhea becomes pronounced, if signs and symptoms of liver dysfunction (unusual fatigue, anorexia, nausea, vomiting, jaundice, dark urine, or pale stools) occur, if unusual bruising or bleeding occur, or if no improvement is seen within a few days of therapy.

● Rep: May cause fetal harm. Advise females of reproductive potential to use effective contraception during and for 1 wk after last dose and to avoid breastfeeding during therapy. Advise patient to notify health care professional if pregnancy is planned or suspected or if breastfeeding.

Evaluation/Desired Outcomes

● Resolution of clinical and laboratory indications of fungal infections. Full course of therapy may require wk or mo of treatment after resolution of symptoms.

● Prevention of candidiasis in patients who have undergone bone marrow transplantation.

● Decrease in skin irritation and vaginal discomfort in patients with vaginal candidiasis. Diagnosis should be reconfirmed with smears or cultures before a second course of therapy to rule out other pathogens associated with vulvovaginitis. Recurrent vaginal infections may be a sign of systemic illness.

fluddrocortisone
(floo-droe-**kor**-ti-sone)
✤ Florinef
Classification
Therapeutic: hormones
Pharmacologic: corticosteroids (mineralocorticoid)

Indications
Sodium loss and hypotension associated with adrenocortical insufficiency (in combination with hydrocortisone or cortisone). Sodium loss due to congenital adrenogenital syndrome (congenital adrenal hyperplasia). **Unlabeled Use:** Idiopathic orthostatic hypotension (with increased sodium intake). Type IV renal tubular acidosis.

Action
Causes sodium reabsorption, hydrogen and potassium excretion, and water retention by its effects on the distal renal tubule. **Therapeutic Effects:** Maintenance of sodium balance and BP in patients with adrenocortical insufficiency.

Pharmacokinetics
Absorption: Well absorbed following oral administration.
Distribution: Widely distributed to tissues.
Metabolism and Excretion: Mostly metabolized by the liver.
Half-life: 3.5 hr.

TIME/ACTION PROFILE (mineralocorticoid activity)

ROUTE	ONSET	PEAK	DURATION
PO	unknown	unknown	1–2 days

Contraindications/Precautions
Contraindicated in: Hypersensitivity.
Use Cautiously in: HF; Addison's disease (patients may have exaggerated response); OB: Safety not established in pregnancy; Lactation: Safety not established in breastfeeding; Pedi: Safety and effectiveness not established in children.

Adverse Reactions/Side Effects
CV: arrhythmias, edema, HF, hypertension. **Endo:** adrenal suppression. **F and E:** hypokalemia, hypokalemic alkalosis. **GI:** anorexia, nausea. **Metab:** weight gain. **MS:** arthralgia, muscular weakness, tendon contractures. **Neuro:** ascending paralysis, dizziness, headache. **Misc:** hypersensitivity reactions.

Interactions
Drug-Drug: Use with **thiazide diuretics**, **loop diuretics**, **piperacillin**, or **amphotericin B** may ↑ risk of hypokalemia. Hypokalemia may ↑ risk of **digoxin**

toxicity. May produce prolonged neuromuscular blockade following the use of **nondepolarizing neuromuscular blocking agents**. **Phenobarbital** or **rifampin** may ↑ metabolism and ↓ effectiveness.
Drug-Food: Large amounts of **salt** or **sodium-containing foods** may cause excessive sodium retention and potassium loss.

Route/Dosage
PO (Adults): *Adrenocortical insufficiency:* 0.1 mg/day (range 0.1 mg 3 times weekly—0.2 mg daily). Doses as small as 0.05 mg daily may be required by some patients. Use with 10–37.5 mg cortisone daily or 10–30 mg hydrocortisone daily. *Adrenogenital syndrome:* 0.1–0.2 mg/day. *Idiopathic hypotension:* 0.05–0.2 mg/day (unlabeled).
PO (Children): 0.05–0.1 mg/day.

Availability (generic available)
Tablets: 0.1 mg.

NURSING IMPLICATIONS

Assessment
- Monitor BP periodically during therapy. Report significant changes. Hypotension may indicate insufficient dose.
- Monitor for fluid retention (weigh daily, assess for edema, and auscultate lungs for rales/crackles).
- Monitor patients with Addison's disease closely and stop treatment if a significant increase in weight or BP, edema, or cardiac enlargement occurs. Patients with Addison's disease are more sensitive to the action of fludrocortisone and may have an exaggerated response.

Lab Test Considerations
- Monitor serum electrolytes periodically during therapy. Fludrocortisone causes ↓ serum potassium levels.

Implementation
- **PO:** Administer without regard to food; take with food if GI upset occurs. Tablets are scored and may be broken if dose adjustment is necessary. May require higher doses when subject to stress.

Patient/Family Teaching
- Instruct patient to take medication as directed. Take missed doses as soon as remembered but not just before next dose is due. Explain that lifelong therapy may be necessary and that abrupt discontinuation may lead to Addisonian crisis. Patient should keep an adequate supply available at all times. Discontinue gradually if needed.
- Advise patient to follow dietary modification prescribed by health care professional. Instruct patient to follow a diet high in potassium (see Appendix J). Amount of sodium allowed in diet varies with pathophysiology.

- Instruct patient to inform health care professional if weight gain or edema, muscle weakness, cramps, nausea, anorexia, or dizziness occurs.
- Rep: Advise females of reproductive potential to notify health care professional if pregnancy is planned or suspected, or if breastfeeding. Monitor newborns of patients taking fludrocortisone during pregnancy for hypoadrenalism.
- Advise patient to carry identification at all times describing disease process and medication regimen.

Evaluation/Desired Outcomes

- Normalization of fluid and electrolyte balance without the development of hypokalemia or hypertension.

flumazenil (flu-maz-e-nil)
~~Romazicon~~
Classification
Therapeutic: antidotes

Indications
Complete/partial reversal of effects of benzodiazepines used as general anesthetics, or during diagnostic or therapeutic procedures. Management of intentional or accidental overdose of benzodiazepines.

Action
Flumazenil is a benzodiazepine derivative that antagonizes the CNS depressant effects of benzodiazepine compounds. It has no effect on CNS depression from other causes, including opioids, alcohol, barbiturates, or general anesthetics. **Therapeutic Effects:** Reversal of benzodiazepine effects.

Pharmacokinetics
Absorption: IV administration results in complete bioavailability.
Distribution: Unknown.
Metabolism and Excretion: Primarily metabolized in the liver. Primarily excreted in feces and urine (<1% as unchanged drug).
Half-life: *Children:* 20–75 min; *Adults:* 41–79 min.

TIME/ACTION PROFILE (reversal of benzodiazepine effects)

ROUTE	ONSET	PEAK	DURATION
IV	1–2 min	6–10 min	1–2 hr†

†Depends on dose/concentration of benzodiazepine and dose of flumazenil.

Contraindications/Precautions
Contraindicated in: Hypersensitivity to flumazenil or benzodiazepines; Patients receiving benzodiazepines for life-threatening medical problems, including status epilepticus or ↑ intracranial pressure; Serious cyclic antidepressant overdose.
Use Cautiously in: Mixed CNS depressant overdose (effects of other agents may emerge when benzodiazepine effect is removed); History of seizures (seizures are more likely to occur in patients who are experienc-

ing sedative/hypnotic withdrawal, who have recently received repeated doses of benzodiazepines, or who have a previous history of seizure activity); Head injury (may ↑ intracranial pressure and risk of seizures); Severe hepatic impairment; OB: Safety not established in pregnancy; Lactation: Safety not established in breastfeeding; Pedi: Children <1 yr (safety and effectiveness not established).

Adverse Reactions/Side Effects
CV: arrhythmias, chest pain, hypertension. **Derm:** flushing, sweating. **EENT:** abnormal hearing, abnormal vision, blurred vision. **GI:** nausea, vomiting, hiccups. **Local:** pain/injection-site reactions, phlebitis. **Neuro:** dizziness, agitation, confusion, drowsiness, emotional lability, fatigue, headache, paresthesia, SEIZURES, sleep disorders. **Misc:** rigors, shivering.

Interactions
Drug-Drug: None reported.

Route/Dosage

Reversal of Conscious Sedation or General Anesthesia
IV (Adults): 0.2 mg. Additional doses may be given at 1-min intervals until desired results are obtained, up to a total dose of 1 mg. If resedation occurs, regimen may be repeated at 20-min intervals, not to exceed 3 mg/hr.
IV (Children): 0.01 mg/kg (up to 0.2 mg); if the desired level of consciousness is not obtained after waiting an additional 45 sec, further injections of 0.01 mg/kg (up to 0.2 mg) can be administered and repeated at 60-sec intervals when necessary (up to a maximum of 4 additional times) to a maximum total dose of 0.05 mg/kg or 1 mg, whichever is lower. The dose should be individualized based on the patient's response.

Suspected Benzodiazepine Overdose
IV (Adults): 0.2 mg. Additional 0.3 mg may be given 30 sec later. Further doses of 0.5 mg may be given at 1-min intervals, if necessary, to a total dose of 3 mg. Usual dose required is 1–3 mg. If resedation occurs, additional doses of 0.5 mg/min for 2 min may be given at 20-min intervals (given no more than 1 mg at a time, not to exceed 3 mg per hr).
IV (Children): *Unlabeled:* 0.01 mg/kg (maximum dose 0.2 mg) with repeat doses every min up to a cumulative dose of 1 mg. As an alternative to repeat doses, continuous infusions of 0.005–0.01 mg/kg/hr have been used.

Availability (generic available)
Solution for injection: 0.1 mg/mL.

NURSING IMPLICATIONS

Assessment
- Assess level of consciousness and respiratory status before and during therapy. Observe patient for at least 2 hr after administration for the appearance of resedation. Hypoventilation may occur.
- **Overdose:** Attempt to determine time of ingestion and amount and type of benzodiazepine taken.

Knowledge of agent ingested allows an estimate of duration of CNS depression.

Implementation

- Do not confuse flumazenil with influenza virus vaccine.
- Ensure that patient has a patent airway before administration of flumazenil.
- Observe IV site frequently for redness or irritation. Administer through a free-flowing IV infusion into a large vein to minimize pain at the injection site.
- Optimal emergence should be undertaken slowly to decrease undesirable effects including confusion, agitation, emotional lability, and perceptual distortion.
- Institute seizure precautions. Seizures are more likely to occur in patients who are experiencing sedative/hypnotic withdrawal, patients who have recently received repeated doses of benzodiazepines, or those who have a previous history of seizure activity. Seizures may be treated with benzodiazepines, barbiturates, or phenytoin. Larger than normal doses of benzodiazepines may be required.
- **Suspected Benzodiazepine Overdose:** If no effects are seen after administration of flumazenil, consider other causes of decreased level of consciousness (alcohol, barbiturates, opioid analgesics).

IV Administration

- **IV Push:** *Dilution:* May be administered undiluted or diluted in syringe with D5W, 0.9% NaCl, or LR. Diluted solution should be discarded after 24 hr. *Concentration:* Up to 0.1 mg/mL. *Rate:* Administer 0.1 mg over 15–30 sec into free-flowing IV in a large vein. Do not exceed 0.2 mg/min in children or 0.5 mg/min in adults.

Patient/Family Teaching

- Flumazenil does not consistently reverse the amnestic effects of benzodiazepines. Provide patient and family with written instructions for postprocedure care. Inform family that patient may appear alert at the time of discharge but the sedative effects of the benzodiazepine may recur. Instruct patient to avoid driving or other activities requiring alertness for at least 24 hr after discharge.
- Instruct patient not to take any alcohol or nonprescription drugs for at least 18–24 hr after discharge.
- Resumption of usual activities should occur only when no residual effects of the benzodiazepine remain.
- Advise patient to notify health care professional if dizziness, headache, upset stomach, vomiting, blurred eyesight, dry mouth, sweating a lot, feeling nervous and excitable, shakiness, or trouble sleeping occur.
- Rep: Flumazenil is not recommended during pregnancy or breastfeeding unless there is a clear indication. Advise females of reproductive potential to notify healthcare professional if pregnancy is planned or suspected and if breastfeeding.

Evaluation/Desired Outcomes

- Improved level of consciousness.
- Decrease in respiratory depression caused by benzodiazepines.

flunisolide, See CORTICOSTEROIDS (NASAL).

fluocinolone, See CORTICOSTEROIDS (TOPICAL/LOCAL).

fluocinonide, See CORTICOSTEROIDS (TOPICAL/LOCAL).

FLUOROQUINOLONES
(floor-oh-**kwin**-oh-lones)
ciprofloxacin† (sip-roe-**flox**-a-sin)
Cipro, ~~Cipro XR~~
delafloxacin (del-a-**floks**-a-sin)
Baxdela
levofloxacin (le-voe-**flox**-a-sin)
~~Levaquin~~
moxifloxacin† (mox-i-**flox**-a-sin)
~~Avelox~~
ofloxacin† (oh-**flox**-a-sin)
~~Floxin~~
Classification
Therapeutic: anti-infectives
Pharmacologic: fluoroquinolones

†See Appendix B for ophthalmic use

Indications

PO, IV: Treatment of the following bacterial infections: Urinary tract infections (UTIs) including cystitis and prostatitis (ciprofloxacin, levofloxacin, ofloxacin) (should be used for acute uncomplicated cystitis only when there are no other alternative treatment options), Gonorrhea (may not be considered first-line agents due to increasing resistance), Gynecologic infections (ciprofloxacin, ofloxacin), Respiratory tract infections including acute sinusitis, acute exacerbations of chronic bronchitis, and pneumonia (should be used for acute sinusitis or acute bacterial exacerbations of chronic bronchitis only when there are no other alternative treatment options), Skin and skin structure infections (delafloxacin, levofloxacin, moxifloxacin, ciprofloxacin, ofloxacin), Bone and joint infections (ciprofloxacin), Infectious diarrhea (ciprofloxacin), Intra-abdominal infections (ciprofloxacin, moxifloxacin). Febrile neutropenia (ciprofloxacin). Postexposure treatment of inhalational anthrax (ciprofloxacin, levofloxacin).

Treatment and prophylaxis of plague (ciprofloxacin, levofloxacin, moxifloxacin).

Action
Inhibit bacterial DNA synthesis by inhibiting DNA gyrase. **Therapeutic Effects:** Death of susceptible bacteria. **Spectrum:** Broad activity includes many gram-positive pathogens: Staphylococci including methicillin-resistant *Staphylococcus aureus*, *Staphylococcus epidermidis*, *Staphylococcus saprophyticus*, *Streptococcus pneumoniae*, *Streptococcus pyogenes*, and *Bacillus anthracis*. Gram-negative spectrum notable for activity against: *Escherichia coli*, *Klebsiella*, *Enterobacter*, *Salmonella*, *Shigella*, *Proteus*, *Providencia*, *Morganella morganii*, *Pseudomonas aeruginosa*, *Serratia*, *Haemophilus*, *Acinetobacter*, *Neisseria gonorrhoeae*, *Moraxella catarrhalis*, *Campylobacter*, and *Yersinia pestis*. Additional spectrum includes: *Chlamydia pneumoniae*, *Legionella pneumoniae*, and *Mycoplasma pneumoniae*.

Pharmacokinetics
Absorption: Well absorbed after oral administration (*ciprofloxacin:* 70%; *delafloxacin:* 59%; *moxifloxacin:* 90%; *levofloxacin:* 99%; *ofloxacin:* 98%).
Distribution: Widely distributed. High tissue and urinary levels are achieved. All agents appear to cross the placenta. *Ciprofloxacin* and *ofloxacin* enter breast milk.
Metabolism and Excretion: *Ciprofloxacin:* 15% metabolized by the liver, 40–50% excreted unchanged by the kidneys; *delafloxacin:* primarily undergoes glucuronidation; 50–65% excreted unchanged by the kidneys; 28–48% excreted in feces; *levofloxacin:* 87% excreted unchanged in urine, small amounts metabolized; *moxifloxacin:* mostly metabolized by the liver, 20% excreted unchanged in urine, 25% excreted unchanged in feces; *ofloxacin:* 70–80% excreted unchanged by the kidneys.
Half-life: *Ciprofloxacin:* 4 hr; *delafloxacin:* 3.7 hr (IV); 4.2–8.5 hr (PO); *levofloxacin:* 8 hr; *moxifloxacin:* 12 hr; *ofloxacin:* 5–7 hr (all are ↑ in renal impairment).

TIME/ACTION PROFILE (blood levels)

ROUTE	ONSET	PEAK	DURATION
Ciprofloxacin—PO	rapid	1–2 hr	12 hr
Ciprofloxacin—IV	rapid	end of infusion	12 hr
Delafloxacin—PO	rapid	1 hr	12 hr
Delafloxacin—IV	rapid	end of infusion	12 hr
Levofloxacin—PO	rapid	1–2 hr	24 hr
Levofloxacin—IV	rapid	end of infusion	24 hr
Moxifloxacin—PO	within 1 hr	1–3 hr	24 hr
Moxifloxacin—IV	rapid	end of infusion	24 hr
Ofloxacin—PO	rapid	1–2 hr	12 hr
Ofloxacin—IV	rapid	end of infusion	12 hr

Contraindications/Precautions
Contraindicated in: Hypersensitivity. Cross-sensitivity among agents within class may occur; History of myasthenia gravis (may worsen symptoms including muscle weakness and breathing problems); Patients with or at ↑ risk for aortic aneurysm (use only if no alternatives); **Moxifloxacin:** Concurrent use of Class IA antiarrhythmics (disopyramide, quinidine, procainamide) or Class III antiarrhythmics (amiodarone, sotalol) (↑ risk of QTc interval prolongation and torsades de pointes); Known QT interval prolongation or concurrent use of agents causing prolongation; **Ciprofloxacin:** Concurrent use with tizanidine; **Delafloxacin:** End-stage renal disease (eGFR <15 mL/min); OB: Do not use unless potential benefit outweighs potential fetal risk (delafloxacin, moxifloxacin, ofloxacin); Lactation: Avoid breastfeeding during treatment and for 2 days after final dose (for ciprofloxacin and levofloxacin, applies for all indications other than post-exposure prophylaxis of inhalational anthrax); Pedi: Use only for treatment of anthrax, plague, and complicated UTIs in children 1–17 yr due to possible arthropathy.
Use Cautiously in: Seizure disorder; Depression; Renal impairment (dose ↓ if CCr ≤50 mL/min for ciprofloxacin, levofloxacin, ofloxacin); Cirrhosis (levofloxacin, moxifloxacin); **Moxifloxacin:** Concurrent use of erythromycin, antipsychotics, and tricyclic antidepressants (↑ risk of QTc prolongation and torsades de pointes); **Moxifloxacin:** Bradycardia; **Moxifloxacin:** Acute myocardial ischemia; **Delafloxacin:** Severe renal impairment (dose ↓ if eGFR 15–29 mL/min) (IV diluent may accumulate and ↑ serum creatinine) (↑ risk of tendon rupture in renal failure); Concurrent use of corticosteroids (↑ risk of tendinitis/tendon rupture); Kidney, heart, or lung transplant patients (↑ risk of tendinitis/tendon rupture); Rheumatoid arthritis (↑ risk of tendon rupture); Diabetes; OB: Use during pregnancy only if potential maternal benefit outweighs potential fetal risk (ciprofloxacin and levofloxacin only); Lactation: Can be used while breastfeeding for post-exposure prophylaxis of anthrax if potential maternal benefit justifies potential risk to infant (ciprofloxacin and levofloxacin only); Geri: ↑ risk of adverse reactions in older adults.

Adverse Reactions/Side Effects
CV: AORTIC ANEURYSM/DISSECTION; *levofloxacin, moxifloxacin:* QT interval prolongation, TORSADES DE POINTES, vasodilation. **Derm:** acute generalized exanthematous pustulosis, photosensitivity, rash, STEVENS-JOHNSON SYNDROME (SJS). **Endo:** hyperglycemia, hypoglycemia. **GI:** diarrhea, nausea, ↑ liver enzymes (ciprofloxacin, moxifloxacin), abdominal pain, CLOSTRIDIOIDES DIFFICILE-ASSOCIATED DIARRHEA (CDAD), HEPATOTOXICITY (ciprofloxacin), vomiting. **GU:** vaginitis. **Local:** phlebitis at IV site. **MS:** arthralgia, myalgia, tendinitis, tendon rupture. **Neuro:** dizziness, headache, insomnia, acute psychoses, agitation, confusion, depression, drowsiness, hallucinations, ↑ INTRACRANIAL PRESSURE (including pseudotumor cerebri), lightheadedness, nightmares,

paranoia, peripheral neuropathy, SEIZURES, SUICIDAL THOUGHTS/BEHAVIORS, toxic psychosis, tremor. **Misc:** HYPERSENSITIVITY REACTIONS (including anaphylaxis).

Interactions

Drug-Drug: Ciprofloxacin may ↑ **tizanidine** levels and risk of hypotension and sedation; concurrent use contraindicated. Concurrent use with **QT interval-prolonging medications** may ↑ risk of QT interval prolongation and torsades de pointes; avoid concurrent use. Ciprofloxacin may ↑ **theophylline** levels and risk of CNS toxicity; avoid concurrent use; if concurrent use cannot be avoided, closely monitor serum theophylline levels. Ciprofloxacin may ↑ levels and risk of toxicity of CYP1A2 substrates, including **ropinirole, clozapine, olanzapine,** and **zolpidem;** avoid concurrent use with **zolpidem.** Administration with **antacids, iron salts, bismuth subsalicylate, sucralfate, sevelemer, lanthanum,** and **zinc salts** ↓ absorption of fluoroquinolones; separate administration of medications. May ↑ the effects of and risk of bleeding from **warfarin.** Ciprofloxacin may alter levels and the effects of **phenytoin.** Levels of fluoroquinolones may be ↓ by **antineoplastics. Probenecid** may ↑ levels and risk of toxicity. May ↑ risk of nephrotoxicity from **cyclosporine.** Concurrent use of ciprofloxacin with **NSAIDs** may ↑ risk of seizures. Concurrent therapy with **corticosteroids** may ↑ the risk of tendon rupture. May ↑ risk of hypoglycemia when used with **antidiabetic agents.**

Drug-Natural Products: Fennel ↓ the absorption of ciprofloxacin.

Drug-Food: Absorption is impaired by **concurrent tube feeding** (because of metal cations). Absorption is ↓ if taken with **dairy products** or calcium-fortified juices.

Route/Dosage

Ciprofloxacin

PO (Adults): *Most infections:* 500–750 mg every 12 hr. *Complicated UTIs:* 500 mg every 12 hr for 7–14 days. *Uncomplicated UTIs:* 250 mg every 12 hr for 3 days. *Gonorrhea:* 250-mg single dose. *Inhalational anthrax (postexposure) or cutaneous anthrax:* 500 mg every 12 hr for 60 days; *Plague:* 500–750 mg every 12 hr for 14 days.

PO (Children 1–17 yr): *Complicated UTIs:* 10–15 mg/kg every 12 hr (max = 750 mg/dose) for 10–21 days. *Inhalational anthrax (postexposure) or cutaneous anthrax:* 10–15 mg/kg every 12 hr (max = 500 mg/dose) for 60 days; *Plague:* 15 mg/kg every 8–12 hr (max = 500 mg/dose) for 14 days.

IV (Adults): *Most infections:* 400 mg every 12 hr. *Complicated UTIs:* 400 mg every 12 hr for 7–14 days. *Uncomplicated UTIs:* 200 mg every 12 hr for 7–14 days. *Inhalational anthrax (post exposure):* 400 mg every 12 hr for 60 days; *Plague:* 400 mg every 8–12 hr for 14 days.

IV (Children 1–17 yr): *Inhalational anthrax (post exposure):* 10 mg/kg every 12 hr (not to exceed 400 mg/dose) for 60 days; *Complicated UTIs:* 6–10 mg/kg every 8 hr (max = 400 mg/dose) for 10–21 days; *Plague:* 10 mg/kg every 8–12 hr (max = 400 mg/dose) for 10–21 days.

Renal Impairment

PO (Adults): *CCr 30–50 mL/min:* 250–500 mg every 12 hr; *CCr 5–29 mL/min:* 250–500 mg every 18 hr.

IV (Adults): *CCr 5–29 mL/min:* 200–400 mg every 18–24 hr.

Delafloxacin

IV (Adults): 300 mg every 12 hr for 5–14 days (for acute bacterial skin and skin structure infections) or 5–10 days (for community-acquired pneumonia [CAP]) *or* 300 mg every 12 hr followed by switching to oral regimen (at dose stated below) for a total of 5–14 days (for acute bacterial skin and skin structure infections) or 5–10 days (for CAP).

PO (Adults): 450 mg every 12 hr for 5–14 days (for acute bacterial skin and skin structure infections) or 5–10 days (for CAP).

Renal Impairment

IV (Adults): *eGFR 15–29 mL/min:* 200 mg every 12 hr for 5–14 days (for acute bacterial skin and skin structure infections) or 5–10 days (for CAP) *or* 200 mg every 12 hr followed by switching to oral regimen (450 mg every 12 hr) for a total of 5–14 days (for acute bacterial skin and skin structure infections) or 5–10 days (for CAP); *eGFR <15 mL/min:* Not recommended.

Levofloxacin

PO, IV (Adults): *Most infections:* 250–750 mg every 24 hr; *Inhalational anthrax (postexposure):* 500 mg once daily for 60 days.

PO, IV (Children >50 kg): *Inhalational anthrax (postexposure):* 500 mg once daily for 60 days; *Plague:* 500 mg once daily for 10–14 days.

PO, IV (Children <50 kg and ≥6 mo): *Inhalational anthrax (postexposure):* 8 mg/kg (max: 250 mg/dose) every 12 hr for 60 days. *Plague:* 8 mg/kg (max: 250 mg/dose) every 12 hr for 10–14 days; *Other infections:* 10 mg/kg/dose every 24 hr (max: 500 mg/dose).

Renal Impairment

PO, IV (Adults): *Normal renal function dosing of 750 mg/day: CCr 20–49 mL/min:* 750 mg every 48 hr; *CCr 10–19 mL/min:* 750 mg initially, then 500 mg every 48 hr; *Normal renal function dosing of 500 mg/day: CCr 20–49 mL/min:* 500 mg initially then 250 mg every 24 hr; *CCr 10–19 mL/min:* 500 mg initially then 250 mg every 48 hr. *Normal renal function dosing of 250 mg/day: CCr 10–19 mL/min:* 250 mg every 48 hr.

Moxifloxacin
PO, IV (Adults): *Bacterial sinusitis:* 400 mg once daily for 10 days; *CAP:* 400 mg once daily for 7–14 days. *Acute bacterial exacerbation of chronic bronchitis:* 400 mg once daily for 5 days. *Complicated intra-abdominal infection:* 400 mg once daily for 5–14 days. *Skin/skin structure infections:* 400 mg/day for 7–21 days. *Treatment/prevention of plague:* 400 mg once daily for 10–14 days.

Ofloxacin
PO (Adults): *Most infections:* 400 mg every 12 hr. *Prostatitis:* 300 mg every 12 hr for 6 wk. *Uncomplicated UTIs:* 200 mg every 12 hr for 3–7 days. *Complicated UTIs:* 200 mg every 12 hr for 10 days. *Gonorrhea:* 400-mg single dose.

Renal Impairment
PO, IV (Adults): *CCr 20–50 mL/min:* 100% of the usual dose every 24 hr; *CCr <20 mL/min:* 50% of the usual dose every 24 hr.

Availability

Ciprofloxacin (generic available)
Immediate-release tablets: 100 mg, 250 mg, 500 mg, 750 mg. **Oral suspension (strawberry flavor):** 250 mg/5 mL, 500 mg/5 mL. **Premixed infusion:** 200 mg/100 mL D5W, 400 mg/200 mL D5W. **Solution for injection:** 10 mg/mL. *In combination with:* fluocinolone (Otovel); hydrocortisone (Cipro HC) (see Appendix N).

Delafloxacin
Tablets: 450 mg. **Lyophilized powder for injection:** 300 mg/vial.

Levofloxacin (generic available)
Tablets: 250 mg, 500 mg, 750 mg. **Oral solution:** 25 mg/mL. **Solution for injection:** 25 mg/mL. **Premixed infusion:** 250 mg/50 mL D5W, 500 mg/100 mL D5W, 750 mg/150 mL D5W.

Moxifloxacin (generic available)
Tablets: 400 mg. **Premixed infusion:** 400 mg/250 mL 0.8% NaCl.

Ofloxacin (generic available)
Tablets: 200 mg, 300 mg, 400 mg.

NURSING IMPLICATIONS

Assessment
- Assess for infection (vital signs; appearance of wound, sputum, urine, and stool; WBC; urinalysis; frequency and urgency of urination; cloudy or foul-smelling urine) prior to and during therapy.
- Obtain specimens for culture and sensitivity before initiating therapy. First dose may be given before receiving results.
- Observe for signs and symptoms of anaphylaxis (rash, pruritus, laryngeal edema, wheezing). Discontinue drug and notify health care professional immediately if these problems occur. Keep epineph-

rine, an antihistamine, and resuscitation equipment close by in case of an anaphylactic reaction.
- Monitor bowel function. Diarrhea, abdominal cramping, fever, and bloody stools should be reported to health care professional promptly as a sign of CDAD. May begin up to several wk following cessation of therapy.
- Assess for rash periodically during therapy. May cause SJS. Discontinue therapy if severe or if accompanied with fever, general malaise, fatigue, muscle or joint aches, blisters, oral lesions, conjunctivitis, hepatitis, and/or eosinophilia.
- Assess for signs and symptoms of peripheral neuropathy (pain, burning, tingling, numbness, and/or weakness or other alterations of sensation including light touch, pain, temperature, position sense, and vibratory sensation) periodically during therapy. Symptoms may be irreversible; discontinue fluoroquinolone if symptoms occur.
- Assess for suicidal tendencies, depression, or changes in behavior periodically during therapy.

Lab Test Considerations
May cause ↑ serum AST, ALT, LDH, bilirubin, and alkaline phosphatase. May also cause ↑ or ↓ serum glucose. Monitor blood glucose in patients with diabetes taking insulin or oral hypoglycemic agents. Medication may cause hyperglycemia or hypoglycemia. Moxifloxacin may cause hyperglycemia, hyperlipidemia, and altered prothrombin time. It may also cause ↑ WBC; ↑ serum calcium, chloride, albumin, and globulin; and ↓ hemoglobin, RBCs, neutrophils, eosinophils, and basophils. Monitor prothrombin time closely in patients receiving fluoroquinolones and warfarin; may enhance the anticoagulant effects of warfarin.

Implementation
- Do not confuse levofloxacin with levetiracetam.
- **PO:** Administer *ofloxacin* on an empty stomach 1 hr before or 2 hr after meals, with a full glass of water. *Moxifloxacin, ciprofloxacin,* and *levofloxacin* may be administered without regard to meals. Should be taken at least 2 hr (4 hr for moxifloxacin) before or 2 hr (6 hr for *ciprofloxacin,* 8 hr for *moxifloxacin*) after antacids or other products containing calcium, iron, zinc, magnesium, or aluminum. *Delafloxacin* may be administered without regard to food and with a full glass of water, at the same time each day. Products or foods containing calcium, magnesium, aluminum, iron, or zinc should not be ingested for 2 hr before and 6 hr after administration.
- If gastric irritation occurs, ciprofloxacin may be administered with meals.
- Ciprofloxacin 5% and 10% oral suspension should not be administered through a feeding tube (may ↓ absorption). Shake solution for 15 sec prior to administration.

FLUOROQUINOLONES 593

Ciprofloxacin

IV Administration

- **Intermittent Infusion: *Dilution:*** Dilute with 0.9% NaCl or D5W. Stable for 14 days at refrigerated or room temperature. ***Concentration:*** 1–2 mg/mL. ***Rate:*** Administer over 60 min into a large vein to minimize venous irritation.

- **Y-Site Compatibility:** alemtuzumab, amifostine, amiodarone, anidulafungin, argatroban, arsenic trioxide, aztreonam, bivalirudin, bleomycin, calcium gluconate, carboplatin, carmustine, caspofungin, ceftaroline, ceftazidime, ceftolozane/tazobactam, cisatracurium, cisplatin, cyclophosphamide, cytarabine, dactinomycin, daptomycin, daunorubicin hydrochloride, dexmedetomidine, dexrazoxane, digoxin, diltiazem, dimenhydrinate, diphenhydramine, dobutamine, docetaxel, dopamine, doxorubicin hydrochloride, doxorubicin liposomal, epirubicin, eptifibatide, eravacycline, etoposide, etoposide phosphate, fludarabine, fosphenytoin, gemcitabine, gentamicin, granisetron, hetastarch, hydrocortisone, hydromorphone, idarubicin, ifosfamide, irinotecan, isavuconazonium, labetalol, leucovorin calcium, lidocaine, linezolid, lorazepam, meperidine, mesna, methadone, methotrexate, metoclopramide, metoprolol, metronidazole, midazolam, milrinone, mitomycin, mitoxantrone, mycophenolate, naloxone, nicardipine, octreotide, ondansetron, oritavancin, oxaliplatin, oxytocin, paclitaxel, palonosetron, pamidronate, plazomicin, posaconazole, potassium acetate, potassium chloride, promethazine, remifentanil, rifampin, rocuronium, tacrolimus, tedizolid, telavancin, thiotepa, tigecycline, tirofiban, tobramycin, topotecan, trastuzumab, vancomycin, vasopressin, vecuronium, verapamil, vinblastine, vincristine, vinorelbine, voriconazole, zoledronic acid.

- **Y-Site Incompatibility:** acyclovir, aminocaproic acid, aminophylline, amphotericin B lipid complex, amphotericin B liposomal, ampicillin/sulbactam, blinatumomab, cangrelor, cefepime, dexamethasone, esmolol, fluorouracil, foscarnet, furosemide, gemtuzumab ozogamicin, heparin, hydrocortisone, magnesium sulfate, meropenem, meropenem/vaborbactam, methylprednisolone, pantoprazole, pemetrexed, phenytoin, piperacillin/tazobactam, potassium phosphate, propofol, rituximab, sodium phosphate, warfarin.

Delafloxacin

- **Intermittent Infusion:** Reconstitute with 10.5 mL D5W or 0.9% NaCl for each 300 mg vial. Shake vigorously to completely dissolve. ***Concentration:*** 25 mg/mL. Solution is clear yellow to amber; do not administer solutions that are discolored or contain particulate matter. Reconstituted solution is stable if refrigerated or at room temperature for 24 hr. ***Dilution:*** Dilute to volume of 250 mL with 0.9% NaCl or D5W. ***Concentration:*** 1.2 mg/mL. Diluted solution is stable if refrigerated or at room temperature for 24 hr. ***Rate:*** Infuse over 60 min.

- **Y-Site Incompatibility:** Do not administer with other drugs; flush line before and after each dose.

Levofloxacin

IV Administration

- **Intermittent Infusion: *Dilution:*** Dilute with 0.9% NaCl, D5W, or dextrose/saline combinations. Also available in premixed bottles and flexible containers with D5W, which need no further dilution. ***Concentration:*** 5 mg/mL. Discard unused solution. Diluted solution is stable for 72 hr at room temperature and 14 days if refrigerated. ***Rate:*** Administer by infusion over at least 60 min for 250 mg or 500 mg doses and over 90 min for 750 mg dose. Avoid rapid bolus injection to prevent hypotension.

- **Y-Site Compatibility:** alemtuzumab, amifostine, amikacin, aminocaproic acid, aminophylline, ampicillin, ampicillin/sulbactam, anidulafungin, argatroban, arsenic trioxide, atracurium, aztreonam, bivalirudin, bleomycin, bumetanide, buprenorphine, busulfan, butorphanol, caffeine citrate, calcium gluconate, cangrelor, carboplatin, carmustine, caspofungin, cefepime, cefotetan, ceftaroline, ceftazidime, ceftolozane/tazobactam, ceftriaxone, cefuroxime, chlorpromazine, cisatracurium, cisplatin, clindamycin, cyclophosphamide, cyclosporine, cytarabine, dacarbazine, dactinomycin, daptomycin, dexamethasone, dexmedetomidine, dexrazoxane, digoxin, diltiazem, diphenhydramine, dobutamine, docetaxel, dopamine, doxorubicin liposomal, doxycycline, droperidol, enalaprilat, ephedrine, epinephrine, epirubicin, eptifibatide, eravacycline, ertapenem, erythromycin, esmolol, etoposide, etoposide phosphate, famotidine, fentanyl, filgrastim, fluconazole, fludarabine, foscarnet, fosphenytoin, gemcitabine, gemtuzumab ozogamicin, gentamicin, granisetron, haloperidol, hetastarch, hydrocortisone, hydromorphone, idarubicin, ifosfamide, imipenem/cilastatin, irinotecan, isavuconazonium, isoproterenol, labetalol, LR, leucovorin calcium, lidocaine, linezolid, mannitol, meperidine, meropenem/vaborbactam, mesna, methadone, methylprednisolone, metoclopramide, metoprolol, metronidazole, midazolam, milrinone, mitomycin, mitoxantrone, mycophenolate, nalbuphine, naloxone, nicardipine, octreotide, ondansetron, oxacillin, oxaliplatin, oxytocin, paclitaxel, palonosetron, pamidronate, pemetrexed, penicillin G sodium, pentamidine, phenylephrine, posaconazole, potassium acetate, potassium chloride, promethazine, propranolol, remifentanil, rocuronium, sargramostim, sodium bicarbonate, succinylcholine, sufentanil, tacrolimus, tedizolid, theophylline, thiotepa, tigecycline, tirofiban, tobramycin, topotecan, trimethoprim/sulfamethoxazole, vanco-

❋ = Canadian drug name. ≋ = Genetic implication. ~~Strikethrough~~ = Discontinued. CAPITALS = life-threatening. <u>Underline</u> = most frequent.

mycin, vasopressin, vecuronium, verapamil, vinblastine, vincristine, vinorelbine, voriconazole, zidovudine, zoledronic acid.

- **Y-Site Incompatibility:** acyclovir, alprostadil, amiodarone, amphotericin B lipid complex, amphotericin B liposomal, cefazolin, cefoxitin, daunorubicin hydrochloride, diazepam, fluorouracil, furosemide, ganciclovir, heparin, indomethacin, ketorolac, methotrexate, micafungin, nitroglycerin, nitroprusside, pantoprazole, pentobarbital, phenytoin, piperacillin/tazobactam, plazomicin, prochlorperazine, propofol, rituximab, telavancin, thiopental, trastuzumab.

Moxifloxacin

IV Administration

- **Intermittent Infusion:** *Dilution:* Premixed bags are diluted in sodium chloride 0.8% and should not be further diluted. Use transfer set whose piercing pin does not require excessive force; insert with a gentle twisting motion until pin is firmly seated. *Concentration:* 1.6 mg/mL. *Rate:* Administer over 60 min. Avoid rapid or bolus infusion.
- **Y-Site Compatibility:** alemtuzumab, amifostine, aminocaproic acid, amiodarone, anidulafungin, argatroban, arsenic trioxide, atracurium, bivalirudin, bleomycin, bumetanide, busulfan, calcium acetate, calcium chloride, calcium gluconate, cangrelor, carboplatin, carmustine, caspofungin, ceftaroline, chlorpromazine, cisatracurium, cisplatin, cyclophosphamide, cyclosporine, cytarabine, dacarbazine, dactinomycin, daptomycin, daunorubicin hydrochloride, dexamethasone, dexmedetomidine, dexrazoxane, digoxin, diltiazem, diphenhydramine, dobutamine, docetaxel, dopamine, doxorubicin hydrochloride, doxorubicin liposomal, droperidol, enalaprilat, epinephrine, epirubicin, ertapenem, esmolol, etoposide, etoposide phosphate, famotidine, fludarabine, gemcitabine, gemtuzumab ozogamicin, glycopyrrolate, granisetron, haloperidol, heparin, hetastarch, hydralazine, hydrocortisone, idarubicin, ifosfamide, insulin, regular, irinotecan, isoproterenol, ketorolac, labetalol, leucovorin calcium, lidocaine, magnesium sulfate, mannitol, melphalan, mesna, methadone, methotrexate, methylprednisolone, metoclopramide, metoprolol, milrinone, mitomycin, mitoxantrone, mycophenolate, naloxone, nicardipine, nitroglycerin, norepinephrine, octreotide, ondansetron, oxaliplatin, oxytocin, paclitaxel, palonosetron, pamidronate, pemetrexed, phentolamine, phenylephrine, potassium acetate, potassium chloride, potassium phosphate, procainamide, prochlorperazine, promethazine, propranolol, rocuronium, sodium acetate, sodium bicarbonate, sodium phosphate, succinylcholine, tacrolimus, theophylline, thiotepa, tigecycline, tirofiban, topotecan, vasopressin, vecuronium, verapamil, vinblastine, vincristine, vinorelbine, zoledronic acid.
- **Y-Site Incompatibility:** allopurinol, aminophylline, amphotericin B lipid complex, dantrolene, fluorouracil, fosphenytoin, furosemide, nitroprusside, pantoprazole, phenytoin, vancomycin, voriconazole.

Patient/Family Teaching

- Instruct patient to take medication as directed at evenly spaced times and to finish drug completely, even if feeling better. Take missed doses as soon as possible, unless almost time (within 6 hr for ciprofloxacin; 8 hr for moxifloxacin) for next dose. Do not double doses. Advise patient that sharing of this medication may be dangerous.
- Advise patient to notify health care professional immediately if they are taking theophylline.
- Encourage patient to maintain a fluid intake of at least 1500–2000 mL/day to prevent crystalluria.
- Advise patient that antacids or medications containing iron or zinc will decrease absorption. *Ciprofloxacin, levofloxacin,* and *ofloxacin* should be taken at least 2 hr before (4 hr for *moxifloxacin*) or 2 hr after (6 hr for *ciprofloxacin,* and *delafloxacin,* 8 hr for *moxifloxacin*) these products.
- May cause dizziness and drowsiness. Caution patient to avoid driving or other activities requiring alertness until response to medication is known.
- Advise patient to notify health care professional of any personal or family history of QTc prolongation or proarrhythmic conditions such as recent hypokalemia, significant bradycardia, or recent myocardial ischemia or if fainting spells or palpitations occur.
- Advise patient to stop taking fluoroquinolone and notify health care professional immediately if signs and symptoms of peripheral neuropathy occur.
- Caution patient to use sunscreen and protective clothing to prevent phototoxicity reactions during and for 5 days after therapy. Notify health care professional if a sunburn-like reaction or skin eruption occurs.
- Instruct patients being treated for gonorrhea that partners also must be treated.
- Advise patient to notify health care professional of all Rx or OTC medications, vitamins, or herbal products being taken and to consult with health care professional before taking other medications.
- Advise patient to report signs of superinfection (furry overgrowth on the tongue, vaginal itching or discharge, loose or foul-smelling stools).
- Instruct patient to notify health care professional if fever and diarrhea develop, especially if stool contains blood, pus, or mucus. Advise patient not to treat diarrhea without consulting health care professional.
- Instruct patient to notify health care professional immediately if rash, jaundice, signs of hypersensitivity, or tendon (shoulder, hand, Achilles, and other) pain, swelling, or inflammation occur. If tendon symptoms occur, avoid exercise and use of the affected area. Increased risk in >65 yr old; kidney, heart, and lung transplant recipients; and patients taking corticosteroids concurrently. Therapy should be discontinued.

- Advise patient, family, and caregivers to look for suicidality, especially during early therapy or dose changes. Notify health care professional immediately if thoughts about suicide or dying, attempts to commit suicide, new or worse depression or anxiety, agitation or restlessness, panic attacks, insomnia, new or worse irritability, aggressiveness, acting on dangerous impulses, mania, or other changes in mood or behavior.
- Inform patient that fluoroquinolones may cause worsening of myasthenia gravis symptoms (muscle weakness, breathing problems). Advise patient to notify health care professional immediately if symptoms occur.
- Rep: Advise females of reproductive potential to use effective contraception during delafloxacin, moxifoxacin, and ofloxacin therapy and to avoid breastfeeding during therapy with delafloxacin, moxifoxacin, ofloxacin and during and for 2 days after last dose of ciprofloxacin or levofloxacin. Advise patient to notify health care professional if pregnancy is planned or suspected.

Evaluation/Desired Outcomes
- Resolution of the signs and symptoms of infection. Time for complete resolution depends on organism and site of infection.
- Post exposure treatment of inhalational anthrax or cutaneous anthrax (ciprofloxacin and levofloxacin).
- Prevention and treatment of plague (ciprofloxacin, levofloxacin, and moxifloxacin).

HIGH ALERT

⚶ fluorouracil
(flure-oh-**yoor**-a-sill)
Carac, Efudex, Tolak
Classification
Therapeutic: antineoplastics
Pharmacologic: antimetabolites

Indications
IV: Used alone and in combination with other modalities (surgery, radiation therapy, other antineoplastics) in the treatment of: Colorectal adenocarcinoma, Breast adenocarcinoma, Gastric adenocarcinoma, Pancreatic adenocarcinoma. **Topical:** Multiple actinic (solar) keratoses and superficial basal cell carcinomas.

Action
Inhibits DNA and RNA synthesis by preventing thymidine production (cell-cycle S-phase–specific). **Therapeutic Effects:** Death of rapidly replicating cells, particularly malignant ones.

Pharmacokinetics
Absorption: Minimal absorption (5–10%) after topical application.

Distribution: Widely distributed; concentrates and persists in tumors.
Metabolism and Excretion: Metabolized by dihydropyrimidine dehydrogenase to a less toxic compound; inactive metabolites are excreted primarily in urine.
Half-life: 20 hr.

TIME/ACTION PROFILE (IV = effects on blood counts, Top = dermatologic effects)

ROUTE	ONSET	PEAK	DURATION
IV	1–9 days	9–21 days (nadir)	30 days
Top	2–3 days	2–6 wk	1–2 mo

Contraindications/Precautions
Contraindicated in: Hypersensitivity; ⚶ Dihydropyrimidine dehydrogenase deficiency (patients at ↑ risk of toxicity); OB: Pregnancy; Lactation: Lactation.
Use Cautiously in: Infections; Depressed bone marrow reserve; Other chronic debilitating illnesses; Obese patients, patients with edema or ascites (dose should be based on ideal body weight); Pedi: Safety and effectiveness not established in children.

Adverse Reactions/Side Effects
More likely to occur with systemic use than with topical use.
CV: CARDIOTOXICITY. **Derm:** alopecia, maculopapular rash, local inflammatory reactions (topical only), melanosis of nails, nail loss, palmar-plantar erythrodysesthesia, phototoxicity. **Endo:** sterility. **GI:** diarrhea, nausea, stomatitis, vomiting. **Hemat:** anemia, leukopenia, thrombocytopenia. **Local:** thrombophlebitis. **Neuro:** acute cerebellar dysfunction. **Misc:** fever.

Interactions
Drug-Drug: Combination chemotherapy with **irinotecan** may produce unacceptable toxicity (dehydration, neutropenia, sepsis). Additive bone marrow depression with other **bone marrow depressants**, including other **antineoplastics** and **radiation therapy**. May ↓ antibody response to **live-virus vaccines** and ↑ risk of adverse reactions.

Route/Dosage
Doses may vary greatly, depending on tumor, patient condition, and protocol used.

Advanced Colorectal Cancer
IV (Adults): *In combination with leucovorin alone or leucovorin + oxaliplatin or irinotecan:* 400 mg/m² as IV bolus on Day 1, then 2400–3000 mg/m² continuous infusion every 2 wk; *In combination with leucovorin:* 500 mg/m² as IV bolus 1 hr after leucovorin on Days 1, 8, 15, 22, 29, and 36 every 8 wk.

Breast Cancer

IV (Adults): *In combination with cyclophosphamide + epirubicin or cyclophosphamide + methotrexate:* 500 mg/m² or 600 mg/m² on Days 1 and 28 every 28 days for 6 cycles.

Gastric Adenocarcinoma

IV (Adults): *As part of platinum-containing regimen:* 200–1000 mg/m² as IV infusion (frequency of administration and number of cycles depends on specific regimen used).

Pancreatic Adenocarcinoma

IV (Adults): *In combination with leucovorin or as part of multidrug regimen:* 400 mg/m² as IV bolus on Day 1, then 2400 mg/m² continuous infusion every 2 wk.

Actinic (Solar) Keratoses

Topical (Adults): *Carac:* Apply 0.5% cream to lesions once daily for up to 4 wk; *Efudex:* Apply 2% or 5% solution or cream to lesions twice daily for 2–4 wk.

Superficial Basal Cell Carcinomas

Topical (Adults): *Efudex:* Apply 5% solution or cream to lesions twice daily for 3–6 wk (up to 12 wk).

Availability (generic available)

Solution for injection: 50 mg/mL. **Topical cream:** 0.5%, 4%, 5%. **Topical solution:** 2%, 5%.

NURSING IMPLICATIONS

Assessment

- Monitor vital signs before and frequently during therapy.
- Assess mucous membranes, number and consistency of stools, and frequency of vomiting. Assess for signs of infection (fever, chills, sore throat, cough, hoarseness, pain in lower back or side, difficult or painful urination). Assess for bleeding (bleeding gums; bruising; petechiae; and guaiac test stools, urine, and emesis). Avoid IM injections and taking rectal temperatures. Apply pressure to venipuncture sites for 10 min. Notify health care professional if Grade 3 or 4 toxicity (stomatitis or esophagopharyngitis, uncontrollable vomiting, diarrhea, GI bleeding, myocardial ischemia, leukocyte count <3500/mm³, platelet count <100,000/mm³, or hemorrhage from any site) occurs; hold fluorouracil until resolution to ≤Grade 1. May be reinitiated at a lower dose when side effects have subsided.
- Assess IV site frequently for inflammation or infiltration. Patient should notify nurse if pain or irritation at injection site occurs. May cause thrombophlebitis. If extravasation occurs, infusion must be stopped and restarted in another vein to avoid damage to SUBQ tissue. Report immediately. Standard treatment includes application of ice compresses.
- Assess skin for palmar-plantar erythrodysesthesia (tingling of hands and feet followed by pain, erythema, swelling, desquamation) throughout therapy. Occurs more frequently with continuous infusion.

Usually occurs after 8–9 wk of therapy, but may occur earlier. Hold fluorouracil for Grades 2 or 3 and resume at lower dose when resolved or Grade 1.

- Monitor intake and output, appetite, and nutritional intake. GI effects usually occur on 4th day of therapy. Adjusting diet as tolerated may help maintain fluid and electrolyte balance and nutritional status and administering antidiarrheal agents. May cause severe diarrhea. Withhold therapy if Grade 3 or 4 diarrhea occurs and until resolved or decreased to Grade 1, then resume at reduced dose.
- Monitor for cerebellar dysfunction (ataxia, confusion, disorientation, visual disturbances). This may persist after discontinuation of therapy.
- Monitor for angina, myocardial infarction/ischemia, arrhythmia, and heart failure in patients with no history of coronary artery disease or myocardial dysfunction. Discontinue therapy if symptoms occur.
- Monitor for signs and symptoms of hyperammonemic encephalopathy (altered mental status, confusion, disorientation, coma, ataxia) with ↑ serum ammonia level within 72 hrs of start of infusion. Discontinue fluorouracil and initiate ammonia-lowering therapy.
- Assess for mucositis, stomatitis, and esophagopharyngitis during therapy. May lead to mucosal sloughing or ulceration. Occurs more frequently with IV bolus doses. If Grade 3 or 4 mucositis occurs, withhold dose and resume at reduced dose when resolved or reduced to Grade 1.
- **Topical:** Inspect involved skin before and throughout therapy.

Lab Test Considerations

- May cause ↓ in plasma albumin.
- Monitor hepatic (AST, ALT, LDH, and serum bilirubin), renal, and hematologic (hematocrit, hemoglobin, leukocyte, platelet count) functions before each treatment and periodically during therapy.
- Monitor CBC daily during IV therapy. Report WBC of <3500/mm³ or platelets <100,000/mm³ immediately; they are criteria for discontinuation. Nadir of leukopenia usually occurs in 9–14 days, with recovery by day 30. May also cause thrombocytopenia. Hold doses if Grade 4 myelosuppression occurs. Resume at reduced dose when resolved or improved to Grade 1.
- May cause ↑ in urine excretion of 5-hydroxyindoleacetic acid (5-HIAA).
- Monitor INR and prothrombin time in patients receiving concomitant warfarin; adjust anticoagulant dose accordingly.

Implementation

- *High Alert:* Fatalities have occurred with incorrect administration of chemotherapeutic agents. Before administering, clarify all ambiguous orders; double-check single, daily, and course-of-therapy dose limits; have second practitioner independently double-check original order, calculations, and infusion pump settings. The number 5 in 5-fluorouracil is part of the drug name and does not refer to the dose.

- Prepare solution in a biologic cabinet. Wear gloves, gown, and mask while handling IV medication. Discard IV equipment in specially designated containers.

- When administering fluorouracil via IV push, 30 min of cryotherapy is recommended to prevent oral mucositis.

IV Administration

- **IV Push:** *Dilution:* May be administered undiluted. *Concentration:* 50 mg/mL. *Rate:* Rapid IV push administration (over 1–2 min) is most effective, but there is a more rapid onset of toxicity.

- **Intermittent Infusion:** *Dilution:* May be diluted with D5W or 0.9% NaCl.

- Use plastic IV tubing and IV bags to maintain greater stability of medication. Solution is stable for 24 hr at room temperature; do not refrigerate. Solution is colorless to faint yellow. Discard highly discolored or cloudy solution. If crystals form, dissolve by warming solution to 140°F, shaking vigorously, and cooling to body temperature. *Concentration:* Up to 50 mg/mL. *Rate:* Onset of toxicity is greatly delayed by administering an infusion over 2–8 hr.

- **Y-Site Compatibility:** acyclovir, allopurinol, amifostine, amikacin, aminophylline, amphotericin B lipid complex, amphotericin B liposomal, ampicillin, ampicillin/sulbactam, anidulafungin, argatroban, azithromycin, aztreonam, bivalirudin, bleomycin, bumetanide, butorphanol, calcium gluconate, carboplatin, carmustine, cefazolin, cefepime, cefotaxime, cefotetan, cefoxitin, ceftazidime, ceftriaxone, cefuroxime, cisatracurium, cisplatin, clindamycin, cyclophosphamide, cyclosporine, dacarbazine, daptomycin, dexamethasone, dexmedetomidine, dexrazoxane, digoxin, docetaxel, dopamine, doxorubicin liposomal, enalaprilat, ephedrine, ertapenem, erythromycin, esmolol, etoposide phosphate, famotidine, fentanyl, fluconazole, fludarabine, foscarnet, fosphenytoin, furosemide, ganciclovir, gemcitabine, gentamicin, granisetron, heparin, hetastarch, hydrocortisone, hydromorphone, ifosfamide, imipenem/cilastatin, isoproterenol, ketorolac, labetalol, leucovorin calcium, lidocaine, linezolid, magnesium sulfate, mannitol, melphalan, meperidine, meropenem, mesna, methohexital, methotrexate, methylprednisolone, metoprolol, metronidazole, milrinone, mitomycin, mitoxantrone, morphine, nalbuphine, naloxone, nitroglycerin, nitroprusside, octreotide, paclitaxel, palonosetron, pamidronate, pantoprazole, pemetrexed, pentobarbital, phenobarbital, phenylephrine, piperacillin/tazobactam, potassium acetate, potassium phosphate, procainamide, propofol, propranolol, remifentanil, rituximab, sargramostim, sodium acetate, sodium bicarbonate, sodium phosphate, succinylcholine, sufentanil, teno-

poside, theophylline, thiopental, thiotepa, tigecycline, tirofiban, tobramycin, trastuzumab, trimethoprim/sulfamethoxazole, vasopressin, vecuronium, vinblastine, vincristine, voriconazole, zidovudine, zoledronic acid.

- **Y-Site Incompatibility:** aldesleukin, amiodarone, amphotericin B deoxycholate, buprenorphine, calcium chloride, caspofungin, chlorpromazine, ciprofloxacin, diazepam, diltiazem, diphenhydramine, dobutamine, doxycycline, droperidol, epinephrine, epirubicin, filgrastim, haloperidol, hydroxyzine, idarubicin, irinotecan, levofloxacin, lorazepam, methadone, midazolam, minocycline, moxifloxacin, nicardipine, pentamidine, phenytoin, prochlorperazine, promethazine, topotecan, vancomycin, verapamil, vinorelbine.

- **Topical:** Consult health care professional before administering topical preparations to determine which skin preparation regimen should be followed. Avoid tight occlusive dressings because of irritation to surrounding healthy tissue. A loose gauze dressing for cosmetic purposes is usually preferred. Wear gloves when applying medication. Do not use metallic applicator.

Patient/Family Teaching

- Explain purpose of fluorouracil to patient.
- Instruct patient to notify health care professional if fever; chills; sore throat; signs of infection; yellowing of skin or eyes; abdominal pain; joint or flank pain; swelling of feet or legs; bleeding gums; bruising; petechiae; or blood in urine, stool, or emesis occurs. Caution patient to avoid crowds and persons with known infections. Instruct patient to use soft toothbrush and electric razor. Patients should be cautioned not to drink alcoholic beverages or take products containing aspirin or NSAIDs.
- Advise patient to rinse mouth with clear water after eating and drinking and to avoid flossing to minimize stomatitis. Viscous lidocaine may be used if mouth pain interferes with eating. Stomatitis pain may require treatment with opioid analgesics.
- Discuss with patient the possibility of hair loss. Explore methods of coping.
- Caution patient to use sunscreen and protective clothing to prevent phototoxicity reactions.
- Instruct patient not to receive any vaccinations without advice of health care professional.
- Instruct patient to notify health care professional of all Rx or OTC medications, vitamins, or herbal products being taken and consult health care professional before taking any new medications. Increase dietary intake of thiamine may be recommended.
- Rep: May cause fetal harm. Advise females of reproductive potential and male patients with female partners of reproductive potential to use effective contraception during therapy and for at least 3 mo

following completion of therapy and to avoid breast-feeding during therapy. Inform patients that fertility may be impaired during therapy.

- Emphasize the importance of routine follow-up lab tests to monitor progress and to check for side effects.
- **Topical:** Instruct patient in correct application of solution or cream. Emphasize importance of avoiding the eyes; caution should also be used when applying medication near mouth and nose. If patient uses clean finger to self-administer, emphasize importance of washing hands thoroughly after application. Explain that erythema, scaling, and blistering with pruritus and burning sensation are expected. Advise patient to avoid sunlight or ultraviolet light (tanning booths) as much as possible; may increase side effects. Therapy is discontinued when erosion, ulceration, and necrosis occur in 2–6 wk (10–12 wk for basal cell carcinomas). Skin heals 4–8 wk later.
- Fluorouracil may be fatal if ingested by pets. Do not allow pets to be in contact with the container or the skin where fluorouracil topical has been applied. Store out of reach of pets. Safely discard or clean any cloth or applicator that may retain fluorouracil and avoid leaving any residues on your hands, clothing, carpeting or furniture.

Evaluation/Desired Outcomes
- Tumor regression.
- Removal of solar keratoses or superficial basal cell skin cancers.

BEERS

▓FLUoxetine (floo-**ox**-uh-teen)
PROzac, ~~Sarafem~~
Classification
Therapeutic: antidepressants
Pharmacologic: selective serotonin reuptake inhibitors (SSRIs)

Indications
Major depressive disorder. Obsessive compulsive disorder (OCD). Bulimia nervosa. Panic disorder. Acute treatment of depressive episodes associated with bipolar I disorder (when used with olanzapine). Treatment-resistant depression (when used with olanzapine). Premenstrual dysphoric disorder (PMDD). **Unlabeled Use:** Anorexia nervosa: Diabetic neuropathy, Fibromyalgia, Obesity, Raynaud's phenomenon, Social anxiety disorder (social phobia), Posttraumatic stress disorder.

Action
Selectively inhibits the reuptake of serotonin in the CNS. **Therapeutic Effects:** Antidepressant action. Decreased behaviors associated with: panic disorder, bulimia. Decreased mood alterations associated with PMDD.

Pharmacokinetics
Absorption: Well absorbed after oral administration.
Distribution: Crosses the blood-brain barrier.
Protein Binding: 94.5%.
Metabolism and Excretion: Converted by the liver to norfluoxetine (primarily by the CYP2D6 isoenzyme), another antidepressant compound; ▓ the CYP2D6 enzyme system exhibits genetic polymorphism (~7% of population may be poor metabolizers and may have significantly ↑ fluoxetine concentrations and an ↑ risk of adverse effects). Fluoxetine and norfluoxetine are mostly metabolized by the liver; 12% excreted by kidneys as unchanged fluoxetine, 7% as unchanged norfluoxetine.
Half-life: 1–3 days (norfluoxetine 5–7 days).

TIME/ACTION PROFILE (antidepressant effect)

ROUTE	ONSET	PEAK	DURATION
PO	1–4 wk	unknown	2 wk

Contraindications/Precautions
Contraindicated in: Hypersensitivity; Concurrent use of MAO inhibitors or MAO-like drugs (linezolid or methylene blue); Concurrent use of pimozide; Concurrent use of thioridazine (fluoxetine should be discontinued at least 5 wk before thioridazine therapy is initiated).
Use Cautiously in: History of seizures; Debilitated patients (↑ risk of seizures); Diabetes mellitus; Patients with concurrent chronic illness or multiple drug therapy (dose adjustments may be necessary); Hepatic impairment (↓ doses/↑ dosing interval may be necessary); May ↑ risk of suicide attempt/ideation especially during early treatment or dose adjustment; Congenital long QT syndrome, history of QT interval prolongation, family history of long QT syndrome or sudden cardiac death, concurrent use of QT interval prolonging drugs, hypokalemia, hypomagnesemia, recent MI, uncompensated HF, or bradycardia; Angle-closure glaucoma; OB: Use during pregnancy only if potential maternal benefit justifies potential fetal risk. Use during first trimester may ↑ risk of cardiovascular malformations in infant. Use during third trimester may result in neonatal serotonin syndrome requiring prolonged hospitalization, respiratory and nutritional support. Use may also be associated with persistent pulmonary hypertension in newborn. May cause sedation in infant; Lactation: Use while breastfeeding only if potential maternal benefit justifies potential risk to infant; Pedi: Risk of suicidal ideation or attempt may be greater in children or adolescents; Pedi: Children <7 yr (safety and effectiveness not established); Geri: Appears on Beers list. May worsen or cause syndrome of inappropriate antidiuretic hormone (SIADH) secretion and/or hyponatremia in older adults. Use with caution in older adults and closely monitor sodium concentrations when starting therapy or ↑ dose.

Adverse Reactions/Side Effects

CV: chest pain, palpitations, QT interval prolongation, TORSADES DE POINTES. **Derm:** ↑ sweating, pruritus, erythema nodosum, flushing, rash. **EENT:** mydriasis, stuffy nose, visual disturbances. **Endo:** SIADH, dysmenorrhea, hot flush. **F and E:** hyponatremia. **GI:** diarrhea, abdominal pain, abnormal taste, anorexia, constipation, dry mouth, dyspepsia, nausea, vomiting, weight loss. **GU:** ↓ libido, delayed/absent orgasm, ejaculatory delay/failure, erectile dysfunction, urinary frequency. **Hemat:** BLEEDING. **MS:** arthralgia, back pain, myalgia. **Neuro:** anxiety, drowsiness, headache, insomnia, nervousness, tremor, abnormal dreams, dizziness, fatigue, hypomania, mania, NEUROLEPTIC MALIGNANT SYNDROME, SEIZURES, SUICIDAL THOUGHTS, weakness. **Resp:** cough. **Misc:** fever, flu-like syndrome, hypersensitivity reactions, SEROTONIN SYNDROME.

Interactions

Drug-Drug: Discontinue use of **MAO inhibitors** for 14 days before fluoxetine therapy; combined therapy may result in confusion, agitation, seizures, hypertension, and hyperpyrexia (serotonin syndrome). Fluoxetine should be discontinued for at least 5 wk before MAO inhibitor therapy is initiated. Concurrent use with **MAO-inhibitor-like drugs,** such as **linezolid** or **methylene blue** may ↑ risk of serotonin syndrome; concurrent use contraindicated; do not start therapy in patients receiving **linezolid** or **methylene blue**; if **linezolid** or **methylene blue** need to be started in a patient receiving fluoxetine, immediately discontinue fluoxetine and monitor for signs/symptoms of serotonin syndrome for 2 wk or until 24 hr after last dose of linezolid or methylene blue, whichever comes first (may resume fluoxetine therapy 24 hr after last dose of linezolid or methylene blue). Concurrent use with **pimozide** may ↑ risk of QT interval prolongation. ↑ levels of **thioridazine** may ↑ risk of QT interval prolongation (concurrent use contraindicated; fluoxetine should be discontinued for at least 5 wk before thioridazine is initiated). **QT interval prolonging drugs** may ↑ the risk of QT interval prolongation with arrhythmias; avoid concurrent use. **Ritonavir** and **efavirenz** may ↑ the risk of developing the serotonin syndrome. For concurrent use with **ritonavir** ↓ fluoxetine dose by 70%; if initiating fluoxetine, start with 10 mg/day dose. ↓ metabolism and ↑ effects of **alprazolam** (decrease alprazolam dose by 50%). Drugs that affect serotonergic neurotransmitter systems, including **tricyclic antidepressants, SNRIs, fentanyl, lithium, buspirone, tramadol, meperidine, methadone, amphetamines,** and **triptans** ↑ risk of serotonin syndrome. ↑ CNS depression with **alcohol, antihistamines,** other **antidepressants, opioid analgesics,** or **sedative/hypnotics.** ↑ risk of side effects and adverse reactions with other **antidepressants, risperidone,** or **phenothiazines.** May ↑ effectiveness/risk of toxicity from **carbamazepine, clozapine, digoxin, haloperidol, phenytoin, lithium,** or **warfarin.** May ↓ the effects of **buspirone. Cyproheptadine** may ↓ or reverse effects of fluoxetine. May ↑ sensitivity to **adrenergics** and increase the risk of serotonin syndrome. May alter the activity of other **drugs that are highly bound to plasma proteins.** ↑ risk of serotonin syndrome with **5HT₁ agonists.** ↑ risk of bleeding with **NSAIDs, aspirin, clopidogrel, prasugrel, ticagrelor, dabigatran, apixaban, edoxaban, rivaroxaban,** or **warfarin.**

Drug-Natural Products: ↑ risk of serotonin syndrome with **St. John's wort** and **SAMe.**

Route/Dosage

PO (Adults): *Depression or OCD:* 20 mg/day in the morning. After several wk, may ↑ by 20 mg/day at weekly intervals. Doses greater than 20 mg/day should be given in 2 divided doses, in the morning and at noon (not to exceed 80 mg/day). Patients who have been stabilized on the 20 mg/day dose may be switched over to delayed-release capsules at dose of 90 mg once weekly, initiated 7 days after the last 20-mg dose. *Panic disorder:* 10 mg/day initially, may ↑ after 1 wk to 20 mg/day (usual dose is 20 mg, but may be ↑ as needed/tolerated up to 60 mg/day). *Bulimia nervosa:* 60 mg/day (may need to titrate up to dosage over several days). *PMDD:* 20 mg/day (not to exceed 80 mg/day) *or* 20 mg/day starting 14 days prior to expected onset on menses, continued through first full day of menstruation, repeated with each cycle. *Depressive episodes associated with bipolar I disorder:* 20 mg/day with olanzapine 5 mg/day (both given in evening); may ↑ fluoxetine dose up to 50 mg/day and olanzapine dose up to 12.5 mg/day; *Treatment-resistant depression:* 20 mg/day with olanzapine 5 mg/day (both given in evening); may ↑ fluoxetine dose up to 50 mg/day and olanzapine dose up to 20 mg/day.

PO (Geriatric Patients): *Depression:* 10 mg/day in the morning initially, may be ↑ (not to exceed 60 mg/day).

PO (Children 7–17 yr): *Depression or OCD (adolescents and higher weight children):* 10 mg/day may be ↑ after 2 wk to 20 mg/day; additional increases may be made after several more wk (range 20–60 mg/day); *Depression or OCD (lower-weight children):* 10 mg/day initially, may be ↑ after several more wk (range 20–30 mg/day).

PO (Children 10–17 yr): *Depressive episodes associated with bipolar I disorder:* 20 mg/day with olanzapine 2.5 mg/day (both given in evening); may ↑ fluoxetine dose up to 50 mg/day and olanzapine dose up to 12 mg/day.

Availability (generic available)

Tablets: 10 mg, 20 mg, 60 mg. **Capsules:** 10 mg, 20 mg, 40 mg, ✦60 mg. **Delayed-release capsules:** 90 mg. **Oral solution (mint flavor):** 20 mg/5 mL. *In*

combination with: olanzapine (Symbyax; see Appendix N).

NURSING IMPLICATIONS

Assessment

- Monitor mood changes. Inform health care professional if patient demonstrates significant increase in anxiety, nervousness, or insomnia.
- Assess for suicidal tendencies, especially during early therapy. Restrict amount of drug available to patient. Risk may be increased in children, adolescents, and adults ≤24 yr. After starting therapy, children, adolescents, and young adults should be seen by health care professional at least weekly for 4 wk, every 3 wk for next 4 wk, and on advice of health care professional thereafter.
- Monitor appetite and nutritional intake. Weigh weekly. Notify health care professional of continued weight loss. Adjust diet as tolerated to support nutritional status.
- Assess for sensitivity reaction (urticaria, fever, arthralgia, edema, carpal tunnel syndrome, rash, hives, lymphadenopathy, respiratory distress) and notify health care professional if present; symptoms usually resolve by stopping fluoxetine but may require administration of antihistamines or corticosteroids.
- Assess sexual function before starting fluoxetine. Assess for changes in sexual function during treatment, including timing of onset; patient may not report.
- Monitor for development of neuroleptic malignant syndrome (fever, respiratory distress, tachycardia, seizures, diaphoresis, arrhythmias, hypertension or hypotension, pallor, tiredness, severe muscle stiffness, loss of bladder control). Report immediately.
- Assess for serotonin syndrome (mental changes [agitation, hallucinations, coma], autonomic instability [tachycardia, labile BP, hyperthermia], neuromuscular aberrations [hyperreflexia, incoordination], and/or GI symptoms [nausea, vomiting, diarrhea]), especially in patients taking other serotonergic drugs (SSRIs, SNRIs, triptans).
- **OCD:** Assess for frequency of obsessive-compulsive behaviors. Note degree to which these thoughts and behaviors interfere with daily functioning.
- **Bulimia Nervosa:** Assess frequency of binge eating and vomiting during therapy.
- **PMDD:** Monitor mood prior to and periodically during therapy.

Lab Test Considerations

- Monitor CBC and differential periodically during therapy. Notify health care professional if leukopenia, anemia, thrombocytopenia, or increased bleeding time occurs.
- Proteinuria and mild ↑ in AST may occur during sensitivity reactions.
- May cause ↑ in serum alkaline phosphatase, ALT, BUN, and CK, as well as hyperuricemia, hypocalcemia, hypoglycemia, hyperglycemia, and hyponatremia.
- May cause hypoglycemia in patient with diabetes.

Implementation

- Do not confuse fluoxetine with duloxetine or paroxetine. Do not confuse Prozac with Prilosec, Prograf, or Provera.
- **PO:** Administer as a single dose in the morning. Some patients may require increased amounts, in divided doses, with a 2nd dose at noon.
- May be administered with food to minimize GI irritation. *DNC:* Do not open, dissolve, chew, or crush delayed-release capsules.
- Delayed release capsules may be started after last dose of *PROzac* 20 mg. Dose may be increased after several wk if improvement not clinically significant.

Patient/Family Teaching

- Instruct patient to take fluoxetine as directed. Take missed doses as soon as remembered unless almost time for next dose, then omit and return to regular schedule. Do not double doses or discontinue without consulting health care professional; discontinuation may cause anxiety, insomnia, nervousness.
- May cause drowsiness, dizziness, impaired judgment, and blurred vision. Caution patient to avoid driving and other activities requiring alertness until response to the drug is known.
- Advise patient, family, and caregivers to watch for suicidality, especially during early therapy or dose changes. Notify health care professional immediately if thoughts about suicide or dying, attempts to commit suicide, new or worse depression or anxiety, agitation or restlessness, panic attacks, insomnia, new or worse irritability, aggressiveness, acting on dangerous impulses, mania, or other changes in mood or behavior, or if symptoms of serotonin syndrome occur.
- Instruct patient to notify health care professional of all Rx or OTC medications, vitamins, or herbal products being taken and consult health care professional before taking any new medications. Advise patient to avoid taking other CNS depressants, including opioids, or alcohol.
- Caution patient to change positions slowly to minimize dizziness.
- Inform patient that frequent mouth rinses, good oral hygiene, and sugarless gum or candy may minimize dry mouth. If dry mouth persists for more than 2 wk, consult health care professional regarding use of saliva substitute.
- Caution patient to wear protective clothing and use sunscreen to prevent photosensitivity reactions.
- Advise patient to notify health care professional if symptoms of sensitivity reaction occur or if headache, nausea, anorexia, anxiety, or insomnia persists.
- Inform patient that fluoxetine may cause symptoms of sexual dysfunction. In males, ejaculatory delay or failure, decreased libido, and erectile dysfunction may occur. In female patients, may result in decreased libido and delayed or absent orgasm. Advise

patient to notify health care professional if symptoms occur.

- Rep: May cause fetal harm. Advise females of reproductive potential to notify health care professional if pregnancy is planned or suspected, or if breastfeeding. Use during first trimester may ↑ risk of cardiovascular malformations in infant. Monitor infants exposed to fluoxetine during 3rd trimester for respiratory distress, cyanosis, apnea, seizures, temperature instability, feeding difficulty, vomiting, hypoglycemia, hypotonia, hypertonia, hyperreflexia, tremors, jitteriness, irritability, and constant crying. May increase risk of postpartum hemorrhage. Monitor infants exposed to fluoxetine via breast milk for agitation, irritability, poor feeding, and poor weight gain. Inform patient of pregnancy exposure registry that monitors pregnancy outcomes in women exposed to antidepressants during pregnancy. Register patient by calling the National Pregnancy Registry for Antidepressants at 1-866-961-2388 or visiting online at https://womensmentalhealth.org/clinical-and-researchprograms/pregnancyregistry/antidepressants/.
- Emphasize the importance of follow-up exams to monitor progress.

Evaluation/Desired Outcomes

- Increased sense of well-being.
- Renewed interest in surroundings. May require 1–4 wk of therapy to obtain antidepressant effects.
- Decrease in obsessive-compulsive behaviors.
- Decrease in binge eating and vomiting in patients with bulimia nervosa.
- Decreased incidence frequency of panic attacks.
- Decreased mood alterations associated with PMDD.

---

flurandrenolide, See CORTICOSTEROIDS (TOPICAL/LOCAL).

fluticasone, See CORTICOSTEROIDS (INHALATION).

fluticasone, See CORTICOSTEROIDS (NASAL).

fluticasone, See CORTICOSTEROIDS (TOPICAL/LOCAL).

fluvastatin, See HMG-CoA REDUCTASE INHIBITORS (statins).

⚕ fluvoxaMINE
(floo-**voks**-a-meen)
✦ Luvox, ~~Luvox CR~~

Classification
Therapeutic: antidepressants, antiobsessive agents
Pharmacologic: selective serotonin reuptake inhibitors (SSRIs)

Indications
Obsessive-compulsive disorder. **Unlabeled Use:** Depression. Generalized anxiety disorder. Social anxiety disorder. Post-traumatic stress disorder.

Action
Inhibits the reuptake of serotonin in the CNS. **Therapeutic Effects:** Decrease in obsessive-compulsive behaviors.

Pharmacokinetics
Absorption: 53% absorbed after oral administration.
Distribution: Enters the CNS. Remainder of distribution not known.
Metabolism and Excretion: Mostly metabolized by the liver via the CYP2D6 isoenzyme; ⚕ the CYP2D6 isoenzyme exhibits genetic polymorphism; ~7% of population may be poor metabolizers and may have significantly ↑ fluvoxamine concentrations and an ↑ risk of adverse effects.
Half-life: 13.6–15.6 hr.

TIME/ACTION PROFILE (improvement on obsessive-compulsive behaviors)

ROUTE	ONSET	PEAK	DURATION
PO	within 2–3 wk	several mo	unknown

Contraindications/Precautions
Contraindicated in: Hypersensitivity to fluvoxamine or other SSRIs; Concurrent use of MAO inhibitors (or within 14 days of discontinuing fluvoxamine), MAO inhibitor-like drugs (linezolid or methylene blue), alosetron, pimozide, thioridazine, or tizanidine.
Use Cautiously in: Hepatic impairment; Risk of suicide (may ↑ risk of suicide attempt/ideation especially during early treatment or dose adjustment); Angle-closure glaucoma; OB: Neonates exposed to SSRI in third trimester may develop drug discontinuation syndrome including respiratory distress, feeding difficulty, and irritability; Lactation: Use while breastfeeding only if potential maternal benefit justifies potential risk to infant; Pedi: Risk of suicidal ideation or attempt may be greater in children or adolescents; Pedi: Safety and effectiveness not established in children <18 yr (controlled release) and <8 yr (immediate-release); Geri: Appears on Beers list. May worsen or cause syndrome

602 fluvoxaMINE

of inappropriate antidiuretic hormone (SIADH) secretion and/or hyponatremia in older adults. Use with caution in older adults and closely monitor sodium concentrations when starting therapy or ↑ dose.

Adverse Reactions/Side Effects

CV: edema, hypertension, palpitations, postural hypotension, tachycardia. **Derm:** ↑ sweating. **EENT:** sinusitis. **Endo:** SIADH. **F and E:** hyponatremia. **GI:** constipation, diarrhea, dry mouth, dyspepsia, nausea, ↑ liver enzymes, anorexia, dysphagia, flatulence, vomiting, weight loss. **GU:** ↓ libido, delayed/absent orgasm, ejaculatory delay/failure, erectile dysfunction. **Hemat:** BLEEDING. **Metab:** weight gain. **MS:** hypertonia, myoclonus/twitching. **Neuro:** dizziness, drowsiness, headache, insomnia, nervousness, weakness, agitation, anxiety, apathy, depression, emotional lability, hypokinesia/hyperkinesia, manic reactions, NEUROLEPTIC MALIGNANT SYNDROME, psychotic reactions, sedation, SUICIDAL THOUGHTS, syncope, tremor. **Resp:** cough, dyspnea. **Misc:** chills, flu-like symptoms, hypersensitivity reactions, SEROTONIN SYNDROME, tooth disorder/caries, yawning.

Interactions

Drug-Drug: Concurrent use with **MAO inhibitors** may result in serious potentially fatal reactions (MAO inhibitors should be stopped at least 14 days before fluvoxamine therapy. Fluvoxamine should be stopped at least 14 days before MAO inhibitor therapy). Concurrent use with **MAO-inhibitor-like drugs**, such as **linezolid** or **methylene blue** may ↑ risk of serotonin syndrome; concurrent use contraindicated; do not start therapy in patients receiving **linezolid** or **methylene blue**; if **linezolid** or **methylene blue** need to be started in a patient receiving fluvoxamine, immediately discontinue fluvoxamine and monitor for signs/symptoms of serotonin syndrome for 2 wk or until 24 hr after last dose of linezolid or methylene blue, whichever comes first (may resume fluvoxamine therapy 24 hr after last dose of linezolid or methylene blue). **Smoking** may ↓ effectiveness of fluvoxamine. Concurrent use with **tricyclic antidepressants** may ↑ plasma levels of fluvoxamine. Drugs that affect serotonergic neurotransmitter systems, including **tricyclic antidepressants**, **SNRIs**, **fentanyl**, **lithium**, **buspirone**, **tramadol**, **meperidine**, **methadone**, **amphetamines**, and **triptans** ↑ risk of serotonin syndrome. ↓ metabolism and may ↑ effects of some **beta blockers (propranolol)**, **alosetron** (avoid concurrent use), some **benzodiazepines** (avoid concurrent **diazepam**), **carbamazepine**, **methadone**, **lithium**, **theophylline** (↓ dose to 33% of usual dose), **ramelteon** (avoid concurrent use), **warfarin**, and L-**tryptophan**. ↑ risk of bleeding with **NSAIDs**, **aspirin**, **clopidogrel**, **prasugrel**, **ticagrelor**, **dabigatran**, **apixaban**, **edoxaban**, **rivaroxaban**, or **warfarin**. ↑ blood levels and risk of toxicity from **clozapine** (dose adjustments may be necessary).
Drug-Natural Products: Use with **St. John's wort** ↑ of serotonin syndrome.

Route/Dosage

PO (Adults): *Immediate release:* 50 mg daily at bedtime; ↑ by 50 mg every 4–7 days until desired effect is achieved. If daily dose >100 mg, give in 2 equally divided doses or give a larger dose at bedtime (not to exceed 300 mg/day); *Controlled release:* 100 mg at bedtime; ↑ by 50 mg every 7 days until desired effect is achieved, not to exceed 300 mg/day.
PO (Children 8–17 yr): *Immediate release:* 25 mg at bedtime, may ↑ by 25 mg/day every 4–7 days (not to exceed 200 mg/day; daily doses >50 mg should be given in divided doses with a larger dose at bedtime).

Hepatic Impairment
PO (Adults): *Immediate release:* 25 mg daily at bedtime initially, slower titration, and longer dosing intervals should be used.

Availability (generic available)
Tablets: 25 mg, 50 mg, 100 mg. **Controlled-release capsules:** 100 mg, 150 mg.

NURSING IMPLICATIONS
Assessment
- Monitor mood changes. Assess patient for frequency of obsessive-compulsive behaviors. Note degree to which these thoughts and behaviors interfere with daily functioning. Inform health care professional if patient demonstrates significant increase in anxiety, nervousness, or insomnia.
- Assess for suicidal tendencies, especially during early therapy. Restrict amount of drug available to patient. Risk may be increased in children, adolescents, and adults ≤24 yr. After starting therapy, children, adolescents, and young adults should be seen by health care professional at least weekly for 4 wk, every 3 wk for next 4 wk, and on advice of health care professional thereafter.
- Monitor appetite and nutritional intake. Weigh weekly. Report significant changes in weight. Adjust diet as tolerated to support nutritional status.
- Assess sexual function before starting fluvoxamine. Assess for changes in sexual function during treatment, including timing of onset; patient may not report.
- Assess for serotonin syndrome (mental changes [agitation, hallucinations, coma], autonomic instability [tachycardia, labile BP, hyperthermia], neuromuscular aberrations [hyperreflexia, incoordination], and/or GI symptoms [nausea, vomiting, diarrhea]), especially in patients taking other serotonergic drugs (SSRIs, SNRIs, triptans).

Toxicity and Overdose
- Common symptoms of toxicity include drowsiness, vomiting, diarrhea, and dizziness. Coma, tachycardia, bradycardia, hypotension, ECG abnormalities, liver function abnormalities, and convulsions may also occur. Treatment is symptomatic and supportive.

Implementation

- Do not confuse fluvoxamine with fluphenazine or flavoxate.
- Taper to avoid withdrawal effects. Reduce dose by 50% for 3 days, then reduce by 50% for 3 days, then discontinue.
- PO: Initial therapy is administered as a single bedtime dose. May be increased every 4–7 days as tolerated.
- Fluvoxamine may be given without regard to meals. *DNC:* Do not open, break, crush, or chew controlled-release capsules.

Patient/Family Teaching

- Instruct patient to take fluvoxamine as directed. Do not skip or double up on missed doses. Improvement in symptoms may be noticed in 2–3 wk, but medication should be continued as directed.
- May cause drowsiness and dizziness. Caution patient to avoid driving and other activities requiring alertness until response to medication is known.
- Advise patient, family, and caregivers to look for suicidality, especially during early therapy or dose changes. Notify health care professional immediately if thoughts about suicide or dying, attempts to commit suicide, new or worse depression or anxiety, agitation or restlessness, panic attacks, insomnia, new or worse irritability, aggressiveness, acting on dangerous impulses, mania, or other changes in mood or behavior or if symptoms of serotonin syndrome occur.
- Advise patient to notify health care professional if rash or hives occur or if headache, nausea, anorexia, anxiety, or insomnia persists.
- Instruct patient to notify health care professional of all Rx or OTC medications, vitamins, or herbal products being taken and consult health care professional before taking any new medications, especially St. John's wort. Advise patient to avoid taking other CNS depressants, including opioids, or alcohol.
- Advise patient to avoid use of caffeine (chocolate, tea, cola).
- Inform patient that fluvoxamine may cause symptoms of sexual dysfunction. In males, ejaculatory delay or failure, decreased libido, and erectile dysfunction may occur. In female patients, may result in decreased libido and delayed or absent orgasm. Advise patient to notify health care professional if symptoms occur.
- Rep: May cause fetal harm. Advise females of reproductive potential to notify health care professional if pregnancy is planned or suspected, or if breastfeeding. Monitor infants exposed to fluvoxamine during 3rd trimester for respiratory distress, cyanosis, apnea, seizures, temperature instability, feeding difficulty, vomiting, hypoglycemia, hypotonia, hypertonia, hyperreflexia, tremors, jitteriness, irritability,

and constant crying. May increase risk of postpartum hemorrhage. Monitor infants exposed to fluvoxamine via breast milk for agitation, irritability, poor feeding, and poor weight gain. Inform patient of pregnancy exposure registry that monitors pregnancy outcomes in women exposed to antidepressants during pregnancy. Register patient by calling the National Pregnancy Registry for Antidepressants at 1-866-961-2388 or visiting online at https://womensmentalhealth.org/clinical-and-research-programs/pregnancyregistry/antidepressants/.
- Emphasize the importance of follow-up exams to monitor progress.

Evaluation/Desired Outcomes

- Decrease in symptoms of obsessive-compulsive disorder.

HIGH ALERT

fondaparinux (fon-da-**par**-i-nux)
Arixtra
Classification
Therapeutic: anticoagulants
Pharmacologic: active factor X inhibitors

Indications
Prevention and treatment of deep vein thrombosis (DVT) and pulmonary embolism (PE). **Unlabeled Use:** Systemic anticoagulation for other diagnoses.

Action
Binds selectively to antithrombin III (AT III). This binding potentiates the neutralization (inactivation) of active factor X (Xa). **Therapeutic Effects:** Interruption of the coagulation cascade resulting in inhibition of thrombus formation. Prevention of thrombus formation decreases the risk of pulmonary emboli.

Pharmacokinetics
Absorption: 100% absorbed following SUBQ administration.
Distribution: Distributes mainly throughout the intravascular space.
Metabolism and Excretion: Eliminated mainly unchanged in urine.
Half-life: 17–21 hr.

TIME/ACTION PROFILE (anticoagulant effect)

ROUTE	ONSET	PEAK	DURATION
SUBQ	rapid	3 hr	24 hr

Contraindications/Precautions
Contraindicated in: Hypersensitivity; Severe renal impairment (CCr <30 mL/min; ↑ risk of bleeding); Body weight <50 kg (for prophylaxis) (markedly ↑ risk of bleeding); Active major bleeding; Bacterial en-

docarditis; Thrombocytopenia due to fondaparinux antibodies.

Use Cautiously in: Mild to moderate renal impairment (CCr 30–50 mL/min); Untreated hypertension; Recent history of ulcer disease; Body weight <50 kg (for treatment of DVT or PE) (may ↑ risk of bleeding); Malignancy; History of heparin-induced thrombocytopenia; OB: Use during pregnancy should be limited to those who have severe allergic reactions to heparin, including heparin-induced thrombocytopenia; Lactation: Safety not established in breastfeeding; Pedi: Safety and effectiveness not established in children; Geri: ↑ risk of bleeding in older adults.

Exercise Extreme Caution in: History of congenital or acquired bleeding disorder; Severe uncontrolled hypertension; Hemorrhagic stroke; Recent CNS or ophthalmologic surgery; Active GI bleeding/ulceration; Retinopathy (hypertensive or diabetic); Neuraxial spinal anesthesia or spinal puncture, especially if concurrent with an indwelling epidural catheter, drugs affecting hemostasis, history of traumatic/repeated spinal puncture or spinal deformity (↑ risk of spinal/epidural hematoma that may lead to long-term or permanent paralysis).

Adverse Reactions/Side Effects

CV: edema, hypotension. **Derm:** bullous eruption, hematoma, purpura, rash. **F and E:** hypokalemia. **GI:** ↑ liver enzymes, constipation, diarrhea, dyspepsia, nausea, vomiting. **GU:** urinary retention. **Hemat:** BLEEDING, thrombocytopenia. **Neuro:** confusion, dizziness, headache, insomnia. **Misc:** fever, HYPERSENSITIVITY REACTIONS (including angioedema).

Interactions

Drug-Drug: Risk of bleeding may be ↑ by concurrent use of **warfarin** or **drugs that affect platelet function**, including **aspirin**, **NSAIDs**, **dipyridamole**, some **cephalosporins**, **valproates**, **clopidogrel**, **prasugrel**, **ticagrelor**, **eptifibatide**, **tirofiban**, and **dextran**.

Drug-Natural Products: ↑ risk of bleeding with **arnica**, **chamomile**, **clove**, **dong quai**, **feverfew**, **garlic**, **ginger**, **gingko**, *Panax ginseng*, and others.

Route/Dosage

Treatment of Deep Vein Thrombosis/Pulmonary Embolism

SUBQ (Adults >100 kg): 10 mg once daily for at least 5 days until therapeutic anticoagulation with warfarin is achieved (INR >2 for 2 consecutive days); warfarin may be started within 72 hr of fondaparinux.

SUBQ (Adults 50–100 kg): 7.5 mg once daily for at least 5 days until therapeutic anticoagulation with warfarin is achieved (INR >2 for 2 consecutive days).

SUBQ (Adults <50 kg): 5 mg once daily for at least 5 days until therapeutic anticoagulation with warfarin is achieved (INR >2 for 2 consecutive days); warfarin may be started within 72 hr of fondaparinux (has been used for up to 26 days).

Prevention of Deep Vein Thrombosis/Pulmonary Embolism

SUBQ (Adults): 2.5 mg once daily, starting 6–8 hr after surgery, continuing for 5–9 days (up to 11 days) following abdominal surgery or knee/hip replacement or continuing for 24 days following hip fracture surgery (up to 32 days).

Availability (generic available)

Solution for injection (prefilled syringes): 2.5 mg/0.5 mL, 5 mg/0.4 mL, 7.5 mg/0.6 mL, 10 mg/0.8 mL.

NURSING IMPLICATIONS

Assessment

- Assess for signs of bleeding and hemorrhage (bleeding gums; nosebleed; unusual bruising; black, tarry stools; hematuria; fall in hematocrit; sudden drop in BP; guaiac positive stools); bleeding from surgical site. Notify health care professional if these occur.
- Assess for evidence of additional or increased thrombosis. Symptoms will depend on area of involvement. Monitor neurological status frequently for signs of impairment, especially in patients with indwelling epidural catheters for administration of analgesia or with concomitant use of drugs affecting hemostasis (NSAIDs, platelet inhibitors, other anticoagulants). Risk is increased by traumatic or repeated epidural or spinal puncture. May require urgent treatment.

Lab Test Considerations

- Monitor platelet count closely; may cause thrombocytopenia. If platelet count is <100,000/mm^3, discontinue fondaparinux.
- Fondaparinux is not accurately measured by PT, activated aPTT, or international standards of heparin or low-molecular-weight heparins. If unexpected changes in coagulation parameters or major bleeding occurs, discontinue fondaparinux.
- Monitor CBC, serum creatinine levels, and stool occult blood tests routinely during therapy.
- May cause asymptomatic ↑ in AST and ALT. Elevations are fully reversible and not associated with ↑ in bilirubin.
- May cause ↑ aPTT temporally associated with bleeding with or without concomitant administration of other anticoagulants and thrombocytopenia with thrombosis similar to heparin-induced thrombocytopenia, with or without exposure to heparin or low-molecular-weight heparins.

Implementation

- *High Alert:* Do not confuse Arixtra with Arista AH (absorbable hemostatic agent).
- Fondaparinux cannot be used interchangeably with heparin, low-molecular-weight heparins, or heparinoids as they differ in manufacturing process, anti-Xa and anti-IIa activity, units, and dose. Each of these medications has its own instructions for use.

- Initial dose should be administered 6–8 hr after surgery. Administration before 6 hr after surgery has been associated with risk of major bleeding.
- **SUBQ:** Administer SUBQ only into fatty tissue, alternating sites between right and left anterolateral or posterolateral abdominal wall. Inject entire length of needle at a 45° or 90° angle into a skin fold held between thumb and forefinger; hold skin fold throughout injection. Do not aspirate or massage. Rotate sites frequently. Do not administer IM because of danger of hematoma formation. Solution should be clear; do not inject solution containing particulate matter. Do not mix with other injections.
- Fondaparinux is provided in a single-dose prefilled syringe with an automatic needle protection system. Do not expel air bubble from prefilled syringe before injection to prevent loss of drug.

Patient/Family Teaching

- Advise patient to report any symptoms of unusual bleeding or bruising, dizziness, itching, rash, fever, swelling, or difficulty breathing to health care professional immediately.
- Instruct patient not to take aspirin or NSAIDs without consulting health care professional during therapy.
- Rep: Advise females of reproductive potential to notify health care professional if pregnancy is planned or suspected or if breastfeeding.

Evaluation/Desired Outcomes

- Prevention and treatment of DVT and PE.

foscarnet (foss-kar-net)
Foscavir, ✦Vocarvi
Classification
Therapeutic: antivirals

Indications
Treatment of cytomegalovirus (CMV) retinitis in patients with HIV (alone or in combination with ganciclovir). Treatment of acyclovir-resistant mucocutaneous herpes simplex virus (HSV) infections in immunocompromised patients.

Action
Prevents viral replication by inhibiting viral DNA-polymerase and reverse transcriptase. **Therapeutic Effects:** Virustatic action against susceptible viruses including CMV.

Pharmacokinetics
Absorption: IV administration results in complete bioavailability.
Distribution: Variable penetration into CSF. May concentrate in and be slowly released from bone.
Metabolism and Excretion: 80–90% excreted unchanged in urine.

Half-life: 3 hr (in patients with normal renal function); longer half-life of 90 hr may reflect release of drug from bone.

TIME/ACTION PROFILE

ROUTE	ONSET	PEAK	DURATION
IV	rapid	end of infusion	8–24 hr

Contraindications/Precautions
Contraindicated in: Hypersensitivity; HF (due to sodium content); Patients on sodium-restricted diets; Hemodialysis; Lactation: Lactation.
Use Cautiously in: Renal impairment (dose ↓ required if CCr ≤1.4–1.6 mL/min/kg); Seizure disorders; QT interval prolongation or cardiovascular disease; Hypokalemia or hypomagnesemia (must be corrected prior to therapy); OB: Safety not established in pregnancy; Pedi: Safety and effectiveness not established in children.

Adverse Reactions/Side Effects
CV: chest pain, edema, palpitations, QT interval prolongation, TORSADES DE POINTES. **Derm:** ↑ sweating, pruritus, rash, skin ulceration. **EENT:** conjunctivitis, eye pain, vision abnormalities. **F and E:** hypocalcemia, hypokalemia, hypomagnesemia, hyperphosphatemia, hypophosphatemia. **GI:** diarrhea, nausea, vomiting, abdominal pain, abnormal taste sensation, anorexia, constipation, dyspepsia. **GU:** renal failure, albuminuria, dysuria, nocturia, polyuria, urinary retention. **Hemat:** anemia, leukopenia, neutropenia. **Local:** pain/inflammation at injection site. **MS:** arthralgia, myalgia, back pain, involuntary muscle contraction. **Neuro:** headache, anxiety, ataxia, confusion, depression, dizziness, fatigue, hypoesthesia, neuropathy, paresthesia, SEIZURES, tremor, weakness. **Resp:** cough, dyspnea. **Misc:** fever, chills, flu-like syndrome, HYPERSENSITIVITY REACTIONS (including anaphylaxis, urticaria, and angioedema), MALIGNANCY.

Interactions
Drug-Drug: QT interval prolonging medications, including **quinidine**, **procainamide**, **amiodarone**, **sotalol**, **chlorpromazine**, **thioridazine**, **moxifloxacin**, **pentamidine**, and **methadone**, may ↑ risk of QT interval prolongation; avoid concurrent use. Concurrent use with parenteral **pentamidine** may result in severe, life-threatening hypocalcemia. Risk of nephrotoxicity may be ↑ by concurrent use of other **nephrotoxic agents**, including **amphotericin B**, **aminoglycosides**, **cyclosporine**, **acyclovir**, **methotrexate**, **tacrolimus**, and **pentamidine (IV)**.

Route/Dosage
Cytomegalovirus Retinitis
IV (Adults): 60 mg/kg every 8 hr or 90 mg/kg every 12 hr for 2–3 wk, then 90–120 mg/kg/day as a single

dose. Dose ↓ required for any degree of renal impairment.

Herpes Simplex Virus

IV (Adults): 40 mg/kg every 8–12 hr for 2–3 wk or until healing occurs.

Availability (generic available)

Solution for injection: 24 mg/mL.

NURSING IMPLICATIONS

Assessment

- Monitor ECG periodically during therapy for QT interval prolongation.
- **CMV Retinitis:** Diagnosis of CMV retinitis should be determined by ophthalmoscopy before treatment with foscarnet. Ophthalmologic examinations should also be performed at the conclusion of induction and every 4 wk during maintenance therapy.
- Culture for CMV (urine, blood, throat) may be taken before administration. However, a negative CMV culture does not rule out CMV retinitis.
- **HSV Infections:** Assess lesions before and daily during therapy.

Lab Test Considerations

- Monitor serum creatinine before and 2–3 times weekly during induction therapy and at least once every 1–2 wk during maintenance therapy. Monitor 24-hr CCr before and periodically throughout therapy. If CCr drops below 0.4 mL/min/kg, discontinue foscarnet.
- Monitor serum calcium, magnesium, potassium, and phosphorus before and 2–3 times weekly during induction therapy and at least weekly during maintenance therapy. May cause ↓ concentrations.
- May cause anemia, granulocytopenia, leukopenia, and thrombocytopenia. May cause ↑ AST and ALT levels and abnormal A-G ratios.

Implementation

- Adequately hydrate patient with 750–1000 mL of 0.9% NaCl or D5W before first infusion to establish diuresis, then administer 750–1000 mL with 120 mg/kg of foscarnet or 500 mL with 40–60 mg/kg of foscarnet with each dose to prevent renal toxicity.

IV Administration

- **Intermittent Infusion:** *Dilution:* May be administered via central line undiluted. If administered via peripheral line, *must* be diluted with D5W or 0.9% NaCl to prevent vein irritation. Do not administer solution that is discolored or contains particulate matter. Do not refrigerate or freeze; stable for 24 hr at room temperature. Use diluted solution within 24 hr. *Concentration:* Undiluted: 24 mg/mL; Diluted: 12 mg/mL.
- Dose is based on patient weight; excess solution may be discarded from bottle before administration to prevent overdosage.
- Patients who experience progression of CMV retinitis during maintenance therapy may be retreated with induction therapy followed by maintenance therapy. *Rate:* Administer at a rate not to exceed 1 mg/kg/min.
- Infuse solution via infusion pump to ensure accurate infusion rate.
- **Y-Site Compatibility:** aldesleukin, alemtuzumab, amifostine, amikacin, aminophylline, amphotericin B liposomal, ampicillin, ampicillin/sulbactam, anidulafungin, argatroban, atracurium, azithromycin, aztreonam, bivalirudin, bleomycin, bumetanide, buprenorphine, busulfan, butorphanol, carboplatin, carmustine, cefazolin, cefotaxime, cefotetan, cefoxitin, ceftazidime, ceftriaxone, cefuroxime, chloramphenicol, cisatracurium, cisplatin, clindamycin, cyclophosphamide, cyclosporine, cytarabine, dacarbazine, dactinomycin, daptomycin, dexamethasone, dexmedetomidine, dexrazoxane, diltiazem, docetaxel, dopamine, enalaprilat, ephedrine, epinephrine, eptifibatide, ertapenem, erythromycin, esmolol, etoposide, etoposide phosphate, famotidine, fentanyl, fluconazole, flucytosine, fludarabine, fluorouracil, fosphenytoin, furosemide, gemcitabine, gentamicin, glycopyrrolate, granisetron, heparin, hetastarch, hydrocortisone, hydromorphone, ifosfamide, imipenem/cilastatin, insulin, regular, irinotecan, isoproterenol, ketorolac, levofloxacin, lidocaine, linezolid, magnesium sulfate, mannitol, melphalan, meperidine, meropenem, mesna, methotrexate, metoclopramide, metoprolol, metronidazole, milrinone, mitomycin, morphine, nafcillin, nalbuphine, naloxone, nitroglycerin, nitroprusside, octreotide, oxacillin, oxaliplatin, oxytocin, paclitaxel, palonosetron, pamidronate, pantoprazole, pemetrexed, penicillin G potassium, pentobarbital, phenylephrine, piperacillin/tazobactam, potassium acetate, potassium chloride, potassium phosphate, procainamide, propranolol, remifentanil, rocuronium, sodium acetate, sodium bicarbonate, sodium phosphate, succinylcholine, sufentanil, tacrolimus, theophylline, thiotepa, tigecycline, tirofiban, tobramycin, vancomycin, vecuronium, vinblastine, vincristine, voriconazole, zidovudine, zoledronic acid.
- **Y-Site Incompatibility:** Manufacturer recommends that foscarnet not be administered concurrently with other drugs or solutions in the same IV catheter except D5W or 0.9% NaCl, acyclovir, allopurinol, amphotericin B deoxycholate, amphotericin B lipid complex, calcium chloride, calcium gluconate, caspofungin, chlorpromazine, ciprofloxacin, dantrolene, daunorubicin hydrochloride, diazepam, digoxin, diphenhydramine, dobutamine, doxorubicin hydrochloride, droperidol, epirubicin, ganciclovir, haloperidol, idarubicin, labetalol, leucovorin, methylprednisolone, midazolam, mitoxantrone, mycophenolate, nicardipine, norepinephrine, ondansetron, pentamidine, prochlorperazine, promethazine, thiopental, topotecan, verapamil, vinorelbine.

Patient/Family Teaching

- Inform patient that foscarnet is not a cure for CMV retinitis. Progression of retinitis may continue in immunocompromised patients during and after therapy. Advise patients to have regular ophthalmologic exams.
- May cause dizziness and seizures. Caution patient to avoid driving or other activities requiring alertness until response to medication is known.
- Advise patient to notify health care professional immediately if perioral tingling or numbness in the extremities or paresthesia occurs during or after infusion. If these signs of electrolyte imbalance occur during administration, infusion should be stopped and lab samples for serum electrolyte concentrations obtained immediately.
- Emphasize the importance of frequent follow-up exams to monitor renal function and electrolytes.

Evaluation/Desired Outcomes

- Management of the symptoms of CMV retinitis in patients with HIV.
- Crusting over and healing of skin lesions in HSV infections.

---

fosinopril, See ANGIOTENSIN-CONVERTING ENZYME (ACE) INHIBITORS.

---

 fosphenytoin (foss-**fen**-i-toyn)
Cerebyx
Classification
Therapeutic: anticonvulsants

Indications

Short-term (<5 day) parenteral management of generalized, tonic-clonic status epilepticus when use of phenytoin is not feasible. Treatment and prevention of seizures during neurosurgery when use of phenytoin is not feasible. Short-term substitution for oral phenytoin in patients ≥2 yr old.

Action

Limits seizure propagation by altering ion transport. May also decrease synaptic transmission. Fosphenytoin is rapidly converted to phenytoin, which is responsible for its pharmacologic effects. **Therapeutic Effects:** Diminished seizure activity.

Pharmacokinetics

Absorption: Rapidly converted to phenytoin after IV administration and completely absorbed after IM administration.

Distribution: Distributes into CSF and other body tissues and fluids. Enters breast milk; crosses the placenta, achieving similar maternal/fetal levels. Preferentially distributes into fatty tissue.

Protein Binding: *Fosphenytoin:* 95–99%; *phenytoin:* 90–95%.

Metabolism and Excretion: Mostly metabolized by the liver via the CYP2C9 isoenzyme, and to a lesser extent by the CYP2C19 isoenzyme; the CYP2C9 isoenzyme exhibits genetic polymorphism (intermediate or poor metabolizers may have significantly ↑ fosphenytoin concentrations and an ↑ risk of adverse reactions).; minimal amounts excreted in the urine.

Half-life: *Fosphenytoin:* 15 min; *phenytoin:* 22 hr (range 7–42 hr).

TIME/ACTION PROFILE (anticonvulsant effect)

ROUTE	ONSET	PEAK	DURATION
IM	unknown	30 min	up to 24 hr
IV	15–45 min	15–60 min	up to 24 hr

Contraindications/Precautions

Contraindicated in: Hypersensitivity; Sinus bradycardia, sinoatrial block, 2nd- or 3rd-degree AV heart block or Adams-Stokes syndrome; Prior acute hepatotoxicity due to fosphenytoin or phenytoin.

Use Cautiously in: Hepatic or renal impairment (↑ risk of adverse reactions; dose ↓ recommended for hepatic impairment); CYP2C9 intermediate or poor metabolizers (↑ risk of phenytoin toxicity); OB: ↑ risk of congenital anomalies; ↑ risk of hemorrhage in newborn if used at term; Lactation: Use while breastfeeding only if potential maternal benefit justifies potential risk to infant.

Exercise Extreme Caution in: Patients positive for HLA-B*1502 allele or carriers of CYP2C9*3 variant (unless benefits clearly outweigh the risks) (↑ risk of serious skin reactions).

Adverse Reactions/Side Effects

CV: hypotension (with rapid IV administration), tachycardia. **Derm:** pruritus, ACUTE GENERALIZED EXANTHEMATOUS PUSTULOSIS, DRUG REACTION WITH EOSINOPHILIA AND SYSTEMIC SYMPTOMS (DRESS), purple glove syndrome, rash, STEVENS-JOHNSON SYNDROME, TOXIC EPIDERMAL NECROLYSIS. **EENT:** amblyopia, deafness, diplopia, tinnitus. **GI:** dry mouth, nausea, taste perversion, tongue disorder, vomiting. **Hemat:** lymphadenopathy, megaloblastic anemia, pure red cell aplasia. **MS:** back pain. **Neuro:** ataxia, dizziness, drowsiness, nystagmus, agitation, brain edema, dysarthria, extrapyramidal syndrome, headache, hypoesthesia, incoordination, paresthesia, stupor, tremor, vertigo. **Misc:** ANGIOEDEMA, pelvic pain.

Interactions

Drug-Drug: Disulfiram, acute ingestion of **alcohol, amiodarone, capecitabine, chloramphenicol, chlordiazepoxide, cimetidine, diazepam, estro-**

---

gens, ethosuximide, felbamate, fluconazole, fluorouracil, fluoxetine, fluvastatin, fluvoxamine, halothane, isoniazid, itraconazole, ketoconazole, methylphenidate, miconazole, omeprazole, oxcarbazepine, phenothiazines, salicylates, sertraline, sulfonamides, topiramate, trazodone, voriconazole, and warfarin may ↑ phenytoin blood levels. Barbiturates, bleomycin, carbamazepine, carboplatin, cisplatin, diazoxide, doxorubicin, folic acid, fosamprenavir, methotrexate, nelfinavir, rifampin, ritonavir, theophylline, vigabatrin, and chronic ingestion of alcohol may ↓ phenytoin blood levels. Phenytoin may ↓ the effects of albendazole, amiodarone, atorvastatin, benzodiazepines, carbamazepine, chloramphenicol, clozapine, corticosteroids, cyclosporine, digoxin, disopyramide, doxycycline, efavirenz, estrogens, felbamate, fluconazole, fluvastatin, folic acid, furosemide, irinotecan, itraconazole, ketoconazole, lamotrigine, lopinavir/ritonavir, methadone, mexiletine, nelfinavir, nifedipine, nimodipine, nisoldipine, oral contraceptives, oxcarbazepine, paclitaxel, paroxetine, posaconazole, propafenone, quetiapine, quinidine, rifampin, ritonavir, sertraline, simvastatin, tacrolimus, theophylline, topiramate, tricyclic antidepressants, verapamil, vitamin D, voriconazole, warfarin, and zonisamide.

Drug-Natural Products: St. John's wort may ↓ levels.

Route/Dosage
Note: Doses of fosphenytoin should be expressed as phenytoin sodium equivalents [PE].

Status Epilepticus
IV (Adults and Children): 15–20 mg PE/kg.

Nonemergent and Maintenance Dosing
IV, IM (Adults and Children >16 yr): *Loading dose:* 10–20 mg PE/kg. *Maintenance dose:* 4–6 mg PE/kg/day (start 12 hr after loading dose; administer in 2–3 divided doses).
IV (Children Birth to 16 yr): *Loading dose:* 10–15 mg PE/kg. *Maintenance dose:* 2–4 mg PE/kg given 12 hr after loading dose, then 4–8 mg PE/kg/day (in 2 divided doses).

Availability (generic available)
Solution for injection: 50 mg PE/mL, ✦ 75 mg PE/mL.

NURSING IMPLICATIONS
Assessment
* Assess location, duration, frequency, and characteristics of seizure activity. EEG may be monitored periodically during therapy.
* Monitor BP, ECG, and respiratory function continuously during administration of fosphenytoin and during period when peak serum phenytoin levels occur (15–30 min after administration).

* Observe patient for development of rash. Discontinue fosphenytoin at the first sign of skin reactions. Serious adverse reactions such as exfoliative, purpuric, or bullous rashes or the development of lupus erythematosus, Stevens-Johnson syndrome, or toxic epidermal necrolysis preclude further use of fosphenytoin. ⚡ Stevens-Johnson syndrome and toxic epidermal necrolysis are significantly more common in patients with a particular HLA allele, HLA-B*1502 (occurs almost exclusively in patients with Asian ancestry, including Han Chinese, Filipinos, Malaysians, South Asian Indians, and Thais). Avoid using fosphenytoin as an alternative to carbamazepine for patients who test positive. If less serious skin eruptions (measles-like or scarlatiniform) occur, fosphenytoin may be resumed after complete clearing of the rash. If rash reappears, avoid further use of fosphenytoin.
* Assess mental status (orientation, mood, behavior) before and periodically during therapy. Monitor closely for notable changes in behavior that could indicate the emergence or worsening of suicidal thoughts or behavior or depression.
* Monitor injection site for edema, discoloration, and pain distal to the site of injection (described as "purple glove syndrome") frequently during therapy. May or may not be associated with extravasation. The syndrome may not develop for several days after injection of fosphenytoin.

Lab Test Considerations
* Fosphenytoin contains 0.0037 mmol phosphate per mg PE. Monitor serum phosphate concentrations in patients with renal insufficiency; may cause ↑ phosphate concentrations.
* May cause ↑ serum alkaline phosphatase, GGT, and glucose levels.
* Fosphenytoin therapy may be monitored using phenytoin levels. Optimal total plasma phenytoin concentrations are typically 10–20 mcg/mL (unbound plasma phenytoin concentrations of 1–2 mcg/mL).

Toxicity and Overdose
* Serum phenytoin levels should not be monitored until complete conversion from fosphenytoin to phenytoin has occurred (2 hr after IV or 4 hr after IM administration).
* Initial signs and symptoms of phenytoin toxicity include nystagmus, ataxia, confusion, nausea, slurred speech, and dizziness.

Implementation
* Do not confuse Cerebyx with Celebrex or Celexa.
* Do not confuse concentration of fosphenytoin with total amount of drug in vial.
* Implement seizure precautions.
* When substituting *fosphenytoin* for oral *phenytoin* therapy, the same total daily dose may be given as a single dose. Unlike parenteral phenytoin, fosphenytoin may be given safely by the IM route.
* The anticonvulsant effect of fosphenytoin is not immediate. Additional measures (including parenteral

benzodiazepines) are usually required in the immediate management of status epilepticus. Loading dose of *fosphenytoin* should be followed with the institution of maintenance anticonvulsant therapy.

IV Administration
- **IV Push: *Dilution:*** D5W or 0.9% NaCl. *Concentration:* 1.5–25 mg PE/mL. May be refrigerated for up to 48 hr. *Rate:* Administer at a rate of <150 mg PE/min in adults and <0.4 mg/kg/min in children 2–17 yrs to minimize risk of hypotension and arrhythmias.
- **Y-Site Compatibility:** acyclovir, alemtuzumab, allopurinol, amifostine, amikacin, aminocaproic acid, aminophylline, amphotericin B lipid complex, amphotericin B liposomal, ampicillin, ampicillin/sulbactam, anidulafungin, argatroban, arsenic trioxide, azithromycin, aztreonam, bivalirudin, bleomycin, bumetanide, buprenorphine, busulfan, butorphanol, carboplatin, carmustine, cefazolin, cefepime, cefotaxime, cefotetan, cefoxitin, ceftazidime, ceftolozane/tazobactam, ceftriaxone, cefuroxime, chloramphenicol, ciprofloxacin, cisatracurium, cisplatin, clindamycin, cyclophosphamide, cyclosporine, cytarabine, dacarbazine, dactinomycin, daptomycin, dexamethasone, dexmedetomidine, dexrazoxane, digoxin, diltiazem, diphenhydramine, docetaxel, doxorubicin liposomal, doxycycline, enalaprilat, ephedrine, epinephrine, eptifibatide, ertapenem, erythromycin, esmolol, etoposide, etoposide phosphate, famotidine, fentanyl, fluconazole, fludarabine, fluorouracil, foscarnet, furosemide, ganciclovir, gemcitabine, gemtuzumab ozogamicin, gentamicin, glycopyrrolate, granisetron, heparin, hetastarch, hydrocortisone, hydromorphone, ifosfamide, imipenem/cilastatin, insulin, regular, isoproterenol, ketotolac, labetalol, leucovorin calcium, levofloxacin, lidocaine, linezolid, lorazepam, magnesium sulfate, mannitol, melphalan, meperidine, meropenem, meropenem/vaborbactam, mesna, methadone, methotrexate, methylprednisolone, metoclopramide, metoprolol, metronidazole, milrinone, mitomycin, morphine, nalbuphine, naloxone, nitroglycerin, nitroprusside, norepinephrine, octreotide, ondansetron, oxaliplatin, oxytocin, paclitaxel, palonosetron, pamidronate, pantoprazole, pemetrexed, pentobarbital, phenobarbital, phentolamine, phenylephrine, piperacillin/tazobactam, plazomicin, potassium acetate, potassium chloride, potassium phosphate, procainamide, propranolol, remifentanil, rocuronium, sodium acetate, sodium bicarbonate, sodium phosphate, succinylcholine, sufentanil, tacrolimus, tedizolid, theophylline, thiotepa, tigecycline, tirofiban, tobramycin, trimethoprim/sulfamethoxazole, vancomycin, vasopressin, vecuronium, vinblastine, vincristine, vinorelbine, voriconazole, zidovudine, zoledronic acid.

- **Y-Site Incompatibility:** amiodarone, calcium chloride, calcium gluconate, caspofungin, chlorpromazine, dantrolene, daunorubicin hydrochloride, diazepam, dobutamine, doxorubicin hydrochloride, droperidol, epirubicin, haloperidol, hydralazine, hydroxyzine, idarubicin, irinotecan, isavuconazonium, midazolam, mitoxantrone, moxifloxacin, mycophenolate, nicardipine, pentamidine, phenytoin, prochlorperazine, thiopental, topotecan, verapamil.

Patient/Family Teaching
- Explain purpose of fosphenytoin to patient.
- May cause drowsiness or dizziness. Caution patient to avoid driving or other activities requiring alertness until response to medication is known. Do not resume driving until physician gives clearance based on control of seizure disorder.
- Instruct patients to notify health care professional immediately if behavioral changes, skin rash, fever, sore throat, mouth ulcers, easy bruising, petechiae, unusual bleeding, abdominal pain, chills, pale stools, dark urine, jaundice, severe nausea or vomiting, drowsiness, slurred speech, unsteady gait, swollen glands, or persistent headache occur. Advise patient and family to notify health care professional if thoughts about suicide or dying, attempts to commit suicide; new or worse depression; new or worse anxiety; feeling very agitated or restless; panic attacks; trouble sleeping; new or worse irritability; acting aggressive; being angry or violent; acting on dangerous impulses; an extreme increase in activity and talking, other unusual changes in behavior or mood occur.
- Advise patient to notify health care professional of all Rx or OTC medications, vitamins, or herbal products being taken and to consult with health care professional before taking other medications, especially St. John's wort.
- Rep: May cause fetal harm. Advise females of reproductive potential to use an additional nonhormonal method of contraception during therapy and until next menstrual period. Instruct patient to notify health care professional if pregnancy is planned or suspected or if breastfeeding. To prevent a potentially life-threatening bleeding disorder related to decreased levels of vitamin K-dependent clotting factors in newborns exposed to phenytoin in utero administer vitamin K to the mother before delivery and to the neonate after birth. Encourage patients who become pregnant to enroll in the North American Antiepileptic Drug Pregnancy Registry by calling 1-888-233-2334 or on the web at www.aedpregnancyregistry.org. Enrollment must be done by patients themselves.
- Advise patient to carry identification describing disease process and medication regimen at all times.
- Emphasize the importance of routine exams to monitor progress. Patient should have routine physical

exams, especially monitoring skin and lymph nodes, and EEG testing.

Evaluation/Desired Outcomes

- Decrease or cessation of seizures without excessive sedation.

---

fremanezumab
(free-ma-**nez**-ue-mab)
Ajovy
Classification
Therapeutic: vascular headache suppressants
Pharmacologic: monoclonal antibodies, calcitonin gene-related peptide receptor antagonists

Indications

Migraine prevention.

Action

Monoclonal antibody that binds to the calcitonin gene-related peptide (CGRP) receptor, which reduces the neuroinflammatory and vasodilatory effects of CGRP. **Therapeutic Effects:** Reduction in frequency of migraines.

Pharmacokinetics

Absorption: Unknown.
Distribution: Minimal distribution to tissues.
Metabolism and Excretion: Degraded by enzymatic proteolysis into small peptides and amino acids.
Half-life: 31 days.

TIME/ACTION PROFILE (plasma concentrations)

ROUTE	ONSET	PEAK	DURATION
SUBQ	unknown	5–7 days	1 mo

Contraindications/Precautions

Contraindicated in: Hypersensitivity.
Use Cautiously in: OB: Safety not established in pregnancy; Lactation: Safety not established in breastfeeding; Pedi: Safety and effectiveness not established in children.

Adverse Reactions/Side Effects

Local: injection site reactions. **Misc:** HYPERSENSITIVITY REACTIONS (including anaphylaxis and angioedema).

Interactions

Drug-Drug: None reported.

Route/Dosage

SUBQ (Adults): 225 mg once monthly *or* 675 mg every 3 mo.

Availability

Solution for injection (prefilled syringes and autoinjectors): 225 mg/1.5 mL.

NURSING IMPLICATIONS

Assessment

- Assess frequency and intensity of migraines.
- Monitor for signs and symptoms of hypersensitivity reactions (rash, pruritus, drug hypersensitivity, urticaria) during therapy. May occur up to 1 mo after administration. If reaction is severe, discontinue fremanezumab and treat as needed.

Implementation

- **SUBQ:** Prior to use allow vial to sit at room temperature for at least 30 min, protect from direct sunlight. Do no use other methods to warm solution (hot water or microwave). Do not shake. Solution is clear to opalescent, colorless to light yellow; do not administer solutions that are discolored, cloudy, or contain particulate matter. Store in refrigerator in original carton to protect from light; do not freeze. May be stored up to 7 days at room temperature; discard if at room temperature >7 days.
- Inject entire contents into abdomen, thigh, or upper arm. Do not inject into areas where the skin is tender, bruised, red, or hard.

Patient/Family Teaching

- Instruct patient to take as directed. Administer missed doses as soon as possible and schedule next dose from date last dose administered. Educate patient and/or caregiver on correct technique for injection and disposal of equipment. Advise patient to read *Patient Information* before starting therapy and with each Rx refill in case of changes.
- Instruct patient to notify health care professional immediately if signs and symptoms of hypersensitivity reaction (itching, rash, hives, swelling of face, mouth, tongue or throat, trouble breathing) occur.
- Advise patient to notify health care professional of all Rx or OTC medications, vitamins, or herbal products being taken and to consult with health care professional before taking other medications.
- Rep: Advise female patients to notify health care professional if pregnancy is planned or suspected or if breastfeeding. Women with migraine may be at increased risk of preeclampsia and gestational hypertension during pregnancy. Inform patient of pregnancy exposure registry that monitors pregnancy outcomes in women exposed to fremanezumab during pregnancy. Enrollment can be done by health care professional or patient by calling 1-833-927-2605 or visiting www.tevamigrainepregnancyregistry.com.

Evaluation/Desired Outcomes

- Decrease in frequency of migraines.

---

frovatriptan (froe-va-**trip**-tan)
Frova
Classification
Therapeutic: vascular headache suppressants
Pharmacologic: 5-HT$_1$ agonists

Indications

Acute treatment of migraine headache.

Action

Acts as an agonist at specific 5-HT receptor sites in intracranial blood vessels and sensory trigeminal nerves. **Therapeutic Effects:** Cranial vessel vasoconstriction with associated decrease in release of neuropeptides and resultant decrease in migraine headache.

Pharmacokinetics

Absorption: 20–30% following oral administration.
Distribution: Well distributed to tissues.
Metabolism and Excretion: Mostly metabolized by the liver via the CYP1A2 isoenzyme; some metabolites eliminated in urine, <10% excreted unchanged.
Half-life: 26 hr.

TIME/ACTION PROFILE (plasma concentrations)

ROUTE	ONSET	PEAK	DURATION
PO	unknown	2–4 hr	unknown

Contraindications/Precautions

Contraindicated in: Hypersensitivity; Ischemic heart disease or vasospastic angina (e.g., Prinzmetal's angina); Wolff-Parkinson-White Syndrome or arrhythmias associated with other cardiac accessory conduction pathway disorders; History of stroke or transient ischemic attack; History of hemiplegic or basilar migraine; Uncontrolled hypertension; Peripheral vascular disease; Ischemic bowel disease; Should not be used within 24 hr of other 5-HT$_1$ agonists or ergot-type compounds (dihydroergotamine).
Use Cautiously in: OB: Safety not established in pregnancy; Lactation: Safety not established in breastfeeding; Pedi: Safety and effectiveness not established in children; Geri: Older adults may be more susceptible to adverse cardiovascular effects.
Exercise Extreme Caution in: Cardiovascular risk factors (hypertension, hypercholesterolemia, cigarette smoking, obesity, diabetes, strong family history, menopausal women or men >40 yr); use only if cardiovascular status has been evaluated and determined to be safe and first dose is administered under supervision.

Adverse Reactions/Side Effects

CV: chest pain, CORONARY ARTERY VASOSPASM, MI, myocardial ischemia, VENTRICULAR ARRHYTHMIAS. **Derm:** flushing. **GI:** dry mouth, dyspepsia, nausea. **MS:** pain. **Neuro:** dizziness, drowsiness, fatigue, paresthesia.

Interactions

Drug-Drug: ↑ risk of serious vasospastic reactions with **dihydroergotamine** or **ergotamine**; concurrent use contraindicated. **Hormonal contraceptives** or **propranolol** may ↑ levels. ↑ risk of serotonin syndrome when used with **fluoxetine, paroxetine, ser-**traline, fluvoxamine, citalopram, escitalopram, venlafaxine, **or** duloxetine.

Route/Dosage

PO (Adults): 2.5 mg; if there has been initial relief, a 2nd tablet may be taken after at least 2 hr (daily dose should not exceed 3 tablets and should not be used to treat more than 4 attacks/30 day period).

Availability (generic available)

Tablets: 2.5 mg.

NURSING IMPLICATIONS

Assessment

- Assess pain location, intensity, duration, and associated symptoms (photophobia, phonophobia, nausea, vomiting) during migraine attack.

Implementation

- **PO:** Tablets may be administered at any time after the headache starts.

Patient/Family Teaching

- Inform patient that frovatriptan should be used only during a migraine attack. It is meant to be used to relieve migraine attack but not to prevent or reduce the number of attacks.
- Instruct patient to administer frovatriptan as soon as symptoms appear, but it may be administered any time during an attack. If migraine symptoms return, a 2nd dose may be used. Allow at least 2 hr between doses, and do not use more than 3 tablets in any 24-hr period.
- If dose does not relieve headache, additional frovatriptan doses are not likely to be effective; notify health care professional.
- Caution patient not to take frovatriptan within 24 hr of another vascular headache suppressant.
- Advise patient that lying down in a darkened room following frovatriptan administration may further help relieve headache.
- May cause dizziness or drowsiness. Caution patient to avoid driving or other activities requiring alertness until response to medication is known.
- Advise patient that overuse (use more than 10 days/ mo) may lead to exacerbation of headache (migraine-like daily headaches, or as a marked increase in frequency of migraine attacks). May require gradual withdrawal of frovatriptan and treatment of symptoms (transient worsening of headache).
- Advise patient to notify health care professional prior to next dose of frovatriptan if pain or tightness in the chest occurs during use. If pain is severe or does not subside, notify health care professional immediately. If wheezing; heart throbbing; swelling of eyelids, face, or lips; skin rash; skin lumps; or hives occur, notify health care professional immediately and do not take more frovatriptan without approval of health care professional. If feelings of tingling, heat,

flushing, heaviness, pressure, drowsiness, dizziness, tiredness, or sickness develop, discuss with health care professional at next visit.

- Advise patient to avoid alcohol, which aggravates headaches, during frovatriptan use.
- Advise patient to notify health care professional of all Rx or OTC medications, vitamins, or herbal products being taken and to consult with health care professional before taking other medications.
- Advise patient to notify health care professional immediately if signs or symptoms of serotonin syndrome occur.
- Rep: Advise females of reproductive potential to notify health care professional if pregnancy is planned or suspected or if breastfeeding.

Evaluation/Desired Outcomes
- Relief of migraine attack.

BEERS

furosemide (fur-oh-se-mide)
Furoscix, Lasix
Classification
Therapeutic: diuretics
Pharmacologic: loop diuretics

Indications
PO, IM, IV: Edema due to HF, hepatic impairment, or renal disease. **SUBQ:** Edema due to New York Heart Association class II-III chronic HF. **PO:** Hypertension.

Action
Inhibits the reabsorption of sodium and chloride from the loop of Henle and distal renal tubule. Increases renal excretion of water, sodium, chloride, magnesium, potassium, and calcium. Effectiveness persists in impaired renal function. **Therapeutic Effects:** Diuresis and subsequent mobilization of excess fluid (edema, pleural effusions). Decreased BP.

Pharmacokinetics
Absorption: 60–67% absorbed after oral administration (↓ in acute HF and in renal failure); also absorbed from IM sites; IV administration results in complete availability; 99.6% absorbed after SUBQ administration.
Distribution: Crosses placenta, enters breast milk.
Protein Binding: 91–99%.
Metabolism and Excretion: Minimally metabolized by liver, some nonhepatic metabolism, some renal excretion as unchanged drug.
Half-life: 30–120 min (↑ in renal impairment).

TIME/ACTION PROFILE (diuretic effect)

ROUTE	ONSET	PEAK	DURATION
PO	30–60 min	1–2 hr	6–8 hr
IM	10–30 min	unknown	4–8 hr
IV	5 min	30 min	2 hr
Subcut	unknown	unknown	8 hr

Contraindications/Precautions
Contraindicated in: Hypersensitivity; Cross-sensitivity with thiazides and sulfonamides may occur; Hepatic coma; Anuria; Hepatic cirrhosis or ascites (SUBQ only); Acute pulmonary edema (SUBQ only); Some liquid products may contain alcohol, avoid in patients with alcohol intolerance.
Use Cautiously in: Severe hepatic impairment (may precipitate hepatic coma; concurrent use with potassium-sparing diuretics may be necessary); Electrolyte depletion; Diabetes mellitus; Hypoproteinemia (↑ risk of ototoxicity); Severe renal impairment (↑ risk of ototoxicity); OB: Use during pregnancy only if potential maternal benefit justifies potential fetal risk; Lactation: Use while breastfeeding only if potential maternal benefit justifies potential risk to infant; Pedi: ↑ risk for renal calculi and patent ductus arteriosis in premature neonates; Geri: Appears on Beers list. May worsen or cause hyponatremia in older adults. Use with caution in older adults and monitor sodium concentrations closely when initiating therapy or ↑ the dose.

Adverse Reactions/Side Effects
CV: hypotension. **Derm:** ERYTHEMA MULTIFORME, photosensitivity, pruritus, rash, STEVENS-JOHNSON SYNDROME, TOXIC EPIDERMAL NECROLYSIS, urticaria. **EENT:** hearing loss, tinnitus. **Endo:** hypercholesterolemia, hyperglycemia, hypertriglyceridemia, hyperuricemia. **F and E:** dehydration, hypocalcemia, hypochloremia, hypokalemia, hypomagnesemia, hyponatremia, hypovolemia, metabolic alkalosis. **GI:** ↑ liver enzymes, anorexia, constipation, diarrhea, dry mouth, dyspepsia, nausea, pancreatitis, vomiting. **GU:** ↑ BUN, excessive urination, nephrocalcinosis. **Hemat:** AGRANULOCYTOSIS, APLASTIC ANEMIA, hemolytic anemia, leukopenia, thrombocytopenia. **MS:** muscle cramps. **Neuro:** blurred vision, dizziness, headache, paresthesia, vertigo. **Misc:** fever.

Interactions
Drug-Drug: ↑ risk of hypotension with **antihypertensives**, **nitrates**, or acute ingestion of **alcohol**. ↑ risk of hypokalemia with other **diuretics**, **amphotericin B**, **stimulant laxatives**, and **corticosteroids**. Hypokalemia may ↑ risk of **digoxin** toxicity and ↑ risk of arrhythmia in patients taking drugs that prolong the QT interval. ↓ **lithium** excretion, may cause **lithium** toxicity. ↑ risk of ototoxicity with **aminoglycosides** or **cisplatin**. ↑ risk of nephrotoxicity with **cisplatin**. **NSAIDs** ↓ effects of furosemide. May ↑ risk of **methotrexate** toxicity. ↓ effects when given at same time as **sucralfate**, **cholestyramine**, or **colestipol**. ↑ risk of **salicylate** toxicity (with use of high-dose **salicylate** therapy). Concurrent use with **cyclosporine** may ↑ risk of gouty arthritis.

Route/Dosage

Edema
PO (Adults): 20–80 mg/day as a single dose initially, may repeat in 6–8 hr; may ↑ dose by 20–40 mg every 6–8 hr until desired response. Maintenance doses may

be given once or twice daily (doses up to 2.5 g/day have been used in patients with HF or renal disease). *Hypertension:* 40 mg twice daily initially (when added to regimen, ↓ dose of other antihypertensives by 50%); adjust further dosing based on response; *Hypercalcemia:* 120 mg/day in 1–3 doses.

PO (Children >1 mo): 2 mg/kg as a single dose; may be ↑ by 1–2 mg/kg every 6–8 hr (maximum dose = 6 mg/kg).

PO (Neonates): 1–4 mg/kg/dose 1–2 times/day.

IM, IV (Adults): 20–40 mg, may repeat in 1–2 hr and ↑ by 20 mg every 1–2 hr until response is obtained, maintenance dose may be given every 6–12 hr; *Continuous infusion:* Bolus 0.1 mg/kg followed by 0.1 mg/kg/hr, double every 2 hr to a maximum of 0.4 mg/kg/hr.

IM, IV (Children): 1–2 mg/kg/dose every 6–12 hr; *Continuous infusion:* 0.05 mg/kg/hr, titrate to clinical effect.

IM, IV (Neonates): 1–2 mg/kg/dose every 12–24 hr.

SUBQ (Adults): 30 mg over the 1st hr, then 12.5 mg per hr over the next 4 hr with the single-use on-body Infusor. Replace with oral diuretic therapy as soon as possible.

Hypertension

PO (Adults): 40 mg twice daily initially (when added to regimen, ↓ dose of other antihypertensives by 50%); adjust further dosing based on response.

Availability (generic available)

Tablets: 20 mg, 40 mg, 80 mg, ✹ 500 mg. **Oral solution (10 mg/mL—orange flavor, 8 mg/mL—pineapple—peach flavor):** 8 mg/mL, 10 mg/mL. **Solution for intravenous/intramuscular injection:** 10 mg/mL. **Solution for SUBQ injection (Furoscix) (Furoscix) (prefilled cartridges):** 80 mg/10 mL.

NURSING IMPLICATIONS

Assessment

● Assess fluid status. Monitor daily weight, intake and output ratios, amount and location of edema, lung sounds, skin turgor, and mucous membranes. Notify health care professional if thirst, dry mouth, lethargy, weakness, hypotension, or oliguria occurs.

● Monitor BP and pulse before and during administration. Monitor frequency of prescription refills to determine compliance in patients treated for hypertension.

● Geri: Diuretic use is associated with increased risk for falls in older adults. Assess falls risk and implement fall prevention strategies.

● Assess patients receiving digoxin for anorexia, nausea, vomiting, muscle cramps, paresthesia, and confusion. Patients taking digoxin are at increased risk of digoxin toxicity because of the potassium-depleting effect of the diuretic. Potassium supplements or

potassium-sparing diuretics may be used concurrently to prevent hypokalemia.

● Assess patient for tinnitus and hearing loss. Audiometry is recommended for patients receiving prolonged high-dose IV therapy. Hearing loss is most common after rapid or high-dose IV administration in patients with decreased renal function or those taking other ototoxic drugs.

● Assess for allergy to sulfonamides.

● Assess patient for skin rash frequently during therapy. Discontinue furosemide at first sign of rash; may be life-threatening. Stevens-Johnson syndrome, toxic epidermal necrolysis, or erythema multiforme may develop. Treat symptomatically; may recur once treatment is stopped.

Lab Test Considerations

● Monitor electrolytes, renal and hepatic function, serum glucose, and uric acid levels before and periodically throughout therapy. Commonly ↓ serum potassium. May cause ↓ serum sodium, calcium, and magnesium concentrations. May also cause ↑ BUN, serum glucose, serum creatinine, and uric acid levels.

Implementation

● If administering twice daily, give last dose no later than 5 PM to minimize disruption of sleep cycle. Do not confuse Lasix with Wakix.

● IV route is preferred over IM route for parenteral administration.

● **PO:** May be taken with food or milk to minimize gastric irritation. Tablets may be crushed if patient has difficulty swallowing.

● Do not administer discolored solution or tablets.

● **SUBQ:** The single-use, on-body *Infusor* with prefilled cartridge is pre-programed to deliver 30 mg of furosemide over the first hr followed by 12.5 mg per hr for the subsequent 4 hrs. Inspect fluid in prefilled cartridge; solution is clear to slightly yellow; do not administer solutions that are discolored or cloudy. Load prefilled cartridge into the on-body infusor and close cartridge holder. Peel away adhesive liner on on-body infusor and apply onto a clean, dry area of the abdomen between top of beltline and bottom of ribcage (at least 2 ½ inches from beltline or bottom of ribcage) that is not tender, bruised, red or indurated. Start injection by firmly pressing and releasing the blue start button. Do not remove until the injection is complete (signaled by the solid green status light, beeping sound, and the white plunger rod filling the cartridge window). Rotate the site of each subcutaneous administration. Patient must limit activity during administration. On-body infusor is not compatible with use in an MRI setting. SUBQ route is not for chronic use; replace with oral diuretics as soon as practical.

IV Administration

● **IV Push:** *Dilution:* Administer undiluted (larger doses may be diluted and administered as intermittent infusion [see below]). *Concentration:* 10 mg/mL. *Rate:* Administer at a rate of 20 mg/min. Pedi: Administer at a maximum rate of 0.5–1 mg/kg/min (for doses <120 mg) with infusion not exceeding 10 min.

- **Intermittent Infusion:** *Dilution:* Dilute larger doses in 50 mL of D5W, D10W, D20W, D5/0.9% NaCl, D5/LR, 0.9% NaCl, 3% NaCl, or LR. Infusion stable for 24 hr at room temperature. Do not refrigerate. Protect from light. *Concentration:* 1 mg/mL. *Rate:* Administer at a rate not to exceed 4 mg/min (for doses >120 mg) in adults to prevent ototoxicity. Pedi: not to exceed 1 mg/kg/min with infusion not exceeding 10 min. Use an infusion pump to ensure accurate dose.

- **Y-Site Compatibility:** acyclovir, allopurinol, alprostadil, amifostine, amikacin, aminocaproic acid, aminophylline, amphotericin B lipid complex, amphotericin B liposomal, anidulafungin, argatroban, arsenic trioxide, ascorbic acid, atropine, azathioprine, aztreonam, bivalirudin, bleomycin, bumetanide, calcium chloride, calcium gluconate, cangrelor, carboplatin, carmustine, cefazolin, cefepime, cefotaxime, cefotetan, cefoxitin, ceftaroline, ceftazidime, ceftazidime/avibactam, ceftolozane/tazobactam, ceftriaxone, cefuroxime, chloramphenicol, cisplatin, cladribine, clindamycin, cyanocobalamin, cyclophosphamide, cyclosporine, cytarabine, dactinomycin, daptomycin, dexamethasone, dexmedetomidine, digoxin, docetaxel, doxorubicin liposomal, enalaprilat, ephedrine, epinephrine, epoetin alfa, ertapenem, esomeprazole, etoposide, etoposide phosphate, fentanyl, fludarabine, fluorouracil, folic acid, foscarnet, fosphenytoin, ganciclovir, granisetron, heparin, hetastarch, hydrocortisone, hydromorphone, ibuprofen, ifosfamide, imipenem/cilastatin, indomethacin, ketorolac, LR, leucovorin calcium, lidocaine, linezolid, lorazepam, mannitol, melphalan, meropenem, meropenem/vaborbactam, mesna, methotrexate, methylprednisolone, metoprolol, metronidazole, micafungin, mitomycin, multivitamins, nafcillin, naloxone, nitroprusside, octreotide, oxacillin, oxaliplatin, oxytocin, paclitaxel, palonosetron, pamidronate, pemetrexed, penicillin G, pentobarbital, phenobarbital, phytonadione, piperacillin/tazobactam, plazomicin, potassium acetate, potassium chloride, procainamide, propofol, propranolol, remifentanil, sargramostim, sodium acetate, sodium bicarbonate, succinylcholine, sufentanil, tedizolid, theophylline, thiotepa, tigecycline, tirofiban, tobramycin, topotecan, trimethoprim/sulfamethoxazole, voriconazole, zoledronic acid.

- **Y-Site Incompatibility:** acetaminophen, alemtuzumab, atracurium, benztropine, blinatumomab, butorphanol, caspofungin, ciprofloxacin, dantrolene, daunorubicin hydrochloride, dexrazoxane, diazepam, diazoxide, diltiazem, diphenhydramine, doxycycline, droperidol, epirubicin, eptifibatide, eravacycline, esmolol, filgrastim, gemcitabine, gemtuzumab ozogamicin, glycopyrrolate, haloperidol, hydroxyzine, idarubicin, irinotecan, isavuconazonium, ketamine, levofloxacin, milrinone, mitoxantrone, moxifloxacin, mycophenolate, nalbuphine, nicardipine, ondansetron, papaverine, pentamidine, phenytoin, prochlorperazine, protamine, pyridoxine, rituximab, rocuronium, telavancin, thiamine, trastuzumab, trimethoprim/sulfamethoxazole, vancomycin, vecuronium, verapamil, vinblastine, vinorelbine.

Patient/Family Teaching

- Instruct patient to take furosemide as directed. Take missed doses as soon as possible; do not double doses.
- Caution patient to change positions slowly to minimize orthostatic hypotension. Caution patient that the use of alcohol, exercise during hot weather, or standing for long periods during therapy may enhance orthostatic hypotension.
- Instruct patient to consult health care professional regarding a diet high in potassium (see Appendix J).
- Advise patient to contact health care professional if weight gain more than 3 lbs in 1 day.
- Instruct patient to notify health care professional of all Rx or OTC medications, vitamins, or herbal products being taken and to consult health care professional before taking any OTC medications concurrently with this therapy.
- Instruct patient to notify health care professional of medication regimen before treatment or surgery.
- Caution patient to use sunscreen and protective clothing to prevent photosensitivity reactions.
- Advise patient to contact health care professional immediately if rash, muscle weakness, cramps, nausea, dizziness, numbness, or tingling of extremities occurs.
- Advise diabetic patients to monitor blood glucose closely; may cause increased blood glucose levels.
- Rep: Advise females of reproductive potential to notify health care professional if pregnancy is planned or suspected, or if breastfeeding. Monitor fetal growth during pregnancy; increased risk for higher birth weights.
- Emphasize the importance of routine follow-up examinations.
- Geri: Caution older patients or their caregivers about increased risk for falls. Suggest strategies for fall prevention.
- **Hypertension:** Advise patients on antihypertensive regimen to continue taking medication even if feeling better. Furosemide controls but does not cure hypertension.
- Reinforce the need to continue additional therapies for hypertension (weight loss, exercise, restricted sodium intake, stress reduction, regular exercise, moderation of alcohol consumption, cessation of smoking).

Evaluation/Desired Outcomes

- Decrease in edema.
- Decrease in abdominal girth and weight.
- Increase in urinary output.
- Decrease in BP.

gabapentin (ga-ba-**pen**-tin)
Gralise, Horizant, Neurontin
Classification
Therapeutic: analgesics, anticonvulsants, mood stabilizers
Pharmacologic: gamma aminobutyric acid (GABA) analogues

Schedule V (only schedule V in some states)

Indications
Partial seizures (adjunct treatment) (immediate-release only). Postherpetic neuralgia. Restless legs syndrome (Horizant only). **Unlabeled Use:** Neuropathic pain. Prevention of migraine headache.

Action
Mechanism of action is not known. May affect transport of amino acids across and stabilize neuronal membranes. **Therapeutic Effects:** Decreased incidence of seizures. Decreased postherpetic pain. Decreased leg restlessness.

Pharmacokinetics
Absorption: Well absorbed after oral administration by active transport. At larger doses, transport becomes saturated and absorption ↓ (bioavailability ranges from 60% for a 300-mg dose to 35% for a 1600-mg dose).
Distribution: Crosses blood-brain barrier; enters breast milk.
Metabolism and Excretion: Eliminated mostly by renal excretion of unchanged drug.
Half-life: *Adults:* 5–7 hr (normal renal function); up to 132 hr in anuria; *Children:* 4.7 hr.

TIME/ACTION PROFILE (blood levels)

ROUTE	ONSET	PEAK	DURATION
PO-IR	rapid	2–4 hr	8 hr
PO-SR	unknown	5–8 hr	24 hr

Contraindications/Precautions
Contraindicated in: Hypersensitivity.
Use Cautiously in: All patients (may ↑ risk of suicidal thoughts/behaviors); Renal impairment (↓ dose and/or ↑ dosing interval if CCr ≤60 mL/min); Respiratory impairment (↑ risk of respiratory depression); OB: Safety not established in pregnancy; Lactation: Use while breastfeeding only if potential maternal benefit justifies potential risk to infant; Pedi: Safety and effectiveness not established in children <18 yr (sustained-/extended-release) or <3 yr (immediate-release); Geri: Older adults may be more susceptible to toxicity due to age-related ↓ in renal function.

Adverse Reactions/Side Effects
Derm: bullous pemphigoid, STEVENS-JOHNSON SYNDROME. **EENT:** abnormal vision, nystagmus. **GI:** ano-rexia, flatulence, gingivitis. **Metab:** weight gain. **MS:** ↑ creatine kinase, arthralgia, RHABDOMYOLYSIS. **Neuro:** ataxia, confusion, depression, dizziness, drowsiness, altered reflexes, anxiety, concentration difficulties (children), emotional lability (children), hostility, hyperkinesia (children), malaise, paresthesia, sedation, SUICIDAL THOUGHTS, vertigo, weakness. **Misc:** HYPERSENSITIVITY REACTIONS (including anaphylaxis or angioedema).

Interactions
Drug-Drug: Antacids may ↓ absorption of gabapentin. ↑ risk of CNS and respiratory depression with other **CNS depressants**, including **alcohol, antihistamines, opioids,** and **sedative/hypnotics.** May ↓ hydrocodone levels.
Drug-Natural Products: Kava-kava, valerian, or chamomile can ↑ CNS depression.

Route/Dosage
The sustained-/extended-release formulations should not be interchanged with the immediate-release products.

Partial Seizures
PO (Adults and Children >12 yr): 300 mg 3 times daily initially. Titration may be continued until desired (range is 900–1800 mg/day in 3 divided doses; doses should not be more than 12 hr apart). Doses up to 2400–3600 mg/day have been well tolerated.
PO (Children ≥5–12 yr): 10–15 mg/kg/day in 3 divided doses initially titrated upward over 3 days to 25–35 mg/kg/day in 3 divided doses; dosage interval should not exceed 12 hr (doses up to 50 mg/kg/day have been used).
PO (Children 3–4 yrs): 10–15 mg/kg/day in 3 divided doses initially titrated upward over 3 days to 40 mg/kg/day in 3 divided doses; dosage interval should not exceed 12 hr (doses up to 50 mg/kg/day have been used).

Renal Impairment
PO (Adults and Children >12 yr): *CCr 30–59 mL/min:* 200–700 mg twice daily; *CCr 15–29 mL/min:* 200–700 mg once daily; *CCr 15 mL/min:* 100–300 mg once daily; *CCr <15 mL/min:* Reduce daily dose in proportion to CCr.

Postherpetic Neuralgia
PO (Adults): *Immediate-release:* 300 mg once daily on first day, then 300 mg 2 times daily on 2nd day, then 300 mg 3 times/day on day 3, may then be titrated upward as needed up to 600 mg 3 times/day; *Sustained-release (Gralise):* 300 mg once daily on first day, then 600 mg once daily on 2nd day, then 900 mg once daily on days 3–6, then 1200 mg once daily on days 7–10, then 1500 mg once daily on days 11–14, then 1800 mg once daily thereafter; *Extended-release (Horizant):* 600 mg once daily in the morning on days 1–3, then 600 mg twice daily thereafter.

Renal Impairment

PO (Adults): *CCr 30–59 mL/min:* 200–700 mg twice daily (immediate-release); 600–1800 mg once daily (sustained-release [Gralise]); 300 mg once daily in the morning on days 1–3, then 300 mg twice daily thereafter (may ↑ to 600 mg twice daily, as needed) (extended-release [Horizant]); *CCr 15–29 mL/min:* 200–700 mg once daily (immediate-release); sustained release (Gralise) not recommended; 300 mg in the morning on days 1 and 3, then 300 mg once daily in the morning thereafter (may ↑ to 300 mg twice daily, as needed) (extended-release [Horizant]); *CCr 15 mL/ min:* 100–300 mg once daily (immediate-release); sustained release (Gralise) not recommended; *CCr <15 mL/min:* ↓ daily dose in proportion to CCr (immediate release); sustained release (Gralise) not recommended; 300 mg every other day in the morning (may ↑ to 300 mg once daily in the morning, as needed) (extended-release [Horizant]); *CCr <15 mL/ min (on hemodialysis):* 300 mg after each dialysis session (may ↑ to 600 mg after each dialysis session, as needed) (extended-release [Horizant]).

Restless Legs Syndrome

PO (Adults): *Extended-release (Horizant):* 600 mg once daily at 5 PM.

Renal Impairment

(Adults): *CCr 30–59 mL/min:* 300 mg once daily at 5 PM; may ↑ to 600 mg once daily at 5 PM as needed; *CCr 15–29 mL/min:* 300 mg once daily at 5 PM; *CCr <15 mL/min:* 300 mg every other day; *CCr <15 mL/min (on hemodialysis):* Not recommended.

Neuropathic Pain (unlabeled use)

PO (Adults): 100 mg 3 times daily initially. Titrate weekly by 300 mg/day up to 900–2400 mg/day (maximum: 3600 mg/day).

PO (Children): 5 mg/kg/dose at bedtime initially then ↑ to 5 mg/kg twice daily on day 2 and 5 mg/kg 3 times daily on day 3. Titrate to effect up to 8–35 mg/kg/day in 3 divided doses.

Availability (generic available)

Immediate-release capsules: 100 mg, 300 mg, 400 mg. **Immediate-release tablets:** 600 mg, 800 mg. **Extended-release tablets (Horizant):** 300 mg, 600 mg. **Sustained-release tablets (Gralise):** 300 mg, 600 mg. **Oral solution (cool strawberry anise flavor):** 250 mg/5 mL.

NURSING IMPLICATIONS

Assessment

● Monitor closely for notable changes in behavior that could indicate the emergence or worsening of suicidal thoughts or behavior or depression.
● If administered with CNS depressants, including opioids, monitor for respiratory depression and sedation. Consider starting gabapentin at a low dose.
● **Seizures:** Assess location, duration, and characteristics of seizure activity.

● **Postherpetic Neuralgia & Neuropathic Pain:** Assess location, characteristics, and intensity of pain periodically during therapy.
● **Migraine Prophylaxis:** Monitor frequency and intensity of pain on pain scale.
● **Restless Leg Syndrome:** Assess frequency and intensity of restless leg syndrome prior to and periodically during therapy.

Lab Test Considerations

● May cause false-positive readings when testing for urinary protein with *Ames N-Multistix SG* dipstick test; use sulfosalicylic acid precipitation procedure.
● May cause leukopenia.

Implementation

● Do not confuse gabapentin with gemfibrozil. Do not confuse Neurontin with Motrin.
● Doses of *Gralise* and *Horizant* are not interchangeable with other dose forms of gabapentin.
● **PO:** May be administered without regard to meals.
● 600-mg and 800-mg tablets are scored and can be broken to administer a half-tablet. If half-tablet is used, administer other half at the next dose. Discard half-tablets not used within several days.
● Administer *Gralise* with evening meal. *DNC:* Swallow tablet whole; do not crush, break, or chew.
● Administer *Horizant for Restless Leg Syndrome* with evening meal at 5 PM. *Horizant for Postherpetic Neuralgia* is administered twice daily. *DNC:* Swallow tablet whole; do not crush, break, or chew.
● Discontinue gabapentin gradually over at least 1 wk. If dose is 600 mg/day, may discontinue without tapering. If >600 mg/day, titrate daily to 600 mg for 1 wk, then discontinue. If patient is taking 600 mg twice daily, taper to once daily before discontinuing. Abrupt discontinuation may cause increase in seizure frequency.

Patient/Family Teaching

● Instruct patient to take medication exactly as directed. Patients on 3 times daily dosing should not exceed 12 hr between doses. Take missed doses as soon as possible; if less than 2 hr until next dose, take dose immediately and take next dose 1–2 hr later, then resume regular dosing schedule. Do not double dose. Do not discontinue abruptly; may cause increase in frequency of seizures. Instruct patient to read the *Medication Guide* before starting and with each Rx refill, as changes may occur.
● Advise patient not to take gabapentin within 2 hr of an antacid.
● Gabapentin may cause dizziness and drowsiness. Caution patient to avoid driving or activities requiring alertness until response to medication is known. Patients with seizure should not resume driving until health care professional gives clearance based on control of seizure disorder.
● Instruct patient to notify health care professional of all Rx or OTC medications, vitamins, or herbal prod-

ucts being taken and consult health care professional before taking any new medications.

- Caution patients about risk of respiratory depression when taken with CNS depressants, including opioids or in patients with underlying respiratory impairment. Teach patients how to recognize respiratory depression and advise them to seek medical attention immediately if it occurs.
- Advise patient and family to notify health care professional if thoughts about suicide or dying, attempts to commit suicide; new or worse depression; new or worse anxiety; feeling very agitated or restless; panic attacks; trouble sleeping; new or worse irritability; acting aggressive; being angry or violent; acting on dangerous impulses; an extreme increase in activity and talking; or other unusual changes in behavior or mood occur.
- Instruct patient to notify health care professional of medication regimen before treatment or surgery.
- Rep: Advise females of reproductive potential to notify health care professional if pregnancy is planned or suspected or if breastfeeding. Encourage patients who become pregnant to enroll in the North American Antiepileptic Drug Pregnancy Registry by calling 1-888-233-2334 or on the web at www.aedpregnancyregistry.org.
- Advise patient to carry identification describing disease process and medication regimen at all times.

Evaluation/Desired Outcomes
- Decreased frequency of or cessation of seizures.
- Decreased postherpetic neuralgia pain.
- Decreased intensity of neuropathic pain.
- Decreased frequency of migraine headaches.
- Decreased effects of restless leg syndrome.

⚇ galantamine (ga-lant-a-meen)
~~Razadyne, Razadyne ER~~
Classification
Therapeutic: anti-Alzheimer's agents
Pharmacologic: cholinergics (cholinesterase inhibitors)

Indications
Mild to moderate dementia/neurocognitive disorder of the Alzheimer's type.

Action
Enhances cholinergic function by reversible inhibition of cholinesterase. **Therapeutic Effects:** Decreased dementia/cognitive decline (temporary) associated with Alzheimer's disease. Cognitive enhancer.

Pharmacokinetics
Absorption: Well absorbed (90%) following oral administration.
Distribution: Unknown.

Metabolism and Excretion: Primarily metabolized by the liver via the CYP2D6 and CYP3A4 isoenzymes; ⚇ the CYP2D6 enzyme system exhibits genetic polymorphism; ~7% of population may be poor metabolizers and may have significantly ↑ galantamine concentrations and an ↑ risk of adverse effects. 20% excreted unchanged in urine.
Half-life: 7 hr.

TIME/ACTION PROFILE (anticholinesterase activity)

ROUTE	ONSET	PEAK	DURATION
PO	unknown	1 hr	12 hr
PO-ER	unknown	1 hr	24 hr

Contraindications/Precautions
Contraindicated in: Hypersensitivity; Severe renal impairment; Severe hepatic impairment.
Use Cautiously in: Supraventricular cardiac conduction defects or concurrent use of drugs that may slow heart rate (↑ risk of bradycardia); History of ulcer disease/GI bleeding/concurrent NSAID use; Severe asthma or obstructive pulmonary disease; Mild to moderate renal impairment (avoid use if CCr <9 mL/min); Mild to moderate hepatic impairment (cautious dose titration recommended); OB: Safety not established in pregnancy; Lactation: Use while breastfeeding only if potential maternal benefit justifies potential risk to infant; Pedi: Safety and effectiveness not established in children.

Adverse Reactions/Side Effects
CV: bradycardia, chest pain. **Derm:** ACUTE GENERALIZED EXANTHEMATOUS PUSTULOSIS, STEVENS-JOHNSON SYNDROME. **GI:** nausea, vomiting, ↓ weight, anorexia, diarrhea, dyspepsia, flatulence. **GU:** bladder outflow obstruction, incontinence. **Neuro:** dizziness, extrapyramidal symptoms, fatigue, headache, syncope, tremor.

Interactions
Drug-Drug: Will ↑ neuromuscular blockade from **succinylcholine-type neuromuscular blocking agents**. May ↑ effects of other **cholinesterase inhibitors** or other **cholinergic agonists**, including **bethanechol**. May ↓ effectiveness of **anticholinergic medications**. Levels and effects may be ↑ by **ketoconazole**, **paroxetine**, **amitriptyline**, **fluvoxamine**, or **quinidine**.

Route/Dosage
PO (Adults): *Immediate-release tablets:* 4 mg twice daily initially, dose increments of 4 mg should be made at 4 wk intervals, up to 12 mg twice daily. Doses up to 16 mg twice daily have been used (range 16–32 mg/day; *Extended-release capsules:* 8 mg/day as a single dose in the morning, may be ↑ to 16 mg/day after 4 wk, then up to 24 mg/day after 4 wk; increments based on benefit/tolerability.

Renal Impairment

PO (Adults): *Moderate renal impairment:* Daily dose should not exceed 16 mg.

Hepatic Impairment

PO (Adults): *Moderate hepatic impairment:* Daily dose should not exceed 16 mg.

Availability (generic available)

Immediate-release tablets: 4 mg, 8 mg, 12 mg. **Extended-release capsules:** 8 mg, 16 mg, 24 mg. **Oral solution:** 4 mg/mL.

NURSING IMPLICATIONS

Assessment

- Assess cognitive function (memory, attention, reasoning, language, ability to perform simple tasks) periodically during therapy.
- Monitor heart rate periodically during therapy. May cause bradycardia.

Implementation

- Patient should be maintained on a stable dose for a minimum of 4 wk prior to increasing dose.
- If dose has been interrupted for ≥3 days, restart at the lowest dose and escalate to the current dose.
- **PO:** Administer preferably with morning and evening meal. Administration with food, the use of antiemetic medications, and ensuring adequate fluid intake may decrease nausea and vomiting.
- Administer extended-release capsules in the morning, preferably with food. *DNC:* Swallow whole; do not open, crush, or chew.
- Measure liquid doses carefully. Use measuring device that comes with drug. Mix dose into 3 to 4 oz. (about 100 mL) of a non-alcoholic liquid. Stir well and drink right away. Do not store for future use.

Patient/Family Teaching

- Emphasize the importance of taking galantamine daily, as directed. Instruct patient and/or caregiver in correct use of pipette if using oral solution; review *Oral Solution Instruction Sheet* included with product prior to use. Skip missed doses and return to regular schedule the following day; do not double doses. If >3 days doses are missed, restart at lowest dose. Do not discontinue abruptly; although no increase in frequency of adverse events may occur, beneficial affects of galantamine are lost when the drug is discontinued.
- Caution patient and caregiver that galantamine may cause dizziness. Monitor and assist with ambulation and caution patient to avoid driving and other activities requiring alertness until response to medication is known.
- Instruct patient to maintain adequate fluid intake during therapy.
- Advise patient and caregiver to stop taking galantamine and notify health care professional immediately if rash occurs.
- Advise patient and caregiver to notify health care professional if nausea or vomiting persists beyond 7 days or if new symptoms occur or previously noted symptoms increase in severity.
- Advise patient and caregiver to notify health care professional of medication regimen prior to treatment or surgery.
- Teach patient and caregivers that improvements in cognitive functioning may take wk to mo to stabilize.
- Caution that disease is not cured and degenerative process is not reversed.
- Rep: Advise females of reproductive potential to notify health care professional if pregnancy is planned or suspected or if breastfeeding.
- Emphasize the importance of follow-up exams to monitor progress.

Evaluation/Desired Outcomes

- Improvement in cognitive function (memory, attention, reasoning, language, ability to perform simple tasks) in patients with Alzheimer's disease.

galcanezumab

(**gal**-ka-**nez**-ue-mab)
Emgality
Classification
Therapeutic: vascular headache suppressants
Pharmacologic: monoclonal antibodies, calcitonin gene-related peptide receptor antagonists

Indications

Migraine prevention. Treatment of episodic cluster headaches.

Action

Monoclonal antibody that binds to the calcitonin gene-related peptide (CGRP) receptor, which reduces the neuroinflammatory and vasodilatory effects of CGRP. **Therapeutic Effects:** Reduction in frequency of migraines and cluster headaches.

Pharmacokinetics

Absorption: Unknown.
Distribution: Some tissue distribution.
Metabolism and Excretion: Degraded into small peptides and amino acids via catabolic pathways.
Half-life: 27 days.

TIME/ACTION PROFILE (plasma concentrations)

ROUTE	ONSET	PEAK	DURATION
SUBQ	unknown	5 days	1 mo

Contraindications/Precautions

Contraindicated in: Hypersensitivity.
Use Cautiously in: OB: Safety not established in pregnancy; Lactation: Use while breastfeeding only if potential maternal benefit justifies potential risk to infant; Pedi: Safety and effectiveness not established in children.

Adverse Reactions/Side Effects

Local: injection site reactions. **Misc:** HYPERSENSITIVITY REACTIONS (including anaphylaxis and angioedema).

Interactions

Drug-Drug: None reported.

Route/Dosage

Migraine Prevention

SUBQ (Adults): 240 mg once initially as loading dose, then 120 mg once monthly.

Episodic Cluster Headache

SUBQ (Adults): 300 mg once at the onset of the cluster period, then 300 mg once monthly until the end of the cluster period.

Availability

Solution for injection (prefilled pens and prefilled syringes): 100 mg/mL, 120 mg/mL.

NURSING IMPLICATIONS

Assessment

● Assess frequency and intensity of migraines and cluster headaches.
● Monitor for signs and symptoms of hypersensitivity reactions (rash, urticaria, dyspnea) during therapy. If reaction is severe, discontinue galcanezumab and treat as needed.

Implementation

● **SUBQ:** Prior to use allow vial to sit at room temperature for at least 30 min, protect from direct sunlight. Do not use other methods to warm solution (hot water or microwave). Do not shake. Solution is clear to opalescent, colorless to light yellow; do not administer solutions that are discolored, cloudy, or contain particulate matter. Store in refrigerator in original carton to protect from light; do not freeze. May be stored in original carton to protect from light up to 7 days at room temperature; discard if at room temperature >7 days. Do not put back in refrigerator.
● Inject entire contents into abdomen, thigh, or upper arm. Do not inject into areas where the skin is tender, bruised, red, or hard.

Migraines

● **SUBQ:** *Loading dose:* 240 mg (2 consecutive SUBQ injections of 120 mg each) once. *Monthly:* follow loading dose with monthly doses of 120 mg.

Cluster Headaches

● **SUBQ:** 300 mg (3 consecutive SUBQ injections of 100 mg each) at onset of cluster period; then monthly until end of cluster period.

Patient/Family Teaching

● Instruct patient to take as directed. Administer missed doses as soon as possible and schedule next dose from date last dose administered. Educate patient and/or caregiver on correct technique for injection and disposal of equipment. Advise patient to read *Patient Information* before starting therapy and with each Rx refill in case of changes.
● Instruct patient to notify health care professional immediately if signs and symptoms of hypersensitivity reaction (itching, rash, hives, swelling of face, mouth, tongue or throat, trouble breathing) occur.
● Advise patient to notify health care professional of all Rx or OTC medications, vitamins, or herbal products being taken and to consult with health care professional before taking other medications.
● Rep: Advise females of reproductive potential to notify health care professional if pregnancy is planned or suspected or if breastfeeding. Inform patient of pregnancy exposure registry that monitors pregnancy outcomes in women exposed to galcanezumab during pregnancy. Health care professionals are encouraged to register pregnant patients, or pregnant women may enroll themselves in the registry by calling 1-833-464-4724 or by contacting the company at www.migrainepregnancyregistry.com.

Evaluation/Desired Outcomes

● Reduction in frequency of migraines and cluster headaches.

---

ganciclovir (gan-sye-kloe-vir)

❋Cytovene

Classification
Therapeutic: antivirals

Indications

Treatment of cytomegalovirus (CMV) retinitis in immunocompromised patients, including patients with HIV (may be used in combination with foscarnet). Prevention of CMV infection in transplant patients at risk. Congenital CMV infection in neonates.

Action

CMV converts ganciclovir to its active form (ganciclovir phosphate) inside the host cell, where it inhibits viral DNA polymerase. **Therapeutic Effects:** Antiviral effect directed preferentially against CMV-infected cells.

Pharmacokinetics

Absorption: IV administration results in complete bioavailability.
Distribution: Widely distributed; enters CSF.
Protein Binding: 1–2%.
Metabolism and Excretion: 90% excreted unchanged by the kidneys.
Half-life: *Adults:* 2.9 hr; *Children 9 mo–12 yr:* 2.4 ±0.7 hr; *Neonates:* 2.4 hr (↑ in renal impairment).

TIME/ACTION PROFILE (antiviral levels)

ROUTE	ONSET	PEAK	DURATION
IV	rapid	end of infu-sion	12–24 hr

Contraindications/Precautions

Contraindicated in: Hypersensitivity to ganciclovir or acyclovir; Bone marrow depression or immunosuppression or thrombocytopenia (do not administer if absolute neutrophil count [ANC] <500/mm³ or platelet count <25,000/mm³); Lactation: Lactation.

Use Cautiously in: Renal impairment (dose ↓ required if CCr <80 mL/min); OB: Use during pregnancy only if potential maternal benefit justifies potential fetal risk; Rep: Women of reproductive potential and men with female partners of reproductive potential; Geri: Dose ↓ recommended in older adults.

Adverse Reactions/Side Effects

CV: arrhythmias, edema, hypertension, hypotension. **Derm:** alopecia, photosensitivity, pruritus, rash, urticaria. **Endo:** hypoglycemia. **GI:** ↑ liver enzymes, abdominal pain, GI BLEEDING, nausea, vomiting. **GU:** ↓ fertility, gonadal suppression, hematuria, renal impairment. **Hemat:** neutropenia, thrombocytopenia, anemia, eosinophilia. **Local:** pain/phlebitis at IV site. **Neuro:** abnormal dreams, ataxia, confusion, dizziness, drowsiness, headache, malaise, nervousness, SEIZURES, tremor. **Resp:** dyspnea. **Misc:** fever.

Interactions

Drug-Drug: Toxicity may be ↑ by **probenecid**. ↑ risk of seizures with **imipenem/cilastatin**; concurrent use not recommended. Concurrent use of **cyclosporine** or **amphotericin B** ↑ risk of nephrotoxicity. ↑ risk of nephrotoxicity and hematological toxicity with **mycophenolate mofetil**. Concurrent use with **dapsone**, **doxorubicin**, **flucytosine**, **hydroxyurea**, **pentamidine**, **tacrolimus**, **trimethoprim/sulfamethoxazole**, **vinblastine**, **vincristine**, or **zidovudine** ↑ risk of nephrotoxicity and myelosuppression.

Route/Dosage

IV (Adults and Children >3 mo): *Induction:* 5 mg/kg every 12 hr for 14–21 days. *Maintenance regimen:* 5 mg/kg/day or 6 mg/kg for 5 days of each wk. If progression occurs, ↑ to every 12 hr regimen. *Prevention:* 5 mg/kg every 12 hr for 7–14 days, then 5 mg/kg/day or 6 mg/kg for 5 days of each wk.
IV (Neonates): *Congenital CMV infection:* 12 mg/kg/day divided every 12 hr for 6 wk.

Renal Impairment

IV (Adults and Children): *Induction:* CCr 50–69 mL/min: 2.5 mg/kg/dose every 12 hr; CCr 25–49 mL/min: 2.5 mg/kg/dose every 24 hr; CCr 10–24 mL/min: 1.25 mg/kg/dose every 24 hr; CCr <10 mL/min: 1.25 mg/kg 3 times/wk after hemodialysis; *Maintenance:* CCr 50–69 mL/min: 2.5 mg/kg/dose every 24 hr; CCr 25–49 mL/min: 1.25 mg/kg/dose every 24 hr; CCr 10–24 mL/min: 0.625 mg/kg/dose every 24 hr; CCr <10 mL/min: 0.625 mg/kg 3 times/wk after hemodialysis.

Availability (generic available)

Lyophilized powder for injection: 500 mg/vial. **Solution for injection:** 50 mg/mL. **Premixed infusion:** 500 mg/250 mL.

NURSING IMPLICATIONS

Assessment

- Diagnosis of CMV retinitis should be determined by ophthalmoscopy before treatment with ganciclovir.
- Culture for CMV (urine, blood, throat) may be taken before administration. However, a negative CMV culture does not rule out CMV retinitis. If symptoms do not respond after several wk, resistance to ganciclovir may have occurred. Ophthalmologic exams should be performed weekly during induction and every 2 wk during maintenance or more frequently if the macula or optic nerve is threatened. Progression of CMV retinitis may occur during or after ganciclovir treatment.
- Assess for signs of infection (fever, chills, cough, hoarseness, lower back or side pain, sore throat, difficult or painful urination). Notify health care professional if these symptoms occur.
- Assess for bleeding (bleeding gums, bruising, petechiae; guaiac stools, urine, and emesis). Avoid IM injections and taking rectal temperatures. Apply pressure to venipuncture sites for 10 min.

Lab Test Considerations

- Verify negative pregnancy test prior to starting therapy.
- Monitor neutrophil and platelet count at least every 2 days during twice daily therapy and weekly thereafter. Granulocytopenia usually occurs during the first 2 wk of treatment but may occur anytime during therapy. Do not administer if ANC <500/mm³ or platelet count <25,000/mm³. Recovery begins within 3–7 days of discontinuation of therapy.
- Monitor BUN and serum creatinine at least once every 2 wk throughout therapy.
- Monitor liver function tests (AST, ALT, serum bilirubin, alkaline phosphatase) periodically during therapy. May cause ↑ levels.
- May cause ↓ blood glucose.

Implementation

- Do not confuse Cytovene (ganciclovir) with Cytosar (cytarabine).
- Do not administer SUBQ or IM; severe tissue irritation may result.
- IV: Observe infusion site for phlebitis. Rotate infusion site to prevent phlebitis.
- Maintain adequate hydration throughout therapy.

IV Administration

- Prepare solution in a biologic cabinet. Wear gloves, gown, and mask while handling medication. Discard IV equipment in specially designated containers.
- **Intermittent Infusion: *Reconstitution:*** Reconstitute 500 mg powder for injection with 10 mL of sterile water for injection for a concentration of 50 mg/mL. Do not reconstitute with bacteriostatic water with parabens; precipitation will occur. Shake well

to dissolve completely. Discard vial if particulate matter or discoloration occurs. Reconstituted solution is stable for 12 hr at room temperature; do not refrigerate.

- **Dilution:** Dilute reconstituted solution or solution for injection in 100 mL of D5W, 0.9% NaCl, Ringer's or LR. Once diluted for infusion, solution should be used within 24 hr. Refrigerate but do not freeze. *Concentration:* 10 mg/mL. *Rate:* Administer slowly, via infusion pump, over 1 hr using an in-line filter. Rapid administration may increase toxicity.

- **Y-Site Compatibility:** alemtuzumab, allopurinol, amphotericin B deoxycholate, amphotericin B lipid complex, anidulafungin, argatroban, arsenic trioxide, atropine, azithromycin, bivalirudin, bleomycin, calcium chloride, calcium gluconate, carboplatin, carmustine, caspofungin, cisplatin, cyanocobalamin, cyclophosphamide, cyclosporine, dactinomycin, daptomycin, defibrotide, dexamethasone, dexmedetomidine, digoxin, docetaxel, doxorubicin liposomal, enalaprilat, epoetin alfa, eptifibatide, ertapenem, etoposide, etoposide phosphate, fentanyl, filgrastim, fluconazole, fluorouracil, folic acid, fosphenytoin, furosemide, glycopyrrolate, granisetron, heparin, hetastarch, hydromorphone, ifosfamide, indomethacin, insulin, regular, labetalol, LR, leucovorin calcium, linezolid, lorazepam, mannitol, melphalan, methotrexate, metoprolol, milrinone, mitoxantrone, nafcillin, naloxone, nitroglycerin, nitroprusside, octreotide, oxytocin, paclitaxel, pamidronate, pantoprazole, pemetrexed, pentobarbital, phenobarbital, phytonadione, potassium chloride, propranolol, protamine, remifentanil, rituximab, rocuronium, sodium acetate, sufentanil, thiotepa, tigecycline, tirofiban, trastuzumab, vasopressin, vinblastine, vincristine, voriconazole, zoledronic acid.

- **Y-Site Incompatibility:** aldesleukin, amifostine, amikacin, aminophylline, amiodarone, ampicillin, ampicillin/sulbactam, ascorbic acid, atracurium, azathioprine, aztreonam, benztropine, bumetanide, butorphanol, cefazolin, cefepime, cefotaxime, cefotetan, cefoxitin, ceftazidime, ceftriaxone, cefuroxime, chloramphenicol, chlorpromazine, clindamycin, cytarabine, dacarbazine, dantrolene, daunorubicin hydrochloride, dexrazoxane, diazepam, diazoxide, diltiazem, diphenhydramine, dobutamine, dopamine, doxorubicin hydrochloride, doxycycline, ephedrine, epinephrine, epirubicin, erythromycin, esmolol, famotidine, fludarabine, foscarnet, gemcitabine, gemtuzumab ozogamicin, gentamicin, haloperidol, hydralazine, hydrocortisone, hydroxyzine, idarubicin, imipenem/cilastatin, irinotecan, isoproterenol, ketorolac, levofloxacin, lidocaine, magnesium sulfate, meperidine, mesna, methadone, methylprednisolone, metoclopramide, metronidazole, midazolam, minocycline, mitomycin, morphine, multivitamins, mycophenolate, nalbu-

phine, nicardipine, norepinephrine, ondansetron, oxacillin, palonosetron, papaverine, penicillin G, pentamidine, phentolamine, phenylephrine, phenytoin, piperacillin, piperacillin/tazobactam, potassium acetate, procainamide, prochlorperazine, promethazine, pyridoxine, sargramostim, sodium bicarbonate, succinylcholine, tacrolimus, theophylline, thiamine, tobramycin, topotecan, trimethoprim/sulfamethoxazole, vancomycin, vecuronium, verapamil, vinorelbine.

Patient/Family Teaching

- Inform patient that ganciclovir is not a cure for CMV retinitis. Progression of retinitis may continue in immunocompromised patients during and after therapy. Advise patients to have regular ophthalmic exams at least every 6 wk. Duration of therapy for CMV prevention is based on the duration and degree of immunosuppression.
- Advise patient to notify health care professional if fever; chills; sore throat; other signs of infection; bleeding gums; bruising; petechiae; or blood in urine, stool, or emesis occurs. Caution patient to avoid crowds and persons with known infections. Instruct patient to use soft toothbrush and electric razor. Patient should be cautioned not to drink alcoholic beverages or take products containing aspirin or NSAIDs.
- Caution patient to use sunscreen and protective clothing to prevent photosensitivity reactions.
- Rep: May cause fetal harm. Advise female patients of reproductive potential to use a nonhormonal method of contraception during and for at least 30 days after last dose and to avoid breastfeeding during therapy. Advise male patients to use condoms during and for at least 90 days after therapy. Inform patients that ganciclovir may cause temporary or permanent female and male infertility.
- Emphasize the importance of frequent follow-up exams to monitor blood counts.

Evaluation/Desired Outcomes

- Treatment of the symptoms of CMV retinitis in immunocompromised patients.
- Prevention of CMV retinitis in transplant patients at risk.

℀ **gefitinib** (je-fit-in-ib)
Iressa

Classification
Therapeutic: antineoplastics
Pharmacologic: enzyme inhibitors

Indications

℀ First-line treatment of patients with metastatic non-small cell lung cancer (NSCLC) whose tumors have epidermal growth factor receptor (EGFR) exon 19 deletions or exon 21 (L858R) substitution mutations.

Action
☒ Inhibits activation of kinases found in transmembrane cell surface receptors, including EGFR. **Therapeutic Effects:** Prolonged progression-free survival.

Pharmacokinetics
Absorption: 60% absorbed following oral administration.
Distribution: Extensively distributed.
Metabolism and Excretion: Primarily metabolized by the liver by the CYP3A4 isoenzyme, with some metabolism via the CYP2D6 isoenzyme; ☒ the CYP2D6 isoenzyme exhibits genetic polymorphism (~7% of population may be poor metabolizers and may have significantly ↑ gefitinib concentrations and an ↑ risk of adverse effects). Primarily excreted in feces, with <4% excreted in urine.
Half-life: 48 hr.

TIME/ACTION PROFILE (plasma levels)

ROUTE	ONSET	PEAK	DURATION
PO	unknown	3–7 hr	unknown

Contraindications/Precautions
Contraindicated in: Hypersensitivity; OB: Pregnancy; Lactation: Lactation.
Use Cautiously in: Idiopathic pulmonary fibrosis (↑ risk of pulmonary toxicity); Rep: Women of reproductive potential; Pedi: Safety and effectiveness not established in children.

Adverse Reactions/Side Effects
Derm: rash, alopecia, ERYTHEMA MULTIFORME, pruritus, STEVENS-JOHNSON SYNDROME, TOXIC EPIDERMAL NECROLYSIS. **EENT:** aberrant eyelash growth, blepharitis, conjunctivitis, corneal erosion/ulcer, dry eye, nose bleeding. **F and E:** dehydration. **GI:** anorexia, diarrhea, nausea, vomiting, dry mouth, GI PERFORATION, HEPATOTOXICITY, mouth ulceration. **GU:** ↓ fertility (females), ↑ serum creatinine, hematuria. **Metab:** weight loss. **Resp:** dyspnea, INTERSTITIAL LUNG DISEASE. **Misc:** fever, HYPERSENSITIVITY REACTIONS (including angioedema).

Interactions
Drug-Drug: **Strong CYP3A4 inducers**, including **rifampin** and **phenytoin**, ↓ blood levels and effects (↑ dose of gefitinib to 500 mg/day). **Strong CYP3A4 inhibitors**, including **ketoconazole** and **itraconazole**, ↑ blood levels and effects. Absorption and effectiveness may be ↓ by **drugs that ↑ gastric pH** including **H₂ receptor antagonists**, **proton pump inhibitors**, and **antacids**; take gefitinib 12 hr after last dose or 12 hr before the next dose of proton pump inhibitor; take gefitinib 6 hr after last dose or 6 hr before next dose H₂ receptor antagonist or antacid. May ↑ risk of bleeding with **warfarin**.

Route/Dosage
PO (Adults): 250 mg once daily; *Concurrent use of rifampin or phenytoin:* 500 mg once daily (resume 250 mg once daily dose 7 days after discontinuing strong CYP3A4 inducer).

Availability (generic available)
Tablets: 250 mg.

NURSING IMPLICATIONS
Assessment
- Assess for signs of pulmonary toxicity (dyspnea, cough, fever). Withhold gefitinib during diagnosis. If interstitial lung disease is confirmed, discontinue gefitinib and treat appropriately.
- Assess patient for eye symptoms such as pain during therapy. May require interruption of therapy and removal of aberrant eyelash. After symptoms and eye changes have resolved, may reinstate therapy.
- Monitor for rash. Interrupt or discontinue therapy if severe bullous, blistering or exfoliating conditions develop.

Lab Test Considerations
- ☒ Patient selection is based on the presence of EGFR exon 19 deletions or exon 21 L858R mutations in their tumor or plasma specimens. If these mutations are not detected in a plasma specimen, test tumor tissue if feasible. Information on FDA-approved tests for the detection of EGFR mutations in NSCLC is available at: http://www.fda.gov/CompanionDiagnostics. Monitor liver function tests periodically. May cause ↑ transaminases, bilirubin, and alkaline phosphatase. Withhold gefitinib in patients with worsening liver function tests; discontinue gefitinib if elevations are severe.
- Monitor for changes in prothrombin time and INR in patients taking warfarin. May cause ↑ levels.

Implementation
- ☒ FDA-approved test must be used to detect EGFR mutations in NSCLC. Patients must have EGFR exon 19 deletions or exon 21 substitutions to use gefitinib.
- **PO:** Administer one tablet daily without regard to food. Tablets can also be dispersed in 4–8 oz of drinking water (noncarbonated). No other liquids should be used. Drop the tablet in the water, without crushing it, stir until the tablet is dispersed (approximately 15 min); drink the liquid immediately. Rinse glass with half a glass of water and drink. Liquid can also be administered through a nasogastric tube.
- May interrupt therapy briefly (14 days) for patients with poorly tolerated diarrhea with dehydration or skin adverse reactions. Follow by restarting 250 mg dose.

Patient/Family Teaching
- Instruct patient to take gefitinib as directed. Take missed doses up to 12 hrs of next dose. Advise patient to read the *Instruction Sheet* with each Rx refill; new information may be available.
- Advise patient to notify health care professional promptly if severe persistent diarrhea, nausea, vomiting, or anorexia occur; if shortness of breath or cough occur or worsen; or if eye irritation or other new symptoms develop.

- Rep: May cause fetal harm. Advise females of reproductive potential to use effective contraception during and for 2 wk after last dose, to avoid breastfeeding during therapy, and to notify health care professional if pregnancy is suspected. May impair fertility in females.

Evaluation/Desired Outcomes

- Decrease in size and spread of tumors in non-small cell lung cancer.

HIGH ALERT

gemcitabine (jem-**site**-a-been)
~~Gemzar~~
Classification
Therapeutic: antineoplastics
Pharmacologic: antimetabolites, nucleoside analogues

Indications

Pancreatic cancer (locally advanced or metastatic). Inoperable locally advanced/metastatic non-small cell lung cancer (with cisplatin). Metastatic breast cancer after failure of prior anthracycline-containing adjuvant chemotherapy (unless anthracycline therapy contraindicated) (with paclitaxel). Advanced ovarian cancer that has relapsed 6 mo after completion of platinum-based therapy (with carboplatin).

Action

Interferes with DNA synthesis (cell-cycle phase specific). **Therapeutic Effects:** Death of rapidly replicating cells, particularly malignant ones.

Pharmacokinetics

Absorption: IV administration results in complete bioavailability.
Distribution: Unknown.
Metabolism and Excretion: Converted in cells to active diphosphate and triphosphate metabolites; these are excreted primarily by the kidneys.
Half-life: 32–94 min.

TIME/ACTION PROFILE (effect on blood counts)

ROUTE	ONSET	PEAK	DURATION
IV	unknown	unknown	unknown

Contraindications/Precautions

Contraindicated in: Hypersensitivity; OB: Pregnancy (may cause fetal harm); Lactation: Lactation.
Use Cautiously in: History of cardiovascular disease; Hepatic or renal impairment (↑ risk of toxicity); Rep: Women of reproductive potential and men with female partners of reproductive potential; Pedi: Safety and effectiveness in children not established.

Adverse Reactions/Side Effects

CV: edema, ARRHYTHMIAS, CAPILLARY LEAK SYNDROME, CEREBROVASCULAR ACCIDENT, hypertension, MI. **Derm:** alopecia, rash. **GI:** ↑ liver enzymes, diarrhea, nausea, stomatitis, vomiting, HEPATOTOXICITY. **GU:** hematuria, proteinuria, ↓ fertility (males), HEMOLYTIC UREMIC SYNDROME, renal failure, thrombotic microangiopathy. **Hemat:** anemia, leukopenia, thrombocytopenia, thrombotic microangiopathy. **Local:** injection site reactions. **Neuro:** paresthesias, POSTERIOR REVERSIBLE ENCEPHALOPATHY SYNDROME (PRES). **Resp:** dyspnea, ADULT RESPIRATORY DISTRESS SYNDROME, bronchospasm, pulmonary edema, PULMONARY FIBROSIS. **Misc:** flu-like symptoms, anaphylactoid reactions, fever.

Interactions

Drug-Drug: ↑ bone marrow depression with other **antineoplastics** or **radiation therapy**. May ↓ antibody response to **live virus vaccines** and ↑ risk of adverse reactions.

Route/Dosage

Pancreatic Cancer

IV (Adults): 1000 mg/m² once weekly for 7 wk, followed by a wk of rest, then on Days 1, 8, and 15 of each 28-day cycle.

Non-Small Cell Lung Cancer

IV (Adults): 1000 mg/m² on Days 1, 8, and 15 of each 28-day cycle (cisplatin is also given on day 1) *or* 1250 mg/m² on Days 1 and 8 of each 21-day cycle (cisplatin is also given on Day 1).

Breast Cancer

IV (Adults): 1250 mg/m² on Days 1 and 8 of each 21-day cycle (paclitaxel is also given on Day 1).

Ovarian Cancer

IV (Adults): 1000 mg/m² on Days 1 and 8 of each 21-day cycle (carboplatin is also given on Day 1).

Availability (generic available)

Powder for injection: 200 mg/vial, 1 g/vial, 2 g/vial.
Solution for injection: 200 mg/5.26 mL, 1 g/26.3 mL, 2 g/52.6 mL, 100 mg/mL.

NURSING IMPLICATIONS

Assessment

- Monitor vital signs before and frequently during therapy.
- Assess injection site during administration. Although gemcitabine is not a vesicant, it is an irritant, and local reactions may occur.
- Monitor for bone marrow depression. Assess for bleeding (bleeding gums, bruising, petechiae; guaiac stools, urine, and emesis) and avoid IM injections and taking rectal temperatures if platelet count is low. Apply pressure to venipuncture sites for 10 min. Assess for signs of infection during neu-

---

tropenia. Anemia may occur. Monitor for increased fatigue, dyspnea, and orthostatic hypotension.

- Monitor intake and output, appetite, and nutritional intake. Mild to moderate nausea and vomiting occur frequently. Antiemetics may be used prophylactically.
- Assess for signs and symptoms of capillary leak syndrome (severe hypotension, hypoalbuminemia, hemoconcentration). Discontinue therapy if symptoms occur.
- Monitor respiratory status during therapy. Discontinue gemcitabine if unexplained dyspnea or other evidence of severe pulmonary toxicity occurs. May occur up to 2 wk after last dose.
- Monitor for signs and symptoms of PRES (headache, seizure, lethargy, hypertension, confusion, blindness, and other visual and neurologic disturbances) during therapy. Confirm diagnosis of PRES with MRI. Discontinue gemcitabine if PRES develops during therapy.

Lab Test Considerations

- Verify negative pregnancy test before starting therapy. Monitor CBC, including differential and platelet count, before each dose. Dose guidelines are based on CBC. **For single-agent use:** *If absolute granulocyte count is >1000 and platelet count is >100,000,* full dose may be administered. *If absolute granulocyte count is 500–999 or platelet count is 50,000–99,000,* 75% of dose may be given. *If absolute granulocyte count is <500 or platelet count is <50,000,* withhold further doses. **For gemcitabine with paclitaxel (breast cancer):** *If absolute granulocyte count is >1200 and platelet count is >75,000,* full dose may be administered. *If absolute granulocyte count is 1000–1199 or platelet count is 50,000–75,000,* 75% of dose may be given. *If absolute granulocyte count is 700–999 or platelet count is ≥50,000,* 50% of dose may be given. *If absolute granulocyte count is <700 or platelet count is <50,000,* withhold further doses. **For gemcitabine with carboplatin (ovarian cancer):** *If absolute granulocyte count is >1500 and platelet count is >100,000,* full dose may be administered. *If the absolute granulocyte count is 1000–1499 or platelet count is 75,000–99,000,* 75% of dose may be given. *If the absolute granulocyte count is <1000 or the platelet count is <75,000,* withhold further doses.
- Monitor serum creatinine, potassium, calcium, and magnesium in patients taking cisplatin with gemcitabine.
- Monitor hepatic and renal function before and periodically during therapy. May cause transient ↑ in serum AST, ALT, alkaline phosphatase, and bilirubin concentrations. Discontinue gemcitabine for severe hepatic toxicity or hemolytic-uremic syndrome.
- May also cause ↑ BUN and serum creatinine concentrations, proteinuria, and hematuria.

Implementation

- **High Alert:** Fatalities have occurred with incorrect administration of chemotherapeutic agents. Before administering, clarify all ambiguous orders; double-check single, daily, and course-of-therapy dose limits; have second practitioner independently double-check original order, calculations, and infusion pump settings.

IV Administration

- Solution should be prepared in a biologic cabinet. Wear gloves, gown, and mask while handling IV medication. Discard IV equipment in specially designated containers.
- **Intermittent Infusion:** *Reconstitution:* To reconstitute, add 5 mL of 0.9% NaCl without preservatives to 200-mg vial, 25 mL of 0.9% NaCl to the 1-g vial of gemcitabine or 50 mL to the 2-g vial. *Concentration:* Concentration of 38 mg/mL. Incomplete dissolution may result in concentrations greater than 40 mg/mL. *Dilution:* May be further diluted with 0.9% NaCl. Solution is colorless to light straw color. Do not administer solutions that are discolored or contain particulate matter. Solution is stable for 24 hr at room temperature. Discard unused portions. Do not refrigerate; crystallization may occur. *Rate:* Administer dose over 30 min. If 2 bags required, infuse total of both bags over 30 min. Infusions longer than 60 min have a greater incidence of toxicity.
- **Y-Site Compatibility:** alemtuzumab, allopurinol, amifostine, amikacin, aminocaproic acid, aminophylline, amiodarone, ampicillin, ampicillin/sulbactam, anidulafungin, argatroban, atracurium, azithromycin, aztreonam, bivalirudin, bleomycin, bumetanide, buprenorphine, butorphanol, calcium acetate, calcium chloride, calcium gluconate, carboplatin, carmustine, caspofungin, cefazolin, cefotetan, cefoxitin, ceftazidime, ceftriaxone, cefuroxime, chlorpromazine, ciprofloxacin, cisatracurium, cisplatin, clindamycin, cyclophosphamide, cyclosporine, cytarabine, dacarbazine, dactinomycin, daunorubicin hydrochloride, dexamethasone, dexmedetomidine, dexrazoxane, digoxin, diltiazem, diphenhydramine, dobutamine, docetaxel, dopamine, doxorubicin hydrochloride, doxycycline, droperidol, enalaprilat, ephedrine, epinephrine, epirubicin, ertapenem, erythromycin, esmolol, etoposide, etoposide phosphate, famotidine, fentanyl, fluconazole, fludarabine, fluorouracil, foscarnet, fosphenytoin, gemtuzumab ozogamicin, gentamicin, glycopyrrolate, granisetron, haloperidol, heparin, hetastarch, hydralazine, hydrocortisone, hydromorphone, idarubicin, ifosfamide, insulin, regular, isoproterenol, labetalol, leucovorin calcium, levofloxacin, lidocaine, linezolid, lorazepam, magnesium sulfate, mannitol, meperidine, meropenem, mesna, methadone, metoclopramide, metoprolol, metronidazole, midazolam, milrinone, mitoxantrone, morphine, moxifloxacin, nalbuphine,

naloxone, nicardipine, nitroglycerin, nitroprusside, norepinephrine, octreotide, ondansetron, oxaliplatin, paclitaxel, paclitaxel protein-bound, palonosetron, pamidronate, pentamidine, pentobarbital, phenobarbital, phentolamine, potassium acetate, potassium chloride, potassium phosphate, procainamide, promethazine, propranolol, remifentanil, rituximab, rocuronium, sodium acetate, sodium bicarbonate, sodium phosphate, succinylcholine, sufentanil, tacrolimus, theophylline, thiotepa, tigecycline, tirofiban, tobramycin, topotecan, trastuzumab, trimethoprim/sulfamethoxazole, vancomycin, vasopressin, vecuronium, verapamil, vinblastine, vincristine, vinorelbine, voriconazole, zidovudine, zoledronic acid.

- **Y-Site Incompatibility:** acyclovir, amphotericin B lipid complex, amphotericin B liposome, cefepime, cefotaxime, chloramphenicol, dantrolene, daptomycin, diazepam, doxorubicin liposomal, furosemide, ganciclovir, imipenem-cilastatin, irinotecan, ketorolac, methotrexate, methylprednisolone, mitomycin, nafcillin, pantoprazole, pemetrexed, phenytoin, piperacillin/tazobactam, prochlorperazine, thiopental.

Patient/Family Teaching
- Explain purpose of gemcitabine to patient.
- Instruct patient to notify health care professional if fever; chills; sore throat; signs of infection; bleeding gums; bruising; petechiae; or blood in urine, stool, or emesis occurs. Caution patient to avoid crowds and persons with known infections. Instruct patient to use soft toothbrush and electric razor. Patient should be cautioned not to drink alcoholic beverages or take products containing aspirin or NSAIDs.
- Instruct patient to inspect oral mucosa for erythema and ulceration. If ulceration occurs, advise patient to use sponge brush and rinse mouth with water after eating and drinking. Stomatitis pain may require management with opioid analgesics.
- Instruct patient to notify health care professional if flu-like symptoms (fever, anorexia, headache, cough, chills, myalgia), swelling of feet or legs, signs and symptoms of pulmonary toxicity (shortness of breath, wheezing, cough), hemolytic-uremic syndrome (changes in color or volume of urine output, increased bruising or bleeding), or hepatic toxicity (jaundice, pain/tenderness in right upper abdominal quadrant) occur.
- Discuss with patient the possibility of hair loss. Explore methods of coping.
- Instruct patient not to receive any vaccinations without advice of health care professional.
- Rep: May cause fetal harm. Advise females of reproductive potential to use effective contraception during and for 6 mo after final dose and to avoid breastfeeding during and for at least 1 wk after last dose. Advise males with female partners of reproductive

potential to use effective contraception during and for 3 mo after last dose. May cause male infertility.
- Emphasize the need for periodic lab tests to monitor for side effects.

Evaluation/Desired Outcomes
- Palliative, symptomatic improvement in patients with pancreatic cancer.
- Decrease in size and spread of malignancy in lung, ovarian, and breast cancer.

gemfibrozil (gem-**fye**-broe-zil)
Lopid
Classification
Therapeutic: lipid-lowering agents
Pharmacologic: fibric acid derivatives

Indications
Management of type II-b hyperlipidemia (decreased high-density lipoprotein cholesterol [HDL-C], increased low-density lipoprotein cholesterol [LDL-C], increased triglycerides) in patients who do not yet have clinical coronary artery disease and have failed therapy with diet, exercise, weight loss, or other agents (niacin, bile acid sequestrants).

Action
Inhibits peripheral lipolysis. Decreases triglyceride production by the liver. Decreases production of the triglyceride carrier protein. Increases HDL-C. **Therapeutic Effects:** Decreased plasma triglycerides and increased HDL-C.

Pharmacokinetics
Absorption: Well absorbed after oral administration.
Distribution: Unknown.
Metabolism and Excretion: Some metabolism by the liver, 70% excreted by the kidneys (mostly unchanged), 6% excreted in feces.
Half-life: 1.3–1.5 hr.

TIME/ACTION PROFILE (triglyceride-lowering effect)

ROUTE	ONSET	PEAK	DURATION
PO	2–5 days	4 wk	several mo

Contraindications/Precautions
Contraindicated in: Hypersensitivity; Severe renal impairment; Hepatic impairment; Primary biliary cirrhosis; Gallbladder disease; Concurrent use of simvastatin, repaglinide, dasabuvir, or selexipag; OB: Avoid use during 1st trimester of pregnancy; Lactation: Lactation.
Use Cautiously in: OB: May be used starting in 2nd trimester of pregnancy, if needed; Pedi: Safety and effectiveness not established in children.

Adverse Reactions/Side Effects

Derm: alopecia, rash, urticaria. **EENT:** blurred vision. **GI:** abdominal pain, diarrhea, epigastric pain, flatulence, gallstones, heartburn, nausea, vomiting. **Hemat:** anemia, leukopenia. **MS:** myositis. **Neuro:** dizziness, headache.

Interactions

Drug-Drug: May ↑ levels of **CYP2C8 substrates**, including **dabrafenib**, **dasabuvir**, **enzalutamide**, **loperamide**, **montelukast**, **paclitaxel**, **pioglitazone**, or **selexipag**; concurrent use with **dasabuvir** or **selexipag** contraindicated. May ↑ levels of **OATP1B1 substrates**, including **atorvastatin**, **bosentan**, **ezetimibe**, **fluvastatin**, **glyburide**, **olmesartan**, **pitavastatin**, **pravastatin**, **repaglinide**, **rifampin**, **rosuvastatin**, **simvastatin**, and **valsartan**; concurrent use with **simvastatin** or **repaglinide** is contraindicated; avoid concurrent use with other **HMG-CoA reductase inhibitors**. May ↑ levels and the risk of bleeding with **warfarin**. Concurrent use with **colchicine** may ↑ risk of rhabdomyolysis, especially in patients with renal dysfunction or older adults. May ↓ the effect of **cyclosporine**. **Cholestyramine** and **colestipol** may ↓ absorption; separate administration by ≥2 hr.

Route/Dosage

PO (Adults): 600 mg twice daily 30 min before breakfast and dinner.

Availability (generic available)

Capsules: ✿ 300 mg. **Tablets:** 600 mg.

NURSING IMPLICATIONS

Assessment

- Obtain patient's diet history, especially regarding fat and alcohol consumption.

Lab Test Considerations

- Monitor serum triglyceride and cholesterol levels before and periodically during therapy. Assess LDL and triglyceride levels before and periodically during therapy. Discontinue gemfibrozil if paradoxical ↑ in lipid levels occurs.
- Assess liver function tests before and periodically during therapy. May cause ↑ serum bilirubin, alkaline phosphatase, CK, LDH, AST, and ALT. If hepatic function tests rise significantly, discontinue therapy and do not resume.
- Evaluate CBC and electrolytes every 3–6 mo and then yearly during therapy. May cause mild ↓ in hemoglobin, hematocrit, and leukocyte counts. May cause ↓ serum potassium concentrations.
- May cause slight ↑ in serum glucose.

Implementation

- Do not confuse gemfibrozil with gabapentin.
- **PO:** Administer 30 min before breakfast or dinner.

Patient/Family Teaching

- Instruct patient to take medication as directed, not to skip doses or double up on missed doses. Take

missed doses as soon as remembered unless almost time for next dose.
- Advise patient that gemfibrozil should be used in conjunction with dietary restrictions (fat, cholesterol, carbohydrates, alcohol), exercise, and cessation of smoking.
- Instruct patient to notify health care professional promptly if severe stomach pains with nausea and vomiting, fever, chills, sore throat, rash, diarrhea, muscle cramping, general abdominal discomfort, or persistent flatulence occur.
- Rep: Advise females of reproductive potential to notify health care professional if pregnancy is planned or suspected or if breastfeeding.

Evaluation/Desired Outcomes

- Decrease in serum triglyceride and cholesterol levels and improved HDL-C to total cholesterol ratios. If response is not seen within 3 mo, medication is usually discontinued.

---

gentamicin, See AMINOGLYCOSIDES.

✖ glecaprevir/pibrentasvir
(glek-**a**-pre-vir/pi-**brent**-as-vir)
❧ Maviret, Mavyret

Classification
Therapeutic: antivirals
Pharmacologic: NS5A inhibitors, protease inhibitors

Indications

✖ Chronic hepatitis C virus (HCV) genotypes 1, 2, 3, 4, 5, or 6 infection without cirrhosis or with compensated cirrhosis. ✖ Chronic HCV genotype 1 infection in patients who have previously received treatment with a regimen containing an HCV NS5A inhibitor or an NS3/4A protease inhibitor, but not both.

Action

Glecaprevir: inhibits the HCV NS3/4A protease, resulting in inhibition of viral replication; *Pibrentasvir:* inhibits the HCV NS5A protein, resulting in inhibition of viral replication. **Therapeutic Effects:** Decreased levels of HCV with sustained virologic response and lessened sequelae of chronic HCV infection.

Pharmacokinetics

Glecaprevir

Absorption: Well absorbed following oral administration; absorption ↑ by high-fat meal.
Distribution: Unknown.
Protein Binding: 97.5%.
Metabolism and Excretion: Partially metabolized by the liver via the CYP3A4 isoenzyme; 92% excreted in feces and <1% eliminated in urine.
Half-life: 6 hr.

Pibrentasvir

Absorption: Well absorbed following oral administration.

Distribution: Unknown.

Protein Binding: >99.9%.

Metabolism and Excretion: Not metabolized; 97% excreted in feces.

Half-life: 13 hr.

TIME/ACTION PROFILE (plasma concentrations)

ROUTE	ONSET	PEAK	DURATION
glecaprevir (PO)	unknown	5 hr	24 hr
pibrentasvir (PO)	unknown	5 hr	24 hr

Contraindications/Precautions

Contraindicated in: Moderate or severe hepatic impairment or any prior history of hepatic decompensation (↑ risk of hepatic decompensation/failure); Concurrent use of atazanavir or rifampin.

Use Cautiously in: Receiving immunosuppressant or chemotherapy medications (↑ risk of hepatitis B virus [HBV] reactivation); OB: Safety not established in pregnancy; Lactation: Safety not established in breastfeeding; Pedi: Children <3 yr (safety and effectiveness not established).

Adverse Reactions/Side Effects

Derm: pruritus. **GI:** diarrhea, HBV reactivation, hyperbilirubinemia, nausea. **Neuro:** fatigue, headache.

Interactions

Drug-Drug: **Atazanavir** may ↑ levels of glecaprevir/pibrentasvir and ↑ risk of liver enzyme elevation; concurrent use contraindicated. **Rifampin** may ↓ levels/effectiveness of glecaprevir/pibrentasvir; concurrent use contraindicated. **Strong CYP3A inducers**, including **carbamazepine** or **efavirenz** may ↓ levels and effectiveness of glecaprevir/pibrentasvir; concurrent use not recommended. **Darunavir, lopinavir,** or **ritonavir** may ↑ levels and risk of toxicity of glecaprevir/pibrentasvir; concurrent use not recommended. May ↑ levels and risk of toxicity of **atorvastatin, fluvastatin, lovastatin, pitavastatin, pravastatin, rosuvastatin,** and **simvastatin** and ↑ risk of myopathy; concurrent use with atorvastatin, lovastatin, and simvastatin not recommended; ↓ dose of pravastatin by 50%; do not exceed rosuvastatin dose of 10 mg/day; use lowest possible dose of fluvastatin or pitavastatin. May ↑ **dabigatran** levels and risk of bleeding; avoid concurrent use. May ↑ **digoxin** levels and risk of toxicity; ↓ digoxin dose by 50% when initiating glecaprevir/pibrentasvir therapy. Concurrent use with **ethinyl estradiol-containing oral contraceptives** may ↑ risk of liver enzyme elevation; concurrent use not recommended. **Cyclosporine** may ↑ levels and risk of toxicity of

glecaprevir/pibrentasvir; concurrent use not recommended if patients require cyclosporine dose >100 mg/day. May cause fluctuations in INR when used with **warfarin**; closely monitor INR. ↑ risk of hypoglycemia with use of certain **antidiabetic agents**.

Drug-Natural Products: **St. John's wort** may ↓ levels and effectiveness of glecaprevir/pibrentasvir; concurrent use not recommended.

Route/Dosage

PO (Adults and Children ≥12 yr or ≥45 kg): *Genotype 1, 2, 3, 4, 5, or 6: Treatment-naive with no cirrhosis or with compensated cirrhosis:* Three 100-mg/40-mg tablets once daily for 8 wk *or* six 50-mg/20-mg pellet packets once daily for 8 wk; *Genotype 1: Treatment-experienced with NS5A inhibitor (with no cirrhosis or with compensated cirrhosis):* Three 100-mg/40-mg tablets once daily for 16 wk *or* six 50-mg/20-mg pellet packets once daily for 16 wk; *Genotype 1: Treatment-experienced with NS3/4A protease inhibitor (with no cirrhosis or with compensated cirrhosis):* Three 100-mg/40-mg tablets once daily for 12 wk *or* six 50-mg/20-mg pellet packets once daily for 12 wk; *Genotype 1, 2, 4, 5, or 6: Treatment-experienced with regimens containing interferon, pegylated interferon, ribavirin, and/or sofosbuvir (no cirrhosis):* Three 100-mg/40-mg tablets once daily for 8 wk *or* six 50-mg/20-mg pellet packets once daily for 8 wk; *Genotype 1, 2, 4, 5, or 6: Treatment-experienced with regimens containing interferon, pegylated interferon, ribavirin, and/or sofosbuvir (with compensated cirrhosis):* Three 100-mg/40-mg tablets once daily for 12 wk *or* six 50-mg/20-mg pellet packets once daily for 12 wk; *Genotype 3: Treatment-experienced with regimens containing interferon, pegylated interferon, ribavirin, and/or sofosbuvir (with no cirrhosis or with compensated cirrhosis):* Three 100-mg/40-mg tablets once daily for 16 wk *or* six 50-mg/20-mg pellet packets once daily for 16 wk; *Liver or kidney transplant recipients:* Three 100-mg/40-mg tablets once daily for 12 wk (16 wk for those with Genotype 1 who are treatment experienced with NS5A inhibitor without prior treatment with an NS3/4A protease inhibitor; 16 wk for those with Genotype 3 who are treatment experienced with regimens containing interferon, pegylated interferon, ribavirin, and/or sofosbuvir) *or* six 50-mg/20-mg pellet packets once daily for 12 wk (16 wk for those with Genotype 1 who are treatment experienced with NS5A inhibitor without prior treatment with an NS3/4A protease inhibitor; 16 wk for those with Genotype 3 who are treatment experienced with regimens containing interferon, pegylated interferon, ribavirin, and/or sofosbuvir).

PO (Children 3–<12 yr and 30–<45 kg): *Genotype 1, 2, 3, 4, 5, or 6: Treatment-naive with no cirrhosis or with compensated cirrhosis:* Five 50-mg/20-mg pellet packets once daily for 8 wk; *Genotype 1:*

Treatment-experienced with NS5A inhibitor (with no cirrhosis or with compensated cirrhosis): Five 50-mg/20-mg pellet packets once daily for 16 wk; *Genotype 1: Treatment-experienced with NS3/4A protease inhibitor (with no cirrhosis or with compensated cirrhosis):* Five 50-mg/20-mg pellet packets once daily for 12 wk; *Genotype 1, 2, 4, 5, or 6: Treatment-experienced with regimens containing interferon, pegylated interferon, ribavirin, and/or sofosbuvir (no cirrhosis):* Five 50-mg/20-mg pellet packets once daily for 8 wk; *Genotype 1, 2, 4, 5, or 6: Treatment-experienced with regimens containing interferon, pegylated interferon, ribavirin, and/or sofosbuvir (with compensated cirrhosis):* Five 50-mg/20-mg pellet packets once daily for 12 wk; *Genotype 3: Treatment-experienced with regimens containing interferon, pegylated interferon, ribavirin, and/or sofosbuvir (with no cirrhosis or with compensated cirrhosis):* Five 50-mg/20-mg pellet packets once daily for 16 wk; *Liver or kidney transplant recipients:* Five 50-mg/20-mg pellet packets once daily for 12 wk (16 wk for those with Genotype 1 who are treatment experienced with NS5A inhibitor without prior treatment with an NS3/4A protease inhibitor; 16 wk for those with Genotype 3 who are treatment experienced with regimens containing interferon, pegylated interferon, ribavirin, and/or sofosbuvir).

PO (Children 3–<12 yr and 20–<30 kg): *Genotype 1, 2, 3, 4, 5, or 6: Treatment-naive with no cirrhosis or with compensated cirrhosis:* Four 50-mg/20-mg pellet packets once daily for 8 wk; *Genotype 1: Treatment-experienced with NS5A inhibitor (with no cirrhosis or with compensated cirrhosis):* Four 50-mg/20-mg pellet packets once daily for 16 wk; *Genotype 1: Treatment-experienced with NS3/4A protease inhibitor (with no cirrhosis or with compensated cirrhosis):* Four 50-mg/20-mg pellet packets once daily for 12 wk; *Genotype 1, 2, 4, 5, or 6: Treatment-experienced with regimens containing interferon, pegylated interferon, ribavirin, and/or sofosbuvir (no cirrhosis):* Four 50-mg/20-mg pellet packets once daily for 8 wk; *Genotype 1, 2, 4, 5, or 6: Treatment-experienced with regimens containing interferon, pegylated interferon, ribavirin, and/or sofosbuvir (with compensated cirrhosis):* Four 50-mg/20-mg pellet packets once daily for 12 wk; *Genotype 3: Treatment-experienced with regimens containing interferon, pegylated interferon, ribavirin, and/or sofosbuvir (with no cirrhosis or with compensated cirrhosis):* Four 50-mg/20-mg pellet packets once daily for 16 wk; *Liver or kidney transplant recipients:* Four 50-mg/20-mg pellet packets once daily for 12 wk (16 wk for those with Genotype 1 who are treatment experienced with NS5A inhibitor without prior treatment with an NS3/4A protease inhibitor; 16 wk for those with Genotype 3 who are treatment experienced with regimens containing interferon, pegylated interferon, ribavirin, and/or sofosbuvir).

PO (Children 3–<12 yr and <20 kg): *Genotype 1, 2, 3, 4, 5, or 6: Treatment-naive with no cirrhosis or* *with compensated cirrhosis:* Three 50-mg/20-mg pellet packets once daily for 8 wk; *Genotype 1: Treatment-experienced with NS5A inhibitor (with no cirrhosis or with compensated cirrhosis):* Three 50-mg/20-mg pellet packets once daily for 16 wk; *Genotype 1: Treatment-experienced with NS3/4A protease inhibitor (with no cirrhosis or with compensated cirrhosis):* Three 50-mg/20-mg pellet packets once daily for 12 wk; *Genotype 1, 2, 4, 5, or 6: Treatment-experienced with regimens containing interferon, pegylated interferon, ribavirin, and/or sofosbuvir (no cirrhosis):* Three 50-mg/20-mg pellet packets once daily for 8 wk; *Genotype 1, 2, 4, 5, or 6: Treatment-experienced with regimens containing interferon, pegylated interferon, ribavirin, and/or sofosbuvir (with compensated cirrhosis):* Three 50-mg/20-mg pellet packets once daily for 12 wk; *Genotype 3: Treatment-experienced with regimens containing interferon, pegylated interferon, ribavirin, and/or sofosbuvir (with no cirrhosis or with compensated cirrhosis):* Three 50-mg/20-mg pellet packets once daily for 16 wk; *Liver or kidney transplant recipients:* Three 50-mg/20-mg pellet packets once daily for 12 wk (16 wk for those with Genotype 1 who are treatment experienced with NS5A inhibitor without prior treatment with an NS3/4A protease inhibitor; 16 wk for those with Genotype 3 who are treatment experienced with regimens containing interferon, pegylated interferon, ribavirin, and/or sofosbuvir).

Availability

Tablets: glecaprevir 100 mg/pibrentasvir 40 mg. **Oral pellets:** glecaprevir 50 mg/pibrentasvir 20 mg per pkt.

NURSING IMPLICATIONS
Assessment

- Monitor for signs and symptoms of HBV reactivation or hepatitis (jaundice, dark urine, light colored stools, fatigue, weakness, loss of appetite, nausea, vomiting, stomach pain) during therapy.

Lab Test Considerations

- Test all patients for current or prior HBV infection before starting HCV therapy; may cause HBV reactivation. Measure hepatitis B surface antigen (HBsAg) and hepatitis core antibody (anti-HBc). Monitor for clinical and laboratory signs of hepatitis flare (↑ AST, ALT, bilirubin, liver failure, death) or HBV reactivation (rapid ↑ in serum HBV DNA level) during HCV treatment and post-treatment follow-up.
- ▓ Test patient with HCV genotype 1a infection for presence of virus with NS5A resistance-associated polymorphisms prior to starting therapy with *Mavyret* to determine dose regimen and duration.

Implementation

- **PO:** Administer once daily with food.
- **Oral Pellets:** Take oral pellets together, with food, once daily. Oral pellets may also be sprinkled on a small amount of soft food with a low water content that will stick to a spoon and should be swallowed

without chewing (peanut butter, chocolate hazelnut spread, cream cheese, thick jam, Greek yogurt). Entire mixture of food and oral pellets should be swallowed within 15 min of preparation; *DNC:* Do not crush or chew oral pellets. Liquids or foods that would drip or slide off the spoon are not recommended as the drug may dissolve quickly and become less effective.

Patient/Family Teaching

- Instruct patient to take medication as directed. Do not skip or miss dose. If dose is missed, take if <18 hr from usual time taken, then take next dose at usual time. If >18 hr from usual time of dose, omit dose and take next dose at usual time. Do not stop medication without consulting health care professional. Advise patient to read *Patient Information* before starting therapy and with each Rx refill in case of changes.
- Advise patient to notify health care professional if they have a history of HBV. May cause reactivation.
- Instruct patient to notify health care professional of all Rx or OTC medications, vitamins, or herbal products being taken and consult health care professional before taking any new medications, especially St. John's wort.
- Rep: Advise females of reproductive potential to notify health care professional if pregnancy is planned or suspected or if breastfeeding.

Evaluation/Desired Outcomes

- Decreased levels of HCV with sustained virologic response and lessened sequelae of chronic HCV infection.

BEERS | HIGH ALERT

⚡glipiZIDE (glip-i-zide)

~~Glucotrol, Glucotrol XL~~

Classification
Therapeutic: antidiabetics
Pharmacologic: sulfonylureas

Indications

PO: Type 2 diabetes mellitus (as adjunct to diet and exercise).

Action

Lowers blood sugar by stimulating the release of insulin from the pancreas and increasing the sensitivity to insulin at receptor sites. May also decrease hepatic glucose production. **Therapeutic Effects:** Lowering of blood sugar in diabetic patients.

Pharmacokinetics

Absorption: Well absorbed following oral administration.
Distribution: Unknown.
Protein Binding: 99%.

Metabolism and Excretion: Mostly metabolized by the liver.
Half-life: 2.1–2.6 hr.

TIME/ACTION PROFILE (hypoglycemic activity)

ROUTE	ONSET	PEAK	DURATION
PO	15–30 min	1–2 hr	up to 24 hr

Contraindications/Precautions

Contraindicated in: Hypersensitivity; Hypersensitivity to sulfonamides (cross-sensitivity may occur); Insulin-dependent diabetics; Diabetic coma or ketoacidosis.
Use Cautiously in: Severe cardiovascular or hepatic disease; ⚡ Glucose 6-phosphate dehydrogenase deficiency (↑ risk of hemolytic anemia); Severe renal impairment (↑ risk of hypoglycemia); Infection, stress, or changes in diet may alter requirements for control of blood sugar; Impaired thyroid, pituitary, or adrenal function; Malnutrition, high fever, prolonged nausea, or vomiting; OB: Crosses the placenta and ↑ risk of neonatal hypoglycemia; should be discontinued ≥2 wk before delivery; insulin recommended during pregnancy; Lactation: May ↑ risk of hypoglycemia in infant; use while breastfeeding only if potential maternal benefit justifies potential risk to infant; Geri: Appears on Beers list. ↑ risk of prolonged hypoglycemia in older adults. Avoid use as first- or second-line monotherapy or as add-on treatment in older adults unless there are significant barriers to the use of safer and more effective agents. If a sulfonylurea must be used, this is the preferred agent.

Adverse Reactions/Side Effects

Derm: <u>photosensitivity</u>, rash. **Endo:** <u>hypoglycemia</u>. **F and E:** hyponatremia. **GI:** constipation, cramps, diarrhea, dyspepsia, hepatitis, nausea, vomiting. **Hemat:** agranulocytosis, APLASTIC ANEMIA, hemolytic anemia, leukopenia, pancytopenia, thrombocytopenia. **Metab:** ↑ appetite. **Neuro:** dizziness, drowsiness, headache, weakness.

Interactions

Drug-Drug: Ingestion of **alcohol** may result in disulfiram-like reaction. Effectiveness may be ↓ by concurrent use of **diuretics, corticosteroids, atypical antipsychotics, danazol, phenothiazines, oral contraceptives, estrogens, progestins, glucagon, protease inhibitors, somatropin, thyroid preparations, phenytoin, niacin, sympathomimetics, calcium channel blockers** and **isoniazid. Alcohol, ACE inhibitors, angiotensin II receptor blockers, chloramphenicol, fibric acid derivatives, fluoxetine, disopyramide, fluoroquinolones, MAO inhibitors, NSAIDs** (except diclofenac), **pentoxifylline, probenecid, salicylates, voriconazole, H₂ receptor antagonists, sulfonamides,** and **warfarin** may ↑ risk of hypoglycemia. Concurrent use with **warfarin** may alter the

G

✦= Canadian drug name. ⚡ = Genetic implication. ~~Strikethrough~~ = Discontinued. CAPITALS = life-threatening. <u>Underline</u> = most frequent.

response to both agents (↑ effects of both initially, then ↓ activity); close monitoring recommended during any changes in dose. **Beta-adrenergic blockers** may mask the signs and symptoms of hypoglycemia. May ↑**cyclosporine** levels. **Colesevelam** may ↓ effects; administer glipizide ≥4 hr before colesevelam.

Route/Dosage
PO (Adults): 5 mg/day initially, ↑ as needed (range 2.5–40 mg/day); extended-release dose form is given once daily. Doses >15 mg/day may be given as 2 divided doses of regular-release product (not extended-release).

PO (Geriatric Patients): 2.5 mg/day initially.

Availability (generic available)
Immediate-release tablets: 5 mg, 10 mg. **Extended-release tablets:** 2.5 mg, 5 mg, 10 mg. *In combination with:* metformin.

NURSING IMPLICATIONS
Assessment
- Observe for signs and symptoms of hypoglycemic reactions (sweating, hunger, weakness, dizziness, tremor, tachycardia, anxiety). Patients on concurrent beta-blocker therapy may have very subtle signs and symptoms of hypoglycemia.
- Assess patient for allergy to sulfonamides.

Lab Test Considerations
- Monitor serum glucose and glycosylated hemoglobin (A_{1C}) periodically during therapy to evaluate effectiveness of treatment.
- Monitor CBC periodically during therapy. Report ↓ in blood counts promptly.
- May cause an ↑ in AST, LDH, BUN, and serum creatinine.

Toxicity and Overdose
- Overdose is manifested by symptoms of hypoglycemia. Mild hypoglycemia may be treated with administration of oral glucose. Treat severe hypoglycemia with IV D50W followed by continuous IV infusion of more dilute dextrose solution at a rate sufficient to keep serum glucose at approximately 100 mg/dL.

Implementation
- *High Alert:* Accidental administration of oral hypoglycemic agents to non-diabetic adults and children has resulted in serious harm or death. Before administering, confirm that patient has Type 2 diabetes.
- *High Alert:* Do not confuse glipizide with glyburide.
- Patients stabilized on a diabetic regimen who are exposed to stress, fever, trauma, infection, or surgery may require administration of insulin.
- To convert from other oral hypoglycemic agents, gradual conversion is not required. For insulin dose of less than 20 units/day, change to glipizide can be made without gradual dose adjustment. Patients taking 20 or more units/day should convert gradually by receiving glipizide and a 25–30% reduction in insulin dose every day or every 2nd day with gradual insulin dose

reduction as tolerated. Monitor serum or glucose and ketones at least 3 times/day during conversion.
- **PO:** Administer 30 min before a meal. *DNC:* Swallow extended-release tablets whole; do not crush, break or chew.

Patient/Family Teaching
- Instruct patient to take medication at same time each day. Take missed doses as soon as remembered unless almost time for next dose. Do not take if unable to eat.
- Explain to patient that this medication controls hyperglycemia but does not cure diabetes. Therapy is long term.
- Review signs of hypoglycemia and hyperglycemia with patient. If hypoglycemia occurs, advise patient to drink a glass of orange juice or ingest 2–3 tsp of sugar, honey, or corn syrup dissolved in water or an appropriate number of glucose tablets and notify health care professional.
- Encourage patient to follow prescribed diet, medication, and exercise regimen to prevent hypoglycemic or hyperglycemic episodes.
- Concurrent use of alcohol may cause a disulfiram-like reaction (abdominal cramps, nausea, flushing, headaches, and hypoglycemia).
- Instruct patient in proper testing of serum glucose and ketones. These tests should be closely monitored during periods of stress or illness and health care professional notified if significant changes occur.
- May occasionally cause dizziness or drowsiness. Caution patient to avoid driving or other activities requiring alertness until response to medication is known.
- Caution patient to avoid other medications, especially aspirin and alcohol, while on this therapy without consulting health care professional.
- Caution patient to use sunscreen and protective clothing to prevent photosensitivity reactions.
- Advise patient to inform health care professional of medication regimen prior to treatment or surgery.
- Advise patient to notify health care professional promptly if unusual weight gain, swelling of ankles, drowsiness, shortness of breath, muscle cramps, weakness, sore throat, rash, or unusual bleeding or bruising occurs.
- Advise patient to carry a form of sugar (sugar packets, candy) and identification describing disease process and medication regimen at all times.
- Rep: May cause fetal harm. Insulin is the recommended method of controlling blood sugar during pregnancy. Counsel female patients to use a form of contraception other than oral contraceptives and to notify health care professional promptly if pregnancy is planned or suspected or if breastfeeding. Discontinue glipizide at least 2 wk before expected delivery. Neonates of women with gestational diabetes who are treated with sulfonylureas during pregnancy may be at increased risk for respiratory distress and hypoglycemia (jitters, cyanosis, apnea, hypothermia, excessive sleepiness, poor feeding, seizures).

- Emphasize the importance of routine follow-up exams.

Evaluation/Desired Outcomes

- Control of blood glucose levels without the appearance of hypoglycemic or hyperglycemic episodes.

glucagon (gloo-ka-gon)
Baqsimi, GlucaGen, Gvoke
Classification
Therapeutic: hormones
Pharmacologic: pancreatics

Indications

Acute management of severe hypoglycemia. Facilitation of radiographic examination of the GI tract. **Unlabeled Use:** Beta-blocker overdose. Calcium channel blocker overdose.

Action

Stimulates hepatic production of glucose from glycogen stores (glycogenolysis). Relaxes the musculature of the GI tract (stomach, duodenum, small bowel, and colon), temporarily inhibiting movement. Has positive inotropic and chronotropic effects. **Therapeutic Effects:** Increase in blood glucose. Relaxation of GI musculature, facilitating radiographic examination.

Pharmacokinetics

Absorption: Well absorbed following IM, intranasal, and SUBQ administration; IV administration results in complete bioavailability.
Distribution: Extensively distributed to tissues.
Metabolism and Excretion: Extensively metabolized by the liver, plasma, and kidneys.
Half-life: 8–18 min.

TIME/ACTION PROFILE

ROUTE	ONSET	PEAK	DURATION
IM (hyperglycemic action)	within 10 min	30 min	12–27 min
IV (hyperglycemic action)	1 min	5 min	9–17 min
SUBQ (hyperglycemic action)	within 10 min	30–45 min	60–90 min
Intranasal (hyperglycemic action)	within 15 min	unknown	unknown
IV (effect on GI musculature)	45 sec (for 0.25–2-mg dose)	unknown	9–17 min (0.25–0.5-mg dose); 22–25 min (2-mg dose)
IM (effect on GI musculature)	8–10 min (1-mg dose); 4–7 min (2-mg dose)	unknown	9–27 min (1-mg dose); 21–32 min (2-mg dose)

Contraindications/Precautions

Contraindicated in: Hypersensitivity; Pheochromocytoma; Insulinoma.
Use Cautiously in: Prolonged fasting, starvation, adrenal insufficiency, or chronic hypoglycemia (low levels of releasable glucose); OB: Use during pregnancy only if potential maternal benefit justifies potential fetal risk; Lactation: Safety not established in breastfeeding; Pedi: Children <4 yr (safety and effectiveness of nasal powder not established).

Adverse Reactions/Side Effects

CV: hypotension. **Derm:** necrolytic migratory erythema. **EENT:** epistaxis, eye redness, itchy eyes, itchy throat, nasal congestion, nasal discomfort, nasal itching, rhinorrhea, sneezing, watery eyes. **GI:** nausea, vomiting. **Neuro:** headache. **Resp:** cough. **Misc:** HYPERSENSITIVITY REACTIONS (including anaphylaxis).

Interactions

Drug-Drug: Large doses may ↑ the effect of **warfarin**. Negates the response to **insulin** or **oral hypoglycemic agents**. **Phenytoin** inhibits the stimulant effect of glucagon on insulin release. Hyperglycemic effect is intensified and prolonged by **epinephrine**. Patients on concurrent **beta blocker** therapy may have a greater ↑ in heart rate and BP.

Route/Dosage

Hypoglycemia

IV, IM, SUBQ (Adults and Children >25 kg): 1 mg; may be repeated in 15 min if necessary.
SUBQ (Adults and Children ≥12 yr): *Gvoke:* 1 mg; may be repeated in 15 min if necessary.
IV, IM, SUBQ (Children <25 kg): 0.5 mg or 0.02–0.03 mg/kg; may be repeated in 15 min if necessary.
IV, IM, SUBQ (Children >6 yr and unknown weight): 1 mg; may be repeated in 15 min if necessary.
IV, IM, SUBQ (Children <6 yr and unknown weight): 0.5 mg or 0.02–0.03 mg/kg; may be repeated in 15 min if necessary.
SUBQ (Children 2–12 yr and ≥45 kg): *Gvoke:* 1 mg; may be repeated in 15 min if necessary.
SUBQ (Children 2–12 yr and <45 kg): *Gvoke:* 0.5 mg; may be repeated in 15 min if necessary.
Intranasal (Adults and Children ≥4 yr): 3 mg (one actuation) in one nostril; may be repeated in 15 min if necessary.

Radiographic Examination of the GI Tract

IM, IV (Adults): 0.25–2 mg; depending on location and duration of examination (0.5 mg IV or 2 mg IM for relaxation of stomach; for examination of the colon 2 mg IM 10 min before procedure).

Beta Blocker or Calcium Channel Blocker Overdose

IV (Adults): *Beta blocker overdose:* 50–150 mcg (0.05–0.15 mg)/kg, followed by 1–5 mg/hr infusion.

Calcium channel blocker overdose: 2 mg; additional doses determined by response.

Availability (generic available)

Nasal powder: 3 mg/device. **Powder for injection:** 1-mg (equivalent to 1 unit) vials as an emergency kit for low blood glucose and as a diagnostic kit. **Solution for SUBQ injection (Gvoke) (prefilled syringes and prefilled autoinjectors):** 0.5 mg/0.1 mL, 1 mg/0.2 mL.

NURSING IMPLICATIONS

Assessment

- Assess for signs of hypoglycemia (sweating, hunger, weakness, headache, dizziness, tremor, irritability, tachycardia, anxiety) prior to and periodically during therapy.
- Assess neurologic status during therapy. Institute safety precautions to protect patient from injury caused by seizures, falling, or aspiration. For insulin shock therapy, 0.5–1 mg is administered after 1 hr of coma; patient usually awakens in 10–25 min. If no response occurs, repeat the dose. Feed patient supplemental carbohydrates orally to replenish liver glycogen and prevent secondary hypoglycemia as soon as possible after awakening, especially pediatric patients.
- Assess nutritional status. Patients who lack liver glycogen stores (starvation, chronic hypoglycemia, adrenal insufficiency) will require glucose instead of glucagon.
- Assess for nausea and vomiting after administration of dose. Protect patients with depressed level of consciousness from aspiration by positioning on side; ensure that a suction unit is available. Notify health care professional if vomiting occurs; patient will require parenteral glucose to prevent recurrent hypoglycemia.

Lab Test Considerations

- Monitor serum glucose levels throughout episode, during treatment, and for 3–4 hr after patient regains consciousness. Use of bedside fingerstick blood glucose determination methods is recommended for rapid results. Follow-up lab results may be ordered to validate fingerstick values, but do not delay treatment while awaiting lab results, as this could result in neurologic injury or death.
- Large doses of glucagon may cause a ↓ in serum potassium concentrations.

Implementation

- May be given SUBQ, IM, or IV. Reconstitute with diluent supplied in kit by manufacturer. Inspect solution prior to use; use only clear, water-like solution. Solution is stable for 48 hr if refrigerated, 24 hr at room temperature. Unmixed medication should be stored at room temperature.
- Administer supplemental carbohydrates IV or orally to facilitate increase of serum glucose levels.

- **SUBQ:** *Gvoke* solution is clear and colorless to pale yellow; do not administer if solution is discolored or contains particulate matter. Inject in lower abdomen, outer thigh, or outer upper arm.
- **Intranasal:** Administer by inserting tip into one nostril and pressing device plunger all the way in until green line is no longer showing. Dose does not need to be inhaled. Call for emergency assistance immediately after administering dose. When patient responds to treatment, give oral carbohydrates.

IV Administration

- **IV Push:** *Reconstitution:* Reconstitute each vial with 1 mL of an appropriate diluent. For doses ≤2 mg, use diluent provided by manufacturer. For doses >2 mg, use sterile water for injection instead of diluent supplied by manufacturer to minimize risk of thrombophlebitis, CNS toxicity, and myocardial depression from phenol preservative in diluent supplied by manufacturer. Reconstituted vials should be used immediately. *Concentration:* Not exceed 1 mg/mL. *Rate:* Administer at a rate not exceeding 1 mg/min. May be administered through IV line containing D5W.
- **Continuous Infusion:** *Reconstitution:* Reconstitute vials as per directions above (use sterile water for injection). *Dilution:* Further dilute 10 mg of glucagon in 100 mL of D5W. *Concentration:* 0.1 mg/mL. *Rate:* See Route/Dosage section.
- **Y-Site Compatibility:** naloxone.

Patient/Family Teaching

- Teach patient and family signs and symptoms of hypoglycemia. Instruct patient to take oral glucose as soon as symptoms of hypoglycemia occur; glucagon is reserved for episodes when patient is unable to swallow because of decreased level of consciousness.
- **Home Care Issues** Instruct family on correct technique to prepare, draw up, and administer injection. Health care professional must be contacted immediately after each dose for orders regarding further therapy or adjustment of insulin dose or diet.
- Advise family that patient should receive oral glucose when alertness returns.
- Instruct family to position patient on side until fully alert. Explain that glucagon may cause nausea and vomiting. Aspiration may occur if patient vomits while lying on back.
- Instruct patient to check expiration date monthly and to replace outdated medication immediately.
- Review hypoglycemic medication regimen, diet, and exercise programs.
- Patients with diabetes mellitus should carry a source of sugar (such as a packet of sugar or candy) and identification describing disease process and treatment regimen at all times.
- Rep: Advise females of reproductive potential to notify health care professional if pregnancy is planned or suspected or if breastfeeding.

Evaluation/Desired Outcomes

- Increase of serum glucose to normal levels with improved level of consciousness.
- Smooth muscle relaxation of the stomach, duodenum, and small and large intestine in patients undergoing radiologic examination of the GI tract.

glycopyrrolate (systemic)
(glye-koe-**pye**-roe-late)
Cuvposa, Glycate, Glyrx-PF, Robinul, Robinul Forte
Classification
Therapeutic: antispasmodics
Pharmacologic: anticholinergics

Indications

Inhibits salivation and excessive respiratory secretions when given preoperatively. Reverses some of the secretory and vagal actions of cholinesterase inhibitors used to treat nondepolarizing neuromuscular blockade (cholinergic adjunct). Adjunctive management of peptic ulcer disease. **Oral solution:** Reduce chronic severe drooling in children with neurologic conditions associated with drooling.

Action

Inhibits the action of acetylcholine at postganglionic sites located in smooth muscle, secretory glands, and the CNS (antimuscarinic activity). Low doses decrease sweating, salivation, and respiratory secretions. Larger doses decrease GI and GU tract motility. **Therapeutic Effects:** Decreased GI and respiratory secretions.

Pharmacokinetics

Absorption: Incompletely absorbed (<10%) after oral administration. Well absorbed after IM administration. IV administration results in complete bioavailability.
Distribution: Distribution not fully known. Does not significantly cross the blood-brain barrier or eye.
Metabolism and Excretion: Eliminated primarily unchanged in the urine and bile.
Half-life: 1.7 hr (0.6–4.6 hr).

TIME/ACTION PROFILE (anticholinergic effects)

ROUTE	ONSET	PEAK	DURATION
PO	1 hr	unknown	8–12 hr
IM	15–30 min	30–45 min	2–7 hr*
IV	1–10 min	unknown	2–7 hr*

*Antisecretory effect lasts up to 7 hr; vagal blockade lasts 2–3 hr.

Contraindications/Precautions

Contraindicated in: Hypersensitivity; Angle-closure glaucoma; Acute hemorrhage; Tachycardia secondary to cardiac insufficiency or thyrotoxicosis; Severe ulcerative colitis; Toxic megacolon; Myasthenia gravis; Obstructive uropathy; Paralytic ileus; Concurrent use of oral potassium chloride dose forms (oral solution only).
Use Cautiously in: Patients who may have intra-abdominal infections; Prostatic hyperplasia; Chronic renal, hepatic, pulmonary, or cardiac disease; Hyperthyroidism; Down syndrome and children with spastic paralysis or brain damage (may be hypersensitive to antimuscarinic effects); OB: Safety not established in pregnancy; Lactation: Use while breastfeeding only if potential maternal benefit justifies potential risk to infant; Pedi: ↑ sensitivity to anticholinergic effects and adverse reactions; Geri: ↑ sensitivity to anticholinergic effects and adverse reactions in children.

Adverse Reactions/Side Effects

CV: tachycardia, orthostatic hypotension, palpitations. **Derm:** flushing. **EENT:** nasal congestion, blurred vision, cycloplegia, dry eyes, mydriasis. **GI:** dry mouth, vomiting, constipation. **GU:** urinary hesitancy, urinary retention. **Neuro:** headache, confusion, drowsiness..

Interactions

Drug-Drug: May ↑ GI mucosal lesions in patients taking oral **potassium chloride** tablets; concurrent use with oral glycopyrrolate solution contraindicated. Additive anticholinergic effects with other **anticholinergics**, including **antihistamines**, **phenothiazines**, **meperidine**, **amantadine**, **tricyclic antidepressants**, **quinidine**, and **disopyramide**. May alter the absorption of other **orally administered drugs** by slowing motility of the GI tract. May ↑ GI transit time of oral **digoxin** and ↑ digoxin levels. **Antacids** or **adsorbent antidiarrheal agents** ↓ absorption of anticholinergics. May ↑ GI mucosal lesions in patients taking oral **potassium chloride** tablets. May ↑ **atenolol** and **metformin** levels. May ↓ levels of **haloperidol** and **levodopa.** Concurrent use may ↓ absorption of **ketoconazole** (administer 2 hr after ketoconazole).

Route/Dosage

Control of Secretions during Surgery
IM (Adults): 4.4 mcg/kg 30–60 min before surgery (not to exceed 0.1 mg).
IM (Children >2 yr): 4.4 mcg/kg 30–60 min before surgery.
IM (Children <2 yr): 4.4–8.8 mcg/kg 30–60 min before surgery.

Control of Secretions (chronic)
IM, IV (Children): 4–10 mcg/kg/dose every 3–4 hr.
PO (Children): 40–100 mcg/kg/dose 3–4 times/day.

Cholinergic Adjunct
IV (Adults and Children): 200 mcg for each 1 mg of neostigmine or 5 mg of pyridostigmine given at the same time.

❦ = Canadian drug name. ⬚ = Genetic implication. ~~Strikethrough~~ = Discontinued. CAPITALS = life-threatening. <u>Underline</u> = most frequent.

Peptic Ulcer

PO (Adults): 1–2 mg 2–3 times daily. An additional 2 mg may be given at bedtime; may be ↓ to 1 mg twice daily (not to exceed 8 mg/day).

IM, IV (Adults): 100–200 mcg every 4 hr up to 4 times daily.

Chronic Severe Drooling

PO (Children 3–16 yr): *Oral solution:* 0.02 mg/kg 3 times daily; may ↑ by 0.02 mg/kg 3 times daily every 5–7 days (not to exceed 0.1 mg/kg 3 times daily or 1.5–3 mg/dose).

Availability (generic available)

Tablets: 1 mg, 1.5 mg, 2 mg. **Oral solution (cherry-flavor):** 1 mg/5 mL. **Solution for injection:** 200 mcg (0.2 mg)/mL. *In combination with:* neostigmine (Prevduo). See Appendix N.

NURSING IMPLICATIONS

Assessment

- Assess heart rate, BP, and respiratory rate before and periodically during parenteral therapy.
- Monitor intake and output ratios in geriatric or surgical patients; glycopyrrolate may cause urinary retention. Instruct patient to void before parenteral administration.
- Assess patient routinely for abdominal distention and auscultate for bowel sounds. If constipation becomes a problem, increasing fluids and adding bulk to the diet may help alleviate the constipating effects of the drug.
- Periodic intraocular pressure determinations should be made for patients receiving long-term therapy.
- Pedi: Monitor amount and frequency of drooling periodically during therapy.
- Assess for hyperexcitability, a paradoxical response that may occur in children.

Lab Test Considerations

- Antagonizes effects of pentagastrin and histamine during the gastric acid secretion test. Avoid administration for 24 hr preceding the test.
- May cause ↓ uric acid levels in patients with gout or hyperuricemia.

Toxicity and Overdose

- If overdose occurs, neostigmine is the antidote.

Implementation

- Do not administer cloudy or discolored solution.
- **PO:** Administer 30–60 min before meals to maximize absorption.
- For drooling: Administer at least 1 hr before or 2 hr after meals.
- Do not administer within 1 hr of antacids or antidiarrheal medications.
- Oral dose is 10 times the parenteral dose.
- **IM:** May be administered undiluted (200 mcg/mL).

IV Administration

- **IV Push:** *Dilution:* May be given undiluted through Y-site. *Concentration:* 200 mcg/mL. *Rate:* Administer at a maximum rate of 20 mcg over 1 min.
- **Y-Site Compatibility:** acyclovir, alemtuzumab, amikacin, aminophylline, amiodarone, anidulafungin, argatroban, arsenic trioxide, ascorbic acid, atracurium, atropine, azathioprine, aztreonam, benztropine, bivalirudin, bleomycin, bumetanide, buprenorphine, butorphanol, calcium chloride, calcium gluconate, carmustine, caspofungin, cefazolin, cefotaxime, cefotetan, cefoxitin, ceftazidime, ceftriaxone, cefuroxime, chloramphenicol, chlorpromazine, cisplatin, clindamycin, cyanocobalamin, cyclosporine, dacarbazine, dactinomycin, daptomycin, daunorubicin hydrochloride, dexamethasone, dexmedetomidine, dexrazoxane, digoxin, diltiazem, diphenhydramine, dobutamine, docetaxel, dopamine, doxorubicin liposomal, doxycycline, enalaprilat, ephedrine, epinephrine, epoetin alfa, ertapenem, erythromycin, esmolol, etoposide, etoposide phosphate, famotidine, fentanyl, fluconazole, fludarabine, folic acid, foscarnet, fosphenytoin, ganciclovir, gemcitabine, gemtuzumab ozogamicin, gentamicin, granisetron, heparin, hetastarch, hydrocortisone, hydromorphone, idarubicin, imipenem/cilastatin, isoproterenol, ketorolac, labetalol, LR, leucovorin calcium, lidocaine, linezolid, lorazepam, magnesium sulfate, mannitol, meperidine, mesna, methadone, methylprednisolone, metoclopramide, metoprolol, metronidazole, midazolam, milrinone, mitoxantrone, morphine, moxifloxcin, multivitamins, mycophenolate, nafcillin, nalbuphine, naloxone, nitroglycerin, nitroprusside, norepinephrine, octreotide, ondansetron, oxacillin, oxaliplatin, oxytocin, paclitaxel, palonosetron, pamidronate, papaverine, pemetrexed, penicillin G, pentamidine, pentobarbital, phenobarbital, phentolamine, phenylephrine, phytonadione, potassium acetate, potassium chloride, procainamide, promethazine, propofol, propranolol, protamine, pyridoxine, sodium bicarbonate, succinylcholine, sufentanil, tacrolimus, theophylline, thiamine, thiotepa, tigecycline, tirofiban, tobramycin, topotecan, vancomycin, vasopressin, vecuronium, verapamil, vinblastine, vinorelbine, voriconazole, zoledronic acid.
- **Y-Site Incompatibility:** amphotericin B lipid complex, dantrolene, diazepam, diazoxide, furosemide, indomethacin, insulin, regular, irinotecan, mitomycin, pantoprazole, phenytoin, piperacillin/tazobactam, trimethoprim/sulfamethoxazole.

Patient/Family Teaching

- Instruct patient to take glycopyrrolate as directed and not to take more than the prescribed amount. Take missed doses as soon as remembered if not just before next dose.
- Medication may cause drowsiness and blurred vision. Caution patient to avoid driving or other activi-

ties requiring alertness until response to the medication is known.

- Inform patient that frequent oral rinses, sugarless gum or candy, and good oral hygiene may help relieve dry mouth. Consult health care professional regarding use of saliva substitute if dry mouth persists for more than 2 wk.
- Advise patient to change positions slowly to minimize the effects of drug-induced orthostatic hypotension.
- Caution patient to avoid extremes of temperature. This medication decreases the ability to sweat and may increase the risk of heat stroke.
- Advise patient to notify health care professional immediately if eye pain or increased sensitivity to light occurs. Emphasize the importance of routine eye exams throughout therapy.
- Advise patient to consult health care professional before taking any OTC medications concurrently with this therapy.
- Rep: Advise females of reproductive potential to notify health care professional if pregnancy is planned or suspected, or if breastfeeding.
- Geri: Advise geriatric patients about increased susceptibility to side effects and to call health care professional immediately if they occur.
- Pedi: Instruct parents to use a calibrated measuring device with solution for accurate dosing.
- Advise parents to stop glycopyrrolate and notify health care professional if constipation; signs of urinary retention (inability to urinate, dry diapers or undergarments, irritability, or crying); or rash, hives, or an allergic reaction occurs.
- Glycopyrrolate reduces sweating. Advise parents to avoid exposure of the patient to hot or very warm environmental temperatures to avoid overheating and heat exhaustion or heat stroke.

Evaluation/Desired Outcomes
- Mouth dryness preoperatively.
- Reversal of cholinergic medications.
- Decrease in GI motility and pain in patients with peptic ulcer disease.
- Reduce chronic severe drooling in children with neurologic conditions associated with drooling.

---

glycopyrrolate/formoterol
(glye-koe-**pye**-roe-late/for-**moe**-te-rol)
Bevespi Aerosphere
Classification
Therapeutic: bronchodilators
Pharmacologic: anticholinergics, long-acting beta₂-adrenergic agonists (LABAs)

Indications
Maintenance treatment of COPD.

Action
Glycopyrrolate: acts as an anticholinergic by inhibiting M3 muscarinic receptors in bronchial smooth muscle resulting in bronchodilation; *Formoterol:* a beta₂-adrenergic agonist that stimulates adenyl cyclase, resulting in accumulation of cyclic adenosine monophosphate at beta₂—adrenergic receptors resulting in bronchodilation. **Therapeutic Effects:** Bronchodilation with decreased airflow obstruction.

Pharmacokinetics
Glycopyrrolate
Absorption: Some systemic absorption from lungs and GI tract (40%).
Distribution: Unknown.
Metabolism and Excretion: Primarily metabolized in the liver via the CYP2D6 isoenzyme; eliminated primarily unchanged in the urine and bile.
Half-life: 33–53 hr.
Formoterol
Absorption: Majority of inhaled drug is swallowed and absorbed.
Distribution: Unknown.
Metabolism and Excretion: Mostly metabolized by the liver via the CYP2D6 and CYP2C9, and CYP2C19 isoenzymes; 10–18% excreted unchanged in urine.
Half-life: 10 hr.

TIME/ACTION PROFILE (bronchodilation)

ROUTE	ONSET	PEAK	DURATION
formoterol—Inhaln	within 3 min	15 min	unknown
glycopyrro-late—Inhaln	unknown	unknown	unknown

Contraindications/Precautions
Contraindicated in: Hypersensitivity; Asthma; Acutely deteriorating COPD or acute respiratory symptoms.
Use Cautiously in: History of cardiovascular disorders (coronary insufficiency, arrhythmias, hypertension); History of seizures; Thyrotoxicosis; Narrow-angle glaucoma; Urinary retention, prostatic hyperplasia, bladder-neck obstruction; Hepatic impairment; OB: Formoterol may interfere with uterine contractility during labor; use during pregnancy only if potential maternal benefit justifies potential fetal risk; Lactation: Use while breastfeeding only if potential maternal benefit justifies potential risk to infant; Pedi: Safety and effectiveness not established in children.
Exercise Extreme Caution in: Concurrent use of MAO inhibitors, tricyclic antidepressants, or drugs that prolong the QTc interval.

Adverse Reactions/Side Effects
CV: chest pain, hypertension, tachycardia. **F and E:** hypokalemia. **GI:** dry mouth, vomiting. **GU:** urinary tract infection. **MS:** arthralgia, muscle spasms. **Neuro:** anx-

iety, dizziness, headache. **Resp:** cough, paradoxical bronchospasm. **Misc:** HYPERSENSITIVITY REACTIONS (including angioedema, urticaria, or rash).

Interactions

Drug-Drug: Concurrent use with other **adrenergics** may ↑ adrenergic adverse reactions (↑ heart rate, BP, jitteriness). ↑ risk of hypokalemia or ECG changes with **xanthine derivatives**, **corticosteroids**, **loop diuretics** or **thiazide diuretics**. ↑ risk of serious adverse cardiovascular effects with **MAO inhibitors**, **tricyclic antidepressants**, **QT-interval prolonging drugs**; use with extreme caution. Effectiveness may be ↓ by **beta-blockers**; use cautiously and only when necessary. ↑ risk of anticholinergic adverse reactions when used concurrently with other **anticholinergics**; avoid concurrent use.

Route/Dosage
Inhaln (Adults): 2 inhalations twice daily.

Availability
Inhalation aerosol: glycopyrrolate 9 mcg/formoterol 4.8 mcg per inhalation in 10.7-g canister (120 inhalations).

NURSING IMPLICATIONS

Assessment
- Assess lung sounds, pulse, and BP before administration and during peak of medication. Note amount, color, and character of sputum produced.
- Monitor pulmonary function tests before initiating and periodically during therapy to determine effectiveness.
- Observe for paradoxical bronchospasm (wheezing, dyspnea, tightness in chest) and hypersensitivity reaction (rash; urticaria; swelling of the face, lips, or eyelids). If condition occurs, withhold medication and notify health care professional immediately.
- Monitor ECG periodically during therapy. May cause prolonged QTc interval.
- Monitor patient for signs of hypersensitivity reactions (difficulties in breathing or swallowing, swelling of tongue, lips and face, urticaria, or skin rash) throughout therapy. Discontinue therapy and consider alternative if reaction occurs.

Lab Test Considerations
- May cause ↑ serum glucose and decreased serum potassium.

Implementation
- **Inhaln:** Administer as 2 inhalations twice daily, morning and evening. Shake well prior to use. Prime by releasing 4 sprays into air away from face before 1st use and by releasing 2 sprays if unused for more than 7 days. See Appendix C for use of metered-dose inhalers.

Patient/Family Teaching
- Instruct patient to use medication as directed. Do not discontinue therapy without discussing with

health care professional, even if feeling better. If a dose is missed skip dose and take next dose at regularly scheduled time. Do not double doses. Use a rapid-acting bronchodilator if symptoms occur before next dose is due. Caution patient not to use more than 2 times a day; may cause adverse effects, paradoxical bronchospasm, or loss of effectiveness of medication. Instruct patient to review *Medication Guide* before starting therapy and with each Rx refill in case of changes.
- Caution patient not to use medication to treat acute symptoms. A rapid-acting inhaled beta-adrenergic bronchodilator should be used for relief of acute asthma attacks. Notify health care professional immediately if symptoms get worse or more inhalations than usual are needed from rescue inhaler.
- Advise patient to clean inhaler each wk so medicine will not build up and block spray through mouthpiece. Take canister out of the actuator, run warm water through actuator, and allowing actuator to air-dry overnight. Shake and reprime with 2 sprays before use.
- Instruct patient to contact health care professional immediately if shortness of breath is not relieved by medication or nausea, vomiting, shakiness, headache, fast or irregular heartbeat, sleeplessness, or signs and symptoms of narrow angle glaucoma (eye pain or discomfort, blurred vision, visual halos or colored images, red eyes) or urinary retention (difficulty passing urine, painful urination) occur.
- Advise patient to consult health care professional before taking any Rx, OTC, or herbal products or alcohol concurrently with this therapy. Caution patient also to avoid smoking and other respiratory irritants.
- Rep: Advise females of reproductive potential to notify health care professional if pregnancy is planned or suspected or if breastfeeding. May interfere with uterine contractility if used during labor or delivery; use during labor only if the potential benefit justifies the potential risk.

Evaluation/Desired Outcomes
- Bronchodilation with decreased airflow obstruction.

---

golimumab (go-li-mu-mab)
Simponi, Simponi Aria, ✸Simponi IV
Classification
Therapeutic: antirheumatics
Pharmacologic: DMARDs, monoclonal antibodies, anti-TNF agents

Indications
Simponi and Simponi Aria: Treatment of the following conditions: Moderately to severely active rheumatoid arthritis (in combination with methotrexate), Active psoriatic arthritis, Active ankylosing spondylitis.
Simponi: Moderately to severely active ulcerative colitis in patients who have demonstrated corticosteroid dependence or have responded inadequately to immunosuppressants such as aminosalicylates, corticoste-

roids, azathioprine, or 6–mercaptopurine. **Simponi Aria:** Active polyarticular juvenile idiopathic arthritis.

Action

Inhibits binding of TNFα to receptors inhibiting activity and resulting in anti-inflammatory and antiproliferative activity. **Therapeutic Effects:** Decreased pain and swelling with decreased joint destruction in patients with rheumatoid arthritis, psoriatic arthritis, ankylosing spondylitis, and polyarticular juvenile idiopathic arthritis. Induction and maintenance of clinical remission of ulcerative colitis.

Pharmacokinetics

Absorption: Well absorbed following SUBQ administration. IV administration results in complete bioavailability.
Distribution: Distributed primarily in the circulatory system with limited extravascular distribution.
Metabolism and Excretion: Unknown.
Half-life: 2 wk.

TIME/ACTION PROFILE (improvement)

ROUTE	ONSET	PEAK	DURATION
SUBQ	within 3 mo	2–7 days†	unknown
IV	within 3 mo	unknown	unknown

† Blood levels.

Contraindications/Precautions

Contraindicated in: Active infection (including localized); Concurrent use of abatacept or anakinra (↑ risk of infections).
Use Cautiously in: History of chronic or recurrent infection or underlying illness/treatment predisposing to infection; History of exposure to tuberculosis; History of opportunistic infection; Patients residing, or who have resided, where tuberculosis, histoplasmosis, coccidioidomycoses, or blastomycosis is endemic; History of HF (may worsen); Pre-existing CNS demyelinating disorders (including multiple sclerosis or Guillain-Barré syndrome); History of cytopenias (may worsen); History of psoriasis (may exacerbate); Hepatitis B virus carriers (risk of reactivation); OB: Use during pregnancy only if potential maternal benefit justifies potential fetal risk; Lactation: Use while breastfeeding only if potential maternal benefit justifies potential risk to infant; Pedi: Safety and effectiveness not established in children <18 yr (rheumatoid arthritis, ankylosing spondylitis, or ulcerative colitis) or <2 yr (psoriatic arthritis or polyarticular juvenile idiopathic arthritis); ↑ risk of lymphoma (including HSTCL), leukemia, and other malignancies in children; Geri: ↑ risk of infection in older adults.

Adverse Reactions/Side Effects

CV: HF, hypertension. **Derm:** psoriasis. **EENT:** nasopharyngitis, optic neuritis. **GI:** ↑ liver enzymes. **Hemat:** agranulocytosis, aplastic anemia, leukopenia, neutro-penia, pancytopenia, thrombocytopenia. **Local:** injection site reactions. **Neuro:** CENTRAL NERVOUS SYSTEM DEMYELINATING DISORDERS, Guillain-Barre syndrome, multiple sclerosis, paresthesia. **Resp:** upper respiratory tract infection. **Misc:** fever, HYPERSENSITIVITY REACTIONS (including anaphylaxis), INFECTION (including reactivation tuberculosis and other opportunistic infections due to bacterial, invasive fungal, viral, mycobacterial, and parasitic pathogens), lupus-like syndrome, MALIGNANCY (including lymphoma, HSTCL, leukemia, and skin cancer).

Interactions

Drug-Drug: Abatacept, anakinra, corticosteroids, or methotrexate ↑ risk of serious infections; concurrent use with anakinra or abatacept is not recommended. Use of **live virus vaccines** or therapeutic infectious agents may ↑ risk of infection; avoid concurrent use. Concurrent use with **azathioprine** and/or 6–mercaptopurine may ↑ risk of HSTCL. May normalize previously suppressed levels of CYP450 enzymes; following initiation or discontinuation of golimumab, effects of substrates of this system may be altered and should be monitored, including **warfarin**, **theophylline**, and **cyclosporine**.

Route/Dosage

Rheumatoid Arthritis and Ankylosing Spondylitis

SUBQ (Adults): 50 mg once monthly.
IV (Adults): 2 mg/kg initially and 4 wk later, then 2 mg/kg every 8 wk.

Psoriatic Arthritis

SUBQ (Adults): 50 mg once monthly.
IV (Adults): 2 mg/kg initially and 4 wk later, then 2 mg/kg every 8 wk.
IV (Children ≥2 yr): 80 mg/m² initially and 4 wk later, then 80 mg/m² every 8 wk.

Ulcerative Colitis

SUBQ (Adults): 200 mg initially, then 100 mg 2 wk later, then 100 mg every 4 wk.

Polyarticular Juvenile Idiopathic Arthritis

IV (Children ≥2 yr): 80 mg/m² initially and 4 wk later, then 80 mg/m² every 8 wk.

Availability

Solution for SUBQ injection (prefilled syringes and autoinjectors): 50 mg/0.5 mL, 100 mg/mL. **Solution for intravenous injection (Simponi Aria):** 12.5 mg/mL.

NURSING IMPLICATIONS

Assessment

● Assess for signs and symptoms of infection (fever, dyspnea, flu-like symptoms, frequent or painful urination, redness or swelling at the site of a wound)

❋= Canadian drug name. ▓▓▓ = Genetic implication. S̶t̶r̶i̶k̶e̶t̶h̶r̶o̶u̶g̶h̶ = Discontinued. CAPITALS= life-threatening. U̲n̲d̲e̲r̲l̲i̲n̲e̲ = most frequent.

prior to, during, and after therapy. Discontinue therapy if serious or opportunistic infection or sepsis occurs. If new infection develops during therapy, assess patient and institute antimicrobial therapy. Patients who tested negative for latent tuberculosis (TB) prior to therapy may develop TB during therapy. Initiate treatment for latent TB prior to initiating therapy.

- Test for HBV prior to therapy and monitor carriers of HBV for signs of reactivation during and for several mo after therapy. If reactivation occurs, discontinue golimumab and institute antiviral therapy.
- Monitor patients with HF for new or worsening symptoms. Discontinue therapy if symptoms occur.
- Assess for exacerbations and new onset psoriasis. Discontinue therapy if these occur.
- Assess patient for latex allergy. Needle cover of syringe contains latex and should not be handled by persons sensitive to latex.
- Assess for signs and symptoms of systemic fungal infections (fever, malaise, weight loss, sweats, cough, dyspnea, pulmonary infiltrates, serious systemic illness with or without concomitant shock). Ascertain if patient lives in or has traveled to areas of endemic mycoses. Consider empiric antifungal treatment for patients at risk of histoplasmosis and other invasive fungal infections until the pathogens are identified. Consult with an infectious diseases specialist. Consider stopping golimumab until the infection has been diagnosed and adequately treated.
- Observe for signs and symptoms of anaphylaxis (rash, pruritus, laryngeal edema, wheezing). Discontinue drug and notify health care professional immediately if these problems occur. Keep epinephrine, an antihistamine, and resuscitation equipment close by in case of an anaphylactic reaction.
- **Rheumatoid Arthritis:** Assess pain and range of motion prior to and periodically during therapy.
- **Ulcerative Colitis:** Assess for signs and symptoms before, during, and after therapy.

Lab Test Considerations
- Monitor liver function tests periodically during therapy. May cause ↑ serum AST and ALT.
- Monitor CBC with differential periodically during therapy. May cause leukopenia, neutropenia, thrombocytopenia, and pancytopenia. Discontinue golimumab if symptoms of blood dyscrasias (persistent fever) occur.
- Monitor for HBV blood tests before starting, during, and for several mo after therapy is completed.

Implementation

- Administer a tuberculin skin test prior to administration of golimumab. Assess if treatment for latent tuberculosis is needed; an induration of 5 mm or greater is a positive tuberculin skin test, even for patients previously vaccinated with Bacille Calmette-Guerin (BCG). Consider antituberculosis therapy prior to therapy in patients with a history of latent or active tuberculosis if an adequate course of treatment cannot be confirmed, and for patients with risk factors for tuberculosis infection.

- Update immunizations before starting therapy following current immunization guidelines for patients receiving immunosuppressive agents.
- Initial injection should be supervised by health care professional.
- Refrigerate solution; do not freeze. Allow prefilled syringe or autoinjector to sit at room temperature for 30 min prior to injection; do not warm in any other way. Do not shake. Solution is clear to slightly opalescent and colorless to light yellow. Do not administer solutions that are discolored, cloudy, or contain particulate matter. Discard unused solution.
- **SUBQ:** Remove the needle cover or autoinjector cap just prior to injection; both caps contain latex. Inject into front of middle thigh or lower part of abdomen 2 inches from navel. Do not inject in areas where skin is tender, bruised, red, scaly, or hard; avoid scars or stretch marks. Press a cotton ball or gauze over injection site for 10 sec; do not rub.
- *Autoinjector:* Press open end of autoinjector against skin at 90° angle. Press button with fingers or thumb; button will stay pressed and does not need to be held. Injection will begin following a loud click. Keep holding the autoinjector against skin until a 2nd loud click is heard (usually 3–6 sec, but may take up to 15 sec). Lift autoinjector from skin following 2nd click. Yellow indicator in viewing window indicates autoinjector worked correctly. If yellow does not appear in viewing window call 1-800-526-7736 for help.
- *Prefilled syringe:* Hold body of syringe between thumb and index finger. Do not pull back on plunger at any time. Pinch skin. Inject all medication by pushing plunger until plunger head is between needle guard wings. Take needle out of skin and let go of skin. Slowly take thumb off plunger to allow empty syringe to move up until entire needle is covered by needle guard.

IV Administration

- **Intermittent Infusion:** Calculate dose and number of vials needed for dose. Solution in vial is colorless to light yellow; may contain a few fine translucent particles of protein. Do not use if opaque particles, discoloration, or other particles present. *Dilution:* Withdraw volume of dose from 100 mL bag of 0.9% NaCl or 0.45% NaCl and discard. Add golimumab dose to infusion bag; mix gently. Solution is stable for 4 hrs at room temperature. *Rate:* Infuse through an in-line, sterile, non-pyrogenic, low protein-binding filter with ≤ 0.22 micrometer pore size over 30 min.

Patient/Family Teaching

- Instruct patient on correct technique for administration. Review patient information sheet, preparation of dose, administration sites and technique, and disposal of equipment into a puncture-resistant con-

tainer. Advise patient of risks and benefits of golimumab therapy. Inject missed doses as soon as
remembered, then return to regular schedule. Instruct patient to read *Medication Guide* before
starting therapy and with each Rx refill; new information may be available.

- Caution patient not to share this medication with others, even with the same symptoms; may be harmful.
- Inform patient of increased risk of infections, malignancies, cardiac and nervous system disorders during therapy.
- Caution patient to notify health care professional
promptly if any signs of infection, including TB, invasive fungal infections (fever, malaise, weight loss,
sweats, cough, dyspnea, pulmonary infiltrates, serious systemic illness with or without concomitant
shock), reactivation of HBV (muscle aches, clay-colored bowel movements, feeling very tired, fever,
dark urine, chills, skin or eyes look yellow, stomach
discomfort, little or no appetite, skin rash, vomiting), hypersensitivity reactions, or nervous system
problems (vision changes, weakness in arms or legs,
numbness or tingling in any part of the body) develop.
- Advise patient to examine skin periodically during
therapy and notify health care professional of any
changes in appearance of skin or growths on skin.
- Advise patient to notify health care professional of all
Rx or OTC medications, vitamins, or herbal products
being taken and to consult with health care professional before taking other medications.
- Inform patient to avoid receiving live vaccinations;
other vaccinations may be given.
- Inform patient of increased risk of cancer. Advise
patient of need for screening for dysplasia (colonos-
copy, skin cancer examinations, biopsy) periodically
during therapy.
- Rep: Advise patient to notify health care professional
if pregnancy is planned or suspected or if breastfeeding. Advise females to notify health care professional if they recently had a baby while taking golimumab. Infants have an increased chance of getting
an infection for up to 6 mo after birth; avoid administration of live vaccines to infants for 6 mo after
mother's last dose.

Evaluation/Desired Outcomes

- Decreased pain and swelling with decreased rate of
joint destruction in patients with rheumatoid arthritis.
- Decreased signs and symptoms, slowed progression
of joint destruction, and improved physical function
in patients with psoriatic arthritis.
- Reduced signs and symptoms of ankylosing spondylitis.
- Decreased symptoms, maintaining remission, and
mucosal healing with decreased corticosteroid use
in ulcerative colitis.

goserelin (goe-se-rel-lin)
Zoladex, ✹Zoladex LA
Classification
Therapeutic: antineoplastics, hormones
Pharmacologic: gonadotropin-releasing hor-
mones

Indications
Palliative treatment of advanced prostate cancer. Locally confined stage T2b−T4 (stage B2−C) prostate
cancer (in combination with flutamide). Palliative treatment of advanced breast cancer in peri menopausal
and postmenopausal women. Endometriosis. Produces
thinning of the endometrium before endometrial ablation for dysfunctional uterine bleeding.

Action
Acts as a synthetic form of luteinizing hormone−releas-
ing hormone (LHRH, GnRH). Inhibits the production of
gonadotropins by the pituitary gland. Initially, levels of
luteinizing hormone (LH), follicle-stimulating hormone
(FSH), and testosterone increase. Continued administration leads to decreased production of testosterone
and estradiol. **Therapeutic Effects:** Decreased spread
of cancer of the prostate or breast. Regression of endometriosis with decreased pain. Thinning of the endometrium.

Pharmacokinetics
Absorption: Well absorbed from SUBQ implant. Absorption is slower in first 8 days, then is faster and continuous for remainder of 28-day dosing cycle.
Distribution: Unknown.
Metabolism and Excretion: Some metabolism by
the liver (<10%), some excretion by kidneys (>90%,
only 20% as unchanged drug).
Half-life: 4.2 hr.

TIME/ACTION PROFILE (↓ in serum testosterone levels)

ROUTE	ONSET	PEAK	DURATION
SUBQ	unknown	2−4 wk	length of ther-apy

Contraindications/Precautions
Contraindicated in: Hypersensitivity; Undiagnosed
vaginal bleeding; OB: Pregnancy; Lactation: Lactation.
Use Cautiously in: Congenital long QT syndrome,
HF, hypokalemia, or hypomagnesemia; Concurrent use
of other drugs known to prolong the QTc interval; Low
BMI (↑ risk of bleeding complications); Concurrent
use of anticoagulant therapy (↑ risk of bleeding complications); Pedi: Safety and effectiveness not established in children.

Adverse Reactions/Side Effects
CV: vasodilation, chest pain, hypertension, MI, palpitations, peripheral edema, QT interval prolongation.

Derm: hot flushing, sweating, acne, rash. **Endo:** ↓ libido, erectile dysfunction, breast swelling, breast tenderness, infertility, ovarian cysts, ovarian hyperstimulation syndrome (with gonadotropins). **GI:** anorexia, constipation, diarrhea, nausea, ulcer, vomiting. **GU:** renal insufficiency, urinary obstruction. **Hemat:** anemia. **Local:** injection site/vascular injury. **Metab:** ↑ weight, gout, hyperglycemia, hyperlipidemia. **MS:** ↑ bone pain, ↓ bone density, arthralgia. **Neuro:** headache, anxiety, depression (women), dizziness, fatigue, insomnia, mood swings, SEIZURES, STROKE, SUICIDAL IDEATION/BEHAVIOR (women), weakness. **Resp:** dyspnea. **Misc:** chills, fever.

Interactions
Drug-Drug: None reported.

Route/Dosage
SUBQ (Adults): 3.6 mg every 4 wk or 10.8 mg every 12 wk. *Endometrial thinning:* 1 or 2 depots given 4 wk apart; if 1 depot used, surgery is performed at 4 wk; if 2 depots used, surgery is performed 2–4 wk after 2nd depot.

Availability
Implant: 3.6 mg, 10.8 mg.

NURSING IMPLICATIONS
Assessment
- Monitor for signs and symptoms of injection site injury/abdominal hemorrhage (abdominal pain, abdominal distension, dyspnea, dizziness, hypotension, and/or any altered levels of consciousness) following administration. Advise patient to report symptoms immediately to health care professional.
- **Cancer:** Monitor patients with vertebral metastases for increased back pain and decreased sensory/motor function.
- Monitor intake and output ratios and assess for bladder distention in patients with urinary tract obstruction during initiation of therapy.
- **Endometriosis:** Assess patient for signs and symptoms of endometriosis before and periodically during therapy. Amenorrhea usually occurs within 8 wk of initial administration and menses usually resume 8 wk after completion.

Lab Test Considerations
- Initially ↑, then ↓ LH and FSH. This leads to castration levels of testosterone in men 2–4 wk after initial increase in concentrations.
- Monitor serum acid phosphatase and prostate-specific antigen concentrations periodically during therapy. May cause transient ↑ in serum acid phosphatase concentrations, which usually return to baseline by the 4th wk of therapy and may ↓ to below baseline or return to baseline if elevated before therapy.
- May cause hypercalcemia in patients with breast or prostate cancer with bony metastases.
- May cause an ↑ in serum HDL, LDL, and triglycerides.

- May cause hyperglycemia. Monitor blood glucose and HbA1c periodically during therapy.

Implementation
- **SUBQ:** Implant is inserted in upper SUBQ tissue of anterior abdominal wall below the navel line every 28 days. Local anesthesia may be used before injection.
- If the implant needs to be removed for any reason, it can be located by ultrasound.

Patient/Family Teaching
- Explain purpose of goserelin to patient. Emphasize importance of adhering to the schedule of monthly or every-3-mo administration.
- Advise patient that bone pain may increase at initiation of therapy. This will resolve with time. Patient should discuss use of analgesics to control pain with health care professional.
- Advise female patients to notify health care professional if regular menstruation persists.
- Inform diabetic patients of potential for hyperglycemia. Encourage close monitoring of serum glucose.
- Advise patient that medication may cause hot flashes. Notify health care professional if these become bothersome. Hormone replacement therapy may be added to decrease vasomotor symptoms and vaginal dryness without compromising beneficial effect.
- Instruct patient to notify health care professional promptly if difficulty urinating or if symptoms of myocardial infarction or stroke (chest pain, difficulty breathing, weakness, loss of consciousness) occur.
- Rep: May cause fetal harm. Advise premenopausal women to notify health care professional if pregnancy is planned or suspected and to avoid breastfeeding. Effective nonhormonal contraception should be used during and for 12 wk after treatment ends.

Evaluation/Desired Outcomes
- Decrease in the spread of prostate cancer.
- Reduction of symptoms of advanced breast cancer in peri- and postmenopausal women.
- Decrease in the signs and symptoms of endometriosis. Symptoms are usually reduced within 4 wk of implantation.
- Thinning of the endometrium before endometrial ablation for dysfunctional uterine bleeding.

granisetron (gra-ni-se-tron)
~~Kytril~~, Sustol

granisetron (transdermal)
Sancuso
Classification
Therapeutic: antiemetics
Pharmacologic: 5-HT₃ antagonists

Indications

PO: Prevention of nausea and vomiting due to emetogenic chemotherapy or radiation therapy. **IV:** Prevention of nausea and vomiting due to emetogenic chemotherapy. **IV:** Prevention and treatment of postoperative nausea and vomiting. **SUBQ:** Prevention of acute and delayed nausea and vomiting due to moderately emetogenic chemotherapy or anthracycline/cyclophosphamide combination chemotherapy (in combination with dexamethasone). **Transdermal:** Prevention of nausea and vomiting due to moderately/highly emetogenic chemotherapy.

Action

Blocks the effects of serotonin at receptor sites (selective antagonist) located in vagal nerve terminals and in the chemoreceptor trigger zone in the CNS. **Therapeutic Effects:** Decreased incidence and severity of nausea and vomiting following emetogenic chemotherapy, radiation therapy, or surgery.

Pharmacokinetics

Absorption: 50% absorbed following oral administration; transdermal enters systemic circulation via passive diffusion through intact skin. IV administration results in complete bioavailability.

Distribution: Distributes into erythrocytes; remainder of distribution is unknown.

Metabolism and Excretion: Mostly metabolized by the liver; 12% excreted unchanged in urine.

Half-life: *Patients with cancer:* 10–12 hr (range 0.9–31.1 hr); *healthy volunteers:* 3–4 hr (range 0.9–15.2 hr); *older adults:* 7.7 hr (range 2.6–17.7 hr); *SUBQ:* 24 hr.

TIME/ACTION PROFILE (plasma concentrations)

ROUTE	ONSET	PEAK	DURATION
PO	rapid	60 min	24 hr
IV	1–3 min	30 min	up to 24 hr
TD	unknown	48 hr	unknown
SUBQ	unknown	12 hr	7 days

Contraindications/Precautions

Contraindicated in: Hypersensitivity; Some products contain benzyl alcohol; avoid use in neonates; Severe renal impairment (SUBQ).

Use Cautiously in: History of arrhythmias or conduction disorders; Recent abdominal surgery (SUBQ); Moderate renal impairment (↓ frequency of administration); Lactation: Safety not established in breastfeeding; Pedi: Safety and effectiveness not established in children <18 yr (oral, SUBQ, or transdermal) or <2 yr (IV).

Adverse Reactions/Side Effects

CV: hypertension, QT interval prolongation. **GI:** <u>constipation</u>, ↑ liver enzymes, abdominal pain, diarrhea, dyspepsia. **Derm:** *Topical:* application site reactions, photosensitivity. **Local:** injection site reactions (SUBQ). **Neuro:** <u>headache</u>, agitation, anxiety, CNS stimulation, dizziness, drowsiness, dysgeusia, headache, insomnia, weakness. **Misc:** fever, HYPERSENSITIVITY REACTIONS (including anaphylaxis).

Interactions

Drug-Drug: ↑ risk of extrapyramidal reactions with other **agents causing extrapyramidal reactions**. ↑ risk of QT interval prolongation with other **agents causing QT interval prolongation**. Drugs that affect serotonergic neurotransmitter systems, including **SSRIs, SNRIs, tricyclic antidepressants, MAO inhibitors, fentanyl, lithium, buspirone, tramadol, methylene blue**, and **triptans** ↑ risk of serotonin syndrome.

Route/Dosage

Prevention of Nausea and Vomiting Due to Emetogenic Chemotherapy

PO (Adults): 1 mg twice daily; 1st dose given at least 60 min prior to chemotherapy and 2nd dose 12 hr later only on days when chemotherapy is administered; may also be given as 2 mg once daily at least 60 min prior to chemotherapy.

IV (Adults and Children 2–16 yr): 10 mcg/kg given within 30 min prior to chemotherapy or 20–40 mcg/kg/day divided once or twice daily (maximum: 3 mg/dose or 9 mg/day).

Transdermal (Adults): One patch applied up to 48 hr prior to chemotherapy, leave in place for at least 24 hr following chemotherapy, may be left in place for a total of 7 days.

Prevention of Nausea and Vomiting Associated with Radiation Therapy

PO (Adults): 2 mg taken once daily within 1 hr of radiation therapy.

Prevention and Treatment of Postoperative Nausea and Vomiting

IV (Adults): *Prevention:* 1 mg prior to induction of anesthesia or just prior to reversal of anesthesia; *Treatment:* 1 mg.

IV (Children ≥4 yr): 20–40 mcg/kg as a single dose (maximum: 1 mg).

Prevention of Acute and Delayed Nausea and Vomiting Due to Emetogenic Chemotherapy

SUBQ (Adults): 10 mg given at least 30 min prior to chemotherapy (with dexamethasone) on Day 1 of chemotherapy; do not administer more frequently than every 7 days.

Renal Impairment

SUBQ (Adults): *CCr 30–59 mL/min:* Do not administer more frequently than every 14 days.

Availability (generic available)

Tablets: 1 mg. **Solution for intravenous injection:** 1 mg/mL. **Solution for SUBQ injection (prefilled syringes):** 10 mg/0.4 mL. **Transdermal patch:** 3.1 mg/24 hr.

NURSING IMPLICATIONS

Assessment

● Assess patient for nausea, vomiting, abdominal distention, and bowel sounds prior to and following administration.
● Assess for extrapyramidal symptoms (involuntary movements, facial grimacing, rigidity, shuffling walk, trembling of hands) during therapy. This occurs rarely and is usually associated with concurrent use of other drugs known to cause this effect.
● Monitor ECG in patients with HF, bradycardia, underlying heart disease, renal impairment, and elderly patients.
● Monitor for signs and symptoms of serotonin syndrome (mental status changes [agitation, hallucinations, delirium, and coma], autonomic instability [tachycardia, labile BP, dizziness, diaphoresis, flushing, hyperthermia], neuromuscular symptoms [tremor, rigidity, myoclonus, hyperreflexia, incoordination], seizures, with or without gastrointestinal symptoms [nausea, vomiting, diarrhea]). If symptoms occur discontinue granisetron and treat symptomatically.
● **Transdermal:** Monitor application site. If allergic, erythematous, macular, or papular rash or pruritus occurs, remove patch.

Lab Test Considerations

● May cause ↑ AST and ALT levels.

Implementation

● Correct hypokalemia and hypomagnesemia before administering.
● For chemotherapy or radiation, granisetron is administered only on the day(s) chemotherapy or radiation is given. Continued treatment when not on chemotherapy or radiation therapy has not been found to be useful.
● **PO:** Administer 1st dose up to 1 hr before chemotherapy or radiation therapy and 2nd dose 12 hr after the first.
● **SUBQ:** Use kit and components provided by manufacturer. Injection should be administered by health care professional. Remove kit from refrigerator and allow to warm to room temperature for 60 min. Activate one syringe warming pouch, and wrap syringe in warming pouch for 5 to 6 min to warm to body temperature. Do not inject solutions that contain particulate matter. Inject in back of upper arm or in skin of abdomen at least 1 inch away from umbilicus. Avoid injecting in areas where skin is burned, hardened, inflamed, or swollen. Topical anesthesia may be used at injection site prior to injection. Solution is viscous and requires a slow, sustained injection over 20 to 30 sec. Pressing the plunger harder will NOT expel medication faster.

IV Administration

● **IV Push:** *Dilution:* May be administered undiluted or diluted in 20–50 mL of 0.9% NaCl or D5W. Solution should be prepared at time of administration but is stable for 24 hr at room temperature. *Concentration:* Up to 1 mg/mL. *Rate:* Administer undiluted granisetron over 30 sec or as a diluted solution over 5 min.
● **Y-Site Compatibility:** acetaminophen, alemtuzumab, allopurinol, amifostine, amikacin, aminocaproic acid, aminophylline, amiodarone, amphotericin B lipid complex, amphotericin B liposomal, ampicillin, ampicillin/sulbactam, anidulafungin, argatroban, arsenic trioxide, atracurium, azithromycin, aztreonam, bivalirudin, bleomycin, bumetanide, buprenorphine, busulfan, butorphanol, calcium acetate, calcium chloride, calcium gluconate, carboplatin, carmustine, caspofungin, cefazolin, cefepime, cefotaxime, cefotetan, cefoxitin, ceftaroline, ceftazidime, ceftriaxone, cefuroxime, chloramphenicol, chlorpromazine, ciprofloxacin, cisatracurium, cisplatin, cladribine, clindamycin, cyclophosphamide, cyclosporine, cytarabine, dacarbazine, dactinomycin, daptomycin, daunorubicin hydrochloride, dexamethasone, dexmedetomidine, dexrazoxane, digoxin, diltiazem, diphenhydramine, dobutamine, docetaxel, dopamine, doxorubicin hydrochloride, doxorubicin liposomal, doxycycline, droperidol, enalaprilat, ephedrine, epinephrine, epirubicin, eptifibatide, ertapenem, erythromycin, esmolol, etoposide, etoposide phosphate, famotidine, fentanyl, filgrastim, floxuridine, fluconazole, fludarabine, fluorouracil, fosaprepitant, foscarnet, fosphenytoin, furosemide, ganciclovir, gemcitabine, gentamicin, glycopyrrolate, haloperidol, heparin, hetastarch, hydralazine, hydrocortisone, hydromorphone, idarubicin, ifosfamide, imipenem/cilastatin, insulin, regular, irinotecan, isoproterenol, ketorolac, labetalol, leucovorin calcium, levofloxacin, lidocaine, linezolid, lorazepam, magnesium sulfate, mannitol, melphalan, meperidine, meropenem, mesna, methotrexate, methylprednisolone, metoclopramide, metoprolol, metronidazole, midazolam, milrinone, mitomycin, mitoxantrone, morphine, moxifloxacin, mycophenolate, nafcillin, nalbuphine, naloxone, nicardipine, nitroglycerin, nitroprusside, norepinephrine, octreotide, oxaliplatin, oxytocin, paclitaxel, pamidronate, pantoprazole, pemetrexed, pentamidine, pentobarbital, phenobarbital, phentolamine, phenylephrine, piperacillin/tazobactam, potassium acetate, potassium chloride, potassium phosphate, procainamide, prochlorperazine, promethazine, propofol, propranolol, remifentanil, rituximab, rocuronium, sargramostim, sodium acetate, sodium bicarbonate, sodium phosphate, succinylcholine, sufentanil, tacrolimus, theophylline, thiopental, thiotepa, tigecycline, tirofiban, tobramycin, topotecan, trastuzumab, trimethoprim/sulfamethoxazole, vancomycin, vasopressin, vecuronium, verapamil, vin-

blastine, vincristine, vinorelbine, voriconazole, zidovudine, zoledronic acid.

- **Y-Site Incompatibility:** amphotericin B deoxycholate, dantrolene, diazepam, gemtuzumab ozogamicin, phenytoin.

- **Transdermal:** Apply system to clear, dry, intact healthy skin on upper outer arm 24–48 hr before chemotherapy. Do not use creams, lotions, or oils that may keep patch from sticking. Do not apply to skin that is red, irritated, or damaged. Apply immediately after removing from package. Do not cut patch into pieces. Remove liner from adhesive layer and press firmly in place with palm of hand for 30 sec, especially around the edges, to make sure contact is complete. Patch should be worn throughout chemotherapy. If patch does not stick, bandages or medical adhesive tape may be applied on edges of patch; do not cover patch with tape or bandages or wrap completely around arm. Patient may shower and wash normally while wearing patch; avoid swimming, strenuous exercise, sauna, or whirlpool during patch use. Remove patch gently at least 24 hr after completion of chemotherapy; may be worn for up to 7 days. Fold so that adhesive edges are together. Throw away in garbage out of reach of children and pets. Do not reuse patch. Use soap and water to remove remaining adhesive; do not use alcohol or acetone.

Patient/Family Teaching
- Instruct patient to take granisetron as directed.
- Advise patient to notify health care professional immediately if involuntary movement of eyes, face, or limbs occurs.
- May cause dizziness and drowsiness. Caution patient to avoid driving and other activities requiring alertness until response to medication is known.
- Advise patient to notify health care professional if symptoms of abnormal heart rate or rhythm (racing heartbeat, shortness of breath, dizziness, fainting) or serotonin syndrome occur.
- Advise patient to notify health care professional of all Rx or OTC medications, vitamins, or herbal products being taken and to consult with health care professional before taking other medications.
- Rep: Advise females of reproductive potential to notify health care professional if pregnancy is planned or suspected or if breastfeeding.
- **Transdermal:** Instruct patient on correct application, removal, and disposal of patch. Advise patient to read *Patient Information* sheet prior to using and with each Rx refill in case of new information. Inform patient that additional granisetron should not be taken during patch application unless directed by health care professional.
- Advise patient referred for MRI test to discuss patch with referring health care professional and MRI facility to determine if removal of patch is necessary prior to test and for directions for replacing patch.
- Advise patient to avoid using a heating pad near or over patch and to cover patch application site with clothing to avoid exposure to sunlight, sunlamp, or tanning beds during and for 10 days following removal of patch.
- Instruct patient to notify health care professional if pain or swelling in the abdomen occurs or if redness at patch removal site remains for more than 3 days.

Evaluation/Desired Outcomes
- Prevention of nausea and vomiting associated with emetogenic cancer chemotherapy or radiation therapy.
- Prevention and treatment of postoperative nausea and vomiting.

BEERS

guanFACINE (gwahn-fa-seen)
Intuniv, ✤ Intuniv XR, ~~Tenex~~
Classification
Therapeutic: antihypertensives, agents for attention deficit disorder
Pharmacologic: alpha adrenergic agonists

Indications
Hypertension (in combination with thiazide-type diuretics) (immediate-release). Attention-deficit hyperactivity disorder (ADHD) (as monotherapy or as adjunctive therapy to stimulants) (extended-release).

Action
Stimulates CNS alpha$_2$-adrenergic receptors, producing a decrease in sympathetic outflow to heart, kidneys, and blood vessels. Result is decreased BP and peripheral resistance, a slight decrease in heart rate, and no change in cardiac output. Mechanism of action in ADHD is unknown. **Therapeutic Effects:** Lowering of BP in hypertension. Increased attention span in ADHD.

Pharmacokinetics
Absorption: Immediate-release is well absorbed (80%); extended-release has lower rate and extent of absorption (↑ absorption with high-fat meals).
Distribution: Appears to be widely distributed.
Metabolism and Excretion: 50% metabolized by the liver, 50% excreted unchanged by the kidneys.
Half-life: 17 hr.

TIME/ACTION PROFILE (antihypertensive effect)

ROUTE	ONSET	PEAK	DURATION
PO (single dose)	unknown	8–12 hr	24 hr
PO (multiple doses)	within 1 wk	1–3 mo	unknown

Contraindications/Precautions
Contraindicated in: Hypersensitivity.

Use Cautiously in: Severe coronary artery disease or recent MI; Cerebrovascular disease; Severe renal impairment; Severe hepatic impairment; History of hypotension, heart block, bradycardia, or cardiovascular disease; OB: Other agents preferred for treatment of hypertension or ADHD in pregnancy; Lactation: Use while breastfeeding only if potential maternal benefit justifies potential risk to infant; Pedi: Children <6 yr (safety and effectiveness not established); Geri: Appears on Beers list. ↑ risk of CNS effects, orthostatic hypotension, and bradycardia in older adults. Avoid use for treatment of hypertension in older adults.

Adverse Reactions/Side Effects
CV: bradycardia, chest pain, hypotension, palpitations, rebound hypertension, syncope. **EENT:** tinnitus. **GI:** constipation, dry mouth, abdominal pain, nausea. **GU:** erectile dysfunction. **Neuro:** drowsiness, headache, weakness, depression, dizziness, fatigue, insomnia, irritability. **Resp:** dyspnea.

Interactions
Drug-Drug: ↑ hypotension with other **antihypertensives**, **nitrates**, and acute ingestion of **alcohol**. ↑ CNS depression may occur with other **CNS depressants**, including **alcohol**, **antihistamines**, **opioid analgesics**, **tricyclic antidepressants**, and **sedative/hypnotics**. **NSAIDs** may ↓ effectiveness. **Adrenergics** may ↓ effectiveness. ↑ risk of hypotension and bradycardia with strong and moderate **CYP3A4 inhibitors**, including **ketoconazole** and **fluconazole** (↓ in dose of guanfacine may be needed). Strong and moderate **CYP3A4 inducers**, including **rifampin**, **efavirenz**, and **carbamazepine** may ↓ effects (an ↑ in dose of guanfacine may be needed). May ↑ levels of **valproic acid**.

Route/Dosage
Immediate-release and extended-release tablets should not be interchanged.

Hypertension
PO (Adults): *Immediate-release:* 1 mg once daily given at bedtime, may be ↑ if necessary at 3−4 wk intervals up to 2 mg/day; may also be given in 2 divided doses.

ADHD
PO (Adults and Children ≥6 yr): *Extended-release:* 1 mg once daily in morning or evening; may be ↑ by 1 mg/day at weekly intervals to achieve dose of 1−4 mg/day (6−12 yr) or 1−7 mg-day (13−17 yr) when used as monotherapy or 1−4 mg/day when used as adjunctive therapy. *Concurrent strong or moderate CYP3A4 inhibitor:* ↓ initial and maintenance dose by 50%; *Concurrent strong or moderate CYP3A4 inducer:* Consider ↑ initial and maintenance dose up to double the recommended level (maintenance dose can be ↑ over period of 1−2 wk).

Availability (generic available)
Immediate-release tablets: 1 mg, 2 mg. **Extended-release tablets (Intuniv):** 1 mg, 2 mg, 3 mg, 4 mg.

NURSING IMPLICATIONS
Assessment
- **Hypertension:** Monitor BP (lying and standing) and pulse frequently during initial dose adjustment and periodically during therapy. Report significant changes.
- Monitor frequency of prescription refills to determine adherence.
- **ADHD:** Assess attention span, impulse control, and interactions with others.
- Monitor BP and heart rate prior to starting therapy, following dose increases, and periodically during therapy. May cause hypotension, orthostatic hypotension, and bradycardia.

Lab Test Considerations
- May cause temporary, clinically insignificant ↑ in plasma growth hormone levels.
- May cause ↓ in urinary catecholamines and vanillylmandelic acid levels.

Implementation
- Do not confuse guanfacine with guaifenesin. Do not confuse Intuniv with Invega.
- Do not substitute extended-release tablets for immediate-release tablets on a mg-mg basis. Doses are not the same.
- **PO:** *For hypertension:* Administer daily dose at bedtime to minimize daytime sedation.
- *For ADHD:* Administer once daily in the morning or evening. *DNC:* Swallow extended-release tablets whole; do not crush, break, or chew. Do not administer with high fat meals, due to increased exposure.

Patient/Family Teaching
- Instruct patient/caregiver to take guanfacine as directed. Advise patient and parents to read the *Medication Guide* prior to starting therapy and with each Rx refill in case of changes. Instruct patients/caregivers not to discontinue guanfacine without consulting health care provider. Monitor blood pressure and pulse when reducing dose or discontinuing the drug. Taper the daily dose in decrements of no >1 mg every 3 to 7 days to minimize risk of rebound hypertension. If two or more doses are missed, may need to decrease dose and titrate to usual dose.
- Advise patient to notify health care professional of all Rx or OTC medications, vitamins, or herbal products being taken and to consult with health care professional before taking other medications, especially cough, cold, or allergy remedies.
- Caution patient to avoid alcohol and other CNS depressants, including opioids, while taking guanfacine.
- Advise patient to notify healthcare professional if dry mouth or constipation persists. Frequent mouth rinses, good oral hygiene, and sugarless gum or candy

may minimize dry mouth. Increase in fluid and fiber intake and exercise may decrease constipation.

- Instruct patient to notify health care professional of medication regimen prior to treatment or surgery.
- Advise patient to notify health care professional if dizziness, prolonged drowsiness, fatigue, weakness, depression, headache, sexual dysfunction, mental depression, or sleep pattern disturbance occurs. Discontinuation may be required if drug-related mental depression occurs.
- Rep: May cause fetal harm. Advise females of reproductive potential to notify health care professional if pregnancy is planned or suspected, or if breastfeeding. Monitor breastfed infants exposed to guanfacine through breast milk for sedation, lethargy, and poor feeding. Inform patient about pregnancy exposure registry that monitors pregnancy outcomes in women exposed to ADHD medications during pregnancy. Healthcare providers are encouraged to register patients by calling the National Pregnancy Registry for ADHD Medications at 1-866-961-2388.
- Emphasize the importance of follow-up exams to evaluate effectiveness of medication.
- **Hypertension:** Emphasize the importance of continuing to take medication as directed, even if feeling well. Medication controls but does not cure hypertension. Instruct patient to take medication at the same time each day. Take missed doses as soon as remembered; do not double doses. If 2 or more doses are missed, consult health care professional. Do not discontinue abruptly; may cause sympathetic overstimulation (nervousness, anxiety, rebound hypertension, chest pain, tachycardia, increased salivation, nausea, trembling, stomach cramps, sweating, difficulty sleeping). These effects may occur 2–7 days after discontinuation, although rebound hypertension is rare and more likely to occur with high doses.
- Advise patient to make sure enough medication is available for weekends, holidays, and vacations. A written prescription may be kept in wallet in case of emergency.
- Encourage patient to comply with additional interventions for hypertension (weight reduction, low-sodium diet, smoking cessation, moderation of alcohol consumption, regular exercise, and stress management).
- Instruct patient and family on proper technique for BP monitoring. Advise them to check BP at least weekly and to report significant changes.
- May cause drowsiness or dizziness. Advise patient to avoid driving or other activities requiring alertness until response to the medication is known.
- **ADHD:** Instruct patient to take medication as directed at the same time each day. Take missed doses as soon as possible, but should not take more than the total daily amount in any 24-hr period. Do not stop taking abruptly; discontinue gradually at no

more than 1 mg every 3–7 days. Monitor heart rate and BP during discontinuation. Advise patient and parents to read the *Medication Guide* prior to starting therapy and with each Rx refill.
- Inform patient that sharing this medication may be dangerous.
- Pedi: Advise parents to notify school nurse of medication regimen.

Evaluation/Desired Outcomes

- Decrease in BP without excessive side effects.
- Improved attention span and social interactions in ADHD. Re-evaluate use if used for >9 wk.

guselkumab (gue-sel-**koo**-mab)
Tremfya
Classification
Therapeutic: antipsoriatics
Pharmacologic: interleukin antagonists, monoclonal antibodies

Indications

Moderate to severe plaque psoriasis in patients who are candidates for phototherapy or systemic therapy. Active psoriatic arthritis (as monotherapy or in combination with a conventional disease-modifying antirheumatic drug).

Action

Binds to the p19 protein subunit of the interleukin (IL)-23 cytokine to prevent its interaction with the IL-23 receptor. This cytokine is normally involved in inflammatory and immune responses. Binding to ILs antagonizes their effects, inhibiting the release of proinflammatory cytokines and chemokines. **Therapeutic Effects:** Decrease in area and severity of psoriatic lesions. Decreased pain and swelling with decreased rate of joint destruction in psoriatic arthritis.

Pharmacokinetics

Absorption: 49% absorbed following SUBQ administration.
Distribution: Well distributed to tissues.
Metabolism and Excretion: Broken down by catabolic processes into peptides and amino acids.
Half-life: 15–18 days.

TIME/ACTION PROFILE (plasma concentrations)

ROUTE	ONSET	PEAK	DURATION
SUBQ	unknown	5.5 days	8 wk

Contraindications/Precautions

Contraindicated in: Hypersensitivity; Active, untreated infection.
Use Cautiously in: History of tuberculosis (TB) (possibility of reactivation); OB: Safety not established

in pregnancy; Lactation: Use while breastfeeding only if potential maternal benefit justifies potential risk to infant; Pedi: Safety and effectiveness not established in children.

Exercise Extreme Caution in: Chronic infection or history of recurrent infection.

Adverse Reactions/Side Effects

GI: ↑ liver enzymes, diarrhea. **Local:** injection site reactions. **MS:** arthralgia. **Neuro:** headache. **Misc:** infection, HYPERSENSITIVITY REACTIONS (including anaphylaxis).

Interactions

Drug-Drug: May ↓ antibody response to and ↑ risk of adverse reactions from **live vaccines**; avoid use during therapy. May affect the activity of CYP450 drug-metabolizing enzymes; appropriate monitoring and dose adjustment should be carried out when treatment is started in patients receiving concurrent treatment with **CYP450 substrate**, especially those with a narrow therapeutic index, including **warfarin** and **cyclosporine**.

Route/Dosage

SUBQ (Adults): 100 mg initially and 4 wk later, then 100 mg every 8 wk.

Availability

Solution for injection (prefilled syringes and patient-controlled injectors): 100 mg/mL.

NURSING IMPLICATIONS

Assessment

- Assess affected area(s) prior to and periodically during therapy.
- Assess patient for latent TB with a tuberculin skin test prior to initiation of therapy. Treatment of latent TB should be started before therapy with guselkumab.
- Assess for signs of infection (fever, dyspnea, flu-like symptoms, frequent or painful urination, redness or swelling at the site of a wound), including tuberculosis, prior to injection. Monitor new infections closely; most common are upper respiratory tract infections, bronchitis, and urinary tract infections.
- Monitor for signs and symptoms of hypersensitivity reactions (rash, hives, dyspnea, swelling of lips, tongue, or throat) during therapy.

Lab Test Considerations
- May cause ↑ liver enzymes.

Implementation

- Update immunizations to current prior to initiating therapy. Patients on guselkumab may receive concurrent vaccinations, except for live vaccines.
- **SUBQ:** Allow syringe and solution to reach room temperature, for 30 min before injecting. Solution is clear and colorless to light yellow solution and may contain small translucent particles; do not administer solutions that are cloudy, discolored or contain large particles. Store solution in refrigerator in original carton to protect from light; do not shake or freeze. Inject full amount (1 mL) of *One Press injector* in front of thigh, abdomen, or upper arm. Avoid areas that are tender, bruised, red, hard, thick, scaly, or affected by psoriasis.

Patient/Family Teaching

- Instruct patient on correct technique for self-injection, care and disposal of equipment. Review *Medication Guide* with patient before starting therapy and with each injection.
- Advise patient to notify health care professional if signs and symptoms of infection (fever, chills, sore throat, painful urination) occur.
- Instruct patient to avoid receiving live vaccines during therapy.
- Advise patient to notify health care professional immediately if signs and symptoms of hypersensitivity reaction (feel faint; swelling of face, eyelids, lips, mouth, tongue or throat; trouble breathing; throat tightness; chest tightness; skin rash; hives) occur.
- Instruct patient to notify health care professional of all Rx or OTC medications, vitamins, or herbal products being taken and consult health care professional before taking any new medications.
- Instruct patient to notify health care professional of medication regimen prior to treatment or surgery.
- Rep: Advise females of reproductive potential to notify health care professional if pregnancy is planned or suspected, or if breastfeeding. Inform patient of pregnancy registry that monitors pregnancy outcomes in women exposed to guselkumab during pregnancy. Encourage patients to enroll by calling 1-877-311-8972.

Evaluation/Desired Outcomes

- Decrease in extent and severity of psoriatic lesions.
- Decreased pain and swelling with decreased rate of joint destruction in psoriatic arthritis.

halcinonide, See CORTICOSTEROIDS (TOPICAL/LOCAL).

halobetasol, See CORTICOSTEROIDS (TOPICAL/LOCAL).

haloperidol (ha-loe-**per**-i-dole)
~~Haldol~~, Haldol Decanoate
Classification
Therapeutic: antipsychotics
Pharmacologic: butyrophenones

Indications
Acute and chronic psychotic disorders including: schizophrenia, manic states, drug-induced psychoses. Patients with schizophrenia who require long-term parenteral (IM) antipsychotic therapy. Agitation or aggressive behavior. Tourette's syndrome. Severe behavioral problems in children which may be accompanied by: unprovoked, combative, explosive hyperexcitability, hyperactivity accompanied by conduct disorders (short-term use when other modalities have failed). **Unlabeled Use:** Nausea and vomiting from surgery or chemotherapy.

Action
Alters the effects of dopamine in the CNS. Also has anticholinergic and alpha-adrenergic blocking activity. **Therapeutic Effects:** Diminished signs and symptoms of psychoses. Improved behavior in children with Tourette's syndrome or other behavioral problems.

Pharmacokinetics
Absorption: Well absorbed following PO/IM administration. Decanoate salt is slowly absorbed and has a long duration of action.
Distribution: Concentrates in liver.
Protein Binding: 92%.
Metabolism and Excretion: Mostly metabolized by the liver.
Half-life: 21–24 hr.

TIME/ACTION PROFILE (antipsychotic activity)

ROUTE	ONSET	PEAK	DURATION
PO	2 hr	2–6 hr	8–12 hr
IM	20–30 min	30–45 min	4–8 hr†
IM (decanoate)	3–9 days	unknown	1 mo

†Effect may persist for several days.

Contraindications/Precautions
Contraindicated in: Hypersensitivity; Angle-closure glaucoma; Bone marrow depression; CNS depression; Parkinsonism; Severe hepatic or cardiovascular disease (↑ risk of QT interval prolongation); Some products contain tartrazine, sesame oil, or benzyl alcohol and should be avoided in patients with known intolerance or hypersensitivity; Lactation: Lactation.
Use Cautiously in: Debilitated patients (↓ dose); Cardiac disease (↑ risk of QT interval prolongation with high doses); Diabetes; Respiratory disease; Prostatic hyperplasia; CNS tumors; Intestinal obstruction; Seizures; Patients at risk for falls; OB: Neonates at ↑ risk for extrapyramidal symptoms and withdrawal after delivery when exposed during the 3rd trimester; use during pregnancy only if potential maternal benefit justifies potential fetal risk; Geri: Appears on Beers list. ↑ risk of stroke, cognitive decline, and mortality in older adults with dementia. Avoid use in older adults, except for schizophrenia, bipolar disorder, or for short-term use as an antiemetic.

Adverse Reactions/Side Effects
CV: hypotension, QT interval prolongation, tachycardia, TORSADES DE POINTES, ventricular arrhythmias. **Derm:** diaphoresis, photosensitivity, rash. **EENT:** blurred vision, dry eyes. **Endo:** amenorrhea, galactorrhea, gynecomastia. **GI:** constipation, dry mouth, anorexia, hepatitis, ileus. **GU:** impotence, urinary retention. **Hemat:** AGRANULOCYTOSIS, anemia, leukopenia, neutropenia. **Metab:** weight gain. **Neuro:** extrapyramidal reactions, confusion, drowsiness, restlessness, SEIZURES, tardive dyskinesia. **Resp:** respiratory depression. **Misc:** hypersensitivity reactions, NEUROLEPTIC MALIGNANT SYNDROME.

Interactions
Drug-Drug: Concurrent use with **QT interval prolonging drugs** may ↑ risk of QT interval prolongation. ↑ hypotension with **antihypertensives**, **nitrates**, or acute ingestion of **alcohol**. ↑ anticholinergic effects with **drugs having anticholinergic properties**, including **antihistamines**, **antidepressants**, **atropine**, **phenothiazines**, **quinidine**, and **disopyramide**. ↑ CNS depression with other **CNS depressants**, including **alcohol**, **antihistamines**, **opioid analgesics**, and **sedative/hypnotics**. Concurrent use with **epinephrine** may result in severe hypotension and tachycardia. May ↓ therapeutic effects of **levodopa**. Acute encephalopathic syndrome may occur when used with **lithium**.
Drug-Natural Products: **Kava-kava**, **valerian**, or **chamomile** can ↑ CNS depression.

Route/Dosage
Haloperidol
PO (Adults): 0.5–5 mg 2–3 times daily. Patients with severe symptoms may require up to 100 mg/day.
PO (Geriatric Patients): 0.5–2 mg twice daily initially; may be gradually ↑ as needed.
PO (Children 3–12 yr or 15–40 kg): 0.25–0.5 mg/day given in 2–3 divided doses; increase by 0.25–

0.5 mg every 5–7 days; maximum dose: 0.15 mg/kg/day (up to 0.75 mg/kg/day for Tourette's syndrome or 0.15 mg/kg/day for psychoses).

IM (Adults): *Haloperidol lactate:* 2–5 mg every 1–8 hr (not to exceed 100 mg/day).

IM (Children 6–12 yr): *Haloperidol lactate:* 1–3 mg/dose every 4–8 hrs to a maximum of 0.15 mg/kg/day.

IV (Adults): *Haloperidol lactate:* 0.5–5 mg, may be repeated every 30 min (unlabeled).

Haloperidol Decanoate

IM (Adults): 10–15 times the previous daily PO dose but not to exceed 100 mg initially, given monthly (not to exceed 300 mg/mo).

Availability (generic available)

Tablets: 0.5 mg, 1 mg, 2 mg, 5 mg, 10 mg, 20 mg. **Oral concentrate:** 2 mg/mL. **Solution for intramuscular injection (decanoate):** 50 mg/mL, 100 mg/mL. **Solution for intravenous injection (lactate):** 5 mg/mL.

NURSING IMPLICATIONS

Assessment

- Assess mental status (orientation, mood, behavior) prior to and periodically during therapy.
- Assess positive (hallucination, delusions) and negative (social isolation) symptoms of schizophrenia.
- Assess weight and BMI initially and during therapy. Refer as appropriate for nutritional/weight and medical management.
- Monitor BP (sitting, standing, lying) and pulse prior to and frequently during the period of dose adjustment. May cause QT interval changes on ECG.
- Observe patient carefully when administering medication, to ensure that medication is actually taken and not hoarded.
- Monitor intake and output ratios and daily weight. Assess patient for signs and symptoms of dehydration (decreased thirst, lethargy, hemoconcentration), especially in geriatric patients.
- Assess fluid intake and bowel function. Increased bulk and fluids in the diet help minimize constipating effects.
- Monitor patient for onset of akathisia (restlessness or desire to keep moving), which may appear within 6 hr of 1st dose and may be difficult to distinguish from psychotic agitation. Benztropine may be used to differentiate agitation from akathisia. Observe closely for extrapyramidal side effects (*parkinsonian:* difficulty speaking or swallowing, loss of balance control, pill rolling of hands, mask-like face, shuffling gait, rigidity, tremors; and *dystonic:* muscle spasms, twisting motions, twitching, inability to move eyes, weakness of arms or legs). Trihexyphenidyl or benzotropine may be used to control these symptoms. Benzodiazepines may alleviate akathisia.
- Monitor for tardive dyskinesia (uncontrolled rhythmic movement of mouth, face, and extremities; lip smacking or puckering; puffing of cheeks; uncontrolled chewing; rapid or worm-like movements of tongue, excessive eye blinking). Report immediately; may be irreversible.
- Monitor for symptoms related to hyperprolactinemia (menstrual abnormalities, galactorrhea, sexual dysfunction).
- Monitor for development of neuroleptic malignant syndrome (fever, respiratory distress, tachycardia, seizures, diaphoresis, hypertension or hypotension, pallor, tiredness, severe muscle stiffness, loss of bladder control). Report symptoms immediately. May also cause leukocytosis, elevated liver function tests, elevated CK.
- Assess for falls risk. Drowsiness, orthostatic hypotension, and motor and sensory instability increase risk. Institute prevention if indicated.

Lab Test Considerations

- Monitor CBC with differential and liver function tests periodically during therapy.
- Monitor serum prolactin prior to and periodically during therapy. May cause ↑ serum prolactin levels.

Implementation

- Avoid skin contact with oral solution; may cause contact dermatitis.
- **PO:** Administer with food or full glass of water or milk to minimize GI irritation.
- Use calibrated measuring device for accurate dose. Do not dilute concentrate with coffee or tea; may cause precipitation. May be given undiluted or mixed with water or juice.
- **IM:** Inject slowly, using 2-in, 21-gauge needle into well-developed muscle via Z-track technique. Do not exceed 3 mL per injection site. Slight yellow color does not indicate altered potency. Keep patient recumbent for at least 30 min following injection to minimize hypotensive effects.

IV Administration

- **IV:** Haloperidol decanoate should not be administered IV.
- **IV Push:** *Dilution:* May be administered undiluted for rapid control of acute psychosis or delirium. *Concentration:* 5 mg/mL. *Rate:* Administer at a rate of 5 mg/min.
- **Intermittent Infusion:** *Dilution:* May be diluted in 30–50 mL of D5W. *Rate:* Infuse over 30 min.
- **Y-Site Compatibility:** acetaminophen, alemtuzumab, amifostine, aminocaproic acid, amphotericin B liposomal, anidulafungin, argatroban, arsenic trioxide, azithromycin, bleomycin, cangrelor, carboplatin, carmustine, caspofungin, ceftaroline, cisatracurium, cisplatin, cladribine, clonidine, cyclophosphamide, cytarabine, dacarbazine, dactinomycin, daptomycin, daunorubicin hydrochloride, dexmedetomidine, dexrazoxane, diltiazem, docetaxel, doxorubicin hydrochloride, doxorubicin liposomal, epirubicin, eptifibatide, ertapenem, etoposide, etoposide phosphate, filgrastim, fludarabine, gemci-

tabine, granisetron, hetastarch, hydromorphone, idarubicin, ifosfamide, irinotecan, ketamine, leucovorin calcium, levofloxacin, linezolid, lorazepam, melphalan, mesna, methadone, metronidazole, milrinone, mitoxantrone, morphine, moxifloxacin, mycophenolate, nicardipine, octreotide, oxaliplatin, paclitaxel, palonosetron, pamidronate, pemetrexed, potassium acetate, propofol, remifentanil, rituximab, rocuronium, sodium acetate, tacrolimus, thiotepa, tigecycline, tirofiban, trastuzumab, vecuronium, vinblastine, vincristine, vinorelbine, voriconazole, zoledronic acid.

- **Y-Site Incompatibility:** acyclovir, allopurinol, aminophylline, amphotericin B deoxycholate, amphotericin B lipid complex, ampicillin, ampicillin/sulbactam, azathioprine, bumetanide, calcium chloride, cefazolin, cefepime, cefotaxime, cefotetan, cefoxitin, ceftazidime, ceftriaxone, cefuroxime, chloramphenicol, clindamycin, dantrolene, dexamethasone, diazepam, epoetin alfa, fluorouracil, folic acid, foscarnet, fosphenytoin, furosemide, ganciclovir, gemtuzumab ozogamicin, heparin, hydralazine, hydrocortisone, imipenem/cilastatin, indomethacin, ketorolac, magnesium sulfate, methylprednisolone, minocycline, mitomycin, nafcillin, oxacillin, pantoprazole, penicillin G, pentobarbital, phenobarbital, phenytoin, piperacillin/tazobactam, potassium chloride, sargramostim, sodium bicarbonate, trimethoprim/sulfamethoxazole.

Patient/Family Teaching

- Advise patient to take medication as directed. Take missed doses as soon as remembered, with remaining doses evenly spaced throughout the day. May require several wk to obtain desired effects. Do not increase dose or discontinue medication without consulting health care professional. Abrupt withdrawal may cause dizziness; nausea; vomiting; GI upset; trembling; or uncontrolled movements of mouth, tongue, or jaw.
- Inform patient of possibility of extrapyramidal symptoms, tardive dyskinesia, and neuroleptic malignant syndrome. Caution patient to report symptoms immediately.
- Advise patient to change positions slowly to minimize orthostatic hypotension. Protect from falls.
- May cause drowsiness. Caution patient to avoid driving or other activities requiring alertness until response to medication is known.
- Instruct patient to notify health care professional of all Rx or OTC medications, vitamins, or herbal products being taken and to consult with health care professional before taking other medications.
- Caution patient to avoid taking alcohol or other CNS depressants, including opioids, concurrently with this medication.
- Advise patient to use sunscreen and protective clothing when exposed to the sun to prevent photosensi-

tivity reactions. Extremes of temperature should also be avoided; drug impairs body temperature regulation.
- Instruct patient to use frequent mouth rinses, good oral hygiene, and sugarless gum or candy to minimize dry mouth.
- Advise patient to notify health care professional of medication regimen prior to treatment or surgery.
- Instruct patient to notify health care professional promptly if weakness, tremors, visual disturbances, dark-colored urine or clay-colored stools, sore throat, fever, menstrual abnormalities, galactorrhea, or sexual dysfunction occur.
- Rep: Advise females of reproductive potential to notify health care professional if pregnancy is planned or suspected and to avoid breastfeeding during therapy. Monitor neonates exposed to haloperidol during the third trimester of pregnancy for extrapyramidal and/or withdrawal symptoms following delivery. There have been reports of agitation, hypertonia, hypotonia, tremor, somnolence, respiratory distress and feeding disorder in these neonates. Inform patient of the National Pregnancy Registry for Psychiatric Medications that monitors the safety of psychiatric medications taken by women during pregnancy. Encourage patient to contact the registry at https://womensmentalhealth.org/clinical-and-research-programs/pregnancyregistry or by phone 1-866-961-2388. Monitor breastfed infants for excessive drowsiness, lethargy, and developmental delays.
- Emphasize the importance of routine follow-up exams to monitor response to medication and detect side effects.

Evaluation/Desired Outcomes

- Decrease in hallucinations, insomnia, agitation, hostility, and delusions.
- Decreased tics and vocalization in Tourette's syndrome.
- Improved behavior in children with severe behavioral problems. If no therapeutic effects are seen in 2–4 wk, dosage may be increased.

HIGH ALERT

heparin (hep-a-rin)
Classification
Therapeutic: anticoagulants
Pharmacologic: antithrombotics

Indications
Prophylaxis and treatment of various thromboembolic disorders including: Deep vein thrombosis (DVT), Pulmonary embolism (PE), Atrial fibrillation with embolization, Acute and chronic consumptive coagulopathies, Peripheral arterial thromboembolism. Used in very low doses (10–100 units) to maintain patency of IV catheters (heparin flush).

Action

Potentiates the inhibitory effect of antithrombin on factor Xa and thrombin. In low doses, prevents the conversion of prothrombin to thrombin by its effects on factor Xa. Higher doses neutralize thrombin, preventing the conversion of fibrinogen to fibrin. **Therapeutic Effects:** Prevention of thrombus formation. Prevention of extension of existing thrombi (full dose).

Pharmacokinetics

Absorption: Erratically absorbed following SUBQ or IM administration.

Distribution: Does not cross the placenta or enter breast milk.

Protein Binding: Very high (to low-density lipoproteins, globulins, and fibrinogen).

Metabolism and Excretion: Probably removed by the reticuloendothelial system (lymph nodes, spleen).

Half-life: 1–2 hr (↑ with increasing dose); affected by obesity, renal and hepatic function, malignancy, presence of PE, and infections.

TIME/ACTION PROFILE (anticoagulant effect)

ROUTE	ONSET	PEAK	DURATION
SUBQ	20–60 min	2 hr	8–12 hr
IV	immediate	5–10 min	2–6 hr

Contraindications/Precautions

Contraindicated in: Hypersensitivity; Uncontrolled bleeding; History of heparin-induced thrombocytopenia (HIT); Severe thrombocytopenia; Open wounds (full dose); Pedi: Avoid use of products containing benzyl alcohol in premature infants.

Use Cautiously in: Severe liver or kidney impairment; Retinopathy (hypertensive or diabetic); Ulcer disease; Spinal cord or brain injury; History of congenital or acquired bleeding disorder; Malignancy; Diabetes mellitus, chronic renal failure, metabolic acidosis, increased serum potassium, or concurrent use of potassium-sparing drugs (↑ risk of hyperkalemia); OB: Use during pregnancy only if potential maternal benefit justifies potential fetal risk; avoid use of products containing benzyl alcohol; Lactation: Use while breastfeeding only if potential maternal benefit justifies potential risk to infant; avoid use of products containing benzyl alcohol; Geri: Women >60 yr have ↑ risk of bleeding.

Exercise Extreme Caution in: Severe uncontrolled hypertension; Bacterial endocarditis, bleeding disorders; GI bleeding/ulceration/pathology; Hemorrhagic stroke; History of thrombocytopenia related to heparin; Recent CNS or ophthalmologic surgery; Active GI bleeding/ulceration;.

Adverse Reactions/Side Effects

Derm: alopecia (long-term use), rash, urticaria. **F and E:** hyperkalemia. **GI:** ↑ liver enzymes. **Hemat:** anemia, BLEEDING, HIT (WITH OR WITHOUT THROMBOSIS). **Local:** pain at injection site. **MS:** osteoporosis (long-term use). **Misc:** fever, hypersensitivity reactions.

Interactions

Heparin is frequently used concurrently or sequentially with other agents affecting coagulation. The risk of potentially serious interactions is greatest with full anticoagulation.

Drug-Drug: Risk of bleeding may be ↑ by concurrent use of **drugs that affect platelet function,** including **aspirin, NSAIDs, clopidogrel, dipyridamole,** some **penicillins, eptifibatide, tirofiban,** and **dextran.** Risk of bleeding may be ↑ by concurrent use of **drugs that cause hypoprothrombinemia,** including **quinidine, cefotetan,** and **valproic acid.** Concurrent use of **thrombolytics** ↑ risk of bleeding. Heparins affect the prothrombin time used in assessing the response to **warfarin. Digoxin, tetracyclines, nicotine,** and **antihistamines** may ↓ anticoagulant effect of heparin.

Drug-Natural Products: ↑ risk of bleeding with **arnica, anise, chamomile, clove, dong quai, feverfew, garlic, ginger,** and **Panax ginseng.**

Route/Dosage

Therapeutic Anticoagulation

IV (Adults): *Intermittent bolus:* 10,000 units, followed by 5000–10,000 units every 4–6 hr. *Continuous infusion:* 5000 units (35–70 units/kg), followed by 20,000–40,000 units infused over 24 hr (approx. 1000 units/hr or 15–18 units/kg/hr).

IV (Children >1 yr): *Intermittent bolus:* 50–100 units/kg, followed by 50–100 units/kg every 4 hr. *Continuous infusion:* Loading dose 75 units/kg, followed by 20 units/kg/hr, adjust to maintain activated partial thromboplastin time (aPTT) of 60–85 sec.

IV (Neonates and Infants <1 yr): *Continuous infusion:* Loading dose 75 units/kg, followed by 28 units/kg/hr, adjust to maintain aPTT of 60–85 sec.

SUBQ (Adults): 5000 units IV, followed by initial SUBQ dose of 10,000–20,000 units, then 8000–10,000 units every 8 hr or 15,000–20,000 units every 12 hr.

Prophylaxis of Thromboembolism

SUBQ (Adults): 5000 units every 8–12 hr (may be started 2 hr prior to surgery).

Cardiovascular Surgery

IV (Adults): At least 150 units/kg (300 units/kg if procedure <60 min; 400 units/kg if >60 min).

Intra-arterial (Neonates, Infants, and Children): 100–150 units/kg via an artery prior to cardiac catheterization.

Line Flushing

IV (Adults and Children): 10–100 units/mL (10 units/mL for infants <10 kg, 100 units/mL for all others) solution to fill heparin lock set to needle hub; replace after each use.

Total Parenteral Nutrition

IV (Adults and Children): 0.5–1 units/mL (final solution concentration) to maintain line patency.

Arterial Line Patency

Intra-arterial (Neonates): 0.5–2 units/mL.

Availability (generic available)

Premixed infusion: 1000 units/500 mL, 2000 units/1000 mL, 12,500 units/250 mL, 25,000 units in 250 and 500 mL. **Solution for injection:** 10 units/mL, 100 units/mL, 1000 units/mL, 5000 units/mL, 7500 units/mL, 10,000 units/mL, 20,000 units/mL, 40,000 units/mL.

NURSING IMPLICATIONS

Assessment

- Assess for signs of bleeding and hemorrhage (bleeding gums; nosebleed; unusual bruising; black, tarry stools; hematuria; fall in hematocrit or BP; guaiac-positive stools). Notify health care professional if these occur.
- Assess patient for evidence of additional or increased thrombosis. Symptoms will depend on area of involvement.
- Monitor patient for hypersensitivity reactions (chills, fever, urticaria).
- **SUBQ:** Observe injection sites for hematomas, ecchymosis, or inflammation.

Lab Test Considerations

- Monitor aPTT and hematocrit prior to and periodically during therapy. When *intermittent IV* therapy is used, draw aPTT levels 30 min before each dose during initial therapy and then periodically. During *continuous* administration, monitor aPTT levels every 4 hr during early therapy. For *SUBQ* therapy, draw blood 4–6 hr after injection.
- Monitor platelet count every 2–3 days during therapy. May cause mild thrombocytopenia, which appears on 4th day and resolves despite continued heparin therapy. HIT, a more severe form which necessitates discontinuing medication, may develop on 8th day of therapy; may reduce platelet count to as low as 5000/mm^3 and lead to increased resistance to heparin therapy. HIT may progress to development of venous and arterial thrombosis and may occur up to several wk after discontinuation. Patients who have received a previous course of heparin may be at higher risk for severe thrombocytopenia for several mo after the initial course.
- May cause hyperkalemia and ↑ AST and ALT levels.

Toxicity and Overdose

- Protamine sulfate is the antidote. Due to short half-life, overdose can often be treated by withdrawing the drug.

Implementation

- ***High Alert:*** Fatal hemorrhages have occurred in pediatric patients due to errors in which heparin sodium injection vials were confused with heparin flush vials. Carefully examine all heparin sodium injection vials to confirm the correct vial choice prior to administration. Have second practitioner independently check original order, dose calculation, and infusion pump settings. Unintended concomitant use of two heparin products (unfractionated heparin and low-molecular weight heparins) has resulted in serious harm or death. Review patients' recent (emergency department, operating room) and current medication administration records before administering any heparin or LMWH product.
- Do not confuse heparin with Hespan. Do not confuse vials of heparin with vials of insulin.
- Inform all personnel caring for patient of anticoagulant therapy. Venipunctures and injection sites require application of pressure to prevent bleeding or hematoma formation. Avoid IM injections of other medications; hematomas may develop.
- In patients requiring long-term anticoagulation, oral anticoagulant therapy should be instituted 4–5 days prior to discontinuing heparin therapy.
- Solution is colorless to slightly yellow.
- **SUBQ:** Administer deep into SUBQ tissue. Alternate injection sites between arm and the left and right abdominal wall above the iliac crest. Inject entire length of needle at a 45°- or 90°-angle into a skin fold held between thumb and forefinger; hold skin fold throughout injection. Do not aspirate or massage. Rotate sites frequently. Do not administer IM because of danger of hematoma formation. Solution should be clear; do not inject solution containing particulate matter.

IV Administration

- **IV Push:** ***Dilution:*** Administer loading dose undiluted. ***Concentration:*** Varies depending upon vial used. ***Rate:*** Administer over at least 1 min. Loading dose given before continuous infusion.
- **Continuous Infusion:** ***Dilution:*** Dilute 25,000 units of heparin in 250–500 mL of 0.9% NaCl or D5W. Premixed infusions are already diluted and ready to use. Admixed solutions stable for 24 hr at room temperature or if refrigerated. Premixed infusion stable for 30 days once overwrap removed. ***Concentration:*** 50–100 units/mL. ***Rate:*** See Route/Dosage section. Adjust to maintain therapeutic aPTT. Use an infusion pump to ensure accuracy.
- **Flush:** To prevent clot formation in intermittent infusion (heparin lock) sets, inject dilute heparin solution of 10–100 units/0.5–1 mL after each medication injection or every 8–12 hr. To prevent incompatibility of heparin with medication, flush lock set with sterile water or 0.9% NaCl for injection before and after medication is administered.

- **Y-Site Compatibility:** acetaminophen, acetylcysteine, acyclovir, alemtuzumab, allopurinol, amifostine, aminocaproic acid, aminophylline, amphotericin B lipid complex, amphotericin B liposomal, anidulafungin, argatroban, arsenic trioxide, ascorbic acid, atropine, azathioprine, azithromycin, aztreonam, benztropine, bivalirudin, bleomycin, buprenorphine, butorphanol, calcium chloride, calcium gluconate, cangrelor, carboplatin, carmustine, cefazolin, cefotaxime, cefotetan, cefoxitin, ceftaroline, ceftazidime, ceftazidime/avibactam, ceftolozane/tazobactam, ceftriaxone, cefuroxime, chloramphenicol, cisplatin, cladribine, clindamycin, cyanocobalamin, cyclophosphamide, cyclosporine, cytarabine, dactinomycin, daptomycin, defibrotide, dexamethasone, dexmedetomidine, dexrazoxane, digoxin, docetaxel, dopamine, doxapram, doxorubicin liposomal, enalaprilat, ephedrine, epinephrine, epoetin alfa, eptifibatide, eravacycline, ertapenem, esmolol, etoposide, etoposide phosphate, famotidine, fentanyl, fluconazole, fludarabine, fluorouracil, folic acid, foscarnet, fosphenytoin, furosemide, ganciclovir, gemcitabine, gemtuzumab ozogamicin, glycopyrrolate, granisetron, hetastarch, hydrocortisone, hydromorphone, ibuprofen lysine, ifosfamide, imipenem/cilastatin, imipenem/cilastatin/relebactam, indomethacin, irinotecan, isoproterenol, ketorolac, LR, leucovorin calcium, lidocaine, linezolid, lorazepam, magnesium sulfate, mannitol, melphalan, meropenem, meropenem/vaborbactam, mesna, methadone, methohexital, methotrexate, methylprednisolone, metoclopramide, metoprolol, metronidazole, micafungin, midazolam, milrinone, mitomycin, morphine, moxifloxacin, multiple vitamins, nafcillin, nalbuphine, naloxone, nitroglycerin, nitroprusside, norepinephrine, octreotide, ondansetron, oxacillin, oxaliplatin, oxytocin, paclitaxel, palonosetron, pamidronate, pemetrexed, penicillin G, pentobarbital, phenobarbital, phentolamine, phenylephrine, phytonadione, piperacillin/tazobactam, potassium acetate, potassium chloride, procainamide, prochlorperazine, propofol, propranolol, pyridostigmine, pyridoxine, remifentanil, rituximab, rocuronium, sargramostim, sodium acetate, sodium bicarbonate, succinylcholine, sufentanil, tacrolimus, tedizolid, theophylline, thiamine, thiopental, thiotepa, tigecycline, tirofiban, topotecan, tranexamic acid, trastuzumab, vasopressin, vecuronium, verapamil, vinblastine, vincristine, voriconazole, warfarin, zidovudine, zoledronic acid.
- **Y-Site Incompatibility:** alteplase, amiodarone, amphotericin B deoxycholate, blinatumomab, caspofungin, ciprofloxacin, dantrolene, daunorubicin hydrochloride, diazepam, diphenhydramine, doxycycline, epirubicin, filgrastim, haloperidol, hydroxyzine, idarubicin, isavuconazonium, ketamine, levofloxacin, minocycline, mitoxantrone, mycophenolate, oritavancin, palifermin, papaverine, pentamidine, phenytoin, plazomicin, protamine, reteplase.

- **Additive Compatibility:** It is recommended that heparin not be mixed in solution with other medications when given for anticoagulation, even those that are compatible, because changes in rate of heparin infusion may be required that would also affect admixtures.

Patient/Family Teaching
- Explain purpose of heparin to patient.
- Advise patient to report any symptoms of unusual bleeding or bruising to health care professional immediately.
- Instruct patient not to take medications containing aspirin or NSAIDs while on heparin therapy.
- Caution patient to avoid IM injections and activities leading to injury and to use a soft toothbrush and electric razor during heparin therapy.
- Advise patient to inform health care professional of medication regimen prior to treatment or surgery.
- Rep: Advise females of reproductive potential to notify health care professional if pregnancy is planned or suspected, or if breastfeeding.
- Patients on anticoagulant therapy should carry an identification card with this information at all times.

Evaluation/Desired Outcomes
- Prolonged aPTT of 1.5–2.5 times the control, without signs of hemorrhage.
- Prevention of DVT and PE.
- Patency of IV catheters.

HIGH ALERT

HEPARINS (LOW MOLECULAR WEIGHT)
dalteparin (dal-**te**-pa-rin)
  Fragmin
enoxaparin (e-nox-a-**pa**-rin)
  ✤Elonox, Enoxiluv Kit, ✤Inclunox, Lovenox, ✤Noromby, ✤Redesca
Classification
Therapeutic: anticoagulants
Pharmacologic: antithrombotics

Indications
Enoxaparin and dalteparin: Prevention of venous thromboembolism (VTE) (deep vein thrombosis [DVT] and/or pulmonary embolism [PE]) in surgical or medical patients. **Dalteparin only:** Extended treatment of symptomatic DVT and/or PE in patients with cancer. **Enoxaparin only:** Treatment of DVT with or without PE (in combination with warfarin). **Enoxaparin and dalteparin:** Prevention of ischemic complications (with aspirin) from unstable angina and non–ST-segment-elevation MI. **Enoxaparin only:** Treatment of acute ST-segment-elevation MI (with thrombolytics or percutaneous coronary intervention).

Action
Potentiate the inhibitory effect of antithrombin on factor Xa and thrombin. **Therapeutic Effects:** Prevention of thrombus formation.

Pharmacokinetics
Absorption: Well absorbed after SUBQ administration (87% for dalteparin, 92% for enoxaparin).
Distribution: Minimally distributed to tissues.
Metabolism and Excretion: *Dalteparin:* unknown; *enoxaparin:* primarily eliminated renally.
Half-life: *Dalteparin:* 2.1–2.3 hr; *enoxaparin:* 3–6 hr (all are ↑ in renal insufficiency).

TIME/ACTION PROFILE (anticoagulant effect)

ROUTE	ONSET	PEAK	DURATION
Dalteparin SUBQ	rapid	4 hr	up to 24 hr
Enoxaparin SUBQ	unknown	3–5 hr	12 hr

Contraindications/Precautions
Contraindicated in: Hypersensitivity to specific agents, unfractionated heparin, or pork products; cross-sensitivity may occur; Some products contain sulfites or benzyl alcohol and should be avoided in patients with known hypersensitivity or intolerance; Active major bleeding; *Enoxaparin:* History of immune-mediated heparin-induced thrombocytopenia (HIT) within the past 100 days or in the presence of circulating antibodies; *Dalteparin:* History of HIT; *Dalteparin:* regional anesthesia during treatment for unstable angina/non–ST-segment elevation MI.
Use Cautiously in: Severe renal impairment (adjust dose of enoxaparin if CCr <30 mL/min); Severe hepatic impairment; Women <45 kg or men <57 kg; Retinopathy (hypertensive or diabetic); Untreated hypertension; *Enoxaparin:* History of HIT >100 days ago and no circulating antibodies present; Recent history of ulcer disease; History of congenital or acquired bleeding disorder; OB: Safety not established in pregnancy; should not be used in pregnant patients with prosthetic heart valves or inherited/acquired thrombophilias without careful monitoring; if enoxaparin used during pregnancy, use preservative-free formulation; Lactation: Use while breastfeeding only if potential maternal benefit justifies potential risk to infant; Pedi: Safety and effectiveness not established in children; enoxaparin multidose vial contains benzyl alcohol, which can cause potentially fatal "gasping syndrome" in neonates; Geri: Older adults may have ↑ risk of bleeding due to age-related ↓ in renal function; Geri: *Dalteparin:* ↑ mortality in patients >70 yr with renal impairment.
Exercise Extreme Caution in: Spinal/epidural anesthesia (↑ risk of spinal/epidural hematomas, especially with concurrent NSAIDs, repeated or traumatic

epidural puncture, or indwelling epidural catheter); Severe uncontrolled hypertension; Bacterial endocarditis; Bleeding disorders.

Adverse Reactions/Side Effects
CV: edema. **Derm:** alopecia, ecchymoses, pruritus, rash, urticaria. **GI:** ↑ liver enzymes, constipation, nausea, vomiting. **GU:** urinary retention. **Hemat:** <u>anemia</u>, BLEEDING, eosinophilia, thrombocytopenia. **Local:** erythema at injection site, hematoma, irritation, pain at injection site. **MS:** osteoporosis. **Neuro:** dizziness, headache, insomnia. **Misc:** fever.

Interactions
Drug-Drug: Risk of bleeding may be ↑ by concurrent use of **drugs that affect platelet function and coagulation**, including **warfarin**, **aspirin**, **NSAIDs**, **dipyridamole**, **clopidogrel**, **prasugrel**, **ticagrelor**, **eptifibatide**, **tirofiban**, and **thrombolytics**.
Drug-Natural Products: ↑ bleeding risk with **arnica**, **chamomile**, **clove**, **feverfew**, **garlic**, **ginger**, **ginkgo**, **Panax ginseng**, and others.

Route/Dosage

Dalteparin
SUBQ (Adults): *Prophylaxis of DVT following abdominal surgery:* 2500 units 1–2 hr before surgery, then once daily for 5–10 days; *Prophylaxis of VTE in high-risk patients undergoing abdominal surgery:* 5000 units evening before surgery, then once daily for 5–10 days *or* in patients with malignancy, 2500 units 1–2 hr before surgery, another 2500 units 12 hr later, then 5000 units once daily for 5–10 days; *Prophylaxis of VTE in patients undergoing hip replacement surgery:* 2500 units within 2 hr before surgery, then 2500 units 4–8 hr after surgery, then 5000 units once daily (start at least 6 hr after postsurgical dose) for 5–10 days *or* 5000 units evening before surgery (10–14 hr before surgery), then 5000 units 4–8 hr after surgery, then 5000 units once daily for 5–10 days *or* 2500 units 4–8 hr after surgery, then 5000 units once daily (start at least 6 hr after postsurgical dose); *Prophylaxis of VTE in medical patients with severely restricted mobility during acute illness:* 5000 units once daily for 12–14 days. *Unstable angina/non–ST-segment-elevation MI:* 120 units/kg (not to exceed 10,000 units) every 12 hr for 5–8 days with concurrent aspirin; *Extended treatment of symptomatic VTE in cancer patients:* 200 units/kg (not to exceed 18,000 units) once daily for first 30 days, followed by 150 units/kg (not to exceed 18,000 units) once daily for mo 2–6.

Renal Impairment
SUBQ (Adults): *Cancer patients receiving extended treatment of symptomatic VTE with CCr <30 mL/min:* Monitor anti-Xa levels (target 0.5–1.5 IU/mL).

Enoxaparin
SUBQ (Adults): *VTE prophylaxis in patients undergoing knee replacement surgery:* 30 mg every 12 hr

starting 12–24 hr postop for 7–10 days; *VTE prophylaxis in patients undergoing hip replacement surgery:* 30 mg every 12 hr starting 12–24 hr postop *or* 40 mg once daily starting 12 hr before surgery (either dose may be continued for 7–14 days; continued prophylaxis with 40 mg once daily may be continued for up to 3 wk); *VTE prophylaxis following abdominal surgery:* 40 mg once daily starting 2 hr before surgery and then continued for 7–12 days or until ambulatory (up to 14 days); *VTE prophylaxis in medical patients with acute illness:* 40 mg once daily for 6–14 days; *Treatment of DVT/PE (outpatient):* 1 mg/kg every 12 hr. Warfarin should be started within 72 hr; enoxaparin may be continued for a minimum of 5 days and until therapeutic anticoagulation with warfarin is achieved (INR >2 for 2 consecutive days); *Treatment of DVT/PE (inpatient):* 1 mg/kg every 12 hr *or* 1.5 mg/kg once daily. Warfarin should be started within 72 hr; enoxaparin may be continued for a minimum of 5 days and until therapeutic anticoagulation with warfarin is achieved (INR >2 for two consecutive days); *Unstable angina/non–ST-segment-elevation MI:* 1 mg/kg every 12 hr for 2–8 days (with aspirin).

IV, SUBQ (Adults <75 yr): *Acute ST-segment-elevation MI:* Administer single IV bolus of 30 mg plus 1 mg/kg SUBQ dose (maximum of 100 mg for first 2 doses only), followed by 1 mg/kg SUBQ every 12 hr. The usual duration of treatment is 2–8 days. In patients undergoing percutaneous coronary intervention, if last SUBQ dose was <8 hr before balloon inflation, no additional dosing needed; if last SUBQ dose was ≥8 hr before balloon inflation, administer single IV bolus of 0.3 mg/kg.

SUBQ (Adults ≥75 yr): *Acute ST-segment-elevation MI:* 0.75 mg/kg every 12 hr (no IV bolus needed) (maximum of 75 mg for first 2 doses only; no initial bolus). The usual duration of treatment is 2–8 days.

Renal Impairment

SUBQ (Adults CCr <30 mL/min): *VTE prophylaxis for abdominal or knee/hip replacement surgery:* 30 mg once daily. *Treatment of DVT/PE:* 1 mg/kg once daily. *Unstable angina/non–ST-segment-elevation MI:* 1 mg/kg once daily. *Acute ST-segment-elevation MI (patients <75 yr):* Single IV bolus of 30 mg plus 1 mg/kg SUBQ dose, followed by 1 mg/kg SUBQ once daily. *Acute ST-segment-elevation MI (patients ≥75 yr):* 1 mg/kg once daily (no initial bolus).

Availability

Dalteparin

Solution for injection (prefilled syringes): 2500 units/0.2 mL, ✸ 3500 units/0.28 mL, 5000 units/0.2 mL, 7500 units/0.3 mL, ✸ 10,000 units/0.4 mL, 10,000 units/1 mL, 12,500 units/0.5 mL, 15,000 units/0.6 mL, ✸ 16,500 units/0.66 mL, 18,000 units/0.72 mL. **Solution for injection (multidose vials):** 25,00 units/mL, ✸ 10,000 units/mL, 25,000 units/mL.

Enoxaparin (generic available)

Solution for injection (prefilled syringes): 30 mg/0.3 mL, 40 mg/0.4 mL, 60 mg/0.6 mL, 80 mg/0.8 mL, 100 mg/1 mL, 120 mg/0.8 mL, 150 mg/mL. **Solution for injection (multidose vials):** 100 mg/mL.

NURSING IMPLICATIONS

Assessment

- Assess for signs of bleeding and hemorrhage (bleeding gums; nosebleed; unusual bruising; black, tarry stools; hematuria; fall in hematocrit or BP; guaiac-positive stools); bleeding from surgical site. Notify health care professional if these occur.
- Assess patient for evidence of additional or increased thrombosis. Symptoms depend on area of involvement.
- Assess for evidence of additional or increased thrombosis. Symptoms depend on area of involvement. Monitor neurological status frequently for signs of neurological impairment. May require urgent treatment.
- Monitor for hypersensitivity reactions (chills, fever, urticaria). Report signs to health care professional.
- Monitor patients with epidural catheters frequently for signs and symptoms of neurologic impairment. Delay placement or removal of catheter for at least 12 hr after administration of lower doses (30 mg once or twice daily or 40 mg once daily) and at least 24 hr after administration of higher doses (0.75 mg/kg twice daily, 1 mg/kg twice daily, or 1.5 mg/kg once daily) of enoxaparin. Do not give 2nd enoxaparin dose in twice daily regimen to patients receiving 0.75 mg/kg twice daily dose or 1 mg/kg twice daily dose to allow a longer delay before catheter placement or removal, then delay next dose for at least 4 hr. *For patients with CCr <30 mL/min,* double timing of removal of catheter, at least 24 hr for lower dose (30 mg once daily) and at least 48 hr for higher dose (1 mg/kg/day). Monitor for signs and symptoms of neurological impairment (midline back pain, sensory and motor deficits [numbness or weakness in lower limbs], bowel and/or bladder dysfunction) frequently if epidural or spinal anesthesia or lumbar puncture is done during therapy.
- **SUBQ:** Observe injection sites for hematomas, ecchymosis, or inflammation.

Lab Test Considerations

- Monitor CBC, platelet count, and stools for occult blood periodically during therapy. *If thrombocytopenia occurs (platelet count <100,000/mm³),* discontinue therapy. *If hematocrit ↓ unexpectedly,* assess patient for potential bleeding sites. For *dalteparin* use for extended treatment of symptomatic VTE in cancer patients, if platelets ↓ to 50,000–100,000/mm³, ↓ dose to 2500 units once daily until recovery to ≥100,000/mm³; if platelets <50,000/mm³, discontinue until count returns to ≥50,000/mm³.

- Special monitoring of aPTT is not necessary. Monitoring of anti-Xa levels may be considered in patients who are obese or have renal dysfunction (for *enoxaparin*, obtain 4 hr after injection).
- Monitoring of antifactor Xa levels may be necessary to titrate doses in pediatric patients (therapeutic range 0.5–1 unit/mL).
- May cause ↑ in AST and ALT levels.

Toxicity and Overdose
- For *enoxaparin* overdose, protamine sulfate 1 mg for each mg of *enoxaparin* should be administered by slow IV injection. For *dalteparin* overdose, protamine sulfate 1 mg for each 100 anti-factor Xa IU of *dalteparin* should be administered by slow IV injection. If the aPTT measured 2–4 hr after protamine administration remains prolonged, a 2nd infusion of protamine 0.5 mg/100 anti-factor Xa IU of *dalteparin* may be administered.

Implementation

- **High Alert:** Unintended concomitant use of two heparin products (unfractionated heparin and low molecular weight heparins) has resulted in serious harm and death. Review patients' recent and current medication administration records before administering any heparin or low-molecular-weight heparin product.
- Do not confuse Lovenox with Levemir.
- Cannot be used interchangeably (unit for unit) with unfractionated heparin or other low-molecular-weight heparins.
- Assess for latex allergy in all persons handling prefilled syringe; dalteparin prefilled syringe needle shield may contain latex.
- **SUBQ:** Administer deep into SUBQ tissue. Alternate injection sites daily between the left and right anterolateral and left and right posterolateral abdominal wall, the upper thigh, or buttocks. Inject entire length of needle at a 45° or 90° angle into a skin fold held between thumb and forefinger; hold skin fold throughout injection. Do not aspirate or massage. Rotate sites frequently. Do not administer IM because of danger of hematoma formation. Solution should be clear and colorless to slightly yellow; do not inject solution containing particulate matter.
- If excessive bruising occurs, ice cube massage of site before injection may lessen bruising.
- **Enoxaparin:** To avoid the loss of drug, do not expel the air bubble from the syringe before the injection.
- **SUBQ:** Per manufacturer's recommendations, to enhance absorption, inject enoxaparin into left or right anterolateral or posterolateral abdominal wall only.
- To minimize risk of bleeding after vascular instrumentation for unstable angina, recommended intervals between doses should be followed closely. Leave vascular access sheath in place for 6–8 hr after enoxaparin dose. Give next enoxaparin dose ≥6–8

hr after sheath removal. Observe site for bleeding or hematoma formation.

IV Administration
- **IV Push:** (for treatment of STEMI only) Inject via IV line. Flush with 0.9% NaCl or D5W prior to and following administration to avoid mixture with other drugs and clear the port of the drug. May be administered with 0.9% NaCl or D5W. *Rate:* Inject as a bolus.
- **Y-Site Incompatibility:** Do not mix or co-administer with other medications.

Patient/Family Teaching

- Instruct patient in correct technique for self injection, care and disposal of equipment.
- Advise patient to report any symptoms of unusual bleeding or bruising, dizziness, itching, rash, fever, swelling, or difficulty breathing to health care professional immediately.
- Instruct patient not to take aspirin or NSAIDs without consulting health care professional while on therapy.
- Rep: Advise females of reproductive potential to notify health care professional if pregnancy is planned or suspected, or if breastfeeding. Use caution when administering dalteparin preserved with benzyl alcohol to pregnant women, benzyl alcohol may cross the placenta. Large amounts of benzyl alcohol (99–404 mg/kg/day) increase risk of "gasping syndrome" (central nervous system depression, metabolic acidosis, gasping respirations) in premature infants. If anticoagulation with dalteparin is needed during pregnancy, use preservative-free formulations where possible.

Evaluation/Desired Outcomes

- Prevention of DVT and PE (enoxaparin and dalteparin).
- Resolution of DVT and PE (enoxaparin only).
- Prevention of ischemic complications (with aspirin) in patients with unstable angina or non–ST-segment-elevation MI (enoxaparin and dalteparin).
- Treatment of acute ST-segment-elevation MI (enoxaparin only).

HISTAMINE H₂ ANTAGONISTS
cimetidine (sye-**me**-ti-deen)
~~Tagamet~~
famotidine (fa-**moe**-ti-deen)
Pepcid, Pepcid AC Maximum Strength
nizatidine (ni-**za**-ti-deen)
~~Axid~~
Classification
Therapeutic: antiulcer agents
Pharmacologic: histamine H₂ antagonists

Indications

Short-term treatment of active duodenal ulcers and benign gastric ulcers. Maintenance therapy for duodenal and gastric ulcers after healing of active ulcers. Management of gastroesophageal reflux disorder (GERD). Treatment of heartburn, acid indigestion, and sour stomach (OTC use). **Cimetidine, famotidine:** Management of gastric hypersecretory states (Zollinger-Ellison syndrome). **Famotidine IV:** Prevention and treatment of stress-induced upper GI bleeding in critically ill patients. **Unlabeled Use:** Management of GI symptoms associated with the use of NSAIDs. Prevention of acid inactivation of supplemental pancreatic enzymes in patients with pancreatic insufficiency. Management of urticaria.

Action

Inhibits the action of histamine at the H$_2$-receptor site located primarily in gastric parietal cells, resulting in inhibition of gastric acid secretion. **Therapeutic Effects:** Healing and prevention of ulcers. Decreased symptoms of gastroesophageal reflux. Decreased secretion of gastric acid.

Pharmacokinetics

Absorption: *Cimetidine:* well absorbed after oral administration. *Famotidine:* 40–45% absorbed after oral administration. *Nizatidine:* 70–95% absorbed after oral administration.

Distribution: All agents enter breast milk and cerebrospinal fluid.

Metabolism and Excretion: *Cimetidine:* 30% metabolized by the liver; remainder is eliminated unchanged by the kidneys. *Famotidine:* up to 70% excreted unchanged by the kidneys, 30–35% metabolized by the liver. *Nizatidine:* 60% excreted unchanged by the kidneys; some hepatic metabolism; at least 1 metabolite has histamine-blocking activity.

Half-life: *Cimetidine:* 2 hr; *famotidine:* 2.5–3.5 hr; *nizatidine:* 1.6 hr (all are ↑ in renal impairment).

TIME/ACTION PROFILE

ROUTE	ONSET	PEAK	DURATION
Cimetidine PO	30 min	45–90 min	4–5 hr
Famotidine PO	within 60 min	1–4 hr	6–12 hr
Famotidine IV	within 60 min	0.5–3 hr	8–15 hr
Nizatidine PO	unknown	unknown	8–12 hr

Contraindications/Precautions

Contraindicated in: Hypersensitivity; Some products contain alcohol and should be avoided in patients with known intolerance; Some products contain aspartame and should be avoided in patients with phenylketonuria.

Use Cautiously in: Renal impairment (more susceptible to adverse CNS reactions; ↑ dose interval recommended for *cimetidine* and *nizatidine* if CCr ≤50 mL/min, and for *famotidine* if CCr <50 mL/min; OB, Lactation: Pregnancy or lactation; Geri: Older adults are

more susceptible to adverse CNS reactions; dose ↓ recommended.

Adverse Reactions/Side Effects

CV: ARRHYTHMIAS. **Endo:** gynecomastia. **GI:** constipation, diarrhea, drug-induced hepatitis (nizatidine, cimetidine), nausea. **GU:** ↓ sperm count, erectile dysfunction (cimetidine). **Hemat:** AGRANULOCYTOSIS, anemia, APLASTIC ANEMIA, neutropenia, thrombocytopenia. **Local:** pain at IM site. **Neuro:** confusion, dizziness, drowsiness, hallucinations, headache. **Misc:** hypersensitivity reactions, vasculitis.

Interactions

Drug-Drug: Cimetidine may ↑ levels and risk of toxicity of **benzodiazepines** (especially **chlordiazepoxide, diazepam,** and **midazolam**), some **beta blockers** (**labetalol, metoprolol, propranolol**), **caffeine, calcium channel blockers, carbamazepine, cyclosporine, dofetilide, lidocaine, metronidazole, mexiletine, nefazodone, pentoxifylline, phenytoin, procainamide, propafenone, quinidine, metformin, risperidone, ritonavir, ropinirole, SSRIs, sildenafil, sulfonylureas, tacrolimus, theophylline, tricyclic antidepressants, venlafaxine,** and **warfarin.** Cimetidine may ↑ myelosuppressive effects of **carmustine;** avoid concurrent use. Cimetidine, famotidine, and nizatidine may ↓ absorption of **ketoconazole, itraconazole, atazanavir,** and **gefitinib.**

Route/Dosage

Cimetidine

PO (Adults): *Short-term treatment of active ulcers:* 300 mg 4 times daily *or* 800 mg at bedtime *or* 400–600 mg twice daily (not to exceed 2.4 g/day) for up to 8 wk. *Duodenal ulcer prophylaxis:* 300 mg twice daily *or* 400 mg at bedtime. *GERD:* 400 mg every 6 hr *or* 800 mg twice daily for 12 wk. *Gastric hypersecretory conditions:* 300–600 mg every 6 hr (up to 2400 mg/day). *OTC use:* up to 200 mg may be taken twice daily (for not more than 2 wk).

PO (Children): *Short-term treatment of active ulcers:* 5–10 mg/kg every 6 hr.

Renal Impairment

PO (Adults): *CCr 10–50 mL/min:* Administer 50% of normal dose; *CCr <10 mL/min:* Administer 25% of normal dose.

Renal Impairment

PO (Children): 10–15 mg/kg/day.

Famotidine

PO (Adults): *Short-term treatment of active duodenal ulcers:* 40 mg/day at bedtime or 20 mg twice daily for up to 8 wk. *Treatment of benign gastric ulcers:* 40 mg/day at bedtime. *Maintenance treatment of duodenal ulcers:* 20 mg once daily at bedtime. *GERD:* 20 mg twice daily for up to 6 wk; up to 40 mg twice daily for up to 12 wk for esophagitis with erosions, ulcerations, and continuing symptoms. *Gastric hypersecretory* *conditions:* 20 mg every 6 hr initially, up to 160 mg every 6 hr. *OTC use:* 10 mg for relief of symptoms; for prevention— 10 mg 60 min before eating or take 10 mg as chewable tablet 15 min before heartburn-inducing foods or beverages (not to exceed 20 mg/24 hr for up to 2 wk).

PO, IV (Children 1–16 yr): *Peptic ulcer:* 0.5 mg/kg/ day as a single bedtime dose or in 2 divided doses (up to 40 mg daily); *GERD:* 1 mg/kg/day in 2 divided doses (up to 80 mg twice daily).

PO (Infants >3 mo–1 yr): *GERD:* 0.5 mg/kg/dose twice daily.

PO (Infants and neonates <3 mo): *GERD:* 0.5 mg/ kg/dose once daily.

IV (Adults): 20 mg every 12 hr.

Renal Impairment

PO (Adults): *CCr <50 mL/min:* administer normal dose every 36–48 hr *or* 50% of normal dose at normal dosing interval. *CCr <10 mL/min:* dosing interval may need to be ↑ to every 36–48 hr.

Nizatidine

PO (Adults): *Short-term treatment of active duodenal or benign gastric ulcers:* 300 mg once daily at bedtime. *Maintenance treatment of duodenal ulcers:* 150 mg once daily at bedtime. *GERD:* 150 mg twice daily.

Renal Impairment

PO (Adults): *Short-term treatment of active ulcers: CCr 20–50 mL/min:* 150 mg once daily; *CCr <20 mL/ min:* 150 mg every other day. *Maintenance treatment of duodenal ulcers: CCr 20–50 mL/min:* 150 mg every other day; *CCr <20 mL/min:* 150 mg every 3 days.

Availability

Cimetidine (generic available)

Tablets: 200 mg^(Rx, OTC), 300 mg, 400 mg, 800 mg.

Famotidine (generic available)

Tablets: 10 mg^(OTC), 20 mg^(Rx, OTC), 40 mg. **Oral suspension** (cherry-banana-mint flavor)**:** 40 mg/5 mL. **Premixed infusion:** 20 mg/50 mL 0.9% NaCl. **Solution for injection:** 10 mg/mL. *In combination with:* calcium carbonate and magnesium hydroxide^(OTC) (Pepcid Complete, see Appendix N).

Nizatidine (generic available)

Capsules: 150 mg, 300 mg. **Oral solution (bubble gum flavor):** 15 mg/mL.

NURSING IMPLICATIONS

Assessment

- Assess for epigastric or abdominal pain and frank or occult blood in the stool, emesis, or gastric aspirate.
- Geri: Assess geriatric and debilitated patients routinely for confusion. Report promptly.

Lab Test Considerations

- Monitor CBC with differential periodically during therapy.
- Antagonize effects of pentagastrin and histamine during gastric acid secretion testing. Avoid administration for 24 hr before the test.
- May cause false-negative results in skin tests using allergenic extracts. Histamine H₂ antagonists should be discontinued 24 hr before the test.
- May cause ↑ in serum transaminases and serum creatinine.
- *Nizatidine* may cause ↑ alkaline phosphatase concentrations.
- *Famotidine* may cause false-positive results for urine protein; test with sulfosalicylic acid.

Implementation

- Do not confuse nizatidine with tizanidine.
- **PO:** Administer with meals or immediately afterward and at bedtime to prolong effect.
- If antacids or sucralfate are used concurrently for relief of pain, avoid administration of antacids within 30 min–1 hr of the H₂ antagonist and take sucralfate 2 hr after H₂ antagonist; may ↓ absorption of H₂ antagonist.
- Doses administered once daily should be administered at bedtime to prolong effect.
- Shake oral suspension before administration. Discard unused suspension after 30 days.

Famotidine

IV Administration

- **IV Push:** *Dilution:* 0.9% NaCl, D5W, D10W, or LR. *Concentration:* 4 mg/mL. *Rate:* Administer at a rate of 10 mg/min. Rapid administration may cause hypotension.
- **Intermittent Infusion:** *Dilution:* Dilute each 20 mg in 100 mL of 0.9% NaCl, D5W, D10W, or LR. Diluted solution is stable for 48 hr at room temperature. Do not use solution that is discolored or contains a precipitate. *Concentration:* 0.2 mg/mL. *Rate:* Administer over 15–30 min.
- **Y-Site Compatibility:** acyclovir, alemtuzumab, allopurinol, amifostine, amikacin, aminocaproic acid, aminophylline, amiodarone, amphotericin B lipid complex, amphotericin B liposomal, anidulafungin, argatroban, ascorbic acid, atracurium, atropine, aztreonam, benztropine, bleomycin, bumetanide, buprenorphine, butorphanol, calcium chloride, calcium gluconate, cangrelor, carboplatin, carmustine, caspofungin, cefotaxime, ceftaroline, ceftazidime, ceftolozane/tazobactam, cefuroxime, chlorpromazine, cisatracurium, cisplatin, cladribine, clindamycin, cyclophosphamide, cyclosporine, cytarabine, dacarbazine, dactinomycin, daptomycin, daunorubicin hydrochloride, dexamethasone, dexmedetomidine, dexrazoxane, digoxin, diltiazem, diphenhydramine, dobutamine, docetaxel, dopamine,

H

doxorubicin hydrochloride, doxorubicin liposomal, doxycycline, droperidol, enalaprilat, ephedrine, epinephrine, epirubicin, epoetin alfa, eptifibatide, ertapenem, erythromycin lactobionate, esmolol, etoposide, etoposide phosphate, fentanyl, filgrastim, fluconazole, fludarabine, fluorouracil, folic acid, foscarnet, fosphenytoin, gemcitabine, gentamicin, glycopyrrolate, granisetron, heparin, hetastarch, hydrocortisone, hydromorphone, idarubicin, ifosfamide, imipenem/cilastatin, irinotecan, isavuconazonium, isoproterenol, ketorolac, labetalol, LR, leucovorin calcium, levofloxacin, lidocaine, linezolid, lorazepam, magnesium sulfate, mannitol, melphalan, meperidine, meropenem/vaborbactam, mesna, methadone, methotrexate, metoclopramide, metoprolol, metronidazole, midazolam, milrinone, mitoxantrone, morphine, moxifloxacin, multivitamins, mycophenolate, nafcillin, nalbuphine, naloxone, nicardipine, nitroglycerin, nitroprusside, norepinephrine, octreotide, ondansetron, oritavancin, oxacillin, oxaliplatin, oxytocin, paclitaxel, palonosetron, pamidronate, papaverine, pemetrexed, penicillin G, pentamidine, pentobarbital, phenobarbital, phentolamine, phenylephrine, phytonadione, plazomicin, posaconazole, potassium acetate, potassium chloride, potassium phosphate, procainamide, prochlorperazine, promethazine, propofol, propranolol, protamine, pyridoxine, remifentanil, rituximab, sargramostim, sodium acetate, sodium bicarbonate, succinylcholine, sufentanil, tacrolimus, tedizolid, telavancin, theophylline, thiamine, thiotepa, tigecycline, tirofiban, tobramycin, topotecan, trastuzumab, vancomycin, vasopressin, vecuronium, verapamil, vinblastine, vincristine, vinorelbine, voriconazole, zoledronic acid.

- **Y-Site Incompatibility:** amphotericin B deoxycholate, azathioprine, cefepime, chloramphenicol, dantrolene, diazepam, ganciclovir, gemtuzumab ozogamicin, indomethacin, mitomycin, pantoprazole, piperacillin/tazobactam, trimethoprim/sulfamethoxazole.

Patient/Family Teaching

- Instruct patient to take medication as directed for the full course of therapy, even if feeling better. Take missed doses as soon as remembered but not if almost time for next dose. Do not double doses.
- Advise patients taking OTC preparations not to take the maximum dose continuously for more than 2 wk without consulting health care professional. Notify health care professional if difficulty swallowing occurs or abdominal pain persists.
- Inform patient that smoking interferes with the action of histamine antagonists. Encourage patient to quit smoking or at least not to smoke after last dose of the day.
- May cause drowsiness or dizziness. Caution patient to avoid driving or other activities requiring alertness until response to the drug is known.

- Advise patient to avoid alcohol, products containing aspirin or NSAIDs, and foods that may cause an increase in GI irritation.
- Inform patient that increased fluid and fiber intake and exercise may minimize constipation.
- Advise patient to report onset of black, tarry stools; fever; sore throat; diarrhea; dizziness; rash; confusion; or hallucinations to health care professional promptly.
- Rep: Advise patient to notify health care professional if pregnancy is planned or suspected or if breastfeeding.

Evaluation/Desired Outcomes

- Decrease in abdominal pain.
- Treatment and prevention of gastric or duodenal irritation and bleeding. Healing of duodenal ulcers can be seen by x-rays or endoscopy. Therapy is continued for at least 6 wk in treatment of ulcers but not usually longer than 8 wk.
- Decreased symptoms of esophageal reflux.
- Treatment of heartburn, acid indigestion, and sour stomach (OTC use).

☒ HMG-CoA REDUCTASE INHIBITORS (statins)

atorvastatin (a-**tore**-va-stat-in)
  Atorvaliq, Lipitor
fluvastatin (**floo**-va-sta-tin)
  ~~Lescol~~, Lescol XL
lovastatin (**loe**-va-sta-tin)
  Altoprev, ~~Mevacor~~
pitavastatin (pi-**tava**-va-sta-tin)
  Livalo, Zypitamag
pravastatin (**pra**-va-sta-tin)
  ~~Pravachol~~
rosuvastatin (roe-**soo**-va-sta-tin)
  Crestor, Ezallor Sprinkle
simvastatin (**sim**-va-sta-tin)
  FloLipid, Zocor
Classification
Therapeutic: lipid-lowering agents
Pharmacologic: HMG-CoA reductase inhibitors

Indications

Adjunctive management of primary hypercholesterolemia and mixed dyslipidemias. **Atorvastatin:** Primary prevention of cardiovascular disease (↓ risk of MI or stroke) in patients with multiple risk factors for coronary heart disease (CHD) or type 2 diabetes mellitus (also ↓ risk of angina or revascularization procedures in patients with multiple risk factors for CHD). **Atorvastatin and pravastatin:** Secondary prevention of cardiovascular disease (↓ risk of MI, stroke, revascularization procedures, angina, and hospitalizations for HF) in patients with clinically evident CHD. **Fluvastatin:** Secondary prevention of coronary revascularization procedures in patients with clinically evident CHD. **Fluvastatin and lovastatin:** Slow progression of coronary atherosclerosis in patients with CHD. **Lovastatin:** Primary prevention of CHD (↓ risk of MI, unstable angina, and coronary revascularization) in patients without symptomatic cardiovascular disease with ↑ total and low-density lipoprotein cholesterol (LDL-C) and ↓ high-density lipoprotein cholesterol (HDL-C). **Pravastatin:** Primary prevention of CHD (↓ risk of MI, coronary revascularization, and cardiovascular mortality) in patients without clinically evident CHD. **Simvastatin:** Secondary prevention of cardiovascular events (↓ risk of MI, coronary revascularization, stroke, and cardiovascular mortality) in patients with clinically evident CHD or those at high-risk for CHD (history of diabetes, peripheral arterial disease, or stroke). **Rosuvastatin:** Slow progression of coronary atherosclerosis. **Rosuvastatin:** Primary prevention of cardiovascular disease (reduces risk of stroke, myocardial infarction, and revascularization) in patients without clinically evident coronary heart disease but with an increased risk of cardiovascular disease because of age (≥50 yr for men; ≥60 yr for women), high-sensitivity C-reactive protein ≥2 mg/L, and the presence of ≥1 risk factor for cardiovascular disease (hypertension, low HDL-C, smoking, or premature family history of coronary heart disease). **Rosuvastatin:** Adjunctive therapy to diet and exercise for the reduction of LDL-C in children 8–17 yr with heterozygous familial hypercholesterolemia if after diet therapy fails the following still exist: LDL-C remains >190 mg/dL or remains >160 mg/dL (with family history of premature cardiovascular disease or ≥2 risk factors for cardiovascular disease).

Action
Inhibit an enzyme, 3-hydroxy-3-methylglutaryl-coenzyme A (HMG-CoA) reductase, which is responsible for catalyzing an early step in the synthesis of cholesterol. **Therapeutic Effects:** Lower total and LDL-C and triglycerides. Slightly increase HDL-C. Slow the progression of coronary atherosclerosis with resultant decrease in CHD-related events (all agents except rosuvastatin have indication for ↓ events).

Pharmacokinetics
Absorption: *Atorvastatin:* rapidly absorbed but undergoes extensive GI and hepatic metabolism, resulting in 14% bioavailability; *fluvastatin:* 98% absorbed after oral administration, but undergoes extensive first-pass metabolism resulting in 24% bioavailability; *lovastatin, pravastatin:* poorly and variably absorbed after oral administration; *pitavastatin:* well absorbed (51%) after oral administration; *rosuvastatin:* 20% absorbed following oral administration; *simvastatin:* 85% absorbed but rapidly metabolized.

Distribution: *Atorvastatin:* probably enters breast milk. *Fluvastatin:* enters breast milk. *Lovastatin:* crosses the blood-brain barrier and placenta. *Prava-*

statin: small amounts enter breast milk. *Pitavastatin, rosuvastatin, and simvastatin:* unknown.

Protein Binding: *Atorvastatin, fluvastatin, pitavastatin, and simvastatin:* >98%.

Metabolism and Excretion: All agents are extensively metabolized by the liver; amount excreted unchanged in urine: *atorvastatin:* <2%, *lovastatin:* 10%, *fluvastatin:* 5%, *pitavastatin:* 15%, *pravastatin:* 20%, and *simvastatin:* 13%.

Half-life: *Atorvastatin:* 14 hr; *fluvastatin:* 1.2 hr; *lovastatin:* 3 hr; *pitavastatin:* 12 hr; *pravastatin:* 1.3–2.7 hr; *rosuvastatin:* 19 hr; *simvastatin:* unknown.

TIME/ACTION PROFILE (cholesterol-lowering effect)

ROUTE	ONSET	PEAK	DURATION*
Atorvastatin	unknown	unknown	20–30 hr
Fluvastatin	1–2 wk	4–6 wk	unknown
Lovastatin	2 wk	4–6 wk	6 wk
Pitavastatin	within 4 wk	4 wk	unknown
Pravastatin	several days	2–4 wk	unknown
Rosuvastatin	unknown	2–4 wk	unknown
Simvastatin	several days	2–4 wk	unknown

*After discontinuation.

Contraindications/Precautions
Contraindicated in: Hypersensitivity; Active liver failure or decompensated cirrhosis; *Simvastatin and lovastatin:* Concurrent use of strong CYP3A4 inhibitors (↑ risk of myopathy/rhabdomyolysis); *Pitavastatin:* Concurrent use of cyclosporine; *Pitavastatin:* severe renal impairment (CCr <30 mL/min); *Simvastatin:* Concurrent use of cyclosporine, gemfibrozil, or danazol (↑ risk of myopathy/rhabdomyolysis); ⚄ *Simvastatin:* Chinese patients receiving ≥1 g/day of niacin (↑ risk of myopathy); Lactation: Lactation.

Use Cautiously in: History of liver disease; Alcoholism; ⚄ *Rosuvastatin:* Patients with Asian ancestry (may have ↑ blood levels and ↑ risk of rhabdomyolysis); *Atorvastatin:* Concurrent use of azole antifungals, clarithromycin, colchicine, cyclosporine, erythromycin, gemfibrozil, glecaprevir/pibrentasvir, ledipasvir/sofosbuvir, letermovir, niacin (>1 g/day), or tipranavir/ritonavir (↑ risk of myopathy); *Lovastatin:* Concurrent use of gemfibrozil, niacin, cyclosporine, amiodarone, danazol, diltiazem, verapamil, colchicine, or ranolazine (higher risk of myopathy/rhabdomyolysis); *Pitavastatin:* Hypothyroidism, concurrent use of fibrates or lipid-lowering doses of niacin (higher risk of myopathy/rhabdomyolysis); *Rosuvastatin:* Concurrent use of gemfibrozil, azole antifungals, protease inhibitors, niacin, cyclosporine, amiodarone, or verapamil (higher risk of myopathy/rhabdomyolysis); *Simvastatin:* Concurrent use of amiodarone, amlodipine, daptomycin, diltiazem, dronedarone, verapamil, lomitapide, or ranolazine (↑ risk of myopathy/rhabdomyolysis); Renal impairment; OB: Use statin therapy during pregnancy

H

only if potential maternal benefit justifies potential fetal risk (if needed, consider using a more water-soluble agent [pravastatin or rosuvastatin] that is less likely to cross the placenta); Rep: Women of reproductive potential; Pedi: Safety and effectiveness not established in children <18 yr (fluvastatin, pitavastatin), <10 yr (atorvastatin, lovastatin, simvastatin), or <8 yr (pravastatin, rosuvastatin); Geri: *Atorvastatin and pitavastatin:* ↑ risk of myopathy in older adults.

Adverse Reactions/Side Effects

CV: chest pain, peripheral edema. **Derm:** rash, pruritus. **EENT:** rhinitis; *lovastatin:* blurred vision. **Endo:** hyperglycemia. **GI:** abdominal cramps, constipation, diarrhea, flatus, heartburn, altered taste, drug-induced hepatitis, dyspepsia, ↑ liver enzymes, nausea, pancreatitis. **GU:** erectile dysfunction. **MS:** arthralgia, arthritis, immune-mediated necrotizing myopathy (IMNM), myalgia, myopathy (↑ with simvastatin 80 mg/day dose), RHABDOMYOLYSIS. **Neuro:** amnesia, confusion, dizziness, headache, insomnia, memory loss, weakness. **Resp:** bronchitis. **Misc:** HYPERSENSITIVITY REACTIONS (including angioedema and urticaria).

Interactions

Atorvastatin, lovastatin, simvastatin, and rosuvastatin are metabolized by the CYP3A4 metabolic pathway. Fluvastatin is metabolized by CYP2C9. Pravastatin is not metabolized by the CYP P450 system.

Drug-Drug: Risk of myopathy with lovastatin is ↑ by concurrent use of **strong CYP3A4 inhibitors**, including **ketoconazole, itraconazole, posaconazole, voriconazole protease inhibitors, clarithromycin, erythromycin, nefazodone**, and **cobicistat-containing products**; concurrent use contraindicated. Risk of myopathy with simvastatin is ↑ by concurrent use of **cyclosporine, gemfibrozil, danazol, erythromycin, clarithromycin, protease inhibitors, nefazodone, ketoconazole, itraconazole, voriconazole, posaconazole,** and **cobicistat-containing products;** concurrent use contraindicated. Risk of myopathy with pitavastatin is ↑ by concurrent use of **cyclosporine;** concurrent use contraindicated. Bioavailability and effectiveness may be ↓ by **cholestyramine** and **colestipol.** Risk of myopathy with atorvastatin is ↑ by concurrent use of **clarithromycin, colchicine, cyclosporine, darunavir/ritonavir, elbasvir/grazoprevir, erythromycin, fosamprenavir, fosamprenavir/ritonavir gemfibrozil, glecaprevir/pibrentasvir, itraconazole, ledipasvir/sofosbuvir, letermovir, lopinavir/ritonavir, nelfinavir, niacin** (>1 g/day), or **tipranavir/ritonavir;** concurrent use with **cyclosporine, gemfibrozil, glecaprevir/pibrentasvir,** or **tipranavir/ritonavir** should be avoided; use lowest dose with **lopinavir/ritonavir;** use ↓ doses with clarithromycin, darunavir/ritonavir, elbasvir/grazoprevir, fosamprenavir, fosamprenavir/ritonavir, itraconazole, letermovir, or nelfinavir. Risk of myopathy with fluvastatin is ↑ by concurrent use of **gemfibrozil, erythromycin, col-**chicine, cyclosporine, azole antifungal agents,** or large doses of **niacin** may ↑ risk of myopathy; concurrent use with gemfibrozil should be avoided; use ↓ doses with cyclosporine and fluconazole. Risk of myopathy with lovastatin is ↑ by concurrent use of **amiodarone cyclosporine, gemfibrozil, diltiazem, verapamil, danazol,** and large doses of **niacin;** concurrent use with gemfibrozil or cyclosporine should be avoided; use ↓ doses with danazol, amiodarone, diltiazem, or verapamil. Risk of myopathy with pitavastatin is ↑ by concurrent use of **erythromycin, rifampin, colchicine, fibrates,** or large doses of **niacin;** use ↓ doses with erythromycin, rifampin, and niacin; concurrent use with gemfibrozil should be avoided. Risk of myopathy with pravastatin is ↑ by concurrent use of **cyclosporine, fibrates, colchicine, erythromycin, clarithromycin, azithromycin,** or large doses of **niacin;** concurrent use with gemfibrozil should be avoided; consider lower dose with niacin. Risk of myopathy with rosuvastatin is ↑ by concurrent use of **atazanavir/ritonavir, colchicine, cyclosporine, darolutamide, dasabuvir/ombitasvir/paritaprevir/ritonavir, elbasvir/grazoprevir, enasidenib, fibrates, glecaprevir/pibrentasvir, ledipasvir/sofosbuvir, lopinavir/ritonavir, niacin** (large doses), **regorafenib, sofosbuvir/velpatasvir, sofosbuvir/velpatasvir/voxilaprevir,** and **teriflunomide;** avoid concurrent use with gemfibrozil, ledipasvir/sofosbuvir, and sofosbuvir/velpatasvir/voxilaprevir; use ↓ doses with atazanavir/ritonavir, cyclosporine, darolutamide, dasabuvir/ombitasvir/paritaprevir/ritonavir, elbasvir/grazoprevir, enasidenib, glecaprevir/pibrentasvir, lopinavir/ritonavir, regorafenib, sofosbuvir/velpatasvir, and teriflunomide. Risk of myopathy with simvastatin is ↑ by concurrent use of **amiodarone, amlodipine, daptomycin, diltiazem, dronedarone, verapamil, ranolazine, lomitapide,** or **niacin;** avoid concurrent use with niacin at doses of ≥1 g/day in Chinese patients; temporarily suspend simvastatin therapy during treatment with daptomycin; use ↓ doses with amiodarone, amlodipine, diltiazem, dronedarone, lomitapide, ranolazine, or verapamil. Atorvastatin, fluvastatin, and simvastatin may slightly ↑ serum **digoxin** levels. Atorvastatin and rosuvastatin may ↑ levels of **hormonal contraceptives.** Atorvastatin, fluvastatin, lovastatin, rosuvastatin, and simvastatin may ↑ risk of bleeding with **warfarin. Alcohol, cimetidine,** and **omeprazole** may ↑ fluvastatin levels. **Rifampin** may ↓ fluvastatin levels. **Antacids** ↓ absorption of rosuvastatin (administer 2 hr after rosuvastatin. **Lopinavir/ritonavir** may ↑ rosuvastatin levels. Fluvastatin ↑ levels of **glyburide.**

Drug-Natural Products: St. John's wort may ↓ levels and effectiveness (lovastatin and simvastatin).

Drug-Food: Large quantities of **grapefruit juice** may ↑ levels and risk of rhabdomyolysis (atorvastatin, lovastatin, and simvastatin); concurrent use contraindicated. **Food** ↑ levels of lovastatin.

Route/Dosage

Atorvastatin

⚇ **PO (Adults):** 10–20 mg once daily initially; (may start with 40 mg/day if LDL-C needs to be ↓ by >45%); may ↑ every 2–4 wk up to 80 mg/day; *Concurrent use of nelfinavir:* Dose should not exceed 40 mg/day; *Concurrent use of clarithromycin, itraconazole, letermovir, darunavir/ritonavir, fosamprenavir, fosamprenavir/ritonavir, or elbasvir/grazoprevir:* Dose should not exceed 20 mg/day.

PO (Children ≥10 yr): 10 mg/day initially, may ↑ every 4 wk up to 20 mg/day; *Concurrent use of nelfinavir:* Dose should not exceed 40 mg/day; *Concurrent use of clarithromycin, itraconazole, darunavir/ritonavir, fosamprenavir, fosamprenavir/ritonavir therapy, or elbasvir/grazoprevir:* Dose should not exceed 20 mg/day.

Fluvastatin

PO (Adults): 20–40 mg (immediate-release) once daily at bedtime. May ↑ to 40 mg twice daily (immediate-release) or 80 mg once daily (extended-release); *Concurrent use of fluconazole or cyclosporine:* Dose should not exceed 20 mg twice daily.

Lovastatin

PO (Adults): 20 mg once daily with evening meal. May ↑ at 4-wk intervals to a maximum of 80 mg/day (immediate-release) or 60 mg/day (extended-release); *Concurrent use of danazol, verapamil, or diltiazem:* Initiate at 10 mg once daily; do not exceed 20 mg/day; *Concurrent use of amiodarone:* Dose should not exceed 40 mg/day.

Renal Impairment

PO (Adults): *CCr <30 mL/min:* Dose should not exceed 20 mg/day unless carefully titrated.

PO (Children ≥10 yr): *Familial heterozygous hypercholesterolemia:* 10–40 mg/day adjusted at 4-wk intervals.

Pitavastatin

PO (Adults): 2 mg once daily initially, may ↑ up to 4 mg once daily depending on response. *Concurrent erythromycin therapy:* Dose should not exceed 1 mg/day; *Concurrent use of rifampin:* Dose should not exceed 2 mg/day.

Renal Impairment

PO (Adults): *CCr 30–<60 mL/min:* 1 mg once daily initially, may ↑ up to 2 mg daily.

Pravastatin

PO (Adults): 40 mg once daily at bedtime, may be ↑ after 4 wk, if needed to 80 mg once daily at bedtime); *Concurrent use of cyclosporine:* Initiate therapy with 10 mg once daily at bedtime; may be ↑ after 4 wk, if needed, to 20 mg once daily at bedtime

(max dose = 20 mg/day); *Concurrent use of clarithromycin:* Dose should not exceed 40 mg/day.

PO (Children 14–18 yr): 40 mg once daily (max dose = 40 mg/day).

PO (Children 8–13 yr): 20 mg once daily (max dose = 20 mg/day).

Renal Impairment

PO (Adults): *CCr <30 mL/min:* Initiate therapy with 10 mg once daily at bedtime; may titrate at 4-wk intervals as needed (max dose = 80 mg/day).

Rosuvastatin

PO (Adults): 10 mg once daily initially (range 5–20 mg initially) (20 mg initial dose may be considered for patients with LDL-C >190 mg/dL or homozygous familial hypercholesterolemia); dose may be adjusted at 2–4 wk intervals, some patients may require up to 40 mg/day, however this dose is associated with ↑ risk of rhabdomyolysis; *Patients with Asian ancestry:* initial dose should be 5 mg; *Concurrent use of cyclosporine or darolutamide:* Dose should not exceed 5 mg/day; *Concurrent use of atazanavir/ritonavir, dasabuvir/ombitasvir/paritaprevir/ritonavir, elbasvir/grazoprevir, enasidenib, glecaprevir/pibrentasvir, lopinavir/ritonavir, regorafenib, sofosbuvir/velpatasvir, or teriflunomide:* Dose should not exceed 10 mg/day; *Concurrent use of gemfibrozil:* Dose should not exceed 10 mg/day (avoid if possible).

PO (Children 10–17 yr): *Heterozygous familial hypercholesterolemia:* 5–20 mg once daily; *Patients with Asian ancestry:* initial dose should be 5 mg;*Concurrent use of cyclosporine:* Dose should not exceed 5 mg/day; *Concurrent use of atazanavir/ritonavir, glecaprevir/pibrentasvir, lopinavir/ritonavir, or sofosbuvir/velpatasvir:* Dose should not exceed 10 mg/day.

PO (Children 8–<10 yr): *Heterozygous familial hypercholesterolemia:* 5–10 mg once daily; *Patients with Asian ancestry:* initial dose should be 5 mg; *Concurrent use of cyclosporine:* Dose should not exceed 5 mg/day; *Concurrent use of atazanavir/ritonavir, lopinavir/ritonavir, or sofosbuvir/velpatasvir:* Dose should not exceed 10 mg/day.

PO (Children 7–17 yr): *Homozygous familial hypercholesterolemia:* 20 mg once daily. *Patients with Asian ancestry:* initial dose should be 5 mg; *Concurrent use of cyclosporine:* Dose should not exceed 5 mg/day; *Concurrent use of atazanavir/ritonavir, lopinavir/ritonavir, or sofosbuvir/velpatasvir:* Dose should not exceed 10 mg/day.

Renal Impairment

PO (Adults): *CCr <30 mL/min:* 5 mg once daily initially; dose may be ↑ but should not exceed 10 mg/day.

Simvastatin

The 80-mg dose should be restricted to patients who have been taking this dose for ≥12 mo without evidence of muscle toxicity.
PO (Adults): 20–40 mg once daily in the evening; if LDL-C goal cannot be achieved with 40 mg/day dose, add another lipid-lowering therapy (do not ↑ simvastatin dose to 80 mg/day). *Concurrent use of verapamil, diltiazem, or dronedarone:* Dose should not exceed 10 mg/day. *Concurrent use of amiodarone, amlodipine, or ranolazine:* Dose should not exceed 20 mg/day; *Concurrent use of lomitapide:* ↓ dose by 50% (dose should not exceed 20 mg/day or 40 mg/day for patients who previously received 80 mg/day chronically [for ≥12 mo] without evidence of myopathy).
PO (Children 10–17 yr): 10 mg once daily in the evening initially, may ↑ at 4-wk intervals up to 40 mg/day. *Concurrent use of verapamil or diltiazem:* Dose should not exceed 10 mg/day. *Concurrent use of amiodarone, amlodipine, or ranolazine:* Dose should not exceed 20 mg/day.

Renal Impairment

PO (Adults): *CCr 15–29 mL/min:* 5 mg once daily in the evening initially, titrate carefully.

Availability

Atorvastatin (generic available)
Tablets: 10 mg, 20 mg, 40 mg, 80 mg. **Oral suspension (orange flavor):** 20 mg/5 mL. *In combination with:* amlodipine (Caduet). See Appendix N.

Fluvastatin (generic available)
Immediate-release capsules: 20 mg, 40 mg. **Extended-release tablets:** 80 mg.

Lovastatin (generic available)
Immediate-release tablets : 10 mg, 20 mg, 40 mg. **Extended-release tablets (Altoprev):** 20 mg, 40 mg, 60 mg.

Pitavastatin (generic available)
Tablets: 1 mg, 2 mg, 4 mg.

Pravastatin (generic available)
Tablets: 10 mg, 20 mg, 40 mg, 80 mg.

Rosuvastatin
Tablets (Crestor): 5 mg, 10 mg, 20 mg, 40 mg. **Sprinkle capsules (Ezallor):** 5 mg, 10 mg, 20 mg, 40 mg. *In combination with:* ezetimibe (Roszet). See Appendix N.

Simvastatin (generic available)
Tablets (Zocor): 5 mg, 10 mg, 20 mg, 40 mg, 80 mg. **Oral suspension (FloLipid):** 20 mg/5 mL, 40 mg/5 mL. *In combination with:* ezetimibe (Vytorin). See Appendix N.

NURSING IMPLICATIONS

Assessment
- Obtain a dietary history, especially with regard to fat consumption.

Lab Test Considerations
- Evaluate serum cholesterol and triglyceride levels before initiating, after 4–6 wk of therapy, and periodically thereafter.
- Monitor liver function tests, including AST and ALT, before initiating therapy and if signs of liver injury (fatigue, anorexia, right upper abdominal discomfort, dark urine, or jaundice) occur. May also cause ↑ alkaline phosphatase and bilirubin levels.
- If patient develops muscle tenderness during therapy, monitor CK levels. If CK levels are >10 times the upper limit of normal or myopathy occurs, therapy should be discontinued. Monitor for signs and symptoms of IMNM (proximal muscle weakness and ↑ serum CK), persisting despite discontinuation of statin therapy. Perform muscle biopsy to diagnose; shows necrotizing myopathy without significant inflammation. Treat with immunosuppressive agents.

Implementation
- Do not confuse Lipitor with Zyrtec. Do not confuse Zocor with Cozaar or Zyrtec. Do not confuse atorvastatin with atomoxetine. Do not confuse HMG-CoA reductase inhibitors ("statins") with nystatin.
- **PO:** Administer *lovastatin* with food. Administration on an empty stomach decreases absorption by approximately 30%. Initial once-daily dose is administered with the evening meal.
- Administer extended-release tablets at bedtime. **DNC:** Extended-release tablets should be swallowed whole, do not break, crush, chew or open capsules.
- Administer *fluvastatin, pravastatin,* and *simvastatin* once daily in the evening. Do not take two 40 mg fluvastatin tablets at one time. *Atorvastatin, pitavastatin,* and *rosuvastatin* can be taken any time of day. May be administered without regard to food.
- Administer *Ezallor Sprinkle* (rosuvastatin) as a single dose at any time of day, with or without food. **DNC:** Swallow capsules whole; do not crush or chew. For patients who cannot swallow capsules, open capsule for administration. When initiating *Ezallor Sprinkle* therapy or switching from another HMG-CoA reductase inhibitor therapy, begin with *Ezallor Sprinkle* starting dose, and then only titrate according to patient's response. Monitor lipid levels within 2–4 wk of starting *Ezallor Sprinkle* and adjust dose as needed. ☒ Consider starting *Ezallor Sprinkle* with 5 mg once daily in Asian patients; may cause increased rosuvastatin plasma concentrations.
- Avoid large amounts of grapefruit juice during therapy; may ↑ risk of toxicity.
- If *fluvastatin* or *pravastatin* is administered in conjunction with bile acid sequestrants (cholestyramine, colestipol), administer at least 4 hr after bile acid sequestrant.
- If *rosuvastatin* is administered in conjunction with magnesium or aluminum-containing antacids, administer antacid at least 2 hr after *rosuvastatin*.

Patient/Family Teaching

● Instruct patient to take medication as directed and not to skip doses or double up on missed doses. Advise patient to avoid drinking more than 200 mL/day of grapefruit juice during therapy. Medication helps control but does not cure elevated serum cholesterol levels.

● Advise patient that this medication should be used in conjunction with diet restrictions (fat, cholesterol, carbohydrates, alcohol), exercise, and cessation of smoking.

● Instruct patient to notify health care professional promptly if signs of liver injury or if unexplained muscle pain, tenderness, or weakness occurs, especially if accompanied by fever or malaise.

● Advise patient to notify health care professional of all Rx or OTC medications, vitamins, or herbal products being taken and to consult with health care professional before taking other medications, especially St. John's wort.

● Advise patient to notify health care professional of medication regimen before treatment or surgery.

● Rep: May cause fetal harm. Advise females of reproductive potential to use effective contraception during therapy and to discuss plans to discontinue statins if trying to conceive. Advise patient to notify health care professional promptly if pregnancy is planned or suspected. Advise patients to avoid breastfeeding during therapy.

● Emphasize the importance of follow-up exams to determine effectiveness and to monitor for side effects.

Evaluation/Desired Outcomes

● Decrease in LDL-C and total cholesterol levels.
● Increase in HDL-C levels.
● Decrease in triglyceride levels.
● Slowing of the progression of CHD.
● Prevention of cardiovascular disease.

☒ hydrALAZINE (hye-dral-a-zeen)

✲ Apresoline
Classification
Therapeutic: antihypertensives
Pharmacologic: vasodilators

Indications

Moderate to severe hypertension. **Unlabeled Use:** New York Heart Associated Class III or IV HF with reduced ejection fraction (in combination with isosorbide dinitrate).

Action

Direct-acting peripheral arteriolar vasodilator. **Therapeutic Effects:** Lowering of BP in hypertensive patients and decreased afterload in patients with HF.

Pharmacokinetics

Absorption: Rapidly absorbed following oral administration; well absorbed from IM sites. IV administration results in complete bioavailability.

Distribution: Widely distributed.

Metabolism and Excretion: Mostly metabolized by the GI mucosa and liver by N-acetyltransferase ☒ (rate of acetylation is genetically determined [slow acetylators have ↑ hydralazine levels and ↑ risk of toxicity; fast acetylators have ↓ hydralazine levels and ↓ response]).

Half-life: 2–8 hr.

TIME/ACTION PROFILE (antihypertensive effect)

ROUTE	ONSET	PEAK	DURATION
PO	45 min	2 hr	2–4 hr
IM	10–30 min	1 hr	3–8 hr
IV	5–20 min	15–30 min	2–6 hr

Contraindications/Precautions

Contraindicated in: Hypersensitivity; Some products contain tartrazine and should be avoided in patients with known intolerance.

Use Cautiously in: Cardiovascular or cerebrovascular disease; Severe renal impairment (dose modification may be necessary); Severe hepatic impairment (dose modification may be necessary).

Adverse Reactions/Side Effects

CV: <u>tachycardia</u>, angina, arrhythmias, edema, orthostatic hypotension. **Derm:** rash. **GI:** diarrhea, nausea, vomiting. **MS:** arthralgias, arthritis. **Neuro:** dizziness, drowsiness, headache, peripheral neuropathy. **Misc:** <u>drug-induced lupus syndrome</u>.

Interactions

Drug-Drug: ↑ hypotension with acute ingestion of alcohol, other **antihypertensives**, or **nitrates**. **MAO inhibitors** may exaggerate hypotension. May ↓ pressor response to **epinephrine**. **NSAIDs** may ↓ antihypertensive response. **Beta blockers** ↓ tachycardia from hydralazine (therapy may be combined for this reason). **Metoprolol** and **propranolol** ↑ levels. ↑ levels of **metoprolol** and **propranolol**.

Route/Dosage

PO (Adults): *Hypertension:* 10 mg 4 times daily initially. After 2–4 days may ↑ to 25 mg 4 times daily for the rest of the 1st wk; may then ↑ to 50 mg 4 times daily (up to 300 mg/day). Once maintenance dose is established, twice-daily dosing may be used. *HF:* 25–37.5 mg 4 times daily; may be ↑ up to 300 mg/day in 3–4 divided doses.

PO (Children >1 mo): 0.75–1 mg/kg/day in 2–4 divided doses (max = 25 mg/dose) initially; may ↑ gradually to 5 mg/kg/day in infants and 7.5 mg/kg/day in children (max = 200 mg/day) in 2–4 divided doses.

H

IM, IV (Adults): *Hypertension:* 5–40 mg repeated as needed. *Eclampsia:* 5 mg every 15–20 min; if no response after a total of 20 mg, consider an alternative agent.

IM, IV (Children >1 mo): 0.1–0.2 mg/kg/dose every 4–6 hr (max = 20 mg/dose) as needed, up to 1.7–3.5 mg/kg/day in 4–6 divided doses.

Availability (generic available)
Tablets: 10 mg, 25 mg, 50 mg, 100 mg. **Injection:** 20 mg/mL. *In combination with:* isosorbide dinitrate (BiDil). See Appendix N.

NURSING IMPLICATIONS
Assessment
● Monitor BP and pulse frequently during initial dose adjustment and periodically during therapy. ✡ About 50–65% of Caucasians, Black, South Indians, and Mexicans are slow acetylators at risk for toxicity, while 80–90% of Inuit, Japanese, and Chinese are rapid acetylators at risk for decreased levels and treatment failure.
● Monitor frequency of prescription refills to determine adherence.

Lab Test Considerations
● Monitor CBC, electrolytes, LE cell prep, and ANA titer prior to and periodically during prolonged therapy.
● May cause a positive direct Coombs' test result.

Implementation
● Do not confuse hydralazine with hydroxyzine, hydromorphone, or hydrochlorothiazide.
● IM or IV route should be used only when drug cannot be given orally.
● May be administered concurrently with diuretics or beta blockers to permit lower doses and minimize side effects.
● **PO:** Administer with meals consistently to enhance absorption.
● Pharmacist may prepare oral solution from hydralazine injection for patients with difficulty swallowing.

IV Administration
● **IV Push:** *Dilution:* Administer undiluted. Use solution as quickly as possible after drawing through needle into syringe. *Concentration:* 20 mg/mL. *Rate:* Administer over at least 1 min. Pedi: Administer at a rate of 0.2 mg/kg/min in children. Monitor BP and pulse in all patients frequently after injection.
● **Y-Site Compatibility:** alemtuzumab, amiodarone, anidulafungin, argatroban, arsenic trioxide, bivalirudin, bleomycin, carmustine, cyclophosphamide, dacarbazine, dactinomycin, daptomycin, daunorubicin hydrochloride, dexrazoxane, diltiazem, docetaxel, etoposide, etoposide phosphate, fludarabine, gemcitabine, granisetron, hetastarch, hydromorphone, idarubicin, irinotecan, LR, leucovorin calcium, linezolid, mesna, methadone, metronidazole, milrinone, mitomycin, mitoxantrone, moxifloxacin, mycophenolate, octreotide, oxaliplatin, paclitaxel, palonose-

tron, pamidronate, prochlorperazine, 0.9% NaCl, 0.45% NaCl, tacrolimus, thiotepa, tirofiban, topotecan, vecuronium, vinblastine, vincristine, vinorelbine, voriconazole, zoledronic acid.
● **Y-Site Incompatibility:** acyclovir, amphotericin B lipid complex, ampicillin/sulbactam, ascorbic acid, azathioprine, aztreonam, cefazolin, cefotaxime, cefotetan, cefoxitin, ceftazidime, ceftriaxone, cefuroxime, D5W, dantrolene, diazepam, doxorubicin liposomal, ertapenem, folic acid, foscarnet, fosphenytoin, ganciclovir, gemtuzumab ozogamicin, haloperidol, indomethacin, lorazepam, meropenem, methylprednisolone, minocycline, multivitamins, nafcillin, nitroprusside, oxacillin, pantoprazole, pemetrexed, pentobarbital, phenytoin, piperacillin/tazobactam, potassium acetate, sodium acetate, tigecycline, trimethoprim/sulfamethoxazole.

Patient/Family Teaching
● Emphasize the importance of continuing to take this medication, even if feeling well. Instruct patient to take medication at the same time each day; last dose of the day should be taken at bedtime. Take missed doses as soon as remembered; do not double doses. If more than 2 doses in a row are missed, consult health care professional. Must be discontinued gradually to avoid sudden increase in BP. Hydralazine controls but does not cure hypertension.
● Encourage patient to comply with additional interventions for hypertension (weight reduction, low-sodium diet, smoking cessation, moderation of alcohol intake, regular exercise, and stress management). Instruct patient and family on proper technique for BP monitoring. Advise them to check BP at least weekly and report significant changes.
● Patients should weigh themselves twice weekly and assess feet and ankles for fluid retention.
● May occasionally cause drowsiness. Advise patient to avoid driving or other activities requiring alertness until response to medication is known.
● Caution patient to avoid sudden changes in position to minimize orthostatic hypotension.
● Advise patient to notify health care professional of all Rx or OTC medications, vitamins, or herbal products being taken and to consult with health care professional before taking other medications, especially cough, cold, or allergy remedies.
● Instruct patient to notify health care professional of medication prior to treatment or surgery.
● Advise patient to notify health care professional immediately if general tiredness; fever; muscle or joint aching; chest pain; skin rash; sore throat; or numbness, tingling, pain, or weakness of hands and feet occurs. Vitamin B_6 (pyridoxine) may be used to treat peripheral neuritis.
● Rep: Advise females of reproductive potential to notify health care professional if pregnancy is planned or suspected or if breastfeeding.
● Emphasize the importance of follow-up exams to evaluate effectiveness of medication.

Evaluation/Desired Outcomes
- Decrease in BP without appearance of side effects.
- Decreased afterload in patients with HF.

hydralazine/isosorbide dinitrate
(hye-**dral**-a-zeen eye-so-**sor**-bide di-**ni**-trate)
   BiDil
   Classification
Therapeutic: vasodilators
Pharmacologic: vasodilators, nitrates

Indications
HF with reduced ejection fraction in black patients.

Action
BiDil is a fixed-dose combination of **isosorbide dinitrate**, a vasodilator with effects on both arteries and veins, and **hydralazine**, a predominantly arterial vasodilator. **Therapeutic Effects:** Improved survival, increased time to hospitalization and decreased symptoms of HF in black patients.

Pharmacokinetics
Hydralazine
Absorption: 10–26% absorbed in patients with HF following oral administration; absorption can be saturated, leading to large ↑ in absorption with higher doses.
Distribution: Widely distributed to tissues.
Metabolism and Excretion: Mostly metabolized by GI mucosa and liver.
Half-life: 4 hr.
Isosorbide Dinitrate
Absorption: Variable absorption (10–90%) following oral administration, reflecting first-pass hepatic metabolism.
Distribution: Accumulates in muscle and venous wall.
Metabolism and Excretion: Undergoes extensive first-pass metabolism in the liver, mostly metabolized by the liver; some metabolites are vasodilators.
Half-life: 2 hr.

TIME/ACTION PROFILE (effect on BP)

ROUTE	ONSET	PEAK	DURATION
hydralazine (PO)	45 min	2 hr	2–4 hr
isosorbide (PO)	15–40 min	unknown	4 hr

Contraindications/Precautions
Contraindicated in: Hypersensitivity to either component; Concurrent use of PDE-5 inhibitor (avanafil, sildenafil, tadalafil, vardenafil) or riociguat.

Use Cautiously in: Severe renal impairment (dose modification may be necessary); Severe hepatic impairment (dose modification may be necessary); Head trauma or cerebral hemorrhage; OB: Safety not established in pregnancy; Lactation: Use while breastfeeding only if potential maternal benefit justifies potential risk to infant; Pedi: Safety and effectiveness not established in children; Geri: Start with lower doses in older adults.

Adverse Reactions/Side Effects
Hydralazine
CV: tachycardia, angina, arrhythmias, edema, orthostatic hypotension. **Derm:** rash. **GI:** diarrhea, nausea, vomiting. **MS:** arthralgias, arthritis. **Neuro:** dizziness, headache, drowsiness, peripheral neuritis, weakness. **Misc:** <u>drug-induced lupus syndrome</u>.

Isosorbide Dinitrate
CV: <u>hypotension</u>, tachycardia, paradoxical bradycardia, syncope. **GI:** abdominal pain, nausea, vomiting. **Misc:** flushing, tolerance.

Interactions
Drug-Drug: Concurrent use of **avanafil**, **sildenafil**, **tadalafil**, or **vardenafil** may result in severe hypotension; concurrent use contraindicated. Concurrent use of **riociguat** may result in severe hypotension; concurrent use contraindicated. ↑ risk of hypotension with other **antihypertensives**, acute ingestion of **alcohol**, and **phenothiazines**. **MAO inhibitors** may exaggerate hypotension. May ↓ the pressor response to **epinephrine**. **Beta blockers** ↓ tachycardia from hydralazine (therapy may be combined for this reason). **Metoprolol** and **propranolol** may ↑ hydralazine levels and risk of toxicity. Hydralazine may ↑ levels and risk of toxicity of **metoprolol** and **propranolol**.

Route/Dosage
PO (Adults): 1 tablet 3 times daily, may be ↑ to 2 tablets 3 times daily.

Availability
Tablets: hydralazine 37.5 mg/isosorbide dinitrate 20 mg.

NURSING IMPLICATIONS
Assessment
- Monitor BP and pulse routinely during period of dose adjustment. Symptomatic hypotension may occur even with small doses. Use caution with patients who are volume depleted or hypotensive.
- Assess for signs and symptoms of peripheral neuritis (paresthesia, numbness, tingling) periodically during therapy. Adding pyridoxine may cause symptoms to decrease.

Lab Test Considerations
- If symptoms of systemic lupus erythematosus (SLE) occur obtain a CBC and ANA titer. If positive for SLE, carefully weigh risks/benefits of continued therapy.

H

Implementation

- Dose may be titrated rapidly over 3–5 days, but may need to decrease if side effects occur. May decrease to one-half tablet 3 times daily if intolerable side effects occur. Titrate up as soon as side effects subside.

Patient/Family Teaching

- Instruct patient to take medication as directed on a regular schedule.
- Caution patient to make position changes slowly to minimize orthostatic hypotension.
- May cause dizziness. Caution patient to avoid driving or other activities requiring alertness until response to medication is known.
- Advise patient to avoid concurrent use of alcohol or medications for erectile dysfunction with this medication. Patient should also consult health care professional before taking Rx, OTC, or herbal products while taking this medication.
- Caution patient that inadequate fluid intake or excessive fluid loss from perspiration, diarrhea, or vomiting may lead to a fall in BP, dizziness, or syncope. If syncope occurs, discontinue medication and notify health care professional promptly.
- Inform patient that headache is a common side effect that should decrease with continuing therapy. Aspirin or acetaminophen may be ordered to treat headache. Notify health care professional if headache is persistent or severe. Do not alter dose to avoid headache.
- Advise patient to notify health care professional if symptoms of systemic lupus erythematosus occur (arthralgia, fever, chest pain, prolonged malaise, or other unexplained symptoms).
- Rep: Advise females of reproductive potential to notify health care professional if pregnancy is planned or suspected or if breastfeeding.

Evaluation/Desired Outcomes

- Improved survival, increased time to hospitalization, and decreased symptoms of HF in black patients.

---

hydroCHLOROthiazide, See DIURETICS (THIAZIDE).

REMS HIGH ALERT

HYDROcodone
(hye-droe-**koe**-done)
Hysingla ER, ~~Zohydro ER~~

HYDROcodone/Acetaminophen
~~Anexsia, Norco, Vicodin~~

HYDROcodone/Ibuprofen
~~Reprexain~~

Classification
Therapeutic: allergy, cold, and cough remedies (antitussive), opioid analgesics
Pharmacologic: opioid agonists/nonopioid analgesic combinations

Schedule II
For information on the acetaminophen and ibuprofen components of these formulations, see the acetaminophen and ibuprofen monographs

Indications
Extended-release product: Management of pain that is severe enough to warrant daily, around-the-clock, long-term opioid treatment where alternative treatment options are inadequate. **Combination products**: Management of moderate to severe pain. Antitussive (usually in combination products with decongestants).

Action
Bind to opiate receptors in the CNS. Alter the perception of and response to painful stimuli while producing generalized CNS depression. Suppress the cough reflex via a direct central action. **Therapeutic Effects:** Decrease in severity of moderate pain. Suppression of the cough reflex.

Pharmacokinetics
Absorption: Well absorbed following oral administration.
Distribution: Unknown.
Metabolism and Excretion: Mostly metabolized by the liver; eliminated in the urine (50–60% as metabolites, 10% as unchanged drug).
Half-life: 2.2 hr; *Extended-release:* 8 hr.

TIME/ACTION PROFILE (analgesic effect)

ROUTE	ONSET	PEAK	DURATION
PO	10–30 min	30–60 min	4–6 hr
PO-ER	unknown	unknown	unknown

Contraindications/Precautions
Noted for hydrocodone only; see acetaminophen/ibuprofen monographs for specific information on individual components
Contraindicated in: Hypersensitivity to hydrocodone (cross-sensitivity may exist to other opioids); Significant respiratory depression; Paralytic ileus; Acute or severe bronchial asthma or hypercarbia; Congenital long QT syndrome (Hysingla only); Products containing alcohol, aspartame, saccharin, sugar, or tartrazine (FDC yellow dye #5) should be avoided in patients who have hypersensitivity or intolerance to these compounds; Lactation: Lactation.
Use Cautiously in: Head trauma; ↑ intracranial pressure; Severe renal, hepatic, or pulmonary disease; Alcoholism; Difficulty swallowing; Patients with undiagnosed abdominal pain; Prostatic hyperplasia; OB: Avoid chronic use during pregnancy. Has been used

during labor but may cause respiratory depression in the newborn; Geri: Older adults are more prone to CNS depression and constipation (initial dose ↓ required).

Adverse Reactions/Side Effects

Noted for hydrocodone only; see acetaminophen/ibuprofen monographs for specific information on individual components.

CV: hypotension, bradycardia, QT interval prolongation (Hysingla only). **Derm:** sweating. **EENT:** blurred vision, diplopia, miosis. **Endo:** adrenal insufficiency. **GI:** constipation, dyspepsia, nausea, choking, dysphagia, esophageal obstruction, vomiting. **GU:** urinary retention. **Neuro:** confusion, dizziness, sedation, euphoria, hallucinations, headache, unusual dreams. **Resp:** RESPIRATORY DEPRESSION (including central sleep apnea and sleep-related hypoxemia). **Misc:** physical dependence, psychological dependence, tolerance.

Interactions

Drug-Drug: Use with extreme caution in patients receiving **MAO inhibitors**; may produce severe, unpredictable reactions—do not use within 14 days of each other. Concurrent use of **CYP3A4 inhibitors** including **ritonavir, ketoconazole, itraconazole, fluconazole, clarithromycin, erythromycin, nefazodone, diltiazem, verapamil, nelfinavir,** and **fosamprenavir** ↑ levels and risk of opioid toxicity; careful monitoring during initiation, dose changes, or discontinuation of the inhibitor is recommended. Concurrent use with **CYP3A4 inducers** including **barbiturates, carbamazcpine, efavirenz, corticosteroids, modafinil, nevirapine, oxcarbazepine, phenobarbital, phenytoin, rifabutin,** or **rifampin** may ↓ fentanyl levels and analgesia; if inducers are discontinued or dosage ↓, patients should be monitored for signs of opioid toxicity and necessary dose adjustments should be made. Use with **benzodiazepines** or other **CNS depressants** including other **opioids, non-benzodiazepine sedative/hypnotics, anxiolytics, general anesthetics, muscle relaxants, antipsychotics,** and **alcohol** may cause profound sedation, respiratory depression, coma, and death; reserve concurrent use for when alternative treatment options are inadequate. **Mixed agonist/antagonist analgesics,** including **nalbuphine** or **butorphanol** and **partial agonist analgesics,** including **buprenorphine,** may ↓ hydrocodone's analgesic effects and/or precipitate opioid withdrawal in physically dependent patients. **Anticholinergic drugs** may ↑ risk of urinary retention and constipation. Drugs that affect serotonergic neurotransmitter systems, including **tricyclic antidepressants, SSRIs, SNRIs, MAO inhibitors, TCAs, tramadol, trazodone, mirtazapine, 5–HT$_3$ receptor antagonists, linezolid, methylene blue,** and **triptans** ↑ risk of serotonin syndrome.

Drug-Natural Products: Concomitant use of **kava-kava, valerian, skullcap, chamomile,** or **hops** can ↑ CNS depression.

Route/Dosage

PO (Adults): *Analgesic (in combo products):* 2.5–10 mg every 3–6 hr as needed; if using combination products, acetaminophen dose should not exceed 4 g/day and should not exceed 5 tablets/day of ibuprofen-containing products; *Antitussive:* 5 mg every 4–6 hr as needed; *Extended-release capsules:* 10 mg every 12 hr; may ↑ as needed in increments of 10 mg every 12 hr every 3–7 days; *Extended-release tablets:* 20 mg once daily; may ↑ as needed in increments of 10–20 mg/day every 3–5 days.

Renal Impairment

PO (Adults): *CCr <45 mL/min:* Extended-release (Hysingla): ↓ initial dose by 50%.

Hepatic Impairment

PO (Adults): *Extended-release tablets:* ↓ initial dose by 50%.

Availability

Hydrocodone (generic available)

Extended-release capsules: 10 mg, 15 mg, 20 mg, 30 mg, 40 mg, 50 mg. **Extended-release tablets (Hysingla ER) (abuse deterrent):** 20 mg, 30 mg, 40 mg, 60 mg, 80 mg, 100 mg, 120 mg. **Syrup:** ✸ 1 mg/mL. *In combination with:* chlorpheniramine,.

Hydrocodone/Acetaminophen (generic available)

Tablets: 5 mg hydrocodone/325 mg acetaminophen 7.5 mg hydrocodone/325 mg acetaminophen, 10 mg hydrocodone/325 mg acetaminophen. **Elixir/oral solution:** 7.5 mg hydrocodone plus 325 mg acetaminophen/15 mL, 10 mg hydrocodone plus 325 mg acetaminophen/15 mL.

Hydrocodone/Ibuprofen (generic available)

Tablets: 5 mg hydrocodone/200 mg ibuprofen, 7.5 mg hydrocodone/200 mg ibuprofen, 10 mg hydrocodone/200 mg ibuprofen.

NURSING IMPLICATIONS

Assessment

- Assess BP, pulse, and respirations before and periodically during administration. If respiratory rate is <10/min, assess level of sedation. Physical stimulation may be sufficient to prevent significant hypoventilation. Dose may need to be decreased by 25–50%. Initial drowsiness will diminish with continued use. Monitor for respiratory depression, especially during initiation or following dose increase; serious, life-threatening, or fatal respiratory depression may occur. May cause sleep-related breathing disorders (central sleep apnea [CSA], sleep-related hypoxemia).

✸ = Canadian drug name. ⚏ = Genetic implication. ~~Strikethrough~~ = Discontinued. CAPITALS = life-threatening. <u>Underline</u> = most frequent.

- Assess bowel function routinely. Prevention of constipation should be instituted with increased intake of fluids and bulk, and laxatives to minimize constipating effects. Stimulant laxatives should be administered routinely if opioid use exceeds 2–3 days, unless contraindicated. Consider drugs for opioid-induced constipation.

- **Pain:** Assess type, location, and intensity of pain prior to and 1 hr (peak) following administration. When titrating opioid doses, increases of 25–50% should be administered until there is either a 50% reduction in the patient's pain rating on a numerical or visual analogue scale or the patient reports satisfactory pain relief. A repeat dose can be safely administered at the time of the peak if previous dose is ineffective and side effects are minimal.

- Patients taking extended-release hydrocodone may require additional short-acting or rapid-onset opioid doses for breakthrough pain. Doses of short-acting opioids should be equivalent to 10–20% of 24 hr total and given every 2 hr as needed.

- An equianalgesic chart (see Appendix I) should be used when changing routes or when changing from one opioid to another.

- Prolonged use may lead to physical and psychological dependence and tolerance. This should not prevent patient from receiving adequate analgesia. Patients who receive opioids for pain rarely develop psychological dependence. If progressively higher doses are required, consider conversion to a stronger opioid. Prolonged use of opioids should be reserved for patients whose pain remains severe enough to require them and alternative treatment options continue to be inadequate. Many acute pain conditions treated in the outpatient setting require no more than a few days of an opioid pain medicine.

- Assess risk for opioid addiction, abuse, or misuse prior to administration. Abuse or misuse of extended-release preparations by crushing, chewing, snorting, or injecting dissolved product will result in uncontrolled delivery of hydrocodone and can result in overdose and death. Hysingla ER is an abuse deterrent formulation that is difficult to crush and, if crushed, results in a gel.

- **Cough:** Assess cough and lung sounds during antitussive use.

Lab Test Considerations
- May cause ↑ plasma amylase and lipase concentrations.

Toxicity and Overdose
- If an opioid antagonist is required to reverse respiratory depression or coma, naloxone is the antidote. Dilute the 0.4-mg ampule of naloxone in 10 mL of 0.9% NaCl and administer 0.5 mL (0.02 mg) by IV push every 2 min. For children and patients weighing <40 kg, dilute 0.1 mg of naloxone in 10 mL of 0.9% NaCl for a concentration of 10 mcg/mL and administer 0.5 mcg/kg every 2 min. Titrate dose to avoid withdrawal, seizures, and severe pain.

Implementation
- ***High Alert:*** Do not confuse hydrocodone with oxycodone.

- Explain therapeutic value of medication prior to administration to enhance the analgesic effect.

- Regularly administered doses may be more effective than prn administration. Analgesic is more effective if given before pain becomes severe.

- Combination with nonopioid analgesics may have additive analgesic effects and permit lower doses. Maximum doses of nonopioid agents limit the titration of hydrocodone doses.

- Medication should be discontinued gradually after long-term use to prevent withdrawal symptoms. For patients on long-acting agents who are physically opioid-dependent, initiate the taper by a small enough increment (e.g., no greater than 10% to 25% of total daily dose) to avoid withdrawal symptoms, and proceed with dose-lowering at an interval of every 2–4 wk. May be necessary to provide patient with a lower dose strength for a successful taper. Monitor frequently to manage pain and withdrawal symptoms (restlessness, lacrimation, rhinorrhea, yawning, perspiration, chills, myalgia, mydriasis, irritability, anxiety, backache, joint pain, weakness, abdominal cramps, insomnia, nausea, anorexia, vomiting, diarrhea, or increased blood pressure, respiratory rate, or heart rate). If withdrawal symptoms occur, pause the taper for a period of time or raise the dose of opioid analgesic to the previous dose, and then proceed with a slower taper. Also, monitor patients for changes in mood, emergence of suicidal thoughts, or use of other substances. A multimodal approach to pain management may optimize the treatment of chronic pain, as well as assist with the successful tapering of the opioid analgesic.

- ***REMS:*** FDA strongly encourages health care professionals to complete a REMS-compliant education program that includes all the elements of the FDA Education *Blueprint for Health Care Providers Involved in the Management or Support of Patients with Pain,* available at www.fda.gov/ OpioidAnalgesicREMSBlueprint. Information on programs can be found at 1-800-503-0784 or www.opioidanalgesicrems.com.

- Discuss availability of naloxone for emergency treatment of opioid overdose with the patient and caregiver and assess the potential need for access to naloxone, both when initiating and renewing therapy, especially if patient has household members (including children) or other close contacts at risk for accidental exposure or overdose. Consider prescribing naloxone, based on the patient's risk factors for overdose, such as concomitant use of CNS depressants, a history of opioid use disorder, or prior opioid overdose. However, the presence of risk factors for overdose should not prevent the proper management of pain in any patient.

- **PO:** May be administered with food or milk to minimize GI irritation.
- *DNC:* Swallow extended-release capsules whole; do not open, crush, dissolve, or chew.

Patient/Family Teaching

- *REMS:* Advise patient to take medication as directed and not to take more than the recommended amount. Severe and permanent liver damage may result from prolonged use or high doses of acetaminophen. Renal damage may occur with prolonged use of acetaminophen or ibuprofen. Doses of nonopioid agents should not exceed the maximum recommended daily dose. Do not stop taking without discussing with health care professional; may cause withdrawal symptoms if discontinued abruptly after prolonged use. Do not increase doses without discussing with health care professional, may lead to overdose. Discuss safe use, risks, and proper storage and disposal of opioid analgesics with patients and caregivers with each Rx. The Patient Counseling Guide (PCG) is available at www.fda.gov/OpioidAnalgesicREMSPCG.
- Instruct patient on how and when to ask for and take pain medication.
- Advise patient that hydrocodone is a drug with known abuse potential. Protect it from theft, and never give to anyone other than the individual for whom it was prescribed. Store out of sight and reach of children, and in a location not accessible by others.
- Educate patients and caregivers on how to recognize respiratory depression and emphasize the importance of calling 911 or getting emergency medical help right away in the event of a known or suspected overdose. Inform patients and caregivers about various ways to obtain naloxone as permitted by individual state naloxone dispensing and prescribing requirements or guidelines (by prescription, directly from a pharmacist, or as part of a community-based program).
- May cause drowsiness or dizziness. Advise patient to call for assistance when ambulating or smoking. Caution patient to avoid driving or other activities requiring alertness until response to the medication is known.
- Advise patient to notify health care professional if pain control is not adequate or if severe or persistent side effects occur.
- Advise patient to change positions slowly to minimize orthostatic hypotension.
- Caution patient to avoid concurrent use of alcohol or other CNS depressants with this medication, may lead to overdose.
- Instruct patient to notify health care professional of all Rx or OTC medications, vitamins, or herbal products being taken and consult health care professional before taking any new medications.

- Emphasize the importance of aggressive prevention of constipation with the use of hydrocodone.
- Encourage patient to turn, cough, and breathe deeply every 2 hr to prevent atelectasis.
- Advise patient that good oral hygiene, frequent mouth rinses, and sugarless gum or candy may decrease dry mouth.
- Rep: Advise females of reproductive potential to notify health care professional if pregnancy is planned or suspected, or if breastfeeding. Inform patient of potential for neonatal opioid withdrawal syndrome with prolonged use during pregnancy. Monitor neonate for signs and symptoms of withdrawal symptoms (irritability, hyperactivity and abnormal sleep pattern, high-pitched cry, tremor, vomiting, diarrhea, and/or failure to gain weight); usually occur the first days after birth. Monitor infants exposed to hydrocodone through breast milk for excess sedation and respiratory depression. Chronic use may reduce fertility in females and males.

Evaluation/Desired Outcomes

- Decrease in severity of pain without a significant alteration in level of consciousness or respiratory status.
- Suppression of nonproductive cough.

---

hydrocortisone, See CORTICOSTEROIDS (SYSTEMIC).

---

hydrocortisone, See CORTICOSTEROIDS (TOPICAL/LOCAL).

REMS HIGH ALERT

HYDROmorphone
(hye-droe-**mor**-fone)
Dilaudid, ~~Dilaudid-HP~~, ~~Exalgo~~, ✤Hydromorph Contin

Classification
Therapeutic: opioid analgesics
Pharmacologic: opioid agonists

Schedule II

Indications

Moderate to severe pain (alone and in combination with nonopioid analgesics). Moderate to severe chronic pain in opioid-tolerant patients requiring use of daily, around-the-clock long-term opioid treatment and for which alternative treatment options are inadequate (extended-release).

Action

Binds to opiate receptors in the CNS. Alters the perception of and response to painful stimuli while producing

---

✤ = Canadian drug name. ▓ = Genetic implication. ~~Strikethrough~~ = Discontinued. CAPITALS = life-threatening. Underline = most frequent.

generalized CNS depression. Suppresses the cough reflex via a direct central action. **Therapeutic Effects:** Decrease in moderate to severe pain.

Pharmacokinetics

Absorption: Well absorbed following oral, rectal, SUBQ, and IM administration. Extended-release product results in an initial release of drug, followed by a 2nd sustained phase of absorption.
Distribution: Widely distributed. Crosses the placenta; enters breast milk.
Metabolism and Excretion: Mostly metabolized by the liver.
Half-life: *Oral (immediate-release), or injection:* 2–4 hr; *Oral (extended-release):* 8–15 hr.

TIME/ACTION PROFILE (analgesic effect)

ROUTE	ONSET	PEAK	DURATION
PO-IR	30 min	30–90 min	4–5 hr
PO-ER	unknown	unknown	unknown
SUBQ	15 min	30–90 min	4–5 hr
IM	15 min	30–60 min	4–5 hr
IV	10–15 min	15–30 min	2–3 hr
Rect	15–30 min	30–90 min	4–5 hr

Contraindications/Precautions

Contraindicated in: Hypersensitivity; Some products contain bisulfites and should be avoided in patients with known hypersensitivity; Severe respiratory depression (in absence of resuscitative equipment) (extended-release only); Acute or severe bronchial asthma (extended-release only); Paralytic ileus (extended-release only); Acute, mild, intermittent, or postoperative pain (extended-release only); Prior GI surgery or narrowing of GI tract (extended-release only); Opioid nontolerant patients (extended-release only); Severe hepatic impairment (extended-release only).
Use Cautiously in: Head trauma; ↑ intracranial pressure; Severe pulmonary disease; Moderate or severe renal disease (extended-release only) (dose ↓ recommended); Moderate hepatic impairment (extended-release only) (dose ↓ recommended); Hypothyroidism; Seizure disorder; Adrenal insufficiency; Alcoholism; Undiagnosed abdominal pain; Prostatic hypertrophy; Biliary tract disease (including pancreatitis); OB: Avoid chronic use during pregnancy. Has been used during labor but may cause respiratory depression in the newborn; Lactation: Use while breastfeeding only if potential maternal benefit justifies potential risk to infant; Geri: Older adults (↑ risk of respiratory depression; dose ↓ suggested).

Adverse Reactions/Side Effects

CV: hypotension, bradycardia. **Derm:** flushing, sweating. **EENT:** blurred vision, diplopia, miosis. **Endo:** adrenal insufficiency. **GI:** constipation, dry mouth, nausea, vomiting. **GU:** urinary retention. **Neuro:** confusion, sedation, dizziness, dysphoria, euphoria, floating feeling, hallucinations, headache, unusual dreams. **Resp:** RESPIRATORY DEPRESSION (including

central sleep apnea and sleep-related hypoxemia). **Misc:** physical dependence, psychological dependence, tolerance.

Interactions

Drug-Drug: Exercise extreme caution with **MAO inhibitors** (may produce severe, unpredictable reactions—reduce initial dose of hydromorphone to 25% of usual dose, discontinue MAO inhibitors 2 wk prior to hydromorphone). Use with **benzodiazepines** or other **CNS depressants** including other **opioids**, **non-benzodiazepine sedative/hypnotics, anxiolytics, general anesthetics, muscle relaxants, antipsychotics,** and **alcohol** may cause profound sedation, respiratory depression, coma, and death; reserve concurrent use for when alternative treatment options are inadequate. **Mixed agonist/antagonist analgesics,** including **nalbuphine** or **butorphanol** and **partial agonist analgesics,** including **buprenorphine,** may ↓ hydromorphone's analgesic effects and/or precipitate opioid withdrawal in physically dependent patients. Drugs that affect serotonergic neurotransmitter systems, including **tricyclic antidepressants, SSRIs, SNRIs, MAO inhibitors, TCAs, tramadol, trazodone, mirtazapine, 5–HT$_3$ receptor antagonists, linezolid, methylene blue,** and **triptans** ↑ risk of serotonin syndrome.
Drug-Natural Products: Concomitant use of **kava-kava, valerian, chamomile,** or **hops** can ↑ CNS depression.

Route/Dosage

Doses depend on level of pain and tolerance. Larger doses may be required during chronic therapy.
PO (Adults ≥50 kg): *Immediate-release:* 4–8 mg every 3–4 hr initially (some patients may respond to doses as small as 2 mg initially); *or* once 24-hr opioid requirement is determined, convert to *extended-release* by administering total daily oral dose once daily.
PO (Adults and Children <50 kg): 0.06 mg/kg every 3–4 hr initially, younger children may require smaller initial doses of 0.03 mg/kg. Maximum dose 5 mg.
IV, IM, SUBQ (Adults ≥50 kg): 1.5 mg every 3–4 hr as needed initially; may be ↑.
IV, IM, SUBQ (Adults and Children <50 kg): 0.015 mg/kg mg every 3–4 hr as needed initially; may be ↑.
IV (Adults): *Continuous infusion (unlabeled):* 0.2–3 mg/hr depending on previous opioid use. An initial bolus of twice the hourly rate in mg may be given with subsequent breakthrough boluses of 50–100% of the hourly rate in mg.
Rect (Adults): 3 mg every 6–8 hr initially as needed.

Hepatic Impairment

PO (Adults): *Moderate hepatic impairment (extended–release):* ↓ initial dose by 75%.

Renal Impairment

PO (Adults): *Moderate renal impairment (extended–release):* ↓ initial dose by 50%; *Severe renal* *impairment (extended–release):* ↓ initial dose by 75%.

Availability (generic available)

Immediate-release tablets: 2 mg, 4 mg, 8 mg. **Controlled-release capsules:** ✿ 3 mg, ✿ 4.5 mg, ✿ 6 mg, ✿ 9 mg, ✿ 12 mg, ✿ 18 mg, ✿ 24 mg, ✿ 30 mg. **Extended-release tablets (abuse-deterrent):** 8 mg, 12 mg, 16 mg, 32 mg. **Oral solution:** 1 mg/mL. **Solution for injection:** 1 mg/mL, 2 mg/mL, 4 mg/mL, 10 mg/mL. **Rectal suppositories:** 3 mg.

NURSING IMPLICATIONS

Assessment

- Assess type, location, and intensity of pain prior to and 1 hr following IM or PO and 5 min (peak) following IV administration. When titrating opioid doses, increases of 25–50% should be administered until there is either a 50% reduction in the patient's pain rating on a numerical or visual analogue scale or the patient reports satisfactory pain relief. When titrating doses of short-acting hydromorphone, a repeat dose can be safely administered at the time of the peak if previous dose is ineffective and side effects are minimal.
- Patients on a continuous infusion should have additional bolus doses provided every 15–30 min, as needed, for breakthrough pain. The bolus dose is usually set to the amount of drug infused each hr by continuous infusion.
- Patients taking extended-release hydromorphone may require additional short-acting or rapid-onset opioid doses for breakthrough pain. Doses of short-acting opioids should be equivalent to 10–20% of 24 hr total and given every 2 hr as needed.
- An equianalgesic chart (see Appendix I) should be used when changing routes or when changing from one opioid to another.
- **High Alert:** Assess level of consciousness, BP, pulse, and respirations before and periodically during administration. If respiratory rate is <10/min, assess level of sedation. Physical stimulation may be sufficient to prevent significant hypoventilation. Subsequent doses may need to be decreased by 25–50%. Initial drowsiness will diminish with continued use. Monitor for respiratory depression, especially during initiation or following dose increase; serious, life-threatening, or fatal respiratory depression may occur. May cause sleep-related breathing disorders (central sleep apnea, sleep-related hypoxemia). Geri, Pedi: Assess geriatric and pediatric patients frequently; more sensitive to the effects of opioid analgesics and may experience side effects and respiratory complications more frequently.
- Prolonged use may lead to physical and psychological dependence and tolerance. This should not prevent patient from receiving adequate analgesia. Patients who receive hydromorphone for pain rarely develop psychological dependence. Progressively higher doses may be required to relieve pain with long-term therapy; may increase risk of overdose. Prolonged use of opioids should be reserved for patients whose pain remains severe enough to require them and alternative treatment options continue to be inadequate. Many acute pain conditions treated in the outpatient setting require no more than a few days of an opioid pain medicine.
- Assess bowel function routinely. Institute prevention of constipation with increased intake of fluids and bulk, and laxatives to minimize constipating effects. Administer stimulant laxatives routinely if opioid use exceeds 2–3 days, unless contraindicated. Consider drugs for opioid induced constipation.
- Assess risk for opioid addiction, abuse, or misuse prior to administration. Abuse or misuse of extended-release preparations by crushing, chewing, snorting, or injecting dissolved product will result in uncontrolled delivery of morphine and can result in overdose and death.

Lab Test Considerations

- May ↑ plasma amylase and lipase levels.

Toxicity and Overdose

- If an opioid antagonist is required to reverse respiratory depression or coma, naloxone (Narcan) is the antidote. Dilute the 0.4-mg ampule of naloxone in 10 mL of 0.9% NaCl and administer 0.5 mL (0.02 mg) by IV push every 2 min. For children and patients weighing <40 kg, dilute 0.1 mg of naloxone in 10 mL of 0.9% NaCl for a concentration of 10 mcg/mL and administer 0.5 mcg every 2 min. Titrate dose to avoid withdrawal, seizures, and severe pain.

Implementation

- **High Alert:** Accidental overdose of opioid analgesics has resulted in fatalities. Before administering, check infusion pump settings. Pedi: Medication errors with opioid analgesics are common in pediatric patients; calculate doses carefully. Use appropriate measuring devices.
- **High Alert:** Do not confuse hydromorphone with buprenorphine, hydralazine, hydroxyzine, morphine, or oxymorphone; fatalities have occurred. Do not confuse high-potency (HP) dose forms with regular dose forms.
- Explain therapeutic value of medication prior to administration to enhance the analgesic effect.
- Regularly administered doses may be more effective than prn administration. Analgesic is more effective if given before pain becomes severe.
- Coadministration with nonopioid analgesics may have additive analgesic effects and permit lower opioid doses.
- When converting from immediate-release to extended-release hydromorphone administer total

daily oral hydromorphone dose once daily; dose of extended-release product can be titrated every 3–4 days (see Appendix I). To convert from another opioid to extended-release hydromorphone, convert to total daily dose of hydromorphone and then administer 50% of this dose as extended-release hydromorphone once daily; can then titrate dose every 3–4 days. When converting from transdermal fentanyl, initiate extended-release hydromorphone 18 hr after removing transdermal fentanyl patch; for each 25 mcg/hr fentanyl transdermal dose, the equianalgesic dose of extended-release hydromorphone is 12 mg once daily (should initiate at 50% of this calculated total daily dose given once daily).

• Medication should be discontinued gradually after long-term use to prevent withdrawal symptoms. For patients on long-acting agents who are physically opioid-dependent, initiate the taper by a small enough increment (no >10% to 25% of total daily dose) to avoid withdrawal symptoms, and proceed with dose-lowering at an interval of every 2–4 wk. May be necessary to provide patient with a lower dose strength for a successful taper. Monitor frequently to manage pain and withdrawal symptoms (restlessness, lacrimation, rhinorrhea, yawning, perspiration, chills, myalgia, mydriasis, irritability, anxiety, backache, joint pain, weakness, abdominal cramps, insomnia, nausea, anorexia, vomiting, diarrhea, or increased blood pressure, respiratory rate, or heart rate). If withdrawal symptoms occur, pause taper for a period of time or raise the dose of opioid analgesic to the previous dose, and then proceed with a slower taper. Monitor patients for changes in mood, emergence of suicidal thoughts, or use of other substances. A multimodal approach to pain management may optimize the treatment of chronic pain, as well as assist with the successful tapering of the opioid analgesic.

• *REMS:* FDA strongly encourages health care professionals to complete a REMS-compliant education program that includes all the elements of the FDA Education *Blueprint for Health Care Providers Involved in the Management or Support of Patients with Pain,* available at www.fda.gov/OpioidAnalgesicREMSBlueprint. Information on programs can be found at 1-800-503-0784 or www.opioidanalgesicrems.com.

• Discuss availability of naloxone for emergency treatment of opioid overdose with the patient and caregiver and assess the potential need for access to naloxone, both when initiating and renewing therapy, especially if patient has household members (including children) or other close contacts at risk for accidental exposure or overdose. Consider prescribing naloxone, based on the patient's risk factors for overdose, such as concomitant use of CNS depressants, a history of opioid use disorder, or prior opioid overdose. However, the presence of risk factors for overdose should not prevent the proper management of pain in any patient.

• **PO:** May be administered with food or milk to minimize GI irritation.

• *DNC:* Swallow extended-release tablets whole; do not break, crush, dissolve, or chew.

IV Administration

• **IV Push:** Administer undiluted. Inspect solution for particulate matter. Slight yellow color does not alter potency. Store at room temperature. *Rate:* Administer slowly over 2–3 min. *High Alert:* Rapid administration may lead to increased respiratory depression, hypotension, and circulatory collapse.

• For other clinical situations (sedation in mechanically ventilated patient), a continuous infusion may also be administered.

• **Y-Site Compatibility:** acetaminophen, acyclovir, alemtuzumab, allopurinol, amifostine, amikacin, aminocaproic acid, aminophylline, amiodarone, amphotericin B deoxycholate, amphotericin B lipid complex, amphotericin B liposomal, ampicillin/sulbactam, anidulafungin, argatroban, arsenic trioxide, atracurium, atropine, azithromycin, aztreonam, bivalirudin, bleomycin, bumetanide, busulfan, calcium chloride, calcium gluconate, cangrelor, carboplatin, carmustine, caspofungin, cefepime, cefotaxime, cefotetan, cefoxitin, ceftaroline, ceftazidime, ceftolozane/tazobactam, ceftriaxone, cefuroxime, chloramphenicol, chlorpromazine, ciprofloxacin, cisatracurium, cisplatin, cladribine, clindamycin, cyclophosphamide, cyclosporine, cytarabine, dacarbazine, dactinomycin, daptomycin, daunorubicin hydrochloride, dexamethasone, dexmedetomidine, dexrazoxane, digoxin, diltiazem, diphenhydramine, dobutamine, docetaxel, dopamine, doxorubicin hydrochloride, doxorubicin liposomal, doxycycline, droperidol, enalaprilat, ephedrine, epinephrine, epirubicin, eptifibatide, eravacycline, ertapenem, erythromycin, esmolol, etoposide, etoposide phosphate, famotidine, fentanyl, filgrastim, fluconazole, fludarabine, fluorouracil, foscarnet, fosphenytoin, furosemide, ganciclovir, gemcitabine, gemtuzumab ozogamicin, gentamicin, glycopyrrolate, granisetron, haloperidol, heparin, hetastarch, hydralazine, hydrocortisone, idarubicin, ifosfamide, imipenem/cilastatin, insulin, regular, irinotecan, isavuconazonium, isoproterenol, ketorolac, labetalol, leucovorin calcium, levofloxacin, lidocaine, linezolid, lorazepam, magnesium sulfate, mannitol, melphalan, meropenem, meropenem/vaborbactam, mesna, methohexital, methotrexate, methylprednisolone, metoclopramide, metoprolol, micafungin, midazolam, milrinone, mitomycin, mitoxantrone, morphine, mycophenolate, nafcillin, naloxone, nicardipine, nitroglycerin, nitroprusside, norepinephrine, octreotide, ondansetron, oxacillin, oxaliplatin, oxytocin, paclitaxel, palonosetron, pamidronate, pemetrexed, penicillin G potassium, pentamidine, pentobarbital, phenylephrine, piperacillin/tazobactam, plazomicin, posaconazole, potassium acetate, potassium chloride, potassium phosphate, procainamide, prochlorperazine, promethazine, propofol, propranolol, remifentanil, rituximab, rocuronium, sodium acetate, sodium phosphate, succinylcholine, tacrolimus, tedizolid, theophylline, thiotepa, tigecycline, tirofiban, tobramycin, topotecan, trastuzumab, trimethoprim/sulfamethoxazole, vancomycin, vasopressin, vecuronium, verapamil, vinblastine, vincristine, vinorelbine, zidovudine, zoledronic acid.

- **Y-Site Incompatibility:** dantrolene, minocycline, phenytoin, sargramostim, thiopental.

Patient/Family Teaching

- **REMS:** Instruct patient on how and when to ask for pain medication. Do not stop taking without discussing with health care professional; may cause withdrawal symptoms if discontinued abruptly after prolonged use. Do not increase doses without discussing with health care professional, may lead to overdose. Discuss safe use, risks, and proper storage and disposal of opioid analgesics with patients and caregivers with each Rx. The Patient Counseling Guide is available at www.fda.gov/ OpioidAnalgesicREMSPCG.
- Advise patient that hydromorphone is a drug with known abuse potential. Protect it from theft, and never give to anyone other than the individual for whom it was prescribed. Store out of sight and reach of children, and in a location not accessible by others.
- Educate patients and caregivers on how to recognize respiratory depression and emphasize the importance of calling 911 or getting emergency medical help right away in the event of a known or suspected overdose. Inform patients and caregivers about ways to obtain naloxone as permitted by individual state naloxone dispensing and prescribing requirements or guidelines (by prescription, directly from a pharmacist, or as part of a community-based program).
- May cause drowsiness or dizziness. Advise patient to call for assistance when ambulating or smoking. Caution patient to avoid driving or other activities requiring alertness until response to medication is known.
- Advise patient to notify health care professional if pain control is not adequate or if side effects occur.
- Advise patient to change positions slowly to minimize orthostatic hypotension.
- Instruct patient to avoid concurrent use of alcohol or other CNS depressants.
- Instruct patient to notify health care professional of all Rx or OTC medications, vitamins, or herbal products being taken and consult health care professional before taking any new medications.
- Encourage patient to turn, cough, and breathe deeply every 2 hr to prevent atelectasis.
- Rep: Advise patient to notify health care professional if pregnancy is planned or suspected, or if breast-

feeding. Inform patient of potential for neonatal opioid withdrawal syndrome with prolonged use during pregnancy. Monitor neonate for signs and symptoms of withdrawal symptoms (irritability, hyperactivity and abnormal sleep pattern, high-pitched cry, tremor, vomiting, diarrhea, and/or failure to gain weight); usually occur the first days after birth. Monitor infants exposed to hydromorphone through breast milk for excess sedation and respiratory depression. Chronic use may reduce fertility in females and males.

- **Home Care Issues:** *High Alert:* Explain to patient and family how and when to administer hydromorphone, discuss safe storage of medication, and how to care for infusion equipment properly. Pedi: Teach parents or caregivers how to accurately measure liquid medication and to use only measuring device dispensed with medication.
- Emphasize the importance of aggressive prevention of constipation with the use of hydromorphone.

Evaluation/Desired Outcomes

- Decrease in severity of pain without a significant alteration in level of consciousness or respiratory status.

---

hydroxocobalamin, See VITAMIN B$_{12}$ PREPARATIONS.

▓ hydroxychloroquine
(hye-drox-ee-**klor**-oh-kwin)
Plaquenil
Classification
Therapeutic: antimalarials, antirheumatics (DMARDs)

Indications
Treatment of uncomplicated malaria in geographic areas where chloroquine resistance is not reported. Prophylaxis of malaria in geographic areas where chloroquine resistance is not reported. Acute and chronic rheumatoid arthritis. Chronic discoid lupus erythematosus and systemic lupus erythematosus.

Action
Inhibits protein synthesis in susceptible organisms by inhibiting DNA and RNA polymerase. **Therapeutic Effects:** Death of plasmodia responsible for causing malaria. Also has anti-inflammatory properties. **Spectrum:** Active against chloroquine-sensitive strains of: *Plasmodium falciparum, Plasmodium malariae, Plasmodium ovale,* and *Plasmodium vivax.*

Pharmacokinetics
Absorption: Highly variable (31–100%) following oral administration.

Distribution: Widely distributed; high concentrations in RBCs; crosses the placenta; excreted into breast milk.

Metabolism and Excretion: Partially metabolized by the liver to active metabolites; partially excreted unchanged by the kidneys.

Half-life: 40 days.

TIME/ACTION PROFILE (plasma concentrations)

ROUTE	ONSET	PEAK	DURATION
PO	rapid†	1–2 hr	days–wk

†Onset of antirheumatic action may take 6 wk.

Contraindications/Precautions

Contraindicated in: Hypersensitivity to hydroxychloroquine or chloroquine; Previous visual damage from hydroxychloroquine or chloroquine.

Use Cautiously in: Concurrent use of hepatotoxic drugs; Hepatic impairment or alcoholism; Use of high doses (>5 mg/kg/day), duration of use >5 yr, renal impairment, concurrent use of tamoxifen or macular disease (↑ risk of retinopathy); ≡ Glucose-6-phosphate dehydrogenase deficiency; Psoriasis; Porphyria; Bone marrow depression; Obesity (determine dose by ideal body weight); Pedi: Safety and effectiveness for treatment of rheumatoid arthritis, chronic discoid lupus erythematosus, or systemic lupus erythematosus not established in children; Geri: ↓ renal function may ↑ risk of adverse reactions in older adults.

Adverse Reactions/Side Effects

CV: heart block, HF, QT interval prolongation, TORSADES DE POINTES. **Derm:** acute generalized exanthematous pustulosis, alopecia, DRUG REACTION WITH EOSINOPHILIA AND SYSTEMIC SYMPTOMS (DRESS), ERYTHEMA MULTIFORME, hair color changes, hyperpigmentation, photosensitivity, pruritus, rash, STEVENS-JOHNSON SYNDROME (SJS), TOXIC EPIDERMAL NECROLYSIS, urticaria. **EENT:** corneal deposits, nystagmus, retinopathy, tinnitus, vertigo, visual disturbances. **Endo:** hypoglycemia. **GI:** ↑ liver enzymes, abdominal pain, anorexia, diarrhea, HEPATOTOXICITY, nausea, vomiting. **GU:** proteinuria. **Hemat:** AGRANULOCYTOSIS, APLASTIC ANEMIA, leukopenia, thrombocytopenia. **Metab:** ↓ weight. **Neuro:** aggressiveness, anxiety, ataxia, dizziness, dyskinesia, dystonia, fatigue, headache, irritability, neuromyopathy, nightmares, peripheral neuritis, personality changes, psychoses, SEIZURES, SUICIDAL THOUGHTS/BEHAVIORS, tremor. **Resp:** bronchospasm, PULMONARY HYPERTENSION. **Misc:** ANGIOEDEMA.

Interactions

Drug-Drug: Concurrent use of other **QT interval-prolonging drugs** may ↑ risk of torsades de pointes. May ↑ the risk of hepatotoxicity when administered with **hepatotoxic drugs**. May ↑ risk of hypoglycemia when used with **antidiabetic agents**. Use with **mefloquine** may ↑ risk of seizures. **Antacids** may bind to and ↓ the absorption of hydroxychloroquine; separate administration by ≥4 hr. **Cimetidine** may ↑ levels; avoid concurrent use. **Urinary acidifiers** may ↑ renal excretion. May ↑ levels of **digoxin** or **cyclosporine**.

Route/Dosage

Malaria

PO (Adults): *Prophylaxis:* 400 mg once weekly; start 2 wk prior to entering malarious area; continue for 4 wk after leaving area. *Treatment:* 800 mg initially, then 400 mg at 6 hr, 24 hr, and 48 hr after initial dose.

PO (Children ≥31 kg): *Prophylaxis:* 6.5 mg/kg (not to exceed 400 mg) once weekly; start 2 wk prior to entering malarious area; continue for 4 wk after leaving area. *Treatment:* 13 mg/kg (not to exceed 800 mg) initially, then 6.5 mg/kg (not to exceed 400 mg) at 6 hr, 24 hr, and 48 hr after initial dose.

Rheumatoid Arthritis

PO (Adults): 400–600 mg per day in 1–2 divided doses; once adequate response obtained, may ↓ dose to maintenance dose of 200–400 mg per day in 1–2 divided doses.

Lupus Erythematosus

PO (Adults): 200–400 mg per day in 1–2 divided doses.

Availability (generic available)

Tablets: 100 mg, 200 mg, 300 mg, 400 mg.

NURSING IMPLICATIONS

Assessment

- Assess deep tendon reflexes periodically to determine muscle weakness. Therapy may be discontinued should this occur.
- Obtain baseline ocular exam within first yr of therapy. Patients on prolonged high-dose therapy should have eye exams prior to and every 3–6 mo during therapy to detect retinal damage. Monitor patients without risk factors every 5 yrs. Retinal changes may progress even after therapy is completed.
- Monitor ECG for cardiomyopathy and QT prolongation periodically during therapy.
- Monitor for signs and symptoms of DRESS (fever, rash, lymphadenopathy, and/or facial swelling), associated with involvement of other organ systems (hepatitis, nephritis, hematologic abnormalities, myocarditis, myositis) during therapy. May resemble an acute viral infection. Eosinophilia is often present. Discontinue therapy if signs occur.
- Assess for rash periodically during therapy. May cause SJS. Discontinue therapy if severe or if accompanied with fever, general malaise, fatigue, muscle or joint aches, blisters, oral lesions, conjunctivitis, hepatitis and/or eosinophilia.
- Assess for suicidal tendencies, depression, or changes in behavior periodically during therapy.
- **Malaria or Lupus Erythematosus:** Assess patient for improvement in signs and symptoms of condition daily throughout course of therapy.

- **Rheumatoid Arthritis:** Assess patient monthly for pain, swelling, and range of motion.

Lab Test Considerations
- Monitor CBC and platelet count periodically during therapy. May cause decreased RBC, WBC, and platelet counts. If severe decreases occur that are not related to the disease process, discontinue hydroxychloroquine.
- Monitor liver function tests periodically during therapy.
- May cause hypoglycemia.

Implementation
- Do not confuse hydroxychloroquine with hydrochlorothiazide or hydroxyurea.
- **PO:** Administer with milk or meals to minimize GI distress.
- Tablets may be crushed and placed inside empty capsules for patients with difficulty swallowing. Contents of capsules may also be mixed with a teaspoonful of jam, jelly, or Jell-O prior to administration.
- **Malaria Prophylaxis:** Hydroxychloroquine therapy should be started 2 wk prior to potential exposure and continued for 4–6 wk after leaving the malarious area.

Patient/Family Teaching
- Instruct patient to take medication as directed and continue full course of therapy even if feeling better. Take missed doses as soon as remembered unless it is almost time for next dose. Do not double doses.
- Advise patients to avoid use of alcohol while taking hydroxychloroquine.
- Caution patient to keep hydroxychloroquine out of reach of children; fatalities have occurred with ingestion of 3 or 4 tablets.

- Explain need for periodic ophthalmic exams for patients on prolonged high-dose therapy. Advise patient that the risk of ocular damage may be decreased by the use of dark glasses in bright light. Protective clothing and sunscreen should also be used to reduce risk of dermatoses.
- Advise patient to notify health care professional promptly if sore throat, fever, unusual bleeding or bruising, blurred vision, visual changes, ringing in the ears, difficulty hearing, or muscle weakness occurs.
- Rep: Advise females of reproductive potential to notify health care professional if pregnancy is planned or suspected, or if breastfeeding. Inform patient of pregnancy exposure registry that monitors pregnancy outcomes in women exposed to hydroxychloroquine during pregnancy. Encourage patients to register by calling 1-877-311-8972.
- **Malaria Prophylaxis:** Review methods of minimizing exposure to mosquitoes with patients receiving hydroxychloroquine prophylactically (use repellent, wear long-sleeved shirt and long trousers, use screen or netting).
- Advise patient to notify health care professional if fever develops while traveling or within 2 mo of leaving an endemic area.
- **Rheumatoid Arthritis:** Instruct patient to contact health care professional if no improvement is noticed within a few days. Treatment for rheumatoid arthritis may require up to 6 mo for full benefit.

Evaluation/Desired Outcomes
- Prevention or resolution of malaria.
- Improvement in signs and symptoms of rheumatoid arthritis.
- Improvement in symptoms of lupus erythematosus.

ibandronate (i-**ban**-dro-nate)
~~Boniva~~
Classification
Therapeutic: bone resorption inhibitors
Pharmacologic: bisphosphonates

Indications
Treatment/prevention of postmenopausal osteoporosis.

Action
Inhibits resorption of bone by inhibiting osteoclast activity. **Therapeutic Effects:** Reversal/prevention of progression of osteoporosis with decreased fractures.

Pharmacokinetics
Absorption: 0.6% absorbed following oral administration (significantly ↓ by food).
Distribution: Rapidly binds to bone.
Protein Binding: 90.9–99.5%.
Metabolism and Excretion: 50–60% excreted in urine; unabsorbed drug is eliminated in feces.
Half-life: *PO:* 10–60 hr; *IV:* 4.6–25.5 hr.

TIME/ACTION PROFILE

ROUTE	ONSET	PEAK	DURATION
PO	unknown	0.5–2 hr	up to 1 mo
IV	unknown	3 hr	up to 3 mo

Contraindications/Precautions
Contraindicated in: Hypersensitivity; Abnormalities of the esophagus that delay esophageal emptying (e.g., strictures, achalasia); Uncorrected hypocalcemia; Inability to stand/sit upright for at least 60 min; Severe renal impairment (CCr <30 mL/min); OB: Pregnancy.
Use Cautiously in: History of upper GI disorders; Concurrent use of NSAIDs or aspirin; Invasive dental procedures, cancer, receiving chemotherapy, corticosteroids, or angiogenesis inhibitors, poor oral hygiene, periodontal disease, dental disease, anemia, coagulopathy, infection, or poorly fitting dentures (may ↑ risk of jaw osteonecrosis); Lactation: Safety not established in breastfeeding; Pedi: Safety and effectiveness not established in children; Geri: Consider age-related ↓ in body mass, renal and hepatic function, concurrent disease states, and drug therapy in older adults.

Adverse Reactions/Side Effects
Derm: ERYTHEMA MULTIFORME, STEVENS-JOHNSON SYNDROME. **GI:** diarrhea, dyspepsia, dysphagia, ESOPHAGEAL CANCER, esophageal/gastric ulcer, esophagitis. **Local:** injection site reactions. **MS:** musculoskeletal pain, pain in arms/legs, femur fractures, osteonecrosis (primarily of jaw). **Resp:** asthma exacerbation. **Misc:** ANAPHYLAXIS.

Interactions
Drug-Drug: Calcium-, aluminum-, magnesium-, and iron- containing products, including antacids ↓ absorption (ibandronate should be taken 60 min before). Concurrent use of **NSAIDs**, including **aspirin**, may ↑ risk of gastric irritation.
Drug-Food: Milk and other foods ↓ absorption.

Route/Dosage
PO (Adults): 150 mg once monthly.
IV (Adults): 3 mg every 3 mo.

Availability (generic available)
Tablets: 150 mg. **Injection (prefilled syringes):** 1 mg/mL.

NURSING IMPLICATIONS
Assessment
- **Osteoporosis:** Assess patients for low bone mass before and periodically during therapy.
- **IV:** Monitor for signs and symptoms of anaphylactic reactions (swelling of face, lips, mouth or tongue; trouble breathing; wheezing; severe itching; skin rash, redness, or swelling; dizziness or fainting; fast heartbeat or pounding in chest; sweating) during therapy. Discontinue injection immediately and begin supportive treatment if symptoms occur.
- Perform a routine oral exam prior to initiation of therapy. Dental exam with appropriate preventative dentistry should be considered prior to therapy. Patients with history of tooth extraction, poor oral hygiene, gingival infections, diabetes, or use of a dental appliance or those taking immunosuppressive therapy, angiogenesis inhibitors, or systemic corticosteroids are at greater risk for osteonecrosis of the jaw.

Lab Test Considerations
- Assess serum calcium before and periodically during therapy. Hypocalcemia and vitamin D deficiency should be treated before initiating ibandronate therapy.
- May cause ↓ total alkaline phosphatase levels.
- May cause hypercholesterolemia.

Implementation
- **PO:** Administer first thing in the morning with 6–8 oz plain water 30 min before other medications, beverages, or food. *DNC:* Tablet should be swallowed whole; do not break, crush, or chew.
- *Once-monthly tablet* should be administered on the same date each mo.

IV Administration
- **IV:** Administer using prefilled syringe. Do not administer solution that is discolored or contains particulate matter. Administer IV only; other routes may cause tissue damage.
- *Rate:* Administer as a 15–30 sec bolus.
- **Y-Site Incompatibility:** Do not administer with calcium-containing solutions or other IV drugs.

Patient/Family Teaching
- Advise patient to eat a balanced diet and consult health care professional about the need for supplemental calcium and vitamin D. Wait at least 60 min after administration before taking supplemental calcium and vitamin D.

- Encourage patient to participate in regular exercise and to modify behaviors that increase the risk of osteoporosis (stop smoking, reduce alcohol consumption).
- Inform patient that severe musculoskeletal pain may occur within days, mo, or yr after starting ibandronate. Symptoms may resolve completely after discontinuation or slow or incomplete resolution may occur. Notify health care professional if severe pain occurs.
- Advise patient to notify health care professional if rash or signs and symptoms of osteonecrosis of the jaw (pain, numbness, swelling of or drainage from the jaw, mouth, or teeth) occur.
- Instruct patient to notify health care professional if swallowing difficulties, chest pain, new or worsening heartburn, or trouble or pain when swallowing occurs; may be signs of problems of the esophagus.
- Advise patient to inform health care professional of ibandronate therapy prior to dental surgery.
- Rep: Advise females of reproductive potential to notify health care professional if pregnancy is planned or suspected or if breastfeeding.
- PO: Instruct patient on the importance of taking as directed, first thing in the morning, 60 min before other medications, beverages, or food. Ibandronate should be taken with 6–8 oz plain water (mineral water, orange juice, coffee, and other beverages decrease absorption). Do not chew or suck on tablet. If a dose is missed, skip dose and resume the next morning; do not double doses or take later in the day. If a once-monthly dose is missed and the next scheduled dose is >7 days away, take in the morning following the date it is remembered. Resume original schedule the following mo. If the next dose is <7 days away, omit dose and take next scheduled dose. Do not discontinue without consulting health care professional.
- Caution patient to remain upright for 60 min following dose to facilitate passage to stomach and minimize risk of esophageal irritation. Advise patient to stop taking ibandronate and contact health care professional if symptoms of esophageal irritation (new or worsening dysphagia, pain on swallowing, retrosternal pain, or heartburn) occur.
- IV: Advise patient that IV doses should not be administered sooner than every 3 mo. If a dose is missed, have health care professional administer as soon as possible; next injection should be scheduled 3 mo from last injection.

Evaluation/Desired Outcomes
- Prevention of or decrease in the progression of osteoporosis in postmenopausal women. Discontinuation after 3–5 yr should be considered for women with low risk for fractures.

ibuprofen (eye-byoo-**proe**-fen)
Advil, Advil Infants, Advil Junior Strength, Advil Migraine, Children's Advil, ✤ Children's Europrofen, Children's Motrin, ✤ Motrin, Motrin IB, Motrin Infants Drops, Motrin Junior Strength, PediaCare IB Ibuprofen

ibuprofen (injection)
Caldolor, NeoProfen (ibuprofen lysine)
Classification
Therapeutic: antipyretics, antirheumatics, nonopioid analgesics
Pharmacologic: nonsteroidal anti-inflammatory drugs (NSAIDs)

Indications
PO, IV: Treatment of: Mild to moderate pain, Fever. **PO:** Treatment of: Inflammatory disorders including rheumatoid arthritis (including juvenile) and osteoarthritis, Dysmenorrhea. **IV:** Moderate to severe pain with opioid analgesics. Closure of a clinically significant patent ductus arteriosus (PDA) in neonates weighing 500–1500 g and ≤32 wk gestational age (ibuprofen lysine only).

Action
Inhibits prostaglandin synthesis. **Therapeutic Effects:** Decreased pain and inflammation. Reduction of fever. Closure of PDA.

Pharmacokinetics
Absorption: Oral formulation is well absorbed (80%) from the GI tract; IV administration results in complete bioavailability.
Distribution: Does not enter breast milk in significant amounts.
Protein Binding: 99%.
Metabolism and Excretion: Mostly metabolized by the liver; small amounts (1%) excreted unchanged by the kidneys.
Half-life: *Neonates:* 26–43 hr; *Children:* 1–2 hr; *Adults:* 2–4 hr.

TIME/ACTION PROFILE

ROUTE	ONSET	PEAK	DURATION
PO (antipyretic)	0.5–2.5 hr	2–4 hr	6–8 hr
PO (analgesic)	30 min	1–2 hr	4–6 hr
PO (anti-inflammatory)	≤7 days	1–2 wk	unknown
IV (analgesic)	unknown	unknown	6 hr
IV (antipyretic)	within 2 hr	10–12 hr†	4–6 hr

†With repeated dosing.

Contraindications/Precautions

Contraindicated in: Hypersensitivity (cross-sensitivity may exist with other NSAIDs, including aspirin); Active GI bleeding or ulcer disease; Chewable tablets contain aspartame and should not be used in patients with phenylketonuria; Coronary artery bypass graft surgery; History of recent MI; Severe HF; OB: Avoid use after 30 wk gestation; Pedi: Ibuprofen lysine: Preterm neonates with untreated infection, congenital heart disease where patency of PDA is necessary for pulmonary or systemic blood flow, bleeding, thrombocytopenia, coagulation defects, necrotizing enterocolitis, significant renal dysfunction.

Use Cautiously in: Cardiovascular disease or risk factors for cardiovascular disease (may ↑ risk of serious cardiovascular thrombotic events, MI, and stroke, especially with prolonged use or use of higher doses); avoid use in patients with recent MI or HF; Renal or hepatic disease, dehydration, or patients on nephrotoxic drugs (may ↑ risk of renal toxicity); Aspirin triad patients (asthma, nasal polyps, and aspirin intolerance); can cause fatal anaphylactoid reactions; Chronic alcohol use/abuse; Coagulation disorders; OB: Use at or after 20 wk gestation may cause fetal or neonatal renal impairment; if treatment is necessary between 20 wk and 30 wk gestation, limit use to the lowest effective dose and shortest duration possible; Lactation: Use while breastfeeding only if potential maternal benefit justifies potential risk to infant; Pedi: Safety and effectiveness not established for children <6 mo (oral) or <3 mo (IV Caldolor); hyperbilirubinemia in neonates (may displace bilirubin from albumin-binding sites); safety and effectiveness of ibuprofen lysine only established in premature infants; Geri: Appears on Beers list. ↑ risk GI bleeding or peptic ulcer disease in older adults. Avoid chronic use unless other alternatives are not effective and the patient can take a gastroprotective agent; avoid short-term use in combination with oral or parenteral corticosteroids, anticoagulants, or antiplatelet agents unless other alternatives are not effective and the patient can take a gastroprotective agent.

Exercise Extreme Caution in: History of GI bleeding or GI ulcer disease.

Adverse Reactions/Side Effects

CV: arrhythmias, edema, HF, hypertension, MI. **Derm:** DRUG REACTION WITH EOSINOPHILIA AND SYSTEMIC SYMPTOMS (DRESS), EXFOLIATIVE DERMATITIS, rash, STEVENS-JOHNSON SYNDROME, TOXIC EPIDERMAL NECROLYSIS. **EENT:** amblyopia, blurred vision, tinnitus. **F and E:** hyperkalemia. **GI:** constipation, dyspepsia, nausea, vomiting, abdominal discomfort, GI BLEEDING, HEPATITIS, necrotizing enterocolitis (ibuprofen lysine). **GU:** cystitis, hematuria, renal failure. **Hemat:** anemia, blood dyscrasias, prolonged bleeding time. **Local:** injection site reaction. **Neuro:** headache, dizziness, drowsiness, intraventricular hemorrhage (ibuprofen lysine), psychic disturbances, STROKE. **Misc:** HYPERSENSITIVITY REACTIONS (including anaphylaxis).

Interactions

Drug-Drug: May limit the cardioprotective (antiplatelet) effects of low-dose **aspirin.** Concurrent use with **aspirin** may ↓ effectiveness of ibuprofen. Additive adverse GI side effects with **aspirin, oral potassium,** other **NSAIDs, corticosteroids,** or **alcohol.** Chronic use with **acetaminophen** may ↑ risk of adverse renal reactions. May ↓ effectiveness of **diuretics, ACE inhibitors,** or other **antihypertensives.** May ↑ hypoglycemic effects of **insulin** or **oral hypoglycemic agents.** May ↑ serum **lithium** levels and risk of toxicity. ↑ risk of toxicity from **methotrexate. Probenecid** ↑ risk of toxicity from ibuprofen. ↑ risk of bleeding with **cefotetan, corticosteroids, valproic acid, thrombolytics, warfarin,** and **drugs affecting platelet function** including **clopidogrel, eptifibatide,** or **tirofiban.** ↑ risk of adverse hematologic reactions with **antineoplastics** or **radiation therapy.** ↑ risk of nephrotoxicity with **cyclosporine.** May ↓ the clearance and ↑ levels of **amikacin.**

Drug-Natural Products: ↑ bleeding risk with **arnica, chamomile, feverfew, garlic, ginger, ginkgo, Panax ginseng,** and others.

Route/Dosage

Analgesia/Anti-inflammatory/Antipyretic

PO (Adults): *Anti-inflammatory:* 400–800 mg 3–4 times daily (not to exceed 3200 mg/day). *Analgesic/antidysmenorrheal/antipyretic:* 200–400 mg every 4–6 hr (not to exceed 1200 mg/day).

PO (Children 6 mo–12 yr): *Anti-inflammatory:* 30–50 mg/kg/day in 3–4 divided doses (maximum dose: 2.4 g/day). *Antipyretic:* 5 mg/kg for temperature <102.5°F or 10 mg/kg for higher temperatures (not to exceed 40 mg/kg/day); may be repeated every 4–6 hr.

PO (Infants and Children): *Analgesic:* 4–10 mg/kg/dose every 6–8 hr.

IV (Adults): *Analgesic (Caldolor):* 400–800 mg every 6 hr as needed (not to exceed 3200 mg/day); *Antipyretic (Caldolor):* 400 mg initially, then 400 mg every 4–6 hr or 100–200 mg every 4 hr as needed (not to exceed 3200 mg/day).

IV (Children 12–17 yr): *Analgesic and antipyretic (Caldolor):* 400 mg every 4–6 hr as needed (not to exceed 2400 mg/day).

IV (Children 6 mo–12 yr): *Analgesic and antipyretic (Caldolor):* 10 mg/kg (not to exceed 400 mg) every 4–6 hr as needed (not to exceed 40 mg/kg/day or 2400 mg/day, whichever is less).

IV (Children 3–<6 mo): *Analgesic and antipyretic (Caldolor):* 10 mg/kg (not to exceed 100 mg) as a single dose.

Pediatric OTC Dosing

PO (Children 11 yr/72–95 lb): 300 mg every 6–8 hr.

PO (Children 9–10 yr/60–71 lb): 250 mg every 6–8 hr.

PO (Children 6–8 yr/48–59 lb): 200 mg every 6–8 hr.

PO (Children 4–5 yr/36–47 lb): 150 mg every 6–8 hr.

PO (Children 2–3 yr/24–35 lb): 100 mg every 6–8 hr.

PO (Children 12–23 mo/18–23 lb): 75 mg every 6–8 hr.

PO (Infants 6–11 mo/12–17 lb): 50 mg every 6–8 hr.

Patent Ductus Arteriosus Closure

IV (Neonates Gestational age ≤32 wk, 500–1500 g): *Neoprofen:* 10 mg/kg followed by two doses of 5 mg/kg at 24 and 48 hr after initial dose.

Availability (generic available)

Tablets: 200 mg^OTC, 400 mg, 600 mg, 800 mg. **Capsules (liquigels):** 200 mg^OTC. **Chewable tablets (fruit, grape, orange, and citrus flavor):** 100 mg^OTC. **Oral solution (berry flavor):** 50 mg/1.25 mL^OTC. **Oral suspension (fruit, berry, grape flavor):** 100 mg/5 mL^OTC. **Solution for injection:** 10 mg/mL (NeoProfen), 100 mg/mL (Caldolor). **Premixed infusion (Caldolor):** 800 mg/200 mL. *In combination with:* decongestants^OTC, hydrocodone.

NURSING IMPLICATIONS

Assessment

● Patients who have asthma, aspirin-induced allergy, and nasal polyps are at increased risk for developing hypersensitivity reactions. Assess for rhinitis, asthma, and urticaria.

● Assess for signs and symptoms of GI bleeding (tarry stools, light-headedness, hypotension), renal dysfunction (elevated BUN and serum creatinine levels, decreased urine output), and hepatic impairment (elevated liver enzymes, jaundice) periodically during therapy. Geri: Higher risk for poor outcomes or death from GI bleeding. Age-related renal impairment increases risk of hepatic and renal toxicity.

● Assess patient for skin rash frequently during therapy. Discontinue ibuprofen at first sign of rash; may be life-threatening. Stevens-Johnson syndrome or toxic epidermal necrolysis may develop. Treat symptomatically; may recur once treatment is stopped.

● Monitor for signs and symptoms of DRESS (fever, rash, lymphadenopathy, facial swelling, eosinophilia) periodically during therapy. If symptoms occur discontinue ibuprofen.

● **Pain:** Assess pain (note type, location, and intensity) prior to and 1–2 hr following administration.

● **Arthritis:** Assess pain and range of motion prior to and 1–2 hr following administration.

● **Fever:** Monitor temperature; note signs associated with fever (diaphoresis, tachycardia, malaise).

● **PDA Closure:** Monitor preterm neonates for signs of bleeding, infection, and decreased urine output.

Monitor IV site for signs of extravasation; ibuprofen lysine is an irritant. If PDA closes or size significantly decreases, 2nd and 3rd doses are unnecessary.

Lab Test Considerations

● BUN, serum creatinine, CBC, and liver function tests should be evaluated periodically in patients receiving prolonged therapy.

● Serum potassium, BUN, serum creatinine, alkaline phosphatase, LDH, AST, and ALT may show ↑ levels. Blood glucose, hemoglobin, and hematocrit concentrations, leukocyte and platelet counts, and CCr may be ↓.

● May cause prolonged bleeding time; may persist for <1 day following discontinuation.

● **PDA Closure:** If urinary output <0.6 mL/kg/hr at time of 2nd or 3rd dose, hold dose until renal function has returned to normal.

Implementation

● Do not confuse Motrin with Neurontin.

● Administration of higher than recommended doses does not provide increased pain relief but may increase incidence of side effects.

● Patient should be well hydrated before administration to prevent renal adverse reactions. Do not give to neonates with urine output <0.6 mL/kg/hr.

● Use lowest effective dose for shortest period of time, especially in the elderly, to minimize risk of cardiovascular thrombotic events.

● Coadministration with opioid analgesics may have additive analgesic effects and may permit lower opioid doses.

● **PO:** For rapid initial effect, administer 30 min before or 2 hr after meals. May be administered with food, milk, or antacids to decrease GI irritation. Tablets may be crushed and mixed with fluids or food; 800-mg tablet can be dissolved in water.

● **Dysmenorrhea:** Administer as soon as possible after the onset of menses. Prophylactic treatment has not been shown to be effective.

IV Administration

● **Intermittent Infusion:** *Ibuprofen injection: Dilution:* 0.9% NaCl, D5W, or LR. *Concentration:* Dilute the 800-mg dose in at least 200 mL and the 100-mg, 200-mg, and 400-mg doses in at least 100 mL for a concentration of 4 mg/mL or less. *Ibuprofen lysine: Dilution:* Dilute in appropriate volume of D5W or 0.9% NaCl. Administer within 30 min of dilution. Do not administer solutions that are discolored or contain particulate matter. Stable for up to 24 hr at room temperature. Discard remaining solution; does not contain preservatives. *Rate:* Infuse *Ibuprofen injection:* over at least 30 min for adults and at least 10 min for children for *Caldolor* or over 15 min for *NeoProfen.* Infuse *Ibuprofen lysine:* over 15 min.

Ibuprofen
- **Y-Site Compatibility:** metoprolol.
- **Y-Site Incompatibility:** esmolol, labetalol.

Ibuprofen Lysine
- **Y-Site Compatibility:** ceftazidime, epinephrine, furosemide, heparin, hydrocortisone, insulin, regular, phenobarbital, potassium chloride, sodium bicarbonate.
- **Y-Site Incompatibility:** amikacin, amino acids, caffeine citrate, dobutamine, dopamine, isoproterenol, midazolam, vancomycin, vecuronium.

Patient/Family Teaching
- Advise patients to take ibuprofen with a full glass of water and to remain in an upright position for 15–30 min after administration.
- Instruct patient to take medication as directed. Take missed doses as soon as remembered but not if almost time for next dose. Do not double doses. Pedi: Teach parents and caregivers to calculate and measure doses accurately and to use measuring device supplied with product.
- May cause drowsiness or dizziness. Advise patient to avoid driving or other activities requiring alertness until response to medication is known.
- Caution patient to avoid the concurrent use of alcohol, aspirin including low dose aspirin, acetaminophen, and other OTC or herbal products without consulting health care professional.
- Advise patient to inform health care professional of medication regimen prior to treatment or surgery.
- Instruct patient not to take OTC ibuprofen preparations for more than 10 days for pain or more than 3 days for fever, and to consult health care professional if symptoms persist or worsen. Many OTC products contain ibuprofen; avoid duplication.
- Caution patient that use of ibuprofen with 3 or more glasses of alcohol per day may increase the risk of GI bleeding.
- Advise patient to consult health care professional if rash, itching, visual disturbances, tinnitus, weight gain, edema, epigastric pain, dyspepsia, black stools, hematemesis, persistent headache, or influenza-like syndrome (chills, fever, muscle aches, pain), or cardiovascular events (chest pain, shortness of breath, weakness, slurring of speech) occurs.
- Pedi: Advise parents or caregivers not to administer ibuprofen to children who may be dehydrated (can occur with vomiting, diarrhea, or poor fluid intake); dehydration increases risk of renal dysfunction.
- Rep: May cause fetal harm. Advise females of reproductive potential to notify health care professional if pregnancy is planned or suspected and to avoid ibuprofen starting at 20 wk gestation due to risk of oligohydramnios and 30 wk gestation because of risk of premature closing of the fetal ductus arteriosus. If NSAIDs are necessary between 20 and 30 wk gestation, limit use to the lowest effective dose and shortest duration possible. Consider ultrasound monitoring of amniotic fluid if NSAID therapy extends beyond 48 hr. Discontinue ibuprofen if oligohydramnios occurs and follow up with infant. Advise women to avoid ibuprofen in the 3rd trimester of pregnancy (after 29 wk), may cause premature closure of the fetal ductus arteriosus. Use during labor or delivery may delay birth and increase risk of stillbirth. Advise patient to notify health care professional if breastfeeding. May cause temporary infertility in women.

Evaluation/Desired Outcomes
- Decrease in severity of pain.
- Improved joint mobility. Partial arthritic relief is usually seen within 7 days, but maximum effectiveness may require 1–2 wk of continuous therapy. Patients who do not respond to one NSAID may respond to another.
- Reduction in fever.
- Closure of PDA.

idaruCIZUmab
(eye-da-roo-**siz**-ue-mab)
　Praxbind
Classification
Therapeutic: antidotes
Pharmacologic: monoclonal antibodies

Indications
To counteract the anticoagulant effect of dabigatran for emergency surgery/urgent procedures or life-threatening uncontrolled bleeding.

Action
Human monoclonal antibody fragment that selectively binds to dabigatran and its metabolites, preventing its binding to thrombin and negating its anticoagulant effects. Does not reverse any other anticoagulants. **Therapeutic Effects:** Reversal of the anticoagulant effect of dabigatran.

Pharmacokinetics
Absorption: IV administration results in complete bioavailability.
Distribution: Minimally distributed to tissues.
Metabolism and Excretion: Biodegraded to smaller molecules. 60% excreted in urine, remainder via protein catabolism primarily in the kidneys.
Half-life: 10.3 hr.

TIME/ACTION PROFILE (plasma concentrations)

ROUTE	ONSET	PEAK	DURATION
IV	immediate	unknown	24 hr

Contraindications/Precautions
Contraindicated in: None reported.
Use Cautiously in: OB: Safety not established in pregnancy; Lactation: Safety not established in breast-

feeding; Pedi: Safety and effectiveness not established in children; Geri: Older adults may be more sensitive to drug effects.

Exercise Extreme Caution in: Hereditary fructose intolerance (risk of serious adverse reactions due to sorbitol excipient); History of serious hypersensitivity (including anaphylactoid reactions) to idarucizumab.

Adverse Reactions/Side Effects
CV: THROMBOEMBOLISM. **F and E:** hypokalemia. **GI:** constipation. **Neuro:** delirium. **Misc:** fever, HYPERSENSITIVITY REACTIONS (including anaphylaxis).

Interactions
Drug-Drug: None reported.

Route/Dosage
IV (Adults): 5 g as single dose.

Availability
Solution for injection (contains sorbitol): 2.5 g/ 50 mL.

NURSING IMPLICATIONS
Assessment
● Reversal of dabigatran exposes patient to thrombotic risk of their underlying disease; may cause thromboembolism. Resume anticoagulant therapy as soon as medically appropriate. Dabigatran therapy can be reinstituted 24 hr after idarucizumab infusion.
● Monitor for signs and symptoms of hypersensitivity reactions (rash, urticaria, fever, pruritus, dyspnea, orofacial swelling). Contains sorbitol; reactions in patients with hereditary fructose intolerance have included hypoglycemia, hypophosphatemia, metabolic acidosis, increase in uric acid, acute liver failure. If symptoms occur discontinue therapy and treat symptomatically.

Lab Test Considerations
● Monitor coagulation parameters (aPTT, ecarin clotting time [ECT]) 12–24 hr after infusion.
● May cause hypokalemia.

Implementation
● Do not confuse idarucizumab with idarubicin.

IV Administration
● **Intermittent Infusion:** Flush IV line with 0.9% NaCl prior to and following infusion. Solution is clear to opalescent, colorless to slightly yellow; do not administer solutions that are discolored or contain precipitates. Administer as 2 consecutive infusion or inject both vials consecutively via syringe. Must be administered within 1 hr when removed from vial. Store at room temperature and use within 6 hr if exposed to light.

Patient/Family Teaching
● Explain purpose of idarucizumab to patient.
● Instruct patient to notify health care professional immediately if bleeding or signs and symptoms of hypersensitivity occur.
● Rep: Advise females of reproductive potential to notify health care professional if pregnancy is planned or suspected or if breastfeeding.

Evaluation/Desired Outcomes
● Reversal of the anticoagulant effect of dabigatran.

ifosfamide (eye-foss-fam-ide)
Ifex
Classification
Therapeutic: antineoplastics
Pharmacologic: alkylating agents

Indications
Germ cell testicular carcinoma (with other chemotherapy agents and with mesna, which prevents ifosfamide-induced hemorrhagic cystitis).

Action
Following conversion to active compounds, interferes with DNA replication and RNA transcription, ultimately disrupting protein synthesis (cell-cycle phase–nonspecific). **Therapeutic Effects:** Death of rapidly replicating cells, particularly malignant ones.

Pharmacokinetics
Absorption: IV administration results in complete bioavailability.
Distribution: Minimally distributed to tissues.
Metabolism and Excretion: Metabolized by the liver to active antineoplastic compounds.
Half-life: 15 hr.

TIME/ACTION PROFILE (effects on blood counts)

ROUTE	ONSET	PEAK	DURATION
IV	unknown	7–14 days	21 days

Contraindications/Precautions
Contraindicated in: Hypersensitivity; OB: Pregnancy; Lactation: Lactation.
Use Cautiously in: Active infections; ↓ bone marrow reserve; Renal impairment; Rep: Women of reproductive potential; Pedi: Safety and effectiveness not established in children; Geri: Drug may accumulate in older adults due to age-related renal impairment.

Adverse Reactions/Side Effects
CV: cardiotoxicity. **Derm:** alopecia. **GI:** nausea, vomiting, anorexia, constipation, diarrhea, hepatotoxicity. **GU:** hemorrhagic cystitis, dysuria, renal impairment, sterility. **Hemat:** ANEMIA, LEUKOPENIA, THROMBOCYTOPENIA. **Local:** phlebitis. **Neuro:** confusion, sedation, dis-

✹ = Canadian drug name. ▓ = Genetic implication. ~~Strikethrough~~ = Discontinued. CAPITALS = life-threatening. Underline = most frequent.

orientation, dizziness. **Misc:** HYPERSENSITIVITY REACTIONS (including anaphylaxis).

Interactions

Drug-Drug: CYP3A4 inhibitors, including **ketoconazole, fluconazole, itraconazole, sorafenib,** and **aprepitant** may ↓ its effectiveness. **CYP3A4 inducers,** including **carbamazepine, phenytoin, phenobarbital,** and **rifampin** may ↑ the formation of a toxic metabolite and may ↑ risk of toxicity. ↑ myelosuppression with other **antineoplastics** or **radiation therapy.** Toxicity may be ↑ by **allopurinol** or **phenobarbital.** May ↓ antibody response to and ↑ risk of adverse reactions from **live-virus vaccines.**

Drug-Food: Grapefruit juice may ↑ levels; avoid concurrent use.

Route/Dosage

IV (Adults): 1.2 g/m²/day for 5 days; coadminister with mesna. May repeat cycle every 3 wk.

Availability (generic available)

Powder for injection: 1 g/vial, 3 g/vial. **Solution for injection:** 50 mg/mL.

NURSING IMPLICATIONS

Assessment

- Monitor BP, pulse, respiratory rate, and temperature frequently during administration. Report significant changes.
- Monitor urinary output frequently during therapy. Notify health care professional if hematuria occurs. To reduce the risk of hemorrhagic cystitis, fluid intake should be at least 3000 mL/day for adults and 1000–2000 mL/day for children. Mesna is given concurrently to prevent hemorrhagic cystitis.
- Monitor neurologic status. Ifosfamide should be discontinued if severe CNS symptoms (agitation, confusion, hallucinations, unusual tiredness) occur. Symptoms usually abate within 3 days of discontinuation of ifosfamide but may persist for longer; fatalities have been reported.
- Assess nausea, vomiting, and appetite. Weigh weekly. Premedication with an antiemetic may be used to minimize GI effects. Adjust diet as tolerated.
- Monitor for bone marrow depression. Assess for bleeding (bleeding gums, bruising, petechiae, guaiac stools, urine, and emesis) and avoid IM injections and taking rectal temperatures if platelet count is low. Apply pressure to venipuncture sites for 10 min. Assess for signs of infection during neutropenia. Anemia may occur. Monitor for increased fatigue, dyspnea, and orthostatic hypotension.

Lab Test Considerations

- Monitor CBC, differential, and platelet count prior to and periodically during therapy. Withhold dose if WBC <2000/mm³ or platelet count is <50,000/mm³. Nadir of leukopenia and thrombocytopenia occurs within 7–14 days and usually recovers within 21 days of therapy.

- Urinalysis should be evaluated before each dose. Withhold dose until recovery if urinalysis shows >10 RBCs per high-power field.
- May cause ↑ in liver enzymes and serum bilirubin.
- Monitor AST, ALT, serum alkaline phosphatase, bilirubin, and LDH prior to and periodically during therapy. May cause ↑ in liver enzymes and serum bilirubin.
- Monitor BUN, serum creatinine, phosphate, and potassium periodically during therapy. May cause hypokalemia.

Implementation

- Prepare solution in a biologic cabinet. Wear gloves, gown, and mask while handling IV medication. Discard IV equipment in specially designated containers.

IV Administration

- **IV:** Prepare solution by diluting each 1-g vial with 20 mL of sterile water or bacteriostatic water for injection containing parabens. Use solution prepared without bacteriostatic water within 6 hr. Solution prepared with bacteriostatic water is stable for 1 wk at 30°C or 6 wk at 5°C.
- **Intermittent Infusion:** *Dilution:* May be further diluted in D5W, 0.9% NaCl, LR, or sterile water for injection. *Concentration:* 0.6 to 20 mg/mL (maximum 40 mg/mL). Dilute solution is stable for 7 days at room temperature or 6 wk if refrigerated. *Rate:* Administer over at least 30 min.
- **Continuous Infusion:** Has also been administered as a continuous infusion over 72 hr.
- **Y-Site Compatibility:** acyclovir, alemtuzumab, allopurinol, amifostine, amikacin, aminocaproic acid, aminophylline, amiodarone, amphotericin B deoxycholate, amphotericin B lipid complex, amphotericin B liposomal, ampicillin, ampicillin/sulbactam, anidulafungin, argatroban, azithromycin, aztreonam, bivalirudin, bleomycin, bumetanide, buprenorphine, butorphanol, calcium chloride, calcium gluconate, carboplatin, caspofungin, cefazolin, cefotaxime, cefotetan, cefoxitin, ceftazidime, ceftriaxone, cefuroxime, chlorpromazine, ciprofloxacin, cisatracurium, cisplatin, clindamycin, cyclosporine, cytarabine, dacarbazine, dactinomycin, daptomycin, dexamethasone, dexmedetomidine, dexrazoxane, digoxin, diltiazem, diphenhydramine, dobutamine, docetaxel, dopamine, doxorubicin hydrochloride, doxorubicin liposomal, doxycycline, droperidol, enalaprilat, ephedrine, epinephrine, epirubicin, ertapenem, erythromycin, esmolol, etoposide, etoposide phosphate, famotidine, fentanyl, filgrastim, fluconazole, fludarabine, fluorouracil, foscarnet, fosphenytoin, furosemide, ganciclovir, gemcitabine, gentamicin, granisetron, haloperidol, heparin, hetastarch, hydrocortisone, hydromorphone, idarubicin, imipenem/cilastatin, insulin, regular, isoproterenol, ketorolac, labetalol, leucovorin calcium, levofloxacin, lidocaine, linezolid, lorazepam, magnesium sulfate,

mannitol, melphalan, meperidine, meropenem, mesna, methylprednisolone, metoclopramide, metoprolol, metronidazole, midazolam, milrinone, minocycline, mitomycin, mitoxantrone, morphine, moxifloxacin, nalbuphine, naloxone, nicardipine, nitroglycerin, nitroprusside, norepinephrine, octreotide, ondansetron, oxaliplatin, paclitaxel, palonosetron, pamidronate, pemetrexed, pentamidine, pentobarbital, phenobarbital, phenylephrine, piperacillin/tazobactam, potassium acetate, potassium chloride, procainamide, prochlorperazine, promethazine, propofol, propranolol, remifentanil, rituximab, rocuronium, sargramostim, sodium acetate, sodium bicarbonate, sodium phosphate, succinylcholine, sufentanil, tacrolimus, theophylline, thiopental, thiotepa, tigecycline, tirofiban, tobramycin, topotecan, trastuzumab, trimethoprim/sulfamethoxazole, vancomycin, vasopressin, vecuronium, verapamil, vinblastine, vincristine, vinorelbine, voriconazole, zidovudine, zoledronic acid.

- **Y-Site Incompatibility:** cefepime, diazepam, methotrexate, pantoprazole, phenytoin, potassium phosphate.

Patient/Family Teaching

- Emphasize need for adequate fluid intake throughout therapy. Patient should void frequently to decrease bladder irritation from metabolites excreted by the kidneys. Notify health care professional immediately if hematuria is noted.
- Instruct patient to drink at least 8 glasses of water/day during and for 3 days after completion of therapy.
- Advise patient to avoid grapefruit and grapefruit juice during therapy.
- Instruct patient to notify health care professional promptly if fever; chills; cough; hoarseness; sore throat; signs of infection; lower back or side pain; painful or difficult urination; bleeding gums; bruising; petechiae; blood in urine, stool, or emesis; or confusion occurs.
- Caution patient to avoid crowds and persons with known infections. Instruct patient to use soft toothbrush and electric razor and to avoid falls. Patient should also be cautioned not to drink alcoholic beverages or to take products containing aspirin or NSAIDs, as these may precipitate GI hemorrhage.
- Discuss with patient the possibility of hair loss. Explore methods of coping.
- Instruct patient to notify health care professional of all Rx or OTC medications, vitamins, or herbal products being taken and to consult with health care professional before taking other medications.
- Instruct patient not to receive any vaccinations without advice of health care professional; ifosfamide may decrease antibody response to and increase risk of adverse reactions from live-virus vaccines.

- Rep: Advise females of reproductive potential to notify health care professional if pregnancy is planned or suspected or if breastfeeding. Review with patient the need for contraception during therapy and for at least 6 mo after therapy. Women should avoid pregnancy and breastfeeding, and men should avoid fathering a child during and for at least 6 mo after end of therapy. Caution patient about the potential for amenorrhea, premature menopause, and sterility from this medication.

Evaluation/Desired Outcomes

- Decrease in size or spread of malignant germ cell testicular carcinoma.

BEERS

⚠ iloperidone
(eye-loe-**per**-i-done)
Fanapt
Classification
Therapeutic: antipsychotics
Pharmacologic: benzisoxazoles

Indications
Schizophrenia.

Action
May act by antagonizing dopamine and serotonin in the CNS. **Therapeutic Effects:** Decreased symptoms of schizophrenia.

Pharmacokinetics
Absorption: Well absorbed (96%) following oral administration.

Distribution: Unknown.

Metabolism and Excretion: Extensively metabolized by the liver primarily by the CYP3A4 and CYP2D6 isoenzymes. ⚠ The CYP2D6 enzyme system exhibits genetic polymorphism (7–10% of Caucasians and 3–8% of Black/African Americans are considered poor metabolizers [PM]). Two major metabolites (P88 and P95) may be partially responsible for pharmacologic activity. 58% excreted in urine as metabolites in extensive metabolizers (EM) and 45% in PM; 20% eliminated in feces in EM and 22.1% in PM.

Half-life: *EMs:* iloperidone–18 hr, P88–26 hr, P95–23 hr; *PMs:* iloperidone–33 hr, P88–37 hr, P95–31 hr.

TIME/ACTION PROFILE (antipsychotic effect)

ROUTE	ONSET	PEAK	DURATION
PO	2–4 wk	2–4 hr†	unknown

†Blood level.

Contraindications/Precautions
Contraindicated in: Hypersensitivity; Bradycardia; recent MI, or uncompensated HF(↑ risk of serious ar-

rhythmias); Congenital long QT syndrome, QTc interval >500 msec or history of cardiac arrhythmias; Electrolyte abnormalities, especially hypomagnesemia or hypokalemia (correct prior to therapy); Severe hepatic impairment; Lactation: Lactation.

Use Cautiously in: Known cardiovascular disease including HF, history of MI/ischemia, conduction abnormalities, cerebrovascular disease, or other conditions known to predispose to hypotension including dehydration, hypovolemia, concurrent antihypertensive therapy (↑ risk of orthostatic hypotension); Known ↓ WBC or history of drug-induced leukopenia/neutropenia; Circumstances that may result in ↑ body temperature, including strenuous exercise, exposure to extreme heat, concurrent anticholinergic activity, or dehydration (may impair thermoregulation); Patients at risk for aspiration or falls; Moderate hepatic impairment; OB: Neonates at ↑ risk for extrapyramidal symptoms and withdrawal after delivery when exposed during the 3rd trimester; use only if potential maternal benefit justifies potential fetal risk; Pedi: Safety and effectiveness not established in children; Geri: Appears on Beers list. ↑ risk of stroke, cognitive decline, and mortality in older adults with dementia. Avoid use in older adults, except for schizophrenia.

Adverse Reactions/Side Effects

CV: orthostatic hypotension, tachycardia, palpitations, QTc interval prolongation. **EENT:** nasal congestion. **Endo:** hyperglycemia, hyperprolactinemia. **GI:** dry mouth, nausea, abdominal discomfort, diarrhea, weight loss. **GU:** priapism, urinary incontinence. **Metab:** weight gain, dyslipidemia. **MS:** ↓ bone density, musculoskeletal stiffness. **Neuro:** dizziness, drowsiness, fatigue, agitation, delusions, extrapyramidal disorders, NEUROLEPTIC MALIGNANT SYNDROME, restlessness, SUICIDAL THOUGHTS, tardive dyskinesia. **Misc:** HYPERSENSITIVITY REACTIONS (including anaphylaxis and angioedema).

Interactions

Drug-Drug: Avoid concurrent use of **QT interval prolonging medications,** including **quinidine, procainamide, amiodarone, sotalol, chlorpromazine, thioridazine, moxifloxacin, pentamidine,** and **methadone.** Concurrent use of **strong CYP2D6 inhibitors,** including **fluoxetine** and **paroxetine** ↑ levels and the risk of toxicity; ↓ dose. Concurrent use of **strong CYP3A4 inhibitors,** including **ketoconazole** and **clarithromycin** ↑ levels and the risk of toxicity; ↓ dose. Concurrent use of **antihypertensives** including **diuretics** may ↑ risk of orthostatic hypotension. Concurrent use of **anticholinergics** may ↑ risk of impaired thermoregulation.

Route/Dosage

PO (Adults): Initiate treatment with 1 mg twice daily on the first day, then 2 mg twice daily the 2nd day, then ↑ by 2 mg/day every day until a target dose of 12–24 mg/day given in two divided doses is reached; *Concur-*

rent use of strong CYP2D6 or CYP3A4 inhibitors: ↓ dose by 50%; if inhibitor is withdrawn ↑ dose to previous amount. Retitration is required if iloperidone is discontinued >300 days; *Poor metabolizers of CYP2D6:* ↓ dose by 50%.

Availability (generic available)

Tablets: 1 mg, 2 mg, 4 mg, 6 mg, 8 mg, 10 mg, 12 mg.

NURSING IMPLICATIONS

Assessment

- Monitor patient's mental status (delusions, hallucinations, and behavior) before and periodically during therapy.
- Monitor mood changes. Assess for suicidal tendencies, especially during early therapy. Restrict amount of drug available to patient.
- Monitor BP (sitting, standing, lying down) and pulse before and periodically during therapy. May cause prolonged QT interval, tachycardia, and orthostatic hypotension. Protect patient from falls.
- Observe patient when administering medication to ensure that medication is actually swallowed and not hoarded.
- Monitor patient for onset of extrapyramidal side effects (*akathisia:* restlessness; *dystonia:* muscle spasms and twisting motions; or *pseudoparkinsonism:* mask-like face, rigidity, tremors, drooling, shuffling gait, dysphagia). Report these symptoms; reduction of dose or discontinuation of medication may be necessary.
- Monitor for tardive dyskinesia (involuntary rhythmic movement of mouth, face, and extremities). Report immediately and discontinue therapy; may be irreversible.
- Monitor for development of neuroleptic malignant syndrome (fever, respiratory distress, tachycardia, seizures, diaphoresis, hypertension or hypotension, pallor, tiredness). Discontinue iloperidone and notify health care professional immediately if these symptoms occur.
- Monitor for symptoms related to hyperprolactinemia (menstrual abnormalities, galactorrhea, sexual dysfunction).
- Assess weight and BMI initially and during therapy. Refer as appropriate for nutritional/weight and medical management.
- Assess for falls risk. Drowsiness, orthostatic hypotension, and motor and sensory instability increase risk. Institute prevention if indicated.

Lab Test Considerations

- Monitor fasting blood glucose before and periodically during therapy in diabetic patients.
- Monitor CBC frequently during initial mo of therapy in patients with pre-existing or history of low WBC. May cause leukopenia, neutropenia, or agranulocytosis. Discontinue therapy if this occurs.
- Monitor serum potassium and magnesium levels in patients at risk for electrolyte disturbances.

- Monitor serum prolactin prior to and periodically during therapy. May cause ↑ serum prolactin levels.

Implementation
- Do not confuse Fanapt with Xanax.
- **PO:** Administer twice daily without regard to food.

Patient/Family Teaching
- Instruct patient to take medication exactly as directed. If doses are missed for >3 days, restart at initiation dose. Advise patient that appearance of tablets in stool is normal and not of concern.
- Inform patient of the possibility of extrapyramidal symptoms, neuroleptic malignant syndrome, and tardive dyskinesia. Instruct patient to report these symptoms immediately to health care professional.
- Advise patient to change positions slowly to minimize orthostatic hypotension. Protect from falls.
- Inform patient of potential for weight gain and hyperglycemia, and the need for monitoring weight and blood glucose periodically during therapy.
- May cause drowsiness. Caution patient to avoid driving or other activities requiring alertness until response to medication is known.
- Extremes in temperature should also be avoided; this drug impairs body temperature regulation.
- Instruct patient to notify health care professional promptly if sore throat, fever, unusual bleeding or bruising, rash, tremors, palpitations, fainting, menstrual abnormalities, galactorrhea, or sexual dysfunction occur.
- Advise patient and family to notify health care professional if thoughts about suicide or dying, attempts to commit suicide; new or worse depression; new or worse anxiety; feeling very agitated or restless; panic attacks; trouble sleeping; new or worse irritability; acting aggressive; being angry or violent; acting on dangerous impulses; an extreme increase in activity and talking; other unusual changes in behavior or mood occur.
- Caution patient to avoid concurrent use of alcohol and other CNS depressants.
- Advise patient to notify health care professional of all Rx or OTC medications, vitamins, or herbal products being taken and to consult with health care professional before taking other medications.
- Advise patient to notify health care professional of medication regimen before treatment or surgery.
- Rep: Advise females of reproductive potential to notify health care professional if pregnancy is planned or suspected, and to avoid breastfeeding during therapy. Monitor neonates exposed to iloperidone during the third trimester of pregnancy for extrapyramidal and/or withdrawal symptoms following delivery. There have been reports of agitation, hypertonia, hypotonia, tremor, somnolence, respiratory distress and feeding disorder in these neonates. Monitor breastfed infants for excessive drowsiness,

lethargy, and developmental delays. Encourage women who become pregnant while taking iloperidone to enroll in the National Pregnancy Registry for Atypical Antipsychotics at 1-866-961-2388 or visit http://womensmentalhealth.org/clinical-and-research-programs/pregnancyregistry/.
- Emphasize the need for continued follow-up for psychotherapy and monitoring for side effects.

Evaluation/Desired Outcomes
- Decrease in excited, paranoid, or withdrawn behavior.

☒ imatinib (i-mat-i-nib)
Gleevec

Classification
Therapeutic: antineoplastics
Pharmacologic: enzyme inhibitors

Indications
☒ Newly diagnosed Philadelphia positive (Ph+) chronic myeloid leukemia (CML). CML in blast crisis, accelerated phase, or in chronic phase after failure of interferon-alpha treatment. ☒ Kit (CD117) positive metastatic/unresectable malignant GI stromal tumors. Adjuvant treatment following resection of Kit (CD117) positive GI stromal tumors. ☒ Pediatric patients with Ph+ CML after failure of bone marrow transplant or resistance to interferon-alpha. ☒ Adult patients with relapsed or refractory Ph+ acute lymphoblastic leukemia (ALL). ☒ Newly diagnosed Ph+ ALL (in combination with chemotherapy). ☒ Myelodysplastic/myeloproliferative disease associated with platelet-derived growth factor receptor gene rearrangements. ☒ Aggressive systemic mastocytosis without the D816V c-Kit mutation or with c-Kit mutational status unknown. Hypereosinophilic syndrome and/or chronic eosinophilic leukemia. Unresectable, recurrent, or metastatic dermatofibrosarcoma protuberans.

Action
Inhibits kinases, which may be produced by malignant cell lines. **Therapeutic Effects:** Inhibits production of malignant cell lines with decreased proliferation of leukemic cells in CML, hypereosinophilic syndrome and/or chronic eosinophilic leukemia, and ALL and malignant cells in GI stromal tumor, myelodysplastic/myeloproliferative disease, aggressive systemic mastocytosis, and dermatofibrosarcoma protuberans.

Pharmacokinetics
Absorption: Well absorbed (98%) following oral administration.
Distribution: Unknown.
Protein Binding: 95%.
Metabolism and Excretion: Primarily metabolized by the liver via the CYP3A4 isoenzyme to N-deme-

thyl imatinib, which is as active as imatinib. Excreted mostly in feces as metabolites. 5% excreted unchanged in urine.

Half-life: *Imatinib:* 18 hr; *N-desmethyl imatinib:* 40 hr.

TIME/ACTION PROFILE (plasma concentrations of imatinib)

ROUTE	ONSET	PEAK	DURATION
PO	unknown	2–4 hr	24 hr

Contraindications/Precautions

Contraindicated in: Hypersensitivity; OB: Pregnancy; Lactation: Lactation.

Use Cautiously in: Hepatic impairment (dose ↓ recommended if bilirubin >3 x upper limit of normal (ULN) or AST/ALT >5 x ULN); Cardiac disease (severe HF and left ventricular dysfunction may occur); Renal impairment, diabetes, hypertension, HF (↑ risk of nephrotoxicity); Rep: Women of reproductive potential; Pedi: Children <1 yr (safety and effectiveness not established); Geri: ↑ risk of edema in older adults.

Adverse Reactions/Side Effects

CV: edema, HF. **Derm:** petechiae, pruritus, rash, DRUG RASH WITH EOSINOPHILIA AND SYSTEMIC SYMPTOMS (DRESS). **EENT:** epistaxis, nasopharyngitis, blurred vision. **Endo:** ↓ growth (in children), hypothyroidism. **GI:** abdominal pain, anorexia, constipation, diarrhea, dyspepsia, nausea, vomiting, HEPATOTOXICITY. **GU:** nephrotoxicity. **Hemat:** BLEEDING, NEUTROPENIA, THROMBOCYTOPENIA. **Metab:** ↑ weight. **MS:** arthralgia, muscle cramps, myalgia, pain. **Neuro:** fatigue, headache, weakness, dizziness, somnolence. **Resp:** cough, dyspnea, pneumonia. **Misc:** fever, night sweats, TUMOR LYSIS SYNDROME.

Interactions

Drug-Drug: **Strong CYP3A4 inhibitors,** including **ketoconazole, itraconazole, clarithromycin, atazanavir, nefazodone, nelfinavir, ritonavir,** or **voriconazole,** may ↑ levels and risk of toxicity. **Strong CYP3A4 inducers,** including **dexamethasone, phenytoin, carbamazepine, rifampin, rifabutin,** and **phenobarbital,** may ↓ levels and effectiveness; if used concurrently, ↑ imatinib dose by 50%. May ↑ levels and risk of toxicity of **benzodiazepines, simvastatin,** and **calcium channel blockers.**

Drug-Food: **Grapefruit juice** may ↑ levels and risk of toxicity; avoid concurrent use.

Route/Dosage

Chronic Myeloid Leukemia

PO (Adults): *Chronic phase:* 400 mg once daily, may be ↑ to 600 mg once daily; *Accelerated phase or blast crisis:* 600 mg once daily; may be ↑ to 800 mg/day given as 400 mg twice daily based on response and circumstances.

PO (Children): *Newly diagnosed Ph+ CML:* 340 mg/m² once daily (not to exceed 600 mg); *CML recurrence*

after failure of bone marrow transplant or resistance to interferon-alpha: 260 mg/m² once daily.

Hepatic Impairment

PO (Adults): *Severe hepatic impairment:* ↓ dose by 25%.

Renal Impairment

PO (Adults): *CCr 40–59 mL/min:* Do not exceed dose of 600 mg/day; *CCr 20–39 mL/min:* ↓ initial dose by 50%; ↑ as tolerated.

Gastrointestinal Stromal Tumors

PO (Adults): *Metastatic or unresectable:* 400 mg once daily; may be ↑ to 400 mg twice daily if well tolerated and response insufficient; *Adjuvant treatment after resection:* 400 mg once daily.

Hepatic Impairment

PO (Adults): *Severe hepatic impairment:* ↓ dose by 25%.

Renal Impairment

PO (Adults): *CCr 40–59 mL/min:* Do not exceed dose of 600 mg/day; *CCr 20–39 mL/min:* ↓ initial dose by 50%; ↑ as tolerated.

Ph+ Acute Lymphoblastic Leukemia

PO (Adults): 600 mg once daily.
PO (Children): 340 mg/m² once daily (not to exceed 600 mg).

Hepatic Impairment

PO (Adults): *Severe hepatic impairment:* ↓ dose by 25%.

Renal Impairment

PO (Adults): *CCr 40–59 mL/min:* Do not exceed dose of 600 mg/day; *CCr 20–39 mL/min:* ↓ initial dose by 50%; ↑ as tolerated.

Myelodysplastic/Myeloproliferative Diseases

PO (Adults): 400 mg once daily.

Hepatic Impairment

PO (Adults): *Severe hepatic impairment:* ↓ dose by 25%.

Renal Impairment

PO (Adults): *CCr 40–59 mL/min:* Do not exceed dose of 600 mg/day; *CCr 20–39 mL/min:* ↓ initial dose by 50%; ↑ as tolerated.

Aggressive Systemic Mastocytosis

PO (Adults): 400 mg once daily. *Patients with eosinophilia:* 100 mg once daily; ↑ to 400 mg once daily if well tolerated and response insufficient.

Hepatic Impairment

PO (Adults): *Severe hepatic impairment:* ↓ dose by 25%.

Renal Impairment

PO (Adults): *CCr 40–59 mL/min:* Do not exceed dose of 600 mg/day; *CCr 20–39 mL/min:* ↓ initial dose by 50%; ↑ as tolerated.

Hypereosinophilic Syndrome and/or Chronic Eosinophilic Leukemia

PO (Adults): 400 mg once daily. *For patients with FIP1L1–PDGFRa fusion kinase:* 100 mg once daily; ↑ to 400 mg once daily if well tolerated and response insufficient.

Hepatic Impairment
PO (Adults): *Severe hepatic impairment:* ↓ dose by 25%.

Renal Impairment
PO (Adults): *CCr 40–59 mL/min:* Do not exceed dose of 600 mg/day; *CCr 20–39 mL/min:* ↓ initial dose by 50%; ↑ as tolerated.

Dermatofibrosarcoma Protuberans
PO (Adults): 400 mg twice daily.

Hepatic Impairment
PO (Adults): *Severe hepatic impairment:* ↓ dose by 25%.

Renal Impairment
PO (Adults): *CCr 40–59 mL/min:* Do not exceed dose of 600 mg/day; *CCr 20–39 mL/min:* ↓ initial dose by 50%; ↑ as tolerated.

Availability (generic available)
Tablets: 100 mg, 400 mg.

NURSING IMPLICATIONS
Assessment
- Monitor for fluid retention. Weigh regularly, and assess for signs of pleural effusion, pericardial effusion, pulmonary edema, ascites (dyspnea, periorbital edema, swelling in feet and ankles, weight gain). Evaluate unexpected weight gain. Edema is usually managed with diuretics. General fluid retention is usually dose related, more common in accelerated phase or blast crisis, and is more common in the elderly. Treatment usually involves diuretics, supportive therapy, and interruption of imatinib.
- Monitor growth rate in children and adolescents; may cause decrease in growth.
- Monitor vital signs; may cause fever.
- Monitor for tumor lysis syndrome (malignant disease progression, high WBC counts, hyperuricemia, hyperkalemia, hyperphosphatemia, hypocalcemia, and/or dehydration). Prevent by maintaining adequate hydration and correcting uric acid levels prior to starting imatinib.
- Monitor for signs and symptoms of DRESS (fever, rash, lymphadenopathy, and/or facial swelling, associated with involvement of other organ systems (hepatitis, nephritis, hematologic abnormalities, myocarditis, myositis) during therapy. May resemble an acute viral infection. Eosinophilia is often present. Discontinue therapy if signs occur.

Lab Test Considerations
- Monitor liver function before and monthly during treatment or when clinically indicated. May cause ↑ AST/ALT and bilirubin, which usually lasts 1 wk and may require dose reduction or interruption. If bilirubin is >3 x ULN or AST/ALT are >5 x ULN, withhold dose until bilirubin levels return to <1.5 x ULN and AST/ALT levels to <2.5 x ULN. Treatment may then be continued at reduced levels (patients on 400 mg/day should receive 300 mg/day and patients receiving 600 mg/day should receive 400 mg/day).
- Monitor CBC weekly for the 1st mo, biweekly for the 2nd mo, and periodically during therapy. May cause neutropenia and thrombocytopenia, usually lasting 2–3 wk or 3–4 wk, respectively, and anemia. Usually requires dose reduction, but may require discontinuation (see Implementation).
- Patients receiving *chronic phase, myelodysplastic/myeloproliferative disease, aggressive systemic mastocytosis, and hypereosinophilic syndrome and/or chronic eosinophilic leukemia* treatment who develop an absolute neutrophil count (ANC) <1.0 × 10⁹/L and/or platelets <50 × 10⁹/L should stop imatinib until ANC ≥1.5 × 10⁹/L and platelets are ≥75 × 10⁹/L. Then resume imatinib treatment at 400 mg or 600 mg/day.
- *Patients receiving accelerated phase and blast crisis treatment or Ph + ALL* treatment who develop an ANC <0.5 × 10⁹/L and/or platelets <10 × 10⁹/L should determine if cytopenia is related to leukemia via marrow aspirate or biopsy. If cytopenia is unrelated to leukemia, reduce dose to 400 mg/day. If cytopenia persists for 2 wk, reduce dose to 300 mg/day. If cytopenia persists for 4 wk and is still unrelated to leukemia, stop imatinib until ANC ≥1 × 10⁹/L and platelets are ≥20 × 10⁹/L. Then resume imatinib treatment at 300 mg/day.
- *Patients receiving aggressive systemic mastocytosis with eosinophilia or hypereosinophilic syndrome and/or chronic eosinophilic leukemia with FIP1L1–PDGFRa fusion kinase* treatment who develop ANC <1.0 × 10⁹/L and platelets <50 × 10⁹/L should stop imatinib until ANC ≥1.5 × 10⁹/L and platelets ≥75 × 10⁹/L. Resume treatment at previous dose.
- May cause hypokalemia.
- Verify pregnancy status in females with reproductive potential before starting therapy.

Implementation
- **High Alert:** Fatalities have occurred with incorrect administration of chemotherapeutic agents. Before administering, clarify all ambiguous orders; double-check single, daily, and course-of-therapy dose limits; have second practitioner independently double-check original order and dose calculations. Therapy should be initiated by physician experienced in the treatment of patients with chronic myeloid leukemia.

✦ = Canadian drug name. ▓ = Genetic implication. ~~Strikethrough~~ = Discontinued. CAPITALS = life-threatening. <u>Underline</u> = most frequent.

- Patients requiring anticoagulation should receive low-molecular-weight or standard heparin, not warfarin.
- Treatment should be continued as long as patient continues to benefit.
- **PO:** Administer with food and a full glass of water to minimize GI irritation.
- Tablets may be dispersed in water or apple juice (50 mL for the 100-mg and 100 mL for the 400-mg tablet) and stirred with a spoon for patients unable to swallow pills. Administer immediately after suspension.
- Doses for children may be given once daily or divided into two doses, one in morning and one in evening.
- Administer doses >800 mg/day as 400 mg twice daily to decrease exposure to iron.

Patient/Family Teaching
- Explain purpose of imatinib to patient. Instruct patient to take imatinib as directed. If a dose is missed, take next dose at regular scheduled time. Do not double doses.
- Advise patient to avoid grapefruit and grapefruit juice during therapy.
- May cause drowsiness or dizziness. Caution patient to avoid driving or other activities requiring alertness until response to medication is known.
- Inform patient of possibility of edema and fluid retention. Advise patient to notify health care professional if unexpected rapid weight gain occurs.
- Advise patient to notify health care professional if signs and symptoms of liver failure (jaundice, anorexia, bleeding or bruising) or DRESS occur.
- Rep: Advise female patient of reproductive potential to use effective contraception during and for at least 14 days after last dose of imatinib. Advise patient to notify health care professional if pregnancy is planned or suspected; avoid breastfeeding for at least 1 mo after last dose of imatinib.

Evaluation/Desired Outcomes
- Decrease in production of leukemic cells in patients with CML, hypereosinophilic syndrome and/or chronic eosinophilic leukemia, and ALL and malignant cells in GI stromal tumor, myelodysplastic/myeloproliferative disease, aggressive systemic mastocytosis, and dermatofibrosarcoma protuberans.

imipenem/cilastatin
(i-me-**pen**-em/sye-la-**stat**-in)
Primaxin
Classification
Therapeutic: anti-infectives
Pharmacologic: carbapenems

Indications
Treatment of: Lower respiratory tract infections, Urinary tract infections, Abdominal infections, Gynecologic infections, Skin and skin structure infections, Bone and joint infections, Bacteremia, Endocarditis, Polymicrobic infections.

Action
Imipenem binds to the bacterial cell wall, resulting in cell death. Combination with cilastatin prevents renal inactivation of imipenem, resulting in high urinary concentrations. Imipenem resists the actions of many enzymes that degrade most other penicillins and penicillin-like anti-infectives. **Therapeutic Effects:** Bactericidal action against susceptible bacteria. **Spectrum:** Spectrum is broad. Active against most gram-positive aerobic cocci: *Streptococcus pneumoniae*, Group A beta-hemolytic streptococci, *Enterococcus*, *Staphylococcus aureus*. Active against many gram-negative bacillary organisms: *Escherichia coli*, *Klebsiella*, *Acinetobacter*, *Proteus*, *Serratia*, *Pseudomonas aeruginosa*. Also displays activity against: *Salmonella*, *Shigella*, *Neisseria gonorrhoeae*, Numerous anaerobes.

Pharmacokinetics
Absorption: IV administration results in complete bioavailability.
Distribution: Widely distributed to tissues.
Metabolism and Excretion: 70% excreted unchanged by the kidneys.
Half-life: 1 hr (↑ in renal impairment).

TIME/ACTION PROFILE (plasma concentrations)

ROUTE	ONSET	PEAK	DURATION
IV	rapid	end of infusion	6–8 hr

Contraindications/Precautions
Contraindicated in: Hypersensitivity; Cross-sensitivity may occur with penicillins and cephalosporins.
Use Cautiously in: Previous history of multiple hypersensitivity reactions; Seizure disorders; Renal impairment (dose ↓ required if CCr ≤90 mL/min); OB: Safety not established in pregnancy; Lactation: Use during breastfeeding only if potential maternal benefit justifies potential risk to infant; Pedi: Children with CNS infections (↑ risk of seizures) or children <30 kg with renal impairment (safety and effectiveness not established); Geri: Older adults may be at ↑ risk for adverse reactions due to age-related ↓ in renal function.

Adverse Reactions/Side Effects
CV: hypotension. Derm: rash, pruritus, sweating, urticaria. GI: diarrhea, nausea, vomiting, CLOSTRIDIOIDES DIFFICILE-ASSOCIATED DIARRHEA (CDAD). Hemat: eosinophilia. Local: phlebitis at IV site. Neuro: dizziness, SEIZURES, somnolence. Misc: fever, HYPERSENSITIVITY REACTIONS (including anaphylaxis), superinfection.

Interactions
Drug-Drug: Do not admix with **aminoglycosides**; inactivation may occur. **Probenecid** ↓ renal excretion

and ↑ levels. ↑ risk of seizures with **ganciclovir** or **cyclosporine**; avoid concurrent use with ganciclovir. May ↓ serum **valproate** levels and ↑ risk of seizures.

Route/Dosage
IV (Adults): *If infection is suspected or proven to be due to a susceptible bacterial species:* 500 mg every 6 hr *or* 1 g every 8 hr; *If infection is suspected or proven to be due to bacterial species with intermediate susceptibility :* 1 g every 6 hr.
IV (Children ≥3 mo): 15–25 mg/kg every 6 hr; higher doses have been used in older children with cystic fibrosis.
IV (Children 4 wk–3 mo): 25 mg/kg every 6 hr.
IV (Children 1–4 wk): 25 mg/kg every 8 hr.
IV (Children <1 wk): 25 mg/kg every 12 hr.

Renal Impairment
IV (Adults): If infection is suspected or proven to be due to a susceptible bacterial species: *CCr 60–89 mL/min:* 400 mg every 6 hr *or* 500 mg every 6 hr; *CCr 30–59 mL/min:* 300 mg every 6 hr *or* 500 mg every 8 hr; *CCr 15–29 mL/min:* 200 mg every 6 hr *or* 500 mg every 12 hr; *CCr <15 mL/min receiving hemodialysis:* 200 mg every 6 hr *or* 500 mg every 12 hr; If infection is suspected or proven to be due to bacterial species with intermediate susceptibility: *CCr 60–89 mL/min:* 750 mg every 8 hr; *CCr 30–59 mL/min:* 500 mg every 6 hr; *CCr 15–29 mL/min:* 500 mg every 12 hr; *CCr <15 mL/min receiving hemodialysis:* 500 mg every 12 hr.

Availability (generic available)
Powder for injection: 250 mg imipenem/250 mg cilastatin, 500 mg imipenem/500 mg cilastatin.

NURSING IMPLICATIONS
Assessment
● Assess patient for infection (vital signs; appearance of wound, sputum, urine, and stool; WBC) at beginning of and throughout therapy.
● Obtain a history before initiating therapy to determine previous use of and reactions to penicillins. Persons with a negative history of penicillin sensitivity may still have an allergic response.
● Obtain specimens for culture and sensitivity before initiating therapy. First dose may be given before receiving results.
● Observe patient for signs and symptoms of anaphylaxis (rash, pruritus, laryngeal edema, wheezing). Discontinue the drug and notify the physician immediately if these occur. Have epinephrine, an antihistamine, and resuscitative equipment close by in the event of an anaphylactic reaction.
● Monitor bowel function. Diarrhea, abdominal cramping, fever, and bloody stools should be reported to health care professional promptly as a sign of CDAD. May begin up to several wk following cessation of therapy.

Lab Test Considerations
● BUN, AST, ALT, LDH, serum alkaline phosphatase, bilirubin, and creatinine may be transiently ↑.
● Hemoglobin and hematocrit concentrations may be ↓.
● May cause positive direct Coombs' test.

Implementation
IV Administration
● **Intermittent Infusion:** Reconstitute each 250- or 500-mg vial with 10 mL of D5W, D5/0.9% NaCl, 0.9% NaCl, or D5/0.45% NaCl and shake well. *Dilution:* Further dilute in 100 mL of D5W or 0.9% NaCl. Solution may range from clear to yellow in color. Infusion is stable for 4 hr at room temperature and 24 hr if refrigerated. *Concentration:* 2.5 mg/mL (with 250-mg vial); 5 mg/mL (with 500-mg vial). *Rate:* Infuse doses ≤500 mg over 20–30 min. Infuse doses ≥750 mg over 40–60 min. Pedi: Infuse doses ≤500 mg over 15–30 min. Infuse doses >500 mg over 40–60 min.
● Rapid infusion may cause nausea and vomiting. If these symptoms develop, slow infusion.
● **Y-Site Compatibility:** acyclovir, amifostine, amikacin, aminocaproic acid, anidulafungin, argatroban, arsenic trioxide, ascorbic acid, atracurium, atropine, benztropine, bivalirudin, bleomycin, bumetanide, buprenorphine, butorphanol, carboplatin, carmustine, caspofungin, cefazolin, cefepime, cefotaxime, cefotetan, cefoxitin, ceftazidime, ceftazidime/avibactam, cefuroxime, chloramphenicol, cisatracurium, cisplatin, clindamycin, cyanocobalamin, cyclophosphamide, cyclosporine, cytarabine, dactinomycin, daunorubicin hydrochloride, dexamethasone, dexmedetomidine, dexrazoxane, digoxin, diltiazem, diphenhydramine, docetaxel, dopamine, doxorubicin hydrochloride, doxorubicin liposomal, doxycycline, enalaprilat, ephedrine, epinephrine, epirubicin, epoetin alfa, eptifibatide, erythromycin, esmolol, etoposide, famotidine, fentanyl, fludarabine, fluorouracil, folic acid, foscarnet, fosphenytoin, furosemide, gemtuzumab, gentamicin, glycopyrrolate, granisetron, heparin, hydrocortisone, hydromorphone, idarubicin, ifosfamide, indomethacin, insulin, regular, irinotecan, isavuconazonium, isoproterenol, ketorolac, labetalol, leucovorin calcium, levofloxacin, lidocaine, linezolid, magnesium sulfate, melphalan, meropenem/vaborbactam, mesna, methotrexate, methylprednisolone, metoclopramide, metoprolol, mitomycin, mitoxantrone, morphine, multivitamins, nafcillin, naloxone, nitroglycerin, norepinephrine, octreotide, ondansetron, oxacillin, oxaliplatin, oxytocin, paclitaxel, pamidronate, pantoprazole, pemetrexed, penicillin G, pentobarbital, phentolamine, phenylephrine, phytonadione, plazomicin, potassium acetate, potassium chloride, propofol, propranolol, protamine, remi-

fentanil, rituximab, rocuronium, sodium acetate, succinylcholine, sufentanil, tacrolimus, tedizolid, theophylline, thiotepa, tigecycline, tirofiban, tobramycin, trastuzumab, vasopressin, verapamil, vinblastine, vincristine, vinorelbine, voriconazole, zidovudine, zoledronic acid.

• **Y-Site Incompatibility:** alemtuzumab, allopurinol, amiodarone, amphotericin B deoxycholate, amphotericin B lipid complex, amphotericin B liposomal, azathioprine, blinatumomab, ceftriaxone, chlorpromazine, dacarbazine, dantrolene, daptomycin, diazepam, diazoxide, etoposide phosphate, ganciclovir, gemcitabine, haloperidol, lorazepam, mannitol, milrinone, mycophenolate, nalbuphine, nicardipine, palonosetron, phenytoin, prochlorperazine, pyridoxine, sargramostim, sodium bicarbonate, thiamine, topotecan, trimethoprim/sulfamethoxazole, vecuronium.

• **Additive Incompatibility:** May be inactivated if administered concurrently with aminoglycosides. If administered concurrently, administer in separate sites, if possible, at least 1 hr apart. If second site is unavailable, flush lines between medications.

Patient/Family Teaching

• Advise patient to report the signs of superinfection (black, furry overgrowth on the tongue; vaginal itching or discharge; loose or foul-smelling stools) and allergy. Consult health care professional before treating with antidiarrheals.

• Caution patient to notify health care professional if fever and diarrhea occur, especially if stool contains blood, pus, or mucus. Advise patient not to treat diarrhea without consulting health care professional. May occur up to several wk after discontinuation of medication.

• Rep: Advise females of reproductive potential to notify health care professional if pregnancy is planned or suspected or if breastfeeding.

Evaluation/Desired Outcomes

• Resolution of the signs and symptoms of infection. Length of time for complete resolution depends on the organism and site of infection.

---

imipenem/cilastatin/relebactam

(i-me-**pen**-em/sye-la-**stat**-in/**rel**-e-**bak**-tam)

Recarbrio

Classification
Therapeutic: anti-infectives
Pharmacologic: carbapenems, beta-lactamase inhibitors

Indications

Complicated urinary tract infections, including pyelonephritis (for patients with limited or no alternative treatment options). Complicated intra-abdominal infections (for patients with limited or no alternative treatment options). Hospital-acquired or ventilator-associated pneumonia.

Action

Imipenem binds to the bacterial cell wall, resulting in cell death. Cilastatin is a renal dehydropeptidase inhibitor that prevents renal inactivation of imipenem (does not have antibacterial properties). Relebactam inhibits beta-lactamase, which is an enzyme that can destroy beta-lactam antibiotics. **Therapeutic Effects:** Bactericidal action against susceptible bacteria. **Spectrum:** Spectrum is broad. Active against many gram-negative aerobic bacteria: *Acinetobacter calcoaceticus-baumannii complex, Citrobacter freundii, Enterobacter cloacae, Escherichia coli, Haemophilus influenzae, Klebsiella aerogenes, Klebsiella oxytoca, Klebsiella pneumoniae, Pseudomonas aeruginosa, Serratia marcescens.* Also active against the following gram-negative anaerobic bacteria: *Bacteroides caccae, Bacteroides fragilis, Bacteroides ovatus, Bacteroides stercoris, Bacteroides thetaiotaomicron, Bacteroides uniformis, Bacteroides vulgatus, Fusobacterium nucleatum.*

Pharmacokinetics

Absorption: IV administration results in complete bioavailability.

Distribution: Widely distributed to tissues.

Metabolism and Excretion: Minimally metabolized. Primarily excreted unchanged by the kidneys (imipenem 63%, cilastatin 77%, relebactam >90%).

Half-life: 1–1.2 hr.

TIME/ACTION PROFILE (plasma concentrations)

ROUTE	ONSET	PEAK	DURATION
IV	unknown	end of infusion	6 hr

Contraindications/Precautions

Contraindicated in: Hypersensitivity (cross-sensitivity may occur with penicillins and cephalosporins).

Use Cautiously in: Seizure disorders; Renal impairment (dose ↓ required if CCr <90 mL/min); OB: Use during pregnancy only if potential maternal benefit justifies potential fetal risk; Lactation: Use while breastfeeding only if potential maternal benefit justifies potential risk to infant; Pedi: Safety and effectiveness not established in children; Geri: Older adults may be at ↑ risk for adverse reactions due to age-related renal impairment.

Adverse Reactions/Side Effects

CV: hypertension. **GI:** ↑ lipase, ↑ liver enzymes, CLOSTRIDIOIDES DIFFICILE-ASSOCIATED DIARRHEA (CDAD), diarrhea, nausea, vomiting. **Hemat:** anemia. **Local:** phlebitis. **Neuro:** headache, SEIZURES. **Misc:** fever, HYPERSENSITIVITY REACTIONS (including anaphylaxis).

Interactions

Drug-Drug: May ↓ serum **valproate** levels and ↑ risk of seizures. ↑ risk of seizures with **ganciclovir**; avoid concurrent use.

Route/Dosage

IV (Adults): 1.25 g every 6 hr.

Renal Impairment

IV (Adults): *CCr 60–89 mL/min:* 1 g every 6 hr; *CCr 30–59 mL/min:* 750 mg every 6 hr; *CCr 15–29 mL/min:* 500 mg every 6 hr; *CCr <15 mL/min on hemodialysis:* 500 mg every 6 hr (on dialysis days, administer doses after hemodialysis).

Availability

Powder for injection: imipenem 500 mg/cilastatin 500 mg/250 mg relebactam.

NURSING IMPLICATIONS

Assessment

- Assess patient for infection (vital signs; appearance of wound, sputum, urine, and stool; WBC) at beginning of and during therapy.
- Obtain a history before initiating therapy to determine previous use of and reactions to penicillins. Persons with a negative history of penicillin sensitivity may still have an allergic response.
- Obtain specimens for culture and sensitivity before initiating therapy. First dose may be given before receiving results.
- Observe patient for signs and symptoms of anaphylaxis (rash, pruritus, laryngeal edema, wheezing). Discontinue the drug and notify the physician immediately if these occur. Have epinephrine, an antihistamine, and resuscitative equipment close by in the event of an anaphylactic reaction.
- Monitor bowel function. Diarrhea, abdominal cramping, fever, and bloody stools should be reported to health care professional promptly as a sign of CDAD. May begin up to several wk following cessation of therapy.

Implementation

- **Intermittent Infusion:** *Reconstitution:* Reconstitute with 0.9% NaCl, D5W, D5/0.9% NaCl, D5/0.45% NaCl, or D5/0.225% NaCl. *Dilution: Step 1:* For diluents available in 100-mL prefilled infusion bags, proceed to step 2. *Step 2:* For diluents not available in 100-mL prefilled infusion bags, withdraw 100 mL of desired diluent and transfer it to an empty infusion bag, then proceed to step 2. Withdraw 20 mL (as two 10-mL aliquots) of diluent from appropriate infusion bag and constitute vial with one 10-mL aliquot of the diluent. Constituted suspension is for intravenous infusion only after dilution in an appropriate infusion solution. *Step 3:* After constitution, shake vial well and transfer suspension into remaining 80 mL of infusion bag. *Step 4:* Add second

10-mL aliquot of infusion diluent to vial and shake well to ensure complete transfer of vial contents; repeat transfer of resulting suspension to infusion solution before administering. Agitate the resulting mixture until clear. Solution is colorless to yellow; do not use solutions that are discolored or contain particulate matter. Stable for 2 hr at room temperature or 24 hr if refrigerated; do not freeze. *Rate:* Infuse over 30 min.
- **Y-Site Compatibility:** dexmedetomidine, dopamine, epinephrine, fentanyl, heparin, midazolam, norepinephrine, phenylephrine.
- **Y-Site Incompatibility:** propofol.

Patient/Family Teaching

- Explain purpose of medication to patient, that it is only for bacterial infections, and that skipping or missing doses can increase risk or resistance to medication.
- Instruct patient to notify health care professional immediately if signs and symptoms of allergic reactions occur.
- Advise patient to report the signs of superinfection (black, furry overgrowth on the tongue; vaginal itching or discharge; loose or foul-smelling stools) and allergy. Consult health care professional before treating with antidiarrheals.
- Instruct patient to notify health care professional of all Rx or OTC medications, vitamins, or herbal products being taken and consult health care professional before taking any new medications, especially valproate.
- Caution patient to notify health care professional if fever and diarrhea occur, especially if stool contains blood, pus, or mucus. Advise patient not to treat diarrhea without consulting health care professional. May occur up to several wk after discontinuation of medication.
- Rep: Advise females of reproductive potential to notify health care professional if pregnancy is planned or suspected or if breastfeeding.

Evaluation/Desired Outcomes

- Resolution of the signs and symptoms of infection. Length of time for complete resolution depends on the organism and site of infection.

BEERS

☒ imipramine (im-ip-ra-meen)
Tofranil
Classification
Therapeutic: antidepressants
Pharmacologic: tricyclic antidepressants

Indications

Major depressive disorder. Enuresis in children. **Unlabeled Use:** Adjunct in the management of chronic pain, incontinence (in adults), vascular headache prophylaxis, cluster headache, insomnia.

Action

Potentiates the effect of serotonin and norepinephrine. Has significant anticholinergic properties. **Therapeutic Effects:** Antidepressant action that develops slowly over several weeks. Diminished incidence of enuresis.

Pharmacokinetics

Absorption: Well absorbed from the GI tract.
Distribution: Widely distributed to tissues.
Protein Binding: 89–95%.
Metabolism and Excretion: Mostly metabolized by the liver (CYP2D6 isoenzyme) to desipramine; ⚥ the CYP2D6 enzyme system exhibits genetic polymorphism; ~7% of population may be poor metabolizers and may have significantly ↑ imipramine concentrations and an ↑ risk of adverse effects.
Half-life: 8–16 hr.

TIME/ACTION PROFILE (antidepressant effect)

ROUTE	ONSET	PEAK	DURATION
PO	hrs	2–6 wk	wk

Contraindications/Precautions

Contraindicated in: Hypersensitivity; Cross-sensitivity with other antidepressants may occur; Angle-closure glaucoma; Hypersensitivity to tartrazine or sulfites (in some preparations); Recent MI, known history of QT interval prolongation, HF; Concurrent use of MAO inhibitors or MAO-like drugs (linezolid or methylene blue); Lactation: Lactation.
Use Cautiously in: Pre-existing cardiovascular disease; Seizures or history of seizure disorder; May ↑ risk of suicide attempt/ideation especially during early treatment or dose adjustment; OB: Use during pregnancy only if potential maternal benefit justifies potential fetal risk; Pedi: Suicide risk may be greater in children or adolescents. Safety and effectiveness not established in children <6 yr; Geri: Appears on Beers list. ↑ risk of adverse reactions in older adults, including falls secondary to sedative and anticholinergic effects and orthostatic hypotension. Avoid use in older adults.

Adverse Reactions/Side Effects

CV: hypotension, ARRHYTHMIAS, ECG changes. **Derm:** photosensitivity. **EENT:** blurred vision, dry eyes. **Endo:** gynecomastia. **GI:** constipation, dry mouth, nausea, paralytic ileus. **GU:** ↓ libido, urinary retention. **Hemat:** blood dyscrasias. **Metab:** weight gain. **Neuro:** drowsiness, fatigue, agitation, confusion, hallucinations, insomnia, SUICIDAL THOUGHTS.

Interactions

Drug-Drug: Concurrent use with **MAO inhibitors** may result in serious potentially fatal reactions (MAO inhibitors should be stopped at least 14 days before imipramine therapy. Imipramine should be stopped at least 14 days before MAO inhibitor therapy). Concurrent use with **MAO-inhibitor like drugs,** such as **linezolid** or **methylene blue,** may ↑ risk of serotonin syndrome; concurrent use contraindicated; do not start therapy in patients receiving **linezolid** or **methylene blue**; if **linezolid** or **methylene blue** need to be started in a patient receiving imipramine, immediately discontinue imipramine and monitor for signs/symptoms of serotonin syndrome for 2 wk or until 24 hr after last dose of linezolid or methylene blue, whichever comes first (may resume imipramine therapy 24 hr after last dose of linezolid or methylene blue). Concurrent use with **SSRIs** may result in ↑ toxicity and should be avoided (**fluoxetine** should be stopped 5 wk before starting imipramine). Hypertensive crisis may occur with **clonidine.** Imipramine is metabolized in the liver by the **CYP2D6 isoenzyme** and its action may be affected by drugs that compete for metabolism by this enzyme including **other antidepressants, phenothiazines, carbamazepine, class IC antiarrhythmics (propafenone, flecainide)**; when used concurrently, dose ↓ of one or the other or both may be necessary. Concurrent use of other drugs that inhibit the activity of the enzyme, including **cimetidine, quinidine, amiodarone,** and **ritonavir,** may result in ↑ effects of imipramine. Concurrent use with **levodopa** may result in delayed/↓ absorption of levodopa or hypertension. Blood levels and effects may be ↓ by **rifamycins.** ↑ CNS depression with other CNS **depressants** including **alcohol, antihistamines, clonidine, opioids,** and **sedative/hypnotics. Barbiturates** may alter blood levels and effects. **Adrenergic** and **anticholinergic** side effects may be ↑ with other **agents having these properties. Phenothiazines** or **hormonal contraceptives** ↑ levels and may cause toxicity. **Cigarette smoking (nicotine**) may ↑ metabolism and alter effects. Drugs that affect serotonergic neurotransmitter systems, including **SSRIs, SNRIs, fentanyl, buspirone, tramadol,** and **triptans** ↑ risk of serotonin syndrome.
Drug-Natural Products: Use with **St. John's wort** ↑ risk of serotonin syndrome. Concomitant use of **kava-kava, valerian,** or **chamomile** can ↑ CNS depression. ↑ anticholinergic effects with **jimson weed** and **scopolia.**

Route/Dosage

Major Depressive Disorder

PO (Adults): 25–50 mg 3–4 times daily (not to exceed 300 mg/day); total daily dose may be given at bedtime.
PO (Geriatric Patients): 25 mg at bedtime initially, up to 100 mg/day in divided doses.
PO (Children >12 yr): 25–50 mg/day in divided doses (not to exceed 100 mg/day).
PO (Children 6–12 yr): 10–30 mg/day in 2 divided doses.

Enuresis

PO (Children ≥6 yr): 25 mg once daily 1 hr before bedtime; ↑ if necessary by 25 mg at weekly intervals to 50 mg in children <12 yr, up to 75 mg in children >12 yr.

Availability (generic available)

Tablets: 10 mg, 25 mg, 50 mg, ✿ 75 mg. **Capsules:** 75 mg, 100 mg, 125 mg, 150 mg.

NURSING IMPLICATIONS
Assessment

- Monitor BP and pulse rate prior to and during initial therapy.
- Monitor plasma levels in treatment-resistant patients.
- Monitor weight and BMI initially and periodically throughout therapy.
- For overweight/obese individuals, obtain fasting blood glucose and cholesterol levels. Refer as appropriate for nutrition/weight management and medical management.
- Obtain weight and BMI initially and regularly throughout therapy.
- Assess for sexual dysfunction (decreased libido; erectile dysfunction).
- Assess for suicidal tendencies, especially during early therapy. Restrict amount of drug available to patient. Risk may be increased in children, adolescents, and adults ≤24 yrs. After starting therapy, children, adolescents, and young adults should be seen by health care professional face-to-face at least weekly for 4 wk, then every other wk for next 4 wk, then at 12 wk, and on advice of health care professional thereafter.
- Pedi, Geri: Monitor baseline and periodic ECGs in older adults or patients with heart disease and before increasing dose with children treated for enuresis. May cause prolonged PR and QT intervals and may flatten T waves.
- **Depression:** Assess mental status (orientation, mood, behavior) frequently. Confusion, agitation, and hallucinations may occur during initiation of therapy and may require dosage reduction. Assess for suicidal tendencies, especially during early therapy. Restrict amount of drug available to patient.
- **Enuresis:** Assess frequency of bedwetting during therapy. Ask patient or caretaker to maintain diary.
- **Pain:** Assess location, duration, and severity of pain periodically during therapy. Use pain scale to monitor effectiveness of therapy.

Lab Test Considerations

- Assess leukocyte and differential blood counts and renal and hepatic functions prior to and periodically during prolonged or high-dose therapy.
- Serum levels may be monitored in patients who fail to respond to usual therapeutic dose. Therapeutic plasma concentration range for depression is 150–300 ng/mL.
- May cause alterations in blood glucose levels.

Toxicity and Overdose

- Symptoms of acute overdose include disturbed concentration, confusion, restlessness, agitation, seizures, drowsiness, mydriasis, arrhythmias, fever, hallucinations, vomiting, and dyspnea.
- Treatment of overdose includes gastric lavage, activated charcoal, and a stimulant cathartic. Maintain respiratory and cardiac function (monitor ECG for at least 5 days) and temperature. Medications may include digoxin for HF, antiarrhythmics, and anticonvulsants.

Implementation

- Dose increases should be made at bedtime because of sedation. Dose titration is a slow process; may take wk to mo. May be given as a single dose at bedtime to minimize sedation during the day.
- Taper to avoid withdrawal effects. Gradually taper dose over 2–4 wk to prevent withdrawal effects.
- **PO:** Administer medication with or immediately following a meal to minimize gastric irritation.
- For enuresis, administer dose 1 hr before bedtime; for early night bedwetters, drug has been shown to be more effective if given earlier and in divided amounts (25 mg in midafternoon and repeated at bedtime).

Patient/Family Teaching

- Instruct patient to take medication as directed. Take missed doses as soon as possible unless almost time for next dose; if regimen is a single dose at bedtime, do not take in the morning because of side effects. Advise patient that drug effects may not be noticed for at least 2 wk. Abrupt discontinuation may cause nausea, vomiting, diarrhea, headache, trouble sleeping with vivid dreams, and irritability.
- May cause drowsiness and blurred vision. Caution patient to avoid driving and other activities requiring alertness until response to drug is known.
- Instruct patient to notify health care professional if visual changes occur. Inform patient that periodic glaucoma testing may be needed during long-term therapy.
- Caution patient to change positions slowly to minimize orthostatic hypotension. Advise patient, family, and caregivers to look for suicidality, especially during early therapy or dose changes. Notify health care professional immediately if thoughts about suicide or dying, attempts to commit suicide, new or worse depression or anxiety, agitation or restlessness, panic attacks, insomnia, new or worse irritability, aggressiveness, acting on dangerous impulses, mania, or other changes in mood or behavior or if symptoms of serotonin syndrome occur.
- Advise patient to avoid alcohol or other CNS depressant drugs during therapy and for at least 3–7 days after therapy has been discontinued.

✿ = Canadian drug name. ⚇ = Genetic implication. ~~Strikethrough~~ = Discontinued. CAPITALS = life-threatening. <u>Underline</u> = most frequent.

- Instruct patient to notify health care professional if urinary retention, dry mouth, or constipation persists. Sugarless candy or gum may diminish dry mouth and an increase in fluid intake or bulk may prevent constipation. If symptoms persist, dose reduction or discontinuation may be necessary. Consult health care professional if dry mouth persists for more than 2 wk.
- Caution patient to use sunscreen and protective clothing to prevent photosensitivity reactions.
- Alert patient that urine may turn blue-green in color.
- Inform patient of need to monitor dietary intake, as possible increase in appetite may lead to undesired weight gain. Inform patient that increased amounts of riboflavin in the diet may be required; consult health care professional.
- Advise patient to notify health care professional of medication regimen prior to treatment or surgery.
- Therapy for depression is usually prolonged. Emphasize the importance of follow-up exams to evaluate progress and improve coping skills.
- Rep: Instruct females of reproductive potential to notify health care professional if pregnancy is planned or suspected, and to avoid breastfeeding.
- Pedi: Inform parents that the side effects most likely to occur include nervousness, insomnia, unusual tiredness, and mild nausea and vomiting. Notify health care professional if these symptoms become pronounced.
- Advise parents to keep medication out of reach of children to prevent inadvertent overdose.

Evaluation/Desired Outcomes
- Increased sense of well-being.
- Renewed interest in surroundings.
- Increased appetite.
- Improved energy level.
- Pain relief.
- Diminished incidence of enuresis.
- Improved sleep in patients treated for depression. Patient may require 2–6 wk of therapy before full therapeutic effects of medication are noticeable.
- Control of bedwetting in children >6 yr.
- Decrease in chronic neurogenic pain.

inclisiran (in-kli-sir-an)
Leqvio
Classification
Therapeutic: lipid-lowering agents
Pharmacologic: small interfering ribonucleic acid agents

Indications
Primary hyperlipidemia, including heterozygous familial hypercholesterolemia (as adjunct to diet and statin therapy).

Action
Acts as a small interfering ribonucleic acid that is taken up by hepatocytes. In hepatocytes, it causes breakdown of mRNA for proprotein convertase subtilisin kexin type 9 (PCSK9), which ultimately increases LDL-C uptake and lowers LDL-C levels. **Therapeutic Effects:** Reduction in LDL-C levels.

Pharmacokinetics
Absorption: Extent of absorption unknown following SUBQ administration.
Distribution: Widely distributed to tissues.
Metabolism and Excretion: Primarily metabolized by nucleases to shorter nucleotides. 16% excreted in the urine.
Half-life: 9 hr.

TIME/ACTION PROFILE (plasma concentrations)

ROUTE	ONSET	PEAK	DURATION
SUBQ	unknown	4 hr	unknown

Contraindications/Precautions
Contraindicated in: OB: Pregnancy.
Use Cautiously in: End-stage renal disease; Severe hepatic impairment; Lactation: Use while breastfeeding only if potential maternal benefit justifies potential risk to infant; Pedi: Safety and effectiveness not established in children.

Adverse Reactions/Side Effects
GI: diarrhea. **GU:** urinary tract infection. **Local:** injection site reactions. **MS:** arthralgia, pain. **Resp:** bronchitis, dyspnea.

Interactions
Drug-Drug: None reported.

Route/Dosage
SUBQ (Adults): 284 mg initially, then in 3 mo, then every 6 mo thereafter.

Availability
Solution for injection: 284 mg/1.5 mL.

NURSING IMPLICATIONS
Assessment
- Obtain a diet history, especially with regard to fat consumption.

Lab Test Considerations
- Monitor LDL-C when indicated. LDL-lowering effect may be measured as early as 30 days after starting and anytime thereafter without regard to timing of the dose.

Implementation
- **SUBQ:** Inject into abdomen, upper arm, or thigh. Do not inject in areas of active skin disease or injury, sunburns, skin rashes, inflammation, or skin infections. Solution is clear and colorless to pale yellow; do not use if cloudy, discolored, or contains particulate matter.

Patient/Family Teaching

- Instruct patient to take inclisiran as directed. If a dose is missed by < 3 mo, administer inclisiran and maintain dosing according to original schedule. If a dose is missed by >3 mo, restart with a new dosing schedule—administer inclisiran initially, again at 3 mo, and then every 6 mo.
- Advise patient that this medication should be used in conjunction with diet restrictions (fat, cholesterol, carbohydrates, alcohol), exercise, and cessation of smoking.
- Advise patient to notify health care professional of all Rx or OTC medications, vitamins, or herbal products being taken and to consult with health care professional before taking other medications.
- Advise patient to notify health care professional of medication regimen before treatment or surgery.
- Rep: May cause fetal harm. Advise females or reproductive potential to notify health care professional if pregnancy is planned or suspected or if breastfeeding. Discontinue inclisiran when pregnancy is recognized.
- Emphasize the importance of follow-up exams to determine effectiveness and to monitor for side effects.

Evaluation/Desired Outcomes

- Reduction in LDL-C levels.

BEERS

indomethacin
(in-doe-**meth**-a-sin)
Indocin, ~~Tivorbex~~
Classification
Therapeutic: antirheumatics, ductus arteriosus patency adjuncts (IV only), nonopioid analgesics
Pharmacologic: nonsteroidal anti-inflammatory drugs (NSAIDs)

Indications

PO: Inflammatory disorders including: Rheumatoid arthritis, Gouty arthritis, Osteoarthritis, Ankylosing spondylitis. Mild-to-moderate acute pain. **IV:** Alternative to surgery in the management of patent ductus arteriosus (PDA) in premature neonates.

Action

Inhibits prostaglandin synthesis. In the treatment of PDA, decreased prostaglandin production allows the ductus to close. **Therapeutic Effects: PO:** Suppression of pain and inflammation. **IV:** Closure of PDA.

Pharmacokinetics

Absorption: Well absorbed after oral administration in adults, incomplete oral absorption in neonates.
Distribution: Crosses the blood-brain barrier.
Protein Binding: 99%.

Metabolism and Excretion: Mostly metabolized by the liver.
Half-life: *Neonates <2 wk:* 20 hr; *Neonates >2 wk:* 11 hr; *Adults:* 2.6–11 hr.

TIME/ACTION PROFILE

ROUTE	ONSET	PEAK	DURATION
PO (analgesic)	30 min	0.5–2 hr	4–6 hr
PO-ER (analgesic)	30 min	unknown	4–6 hr
PO (anti-inflammatory)	up to 7 days	1–2 wk	4–6 hr
PO-ER (anti-inflammatory)	up to 7 days	1–2 wk	4–6 hr
IV (closure of PDA)	up to 48 hr	unknown	unknown

Contraindications/Precautions

Contraindicated in: Hypersensitivity; Known alcohol intolerance (suspension); Cross-sensitivity may exist with other NSAIDs, including aspirin; Active GI bleeding; Ulcer disease; Proctitis or recent history of rectal bleeding; Intraventricular hemorrhage; Thrombocytopenia; Coronary artery bypass graft surgery; OB: Avoid use after 30 wk gestation (may cause premature closure of fetal ductus arteriosus); Pedi: ↑ risk of necrotizing enterocolitis and bowel perforation in premature infants with PDA.

Use Cautiously in: Severe renal impairment; Severe hepatic impairment; Cardiovascular disease or risk factors for cardiovascular disease (may ↑ risk of serious cardiovascular thrombotic events, MI, and stroke, especially with prolonged use or use of higher doses); Avoid use in patients with recent MI or HF; History of ulcer disease; Seizure disorders; Hypertension; OB: Use at or after 20 wk gestation may cause fetal renal impairment leading to oligohydramnios and, possibly neonatal renal impairment; if treatment is necessary between 20 wk and 30 wk gestation, limit use to the lowest effective dose and shortest duration possible; Geri: Appears on Beers list. ↑ risk GI bleeding or peptic ulcer disease in older adults. Avoid chronic use unless other alternatives are not effective and the patient can take a gastroprotective agent; avoid short-term use in combination with oral or parenteral corticosteroids, anticoagulants, or antiplatelet agents unless other alternatives are not effective and the patient can take a gastroprotective agent.

Adverse Reactions/Side Effects

CV: edema, HF, hypertension, MI. **Derm:** rash. **EENT:** blurred vision, tinnitus. **Endo:** *IV:* hypoglycemia. **F and E:** hyperkalemia; *IV:* dilutional hyponatremia. **GI:** constipation, dyspepsia, nausea, vomiting, discomfort;

PO: GI BLEEDING, HEPATOTOXICITY, necrotizing enterocolitis, PANCREATITIS. **GU:** cystitis, hematuria, renal failure. **Hemat:** blood dyscrasias, prolonged bleeding time, thrombocytopenia. **Local:** phlebitis at IV site. **Neuro:** dizziness, drowsiness, headache, psychic disturbances, STROKE. **Misc:** HYPERSENSITIVITY REACTIONS (including anaphylaxis).

Interactions

Drug-Drug: Concurrent use with **aspirin** may ↓ effectiveness. Additive adverse GI effects with **aspirin**, other **NSAIDs, corticosteroids,** or **alcohol.** Chronic use of **acetaminophen** ↑ risk of adverse renal reactions. May ↓ effectiveness of **diuretics** or **antihypertensives.** May ↑ hypoglycemia from **insulins** or **oral hypoglycemic agents.** May ↑ risk of toxicity from **lithium** or **zidovudine** (avoid concurrent use with zidovudine). ↑ risk of toxicity from **methotrexate. Probenecid** ↑ risk of toxicity from indomethacin. ↑ risk of bleeding with **anticoagulants, aspirin, clopidogrel, ticagrelor, prasugrel, corticosteroids, fibrinolytics, SNRIs,** or **SSRIs.** ↑ risk of adverse hematologic reactions with **antineoplastics** or **radiation therapy.** ↑ risk of nephrotoxicity with **cyclosporine.** Concurrent use with **potassium-sparing diuretics** may result in hyperkalemia. May ↑ levels of **digoxin, methotrexate, lithium,** and **aminoglycosides** when used IV in neonates.
Drug-Natural Products: ↑ bleeding risk with **anise, arnica, chamomile, clove, dong quai, feverfew, garlic, ginger, ginkgo, Panax ginseng.**

Route/Dosage

Anti-inflammatory

PO (Adults): *Arthritis (immediate–release):* 25–50 mg 2–4 times daily (max dose = 200 mg/day). A single bedtime dose of 100 mg may alternatively be used; *Arthritis (extended–release):* 75 mg once or twice daily (max dose = 150 mg/day). *Gout:* 100 mg initially, followed by 50 mg 3 times daily for relief of pain, then ↓ further.
PO (Children >2 yr): 1–2 mg/kg/day in 2–4 divided doses (not to exceed 4 mg/kg/day or 150–200 mg/day).

PDA Closure

IV (Neonates): *Treatment:* 0.2 mg/kg initially, then 2 subsequent doses at 12–24 hr intervals of 0.1 mg/kg if age <48 hr at time of initial dose; 0.2 mg/kg if 2–7 days at initial dose; 0.25 mg/kg if age >7 days at initial dose. *Prophylaxis:* 0.1–0.2 mg/kg initially, then 0.1 mg/kg every 12–24 hr for 2 doses.

Availability (generic available)

Capsules: 25 mg, 50 mg. **Extended-release capsules:** 75 mg. **Oral suspension (fruit mint, pineapple, coconut, mint flavors):** 25 mg/5 mL. **Powder for injection:** 1 mg/vial. **Rectal suppository:** 50 mg, ✤ 100 mg.

NURSING IMPLICATIONS

Assessment

● Patients who have asthma, aspirin-induced allergy, and nasal polyps are at increased risk for developing hypersensitivity reactions. Monitor for rhinitis, asthma, and urticaria.

● Assess patient for skin rash frequently during therapy. Discontinue indomethacin at first sign of rash; may be life-threatening. Stevens-Johnson syndrome or toxic epidermal necrolysis may develop. Treat symptomatically; may recur once treatment is stopped.

● Monitor BP during initiation and periodically during therapy. May cause fluid retention and edema, leading to new onset or worsening hypertension.

● **Arthritis:** Assess limitation of movement and pain—note type, location, and intensity before and 1–2 hr after administration.

● **PDA:** Monitor respiratory status, heart rate, BP, echocardiogram, and heart sounds routinely throughout therapy.

● Monitor intake and output. Fluid restriction is usually instituted throughout therapy.

● **Acute pain:** Assess type, location, and intensity of pain prior to and 2 hrs (peak) following administration.

Lab Test Considerations

● Evaluate BUN, serum creatinine, CBC, serum potassium levels, and liver function tests periodically in patients receiving prolonged therapy.

● Serum potassium, BUN, serum creatinine, AST, and ALT tests may show ↑ levels. Blood glucose concentrations may be altered. Hemoglobin and hematocrit concentrations, leukocyte and platelet counts, and CCr may be ↓.

● Urine glucose and urine protein concentrations may be ↑.

● Leukocyte and platelet count may be ↓. Bleeding time may be prolonged for several days after discontinuation.

Implementation

● If prolonged therapy is used, dose should be reduced to the lowest level that controls symptoms to minimize risk of cardiovascular thrombotic events.

● **PO:** Administer after meals, with food, or with antacids to decrease GI irritation. *DNC:* Do not break, crush, or chew sustained-release capsules.

● Shake suspension before administration. Do not mix with antacid or any other liquid.

IV Administration

● **IV Push:** *Reconstitution:* Preservative-free 0.9% NaCl or preservative-free sterile water. Reconstitute with 1 or 2 mL of diluent. *Concentration:* 0.5–1 mg/mL. Reconstitute immediately before use and discard any unused solution. Do not dilute further or admix. Do not administer via umbilical catheter into vessels near the superior mesenteric artery, as these can cause vasoconstriction and compromise blood flow to the intestines. Do not administer intra-arterially. *Rate:* Administer over 20–30 min. Avoid extravasation, as solution is irritating to tissues.

- **Y-Site Compatibility:** aminophylline, ascorbic acid, atropine, bumetanide, cefazolin, cefotaxime, cefoxitin, ceftazidime, ceftriaxone, cefuroxime, chloramphenicol, cisplatin, clindamycin, cyanocobalamin, cyclosporine, dexamethasone, digoxin, enalaprilat, ephedrine, epoetin alfa, fentanyl, fluconazole, folic acid, furosemide, ganciclovir, heparin, hydrocortisone, imipenem/cilastatin, insulin regular, ketorolac, lactated Ringer's, lidocaine, mannitol, metoclopramide, metoprolol, multivitamins, nafcillin, nitroglycerin, nitroprusside, penicillin G, pentobarbital, phenobarbital, phytonadione, potassium chloride, procainamide, Ringer's injection, sodium bicarbonate, theophylline.
- **Y-Site Incompatibility:** amikacin, amino acid injection, atracurium, aztreonam, benztropine, buprenorphine, butorphanol, calcium chloride, calcium gluconate, cefotetan, chlorpromazine, dactinomycin, dantrolene, daunorubicin hydrochloride, diazepam, diphenhydramine, dobutamine, dopamine, doxycycline, epinephrine, erythromycin, esmolol, etoposide, famotidine, gentamicin, glycopyrrolate, haloperidol, hydralazine, isoproterenol, labetalol, levofloxacin, magnesium sulfate, meperidine, midazolam, minocycline, morphine, nalbuphine, norepinephrine, ondansetron, oxytocin, paclitaxel, pantoprazole, papaverine, pentamidine, phenylephrine, phenytoin, prochlorperazine, promethazine, propranolol, protamine, pyridoxine, succinylcholine, sufentanil, thiamine, tobramycin, trimethoprim/sulfamethoxazole, vancomycin, vasopressin, verapamil.

Patient/Family Teaching

- Advise patient to take this medication with a full glass of water and to remain in an upright position for 15–30 min after administration.
- Instruct patient to take medication as directed. Take missed doses as soon as remembered if not almost time for next dose. Do not double doses.
- May cause drowsiness or dizziness. Advise patient to avoid driving or other activities requiring alertness until response to medication is known.
- Caution patient to avoid the concurrent use of alcohol, aspirin, other NSAIDs, acetaminophen, or other OTC medications without consulting health care professional.
- Caution patient to wear sunscreen and protective clothing to prevent photosensitivity reactions.
- Advise patient to inform health care professional of medication regimen before treatment or surgery.
- Instruct patient to notify health care professional immediately if signs and symptoms of cardiovascular

thrombotic events (shortness of breath or trouble breathing, chest pain, weakness in one part or side of body, slurred speech); hepatotoxicity (nausea, fatigue, lethargy, diarrhea, pruritus, jaundice, right upper quadrant tenderness, "flu-like" symptoms) occur or if rash, itching, chills, fever, muscle aches, visual disturbances, weight gain, edema, abdominal pain, black stools, or persistent headache occurs.
- Rep: May cause fetal harm. Advise females of reproductive potential to notify health care professional if pregnancy is planned or suspected or if breastfeeding. Advise women to avoid indomethacin in the 3rd trimester of pregnancy (after 29 wk), may cause premature closure of the fetal ductus arteriosus. Use of indomethacin after 20 wk may cause fetal renal dysfunction leading to oligohydramnios. May cause temporary infertility in women.
- **PDA:** Explain to parents the purpose of medication and the need for frequent monitoring.

Evaluation/Desired Outcomes

- Decrease in severity of mild to moderate pain.
- Improved joint mobility. Partial arthritic relief is usually seen within 2 wk, but maximum effectiveness may require up to 1 mo of continuous therapy. Patients who do not respond to one NSAID may respond to another.
- Successful PDA closure.

inFLIXimab (in-flix-i-mab)
Avsola, Inflectra, Remicade, Renflexis, ✦Remsima
Classification
Therapeutic: antirheumatics (DMARDs), gastrointestinal anti-inflammatories
Pharmacologic: monoclonal antibodies

Indications
Moderately to severely active rheumatoid arthritis (in combination with methotrexate). Moderately to severely active Crohn's disease in patients with an inadequate response to conventional therapy. Active psoriatic arthritis. Active ankylosing spondylitis. Moderately to severely active ulcerative colitis in patients with an inadequate response to conventional therapy. Chronic severe plaque psoriasis in patients who are candidates for systemic therapy and when other systemic therapies are less appropriate.

Action
Neutralizes and prevents the activity of tumor necrosis factor-alpha (TNF-alpha), resulting in anti-inflammatory and antiproliferative activity. **Therapeutic Effects:** Decreased signs and symptoms, decreased rate of joint destruction, and improved physical function in rheumatoid arthritis and psoriatic arthritis. Decreased signs and symptoms and induction and maintenance of clini-

cal remission in Crohn's disease. Reduction in number of fistulas and maintenance of closure of fistulae in Crohn's disease. Decreased signs and symptoms in ankylosing spondylitis. Decreased signs and symptoms, maintenance of clinical remission and mucosal healing, and eliminating corticosteroid use in ulcerative colitis. Decreased induration, scaling, and erythema of psoriatic lesions.

Pharmacokinetics

Absorption: IV administration results in complete bioavailability.

Distribution: Predominantly distributed within the vascular compartment.

Metabolism and Excretion: Unknown.

Half-life: 9.5 days.

TIME/ACTION PROFILE (symptoms of Crohn's disease)

ROUTE	ONSET	PEAK	DURATION
IV	1–2 wk	unknown	12–48 wk†

†After infusion.

Contraindications/Precautions

Contraindicated in: Hypersensitivity to infliximab, murine (mouse) proteins, or other components in the formulation; Moderate to severe HF (doses >5 mg/kg); Concurrent anakinra or abatacept.

Use Cautiously in: History of chronic or recurrent infection or underlying illness/treatment predisposing to infection; Patients being retreated after 2 yr without treatment (↑ risk of adverse reactions); History of tuberculosis or exposure (latent tuberculosis should be treated prior to infliximab therapy); History of opportunistic infection; Moderate to severe HF (doses ≤5 mg/kg); Patients residing, or who have resided, where tuberculosis, histoplasmosis, coccidioidomycoses, or blastomycosis is endemic; Chronic obstructive pulmonary disease (↑ risk of malignancy); OB: Use only if potential maternal benefit justifies potential fetal risk; infants exposed in utero may be at ↑ risk for infection or agranulocytosis; Lactation: Use while breastfeeding only if potential maternal benefit justifies potential risk to infant; Pedi: Children <6 yr (safety not established); ↑ risk of lymphoma (including hepatosplenic T-cell lymphoma [HSTCL] in patients with Crohn's disease or ulcerative colitis), leukemia, and other malignancies; Geri: ↑ risk of adverse reactions, including serious infections, in older adults.

Adverse Reactions/Side Effects

CV: ARRHYTHMIAS, chest pain, edema, HF, hypertension, hypotension, MYOCARDIAL ISCHEMIA/INFARCTION, pericardial effusion, tachycardia, vasculitis. **Derm:** acne, ACUTE GENERALIZED EXANTHEMATOUS PUSTULOSIS (AGEP), alopecia, dry skin, ecchymosis, eczema, erythema, flushing, hematoma, hot flushing, pruritus, psoriasis, rash, STEVENS-JOHNSON SYNDROME, sweating, TOXIC EPIDERMAL NECROLYSIS, urticaria. **EENT:** conjunctivitis, vision loss. **GI:** abdominal pain, nausea, vomiting, constipation, diarrhea, dyspepsia, flatulence, hepatotoxicity, intestinal obstruction, oral pain, tooth pain, ulcerative stomatitis. **GU:** dysuria, urinary frequency, urinary tract infection. **Hemat:** neutropenia. **MS:** arthralgia, arthritis, back pain, involuntary muscle contractions, myalgia. **Neuro:** fatigue, headache, anxiety, depression, dizziness, insomnia, paresthesia, STROKE. **Resp:** upper respiratory tract infection, bronchitis, cough, dyspnea, laryngitis, pharyngitis, respiratory tract allergic reaction, rhinitis, sinusitis. **Misc:** fever, infusion reactions, chills, flu-like syndrome, HYPERSENSITIVITY REACTIONS (including anaphylaxis), INFECTION (including reactivation tuberculosis and other opportunistic infections due to bacterial, invasive fungal, viral, mycobacterial, and parasitic pathogens), lupus-like syndrome, MALIGNANCY (including lymphoma, HSTCL, leukemia, skin cancer, and cervical cancer), pain, SARCOIDOSIS.

Interactions

Drug-Drug: Concurrent use with **anakinra** or **abatacept** ↑ risk of serious infections (not recommended). Concurrent use with **azathioprine** and/or **methotrexate** may ↑ risk of HSTCL. Use of **live virus vaccines** or therapeutic infectious agents may ↑ risk of infection; avoid concurrent use; wait for ≥6 mo before administering any live vaccines to infants exposed in utero.

Route/Dosage

Rheumatoid Arthritis

IV (Adults): 3 mg/kg initially, then repeat at 2 and 6 wk after initial infusion, then repeat every 8 wk; dose may be adjusted in partial responders up to 10 mg/kg or treatment as often as every 4 wk (to be used with methotrexate).

Crohn's Disease

IV (Adults): 5 mg/kg initially, then repeat at 2 and 6 wk after initial infusion, then maintenance dose of 5 mg/kg every 8 wk; dose may be adjusted up to 10 mg/kg in patients who initially respond and then lose their response.

IV (Children): 5 mg/kg initially, then repeat at 2 and 6 wk after initial infusion, then maintenance dose of 5 mg/kg every 8 wk.

Ankylosing Spondylitis

IV (Adults): 5 mg/kg initially, then repeat at 2 and 6 wk after initial infusion, then maintenance dose of 5 mg/kg every 6 wk.

Psoriatic Arthritis

IV (Adults): 5 mg/kg initially, then repeat at 2 and 6 wk after initial infusion, then maintenance dose of 5 mg/kg every 8 wk (to be used with or without methotrexate).

Ulcerative Colitis

IV (Adults and Children ≥6 yr): 5 mg/kg initially, then repeat at 2 and 6 wk after initial infusion, then maintenance dose of 5 mg/kg every 8 wk.

Plaque Psoriasis
IV (Adults): 5 mg/kg initially, then repeat at 2 and 6 wk after initial infusion, then maintenance dose of 5 mg/kg every 8 wk.

Availability (generic available)
Lyophilized powder for injection: 100 mg/vial.

NURSING IMPLICATIONS
Assessment
- Assess for infusion-related reactions (fever, chills, urticaria, pruritus) during and for 2 hr after infusion. Symptoms usually resolve when infusion is discontinued. Reactions are more common after 1st or 2nd infusion. Frequency of reactions may be reduced with immunosuppressant agents.
- Monitor patients who develop a new infection while taking infliximab closely. Discontinue therapy in patients who develop a serious infection or sepsis. Do not initiate therapy in patients with active infections.
- Assess for signs and symptoms of systemic infections (fever, malaise, weight loss, sweats, cough, dyspnea, pulmonary infiltrates, serious systemic illness with or without concomitant shock). Ascertain if patient lives in or has traveled to areas of endemic mycoses. Consider empiric antifungal treatment for patients at risk of histoplasmosis and other invasive fungal infections until the pathogens are identified. Consult with an infectious diseases specialist. Consider stopping infliximab until the infection has been diagnosed and adequately treated.
- Assess for latent tuberculosis with a tuberculin skin test prior to initiation of and during therapy. Treatment of latent tuberculosis should be initiated prior to therapy with infliximab.
- Monitor patient for hypersensitivity reactions (urticaria, dyspnea, hypotension) during infusion. Discontinue infliximab if severe reaction occurs. Have medications (antihistamines, acetaminophen, corticosteroids, epinephrine) and equipment readily available in the event of a severe reaction.
- **Rheumatoid Arthritis:** Assess pain and range of motion prior to and periodically during therapy.
- **Crohn's Disease and Ulcerative Colitis:** Assess for signs and symptoms before, during, and after therapy.
- **Psoriasis:** Assess lesions periodically during therapy.

Lab Test Considerations
- May cause ↑ in positive ANA. Frequency may be decreased with baseline immunosuppressant therapy.
- Monitor liver function tests periodically during therapy. May cause mild to moderate AST and ALT ↑ without progressing to liver dysfunction. If patient develops jaundice or liver enzyme elevations ≥5 times the upper limits of normal, discontinue infliximab.

- Monitor CBC with differential periodically during therapy. May cause leukopenia, neutropenia, thrombocytopenia, and pancytopenia. Discontinue infliximab if symptoms of blood dyscrasias (persistent fever) occur.

Implementation
- Do not confuse infliximab with rituximab.
- Ensure vaccinations are brought up to date in adult and pediatric patients before starting therapy.

IV Administration
- **Intermittent Infusion:** Calculate the total number of vials needed. **Reconstitution:** Reconstitute each vial with 10 mL of sterile water for injection using a syringe with a 21-gauge needle or smaller. Direct stream to sides of vial. Do not use if vacuum is not present in vial. Gently swirl solution by rotating vial to dilute; do not shake. May foam on reconstitution; allow to stand for 5 min. Solution is colorless to light yellow and opalescent; a few translucent particles may develop because infliximab is a protein. Do not use if opaque particles, discoloration, or other particles occur. **Dilution:** Withdraw volume of total infliximab dose from infusion container containing 250 mL with 0.9% NaCl. Slowly add total dose of infliximab. Do not dilute with other solutions. **Concentration:** 0.4 to 4 mg/mL. Mix gently. Infusion should begin within 3 hr (4 hr for *Renflexis*) of preparation. Solution is incompatible with polyvinyl chloride equipment. Prepare in glass infusion bottle or polypropylene or polyolefin bags. Do not reuse or store any portion of infusion solution. Unopened vials are stable for 6 mo at room temperature; once removed from refrigerator, cannot be returned to the refrigerator. Diluted solution is stable for 4 hr at room temperature, 34 days if refrigerated, and 6 hr at room temperature when removed from refrigerator. **Rate:** Administer over at least 2 hr through polyethylene-lined administration set with an in-line, sterile, nonpyrogenic, low protein-building filter with ≤1.2-micron pore size.
- **Y-Site Incompatibility:** Do not administer concurrently in the same line with any other agents.

Patient/Family Teaching
- Explain purpose of infliximab to patient.
- Advise patient that adverse reactions (myalgia, rash, fever, polyarthralgia, pruritus) may occur 3–12 days after delayed (>2 yr) retreatment with infliximab. Symptoms usually decrease or resolve within 1–3 days. Instruct patient to notify health care professional if symptoms occur.
- May cause dizziness. Caution patient to avoid driving or other activities requiring alertness until response to medication is known.
- Advise patient to notify health care professional promptly if symptoms of fungal infection occur.

- Instruct patient to notify health care professional of all Rx or OTC medications, vitamins, or herbal products being taken and consult health care professional before taking any new medications.
- Advise patient of risk of malignancies such as hepatosplenic T-cell lymphoma. Instruct patient to report signs and symptoms (splenomegaly, hepatomegaly, abdominal pain, persistent fever, night sweats, weight loss) to health care professional promptly.
- Advise patient to examine skin periodically during therapy and notify health care professional of any changes in appearance of skin or growths on skin.
- Instruct patient not to receive live vaccines during therapy.
- Advise females to continue regular PAP smears for cervical cancer screening.
- Rep: Advise females of reproductive potential to notify health care professional if pregnancy is planned or suspected and or if breastfeeding. Infants exposed to infliximab in utero should wait at least 6 mo before receiving any live vaccine; may be at increased risk of infection.

Evaluation/Desired Outcomes
- Decreased pain and swelling with decreased rate of joint destruction and improved physical function in patients with ankylosing spondylitis, psoriatic, or rheumatoid arthritis.
- Decrease in the signs and symptoms of Crohn's disease and a decrease in the number of draining enterocutaneous fistulas. Decreased symptoms, maintaining remission, and mucosal healing with decreased corticosteroid use in ulcerative colitis.
- Decrease in induration, scaling, and erythema of psoriatic lesions.

HIGH ALERT

INSULIN (mixtures) (in-su-lin)
insulin aspart protamine suspension/insulin aspart injection mixtures, rDNA origin
NovoLOG Mix 70/30, NovoLOG Mix 70/30 FlexPen
insulin lispro protamine suspension/insulin lispro injection mixtures, rDNA origin
HumaLOG Mix 75/25, HumaLOG Mix 50/50
NPH/regular insulin mixtures
HumuLIN 70/30, NovoLIN 70/30
Classification
Therapeutic: antidiabetics, hormones
Pharmacologic: pancreatics

See Appendix K for more information concerning insulins

Indications
Control of hyperglycemia in patients with type 1 or type 2 diabetes mellitus.

Action
Lower blood glucose by: stimulating glucose uptake in skeletal muscle and fat, inhibiting hepatic glucose production. Other actions: inhibition of lipolysis and proteolysis, enhanced protein synthesis. **Therapeutic Effects:** Control of hyperglycemia in diabetic patients.

Pharmacokinetics
Absorption: Well absorbed from SUBQ administration sites.
Distribution: Widely distributed.
Metabolism and Excretion: Metabolized by liver, spleen, kidney, and muscle.
Half-life: 5–6 min (prolonged in patients with diabetes; biologic half-life is 1–1.5 hr).

TIME/ACTION PROFILE (hypoglycemic effect)

ROUTE	ONSET	PEAK	DURATION
Insulin aspart protamine suspension/ insulin aspart injection mixture SUBQ	15 min	1–4 hr	18–24 hr
Insulin lispro protamine suspension/ insulin lispro injection mixture SUBQ	15–30 min	2.8 hr	24 hr
NPH/regular insulin mixture SUBQ	30 min	2–12 hr	24 hr

Contraindications/Precautions
Contraindicated in: Hypoglycemia; Allergy or hypersensitivity to a particular type of insulin, preservatives, or other additives.
Use Cautiously in: Stress and infection (may temporarily ↑ insulin requirements); Renal/hepatic impairment (may ↓ insulin requirements); Concomitant use with pioglitazone (↑ risk of fluid retention and worsening HF); OB: Pregnancy may temporarily ↑ insulin requirements; Lactation: Use while breastfeeding only if potential maternal benefit justifies potential risk to infant; Pedi: Safety of Humalog not established.

Adverse Reactions/Side Effects
Endo: HYPOGLYCEMIA. **F and E:** hypokalemia. **Local:** cutaneous amyloidosis, erythema, lipodystrophy, pruritus, swelling. **Misc:** HYPERSENSITIVITY REACTIONS (including anaphylaxis).

Interactions
Drug-Drug: **Beta blockers** and **clonidine** may mask some of the signs and symptoms of hypoglycemia.

Corticosteroids, thyroid supplements, estrogens, isoniazid, niacin, phenothiazines, and rifampin may ↑ insulin requirements. Alcohol, ACE inhibitors, MAO inhibitors, octreotide, oral hypoglycemic agents, and salicylates may ↓ insulin requirements. Concurrent use with pioglitazone may ↑ risk of fluid retention and worsening HF.

Drug-Natural Products: Glucosamine may worsen blood glucose control. Fenugreek, chromium, and coenzyme Q-10 may produce additive hypoglycemic effects.

Route/Dosage
Dose depends on blood glucose, response, and many other factors.

SUBQ (Adults and Children): 0.5–1 unit/kg/day. *Adolescents during rapid growth:* 0.8–1.2 units/kg/day.

Availability
Insulin aspart protamine suspension/insulin aspart injection mixture: 70% insulin aspart protamine suspension and 30% insulin aspart inection— NovoLog Mix 70/30 100 units/mL (vials and prefilled pens). **Insulin lispro protamine suspension/insulin lispro injection mixture:** 75% insulin lispro protamine suspension and 25% insulin lispro injection— Humalog Mix 75/25 100 units/mL (vials and prefilled pens), 50% insulin lispro protamine suspension and 50% insulin lispro injection— Humalog Mix 50/50 100 units/mL (vials and prefilled pens). **NPH insulin/regular insulin suspension mixture:** 70 units NPH/30 units regular insulin/mL— Novolin 70/30, Humulin 70/30 (100 units/mL total) (vials and prefilled pens).

NURSING IMPLICATIONS

Assessment
- Assess for symptoms of hypoglycemia (anxiety; restlessness; tingling in hands, feet, lips, or tongue; chills; cold sweats; confusion; cool, pale skin; difficulty in concentration; drowsiness; excessive hunger; headache; irritability; nightmares or trouble sleeping; nausea; nervousness; tachycardia; tremor; weakness; unsteady gait) and hyperglycemia (confusion, drowsiness; flushed, dry skin; fruit-like breath odor; rapid, deep breathing, polyuria; loss of appetite; nausea; vomiting; unusual thirst) periodically during therapy.
- Monitor body weight periodically. Changes in weight may necessitate changes in insulin dose.

Lab Test Considerations
- Monitor blood glucose every 6 hr during therapy, more frequently in ketoacidosis and times of stress. Hemoglobin A$_{1C}$ may also be monitored every 3–6 mo to determine effectiveness.
- Monitor serum potassium in patients at risk for hypokalemia (those using potassium-lowering agents,

those receiving IV insulin) periodically during therapy.

Toxicity and Overdose
- Overdose is manifested by symptoms of hypoglycemia. Mild hypoglycemia may be treated by ingestion of oral glucose. Severe hypoglycemia is a life-threatening emergency; treatment consists of IV glucose, glucagon, or epinephrine.

Implementation
- *High Alert:* Insulin-related medication errors have resulted in patient harm and death. Clarify ambiguous orders; do not accept orders using the abbreviation "u" for units (can be misread as a zero or the numeral 4; has resulted in tenfold overdoses).
- Insulins are available in different types and strengths. Check type, dose, and expiration date with another licensed nurse. Do not interchange insulins without consulting health care professional.
- Do not confuse Humulin 70/30 with Humalog Mix 75/25. Do not confuse Novolin 70/30 with Novolog Mix 70/30. Do not confuse Novolog Mix 70/30 Flexpen with Novolog Flexpen.
- Use *only* insulin syringes to draw up dose. The unit markings on the insulin syringe must match the insulin's units/mL.
- Insulin should be stored in a cool place but does not need to be refrigerated. Follow manufacturer's instructions regarding storage of insulin and insulin pens before and after use. Do not use if cloudy, discolored, or unusually viscous.
- NPH insulins should not be used in the management of ketoacidosis.
- **SUBQ:** Rotate injection sites to prevent lipodystrophy and cutaneous amyloidosis. Repeated insulin injections into areas of localized cutaneous amyloidosis may cause hyperglycemia; a sudden change to an unaffected injection site may cause hypoglycemia.
- Administer into abdominal wall, thigh, or upper arm SUBQ.

Patient/Family Teaching
- Instruct patient on proper technique for administration. Include type of insulin, equipment (syringe, cartridge pens, alcohol swabs), storage, and place to discard syringes. Discuss the importance of not changing brands of insulin or syringes, selection and rotation of injection sites, and compliance with therapeutic regimen. Caution patient that insulin pens should not be shared with others, even if clean needles are used.
- Caution patient not to share pen device with another person, even if needle is changed; may risk transmission of bloodborne pathogens.
- Explain to patient that this medication controls hyperglycemia but does not cure diabetes. Therapy is long term.

I

✦ = Canadian drug name. ≋ = Genetic implication. ~~Strikethrough~~ = Discontinued. CAPITALS = life-threatening. <u>Underline</u> = most frequent.

- Instruct patient in proper testing of serum glucose and ketones. These tests should be closely monitored during periods of stress or illness and health care professional notified of significant changes.
- Emphasize the importance of compliance with nutritional guidelines and regular exercise as directed by health care professional.
- Instruct patient to notify health care professional of all Rx or OTC medications, vitamins, or herbal products being taken and to consult health care professional before taking other Rx, OTC, herbal products, or alcohol.
- Advise patient to notify health care professional of medication regimen prior to treatment or surgery.
- Advise patient to notify health care professional if nausea, vomiting, or fever develops, if unable to eat regular diet, or if blood glucose levels are not controlled.
- Instruct patient on signs and symptoms of hypoglycemia and hyperglycemia and what to do if they occur.
- Patients with diabetes mellitus should carry a source of sugar (candy, glucose gel) and identification describing their disease and treatment regimen at all times.
- Rep: Advise patient to notify health care professional if pregnancy is planned or suspected, or if breastfeeding.
- Emphasize the importance of regular follow-up, especially during first few wk of therapy.

Evaluation/Desired Outcomes

- Control of blood glucose levels in diabetic patients without the appearance of hypoglycemic or hyperglycemic episodes.

HIGH ALERT

NPH insulin (isophane insulin suspension)
HumuLIN N, HumuLIN N KwikPen, NovoLIN N, NovoLIN N FlexPen

Classification
Therapeutic: antidiabetics, hormones
Pharmacologic: pancreatics

See Appendix K for more information concerning insulins

Indications
Control of hyperglycemia in patients with diabetes mellitus.

Action
Lowers blood glucose by: stimulating glucose uptake in skeletal muscle and fat, inhibiting hepatic glucose production. Other actions of insulin: inhibition of lipolysis and proteolysis, enhanced protein synthesis. **Therapeutic Effects:** Control of hyperglycemia in diabetic patients.

Pharmacokinetics
Absorption: Rapidly absorbed from SUBQ administration sites. Presence of protamine delays peak effect and prolongs action.
Distribution: Identical to endogenous insulin.
Metabolism and Excretion: Metabolized by liver, spleen, kidney, and muscle.
Half-life: Unknown.

TIME/ACTION PROFILE (hypoglycemic effect)

ROUTE	ONSET	PEAK	DURATION
NPH SUBQ	2–4 hr	4–10 hr	10–16 hr
70% NPH/ 30% regular insulin mixture	30 min	2–12 hr	24 hr

Contraindications/Precautions
Contraindicated in: Hypoglycemia; Allergy or hypersensitivity to a particular type of insulin, preservatives, or other additives.
Use Cautiously in: Stress or infection (may temporarily ↑ insulin requirements); Renal impairment (may ↓ insulin requirements); Hepatic impairment (may ↓ insulin requirements); OB: Pregnancy may temporarily ↑ insulin requirements; Lactation: Use while breastfeeding only if potential maternal benefit justifies potential risk to infant.

Adverse Reactions/Side Effects
Endo: HYPOGLYCEMIA. **F and E:** hypokalemia. **Local:** cutaneous amyloidosis, erythema, lipodystrophy, pruritus, swelling. **Misc:** HYPERSENSITIVITY REACTIONS (including anaphylaxis).

Interactions
Drug-Drug: Beta blockers and clonidine may mask some of the signs and symptoms of hypoglycemia. **Corticosteroids, thyroid supplements, estrogens, isoniazid, niacin, phenothiazines,** and **rifampin** may ↑ insulin requirements. **Alcohol, ACE inhibitors, MAO inhibitors, octreotide, oral hypoglycemic agents,** and **salicylates** may ↓ insulin requirements. Concurrent use with **pioglitazone** may ↑ risk of fluid retention and worsening HF.
Drug-Natural Products: Glucosamine may worsen blood glucose control. **Fenugreek, chromium,** and **coenzyme Q-10** may produce additive hypoglycemic effects.

Route/Dosage
Dose depends on blood glucose, response, and many other factors.
SUBQ (Adults and Children): 0.5–1 unit total insulin/kg/day. *Adolescents during rapid growth:* 0.8–1.2 units total insulin/kg/day.

Availability
Solution for injection (vials and prefilled pens): 100 units/mL.

NURSING IMPLICATIONS

Assessment

- Assess patient periodically for symptoms of hypoglycemia (anxiety; restlessness; tingling in hands, feet, lips, or tongue; chills; cold sweats; confusion; cool, pale skin; difficulty in concentration; drowsiness; nightmares or trouble sleeping; excessive hunger; headache; irritability; nausea; nervousness; tachycardia; tremor; weakness; unsteady gait) and hyperglycemia (confusion, drowsiness; flushed, dry skin; fruit-like breath odor; rapid, deep breathing, polyuria; loss of appetite; unusual thirst) during therapy.
- Monitor body weight periodically. Changes in weight may necessitate changes in insulin dose.

Lab Test Considerations

- Monitor blood glucose every 6 hr during therapy, more frequently in changes to insulin regimen, ketoacidosis, and times of stress. A1C may be monitored every 3–6 mo to determine effectiveness.
- Monitor serum potassium in patients at risk for hypokalemia (those using potassium-lowering agents, those receiving IV insulin) periodically during therapy.

Toxicity and Overdose

- Overdose is manifested by symptoms of hypoglycemia. Mild hypoglycemia may be treated by ingestion of oral glucose. Severe hypoglycemia is a life-threatening emergency; treatment consists of IV glucose, glucagon, or epinephrine.

Implementation

- **High Alert:** Medication errors involving insulins have resulted in serious patient harm and death. Clarify all ambiguous orders and do not accept orders using the abbreviation "u" for units, which can be misread as a zero or the numeral 4 and has resulted in tenfold overdoses. Insulins are available in different types and strengths. Check type, dose, and expiration date with another licensed nurse. Do not interchange insulins without consulting other health care professional.
- Do not confuse Humulin with Humalog or Novolin. Do not confuse Novolin N with Novolog.
- Use *only* insulin syringes to draw up dose. The unit markings on the insulin syringe must match the insulin's units/mL. Special syringes for doses <50 units are available. Prior to withdrawing dose, rotate vial between palms to ensure uniform solution; do not shake.
- When mixing insulins, draw regular insulin or insulin lispro into syringe first to avoid contamination of regular insulin vial.
- Insulin should be stored in a cool place but does not need to be refrigerated. Once opened, store at room temperature. Follow manufacturer's instructions regarding storage of insulin and insulin pens before and after use.
- When transferring from once-daily NPH human insulin to *insulin glargine*, the dose usually remains unchanged. When transferring from twice-daily NPH human insulin to insulin glargine, the initial dose of insulin glargine is usually reduced by 20%.
- NPH insulin should not be used in the management of ketoacidosis.
- **SUBQ:** Administer NPH insulin within 30–60 min before a meal. Inject SUBQ in abdomen, thigh, upper arm, or buttocks. Rotate injection sites to reduce risk of lipodystrophy or localized cutaneous amyloidosis. Repeated insulin injections into areas of lipodystrophy or localized cutaneous amyloidosis may result in hyperglycemia; and a sudden change in the injection site (to an unaffected area) may result in hypoglycemia.

Patient/Family Teaching

- Instruct patient on proper technique for administration. Include type of insulin, equipment (syringe, cartridge pens, alcohol swabs), storage, and place to discard syringes. Discuss the importance of not changing brands of insulin or syringes, selection and rotation of injection sites, and compliance with therapeutic regimen. Caution patient that insulin pens should not be shared with others, even if clean needles are used.
- Demonstrate technique for mixing insulins by drawing up regular insulin or insulin lispro first and rolling intermediate-acting insulin vial between palms to mix, rather than shaking (may cause inaccurate dose).
- Caution patient not to share pen device with another person, even if needle is changed; may risk transmission of bloodborne pathogens.
- Explain to patient that this medication controls hyperglycemia but does not cure diabetes. Therapy is long term.
- Instruct patient in proper testing of serum glucose and ketones. These tests should be closely monitored during periods of stress or illness and health care professional notified of significant changes.
- Emphasize the importance of compliance with nutritional guidelines and regular exercise as directed by health care professional.
- Instruct patient to notify health care professional of all Rx or OTC medications, vitamins, or herbal products being taken and to consult health care professional before taking other Rx, OTC, herbal products, or alcohol.
- Advise patient to notify health care professional of medication regimen prior to treatment or surgery.
- Advise patient to notify health care professional if nausea, vomiting, or fever develops, if unable to eat regular diet, or if blood glucose levels are not controlled.

- Instruct patient on signs and symptoms of hypoglycemia and hyperglycemia and what to do if they occur.
- Patients with diabetes mellitus should carry a source of sugar (candy, glucose gel) and identification describing their disease and treatment regimen at all times.
- Rep: Advise females of reproductive potential to notify health care professional if pregnancy is planned or suspected, or if breastfeeding.
- Emphasize the importance of regular follow-up, especially during first few wk of therapy.

Evaluation/Desired Outcomes

- Control of blood glucose levels in diabetic patients without the appearance of hypoglycemic or hyperglycemic episodes.

BEERS   HIGH ALERT

insulin regular (in-su-lin)

✦ Entuzity Kwikpen, HumuLIN R, HumuLIN R U-500 (Concentrated), HumuLIN R U-500 KwikPen (Concentrated), Myxredlin, NovoLIN R, NovoLIN R FlexPen

Classification
Therapeutic: antidiabetics, hormones
Pharmacologic: pancreatics

See Appendix K for more information concerning insulins

Indications

Type 1 or type 2 diabetes mellitus. **Concentrated regular insulin U-500:** Only for use in patients with insulin requirements >200 units/day. **Unlabeled Use:** Hyperkalemia.

Action

Lowers blood glucose by: stimulating glucose uptake in skeletal muscle and fat, inhibiting hepatic glucose production. Other actions of insulin: inhibition of lipolysis and proteolysis, enhanced protein synthesis. **Therapeutic Effects:** Control of hyperglycemia in diabetic patients.

Pharmacokinetics

Absorption: Rapidly absorbed from SUBQ administration sites. U-100 regular insulin is absorbed slightly more quickly than U-500. IV administration results in complete bioavailability.
Distribution: Identical to endogenous insulin.
Metabolism and Excretion: Metabolized by liver, spleen, kidney, and muscle.
Half-life: 30–60 min.

TIME/ACTION PROFILE (hypoglycemic effect)

ROUTE	ONSET	PEAK	DURATION
IV	10–30 min	15–30 min	30–60 min
SUBQ	30–60 min	2–4 hr	5–7 hr

Contraindications/Precautions

Contraindicated in: Hypoglycemia; Allergy or hypersensitivity to a particular type of insulin, preservatives, or other additives.
Use Cautiously in: Stress or infection—may temporarily ↑ insulin requirements; Renal impairment (may ↓ insulin requirements); Hepatic impairment (may ↓ insulin requirements); OB: Pregnancy may temporarily ↑ insulin requirements; Geri: Appears on Beers list. ↑ risk of hypoglycemia in older adults. Avoid use of regimens containing only short- or rapid-acting insulin without concurrent use of basal or long-acting insulin.

Adverse Reactions/Side Effects

Endo: HYPOGLYCEMIA. **F and E:** hypokalemia. **Local:** cutaneous amyloidosis, erythema, lipodystrophy, pruritus, swelling. **Misc:** HYPERSENSITIVITY REACTIONS (including anaphylaxis).

Interactions

Drug-Drug: **Beta blockers** and **clonidine** may mask some of the signs and symptoms of hypoglycemia. **Corticosteroids, thyroid supplements, estrogens, isoniazid, niacin, phenothiazines,** and **rifampin** may ↑ insulin requirements. **Alcohol, ACE inhibitors, MAO inhibitors, octreotide, oral hypoglycemic agents,** and **salicylates** may ↓ insulin requirements. Concurrent use with **pioglitazone** may ↑ risk of fluid retention and worsening HF.
Drug-Natural Products: Glucosamine may worsen blood glucose control. **Fenugreek, chromium,** and **coenzyme Q-10** may produce additive hypoglycemic effects.

Route/Dosage

Dose depends on blood glucose, response, and many other factors.

Ketoacidosis—Regular (100 units/mL) Insulin Only

IV (Adults): 0.1 unit/kg/hr as a continuous infusion.
IV (Children): Loading dose—0.1 unit/kg, then maintenance continuous infusion 0.05–0.2 unit/kg/hr, titrate to optimal rate of ↓ of serum glucose of 80–100 mg/dL/hr.

Maintenance Therapy

SUBQ (Adults and Children): 0.5–1 unit/kg/day in divided doses. *Adolescents during rapid growth:* 0.8–1.2 unit/kg/day in divided doses.

Treatment of Hyperkalemia

SUBQ, IV (Adults and Children): Dextrose 0.5–1 g/kg combined with insulin 1 unit for every 4–5 g dextrose given.

Availability

Premixed infusion: 100 units/100 mL 0.9% NaCl. **Solution for injection (vials and prefilled pens):** 100 units/mL.^OTC. **Solution for injection (concentrated) (vials and prefilled pens):** 500 units/mL. *In*

combination with: NPH insulins (Humulin 70/30, Novolin 70/30).

NURSING IMPLICATIONS
Assessment
- Assess patient periodically for symptoms of hypoglycemia (anxiety; restlessness; tingling in hands, feet, lips, or tongue; chills; cold sweats; confusion; cool, pale skin; difficulty in concentration; drowsiness; nightmares or trouble sleeping; excessive hunger; headache; irritability; nausea; nervousness; tachycardia; tremor; weakness; unsteady gait) and hyperglycemia (confusion, drowsiness; flushed, dry skin; fruit-like breath odor; rapid, deep breathing, polyuria; loss of appetite; unusual thirst) during therapy.
- Monitor body weight periodically. Changes in weight may necessitate changes in insulin dose.

Lab Test Considerations
- Monitor blood glucose every 6 hr during therapy, more frequently in ketoacidosis and times of stress. A1C may be monitored every 3–6 mo to determine effectiveness.
- Monitor serum potassium in patients at risk for hypokalemia (those using potassium-lowering agents, those receiving IV insulin) periodically during therapy.

Toxicity and Overdose
- Overdose is manifested by symptoms of hypoglycemia. Mild hypoglycemia may be treated by ingestion of oral glucose. Severe hypoglycemia is a life-threatening emergency; treatment consists of IV glucose, glucagon, or epinephrine.

Implementation
- *High Alert:* Medication errors involving insulins have resulted in serious patient harm and death. Clarify all ambiguous orders and do not accept orders using the abbreviation "u" for units, which can be misread as a zero or the numeral 4 and has resulted in tenfold overdoses. Insulins are available in different types and strengths. Check type, dose, and expiration date with another licensed nurse. Do not interchange insulins without consulting health care professional. Do not confuse regular **concentrated (U-500)** insulin with regular insulin.To prevent errors between regular U-100 insulin and concentrated U-500 insulin, concentrated U-500 insulin is marked with a band of diagonal brown strips and "U-500" is highlighted in red on the label and a conversion chart should always be available.
- Do not confuse Humulin with Humalog or Novolin. Do not confuse Novolin with Novolog.
- Use *only* insulin syringes to draw up dose. The unit markings on the insulin syringe must match the insulin's units/mL. Special syringes for doses <50 units and U-500 insulin are available. Prior to withdrawing dose, rotate vial between palms to ensure uniform solution; do not shake.
- When mixing insulins, draw regular insulin into syringe first to avoid contamination of regular insulin vial.
- Insulin should be stored in a cool place but does not need to be refrigerated. Once opened, store at room temperature. Follow manufacturer's instructions regarding storage of insulin and insulin pens before and after use.
- **SUBQ:** Administer regular insulin within 30 min before a meal into the thigh, upper arm, abdomen, or buttocks. Rotate sites with each injection to prevent lipodystrophy and cutaneous amyloidosis. Repeated insulin injections into areas of localized cutaneous amyloidosis may cause hyperglycemia; a sudden change to an unaffected injection site may cause hypoglycemia.

IV Administration
- **IV:** Do not use if cloudy, discolored, or unusually viscous. *High Alert:* Do not administer regular (concentrated) insulin U-500 IV.
- **IV Push: *Dilution:*** May be administered IV undiluted directly into vein or through Y-site. *Rate:* Administer up to 50 units over 1 min.
- **Continuous Infusion: *Dilution:*** May be diluted in 0.9% NaCl using polyvinyl chloride infusion bags. *Concentration:* 0.1 unit/mL to 1 unit/mL in infusion systems with the infusion fluids. *Rate:* Place on an IV pump for accurate administration.
- Rate of administration should be decreased when serum glucose level reaches 250 mg/dL.
- **Y-Site Compatibility:** acetaminophen, acyclovir, aminophylline, amphotericin B lipid complex, anidulafungin, argatroban, arsenic trioxide, ascorbic acid, atropine, azathioprine, aztreonam, benztropine, bivalirudin, bleomycin, bumetanide, buprenorphine, calcium chloride, calcium gluconate, carboplatin, carmustine, caspofungin, cefazolin, cefepime, ceftaroline, ceftazidime, ceftolozane/tazobactam, ceftriaxone, cefuroxime, chloramphenicol, clindamycin, cyanocobalamin, cyclophosphamide, cytarabine, dacarbazine, dactinomycin, daptomycin, daunorubicin hydrochloride, dexamethasone, dexmedetomidine, dexrazoxane, docetaxel, doxorubicin liposomal, doxycycline, enalapril, ephedrine, epirubicin, epoetin alfa, eravacycline, ertapenem, erythromycin, esmolol, esomeprazole, etoposide, etoposide phosphate, fentanyl, fluconazole, fludarabine, folic acid, foscarnet, fosphenytoin, ganciclovir, gemcitabine, granisetron, hetastarch, hydrocortisone, hydromorphone, ibuprofen lysine, idarubicin, ifosfamide, imipenem/cilastatin, indomethacin, irinotecan, isavuconazonium, ketorolac, LR, leucovorin calcium, lidocaine, linezolid, lorazepam, magnesium sulfate, mannitol, meperidine, meropenem, meropenem/vaborbactam, mesna, methadone, metho-

trexate, methylprednisolone, metoclopramide, metoprolol, metronidazole, milrinone, mitoxantrone, moxifloxacin, mycophenolate, nalbuphine, naloxone, nitroglycerin, nitroprusside, octreotide, oritavancin, oxacillin, oxaliplatin, paclitaxel, palonosetron, pamidronate, papaverine, pemetrexed, penicillin G, pentobarbital, phenobarbital, phytonadione, plazomicin, potassium acetate, potassium chloride, procainamide, promethazine, propofol, pyridoxine, remifentanil, sodium bicarbonate, sufentanil, tacrolimus, tedizolid, terbutaline, theophylline, thiamine, thiotepa, tigecycline, tirofiban, topotecan, vancomycin, vecuronium, verapamil, vinblastine, vincristine, vinorelbine, voriconazole, zoledronic acid.

- **Y-Site Incompatibility:** alemtuzumab, butorphanol, cefoxitin, chlorpromazine, cisplatin, dantrolene, diazepam, diphenhydramine, gemtuzumab ozogamicin, glycopyrrolate, hydroxyzine, isoproterenol, ketamine, labetalol, micafungin, minocycline, mitomycin, pentamidine, phentolamine, phenylephrine, phenytoin, piperacillin/tazobactam, prochlorperazine, propranolol, protamine, rocuronium, trimethoprim/sulfamethoxazole.
- **Additive Compatibility:** May be added to total parenteral nutrition solutions.

Patient/Family Teaching

- Instruct patient on proper technique for administration. Include type of insulin, equipment (syringe, cartridge pens, alcohol swabs), storage, and place to discard syringes. Discuss the importance of not changing brands of insulin or syringes, selection and rotation of injection sites, and compliance with therapeutic regimen. Opened, unused insulin vials should be discarded 1 mo after opening.
- Demonstrate technique for mixing insulins by drawing up regular insulin first and rolling intermediate-acting insulin vial between palms to mix, rather than shaking (may cause inaccurate dose).
- Caution patient not to share pen device with another person, even if needle is changed; may risk transmission of bloodborne pathogens.
- Explain to patient that this medication controls hyperglycemia but does not cure diabetes. Therapy is long term.
- Instruct patient in proper testing of serum glucose and ketones. These tests should be closely monitored during periods of stress or illness and health care professional notified of significant changes.
- Emphasize the importance of compliance with nutritional guidelines and regular exercise as directed by health care professional.
- Instruct patient to notify health care professional of all Rx or OTC medications, vitamins, or herbal products being taken and to consult health care professional before taking other Rx, OTC, herbal products, or alcohol.
- Advise patient to notify health care professional of medication regimen prior to treatment or surgery.

- Advise patient to notify health care professional if nausea, vomiting, or fever develops, if unable to eat regular diet, or if blood glucose levels are not controlled.
- Instruct patient on signs and symptoms of hypoglycemia and hyperglycemia and what to do if they occur.
- Rep: Advise females of reproductive potential to notify health care professional if pregnancy is planned or suspected or if breastfeeding.
- Patients with diabetes mellitus should carry a source of sugar (candy, glucose gel) and identification describing their disease and treatment regimen at all times.
- Emphasize the importance of regular follow-up, especially during first few wk of therapy.

Evaluation/Desired Outcomes

- Control of blood glucose levels in diabetic patients without the appearance of hypoglycemic or hyperglycemic episodes.

HIGH ALERT

INSULINS (long-acting)
(in-su-lin)
insulin degludec
Tresiba, Tresiba FlexTouch
insulin detemir
Levemir, Levemir FlexPen
insulin glargine
Basaglar KwikPen, Basaglar Tempo Pen, Lantus, Lantus SoloStar, Rezvoglar KwikPen, Semglee, Toujeo Max SoloStar, Toujeo SoloStar
Classification
Therapeutic: antidiabetics, hormones
Pharmacologic: pancreatics

See Appendix K for more information concerning insulins

Indications
Control of hyperglycemia in patients with type 1 or type 2 diabetes mellitus.

Action
Lower blood glucose by: stimulating glucose uptake in skeletal muscle and fat, inhibiting hepatic glucose production. Other actions: inhibition of lipolysis and proteolysis, enhanced protein synthesis. **Therapeutic Effects:** Control of hyperglycemia in diabetic patients.

Pharmacokinetics
Absorption: Physiochemical characteristics of long-acting insulins result in delayed and prolonged absorption.
Distribution: Widely distributed.
Metabolism and Excretion: Metabolized by liver, spleen, kidney, and muscle.

Half-life: 5–6 min (prolonged in patients with diabetes); biologic half-life is 1–1.5 hr; *insulin degludec* 25 hr; *insulin detemir* 5–7 hr (dose-dependent).

TIME/ACTION PROFILE (hypoglycemic effect)

ROUTE	ONSET	PEAK	DURATION
Insulin degludec	within 2 hr	12 hr	up to 42 hr*
Insulin detemir	3–4 hr	3–14 hr†	6–24 hr‡
Insulin glargine	3–4 hr	none†	24 hr

*Following discontinuation after chronic use.
†Small amounts of insulin glargine and insulin detemir are slowly released resulting in a relatively constant effect over time.
‡Duration is dose dependent; duration ↑ as dose ↑.

Contraindications/Precautions
Contraindicated in: Hypoglycemia; Allergy or hypersensitivity to a particular type of insulin, preservatives, or other additives.
Use Cautiously in: Stress and infection (may temporarily ↑ insulin requirements); Renal/hepatic impairment (may ↓ insulin requirements); Concomitant use with pioglitazone (↑ risk of fluid retention and worsening HF); Patients with visual impairment who may rely on audible clicks to dial their dose (Toujeo and Tresiba); OB: Pregnancy may temporarily ↑ insulin requirements; Pedi: Children <18 yr (Toujeo), <6 yr (Basaglar, Lantus, Rezvoglar, or Semglee), <2 yr (detemir), or <1 yr (degludec) (safety not established).

Adverse Reactions/Side Effects
Endo: HYPOGLYCEMIA. **F and E:** hypokalemia. **Local:** cutaneous amyloidosis, erythema, lipodystrophy, pruritus, swelling. **Misc:** HYPERSENSITIVITY REACTIONS (including anaphylaxis).

Interactions
Drug-Drug: Beta blockers and **clonidine** may mask some of the signs and symptoms of hypoglycemia. **Corticosteroids, thyroid supplements, estrogens, isoniazid, niacin, phenothiazines,** and **rifampin** may ↑ insulin requirements. **Alcohol, ACE inhibitors, MAO inhibitors, octreotide, oral hypoglycemic agents,** and **salicylates** may ↓ insulin requirements. Concurrent use with **pioglitazone** may ↑ risk of fluid retention and worsening HF.
Drug-Natural Products: Glucosamine may worsen blood glucose control. **Fenugreek, chromium,** and **coenzyme Q-10** may produce additive hypoglycemic effects.

Route/Dosage
Toujeo has a lower glucose-lowering effect than Basaglar, Lantus, Rezvoglar, or Semglee on a unit-to-unit basis.

Insulin Degludec
SUBQ (Adults): *Type 1 diabetes (insulin naïve):* ⅓–½ of the total daily insulin dose given once daily, then adjust on the basis of patient's needs (remainder of insulin dose should be given as a short-acting insulin and divided between each daily meal) (usual starting total daily insulin dose = 0.2–0.4 units/kg); *Type 2 diabetes (insulin naïve):* 10 units once daily, then adjust on the basis of patient's needs; *Type 1 or 2 diabetes (and already on insulin):* Give the same dose as the total daily dose of the long-acting or intermediate-acting insulin once daily, then adjust on the basis of patient's needs.
SUBQ (Children ≥1 yr): *Type 1 or 2 diabetes (and already on insulin):* Give 80% of the total daily dose of the long-acting or intermediate-acting insulin once daily, then adjust on the basis of patient's needs.

Insulin Detemir
SUBQ (Adults and Children ≥6 yr): *Type 2 diabetes patients who are insulin-naive:* 0.1–0.2 units/kg once daily in the evening (or divided into a twice daily regimen) *or* 10 units once daily in the evening (or divided into a twice daily regimen). *Patients with type 1 or 2 diabetes receiving basal insulin or basal bolus therapy:* May substitute on an equivalent unit-per-unit basis.

Insulin Glargine (Basaglar, Lantus, Rezvoglar, or Semglee)
SUBQ (Adults and Children ≥6 yr): *Type 1 diabetes (insulin naïve):* ⅓ of the total daily insulin dose given once daily, then adjust on the basis of patient's needs (remainder of insulin dose should be given as a short-acting insulin) (usual starting total daily insulin dose = 0.2–0.4 units/kg); *Type 2 diabetes (insulin naïve):* 0.2 units/kg or up to 10 units once daily; then adjust on the basis of patient's needs; *Type 1 or 2 diabetes (and converting from Toujeo):* Give 80% of Toujeo dose as Basaglar, Lantus, or Semglee once daily, then adjust on the basis of patient's needs; *Type 1 or 2 diabetes (and converting from once daily NPH):* Give the same dose once daily, then adjust on the basis of patient's needs; *Type 1 or 2 diabetes (and converting from twice daily NPH):* Give 80% of the total daily NPH dose once daily, then adjust on the basis of patient's needs.

Insulin Glargine (Toujeo)
SUBQ (Adults): *Type 1 diabetes (insulin naïve):* ⅓–½ of the total daily insulin dose given once daily, then adjust on the basis of patient's needs (range = 1–80 units/day), (remainder of insulin dose should be given as a short-acting insulin) (usual starting total daily insulin dose = 0.2–0.4 units/kg); *Type 2 diabetes (insulin naïve):* 0.2 units/kg once daily, then adjust on

the basis of patient's needs; *Type 1 or 2 diabetes (and converting from intermediate or long-acting insulin):* Use same total daily dose and give once daily, then adjust on the basis of patient's needs; *Type 1 or 2 diabetes (and converting from NPH insulin):* Use 80% of the total daily NPH and give once daily, then adjust on the basis of patient's needs.

Availability

Insulin Degludec
Solution for injection: 100 units/mL (prefilled pens and vials), 200 units/mL (prefilled pens). *In combination with:* liraglutide (Xultophy). See Appendix N.

Insulin Detemir
Solution for injection: 100 units/mL (prefilled pens and vials).

Insulin Glargine
Solution for injection (Basaglar, Rezvoglar): 100 units/mL (prefilled pens). **Solution for injection (Lantus, Semglee):** 100 units/mL (prefilled pens and vials). **Solution for injection (Toujeo):** 300 units/mL (prefilled pens). *In combination with:* lixisenatide (Soliqua). See Appendix N.

NURSING IMPLICATIONS

Assessment
- Assess patient for signs and symptoms of hypoglycemia (anxiety; restlessness; mood changes; tingling in hands, feet, lips, or tongue; chills; cold sweats; confusion; cool, pale skin; difficulty in concentration; drowsiness; nightmares or trouble sleeping; excessive hunger; headache; irritability; nausea; nervousness; tachycardia; tremor; weakness; unsteady gait) and hyperglycemia (confusion, drowsiness; flushed, dry skin; fruit-like breath odor; rapid, deep breathing, polyuria; loss of appetite; nausea; vomiting; tiredness; unusual thirst) periodically during therapy.
- Monitor body weight periodically. Changes in weight may necessitate changes in insulin dose.

Lab Test Considerations
- Monitor blood glucose every 6 hr during therapy, more frequently in ketoacidosis and times of stress. Hemoglobin A_{1C} may also be monitored every 3–6 mo to determine effectiveness.
- Monitor serum potassium in patients at risk for hypokalemia (those using potassium-lowering agents, those receiving IV insulin) periodically during therapy.

Toxicity and Overdose
- Overdose is manifested by symptoms of hypoglycemia. Mild hypoglycemia may be treated by ingestion of oral glucose. Severe hypoglycemia is a life-threatening emergency; treatment consists of IV glucose, glucagon, or epinephrine. Recovery from hypoglycemia may be delayed due to the prolonged effect of long-acting insulins.

Implementation
- *High Alert:* Insulin-related medication errors have resulted in patient harm and death. Clarify ambiguous orders; do not accept orders using the abbreviation "u" for units (can be misread as a zero or the numeral 4; has resulted in tenfold overdoses).
- Insulins are available in different types and strengths. Check type, dose, and expiration date with another licensed nurse. Do not interchange insulins without consulting health care professional.
- Do not confuse Levemir with Lovenox. Do not confuse Lantus with Latuda. Do not confuse Toujeo with Tradjenta, Tresiba, or Trulicity. Do not confuse Tresiba with Tarceva, Toujeo, Tradjenta, or Trulicity.
- Use *only* insulin syringes to draw up dose. The unit markings on the insulin syringe must match the insulin's units/mL. Special syringes for doses <50 units are available. Prior to withdrawing dose, rotate vial between palms to ensure uniform solution; do not shake.
- Use U-100 vial for pediatric patients requiring <5 units of insulin degludec each day.
- *High Alert:* Do not mix *insulin glargine or insulin detemir* with any other insulin or solution, or use syringes containing any other medicinal product or residue. If giving with a short-acting insulin, use separate syringes and different injection sites. Solution should be clear and colorless with no particulate matter.
- Do not use if cloudy, discolored, or unusually viscous. Store unopened vials and cartridges of *insulin glargine and insulin detemir* in the refrigerator; do not freeze. If unable to refrigerate, the 10-mL vial of *insulin glargine* can be kept in a cool place unrefrigerated for up to 28 days. Once the cartridge is placed in a pen, do not refrigerate. After initial use, *insulin detemir* vials, cartridges, or a prefilled syringe may be stored in a cool place for up to 42 days. *Insulin degludec* pens may be stored in the refrigerator or kept at room temperature for up to 56 days. Do not store in-use cartridges and prefilled syringes in refrigerator or with needle in place. Keep away from direct heat and sunlight.
- When transferring from once-daily NPH human insulin to *insulin glargine*, the dose usually remains unchanged. When transferring from twice-daily NPH human insulin to insulin glargine, the initial dose of insulin glargine is usually reduced by 20%.
- **SUBQ:** Inject in abdominal area, thigh, buttocks or upper arms, and rotate injection sites with each injection to reduce the risk of lipodystrophy and localized cutaneous amyloidosis. Repeated insulin injections into areas of localized cutaneous amyloidosis may cause hyperglycemia; a sudden change to an unaffected injection site may cause hypoglycemia.
- Administer *insulin glargine* and *insulin degludec* once daily at the same time each day.
- Administer *daily insulin detemir* with evening meal or at bedtime. With *twice daily insulin detemir*, ad-

minister evening dose with evening meal, at bedtime, or 12 hr after morning dose.

● Do not administer *insulin detemir, insulin degludec,* or *insulin glargine* IV or in insulin pumps.

Patient/Family Teaching

● Instruct patient on proper technique for administration. Include type of insulin, equipment (syringe, cartridge pens, alcohol swabs), storage, and place to discard syringes. Discuss the importance of not changing brands of insulin or syringes, selection and rotation of injection sites, and compliance with therapeutic regimen. Patients taking insulin detemir and *insulin degludec* should be given the *Patient Information* circular for this product.

● Caution patient not to share pen device with another person, even if needle is changed; may risk transmission of bloodborne pathogens.

● Explain to patient that this medication controls hyperglycemia but does not cure diabetes. Therapy is long term.

● Instruct patient in proper testing of serum glucose and ketones. These tests should be closely monitored during periods of stress or illness and health care professional notified of significant changes.

● Emphasize the importance of compliance with nutritional guidelines and regular exercise as directed by health care professional.

● Instruct patient to notify health care professional of all Rx or OTC medications, vitamins, or herbal products being taken and to consult health care professional before taking other Rx, OTC, herbal products, or alcohol.

● Advise patient to notify health care professional of medication regimen prior to treatment or surgery.

● Advise patient to notify health care professional if nausea, vomiting, or fever develops; if unable to eat regular diet; or if blood glucose levels are not controlled.

● Instruct patient on signs and symptoms of hypoglycemia and hyperglycemia and what to do if they occur.

● Patients with diabetes mellitus should carry a source of sugar (candy, glucose gel) and identification describing their disease and treatment regimen at all times.

● Rep: Advise patient to notify health care professional if pregnancy is planned or suspected or if breastfeeding.

● Emphasize the importance of regular follow-up, especially during first few wk of therapy.

Evaluation/Desired Outcomes

● Control of blood glucose levels in diabetic patients without the appearance of hypoglycemic or hyperglycemic episodes.

INSULINS (rapid-acting)
(in-su-lin)
insulin aspart
Fiasp, Fiasp FlexTouch, Fiasp PenFill, NovoLOG, NovoLOG FlexPen, NovoLOG PenFill, ✲ NovoRapid
insulin glulisine
Apidra, Apidra SoloStar
insulin lispro
Admelog, Admelog SoloStar, HumaLOG, HumaLOG Junior KwikPen, HumaLOG KwikPen, HumaLOG Tempo Pen, Lyumjev, Lyumjev KwikPen, Lyumjev Tempo Pen

Classification
Therapeutic: antidiabetics, hormones
Pharmacologic: pancreatics

See Appendix K for more information concerning insulins

Indications
Control of hyperglycemia in patients with type 1 or type 2 diabetes mellitus.

Action
Lower blood glucose by: stimulating glucose uptake in skeletal muscle and fat, inhibiting hepatic glucose production. Other actions: inhibition of lipolysis and proteolysis, enhanced protein synthesis. These are rapid-acting insulins with a more rapid onset and shorter duration than regular insulin; should be used with an intermediate- or long-acting insulin. **Therapeutic Effects:** Control of hyperglycemia in diabetic patients.

Pharmacokinetics
Absorption: Very rapidly absorbed from SUBQ administration sites.
Distribution: Widely distributed.
Metabolism and Excretion: Metabolized by liver, spleen, kidney, and muscle.
Half-life: *Insulin aspart:* 1–1.5 hr; *Insulin lispro:* 1 hr; *insulin glulisine:* 42 min.

TIME/ACTION PROFILE (hypoglycemic effect)

ROUTE	ONSET	PEAK	DURATION
Insulin aspart	within 15 min	1–2 hr	3–4 hr
Insulin glulisine	within 15 min	1–2 hr	3–4 hr
Insulin lispro	within 15 min	1–2 hr	3–4 hr

Contraindications/Precautions
Contraindicated in: Hypoglycemia; Allergy or hypersensitivity to a particular type of insulin, preservatives, or other additives.

✲= Canadian drug name. ▒▒ = Genetic implication. S̶t̶r̶i̶k̶e̶t̶h̶r̶o̶u̶g̶h̶ = Discontinued. CAPITALS = life-threatening. <u>Underline</u> = most frequent.

Use Cautiously in: Stress and infection (may temporarily ↑ insulin requirements); Renal/hepatic dysfunction (may ↓ insulin requirements); Concomitant use with pioglitazone (↑ risk of fluid retention and worsening HF); OB: Pregnancy may temporarily ↑ insulin requirements; Pedi: Safety not established in children <1 yr (Lyumjev), <3 yr (Admelog and Humalog), <4 yr (insulin glulisine), or <6 yr (for insulin aspart).

Adverse Reactions/Side Effects

Endo: HYPOGLYCEMIA. **F and E:** hypokalemia. **Local:** cutaneous amyloidosis, erythema, lipodystrophy, pruritus, swelling. **Misc:** HYPERSENSITIVITY REACTIONS (including anaphylaxis).

Interactions

Drug-Drug: Beta blockers and clonidine may mask some of the signs and symptoms of hypoglycemia. **Corticosteroids, thyroid supplements, estrogens, isoniazid, niacin, phenothiazines,** and **rifampin** may ↑ insulin requirements. **Alcohol, ACE inhibitors, MAO inhibitors, octreotide, oral hypoglycemic agents,** and **salicylates** may ↓ insulin requirements. Concurrent use with **pioglitazone** may ↑ risk of fluid retention and worsening HF.
Drug-Natural Products: Glucosamine may worsen blood glucose control. **Fenugreek, chromium,** and **coenzyme Q-10** may produce additive hypoglycemic effects.

Route/Dosage

Dose depends on blood glucose, response, and many other factors. Only insulin aspart and insulin glulisine can be administered IV. Lyumjev has faster onset of action and greater blood glucose-lowering effect than Admelog or Humalog on a unit-to-unit basis.
SUBQ (Adults and Children): Total insulin dose determined by needs of patient; generally 0.5–1 unit/kg/day; 50–70% of this dose may be given as meal-related boluses of rapid-acting insulin, and the remainder as an intermediate or long-acting insulin. *SUBQ infusion pump:* ~50% of total dose can be given as meal-related boluses and ~50% of total dose can be given as basal infusion.

Availability

Insulin Aspart
Solution for injection: 100 units/mL (vials, prefilled cartridges, and prefilled pens).

Insulin Glulisine
Solution for injection: 100 units/mL (vials and prefilled pens).

Insulin Lispro
Solution for injection (Admelog): 100 units/mL (vials, prefilled cartridges, and prefilled pens). **Solution for injection (Humalog, Lyumjev):** 100 units/mL (vials, prefilled cartridges, and prefilled pens), 200 units/mL (prefilled pens).

NURSING IMPLICATIONS

Assessment

- Assess for symptoms of hypoglycemia (anxiety; restlessness; tingling in hands, feet, lips, or tongue; chills; cold sweats; confusion; cool, pale skin; difficulty in concentration; drowsiness; nightmares or trouble sleeping; excessive hunger; headache; irritability; nausea; nervousness; tachycardia; tremor; weakness; unsteady gait) and hyperglycemia (confusion, drowsiness; flushed, dry skin; fruit-like breath odor; rapid, deep breathing; polyuria; loss of appetite; nausea; vomiting; unusual thirst) periodically during therapy.
- Monitor body weight periodically. Changes in weight may necessitate changes in insulin dose.
- Assess patient for signs of allergic reactions (rash, shortness of breath, wheezing, rapid pulse, sweating, low BP) during therapy.

Lab Test Considerations
- Monitor blood glucose every 6 hr during therapy, more frequently in ketoacidosis and times of stress. HbA₁c may also be monitored every 3–6 mo to determine effectiveness.
- Monitor serum potassium in patients at risk for hypokalemia (those using potassium-lowering agents, those receiving IV insulin) periodically during therapy.

Toxicity and Overdose
- Overdose is manifested by symptoms of hypoglycemia. Mild hypoglycemia may be treated by ingestion of oral glucose. Severe hypoglycemia is a life-threatening emergency; treatment consists of IV glucose, glucagon, or epinephrine. Early signs of hypoglycemia may be less pronounced by long duration of diabetes, diabetic nerve disease, and use of beta blockers; may result in loss of consciousness prior to patient's awareness of hypoglycemia.

Implementation
- *High Alert:* Insulin-related medication errors have resulted in patient harm and death. Clarify ambiguous orders; do not accept orders using the abbreviation "u" for units (can be misread as a zero or the numeral 4; has resulted in tenfold overdoses).
- Insulins are available in different types and strengths. Check type, dose, and expiration date with another licensed nurse. Do not interchange insulins without consulting health care professional.
- Do not confuse Humalog with Humulin or Novolog. Do not confuse Novolog with Novolin. Do not confuse Apidra with Spiriva.
- Use *only* insulin syringes to draw up dose. The unit markings on the insulin syringe must match the insulin's units/mL. Special syringes for doses <50 units are available. Do not draw up dose into a syringe from the Kwik Pens; syringe markings do not match-up and could lead to a medication error. Use *only* U-100 insulin syringes to draw up *insulin lis-*

pro dose. Prior to withdrawing dose, rotate vial between palms to ensure uniform solution; do not shake.

• *Insulin aspart, insulin glulisine,* and *insulin lispro* may be mixed with NPH insulin. When mixing insulins, draw insulin aspart, insulin glulisine, or insulin lispro into syringe first to avoid contamination of rapid-acting insulin vial. Mixed insulins should never be used in a pump or for IV infusion.

• Store vials in refrigerator. Vials may also be kept at room temperature for up to 28 days. Do not use if cloudy, discolored, or unusually viscous. Store cartridges and pens at room temperature and use within 28 days. Never use the *PenFill* cartridge after the expiration date on the *PenFill* cartridge or on the box.

• Because of their short duration, *insulin lispro, insulin glulisine,* and *insulin aspart* must be used with a longer-acting insulin or insulin infusion pump. In patients with type 2 diabetes, *insulin lispro* may be used without a longer-acting insulin when used in combination with an oral sulfonylurea agent.

• Humalog U-200 and Lyumjev U-200 should not be mixed with other insulins, administered IV, or used in insulin pumps.

• **SUBQ:** Administer into abdominal wall, thigh, or upper arm SUBQ. Rotate injection sites to prevent lipodystrophy and cutaneous amyloidosis. Repeated insulin injections into areas of localized cutaneous amyloidosis may cause hyperglycemia; a sudden change to an unaffected injection site may cause hypoglycemia.

• Administer *insulin aspart* within 5–10 min before a meal.

• When used as meal-time insulin, administer *insulin glulisine* 15 min before or within 20 min after starting a meal.

• Administer *insulin lispro: Admelog* and *Humalog* within 15 min before or immediately after a meal. Administer *Lyumjev* at the start of a meal or within 20 minutes after starting a meal.

• May also be administered SUBQ via external insulin pump. Do not mix with other insulins or solution when used with a pump. Change the solution in the reservoir at least every 6 days (Lyumjev at least every 9 days), change the infusion set, and the infusion set insertion site at least every 3 days. Do not mix with other insulins or with a diluent when used in the pump.

• **IV:** *Insulin aspart* and *insulin glulisine* may be administered IV in selected situations under appropriate medical supervision. *Dilution:* Dilute *insulin aspart* with 0.9% NaCl or D5W in infusion systems using polypropylene infusion bags. Dilute *insulin glulisine* with 0.9% NaCl, using polyvinyl chloride (PVC) Viaflex infusion bags and PVC tubing (Clear-link System Continu-Flo solution set) with a dedicated infusion line. *Concentration:* 0.05–1 unit/mL. *Insulin lispro (Humalog U-100)* can be administered IV under medical supervision ONLY with close monitoring of blood glucose and potassium levels to avoid hypoglycemia and hypokalemia. . *Concentration:* 0.1 unit/mL to 1 unit/mL. *Dilution:* 0.9% NaCl. Solutions of insulin lispro and 0.9% NaCl can be stored for 48 hr in refrigerator, then used at room temperature for another 48 hr.

Patient/Family Teaching

• Instruct patient on proper technique for administration. Include type of insulin, equipment (syringe, cartridge pens, external pump, alcohol swabs), storage, and place to discard syringes. Discuss the importance of not changing brands of insulin or syringes, selection and rotation of injection sites, and compliance with therapeutic regimen. Caution patient that insulin pens should not be shared with others, even if clean needles are used.

• Demonstrate technique for mixing insulins by drawing up insulin aspart, insulin glulisine, or insulin lispro first. Roll intermediate-acting insulin vial between palms to mix, rather than shaking (may cause inaccurate dose).

• Caution patient not to share pen device with another person, even if needle is changed; may risk transmission of bloodborne pathogens.

• Instruct patient in prompt identification and correction of the cause of hyperglycemia or ketosis. Pump or infusion set malfunctions can lead to a rapid onset of hyperglycemia and ketoacidosis. Interim therapy with SUBQ injection may be required. Patients using continuous SUBQ insulin infusion pump therapy must be trained to administer insulin by injection and have alternate insulin therapy available in case of pump failure.

• Explain to patient that this medication controls hyperglycemia but does not cure diabetes. Therapy is long term.

• Instruct patient in proper testing of serum glucose and ketones. These tests should be closely monitored during periods of stress or illness and health care professional notified of significant changes.

• Emphasize the importance of compliance with nutritional guidelines and regular exercise as directed by health care professional.

• Advise patient to notify health care professional of all Rx or OTC medications, vitamins, or herbal products being taken and to consult with health care professional before taking other medications or alcohol.

• Advise patient to notify health care professional of medication regimen prior to treatment or surgery.

• Advise patient to notify health care professional if nausea, vomiting, or fever develops, if unable to eat regular diet, or if blood glucose levels are not controlled.

- Instruct patient on signs and symptoms of hypoglycemia and hyperglycemia and what to do if they occur.
- Rep: Advise patient to notify health care professional if pregnancy is planned or suspected or if breastfeeding.
- Patients with diabetes mellitus should carry a source of sugar (candy, glucose gel) and identification describing their disease and treatment regimen at all times.
- Emphasize the importance of regular follow-up, especially during first few wk of therapy.

Evaluation/Desired Outcomes
- Control of blood glucose levels without the appearance of hypoglycemic or hyperglycemic episodes.

⚕ ipilimumab (i-pil-li-moo-mab)
Yervoy

Classification
Therapeutic: antineoplastics
Pharmacologic: monoclonal antibodies, cytotoxic lymphocyte antigen 4 inhibitors

Indications
Unresectable/metastatic melanoma (as monotherapy or in combination with nivolumab). Adjuvant treatment of cutaneous melanoma with pathologic involvement of regional lymph nodes >1 mm in patients who have undergone complete resection, including total lymphadenectomy. Previously untreated, advanced renal cell carcinoma in patients who are at intermediate or poor risk (in combination with nivolumab). ⚕ Microsatellite instability-high (MSI-H) or mismatch repair deficient (dMMR) metastatic colorectal cancer that has progressed following treatment with a fluoropyrimidine, oxaliplatin, and irinotecan. Hepatocellular carcinoma in patients who have been previously treated with sorafenib (in combination with nivolumab). ⚕ First-line treatment of metastatic non-small cell lung cancer (NSCLC) in patients whose tumors express PD-L1 (≥1%) and have no epidermal growth factor receptor (EGFR) or anaplastic lymphoma kinase (ALK) genomic tumor aberrations (in combination with nivolumab). ⚕ First-line treatment of metastatic or recurrent NSCLC in patients whose tumors have no EGFR or ALK genomic tumor aberrations (in combination with nivolumab and two cycles of platinum-based chemotherapy). First-line treatment of unresectable malignant pleural mesothelioma (in combination with nivolumab). First-line treatment of unresectable advanced or metastatic esophageal squamous cell carcinoma (in combination with nivolumab).

Action
Binds to cytotoxic T-lymphocyte-associated antigen 4 (CTLA-4) and prevents it from binding to CD80/CD86 ligands. CTLA-4 is a negative regulator of T-cell activation; binding results in augmented T-cell activation and proliferation as well as enhanced T-cell responsiveness. **Therapeutic Effects:** ↓ spread or recurrence of melanoma and improved survival. Improved survival with renal cell carcinoma, NSCLC, malignant pleural mesothelioma, and esophageal squamous cell carcinoma. ↓ progression of MSI-H or dMMR metastatic colorectal cancer. ↓ progression of hepatocellular carcinoma.

Pharmacokinetics
Absorption: IV administration results in complete bioavailability.
Distribution: Crosses the placenta.
Metabolism and Excretion: Unknown.
Half-life: 14.7 days.

TIME/ACTION PROFILE

ROUTE	ONSET	PEAK	DURATION
IV	unknown	unknown	unknown

Contraindications/Precautions
Contraindicated in: Lactation: Lactation.
Use Cautiously in: Patients undergoing allogeneic hematopoietic stem cell transplantation (↑ risk of graft-versus-host disease; OB: Use only if potential maternal benefit justifies potential risk to the fetus; Rep: Women of reproductive potential; Pedi: Children <12 yr (safety and effectiveness not established).

Adverse Reactions/Side Effects
CV: MYOCARDITIS, pericarditis, vasculitis. **Derm:** pruritus, rash, DRUG REACTION WITH EOSINOPHILIA AND SYSTEMIC SYMPTOMS (DRESS), STEVENS-JOHNSON SYNDROME (SJS), TOXIC EPIDERMAL NECROLYSIS (TEN). **EENT:** hearing loss, immune-mediated iritis, immune-mediated uveitis. **Endo:** immune-mediated hypothyroidism, IMMUNE-MEDIATED ADRENAL INSUFFICIENCY, immune-mediated hyperthyroidism, immune-mediated hypoparathyroidism, immune-mediated hypophysitis, immune-mediated type 1 diabetes. **GI:** diarrhea, IMMUNE-MEDIATED COLITIS, immune-mediated gastritis, IMMUNE-MEDIATED HEPATITIS, immune-mediated pancreatitis. **GU:** immune-mediated nephritis. **Hemat:** immune-mediated hemolytic anemia. **MS:** immune-mediated myositis, IMMUNE-MEDIATED RHABDOMYOLYSIS. **Neuro:** fatigue, autoimmune neuropathy, Guillain-Barré syndrome, IMMUNE-MEDIATED ENCEPHALITIS, IMMUNE-MEDIATED MENINGITIS, immune-mediated myasthenic syndrome, immune-mediated myelitis. **Resp:** IMMUNE-MEDIATED PNEUMONITIS. **Misc:** INFUSION REACTIONS.

Interactions
Drug-Drug: Concurrent use with **vemurafenib** may ↑ risk of hepatic dysfunction.

Route/Dosage
Unresectable/Metastatic Melanoma
IV (Adults and Children ≥12 yr): *As monotherapy:* 3 mg/kg every 3 wk for up to 4 doses. *In combination*

with nivolumab: 3 mg/kg every 3 wk for up to 4 doses or unacceptable toxicity (administer after nivolumab on same day); after completing 4 doses of the combination, give nivolumab alone until disease progression or unacceptable toxicity.

Adjuvant Treatment of Melanoma

IV (Adults and Children ≥12 yr): 10 mg/kg every 3 wk for up to 4 doses, then 10 mg/kg every 12 wk for up to 3 yr.

Advanced Renal Cell Carcinoma

IV (Adults): 1 mg/kg every 3 wk for up to 4 doses (administer after nivolumab on same day); after completing 4 doses of the combination, give nivolumab alone until disease progression or unacceptable toxicity.

Colorectal Cancer

IV (Adults): 1 mg/kg every 3 wk for 4 doses (administer after nivolumab on same day); after completing 4 doses of the combination, give nivolumab alone until disease progression or unacceptable toxicity.

Hepatocellular Carcinoma

IV (Adults): 3 mg/kg every 3 wk for 4 doses (administer after nivolumab on same day); after completing 4 doses of the combination, give nivolumab alone until disease progression or unacceptable toxicity.

Metastatic or Recurrent Non-Small Cell Lung Cancer

IV (Adults): 1 mg/kg every 6 wk until disease progression, unacceptable toxicity or for up to 2 yr (if no disease progression) (administer after nivolumab, but before platinum-based chemotherapy [if being given] on same day) .

Malignant Pleural Mesothelioma

IV (Adults): 1 mg/kg every 6 wk until disease progression, unacceptable toxicity or for up to 2 yr (if no disease progression) (administer after nivolumab on same day).

Esophageal Squamous Cell Carcinoma

IV (Adults): 1 mg/kg every 6 wk until disease progression, unacceptable toxicity or for up to 2 yr (administer after nivolumab on same day).

Availability

Solution for injection: 5 mg/mL.

NURSING IMPLICATIONS

Assessment

● Monitor for signs and symptoms of colitis (diarrhea, abdominal pain, mucus or blood in stool, with or without fever) and bowel perforation (peritoneal signs, ileus). Rule out infection and consider endoscopic evaluation. *If Grade 2 colitis occurs,* hold therapy and administer corticosteroids (initial dose of 1–2 mg/kg/day prednisone or equivalent, followed by a corticosteroid taper. Resume therapy at

Grade 0 or 1 after corticosteroid taper. Permanently discontinue if no complete or partial resolution within 12 wk of last dose or inability to reduce prednisone to ≤10 mg per day (or equivalent) within 12 wk of initiating steroids. *If Grade 3 or 4 colitis occurs,* permanently discontinue ipilimumab.

● Assess for skin reactions including SJS, TEN, and DRESS (prodrome of fever, flu-like symptoms, mucosal lesions, progressive skin rash) during therapy. Treat mild to moderate nonexfoliative rashes with topical emollients and/or topical corticosteroids. *If SJS, TEN, or DRESS is suspected,* hold ipilimumab; if confirmed, permanently discontinue ipilimumab.

● Monitor for signs and symptoms of pneumonitis (new or worsening cough, chest pain, shortness of breath) during therapy. Evaluate with x ray. Administer corticosteroids (initial dose of 1–2 mg/kg/day prednisone or equivalent, followed by a corticosteroid taper. *For Grade 2 pneumonitis:* hold ipilimumab and resume with complete or partial resolution (Grade 0–1) after corticosteroid taper. *For Grade 3 or 4 or recurrent Grade 2 pneumonitis:* permanently discontinue ipilimumab.

● Monitor for signs and symptoms of neurologic toxicity (headache, neck stiffness, change in consciousness, weakness) periodically during therapy. *If Grade 2 symptoms occur,* hold ipilimumab. *If Grade 3 or 4 symptoms occur,* discontinue ipilimumab permanently.

● Monitor for signs and symptoms of hypophysitis (headache, photophobia, visual field defects) during therapy. May cause hypopituitarism. Begin hormone replacement therapy. Hold or permanently discontinue ipilimumab based on severity.

● Assess eyes for signs and symptoms of uveitis, iritis, or episcleritis. Administer corticosteroid eye drops if these occur. Consider Vogt Koyanagi-Harada-like syndrome if uveitis occurs with other immune-mediated adverse reactions. May require treatment with systemic steroids to reduce the risk of permanent vision loss. *If Grade 2, 3, or 4 ophthalmologic symptoms occur that do not improve to Grade 1 within 2 wk while receiving topical therapy or that requires systemic treatment:* permanently discontinue ipilimumab.

● Monitor for signs and symptoms of infusion-related reactions (pyrexia, chills, flushing, hypotension, dyspnea, wheezing, back pain, abdominal pain, urticaria) during infusion. *For Grade 1 or 2 infusion-related reactions:* interrupt or slow rate of infusion. *For severe (Grade 3) or life-threatening (Grade 4) infusion-related reactions:* stop infusion and permanently discontinue ipilimumab.

● Monitor for signs and symptoms of cardiovascular events during therapy. Assess left ventricular ejection fraction at baseline and periodically during therapy. Manage cardiovascular risk factors (hypertension, diabetes, dyslipidemia). Discontinue ipilimumab for Grade 2, 3, or 4 cardiovascular events.

Lab Test Considerations
- ✂ Patient selection with metastatic NSCLC for treatment with ipilimumab in combination with nivolumab is based on PD-L1 expression. Information on FDA-approved tests for the determination of PD-L1 expression in NSCLC is available at: http://www.fda.gov/CompanionDiagnostics.
- Verify negative pregnancy status before starting therapy.
- May cause hepatitis; monitor liver function tests prior to and periodically during therapy. *If levels increase:* administer corticosteroids (initial dose of 1–2 mg/kg/day prednisone or equivalent, followed by a corticosteroid taper). For hepatitis with no tumor involvement of the liver or hepatitis with tumor involvement of liver/non-hepatocellular carcinoma: *If AST or ALT ↑ >3 times to <5 times upper limit of normal (ULN) or total bilirubin ↑ >1.5 times to <3 times ULN:* hold ipilimumab and resume with complete or partial resolution (Grade 0–1) after corticosteroid taper. *If AST or ALT >5 times ULN or total bilirubin >3 times ULN:* discontinue ipilimumab permanently. For hepatitis with tumor involvement of the liver/hepatocellular carcinoma: *If baseline AST or ALT >1– <3 times ULN and increases to >5– <10 times ULN or if baseline AST or ALT >3– <5 times ULN and increases to >8 to <10 times ULN:* hold ipilimumab and resume with complete or partial resolution (Grade 0 to 1) after corticosteroid taper. *If AST or ALT >10 times ULN or if total bilirubin >3 times ULN:* permanently discontinue ipilimumab.
- Monitor for signs and symptoms of adrenal insufficiency, including but not limited to hypothyroidism, hyperthyroidism, adrenal insufficiency, and hyperglycemia during and after treatment. Administer corticosteroids as appropriate, followed by a corticosteroid taper. *If Grade 3 or 4 endocrinopathies occur:* hold ipilimumab until clinically stable or permanently discontinue base on severity, treat low levels, and resume with complete or partial resolution (Grade 0–1) after corticosteroid taper.
- May cause nephritis; monitor for ↑ serum creatinine prior to and periodically during therapy. Administer corticosteroids (initial dose of 1–2 mg/kg/day prednisone or equivalent, followed by a corticosteroid taper. *If Grade 2 or 3 increased blood creatinine occurs:* hold ipilimumab and resume with complete or partial resolution (Grade 0–1) of nephritis and renal dysfunction after corticosteroid taper. *If Grade 4 increased blood creatinine occurs:* permanently discontinue ipilimumab.

Implementation
- For unresectable/metastatic melanoma, doses may be delayed in the event of toxicity, but must be administered within 16 wk from 1st dose. For adjuvant

treatment of melanoma, doses can be omitted, but not delayed in the event of toxicity.
- Hold dose for any moderate immune-mediated adverse reactions or for symptomatic endocrinopathy. For patients with complete or partial resolution of adverse reactions (Grade 0–1), who are receiving equivalents of <7.5 mg prednisone/day, resume ipilimumab therapy.
- Permanently discontinue if persistent moderate adverse reactions or inability to reduce corticosteroid dose to equivalent of prednisone 7.5 mg/day, failure to complete full treatment course within 16 wk from infusion of 1st dose, or severe or life-threatening adverse reactions occur including: Colitis with abdominal pain, fever, or peritoneal signs; ↑ in stool frequency of 7 or more over baseline, stool incontinence. Need for IV hydration for >24 hrs, GI hemorrhage and GI perforation; AST or ALT >5 times the upper limits of normal or total bilirubin >3 times the upper limit of normal; Stevens-Johnson syndrome, toxic epidermal necrolysis, or rash complicated by full-thickness dermal ulceration, or necrotic, bullous, or hemorrhagic manifestations; Severe motor or sensory neuropathy, Guillain-Barré syndrome, or myasthenia gravis; Severe immune-mediated reactions involving any organ system (nephritis, pneumonitis, pancreatitis, noninfectious myocarditis); and immune-mediated ocular disease that is unresponsive to topical immunosuppressive therapy.
- Allow vial to stand at room temperature for 5 min prior to preparation of infusion. Withdraw amount of ipilimumab required and transfer to IV bag. *Dilution:* Dilute with 0.9% NaCl or D5W. *Concentration:* 1 mg/mL–2 mg/mL. Mix slowly by gentle inversion; do not shake. Solution is clear, pale yellow, and may contain translucent-to-white amorphous particles; do not administer if cloudy, discolored, or contains particulate matter. Store for up to 24 hr at room temperature or refrigerated; do not freeze, protect from light. Discard partially used vials.
- **Melanoma:** *For unresectable or metastatic melanoma:* infuse over 30 min and *for adjuvant treatment of melanoma:* infuse over 90 min, through a sterile, nonpyrogenic, low-protein-binding in-line filter. Flush the IV line with 0.9% NaCl or D5W after each dose.
- **Renal cell carcinoma, hepatocellular carcinoma, NSCLC, malignant pleural mesothelioma, esophageal squamous cell carcinoma, or colorectal cancer:** Infuse over 30 min immediately following nivolumab infusion through a sterile, nonpyrogenic, low-protein-binding in-line filter. Flush the IV line with 0.9% NaCl or D5W after each dose.
- **Y-Site Incompatibility:** Do not mix with or infuse with other solutions or products.

Patient/Family Teaching

- Explain purpose and potential adverse effects of ipilimumab to patient.
- Inform patient of the risk of immune-mediated reactions due to T-cell activation and proliferation. Advise patients these may be severe and fatal. Instruct patient to notify health care professional immediately if signs and symptoms occur.
- Instruct patient to read the *Medication Guide* before starting therapy and with each Rx refill in case of changes.
- Advise patient to notify health care professional if signs and symptoms of colitis (diarrhea; black, tarry, sticky, bloody, or mucus in stools; severe abdominal pain or tenderness), hepatitis (yellowing of skin or the whites of eyes, severe nausea or vomiting, pain on right side of abdomen), skin reactions (rash, itching, skin blistering or peeling, painful sores in mouth or nose, throat, or genital area), endocrinopathies (persistent or unusual headache, eye sensitivity to light, eye problems, rapid heartbeat, increased sweating, extreme tiredness, weight gain or weight loss, feeling more hungry or thirsty than usual, urinating more often than usual, hair loss, feeling cold, constipation, deepening of voice, dizziness or fainting, changes in mood or behavior, decreased sex drive, irritability, or forgetfulness), pneumonitis (new or worsening cough, shortness of breath, chest pain), nephritis (decrease in amount of urine, blood in urine, swelling of ankles, loss of appetite), or eye problems (blurry vision, double vision, or other vision problems, eye pain or redness) occur.
- Instruct patient to notify health care professional of all Rx or OTC medications, vitamins, or herbal products being taken and to consult health care professional before taking other Rx, OTC, herbal products.
- Rep: May cause fetal harm. Advise females of reproductive potential to use effective contraception and avoid breastfeeding during and for 3 mo following last dose. Women must choose to discontinue breastfeeding or ipilimumab. Advise female patients to notify health care professional if pregnancy is planned or suspected. Encourage women who become pregnant during therapy to contact Bristol-Myers Squibb by calling 1-844-593-7869.

Evaluation/Desired Outcomes

- ↓ spread or recurrence of melanoma.
- Improved survival with renal cell carcinoma, NSCLC, malignant pleural mesothelioma, and esophageal squamous cell carcinoma.
- ↓ progression of MSI-H or dMMR metastatic colorectal cancer.
- ↓ progression of hepatocellular carcinoma.

ipratropium (i-pra-**troe**-pee-um)
Atrovent HFA
Classification
Therapeutic: allergy, cold, and cough remedies, bronchodilators
Pharmacologic: anticholinergics

Indications
Inhaln: Maintenance therapy of reversible airway obstruction due to COPD, including chronic bronchitis and emphysema. **Intranasal:** Rhinorrhea associated with allergic and nonallergic perennial rhinitis (0.03% solution) or the common cold (0.06% solution). **Unlabeled Use: Inhaln:** Adjunctive management of bronchospasm caused by asthma.

Action
Inhaln: Inhibits cholinergic receptors in bronchial smooth muscle, resulting in decreased concentrations of cyclic guanosine monophosphate (cGMP). Decreased levels of cGMP produce local bronchodilation. **Intranasal:** Local application inhibits secretions from glands lining the nasal mucosa. **Therapeutic Effects: Inhaln:** Bronchodilation without systemic anticholinergic effects. **Intranasal:** Decreased rhinorrhea.

Pharmacokinetics
Absorption: Minimal systemic absorption (2% for inhalation solution; 20% for inhalation aerosol; <20% following nasal use).
Distribution: 15% of dose reaches lower airways after inhalation.
Metabolism and Excretion: Small amounts absorbed are metabolized by the liver.
Half-life: 2 hr.

TIME/ACTION PROFILE (bronchodilation)

ROUTE	ONSET	PEAK	DURATION
Inhalation	1–3 min	1–2 hr	4–6 hr
Intranasal	15 min	unknown	6–12 hr

Contraindications/Precautions
Contraindicated in: Hypersensitivity to ipratropium, atropine, belladonna alkaloids, or bromide; Acute bronchospasm.
Use Cautiously in: Bladder-neck obstruction, prostatic hyperplasia, glaucoma, or urinary retention; Lactation: Safety not established in breastfeeding; Geri: Older adults may be more sensitive to effects.

Adverse Reactions/Side Effects
CV: hypotension, palpitations. **Derm:** rash. **EENT:** blurred vision, sore throat; *nasal only:* epistaxis, nasal dryness/irritation. **GI:** GI irritation, nausea. **Neuro:** dizziness, headache, nervousness. **Resp:** bronchospasm, cough. **Misc:** HYPERSENSITIVITY REACTIONS (including anaphylaxis).

Interactions

Drug-Drug: ↑ anticholinergic effects with other **drugs having anticholinergic properties**, including **antihistamines, phenothiazines**, and **disopyramide**.

Route/Dosage

Inhaln (Adults and Children >12 yr): *Metered-dose inhaler (nonacute):* 2 inhalations 4 times daily (not to exceed 12 inhalations/24 hr or more frequently than every 4 hr). *Acute exacerbations:* 4–8 puffs using a spacer device as needed. *Via nebulization (nonacute):* 500 mcg 3–4 times daily. *Via nebulization (acute exacerbations):* 500 mcg every 30 min for 3 doses, then every 2–4 hr as needed.
Inhaln (Adults and Children 5–12 yr): *Metered-dose inhaler (nonacute):* 1–2 inhalations every 6 hr as needed (not to exceed 12 inhalations/24 hr). *Acute exacerbations:* 4–8 puffs as needed. *Via nebulization (nonacute):* 250–500 mcg 4 times daily given every 6 hr. *Acute exacerbations:* 250 mcg every 20 min for 3 doses, then every 2–4 hr as needed.
Inhaln (Infants): *Nebulization:* 125–250 mcg 3 times a day.
Inhaln (Neonates): *Nebulization:* 25 mcg/kg/dose 3 times a day.
Intranasal (Adults and Children >6 yr): *0.03% solution:* 2 sprays in each nostril 2–3 times daily (21 mcg/spray).
Inhaln (Adults and Children >5 yr): *0.06% solution:* 2 sprays in each nostril 3–4 times daily (42 mcg/spray).

Availability (generic available)

Aerosol inhaler (HFA) (chlorofluorocarbon-free): 17 mcg/inhalation in 12.9-g canister (200 inhalations). **Inhalation solution:** ❀ 0.0125%, 0.02%, ❀ 0.025%. **Nasal spray:** 0.03% solution— 21 mcg/spray in 30-mL bottle (345 sprays/bottle), 0.06% solution— 42 mcg/spray in 15-mL bottle (165 sprays). *In combination with:* albuterol (Combivent Respimat). See Appendix N.

NURSING IMPLICATIONS

Assessment

- Assess for allergy to atropine and belladonna alkaloids; patients with these allergies may also be sensitive to ipratropium.
- **Inhaln:** Assess respiratory status (rate, breath sounds, degree of dyspnea, pulse) before administration and at peak of medication. Consult health care professional about alternative medication if severe bronchospasm is present; onset of action is too slow for patients in acute distress. If paradoxical bronchospasm (wheezing) occurs, withhold medication and notify health care professional immediately.
- **Nasal Spray:** Assess patient for rhinorrhea.

Implementation

- **Inhaln:** See Appendix C for administration of inhalation medications.
- When ipratropium is administered concurrently with other inhalation medications, administer adrenergic bronchodilators first, followed by ipratropium, then corticosteroids. Wait 5 min between medications.
- Solution for *nebulization* can be diluted with preservative-free 0.9% NaCl. Diluted solution should be used within 24 hr at room temperature or 48 hr if refrigerated. Solution can be mixed with preservative-free albuterol or cromolyn if used within 1 hr of mixing.

Patient/Family Teaching

- Instruct patient in proper use of inhaler, nebulizer, or nasal spray and to take medication as directed. Take missed doses as soon as remembered unless almost time for the next dose; space remaining doses evenly during day. Do not double doses.
- Advise patient that rinsing mouth after using inhaler, good oral hygiene, and sugarless gum or candy may minimize dry mouth. Health care professional should be notified if stomatitis occurs or if dry mouth persists for more than 2 wk.
- Rep: Advise females of reproductive potential to notify health care professional if pregnancy is planned or suspected or if breastfeeding.
- **Inhalation:** Caution patient not to exceed 12 doses within 24 hr. Patient should notify health care professional if symptoms do not improve within 30 min after administration of medication or if condition worsens.
- Explain need for pulmonary function tests prior to and periodically during therapy to determine effectiveness of medication.
- Caution patient to avoid spraying medication in eyes; may cause blurring of vision or irritation.
- Advise patient to inform health care professional if cough, nervousness, headache, dizziness, nausea, or GI distress occurs.
- **Nasal Spray:** Instruct patient in proper use of nasal spray. Clear nasal passages gently before administration. Do not inhale during administration, so medication remains in nasal passages. Prime pump initially with 7 actuations. If used regularly, no further priming is needed. If not used in 24 hr, prime with 2 actuations. If not used for >7 days, prime with 7 actuations.
- Advise patient to contact health care professional if symptoms do not improve within 1–2 wk or if condition worsens.

Evaluation/Desired Outcomes

- Decreased dyspnea.
- Improved breath sounds.
- Decrease in rhinorrhea from perennial rhinitis or the common cold.

irbesartan, See ANGIOTENSIN II
RECEPTOR ANTAGONISTS.

⅀ irinotecan (eye-ri-noe-**tee**-kan)
Camptosar
Classification
Therapeutic: antineoplastics
Pharmacologic: enzyme inhibitors

Indications
First-line therapy of metastatic colorectal cancer (in combination with 5-fluorouracil and leucovorin). Metastatic colorectal cancer that has recurred or progressed following initial fluorouracil-based therapy.

Action
Interferes with DNA synthesis by inhibiting the enzyme topoisomerase. **Therapeutic Effects:** Death of rapidly replicating cells, particularly malignant ones.

Pharmacokinetics
Absorption: IV administration results in complete bioavailability.
Distribution: Unknown.
Protein Binding: *Irinotecan:* 30–68%; *SN–38 (active metabolite):* 95%.
Metabolism and Excretion: Converted by the liver to SN–38, its active metabolite, which is metabolized by the liver by UDP-glucuronosyl 111 transferase 1A1 (UGT1A1) and CYP3A4. Small amounts excreted by kidneys.
Half-life: 6 hr.

TIME/ACTION PROFILE (hematologic effects)

ROUTE	ONSET	PEAK	DURATION
IV	unknown	21–29 days	27–34 days

Contraindications/Precautions
Contraindicated in: Hypersensitivity; Hereditary fructose intolerance (contains sorbitol); Concurrent use of ketoconazole or St. John's wort; OB: Pregnancy; Lactation: Lactation.
Use Cautiously in: Previous pelvic or abdominal irradiation or age ≥65 yr (↑ risk of myelosuppression); Presence of infection, underlying bone marrow depression, or concurrent chronic illness; History of prior pelvic/abdominal irradiation and serum bilirubin >1–2 mg/dL (initial dose ↓ recommended); Hepatic impairment; Previous severe myelosuppression or diarrhea (reinstitute at lower dose following resolution); ⅀ Homozygous for UGT1A1*28 [*28/*28] or UGT1A1*6 [*6/*6] alleles or compound heterozygous for UGT1A1*28 or UGT1A1*6 [*6/*28] alleles (poor

UGT1A1 metabolizers) or heterozygous for either the UGT1A1*28 or UGT1A1*6 alleles (*1/*28, *1/*6) (intermediate UGT1A1 metabolizers) (↑ risk of severe or life-threatening neutropenia); Rep: Women of reproductive potential and men with female partners of reproductive potential; Pedi: Safety and effectiveness not established in children; Geri: ↑ sensitivity to adverse effects (myelosuppression) in older adults; initiate at lower dose.

Adverse Reactions/Side Effects
CV: edema, vasodilation. **Derm:** alopecia, rash, sweating. **EENT:** rhinitis. **F and E:** dehydration. **GI:** abdominal pain/cramping, anorexia, constipation, DIARRHEA, dyspepsia, flatulence, nausea, stomatitis, vomiting, ↑ liver enzymes, abdominal enlargement, colonic ulceration. **GU:** ↓ fertility, menstrual abnormalities. **Hemat:** anemia, leukopenia, NEUTROPENIA, thrombocytopenia. **Local:** injection site reactions. **Metab:** weight loss. **MS:** back pain. **Neuro:** dizziness, headache, insomnia, weakness.. **Resp:** coughing, dyspnea, INTERSTITIAL LUNG DISEASE. **Misc:** chills, fever, INFECTION.

Interactions
Drug-Drug: Combination with **fluorouracil** may result in serious toxicity (dehydration, neutropenia, sepsis). ↑ bone marrow depression may occur with other **antineoplastics** or **radiation therapy**. Strong **CYP3A4 inhibitors** (**ketoconazole, clarithromycin, itraconazole, lopinavir, nefazodone, nelfinavir, ritonavir,** and **voriconazole**) and strong **UGT1A1 inhibitors** (**atazanavir,** and **gemfibrozil**) may ↑ levels of irinotecan and its active metabolite; should be discontinued ≥1 wk before initiating irinotecan. **Phenobarbital, phenytoin, carbamazepine, rifampin,** or **rifabutin** may ↓ levels of irinotecan and its active metabolite; consider using an alternative anticonvulsant at least 2 wk before initiating irinotecan. **Laxatives** should be avoided (diarrhea may be ↑). **Diuretics** ↑ risk of dehydration (may discontinue during therapy). **Dexamethasone** may ↑ risk of hyperglycemia and lymphocytopenia. **Prochlorperazine** given on the same day as irinotecan ↑ risk of akathisia. May ↓ antibody response to and ↑ risk of adverse reactions from **live virus vaccines**.
Drug-Natural Products: St. John's wort ↓ levels of the active metabolite; concurrent use is contraindicated; should be discontinued at least 2 wk before initiating irinotecan.

Route/Dosage
Other regimens are used; careful modification required for all levels of toxicity/tolerance.

Single Agent
⅀ **IV (Adults):** *Weekly dosage schedule:* 125 mg/m² once weekly for 4 wk, followed by a 2-wk rest period. Cycle may be repeated using doses which depend on

patient tolerance and degree of toxicity encountered. *Once-every-3-wk schedule:* 350 mg/m² once every 3 wk. Cycle may be repeated using doses which depend on patient tolerance and degree of toxicity encountered.

IV (Geriatric Patients >70 yr): *Weekly dosage schedule:* 125 mg/m² once weekly for 4 wk, followed by a 2-wk rest period. Cycle may be repeated using doses which depend on patient tolerance and degree of toxicity encountered. *Once-every-3-wk schedule:* 300 mg/m² once every 3 wk. Cycle may be repeated using doses which depend on patient tolerance and degree of toxicity encountered.

⚠ IV (Adults Homozygous for UGT1A1*28 [*28/ *28] or UGT1A1*6 [*6/*6] Alleles or Compound Heterozygous for UGT1A1*28 or UGT1A1*6 [*6/ *28] Alleles): *Weekly dosage schedule:* 100 mg/m² once weekly for 4 wk, followed by a 2-wk rest period. Cycle may be repeated using doses which depend on patient tolerance and degree of toxicity encountered. *Once-every-3-wk schedule:* 300 mg/m² once every 3 wk. Cycle may be repeated using doses which depend on patient tolerance and degree of toxicity encountered.

Hepatic Impairment

IV (Adults): *Bilirubin 1–2 mg/dL and history of prior pelvic/abdominal irradiation: Weekly dosage schedule:* Initiate therapy at lower dose (100 mg/m²); once weekly for 4 wk, followed by a 2-wk rest period. Cycle may be repeated with dose adjusted as tolerated. *Once-every-3-wk schedule:* 300 mg/m² once every 3 wk. Cycle may be repeated with dose adjusted as tolerated.

As Part of Combination Therapy With Leucovorin and 5-Fluorouracil

IV (Adults): *Regimen 1 (Bolus regimen):* 125 mg/m² once weekly for 4 wk, followed by a 2-wk rest period. Cycle may be repeated using doses that depend on patient tolerance and degree of toxicity encountered; *Regimen 2 (Infusional regimen):* 180 mg/m² every 2 wk for 3 doses, followed by a 3-wk rest period. Cycle may be repeated using doses that depend on patient tolerance and degree of toxicity encountered.

⚠ IV (Adults Homozygous for UGT1A1*28 [*28/ *28] or UGT1A1*6 [*6/*6] Alleles or Compound Heterozygous for UGT1A1*28 or UGT1A1*6 [*6/ *28] Alleles): *Regimen 1 (Bolus regimen):* 100 mg/ m² once weekly for 4 wk, followed by a 2-wk period. Cycle may be repeated using doses that depend on patient tolerance and degree of toxicity encountered; *Regimen 2 (Infusional regimen):* 150 mg/m² every 2 wk for 3 doses, followed by a 3-wk rest period. Cycle may be repeated using doses that depend on patient tolerance and degree of toxicity encountered.

Availability (generic available)
Solution for injection: 20 mg/mL.

NURSING IMPLICATIONS
Assessment
- Monitor vital signs frequently during administration.
- Monitor for bone marrow depression. Assess for bleeding (bleeding gums, bruising, petechiae, guaiac stools, urine, and emesis) and avoid IM injections and taking rectal temperatures if platelet count is low. Apply pressure to venipuncture sites for 10 min. Assess for signs of infection during neutropenia. Anemia may occur. Monitor for increased fatigue, dyspnea, and orthostatic hypotension.
- Monitor closely for the development of diarrhea. Two types may occur. The early type occurs within 24 hr of administration and may be preceded by cramps and sweating. Atropine 0.25–1 mg IV or SUBQ may be given to decrease symptoms. Potentially life-threatening diarrhea may occur >24 hr after a dose; may be accompanied by severe dehydration and electrolyte imbalance. Loperamide 4 mg initially, followed by 2 mg every 2 hr until diarrhea ceases for at least 12 hr (or 4 mg every 4 hr if given during sleeping hours) should be administered promptly to treat late-occurring diarrhea. Do not administer loperamide at these doses for >48 hr. Careful fluid and electrolyte replacement should be instituted to prevent complications. *If diarrhea of 2–3 stools/day pretreatment occurs,* maintain dose. *If diarrhea of 4–6 stools/day pretreatment occurs during a cycle,* ↓ by 25 mg/m². *If diarrhea of 4–6 stools/day pretreatment occurs at the beginning of a weekly cycle or at the beginning of a once every 3-wk cycle,* maintain dose. *If diarrhea of 7– 9 stools/day pretreatment occurs during a cycle,* hold dose until resolved to ≤Grade 2, then ↓ by 25 mg/m². *If diarrhea of 7–9 stools/day pretreatment occurs at the beginning of a weekly cycle,* ↓ by 25 mg/m². *If diarrhea of 7–9 stools/day pretreatment occurs at the beginning of a once every 3-wk cycle,* ↓ by 50 mg/m². *If diarrhea ≥10 stools/ day pretreatment occurs during a cycle,* hold dose until resolved to ≤Grade 2, then ↓ by 50 mg/m². *If diarrhea ≥10 stools/day pretreatment occurs at the beginning of a weekly cycle or at the beginning of a once every 3-wk cycle,* ↓ by 50 mg/m².
- Assess IV site frequently for inflammation. Avoid extravasation. If extravasation occurs, infusion must be stopped and restarted in another vein to avoid damage to SUBQ tissue. Flushing site with sterile water and application of ice over the extravasated site are recommended.
- If signs of pulmonary toxicity (dyspnea, cough, fever) occur, interrupt therapy. If interstitial pulmonary disease is determined, discontinue irinotecan.
- Assess for cholinergic symptoms (rhinitis, increased salivation, miosis, lacrimation, diaphoresis, flushing, abdominal cramping, diarrhea) during therapy. Atropine 0.25–1 mg SUBQ or IV may be used to prevent or treat symptoms.

Lab Test Considerations

- ⚇ Consider laboratory test to determine the UGT1A1 status. Testing can detect the UGT1A1 *6 and *28 genotypes.Verify negative pregnancy test before starting therapy. Monitor CBC with differential and platelet count prior to each dose. *If neutropenia, ANC 1500–1999/mm³ occurs,* maintain dose. *If ANC 1000–1499/mm³ occurs during a cycle,* ↓ dose by 25 mg/m². *If ANC 1000–1499/mm³ occurs at beginning of cycle,* maintain dose. *If ANC 500–999/ mm³ occurs during a cycle,* hold dose until resolved to ≤Grade 2, then ↓ by 25 mg/m². *If ANC 500–999/mm³ occurs at the beginning of a weekly cycle,* ↓ dose by 25 mg/m². *If ANC 500– 999/mm³ occurs at the beginning of a once every 3-wk cycle,* ↓ dose by 50 mg/m². *If ANC <500/mm³ occurs during a cycle,* hold dose until resolved to ≤Grade 2, then ↓ by 50 mg/m². *If ANC 500–999/ mm³ occurs at the beginning of a weekly cycle or at the beginning of a once every 3-wk cycle,* ↓ dose by 50 mg/m². *If neutropenic fever occurs during a cycle,* hold dose until resolved, then ↓ by 50 mg/m² when resolved. *If neutropenic fever occurs at the beginning of a weekly cycle or at the beginning of a once every 3-wk cycle,* ↓ by 50 mg/ m². Administration of a colony-stimulating factor may be considered if clinically significant decreases in WBC (<2000/mm³), neutrophil count (<1000/ mm³), hemoglobin (<9 g/dL), or platelet count (<100,000 cells/mm³) occur.
- May cause ↑ serum alkaline phosphatase and AST concentrations.

Implementation

IV Administration

- Prepare solution in a biologic cabinet. Wear gloves, gown, and mask while handling IV medication. Discard IV equipment in specially designated containers.
- Nausea and vomiting are common. Pretreatment with dexamethasone 10 mg along with agents such as ondansetron or granisetron should be started on the same day as irinotecan at least 30 min before administration. Prochlorperazine may be used on subsequent days but may increase risk of akathisia if given on the same day as irinotecan.
- **Intermittent Infusion:** *Dilution:* Dilute before infusion with D5W or 0.9% NaCl. Usual diluent is 500 mL of D5W. *Concentration:* 0.12–2.8 mg/ mL. Solution is pale yellow. Do not administer solutions that are cloudy, discolored, or contain particulate matter. Solution is stable for 24 hr if refrigerated. To prevent microbial contamination, solutions should be prepared immediately prior to use and begin infusion as soon as possible after preparation. *Rate:* Administer dose over 90 min.
- **Y-Site Compatibility:** alemtuzumab, amifostine, amikacin, aminocaproic acid, aminophylline, amiodarone, ampicillin, ampicillin/sulbactam, anidulafungin, argatroban, atracurium, azithromycin, aztreonam, bivalirudin, bleomycin, bumetanide, buprenorphine, butorphanol, calcium chloride, calcium gluconate, carboplatin, caspofungin, cefazolin, cefotetan, cefoxitin, ceftazidime, cefuroxime, ciprofloxacin, cisatracurium, cisplatin, clindamycin, cyclophosphamide, cyclosporine, cytarabine, dacarbazine, daptomycin, daunorubicin hydrochloride, dexamethasone, dexrazoxane, digoxin, diltiazem, diphenhydramine, dobutamine, docetaxel, dopamine, doxorubicin hydrochloride, doxorubicin liposomal, doxycycline, enalaprilat, ephedrine, epinephrine, ertapenem, erythromycin, esmolol, etoposide, etoposide phosphate, famotidine, fentanyl, fluconazole, foscarnet, gemtuzumab ozogamicin, gentamicin, granisetron, haloperidol, heparin, hetastarch, hydralazine, hydrocortisone, hydromorphone, idarubicin, imipenem/cilastatin, insulin, regular, isoproterenol, ketorolac, labetalol, leucovorin calcium, levofloxacin, levoleucovorin, lidocaine, linezolid, lorazepam, magnesium sulfate, mannitol, meperidine, meropenem, mesna, methadone, metoclopramide, metoprolol, metronidazole, midazolam, milrinone, mitoxantrone, morphine, moxifloxacin, nalbuphine, naloxone, nicardipine, nitroglycerin, norepinephrine, octreotide, ondansetron, oxaliplatin, paclitaxel, palonosetron, pantoprazole, pentamidine, pentobarbital, phenobarbital, phentolamine, phenylephrine, potassium acetate, potassium chloride, potassium phosphate, procainamide, prochlorperazine, promethazine, propranolol, remifentanil, rituximab, rocuronium, sodium acetate, sodium bicarbonate, sodium phosphate, succinylcholine, sufentanil, tacrolimus, theophylline, thiotepa, tigecycline, tirofiban, tobramycin, trimethoprim/ sulfamethoxazole, vancomycin, vasopressin, vecuronium, verapamil, vinblastine, vinorelbine, voriconazole, zidovudine, zoledronic acid.
- **Y-Site Incompatibility:** acyclovir, allopurinol, amphotericin B lipid complex, amphotericin B liposome, cefepime, cefotaxime, ceftriaxone, chloramphenicol, chlorpromazine, dantrolene, dexmedetomidine, diazepam, droperidol, fluorouracil, fosphenytoin, furosemide, ganciclovir, gemcitabine, glycopyrrolate, methohexital, methylprednisolone, mitomycin, nafcillin, nitroprusside, pemetrexed, phenytoin, piperacillin/tazobactam, thiopental, trastuzumab.

Patient/Family Teaching

- Explain purpose of irinotecan to patient.
- Instruct patient to report occurrence of diarrhea to health care professional immediately if diarrhea occurs for first time during treatment; black or bloody stools; symptoms of dehydration such as lightheadedness, dizziness, or faintness; inability to take fluids

by mouth due to nausea or vomiting; or inability to get diarrhea under control within 24 hr. Diarrhea may be accompanied by severe dehydration and electrolyte imbalance. It may be life-threatening; treat promptly. Loperamide may be used for treatment up to 48 hr.

• Instruct patient to monitor their temperature and to notify health care professional promptly if fever; chills; sore throat; signs of infection; bleeding gums; bruising; petechiae; blood in urine, stool, or emesis occurs. Caution patient to avoid crowds and persons with known infections. Instruct patient to monitor temperature frequently, use soft toothbrush and electric razor. Caution patient not to drink alcoholic beverages or take products containing aspirin or other NSAIDs.

• Instruct patient to notify nurse of pain at injection site immediately.

• Instruct patient to notify health care professional if vomiting, fainting, or dizziness occurs.

• Discuss with patient possibility of hair loss. Explore methods of coping.

• Instruct patient not to receive any vaccinations without consulting health care professional.

• Rep: May cause fetal harm. Advise females of reproductive potential to use highly effective contraception during and for 6 mo after last dose of therapy and to avoid breastfeeding during and for 7 days after final dose. Advise males with female partners of reproductive potential to use condoms during and for 3 mo after last dose. May impair female and male infertility.

• Emphasize the need for periodic lab tests to monitor for side effects.

Evaluation/Desired Outcomes

• Decrease in size and spread of malignancy.

---

iron sucrose (eye-ern su-krose)
Venofer
Classification
Therapeutic: antianemics
Pharmacologic: iron supplements

Indications
Iron deficiency anemia in chronic kidney disease.

Action
Enters the bloodstream and is transported to the organs of the reticuloendothelial system (liver, spleen, bone marrow) where it becomes separated from the sucrose complex and becomes part of iron stores. **Therapeutic Effects:** Resolution of iron deficiency anemia associated with chronic kidney disease.

Pharmacokinetics
Absorption: Following IV administration, the uptake of iron by the reticuloendothelial system is constant at about 40–60 mg/hr. Following IM doses, 60% is absorbed after 3 days; 90% after 1–3 weeks, the balance is absorbed slowly over mo.

Distribution: Taken up by the reticuloendothelial system.
Metabolism and Excretion: Most sucrose is eliminated in urine. Most of the iron remains stored and used on demand. Small amounts eliminated in urine.
Half-life: 6 hr.

TIME/ACTION PROFILE (effects on erythropoiesis)

ROUTE	ONSET	PEAK	DURATION
IV	days	1–2 wk	wks–mos

Contraindications/Precautions
Contraindicated in: Anemia not due to iron deficiency; Hemochromatosis, hemosiderosis, or other evidence of iron overload; Hypersensitivity to iron sucrose.

Use Cautiously in: Any evidence of tissue iron overload; OB: Severe hypersensitivity reactions may occur that can lead to bradycardia in fetus, especially during second and third trimesters; safety not established during first trimester; Lactation: Use during breastfeeding only if potential maternal benefit justifies potential risk to infant; Pedi: Children <2 yr (safety and effectiveness not established).

Adverse Reactions/Side Effects
CV: chest pain, HF, hypertension, hypotension. **Derm:** pruritus. **F and E:** hypervolemia. **GI:** diarrhea, nausea, vomiting, ↑ liver enzymes, abdominal pain. **Local:** injection site reactions. **MS:** leg cramps, musculoskeletal pain. **Neuro:** headache, dizziness, dysgeusia, weakness. **Resp:** cough, dyspnea. **Misc:** fever, HYPERSENSITIVITY REACTIONS (including anaphylaxis), sepsis.

Interactions
Drug-Drug: Chloramphenicol and **vitamin E** may ↓ hematologic response to iron therapy.

Route/Dosage
IV (Adults): *Hemodialysis dependent patients:* 100 mg during each dialysis session for 10 doses (total of 1000 mg); may repeat if iron deficiency recurs; *Non-dialysis dependent patients:* 200 mg on 5 different days within a 14 day period to a total of 1000 mg; may also be given as infusion of 500 mg on day 1 and day 14; may repeat if iron deficiency recurs; *Peritoneal dialysis patients:* administered in a total cumulative dose of 1000 mg in 3 divided doses, 14 days apart within a 28 day period with first 2 doses of 300 mg and third dose of 400 mg; may repeat if iron deficiency recurs. **IV (Children ≥2 yr):** *Hemodialysis dependent patients (for iron maintenance therapy):* 0.5 mg/kg (max = 100 mg/dose) every 2 wk for 12 wk; may repeat if necessary; *Non-dialysis dependent patients or peritoneal dialysis patients who are receiving erythropoietin for iron maintenance therapy:* 0.5 mg/kg (max = 100 mg/dose) every 4 wk for 12 wk; may repeat if necessary.

Availability
Solution for injection: 20 mg/mL.

NURSING IMPLICATIONS

Assessment
- Monitor BP during infusion. May cause hypotension; usually related to rate of administration and total dose administered.
- Assess for hypersensitivity reactions and anaphylaxis (rash, dyspnea, loss of consciousness, hypotension, collapse, convulsions) for at least 30 min following injection. Equipment for resuscitation should be readily available.

Lab Test Considerations
- Monitor hemoglobin, hematocrit, serum ferritin, and transferrin saturation prior to and periodically during therapy. Transferrin saturation values ↑ rapidly after IV administration; therefore, serum iron values may be reliably obtained 48 hr after IV administration. Withhold iron therapy if evidence of iron overload occurs.
- May cause ↑ liver enzymes.

Toxicity and Overdose
- Symptoms of iron overdose or too rapid infusion are hypotension, headache, vomiting, nausea, dizziness, joint aches, paresthesia, abdominal and muscle pain, edema, and cardiovascular collapse. Treatment includes IV fluids, corticosteroids, and/or antihistamines. Administering at a slower rate usually relieves symptoms.

Implementation
- Do not confuse Venofer with Vfend or Vimpat.
- Do not administer iron sucrose concurrently with oral iron, as the absorption of oral iron is reduced. Each mL vial contains 20 mg of elemental iron.
- Solution is brown. Inspect for particulate matter or discoloration. Do not administer solutions that contain particulate matter or are discolored. Solution is stable for 7 days at room temperature or if refrigerated in syringe or 7 days at room temperature diluted in IV bag.
- Pedi: Exercise caution when administering and calculating doses; overdose can be fatal.

IV Administration
Hemodialysis Dependent Patients
- Most patients require a minimum cumulative dose of 1000 mg of elemental iron, administered over 10 sequential dialysis sessions, to achieve a favorable hemoglobin or hematocrit response.
- IV Push: May be administered undiluted by slow injection. *Rate:* Inject at a rate of 100 mg over 2–5 min into dialysis line early during the dialysis session (generally within the first hour), not to exceed one vial per injection. Discard any unused portion.

- **Intermittent Infusion:** May be administered as an infusion of 100 mg diluted in a maximum of 100 mL of 0.9% NaCl. *Rate:* Infuse over at least 15 minutes, per consecutive hemodialysis session.

Non-dialysis Dependent Patients
- **IV Push:** May be administered as a slow injection of 200 mg undiluted. *Rate:* Administer over 2–5 min.
- **Intermittent Infusion:** Dilute 200 mg in 100 mL 0.9% NaCl. Has also been given as 500 mg diluted in 250 mL 0.9% NaCl. *Rate:* Infuse over 15 min. Infuse 500 mg dose over 3.5–4 hr on days 1 and 14. May cause hypotension; monitor closely.
- **Additive Incompatibility:** Iron sucrose should not be admixed with any other medications or parenteral nutrition solutions.

Peritoneal Dialysis Patients
- **Intermittent Infusion:** *Dilution:* Dilute each dose in a maximum of 250 mL of 0.9% NaCl. *Rate:* Administer doses of 300 mg over 1.5 hr and doses of 400 mg over 2.5 hr.

Pediatric Patients
- **IV Push:** May be administered undiluted as 0.5 mg/kg, not to exceed 100 mg per dose. *Rate:* Inject over 5 min.
- **Intermittent Infusion:** Dilute in 0.9% NaCl at a concentration of 1 to 2 mg/mL. Do not dilute to concentrations below 1 mg/mL. *Rate:* Infuse over 5–60 min.

Patient/Family Teaching
- Explain purpose of iron therapy to patient.
- Instruct patient to report symptoms of hypersensitivity reaction to health care professional immediately.
- Rep: Advise females of reproductive potential to notify health care professional if pregnancy is planned or suspected, or if breastfeeding. Maternal hypersensitivity reactions (anaphylaxis, hypotension, shock) following use of parenteral iron may result in fetal bradycardia, especially during the second and third trimesters. Monitor breastfed infants for gastrointestinal toxicity (constipation, diarrhea).

Evaluation/Desired Outcomes
- Improvement in anemia of chronic kidney disease.

---

isavuconazonium
(eye-sa-vue-kon-a-**zoe**-nee-um)
Cresemba
Classification
Therapeutic: antifungals
Pharmacologic: azoles

Indications
Invasive aspergillosis. Mucormycosis.

Action
A prodrug that is converted (rapidly hydrolyzed) to isavuconazole. Inhibits the synthesis of ergosterol, a key

component of fungal cell walls. **Therapeutic Effects:** Resolution of invasive fungal infections. **Spectrum:** Active against *Aspergillus flavus*, *Aspergillus fumigatus*, *Aspergillus niger*, and Mucormycetes species including *Rhizopus oryzae*.

Pharmacokinetics

Absorption: Prodrug is rapidly converted to isavuconazole, the active component. 98% absorbed following oral administration. Similar conversion follows intravenous administration, resulting in complete bioavailability.

Distribution: Extensively distributed.

Protein Binding: >99%.

Metabolism and Excretion: Extensively metabolized (mostly by CYP3A4 and CYP3A5); inactive metabolites are mostly renally eliminated, <1% excreted unchanged in urine.

Half-life: 130 hr.

TIME/ACTION PROFILE (plasma concentrations)

ROUTE	ONSET	PEAK	DURATION
PO	unknown	2 hr	unknown
IV	unknown	end of infusion	unknown

Contraindications/Precautions

Contraindicated in: Hypersensitivity; Strong CYP3A4 inhibitors; Familial short QT syndrome; Strong CYP3A4 inducers; OB: Pregnancy; Lactation: Lactation.

Use Cautiously in: Severe hepatic impairment (use only if benefits outweigh risks, monitor carefully for adverse reactions); Rep: Women of reproductive potential; Pedi: Safety and effectiveness not established in children.

Adverse Reactions/Side Effects

CV: peripheral edema, chest pain, hypotension. **Derm:** pruritus, rash, STEVENS-JOHNSON SYNDROME. **F and E:** hypokalemia, hypomagnesemia. **GI:** ↑ liver enzymes, constipation, diarrhea, nausea, vomiting, ↓ appetite, dyspepsia. **GU:** renal failure. **Local:** injection site reactions. **MS:** back pain. **Neuro:** fatigue, headache, insomnia, anxiety, delirium. **Resp:** cough, dyspnea, respiratory failure. **Misc:** HYPERSENSITIVITY REACTIONS (including anaphylaxis), infusion-related reactions.

Interactions

Drug-Drug: ↑ levels and risk of toxicity with **strong inhibitors of CYP3A4**, including **ketoconazole** or high-dose **ritonavir**; concurrent use is contraindicated. **Lopinavir/ritonavir** significantly ↑ levels and risk of toxicity; concurrent use should be undertaken with caution. Isavuconazonium ↓ levels and effectiveness of **lopinavir/ritonavir**. Isavuconazonium ↑ levels and risk of toxicity with **atorvastatin**, **cyclosporine**, **digoxin**, **midazolam**, **mycophenolate**, **sirolimus**, **tacrolimus**; undertake concurrent use with caution, monitoring drug effects and making adjustments if nec-

essary. **Strong inducers of CYP3A4** including long-acting **barbiturates, carbamazepine**, or **rifampin** ↓ levels and effectiveness; concurrent use is contraindicated. ↓ levels and effectiveness of **bupropion**; bupropion dose may need to be ↑ but should not exceed maximum recommended dose.

Drug-Natural Products: St. John's wort ↓ blood levels and effectiveness; concurrent use is contraindicated.

Route/Dosage

PO, IV (Adults ≥18 yr): *Loading dose:* 372 mg isavuconazonium (equivalent to 200 mg isavuconazole) every 8 hr for six doses; *Maintenance dose:* 372 mg isavuconazonium (equivalent to 200 mg isavuconazole) once daily starting 12–24 hr after last loading dose.

Availability

Capsules: 186 mg isavuconazonium (equivalent to 100 mg isavuconazole). **Lyophilized powder for injection:** 372 mg isavuconazonium (equivalent to 200 mg isavuconazole)/vial.

NURSING IMPLICATIONS

Assessment

- Monitor signs and symptoms of infection periodically during therapy.
- Obtain specimens for culture and sensitivity prior to therapy. First dose may be given before receiving results.
- Monitor for signs and symptoms of infusion-related reactions (hypotension, dyspnea, chills, dizziness, paresthesia, hypoesthesia) periodically during therapy. Discontinue infusion if symptoms occur.
- Monitor skin for hypersensitivity reactions during therapy.

Lab Test Considerations
- Monitor liver function tests prior to and periodically during therapy. Discontinue therapy if clinical signs of liver disease occur.
- May cause hypokalemia and hypomagnesemia.

Implementation

- Oral and IV formulations are bioequivalent; may be used interchangeably. Loading dose is not needed when switching.
- **PO:** Administer without regard to food. *DNC:* Swallow capsule whole; do not open, dissolve, crush or chew.
- To administer via NG tube, reconstitute one vial isavuconazonium for injection (equivalent to 200 mg isavuconazonium) with 5 mL of water for injection. Withdraw the entire contents (5 mL) of vial using a syringe and needle. Discard the needle and cap the syringe. To administer, remove cap from syringe containing the reconstituted solution and connect the syringe to NG tube to deliver dose. After administering, administer three 5 mL rinses to NG tube with water. Administer reconstituted solution via NG tube within 1 hr of reconstitution.

IV Administration

- **Reconstitution:** Reconstitute by adding 5 mL sterile water to vial. Shake gently to dissolve powder completely. Solution should be clear and colorless; do not administer solutions that are discolored or contain particulate matter. Solution is stable for 1 hr at room temperature.
- **Intermittent Infusion:** *Dilution:* Remove 5 mL of reconstituted solution from vial and add to 250 mL 0.9% NaCl or D5W. *Concentration:* 1.5 mg isavuconazonium/mL. Diluted solution may show visible translucent to white particulates; removed with in-line filter. Roll bag to mix gently; avoid shaking. Solution is stable if infused at room temperature within 6 hr; may refrigerate for up to 24 hr; do not freeze. Flush line with 0.9% NaCl or D5W prior to and following infusion. *Rate:* Infuse over at least 1 hr to minimize infusion-related reactions. Infuse through a 0.2–1.2 micron in-line filter. Do not administer as a bolus injection.
- **Y-Site Compatibility:** amikacin, amiodarone, anidulafungin, aztreonam, calcium chloride, calcium gluconate, caspofungin, ceftolozane/tazobactam, ciprofloxacin, cisatracurium, daptomycin, dexamethasone, dexmedetomidine, digoxin, diltiazem, diphenhydramine, dobutamine, dopamine, doxycycline, epinephrine, eptifibatide, esmolol, famotidine, fentanyl, gentamicin, hydrocortisone, hydromorphone, imipenem/cilastatin, insulin, regular, labetalol, levofloxacin, lidocaine, linezolid, lorazepam, magnesium sulfate, mannitol, meperidine, mesna, metoclopramide, midazolam, milrinone, morphine, mycophenolate, naloxone, nicardipine, nitroglycerin, nitroprusside, norepinephrine, octreotide, ondansetron, pantoprazole, phenylephrine, plazomicin, potassium chloride, rocuronium, tacrolimus, tigecycline, tobramycin, vancomycin, vasopressin, vecuronium.
- **Y-Site Incompatibility:** albumin, human, amphotericin B deoxycholate, amphotericin B lipid complex, amphotericin B liposome, ampicillin/sulbactam, cefazolin, cefepime, ceftaroline, ceftazidime, ceftriaxone, cefuroxime, cyclosporine, ertapenem, esomeprazole, filgrastim, fosphenytoin, furosemide, heparin, meropenem, meropenem/vaborbactam, methylprednisolone, micafungin, phenytoin, potassium phosphate, propofol, sodium bicarbonate, sodium phosphate, tedizolid.

Patient/Family Teaching

- Instruct patient to take isavuconazonium as directed. Do not stop taking isavuconazonium without consulting heath care professional. Advise patient to read *Patient Information* before starting and with each Rx refill in case of changes.
- Advise patient to notify health care professional promptly of signs and symptoms of liver disease

(itchy skin, nausea, vomiting, yellowing of eyes, feeling very tired, flu-like symptoms), infusion-related reactions, or rash occur.
- Instruct patient to notify health care professional of all Rx or OTC medications, vitamins, or herbal products being taken and consult health care professional before taking any new medications.
- Rep: May cause fetal harm. Advise females of reproductive potential to use effective contraception during and for 28 days after final dose and to avoid breastfeeding during therapy. Advise patient to notify health care professional if pregnancy is planned or suspected.
- Emphasize the importance of lab tests to monitor for side effects during therapy.

Evaluation/Desired Outcomes

- Resolution of signs and symptoms of invasive aspergillosis.
- Resolution of signs and symptoms of mucormycosis.

⊠ isoniazid (eye-soe-**nye**-a-zid)

🍁 Isotamine

Classification
Therapeutic: antituberculars

Indications

First-line therapy of active tuberculosis (TB) (in combination with other agents). Prevention of TB in patients exposed to active disease (as monotherapy).

Action

Inhibits mycobacterial cell wall synthesis and interferes with metabolism. **Therapeutic Effects:** Bacteriostatic or bactericidal action against susceptible mycobacteria.

Pharmacokinetics

Absorption: Well absorbed following PO/IM administration.

Distribution: Widely distributed; readily crosses the blood-brain barrier.

Metabolism and Excretion: 50% metabolized by the liver by N-acetyltransferase ⊠ (rate of acetylation is genetically determined [slow acetylators have ↑ isoniazid levels and ↑ risk of toxicity; fast acetylators have ↓ isoniazid levels and ↑ risk for treatment failure]); 50% excreted unchanged by the kidneys.

Half-life: 1–4 hr in patients with normal renal and hepatic function; ⊠ 0.5–1.6 hr in fast acetylators; 2–5 hr in slow acetylators.

TIME/ACTION PROFILE (plasma concentrations)

ROUTE	ONSET	PEAK	DURATION
PO	rapid	1–2 hr	up to 24 hr
IM	rapid	1–2 hr	up to 24 hr

Contraindications/Precautions

Contraindicated in: Hypersensitivity; Acute liver disease; History of hepatitis from previous use.

Use Cautiously in: History of liver damage or chronic alcohol ingestion; Black and Hispanic women, women in the postpartum period, or patients >50 yr (↑ risk of drug-induced hepatitis); Severe renal impairment (dose ↓ may be necessary); Malnourished patients, patients with diabetes, or chronic alcoholics (↑ risk of neuropathy).

Adverse Reactions/Side Effects

Derm: DRUG REACTION WITH EOSINOPHILIA AND SYSTEMIC SYMPTOMS (DRESS), rash, TOXIC EPIDERMAL NECROLYSIS. **EENT:** visual disturbances. **Endo:** gynecomastia. **GI:** HEPATOTOXICITY, nausea, vomiting. **Hemat:** blood dyscrasias. **Neuro:** peripheral neuropathy, psychosis, seizures. **Misc:** fever.

Interactions

Drug-Drug: Additive CNS toxicity with other **antituberculars**. **BCG vaccine** may not be effective during isoniazid therapy. Isoniazid may ↑ levels and risk of toxicity of **phenytoin**. **Aluminum-containing antacids** may ↓ absorption. Psychotic reactions and coordination difficulties may result with **disulfiram**. Concurrent administration of **pyridoxine** may prevent neuropathy. ↑ risk of hepatotoxicity with other **hepatotoxic agents**, including **alcohol**, **acetaminophen**, and **rifampin**. Isoniazid may ↓ levels and effectiveness of **ketoconazole**. May ↑ **carbamazepine** levels and risk of hepatotoxicity. May ↓ effectiveness of **clopidogrel**; avoid concurrent use.

Drug-Food: Severe reactions may occur with ingestion of foods containing high concentrations of **tyramine** (see Appendix J).

Route/Dosage

PO, IM (Adults): 5 mg/kg/day (max dose = 300 mg once daily) *or* 15 mg/kg (max dose = 900 mg) 2–3 times weekly.

PO, IM (Children <40 kg): *Latent TB infection:* 10–20 mg/kg/day (max dose = 300 mg once daily) *or* 20–40 mg/kg (max dose = 900 mg) 2 times weekly; *Active TB infection:* 10–15 mg/kg/day (max dose = 300 mg once daily) *or* 20–40 mg/kg (max dose = 900 mg) 2 times weekly.

Availability (generic available)

Tablets: 100 mg, 300 mg. **Oral solution (orange, raspberry flavor):** 50 mg/5 mL. **Solution for injection:** 100 mg/mL.

NURSING IMPLICATIONS

Assessment

- ⌷ Mycobacterial studies and susceptibility tests should be performed prior to and periodically during therapy to detect possible resistance. About 50–65% of Caucasians, Blacks, South Indians, and Mexicans are slow acetylators at risk for toxicity, while 80–90% of Inuit, Japanese, and Chinese are rapid acetylators at risk for decreased levels and treatment failure.
- Monitor for signs and symptoms of DRESS (fever, rash, lymphadenopathy, and/or facial swelling, associated with involvement of other organ systems (hepatitis, nephritis, hematologic abnormalities, myocarditis, myositis) during therapy. May resemble an acute viral infection. Eosinophilia is often present. Discontinue therapy if signs occur.

Lab Test Considerations

- ⌷ Hepatic function should be evaluated prior to and monthly throughout therapy. Increased AST, ALT, and serum bilirubin may indicate drug-induced hepatitis. Black and Hispanic women, pregnant women, postpartal women, and patients >50 yr are at highest risk. Risk is lower in children; therefore, liver function tests are usually ordered less frequently for children. If AST, ALT, or serum bilirubin are >3–5 × upper limit of normal, temporarily discontinue isoniazid and consider restarting therapy.

Toxicity and Overdose

- If isoniazid overdose occurs, treatment with pyridoxine (vitamin B) is instituted.

Implementation

- **PO:** Administer on an empty stomach.
- **IM:** Medication may cause discomfort at injection site. Massage site after administration and rotate injection sites.
- Solution may form crystals at low temperatures; crystals will redissolve upon warming to room temperature.

Patient/Family Teaching

- Advise patient to take medication as directed. Take missed doses as soon as possible unless almost time for next dose; do not double up on missed doses. Emphasize the importance of continuing therapy even after symptoms have subsided. Therapy may be continued for 6 mo–2 yr.
- Advise patient to notify health care professional promptly if signs and symptoms of hepatitis (yellow eyes and skin, nausea, vomiting, anorexia, dark urine, unusual tiredness, or weakness) or peripheral neuritis (numbness, tingling, paresthesia) occur. Pyridoxine may be used concurrently to prevent neuropathy. Any changes in visual acuity, eye pain, or blurred vision should also be reported immediately.
- Caution patient to avoid the use of alcohol during this therapy, as this may increase the risk of hepatotoxicity. Avoid ingestion of Swiss or Cheshire cheeses, fish (tuna, skipjack, and sardines), and tyramine-containing foods (see Appendix J); may result in redness or itching of the skin; hot feeling; rapid or pounding heartbeat; sweating; chills; cold, clammy feeling; headache; or light-headedness.
- Rep: May be used as treatment for active TB during pregnancy. Begin preventative therapy after delivery.

May increase the risk of isoniazid-associated peripheral neurotoxicity in the mother; pyridoxine supplementation is recommended in pregnant patients during therapy. May be used during breastfeeding, as the small concentrations in breast milk do not produce toxicity in the nursing newborn; breastfeeding should not be discouraged. Low levels of isoniazid in breast milk can not be relied upon for prophylaxis or therapy in nursing infants. Monitor breastfed infants for jaundice; discontinue breastfeeding or consider changing to a different maternal medication if jaundice develops. Pyridoxine supplementation is recommended for the mother and infant.

- Emphasize the importance of regular follow-up physical and ophthalmologic exams to monitor progress and to check for side effects.

Evaluation/Desired Outcomes

- Resolution of signs and symptoms of TB.
- Negative sputum cultures.
- Prevention of activation of TB in persons known to have been exposed.

ISOSORBIDE
isosorbide dinitrate
(eye-soe-**sor**-bide dye-**nye**-trate)
~~Dilatrate-SR~~, Isordil
isosorbide mononitrate
(eye-soe-**sor**-bide mo-noe-**nye**-trate)
~~Imdur~~, ✸Imdur, ~~Ismo~~, Monoket
Classification
Therapeutic: antianginals
Pharmacologic: nitrates

Indications
Prophylactic management of angina pectoris. **Unlabeled Use:** Treatment of chronic heart failure (unlabeled).

Action
Produce vasodilation (venous greater than arterial). Decrease left ventricular end-diastolic pressure and left ventricular end-diastolic volume (preload). Net effect is reduced myocardial oxygen consumption. Increase coronary blood flow by dilating coronary arteries and improving collateral flow to ischemic regions. **Therapeutic Effects:** Prevention of anginal attacks.

Pharmacokinetics
Absorption: Isosorbide dinitrate undergoes extensive first-pass metabolism by the liver, resulting in 25% bioavailability; isosorbide mononitrate has 100% bioavailability (does not undergo first-pass metabolism).
Distribution: Unknown.
Metabolism and Excretion: Isosorbide dinitrate is metabolized by the liver to 2 active metabolites (5-mononitrate and 2-mononitrate). Isosorbide mononi-

trate is primarily metabolized by the liver to inactive metabolites; primarily excreted in urine as metabolites.
Half-life: *Isosorbide dinitrate:* 1 hr; *isosorbide mononitrate:* 5 hr.

TIME/ACTION PROFILE (cardiovascular effects)

ROUTE	ONSET	PEAK	DURATION
ISDN-PO	45–60 min	unknown	4 hr
ISMN-PO	30–60 min	unknown	7 hr
ISMN-ER	unknown	unknown	12 hr

Contraindications/Precautions
Contraindicated in: Hypersensitivity; Concurrent use of PDE-5 inhibitor or riociguat.
Use Cautiously in: Volume depleted patients; Right ventricular infarction; Hypertrophic cardiomyopathy; OB: Safety not established in pregnancy; Lactation: Safety not established in breastfeeding; Pedi: Safety and effectiveness not established in children; Geri: Initial dose ↓ required in older adults due to ↑ potential for hypotension.

Adverse Reactions/Side Effects
CV: <u>hypotension</u>, <u>tachycardia</u>, paradoxic bradycardia, syncope. **Derm:** flushing. **GI:** nausea, vomiting. **Neuro:** <u>dizziness</u>, <u>headache</u>. **Misc:** tolerance.

Interactions
Drug-Drug: Concurrent use of **avanafil**, **sildenafil**, **tadalafil**, or **vardenafil** may result in severe hypotension (do not use within 24 hr of isosorbide dinitrate or mononitrate); concurrent use contraindicated. Concurrent use of **riociguat** may result in severe hypotension; concurrent use contraindicated. Additive hypotension with **antihypertensives**, acute ingestion of **alcohol**, **beta blockers**, **calcium channel blockers**, and **phenothiazines**.

Route/Dosage
Isosorbide Dinitrate
PO (Adults): *Prophylaxis of angina pectoris:* 5–20 mg 2–3 times daily; usual maintenance dose is 10–40 mg every 6 hr.

Isosorbide Mononitrate
PO (Adults): *ISMO, Monoket:* 5–20 mg twice daily with the 2 doses given 7 hr apart. *Imdur:* 30–60 mg once daily; may ↑ to 120 mg once daily (maximum dose = 240 mg/day).

Availability
Isosorbide Dinitrate (generic available)
Tablets: 5 mg, 10 mg, 20 mg, 30 mg, 40 mg. *In combination with:* hydralazine (BiDil). See Appendix N.

Isosorbide Mononitrate (generic available)
Tablets (Monoket): 10 mg, 20 mg. **Extended-release tablets:** 30 mg, 60 mg, 120 mg.

✸= Canadian drug name. ⅏ = Genetic implication. ~~Strikethrough~~ = Discontinued. CAPITALS = life-threatening. <u>Underline</u> = most frequent.

NURSING IMPLICATIONS
Assessment
- Assess location, duration, intensity, and precipitating factors of anginal pain.
- Monitor BP and pulse routinely during period of dose adjustment.

Lab Test Considerations
- Excessive doses may ↑ methemoglobin concentrations.

Implementation
Isosorbide Dinitrate
- **PO:** Do not administer around the clock to prevent tolerance to nitrate effect; allow nitrate-free interval for ≥14 hr. Twice-daily dosing may be administered at 8 AM and 1 PM and 3 times daily dosing may be given at 8 AM, 1 PM, and 6 PM.

Isosorbide Mononitrate
- **PO:** Do not administer around the clock. Administer immediate release tablets twice daily with doses 7 hr apart (8 AM and 3 PM); administer extended release tablet once daily in the morning upon rising with a half-glassful of fluid. *DNC:* Swallow extended-release tablets whole; do not break, crush, or chew. Extended release tablets that are scored may be split.

Patient/Family Teaching
- Instruct patient to take medication as directed, even if feeling better. Take missed doses as soon as remembered; doses of isosorbide dinitrate should be taken at least 2 hr apart; daily doses of isosorbide mononitrate should be taken 7 hr apart. Do not double doses. Do not discontinue abruptly.
- Instruct patient to take last dose of day (when taking 2–4 doses/day) no later than 7 PM to prevent the development of tolerance.
- Caution patient to make position changes slowly to minimize orthostatic hypotension.
- May cause dizziness. Caution patient to avoid driving or other activities requiring alertness until response to medication is known.
- Advise patient to avoid concurrent use of alcohol with this medication. Instruct patient to notify health care professional of all Rx or OTC medications, vitamins, or herbal products being taken and to consult health care professional before taking other Rx, OTC, or herbal products.
- Inform patient that headache is a common side effect that should decrease with continuing therapy. Aspirin or acetaminophen may be ordered to treat headache. Notify health care professional if headache is persistent or severe. Do not alter dose to avoid headache.
- Advise patient to notify health care professional if dry mouth or blurred vision occurs.
- Advise females of reproductive potential to notify health care professional if pregnancy is planned or suspected, or if breastfeeding.

Evaluation/Desired Outcomes
- Decrease in frequency and severity of anginal attacks.
- Increase in activity tolerance.

REMS

ISOtretinoin
(eye-soe-**tret**-i-noyn)
Absorica, Absorica LD, Accutane, Amnesteem, Claravis, ✳Clarus, ✳Epuris, Myorisan, Zenatane
Classification
Therapeutic: antiacne agents
Pharmacologic: retinoids

Indications
Severe recalcitrant nodular acne in patients with multiple inflammatory nodules having a diameter of ≥5 mm and that are unresponsive to more conventional therapy, including systemic antibiotics.

Action
A metabolite of vitamin A (retinol); reduces sebaceous gland size and differentiation. **Therapeutic Effects:** Diminution and resolution of severe acne. May also prevent abnormal keratinization.

Pharmacokinetics
Absorption: Rapidly absorbed following (23–25%) oral administration (bioavailability of Absorica LD higher than that of Absorica); absorption ↑ when taken with a high-fat meal.
Distribution: Appears to be widely distributed.
Protein Binding: 99.9%.
Metabolism and Excretion: Metabolized by the liver and excreted in the urine and feces.
Half-life: 10–20 hr.

TIME/ACTION PROFILE (diminution of acne)

ROUTE	ONSET	PEAK	DURATION
PO	unknown	up to 8 wk	unknown

Contraindications/Precautions
Contraindicated in: Hypersensitivity to retinoids, glycerin, soybean oil, or parabens; Patients planning to donate blood; OB: Pregnancy; Lactation: Lactation; Rep: Women of childbearing age who may become or who intend to become pregnant;.
Use Cautiously in: Pre-existing hypertriglyceridemia; Diabetes mellitus; History of alcohol abuse, psychosis, depression, or suicide attempt; Obese patients; Inflammatory bowel disease; Pedi: Children <12 yr (safety and effectiveness not established).

Adverse Reactions/Side Effects
CV: edema. **Derm:** pruritus, palmar desquamation, photosensitivity, skin infections, STEVENS-JOHNSON SYNDROME (SJS), thinning of hair, TOXIC EPIDERMAL NE-

CROLYSIS (TEN). **EENT:** conjunctivitis, epistaxis, ↓ night vision, blurred vision, contact lens intolerance, corneal opacities, dry eyes. **Endo:** hyperglycemia. **F and E:** ↑ thirst. **GI:** cheilitis, dry mouth, nausea, vomiting, abdominal pain, anorexia, hepatitis, pancreatitis. **Hemat:** anemia. **Metab:** ↓ high-density lipoprotein cholesterol (HDL-C), hypercholesterolemia, hypertriglyceridemia, ↑ appetite, hyperuricemia. **MS:** arthralgia, back pain, muscle/bone pain (↑ in adolescents), hyperostosis. **Neuro:** behavior changes, depression, PSEUDOTUMOR CEREBRI, psychosis, SUICIDAL THOUGHTS/BEHAVIORS.

Interactions
Drug-Drug: Additive toxicity with **vitamin A** and **drugs having anticholinergic properties.** ↑ risk of pseudotumor cerebri with **tetracycline** or **minocycline.** Concurrent use with **alcohol** ↑ risk of hypertriglyceridemia. Drying effects ↑ by concurrent use of **benzoyl peroxide, sulfur, tretinoin,** and **other topical agents.**
Drug-Food: Excessive ingestion of **foods high in vitamin A** may result in additive toxicity.

Route/Dosage
Absorica and Absorica LD are not interchangeable.
PO (Adults and Children ≥12 yr): 0.5–1 mg/kg/day (may use up to 2 mg/kg/day for very severe disease) in 2 divided doses for 15–20 wk. Once discontinued, if relapse occurs, therapy may be reinstituted after an 8-wk rest period. *Absorica LD:* 0.4–0.8 mg/kg/day (may use up to 1.6 mg/kg/day for very severe disease) in 2 divided doses for 15–20 wk. Once discontinued, if relapse occurs, therapy may be reinstituted after an 8-wk rest period.

Availability (generic available)
Capsules: 10 mg, 20 mg, 25 mg, 30 mg, 35 mg, 40 mg. **Capsules (Absorica LD):** 8 mg, 16 mg, 24 mg, 32 mg.

NURSING IMPLICATIONS
Assessment
* *REMS:* Verify that patient receiving isotretinoin is registered with the *iPLEDGE REMS* and is completing all required interactions with their health care provider.
* Assess skin prior to and periodically during therapy. Transient worsening of acne may occur at initiation of therapy. Note number and severity of cysts, degree of skin dryness, erythema, and itching.
* Assess for allergy to parabens; capsules contain parabens as a preservative.
* Monitor patient for behavioral changes throughout therapy. May cause depression, psychosis, and suicide ideation. If behavioral changes occur, they usually resolve with discontinuation of therapy.
* Assess for rash periodically during therapy. May cause SJS or TEN. Discontinue therapy if severe or if

accompanied with fever, general malaise, fatigue, muscle or joint aches, blisters, oral lesions, conjunctivitis, hepatitis, and/or eosinophilia.

Lab Test Considerations
* Verify two negative sequential serum or urine pregnancy tests with a sensitivity ≥25 mIU/mL before receiving initial prescription and monthly before each new Rx.
* Monitor liver function (AST, ALT, and LDH) prior to therapy, after 1 mo of therapy, and periodically thereafter. Inform health care professional if these values become ↑ therapy; may need to be discontinued.
* Monitor blood lipids (cholesterol, HDL-C, triglycerides) under fasting conditions prior to beginning therapy, at 1–2 wk intervals until lipid response to isotretinoin is established (usually within 1 mo), and periodically thereafter. Report ↑ cholesterol and triglyceride levels or ↓ HDL-C.
* Obtain baseline and periodic CBC, urinalysis, and metabolic panel. May cause ↑ blood glucose, CK, platelet counts, and sedimentation rate. May ↓ RBC and WBC parameters. May cause proteinuria, RBCs and WBCs in urine, and ↑ uric acid.

Implementation
* Do not confuse isotretinoin with tretinoin.
* *REMS:* Isotretinoin is approved for marketing only under the *iPLEDGE REMS*, a special restricted distribution program approved by the FDA.
* *REMS:* Only patients who meet all requirements of the *iPLEDGE REMS* may receive isotretinoin.
* *REMS:* Isotretinoin may only be prescribed by health care providers registered and activated with the *iPLEDGE REMS.*
* *REMS:* Isotretinoin may only be dispensed by pharmacies registered with the *iPLEDGE REMS.*
* **PO:** Administer without regard to meals. Administer with a full glass of liquid to decrease the risk of esophageal irritation. *DNC:* Do not crush or open capsules.

Patient/Family Teaching
* *REMS:* Explain the *iPLEDGE REMS* and its requirements to patient and parent.
* Instruct patient to take isotretinoin as directed. Do not take more than the amount prescribed. If a dose is missed omit dose; do not double doses. Patients must read *Medication Guide* and sign consent form prior to initiation of therapy.
* Explain to patient that a temporary worsening of acne may occur at beginning of therapy.
* Advise patient and family to notify health care professional if rash or thoughts about suicide or dying, attempts to commit suicide; new or worse depression; new or worse anxiety; feeling very agitated or restless; panic attacks; trouble sleeping; new or worse

irritability; acting aggressive; being angry or violent; acting on dangerous impulses; an extreme increase in activity and talking; other unusual changes in behavior or mood occur.

- May cause sudden decrease in night vision. Caution patient to avoid driving at night until response to the medication is known.
- Advise patient to consult with health care professional before using other acne preparations while taking isotretinoin. Soaps, cosmetics, and shaving lotion may also worsen dry skin.
- Advise patient to notify health care professional of all Rx or OTC medications, vitamins, or herbal products being taken and to consult with health care professional before taking other medications, especially St. John's wort.
- Instruct patient not to take vitamin A supplements and to avoid excessive ingestion of foods high in vitamin A (liver; fish liver oils; egg yolks; yellow-orange fruits and vegetables; dark green, leafy vegetables; whole milk; vitamin A—fortified skim milk; butter; margarine) while taking isotretinoin; this may result in hypervitaminosis.
- Advise patient to avoid alcoholic beverages while taking isotretinoin, as this may further increase triglyceride levels.
- Inform patient that dry skin and chapped lips will occur. Lubricant to lips may help cheilitis.
- Instruct patient that oral rinses, good oral hygiene, and sugarless gum or candy may help minimize dry mouth. Notify health care professional if dry mouth persists for more than 2 wk.
- Discuss possibility of excessively dry eyes with patients who wear contact lenses. Patient should contact health care professional about eye lubricant. Patient may need to switch to glasses during course of therapy and for up to 2 wk following discontinuation.
- Caution patient to use sunscreen and protective clothing to prevent photosensitivity reactions. Consult health care professional about sunscreen, as some sunscreens may worsen acne.
- Inform diabetic patients that difficulty controlling blood glucose may occur.
- Instruct patient to report burning of eyes, visual changes, rash, abdominal pain, diarrhea, headache, nausea, and vomiting to health care professional.
- Advise patient not to donate blood while receiving this medication. After discontinuing isotretinoin, wait at least 1 mo before donating blood to prevent the possibility of a pregnant patient receiving the blood.
- Rep: May cause fetal harm. Instruct female patients of reproductive potential to use 2 forms of contraception 1 mo before therapy, during therapy, and for at least 1 mo after discontinuation of isotretinoin. Patient who can become pregnant must have 2 negative serum or urine pregnancy tests with a sensitivity ≥25 mIU/mL before receiving initial prescription.

First test is obtained by prescriber when decision is made to prescribe isotretinoin. Second pregnancy test should be done after patient has used 2 forms of contraception for 1 mo and during first 5 days of menstrual period immediately preceding beginning of therapy. For patients with amenorrhea, second test should be done 11 days after last act of unprotected sexual intercourse. Each mo of therapy patient must have a negative result from a urine or serum pregnancy test. Pregnancy test must be repeated every mo prior to receiving prescription in patients who can become pregnant. Patient should discontinue medication and inform health care professional immediately if pregnancy is suspected during or 1 month after therapy. If pregnancy occurs, must be reported immediately to the FDA via the MedWatch telephone number 1-800-FDA-1088, and also to the iPLEDGE pregnancy registry at 1-866-495-0654 or via the internet (www.ipledgeprogram.com). Recommended consent form prepared by manufacturer stresses fetal risk. Parents of minors should also read and sign form. Yellow self-adhesive qualification stickers completed by prescriber must accompany prescription. Advise patient to avoid breastfeeding during and for at least 8 days after last dose.

- Inform patient of need for medical follow-up. Periodic lab tests may be required.

Evaluation/Desired Outcomes

- Decrease in the number and severity of cysts in severe acne. Therapy may take 4–5 mo before full effects are seen. Therapy is discontinued when the number of cysts is reduced by 70% or after 5 mo. Improvement may occur after discontinuation of therapy; therefore, a delay of at least 8 wk is recommended before a second course of therapy is considered.

istradefylline (is-tra-def-i-lin)
Nourianz
Classification
Therapeutic: antiparkinson agents
Pharmacologic: adenosine receptor antagonist

Indications
Adjunctive treatment to levodopa/carbidopa in patients with Parkinson's disease experiencing "off" episodes.

Action
Acts as an adenosine receptor antagonist; the mechanism by which these effects exert beneficial effects in patients with Parkinson's disease is unknown. **Therapeutic Effects:** Reduction in "off" time.

Pharmacokinetics
Absorption: Unknown.
Distribution: Extensively distributed to tissues.
Protein Binding: 98%.

Metabolism and Excretion: Primarily metabolized in the liver via the CYP1A1 and CYP3A4 isoenzymes. 48% excreted in feces, 39% in urine.
Half-life: 83 hr.

TIME/ACTION PROFILE (plasma concentrations)

ROUTE	ONSET	PEAK	DURATION
PO	unknown	4 hr	24 hr

Contraindications/Precautions
Contraindicated in: Severe psychotic disorders (may worsen psychosis); Severe hepatic impairment; OB: Pregnancy.
Use Cautiously in: End-stage renal disease; Moderate hepatic impairment; Lactation: Use while breastfeeding only if potential maternal benefit justifies potential risk to infant; Rep: Women of reproductive potential; Pedi: Safety and effectiveness not established in children.

Adverse Reactions/Side Effects
Derm: rash. **Endo:** hyperglycemia. **GI:** ↓ appetite, constipation, diarrhea, nausea. **Metab:** hyperuricemia. **Neuro:** dyskinesia, aggression, agitation, confusion, delirium, delusions, disorientation, dizziness, hallucinations, impulse control disorders (gambling, sexual), insomnia, mania, paranoid ideation.

Interactions
Drug-Drug: Concurrent use with **levodopa** may cause or exacerbate dyskinesia. **Cigarette smoking** may ↓ levels; if patient smokes ≥20 cigarettes/day, ↑ dose to 40 mg once daily. **Strong CYP3A4 inhibitors**, including **clarithromycin**, **itraconazole**, and **ketoconazole**, may ↑ levels and risk of toxicity. **Strong CYP3A4 inducers**, including **carbamazepine**, **phenytoin**, and **rifampin**, may ↓ levels and effectiveness; avoid concurrent use. Higher doses (40 mg/day) may ↑ levels and risk of toxicity of **CYP3A4 substrates**, including **atorvastatin**. May ↑ levels and risk of toxicity of **P-glycoprotein substrates**, including **digoxin**.
Drug-Natural Products: St. John's wort may ↓ levels and effectiveness; avoid concurrent use.

Route/Dosage
PO (Adults): 20 mg once daily; may ↑ to 40 mg once daily, if needed, based on clinical response. *Concurrent use of strong CYP3A4 inhibitors:* Do not exceed 20 mg/day.

Hepatic Impairment
PO (Adults): *Moderate hepatic impairment:* Do not exceed 20 mg/day.

Availability
Tablets: 20 mg, 40 mg.

NURSING IMPLICATIONS
Assessment
- Assess parkinsonian symptoms (akinesia, rigidity, tremors, pill rolling, shuffling gait, mask-like face, twisting motions, and drooling) during therapy. "On-off phenomenon" may cause symptoms to appear or improve suddenly.
- Assess for signs and symptoms of dyskinesia (abnormal movements, uncontrolled sudden movements) before and during therapy.
- Monitor for signs and symptoms of behavior changes (hallucinations, psychotic behavior, paranoid ideation, delusions, confusion, mania, disorientation, aggressive behavior, agitation, delirium) during therapy. Consider reducing dose or discontinuing therapy.

Implementation
- **PO:** Administer once daily without regard for food.

Patient/Family Teaching
- Instruct patient to take medication at regular intervals as directed. Advise patient to read *Patient Information* before starting therapy and with each Rx refill in case of changes.
- Advise patient to notify health care professional of all Rx or OTC medications, vitamins, or herbal products being taken and to consult with health care professional before taking other medications.
- Advise patient and family to notify health care professional if signs and symptoms of hallucinations or psychosis (being overly suspicious or feeling people want to harm you, disorientation, believing things that are not real, aggressive behavior, seeing or hearing things that are not real, agitation, confusion, delirium, increased activity or talking, or if new or increased gambling, sexual, or other intense urges occur). Dose reduction may be required.
- Rep: Advise females of reproductive potential to use effective contraception and avoid breastfeeding during therapy. Advise patient to notify health care professional if pregnancy is planned or suspected, or if breastfeeding.

Evaluation/Desired Outcomes
- Decreased "off" time in patients with Parkinson's disease.

ivabradine (eye-**vab**-ra-deen)
Corlanor, ♣Lancora
Classification
Therapeutic: heart failure agents
Pharmacologic: hyperpolarization-activated cyclic nucleotide-gated channel blockers

Indications
To decrease the need for hospitalization due to worsening HF in patients with stable, but symptomatic chronic

HF (ejection fraction <35%, sinus rhythm ≥70 bpm, receiving highest tolerated doses of beta-blockers or are unable to tolerate beta-blockers). Stable, symptomatic HF due to dilated cardiomyopathy in pediatric patients ≥6 mo old who are in sinus rhythm with an elevated heart rate.

Action

Inhibits the cardiac pacemaker I_f-current by acting as a hyperpolarization-activated cyclic nucleoside-gated channel blocker, resulting in ↓ spontaneous pacemaker activity of sinus node. Decreases heart rate without affecting contractility or ventricular repolarization. **Therapeutic Effects:** Lowering of heart rate with reduced need for hospitalization in patients with HF.

Pharmacokinetics

Absorption: 40% absorbed following oral administration (undergoes first pass metabolism); food delays absorption and ↑ blood levels.
Distribution: Unknown.
Metabolism and Excretion: Extensively metabolized, primarily by the CYP3A4 enzyme system. The major metabolite is pharmacologically active and has the same potency as ivabradine. Metabolites excreted equally in urine and feces; 4% excreted unchanged in urine.
Half-life: 6 hr.

TIME/ACTION PROFILE (blood levels)

ROUTE	ONSET	PEAK	DURATION
PO	unknown	1 hr	12 hr

Contraindications/Precautions

Contraindicated in: Acute decompensated heart failure; Clinically significant hypotension; Sick sinus syndrome, sinoatrial block, or 2nd or 3rd degree heart block (unless a functioning demand pacemaker is in place, ↑ risk of bradycardia); Clinically significant bradycardia; Severe hepatic impairment; Pacemaker dependence; Concurrent use of strong CYP3A4 inhibitors; OB: Pregnancy; Lactation: Lactation.
Use Cautiously in: Rep: Women of reproductive potential; Pedi: Children <6 mo (safety and effectiveness not established).

Adverse Reactions/Side Effects

CV: atrial fibrillation, bradycardia, heart block, hypertension, QT interval prolongation, sinus arrest, TORSADES DE POINTES. **EENT:** phosphenes (luminous phenomena).

Interactions

Drug-Drug: **Strong CYP3A4 inhibitors**, including **azole antifungals**, **macolide anti-infectives**, **HIV protease inhibitors**, and **nefazodone** may ↑ levels; concurrent use contraindicated. **Moderate CYP3A4 inhibitors**, including **diltiazem** and **verapamil**, may ↑ levels and ↑ risk of bradycardia; avoid concurrent use. **CYP3A4 inducers**, including **barbiturates**, **phenytoin**, and **rifampicin** may ↓ levels; avoid concurrent

use. ↑ risk of bradycardia with concurrent use of **negative chronotropes** including **amiodarone**, **beta-blockers**, and **digoxin**; monitor heart rate. Concurrent use of **QT-interval prolonging drugs** may ↑ risk of QT interval prolongation and torsades de pointes.
Drug-Natural Products: Concurrent use of **St. John's wort** may ↓ blood levels and effectiveness and should be avoided.
Drug-Food: Concurrent ingestion of **grapefruit juice** may ↑ blood levels and the risk of adverse effects and should be avoided.

Route/Dosage

PO (Adults): 5 mg twice daily for 2 wk; dose may then be adjusted based on heart rate, not to exceed 7.5 mg twice daily; *Patients with conduction defects or bradycardia:* 2.5 mg twice daily initially.
PO (Children ≥6 mo and ≥40 kg): *Tablets:* 2.5 mg twice daily; adjust dose at 2-wk intervals by 2.5 mg twice daily to achieve a heart rate reduction of ≥20%; not to exceed 7.5 mg twice daily.
PO (Children ≥6 mo and <40 kg): *Oral solution:* 0.05 mg/kg twice daily; adjust dose at 2-wk intervals by 0.05 mg/kg twice daily to achieve a heart rate reduction of ≥20%; not to exceed 0.2 mg/kg twice daily (6 mo– <1 yr) or 0.3 mg/kg twice daily (≥1 yr) up to max of 7.5 mg twice daily.

Availability (generic available)

Oral solution: 1 mg/mL. **Tablets:** 5 mg, 7.5 mg.

NURSING IMPLICATIONS

Assessment

- Assess heart rate prior to, after 2 wk, and periodically during therapy. Adjust dose for a resting heart rate 50–60 bpm. *If heart rate >60 bpm,* increase dose by 2.5 mg given twice daily up to 7.5 mg twice daily. *If heart rate 50–60 bpm,* maintain dose. *If heart rate <50 bpm or signs and symptoms of bradycardia (dizziness, fatigue, hypotension) occur,* decrease dose by 2.5 mg given twice daily; if current dose is 2.5 mg given twice daily, discontinue ivabradine.
- Monitor ECG periodically during therapy. May cause atrial fibrillation and torsades de pointes. Discontinue ivabradine if atrial fibrillation occurs.

Implementation

- **PO:** Administer twice daily with meals.
- For oral solution, empty entire contents of ampule(s) into a medication cup. With a calibrated oral syringe, measure prescribed dose and administer orally. Discard unused oral solution; do not store or reuse. Solution is colorless.

Patient/Family Teaching

- Instruct patient to take ivabradine as directed. If dose is missed or patient spits out drug omit dose; do not double doses.
- Advise patient to avoid taking grapefruit juice during therapy; may increase risk of side effects.

- Advise patient to notify health care professional if signs and symptoms of irregular or rapid heartbeat (heart pounding or racing, chest pressure, worsened shortness of breath, near fainting or fainting) or slower than normal heart rate (dizziness, fatigue, lack of energy) occur. In young children signs and symptoms of slow heart rate (poor feeding, difficulty breathing, turning blue).
- Inform patient that ivabradine may cause phosphenes or luminous phenomena, a transiently enhanced brightness in a limited area of the visual field, halos, image decomposition, colored bright lights, or multiple images. Phosphenes are usually triggered by sudden variations in light intensity. Usually begin within first 2 mo of therapy, may occur repeatedly of mild to moderate intensity, and resolve after therapy is discontinued.
- Instruct patient to notify health care professional of all Rx or OTC medications, vitamins, or herbal products being taken and to consult health care professional before taking any other Rx, OTC, or herbal products, especially St. John's wort.
- Rep: May cause fetal harm. Advise females of reproductive potential to use effective contraception during therapy and to avoid breastfeeding during therapy. Advise patient to notify health care professional immediately if pregnancy is suspected.

Evaluation/Desired Outcomes
- Lowering of heart rate to prevent hospitalization in patients with HF.

---

ixazomib (ix-az-oh-mib)
Ninlaro
Classification
Therapeutic: antineoplastics
Pharmacologic: proteasome inhibitors

Indications
Multiple myeloma in patients whose disease has relapsed despite receiving ≥1 previous drug therapy (in combination with lenalidomide and dexamethasone).

Action
Acts as a proteasome inhibitor by binding to sites on the 20s proteasome. Has antiproliferative and proapoptotic activity. **Therapeutic Effects:** Delayed progression of multiple myeloma.

Pharmacokinetics
Absorption: 58% absorbed following oral administration; bioavailability ↓ by high-fat foods.
Distribution: Extensively distributed to tissues.
Protein Binding: 99%.
Metabolism and Excretion: Metabolized by multiple CYP450 enzymes (including CYP1A2, CYP2B6, CYP2C8, CYP2C9, CYP2C19, CYP2D6, and CYP3A4).

62% excreted in urine (<3.5% as unchanged drug), 22% excreted in feces.
Half-life: 9.5 days.

TIME/ACTION PROFILE (plasma concentrations)

ROUTE	ONSET	PEAK	DURATION
PO	unknown	1 hr	unknown

Contraindications/Precautions
Contraindicated in: Maintenance setting (may ↑ risk of mortality); OB: Pregnancy; Lactation: Lactation.
Use Cautiously in: Moderate or severe hepatic impairment (↓ dose recommended); Severe renal impairment or end stage renal disease (↓ dose recommended); Rep: Women and men of reproductive potential; Pedi: Safety and effectiveness not established in children.

Adverse Reactions/Side Effects
CV: edema. **Derm:** rash, STEVENS-JOHNSON SYNDROME. **EENT:** blurred vision, conjunctivitis, dry eye. **GI:** constipation, diarrhea, nausea, vomiting, HEPATOTOXICITY. **Hemat:** HEMOLYTIC UREMIC SYNDROME, NEUTROPENIA, THROMBOCYTOPENIA, THROMBOTIC MICROANGIOPATHY, THROMBOTIC THROMBOCYTOPENIC PURPURA. **MS:** back pain. **Neuro:** peripheral neuropathy. **Misc:** herpes zoster infection.

Interactions
Drug-Drug: Strong CYP3A4 inducers, including **carbamazepine**, **phenytoin**, and **rifampin**, may ↓ levels and effectiveness; avoid concurrent use.
Drug-Natural Products: St. John's wort may ↓ levels and effectiveness; avoid concurrent use.

Route/Dosage
PO (Adults): 4 mg on Days 1, 8, and 15 of a 28-day treatment cycle.

Renal Impairment
(Adults): *CCr <30 mL/min or requiring dialysis:* 3 mg on Days 1, 8, and 15 of a 28-day treatment cycle.

Hepatic Impairment
(Adults): *Moderate or severe hepatic impairment (total bilirubin >1.5 × upper limit of normal):* 3 mg on Days 1, 8, and 15 of a 28-day treatment cycle.

Availability
Capsules: 2.3 mg, 3 mg, 4 mg.

NURSING IMPLICATIONS
Assessment
- Assess for rash (usually maculopapular or macular) periodically during therapy. *If Grade 2 or 3 rash occurs,* withhold lenalidomide until rash recovers to ≤Grade 1, then resume lenalidomide at next lower dose. *If Grade 2 or 3 rash occurs again,* withhold ixazomib and lenalidomide until rash ≤Grade 1,

then resume ixazomib at next lower dose and resume lenalidomide at most recent dose. *If Grade 4 rash occurs,* discontinue therapy.

- Assess for signs and symptoms of peripheral neuropathy (numbness, tingling, burning, pain in feet or hands, or weakness in arms or legs) periodically during therapy. *If Grade 1 peripheral neuropathy with pain or Grade 2 peripheral neuropathy occurs,* withhold ixazomib until peripheral neuropathy recovers to ≤Grade 1 without pain or patient's baseline, then resume ixazomib at most recent dose. *If Grade 2 peripheral neuropathy with pain or Grade 3 peripheral neuropathy occurs,* withhold ixazomib until return to patient's baseline condition or ≤Grade 1 peripheral neuropathy, then resume ixazomib at next lower dose. *If Grade 4 peripheral neuropathy occurs,* discontinue therapy.
- Monitor for signs and symptoms of thrombotic microangiopathy (fever, bruising, nose bleeds, tiredness, decreased urination) during therapy. If symptoms occur, hold ixazomib and evaluate. If diagnosis is excluded, may consider restarting therapy.

Lab Test Considerations
- Verify negative pregnancy test before starting therapy.
- Prior to each 28-day cycle, absolute neutrophil count (ANC) should be ≥1,000/mm³, platelet count should be ≥75,000/mm³, and nonhematologic toxicities should be recovered to patient's baseline condition or ≤Grade 1.
- For patients taking ixazomib, lenalidomide, and dexamethasone, *if ANC <500/mm³,* withhold ixazomib and lenalidomide until ANC ≥500/mm³, then resume lenalidomide at next lower dose and resume ixazomib at most recent dose. Consider adding granulocyte stimulating factor (G-CSF) as per clinical guidelines. *If ANC <500/mm³ again,* withhold ixazomib and lenalidomide until ANC ≥500/mm³, then resume ixazomib at next lower dose and resume lenalidomide at most recent dose.
- Monitor platelet counts at least monthly during therapy and more frequently during 1st three cycles. Nadir of thrombocytopenia usually occurs Days 14–21 of each 28-day cycle and recovery to baseline by start of next cycle. *If platelet count ≤30,000/mm³,* withhold ixazomib and lenalidomide until platelet count is ≥30,000/mm³, then resume lenalidomide at next lower dose and resume ixazomib at most recent dose. *If platelet count <30,000/mm³ again,* withhold ixazomib and lenalidomide until platelet count is ≥30,000/mm³, then resume ixazomib at next lower dose and resume lenalidomide at most recent dose.
- Monitor hepatic enzymes periodically during therapy and adjust dosing for Grade 3 or 4 symptoms.

Implementation
- Consider starting antiviral prophylaxis prior therapy to decrease risk of herpes zoster infection.

- **PO:** Administer once weekly on same day and at same time for first 3 wk of four-wk cycle. Take capsules at least 1 hr before or at least 2 hr after food. *DNC:* Swallow capsule whole with water; do not open, crush, or chew.
- Avoid direct contact with capsule contents. If powder from the capsule comes in contact with skin, wash area well with soap and water. If powder from capsule gets in the eyes, flush eyes well with water.
- Dexamethasone should be taken with food and not with ixazomib.

Patient/Family Teaching
- Instruct patient to take ixazomib as directed and to avoid contact with capsule contents. Take delayed or missed doses only if next scheduled dose is ≥72 hr away. Do not take within 72 hr of next scheduled dose and do not double doses. If vomiting occurs after taking dose, omit dose and resume dosing at time of next scheduled dose. Advise patient to read *Patient Information* sheet prior to starting therapy and with each Rx refill in case of changes.
- Caution patient to avoid direct contact with capsule contents. If powder accidentally gets on skin, wash area well with soap and water. If in eyes, flush eyes well with water.
- Advise patient to notify health care professional if signs and symptoms of thrombocytopenia (bleeding, easy bruising), thrombotic microangiopathy, GI problems (diarrhea, constipation, nausea, vomiting), peripheral neuropathy (tingling, numbness, pain, burning in feet or hands, weakness in arms or legs), liver problems (yellowing of skin or whites of eyes, pain in right upper abdomen), swelling in arms, hands, legs, ankles, or feet, or weight gain from swelling, new or worsening rash, or back pain occurs.
- Advise patient to notify health care professional of all Rx or OTC medications, vitamins, or herbal products being taken and to consult with health care professional before taking other medications, especially St. John's wort.
- **Rep:** May cause fetal harm. Advise females of reproductive potential and males with female partners of reproductive potential to use effective nonhormonal contraception during and for 90 days after last dose and to avoid breastfeeding during and for 90 days after last dose. Advise patient to notify health care professional immediately if pregnancy is suspected.

Evaluation/Desired Outcomes
- Delayed progression of multiple myeloma signs and symptoms.

ixekizumab (ix-ee-kiz-ue-mab)
Taltz
Classification
Therapeutic: antipsoriatics
Pharmacologic: interleukin antagonists

Indications
Moderate-to-severe plaque psoriasis in patients who are candidates for systemic therapy or phototherapy. Active psoriatic arthritis (as monotherapy or in combination with a nonbiologic DMARD). Active ankylosing spondylitis. Active nonradiographic axial spondyloarthritis in patients with objective signs of inflammation.

Action
A monoclonal antibody that acts as an antagonist of interleukin (IL)−17A by selectively binding to it and preventing its interaction with the IL−17 receptor. Antagonism prevents the production of inflammatory cytokines and chemokines. **Therapeutic Effects:** Decreased plaque formation and spread in plaque psoriasis. Decreased pain and swelling with decreased joint destruction in psoriatic arthritis. Decreased disease activity in ankylosing spondylitis and nonradiographic axial spondyloarthritis.

Pharmacokinetics
Absorption: Well absorbed (60−81%) following SUBQ administration.
Distribution: Minimally distributed to tissues.
Metabolism and Excretion: Catabolized into small peptides and amino acids.
Half-life: 13 days.

TIME/ACTION PROFILE (plasma concentrations)

ROUTE	ONSET	PEAK	DURATION
SUBQ	unknown	4 days	unknown

Contraindications/Precautions
Contraindicated in: Hypersensitivity; Active tuberculosis.
Use Cautiously in: Inflammatory bowel disease (may lead to exacerbations); OB: Safety not established in pregnancy; Lactation: Use while breastfeeding only if potential maternal benefit justifies potential risk to infant; Pedi: Children <6 yr (safety and effectiveness not established).

Adverse Reactions/Side Effects
GI: inflammatory bowel disease, nausea. **Hemat:** neutropenia, thrombocytopenia. **Local:** injection site reactions. **Misc:** INFECTION (including reactivation tuberculosis), HYPERSENSITIVITY REACTIONS (including anaphylaxis, angioedema, and urticaria).

Interactions
Drug-Drug: May ↓ antibody response to **live-virus vaccine** and ↑ risk of adverse reactions (do not administer concurrently).

Route/Dosage

Plaque Psoriasis
SUBQ (Adults): 160 mg (as two 80-mg injections) at Wk 0, then 80 mg at Wk 2, 4, 6, 8, 10, and 12, then 80 mg every 4 wk.

SUBQ (Children ≥6 yr and >50 kg): 160 mg (as two 80-mg injections) at Wk 0, then 80 mg every 4 wk.
SUBQ (Children ≥6 yr and 25−50 kg): 80 mg at Wk 0, then 40 mg every 4 wk.
SUBQ (Children ≥6 yr and <25 kg): 40 mg at Wk 0, then 20 mg every 4 wk.

Psoriatic Arthritis and Ankylosing Spondylitis
SUBQ (Adults): 160 mg (as two 80-mg injections) initially, then 80 mg every 4 wk.

Nonradiographic Axial Spondyloarthritis
SUBQ (Adults): 80 mg every 4 wk.

Availability
Solution for injection (prefilled autoinjectors and prefilled syringes): 80 mg/mL.

NURSING IMPLICATIONS
Assessment
- Assess for tuberculosis infection before starting therapy; do not administer to patient with active TB infection. Initiate treatment of latent TB before administering ixekizumab. In patient with previous history of TB in whom an adequate course cannot be confirmed, consider anti-TB therapy before starting ixekizumab.
- Monitor for signs and symptoms of infection (fever, sweats, chills, muscle aches, cough, dyspnea, blood in mucus, weight loss, warm, red, or painful skin or sores, diarrhea or stomach pain, burning or frequency of urination) before and periodically during therapy.
- Monitor for signs and symptoms of hypersensitivity (urticaria, feeling faint, swelling of face, eyelids, lips, mouth, tongue, or throat, dyspnea, throat tightness, chest tightness, rash) during therapy. If hypersensitivity reaction occurs, discontinue ixekizumab immediately and begin supportive therapy.
- Monitor for onset or exacerbation of inflammatory bowel disease (abdominal pain, diarrhea with or without blood, weight loss) during therapy.

Lab Test Considerations
- May cause neutropenia and thrombocytopenia.

Implementation
- Complete all age-appropriate vaccinations as recommended by current immunization guidelines before starting therapy.
- **SUBQ:** Allow to reach room temperature (30 min) before injection; do not microwave, run under hot water, or leave in sunlight to warm. Solution is clear and colorless to slightly yellow; do not administer solutions that are cloudy, discolored, or contain a precipitate. For *prefilled syringe,* pinch skin and inject into upper arm, thigh, or abdomen at a 45° angle; let go of skin pinch before injecting. Place *au-*

toinjector flat against skin at injection site before injecting. Avoid areas where skin is bruised, tender, erythematous, indurated, or affected by psoriasis. Rotate injection sites. Store in refrigerator in original box to protect from light; may be stored at room temperature for up to 5 days. Do not return to refrigerator once stored at room temperature.

- For children ≤50 kg, after withdrawing dose from vial, change to a 27–gauge needle for administration.

Patient/Family Teaching

- Instruct patient and caregiver in proper technique for self-injection and care and disposal of equipment. Administer missed doses as soon as possible and resume regular dosing schedule. Advise patient to read *Medication Guide and Instructions for Use* prior to starting therapy and with each Rx refill in case of changes.
- Advise patient to notify health care professional if signs and symptoms of allergic reaction, infection, or inflammatory bowel disease occur.
- Advise patient to avoid use of live vaccines during therapy.

- Instruct patient to notify health care professional of all Rx or OTC medications, vitamins, or herbal products being taken and consult health care professional before taking any new medications.
- Rep: Advise female patients of reproductive potential to notify health care professional if pregnancy is planned or suspected, or if breastfeeding. There is a pregnancy exposure registry that monitors pregnancy outcomes in women exposed to *Taltz* during pregnancy. Pregnant women exposed to ixekizumab are encouraged to enroll in the pregnancy exposure registry that monitors pregnancy outcomes in women exposed to ixekizumab during pregnancy, by calling the *Taltz* Pregnancy Registry at 1-800-284-1695 or contacting the registry at https://www.taltz.com.

Evaluation/Desired Outcomes

- Decreased plaque formation and spread in patients with plaque psoriasis.
- Decreased pain and swelling with decreased joint destruction in psoriatic arthritis.
- Decreased disease activity in ankylosing spondylitis and non-radiographic axial spondyloarthritis.

ketoconazole, See ANTIFUNGALS (TOPICAL).

---

ketorolac† (kee-toe-role-ak)
Sprix, ~~Toradol~~, ✽ Toradol

Classification
Therapeutic: nonopioid analgesics
Pharmacologic: nonsteroidal anti-inflammatory drugs (NSAIDs)

†See Appendix B for ophthalmic use

Indications
Short-term management of pain.

Action
Inhibits prostaglandin synthesis, producing peripherally mediated analgesia. Also has antipyretic and anti-inflammatory properties. **Therapeutic Effects:** Decreased pain.

Pharmacokinetics
Absorption: Rapidly and completely absorbed following all routes of administration.
Distribution: Well distributed to tissues.
Protein Binding: 99%.
Metabolism and Excretion: Primarily metabolized by the liver. Primarily by the kidneys (92%); 6% excreted in feces.
Half-life: 4.5 hr (range 3.8–6.3 hr; ↑ in geriatric patients and patients with impaired renal function).

TIME/ACTION PROFILE (analgesic effects)

ROUTE	ONSET	PEAK	DURATION
PO	unknown	2–3 hr	4–6 hr or longer
IM, IV	10 min	1–2 hr	6 hr or longer
IN	unknown	unknown	6–8 hr or longer

Contraindications/Precautions
Contraindicated in: Hypersensitivity; Cross-sensitivity with other NSAIDs may exist; Preoperative use; Active or history of peptic ulcer disease or GI bleeding; Known alcohol intolerance (injection only); Coronary artery bypass graft surgery; Cerebrovascular bleeding; Advanced renal impairment or at risk for renal failure due to volume depletion; Concurrent use of pentoxifylline or probenecid; OB: Avoid use of after 30 wk gestation; may inhibit labor and ↑ maternal bleeding at delivery.
Use Cautiously in: Cardiovascular disease or risk factors for cardiovascular disease (may ↑ risk of serious cardiovascular thrombotic events, MI, and stroke, especially with prolonged use or use of higher doses);

avoid use in patients with recent MI or HF; HF; Coagulation disorders; Mild-to-moderate renal impairment (↓ dose may be required); Hepatic impairment; OB: Use at or after 20 wk gestation may cause fetal or neonatal renal impairment; if treatment is necessary between 20 wk and 30 wk gestation, limit use to the lowest effective dose and shortest duration possible; Lactation: Use while breastfeeding only if potential maternal benefit justifies potential risk to infant; Pedi: Safety and effectiveness not established in neonates; Geri: Appears on Beers list. ↑ risk GI bleeding or peptic ulcer disease in older adults. Avoid chronic use unless other alternatives are not effective and the patient can take a gastroprotective agent; avoid short-term use in combination with oral or parenteral corticosteroids, anticoagulants, or antiplatelet agents unless other alternatives are not effective and the patient can take a gastroprotective agent.

Adverse Reactions/Side Effects
CV: edema, HF, MI. **Derm:** DRUG REACTION WITH EOSINOPHILIA AND SYSTEMIC SYMPTOMS (DRESS), EXFOLIATIVE DERMATITIS, pruritus, purpura, STEVENS-JOHNSON SYNDROME, sweating, TOXIC EPIDERMAL NECROLYSIS, urticaria. **EENT:** ↑ lacrimation (spray), nasal discomfort (spray), throat irritation (spray). **F and E:** hyperkalemia. **GI:** ↑ liver enzymes, abdominal pain, abnormal taste, diarrhea, dry mouth, dyspepsia, GI BLEEDING, nausea. **GU:** oliguria, renal toxicity, urinary frequency. **Hemat:** prolonged bleeding time. **Local:** injection site pain. **Neuro:** drowsiness, abnormal thinking, dizziness, euphoria, headache, paresthesia, STROKE. **Resp:** asthma, dyspnea. **Misc:** HYPERSENSITIVITY REACTIONS (including anaphylaxis).

Interactions
Drug-Drug: Probenecid ↑ levels and the risk of adverse reactions; concurrent use is contraindicated. ↑ risk of bleeding when used with **pentoxifylline**; concurrent use is contraindicated. Concurrent use with **aspirin** may ↓ effectiveness. ↑ adverse GI effects with **aspirin**, other **NSAIDs**, **potassium supplements**, **corticosteroids**, or **alcohol**. May ↓ effectiveness of **diuretics** or **antihypertensives**. May ↑ serum **lithium** levels and ↑ risk of toxicity. ↑ risk of toxicity from **methotrexate**. ↑ risk of bleeding with **anticoagulants**, **aspirin**, **clopidogrel**, **ticagrelor**, **prasugrel**, **corticosteroids**, **fibrinolytics**, **SNRIs**, or **SSRIs**. ↑ risk of adverse hematologic reactions with **antineoplastics** or **radiation therapy**. May ↑ risk of nephrotoxicity from **cyclosporine**.
Drug-Natural Products: ↑ bleeding risk with **arnica, chamomile, clove, dong quai, feverfew, garlic, ginger, ginkgo, Panax ginseng**.

Route/Dosage
Oral therapy is indicated only as a continuation of parenteral therapy. Total duration of therapy by all routes should not exceed 5 days.

✽ = Canadian drug name. ⚇ = Genetic implication. ~~Strikethrough~~ = Discontinued. CAPITALS = life-threatening. Underline = most frequent.

PO (Adults <65 yr): 20 mg initially, followed by 10 mg every 4–6 hr (not to exceed 40 mg/day).
PO (Adults ≥65 yr, <50 kg, or with renal impairment): 10 mg every 4–6 hr (not to exceed 40 mg/day).
PO (Children 2–16 yr, <50 kg): 1 mg/kg as a single dose. No data available for multiple doses.
IM (Adults <65 yr): *Single dose:* 60 mg. *Multiple dosing:* 30 mg every 6 hr (not to exceed 120 mg/day).
IM (Adults ≥65 yr, <50 kg, or with renal impairment): *Single dose:* 30 mg. *Multiple dosing:* 15 mg every 6 hr (not to exceed 60 mg/day).
IM (Children 2–16 yr, <50 kg): *Single dose:* 0.4–1 mg/kg (maximum: 30 mg/dose). *Multiple dosing:* 0.5 mg/kg every 6 hr.
IV (Adults <65 yr): *Single dose:* 30 mg. *Multiple dosing:* 30 mg every 6 hr (not to exceed 120 mg/day).
IV (Adults ≥65 yr, <50 kg, or with renal impairment): *Single dose:* 15 mg. *Multiple dosing:* 15 mg every 6 hr (not to exceed 60 mg/day).
IV (Children 2–16 yr, <50 kg): *Single dose:* 0.4–1 mg/kg (maximum: 15 mg/dose). *Multiple dosing:* 0.5 mg/kg every 6 hr.
Intranasal (Adults <65 yr): 1 spray in each nostril every 6–8 hr (not to exceed 4 sprays in each nostril/day).
Intranasal (Adults ≥65 yr, <50 kg, or with renal impairment): 1 spray in only one nostril every 6–8 hr (not to exceed 4 sprays in one nostril/day).

Availability (generic available)
Tablets: 10 mg. **Nasal spray (Sprix):** 15.75 mg/spray in 1.7-g bottle (delivers 8 sprays). **Solution for injection:** 15 mg/mL, 30 mg/mL.

NURSING IMPLICATIONS
Assessment
● Assess pain (note type, location, and intensity) prior to and 1–2 hr following administration.
● Patients who have asthma, aspirin-induced allergy, and nasal polyps are at increased risk for developing hypersensitivity reactions. Assess for rhinitis, asthma, and urticaria.
● Assess for rash periodically during therapy. May cause Stevens-Johnson syndrome or toxic epidermal necrolysis. Discontinue therapy if severe or if accompanied with fever, general malaise, fatigue, muscle or joint aches, blisters, oral lesions, conjunctivitis, hepatitis, and/or eosinophilia.
● Monitor BP during initiation and periodically during therapy. May cause fluid retention and edema leading to new onset or worsening hypertension.
● Monitor for signs and symptoms of DRESS (fever, rash, lymphadenopathy, facial swelling) periodically during therapy. Discontinue therapy if symptoms occur.

Lab Test Considerations
● Evaluate liver function tests, especially AST and ALT, periodically in patients receiving prolonged therapy. May cause ↑ levels.

● May cause prolonged bleeding time that may persist for 24–48 hr following discontinuation of therapy.
● May cause ↑ BUN, serum creatinine, or potassium concentrations.

Implementation
● Do not confuse ketorolac with Ketalar, ketamine, or methadone.
● Administration in higher-than-recommended doses does not provide increased effectiveness but may cause increased side effects. Duration of ketorolac therapy, by all routes combined, should not exceed 5 days. Use lowest effective dose for shortest period of time to minimize risk of cardiovascular thrombotic events.
● Coadministration with opioid analgesics may have additive analgesic effects and may permit lower opioid doses.
● Avoid concurrent administration with other NSAIDs.
● **PO:** Ketorolac therapy should always be given initially by the IM or IV route. Use oral therapy *only* as a continuation of parenteral therapy.

IV Administration
● **IV Push:** Administer undiluted. *Concentration:* 15–30 mg/mL. *Rate:* Administer over at least 15 sec.
● **Y-Site Compatibility:** amikacin, aminocaproic acid, aminophylline, amphotericin B lipid complex, amphotericin B liposomal, anidulafungin, argatroban, ascorbic acid, atracurium, atropine, aztreonam, benztropine, bivalirudin, bleomycin, bumetanide, buprenorphine, butorphanol, carboplatin, carmustine, cefazolin, cefotaxime, cefotetan, cefoxitin, ceftazidime, ceftriaxone, cefuroxime, chloramphenicol, cisatracurium, cisplatin, clindamycin, cyanocobalamin, cyclophosphamide, cyclosporine, cytarabine, dactinomycin, daptomycin, dexamethasone, dexmedetomidine, dexrazoxane, digoxin, docetaxel, dopamine, doxorubicin hydrochloride, doxorubicin liposomal, enalaprilat, ephedrine, epinephrine, epoetin alfa, eptifibatide, ertapenem, etoposide, etoposide phosphate, famotidine, fentanyl, fluconazole, fludarabine, fluorouracil, folic acid, foscarnet, fosphenytoin, furosemide, gentamicin, glycopyrrolate, granisetron, heparin, hetastarch, hydrocortisone, hydromorphone, ifosfamide, imipenem/cilastatin, indomethacin, insulin regular, irinotecan, isoproterenol, LR, leucovorin calcium, lidocaine, linezolid, lorazepam, magnesium sulfate, mannitol, meperidine, mesna, methotrexate, methylprednisolone, metoclopramide, metoprolol, metronidazole, milrinone, mitoxantrone, mivacurium, morphine, moxifloxacin, multivitamins, nafcillin, naloxone, nitroglycerin, nitroprusside, norepinephrine, octreotide, ondansetron, oxacillin, oxaliplatin, oxytocin, paclitaxel, palonosetron, pamidronate, pemetrexed, penicillin G, phenobarbital, phenylephrine, phytonadione, piperacillin/tazobactam, potassium acetate, potassium chloride, procainamide,

propranolol, remifentanil, sodium acetate, sodium bicarbonate, succinylcholine, sufentanil, tacrolimus, theophylline, thiotepa, tigecycline, tirofiban, tobramycin, vasopressin, verapamil, vinblastine, vincristine, voriconazole, zoledronic acid.

- **Y-Site Incompatibility:** acyclovir, alemtuzumab, amiodarone, azithromycin, calcium chloride, caspofungin, chlorpromazine, dacarbazine, dantrolene, daunorubicin hydrochloride, diazepam, diltiazem, diphenhydramine, dobutamine, doxycycline, epirubicin, erythromycin, esmolol, ganciclovir, gemcitabine, gemtuzumab ozogamicin, haloperidol, hydroxyzine, idarubicin, labetalol, levofloxacin, midazolam, minocycline, mycophenolate, nalbuphine, nicardipine, pantoprazole, papaverine, pentamidine, phentolamine, phenytoin, prochlorperazine, promethazine, protamine, pyridoxine, rocuronium, topotecan, trimethoprim/sulfamethoxazole, vancomycin, vecuronium, vinorelbine.
- **Intranasal:** Activate pump before first use by holding bottle arm's length away with index finger and middle finger resting on top of finger flange and thumb supporting base. Press down evenly and release pump 5 times to activate. Prior to each use, blow nose gently to clear nostrils. Sit up straight or stand. Tilt head slightly forward. Insert tip of container into nostril. Point container away from center of nose. Push down to spray. Bottles are for 24 hr use; discard bottle no more than 24 hr after taking first dose, even if the bottle still contains some liquid.

Patient/Family Teaching

- Instruct patient on how and when to ask for and take pain medication. Advise patient to read *Medication Guide* and *Instructions for Use* before starting and with each Rx refill in case of changes.
- Instruct patient to take medication exactly as directed. Take missed doses as soon as remembered if not almost time for next dose. Do not double doses.

Do not take more than prescribed or for longer than 5 days.

- May cause drowsiness or dizziness. Advise patient to avoid driving or other activities requiring alertness until response to the medication is known.
- Instruct patient to notify health care professional of all Rx or OTC medications, vitamins, or herbal products being taken and consult health care professional before taking any new medications.
- Caution patient to avoid the concurrent use of alcohol, aspirin, NSAIDs, acetaminophen, or other OTC medications without consulting health care professional.
- Advise patient to inform health care professional of medication regimen prior to treatment or surgery.
- Advise patient to consult health care professional if rash, itching, visual disturbances, tinnitus, weight gain, edema, black stools, persistent headache, or influenza-like syndrome (chills, fever, muscle aches, pain) occurs.
- Rep: May cause fetal harm. Advise females of reproductive potential to notify health care professional if pregnancy is planned or suspected or if breastfeeding. Advise women to avoid ketorolac in the 3rd trimester of pregnancy (after 29 wk), may cause premature closure of the fetal ductus arteriosus. Use of ketorolac after 20 wk may cause fetal renal dysfunction leading to oligohydramnios. Avoid use of ketorolac in labor and delivery; may adversely affect fetal circulation and inhibit uterine contractions. The risk of uterine hemorrhage may be increased. May cause reversible infertility in women attempting to conceive; may consider discontinuing ketorolac.
- **Intranasal:** Instruct patient on correct technique for administration, need to open a new bottle every 24 hr, and the 5-day limit for use.

Evaluation/Desired Outcomes

- Decrease in severity of pain. Patients who do not respond to one NSAID may respond to another.

HIGH ALERT

labetalol (la-bet-a-lole)

✤Trandate

Classification

Therapeutic: antianginals, antihypertensives
Pharmacologic: beta blockers

Indications

Hypertension.

Action

Blocks stimulation of beta$_1$ (myocardial)- and beta$_2$ (pulmonary, vascular, and uterine)-adrenergic receptor sites. Also has alpha$_1$-adrenergic blocking activity, which may result in more orthostatic hypotension. **Therapeutic Effects:** Decreased BP.

Pharmacokinetics

Absorption: Well absorbed but rapidly undergoes extensive first-pass hepatic metabolism, resulting in 25% bioavailability.

Distribution: Widely distributed to tissues.

Metabolism and Excretion: Undergoes extensive hepatic metabolism.

Half-life: 3–8 hr.

TIME/ACTION PROFILE (cardiovascular effects)

ROUTE	ONSET	PEAK	DURATION
PO	20 min–2 hr	1–4 hr	8–12 hr
IV	2–5 min	5 min	16–18 hr

Contraindications/Precautions

Contraindicated in: Decompensated HF; Pulmonary edema; Cardiogenic shock; Bradycardia or heart block.

Use Cautiously in: Renal impairment; Hepatic impairment; Pulmonary disease (including asthma); Diabetes mellitus (may mask signs of hypoglycemia); Thyrotoxicosis (may mask symptoms); History of severe allergic reactions (intensity of reactions may be ↑); OB: Recommended for treatment of chronic hypertension (PO) or hypertensive emergency in pregnancy (IV); may cause fetal/neonatal bradycardia, hypotension, hypoglycemia, or respiratory depression; Pedi: Safety and effectiveness not established in children; Geri: Older adults may have ↑ sensitivity (↑ risk of orthostatic hypotension); initial dosage ↓ recommended.

Adverse Reactions/Side Effects

CV: orthostatic hypotension, ARRHYTHMIAS, BRADYCARDIA, HF. **Derm:** rash. **EENT:** blurred vision, dry eyes, intraoperative floppy iris syndrome, nasal stuffiness. **Endo:** hyperglycemia, hypoglycemia. **GI:** constipation, diarrhea, nausea. **GU:** erectile dysfunction, ↓ libido. **MS:** arthralgia, back pain, muscle cramps. **Neuro:** fatigue, weakness, anxiety, depression, dizziness, drowsiness, insomnia, memory loss, mental status changes, nightmares, paresthesia. **Resp:** bronchospasm, PULMONARY EDEMA, wheezing.

Interactions

Drug-Drug: General anesthesia and **verapamil** may cause additive myocardial depression. Additive bradycardia may occur with **digoxin**, **verapamil**, **diltiazem**, **clonidine**, or **ivabradine**. Additive hypotension may occur with other **antihypertensives**, acute ingestion of **alcohol**, or **nitrates**. Concurrent **thyroid** administration may ↓ effectiveness. May alter the effectiveness of **insulin** or **oral hypoglycemic agents** (dose adjustments may be necessary). May ↓ the effectiveness of **adrenergic bronchodilators** and **theophylline**. May ↓ beneficial beta cardiovascular effects of **dopamine** or **dobutamine**. Use cautiously within 14 days of **MAO inhibitor** therapy (may result in hypertension). Effects may be ↑ by **propranolol** or **cimetidine**. Concurrent **NSAIDs** may ↓ antihypertensive action.

Route/Dosage

PO (Adults): 100 mg twice daily initially, may ↑ by 100 mg twice daily every 2–3 days as needed (usual range 400–800 mg/day in 2–3 divided doses; doses up to 1.2–2.4 g/day have been used).

IV (Adults): 20 mg (0.25 mg/kg) initially, additional doses of 40–80 mg may be given every 10 min as needed (not to exceed 300 mg total dose) *or* 2 mg/min infusion (range 50–300 mg total dose required).

Availability (generic available)

Tablets: 100 mg, 200 mg, 300 mg. **Premixed infusion:** 100 mg/100 mL 0.72% NaCl, 200 mg/200 mL D5W, 200 mg/200 mL 0.72% NaCl, 300 mg/300 mL 0.72% NaCl. **Solution for injection:** 5 mg/mL.

NURSING IMPLICATIONS

Assessment

- Monitor BP and pulse frequently during dose adjustment and periodically during therapy. Assess for orthostatic hypotension when assisting patient up from supine position.
- Check frequency of refills to determine compliance.
- Patients receiving IV labetalol must be supine during and for 3 hr after administration. Vital signs should be monitored every 5–15 min during and for several hrs after administration.
- Monitor intake and output ratios and daily weight. Assess patient routinely for evidence of fluid overload (peripheral edema, dyspnea, rales/crackles, fatigue, weight gain, jugular venous distention).

Lab Test Considerations

- May cause ↑ BUN, serum potassium, triglyceride, and uric acid levels.
- May cause ↑ ANA titers.
- May cause ↑ in blood glucose levels.
- May cause ↑ serum alkaline phosphatase, LDH, AST, and ALT levels. Discontinue if jaundice or laboratory signs of hepatic function impairment occur.

Toxicity and Overdose

- Monitor patients receiving beta blockers for signs of overdose (bradycardia, severe dizziness or fainting, severe drowsiness, dyspnea, bluish fingernails or palms, seizures). Notify health care professional immediately if these signs occur.

- Glucagon has been used to treat bradycardia and hypotension.

Implementation

- **High Alert:** Before administering IV, have second practitioner independently check original order, dosage calculations, and infusion pump settings.
- Do not confuse labetalol with Lamictal or lamotrigine.
- Discontinuation of concurrent clonidine should take place gradually, with beta blocker discontinued first. Then, after several days, discontinue clonidine.
- **PO:** Take apical pulse prior to administering. If <50 bpm or if arrhythmia occurs, withhold medication and notify health care professional.
- Administer with meals or directly after eating to enhance absorption.

IV Administration

- **IV Push:** *Dilution:* Administer undiluted. *Concentration:* 5 mg/mL. *Rate:* Administer slowly over 2 min.
- **Continuous Infusion:** *Dilution:* Add 200 mg of labetalol to 160 mL of diluent. May also be administered as undiluted drug. Compatible diluents include D5W, 0.9% NaCl, D5/0.9% NaCl, and LR. *Concentration:* Diluted: 1 mg/mL; Undiluted: 5 mg/mL. *Rate:* Administer at a rate of 2 mg/min. Titrate for desired response. Infuse via infusion pump to ensure accurate dose.
- **Y-Site Compatibility:** acetaminophen, alemtuzumab, amikacin, aminocaproic acid, aminophylline, amiodarone, anidulafungin, argatroban, arsenic trioxide, ascorbic acid, atracurium, atropine, azithromycin, aztreonam, benztropine, bleomycin, bumetanide, buprenorphine, butorphanol, calcium chloride, calcium gluconate, carboplatin, carmustine, caspofungin, ceftazidime, ceftolozane/tazobactam, chlorpromazine, ciprofloxacin, cisplatin, clonidine, cyanocobalamin, cyclophosphamide, cyclosporine, dacarbazine, dactinomycin, daptomycin, daunorubicin hydrochloride, dexmedetomidine, digoxin, diltiazem, diphenhydramine, dobutamine, docetaxel, dopamine, doxorubicin hydrochloride, doxorubicin liposomal, doxycycline, enalaprilat, ephedrine, epinephrine, epirubicin, epoetin alfa, eptifibatide, ertapenem, erythromycin, esmolol, etoposide, etoposide phosphate, famotidine, fentanyl, fluconazole, fludarabine, fluorouracil, folic acid, fosphenytoin, ganciclovir, gemcitabine, gentamicin, glycopyrrolate, granisetron, hetastarch, hydromorphone, idarubicin, ifosfamide, imipenem/cilastatin, irinotecan, isavuconazonium, isoproterenol, LR, leucovorin calcium, levofloxacin, levothyroxine, lidocaine, linezolid, lorazepam, magnesium sulfate, mannitol, meperidine, meropenem, meropenem/vaborbactam, mesna, methylprednisolone, metoclopramide, metoprolol, metronidazole, midazolam, milrinone, mitoxantrone, morphine, multivitamins, mycophenolate, nalbuphine, naloxone, nicardipine, nitroglycerin, nitroprusside, norepinephrine, octreotide, ondansetron, oxacillin, oxaliplatin, oxytocin, palonosetron, pamidronate, papaverine, pemetrexed, pentamidine, pentobarbital, phenobarbital, phentolamine, phenylephrine, phytonadione, plazomicin, potassium acetate, potassium chloride, potassium phosphate, procainamide, prochlorperazine, promethazine, propofol, propranolol, protamine, pyridoxine, rocuronium, sodium acetate, sodium bicarbonate, succinylcholine, sufentanil, tacrolimus, tedizolid, telavancin, theophylline, thiamine, thiotepa, tigecycline, tirofiban, tobramycin, topotecan, vancomycin, vasopressin, vecuronium, verapamil, vincristine, vinorelbine, voriconazole, zoledronic acid.

- **Y-Site Incompatibility:** acyclovir, albumin, amphotericin B deoxycholate, amphotericin B lipid complex, amphotericin B liposomal, azathioprine, cangrelor, cefepime, cefotaxime, cefotetan, cefoxitin, ceftaroline, ceftriaxone, cefuroxime, dantrolene, dexamethasone, diazepam, diazoxide, foscarnet, gemtuzumab ozogamicin, hydrocortisone, ibuprofen, indomethacin, insulin regular, ketorolac, micafungin, mitomycin, paclitaxel, pantoprazole, penicillin G, phenytoin, piperacillin/tazobactam, thiopental.

Patient/Family Teaching

- Instruct patient to take medication as directed, at the same time each day, even if feeling well; do not skip or double up on missed doses. Take missed doses as soon as possible up to 8 hr before next dose. Abrupt withdrawal may precipitate life-threatening arrhythmias, hypertension, or myocardial ischemia.
- Advise patient to make sure enough medication is available for weekends, holidays, and vacations. A written prescription may be kept in wallet in case of emergency.
- Teach patient and family how to check pulse and BP. Instruct them to check pulse daily and BP biweekly. Advise patient to hold dose and contact health care professional if pulse is <50 bpm or BP changes significantly.
- May cause drowsiness or dizziness. Caution patients to avoid driving or other activities that require alertness until response to the drug is known. Caution patients receiving labetalol IV to call for assistance during ambulation or transfer.
- Advise patients to make position changes slowly to minimize orthostatic hypotension, especially during initiation of therapy or when dose is increased. Patients taking oral labetalol should be especially cautious when drinking alcohol, standing for long peri-

ods, or exercising, and during hot weather, because orthostatic hypotension is enhanced.

• Caution patient that this medication may increase sensitivity to cold.

• Instruct patient to notify health care professional of all Rx or OTC medications, vitamins, or herbal products being taken and to consult health care professional before taking any Rx, OTC, or herbal products, especially NSAIDs and cold preparations, concurrently with this medication. Patients on antihypertensive therapy should also avoid excessive amounts of coffee, tea, and cola.

• Advise patients with diabetes to closely monitor blood glucose, especially if weakness, malaise, irritability, or fatigue occurs. Medication may mask tachycardia and increased BP as signs of hypoglycemia, but dizziness and sweating may still occur.

• Advise patient to notify health care professional if slow pulse, difficulty breathing, wheezing, cold hands and feet, dizziness, light-headedness, confusion, depression, rash, fever, sore throat, unusual bleeding, or bruising occurs.

• Instruct patient to inform health care professional of medication regimen prior to treatment or surgery.

• Rep: Advise females of reproductive potential to notify health care professional if pregnancy is planned or suspected, or if breastfeeding. Appropriate for treatment of chronic hypertension in pregnancy and breastfeeding. Monitor fetal growth during pregnancy and the newborn should be monitored for 48 hr after delivery for bradycardia, hypoglycemia, and respiratory depression.

• Advise patient to carry identification describing disease process and medication regimen at all times.

• **Hypertension:** Reinforce the need to continue additional therapies for hypertension (weight loss, sodium restriction, stress reduction, regular exercise, moderation of alcohol consumption, and smoking cessation). Medication controls but does not cure hypertension.

Evaluation/Desired Outcomes
• Decrease in BP.

lacosamide (la-**kose**-a-mide)
Motpoly XR, Vimpat
Classification
Therapeutic: anticonvulsants

Schedule V

Indications
Partial-onset seizures (as either monotherapy or adjunctive therapy) (immediate-release/extended-release PO or IV). Primary generalized tonic-clonic seizures (as adjunctive therapy) (immediate-release PO or IV).

Action
Mechanism is not known, but may involve enhancement of slow inactivation of sodium channels with resultant membrane stabilization. **Therapeutic Effects:** Decreased incidence and severity of partial-onset seizures generalized tonic-clonic seizures.

Pharmacokinetics
Absorption: 100% absorbed following oral administration; IV administration results in complete bioavailability.
Distribution: Unknown.
Protein Binding: <15%.
Metabolism and Excretion: Partially metabolized by the liver; 40% excreted in urine as unchanged drug, 30% as a metabolite.
Half-life: 13 hr.

TIME/ACTION PROFILE (plasma concentrations)

ROUTE	ONSET	PEAK	DURATION
PO-IR	unknown	1–4 hr	12 hr
PO-XR	unknown	7 hr	24 hr
IV	unknown	end of infusion	12 hr

Contraindications/Precautions
Contraindicated in: Hypersensitivity; Severe hepatic impairment.
Use Cautiously in: CCr <30 mL/min (use lower daily dose); All patients (may ↑ risk of suicidal thoughts/behaviors); Hepatic or renal impairment and taking strong CYP3A4 or CYP2C9 inhibitor (dose ↓ may be needed); Mild to moderate hepatic impairment; Severe renal impairment; Known cardiac conduction problems (heart block or sick sinus syndrome without a pacemaker), severe cardiac disease (MI or HF), Brugada syndrome, or taking medications that affect cardiac conduction; Diabetic neuropathy or cardiac disease (↑ risk for atrial fibrillation/flutter); OB: Use during pregnancy only if potential maternal benefit justifies potential fetal risk; Lactation: Use while breastfeeding only if potential maternal benefit justifies potential risk to infant; Pedi: Children <1 mo (safety and effectiveness not established); Geri: Titrate dose carefully in older adults.

Adverse Reactions/Side Effects
CV: atrial fibrillation/flutter, bradycardia, heart block, syncope, VENTRICULAR ARRHYTHMIAS. **Derm:** DRUG REACTION WITH EOSINOPHILIA AND SYSTEMIC SYMPTOMS (DRESS), rash, STEVENS-JOHNSON SYNDROME, TOXIC EPIDERMAL NECROLYSIS. **EENT:** diplopia. **GI:** nausea, vomiting. **Hemat:** AGRANULOCYTOSIS. **Neuro:** dizziness, headache, ataxia, hallucinations, SUICIDAL THOUGHTS, syncope, vertigo. **Misc:** physical dependence, psychological dependence.

Interactions
Drug-Drug: Use cautiously with other drugs that affect cardiac conduction, including **sodium channel blockers**, **beta blockers**, **diltiazem**, **verapamil**, **potassium channel blockers**, and **PR-interval prolonging medications**.

Route/Dosage

Partial-Onset Seizures

PO, IV (Adults): *Monotherapy (immediate-release PO or IV):* 100 mg twice daily; may ↑ weekly by 100 mg/day in 2 divided doses up to a maintenance dose of 150–200 mg twice daily; may also initiate therapy with 200-mg single loading dose followed 12 hr later by 100 mg twice daily for 1 wk; may then ↑ weekly by 100 mg/day in 2 divided doses up to a maintenance dose of 150–200 mg twice daily. *Monotherapy (extended-release PO)* 200 mg once daily; may ↑ weekly by 100 mg once daily up to a maintenance dose of 300–400 mg once daily; *Adjunctive therapy (immediate–release PO or IV):* 50 mg twice daily; may ↑ weekly by 100 mg/day in 2 divided doses up to a maintenance dose of 100–200 mg twice daily; may also initiate therapy with 200-mg single loading dose followed 12 hr later by 100 mg twice daily for 1 wk; may then ↑ weekly by 100 mg/day in 2 divided doses up to a maintenance dose of 100–200 mg twice daily. *Adjunctive therapy (extended–release PO):* 100 mg once daily; may ↑ weekly by 100 mg once daily up to a maintenance dose of 200–400 mg once daily.

PO, IV (Children ≥1 mo and ≥50 kg): *Monotherapy (immediate–release PO or IV):* 50 mg twice daily; may ↑ weekly by 100 mg/day in 2 divided doses up to a maintenance dose of 150–200 mg twice daily; may also initiate therapy with 200-mg single loading dose followed 12 hr later by 100 mg twice daily for 1 wk; may then ↑ weekly by 100 mg/day in 2 divided doses up to a maintenance dose of 150–200 mg twice daily. *Monotherapy (extended–release PO):* 100 mg once daily; may ↑ weekly by 100 mg once daily up to a maintenance dose of 300–400 mg once daily. *Adjunctive therapy (immediate–release PO or IV):* 50 mg twice daily; may ↑ weekly by 100 mg/day in 2 divided doses up to a maintenance dose of 100–200 mg twice daily; may also initiate therapy with 200-mg single loading dose followed 12 hr later by 100 mg twice daily for 1 wk; may then ↑ weekly by 100 mg/day in 2 divided doses up to a maintenance dose of 100–200 mg twice daily. *Adjunctive therapy (extended–release PO):* 100 mg once daily; may ↑ weekly by 100 mg once daily up to a maintenance dose of 200–400 mg once daily.

PO, IV (Children ≥1 mo and 30–<50 kg): *Monotherapy or adjunctive therapy:* 1 mg/kg twice daily; may ↑ weekly by 2 mg/kg/day in 2 divided doses up to a maintenance dose of 2–4 mg/kg twice daily; may also initiate therapy with 4 mg/kg single loading dose followed 12 hr later by 2 mg/kg twice daily for 1 wk; may then ↑ weekly by 2 mg/kg/day in 2 divided doses up to a maintenance dose of 2–4 mg/kg twice daily.

PO, IV (Children ≥1 mo and 6–<30 kg): *Monotherapy or adjunctive therapy:* 1 mg/kg twice daily; may ↑ weekly by 2 mg/kg/day in 2 divided doses up to a maintenance dose of 3–6 mg/kg twice daily; may also initiate therapy with 4.5 mg/kg single loading dose followed 12 hr later by 3 mg/kg twice daily for 1 wk; may then ↑ weekly by 2 mg/kg/day in 2 divided doses up to a maintenance dose of 3–6 mg/kg twice daily.

PO (Children ≥1 mo and <6 kg): *Monotherapy or adjunctive therapy:* 1 mg/kg twice daily; may ↑ weekly by 2 mg/kg/day in 2 divided doses up to a maintenance dose of 3.75–7.5 mg/kg twice daily; may also initiate therapy with 3.75 mg/kg twice daily for 1 wk; may then ↑ weekly by 2 mg/kg/day in 2 divided doses up to a maintenance dose of 3.75–7.5 mg/kg twice daily.

IV (Children ≥1 mo and <6 kg): *Monotherapy or adjunctive therapy:* 0.66 mg/kg 3 times daily; may ↑ weekly by 2 mg/kg/day in 3 divided doses up to a maintenance dose of 2.5–5 mg/kg 3 times daily; may also initiate therapy with 2.5 mg/kg 3 times daily for 1 wk; may then ↑ weekly by 2 mg/kg/day in 3 divided doses up to a maintenance dose of 2.5–5 mg/kg 3 times daily.

Renal Impairment

PO, IV (Adults and Children ≥1 mo): *CCr ≤30 mL:* Monotherapy or adjunctive therapy (immediate-release PO or IV): ↓ maximum dose by 25%. Monotherapy or adjunctive therapy (extended-release PO): Not to exceed maximum dose of 300 mg once daily.

Hepatic Impairment

PO, IV (Adults and Children ≥1 mo): *Mild or moderate hepatic impairment:* Monotherapy or adjunctive therapy (immediate-release PO or IV): ↓ maximum dose by 25%. Monotherapy or adjunctive therapy (extended-release PO): Not to exceed maximum dose of 300 mg once daily.

Primary Generalized Tonic-Clonic Seizures

PO, IV (Adults): *Adjunctive therapy:* 50 mg twice daily; may ↑ weekly by 100 mg/day in 2 divided doses up to a maintenance dose of 100–200 mg twice daily; may also initiate therapy with 200-mg single loading dose followed 12 hr later by 100 mg twice daily; may ↑ weekly by 100 mg/day in 2 divided doses up to a maintenance dose of 100–200 mg twice daily.

PO, IV (Children ≥4 yr and ≥50 kg): *Adjunctive therapy:* 50 mg twice daily; may ↑ weekly by 100 mg/day in 2 divided doses up to a maintenance dose of 100–200 mg twice daily; may also initiate therapy with 200-mg single loading dose followed 12 hr later by 100 mg twice daily; may ↑ weekly by 100 mg/day in 2 divided doses up to a maintenance dose of 100–200 mg twice daily.

PO, IV (Children ≥4 yr and 30–<50 kg): *Adjunctive therapy:* 1 mg/kg twice daily; may ↑ weekly by 2 mg/kg/day in 2 divided doses up to a maintenance dose of 2–4 mg/kg twice daily; may also initiate therapy with 4 mg/kg single loading dose followed 12 hr later by 2 mg/kg twice daily; may ↑ weekly by 2 mg/kg/day in 2 divided doses up to a maintenance dose of 2–4 mg/kg twice daily.

L

PO, IV (Children ≥4 yr and 11–<30 kg): *Adjunctive therapy:* 1 mg/kg twice daily; may ↑ weekly by 2 mg/kg/day in 2 divided doses up to a maintenance dose of 3–6 mg/kg twice daily; may also initiate therapy with 4.5 mg/kg single loading dose followed 12 hr later by 3 mg/kg twice daily; may ↑ weekly by 2 mg/kg/day in 2 divided doses up to a maintenance dose of 3–6 mg/kg twice daily.

Renal Impairment
PO, IV (Adults and Children ≥4 yr): *CCr ≤30 mL/min:* Adjunctive therapy (immediate-release PO or IV): ↓ maximum dose by 25%.

Hepatic Impairment
PO, IV (Adults and Children ≥4 yr): *Mild or moderate hepatic impairment:* Adjunctive therapy (immediate-release PO or IV): ↓ maximum dose by 25%.

Availability (generic available)
Immediate-release tablets: 50 mg, 100 mg, 150 mg, 200 mg. **Extended-release capsules:** 100 mg, 150 mg, 200 mg. **Oral solution:** 10 mg/mL. **Solution for injection:** 10 mg/mL.

NURSING IMPLICATIONS
Assessment
- Assess location, duration, and characteristics of seizure activity. Institute seizure precautions.
- Monitor for changes in behavior that could indicate the emergence or worsening of suicidal thoughts or behavior or depression.
- Assess patient for skin rash frequently during therapy. Discontinue at first sign of rash; may be life-threatening. Stevens-Johnson syndrome may develop. Treat symptomatically; may recur once treatment is stopped.
- Monitor for signs and symptoms of DRESS (fever, rash, lymphadenopathy, and/or facial swelling, associated with involvement of other organ systems (hepatitis, nephritis, hematologic abnormalities, myocarditis, myositis) during therapy. May resemble an acute viral infection. Eosinophilia is often present. Discontinue therapy if signs occur.
- **IV:** Assess ECG prior to therapy in patients with pre-existing cardiac disease before starting after titration to steady-state maintenance. Monitor patients with cardiac conduction problems, on medications that prolong PR interval, or with severe cardiac disease (myocardial ischemia, heart failure) closely, as IV lacosamide may cause bradycardia or AV block.

Lab Test Considerations
- May cause ↑ ALT, which may return to normal without treatment.
- Monitor CBC and platelets periodically during therapy.

Implementation
- Do not confuse Vimpat with Venofer or Vfend.
- IV administration is indicated for short term replacement (up to 5 days) when PO administration is not

feasible. When switching from PO to IV, initial total daily dose should be equivalent to total daily dose and frequency of PO therapy. At end of IV period, may switch to PO at equivalent daily dose and frequency of IV therapy.

- When switching from another antiepileptic drug to lacosamide, administer 150 mg–200 mg twice daily for at least 3 days before beginning withdrawal of other antiepileptic drug. Gradually decrease other antiepileptic drug over 6 wk.
- When administering loading dose, monitor for CNS adverse reactions (dizziness, headache, nausea, somnolence, fatigue). May occur more frequently.
- When discontinuing lacosamide, gradually decrease dose over 1 wk.
- **PO:** May be administered with or without food. *DNC:* Swallow tablets whole with liquid; do not crush, break, or chew.
- Use a calibrated measuring device for accurate dosing of oral solution; household measures are not accurate. Discard any unused solution 6 mo after opening bottle.
- Oral solution may also be given via nasogastric tube or gastrostomy tube.

IV Administration
- **Intermittent Infusion:** *Dilution:* May be administered undiluted or diluted with 0.9% NaCl, D5W, or LR. *Concentration:* 10 mg/mL. Solution is clear and colorless; do not administer solutions that are cloudy, discolored or contain a precipitate. Solution is stable for 4 hr at room temperature. Discard unused portion. *Rate:* Infuse over 15–60 min, preferably 30–60 min. Do not infuse over less than 30 min in children.

Patient/Family Teaching
- Instruct patient to take lacosamide around the clock, as directed. Medication should be gradually discontinued over at least 1 wk to prevent seizures. Advise patient to read the *Medication Guide* before starting therapy and with each Rx refill.
- May cause dizziness, ataxia, and syncope. Caution patient to avoid driving or other activities requiring alertness until response to medication is known. Tell patient not to resume driving until health care professional gives clearance based on control of seizure disorder. If syncope occurs, advise patient to lay down with legs raised until recovered and notify health care professional.
- Inform patients and families of risk of suicidal thoughts and behavior and advise that behavioral changes, emergency or worsening signs and symptoms of depression, unusual changes in mood, or emergence of suicidal thoughts, behavior, or thoughts of self-harm, rash, or signs and symptoms of DRESS should be reported to health care professional immediately.
- Instruct patient to notify health care professional if signs of multiorgan hypersensitivity reactions (fever, rash, fatigue, jaundice, dark urine) occur.

- Advise patient to consult health care professional before taking other Rx, OTC, or herbal preparation and to avoid taking alcohol or other CNS depressants, including opioids, concurrently with lacosamide.
- Rep: Advise females of reproductive potential to notify health care professional if pregnancy is planned or suspected or if breastfeeding. Monitor infants exposed to lacosamide through breast milk for excess sedation. Encourage pregnant patients to enroll in the North American Antiepileptic Drug pregnancy registry by calling 1-888-233-2334, call must be made by patient. Information on registry can be found at the website http://www.aedpregnancyregistry.org/.

Evaluation/Desired Outcomes
- Decreased seizure activity.

lactic acid/citric acid/potassium bitartrate
(lak-tik as-id/sit-rik as-id/poe-**tas**-ee-um bye-**tar**-trate)
Phexxi
Classification
Therapeutic: contraceptive nonhormonals

Indications
Rep: Prevention of pregnancy in women of reproductive potential as an on-demand form of contraception.

Action
Lowers the pH in the vagina, which subsequently reduces sperm motility. **Therapeutic Effects:** Prevention of pregnancy.

Pharmacokinetics
Absorption: Systemic absorption not expected following vaginal administration.
Distribution: Systemic absorption not expected following vaginal administration.
Metabolism and Excretion: Unknown.
Half-life: Unknown.

TIME/ACTION PROFILE

ROUTE	ONSET	PEAK	DURATION
Vag	unknown	unknown	unknown

Contraindications/Precautions
Contraindicated in: Hypersensitivity; OB: Pregnancy; Rep: History of recurrent urinary tract infection or urinary tract abnormalities.
Use Cautiously in: Lactation: Safety not established in breastfeeding.

Adverse Reactions/Side Effects
GU: <u>vulvovaginal burning</u>, <u>vulvovaginal pruritus</u>, bacterial vaginosis, cystitis, dysuria, genital discomfort, py-

elonephritis, urinary tract infection, vagina discharge, vulvovaginal candidiasis, vulvovaginal pain. **Misc:** hypersensitivity reactions.

Interactions
Drug-Drug: Avoid use with **vaginal rings**.

Route/Dosage
Vag (Adults and Children [females of reproductive potential]): One prefilled applicator (5 g) immediately before or up to 1 hr before each act of vaginal intercourse. If ≥1 act of vaginal intercourse occurs within 1 hr, must insert another prefilled applicator.

Availability
Vaginal gel: lactic acid 90 mg/citric acid 50 mg/potassium bitartrate 20 mg in each 5-g prefilled applicator.

NURSING IMPLICATIONS
Assessment
- Assess patient for history of recurrent urinary tract infections or urinary tract abnormalities. May cause cystitis and pyelonephritis.

Implementation
- **Vag:** Administer one prefilled applicator vaginally immediately before or up to 1 hr before each act of vaginal intercourse. If >1 act of vaginal intercourse occurs within 1 hr, apply an additional dose.

Patient/Family Teaching
- Instruct patient in correct timing and technique for vaginal administration **before** vaginal sex. May be used during any part of menstrual cycle and as soon as it is safe to resume vaginal intercourse after childbirth, abortion, or miscarriage. Advise patient to read *Patient Information* before starting and with each Rx refill in case of changes.
- Advise patient that *Phexxi* is not effective at preventing pregnancy when used **after** vaginal sex.
- Inform patient that *Phexxi* may be used with hormonal contraceptives; latex, polyurethane, and polyisoprene condoms; and vaginal diaphragms. Avoid use with vaginal rings. May also be used concomitantly with other products for vaginal infections (miconazole, metronidazole, tioconazole).
- Advise patient to notify health care professional if severe or prolonged genital irritation or symptoms of urinary tract infection (burning feeling when passing urine, cloudy urine, pain in the pelvis, back pain) occur. May also cause burning, itching, and pain in male partner.
- Inform patient that *Phexxi* does not protect against HIV or other sexually transmitted infections.
- Advise parents to notify health care professional of all Rx or OTC medications, vitamins, or herbal products being taken and to consult with health care professional before taking other medications.
- Rep: Advise females of reproductive potential to notify health care professional if pregnancy is planned

or suspected or if breastfeeding. There is no use for *Phexxi* in pregnancy; discontinue use.

Evaluation/Desired Outcomes
● Prevention of pregnancy.

---

lactulose (lak-tyoo-lose)
Constulose, Enulose, Generlac, Kristalose
Classification
Therapeutic: laxatives
Pharmacologic: osmotics

Indications
Chronic constipation. Adjunct in the management of portal-systemic (hepatic) encephalopathy.

Action
Increases water content and softens the stool. Lowers the pH of the colon, which inhibits the diffusion of ammonia from the colon into the blood, thereby reducing blood ammonia levels. **Therapeutic Effects:** Relief of constipation. Decreased blood ammonia levels with improved mental status in portal-systemic encephalopathy.

Pharmacokinetics
Absorption: Less than 3% absorbed after oral administration.
Distribution: Unknown.
Metabolism and Excretion: Absorbed lactulose is excreted unchanged in the urine. Unabsorbed lactulose is metabolized by colonic bacteria to lactic, acetic, and formic acids.
Half-life: Unknown.

TIME/ACTION PROFILE (relief of constipation)

ROUTE	ONSET	PEAK	DURATION
PO	24-48 hr	unknown	unknown

Contraindications/Precautions
Contraindicated in: Patients on low-galactose diets.
Use Cautiously in: Diabetes mellitus; Excessive or prolonged use (may lead to dependence); Lactation: Safety not established in breastfeeding.

Adverse Reactions/Side Effects
Endo: hyperglycemia (patients with diabetes). **GI:** belching, cramps, distention, flatulence, diarrhea.

Interactions
Drug-Drug: Should not be used with other **laxatives** in the treatment of hepatic encephalopathy (leads to inability to determine optimal dose of lactulose). **Antiinfectives** may ↓ effectiveness in treatment of hepatic encephalopathy.

Route/Dosage
Constipation
PO (Adults): 15-30 mL/day up to 60 mL/day as liquid or 10-20 g as powder for oral solution (up to 40 g/day has been used).
PO (Children): 7.5 mL once daily after breakfast (unlabeled).

Portal-Systemic Encephalopathy
PO (Adults): 30-45 mL 3-4 times/day; may be given every 1-2 hr initially to induce laxation.
PO (Infants): 2.5-10 mL/day in 3-4 divided doses (unlabeled).
PO (Children and Adolescents): 40-90 mL/day in 3-4 divided doses (unlabeled).
Rect (Adults): 300 mL diluted and administered as a retention enema every 4-6 hr.

Availability (generic available)
Oral solution: 10 g/15 mL. **Single-use packets (Kristalose):** 10 g (equal to 15 mL liquid lactulose), 20 g (equal to 30 mL liquid lactulose).

NURSING IMPLICATIONS
Assessment
● Assess patient for abdominal distention, presence of bowel sounds, and normal pattern of bowel function.
● Assess color, consistency, and amount of stool produced.
● **Portal-Systemic Encephalopathy:** Assess mental status (orientation, level of consciousness) before and periodically throughout course of therapy.

Lab Test Considerations
● Should ↓ blood ammonia concentrations by 25-50%.
● May cause ↑ blood glucose levels in patients with diabetes.
● Monitor serum electrolytes periodically when used chronically. May cause diarrhea with resulting hypokalemia and hypernatremia.

Implementation
● When used in hepatic encephalopathy, adjust dose until patient averages 2-3 soft bowel movements per day. During initial therapy, 30-45 mL may be given hourly to induce rapid laxation.
● Darkening of solution does not alter potency.
● **PO:** Mix with fruit juice, water, milk, or carbonated citrus beverage to improve flavor. Administer with a full glass (240 mL) of water or juice. May be administered on an empty stomach for more rapid results.
● Dissolve single dose packets (Kristalose) in 4 oz of water. Solution should be colorless to slightly pale yellow.
● **Rect:** To administer enema, use rectal balloon catheter. Mix 300 mL of lactulose with 700 mL of water or 0.9% NaCl. Enema should be retained for 30-60 min. If inadvertently evacuated, may repeat administration.

Patient/Family Teaching

- Explain purpose of lactulose to patient. Instruct patient to take lactulose as directed.
- Encourage patients to use other forms of bowel regulation, such as increasing bulk in the diet, increasing fluid intake, and increasing mobility. Normal bowel habits are individualized and may vary from 3 times/day to 3 times/wk.
- Caution patients that this medication may cause belching, flatulence, or abdominal cramping. Health care professional should be notified if this becomes bothersome or if diarrhea occurs.
- Rep: Advise females of reproductive potential to notify health care professional if pregnancy is planned or suspected or if breastfeeding.

Evaluation/Desired Outcomes

- Passage of a soft, formed bowel movement, usually within 24–48 hr.
- Clearing of confusion, apathy, and irritation, and improved mental status in portal-systemic encephalopathy. Improvement may occur within 2 hr after enema and 24–48 hr after oral administration.

---

lamiVUDine (la-**mi**-vyoo-deen)
Epivir, Epivir-HBV
Classification
Therapeutic: antiretrovirals, antivirals
Pharmacologic: nucleoside reverse transcriptase inhibitors

Indications

Epivir: HIV infection (in combination with other antiretrovirals). **Epivir HBV:** Chronic hepatitis B virus (HBV) infection. **Unlabeled Use:** HIV-postexposure prophylaxis (in combination with other antiretrovirals).

Action

After intracellular conversion to its active form (lamivudine-5-triphosphate), inhibits viral DNA synthesis by inhibiting the enzyme reverse transcriptase. **Therapeutic Effects:** Slows the progression of HIV infection and decreases the occurrence of its sequelae. Increases CD4 cell counts and decreases viral load. Protection from liver damage caused by chronic HBV infection; decreases viral load.

Pharmacokinetics

Absorption: Well absorbed after oral administration (86% in adults, 66% in infants and children).
Distribution: Distributes into the extravascular space. Some penetration into CSF; remainder of distribution unknown.
Metabolism and Excretion: Mostly excreted unchanged in urine; <5% metabolized by the liver.
Half-life: *Epivir:* 5–7 hr; *Epivir HBV:* 13–19 hr.

TIME/ACTION PROFILE (blood levels)

ROUTE	ONSET	PEAK	DURATION
PO	unknown	0.9 hr†	12 hr

†On an empty stomach; peak levels occur at 3.2 hr if lamivudine is taken with food. Food does not affect total amount of drug absorbed.

Contraindications/Precautions

Contraindicated in: Hypersensitivity; Concurrent use of antiretroviral combination products containing lamivudine or emtricitabine; Lactation: Breastfeeding not recommended for mothers with HIV.

Use Cautiously in: Renal impairment (↑ dosing interval/↓ dose if CCr <50 mL/min); Women and obesity (↑ risk of lactic acidosis and severe hepatomegaly with steatosis); Coinfection with HBV (hepatitis may recur after discontinuation of lamivudine; Epivir HBV is not indicated for treatment of HIV because lamivudine dosage is subtherapeutic); OB: Considered a preferred nucleoside reverse transcriptase inhibitor (NRTI) for pregnant patients with HIV infection who are antiretroviral-naïve, who have had antiretroviral therapy in the past but are restarting, or who require a new antiretroviral regimen; use has also been studied in pregnant women with HBV; Pedi: Safety and effectiveness not established in children <3 mo (HIV) or <2 yr (HBV); Geri: ↓ dose may be necessary in older adults due to age-related ↓ in renal function.

Exercise Extreme Caution in: Pedi: Pediatric patients with a history of or significant risk factors for pancreatitis (use only if no alternative).

Adverse Reactions/Side Effects

Derm: alopecia, erythema multiforme, rash, urticaria. **Endo:** hyperglycemia. **F and E:** lactic acidosis. **GI:** anorexia, diarrhea, nausea, vomiting, ↑ liver enzymes, abdominal discomfort, dyspepsia, HEPATOMEGALY WITH STEATOSIS, PANCREATITIS (↑ in pediatric patients). **Hemat:** anemia, neutropenia, pure red cell aplasia. **MS:** musculoskeletal pain, arthralgia, muscle weakness, myalgia, rhabdomyolysis. **Neuro:** fatigue, headache, insomnia, malaise, neuropathy, depression, dizziness, SEIZURES. **Resp:** cough. **Misc:** HYPERSENSITIVITY REACTIONS (including anaphylaxis), immune reconstitution syndrome.

Interactions

Drug-Drug: **Trimethoprim/sulfamethoxazole** may ↑ levels (dose alteration may be necessary in renal impairment). ↑ risk of pancreatitis with concurrent use of other **drugs causing pancreatitis.** ↑ risk of neuropathy with concurrent use of other **drugs causing neuropathy.** Combination therapy with **tenofovir** and **abacavir** may lead to virologic nonresponse and should not be used. **Sorbitol** may ↓ levels; avoid concurrent use.

Route/Dosage

HIV–1 Infection (Epivir)

PO (Adults): 150 mg twice daily or 300 mg once daily.
PO (Children ≥3 mo): *Oral solution:* 5 mg/kg twice daily or 10 mg/kg once daily (max dose = 300 mg/day); *Tablets:* 14–19 kg: 75 mg twice daily or 150 mg once daily; 20–24 kg: 75 mg in AM, 150 mg in PM or 225 mg once daily; ≥25 kg: 150 mg twice daily or 300 mg once daily.

Renal Impairment

(Adults and Children ≥25 kg): *CCr 30–49 mL/min:* 150 mg once daily; *CCr 15–29 mL/min:* 150 mg initially, then 100 mg once daily; *CCr 5–14 mL/min:* 150 mg initially, then 50 mg once daily; *CCr <5 mL/min:* 50 mg initially, then 25 mg once daily.

Chronic Hepatitis B (Epivir HBV)

PO (Adults): 100 mg once daily.
PO (Children 2–17 yr): 3 mg/kg once daily (up to 100 mg/day).

Renal Impairment

PO (Adults): *CCr 30–49 mL/min:* 100 mg first dose, then 50 mg once daily; *CCr 15–29 mL/min:* 100 mg first dose, then 25 mg once daily; *CCr 5–14 mL/min:* 35 mg first dose, then 15 mg once daily; *CCr <5 mL/min:* 35 mg first dose, then 10 mg once daily.

Availability (generic available)

Epivir

Tablets: 150 mg, 300 mg. **Oral solution (strawberry-banana flavor):** 10 mg/mL. *In combination with:* abacavir (generic only); abacavir and dolutegravir (Triumeq); abacavir and zidovudine (generic only); efavirenz and tenofovir disoproxil fumarate (Symfi); lamivudine (Dovato); tenofovir disoproxil fumarate (Cimduo, Temixys); zidovudine (Combivir). See Appendix N.

Epivir-HBV

Tablets: 100 mg. **Oral solution (strawberry-banana flavor):** 5 mg/mL.

NURSING IMPLICATIONS

Assessment

- Assess patient, especially pediatric patients, for signs of pancreatitis (nausea, vomiting, abdominal pain) periodically during therapy. May require discontinuation of therapy.
- **HIV:** Assess patient for change in severity of symptoms of HIV infection and for symptoms of opportunistic infection during therapy.
- Monitor patient for signs and symptoms of peripheral neuropathy (tingling, burning, numbness, or pain in hands or feet); may be difficult to differentiate from peripheral neuropathy of severe HIV disease. May require discontinuation of therapy.
- **Chronic Hepatitis B Infection:** Monitor signs of hepatitis (jaundice, fatigue, anorexia, pruritus) during therapy.

Lab Test Considerations

- Monitor viral load and CD4 levels before and periodically during therapy.
- Monitor serum amylase, lipase, and triglycerides periodically during therapy. Elevated serum levels may indicate pancreatitis and require discontinuation.
- Monitor liver function. May cause ↑ levels of AST, ALT, CK, bilirubin, and alkaline phosphatase, which usually resolve after interruption of therapy. Lactic acidosis may occur with hepatic toxicity causing hepatic steatosis; may be fatal, especially in women.
- May rarely cause neutropenia and anemia.

Implementation

- Do not confuse lamivudine with lamotrigine. Do not confuse Epivir tablets and oral solution with Epivir-HBV tablets and oral solutions. Epivir Tablets and Oral Solution contain a higher dose of the same active ingredient (lamivudine) as Epivir-HBV Tablets and Oral Solution. Epivir-HBV was developed for patients with hepatitis B; do not use for patients dually infected with HIV and hepatitis B; use may lead to lamivudine-resistant HIV due to subtherapeutic dose.
- **PO:** May be administered without regard to food.
- Epivir scored tablet is preferred for HIV-1-infected pediatric patients weighing at least 14 kg and able to swallow pill; solution is associated with higher resistance rates. Before prescribing, assess for ability to swallow tablets. For patients unable to safely and reliably swallow tablets, oral solution may be used.

Patient/Family Teaching

- Instruct patient to take lamivudine as directed, every 12 hr. Explain the difference between Epivir and Epivir-HBV to patients. Emphasize the importance of compliance with full course of therapy, not taking more than the prescribed amount, and not discontinuing without consulting health care professional; discontinuation may lead to deterioration of liver disease. Take missed doses as soon as possible unless almost time for next dose. Do not double doses. Caution patient not to share medication with others. Advise patient to read *Patient Information* before starting and with each Rx refill in case of changes.
- Inform patient that lamivudine does not cure HIV disease or prevent associated or opportunistic infections. Lamivudine may reduce the risk of transmission of HIV to others through sexual contact or blood contamination. Caution patient to use a condom during sexual contact and avoid sharing needles or donating blood to prevent spreading HIV to others. Advise patient that the long-term effects of lamivudine are unknown at this time.
- Instruct patient to notify health care professional promptly if signs of peripheral neuropathy, pancreatitis, lactic acidosis (feel very weak or tired; feel cold, especially in arms and legs; unusual muscle pain; feel dizzy or lightheaded; trouble breathing; fast or irregular heartbeat; stomach pain with nausea and vomiting), liver problems (yellowing of skin or

white part of eyes; loss of appetite; nausea; dark or "tea-colored" urine; pain, aching, or tenderness on right side of abdomen; light-colored stools) or Immune Reconstitution Syndrome (signs and symptoms of an infection, *Mycobacterium avium* infection, cytomegalovirus, Pneumocystis jirovecii pneumonia, tuberculosis) occur.

- Inform patient that redistribution and accumulation of body fat may occur, causing central obesity, dorsocervical fat enlargement (buffalo hump), peripheral wasting, breast enlargement, and cushingoid appearance. The cause and long-term effects are not known.
- Instruct patient to notify health care professional of all Rx or OTC medications, vitamins, or herbal products being taken and to consult health care professional before taking other Rx, OTC, or herbal products.
- Rep: Advise females of reproductive potential using hormonal contraceptives to use an alternative non-hormonal method of contraception. Advise patient to notify health care professional if pregnancy is planned or suspected and to avoid breastfeeding. If pregnant patient is exposed to lamivudine, register patient in *Antiretroviral Pregnancy Registry* by calling 1-800-258-4263.
- Emphasize the importance of regular follow-up exams and blood tests to determine progress and monitor for side effects.

Evaluation/Desired Outcomes

- Slowing of the progression of HIV infection and its sequelae.
- Decrease in viral load and improvement in CD4 levels in patients with advanced HIV infection.
- Protection from liver damage caused by chronic hepatitis B infection; decreases viral load.

lamoTRIgine (la-moe-tri-jeen)
LaMICtal, LaMICtal ODT, LaMICtal XR, Subvenite
Classification
Therapeutic: anticonvulsants

Indications

Adjunct treatment of partial seizures in adults and children with epilepsy (immediate-release, extended-release, chewable, and orally disintegrating tablets). Lennox-Gastaut syndrome (immediate-release, chewable, and orally disintegrating tablets only). Adjunct treatment of primary generalized tonic-clonic seizures in adults and children (immediate-release, extended-release, chewable, and orally disintegrating tablets). Conversion to monotherapy in adults with partial seizures receiving carbamazepine, phenytoin, phenobarbital, primidone, or valproate as the single antiepileptic drug (immediate-release, extended-release, chewable, and orally disintegrating tablets only). Maintenance treat-

ment of bipolar disorder (immediate-release, chewable, and orally disintegrating tablets only).

Action

Stabilizes neuronal membranes by inhibiting sodium transport. **Therapeutic Effects:** Decreased incidence of seizures. Delayed time to recurrence of mood episodes in bipolar disorder.

Pharmacokinetics

Absorption: 98% absorbed following oral administration.

Distribution: Highly bound to melanin-containing tissues (eyes, pigmented skin).

Metabolism and Excretion: Mostly metabolized by the liver via glucuronidation to inactive metabolites; 10% excreted unchanged by the kidneys.

Half-life: *Children taking enzyme-inducing anticonvulsants:* 7–10 hr; *Children taking enzyme inducers and valproic acid:* 15–27 hr; *Children taking valproic acid:* 44–94 hr; *Adults:* 25.4 hr (during chronic therapy of lamotrigine alone).

TIME/ACTION PROFILE (plasma concentrations)

ROUTE	ONSET	PEAK	DURATION
PO	unknown	1.4–4.8 hr; 4–10 hr (XR)	unknown

Contraindications/Precautions

Contraindicated in: Hypersensitivity; Acute manic or mixed episodes; Second- or third-degree heart block, ventricular arrhythmias, ischemic heart disease, HF, valvular heart disease, congenital heart disease, or Brugada syndrome.

Use Cautiously in: All patients (may ↑ risk of suicidal thoughts/behaviors); Renal impairment (lower maintenance doses may be required); Hepatic impairment (lower maintenance doses may be required); Prior history of rash to lamotrigine; OB: Exposure during first trimester may ↑ risk of cleft lip/palate; Lactation: Use while breastfeeding only if potential maternal benefit justifies potential risk to infant; Pedi: Safety and effectiveness not established in children <13 yr (extended-release tablets) and <2 yr (immediate-release, chewable, and orally disintegrating tablets).

Adverse Reactions/Side Effects

CV: arrhythmias, bradycardia, CARDIAC ARREST, heart block, QRS interval prolongation. **Derm:** photosensitivity, rash (higher incidence in children, patients taking valproic acid, high initial doses, or rapid dose increases), DRUG REACTION WITH EOSINOPHILIA AND SYSTEMIC SYMPTOMS (DRESS), STEVENS-JOHNSON SYNDROME (SJS), TOXIC EPIDERMAL NECROLYSIS (TEN). **EENT:** blurred vision, double vision, rhinitis. **GI:** nausea, vomiting, HEPATIC FAILURE. **GU:** vaginitis. **Hemat:** HEMO-

L

PHAGOCYTIC LYMPHOHISTIOCYTOSIS. **MS:** arthralgia.
Neuro: ataxia, dizziness, headache, ASEPTIC MENINGITIS, behavior changes, depression, drowsiness, insomnia, SUICIDAL THOUGHTS, tremor.

Interactions

Drug-Drug: Concurrent use with **carbamazepine** may ↑ levels of an active metabolite of carbamazepine. Concurrent use with drugs that induce glucuronidation, including **phenobarbital, phenytoin, primidone, carbamazepine, estrogen-containing oral contraceptives, rifampin, lopinavir/ritonavir,** or **atazanavir/ritonavir** may ↓ levels; lamotrigine dose adjustments may be necessary when starting and stopping oral contraceptive or atazanavir/ritonavir therapy. Concurrent use with drugs that inhibit glucuronidation, including **valproic acid,** may ↑ levels and ↑ incidence of rash; may also ↓ valproic acid levels (↓ lamotrigine dose by at least 50%). **Amiodarone, disopyramide, dronedarone, flecainide, lidocaine, mexiletine, procainamide, propafenone,** or **quinidine** may ↑ risk of proarrhythmia; avoid concurrent use.

Route/Dosage

Epilepsy

In Combination with Other Antiepileptic Agents

PO (Adults and Children >12 yr; Immediate-release, chewable, or orally disintegrating tablets): *Patients taking anticonvulsant drugs other than carbamazepine, phenobarbital, phenytoin, primidone, or valproate:* 25 mg once daily for first 2 wk, then 50 mg once daily for next 2 wk; then ↑ by 50 mg/day every 1–2 wk to maintenance dose of 225–375 mg/day (in 2 divided doses); *Patients taking carbamazepine, phenobarbital, phenytoin, or primidone (and not valproate):* 50 mg once daily for first 2 wk, then 50 mg twice daily for next 2 wk; then ↑ by 100 mg/day every 1–2 wk to maintenance dose of 300–500 mg/day (in 2 divided doses); *Patients taking regimen containing valproate:* 25 mg every other day for first 2 wk, then 25 mg once daily for next 2 wk; then ↑ by 25–50 mg/day every 1–2 wk to maintenance dose of 100–400 mg/day (in 1–2 divided doses) (maintenance dose of 100–200 mg/day if receiving valproate alone).

PO (Adults and Children ≥13 yr; Extended-release tablets): *Patients taking anticonvulsant drugs other than carbamazepine, phenobarbital, phenytoin, primidone, or valproate:* 25 mg once daily for first 2 wk, then 50 mg once daily for next 2 wk; then 100 mg once daily for 1 wk, then 150 mg once daily for 1 wk, then 200 mg once daily for 1 wk, then ↑ by 100 mg/day every wk to maintenance dose of 300–400 mg once daily; *Patients taking carbamazepine, phenobarbital, phenytoin, or primidone (and not valproate):* 50 mg once daily for first 2 wk, then 100 mg once daily for next 2 wk, then 200 mg once daily for 1 wk, then 300 mg once daily for 1 wk, then 400 mg once

daily for 1 wk, then ↑ by 100 mg/day every wk to maintenance dose of 400–600 mg once daily; *Patients taking regimen containing valproate:* 25 mg every other day for first 2 wk, then 25 mg once daily for next 2 wk, then 50 mg once daily for 1 wk, then 100 mg once daily for 1 wk, then 150 mg once daily for 1 wk, then maintenance dose of 200–250 mg once daily.

PO (Children 2–12 yr; Immediate-release, chewable, or orally disintegrating tablets): *Patients taking anticonvulsant drugs other than carbamazepine, phenobarbital, phenytoin, primidone, or valproate:* 0.3 mg/kg/day in 1–2 divided doses (rounded down to nearest whole tablet) for first 2 wk, then 0.6 mg/kg/day in 2 divided doses (rounded down to nearest whole tablet) for next 2 wk; then ↑ by 0.6 mg/kg/day (rounded down to nearest whole tablet) every 1–2 wk to maintenance dose of 4.5–7.5 mg/kg/day (not to exceed 300 mg/day in 2 divided doses); *Patients taking carbamazepine, phenobarbital, phenytoin, or primidone (and not valproate):* 0.6 mg/kg/day in 2 divided doses (rounded down to nearest whole tablet) for first 2 wk, then 1.2 mg/kg/day in 2 divided doses (rounded down to nearest whole tablet) for next 2 wk; then ↑ by 1.2 mg/kg/day (rounded down to nearest whole tablet) every 1–2 wk to maintenance dose of 5–15 mg/kg/day (not to exceed 400 mg/day in 2 divided doses). *Patients taking regimen containing valproate:* 0.15 mg/kg/day in 1–2 divided doses (rounded down to nearest whole tablet) for first 2 wk, then 0.3 mg/kg in 1–2 divided doses (rounded down to nearest whole tablet) for next 2 wk; then ↑ by 0.3 mg/kg/day (rounded down to nearest whole tablet) every 1–2 wk to maintenance dose of 1–5 mg/kg/day (not to exceed 200 mg/day in 1–2 divided doses) (maintenance dose of 1–3 mg/kg/day if receiving valproate alone).

Conversion to Monotherapy

PO (Adults and Children ≥16 yr; Immediate-release, chewable, or orally disintegrating tablets): *Patients taking carbamazepine, phenobarbital, phenytoin, or primidone (and not valproate):* After achieving a dose of 500 mg/day (as per dosing guidelines above), ↓ dose of other antiepileptic by 20% weekly over 4 wk; *Patients taking regimen containing valproate:* After achieving a dose of 200 mg/day (as per dosing guidelines above), ↓ valproate dose by 500 mg/day on a weekly basis until a dose of 500 mg/day is achieved. Maintain the valproate dose of 500 mg/day and the lamotrigine dose of 500 mg/day for 1 wk. Then ↑ lamotrigine dose to 300 mg/day and ↓ valproate dose to 250 mg/day, and maintain these doses for 1 wk. Then discontinue valproate and ↑ lamotrigine dose by 100 mg/day every wk until maintenance dose of 500 mg/day is achieved.

PO (Adults and Children ≥13 yr; Extended-release tablets): *Patients taking carbamazepine, phenobarbital, phenytoin, or primidone (and not valproate):* After achieving a dose of 500 mg/day (as per dosing guidelines above), ↓ dose of other antiepileptic by 20% weekly over 4 wk. Two wk later, ↓ dose of lamotrigine by 100 mg/day every wk to achieve maintenance dose of 250–300 mg/day; *Patients taking regimen containing valproate:* After achieving a dose of 150 mg/day (as per dosing guidelines above), ↓ valproate dose by 500 mg/day on a weekly basis until a dose of 500 mg/day is achieved. Maintain the valproate dose of 500 mg/day and the lamotrigine dose of 150 mg/day for 1 wk. Then ↑ lamotrigine dose to 200 mg/day and ↓ valproate dose to 250 mg/day, and maintain these doses for 1 wk. Then discontinue valproate and ↑ lamotrigine dose to 250–300 mg/day; *Patients taking anticonvulsant drugs other than carbamazepine, phenobarbital, phenytoin, primidone, or valproate:* After achieving a dose of 250–300 mg/day (as per dosing guidelines above), ↓ dose of other antiepileptic by 20% weekly over 4 wk.

Bipolar Disorder
Escalation Regimen
PO (Adults): *Patients not taking carbamazepine, phenobarbital, phenytoin, primidone, rifampin, or valproate:* 25 mg once daily for first 2 wk, then 50 mg once daily for next 2 wk, then 100 mg once daily for 1 wk, then 200 mg once daily; *Patients taking valproate:* 25 mg every other day for first 2 wk, then 25 mg once daily for next 2 wk, then 50 mg once daily for 1 wk, then 100 mg once daily; *Patients taking carbamazepine, phenobarbital, phenytoin, primidone, or rifampin (and not valproate):* 50 mg once daily for first 2 wk, then 100 mg/day (in divided doses) for next 2 wk, then 200 mg/day (in divided doses) for one wk, then 300 mg/day (in divided doses) for 1 wk, then up to 400 mg/day (in divided doses).

Dosage Adjustment Following Discontinuation of Other Psychotropics
PO (Adults): *Following discontinuation of valproate (if current dose 100 mg/day):* ↑ to 150 mg/day for 1 wk, then 200 mg/day; *Following discontinuation of carbamazepine, phenobarbital, phenytoin, primidone, or rifampin (if current dose 400 mg/day):* 400 mg/day for 1 wk, then 300 mg/day for 1 wk, then 200 mg/day; *Following discontinuation of other psychotropics:* maintain previous dose.

Availability (generic available)
Immediate-release tablets: 25 mg, 100 mg, 150 mg, 200 mg. **Extended-release tablets:** 25 mg, 50 mg, 100 mg, 200 mg, 250 mg, 300 mg. **Orally disintegrating tablets:** 25 mg, 50 mg, 100 mg, 200 mg. **Tablets for oral suspension:** 2 mg, 5 mg, 25 mg.

NURSING IMPLICATIONS
Assessment
- Monitor closely for changes in behavior that could indicate the emergence or worsening of suicidal thoughts or behavior or depression.

- Assess patient for skin rash frequently during therapy. Discontinue lamotrigine at first sign of rash; may be life-threatening. SJS or TEN may develop. Rash usually occurs during the initial 2–8 wk of therapy and is more frequent in patients taking multiple antiepileptic agents, especially valproic acid, and much more frequent in patients <16 yr.
- Monitor for signs and symptoms of multiorgan hypersensitivity reactions—DRESS (rash, fever, lymphadenopathy). May be associated with other organ involvement (hepatitis, hepatic failure, blood dyscrasias, acute multiorgan failure). If cause cannot be determined, discontinue lamotrigine immediately.
- **Seizures:** Assess location, duration, and characteristics of seizure activity.
- **Bipolar disorders:** Assess mood, ideation, and behaviors frequently. Initiate suicide precautions if indicated.

Lab Test Considerations
- Lamotrigine plasma concentrations may be monitored periodically during therapy, especially in patients concurrently taking other anticonvulsants. Therapeutic plasma concentration range has not been established, proposed therapeutic range: 1–5 mcg/mL.
- May cause false-positive results for phencyclidine in some rapid urine drug screens. Use a more specific analytical method to confirm results.

Implementation
- Do not confuse lamotrigine with labetalol, lamivudine, levetiracetam, or levothyroxine. Do not confuse Lamictal with labetalol.
- When converting from immediate-release to XR form, initial dose of XR should match the total daily dose of immediate-release lamotrigine; monitor closely and adjust as needed.
- **PO:** May be administered without regard to meals. *DNC:* Swallow XR tablets whole; do not break, crush, or chew.
- Lamotrigine should be discontinued gradually over at least 2 wk, unless safety concerns require a more rapid withdrawal. Abrupt discontinuation may cause increase in seizure frequency.
- **Orally Disintegrating Tablets:** Place on the tongue and move around the mouth. Tablet will rapidly disintegrate, can be swallowed with or without water, and can be taken with or without food.
- **Tablets for Oral Suspension:** May be swallowed whole, chewed, or dispersed in water or dispersed in fruit juice. If chewed, follow with water or fruit juice to aid in swallowing. Only use whole tablets, do not attempt to administer partial quantities of dispersible tablets.

Patient/Family Teaching
- Instruct patient to take medication as directed. Take missed doses as soon as possible unless almost time

for next dose. Do not double doses. Do not discontinue abruptly; may cause increase in frequency of seizures. Instruct patient to read the *Medication Guide* before starting and with each Rx refill, changes may occur.

- Advise patient to notify health care professional immediately if skin rash, fever, or swollen lymph glands occur or if frequency of seizures increases.
- May cause dizziness, drowsiness, and blurred vision. Caution patient to avoid driving or activities requiring alertness until response to medication is known. Do not resume driving until physician gives clearance based on control of seizure disorder.
- Caution patient to wear sunscreen and protective clothing to prevent photosensitivity reactions.
- Advise patient and family to notify health care professional if thoughts about suicide or dying, attempts to commit suicide; new or worse depression; new or worse anxiety; feeling very agitated or restless; panic attacks; trouble sleeping; new or worse irritability; acting aggressive; being angry or violent; acting on dangerous impulses; an extreme increase in activity and talking; other unusual changes in behavior or mood or if symptoms of aseptic meningitis (headache, fever, nausea, vomiting, and nuchal rigidity, rash, photophobia, myalgia, chills, altered consciousness, somnolence) or cardiac symptoms (fast, slow, or pounding heartbeat; heart skipping beats; shortness of breath; chest pain; feeling lightheaded) occur.
- Advise patient to notify health care professional of all Rx or OTC medications, vitamins, or herbal products being taken and to consult with health care professional before taking other medications.
- Instruct patient to notify health care professional of medication regimen prior to treatment or surgery.
- Advise patient to notify health care professional immediately if signs and symptoms of hemophagocytic lymphohistiocytosis (fever, hepatosplenomegaly, rash, lymphadenopathy, neurologic symptoms, cytopenias, high serum ferritin, hypertriglyceridemia, liver function, coagulation abnormalities) occur. Symptoms usually occur between 8 and 24 days. May be fatal.
- Rep: Advise females of reproductive potential to use a nonhormonal form of contraception while taking lamotrigine, to avoid breastfeeding, and to notify health care professional if pregnancy is planned or suspected. Encourage patients who become pregnant to enroll in the North American Antiepileptic Drug Pregnancy Registry. Must be done by patients themselves by calling 1-888-233-2334 or on the website http://www.aedpregnancyregistry.org. Enrollment in the registry must be done prior to any prenatal diagnostic tests and before fetal outcome is known.
- Advise patient to carry identification at all times describing disease process and medication regimen.

Evaluation/Desired Outcomes

- Decrease in the frequency of or cessation of seizures.
- Delay in time to occurrence of mood episodes (depression, mania, hypomania, mixed episodes) in patients with bipolar I disorder.

BEERS

lansoprazole (lan-**soe**-pra-zole)
Prevacid, Prevacid 24 Hr, Prevacid SoluTab
Classification
Therapeutic: antiulcer agents
Pharmacologic: proton-pump inhibitors

Indications
Erosive esophagitis. Duodenal ulcers (with or without anti-infectives for *Helicobacter pylori*). Active benign gastric ulcer. Short-term treatment of symptomatic GERD. Healing and risk reduction of NSAID-associated gastric ulcer. Pathologic hypersecretory conditions, including Zollinger-Ellison syndrome. **OTC:** Heartburn occurring ≥twice/wk.

Action
Binds to an enzyme in the presence of acidic gastric pH, preventing the final transport of hydrogen ions into the gastric lumen. **Therapeutic Effects:** Diminished accumulation of acid in the gastric lumen, with lessened acid reflux. Healing of duodenal ulcers and esophagitis.

Pharmacokinetics
Absorption: 80% absorbed after oral administration.
Distribution: Unknown.
Protein Binding: 97%.
Metabolism and Excretion: Extensively metabolized by the liver into inactive compounds. Converted intracellularly to at least two other antisecretory compounds.
Half-life: *Children:* 1.2–1.5 hr; *Adults:* 1.3–1.7 hr (↑ in geriatric patients and patients with impaired hepatic function).

TIME/ACTION PROFILE (acid suppression)

ROUTE	ONSET	PEAK	DURATION
PO	rapid	1.7 hr	more than 24 hr

Contraindications/Precautions
Contraindicated in: Hypersensitivity to lansoprazole or related drugs (benzimidazoles); Concurrent use of rilpivirine-containing products.
Use Cautiously in: Phenylketonuria (solutabs contain aspartame); Severe hepatic impairment (do not exceed 30 mg/day); Patients using high-doses for >1 yr (↑ risk of hip, wrist, or spine fractures and fundic gland polyps); Patients using therapy for >3 yr (↑ risk of vitamin B_{12} deficiency); Pre-existing risk of hypocalcemia; Lactation: Safety not established in breastfeed-

ing; Pedi: Children <1 yr (↑ risk of heart valve thickening); Geri: Appears on Beers list. ↑ risk of *Clostridioides difficile* infection, pneumonia, GI malignancies, bone loss, and fractures in older adults. Avoid scheduled use for >8 wk in older adults unless for high-risk patients [e.g. oral corticosteroid or chronic NSAID use] or patients with erosive esophagitis, Barrett's esophagitis, pathological hypersecretory condition, or demonstrated need for maintenance therapy [e.g. failure of H_2 antagonist]).

Adverse Reactions/Side Effects
Derm: ACUTE GENERALIZED EXANTHEMATOUS PUSTULOSIS, cutaneous lupus erythematosus, DRUG REACTION WITH EOSINOPHILIA AND SYSTEMIC SYMPTOMS (DRESS), rash, STEVENS-JOHNSON SYNDROME (SJS), TOXIC EPIDERMAL NECROLYSIS (TEN). **F and E:** hypocalcemia (especially if treatment duration ≥3 mo), hypokalemia (especially if treatment duration ≥3 mo), hypomagnesemia (especially if treatment duration ≥3 mo). **GI:** diarrhea, abdominal pain, CLOSTRIDIOIDES DIFFICILE-ASSOCIATED DIARRHEA (CDAD), fundic gland polyps, nausea. **GU:** acute tubulointerstitial nephritis. **Hemat:** vitamin B_{12} deficiency. **MS:** bone fracture. **Neuro:** dizziness, headache. **Misc:** HYPERSENSITIVITY REACTIONS (including anaphylaxis, angioedema, or acute tubulointerstitial nephritis), systemic lupus erythematosus.

Interactions
Drug-Drug: May ↓ **rilpivirine** levels and ↑ risk of resistance; concurrent use contraindicated. **Sucralfate** ↓ absorption of lansoprazole (take 30 min before sucralfate). May ↓ absorption of drugs requiring acid pH, including **ketoconazole**, **itraconazole**, **atazanavir**, **nelfinavir**, **ampicillin esters**, **iron salts**, **erlotinib**, and **mycophenolate mofetil**; avoid concurrent use with **atazanavir** and **nelfinavir**. May ↑ levels of **digoxin tacrolimus**, and **methotrexate**. May ↑ risk of bleeding with **warfarin** (monitor INR/PT). Hypomagnesemia and hypokalemia ↑ risk of **digoxin** toxicity.

Route/Dosage
PO (Adults): *Short-term treatment of duodenal ulcer:* 15 mg once daily for 4 wk; *H. pylori eradication to reduce the risk of duodenal ulcer recurrence:* 30 mg twice daily with clarithromycin 500 mg twice daily and amoxicillin 1000 mg twice daily for 10–14 days (triple therapy) or 30 mg 3 times daily with 1000 mg amoxicillin 3 times daily for 14 days (dual therapy); *Maintenance of healed duodenal ulcers:* 15 mg once daily; *Short-term treatment of gastric ulcers/healing of NSAID-associated gastric ulcer:* 30 mg once daily for up to 8 wk; *Risk reduction of NSAID-associated gastric ulcer:* 15 mg once daily for up to 12 wk; *Short-term treatment of symptomatic GERD:* 15 mg once daily for up to 8 wk; *Short-term treatment of erosive esophagitis:* 30 mg once daily for up to 8 wk (8 additional wk may be necessary); *Maintenance of healing*

of erosive esophagitis: 15 mg once daily; *Pathologic hypersecretory conditions:* 60 mg once daily initially, up to 90 mg twice daily (daily dose >120 mg should be given in divided doses).
PO (Adults): *OTC:* 15 mg once daily for up to 14 days (14 day course may be repeated every 4 mo).
PO (Children 12–17 yr): *Non-erosive GERD:* 15 mg once daily for up to 8 wk; *Erosive esophagitis:* 30 mg once daily for up to 8 wk.
PO (Children 1–11 yr and >30 kg): *GERD and Erosive Esophagitis:* 30 mg once daily for up to 12 wk.
PO (Children 1–11 yr and ≤30 kg): *GERD and Erosive Esophagitis:* 15 mg once daily for up to 12 wk.

Availability (generic available)
Delayed-release capsules: 15 mg$^{Rx, OTC}$, 30 mg. **Delayed-release orally disintegrating tablets (SoluTabs):** 15 mg$^{Rx, OTC}$, 30 mg. *In combination with:* amoxicillin and clarithromycin as part of a compliance package (Prevpac). See Appendix N.

NURSING IMPLICATIONS
Assessment
- Assess patient routinely for epigastric or abdominal pain and for frank or occult blood in stool, emesis, or gastric aspirate.
- Monitor bowel function. Diarrhea, abdominal cramping, fever, and bloody stools should be reported to health care professional promptly as a sign of CDAD. May begin up to several wk following cessation of therapy.
- Monitor for severe cutaneous reactions (SJS, TEN, DRESS, acute generalized exanthematous pustulosis). Discontinue lansoprazole at first signs of severe cutaneous reactions or hypersensitivity.

Lab Test Considerations
- May cause abnormal liver function tests, including ↑ AST, ALT, alkaline phosphatase, LDH, and bilirubin.
- May cause ↑ serum creatinine and ↑ or ↓ electrolyte levels.
- May alter RBC, WBC, and platelet levels.
- May also cause ↑ gastrin levels, abnormal A/G ratio, hyperlipidemia, and ↑ or ↓ cholesterol.
- Monitor INR and prothrombin time in patients taking warfarin.
- May cause hypomagnesemia. Monitor serum magnesium prior to and periodically during therapy.
- May cause vitamin B_{12} deficiency with long term use (>3 yrs).
- May ↑ serum chromogranin levels which may interfere with diagnosis of neuroendocrine tumors.

Implementation
- **PO:** *Delayed-release capsules:* Administer before meals. *DNC:* Swallow whole; do not crush or chew capsule contents. Capsules may be opened and sprinkled on 1 tbsp of applesauce, *Ensure*, pudding,

cottage cheese, yogurt, or strained pears and swallowed immediately for patients with difficulty swallowing. Capsule contents may also be sprinkled with intact granules into a small volume of either apple juice, orange juice or tomato juice (60 mL – 2 oz.). Mix briefly and administer immediately.

- For patients with a nasogastric (NG) tube, capsules may be opened and intact granules may be mixed in 40 mL of apple juice and injected through the NG tube into stomach. Flush NG tube with additional apple juice to clear tube.

- *Orally disintegrating tablets* may be placed on tongue, allowed to disintegrate and swallowed with or without water. Do not cut or break tablet. For administration via oral syringe or NG tube, *Prevacid SoluTab* can be administered by placing a 15-mg tablet in oral syringe and drawing up 4 mL of water, or a 30-mg tablet in oral syringe and drawing up 10 mL of water. Shake gently to allow for a quick dispersal. After tablet has dispersed, administer the contents within 15 min. Refill syringe with 2 mL (5 mL for the 30-mg tablet) of water, shake gently, and administer any remaining contents and flush NG tube.

- Antacids may be used concurrently.

Patient/Family Teaching

- Instruct patient to take medication as directed for the full course of therapy, even if feeling better. Take missed doses as soon as remembered unless almost time for next dose; do not double doses. Advise patient to read *Medication Guide* before starting and with each Rx refill in case of changes.

- May occasionally cause dizziness. Caution patient to avoid driving and other activities that require alertness until response to medication is known.

- Advise patient to avoid alcohol, products containing aspirin or NSAIDs, and foods that may cause an increase in GI irritation.

- Advise patient to report onset of black, tarry stools; diarrhea; or abdominal pain to health care professional promptly. Instruct patient to notify health care professional immediately if rash, diarrhea, abdominal cramping, fever, or bloody stools occur and not to treat with antidiarrheals without consulting health care professional.

- Instruct patient to notify health care professional of all Rx or OTC medications, vitamins, or herbal products being taken and consult health care professional before taking any new medications.

- Rep: Advise females of reproductive potential to notify health care professional if pregnancy is planned or suspected or if breastfeeding.

Evaluation/Desired Outcomes

- Decrease in abdominal pain or prevention of gastric irritation and bleeding. Healing of duodenal ulcers can be seen on x-ray examination or endoscopy. Therapy is continued for at least 2–4 wk. Therapy for pathologic hypersecretory conditions may be long term.

- Healing in patients with erosive esophagitis. Therapy is continued for up to 8 wk, and an additional 8-wk course may be used for patients who do not heal in 8 wk or whose ulcer recurs.

lanthanum (lan-than-um)
Fosrenol
Classification
Therapeutic: hypophosphatemics
Pharmacologic: phosphate binders

Indications
Hyperphosphatemia in end-stage kidney disease.

Action
Dissociates in the upper GI tract forming lanthanate ions, which form an insoluble complex with phosphate. **Therapeutic Effects:** Decreased serum phosphate levels.

Pharmacokinetics
Absorption: Negligible absorption.
Distribution: Stays within the GI tract.
Metabolism and Excretion: Eliminated almost entirely in feces.
Half-life: 53 hr (in plasma).

TIME/ACTION PROFILE (effect on phosphate levels)

ROUTE	ONSET	PEAK	DURATION
PO	unknown	2–3 wk	unknown

Contraindications/Precautions
Contraindicated in: Bowel obstruction; Ileus; Fecal impaction; OB: Pregnancy; Lactation: Lactation; Pedi: Use in children not recommended (potential negative effect on developing bone).
Use Cautiously in: Patients with risk factors for GI obstruction or perforation, including history of GI surgery, colon cancer, or GI ulceration, diverticular disease, peritonitis, constipation, ileus, diabetic gastroparesis, or taking medications that cause constipation.

Adverse Reactions/Side Effects
F and E: hypocalcemia. **GI:** nausea, vomiting, diarrhea, fecal impaction, GI obstruction, GI perforation, ileus.

Interactions
Drug-Drug: May ↓ absorption of **fluoroquinolones, tetracyclines,** and **levothyroxine**; administer ≥1 hr before or 3 hr after lanthanum.

Route/Dosage
PO (Adults): 1500 mg/day in divided doses; may be titrated upward every 2–3 wk in increments of 750 mg/day up to 4500 mg/day (usual range 1500–3000 mg/day).

Availability (generic available)
Chewable tablets: ✿ 250 mg, 500 mg, 750 mg, 1000 mg. **Oral powder:** 750 mg/pkt, 1000 mg/pkt.

NURSING IMPLICATIONS
Assessment
- Assess for GI adverse reactions (gastrointestinal obstruction, ileus, subileus, gastrointestinal perforation, fecal impaction). May require discontinuation of therapy in patients without another explanation for severe GI symptoms.
- Assess for nausea and vomiting during therapy.

Lab Test Considerations
- Monitor serum phosphate levels prior to and periodically during therapy.

Implementation
- Do not confuse lanthanum carbonate with lithium carbonate.
- Divide total daily dose and administer with meals.
- **PO:** Administer with or immediately after meals. Tablets should be crushed or chewed completely before swallowing; intact tablets should not be swallowed.
- Sprinkle powder on small quantity of applesauce or other similar food; consume immediately. Consider powder formulation for patients with poor dentition or who have difficulty chewing tablets.

Patient/Family Teaching
- Instruct patient to take lanthanum as directed. Advise patient to read *Medication Guide* before starting therapy and with each Rx refill in case of changes.
- Advise patient to take antacids or thyroid medicine (levothyroxine), 2 hr before or after lanthanum carbonate and antibiotics 1 hr before or 4 hr after lanthanum carbonate.
- Advise patient to notify health care professional of all Rx or OTC medications, vitamins, or herbal products being taken and to consult with health care professional before taking other medications.
- Advise patient to notify health care professional of medication regimen before an abdominal x-ray or if they have a history of gastrointestinal disease.
- Rep: May cause fetal harm. Advise females of reproductive potential to notify health care professional if pregnancy is planned or suspected and to avoid breastfeeding during therapy.

Evaluation/Desired Outcomes
- Decrease in serum phosphate to below than 6 mg/dL in patients with end stage renal disease.

▒ lapatinib (la-pat-i-nib)
Tykerb
Classification
Therapeutic: antineoplastics
Pharmacologic: enzyme inhibitors, kinase inhibitors

Indications
▒ Advanced or metastatic breast cancer with tumor overexpression of the human epidermal receptor type 2 (HER2) and past therapy with an anthracycline, a taxane and trastuzumab (in combination with capecitabine). ▒ Hormone-receptor positive metastatic breast cancer that overexpresses HER2 in postmenopausal women for whom hormonal therapy is indicated (in combination with letrozole).

Action
▒ Acts as an inhibitor of intracellular tyrosine kinase affecting epidermal growth factor (EGFR, ErbB1) and HER2 (ErbB2). Inhibits the growth of ErbB-driven tumors. Effect is additive with capecitabine. **Therapeutic Effects:** Decreased/slowed spread of metastatic breast cancer.

Pharmacokinetics
Absorption: Incompletely and variably absorbed following oral administration; levels ↑ by food.
Distribution: Unknown.
Protein Binding: >99%.
Metabolism and Excretion: Extensively metabolized by the liver via the CYP3A4 and CYP3A5 isoenzymes; <2% excreted by kidneys.
Half-life: 24 hr.

TIME/ACTION PROFILE (plasma concentrations)

ROUTE	ONSET	PEAK	DURATION
PO	unknown	4 hr	24 hr

Contraindications/Precautions
Contraindicated in: Hypersensitivity; ↓ left ventricular ejection fraction (LVEF) (Grade 2 or greater); OB: Pregnancy; Lactation: Lactation.
Use Cautiously in: Severe hepatic impairment (dose ↓ recommended); Known QTc interval prolongation or coexisting risk factors for QTc interval prolongation including hypokalemia, hypomagnesemia, concurrent antiarrhythmics or medications that are known to prolong the QTc interval; Rep: Women of reproductive potential and men with female partners of reproductive potential; Pedi: Safety and effectiveness not established in children; Geri: Older adults may be more sensitive to effects.

Adverse Reactions/Side Effects
CV: ↓ LVEF, QT interval prolongation. **Derm:** palmar-plantar erythrodysesthesia, rash, dry skin, ERYTHEMA MULTIFORM (EM), nail disorders, STEVENS-JOHNSON SYNDROME (SJS), TOXIC EPIDERMAL NECROLYSIS (TEN). **GI:** nausea, vomiting, ↑ liver enzymes, DIARRHEA, dyspepsia, HEPATOTOXICITY, stomatitis. **Hemat:** neutropenia. **MS:** pain. **Neuro:** fatigue, insomnia. **Resp:** dyspnea, INTERSTITIAL LUNG DISEASE (ILD).

Interactions

Drug-Drug: May ↑ effects of **midazolam**, **paclitaxel**, and **digoxin**. **Strong CYP3A4 inhibitors**, including **ketoconazole**, **itraconazole**, **clarithromycin**, **atazanavir**, **nefazodone**, **nelfinavir**, **ritonavir**, and **voriconazole** may ↑ levels and risk of toxicity; avoid concurrent use; if concurrent use unavoidable, ↓ lapatinib dose. **Strong CYP3A4 inducers**, including **dexamethasone**, **phenytoin**, **carbamazepine**, **rifampin**, **rifabutin**, **rifapentin**, and **phenobarbital**, may ↓ levels and effectiveness; avoid concurrent use; if concurrent use unavoidable, ↑ lapatinib dose.

Drug-Natural Products: St. John's wort may ↓ levels and effectiveness; avoid concurrent use; if concurrent use unavoidable, ↑ lapatinib dose.

Drug-Food: Grapefruit juice may ↑ levels and risk of toxicity; avoid concurrent use.

Route/Dosage

HER2–Positive Metastatic Breast Cancer (Past Therapy with an Anthracycline, a Taxane and Trastuzumab)

PO (Adults): 1250 mg once daily on Days 1–21 of 21-day cycle; continue until disease progression or unacceptable toxicity; *Concurrent use of strong CYP3A4 inhibitors:* 500 mg once daily on Days 1–21 of 21-day cycle; continue until disease progression or unacceptable toxicity; *Concurrent use of strong CYP3A4 inducers:* Gradually titrate dose from 1250 mg once daily up to 4500 mg once daily as tolerated; administer dose on Days 1–21 of 21-day cycle and continue until disease progression or unacceptable toxicity.

Hepatic Impairment

PO (Adults): *Severe hepatic impairment:* 750 mg once daily on Days 1–21 of 21-day cycle; continue until disease progression or unacceptable toxicity.

Hormone Receptor-Positive, HER2–Positive Metastatic Breast Cancer (Hormone Therapy Indicated)

PO (Adults): 1500 mg once daily on Days 1–21 of 21-day cycle; continue until disease progression or unacceptable toxicity; *Concurrent use of strong CYP3A4 inhibitors:* 500 mg once daily on Days 1–21 of 21-day cycle; continue until disease progression or unacceptable toxicity; *Concurrent use of strong CYP3A4 inducers:* Gradually titrate dose from 1500 mg once daily up to 5500 mg once daily as tolerated; administer dose on Days 1–21 of 21-day cycle and continue until disease progression or unacceptable toxicity.

Hepatic Impairment

PO (Adults): *Severe hepatic impairment:* 1000 mg once daily on Days 1–21 of 21-day cycle; continue until disease progression or unacceptable toxicity.

Availability (generic available)

Tablets: 250 mg.

NURSING IMPLICATIONS

Assessment

● Evaluate LVEF prior to therapy to determine if within institution's normal limits. Continue to monitor periodically during therapy to ensure it does not fall below limits. If LVEF ↓ to Grade 2 or greater, discontinue therapy. If returns to normal and patient is asymptomatic after 2 wk, may restart therapy at a reduced dose of 1000 mg/day (with capecitabine) or 1250 mg/day (with letrozole).

● Monitor for diarrhea; usually occurs within first 6 days of therapy and lasts 4–5 days. Treat with antidiarrheals (loperamide) after first loose stool. If diarrhea is severe, treat with oral or intravenous fluids, antibiotics (fluoroquinolones) especially if diarrhea persists >24 hr or accompanied by fever; may require interruption or discontinuation of therapy. If accompanied by moderate to severe abdominal cramping, nausea or vomiting, decreased performance status, fever, sepsis, neutropenia, frank bleeding, or dehydration, interrupt therapy and reintroduce at lower dose (from 1,250 mg/day to 1,000 mg/day or from 1,500 mg/day to 1,250 mg/day) when diarrhea <Grade 1. If Grade 4 diarrhea occurs, discontinue therapy.

● Monitor ECG prior to and periodically during therapy to monitor the QT interval. Monitor patients who have or may develop QTc interval prolongation (hypokalemia, hypomagnesemia, congenital long QT syndrome, patients taking antiarrhythmics or other medication with known risk for QT interval prolongation/torsades de pointes, and cumulative high-dose anthracycline therapy) during therapy.

● Monitor for respiratory status for symptoms of ILD and pneumonitis (dyspnea, cough); may require discontinuation of therapy.

● Monitor for signs and symptoms of skin reactions (progressive skin rash often with blisters or mucosal lesions). Discontinue lapatinib if EM, SJS, or TEN are suspected.

Lab Test Considerations

● Verify negative pregnancy test before starting therapy. Monitor liver function tests prior to initiation and every 4–6 wk during therapy and as clinically indicated. Discontinue and do not restart lapatinib if patients experience severe changes in liver function tests.

● Monitor serum potassium and magnesium prior to and periodically during therapy. Correct hypokalemia or hypomagnesemia before starting therapy.

Implementation

● Correct hypokalemia and hypomagnesemia prior to therapy.

● **PO:** Administer tablets once daily at least 1 hr before or 1 hr after a meal for 21 days. Do not divide daily dose.

Patient/Family Teaching

- Instruct patient to take lapatinib as directed and to review the *Patient Information Sheet* prior to therapy and with each refill for new information. If a dose is missed take as soon remembered that day. If a day is missed, skip the dose; do not double doses. Caution patient not to share this medication with others, even with same condition; may be harmful.
- Advise patient to avoid drinking grapefruit juice or eating grapefruit during therapy.
- Advise patient to report signs or decreased LVEF (shortness of breath, palpitations, fatigue) and skin rash to health care professional promptly.
- Instruct patient to notify health care professional of all Rx or OTC medications, vitamins, or herbal products being taken and consult health care professional before taking any new medications, especially St. John's wort.
- Advise patient that lapatinib may cause diarrhea, which may become severe. Instruct patient in how to prevent and manage diarrhea and to notify health care professional if severe.
- Rep: May cause fetal harm. Advise females of reproductive potential and males with female partners of reproductive potential to use effective contraception during and for 1 wk after last dose and to avoid breastfeeding for 1 wk after last dose. Advise patient to notify health care professional if pregnancy is planned or suspected.

Evaluation/Desired Outcomes

- Decreased/slowed spread of metastatic breast cancer.

lecanemab (lek-an-e-mab)
Leqembi
Classification
Therapeutic: anti-Alzheimer's agents
Pharmacologic: monoclonal antibodies, anti-amyloid monoclonal antibodies

Indications
Alzheimer's disease (with mild cognitive impairment or mild dementia).

Action
Acts as a monoclonal antibody directed against aggregated soluble and insoluble forms of amyloid beta. **Therapeutic Effects:** Reduction in clinical decline. Reduction in amyloid beta plaques in the brain.

Pharmacokinetics
Absorption: IV administration results in complete bioavailability.
Distribution: Not widely distributed to extravascular tissues.
Metabolism and Excretion: Degraded into small peptides and amino acids via catabolic pathways.

Half-life: 5–7 days.

TIME/ACTION PROFILE (plasma concentrations)

ROUTE	ONSET	PEAK	DURATION
IV	rapid	unknown	2 wk

Contraindications/Precautions
Contraindicated in: Previous localized superficial siderosis, >4 brain microhemorrhages, and/or brain hemorrhage (↑ risk of intracerebral hemorrhage).
Use Cautiously in: OB: Safety not established in pregnancy; Lactation: Safety not established in breastfeeding; Pedi: Safety and effectiveness not established in children.

Adverse Reactions/Side Effects
CV: atrial fibrillation. **GI:** diarrhea. **Hemat:** lymphopenia. **Neuro:** amyloid-related imaging abnormalities (including edema and hemosiderin deposition), headache, SEIZURES. **Resp:** cough. **Misc:** infusion-related reactions.

Interactions
Drug-Drug: Antithrombotic drugs and thrombolytics may ↑ risk of intracerebral hemorrhage.

Route/Dosage
IV (Adults): 10 mg/kg every 2 wk.

Availability
Solution for injection: 100 mg/mL.

NURSING IMPLICATIONS
Assessment
- Baseline brain MRI and periodic monitoring with MRI are recommended. Enhanced clinical vigilance for ARIA is recommended during the first 14 wks of therapy.
- May cause amyloid related imaging abnormalities -edema (ARIA-E) and -hemosiderin deposition (ARIA-H). For patients with ARIA-E severity on MRI: *If asymptomatic and mild severity,* continue dosing. *If asymptomatic and moderate or severe severity,* suspend dosing. *If symptoms are mild (discomfort noticed, but no disruption of normal daily activity) with mild severity,* May continue dosing based on clinical judgment. *If symptoms are mild with moderate or severe severity,* suspend dosing. *If symptoms are moderate (discomfort sufficient to reduce or affect normal daily activity) or severe (incapacitating, with inability to work or to perform normal daily activity),* suspend dosing. Suspend until MRI demonstrates radiographic resolution and symptoms, if present, resolve; consider a follow-up MRI to assess for resolution 2 to 4 mo after initial identification. Use clinical judgement when considering resumption of dosing.

- For patients with ARIA-H severity on MRI: *If asymptomatic and mild severity,* continue dosing. *If asymptomatic and moderate or severe severity,* suspend dosing. *If symptomatic,* suspend dosing. *For mild or moderate severity,* Suspend until MRI demonstrates radiographic stabilization and symptoms resolve; use clinical judgement regarding resumption of dosing; consider a follow-up MRI to assess for stabilization 2 to 4 months after initial identification. *For severe ARIA-H severity on MRI,* Suspend until MRI demonstrates radiographic stabilization and symptoms resolve; use clinical judgment in considering whether to continue or permanently discontinue therapy.
- If patient develops an intracerebral hemorrhage >1 cm in diameter during therapy, suspend dosing until MRI demonstrates radiographic stabilization and symptoms resolve. Use clinical judgment in considering whether to continue or permanently discontinue therapy.
- Monitor for any signs or symptoms of an infusion-related reaction (fever and flu-like symptoms [chills, generalized aches, feeling shaky, and joint pain], nausea, vomiting, hypotension, hypertension, and oxygen desaturation) during therapy. The infusion rate may be reduced, or the infusion may be discontinued, and appropriate therapy administered. Consider pre-medication at subsequent dosing with antihistamines, non-steroidal anti-inflammatory drugs, or corticosteroids.

Lab Test Considerations
- Confirm the presence of amyloid beta pathology before starting therapy.

Implementation
- Obtain a recent (within one year) brain magnetic resonance imaging (MRI) prior to starting therapy. Obtain an MRI prior to the 5th, 7th, and 14th infusions.
- *Dilution:* Dilute in 250 mL of 0.9% NaCl. Solution is clear to opalescent and colorless to pale yellow; do not administer solution that are discolored, cloudy, or contain particulate matter. Gently invert to mix; do not shake. Solution is stable for 4 hr at room temperature or if refrigerated; do not freeze. Allow solution to warm to room temperature before infusing. *Rate:* Infuse over 1 hr through a terminal low-protein binding 0.2 micron in-line filter. Flush infusion line to ensure all medication is administered.

Patient/Family Teaching
- Explain purpose of lecanemab to patient and family. Advise patient and caregiver to read the *Medication Guide* before and periodically during therapy in case of changes. If an infusion is missed, schedule next infusion as soon as possible.
- Advise patient to notify health care professional if signs an symptoms of ARIA (headache, confusion,

dizziness, vision changes, nausea, difficulty walking, seizures) or infusion-related reaction occur.
- Instruct patient to notify health care professional of all Rx or OTC medications, vitamins, or herbal products being taken and consult health care professional before taking any new medications.
- Advise patients that the Alzheimer's Network for Treatment and Diagnostics (ALZ-NET) is a voluntary provider-enrolled patient registry that collects information on treatments for Alzheimer's disease, including *Leqembi*. Encourage patients to participate in the ALZ-NET registry.
- Advise patient to notify health care professional if pregnancy is planned or suspected or if breastfeeding.

Evaluation/Desired Outcomes
- Reduction in amyloid beta plaques in the brain.

lefamulin (le-fam-ue-lin)
Xenleta
Classification
Therapeutic: anti-infectives
Pharmacologic: pleuromutilins

Indications
Community-acquired bacterial pneumonia.

Action
Acts as a pleuromutilin that ultimately interferes with bacterial protein synthesis at the level of the 50S ribosome. **Therapeutic Effects:** Resolution of pneumonia. **Spectrum:** Active against gram-positive pathogens, including: *Staphylococcus aureus* (methicillin-sensitive strains only), *Streptococcus pneumoniae*. Also active against the following gram-negative pathogen: *Haemophilus influenzae*. Also active against several other pathogens, including: *Legionella pneumophilia*, *Chlamydia pneumoniae*, *Mycoplasma pneumoniae*.

Pharmacokinetics
Absorption: 25% absorbed following oral administration; IV administration results in complete bioavailability.
Distribution: Extensively distributed to tissues.
Protein Binding: 94–97%.
Metabolism and Excretion: Primarily metabolized in the liver via the CYP3A4 isoenzyme. Primarily excreted in feces (77%; 4–9% as unchanged drug), with 15% excreted in urine (9–14% as unchanged drug).
Half-life: 8 hr.

TIME/ACTION PROFILE (plasma concentrations)

ROUTE	ONSET	PEAK	DURATION
IV	unknown	at end of infusion	12 hr
PO	unknown	0.88–2 hr	12 hr

Contraindications/Precautions

Contraindicated in: Hypersensitivity to lefamulin or retapamulin; Concurrent use of CYP3A4 substrates that prolong the QT interval; QT interval prolongation or a history of ventricular arrhythmias (including torsades de pointes); Moderate or severe hepatic impairment (oral tablets only); OB: Pregnancy; Lactation: Lactation.

Use Cautiously in: Severe hepatic impairment (↑ dosing interval for IV injection); Rep: Women of reproductive potential; Pedi: Safety and effectiveness not established in children.

Adverse Reactions/Side Effects

CV: QT interval prolongation. **F and E:** hypokalemia. **GI:** diarrhea, ↑ liver enzymes, CLOSTRIDIOIDES DIFFICILE ASSOCIATED DIARRHEA (CDAD), nausea, vomiting. **Local:** injection site reactions. **Neuro:** headache, insomnia.

Interactions

Drug-Drug: **CYP3A4 substrates** that prolong the QT interval, including **pimozide**, may ↑ the risk of QT interval prolongation and torsades de pointes; concurrent use contraindicated. **Class Ia antiarrhythmics** or **Class III antiarrhythmics** may ↑ the risk of QT interval prolongation and torsades de pointes; avoid concurrent use. **QT interval prolonging medications**, including **antipsychotics, erythromycin, moxifloxacin,** or **tricyclic antidepressants**, may ↑ the risk of QT interval prolongation and torsades de pointes; avoid concurrent use. **Strong CYP3A4 inhibitors** or **P-glycoprotein (P-gp) inhibitors** may ↑ levels and risk of toxicity of oral lefamulin; avoid concurrent use. **Moderate or strong CYP3A4 inducers** or **P-gp inducers** may ↓ levels and effectiveness of either oral or IV lefamulin; avoid concurrent use. Lefamulin tablets may ↑ levels of **CYP3A4 substrates**, including **benzodiazepines, diltiazem, lovastatin, PDE5 inhibitors, simvastatin,** and **verapamil**; monitor closely for adverse reactions.

Route/Dosage

IV (Adults): 150 mg every 12 hr for 5–7 days; may switch at any time to oral regimen to complete the treatment course.
PO (Adults): 600 mg every 12 hr for 5 days.

Hepatic Impairment

IV (Adults): *Severe hepatic impairment:* 150 mg every 24 hr for 5–7 days.

Availability

Film-coated tablets: 600 mg. **Solution for injection:** 10 mg/mL.

NURSING IMPLICATIONS

Assessment

- Assess for infection (vital signs; appearance of wound, sputum, urine, and stool; WBC) at beginning

of and during therapy, especially in geriatric patients.
- Obtain specimens for culture and sensitivity before initiating therapy. First dose may be given before receiving results.
- Monitor bowel function. Diarrhea, abdominal cramping, fever, and bloody stools should be reported to health care professional promptly as a sign of CDAD. May begin up to several wk following cessation of therapy.
- Monitor ECG for QT interval prolongation in patients with ventricular arrhythmias or those on other drugs that prolong QT interval.
- Monitor for signs and symptoms of hypersensitivity reactions (rash, hives, swelling of face or throat) during therapy.

Lab Test Considerations
- Obtain a negative pregnancy test before starting therapy.

Implementation

- **PO:** Administer at least 1 hr before or 2 hr after a meal. Swallow tablets whole with 6–8 oz of water; ***DNC:*** Do not crush, break, or chew film-coated tablets.
- **Intermittent Infusion:** Dilute entire 15 mL vial into diluent bag supplied containing 250 mL of 10 mM citrate buffered 0.9% NaCl. Mix thoroughly. Solution is clear and colorless; do not administer solutions that are discolored or contain particulate matter. Solution is stable for 24 hr at room temperature or 48 hr if refrigerated. ***Rate:*** Infuse over 60 min.

Patient/Family Teaching

- Instruct patient to take lefamulin as directed. Take missed doses as soon as remembered up to 8 hr before next dose. If less than 8 hr before next dose, omit dose, and resume dosing at next scheduled dose.
- Instruct patient to notify health care professional immediately if rash, diarrhea, abdominal cramping, fever, or bloody stools occur and not to treat with antidiarrheals without consulting health care professionals.
- Advise patient to report the signs of superinfection (black, furry overgrowth on the tongue, vaginal itching or discharge, loose or foul-smelling stools) to health care professional.
- Advise patient to notify health care professional of all Rx or OTC medications, vitamins, or herbal products being taken and to consult with health care professional before taking other medications.
- Rep: Advise females of reproductive potential to use effective contraception and avoid breastfeeding during and for 2 days after final dose. If patient becomes pregnant while taking lefamulin, encourage patient to enrol in registry to monitor pregnancy outcomes by calling 1-855-5NABRIVA to enrol.

L

Evaluation/Desired Outcomes
● Resolution of the signs and symptoms of infection. Length of time for complete resolution depends on the organism and site of infection.

leflunomide (le-flu-noe-mide)
Arava
Classification
Therapeutic: antirheumatics (DMARDs)
Pharmacologic: immune response modifiers, pyrimidine synthesis inhibitors

Indications
Rheumatoid arthritis (disease-modifying agent).

Action
Inhibits an enzyme required for pyrimidine synthesis; has antiproliferative and anti-inflammatory effects.
Therapeutic Effects: Decreased pain and inflammation, slowed structural progression and improved physical function.

Pharmacokinetics
Absorption: 80% absorbed following oral administration.
Distribution: Crosses the placenta.
Protein Binding: 99%.
Metabolism and Excretion: Extensively metabolized in the liver to teriflunomide, which is responsible for pharmacologic activity; metabolites excreted in urine (43%) and feces (48%). Also undergoes biliary recycling.
Half-life: 14–18 days.

TIME/ACTION PROFILE (antirheumatic effect)

ROUTE	ONSET	PEAK	DURATION
PO	1 mo	3–6 mo	wk–mos†

†Due to persistence of active metabolite.

Contraindications/Precautions
Contraindicated in: Hypersensitivity to leflunomide or teriflunomide; Compromised immune function, including bone marrow dysplasia or severe uncontrolled infection; Concurrent vaccination with live vaccines; Hepatic impairment; OB: Pregnancy; Lactation: Lactation.
Use Cautiously in: Renal impairment; History of interstitial lung disease; Patients >60 yr, with diabetes, or taking neurotoxic medications (↑ risk of peripheral neuropathy); Rep: Women of reproductive potential; Pedi: Safety and effectiveness not established in children.
Exercise Extreme Caution in: Concurrent use of other hepatotoxic agents (↑ risk of hepatotoxicity).

Adverse Reactions/Side Effects
CV: chest pain, hypertension. **Derm:** alopecia, rash, DRUG REACTION WITH EOSINOPHILIA AND SYSTEMIC SYMP-

TOMS (DRESS), dry skin, eczema, pruritus, STEVENS-JOHNSON SYNDROME (SJS), TOXIC EPIDERMAL NECROLYSIS (TEN). **EENT:** pharyngitis, rhinitis, sinusitis. **F and E:** hypokalemia. **GI:** diarrhea, nausea, ↑ liver enzymes, abdominal pain, anorexia, dyspepsia, gastroenteritis, HEPATOTOXICITY, HEPATOTOXICITY, mouth ulcers, vomiting. **GU:** urinary tract infection. **Metab:** ↓ weight. **MS:** arthralgia, back pain, joint disorder, leg cramps, synovitis, tenosynovitis. **Neuro:** headache, dizziness, paresthesia, peripheral neuropathy, weakness. **Resp:** bronchitis, cough, INTERSTITIAL LUNG DISEASE (ILD), pneumonia. **Misc:** INFECTION (including sepsis and tuberculosis [TB] reactivation).

Interactions
Drug-Drug: Cholestyramine and **activated charcoal** cause a rapid and significant ↓ in levels of the active metabolite. Concurrent use of **methotrexate** and other **hepatotoxic drugs** ↑ risk of hepatotoxicity. Concurrent administration of **rifampin** ↑ levels of the active metabolite. May ↑ risk of bleeding with **warfarin**.

Route/Dosage
PO (Adults): *Loading dose:* 100 mg daily for 3 days; *Maintenance dose:* 20 mg once daily (if intolerance occurs, dose may be ↓ to 10 mg once daily).

Availability (generic available)
Tablets: 10 mg, 20 mg.

NURSING IMPLICATIONS
Assessment
● Assess range of motion and degree of swelling and pain in affected joints before and periodically during therapy.
● Monitor for signs and symptoms of ILD (new onset or worsening cough or dyspnea, associated with fever). May require discontinuation of therapy; consider drug elimination procedure if needed.
● Assess for rash periodically during therapy. May cause SJS or toxic epidermal necrolysis. Discontinue therapy if severe or if accompanied with fever, general malaise, fatigue, muscle or joint aches, blisters, oral lesions, conjunctivitis, hepatitis, and/or eosinophilia.
● Monitor for signs and symptoms of DRESS (fever, rash, lymphadenopathy, and/or facial swelling), associated with involvement of other organ systems (hepatitis, nephritis, hematologic abnormalities, myocarditis, myositis) during therapy. May resemble an acute viral infection. Eosinophilia is often present. Discontinue therapy if signs occur.

Lab Test Considerations
● Monitor liver function throughout therapy. Assess ALT at baseline, then monthly during initial 6 mo of therapy, then every 6–8 wk. If given concurrently with methotrexate, monitor ALT, AST, and serum albumin monthly. May cause ↑ ALT and AST, which are usually reversible with reduction in dose or discontinuation, but may be fatal. If ALT is 2–3 x the upper limit of

normal (ULN), ↓ dose to 10 mg/day and continue therapy. Monitor closely after dose reduction; plasma concentrations may not ↓ for several wk due to long half-life. If ALT ↑ of 2–3 x ULN persists despite dose reduction or if ALT >3 x ULN occurs, discontinue leflunomide and administer cholestyramine (see Toxicity and Overdose). Monitor closely and readminister cholestyramine as indicated.

● Monitor CBC with platelets monthly for 6 mo following initiation of therapy and every 6–8 wk thereafter. If used with methotrexate or other immunosuppressive therapy continue monitoring monthly. If bone marrow depression occurs, discontinue leflunomide and begin ↓ levels with cholestyramine (see Implementation).

● May rarely cause ↑ of alkaline phosphatase and bilirubin.

Toxicity and Overdose

● If overdose or significant toxicity occurs, cholestyramine 8 g 3 times a day for 24 hr, or activated charcoal orally or via nasogastric tube, 50 g every 6 hr for 24 hr, is recommended to accelerate elimination.

Implementation

● Administer a tuberculin skin test prior to administration of leflunomide. Patients with active latent TB should be treated for TB prior to therapy.

● **PO:** Initiate therapy with loading dose of 100 mg/day for 3 days, followed by 20 mg/day dose. May ↓ to 10 mg/day if not well tolerated.

● **Drug Elimination Procedure:** Recommended to achieve nondetectable plasma teriflunomide concentrations <0.02 mg/L after stopping treatment with leflunomide. Administer cholestyramine 8 g 3 times daily for 11 days (days do not need to be consecutive unless rapid lowering of levels is desired). Verify plasma teriflunomide concentrations <0.02 mg/L by two separate tests at least 14 days apart. If plasma teriflunomide concentrations >0.02 mg/L, consider additional cholestyramine treatment. Plasma teriflunomide concentrations may take up to 2 yr to reach nondetectable levels without drug elimination procedure.

Patient/Family Teaching

● Instruct patient to take leflunomide as directed.

● May cause dizziness. Caution patient to avoid driving or other activities requiring alertness until response to medication is known.

● Advise patient to consult health care professional prior to taking other Rx, OTC, or herbal products concurrently with leflunomide. Aspirin, NSAIDs, or low-dose corticosteroids may be continued during therapy, but other agents for treatment of rheumatoid arthritis may require discontinuation.

● Discuss the possibility of hair loss with patient. Explore methods of coping.

● Advise patient to notify health care professional if rash, mucous membrane lesions, unusual tiredness, abdominal pain, jaundice, or symptoms of ILD occur.

● Instruct patient to avoid vaccinations with live vaccines during and following therapy without consulting health care professional.

● Rep: May cause fetal harm. Women wishing to become pregnant must undergo the drug elimination procedure (see Implementation) and verify that the plasma teriflunomide concentrations are <0.02 mg/L.

● Emphasize the importance of routine lab tests to monitor for side effects.

Evaluation/Desired Outcomes

● Decrease in signs and symptoms of rheumatoid arthritis and slowing of structural damage as evidenced by x-ray erosions and joint narrowings.

● Improved physical function.

L

REMS

▓ lenalidomide
(le-na-**lid**-o-mide)
Revlimid
Classification
Therapeutic: antineoplastics
Pharmacologic: immunomodulatory agents

Indications

▓ Transfusion-dependent anemia due to specific myelodysplastic syndromes associated with deletion 5q cytogenetic abnormality. Multiple myeloma (in combination with dexamethasone). Maintenance therapy in patients with multiple myeloma after autologous hematopoietic stem cell transplantation. Mantle cell lymphoma patients whose disease has relapsed or progressed after 2 prior therapies including bortezomib. Previously treated follicular lymphoma (in combination with rituximab). Previously treated marginal zone lymphoma (in combination with rituximab).

Action

Lenalidomide is a structural analog of thalidomide. Inhibits secretion of pro-inflammatory cytokines and increases secretion of anti-inflammatory cytokines. **Therapeutic Effects:** Decreased anemia in certain myelodysplastic syndromes with a decreased requirement for transfusions. Slowed progression of multiple myeloma and mantle cell lymphoma. Improved progression-free survival in follicular lymphoma and marginal zone lymphoma.

Pharmacokinetics

Absorption: Well absorbed following oral administration. Levels are higher in patients with multiple myeloma.
Distribution: Crosses the placenta.

Metabolism and Excretion: 66% excreted unchanged in urine, some renal excretion involves active secretion.

Half-life: 3 hr.

TIME/ACTION PROFILE (↓ need for transfusions)

ROUTE	ONSET	PEAK	DURATION
PO	within 3 mo	unknown	unknown

Contraindications/Precautions

Contraindicated in: Hypersensitivity; Chronic lymphocytic leukemia (↑ risk of mortality); Concurrent use of pembrolizumab in patients with multiple myeloma (↑ risk of mortality); OB: Pregnancy; Lactation: Lactation.

Use Cautiously in: Renal impairment (may ↑ risk of adverse reactions; dose ↓ recommended if CCr <60 mL/min); Patients with mantle cell lymphoma with high tumor burden, high mantle cell lymphoma International Prognostic Index at diagnosis, and high white blood cell count at baseline (↑ risk of early mortality); Rep: Women of reproductive potential and men with female partners of reproductive potential; Pedi: Safety and effectiveness not established in children; Geri: Consider age-related ↓ in renal function in older adults.

Adverse Reactions/Side Effects

CV: edema, chest pain, DEEP VEIN THROMBOSIS, MI, palpitations. **Derm:** pruritus, rash, DRUG REACTION WITH EOSINOPHILIA AND SYSTEMIC SYMPTOMS (DRESS), dry skin, STEVENS-JOHNSON SYNDROME (SJS), sweating, TOXIC EPIDERMAL NECROLYSIS (TEN). **Endo:** hyperthyroidism, hypothyroidism. **F and E:** hypokalemia, hypomagnesemia. **GI:** abdominal pain, constipation, diarrhea, nausea, vomiting, abnormal taste, anorexia, dry mouth, HEPATOTOXICITY. **Hemat:** NEUTROPENIA, THROMBOCYTOPENIA. **MS:** arthralgia, myalgia. **Neuro:** dizziness, fatigue, headache, depression, insomnia, STROKE. **Resp:** cough, pharyngitis, PULMONARY EMBOLISM. **Misc:** fever, TUMOR FLARE REACTION, chills, HYPERSENSITIVITY REACTIONS (including anaphylaxis and angioedema), MALIGNANCY, tumor lysis syndrome.

Interactions

Drug-Drug: Risk of neutropenia and thrombocytopenia may ↑ with **antineoplastics, immunosuppressants,** and **radiation therapy.** May ↑ **digoxin** levels. **Erythropoeitin, darbepoeitin,** and **estrogens** may ↑ risk of thromboembolic events.

Route/Dosage

Myelodysplastic Syndromes
PO (Adults): 10 mg once daily.

Renal Impairment
PO (Adults): *CCr 30–60 mL/min:* 5 mg once daily; *CCr <30 mL/min (not on dialysis):* 2.5 mg once daily; *CCr <30 mL/min (requiring dialysis):* 2.5 mg once daily (give after dialysis on dialysis days).

Multiple Myeloma
PO (Adults): 25 mg once daily on days 1–21 of repeated 28-day cycles (with dexamethasone); if patients not eligible for auto-HSCT, continue treatment until disease progression or unacceptable toxicity; for patients eligible for auto-HSCT, hematopoietic stem cell mobilization should take place within 4 cycles.

Renal Impairment
PO (Adults): *CCr 30–60 mL/min:* 10 mg once daily; if patient tolerates initial dose, may ↑ to 15 mg once daily after 2 cycles; *CCr <30 mL/min (not on dialysis):* 15 mg every 48 hr; *CCr <30 mL/min (requiring dialysis):* 5 mg once daily (give after dialysis on dialysis days).

Maintenance Therapy for Multiple Myeloma Following Autologous Hematopoietic Stem Cell Transplantation
PO (Adults): After adequate hematologic recovery (ANC ≥ 1000/mcL and/or platelet counts ≥75,000/mcL), initiate therapy with 10 mg once daily continuously on Days 1–28 of repeated 28–day cycles); after 3 cycles, dose may be ↑ to 15 mg once daily, if tolerated; continue treatment until disease progression or unacceptable toxicity.

Renal Impairment
PO (Adults): *CCr 30–60 mL/min:* 5 mg once daily; *CCr <30 mL/min (not on dialysis):* 2.5 mg once daily; *CCr <30 mL/min (requiring dialysis):* 2.5 mg once daily (give after dialysis on dialysis days).

Mantle Cell Lymphoma
PO (Adults): 25 mg once daily on days 1–21 of repeated 28–day cycles; continue treatment until disease relapse or unacceptable toxicity develops.

Renal Impairment
PO (Adults): *CCr 30–60 mL/min:* 10 mg once daily; *CCr <30 mL/min (not on dialysis):* 15 mg every 48 hr; *CCr <30 mL/min (requiring dialysis):* 5 mg once daily (give after dialysis on dialysis days).

Follicular Lymphoma or Marginal Zone Lymphoma
PO (Adults): 20 mg once daily on days 1–21 of repeated 28–day cycles for up to 12 cycles (with rituximab).

Renal Impairment
PO (Adults): *CCr 30–60 mL/min:* 10 mg once daily; if patient tolerates initial dose, may ↑ to 15 mg once daily after 2 cycles; *CCr <30 mL/min (not on dialysis):* 5 mg once daily; *CCr <30 mL/min (requiring dialysis):* 5 mg once daily (give after dialysis on dialysis days).

Availability (generic available)
Capsules: 2.5 mg, 5 mg, 10 mg, 15 mg, 20 mg, 25 mg.

NURSING IMPLICATIONS

Assessment
● Assess for signs of deep venous thrombosis and pulmonary edema (dyspnea, chest pain, arm or leg swelling) periodically during therapy; risk is greater

when lenalidomide is administered with dexamethasone.

● Assess for skin rash. Discontinue lenalidomide if rash occurs; may cause SJS, DRESS, or TEN. Consider interruption or discontinuation for Grade 2-3 skin rash. Permanently discontinue lenalidomide for Grade 4 rash, exfoliative or bullous rash, or for other severe cutaneous reactions such as SJS, TEN or DRESS.

● Monitor for signs and symptoms of tumor flare reaction (tender lymph node swelling, low-grade fever, pain rash) in patients with MCL; may mimic disease progression. *Grade 1 and 2 tumor flare reaction (TFR):* Lenalidomide may be continued in patients without interruption or modification, at health care professional's discretion. May also be treated with corticosteroids, nonsteroidal anti-inflammatory drugs (NSAIDs) and/or opioid analgesics. *Grade 3 or 4 TFR:* withhold treatment with lenalidomide until TFR resolves to ≤ Grade 1. May be treated for management of symptoms per the guidance for treatment of Grade 1 and 2 TFR.

Lab Test Considerations

● Verify negative pregnancy status before starting therapy. Pregnancy tests with a sensitivity of at least 50 mIU/mL must be done within 10–14 days and within 24 hrs of starting therapy. Once treatment has started, verify negative pregnancy tests weekly during first 4 wk of use, then every 4 wk in females with a regular menstrual cycle and every 2 wk in females with an irregular cycle.

● *Patients taking lenalidomide for multiple myeloma with dexamethasone or as maintenance therapy:* Monitor CBC every 7 days for first 2 cycles, on days 1 and 15 of Cycle 3, and every 28 days thereafter. *Patients taking lenalidomide for myelodysplastic syndrome:* Monitor CBC with differential, platelet count, hemoglobin, and hematocrit weekly for first 8 wk of therapy and at least monthly thereafter. *Patients taking lenalidomide for mantle cell lymphoma:* Monitor CBC weekly for first 28 days, every 2 wk during Cycles 2–4, and monthly thereafter. May require dose interruption and/or reduction and use of blood support and/or growth factors.

● May cause neutropenia with an onset of 42 days (range 4–411 days) and recovery time of 17 days (range 2–170 days). *For multiple myeloma:* starting dose is 25 mg/day—If neutropenia develops and neutrophils fall to <1000/mcL interrupt therapy, follow CBC weekly. When neutrophils return to ≥1000/mcL and neutropenia is the only toxicity, resume lenalidomide at 25 mg daily. If neutrophils return to ≥1000/mcL and if other toxicity, resume lenalidomide at next lower dose. For each subsequent drop <1000/mcL interrupt therapy. If neutrophils return to ≥1000/mcL, resume at next lower dose.

Do not administer doses below 2.5 mg. *For myelodysplastic syndromes:* starting dose is 10 mg/day— if neutropenia develops within 4 wk of starting at a 10 mg/day dose in a patient with a baseline neutrophil count (ANC) ≥1000/mcL and ANC falls to <750/mcL interrupt lenalidomide therapy and resume at 5 mg/day dose when ANC returns to ≥1000/mcL. If baseline ANC is <1000/mcL and ANC falls to <500/mcL, interrupt therapy and resume at 5 mg/day dose when ANC returns to ≥500/mcL. If neutropenia develops after 4 wk of therapy at 10 mg/day dose, and ANC <500/mcL for ≥7 days or <500/mcL associated with fever ≥38.5°C, interrupt therapy and resume at 5 mg/day when ANC returns to ≥500/mcL. If neutropenia develops at 5 mg/day dose and ANC <500/mcL for ≥7 days or <500/mcL associated with fever ≥38.5°C, interrupt therapy and resume at 2.5 mg daily when ANC returns to ≥500/mcL. *For mantle cell lymphoma:* starting dose is 25 mg/day on days 1–21 of repeated 28-day cycles—If neutrophils fall to <1000/mcL for at least 7 days or fall to <1000/mcL with fever ≥38.5°C or fall to <500/mcL, interrupt therapy and follow CBC weekly. If neutrophils return to ≥1000/mcL resume at 5 mg less than previous dose. Do not administer doses below 5 mg. *For marginal zone lymphoma or follicular lymphoma:* If neutrophils <1000/mcL for at least 7 days OR <1000/mcL with associated temperature at least 38.5° C OR <500/mcL hold lenalidomide and follow with weekly CBC. If neutrophils return to ≥1000/mcL and patient starting dose was 20 mg daily, resume at 5 mg less than previous dose. Do not administer doses below 5 mg. If neutrophils return to ≥1000/mcL patient starting dose was 10 mg daily, resume at 5 mg less than previous dose. Do not administer doses below 2.5 mg.

● May cause thrombocytopenia with an onset of 28 days (range 8–290 days) and a recovery in 22 days (range 5–224 days). *For multiple myeloma:* starting dose is 25 mg/day— If platelets fall to <30,000/mcL interrupt therapy and follow CBC weekly. When platelets return to ≥30,000/mcL restart lenalidomide at next lower dose. For each subsequent drop <30,000/mcL interrupt therapy. When platelets return to ≥30,000/mcL resume at next lower dose. Do not administer doses below 2.5 mg. *For myelodysplastic syndrome:* starting dose is 10 mg/day— If thrombocytopenia develops within 4 wk of starting a 10 mg dose in a patient with a baseline of ≥100,000/mcL, and platelets fall to <50,000/mcL interrupt lenalidomide therapy and resume at 5 mg/day dose when platelets return to >50,000/mcL. If baseline was <100,000/mcL and platelets fall to 50% of baseline value interrupt therapy. If baseline ≥60,000/mcL and returns to ≥50,000/mcL or if baseline is <60,000/mcL and returns to ≥30,000/mcL resume therapy at 5 mg/day. If thrombocytopenia develops after 4 wk of treatment at 10 mg/day and platelets are <30,000/mcL or <50,000/mcL with platelet transfusions, interrupt therapy. When platelets return to ≥30,000/mcL without hemostatic failure resume therapy at 2.5 mg/day. *For mantle cell lymphoma:* starting dose is 25 mg/day on days 1–21 of repeated 28–day cycles— If platelets fall to <50,000/mcL interrupt therapy and follow CBC weekly. If platelets return to ≥50,000/mcL resume at 5 mg less than previous dose. Do not administer doses below 5 mg. *For follicular lymphoma or marginal cell lymphoma:* if platelets <50,000/mcL, hold lenalidomide and follow with weekly CBC. When platelets return to ≥50,000/mcL, if starting dose was 20 mg daily, resume lenalidomide at 5 mg less than the previous dose. Do not dose below 5 mg daily. If starting dose was 10 mg daily, resume at 5 mg less than previous dose. Do not dose below 2.5 mg daily.

- Monitor liver enzymes periodically during therapy. Stop therapy if enzymes are elevated; may resume when return to normal or decrease dose.
- May cause anemia and leukopenia.
- May cause hypokalemia, hypomagnesemia, and ↑ ALT levels.
- Monitor thyroid function before starting and periodically during therapy.

Implementation

- *REMS:* Patients must sign a Patient-Physician agreement form and must meet the following conditions before receiving therapy: they must understand the risks and be able to carry out instructions, must be capable of complying with patient registration and patient survey in the *Lenalidomide REMS program*, must comply with contraceptive measures, have received both oral and written warnings of the risks of contraception failure and the need for two reliable forms of contraception (females) or the risks of exposing a fetus to the drug and the need to use a latex condom during sexual conduct with a female with childbearing potential (male), acknowledge understanding of these warnings in writing, and if the patient is between 12 and 18 yr of age, their parent or legal guardian is to read the educational materials and agree to try to ensure compliance with conditions.
- *REMS:* Lenalidomide can only be prescribed by health care providers registered in the *Lenalidomide REMS program* and only be dispensed by a pharmacy that is registered in the *Lenalidomide REMS program*. Patients with multiple myeloma who are eligible for autologous stem cell transplantation should have stem cell mobilization performed within 4 cycles of therapy.
- *PO:* Administer once daily without regard to food, at the same time each day, with water. *DNC:* Swallow capsules whole; do not open, break, or chew.

Patient/Family Teaching

- *REMS:* Lenalidomide is only available through a restricted program, the *Lenalidomide REMS program*. Instruct patient to take lenalidomide as directed and to comply with all aspects of the *Lenalidomide REMS program*. Take missed doses as soon as remembered within 12 hr of dose missed. If more than 12 hrs, skip dose and return to next scheduled dose; do not administer 2 doses within 12 hrs. Inform patient that they are required to participate in a telephone survey and patient registry while taking lenalidomide. Details are available at www.lenalidomiderems.com. Advise patient to read *Medication Guide* before starting and with each Rx refill in case of changes.
- Caution patient not to share lenalidomide with anyone, even someone who has similar symptoms.
- Advise patient to notify health care professional if rash, shortness of breath, chest pain, or arm or leg swelling, signs of infection (fever, dyspnea), rash, signs and symptoms of liver failure (yellowing of skin or white part of eyes; dark or brown (tea-colored) urine; pain on upper right side of your abdomen; feeling tired; unusual bleeding or bruising), hypersensitivity (swelling of lips, mouth, tongue, or throat; trouble breathing or swallowing; hives; very fast heartbeat; feeling dizzy or faint) occur.
- May cause dizziness. Caution patient to avoid driving and other activities requiring alertness until response to medication is known.
- Inform patient that lenalidomide may cause an increased risk of death in patients with mantle cell lymphoma and may increase risk of new cancers.
- Instruct patient to notify health care professional of all Rx or OTC medications, vitamins, or herbal products being taken and consult health care professional before taking any new medications.
- Advise patient that they cannot donate blood during and for 1 mo following therapy and male patients cannot donate sperm while taking lenalidomide.
- Inform patient of risk of new cancers during therapy.
- Rep: May cause fetal harm. Inform females of reproductive potential that they must use one highly effective method (IUD, hormonal contraceptive, tubal ligation, partner's vasectomy) and one additional method (latex or synthetic condom, diaphragm, cervical cap) AT THE SAME TIME for ≥4 wk before, during therapy and interruptions of therapy, and for 4 wk following discontinuation of therapy, even with a history of infertility unless due to a hysterectomy or patient has been postmenopausal naturally for 24 consecutive mo. Advise female patients to avoid breastfeeding during therapy. Males with female partners of reproductive potential receiving lenalidomide must always use a latex or synthetic condom during and for up to 4 wk following discontinuation,

even if they have undergone a successful vasectomy. Male patients taking lenalidomide must not donate sperm during and for 4 wks after last dose. Lenalidomide must be discontinued if pregnancy is suspected or confirmed. Suspected fetal exposure must be reported to FDA via MedWatch at 1-800-FDA-1088 and to Celgene Corporation at 1-888-423-5436. Inform females there is a Pregnancy Exposure Registry that monitors pregnancy outcomes in females exposed to lenalidomide during pregnancy and that they can contact the Pregnancy Exposure Registry by calling 1-888-423-5436 or at www.lenalidomiderems.com.

Evaluation/Desired Outcomes

• Decreased anemia in myelodysplastic syndromes with a decreased requirement for transfusions.
• Slowing of multiple myeloma progression.
• Slowing progression of mantle cell lymphoma.
• Improved progression-free survival in follicular lymphoma and marginal zone lymphoma.

⧚ lenvatinib (len-va-ti-nib)
Lenvima
Classification
Therapeutic: antineoplastics
Pharmacologic: kinase inhibitors

Indications
Locally recurrent or metastatic/progressive, radioactive-iodine-refractory differentiated thyroid cancer. Advanced renal cell carcinoma following one previous anti-angiogenic therapy (in combination with everolimus). First-line treatment of advanced renal cell carcinoma (in combination with pembrolizumab). Unresectable hepatocellular carcinoma. ⧚ Advanced endometrial carcinoma that is mismatch repair proficient (pMMR) or not microsatellite instability-high (MSI-H), in patients who have disease progression following prior systemic therapy in any setting and are not candidates for curative surgery or radiation (in combination with pembrolizumab).

Action
Acts as a receptor tyrosine kinase inhibitor; inhibits kinase activities of various vascular endothelial growth factor receptors, resulting in decreased pathogenic angiogenesis, tumor growth and spread. **Therapeutic Effects:** Decreased progression and improved survival of differentiated thyroid cancer, endometrial cancer, renal cell carcinoma, and hepatocellular carcinoma.

Pharmacokinetics
Absorption: Well absorbed following oral administration.
Distribution: Unknown.
Protein Binding: 98–99%.

Metabolism and Excretion: Metabolized primarily by the CYP3A isoenzyme and aldehyde oxidase; 64% eliminated in feces, 25% in urine.
Half-life: 28 hr.

TIME/ACTION PROFILE (improvement in progression-free survival)

ROUTE	ONSET	PEAK	DURATION
PO	within 2 mo	8 mo	throughout treatment

Contraindications/Precautions
Contraindicated in: OB: Pregnancy; Lactation: Lactation.

Use Cautiously in: Hypertension (control BP before initiating treatment, may need to withhold/discontinue for life-threatening elevation); History of HF (may need to withhold/discontinue for worsening HF); History of congenital long QTc syndrome, HF, bradyarrhythmias, concurrent use of drugs that prolong QTc, including Class Ia and III antiarrhythmics (↑ risk of further QTc prolongation and serious arrhythmias, may require interruption/discontinuation of lenvatinib); Severe hepatic or renal impairment (↓ dose); Dehydration/volume depletion (↑ risk of renal impairment, may need to withhold/discontinue for worsening renal function); Hypocalcemia (replace calcium; if persistent may require dose adjustment/interruption); History of reversible posterior leukoencephalopathy syndrome (may require dose adjustment/interruption); Invasive dental procedures, concurrent use of bisphosphonates or denosumab, or dental disease (may ↑ risk of osteonecrosis of the jaw [ONJ]); Rep: Women and men of reproductive potential; Pedi: Safety and effectiveness not established in children.

Adverse Reactions/Side Effects
CV: hypertension, HF, hypotension, MI, QT interval prolongation. **Derm:** alopecia, palmar-plantar erythrodysesthesia syndrome, rash, hyperkeratosis, impaired wound healing. **EENT:** dysphonia, epistaxis. **Endo:** hypothyroidism. **F and E:** dehydration, hypocalcemia, hypokalemia. **GI:** ↓ appetite, abdominal pain, diarrhea, dry mouth, nausea, stomatitis, vomiting, ↑ liver enzymes, GI PERFORATION/FISTULA FORMATION, HEPATOTOXICITY. **GU:** proteinuria, renal impairment, ↓ fertility, NEPHROTIC SYNDROME. **Hemat:** BLEEDING, thrombocytopenia. **Metab:** ↓ weight. **MS:** arthralgia/myalgia, osteonecrosis (primarily of jaw). **Neuro:** dysgeusia, fatigue, headache, insomnia, CAROTID ARTERY HEMORRHAGE, REVERSIBLE POSTERIOR LEUKOENCEPHALOPATHY SYNDROME (RPLS), STROKE. **Resp:** cough.

Interactions
Drug-Drug: Concurrent use of **QT interval prolonging drugs,** including **Class Ia and III antiarrhythmics** may ↑ risk of further QTc prolongation and serious arrhythmias (may require interruption/discon-

---

⧩ = Canadian drug name. ⧚ = Genetic implication. ~~Strikethrough~~ = Discontinued. CAPITALS = life-threatening. Underline = most frequent.

tinuation of lenvatinib). Concurrent use of **alendronate**, **denosumab**, **ibandronate**, **pamidronate**, **risedronate**, or **zoledronic acid** may ↑ risk of ONJ.

Route/Dosage

Differentiated Thyroid Cancer
PO (Adults): 24 mg once daily until disease progression or unacceptable toxicity.

Renal Impairment
PO (Adults): *CCr <30 mL/min:* 14 mg once daily until disease progression or unacceptable toxicity.

Hepatic Impairment
PO (Adults): *Severe hepatic impairment:* 14 mg once daily until disease progression or unacceptable toxicity.

Renal Cell Carcinoma
PO (Adults): *First-line treatment of advanced renal cell carcinoma:* 20 mg once daily (in combination with pembrolizumab) until disease progression or unacceptable toxicity or up to 2 yr. After 2 yr of combination therapy, continue 20 mg once daily (as monotherapy) until disease progression or unacceptable toxicity. *Previously treated renal cell carcinoma:* 18 mg once daily until disease progression or unacceptable toxicity.

Renal Impairment
PO (Adults): *CCr <30 mL/min:* First-line treatment of advanced renal cell carcinoma: 10 mg once daily (in combination with pembrolizumab) until disease progression or unacceptable toxicity or up to 2 yr. After 2 yr of combination therapy, continue 10 mg once daily (as monotherapy) until disease progression or unacceptable toxicity. Previously treated renal cell carcinoma: 10 mg once daily until disease progression or unacceptable toxicity.

Hepatic Impairment
PO (Adults): *Severe hepatic impairment:* 10 mg once daily until disease progression or unacceptable toxicity.

Hepatocellular Carcinoma
PO (Adults ≥60 kg): 12 mg once daily until disease progression or unacceptable toxicity.
PO (Adults <60 kg): 8 mg once daily until disease progression or unacceptable toxicity.

Endometrial Carcinoma
PO (Adults): 20 mg once daily until disease progression or unacceptable toxicity.

Renal Impairment
PO (Adults): *CCr <30 mL/min:* 10 mg once daily until disease progression or unacceptable toxicity.

Hepatic Impairment
PO (Adults): *Severe hepatic impairment:* 10 mg once daily until disease progression or unacceptable toxicity.

Availability
Capsules: 4 mg, 10 mg.

NURSING IMPLICATIONS

Assessment
- Assess BP prior to and after 1 wk, then every 2 wk for first 2 mo, and then at least monthly thereafter during therapy. Initiate or adjust medication management to control BP. Hold lenvatinib for Grade 3 hypertension that persists despite antihypertensive therapy. Resume at a reduced dose (*1st occurrence:* 20 mg/day; *2nd occurrence:* 14 mg/day; *3rd occurrence:* 10 mg/day) when hypertension is controlled or ≤Grade 2). Discontinue lenvatinib for life-threatening hypertension.
- Monitor for clinical signs and symptoms of cardiac dysfunction (shortness of breath, swollen ankles) during therapy. Hold lenvatinib for Grade 3 cardiac dysfunction until improved to Grade 0 or baseline. Resume at reduced dose (*1st occurrence:* 20 mg/day; *2nd occurrence:* 14 mg/day; *3rd occurrence:* 10 mg/day) or discontinue depending on severity and persistence of cardiac dysfunction.
- Monitor for signs and symptoms of arterial thromboembolic events (chest pain, acute neurologic symptoms of MI or stroke) during therapy. Discontinue lenvatinib if event occurs.
- Assess for signs and symptoms of gastrointestinal perforation or fistula formation (severe abdominal pain) during therapy. Discontinue lenvatinib if gastrointestinal perforation or fistula occurs.
- Monitor ECG for patients with congenital long QT syndrome, congestive heart failure, bradyarrhythmias, or those taking drugs known to prolong QT interval. Hold lenvatinib for development of QT interval prolongation >500 msec or >60 msec increase from baseline. Hold until improves to ≤480 msec or baseline. Resume at reduced dose (*1st occurrence:* 20 mg/day; *2nd occurrence:* 14 mg/day; *3rd occurrence:* 10 mg/day) when QT prolongation resolves to Grade 0 or 1.
- Monitor for signs and symptoms of RPLS (severe headache, seizures, weakness, confusion, blindness or change in vision) during therapy. If symptoms occur, confirm diagnosis with MRI. Hold lenvatinib for RPLS until fully resolved. Resume at reduced dose (*1st occurrence:* 20 mg/day; *2nd occurrence:* 14 mg/day; *3rd occurrence:* 10 mg/day) or discontinue depending on severity and persistence of neurologic symptoms.
- Monitor for bleeding (severe and persistent nose bleeds, vomiting blood, red or black stools, coughing up blood or blood clots, heavy or new onset vaginal bleeding) during therapy. Hold lenvatinib for Grade 3 hemorrhage until resolved to Grade 0 or 1. Resume at reduced dose (*1st occurrence:* 20 mg/day; *2nd occurrence:* 14 mg/day; *3rd occurrence:* 10 mg/day) or discontinue depending on severity and persistence of hemorrhage. Discontinue lenvatinib if Grade 4 hemorrhage occurs.
- Obtain an oral exam prior to and periodically during therapy. Hold lenvatinib for at least 1 wk before

scheduled dental surgery or invasive dental procedures, if possible. Discontinuation of bisphosphonate therapy may reduce the risk of ONJ. Hold lenvatinib if ONJ develops and restart after adequate resolution.

Lab Test Considerations
● Verify negative pregnancy test before starting therapy. For the pMMR/not MSI-H advanced endometrial carcinoma indication, select patients for therapy with lenvatinib in combination with pembrolizumab based on MSI or MMR status in tumor specimens. Information on FDA-approved tests for patient selection is available at: http://www.fda.gov/CompanionDiagnostics. An FDA-approved test for selection of patients who are not MSI-H is not currently available. Monitor serum ALT and AST levels for hepatotoxicity prior to and every 2 wk for first 2 mo, and at least monthly thereafter during therapy. Hold lenvatinib for Grade 3 cardiac dysfunction until improved to Grade 0 or 1 or baseline. Resume at reduced dose (*1st occurrence:* 20 mg/day; *2nd occurrence:* 14 mg/day; *3rd occurrence:* 10 mg/day) or discontinue depending on severity and persistence of hepatotoxicity. May cause hypoalbuminemia, ↑ alkaline phosphatase, and hyperbilirubinemia.
● Monitor for proteinuria prior to and periodically during therapy. If urine dipstick proteinuria ≥2+ is detected, obtain 24 hr urine protein. Hold lenvatinib for ≥2 g proteinuria/24 hr and resume at reduced dose (*1st occurrence:* 20 mg/day; *2nd occurrence:* 14 mg/day; *3rd occurrence:* 10 mg/day) when proteinuria <2 g/24 hr. Discontinue lenvatinib for nephrotic syndrome.
● Monitor BUN and serum creatinine prior to and periodically during therapy. Hold lenvatinib for Grade 3 or 4 renal failure/impairment until resolved to Grade 0 or 1 or baseline. Resume at reduced dose (*1st occurrence:* 20 mg/day; *2nd occurrence:* 14 mg/day; *3rd occurrence:* 10 mg/day) or discontinue depending on severity and persistence of renal impairment.
● Monitor and correct electrolyte abnormalities. Monitor serum calcium levels at least monthly and replace calcium as needed during therapy. Interrupt and adjust lenvatinib dose based on severity, presence of ECG changes, and persistence of hypocalcemia. May cause hypokalemia, hypomagnesemia, hypoglycemia, hypercalcemia, and hyperkalemia.
● Monitor TSH levels monthly and adjust thyroid replacement medication as needed in patients with ↓ thyroid levels.
● May cause ↑ serum lipase and amylase, hypercholesterolemia, and ↓ platelet count.

Implementation
● Hold therapy for at least 1 wk before elective surgery and for at least 2 wk after major surgery and until adequate wound healing occurs.

● **PO:** Administer two 10-mg capsules and one 4-mg capsule to make 24 mg at the same time each day without regard to food. *DNC:* Swallow capsules whole; do not open, crush, or chew. For patients with difficulty swallowing, measure 1 tablespoon of water or apple juice and put capsule in liquid without breaking or crushing. Leave capsule in liquid for at least 10 min. Stir for at least 3 min, then drink mixture. After drinking, add same amount (1 tablespoon) of water or apple juice to glass. Swirl contents and swallow additional liquid. *For administration via feeding tube:* Place required number of capsules, up to a maximum of 5, in a small container (20 mL capacity) or syringe (20 mL). Do not break or crush capsules. Add 3 mL of liquid to container or syringe. Wait 10 minutes for the capsule shell (outer surface) to disintegrate, then stir or shake mixture for 3 min until capsules are fully disintegrated and administer the entire contents. Add an additional 2 mL of liquid to container or syringe using a second syringe or dropper, swirl or shake, and administer. Repeat this step at least once and until there is no visible residue to ensure all of the medication is taken. Suspension is stable for 24 hr if covered and refrigerated; discard suspension after 24 hr.

Patient/Family Teaching
● Instruct patient to take lenvatinib as directed at the same time each day. Take missed dose within 12 hr or omit and take next dose at usual time; do not double doses. Advise patient to read *Patient Information* before starting therapy and with each Rx refill in case of changes.
● Advise patient to notify health care professional promptly if signs and symptoms of high BP, heart problems, blood clots (severe chest pain or pressure; pain in arms, back, or jaw; shortness of breath; numbness or weakness on 1 side of body; trouble talking; sudden severe headache; sudden vision changes), liver problems (yellow skin or whites of eyes, dark tea colored urine, light-colored bowel movements), severe stomach pain, RPLS, or bleeding occur.
● Instruct patient to notify health care professional of therapy before any elective surgery or dental procedure. Lenvatinib must be stopped at least 1 wk before and for at least 2 wk after major surgery and until wound healing occurs.
● Advise patient to practice good mouth care during therapy and to notify health care professional if signs and symptoms of ONJ (jaw pain, toothache, sores on gums) occur.
● Advise patient to notify health care professional of all Rx or OTC medications, vitamins, or herbal products being taken and to consult with health care professional before taking other medications.

- Rep: May cause fetal harm. Advise females of reproductive potential to use effective contraception during and for at least 30 days following last dose of therapy and to notify health care professional if pregnancy is suspected. Advise patient to avoid breastfeeding during and for at least 1 wk after last dose. May impair fertility in males and females.
- Emphasize importance of lab tests to monitor for adverse reactions.

Evaluation/Desired Outcomes

- Decreased progression and improved survival of differentiated thyroid cancer, endometrial cancer, renal cell carcinoma, and hepatocellular carcinoma.

※ letrozole (let-roe-zole)
Femara
Classification
Therapeutic: antineoplastics
Pharmacologic: aromatase inhibitors

Indications
※ First-line or second-line treatment of postmenopausal women with hormone receptor positive or hormone receptor unknown advanced breast cancer. ※ Adjuvant treatment of postmenopausal women with hormone receptor positive early breast cancer. Extended adjuvant treatment of postmenopausal early breast cancer already treated with 5 yr of tamoxifen.

Action
Inhibits the enzyme aromatase, which is partially responsible for conversion of precursors to estrogen. **Therapeutic Effects:** Lowers levels of circulating estrogen, which may halt progression of estrogen-sensitive breast cancer. Decreased risk of recurrence/metastatic disease.

Pharmacokinetics
Absorption: Rapidly and completely absorbed. **Distribution:** Well distributed to tissues. **Metabolism and Excretion:** Mostly metabolized by the liver. Primarily excreted in the urine (90%), with 6% being excreted as unchanged drug. **Half-life:** 2 days.

TIME/ACTION PROFILE (effect on lowering of serum estradiol concentrations)

ROUTE	ONSET	PEAK	DURATION
PO	unknown	2–3 days	unknown

Contraindications/Precautions
Contraindicated in: Hypersensitivity; Premenopausal women; OB: Pregnancy; Lactation: Lactation. **Use Cautiously in:** Severe hepatic impairment; Rep: Women of reproductive potential; Pedi: Safety and effectiveness not established in children.

Adverse Reactions/Side Effects
CV: chest pain, DEEP VEIN THROMBOSIS, edema, hypertension. **Derm:** ↑ sweating, alopecia, hot flush, pruritus, rash. **F and E:** hypercalcemia. **GI:** nausea, abdominal pain, anorexia, constipation, diarrhea, dyspepsia, vomiting. **GU:** ↓ fertility. **Metab:** hypercholesterolemia, weight gain. **MS:** musculoskeletal pain, ↓ bone density, arthralgia, fracture. **Neuro:** anxiety, depression, dizziness, drowsiness, fatigue, headache, STROKE/TIA, vertigo, weakness. **Resp:** cough, dyspnea, pleural effusion, PULMONARY EMBOLISM.

Interactions
Drug-Drug: None reported.

Route/Dosage
PO (Adults): 2.5 mg once daily.

Hepatic Impairment
PO (Adults): *Severe hepatic impairment:* 2.5 mg every other day.

Availability (generic available)
Tablets: 2.5 mg.

NURSING IMPLICATIONS
Assessment
- Assess patient for pain and other side effects periodically during therapy.
- Monitor bone mineral density periodically during therapy.

Lab Test Considerations
- Verify negative pregnancy test before starting therapy.May cause elevated AST, ALT, alkaline phosphatase, bilirubin, GGT and cholesterol levels.

Implementation
- **PO:** May be taken without regard to food.

Patient/Family Teaching
- Instruct patient to take medication as directed.
- May cause dizziness and fatigue. Caution patient to avoid driving and other activities requiring awareness until response to medication is known.
- Inform patient of potential for adverse reactions and advise her to notify health care professional if side effects are problematic.
- Rep: May cause fetal harm. Advise females of reproductive potential to use effective contraception and to avoid breastfeeding during and for at least 3 wk after last dose of letrozole. May impair fertility in males and females. Caution women who are perimenopausal or who recently became menopausal to use adequate contraception during therapy.

Evaluation/Desired Outcomes
- Slowing of disease progression in women with advanced breast cancer.
- Decreased risk of recurrence/metastatic disease.

leucovorin calcium
(loo-koe-**vor**-in)
Classification
Therapeutic: antidotes (for methotrexate), vitamins
Pharmacologic: folic acid analogues

Indications
Minimizes hematologic effects of high-dose methotrexate therapy (leucovorin rescue). Advanced colorectal carcinoma (with 5-fluorouracil). Management of overdoses/prevention of toxicity from folic acid antagonists (pyrimethamine, trimethoprim). Folic acid deficiency (megaloblastic anemia) unresponsive to oral replacement.

Action
The reduced form of folic acid that serves as a cofactor in the synthesis of DNA and RNA. **Therapeutic Effects:** Reversal of toxic effects of folic acid antagonists. Reversal of folic acid deficiency.

Pharmacokinetics
Absorption: Well absorbed (38%) following PO administration. ↓ bioavailability with larger doses. Oral absorption is saturated at doses >25 mg. Well absorbed following IM administration. IV administration results in complete bioavailability.
Distribution: Widely distributed to tissues. Concentrates in the CNS and liver.
Metabolism and Excretion: Extensively converted to tetrahydrofolic derivatives, including 5-methyltetrahydrofolate, a major storage form.
Half-life: 3.5 hr.

TIME/ACTION PROFILE (serum folate concentrations)

ROUTE	ONSET	PEAK	DURATION
PO	20–30 min	unknown	3–6 hr
IM	10–20 min	unknown	3–6 hr
IV	<5 min	unknown	3–6 hr

Contraindications/Precautions
Contraindicated in: Hypersensitivity; Pedi: Preparations containing benzyl alcohol should not be used in neonates.
Use Cautiously in: Undiagnosed anemia (may mask the progression of pernicious anemia); Ascites; Renal failure; Dehydration; Pleural effusions; Urine pH <7; OB: Safety not established in pregnancy; Lactation: Safety not established in breastfeeding.

Adverse Reactions/Side Effects
Hemat: thrombocytosis. **Misc:** allergic reactions (rash, urticaria, wheezing).

Interactions
Drug-Drug: May ↓ anticonvulsant effect of **barbiturates**, **phenytoin**, or **primidone**. High doses of the liquid contain significant **alcohol** and may cause ↑ CNS depression when used with **CNS depressants**. Concurrent use with **trimethoprim/sulfamethoxazole** may result in ↓ anti-infective efficacy and poor therapeutic outcome when used to treat *Pneumocystis jirovecii* pneumonia in patients with HIV. May ↑ therapeutic effects and toxicity of **fluorouracil**; therapy may be combined for this purpose.

Route/Dosage
High-Dose Methotrexate—Leucovorin Rescue. Must start within 24 hr of methotrexate.
PO, IM, IV (Adults and Children): *Normal methotrexate elimination:* 10 mg/m^2 every 6 hr (1st dose IV/IM, then change to PO) until methotrexate level is <5 × 10^{-8} M (0.05 micromolar). Larger doses/longer duration may be required in patients with aciduria, ascites, dehydration, renal impairment, GI obstruction, pleural/peritoneal effusions. Dose of leucovorin should be determined on the basis of plasma methotrexate levels.

Advanced Colorectal Cancer
IV (Adults): 200 mg/m^2 followed by 5-fluorouracil 370 mg/m^2 or leucovorin 20 mg/m^2 is followed by 5-fluorouracil 425 mg/m^2. Regimen is given daily for 5 days every 4–5 wk.

Prevention of Hematologic Toxicity from Pyrimethamine
PO, IV (Adults and Children): 5–15 mg/day.

Inadvertent Overdose of Folic Acid Antagonists
IM, IV (Adults and Children): *Methotrexate–large doses:* 75 mg IV followed by 12 mg IM every 6 hr for 4 doses; *methotrexate–average doses:* 6–12 mg IM every 6 hr for 4 doses; *other folic acid antagonists:* amount equal in mg to folic acid antagonist.

Megaloblastic Anemia
PO, IM, IV (Adults and Children): Up to 1 mg/day (up to 6 mg/day for dihydrofolate reductase deficiency).

Availability (generic available)
Tablets: 5 mg, 10 mg, 15 mg, 25 mg. **Powder for injection:** 50 mg/vial, 100 mg/vial, 200 mg/vial, 350 mg/vial, 500 mg/vial. **Solution for injection (preservative-free):** 10 mg/mL.

NURSING IMPLICATIONS
Assessment
- Assess patient for nausea and vomiting secondary to methotrexate therapy or folic acid antagonists

L

✦ = Canadian drug name. **ⵣ** = Genetic implication. ~~Strikethrough~~ = Discontinued. CAPITALS = life-threatening. <u>Underline</u> = most frequent.

(pyrimethamine and trimethoprim) overdose. Parenteral route may be necessary to ensure that patient receives dose.

● Monitor for development of allergic reactions (rash, urticaria, wheezing). Notify health care professional if these occur.

● **Megaloblastic Anemia:** Assess degree of weakness and fatigue.

Lab Test Considerations

● **Leucovorin rescue:** Monitor serum methotrexate levels to determine dose and effectiveness of therapy. Leucovorin calcium levels should be equal to or greater than methotrexate level. Rescue continues until serum methotrexate level is $<5 \times 10$ M.

● Monitor CCr and serum creatinine prior to and every 24 hr during therapy to detect methotrexate toxicity. An increase >50% over the pretreatment concentration at 24 hr is associated with severe renal toxicity.

● Monitor urine pH every 6 hr during therapy; pH should be maintained >7 to decrease nephrotoxic effects of high-dose methotrexate. Sodium bicarbonate or acetazolamide may be ordered to alkalinize urine.

● *Megaloblastic anemia:* Monitor plasma folic acid levels, hemoglobin, hematocrit, and reticulocyte count prior to and periodically during therapy.

Implementation

● Do not confuse leucovorin calcium with levoleucovorin. Do not confuse leucovorin calcium with Leukeran.

● Make sure leucovorin calcium is available before administering high-dose methotrexate. Administration must be initiated within 24 hr of methotrexate therapy.

● Administer as soon as possible after toxic dose of folic acid antagonists (pyrimethamine and trimethoprim). Effectiveness of therapy begins to decrease 1 hr after overdose.

● **PO:** Parenteral therapy should be used in patients with GI toxicity, with nausea and vomiting, or with doses >25 mg.

● **IM:** IM route is preferred for treatment of megaloblastic anemia. Ampules of leucovorin calcium injection for IM use do not require reconstitution.

IV Administration

● **IV Push:** *Reconstitution:* Reconstitute with bacteriostatic water or sterile water. Do not use product containing benzyl alcohol. Use immediately if reconstituted with sterile water for injection. Stable for 7 days when reconstituted with bacteriostatic water. *Concentration:* Reconstitute 50-mg, 100-mg, and 200-mg vials to a concentration of 10 mg/mL; reconstitute 350-mg vial to a concentration of 20 mg/mL. Do not administer with methotrexate; start leucovorin calcium 24 hr after start of methotrexate. *Rate:*

Administer by slow injection over a minimum of 3 min; not to exceed 160 mg/min.

● **Intermittent Infusion:** *Dilution:* May be diluted in 100–500 mL of D5W, D10W, 0.9% NaCl, Ringer's, or LR. Stable for 24 hr.

● **Y-Site Compatibility:** acyclovir, alemtuzumab, allopurinol, amifostine, amikacin, aminocaproic acid, aminophylline, ampicillin, ampicillin/sulbactam, anidulafungin, argatroban, arsenic trioxide, azithromycin, aztreonam, bivalirudin, bleomycin, bumetanide, buprenorphine, busulfan, butorphanol, calcium chloride, calcium gluconate, carmustine, caspofungin, cefepime, cefotaxime, cefotetan, cefoxitin, ceftazidime, cefuroxime, chloramphenicol, ciprofloxacin, cisatracurium, cisplatin, cladribine, clindamycin, cyclophosphamide, cyclosporine, cytarabine, dacarbazine, dactinomycin, daptomycin, daunorubicin hydrochloride, dexamethasone, dexamedetomidine, dexrazoxane, digoxin, diltiazem, diphenhydramine, dobutamine, docetaxel, dopamine, doxorubicin hydrochloride, doxorubicin liposomal, doxycycline, enalaprilat, ephedrine, epinephrine, eptifibatide, ertapenem, erythromycin, esmolol, etoposide, etoposide phosphate, famotidine, fentanyl, filgrastim, fluconazole, fludarabine, fluorouracil, fosphenytoin, furosemide, ganciclovir, gemcitabine, gentamicin, glycopyrrolate, granisetron, haloperidol, heparin, hetastarch, hydralazine, hydrocortisone, hydromorphone, idarubicin, ifosfamide, imipenem/cilastatin, insulin regular, isoproterenol, ketorolac, labetalol, levofloxacin, lidocaine, linezolid, lorazepam, magnesium sulfate, mannitol, melphalan, meperidine, meropenem, mesna, methadone, methotrexate, metoclopramide, metoprolol, metronidazole, midazolam, milrinone, mitomycin, mitoxantrone, morphine, moxifloxacin, mycophenolate, nafcillin, nalbuphine, nicardipine, nitroglycerin, nitroprusside, norepinephrine, octreotide, ondansetron, oxaliplatin, oxytocin, paclitaxel, palonosetron, pemetrexed, pentobarbital, phenobarbital, phentolamine, phenylephrine, piperacillin/tazobactam, potassium acetate, potassium chloride, procainamide, prochlorperazine, promethazine, propranolol, remifentanil, rituximab, rocuronium, sodium acetate, sodium phosphate, succinylcholine, sufentanil, tacrolimus, theophylline, thiotepa, tigecycline, tirofiban, tobramycin, topotecan, trastuzumab, trimethoprim/sulfamethoxazole, vasopressin, vecuronium, verapamil, vinblastine, vincristine, vinorelbine, voriconazole, zidovudine.

● **Y-Site Incompatibility:** amiodarone, amphotericin B deoxycholate, amphotericin B lipid complex, amphotericin B liposomal, carboplatin, ceftriaxone, chlorpromazine, dantrolene, diazepam, droperidol, epirubicin, foscarnet, gemtuzumab ozogamicin, methylprednisolone, minocycline, naloxone, pamidronate, pantoprazole, pentamidine, phenytoin, potassium phosphate, sodium bicarbonate, thiopental, vancomycin.

Patient/Family Teaching

- Explain purpose of medication to patient. Emphasize need to take exactly as ordered. Advise patient to contact health care professional if a dose is missed.
- Rep: Advise females of reproductive potential to notify health care professional if pregnancy is planned or suspected, or if breastfeeding.
- **Leucovorin Rescue:** Instruct patient to drink at least 3 liters of fluid each day during leucovorin rescue.
- **Folic Acid Deficiency:** Encourage patient to eat a diet high in folic acid (meat proteins; bran; dried beans; and green, leafy vegetables).

Evaluation/Desired Outcomes

- Reversal of bone marrow and GI toxicity in patients receiving methotrexate or in overdose of folic acid antagonists.
- Increased sense of well-being and increased production of normoblasts in patients with megaloblastic anemia.

leuprolide (loo-proe-lide)

Camcevi, Eligard, Fensolvi, ~~Lupron~~, Lupron Depot, Lupron Depot-Ped, ✹ Zeulide Depot

Classification

Therapeutic: antineoplastics
Pharmacologic: hormones, gonadotropin-releasing hormones

Indications

Advanced prostate cancer. Central precocious puberty. Endometriosis (as monotherapy or in combination with norethindrone). Uterine fibroids (in combination with iron).

Action

Acts as an agonist of gonadotropin releasing hormone (GnRH) receptors. Initially causes a transient increase in testosterone; however, with continuous administration, testosterone levels are decreased. Reduces gonadotropins, testosterone, and estradiol. **Therapeutic Effects:** Decreased testosterone levels and resultant decrease in spread of prostate cancer. Reduction of pain/lesions in endometriosis. Decreased growth of fibroids. Delayed puberty.

Pharmacokinetics

Absorption: Rapidly and almost completely absorbed following SUBQ administration. More slowly absorbed following IM administration of depot form.
Distribution: Unknown.
Metabolism and Excretion: Unknown.
Half-life: 3 hr.

TIME/ACTION PROFILE (effect on hormone levels)

ROUTE	ONSET†	PEAK‡	DURATION§
SUBQ	within 1st wk	2–4 wk	4–12 wk
IM	within 1st wk	2–4 wk	4–12 wk
IM-depot	within 1st wk	2–4 wk	4–12 wk

†Initial transient ↑ in testosterone and estradiol levels.
‡Maximum decline in testosterone and estradiol levels.
§Restoration of normal pituitary-gonadal function; in amenorrheic patients, normal menses usually returns 60–90 days after treatment is discontinued.

Contraindications/Precautions

Contraindicated in: Hypersensitivity to GnRH agonists; OB: Pregnancy; Lactation: Lactation.
Use Cautiously in: Hypersensitivity to benzyl alcohol (results in induration and erythema at SUBQ site); Congenital long QT syndrome, HF, electrolyte abnormalities, or concurrent use of other drugs known to prolong the QT interval; Seizures, cerebrovascular disorders, CNS tumor, or concurrent use of bupropion or SSRIs; Rep: Women of reproductive potential ; Pedi: Children <1 yr (safety and effectiveness not established).

Adverse Reactions/Side Effects

CV: angina, arrhythmias, MI; *Depot:* QT interval prolongation, vasodilation. **Derm:** hot flushing; *Depot:* hair growth, rash; *SUBQ:* dry skin, hair loss, pigmentation, skin cancer, skin lesions. **EENT:** blurred vision; *Depot:* epistaxis, throat nodules; *SUBQ:* hearing disorder. **Endo:** breast swelling, breast tenderness, hyperglycemia. **F and E:** hypercalcemia, lower extremity edema. **GI:** anorexia, diarrhea, dysphagia, nausea, vomiting; *Depot:* gingivitis, HEPATOTOXICITY; *SUBQ:* GI BLEEDING, hepatic impairment, peptic ulcer, rectal polyps. **GU:** ↓ fertility (males), ↓ libido, ↓ testicular size, dysuria, incontinence, testicular pain; *Depot:* cervix disorder; *SUBQ:* bladder spasm, penile swelling, prostate pain, urinary obstruction. **Local:** burning, itching, swelling at injection site. **Metab:** *Depot:* ↓ bone density, hyperuricemia. **MS:** fibromyalgia, transient ↑ in bone pain (prostate cancer only); *SUBQ:* ankylosing spondylitis, joint pain, pelvic fibrosis, temporal bone pain. **Neuro:** *SUBQ:* aggression, anger, anxiety, dizziness, dysgeusia, headache, impatience, intracranial hypertension (children), irritability, lethargy, memory disorder, mood swings, peripheral neuropathy, SEIZURES, STROKE, syncope; *Depot:* depression, drowsiness, intracranial hypertension (children), personality disorder. **Resp:** hemoptysis, PULMONARY EMBOLISM; *SUBQ:* cough, pleural rub, pulmonary fibrosis, pulmonary infiltrate. **Misc:** chills, fever; *Depot:* body odor.

Interactions

Drug-Drug: ↑ antineoplastic effects with **antiandrogens** (**megestrol, flutamide**). Concurrent use with **bupropion** or **SSRIs** may ↑ risk of seizures. **QT in-**

terval prolonging drugs may ↑ risk of QT interval prolongation.

Route/Dosage

Advanced Prostate Cancer

SUBQ (Adults): *Leuprolide acetate:* 1 mg/day; *Eligard:* 7.5 mg once monthly, 22.5 mg every 3 mo, 30 mg every 4 mo, or 45 mg every 6 mo. *Camcevi:* 42 mg every 6 mo.

IM (Adults): *Lupron Depot:* 7.5 mg once monthly *or* 22.5 mg every 3 mo *or* 30 mg every 4 mo *or* 45 mg every 6 mo.

Endometriosis

IM (Adults): *Lupron Depot:* 3.75 mg once monthly for up to 6 mo *or* 11.25 mg every 3 mo for up to 2 doses; if symptoms recur after initial course of therapy, may administer a 2nd course of therapy.

Uterine Fibroids

IM (Adults): *Lupron Depot:* 3.75 mg once monthly for up to 3 mo *or* 11.25 mg single injection.

Central Precocious Puberty

SUBQ (Children ≥2 yr): *Leuprolide acetate:* 50 mcg/kg/day, may ↑ by 10 mcg/kg/day as required. *Fensolvi:* 45 mg every 6 mo.

IM (Children ≥1 yr and >37.5 kg): *Lupron Depot-Ped (monthly formulation):* 15 mg every 4 wk; may ↑ by 3.75 mg every 4 wk as required.

IM (Children ≥1 yr and 26–37.5 kg): *Lupron Depot-Ped (monthly formulation):* 11.25 mg every 4 wk; may ↑ by 3.75 mg every 4 wk as required.

IM (Children ≥1 yr and ≤25 kg): *Lupron Depot-Ped (monthly formulation):* 7.5 mg every 4 wk; may ↑ by 3.75 mg every 4 wk as required.

IM (Children ≥1 yr): *Lupron Depot-Ped (3-month formulation)* 11.25 or 30 mg every 3 mo.

IM (Children ≥1 yr): *Lupron Depot-Ped (6-month formulation)* 45 mg every 6 mo.

Availability (generic available)

Emulsion for injection (Camcevi) (prefilled syringe): 42 mg. Lyophilized microspheres for depot injection (Lupron Depot): 3.75 mg, 7.5 mg, 11.25 mg, 22.5 mg, 30 mg, 45 mg. Lyophilized microspheres for depot injection (Lupron Depot-Ped): 7.5 mg, 11.25 mg, 15 mg, 30 mg, 45 mg. Lyophilized powder for injection (Fensolvi): 45 mg/vial. Polymeric matrix injectable formulation for injection (Eligard): 7.5 mg, 22.5 mg, 30 mg, 45 mg. Solution for injection (leuprolide acetate): 1 mg/0.2 mL.

NURSING IMPLICATIONS

Assessment

● Monitor ECG periodically in patients at risk for QT interval prolongation.
● **Prostate Cancer:** Assess for an increase in bone pain, especially during the first few wk of therapy. Monitor patients with vertebral metastases for in-

creased back pain and decreased sensory/motor function.
● Monitor intake and output ratios; assess for bladder distention in patients with urinary tract obstruction during initiation of therapy.
● **Fibroids:** Assess for severity of symptoms (bloating, pelvic pain, pressure, excessive vaginal bleeding) periodically during therapy.
● **Endometriosis:** Assess for endometrial pain prior to and periodically during therapy.
● **Central Precocious Puberty:** Prior to therapy, confirm diagnosis of central precocious puberty by onset of secondary sex characteristics in girls <8 yr or boys <9 yr; a complete physical and endocrinologic examination, including height, weight, hand and wrist x-ray; total sex steroid level (estradiol or testosterone); adrenal steroid level; beta human chorionic gonadotropin level; GnRH stimulation test; and computerized tomography of the head must be performed. These parameters are monitored after 1–2 mo and every 3–6 mo during therapy.
● Assess for signs of precocious puberty (menses, breast development, testicular growth) periodically during therapy. Dose is increased until no progression of the disease is noted either clinically or by lab test parameters, then usually maintained throughout therapy. Discontinuation of therapy should be considered before age 11 in girls and age 12 in boys.

Lab Test Considerations
● Verify negative pregnancy test before starting therapy. Initially ↑, then ↓ luteinizing hormone and follicle-stimulating hormone). This leads to castration levels of testosterone in boys 2–4 wk after initial increase in concentrations.
● Monitor testosterone, prostatic acid phosphate, and prostate-specific antigen levels to evaluate response to therapy. Transient ↑ in levels may occur during the 1st mo of therapy for prostate cancer.
● Monitor electrolytes before starting and periodically during therapy. May cause ↑ BUN, serum calcium, uric acid, hypoproteinemia, LDH, alkaline phosphatase, AST, hyperglycemia, hyperlipidemia, hyperphosphatemia, WBC, PT, or aPTT. May also cause ↓ platelets and serum potassium.
● Monitor blood sugar and A1c periodically during therapy.

Implementation

● Do not confuse Lupron Depot with Lupron Depot-Ped.
● Norethindrone acetate 5 mg daily may be used to prevent bone density loss from leuprolide.
● Correct electrolyte abnormalities before starting therapy.
● **SUBQ** *Camcevi:* **Must be administered by a health care professional. Allow prefilled syringe to stand at room temperature for 30 min before injection. Wear gloves during preparation and administration. Inject into**

upper- or mid-abdominal area with sufficient soft or loose SUBQ tissue that has not recently been used. Clean the injection site with an alcohol swab. Do NOT inject in areas with brawny or fibrous SUBQ tissue or locations that can be rubbed or compressed (with a belt or clothing waistband). Avoid applying heat directly to the site of injection. Pinch skin and inject at 90° angle, release skin and inject full contents of syringe. *Eligard SUBQ formulation:* Bring to room temperature before mixing. *Reconstitution:* Assemble the *Eligard* kit and reconstitute solution using syringes provided, as directed by manufacturer. Wearing gloves, mix in syringes as directed by manufacturer, do not shake. Solution must reach room temperature before administration and must be administered within 30 min of mixing, or discard. Solution is light tan to tan in color. Inject into abdomen, upper buttocks, or anywhere that has adequate amounts of SUBQ tissue without excessive pigment, nodules, lesions, or hair. Vary site with each injection. Store in refrigerator; may also be stored at room temperature in original packing for up to 8 wk before mixing. *Fensolvi:* Must be administered by a health care professional. Allow to reach room temperature before reconstitution. *Reconstitution:* Follow manufacturer's instructions for assembling syringes and mixing. *Concentration:* 45 mg/0.375 mL. Administer within 30 min or discard. Inject into abdomen or upper buttocks. Avoid areas that have excessive pigment, nodules, lesions, or hair. Pinch skin and inject at 90° angle. Release skin and inject slowly. Rotate injection sites.

- **IM:** Use syringe supplied by manufacturer. Rotate sites.
- Leuprolide depot is *only* for IM injection.
- *Lupron Depot formulation*and *Lupron Depot-Ped* must be administered by a health care professional. *Reconstitution:* To prepare for injection screw white plunger into end stopper until stopper begins to turn. Hold syringe upright; release diluent by slowly pushing, over 6–8 sec, until the first stopper is at the blue line in the middle of the barrel. Keep syringe upright. Mix microspheres by shaking syringe until power forms a unified suspension. Tap syringe if caking or clumping occurs. Do not combine syringes or partial syringes to arrive at a dose of *Lupron Depot-Ped.* Suspension will appear milky. Do not use if powder does not go into suspension. Keep syringe upright, remove cap and expel air. Inject at 90° angle in gluteal area, anterior thigh, or deltoid, aspirate and discard if blood in syringe. Suspension settles very quickly; mix and administer immediately. Administer within 2 hr or discard. Rotate injection sites.

Patient/Family Teaching
- Explain purpose of leuprolide to patient.
- Advise patient that medication may cause hot flashes. Notify health care professional if these become bothersome.
- Leuprolide depot usually causes a temporary discontinuation of menstruation. Advise patient to notify health care professional if menstruation persists or if intermittent bleeding occurs.
- Inform patient of the possibility of the development or worsening of depression and occurrence of memory disorders.
- Rep: May cause fetal harm. Advise females of reproductive potential to use effective contraception during therapy. Advise patient to notify health care professional if pregnancy is planned or suspected or if breastfeeding. Advise patient that leuprolide may impair fertility.
- **Prostate Cancer:** Instruct patient and family on SUBQ injection technique. Review patient insert provided with leuprolide patient-administration kit.
- Instruct patient to take medication exactly as directed. Take missed doses as soon as remembered unless not remembered until next day.
- Inform patient that bone pain may increase at initiation of therapy, but will resolve with time. Advise patient to discuss use of analgesics to control pain with health care professional.
- Instruct patient to notify health care professional promptly if difficulty urinating, weakness, or numbness occurs.
- **Endometriosis:** Advise patient to use a form of contraception other than oral contraceptives during therapy. Inform patient that amenorrhea is expected but does not guarantee contraception. Advise patient that breastfeeding should be avoided during therapy.
- **Central Precocious Puberty:** Instruct patient and family on the proper technique for SUBQ injection. Emphasize the importance of administering the medication at the same time each day. Rotate injection sites periodically.
- Inform patient and parents that if injections are not given daily, pubertal process may be reactivated.
- Advise patient and parents that during the first 2 mo of therapy patient may experience a light menstrual flow or spotting. Health care professional should be notified if this continues beyond 2nd mo.
- Instruct patient and parents to notify health care professional immediately if irritation at the injection site or unusual signs or symptoms occur.

Evaluation/Desired Outcomes
- Decrease in the spread of prostate cancer.
- Decrease in lesions and pain in endometriosis.
- Resolution of the signs of central precocious puberty.
- Improvement in preoperative hematologic parameters in patients with anemia from uterine fibroids.

levalbuterol (lev-al-**byoo**-ter-ole)
Xopenex, Xopenex HFA
Classification
Therapeutic: bronchodilators
Pharmacologic: adrenergics

Indications
Bronchospasm due to reversible airway disease (short-term control agent).

Action
R-enantiomer of racemic albuterol. Binds to beta-2 adrenergic receptors in airway smooth muscle leading to activation of adenylcyclase and increased levels of cyclic-3′, 5′-adenosine monophosphate (cAMP). Increases in cAMP activate kinases, which inhibit the phosphorylation of myosin and decrease intracellular calcium. Decreased intracellular calcium relaxes bronchial smooth muscle. **Therapeutic Effects:** Relaxation of airway smooth muscle with subsequent bronchodilation. Relatively selective for beta-2 (pulmonary) receptors.

Pharmacokinetics
Absorption: Some absorption occurs following inhalation.
Distribution: Unknown.
Metabolism and Excretion: Metabolized in the liver to an inactive sulfate; 3–6% excreted unchanged in the urine.
Half-life: 3.3–4 hr.

TIME/ACTION PROFILE (bronchodilation)

ROUTE	ONSET	PEAK	DURATION
Inhaln	10–17 min	90 min	5–6 hr

Contraindications/Precautions
Contraindicated in: Hypersensitivity to levalbuterol or albuterol.
Use Cautiously in: Cardiovascular disorders (including coronary insufficiency, hypertension, and arrhythmias); History of seizures; Hypokalemia; Hyperthyroidism; Diabetes mellitus; Unusual sensitivity to adrenergic amines; OB: Safety not established in pregnancy; Lactation: Use while breastfeeding only if potential maternal benefit justifies potential risk to infant; Pedi: Safety and effectiveness not established in children <6 yr (nebulized solution) or <4 yr (metered-dose inhaler).
Exercise Extreme Caution in: Concurrent use or use within 2 wk of **tricyclic antidepressants** or **MAO inhibitors** may ↑ risk of adverse cardiovascular reactions.

Adverse Reactions/Side Effects
CV: tachycardia. **EENT:** turbinate edema. **Endo:** hyperglycemia. **F and E:** hypokalemia. **GI:** dyspepsia, vomiting. **Neuro:** anxiety, dizziness, headache, nervousness, tremor. **Resp:** cough, PARADOXICAL BRONCHOSPASM (excessive use of inhalers).

Interactions
Drug-Drug: Concurrent use or use within 2 wk of **tricyclic antidepressants** or **MAO inhibitors** may ↑ risk of adverse cardiovascular reactions (use with extreme caution). **Beta blockers** block the beneficial pulmonary effects of adrenergic bronchodilators; choose cardioselective beta blockers if necessary and with caution. May ↑ risk of hypokalemia from **thiazide diuretics** and **loop diuretics**. May ↓ **digoxin** levels. May ↑ risk of arrhythmias with **hydrocarbon inhalation anesthetics** or **cocaine**.
Drug-Natural Products: Use with caffeine-containing herbs (**guarana**, **tea**, **coffee**) ↑ stimulant effect.

Route/Dosage
Inhaln (Adults and Children ≥4 yr): 2 inhalations every 4–6 hr; some patients may respond to 1 inhalation every 4 hr.
Inhaln (Adults and Children >12 yr): 0.63 mg via nebulization 3 times daily (every 6–8 hr); may be ↑ to 1.25 mg 3 times daily (every 6–8 hr).
Inhaln (Children 6–11 yr): 0.31 mg via nebulization 3 times daily (not to exceed 0.63 mg 3 times daily).

Availability (generic available)
Inhalation aerosol: 45 mcg/actuation in 15-g canisters (200 metered actuations). **Inhalation solution:** 0.31 mg/3 mL, 0.63 mg/3 mL, 1.25 mg/3 mL, 1.25 mg/0.5 mL.

NURSING IMPLICATIONS
Assessment
- Assess lung sounds, pulse, and BP before administration and during peak of medication. Note amount, color, and character of sputum produced. Closely monitor patients on higher dose for adverse effects.
- Monitor pulmonary function tests before initiating therapy and periodically during course to determine effectiveness of medication.
- Observe for paradoxical bronchospasm (wheezing, dyspnea, tightness in chest). If condition occurs, withhold medication and notify health care provider immediately.

Lab Test Considerations
- May cause ↑ serum glucose and ↓ serum potassium.

Implementation
- **Inhaln:** Allow at least 1 min between inhalations of aerosol medication.
- For nebulization, levalbuterol solution does not require dilution prior to administration. Once the foil pouch is opened, vials must be used within 2 wk; open vials may be stored for 1 wk. Discard vial if solution is not clear or colorless.

Patient/Family Teaching
- Instruct patient in the proper use of inhalation aerosol nebulizer (see Appendix C) and to take levalbuterol as directed. Caution patient not to exceed rec-

ommended dose; may cause adverse effects, paradoxical bronchospasm, or loss of effectiveness of medication.

- Instruct patient to notify health care professional of all Rx or OTC medications, vitamins, or herbal products being taken and to consult health care professional before taking any OTC medications or alcoholic beverages concurrently with this therapy. Caution patient also to avoid smoking and other respiratory irritants.
- Instruct patient to contact health care professional immediately if shortness of breath is not relieved by medication or is accompanied by diaphoresis, dizziness, palpitations, or chest pain.
- Advise patients to use levalbuterol first if using other inhalation medications, and allow 5 min to elapse before administering other inhalant medications unless otherwise directed.
- Advise patient to rinse mouth with water after each inhalation dose to minimize dry mouth.
- Rep: Advise females of reproductive potential to notify health care professional if pregnancy is planned or suspected, or if breastfeeding. Encourage women who become pregnant while taking levalbuterol to enroll in the Asthma & Pregnancy Study to monitor pregnancy outcomes in women exposed to asthma medications by calling 1-877-311-8972 or visiting www.mothertobaby.org/ongoing-study/asthma.
- Instruct patient to notify health care professional if no response to the usual dose of levalbuterol.

Evaluation/Desired Outcomes

- Prevention or relief of bronchospasm.

levETIRAcetam

(le-ve-teer-**a**-se-tam)

Elepsia XR, Keppra, Keppra XR, Roweepra, Spritam

Classification

Therapeutic: anticonvulsants
Pharmacologic: pyrrolidines

Indications

Partial onset seizures (as monotherapy or adjunctive therapy). Primary generalized tonic-clonic seizures (adjunct) (immediate-release and injection only). Myoclonic seizures in patients with juvenile myoclonic epilepsy (adjunct) (immediate-release and injection only). **Unlabeled Use:** Status epilepticus.

Action

Appears to inhibit burst firing without affecting normal neuronal excitability and may selectively prevent hypersynchronization of epileptiform burst firing and propagation of seizure activity. **Therapeutic Effects:** Decreased incidence and severity of seizures.

Pharmacokinetics

Absorption: Rapidly and completely absorbed following oral administration. IV administration results in complete bioavailability.

Distribution: Well distributed to tissues.

Metabolism and Excretion: 66% excreted unchanged by the kidneys; some metabolism by the liver (metabolites inactive).

Half-life: 7.1 hr (↑ in renal impairment).

TIME/ACTION PROFILE (plasma concentrations)

ROUTE	ONSET	PEAK	DURATION
PO	rapid	1–1.5 hr†‡	12 hr
IV	rapid	end of infusion	unknown

†1 hr in the fasting state, 1.5 hr when taken with food.
‡4 hr with extended-release.

Contraindications/Precautions

Contraindicated in: Hypersensitivity.

Use Cautiously in: All patients (may ↑ risk of suicidal thoughts/behaviors); Renal impairment (dose ↓ recommended if CCr ≤80 mL/min); OB: Use during pregnancy only if potential maternal benefit justifies potential fetal risk; blood levels may be ↓ during pregnancy (especially during 3rd trimester); Lactation: Safety not established in breastfeeding; Pedi: Safety and effectiveness not established in children <1 mo (immediate-release tablets, tablets for oral suspension, oral solution, and injection), <12 yr (extended-release tablets); Geri: Older adults may have ↓ renal elimination (dose ↓ may be necessary).

Adverse Reactions/Side Effects

CV: <u>hypertension</u>. **Derm:** DRUG REACTION WITH EOSINOPHILIA AND SYSTEMIC SYMPTOMS (DRESS), STEVENS-JOHNSON SYNDROME (SJS), TOXIC EPIDERMAL NECROLYSIS. **Hemat:** AGRANULOCYTOSIS, anemia, eosinophilia, neutropenia, thrombocytopenia. **Neuro:** <u>aggression</u>, <u>agitation</u>, <u>anger</u>, <u>anxiety</u>, <u>apathy</u>, <u>depersonalization</u>, <u>depression</u>, <u>dizziness</u>, <u>drowsiness</u>, <u>fatigue</u>, <u>hostility</u>, <u>irritability</u>, personality disorder, psychosis, weakness, coordination difficulties (adults only), hyperkinesia, SUICIDAL THOUGHTS. **Misc:** HYPERSENSITIVITY REACTIONS (including anaphylaxis and angioedema).

Interactions

Drug-Drug: None reported.

Route/Dosage

Only the oral solution should be used in patients ≤20 kg.

Partial Onset Seizures

PO, IV (Adults and Children ≥16 yr): 500 mg twice daily initially; may ↑ by 1000 mg/day at 2-wk intervals up to 3000 mg/day in 2 divided doses.

PO (Adults and Children 4–15 yr): *Oral solution:* 10 mg/kg twice daily; ↑ by 20 mg/kg/day at 2-wk intervals to recommended dose of 30 mg/kg twice daily (not to exceed 1500 mg twice daily). *Immediate-release tablets or tablets for oral suspension (for patients >40 kg):* 500 mg twice daily; may ↑ by 1000 mg/day at 2-wk intervals up to 3000 mg/day in 2 divided doses. *Immediate-release tablets or tablets for oral suspension (for patients 20–40 kg):* 250 mg twice daily; may ↑ by 500 mg/day at 2-wk intervals up to 1500 mg/day in 2 divided doses.

PO (Adults and Children ≥12 yr and ≤50 kg): *Extended-release:* 1000 mg once daily; may ↑ by 1000 mg/day at 2-wk intervals up to 3000 mg once daily.

IV (Children 4–15 yr): 10 mg/kg twice daily; ↑ by 20 mg/kg/day at 2-wk intervals to recommended dose of 30 mg/kg twice daily (not to exceed 1500 mg twice daily).

PO, IV (Children 6 mo–3 yr): 10 mg/kg twice daily; ↑ by 20 mg/kg/day at 2-wk intervals to recommended dose of 25 mg/kg twice daily.

PO, IV (Children 1–5 mo): 7 mg/kg twice daily; ↑ by 14 mg/kg/day at 2-wk intervals to recommended dose of 21 mg/kg twice daily.

Renal Impairment

PO, IV (Adults): *CCr 50–80 mL/min:* 500–1000 mg twice daily (1000–2000 mg once daily for extended-release); *CCr 30–50 mL/min:* 250–750 mg twice daily (500–1500 mg once daily for extended-release); *CCr <30 mL/min:* 250–500 mg twice daily (500–1000 mg once daily for extended-release); *Dialysis (immediate-release and injection):* 500–1000 mg once daily with a 250–500-mg supplemental dose after dialysis.

Primary Generalized Tonic-Clonic Seizures

PO, IV (Adults and Children ≥16 yr): 500 mg twice daily initially; ↑ by 1000 mg/day at 2-wk intervals to recommended dose of 3000 mg/day.

PO (Adults and Children ≥6 yr and >40 kg): *Tablets for oral suspension:* 500 mg twice daily; may ↑ by 1000 mg/day at 2-wk intervals up to 3000 mg/day in 2 divided doses.

PO, IV (Children 6–15 yr): 10 mg/kg twice daily; ↑ by 20 mg/kg/day at 2-wk intervals to recommended dose of 30 mg/kg twice daily.

PO (Children ≥6 yr and 20–40 kg): *Tablets for oral suspension:* 250 mg twice daily; may ↑ by 500 mg/day at 2-wk intervals up to 1500 mg/day in 2 divided doses.

Renal Impairment

PO, IV (Adults): *CCr 50–80 mL/min (immediate release and injection):* 500–1000 mg twice daily; *CCr 30–50 mL/min (immediate release and injection):* 250–750 mg twice daily; *CCr <30 mL/min (immediate release and injection):* 250–500 mg twice daily; *Dialysis (immediate-release and injection):* 500–1000 mg once daily with a 250–500-mg supplemental dose after dialysis.

Myoclonic Seizures

PO, IV (Adults and Children ≥12 yr): 500 mg twice daily initially; ↑ by 1000 mg/day at 2-wk intervals to recommended dose of 3000 mg/day (in 2 divided doses).

Renal Impairment

PO, IV (Adults): *CCr 50–80 mL/min (immediate release and injection):* 500–1000 mg twice daily; *CCr 30–50 mL/min (immediate release and injection):* 250–750 mg twice daily; *CCr <30 mL/min (immediate release and injection):* 250–500 mg twice daily; *Dialysis (immediate-release and injection):* 500–1000 mg once daily with a 250–500-mg supplemental dose after dialysis.

Status Epilepticus

IV (Infants and Children <16 yr): 50 mg/kg as a loading dose followed by maintenance dose of 30–55 mg/kg/day IV/PO in 2 divided doses.

IV (Neonates): 20–30 mg/kg as a loading dose followed by neonatal seizure dosing.

Availability (generic available)

Immediate-release tablets: 250 mg, 500 mg, 750 mg, 1000 mg. **Extended-release tablets:** 500 mg, 750 mg, 1000 mg, 1500 mg. **Oral solution (grape-flavored):** 100 mg/mL. **Tablets for oral suspension (Spritam) (spearmint-flavored):** 250 mg, 500 mg, 750 mg, 1000 mg. **Premixed infusion:** 250 mg/50 mL 0.82% NaCl, 500 mg/100 mL 0.82% NaCl, 1000 mg/100 mL 0.75% NaCl, 1500 mg/100 mL 0.54% NaCl. **Solution for injection (requires dilution):** 100 mg/mL.

NURSING IMPLICATIONS

Assessment

- Assess location, duration, and characteristics of seizure activity.
- Assess patient for CNS adverse effects during therapy. Adverse effects are categorized as somnolence and fatigue (asthenia), coordination difficulties (ataxia, abnormal gait, or incoordination), and behavioral abnormalities (agitation, hostility, anxiety, apathy, emotional lability, depersonalization, depression) and usually occur during the first 4 wk of therapy.
- Monitor mood changes. Assess for suicidal tendencies, especially during early therapy. Restrict amount of drug available to patient.
- Assess for rash periodically during therapy. May cause SJS. Discontinue therapy if severe or if accompanied with fever, general malaise, fatigue, muscle or joint aches, blisters, oral lesions, conjunctivitis, hepatitis, and/or eosinophilia.
- Monitor for signs and symptoms of DRESS (fever, rash, lymphadenopathy, and/or facial swelling, associated with involvement of other organ systems (hepatitis, nephritis, hematologic abnormalities, myocarditis, myositis) during therapy. May resemble an acute viral infection. Eosinophilia is often present. Discontinue therapy if signs occur.

- Monitor for signs and symptoms of anaphylaxis (dyspnea, wheezing, facial swelling). Discontinue levetiracetam if symptoms occur.
- Pedi: Monitor patients 1 mo to <4 yr of age for increases in diastolic BP.

Lab Test Considerations
- May cause ↓ RBC and WBC and abnormal liver function tests.

Implementation

- Do not confuse Keppra with Kaletra. Do not confuse levetiracetam with lamotrigine, levocarnitine, or levofloxacin.
- IV doses should be used temporarily when oral route is not feasible. To convert IV to PO, equivalent dose and frequency may be used.
- PO: May be administered without regard to meals.
- *DNC:* Administer tablets whole; do not administer partial tablets. Do not break, crush, or chew XR tablets.
- *Tablets for oral suspension (Spritam)* can be administered by placing tablet on tongue with a dry hand, follow with a sip of liquid and swallow only after tablet disintegrates; do not swallow tablet intact. Do not administer partial tablets. *Spritam* disintegrates in about 11 seconds in the mouth when taken with a sip of liquid. May also add whole tablet to a small volume of liquid in a cup (one tablespoon or enough to cover tablets). Allow the tablet to disperse before consuming the entire contents immediately. After administration of suspension, resuspend any residue by adding an additional small volume of liquid and swallow the full amount. Do not administer partial quantities of dispersed tablets. Peel foil to access tablet, do not push through foil.
- Pedi: Patients <20 kg should receive oral solution. Administer with calibrated measuring device for accurate dose.
- Discontinue gradually to minimize the risk of increase in seizure frequency.

IV Administration
- **Intermittent Infusion:** *Dilution:* Dilute dose in 100 mL of 0.9% NaCl, D5W, or LR. If a smaller volume is required (e.g. pediatric patients), concentration should not exceed 15 mg/mL. Do not administer solutions that are cloudy or contain particulate matter. *Rate:* Infuse over 15 min.
- **Y-Site Compatibility:** diazepam, lorazepam, valproate.

Patient/Family Teaching

- Instruct patient to take medication as directed. Pedi: Explain to parents the importance of using calibrated measuring device for accurate dosing. Take missed doses as soon as possible unless almost time for next dose. Do not double doses. Do not discontinue abruptly; may cause increase in frequency of

seizures. Advise patient and parents to read the *Medication Guide* prior to starting therapy and with each Rx refill in case of changes.
- May cause dizziness and somnolence. Caution patient to avoid driving or activities requiring alertness until response to medication is known. Do not resume driving until physician gives clearance based on control of seizure disorder.
- Advise patient and family to notify health care professional if thoughts about suicide or dying, attempts to commit suicide; new or worse depression; new or worse anxiety; feeling very agitated or restless; panic attacks; trouble sleeping; new or worse irritability; acting aggressive; being angry or violent; acting on dangerous impulses; an extreme increase in activity and talking; other unusual changes in behavior or mood, or if skin rash occur.
- Advise patient to notify health care professional of all Rx or OTC medications, vitamins, or herbal products being taken and to consult with health care professional before taking other medications.
- Instruct patient to notify health care professional of medication regimen prior to treatment or surgery.
- Rep: Advise females of reproductive potential to notify health care professional if pregnancy is planned or suspected or if breastfeeding. Encourage pregnant patients to enroll in the North American Antiepileptic Drug Pregnancy Registry by calling 1-888-233-2334; information is available at www.aedpregnancyregistry.org. Levetiracetam levels may decrease during pregnancy, especially in the 3rd trimester. Dose adjustments may be necessary to maintain clinical response.
- Advise patient to carry identification describing disease process and medication regimen at all times.

Evaluation/Desired Outcomes

- Decrease in the frequency of or cessation of seizures.

---

levocetirizine
(lee-vo-se-**teer**-i-zeen)
~~Xyzal~~, Xyzal Allergy 24HR
Classification
Therapeutic: allergy, cold, and cough remedies
Pharmacologic: antihistamines

Indications
Seasonal/perennial allergic rhinitis. Chronic idiopathic urticaria.

Action
Antagonizes the effects of histamine at H_1 receptor sites; does not bind to or inactivate histamine. **Therapeutic Effects:** Decreased symptoms of histamine excess (rhinitis, itching).

Pharmacokinetics

Absorption: Well absorbed following oral administration.

Distribution: Unknown.

Metabolism and Excretion: Excreted mostly unchanged by the kidneys (85%).

Half-life: 8 hr.

TIME/ACTION PROFILE

ROUTE	ONSET	PEAK	DURATION
PO	rapid	0.9 hr	24 hr

Contraindications/Precautions

Contraindicated in: Hypersensitivity to levocetirizine or cetirizine; Severe renal impairment (CCr <10 mL/min).

Use Cautiously in: OB: Other 2nd-generation antihistamines preferred in pregnancy; Lactation: Other 2nd-generation antihistamines preferred in breastfeeding; Pedi: Children <6 mo (safety and effectiveness not established); Geri: Consider age related ↓ in renal function and concurrent disease states in older adults.

Adverse Reactions/Side Effects

Derm: acute generalized exanthematous pustulosis. **GI:** dry mouth. **GU:** urinary retention. **Neuro:** drowsiness, fatigue, weakness.

Interactions

Drug-Drug: ↑ levels of **ritonavir**. ↑ CNS depression may occur with **alcohol, opioid analgesics,** or **sedative hypnotics**.

Route/Dosage

PO (Adults and Children ≥12 yr): 5 mg once daily in the evening; some patients may respond to 2.5 mg once daily.

PO (Children 6–11 yr): 2.5 mg once daily in the evening.

PO (Children 6 mo–5 yr): 1.25 mg (oral solution) once daily in the evening.

Renal Impairment

(Adults and Children ≥12 yr): *CCr 50–80 mL/min:* 2.5 mg once daily; *CCr 30–50 mL/min:* 2.5 mg every other day; *CCr 10–30 mL/min:* 2.5 mg twice weekly (every 3–4 days).

Availability (generic available)

Tablets: 5 mg ^{OTC}. **Oral solution (tutti-frutti, grape, and bubble gum flavors):** 2.5 mg/5 mL^{OTC}.

NURSING IMPLICATIONS

Assessment

- Assess allergy symptoms (rhinitis, conjunctivitis, hives) before and periodically during therapy.
- Assess lung sounds and character of bronchial secretions. Maintain fluid intake of 1500–2000 mL/day to decrease viscosity of secretions.

Lab Test Considerations

- May cause false-negative result in allergy skin testing.
- May cause transient ↑ in serum bilirubin and transaminases.

Implementation

- **PO:** Administer once daily in the evening without regard to food. Oral solution is clear and colorless; administer undiluted.

Patient/Family Teaching

- Instruct patient to take medication as directed. Do not increase doses; may cause increased drowsiness.
- May cause drowsiness. Caution patient to avoid driving or other activities requiring alertness until response to medication is known.
- Advise patient to avoid taking alcohol or other CNS depressants concurrently with this drug.
- Advise patient that good oral hygiene, frequent rinsing of mouth with water, and sugarless gum or candy may minimize dry mouth. Patient should notify dentist if dry mouth persists >2 wk.
- Rep: Advise females of reproductive potential to notify health care professional if pregnancy is planned or suspected or if breastfeeding.

Evaluation/Desired Outcomes

- Decrease in allergic symptoms.
- Resolution of uncomplicated skin manifestations of chronic idiopathic urticaria.

levofloxacin, See FLUOROQUINOLONES.

levonorgestrel, See CONTRACEPTIVES, HORMONAL.

levothyroxine
(lee-voe-thye-**rox**-een)

✦ Eltroxin, Ermeza, Euthyrox, Levo-T, Levoxyl, Synthroid, Thyquidity, Tirosint, Tirosint-SOL, Unithroid

Classification
Therapeutic: hormones
Pharmacologic: thyroid preparations

Indications

Thyroid supplementation in hypothyroidism. Treatment or suppression of euthyroid goiters. Adjunctive treatment for thyrotropin-dependent thyroid cancer.

Action

Synthetic form of thyroxine (T$_4$). Replacement of or supplementation to endogenous thyroid hormones.

Principal effect is increasing metabolic rate of body tissues: Promote gluconeogenesis, Increase utilization and mobilization of glycogen stores, Stimulate protein synthesis, Promote cell growth and differentiation, Aid in the development of the brain and CNS. **Therapeutic Effects:** Replacement in hypothyroidism to restore normal hormonal balance. Suppression of thyroid cancer.

Pharmacokinetics

Absorption: Levothyroxine is variably (40–80%) absorbed from the GI tract.
Distribution: Distributed into most body tissues. Thyroid hormones do not readily cross the placenta; minimal amounts enter breast milk.
Protein Binding: >99%.
Metabolism and Excretion: Metabolized by the liver and other tissues to active T3. Thyroid hormone undergoes enterohepatic recirculation and is excreted in the feces via the bile.
Half-life: 6–7 days.

TIME/ACTION PROFILE

ROUTE	ONSET	PEAK	DURATION
PO	unknown	1–3 wk	1–3 wk
IV	6–8 hr	24 hr	unknown

Contraindications/Precautions

Contraindicated in: Hypersensitivity; Recent MI; Hyperthyroidism.
Use Cautiously in: Cardiovascular disease (initiate therapy with lower doses); Severe renal impairment; Uncorrected adrenocortical disorders; Pedi: Monitor neonates and infants for cardiac overload, arrhythmias, and aspiration during first 2 wk of therapy; Geri: Older adults are extremely sensitive to thyroid hormones; initial dose should be ↓.

Adverse Reactions/Side Effects

Usually only seen when excessive doses cause iatrogenic hyperthyroidism.
CV: angina, arrhythmias, tachycardia. **Derm:** sweating. **Endo:** heat intolerance, hyperthyroidism, menstrual irregularities. **GI:** abdominal cramps, diarrhea, vomiting. **Metab:** weight loss. **MS:** accelerated bone maturation in children. **Neuro:** headache, insomnia, irritability.

Interactions

Drug-Drug: Cholestyramine, colesevelam, colestipol, and **sodium polystyrene sulfonate** may bind to and ↓ absorption of orally administered levothyroxine; administer levothyroxine ≥4 hr prior to these medications or monitor TSH levels. **Phosphate binders,** including **calcium carbonate, ferrous sulfate, lanthanum carbonate,** and **sevelemer** may bind to and ↓ absorption of orally administered levothyroxine; administer levothyroxine ≥4 hr apart from these medications. Absorption may be ↓ by **orlistat,**

proton pump inhibitors, sucralfate, antacids, and **simethicone. Phenobarbital** and **rifampin** may ↑ metabolism of and ↓ efficacy of levothyroxine; may need to ↑ levothyroxine dosage. May ↑ the effects of **warfarin.** May ↑ requirement for **insulin** or **oral hypoglycemic agents** in diabetics. May ↓ the therapeutic effects of **digoxin**; may need to ↑ digoxin dosage. Concurrent use with **ketamine** may lead to significant hypertension and tachycardia. ↑ cardiovascular effects with **adrenergics** (sympathomimetics).
Drug-Food: Foods or supplements containing calcium, iron, magnesium, or zinc may bind levothyroxine and prevent complete absorption. Absorption may be delayed when used with **grapefruit juice.**

Route/Dosage

PO (Adults): *Hypothyroidism:* 1.6 mcg/kg once daily; may ↑ by 12.5–25 mcg/day every 4–6 wk until patient clinically euthyroid based on signs/symptoms and TSH levels.
PO (Geriatric Patients and Patients with Cardiac Disease): 12.5–25 mcg once daily; may ↑ by 12.5–25 mcg/day every 6–8 wk until patient clinically euthyroid based on signs/symptoms and TSH levels.
PO (Children >12 yr): 2–3 mcg/kg/day (≥150 mcg/day).
PO (Children 6–12 yr): 4–5 mcg/kg/day (100–125 mcg/day).
PO (Children 1–5 yr): 5–6 mcg/kg/day (75–100 mcg/day).
PO (Children 6–12 mo): 6–8 mcg/kg/day (50–75 mcg/day).
PO (Infants 3–6 mo): 8–10 mcg/kg/day (25–50 mcg/day).
PO (Infants 0–3 mo or Infants at Risk for Cardiac Failure): 10–15 mcg/kg/day or 25 mcg/day; may be ↑ after 4–6 wk to 50 mcg.
IM, IV (Adults): *Hypothyroidism:* 50–100 mcg/day as a single dose. *Myxedema coma/stupor:* 300–500 mcg IV; additional 100–300 mcg may be given on 2nd day, followed by daily administration of smaller doses.
IM, IV (Children): *Hypothyroidism:* 50–80% of the oral dose.

Availability (generic available)

Tablets: 25 mcg, 50 mcg, 75 mcg, 88 mcg, 100 mcg, 112 mcg, 125 mcg, 137 mcg, 150 mcg, 175 mcg, 200 mcg, 300 mcg. **Capsules (Tirosint):** 13 mcg, 25 mcg, 50 mcg, 75 mcg, 88 mcg, 100 mcg, 112 mcg, 125 mcg, 137 mcg, 150 mcg, 175 mcg, 200 mcg. **Oral solution:** 13 mcg/mL, 20 mcg/mL, 25 mcg/mL, 50 mcg/mL, 75 mcg/mL, 88 mcg/mL, 100 mcg/mL, 112 mcg/mL, 125 mcg/mL, 137 mcg/mL, 150 mcg/mL, 175 mcg/mL, 200 mcg/mL. **Powder for injection:** 100 mcg/vial, 200 mcg/vial, 500 mcg/vial. **Solution for injection:** 20 mcg/mL, 40 mcg/mL, 100 mcg/mL.

NURSING IMPLICATIONS
Assessment
- Assess apical pulse and BP prior to and periodically during therapy. Assess for tachyarrhythmias and chest pain.
- **Children:** Monitor height, weight, and psychomotor development.

Lab Test Considerations
- Monitor thyroid function studies prior to and during therapy. Monitor thyroid-stimulating hormone (TSH) serum levels in adults 6–8 wk after change in dose or changing from one brand to another in adults. For pediatric patients, monitor TSH and total or free-T4 in children 2 and 4 wk after start of therapy, 2 wk after any change in dose, and then every 3–12 mo thereafter after dose stabilization until growth is completed.
- Monitor blood and urine glucose in diabetic patients. Insulin or oral hypoglycemic dose may need to be increased.

Toxicity and Overdose
- Overdose is manifested as hyperthyroidism (tachycardia, chest pain, nervousness, insomnia, diaphoresis, tremors, weight loss). Usual treatment is to withhold dose for 2–6 days then resume at a lower dose. Acute overdose is treated by induction of emesis or gastric lavage, followed by activated charcoal. Sympathetic overstimulation may be controlled by antiadrenergic drugs (beta blockers), such as propranolol. Oxygen and supportive measures to control symptoms are also used.

Implementation
- **High Alert:** Do not confuse levothyroxine with lamotrigine, Lanoxin, or liothyronine.
- **PO:** Administer with a full glass of water, on an empty stomach, 30–60 min before breakfast, to prevent insomnia.
- Initial dose is low, especially in geriatric and cardiac patients. Dose is increased gradually, based on thyroid function tests.
- For patients with difficulty swallowing, tablets can be crushed and placed in 5–10 mL of water and administered immediately via dropper or spoon; do not store suspension.

IV Administration
- **IV Push: *Reconstitution:*** Reconstitute the 200-mcg and 500-mcg vials with 2 or 5 mL, respectively, of 0.9% NaCl without preservatives (diluent usually provided). ***Concentration:*** 100 mcg/mL. Shake well to dissolve completely. Administer solution immediately after preparation; discard unused portion. *Rate:* Administer at a rate of 100 mcg over 1 min. Do not add to IV infusions; may be administered through Y-tubing.
- **Y-Site Incompatibility:** Do not admix with other IV solutions.

Patient/Family Teaching
- Instruct patient to take medication as directed at the same time each day. Take missed doses as soon as remembered unless almost time for next dose. If more than 2–3 doses are missed, notify health care professional. Do not discontinue without consulting health care professional.
- Explain to patient that medication does not cure hypothyroidism; it provides a thyroid hormone supplement. Therapy is lifelong.
- Advise patient to notify health care professional if headache, nervousness, diarrhea, excessive sweating, heat intolerance, chest pain, increased pulse rate, palpitations, weight loss >2 lb/wk, or any unusual symptoms occur.
- Caution patient to avoid taking other medications concurrently with thyroid preparations unless instructed by health care professional. Advise patient to take 4 hrs apart from antacids, iron, and calcium supplements.
- Instruct patient to inform health care professionals of thyroid therapy.
- Rep: Advise females of reproductive potential to notify health care professional if pregnancy is planned or suspected, or if breastfeeding. Pregnancy may increase thyroid requirements. Monitor serum TSH levels and adjust levothyroxine dose accordingly during pregnancy. Since postpartum TSH levels are similar to preconception values, levothyroxine dose should return to pre-pregnancy dose immediately after delivery.
- Emphasize importance of follow-up exams to monitor effectiveness of therapy. Thyroid function tests are performed at least yearly.
- Pedi: Discuss with parents the need for routine follow-up studies to ensure correct development. Inform patient that partial hair loss may be experienced by children on thyroid therapy. This is usually temporary.

Evaluation/Desired Outcomes
- Resolution of symptoms of hypothyroidism and normalization of hormone levels.

HIGH ALERT

LIDOCAINE
lidocaine (parenteral)
(lye-doe-kane)
Xylocaine, ✤ Xylocard
lidocaine (local anesthetic)
Xylocaine
lidocaine (mucosal)
✤ Jampocaine Viscous, Xylocaine Viscous
lidocaine (topical)
✤ Betacaine, ✤ Cathejell, Glydo, ✤ Lidodan, Lidoderm, L-M-X 4, L-M-X 5, ✤ Lyracaine, ✤ Maxilene,

✤Stallion, ✤Topicaine, Xylocaine, ZTLido

Classification
Therapeutic: anesthetics (topical/local), antiarrhythmics (class IB)

Indications
IV: Ventricular arrhythmias. **Local:** Infiltration/mucosal/topical anesthetic. **Topical:** Pain due to post-herpetic neuralgia.

Action
IV: Suppresses automaticity and spontaneous depolarization of the ventricles during diastole by altering the flux of sodium ions across cell membranes with little or no effect on heart rate. **Local:** Produces local anesthesia by inhibiting transport of ions across neuronal membranes, thereby preventing initiation and conduction of normal nerve impulses. **Therapeutic Effects:** Control of ventricular arrhythmias. Local anesthesia.

Pharmacokinetics
Absorption: IV administration results in complete bioavailability; some absorption follows local use.
Distribution: Widely distributed. Concentrates in adipose tissue. Crosses the blood-brain barrier.
Metabolism and Excretion: Mostly metabolized by the liver; <10% excreted in urine as unchanged drug.
Half-life: Biphasic—initial phase, 7–30 min; terminal phase, 90–120 min; ↑ in HF and hepatic impairment.

TIME/ACTION PROFILE (IV = antiarrhythmic effects; local = anesthetic effects)

ROUTE	ONSET	PEAK	DURATION
IV	immediate	immediate	10–20 min (up to several hr after continuous infusion)
Local	rapid	unknown	1–3 hr

Contraindications/Precautions
Contraindicated in: Hypersensitivity; cross-sensitivity may occur; Third-degree heart block; Wolff-Parkinson-White syndrome; Pedi: Children <3 yr (↑ risk of seizures, cardiac arrest and death with viscous lidocaine); viscous lidocaine should not be used for teething pain; should only be used for other indications when safer alternatives are not available or have failed.
Use Cautiously in: Glucose–6–phosphate dehydrogenase deficiency, history of methemoglobinemia, cardiac or pulmonary disease, or concurrent exposure to oxidizing agents (or metabolites of these agents) (↑ risk of methemoglobinemia); Liver disease, HF, patients weighing <50 kg, and geriatric patients (↓ bolus and/

or maintenance dose); Respiratory depression; Shock; Heart block; OB, Lactation: Use only if the potential benefit justifies the potential risk to the fetus; Pedi: Infants <6 mo (↑ risk of methemoglobinemia); safety of topical patch not established in children.

Adverse Reactions/Side Effects
CV: arrhythmias, bradycardia, CARDIAC ARREST, heart block, hypotension. **EENT:** *mucosal use:* ↓ or absent gag reflex. **GI:** nausea, vomiting. **Hemat:** methemoglobinemia. **Local:** stinging, burning, contact dermatitis, erythema. **MS:** chondrolysis. **Neuro:** confusion, drowsiness, agitation, blurred vision, dizziness, paresthesia, SEIZURES, slurred speech, tremor. **Resp:** bronchospasm. **Misc:** HYPERSENSITIVITY REACTIONS (including anaphylaxis).

Interactions
Drug-Drug: Concurrent use of **acetaminophen**, **benzocaine**, **bupivacaine**, **chloroquine**, **cyclophosphamide**, **dapsone**, **flutamide**, **hydroxyurea**, **ifosfamide**, **metoclopramide**, **nitrofurantoin**, **nitroglycerin**, **nitroprusside**, **nitrous oxide**, **phenobarbital**, **phenytoin**, **prilocaine**, **primaquine**, **procaine**, **quinine**, **rasburicase**, **ropivacaine**, **sulfonamides**, **tetracaine**, and **valproate** may ↑ risk of methemoglobinemia; monitor closely. ↑ cardiac depression and toxicity with **phenytoin**, **amiodarone**, **quinidine**, **procainamide**, or **propranolol**. **Cimetidine**, **azole antifungals**, **clarithromycin**, **erythromycin**, **fluoxetine**, **fluvoxamine**, **nefazodone**, **paroxetine**, **protease inhibitors**, **propofol**, **ritonavir**, **verapamil**, and **propranolol** may ↓ metabolism and ↑ risk of toxicity. Lidocaine may ↑ levels of **calcium channel blockers**, certain **benzodiazepines**, **cyclosporine**, **fluoxetine**, **lovastatin**, **simvastatin**, **mirtazapine**, **paroxetine**, **ritonavir**, **tacrolimus**, **theophylline**, **tricyclic antidepressants**, and **venlafaxine**. Effects of lidocaine may be ↓ by **carbamazepine**, **phenobarbital**, **phenytoin**, and **rifampin**.

Route/Dosage
Ventricular Tachycardia (with a Pulse) or Pulseless Ventricular Tachycardia/Ventricular Fibrillation
IV (Adults): 1–1.5 mg/kg bolus; may repeat doses of 0.5–0.75 mg/kg every 5–10 min up to a total dose of 3 mg/kg; may then start continuous infusion of 1–4 mg/min.
Endotracheal (Adults): Give 2–2.5 times the IV loading dose down the endotracheal tube, followed by a 10 mL saline flush.
IV (Children): 1 mg/kg bolus (not to exceed 100 mg), followed by 20–50 mcg/kg/min continuous infusion (range 20–50 mcg/kg/min); may administer 2nd bolus of 0.5–1 mg/kg if delay between bolus and continuous infusion.

L

✤ = Canadian drug name. ≋ = Genetic implication. S̶t̶r̶i̶k̶e̶t̶h̶r̶o̶u̶g̶h̶ = Discontinued. CAPITALS = life-threatening. <u>Underline</u> = most frequent.

Endotracheal (Children): Give 2–3 mg/kg down the endotracheal tube followed by a 5 mL saline flush.

Local

Infiltration (Adults and Children): Infiltrate affected area as needed (increased amount and frequency of use increases likelihood of systemic absorption and adverse reactions).

Topical (Adults): *Cream/ointment/gel/solution/jelly:* Apply to affected area 2–3 times daily. *Patch:* Up to 3 patches may be applied once for up to 12 hr in any 24-hr period; consider smaller areas of application in geriatric or debilitated patients.

Mucosal (Adults): *For anesthetizing oral surfaces:* 20 mg as 2 sprays/quadrant (not to exceed 30 mg/quadrant) may be used. 15 mL of the viscous solution may be used every 3 hr for oral or pharyngeal pain. *For anesthetizing the female urethra:* 3–5 mL of the jelly or 20 mg as 2% solution may be used. *For anesthetizing the male urethra:* 5–10 mL of the jelly or 5–15 mL of 2% solution may be used before catheterization or 30 mL of jelly before cystoscopy or similar procedures. Topical solutions may be used to anesthetize mucous membranes of the larynx, trachea, or esophagus.

Mucosal (Children ≥3 yr): Do not exceed 4.5 mg/kg/dose (or 300 mg/dose) of viscous solution; swish in the mouth and spit out no more frequently than every 3 hr (maximum: 4 doses per 12-hr period).

Mucosal (Children <3 yr): ≤1.2 mL applied to area with a cotton-tipped applicator no more frequently than every 3 hr (maximum: 4 doses per 12-hr period); use only if the underlying condition requires treatment with product volume of ≤1.2 mL.

Availability (generic available)

Solution for injection: 5 mg/mL (0.5%), 10 mg/mL (1%), 15 mg/mL (1.5%), 20 mg/mL (2%). **Premixed infusion:** 1000 mg/250 mL D5W (0.4%), 2000 mg/500 mL D5W (0.4%), 2000 mg/250 mL D5W (0.8%). **Injection for local infiltration/nerve block:** 0.5%, 1%, 2%, 4%. **Topical cream:** 4%^{OTC}, 5%. **Topical gel:** 2%^{OTC}, 3%, 4%, 5%^{OTC}. **Topical jelly:** 2%. **Topical liquid:** 2.5%. **Topical ointment:** 4%, 5%. **Topical patch:** 1.8%, 3.5%, 4%, 5%. **Topical solution:** 2%, 4%. **Topical spray:** 2%, 4%. **Viscous solution:** 2%. *In combination with:* diclofenac (Diclona); epinephrine (Xylocaine with Epinephrine); prilocaine (Oraquix).

NURSING IMPLICATIONS

Assessment

- **Antiarrhythmic:** Monitor ECG continuously and BP and respiratory status frequently during administration.
- **Anesthetic:** Assess degree of numbness of affected part.
- **Topical:** Monitor for pain intensity in affected area periodically during therapy.

Lab Test Considerations

- Serum electrolyte levels should be monitored periodically during prolonged therapy.

Toxicity and Overdose

- Monitor serum lidocaine levels periodically during prolonged or high-dose IV therapy. Therapeutic serum lidocaine levels range from 1.5–5 mcg/mL.
- Signs and symptoms of toxicity include confusion, excitation, blurred or double vision, nausea, vomiting, ringing in ears, tremors, twitching, seizures, difficulty breathing, severe dizziness or fainting, and unusually slow heart rate.
- If symptoms of overdose occur, stop infusion and monitor patient closely.

Implementation

- **High Alert:** Lidocaine is readily absorbed through mucous membranes. Inadvertent overdose of lidocaine jelly and spray has resulted in patient harm or death from neurologic and/or cardiac toxicity. Do not exceed recommended doses.
- **Throat Spray:** Ensure that gag reflex is intact before allowing patient to drink or eat.

IV Administration

- **IV Push:** Only 1% and 2% solutions are used for IV push injection. *Dilution:* Administer undiluted. *Rate:* Administer loading dose over 2–3 min. Follow by IV continuous infusion.
- **Continuous Infusion:** *Dilution:* Lidocaine vials need to be further diluted. Dilute 2 g of lidocaine in 250 mL or 500 mL of D5W or 0.9% NaCl. Admixed infusion stable for 24 hr at room temperature. Premixed infusions are already diluted and ready to use. *Concentration:* 4–8 mg/mL. *Rate:* See Route/Dosage section. Administer via infusion pump for accurate dose.
- **Y-Site Compatibility:** acetaminophen, alemtuzumab, alteplase, amikacin, aminocaproic acid, aminophylline, amiodarone, amphotericin B lipid complex, amphotericin B liposomal, anidulafungin, argatroban, arsenic trioxide, ascorbic acid, atropine, azithromycin, aztreonam, benztropine, bivalirudin, bleomycin, bumetanide, buprenorphine, butorphanol, calcium chloride, calcium gluconate, cangrelor, carboplatin, carmustine, caspofungin, cefazolin, cefotaxime, cefoxitin, ceftaroline, ceftazidime, ceftolozane/tazobactam, ceftriaxone, cefuroxime, chloramphenicol, chlorpromazine, ciprofloxacin, cisatracurium, cisplatin, clindamycin, cyanocobalamin, cyclophosphamide, cyclosporine, cytarabine, dacarbazine, dactinomycin, daptomycin, daunorubicin hydrochloride, dexamethasone, dexmedetomidine, dexrazoxane, digoxin, diltiazem, diphenhydramine, dobutamine, docetaxel, dopamine, doxorubicin hydrochloride, doxorubicin liposomal, doxycycline, enalaprilat, ephedrine, epinephrine, epirubicin, epoetin alfa, eptifibatide, ertapenem, erythromycin, esmolol, etomidate, etoposide, etoposide phosphate, famotidine, fentanyl, fluconazole,

---

fludarabine, fluorouracil, folic acid, foscarnet, fosphenytoin, furosemide, gemcitabine, gentamicin, glycopyrrolate, granisetron, heparin, hetastarch, hydrocortisone, hydromorphone, idarubicin, ifosfamide, imipenem/cilastatin, indomethacin, insulin regular, irinotecan, isavuconazonium, isoproterenol, ketorolac, labetalol, LR, leucovorin calcium, levofloxacin, linezolid, lorazepam, magnesium sulfate, mannitol, meperidine, meropenem/vaborbactam, mesna, methotrexate, methylprednisolone, metoclopramide, metronidazole, micafungin, midazolam, mitomycin, mitoxantrone, morphine, moxifloxacin, multivitamins, mycophenolate, nafcillin, nalbuphine, naloxone, nicardipine, nitroglycerin, nitroprusside, norepinephrine, octreotide, ondansetron, oxacillin, oxaliplatin, oxytocin, paclitaxel, palonosetron, pamidronate, papaverine, pemetrexed, penicillin G, pentamidine, phentolamine, phenylephrine, phytonadione, piperacillin/tazobactam, plazomicin, potassium acetate, potassium chloride, procainamide, prochlorperazine, promethazine, propofol, propranolol, protamine, pyridoxine, remifentanil, rocuronium, sodium acetate, sodium bicarbonate, succinylcholine, sufentanil, tacrolimus, tedizolid, theophylline, thiamine, thiotepa, tigecycline, tirofiban, tobramycin, topotecan, vancomycin, vasopressin, vecuronium, verapamil, vinblastine, vincristine, vinorelbine, voriconazole, zoledronic acid.

- **Y-Site Incompatibility:** acyclovir, amphotericin B deoxycholate, azathioprine, caspofungin, dantrolene, diazepam, ganciclovir, gemtuzumab ozogamicin, milrinone, pantoprazole, pentobarbital, phenobarbital, phenytoin, thiopental, trimethoprim/sulfamethoxazole.
- **Infiltration:** Lidocaine with epinephrine may be used to minimize systemic absorption and prolong local anesthesia.
- **Topical:** When used concomitantly with other products containing local anesthetic agents, consider amount absorbed from all formulations.
- *Lidoderm* and *ZTLido* are not interchangeable.

Patient/Family Teaching
- Explain purpose of lidocaine to patient.
- May cause drowsiness and dizziness. Advise patient to call for assistance during ambulation and transfer.
- Rep: Advise females of reproductive potential to notify health care professional if pregnancy is planned or suspected, or if breastfeeding.
- **Topical:** Apply *Lidoderm Patch* to intact skin to cover the most painful area. Patch may be cut to smaller sizes with scissors before removing release liner. Clothing may be worn over patch. Avoid contact with water (bathing, swimming, showering), may not stick if it gets wet. If irritation or burning sensation occurs during application, remove patch

until irritation subsides. Wash hands after application; avoid contact with eyes. Dispose of used patch to avoid access by children or pets.
- Apply *ZTLido* to intact skin to cover the most painful area. Apply immediately after removing from envelope. System may be cut to smaller sizes with scissors before removing release liner. Clothing may be worn over patch. May be used during moderate exercise (biking for 30 min). May be exposed to water (showering for 10 min or immersion for 15 min). Dry by gently patting the skin, not by rubbing skin or topical system. If edges have lifted, press firmly on edges. If system detaches, may be reapplied as originally directed. If system will not stick, dispose by folding adhesive sides together and discard where children or pets cannot get to them. Apply a new system for total duration of 12 hr of used and new system together. If irritation or a burning sensation occurs during application, remove and reapply when irritation subsides.
- Caution women to consult health care professional before using a topical anesthetic for a mammogram or other procedures. If recommended, use lowest drug concentration, and apply sparingly. Do not apply to broken or irritated skin, do not wrap skin, and do not apply heat to area (heating pad/electric blanket), to decrease chance that drug may be absorbed into the body. May result in seizures, cardiac arrhythmias, respiratory failure, coma, and death.
- Advise patient referred for MRI test to discuss patch with referring health care professional and MRI facility to determine if removal of patch is necessary prior to test and for directions for replacing patch.
- **Mucosal:** Caution parent to administer as directed, not to use more or more often than directed, and to use measuring device for accurate dose in children younger than 3 yr. Advise parent that if signs and symptoms of toxicity (lethargy, shallow breathing, seizure activity) occur to seek emergency attention and not to administer more lidocaine.
- Caution parents that oral lidocaine causes numbness and may impair swallowing; do not administer food and/or chewing gum for at least 60 min after administration.

Evaluation/Desired Outcomes
- Decrease in ventricular arrhythmias.
- Local anesthesia.

linaGLIPtin (lin-a-glip-tin)
Tradjenta, ✦ Trajenta
Classification
Therapeutic: antidiabetics
Pharmacologic: dipeptidyl peptidase-4 (DPP-4) inhibitors, enzyme inhibitors

Indications

Type 2 diabetes mellitus (as adjunct to diet and exercise.

Action

Inhibits the enzyme dipeptidyl peptidase-4 (DPP-4), which slows the inactivation of incretin hormones, resulting in increased levels of active incretin hormones. These hormones are released by the intestine throughout the day, and are involved in regulation of glucose. Increased/prolonged incretin levels increase insulin release and decrease glucagon levels. **Therapeutic Effects:** Improved control of blood glucose.

Pharmacokinetics

Absorption: 30% absorbed following oral administration.

Distribution: Extensively distributed to tissues.

Metabolism and Excretion: Minimally metabolized; primarily excreted in feces (80%) and urine (5%) as unchanged drug.

Half-life: >100 hr (due to saturable binding to DPP-4).

TIME/ACTION PROFILE

ROUTE	ONSET	PEAK	DURATION
PO	unknown	1.5 hr†	24 hr

†Blood level.

Contraindications/Precautions

Contraindicated in: Hypersensitivity. Cross-sensitivity may exist with sitagliptin, alogliptin, or saxagliptin; Type 1 diabetes mellitus; Diabetic ketoacidosis.

Use Cautiously in: History of pancreatitis; History of HF or renal impairment (↑ risk of HF); OB: Use during pregnancy only if potential maternal benefit justifies potential fetal risk; Lactation: Use while breastfeeding only if potential maternal benefit justifies potential risk to infant; Pedi: Safety and effectiveness not established in children; Geri: Older adults may have ↑ risk of hypoglycemia.

Adverse Reactions/Side Effects

CV: HF. **Derm:** bullous pemphigoid, localized exfoliation, urticaria. **Endo:** hypoglycemia. **GI:** ↑ lipase, PANCREATITIS. **Metab:** hypertriglyceridemia. **MS:** arthralgia, RHABDOMYOLYSIS. **Resp:** bronchial hyperreactivity. **Misc:** HYPERSENSITIVITY REACTIONS (including anaphylaxis, angioedema, and exfoliative skin conditions).

Interactions

Drug-Drug: ↑ risk of hypoglycemia with **sulfonylureas** or **insulin**; dose ↓ of sulfonylurea or insulin may be necessary. Concurrent use of P-glycoprotein or CYP3A4 inducers, including **rifampin**, may ↓ levels and effectiveness and should be avoided.

Route/Dosage

PO (Adults): 5 mg once daily.

Availability (generic available)

Tablets: 5 mg. *In combination with:* empagliflozin (Glyxambi); empagliflozin and metformin XR (Trijardy XR); metformin (Jentadueto); metformin XR (Jentadueto XR). See Appendix N.

NURSING IMPLICATIONS

Assessment

- Assess for signs and symptoms of hypoglycemic reactions (abdominal pain, sweating, hunger, weakness, dizziness, headache, tremor, tachycardia, anxiety).
- Monitor for signs of pancreatitis (nausea, vomiting, anorexia, persistent severe abdominal pain, sometimes radiating to the back) during therapy. If pancreatitis occurs, discontinue linagliptin and monitor serum and urine amylase, amylase/CCr ratio, electrolytes, serum calcium, glucose, and lipase.
- Monitor for arthralgia. Severe joint pain usually disappears with discontinuation of linagliptin.

Lab Test Considerations
- Monitor hemoglobin A1C prior to and periodically during therapy.
- May cause ↑ uric acid levels.

Implementation

- Do not confuse linagliptin with linaclotide. Do not confuse Tradjenta with Toujeo, Tresiba, or Trulicity.
- Patients stabilized on a diabetic regimen who are exposed to stress, fever, trauma, infection, or surgery may require administration of insulin.
- **PO:** May be administered without regard to food.

Patient/Family Teaching

- Instruct patient to take linagliptin as directed. Take missed doses as soon as remembered, unless it is almost time for next dose; do not double doses. Advise patient to read the *Medication Guide* before starting and with each Rx refill in case of changes.
- Explain to patient that linagliptin helps control hyperglycemia but does not cure diabetes. Therapy is usually long term.
- Instruct patient not to share this medication with others, even if they have the same symptoms; it may harm them.
- Encourage patient to follow prescribed diet, medication, and exercise regimen to prevent hyperglycemic or hypoglycemic episodes.
- Review signs of hypoglycemia and hyperglycemia with patient. If hypoglycemia occurs, advise patient to take a glass of orange juice or 2–3 tsp of sugar, honey, or corn syrup dissolved in water, and notify health care professional.
- Instruct patient in proper testing of blood glucose and urine ketones. These tests should be monitored closely during periods of stress or illness and health care professional notified if significant changes occur.
- Advise patient to notify health care professional promptly if signs and symptoms of pancreatitis or if rash; hives; blisters; or swelling of face, lips, or throat occur.

- Advise patient to notify health care professional of all Rx or OTC medications, vitamins, or herbal products being taken and to consult with health care professional before taking other medications, especially other oral hypoglycemic medications.
- Rep: Insulin is the recommended method of controlling blood sugar during pregnancy. Advise females of reproductive potential to notify health care professional if pregnancy is planned or suspected, or if breastfeeding.

Evaluation/Desired Outcomes
- Improved hemoglobin A1C, fasting plasma glucose and 2-hr postprandial glucose levels.

---

linezolid (li-nez-o-lid)
Zyvox, ✲ Zyvoxam
Classification
Therapeutic: anti-infectives
Pharmacologic: oxazolidinones

Indications
Nosocomial pneumonia. Community-acquired pneumonia. Complicated skin and skin structure infections. Uncomplicated skin and skin structure infections. Infections caused by vancomycin-resistant *Enterococcus faecium*.

Action
Inhibits bacterial protein synthesis at the level of the 23S ribosome of the 50S subunit. **Therapeutic Effects:** Bactericidal action against streptococci; bacteriostatic action against enterococci and staphylococci. **Spectrum:** Active against gram-positive pathogens, including: *Staphylococcus aureus* (methicillin-susceptible and methicillin-resistant), *Streptococcus agalactiae*, *Streptococcus pneumoniae*, *Streptococcus pyogenes*, *Enterococcus faecium*.

Pharmacokinetics
Absorption: Rapidly and extensively (100%) absorbed following oral administration. IV administration results in complete bioavailability.

Distribution: Readily distributes to well-perfused tissues.

Metabolism and Excretion: 65% metabolized, mostly by the liver; 30% excreted unchanged by the kidneys.

Half-life: 6.4 hr.

TIME/ACTION PROFILE

ROUTE	ONSET	PEAK	DURATION
PO	rapid	1–2 hr	12 hr
IV	rapid	end of infusion	12 hr

Contraindications/Precautions
Contraindicated in: Hypersensitivity; Phenylketonuria (suspension contains phenylalanine); Uncon-

trolled HTN, pheochromocytoma, thyrotoxicosis, or concurrent use of sympathomimetic agents, vasopressors, or dopaminergic agents (↑ risk of hypertensive response); Concurrent or recent (<2 wk) use of MAO inhibitors (↑ risk of hypertensive response); Carcinoid syndrome or concurrent use of SSRIs, SNRIs, TCAs, triptans, opioids, bupropion, or buspirone (↑ risk of serotonin syndrome).

Use Cautiously in: Thrombocytopenia, concurrent use of antiplatelet agents or bleeding diathesis (platelet counts should be monitored more frequently); Diabetes (↑ risk of hypoglycemia); OB: Use during pregnancy only if potential maternal benefit justifies potential fetal risk; Lactation: Use while breastfeeding only if potential maternal benefit justifies potential risk to infant.

Adverse Reactions/Side Effects
CV: headache, insomnia. **Derm:** TOXIC EPIDERMAL NECROLYSIS. **EENT:** teeth discoloration, tongue discoloration. **Endo:** hypoglycemia, syndrome of inappropriate diuretic hormone (SIADH) secretion. **F and E:** hyponatremia, lactic acidosis. **GI:** ↑ liver enzymes, CLOSTRIDIOIDES DIFFICILE-ASSOCIATED DIARRHEA (CDAD), diarrhea, nausea, vomiting. **Hemat:** anemia, leukopenia, thrombocytopenia. **Neuro:** dysgeusia, optic neuropathy, peripheral neuropathy. **Misc:** SEROTONIN SYNDROME.

Interactions
Drug-Drug: ↑ risk of hypertensive crisis with **MAO inhibitors**, **sympathomimetics** (e.g., **pseudoephedrine**), **vasopressors** (e.g., **epinephrine**, **norepinephrine**), and **dopaminergic agents** (e.g., **dopamine**, **dobutamine**); concurrent or recent use should be avoided. ↑ risk of serotonin syndrome with **SSRIs, SNRIs, TCAs, triptans, opioids, bupropion**, or **buspirone**; avoid concurrent use. **Rifampin, carbamazepine, phenytoin**, and **phenobarbital** may ↓ levels. Concurrent use with **oral hypoglycemics** or **insulin** may ↑ risk of hypoglycemia.

Drug-Food: Because of monoamine oxidase inhibitory properties, consumption of large amounts of foods or beverages containing tyramine should be avoided (↑ risk of pressor response. See Appendix J).

Route/Dosage

Vancomycin-Resistant *Enterococcus faecium* Infections
PO, IV (Adults): 600 mg every 12 hr for 14–28 days.
PO, IV (Children birth–11 yr): In the first wk of life, pre-term neonates may initially receive 10 mg/kg every 12 hr.

Pneumonia or Complicated Skin/Skin Structure Infections
PO, IV (Adults): 600 mg every 12 hr for 10–14 days.
PO, IV (Children birth–11 yr): 10 mg/kg every 8 hr for 10–14 days (in the first wk of life, preterm neonates may initially receive 10 mg/kg every 12 hr).

L

✲ = Canadian drug name. 🔛 = Genetic implication. S̶t̶r̶i̶k̶e̶t̶h̶r̶o̶u̶g̶h̶ = Discontinued. CAPITALS = life-threatening. <u>Underline</u> = most frequent.

Uncomplicated Skin/Skin Structure Infections

PO (Adults): 400 mg every 12 hr for 10–14 days.
PO, IV (Children 5–11 yr): 10 mg/kg every 12 hr for 10–14 days.
PO, IV (Children <5 yr): 10 mg/kg every 8 hr for 10–14 days (in the first wk of life, pre-term neonates may initially receive 10 mg/kg every 12 hr).

Availability (generic available)

Tablets: 600 mg. **Oral suspension: (orange-flavored):** 100 mg/5 mL (each 5 mL contains phenylalanine 20 mg). **Premixed infusion:** 200 mg/100 mL, 600 mg/300 mL.

NURSING IMPLICATIONS

Assessment

- Assess for infection (vital signs; appearance of wound, sputum, urine, and stool; WBC) at beginning of and during therapy.
- Obtain specimens for culture and sensitivity prior to initiating therapy. First dose may be given before receiving.
- May cause lactic acidosis. Notify health care professional if recurrent nausea and vomiting, unexplained acidosis, or low bicarbonate levels occur.
- Monitor visual function in patients receiving linezolid for ≥3 mo or who report visual symptoms (changes in acuity or color vision, blurred vision, visual field defect) regardless of length of therapy. If optic neuropathy occurs, therapy should be reconsidered.
- Monitor bowel function. Diarrhea, abdominal cramping, fever, and bloody stools should be reported to health care professional promptly as a sign of CDAD. May begin up to several wk following cessation of therapy.
- Monitor patient taking serotonergic drugs for signs of serotonin syndrome (hyperthermia, rigidity, myoclonus, autonomic instability, mental status changes, extreme agitation progressing to delirium and coma) for 2 wk (5 wk if fluoxetine was taken) or until 24 hrs after the last dose of linezolid, whichever comes first.

Lab Test Considerations

- May cause bone marrow suppression, anemia, leukopenia, pancytopenia. Monitor CBC and platelet count weekly, especially in patients at risk for increased bleeding, having pre-existing bone marrow suppression, having severe renal impairment or moderate/severe hepatic impairment, receiving concurrent medications that may cause myelosuppression, or requiring >2 wk of therapy. Discontinue therapy if bone marrow suppression occurs or worsens.
- May cause ↑ AST, ALT, LDH, alkaline phosphatase, and BUN.
- May cause hypoglycemia requiring decrease in dose of antidiabetic agent or discontinuation of linezolid.
- Monitor serum sodium levels regularly in the elderly, in patients taking diuretics, and in other patients at risk of hyponatremia and/or SIADH. If signs and symptoms of hyponatremia and/or SIADH (confusion, somnolence, generalized weakness, respiratory failure, death) occur, discontinue linezolid, and institute supportive measures.

Implementation

- **High Alert:** Do not confuse Zyvox with Zovirax.
- Dose adjustment is not necessary when switching from IV to oral dose.
- **PO:** May be administered with or without food.
- Before using oral solution gently invert 3–5 times to mix; do not shake. Store at room temperature; use within 21 days of constitution.

IV Administration

- **Intermittent Infusion:** *Dilution:* Premixed infusions are already diluted and ready to use. Solution is yellowish in color which may intensify over time without affecting its potency. *Concentration:* 2 mg/mL. Do not use in series connections. *Rate:* Infuse over 30–120 min. Flush line before and after infusion.
- **Y-Site Compatibility:** acetaminophen, acyclovir, alemtuzumab, allopurinol, amifostine, amikacin, aminocaproic acid, aminophylline, amiodarone, amphotericin B lipid complex, amphotericin B liposomal, ampicillin, ampicillin/sulbactam, anidulafungin, argatroban, arsenic trioxide, azithromycin, aztreonam, bivalirudin, bleomycin, bumetanide, buprenorphine, busulfan, butorphanol, calcium chloride, calcium gluconate, cangrelor, carboplatin, carmustine, caspofungin, cefazolin, cefepime, cefotaxime, cefotetan, cefoxitin, ceftazidime, ceftazidime/avibactam, ceftolozane/tazobactam, ceftriaxone, cefuroxime, chloramphenicol, ciprofloxacin, cisatracurium, cisplatin, clindamycin, cyclophosphamide, cyclosporine, cytarabine, D5W, dacarbazine, dactinomycin, daptomycin, daunorubicin hydrochloride, dexamethasone, dexmedetomidine, dexrazoxane, D5/0.45% NaCl, D5/0.9% NaCl, digoxin, diltiazem, diphenhydramine, dobutamine, docetaxel, dopamine, doxorubicin hydrochloride, doxorubicin liposomal, doxycycline, droperidol, enalaprilat, ephedrine, epinephrine, epirubicin, eptifibatide, eravacycline, ertapenem, esmolol, etoposide, etoposide phosphate, famotidine, fentanyl, fluconazole, fludarabine, fluorouracil, foscarnet, fosphenytoin, furosemide, ganciclovir, gemcitabine, gemtuzumab ozogamicin, gentamicin, glycopyrrolate, granisetron, haloperidol, heparin, hetastarch, hydralazine, hydrocortisone, hydromorphone, idarubicin, ifosfamide, imipenem/cilastatin, insulin regular, irinotecan, isavuconazonium, isoproterenol, ketorolac, labetalol, LR, leucovorin calcium, levofloxacin, lidocaine, lorazepam, magnesium sulfate, mannitol, melphalan, meperidine, meropenem, meropenem/vaborbactam, mesna, methadone, methotrexate, methylprednisolone, metoclopramide, metoprolol, metronidazole, midazolam, milrinone, mitomycin,

mitoxantrone, morphine, mycophenolate, nafcillin, nalbuphine, naloxone, nicardipine, nitroglycerin, nitroprusside, norepinephrine, 0.9% NaCl, octreotide, ondansetron, oxaliplatin, oxytocin, paclitaxel, palonosetron, pamidronate, pemetrexed, pentobarbital, phenobarbital, phenylephrine, piperacillin/tazobactam, plazomicin, potassium acetate, potassium chloride, potassium phosphate, procainamide, prochlorperazine, promethazine, propranolol, remifentanil, rocuronium, sodium acetate, sodium bicarbonate, sodium phosphate, succinylcholine, sufentanil, tacrolimus, theophylline, thiotepa, tigecycline, tirofiban, tobramycin, topotecan, trimethoprim/sulfamethoxazole, vancomycin, vasopressin, vecuronium, verapamil, vinblastine, vincristine, vinorelbine, voriconazole, zidovudine, zoledronic acid.

- **Y-Site Incompatibility:** chlorpromazine, dantrolene, diazepam, erythromycin, pantoprazole, pentamidine, phenytoin, thiopental.

Patient/Family Teaching

- Instruct patients taking oral linezolid to take as directed, for full course of therapy, even if feeling better. Take missed doses as soon as remembered unless almost time for next dose; do not double dose.
- Instruct patient to avoid large quantities of foods or beverages containing tyramine (See Appendix J). May cause hypertensive response.
- Instruct patient to notify health care professional if patient has a history of hypertension or seizures.
- Advise patient to notify health care professional of all Rx or OTC medications, vitamins, or herbal products being taken and to consult with health care professional before taking other medications, especially cold remedies, decongestants, or antidepressants.
- Instruct patient to notify health care professional if changes in vision occur or immediately if diarrhea, abdominal cramping, fever, or bloody stools occur and not to treat with antidiarrheals without consulting health care professionals.
- Advise patient to notify health care professional promptly if signs and symptoms of SIADH (confusion, somnolence, generalized weakness, respiratory failure). May be fatal.
- Rep: Advise females of reproductive potential to notify health care professional if pregnancy is planned or suspected or if breastfeeding. Advise lactating women to monitor breastfed infant for diarrhea and vomiting. May reversibly impair fertility in male patients.
- Advise patient to notify health care professional if no improvement is seen in a few days.

Evaluation/Desired Outcomes

- Resolution of signs and symptoms of infection. Length of time for complete resolution depends on organism and site of infection.

liraglutide (lir-a-**gloo**-tide)
Saxenda, Victoza
Classification
Therapeutic: antidiabetics
Pharmacologic: glucagon-like peptide-1
(GLP-1) receptor agonists

Indications
Victoza: Type 2 diabetes mellitus (as adjunct to diet and exercise). To reduce the risk of major adverse cardiovascular events (cardiovascular death, nonfatal MI, or nonfatal stroke) in patients with type 2 diabetes mellitus and established cardiovascular disease. **Saxenda:** Chronic weight management in adults who are obese (body mass index [BMI] ≥30 kg/m²) or are overweight (BMI ≥27 kg/m²) with ≥1 weight-related comorbid condition (e.g. hypertension, dyslipidemia, type 2 diabetes) (as adjunct to reduced-calorie diet and increased physical activity). **Saxenda:** Chronic weight management in children ≥12 yrs old with a body weight >60 kg and an initial BMI corresponding to ≥30 kg/m² for adults (obese) by international cutoffs (Cole Criteria) (as adjunct to reduced-calorie diet and increased physical activity).

Action
Acts as an acylated human glucagon-like peptide-1 (GLP-1, an incretin) receptor agonist; increases intracellular cyclic AMP (cAMP) leading to insulin release when glucose is elevated, which then subsides as blood glucose decreases toward euglycemia. Also decreases glucagon secretion and delays gastric emptying. Also helps to suppress appetite, leading to decreased caloric intake. **Therapeutic Effects:** Improved glycemic control. Reduction in body weight. Reduction in cardiovascular death, nonfatal myocardial infarction, or nonfatal stroke.

Pharmacokinetics
Absorption: 55% absorbed following SUBQ injection.
Distribution: Unknown.
Protein Binding: >98%.
Metabolism and Excretion: Endogenously metabolized.
Half-life: 13 hr.

TIME/ACTION PROFILE

ROUTE	ONSET	PEAK	DURATION
SUBQ	within 4 wk† within 2 wk‡	8 wk† 40 wk‡	unknown†‡

†↓ in A1c.
‡↓ in body weight.

Contraindications/Precautions
Contraindicated in: Hypersensitivity; Personal or family history of medullary thyroid carcinoma; Multiple

Endocrine Neoplasia syndrome type 2; Type 1 diabetes (Victoza only); Diabetic ketoacidosis (Victoza only); Concurrent use with other weight-loss products (Saxenda only); History of suicidal attempts or suicidal thoughts (Saxenda only); OB: Weight loss not recommended during pregnancy (Saxenda only); Lactation: Lactation; Pedi: Children ≥12 yr with type 2 diabetes (safety and effectiveness not established) (Saxenda only).

Use Cautiously in: History of pancreatitis; History of angioedema or anaphylaxis to another GLP-1 receptor agonist; Hepatic impairment; Renal impairment; OB: Use during pregnancy only if potential maternal benefit justifies potential fetal risk (Victoza only); Pedi: Safety and effectiveness not established in children <12 yr (Saxenda) and children <10 yr (Victoza); ↑ risk of hypoglycemia with use of either Saxenda or Victoza in children.

Adverse Reactions/Side Effects

CV: tachycardia. **Derm:** cutaneous amyloidosis, pruritus, rash. **Endo:** hypoglycemia, THYROID C-CELL TUMORS. **GI:** diarrhea, nausea, vomiting, cholecystitis, cholelithiasis, constipation, PANCREATITIS. **GU:** acute renal failure. **Local:** injection site reactions. **Neuro:** headache, SUICIDAL BEHAVIOR/IDEATION (Saxenda only). **Misc:** HYPERSENSITIVITY REACTIONS (including anaphylaxis and angioedema).

Interactions

Drug-Drug: Concurrent use with **agents that increase insulin secretion**, including **sulfonylureas** and **insulin** may ↑ the risk of serious hypoglycemia; use cautiously and consider ↓ dose of agent increasing insulin secretion. May alter absorption of concomitantly administered **oral medications** due to delayed gastric emptying.

Route/Dosage

Victoza

Type 2 Diabetes Mellitus

SUBQ (Adults): 0.6 mg once daily for 1 wk, then 1.2 mg once daily for 1 wk; may then ↑ dose, if needed, up to 1.8 mg once daily.
SUBQ (Children ≥10 yr): 0.6 mg once daily for 1 wk; may then ↑ dose, if needed, to 1.2 mg once daily; after 1 wk, if additional glycemic control needed, may then ↑ dose to 1.8 mg once daily.

Reduction in Risk of Major Adverse Cardiovascular Events

SUBQ (Adults): 0.6 mg once daily for 1 wk, then 1.2 mg once daily for 1 wk; may then ↑ dose, if needed, up to 1.8 mg once daily.

Saxenda

SUBQ (Adults): 0.6 mg once daily for 1 wk (Wk 1), then 1.2 mg once daily for 1 wk (Wk 2), then 1.8 mg once daily for 1 wk (Wk 3), then 2.4 mg once daily for 1 wk (Wk 4), then 3 mg once daily. Discontinue if patient cannot tolerate dose of 3 mg once daily.

SUBQ (Children ≥12 yr): 0.6 mg once daily for 1 wk (Wk 1), then 1.2 mg once daily for 1 wk (Wk 2), then 1.8 mg once daily for 1 wk (Wk 3), then 2.4 mg once daily for 1 wk (Wk 4), then 3 mg once daily. If patient cannot tolerate dose of 3 mg once daily, ↓ to 2.4 mg once daily; discontinue if patient cannot subsequently tolerate dose of 2.4 mg once daily.

Availability

Solution for injection (Saxenda) (prefilled pens): 18 mg/3 mL (delivers doses of 0.6 mg, 1.2 mg, 1.8 mg, 2.4 mg, or 3 mg). **Solution for injection (Victoza) (prefilled pens):** 18 mg/3 mL (delivers doses of 0.6 mg, 1.2 mg, or 1.8 mg). *In combination with:* insulin degludec (Xultophy). See Appendix N.

NURSING IMPLICATIONS

Assessment

- If thyroid nodules or elevated serum calcitonin are noted, refer patient to an endocrinologist.
- Monitor for pancreatitis during therapy (persistent severe abdominal pain, sometimes radiating to the back, with or without vomiting). If pancreatitis is suspected, discontinue liraglutide; if confirmed, do not restart liraglutide.
- **Victoza:** Observe patient taking concurrent insulin for signs and symptoms of hypoglycemic reactions (sweating, hunger, weakness, dizziness, tremor, tachycardia, anxiety).
- **Saxenda:** Monitor patient for weight loss and adjust concurrent medications (antihypertensives, antidiabetics, lipid-lowering agents) as needed.

Lab Test Considerations

- Monitor serum A1c periodically during therapy to evaluate effectiveness.

Implementation

- Patients stabilized on a diabetic regimen who are exposed to stress, fever, trauma, infection, or surgery may require administration of insulin.
- **SUBQ:** Administer once daily at any time of the day, without regard to food. Inject at a 90° angle into abdomen, thigh, or upper arm. Apply light pressure but do not rub injection site. Solution should be clear and colorless; do not administer solutions that are discolored or contain particulate matter. Rotate injection sites within the same region to reduce risk of cutaneous amyloidosis. Use a new needle for each injection. Store in refrigerator before first dose; after first dose, may be stored for 30 days at room temperature or in refrigerator.
- Initial dose of 0.6 mg/day is increased after 1 wk to 1.2 mg/day. If glycemic control is not acceptable, increase to 1.8 mg/day. Available in a prefilled pen without needle; patient may require Rx for needles.

Patient/Family Teaching

- Instruct patient on use of pen injector and to take liraglutide as directed. If a dose is missed, omit and take next dose as scheduled; do not double doses. If >3 days dosing missed, reinitiate with 0.6 mg dose; titrate at direction of health care professional. Pen should never be shared between patients, even if needle is changed. Store pen in refrigerator; do not freeze. After initial use, pen may be stored at room temperature or refrigerated up to 30 days. Keep pen cap on when not in use. Protect from excessive heat and sunlight. Remove and safely discard needle after each injection and store pen without needle attached. Advise patient to read the *Patient Medication Guide* before starting liraglutide and with each Rx refill.

- Inform patient that nausea is the most common side effect, but usually decreases over time.
- Advise patient taking insulin and liraglutide to never mix insulin and liraglutide together. Give as 2 separate injections. Both injections may be given in the same body area, but should not be given right next to each other.
- Explain to patient that this medication controls hyperglycemia but does not cure diabetes. Therapy is long-term.
- Review signs of hypoglycemia and hyperglycemia with patient. If hypoglycemia occurs, advise patient to take a glass of orange juice or 2−3 tsp of sugar, honey, or corn syrup dissolved in water and notify health care professional.
- Encourage patient to follow prescribed diet, medication, and exercise regimen to prevent hypoglycemic or hyperglycemic episodes.
- Instruct patient in proper testing of serum glucose and ketones. These tests should be closely monitored during periods of stress or illness, and health care professional should be notified if significant changes occur.
- Advise patient to notify health care professional of all Rx or OTC medications, vitamins, or herbal products being taken and to consult with health care professional before taking other medications.
- Advise patient to discontinue liraglutide and notify health care professional immediately if signs of pancreatitis (nausea, vomiting, abdominal pain) occur.
- Advise patient to inform health care professional of medication regimen before treatment or surgery.
- Inform patient of risk of benign and malignant thyroid C-cell tumors. Advise patient to notify health care professional if symptoms of thyroid tumors (lump in neck, hoarseness, trouble swallowing, shortness of breath) or if signs of allergic reaction (swelling of face, lips, tongue, or throat; fainting or feeling dizzy; very rapid heartbeat; problems breathing or swallowing; severe rash or itching) occur.
- Rep: Insulin is the preferred method of controlling blood glucose during pregnancy. Counsel females of reproductive potential to notify health care professional if pregnancy is planned or suspected, or if breastfeeding. *Saxenda* is contraindicated in pregnancy, as weight loss during pregnancy may cause fetal harm.
- Advise patient to carry a form of sugar (sugar packets, candy) and identification describing disease process and medication regimen at all times.
- Emphasize the importance of routine follow-up exams.

Evaluation/Desired Outcomes
- Improved glycemic control.
- Reduction in body weight. If patient has not lost at least 4% of body weight after 16 wk of therapy, it is unlikely that patient will achieve and sustain clinically meaningful weight loss with continued treatment.
- Reduction in cardiovascular death, nonfatal myocardial infarction, or nonfatal stroke.

lisdexamfetamine
(lis-dex-am-**fet**-a-meen)
Vyvanse
Classification
Therapeutic: central nervous system stimulants
Pharmacologic: sympathomimetics

Schedule II

Indications
Attention deficit hyperactivity disorder (ADHD). Moderate to severe binge eating disorder.

Action
Blocks reuptake and increases release of norepinephrine and dopamine resulting in increased levels in extraneuronal space. **Therapeutic Effects:** Improved attention span in ADHD. Reduction in number of binge eating days per wk.

Pharmacokinetics
Absorption: Rapidly absorbed and converted to dextroamphetamine, the active drug.
Distribution: Unknown.
Metabolism and Excretion: 42% excreted in urine as amphetamine.
Half-life: less than 1 hr for lisdexamfetamine.

TIME/ACTION PROFILE

ROUTE	ONSET	PEAK	DURATION
PO	rapid	1 hr	24 hr

Contraindications/Precautions
Contraindicated in: Hypersensitivity to lisdexamfetamine or other sympathomimetic amines; Advanced arteriosclerosis; Symptomatic cardiovascular disease including known structural cardiac abnormalities (may ↑ the risk of sudden death); Moderate to severe hypertension; Glaucoma; Agitation; History of substance abuse; Concurrent use or use within 14 days of MAO in-

hibitors or MAO-like drugs (linezolid or methylene blue); Lactation: Lactation.

Use Cautiously in: History of pre-existing psychosis, bipolar disorder, aggression, tics, Tourette's syndrome or seizures (may exacerbate condition); Severe renal impairment (↓ maximum daily dose); OB: Use during pregnancy only if potential maternal benefit outweighs potential fetal risk; Pedi: Children <6 yr (safety and effectiveness not established).

Adverse Reactions/Side Effects
CV: Raynaud's phenomenon, SUDDEN DEATH. **Derm:** alopecia, rash. **EENT:** blurred vision, poor accommodation. **GI:** ↓ appetite, abdominal pain, dry mouth, intestinal ischemia, nausea, vomiting. **GU:** ↓ libido, priapism. **Metab:** ↓ weight. **MS:** RHABDOMYOLYSIS. **Neuro:** behavioral disturbances, dizziness, hallucinations, insomnia, irritability, mania, paresthesia, psychomotor hyperactivity, thought disorder, tics. **Misc:** long-term growth suppression, SEROTONIN SYNDROME.

Interactions
Drug-Drug: Concurrent use with **MAO inhibitors** or **MAO-inhibitor-like drugs**, such as **linezolid** or **methylene blue** may result in serious, potentially fatal reactions; wait at least 14 days following discontinuation of MAO inhibitor before initiation of amphetamine mixtures. Drugs that affect serotonergic neurotransmitter systems, including **MAO inhibitors, tricyclic antidepressants, SSRIs, SNRIs, fentanyl, buspirone, tramadol, lithium,** and **triptans** ↑ risk of serotonin syndrome. Concurrent use of other **sympathomimetic amines** may result in additive effects and ↑ risk of adverse reactions. **Urinary acidifying agents** including **sodium acid phosphate** ↑ excretion and ↓ blood levels and may result in ↓ effectiveness. May ↓ effectiveness of **adrenergic blockers**. ↑ risk of adverse cardiovascular reactions with **tricyclic antidepressants**. May ↓ sedating effects of **antihistamines**. May ↓ effectiveness of **antihypertensives**. Effects may be ↓ by **haloperidol, lithium,** or **chlorpromazine**. May ↓ absorption of **phenobarbital** or **phenytoin**.

Route/Dosage
Attention Deficit Hyperactivity Disorder
PO (Adults and Children ≥6 yr): 30 mg once daily; may ↑ by 10–20 mg/day at weekly intervals, up to 70 mg/day.

Renal Impairment
PO (Adults and Children ≥6 yr): *CCr 15–29 mL/min:* Do not exceed 50 mg/day; *CCr <15 mL/min:* Do not exceed 30 mg/day.

Binge Eating Disorder
PO (Adults): 30 mg once daily; may ↑ by 20 mg/day at weekly intervals, up to target dose of 50–70 mg/day.

Availability (generic available)
Capsules: 10 mg, 20 mg, 30 mg, 40 mg, 50 mg, 60 mg, 70 mg. **Chewable tablets:** 10 mg, 20 mg, 30 mg, 40 mg, 50 mg, 60 mg.

NURSING IMPLICATIONS
Assessment
- Monitor BP, pulse, and respiration before administering and periodically during therapy. Obtain a history (including assessment of family history of sudden death or ventricular arrhythmia), physical exam to assess for cardiac disease, and further evaluation (ECG and echocardiogram), if indicated. If exertional chest pain, unexplained syncope, or other cardiac symptoms occur, evaluate promptly.
- Assess risk of abuse prior to prescribing. After prescribing, keep accurate prescription records, educate patient and family about risk of abuse, monitor for signs of abuse and overdose, and evaluate need for use periodically during therapy.
- Screen patients with bipolar disorder for risk of manic episode (comorbid or history of depressive symptoms or a family history of suicide, bipolar disorder, depression) prior to starting therapy.
- Monitor growth, both height and weight, in children on long-term therapy. May need to interrupt therapy in patients who are not growing or gaining height or weight as expected.
- Monitor closely for behavior change.
- Assess for signs and symptoms of serotonin syndrome (mental changes [agitation, hallucinations, coma], autonomic instability [tachycardia, labile BP, hyperthermia], neuromuscular aberrations [hyperreflexia, incoordination], and/or GI symptoms [nausea, vomiting, diarrhea]), especially in patients taking other serotonergic drugs (SSRIs, SNRIs, triptans).
- **ADHD:** Assess child's attention span, impulse control, and interactions with others. Therapy may be interrupted at intervals to determine whether symptoms are sufficient to continue therapy.
- **Binge Eating Disorder:** Monitor frequency and amount of binge eating.

Lab Test Considerations
- May cause ↑ plasma corticosteroid levels interfering with urinary steroid determinations.

Implementation
- **PO:** Administer in the morning without regard to meals. Avoid afternoon doses due to potential for insomnia. Capsules may be swallowed whole or opened and the entire contents dissolved in yogurt, water, or orange juice. If solution method is used, consume immediately; do not store for future use. Do not divide capsules or take less than one capsule per day. Chewable tablets must be chewed thoroughly. Tablets and chewable tablets can be substituted on a unit per unit/mg per mg basis.

Patient/Family Teaching
- Instruct patient to take medication as directed. Advise patient and parents to read *Medication Guide* prior to initiation of therapy and with each renewal of Rx refill. If more than prescribed amount is taken notify health care professional immediately. Instruct patient not to alter dose without consulting health care professional.

- Inform patient that sharing this medication may be dangerous.
- Advise patient to check weight 2–3 times weekly and report weight loss to health care professional. Pedi: If reduced appetite and weight loss are a problem, advise parents to provide high calorie meals when drug levels are low (at breakfast and or bedtime).
- Inform patients starting therapy of risk of peripheral vasculopathy. Instruct patients to notify health care professional of any new numbness; pain; skin color change from pale, to blue, to red; or coolness or sensitivity to temperature in fingers or toes, and call if unexplained wounds appear on fingers or toes. May require rheumatology consultation.
- Advise parents to notify health care professional immediately if child has signs of heart problems (chest pain, shortness of breath, fainting) or if new or worsening mental symptoms or problems, especially seeing or hearing things that are not real, or are suspicious occur.
- May cause dizziness or blurred vision. Caution patient to avoid driving or activities requiring alertness until response to medication is known.
- Advise patient to notify health care professional if nervousness, restlessness, insomnia, dizziness, anorexia, or dry mouth becomes severe.
- Advise patient to notify health care professional of all Rx or OTC medications, vitamins, or herbal products being taken and to consult with health care professional before taking other medications.
- Inform patient that health care professional may order periodic holidays from the drug to assess progress and to decrease dependence.
- Rep: May cause fetal harm. Advise patient to notify health care professional if pregnancy is planned or suspected, and to avoid breastfeeding. May cause premature delivery. Monitor infants born to mothers taking lisdexamfetamine for symptoms of withdrawal (feeding difficulties, irritability, agitation, excessive drowsiness). Inform patient of pregnancy exposure registry that monitors pregnancy outcomes in women exposed to ADHD medications during pregnancy. Register patient by calling the National Pregnancy Registry for Psychostimulants at 1-866-961-2388 or visiting online at https://womensmentalhealth.org/clinical-and-researchprograms/pregnancyregistry/adhdmedications/.
- Emphasize the importance of routine follow-up exams to monitor progress.
- **Home Care Issues:** Advise parents to notify school nurse of medication regimen.

Evaluation/Desired Outcomes
- Improved attention span, decreased impulsiveness and hyperactivity in ADHD.
- Reduction in number of binge eating days per wk.

lisinopril, See ANGIOTENSIN-CONVERTING ENZYME (ACE) INHIBITORS.

lithium (lith-ee-um)
✳ Carbolith, ✳ Lithane, ✳ Lithmax, Lithobid
Classification
Therapeutic: mood stabilizers

Indications
Acute manic and mixed episodes associated with bipolar I disorder. Maintenance treatment of bipolar I disorder.

Action
Alters cation transport in nerve and muscle. May also influence reuptake of neurotransmitters. **Therapeutic Effects:** Prevents/decreases incidence of acute manic episodes.

Pharmacokinetics
Absorption: Completely absorbed after oral administration.
Distribution: Widely distributed into many tissues and fluids; CSF levels are 50% of plasma levels. Crosses the placenta; enters breast milk.
Metabolism and Excretion: Excreted almost entirely unchanged by the kidneys.
Half-life: 20–27 hr.

TIME/ACTION PROFILE (antimanic effects)

ROUTE	ONSET	PEAK	DURATION
PO, PO–ER	5–7 days	10–21 days	days

Contraindications/Precautions
Contraindicated in: Hypersensitivity; Brugada syndrome; Some products contain alcohol or tartrazine and should be avoided in patients with known hypersensitivity or intolerance; OB: Pregnancy; Lactation: Lactation.
Use Cautiously in: Significant cardiovascular disease, renal impairment, dehydration, fever, or hyponatremia (↑ risk of lithium toxicity); Diabetes mellitus; Pedi: Children <7 yr (safety and effectiveness not established); Geri: Initial dosage ↓ recommended in older adults.

Adverse Reactions/Side Effects
CV: ECG changes, arrhythmias, edema, hypotension, unmasking of Brugada syndrome. **Derm:** acneiform eruption, folliculitis, alopecia, diminished sensation, DRUG REACTION WITH EOSINOPHILIA AND SYSTEMIC SYMPTOMS (DRESS), pruritus. **EENT:** aphasia, blurred vision, dysarthria, tinnitus. **Endo:** hypothyroidism, goiter, hy-

perglycemia, hyperparathyroidism, hyperthyroidism. **F and E:** hypercalcemia, hyponatremia. **GI:** <u>abdominal pain</u>, anorexia, bloating, diarrhea, nausea, dry mouth, metallic taste. **GU:** <u>polyuria</u>, glycosuria, nephrogenic diabetes insipidus, renal impairment. **Hemat:** <u>leukocytosis</u>. **Metab:** weight gain. **MS:** muscle weakness, hyperirritability, rigidity. **Neuro:** <u>fatigue</u>, <u>headache</u>, impaired memory, <u>tremors</u>, ataxia, confusion, dizziness, drowsiness, PSEUDOTUMOR CEREBRI, psychomotor retardation, restlessness, sedation, SEIZURES, stupor. **Misc:** SEROTONIN SYNDROME.

Interactions

Drug-Drug: May prolong the action of **neuromuscular blocking agents**. ↑ risk of neurologic toxicity with **calcium channel blockers**, **phenytoin**, or **carbamazepine**. **Diuretics, NSAIDs, ACE inhibitors, angiotensin II receptor blockers**, and **metronidazole** may ↑ levels and risk of toxicity. Hypothyroid effects may be additive with **potassium iodide** or **antithyroid agents**. **Aminophylline**, **acetazolamide**, **theophylline**, and **sodium bicarbonate** ↑ renal elimination and ↓ effectiveness. **Psyllium** can ↓ **lithium** levels. Drugs that affect serotonergic neurotransmitter systems, including **tricyclic antidepressants**, **SSRIs, SNRIs, fentanyl, buspirone, tramadol, amphetamines**, and **triptans** ↑ risk of serotonin syndrome. Concurrent use with **antipsychotics** may ↑ risk of developing an encephalopathic syndrome (i.e., weakness, lethargy, fever, tremulousness and confusion, extrapyramidal symptoms, leukocytosis, ↑ BUN, and ↑ fasting blood glucose); monitor closely. **SGLT2 inhibitors** may ↓ levels and effectiveness.

Drug-Natural Products: Caffeine-containing herbs (**cola nut, guarana, mate, tea, coffee**) may ↓ **lithium** serum levels and efficacy. ↑ risk of serotonergic side effects including serotonin syndrome with **St. John's wort**.

Drug-Food: Large changes in **sodium** intake may alter the renal elimination of lithium. ↑ sodium intake will ↑ renal excretion.

Route/Dosage

Precise dosing is based on serum lithium levels. 300 mg lithium carbonate contains ≥8–12 mEq lithium.

PO (Adults and Children ≥7 yr and >30 kg): *Tablets/capsules/liquid:* 300 mg 3 times daily initially; ↑ by 300 mg/day every 3 days; usual dose for treatment of acute manic and mixed episodes = 600 mg 2–3 times daily; usual maintenance dose = 300–600 mg 2–3 times daily.

PO (Adults and Children >12 yr): *Extended-release tablets:* 450–900 mg twice daily *or* 300–600 mg 3 times daily initially; usual maintenance dose is 450 mg twice daily *or* 300 mg 3 times daily.

PO (Children ≥7 yr and 20–30 kg): *Tablets/capsules/liquid:* 300 mg twice daily initially; ↑ by 300 mg/wk; usual dose for treatment of acute manic and mixed episodes = 600–1500 mg/day in divided doses; usual

maintenance dose = 600–1200 mg/day in divided doses.

Availability (generic available)

Immediate-release tablets: 300 mg. **Immediate-release capsules:** 150 mg, 300 mg, 600 mg. **Extended-release tablets:** 300 mg, 450 mg. **Oral solution:** 300 mg (8 mEq lithium)/5 mL.

NURSING IMPLICATIONS

Assessment

- Assess mental status (orientation, mood, behavior) initially and periodically. Initiate suicide precautions if indicated.
- Monitor intake and output ratios. Report significant changes in totals. Unless contraindicated, fluid intake of at least 2000–3000 mL/day should be maintained. Weight should also be monitored at least every 3 mo.

Lab Test Considerations

- Evaluate renal and thyroid function, WBC with differential, serum electrolytes, and glucose periodically during therapy.

Toxicity and Overdose

- Monitor serum lithium levels twice weekly during initiation of therapy and every 2 mo during chronic therapy. Draw blood samples in the morning immediately before next dose. Therapeutic levels range from 0.5–1.5 mEq/L for acute mania and 0.6–1.2 mEq/L for long term control. Serum concentrations should not exceed 2.0 mEq/L.
- Assess patient for signs and symptoms of lithium toxicity (vomiting, diarrhea, slurred speech, lightheadedness, decreased coordination, drowsiness, muscle weakness, tremor, or twitching). If these occur, report before administering next dose.

Implementation

- Do not confuse lithium carbonate with lanthanum carbonate.
- **PO:** Administer with food or milk to minimize GI irritation. *DNC:* Extended-release preparations should be swallowed whole; do not break, crush, or chew.

Patient/Family Teaching

- Instruct patient to take medication as directed, even if feeling well. Take missed doses as soon as remembered unless within 2 hr of next dose (6 hr if extended release).
- Lithium may cause dizziness or drowsiness. Caution patient to avoid driving or other activities requiring alertness until response to medication is known.
- Low sodium levels may predispose patient to toxicity. Advise patient to drink 2000–3000 mL fluid each day and eat a diet with consistent and moderate sodium intake. Excessive amounts of coffee, tea, and cola should be avoided because of diuretic effect. Avoid activities that cause excess sodium loss (heavy exertion, exercise in hot weather, saunas). Notify

health care professional of fever, vomiting, and diarrhea, which also cause sodium loss.
- Advise patient that weight gain may occur. Review principles of a low-calorie diet.
- Advise patient to notify health care professional of all Rx or OTC medications, vitamins, or herbal products being taken and to consult with health care professional before taking other medications, especially NSAIDs and St. John's wort.
- Review side effects and symptoms of toxicity with patient. Instruct patient to stop medication and report signs of toxicity to health care professional promptly.
- Advise patient to notify health care professional if fainting, irregular pulse, or difficulty breathing occurs.
- Rep: May cause fetal harm. Advise females of reproductive potential to use contraception during therapy, to consult health care professional if pregnancy is planned or suspected, and to avoid breastfeeding. Monitor breastfed infants for signs and symptoms of lithium toxicity (hypertonia, hypothermia, cyanosis, ECG changes).
- Emphasize the importance of periodic lab tests to monitor for lithium toxicity.

Evaluation/Desired Outcomes
- Resolution of the symptoms of mania (hyperactivity, pressured speech, poor judgment, need for little sleep).
- Decreased incidence of mood swings in bipolar disorders.
- Improved affect in unipolar disorders. Improvement in condition may require 1–3 wk.
- Decreased incidence of acute manic episodes.

℥ lofexidine (loe-fex-i-deen)
Lucemyra
Classification
Therapeutic: none assigned
Pharmacologic: adrenergics (centrally acting)

Indications
Mitigation of opioid withdrawal symptoms to facilitate abrupt opioid discontinuation in adults.

Action
Stimulates alpha$_2$-adrenergic receptors in the CNS, which results in decreased sympathetic outflow. **Therapeutic Effects:** Reduction in severity of opioid withdrawal symptoms.

Pharmacokinetics
Absorption: 72% absorbed following oral administration.
Distribution: Extensively distributed to tissues, including CNS.
Metabolism and Excretion: Primarily metabolized by the liver via the CYP2D6 isoenzyme and to a

lesser extent by the CYP1A2 and CYP2C19 isoenzymes to inactive metabolites; primarily excreted in urine (15–20% as unchanged drug); ℥ the CYP2D6 isoenzyme exhibits genetic polymorphism; ~7% of population may be poor metabolizers and may have significantly ↑ lofexidine concentrations and an ↑ risk of adverse effects.
Half-life: 17–22 hr.

TIME/ACTION PROFILE (plasma concentrations)

ROUTE	ONSET	PEAK	DURATION
PO	unknown	3–5 hr	unknown

Contraindications/Precautions
Contraindicated in: Congenital long QT syndrome.
Use Cautiously in: Severe cardiac or cerebrovascular disease, recent MI, chronic kidney disease, or severe bradycardia (↑ risk of hypotension, bradycardia, and/or syncope); HF, bradyarrhythmias, hepatic impairment, renal impairment, hypokalemia, hypomagnesemia, or concurrent use of QT-interval prolonging medications (↑ risk of QT interval prolongation); ℥ CYP2D6 poor metabolizers; OB: Safety not established in pregnancy; Lactation: Safety not established in breastfeeding; Pedi: Safety and effectiveness not established in children; Geri: ↑ risk of orthostatic hypotension and adverse CNS effects in older adults (↓ dose recommended).

Adverse Reactions/Side Effects
CV: bradycardia, hypotension, palpitations, QT interval prolongation, syncope, TORSADES DE POINTES. **EENT:** tinnitus. **GI:** dry mouth. **Neuro:** dizziness, drowsiness, insomnia.

Interactions
Drug-Drug: Additive hypotension with other **antihypertensives** and **nitrates**; avoid concurrent use. Additive bradycardia with **beta blockers**, **diltiazem**, **verapamil**, **digoxin**, **clonidine**, or **ivabradine**; avoid concurrent use. Additive sedation with **CNS depressants**, including **alcohol**, **antihistamines**, **opioid analgesics**, and **sedative/hypnotics**. Concurrent use with **QT interval-prolonging medications**, including **methadone**, may ↑ risk of QT interval prolongation and torsades de pointes. May ↓ **naltrexone** (PO) levels; separate administration by >2 hr. **CYP2D6 inhibitors**, including **paroxetine** may ↑ levels and risk of toxicity.

Route/Dosage
PO (Adults): 0.54 mg 4 times daily (with 5–6 hr between each dose) during the period of peak withdrawal symptoms (usually the first 5–7 days after the last opioid dose); may adjust dose based on symptoms (max dose = 2.88 mg/day or 0.72 mg/dose); may be continued for up to 14 days. Must taper therapy upon discontinuation (gradually ↓ dose over 2–4-day period).

Hepatic Impairment
PO (Adults): *Moderate hepatic impairment:* 0.36 mg 4 times daily (with 5–6 hr between each dose) during the period of peak withdrawal symptoms (usually the first 5–7 days after the last opioid dose); *Severe hepatic impairment:* 0.18 mg 4 times daily (with 5–6 hr between each dose) during the period of peak withdrawal symptoms (usually the first 5–7 days after the last opioid dose).

Renal Impairment
PO (Adults): *CCr 30– <90 mL/min:* 0.36 mg 4 times daily (with 5–6 hr between each dose) during the period of peak withdrawal symptoms (usually the first 5–7 days after the last opioid dose); *CCr <30 mL/min:* 0.18 mg 4 times daily (with 5–6 hr between each dose) during the period of peak withdrawal symptoms (usually the first 5–7 days after the last opioid dose).

Availability
Tablets: 0.18 mg.

NURSING IMPLICATIONS

Assessment
- Assess vital signs and symptoms of bradycardia and orthostatic hypotension (low BP, slow HR, dizziness, light-headedness, feeling faint at rest or when standing up) before dose and as needed during therapy.
- Monitor ECG when starting therapy and in patients with HF, bradyarrhythmias, hepatic impairment, renal impairment, or those taking medications (methadone) that lead to QT prolongation.

Lab Test Considerations
- Monitor electrolytes before starting and during therapy. Correct electrolyte abnormalities (hypokalemia, hypomagnesemia) before starting therapy.

Implementation
- **PO:** Administer 3 tablets four times daily without regard to food, with 5–6 hr between doses.

Patient/Family Teaching
- Instruct patient to take lofexidine as directed and not to stop without consulting health care professional. Abrupt discontinuation can cause diarrhea, insomnia, anxiety, chills, hyperhidrosis, and extremity pain. Reduce dose gradually.
- Caution patients that after a period of not using opioids, they may be more sensitive to the effects of opioids and at greater risk of overdosing.
- May cause dizziness and sedation. Caution patient to avoid driving and activities requiring alertness until response to medication is known.
- Caution patient to avoid sudden changes in position to decrease orthostatic hypotension. Use of alcohol, standing for long periods, exercising, dehydration, and hot weather may increase orthostatic hypotension.
- Instruct patient to notify health care professional of all Rx or OTC medications, vitamins, or herbal products being taken and to consult health care professional before taking any other Rx, OTC, or herbal

products, especially benzodiazepines, barbiturates, tranquilizers, or sleeping pills.
- Caution patient to avoid concurrent use of alcohol or other CNS depressants with lofexidine.
- Rep: Advise females of reproductive potential to notify health care professional if pregnancy is planned or suspected or if breastfeeding.

Evaluation/Desired Outcomes
- Reduction in severity of opioid withdrawal symptoms.

---

loperamide (loe-**per**-a-mide)
Imodium A-D
Classification
Therapeutic: antidiarrheals

Indications
Adjunctive therapy of acute diarrhea. Chronic diarrhea associated with inflammatory bowel disease. Decreases the volume of ileostomy drainage.

Action
Inhibits peristalsis and prolongs transit time by a direct effect on nerves in the intestinal muscle wall. Reduces fecal volume, increases fecal viscosity and bulk while diminishing loss of fluid and electrolytes. **Therapeutic Effects:** Relief of diarrhea.

Pharmacokinetics
Absorption: Not well absorbed following oral administration.
Distribution: Does not cross the blood-brain barrier.
Protein Binding: 97%.
Metabolism and Excretion: Metabolized partially by the liver, undergoes enterohepatic recirculation; 30% eliminated in the feces. Minimal excretion in the urine.
Half-life: 10.8 hr.

TIME/ACTION PROFILE (relief of diarrhea)

ROUTE	ONSET	PEAK	DURATION
PO	1 hr	2.5–5 hr	10 hr

Contraindications/Precautions
Contraindicated in: Hypersensitivity; Patients in whom constipation must be avoided; Abdominal pain of unknown cause, especially if associated with fever; Alcohol intolerance (liquid only).
Use Cautiously in: Hepatic impairment; OB: Safety not established in pregnancy; Pedi: Children <2 yr (safety and effectiveness not established); Geri: Older adults may have ↑ sensitivity to effects.

Adverse Reactions/Side Effects
CV: CARDIAC ARREST, QT interval prolongation, syncope, TORSADES DE POINTES, VENTRICULAR ARRHYTHMIAS. **GI:** constipation, abdominal pain/distention/discomfort,

dry mouth, nausea, vomiting. **Neuro:** drowsiness, dizziness. **Misc:** HYPERSENSITIVITY REACTIONS (including anaphylaxis).

Interactions

Drug-Drug: ↑ CNS depression with other **CNS depressants**, including **alcohol, antihistamines, opioid analgesics,** and **sedative/hypnotics.** ↑ anticholinergic properties with other **drugs having anticholinergic properties,** including **antidepressants** and **antihistamines.** Concurrent use of **cimetidine, clarithromycin, erythromycin, gemfibrozil, itraconazole, ketoconazole, quinidine, quinine,** or **ritonavir** may ↑ levels and risk of cardiac arrhythmias. **Drug-Natural Products:** Kava-kava, valerian, skullcap, chamomile, or hops can ↑ CNS depression.

Route/Dosage

Acute Diarrhea

PO (Adults and Children ≥12 yr): 4 mg initially, then 2 mg after each loose stool. Maintenance dose usually 4–8 mg/day in divided doses (not to exceed 8 mg/day for OTC use or 16 mg/day for Rx use).
PO (Children 9–11 yr or 30–47 kg): 2 mg initially, then 1 mg after each loose stool (not to exceed 6 mg/24 hr; OTC use should not exceed 2 days).
PO (Children 6–8 yr or 24–30 kg): 1 mg initially, then 1 mg after each loose stool (not to exceed 4 mg/24 hr; OTC use should not exceed 2 days).
PO (Children 2–5 yr or 13–20 kg): 1 mg initially, then 0.1 mg/kg after each loose stool (not to exceed 3 mg/24 hr; OTC use should not exceed 2 days).

Chronic Diarrhea

PO (Adults): 4 mg initially, then 2 mg after each loose stool. Maintenance dose usually 4–8 mg/day in divided doses (not to exceed 16 mg/day for Rx use).
PO (Children): 0.08–0.24 mg/kg/day divided 2–3 times/day (not to exceed 2 mg/dose).

Reduction of Ileostomy Output

PO (Adults): 2 mg 2–3 times daily (tablets or capsules only); may ↑ dose in 2 mg/day increments if output remains elevated (not to exceed 16 mg/day for Rx use).

Availability (generic available)

Tablets: 2 mg^OTC. **Capsules:** 2 mg. **Oral liquid (mint):** 1 mg/7.5 mL^OTC. *In combination with:* simethicone (Imodium Multi-Symptom Relief), see Appendix N).

NURSING IMPLICATIONS

Assessment

- Assess frequency and consistency of stools and bowel sounds prior to and during therapy.
- Assess fluid and electrolyte balance and skin turgor for dehydration.

Implementation

- **PO:** Administer with clear fluids to help prevent dehydration, which may accompany diarrhea.

Patient/Family Teaching

- Instruct patient to take medication as directed. Do not take missed doses, and do not double doses. In acute diarrhea, medication may be ordered after each unformed stool. Advise patient not to exceed the maximum number of doses.
- May cause drowsiness. Advise patient to avoid driving or other activities requiring alertness until response to drug is known.
- Advise patient that frequent mouth rinses, good oral hygiene, and sugarless gum or candy may relieve dry mouth.
- Caution patient to avoid using alcohol and other CNS depressants concurrently with this medication.
- Instruct patient to notify health care professional if diarrhea persists or if fever, abdominal pain, or distention occurs.
- Rep: Advise females of reproductive potential to notify health care professional if breastfeeding.

Evaluation/Desired Outcomes

- Decrease in diarrhea.
- In acute diarrhea, treatment should be discontinued if no improvement is seen in 48 hr.
- In chronic diarrhea, if no improvement has occurred after at least 10 days of treatment with maximum dose, loperamide is unlikely to be effective.

---

loratadine (lor-a-ta-deen)

Alavert, Claritin, Claritin Allergy Childrens, Claritin Childrens, Claritin Reditabs, Loradamed
Classification
Therapeutic: allergy, cold, and cough remedies
Pharmacologic: antihistamines

Indications

Seasonal allergies. Chronic idiopathic urticaria. Hives.

Action

Blocks peripheral effects of histamine released during allergic reactions. **Therapeutic Effects:** Decreased symptoms of allergic reactions (nasal stuffiness; red, swollen eyes; itching).

Pharmacokinetics

Absorption: Rapidly absorbed after oral administration (80%).
Distribution: Unknown.
Protein Binding: *Loratadine:* 97%; *descarboethoxyloratadine:* 73–77%.
Metabolism and Excretion: Rapidly and extensively metabolized during first pass through the liver.

✳ = Canadian drug name. ✂ = Genetic implication. ~~Strikethrough~~ = Discontinued. CAPITALS = life-threatening. <u>Underline</u> = most frequent.

Much is converted to descarboethoxyloratadine, an active metabolite.
Half-life: *Loratadine:* 8.4 hr; *descarboethoxyloratadine:* 28 hr.

TIME/ACTION PROFILE (antihistaminic effects)

ROUTE	ONSET	PEAK	DURATION
PO	1–3 hr	8–12 hr	>24 hr

Contraindications/Precautions
Contraindicated in: Hypersensitivity.
Use Cautiously in: Hepatic impairment or CCr <30 mL/min (↓ dose to 10 mg every other day); Pedi: Children <2 yr (safety and effectiveness not established); Syrup contains sodium benzoate; avoid use in neonates; Geri: ↑ risk of adverse reactions in older adults.

Adverse Reactions/Side Effects
Derm: photosensitivity, rash. **EENT:** blurred vision. **GI:** dry mouth, GI upset. **Metab:** weight gain. **Neuro:** confusion, drowsiness (rare), paradoxical excitation.

Interactions
Drug-Drug: The following interactions may occur, but are less likely to occur with loratadine than with more sedating antihistamines. **MAO inhibitors** may intensify and prolong effects of antihistamines. ↑ CNS depression may occur with other **CNS depressants**, including **alcohol, antidepressants, opioid analgesics,** and **sedative/hypnotics. Amiodarone** may ↑ loratadine levels and ↑ risk of QTc interval prolongation.
Drug-Natural Products: Kava-kava, valerian, or **chamomile** can ↑ CNS depression.

Route/Dosage
PO (Adults and Children ≥6 yr): 10 mg once daily.
PO (Children ≥2–5 yr): 5 mg once daily.

Renal Impairment
PO (Adults): *CCr <30 mL/min:* 10 mg every other day.

Hepatic Impairment
PO (Adults): 10 mg every other day.

Availability (generic available)
Tablets: 10 mg^OTC. **Capsules:** 10 mg^OTC. **Chewable tablets (cool-mint-flavor, grape-flavor, bubble-gum-flavor):** 5 mg^OTC, 10 mg^OTC. **Orally disintegrating tablets (mint):** 5 mg^OTC, 10 mg^OTC. **Oral solution (grape-flavor, fruit-flavor):** 5 mg/5 mL^OTC. *In combination with:* pseudoephedrine (Claritin-D)^OTC. See Appendix N.

NURSING IMPLICATIONS
Assessment
- Assess allergy symptoms (rhinitis, conjunctivitis, hives) before and periodically during therapy.
- Assess lung sounds and character of bronchial secretions. Maintain fluid intake of 1500–2000 mL/day to decrease viscosity of secretions.

Lab Test Considerations
- May cause false-negative result on allergy skin testing.

Implementation
- **PO:** Administer once daily.
- *For rapidly disintegrating tablets (Alavert, Claritin Reditabs):* place on tongue. Tablet disintegrates rapidly. May be taken with or without water.

Patient/Family Teaching
- Instruct patient to take medication as directed.
- May cause dizziness or drowsiness. Caution patient to avoid driving or other activities requiring alertness until response to medication is known.
- Caution patient to use sunscreen and protective clothing to prevent photosensitivity reactions.
- Advise patient to avoid taking alcohol or other CNS depressants concurrently with this drug.
- Advise patient that good oral hygiene, frequent rinsing of mouth with water, and sugarless gum or candy may minimize dry mouth. Patient should notify dentist if dry mouth persists >2 wk.
- Instruct patient to contact health care professional immediately if dizziness, fainting, or fast or irregular heartbeat occurs or if symptoms persist.
- Rep: Advise females of reproductive potential to notify health care professional if pregnancy is planned or suspected, or if breastfeeding.

Evaluation/Desired Outcomes
- Decrease in allergic symptoms.
- Management of chronic idiopathic urticaria.
- Management of hives.

BEERS

LORazepam (lor-az-e-pam)
Ativan, Loreev XR
Classification
Therapeutic: anesthetic adjuncts, antianxiety agents, sedative/hypnotics
Pharmacologic: benzodiazepines

Schedule IV

Indications
PO: Anxiety disorder. IM, IV: Status epilepticus, Preanesthetic to produce sedation, decrease preoperative anxiety and induce amnesia.

Action
Depresses the CNS, probably by potentiating GABA, an inhibitory neurotransmitter. **Therapeutic Effects:** Sedation. Decreased anxiety. Decreased seizures.

Pharmacokinetics
Absorption: Well absorbed following oral administration. Rapidly and completely absorbed following IM administration. Sublingual absorption is more rapid than oral and is similar to IM. IV administration results in complete bioavailability.
Distribution: Widely distributed. Crosses the blood-brain barrier. Crosses the placenta; enters breast milk.

Metabolism and Excretion: Highly metabolized by the liver.

Half-life: *Full-term neonates:* 18–73 hr; *Older children:* 6–17 hr; *Adults:* 10–16 hr.

TIME/ACTION PROFILE (sedation)

ROUTE	ONSET	PEAK	DURATION
PO	15–60 min	1–6 hr	8–12 hr
PO-XR	unknown	unknown	unknown
IM	30–60 min	1–2 hr†	8–12 hr
IV	15–30 min	15–20 min	8–12 hr

†Amnestic response.

Contraindications/Precautions

Contraindicated in: Hypersensitivity; Cross-sensitivity with other benzodiazepines may exist; Comatose patients or those with pre-existing CNS depression; Uncontrolled severe pain; Angle-closure glaucoma; Severe hypotension; Sleep apnea.

Use Cautiously in: Severe hepatic/renal/pulmonary impairment; Myasthenia gravis; Depression; Psychosis; History of suicide attempt or drug abuse/substance use disorder; COPD; Sleep apnea; OB: Use late in pregnancy can result in sedation (respiratory depression, lethargy, hypotonia) and/or withdrawal symptoms (hyperreflexia, irritability, restlessness, tremors, inconsolable crying, and feeding difficulties) in neonates; Lactation: Use while breastfeeding only if potential maternal benefit outweighs potential risk to infant; Pedi: Safety and effectiveness not established in children <18 yr (IV) or <12 yr (PO); in ↑ doses, benzyl alcohol in injection may cause potentially fatal "gasping syndrome" in neonates; IV use may affect brain development in children <3 yr; Geri: Appears on Beers list. ↑ risk of cognitive impairment, delirium, falls, fractures, and motor vehicle accidents in older adults. If possible, avoid use in older adults.

Adverse Reactions/Side Effects

CV: bradycardia hypotension; *rapid IV use only:* APNEA, CARDIAC ARREST. **Derm:** rash. **EENT:** blurred vision. **GI:** constipation, diarrhea, nausea, vomiting. **Neuro:** dizziness, drowsiness, lethargy, ataxia, confusion, forgetfulness, hangover, headache, mental depression, rhythmic myoclonic jerking in pre-term infants, paradoxical excitation, slurred speech. **Resp:** respiratory depression. **Misc:** physical dependence, psychological dependence, tolerance.

Interactions

Drug-Drug: Use with **opioids** or other **CNS depressants**, including other **benzodiazepines, nonbenzodiazepine sedative/hypnotics, anxiolytics, general anesthetics, muscle relaxants, antipsychotics,** and **alcohol** may cause profound sedation, respiratory depression, coma, and death; reserve concurrent use for when alternative treatment options are inadequate. May ↓ the efficacy of **levodopa. Smoking** may ↑ metabolism and ↓ effectiveness. **Valproate** and **probenecid** can ↑ levels; ↓ dose by 50%. **Oral contraceptives** may ↓ levels.

Drug-Natural Products: Concomitant use of **kava-kava, valerian,** or **chamomile** can ↑ CNS depression.

Route/Dosage

Status Epilepticus

IV, IM (Adults): 4 mg; may be repeated after 10–15 min.

Preanesthetic

IM (Adults): 0.05 mg/kg (not to exceed 4 mg) ≥2 hr before surgery.

IV (Adults): 0.044 mg/kg (not to exceed 2 mg) 15–20 min before surgery.

Anxiety

PO (Adults): *Immediate-release tablets:* 1–3 mg 2–3 times daily (up to 10 mg/day). *Extended-release capsules:* Give total daily dose of lorazepam immediate-release tablets (at the previous three times daily dose) and administer once daily in the morning. If dose ↑ needed, switch to lorazepam immediate-release tablets to ↑ the dose; once stable response achieved, may switch back to equivalent daily dose of lorazepam extended-release capsules.

PO (Geriatric Patients or Debilitated Patients): 0.5–2 mg/day in divided doses initially.

Availability (generic available)

Immediate-release tablets: 0.5 mg, 1 mg, 2 mg. **Extended-release capsules (Loreev XR):** 1 mg, 2 mg, 3 mg. **Sublingual tablets :** ✳ 0.5 mg, ✳ 1 mg, ✳ 2 mg. **Concentrated oral solution:** 2 mg/mL. **Solution for injection:** 2 mg/mL, 4 mg/mL.

NURSING IMPLICATIONS

Assessment

- Conduct regular assessment of continued need for treatment.
- Assess risk for addiction, abuse, or misuse prior to administration and periodically during therapy.
- Geri: Assess geriatric patients carefully for CNS reactions as they are more sensitive to these effects. Assess falls risk.
- Anxiety: Assess degree and manifestations of anxiety and mental status (orientation, mood, behavior) prior to and periodically during therapy.
- Prolonged high-dose therapy may lead to psychological or physical dependence. Restrict amount of drug available to patient.
- Status Epilepticus: Assess location, duration, characteristics, and frequency of seizures. Institute seizure precautions.

✳ = Canadian drug name. ☷ = Genetic implication. ~~Strikethrough~~ = Discontinued. CAPITALS = life-threatening. <u>Underline</u> = most frequent.

Lab Test Considerations
● Patients on high-dose therapy should receive routine evaluation of renal, hepatic, and hematologic function.

Toxicity and Overdose
● If overdose occurs, flumazenil is the antidote. Do not use with patients with seizure disorder. May induce seizures.

Implementation
● Do not confuse lorazepam with alprazolam, clonazepam, or Lovaza.
● Gradually taper to discontinue or reduce the dose to reduce risk of withdrawal reactions, increased seizure frequency, and status epilepticus. If a patient develops withdrawal reactions, consider pausing taper or increasing the dose to the previous tapered dose level. Subsequently decrease the dose more slowly. Some patients may require longer tapering period (weeks to >12 mo).
● Following parenteral administration, keep patient supine for at least 8 hr and observe closely.
● PO: Tablet may also be given sublingually (unlabeled) for more rapid onset.
● Administer XR capsules with or without food. *DNC:* Do not crush or chew. Swallow whole or open and sprinkle the entire contents of capsule over a tablespoon of applesauce, then drink water after consuming the applesauce (without chewing). Consume entire contents of capsule within 2 hrs of opening capsule.
● Take concentrated liquid solution with water, soda, pudding, or applesauce. Use calibrated dropper provided to ensure accurate dose.
● IM: Administer IM doses deep into muscle mass at least 2 hr before surgery for optimum effect.

IV Administration
● IV Push: *Dilution:* Dilute immediately before use with an equal amount of sterile water for injection, D5W, or 0.9% NaCl for injection. Pedi: To decrease the amount of benzyl alcohol delivered to neonates, dilute the 4 mg/mL injection with preservative-free sterile water for injection to make a 0.4 mg/mL dilution for IV use. Do not use if solution is colored or contains a precipitate. *Rate:* Administer at a rate not to exceed 2 mg/min or 0.05 mg/kg over 2–5 min. Rapid IV administration may result in apnea, hypotension, bradycardia, or cardiac arrest.
● Y-Site Compatibility: acetaminophen, acyclovir, albumin, alemtuzumab, allopurinol, amifostine, amikacin, aminocaproic acid, aminophylline, amiodarone, amphotericin B deoxycholate, amphotericin B lipid complex, anakinra, anidulafungin, argatroban, arsenic trioxide, atracurium, azithromycin, bleomycin, bumetanide, buprenorphine, busulfan, butorphanol, calcium chloride, calcium gluconate, cangrelor, carboplatin, carmustine, cefazolin, cefepime, cefotaxime, cefotetan, cefoxitin, ceftaroline, ceftazidime, ceftolozane/tazobactam, ceftriaxone, cefuroxime, chloramphenicol, ciprofloxacin, cisatracurium, cisplatin, cladribine, clindamycin, cyclophosphamide, cyclosporine, cytarabine, dacarbazine, dactinomycin, daptomycin, dexamethasone, dexmedetomidine, dexrazoxane, digoxin, diltiazem, diphenhydramine, dobutamine, docetaxel, dopamine, doxorubicin hydrochloride, doxorubicin liposomal, doxycycline, droperidol, enalaprilat, ephedrine, epinephrine, epirubicin, eptifibatide, ertapenem, erythromycin lactobionate, esmolol, etomidate, etoposide phosphate, famotidine, fentanyl, filgrastim, fluconazole, fludarabine, fosphenytoin, furosemide, ganciclovir, gemcitabine, gentamicin, glycopyrrolate, granisetron, haloperidol, heparin, hetastarch, hydrocortisone sodium succinate, hydromorphone, ifosfamide, insulin regular, irinotecan, isavuconazonium, isoproterenol, ketorolac, labetalol, leucovorin calcium, lidocaine, linezolid, magnesium sulfate, mannitol, melphalan, meropenem, meropenem/vaborbactam, mesna, methadone, methotrexate, methylprednisolone, metoclopramide, metoprolol, metronidazole, micafungin, midazolam, milrinone, mitoxantrone, morphine, mycophenolate, nafcillin, nalbuphine, naloxone, nicardipine, nitroglycerin, nitroprusside, norepinephrine, octreotide, oritavancin, oxaliplatin, oxytocin, paclitaxel, palonosetron, pamidronate, pemetrexed, pentamidine, pentobarbital, phentolamine, phenobarbital, phenylephrine, piperacillin/tazobactam, plazomicin, potassium acetate, potassium chloride, procainamide, prochlorperazine, promethazine, propofol, propranolol, remifentanil, rituximab, sodium acetate, sodium bicarbonate, sodium phosphate, succinylcholine, tacrolimus, tedizolid, theophylline, thiotepa, tigecycline, tirofiban, tobramycin, trastuzumab, trimethoprim/sulfamethoxazole, vancomycin, vasopressin, vecuronium, verapamil, vinblastine, vincristine, vinorelbine, voriconazole, zidovudine, zoledronic acid.
● Y-Site Incompatibility: aldesleukin, amphotericin B liposomal, ampicillin, ampicillin/sulbactam, aztreonam, dantrolene, fluorouracil, gemtuzumab ozogamicin, hydralazine, idarubicin, imipenem/cilastatin, meperidine, mitomycin, ondansetron, pantoprazole, phenytoin, potassium phosphate, rocuronium, sargramostim, sufentanil.

Patient/Family Teaching
● Instruct patient to take medication exactly as directed and not to skip or double up on missed doses. If medication is less effective after a few wk, check with health care professional; do not increase dose. Must be discontinued gradually. Do not suddenly stop taking lorazepam without consulting health care professional; may cause unusual movements, responses or expressions, seizures, sudden and severe mental or nervous system changes,

depression, seeing or hearing things that others do not see or hear, an extreme increase in activity or talking, losing touch with reality, and suicidal thoughts or actions. Instruct patient to ready *Medication Guide* before starting therapy and with each Rx refill in case of changes.

- Advise patient that lorazepam is a drug with known abuse potential. Protect it from theft, and never give to anyone other than the individual for whom it was prescribed. Store out of sight and reach of children, and in a location not accessible by others.
- Advise patient that lorazepam is usually prescribed for short-term use and does not cure underlying problem.
- May cause drowsiness or dizziness. Advise patient to avoid driving or other activities requiring alertness until response to medication is known.
- Instruct patient to notify health care professional of all Rx or OTC medications, vitamins, or herbal products being taken and consult health care professional before taking any new medications.
- Caution patient to avoid taking alcohol or other CNS depressants, including opioids and cannabidiol, concurrently with this medication without consulting health care professional to prevent overdose.
- Rep: May cause fetal harm. Advise females of reproductive potential to contact health care professional immediately if pregnancy is planned or suspected. Monitor infants exposed to lorazepam during pregnancy or labor for several wks or more prior to delivery for signs and symptoms of withdrawal (hypoactivity, hypotonia, hypothermia, respiratory depression, apnea, feeding problems, impaired metabolic response to cold stress). Monitor infants exposed to lorazepam during breastfeeding for excessive sedation, poor feeding and poor weight gain, and to seek medical attention if they notice these signs. There is a pregnancy registry that monitors pregnancy outcomes in women exposed to psychiatric medications, including lorazepam, during pregnancy. Health care providers are encouraged to register patients by calling the National Pregnancy Registry for Psychiatric Medications at 1-866-961-2388 or online at https://womensmentalhealth.org/pregnancyregistry/.
- Emphasize the importance of follow-up exams to determine effectiveness of the medication.

Evaluation/Desired Outcomes
- Increase in sense of well-being.
- Decrease in subjective feelings of anxiety without excessive sedation.
- Reduction of preoperative anxiety.
- Postoperative amnesia.
- Improvement in sleep patterns.

losartan, See ANGIOTENSIN II RECEPTOR ANTAGONISTS.

lovastatin, See HMG-CoA REDUCTASE INHIBITORS (statins).

luliconazole, See ANTIFUNGALS (TOPICAL).

⚅ lumacaftor/ivacaftor
(loo-ma-**kaf**-tor/**eye**-va-**kaf**-tor)
Orkambi
Classification
Therapeutic: cystic fibrosis therapy adjuncts
Pharmacologic: transmembrane conductance regulator potentiators

L

Indications
⚅ Cystic fibrosis (CF) in patients who are homozygous for the *F508del* mutation in the *CFTR* gene.

Action
Ivacaftor: acts as a potentiator of the CFTR protein (a chloride channel on the surface of endothelial cells) facilitating chloride transport by increasing the channel-open probability (gating). *Lumacaftor:* improves the conformational stability of *F508del-CFTR* which results in increased processing and trafficking of mature protein to the cell surface. **Therapeutic Effects:** Improved lung function with increased weight, decreased exacerbations and CF symptoms.

Pharmacokinetics
Lumacaftor
Absorption: Some absorption follows oral administration; absorption is enhanced 2-fold by fat-containing foods.
Distribution: Widely distributed.
Protein Binding: >99%.
Metabolism and Excretion: Minimally metabolized via oxidation and glucuronidation; 51% excreted unchanged in feces; <1% excreted unchanged in urine.
Half-life: 26 hr.
Ivacaftor
Absorption: Some absorption follows oral administration; absorption is enhanced 3-fold by fat-containing foods.
Distribution: Unknown.
Protein Binding: >99%.
Metabolism and Excretion: Extensively metabolized by the liver, mostly by the CYP3A isoenzyme; one

metabolite (M1) is pharmacologically active; 87.8% eliminated in feces; negligible urinary elimination.
Half-life: 9 hr.

TIME/ACTION PROFILE (plasma concentrations)

ROUTE	ONSET	PEAK	DURATION
Lumacaftor (PO)	within 1 wk	4 hr	12 hr
Ivacaftor (PO)	within 1 wk	4 hr	12 hr

Contraindications/Precautions

Contraindicated in: None.
Use Cautiously in: Moderate or severe hepatic impairment (dose ↓ recommended); Severe renal impairment (CCr <30 mL/min) or end stage renal disease; Advanced lung disease (↑ risk of respiratory events); OB: Use in pregnancy only if clearly needed; Lactation: Use while breastfeeding only if potential maternal benefit outweighs potential risk to infant; Pedi: Children <1 yr (safety and effectiveness not established).

Adverse Reactions/Side Effects

CV: ↑ blood pressure. **Derm:** rash. **EENT:** cataracts, rhinorrhea. **GI:** diarrhea, nausea, ↑ liver enzymes, flatulence, hyperbilirubinemia. **GU:** amenorrhea, dysmenorrhea, menorrhagia. **MS:** ↑ creatine kinase. **Neuro:** fatigue. **Resp:** dyspnea, chest discomfort. **Misc:** HYPERSENSITIVITY REACTIONS (including anaphylaxis and angioedema).

Interactions

Drug-Drug: Strong CYP3A inducers including **rifampin, rifabutin, phenobarbital, carbamazepine** and **phenytoin** may ↓ ivacaftor levels and effectiveness; avoid concurrent use. Lumacaftor may ↓ levels of **CYP3A substrates**, including **hormonal contraceptive agents**; avoid concurrent use with sensitive CYP3A substrates or those with a narrow therapeutic index, including **cyclosporine, everolimus, midazolam, sirolimus, tacrolimus,** or **triazolam**. Strong CYP3A inhibitors including **ketoconazole, itraconazole, posaconazole, voriconazole,** and **clarithromycin** may ↑ ivacaftor levels; no dose adjustment required when initiating CYP3A inhibitor in patients currently receiving ivacaftor/lumacaftor; ↓ initial ivacaftor/lumacaftor dose for 1 wk when starting therapy in patient currently receiving strong CYP3A4 inhibitor and then proceed with recommended dose. Lumacaftor may ↓ levels of **CYP2B6 substrates, CYP2C8 substrates, CYP2C9 substrates,** and **CYP2C19 substrates.** Ivacaftor may ↑ levels of **CYP2C9 substrates.** May ↑ or ↓ **digoxin** or **warfarin** levels. May ↓ levels of **citalopram, clarithromycin, corticosteroids, erythromycin, escitalopram, ibuprofen, itraconazole, ketoconazole, montelukast, posaconazole, proton pump inhibitors, repaglinide, sertraline, sulfonylureas, voriconazole.**
Drug-Natural Products: St. John's wort may ↓ ivacaftor levels and effectiveness; avoid concurrent use.

Route/Dosage

PO (Adults and Children ≥12 yr): Two lumacaftor 200 mg/ivacaftor 125 mg tablets every 12 hr with fat-containing food; *Initiation of therapy in patients receiving strong CYP3A inhibitor:* One lumacaftor 200 mg/ivacaftor 125 mg tablet once daily for 1 wk, then ↑ to two lumacaftor 200 mg/ivacaftor 125 mg tablets every 12 hr.

PO (Children 6–11 yr): Two lumacaftor 100 mg/ivacaftor 125 mg tablets every 12 hr with fat-containing food; *Initiation of therapy in patients receiving strong CYP3A inhibitor:* One lumacaftor 100 mg/ivacaftor 125 mg tablet once daily for 1 wk, then ↑ to two lumacaftor 200 mg/ivacaftor 125 mg tablets every 12 hr.

PO (Children 2–5 yr and ≥14 kg): One lumacaftor 150 mg/ivacaftor 188 mg granule packet every 12 hr with fat-containing food; *Initiation of therapy in patients receiving strong CYP3A inhibitor:* One lumacaftor 150 mg/ivacaftor 188 mg granule packet every other day for 1 wk, then ↑ to one lumacaftor 150 mg/ivacaftor 188 mg granule packet every 12 hr.

PO (Children 2–5 yr and <14 kg): One lumacaftor 100 mg/ivacaftor 125 mg granule packet every 12 hr with fat-containing food; *Initiation of therapy in patients receiving strong CYP3A inhibitor:* One lumacaftor 100 mg/ivacaftor 125 mg granule packet every other day for 1 wk, then ↑ to one lumacaftor 100 mg/ivacaftor 125 mg granule packet every 12 hr.

PO (Children 1–<2 yr and ≥14 kg): One lumacaftor 150 mg/ivacaftor 188 mg granule packet every 12 hr with fat-containing food; *Initiation of therapy in patients receiving strong CYP3A inhibitor:* One lumacaftor 150 mg/ivacaftor 188 mg granule packet every other day for 1 wk, then ↑ to one lumacaftor 150 mg/ivacaftor 188 mg granule packet every 12 hr.

PO (Children 1–<2 yr and 9–<14 kg): One lumacaftor 100 mg/ivacaftor 125 mg granule packet every 12 hr with fat-containing food; *Initiation of therapy in patients receiving strong CYP3A inhibitor:* One lumacaftor 100 mg/ivacaftor 125 mg granule packet every other day for 1 wk, then ↑ to one lumacaftor 100 mg/ivacaftor 125 mg granule packet every 12 hr.

PO (Children 1–<2 yr and 7–<9 kg): One lumacaftor 75 mg/ivacaftor 94 mg granule packet every 12 hr with fat-containing food; *Initiation of therapy in patients receiving strong CYP3A inhibitor:* One lumacaftor 75 mg/ivacaftor 94 mg granule packet every other day for 1 wk, then ↑ to one lumacaftor 75 mg/ivacaftor 94 mg granule packet every 12 hr.

Hepatic Impairment

(Adults and Children ≥12 yr): *Moderate hepatic impairment:* Two lumacaftor 200 mg/ivacaftor 125 mg tablets in AM and one lumacaftor 200 mg/ivacaftor 125 mg tablet in PM; *Severe hepatic impairment:* One lumacaftor 200 mg/ivacaftor 125 mg tablet in AM and one lumacaftor 200 mg/ivacaftor 125 mg tablet in PM.

Hepatic Impairment

(Children 6–11 yr): *Moderate hepatic impairment:* Two lumacaftor 100 mg/ivacaftor 125 mg tablets in AM and one lumacaftor 100 mg/ivacaftor 125 mg tablet in PM; *Severe hepatic impairment:* One lumacaftor 100 mg/ivacaftor 125 mg tablet in AM and one lumacaftor 100 mg/ivacaftor 125 mg tablet in PM.

Hepatic Impairment

(Children 2–5 yr and ≥14 kg): *Moderate hepatic impairment:* One lumacaftor 150 mg/ivacaftor 188 mg granule packet in AM and one lumacaftor 150 mg/ivacaftor 188 mg granule packet every other PM; *Severe hepatic impairment:* One lumacaftor 150 mg/ivacaftor 188 mg granule packet in AM.

Hepatic Impairment

(Children 2–5 yr and <14 kg): *Moderate hepatic impairment:* One lumacaftor 100 mg/ivacaftor 125 mg granule packet in AM and one lumacaftor 100 mg/ivacaftor 125 mg granule packet every other PM; *Severe hepatic impairment:* One lumacaftor 100 mg/ivacaftor 125 mg granule packet in AM.

Hepatic Impairment

(Children 1–<2 yr and ≥14 kg): *Moderate hepatic impairment:* One lumacaftor 150 mg/ivacaftor 188 mg granule packet in AM and one lumacaftor 150 mg/ivacaftor 188 mg granule packet every other PM; *Severe hepatic impairment:* One lumacaftor 150 mg/ivacaftor 188 mg granule packet in AM.

Hepatic Impairment

(Children 1–<2 yr and 9–<14 kg): *Moderate hepatic impairment:* One lumacaftor 100 mg/ivacaftor 125 mg granule packet in AM and one lumacaftor 100 mg/ivacaftor 125 mg granule packet every other PM; *Severe hepatic impairment:* One lumacaftor 100 mg/ivacaftor 125 mg granule packet in AM.

Hepatic Impairment

(Children 1–<2 yr and 7–<9 kg): *Moderate hepatic impairment:* One lumacaftor 75 mg/ivacaftor 94 mg granule packet in AM and one lumacaftor 75 mg/ivacaftor 94 mg granule packet every other PM; *Severe hepatic impairment:* One lumacaftor 75 mg/ivacaftor 94 mg granule packet in AM.

Availability

Oral granules: lumacaftor 75 mg/ivacaftor 94 mg/pkt, lumacaftor 100 mg/ivacaftor 125 mg/pkt, lumacaftor 150 mg/ivacaftor 188 mg/pkt. **Tablets:** lumacaftor 100 mg/ivacaftor 125 mg, lumacaftor 200 mg/ivacaftor 125 mg.

NURSING IMPLICATIONS

Assessment

- Assess respiratory status (chest discomfort, dyspnea, abnormal respiration) prior to and periodically during therapy.

- Monitor BP periodically during therapy; may cause hypertension.
- Obtain baseline and periodic ophthalmological exams on pediatric patients starting therapy; may cause cataracts.
- Monitor for hypersensitivity reactions (angioedema, anaphylaxis). If signs or symptoms of serious hypersensitivity reactions (hives, rash, swelling of lips, face, dyspnea) occur, discontinue *Orkambi* and institute appropriate therapy.

Lab Test Considerations

- ⚏ Determine patient's genotype prior to starting therapy. If genotype is unknown, use an FDA-cleared CF mutation test to detect presence of the F508del mutation on both alleles of the CFTR gene.
- Monitor ALT, AST, and bilirubin prior to starting therapy, every 3 mo during 1st yr of therapy, and annually thereafter. Monitor patients with a history of ALT, AST, or bilirubin ↑ more frequently. If ↑ ALT, AST, or bilirubin occur, monitored closely until resolved. *If ALT or AST >5 × upper limit of normal (ULN) when not associated* ↑ *bilirubin,* withhold therapy. *If ALT or AST >3 × ULN when associated with bilirubin >2 × ULN,* withhold therapy. Consider benefits and risks of resuming dosing, once ↑ levels resolve.

Implementation

- **PO:** Administer 2 tablets every 12 hrs with fat-containing food (eggs, avocados, nuts, butter, peanut butter, cheese pizza, whole-milk dairy products [whole milk, cheese, yogurt], etc).
- To administer granules, mix entire content of single-use packet with 1 tsp (5 mL) of age-appropriate soft food or liquid (puréed fruits, flavored yogurt or pudding, milk or juice). Food should be at room temperature or below. Mixture is stable for 1 hr.

Patient/Family Teaching

- Instruct patient to take medication as directed. Take missed doses within 6 hrs with fat-containing food. If >6 hrs after usual dosing time, omit dose and resume normal schedule for following dose; do not double doses. Advise patient to read *Patient Information* prior to starting and with each Rx refill in case of changes.
- May cause dizziness. Avoid driving and other activities requiring alertness until response to medication is known.
- Advise patient to notify health care professional if signs and symptoms of liver problems (pain or discomfort in upper right abdomen, yellowing of skin or white of eyes, loss of appetite, nausea or vomiting, dark, amber-colored urine, confusion) or respiratory problems (shortness of breath, chest tightness) occur.
- Advise patient to notify health care professional of all Rx or OTC medications, vitamins, or herbal products

being taken and to consult with health care professional before taking other medications, especially St. John's wort.

- Rep: Advise females of reproductive potential to use a nonhormonal contraceptive during therapy and to notify health care professional if pregnancy is planned or suspected, or if breastfeeding. Ivacaftor/lumacaftor may ↓ hormonal contraceptive exposure (oral, injectable, transdermal, implantable) and ↓ effectiveness; do not rely upon as effective method of contraception.

Evaluation/Desired Outcomes

- Improved lung function with ↑ weight, decreased exacerbations and fewer CF symptoms.

BEERS

lurasidone (loo-ras-i-done)
Latuda
Classification
Therapeutic: antipsychotics
Pharmacologic: benzoisothiazole

Indications
Schizophrenia. Depressive episodes associated with bipolar I disorder (as monotherapy or in combination with lithium or valproate).

Action
Effect may be mediated via effects on central dopamine Type 2 (D_2) and serotonin Type 2 ($5HT_{2A}$) receptor antagonism. **Therapeutic Effects:** Reduction in schizophrenic behavior. Reduction in depressive episodes in bipolar I disorder.

Pharmacokinetics
Absorption: 9–19% absorbed following oral administration.
Distribution: Unknown.
Protein Binding: >99%.
Metabolism and Excretion: Primarily metabolized by the liver via the CYP3A4 isoenzyme. Two metabolites are pharmacologically active; 80% eliminated in feces, 8% in urine primarily as metabolites.
Half-life: 18 hr.

TIME/ACTION PROFILE (plasma concentrations)

ROUTE	ONSET	PEAK	DURATION
PO	unknown	1–3 hr	24 hr

Contraindications/Precautions
Contraindicated in: Hypersensitivity; Concurrent use of strong CYP3A4 inhibitors or inducers.
Use Cautiously in: Moderate or severe renal impairment (dose adjustment recommended); Moderate or severe hepatic impairment (dose adjustment recommended); History of suicide attempt; Diabetes mellitus; Overheating/dehydration (may ↑ risk of serious adverse

reactions); Patients at risk for falls; History of leukopenia or previous drug-induced leukopenia/neutropenia; OB: Use in pregnancy only if potential maternal benefit justifies potential fetal risk; Lactation: Use while breastfeeding only if potential maternal benefit justifies potential risk to infant; Pedi: May ↑ risk of suicide attempt/ideation especially during dose early treatment or dose adjustment; risk may be greater in children, adolescents, and young adults taking antidepressants; safety and effectiveness not established in children <10 yr; Geri: Appears on Beers list. ↑ risk of stroke, cognitive decline, and mortality in older adults with dementia. Avoid use in older adults, except for schizophrenia or bipolar disorder.

Adverse Reactions/Side Effects
CV: bradycardia, orthostatic hypotension, syncope, tachycardia. **Derm:** pruritus, rash. **EENT:** blurred vision. **Endo:** hyperglycemia, hyperprolactinemia. **GI:** nausea, esophageal dysmotility. **Hemat:** AGRANULOCYTOSIS, anemia, leukopenia. **Metab:** dyslipidemia, weight gain. **Neuro:** akathisia, drowsiness, parkinsonism, agitation, anxiety, cognitive/motor impairment, dizziness, dystonia, NEUROLEPTIC MALIGNANT SYNDROME, SEIZURES, SUICIDAL THOUGHTS, tardive dyskinesia.

Interactions
Drug-Drug: **Strong CYP3A4 inhibitors**, including **ketoconazole**, **clarithromycin**, **ritonavir**, and **voriconazole** ↑ levels and risk of toxicity; concurrent use contraindicated. **Strong CYP3A4 inducers**, including **rifampin**, **phenytoin**, and **carbamazepine** ↓ levels and effectiveness; concurrent use contraindicated. **Moderate CYP3A4 inhibitors**, including **diltiazem**, **atazanavir**, **erythromycin**, **fluconazole**, and **verapamil** ↑ levels and risk of toxicity; if used concurrently, lurasidone dose should not exceed 40 mg/day. ↑ sedation may occur with other **CNS depressants**, including **alcohol**, **sedative/hypnotics**, **opioids**, some **antidepressants** and **antihistamines**.
Drug-Natural Products: St. John's wort ↓ levels and effectiveness; concurrent use contraindicated.
Drug-Food: Grapefruit juice ↑ levels and risk of toxicity; concurrent use contraindicated.

Route/Dosage
Schizophrenia
PO (Adults): 40 mg once daily (not to exceed 160 mg once daily); *Addition of moderate CYP3A4 inhibitor to existing lurasidone therapy:* ↓ lurasidone dose by 50%; *Addition of lurasidone to existing moderate CYP3A4 inhibitor therapy:* 20 mg once daily (not to exceed 80 mg once daily).
PO (Children 13–17 yr): 40 mg once daily (not to exceed 80 mg once daily); *Addition of moderate CYP3A4 inhibitor to existing lurasidone therapy:* ↓ lurasidone dose by 50%; *Addition of lurasidone to existing moderate CYP3A4 inhibitor therapy:* 20 mg once daily (not to exceed 80 mg once daily).

Renal Impairment
PO (Adults and Children 13–17 yr): *CCr <50 mL/ min:* 20 mg once daily (not to exceed 80 mg once daily).

Hepatic Impairment
(Adults and Children 13–17 yr): *Moderate hepatic impairment:* 20 mg once daily (not to exceed 80 mg once daily); *Severe hepatic impairment:* 20 mg once daily (not to exceed 40 mg once daily).

Depressive Episodes Associated with Bipolar I Disorder
PO (Adults): 20 mg once daily (not to exceed 120 mg once daily); *Addition of moderate CYP3A4 inhibitor to existing lurasidone therapy:* ↓ lurasidone dose by 50%; *Addition of lurasidone to existing moderate CYP3A4 inhibitor therapy:* 20 mg once daily (not to exceed 80 mg once daily).

PO (Children 10–17 yr): 20 mg once daily (not to exceed 80 mg once daily); *Addition of moderate CYP3A4 inhibitor to existing lurasidone therapy:* ↓ lurasidone dose by 50%; *Addition of lurasidone to existing moderate CYP3A4 inhibitor therapy:* 20 mg once daily (not to exceed 80 mg once daily).

Renal Impairment
PO (Adults and Children 10–17 yr): *CCr <50 mL/ min:* 20 mg once daily (not to exceed 80 mg once daily).

Hepatic Impairment
PO (Adults and Children 10–17 yr): *Moderate hepatic impairment:* 20 mg once daily (not to exceed 80 mg once daily); *Severe hepatic impairment:* 20 mg once daily (not to exceed 40 mg once daily).

Availability (generic available)
Tablets: 20 mg, 40 mg, 60 mg, 80 mg, 120 mg.

NURSING IMPLICATIONS

Assessment
- Monitor patient's mental status (orientation, mood, behavior) before and periodically during therapy.
- Assess weight and BMI initially and during therapy. Refer as appropriate for nutritional/weight and medical management.
- Monitor mood changes. Assess for suicidal tendencies, especially during early therapy. Restrict amount of drug available to patient.
- Monitor BP (sitting, standing, lying down) and pulse before and frequently during initial dose titration. May cause tachycardia and orthostatic hypotension. If hypotension occurs, dose may need to be ↓.
- Observe patient when administering medication to ensure medication is swallowed and not hoarded or cheeked.
- Monitor patient for onset of extrapyramidal side effects (*akathisia:* restlessness; *dystonia:* muscle spasms and twisting motions; or *pseudoparkinson-*

ism: mask-like face, rigidity, tremors, drooling, shuffling gait, dysphagia). Report these symptoms; reduction of dose or discontinuation may be necessary. Trihexyphenidyl or benztropine may be used to control symptoms.
- Monitor for tardive dyskinesia (involuntary rhythmic movement of mouth, face, and extremities). Report immediately; may be irreversible.
- Monitor for symptoms related to hyperprolactinemia (menstrual abnormalities, galactorrhea, sexual dysfunction).
- Monitor for development of neuroleptic malignant syndrome (fever, respiratory distress, tachycardia, seizures, diaphoresis, hypertension or hypotension, pallor, tiredness). Notify health care professional immediately if these symptoms occur.
- Monitor for symptoms of hyperglycemia (polydipsia, polyuria, polyphagia, weakness) periodically during therapy.
- Assess for falls risk. Drowsiness, orthostatic hypotension, and motor and sensory instability increase risk. Institute prevention if indicated.

Lab Test Considerations
- May cause ↑ serum prolactin levels.
- May cause ↑ CK.
- Obtain fasting blood glucose and cholesterol levels initially and periodically during therapy.
- Monitor CBC frequently during initial mo of therapy in patients with pre-existing or history of low WBC. May cause leukopenia, neutropenia, or agranulocytosis. Discontinue therapy if this occurs.

Implementation
- **High Alert:** Do not confuse Latuda with Lantus.
- **PO:** Administer once daily with food of at least 350 calories. Use beyond 6 wk has not been studied.

Patient/Family Teaching
- Instruct patient to take medication as directed. Emphasize the caloric food needs for taking medication.
- Inform patient of the possibility of extrapyramidal symptoms. Instruct patient to report these symptoms immediately to health care professional.
- Advise patient to change positions slowly to minimize orthostatic hypotension. Protect from falls.
- May cause drowsiness and cognitive and motor impairment. Caution patient to avoid driving or other activities requiring alertness until response to medication is known.
- Advise patient and family to notify health care professional if thoughts about suicide or dying, attempts to commit suicide; new or worse depression; new or worse anxiety; feeling very agitated or restless; panic attacks; trouble sleeping; new or worse irritability; acting aggressive; being angry or violent; acting on dangerous impulses; an extreme ↑ in activity and

talking, other unusual changes in behavior or mood occur.

- Advise patient to avoid extremes in temperature; this drug impairs body temperature regulation.
- Advise patient to tell health care professional what medications they are taking and to avoid taking new Rx, OTC, vitamins, or herbal products without consulting health care professional, especially alcohol and other CNS depressants.
- Advise patient to notify health care professional of medication regimen before treatment or surgery.
- Instruct patient to notify health care professional promptly if sore throat, fever, unusual bleeding or bruising, rash, or tremors occur.
- Rep: Advise females of reproductive potential to notify health care professional if pregnancy is planned or suspected, and to avoid breastfeeding during therapy. Monitor neonates exposed to lurasidone during the third trimester of pregnancy for extrapyramidal and/or withdrawal symptoms following delivery. There have been reports of agitation, hypertonia, hypotonia, tremor, somnolence, respiratory distress and feeding disorder in these neonates. Monitor breastfed infants for excessive drowsiness, lethargy, and developmental delays. Encourage women who become pregnant while taking lurasidone to enroll in the National Pregnancy Registry for Atypical Antipsychotics at 1-866-961-2388 or visit http://womensmentalhealth.org/clinical-and-research-programs/pregnancyregistry/. Monitor neonates for extrapyramidal and/or withdrawal symptoms and manage symptoms appropriately.
- Emphasize the importance of routine follow up exams to monitor side effects.

Evaluation/Desired Outcomes

- ↓ in symptoms of schizophrenia (delusions, hallucinations, social withdrawal, flat, blunted affects).
- ↓ depressive episodes in bipolar I disorder.

luspatercept (lus-pat-er-sept)
Reblozyl
Classification
Therapeutic: antianemics
Pharmacologic: fusion proteins

Indications

Anemia in patients with beta thalassemia who require regular red blood cell (RBC) transfusions. Anemia in patients with very low- to intermediate-risk myelodysplastic syndromes with ring sideroblasts or with myelodysplastic/myeloproliferative neoplasm with ring sideroblasts and thrombocytosis who have failed an erythropoiesis stimulating agent and require ≥2 RBC units over 8 wk. Anemia in patients who have not previously used erythropoiesis-stimulating agents, have very low- to intermediate-risk myelodysplastic syndromes, and may require regular RBC transfusions.

Action

A fusion protein that binds several endogenous transforming growth factor-beta (TGF-β) superfamily ligands. Inhibition of TGF-β superfamily results in increased differentiation and proliferation of erythroid precursors. **Therapeutic Effects:** Reduction in RBC transfusions. Increase in hemoglobin.

Pharmacokinetics

Absorption: Unknown.
Distribution: Not significantly distributed to tissues.
Metabolism and Excretion: Broken down into amino acids.
Half-life: 11–13 days.

TIME/ACTION PROFILE (↑ in hemoglobin levels)

ROUTE	ONSET	PEAK	DURATION
SUBQ	Within 7 days	Unknown	8 wk

Contraindications/Precautions

Contraindicated in: OB: Pregnancy; Lactation: Lactation; Pedi: Not recommended for use in children (may ↑ risk of hematologic malignancies).
Use Cautiously in: Risk factors for thromboembolism; Hypertension; History of extramedullary hematopoietic masses, splenectomy, hepatomegaly, or low baseline hemoglobin (<8.5 g/dL) (↑ risk of extramedullary hematopoietic masses); Rep: Women of reproductive potential.

Adverse Reactions/Side Effects

CV: hypertension, DEEP VEIN THROMBOSIS, syncope. **EENT:** vertigo. **GI:** ↑ liver enzymes, abdominal pain, diarrhea, nausea. **GU:** ↓ fertility (females). **Hemat:** extramedullary hematopoietic masses. **Local:** injection site reactions. **Metab:** hyperuricemia. **MS:** arthralgia, bone pain. **Neuro:** dizziness, fatigue, headache, STROKE. **Resp:** cough, PULMONARY EMBOLISM, upper respiratory tract infection. **Misc:** hypersensitivity reactions.

Interactions

Drug-Drug: None reported.

Route/Dosage

Anemia in Beta Thalassemia

SUBQ (Adults): 1 mg/kg every 3 wk. If no reduction in RBC transfusion burden occurs after 2 consecutive doses (6 wk), ↑ dose to 1.25 mg/kg every 3 wk. Discontinue therapy if no reduction in RBC transfusion burden occurs after 3 consecutive doses (9 wk) at maximum dose (1.25 mg/kg) or if unacceptable toxicity occurs.

Anemia in Myelodysplastic Syndromes

SUBQ (Adults): 1 mg/kg every 3 wk. If patient is not RBC transfusion-free after ≥2 consecutive doses (6 wk), ↑ dose to 1.33 mg/kg every 3 wk. Then, if patient is not RBC transfusion-free after ≥2 consecutive doses (6 wk) at 1.33 mg/kg dose, ↑ dose to 1.75 mg/kg every

3 wk. Discontinue therapy if no reduction in RBC transfusion burden occurs after 3 consecutive doses (9 wk) at maximum dose (1.75 mg/kg) or if unacceptable toxicity occurs.

Availability
Lyophilized powder for injection: 25 mg/vial, 75 mg/vial.

NURSING IMPLICATIONS
Assessment
● Monitor patient for signs and symptoms of thromboembolic events during therapy.
● Monitor BP before each administration. Manage hypertension or exacerbations.

Lab Test Considerations
● Verify negative pregnancy test before starting therapy.
● Review hemoglobin level and transfusion record before each dose. If an RBC transfusion occurred before dosing, use pretransfusion hemoglobin for dose evaluation. **Dose modification for predose hemoglobin levels or rapid hemoglobin rise in beta thalassemia:** *If predose hemoglobin ≥11.5 g/dL in the absence of transfusions,* interrupt therapy and restart when hemoglobin is ≤11 g/dL. *If increase in hemoglobin >2 g/dL within 3 wk in the absence of transfusion and current dose is 1.25 mg/kg,* reduce dose to 1 mg/kg. *If current dose is 1 mg/kg,* reduce dose to 0.8 mg/kg. *If current dose is 0.8 mg/kg,* reduce dose to 0.6 mg/kg. *If current dose is 0.6 mg/kg,* discontinue therapy. **Dose modification for predose hemoglobin levels or rapid hemoglobin rise in myelodysplastic syndromes with ring sideroblasts or with myelodysplastic/myeloproliferative neoplasm with ring sideroblasts and thrombocytosis:** *If predose hemoglobin ≥11.5 g/dL in the absence of transfusions,* interrupt therapy and restart when hemoglobin is ≤11 g/dL. *If increase in hemoglobin >2 g/dL within 3 wk in the absence of transfusion and current dose is 1.75 mg/kg,* reduce dose to 1.33 mg/kg. *If current dose is 1.33 mg/kg,* reduce dose to 1 mg/kg. *If current dose is 1 mg/kg,* reduce dose to 0.8 mg/kg. *If current dose is 0.8 mg/kg,* reduce dose to 0.6 mg/kg. *If current dose is 0.6 mg/kg,* discontinue therapy. May cause ↑ AST, ALT, alkaline phosphatase, total and direct bilirubin.

Implementation
● Luspatercept should be reconstituted and administered by a health care professional.
● If a dose is missed administer as soon as possible and continue dosing with at least 3 wk between doses.

● **Reconstitution:** Reconstitute 25 mg vial with 0.68 mL and 75 mg vial with 1.6 mL Sterile Water for Injection, directing stream onto powder. *Concentration:* 25 mg/0.5 mL and 75 mg/1.5 mL, respectively. Allow to stand for 1 min. Discard needle and syringe; do not use for injection. Swirl gently for 30 sec, then allow vial to sit upright for 30 sec. If undissolved powder is observed, repeat step 3 until the powder is completely dissolved. *Invert vial and swirl gently in inverted position for 30 sec. Return vial to upright position and let sit for 30 sec.* Repeat procedure in italics 7 more times to ensure complete reconstitution of material on sides of vial. Solution is colorless to slightly yellow, clear to slightly opalescent; do not inject solutions that are cloudy, discolored, or contain particulate matter. Store reconstituted solution in original vial at room temperature for up to 8 hr; discard if not used in 8 hr. May be stored in refrigerator for up to 24 hr in original vial; do not freeze. Remove from refrigerator 15–30 min before injection to allow to reach room temperature. Discard if not used in 24 hr. Vials are for single dose only.
● **SUBQ:** Withdraw dose into syringe; divide doses >1.2 mL into 2 syringes and inject into 2 different sites. Administer into upper arm, thigh, or abdomen.

Patient/Family Teaching
● Explain purpose of luspatercept to patient. Advise patient to read *Patient Information* before starting and periodically during therapy in case of changes.
● Advise patient to notify health care professional immediately if signs and symptoms of blood clots (chest pain; trouble breathing or shortness of breath; pain in leg, with or without swelling; a cold or pale arm or leg; sudden numbness or weakness that are both short-term or continue to happen over a long period of time, especially on one side of the body; severe headache or confusion; sudden problems with vision, speech, or balance) occur.
● Inform patient that BP will be monitored before each dose. May require antihypertensive medication to treat elevated BP.
● Instruct patient to notify health care professional of all Rx or OTC medications, vitamins, or herbal products being taken and consult health care professional before taking any new medications.
● Rep: May cause fetal harm. Advise females of reproductive potential to use effective contraception and avoid breastfeeding during and for at least 3 mo after last dose. May impair female fertility.

Evaluation/Desired Outcomes
● Reduction in RBC transfusions.
● Increase in hemoglobin.

MAGNESIUM SALTS (ORAL)
magnesium chloride (12% Mg; 9.8 mEq Mg/g)
(mag-**nee**-zhum **klor**-ide)
Slo-Mag
magnesium citrate (16.2% Mg; 4.4 mEq Mg/g)
(mag-**nee**-zhum **si**-trate)
Citroma
magnesium gluconate (5.4% Mg; 4.4 mEq/g)
(mag-**nee**-zhum **gloo**-con-ate)
magnesium hydroxide (41.7% Mg; 34.3 mEq Mg/g)
(mag-**nee**-zhum hye-**drox**-ide)
Milk of Magnesia
magnesium oxide (60.3% Mg; 49.6 mEq Mg/g)
(mag-**nee**-zhum **ox**-ide)
Mag-Oxide

Classification
Therapeutic: mineral and electrolyte replacements/supplements, laxatives
Pharmacologic: salines

Indications
Treatment/prevention of hypomagnesemia. As a: Laxative, Bowel evacuant in preparation for surgical/radiographic procedures. Milk of magnesia has also been used as an antacid.

Action
Essential for the activity of many enzymes. Play an important role in neurotransmission and muscular excitability. Are osmotically active in GI tract, drawing water into the lumen and causing peristalsis. **Therapeutic Effects:** Replacement in deficiency states. Evacuation of the colon.

Pharmacokinetics
Absorption: Up to 30% may be absorbed orally.
Distribution: Widely distributed to tissues.
Metabolism and Excretion: Excreted primarily by the kidneys.
Half-life: Unknown.

TIME/ACTION PROFILE (laxative effect)

ROUTE	ONSET	PEAK	DURATION
PO	3–6 hr	unknown	unknown

Contraindications/Precautions
Contraindicated in: Hypermagnesemia; Hypocalcemia; Anuria; Heart block; OB: Unless used for preterm labor, use during active labor or within 2 hr of delivery may ↑ potential for magnesium toxicity in newborn.
Use Cautiously in: Renal impairment.

Adverse Reactions/Side Effects
Derm: flushing, sweating. **GI:** diarrhea.

Interactions
Drug-Drug: Potentiates **neuromuscular blocking agents**. May ↓ absorption of **fluoroquinolones**, **nitrofurantoin**, and **tetracyclines** and **penicillamine**.

Route/Dosage
Prevention of Deficiency (in mg of Magnesium)
PO (Adults and Children >10 yr): *Adolescent and adult men:* 270–400 mg/day; *Adolescent and adult women:* 280–300 mg/day; *Pregnant women:* 320 mg/day; *Breastfeeding women:* 340–355 mg/day.
PO (Children 7–10 yr): 170 mg/day.
PO (Children 4–6 yr): 120 mg/day.
PO (Children birth–3 yr): 40–80 mg/day.

Treatment of Deficiency (in mg of Magnesium)
PO (Adults): 200–400 mg/day in 3–4 divided doses.
PO (Children 6–11 yr): 3–6 mg/kg/day in 3–4 divided doses.

Laxative
PO (Adults): *Magnesium citrate:* 240 mL; *Magnesium hydroxide:* 30–60 mL single or divided dose or 10–20 mL as concentrate.
PO (Children 6–12 yr): *Magnesium citrate:* 100 mL; *Magnesium hydroxide:* 15–30 mL single or divided dose.
PO (Children 2–5 yr): *Magnesium hydroxide:* 5–15 mL single or divided dose.

Availability
Magnesium Chloride (generic available)
Sustained-release tablets: 535 mg (64 mg magnesium)^{OTC}.

Magnesium Citrate (generic available)
Oral solution: 240-, 296-, and 300-mL bottles (77 mEq magnesium/100 mL)^{OTC}.

Magnesium Gluconate (generic available)
Tablets: 500 mg^{OTC}.

Magnesium Hydroxide (generic available)
Liquid: 400 mg/5 mL (164 mg magnesium/5 mL)^{OTC}. **Concentrated liquid:** 800 mg/5 mL (328 mg magnesium/5 mL)^{OTC}. **Chewable tablets:** 400 mg (173 mg magnesium)^{OTC}.

Magnesium Oxide (generic available)
Tablets: 400 mg (241.3 mg magnesium)^{OTC}.

NURSING IMPLICATIONS
Assessment
- **Laxative:** Assess patient for abdominal distention, presence of bowel sounds, and usual pattern of bowel function.
- Assess color, consistency, and amount of stool produced.

- **Antacid:** Assess for heartburn and indigestion as well as location, duration, character, and precipitating factors of gastric pain.

Implementation

- **PO:** To prevent tablets entering small intestine in undissolved form, they must be chewed thoroughly before swallowing. Follow with ½ glass of water.
- *Magnesium citrate:* Refrigerate solutions to ensure they retain potency and palatability. May be served over ice. Magnesium citrate in an open container will lose carbonation upon standing; this will not affect potency but may reduce palatability.
- *Magnesium hydroxide:* Shake solution well before administration.
- **Antacid:** Administer 1–3 hr after meals and at bedtime.
- Powder and liquid forms are considered more effective than tablets.
- **Laxative:** Administer on empty stomach for more rapid results. Follow all oral laxative doses with a full glass of liquid to prevent dehydration and for faster effect. Do not administer at bedtime or late in the day.

Patient/Family Teaching

- Advise patient not to take this medication within 2 hr of taking other medications, especially fluoroquinolones, nitrofurantoin, and tetracyclines.
- **Antacids:** Caution patient to consult health care professional before taking antacids for more than 2 wk if problem is recurring, if relief is not obtained, or if symptoms of gastric bleeding (black, tarry stools; coffee-ground emesis) occur.
- **Laxatives:** Advise patient that laxatives should be used only for short-term therapy. Long-term therapy may cause electrolyte imbalance and dependence.
- Encourage patient to use other forms of bowel regulation, such as increasing bulk in the diet, fluid intake, and mobility. Normal bowel habits are individualized; frequency of bowel movement may vary from 3 times/day to 3 times/wk.
- Advise patient to notify health care professional if unrelieved constipation, rectal bleeding, or symptoms of electrolyte imbalance (muscle cramps or pain, weakness, dizziness) occur.

Evaluation/Desired Outcomes

- Relief of gastric pain and irritation.
- Passage of a soft, formed bowel movement, usually within 3–6 hr.
- Prevention and treatment of magnesium deficiency.

HIGH ALERT

magnesium sulfate (parenteral)
(mag-**nee**-zhum **sul**-fate)

Classification
Therapeutic: mineral and electrolyte replacements/supplements
Pharmacologic: minerals/electrolytes

Indications
Treatment/prevention of hypomagnesemia. Prevention and treatment of seizures associated with severe eclampsia or pre-eclampsia. **Unlabeled Use:** Treatment of torsades de pointes. Adjunctive treatment for bronchodilation in moderate to severe acute asthma.

Action
Essential for the activity of many enzymes. Plays an important role in neurotransmission and muscular excitability. **Therapeutic Effects:** Replacement in deficiency states. Resolution of eclampsia.

Pharmacokinetics
Absorption: IV administration results in complete bioavailability; well absorbed from IM sites.
Distribution: Widely distributed to tissues.
Metabolism and Excretion: Excreted primarily by the kidneys.
Half-life: Unknown.

TIME/ACTION PROFILE (anticonvulsant effect)

ROUTE	ONSET	PEAK	DURATION
IM	60 min	unknown	3–4 hr
IV	immediate	unknown	30 min

Contraindications/Precautions
Contraindicated in: Hypermagnesemia; Hypocalcemia; Anuria; Heart block.
Use Cautiously in: Renal impairment; OB: Avoid using for more than 5–7 days for preterm labor (may ↑ risk of hypocalcemia and bone changes in newborn); avoid continuous use during active labor or within 2 hr of delivery due to potential for magnesium toxicity in newborn; Geri: Older adults may require ↓ dosage due to age-related ↓ in renal function.

Adverse Reactions/Side Effects
CV: arrhythmias, bradycardia, hypotension. **Derm:** flushing, sweating. **GI:** diarrhea. **Metab:** hypothermia. **MS:** muscle weakness. **Neuro:** drowsiness. **Resp:** ↓ respiratory rate.

Interactions
Drug-Drug: May potentiate **calcium channel blockers** and **neuromuscular blocking agents**.

Route/Dosage
Treatment of Deficiency
IM, IV (Adults): *Severe deficiency:* 8–12 g/day in divided doses; *Mild deficiency:* 1 g every 6 hr for 4 doses or 250 mg/kg over 4 hr.

M

✳= Canadian drug name. ⬚ = Genetic implication. ~~Strikethrough~~ = Discontinued. CAPITALS = life-threatening. <u>Underline</u> = most frequent.

IM, IV (Children >1 mo): 25–50 mg/kg/dose every 4–6 hr for 3–4 doses (max single dose = 2 g).
IV (Neonates): 25–50 mg/kg/dose every 8–12 hr for 2–3 doses.

Seizures Associated with Eclampsia/Pre-Eclampsia

IV (Adults): 4–6 g loading dose over 15–30 min at onset of labor or induction/cesarean delivery, followed by 1–2 g/hr continuous infusion for ≥24 hr after delivery (max infusion rate = 3 g/hr). If seizure occurs while receiving magnesium, an additional bolus of 2–4 g may be administered over ≥5 minutes. Max dose = 40 g/24 hr.
IM (Adults): 10 g loading dose administered as 5 g in each buttock at onset of labor or induction/cesarean delivery, followed by 5 g every 4 hr for ≥24 hr after delivery.

Torsades de Pointes

IV (Adults): 1–2 g over 15 minutes. If no response or torsades de pointes recurs, may repeat dose up to a total of 4 g in 1 hour; may follow with a continuous IV infusion of 0.5–1 g/hr.
IV (Infants and Children): 25–50 mg/kg/dose (max dose = 2 g).

Bronchodilation

IV (Adults): 2 g single dose.
IV (Children): 25 mg/kg/dose (max dose = 2 g).

Parenteral Nutrition

IV (Adults): 4–24 mEq/day.
IV (Children): 0.25–0.5 mEq/kg/day.

Availability (generic available)

Solution for injection (8.1 mEq Mg/g): 500 mg/mL (50%). Premixed infusion: 1 g/100 mL, 2 g/50 mL, 4 g/50 mL, 4 g/100 mL, 20 g/500 mL, 40 g/1000 mL.

NURSING IMPLICATIONS

Assessment

● **Hypomagnesemia/Anticonvulsant:** Monitor pulse, BP, respirations, and ECG frequently during administration of parenteral magnesium sulfate. Respirations should be at least 16/min before each dose.
● Monitor neurologic status before and throughout therapy. Institute seizure precautions. Patellar reflex (knee jerk) should be tested before each parenteral dose of magnesium sulfate. If response is absent, no additional doses should be administered until positive response is obtained.
● Monitor newborn for hypotension, hyporeflexia, and respiratory depression if mother has received magnesium sulfate.
● Monitor intake and output ratios. Urine output should be maintained at a level of at least 100 mL/4 hr.

Lab Test Considerations
● Monitor serum magnesium levels and renal function periodically during administration of parenteral magnesium sulfate.

Implementation

● **High Alert:** Accidental overdose of IV magnesium has resulted in serious patient harm and death. Have second practitioner independently double-check original order, dose calculations, and infusion pump settings. Do not confuse milligram (mg), gram (g), or milliequivalent (mEq) doses.
● **IM:** IM route should only be used when unable to establish venous access. Administer deep IM into gluteal sites. Administer subsequent injections in alternate sides. Dilute to a concentration of 200 mg/mL prior to injection.

IV Administration
● **IV Push: *Dilution:*** 50% solution must be diluted in 0.9% NaCl or D5W to a concentration of ≤20% prior to administration. ***Concentration:*** ≤20%. ***Rate:*** Administer over several min at a rate not to exceed 150 mg/min. In patients not in cardiac arrest, rapid administration may cause hypotension and asystole.
● **Intermittent Infusion: *Dilution:*** 50% solution must be diluted in 0.9% NaCl or D5W to a concentration of ≤20% prior to administration. ***Concentration:*** ≤20%. ***Rate: For ventricular tachycardia/torsades:*** Infuse over 10–20 min; rapid infusion may cause hypotension. *For severe asthma exacerbation:* Infuse over 15–60 min.
● **Continuous Infusion: *Dilution:*** Dilute in D5W, 0.9% NaCl, or LR. ***Concentration:*** 0.5 mEq/mL (60 mg/mL) (may use maximum concentration of 1.6 mEq/mL) (200 mg/mL) in fluid-restricted patients. ***Rate:*** Infuse over 2–4 hr. Do not exceed a rate of 1 mEq/kg/hr (125 mg/kg/hr). When rapid infusions are needed (severe asthma or torsades de pointes) may infuse over 10–20 min.
● **Y-Site Compatibility:** acetaminophen, acyclovir, aldesleukin, alemtuzumab, amifostine, amikacin, aminocaproic acid, argatroban, arsenic trioxide, ascorbic acid, atropine, azithromycin, aztreonam, benztropine, bivalirudin, bleomycin, bumetanide, buprenorphine, butorphanol, calcium gluconate, cangrelor, carboplatin, carmustine, caspofungin, cefotaxime, cefotetan, cefoxitin, ceftazidime, ceftazidime/avibactam, ceftolozane/tazobactam, chloramphenicol, chlorpromazine, cisatracurium, cisplatin, clindamycin, cyanocobalamin, cyclophosphamide, cytarabine, dacarbazine, dactinomycin, daptomycin, daunorubicin hydrochloride, dexmedetomidine, dexrazoxane, digoxin, diltiazem, diphenhydramine, dobutamine, docetaxel, dopamine, doxorubicin liposomal, doxycycline, enalaprilat, ephedrine, epinephrine, epoetin alfa, eptifibatide, eravacycline, ertapenem, esmolol, etoposide, etoposide phosphate, famotidine, fentanyl, fluconazole, fludarabine, fluo-

rouracil, folic acid, foscarnet, fosphenytoin, gemcitabine, gemtuzumab ozogamicin, gentamicin, glycopyrrolate, granisetron, heparin, hetastarch, hydromorphone, idarubicin, ifosfamide, imipenem/cilastatin, insulin regular, irinotecan, isavuconazonium, isoproterenol, ketamine, ketorolac, labetalol, LR, leucovorin calcium, lidocaine, linezolid, lorazepam, mannitol, meropenem/vaborbactam, mesna, methotrexate, metoclopramide, metoprolol, metronidazole, micafungin, midazolam, milrinone, mitomycin, mitoxantrone, morphine, moxifloxacin, multivitamins, mycophenolate, nafcillin, nalbuphine, nicardipine, nitroglycerin, nitroprusside, norepinephrine, octreotide, ondansetron, oxaliplatin, oxytocin, paclitaxel, palonosetron, pamidronate, papaverine, pemetrexed, penicillin G, pentobarbital, phenobarbital, phentolamine, phenylephrine, piperacillin/tazobactam, plazomicin, potassium acetate, potassium chloride, procainamide, prochlorperazine, promethazine, propranolol, protamine, pyridoxine, remifentanil, rituximab, rocuronium, sargramostim, sodium acetate, sodium bicarbonate, succinylcholine, sufentanil, tacrolimus, telavancin, theophylline, thiamine, thiotepa, tigecycline, tirofiban, tobramycin, topotecan, trastuzumab, vancomycin, vasopressin, vecuronium, verapamil, vinblastine, vincristine, vinorelbine, voriconazole, zoledronic acid.

- **Y-Site Incompatibility:** aminophylline, amphotericin B deoxycholate, amphotericin B lipid complex, amphotericin B liposomal, anidulafungin, azathioprine, calcium chloride, cefepime, cefuroxime, ciprofloxacin, dantrolene, dexamethasone, diazepam, diazoxide, doxorubicin hydrochloride, epirubicin, ganciclovir, haloperidol, indomethacin, methylprednisolone, pentamidine, phenytoin, phytonadione, tedizolid.

Patient/Family Teaching
- Explain purpose of medication to patient and family.
- Rep: Monitor vital signs, oxygen saturation, respiration, deep tendon reflexes, level of consciousness, fetal heart rate, maternal uterine activity, and renal function when used during pregnancy. Monitor magnesium concentrations every 4 hr in patients with renal dysfunction (every 2 hr if serum magnesium is elevated). Breast milk concentrations are increased for only 24 hr after end of therapy. When used for prevention of seizures, magnesium sulfate is considered compatible with breastfeeding.

Evaluation/Desired Outcomes
- Normal serum magnesium concentrations.
- Control of seizures associated with toxemias of pregnancy.

BEERS

ℨ meclizine (mek-li-zeen)
Antivert, Bonine
Classification
Therapeutic: antiemetics, antihistamines

Indications
Motion sickness. Vertigo associated with diseases of the vestibular system.

Action
Has central anticholinergic, CNS depressant, and antihistaminic properties. Decreases excitability of the middle ear labyrinth and depresses conduction in middle ear vestibular-cerebellar pathways. **Therapeutic Effects:** Decreased motion sickness. Decreased vertigo from vestibular pathology.

Pharmacokinetics
Absorption: Absorbed after oral administration.
Distribution: Unknown.
Metabolism and Excretion: Primarily metabolized by liver via the CYP2D6 isoenzyme; ℨ the CYP2D6 isoenzyme exhibits genetic polymorphism (~7% of population may be poor metabolizers and may have significantly ↑ meclizine concentrations and an ↑ risk of adverse effects).
Half-life: 6 hr.

TIME/ACTION PROFILE (antihistaminic effects)

ROUTE	ONSET	PEAK	DURATION
PO	1 hr	unknown	8–24 hr

Contraindications/Precautions
Contraindicated in: Hypersensitivity.
Use Cautiously in: Prostatic hyperplasia; Angle-closure glaucoma; Lactation: Use while breastfeeding only if potential maternal benefit justifies potential risk to infant; Pedi: Children <12 yr (safety and effectiveness not established); Geri: Appears on Beers list. ↑ risk of anticholinergic adverse reactions in older adults, including falls, delirium, and dementia. Avoid use in older adults.

Adverse Reactions/Side Effects
EENT: blurred vision. **GI:** dry mouth. **Neuro:** <u>drowsiness</u>, fatigue.

Interactions
Drug-Drug: Additive CNS depression with other **CNS depressants**, including **alcohol**, other **antihistamines**, **opioid analgesics**, and **sedative/hypnotics**. Additive anticholinergic effects with other **drugs possessing anticholinergic properties**, including some **antihistamines**, **antidepressants**, **atropine**, **haloperidol**, **phenothiazines**, **quinidine**, and **disopyramide**. **CYP2D6 inhibitors** may ↑ levels and risk of toxicity.

✹ = Canadian drug name. ℨ = Genetic implication. S̶t̶r̶i̶k̶e̶t̶h̶r̶o̶u̶g̶h̶ = Discontinued. CAPITALS = life-threatening. <u>Underline</u> = most frequent.

Route/Dosage

PO (Adults and Children ≥12 yr): *Motion sickness:* 25–50 mg 1 hr before exposure; may repeat in 24 hr; *Vertigo:* 25–100 mg/day in divided doses.

Availability (generic available)

Tablets: 12.5 mg, 25 mg^Rx, OTC, 50 mg. **Chewable tablets (raspberry flavor):** 25 mg^OTC.

NURSING IMPLICATIONS

Assessment

● Assess patient for level of sedation after administration.
● **Motion Sickness:** Assess patient for nausea and vomiting before and 60 min after administration.
● **Vertigo:** Assess degree of vertigo periodically in patients receiving meclizine for labyrinthitis.

Lab Test Considerations

● May cause false-negative results in skin tests using allergen extracts. Discontinue meclizine 72 hr before testing.

Implementation

● **PO:** Administer oral doses with food, water, or milk to minimize GI irritation. *DNC:* Swallow tablets whole; do not crush, break, or chew.
● Chewable tablets must be chewed or crushed completely before swallowing. Do not swallow chewable tablets whole.

Patient/Family Teaching

● Instruct patient to take meclizine exactly as directed. If a dose is missed, take as soon as possible unless almost time for next dose. Do not double dose.
● May cause drowsiness. Caution patient to avoid driving or other activities requiring alertness until response to the medication is known.
● Advise patient that frequent mouth rinses, good oral hygiene, and sugarless gum or candy may decrease dryness of mouth.
● Caution patient to avoid concurrent use of alcohol and other CNS depressants, including opioids, with this medication.
● Rep: Advise females of reproductive potential to notify health care professional if pregnancy is planned or suspected, or if breastfeeding.
● **Motion Sickness:** When used as prophylaxis for motion sickness, advise patient to take medication at least 1 hr before exposure to conditions that may cause motion sickness.

Evaluation/Desired Outcomes

● Prevention and relief of symptoms in motion sickness.
● Prevention and treatment of vertigo due to vestibular pathology.

---

medroxyPROGESTERone†

(me-**drox**-ee-proe-**jess**-te-rone)
Depo-Provera, Depo-SubQ Provera 104, Provera

Classification

Therapeutic: antineoplastics, contraceptive hormones
Pharmacologic: hormones, progestins

Indications

Prevention of pregnancy. To decrease endometrial hyperplasia in postmenopausal women receiving concurrent estrogen (0.625 mg/day conjugated estrogens). Treatment of secondary amenorrhea and abnormal uterine bleeding caused by hormonal imbalance. **IM:** Treatment of advanced unresponsive endometrial or renal carcinoma. †Prevention of pregnancy. Management of endometriosis-associated pain (Depo-Sub Q Provera 104 only).

Action

A synthetic form of progesterone—actions include secretory changes in the endometrium, increases in basal body temperature, histologic changes in vaginal epithelium, relaxation of uterine smooth muscle, mammary alveolar tissue growth, pituitary inhibition, and withdrawal bleeding in the presence of estrogen. **Therapeutic Effects:** Decreased endometrial hyperplasia in postmenopausal women receiving concurrent estrogen (combination with estrogen decreases vasomotor symptoms and prevents osteoporosis). Restoration of hormonal balance with control of uterine bleeding. Management of endometrial or renal cancer. Prevention of pregnancy.

Pharmacokinetics

Absorption: 0.6–10% absorbed after oral administration.
Distribution: Unknown.
Metabolism and Excretion: Metabolized by the liver. Primarily excreted in the urine as metabolites.
Half-life: *1st phase:* 52 min; *2nd phase:* 230 min; *biological:* 14.5 hr.

TIME/ACTION PROFILE (IM = antineoplastic effects)

ROUTE	ONSET	PEAK	DURATION
PO	unknown	unknown	unknown
IM	wk–mos	mo	unknown†
SC	unknown	1 wk	3 mo

†Contraceptive effect lasts 3 mo.

Contraindications/Precautions

Contraindicated in: Hypersensitivity; Hypersensitivity to parabens (IM suspension only); Missed abortion; Thromboembolic disease; Cerebrovascular disease; Severe hepatic impairment; Breast or genital cancer; Porphyria; OB: Pregnancy; Lactation: Lactation. **Use Cautiously in:** History of liver disease; Renal impairment; Cardiovascular disease; Seizure disorders; Depression.

Adverse Reactions/Side Effects

CV: DEEP VEIN THROMBOSIS, edema, thrombophlebitis.
Derm: chloasma, melasma, rash. **EENT:** retinal throm-

bosis. **Endo:** breast tenderness, galactorrhea, hyperglycemia. **GI:** ↓ weight, drug-induced hepatitis, gingival bleeding. **GU:** amenorrhea, breakthrough bleeding, cervical erosions, changes in menstrual flow, dysmenorrhea. **Local:** injection site reactions. **Metab:** ↑ weight. **MS:** bone loss. **Neuro:** depression. **Resp:** PULMONARY EMBOLISM. **Misc:** BREAST CANCER, HYPERSENSITIVITY REACTIONS (including anaphylaxis or angioedema).

Interactions

Drug-Drug: Strong **CYP3A4 inhibitors**, including **ketoconazole**, **itraconazole**, **clarithromycin**, **atazanavir**, **nefazodone**, **nelfinavir**, **ritonavir**, and **voriconazole** may ↑ levels; avoid concurrent use. Strong **CYP3A4 inducers**, including **phenytoin**, **carbamazepine**, **rifampin**, **rifabutin**, **rifapentin**, and **phenobarbital** may ↓ levels; avoid concurrent use. May ↓ effectiveness of **bromocriptine** when used concurrently for galactorrhea/amenorrhea. Contraceptive effectiveness may be ↓ by **carbamazepine**, **phenobarbital**, **phenytoin**, **rifampin**, or **rifabutin**. **Drug-Natural Products:** St. John's wort may ↓ levels; avoid concurrent use.

Route/Dosage

Postmenopausal Women Receiving Concurrent Estrogen

PO (Adults): 2.5–5 mg daily concurrently with 0.625 mg conjugated estrogens (monophasic regimen) *or* 5 mg daily on days 15–28 of the cycle with 0.625 mg conjugated estrogens taken daily throughout cycle (biphasic regimen).

Secondary Amenorrhea

PO (Adults): 5–10 mg/day for 5–10 days; start at any time in cycle.

Dysfunctional Uterine Bleeding/Induction of Menses

PO (Adults): 5–10 mg/day for 5–10 days, starting on day 16 or day 21 of menstrual cycle.

Renal or Endometrial Carcinoma

IM (Adults): 400–1000 mg, may be repeated weekly; if improvement occurs, attempt to ↓ dose to 400 mg monthly.

Endometriosis-Associated Pain

SUBQ (Adults): 104 mg every 12–14 wk (3 mo), beginning on day 5 of normal menses (not recommended for more than 2 yr).

Prevention of Pregnancy

IM (Adults): 150 mg within first 5 days of menses or within 5 days postpartum, if not breastfeeding. If breastfeeding, give 6 wk postpartum; repeat every 3 mo. **SUBQ (Adults):** 104 mg within first 5 days of menses or within 5 days postpartum, if not breastfeeding. If breastfeeding, give 6 wk postpartum; repeat every 12–14 wk.

Availability (generic available)

Tablets: 2.5 mg, 5 mg, 10 mg, ✽ 100 mg. **Suspension for intramuscular injection:** ✽ 50 mg/mL, 150 mg/mL. **Suspension for SUBQ injection (DepoSubQ Provera 104):** 104 mg/0.65 mL. *In combination with:* conjugated estrogens as Prempro (single combination tablet of 0.626 mg conjugated estrogens plus 2.5 or 5 mg medroxyprogesterone) or Premphase (0.625 mg conjugated estrogens tablet for 14 days followed by combination tablet of 0.625 mg conjugated estrogens plus 5 mg medroxyprogesterone for days 15–28) in convenience packages. See Appendix N.

NURSING IMPLICATIONS

Assessment

- Monitor BP periodically during therapy.
- Monitor intake and output ratios and weekly weight. Report significant discrepancies or steady weight gain.

Lab Test Considerations

- Monitor hepatic function before and periodically during therapy.
- May cause ↑ alkaline phosphatase levels. May ↓ pregnanediol excretion concentrations.
- May cause ↑ serum LDL concentrations or ↓ HDL concentrations.
- May alter thyroid hormone assays.
- May ↓ glucose tolerance; monitor diabetic patients closely.

Implementation

- Do not confuse Depo-Provera with Depo-SubQ Provera 104. Do not confuse Provera with Proscar or Prozac. Do not confuse medroxyprogesterone with methylprednisolone, or methyltestosterone.
- *Contraception:* To ensure patient is not pregnant at time of 1st injection, administer ONLY during first 5 days of a normal menstrual period; ONLY within first 5-days postpartum if not breastfeeding; and if exclusively breastfeeding, ONLY at the sixth postpartum week. If interval between injections >13 weeks, use pregnancy test to ensure patient is not pregnant before administration. Only the 150 mg/mL vial or prefilled syringe should be used for contraception.
- When switching from other hormonal contraceptives, administer within dosing period (7 days after taking last active pill, removing patch or ring, or within dosing period for IM injection).
- Injectable medroxyprogesterone may lead to bone loss, especially in women younger than 21 yr. Injectable medroxyprogesterone should be used for <2 yr only if other methods of contraception are inadequate. If used long term, women should use supplemental calcium and vitamin D, and monitor bone mineral density.
- IM and SUBQ injections are to be administered by a health care professional.

- **SUBQ:** Shake vigorously before use to form a uniform suspension. Inject slowly (over 5–7 sec) at a 45° angle into fatty area of anterior thigh or abdomen every 12 to 14 wk. If more than 14 wk elapse between injections, rule out pregnancy prior to administration. **Do not rub area after injection.**
- **IM:** Shake vial or prefilled syringe vigorously before preparing IM dose. Administer deep IM into gluteal or deltoid muscle. Rotate sites with each injection. If period between injections is >14 wk, determine that patient is not pregnant before administering the drug.
- In patients with cancer, IM dose may initially be required weekly. Once stabilized, IM dose may be required only monthly.
- Dose for contraception lasts 3 mo and should not be used longer than 2 yr.

Patient/Family Teaching

- Explain the dose schedule. Instruct patient to take medication at the same time each day. Take missed doses as soon as remembered, but do not double doses. Advise patient to read *Patient Information* before starting therapy and with each Rx refill or injection in case of changes.
- Explain the importance of adhering to every 3-mo schedule to patients using medroxyprogesterone for contraception.
- Advise patients receiving medroxyprogesterone for menstrual dysfunction to anticipate withdrawal bleeding 3–7 days after discontinuing medication.
- Emphasize the importance of notifying health care professional if visual changes, sudden weakness, incoordination, difficulty with speech, headache, leg or calf pain, shortness of breath, chest pain, changes in vaginal bleeding pattern, yellow skin, swelling of extremities, depression, or rash occur.
- Advise patient to keep a 1-mo supply of medroxyprogesterone available at all times.
- Instruct patient in correct method of monthly breast self-examination. Increased breast tenderness may occur.
- Advise patient that gingival bleeding may occur. Instruct patient to use good oral hygiene and to receive regular dental care and examinations.
- Inform patient that medroxyprogesterone does not protect against HIV infection and other sexually transmitted infections.
- Medroxyprogesterone may cause melasma (brown patches of discoloration) on face when patient is exposed to sunlight. Advise patient to avoid sun exposure and to wear sunscreen or protective clothing when outdoors.
- Advise patient to notify health care professional of all Rx or OTC medications, vitamins, or herbal products being taken and to consult with health care professional before taking other medications.
- Rep: Advise females of reproductive potential to notify health care professional if menstrual period is missed or if pregnancy is suspected or if breastfeed-

ing. Patient should not attempt conception for 3 mo after discontinuing medication in order to decrease risk to fetus. Once discontinued may delay conception for 10 mo or more.
- Emphasize the importance of routine follow-up physical exams, including BP; breast, abdomen, and pelvic exams; and Papanicolaou smears every 6–12 mo.
- **IM SUBQ:** Advise patient to maintain adequate amounts of dietary calcium and vitamin D to help prevent bone loss.

Evaluation/Desired Outcomes

- Regular menstrual periods.
- Decrease in endometrial hyperplasia in postmenopausal women receiving concurrent estrogen.
- Management of the spread of endometrial or renal cancer.
- Prevention of pregnancy.

---

medroxyprogesterone, See CONTRACEPTIVES, HORMONAL.

BEERS

megestrol (me-**jess**-trole)
~~Megace~~
Classification
Therapeutic: antineoplastics, hormones
Pharmacologic: progestins

Indications
Palliative treatment of endometrial and breast carcinoma, either alone or with surgery or radiation (tablets only). Treatment of anorexia, weight loss, and cachexia associated with AIDS (oral suspension only).

Action
Antineoplastic effect may result from inhibition of pituitary function. **Therapeutic Effects:** Regression of tumor. Increased appetite and weight gain in patients with AIDS.

Pharmacokinetics
Absorption: Well absorbed from the GI tract.
Distribution: Unknown.
Protein Binding: ≥90%.
Metabolism and Excretion: Completely metabolized by the liver.
Half-life: 38 hr (range 13–104 hr).

TIME/ACTION PROFILE (antineoplastic activity)

ROUTE	ONSET	PEAK	DURATION
PO	wk–mos	2 mo	unknown

Contraindications/Precautions
Contraindicated in: Hypersensitivity; Undiagnosed vaginal bleeding; Severe hepatic impairment; Suspension

contains alcohol and should be avoided in patients with known intolerance; OB: Pregnancy; Lactation: Lactation.
Use Cautiously in: Diabetes; Mental depression; Renal impairment; History of thrombophlebitis; Cardiovascular disease; Seizures; Rep: Women of reproductive potential; Pedi: Safety and effectiveness not established in children; Geri: Appears on Beers list. ↑ risk of thrombotic events and possibly death in older adults. Avoid use in older adults.

Adverse Reactions/Side Effects
CV: edema, THROMBOEMBOLISM. **Derm:** alopecia. **Endo:** asymptomatic adrenal suppression (chronic therapy). **GI:** GI irritation. **GU:** vaginal bleeding. **MS:** carpal tunnel syndrome.

Interactions
Drug-Drug: May ↑ INR and risk of bleeding when used with **warfarin**.

Route/Dosage
PO (Adults): *Breast carcinoma:* 160 mg/day as a single dose or divided doses; *Endometrial/ovarian carcinoma:* 40–320 mg/day in divided doses; *Anorexia associated with AIDS:* 40 mg/mL suspension: 800 mg once daily; may ↓ to 400 mg/day after 1 mo (range 400–800 mg/day); 125 mg/mL suspension: 625 mg once daily.

Availability (generic available)
Oral suspension (lemon-lime flavor): 40 mg/mL, 125 mg/mL. **Tablets:** 20 mg, 40 mg, ✹ 160 mg.

NURSING IMPLICATIONS

Assessment
- Assess for swelling, pain, or tenderness in legs. Report these signs of deep vein thrombophlebitis.
- **Anorexia:** Monitor weight, appetite, and nutritional intake in patients with AIDS.

Lab Test Considerations
- Verify negative pregnancy test before starting therapy.

Implementation
- Because of high dose, suspension is most convenient form for patients with AIDS.
- **PO:** May be administered with meals if GI irritation becomes a problem.
- Shake suspension well before administering.

Patient/Family Teaching
- Instruct patient to take megestrol as directed; do not skip or double up on missed doses. Missed doses may be taken as long as not right before next dose. Gradually decrease dose prior to discontinuation.
- Advise patient to report to health care professional any unusual vaginal bleeding or signs of deep vein thrombophlebitis.
- Discuss with patient the possibility of hair loss. Explore methods of coping.

- Rep: May cause fetal harm. Advise females of reproductive potential to use effective contraception during and for at least 4 mo after therapy is completed. Advise patient to notify health care professional immediately if pregnancy is planned or suspected, and to avoid breastfeeding during therapy.

Evaluation/Desired Outcomes
- Slowing or arresting the spread of endometrial or breast malignancy. Therapeutic effects usually occur within 2 mo of initiating therapy.
- Increased appetite and weight gain in patients with AIDS.

BEERS

℥ meloxicam (me-lox-i-kam)
~~Mobic~~

Classification
Therapeutic: nonopioid analgesics
Pharmacologic: nonsteroidal anti-inflammatory drugs (NSAIDs)

Indications
Relief of signs and symptoms of osteoarthritis and rheumatoid arthritis (including juvenile rheumatoid arthritis).

Action
Inhibits prostaglandin synthesis, probably by inhibiting the enzyme cyclooxygenase. **Therapeutic Effects:** Decreased pain and inflammation.

Pharmacokinetics
Absorption: Well absorbed following oral administration.
Distribution: Not widely distributed to tissues.
Protein Binding: 99.4%.
Metabolism and Excretion: Mostly metabolized to inactive metabolites by the liver via the CYP2C9 isoenzyme (and to a lesser extent by the CYP3A4 isoenzyme); ℥ the CYP2C9 isoenzyme exhibits genetic polymorphism (intermediate or poor metabolizers may have significantly ↑ meloxicam concentrations and an ↑ risk of adverse reactions). Metabolites are excreted in urine and feces.
Half-life: 20.1 hr.

TIME/ACTION PROFILE (plasma concentrations)

ROUTE	ONSET	PEAK	DURATION
PO	unknown	5–6 hr	24 hr

Contraindications/Precautions
Contraindicated in: Hypersensitivity; Cross-sensitivity may occur with other NSAIDs, including aspirin; Severe renal impairment (CCr ≤15 mL/min); Concurrent use of aspirin (↑ risk of adverse reactions); Coro-

---

✹ = Canadian drug name. ℥ = Genetic implication. ~~Strikethrough~~ = Discontinued. CAPITALS = life-threatening. <u>Underline</u> = most frequent.

nary artery bypass graft surgery; OB: Avoid use after 30 wk gestation.

Use Cautiously in: Cardiovascular disease or risk factors for cardiovascular disease (may ↑ risk of serious cardiovascular thrombotic events, myocardial infarction, and stroke, especially with prolonged use or use of higher doses); avoid use in patients with recent MI or HF; Dehydration (correct deficits before initiating therapy); Renal impairment, HF, hepatic impairment, concurrent ACE inhibitor or diuretic therapy (↑ risk of renal impairment); Hypertension; Coagulation disorders or concurrent anticoagulant therapy (may ↑ risk of bleeding); OB: Use at or after 20 wk gestation may cause fetal or neonatal renal impairment; if treatment is necessary between 20 wk and 30 wk gestation, limit use to the lowest effective dose and shortest duration possible; Lactation: Safety not established in breastfeeding; Pedi: Children <2 yr or <60 kg (safety and effectiveness of tablets not established); safety and effectiveness of capsules and injection not established in children; Geri: Appears on Beers list. ↑ risk GI bleeding or peptic ulcer disease in older adults. Avoid chronic use unless other alternatives are not effective and the patient can take a gastroprotective agent; avoid short-term use in combination with oral or parenteral corticosteroids, anticoagulants, or antiplatelet agents unless other alternatives are not effective and the patient can take a gastroprotective agent.

Adverse Reactions/Side Effects

CV: edema, HF, hypertension, MI. **Derm:** DRUG REACTION WITH EOSINOPHILIA AND SYSTEMIC SYMPTOMS (DRESS), EXFOLIATIVE DERMATITIS, pruritus, STEVENS-JOHNSON SYNDROME (SJS), TOXIC EPIDERMAL NECROLYSIS (TEN). **F and E:** hyperkalemia. **GI:** ↑ liver enzymes, BLEEDING, diarrhea, dyspepsia, HEPATOTOXICITY, nausea. **GU:** delayed ovulation. **Hemat:** anemia, leukopenia, thrombocytopenia. **Neuro:** STROKE.

Interactions

Drug-Drug: May ↓ antihypertensive effects of **ACE inhibitors.** May ↓ diuretic effects of **furosemide** or **thiazide diuretics.** Concurrent use with **aspirin** ↑ meloxicam blood levels and may ↑ risk of adverse reactions. Concurrent use with **cholestyramine** ↓ blood levels. ↑ plasma **lithium** levels (close monitoring recommended when meloxicam is introduced or withdrawn). ↑ risk of bleeding with **anticoagulants, aspirin, clopidogrel, ticagrelor, prasugrel, corticosteroids, fibrinolytics, SNRIs,** or **SSRIs.** Concurrent use with **sodium polystyrene sulfonate** may ↑ risk of colonic necrosis; concurrent use should be avoided.

Route/Dosage

PO (Adults): *Capsules:* 5 mg once daily; may ↑ to 10 mg once daily, if needed; *Tablets:* 7.5 mg once daily; may ↑ to 15 mg once daily, if needed.
PO (Children 2–17 yr and ≥60 kg): *Tablets:* 7.5 mg once daily.

Availability (generic available)

Tablets: 7.5 mg, 15 mg. **Capsules:** 5 mg, 10 mg. **Oral suspension (raspberry flavor):** 7.5 mg/5 mL. *In combination with:* bupivacaine (Zynrelef Kit). See Appendix N.

NURSING IMPLICATIONS

Assessment

* Patients who have asthma, aspirin-induced allergy, and nasal polyps are at increased risk for developing hypersensitivity reactions. Assess for rhinitis, asthma, and urticaria.
* Analgesic effect is delayed. Assess pain and range of motion prior to and 2–3 hr following administration. Patient may not experience adequate analgesia for entire 24-hr dosing interval and may require administration of a short-acting, non-NSAID, immediate-release analgesic.
* Assess for rash periodically during therapy. May cause SJS or TEN. Discontinue therapy if severe or if accompanied with fever, general malaise, fatigue, muscle or joint aches, blisters, oral lesions, conjunctivitis, hepatitis, and/or eosinophilia.
* Monitor BP during initiation and periodically during therapy. May cause fluid retention and edema leading to new onset or worsening hypertension.
* Monitor for signs and symptoms of DRESS (fever, rash, lymphadenopathy, facial swelling) periodically during therapy. Discontinue therapy if symptoms occur.

Lab Test Considerations

* Evaluate BUN, serum creatinine, CBC, and liver function periodically in patients receiving prolonged therapy. May cause anemia, thrombocytopenia, leukopenia, and abnormal liver or renal function tests.
* Bleeding time may be prolonged.

Implementation

* Administration in higher than recommended doses does not provide increased effectiveness but may cause increased side effects. Use lowest effective dose for shortest period of time to minimize risk of cardiovascular thrombotic events.
* To reduce risk of renal toxicity, ensure patient is well hydrated prior to administration.
* PO: May be administered without regard to food. Administer with food or milk to minimize GI irritation.
* Shake oral suspension gently before using.

Patient/Family Teaching

* Advise patient to take this medication with a full glass of water and to remain in an upright position for 15–30 min after administration.
* Instruct patient to take medication as directed. Take missed doses as soon as remembered but not if almost time for the next dose. Do not double doses. Instruct parent/caregiver to read the *Medication Guide* prior to use and with each Rx refill in case of changes.

- Caution patient to avoid the concurrent use of alcohol, aspirin, acetaminophen, or other OTC medications without consulting health care professional.
- Inform patient that meloxicam may increase the risk for heart attack and stroke; risk increases with longer use or in patients with heart disease.
- Advise patient to inform health care professional of medication regimen prior to treatment or surgery, especially right before or after coronary artery bypass graft surgery.
- Advise patient to consult health care professional if rash, itching, visual disturbances, weight gain, edema, black stools, or signs of hepatotoxicity (nausea, fatigue, lethargy, jaundice, upper right quadrant tenderness, flu-like symptoms) occur.
- Rep: May cause fetal harm. Advise females of reproductive potential to notify health care professional if pregnancy is planned or suspected or if breastfeeding. Advise women to avoid meloxicam in the 3rd trimester of pregnancy (after 29 wks), may cause premature closure of the fetal ductus arteriosus. Use of meloxicam after 20 wks may cause fetal renal dysfunction leading to oligohydramnios. May cause reversible infertility in females and males attempting to conceive; may consider discontinuing meloxicam.

Evaluation/Desired Outcomes
- Relief of pain.
- Improved joint mobility. Patients who do not respond to one NSAID may respond to another.

REMS

melphalan (mel-fa-lan)
Alkeran, Evomela, Hepzato
Classification
Therapeutic: antineoplastics
Pharmacologic: alkylating agents

Indications
IV: High-dose conditioning treatment prior to hematopoietic stem cell transplantation (Evomela only). IV: Palliative treatment of multiple myeloma. Intra-arterial: Patients with uveal melanoma with unresectable hepatic metastases affecting <50% of the liver and no extrahepatic disease or extrahepatic disease limited to the bone, lymph nodes, subcutaneous tissues, or lung that is amenable to resection or radiation (Hepzato only).

Action
Inhibits DNA and RNA synthesis by alkylation (cell-cycle phase–nonspecific). Therapeutic Effects: Death of rapidly replicating cells, particularly malignant ones. Also has immunosuppressive properties.

Pharmacokinetics
Absorption: IV and intra-arterial administration results in complete bioavailability.
Distribution: Rapidly distributed to tissues.

Metabolism and Excretion: Rapidly metabolized in the bloodstream. Small amounts (10%) excreted unchanged by the kidneys.
Half-life: IV: 1.5 hr; Intra-arterial: 1.1 hr.

TIME/ACTION PROFILE (effects on blood counts)

ROUTE	ONSET	PEAK	DURATION
IV	unknown	2–3 wk	4–5 wk
Intra-arterial	unknown	10–13 days	2–3 wk

Contraindications/Precautions
Contraindicated in: Hypersensitivity to melphalan; History of allergy to natural rubber latex or heparin (Hepzato only); Heparin-induced thrombocytopenia (Hepzato only); History of severe allergic reaction to iodinated contrast not controlled by premedication with antihistamines and steroids (Hepzato only); Active intracranial metastases or brain lesion at risk for bleeding (Hepzato only); Liver failure, portal hypertension, or known varices at risk for bleeding (Hepzato only); Surgical or medical treatment of the liver in the past 4 wk (Hepzato only); Uncorrectable coagulopathy (Hepzato only); Unable to safely undergo general anesthesia, including active cardiac conditions (e.g., unstable coronary syndromes [unstable or severe angina or MI], worsening or new-onset HF, significant arrhythmias, or severe valvular disease) (Hepzato only); Platelets ≤100,000 cells/mm³ (Hepzato only); Hgb <10 g/dL (Hepzato only); Neutrophils ≤2,000 cells/mm³ (Hepzato only); OB: Pregnancy; Lactation: Lactation.
Use Cautiously in: Active infections; ↓ bone marrow reserve; Renal impairment (dose ↓ recommended for palliative treatment only if BUN ≥30 mg/dL); Abnormal hepatic vascular or biliary anatomy or gastric acid hypersecretion syndromes (↑ risk of peri-procedural complications with intra-arterial administration); Rep: Women of reproductive potential and men with female sexual partners of reproductive potential; Pedi: Safety and effectiveness not established in children; Geri: Begin at lower end of dosing range in older adults due to potential for age-related ↓ in renal, hepatic, or cardiac function.

Adverse Reactions/Side Effects
CV: hypotension (Hepzato only), peripheral edema, THROMBOEMBOLIC EVENTS (Hepzato only). Derm: alopecia, pruritus, rash. Endo: menstrual irregularities. F and E: hypokalemia, hypophosphatemia. GI: ↓ appetite, ↑ liver enzymes (Hepzato Kit only), abdominal pain, constipation, diarrhea, hyperbilirubinemia, mucositis, nausea, vomiting, hepatotoxicity. GU: infertility. Hemat: ↑ activated partial thromboplastin time, ↑ international normalized ratio, anemia, leukopenia, neutropenia, thrombocytopenia, HEMORRHAGE (Hepzato only). Metab: hyperuricemia. MS: ↑ troponin I, pain. Neuro: dizziness, fatigue, headache, lethargy. Resp:

cough, dyspnea. **Misc:** fever, HYPERSENSITIVITY REACTIONS (including anaphylaxis), SECONDARY MALIGNANCY.

Interactions

Drug-Drug: ↑ bone marrow depression with other **antineoplastics** or **radiation therapy.** May ↓ antibody response to **live-virus vaccines** and ↑ risk of adverse reactions. Concurrent use with **cyclosporine** may ↑ risk of renal failure. **Apixaban, aspirin, clopidogrel, dabigatran, edoxaban, NSAIDs, prasugrel, rivaroxaban, ticagrelor,** and **warfarin** may ↑ risk of bleeding during administration of intra-arterial infusion; discontinue prior to procedure. Use of **ACE inhibitors, calcium channel blockers,** or **alpha-1 receptor blockers** may ↑ risk of hypotension during administration of intra-arterial infusion; discontinue antihypertensives ≥5 half-lives before administration of intra-arterial infusion.

Route/Dosage

Multiple Myeloma (Palliative Treatment)

IV (Adults): 16 mg/m² every 2 wk for 4 doses, then every 4 wk.

Renal Impairment

IV (Adults): *BUN ≥30 mg/dL:* ↓ dose by up to 50%.

Multiple Myeloma (Conditioning Treatment)

IV (Adults): 100 mg/m²/day on Day 3 and Day 2 prior to autologous stem cell transplantation on Day 0.

Unresectable Hepatic Metastases in Patients with Uveal Melanoma

Intra-arterial (Adults): 3 mg/kg (based on ideal body weight) (max dose = 220 mg) every 6–8 wk for a total of 6 infusions.

Availability (generic available)

Powder for injection: 50 mg/vial.

NURSING IMPLICATIONS

Assessment

- Assess for signs of infection (fever, chills, sore throat, cough, hoarseness, lower back or side pain, difficult or painful urination). Notify health care professional if these symptoms occur.
- Assess for bleeding (bleeding gums, bruising, petechiae, guaiac stools, urine, and emesis). Avoid IM injections and taking rectal temperatures. Apply pressure to venipuncture sites for 10 min.
- May cause nausea and vomiting. Monitor intake and output, appetite, and nutritional intake. Prophylactic antiemetics may be used. Adjust diet as tolerated.
- Monitor for symptoms of gout (increased uric acid, joint pain, edema). Encourage patient to drink at least 2 L of fluid per day. Allopurinol may be given to decrease uric acid levels.
- Anemia may occur. Monitor for increased fatigue and dyspnea.
- Assess patient for allergy to chlorambucil. Patients may have cross-sensitivity.

- **Evomela:** For patients receiving *Evomela* as part of a conditioning regimen, nausea, vomiting, mucositis, and diarrhea may occur in over 50% of patients. Use prophylactic antiemetic medication and provide supportive care. Provide nutritional support and analgesics for patients with severe mucositis.

Lab Test Considerations

- Monitor CBC and differential weekly during therapy. The nadir of leukopenia occurs in 2–3 wk. Notify health care professional if leukocyte count is <3000/mm³. The nadir of thrombocytopenia occurs in 2–3 wk. Notify health care professional if platelet count is <100,000/mm³. Recovery of leukopenia and thrombocytopenia occurs in 5–6 wk.
- Monitor liver function studies (AST, ALT, LDH, bilirubin) and renal function studies (BUN, serum creatinine) prior to and periodically during therapy to detect hepatotoxicity and nephrotoxicity.
- May cause ↑ uric acid. Monitor periodically during therapy.
- May cause ↑ 5-hydroxyindoleacetic acid concentrations as a result of tumor breakdown.
- Intra-hepatic *Hepzato* can only be used in patients with Hgb ≥10 g/dL, platelets ≥100,000/mm³, and neutrophils >2000/mm³ who weigh ≥35 kg.

Implementation

IV Administration

- Solution should be prepared in a biologic cabinet. Wear gloves, gown, and mask while handling medication. Discard IV equipment in specially designated container.
- If solution contacts skin or mucosa, immediately wash skin or mucosa with soap and water.
- **Intermittent Infusion:** *Reconstitution:* Reconstitute with 10 mL of diluent supplied. *Concentration:* 5 mg/mL. Shake vigorously until solution is clear. *Dilution:* Dilute dose immediately with 0.9% NaCl. *Concentration:* Not to exceed 0.45 mg/mL. Administer within 60 min of reconstitution. Store at room temperature and protect from light; do not refrigerate reconstituted solution. *Rate:* Administer over 15–30 min. Keep time between reconstitution/ dilution and administration to a minimum; reconstituted and diluted solutions are unstable.
- **Evomela Intermittent Infusion:** For patients receiving *Evomela* as part of a conditioning regimen, myeloablation occurs in all patients. Do not begin the conditioning regimen if a stem cell product is not available for rescue.
- *Reconstitution:* Reconstitute with 8.6 mL 0.9% NaCl. *Concentration:* 5 mg/mL. Reconstituted solution is stable for 1 hr at room temperature and 24 hr if refrigerated. Solution is clear and colorless to light yellow; do not administer solutions that are discolored or contain particulate matter. *Dilution:* Dilute further in 0.9% NaCl. *Concentration:* 0.45 mg/mL. Diluted solution is stable for an additional 4 hr at room temperature. *Rate:* Infuse over 30 min

via injection port or central venous catheter; may cause local tissue damage if extravasation occurs. Do not administer IV push into a peripheral vein. Administer *Evomela* by injecting slowly into a fast-running IV infusion via a central venous access line.

- **Y-Site Compatibility:** acyclovir, alemtuzumab, amikacin, aminophylline, amphotericin B lipid complex, ampicillin, anidulafungin, argatroban, arsenic trioxide, aztreonam, bivalirudin, bleomycin, bumetanide, buprenorphine, butorphanol, calcium gluconate, carboplatin, carmustine, caspofungin, cefazolin, cefepime, cefotaxime, cefotetan, ceftazidime, ceftriaxone, cefuroxime, cisplatin, clindamycin, cyclophosphamide, cytarabine, dacarbazine, dactinomycin, daptomycin, daunorubicin hydrochloride, dexamethasone, dexrazoxane, diltiazem, diphenhydramine, doxorubicin hydrochloride, doxycycline, droperidol, enalaprilat, ertapenem, etoposide, famotidine, filgrastim, floxuridine, fluconazole, fludarabine, fluorouracil, foscarnet, fosphenytoin, furosemide, ganciclovir, gemtuzumab ozogamicin, gentamicin, granisetron, haloperidol, heparin, hetastarch, hydrocortisone, hydromorphone, idarubicin, ifosfamide, imipenem/cilastatin, leucovorin calcium, linezolid, lorazepam, mannitol, meperidine, mesna, methadone, methotrexate, methylprednisolone, metoclopramide, metronidazole, milrinone, mitomycin, mitoxantrone, morphine, moxifloxacin, nalbuphine, octreotide, ondansetron, palonosetron, pamidronate, pentostatin, piperacillin/tazobactam, potassium acetate, potassium chloride, prochlorperazine, promethazine, sodium bicarbonate, thiotepa, tigecycline, tirofiban, tobramycin, trimethoprim/sulfamethoxazole, vancomycin, vasopressin, vecuronium, vinblastine, vincristine, vinorelbine, voriconazole, zidovudine, zoledronic acid.
- **Y-Site Incompatibility:** amiodarone, chlorpromazine, pantoprazole.
- *Hepzato:* **REMS:** *Hepzato* is part of the *Hepzato Kit Hepatic Delivery System [HDS],* which is only available through the *Hepzato Kit Hepatic Delivery System REMS.* Health care professionals must complete required *Hepzato Kit REMS* training before administering *Hepzato Kit,* and health care facilities must be certified to offer the program. Oral anticoagulation, drugs affecting platelet function, ACE inhibitors, calcium channel blockers, and alpha-1-adrenergic blockers must be discontinued before the procedure..
- Assess for latex allergies. The double balloon catheter component of the HDS contains natural rubber latex, which may cause allergic reactions.
- If Grade 4 neutropenia of >5 days duration despite growth factor support or associated with neutropenic fever OR Grade 4 thrombocytopenia of >5 days duration or associated with a hemorrhage that required a transfusion occurs, a dose reduction to 2

mg/kg is recommended for subsequent treatments. Discontinue *Hepzato* if patients have life-threatening or *Hepzato*-related persistent toxicity that has not resolved to Grade ≤ 2 by 8 wk following treatment.

- **Intra-arterial:** Rapidly (in ≤5 seconds) inject 10 mL of the supplied sterile diluent into the *Hepzato* 50 mg vial using a sterile needle (≥20-gauge) and syringe. Resulting solution will contain melphalan 5 mg/mL. Immediately shake vial vigorously until a clear solution is obtained. No >5 seconds should elapse between discharge of the syringe and shaking. Immediately further dilute the required dose with the provided 0.9% NaCl, to a concentration <0.45 mg/mL. *For Hepzato doses <110 mg:* dilute in 250 mL of 0.9% NaCl. *For Hepzato doses 111 mg–220 mg:* divide total dose equally into 2 and dilute each in 250 mL of 0.9% NaCl. Solution is clear; do not administer solutions that are discolored or contain particulate matter. Administer diluted *Hepzato* intra-arterially with the Hepzato kit hepatic delivery system. Complete infusion within 30 min, followed by a 30-min washout period. Reconstituted and diluted solutions of *Hepzato* are unstable. No more than 60 min should elapse from reconstitution and completion of the intra-hepatic infusion of the diluted *Hepzato* solution. Do not refrigerate *Hepzato* once reconstituted.
- Administration of *Hepzato* requires general anesthesia and extracorporeal bypass of circulation. Ensure patient is euvolemic, but do not overhydrate. Monitor for hemorrhage, hepatocellular injury, and thromboembolic events during the procedure and for at least 72 hr following the procedure. Closely monitor blood pressure during procedure; patients may require fluid support and vasopressors.

Patient/Family Teaching

- Explain purpose of melphalan to patient.
- Advise patient to notify health care professional if fever; chills; dyspnea; persistent cough; sore throat; signs of infection; bleeding gums; bruising; petechiae; or blood in urine, stool, or emesis occurs. Caution patient to avoid crowds and persons with known infections. Instruct patient to use soft toothbrush and electric razor. Caution patient not to drink alcoholic beverages or take products containing aspirin or other NSAIDs.
- Instruct patient to notify health care professional if skin rash, vasculitis, bleeding, fever, persistent cough, nausea, vomiting, amenorrhea, weight loss, or unusual lumps/masses occur.
- Instruct patient to inspect oral mucosa for redness and ulceration. If ulceration occurs, advise patient to use sponge brush and to rinse mouth with water after eating and drinking. Consult health care professional if pain interferes with eating. Stomatitis pain may require treatment with opioid analgesics.

- Advise patient to notify health care professional immediately if signs and symptoms of allergic reactions (skin reactions, including welts, rash, itching, and redness; fast heartbeat; shortness of breath or trouble breathing; feel lightheaded or dizzy; blurry vision; swelling of face, tongue, or throat) occur.
- Instruct patient not to receive any vaccinations without advice of health care professional.
- Inform patient that melphalan may cause new cancers.
- Rep: May cause fetal harm. Advise females of reproductive potential to use effective contraception during and for 6 mo after last dose of melphalan and avoid breastfeeding during and for 1 wk after last dose. Advise males with a female partner of reproductive potential to use effective contraception during and for 3 mo after last dose. May cause female and male infertility.
- Emphasize need for periodic lab tests to monitor for side effects.

Evaluation/Desired Outcomes
- Decrease in size and spread of malignant tissue.

---

memantine (me-man-teen)
★ Ebixa, ~~Namenda~~, ~~Namenda XR~~
Classification
Therapeutic: anti-Alzheimer's agents
Pharmacologic: N-methyl-D-aspartate antagonist

Indications
Moderate to severe dementia/neurocognitive disorder associated with Alzheimer's disease.

Action
Binds to CNS N-methyl-D-aspartate (NMDA) receptor sites, preventing binding of glutamate, an excitatory neurotransmitter. **Therapeutic Effects:** Decreased symptoms of dementia/cognitive decline. Does not slow progression. Cognitive enhancement.

Pharmacokinetics
Absorption: Well absorbed after oral administration. **Distribution:** Unknown.
Metabolism and Excretion: 57–82% excreted unchanged in urine by active tubular secretion moderated by pH dependent tubular reabsorption. Remainder metabolized; metabolites are not pharmacologically active.
Half-life: 60–80 hr.

TIME/ACTION PROFILE (plasma concentrations)

ROUTE	ONSET	PEAK	DURATION
PO	unknown	3–7 hr	12 hr
PO-ER	unknown	9–12 hr	24 hr

Contraindications/Precautions
Contraindicated in: Hypersensitivity.
Use Cautiously in: Severe renal impairment (↓ dose); Severe hepatic impairment; Concurrent use of other NMDA antagonists (amantadine, rimantadine, ketamine, dextromethorphan); Concurrent use of drugs or diets that cause alkaline urine; Conditions that ↑ urine pH including severe urinary tract infections or renal tubular acidosis (lead to ↓ excretion and ↑ levels); OB: Safety not established in pregnancy; Lactation: Use while breastfeeding only if potential maternal benefit justifies potential risk to infant; Pedi: Safety and effectiveness not established in children.

Adverse Reactions/Side Effects
CV: hypertension. **Derm:** rash. **GI:** diarrhea. **GU:** urinary frequency. **Hemat:** anemia. **Metab:** weight gain. **Neuro:** dizziness, fatigue, headache, sedation.

Interactions
Drug-Drug: Medications that ↑ urine pH (e.g. **carbonic anhydrase inhibitors**, **sodium bicarbonate**) may↓ excretion and ↑ levels and risk of toxicity.

Route/Dosage
PO (Adults): *Immediate-release:* 5 mg once daily initially, ↑ at weekly intervals to 10 mg/day (5 mg twice daily), then 15 mg/day (5 mg once daily, 10 mg once daily as separate doses), then to target dose of 20 mg/day (10 mg twice daily); *Extended-release:* 7 mg once daily, ↑ at weekly intervals by 7 mg/day to target dose of 28 mg once daily.

Renal Impairment
(Adults): *CCr 5–29 mL/min:* Immediate-release (solution): Target dose is 10 mg/day (5 mg twice daily); Extended-release: Target dose is 14 mg once daily.

Availability (generic available)
Immediate-release tablets: 5 mg, 10 mg. **Extended-release capsules:** 7 mg, 14 mg, 21 mg, 28 mg. **Oral solution, sugar-free, alcohol-free (peppermint):** 2 mg/mL. *In combination with:* donepezil (Namzaric). See Appendix N.

NURSING IMPLICATIONS
Assessment
- Assess cognitive function (memory, attention, reasoning, language, ability to perform simple tasks) periodically during therapy.

Lab Test Considerations
- May cause anemia.

Implementation
- Do not confuse memantine with methadone.
- Dose increases should occur no more frequently than weekly.
- To switch from *immediate release* to *extended release*, patients taking 10 mg twice daily of *immediate release* tablets may be switched to *extended release* 28 mg once daily capsules the day follow-

ing the last dose of a 10 mg *immediate release* tablet. Patients with renal impairment may use the same procedure to switch from *immediate release* 5 mg twice daily to *extended release* 14 mg once daily.

- Discontinuation of therapy may result in worsening of cognitive function. Avoid abrupt discontinuation to minimize withdrawal symptoms (altered mental status, hallucinations, delusions, insomnia, increased anxiety, agitation). To taper memantine, use a 50% dose reduction or stepwise reduction via available dose formulations every 4 wks to lowest dose prior to discontinuation. Consider reinitiation if clear worsening of the condition occurs after withdrawal.
- **PO:** May be administered without regard to food.
- Administer oral solution using syringe provided. Do not dilute or mix with other fluids. Slowly squirt into corner of patient's mouth.
- *DNC:* Swallow extended release capsules whole; do not crush, chew, or divide. Capsules may be opened, sprinkled on applesauce, and swallowed. Entire contents of each capsule should be consumed; do not divide dose.

Patient/Family Teaching
- Instruct patient and caregiver on how and when to administer memantine and how to titrate dose. Take missed doses as soon as remembered but not just before next dose; do not double doses. If several days doses are missed, may need to resume at a lower dose and re-titrate up to previous dose; consult health care professional. Advise patient and caregiver to read *Patient Instructions* before starting and with each Rx refill in case of changes.
- Caution patient and caregiver that memantine may cause dizziness. Monitor and assist with ambulation and caution patient to avoid driving and other activities requiring alertness until response to medication is known.
- Advise patient and caregiver to notify health care professional of all Rx or OTC medications, vitamins, or herbal products being taken and to consult with health care professional before taking other medications.
- Teach patient and caregivers that improvement in cognitive functioning may take months; degenerative process is not reversed.
- Rep: Advise females of reproductive potential to notify health care professional if pregnancy is planned or suspected, or if breastfeeding.

Evaluation/Desired Outcomes
- Improvement in neurocognitive decline (memory, attention, reasoning, language, ability to perform simple tasks) in patients with Alzheimer's disease.

mepolizumab
(me-poe-**liz**-ue-mab)
Nucala
Classification
Therapeutic: anti-asthmatics
Pharmacologic: monoclonal antibodies, interleukin antagonists

Indications
Severe asthma that is of an eosinophilic phenotype (as add-on maintenance treatment). Eosinophilic granulomatosis with polyangiitis. Hypereosinophilic syndrome with a duration of ≥6 mo that has no identifiable, non-hematologic, secondary cause. Chronic rhinosinusitis with nasal polyps in patients with an inadequate response to nasal corticosteroids (as add-on maintenance treatment).

Action
Interleukin-5 (IL-5) antagonist that inhibits binding of IL-5 to the surface of the eosinophil, which reduces the production and survival of eosinophils. **Therapeutic Effects:** Decreased incidence of asthma exacerbations and reduction in use of maintenance oral corticosteroid therapy. Prolonged duration of remission and reduction in use of maintenance oral corticosteroid therapy in eosinophilic granulomatosis with polyangiitis. Reduction in hypereosinophilic syndrome flares. Reduction in nasal polyps and nasal obstruction.

Pharmacokinetics
Absorption: 80% absorbed following SUBQ administration.
Distribution: Minimally distributed to tissues.
Metabolism and Excretion: Degraded by proteolytic enzymes located throughout the body.
Half-life: 16–22 days.

TIME/ACTION PROFILE (plasma concentrations)

ROUTE	ONSET	PEAK	DURATION
SUBQ	unknown	unknown	unknown

Contraindications/Precautions
Contraindicated in: Hypersensitivity; Acute bronchospasm or status asthmaticus.
Use Cautiously in: OB: Safety not established in pregnancy; expected to cross the placenta (potential effects likely to be greater during 2nd and 3rd trimesters); Lactation: Safety not established in breastfeeding; Pedi: Safety and effectiveness not established in children <18 yr (eosinophilic granulomatosis with polyangiitis), <12 yr (hypereosinophilic syndrome), or <6 yr (severe asthma of an eosinophilic phenotype).

Adverse Reactions/Side Effects
Derm: flushing, rash. **Local:** injection site reactions. **MS:** back pain, myalgia. **Neuro:** <u>headache</u>, fatigue.

Misc: herpes zoster infection, HYPERSENSITIVITY REACTIONS (including anaphylaxis and angioedema).

Interactions
Drug-Drug: None reported.

Route/Dosage

Severe Asthma
SUBQ (Adults and Children ≥12 yr): 100 mg every 4 wk.
SUBQ (Children 6–11 yr): 40 mg every 4 wk.

Eosinophilic Granulomatosis with Polyangiitis
SUBQ (Adults): 300 mg every 4 wk.

Hypereosinophilic Syndrome
SUBQ (Adults and Children ≥12 yr): 300 mg every 4 wk.

Chronic Rhinosinusitis with Nasal Polyps
SUBQ (Adults): 100 mg every 4 wk.

Availability
Lyophilized powder for injection: 100 mg/vial. **Solution for injection:** 40 mg/0.4 mL (prefilled syringes), 100 mg/mL (prefilled autoinjectors and prefilled syringes).

NURSING IMPLICATIONS

Assessment
● Assess respiratory status (rate, breath sounds, degree of dyspnea, pulse) periodically during therapy.
● Monitor for signs and symptoms of hypersensitivity reactions (anaphylaxis, angioedema, bronchospasm, urticaria, rash) following injection. Reactions usually occur within hrs, but may have a delayed onset (days). Discontinue mepolizumab if hypersensitivity reaction occurs.
● Assess for and treat parasitic infections prior to therapy. If infected during therapy and unresponsive to antihelminth treatment, discontinue mepolizumab until infection resolves.

Implementation
● Only administer in a health care setting by a health care professional able to manage anaphylaxis. Mepolizumab is for prevention; do not use to treat acute bronchospasm or status asthmaticus.
● Consider administration of varicella vaccination prior to starting therapy.
● Do not abruptly stop systemic or inhaled corticosteroids when starting therapy. May ↓ corticosteroid doses gradually under direct supervision of health care professional. Corticosteroid ↓ may lead to systemic withdrawal symptoms and/or unmask conditions previously suppressed.
● *Reconstitution:* Reconstitute with 1.2 mL of sterile water for injection using a 2- or 3-mL syringe and a 21-gauge needle. *Concentration:* 100 mg/mL. Direct stream into center of cake. Swirl gently for

10 sec until powder is dissolved; do not shake. Reconstitution takes 5 min or more. Solution is clear to opalescent and colorless to pale yellow or pale brown; do not administer if solution is discolored, cloudy, or contains particles. Stable for 8 hr if refrigerated.
● **SUBQ:** Using a 21- to 27-gauge needle, administer 1 mL for the 100 mg dose or 0.4 mL for the 40 mg dose once every 4 wk into upper arm, thigh, or abdomen. 100 mg/mL prefilled autoinjector and prefilled syringe are for use by adults and children 12 yr and older. The 40 mg/0.4 mL prefilled syringe is for children 6-11 yr (must be administered by health care professional or parent caregiver).
● Remove prefilled autoinjector from refrigerator 30 min before injection and allow to sit to warm to room temperature; do not warm in any other way.
● 300 mg dose must be given as three separate 100-mg injections at least 2 inches apart.

Patient/Family Teaching
● Explain purpose of mepolizumab to patient. Administer missed doses as soon as possible; if next dose is already due administer as planned. Instruct patient to read *Patient Information* before starting therapy.
● May be self-administered by adults and adolescents 12 yrs or older using the prefilled auto-injector and prefilled syringe. Remove autoinjector from refrigerator 30 min before injection; do not warm in any other way. Inspect window of autoinjector; solution is clear to opalescent, colorless to pale yellow to pale brown in color. Do not administer solutions that are discolored or contain particulate matter. Inject into thigh or abdomen, 2 inches from navel, or upper arm if administered by caregiver. If multiple injections are needed, separate each injection by at least 2 inches. Avoid areas that are tender, bruised, red, or hard.
● Inform patient of risk and signs and symptoms of anaphylaxis. Instruct patient to notify health care professional immediately if signs and symptoms of hypersensitivity reactions (swelling of face, mouth, tongue, fainting, dizziness, feeling lightheaded, hives, breathing problems, rash) occur.
● Advise patient to notify health care professional if asthma remains uncontrolled or worsens after starting therapy.
● Caution patient not to reduce corticosteroid dose unless instructed by health care professional.
● Instruct patient to notify health care professional of all Rx or OTC medications, vitamins, or herbal products being taken and consult health care professional before taking any new medications.
● Rep: Advise females of reproductive potential to notify health care professional if pregnancy is planned or suspected or if breastfeeding. Avoid breastfeeding during therapy.

Evaluation/Desired Outcomes

- Decreased incidence of asthma exacerbations and reduction in use of maintenance oral corticosteroid therapy.
- Reduction in hypereosinophilic syndrome flares.
- Reduction in nasal polyps and nasal obstruction.

meropenem (mer-oh-**pen**-nem)
~~Merrem~~

Classification
Therapeutic: anti-infectives
Pharmacologic: carbapenems

Indications

Complicated skin and skin structure infections. Complicated intra-abdominal infections. Bacterial meningitis. **Unlabeled Use:** Febrile neutropenia. Hospital-acquired pneumonia and sepsis.

Action

Binds to bacterial cell wall, resulting in cell death. Meropenem resists the actions of many enzymes that degrade most other penicillins and penicillin-like anti-infectives. **Therapeutic Effects:** Bactericidal action against susceptible bacteria. **Spectrum:** Active against the following gram-positive organisms: *Staphylococcus aureus, Streptococcus agalactiae, Streptococcus pneumoniae, Streptococcus pyogenes,* viridans group streptococci, *Enterococcus faecalis.* Also active against the following gram-negative pathogens: *Escherichia coli, Haemophilus influenzae, Klebsiella pneumoniae, Neisseria meningitidis, Proteus mirabilis, Pseudomonas aeruginosa.* Active against the following anaerobes: *Bacteroides fragilis, Bacteroides thetaiotaomicron, Peptostreptococcus spp.*

Pharmacokinetics

Absorption: IV administration results in complete bioavailability.

Distribution: Widely distributed to tissues; enters CSF when meninges are inflamed.

Metabolism and Excretion: Primarily metabolized by the liver; 50–75% excreted unchanged by the kidneys.

Half-life: *Premature neonates:* 3 hr; *Term neonates:* 2 hr; *Infants (3 mo–2 yr)* 1.4 hr; *Children >2 yr and Adults:* 1 hr (↑ in renal impairment).

TIME/ACTION PROFILE (plasma concentrations)

ROUTE	ONSET	PEAK	DURATION
IV	rapid	end of infusion	8 hr

Contraindications/Precautions

Contraindicated in: Hypersensitivity to meropenem or imipenem; Serious hypersensitivity to other beta-lactams (penicillins or cephalosporins; cross-sensitivity may occur).

Use Cautiously in: Renal impairment (↑ risk of thrombocytopenia and seizures; dose ↓ recommended if CCr <50 mL/min); History of seizures, brain lesions, or meningitis; OB: Safety not established in pregnancy; Lactation: Use during breastfeeding only if potential maternal benefit outweighs potential risk to infant; Pedi: Children <3 mo (safety and effectiveness not established for complicated skin/skin structure infections and meningitis).

Adverse Reactions/Side Effects

Derm: acute generalized exanthematous pustulosis, DRUG REACTION WITH EOSINOPHILIA AND SYSTEMIC SYMPTOMS (DRESS), ERYTHEMA MULTIFORME, moniliasis (children only), pruritus, rash, STEVENS-JOHNSON SYNDROME (SJS), TOXIC EPIDERMAL NECROLYSIS (TEN). **GI:** diarrhea, nausea, vomiting, CLOSTRIDIOIDES DIFFICILE-ASSOCIATED DIARRHEA (CDAD), constipation, glossitis (↑ in children), thrush (↑ in children). **Hemat:** thrombocytopenia (↑ in renal impairment). **Local:** inflammation at injection site, phlebitis. **Neuro:** dizziness, headache, paresthesias, SEIZURES. **Resp:** APNEA. **Misc:** HYPERSENSITIVITY REACTIONS (including anaphylaxis).

Interactions

Drug-Drug: **Probenecid** ↓ renal excretion and ↑ levels; concurrent use not recommended. May ↓ serum **valproate** levels and ↑ the risk of seizures.

Route/Dosage

Complicated Skin/Skin Structure Infections

IV (Adults): 500 mg every 8 hr or 1 g every 8 hr (if caused by *Pseudomonas aeruginosa*).

IV (Children ≥3 mo–12 yr): 10 mg/kg (max dose = 500 mg) every 8 hr or 20 mg/kg (max dose = 1 g) every 8 hr (if caused by *Pseudomonas aeruginosa*).

Renal Impairment

IV (Adults): *CCr 26–50 mL/min:* 500 mg every 12 hr; *CCr 10–25 mL/min:* 250 mg every 12 hr; *CCr <10 mL/min:* 250 mg every 24 hr.

Intra-abdominal Infections

IV (Adults): 1 g every 8 hr.

IV (Children ≥3 mo–12 yr): 20 mg/kg (max dose = 1 g) every 8 hr.

IV (Children <3 mo): *<32 wk gestational age (GA) and postnatal age (PNA) <2 wk:* 20 mg/kg every 12 hr; *<32 wk GA and PNA ≥2 wk:* 20 mg/kg every 8 hr; *≥32 wk GA and PNA <2 wk:* 20 mg/kg every 8 hr; *≥32 wk GA and PNA ≥2 wk:* 30 mg/kg every 8 hr.

Renal Impairment

IV (Adults): *CCr 26–50 mL/min:* 1 g every 12 hr; *CCr 10–25 mL/min:* 500 mg every 12 hr; *CCr <10 mL/min:* 500 mg every 24 hr.

M

Bacterial Meningitis

IV (Children ≥3 mo): 40 mg/kg (max dose = 2 g) every 8 hr.

Availability (generic available)

Powder for injection (requires reconstitution): 500 mg/vial, 1 g/vial, 2 g/vial. **Premixed infusion:** 500 mg/50 mL 0.9% NaCl, 1 g/50 mL 0.9% NaCl.

NURSING IMPLICATIONS

Assessment

● Assess for infection (vital signs; appearance of wound, sputum, urine, and stool; WBC) at beginning of and throughout therapy.

● Obtain a history before initiating therapy to determine previous use of and reactions to penicillins. Persons with a negative history of penicillin sensitivity may still have an allergic response.

● Obtain specimens for culture and sensitivity prior to initiating therapy. First dose may be given before receiving results.

● Monitor bowel function. Diarrhea, abdominal cramping, fever, and bloody stools should be reported to health care professional promptly as a sign of CDAD. May begin up to several wk following cessation of therapy.

● Observe for signs and symptoms of anaphylaxis (rash, pruritus, laryngeal edema, wheezing). Discontinue the drug and notify health care professional immediately if these symptoms occur. Have epinephrine, an antihistamine, and resuscitative equipment close by in the event of an anaphylactic reaction.

● **Assess injection site for phlebitis, pain, and swelling periodically during administration.**

● Monitor for signs and symptoms of DRESS (fever, rash, lymphadenopathy, and/or facial swelling, associated with involvement of other organ systems (hepatitis, nephritis, hematologic abnormalities, myocarditis, myositis) during therapy. May resemble an acute viral infection. Eosinophilia is often present. Discontinue therapy if signs occur.

● Assess patient for skin rash frequently during therapy. Discontinue meropenem at first sign of rash; may be life-threatening. SJS or TEN may develop. Treat symptomatically; may recur once treatment is stopped.

Lab Test Considerations

● Monitor hematologic, hepatic, and renal functions periodically during therapy.

● BUN, AST, ALT, LDH, serum alkaline phosphatase, bilirubin, and creatinine may be transiently ↑.

● Hemoglobin and hematocrit concentrations may be ↓.

● May cause positive direct or indirect Coombs' test.

Implementation

IV Administration

● **IV Push:** *Reconstitution:* Reconstitute 500-mg and 1-g vials with 10 mL and 20 mL, respectively, of sterile water for injection. *Concentration:* 50 mg/mL. *Rate:* Administer over 3–5 min.

● **Intermittent Infusion:** *Reconstitution:* Reconstitute 500-mg and 1-g vials with 10 mL and 20 mL, respectively, of sterile water for injection, 0.9% NaCl, or D5W. Vials reconstituted with sterile water for injection are stable for 3 hr at room temperature and 13 hr if refrigerated; if reconstituted with 0.9% NaCl, stable for 1 hr at room temperature and 15 hr if refrigerated; if reconstituted with D5W, should be used immediately. *Dilution:* Further dilute in 0.9% NaCl or D5W to achieve concentration below. Infusions further diluted in 0.9% NaCl are stable for 4 hr at room temperature and 24 hr if refrigerated. Infusions further diluted in D5W are stable for 1 hr at room temperature and 4 hr if refrigerated. *Concentration:* 1–20 mg/mL. *Rate:* Infuse over 15–30 min.

● **Y-Site Compatibility:** acetaminophen, acetylcysteine, albumin, human, alemtuzumab, amikacin, aminocaproic acid, aminophylline, ampicillin, anidulafungin, argatroban, arsenic trioxide, atropine, azithromycin, aztreonam, benztropine, bivalirudin, bleomycin, calcium gluconate, cangrelor, carboplatin, carmustine, caspofungin, cefazolin, cefotaxime, cefoxitin, ceftazidime, ceftazidime/avibactam, ceftolozane/tazobactam, ceftriaxone, cefuroxime, cisplatin, clindamycin, cyclophosphamide, cytarabine, dactinomycin, daptomycin, daunorubicin hydrochloride, dexamethasone, dexmedetomidine, dexrazoxane, D5W, digoxin, diltiazem, dimenhydrinate, diphenhydramine, docetaxel, doxorubicin liposomal, enalaprilat, epinephrine, eptifibatide, erythromycin, etoposide, etoposide phosphate, fluconazole, fludarabine, fluorouracil, foscarnet, fosphenytoin, furosemide, gemcitabine, gemtuzumab ozogamicin, gentamicin, granisetron, heparin, hetastarch, hydrocortisone, hydromorphone, ifosfamide, insulin regular, irinotecan, isoproterenol, labetalol, LR, leucovorin calcium, lidocaine, linezolid, magnesium sulfate, mannitol, mesna, methadone, methotrexate, metoclopramide, metoprolol, metronidazole, milrinone, mitomycin, mitoxantrone, morphine, naloxone, nitroprusside, norepinephrine, octreotide, oxaliplatin, oxytocin, paclitaxel, palonosetron, pamidronate, pemetrexed, penicillin G, phenobarbital, piperacillin/tazobactam, plazomicin, posaconazole, potassium acetate, potassium chloride, potassium phosphate, rocuronium, sodium bicarbonate, sufentanil, tacrolimus, tedizolid, telavancin, thiotepa, tigecycline, tirofiban, tobramycin, valproate sodium, vasopressin, vecuronium, vinblastine, vincristine, vinorelbine, voriconazole, zoledronic acid.

● **Y-Site Incompatibility:** amiodarone, amphotericin B lipid complex, blinatumomab, ciprofloxacin, dacarbazine, diazepam, dobutamine, doxorubicin hydrochloride, epirubicin, eravacycline, hydralazine, hydroxyzine, idarubicin, isavuconazonium, ketamine, midazolam, mycophenolate, nicardipine, nitroglycerin, oritavancin, phenytoin, sodium phosphate, topotecan.

Patient/Family Teaching

- Explain purpose of meropenem to patient.
- Advise patient to report the signs of superinfection (black, furry overgrowth on the tongue; vaginal itching or discharge; loose or foul-smelling stools) and allergy.
- May cause dizziness. Caution patient to avoid driving or other activities requiring alertness until response to drug is known.
- Caution patient to notify health care professional if rash or fever and diarrhea occur, especially if stool contains blood, pus, or mucus. Advise patient not to treat diarrhea without consulting health care professional. May occur up to several wk after discontinuation of medication.
- Advise patient to notify health care professional of all Rx or OTC medications, vitamins, or herbal products being taken and to consult with health care professional before taking other medications.
- Rep: Advise female patient to notify health care professional if pregnancy is planned or suspected, or if breastfeeding. Monitor breastfed infants for disturbances (thrush, diarrhea).

Evaluation/Desired Outcomes

- Resolution of the signs and symptoms of infection. Length of time for complete resolution depends on the organism and site of infection.

---

meropenem/vaborbactam
(mer-oh-**pen**-nem/va-bor-**bak**-tam)
Vabomere
Classification
Therapeutic: anti-infectives
Pharmacologic: carbapenems beta-lactamase inhibitors

Indications

Complicated urinary tract infections, including pyelonephritis.

Action

Binds to bacterial cell wall, resulting in cell death. Addition of vaborbactam protects meropenem from being degraded by certain serine beta-lactamases such as *Klebsiella pneumoniae* carbapenemase. **Therapeutic Effects:** Bactericidal action against susceptible bacteria. **Spectrum:** Active against the following gram-negative pathogens: *Escherichia coli*, *Enterobacter cloacae*, *Klebsiella pneumoniae*.

Pharmacokinetics

Absorption: IV administration results in complete bioavailability.
Distribution: Well distributed to tissues.

Metabolism and Excretion: Meropenem undergoes hydrolysis; vaborbactam is not metabolized. Both meropenem and vaborbactam are primarily excreted by the kidneys (40–60% of meropenem and 75–95% of vaborbactam excreted unchanged in the urine).
Half-life: *Meropenem:* 1.22 hr; *Vaborbactam:* 1.68 hr.

TIME/ACTION PROFILE (plasma concentrations)

ROUTE	ONSET	PEAK	DURATION
IV	rapid	end of infusion	8 hr

Contraindications/Precautions

Contraindicated in: Hypersensitivity to any of the carbapenems (ertapenem, imipenem, meropenem); Anaphylactic reactions to other beta-lactams (cross-sensitivity may occur); OB: Pregnancy.
Use Cautiously in: Renal impairment (↑ risk of thrombocytopenia and seizures; ↓ dose if eGFR <50 mL/min/1.73 m²); History of seizures, brain lesions, or meningitis; Lactation: Use while breastfeeding only if potential maternal benefit justifies potential risk to infant; Pedi: Safety and effectiveness not established in children; Geri: Older adults may be at ↑ risk for adverse reactions due to age-related ↓ in renal function.

Adverse Reactions/Side Effects

GI: CLOSTRIDIOIDES DIFFICILE-ASSOCIATED DIARRHEA (CDAD), diarrhea. **Local:** infusion site reactions, phlebitis. **Neuro:** delirium, headache, paresthesias, SEIZURES. **Misc:** HYPERSENSITIVITY REACTIONS (including anaphylaxis).

Interactions

Drug-Drug: Probenecid ↓ renal excretion of meropenem and ↑ its levels; concurrent use not recommended. May ↓ **valproate** levels and ↑ risk of seizures; concurrent use not recommended.

Route/Dosage

IV (Adults): 4 g (meropenem 2 g/vaborbactam 2 g) every 8 hr for up to 14 days.

Renal Impairment

IV (Adults): *eGFR 30–49 mL/min/1.73 m²:* 2 g (meropenem 1 g/vaborbactam 1 g) every 8 hr for up to 14 days; *eGFR 15–29 mL/min/1.73 m²:* 2 g (meropenem 1 g/vaborbactam 1 g) every 12 hr for up to 14 days; *eGFR <15 mL/min/1.73 m²:* 1 g (meropenem 0.5 g/vaborbactam 0.5 g) every 12 hr for up to 14 days.

Availability

Powder for injection: 2 g/vial (1 g meropenem/1 g vaborbactam).

✤ = Canadian drug name. ⬚ = Genetic implication. S̶t̶r̶i̶k̶e̶t̶h̶r̶o̶u̶g̶h̶ = Discontinued. CAPITALS = life-threatening. Underline = most frequent.

NURSING IMPLICATIONS

Assessment

- Assess for infection (vital signs; appearance of wound, sputum, urine, and stool; WBC) at beginning of and throughout therapy.
- Obtain a history before initiating therapy to determine previous use of and reactions to penicillins. Persons with a negative history of penicillin sensitivity may still have an allergic response.
- Obtain specimens for culture and sensitivity prior to initiating therapy. First dose may be given before receiving results.
- Monitor bowel function. Diarrhea, abdominal cramping, fever, and bloody stools should be reported to health care professional promptly as a sign of CDAD. May begin up to several wk following cessation of therapy.
- Observe for signs and symptoms of anaphylaxis (rash, pruritus, laryngeal edema, wheezing). Discontinue the drug and notify health care professional immediately if these symptoms occur. Have epinephrine, an antihistamine, and resuscitative equipment close by in the event of an anaphylactic reaction.

Lab Test Considerations
- May cause hyperkalemia, hyperglycemia, and hypoglycemia.

Implementation

- **Intermittent Infusion:** *Reconstitution:* Reconstitute each vial with 20 mL 0.9% NaCl withdrawn from infusion bag. Mix gently to dissolve. *Dilution:* Dilute further in 250 mL to 1000 mL infusion bag of 0.9% NaCl. *Concentration:* 2 mg/mL to 16 mg/mL. Solution is clear to light yellow; do not infuse solutions that are discolored or contain particulate matter. Infusion must be completed within 4 hr if stored at room temperature or 22 hr if refrigerated. *Rate:* Infuse over 3 hr.

Patient/Family Teaching

- Advise patient to report the signs of superinfection (black, furry overgrowth on the tongue; vaginal itching or discharge; loose or foul-smelling stools) and allergy.
- May cause seizures, delirium, headaches, and/or paresthesias. Caution patient to avoid driving or other activities requiring alertness until response to medication is known.
- Caution patient to notify health care professional if fever and diarrhea occur, especially if stool contains blood, pus, or mucus. Advise patient not to treat diarrhea without consulting health care professional. May occur up to several wk after discontinuation of medication.
- Advise patient to notify health care professional of all Rx or OTC medications, vitamins, or herbal products being taken and to consult with health care professional before taking other medications.
- Rep: Advise females of reproductive potential to notify health care professional if pregnancy is planned or suspected or if breastfeeding.

Evaluation/Desired Outcomes

- Resolution of the signs and symptoms of infection. Length of time for complete resolution depends on the organism and site of infection.

---

mesalamine (me-sal-a-meen)

Apriso, ~~Asacol~~, ~~Asacol HD~~, Canasa, Delzicol, Lialda, ✸Mezavant, ✸Mezera, ✸Octasa, Pentasa, Rowasa, ✸Salofalk, ✸Teva 5−ASA

Classification
Therapeutic: gastrointestinal anti-inflammatories

Indications

Delzicol, Lialda, and Pentasa: Treatment and maintenance of remission of mildly-to-moderately-active ulcerative colitis. **Apriso:** Maintenance of remission of ulcerative colitis. **Canasa:** Treatment of active ulcerative proctitis. **Rowasa:** Treatment of active mild-to-moderate distal ulcerative colitis, proctosigmoiditis, or proctitis.

Action

Locally acting anti-inflammatory action in the colon, where activity is probably due to inhibition of prostaglandin synthesis. **Therapeutic Effects:** Reduction in the symptoms of ulcerative colitis, proctosigmoiditis, and proctitis.

Pharmacokinetics

Absorption: 28% absorbed following oral administration; 10−30% absorbed from the colon, depending on retention time, following rectal administration.
Distribution: Unknown.
Metabolism and Excretion: Some metabolism occurs, site unknown; mostly eliminated unchanged in the feces.
Half-life: *Oral:* 12 hr (range 2−15 hr); *Rectal:* 0.5−1.5 hr.

TIME/ACTION PROFILE (clinical improvement)

ROUTE	ONSET	PEAK	DURATION
PO	unknown	unknown	6−8 hr
ER	2 hr	9−12 hr	24 hr
Rectal	3−21 days	unknown	24 hr

Contraindications/Precautions

Contraindicated in: Hypersensitivity reactions to sulfonamides, salicylates, mesalamine, or sulfasalazine; Cross-sensitivity with furosemide, sulfonylureas, or carbonic anhydrase inhibitors may exist; Hypersensitivity to bisulfites (mesalamine enema only); Urinary tract or intestinal obstruction; Porphyria.

Use Cautiously in: Renal impairment; Hepatic impairment; Atopic dermatitis or atopic eczema (↑ risk of photosensitivity); Phenylketonuria (Apriso contains phenylalanine); OB: Use tablets only if potential benefits justify potential fetal risks (enteric coating contains dibutyl phthalate, which has been shown to cause congenital malformations in animals); Lactation: Use while breastfeeding only if potential maternal benefits justify potential risk to infant; Geri: Older adults may have ↑ risk of agranulocytosis, neutropenia, and pancytopenia.

Adverse Reactions/Side Effects

CV: pericarditis. **Derm:** ACUTE GENERALIZED EXANTHEMATOUS PUSTULOSIS, DRUG REACTION WITH EOSINOPHILIA AND SYSTEMATIC SYMPTOMS (DRESS), hair loss, photosensitivity, rash, STEVENS-JOHNSON SYNDROME, TOXIC EPIDERMAL NECROLYSIS. **EENT:** pharyngitis, rhinitis. **GI:** diarrhea, eructation (PO), flatulence, HEPATOTOXICITY, nausea, pancreatitis, vomiting. **GU:** interstitial nephritis, nephrolithiasis, renal impairment. **Local:** anal irritation (enema, suppository). **MS:** back pain, myalgia. **Neuro:** headache, dizziness, malaise, weakness. **Misc:** acute intolerance syndrome, fever, HYPERSENSITIVITY REACTIONS (including anaphylaxis and angioedema).

Interactions

Drug-Drug: May ↑ myelosuppressive effects of **mercaptopurine** or **azathioprine**; avoid concurrent use, if possible. Concurrent use with **NSAIDs** may ↑ risk of nephrotoxicity.

Route/Dosage

One 800-mg tablet is NOT bioequivalent to two Delzicol 400-mg capsules.

Treatment of Ulcerative Colitis

PO (Adults): 1.6 g (two 800-mg tablets) 3 times daily for 6 wk; *Delzicol:* 800 mg (two 400-mg capsules) 3 times daily for 6 wk; *Lialda:* 2.4–4.8 g (two to four 1.2-g tablets) once daily for up to 8 wk; *Pentasa:* 1 g (four 250-mg capsules or two 500-mg capsules) 4 times daily for up to 8 wk.

Rect (Adults): *Rowasa:* 4-g enema (60 mL) at bedtime, retained for 8 hr for 3–6 wk.

PO (Children ≥12 yr and 54–90 kg): *Delzicol:* 27–44 mg/kg/day in 2 divided doses (max dose = 2.4 g/day) for 6 wk.

PO (Children ≥12 yr and 33–53 kg): *Delzicol:* 37–61 mg/kg/day in 2 divided doses (max dose = 2 g/day) for 6 wk.

PO (Children ≥12 yr and 17–32 kg): *Delzicol:* 36–71 mg/kg/day in 2 divided doses (max dose = 1.2 g/day) for 6 wk.

PO (Children >50 kg): *Lialda:* 4.8 g (four 1.2-g tablets) once daily for 8 wk, then 2.4 g (two 1.2–g tablets) once daily.

PO (Children 36–50 kg): *Lialda:* 3.6 g (three 1.2-g tablets) once daily for 8 wk, then 2.4 g (two 1.2–g tablets) once daily.

PO (Children 24–35 kg): *Lialda:* 2.4 g (two 1.2-g tablets) once daily for 8 wk, then 1.2 g once daily.

Maintenance of Remission of Ulcerative Colitis

PO (Adults): *Apriso:* 1.5 g (four 375-mg capsules) once daily in the morning; *Delzicol:* 800 mg (two 400-mg capsules) 2 times daily; *Lialda:* 2.4 g (two 1.2-g tablets) once daily; *Pentasa:* 1 g (four 250-mg capsules or two 500-mg capsules) 4 times daily.

Treatment of Ulcerative Proctosigmoiditis

Rect (Adults): *Rowasa:* 4-g enema (60 mL) at bedtime, retained for 8 hr (treatment duration = 3–6 wk).

Treatment of Ulcerative Proctitis

Rect (Adults): *Rowasa:* 4-g enema (60 mL) at bedtime, retained for 8 hr (treatment duration = 3–6 wk); *Canasa:* Insert a 1-g suppository at bedtime, retain for at least 1–3 hr (treatment duration = 3–6 wk).

Availability (generic available)

Delayed-release tablets: ✸ 400 mg, ✸ 500 mg, 800 mg, ✸ 1 g, 1.2 g (Lialda). **Delayed-release capsules (Delzicol):** 400 mg. **Extended-release capsules (Apriso) (contain phenylalanine):** 375 mg. **Extended-release capsules (Pentasa):** 250 mg, 500 mg. **Rectal enema (Rowasa):** ✸ 1 g/100 mL, ✸ 2 g/60 mL, 4 g/60 mL, ✸ 4 g/100 mL. **Rectal foam:** ✸ 1 g/actuation. **Rectal suppository (Canasa):** ✸ 500 mg, 1 g.

NURSING IMPLICATIONS

Assessment

- Assess abdominal pain and frequency, quantity, and consistency of stools at the beginning of and during therapy.
- Assess for allergy to sulfonamides and salicylates. Patients allergic to sulfasalazine may take mesalamine or olsalazine without difficulty, but therapy should be discontinued if rash or fever occurs.
- Monitor intake and output ratios. Fluid intake should be sufficient to maintain a urine output of at least 1200–1500 mL daily to prevent crystalluria and stone formation.
- Monitor for signs and symptoms of acute intolerance syndrome (cramping, acute abdominal pain and bloody diarrhea, sometimes fever, headache, rash) during therapy; may be difficult to distinguish from an exacerbation of ulcerative colitis. If syndrome occurs, promptly discontinue therapy.

Lab Test Considerations

- Monitor urinalysis, BUN, and serum creatinine prior to and periodically during therapy. Mesalamine may cause renal toxicity. Discontinue mesalamine if renal functions declines.

✸ = Canadian drug name. ⚏ = Genetic implication. ~~Strikethrough~~ = Discontinued. CAPITALS = life-threatening. Underline = most frequent.

- Mesalamine may cause ↑ AST and ALT levels, serum alkaline phosphatase, GGT, LDH, amylase, and lipase.

Implementation

- **PO:** Administer with a full glass of water. *DNC:* Swallow tablets whole; do not break the outer coating, which is designed to remain intact. Take *Lialda* tablets with a meal. Take *Apriso* capsules in the morning without regard to meals. Do not coadminister with antacids; may affect dissolution of the coating of the granules in *Apriso* capsules. Intact or partially intact tablets may occasionally be found in the stool. If this occurs repeatedly, advise patient to notify health care professional. *DNC:* Swallow *Delzicol* capsules whole; do not break, crush, or chew. Administer without regard to meals. If unable to swallow capsules, may open capsule and swallow inner tablets. Intact or partially intact tablets may occasionally be found in the stool. If this occurs repeatedly, advise patient to notify health care professional. Two *Delzicol* 400-mg capsules are not equal to one *Asacol HD* (mesalamine) delayed-release 800-mg tablet. *Pentasa* capsules may be swallowed whole or opened and sprinkled onto applesauce or yogurt. Consume entire contents immediately. *DNC:* Avoid crushing or chewing capsules and capsule contents.
- **Rect:** Patient should empty bowel prior to administration of rectal dose forms.
- Avoid excessive handling of *suppository*. Remove foil wrapper and insert pointed end first into rectum with gentle pressure. Do not cut or break suppository. Retain suppository for 1–3 hr or more for maximum benefit.
- Administer 60-mL retention enema once daily at bedtime. Solution should be retained for approximately 8 hr. Prior to administration of *rectal suspension*, shake bottle well and remove the protective cap. Have patient lie on left side with the lower leg extended and the upper leg flexed for support or place the patient in knee-chest position. Gently insert the applicator tip into the rectum, pointing toward the umbilicus. Squeeze the bottle steadily to discharge most of the preparation.

Patient/Family Teaching

- Instruct patient on the correct method of administration. Advise patient to take medication as directed, even if feeling better. Take missed doses as soon as remembered unless almost time for next dose. Advise patient to read *Patient Information* before starting therapy and with each Rx refill in case of changes.
- Advise patient not to change brands of mesalamine without consulting health care professional.
- Encourage patient to drink an adequate amount of fluids to minimize risk of kidney stones and to notify health care professional if signs and symptoms of kidney stones (severe side or back pain, blood in urine) occur.

- May cause dizziness. Caution patient to avoid driving or other activities that require alertness until response to medication is known.
- Advise patient to notify health care professional if skin rash, sore throat, fever, mouth sores, unusual bleeding or bruising, wheezing, fever, or hives occur.
- Advise patient to avoid sun exposure, wear protective clothing, and use a broad-spectrum sunscreen when outdoors to decrease risk of photosensitivity.
- Instruct patient to notify health care professional if symptoms do not improve after 1–2 mo of therapy.
- Instruct patient to notify health care professional if symptoms worsen or do not improve. If symptoms of acute intolerance (cramping, acute abdominal pain, bloody diarrhea, fever, headache, rash) occur, discontinue therapy and notify health care professional immediately.
- Inform patient that proctoscopy and sigmoidoscopy may be required periodically during treatment to determine response.
- Rep: Advise females of reproductive potential to notify health care professional if pregnancy is planned or suspected, or if breastfeeding. Monitor breastfed infants for diarrhea.
- **Rect:** Instruct patient to use *rectal suspension* at bedtime and retain suspension all night for best results.

Evaluation/Desired Outcomes

- Decrease in diarrhea and abdominal pain.
- Return to normal bowel pattern in patients with inflammatory bowel disease. Effects may be seen within 3–21 days. The usual course of therapy is 3–6 wk.
- Maintenance of remission in patients with inflammatory bowel disease.

---

mesna (mes-na)

Mesnex, ✦Uromitexan
Classification
Therapeutic: antidotes
Pharmacologic: ifosfamide detoxifying agents

Indications

Prevention of ifosfamide-induced hemorrhagic cystitis. **Unlabeled Use:** Prevention of cyclophosphamide-induced hemorrhagic cystitis.

Action

Binds to the toxic metabolites of ifosfamide in the kidneys. **Therapeutic Effects:** Prevents hemorrhagic cystitis from ifosfamide.

Pharmacokinetics

Absorption: IV administration results in complete bioavailability; 45–79% absorbed after oral administration. Following IV with PO dosing ↑ systemic exposure.

Distribution: Minimally distributed to tissues.

Metabolism and Excretion: Rapidly converted to mesna disulfide, then back to mesna in the kidneys, where it binds to toxic metabolites of ifosfamide (18–26% excreted as free mesna in urine after IV and PO dosing).

Half-life: *Mesna:* 0.36 hr (IV); 1.2—8.3 hr (IV followed by PO); *Mesna disulfide:* 1.17 hr.

TIME/ACTION PROFILE (detoxifying action)

ROUTE	ONSET	PEAK	DURATION
PO, IV	rapid	unknown	4 hr

Contraindications/Precautions

Contraindicated in: Hypersensitivity to mesna or other thiol (rubber) compounds; Lactation: Lactation.
Use Cautiously in: OB: Safety not established in pregnancy; Pedi: Injection contains benzyl alcohol, which can cause potentially fatal "gasping syndrome" in neonates.

Adverse Reactions/Side Effects

Derm: flushing. **GI:** anorexia, diarrhea, nausea, unpleasant taste, vomiting. **Local:** injection site reactions. **Neuro:** dizziness, drowsiness, headache. **Misc:** flu-like symptoms.

Interactions

Drug-Drug: None reported.

Route/Dosage

IV (Adults): Give a dose of mesna equal to 20% of the ifosfamide dose at the same time as ifosfamide and 4 and 8 hr after.
PO, IV (Adults): Give a dose of IV mesna equal to 20% of the ifosfamide dose at the same time as ifosfamide; then give PO mesna equal to 40% of the ifosfamide dose 2 and 6 hr after ifosfamide (total mesna dose is 100% of ifosfamide dose).

Availability (generic available)

Solution for injection: 100 mg/mL. **Tablets:** 400 mg.

NURSING IMPLICATIONS

Assessment

- Monitor for development of hemorrhagic cystitis in patients receiving ifosfamide.

Lab Test Considerations

- Obtain a negative pregnancy test before starting when mesna is given with ifosfamide. Causes a false-positive result when testing urinary ketones.

Implementation

- Initial IV bolus is to be given at time of ifosfamide administration.
- PO: If second and third doses are given orally, administer 2 and 6 hr after IV dose.

- If PO mesna is vomited within 2 hr of administration, repeat dose or use IV mesna.

IV Administration

- **Intermittent Infusion:** 2nd IV dose is given 4 hr later, 3rd dose is given 8 hr after initial dose. This schedule must be repeated with each subsequent dose of ifosfamide. *Dilution:* Dilute 2-, 4-, and 10-mL ampules, containing a concentration of 100 mg/mL in 8 mL, 16 mL, or 50 mL, respectively, of D5W, 0.9% NaCl, D5/0.9% NaCl, D5/0.2% NaCl, D5/0.33% NaCl, or LR. *Concentration:* 20 mg/mL. Refrigerate to store. Use within 6 hr. Discard unused solution. *Rate:* Administer over 15–30 min or as a continuous infusion.
- **Syringe Compatibility:** ifosfamide.
- **Y-Site Compatibility:** alemtuzumab, allopurinol, amifostine, amikacin, aminocaproic acid, aminophylline, amiodarone, amphotericin B liposomal, ampicillin, ampicillin/sulbactam, anidulafungin, argatroban, azithromycin, aztreonam, bivalirudin, bleomycin, bumetanide, buprenorphine, butorphanol, calcium acetate, calcium chloride, calcium gluconate, carmustine, caspofungin, cefazolin, cefepime, cefotaxime, cefotetan, cefoxitin, ceftriaxone, cefuroxime, chloramphenicol, chlorpromazine, ciprofloxacin, cisatracurium, cladribine, clindamycin, cyclophosphamide, cytarabine, dactinomycin, dexamethasone, dexmedetomidine, dexrazoxane, digoxin, diltiazem, diphenhydramine, dobutamine, docetaxel, dopamine, doxorubicin hydrochloride, doxorubicin liposomal, doxycycline, droperidol, enalaprilat, ephedrine, epinephrine, epirubicin, ertapenem, erythromycin, esmolol, etoposide, etoposide phosphate, famotidine, fentanyl, filgrastim, fluconazole, fludarabine, fluorouracil, foscarnet, fosphenytoin, furosemide, gemcitabine, gentamicin, glycopyrrolate, granisetron, haloperidol, heparin, hetastarch, hydralazine, hydrocortisone, hydromorphone, idarubicin, ifosfamide, imipenem/cilastatin, insulin regular, irinotecan, isoproterenol, ketorolac, labetalol, leucovorin, levofloxacin, lidocaine, linezolid, lorazepam, magnesium sulfate, mannitol, melphalan, meperidine, meropenem, methotrexate, methylprednisolone, metoclopramide, metoprolol, metronidazole, micafungin, midazolam, milrinone, mitomycin, mitoxantrone, morphine, moxifloxacin, mycophenolate, nafcillin, nalbuphine, naloxone, nitroglycerin, norepinephrine, octreotide, ondansetron, oxaliplatin, paclitaxel, palonosetron, pamidronate, pantoprazole, pemetrexed, pentamidine, pentobarbital, phenobarbital, phenylephrine, piperacillin/tazobactam, potassium acetate, potassium chloride, potassium phosphate, procainamide, prochlorperazine, promethazine, propranolol, remifentanil, rituximab, rocuronium, sargramostim, sodium acetate, sodium bicarbonate, sodium phosphate, succinylcholine, sufentanil, tacrolimus, theophylline, thiotepa, tige-

cycline, tirofiban, tobramycin, topotecan, trastuzumab, vancomycin, vasopressin, vecuronium, verapamil, vinblastine, vincristine, vinorelbine, voriconazole, zidovudine, zoledronic acid.

- **Y-Site Incompatibility:** acyclovir, amphotericin B deoxycholate, amphotericin B lipid complex, dacarbazine, dantrolene, diazepam, ganciclovir, nicardipine, nitroprusside, phenytoin, thiopental.

Patient/Family Teaching

- Inform patient that unpleasant taste may occur during administration.
- Advise patient to notify health care professional if nausea, vomiting, or diarrhea persists or is severe.
- Rep: Advise female patients of reproductive potential to use effective contraception during mesna/ifosfamide treatment and for 6 mo after last dose of mesna/ifosfamide and to avoid breastfeeding during mesna/ifosfamide treatment and for 1 wk after last dose of mesna/ifosfamide. Advise males with female partners of reproductive potential to use effective contraception during mesna/ifosfamide treatment and for 3 mo after last dose of mesna/ifosfamide. Advise patient to notify health care professional immediately if pregnancy is suspected.

Evaluation/Desired Outcomes

- Prevention of hemorrhagic cystitis associated with ifosfamide therapy.

---

metFORMIN (met-for-min)

✦ Glucophage, ~~Glucophage XR~~, Glumetza, ✦ Glycon, Riomet, ~~Riomet ER~~

Classification
Therapeutic: antidiabetics
Pharmacologic: biguanides

Indications

Type 2 diabetes mellitus.

Action

Decreases hepatic glucose production. Decreases intestinal glucose absorption. Increases sensitivity to insulin. **Therapeutic Effects:** Maintenance of blood glucose.

Pharmacokinetics

Absorption: 50–60% absorbed after oral administration.

Distribution: Extensively distributed to tissues.

Metabolism and Excretion: Eliminated almost entirely unchanged by the kidneys.

Half-life: 17.6 hr.

TIME/ACTION PROFILE (plasma concentrations)

ROUTE	ONSET	PEAK	DURATION
PO-IR	unknown	unknown	12 hr
PO-ER	unknown	4–8 hr	24 hr

Contraindications/Precautions

Contraindicated in: Hypersensitivity; Metabolic acidosis (including diabetic ketoacidosis); Severe renal impairment (CCr <30 mL/min); Iodinated contrast imaging procedure in patients with CCr 30–60 mL/min, a history of liver disease, alcoholism, or heart failure, or those who will be administered intra-arterial iodinated contrast (discontinue metformin and reevaluate renal function 48 hr after imaging procedure; may restart therapy if renal function stable); Hepatic impairment; Lactation: Lactation.

Use Cautiously in: Mild to moderate renal impairment (initiation of therapy not recommended if CCr 30–45 mL/min; if CCr becomes <45 mL/min during therapy, assess risk-to-benefit of continuing therapy); Chronic alcohol use/abuse; Hypoxic states (acute HF, shock, MI, sepsis; discontinue metformin); Surgery (temporarily discontinue metformin when food and/or fluid intake is restricted); Pituitary deficiency or hyperthyroidism; OB: Insulin recommended during pregnancy; Pedi: Safety and effectiveness not established in children <18 yr (extended release) or <10 yr (immediate release); Geri: Older adults may be at ↑ risk of lactic acidosis.

Adverse Reactions/Side Effects

F and E: LACTIC ACIDOSIS. **GI:** abdominal bloating, diarrhea, nausea, vomiting, unpleasant metallic taste. **Hemat:** ↓ vitamin B$_{12}$ levels.

Interactions

Drug-Drug: Acute or chronic **alcohol** ingestion or **iodinated contrast media** ↑ risk of lactic acidosis. **Amiloride, digoxin, morphine, procainamide, quinidine, triamterene, trimethoprim, calcium channel blockers,** and **vancomycin** may compete for elimination pathways with metformin. Altered responses may occur. **Cimetidine** and **furosemide** may ↑ effects of metformin. **Nifedipine** ↑ absorption and effects.

Drug-Natural Products: Glucosamine may worsen blood glucose control. **Chromium** and **coenzyme Q-10** may produce ↑ hypoglycemic effects.

Route/Dosage

PO (Adults): *Immediate-release tablets:* 500 mg twice daily; may ↑ by 500 mg at weekly intervals up to 2000 mg/day. If doses >2000 mg/day are required, give in 3 divided doses (not to exceed 2500 mg/day) or 850 mg once daily; may ↑ by 850 mg at 2-wk intervals (in divided doses) up to 2550 mg/day in divided doses (up to 850 mg 3 times daily); *Extended-release tablets:* 500 mg once daily with evening meal, may ↑ by 500 mg at weekly intervals up to 2000 mg once daily.

PO (Children 10–17 yr): *Immediate-release tablets:* 500 mg twice daily, may be ↑ by 500 mg/day at 1-wk intervals, up to 2000 mg/day in 2 divided doses.

Availability (generic available)

Immediate-release tablets: 500 mg, 625 mg, 850 mg, 1000 mg. **Extended-release tablets (Glucophage XR, Glumetza):** 500 mg, 750 mg, 1000 mg. **Oral solution (Riomet) (cherry flavor):** 500 mg/5 mL. *In combination with:* alogliptin (Kazano); canagliflozin (Invokamet, Invokamet XR); dapagliflozin (Xigduo XR); empagliflozin (Synjardy, Synjardy XR); empagliflozin and linagliptin (Trijardy XR); ertugliflozin (Segluromet); glipizide (generic only); glyburide (generic only); linagliptin (Jentadueto, Jentadueto XR); pioglitazone (Actoplus Met); saxagliptin (Kombiglyze XR); and sitagliptin (Janumet, Janumet XR). See Appendix N.

NURSING IMPLICATIONS

Assessment

- When combined with oral sulfonylureas, observe for signs and symptoms of hypoglycemic reactions (abdominal pain, sweating, hunger, weakness, dizziness, headache, tremor, tachycardia, anxiety).
- Patients whose blood sugar has been well controlled on metformin who develop illness or laboratory abnormalities should be assessed for ketoacidosis or lactic acidosis. Assess serum electrolytes, ketones, glucose, and, if indicated, blood pH, lactate, pyruvate, and metformin levels. If either form of acidosis is present, discontinue metformin immediately and treat the acidosis. Patients with severe renal impairment are at greatest risk for lactic acidosis.

Lab Test Considerations

- Monitor serum glucose and glycosylated hemoglobin (A1c) periodically during therapy to evaluate effectiveness of therapy. May cause false-positive results for urine ketones.
- Assess renal function before starting and at least annually during therapy. Monitor patients at risk for renal impairment (elderly) more frequently. Discontinue metformin if renal impairment occurs.
- Monitor serum folic acid and vitamin B$_{12}$ every 1–2 yr in long-term therapy. Metformin may interfere with absorption.

Implementation

- Do not confuse metformin with metronidazole.
- Patients stabilized on a diabetic regimen who are exposed to stress, fever, trauma, infection, or surgery may require administration of insulin. Withhold metformin and reinstitute after resolution of acute episode.
- Temporarily discontinue metformin in patients requiring surgery involving restricted intake of food and fluids. Resume metformin when oral intake has resumed and renal function is normal.

- Hold metformin before or at the time of studies requiring IV administration of iodinated contrast media and for 48 hr after study.
- **PO:** Administer metformin with meals to minimize GI effects.
- *DNC:* XR tablets must be swallowed whole; do not crush, dissolve, or chew. Administer *Glumetza* with the evening meal.

Patient/Family Teaching

- Instruct patient to take metformin at the same time each day, as directed. Take missed doses as soon as possible unless almost time for next dose. Do not double doses. Instruct parent/caregiver to read the *Medication Guide* prior to use and with each Rx refill as changes may occur.
- Explain to patient that metformin helps control hyperglycemia but does not cure diabetes. Therapy is usually long term.
- Encourage patient to follow prescribed diet, medication, and exercise regimen to prevent hyperglycemic or hypoglycemic episodes.
- Review signs of hypoglycemia and hyperglycemia with patient. If hypoglycemia occurs, advise patient to take a glass of orange juice or 2–3 tsp of sugar, honey, or corn syrup dissolved in water, and notify health care professional.
- Instruct patient in proper testing of blood glucose and urine ketones. These tests should be monitored closely during periods of stress or illness and health care professional notified if significant changes occur.
- Explain to patient the risk of lactic acidosis and the potential need for discontinuation of metformin therapy if a severe infection, dehydration, or severe or continuing diarrhea occurs or if medical tests or surgery is required. Symptoms of lactic acidosis (chills, diarrhea, dizziness, low BP, muscle pain, abdominal pain, sleepiness, slow heartbeat or pulse, dyspnea, or weakness) should be reported to health care professional immediately.
- Advise patient to notify health care professional of all Rx or OTC medications, vitamins, or herbal products being taken and to consult with health care professional before taking other medications or alcohol.
- Inform patient that metformin may cause an unpleasant or metallic taste that usually resolves spontaneously.
- Inform patients taking XR tablets that inactive ingredients resembling XR tablet may appear in stools.
- Advise patient to inform health care professional of medication regimen before treatment or surgery.
- Advise patient to report the occurrence of diarrhea, nausea, vomiting, and stomach pain or fullness to health care professional.
- Advise patient to carry a form of sugar (sugar packets, candy) and identification describing disease process and medication regimen at all times.

✦ = Canadian drug name. ⚎ = Genetic implication. ~~Strikethrough~~ = Discontinued. CAPITALS = life-threatening. <u>Underline</u> = most frequent.

- Rep: Insulin is the recommended method of controlling blood glucose during pregnancy. Advise females of reproductive potential to notify health care professional promptly if pregnancy is planned or suspected, or if breastfeeding. Caution patient that metformin may result in ovulation in some anovulatory women leading to unintended pregnancy.
- Emphasize the importance of routine follow-up exams and regular testing of blood glucose, A1c, renal function, and hematologic parameters.

Evaluation/Desired Outcomes

- Control of blood glucose levels without the appearance of hypoglycemic or hyperglycemic episodes.

REMS | HIGH ALERT

methadone (meth-a-done)

~~Dolophine~~, ✦Metadol, ✦Metadol-D, Methadose

Classification
Therapeutic: opioid analgesics
Pharmacologic: opioid agonists

Schedule II

Indications
Moderate to severe chronic pain in opioid-tolerant patients requiring use of daily, around-the-clock long-term opioid treatment and for which alternative treatment options are inadequate (extended-release). Detoxification and maintenance therapy for opioid use disorder. **Unlabeled Use:** Neonatal abstinence syndrome.

Action
Binds to opiate receptors in the CNS. Alters the perception of and response to painful stimuli, while producing generalized CNS depression. **Therapeutic Effects:** Decrease in severity of pain. Suppression of withdrawal symptoms during detoxification and maintenance from heroin and other opioids.

Pharmacokinetics
Absorption: 50% absorbed following oral administration. IV administration results in complete bioavailability.
Distribution: Widely distributed to tissues.
Protein Binding: 85–90%.
Metabolism and Excretion: Mostly metabolized by the liver; some metabolites are active and may accumulate with chronic administration. Primarily excreted in the urine (<10% as unchanged drug).
Half-life: 15–25 hr (↑ with chronic use).

TIME/ACTION PROFILE (analgesic effect)

ROUTE	ONSET	PEAK	DURATION
PO	30–60 min	90–120 min	4–12 hr
IM, IV, SUBQ	10–20 min	60–120 min	8–12 hr

Contraindications/Precautions
Contraindicated in: Hypersensitivity; Significant respiratory depression; Acute or severe bronchial asthma; Paralytic ileus; Known alcohol intolerance (some oral solutions); Concurrent MAO inhibitor therapy.
Use Cautiously in: Structural heart disease, concomitant diuretic use, hypokalemia, hypomagnesemia, history of arrhythmia/syncope, or other risk factors for arrhythmias; Concurrent use of drugs that prolong the QT interval or are CYP3A4 inhibitors; Head trauma; Seizure disorders; ↑ intracranial pressure; Severe renal impairment; Severe hepatic impairment; Severe pulmonary disease; Hypothyroidism; Adrenal insufficiency; Alcoholism; Undiagnosed abdominal pain; Prostatic hyperplasia or ureteral stricture; OB: Use during pregnancy only if the potential maternal benefit justifies the potential fetal risk. Prolonged use of methadone during pregnancy can result in neonatal opioid withdrawal syndrome; Lactation: Use while breastfeeding only if potential maternal benefit justifies potential risk to infant; Geri: ↑ risk of respiratory depression in older adults (dose ↓ suggested).

Adverse Reactions/Side Effects
CV: hypotension, bradycardia, QT interval prolongation, TORSADES DE POINTES. **Derm:** flushing, sweating. **EENT:** blurred vision, diplopia, miosis. **Endo:** adrenal insufficiency. **GI:** constipation, nausea, vomiting. **GU:** urinary retention. **Neuro:** confusion, sedation, dizziness, dysphoria, euphoria, floating feeling, hallucinations, headache, unusual dreams. **Resp:** RESPIRATORY DEPRESSION (including central sleep apnea and sleep-related hypoxemia). **Misc:** physical dependence, psychological dependence, tolerance.

Interactions
Drug-Drug: Use with extreme caution in patients receiving **MAO inhibitors** (may result in severe, unpredictable reactions— ↓ initial dose of methadone to 25% of usual dose). Use with extreme caution with any drug known to potentially prolong QT interval, including **class I and III antiarrhythmics**, some **neuroleptics** and **tricyclic antidepressants**, and **calcium channel blockers**. Use with extreme caution with CYP3A4 inhibitors, including **ketoconazole, itraconazole, erythromycin, clarithromycin, calcium channel blockers,** or **voriconazole**. Concurrent use with **laxatives, diuretics,** or **mineralocorticoids** may ↑ risk of hypomagnesemia or hypokalemia and ↑ risk of arrhythmias. Drugs that affect serotonergic neurotransmitter systems, including **tricyclic antidepressants, SSRIs, SNRIs, MAO inhibitors, TCAs, tramadol, trazodone, mirtazapine, 5–HT₃ receptor antagonists, linezolid, methylene blue,** and **triptans** ↑ risk of serotonin syndrome. Concurrent use of **CYP3A4 inhibitors, CYP2C9 inhibitors, CYP2C19 inhibitors,** or **CYP2D6 inhibitors** including **ritonavir, ketoconazole, itraconazole, fluconazole, clarithromycin, erythromycin, nefazodone, dilti-**

azem, **verapamil, nelfinavir, fosamprenavir**, and **fluvoxamine** ↑ levels and risk of opioid toxicity; careful monitoring during initiation, dose changes, or discontinuation of the inhibitor is recommended. Concurrent use with **CYP3A4 inducers, CYP2C9 inducers,** or **CYP2C19 inducers** including **barbiturates, carbamazepine, efavirenz, corticosteroids, modafinil, nevirapine, oxcarbazepine, phenobarbital, phenytoin, rifabutin,** or **rifampin** may ↓ levels and analgesia; if inducers are discontinued or dosage ↓, patients should be monitored for signs of opioid toxicity and necessary dose adjustments should be made. Use with **benzodiazepines** or other **CNS depressants** including other **opioids, non-benzodiazepine sedative/hypnotics, anxiolytics, general anesthetics, muscle relaxants, antipsychotics,** and **alcohol** may cause profound sedation, respiratory depression, coma, and death; reserve concurrent use for when alternative treatment options are inadequate. Administration of **agonist/antagonist opioids** may precipitate opioid withdrawal in physically dependent patients. **Nalbuphine** may ↓ analgesia. **Interferons (alpha)** may ↓ metabolism and ↑ effects. May ↑ blood levels and effects of **zidovudine** and **desipramine**. Concurrent abuse of methadone with **benzodiazepines** has resulted in death. **Mixed agonist/antagonist analgesics,** including **nalbuphine** or **butorphanol** and **partial agonist analgesics,** including **buprenorphine,** may ↓ methadone's analgesic effects and/or precipitate opioid withdrawal in physically dependent patients.

Drug-Natural Products: St. John's wort ↑ metabolism and ↓ blood levels, concurrent use may result in withdrawal. **Kava-kava, valerian,** or **chamomile** can ↑ CNS depression.

Route/Dosage
Moderate-to-Severe Pain
PO (Adults and Children ≥50 kg): *Usual starting dose for moderate to severe pain in opioid-naive patients:* 2.5 mg every 8–12 hr.
PO (Adults and Children <50 kg): 0.1 mg/kg/dose every 4 hr for 2–3 doses then every 6–8 hr prn; maximum: 10 mg/dose.
PO, IV (Neonates): Initial 0.05–0.2 mg/kg/dose every 12–24 hr or 0.5 mg/kg/day divided every 8 hr; taper dose by 10–20% per wk over 1–1.5 mo.
IV, IM, SUBQ (Adults and Children ≥50 kg): 10 mg every 6–8 hr.
IV, IM, SUBQ (Adults and Children <50 kg): 0.1 mg/kg every 6–8 hr; maximum: 10 mg/dose.

Opioid Detoxification
PO (Adults and Children ≥50 kg): 15–40 mg once daily or amount needed to prevent withdrawal. Dose may be ↓ every 1–2 days; maintenance dose is determined on an individual basis.

PO (Adults and Children <50 kg): 0.05–0.1 mg/kg/dose every 6 hr; ↑ by 0.05 mg/kg/dose until withdrawal symptoms controlled; after 1–2 days lengthen dosing interval to every 12–24 hr; taper by ↓ dose by 0.05 mg/kg/day.
IV, IM, SUBQ (Adults and Children ≥50 kg): 15–40 mg once daily or amount needed to prevent withdrawal. Dose may be ↓ every 1–2 days; maintenance dose is determined on an individual basis.

Availability (generic available)
Tablets: ✣1 mg, 5 mg, 10 mg, ✣25 mg. **Tablets for oral suspension:** 40 mg (available only to licensed detoxification/maintenance programs). **Oral concentrate (cherry and unflavored):** 10 mg/mL. **Oral solution (contains alcohol) (citrus):** 5 mg/5 mL, 10 mg/5 mL. **Solution for injection:** 10 mg/mL.

NURSING IMPLICATIONS
Assessment
- **Pain:** Assess type, location, and intensity of pain prior to and 1–2 hr (peak) following administration. When titrating opioid doses, increases of 25–50% should be administered until there is either a 50% reduction in the patient's pain rating on a numeric or visual analogue scale or the patient reports satisfactory pain relief. Dose increases should be made no more frequently than every 3–5 days because of variability in half-life between patients. Cumulative effects of this medication may require periodic dose adjustments.
- Doses of methadone for patients on methadone maintenance only prevent withdrawal symptoms; *no analgesia is provided.* Additional opioid doses are required for treatment of pain.
- An equianalgesic chart (see Appendix I) should be used when changing routes or when changing from one opioid to another.
- Assess BP, pulse, and respirations before and periodically during administration. If respiratory rate is <10/min, assess level of sedation. Dose may need to be decreased by 25–50%. Initial drowsiness will diminish with continued use. Monitor for respiratory depression, especially during initiation or following dose increase; serious, life-threatening, or fatal respiratory depression may occur. May cause sleep-related breathing disorders (central sleep apnea, sleep-related hypoxemia).
- Assess bowel function routinely. Prevention of constipation should be instituted with increased intake of fluids and bulk and with laxatives to minimize constipating effects. Stimulant laxatives should be administered routinely if opioid use exceeds 2–3 days, unless contraindicated. Consider drugs for opioid induced constipation.
- Prolonged use may lead to physical and psychological dependence and tolerance. This should not pre-

vent patient from receiving adequate analgesia. Patients who receive methadone for pain rarely develop psychological dependence. Progressively higher doses may be required to relieve pain with long-term therapy.

- Assess for history of structural heart disease, arrhythmia, and syncope. Obtain a pretreatment ECG to measure QTc interval and follow-up ECG within 30 days and annually. Additional ECGs recommended if dose >100 mg/day or if patients have unexplained syncope or seizures. If QTc interval is >450 msec but <500 msec, discuss potential risks and benefits with patients and monitor more frequently. If the QTc interval >500 msec, consider discontinuing or reducing dose; eliminating contributing factors (drugs that promote hypokalemia) or using an alternative therapy.
- Assess risk for opioid addiction, abuse, or misuse prior to administration. Abuse or misuse by crushing, chewing, snorting, or injecting dissolved product will result in uncontrolled delivery of methadone and can result in overdose and death.
- **Opioid Detoxification:** Assess patient for signs of opioid withdrawal (irritability, runny nose and eyes, abdominal cramps, body aches, sweating, loss of appetite, shivering, unusually large pupils, trouble sleeping, weakness, yawning). Methadone maintenance is undertaken only by federally approved treatment centers. This does not preclude maintenance for addicts hospitalized for other conditions and who require temporary maintenance during their care.

Lab Test Considerations
- May ↑ plasma amylase and lipase levels.

Toxicity and Overdose
- If an opioid antagonist is required to reverse respiratory depression or coma, naloxone is the antidote. Dilute the 0.4-mg ampule of naloxone in 10 mL of 0.9% NaCl and administer 0.5 mL (0.02 mg) by IV push every 2 min. For children and patients weighing <40 kg, dilute 0.1 mg of naloxone in 10 mL of 0.9% NaCl for a concentration of 10 mcg/mL and administer 0.5 mcg/kg every 2 min. Titrate dose to avoid withdrawal, seizures, and severe pain.

Implementation

- *High Alert:* Do not confuse methadone with dexmethylphenidate, ketorolac, memantine, methylphenidate, or metolazone.
- When used for the treatment of opioid addiction in detoxification or maintenance programs, methadone is dispensed only by opioid treatment programs certified by the Substance Abuse and Mental Health Services Administration approved by the designated state authority.
- Explain therapeutic value of medication prior to administration to enhance the analgesic effect.
- Regularly administered doses may be more effective than prn administration. Analgesic is more effective

if administered before pain becomes severe. For patients in chronic severe pain, the oral solution containing 5 or 10 mg/5 mL is recommended on a fixed dose schedule.

- Coadministration with nonopioid analgesics may have additive analgesic effects and may permit lower doses.
- Avoid the use of mixed agonist/antagonist (nalbuphine, butorphanol) or partial agonist (buprenorphine) analgesics in patients taking methadone; may cause withdrawal.
- Medication should be discontinued gradually after long-term use to prevent withdrawal symptoms. For patients on long-acting agents who are physically opioid-dependent, initiate the taper by a small enough increment (less than 10% of total daily dose) to avoid withdrawal symptoms, and proceed with dose-lowering at an interval of every 2 to 4 wk. Patients who have been taking opioids for briefer periods of time may tolerate a more rapid taper. Monitor frequently to manage pain and withdrawal symptoms (restlessness, lacrimation, rhinorrhea, yawning, perspiration, chills, myalgia, mydriasis, irritability, anxiety, backache, joint pain, weakness, abdominal cramps, insomnia, nausea, anorexia, vomiting, diarrhea, or increased blood pressure, respiratory rate, or heart rate). If withdrawal symptoms occur, pause the taper for a period of time or raise the dose of opioid analgesic to the previous dose, and then proceed with a slower taper. Also, monitor patients for changes in mood, emergence of suicidal thoughts, or use of other substances. A multimodal approach to pain management may optimize the treatment of chronic pain, as well as assist with the successful tapering of the opioid analgesic.
- *REMS:* FDA strongly encourages health care professionals to complete a REMS-compliant education program that includes all the elements of the FDA Education *Blueprint for Health Care Providers Involved in the Management or Support of Patients with Pain,* available at www.fda.gov/OpioidAnalgesicREMSBlueprint. Information on programs can be found at 1-800-503-0784 or www.opioidanalgesicrems.com.
- Discuss availability of naloxone for emergency treatment of opioid overdose with the patient and caregiver and assess the potential need for access to naloxone, both when initiating and renewing therapy, especially if patient has household members (including children) or other close contacts at risk for accidental exposure or overdose. Consider prescribing naloxone, based on the patient's risk factors for overdose, such as concomitant use of CNS depressants, a history of opioid use disorder, or prior opioid overdose. However, the presence of risk factors for overdose should not prevent the proper management of pain in any patient.
- **PO:** Doses may be administered with food or milk to minimize GI irritation.

- Dilute each dose of 10 mg/mL oral concentrate with at least 30 mL of water or other liquid prior to administration.
- Diskettes (dispersible tablets) are to be dissolved and used for detoxification and maintenance treatment only. Available only to licensed detoxification/maintenance programs.
- **SUBQ, IM:** IM is the preferred parenteral route for repeated doses. SUBQ administration may cause tissue irritation.
- **IV Push:** Administer undiluted. *Rate:* Inject slowly.
- **Y-Site Compatibility:** amifostine, amikacin, aminocaproic acid, aminophylline, amiodarone, amphotericin B lipid complex, amphotericin B liposomal, ampicillin, ampicillin/sulbactam, anidulafungin, argatroban, arsenic trioxide, atropine, azithromycin, aztreonam, bleomycin, bumetanide, busulfan, calcium chloride, calcium gluconate, carboplatin, carmustine, caspofungin, cefazolin, cefepime, cefotaxime, cefotetan, cefoxitin, ceftazidime, ceftriaxone, cefuroxime, chloramphenicol, chlorpromazine, ciprofloxacin, cisatracurium, cisplatin, clindamycin, cyclophosphamide, cyclosporine, cytarabine, dacarbazine, dactinomycin, daptomycin, daunorubicin hydrochloride, dexamethasone, dexmedetomidine, dexrazoxane, diazepam, digoxin, diltiazem, diphenhydramine, dobutamine, docetaxel, dopamine, doxorubicin hydrochloride, doxorubicin liposomal, doxycycline, droperidol, enalaprilat, ephedrine, epinephrine, epirubicin, eptifibatide, ertapenem, erythromycin, esmolol, esomeprazole, etoposide, etoposide phosphate, famotidine, fluconazole, fludarabine, foscarnet, fosphenytoin, gemcitabine, gentamicin, glycopyrrolate, granisetron, haloperidol, heparin, hydralazine, hydrocortisone, idarubicin, ifosfamide, imipenem/cilastatin, insulin regular, irinotecan, isoproterenol, ketorolac, labetalol, leucovorin calcium, levofloxacin, lidocaine, linezolid, lorazepam, magnesium sulfate, mannitol, melphalan, meropenem, mesna, methotrexate, methylprednisolone, metoclopramide, metoprolol, metronidazole, midazolam, milrinone, mitomycin, mitoxantrone, morphine, moxifloxacin, mycophenolate, nafcillin, naloxone, nicardipine, nitroglycerin, nitroprusside, norepinephrine, octreotide, ondansetron, oxaliplatin, oxytocin, paclitaxel, palonosetron, pamidronate, pantoprazole, pemetrexed, phenobarbital, phenylephrine, potassium acetate, potassium chloride, potassium phosphate, procainamide, prochlorperazine, promethazine, propranolol, rocuronium, sodium acetate, sodium bicarbonate, sodium phosphate, succinylcholine, tacrolimus, theophylline, thiotepa, tirofiban, tobramycin, topotecan, vancomycin, vasopressin, vecuronium, verapamil, vinblastine, vincristine, vinorelbine, voriconazole, zidovudine, zoledronic acid.

- **Y-Site Incompatibility:** acyclovir, allopurinol, dantrolene, fluorouracil, ganciclovir, methohexital, pentobarbital, phenytoin, piperacillin/tazobactam, thiopental, trimethoprim/sulfamethoxazole.

Patient/Family Teaching

- Instruct patient on how and when to ask for and take pain medication.
- *REMS:* Instruct patient to take methadone exactly as directed. If dose is less effective after a few wk, do not increase dose without consulting health care professional. Discuss safe use, risks, and proper storage and disposal of opioid analgesics with patients and caregivers with each Rx. The Patient Counseling Guide is available at www.fda.gov/OpioidAnalgesicREMSPCG.
- Advise patient that methadone is a drug with known abuse potential. Protect it from theft, and never give to anyone other than the individual for whom it was prescribed. Store out of sight and reach of children, and in a location not accessible by others.
- Educate patients and caregivers on how to recognize respiratory depression and emphasize the importance of calling 911 or getting emergency medical help right away in the event of a known or suspected overdose. Inform patients and caregivers about various ways to obtain naloxone as permitted by individual state naloxone dispensing and prescribing requirements or guidelines (by prescription, directly from a pharmacist, or as part of a community-based program).
- May cause drowsiness or dizziness. Advise patient to call for assistance when ambulating or smoking and to avoid driving or other activities requiring alertness until response to medication is known.
- Inform patient of the potential for arrhythmias and emphasize the importance of regular ECGs.
- Advise patient to notify health care professional if pain control is not adequate or if side effects occur.
- Caution patient to notify health care professional if signs of overdose (difficult or shallow breathing, extreme tiredness or sleepiness, blurred vision, inability to think, talk, or walk normally, and feelings of faintness, dizziness, or confusion) occur. Methadone has a prolonged action causing increased risk of overdose.
- Advise patient to change positions slowly to minimize orthostatic hypotension.
- Advise patient to tell health care professional what medications they are taking and to avoid taking new Rx, OTC, vitamins, or herbal products without consulting health care professional. Caution patient to avoid concurrent use of alcohol or other CNS depressants, including other opioids, with this medication.
- Encourage patient to turn, cough, and breathe deeply every 2 hr to prevent atelectasis.

M

✦ = Canadian drug name. ▒ = Genetic implication. S̶t̶r̶i̶k̶e̶t̶h̶r̶o̶u̶g̶h̶ = Discontinued. CAPITALS = life-threatening. <u>Underline</u> = most frequent.

- Emphasize the importance of aggressive prevention of constipation with the use of methadone.
- Rep: Advise patient to notify health care professional if pregnancy is planned or suspected, or if breastfeeding. Inform patient of potential for neonatal opioid withdrawal syndrome with prolonged use during pregnancy. Monitor neonate for signs and symptoms of withdrawal (irritability, hyperactivity and abnormal sleep pattern, high pitched cry, tremor, vomiting, diarrhea, and/or failure to gain weight); usually occur the first days after birth. Monitor infants exposed to methadone through breast milk for excess sedation and respiratory depression. Chronic use may reduce fertility in females and males. During pregnancy, a woman's methadone dose may need to be increased or the dosing interval decreased due to increased clearance.

Evaluation/Desired Outcomes

- Decrease in severity of pain without a significant alteration in level of consciousness or respiratory status.
- Prevention of withdrawal symptoms in detoxification from heroin and other opioid analgesics.

---

methIMAzole (meth-**im**-a-zole)

❋ Tapazole
Classification
Therapeutic: antithyroid agents

Indications

Palliative treatment of hyperthyroidism. Used as an adjunct to control hyperthyroidism in preparation for thyroidectomy or radioactive iodine therapy.

Action

Inhibits the synthesis of thyroid hormones. **Therapeutic Effects:** Decreased signs and symptoms of hyperthyroidism.

Pharmacokinetics

Absorption: Rapidly absorbed following oral administration.
Distribution: Concentrated in the thyroid gland.
Metabolism and Excretion: Mostly metabolized by the liver; <10% eliminated unchanged by the kidneys.
Half-life: 3–5 hr.

TIME/ACTION PROFILE (effect on thyroid function)

ROUTE	ONSET	PEAK	DURATION
PO	1 wk	4–10 wk	1–2 wk

Contraindications/Precautions

Contraindicated in: Hypersensitivity.
Use Cautiously in: Patients with ↓ bone marrow reserve; Patients >40 yr (↑ risk of agranulocytosis); OB: Use during pregnancy only if potential maternal benefit

justifies potential fetal risk. May cause congenital malformations (especially if used during 1st trimester).

Adverse Reactions/Side Effects

Derm: rash, skin discoloration, urticaria. **GI:** diarrhea, HEPATOTOXICITY, loss of taste, nausea, parotitis, vomiting. **Hemat:** AGRANULOCYTOSIS, anemia, leukopenia, thrombocytopenia. **MS:** arthralgia. **Neuro:** drowsiness, headache, vertigo. **Misc:** fever, lymphadenopathy.

Interactions

Drug-Drug: Additive bone marrow depression with **antineoplastics** or **radiation therapy**. Antithyroid effect may be ↓ by **potassium iodide** or **amiodarone**. ↑ risk of agranulocytosis with **phenothiazines**. May alter response to **warfarin** and **digoxin**.

Route/Dosage

PO (Adults): *Initial:* 15–60 mg/day in 3 divided doses. *Maintenance:* 5–15 mg once daily.
PO (Children): *Initial:* 0.4 mg/kg/day in 3 divided doses. *Maintenance:* 0.2 mg/kg/day in single dose or 2 divided doses.

Availability (generic available)

Tablets: 5 mg, 10 mg.

NURSING IMPLICATIONS

Assessment

- Monitor response for symptoms of hyperthyroidism or thyrotoxicosis (tachycardia, palpitations, nervousness, insomnia, fever, diaphoresis, heat intolerance, tremors, weight loss, diarrhea).
- Assess for development of hypothyroidism (intolerance to cold, constipation, dry skin, headache, listlessness, tiredness, or weakness). Dose adjustment may be required.
- Assess for skin rash or swelling of cervical lymph nodes. Treatment may be discontinued if this occurs.

Lab Test Considerations

- Monitor thyroid function studies prior to therapy, monthly during initial therapy, and every 2–3 mo during therapy.
- Monitor WBC and differential counts periodically during therapy. Agranulocytosis may develop rapidly; usually occurs during the first 2 mo and is more common in patients over 40 yr and those receiving >40 mg/day. This necessitates discontinuation of therapy.
- May cause ↑ AST, ALT, LDH, alkaline phosphatase, serum bilirubin, and PT.

Implementation

- Do not confuse methimazole with metolazone or methazolamide.
- **PO:** Administer at same time in relation to meals every day. Food may either increase or decrease absorption.

Patient/Family Teaching

- Instruct patient to take medication as directed, around the clock. Take missed doses as soon as remembered; take both doses together if almost time for next dose; check with health care professional if more than 1 dose is missed. Consult health care professional prior to discontinuing medication.

- Instruct patient to monitor weight 2–3 times weekly. Notify health care professional of significant changes.
- May cause drowsiness. Caution patient to avoid driving or other activities requiring alertness until response to medication is known.
- Advise patient to consult health care professional regarding dietary sources of iodine (iodized salt, shellfish).
- Advise patient to report sore throat, fever, chills, headache, malaise, weakness, yellowing of eyes or skin, unusual bleeding or bruising, rash, or symptoms of hyperthyroidism or hypothyroidism promptly.
- Instruct patient to notify health care professional of all Rx or OTC medications, vitamins, or herbal products being taken and to consult with health care professional before taking other medications.
- Advise patient to carry identification describing medication regimen at all times.
- Advise patient to notify health care professional of medication regimen prior to treatment or surgery.
- Rep: Advise female patients of reproductive potential to notify health care professional if pregnancy is planned or suspected or if breastfeeding. May cause fetal harm, especially during 1st trimester. If breastfeeding, monitor infant thyroid levels weekly or biweekly.
- Emphasize the importance of routine exams to monitor progress and to check for side effects.

Evaluation/Desired Outcomes
- Decrease in severity of symptoms of hyperthyroidism (lowered pulse rate and weight gain).
- Return of thyroid function studies to normal.
- May be used as short-term adjunctive therapy to prepare patient for thyroidectomy or radiation therapy or may be used in treatment of hyperthyroidism. Treatment from 6 mo to several yr may be necessary, usually averaging 1 yr.

HIGH ALERT

methotrexate (meth-o-**trex**-ate)
Jylamvo, ✦ Metoject, Otrexup, Rasuvo, ~~Rheumatrex~~, Trexall, Xatmep

Classification
Therapeutic: antineoplastics, antirheumatics (DMARDs), immunosuppressants
Pharmacologic: antimetabolites

Indications
Acute lymphoblastic leukemia (in combination with other chemotherapy drugs). Treatment and prophylaxis

of meningeal leukemia. Non-Hodgkin's lymphoma (in combination with other chemotherapy drugs). Osteosarcoma (in combination with other chemotherapy drugs). Breast cancer (in combination with other chemotherapy drugs). Squamous cell carcinoma of the head and neck. Gestational trophoblastic neoplasia (in combination with other chemotherapy drugs). Severe, active rheumatoid arthritis and polyarticular juvenile idiopathic arthritis in patients with intolerance or an inadequate response to first-line therapy. Severe, recalcitrant, disabling psoriasis in patients with an inadequate response to other therapies. Mycosis fungoides (cutaneous T-cell lymphoma) (as monotherapy or in combination with other chemotherapy drugs).

Action
Interferes with folic acid metabolism. Result is inhibition of DNA synthesis and cell reproduction (cell-cycle S-phase–specific). Also has immunosuppressive activity. **Therapeutic Effects:** Death of rapidly replicating cells, particularly malignant ones, and immunosuppression.

Pharmacokinetics
Absorption: Small doses are well absorbed from the GI tract. Larger doses incompletely absorbed.
Distribution: Actively transported across cell membranes, widely distributed. Does not reach therapeutic concentrations in the CSF. Absorption in children is variable (23–95%) and dose-dependent.
Metabolism and Excretion: Excreted mostly unchanged by the kidneys.
Half-life: *Low dose:* 3–10 hr; *high dose:* 8–15 hr (↑ in renal impairment).

TIME/ACTION PROFILE (effects on blood counts)

ROUTE	ONSET	PEAK	DURATION
PO, IM, IV	4–7 days	7–14 days	21 days
SUBQ	unknown	unknown	unknown

Contraindications/Precautions
Contraindicated in: Hypersensitivity; Alcoholism or hepatic impairment; Immunosuppression; ↓ bone marrow reserve; OB: Pregnancy; Lactation: Lactation; Pedi: Products containing benzyl alcohol should not be used in neonates.
Use Cautiously in: Cranial radiation (↑ risk of leukoencephalopathy); Peptic ulcer disease or ulcerative colitis; Renal impairment (CCr must be ≥60 mL/min prior to therapy); Active infections; Rep: Women of reproductive potential and men with female partners of reproductive potential; Geri: Older adults may be more sensitive to toxicity and adverse events.

Adverse Reactions/Side Effects
Derm: alopecia, ERYTHEMA MULTIFORME, painful plaque erosions (during psoriasis treatment), photosensitivity,

pruritus, rash, skin ulceration, soft tissue necrosis, STEVENS-JOHNSON SYNDROME, TOXIC EPIDERMAL NECROLYSIS, urticaria. **EENT:** blurred vision, transient blindness. **GI:** anorexia, diarrhea, nausea, stomatitis, vomiting, GI PERFORATION, HEPATOTOXICITY. **GU:** nephropathy, ↓ fertility, acute renal failure, menstrual abnormalities, oligospermia. **Hemat:** anemia, leukopenia, thrombocytopenia, APLASTIC ANEMIA. **Metab:** hyperuricemia. **MS:** hemiparesis, osteonecrosis, stress fracture. **Neuro:** arachnoiditis (IT use only), confusion, dizziness, drowsiness, dysarthria, headache, leukoencephalopathy, malaise, SEIZURES. **Resp:** INTERSTITIAL PNEUMONITIS. **Misc:** chills, fever, HYPERSENSITIVITY REACTIONS (including anaphylaxis), INFECTION, SECONDARY MALIGNANCY, tumor lysis syndrome.

Interactions

Drug-Drug: The following drugs may ↑ hematologic toxicity of methotrexate: high-dose **salicylates**, **dapsone**, **pemetrexed**, **mercaptopurine**, **NSAIDs**, **phenytoin**, **tetracyclines**, **probenecid**, **trimethoprim/sulfamethoxazole**, **penicillins**, **pyrimethamine**, **sulfonylureas**, and **warfarin**. ↑ risk of hepatotoxicity with other **hepatotoxic drugs** including **azathioprine**, **sulfasalazine**, and **retinoids**. ↑ risk of nephrotoxicity with other **nephrotoxic drugs**. ↑ risk of bone marrow depression with other **antineoplastics** or **radiation therapy**. **Radiation therapy** ↑ risk of soft tissue necrosis and osteonecrosis. May ↓ antibody response to **live-virus vaccines** and ↑ risk of adverse reactions. ↑ risk of neurologic reactions with **acyclovir** (IT methotrexate only). **Nitrous oxide** may ↑ risk of toxicity; avoid concurrent use. **Folic acid** may ↓ antineoplastic effects; avoid concurrent use. May ↑ levels and risk of toxicity of **theophylline**.

Drug-Natural Products: Concomitant use with **echinacea** and **melatonin** may interfere with immunosuppression. **Caffeine** may ↓ efficacy of methotrexate, similar effect may occur with **guarana**.

Route/Dosage

Acute Lymphoblastic Leukemia

IV (Adults and Children): 10–5,000 mg/m² followed by leucovorin rescue (for doses >500 mg/m²). Lower doses (20–30 mg/m²/wk may be used IM.
PO (Adults): 20 mg/m² once weekly.

Meningeal Leukemia

IT (Adults and Children ≥9 yr): 12–15 mg given at intervals of 2 or more days up to twice weekly (for treatment) and no more than once weekly (for prophylaxis).
IT (Children 3–<9 yr): 12 mg given at intervals of 2 or more days up to twice weekly (for treatment) and no more than once weekly (for prophylaxis).
IT (Children 2–<3 yr): 10 mg given at intervals of 2 or more days up to twice weekly (for treatment) and no more than once weekly (for prophylaxis).
IT (Children 1–<2 yr): 8 mg given at intervals of 2 or more days up to twice weekly (for treatment) and no more than once weekly (for prophylaxis).

IT (Children <1 yr): 6 mg given at intervals of 2 or more days up to twice weekly (for treatment) and no more than once weekly (for prophylaxis).

Non-Hodgkin's Lymphoma

IV (Adults and Children): *In combination with other chemotherapy agents:* 1000 mg/m² *or* 3000 mg/m² over 24 hours followed by leucovorin rescue. *CNS-directed therapy:* 8000 mg/m² over 4 hr followed by leucovorin rescue (as monotherapy) *or* 3000–8000 mg/m² followed by leucovorin rescue (in combination with immunochemotherapy).
PO (Adults): 2.5 mg 2–4 times weekly.

Osteosarcoma

IV (Adults and Children): 12 g/m² (max = 20 g/dose) over 4 hr followed by leucovorin rescue, usually as part of a combination chemotherapeutic regimen (or ↑ dose until peak serum methotrexate level is 1 × 10⁻³ M/L but not to exceed 15 g/m²); 12 courses are given starting 4 wk after surgery and repeated at scheduled intervals.

Breast Cancer

IV (Adults): 40 mg/m² on days 1 and 8 (with other agents; many regimens are used).

Squamous Cell Carcinoma of Head and Neck

IV (Adults): 40–60 mg/m² once weekly.

Gestational Trophoblastic Neoplasia

IV, IM (Adults): *Low-risk gestational trophoblastic neoplasia:* 30–200 mg/m².
IV (Adults): *High-risk gestational trophoblastic neoplasia:* 300 mg/m² over 12 hr (with other agents).

Mycosis Fungoides

PO (Adults): *Monotherapy:* 25–75 mg once weekly; *As part of combination regimen:* 10 mg/m² twice weekly.
IM (Adults): *Early stage:* 5–50 mg once weekly; *If poor response to weekly therapy:* 15–37.5 mg twice weekly.

Rheumatoid Arthritis

PO, IM, SUBQ (Adults): 7.5 mg once weekly (not to exceed 20 mg/wk); when optimal clinical response is obtained, dose should be ↓. Otrexup may be used when dose is 10–20 mg/wk.

Polyarticular Juvenile Idiopathic Arthritis

PO, IM, SUBQ (Children): 10 mg/m² once weekly initially, may be ↑ up to 20–30 mg/m²; however, response may be better if doses >20 mg/m² are given IM or SUBQ; Otrexup may be used when dose is 10–25 mg/wk.

Psoriasis

Therapy may be preceded by a 5–10-mg test dose.
PO, IM, SUBQ, IV (Adults): 10–25 mg once weekly (not to exceed 25 mg/wk); when optimal clinical response is obtained, dose should be ↓. Otrexup may be used when dose is 10–25 mg/wk.

Availability (generic available)

Tablets: 2.5 mg, 5 mg, 7.5 mg, 10 mg, 15 mg. **Oral solution (Jylamvo) (orange flavor):** 2 mg/mL. **Oral solution (Xatmep) (orange flavor):** 2.5 mg/mL. **Solution for SUBQ injection (Otrexup):** 10 mg/0.4 mL, 12.5 mg/0.4 mL, 15 mg/0.4 mL, 17.5 mg/0.4 mL, 20 mg/0.4 mL, 22.5 mg/0.4 mL, 25 mg/0.4 mL. **Solution for SUBQ injection (Rasuvo):** 7.5 mg/0.15 mL, 10 mg/0.2 mL, 12.5 mg/0.25 mL, 15 mg/0.3 mL, 17.5 mg/0.35 mL, 20 mg/0.4 mL, 22.5 mg/0.45 mL, 25 mg/ 0.5 mL, 30 mg/0.6 mL. **Powder for injection:** 1 g/ vial. **Solution for injection:** 25 mg/mL. **Solution for injection (preservative free):** 25 mg/mL.

NURSING IMPLICATIONS

Assessment

- Monitor vital signs periodically during administration. Report significant changes.
- Monitor for abdominal pain, diarrhea, or stomatitis; therapy may need to be discontinued.
- Monitor for bone marrow depression. Assess for bleeding (bleeding gums, bruising, petechiae, guaiac stools, urine, and emesis) and avoid IM injections and taking rectal temperatures if platelet count is low. Apply pressure to venipuncture sites for 10 min. Assess for signs of infection during neutropenia. Anemia may occur. Monitor for increased fatigue, dyspnea, and orthostatic hypotension.
- Monitor intake and output ratios and daily weights. Report significant changes in totals.
- Monitor for symptoms of interstitial pneumonitis, which may manifest early as a dry, nonproductive cough.
- Monitor for symptoms of gout (increased uric acid, joint pain, edema). Encourage patient to drink at least 2 L of fluid each day. Allopurinol and alkalinization of urine may be used to decrease uric acid levels.
- Assess nutritional status. Administering an antiemetic prior to and periodically during therapy and adjusting diet as tolerated may help maintain fluid and electrolyte balance and nutritional status.
- Assess for rash periodically during therapy. May cause Stevens-Johnson syndrome. Discontinue therapy if severe or if accompanied with fever, general malaise, fatigue, muscle or joint aches, blisters, oral lesions, conjunctivitis, hepatitis, and/or eosinophilia.
- **IT:** Assess for development of nuchal rigidity, headache, fever, confusion, drowsiness, dizziness, weakness, or seizures.
- **Rheumatoid Arthritis:** Assess patient for pain and range of motion prior to and periodically during therapy.
- **Psoriasis:** Assess skin lesions prior to and periodically during therapy.

Lab Test Considerations

- Verify negative pregnancy test prior to starting therapy. Monitor CBC and differential prior to and at least monthly during therapy and at least daily for high-dose regimens. The nadir of leukopenia and thrombocytopenia occurs in 7–14 days. Leukocyte and thrombocyte counts usually recover 7 days after the nadirs. Discontinue methotrexate immediately for any sudden drop in values.
- Monitor renal (BUN and serum creatinine) and hepatic function (AST, ALT, bilirubin, and LDH) prior to and every 1–2 mo during therapy. Urine pH should be monitored prior to high-dose methotrexate therapy and every 6 hr during leucovorin rescue. Urine pH should be kept above 7.0 from before 1st dose through therapy to prevent renal damage.
- May cause ↑ serum uric acid concentrations, especially during initial treatment of leukemia and lymphoma.

Toxicity and Overdose

- Monitor serum methotrexate levels at least daily during high-dose therapy and adjust hydration and leucovorin dosing as needed. This monitoring is essential to plan correct leucovorin dose and determine duration of rescue therapy.
- With high-dose therapy (doses of $\geq$500 mg/m^2), patient must receive leucovorin rescue within 24–48 hr to prevent fatal toxicity. May be considered for intermediate doses of 100 mg/m^2 to <500 mg/m^2. Administer IV fluids starting before 1st dose and continuing through therapy to maintain adequate hydration and urine output. Administer glucarpidase in patients who have toxic plasma methotrexate concentrations (>1 micromole per liter) and delayed methotrexate clearance due to impaired renal function. Glucarpidase may be used for patients with impaired renal function. If glucarpidase is used, do not administer leucovorin within 2 hrs before or after glucarpidase because leucovorin is a substrate for glucarpidase. In cases of massive overdose, hydration and urinary alkalinization with sodium bicarbonate are required to prevent renal tubule damage. Leucovorin and levoleucovorin are indicated to diminish the toxicity and counteract the effect of inadvertently administered overdoses of methotrexate. Monitor fluid and electrolyte status; patients must be well hydrated. Intermittent hemodialysis using a high-flux dialyzer may be used for clearance until levels are <0.05 micromolar. Methotrexate should be delayed until recovery if WBC <1500/mcL, neutrophil count <200/mcL, platelet count <75,000/mcL, serum bilirubin level >1.2 mg/dL, AST level >450 IU/L, mucositis is present, until evidence of healing, persistent pleural effusion is present, should be drained dry prior to infusion. Adequate renal function is required. Serum creatinine must be normal, CCr must be >60 mL/min, before initiation

M

of therapy. Serum creatinine must be measured before each course of therapy. If ↑ by ≥50% of a prior value, CCr must be >60 mL/min, even if serum creatinine is within normal range.

Implementation

- **High Alert:** Fatalities have occurred with chemotherapeutic agents. Before administering, clarify all ambiguous orders; double-check single, daily, and course-of-therapy dose limits; have second practitioner independently double-check original order, calculations, and infusion pump settings. Methotrexate for nononcologic use is given at a much lower dose and frequency—often just once a wk. Do not confuse nononcologic dosing regimens with dosing regimens for cancer patients. Do not confuse methotrexate with metolazone or MTX Patch (lidocaine/menthol). Do not confuse Trexall with Paxil.
- Administer IV fluids starting before 1st dose and continuing through therapy to maintain adequate hydration and urine output.
- Solutions for injection should be prepared in a biologic cabinet. Wear gloves, gown, and mask while handling medication. Discard equipment in specially designated containers.
- **PO:** Use only the copackaged syringe to measure *Jylamvo*; a teaspoon is not an accurate measuring device. Solution is clear yellow; do not administer solutions that are discolored, cloudy, or contain particulate matter.
- *Otrexup* and *Rasuvo* are not indicated for treatment of neoplastic diseases. Not for patients requiring oral, IM, IV, intra-arterial, or IT dosing, doses <10 mg/wk, doses >25 mg/wk, high-dose regimens, or dose adjustments of less than 5 mg increments.
- **SUBQ:** *Otrexup* and *Rasuvo* are single-dose auto-injectors. Inject once weekly in abdomen or upper thigh. Avoid areas where skin is tender, bruised, red, scaly, hard, or has scars or stretch marks. Solution is clear and yellow; do not inject solutions that are discolored or contain particulate matter.

IV Administration

- **IV Push:** *Reconstitution:* Reconstitute each vial with 25 mL of 0.9% NaCl. Use sterile preservative-free diluents for high-dose regimens, neonates, low-birth weight infants, and intrathecal use to prevent complications from large amounts of benzyl alcohol. Solution is clear yellow; do not use preparations that are cloudy, discolored or that contain a precipitate. Reconstitute immediately before use. Discard unused portion. *Concentration:* <25 mg/mL for IV push and intermittent/continuous infusions. *Rate:* Administer at a rate of 10 mg/min into Y-site of a free-flowing IV.
- **Intermittent/Continuous Infusion:** *Dilution:* Doses >100–300 mg/m² may also be diluted in D5W, D5/0.9% NaCl, or 0.9% NaCl and infused as intermittent or continuous infusion. *Rate:* Administration rates of 4–20 mg/hr have been used.

- **Y-Site Compatibility:** acyclovir, alemtuzumab, allopurinol, amifostine, amikacin, aminophylline, amiodarone, amphotericin B lipid complex, amphotericin B liposomal, ampicillin, ampicillin/sulbactam, anidulafungin, argatroban, azithromycin, aztreonam, bivalirudin, bleomycin, bumetanide, buprenorphine, butorphanol, calcium chloride, calcium gluconate, carboplatin, carmustine, cefazolin, cefepime, cefotaxime, cefotetan, cefoxitin, ceftazidime, ceftriaxone, cefuroxime, ciprofloxacin, cisatracurium, cisplatin, clindamycin, cyclophosphamide, cyclosporine, cytarabine, dactinomycin, daunorubicin hydrochloride, dexmedetomidine, digoxin, diphenhydramine, docetaxel, doxorubicin hydrochloride, doxorubicin liposomal, enalaprilat, ephedrine, epinephrine, epirubicin, ertapenem, erythromycin, esmolol, etoposide, etoposide phosphate, famotidine, fentanyl, filgrastim, fluconazole, fludarabine, fluorouracil, foscarnet, fosphenytoin, furosemide, ganciclovir, gemtuzumab ozogamicin, granisetron, heparin, hetastarch, hydrocortisone, hydromorphone, imipenem/cilastatin, insulin regular, isoproterenol, ketorolac, leucovorin calcium, lidocaine, linezolid, lorazepam, magnesium sulfate, mannitol, melphalan, meperidine, meropenem, mesna, methadone, methohexital, methylprednisolone, metoclopramide, metoprolol, metronidazole, milrinone, mitomycin, mitoxantrone, morphine, moxifloxacin, naloxone, nitroglycerin, norepinephrine, octreotide, ondansetron, oxacillin, oxaliplatin, paclitaxel, palonosetron, pamidronate, pentobarbital, phenobarbital, phenylephrine, piperacillin/tazobactam, potassium acetate, potassium chloride, potassium phosphate, procainamide, prochlorperazine, propranolol, remifentanil, rituximab, rocuronium, sargramostim, sodium acetate, sodium bicarbonate, sodium phosphate, succinylcholine, sufentanil, tacrolimus, theophylline, thiopental, thiotepa, tigecycline, tirofiban, tobramycin, trastuzumab, trimethoprim/sulfamethoxazole, vasopressin, vecuronium, verapamil, vinblastine, vincristine, vinorelbine, voriconazole, zidovudine, zoledronic acid.
- **Y-Site Incompatibility:** amiodarone, caspofungin, chlorpromazine, dacarbazine, daptomycin, dexrazoxane, diazepam, diltiazem, dobutamine, dopamine, doxycycline, gemcitabine, gentamicin, idarubicin, ifosfamide, levofloxacin, midazolam, mycophenolate, nalbuphine, nicardipine, pantoprazole, pentamidine, phenytoin, propofol.
- **IT:** Reconstitute preservative-free methotrexate with preservative-free 0.9% NaCl, Elliot's B solution, or patient's CSF to a concentration not greater than 2 mg/mL. May be administered via lumbar puncture or Ommaya reservoir. To prevent bacterial contamination, use immediately.

Patient/Family Teaching

- Instruct patient to take medication as directed. If a dose is missed, it should be omitted. Consult health care professional if vomiting occurs shortly after a dose is taken. Advise patients taking PO or SUBQ therapy to read *Patient Information* before starting therapy and with each Rx refill in case of changes.

- Instruct patient to notify health care professional promptly if rash, fever; chills; cough; hoarseness; sore throat; signs of infection; lower back or side pain; painful or difficult urination; bleeding gums; bruising; petechiae; blood in stools, urine, or emesis; increased fatigue; dyspnea; or orthostatic hypotension occurs. Caution patient to avoid crowds and persons with known infections. Instruct patient to use soft toothbrush and electric razor and to avoid falls. Caution patient not to drink alcoholic beverages or take medication containing aspirin or other NSAIDs; may precipitate gastric bleeding.
- Instruct patient to inspect oral mucosa for erythema and ulceration. If ulceration occurs, advise patient to use sponge brush and to rinse mouth with water after eating and drinking. Topical therapy may be used if mouth pain interferes with eating. Stomatitis pain may require treatment with opioid analgesics.
- Advise patient to notify health care professional of all Rx or OTC medications, vitamins, or herbal products being taken and to consult with health care professional before taking other medications.
- Discuss the possibility of hair loss with patient. Explore methods of coping.
- Instruct patient not to receive any vaccinations without advice of health care professional.
- Caution patient to use sunscreen and protective clothing to prevent photosensitivity reactions.
- Rep: May cause fetal harm. Advise females of reproductive potential to use effective contraception during and for 6 mo after last dose and avoid breastfeeding during and for 1 wk after last dose of therapy. Advise males with female partners of reproductive potential to use effective contraception during and for 3 mo after therapy. Advise patient to notify health care professional if pregnancy is planned or suspected. May impair fertility in both men and women.
- Emphasize the need for periodic lab tests to monitor for side effects.
- SUBQ: Instruct patient on correct technique for injection and care and disposal of equipment.

Evaluation/Desired Outcomes

- Improvement of hematopoietic values in leukemia.
- Decrease in symptoms of meningeal involvement in leukemia.
- Decrease in size and spread of non-Hodgkin's lymphomas and other solid cancers.
- Resolution of skin lesions in severe psoriasis.
- Decreased joint pain and swelling.
- Improved mobility in patients with rheumatoid arthritis.
- Regression of lesions in mycosis fungoides.

methylergonovine
(meth-ill-er-goe-**noe**-veen)
Methergine
Classification
Therapeutic: oxytocic
Pharmacologic: ergot alkaloids

M

Indications
Prevention and treatment of postpartum or postabortion hemorrhage caused by uterine atony or subinvolution.

Action
Directly stimulates uterine and vascular smooth muscle.
Therapeutic Effects: Uterine contraction.

Pharmacokinetics
Absorption: Well absorbed following oral or IM administration.
Distribution: Widely distributed to tissues.
Metabolism and Excretion: Probably metabolized by the liver.
Half-life: 30–120 min.

TIME/ACTION PROFILE (effects on uterine contractions)

ROUTE	ONSET	PEAK	DURATION
PO	5–15 min	unknown	3 hr
IM	2–5 min	unknown	3 hr
IV	immediate	unknown	45 min–3 hr

Contraindications/Precautions
Contraindicated in: Hypersensitivity; Concurrent use of strong CYP3A4 inhibitors; OB: Should not be used to induce labor; Lactation: Lactation.
Use Cautiously in: Hypertensive or eclamptic patients (more susceptible to hypertensive and arrhythmogenic side effects); History of or risk factors for coronary artery disease; Severe renal impairment; Severe hepatic impairment; Sepsis.
Exercise Extreme Caution in: OB: Third stage of labor.

Adverse Reactions/Side Effects
CV: arrhythmias, chest pain, heart block, HYPERTENSION, palpitations. **Derm:** ↑ sweating. **EENT:** tinnitus. **GI:** nausea, vomiting. **GU:** cramps. **Neuro:** dizziness, headache, paresthesia, STROKE. **Resp:** dyspnea.

Interactions
Drug-Drug: Strong CYP3A4 inhibitors, including **erythromycin, clarithromycin, ritonavir, nelfinavir, ketoconazole, itraconazole,** or **voriconazole,** may ↑ levels and ↑ risk of ischemia; concurrent use contraindicated. Excessive vasoconstriction may result when used with heavy cigarette smoking (**nicotine**), other **vasopressors,** such as **dopamine,** or **beta-**

blockers. **Moderate CYP3A4 inhibitors**, including **nefazodone, fluconazole, fluoxetine, fluvoxamine, zileuton,** or **clotrimazole,** may ↑ levels and risk of toxicity; use concurrently with caution. **CYP3A4 inducers**, including **nevirapine** and **rifampin,** may ↓ levels and effectiveness. **Anesthetics** may ↓ its oxytocic properties. May ↓ the antianginal effects of **nitrates**.

Drug-Food: Grapefruit juice may ↑ levels and risk of toxicity; use concurrently with caution.

Route/Dosage

PO (Adults): 0.2–0.4 mg every 6–12 hr for 2–7 days.

IM, IV (Adults): 0.2 mg every 2–4 hr for up to 5 doses.

Availability (generic available)
Tablets: 0.2 mg. **Injection:** 0.2 mg/mL.

NURSING IMPLICATIONS

Assessment
- Monitor BP, heart rate, and uterine response frequently during medication administration. Notify health care professional promptly if uterine relaxation becomes prolonged or if character of vaginal bleeding changes.
- Assess for signs of ergotism (cold, numb fingers and toes, chest pain, nausea, vomiting, headache, muscle pain, weakness).

Lab Test Considerations
- If no response to methylergonovine, calcium levels may need to be assessed. Effectiveness of medication is ↓ with hypocalcemia.
- May cause ↓ serum prolactin levels.

Implementation

IV Administration
- **IV:** IV administration is used for emergencies only. Oral and IM routes are preferred.
- **IV Push: *Dilution:*** May be given undiluted or diluted in 5 mL of 0.9% NaCl and administered through Y-site. Do not add to IV solutions. Do not mix in syringe with any other drug. Refrigerate; stable for storage at room temperature for 60 days; deteriorates with age. Use only solution that is clear and colorless and that contains no precipitate. *Concentration:* 0.2 mg/mL. *Rate:* Administer at a rate of 0.2 mg over at least 1 min.
- **Y-Site Compatibility:** heparin, hydrocortisone, potassium chloride.

Patient/Family Teaching
- Instruct patient to take medication as directed; do not skip or double up on missed doses. If a dose is missed, omit it and return to regular dose schedule.
- Advise patient that medication may cause menstrual-like cramps.
- Caution patient to avoid smoking, because nicotine constricts blood vessels.

- Instruct patient to notify health care professional if infection develops, as this may cause increased sensitivity to the medication.
- Advise patient to notify health care professional of all Rx or OTC medications, vitamins, or herbal products being taken and to consult with health care professional before taking other medications.

Evaluation/Desired Outcomes
- Contractions that maintain uterine tone and prevent postpartum hemorrhage.

methylnaltrexone
(me-thil-nal-**trex**-one)
Relistor
Classification
Therapeutic: laxatives
Pharmacologic: opioid antagonists

Indications
SUBQ: Treatment of opioid-induced constipation (OIC) in patients with advanced illness or pain caused by active cancer who require opioid dose escalation for palliative care. **SUBQ, PO:** Treatment of OIC in patients with chronic, non-cancer pain, including those with chronic pain related to prior cancer or its treatment who do not require frequent (e.g. weekly) opioid dose escalation.

Action
Acts peripherally as mu-opioid receptor antagonist, blocking opioid effects on the GI tract. **Therapeutic Effects:** Blocks constipating effects of opioids on the GI tract without loss of analgesia.

Pharmacokinetics
Absorption: Rapidly absorbed after SUBQ and oral administration; oral absorption delayed by high-fat meal by 2 hr.

Distribution: Moderate tissue distribution, does not cross the blood-brain barrier.

Metabolism and Excretion: Some metabolism; 85% excreted unchanged in urine.

Half-life: 15 hr (oral).

TIME/ACTION PROFILE (plasma concentrations)

ROUTE	ONSET	PEAK	DURATION
SUBQ	rapid	0.5 hr	24–48 hr
PO	rapid	1.5 hr	unknown

Contraindications/Precautions
Contraindicated in: Known/suspected mechanical GI obstruction; Lactation: Lactation.

Use Cautiously in: Known/suspected lesions of GI tract (↑ risk for GI perforation); Moderate or severe renal impairment (dose ↓ required); Moderate or severe hepatic impairment (dose ↓ may be required); OB: Use during pregnancy only if potential maternal benefit justifies potential fetal risk; Pedi: Safety and effectiveness not established in children.

Adverse Reactions/Side Effects

Derm: ↑ sweating. **GI:** <u>abdominal pain</u>, <u>flatulence</u>, <u>nausea</u>, diarrhea. **Neuro:** dizziness. **Misc:** opioid withdrawal.

Interactions

Drug-Drug: None reported.

Route/Dosage

Opioid-Induced Constipation in Patients with Advanced Illness

SUBQ (Adults >114 kg): 0.15 mg/kg every other day, as needed (not to exceed 1 dose every 24 hr).

Renal Impairment
(Adults): *CCr <60 mL/min:* use 50% of recommended dose based on weight.
SUBQ (Adults 62–114 kg): 12 mg every other day, as needed (not to exceed 1 dose every 24 hr).
SUBQ (Adults 38–62 kg): 8 mg every other day, as needed (not to exceed 1 dose every 24 hr).
SUBQ (Adults <38 kg): 0.15 mg/kg every other day, as needed (not to exceed 1 dose every 24 hr).

Renal Impairment
SUBQ (Adults >114 kg): *CCr <60 mL/min:* 0.075 mg/kg every other day, as needed (not to exceed 1 dose every 24 hr).

Renal Impairment
SUBQ (Adults 62–114 kg): *CCr <60 mL/min:* 6 mg every other day, as needed (not to exceed 1 dose every 24 hr).

Renal Impairment
SUBQ (Adults 38–<62 kg): *CCr <60 mL/min:* 4 mg every other day, as needed (not to exceed 1 dose every 24 hr).

Renal Impairment
SUBQ (Adults <38 kg): *CCr <60 mL/min:* 0.15 mg/kg every other day, as needed (not to exceed 1 dose every 24 hr).

Opioid-Induced Constipation in Patients with Non-Cancer Pain

SUBQ (Adults): 12 mg once daily.
PO (Adults): 450 mg once daily.

Renal Impairment
SUBQ (Adults): *CCr <60 mL/min:* 6 mg once daily.

Renal Impairment
PO (Adults): *CCr <60 mL/min:* 150 mg once daily.

Hepatic Impairment
SUBQ (Adults >114 kg): *Severe hepatic impairment:* 0.075 mg/kg once daily.

Hepatic Impairment
SUBQ (Adults 62–114 kg): *Severe hepatic impairment:* 6 mg once daily.

Hepatic Impairment
SUBQ (Adults 38–<62 kg): *Severe hepatic impairment:* 4 mg once daily.

Hepatic Impairment
SUBQ (Adults <38 kg): *Severe hepatic impairment:* 0.075 mg/kg once daily.

Hepatic Impairment
PO (Adults): *Moderate or severe hepatic impairment:* 150 mg once daily.

Availability

Tablets: 150 mg. **Solution for injection (prefilled syringes):** 8 mg/0.4 mL, 12 mg/0.6 mL. **Solution for injection (single-use vials):** 12 mg/0.6 mL.

NURSING IMPLICATIONS

Assessment

- Assess bowel sounds and frequency, quantity, and consistency of stools periodically during therapy.
- Monitor pain intensity during therapy. Methylnaltrexone does not affect pain or effects of opioid analgesics on pain control.

Implementation

- Maintenance laxative must be stopped prior to administration of methylnaltrexone. If response is not sufficient after 3 days, laxatives may be restarted.
- **PO:** Administer with water on an empty stomach at least 30 min before first meal of the day.
- **SUBQ:** Pinch skin and administer in upper arm, abdomen, or thigh at a 45° angle using a 1-mL syringe with a 27-gauge needle inserted the full length of the needle. Do not rub the injection site. Solution is clear and colorless to pale yellow. Do not administer solutions that are discolored or contain a precipitate. Solution is stable for 24 hr at room temperature. Protect vials from light. Do not freeze. Do not use single-use vials for more than 1 dose.

Patient/Family Teaching

- Instruct patient to take methylnaltrexone as directed and on correct technique for administration of methylnaltrexone and disposal of supplies. Usual schedule is one dose every other day, as needed, but no more than one dose in a 24-hr period. Advise patient to read the *Patient Information* prior to starting therapy and with each Rx refill in case of changes.
- Advise patient that laxation may occur within 30 min of SUBQ injection, so toilet facilities should be available following administration.
- Advise patient to discontinue all maintenance laxatives; can be added if inadequate response to methylnaltrexone.

- May cause dizziness. Caution patient to avoid driving and other activities requiring alertness until response to medication is known.
- Advise patient to notify health care professional and discontinue therapy if severe or persistent diarrhea occurs or if abdominal pain, nausea, or vomiting persists or worsens.
- Instruct patient to stop taking methylnaltrexone if they stop taking opioid medications.
- Advise patient to consult health care professional prior to taking other Rx, OTC, or herbal products.
- Rep: Advise females of reproductive potential to notify health care professional if pregnancy is planned or suspected or if breastfeeding.

Evaluation/Desired Outcomes
- Laxation and relief of OIC.

METHYLPHENIDATE
methylphenidate (oral)
(meth-ill-**fen**-i-date)
~~Adhansia XR~~, Aptensio XR, ✦ Biphentin, Concerta, Cotempla XR-ODT, ✦ Foquest, Jornay PM, ~~Metadate CD~~, Methylin, Quillichew ER, Quillivant XR, Relexxii, Ritalin, Ritalin LA
methylphenidate (transdermal)
Daytrana
Classification
Therapeutic: central nervous system stimulants

Schedule II

Indications
Oral, orally disintegrating tablets, and transdermal: Attention-deficit/hyperactivity disorder (ADHD) (adjunct). **Oral only**: Narcolepsy.

Action
Produces CNS and respiratory stimulation with weak sympathomimetic activity. **Therapeutic Effects:** Increased attention span in ADHD. Increased motor activity, mental alertness, and diminished fatigue in narcolepsy.

Pharmacokinetics
Absorption: Slow and incomplete after oral administration; absorption of sustained or extended-release tablet (SR) is delayed and provides continuous release; well absorbed from skin. *Aptensio XR, Concerta, Relexxii, Ritalin LA:* provides initial rapid release followed by a second continuous release (biphasic release).
Distribution: Unknown.
Metabolism and Excretion: Mostly metabolized (80%) by the liver.
Half-life: 2–4 hr.

TIME/ACTION PROFILE (CNS stimulation)

ROUTE	ONSET	PEAK	DURATION
PO	unknown	1–3 hr	4–6 hr
PO-ER	unknown	4–7 hr	3–12 hr†
Transdermal	unknown	unknown	12 hr

†Depends on formulation.

Contraindications/Precautions
Contraindicated in: Hypersensitivity; Hyperexcitable states; Hyperthyroidism; Patients with psychotic personalities or suicidal or homicidal tendencies; Personal or family history of Tourette's syndrome; Glaucoma; Motor tics; Concurrent use or use within 14 days of MAO inhibitors or MAO inhibitor-like drugs (linezolid or methylene blue); Fructose intolerance, glucose-galactose malabsorption, or sucrose-isomaltase insufficiency; Surgery.
Use Cautiously in: History of cardiovascular disease (sudden death has occurred in children with structural cardiac abnormalities or other serious heart problems); Hypertension; Diabetes mellitus; History of contact sensitization with transdermal product (may be at ↑ risk for systemic sensitization reactions with oral products); History or family history of vitiligo (may be at ↑ risk for loss of skin pigmentation with transdermal product); Continual use (may result in psychological or physical dependence); Seizure disorders (may lower seizure threshold); Concerta product should be used cautiously in patients with esophageal motility disorders or severe GI narrowing (may ↑ the risk of obstruction); OB: Use during pregnancy only if potential maternal benefit outweighs potential fetal risk; may lead to premature delivery and low birth weight infants; Lactation: Use while breastfeeding only if potential maternal benefit outweighs potential risk to infant; Pedi: Growth suppression may occur in children with long-term use; children <6 yr (↑ risk of adverse reactions, particularly weight loss in children 4–<6 yr); Geri: Safety and effectiveness of many of the products have not been evaluated in older adults.

Adverse Reactions/Side Effects
CV: hypertension, palpitations, tachycardia, hypotension, peripheral vasculopathy, SUDDEN DEATH. **Derm:** contact sensitization (erythema, edema, papules, vesicles) (transdermal), erythema, loss of skin pigmentation (transdermal), rash. **EENT:** blurred vision, teeth grinding. **GI:** anorexia, constipation, cramps, diarrhea, dry mouth, metallic taste, nausea, vomiting. **GU:** priapism. **Metab:** growth suppression (especially with prolonged use), weight loss (especially with prolonged use). **MS:** RHABDOMYOLYSIS. **Neuro:** hyperactivity, insomnia, restlessness, tremor, akathisia, behavioral disturbances, dizziness, dyskinesia, hallucinations, headache, irritability, mania, thought disorder, tics. **Misc:** fever, HYPERSENSITIVITY REACTIONS (including anaphylaxis and angioedema), physical dependence, psychological dependence, tolerance.

Interactions

Drug-Drug: Concurrent use with **MAO inhibitors** or **MAO-inhibitor-like drugs**, such as **linezolid** or **methylene blue** may result in serious, potentially fatal reactions; wait at least 14 days following discontinuation of MAO inhibitor before initiation of amphetamine mixtures. Drugs that affect serotonergic neurotransmitter systems, including **MAO inhibitors**, **tricyclic antidepressants**, **SSRIs**, **SNRIs**, **fentanyl**, **buspirone**, **tramadol**, **lithium**, and **triptans** ↑ risk of serotonin syndrome. ↑ sympathomimetic effects with other **adrenergics**, including **vasoconstrictors**, **decongestants**, and **halogenated anesthetics**. Metabolism of **warfarin**, **phenytoin**, **phenobarbital**, **primidone**, **SSRIs**, and **tricyclic antidepressants** may be ↓ and effects ↑. Avoid concurrent use with **pimozide** (may mask cause of tics). May ↓ the effectiveness of **antihypertensives**. **Alcohol** may ↑ rate of release of drug from some methylphenidate formulations (Metadate CD, Ritalin LA). Concurrent use with **risperidone** may ↑ risk of extrapyramidal symptoms.

Drug-Natural Products: Use with caffeine-containing herbs (**guarana**, **tea**, **coffee**) ↑ stimulant effect. **St. John's wort** may ↑ risk of serotonin syndrome.

Drug-Food: Excessive use of **caffeine**-containing foods or beverages (**coffee**, **cola**, **tea**) may cause ↑ CNS stimulation.

Route/Dosage

Attention-Deficit/Hyperactivity Disorder

PO (Adults <65 yr): *Immediate-release tablets:* 5–20 mg 2–3 times daily. When maintenance dose is determined, may change to extended-release formulation. *Methylphenidate SR:* may be used in place of the immediate-release tablets when the 8-hr dose corresponds to the titrated 8-hr dosage of the immediate-release tablets; *Concerta and Relexxii (patients who have not taken methylphenidate previously):* 18–36 mg once daily in the morning initially, may be titrated as needed up to 72 mg/day. *Concerta and Relexxii (patients are currently taking other forms of methylphenidate):* 18 mg once daily in the morning if previous dose was 5 mg 2–3 times daily; 36 mg once daily in the morning if previous dose was 10 mg 2–3 times daily; 54 mg once daily in the morning if previous dose was 15 mg 2–3 times daily; 72 mg once daily in the morning if previous dose was 20 mg 2–3 times daily. *Aptensio XR:* 10 mg once daily; may ↑ dose in 10-mg increments at weekly intervals (maximum dose = 60 mg/day). *Quillivant XR and Quillichew ER:* 20 mg once daily; may ↑ dose in 10–20-mg increments at weekly intervals (maximum dose = 60 mg/day). *Jornay PM:* 20 mg once daily in the evening; may ↑ dose in 20-mg increments at weekly intervals (maximum dose = 100 mg/day).

PO (Children ≥6 yr [Ritalin LA for children 6–12 yr]): *Immediate-release tablets:* 0.3 mg/kg/dose or 2.5–5 mg before breakfast and lunch; may ↑ dose by 0.1 mg/kg/dose or by 5–10 mg/day at weekly intervals (not to exceed 60 mg/day or 2 mg/kg/day). When maintenance dose is determined, may change to extended-release formulation. *Methylphenidate SR:* may be used in place of the immediate-release tablets when the 8-hr dose corresponds to the titrated 8-hr dosage of the immediate-release tablets; *Ritalin LA (patients who have not taken methylphenidate previously):* 20 mg once daily; may ↑ by 10 mg/day at weekly intervals (max = 60 mg/day); *Ritalin LA (patients currently taking other forms of methylphenidate):* can be used in place of immediate-release twice daily regimen given once daily at same total dose, or in place of SR product at same dose; *Concerta (patients who have not taken methylphenidate previously):* 18 mg once daily in the morning initially, may be titrated as needed up to 54 mg/day (children 6–12 yr old) or up to 72 mg/day (children 13–17 yr old). *Concerta (patients are currently taking other forms of methylphenidate):* 18 mg once daily in the morning if previous dose was 5 mg 2–3 times daily; 36 mg once daily in the morning if previous dose was 10 mg 2–3 times daily; 54 mg once daily in the morning if previous dose was 15 mg 2–3 times daily; 72 mg once daily in the morning if previous dose was 20 mg 2–3 times daily. *Aptensio XR:* 10 mg once daily; may ↑ dose in 10-mg increments at weekly intervals (maximum dose = 60 mg/day). *Quillivant XR and Quillichew ER:* 20 mg once daily; may ↑ dose in 10–20-mg increments at weekly intervals (maximum dose = 60 mg/day). *Jornay PM:* 20 mg once daily in the evening; may ↑ dose in 20-mg increments at weekly intervals (maximum dose = 100 mg/day). *Cotempla XR-ODT:* 17.3 mg once daily in the morning; may ↑ dose in 8.6–17.3-mg increments at weekly intervals (maximum dose = 51.8 mg/day).

Transdermal (Children ≥6 yr): Apply one 10-mg patch initially (should be applied 2 hr before desired effect and removed 9 hr after application); may be titrated based on response and tolerability; may ↑ to 15-mg patch after 1 wk, and then to 20-mg patch after another wk, and then to 30-mg patch after another wk.

Narcolepsy

PO (Adults): *Immediate-release tablets:* 10 mg 2–3 times/day; maximum dose 60 mg/day.

Availability (generic available)

Immediate-release tablets (Ritalin): 5 mg, 10 mg, 20 mg. **Extended-release capsules (Aptensio XR):** 10 mg, 15 mg, 20 mg, 30 mg, 40 mg, 50 mg, 60 mg. **Extended-release capsules (Jornay PM):** 20 mg, 40 mg, 60 mg, 80 mg, 100 mg. **Extended-release capsules (Ritalin LA):** 10 mg, 20 mg, 30 mg, 40 mg. **Extended-release tablets (Concerta):** 18 mg, 27 mg, 36 mg, 54 mg. **Extended-release tablets (Rele-**

xxii): 18 mg, 27 mg, 36 mg, 45 mg, 54 mg, 63 mg, 72 mg. **Sustained-release tablets (Ritalin SR):** ✸ 20 mg. **Extended-release orally-disintegrating tablets (Cotempla XR-ODT):** 8.6 mg, 17.3 mg, 25.9 mg. **Chewable tablets (Methylin) (grape flavor):** 2.5 mg, 5 mg, 10 mg. **Extended-release chewable tablets (Quillichew ER):** 20 mg, 30 mg, 40 mg. **Oral solution (Methylin) (grape flavor):** 5 mg/5 mL, 10 mg/5 mL. **Extended-release oral suspension (Quillivant XR) (banana flavor):** 25 mg/5 mL. **Transdermal patch:** 10 mg/9 hr, 15 mg/9 hr, 20 mg/9 hr, 30 mg/9 hr.

NURSING IMPLICATIONS

Assessment

- Monitor BP, pulse, and respiration before administering and periodically during therapy. Obtain a history (including assessment of family history of sudden death or ventricular arrhythmia), physical exam to assess for cardiac disease, and further evaluation (ECG and echocardiogram), if indicated. If exertional chest pain, unexplained syncope, or other cardiac symptoms occur, evaluate promptly.
- Monitor closely for behavior change.
- Assess risk of abuse prior to prescribing. After prescribing, keep accurate prescription records, educate patient and family about risk of abuse, monitor for signs of abuse and overdose, and evaluate need for use periodically during therapy.
- Screen patients with bipolar disorder for risk of manic episode (comorbid or history of depressive symptoms or a family history of suicide, bipolar disorder, depression) prior to starting therapy.
- Monitor for signs and symptoms of peripheral vasculopathy (numbness and burning in fingers, digital changes). May require reduction in dose or discontinuation.
- Pedi: Monitor growth, both height and weight, in children on long-term therapy. May need to interrupt therapy in patients who are not growing or gaining height or weight as expected.
- May produce a false sense of euphoria and well-being. Provide frequent rest periods and observe patient for rebound depression after the effects of the medication have worn off.
- **ADHD:** Assess children for attention span, impulse control, and interactions with others. Therapy may be interrupted at intervals to determine whether symptoms are sufficient to continue therapy.
- **Narcolepsy:** Observe and document frequency of episodes.
- **Transdermal:** Assess skin for signs of contact sensitization (erythema with edema, papules, or vesicles that does not improve within 48 hr or spreads beyond patch site) during therapy. May lead to systemic sensitization to other forms of methylphenidate (flare-up of previous dermatitis or prior positive patch-test sites, generalized skin eruptions, headache, fever, malaise, arthralgia, diarrhea, vomiting). If contact sensitization develops and oral methylphenidate is instituted, monitor closely.
- Monitor for signs of skin depigmentation. May cause persistent loss of skin pigmentation at and around the application site and at other sites distant from application site. Discontinue transdermal if depigmentation occurs.

Lab Test Considerations

- Monitor CBC, differential, and platelet count periodically in patients receiving prolonged therapy.

Implementation

- Do not confuse methylphenidate with methadone.
- **PO:** Administer immediate and sustained-release tablets on an empty stomach (30–45 min before a meal). *DNC:* Sustained-release tablets should be swallowed whole; do not break, crush, or chew. *Quillichew ER* chewable tablets may be broken in half. *Aptensio XL, Metadate CD* and *Ritalin LA* capsules may be opened and sprinkled on cool applesauce; entire mixture should be ingested immediately and followed by a drink of water. Do not store for future use. *Concerta* may be administered without regard to food, but must be taken with water, milk, or juice.
- Shake extended-release oral suspension for 10 sec before administering. May be given with or without food.
- **Transdermal:** Apply patch to a clean, dry site on the hip which is not oily, damaged, or irritated; do not apply to waistline where tight clothing may rub it. Press firmly in place with palm of hand for 30 sec to make sure of good contact with skin, especially around edges. Alternate site daily. Apply patch 2 hr before desired effect and remove 9 hr after applied; effects last several more hr. Do not apply or reapply with dressings, tape, or other adhesives. Do not cut patches.
- If difficulty in separating patch from release liner, tearing, or other damage occurs during removal from liner, discard patch and apply a new patch. Inspect release liner to ensure no adhesive containing medication was transferred to liner; if transfer has occurred, discard patch. Avoid touching adhesive during application; wash hands immediately after application.
- If patch does not fully adhere or partially detaches, remove and replace with another patch. Wear patch for a total of 9 hr, regardless of number used. Exposure to water during bathing, swimming, or showering may affect patch adherence.
- Patches may be removed earlier before decreasing dose if an unacceptable loss of appetite or insomnia occurs.
- Store patches at room temperature in a safe place to prevent abuse and misuse; do not refrigerate or freeze.
- To remove patch, peel off slowly. An oil-based product (petroleum jelly, olive oil, mineral oil) may be

applied gently to facilitate removal. Upon removal, fold so that adhesive side of patch adheres to itself and flush down toilet or dispose of in an appropriate lidded container.

Patient/Family Teaching

- Instruct patient to take medication as directed. If an oral dose is missed, take the remaining doses for that day at regularly spaced intervals; do not double doses. Take the last dose before 6 PM to minimize the risk of insomnia. Instruct patient not to alter dose without consulting health care professional. Abrupt cessation of high doses may cause extreme fatigue and mental depression. Instruct parent/caregiver to read the *Medication Guide* prior to use and with each Rx refill as changes may occur.
- Advise patient to check weight 2–3 times weekly and report weight loss to health care professional.
- Advise patient that methylphenidate is a drug with known abuse potential. Protect it from theft, and never give to anyone other than the individual for whom it was prescribed. Store out of sight and reach of children, and in a location not accessible by others.
- May cause dizziness or blurred vision. Caution patient to avoid driving or activities requiring alertness until response to medication is known.
- Inform patient and/or parents that shell of *Concerta* tablet may appear in the stool. This is no cause for concern.
- Advise patient to avoid using caffeine-containing beverages concurrently with this therapy.
- Advise patient to notify health care professional if nervousness, insomnia, palpitations, vomiting, skin rash, fever, painful and prolonged erections, or circulation problems (fingers or toes feel numb, cool, painful; fingers or toes change color from pale, to blue, to red) occur.
- Advise patient and/or parents to notify health care professional of behavioral changes.
- Advise patient to notify health care professional of all Rx or OTC medications, vitamins, or herbal products being taken and to consult with health care professional before taking other medications, especially St. John's wort.
- Inform patient that health care professional may order periodic holidays from the drug to assess progress and to decrease dependence.
- Rep: Advise females of reproductive potential to notify health care professional if pregnancy is planned or suspected or if breastfeeding. May lead to premature delivery and low birth weight infants. Inform patients who become pregnant while taking methylphenidate of National Pregnancy Registry of ADHD Medications that monitors pregnancy outcomes in women exposed to ADHD medications during pregnancy. Enroll patient by calling 1-866-961-2388 or

visit online at https://womensmentalhealth.org/adhd-medications/. Monitor breastfed infants for agitation, insomnia, anorexia, and reduced weight gain.
- Emphasize the importance of routine follow-up exams to monitor progress.
- **Transdermal:** Encourage parent or caregiver to use the administration chart included in package to monitor application and removal time and disposal method.
- Caution patient to avoid exposing patch to direct external heat sources (hair dryers, heating pads, electric blankets, heated water beds, etc.). May increase rate and extent of absorption.
- Inform parent/caregiver that skin redness, itching and small bumps on the skin are common. If swelling or blistering occurs, the patch should not be worn and health care professional notified. Caution parent/caregiver not to apply hydrocortisone or other solutions, creams, ointments, or emollients prior to application.
- Advise patient referred for MRI test to discuss patch with referring health care professional and MRI facility to determine if removal of patch is necessary prior to test and for directions for replacing patch.
- **Home Care Issues:** Pedi: Advise parents to notify school nurse of medication regimen.

Evaluation/Desired Outcomes

- Improved attention span and social interactions in ADHD.
- Decreased frequency of narcoleptic symptoms.

methylPREDNISolone, See CORTICOSTEROIDS (SYSTEMIC).

BEERS

⚠ metoclopramide
(met-oh-**kloe**-pra-mide)
Gimoti, ✦Metonia, Reglan
Classification
Therapeutic: antiemetics

Indications

PO: Gastroesophageal reflux. **PO, IV, Intranasal:** Acute and recurrent diabetic gastroparesis. **IV:** Used for the following conditions: Prevention of nausea and vomiting associated with emetogenic chemotherapy, Prevention of postoperative nausea and vomiting when nasogastric suctioning is undesirable. Facilitation of small bowel intubation in radiographic procedures. **Unlabeled Use:** Treatment of hiccups.

Action

Blocks dopamine receptors in chemoreceptor trigger zone of the CNS. Stimulates motility of the upper GI tract and accelerates gastric emptying. **Therapeutic Effects:** Decreased nausea and vomiting. Decreased symptoms of gastric stasis. Easier passage of nasogastric tube into small bowel.

Pharmacokinetics

Absorption: Well absorbed from the GI tract, from rectal mucosa, and from IM sites. 47% absorbed following intranasal administration. IV administration results in complete bioavailability.

Distribution: Widely distributed into body tissues and fluids. Crosses blood-brain barrier.

Metabolism and Excretion: Partially metabolized by the liver via the CYP2D6 isoenzyme; ⚥ the CYP2D6 isoenzyme exhibits genetic polymorphism (~7% of population may be poor metabolizers and may have significantly ↑ metoclopramide concentrations and an ↑ risk of adverse effects). 25% eliminated unchanged in the urine.

Half-life: 2.5–6 hr.

TIME/ACTION PROFILE (effects on peristalsis)

ROUTE	ONSET	PEAK	DURATION
PO	30–60 min	unknown	1–2 hr
IM	10–15 min	unknown	1–2 hr
Intranasal	unknown	unknown	unknown
IV	1–3 min	immediate	1–2 hr

Contraindications/Precautions

Contraindicated in: Hypersensitivity; Possible GI obstruction, perforation, or hemorrhage; Seizure disorders; Hypertension; Pheochromocytoma; History of tardive dyskinesia; Parkinson's disease; Concurrent use of MAO inhibitors; Moderate or severe renal or hepatic impairment (intranasal only); ⚥ CYP2D6 poor metabolizers (↑ risk for tardive dyskinesia) (intranasal only); Concurrent use of strong CYP2D6 inhibitors (intranasal only).

Use Cautiously in: History of depression; Diabetes (may alter response to insulin); Cirrhosis or HF (↑ risk of fluid retention); Renal impairment (↓ dose in CCr <50 mL/min) (oral and IV/IM only); Chronic use >12 wk (↑ risk for tardive dyskinesia); Moderate or severe hepatic impairment; ⚥ CYP2D6 poor metabolizers (↑ risk for tardive dyskinesia) (oral and IV/IM only); OB: May cause extrapyramidal symptoms or methemoglobinemia in neonate when used during pregnancy; Lactation: May lead to diarrhea, extrapyramidal symptoms, or methemoglobinemia in infant when used during breastfeeding; Pedi: Prolonged clearance in neonates can result in high serum concentrations and ↑ the risk for methemoglobinemia. Side effects are more common in children, especially extrapyramidal reactions. Avoid use of tablets and intranasal because of ↑ risk of tardive dyskinesia and methemoglobinemia (in neonates); Geri: Appears on Beers list. ↑ risk of extrapyramidal effects, including tardive dyskinesia, in older adults. Avoid use in older adults, except for gastroparesis (duration for this indication should generally not exceed

12 wk). Intranasal therapy not recommended as initial therapy in older adults (can be transitioned to intranasal therapy once stabilized on oral therapy).

Adverse Reactions/Side Effects

CV: bradycardia, hypertension, hypotension, supraventricular tachycardia. **Endo:** gynecomastia, hyperprolactinemia. **GI:** constipation, diarrhea, dry mouth, nausea. **Hemat:** agranulocytosis, leukopenia, methemoglobinemia, neutropenia. **Neuro:** drowsiness, dysgeusia (intranasal), extrapyramidal reactions, restlessness, anxiety, bradykinesia, cog-wheel rigidity, depression, irritability, NEUROLEPTIC MALIGNANT SYNDROME, tardive dyskinesia, tremor.

Interactions

Drug-Drug: MAO inhibitors may cause release of catecholamines which may ↑ BP; avoid concurrent use. Additive CNS depression with other **CNS depressants**, including **alcohol, antidepressants, antihistamines, opioid analgesics,** and **sedative/hypnotics**. May ↑ absorption and risk of toxicity from **cyclosporine**. May affect the GI absorption of other **orally administered drugs** as a result of effect on GI motility. May exaggerate hypotension during **general anesthesia**. ↑ risk of tardive dyskinesia, extrapyramidal reactions, or neuroleptic malignant syndrome with **antipsychotic agents**; avoid concurrent use. **Strong CYP2D6 inhibitors**, including **bupropion, fluoxetine, paroxetine,** or **quinidine** may ↑ levels and risk of extrapyramidal reactions; avoid concurrent use with intranasal metoclopramide; ↓ PO or IV/IM metoclopramide dose. **Opioids** and **anticholinergics** may antagonize the GI effects of metoclopramide. May ↑ neuromuscular blockade from **succinylcholine**. May ↓ effectiveness of **levodopa**. May ↑ **tacrolimus** serum levels.

Route/Dosage

Prevention of Chemotherapy-Induced Nausea and Vomiting

IV (Adults and Children): 1–2 mg/kg 30 min before chemotherapy. Additional doses of 1–2 mg/kg may be given every 2–4 hr, pretreatment with diphenhydramine will ↓ the risk of extrapyramidal reactions to this dose.

Facilitation of Small Bowel Intubation

IV (Adults and Children >14 yr): 10 mg over 1–2 min.

IV (Children 6–14 yr): 2.5–5 mg (dose should not exceed 0.5 mg/kg) over 1–2 min.

IV (Children <6 yr): 0.1 mg/kg over 1–2 min.

Diabetic Gastroparesis

PO, IV, IM (Adults): 10 mg 30 min before meals and at bedtime for 2–8 wk (not to exceed 40 mg/day). *CYP2D6 poor metabolizers:* 5 mg 30 min before meals and at bedtime for 2–8 wk (not to exceed 20 mg/day). *Concurrent use of strong CYP2D6 inhibitor:* 5 mg 30 min before meals and at bedtime for 2–8 wk (not to exceed 20 mg/day).

Intranasal (Adults): One spray (15 mg) in one nostril 30 min before each meal and at bedtime (not to exceed 60 mg/day) for 2–8 wk (not to exceed 12 wk).

PO, IV, IM (Geriatric Patients): 5 mg 30 min before meals and at bedtime for 2–8 wk; may titrate up to 10 mg 30 min before each meal and at bedtime based on response and tolerability (not to exceed 40 mg/day).

Intranasal (Geriatric Patients): *Patients receiving alternative metoclopramide product at stable dose of 10 mg four times daily:* One spray (15 mg) in one nostril 30 min before each meal and at bedtime (not to exceed 60 mg/day) for 2–8 wk (not to exceed 12 wk).

Renal Impairment

PO (Adults): *CCr ≤60 mL/min:* 5 mg 30 min before meals and at bedtime for 2–8 wk (not to exceed 20 mg/day). *End-stage renal disease (including hemodialysis and peritoneal dialysis):* 5 mg twice daily for 2–8 wk (not to exceed 10 mg/day).

Hepatic Impairment

PO, IV, IM (Adults): *Mild hepatic impairment:* 10 mg 30 min before meals and at bedtime for 2–8 wk (not to exceed 40 mg/day). *Moderate or severe hepatic impairment:* 5 mg 30 min before meals and at bedtime for 2–8 wk (not to exceed 20 mg/day).

Gastroesophageal Reflux

PO (Adults): 10–15 mg 30 min before each meal and at bedtime (not to exceed 60 mg/day). *CYP2D6 poor metabolizers:* 5 mg 30 min before each meal and at bedtime or 10 mg 3 times daily (not to exceed 30 mg/day). *Concurrent use of strong CYP2D6 inhibitor:* 5 mg 30 min before each meal and at bedtime or 10 mg 3 times daily (not to exceed 30 mg/day).

PO (Geriatric Patients): 5 mg 30 min before each meal and at bedtime; may titrate up to 10–15 mg 30 min before each meal and at bedtime based on response and tolerability (not to exceed 60 mg/day).

Renal Impairment

PO (Adults): *CCr ≤60 mL/min:* 5 mg 30 min before each meal and at bedtime or 10 mg 3 times daily (not to exceed 30 mg/day). *End-stage renal disease (including hemodialysis and peritoneal dialysis):* 5 mg 30 min before each meal and at bedtime or 10 mg twice daily (not to exceed 20 mg/day).

Hepatic Impairment

PO (Adults): *Mild hepatic impairment:* 10–15 mg 30 min before each meal and at bedtime (not to exceed 60 mg/day). *Moderate or severe hepatic impairment:* 5 mg 30 min before each meal and at bedtime or 10 mg 3 times daily (not to exceed 30 mg/day).

Prevention of Postoperative Nausea and Vomiting

IM, IV (Adults): 10 mg at the end of surgical procedure, repeat in 6–8 hr if needed.

Treatment of Hiccups

PO, IM (Adults): 10–20 mg 4 times daily PO; may be preceded by a single 10-mg dose IM.

Availability (generic available)

Tablets: 5 mg, 10 mg. Orally disintegrating tablets: 5 mg, 10 mg. Oral solution (apricot-peach flavor): 5 mg/5 mL. Nasal spray: 15 mg/metered spray in 9.8–mL bottle (delivers 112 metered sprays). Solution for injection: 5 mg/mL.

NURSING IMPLICATIONS

Assessment

- Assess for nausea, vomiting, abdominal distention, and bowel sounds before and after administration.
- Assess for extrapyramidal side effects (*parkinsonian:* difficulty speaking or swallowing, loss of balance control, pill rolling, mask-like face, shuffling gait, rigidity, tremors; and *dystonic:* muscle spasms, twisting motions, twitching, inability to move eyes, weakness of arms or legs) periodically throughout course of therapy. May occur wk to mo after initiation of therapy and are reversible on discontinuation. Dystonic reactions may occur within min of IV infusion and stop within 24 hr of discontinuation of metoclopramide. May be treated with 50 mg of IM diphenhydramine or diphenhydramine 1 mg/kg IV may be administered prophylactically 15 min before metoclopramide IV infusion.
- Monitor for tardive dyskinesia (uncontrolled rhythmic movement of mouth, face, and extremities; lip smacking or puckering; puffing of cheeks; uncontrolled chewing; rapid or worm-like movements of tongue). Avoid treatment with metoclopramide (all dose forms and routes of administration) for longer than 12 wk due to increased risk of developing tardive dyskinesia with longer-term use. Report immediately and discontinue metoclopramide; may be irreversible.
- Monitor for neuroleptic malignant syndrome (hyperthermia, muscle rigidity, altered consciousness, irregular pulse or BP, tachycardia, and diaphoresis). Report immediately.
- Assess for signs of depression periodically throughout therapy.
- Monitor for symptoms related to hyperprolactinemia (menstrual abnormalities, galactorrhea, sexual dysfunction).

Lab Test Considerations

- May alter hepatic function test results.
- May cause ↑ serum prolactin and aldosterone concentrations.

Implementation

- PO: Administer doses 30 min before meals and at bedtime.
- Do not remove *orally disintegrating tablets* from the bottle until just prior to dosing. Remove tablet

M

from bottle with dry hands and immediately place on tongue to disintegrate and swallow with saliva. Tablet typically disintegrates in 1–1.5 min. Administration with liquid is not necessary.

- **IM:** For prevention of postoperative nausea and vomiting, inject IM near the end of surgery.
- **Intranasal:** Administer 1 spray in one nostril. Before administering 1st dose from a bottle, prime the pump by pressing down on the finger flange and releasing 10 sprays in the air. Place the spray nozzle tip under one nostril and lean the head slightly forward so the tip of spray nozzle is aimed away from the septum and toward the back of the nose. Close the other nostril with the other index finger. Move spray pump upwards so the tip of the nozzle is in the nostril. To ensure a full dose, hold the bottle upright while pressing down firmly and completely on finger flange and release while inhaling slowly through the open nostril. Remove spray pump nozzle tip from nostril and exhale slowly through the mouth. Wipe the spray nozzle with a clean tissue. If uncertain that spray entered the nose, do not repeat dose. Take next dose at scheduled time.

IV Administration

- **IV Push:** Administer IV dose 30 min before administration of chemotherapeutic agent. *Rate:* Doses may be given slowly over 1–2 min. Rapid administration causes a transient but intense feeling of anxiety and restlessness followed by drowsiness.
- **Intermittent Infusion:** *Dilution:* May be diluted for IV infusion in 50 mL of D5W, 0.9% NaCl, D5/0.45% NaCl, Ringer's solution, or LR. Diluted solution is stable for 48 hr if protected from light or 24 hr under normal light. *Concentration:* May dilute to 0.2 mg/mL or give undiluted at 5 mg/mL. *Rate:* Infuse slowly (maximum rate 5 mg/min) over at least 15–30 min.
- **Y-Site Compatibility:** acetaminophen, aldesleukin, alemtuzumab, amifostine, amikacin, aminocaproic acid, aminophylline, amiodarone, amphotericin B lipid complex, anidulafungin, argatroban, arsenic trioxide, ascorbic acid, atropine, azathioprine, azithromycin, aztreonam, benztropine, bivalirudin, bleomycin, bumetanide, buprenorphine, butorphanol, calcium chloride, calcium gluconate, cangrelor, carboplatin, caspofungin, cefazolin, cefotaxime, cefotetan, cefoxitin, ceftaroline, ceftazidime, ceftolozane/tazobactam, ceftriaxone, cefuroxime, chloramphenicol, chlorpromazine, ciprofloxacin, cisatracurium, cisplatin, cladribine, clindamycin, cyanocobalamin, cyclophosphamide, cyclosporine, cytarabine, dacarbazine, dactinomycin, daptomycin, daunorubicin hydrochloride, dexamethasone, dexmedetomidine, dexrazoxane, digoxin, diltiazem, diphenhydramine, dobutamine, docetaxel, dopamine, doxorubicin hydrochloride, doxycycline, droperidol, enalaprilat, ephedrine, epinephrine, epirubicin, epoetin alfa, eptifibatide, ertapenem, erythromycin, esmolol, etoposide, etoposide phosphate, famotidine, fentanyl, fil-

grastim, fluconazole, fludarabine, folic acid, foscarnet, fosphenytoin, gemcitabine, gentamicin, glycopyrrolate, granisetron, heparin, hetastarch, hydrocortisone, hydromorphone, idarubicin, ifosfamide, imipenem/cilastatin, indomethacin, insulin regular, irinotecan, isavuconazonium, isoproterenol, ketamine, ketorolac, labetalol, LR, leucovorin calcium, levofloxacin, lidocaine, linezolid, lorazepam, magnesium sulfate, mannitol, melphalan, meperidine, meropenem, meropenem/vaborbactam, mesna, methadone, methotrexate, methylprednisolone, metoprolol, metronidazole, midazolam, milrinone, mitomycin, mitoxantrone, morphine, moxifloxacin, multiple vitamins, mycophenolate, nafcillin, nalbuphine, naloxone, nicardipine, nitroglycerin, nitroprusside, norepinephrine, octreotide, ondansetron, oxacillin, oxaliplatin, oxytocin, paclitaxel, palonosetron, pamidronate, papaverine, pemetrexed, penicillin G, pentamidine, pentobarbital, phenobarbital, phentolamine, phenylephrine, phytonadione, piperacillin/tazobactam, plazomicin, potassium acetate, potassium chloride, procainamide, prochlorperazine, promethazine, propranolol, protamine, pyridoxine, remifentanil, rituximab, rocuronium, sargramostim, sodium acetate, sodium bicarbonate, succinylcholine, sufentanil, tacrolimus, tedizolid, telavancin, theophylline, thiamine, thiotepa, tigecycline, tirofiban, tobramycin, topotecan, trastuzumab, vancomycin, vasopressin, vecuronium, verapamil, vinblastine, vincristine, vinorelbine, voriconazole, zidovudine, zoledronic acid.

- **Y-Site Incompatibility:** amphotericin B deoxycholate, amphotericin B liposomal, carmustine, cefepime, dantrolene, diazepam, doxorubicin liposomal, ganciclovir, gemtuzumab ozogamicin, phenytoin, propofol, trimethoprim/sulfamethoxazole.

Patient/Family Teaching

- Instruct patient to take metoclopramide as directed. Explain how to administer intranasal doses. Take oral missed doses as soon as remembered if not almost time for next dose. If an intranasal dose is missed, omit and take the next dose at regularly scheduled time; do not double doses. Advise patient to read the *Medication Guide* before starting therapy and with each Rx refill in case of changes.
- Pedi: Unintentional overdose has been reported in infants and children with the use of metoclopramide oral solution. Teach parents how to accurately read labels and administer medication.
- May cause drowsiness. Caution patient to avoid driving or other activities requiring alertness until response to medication is known.
- Advise patient to avoid concurrent use of alcohol and other CNS depressants while taking this medication.
- Inform patient of risk of extrapyramidal symptoms, tardive dyskinesia, and neuroleptic malignant syndrome. Advise patient to notify health care profes-

sional immediately if involuntary or repetitive movements of eyes, face, or limbs occur.

- Rep: Advise females of reproductive potential to notify health care professional if pregnancy is planned or suspected, or if breastfeeding. Monitor neonates for extrapyramidal signs and methemoglobinemia.

Evaluation/Desired Outcomes

- Prevention or relief of nausea and vomiting.
- Decreased symptoms of gastric stasis.
- Facilitation of small bowel intubation.
- Decreased symptoms of esophageal reflux.
- Metoclopramide should not be used for more than 12 wk due to risk of tardive dyskinesia.

---

metOLazone (me-tole-a-zone)
❦ Zaroxolyn

Classification
Therapeutic: antihypertensives, diuretics
Pharmacologic: thiazide-like diuretics

Indications
Mild to moderate hypertension. Edema associated with HF or the nephrotic syndrome.

Action
Increases excretion of sodium and water by inhibiting sodium reabsorption in the distal tubule. Promotes excretion of chloride, potassium, magnesium, and bicarbonate. May produce arteriolar dilation. **Therapeutic Effects:** Lowering of BP in hypertensive patients. Diuresis with subsequent mobilization of edema. Effect may continue in renal impairment.

Pharmacokinetics
Absorption: Absorption is variable.
Distribution: Extensively distributed to tissues.
Protein Binding: 95%.
Metabolism and Excretion: Excreted mainly unchanged by the kidneys.
Half-life: 6–20 hr.

TIME/ACTION PROFILE (diuretic effect†)

ROUTE	ONSET	PEAK	DURATION
PO	1 hr	2 hr	12–24 hr

†Full antihypertensive effect may take days–wk.

Contraindications/Precautions
Contraindicated in: Hypersensitivity; Cross-sensitivity with other sulfonamides may exist; Anuria; Lactation: Lactation.
Use Cautiously in: Severe hepatic impairment; OB: Use during pregnancy only if potential maternal benefit justifies potential fetal risk; may ↑ risk of hypoglycemia, hypokalemia, hyponatremia, jaundice, and thrombocytopenia in fetus; Geri: Older adults may have ↑ sensitivity to drug effects.

Adverse Reactions/Side Effects
CV: chest pain, hypotension, palpitations. **Derm:** photosensitivity, rash. **Endo:** hyperglycemia. **F and E:** hypokalemia, dehydration, hypercalcemia, hypochloremic alkalosis, hypomagnesemia, hyponatremia, hypophosphatemia, hypovolemia. **GI:** anorexia, bloating, cramping, drug-induced hepatitis, nausea, pancreatitis, vomiting. **Hemat:** blood dyscrasias. **Metab:** hyperuricemia. **MS:** muscle cramps. **Neuro:** drowsiness, lethargy.

Interactions
Drug-Drug: ↑ risk of hypotension with **nitrates**, acute ingestion of **alcohol**, or other **antihypertensives**. ↑ risk of hypokalemia with **corticosteroids**, **amphotericin B**, or **piperacillin/tazobactam**. May ↑ the risk of **digoxin** toxicity. ↓ the excretion of **lithium**; may cause toxicity. May ↓ the effectiveness of **methenamine**. Stimulant laxatives (including **aloe**, **senna**) may ↑ risk of potassium depletion.
Drug-Food: Food may ↑ extent of absorption.

Route/Dosage
PO (Adults): *Hypertension:* 2.5–5 mg/day; *edema:* 5–20 mg/day.
PO (Children): 0.2–0.4 mg/kg/day divided every 12–24 hr.

Availability (generic available)
Tablets: 2.5 mg, 5 mg, 10 mg.

NURSING IMPLICATIONS
Assessment
- Monitor BP, intake and output, and daily weight, and assess feet, legs, and sacral area for edema daily.
- Assess patient, especially if taking digoxin, for anorexia, nausea, vomiting, muscle cramps, paresthesia, and confusion. Notify health care professional if these signs of electrolyte imbalance occur. Patients taking digoxin are at risk of digoxin toxicity because of the potassium-depleting effect of the diuretic.
- Assess patient for allergy to sulfonamides.
- **Hypertension:** Monitor BP before and periodically during therapy.
- Monitor frequency of prescription refills to determine compliance.

Lab Test Considerations
- Monitor electrolytes (especially potassium), blood glucose, BUN, and serum creatinine and uric acid levels before and periodically during therapy.
- May cause ↑ in serum and urine glucose in diabetic patients.
- May cause an ↑ in serum bilirubin, calcium, creatinine, and uric acid, and a ↓ in serum magnesium, potassium, and sodium and urinary calcium concentrations.

❦ = Canadian drug name. ✕✕✕ = Genetic implication. S̶t̶r̶i̶k̶e̶t̶h̶r̶o̶u̶g̶h̶ = Discontinued. CAPITALS = life-threatening. Underline = most frequent.

- May cause ↑ serum cholesterol, low-density lipoprotein cholesterol, and triglyceride concentrations.

Implementation
- Do not confuse metolazone with methimazole, methazolamide, methadone, or methotrexate.
- Administer in the morning to prevent disruption of sleep cycle.
- Intermittent dose schedule may be used for continued control of edema.
- **PO:** May give with food or milk to minimize GI irritation.

Patient/Family Teaching
- Instruct patient to take metolazone at the same time each day. Take missed doses as soon as remembered but not just before next dose is due. Do not double doses.
- Instruct patient to monitor weight biweekly and notify health care professional of significant changes.
- Caution patient to change positions slowly to minimize orthostatic hypotension; may be potentiated by alcohol.
- Advise patient to use sunscreen and protective clothing in the sun to prevent photosensitivity reactions.
- Instruct patient to discuss dietary potassium requirements with health care professional (see Appendix J).
- Instruct patient to notify health care professional of medication regimen before treatment or surgery.
- Advise patient to report muscle weakness, cramps, nausea, vomiting, diarrhea, or dizziness to health care professional.
- Rep: Advise females of reproductive potential to notify health care professional if pregnancy is planned or suspected, and to avoid breastfeeding during therapy. Monitor for hypoglycemia, hypokalemia, hyponatremia, jaundice, and thrombocytopenia in the fetus or newborn following maternal use.
- Emphasize the importance of routine follow-up exams.
- **Hypertension:** Advise patient to continue taking the medication even if feeling better. Medication controls but does not cure hypertension.
- Encourage patient to comply with additional interventions for hypertension (weight reduction, low-sodium diet, regular exercise, smoking cessation, moderation of alcohol consumption, and stress management).
- Instruct patient and family in correct technique for monitoring weekly BP.
- Advise patient to notify health care professional of all Rx or OTC medications, vitamins, or herbal products being taken and to consult with health care professional before taking other medications, especially cough or cold preparations, concurrently with this therapy.

Evaluation/Desired Outcomes
- Decrease in BP.
- Increase in urine output.
- Decrease in edema.

⚠ metoprolol (me-toe-proe-lole)
Kapspargo Sprinkle, Lopressor, Toprol XL
Classification
Therapeutic: antianginals, antihypertensives
Pharmacologic: beta blockers

Indications
Hypertension. Angina pectoris. Prevention of MI and decreased mortality in patients with recent MI. Stable, symptomatic (class II or III) heart failure due to ischemic, hypertensive, or cardiomyopathic origin (Toprol XL only). **Unlabeled Use:** Ventricular arrhythmias/tachycardia. Migraine prophylaxis. Tremors. Aggressive behavior. Drug-induced akathisia. Anxiety.

Action
Blocks stimulation of beta$_1$ (myocardial)-adrenergic receptors. Does not usually affect beta$_2$ (pulmonary, vascular, uterine)-adrenergic receptor sites. **Therapeutic Effects:** Decreased BP and heart rate. Decreased frequency of attacks of angina pectoris. Decreased rate of cardiovascular mortality and hospitalization in patients with heart failure.

Pharmacokinetics
Absorption: Well absorbed after oral administration.
Distribution: Crosses the blood-brain barrier, crosses the placenta; small amounts enter breast milk.
Metabolism and Excretion: Mostly metabolized by the liver via the CYP2D6 isoenzyme; ⚠ the CYP2D6 isoenzyme exhibits genetic polymorphism; ~7% of population may be poor metabolizers and may have significantly ↑ metoprolol concentrations and an ↑ risk of adverse effects.
Half-life: 3–7 hr.

TIME/ACTION PROFILE (cardiovascular effects)

ROUTE	ONSET	PEAK	DURATION
PO†	15 min	unknown	6–12 hr
PO–ER	unknown	6–12 hr	24 hr
IV	immediate	20 min	5–8 hr

†Maximal effects on BP (chronic therapy) may not occur for 1 wk. Hypotensive effects may persist for up to 4 wk after discontinuation.

Contraindications/Precautions
Contraindicated in: Uncompensated HF; Pulmonary edema; Cardiogenic shock; Bradycardia, heart block, or sick sinus syndrome (in absence of a pacemaker).
Use Cautiously in: Renal impairment; Hepatic impairment; Pulmonary disease (including asthma; beta$_1$ selectivity may be lost at higher doses); Diabetes mellitus or patients with ↓ nutritional intake (may mask signs of hypoglycemia); Thyrotoxicosis (may mask symptoms); History of severe allergic reactions (inten-

sity of reactions may be ↑); Untreated pheochromocytoma (initiate only after alpha blocker therapy started); OB: Use during pregnancy only if potential maternal benefit justifies potential fetal risk; Lactation: ፠ Use while breastfeeding only if potential maternal benefit justifies potential risk to infant; may result in bradycardia, constipation, diarrhea, and dry mouth/skin/eyes in infant, especially in mothers who are CYP2D6 poor metabolizers.; Pedi: Safety and effectiveness not established in children <18 yr (tablets, extended-release tablets, and injection) or <6 yr (extended-release capsules); Geri: Older adults may have ↑ sensitivity to beta blockers; initial dose ↓ recommended.

Adverse Reactions/Side Effects

CV: BRADYCARDIA, heart block, HF, hypotension, peripheral vasoconstriction. **Derm:** rash. **EENT:** blurred vision, stuffy nose. **Endo:** hyperglycemia, hypoglycemia. **GI:** ↑ liver enzymes, constipation, diarrhea, drug-induced hepatitis, dry mouth, flatulence, gastric pain, heartburn, nausea, vomiting. **GU:** erectile dysfunction, ↓ libido, urinary frequency. **MS:** arthralgia, back pain, joint pain. **Neuro:** fatigue, weakness, anxiety, depression, dizziness, drowsiness, insomnia, memory loss, mental status changes, nervousness, nightmares. **Resp:** bronchospasm, PULMONARY EDEMA, wheezing. **Misc:** drug-induced lupus syndrome.

Interactions

Drug-Drug: General anesthesia, IV phenytoin, and **verapamil** may cause ↑ myocardial depression. ↑ risk of bradycardia when used with **digoxin, verapamil, diltiazem,** or **clonidine.** ↑ hypotension may occur with other **antihypertensives,** acute ingestion of **alcohol,** or **nitrates.** Concurrent use with **amphetamines, cocaine, ephedrine, epinephrine, norepinephrine, phenylephrine,** or **pseudoephedrine** may result in unopposed alpha-adrenergic stimulation (excessive hypertension, bradycardia). Concurrent administration of **thyroid** administration may ↓ effectiveness. May alter the effectiveness of **insulins** or **oral hypoglycemic agents** (dose adjustments may be necessary). May ↓ the effectiveness of **theophylline.** May ↓ the beneficial beta₁-cardiovascular effects of **dopamine** or **dobutamine.** Use cautiously within 14 days of **MAO inhibitor** therapy (may result in hypertension).

Route/Dosage

When switching from immediate-release to extended-release product, the same total daily dose can be used

PO (Adults): *Hypertension/angina:* 25–100 mg/day as a single dose initially or 2 divided doses; may be ↑ every 7 days as needed up to 450 mg/day (immediate-release) or 400 mg/day (extended-release) (for angina, give in divided doses). Extended-release products are given once daily. *MI:* 25–50 mg (starting 15 min after last IV dose) every 6 hr for 48 hr, then 100 mg twice

daily. *Heart failure:* 12.5–25 mg once daily (of extended-release), can be doubled every 2 wk up to 200 mg/day. *Migraine prevention:* 50–100 mg 2–4 times daily (unlabeled).

IV (Adults): *MI:* 5 mg every 2 min for 3 doses, followed by oral dosing.

PO (Children ≥6 yr): *Hypertension:* 1 mg/kg once daily (extended-release capsules); may be titrated, as needed (not to exceed 50 mg/day).

Availability (generic available)

Tablets (tartrate): 25 mg, 37.5 mg, 50 mg, 75 mg, 100 mg. **Extended-release capsules (succinate; Kapspargo Sprinkle):** 25 mg, 50 mg, 100 mg, 200 mg. **Extended-release tablets (succinate; Toprol XL):** 25 mg, 50 mg, 100 mg, 200 mg. **Solution for injection:** 1 mg/mL. *In combination with:* hydrochlorothiazide (Lopressor HCT). See Appendix N.

NURSING IMPLICATIONS

Assessment

- Monitor BP, ECG, and pulse frequently during dose adjustment and periodically during therapy.
- Monitor frequency of prescription refills to determine compliance.
- Monitor vital signs and ECG every 5–15 min during and for several hrs after parenteral administration. If heart rate <40 bpm, especially if cardiac output is also decreased, administer atropine 0.25–0.5 mg IV.
- Monitor intake and output ratios and daily weights. Assess routinely for signs and symptoms of HF (dyspnea, rales/crackles, weight gain, peripheral edema, jugular venous distention).
- **Angina:** Assess frequency and characteristics of anginal attacks periodically during therapy.

Lab Test Considerations

- May cause ↑ BUN, serum lipoprotein, potassium, triglyceride, and uric acid levels.
- May cause ↑ ANA titers.
- May cause ↑ in blood glucose levels.
- May cause ↑ serum alkaline phosphatase, LDH, AST, and ALT levels.

Implementation

- **High Alert:** IV vasoactive medications are inherently dangerous. Before administering intravenously, have second practitioner independently check original order and dose calculations.
- **High Alert:** Do not confuse Toprol-XL with Topamax. Do not confuse Lopressor with Lyrica. Do not confuse metoprolol tartrate with metoprolol succinate.
- **PO:** Take apical pulse before administering. If <50 bpm or if arrhythmia occurs, withhold medication and notify health care professional.
- Administer metoprolol with meals or directly after eating.

M

- *DNC:* Extended-release tablets may be broken in half; do not crush or chew.
- Swallow *Kapspargo Sprinkle* whole. If unable to swallow a capsule, may be opened and contents sprinkled over soft food (applesauce, pudding, yogurt). Swallow contents of capsule along with a small amount (tsp) of soft food. Swallow drug/food mixture within 60 min; do not store for future use. May also be administered via NG tube by opening and adding capsule contents to an all plastic oral tip syringe and adding 15 mL of water. Gently shake syringe for about 10 sec. Promptly administer through a 12 French or larger NG tube. Rinse with additional water to ensure no granules are left in syringe.

IV Administration

- **IV Push:** *Dilution:* Administer undiluted. *Concentration:* 1 mg/mL. *Rate:* Administer over 1 min.
- **Y-Site Compatibility:** acetaminophen, acyclovir, albumin, human, alemtuzumab, amikacin, aminocaproic acid, aminophylline, amiodarone, amphotericin B liposomal, anidulafungin, argatroban, arsenic trioxide, ascorbic acid, atropine, aztreonam, benztropine, bivalirudin, bleomycin, bumetanide, buprenorphine, butorphanol, calcium chloride, calcium gluconate, cangrelor, carboplatin, carmustine, caspofungin, cefazolin, cefepime, cefotaxime, cefotetan, cefoxitin, ceftaroline, ceftazidime, ceftriaxone, cefuroxime, chloramphenicol, chlorpromazine, ciprofloxacin, cisplatin, clindamycin, cyanocobalamin, cyclophosphamide, cyclosporine, cytarabine, dacarbazine, dactinomycin, daptomycin, daunorubicin hydrochloride, dexamethasone, dexmedetomidine, dexrazoxane, digoxin, diltiazem, diphenhydramine, dobutamine, docetaxel, dopamine, doxorubicin hydrochloride, doxorubicin liposomal, doxycycline, enalaprilat, ephedrine, epinephrine, epirubicin, epoetin alfa, eptifibatide, erythromycin, esmolol, esomeprazole, etoposide, etoposide phosphate, famotidine, fentanyl, fluconazole, fludarabine, fluorouracil, folic acid, foscarnet, fosphenytoin, furosemide, ganciclovir, gemcitabine, gentamicin, glycopyrrolate, granisetron, heparin, hetastarch, hydrocortisone, hydromorphone, ibuprofen, idarubicin, ifosfamide, imipenem/cilastatin, indomethacin, insulin regular, irinotecan, isoproterenol, ketorolac, labetalol, LR, leucovorin calcium, levofloxacin, levothyroxine, linezolid, lorazepam, magnesium sulfate, mannitol, meperidine, meropenem, mesna, methadone, methotrexate, methylprednisolone, metoclopramide, metronidazole, midazolam, milrinone, mitomycin, mitoxantrone, morphine, moxifloxacin, multivitamins, mycophenolate, nafcillin, nalbuphine, naloxone, nicardipine, nitroprusside, norepinephrine, 0.9% NaCl, octreotide, ondansetron, oxacillin, oxaliplatin, oxytocin, paclitaxel, palonosetron, pamidronate, papaverine, pemetrexed, penicillin G, pentamidine, pentobarbital, phenobarbital, phentolamine, phenylephrine, phytonadione, piperacillin/tazobactam, potassium acetate, potassium chloride, procainamide, prochlorperazine, promethazine, propranolol, protamine, pyridoxine, rocuronium, sodium bicarbonate, succinylcholine, sufentanil, tacrolimus, theophylline, thiamine, thiotepa, tigecycline, tirofiban, tobramycin, topotecan, vancomycin, vasopressin, vecuronium, verapamil, vinblastine, vincristine, vinorelbine, voriconazole, zoledronic acid.
- **Y-Site Incompatibility:** allopurinol, amphotericin B deoxycholate, amphotericin B lipid complex, dantrolene, diazepam, gemtuzumab ozogamicin, pantoprazole, phenytoin, trimethoprim/sulfamethoxazole.

Patient/Family Teaching

- Instruct patient to take medication as directed, at the same time each day, even if feeling well; do not skip or double up on missed doses. Take missed doses as soon as possible up to 8 hr before next dose. Abrupt withdrawal may precipitate life-threatening arrhythmias, hypertension, or myocardial ischemia.
- Teach patient and family how to check pulse daily and BP biweekly and to report significant changes to health care professional.
- May cause drowsiness. Caution patient to avoid driving or other activities that require alertness until response to the drug is known.
- Advise patient to change positions slowly to minimize orthostatic hypotension.
- Caution patient that this medication may increase sensitivity to cold.
- Instruct patient to notify health care professional of all Rx or OTC medications, vitamins, or herbal products being taken and to consult health care professional before taking any Rx, OTC, or herbal products, especially cold preparations, concurrently with this medication. Patients on antihypertensive therapy should also avoid excessive amounts of coffee, tea, and cola.
- Diabetics should closely monitor blood glucose, especially if weakness, malaise, irritability, or fatigue occurs. Medication does not block sweating as a sign of hypoglycemia.
- Advise patient to notify health care professional if slow pulse, difficulty breathing, wheezing, cold hands and feet, dizziness, light-headedness, confusion, depression, rash, fever, sore throat, unusual bleeding, or bruising occurs.
- Instruct patient to inform health care professional of medication regimen before treatment or surgery.
- Rep: Advise females of reproductive potential to notify health care professional if pregnancy is planned or suspected, or if breastfeeding. Monitor neonates of women taking metoprolol for symptoms of hypotension, bradycardia, hypoglycemia, and respiratory depression and manage accordingly. Monitor breastfed infants for bradycardia, dry mouth, skin or eyes, and diarrhea or constipation.
- Advise patient to carry identification describing disease process and medication regimen at all times.

- **Hypertension:** Reinforce the need to continue additional therapies for hypertension (weight loss, sodium restriction, stress reduction, regular exercise, moderation of alcohol consumption, and smoking cessation). Medication controls but does not cure hypertension.

Evaluation/Desired Outcomes

- Decrease in BP.
- Reduction in frequency of anginal attacks.
- Increase in activity tolerance.
- Prevention of MI.

metroNIDAZOLE
(me-troe-**ni**-da-zole)
Flagyl, MetroCream, MetroGel, MetroLotion, ✳Nidagel, Noritate, Nuvessa, Vandazole
Classification
Therapeutic: anti-infectives, antiprotozoals, antiulcer agents

Indications

PO, IV: Treatment of the following anaerobic infections: Intra-abdominal infections (may be used with a cephalosporin), Gynecologic infections, Skin and skin structure infections, Lower respiratory tract infections, Bone and joint infections, CNS infections, Septicemia, Endocarditis. **IV:** Perioperative prophylactic agent in colorectal surgery. **PO:** Treatment of the following infections: Amebic dysentery, amebic liver abscess, and trichomoniasis, Peptic ulcer disease caused by *Helicobacter pylori*. **Topical:** Acne rosacea. **Vag:** Bacterial vaginosis. **Unlabeled Use:** Giardiasis. Anti-infective associated *Clostridioides difficile*-associated diarrhea (CDAD).

Action

Disrupts DNA and protein synthesis in susceptible organisms. **Therapeutic Effects:** Bactericidal, trichomonacidal, or amebicidal action. **Spectrum:** Most notable for activity against anaerobic bacteria, including: *Bacteroides spp., Clostridioides difficile, Gardnerella vaginalis, Mobiluncus spp., Peptostreptococcus spp.* In addition, is active against: *Trichomonas vaginalis, Entamoeba histolytica, Giardia lamblia, H. pylori*.

Pharmacokinetics

Absorption: 80% absorbed after oral administration. Minimal absorption after topical or vaginal application.
Distribution: Widely distributed into most tissues and fluids, including CSF.
Metabolism and Excretion: Partially metabolized by the liver (30–60%), partially excreted unchanged in the urine, 6–15% eliminated in the feces.
Half-life: Neonates: 25–75 hr; Children and adults: 6–12 hr.

TIME/ACTION PROFILE (PO, IV = blood levels; topical = improvement in rosacea)

ROUTE	ONSET	PEAK	DURATION
PO	rapid	1–3 hr	8 hr
PO-ER	rapid	unknown	up to 24 hr
IV	rapid	end of infusion	6–8 hr
Topical	3 wk	9 wk	12 hr
Vaginal	unknown	6–12 hr	12 hr

Contraindications/Precautions

Contraindicated in: Hypersensitivity; Hypersensitivity to parabens (topical only); Cockayne syndrome (↑ risk of hepatotoxicity and death); OB: First trimester of pregnancy.
Use Cautiously in: History of blood dyscrasias; History of seizures or neurologic problems; Severe hepatic impairment (dose ↓ suggested); Patients receiving corticosteroids or predisposed to edema (injection contains 28 mEq sodium/g metronidazole); OB: Although safety has not been established, has been used to treat trichomoniasis in 2nd- and 3rd-trimester pregnancy—but not as single-dose regimen; Lactation: If needed, use single dose and interrupt nursing for 24 hr thereafter.

Adverse Reactions/Side Effects

Derm: rash, STEVENS-JOHNSON SYNDROME (SJS), urticaria; *topical only:* burning, mild dryness, skin irritation, transient redness. **EENT:** optic neuropathy, tearing (topical only). **GI:** abdominal pain, anorexia, nausea, diarrhea, dry mouth, furry tongue, glossitis, unpleasant taste, vomiting. **Hemat:** leukopenia. **Local:** phlebitis at IV site. **Neuro:** dizziness, headache, aseptic meningitis (IV), encephalopathy (IV), peripheral neuropathy, psychosis, SEIZURES. **Misc:** superinfection.

Interactions

Drug-Drug: **Cimetidine** may ↑ levels and risk of toxicity. **Phenobarbital** and **rifampin** may ↓ levels and effectiveness. May ↑ levels and the risk of toxicity of **phenytoin, lithium,** and **warfarin**. Disulfiram-like reaction may occur with **alcohol** ingestion. May cause acute psychosis and confusion with **disulfiram**. ↑ risk of leukopenia with **fluorouracil** or **azathioprine**. Use with **QT interval prolonging medications** may ↑ risk of QT interval prolongation.

Route/Dosage

PO (Adults): *Anaerobic infections:* 7.5 mg/kg every 6 hr (not to exceed 4 g/day). *Trichomoniasis:* 250 mg every 8 hr for 7 days *or* single 2-g dose *or* 1 g twice daily for 1 day. *Amebiasis:* 500–750 mg every 8 hr for 5–10 days. *H. pylori:* 250 mg 4 times daily *or* 500 mg twice daily for 1–2 wk (with other agents). *Antibiotic associated Clostridioides difficile-associated diarrhea (CDAD):* 250–500 mg 3–4 times/day for 10–14 days.

PO (Infants and Children): *Anaerobic infections:* 30 mg/kg/day divided every 6 hr, maximum dose: 4 g/day *Trichomoniasis:* 15–30 mg/kg/day divided every 8 hr for 7–10 days. *Amebiasis:* 35–50 mg/kg/day divided every 8 hr for 5–10 days (not to exceed 750 mg/dose). *Clostridioides difficile-associated diarrhea (CDAD):* 30 mg/kg/day divided every 6 hr for 7–10 days. *H. pylori:* 15–20 mg/kg/day divided twice daily for 4 wk.

IV, PO (Neonates 0–4 wk, <1200 g): 7.5 mg/kg every 48 hr. *Postnatal age <7 days, 1200–2000 g:* 7.5 mg/kg/day every 24 hr. *Postnatal age <7 days, >2000 g:* 15 mg/kg/day divided every 12 hr. *Postnatal age >7 days, 1200–2000 g:* 15 mg/kg/day divided every 12 hr. *Postnatal age >7 days, >2000 g:* 30 mg/kg/day divided every 12 hr.

IV (Adults): *Anaerobic infections:* Initial dose 15 mg/kg, then 7.5 mg/kg every 6–8 hr *or* 500 mg every 6–8 hr (not to exceed 4 g/day). *Perioperative prophylaxis:* Initial dose 15 mg/kg 1 hr before surgery, then 7.5 mg/kg 6 and 12 hr later. *Amebiasis:* 500–750 mg every 8 hr for 5–10 days.

IV (Children): *Anaerobic infections:* 30 mg/kg/day divided every 6 hr, maximum dose: 4 g/day.

Topical (Adults): *Acne rosacea:* Apply thin film to affected area bid.

Vag (Adults): *0.75% vaginal gel:* One applicatorful (37.5 mg) of 0.75% gel 1–2 times daily for 5 days; *Nuvessa:* One applicatorful (65 mg) of 1.3% gel as a single dose at bedtime; *Vandazole:* One applicatorful (37.5 mg) of 0.75% gel once daily for 5 days.

Vag (Children ≥12 yr): *Nuvessa:* One applicatorful (65 mg) of 1.3% gel as a single dose at bedtime.

Vag (Children Post-menarchal): *Vandazole:* One applicatorful (37.5 mg) of 0.75% gel once daily for 5 days.

Availability (generic available)

Tablets: 250 mg, 500 mg. **Capsules:** 375 mg, ✿ 500 mg. **Premixed infusion:** 500 mg/100 mL. **Topical cream:** 0.75%, 1%. **Topical gel:** 0.75%, 1%. **Topical lotion:** 0.75%. **Vaginal cream:** ✿ 10% (500 mg/applicatorful). **Vaginal gel:** 0.75% (37.5 mg/5 g applicatorful), 1.3% (65 mg/5 g applicatorful). *In combination with:* bismuth subcitrate potassium and tetracycline (Pylera). See Appendix N.

NURSING IMPLICATIONS

Assessment

- Assess for infection (vital signs; appearance of wound, sputum, urine, and stool; WBC) at beginning of and during therapy.
- Obtain specimens for culture and sensitivity before initiating therapy. First dose may be given before receiving results.
- Monitor neurologic status during and after IV infusions. Inform health care professional if numbness, paresthesia, weakness, ataxia, or seizures occur.
- Monitor intake, output, and daily weight, especially for patients on sodium restriction. Each 500 mg of

premixed injection for dilution contains 14 mEq of sodium.
- Assess for rash periodically during therapy. May cause SJS. Discontinue therapy if severe or if accompanied with fever, general malaise, fatigue, muscle or joint aches, blisters, oral lesions, conjunctivitis, hepatitis, and/or eosinophilia.
- **Giardiasis:** Monitor three stool samples taken several days apart, beginning 3–4 wk after treatment.

Lab Test Considerations
- May alter results of serum AST, ALT, and LDH tests.
- Monitor CBC before, during, and after prolonged or repeated courses of metronidazole.

Implementation

- Do not confuse metronidazole with metformin.
- **PO:** Administer on an empty stomach, or may administer with food or milk to minimize GI irritation. Tablets may be crushed for patients with difficulty swallowing. *DNC:* Swallow extended-release tablets whole; do not break, crush, or chew.

IV Administration
- **Intermittent Infusion:** *Dilution:* Administer premixed injection (500 mg/100 mL) undiluted. Do not refrigerate. Once taken out of overwrap, premixed infusion stable for 30 days at room temperature. *Concentration:* 5 mg/mL. *Rate:* Infuse over 30–60 min.
- **Y-Site Compatibility:** acyclovir, alemtuzumab, allopurinol, amifostine, amikacin, aminocaproic acid, aminophylline, amiodarone, ampicillin, ampicillin/sulbactam, anidulafungin, argatroban, arsenic trioxide, azithromycin, bivalirudin, bleomycin, bumetanide, buprenorphine, busulfan, butorphanol, calcium acetate, calcium chloride, calcium gluconate, cangrelor, carboplatin, carmustine, cefazolin, cefepime, cefotaxime, cefotetan, cefoxitin, ceftaroline, ceftazidime, ceftozolane/tazobactam, ceftriaxone, cefuroxime, chloramphenicol, chlorpromazine, ciprofloxacin, cisatracurium, cisplatin, clindamycin, cyclophosphamide, cyclosporine, cytarabine, dacarbazine, dactinomycin, daunorubicin hydrochloride, defibrotide, dexamethasone, dexmedetomidine, dexrazoxane, digoxin, diltiazem, diphenhydramine, dobutamine, docetaxel, dopamine, doxorubicin hydrochloride, doxorubicin liposomal, doxycycline, droperidol, enalaprilat, ephedrine, epinephrine, epirubicin, eptifibatide, eravacycline, ertapenem, erythromycin, esmolol, etoposide, etoposide phosphate, famotidine, fentanyl, fluconazole, fludarabine, fluorouracil, foscarnet, fosphenytoin, furosemide, gemcitabine, gemtuzumab ozogamicin, gentamicin, glycopyrrolate, granisetron, haloperidol, heparin, hetastarch, hydralazine, hydrocortisone, idarubicin, ifosfamide, imipenem/cilastatin, insulin regular, irinotecan, isoproterenol, ketamine, ketorolac, labetalol, LR, leucovorin calcium, levofloxacin, lidocaine, linezolid, lorazepam, magnesium sulfate, mannitol, melphalan, meperidine, meropenem, meropenem/

vaborbactam, mesna, methadone, methotrexate, methylprednisolone, metoclopramide, metoprolol, midazolam, milrinone, mitoxantrone, morphine, mycophenolate, nafcillin, nalbuphine, naloxone, nicardipine, nitroglycerin, nitroprusside, norepinephrine, octreotide, ondansetron, oxaliplatin, oxytocin, paclitaxel, palonosetron, pamidronate, pentamidine, pentobarbital, phenobarbital, phentolamine, phenylephrine, piperacillin/tazobactam, plazomicin, potassium acetate, potassium chloride, potassium phosphate, prochlorperazine, promethazine, propranolol, remifentanil, rituximab, rocuronium, sargramostim, sodium acetate, sodium bicarbonate, sodium phosphate, succinylcholine, sufentanil, tacrolimus, tedizolid, theophylline, thiopental, thiotepa, tigecycline, tirofiban, tobramycin, topotecan, trastuzumab, trimethoprim/sulfamethoxazole, vancomycin, vasopressin, vecuronium, verapamil, vincristine, vinorelbine, voriconazole, zidovudine, zoledronic acid.

- **Y-Site Incompatibility:** amphotericin B deoxycholate, amphotericin B lipid complex, amphotericin B liposome, aztreonam, blinatumomab, dantrolene, daptomycin, diazepam, filgrastim, ganciclovir, minocycline, pantoprazole, pemetrexed, phenytoin, procainamide, propofol.
- **Topical:** Cleanse affected area before application. Apply and rub in a thin film twice daily, morning and evening. Avoid contact with eyes.
- **Vag:** Administer once daily dosing at bedtime.

Patient/Family Teaching

- Instruct patient to take medication as directed with evenly spaced times between doses, even if feeling better. Do not skip doses or double up on missed doses. Take missed doses as soon as remembered if not almost time for next dose.
- Advise patients treated for trichomoniasis that sexual partners may be asymptomatic sources of reinfection and should be treated concurrently. Patient should also refrain from intercourse or use a condom to prevent reinfection.
- Caution patient to avoid intake of alcoholic beverages or preparations containing alcohol during and for at least 3 days after treatment with metronidazole, including vaginal gel. May cause a disulfiram-like reaction (flushing, nausea, vomiting, headache, abdominal cramps).
- May cause dizziness or light-headedness. Caution patient to avoid driving or other activities requiring alertness until response to medication is known.
- Instruct patient to notify health care professional promptly if rash occurs.
- Inform patient that medication may cause an unpleasant metallic taste.
- Advise patient to notify health care professional of all Rx or OTC medications, vitamins, or herbal products

being taken and to consult with health care professional before taking other medications.
- Advise patient that frequent mouth rinses, good oral hygiene, and sugarless gum or candy may minimize dry mouth. Notify health care professional if dry mouth persists for more than 2 wk.
- Inform patient that medication may cause urine to turn dark.
- Advise patient to consult health care professional if no improvement in a few days or if signs and symptoms of superinfection (black, furry overgrowth on tongue; vaginal itching or discharge; loose or foul-smelling stools) develop.
- Rep: Advise females of reproductive potential to inform health care professional if pregnancy is planned or suspected and to avoid breastfeeding during therapy.
- **Vag:** Instruct patient in correct technique for intravaginal instillation. Advise patient to avoid intercourse during treatment with vaginal gel.
- **Topical:** Instruct patient on correct technique for application of topical gel. Cosmetics may be used after application of gel.

Evaluation/Desired Outcomes

- Resolution of the signs and symptoms of infection. Length of time for complete resolution depends on organism and site of infection.
- Significant results should be seen within 3 wk of application of topical gel. Application may be continued for 9 wk.

---

micafungin (my-ka-**fun**-gin)
Mycamine
Classification
Therapeutic: antifungals
Pharmacologic: echinocandins

Indications

Treatment of esophageal candidiasis. Treatment of candidemia/acute disseminated candidiasis/*Candida* peritonitis and abscesses (in adults and pediatric patients ≥4 mo). Treatment of candidemia/acute disseminated candidiasis/*Candida* peritonitis and abscesses without meningoencephalitis and/or ocular dissemination (in pediatric patients <4 mo). Prophylaxis of *Candida* infections during hematopoietic stem cell transplantation.

Action

Inhibits synthesis of glucan required for the formation of fungal cell wall. **Therapeutic Effects:** Death of susceptible fungi. **Spectrum:** Active against the following *Candida* spp.: *C. albicans, C. glabrata, C. krusei, C. parapsilosis, C. tropicalis.*

Pharmacokinetics

Absorption: IV administration results in complete bioavailability.

Distribution: Primarily distributed into lung, liver, and spleen; minimal distribution to CNS and eyes.
Protein Binding: >99%.
Metabolism and Excretion: Mostly metabolized in the liver; 71% fecal elimination.
Half-life: 15 hr.

TIME/ACTION PROFILE (plasma concentrations)

ROUTE	ONSET	PEAK	DURATION
IV	rapid	end of infusion	24 hr

Contraindications/Precautions

Contraindicated in: Hypersensitivity.
Use Cautiously in: Severe hepatic impairment; OB: Use during pregnancy only if potential maternal benefit justifies potential fetal risk; Lactation: Use while breastfeeding only if potential maternal benefit justifies potential risk to infant; Pedi: Children <4 mo with meningoencephalitis and/or ocular dissemination (safety and effectiveness not established).

Adverse Reactions/Side Effects

GI: worsening hepatic function/hepatitis. **GU:** renal impairment. **Hemat:** hemolysis/hemolytic anemia. **Local:** injection site reactions. **Misc:** infusion reactions, HYPERSENSITIVITY REACTIONS (including anaphylaxis).

Interactions

Drug-Drug: ↑ levels and risk of toxicity with **sirolimus** and **nifedipine** (dose adjustments may be necessary).

Route/Dosage

Treatment of Esophageal Candidiasis

IV (Adults): 150 mg once daily for 15 days (range 10–30 days).
IV (Children ≥4 mo and >30 kg): 2.5 mg/kg once daily (max daily dose = 150 mg).
IV (Children ≥4 mo and ≤30 kg): 3 mg/kg once daily.

Treatment of Candidemia/Acute Disseminated Candidiasis/Candida Peritonitis and Abscesses

IV (Adults): 100 mg once daily for 15 days (range 10–47 days).
IV (Children ≥4 mo and >30 kg): 2 mg/kg once daily (max daily dose = 100 mg).
IV (Children ≥4 mo and ≤30 kg): 2 mg/kg once daily.

Treatment of Candidemia/Acute Disseminated Candidiasis/Candida Peritonitis and Abscesses Without Meningoencephalitis and/or Ocular Dissemination

IV (Children <4 mo): 4 mg/kg once daily.

Prophylaxis of Candida Infections During Hematopoetic Stem Cell Transplantation

IV (Adults): 50 mg once daily (duration range 6–51 days).
IV (Children ≥4 mo and >30 kg): 1 mg/kg once daily (max daily dose = 50 mg).
IV (Children ≥4 mo and ≤30 kg): 1 mg/kg once daily.

Availability (generic available)

Lyophilized powder for injection: 50 mg/vial, 100 mg/vial.

NURSING IMPLICATIONS

Assessment

- Assess symptoms of esophageal candidiasis (dysphagia, odynophagia, retrosternal pain) prior to and during therapy.
- Monitor for signs of anaphylaxis (rash, pruritus, wheezing, laryngeal edema, abdominal pain). Discontinue micafungin and notify health care professional immediately if these occur.
- Monitor for signs and symptoms of histamine-mediated reactions (rash, pruritus, facial swelling, vasodilation) during infusion. If symptoms occur, slow infusion rate.
- Assess for injection site reactions (phlebitis, thrombophlebitis) during therapy. These occur more frequently in patients receiving micafungin via peripheral IV infusion.

Lab Test Considerations

- May cause ↑ serum alkaline phosphatase, bilirubin, ALT, AST, and LDH levels. If elevations occur, monitor for worsening liver function; may require discontinuation of therapy.
- May cause ↑ BUN and serum creatinine.
- May cause leukopenia, neutropenia, thrombocytopenia, and anemia. Monitor for worsening levels; may require discontinuation of therapy.
- May cause hypokalemia, hypocalcemia, and hypomagnesemia.

Implementation

IV Administration

- **Intermittent Infusion:** *Reconstitution: For Adults:* Reconstitute each 50-mg vial with 5 mL of 0.9% NaCl or D5W to achieve concentration of 10 mg/mL. Reconstitute each 100-mg vial with 5 mL of 0.9% NaCl or D5W to achieve concentration of 20 mg/mL. Dissolve by gently swirling vial; do not shake vigorously. *Dilution:* Directions for further dilution based on indication for use. For prophylaxis of *Candida* infections, add 50 mg of micafungin to 100 mL of 0.9% NaCl or D5W. For treatment of esophageal candidiasis, add 150 mg of micafungin to 100 mL of 0.9% NaCl or D5W. Reconstituted vials and infusion are stable for 24 hr at room temperature. Protect diluted solution from light. *Concentration:* 0.5–1.5 mg/mL.

- *For Children: Dilution:* Determine dose and divide by final concentration (10 or 20 mg/mL). Add withdrawn volume to 0.9% NaCl or D5W in IV bag or syringe. *Concentration:* 0.5–4 mg/mL. Concentrations >1.5 mg/mL should be administered via central venous catheter to minimize infusion reactions. Discard unused vials. *Rate:* Flush line with 0.9% NaCl prior to administration. Infuse over 1 hr. More rapid infusions may result in more frequent histamine mediated reactions.

- **Y-Site Compatibility:** aminophylline, bumetanide, calcium chloride, calcium gluconate, cangrelor, carboplatin, ceftolozane/tazobactam, cyclosporine, dopamine, eptifibatide, esmolol, etoposide, furosemide, heparin, hydromorphone, lidocaine, lorazepam, magnesium sulfate, meropenem/vaborbactam, mesna, milrinone, nitroglycerin, nitroprusside, norepinephrine, phenylephrine, posaconazole, potassium chloride, potassium phosphate, sodium phosphate, tacrolimus, tedizolid, theophylline, vasopressin.

- **Y-Site Incompatibility:** albumin, human, amiodarone, cisatracurium, diltiazem, dobutamine, epinephrine, eravacycline, insulin regular, isavuconazonium, labetalol, levofloxacin, meperidine, midazolam, morphine, mycophenolate, nicardipine, octreotide, ondansetron, phenytoin, plazomicin, rocuronium, telavancin, vecuronium.

Patient/Family Teaching

- Inform patient of the purpose of micafungin.
- Advise patient to notify health care professional immediately if signs of anaphylaxis occur. Infusion should be discontinued if symptoms occur.
- Instruct patient to notify health care professional of all Rx or OTC medications, vitamins, or herbal products being taken and to consult health care professional before taking any other Rx, OTC, or herbal products.
- Rep: May cause fetal harm. Advise females of reproductive potential to notify health care professional if pregnancy is planned or suspected or if breastfeeding.

Evaluation/Desired Outcomes

- Resolution of signs and symptoms of esophageal candidiasis, candidemia, acute disseminated candidiasis, candidal peritonitis, and abscesses.
- Prevention of *Candida* infections during hematopoetic stem cell transplantation.

---

miconazole, See ANTIFUNGALS (TOPICAL).

---

miconazole, See ANTIFUNGALS (VAGINAL).

BEERS   HIGH ALERT

midazolam (mid-ay-zoe-lam)
Nayzilam, Seizalam, ~~Versed~~

Classification
Therapeutic: antianxiety agents, anticonvulsants, sedative/hypnotics
Pharmacologic: benzodiazepines

Schedule IV

Indications

PO: Preprocedural sedation and anxiolysis in pediatric patients. **IM, IV:** Preoperative sedation/anxiolysis/amnesia: Status epilepticus. **IV:** Provides sedation/anxiolysis/amnesia during therapeutic, diagnostic, or radiographic procedures (conscious sedation). Aids in the induction of anesthesia and as part of balanced anesthesia. As a continuous infusion, provides sedation of mechanically ventilated patients during anesthesia or in a critical care setting. **Intranasal:** Acute treatment of intermittent, stereotypic episodes of frequent seizure activity (i.e., seizure clusters, acute repetitive seizures) that are distinct from a patient's usual seizure pattern in patients with epilepsy.

Action

Acts at many levels of the CNS to produce generalized CNS depression. Effects may be mediated by GABA, an inhibitory neurotransmitter. **Therapeutic Effects:** Short-term sedation. Postoperative amnesia. Termination of seizure activity.

Pharmacokinetics

Absorption: Rapidly absorbed following oral and nasal administration; undergoes substantial intestinal and first-pass hepatic metabolism. Well absorbed following IM administration; IV administration results in complete bioavailability.

Distribution: Crosses the blood-brain barrier and placenta; excreted in breast milk.

Protein Binding: 97%.

Metabolism and Excretion: Almost exclusively metabolized by the liver by the CYP3A4 isoenzyme, resulting in conversion to hydroxymidazolam, an active metabolite, and 2 other inactive metabolites; metabolites are excreted in urine.

Half-life: *Preterm neonates:* 2.6–17.7 hr; *Neonates:* 4–12 hr; *Children:* 3–7 hr; *Adults:* 2–6 hr (↑ in renal impairment, HF, or cirrhosis).

TIME/ACTION PROFILE (sedation)

ROUTE	ONSET	PEAK	DURATION
IN	5 min	10 min	30–60 min
IM	15 min	30–60 min	2–6 hr
IV	1.5–5 min	rapid	2–6 hr

✦ = Canadian drug name. ▒ = Genetic implication. ~~Strikethrough~~ = Discontinued. CAPITALS = life-threatening. Underline = most frequent.

Contraindications/Precautions

Contraindicated in: Hypersensitivity; Cross-sensitivity with other benzodiazepines may occur; Shock; Comatose patients or those with pre-existing CNS depression; Uncontrolled severe pain; Acute angle-closure glaucoma; Pedi: Products containing benzyl alcohol should not be used in neonates.

Use Cautiously in: All patients (may ↑ risk of suicidal thoughts/behaviors); Pulmonary disease; HF; Renal impairment; Severe hepatic impairment; Obese pediatric patients (calculate dose on the basis of ideal body weight); Open-angle glaucoma; OB: Use late in pregnancy can result in sedation (respiratory depression, lethargy, hypotonia) and/or withdrawal symptoms (hyperreflexia, irritability, restlessness, tremors, inconsolable crying, and feeding difficulties) in neonates; Lactation: Use while breastfeeding only if potential maternal benefit justifies potential risk to infant; Pedi: Rapid injection in neonates has caused severe hypotension and seizures, especially when used with fentanyl; may affect brain development in children <3 yr; safety and effectiveness of nasal spray has not been established in children <12 yr; Geri: Appears on Beers list. ↑ risk of cognitive impairment, delirium, falls, fractures, and motor vehicle accidents in older adults. If possible, avoid use in older adults.

Adverse Reactions/Side Effects

CV: arrhythmias, CARDIAC ARREST. **Derm:** rash. **EENT:** blurred vision. **GI:** hiccups, nausea, vomiting. **Local:** phlebitis at IV site, pain at IM site. **Neuro:** agitation, drowsiness, excess sedation, headache, SUICIDAL THOUGHTS. **Resp:** APNEA, bronchospasm, cough, LARYNGOSPASM, RESPIRATORY DEPRESSION.

Interactions

Drug-Drug: ↑ CNS depression with **alcohol**, **antihistamines**, **opioid analgesics**, and other **sedative/hypnotics** (↓ midazolam dose by 30–50% if used concurrently). ↑ risk of hypotension with **antihypertensives**, **opioid analgesics**, acute ingestion of **alcohol**, or **nitrates**. **Moderate CYP3A4 inhibitors** and **strong CYP3A4 inhibitors**, including **clarithromycin**, **diltiazem**, **erythromycin**, **itraconazole**, **ketoconazole**, and **verapamil** may ↑ levels and the risk of toxicity; avoid concurrent use. **Strong CYP3A4 inducers**, including **carbamazepine**, **phenobarbital**, **phenytoin**, **rifampin**, and **rifabutin** may ↓ levels.
Drug-Natural Products: Concomitant use of **kava-kava**, **valerian**, or **chamomile** can ↑ CNS depression. Long-term use of **St. John's wort** may significantly ↓ levels.
Drug-Food: **Grapefruit juice** ↓ metabolism and may ↑ risk of toxicity.

Route/Dosage

Preoperative Sedation/Anxiolysis/Amnesia

PO (Children 6 mo–16 yr): 0.25–0.5 mg/kg, may require up to 1 mg/kg (dose should not exceed 20 mg); *patients with cardiac/respiratory compromise or concurrent CNS depressants:* 0.25 mg/kg.
IM (Adults Otherwise Healthy and <60 yr): 0.07–0.08 mg/kg 1 hr before surgery (usual dose 5 mg).
IM (Adults ≥60 yr, Debilitated or Chronically Ill): 0.02–0.03 mg/kg 1 hr before surgery (usual dose 1–3 mg).
IM (Children): 0.1–0.15 mg/kg up to 0.5 mg/kg 30–60 min prior to procedure; not to exceed 10 mg/dose.

Conscious Sedation for Short Procedures

IV (Adults and Children Otherwise Healthy >12 yr and <60 yr): 1–2.5 mg initially; dosage may be ↑ further as needed. Total doses >5 mg are rarely needed (↓ dose by 50% if other CNS depressants are used). Maintenance doses of 25% of the dose required for initial sedation may be given as necessary.
IV (Children 6–12 yr): 0.025–0.05 mg/kg initially, then titrate dose carefully, may need up to 0.4 mg/kg total, maximum dose 10 mg.
IV (Children 6 mo–5 yr): 0.05 mg/kg initially, then titrate dose carefully, may need up to 0.6 mg/kg total, maximum dose 6 mg.
IV (Geriatric Patients ≥60 yr, Debilitated or Chronically Ill): 1–1.5 mg initially; dose may be ↑ further as needed. Total doses >3.5 mg are rarely needed (↓ dose by 30% if other CNS depressants are used). Maintenance doses of 25% of the dose required for initial sedation may be given as necessary.
Intranasal (Children): 0.2–0.3 mg/kg, may repeat in 5–15 min.

Status Epilepticus

IM (Adults): 10 mg single dose.
IV (Children >2 mo): 0.15 mg/kg load followed by a continuous infusion of 1 mcg/kg/min. Titrate dose upward every 5 min until seizure controlled; range: 1–18 mcg/kg/min.

Seizure Clusters

Intranasal (Adults and Children ≥12 yr): One spray (5 mg) into one nostril initially; if inadequate response after 10 min, administer one spray (5 mg) into other nostril. Not to exceed 2 doses for a single seizure episode. Should not be used to treat more than one episode every 3 days and no more than 5 episodes per mo.

Induction of Anesthesia (Adjunct)

IV (Adults Otherwise Healthy and <55 yr): 300–350 mcg/kg initially (up to 600 mcg/kg total). May give additional dose of 25% of initial dose if needed. If patient is premedicated, initial dose should be further ↓.
IV (Geriatric Patients >55 yr): 150–300 mcg/kg as initial dose. May give additional dose of 25% of initial dose if needed. If patient is premedicated, initial dose should be further ↓.
IV (Adults —Debilitated): 150–250 mcg/kg initial dose. May give additional dose of 25% of initial dose if needed. If patient is premedicated, initial dose should be further ↓.

Sedation in Critical Care Settings

IV (Adults): 0.01–0.05 mg/kg (0.5–4 mg in most adults) initially if a loading dose is required; may repeat every 10–15 min until desired effect is obtained; may be followed by infusion at 0.02–0.1 mg/kg/hr (1–7 mg/hr in most adults).

IV (Children): *Intubated patients only:* 0.05–0.2 mg/kg initially as a loading dose; follow with infusion at 0.06–0.12 mg/kg/hr (1–2 mcg/kg/min), titrate to effect, range: 0.4–6 mcg/kg/min.

IV (Neonates >32 wk): *Intubated patients only:* 0.06 mg/kg/hr (1 mcg/kg/min).

IV (Neonates <32 wk): *Intubated patients only:* 0.03 mg/kg/hr (0.5 mcg/kg/min).

Availability (generic available)

Oral syrup (cherry flavor): 2 mg/mL. **Nasal spray (Nayzilam):** 5 mg/0.1 mL single-dose unit. **Premixed infusion:** 50 mg/50 mL 0.8% NaCl, 100 mg/100 mL 0.8% NaCl, 50 mg/50 mL 0.9% NaCl, 100 mg/100 mL 0.9% NaCl. **Solution for injection:** 1 mg/mL, 5 mg/mL. **Solution for intramuscular injection:** 10 mg/0.7 mL (prefilled autoinjector).

NURSING IMPLICATIONS

Assessment

- Assess level of sedation and level of consciousness during and for 2–6 hr following administration.
- Monitor BP, pulse, and respiration continuously during administration, especially if co-administering opioid analgesics. Oxygen and resuscitative equipment should be immediately available during IV administration.
- Assess risk for addiction, abuse, or misuse before starting and periodically during therapy.

Toxicity and Overdose
- If overdose occurs, monitor pulse, respiration, and BP continuously. Maintain patent airway and assist ventilation as needed. If hypotension occurs, treatment includes IV fluids, repositioning, and vasopressors.
- The effects of midazolam can be reversed with flumazenil.

Implementation

- **High Alert:** Accidental overdose of oral midazolam syrup in children has resulted in serious harm or death. Do not accept orders prescribed by volume (5 mL or 1 tsp); instead, request dose be expressed in milligrams. Have second practitioner independently check original order and dose calculations. Midazolam syrup should only be administered by health care professionals authorized to administer conscious sedation.
- Supervise ambulation and transfer of patients after administration. Two side rails should be raised and call bell within reach at all times.

- Gradually taper to discontinue or reduce the dose to reduce risk of withdrawal reactions, increased seizure frequency, and status epilepticus. If withdrawal symptoms develop, pause taper or increase dose to previous tapered dose level; decrease dose more slowly. Some patients may require longer tapering period (weeks to >12 mo).
- **PO:** To use the *Press-in Bottle Adaptor (PIBA)*, remove the cap and push bottle adaptor into neck of bottle. Close bottle tightly with cap. Solution is a clear red to purplish-red, cherry-flavored syrup. Then remove cap and insert tip of oral dispenser in bottle adaptor. Push the plunger completely down toward tip of oral dispenser and insert firmly into bottle adaptor. Turn entire unit (bottle and oral dispenser) upside down. Pull plunger out slowly until desired amount of medication is withdrawn into oral dispenser. Turn entire unit right side up and slowly remove oral dispenser from the bottle. Tip of dispenser may be covered with tip of cap until time of use. Close bottle with cap after each use.
- Dispense directly into mouth. Do not mix with any liquid prior to dispensing.
- **Intranasal:** Administer 1 spray into one nostril. If no response to initial dose after 10 min, may administer 1 spray into other nostril.
- **IM:** Administer IM doses deep into mid-outer thigh (vastus lateralis muscle), maximum concentration 1 mg/mL. Solution is clear, colorless to light yellow. Do not administer solutions that are discolored or contain particulate matter.

IV Administration
- **IV Push:** *Dilution:* Administer undiluted or diluted with D5W or 0.9% NaCl. *Concentration:* Undiluted: 1 mg/mL or 5 mg/mL. Diluted: 0.03–3 mg/mL. *Rate:* Administer slowly over at least 2–5 min. Titrate dose to patient response. Rapid injection, especially in neonates, has caused severe hypotension.
- **Continuous Infusion:** *Dilution:* Dilute with 0.9% NaCl or D5W. *Concentration:* 0.5–1 mg/mL. *Rate:* Based on patient's weight (see Route/Dosage section). Titrate to desired level of sedation. Assess sedation at regular intervals and adjust rate up or down by 25–50% as needed. Dose should also be decreased by 10–25% every few hrs to find minimum effective infusion rate, which prevents accumulation of midazolam and provides more rapid recovery upon termination.
- **Y-Site Compatibility:** acetaminophen, alemtuzumab, amikacin, amiodarone, anidulafungin, argatroban, arsenic trioxide, atracurium, atropine, aztreonam, benztropine, bivalirudin, bleomycin, buprenorphine, calcium chloride, calcium gluconate, carboplatin, carmustine, caspofungin, cefazolin, cefotaxime, cefoxitin, ceftaroline, ceftolozane/tazobactam, ceftriaxone, ciprofloxacin, cisatracurium, cisplatin, cyanocobalamin, cyclophosphamide, cy-

closporine, cytarabine, dacarbazine, dactinomycin, daptomycin, daunorubicin hydrochloride, dexmedetomidine, dexrazoxane, digoxin, diltiazem, diphenhydramine, docetaxel, dopamine, doxorubicin hydrochloride, doxorubicin liposomal, doxycycline, enalaprilat, ephedrine, epinephrine, epirubicin, eptifibatide, eravacycline, erythromycin lactobionate, esmolol, etomidate, etoposide, etoposide phosphate, famotidine, fentanyl, fluconazole, fludarabine, folic acid, gemcitabine, gentamicin, glycopyrrolate, granisetron, heparin, hetastarch, hydromorphone, idarubicin, ifosfamide, imipenem/cilastatin/relebactam, irinotecan, isavuconazonium, isoproterenol, ketamine, labetalol, LR, leucovorin calcium, levofloxacin, lidocaine, linezolid, lorazepam, magnesium sulfate, mannitol, meperidine, mesna, methadone, metoclopramide, metoprolol, metronidazole, milrinone, mitoxantrone, morphine, multivitamins, mycophenolate, nalbuphine, naloxone, nicardipine, nitroglycerin, nitroprusside, norepinephrine, octreotide, ondansetron, oritavancin, oxacillin, oxaliplatin, oxytocin, paclitaxel, palonosetron, pamidronate, papaverine, pemetrexed, penicillin G, pentamidine, phentolamine, phenylephrine, phytonadione, plazomicin, potassium chloride, procainamide, promethazine, propranolol, protamine, pyridoxine, remifentanil, rifampin, rocuronium, succinylcholine, sufentanil, tacrolimus, tedizolid, theophylline, thiotepa, tigecycline, tirofiban, tobramycin, topotecan, vancomycin, vasopressin, vecuronium, verapamil, vinblastine, vincristine, vinorelbine, voriconazole, zoledronic acid.

● **Y-Site Incompatibility:** acyclovir, albumin, human, aminocaproic acid, aminophylline, amphotericin B deoxycholate, amphotericin B lipid complex, amphotericin B liposomal, ampicillin, ampicillin/sulbactam, ascorbic acid, azathioprine, azithromycin, blinatumomab, cefepime, ceftazidime, cefuroxime, chloramphenicol, dantrolene, dexamethasone, diazepam, epoetin alfa, ertapenem, esomeprazole, fluorouracil, foscarnet, fosphenytoin, ganciclovir, gemtuzumab ozogamicin, hydrocortisone, ibuprofen lysine, indomethacin, ketorolac, meropenem, meropenem/vaborbactam, methotrexate, micafungin, mitomycin, pentobarbital, phenobarbital, phenytoin, piperacillin/tazobactam, potassium acetate, prochlorperazine, sodium bicarbonate, thiopental, trimethoprim/sulfamethoxazole.

Patient/Family Teaching

● Inform patient that this medication will decrease mental recall of the procedure.
● Advise patient to avoid grapefruit juice during therapy.
● May cause drowsiness or dizziness. Advise patient to request assistance prior to ambulation and transfer and to avoid driving or other activities requiring alertness for 24 hr following administration.
● Instruct patient to notify health care professional of all Rx or OTC medications, vitamins, or herbal products being taken and to consult health care professional before taking any Rx, OTC, or herbal products, especially blood pressure medicine, antibiotics, and St. John's wort.
● Advise patient to avoid alcohol or other CNS depressants, including opioids, for 24 hr following administration of midazolam; may cause overdose.
● Advise patient and family to notify health care professional if thoughts about suicide or dying, attempts to commit suicide; new or worse depression; new or worse anxiety; feeling very agitated or restless; panic attacks; trouble sleeping; new or worse irritability; acting aggressive; being angry or violent; acting on dangerous impulses; an extreme increase in activity and talking; other unusual changes in behavior or mood, or skin rash occur.
● Advise patient that midazolam is a drug with known abuse potential. Protect it from theft, and never give to anyone other than the individual for whom it was prescribed. Store out of sight and reach of children, and in a location not accessible by others.
● Rep: May cause fetal harm. Advise patient to notify health care professional if pregnancy is planned or suspected or if breastfeeding. Use in late pregnancy can result in sedation (respiratory depression, lethargy, hypotonia) and/or withdrawal symptoms (hyperreflexia, irritability, restlessness, tremors, inconsolable crying, and feeding difficulties) in the neonate. Monitor neonates exposed to midazolam during pregnancy or labor for signs of sedation and monitor neonates exposed to midazolam during pregnancy for signs of withdrawal. Monitor infants exposed to midazolam through breast milk for sedation, poor feeding, and poor weight gain. Encourage women who take midazolam during pregnancy to enroll in the North American Antiepileptic Drug Pregnancy Registry by calling 1-888-233-2334 or visiting http://www.aedpregnancyregistry.org to monitor pregnancy outcomes in women exposed to antiepileptic drugs.
● **Nayzilam:** Instruct individual administering *Nayzilam* on how to identify seizure clusters and use product appropriately. Advise patients and caregivers to read *Medication Guide* before starting and with each Rx refill in case of changes. Discuss safe use, risks, and proper storage and disposal of midazolam with patients and caregivers with each Rx refill.
● Advise patient that midazolam is a drug with known abuse potential. Protect it from theft, and never give to anyone other than the individual for whom it was prescribed. Store out of sight and reach of children, and in a location not accessible by others.

Evaluation/Desired Outcomes

● Sedation during and amnesia following surgical, diagnostic, and radiologic procedures.
● Sedation and amnesia for mechanically ventilated patients in a critical care setting.
● Termination of seizure activity.

miFEPRIStone (mi-fe-**priss**-tone)
Korlym, Mifeprex
Classification
Therapeutic: abortifacients, antidiabetics
Pharmacologic: antiprogestational agents

Indications
Mifeprex: Medical termination of intrauterine pregnancy up to day 70 of pregnancy (in combination with misoprostol). **Korlym**: Hyperglycemia secondary to hypercortisolism in patients with endogenous Cushing's syndrome who have type 2 diabetes or glucose intolerance and have failed or are not candidates for surgery.

Action
Antagonizes endometrial and myometrial effects of progesterone. Sensitizes the myometrium to contraction-inducing activity of prostaglandins. Antagonizes the glucocorticoid receptor. **Therapeutic Effects:** Termination of pregnancy. Improved control of blood glucose.

Pharmacokinetics
Absorption: Rapidly absorbed following oral administration (69% bioavailability); absorption enhanced with food.
Distribution: Unknown.
Protein Binding: 98%.
Metabolism and Excretion: Primarily metabolized by the liver via the CYP3A4 isoenzyme; primarily excreted in the feces.
Half-life: 18 hr.

TIME/ACTION PROFILE (termination of pregnancy)

ROUTE	ONSET	PEAK	DURATION
PO	unknown	within 2 days	unknown

Contraindications/Precautions
Contraindicated in: Hypersensitivity; Presence of an intrauterine device (IUD) (Mifeprex); Undiagnosed adnexal mass (Mifeprex); Chronic adrenal failure (Mifeprex); Concurrent long-term corticosteroid therapy; Bleeding disorders or concurrent anticoagulant therapy (Mifeprex); Inherited porphyrias (Mifeprex); Severe hepatic impairment (Korlym); Concurrent use with simvastatin, lovastatin, cyclosporine, dihydroergotamine, ergotamine, fentanyl, pimozide, quinidine, sirolimus, or tacrolimus (Korlym); Vaginal bleeding; Endometrial hyperplasia with atypia or endometrial carcinoma (Korlym); OB: Confirmed or suspected ectopic pregnancy (Mifeprex); OB: Pregnancy (Korlym).
Use Cautiously in: Chronic medical conditions such as cardiovascular, hypertensive, hepatic, renal, or respiratory disease (Mifeprex); Women >35 yrs old or who smoke ≥10 cigarettes/day (Mifeprex); Bleeding disorders or concurrent anticoagulant therapy (Korlym).

Adverse Reactions/Side Effects
CV: hypertension (Korlym), peripheral edema (Korlym), QT interval prolongation (Korlym). **Derm:** rash (Korlym). **Endo:** hypothyroidism (Korlym), ↓ HDL cholesterol (Korlym), adrenal insufficiency (Korlym). **F and E:** hypokalemia (Korlym). **GI:** abdominal pain (Mifeprex), anorexia (Korlym), constipation (Korlym), diarrhea, dry mouth (Korlym), nausea, vomiting. **GU:** uterine bleeding, uterine cramping (Mifeprex), pelvic pain (Mifeprex), ruptured ectopic pregnancy (Mifeprex). **MS:** arthralgia (Korlym), myalgia (Korlym). **Neuro:** anxiety (Korlym), dizziness, fatigue (Korlym), headache, fainting (Mifeprex), weakness (Mifeprex). **Resp:** dyspnea (Korlym), *Pneumocystis jiroveci* pneumonia. **Misc:** ANGIOEDEMA.

Interactions
Drug-Drug: ↑ blood levels and risk of toxicity from **dihydroergotamine, ergotamine, lovastatin, simvastatin, cyclosporine, fentanyl, pimozide, quinidine, sirolimus,** or **tacrolimus;** concurrent use with Korlym is contraindicated. **Strong CYP3A4 inhibitors,** including **ketoconazole, itraconazole, nefazodone, ritonavir, nelfinavir, atazanavir, fosamprenavir, clarithromycin, conivaptan, lopinavir/ritonavir, posaconazole,** or **voriconazole** may ↑ levels; adjust dose of Korlym. **Moderate CYP3A4 inhibitors,** including **aprepitant, diltiazem, fluconazole, imatinib,** or **verapamil** may ↑ levels; caution with concurrent use of Korlym. Blood levels and effects may be ↓ by **rifampin, rifabutin dexamethasone, phenytoin, phenobarbital,** and **carbamazepine;** avoid concurrent use with Korlym.
Drug-Natural Products: Levels and effects may be ↓ by **St. John's wort;** avoid concurrent use with Korlym.
Drug-Food: Levels and effects may be ↑ by **grapefruit juice;** caution with concurrent use of Korlym.

Route/Dosage
Mifeprex
PO (Adults): *Day 1:* 200 mg as a single dose, followed on *Day 2 or Day 3 (within 24–48 hr of taking Mifeprex)* by misoprostol 800 mcg (given as four 200–mcg tablets) given buccally.

Korlym
PO (Adults): 300 mg once daily; may ↑ by 300 mg/day every 2–4 wk (maximum dose = 1200 mg/day or 20 mg/kg/day); *Initiation of Korlym in patients already being treated with strong CYP3A4 inhibitor:* 300 mg once daily; may titrate up to 900 mg once daily, if needed; *Initiation of strong CYP3A4 inhibitor in patients already being treated with Korlym:* Current

M

dose of Korlym = 300 mg once daily: No change; Current dose of Korlym = 600 mg once daily: ↓ dose to 300 mg once daily (may titrate up to 600 mg once daily, if needed); Current dose of Korlym = 900 mg once daily: ↓ dose to 600 mg once daily; Current dose of Korlym = 1200 mg once daily: ↓ dose to 900 mg once daily.

Renal Impairment
PO (Adults): 300 mg once daily; may ↑ by 300 mg/day every 2–4 wk (maximum dose = 600 mg/day).

Hepatic Impairment
PO (Adults): 300 mg once daily; may ↑ by 300 mg/day every 2–4 wk (maximum dose = 600 mg/day).

Availability (generic available)
Tablets (Korlym): 300 mg. **Tablets (Mifeprex):** 200 mg.

NURSING IMPLICATIONS
Assessment
- **Mifeprex**: Determine duration of pregnancy. Pregnancy is dated from the first day of the last menstrual period in a presumed 28-day cycle with ovulation occurring at mid-cycle and can be determined by menstrual history and clinical examination; use ultrasound if duration is uncertain or if ectopic pregnancy is suspected. Assess women who became pregnant with an IUD in place for ectopic pregnancy.
- Assess amount of bleeding and cramping during treatment. Determine if termination is complete on day 14.
- **Korlym:** Monitor for changes in cushingoid appearance (acne, hirsutism, striae, body weight) during therapy.
- Monitor for signs and symptoms of adrenal insufficiency (weakness, nausea, increased fatigue, hypotension, hypoglycemia) during therapy. If adrenal insufficiency is suspected, discontinue Korlym and administer glucocorticoids immediately.

Lab Test Considerations
- **Mifeprex:** ↓ hemoglobin, hematocrit, and RBCs may occur in women who bleed heavily.
- Changes in quantitative human chorionic gonadotropin (hCG) levels are not accurate until at least 10 days after mifepristone administration; complete termination of pregnancy must be confirmed by clinical examination.
- **Korlym:** Verify negative pregnancy test in women prior to starting therapy or before restarting therapy if stopped for more than 14 days. Correct hypokalemia prior to starting therapy. Assess serum potassium 1–2 wk after starting or increasing dose of Korlym and periodically thereafter.
- Monitor A1c periodically during therapy.

Implementation
- Do not confuse mifepristone with misoprostol.
- *REMS:* Mifeprex is only available through a restricted program, mifepristone REMS program. Pre-scribers and pharmacies that dispense mifepristone must be certified by the program and patients must sign an agreement form.
- **Mifeprex:** Mifepristone should be administered only by health care professionals who have read and understood the prescribing information, are able to assess gestational age of an embryo and diagnose ectopic pregnancies, and who are able to provide surgical intervention in cases of incomplete abortion or severe bleeding.
- Remove any IUD prior to mifepristone administration.
- Measures to prevent rhesus immunization, similar to those of surgical abortion, should be taken.
- **PO:** On *day 1*, after the patient has read the *Medication Guide* and signed the Patient Agreement, administer one 200–mg tablet of mifepristone as a single dose. On *day 2 or 3*, unless abortion has occurred and been confirmed by clinical examination or ultrasound, administer four 200-mcg tablets of misoprostol buccally between 24 and 48 hrs after taking mifepristone. Expulsion of pregnancy usually happens within 2–24 hrs of taking misoprostol. On *day 7–14*, confirm that termination of pregnancy has occurred by clinical examination or ultrasound. If complete expulsion has not occurred, administer another dose of misoprostol 800 mcg buccally.
- **Korlym:** Administer with a meal. *DNC:* Swallow tablet whole; do not crush, break, or chew.
- If Korlym therapy is interrupted, reinitiate at lowest dose (300 mg).

Patient/Family Teaching
- **Mifeprex:** Advise patient of the treatment and its effects. Patients must be given a copy of the *Medication Guide and Patient Agreement*. Patient must understand the necessity of completing the treatment schedule of three office visits (day 1, day 2–3, and day 7–14).
- Inform patient that vaginal bleeding and uterine cramping will probably occur and that prolonged or heavy vaginal bleeding is not proof of complete expulsion. Bleeding or spotting occurs for an average of 9–16 days; but may continue for more than 30 days. Advise patient that if the treatment fails, there is a risk of fetal malformation; medical abortion failures are managed by surgical termination.
- Caution patient to notify health care professional immediately if heavy bleeding (soak through 2 thick full-size sanitary pads per hr for 2 consecutive hrs or are concerned about heavy bleeding); abdominal pain or feeling sick (weakness, nausea, vomiting, diarrhea, with or without abdominal pain or fever more than 24 hr after taking mifepristone); or fever (≥100.4°F that lasts >4 hrs, may indicate life-threatening sepsis) occurs.
- Instruct patient in the steps to take in an emergency situation, including precise instructions and a telephone number to call if she has problems or concerns.

- May cause dizziness or fainting. Caution patient to avoid driving or other activities requiring alertness until response to medication is known.
- Advise patient to notify health care professional if she smokes at least 10 cigarettes a day.
- Rep: Caution patient that pregnancy can occur following termination of pregnancy and before resumption of normal menses. Contraception can be initiated as soon as pregnancy termination is confirmed, or before sexual intercourse is resumed.
- Korlym: Instruct patient to take Korlym as directed. Advise patient to read *Medication Guide* prior to starting therapy and with each refill in case of changes.
- Caution patient to avoid drinking grapefruit juice during therapy; may increase risk of side effects.
- Instruct patient to notify health care professional if signs and symptoms of adrenal insufficiency, abnormal vaginal bleeding, or low potassium (muscle weakness, aches, cramps, palpitations) occur.
- Advise patient to notify health care professional of all Rx or OTC medications, vitamins, or herbal products being taken and to consult with health care professional before taking other medications.
- Rep: May cause fetal harm. Advise female patient to use a nonhormonal form of contraception during and for at least 1 mo after last dose of therapy. Notify health care professional immediately if pregnancy is suspected. Advise female patient to avoid breastfeeding during therapy. To minimize exposure to a breastfed infant, women who discontinue or interrupt Korlym therapy may consider pumping and discarding milk during therapy and for 18–21 days (5–6 half-lives) after last dose, before breastfeeding.

Evaluation/Desired Outcomes

- **Mifeprex:** Termination of an intrauterine pregnancy of less than 70 days duration.
- **Korlym:** Improved control of blood glucose.

BEERS

milnacipran (mil-na-**sip**-ran)
Savella
Classification
Therapeutic: antifibromyalgia agents
Pharmacologic: selective norepinephrine reuptake inhibitors

Indications
Fibromyalgia.

Action
Inhibits neuronal reuptake of norepinephrine and serotonin. **Therapeutic Effects:** Decreased pain associated with fibromyalgia.

Pharmacokinetics
Absorption: 85–90% absorbed following oral administration.
Distribution: Unknown.
Metabolism and Excretion: Mostly excreted in urine as unchanged drug (55%) and inactive metabolites.
Half-life: *D:* isomer 8–10 hr; *L:* isomer 4–6 hr.

TIME/ACTION PROFILE (↓ in pain)

ROUTE	ONSET	PEAK	DURATION
PO	1 wk	unknown	unknown

Contraindications/Precautions
Contraindicated in: Concurrent use of MAO inhibitors or MAO-like drugs (linezolid or methylene blue); End-stage renal disease; Significant history of alcohol use/abuse; Chronic liver disease; Lactation: Lactation.
Use Cautiously in: History of suicide risk or attempt; History of seizures; Moderate to severe renal impairment (↓ dose if CCr <30 mL/min); Hypertension; Severe hepatic impairment; Obstructive uropathy (↑ risk of adverse genitourinary effects); Angle-closure glaucoma; OB: Use during pregnancy only if potential maternal benefit justifies potential fetal risk; Pedi: ↑ risk of suicidal thinking and behavior (suicidality) in adolescents and young adults up to 24 yr with major depressive disorder and other psychiatric disorders; Geri: Appears on Beers list. May worsen or cause syndrome of inappropriate antidiuretic hormone (SIADH) secretion and/or hyponatremia in older adults. Use with caution in older adults and closely monitor sodium concentrations when starting therapy or ↑ dose.

Adverse Reactions/Side Effects
CV: hypertension, tachycardia. **Derm:** ↑ sweating, hot flush. **Endo:** SIADH. **F and E:** hyponatremia. **GI:** ↑ liver enzymes, constipation, dry mouth, nausea, PANCREATITIS, vomiting. **GU:** ↓ libido, delayed/absent orgasm, ejaculatory delay/failure, erectile dysfunction. **Hemat:** BLEEDING. **Neuro:** dizziness, headache, insomnia, NEUROLEPTIC MALIGNANT SYNDROME, SUICIDAL THOUGHTS. **Misc:** SEROTONIN SYNDROME.

Interactions
Drug-Drug: Concurrent use with **MAO inhibitors** may result in serious, potentially fatal reactions; wait at least 14 days following discontinuation of MAO inhibitor before initiation of milnacipran. Wait at least 5 days after discontinuing milnacipran before initiation of MAO inhibitor. Concurrent use with **MAO-inhibitor-like drugs**, such as **linezolid** or **methylene blue** may ↑ risk of serotonin syndrome; concurrent use contraindicated; do not start therapy in patients receiving linezolid or methylene blue; if linezolid or methylene blue need to be started in a patient receiving milnacipran, immediately discontinue milnacipran and

monitor for signs/symptoms of serotonin syndrome for 5 days or until 24 hr after last dose of linezolid or methylene blue, whichever comes first (may resume milnacipran therapy 24 hr after last dose of linezolid or methylene blue). Drugs that affect serotonergic neurotransmitter systems, including **tricyclic antidepressants**, **SNRIs**, **fentanyl**, **lithium**, **buspirone**, **tramadol**, **meperidine**, **methadone**, **amphetamines**, and **triptans** ↑ risk of serotonin syndrome. ↑ risk of bleeding with **NSAIDs**, **aspirin**, **clopidogrel**, **prasugrel**, **ticagrelor**, **dabigatran**, **apixaban**, **edoxaban**, **rivaroxaban**, or **warfarin**. May ↓ antihypertensive effectiveness of **clonidine**. ↑ risk of hypertension and arrhythmias with **epinephrine** or **norepinephrine**. ↑ risk of euphoria and hypotension when switching from **clomipramine**. Concurrent use with **digoxin** may result in adverse hemodynamics, including hypotension and tachycardia; avoid concurrent use with IV digoxin. **Drug-Natural Products:** Use with **St. John's wort** ↑ serotonin syndrome.

Route/Dosage
PO (Adults): *Day 1:* 12.5 mg; *Day 2–3:* 12.5 mg twice daily; *Day 4–7:* 25 mg twice daily; *After Day 7:* 50 mg twice daily. Some patients may require up to 100 mg twice daily depending on response.

Renal Impairment
PO (Adults): *CCr 5–29 mL/min:* maintenance dose is 25 mg twice daily; some patients may require up to 50 mg twice daily depending on response.

Availability (generic available)
Tablets (contain tartrazine): 12.5 mg, 25 mg, 50 mg, 100 mg.

NURSING IMPLICATIONS
Assessment
- Assess intensity, quality, and location of pain periodically during therapy. May require several wk for effects to be seen.
- Monitor BP and heart rate before and periodically during therapy. Treat pre-existing hypertension and cardiac disease prior to therapy. Sustained hypertension may be dose related; decrease dose or discontinue therapy if this occurs.
- Monitor closely for changes in behavior that could indicate the emergence or worsening of suicidal thoughts or behavior or depression.
- Monitor for development of neuroleptic malignant syndrome (fever, respiratory distress, tachycardia, convulsions, diaphoresis, hypertension or hypotension, pallor, tiredness, severe muscle stiffness, loss of bladder control). Report symptoms immediately.
- Assess sexual function before starting milnacipran. Assess for changes in sexual function during treatment, including timing of onset; patient may not report.

Lab Test Considerations
- May cause ↑ ALT, AST, and bilirubin.
- May cause hyponatremia.

Implementation
- **PO:** May be administered without regard to meals; may be more tolerable if taken with food.

Patient/Family Teaching
- Instruct patient to take milnacipran as directed at the same time each day. Take missed doses as soon as possible unless time for next dose. Do not stop abruptly; must be decreased gradually. Advise patient to read the *Medication Guide* prior to therapy and with each Rx refill in case of changes.
- Encourage patient and family to be alert for emergence of anxiety, agitation, panic attacks, insomnia, irritability, hostility, impulsivity, akathisia, hypomania, mania, worsening of depression and suicidal ideation, especially during early antidepressant therapy. Assess symptoms on a day-to-day basis as changes may be abrupt. If these symptoms occur, notify health care professional.
- May cause dizziness. Caution patient to avoid driving or other activities requiring alertness until response to medication is known.
- Advise patient to notify health care professional of all Rx or OTC medications, vitamins, or herbal products being taken and to consult with health care professional before taking other medications, especially St. John's wort. Avoid use of aspirin, NSAIDs, and warfarin due to increased risk for bleeding.
- Instruct patient to notify health care professional if signs of liver damage (pruritus, dark urine, jaundice, right upper quadrant tenderness, unexplained "flu-like" symptoms) or hyponatremia (headache, difficulty concentrating, memory impairment, confusion, weakness, unsteadiness, falls), rash, or serotonin syndrome (mental status changes: agitation, hallucinations, coma; autonomic instability: tachycardia, labile BP, hyperthermia; neuromuscular aberrations: hyperreflexia, incoordination; and/or GI symptoms: nausea, vomiting, diarrhea) occur.
- Advise patient to avoid taking alcohol during milnacipran therapy.
- Inform patient that milnacipran may cause symptoms of sexual dysfunction. In males, ejaculatory delay or failure, decreased libido, and erectile dysfunction may occur. In female patients, may result in decreased libido and delayed or absent orgasm. Advise patient to notify health care professional if symptoms occur.
- Rep: May cause fetal harm. Instruct patient to notify health care professional if pregnancy is planned or suspected or if breastfeeding. May be associated with an increased risk of postpartum hemorrhage. Neonates exposed to milnacipran late in the third trimester have developed complications requiring prolonged hospitalization, respiratory support, and tube feeding; can arise immediately upon delivery. Symptoms may include respiratory distress, cyanosis, apnea, seizures, temperature instability, feeding difficulty, vomiting, hypoglycemia, hypotonia, hypertonia, hyperreflexia, tremor, jitteriness, irrita-

bility, and constant crying. Monitor infants exposed to milnacipran for agitation, irritability, poor feeding and poor weight gain. Encourage patients who become pregnant while taking milnacipran to enroll in the Savella pregnancy registry by calling 1-800-643-3010 or at www.savellapregnancyregistry.com.

- Encourage patient to maintain routine follow-up visits with health care provider to determine effectiveness.

Evaluation/Desired Outcomes
- Reduction in pain and soreness associated with fibromyalgia.

HIGH ALERT

milrinone (mill-ri-none)
~~Primacor~~
Classification
Therapeutic: inotropics

Indications
Short-term treatment of HF unresponsive to conventional therapy with digoxin, diuretics, and vasodilators.

Action
Increases myocardial contractility. Decreases preload and afterload by a direct dilating effect on vascular smooth muscle. **Therapeutic Effects:** Increased cardiac output (inotropic effect).

Pharmacokinetics
Absorption: IV administration results in complete bioavailability.
Distribution: Moderately distributed to tissues.
Metabolism and Excretion: 80–90% excreted unchanged by the kidneys.
Half-life: 2.3 hr (↑ in renal impairment).

TIME/ACTION PROFILE (hemodynamic effects)

ROUTE	ONSET	PEAK	DURATION
IV	5–15 min	unknown	3–6 hr

Contraindications/Precautions
Contraindicated in: Hypersensitivity; Severe aortic or pulmonic valvular heart disease; Hypertrophic subaortic stenosis (may ↑ outflow tract obstruction).
Use Cautiously in: History of arrhythmias, electrolyte abnormalities, abnormal digoxin levels, or insertion of vascular catheters (↑ risk of ventricular arrhythmias); Renal impairment (↓ infusion rate if CCr is <50 mL/min); OB: Safety not established in pregnancy; Lactation: Safety not established in breastfeeding.

Adverse Reactions/Side Effects
CV: angina pectoris, chest pain, hypotension, supraventricular arrhythmias, VENTRICULAR ARRHYTHMIAS. **Derm:**

rash. **GI:** ↑ liver enzymes. **Hemat:** thrombocytopenia. **Neuro:** headache, tremor.

Interactions
Drug-Drug: None reported.

Route/Dosage
IV (Adults): *Loading dose:* 50 mcg/kg followed by *Continuous infusion* at 0.5 mcg/kg/min (range 0.375–0.75 mcg/kg/min).
IV (Infants and Children): *Loading dose:* 50 mcg/kg over 10 min followed by *Continuous infusion* at 0.5 mcg/kg/min (range 0.25–0.75 mcg/kg/min).

Availability (generic available)
Solution for injection: 1 mg/mL. **Premixed infusion:** 20 mg/100 mL, 40 mg/200 mL.

NURSING IMPLICATIONS
Assessment
- Monitor heart rate and BP continuously during administration. Slow or discontinue if BP drops excessively.
- Monitor intake and output and daily weight. Assess patient for resolution of signs and symptoms of HF (peripheral edema, dyspnea, rales/crackles, weight gain) and improvement in hemodynamic parameters (increase in cardiac output and cardiac index, decrease in pulmonary capillary wedge pressure). Correct effects of previous aggressive diuretic therapy to allow for optimal filling pressure.
- Monitor ECG continuously during infusion. Arrhythmias are common and may be life threatening. The risk of ventricular arrhythmias is increased in patients with a history of arrhythmias, electrolyte abnormalities, abnormal digoxin levels, or insertion of vascular catheters.

Lab Test Considerations
- Monitor electrolytes and renal function frequently during administration. Correct hypokalemia prior to administration to decrease the risk of arrhythmias.
- Monitor platelet count during therapy.

Toxicity and Overdose
- *High Alert:* Overdose manifests as hypotension. Dose should be decreased or discontinued. Supportive measures may be necessary.

Implementation
- *High Alert:* Accidental overdose of milrinone can cause patient harm or death. Have second practitioner independently check original order, dose calculations, and infusion pump settings.

IV Administration
- IV Push: *Dilution:* Loading dose may be administered undiluted. May also be diluted in 0.9% NaCl, 0.45% NaCl, or D5W for ease of administration. *Concentration:* 1 mg/mL. *Rate:* Administer the loading dose over 10 min.

M

- **Continuous Infusion:** *Dilution:* Milrinone drawn from vials must be diluted. Dilute 10 mg (10 mL) of milrinone in 40 mL of diluent or 20 mg (20 mL) of milrinone in 80 mL of diluent. Compatible diluents include 0.45% NaCl, 0.9% NaCl, and D5W. Premixed infusions are already diluted and ready to use. Admixed solutions are stable for 72 hr at room temperature. Stability of premixed infusions based on manufacturer's expiration date. Do not use solutions that are discolored or contain particulate matter. *Concentration:* 200 mcg/mL. *Rate:* Based on patient's weight (see Route/Dosage section). Titrate according to hemodynamic and clinical response.
- **Y-Site Compatibility:** acyclovir, allopurinol, amifostine, amikacin, aminophylline, amiodarone, amphotericin B liposomal, ampicillin, anidulafungin, argatroban, atracurium, aztreonam, bivalirudin, bleomycin, bumetanide, buprenorphine, busulfan, butorphanol, calcium chloride, calcium gluconate, carboplatin, carmustine, caspofungin, cefazolin, cefepime, cefotaxime, cefotetan, cefoxitin, ceftaroline, ceftazidime, ceftriaxone, cefuroxime, chloramphenicol, chlorpromazine, ciprofloxacin, cisatracurium, cisplatin, clindamycin, cyclophosphamide, cyclosporine, cytarabine, dactinomycin, daptomycin, dexamethasone, dexmedetomidine, digoxin, diltiazem, dobutamine, docetaxel, dopamine, doxorubicin hydrochloride, doxycycline, droperidol, enalaprilat, ephedrine, epinephrine, epirubicin, eptifibatide, ertapenem, erythromycin, etoposide, etoposide phosphate, fentanyl, fluconazole, fludarabine, fluorouracil, ganciclovir, gemcitabine, gentamicin, glycopyrrolate, granisetron, haloperidol, heparin, hetastarch, hydralazine, hydrocortisone, hydromorphone, idarubicin, ifosfamide, insulin regular, irinotecan, isoproterenol, ketamine, ketorolac, labetalol, levofloxacin, linezolid, lorazepam, magnesium sulfate, mannitol, melphalan, meperidine, meropenem, methohexital, methotrexate, methylprednisolone, metoclopramide, metoprolol, metronidazole, micafungin, midazolam, mitoxantrone, morphine, mycophenolate, nafcillin, nalbuphine, naloxone, nicardipine, nitroglycerin, nitroprusside, norepinephrine, octreotide, oxacillin, oxaliplatin, oxytocin, paclitaxel, palonosetron, pamidronate, pemetrexed, pentobarbital, phenobarbital, phenylephrine, piperacillin/tazobactam, potassium acetate, potassium chloride, potassium phosphate, prochlorperazine, promethazine, propofol, propranolol, remifentanil, rocuronium, sodium acetate, sodium bicarbonate, sodium phosphate, succinylcholine, sufentanil, tacrolimus, telavancin, theophylline, thiopental, thiotepa, tigecycline, tirofiban, tobramycin, torsemide, vancomycin, vasopressin, vecuronium, verapamil, vincristine, vinorelbine, voriconazole, zidovudine, zoledronic acid.
- **Y-Site Incompatibility:** amphotericin B deoxycholate, amphotericin B lipid complex, dantrolene, diazepam, diphenhydramine, esmolol, furosemide, hydroxyzine, imipenem/cilastatin, lidocaine, ondansetron, pantoprazole, phenytoin, procainamide.

Patient/Family Teaching
- Inform patient and family of reasons for administration. Milrinone is not a cure but is a temporary measure to control the symptoms of HF.
- Rep: Advise females of reproductive potential to notify health care professional if pregnancy is planned or suspected or if breastfeeding.

Evaluation/Desired Outcomes
- Decrease in the signs and symptoms of HF.
- Improvement in hemodynamic parameters.

---

minocycline, See TETRACYCLINES.

---

mirabegron (mye-ra-**beg**-ron)
Myrbetriq
Classification
Therapeutic: urinary tract antispasmodics
Pharmacologic: beta-adrenergic agonists

Indications
Overactive bladder (OAB), including urge urinary incontinence, urgency, and frequency (either as monotherapy or in combination with solifenacin). Pediatric neurogenic detrusor overactivity.

Action
Acts as a selective beta-3 adrenergic agonist. Increases bladder capacity by relaxing detrusor smooth muscle during storage phase of bladder fill-void cycle. **Therapeutic Effects:** Decreased symptoms of OAB. Improved bladder capacity in neurogenic detrusor overactivity.

Pharmacokinetics
Absorption: 29–35% absorbed following oral administration.
Distribution: Widely distributed.
Metabolism and Excretion: Extensively metabolized, 6% excreted unchanged in urine (25 mg dose), remainder excreted in urine and feces as metabolites.
Half-life: *Adults:* 50 hr; *Children:* 26–31 hr.

TIME/ACTION PROFILE (effects on bladder)

ROUTE	ONSET	PEAK	DURATION
PO	unknown	3–4 hr†	24 hr

†Blood level.

Contraindications/Precautions
Contraindicated in: Hypersensitivity; Severe uncontrolled hypertension; End-stage renal disease (eGFR <15 mL/min/1.73 m² or requiring dialysis); Severe hepatic impairment.

Use Cautiously in: Hypertension; Bladder outlet obstruction/concurrent antimuscarinics (↑ risk of urinary retention); Concurrent use of antimuscarinics used to treat OAB; OB: Safety not established in pregnancy; Lactation: Safety not established in breastfeeding; Pedi: Children <3 yr (safety and effectiveness not established).

Adverse Reactions/Side Effects
CV: ↑ BP, tachycardia. **EENT:** nasopharyngitis. **GI:** constipation, diarrhea, nausea. **GU:** urinary tract infection. **Neuro:** dizziness, headache. **Misc:** ANGIOEDEMA.

Interactions
Drug-Drug: May ↑ levels and risk of toxicity of **CYP2D6 substrates**, including **desipramine, flecainide, metoprolol, propafenone**, and **thioridazine**. May ↑ levels and risk of toxicity with **digoxin**; use lowest effective level of digoxin/monitor serum levels).

Route/Dosage
The extended-release tablets and extended-release oral suspension are NOT interchangeable and should NOT be combined.

Overactive Bladder
PO (Adults): 25 mg once daily; may ↑ to 50 mg once daily, if needed, after 4–8 wk.

Renal Impairment
PO (Adults): *eGFR 15–29 mL/min/m²:* 25 mg once daily (max dose = 25 mg/day).

Hepatic Impairment
PO (Adults): *Moderate hepatic impairment:* 25 mg once daily (max dose = 25 mg/day).

Neurogenic Detrusor Overactivity
PO (Children ≥3 yr and ≥35 kg): *Extended-release tablets:* 25 mg once daily; may ↑ to 50 mg once daily, if needed, after 4–8 wk. *Extended-release oral suspension (granules):* 48 mg once daily; may ↑ to 80 mg once daily, if needed after 4–8 wk.
PO (Children ≥3 yr and 22–<35 kg): *Extended-release oral suspension (granules):* 32 mg once daily; may ↑ to 64 mg once daily, if needed after 4–8 wk.
PO (Children ≥3 yr and 11–<22 kg): *Extended-release oral suspension (granules):* 24 mg once daily; may ↑ to 48 mg once daily, if needed after 4–8 wk.

Renal Impairment
PO (Children ≥3 yr and ≥35 kg): *eGFR 15–29 mL/min/m²:* Extended-release tablets: 25 mg once daily (max dose = 25 mg/day); Extended-release oral suspension (granules): 48 mg once daily (max dose = 48 mg/day).

Renal Impairment
PO (Children ≥3 yr and 22–<35 kg): *eGFR 15–29 mL/min/m²:* Extended-release oral suspension (granules): 32 mg once daily (max dose = 32 mg/day).

Renal Impairment
PO (Children ≥3 yr and 11–<22 kg): *eGFR 15–29 mL/min/m²:* Extended-release oral suspension (granules): 24 mg once daily (max dose = 24 mg/day).

Hepatic Impairment
PO (Children ≥3 yr and ≥35 kg): *Moderate hepatic impairment:* Extended-release tablets: 25 mg once daily (max dose = 25 mg/day); Extended-release oral suspension (granules): 48 mg once daily (max dose = 48 mg/day).

Hepatic Impairment
PO (Children ≥3 yr and 22–<35 kg): *Moderate hepatic impairment:* Extended-release oral suspension (granules): 32 mg once daily (max dose = 32 mg/day).

Hepatic Impairment
PO (Children ≥3 yr and 11–<22 kg): *Moderate hepatic impairment:* Extended-release oral suspension (granules): 24 mg once daily (max dose = 24 mg/day).

Availability (generic available)
Extended-release tablets: 25 mg, 50 mg. **Extended-release oral suspension (granules):** 8 mg/mL.

NURSING IMPLICATIONS
Assessment
- Assess patient for urinary urgency, frequency, and urge incontinence periodically during therapy.
- Monitor BP prior to starting and periodically during therapy; may cause ↑ BP.
- Monitor for signs and symptoms of angioedema (swelling of face, lips, tongue and/or larynx). Discontinue mirabegron and treat symptomatically.

Implementation
- Tablets and granules are different products. Do not interchange, substitute, or combine.

Overactive Bladder
- **PO:** Administer without regard to food.
- *DNC:* Swallow tablets whole with water; do not break, crush, or chew.

Neurogenic Detrusor Overactivity
- Pediatric patients weighing ≥35 kg may use tablets or granules. Administer as an extended-release oral suspension once daily.
- *DNC:* Swallow tablets whole with water; do not break, crush, or chew.
- Administer granules for patients weighing <35 kg. Granules are prepared as an extended-release oral suspension with a concentration of 8 mg/mL. Shake bottle for 1 min then let stand until foam on top of suspension is gone (about 1–2 min). Administer

within 1 hr after preparation with food once daily; do not save dose for later.

Patient/Family Teaching

- Instruct patient to take mirabegron as directed. If a dose is missed, take as soon as remembered unless >12 hrs since missed dose. If >12 hrs since missed dose, omit dose and take next dose at scheduled time. Advise patient to read *Patient Information* sheet prior to starting and with each Rx refill, in case of changes.
- Inform patient that mirabegron may cause an increase in BP. Advise patient to have BP checked periodically during therapy.
- May cause dizziness. Caution patient to avoid driving or other activities requiring alertness until response to medication is known.
- Advise patient to notify health care professional if difficulty emptying bladder occurs.
- Advise patient to notify health care professional of all Rx or OTC medications, vitamins, or herbal products being taken and to consult with health care professional before taking other medications.
- Rep: Advise females of reproductive potential to notify health care professional if pregnancy is planned or suspected or if breastfeeding.

Evaluation/Desired Outcomes

- Decreased urinary frequency, urgency, and urge incontinence.

BEERS

mirtazapine (meer-taz-a-peen)
Remeron, ❋ Remeron RD, Remeron SolTab
Classification
Therapeutic: antidepressants
Pharmacologic: tetracyclic antidepressants

Indications

Major depressive disorder. **Unlabeled Use:** Panic disorder. Generalized anxiety disorder. Post-traumatic stress disorder.

Action

Potentiates the effects of norepinephrine and serotonin. **Therapeutic Effects:** Antidepressant action, which may develop only after several wk.

Pharmacokinetics

Absorption: Well absorbed but rapidly metabolized, resulting in 50% bioavailability.
Distribution: Unknown.
Protein Binding: 85%.
Metabolism and Excretion: Extensively metabolized by the liver by the CYP1A2, CYP2D6, and CYP3A isoenzymes; metabolites excreted in urine (75%) and feces (15%).
Half-life: 20–40 hr.

TIME/ACTION PROFILE (antidepressant effect)

ROUTE	ONSET	PEAK	DURATION
PO	1–2 wk	6 wk or more	unknown

Contraindications/Precautions

Contraindicated in: Hypersensitivity; Concurrent use of MAO inhibitors or MAO-like drugs (linezolid or methylene blue).
Use Cautiously in: History of seizures; History of suicide attempt; May ↑ risk of suicide attempt/ideation especially during early treatment or dose adjustment; History of mania/hypomania; Patients with hepatic or renal impairment; Angle-closure glaucoma; OB: Other antidepressants are preferred in pregnancy; Lactation: Other antidepressants are preferred when breastfeeding; Pedi: Safety and effectiveness in children not established. Suicide risk may be greater in children or adolescents; Geri: Appears on Beers list. May worsen or cause syndrome of inappropriate antidiuretic hormone (SIADH) secretion and/or hyponatremia in older adults. Use with caution in older adults and closely monitor sodium concentrations when starting therapy or ↑ dose.

Adverse Reactions/Side Effects

CV: edema, hypotension. **Derm:** BULLOUS DERMATITIS, DRUG REACTION WITH EOSINOPHILIA AND SYSTEMIC SYMPTOMS (DRESS), ERYTHEMA MULTIFORME, pruritus, rash, STEVENS-JOHNSON SYNDROME, TOXIC EPIDERMAL NECROLYSIS. **EENT:** sinusitis. **Endo:** SIADH. **F and E:** ↑ thirst, hyponatremia. **GI:** ↑ appetite, constipation, dry mouth, ↑ liver enzymes, abdominal pain, anorexia, nausea, vomiting. **GU:** urinary frequency. **Hemat:** AGRANULOCYTOSIS. **Metab:** weight gain, hypercholesterolemia, hypertriglyceridemia. **MS:** arthralgia, back pain, myalgia. **Neuro:** drowsiness, abnormal dreams, abnormal thinking, agitation, akathisia, anxiety, apathy, confusion, dizziness, hyperkinesia, hypoesthesia, malaise, NEUROLEPTIC MALIGNANT SYNDROME, SUICIDAL THOUGHTS, twitching, weakness. **Resp:** cough, dyspnea. **Misc:** flu-like syndrome, SEROTONIN SYNDROME.

Interactions

Drug-Drug: May cause hypertension, seizures, and death when used with **MAO inhibitors**; do not use within 14 days of MAO inhibitor therapy. Concurrent use with **MAO-inhibitor like drugs**, such as **linezolid** or **methylene blue** may ↑ risk of serotonin syndrome; concurrent use contraindicated; do not start therapy in patients receiving **linezolid** or **methylene blue**; if **linezolid** or **methylene blue** need to be started in a patient receiving mirtazapine, immediately discontinue mirtazapine and monitor for signs/symptoms of serotonin syndrome for 2 wk or until 24 hr after last dose of linezolid or methylene blue, whichever comes first (may resume mirtazapine therapy 24 hr after last dose of linezolid or methylene blue). **Drugs that affect serotonergic neurotransmitter systems, including**

tricyclic antidepressants, SNRIs, fentanyl, buspirone, tramadol, and triptans ↑ risk of serotonin syndrome. ↑ CNS depression with other CNS depressants, including alcohol and benzodiazepines. Ketoconazole, cimetidine, clarithromycin, erythromycin, itraconazole, nefazodone, nelfinavir, or ritonavir may ↑ levels. Phenobarbital, phenytoin, carbamazepine, rifampin, or rifabutin may ↓ levels; may need to ↑ mirtazapine dose. May ↑ the effects and risk of bleeding from warfarin.

Drug-Natural Products: Concomitant use of kava-kava, valerian, skullcap, chamomile, or hops can ↑ CNS depression. ↑ risk of serotonin syndrome with St. John's wort and SAMe.

Route/Dosage
PO (Adults): 15 mg/day as a single bedtime dose initially; may be ↑ every 1–2 wk up to 45 mg/day.

Availability (generic available)
Tablets: 7.5 mg, 15 mg, 30 mg, 45 mg. Orally disintegrating tablets (orange flavor): 15 mg, 30 mg, 45 mg.

NURSING IMPLICATIONS

Assessment
- Assess mental status (orientation, mood, behavior) frequently. Assess for suicidal tendencies, especially during early therapy. Restrict amount of drug available to patient.
- Monitor closely for changes in behavior that could indicate the emergence or worsening of suicidal thoughts or behavior or depression.
- Assess weight and BMI initially and throughout therapy. For overweight/obese individuals, obtain fasting blood glucose and cholesterol levels. Refer as appropriate for nutritional/weight management and medical management.
- Monitor BP and pulse rate periodically during initial therapy. Report significant changes.
- Monitor for seizure activity in patients with a history of seizures or alcohol abuse. Institute seizure precautions.
- Assess skin periodically during therapy. Severe skin reactions, including drug reaction with eosinophilia and systemic symptoms (DRESS), Stevens-Johnson syndrome, bullous dermatitis, erythema multiforme and toxic epidermal necrolysis may occur. Discontinue mirtazapine immediately if signs of severe skin reactions occur.
- Assess for serotonin syndrome (mental changes [agitation, hallucinations, coma], autonomic instability [tachycardia, labile BP, hyperthermia], neuromuscular aberrations [hyper reflexia, incoordination], and/or GI symptoms [nausea, vomiting, diarrhea]), especially in patients taking other serotonergic drugs (SSRIs, SNRIs, triptans).
- Monitor for development of neuroleptic malignant syndrome (fever, respiratory distress, tachycardia, seizures, diaphoresis, hypertension or hypotension, pallor, tiredness). Discontinue mirtazapine and notify health care professional immediately if these symptoms occur.

Lab Test Considerations
- Assess CBC and hepatic function before and periodically during therapy.

Implementation
- Do not confuse Remeron with Rozerem.
- May be given as a single dose at bedtime to minimize excessive drowsiness or dizziness.
- May be taken without regard to food.
- For *orally disintegrating tablets*, do not attempt to push through foil backing; with dry hands, peal back backing and remove tablet. Immediately place tablet on tongue; tablet will dissolve in sec, then swallow with saliva. Administration with liquid is not necessary.

Patient/Family Teaching
- Instruct patient to take mirtazapine as directed. Take missed doses as soon as remembered; if almost time for next dose, skip missed dose and return to regular schedule. If single bedtime dose regimen is used, do not take missed dose in morning, but consult health care professional. Do not discontinue abruptly; gradual dose reduction may be required. Advise patient to read *Medication Guide* before starting therapy and with each Rx refill in case of changes.
- May cause drowsiness and dizziness. Caution patient to avoid driving and other activities requiring alertness until response to drug is known.
- Encourage patient and family to be alert for emergence of anxiety, agitation, panic attacks, insomnia, irritability, hostility, impulsivity, akathisia, hypomania, mania, worsening of depression and suicidal ideation, especially during early antidepressant therapy. Assess symptoms on a day-to-day basis as changes may be abrupt. If these symptoms occur, notify health care professional.
- Caution patient to change positions slowly to minimize orthostatic hypotension.
- Advise patient to avoid alcohol or other CNS depressant drugs during and for at least 3–7 days after therapy has been discontinued.
- Instruct patient to notify health care professional of signs and symptoms of serotonin syndrome (mental status changes: agitation, hallucinations, coma; autonomic instability: tachycardia, labile BP, hyperthermia; neuromuscular aberrations: hyperreflexia, incoordination; and/or gastrointestinal symptoms: nausea, vomiting, diarrhea) or rash occur.
- Advise patient to notify health care professional if dry mouth, urinary retention, or constipation occurs.

M

Frequent rinses, good oral hygiene, and sugarless candy or gum may diminish dry mouth. An increase in fluid intake, fiber, and exercise may prevent constipation.

- Inform patient of need to monitor dietary intake. Increase in appetite may lead to undesired weight gain.
- Advise patient to notify health care professional of all Rx or OTC medications, vitamins, or herbal products being taken and to consult with health care professional before taking other medications, especially St. John's wort.
- Advise patient to notify health care professional of medication regimen before treatment or surgery.
- Rep: Advise females of reproductive potential to notify health care professional if pregnancy is planned or suspected or if breastfeeding. Inform patient of National Pregnancy Registry for Antidepressants that monitors pregnancy outcomes in women exposed to antidepressants during pregnancy. Register patients by calling 1-844-405-6185 or visiting online at https://womensmentalhealth.org/clinical-and-research-programs/pregnancyregistry/antidepressants/.
- Therapy for depression may be prolonged. Emphasize the importance of follow-up exam to monitor effectiveness and side effects.

Evaluation/Desired Outcomes
- Resolution of the symptoms of depression.
- Increased sense of well-being.
- Renewed interest in surroundings.
- Increased appetite.
- Improved energy level.
- Improved sleep.
- Therapeutic effects may be seen within 1 wk, although several wk are usually necessary before improvement is observed.

miSOPROStol
(mye-soe-**prost**-ole)
Cytotec
Classification
Therapeutic: antiulcer agents, cytoprotective agents, abortifacients
Pharmacologic: prostaglandins

Indications
Prevention of gastric mucosal injury from NSAIDs, including aspirin, in high-risk patients (older adults, debilitated patients, or those with a history of ulcers). Termination of pregnancy (in combination with mifepristone). **Unlabeled Use:** Treatment of duodenal ulcers. Cervical ripening and labor induction.

Action
Acts as a prostaglandin analogue, decreasing gastric acid secretion (antisecretory effect) and increasing the production of protective mucus (cytoprotective effect).

Causes uterine contractions. **Therapeutic Effects:** Prevention of gastric ulceration from NSAIDs. With mifepristone, terminates pregnancy of less than 49 days.

Pharmacokinetics
Absorption: Well absorbed following oral administration.
Distribution: Unknown.
Protein Binding: 85%.
Metabolism and Excretion: Metabolized in liver to its active form (misoprostol acid); 80% excreted by the kidneys.
Half-life: 20–40 min.

TIME/ACTION PROFILE (effect on gastric acid secretion)

ROUTE	ONSET	PEAK	DURATION
PO	30 min	unknown	3–6 hr

Contraindications/Precautions
Contraindicated in: Hypersensitivity to prostaglandins; OB: Should not be used to prevent NSAID-induced gastric injury in pregnancy due to potential for fetal harm or death; Lactation: Lactation.
Use Cautiously in: Rep: Women of reproductive potential; Pedi: Safety and effectiveness not established in children.
Exercise Extreme Caution in: Late trimester pregnancy, previous Caesarian section or uterine surgery, advanced gestational age, or ≥5 previous pregnancies (when used for cervical ripening or to induce abortion, may cause uterine rupture).

Adverse Reactions/Side Effects
GI: abdominal pain, diarrhea, constipation, dyspepsia, flatulence, nausea, vomiting. **GU:** miscarriage, menstrual disorders. **Neuro:** headache.

Interactions
Drug-Drug: ↑ risk of diarrhea with **magnesium-containing antacids**.

Route/Dosage
Prevention of NSAID-Induced Ulcers
PO (Adults): 200 mcg 4 times daily with or after meals and at bedtime, *or* 400 mcg twice daily, with the last dose at bedtime. If intolerance occurs, dose may be ↓ to 100 mcg 4 times daily.

Pregnancy Termination
PO (Adults): 400 mcg single dose 2 days after mifepristone if abortion has not occurred.

Cervical Ripening and Labor Induction
Intravaginally (Adults): 25 mcg (¼ of 100-mcg tablet); may repeat every 3–6 hr, if needed.

Availability (generic available)
Tablets: 100 mcg, 200 mcg. *In combination with:* diclofenac (Arthrotec). See Appendix N.

NURSING IMPLICATIONS
Assessment
- Assess patient routinely for epigastric or abdominal pain and for frank or occult blood in the stool, emesis, or gastric aspirate.
- Assess women of reproductive potential for pregnancy. Misoprostol is usually begun on 2nd or 3rd day of menstrual period following a negative pregnancy test result.
- **Termination of pregnancy:** Monitor uterine cramping and bleeding during therapy.
- **Cervical Ripening:** Assess dilation of cervix periodically during therapy.

Implementation
- Do not confuse misoprostol with mifepristone.
- Misoprostol therapy should be started at the onset of treatment with NSAIDs.
- **PO:** Administer medication with meals and at bedtime to reduce severity of diarrhea.
- Antacids may be administered before or after misoprostol for relief of pain. Avoid those containing magnesium, because of increased diarrhea with misoprostol.

Patient/Family Teaching
- Instruct patient to take medication as directed for the full course of therapy, even if feeling better. Take missed doses as soon as possible unless next dose is due within 2 hr; do not double doses. Emphasize that sharing of this medication may be dangerous.
- Advise patient not to share misoprostol with others, even if they have similar symptoms; may be dangerous.
- Rep: Inform patient that misoprostol will cause spontaneous abortion. Women of reproductive potential must be informed of this effect through verbal and written information and must use contraception throughout therapy. If pregnancy is suspected, the woman should stop taking misoprostol and immediately notify her health care professional.
- Inform patient that diarrhea may occur. Health care professional should be notified if diarrhea persists for more than 1 wk. Also advise patient to report onset of black, tarry stools or severe abdominal pain.
- Advise patient to avoid alcohol and foods that may cause an increase in GI irritation.

Evaluation/Desired Outcomes
- The prevention of gastric ulcers in patients receiving chronic NSAID therapy.
- Termination of pregnancy.
- Cervical ripening and induction of labor.

---

mitoXANTRONE
(mye-toe-**zan**-trone)
~~Novantrone~~

Classification
Therapeutic: antineoplastics, immune modifiers
Pharmacologic: antitumor antibiotics

Indications
Acute nonlymphocytic leukemia (in combination with other antineoplastics). Initial chemotherapy for patients with pain associated with advanced hormone-refractory prostate cancer. Secondary (chronic) progressive, progressive relapsing, or worsening relapsing-remitting multiple sclerosis (MS).

Action
Inhibits DNA synthesis (cell-cycle phase–nonspecific). **Therapeutic Effects:** Death of rapidly replicating cells, particularly malignant ones. Decreased pain in patients with advanced prostate cancer. Decreased disability and slowed progression of MS.

Pharmacokinetics
Absorption: IV administration results in complete bioavailability.
Distribution: Widely distributed to tissues; limited penetration of CSF.
Metabolism and Excretion: Mostly eliminated by hepatobiliary clearance; <10% excreted unchanged by the kidneys.
Half-life: 5.8 days.

TIME/ACTION PROFILE (effects on blood counts)

ROUTE	ONSET	PEAK	DURATION
IV	unknown	10 days	21 days

Contraindications/Precautions
Contraindicated in: Hypersensitivity; OB: Pregnancy; Lactation: Lactation.
Use Cautiously in: Cardiovascular disease (↑ risk of HF); Active infection; ↓ bone marrow reserve; Previous mediastinal radiation or use of anthracyclines (↑ risk of HF); Impaired hepatobiliary function; Rep: Women of reproductive potential; Pedi: Safety and effectiveness not established in children; Geri: Older adults may have ↑ sensitivity to drug effects.

Adverse Reactions/Side Effects
CV: arrhythmias, ECG changes, HF. **Derm:** alopecia, rash. **EENT:** blue-green sclera, conjunctivitis. **GI:** abdominal pain, diarrhea, HEPATOTOXICITY, nausea, stomatitis, vomiting. **GU:** blue-green urine, gonadal suppression, renal failure. **Hemat:** anemia, leukopenia, thrombocytopenia, SECONDARY LEUKEMIA. **Metab:** hyperuricemia. **Neuro:** headache, SEIZURES. **Resp:** cough, dyspnea. **Misc:** fever, HYPERSENSITIVITY REACTIONS.

Interactions
Drug-Drug: ↑ bone marrow depression with other **antineoplastics** or **radiation therapy**. Risk of car-

diomyopathy ↑ by previous **anthracycline antineo-plastics (daunorubicin, doxorubicin, idarubicin)** or **mediastinal radiation**. May ↓ antibody response to **live-virus vaccines** and ↑ risk of adverse reactions.

Route/Dosage
Acute Nonlympocytic Leukemia
IV (Adults): *Induction:* 12 mg/m²/day for 3 days (usually given with cytosine arabinoside 100 mg/m²/day for 7 days); if incomplete remission occurs, a 2nd induction may be given. *Consolidation:* 12 mg/m²/day for 2 days (usually given with cytosine arabinoside 100 mg/m²/day for 5 days), given 6 wk after induction with another course 4 wk later.

Advanced Prostate Cancer
IV (Adults): 12–14 mg/m² as single dose (with corticosteroids).

Multiple Sclerosis
IV (Adults): 12 mg/m² every 3 mo.

Availability (generic available)
Solution for injection: 2 mg/mL.

NURSING IMPLICATIONS
Assessment
- Monitor for hypersensitivity reaction (rash, urticaria, bronchospasm, tachycardia, hypotension, wheezing, tightness in chest or throat, swelling of mouth, face, lips, tongue, or throat). If these occur, stop infusion and notify health care professional. Keep epinephrine, an antihistamine, and resuscitation equipment close by in the event of an anaphylactic reaction.
- Monitor for bone marrow depression. Assess for bleeding (bleeding gums, bruising, petechiae, guaiac stools, urine, and emesis) and avoid IM injections and taking rectal temperatures if platelet count is low. Apply pressure to venipuncture sites for 10 min. Assess for signs of infection during neutropenia. Anemia may occur. Monitor for increased fatigue, dyspnea, and orthostatic hypotension.
- Monitor intake and output, appetite, and nutritional intake. Assess patient for nausea and vomiting. Antiemetics may be administered prophylactically. Adjust diet as tolerated to help maintain fluid and electrolyte balance and nutritional status.
- Monitor chest x-ray, ECG, echocardiography or MUGA, and radionuclide angiography to determine ejection fraction prior to and periodically during therapy. Multiple sclerosis patients with baseline left ventricular ejection fraction (LVEF)<50% should not receive mitoxantrone. May cause cardiotoxicity, especially in patients who have received daunorubicin or doxorubicin. Assess for rales/crackles, dyspnea, edema, jugular vein distention, ECG changes, arrhythmias, and chest pain. Monitor LVEF with echocardiogram or MUGA if signs of HF occur, prior to each dose, and yearly after stopping therapy in patients with multiple sclerosis. Potentially fatal HF may

occur during or for mo or years after therapy. Risk is greater in patients receiving a cumulative dose >140 mg/m².
- Monitor for symptoms of gout (↑ uric acid levels and joint pain and swelling). Encourage patient to drink at least 2 L of fluid per day. Allopurinol may be given to decrease serum uric acid levels.
- **Multiple sclerosis:** Asses frequency of exacerbations of symptoms of multiple sclerosis periodically during therapy.

Lab Test Considerations
- Verify negative pregnancy test before starting therapy.
- Monitor CBC with differential and platelet count prior to and periodically during therapy. The nadir of leukopenia usually occurs within 10 days, and recovery usually occurs within 21 days.
- Monitor liver function studies (AST, ALT, LDH, bilirubin) and renal function studies (BUN, serum creatinine) prior to and periodically during therapy to detect hepatotoxicity and nephrotoxicity.
- May cause ↑ uric acid concentrations. Monitor periodically during therapy.

Implementation
- Do not confuse mitoxantrone with mitomycin or MTX Patch (lidocaine/menthol).
- There are lifetime maximum doses for mitoxantrone. Check manufacturer's information and patient history before administering.
- Solution should be prepared in a biologic cabinet. Wear gloves, gown, and mask while handling medication. Discard equipment in designated containers.
- Avoid contact with skin. Use Luer-Lok tubing to prevent accidental leakage. If contact with skin occurs, immediately wash skin with soap and water.
- Clean all spills with an aqueous solution of calcium hypochlorite. Mix solution by adding 5.5 parts (per weight) of calcium hypochlorite to 13 parts water.

IV Administration
- **IV:** Monitor IV site. Mitoxantrone is an irritant with vesicant-like properties. Administer only into a free-flowing IV; may cause severe local tissue damage if extravasation occurs. Ensure proper needle or catheter placement prior to and during infusion. Avoid extravasation. If extravasation occurs, discontinue IV and restart at another site. Elevate extremity with extravasation and place ice packs over area. Monitor closely and obtain surgical consultation if local reaction occurs.
- **IV Push:** *Dilution:* Dilute dark blue mitoxantrone solution in at least 50 mL of 0.9% NaCl or D5W. Discard unused solution appropriately. *Rate:* Administer slowly over at least 3 min into the tubing of a free-flowing IV of 0.9% NaCl or D5W.
- **Intermittent Infusion:** May be further diluted in D5W, 0.9% NaCl, or D5/0.9% NaCl and used immediately. *Concentration:* 0.02–0.5 mg/mL. Open vials may be stored at room temperature for 7 days

or under refrigeration for up to 14 days. Solutions diluted in D5W or 0.9% NaCl are stable for up to 7 days at room temperature or under refrigeration; manufacturer recommends immediate use. *Rate:* Administer over 15–30 min.

- **Continuous Infusion:** May also be administered over 24 hr.

- **Y-Site Compatibility:** acyclovir, alemtuzumab, allopurinol, amikacin, aminocaproic acid, aminophylline, amiodarone, anidulafungin, argatroban, atracurium, bivalirudin, bleomycin, bumetanide, buprenorphine, butorphanol, calcium chloride, calcium gluconate, carboplatin, carmustine, caspofungin, cefotetan, chloramphenicol, chlorpromazine, ciprofloxacin, cisatracurium, cisplatin, cladribine, cyclophosphamide, cyclosporine, cytarabine, dacarbazine, dactinomycin, daptomycin, dexmedetomidine, dexrazoxane, diltiazem, diphenhydramine, dobutamine, docetaxel, dopamine, doxycycline, droperidol, enalaprilat, ephedrine, epinephrine, erythromycin, esmolol, etoposide, etoposide phosphate, famotidine, fentanyl, filgrastim, fluconazole, fludarabine, fluorouracil, ganciclovir, gemcitabine, gentamicin, glycopyrrolate, granisetron, haloperidol, hetastarch, hydralazine, hydrocortisone, hydromorphone, ifosfamide, imipenem/cilastatin, insulin regular, irinotecan, isoproterenol, ketorolac, labetalol, leucovorin calcium, levofloxacin, lidocaine, linezolid, lorazepam, magnesium sulfate, mannitol, melphalan, meperidine, meropenem, mesna, methadone, methohexital, methotrexate, metoclopramide, metoprolol, metronidazole, midazolam, milrinone, morphine, moxifloxacin, nalbuphine, naloxone, nicardipine, nitroglycerin, norepinephrine, octreotide, ondansetron, oxaliplatin, palonosetron, pamidronate, pentamidine, pentobarbital, phenobarbital, phentolamine, phenylephrine, potassium acetate, potassium chloride, procainamide, prochlorperazine, promethazine, propranolol, remifentanil, rituximab, rocuronium, sargramostim, sodium acetate, sodium bicarbonate, succinylcholine, sufentanil, tacrolimus, theophylline, thiopental, thiotepa, tigecycline, tirofiban, tobramycin, topotecan, trastuzumab, trimethoprim/sulfamethoxazole, vancomycin, vasopressin, vecuronium, verapamil, vinblastine, vincristine, vinorelbine, zidovudine, zoledronic acid.

- **Y-Site Incompatibility:** amphotericin B deoxycholate, amphotericin B lipid complex, amphotericin B liposomal, ampicillin, ampicillin/sulbactam, azithromycin, aztreonam, cefazolin, cefepime, cefotaxime, cefoxitin, ceftazidime, ceftriaxone, cefuroxime, clindamycin, dantrolene, daunorubicin hydrochloride, dexamethasone, diazepam, digoxin, doxorubicin liposomal, ertapenem, foscarnet, fosphenytoin, furosemide, gemtuzumab ozogamicin, heparin, idarubicin, methylprednisolone, nafcillin, nitroprusside,

paclitaxel, pantoprazole, pemetrexed, phenytoin, piperacillin/tazobactam, potassium phosphate, propofol, sodium phosphate, voriconazole.

Patient/Family Teaching

- Advise patient to read the *Patient Package Insert* before starting therapy and before each dose in case of changes. Explain purpose of mitoxantrone to patient.
- Instruct patient to notify health care professional promptly if fever; chills; cough; hoarseness; sore throat; signs of infection; lower back or side pain; painful or difficult urination; bleeding gums; bruising; petechiae; blood in stools, urine, or emesis; increased fatigue; dyspnea; or orthostatic hypotension occurs. Caution patient to avoid crowds and persons with known infections. Instruct patient to use soft toothbrush and electric razor and to avoid falls. Caution patient not to drink alcoholic beverages or take medication containing aspirin or NSAIDs; may precipitate gastric bleeding.
- Instruct patient to notify health care professional if abdominal pain, yellow skin, cough, diarrhea, or decreased urine output occurs.
- Inform patient that medication may cause the urine and sclera to turn blue-green.
- Instruct patient to inspect oral mucosa for redness and ulceration. If mouth sores occur, advise patient to use sponge brush and rinse mouth with water after eating and drinking. Topical agents may be used if pain interferes with eating. Stomatitis pain may require treatment with opioid analgesics.
- Discuss with patient the possibility of hair loss. Explore coping strategies.
- Instruct patient not to receive any vaccinations without advice of health care professional.
- Rep: May cause fetal harm. Refer patient to a facility with expertise in cancer during pregnancy. Advise patient that although mitoxantrone may cause infertility, contraception during therapy is necessary because of possible fetal harm. Discontinue breastfeeding before starting mitoxantrone.
- Emphasize need for periodic lab tests to monitor for side effects.

Evaluation/Desired Outcomes

- Decrease in the production and spread of leukemic cells.
- Decreased pain in patients with prostate cancer.
- Decrease disability and slowed progression of MS.

---

modafinil (mo-daf-i-nil)

✤ Alertec, Provigil

Classification
Therapeutic: central nervous system stimulants

Schedule IV

M

Indications

Excessive daytime drowsiness due to narcolepsy, obstructive sleep apnea, or shift work sleep disorder.

Action

Produces CNS stimulation. **Therapeutic Effects:** Decreased daytime drowsiness in patients with narcolepsy and obstructive sleep apnea. Decreased drowsiness during work in patients with shift work sleep disorder.

Pharmacokinetics

Absorption: Rapidly absorbed; bioavailability unknown.

Distribution: Well distributed to tissues.

Metabolism and Excretion: Highly (90%) metabolized by the liver; <10% eliminated unchanged in the urine.

Half-life: 15 hr.

TIME/ACTION PROFILE (plasma concentrations)

ROUTE	ONSET	PEAK	DURATION
PO	rapid	2–4 hr	24 hr

Contraindications/Precautions

Contraindicated in: Hypersensitivity; History of left ventricular hypertrophy or ischemic ECG changes, chest pain, arrhythmia, or other significant manifestations of mitral valve prolapse in association with CNS stimulant use; OB: Pregnancy.

Use Cautiously in: History of MI or unstable angina; Severe hepatic impairment with or without cirrhosis (dosage ↓ recommended); Lactation: Use while breastfeeding only if potential maternal benefit justifies potential risk to infant; Pedi: Safety and effectiveness not established in children; Geri: Lower doses may be necessary in older adults due to ↑ sensitivity to drug effects.

Adverse Reactions/Side Effects

CV: arrhythmias, chest pain, hypertension, hypotension, syncope. **Derm:** dry skin, rash, STEVENS-JOHNSON SYNDROME (SJS). **EENT:** rhinitis, abnormal vision, amblyopia, epistaxis, pharyngitis. **Endo:** hyperglycemia. **F and E:** ↑ thirst. **GI:** ↑ liver enzymes, nausea, anorexia, diarrhea, gingivitis, mouth ulcers, vomiting. **GU:** abnormal ejaculation, albuminuria, urinary retention. **Hemat:** eosinophilia. **MS:** joint disorder, neck pain. **Neuro:** headache, aggression, amnesia, anxiety, ataxia, cataplexy, confusion, delusions, depression, dizziness, dyskinesia, hallucinations, hypertonia, insomnia, mania, paresthesia, SEIZURES, SUICIDAL IDEATION, tremor. **Resp:** dyspnea. **Misc:** HYPERSENSITIVITY REACTIONS (including anaphylaxis and angioedema), infection.

Interactions

Drug-Drug: May ↓ the metabolism and ↑ the effects of **diazepam**, **phenytoin**, **propranolol**, or **tricyclic antidepressants**; dosage adjustments may be necessary. May ↑ the metabolism and ↓ the effects of **hormonal contraceptives**, **cyclosporine**, and **theoph-**ylline; dosage adjustments or additional methods of contraception may be necessary.

Drug-Natural Products: Use with caffeine-containing herbs (**cola nut**, **guarana**, **mate**, **tea**, **coffee**) may ↑ stimulant effect.

Route/Dosage

PO (Adults): 200 mg once daily.

Hepatic Impairment

PO (Adults): *Severe hepatic impairment:* 100 mg once daily.

Availability (generic available)

Tablets: 100 mg, 200 mg.

NURSING IMPLICATIONS

Assessment

- Observe and document frequency of narcoleptic episodes.
- Monitor closely for changes in behavior that could indicate the emergence or worsening of suicidal thoughts or behavior or depression.
- Assess for rash periodically during therapy. May cause SJS. Discontinue therapy if severe or if accompanied with fever, general malaise, fatigue, muscle or joint aches, blisters, oral lesions, conjunctivitis, hepatitis and/or eosinophilia.
- Monitor for signs and symptoms of angioedema or anaphylaxis (rash, swelling of face, eyes, lips, tongue or larynx; difficulty in swallowing or breathing; hoarseness).

Lab Test Considerations
- May cause elevated liver enzymes.

Implementation

- **PO:** Administer as a single dose in the morning for patients with narcolepsy or obstructive sleep apnea. Administer 1 hr before the start of work shift for patients with shift work sleep disorder.

Patient/Family Teaching

- Instruct patient to take medication as directed. Advise patient to read the *Medication Guide* prior to starting therapy and with each Rx refill, in case of changes.
- Medication may impair judgment. Advise patient to use caution when driving or during other activities requiring alertness.
- Advise patient that modafinil is a drug with known abuse potential. Advise patient that sharing this medication with others, even those with the same symptoms, is dangerous and illegal. Protect it from theft; store out of sight and reach of children, and in a location not accessible by others.
- Encourage patient and family to be alert for emergence of anxiety, agitation, panic attacks, insomnia, irritability, hostility, impulsivity, akathisia, hypomania, mania, worsening of depression and suicidal ideation, especially during early antidepressant therapy. Assess symptoms on a day-to-day basis as

changes may be abrupt. If these symptoms occur, notify health care professional.
- Advise patient to notify health care professional immediately if rash or symptoms of anaphylaxis occur.
- Advise patient to notify health care professional of all Rx or OTC medications, vitamins, or herbal products being taken and to consult with health care professional before taking other medications. If alcohol is used during therapy, intake should be limited to moderate amounts.
- Rep: Advise females of reproductive potential to use effective nonhormonal methods of contraception during and for 1 mo following discontinuation of therapy. Instruct patient to notify health care professional promptly if pregnancy is planned or suspected, or if breastfeeding. Encourage women who become pregnant to enroll in the registry by calling 1-866-404-4106. Registry collects information about the safety of modafinil during pregnancy.

Evaluation/Desired Outcomes
- Decrease in narcoleptic symptoms and an enhanced ability to stay awake.

---

moexipril, See ANGIOTENSIN-CONVERTING ENZYME (ACE) INHIBITORS.

---

molnupiravir
(mol-noo-**peer**-a-veer)
Lagevrio
Classification
Therapeutic: antivirals
Pharmacologic: nucleoside analogues

Indications
Mild-to-moderate COVID-19 infection in non-hospitalized patients with positive results of direct SARS-CoV-2 viral testing, and who are at high risk for progression to severe COVID-19, including hospitalization or death, and for whom alternative COVID-19 treatment options authorized by FDA are not accessible or clinically appropriate. An Emergency Use Authorization (EUA) has been issued for this use of molnupiravir; this drug is not FDA-approved for the above indication.

Action
As a prodrug, molnupiravir is metabolized to the active cytidine nucleoside analogue, NHC, which distributes into cells where NHC is phosphorylated to the active ribonucleoside triphosphate (NHC-TP). NHC-TP is incorporated as NHC-monophosphate into SARS-CoV-2 RNA by the viral RNA polymerase which results in inhibition of viral RNA replication. **Therapeutic Effects:** Reduction in hospitalization or mortality.

Pharmacokinetics
Absorption: Well absorbed.
Distribution: Widely distributed to extravascular tissues.
Metabolism and Excretion: Molnupiravir is a prodrug that is metabolized intracellularly to the active metabolite, NHC-TP. 3% excreted in urine.
Half-life: 3.3 hr.

TIME/ACTION PROFILE (plasma concentrations)

ROUTE	ONSET	PEAK	DURATION
PO	unknown	1.5 hr	12 hr

Contraindications/Precautions
Contraindicated in: Pedi: Children <18 yr (may affect bone and cartilage growth); Lactation: Lactation.
Use Cautiously in: Rep: Women and men of reproductive potential; OB: Use during pregnancy only if the potential maternal benefit outweighs potential fetal risk (has caused fetal harm in animal studies).

Adverse Reactions/Side Effects
GI: diarrhea, nausea. **Neuro:** dizziness.

Interactions
Drug-Drug: None reported.

Route/Dosage
PO (Adults): 800 mg every 12 hr for 5 days. Should be started as soon as possible after diagnosis of COVID-19 and within 5 days of symptom onset.

Availability
Capsules: 200 mg.

NURSING IMPLICATIONS
Assessment
- Assess COVID-19 symptoms (fever or chills, cough, shortness of breath or difficulty breathing, fatigue, muscle or body aches, headache, new loss of taste or smell, sore throat, congestion or runny nose, nausea or vomiting, diarrhea) during therapy.

Lab Test Considerations
- Verify negative pregnancy test before starting therapy.

Implementation
- **PO:** Administer twice daily without regard to food for 5 days.
- Administration via nasogastric (NG) or orogastric (OG) tube (≥12F), open four (4) capsules and transfer contents into a clean container with a lid. Add 40 mL of water to container. Put lid on container and shake to mix the capsule contents and water thoroughly for 3 minutes. Capsule contents may not dissolve completely; prepared mixture may have visible undissolved particulates and are

acceptable for administration. Flush NG/OG tube with 5 mL of water before administration. Using a catheter tip syringe, draw up entire contents from container and administer immediately through the NG/OG tube. Do not keep mixture for future use. If any portion of capsule contents are left in container, add 10 mL of water to container, mix, and using the same syringe draw up entire contents of the container and administer through the NG/OG. Repeat as needed until no capsule contents are left in container or syringe. Flush NG/OG tube with 5 mL of water twice (10 mL total) after administration of mixture.

- If patient requires hospitalization after starting therapy, patient may complete the full 5 day course per the health care professional's discretion.

Patient/Family Teaching

- Instruct patient to take molnupiravir as directed for full course of therapy. If dose is missed within 10 hr of usual time take it as soon as possible and resume normal dosing schedule. If dose is missed by >10 hours, omit dose and take next dose at the regularly scheduled time. Do not double dose to make up for a missed dose.
- Advise patient to discontinue therapy and notify health care professional promptly at first sign of hypersensitivity reaction (skin rash, hives or other skin reactions, rapid heartbeat, difficulty swallowing or breathing, swelling of the lips, tongue, face, tightness of the throat, hoarseness).
- Advise patient to continue isolation in accordance with public health recommendations to maximize viral clearance and minimize transmission of SARS-CoV-2.
- Rep: May cause fetal harm. Advise females of reproductive potential to use effective contraception during therapy and avoid breastfeeding during and for 4 days after last dose. Advise males with female partners of reproductive potential to use effective contraception during and for 3 months after last dose. If patient decides to take molnupiravir during pregnancy, prescribing health care professional must document that the known and potential benefits and potential risks of using molnupiravir during pregnancy were communicated to the pregnant individual. Pregnancy registry monitors pregnancy outcomes in individuals exposed to molnupiravir during pregnancy. Encourage patient to enroll in pregnancy registry at https://covid-pr.pregistry.com or 1-800-616-3791.

Evaluation/Desired Outcomes

- Reduction in hospitalization or mortality.

mometasone, See CORTICOSTEROIDS (INHALATION).

mometasone, See CORTICOSTEROIDS (NASAL).

mometasone, See CORTICOSTEROIDS (TOPICAL/LOCAL).

montelukast (mon-te-loo-kast)
Singulair
Classification
Therapeutic: allergy, cold, and cough remedies, bronchodilators
Pharmacologic: leukotriene antagonists

Indications
Prevention and chronic treatment of asthma. Seasonal or perennial allergic rhinitis (should only be used in patients with inadequate response or intolerance to other therapies). Prevention of exercise-induced bronchoconstriction.

Action
Antagonizes the effects of leukotrienes, which mediate the following: Airway edema, Smooth muscle constriction, Altered cellular activity. Result is decreased inflammatory process, which is part of asthma and allergic rhinitis. **Therapeutic Effects:** Decreased frequency and severity of acute asthma attacks. Decreased severity of allergic rhinitis. Decreased attacks of exercise-induced bronchoconstriction.

Pharmacokinetics
Absorption: Rapidly absorbed (63–73%) following oral administration.
Distribution: Minimally distributed to tissues.
Protein Binding: 99%.
Metabolism and Excretion: Mostly metabolized by the liver by the CYP3A4 and CYP2C9 isoenzymes; metabolites eliminated in feces via bile; negligible renal excretion.
Half-life: 2.7–5.5 hr.

TIME/ACTION PROFILE (improved symptoms of asthma)

ROUTE	ONSET	PEAK†	DURATION
PO (swallow)	within 24 hr	3–4 hr	24 hr
PO (chew)	within 24 hr	2–2.5 hr	24 hr

†Plasma concentrations.

Contraindications/Precautions
Contraindicated in: Hypersensitivity; Acute attacks of asthma.
Use Cautiously in: Phenylketonuria (chewable tablets contain aspartame); Hepatic impairment (may need ↓ doses); Reduction of corticosteroid therapy (may ↑ the risk of eosinophilic conditions); Pedi: Chil-

dren <6 yr (exercise-induced bronchoconstriction), <2 yr (seasonal allergic rhinitis), <12 mo (asthma), <6 mo (perennial allergic rhinitis) (safety and effectiveness not established).

Adverse Reactions/Side Effects

Derm: rash, STEVENS-JOHNSON SYNDROME (SJS), TOXIC EPIDERMAL NECROLYSIS. **EENT:** epistaxis, otitis (children), rhinorrhea, sinusitis (children). **GI:** ↑ liver enzymes, abdominal pain, diarrhea (children), dyspepsia, nausea (children). **Neuro:** aggression, agitation, anxiety, attention disturbance, depression, disorientation, dream abnormalities, fatigue, hallucinations, headache, insomnia, irritability, memory impairment, obsessive-compulsive symptoms, restlessness, sleep walking, stuttering, SUICIDAL BEHAVIORS/THOUGHTS, tics, tremor, weakness. **Resp:** cough. **Misc:** EOSINOPHILIC CONDITIONS (including Churg-Strauss syndrome), fever.

Interactions

Drug-Drug: Levels and effectiveness may be ↓ by **CYP3A4 or CYP2C9 inducers**, including **phenobarbital** and **rifampin**.

Route/Dosage

Asthma

PO (Adults and Children ≥15 yr): 10 mg once daily.
PO (Children 6–14 yr): 5 mg once daily (as chewable tablet).
PO (Children 2–5 yr): 4 mg once daily (as chewable tablet or granules).
PO (Children 12–23 mo): 4 mg once daily (as granules).

Exercise-Induced Bronchoconstriction

PO (Adults and Children ≥15 yr): 10 mg ≥2 hr before exercise. Do not take within 24 hr of another dose; if taking daily doses, do not take dose for exercise-induced bronchoconstriction.
PO (Children 6–14 yr): 5 mg (as chewable tablet) ≥2 hr before exercise. Do not take within 24 hr of another dose; if taking daily doses, do not take dose for exercise-induced bronchoconstriction.

Allergic Rhinitis

PO (Adults and Children ≥15 yr): *Seasonal or perennial:* 10 mg once daily.
PO (Children 6–14 yr): *Seasonal or perennial:* 5 mg once daily (as chewable tablet).
PO (Children 2–5 yr): *Seasonal or perennial:* 4 mg once daily (as chewable tablet or granules).
PO (Children 6–23 mo): *Perennial only:* 4 mg once daily (as granules).

Availability (generic available)

Tablets: 10 mg. **Chewable tablets (cherry flavor):** 4 mg, 5 mg. **Oral granules:** 4 mg/pkt.

NURSING IMPLICATIONS

Assessment

● Assess lung sounds and respiratory function prior to and periodically during therapy.
● Assess allergy symptoms (rhinitis, conjunctivitis, hives) before and periodically during therapy.
● Monitor closely for changes in behavior that could indicate the emergence or worsening of depression or suicidal thoughts.
● Assess for rash periodically during therapy. May cause SJS. Discontinue therapy if severe or if accompanied with fever, general malaise, fatigue, muscle or joint aches, blisters, oral lesions, conjunctivitis, hepatitis, and/or eosinophilia.

Lab Test Considerations
● May cause ↑ AST and ALT.

Implementation

● Doses of inhaled corticosteroids may be gradually decreased with supervision of health care professional; do not discontinue abruptly.
● **PO:** For asthma, administer once daily in the evening. For allergic rhinitis, may be administered at any time of day.
● Administer granules directly into mouth or mixed in a spoonful of cold or room temperature foods (use only applesauce, mashed carrots, rice, or ice cream). Do not open packet until ready to use. After opening packet, administer full dose within 15 min. Do not store mixture. Discard unused portion. Do not dissolve granules in fluid, but fluid may be taken following administration. Granules may be administered without regard to meals.
● *For Exercise-Induced Bronchoconstriction:* Administer one tablet at least 2 hr before exercise; do not take within 24 hr of another dose.

Patient/Family Teaching

● Instruct patient to take medication daily in the evening or at least 2 hr before exercise, even if not experiencing symptoms of asthma. If dose is missed, omit and take next dose at regularly scheduled time; do not double doses. Do not discontinue therapy without consulting health care professional. Advise patient to read *Patient Information* before starting therapy and with each Rx refill in case of changes.
● Instruct patient not to discontinue or reduce other asthma medications without consulting health care professional.
● Advise patient that montelukast is not used to treat acute asthma attacks, but may be continued during an acute exacerbation. Patient should carry rapid-acting therapy for bronchospasm at all times. Advise patient to notify health care professional if more than the maximum number of short-acting bronchodilator treatments prescribed for a 24-hr period are needed.

M

🍁 = Canadian drug name. ⚄ = Genetic implication. ~~Strikethrough~~ = Discontinued. CAPITALS = life-threatening. <u>Underline</u> = most frequent.

- Advise patient to notify health care professional of all Rx or OTC medications, vitamins, or herbal products being taken and to consult health care professional before taking any new medications.
- Encourage patient and family to be alert for emergence of anxiety, agitation, panic attacks, insomnia, irritability, hostility, impulsivity, akathisia, hypomania, mania, worsening of depression and suicidal ideation, especially during early antidepressant therapy. Assess symptoms on a day-to-day basis as changes may be abrupt. If these symptoms or rash occurs, notify health care professional.
- Rep: Advise females of reproductive potential to notify health care professional if pregnancy is planned or suspected or if breastfeeding.

Evaluation/Desired Outcomes

- Prevention of and reduction in symptoms of asthma.
- Decrease in severity of allergic rhinitis.
- Prevention of exercise-induced bronchoconstriction.

| REMS | HIGH ALERT |

morphine (mor-feen)
AVINza, ✳Doloral, Duramorph, ~~Embeda~~, Infumorph, ✳Kadian, ✳M-Eslon, Mitigo, ~~Morphabond ER~~, ✳Morphine LP Epidural, MS Contin, ~~Roxanol~~

Classification
Therapeutic: opioid analgesics
Pharmacologic: opioid agonists

Schedule II

Indications
Severe pain (the 20 mg/mL oral solution concentration should only be used in opioid-tolerant patients). Pain severe enough to require daily, around-the-clock long-term opioid treatment and for which alternative treatment options are inadequate (extended-release). Pulmonary edema. Pain associated with MI.

Action
Binds to opiate receptors in the CNS. Alters the perception of and response to painful stimuli while producing generalized CNS depression. **Therapeutic Effects:** Decrease in severity of pain.

Pharmacokinetics
Absorption: Variably absorbed (about 30%) following oral administration. More reliably absorbed from rectal, SUBQ, and IM sites. Following epidural administration, systemic absorption and absorption into the intrathecal space via the meninges occurs.
Distribution: Widely distributed to tissues.
Metabolism and Excretion: Mostly metabolized by the liver. Active metabolites excreted renally.
Half-life: *Premature neonates:* 10–20 hr; *Neonates:* 7.6 hr; *Infants 1–3 mo:* 6.2 hr; *Children 6*

mo–2.5 yr: 2.9 hr; *Children 3–6 yr:* 1–2 hr; *Children 6–19 yr with sickle cell disease:* 1.3 hr; *Adults:* 2–4 hr.

TIME/ACTION PROFILE (analgesia)

ROUTE	ONSET	PEAK	DURATION
PO	unknown	60 min	4–5 hr
PO-ER	unknown	3–4 hr	8–24 hr
IM	10–30 min	30–60 min	4–5 hr
SUBQ	20 min	50–90 min	4–5 hr
Rect	unknown	20–60 min	3–7 hr
IV	rapid	20 min	4–5 hr
Epidural	6–30 min	1 hr	up to 24 hr
IT	rapid (min)	unknown	up to 24 hr

Contraindications/Precautions
Contraindicated in: Hypersensitivity; Some products contain tartrazine, bisulfites, or alcohol and should be avoided in patients with known hypersensitivity; Acute, mild, intermittent, or postoperative pain (extended/sustained-release); Significant respiratory depression (extended-release); Acute or severe bronchial asthma (extended-release); Paralytic ileus (extended-release).
Use Cautiously in: Head trauma; ↑ intracranial pressure; Severe renal impairment; Severe hepatic impairment; Severe pulmonary disease; Hypothyroidism; Seizure disorder; Adrenal insufficiency; History of substance abuse; Undiagnosed abdominal pain; Prostatic hyperplasia; Patients undergoing procedures that rapidly ↓ pain (cordotomy, radiation); long-acting agents should be discontinued 24 hr before and replaced with short-acting agents; OB: Avoid chronic use; prolonged use of opioids during pregnancy can result in neonatal opioid withdrawal syndrome; Lactation: Use while breastfeeding only if potential maternal benefit justifies potential risk to infant ; Pedi: Neonates and infants <3 mo (more susceptible to respiratory depression); Pedi: Neonates (oral solution contains sodium benzoate which can cause potentially fatal gasping syndrome); Geri: ↑ risk of respiratory depression in older adults; dose ↓ suggested.

Adverse Reactions/Side Effects
CV: hypotension, bradycardia. **Derm:** flushing, itching, sweating. **EENT:** blurred vision, diplopia, miosis. **Endo:** adrenal insufficiency. **GI:** constipation, nausea, vomiting. **GU:** urinary retention. **Neuro:** confusion, sedation, dizziness, dysphoria, euphoria, floating feeling, hallucinations, headache, unusual dreams. **Resp:** RESPIRATORY DEPRESSION (including central sleep apnea and sleep-related hypoxemia). **Misc:** physical dependence, psychological dependence, tolerance.

Interactions
Drug-Drug: Use with **extreme caution** in patients receiving **MAO inhibitors** within 14 days prior (may result in unpredictable, severe reactions— ↓ initial dose of morphine to 25% of usual dose). Use with **benzodiazepines** or other **CNS depressants** including other **opioids, nonbenzodiazepine sedative/hyp-**

notics, **anxiolytics**, **general anesthetics**, **muscle relaxants**, **antipsychotics**, and **alcohol** may cause profound sedation, respiratory depression, coma, and death; reserve concurrent use for when alternative treatment options are inadequate. Drugs that affect serotonergic neurotransmitter systems, including **tricyclic antidepressants**, **SSRIs**, **SNRIs**, **MAO inhibitors**, **TCAs**, **tramadol**, **trazodone**, **mirtazapine**, 5−HT$_3$ **receptor antagonists**, **linezolid**, **methylene blue**, and **triptans** ↑ risk of serotonin syndrome. **Mixed agonist/antagonist analgesics**, including **nalbuphine** or **butorphanol** and **partial agonist analgesics**, including **buprenorphine**, may ↓ morphine's analgesic effects and/or precipitate opioid withdrawal in physically dependent patients. May ↑ the anticoagulant effect of **warfarin**. **Cimetidine** ↓ metabolism and may ↑ effects. IV morphine may ↓ levels and antiplatelet effects of **clopidogrel**, **prasugrel**, and **ticagrelor**; consider IV antiplatelet agent as alternative in patients with acute coronary syndrome if morphine concomitantly used.
Drug-Natural Products: Concomitant use of **kava-kava**, **valerian**, or **chamomile** can ↑ CNS depression.

Route/Dosage
Larger doses may be required during chronic therapy.
PO, Rect (Adults ≥50 kg): *Usual starting dose for moderate to severe pain in opioid-naive patients:* 30 mg every 3−4 hr initially *or* once 24-hr opioid requirement is determined, convert to extended-release morphine by administering total daily oral morphine dose every 24 hr (as ER capsules), 50% of the total daily oral morphine dose every 12 hr (as *MS Contin*), or 33% of the total daily oral morphine dose every 8 hr (as *MS Contin*). See equianalgesic chart, Appendix I. Dose of ER capsules should not exceed 1600 mg/day because of fumaric acid in formulation.
PO, Rect (Adults and Children <50 kg): *Usual starting dose for moderate to severe pain in opioid-naive patients:* 0.3 mg/kg every 3−4 hr initially.
PO (Children >1 mo): *Prompt-release tablets and solution:* 0.2−0.5 mg/kg every 4−6 hr as needed. *Controlled-release tablet:* 0.3−0.6 mg/kg every 12 hr.
IM, IV, SUBQ (Adults ≥50 kg): *Usual starting dose for moderate to severe pain in opioid-naive patients:* 4−10 mg every 3−4 hr. *MI:* 8−15 mg, for very severe pain additional smaller doses may be given every 3−4 hr.
IM, IV, SUBQ (Adults and Children <50 kg): *Usual starting dose for moderate to severe pain in opioid-naive patients:* 0.05−0.2 mg/kg every 3−4 hr, maximum: 15 mg/dose.
IM, IV, SUBQ (Neonates): 0.05 mg/kg every 4−8 hr, maximum dose: 0.1 mg/kg. Use preservative-free formulation.
IV, SUBQ (Adults): *Continuous infusion:* 0.8−10 mg/hr; may be preceded by a bolus of 15 mg (infusion rates vary greatly; up to 80 mg/hr have been used).

IV, SUBQ (Children >1 mo): *Continuous infusion, postoperative pain:* 0.01−0.04 mg/kg/hr. *Continuous infusion, sickle cell or cancer pain:* 0.02−2.6 mg/kg/hr.
IV (Neonates): *Continuous infusion:* 0.01−0.03 mg/kg/hr.
Epidural (Adults): *Intermittent injection:* 5 mg/day (initially); if relief is not obtained at 60 min, 1−2 mg increments may be made (total dose not to exceed 10 mg/day). *Continuous infusion:* 2−4 mg/24 hr; may ↑ by 1−2 mg/day (up to 30 mg/day).
Epidural (Children >1 mo): 0.03−0.05 mg/kg, maximum dose: 0.1 mg/kg or 5 mg/24 hr. Use preservative-free formulation.
IT (Adults): 0.2−1 mg. Use preservative-free formulation.

Availability (generic available)
Immediate-release tablets: 15 mg, 30 mg. **Extended-release tablets (MS Contin):** 15 mg, 30 mg, 60 mg, 100 mg, 200 mg. **Extended-release capsules:** 10 mg, 20 mg, 30 mg, 45 mg, 50 mg, 60 mg, 75 mg, 80 mg, 90 mg, 100 mg, 120 mg. **Oral solution:** ✽ 1 mg/mL, 10 mg/5 mL, 20 mg/5 mL, ✽ 5 mg/mL, 100 mg/5 mL. **Rectal suppositories:** 5 mg, 10 mg, 20 mg, 30 mg. **Solution for epidural, IV injection (preservative-free):** 0.5 mg/mL, 1 mg/mL. **Solution for epidural or IT use (continuous microinfusion device; preservative-free):** 10 mg/mL, 25 mg/mL. **Solution for IM, SUBQ, IV injection:** 1 mg/mL, 2 mg/mL, 4 mg/mL, 5 mg/mL, 8 mg/mL, 10 mg/mL, 25 mg/mL, 50 mg/mL. **Solution for IV injection (PCA device):** 1 mg/mL, 2 mg/mL, 3 mg/mL, 5 mg/mL.

NURSING IMPLICATIONS
Assessment
- Assess type, location, and intensity of pain prior to and 1 hr following PO, SUBQ, IM, and 20 min (peak) following IV administration. When titrating opioid doses, increases of 25−50% should be administered until there is either a 50% reduction in the patient's pain rating on a numerical or visual analogue scale or the patient reports satisfactory pain relief. When titrating doses of short-acting morphine, a repeat dose can be safely administered at the time of the peak if previous dose is ineffective and side effects are minimal.
- Patients on a continuous infusion should have additional bolus doses provided every 15−30 min, as needed, for breakthrough pain. The bolus dose is usually set to the amount of drug infused each hr by continuous infusion.
- Patients taking extended-release morphine may require additional short-acting opioid doses for breakthrough pain. Doses of short-acting opioids should be equivalent to 10−20% of 24 hr total and given every 2 hr as needed.

- An equianalgesic chart (see Appendix I) should be used when changing routes or when changing from one opioid to another.
- *High Alert:* Assess level of consciousness, BP, pulse, and respirations before and periodically during administration. If respiratory rate is <10/min, assess level of sedation. Physical stimulation may be sufficient to prevent significant hypoventilation. Subsequent doses may need to be decreased by 25–50%. Initial drowsiness will diminish with continued use. Monitor for respiratory depression, especially during initiation or following dose increase; serious, life-threatening, or fatal respiratory depression may occur. May cause sleep-related breathing disorders (central sleep apnea [CSA], sleep-related hypoxemia). Geri: Assess geriatric patients frequently; older adults are more sensitive to the effects of opioid analgesics and may experience side effects and respiratory complications more frequently. Pedi: Assess pediatric patient frequently; children are more sensitive to the effects of opioid analgesics and may experience respiratory complications, excitability, and restlessness more frequently.
- Prolonged use may lead to physical and psychological dependence and tolerance. This should not prevent patient from receiving adequate analgesia. Patients who receive morphine for pain rarely develop psychological dependence. Progressively higher doses may be required to relieve pain with long-term therapy; may increase risk of overdose. Prolonged use of opioids should be reserved for patients whose pain remains severe enough to require them and when alternative treatment options continue to be inadequate. Many acute pain conditions treated in the outpatient setting require no more than a few days of an opioid pain medicine.
- Assess bowel function routinely. Institute prevention of constipation with increased intake of fluids and bulk and with laxatives to minimize constipating effects. Administer stimulant laxatives routinely if opioid use exceeds 2–3 days, unless contraindicated. Consider drugs for opioid-induced constipation.
- Assess risk for opioid addiction, abuse, or misuse prior to administration. Abuse or misuse of extended-release preparations by crushing, chewing, snorting, or injecting dissolved product will result in uncontrolled delivery of morphine and can result in overdose and death.

Lab Test Considerations
- May ↑ plasma amylase and lipase levels.

Toxicity and Overdose
- If an opioid antagonist is required to reverse respiratory depression or coma, naloxone is the antidote. Dilute the 0.4-mg ampule of naloxone in 10 mL of 0.9% NaCl and administer 0.5 mL (0.02 mg) by IV push every 2 min. For children and adults weighing <40 kg, dilute 0.1 mg of naloxone in 10 mL of 0.9% NaCl for a concentration of 10 mcg/mL and administer 0.5 mcg/kg every 2 min. Titrate dose to avoid withdrawal, seizures, and severe pain.

Implementation
- *High Alert:* Do not confuse MS Contin with Oxycontin. Do not confuse morphine with hydromorphone. Do not confuse morphine (nonconcentrated oral liquid) with morphine (concentrated oral liquid).
- Use only preservative-free formulations for neonates, and for epidural and intrathecal routes in all patients.
- Explain therapeutic value of medication prior to administration to enhance the analgesic effect.
- Regularly administered doses may be more effective than prn administration. Analgesic is more effective if given before pain becomes severe.
- Coadministration with nonopioid analgesics may have additive analgesic effects and may permit lower doses.
- When transferring from other opioids or other forms of morphine to extended-release tablets, administer a total daily dose of oral morphine equivalent to previous daily dose (see Appendix I) and divided every 8 hr (MS Contin), every 12 hr (MS Contin), or every 24 hr.
- Morphine should be discontinued gradually to prevent withdrawal symptoms after long-term use. For patients on long-acting agents who are physically opioid-dependent, initiate the taper by a small enough increment (no greater than 10% to 25% of total daily dose) to avoid withdrawal symptoms, and proceed with dose-lowering at an interval of every 2 to 4 wk. Patients who have been taking opioids for briefer periods of time may tolerate a more rapid taper. Monitor frequently to manage pain and withdrawal symptoms (restlessness, lacrimation, rhinorrhea, yawning, perspiration, chills, myalgia, mydriasis, irritability, anxiety, backache, joint pain, weakness, abdominal cramps, insomnia, nausea, anorexia, vomiting, diarrhea, or increased blood pressure, respiratory rate, or heart rate). If withdrawal symptoms occur, pause the taper for a period of time or raise the dose of opioid analgesic to the previous dose, and then proceed with a slower taper. Also, monitor patients for changes in mood, emergence of suicidal thoughts, or use of other substances. A multimodal approach to pain management may optimize the treatment of chronic pain, as well as assist with the successful tapering of the opioid analgesic.
- *REMS:* FDA strongly encourages health care professionals to complete a REMS-compliant education program that includes all the elements of the FDA Education *Blueprint for Health Care Providers Involved in the Management or Support of Patients with Pain,* available at www.fda.gov/OpioidAnalgesicREMSBlueprint. Information on programs can be found at 1-800-503-0784 or www.opioidanalgesicrems.com.
- Discuss availability of naloxone for emergency treatment of opioid overdose with the patient and care-

M

giver and assess the potential need for access to naloxone, both when initiating and renewing therapy, especially if patient has household members (including children) or other close contacts at risk for accidental exposure or overdose. Consider prescribing naloxone, based on the patient's risk factors for overdose, such as concomitant use of CNS depressants, a history of opioid use disorder, or prior opioid overdose. However, the presence of risk factors for overdose should not prevent the proper management of pain in any patient.
- **PO:** Doses may be administered with food or milk to minimize GI irritation.
- Administer oral solution with properly calibrated measuring device; may be diluted in a glass of fruit juice just prior to administration to improve taste. Verify correct dose (mg) and correct volume (mL) prior to administration. Use an oral syringe when using 20 mg/mL concentration of oral solution.
- *DNC:* Swallow extended-release tablets whole; do not break, crush, dissolve, or chew (could result in rapid release and absorption of a potentially toxic dose).
- Extended release capsules may be opened and the pellets sprinkled onto applesauce immediately prior to administration. Patients should rinse mouth and swallow to assure ingestion of entire dose. *DNC:* Pellets should not be chewed, crushed, or dissolved. Capsules may also be opened and sprinkled on approximately 10 mL of water and flushed while swirling through a pre-wetted 16 French gastrostomy tube fitted with a funnel at the port end. Additional water should be used to transfer and flush any remaining pellets. Do not administer extended release capsules via a nasogastric tube.
- **Rect:** *MS Contin* has been administered rectally.
- **IM, SUBQ:** Use IM route for repeated doses, because morphine is irritating to SUBQ tissues.

IV Administration
- **IV:** Solution is colorless; do not administer discolored solution.
- **IV Push:** *Dilution:* Do not dilute prior to injection. *Rate: High Alert:* Administer slowly at 2.5–15 mg over 5 min. Rapid administration may lead to increased respiratory depression, hypotension, and circulatory collapse.
- **Continuous Infusion:** *Dilution:* May be added to D5W, D10W, 0.9% NaCl, 0.45% NaCl, Ringer's or LR, dextrose/saline solution, or dextrose/Ringer's or LR. *Concentration:* 0.1–1 mg/mL or greater for continuous infusion. *Rate:* Administer via infusion pump to control the rate. Dose should be titrated to ensure adequate pain relief without excessive sedation, respiratory depression, or hypotension. May be administered via patient-controlled analgesia (PCA) pump.

- **Y-Site Compatibility:** acetaminophen, aldesleukin, allopurinol, amifostine, amikacin, aminocaproic acid, aminophylline, amiodarone, anidulafungin, argatroban, arsenic trioxide, ascorbic acid, atropine, aztreonam, benztropine, bivalirudin, bleomycin, bumetanide, buprenorphine, butorphanol, calcium chloride, calcium gluconate, cangrelor, carboplatin, carmustine, caspofungin, cefazolin, cefotaxime, cefotetan, cefoxitin, ceftaroline, ceftazidime, ceftolozane/tazobactam, ceftriaxone, cefuroxime, chloramphenicol, chlorpromazine, cisatracurium, cladribine, clindamycin, cyclophosphamide, cyclosporine, cytarabine, dacarbazine, dactinomycin, daptomycin, daunorubicin hydrochloride, dexamethasone, dexmedetomidine, dexrazoxane, digoxin, diltiazem, diphenhydramine, dobutamine, docetaxel, dopamine, doxorubicin hydrochloride, doxycycline, enalaprilat, ephedrine, epinephrine, epirubicin, epoetin alfa, eptifibatide, ertapenem, erythromycin, esmolol, etomidate, etoposide, etoposide phosphate, famotidine, fentanyl, filgrastim, fluconazole, fludarabine, fluorouracil, foscarnet, fosphenytoin, gemcitabine, gentamicin, glycopyrrolate, granisetron, heparin, hetastarch, hydrocortisone, hydromorphone, idarubicin, ifosfamide, imipenem/cilastatin, irinotecan, isavuconazonium, isoproterenol, ketorolac, labetalol, LR, leucovorin calcium, lidocaine, linezolid, lorazepam, magnesium sulfate, mannitol, melphalan, meperidine, meropenem, meropenem/vaborbactam, mesna, methotrexate, methylprednisolone, metoclopramide, metoprolol, metronidazole, midazolam, milrinone, mitoxantrone, multivitamins, mycophenolate, nafcillin, nalbuphine, naloxone, nicardipine, nitroglycerin, nitroprusside, norepinephrine, octreotide, ondansetron, oritavancin, oxacillin, oxaliplatin, oxytocin, paclitaxel, palonosetron, pamidronate, papaverine, pemetrexed, penicillin G, phenobarbital, phentolamine, phenylephrine, phytonadione, piperacillin/tazobactam, plazomicin, posaconazole, potassium acetate, potassium chloride, procainamide, prochlorperazine, promethazine, propranolol, protamine, pyridoxine, remifentanil, rituximab, rocuronium, sodium acetate, sodium bicarbonate, succinylcholine, sufentanil, tacrolimus, tedizolid, theophylline, thiamine, thiotepa, tigecycline, tirofiban, tobramycin, topotecan, vancomycin, vasopressin, vecuronium, verapamil, vinblastine, vincristine, vinorelbine, voriconazole, zidovudine, zoledronic acid.
- **Y-Site Incompatibility:** alemtuzumab, amphotericin B deoxycholate, amphotericin B lipid complex, amphotericin B liposomal, azathioprine, dantrolene, doxorubicin liposomal, folic acid, ganciclovir, gemtuzumab ozogamicin, indomethacin, micafungin, minocycline, mitomycin, pentamidine, pentobarbital, phenytoin, sargramostim, trastuzumab.

- **Epidural:** Administer undiluted. Do not use an in-line filter. Do not admix or administer other medications in epidural space for 48 hr after administration. Administer within 4 hr after removing from vial. Store in refrigerator; do not freeze.

Patient/Family Teaching

- **REMS:** Instruct patient how and when to ask for pain medication. Do not stop taking without discussing with health care professional; may cause withdrawal symptoms if discontinued abruptly after prolonged use. Do not increase doses without discussing with health care professional; may lead to overdose. Discuss safe use, risks, and proper storage and disposal of opioid analgesics with patients and caregivers with each Rx. The Patient Counseling Guide is available at www.fda.gov/OpioidAnalgesicREMSPCG.
- Instruct patient on how and when to ask for and take pain medication.
- May cause drowsiness or dizziness. Caution patient to call for assistance when ambulating or smoking and to avoid driving or other activities requiring alertness until response to medication is known.
- Advise patient that morphine is a drug with known abuse potential. Protect it from theft, and never give to anyone other than the individual for whom it was prescribed. Store out of sight and reach of children, and in a location not accessible by others.
- Educate patients and caregivers on how to recognize respiratory depression and emphasize the importance of calling 911 or getting emergency medical help right away in the event of a known or suspected overdose. Inform patients and caregivers about ways to obtain naloxone as permitted by individual state naloxone dispensing and prescribing requirements or guidelines (by prescription, directly from a pharmacist, or as part of a community-based program).
- Advise patient to notify health care professional if pain control is not adequate or if severe or persistent side effects occur.
- Advise patient to change positions slowly to minimize orthostatic hypotension.
- Instruct patient to notify health care professional of all Rx or OTC medications, vitamins, or herbal products being taken and consult health care professional before taking any new medications.
- Emphasize the importance of aggressive prevention of constipation with the use of morphine.
- Caution patient to avoid concurrent use of alcohol or other CNS depressants with this medication.
- Encourage patients who are immobilized or on prolonged bedrest to turn, cough, and breathe deeply every 2 hr to prevent atelectasis.
- Advise patient that good oral hygiene, frequent mouth rinses, and sugarless gum or candy may decrease dry mouth.
- Rep: Advise patient to notify health care professional if pregnancy is planned or suspected, or if breast-feeding. Inform patient of potential for neonatal opioid withdrawal syndrome with prolonged use during pregnancy. Monitor neonate for signs and symptoms of withdrawal (irritability, hyperactivity and abnormal sleep pattern, high pitched cry, tremor, vomiting, diarrhea, and/or failure to gain weight); usually occur the first days after birth. Monitor infants exposed to morphine through breast milk for excess sedation and respiratory depression. Chronic use may reduce fertility in females and males.
- **Home Care Issues:** *High Alert:* Explain to patient and family how and when to administer morphine and how to care for infusion equipment properly. Pedi: Teach parents or caregivers how to accurately measure liquid medication and to use only the measuring device dispensed with the medication.

Evaluation/Desired Outcomes

- Decrease in severity of pain without a significant alteration in level of consciousness or respiratory status.
- Decrease in symptoms of pulmonary edema.

---

moxifloxacin, See FLUOROQUINOLONES.

---

mupirocin (myoo-**peer**-oh-sin)
~~Bactroban~~
Classification
Therapeutic: anti-infectives

Indications

Topical: Treatment of: Impetigo, Secondarily infected traumatic skin lesions (up to 10 cm in length or 100 cm² area) caused by *Staphylococcus aureus* and *Streptococcus pyogenes*.

Action

Inhibits bacterial protein synthesis. **Therapeutic Effects:** Inhibition of bacterial growth and reproduction. **Spectrum:** Greatest activity against gram-positive organisms, including: *S. aureus*, Beta-hemolytic streptococci. Resolution of impetigo. Eradication of *S. aureus* carrier state.

Pharmacokinetics

Absorption: Minimal systemic absorption.
Distribution: Remains in the stratum corneum after topical use for prolonged periods of time (72 hr).
Metabolism and Excretion: Metabolized in the skin, removed by desquamation.
Half-life: 17–36 min.

TIME/ACTION PROFILE (anti-infective effect)

ROUTE	ONSET	PEAK	DURATION
Topical†	unknown	3–5 days	72 hr

†Resolution of lesions.

Contraindications/Precautions
Contraindicated in: Hypersensitivity to mupirocin or polyethylene glycol.
Use Cautiously in: Renal impairment; Burn patients.

Adverse Reactions/Side Effects
Derm: burning, itching, pain, stinging.

Interactions
Drug-Drug: None reported.

Route/Dosage
Topical (Adults and Children ≥2 mo): *Ointment:* Apply 3–5 times daily for 5–14 days.
Topical (Adults and Children ≥3 mo): *Cream:* Apply small amount 3 times/day for 10 days.

Availability (generic available)
Cream: 2%. **Ointment:** 2%.

NURSING IMPLICATIONS

Assessment
* Assess lesions before and daily during therapy.

Implementation
* **Topical:** Wash affected area with soap and water and dry thoroughly. Apply a small amount of mupirocin to the affected area 3 times daily and rub in gently. Treated area may be covered with gauze if desired.

Patient/Family Teaching
* Instruct patient on the correct application of mupirocin. Advise patient to apply medication exactly as directed for the full course of therapy. If a dose is missed, apply as soon as possible unless almost time for next dose. Avoid contact with eyes.
* **Topical:** Teach patient and family appropriate hygienic measures to prevent spread of impetigo.
* Instruct parents to notify school nurse for screening and prevention of transmission.
* Patient should consult health care professional if symptoms have not improved in 3–5 days.

Evaluation/Desired Outcomes
* Healing of skin lesions. If no clinical response is seen in 3–5 days, condition should be re-evaluated.

REMS

mycophenolate mofetil
(mye-koe-**fee**-noe-late **moe**-fe-til)
CellCept

mycophenolic acid
(mye-koe-**fee**-noe-lik)
Myfortic
Classification
Therapeutic: immunosuppressants

Indications
Mycophenolate mofetil: Prevention of rejection in allogeneic kidney, liver, and heart transplantation (used concurrently with cyclosporine and corticosteroids).
Mycophenolic acid: Prevention of rejection in allogenic renal transplantation (used concurrently with cyclosporine and corticosteroids).

Action
Inhibits the enzyme inosine monophosphate dehydrogenase, which is involved in purine synthesis. This inhibition results in suppression of T- and B-lymphocyte proliferation. **Therapeutic Effects:** Prevention of heart, kidney, or liver transplant rejection.

Pharmacokinetics
Absorption: Following oral and IV administration, mycophenolate mofetil is rapidly hydrolyzed to mycophenolic acid (MPA), the active metabolite. Absorption of enteric-coated mycophenolic acid (Myfortic) is delayed compared with mycophenolate mofetil (CellCept).
Distribution: Cross the placenta and enter breast milk.
Protein Binding: *MPA:* 97%.
Metabolism and Excretion: MPA is extensively metabolized; <1% excreted unchanged in urine. Some enterohepatic recirculation of MPA occurs.
Half-life: *MPA:* 8–18 hr.

TIME/ACTION PROFILE (blood levels of MPA)

ROUTE	ONSET	PEAK	DURATION
mycophen-olate mofe-til-PO	rapid	0.25–1.25 hr	N/A
mycophenolic acid	rapid	1.5–2.75 hr	N/A

Contraindications/Precautions
Contraindicated in: Hypersensitivity; Hypersensitivity to polysorbate 80 (for IV mycophenolate mofetil); OB: Pregnancy (↑ risk of congenital anomalies or spontaneous abortion).
Use Cautiously in: Active serious pathology of the GI tract (including history of ulcer disease or GI bleeding); Phenylketonuria (oral suspension contains aspartame); Severe chronic renal impairment (dose not to exceed 1 g twice daily [CellCept] if CCr <25 mL/min/1.73 m²); careful monitoring recommended; Delayed graft function following transplantation (observe for ↑ toxicity); Lactation: Use while breastfeeding only if potential maternal benefit justifies potential risk to infant; Rep: Women of reproductive potential and men with female partners of reproductive potential; Pedi: Safety and effectiveness not established in children <3 mo (mycophenolate mofetil) or <5 yr (mycophenolic

M

acid); Geri: ↑ risk of adverse reactions related to immunosuppression in older adults.

Adverse Reactions/Side Effects

CV: edema, hypertension, hypotension, tachycardia. **Derm:** rash. **Endo:** hyperglycemia. **F and E:** hyperkalemia, hypocalcemia, hypokalemia, hypomagnesemia. **GI:** anorexia, constipation, diarrhea, nausea, vomiting, abdominal pain, GI BLEEDING. **GU:** renal impairment. **Hemat:** leukocytosis, leukopenia, thrombocytopenia, anemia, pure red cell aplasia. **Metab:** hypercholesterolemia. **Neuro:** anxiety, confusion, dizziness, headache, insomnia, paresthesia, sedation, tremor, PROGRESSIVE MULTIFOCAL LEUKOENCEPHALOPATHY (PML). **Resp:** cough, dyspnea. **Misc:** fever, infection (including activation of latent viral infections such as Polyomavirus-associated nephropathy or Hepatitis B/C), acute inflammatory syndrome, MALIGNANCY.

Interactions

Drug-Drug: Combined use with **azathioprine** is not recommended (effects unknown). **Acyclovir** and **ganciclovir** compete with MPA for renal excretion and, in patients with renal dysfunction, may ↑ each other's toxicity. **Magnesium and aluminum hydroxide** antacids ↓ the absorption of MPA (avoid simultaneous administration). **Proton pump inhibitors,** including **dexlansoprazole, esomeprazole, lansoprazole, omeprazole, pantoprazole,** and **rabeprazole** may ↓ levels. **Cholestyramine** and **colestipol** ↓ the absorption of MPA (avoid concurrent use). May ↓ the effectiveness of **oral contraceptives** (additional contraceptive method should be used). May ↓ the antibody response to and ↑ risk of adverse reactions from **live attenuated vaccines. Amoxicillin/clavulanic acid** or **ciprofloxacin** may ↓ MPA trough levels. **Cyclosporine** may ↓ levels; use caution when discontinuing cyclosporine (may ↑ mycophenolate levels) or when switching from cyclosporine to another immunosuppressant, such as tacrolimus or belatacept. **Telmisartan** may ↓ levels.

Route/Dosage

Mycophenolate Mofetil

Kidney Transplantation

PO, IV (Adults): 1 g twice daily; IV should be started ≤24 hr after transplantation and switched to PO as soon as possible (IV not recommended for ≥14 days). **PO (Children ≥3 mo):** 600 mg/m² twice daily (not to exceed 2 g/day).

Liver Transplantation

PO, IV (Adults): 1 g twice daily IV, or 1.5 g twice daily PO. IV should be started ≤24 hr after transplantation and switched to PO as soon as possible (IV not recommended for ≥14 days). **PO (Children ≥3 mo):** 600 mg/m² twice daily; if well tolerated, can ↑ to 900 mg/m² twice daily (not to exceed 3 g/day).

Heart Transplantation

PO, IV (Adults): 1.5 g twice daily; IV should be started ≤24 hr after transplantation and switched to PO as soon as possible (IV not recommended for ≥14 days). **PO (Children ≥3 mo):** 600 mg/m² twice daily; if well tolerated, can ↑ to 900 mg/m² twice daily (not to exceed 3 g/day).

Renal Impairment

PO, IV (Adults): *CCr <25 mL/min:* daily dose should not exceed 2 g.

Mycophenolic Acid

Mycophenolate mofetil and mycophenolic acid should not be used interchangeably without the advice of a health care professional.

Kidney Transplantation

PO (Adults): 720 mg twice daily. **PO (Children 5–16 yr and ≥1.19 m²):** 400–450 mg/m² twice daily (not to exceed 720 mg twice daily).

Availability (generic available)

Mycophenolate Mofetil

Tablets: 500 mg. **Capsules:** 250 mg. **Oral suspension (fruit flavor):** 200 mg/mL. **Powder for injection :** 500 mg/vial.

Mycophenolic Acid

Delayed-release tablets: 180 mg, 360 mg.

NURSING IMPLICATIONS

Assessment

- Assess for symptoms of organ rejection throughout therapy.
- Assess for signs of PML (hemiparesis, apathy, confusion, cognitive deficiencies, and ataxia) periodically during therapy.
- Monitor for symptoms and laboratory parameters of Acute Inflammatory Syndrome when starting treatment with mycophenolate products or when increasing the dose. Discontinue treatment and consider other treatment alternatives based on risk and benefit for the patient.

Lab Test Considerations

- Verify negative urine pregnancy test with a specificity of 25 mIU/mL immediately prior to beginning therapy and again 8–10 days later. Repeat pregnancy tests should be preformed during routine follow-up visits.
- Monitor CBC with differential weekly during the 1st mo, twice monthly for the 2nd and 3rd mo of therapy, and then monthly during the 1st yr. Neutropenia occurs most frequently from 31–180 days posttransplant. If ANC is <1000/mm³, dose should be reduced or discontinued.
- Monitor hepatic and renal status and electrolytes periodically during therapy. May cause ↑ alkaline phosphatase, AST, ALT, LDH, BUN, and serum creatinine. May also cause hyperkalemia, hypokalemia, hypocalcemia, hypomagnesemia, hyperglycemia, and hyperlipidemia.

Implementation

- The initial dose of mycophenolate should be given within 24 hr of transplant.
- Mycophenolate mofetil (Cellcept) and mycophenolic acid (Myfortic) are not interchangeable; rate of absorption is different.
- *REMS:* Mycophenolate is administered under REMS requirements. Prescribers are encouraged to complete Prescriber Training program and patients are encouraged to complete the *Information for Patients* to mitigate the risk of embryofetal toxicity associated with the use of mycophenolate during pregnancy.
- **PO:** Administer on an empty stomach, 1 hr before or 2 hr after meals. *DNC:* Swallow capsules and delayed-release tablets whole; do not open, crush, or chew. Mycophenolate may be teratogenic; wear gloves and avoid contact with skin or mucous membranes or inhalation of contents of capsules or oral suspension powder. Oral suspension can be administered by nasogastric tube (minimum size of 8 French). Oral solution is stable for 60 days if refrigerated.
- Do not administer mycophenolate concurrently with antacids containing magnesium or aluminum.

IV Administration

- **IV:** IV route should only be used for patients unable to take oral medication and should be switched to oral dose form as soon as patient can tolerate capsules or tablets.
- **Intermittent Infusion:** *Dilution:* Reconstitute each vial with 14 mL of D5W. Shake gently to dissolve. Solution is slightly yellow; discard if solution is discolored or contains particulate matter. Dilute contents of 2 vials (1-g dose) further with 140 mL of D5W or 3 vials (1.5-g dose) with 210 mL of D5W. *Concentration:* 6 mg/mL. Solution is stable for 4 hr. *Rate:* Administer via slow IV infusion over at least 2 hr. Do not administer as a bolus or via rapid infusion; increases risk of phlebitis and thrombosis.
- **Y-Site Compatibility:** alemtuzumab, amikacin, amiodarone, anidulafungin, argatroban, atracurium, bivalirudin, bumetanide, buprenorphine, butorphanol, calcium chloride, caspofungin, ceftolozane/tazobactam, chlorpromazine, ciprofloxacin, cisatracurium, daptomycin, dexmedetomidine, dexrazoxane , digoxin, diltiazem, diphenhydramine, dobutamine, dopamine, doxorubicin liposomal, doxycycline, droperidol, enalaprilat, ephedrine, epinephrine, erythromycin, esmolol, famotidine, fentanyl, fluconazole, gentamicin, glycopyrrolate, granisetron, haloperidol, hydralazine, hydromorphone, insulin regular, isavuconazonium, isoproterenol, labetalol, leucovorin calcium, levofloxacin, lidocaine, linezolid, lorazepam, magnesium sulfate, mannitol, meperidine, mesna, methadone, metoclopramide, metoprolol, metronidazole, midazolam, milrinone, minocycline, morphine, moxifloxacin, nalbuphine, naloxone, nicardipine, nitroglycerin, norepinephrine, 0.9% NaCl, octreotide, ondansetron, oxytocin, pamidronate, pentamidine, phentolamine, phenylephrine, potassium chloride, procainamide, prochlorperazine, promethazine, propranolol, remifentanil, rocuronium, succinylcholine, sufentanil, tacrolimus, theophylline, tigecycline, tirofiban, tobramycin, vancomycin, vasopressin, vecuronium, verapamil, voriconazole, zidovudine, zoledronic acid.

- **Y-Site Incompatibility:** acyclovir, allopurinol, amifostine, aminocaproic acid, aminophylline, amphotericin B deoxycholate, amphotericin B lipid complex, amphotericin B liposomal, ampicillin, ampicillin/sulbactam, azithromycin, aztreonam, calcium gluconate, cangrelor, cefazolin, cefotaxime, cefotetan, cefoxitin, ceftazidime, ceftriaxone, cefuroxime, chloramphenicol, clindamycin, dantrolene, defibrotide, dexamethasone, diazepam, eptifibatide, foscarnet, fosphenytoin, furosemide, ganciclovir, gemtuzumab ozogamicin, heparin, hydrocortisone, imipenem/cilastatin, ketorolac, meropenem, methotrexate, methylprednisolone, micafungin, nafcillin, nitroprusside, pantoprazole, pentobarbital, phenobarbital, phenytoin, piperacillin/tazobacatam, potassium acetate, potassium phosphate, sodium acetate, sodium bicarbonate, sodium phosphate, trimethoprim/sulfamethoxazole.

Patient/Family Teaching

- Instruct patient to take medication as directed, at the same time each day. Take missed dose as soon as remembered, but not if within 2 hrs before next dose. Do not skip or double up on missed doses. Do not discontinue without consulting health care professional. Advise patient to read *Medication Guide* before starting therapy and with each Rx refill in case of changes.
- *REMS:* Explain REMS program to patient.
- Reinforce the need for lifelong therapy to prevent transplant rejection. Review symptoms of rejection for the transplanted organ, and stress need to notify health care professional immediately if signs of rejection or infection occur.
- May cause somnolence, confusion, dizziness, tremor, or hypotension. Caution patient to avoid driving and other activities requiring alertness until response from medication is known.
- Instruct patient to notify health care professional immediately if signs and symptoms of infection (temperature ≥100.5°F, cold symptoms [runny nose, sore throat], flu symptoms [upset stomach, stomach pain, vomiting, diarrhea], earache or headache, pain during urination, frequent urination, white patches in mouth or throat, unexpected bruising or

bleeding, cuts, scrapes, or incisions that are red, warm, and oozing pus) or PML.

- Advise patient to avoid contact with persons with contagious diseases.
- Advise patient to avoid vaccinations with live attenuated virus during therapy.
- Inform patient of the increased risk of lymphoma and other malignancies. Advise patient to use sunscreen and wear protective clothing to decrease risk of skin cancer.
- Advise patient to notify health care professional of all Rx or OTC medications, vitamins, or herbal products being taken and to consult with health care professional before taking other medications.
- Instruct patient to avoid donating blood during and for at least 6 wk after discontinuation of therapy.
- Rep: May cause fetal harm. Inform females of reproductive potential of the potential for pregnancy loss and fetal harm. Discuss importance of simultaneously using two reliable nonhormonal forms of contraception, unless abstinence is the chosen method, prior to beginning, during, and for 6 wk following discontinuation of therapy and to avoid breastfeeding. Discuss acceptable forms of contraception with health care professional. Mycophenolate may decrease effectiveness of hormonal contraceptives. Encourage patients who become pregnant during or within 6 wk after therapy to enroll in the Pregnancy Registry by calling 1-800-617-8191 or www.mycophenolateREMS.com to monitor pregnancy outcomes in women exposed to mycophenolate during pregnancy. Instruct male patients with female partners of reproductive potential to use effective contraception during and for at least 90 days after discontinuing therapy. Advise male patients to avoid semen donation during and for at least 90 days after discontinuing therapy.
- Emphasize the importance of routine follow-up laboratory tests.

Evaluation/Desired Outcomes
- Prevention of rejection of transplanted organs.

nafarelin (na-fare-e-lin)
Synarel
Classification
Therapeutic: hormones
Pharmacologic: gonadotropin-releasing hormones

Indications
Endometriosis. Central precocious puberty (gonadotropin-dependent) in children.

Action
Acts as a synthetic analogue of gonadotropin-releasing hormone (GnRH). Initially increases pituitary production of luteinizing hormone and follicle-stimulating hormone, which cause ovarian steroid production. Chronic administration leads to decreased production of gonadotropins. Endometriotic lesions are sensitive to ovarian hormones. **Therapeutic Effects:** Reduction in lesions and associated pain in endometriosis. Arrest and regression of puberty in children with central precocious puberty.

Pharmacokinetics
Absorption: Well absorbed following intranasal administration.
Distribution: Unknown.
Metabolism and Excretion: 20–40% excreted in feces; 3% excreted unchanged by the kidneys.
Half-life: 3 hr.

TIME/ACTION PROFILE (↓ ovarian steroid production)

ROUTE	ONSET	PEAK	DURATION
Intranasal	within 4 wk	3–4 wk	3–6 mo†

†Relief of symptoms of endometriosis following discontinuation.

Contraindications/Precautions
Contraindicated in: Hypersensitivity to GnRH, its analogues, or sorbitol; OB: Pregnancy ; Lactation: Lactation.
Use Cautiously in: Rhinitis; Seizures, cerebrovascular disorders, CNS tumor, or concurrent use of bupropion or selective serotonin reuptake inhibitors.

Adverse Reactions/Side Effects
CV: edema, MI. **Derm:** acne, hot flushing, hirsutism, seborrhea. **EENT:** nasal irritation. **Endo:** ↓ breast size, hyperglycemia. **GU:** ↓ fertility, ↓ libido, cessation of menses, vaginal dryness. **Metab:** weight gain. **MS:** ↓ bone density, myalgia. **Neuro:** headache, aggression, anger, depression, impatience, insomnia, intracranial hypertension (children), irritability, SEIZURES, STROKE, SUICIDAL ATTEMPT/IDEATION (in children). **Misc:** hypersensitivity reactions.

Interactions
Drug-Drug: Concurrent **topical nasal decongestants** may ↓ absorption (administer decongestant at least 2 hr after nafarelin). Concurrent use with **bupropion** or **SSRIs** may ↑ risk of seizures.

Route/Dosage
Endometriosis
Intranasal (Adults): 1 spray (200 mcg) in one nostril in the morning and 1 spray in the other nostril in the evening (400 mcg/day). May ↑ to 1 spray in each nostril in the morning and evening (800 mcg/day).

Central Precocious Puberty
Intranasal (Children): 2 sprays in each nostril in the morning and in the evening (1600 mcg/day); may ↑ up to 1800 mcg/day (3 sprays in alternating nostrils 3 times daily).

Availability
Nasal spray: 2 mg/mL (200 mcg/spray).

NURSING IMPLICATIONS
Assessment
- **Endometriosis:** Assess patient for endometriotic pain periodically during therapy.
- **Central Precocious Puberty:** Prior to therapy, a complete physical and endocrinologic examination including height, weight, hand and wrist x-ray, total sex steroid level (estradiol or testosterone), adrenal steroid level, beta human chorionic gonadotropin level, GnRH stimulation test, pelvic/adrenal/testicular ultrasound, and CT of the head must be performed. These parameters are monitored after 6–8 wk and every 3–6 mo during therapy.
- Assess patient for signs of precocious puberty (menses, breast development, testicular growth) periodically during therapy.
- Nafarelin is discontinued when the onset of normal puberty is desired. Monitor the onset of normal puberty and assess menstrual cycle, reproductive function, and final adult height.

Implementation
- **Endometriosis:** Treatment should be started between days 2 and 4 of the menstrual cycle and continued for up to 6 mo.

Patient/Family Teaching
- Instruct patient on the correct technique for nasal spray: The head should be tilted back slightly; wait 30 sec between sprays.
- Advise patient to consult health care professional if rhinitis occurs during therapy. If a topical decongestant is needed, do not use decongestant until 2 hr after nafarelin dosing. If possible, avoid sneezing during and immediately after nafarelin dose.

- Rep: May cause fetal harm. Advise females of reproductive potential to use effective contraception and to avoid breastfeeding during therapy.
- **Endometriosis:** Inform patient that 1 spray should be administered into one nostril in the morning and 1 spray into the other nostril in the evening for the 400-mcg/day dose. If dose is increased to 800 mcg/day, administer 1 spray to each nostril (2 sprays) morning and evening; 1 bottle should provide a 30-day supply at the 400 mcg/day dose.
- Advise patient to use a form of contraception other than oral contraceptives during therapy. Inform patient that amenorrhea is expected. Instruct patient to notify health care professional if regular menstruation persists or if successive doses are missed.
- Advise patient that medication may cause hot flashes. Notify health care professional if these become bothersome.
- **Central Precocious Puberty:** Instruct patient on correct timing and number of sprays. The 1600-mcg/day dose is achieved by 2 sprays to each nostril in the morning (4 sprays) and 2 sprays to each nostril in the evening (4 sprays), for a total of 8 sprays. The 1800 mcg/day dose is achieved by 3 sprays into alternating nostrils 3 times per day, for a total of 9 sprays. Inform patient and parents that if doses are not taken as directed pubertal process may be reactivated. One bottle should provide a 7-day supply at the 1600-mcg/day dose.
- Advise patient and parents that during 1st mo of therapy some signs of puberty (vaginal bleeding, breast enlargement) may occur. These should resolve after the 1st mo of therapy. If these signs persist after the 2nd mo of therapy, notify health care professional.

Evaluation/Desired Outcomes

- Reduction in lesions and associated pain in endometriosis.
- Regression of the signs of precocious puberty.

---

nafcillin, See PENICILLINS, PENICILLINASE RESISTANT.

---

naftifine, See ANTIFUNGALS (TOPICAL).

HIGH ALERT

nalbuphine (nal-byoo-feen)
✥Nubain
Classification
Therapeutic: opioid analgesics
Pharmacologic: opioid agonists/analgesics

Indications
Moderate to severe pain. Supplement to balanced anesthesia. Pain control during labor. Sedation before surgery.

Action
Binds to opiate receptors in the CNS. Alters the perception of and response to painful stimuli while producing generalized CNS depression. In addition, has partial antagonist properties, which may result in opioid withdrawal in physically dependent patients. **Therapeutic Effects:** Decreased pain.

Pharmacokinetics
Absorption: Well absorbed after IM and SUBQ administration. IV administration results in complete bioavailability.
Distribution: Unknown.
Metabolism and Excretion: Mostly metabolized by the liver and eliminated in the feces via biliary excretion. Minimal amounts excreted unchanged by the kidneys.
Half-life: *Children (1–8 yr):* 0.9 hr; *Adults:* 3.5–5 hr.

TIME/ACTION PROFILE (analgesia)

ROUTE	ONSET	PEAK	DURATION
IM	<15 min	60 min	3–6 hr
SUBQ	<15 min	unknown	3–6 hr
IV	2–3 min	30 min	3–6 hr

Contraindications/Precautions
Contraindicated in: Hypersensitivity to nalbuphine or bisulfites; Patients physically dependent on opioids and who have not been detoxified (may precipitate withdrawal).
Use Cautiously in: Head trauma; ↑ intracranial pressure; Severe renal impairment; Severe hepatic impairment; Severe pulmonary disease; Hypothyroidism; Adrenal insufficiency; Alcoholism; Undiagnosed abdominal pain; Prostatic hyperplasia; Patients who have recently received opioid agonists; OB: Use during pregnancy only if potential maternal benefit justifies potential fetal risk. Has been used during labor but may cause respiratory depression in the newborn; prolonged use of opioids during pregnancy can result in neonatal opioid withdrawal syndrome; Lactation: Use while breastfeeding only if potential maternal benefit justifies potential risk to infant. May cause respiratory depression and excessive sedation in infant; Pedi: Safety and effectiveness not established in children; Geri: Dose ↓ suggested in older adults.

Adverse Reactions/Side Effects
CV: hypertension, orthostatic hypotension, palpitations. **Derm:** ↑ sweating, clammy feeling. **EENT:** blurred vision, diplopia, miosis (high doses). **Endo:** adrenal insufficiency. **GI:** dry mouth, nausea, vomiting, constipation, ileus. **GU:** urinary urgency. **Neuro:** dizziness, headache, sedation, confusion, dysphoria, euphoria,

floating feeling, hallucinations, unusual dreams. **Resp:** RESPIRATORY DEPRESSION (including central sleep apnea and sleep-related hypoxemia). **Misc:** physical dependence, psychological dependence, tolerance.

Interactions

Drug-Drug: Use with extreme caution in patients receiving **MAO inhibitors** (may result in unpredictable, severe reactions—↓ initial dose of nalbuphine to 25% of usual dose). Use with **benzodiazepines** or other **CNS depressants** including other **opioids, non-benzodiazepine sedative/hypnotics, anxiolytics, general anesthetics, muscle relaxants, antipsychotics,** and **alcohol**; may cause profound sedation, respiratory depression, coma, and death; reserve concurrent use for when alternative treatment options are inadequate. May precipitate withdrawal in patients who are physically dependent on **opioid agonists.** Avoid concurrent use with other **opioid agonists**; may diminish analgesic effect. Drugs that affect serotonergic neurotransmitter systems, including **tricyclic antidepressants, SSRIs, SNRIs, MAO inhibitors, tramadol, trazodone, mirtazapine, 5HT₃ receptor antagonists, linezolid, methylene blue,** and **triptans,** may ↑ risk of serotonin syndrome.

Drug-Natural Products: Concomitant use of **kava-kava, valerian, skullcap, chamomile,** or **hops** can ↑ CNS depression.

Route/Dosage

Analgesia

IM, SUBQ, IV (Adults): Usual dose is 10 mg every 3–6 hr (maximum: 20 mg/dose or 160 mg/day).
IM, SUBQ, IV (Children): 0.1–0.15 mg/kg every 3–6 hr (maximum: 20 mg/dose or 160 mg/day).

Supplement to Balanced Anesthesia

IV (Adults): *Initial:* 0.3–3 mg/kg over 10–15 min. *Maintenance:* 0.25–0.5 mg/kg as needed.

Availability (generic available)

Solution for injection: 10 mg/mL, 20 mg/mL.

NURSING IMPLICATIONS

Assessment

- Assess type, location, and intensity of pain before and 1 hr after IM or 30 min (peak) after IV administration. When titrating opioid doses, increases of 25–50% should be administered until there is either a 50% reduction in the patient's pain rating on a numeric or visual analogue scale or the patient reports satisfactory pain relief. A repeat dose can be safely administered at the time of the peak if previous dose is ineffective and side effects are minimal. Patients requiring doses higher than 20 mg should be converted to an opioid agonist. Nalbuphine is not recommended for prolonged use or as first-line therapy for acute or cancer pain.

- An equianalgesic chart (see Appendix I) should be used when changing routes or when changing from one opioid to another.

- Assess BP, pulse, and respirations before and periodically during administration. If respiratory rate is <10/min, assess level of sedation. Physical stimulation may be sufficient to prevent significant hypoventilation. Dose may need to be decreased by 25–50%. Monitor for respiratory depression, especially during initiation or following dose increase; serious, life-threatening, or fatal respiratory depression may occur. May cause sleep-related breathing disorders (central sleep apnea, sleep-related hypoxemia). Nalbuphine produces respiratory depression, but this does not markedly increase with increased doses.

- Assess previous analgesic history. Antagonistic properties may induce withdrawal symptoms (vomiting, restlessness, abdominal cramps, and increased BP and temperature) in patients physically dependent on opioids.

- Although this drug has a low potential for dependence, prolonged use may lead to physical and psychological dependence and tolerance. This should not prevent patient from receiving adequate analgesia. Most patients who receive nalbuphine for pain do not develop psychological dependence. If tolerance develops, changing to an opioid agonist may be required to relieve pain.

- Assess risk for opioid addiction, abuse, or misuse prior to administration.

Lab Test Considerations
- May cause ↑ serum amylase and lipase.

Toxicity and Overdose
- If an opioid antagonist is required to reverse respiratory depression or coma, naloxone is the antidote. Dilute the 0.4-mg ampule of naloxone in 10 mL of 0.9% NaCl and administer 0.5 mL (0.02 mg) by IV push every 2 min. For children and patients weighing <40 kg, dilute 0.1 mg of naloxone in 10 mL of 0.9% NaCl for a concentration of 10 mcg/mL and administer 0.5 mcg/kg every 2 min. Titrate dose to avoid withdrawal, seizures, and severe pain.

Implementation

- **_High Alert:_** Do not confuse nalbuphine with naloxone.
- Explain therapeutic value of medication before administration to enhance the analgesic effect.
- Regularly administered doses may be more effective than prn administration. Analgesic is more effective if administered before pain becomes severe.
- Coadministration with nonopioid analgesics may have additive effects and permit lower opioid doses.
- Nalbuphine should be discontinued gradually to prevent withdrawal symptoms after long-term use. Monitor frequently to manage pain and withdrawal symptoms (restlessness, lacrimation, rhinorrhea,

N

yawning, perspiration, chills, myalgia, mydriasis, irritability, anxiety, backache, joint pain, weakness, abdominal cramps, insomnia, nausea, anorexia, vomiting, diarrhea, or increased blood pressure, respiratory rate, or heart rate). If withdrawal symptoms occur, pause the taper for a period of time or raise the dose of opioid analgesic to the previous dose, and then proceed with a slower taper. Also, monitor patients for changes in mood, emergence of suicidal thoughts, or use of other substances. A multimodal approach to pain management may optimize the treatment of chronic pain, as well as assist with the successful tapering of the opioid analgesic.

- **REMS:** FDA strongly encourages health care professionals to complete a REMS-compliant education program that includes all the elements of the FDA Education *Blueprint for Health Care Providers Involved in the Management or Support of Patients with Pain,* available at www.fda.gov/OpioidAnalgesicREMSBlueprint. Information on programs can be found at 1-800-503-0784 or www.opioidanalgesicrems.com.
- Discuss availability of naloxone for emergency treatment of opioid overdose with the patient and caregiver and assess the potential need for access to naloxone, both when initiating and renewing therapy, especially if patient has household members (including children) or other close contacts at risk for accidental exposure or overdose. Consider prescribing naloxone, based on the patient's risk factors for overdose, such as concomitant use of CNS depressants, a history of opioid use disorder, or prior opioid overdose. However, the presence of risk factors for overdose should not prevent the proper management of pain in any patient.
- **IM:** Administer deep into well-developed muscle. Rotate sites of injections.

IV Administration
- **IV Push:** May give IV undiluted.
- **Concentration:** 10–20 mg/mL. *Rate:* Administer slowly, each 10 mg over 3–5 min.
- **Y-Site Compatibility:** acetaminophen, amifostine, amikacin, aminocaproic acid, aminophylline, amiodarone, argatroban, arsenic trioxide, ascorbic acid, atropine, azithromycin, aztreonam, benztropine, bivalirudin, bleomycin, bumetanide, buprenorphine, butorphanol, calcium chloride, calcium gluconate, cangrelor, carboplatin, carmustine, caspofungin, cefazolin, cefotaxime, cefotetan, cefoxitin, ceftazidime, ceftriaxone, cefuroxime, chlorpromazine, cisatracurium, cladribine, clindamycin, cyanocobalamin, cyclophosphamide, cytarabine, dacarbazine, dactinomycin, daptomycin, daunorubicin hydrochloride, dexamethasone, dexmedetomidine, dexrazoxane, digoxin, diltiazem, diphenhydramine, dobutamine, dopamine, doxorubicin hydrochloride, doxorubicin liposomal, doxycycline, enalaprilat, ephedrine, epinephrine, epirubicin, epoetin alfa, eptifibatide, ertapenem, erythromycin, esmolol, etoposide, eto-

poside phosphate, famotidine, fentanyl, filgrastim, fluconazole, fludarabine, fluorouracil, foscarnet, fosphenytoin, gemcitabine, gentamicin, glycopyrrolate, granisetron, heparin, hetastarch, idarubicin, ifosfamide, insulin regular, irinotecan, isoproterenol, labetalol, LR, leucovorin calcium, levofloxacin, lidocaine, linezolid, lorazepam, magnesium sulfate, mannitol, melphalan, meperidine, mesna, metoclopramide, metoprolol, midazolam, milrinone, mitoxantrone, morphine, multivitamins, mycophenolate, naloxone, nicardipine, nitroglycerin, nitroprusside, norepinephrine, octreotide, ondansetron, oxaliplatin, oxytocin, paclitaxel, palonosetron, pamidronate, papaverine, penicillin G, phentolamine, phenylephrine, phytonadione, potassium acetate, potassium chloride, procainamide, prochlorperazine, promethazine, propofol, propranolol, protamine, pyridoxine, remifentanil, rituximab, rocuronium, sodium acetate, succinylcholine, sufentanil, tacrolimus, theophylline, thiamine, thiotepa, tigecycline, tirofiban, tobramycin, topotecan, vancomycin, vasopressin, vecuronium, verapamil, vinblastine, vincristine, vinorelbine, voriconazole, zoledronic acid.

- **Y-Site Incompatibility:** alemtuzumab, allopurinol, amphotericin B deoxycholate, amphotericin B lipid complex, amphotericin B liposomal, anidulafungin, azathioprine, cefepime, chloramphenicol, cyclosporine, dantrolene, diazepam, docetaxel, folic acid, furosemide, ganciclovir, gemtuzumab ozogamicin, hydrocortisone, imipenem/cilastatin, indomethacin, ketorolac, methotrexate, methylprednisolone, mitomycin, pantoprazole, pemetrexed, pentamidine, pentobarbital, phenobarbital, phenytoin, piperacillin/tazobactam, sargramostim, sodium bicarbonate, trastuzumab, trimethoprim/sulfamethoxazole.

Patient/Family Teaching
- Instruct patient on how and when to ask for pain medication.
- May cause drowsiness or dizziness. Advise patient to call for assistance when ambulating and to avoid driving or other activities requiring alertness until response to the medication is known.
- Advise patient to notify health care professional if pain control is not adequate or if severe or persistent side effects occur.
- Caution patient to change positions slowly to minimize orthostatic hypotension.
- Advise patient that frequent mouth rinses, good oral hygiene, and sugarless gum or candy may decrease dry mouth.
- Encourage patient to turn, cough, and breathe deeply every 2 hr to prevent atelectasis.
- Advise patient to avoid concurrent use of alcohol or other CNS depressants with this medication.
- Rep: Advise patient to notify health care professional if pregnancy is planned or suspected, or if breastfeeding. Inform patient of potential for neonatal opioid withdrawal syndrome with prolonged use

during pregnancy. Monitor neonate for signs and symptoms of withdrawal (irritability, hyperactivity and abnormal sleep pattern, high pitched cry, tremor, vomiting, diarrhea, and/or failure to gain weight); usually occur the first days after birth. Monitor infants exposed to nalbuphine through breast milk for excess sedation and respiratory depression. Chronic use may reduce fertility in females and males.

Evaluation/Desired Outcomes
● Decrease in severity of pain without significant alteration in level of consciousness or respiratory status.

naldemedine (nal-dem-e-deen)
Symproic
Classification
Therapeutic: laxatives
Pharmacologic: opioid antagonists

Indications
Treatment of opioid-induced constipation in patients with chronic noncancer pain, including those with chronic pain related to prior cancer or its treatment who do not require frequent (e.g., weekly) opioid dosage escalation.

Action
Acts peripherally as a mu-opioid receptor antagonist, blocking opioid effects on the GI tract. **Therapeutic Effects:** Blocks constipating effects of opioids on the GI tract without loss of analgesia.

Pharmacokinetics
Absorption: Rapidly absorbed; absorption delayed by high-fat meal by 2 hr.
Distribution: Moderate tissue distribution, does not cross the blood-brain barrier.
Protein Binding: 93–94%.
Metabolism and Excretion: Primarily metabolized by liver via the CYP3A isoenzyme to an active metabolite (nor-naldemedine); 57% excreted in urine (16–18% as unchanged drug), 35% excreted in feces.
Half-life: 11 hr.

TIME/ACTION PROFILE (plasma concentrations)

ROUTE	ONSET	PEAK	DURATION
PO	unknown	0.75 hr	unknown

Contraindications/Precautions
Contraindicated in: Hypersensitivity; Known/suspected mechanical GI obstruction; ↑ risk of recurrent GI obstruction; Severe hepatic impairment; Lactation: Lactation.
Use Cautiously in: Known/suspected lesions of GI tract (↑ risk for GI perforation); Receiving opioids for

<4 wk (may be less responsive to naldemedine); OB: Use during pregnancy only if potential maternal benefit justifies potential fetal risk; Pedi: Safety and effectiveness not established in children.

Adverse Reactions/Side Effects
GI: abdominal pain, diarrhea, gastroenteritis, GI PERFORATION, nausea, vomiting. **Misc:** opioid withdrawal.

Interactions
Drug-Drug: Strong CYP3A inducers, including **carbamazepine, phenytoin,** or **rifampin,** may ↓ levels and effectiveness; avoid concurrent use. Other **opioid antagonists** may cause additive effects and ↑ risk of opioid withdrawal. **Moderate CYP3A inhibitors** and **strong CYP3A inhibitors,** including **aprepitant, atazanavir, clarithromycin, diltiazem, erythromycin, fluconazole, itraconazole, ketoconazole,** or **ritonavir,** may ↑ levels and risk of toxicity. **P-glycoprotein inhibitors,** including **amiodarone, captopril, cyclosporine, quinidine,** or **verapamil,** may ↑ levels and risk of toxicity.
Drug-Natural Products: St. John's wort may ↓ levels and its effectiveness; avoid concurrent use.

Route/Dosage
PO (Adults): 0.2 mg once daily.

Availability
Tablets: 0.2 mg.

NURSING IMPLICATIONS
Assessment
● Assess bowel sounds and frequency, quantity, and consistency of stools periodically during therapy.
● Monitor pain intensity during therapy. Naldemedine does not affect pain or effects of opioid analgesics on pain control. Discontinue naldemedine if opioid analgesic is discontinued. Patients receiving opioids for <4 wk may be less responsive to naldemedine.
● Monitor for signs and symptoms of GI perforation (severe, persistent, or worsening abdominal pain) periodically during therapy. Discontinue naldemedine if symptoms occur.

Implementation
● **PO:** Administer once daily without regard to food.

Patient/Family Teaching
● Instruct patient to take naldemedine as directed. Advise patient to read *Medication Guide* prior to starting therapy and with each refill in case of changes.
● Advise patient to notify health care professional immediately if stomach pain that does not go away occurs.
● Advise patient to notify health care professional if signs and symptoms of opioid withdrawal (sweating, chills, diarrhea, stomach pain, anxiety, irritability, yawning) occur. Patients taking methadone for pain are at increased risk for stomach pain and diarrhea.

✱ = Canadian drug name. ▓ = Genetic implication. ~~Strikethrough~~ = Discontinued. CAPITALS = life-threatening. Underline = most frequent.

- Instruct patient to stop taking naldemedine if they stop taking opioid medications.
- Instruct patient to notify health care professional of all Rx or OTC medications, vitamins, or herbal products being taken and consult health care professional before taking any new medications.
- Rep: Advise females of reproductive potential to notify health care professional if pregnancy is planned or suspected and to avoid breastfeeding during and for 3 days after last dose of therapy.

Evaluation/Desired Outcomes
- Relief of opioid induced constipation, especially if opioid therapy has been for 4 wk or more.

※ naloxegol (nal-ox-ee-gol)
Movantik
Classification
Therapeutic: laxatives
Pharmacologic: opioid antagonists

Indications
Treatment of opioid-induced constipation in patients with chronic noncancer pain, including those with chronic pain related to prior cancer or its treatment who do not require frequent (e.g., weekly) opioid dose escalation.

Action
Acts peripherally as a mu receptor antagonist, blocking opioid receptors in the GI tract. **Therapeutic Effects:** Blocks constipating effects of opioids on the GI tract without loss of analgesia.

Pharmacokinetics
Absorption: Systemic absorption follows oral administration. A high-fat meal ↑ absorption.
Distribution: Does not cross the blood-brain barrier.
Metabolism and Excretion: Primarily metabolized by the liver via the CYP3A4 isoenzyme; 68% excreted in feces, 16% in urine mostly as metabolites.
Half-life: 6–11 hr.

TIME/ACTION PROFILE (spontaneous bowel movement)

ROUTE	ONSET	PEAK	DURATION
PO	within 24 hr	unknown	unknown

Contraindications/Precautions
Contraindicated in: Hypersensitivity; Known/suspected/history of GI obstruction; Severe hepatic impairment; Concurrent use of strong CYP3A4 inhibitors, strong CYP3A4 inducers, or other opioid antagonists; Severe hepatic impairment; Lactation: Lactation.
Use Cautiously in: Infiltrative GI tract malignancy, recent GI tract surgery, diverticular disease, ischemic colitis, or concurrent use of bevacizumab (↑ risk of GI perforation); Patients with disruption of the blood-

brain barrier (may precipitate opioid withdrawal); OB: Use during pregnancy only if potential maternal benefit justifies potential fetal risk; Pedi: Safety and effectiveness not established in children; Geri: ※ Blood levels are ↑ in elderly Japanese patients.

Adverse Reactions/Side Effects
Derm: ↑ sweating. **GI:** <u>abdominal pain</u>, diarrhea, flatulence, GI PERFORATION, nausea, vomiting. **Neuro:** headache. **Misc:** HYPERSENSITIVITY REACTIONS (including angioedema), opioid withdrawal.

Interactions
Drug-Drug: **Strong CYP3A4 inhibitors**, including **clarithromycin** and **ketoconazole**, may significantly ↑ levels and risk of toxicity; concurrent use contraindicated. **Strong CYP3A4 inducers**, including **rifampin**, may significantly ↓ levels and effectiveness; concurrent use contraindicated. Other **opioid antagonists** may precipitate opioid withdrawal; concurrent use contraindicated. **Moderate CYP3A4 inhibitors**, including **diltiazem**, **erythromycin**, and **verapamil**, may ↑ levels and risk of toxicity; ↓ naloxegol dose. Concurrent use of **methadone** for pain ↑ risk of stomach pain and diarrhea. Concurrent use of **bevacizumab** may ↑ risk of GI perforation.
Drug-Food: **Grapefruit/grapefruit juice** may ↑ levels and the risk of toxicity/adverse reactions; avoid concurrent use.

Route/Dosage
PO (Adults): 25 mg once daily; if poorly tolerated, ↓ dose to 12.5 mg once daily; *Concurrent use of moderate CYP3A4 inhibitors:* 12.5 mg once daily (careful monitoring recommended).

Renal Impairment
PO (Adults): *CCr <60 mL/min:* 12.5 mg once daily initially; may cautiously ↑ to 25 mg once daily, if necessary, with careful monitoring.

Availability
Tablets: 12.5 mg, 25 mg.

NURSING IMPLICATIONS
Assessment
- Assess bowel sounds and frequency, quantity, and consistency of stools periodically during therapy.
- Monitor pain intensity during therapy. Naloxegol does not affect pain or effects of opioid analgesics on pain control. Discontinue naloxegol if opioid analgesic is discontinued.
- Monitor for signs and symptoms of GI perforation (severe, persistent, or worsening abdominal pain) periodically during therapy. Discontinue naloxegol if symptoms occur.

Implementation
- Discontinue all maintenance laxative therapy before starting naloxegol. If a suboptimal response occurs with naloxegol, laxatives may be used after 3 days.

- **PO:** Administer on an empty stomach at least 1 hr before first meal in morning or 2 hr after meal. Tablet may be crushed to a powder, mixed with 4 oz of water (120 mL) for patients with difficulty swallowing. Drink mixture immediately; refill glass with 120 mL water, stir and drink contents.
- May be administered by nasogastric (NG) tube. Flush the NG tube with 1 oz (30 mL) of water using a 60 mL syringe. Crush tablet to a powder and mix with 2 oz (60 mL) of water. Draw up mixture using the 60 mL syringe and administer through the NG tube. Add 2 oz (60 mL) of water to rinse container and administer to flush NG tube and any remaining medicine from NG tube into stomach.
- Avoid grapefruit and grapefruit juice during therapy.

Patient/Family Teaching
- Instruct patient to take naloxegol on an empty stomach as directed. Laxatives should be stopped before starting naloxegol, but may be restarted after 3 days if needed. Advise patient to read the *Medication Guide* prior to starting therapy and with each Rx refill in case of changes.
- Caution patient to avoid grapefruit and grapefruit juice during therapy.
- Advise patient to notify health care professional immediately if stomach pain that does not go away occurs.
- Advise patient to notify health care professional if signs and symptoms of opioid withdrawal (sweating, chills, diarrhea, stomach pain, anxiety, irritability, yawning) occur. Patients taking methadone for pain are at increased risk for stomach pain and diarrhea.
- Instruct patient to stop taking naloxegol if they stop taking opioid medications.
- Instruct patient to notify health care professional of all Rx or OTC medications, vitamins, or herbal products being taken and consult health care professional before taking any new medications.
- Rep: Advise females of reproductive potential to notify health care professional if pregnancy is planned or suspected and avoid breastfeeding during therapy; may cause opioid withdrawal in infant.

Evaluation/Desired Outcomes
- Relief of opioid-induced constipation, especially if opioid therapy has been for 4 wk or more.

naloxone (nal-**ox**-one)
~~Evzio~~, Kloxxado, Narcan, Rivive, Zimhi
Classification
Therapeutic: antidotes (for opioids)
Pharmacologic: opioid antagonists

Indications
Reversal of CNS depression and respiratory depression because of suspected opioid overdose. **Unlabeled Use:**

Opioid-induced pruritus (low-dose IV infusion). Management of refractory circulatory shock.

Action
Competitively blocks the effects of opioids, including CNS and respiratory depression, without producing any agonist (opioid-like) effects. **Therapeutic Effects:** Reversal of signs of opioid excess.

Pharmacokinetics
Absorption: Well absorbed after IM or SUBQ administration. IV administration results in complete bioavailability. Rapidly absorbed from nasal mucosa.
Distribution: Rapidly distributed to tissues. Crosses the placenta.
Metabolism and Excretion: Metabolized by the liver.
Half-life: *IM, IV, or SUBQ:* 30–90 min (up to 3 hr in neonates); *Intranasal:* 2 hr.

TIME/ACTION PROFILE (reversal of opioid effects)

ROUTE	ONSET	PEAK	DURATION
IV	1–2 min	unknown	45 min
IM, SUBQ	2–5 min	unknown	>45 min
Intranasal	8–13 min	unknown	unknown

Contraindications/Precautions
Contraindicated in: Hypersensitivity.
Use Cautiously in: Cardiovascular disease; Patients physically dependent on opioids (may precipitate severe withdrawal); OB: May cause acute withdrawal syndrome in mother and fetus if mother is opioid dependent; Lactation: Safety not established in breastfeeding; Pedi: May cause acute withdrawal syndrome in neonates of opioid-dependent mothers.

Adverse Reactions/Side Effects
CV: hypertension, hypotension, VENTRICULAR ARRHYTHMIA. **GI:** nausea, vomiting.

Interactions
Drug-Drug: Can precipitate withdrawal in patients physically dependent on **opioid analgesics**. Larger doses may be required to reverse the effects of **buprenorphine**, **butorphanol**, or **nalbuphine**. Antagonizes postoperative **opioid analgesics**.

Route/Dosage
Postoperative Opioid-Induced Respiratory Depression
IV (Adults): 0.02–0.2 mg every 2–3 min until response obtained; repeat every 1–2 hr if needed.
IV (Children): 0.01 mg/kg; may repeat every 2–3 min until response obtained. Additional doses may be given every 1–2 hr if needed.
IM, IV, SUBQ (Neonates): 0.01 mg/kg; may repeat every 2–3 min until response obtained. Additional doses may be given every 1–2 hr if needed.

Opioid-Induced Respiratory Depression During Chronic (>1 wk) Opioid Use

IV, IM, SUBQ (Adults >40 kg): 20–40 mcg (0.02–0.04 mg) given as small, frequent (every min) boluses or as an infusion titrated to improve respiratory function without reversing analgesia.

IV, IM, SUBQ (Adults and Children <40 kg): 0.005–0.02 mg/dose given as small, frequent (every min) boluses or as an infusion titrated to improve respiratory function without reversing analgesia.

Overdose of Opioids

IV, IM, SUBQ (Adults): *Patients not suspected of being opioid dependent:* 0.4 mg (10 mcg/kg); may repeat every 2–3 min (IV route is preferred). Some patients may require up to 2 mg. *Patients suspected to be opioid dependent:* Initial dose should be ↓ to 0.1–0.2 mg every 2–3 min. May also be given by IV infusion at rate adjusted to patient's response.

IV, IM, SUBQ (Children >5 yr or >20 kg): 2 mg/dose, may repeat every 2–3 min.

IV, IM, SUBQ (Infants up to 5 yr or 20 kg): 0.1 mg/kg, may repeat every 2–3 min.

IM, SUBQ (Adults and Children): *Zimbi:* 5 mg, may repeat every 2–3 min.

Intranasal (Adults and Children): 1 spray (3 mg, 4 mg, or 8 mg) in one nostril; may repeat dose every 2–3 min (with each subsequent dose being administered in alternate nostril).

Opioid-Induced Pruritus

IV (Children): 2 mcg/kg/hr continuous infusion, may ↑ by 0.5 mcg/kg/hr every few hrs if pruritus continues.

Availability (generic available)

Nasal spray: 3 mg/0.1 mL ᴼᵀᶜ, 4 mg/0.1 mL ᴼᵀᶜ, 8 mg/0.1 mL. **Solution for injection:** 0.4 mg/mL, 2 mg/2 mL (prefilled syringe), 5 mg/0.5 mL (prefilled syringe). *In combination with:* buprenorphine (Suboxone, Zubsolv). See Appendix N.

NURSING IMPLICATIONS

Assessment

- Monitor respiratory rate, rhythm, and depth; pulse, ECG, BP; and level of consciousness frequently for 3–4 hr after the expected peak of blood concentrations. After a moderate overdose of a short half-life opioid, physical stimulation may be enough to prevent significant hypoventilation. The effects of some opioids may last longer than the effects of naloxone, and repeat doses may be necessary.
- Patients who have been receiving opioids for >1 wk are extremely sensitive to the effects of naloxone. Dilute and administer in slow increments.
- Assess patient for level of pain after administration when used to treat postoperative respiratory depression. Naloxone decreases respiratory depression but also reverses analgesia.
- Assess patient for signs and symptoms of opioid withdrawal (restlessness, lacrimation, rhinorrhea, yawning, perspiration, chills, myalgia, mydriasis, irritability, anxiety, backache, joint pain, weakness, abdominal cramps, insomnia, nausea, anorexia, vomiting, diarrhea, or increased blood pressure, respiratory rate, or heart rate). Symptoms may occur within a few min to 2 hr. Severity depends on dose of naloxone, the opioid involved, and degree of physical dependence.
- Lack of significant improvement indicates that symptoms are caused by a disease process or other non-opioid CNS depressants not affected by naloxone.

Toxicity and Overdose
- Naloxone is a pure antagonist with no agonist properties and minimal toxicity.

Implementation

- Do not confuse naloxone with Lanoxin or nalbuphine.
- Larger doses of naloxone may be necessary when used to antagonize the effects of buprenorphine, butorphanol, and nalbuphine.
- Resuscitation equipment, oxygen, vasopressors, and mechanical ventilation should be available to supplement naloxone therapy as needed.
- Doses should be titrated carefully in postoperative patients to avoid interference with control of postoperative pain.
- **Intranasal:** Administer a single spray into one nostril. If patient does not respond or responds and relapses into respiratory depression, additional doses may be given every 2–3 min in alternating nostrils until emergency medical assistance arrives. Naloxone is not a substitute for emergency medical care.

IV Administration
- **IV Push:** *Dilution:* Administer undiluted for *suspected opioid overdose.* For *opioid-induced respiratory depression,* dilute with sterile water for injection. For children or adults weighing <40 kg, dilute 0.1 mg of naloxone in 10 mL of sterile water or 0.9% NaCl for injection. *Concentration:* 0.4 mg/mL, 1 mg/mL, or 10 mcg/mL (depending on preparation used). *Rate:* Administer over 30 sec for patients with a *suspected opioid overdose.* For patients who develop *opioid-induced respiratory depression,* administer dilute solution of 0.4 mg/10 mL at a rate of 0.5 mL (0.02 mg) IV push every 2 min. Titrate to avoid withdrawal and severe pain. Excessive dose in postoperative patients may cause excitement, pain, hypotension, hypertension, pulmonary edema, ventricular tachycardia and fibrillation, and seizures. For children and adults weighing <40 kg, administer 10 mcg/mL solution at a rate of 0.5 mcg/kg every 1–2 min.
- **Continuous Infusion:** *Dilution:* Dilute 2 mg of naloxone in 500 mL of 0.9% NaCl or D5W. Infusion is stable for 24 hr. *Concentration:* 4 mcg/mL. *Rate:* Titrate dose according to patient response.
- **Y-Site Compatibility:** acetylcysteine, amikacin, aminocaproic acid, amiodarone, anidulafungin, ar-

gatroban, arsenic trioxide, ascorbic acid, atropine, azithromycin, aztreonam, benztropine, bivalirudin, bleomycin, bumetanide, buprenorphine, butorphanol, calcium chloride, calcium gluconate, carboplatin, carmustine, caspofungin, cefotaxime, cefotetan, cefoxitin, ceftazidime, ceftolozane/tazobactam, ceftriaxone, cefuroxime, chloramphenicol, chlorpromazine, ciprofloxacin, cisplatin, clindamycin, cyanocobalamin, cyclophosphamide, cytarabine, dacarbazine, dactinomycin, daptomycin, daunorubicin hydrochloride, defibrotide, desmopressin, dexamethasone, dexmedetomidine, dexrazoxane, digoxin, diltiazem, diphenhydramine, dobutamine, docetaxel, dopamine, doxorubicin hydrochloride, doxorubicin liposomal, doxycycline, droperidol, enalaprilat, ephedrine, epinephrine, epirubicin, epoetin alfa, eptifibatide, ertapenem, erythromycin, esmolol, etoposide, etoposide phosphate, famotidine, fentanyl, fluconazole, fludarabine, fluorouracil, folic acid, foscarnet, fosphenytoin, furosemide, ganciclovir, gemcitabine, gentamicin, glucagon, glycopyrrolate, granisetron, heparin, hetastarch, hydrocortisone, hydromorphone, idarubicin, ifosfamide, imipenem/cilastatin, indomethacin, insulin regular, irinotecan, isavuconazonium, isoproterenol, ketamine, ketorolac, labetalol, LR, levofloxacin, lidocaine, linezolid, mannitol, meperidine, meropenem, meropenem/vaborbactam, mesna, methadone, methotrexate, methylprednisolone, metoclopramide, metoprolol, metronidazole, midazolam, milrinone, mitoxantrone, morphine, moxifloxacin, multivitamins, mycophenolate, nafcillin, nalbuphine, nicardipine, nitroprusside, norepinephrine, octreotide, ondansetron, oxacillin, oxaliplatin, oxytocin, paclitaxel, palonosetron, pamidronate, papaverine, pemetrexed, penicillin G, pentamidine, pentobarbital, phenobarbital, phentolamine, phenylephrine, phytonadione, piperacillin/tazobactam, plazomicin, potassium acetate, potassium chloride, potassium phosphate, procainamide, prochlorperazine, promethazine, propofol, propranolol, protamine, pyridoxine, rocuronium, sodium acetate, sodium bicarbonate, succinylcholine, sufentanil, tacrolimus, tedizolid, theophylline, thiamine, tigecycline, tirofiban, tobramycin, topotecan, vancomycin, vasopressin, vecuronium, verapamil, vinblastine, vincristine, vinorelbine, voriconazole, zoledronic acid.
- **Y-Site Incompatibility:** alemtuzumab, amphotericin B lipid complex, amphotericin B liposomal, blinatumomab, dantrolene, diazepam, gemtuzumab ozogamicin, leucovorin calcium, mitomycin, pantoprazole, phenytoin, thiopental, thiotepa.

Patient/Family Teaching
- As medication becomes effective, explain purpose and effects of naloxone to patient.
- Rep: Advise females of reproductive potential to notify health care professional if pregnancy is planned

or suspected or if breastfeeding. Monitor mother and fetus for withdrawal syndrome if mother is opioid dependent.
- **Intranasal:** Instruct parents and caregivers in the correct technique for use.

Evaluation/Desired Outcomes
- Adequate ventilation following opioid excess.
- Alertness without significant pain or withdrawal symptoms.

BEERS

naproxen (na-**prox**-en)
Aleve, ✹Anaprox, Anaprox DS, EC-Naprosyn, Naprelan, Naprosyn
Classification
Therapeutic: antipyretics, antirheumatics, nonopioid analgesics
Pharmacologic: nonsteroidal anti-inflammatory drugs (NSAIDs)

Indications
Mild to moderate pain. Dysmenorrhea. Fever. Inflammatory disorders, including: Rheumatoid arthritis, Osteoarthritis.

Action
Inhibits prostaglandin synthesis. **Therapeutic Effects:** Decreased pain. Reduction of fever. Suppression of inflammation.

Pharmacokinetics
Absorption: Completely absorbed from the GI tract. Sodium salt is more rapidly absorbed.
Distribution: Crosses the placenta; enters breast milk in low concentrations.
Protein Binding: >99%.
Metabolism and Excretion: Mostly metabolized by the liver.
Half-life: *Children <8 yr:* 8–17 hr; *Children 8–14 yr:* 8–10 hr; *Adults:* 10–20 hr.

TIME/ACTION PROFILE

ROUTE	ONSET	PEAK	DURATION
PO (analgesic)	1 hr	unknown	8–12 hr
PO (anti-inflammatory)	14 days	2–4 wk	unknown

Contraindications/Precautions
Contraindicated in: Hypersensitivity; Cross-sensitivity may occur with other NSAIDs, including aspirin; Active GI bleeding; Ulcer disease; Coronary artery bypass graft surgery; OB: Avoid use after 30 wk gestation; Lactation: Lactation.
Use Cautiously in: Severe renal impairment; Severe hepatic impairment; Cardiovascular disease or risk fac-

tors for cardiovascular disease (may ↑ risk of serious cardiovascular thrombotic events, MI, and stroke, especially with prolonged use or use of higher doses); avoid use in patients with recent MI or HF; History of ulcer disease or any other history of gastrointestinal bleeding (may ↑ risk of GI bleeding); Chronic alcohol use/abuse; OB: Use at or after 20 wk gestation may cause fetal or neonatal renal impairment; if treatment is necessary between 20 wk and 30 wk gestation, limit use to the lowest effective dose and shortest duration possible; Pedi: Children <2 yr (safety and effectiveness not established); Geri: Appears on Beers list. ↑ risk GI bleeding or peptic ulcer disease in older adults. Avoid chronic use unless other alternatives are not effective and the patient can take a gastroprotective agent; avoid short-term use in combination with oral or parenteral corticosteroids, anticoagulants, or antiplatelet agents unless other alternatives are not effective and the patient can take a gastroprotective agent.

Adverse Reactions/Side Effects

CV: edema, HF, hypertension, MI, palpitations, tachycardia. **Derm:** ↑ sweating, DRUG REACTION WITH EOSINOPHILIA AND SYSTEMIC SYMPTOMS (DRESS), photosensitivity, pseudoporphyria (12% incidence in children with juvenile rheumatoid arthritis—discontinue therapy if this occurs), rash, STEVENS-JOHNSON SYNDROME, TOXIC EPIDERMAL NECROLYSIS. **EENT:** tinnitus, visual disturbances. **F and E:** hyperkalemia. **GI:** constipation, dyspepsia, nausea, anorexia, diarrhea, discomfort, flatulence, GI BLEEDING, HEPATITIS, vomiting. **GU:** cystitis, hematuria, renal failure. **Hemat:** blood dyscrasias, prolonged bleeding time. **Neuro:** dizziness, drowsiness, headache, STROKE. **Resp:** dyspnea. **Misc:** HYPERSENSITIVITY REACTIONS (including anaphylaxis).

Interactions

Drug-Drug: May limit the cardioprotective (antiplatelet) effects of **aspirin**. ↑ risk of bleeding with **anticoagulants, aspirin, clopidogrel, ticagrelor, prasugrel, corticosteroids, fibrinolytics, SNRIs,** or **SSRIs.** Additive adverse GI side effects with **aspirin, corticosteroids, alcohol,** and other **NSAIDs. Probenecid** ↑ blood levels and may ↑ toxicity. May ↑ risk of toxicity from **methotrexate, antineoplastics,** or **radiation therapy.** May ↑ serum levels and risk of toxicity from **lithium.** ↑ risk of adverse renal effects with **cyclosporine, ACE inhibitors, angiotensin II antagonists,** or chronic use of **acetaminophen.** May ↓ response to **antihypertensives** or **diuretics.** May ↑ risk of hypoglycemia with **insulin** or **oral hypoglycemic agents. Oral potassium supplements** may ↑ GI adverse effects.
Drug-Natural Products: ↑ anticoagulant effect and bleeding risk with **anise, arnica, chamomile, clove, dong quai, feverfew, garlic, ginger, ginkgo, Panax ginseng, licorice,** and others.

Route/Dosage

275 mg naproxen sodium is equivalent to 250 mg naproxen.

Anti-inflammatory/Analgesic/Antidysmenorrheal

PO (Adults): *Naproxen:* 250–500 mg twice daily (up to 1.5 g/day). *Delayed-release naproxen:* 375–500 mg twice daily. *Naproxen sodium:* 275–550 mg twice daily (up to 1.65 g/day).
PO (Children >2 yr): *Analgesia:* 5–7 mg/kg/dose every 8–12 hr. *Inflammatory disease:* 10–15 mg/kg/day divided every 12 hr, maximum: 1000 mg/day.

Gout

PO (Adults): *Naproxen:* 750 mg initially, then 250 mg every 8 hr. *Naproxen sodium:* 825 mg initially, then 275 mg every 8 hr.

OTC Use (naproxen sodium)

PO (Adults): 200 mg every 8–12 hr or 400 mg followed by 200 mg every 12 hr (not to exceed 600 mg/24 hr).
PO (Geriatric Patients >65 yr): Not to exceed 200 mg every 12 hr.

Availability

Naproxen (generic available)
Immediate-release tablets (Naprosyn): ✹ 125 mg, 250 mg, 375 mg, 500 mg. **Delayed-release tablets (EC-Naprosyn):** 375 mg, 500 mg. **Extended-release tablets:** ✹ 750 mg. **Oral suspension (Naprosyn):** 125 mg/5 mL. *In combination with:* esomeprazole (Vimovo).

Naproxen Sodium (generic available)
Immediate-release tablets (Aleve, Anaprox DS): 220 mg^OTC, 275 mg, 550 mg. **Immediate-release capsules (Maxidol):** ✹ 220 mg^OTC. **Extended-release tablets (Naprelan):** 375 mg, 500 mg, 750 mg. *In combination with:* pseudoephedrine (Aleve-D Sinus and Cold), sumatriptan (Treximet). See Appendix N.

NURSING IMPLICATIONS

Assessment

● Patients who have asthma, aspirin-induced allergy, and nasal polyps are at increased risk for developing hypersensitivity reactions. Assess for rhinitis, asthma, and urticaria.
● Monitor BP during initiation and periodically during therapy. May cause fluid retention and edema leading to new onset or worsening hypertension.
● Assess for rash periodically during therapy. May cause Stevens-Johnson syndrome. Discontinue therapy if severe or if accompanied with fever, general malaise, fatigue, muscle or joint aches, blisters, oral lesions, conjunctivitis, hepatitis, and/or eosinophilia.
● Monitor for signs and symptoms of DRESS (fever, rash, lymphadenopathy, facial swelling) periodically during therapy. Discontinue therapy if symptoms occur.
● **Pain:** Assess pain (note type, location, and intensity) prior to and 1–2 hr following administration.

- **Arthritis:** Assess pain and range of motion prior to and 1–2 hr following administration.
- **Fever:** Monitor temperature; note signs associated with fever (diaphoresis, tachycardia, malaise).

Lab Test Considerations
- Evaluate BUN, serum creatinine, CBC, and liver function tests periodically in patients receiving prolonged therapy.
- May ↑ serum potassium, BUN, serum creatinine, alkaline phosphatase, LDH, AST, and ALT tests levels. May ↓ blood glucose, hemoglobin, and hematocrit concentrations, leukocyte and platelet counts, and CCr.
- Bleeding time may be prolonged up to 4 days following discontinuation of therapy.
- May alter test results for urine 5-HIAA and urine steroid determinations.

Implementation
- Administration in higher than recommended doses does not provide increased effectiveness but may cause increased side effects. Use lowest effective dose for the shortest duration possible to minimize risk of cardiovascular thrombotic events.
- Coadministration with opioid analgesics may have additive analgesic effects and may permit lower opioid doses.
- Naproxen is more effective if given before pain becomes severe.
- **PO:** For rapid initial effect, administer 30 min before or 2 hr after meals. May be administered with food, milk, or antacids to decrease GI irritation. Food slows but does not reduce the extent of absorption. Do not mix suspension with antacid or other liquid prior to administration. *DNC:* Swallow extended-release, delayed-release, and controlled-release tablets whole; do not break, crush, or chew.
- **Dysmenorrhea:** Administer as soon as possible after the onset of menses. Prophylactic treatment has not been shown to be effective.

Patient/Family Teaching
- Instruct patient to take medication as directed. Take missed doses as soon as remembered but not if almost time for the next dose. Do not double doses.
- Advise patient to take this medication with a full glass of water and to remain in an upright position for 15–30 min after administration.
- May cause drowsiness or dizziness. Advise patient to avoid driving or other activities requiring alertness until response to the medication is known.
- Caution patient to avoid the concurrent use of alcohol, aspirin, acetaminophen, or other OTC medications without consulting health care professional. Use of naproxen with 3 or more glasses of alcohol per day may increase risk of GI bleeding.
- Advise patient to inform health care professional of medication regimen prior to treatment or surgery.

- Caution patient to wear sunscreen and protective clothing to prevent photosensitivity reactions (especially in children with juvenile rheumatoid arthritis).
- Instruct patient not to take OTC naproxen preparations for more than 3 days for fever and to consult health care professional if symptoms persist or worsen.
- Advise patient to consult health care professional if rash, itching, visual disturbances, tinnitus, weight gain, edema, black stools, persistent headache, or influenza-like syndrome (chills, fever, muscle aches, pain) occurs.
- Rep: May cause fetal harm. Advise females of reproductive potential to notify health care professional if pregnancy is planned or suspected or if breastfeeding. Advise women to avoid naproxen in the 3rd trimester of pregnancy (after 29 wk); may cause premature closure of the fetal ductus arteriosus. Use of naproxen after 20 wk may cause fetal renal dysfunction leading to oligohydramnios. May cause reversible infertility in women attempting to conceive; may consider discontinuing naproxen.

Evaluation/Desired Outcomes
- Relief of pain.
- Improved joint mobility. Partial arthritic relief is usually seen within 2 wk, but maximum effectiveness may require 2–4 wk of continuous therapy. Patients who do not respond to one NSAID may respond to another.
- Reduction of fever.

naratriptan (nar-a-trip-tan)
~~Amerge~~
Classification
Therapeutic: vascular headache suppressants
Pharmacologic: 5-HT₁ agonists

Indications
Acute treatment of migraine headache.

Action
Acts as an agonist at specific 5-HT₁ receptor sites in intracranial blood vessels and sensory trigeminal nerves. **Therapeutic Effects:** Cranial vessel vasoconstriction with resultant decrease in migraine headache.

Pharmacokinetics
Absorption: Well absorbed (70%) following oral administration.
Distribution: Extensively distributed to tissues.
Metabolism and Excretion: Primarily metabolized in the liver. 60% excreted unchanged in urine; 30% metabolized by the liver.
Half-life: 6 hr (↑ in renal impairment).

TIME/ACTION PROFILE (↓ migraine pain)

ROUTE	ONSET	PEAK	DURATION
PO	30–60 min	2–3 hr†	up to 24 hr

†3–4 hr during migraine attack.

Contraindications/Precautions

Contraindicated in: Hypersensitivity; Ischemic heart disease or Prinzmetal's angina; Uncontrolled hypertension; Wolff-Parkinson-White syndrome or other arrhythmias involving conduction pathways; Hemiplegic or basilar migraine; Stroke or transient ischemic attack; Peripheral vascular disease; Ischemic bowel disease; Severe renal impairment (CCr <15 mL/min); Severe hepatic impairment.

Use Cautiously in: Mild to moderate renal impairment (dose should not exceed 2.5 mg/24 hr; initial dose should be ↓); Mild to moderate hepatic impairment (dose should not exceed 2.5 mg/24 hr; initial dose should be ↓); OB: Safety not established in pregnancy; Lactation: Safety not established in breastfeeding; Pedi: Safety and effectiveness not established in children; Geri: Age-related ↓ in renal function and ↑ likelihood of CAD greatly ↑ risk of fatal adverse events in older adults.

Exercise Extreme Caution in: Cardiovascular risk factors (hypertension, hypercholesterolemia, cigarette smoking, obesity, diabetes, strong family history, menopausal women, or men >40 yr); use only if cardiovascular status has been evaluated and determined to be safe and 1st dose is administered under supervision.

Adverse Reactions/Side Effects

CV: CORONARY ARTERY VASOSPASM, MI, myocardial ischemia, VENTRICULAR FIBRILLATION, VENTRICULAR TACHYCARDIA. **GI:** nausea. **Neuro:** dizziness, drowsiness, fatigue, paresthesia. **Misc:** pain/pressure sensation in throat/neck.

Interactions

Drug-Drug: ↑ risk of serotonin syndrome when used with **SSRIs** or **SNRIs**. **Cigarette smoking** ↑ the metabolism and ↓ levels of naratriptan. Levels and risk of toxicity are ↑ by **hormonal contraceptives**. Avoid concurrent use (within 24 hr of each other) with **ergot-containing drugs (dihydroergotamine)**; may result in prolonged vasospastic reactions. Avoid concurrent (within 2 wk) use with **MAO inhibitors**; produces ↑ systemic exposure and risk of adverse reactions to naratriptan.

Drug-Natural Products: ↑ risk of serotonergic side effects including serotonin syndrome with **St. John's wort** and **SAMe**.

Route/Dosage

PO (Adults): 1 or 2.5 mg; dose may be repeated in 4 hr if response is inadequate (not to exceed 5 mg/24 hr or treatment of more than 4 headaches/mo).

Availability (generic available)

Tablets: 1 mg, 2.5 mg.

NURSING IMPLICATIONS

Assessment

- Assess pain location, character, intensity, and duration and associated symptoms (photophobia, phonophobia, nausea, vomiting) during migraine attack.
- Monitor for serotonin syndrome in patients taking SSRIs or SNRIs concurrently with naratriptan.

Implementation

- **PO:** Tablets may be administered at any time after the headache starts.

Patient/Family Teaching

- Inform patient that naratriptan should be used only during a migraine attack. It is meant to be used for relief of migraine attacks but not to prevent or reduce the number of attacks.
- Instruct patient to administer naratriptan as soon as symptoms of a migraine attack appear, but it may be administered any time during an attack. If migraine symptoms return, a 2nd dose may be used. Allow at least 4 hr between doses, and do not use more than 2 tablets in any 24-hr period. Do not use to treat more than 4 headaches per mo.
- Advise patient that lying down in a darkened room following naratriptan administration may further help relieve headache.
- Advise patient that overuse (use more than 10 days/mo) may lead to exacerbation of headache (migraine-like daily headaches, or as a marked increase in frequency of migraine attacks). May require gradual withdrawal of naratriptan and treatment of symptoms (transient worsening of headache).
- Advise patient to notify health care professional prior to next dose of naratriptan if pain or tightness in the chest occurs during use. If pain is severe or does not subside, notify health care professional immediately. If wheezing; heart throbbing; swelling of eyelids, face, or lips; skin rash; skin lumps; or hives occur, notify health care professional immediately and do not take more naratriptan without approval of health care professional. If feelings of tingling, heat, flushing, heaviness, pressure, drowsiness, dizziness, tiredness, or sickness develop, discuss with health care professional at next visit.
- Instruct patient not to take additional naratriptan if no response is seen with initial dose without consulting health care professional. There is no evidence that 5 mg provides greater relief than 2.5-mg dose. Additional naratriptan doses are not likely to be effective, and alternative medications, as previously discussed with health care professional, may be used.
- Naratriptan may cause dizziness or drowsiness. Caution patient to avoid driving or other activities requiring alertness until response to medication is known.
- Advise patient to avoid alcohol, which aggravates headaches, during naratriptan use.

- Advise patient to notify health care professional of all Rx or OTC medications, vitamins, or herbal products being taken and to consult with health care professional before taking other medications. Patients concurrently taking SSRI or SNRI antidepressants should notify health care professional promptly if signs of serotonin syndrome (mental status changes: agitation, hallucinations, coma; autonomic instability: tachycardia, labile BP, hyperthermia; neuromuscular aberrations: hyperreflexia, incoordination; and/or gastrointestinal symptoms: nausea, vomiting, diarrhea) occur.
- Rep: Advise females of reproductive potential to notify health care professional if pregnancy is planned or suspected or if breastfeeding.

Evaluation/Desired Outcomes

- Relief of migraine attack.

---

neomycin, See AMINOGLYCOSIDES.

⚕ neratinib (ne-ra-ti-nib)
Nerlynx
Classification
Therapeutic: antineoplastics
Pharmacologic: enzyme inhibitors, kinase inhibitors

Indications

⚕ Extended adjuvant treatment of early stage human epidermal receptor type 2 (HER2)-overexpressed/amplified breast cancer following adjuvant trastuzumab-based therapy. ⚕ Advanced or metastatic HER2-positive breast cancer in patients who have received ≥2 prior anti-HER2–based regimens in the metastatic setting (in combination with capecitabine).

Action

⚕ Irreversibly binds to epidermal growth factor receptor (EGFR), HER2, and HER4 to inhibit growth of tumors that express HER2 and EGFR. **Therapeutic Effects:** Decreased progression of breast cancer and improved survival.

Pharmacokinetics

Absorption: Blood levels ↑ by high-fat foods.
Distribution: Extensively distributed to tissues.
Protein Binding: >99%.
Metabolism and Excretion: Primarily metabolized in liver via the CYP3A4 isoenzyme into active metabolites (M3, M6, M7, and M11); 97% excreted in feces, <2% excreted by kidneys.
Half-life: 7–17 hr.

TIME/ACTION PROFILE (plasma concentrations)

ROUTE	ONSET	PEAK	DURATION
PO	unknown	2–8 hr	24 hr

Contraindications/Precautions

Contraindicated in: OB: Pregnancy; Lactation: Lactation.
Use Cautiously in: Severe hepatic impairment (↓ dose); Rep: Women of reproductive potential and men with female partners of reproductive potential; Pedi: Safety and effectiveness not established in children; Geri: ↑ risk of adverse reactions/side effects in older adults.

Adverse Reactions/Side Effects

CV: hypotension. **Derm:** <u>rash</u>, dry skin, nail disorder. **EENT:** epistaxis. **GI:** ↓ <u>appetite</u>, <u>abdominal pain</u>, DIARRHEA, dyspepsia, <u>nausea</u>, stomatitis, vomiting, ↓ weight, abdominal distention, dry mouth, HEPATOTOXICITY. **GU:** renal failure, urinary tract infection. **MS:** <u>muscle spasms</u>. **Neuro:** <u>fatigue</u>.

Interactions

Drug-Drug: ↓ levels with **proton pump inhibitors**, **H₂ blockers**, and **antacids**; avoid concurrent use with **proton pump inhibitors**; take ≥2 hr before next dose of **H₂ antagonist** or 10 hr after the **H₂ antagonist**; take 3 hr after **antacids**. **Strong or moderate CYP3A4 inhibitors**, including **aprepitant, cimetidine, ciprofloxacin, clarithromycin, clotrimazole, cobicistat, conivaptan, crizotinib, cyclosporine, diltiazem, dronedarone, erythromycin, fluconazole, fluvoxamine, idelalisib, imatinib, itraconazole, ketoconazole, lopinavir, nefazodone, nelfinavir, posaconazole, ritonavir, tipranavir, verapamil,** and **voriconazole,** may ↑ levels and risk of toxicity; avoid concurrent use. **Strong or moderate CYP3A4 inducers,** including **bosentan, carbamazepine, efavirenz, enzalutamide, mitotane, modafanil, phenytoin,** and **rifampin,** may ↓ levels and effectiveness; avoid concurrent use. May ↑ levels and risk of toxicity of **digoxin**.
Drug-Natural Products: St. John's wort may ↓ levels and effectiveness; avoid concurrent use.

Route/Dosage

Extended Adjuvant Treatment of Early Stage Breast Cancer

PO (Adults): *Non-dose escalation strategy (administer antidiarrheal prophylaxis for the first 56 days of treatment on scheduled basis):* 240 mg once daily until disease recurrence or for up to 1 yr *OR Dose escalation strategy (use antidiarrheals only as needed for diarrhea):* 120 mg once daily for 7 days, then 160 mg once daily for 7 days, then 240 mg once daily thereafter until disease recurrence or for up to 1 yr.

N

✦ = Canadian drug name. ⚕ = Genetic implication. ~~Strikethrough~~ = Discontinued. CAPITALS = life-threatening. <u>Underline</u> = most frequent.

Hepatic Impairment
PO (Adults): *Severe hepatic impairment:* 80 mg once daily until disease recurrence or for up to 1 yr.

Advanced or Metastatic Breast Cancer
PO (Adults): *Non-dose escalation strategy (administer antidiarrheal prophylaxis for the first 56 days of treatment on scheduled basis):* 240 mg once daily on days 1–21 of a 21-day cycle; continue until disease recurrence or unacceptable toxicity. *OR Dose escalation strategy (use antidiarrheals only as needed for diarrhea):* 120 mg once daily for 7 days, then 160 mg once daily for 7 days, then 240 mg once daily for 7 days, then 240 mg once daily on days 1–21 of a 21-day cycle; continue until disease recurrence of unacceptable toxicity.

Hepatic Impairment
PO (Adults): *Severe hepatic impairment:* 80 mg once daily on days 1–21 of a 21-day cycle; continue until disease recurrence or unacceptable toxicity.

Availability
Tablets: 40 mg.

NURSING IMPLICATIONS
Assessment
● Monitor for diarrhea. Use antidiarrheal prophylaxis with first dose and for first 2 cycles (56 days). *If Grade 1 diarrhea (increase of < 4 stools per day over baseline), Grade 2 diarrhea (increase of 4–6 stools per day over baseline) lasting < 5 days, Grade 3 diarrhea (increase of ≥ 7 stools per day over baseline; incontinence; hospitalization indicated; limiting self-care activities of daily living) lasting < 2 days occurs,* modify antidiarrheal therapy, modify diet, and maintain fluid intake of 2 L to avoid dehydration. Once event resolves to ≤ Grade 1 or baseline, start loperamide 4 mg with each subsequent neratinib administration. *If any grade diarrhea with dehydration, fever, hypotension, renal failure, neutropenia, Grade 2 diarrhea lasting ≥ 5 days, Grade 3 diarrhea lasting >2 days despite medical therapy occurs,* hold therapy, modify diet, and maintain fluid intake of 2 L to avoid dehydration. If diarrhea resolves to Grade 0–1 in ≤1 wk, resume therapy at same dose. If diarrhea resolves to Grade 0–1 in >1 wk, resume therapy at reduced dose. Once diarrhea resolves to ≤Grade 1 or baseline, start loperamide 4 mg with each subsequent neratinib administration. *If Grade 4 diarrhea (life-threatening consequences; urgent intervention indicated) occurs,* permanently discontinue neratinib. *If diarrhea recurs to ≥Grade 2 at 120 mg neratinib per day,* permanently discontinue neratinib. Obtain stool cultures to determine infectious causes of Grade 3 or 4 or with dehydration, fever, or neutropenia.
● Monitor for signs and symptoms of hepatotoxicity (worsening of fatigue, nausea, vomiting, right upper quadrant tenderness, fever, rash, eosinophilia, Grade 3 diarrhea) periodically during therapy. If symptoms occur, obtain liver function test levels to measure changes.

Lab Test Considerations
● Verify negative pregnancy test in women of reproductive potential before starting therapy.
● Monitor total bilirubin, AST, ALT, and alkaline phosphatase before starting therapy, monthly for first 3 mo, and every 3 mo during therapy. If evaluating hepatotoxicity, also obtain fractionated bilirubin and prothrombin time. *If Grade 3 ALT (>5–20 × upper limit of normal [ULN]) or Grade 3 bilirubin (>3–10 × ULN),* withhold dose until recovery to ≤ Grade 1, evaluate alternative causes, resume neratinib at next lower dose if recovery to ≤Grade 1 occurs within 3 wk. If Grade 3 ALT or bilirubin occurs again despite one dose reduction, permanently discontinue neratinib. If Grade 4 ALT (>20 × ULN) or Grade 4 bilirubin (>10 × ULN), discontinue neratinib permanently and evaluate alternative causes.

Implementation
● Do not confuse neratinib with nilotinib or niraparib.
● **Premedication for Diarrhea:** When not using dose escalation, use antidiarrheal prophylaxis for first 56 days of therapy, starting with first dose of neratinib. *For weeks 1–2 (days 1–14),* administer loperamide 4 mg three times daily. *For weeks 3–8 (days 15–56),* administer loperamide 4 mg twice daily. *For week 9– discontinuation of neratinib,* administer 4 mg loperamide as needed, not to exceed 16 mg/day; titrate to achieve 1–2 bowel movements/day. If diarrhea occurs despite prophylaxis, treat with additional antidiarrheals, fluids and electrolytes as indicated. Neratinib interruptions and dose reductions may also be required to manage diarrhea.
● **PO:** Administer once daily, at same time each day, with food, continuously for 1 yr; 240-mg dose = 6 tablets. *DNC:* Swallow tablets whole; do not crush, break, or chew.

Patient/Family Teaching
● Instruct patient to take neratinib as directed. If dose is missed, omit and take next scheduled dose next day. Advise patient to read *Patient Information* before starting therapy and with each Rx refill in case of changes.
● Advise patient to avoid taking grapefruit or grapefruit juice during therapy.
● Instruct patient to take loperamide according to schedule and titrate to 1–2 bowel movements/day: *For days 1–14 (wk 1–2),* take 4 mg three times daily. *Days 15–56 (wk 3–8),* take 4 mg twice daily. *Days 57–365 (wk 9–52),* take 4 mg as needed up to 16 mg/day. May require additional antidiarrheal agents and dose reduction.

- Caution patient to avoid proton pump inhibitors and H_2 antagonists during therapy and to avoid taking antacids within 3 hr of neratinib.
- Instruct patient to notify health care professional of all Rx or OTC medications, vitamins, or herbal products being taken and consult health care professional before taking any new medications, especially St. John's wort.
- Advise patient to notify health care professional immediately if severe ($\geq$ Grade 3) diarrhea or diarrhea associated with weakness, dizziness, or fever, or if signs and symptoms of liver dysfunction occur.
- Rep: May cause fetal harm. Advise females of reproductive potential to use effective contraception and avoid breastfeeding during and for at least 1 mo after last dose. Advise male patients with partners of reproductive potential to use effective contraception during and for 3 mo after last dose.

Evaluation/Desired Outcomes
- Decreased progression of breast cancer.

netupitant/palonosetron (oral)
(ne-**too**-pi-tant/pa-lone-**o**-se-tron)
  Akynzeo

fosnetupitant/palonosetron (injection)
(fos-ne-**too**-pi-tant/pa-lone-**o**-se-tron)
  Akynzeo
Classification
Therapeutic: antiemetics
Pharmacologic: neurokinin antagonists, 5-HT_3 antagonists

Indications
PO: Prevention of acute and delayed nausea and vomiting associated with initial and repeat courses of cancer chemotherapy, including, but not limited to, highly emetogenic chemotherapy (in combination with dexamethasone). **IV:** Prevention of acute and delayed nausea and vomiting associated with initial and repeat courses of highly emetogenic chemotherapy (in combination with dexamethasone).

Action
Netupitant: Acts as a selective antagonist at substance P/neurokinin 1 (NK1) receptors in the CNS; prevents nausea and vomiting in the acute and delayed phases after chemotherapy. *Palonosetron:* Blocks the effects of serotonin at receptor sites (selective antagonist) located in vagal nerve terminals and in the chemoreceptor trigger zones in the CNS; prevents nausea and vomiting in the acute phase. **Therapeutic Effects:** Decreased incidence and severity of nausea and vomiting following emetogenic chemotherapy.

Pharmacokinetics
Netupitant
Absorption: Extent of absorption following oral administration unknown.
Distribution: Extensively distributed to tissues.
Protein Binding: >99.5%.
Metabolism and Excretion: Primarily metabolized in the liver via the CYP3A4 isoenzyme, and to a lesser extent by the CYP2C9 and CYP2D6 isoenzymes to three metabolites that have antiemetic activity; <1% excreted unchanged in urine.
Half-life: 80 hr.

Fosnetupitant
Absorption: Following IV administration, fosnetupitant is rapidly converted to netupitant, the active component. IV administration results in complete bioavailability.
Distribution: Extensively distributed to tissues.
Protein Binding: 92–95%.
Metabolism and Excretion: Netupitant is primarily metabolized in the liver via the CYP3A4 isoenzyme, and to a lesser extent by the CYP2C9 and CYP2D6 isoenzymes to three metabolites that have antiemetic activity; <1% excreted unchanged in urine.
Half-life: *Netupitant:* 80 hr.

Palonosetron
Absorption: 97% absorbed following oral administration. IV administration results in complete bioavailability.
Distribution: Extensively distributed to tissues.
Metabolism and Excretion: 50% metabolized by the liver, (mostly by the CYP2D6 isoenzyme, and to a lesser extent by the CYP3A4 and CYP1A2 isoenzymes; 40% excreted unchanged in urine.
Half-life: 40 hr.

TIME/ACTION PROFILE (plasma concentrations)

ROUTE	ONSET	PEAK	DURATION
PO	within 1 hr	5 hr	unknown
IV	rapid	30 min	unknown

Contraindications/Precautions
Contraindicated in: Cross-sensitivity may occur with other 5-HT_3 antagonists; Severe hepatic or renal impairment.
Use Cautiously in: OB: Safety not established in pregnancy; Lactation: Safety not established in breastfeeding; Pedi: Safety and effectiveness not established in children; Geri: Consider age-related $\downarrow$ in renal, hepatic, and cardiac function, concurrent disease states and drug therapies in older adults.

Adverse Reactions/Side Effects
Derm: erythema. **GI:** constipation, dyspepsia. **Neuro:** fatigue, headache, weakness. **Misc:** HYPERSENSITIVITY

✲ = Canadian drug name. ⚇ = Genetic implication. ~~Strikethrough~~ = Discontinued. CAPITALS = life-threatening. <u>Underline</u> = most frequent.

REACTIONS (including anaphylaxis), SEROTONIN SYNDROME.

Interactions

Drug-Drug: Netupitant is a moderate inhibitor of CYP3A4 and can ↑ levels of drugs that are **CYP3A4 substrates**, including **alprazolam, cyclophosphamide, dexamethasone, docetaxel, etoposide, ifosfamide, imatinib, irinotecan, midazolam, erythromycin, paclitaxel, triazolam, vinorelbine, vinblastine**, and **vincristine**; avoid concomitant use for one wk; if avoiding use not feasible, ↓ dose of CYP3A4 substrate. **CYP3A4 inducers** including **rifampin** may ↓ netupitant levels and effectiveness; avoid concurrent use. Drugs that affect serotonergic neurotransmitter systems, including **tricyclic antidepressants, SNRIs, fentanyl, buspirone, tramadol, amphetamines**, and **triptans**, ↑ risk of serotonin syndrome.

Route/Dosage

Netupitant/Palonosetron

PO (Adults): *Highly emetogenic chemotherapy (included cisplatin-based):* One capsule (netupitant 300 mg/palonosetron 0.5 mg) 1 hr before chemotherapy on day 1. *Anthracycline and cyclophosphamide–based chemotherapy and other chemotherapy not considered highly emetogenic:* One capsule (netupitant 300 mg/palonosetron 0.5 mg) 1 hr before chemotherapy on day 1.

Fosnetupitant/Palonosetron

IV (Adults): *Highly emetogenic chemotherapy (included cisplatin-based):* Fosnetupitant 235 mg/palonosetron 0.25 mg administered 30 min before chemotherapy on day 1.

Availability

Capsules: netupitant 300 mg/palonosetron 0.5 mg. **Lyophilized powder for injection:** fosnetupitant 235 mg/palonosetron 0.25 mg/vial. **Solution for injection:** fosnetupitant 235 mg/palonosetron 0.25 mg/20 mL.

NURSING IMPLICATIONS

Assessment

- Assess patient for nausea, vomiting, abdominal distention, and bowel sounds prior to and following administration.
- Assess for serotonin syndrome (mental changes [agitation, hallucinations, delirium, coma], autonomic instability [tachycardia, labile BP, dizziness, diaphoresis, flushing, hyperthermia], neuromuscular aberrations [tremor, rigidity, myoclonus, hyperreflexia, incoordination], seizure, and/or GI symptoms [nausea, vomiting, diarrhea]), especially in patients taking other serotonergic drugs (SSRIs, SNRIs, triptans).

Lab Test Considerations

- May cause transient ↑ in serum bilirubin, AST, and ALT levels.

Implementation

- *For highly emetogenic chemotherapy,* administer with dexamethasone PO 12 mg 30 min prior to chemotherapy on day 1 and 8 mg PO on days 2 and 4. *For chemotherapy not considered highly emetogenic,* administer dexamethasone 30 min prior to chemotherapy on day 1 (day 2 and 4 not needed).
- **PO:** Administer netupitant/palonosetron 1 hr prior to start of chemotherapy without regard to food.

IV Administration

- **Intermittent Infusion:** *Reconstitution:* Reconstitute with 20 mL D5W or 0.9% NaCl into vial along vial wall to prevent foaming; swirl gently to mix. Prepare an infusion vial or bag filled with 30 mL D5W or NaCl. Withdraw entire volume of reconstituted solution and transfer it into infusion vial or bag containing 30 mL of D5W or 0.9% NaCl for a total volume of 50 mL. Gently invert bag until complete dissolution. Solution is clear; do not administer solutions that are cloudy, discolored, or contain particulate matter. Total time from reconstitution to the start of infusion should not exceed 24 hr. Store reconstituted solution and final diluted solution at room temperature. Dexamethasone can be given concomitantly or added to solution.
- Ready-to-use solution does not require reconstitution. *Rate:* Infuse over 30 min starting 30 min before chemotherapy. Flush line with 0.9% NaCl at end of infusion.
- **Y-Site Compatibility:** dexamethasone.
- **Y-Site Incompatibility:** solutions containing calcium, solutions containing magnesium, LR, Hartmann's solution.

Patient/Family Teaching

- Instruct patient to take netupitant/palonosetron as directed. Advise patient to read *Patient Information* prior to starting therapy and with each Rx refill in case of changes.
- Advise patient to notify health care professional promptly if signs and symptoms of anaphylaxis (shortness of breath, rash, hives, swelling of mouth, throat, and lips) or serotonin syndrome occur.
- Instruct patient to notify health care professional of all Rx or OTC medications, vitamins, or herbal products being taken and consult health care professional before taking any new medications.
- Rep: May cause fetal harm. Advise females of reproductive potential to notify health care professional if pregnancy is planned or suspected, and to avoid breastfeeding during therapy.

Evaluation/Desired Outcomes

- Decrease in frequency and severity of nausea and vomiting.

NICOTINE (nik-o-teen)
nicotine chewing gum
Nicorette
nicotine lozenge
Nicorette
nicotine nasal spray
Nicotrol NS
nicotine transdermal patch
Habitrol, Nicoderm CQ
Classification
Therapeutic: smoking deterrents

Indications
Adjunct therapy (with behavior modification) in the management of nicotine withdrawal in patients desiring to give up cigarette smoking.

Action
Provides a source of nicotine during controlled withdrawal from cigarette smoking. **Therapeutic Effects:** Lessened sequelae of nicotine withdrawal (irritability, insomnia, somnolence, headache, and increased appetite).

Pharmacokinetics
Absorption: *Gum, lozenge:* Slowly absorbed from buccal mucosa during chewing/sucking. *Nasal spray:* 53% absorbed from nasal mucosa. *Transdermal:* 70% of nicotine released from the system is absorbed through the skin.
Distribution: Enter breast milk.
Metabolism and Excretion: Mostly metabolized by the liver. Small amounts are metabolized by kidneys and lungs; 10–20% excreted unchanged by kidneys.
Half-life: 1–2 hr.

TIME/ACTION PROFILE (plasma concentrations)

ROUTE	ONSET	PEAK	DURATION
Gum	rapid	15–30 min	unknown
Lozenge	unknown	unknown	unknown
Nasal spray	rapid	4–15 min	unknown
Transdermal	rapid	2–4 hr	unknown

Contraindications/Precautions
Contraindicated in: Hypersensitivity; Recent history of MI (nasal spray); Arrhythmias (nasal spray); Severe or worsening angina (nasal spray); Severe cardiovascular disease; OB: Pregnancy.

Use Cautiously in: Cardiovascular disease (including hypertension); Recent history of MI (gum, lozenge, patch); Arrhythmias (gum, lozenge, patch); Severe or worsening angina (gum, lozenge, patch); Diabetes mellitus; Pheochromocytoma; Peripheral vascular diseases; Hyperthyroidism; Continued smoking; Peptic ulcer disease; Seizures; Hepatic disease; Bronchospastic lung disease (nasal spray); Allergic reaction to adhesive tape (patch); Lactation: Use while breastfeeding only if potential maternal benefit justifies potential risk to infant; Pedi: Safety and effectiveness not established in children; Geri: Begin at lower dosages in older adults.

Adverse Reactions/Side Effects
CV: tachycardia, chest pain, hypertension. **Derm:** *transdermal:* burning at patch site, erythema, pruritus, cutaneous hypersensitivity, rash, sweating. **EENT:** sinusitis; *gum:* pharyngitis; *nasal spray:* nasopharyngeal irritation, sneezing, watering eyes, change in smell, earache, epistaxis, eye irritation, hoarseness. **Endo:** dysmenorrhea. **GI:** abdominal pain, abnormal taste, constipation, diarrhea, dry mouth, dyspepsia, hiccups, nausea, vomiting; *gum:* belching, ↑ appetite, ↑ salivation, oral injury, sore mouth. **MS:** arthralgia, back pain, myalgia; *gum:* jaw muscle ache. **Neuro:** paresthesia, headache, insomnia, abnormal dreams, dizziness, drowsiness, impaired concentration, nervousness, seizures, weakness. **Resp:** *Nasal spray:* cough, dyspnea.

Interactions
Drug-Drug: Effects of **acetaminophen, caffeine, imipramine, insulin, oxazepam, propranolol,** or other **beta blockers, adrenergic antagonists (prazosin, labetalol),** and **theophylline** may be ↑ upon smoking cessation; dose ↓ at cessation may be necessary. Effects of adrenergic agonists (e.g., **isoproterenol, phenylephrine**) may be ↓ upon smoking cessation; dose ↑ at cessation may be necessary. Concurrent treatment with **bupropion** may cause treatment-emergent hypertension.

Route/Dosage
Gum (Adults): If first cigarette is desired >30 min after awakening, start with 2 mg gum; if first cigarette is desired <30 min after awakening, start with 4 mg gum. Patients should chew one piece of gum every 1–2 hr for 6 wk, then one piece of gum every 2–4 hr for 3 wk, then one piece of gum every 4–8 hr for 3 wk, then discontinue. Should not exceed 24 pieces of gum/day.
Lozenge (Adults): If first cigarette is desired >30 min after awakening, start with 2 mg lozenge; if first cigarette is desired <30 min after awakening, start with 4 mg lozenge. Patients should use one lozenge every 1–2 hr for 6 wk, then one lozenge every 2–4 hr for 3 wk, then one lozenge every 4–8 hr for 3 wk, then discontinue. Should not exceed 20 lozenges/day or more than 5 lozenges in 6 hr.
Intranasal (Adults): One spray in each nostril 1–2 times/hr (up to 5 times/hr); may be ↑ up to maximum of 40 times/day (should not exceed 3 mo of therapy).
Transdermal (Adults): *Patients smoking >10 cigarettes/day:* Begin with Step 1 (21 mg/day) for 6 wk, followed by Step 2 (14 mg/day) for 2 wk, and then Step 3 (7 mg/day) for 2 wk, then stop (total of 10 wk) (new patch should be applied every 24 hr); *Patients smok-*

N

ing ≤10 cigarettes/day: Begin with Step 2 (14 mg/day) for 6 wk, followed by Step 3 (7 mg/day) for 2 wk, then stop (total of 8 wk) (new patch should be applied every 24 hr).

Availability (generic available)

Chewing gum (cinnamon, mint, spearmint, white ice, and fruit chill flavors): 2 mg^OTC, 4 mg^OTC. **Lozenges (original, mint, cherry, and cappuccino flavors):** 2 mg^OTC, 4 mg^OTC. **Nasal spray:** 0.5 mg/spray in 10-mL bottles (200 sprays). **Transdermal patch:** 7 mg/day^OTC, 14 mg/day^OTC, 21 mg/day^OTC.

NURSING IMPLICATIONS

Assessment

- Prior to therapy, assess smoking history (number of cigarettes smoked daily, smoking patterns, nicotine content of preferred brand, degree to which patient inhales smoke).
- Assess patient for symptoms of smoking withdrawal (irritability, drowsiness, fatigue, headache, nicotine craving) periodically during nicotine replacement therapy (NRT).
- Evaluate progress in smoking cessation periodically during therapy.

Toxicity and Overdose

- Monitor for nausea, vomiting, diarrhea, increased salivation, abdominal pain, headache, dizziness, auditory and visual disturbances, weakness, dyspnea, hypotension, and irregular pulse.

Implementation

- **Gum:** Protect gum from light; exposure to light causes gum to turn brown.
- **Lozenge:** Lozenge should be allowed to dissolve slowly in the mouth; it should not be chewed or swallowed.
- **Transdermal:** Patch can be worn for 16 or 24 hr; the patch can be removed before the patient goes to bed (especially if patient has vivid dreams or sleep disturbances) or can remain on while the patient sleeps (especially if patient craves cigarettes upon awakening).
- **Nasal Spray:** Regular use of the spray during the first wk of therapy may help patient adjust to irritant effects of the spray.

Patient/Family Teaching

- Encourage patient to participate in a smoking cessation program while using this product.
- Review the patient instruction sheet enclosed in the package.
- Instruct patient in proper method of disposal of unit. Emphasize need to keep out of the reach of children or pets.
- Rep: Nicotine in any form can be harmful to a pregnant woman and/or the fetus. Assist patient in determining risk/benefit of NRT and harm to the fetus versus the likelihood of stopping smoking without NRT. Maternal smoking and nicotine increase risk of sudden infant death syndrome.

- Emphasize the importance of regular visits to health care professional to monitor progress of smoking cessation.
- **Gum:** Explain purpose of nicotine gum to patient. Patient should chew 1 piece of gum whenever a craving for nicotine occurs or according to a fixed schedule (every 1–2 hr while awake) as directed. Chew gum slowly until a tingling sensation is felt (about 15 chews). Then, patient should stop chewing and store the gum between the cheek and gums until the tingling sensation disappears (about 1 min). Process of stopping, then resuming chewing should be repeated for approximately 30 min until most of the tingle has disappeared. Rapid, vigorous chewing may result in side effects similar to those of smoking too many cigarettes (headache, dizziness, nausea, increased salivation, heartburn, and hiccups). For best chances of quitting, chew at least 9 pieces of gum/day during 1st 6 wk.
- Inform patient that the gum has a slight tobacco/pepper-like taste. Many patients initially find it unpleasant and slightly irritating to the mouth. This usually resolves after several days of therapy.
- Advise patient to carry gum at all times during therapy.
- Advise patient to avoid eating or drinking for 15 min before and during chewing of nicotine gum; these interfere with buccal absorption of nicotine.
- The gum usually can be chewed by denture wearers. Contact dentist if the gum adheres to bridgework.
- Inform patient that if they still feel need to use gum after completion of treatment period, advise them to contact a health care professional.
- Instruct patient not to swallow gum.
- Dispose of the gum by wrapping in wrapper to prevent ingestion by children and animals. Call the poison control center, emergency department, or health care professional immediately if a child ingests the gum.
- Rep: Emphasize the need to discontinue the gum and to inform health care professional if pregnancy occurs.
- **Transdermal:** Instruct patient in application and use of patch. Apply patch at the same time each day. Keep patch in sealed pouch until ready to apply. Apply to clean, dry skin of upper arm or torso free of oil, hair, scars, cuts, burns, or irritation. Press patch firmly in place with palm for 10 sec, making sure there is good contact, especially around the edges. Keep patch in place during showering, bathing, or swimming; replace patches that have fallen off. Wash hands with soap and water after handling patches. Do not trim or cut patch. No more than 1 patch should be worn at a time. Alternate application sites. Dispose of used patches by folding adhesive sides together and replacing in protective pouch or aluminum foil; keep out of reach of children.
- Advise patient that redness, itching, and burning at application site usually subside within 1 hr. Instruct

patient to notify health care professional and not apply new patch if signs of allergic reaction (urticaria, generalized rash, hives) or persistent local skin reactions (severe erythema, pruritus, edema) occur.

- May cause drowsiness or dizziness. Caution patient to avoid driving or other activities requiring alertness until response to medication is known.

- Advise patient referred for MRI test to discuss patch with referring health care professional and MRI facility to determine if removal of patch is necessary prior to test and for directions for replacing patch.

- **Nasal Spray:** Instruct patient in proper use of spray. Tilt head back slightly. Do not sniff, swallow, or inhale through nose as spray is being administered. Patients who have successfully stopped smoking should continue to use the same dose for up to 8 wk, after which the spray should be discontinued over the next 4–6 wk.

- Discontinue nasal spray by using ½ dose (1 spray at a time), using the spray less frequently, skipping a dose by not using every hr, or setting a planned stop date for use of the spray.

- Treatment should be discontinued in patients who are unable to stop smoking by the 4th wk of therapy (patient is unlikely to quit on that attempt).

- Patients who fail to stop smoking should be given a therapy holiday before another attempt.

- Instruct patient to replace childproof cap after using and before disposal.

- **Lozenge:** Instruct patient to place lozenge in mouth and allow it to slowly dissolve (20–30 min). Minimize swallowing; advise patient not to chew or swallow lozenge. May cause a warm tingling sensation in mouth. Advise patient to occasionally move lozenge from side to side of mouth until completely dissolved. Instruct patient not to eat or drink 15 min before or while lozenge is in mouth. For best chances of quitting, use at least 9 lozenges/day during 1st 6 wk. Do not use more than 1 lozenge at a time or use continuously one after the another. Lozenge should not be used after 12 wk without consulting health care professional.

Evaluation/Desired Outcomes

- Lessened sequelae of nicotine withdrawal (irritability, insomnia, somnolence, headache, and increased appetite) during smoking cessation.

BEERS

NIFEdipine (nye-fed-i-peen)
~~Adalat CC~~, ✦ Adalat XL, ~~Afeditab CR~~, ~~Procardia~~, Procardia XL
Classification
Therapeutic: antianginals, antihypertensives
Pharmacologic: calcium channel blockers

Indications
Management of: Hypertension (extended-release only), Angina pectoris, Vasospastic (Prinzmetal's) angina. **Unlabeled Use:** Prevention of migraine headache.

Action
Inhibits calcium transport into myocardial and vascular smooth muscle cells, resulting in inhibition of excitation-contraction coupling and subsequent contraction. **Therapeutic Effects:** Systemic vasodilation, resulting in decreased BP. Coronary vasodilation, resulting in decreased frequency and severity of attacks of angina.

Pharmacokinetics
Absorption: Well absorbed after oral administration, but large amounts are rapidly metabolized, resulting in ↓ bioavailability (45–70%); bioavailability is ↑ (80%) with extended-release forms.
Distribution: Unknown.
Protein Binding: 92–98%.
Metabolism and Excretion: Mostly metabolized by the liver by the CYP3A4 isoenzyme.
Half-life: 2–5 hr.

TIME/ACTION PROFILE

ROUTE	ONSET	PEAK	DURATION
PO	20 min	unknown	6–8 hr
PO–ER	unknown	6 hr	24 hr

Contraindications/Precautions
Contraindicated in: Hypersensitivity; Sick sinus syndrome; 2nd- or 3rd-degree AV block (unless an artificial pacemaker is in place); Systolic BP <90 mm Hg; Coadministration with grapefruit juice, rifampin, rifabutin, phenobarbital, phenytoin, carbamazepine, or St. John's wort.
Use Cautiously in: Severe hepatic impairment (↓ dose); History of porphyria; Severe renal impairment (↓ dose may be necessary); History of serious ventricular arrhythmias or HF; Pedi: Safety and effectiveness not established in children; Geri: Immediate-release formulation appears on Beers list. ↑ risk of hypotension and myocardial ischemia in older adults. Avoid use of immediate-release formulation in older adults.

Adverse Reactions/Side Effects
CV: peripheral edema, bradycardia, chest pain, HF, hypotension, palpitations, syncope, tachycardia. **Derm:** flushing, ↑ sweating, dermatitis, erythema multiforme, photosensitivity, pruritus/urticaria, rash, STEVENS-JOHNSON SYNDROME. **EENT:** blurred vision, disturbed equilibrium, epistaxis, tinnitus. **Endo:** gynecomastia, hyperglycemia. **GI:** ↑ liver enzymes, GI obstruction, anorexia, constipation, diarrhea, dry mouth, dyspepsia, nausea, vomiting. **GU:** dysuria, nocturia, polyuria, sexual dysfunction, urinary frequency. **Hemat:** anemia, leukopenia, thrombocytopenia. **Metab:** weight gain. **MS:** joint stiffness, muscle cramps. **Neuro:** paresthesia,

N

tremor. **Resp:** cough, dyspnea, shortness of breath.
Misc: gingival hyperplasia.

Interactions

Drug-Drug: Rifampin, rifabutin, phenobarbital,
phenytoin, or carbamazepine may significantly ↓
levels and effects; concurrent use is contraindicated.
**Ketoconazole, fluconazole, itraconazole, clarith-
romycin, erythromycin, nefazodone, nelfinavir,**
or **ritonavir** may ↑ levels and effects; consider initiating nifedipine at lowest dose. Additive hypotension may
occur when used concurrently with **fentanyl**, other
antihypertensives, nitrates, acute ingestion of **alcohol,** or **quinidine.** Antihypertensive effects may be ↓
by concurrent use of **NSAIDs.** May ↑ serum levels and
risk of toxicity from **digoxin.** Concurrent use with **beta
blockers, digoxin,** or **disopyramide** may result in
bradycardia, conduction defects, or HF. **Cimetidine**
and **propranolol** may ↓ metabolism and ↑ risk of toxicity. May ↓ metabolism of and ↑ risk of toxicity from
cyclosporine, tacrolimus, prazosin, quinidine, or
carbamazepine. ↑ risk of GI obstruction when used
concurrently with **H₂ blockers, opioids, NSAIDs,
laxatives, anticholinergic drugs, levothyroxine,**
or **neuromuscular blockers.**
Drug-Natural Products: St. John's wort may significantly ↓ levels and effects; concurrent use is contraindicated.
Drug-Food: Grapefruit and grapefruit juice ↑ serum levels and effect; avoid concurrent use.

Route/Dosage

PO (Adults): *Immediate-release:* 10–30 mg 3 times
daily (not to exceed 180 mg/day); *Extended-release:*
30–90 mg once daily (not to exceed 90–120 mg/day).

Availability (generic available)

Capsules: ✿ 5 mg, 10 mg, 20 mg. **Extended-release
tablets:** 30 mg, 60 mg, 90 mg.

NURSING IMPLICATIONS

Assessment

- Monitor BP and pulse before therapy, during dose titration, and periodically during therapy. Monitor
ECG periodically during prolonged therapy.
- Monitor intake and output ratios and daily weight.
Assess for signs of HF (peripheral edema, rales/
crackles, dyspnea, weight gain, jugular venous distention).
- Patients receiving digoxin concurrently with nifedipine should have routine tests of serum digoxin levels and be monitored for signs and symptoms of digoxin toxicity.
- Assess for rash periodically during therapy. May
cause Stevens-Johnson syndrome. Discontinue therapy if severe or if accompanied with fever, general
malaise, fatigue, muscle or joint aches, blisters, oral
lesions, conjunctivitis, hepatitis, and/or eosinophilia.
- **Angina:** Assess location, duration, intensity, and
precipitating factors of patient's anginal pain.

Lab Test Considerations
- Total serum calcium concentrations are not affected
by calcium channel blockers.
- Monitor serum potassium periodically. Hypokalemia
increases risk of arrhythmias; should be corrected.
- Monitor renal and hepatic functions periodically
during long-term therapy. Several days of therapy
may cause ↑ hepatic enzymes, which return to normal upon discontinuation of therapy.
- Nifedipine may cause positive ANA and direct
Coombs' test results.

Implementation

- Do not confuse nifedipine with nicardipine or nimodipine.
- **PO:** May be administered without regard to meals.
May be administered with meals if GI irritation becomes a problem.
- *DNC:* Swallow tablets whole; do not open, break,
crush, or chew extended-release tablets. Empty tablets that appear in stool are not significant.
- Avoid administration with grapefruit juice.
- Sublingual use is not recommended due to serious
adverse drug reactions.

Patient/Family Teaching

- Advise patient to take medication as directed, even if
feeling well. Take missed doses as soon as possible
unless almost time for next dose; do not double
doses. May need to be discontinued gradually.
- Instruct patient on technique for monitoring pulse.
Instruct patient to contact health care professional if
heart rate is <50 bpm.
- Advise patient to avoid grapefruit or grapefruit juice
during therapy.
- Caution patient to change positions slowly to minimize orthostatic hypotension.
- May cause drowsiness or dizziness. Advise patient to
avoid driving or other activities requiring alertness
until response to the medication is known.
- Geri: Teach patient and family about risk for falls
and how to reduce risk in the home.
- Instruct patient on importance of maintaining good
dental hygiene and seeing dentist frequently for teeth
cleaning to prevent tenderness, bleeding, and gingival hyperplasia (gum enlargement).
- Instruct patient to notify health care professional of
all Rx or OTC medications, vitamins, or herbal products being taken and to avoid concurrent use of alcohol or OTC medications and herbal products, especially cold preparations and St. John's wort,
without consulting health care professional.
- Advise patient to notify health care professional if
rash, irregular heartbeat, dyspnea, swelling of hands
and feet, pronounced dizziness, nausea, constipation, or hypotension occurs or if headache is severe
or persistent.
- Caution patient to wear protective clothing and use
sunscreen to prevent photosensitivity reactions.

- Rep: Advise females of reproductive potential to notify health care professional if pregnancy is planned or suspected or if breastfeeding.
- **Angina:** Instruct patient on concurrent nitrate or beta-blocker therapy to continue taking both medications as directed and use SL nitroglycerin as needed for anginal attacks.
- Inform patient that anginal attacks may occur 30 min after administration because of reflex tachycardia. This is usually temporary and is not an indication for discontinuation.
- Advise patient to contact health care professional if chest pain does not improve, worsens after therapy, or occurs with diaphoresis; if shortness of breath occurs; or if persistent headache occurs.
- Caution patient to discuss exercise restrictions with health care professional before exertion.
- **Hypertension:** Encourage patient to comply with other interventions for hypertension (weight reduction, low-sodium diet, smoking cessation, moderation of alcohol consumption, regular exercise, and stress management). Medication controls but does not cure hypertension.
- Instruct patient and family in proper technique for monitoring BP. Advise patient to take BP weekly and to report significant changes to health care professional.

Evaluation/Desired Outcomes
- Decrease in BP.
- Decrease in frequency and severity of anginal attacks.
- Decrease in need for nitrate therapy.

⚇ nilotinib (ni-lo-ti-nib)
Tasigna
Classification
Therapeutic: antineoplastics
Pharmacologic: enzyme inhibitors, kinase inhibitors

Indications
⚇ Newly diagnosed Philadelphia chromosome positive (Ph+) chronic myelogenous leukemia (CML) in chronic phase. ⚇ Chronic or accelerated phase Ph+ CML in adult patients who are resistant or intolerant to prior treatment, including imatinib. ⚇ Chronic or accelerated phase Ph+ CML in pediatric patients ≥1 yr who are resistant or intolerant to prior tyrosine-kinase inhibitor treatment.

Action
Inhibits kinases, which may be produced by malignant cell lines. **Therapeutic Effects:** Inhibits production of malignant cells lines with decreased proliferation of leukemic cells.

Pharmacokinetics
Absorption: Well absorbed following oral administration. Levels are significantly ↑ by food.
Distribution: Unknown.
Metabolism and Excretion: Mostly metabolized by the liver via the CYP3A4 isoenzyme to inactive metabolites. Primarily excreted in the feces (93%), with 69% being excreted unchanged.
Half-life: 17 hr.

TIME/ACTION PROFILE (plasma concentrations)

ROUTE	ONSET	PEAK	DURATION
PO	unknown	3 hr	12 hr

Contraindications/Precautions
Contraindicated in: Hypokalemia or hypomagnesemia; Long QT syndrome; Galactose intolerance, severe lactase deficiency, or glucose-galactose malabsorption (capsules contain lactose); OB: Pregnancy; Lactation: Lactation.
Use Cautiously in: Electrolyte abnormalities; correct prior to administration to ↓ risk of arrhythmias; Hepatic impairment (↓ dose required for Grade 3 elevated bilirubin, transaminases or lipase); Total gastrectomy (may need to ↑ dose or use alterative therapy); History of pancreatitis; ⚇ Patients with genetically reduced UGT1A1 activity (presence of UGT1A1*28 allele) (↑ risk of hyperbilirubinemia); Rep: Women of reproductive potential; Pedi: May affect growth and development of children; safety and effectiveness not established in children <1 yr.

Adverse Reactions/Side Effects
CV: hypertension, MI, palpitations, pericardial effusion, peripheral arterial disease, QT interval prolongation, TORSADES DE POINTES. **Derm:** pruritus, rash, alopecia, flushing. **EENT:** vertigo. **F and E:** hyperkalemia, hypocalcemia, hypokalemia, hyponatremia, hypophosphatemia. **GI:** ↑ lipase, constipation, diarrhea, nausea, vomiting, abdominal discomfort, anorexia, ascites, dyspepsia, flatulence, hepatitis B virus reactivation, HEPATOTOXICITY. **Hemat:** BLEEDING, MYELOSUPPRESSION. **Metab:** hyperglycemia. **MS:** ↓ growth, musculoskeletal pain. **Neuro:** fatigue, headache, dizziness, paresthesia, STROKE. **Resp:** pleural effusion, pulmonary edema. **Misc:** fever, night sweats, tumor lysis syndrome.

Interactions
Drug-Drug: **Strong CYP3A4 inhibitors**, including **ketoconazole, itraconazole, voriconazole, clarithromycin, atazanavir, nelfinavir, ritonavir,** and **nefazodone**, may ↑ levels and the risk of toxicity; avoid concurrent use, if possible; if concurrent use is necessary, ↓ nilotinib dose. **Strong CYP3A4 inducers**, including **carbamazepine, dexamethasone,**

phenobarbital, phenytoin, rifabutin, rifampin, and **rifapentine,** may ↓ levels and effectiveness; avoid concurrent use. May ↑ levels and the risk of toxicity of **CYP3A4 substrates,** including **atorvastatin, cyclosporine, dihydroergotamine, ergotamine, fentanyl, lovastatin, midazolam, simvastatin, sirolimus,** and **tacrolimus.** Concurrent use of other **drugs that prolong QT interval;** may ↑ risk of serious arrhythmias; avoid concurrent use. **Proton pump inhibitors, H₂ receptor antagonists,** and **antacids** may ↓ the bioavailability of nilotinib; avoid concurrent use of proton pump inhibitors; doses of H₂ receptor antagonists may be administered 10 hr before or 2 hr after nilotinib; doses of antacids may be administered 2 hr before or after nilotinib.

Drug-Natural Products: St. John's wort may ↓ levels and effectiveness; avoid concurrent use.

Drug-Food: Grapefruit juice may ↑ levels and the risk of toxicity; avoid concurrent use.

Route/Dosage

Newly Diagnosed Chronic Phase Ph+ Chronic Myelogenous Leukemia

PO (Adults): 300 mg twice daily; treatment discontinuation may be considered in patients who have received nilotinib for ≥3 yr and achieved a sustained molecular response; if patients lose molecular response after discontinuing therapy, restart nilotinib within 4 wk at the dose level prior to discontinuation; *Concurrent use of strong CYP3A4 inhibitors (ketoconazole, itraconazole, clarithromycin, atazanavir, nefazodone, nelfinavir, ritonavir, or voriconazole):* 200 mg once daily.

PO (Children ≥1 yr): 230 mg/m² twice daily (max single dose = 400 mg) until disease progression or unacceptable toxicity; treatment discontinuation may be considered in patients who have received nilotinib for ≥3 yr and achieved a sustained molecular response; if patients lose molecular response after discontinuing therapy, restart nilotinib within 4 wk at the dose level prior to discontinuation; *Concurrent use of strong CYP3A4 inhibitors (ketoconazole, itraconazole, clarithromycin, atazanavir, nefazodone, nelfinavir, ritonavir, or voriconazole):* 200 mg once daily.

Hepatic Impairment

PO (Adults and Children ≥1 yr): *Mild, moderate, or severe hepatic impairment:* 200 mg twice daily; may ↑ to 300 mg twice daily if tolerates.

Resistant or Intolerant Chronic or Accelerated Phase Ph+ Chronic Myelogenous Leukemia

PO (Adults): 400 mg twice daily; treatment discontinuation may be considered in patients who have received nilotinib for ≥3 yr and achieved a sustained molecular response; if patients lose molecular response after discontinuing therapy, restart nilotinib within 4 wk at the dose level prior to discontinuation; *Concurrent use of strong CYP3A4 inhibitors (ketoconazole, itraconazole, clarithromycin, atazanavir, nefazodone, nelfinavir, ritonavir, or voriconazole):* 300 mg once daily.

PO (Children ≥1 yr): 230 mg/m² twice daily (max single dose = 400 mg) until disease progression or unacceptable toxicity; treatment discontinuation may be considered in patients who have received nilotinib for ≥3 yr and achieved a sustained molecular response; if patients lose molecular response after discontinuing therapy, restart nilotinib within 4 wk at the dose level prior to discontinuation; *Concurrent use of strong CYP3A4 inhibitors (ketoconazole, itraconazole, clarithromycin, atazanavir, nefazodone, nelfinavir, ritonavir, or voriconazole):* 200 mg once daily.

Hepatic Impairment

PO (Adults and Children ≥1 yr): *Mild or moderate hepatic impairment:* 300 mg twice daily; may ↑ to 400 mg twice daily if tolerates; *Severe hepatic impairment:* 200 mg twice daily; may ↑ to 300 mg twice daily, and eventually to 400 mg twice daily if tolerates.

Availability

Capsules: 50 mg, 150 mg, 200 mg.

NURSING IMPLICATIONS

Assessment

- Monitor ECG to assess the QTc interval at baseline, 7 days after initiation of therapy, after any dose adjustment, and periodically thereafter. For ECGs with QTc interval >480 msec, withhold nilotinib and check serum potassium and magnesium. If below lower limit of normal, correct to normal with supplements. Review concomitant medications for effects on electrolytes. If QTc interval returns to <450 msec and within 20 msec of baseline within 2 wk, return to prior dose. If QTc interval is <480 msec and >450 msec after 2 wk, reduce nilotinib dose to 400 mg once daily. Following dose reduction to 400 mg once daily, if QTc interval returns to >480 msec, discontinue nilotinib. Repeat ECG approximately 7 days after any dose adjustment.

- Monitor for myelosuppression. Assess for bleeding (bleeding gums, bruising, petechiae, blood in stools, urine, emesis) and avoid IM injections and taking rectal temperatures if platelet count is low. Apply pressure to venipuncture sites for at least 10 min. Assess for signs of infection during neutropenia. Anemia may occur. Monitor for fatigue, dyspnea, and orthostatic hypotension.

- Monitor for tumor lysis syndrome (malignant disease progression, high WBC counts, hyperuricemia, hyperkalemia, hyperphosphatemia, hypocalcemia, and/or dehydration). Prevent by maintaining adequate hydration and correcting uric acid levels prior to starting nilotinib.

- Monitor for signs of severe fluid retention (unexpected rapid weight gain or swelling) and for symptoms of respiratory or cardiac compromise (shortness of breath) periodically during therapy; evaluate cause and treat patients as needed.

- Monitor growth and development in pediatric patients receiving nilotinib.

Lab Test Considerations

- Verify negative pregnancy test before starting therapy.
- Monitor serum electrolytes prior to and periodically during therapy. May cause hypokalemia, hypomagnesemia, hypophosphatemia, hyperkalemia, hypocalcemia, hyperglycemia, and hyponatremia.
- Monitor CBC every 2 wk for first 2 mo and monthly thereafter or as indicated. May cause Grade 3–4 thrombocytopenia, neutropenia, and anemia. If ANC is <1.0 × 10⁹/L and/or platelet counts <50 × 10⁹/L, stop nilotinib and monitor blood counts. Resume within 2 wk at prior dose if ANC >1.0 × 10⁹/L and platelets >50 × 10⁹/L. If blood counts remain low for >2 wk, reduce dose to 400 mg once daily. Myelosuppression is generally reversible.
- May cause ↑ serum lipase or amylase. If ↑ to ≥Grade 3, withhold nilotinib and monitor serum levels. Resume treatment at 400 mg once daily (230 mg/m² once daily if prior dose was 230 mg/m² twice daily; if serum lipase or amylase return to ≤Grade 1. For pediatric patients, hold nilotinib until serum lipase or amylase return to ≤Grade 1. Resume therapy at 230 mg/m² once daily if prior dose was 230 mg/m² twice daily; discontinue therapy if prior dose was 230 mg/m² once daily.
- Monitor liver function tests monthly. May cause ↑ serum ALT, AST, alkaline phosphatase, and serum bilirubin. If ↑ to ≥Grade 3, withhold nilotinib and monitor bilirubin. Resume treatment at 400 mg once daily if serum lipase or amylase return to ≤Grade 1. For pediatric patients, hold nilotinib until serum bilirubin returns to ≤Grade 1. Resume therapy at 230 mg/m² once daily if prior dose was 230 mg/m² twice daily; discontinue therapy if prior dose was 230 mg/m² once daily, and recovery to ≤Grade 1 takes >28 days.
- Monitor lipid panel and glucose prior to and periodically during first yr of therapy, and then yearly during chronic therapy.
- Upon discontinuation, monitor BCR-ABL transcript levels and CBC with differential monthly for 1 yr, then every 6 wk for 2nd yr, and every 12 wk thereafter.

Implementation

- Do not confuse nilotinib with neratinib or niraparib.
- Correct hypokalemia and hypomagnesemia prior to beginning therapy.
- **PO:** Administer twice daily at 12-hr intervals on an empty stomach, at least 1 hr before and 2 hr after food. *DNC:* Swallow capsule whole with water; do not open capsule.
- Patients unable to swallow capsule may open capsule and sprinkle contents of each capsule in 1 teaspoon of applesauce. Swallow mixture within 15 min. Do not use more than 1 teaspoon of applesauce and use only applesauce.
- Avoid antacids less than 2 hr before or after and H₂ antagonists less than 10 hr before or less than 2 hr after administration.

Patient/Family Teaching

- Instruct patient to take nilotinib as directed, approximately 12 hr apart. If a dose is missed, skip dose and resume taking next prescribed dose. Nilotinib is a long-term treatment; do not stop medication or change dose without consulting health care professional. Advise patient to read the *Medication Guide* before starting and with each Rx refill, in case of changes.
- Advise patient to avoid grapefruit, grapefruit juice, or products with grapefruit extract during therapy; may cause toxicity.
- May cause dizziness. Caution patient to avoid driving or other activities requiring alertness until response to medication is known.
- Advise patient to notify health care professional of all Rx or OTC medications, vitamins, or herbal products being taken and to consult with health care professional before taking other medications, especially St. John's wort, during therapy.
- Instruct patient to notify health care professional promptly if fever; chills; cough; hoarseness; sore throat; signs of infection; lower back or side pain; painful or difficult urination; bleeding gums; bruising; petechiae; blood in stools, urine, or emesis; increased fatigue; dyspnea; signs of fluid retention; or orthostatic hypotension occurs. Caution patient to avoid crowds and persons with known infections. Instruct patient to use a soft toothbrush and electric razor and to avoid falls. Caution patient not to drink alcoholic beverages or take medication containing aspirin or NSAIDs; may precipitate bleeding.
- Instruct patient not to receive any vaccinations without advice of health care professional.
- Discuss the possibility of hair loss with patient. Explore methods of coping. Regrowth usually occurs 2–3 mo after discontinuation of therapy.
- Rep: May cause fetal harm. Advise women of reproductive potential to use highly effective contraception during therapy and for at least 14 days following last dose and to avoid breastfeeding for at least 14 days following last dose. Advise patient to notify health care professional immediately if pregnancy is suspected.

Evaluation/Desired Outcomes

- Decrease in production of leukemic cells.

---

niMODipine (nye-moe-di-peen)
✳Nimotop, Nymalize

Classification
Therapeutic: subarachnoid hemorrhage therapy agents
Pharmacologic: calcium channel blockers

Indications
Subarachnoid hemorrhage.

N

Action

Inhibits the transport of calcium into vascular smooth muscle cells, resulting in inhibition of excitation-contraction coupling and subsequent contraction. Potent peripheral vasodilator. **Therapeutic Effects:** Prevention of vascular spasm after subarachnoid hemorrhage, resulting in decreased neurologic impairment.

Pharmacokinetics

Absorption: Well absorbed following oral administration but undergoes first-pass metabolism, resulting in ↓ bioavailability.
Distribution: Crosses the blood-brain barrier; remainder of distribution unknown.
Protein Binding: >95%.
Metabolism and Excretion: Mostly metabolized by the liver; ≤10% excreted unchanged by kidneys.
Half-life: 1–2 hr.

TIME/ACTION PROFILE (vasodilation)

ROUTE	ONSET	PEAK	DURATION
PO	unknown	1 hr	4 hr

Contraindications/Precautions

Contraindicated in: Hypersensitivity; Systolic BP <90 mm Hg.
Use Cautiously in: Severe hepatic impairment (dose ↓ recommended); Severe renal impairment; History of serious ventricular arrhythmias or HF; OB: Safety not established in pregnancy; Lactation: Safety not established in breastfeeding; Pedi: Safety and effectiveness not established in children; Geri: Dose ↓ recommended in older adults due to↑ risk of hypotension.

Adverse Reactions/Side Effects

CV: ARRHYTHMIAS, chest pain, HF, hypotension, palpitations, peripheral edema, syncope, tachycardia. **Derm:** ↑ sweating, dermatitis, ERYTHEMA MULTIFORME, flushing, photosensitivity, pruritus/urticaria, rash, STEVENS-JOHNSON SYNDROME (SJS). **EENT:** blurred vision, disturbed equilibrium, epistaxis, tinnitus. **Endo:** gynecomastia, hyperglycemia. **GI:** ↑ liver enzymes, anorexia, constipation, diarrhea, dry mouth, dyspepsia, nausea, vomiting. **GU:** dysuria, nocturia, polyuria, sexual dysfunction, urinary frequency. **Hemat:** anemia, leukopenia, thrombocytopenia. **Metab:** ↑ weight. **MS:** joint stiffness, muscle cramps. **Neuro:** abnormal dreams, anxiety, confusion, dizziness, drowsiness, dysgeusia, headache, nervousness, paresthesia, psychiatric disturbances, tremor, weakness. **Resp:** cough, dyspnea. **Misc:** gingival hyperplasia.

Interactions

Drug-Drug: Strong CYP3A4 inhibitors, including **clarithromycin**, **nelfinavir**, **ritonavir**, **ketoconazole**, **itraconazole**, **posaconazole**, **voriconazole**, **conivaptan**, and **nefazodone**, may ↑ levels and the risk of hypotension; avoid concurrent use. **Strong CYP3A4 inducers**, including **carbamazepine**, **phenobarbital**, **phenytoin**, and **rifampin**, may ↓ levels and effectiveness; avoid concurrent use. Additive hypotension may occur when used concurrently with **fentanyl**, other **antihypertensives**, **nitrates**, acute ingestion of **alcohol**, or **quinidine**.
Drug-Natural Products: St. John's wort may ↓ levels and effectiveness; avoid concurrent use.
Drug-Food: Grapefruit and **grapefruit juice** may ↑ levels and the risk of toxicity; avoid concurrent use.

Route/Dosage

PO (Adults): 60 mg every 4 hr for 21 days; therapy should be started within 96 hr of subarachnoid hemorrhage.

Hepatic Impairment

PO (Adults): *Severe hepatic impairment:* 30 mg every 4 hr for 21 days; therapy should be started within 96 hr of subarachnoid hemorrhage.

Availability (generic available)

Capsules: 30 mg. **Oral solution:** 6 mg/mL.

NURSING IMPLICATIONS

Assessment

- Assess patient's neurologic status (level of consciousness, movement) prior to and periodically following administration.
- Monitor BP and pulse prior to therapy and periodically during therapy.
- Monitor intake and output ratios and daily weight. Assess for signs of HF (peripheral edema, rales/crackles, dyspnea, weight gain, jugular venous distention).
- Assess for rash periodically during therapy. May cause SJS. Discontinue therapy if severe or if accompanied with fever, general malaise, fatigue, muscle or joint aches, blisters, oral lesions, conjunctivitis, hepatitis, and/or eosinophilia.

Lab Test Considerations

- Total serum calcium concentrations are not affected by calcium channel blockers.
- Monitor serum potassium periodically. Hypokalemia ↑ risk of arrhythmias; should be corrected.
- Monitor renal and hepatic functions periodically. Several days of therapy may cause ↑ hepatic enzymes, which return to normal upon discontinuation of therapy.
- May occasionally cause ↓ platelet count.

Implementation

- Do not confuse nimodipine with nicardipine or nifedipine.
- Begin administration within 96 hr of subarachnoid hemorrhage and continue every 4 hr for 21 consecutive days.
- Administer by PO route ONLY; administration via IV or parenterally, may cause serious adverse events, including death.
- PO: If patient is unable to swallow capsule, make a hole in both ends of the capsule with a sterile 18-gauge needle and extract the contents into a syringe.

Empty contents into water or nasogastric tube and flush with 30 mL normal saline.

- Administer oral solution 1 hr before or 2 hr after meals. For administration via nasogastric (NG) or gastric tube, administer via syringe included, then refill syringe with 20 mL of 0.9% saline water solution; flush remaining contents from NG or gastric tube into stomach.

Patient/Family Teaching

- Advise patient to take medication as directed, even if feeling well. Take missed doses as soon as possible unless almost time for next dose; do not double doses. May need to be discontinued gradually.
- Advise patient to avoid grapefruit or grapefruit juice during therapy.
- Caution patient to change positions slowly to minimize orthostatic hypotension.
- May cause drowsiness or dizziness. Advise patient to avoid driving or other activities requiring alertness until response to the medication is known.
- Instruct patient to notify health care professional of all Rx or OTC medications, vitamins, or herbal products being taken and to avoid concurrent use of alcohol or OTC medications and herbal products, especially cold preparations, without consulting health care professional.
- Advise patient to notify health care professional if rash, irregular heartbeat, dyspnea, swelling of hands and feet, pronounced dizziness, nausea, constipation, or hypotension occurs or if headache is severe or persistent.
- Caution patient to wear protective clothing and use sunscreen to prevent photosensitivity reactions.
- Rep: Advise females of reproductive potential to notify health care professional if pregnancy is planned or suspected or if breastfeeding.

Evaluation/Desired Outcomes

- Improvement in neurologic deficits due to vasospasm following subarachnoid hemorrhage.

🞖 niraparib (nye-rap-a-rib)
Zejula
Classification
Therapeutic: antineoplastics
Pharmacologic: enzyme inhibitors

Indications
🞖 Maintenance treatment of deleterious or suspected deleterious germline *BRCA*-mutated recurrent epithelial ovarian, fallopian tube, or primary peritoneal cancer in patients who are in a complete or partial response to platinum-based chemotherapy. Maintenance treatment of advanced epithelial ovarian, fallopian tube, or primary peritoneal cancer in patients who are in a complete or partial response to first-line platinum-based chemotherapy.

Action
Acts as a poly (ADP-ribose) polymerase (PARP-1 and PARP-2) inhibitor; results in DNA damage, apoptosis, and cell death. **Therapeutic Effects:** Decreased progression of ovarian, fallopian tube, or primary peritoneal cancer and improved survival.

Pharmacokinetics
Absorption: 73% absorbed following oral administration.
Distribution: Extensively distributed to tissues.
Metabolism and Excretion: Primarily metabolized by carboxylesterases to an inactive metabolite; 48% excreted in urine (11% as unchanged drug), 39% in feces (19% as unchanged drug).
Half-life: 36 hr.

TIME/ACTION PROFILE (plasma concentrations)

ROUTE	ONSET	PEAK	DURATION
PO	unknown	3 hr	24 hr

Contraindications/Precautions
Contraindicated in: OB: Pregnancy; Lactation: Lactation.
Use Cautiously in: Ischemic heart disease, arrhythmias, or hypertension; Severe renal impairment (CCr <30 mL/min); Previous use of platinum chemotherapy agents or radiation (↑ risk of secondary myelodysplastic syndrome or acute myeloid leukemia); Moderate or severe hepatic impairment (↓ dose in moderate hepatic impairment); Aspirin hypersensitivity (contains tartrazine); Rep: Women of reproductive potential; Pedi: Safety and effectiveness not established in children.

Adverse Reactions/Side Effects
CV: palpitations, hypertension. Derm: rash. GI: ↑ liver enzymes, abdominal pain/distention, constipation, diarrhea, dry mouth, dyspepsia, nausea, stomatitis, vomiting. GU: urinary tract infection, ↓ fertility (males). Hemat: anemia, leukopenia, NEUTROPENIA, thrombocytopenia, MYELODYSPLASTIC SYNDROME (MDS)/ACUTE MYELOID LEUKEMIA (AML), pancytopenia. Metab: ↓ appetite. MS: arthralgia, myalgia. Neuro: anxiety, dizziness, dysgeusia, fatigue, headache, insomnia, POSTERIOR REVERSIBLE ENCEPHALOPATHY SYNDROME (PRES). Resp: cough, dyspnea.

Interactions
Drug-Drug: None reported.

Route/Dosage
Maintenance Treatment of Recurrent Germline *BRCA*-Mutated Epithelial Ovarian, Fallopian Tube, or Primary Peritoneal Cancer
PO (Adults): 300 mg once daily until disease progression or unacceptable toxicity. Treatment should be

started within 8 wk after most-recent platinum-containing regimen.

Hepatic Impairment

PO (Adults): *Moderate hepatic impairment:* 200 mg once daily until disease progression or unacceptable toxicity. Treatment should be started within 8 wk after most-recent platinum-containing regimen.

Maintenance Treatment of Advanced Epithelial Ovarian, Fallopian Tube, or Primary Peritoneal Cancer

PO (Adults ≥77 kg AND platelet count ≥150,000/mm³): 300 mg once daily until disease progression or unacceptable toxicity. Treatment should be started within 12 wk after most-recent platinum-containing regimen.

PO (Adults <77 kg OR platelet count <150,000/mm³): 200 mg once daily until disease progression or unacceptable toxicity. Treatment should be started within 12 wk after most-recent platinum-containing regimen.

Hepatic Impairment

PO (Adults): *Moderate hepatic impairment:* 200 mg once daily until disease progression or unacceptable toxicity. Treatment should be started within 12 wk after most-recent platinum-containing regimen.

Availability

Capsules (contain tartrazine): 100 mg. **Tablets:** 100 mg, 200 mg, 300 mg.

NURSING IMPLICATIONS

Assessment

* Monitor for signs and symptoms of MDS or AML (weakness, feeling tired, fever, weight loss, frequent infections, bruising, bleeding easily, breathlessness, blood in urine or stool, and/or low blood cell counts, or need for blood transfusions) periodically during therapy.
* Monitor BP and HR weekly for first 2 mo, then monthly for first year and periodically during therapy. Closely monitor patients with cardiovascular disorders, especially coronary insufficiency, cardiac arrhythmias, and hypertension. Manage hypertension with antihypertensive medications and adjustment of niraparib dose, if necessary.
* Monitor for signs and symptoms of PRES (seizure, headache, altered mental status, visual disturbance, cortical blindness, with or without associated hypertension). If symptoms occur, promptly discontinue niraparib.

Lab Test Considerations

* ※ Patient selection is based on either deleterious or suspected deleterious BRCA mutation and/or genomic instability score. Information on FDA-approved tests for the detection of either deleterious or suspected deleterious BRCA mutation or genomic instability for this indication is available at https://

www.fda.gov/companiondiagnostics.Verify negative pregnancy test before starting therapy.

* Monitor CBC weekly for first mo, monthly for next 11 mo, and periodically during therapy. Do not start niraparib until recovery of hematological toxicity from previous chemotherapy has recovered. **If platelet count <100,000 /mm³/L: *First occurrence:*** Hold niraparib for a maximum of 28 days and monitor blood counts weekly until platelet counts return to ≥100,000 /mm³/L. Resume at same or reduced dose. If platelet count is <75,000/ mm³/L, resume at a reduced dose. *Second occurrence:* Hold niraparib for a maximum of 28 days and monitor blood counts weekly until platelet counts return to ≥100,000/mm³. Resume at a reduced dose. Discontinue niraparib if platelet count has not returned to acceptable levels within 28 days of the dose interruption period, or if dose already reduced to 100 mg once daily. *For platelet count ≤10,000/mm³/L,* consider platelet transfusion. If other risk factors such as coadministration of anticoagulation or antiplatelet drugs exist, consider interrupting these drugs and/or transfusion. Resume therapy at a reduced dose.
* *If neutrophil <1,000/mm³ or hemoglobin <8 g/ dL:* Hold niraparib for a maximum of 28 days and monitor blood counts weekly until neutrophil counts return to ≥1,500/mm³ or hemoglobin returns to ≥9 g/dL. Resume at a reduced dose. Discontinue therapy if neutrophils and/or hemoglobin have not returned to acceptable levels within 28 days of dose interruption, or if dose already reduced to 100 mg once daily.
* May cause anemia.
* May cause ↑ AST and ALT.

Implementation

* Do not confuse niraparib with neratinib or nilotinib.
* For the maintenance treatment of advanced ovarian cancer, start therapy with no later than 12 wk after most recent platinum-containing regimen.
* **Dose Modification Recommendations:** *First dose reduction:* If taking 200 mg, decrease to 100 mg/day. If taking 300 mg, decrease to 200 mg/day. *Second dose reduction:* If taking 200 mg, discontinue niraparib. If taking 300 mg decrease to 100 mg/day. If further dose reduction below 100 mg/day is required, discontinue niraparib.
* *For nonhematologic adverse reactions:* If nonhematologic CTCAE ≥Grade 3 adverse reaction that persists despite medical management, hold niraparib for a maximum of 28 days or until resolution of adverse reaction. Resume niraparib at a reduced dose. If CTCAE ≥Grade 3 treatment-related adverse reaction lasting >28 days while patient is administered niraparib 100 mg/day, discontinue niraparib.
* **PO:** Administer once daily, at the same time each day, without regard to food. Nausea may be minimized by administering at bedtime. *DNC:* Swallow

capsules and tablets whole; do not open, crush, or chew.

Patient/Family Teaching

- Instruct patient to take niraparib as directed at the same time each day. Do not stop therapy without consulting health care professional. If dose missed or patient vomits after dose, omit and take next dose at scheduled time; do not double doses. Advise patient to read *Patient Information* before starting therapy and with each Rx refill in case of changes.
- Advise patient to notify health care professional if symptoms of MDS or AML (weakness, fever, feeling tired, weight loss, shortness of breath, blood in urine or stool, frequent infections, unusual bruising or bleeding) occur.
- Advise patient to notify health care professional of all Rx or OTC medications, vitamins, or herbal products being taken and consult health care professional before taking any new medications.
- Rep: May cause fetal harm. Advise females of reproductive potential to use effective contraception during and for 6 mo after last dose and to avoid breastfeeding during and for 1 mo after last dose of therapy. Inform male patients niraparib may impair fertility.

Evaluation/Desired Outcomes

- Decreased progression of ovarian, fallopian tube, or primary peritoneal cancer and improved survival.

---

nirmatrelvir/ritonavir
(nur-ma**trel**-veer/ri-**toe**-na-veer)
Paxlovid
Classification
Therapeutic: antivirals
Pharmacologic: protease inhibitors

Indications

Treatment of mild-to-moderate COVID-19 infection in patients who are at high risk for progression to severe COVID-19, including hospitalization or death.

Action

Nirmatrelvir acts as an inhibitor of the SARS-CoV-2 main protease (Mpro) which ultimately prevents viral replication. While ritonavir is also a protease inhibitor, this drug has no activity against Mpro. Ritonavir inhibits the CYP3A4-mediated metabolism of nirmatrelvir, resulting in increased plasma concentrations of nirmatrelvir. **Therapeutic Effects:** Reduction in COVID-19 related hospitalization or death from any cause.

Pharmacokinetics

Nirmatrelvir
Absorption: Well absorbed.
Distribution: Extensively distributed to extravascular tissues.

Metabolism and Excretion: CYP3A4 substrate; minimal metabolism by this isoenzyme when coadministered with ritonavir. Excreted in feces (49.6%) and urine (35.3%);.
Half-life: 6 hr.

Ritonavir
Absorption: Well absorbed.
Distribution: Extensively distributed to extravascular tissues.
Protein Binding: 98–99%.
Metabolism and Excretion: Primarily metabolized in the liver via the CYP3A isoenzyme, and to a lesser extent by the CYP2D6 isoenzyme. Primarily excreted in feces (86.4%), with 11.3% excreted in urine.
Half-life: 6 hr.

TIME/ACTION PROFILE (plasma concentrations)

ROUTE	ONSET	PEAK	DURATION
PO (nirmatrelvir)	unknown	3 hr	12 hr
PO (ritonavir)	unknown	4 hr	12 hr

Contraindications/Precautions

Contraindicated in: Hypersensitivity; Concurrent use of alfuzosin, amiodarone, apalutamide, carbamazepine, clozapine, colchicine, dihydroergotamine, dronedarone, ergotamine, flecainide, lovastatin, lurasidone, methylergonovine, midazolam (PO), phenobarbital, phenytoin, piroxicam, pimozide, propafenone, quinidine, ranolazine, rifampin, simvastatin, sildenafil (Revatio), St. John's wort, or triazolam; Severe renal impairment (CCr <30 mL/min); Severe hepatic impairment.

Use Cautiously in: Moderate renal impairment (↓ dose); OB: Use during pregnancy only if potential maternal benefit justifies potential fetal risk; Lactation: Safety not established in breastfeeding; Pedi: Safety and effectiveness not established in children.

Adverse Reactions/Side Effects

CV: hypertension. **Derm:** STEVENS-JOHNSON SYNDROME, TOXIC EPIDERMAL NECROLYSIS. **GI:** ↑ liver enzymes, abdominal pain, diarrhea, nausea, vomiting. **MS:** myalgia. **Neuro:** dysgeusia, headache. **Misc:** HYPERSENSITIVITY REACTIONS (including anaphylaxis).

Interactions

Drug-Drug: May ↑ levels and risk of toxicity of some antiarrhythmics (**amiodarone, dronedarone, flecainide, propafenone, quinidine**), some antipsychotics (**clozapine, pimozide, lurasidone**), **alfuzosin**, ergot derivatives (**dihydroergotamine, ergotamine, methylergonovine**), **colchicine, piroxicam, ranolazine, sildenafil (Revatio)**, **midazolam (oral)**, and **triazolam**; concurrent use con-

N

---

traindicated. May ↑ levels and risk of toxicity of **lovastatin** and **simvastatin**; concurrent use contraindicated; discontinue lovastatin and simvastatin ≥12 hr before starting nirmatrelvir/ritonavir. **Apalutamide, carbamazepine, phenobarbital, phenytoin, rifampin** may ↓ levels and effectiveness and promote resistance; concurrent use contraindicated. May ↑ levels and risk of toxicity of **lidocaine**; monitor lidocaine levels closely. May ↑ levels and risk of toxicity of **digoxin**; monitor digoxin levels closely. May ↑ levels and risk of toxicity of **cyclosporine, sirolimus**, and **tacrolimus**; avoid concurrent use with sirolimus; monitor cyclosporine and tacrolimus levels closely. May ↑ levels and risk of toxicity of **abemaciclib, ceritinib, dasatinib, encorafenib, ibrutinib, ivosidenib, neratinib, nilotinib, venetoclax, vinblastine**, and **vincristine**; avoid concurrent use with encorafenib ibrutinib, ivosidenib, neratinib, and venetoclax. May ↑ or ↓ **warfarin** levels; closely monitor INR. May ↑ levels of and risk of bleeding with **rivaroxaban**; avoid concurrent use. May ↓ levels and effectiveness of **bupropion**. May ↑ levels and risk of toxicity of **trazodone**; consider ↓ trazodone dose. May ↑ levels and risk of toxicity of **quetiapine**; consider ↓ quetiapine dose. May ↑ levels and risk of toxicity of **amlodipine, diltiazem, felodipine, nicardipine**, and **nifedipine**; consider ↓ calcium channel blocker dose. May ↓ levels and effectiveness of **voriconazole**; avoid concurrent use. May ↑ levels and risk of toxicity of **atazanavir, bedaquiline, bictegravir, clarithromycin, darunavir, efavirenz, erythromycin, fentanyl, fosamprenavir, isavuconazonium, itraconazole, ketoconazole, maraviroc, midazolam (parenteral) nelfinavir, nevirapine, rifabutin, tenofovir**, and **tipranavir. Isavuconazonium, itraconazole**, and **ketoconazole** may ↑ levels and risk of toxicity. May ↓ levels and effects of **raltegravir** and **zidovudine**. May ↑ levels and risk of toxicity of **bosentan**; discontinue bosentan ≥36 hr prior to starting nirmatrelvir/ritonavir. May ↑ levels and risk of toxicity of **elbasvir/grazoprevir, glecaprevir/pibrentasvir, ombitasvir/partiaprevir/ritonavir/dasabuvir**, and **sofosbuvir/velpatasvir/voxilaprevir**; avoid concurrent use with glecaprevir/pibrentasvir. May ↑ levels and risk of toxicity of **atorvastatin** and **rosuvastatin**; consider temporarily discontinuing atorvastatin and rosuvastatin during treatment. May ↓ levels and effectiveness of oral contraceptives containing **ethinyl estradiol**; use an additional non-hormonal contraceptive during treatment. May ↑ levels and risk of toxicity of **salmeterol**; concurrent use not recommended. May ↓ levels and effectiveness of **methadone**; monitor patients closely for signs/symptoms of withdrawal. May ↑ levels and risk of toxicity of **betamethasone, budesonide, ciclesonide, dexamethasone, fluticasone, methylprednisolone, mometasone, prednisone**, or **triamcinolone**; consider alternative corticosteroid such as beclomethasone or prednisolone.

Drug-Natural Products: St. John's wort may ↓ levels and effectiveness and promote resistance; concurrent use contraindicated.

Route/Dosage

PO (Adults): Two nirmatrelvir 150–mg tablets and one ritonavir 100–mg tablet twice daily for 5 days. Should be started as soon as possible after diagnosis of COVID-19 and within 5 days of symptom onset.

Renal Impairment

PO (Adults): *CCr 30–59 mL/min:* One nirmatrelvir 150–mg tablet and one ritonavir 100–mg tablet twice daily for 5 days. Should be started as soon as possible after diagnosis of COVID-19 and within 5 days of symptom onset.

Availability

Tablets: nirmatrelvir 150 mg + ritonavir 100 mg (separate tablets).

NURSING IMPLICATIONS

Assessment

- Assess signs and symptoms of COVID-19 before starting and during therapy.

Implementation

- Prior to prescribing *Paxlovid*: Review all medications taken by the patient to assess potential drug-drug interactions with a strong CYP3A inhibitors and determine if concomitant medications require a dose adjustment, interruption, and/or additional monitoring.
- *Paxlovid* is not approved for use as pre-exposure or post-exposure prophylaxis for prevention of COVID-19.
- Start 5-day course of *Paxlovid* as soon as possible after a diagnosis of COVID-19 has been made, and within 5 days of symptom onset even if baseline COVID-19 symptoms are mild. If the patient requires hospitalization due to severe or critical COVID-19 after starting treatment with *Paxlovid*, patient should complete the full 5-day course.
- **PO:** Administer tablets twice daily without regard to food. Dose packs contain two nirmatrelvir tablets and one ritonavir tablet. Dose for renal impairment contains one nirmatrelvir tablet and one ritonavir tablet. Nirmatrelvir must be co-administered with ritonavir. *DNC:* Swallow tablets whole; do not break, crush, or chew. Completion of the full 5-day course of therapy and continued isolation in accordance with public health recommendations are important to maximize viral clearance and minimize transmission of SARS-Co-2.

Patient/Family Teaching

- Instruct patient to take *Paxlovid* as directed. If a dose is missed within 8 hr of the time it is usually taken, patient should take it as soon as possible and resume the normal dosing schedule. If the dose is missed by >8 hrs, omit dose and take next dose at regularly scheduled time. Do not double dose to make up for a missed dose. Advise patient to read *Patient Information* before starting therapy.

- Advise patient to notify health care professional if signs and symptoms of hypersensitivity reactions (skin rash, hives or other skin reactions, difficulty in swallowing or breathing, swelling of the lips, tongue, face, tightness of the throat, hoarseness, or other symptoms of an allergic reaction) occur. Advise patient to immediately discontinue *Paxlovid* and to notify health care professional at the first sign of a reaction.
- Instruct patient to notify health care professional of all Rx or OTC medications, vitamins, or herbal products being taken and to consult with health care professional before taking other medications, especially St. John's wort.
- Rep: Advise females of reproductive potential to notify health care professional is pregnancy is planned or suspected or if breastfeeding. Ritonavir may reduce the efficacy of hormonal contraceptives. Advise patients using hormonal contraceptives to use an effective alternative contraceptive method or an additional barrier method of contraception.

Evaluation/Desired Outcomes
- Reduction in COVID-19 related hospitalization or death.

BEERS

⚅ nitrofurantoin
(nye-troe-fyoor-**an**-toyn)
Furadantin, Macrobid, Macrodantin
Classification
Therapeutic: anti-infectives

Indications
Prevention and treatment of urinary tract infections caused by susceptible organisms.

Action
Interferes with bacterial enzymes. **Therapeutic Effects:** Bactericidal or bacteriostatic action against susceptible organisms. **Spectrum:** Many gram-negative and some gram-positive organisms, specifically: *Citrobacter, Corynebacterium, Enterobacter, Escherichia coli, Klebsiella, Neisseria, Salmonella, Shigella, Staphylococcus aureus, Staphylococcus epidermidis, Enterococcus.*

Pharmacokinetics
Absorption: Readily absorbed after oral administration. Absorption is slower but more complete with macrocrystals (Macrodantin).
Distribution: Minimally distributed to tissues (concentrated in urine).

Metabolism and Excretion: Partially metabolized by the liver; 30–50% excreted unchanged by the kidneys.
Half-life: 20 min (↑ in renal impairment).

TIME/ACTION PROFILE (urine levels)

ROUTE	ONSET	PEAK	DURATION
PO	unknown	30 min	6–12 hr

Contraindications/Precautions
Contraindicated in: Hypersensitivity; Hypersensitivity to parabens (suspension); Oliguria, anuria, or significant renal impairment (CCr <60 mL/min); History of cholestatic jaundice or hepatic impairment with previous use of nitrofurantoin; OB: Pregnancy near term (38–42 wk gestation) and during labor/delivery (↑ risk of hemolytic anemia); Pedi: Infants <1 mo (↑ risk of hemolytic anemia).

Use Cautiously in: ⚅ Glucose–6–phosphate dehydrogenase (G6PD) deficiency (↑ risk of hemolytic anemia, especially in Blacks and Mediterranean and Near-Eastern ethnic groups); Diabetes (↑ risk of neuropathy); OB: Has been used safely in pregnancy. Lactation: May cause hemolysis in infants with G6PD deficiency who are breastfed; Geri: Appears on Beers list. ↑ risk of pulmonary toxicity, hepatotoxicity, and peripheral neuropathy, especially with long-term use, in older adults. Avoid use in older adults if CCr <30 mL/min or for long-term suppression of urinary tract infections.

Adverse Reactions/Side Effects
CV: chest pain. **Derm:** photosensitivity. **EENT:** nystagmus. **GI:** anorexia, nausea, vomiting, abdominal pain, CLOSTRIDIOIDES DIFFICILE-ASSOCIATED DIARRHEA (CDAD), diarrhea, HEPATOTOXICITY. **GU:** rust/brown discoloration of urine. **Hemat:** blood dyscrasias, hemolytic anemia. **Neuro:** dizziness, drowsiness, headache, peripheral neuropathy. **Resp:** PNEUMONITIS, PULMONARY FIBROSIS. **Misc:** hypersensitivity reactions.

Interactions
Drug-Drug: Probenecid prevents high urinary concentrations; may ↓ effectiveness. **Antacids** may ↓ absorption. ↑ risk of neurotoxicity with **neurotoxic drugs.** ↑ risk of hepatotoxicity with **hepatotoxic drugs.** ↑ risk of pneumonitis with **drugs having pulmonary toxicity.**

Route/Dosage
PO (Adults): *Treatment of active infection:* 50–100 mg every 6–8 hr *or* 100 mg every 12 hr as extended-release product. *Chronic suppression:* 50–100 mg single evening dose.
PO (Children >1 mo): *Treatment of active infection:* 5–7 mg/kg/day divided every 6 hr; maximum dose: 400 mg/day. *Chronic suppression:* 1–2 mg/kg/day as a single dose at bedtime; maximum dose: 100 mg/day (unlabeled).

✦= Canadian drug name. ⚅ = Genetic implication. ~~Strikethrough~~ = Discontinued. CAPITALS = life-threatening. <u>Underline</u> = most frequent.

Availability (generic available)

Capsules: 25 mg, 50 mg, 100 mg. **Extended-release capsules:** 100 mg. **Oral suspension:** 25 mg/5 mL.

NURSING IMPLICATIONS

Assessment

- Assess for signs and symptoms of urinary tract infection (frequency, urgency, pain, and burning on urination; fever; cloudy or foul-smelling urine) before and periodically during therapy.
- Obtain specimens for culture and sensitivity before and during drug administration.
- Monitor intake and output ratios. Report significant discrepancies in totals.
- Monitor bowel function. Diarrhea, abdominal cramping, fever, and bloody stools should be reported to health care professional promptly as a sign of CDAD. May begin up to several wk following cessation of therapy.
- Assess for signs and symptoms of pulmonary reactions periodically during therapy. Acute reactions (fever, chills, cough, chest pain, dyspnea, pulmonary infiltration with consolidation or pleural effusion on x ray, eosinophilia) usually occur within first wk of treatment and resolve when therapy is discontinued. Chronic reactions (malaise, dyspnea on exertion, cough, altered pulmonary function) may indicate pneumonitis or pulmonary fibrosis and are more common in patients taking nitrofurantoin for 6 mo or longer.

Lab Test Considerations

- Monitor CBC routinely with patients on prolonged therapy.
- Monitor liver function tests periodically during therapy. May cause ↑ serum glucose, bilirubin, alkaline phosphatase, BUN, and creatinine. If hepatotoxicity occurs, discontinue therapy.
- Monitor renal function periodically during therapy.

Implementation

- **PO:** Administer with food or milk to minimize GI irritation, to delay and increase absorption, to increase peak concentration, and to prolong duration of therapeutic concentration in the urine.
- **DNC:** Do not crush tablets or open capsules.
- Administer liquid preparations with calibrated measuring device. Shake well before administration. Oral suspension may be mixed with water, milk, fruit juices, or infant formula. Rinse mouth with water after administration of oral suspension to avoid staining teeth.

Patient/Family Teaching

- Instruct patient to take medication around the clock, as directed. Take missed doses as soon as remembered and space next dose 2–4 hr apart. Do not skip or double up on missed doses.
- May cause dizziness or drowsiness. Caution patient to avoid driving or other activities requiring alertness until response to medication is known.
- Inform patient that medication may cause a rust-yellow to brown discoloration of urine, which is not significant.
- Advise patient to notify health care professional if fever, chills, cough, chest pain, dyspnea, skin rash, numbness or tingling of the fingers or toes, or intolerable GI upset occurs. Signs of superinfection (milky, foul-smelling urine; perineal irritation; dysuria) should also be reported.
- Instruct patient to notify health care professional if fever and diarrhea develop, especially if stool contains blood, pus, or mucus. Advise patient not to treat diarrhea without consulting health care professional.
- Rep: May cause fetal harm. Advise females of reproductive potential to notify health care professional if pregnancy is planned or suspected and to avoid breastfeeding during therapy and for 1 mo after last dose of therapy. May cause hemolytic anemia in pregnant patients at term (38 to 42 weeks' gestation), during labor and delivery, or when the onset of labor is imminent.
- Instruct patient to consult health care professional if no improvement is seen within a few days after initiation of therapy.

Evaluation/Desired Outcomes

- Resolution of the signs and symptoms of infection. Therapy should be continued for a minimum of 7 days and for at least 3 days after the urine has become sterile.
- Decrease in the frequency of infections in chronic suppressive therapy.

NITROGLYCERIN

(nye-tro-**gli**-ser-in)

nitroglycerin extended-release capsules

Nitro-Time

nitroglycerin intravenous

~~Nitro-Bid IV~~, ✿ Nitroject, ~~Tridil~~

nitroglycerin sublingual tablets

Nitrostat

nitroglycerin transdermal ointment

Nitro-Bid

nitroglycerin transdermal patch

Nitro-Dur, ✿ Trinipatch

nitroglycerin translingual spray

Nitrolingual, Nitromist, ✿ Rho-Nitro

Classification

Therapeutic: antianginals
Pharmacologic: nitrates

Indications

Acute (**translingual, SL, ointment**) and long-term prophylactic (**oral, transdermal**) management of angina pectoris. **PO:** Adjunct treatment of HF. **IV:** Adjunct treatment of acute MI. Production of controlled hypotension during surgical procedures. Treatment of HF.

Action

Increases coronary blood flow by dilating coronary arteries and improving collateral flow to ischemic regions. Produces vasodilation (venous greater than arterial). Decreases left ventricular end-diastolic pressure and left ventricular end-diastolic volume (preload). Reduces myocardial oxygen consumption. **Therapeutic Effects:** Relief or prevention of anginal attacks. Increased cardiac output. Reduction of BP.

Pharmacokinetics

Absorption: Well absorbed after oral, buccal, and sublingual administration. Also absorbed through skin. Orally administered nitroglycerin is rapidly metabolized, leading to ↓ bioavailability.
Distribution: Unknown.
Metabolism and Excretion: Undergoes rapid and almost complete metabolism by the liver; also metabolized by enzymes in bloodstream.
Half-life: 1–4 min.

TIME/ACTION PROFILE (cardiovascular effects)

ROUTE	ONSET	PEAK	DURATION
SL/Translingual	1–3 min	unknown	30–60 min
PO-ER	40–60 min	unknown	8–12 hr
Oint	20–60 min	unknown	4–8 hr
Patch	40–60 min	unknown	8–24 hr
IV	immediate	unknown	several min

Contraindications/Precautions

Contraindicated in: Hypersensitivity; ↑ intracranial pressure; Severe anemia; Pericardial tamponade; Constrictive pericarditis; Uncorrected hypovolemia; Alcohol intolerance (large IV doses only); Acute circulatory failure/shock; Concurrent use of PDE-5 inhibitor (avanafil, sildenafil, tadalafil, vardenafil) or riociguat.
Use Cautiously in: Head trauma or cerebral hemorrhage; Glaucoma; Hypertrophic cardiomyopathy; Severe liver impairment; Malabsorption or hypermotility (PO); Cardioversion (remove transdermal patch before procedure); OB: May compromise maternal/fetal circulation; Lactation: Safety not established in breastfeeding; Pedi: Safety and effectiveness not established in children.

Adverse Reactions/Side Effects

CV: hypotension, tachycardia, syncope. **Derm:** contact dermatitis (transdermal), flushing. **EENT:** blurred vision. **GI:** abdominal pain, nausea, vomiting. **Neuro:** dizziness, headache, apprehension, restlessness, weakness. **Misc:** alcohol intoxication (large IV doses only), tolerance.

Interactions

Drug-Drug: Concurrent use of avanafil, sildenafil, tadalafil, or vardenafil may result in severe hypotension (do not use within 24 hr of isosorbide dinitrate or mononitrate); concurrent use contraindicated. Concurrent use of riociguat may result in severe hypotension; concurrent use contraindicated. Additive hypotension with antihypertensives, acute ingestion of alcohol, beta blockers, calcium channel blockers, haloperidol, or phenothiazines. Agents having anticholinergic properties (tricyclic antidepressants, antihistamines, phenothiazines) may ↓ absorption of translingual or sublingual nitroglycerin.

Route/Dosage

SL (Adults): *Tablets:* 0.3–0.6 mg; may repeat every 5 min for 2 additional doses for acute attack; may also be used prophylactically 5–10 min before activities that may precipitate an acute attack.
Translingual Spray (Adults): 1–2 sprays; may be repeated every 5 min for 2 additional doses for acute attack; may also be used prophylactically 5–10 min before activities that may precipitate an acute attack.
PO (Adults): 2.5–9 mg every 8–12 hr.
IV (Adults): 5 mcg/min; ↑ by 5 mcg/min every 3–5 min to 20 mcg/min; if no response, ↑ by 10–20 mcg/min every 3–5 min (dosing determined by hemodynamic parameters; max: 200 mcg/min).
Transdermal (Adults): *Ointment:* 1–2 in. every 6–8 hr. *Transdermal patch:* 0.2–0.4 mg/hr initially; may titrate up to 0.4–0.8 mg/hr. Patch should be worn 12–14 hr/day and then taken off for 10–12 hr/day.

Availability (generic available)

Extended-release capsules: 2.5 mg, 6.5 mg, 9 mg. **Sublingual tablets:** 0.3 mg, 0.4 mg, 0.6 mg. **Translingual spray:** 0.4 mg/spray in 4.9-g bottle (60 doses) or 14.6-g bottle (200 doses) (Nitrolingual), 0.4 mg/spray in 8.5-g bottle (230 doses) (Nitromist). **Transdermal patch:** 0.1 mg/hr, 0.2 mg/hr, 0.3 mg/hr, 0.4 mg/hr, 0.6 mg/hr, 0.8 mg/hr. **Transdermal ointment:** 2%. **Solution for injection:** 5 mg/mL. **Premixed infusion:** 25 mg/250 mL D5W, 50 mg/250 mL D5W, 100 mg/250 mL D5W.

NURSING IMPLICATIONS

Assessment

- Assess location, duration, intensity, and precipitating factors of patient's anginal pain.
- Monitor BP and pulse before and after administration. Patients receiving IV nitroglycerin require continuous ECG and BP monitoring. Additional hemodynamic parameters may be monitored.

Lab Test Considerations
- May cause ↑ urine catecholamine and urine vanillylmandelic acid concentrations.

- Excessive doses may cause ↑ methemoglobin concentrations.
- May cause falsely ↑ serum cholesterol levels.

Implementation

- **PO:** Administer dose 1 hr before or 2 hr after meals with a full glass of water for faster absorption. *DNC:* Sustained-release preparations should be swallowed whole; do not break, crush, or chew.
- **SL:** Tablet should be held under tongue until dissolved. Avoid eating, drinking, or smoking until tablet is dissolved.
- **Translingual spray:** Spray *Nitrolingual* under tongue. Spray *Nitromist* on or under tongue.

IV Administration

- **IV:** Doses must be diluted and administered as an infusion. Standard infusion sets made of polyvinyl chloride (PVC) plastic may absorb up to 80% of the nitroglycerin in solution. Use glass bottles only and special tubing provided by manufacturer.
- **Continuous Infusion:** *Dilution:* Vials must be diluted in D5W or 0.9% NaCl. Premixed infusions already diluted in D5W and are ready to be administered (no further dilution needed). Admixed solutions stable for 48 hr at room temperature or 7 days if refrigerated. Stability of premixed solutions based on manufacturer's expiration date. *Concentration:* Should not exceed 400 mcg/mL. *Rate:* See Route/Dosage section. Administer via infusion pump to ensure accurate rate. Titrate rate according to patient response.
- **Y-Site Compatibility:** acyclovir, alemtuzumab, amikacin, aminocaproic acid, aminophylline, amiodarone, amphotericin B deoxycholate, amphotericin B lipid complex, amphotericin B liposome, anidulafungin, argatroban, arsenic trioxide, ascorbic acid, atracurium, atropine, azathioprine, azithromycin, aztreonam, benztropine, bivalirudin, bleomycin, bumetanide, buprenorphine, butorphanol, calcium chloride, calcium gluconate, cangrelor, carboplatin, carmustine, caspofungin, cefazolin, cefotaxime, cefotetan, cefoxitin, ceftazidime, ceftolozane/tazobactam, ceftriaxone, cefuroxime, chloramphenicol, chlorpromazine, cisatracurium, cisplatin, clindamycin, cyanocobalamin, cyclophosphamide, cyclosporine, cytarabine, dacarbazine, dactinomycin, daunorubicin hydrochloride, dexamethasone, dexmedetomidine, dexrazoxane, digoxin, diltiazem, diphenhydramine, dobutamine, docetaxel, dopamine, doxorubicin hydrochloride, doxorubicin liposomal, doxycycline, enalaprilat, ephedrine, epinephrine, epirubicin, epoetin alfa, eptifibatide, ertapenem, erythromycin, esmolol, esomeprazole, etoposide, etoposide phosphate, famotidine, fentanyl, fluconazole, fludarabine, fluorouracil, folic acid, foscarnet, fosphenytoin, ganciclovir, gemcitabine, gemtuzumab ozogamicin, gentamicin, glycopyrrolate, granisetron, heparin, hetastarch, hydro-

cortisone, hydromorphone, idarubicin, ifosfamide, imipenem/cilastatin, indomethacin, insulin regular, irinotecan, isavuconazonium, isoproterenol, ketorolac, labetalol, LR, leucovorin calcium, lidocaine, linezolid, lorazepam, magnesium sulfate, mannitol, meperidine, meropenem/vaborbactam, mesna, methadone, methotrexate, methylprednisolone, metoclopramide, metronidazole, micafungin, midazolam, milrinone, minocycline, mitoxantrone, morphine, moxifloxacin, multivitamins, mycophenolate, nafcillin, nalbuphine, naloxone, nicardipine, nitroprusside, norepinephrine, octreotide, ondansetron, oritavancin, oxacillin, oxaliplatin, oxytocin, paclitaxel, palonosetron, pamidronate, papaverine, pemetrexed, penicillin G, pentamidine, pentobarbital, phenobarbital, phentolamine, phenylephrine, phytonadione, piperacillin/tazobactam, plazomicin, potassium acetate, potassium chloride, procainamide, prochlorperazine, promethazine, propranolol, protamine, pyridoxine, remifentanil, rocuronium, sodium bicarbonate, sodium citrate, succinylcholine, sufentanil, tacrolimus, tedizolid, theophylline, thiamine, thiopental, thiotepa, tigecycline, tirofiban, tobramycin, topotecan, vancomycin, vasopressin, vecuronium, verapamil, vinblastine, vincristine, vinorelbine, voriconazole, zoledronic acid.

- **Y-Site Incompatibility:** alteplase, dantrolene, daptomycin, diazepam, levofloxacin, meropenem, phenytoin, trimethoprim/sulfamethoxazole.
- **Topical:** Rotate sites of topical application to prevent skin irritation. Remove patch or ointment from previous site before application.
- Doses may be increased to the highest dose that does not cause symptomatic hypotension.
- Apply ointment by using dose-measuring application papers supplied with ointment. Squeeze ointment onto measuring scale printed on paper. Use paper to spread ointment onto nonhairy area of skin (chest, abdomen, thighs; avoid distal extremities) in a thin, even layer, covering a 2–3-in. area. Do not allow ointment to come in contact with hands. Do not massage or rub in ointment; this will increase absorption and interfere with sustained action. Apply occlusive dressing if ordered.
- Transdermal patches may be applied to any hairless site (avoid distal extremities or areas with cuts or calluses). Apply firm pressure over patch to ensure contact with skin, especially around edges. Apply a new dose unit if the first one becomes loose or falls off. Units are waterproof and not affected by showering or bathing. Do not cut or trim system to adjust dosage. Do not alternate between brands of transdermal products; dose may not be equivalent. Remove patches before MRI, cardioversion or defibrillation to prevent patient burns. Patch may be worn for 12–14 hr and removed for 10–12 hr at night to prevent development of tolerance.

Patient/Family Teaching

- Instruct patient to take medication as directed, even if feeling better. Take missed doses as soon as remembered unless next dose is scheduled within 2 hr (6 hr with extended-release preparations). Do not double doses. Do not discontinue abruptly; gradual dose reduction may be necessary to prevent rebound angina.
- Caution patient to change positions slowly to minimize orthostatic hypotension. First dose should be taken while in a sitting or reclining position, especially in geriatric patients.
- Advise patient to avoid concurrent use of alcohol with this medication. Patient should also consult health care professional before taking OTC medications while taking nitroglycerin.
- Inform patient that headache is a common side effect that should decrease with continuing therapy. Aspirin or acetaminophen may be ordered to treat headache. Notify health care professional if headache is persistent or severe.
- Advise patient to notify health care professional if dry mouth or blurred vision occurs.
- Rep: Advise females of reproductive potential to notify health care professional if pregnancy is planned or suspected or if breastfeeding.
- **Acute Anginal Attacks:** Advise patient to sit down and use medication at first sign of attack. Relief usually occurs within 5 min. Dose may be repeated if pain is not relieved in 5–10 min. Call health care professional or go to nearest emergency room if anginal pain is not relieved by 3 tablets in 15 min.
- **SL:** Inform patient that tablets should be kept in original glass container or in specially made metal containers, with cotton removed to prevent absorption. Tablets lose potency in containers made of plastic or cardboard or when mixed with other capsules or tablets. Exposure to air, heat, and moisture also causes loss of potency. Instruct patient not to open bottle frequently, handle tablets, or keep bottle of tablets next to body (i.e., shirt pocket) or in automobile glove compartment. Advise patient that tablets should be replaced 6 mo after opening to maintain potency.
- **Lingual Spray:** Instruct patient to lift tongue and spray dose under tongue (*Nitrolingual, NitroMist*) or on tongue (*NitroMist*).

Evaluation/Desired Outcomes

- Decrease in frequency and severity of anginal attacks.
- Increase in activity tolerance. During long-term therapy, tolerance may be minimized by intermittent administration in 12–14 hr or 10–12 hr off intervals.
- Controlled hypotension during surgical procedures.
- Treatment of HF associated with acute MI.

HIGH ALERT

nitroprusside
(nye-troe-**pruss**-ide)
❋Nipride, Nipride RTU, ~~Nitropress~~
Classification
Therapeutic: antihypertensives
Pharmacologic: vasodilators

Indications
Hypertensive crises. Controlled hypotension during anesthesia. Cardiac pump failure or cardiogenic shock (alone or in combination with dopamine).

Action
Produces peripheral vasodilation by a direct action on venous and arteriolar smooth muscle. **Therapeutic Effects:** Rapid lowering of BP. Decreased cardiac preload and afterload.

Pharmacokinetics
Absorption: IV administration results in complete bioavailability.
Distribution: Unknown.
Metabolism and Excretion: Rapidly metabolized in RBCs and tissues to cyanide and subsequently by the liver to thiocyanate.
Half-life: 2 min.

TIME/ACTION PROFILE (hypotensive effect)

ROUTE	ONSET	PEAK	DURATION
IV	immediate	rapid	1–10 min

Contraindications/Precautions
Contraindicated in: Hypersensitivity; ↓ cerebral perfusion.
Use Cautiously in: Renal impairment (↑ risk of thiocyanate accumulation); Hepatic impairment (↑ risk of cyanide accumulation); Hypothyroidism; Hyponatremia; Vitamin B deficiency; OB: Safety not established in pregnancy; Lactation: Safety not established in breastfeeding; Geri: Older adults may have ↑ sensitivity to drug effects.

Adverse Reactions/Side Effects
CV: dyspnea, hypotension, palpitations. EENT: blurred vision, tinnitus. F and E: acidosis. GI: abdominal pain, nausea, vomiting. **Local:** phlebitis at IV site. **Neuro:** dizziness, headache, restlessness. **Misc:** CYANIDE TOXICITY, thiocyanate toxicity.

Interactions
Drug-Drug: ↑ hypotensive effect with **ganglionic blocking agents**, **general anesthetics**, and other **antihypertensives**. **Estrogens** and **sympathomimetics** may ↓ the response to nitroprusside.

Route/Dosage

IV (Adults and Children): 0.3 mcg/kg/min initially; may be ↑ as needed up to 10 mcg/kg/min (usual dose is 3 mcg/kg/min; not to exceed 10 min of therapy at 10 mcg/kg/min infusion rate).

Availability (generic available)

Premixed infusion: 20 mg/100 mL 0.9% NaCl, 50 mg/100 mL 0.9% NaCl. **Solution for injection:** 25 mg/mL.

NURSING IMPLICATIONS

Assessment

- Monitor BP, heart rate, and ECG frequently throughout therapy; continuous monitoring is preferred. Consult physician for parameters. Monitor for rebound hypertension following discontinuation of nitroprusside.
- Pulmonary capillary wedge pressure (PCWP) may be monitored in patients with MI or HF.

Lab Test Considerations

- May cause ↓ bicarbonate concentrations, pCO_2, and pH.
- May cause ↑ lactate concentrations.
- May cause ↑ serum cyanide and thiocyanate concentrations.
- Monitor serum methemoglobin concentrations in patients receiving >10 mg/kg and exhibiting signs of impaired oxygen delivery despite adequate cardiac output and arterial pCO_2 (blood is chocolate brown without change on exposure to air). Treatment of methemoglobinemia is 1–2 mg/kg of methylene blue IV administered over several min.

Toxicity and Overdose

- If severe hypotension occurs, drug effects are quickly reversed, within 1–10 min, by decreasing rate or temporarily discontinuing infusion. May place patient in Trendelenburg position to maximize venous return.
- Monitor plasma thiocyanate levels daily in patients receiving prolonged infusions at a rate >3 mcg/kg/min or 1 mcg/kg/min in patients with anuria. Thiocyanate levels should not exceed 1 mmol/L.
- Signs and symptoms of thiocyanate toxicity include tinnitus, toxic psychoses, hyperreflexia, confusion, weakness, seizures, and coma.
- Cyanide toxicity may manifest as lactic acidosis, hypoxemia, tachycardia, altered consciousness, seizures, and characteristic breath odor similar to almonds.
- Acute treatment of cyanide toxicity includes 4–6 mg/kg of *sodium nitrite* (as a 3% solution) over 2–4 min. This acts as a buffer for cyanide by converting 10% of hemoglobin to methemoglobin. If administration of sodium nitrite is delayed, inhalation of crushed ampule of *amyl nitrite* for 15–30 sec of every min should be started until sodium nitrite is running. Following completion of sodium nitrite infusion, administer *sodium thiosulfate* 150–200

mcg/kg (available as 25% and 50% solutions). This will convert cyanide to thiocyanate, which may then be eliminated. If required, entire regimen may be repeated in 2 hr at 50% of the initial doses.

Implementation

- If infusion of 10 mcg/kg/min for 10 min does not produce adequate reduction in BP, manufacturer recommends nitroprusside be discontinued.
- May be administered in left ventricular HF concurrently with an inotropic agent (dopamine, dobutamine) when effective doses of nitroprusside restore pump function and cause excessive hypotension.

IV Administration

- **Continuous Infusion:** *Dilution:* Dilute 50 mg of nitroprusside in 250–1000 mL of D5W. Wrap infusion in aluminum foil to protect from light; administration set tubing need not be covered. Amber plastic bags do not offer sufficient protection from light; wrap must be opaque. Freshly prepared solution has a slight brownish tint; discard if solution is dark brown, orange, blue, green, or dark red. Solution must be used within 24 hr of preparation. *Concentration:* 50–200 mcg/mL. *Rate:* Based on patient's weight (see Route/Dosage section). Administer via volumetric infusion pump to ensure accurate dosage rate.
- **Y-Site Compatibility:** alemtuzumab, alprostadil, amikacin, aminocaproic acid, aminophylline, amphotericin B lipid complex, amphotericin B liposomal, anidulafungin, argatroban, atropine, azithromycin, aztreonam, benztropine, bivalirudin, bleomycin, bumetanide, buprenorphine, butorphanol, calcium chloride, calcium gluconate, cangrelor, carboplatin, carmustine, cefazolin, cefotaxime, cefotetan, cefoxitin, ceftolozane/tazobactam, ceftriaxone, cefuroxime, chloramphenicol, cisplatin, clindamycin, cyanocobalamin, cyclophosphamide, cyclosporine, cytarabine, dacarbazine, dactinomycin, daptomycin, dexamethasone, dexmedetomidine, dexrazoxane, digoxin, diltiazem, docetaxel, dopamine, doxorubicin hydrochloride, doxorubicin liposomal, doxycycline, enalaprilat, ephedrine, epinephrine, epirubicin, epoetin alfa, eptifibatide, ertapenem, esmolol, etoposide, etoposide phosphate, famotidine, fentanyl, fluconazole, fludarabine, fluorouracil, folic acid, foscarnet, fosphenytoin, furosemide, ganciclovir, gemcitabine, gemtuzumab ozogamicin, gentamicin, glycopyrrolate, granisetron, heparin, hetastarch, hydrocortisone, hydromorphone, idarubicin, ifosfamide, indomethacin, insulin regular, isavuconazonium, isoproterenol, ketorolac, labetalol, LR, leucovorin calcium, lidocaine, linezolid, lorazepam, magnesium sulfate, mannitol, meperidine, meropenem, methadone, methylprednisolone, metoclopramide, metoprolol, metronidazole, micafungin, midazolam, milrinone, morphine, multivitamins, nafcillin, nalbuphine, naloxone, nicardipine, nitroglycerin, norepinephrine, octreotide, ondansetron,

oxacillin, oxaliplatin, oxytocin, paclitaxel, palonosetron, pamidronate, pantoprazole, penicillin G, pentamidine, pentobarbital, phenobarbital, phentolamine, phenylephrine, phytonadione, piperacillin/tazobactam, plazomicin, potassium acetate, potassium chloride, potassium phosphates, procainamide, propofol, propranolol, protamine, pyridoxine, rocuronium, sodium acetate, sodium bicarbonate, succinylcholine, sufentanil, tacrolimus, theophylline, thiamine, tigecycline, tirofiban, tobramycin, topotecan, vancomycin, vasopressin, vecuronium, verapamil, vinblastine, vincristine, zoledronic acid.
- **Y-Site Incompatibility:** acyclovir, ascorbic acid, azathioprine, caspofungin, ceftazidime, chlorpromazine, dantrolene, daunorubicin hydrochloride, diazepam, diphenhydramine, erythromycin, hydralazine, hydroxyzine, irinotecan, levofloxacin, mesna, mitomycin, mitoxantrone, moxifloxacin, mycophenolate, oritavancin, papaverine, pemetrexed, phenytoin, prochlorperazine, promethazine, thiotepa, trimethoprim/sulfamethoxazole, vinorelbine, voriconazole.

Patient/Family Teaching
- Explain purpose of nitroprusside to patient.
- Advise patient to report the onset of tinnitus, dyspnea, dizziness, headache, or blurred vision immediately.
- Rep: May cause fetal harm. Prolonged or large doses may cause fetal harm. Advise females of reproductive potential to notify health care professional if pregnancy is planned or suspected or if breastfeeding.

Evaluation/Desired Outcomes
- Decrease in BP without the appearance of side effects.
- Treatment of cardiac pump failure or cardiogenic shock by decreasing cardiac preload and afterload.

---

nivolumab (nye-vol-ue-mab)
Opdivo
Classification
Therapeutic: antineoplastics
Pharmacologic: monoclonal antibodies, programmed death-1 inhibitors

Indications
Unresectable/metastatic melanoma (as monotherapy or in combination with ipilimumab). Adjuvant treatment of melanoma in patients that have involvement of lymph nodes or metastatic disease and have undergone complete resection. Metastatic non–small-cell lung cancer (NSCLC) with progression on or after platinum-based chemotherapy. Patients with epidermal growth factor receptor (EGFR) or anaplastic lymphoma kinase (ALK) genomic tumor aberrations should have disease progression on an FDA-approved therapy for these aberrations prior to receiving nivolumab. First-line treatment of metastatic NSCLC in patients whose tumors express PD-L1 ($\geq$1%) and have no epidermal growth factor receptor (EGFR) or anaplastic lymphoma kinase (ALK) genomic tumor aberrations (in combination with ipilimumab). First-line treatment of metastatic or recurrent NSCLC in patients whose tumors have no EGFR or ALK genomic tumor aberrations (in combination with ipilimumab and two cycles of platinum-based chemotherapy). Neoadjuvant treatment of resectable (tumors $\geq$4 cm or node positive) NSCLC (in combination with platinum-doublet chemotherapy). Advanced renal cell carcinoma (RCC) in patients who have previously received anti-angiogenic therapy (as monotherapy). Immediate or poor risk, previously untreated advanced RCC (in combination with ipilimumab). First-line treatment of advanced RCC (in combination with cabozantinib). Classic Hodgkin's lymphoma that has relapsed or progressed after either autologous hematopoietic stem cell transplantation (HSCT) and brentuximab or $\geq$3 lines of systemic therapy that includes autologous HSCT. Recurrent or metastatic squamous cell carcinoma of the head and neck with progression on or after platinum-based therapy. Adjuvant treatment of urothelial carcinoma in patients who are at high risk of recurrence after undergoing radical resection of urothelial carcinoma. Locally advanced or metastatic urothelial carcinoma in patients who either have progression during or following platinum-based therapy or progression within 12 mo of neoadjuvant or adjuvant treatment with platinum-based therapy. Microsatellite instability-high (MSI-H) or mismatch repair deficient (dMMR) metastatic colorectal cancer that has progressed following treatment with a fluoropyrimidine, oxaliplatin, and irinotecan (as monotherapy or in combination with ipilimumab). Hepatocellular carcinoma in patients who have been previously treated with sorafenib (in combination with ipilimumab). Unresectable advanced, recurrent, or metastatic esophageal squamous cell carcinoma after prior fluoropyrimidine- and platinum-based chemotherapy. First-line treatment of unresectable advanced or metastatic esophageal squamous cell carcinoma (in combination with fluoropyrimidine- and platinum-containing chemotherapy). First-line treatment of unresectable advanced or metastatic esophageal squamous cell carcinoma (in combination with ipilimumab). Adjuvant treatment of completely resected esophageal or gastroesophageal junction cancer with residual pathologic disease in patients who have received neoadjuvant chemoradiotherapy. Advanced or metastatic gastric cancer, gastroesophageal junction cancer, and esophageal adenocarcinoma (in combination with fluoropyrimidine- and platinum-containing chemotherapy). First-line treatment of unresectable malignant pleural mesothelioma (in combination with ipilimumab).

Action

Programmed death receptor-1 (PD-1) blocking antibody (an IgG4 kappa immunoglobulin) that binds to PD-1 and blocks its interaction with its ligands, PD-L1 and PD-L2, resulting in activation of the immune system and decreased tumor growth. **Therapeutic Effects:** Decreased progression of melanoma, Hodgkin's lymphoma, urothelial carcinoma, colorectal cancer, and hepatocellular carcinoma. Decreased progression of and improved survival with NSCLC and advanced RCC. Improved survival in squamous cell carcinoma of head and neck, esophageal cancer, gastric cancer, gastroesophageal junction cancer, esophageal adenocarcinoma, and malignant pleural mesothelioma.

Pharmacokinetics

Absorption: IV administration results in complete bioavailability.
Distribution: Unknown.
Metabolism and Excretion: Unknown.
Half-life: 26.7 days.

TIME/ACTION PROFILE

ROUTE	ONSET	PEAK	DURATION
IV	unknown	unknown	unknown

Contraindications/Precautions

Contraindicated in: OB: Pregnancy; Lactation: Lactation.
Use Cautiously in: Patients undergoing allogeneic HSCT before or after nivolumab therapy (↑ risk of complications); Patients with multiple myeloma receiving a thalidomide analogue and dexamethasone (↑ risk of mortality); Rep: Women of reproductive potential; Pedi: Safety and effectiveness not established in children <12 yr (MSI-H dMMR colorectal cancer and melanoma) or children <18 yr (all other indications).

Adverse Reactions/Side Effects

CV: MYOCARDITIS, pericarditis, peripheral edema, vasculitis. **Derm:** rash, DRUG REACTION WITH EOSINOPHILIA AND SYSTEMIC SYMPTOMS (DRESS), STEVENS-JOHNSON SYNDROME (SJS), TOXIC EPIDERMAL NECROLYSIS (TEN). **EENT:** iritis, uveitis. **Endo:** hypothyroidism, ADRENAL INSUFFICIENCY, hyperthyroidism, hypoparathyroidism, hypophysitis, type 1 diabetes. **F and E:** hyperkalemia. **GI:** COLITIS, gastritis, HEPATITIS, pancreatitis. **GU:** nephritis. **Hemat:** hemolytic anemia. **MS:** myositis, RHABDOMYOLYSIS. **Neuro:** autoimmune neuropathy, ENCEPHALITIS, Guillain-Barré syndrome, MENINGITIS, myasthenic syndrome, myelitis. **Resp:** cough, PNEUMONITIS. **Misc:** INFUSION-RELATED REACTIONS.

Interactions

Drug-Drug: None reported.

Route/Dosage

Unresectable or Metastatic Melanoma

IV (Adults and Children ≥12 yr and ≥40 kg): *As monotherapy:* 240 mg every 2 wk until disease progression or unacceptable toxicity *or* 480 mg every 4 wk until disease progression or unacceptable toxicity; *In combination with ipilimumab:* 1 mg/kg every 3 wk for 4 doses or until unacceptable toxicity (whichever occurs first) (administer before ipilimumab on same day), then either 240 mg as monotherapy every 2 wk until disease progression or unacceptable toxicity *or* 480 mg as monotherapy every 4 wk until disease progression or unacceptable toxicity.
IV (Children ≥12 yr and <40 kg): *As monotherapy:* 3 mg/kg every 2 wk until disease progression or unacceptable toxicity *or* 6 mg/kg every 4 wk until disease progression or unacceptable toxicity; *In combination with ipilimumab:* 1 mg/kg every 3 wk for 4 doses or until unacceptable toxicity (whichever occurs first) (administer before ipilimumab on same day), then either 3 mg/kg as monotherapy every 2 wk until disease progression or unacceptable toxicity *or* 6 mg/kg as monotherapy every 4 wk until disease progression or unacceptable toxicity.

Adjuvant Treatment of Melanoma

IV (Adults and Children ≥12 yr and ≥40 kg): 240 mg every 2 wk until disease progression or unacceptable toxicity for up to 1 yr *or* 480 mg every 4 wk until disease progression or unacceptable toxicity for up to 1 yr.
IV (Children ≥12 yr and <40 kg): 3 mg/kg every 2 wk until disease progression or unacceptable toxicity *or* 6 mg/kg every 4 wk until disease progression or unacceptable toxicity.

Hepatocellular Carcinoma

IV (Adults): 1 mg/kg every 3 wk for 4 doses (administer before ipilimumab on same day), then 240 mg as monotherapy every 2 wk *or* 480 mg as monotherapy every 4 wk until disease progression or unacceptable toxicity.

Adjuvant Treatment of Urothelial Carcinoma

IV (Adults): 240 mg every 2 wk until disease progression or unacceptable toxicity for up to 1 yr *or* 480 mg every 4 wk until disease progression or unacceptable toxicity for up to 1 yr.

Classical Hodgkin's Lymphoma, Urothelial Carcinoma, or Squamous Cell Carcinoma of Head and Neck

IV (Adults): 240 mg every 2 wk until disease progression or unacceptable toxicity *or* 480 mg every 4 wk until disease progression or unacceptable toxicity.

Esophageal Squamous Cell Carcinoma

IV (Adults): *As monotherapy:* 240 mg every 2 wk until disease progression or unacceptable toxicity *or* 480 mg every 4 wk until disease progression or unacceptable toxicity. *In combination with fluoropyrimidine- and platinum-containing chemotherapy:* 240 mg every 2 wk until disease progression, unacceptable toxicity, or for up to 2 yr *or* 480 mg every 4 wk until disease progression, unacceptable toxicity, or for up to 2 yr. *In combination with ipilimumab:* 3 mg/kg every 2 wk until disease progression, unacceptable toxicity, or for up to 2 yr (administer before ipilimumab on same day) *or* 360 mg every 3 wk until disease progression, unacceptable toxicity, or for up to 2 yr (administer before ipilimumab on same day).

Adjuvant Treatment of Resected Esophageal or Gastroesophageal Junction Cancer

IV (Adults): 240 mg every 2 wk until disease progression or unacceptable toxicity for a total treatment duration of 1 yr *or* 480 mg every 4 wk until disease progression or unacceptable toxicity for a total treatment duration of 1 yr.

Metastatic Non–Small-Cell Lung Cancer

IV (Adults): *As monotherapy:* 240 mg every 2 wk until disease progression or unacceptable toxicity *or* 480 mg every 4 wk until disease progression or unacceptable toxicity; *In combination with ipilimumab (for metastatic tumors expressing PD-L1):* 3 mg/kg every 3 wk until disease progression, unacceptable toxicity or for up to 2 yr (if no disease progression) (administer before ipilimumab on same day). *In combination with ipilimumab (for metastatic or recurrent tumors not expressing PD-L1):* 360 mg every 3 wk until disease progression, unacceptable toxicity or for up to 2 yr (if no disease progression) (when given just with platinum-based chemotherapy on same day, administer nivolumab then platinum-based chemotherapy; when given with ipilimumab and platinum-based chemotherapy on same day, administer nivolumab, then ipilimumab, then platinum-based chemotherapy).

Neoadjuvant Treatment of Resectable Non-Small-Cell Lung Cancer

IV (Adults): 360 mg every 3 wk (when given with platinum-doublet chemotherapy on same day) for 3 cycles.

Advanced Renal Cell Carcinoma

IV (Adults): *As monotherapy:* 240 mg every 2 wk until disease progression or unacceptable toxicity *or* 480 mg every 4 wk until disease progression or unacceptable toxicity; *In combination with ipilimumab:* 3 mg/kg every 3 wk for 4 doses (administer before ipilimumab on same day), then 240 mg as monotherapy every 2 wk until disease progression or unacceptable toxicity *or* 480 mg as monotherapy every 4 wk until disease progression or unacceptable toxicity. *In combination with cabozantinib:* 240 mg every 2 wk until disease progression, unacceptable toxicity, or up to 2 yr *or* 480 mg every 4 wk until disease progression, unacceptable toxicity, or up to 2 yr.

Microsatellite Instability-High or Mismatch Repair Deficient Metastatic Colorectal Cancer

IV (Adults and Children ≥12 yr and ≥40 kg): *As monotherapy:* 240 mg every 2 wk until disease progression or unacceptable toxicity *or* 480 mg every 4 wk until disease progression or unacceptable toxicity; *In combination with ipilimumab:* 3 mg/kg every 3 wk for 4 doses (administer before ipilimumab on same day), then 240 mg as monotherapy every 2 wk until disease progression or unacceptable toxicity *or* 480 mg as monotherapy every 4 wk until disease progression or unacceptable toxicity.

IV (Children ≥12 yr and <40 kg): *As monotherapy:* 3 mg/kg every 2 wk until disease progression or unacceptable toxicity; *In combination with ipilimumab:* 3 mg/kg every 3 wk for 4 doses (administer before ipilimumab on same day), then 3 mg/kg as monotherapy every 2 wk until disease progression or unacceptable toxicity.

Gastric Cancer, Gastroesophageal Junction Cancer, and Esophageal Adenocarcinoma

IV (Adults): 240 mg every 2 wk until disease progression, unacceptable toxicity or for up to 2 yr (administer before fluoropyrimidine- and platinum-containing chemotherapy on same day) *or* 360 mg every 3 wk until disease progression, unacceptable toxicity or for up to 2 yr (administer before fluoropyrimidine- and platinum-containing chemotherapy on same day).

Malignant Pleural Mesothelioma

IV (Adults): 360 mg/kg every 3 wk until disease progression, unacceptable toxicity or for up to 2 yr (if no disease progression) (administer before ipilimumab on same day).

Availability

Solution for injection: 10 mg/mL.

NURSING IMPLICATIONS
Assessment

- Monitor for signs and symptoms of immune-mediated pneumonitis (shortness of breath, chest pain, new or worse cough) periodically during therapy. Treat with corticosteroids 1–2 mg/kg/day prednisone equivalents for ≥Grade 2 pneumonitis followed by corticosteroid taper. *If Grade 2 pneumonitis occurs,* hold nivolumab; resume therapy when recovery to Grade 0–1. *If Grade 3 or 4 pneumonitis occurs,* permanently discontinue nivolumab.
- Assess for signs and symptoms of infusion reactions (chills or shaking, itching or rash, flushing, difficulty breathing, dizziness, fever, feeling faint) periodically during therapy. If Grade 1 or 2 infusion reactions occur, hold or slow infusion. *If Grade 3 or 4 infusion reactions occur,* discontinue therapy.
- Monitor for signs and symptoms of immune-mediated colitis (diarrhea, abdominal pain, mucus or blood in stool, with or without fever). Treat with corticosteroids at doses of 1–2 mg/kg/day of prednisone or equivalents followed by corticosteroid taper for severe (Grade 3) or life-threatening (Grade 4) colitis. *If Grade 2 or 3 colitis occurs,* hold nivolu-

mab. Resume with complete or partial resolution (Grade 0–1) after corticosteroid taper. Permanently discontinue if no complete or partial resolution within 12 wk of last dose or inability to reduce prednisone to ≤10 mg per day (or equivalent) within 12 wk of initiating steroids. *If Grade 4 colitis occurs,* permanently discontinue nivolumab. *If administered with ipilimumab,* hold for Grade 2 colitis. For moderate or severe (Grade 3 or 4) or recurrent colitis, permanently discontinue nivolumab and ipilimumab.

- Monitor for signs and symptoms of hepatitis (yellowing of skin or whites of eyes, severe nausea or vomiting, right-sided abdominal pain, drowsiness, dark urine, unusual bleeding or bruising, anorexia) periodically during therapy.
- Assess for rash periodically during therapy. Topical emollients and/or topical corticosteroids may be adequate to treat mild to moderate nonexfoliative rashes. May cause SJS and TEN. *If rash, itching, blistering, or ulcers in mouth or other mucous membranes occur and SJS, TEN, or DRESS are suspected,* hold dose and refer for assessment and treatment. *If SJS, TEN, or DRESS are confirmed,* permanently discontinue therapy. Discontinue therapy if severe or if accompanied with fever, general malaise, fatigue, muscle or joint aches, blisters, oral lesions, conjunctivitis, hepatitis and/or eosinophilia. For immune-mediated rash, administer corticosteroids at doses of 1–2 mg/kg/day of prednisone or equivalents followed by corticosteroid taper for severe (Grade 3) or life-threatening (Grade 4) rash. Withhold for severe rash; permanently discontinue for life-threatening rash.
- Monitor for signs and symptoms of hypophysitis (headaches, photophobia, visual field defects, extreme tiredness, weight gain or loss, dizziness or fainting, mood changes, hair loss, feeling cold, constipation, deepening voice, excessive thirst and urination) periodically during therapy. Administer hormone replacement and corticosteroids at a dose of 1 mg/kg/day prednisone equivalents followed by corticosteroid taper for moderate or severe hypophysitis. Withhold therapy for moderate or severe hypophysitis. Discontinue for life-threatening Grade 4.
- Monitor for signs and symptoms of adrenal insufficiency. Administer corticosteroids at a dose of 1–2 mg/kg/day prednisone equivalents followed by corticosteroid taper for severe (Grade 3) or life-threatening (Grade 4) symptoms. Withhold for moderate (Grade 2) and permanently discontinue therapy for severe or life-threatening adrenal insufficiency.
- Monitor for signs and symptoms of encephalitis (headache, fever, tiredness or weakness, confusion, memory problems, sleepiness, hallucinations, seizures, stiff neck) periodically during therapy. *If Grade 2 neurological toxicities occur,* hold therapy for patients with new-onset moderate to severe neurologic symptoms during diagnosis. *If Grade 3*

or 4 neurological toxicities occur, permanently discontinue nivolumab and administer corticosteroids at dose of 1–2 mg/kg/day prednisone equivalents for immune-mediated encephalitis, followed by corticosteroid taper.

- Monitor for signs and symptoms of kidney dysfunction (decrease in amount of urine, blood in urine, swelling in ankles, anorexia) periodically during therapy.
- Monitor for signs and symptoms of myocarditis (chest pain, dyspnea) during therapy. If Grade 2, 3 or 4 myocarditis occurs, permanently discontinue nivolumab.

Lab Test Considerations

- Verify negative pregnancy test before starting therapy. ⚇ Patient selection for NSCLC in combination with ipilimumab is based on PD-L1 expression. Information on FDA-approved tests for the determination of PD-L1 expression in NSCLC is available at: http://www.fda.gov/CompanionDiagnostics. Monitor for abnormal liver tests prior to and periodically during therapy. *For hepatitis with no tumor involvement: If AST/ALT >3 and ≤8 times (or ≤5 if given with ipilimumab) upper limit of normal (ULN) or total bilirubin >1.5 and ≤3 times ULN,* hold nivolumab. Resume with complete or partial resolution (Grade 0–1) after corticosteroid taper. Permanently discontinue if no complete or partial resolution within 12 wk of last dose or inability to reduce prednisone to ≤10 mg per day (or equivalent) within 12 wk of starting steroids. *If AST or ALT >8 times (or >5 if given with ipilimumab) ULN or total bilirubin >3 times ULN,* permanently discontinue nivolumab. For hepatitis with tumor involvement of the liver: *If baseline AST/ALT is >1 and ≤3 times ULN and increases to >5 and ≤10 times ULN or baseline AST/ALT is >3 and ≤5 times ULN and increases to >8 and ≤10 times ULN,* hold nivolumab. *If AST/ALT >10 times ULN or total bilirubin >3 times ULN,* discontinue nivolumab permanently. *If given with cabozantinib and ALT or AST >3 times ULN but ≤10 times ULN with concurrent total bilirubin <2 times ULN,* hold nivolumab and cabozantinib until recovery to Grade 0–1. *If given with cabozantinib and AST or ALT >10 times ULN or >3 times with concurrent bilirubin ≥2 times ULN,* permanently discontinue nivolumab and cabozantinib.
- Monitor for ↑ serum creatinine prior to and periodically during therapy. If Grade 2 or 3 increases in blood creatinine occur, hold nivolumab. Resume in patients with complete or partial resolution (Grade 0–1) after corticosteroid taper. Permanently discontinue if no complete or partial resolution within 12 wk of last dose or inability to reduce prednisone to ≤10 mg per day (or equivalent) within 12 wk of starting steroids. *If Grade 4 increases in blood creatinine occur,* permanently discontinue nivolumab.
- Monitor thyroid function prior to and periodically during therapy. Treat hypothyroidism with replace-

ment therapy. Use medical management for hyperthyroidism. Immune-mediated thyroid dysfunction does not require dose modification of nivolumab.
- Monitor for hyperglycemia. If severe, withhold therapy until metabolic control achieved. If life-threatening, permanently discontinue nivolumab.

Implementation
IV Administration
- **Intermittent Infusion:** *Dilution:* 0.9% NaCl or D5W. *Concentration:* 1–10 mg/mL. Mix by gentle inversion; do not shake. Solution is clear to slightly opalescent, colorless to slightly yellow; do not administer solution if discolored or contains particulate matter other than translucent to white proteinaceous particles. Solution is stable at room temperature for up to 4 hr and 24 hr if refrigerated. *Rate:* Infuse through a sterile, nonpyrogenic, low-protein binding 0.2–1.2 micrometer in-line filter over 60 min. Flush line at end of infusion.
- **Y-Site Incompatibility:** Do not administer other drugs through same infusion line.

Patient/Family Teaching
- Explain purpose of nivolumab to patient.
- Advise patient to notify health care professional immediately if signs and symptoms of pneumonitis, colitis, hepatitis (jaundice, severe nausea or vomiting, pain on right side of abdomen, lethargy, easy bruising or bleeding), kidney problems (decreased urine output, blood in urine, swollen ankles, loss of appetite), hormone gland problems (rapid heartbeat, weight loss, increased sweating, weight gain, hair loss, feeling cold, constipation, deepening of voice, muscle aches, dizziness or fainting, persistent or unusual headache) occur.
- Instruct patient to notify health care professional of all Rx or OTC medications, vitamins, or herbal products being taken and to consult with health care professional before taking other medications.
- Rep: May cause fetal harm. Advise females of reproductive potential to use highly effective contraception and avoid breastfeeding during and for 5 mo after last dose. Advise patient to notify healthcare professional immediately if pregnancy is planned or suspected.
- Emphasize importance of keeping scheduled appointments for blood work or other laboratory tests.

Evaluation/Desired Outcomes
- Decreased progression of melanoma, Hodgkin's lymphoma, urothelial carcinoma, colorectal cancer, and hepatocellular carcinoma.
- Decreased progression of and improved survival with NSCLC and advanced RCC.
- Improved survival in squamous cell carcinoma of head and neck, esophageal cancer, gastric cancer, gastroesophageal junction cancer, esophageal adenocarcinoma, and malignant pleural mesothelioma.

nizatidine, See HISTAMINE H₂ ANTAGONISTS.

`HIGH ALERT`

norepinephrine
(nor-ep-i-nef-rin)
Levophed
Classification
Therapeutic: vasopressors

Indications
Produces vasoconstriction and myocardial stimulation, which may be required after adequate fluid replacement in the treatment of severe hypotension and shock.

Action
Stimulates alpha-adrenergic receptors located mainly in blood vessels, causing constriction of both capacitance and resistance vessels. Also has minor beta-adrenergic activity (myocardial stimulation). **Therapeutic Effects:** Increased BP. Increased cardiac output.

Pharmacokinetics
Absorption: IV administration results in complete bioavailability.
Distribution: Concentrates in sympathetic nervous tissue. Does not cross the blood-brain barrier but readily crosses the placenta.
Metabolism and Excretion: Taken up and metabolized rapidly by sympathetic nerve endings.
Half-life: Unknown.

TIME/ACTION PROFILE (effects on BP)
ROUTE	ONSET	PEAK	DURATION
IV	immediate	rapid	1–2 min

Contraindications/Precautions
Contraindicated in: Vascular, mesenteric, or peripheral thrombosis; Hypoxia; Hypercarbia; Hypotension secondary to hypovolemia (without appropriate volume replacement); Hypersensitivity to bisulfites.
Use Cautiously in: Hypertension; Concurrent use of MAO inhibitors, tricyclic antidepressants, or cyclopropane or halothane anesthetics; Hyperthyroidism; Cardiovascular disease; OB: May ↓ uterine blood flow in pregnancy; Lactation: Safety not established in breastfeeding.

Adverse Reactions/Side Effects
CV: arrhythmia, bradycardia, chest pain, hypertension. **Endo:** hyperglycemia. **F and E:** metabolic acidosis. **GU:** ↓ urine output, renal failure. **Local:** phlebitis at IV site. **Neuro:** anxiety, dizziness, headache, insomnia, restlessness, tremor, weakness. **Resp:** dyspnea. **Misc:** fever.

Interactions

Drug-Drug: Use with **cyclopropane** or **halothane anesthesia**, **digoxin**, **doxapram**, or local use of **cocaine** may result in ↑ myocardial irritability. Use with **MAO inhibitors**, **doxapram**, or **tricyclic antidepressants** may result in severe hypertension. **Alphaadrenergic blockers** can prevent pressor response. **Beta blockers** may exaggerate hypertension or block cardiac stimulation. Concurrent use with **ergot alkaloids** (**ergotamine**, **methylergonovine**, or **oxytocin**) may result in enhanced vasoconstriction and hypertension.

Route/Dosage

IV (Adults): 0.5–1 mcg/min initially, followed by maintenance infusion of 2–12 mcg/min titrated by BP response (average rate 2–4 mcg/min, up to 30 mcg/min for refractory shock have been used).

IV (Children): 0.1 mcg/kg/min initially; may be followed by infusion titrated to BP response, up to 1 mcg/kg/min.

Availability (generic available)

Premixed infusion: 4 mg/250 mL D5W or 0.9% NaCl, 8 mg/250 mL D5W or 0.9% NaCl, 16 mg/250 mL 0.9% NaCl. **Solution for injection:** 1 mg/mL.

NURSING IMPLICATIONS

Assessment

- Monitor BP every 2–3 min until stabilized and every 5 min thereafter. Systolic BP is usually maintained at 80–100 mm Hg or 30–40 mm Hg below the previously existing systolic pressure in previously hypertensive patients. Consult health care professional for parameters. Continue to monitor BP frequently for hypotension following discontinuation of norepinephrine.
- ECG should be monitored continuously. CVP, intraarterial pressure, pulmonary artery diastolic pressure, pulmonary capillary wedge pressure (PCWP), and cardiac output may also be monitored.
- Monitor urine output and notify health care professional if it decreases to <30 mL/hr.
- Assess IV site frequently during infusion. A large vein should be used to minimize risk of extravasation, which may cause tissue necrosis. If prolonged therapy is required or if blanching along the course of the vein occurs, change injection sites to provide relief from vasoconstriction.

Toxicity and Overdose

- If overdose occurs, discontinue norepinephrine and administer fluid and electrolyte replacement therapy. An alpha-adrenergic blocking agent may be administered intravenously to treat hypertension.

Implementation

- *High Alert:* Vasoactive medications are inherently dangerous. Have second practitioner independently check original order, dose calculations, and infusion pump programming. Establish maximum dose

limits. Norepinephrine overdose can result in severe peripheral vasoconstriction with resultant ischemia and necrosis of peripheral tissue. Assess peripheral circulation frequently.

- Correct volume depletion, if possible, prior to initiation of norepinephrine.
- Norepinephrine may deplete plasma volume and cause ischemia of vital organs, resulting in hypotension when discontinued, if used for prolonged periods. Prolonged or large doses may also decrease cardiac output.
- Infusion should be discontinued gradually, upon adequate tissue perfusion and maintenance of BP, to prevent hypotension. Do not resume therapy unless BP falls to 70–80 mm Hg.

IV Administration

- **Continuous Infusion:** *Dilution:* Dilute 4 mg in 1000 mL of D5W or D5/0.9% NaCl. Do not dilute in 0.9% NaCl without dextrose. *Concentration:* 4 mcg/mL. Solution is colorless. Do not use discolored solutions (pink, yellow, brown) or those containing a precipitate. Solution is stable for 24 hr at room temperature. Protect from light. *Rate:* Titrate infusion rate according to patient response, using slowest possible rate to correct hypotension. Administer via infusion pump to ensure accurate dose. Typical maintenance IV dose is 2 to 4 mcg per min.
- **Y-Site Compatibility:** alemtuzumab, amikacin, anidulafungin, argatroban, arsenic trioxide, ascorbic acid, atracurium, atropine, aztreonam, benztropine, bivalirudin, bleomycin, bumetanide, buprenorphine, butorphanol, calcium chloride, calcium gluconate, cangrelor, carboplatin, carmustine, caspofungin, cefazolin, cefotaxime, cefotetan, cefoxitin, ceftaroline, ceftazidime, ceftazidime/avibactam, ceftolozane/tazobactam, ceftriaxone, cefuroxime, chloramphenicol, chlorpromazine, cisatracurium, cisplatin, clindamycin, cyanocobalamin, cyclophosphamide, cyclosporine, cytarabine, dactinomycin, daptomycin, daunorubicin hydrochloride, dexamethasone, dexmedetomidine, dexrazoxane, digoxin, diltiazem, diphenhydramine, dobutamine, docetaxel, dopamine, doxycycline, doxorubicin liposomal, enalaprilat, ephedrine, epinephrine, epirubicin, epoetin alfa, eravacycline, ertapenem, erythromycin, esmolol, etoposide, etoposide phosphate, famotidine, fentanyl, fluconazole, fludarabine, fosphenytoin, gemcitabine, gentamicin, glycopyrrolate, granisetron, heparin, hetastarch, hydrocortisone, hydromorphone, idarubicin, ifosfamide, imipenem/cilastatin/relebactam, imipenem/cilastatin, irinotecan, isavuconazonium, isoproterenol, ketorolac, labetalol, LR, leucovorin calcium, lidocaine, linezolid, lorazepam, magnesium sulfate, mannitol, meperidine, meropenem, meropenem/vaborbactam, mesna, methotrexate, methylprednisolone, metoclopramide, metoprolol, metronidazole, micafungin, midazolam, milrinone, mitoxantrone, morphine, moxifloxacin, multivitamins, mycophenolate, nafcillin, nalbuphine, nalox-

one, nicardipine, nitroglycerin, nitroprusside, octreotide, ondansetron, oritavancin, oxacillin, oxaliplatin, oxytocin, paclitaxel, palonosetron, pamidronate, papaverine, pemetrexed, penicillin G, pentamidine, phentolamine, phenylephrine, phytonadione, piperacillin/tazobactam, plazomicin, posaconazole, potassium acetate, potassium chloride, procainamide, prochlorperazine, promethazine, propofol, propranolol, protamine, pyridoxine, remifentanil, succinylcholine, sufentanil, tacrolimus, tedizolid, telavancin, theophylline, thiamine, thiotepa, tigecycline, tirofiban, tobramycin, topotecan, vancomycin, vasopressin, vecuronium, verapamil, vinblastine, vincristine, vinorelbine, voriconazole, zoledronic acid.

- **Y-Site Incompatibility:** aminophylline, amphotericin B deoxycholate, amphotericin B lipid complex, azathioprine, dacarbazine, dantrolene, diazepam, folic acid, foscarnet, ganciclovir, gemtuzumab ozogamicin, indomethacin, mitomycin, pentobarbital, phenobarbital, phenytoin, sodium bicarbonate, thiopental, trimethoprim/sulfamethoxazole.

Patient/Family Teaching
- Explain purpose of norepinephrine to patient.
- Instruct patient to report headache, dizziness, dyspnea, chest pain, or pain at infusion site promptly.
- Rep: Advise females of reproductive potential to notify health care professional if pregnancy is planned or suspected or if breastfeeding.

Evaluation/Desired Outcomes
- Increase in BP to normal range.
- Increased tissue perfusion.

norethindrone, See CONTRACEPTIVES, HORMONAL.

BEERS

☒ nortriptyline (nor-trip-ti-leen)
❋Aventyl, Pamelor
Classification
Therapeutic: antidepressants
Pharmacologic: tricyclic antidepressants

Indications
Major depressive disorder. **Unlabeled Use:** Chronic neuropathic pain.

Action
Potentiates the effect of serotonin and norepinephrine. Has significant anticholinergic properties. **Therapeutic Effects:** Antidepressant action that develops slowly over several wk.

Pharmacokinetics
Absorption: Well absorbed after oral administration.
Distribution: Widely distributed to tissues.
Protein Binding: 92%.
Metabolism and Excretion: Mostly metabolized by the liver by the CYP2D6 isoenzyme; ☒ the CYP2D6 enzyme system exhibits genetic polymorphism; ~7% of population may be poor metabolizers and may have significantly ↑ nortriptyline concentrations and an ↑ risk of adverse effects.
Half-life: 18–28 hr.

TIME/ACTION PROFILE (antidepressant effect)

ROUTE	ONSET	PEAK	DURATION
PO	2–3 wk	6 wk	unknown

Contraindications/Precautions
Contraindicated in: Hypersensitivity; Angle-closure glaucoma; Alcohol intolerance (solution only); Brugada syndrome; Concurrent use of MAO inhibitors or MAO-like drugs (linezolid or methylene blue); Lactation: Lactation.
Use Cautiously in: Pre-existing cardiovascular disease; History of seizures; Asthma; May ↑ risk of suicide attempt/ideation especially during early treatment or dose adjustment; OB: Use during pregnancy only if potential maternal benefit justifies potential fetal risk; Pedi: Suicide risk may be greater in children or adolescents. Safety and effectiveness not established in children; Geri: Appears on Beers list. ↑ risk of adverse reactions in older adults, including falls secondary to sedative and anticholinergic effects and orthostatic hypotension. Avoid use in older adults.

Adverse Reactions/Side Effects
CV: hypotension, ARRHYTHMIAS, ECG changes. **Derm:** photosensitivity. **EENT:** blurred vision, dry eyes. **Endo:** gynecomastia. **GI:** constipation, dry mouth, nausea, paralytic ileus, unpleasant taste. **GU:** urinary retention. **Hemat:** blood dyscrasias. **Metab:** weight gain. **Neuro:** drowsiness, fatigue, lethargy, agitation, confusion, extrapyramidal reactions, hallucinations, headache, insomnia, SUICIDAL THOUGHTS.

Interactions
Drug-Drug: Concurrent use with **MAO inhibitors** may result in serious potentially fatal reactions (MAO inhibitors should be stopped at least 14 days before nortriptyline therapy. Nortriptyline should be stopped at least 14 days before MAO inhibitor therapy). Concurrent use with **MAO-inhibitor like drugs**, such as linezolid or methylene blue, may ↑ risk of serotonin syndrome; concurrent use contraindicated; do not start therapy in patients receiving linezolid or methylene blue; if linezolid or methylene blue need to be started in a patient receiving nortriptyline, immediately

discontinue nortriptyline and monitor for signs/symptoms of serotonin syndrome for 2 wk or until 24 hr after last dose of linezolid or methylene blue, whichever comes first (may resume nortriptyline therapy 24 hr after last dose of linezolid or methylene blue). **May prevent the therapeutic response to most antihypertensives.** Hypertensive crisis may occur with **clonidine.** ↑ CNS depression with other **CNS depressants,** including **alcohol, antihistamines, opioids,** and **sedative/hypnotics.** Adrenergic effects may be ↑ with other **adrenergic agents,** including **vasoconstrictors** and **decongestants.** ↑ anticholinergic effects with other **drugs possessing anticholinergic properties,** including **antihistamines, antidepressants, atropine, haloperidol, phenothiazines, quinidine,** and **disopyramide. Cimetidine, fluoxetine,** or **hormonal contraceptives** ↑ blood levels and risk of toxicity. ↑ risk of agranulocytosis with **antithyroid agents.** Drugs that affect serotonergic neurotransmitter systems, including **SSRIs, SNRIs, fentanyl, buspirone, tramadol,** and **triptans,** ↑ risk of serotonin syndrome.

Drug-Natural Products: Concomitant use of **kava-kava, valerian,** or **chamomile** can ↑ CNS depression. Use with **St. John's wort** ↑ serotonin syndrome. ↑ anticholinergic effects with **jimson weed** and **scopolia.**

Route/Dosage
PO (Adults): 25 mg 3–4 times daily, up to 150 mg/day.
PO (Geriatric Patients or Adolescents): 30–50 mg/day in divided doses or as a single dose.

Availability (generic available)
Capsules: 10 mg, 25 mg, 50 mg, 75 mg. **Oral solution:** 10 mg/5 mL.

NURSING IMPLICATIONS
Assessment
- Monitor mental status (orientation, mood, behavior).
- Assess weight and BMI initially and throughout treatment. For overweight/obese individuals, monitor fasting blood glucose and cholesterol levels.
- Monitor BP and pulse rate before and during initial therapy. Report significant decreases in BP or a sudden increase in pulse rate.
- Monitor baseline and periodic ECGs in geriatric patients or patients with heart disease. May cause prolonged PR and QT intervals and may flatten T waves.
- Assess for suicidal tendencies, especially during early therapy. Restrict amount of drug available to patient. Risk may be increased in children, adolescents, and adults ≤24 yrs. After starting therapy, children, adolescents, and young adults should be seen by health care professional face-to-face at least weekly for 4 wk, then every other wk for next 4 wk, then at 12 wk, and then on advice of health care professional thereafter.
- **Pain:** Assess type, location, and severity of pain before and periodically during therapy. Use pain scale to monitor effectiveness of medication.

Lab Test Considerations
- Assess leukocyte and differential blood counts, liver function, and serum glucose periodically. May cause ↑ serum bilirubin and alkaline phosphatase. May cause bone marrow depression. Serum glucose may be ↑ or ↓.
- Serum levels may be monitored in patients who fail to respond to usual therapeutic dose. Therapeutic plasma concentration range is 50–150 ng/mL.
- May cause alterations in blood glucose levels.

Toxicity and Overdose
- Symptoms of acute overdose include disturbed concentration, confusion, restlessness, agitation, seizures, drowsiness, mydriasis, arrhythmias, fever, hallucinations, vomiting, and dyspnea.
- Treatment of overdose includes gastric lavage, activated charcoal, and a stimulant cathartic. Maintain respiratory and cardiac function (monitor ECG for at least 5 days) and temperature. Medications may include digoxin for HF, antiarrhythmics, and anticonvulsants.

Implementation
- Taper to avoid withdrawal effects. Reduce dose 50% for 3 days, then by 50% for 3 more days, then discontinue.
- **PO:** Administer medication with meals to minimize gastric irritation.
- May be given as a single dose at bedtime to minimize sedation during the day. Dose increases should be made at bedtime because of sedation.

Patient/Family Teaching
- Instruct patient to take medication as directed. Take missed doses as soon as possible unless almost time for next dose; if regimen is a single dose at bedtime, do not take in the morning because of side effects. Advise patient that drug effects may not be noticed for at least 2 wk. Abrupt discontinuation may cause nausea, vomiting, diarrhea, headache, trouble sleeping with vivid dreams, and irritability.
- May cause drowsiness and blurred vision. Caution patient to avoid driving and other activities requiring alertness until response to drug is known.
- Instruct patient to notify health care professional if visual changes occur. Inform patient that periodic glaucoma testing may be required during long-term therapy.
- Caution patient to make position changes slowly to minimize orthostatic hypotension. (This side effect is less pronounced with this medication than with other tricyclic antidepressants.).
- Advise patient, family, and caregivers to look for suicidality, especially during early therapy or dose changes. Notify health care professional immediately if thoughts about suicide or dying, attempts to commit suicide, new or worse depression or anxiety, agitation or restlessness, panic attacks, insomnia, new or worse irritability, aggressiveness, acting on dangerous impulses, mania, or other changes in mood

or behavior or if symptoms of serotonin syndrome occur.

- Advise patient to avoid alcohol or other CNS depressant drugs, including opioids, during therapy and for at least 3–7 days after therapy has been discontinued.
- Instruct patient to notify health care professional if urinary retention occurs or if dry mouth or constipation persists. Sugarless candy or gum may diminish dry mouth, and an increase in fluid intake or bulk may prevent constipation. If symptoms persist, dose reduction or discontinuation may be necessary. Consult health care professional if dry mouth persists for more than 2 wk.
- Caution patient to use sunscreen and protective clothing to prevent photosensitivity reactions.
- Alert patient that urine may turn blue-green in color.
- Inform patient of need to monitor dietary intake. Increase in appetite may lead to undesired weight gain. Refer as appropriate for nutritional, weight, or medical management.
- Advise patient to notify health care professional of medication regimen before treatment or surgery.
- Rep: May cause fetal harm. Advise females of reproductive potential to use effective contraception during and for at least 5 mo after last dose and to avoid breastfeeding during therapy. Advise patient to notify health care professional immediately if pregnancy is planned or suspected.
- Therapy for depression is usually prolonged. Emphasize the importance of follow-up exams.

Evaluation/Desired Outcomes

- Increased sense of well-being.
- Renewed interest in surroundings.
- Increased appetite.
- Improved energy level.
- Improved sleep.
- Decrease in severity of chronic neurogenic pain.
- May require 2–6 wk of therapy before full therapeutic effects of medication are seen.

nystatin, See ANTIFUNGALS (TOPICAL).

nystatin (oral) (nye-stat-in)
~~Mycostatin~~
Classification
Therapeutic: antifungals

For other nystatin dosage forms, see antifungals (topical) and antifungals (vaginal)

Indications
Oral suspension: Local treatment of oropharyngeal candidiasis. **Oral tablet:** Treatment of nonesophageal mucus membrane gastrointestinal candidiasis.

Action
Binds to fungal cell membrane, allowing leakage of cellular contents. **Therapeutic Effects:** Fungistatic or fungicidal action. **Spectrum:** Active against most pathogenic *Candida* species, including *C. albicans*.

Pharmacokinetics
Absorption: Poorly absorbed; action is primarily local.
Distribution: Unknown.
Metabolism and Excretion: Excreted unchanged in the feces after oral administration.
Half-life: Unknown.

TIME/ACTION PROFILE (antifungal effects)

ROUTE	ONSET	PEAK	DURATION
PO	24–72 hr	unknown	unknown

Contraindications/Precautions
Contraindicated in: Hypersensitivity; Some products may contain ethyl alcohol or benzyl alcohol—avoid use in patients who may be hypersensitive to or intolerant of these additives.
Use Cautiously in: Denture wearers (dentures require soaking in nystatin suspension).

Adverse Reactions/Side Effects
Derm: contact dermatitis, STEVENS-JOHNSON SYNDROME.
GI: diarrhea, nausea, stomach pain (large doses), vomiting.

Interactions
Drug-Drug: None significant.

Route/Dosage
Oropharyngeal Candidiasis
PO (Adults and Children): 400,000–600,000 units 4 times daily as oral suspension.
PO (Infants): 200,000 units 4 times daily or 100,000 units to each side of the mouth 4 times daily.
PO (Neonates, Premature, and Low Birth Weight): 100,000 units 4 times daily or 50,000 units to each side of the mouth 4 times a day.

Gastrointestinal Candidiasis
PO (Adults): 500,000–1,000,000 units 3 times daily. Continue for ≥48 hr after clinical cure to prevent relapse.

Availability (generic available)
Oral suspension: 100,000 units/mL. **Oral tablets:** 500,000 units.

NURSING IMPLICATIONS

Assessment

- Inspect oral mucous membranes before and frequently during therapy. Increased irritation of mucous membranes may indicate need to discontinue medication.

Implementation

- Do not confuse nystatin with HMG-CoA reductase inhibitors ("statins").
- **PO:** Administer suspension by placing ½ of dose in each side of mouth. Patient should hold suspension in mouth or swish throughout mouth for several min before swallowing, then gargle and swallow. Use calibrated measuring device for liquid doses. Shake well before administration. Pedi: For neonates and infants, paint suspension into recesses of the mouth. Avoid feedings for 5–10 min following administration or administer after meals.

Patient/Family Teaching

- Instruct patient to take medication as directed. If a dose is missed, take as soon as remembered but not if almost time for next dose. Do not double doses. Therapy should be continued for at least 2 days after symptoms subside.
- Pedi: Instruct parents or caregivers of infants and children on correct dose and administration. Remind them to use only the measuring device dispensed with the product.
- Advise patient to report increased irritation of mucous membranes or lack of therapeutic response to health care professional.
- Rep: Advise females of reproductive potential to notify health care professional if pregnancy is planned or suspected or if breastfeeding.

Evaluation/Desired Outcomes

- Decrease in stomatitis.
- Treatment of intestinal candidiasis.

ocrelizumab (ok-re-liz-ue-mab)
Ocrevus

Classification
Therapeutic: anti-multiple sclerosis agents
Pharmacologic: monoclonal antibodies

Indications
Relapsing forms of multiple sclerosis (MS), including clinically isolated syndrome, relapsing-remitting disease, and active secondary progressive disease. Primary progressive MS.

Action
Binds to the CD20 antigen on pre-B and mature B lymphocytes, which results in antibody-dependent and complement-mediated cell lysis. **Therapeutic Effects:** Reduction in relapse rate and decreased progression toward disability.

Pharmacokinetics
Absorption: IV administration results in complete bioavailability.
Distribution: Binds specifically to CD20 binding sites on B lymphocytes.
Metabolism and Excretion: Unknown.
Half-life: 26 days.

TIME/ACTION PROFILE

ROUTE	ONSET	PEAK	DURATION
IV	unknown	unknown	unknown

Contraindications/Precautions
Contraindicated in: Active hepatitis B virus (HBV) infection (may reactivate infection during and for several mo after treatment); History of life-threatening infusion reaction to ocrelizumab.
Use Cautiously in: Patients who are immunocompromised or receiving other immunosuppressants; OB: Safety not established in pregnancy (may cause fetal B-cell depletion); Lactation: Safety not established in breastfeeding; Rep: Women of reproductive potential; Pedi: Safety and effectiveness not established in children.

Adverse Reactions/Side Effects
CV: peripheral edema. GI: diarrhea, HEPATITIS B VIRUS REACTIVATION, IMMUNE-MEDIATED COLITIS. **Hemat:** neutropenia. MS: back pain. **Neuro:** depression, PROGRESSIVE MULTIFOCAL LEUKOENCEPHALOPATHY (PML). **Resp:** cough. **Misc:** INFECTION, INFUSION REACTIONS (including anaphylaxis), MALIGNANCY (primarily breast cancer).

Interactions
Drug-Drug: Concurrent use with **immunosuppressive therapies** may ↑ risk of immunosuppression. May ↓ antibody response to or ↑ risk of adverse reactions to **non-live vaccines** and **live vaccines**.

Route/Dosage
IV (Adults): 300 mg initially, then 300 mg in 2 wk, then 600 mg every 6 mo.

Availability
Solution for injection: 30 mg/mL.

NURSING IMPLICATIONS

Assessment
- Assess for active infection prior to each infusion. Delay infusion until infection resolves.
- Monitor for signs and symptoms of infusion reaction (pruritus, rash, urticaria, erythema, bronchospasm, throat irritation, oropharyngeal pain, dyspnea, pharyngeal or laryngeal edema, flushing, hypotension, pyrexia, fatigue, headache, dizziness, nausea, tachycardia) during and for at least 1 hr after completion of infusion. *If mild to moderate infusion reaction occurs,* reduce infusion rate by half at onset of reaction and for at least 30 min. If rate tolerated, increase rate (see Rate below). Will increase duration of infusion, but not total dose. *If severe reaction occurs,* immediately stop infusion and administer supportive treatment. Restart infusion only after all symptoms resolved. Restart at half rate at time of onset of reaction. If tolerated, increase (see Rate below). Will increase duration of infusion, but not total dose. *If life-threatening infusion reaction occurs,* immediately stop infusion and permanently discontinue ocrelizumab. Provide supportive treatment.
- Assess for signs and symptoms of PML (progressive weakness on one side of body or clumsiness of limbs, disturbance of vision, and changes in thinking, memory, and orientation leading to confusion and personality changes) periodically during therapy. Symptoms are diverse and progress over days to wks. At first sign of PML, suspend ocrelizumab and perform diagnostic evaluation. MRI findings may be apparent before clinical signs or symptoms. If PML is confirmed, discontinue ocrelizumab.
- Monitor for signs and symptoms of immune-mediated colitis (diarrhea, abdominal pain, blood in stool) during therapy. May require systemic corticosteroids and hospitalization.

Lab Test Considerations
- Determine current or prior HBV infection by measuring hepatitis B surface antigen (HBsAg) and hepatitis B core antibody (anti-HBc) before starting therapy. Do not administer to patients with active HBV infection.
- Perform testing for quantitative serum immunoglobulins before starting therapy. May require immunology consult if serum immunoglobulins are low.

Implementation
- Administer all necessary immunizations at least 6 wk before starting therapy. Avoid immunizations during

therapy and after discontinuation until B-cell reple-
tion.
- Premedicate to reduce frequency and severity of infusion reactions with methylprednisolone 100 mg IV
or equivalent 30 min and an antihistamine, diphenhydramine, 30–60 min before each infusion. May
add an antipyretic, acetaminophen.
- **Intermittent Infusion: *Dilution:*** Dilute each
dose with 250 mL or 500 mL 0.9% NaCl. Do not use
other diluents. Do not shake. Allow infusion bag to
come to room temperature before infusion. *Concentration:* 1.2 mg/mL. Solution is clear or slightly
opalescent, and colorless to pale brown; do not administer solutions that are discolored or contain
particulate matter. Solution is stable for 24 hr if refrigerated or up to 8 hr (including infusion time) at
room temperature. *Rate:* Administer using a dedicated line with a 0.2 or 0.22 micron in-line filter.
For first 2 infusions (300 mg in 250 mL), begin at
30 mL/hr. Increase by 30 mL/hr every 30 min to 180
mL/hr over 2.5 hr or longer. *For subsequent infusions (600 mg in 500 mL),* begin at 40 mL/hr. Increase by 40 mL/hr every 30 min to 200 mL/hr over
3.5 hr or longer OR start at 100 mL/hr for first 15
min. Increase to 200 mL/hr for next 15 min. Increase to 250 mL/hr for next 30 min. Increase to
300 mL/hr for last 60 min. Duration 2 hr or longer.

Patient/Family Teaching

- Explain purpose of infusions and importance of
maintaining schedule to patient. If infusion is
missed, administer as soon as possible; do not wait
for next scheduled dose. Reset schedule for 6 mo after missed dose is given. Separate doses by at least 5
mo. Advise patient to read *Medication Guide* before
starting therapy and with each dose in case of
changes.
- Inform patient that infusion reactions may occur up
to 24 hr after infusion. Advise patient to notify health
care professional immediately if infusion reaction
symptoms occur.
- Advise patient to notify health care professional if
signs and symptoms of infection (fever, chills, constant cough, cold sore, shingles, genital sores), immune-mediated colitis (new or persistent diarrhea,
abdominal pain, blood in stool) or PML (problems
with thinking, balance, eyesight, weakness on 1 side
of body, strength, using arms or legs) occur.
- Instruct patient to notify health care professional of
all Rx or OTC medications, vitamins, or herbal products being taken and to consult health care professional before taking other Rx, OTC, or herbal products.
- Instruct patient to avoid live vaccines during therapy.
Administer any live or live-attenuated vaccines ≥4
wk prior to start of therapy and administer any non-
live vaccines ≥2 wk prior to start of therapy.
- Inform patient of increased risk of malignancy. Advise patient to receive regular breast cancer screening.

- Rep: May cause fetal harm. Advise females of reproductive potential to use effective contraception during and for 6 mo after last infusion and to notify
health care professional if breastfeeding. Do not administer live or live-attenuated vaccines to infants
born to mothers taking ocrelizumab until recovery
of B-cell counts is confirmed; may administer non-
live vaccines to these infants, but should consider assessing vaccine immune responses to determine
whether protective immune response developed. Inform patient of pregnancy exposure registry that
monitors pregnancy and fetal/neonatal/infant outcomes in women exposed to ocrelizumab during
pregnancy. Encourage patient to register themselves
by calling 1-833-872-4370 or visiting
www.ocrevuspregnancyregistry.com.

Evaluation/Desired Outcomes

- Reduction in relapse rate and decreased progression toward disability in patients with MS.

---

octreotide (ok-**tree**-oh-tide)
Mycapssa, SandoSTATIN,
✦ SandoSTATIN LAR, SandoSTATIN
LAR Depot
Classification
Therapeutic: antidiarrheals, hormones

Indications

IV, IM, SUBQ: Treatment of the following: Symptoms
(flushing and diarrhea) associated with metastatic carcinoid tumors; Profuse, watery diarrhea associated with
vasoactive intestinal peptide tumors (VIPomas); Acromegaly in patients who have had inadequate response
to or cannot be treated with surgical resection, pituitary
irradiation, and bromocriptine at maximally tolerated
doses. **PO:** Long-term maintenance treatment of acromegaly in patients who have responded to and tolerated
treatment with octreotide or lanreotide. **Unlabeled
Use:** Management of diarrhea associated with chemotherapy or graft-versus-host disease. Gastroesophageal
variceal hemorrhage.

Action

Suppresses secretion of serotonin and gastroenterohe-
patic peptides. Increases absorption of fluid and electrolytes from the GI tract and increases transit time. Decreases levels of serotonin metabolites. Also suppresses
growth hormone, insulin, and glucagon. **Therapeutic
Effects:** Normalization of growth hormone and insulin-
like growth factor–1 (IGF-1) levels and maintenance of
these levels. Control of severe flushing and diarrhea associated with metastatic carcinoid tumors and VIPomas.

Pharmacokinetics

Absorption: IV administration results in complete
bioavailability. Well absorbed following SUBQ administration and IM administration of depot form. Food reduces rate and extent of oral absorption.

Distribution: Some distribution to extravascular tissues.

Metabolism and Excretion: Extensive hepatic metabolism; 32% excreted unchanged in urine.

Half-life: 1.5 hr.

TIME/ACTION PROFILE (control of symptoms)

ROUTE	ONSET	PEAK	DURATION
SUBQ, IV	unknown	unknown	up to 12 hr
IM (LAR depot)	unknown	2 wk	up to 4 wk
PO	unknown	unknown	unknown

Contraindications/Precautions

Contraindicated in: Hypersensitivity.

Use Cautiously in: Gallbladder disease (↑ risk of stone formation); Renal impairment (dose ↓ may be necessary); Hyperglycemia or hypoglycemia (changes in blood glucose may occur); Fat malabsorption (may be aggravated); OB: Safety not established in pregnancy; Lactation: Safety not established in breastfeeding; Rep: Premenopausal women (may ↑ fertility and ↑ risk of pregnancy); Pedi: Safety and effectiveness of depot injection and oral formulation not established in children.

Adverse Reactions/Side Effects

CV: edema, QT interval prolongation, atrioventricular block, bradycardia, hypertension, orthostatic hypotension, palpitations. **Derm:** ↑ sweating, flushing. **EENT:** sinusitis, visual disturbances. **Endo:** hyperglycemia, hypoglycemia, hypothyroidism. **GI:** abdominal pain, cholelithiasis, diarrhea, nausea, vomiting, cholecystitis, fat malabsorption, flatulence, ILEUS, PANCREATITIS. **GU:** urinary tract infection. **Local:** injection-site pain. **MS:** arthralgia. **Neuro:** headache, dizziness, drowsiness, fatigue, weakness.. **Misc.:** ↓ vitamin B$_{12}$ levels.

Interactions

Drug-Drug: May alter requirements for **insulin** or **oral hypoglycemic agents.** May ↓ levels of **cyclosporine** and **digoxin**; closely monitor levels and adjust dose of cyclosporine and digoxin as needed. **Beta blockers, digoxin, diltiazem, ivabradine,** and **verapamil** may ↑ risk of bradycardia. **Proton pump inhibitors, H$_2$ receptor antagonists,** and **antacids** may ↓ absorption and levels of orally administered octreotide; may need to ↑ dosage of oral octreotide. May ↑ levels of **lisinopril**; closely monitor BP. May ↓ levels of **levonorgestrel**; advise patient to use nonhormonal contraceptive or a backup method while receiving octreotide. May ↑ levels of **bromocriptine**; may need to ↓ dose of bromocriptine. May ↓ effectiveness of **lutetium Lu 177 dotatate**; discontinue long-acting octreotide ≥4 wk and short-acting octreotide ≥24 hr prior to each dose of lutetium Lu 177 dotatate.

Route/Dosage

Carcinoid Tumors

SUBQ, IV (Adults): 100–600 mcg/day in 2–4 divided doses during first 2 wk of therapy (range 50–1500 mcg/day).

IM (Adults): *Sandostatin LAR:* 20 mg every 4 wk for 2 mo; dose may be further adjusted.

VIPomas

SUBQ, IV (Adults): 200–300 mcg/day in 2–4 divided doses during first 2 wk of therapy (range 150–750 mcg/day).

IM (Adults): *Sandostatin LAR:* 20 mg every 2 wk for 2 mo; dose may be further adjusted.

Acromegaly

SUBQ, IV (Adults): 50–100 mcg 3 times daily; titrate to achieve growth hormone levels <5 ng/mL or IGF-1 levels <1.9 units/mL (males) or <2.2 units/mL (females) (usual effective dose = 100–200 mcg 3 times daily).

IM (Adults): *Sandostatin LAR:* 20 mg every 4 wk for 3 mo, then adjusted on the basis of growth hormone levels.

PO (Adults): 20 mg twice daily initially; titrate based on IGF-1 levels obtained every 2 wk by 20 mg/day. If maintenance dose = 60 mg/day, administer as 40 mg in AM and 20 mg in PM; if maintenance dose = 80 mg/day, administer as 40 mg twice daily (not to exceed 80 mg/day).

Renal Impairment

PO (Adults): *End-stage renal disease:* 20 mg once daily initially; titrate based on IGF-1 levels obtained every 2 wk by 20 mg/day. If maintenance dose = 40 mg/day, administer as 20 mg twice daily; if maintenance dose = 60 mg/day, administer as 40 mg in AM and 20 mg in PM; if maintenance dose = 80 mg/day, administer as 40 mg twice daily (not to exceed 80 mg/day).

Diarrhea Associated With Chemotherapy (off-label)

SUBQ, IV (Adults): 100–150 mcg SUBQ every 8 hr; may ↑ to 500–1500 mcg SUBQ or IV every 8 hr for severe diarrhea.

SUBQ (Children): 1–10 mcg/kg every 8–12 hr.

Diarrhea Associated With Graft-Versus-Host Disease (off-label)

IV (Adults): 500 mcg every 8 hr; do not continue for longer than 7 days (discontinue within 24 hr of diarrhea resolution).

SUBQ (Children): 1–10 mcg/kg every 8–12 hr.

Gastroesophageal Variceal Hemorrhage (off-label)

IV (Adults): 25–100 mcg bolus (may repeat in 1st hr if hemorrhage uncontrolled), followed by continuous infusion of 25–50 mcg/hr for 2–5 days.

✦= Canadian drug name. ░ = Genetic implication. S̶t̶r̶i̶k̶e̶t̶h̶r̶o̶u̶g̶h̶ = Discontinued. CAPITALS = life-threatening. Underline = most frequent.

IV (Children): 1–2 mcg/kg bolus, followed by continuous infusion of 1–2 mcg/kg/hr; taper dose by 50% every 12 hr when no active bleeding for 24 hr; discontinue when dose is 25% of initial dose.

Availability (generic available)

Delayed release capsules: 20 mg. **Solution for injection:** 50 mcg/mL, 100 mcg/mL, 200 mcg/mL, 500 mcg/mL, 1000 mcg/mL. **Suspension for injection (depot):** 10 mg/6 mL, 20 mg/6 mL, 30 mg/6 mL.

NURSING IMPLICATIONS

Assessment

● Assess frequency and consistency of stools and bowel sounds during therapy.
● Monitor pulse and BP prior to and periodically during therapy.
● Assess patient's fluid and electrolyte balance and skin turgor for dehydration.
● Monitor diabetic patients for signs of hypoglycemia. May require reduction in requirements for insulin and sulfonylureas and treatment with diazoxide.
● Assess for gallbladder disease; assess for pain and monitor ultrasound examinations of gallbladder and bile ducts prior to and periodically during prolonged therapy.

Lab Test Considerations
● Monitor growth hormone, IGF-1 in patients with acromegaly, 5-HIAA (urinary 5-hydroxyindoleacetic acid), plasma serotonin, and plasma substance P in patients with carcinoid tumors; plasma VIP in patients with VIPoma; and free T_4 and serum glucose concentrations prior to and periodically during therapy in all patients taking octreotide.
● Monitor quantitative 72-hr fecal fat and serum carotene determinations periodically for possible drug-induced aggravations of fat malabsorption.
● May cause a slight ↑ in liver enzymes.
● Monitor glycemic control for all patients with diabetes and adjust antidiabetic treatment as necessary for hyperglycemia and hypoglycemia.

Implementation

● Do not confuse Sandostatin with Sandimmune.
● **PO:** Administer with water on an empty stomach, at least 1 hr before a meal or at least 2 hr after a meal. *DNC:* Swallow capsules whole; do not open, crush or chew.
● Solution is clear and colorless; do not use solution that is cloudy, discolored, or contains particulate matter. Ampules should be refrigerated but may be stored at room temperature for the days they will be used. Discard unused solution.
● **SUBQ:** Administer the smallest volume needed to achieve required dose to prevent pain at injection site. Rotate injection sites; avoid multiple injections in same site within short periods of time. Preferred injection sites are the hip, thigh, or abdomen.
● Administer injections between meals and at bedtime to avoid GI side effects.

● Allow medication to reach room temperature prior to injection to minimize local reactions at injection site. Rotate injection sites at least 2 in. away from last injection site.
● **IM:** Should be administered by a health care professional. Mix IM solution by adding diluent included in kit. Administer immediately after mixing into the gluteal muscle. Avoid using deltoid site due to pain of injection.
● Patients with carcinoid tumors and VIPomas should continue to receive SUBQ dose for 2 wk following switch to IM depot form to maintain therapeutic level.

IV Administration
● **IV Push:** *Dilution:* May be administered undiluted. *Rate:* Administer over 3 min.
● **Intermittent Infusion:** *Dilution:* Dilute in 50–200 mL of 0.9% NaCl or D5W. *Concentration:* 1.5–250 mcg/mL. Store ampules in refrigerator and keep in outer carton to protect from light. *Rate:* Infuse over 15–30 min.
● **Y-Site Compatibility:** acyclovir, allopurinol, amifostine, amikacin, aminocaproic acid, aminophylline, amiodarone, amphotericin B lipid complex, amphotericin B liposomal, ampicillin, ampicillin/sulbactam, anidulafungin, argatroban, arsenic trioxide, atracurium, azithromycin, aztreonam, bivalirudin, bleomycin, bumetanide, buprenorphine, busulfan, butorphanol, calcium chloride, calcium gluconate, carboplatin, carmustine, caspofungin, cefazolin, cefepime, cefotaxime, cefotetan, cefoxitin, ceftazidime, ceftolozane/tazobactam, ceftriaxone, cefuroxime, chloramphenicol, chlorpromazine, ciprofloxacin, cisatracurium, cisplatin, clindamycin, cyclophosphamide, cyclosporine, cytarabine, dacarbazine, dactinomycin, daptomycin, daunorubicin hydrochloride, dexamethasone, dexmedetomidine, dexrazoxane, digoxin, diltiazem, diphenhydramine, dobutamine, docetaxel, dopamine, doxorubicin hydrochloride, doxorubicin liposomal, doxycycline, droperidol, enalaprilat, ephedrine, epinephrine, epirubicin, eptifibatide, eravacycline, ertapenem, erythromycin, esmolol, etoposide, etoposide phosphate, famotidine, fentanyl, fluconazole, fludarabine, fluorouracil, foscarnet, fosphenytoin, furosemide, ganciclovir, gemcitabine, gentamicin, glycopyrrolate, granisetron, haloperidol, heparin, hydralazine, hydrocortisone, hydromorphone, idarubicin, ifosfamide, imipenem/cilastatin, insulin regular, irinotecan, isavuconazonium, isoproterenol, ketorolac, labetalol, LR, leucovorin calcium, levofloxacin, lidocaine, linezolid, lorazepam, magnesium hydroxide, mannitol, melphalan, meperidine, meropenem, meropenem/vaborbactam, mesna, methadone, methohexital, methotrexate, methylprednisolone, metoclopramide, metoprolol, metronidazole, midazolam, milrinone, mitomycin, mitoxantrone, morphine, moxifloxacin, mycophenolate, nafcillin, nalbuphine, naloxone, nicardipine, nitroglycerin,

nitroprusside, norepinephrine, ondansetron, oxaliplatin, paclitaxel, palonosetron, pamidronate, pemetrexed, pentamidine, pentobarbital, phenobarbital, phentolamine, phenylephrine, piperacillin/tazobactam, plazomicin, potassium acetate, potassium chloride, potassium phosphates, procainamide, prochlorperazine, promethazine, propranolol, remifentanil, rocuronium, sodium acetate, sodium bicarbonate, sodium phosphates, succinylcholine, sufentanil, tacrolimus, thiopental, thiotepa, tigecycline, tirofiban, tobramycin, topotecan, trimethoprim/sulfamethoxazole, vancomycin, vasopressin, vecuronium, verapamil, vinblastine, vincristine, vinorelbine, voriconazole, zidovudine, zoledronic acid.

- **Y-Site Incompatibility:** dantrolene, diazepam, micafungin, phenytoin, total parenteral nutrition (TPN) solutions.

Patient/Family Teaching

- Explain purpose of octreotide to patient. Instruct patient to take octreotide as directed. Advise patient taking PO form to read *Patient Information* before starting therapy and with each Rx refill in case of changes.
- May cause dizziness, drowsiness, or visual disturbances. Caution patient to avoid driving or other activities requiring alertness until response to medication is known.
- Advise patient to change positions slowly to minimize orthostatic hypotension.
- Advise patient to notify health care professional if signs and symptoms of gallstones, hyperglycemia, hypoglycemia, thyroid function abnormalities, or irregular heartbeat occur.
- Rep: Inform females of reproductive potential that therapy with octreotide may result in improved fertility. Caution patient to use nonhormonal contraception to prevent unintended pregnancy. Advise patient to notify health care professional if pregnancy is planned or suspected or if breastfeeding.
- Home Care Issues: Instruct patient administering octreotide at home on correct technique for injection, storage, and disposal of equipment. Advise patient to read *Instructions for Use* before starting therapy and with each Rx refill in case of changes.
- Instruct patient to administer octreotide exactly as directed. If a dose is missed, administer as soon as possible, then return to regular schedule. Do not double doses.

Evaluation/Desired Outcomes

- Decrease in severity of diarrhea and improvement of electrolyte imbalances in patients with carcinoid or VIP-secreting tumors.
- Relief of symptoms and suppressed tumor growth in patients with pituitary tumors associated with acromegaly.

- Growth hormone levels <5 ng/mL or IGF-1 levels within normal reference ranges for age and sex in patients treated for acromegaly.

ofloxacin, See FLUOROQUINOLONES.

BEERS REMS

OLANZapine (oh-**lan**-za-peen)
ZyPREXA, ZyPREXA Relprevv, ZyPREXA Zydis
Classification
Therapeutic: antipsychotics, mood stabilizers
Pharmacologic: thienobenzodiazepines

Indications
PO, IM: Schizophrenia. **PO:** Management of the following: Acute therapy of manic or mixed episodes associated with bipolar I disorder (as monotherapy [adults and adolescents] or in combination with lithium or evaporate [adults only]); Maintenance therapy of bipolar I disorder; Depressive episodes associated with bipolar I disorder (in combination with fluoxetine); Treatment-resistant depression (in combination with fluoxetine). **IM:** Acute agitation due to schizophrenia or bipolar I mania. **Unlabeled Use:** Anorexia nervosa. Treatment of nausea and vomiting related to highly emetogenic chemotherapy.

Action
Antagonizes dopamine and serotonin type 2 in the CNS. Also has anticholinergic, antihistaminic, and anti–alpha₁-adrenergic effects. **Therapeutic Effects:** Decreased manifestations of psychoses.

Pharmacokinetics
Absorption: Well absorbed but rapidly metabolized by first-pass effect, resulting in 60% bioavailability. Conventional tablets and orally disintegrating tablets (Zydis) are bioequivalent. IM administration results in significantly higher blood levels (5 times that of oral).
Distribution: Extensively distributed.
Protein Binding: 93%.
Metabolism and Excretion: Primarily metabolized by the liver by the CYP1A2 isoenzyme; 7% excreted unchanged in urine.
Half-life: 21–54 hr.

TIME/ACTION PROFILE (antipsychotic effects)

ROUTE	ONSET	PEAK*	DURATION
PO	unknown	6 hr	unknown
IM	rapid	15–45 min	2–4 hr

*Blood levels.

Contraindications/Precautions

Contraindicated in: Hypersensitivity; Phenylketonuria (orally disintegrating tablets contain aspartame). **Use Cautiously in:** Hepatic impairment; Patients at risk for aspiration or falls; Cardiovascular or cerebrovascular disease; History of seizures; History of attempted suicide; Diabetes or risk factors for diabetes (may worsen glucose control); Presence/history of constipation, urinary retention, prostatic hypertrophy, or paralytic ileus; Low WBC or ANC or history of drug-induced neutropenia/leukopenia; Angle-closure glaucoma; OB: Use during pregnancy only if potential maternal benefit justifies potential fetal risk; neonates at ↑ risk for extrapyramidal symptoms and withdrawal after delivery when exposed during the 3rd trimester; Lactation: Use while breastfeeding only if potential maternal benefit justifies potential fetal risk; Pedi: Children <13 yr (safety and effectiveness not established); adolescents at ↑ risk for weight gain and hyperlipidemia; Geri: Appears on Beers list. ↑ risk of stroke, cognitive decline, and mortality in older adults with dementia. Avoid use in older adults, except for schizophrenia, bipolar disorder, or adjunctive treatment of major depressive disorder.

Adverse Reactions/Side Effects

CV: orthostatic hypotension, bradycardia, chest pain, syncope, tachycardia. **Derm:** DRUG REACTION WITH EOSINOPHILIA AND SYSTEMIC SYMPTOMS (DRESS), photosensitivity. **EENT:** amblyopia, rhinitis, ↑ salivation, pharyngitis. **Endo:** galactorrhea, goiter, gynecomastia, hyperglycemia, hyperprolactinemia. **F and E:** ↑ thirst. **GI:** ↑ liver enzymes, constipation, dry mouth, weight loss, abdominal pain, dysphagia, nausea. **GU:** ↓ fertility (females), ↓ libido, amenorrhea, impotence, urinary incontinence. **Hemat:** AGRANULOCYTOSIS, leukopenia, neutropenia. **Metab:** weight gain, ↑ appetite, dyslipidemia. **MS:** hypertonia, joint pain. **Neuro:** agitation, delirium, dizziness, headache, restlessness, sedation, tremor, weakness, dystonia, falls, insomnia, mood changes, NEUROLEPTIC MALIGNANT SYNDROME, personality disorder, SEIZURES, speech impairment, SUICIDAL THOUGHTS, tardive dyskinesia. **Resp:** aspiration, cough, dyspnea. **Misc:** body temperature dysregulation, fever, flu-like syndrome.

Interactions

Drug-Drug: ↑ anticholinergic effects with other **anticholinergic drugs**, including **antihistamines, quinidine, disopyramide,** and **antidepressants**; avoid concurrent use. Effects may be ↓ by concurrent **carbamazepine, omeprazole,** or **rifampin. Antihypertensives** and **CNS depressants** may ↑ risk of orthostatic hypotension. ↑ CNS depression may occur with concurrent use of **alcohol** or other **CNS depressants**; concurrent use of IM olanzapine and parenteral benzodiazepines should be avoided. May antagonize the effects of **levodopa** or other **dopamine agonists. Fluvoxamine** may ↑ levels. **Nicotine** can ↓ olanzapine levels.

Route/Dosage

Schizophrenia

PO (Adults —Most Patients): 5–10 mg/day initially; may ↑ at weekly intervals by 5 mg/day (target dose = 10 mg/day; not to exceed 20 mg/day).
PO (Adults —Debilitated or Nonsmoking Female Patients ≥65 yr): Initiate therapy at 5 mg/day.
PO (Children 13–17 yr): 2.5–5 mg/day initially; may ↑ at weekly intervals by 2.5–5 mg/day (target dose = 10 mg/day; not to exceed 20 mg/day).
IM (Adults): *Oral olanzapine dose = 10 mg/day:* 210 mg every 2 wk or 410 mg every 4 wk for the first 8 wk, then 150 mg every 2 wk or 300 mg every 4 wk as maintenance therapy; *Oral olanzapine dose = 15 mg/day:* 300 mg every 2 wk for the first 8 wk, then 210 mg every 2 wk or 405 mg every 4 wk as maintenance therapy; *Oral olanzapine dose = 20 mg/day:* 300 mg every 2 wk for the first 8 wk, then 300 mg every 2 wk as maintenance therapy.
IM (Adults —Debilitated or Nonsmoking Female Patients ≥65 yr): Initiate therapy at 150 mg every 4 wk.

Acute Manic or Mixed Episodes Associated With Bipolar I Disorder

PO (Adults): 10–15 mg/day initially (use 10 mg/day when used with lithium or evaporate); may ↑ every 24 hr by 5 mg/day (not to exceed 20 mg/day).
PO (Children 13–17 yr): 2.5–5 mg/day initially; may ↑ by 2.5–5 mg/day (target dose = 10 mg/day; not to exceed 20 mg/day).

Maintenance Treatment of Bipolar I Disorder

PO (Adults): Continue at the dose required to maintain symptom remission (usual dose: 5–20 mg/day).
PO (Children 13–17 yr): Continue at the lowest dose required to maintain symptom remission.

Acute Agitation due to Schizophrenia or Bipolar I Mania

IM (Adults): 10 mg, may repeat in 2 hr, then 4 hr later.
IM (Adults >65 yr): Initiate therapy with 5 mg.

Depressive Episodes Associated With Bipolar I Disorder

PO (Adults): 5 mg/day with fluoxetine 20 mg/day (both given in evening); may ↑ fluoxetine dose up to 50 mg/day and olanzapine dose up to 12.5 mg/day.
PO (Children 10–17 yr): 20 mg/day with olanzapine 2.5 mg/day (both given in evening); may ↑ fluoxetine dose up to 50 mg/day and olanzapine dose up to 12 mg/day.

Treatment-Resistant Depression

PO (Adults): 5 mg/day with fluoxetine 20 mg/day (both given in evening); may ↑ fluoxetine dose up to 50 mg/day and olanzapine dose up to 20 mg/day.

Availability (generic available)

Tablets: 2.5 mg, 5 mg, 7.5 mg, 10 mg, 15 mg, 20 mg. **Orally disintegrating tablets (Zyprexa Zydis):** 5 mg, 10 mg, 15 mg, 20 mg. **Powder for injection:** 10 mg/vial. **Extended-release powder for suspension for injection (Zyprexa Relprevv):** 210 mg/vial, 300 mg/vial, 405 mg/vial. *In combination with:* fluoxetine (Symbyax); samidorphan (Lybalvi). See Appendix N.

NURSING IMPLICATIONS
Assessment

- Assess mental status (orientation, mood, behavior) before and periodically during therapy. Monitor closely for notable changes in behavior that could indicate the emergence or worsening of suicidal thoughts or behavior or depression.
- Monitor BP (sitting, standing, lying), ECG, pulse, and respiratory rate before and frequently during dose adjustment.
- Assess weight and BMI initially and throughout therapy.
- Observe patient carefully when administering medication to ensure that medication is taken and not hoarded or cheeked.
- Assess fluid intake and bowel function. Increased bulk and fluids in the diet may help minimize constipation.
- Monitor patient for onset of akathisia (restlessness or desire to keep moving) and extrapyramidal side effects (*parkinsonian:* difficulty speaking or swallowing, loss of balance control, pill rolling of hands, mask-like face, shuffling gait, rigidity, tremors; and *dystonic:* muscle spasms, twisting motions, twitching, inability to move eyes, weakness of arms or legs) every 2 mo during therapy and 8–12 wk after therapy has been discontinued. Report these symptoms if they occur, as reduction in dose or discontinuation of medication may be necessary. Trihexyphenidyl or benztropine may be used to control symptoms.
- Monitor for tardive dyskinesia (uncontrolled rhythmic movement of mouth, face, and extremities; lip smacking or puckering; puffing of cheeks; uncontrolled chewing; rapid or worm-like movements of tongue, excessive blinking of eyes). Discontinue olanzapine and report immediately; may be irreversible.
- Monitor for development of neuroleptic malignant syndrome (fever, respiratory distress, tachycardia, seizures, diaphoresis, hypertension or hypotension, pallor, tiredness, severe muscle stiffness, loss of bladder control). Notify health care professional immediately if these symptoms occur.
- Monitor for symptoms related to hyperprolactinemia (menstrual abnormalities, galactorrhea, sexual dysfunction).

- Assess for falls risk. Drowsiness, orthostatic hypotension, and motor and sensory instability increase risk. Institute prevention if indicated.
- Monitor for signs and symptoms of DRESS (fever, rash, lymphadenopathy, and/or facial swelling), associated with involvement of other organ systems (hepatitis, nephritis, hematologic abnormalities, myocarditis, myositis) during therapy. May resemble an acute viral infection. Eosinophilia is often present. Discontinue therapy if signs occur.
- *Zyprexa Relprevv*: Observe for signs and symptoms of Post-injection Delirium/Sedation Syndrome (dizziness, confusion, disorientation, slurred speech, altered gait, difficulty ambulating, weakness, agitation, extrapyramidal symptoms, hypertension, convulsion, reduced level of consciousness ranging from mild sedation to coma) for at least 3 hr after injection.

Lab Test Considerations

- Evaluate CBC, liver function tests, and ocular examinations periodically during therapy. May cause ↓ platelets. May cause ↑ bilirubin, AST, ALT, GGT, CK, and alkaline phosphatase.
- Monitor blood glucose prior to and periodically during therapy.
- Monitor serum prolactin prior to and periodically during therapy. May cause ↑ serum prolactin levels.
- Monitor CBC frequently during initial mo of therapy in patients with pre-existing or history of low WBC. May cause leukopenia, neutropenia, or agranulocytosis. Discontinue therapy if this occurs.
- May cause hyperlipidemia; monitor serum lipids prior to and periodically during therapy.

Implementation

- Do not confuse Zyprexa with Celexa, Zyrtec, Zestril, or Zelapar. Do not confuse olanzapine with quetiapine.
- *REMS: Zyprexa Relprevv* is only prescribed through the *Zyprexa Relprevv Patient Care Program*. Prescribers, pharmacies, and patients must be educated about the program and must comply with the program requirements.
- **PO:** May be administered without regard to meals.
- For orally disintegrating tablets, peel back foil on blister, do not push tablet through foil. Using dry hands, remove from foil and place entire tablet in mouth. Tablet will disintegrate with or without liquid.
- **IM:** *Reconstitution:* Reconstitute with 2.1 mL of sterile water for injection for a concentration of 5 mg/mL. Solution should be clear and yellow; do not administer solutions that are discolored or contain particulate matter. Inject slowly, deep into muscle. Do not administer IV or SUBQ. Administer within 1 hr of reconstitution. Discard unused solution.
- For *Zyprexa Relprevv*: Use gloves when preparing; solution may be irritating to skin. *Reconstitution:*

Use only diluent provided by manufacturer. Reconstitute 150-mg or 210-mg dose with 1.3 mL, 300 mg with 1.8 mL, and 405 mg with 2.3 mL of diluent. Loosen powder by tapping vial; inject diluent into powder. Remove needle from vial holding vial upright to prevent loss of solution. Engage needle safety device as explained by manufacturer. Pad a hard surface and tap vial repeatedly until no powder or yellow, dry clumps are visible. Shake vial vigorously until suspension appears smooth and consistent in color and texture. Solution will be yellow and opaque. Allow foam to dissipate. Suspension is stable for 24 hr at room temperature; if not used immediately, shake to resuspend. *Concentration:* 150 mg/mL. Replace needle with 19 gauge, 1.5 in. or 2 in. for obese patients. Slowly withdraw desired amount from vial; 150 mg = 1 mL, 210 mg = 1.4 mL, 300 mg = 2 mL, 405 mg = 2.7 mL. Administer immediately deep IM gluteal after withdrawing. Do not massage injection site. Patient must be observed for at least 3 hr after injection for Post-Injection Delirium/Sedation Syndrome.

Patient/Family Teaching

● *REMS:* Advise patient to take medication as directed and not to skip doses or double up on missed doses. May need to discontinue gradually. Advise patient to read the *Medication Guide* prior to starting therapy and with each Rx refill in case of changes. Explain the *Zyprexa Relprevv Patient Care Program* to patient and encourage patient to enroll in the *Zyprexa Relprevv Patient Care Program* registry.
● Inform patient of possibility of extrapyramidal symptoms and tardive dyskinesia. Instruct patient to report these symptoms immediately to health care professional.
● Advise patient to change positions slowly to minimize orthostatic hypotension. Protect from falls.
● Medication may cause drowsiness. Caution patient to avoid driving or other activities requiring alertness until response to the medication is known. Patients receiving *Zyprexa Relprevv* should not drive for 24 hr following injection.
● Advise patient and family to notify health care professional if thoughts about suicide or dying, attempts to commit suicide; new or worse depression; new or worse anxiety; feeling very agitated or restless; panic attacks; trouble sleeping; new or worse irritability; acting aggressive; being angry or violent; acting on dangerous impulses; an extreme increase in activity and talking, other unusual changes in behavior or mood occur.
● Advise patient to notify health care professional of all Rx or OTC medications, vitamins, or herbal products being taken and to consult with health care professional before taking other medications and alcohol.
● Advise patient to use sunscreen and protective clothing when exposed to the sun. Extremes of temperature (exercise, hot weather, hot baths, or showers)

should also be avoided; this drug impairs body temperature regulation.
● Instruct patient to use saliva substitute, frequent mouth rinses, good oral hygiene, and sugarless gum or candy to minimize dry mouth. Consult dentist if dry mouth continues for >2 wk.
● Advise patient to notify health care professional of medication regimen before treatment or surgery.
● Instruct patient to notify health care professional promptly if sore throat, fever, unusual bleeding or bruising, rash, symptoms of Post-Injection Delirium/Sedation Syndrome, or weakness, tremors, visual disturbances, dark-colored urine, clay-colored stools, menstrual abnormalities, galactorrhea, or sexual dysfunction occur.
● Rep: Advise females of reproductive potential to notify health care professional if pregnancy is planned or suspected, and to avoid breastfeeding during therapy. Encourage women who become pregnant while taking olanzapine to enroll in the National Pregnancy Registry for Atypical Antipsychotics at 1-866-961-2388 or visit https://womensmentalhealth.org/research/pregnancyregistry/. Monitor neonates for extrapyramidal and/or withdrawal symptoms and manage symptoms appropriately. Monitor infants exposed through breastfeeding for excess sedation, irritability, poor feeding, and extrapyramidal symptoms (tremors and abnormal muscle movements).
● Emphasize the importance of routine follow-up exams and continued participation in psychotherapy.

Evaluation/Desired Outcomes
● Decrease in excitable, manic behavior.
● Decrease in positive symptoms (delusions, hallucinations) of schizophrenia.
● Decrease in negative symptoms (social withdrawal, flat, blunted affect) of schizophrenia.
● Increased sense of well-being.
● Decreased agitation.

℀ **olaparib** (oh-**lap**-a-rib)
Lynparza
Classification
Therapeutic: antineoplastics
Pharmacologic: enzyme inhibitors

Indications
Maintenance treatment of recurrent epithelial ovarian, fallopian tube, or primary peritoneal cancer in patients who are in a complete or partial response to platinum-based chemotherapy. ℀ First-line maintenance treatment of deleterious/suspected deleterious germline or somatic *BRCA*-mutated advanced epithelial ovarian, fallopian tube, or primary peritoneal cancer in patients who are in a complete or partial response to first-line platinum-based chemotherapy. ℀ First-line maintenance treatment of advanced epithelial ovarian, fallopian tube, or primary peritoneal cancer in patients who

are in a complete or partial response to first-line platinum-based chemotherapy and whose cancer is associated with homologous recombination deficiency positive status defined by either a deleterious/suspected deleterious *BRCA* mutation and/or genomic instability (in combination with bevacizumab). ☒ Adjuvant treatment of deleterious or suspected deleterious germline *BRCA*-mutated human epidermal growth factor receptor 2 (HER2)-negative high risk early breast cancer in patients who have been treated with neoadjuvant or adjuvant chemotherapy. ☒ Deleterious/suspected deleterious germline *BRCA*-mutated HER2–negative metastatic breast cancer in patients who have been treated with chemotherapy in the neoadjuvant, adjuvant, or metastatic setting (should have been previously treated with or considered intolerant to an endocrine therapy). ☒ First-Line maintenance treatment of deleterious/suspected deleterious germline *BRCA*-mutated metastatic pancreatic adenocarcinoma in patients whose disease has not progressed on ≥16 wks of a first-line platinum-based chemotherapy regimen. ☒ Deleterious/suspected deleterious germline or somatic homologous recombination repair (HRR) gene-mutated metastatic castration-resistant prostate cancer in patients who have progressed following previous treatment with enzalutamide or abiraterone. ☒ Deleterious/suspected deleterious *BRCA*-mutated metastatic castration-resistant prostate cancer (in combination with abiraterone and prednisolone [or prednisone]).

Action

Acts as a poly (ADP-ribose) polymerase (PARP) inhibitor; disrupts DNA transcription, cell cycle regulation, and DNA repair. **Therapeutic Effects:** Improved progression-free survival in ovarian, fallopian tube, primary peritoneal, breast, pancreatic, and prostate cancer.

Pharmacokinetics

Absorption: Well absorbed following oral administration.

Distribution: Unknown.

Metabolism and Excretion: Extensively metabolized (mostly by the CYP3A isoenzyme); 15% excreted unchanged in urine, 6% in feces.

Half-life: 14.9 hr.

TIME/ACTION PROFILE (plasma concentrations)

ROUTE	ONSET	PEAK	DURATION
PO	unknown	1–3 hr	12 hr

Contraindications/Precautions

Contraindicated in: OB: Pregnancy; Lactation: Lactation.

Use Cautiously in: Moderate or severe hepatic impairment; Moderate or severe renal impairment (CCr

<50 mL/min) (dose ↓ may be needed); Rep: Women of reproductive potential and men with female partners of reproductive potential; Pedi: Safety and effectiveness not established in children.

Adverse Reactions/Side Effects

CV: DEEP VEIN THROMBOSIS. **Derm:** dermatitis/rash. **GI:** abdominal pain, diarrhea, dyspepsia, nausea, vomiting. **Hemat:** anemia, lymphopenia, neutropenia, thrombocytopenia, MYELODYSPLASTIC SYNDROME (MDS)/ACUTE MYELOID LEUKEMIA (AML). **Metab:** ↓ appetite. **MS:** arthralgia, back pain, myalgia. **Neuro:** fatigue, headache, dysgeusia, weakness. **Resp:** cough, PNEUMONITIS, PULMONARY EMBOLISM.

Interactions

Drug-Drug: ↑ risk of prolonged myelosuppression with other **antineoplastics**. Concurrent use with **strong CYP3A4 inhibitors**, including **clarithromycin, itraconazole, ketoconazole, lopinavir/ritonavir, nefazodone, nelfinavir, posaconazole, ritonavir,** or **voriconazole,** ↑ levels and risk of toxicity; avoid concurrent use if possible but if necessary, ↓ olaparib dose. Concurrent use with **moderate CYP3A4 inhibitors,** including **aprepitant, atazanavir, ciprofloxacin, crizotinib, darunavir/ritonavir, diltiazem, erythromycin, fluconazole, fosamprenavir, imatinib,** or **verapamil** ↑ levels and risk of toxicity; avoid concurrent use if possible but if necessary, ↓ olaparib dose. Concurrent use with **strong CYP3A inducers** including **carbamazepine, phenytoin,** and **rifampin** ↓ blood levels and effectiveness and should be avoided. Concurrent use with **moderate CYP3A inducers** including **bosentan, efavirenz, etravirine, modafinil,** and **nafcillin** ↓ blood levels and effectiveness; avoid if possible.

Drug-Natural Products: St. John's wort may ↓ blood levels and effectiveness and should be avoided.

Drug-Food: Concurrent ingestion of **grapefruit** and **Seville oranges** may ↑ blood levels and the risk of toxicity and should be avoided.

Route/Dosage

First-Line Maintenance Treatment of *BRCA*-Mutated Advanced Ovarian Cancer or Advanced Ovarian Cancer (in Combination with Bevacizumab)

PO (Adults): 300 mg twice daily until disease progression, unacceptable toxicity, or completion of 2 yr of treatment. If complete response achieved after 2 yr of treatment (i.e., no radiological evidence of disease), can stop therapy. If evidence of disease at 2 yr, may continue therapy. *Concurrent use of strong CYP3A4 inhibitor:* 100 mg twice daily until disease progression, unacceptable toxicity, or completion of 2 yr of treatment. If complete response achieved after 2 yr of treatment (i.e., no radiological evidence of disease), can stop therapy. If evidence of disease at 2 yr, may continue therapy. *Concurrent use of moderate CYP3A4 inhibitor:* 150 mg twice daily until disease progression, unacceptable toxicity, or completion of 2 yr of treatment. If complete response achieved after 2 yr of treatment (i.e., no radiological evidence of disease), can stop therapy. If evidence of disease at 2 yr, may continue therapy.

Renal Impairment
PO (Adults): *CCr 31–50 mL/min:* 200 mg twice daily until disease progression, unacceptable toxicity, or completion of 2 yr of treatment. If complete response achieved after 2 yr of treatment (i.e., no radiological evidence of disease), can stop therapy. If evidence of disease at 2 yr, may continue therapy.

Adjuvant Treatment of Germline *BRCA*-Mutated HER2-Negative High Risk Early Breast Cancer
PO (Adults): 300 mg twice daily for 1 yr or until disease recurrence or unacceptable toxicity, whichever occurs first. *Concurrent use of strong CYP3A4 inhibitor:* 100 mg twice daily for 1 yr or until disease recurrence or unacceptable toxicity, whichever occurs first. *Concurrent use of moderate CYP3A4 inhibitor:* 150 mg twice daily for 1 yr or until disease recurrence or unacceptable toxicity, whichever occurs first.

Renal Impairment
PO (Adults): *CCr 31–50 mL/min:* 200 mg twice daily for 1 yr or until disease recurrence or unacceptable toxicity, whichever occurs first.

Recurrent Ovarian Cancer, Germline *BRCA*-Mutated HER2–Negative Metastatic Breast Cancer, Germline *BRCA*-Mutated Metastatic Pancreatic Adenocarcinoma, HRR Gene-mutated Metastatic Castration-Resistant Prostate Cancer, *BRCA*-Mutated Metastatic Castration-Resistant Prostate Cancer
PO (Adults): 300 mg twice daily until disease progression or unacceptable toxicity. *Concurrent use of strong CYP3A4 inhibitor:* 100 mg twice daily until disease progression or unacceptable toxicity. *Concurrent use of moderate CYP3A4 inhibitor:* 150 mg twice daily until disease progression or unacceptable toxicity.

Renal Impairment
PO (Adults): *CCr 31–50 mL/min:* 200 mg twice daily until disease progression or unacceptable toxicity.

Availability
Tablets: 100 mg, 150 mg.

NURSING IMPLICATIONS
Assessment
- Monitor for signs and symptoms of pneumonitis (new or worsening respiratory symptoms, dyspnea, fever, cough, wheezing, radiological abnormality) during therapy. Interrupt therapy; if pneumonitis confirmed, discontinue therapy.

- Monitor for signs and symptoms of venous thrombosis and pulmonary embolism and treat as medically appropriate. May require long-term anticoagulation.

Lab Test Considerations
- ✡ Patient selection is based on the presence of deleterious or suspected deleterious HRR gene mutations, including BRCA mutations, or genomic instability based on the indication, biomarker, and sample type. Information on FDA-approved tests for the detection of genetic mutations is available at http://www.fda.gov/companiondiagnostics.
- Verify negative pregnancy test prior to starting therapy.
- Monitor CBC at baseline and monthly during therapy. Do not start olaparib until patient has recovered from hematological toxicities from previous chemotherapy (≤CTCAE Grade 1). For prolonged hematological toxicities, interrupt olaparib and monitor CBC weekly until recovery. If levels have not recovered to Grade ≤1 after 4 wk, refer to hematologist. Discontinue olaparib if MDS or AML is confirmed.
- May cause ↓ hemoglobin, neutrophils, platelets, and lymphocytes. May cause ↑ mean corpuscular volume and serum creatinine.

Implementation
- **PO:** Administer twice daily, about 12 hr apart, without regard to food. *DNC:* Swallow tablets whole; do not break, chew, or dissolve tablets.

Patient/Family Teaching
- Instruct patient to take olaparib as directed. If a dose is missed, do not take another to make up; omit dose and take next scheduled dose.
- Inform patient that mild to moderate nausea and/or vomiting is common when taking olaparib. Notify healthcare professional for antiemetic options if this is problematic.
- Advise patient to avoid grapefruit, grapefruit juice, Seville oranges, and Seville orange juice during therapy.
- Advise patient to notify healthcare professional if signs and symptoms of pneumonitis or hematological toxicity (weakness, feeling tired, fever, weight loss, frequent infections, bruising, bleeding easily, shortness of breath, blood in urine or stool, low blood cell counts on laboratory findings, need for blood transfusions) occur. May also be MDS or AML.
- Instruct patient to notify healthcare professional of all Rx or OTC medications, vitamins, or herbal products being taken and to consult with healthcare professional before taking other medications, especially St. John's wort.
- Rep: May cause fetal harm and increased risk for loss of pregnancy. Advise females of reproductive potential to use effective contraception during and for at least 6 mo after last dose and to avoid breastfeeding for 1 mo after last dose. Advise patient to notify healthcare professional if pregnancy is planned

or suspected. Advise males with female partners of reproductive potential to use effective contraception during and for 3 mo after last dose. Advise male patients not to donate sperm during therapy and for 3 mo following the last dose.

- Emphasize importance of lab test to monitor for side effects.

Evaluation/Desired Outcomes

- Improved progression-free survival in ovarian, fallopian tube, primary peritoneal, breast, pancreatic, and prostate cancer.

---

olmesartan, See ANGIOTENSIN II RECEPTOR ANTAGONISTS.

---

olodaterol (oh-loh-dat-er-ole)
Striverdi Respimat
Classification
Therapeutic: bronchodilators
Pharmacologic: beta-adrenergic agonists

Indications
Maintenance treatment of airflow obstruction in patients with COPD, including chronic bronchitis and emphysema.

Action
A long-acting beta$_2$-adrenergic agonist (LABA) that stimulates adenyl cyclase, resulting in accumulation of cyclic adenosine monophosphate (cAMP) at beta$_2$-adrenergic receptors resulting in bronchodilation. **Therapeutic Effects:** Bronchodilation with decreased airflow obstruction.

Pharmacokinetics
Absorption: 30% absorbed following oral inhalation (from lung surface); swallowed drug is minimally absorbed.
Distribution: Extensively distributed to tissues.
Metabolism and Excretion: Extensively metabolized by the liver, some by the CYP3A4 isoenzyme; only one metabolite binds to beta$_2$ adrenergic receptors. 5–7% excreted unchanged in urine, remainder in feces as drug and metabolites (84%).
Half-life: 45 hr.

TIME/ACTION PROFILE (improvement in FEV$_1$)

ROUTE	ONSET	PEAK	DURATION
Inhaln	within 1 hr	1–5 hr	24 hr

Contraindications/Precautions
Contraindicated in: Acutely deteriorating COPD or acute respiratory symptoms; Asthma.

Use Cautiously in: History of seizures; Thyrotoxicosis; History of cardiovascular disorders (coronary insufficiency, arrhythmias, hypertension); Sensitivity to sympathomimetics (adrenergics); Severe hepatic impairment; OB: Use during pregnancy only if potential maternal benefit justifies potential fetal risk; may interfere with uterine contractility during labor; Lactation: Use while breastfeeding only if potential maternal benefit justifies potential risk to infant; Pedi: Safety and effectiveness not established in children.

Exercise Extreme Caution in: Concurrent use with MAO inhibitors, tricyclic antidepressants, or drugs that prolong the QTc interval (↑ risk of adverse cardiovascular reactions).

Adverse Reactions/Side Effects
CV: ↑ BP, ECG changes, tachycardia. **EENT:** nasopharyngitis. **Endo:** hyperglycemia. **F and E:** hypokalemia. **GI:** diarrhea. **MS:** arthralgia, back pain. **Neuro:** dizziness.. **Resp:** cough, PARADOXICAL BRONCHOSPASM. **Misc:** HYPERSENSITIVITY REACTIONS (including angioedema).

Interactions
Drug-Drug: Concurrent use with **MAO inhibitors**, **tricyclic antidepressants**, or **QT interval prolonging medications** ↑ risk of adverse cardiovascular reactions; use with extreme caution. Concurrent use of other **adrenergics** ↑ risk of adrenergic adverse reactions (tachycardia, ↑ BP). Concurrent use with **corticosteroids**, **non-potassium sparing diuretics**, or **theophylline** may ↑ risk of hypokalemia and adverse cardiovascular reactions; use cautiously. Concurrent use with **beta blockers** may ↓ effectiveness and cause severe bronchospasm; use cautiously. Should not be used concurrently with any other **long-acting beta$_2$-adrenergic blockers**. **Ketoconazole** may ↑ levels and risk of toxicity.

Route/Dosage
Inhaln (Adults): 2 inhalations once daily.

Availability
Inhalation spray: 2.7 mcg (delivers 2.5 mcg) per actuation in cartridges containing 14 doses/cartridge (one actuation lost in priming) for use with Respimat inhaler. *In combination with:* tiotropium (Stiolto Respimat). See Appendix N.

NURSING IMPLICATIONS
Assessment
- Assess respiratory status (rate, breath sounds, degree of dyspnea, pulse) before administration and at peak of medication. Consult health care professional about alternative medication if severe bronchospasm is present; onset of action is too slow for patients in acute distress. If paradoxical bronchospasm (wheezing) occurs, withhold medication and notify health care professional immediately.

- Monitor for signs and symptoms of allergic reactions (difficulties in breathing or swallowing, swelling of tongue, lips and face, urticaria, skin rash). Discontinue therapy if symptoms occur.

Lab Test Considerations
- May cause transient hypokalemia and hyperglycemia.

Implementation

- **Inhaln:** Prior to first use, prime the inhaler by actuating toward ground until aerosol cloud is visible, then repeat procedure 3 more times. If not used for 3 days, actuate inhaler once to prepare for use. *Striverdi Respimat* has a slow-moving mist to assist with inhalation. Use once (2 puffs), at the same time daily.
- A rescue inhaler of short-acting beta$_2$-agonists should always be available to treat sudden bronchospasm.

Patient/Family Teaching

- Instruct patient in the correct use of *Striverdi Respimat*. Take missed doses as soon as remembered. Do not take more than 1 dose (2 puffs) in 24 hr. Advise patient not to discontinue without consulting health care professional; symptoms may recur.
- Inform patient that olodaterol is a long-acting bronchodilator and should not be used for treating sudden breathing problems of COPD or asthma.
- Advise patient to notify health care professional if signs and symptoms of allergic reaction, worsening symptoms; decreasing effectiveness of inhaled, short-acting beta$_2$-agonists; need for more inhalations than usual of inhaled, short-acting beta$_2$-agonists; or significant decrease in lung function occur.
- Instruct patient to notify health care professional of all Rx or OTC medications, vitamins, or herbal products being taken and to avoid concurrent use of Rx, OTC, and herbal products without consulting health care professional.
- Rep: Advise females of reproductive potential to notify health care professional if pregnancy is planned or suspected or if breastfeeding.

Evaluation/Desired Outcomes

- Bronchodilation with decreased airflow obstruction.

☒ olsalazine (ole-sal-a-zeen)
Dipentum
Classification
Therapeutic: gastrointestinal anti-inflammatories

Indications
Ulcerative colitis (when patients cannot tolerate sulfasalazine).

Action
Locally acting anti-inflammatory action in the colon, where activity is probably due to inhibition of prosta-

glandin synthesis. **Therapeutic Effects:** Reduction in the symptoms of inflammatory bowel disease.

Pharmacokinetics
Absorption: Acts locally in colon, where 98–99% is converted to mesalamine (5-aminosalicylic acid).
Distribution: Action is primarily local and remains in the colon.
Metabolism and Excretion: 2% absorbed into systemic circulation is rapidly metabolized; mostly eliminated as mesalamine in the feces.
Half-life: 0.9 hr.

TIME/ACTION PROFILE (plasma concentrations)

ROUTE	ONSET	PEAK	DURATION
PO	unknown	1 hr; 4–8 hr	12 hr

Contraindications/Precautions
Contraindicated in: Hypersensitivity reaction to salicylates; Cross-sensitivity with furosemide, sulfonylureas, or carbonic anhydrase inhibitors may exist; ☒ Glucose-6–phosphate dehydrogenase (G6PD) deficiency; Urinary tract or intestinal obstruction; Porphyria; Lactation: Lactation.
Use Cautiously in: Severe hepatic or renal impairment; Renal impairment (↑ risk of renal tubular damage); OB: Safety not established in pregnancy; Pedi: Children <2 yr (safety and effectiveness not established); Geri: ↑ risk of blood dyscrasias (agranulocytosis, neutropenia, pancytopenia) in older adults. Consider ↓ hepatic/renal/cardiac function, concomitant illnesses, and drug therapies.

Adverse Reactions/Side Effects
Derm: ACUTE GENERALIZED EXANTHEMATOUS PUSTULOSIS (AGEP), DRUG REACTION WITH EOSINOPHILIA AND SYSTEMIC SYMPTOMS (DRESS), itching, photosensitivity, rash, STEVENS-JOHNSON SYNDROME (SJS), TOXIC EPIDERMAL NECROLYSIS (TEN). **GI:** diarrhea, abdominal pain, anorexia, exacerbation of colitis, HEPATOTOXICITY, nausea, vomiting. **GU:** interstitial nephritis, nephrolithiasis, renal impairment. **Hemat:** blood dyscrasias. **Neuro:** ataxia, confusion, depression, dizziness, drowsiness, headache, psychosis, restlessness. **Misc:** acute intolerance syndrome, hypersensitivity reactions.

Interactions
Drug-Drug: ↑ risk of bleeding after neuraxial anesthesia with **low molecular weight heparins** and **heparin**; discontinue olsalazine before initiation of therapy or monitor closely if discontinuation not possible. May ↑ levels of and risk of bleeding from **warfarin**; closely monitor INR. May ↑ myelosuppressive effects of **mercaptopurine** or **azathioprine**; avoid concurrent use, if possible. Concurrent use with **NSAIDs** may ↑ risk of nephrotoxicity. ↑ risk of developing Reye's syndrome; avoid olsalazine during 6 wk after **varicella vaccine**.

Route/Dosage
PO (Adults): 500 mg twice daily.

Availability
Capsules: 250 mg.

NURSING IMPLICATIONS
Assessment
- Assess abdominal pain and frequency, quantity, and consistency of stools at the beginning of and during therapy.
- Monitor for hypersensitivity reactions may present as internal organ involvement (myocarditis, pericarditis, nephritis, hepatitis, pneumonitis, hematologic abnormalities). Discontinue olsalazine if hypersensitivity reactions occur.
- Assess patient for allergy to sulfonamides and salicylates. Patients allergic to sulfasalazine may take mesalamine or olsalazine without difficulty, but therapy should be discontinued if rash or fever occur.
- Monitor intake and output ratios. Fluid intake should be sufficient to maintain a urine output of at least 1200–1500 mL daily to prevent crystalluria and stone formation.
- Assess for severe cutaneous adverse reactions (SJS, TEN, DRESS, and AGEP). Discontinue olsalazine at first sign of severe cutaneous reactions.

Lab Test Considerations
- Monitor urinalysis, BUN, and serum creatinine prior to and periodically during therapy. If renal function declines during therapy, discontinue olsalazine.
- Olsalazine may cause ↑ AST and ALT levels.
- Monitor CBC prior to and every 3–6 mo during prolonged therapy. Discontinue olsalazine if blood dyscrasias occur.

Implementation
- Maintain adequate hydration during therapy.
- **PO:** Administer with food in evenly divided doses every 12 hr.

Patient/Family Teaching
- Instruct patient to take medication as directed, even if feeling better. Take missed doses as soon as remembered unless almost time for next dose.
- May cause dizziness. Caution patient to avoid driving or other activities that require alertness until response to medication is known.
- Advise patient to notify health care professional if skin rash, sore throat, fever, mouth sores, unusual bleeding or bruising, wheezing, fever, or hives occurs.
- Advise patient to avoid sun exposure, wear sunscreen and protective clothing to minimize risk of photosensitivity reactions.
- Instruct patient to notify healthcare professional if symptoms do not improve after 1–2 mo of therapy.

- Instruct patient to notify healthcare professional if symptoms worsen or do not improve. If symptoms of acute intolerance (cramping, acute abdominal pain, bloody diarrhea, fever, headache, rash) occur, discontinue therapy and notify health care professional immediately.
- Rep: May cause fetal harm. Advise females of reproductive potential to use effective contraception and to notify healthcare professional if pregnancy is planned or suspected and to avoid breastfeeding during therapy. Monitor breastfed infants for diarrhea.
- Inform patient that proctoscopy and sigmoidoscopy may be required periodically during treatment to determine response.

Evaluation/Desired Outcomes
- Decrease in diarrhea and abdominal pain.
- Return to normal bowel pattern in patients with inflammatory bowel disease. Effects may be seen within 3–21 days. The usual course of therapy is 3–6 wk.
- Maintenance of remission in patients with inflammatory bowel disease.

omega-3-acid ethyl esters
(oh-**me**-ga three **as**-id **eth**-il **es**-ters)
Lovaza
Classification
Therapeutic: lipid-lowering agents
Pharmacologic: fatty acids

Indications
Hypertriglyceridemia (triglycerides ≥500 mg/dL).

Action
Inhibits synthesis of triglycerides. **Therapeutic Effects:** Reduction of triglycerides.

Pharmacokinetics
Absorption: Well absorbed.
Distribution: Widely distributed to tissues.
Metabolism and Excretion: Incorporated into phospholipids.
Half-life: Unknown.

TIME/ACTION PROFILE (lowering of triglycerides)

ROUTE	ONSET	PEAK	DURATION
PO	unknown	2 mo	unknown

Contraindications/Precautions
Contraindicated in: Hypersensitivity.
Use Cautiously in: Allergy/hypersensitivity to fish; OB: Safety not established in pregnancy; Lactation: Safety not established in breastfeeding; Pedi: Safety and effectiveness not established in children.

✱= Canadian drug name. ▨ = Genetic implication. ~~Strikethrough~~ = Discontinued. CAPITALS = life-threatening. <u>Underline</u> = most frequent.

Adverse Reactions/Side Effects
Derm: rash. **GI:** ↑ liver enzymes, altered taste, eructation.

Interactions
Drug-Drug: May ↑ risk of bleeding with **aspirin** or **warfarin**.

Route/Dosage
PO (Adults): 4 g once daily *or* 2 g twice daily.

Availability (generic available)
Gelatin capsules (oil-filled): 1 g.

NURSING IMPLICATIONS
Assessment
- Obtain a diet history, especially with regard to fat consumption.

Lab Test Considerations
- Monitor serum triglyceride levels prior to and periodically during therapy.
- Monitor serum ALT periodically during therapy. May cause ↑ serum ALT without concurrent ↑ in AST levels.
- Monitor serum LDL cholesterol levels periodically during therapy. May cause ↑ in serum LDL levels.

Implementation
- Do not confuse Lovaza with lorazepam.
- An appropriate lipid-lowering diet should be followed before therapy and should continue during therapy.
- **PO:** May be taken as a single 4-g dose or as 2 g twice daily. May be administered with meals. *DNC:* Swallow capsules whole; do not break, dissolve, or chew.

Patient/Family Teaching
- Instruct patient to take medication as directed, not to skip doses or double up on missed doses. Take missed doses as soon as remembered, but if a day is missed, do not double doses the next day. Medication helps control but does not cure elevated serum triglyceride levels.
- Advise patient that this medication should be used in conjunction with diet restrictions (fat, cholesterol, carbohydrates, alcohol), exercise, weight loss in overweight patients, and control of medical problems (such as diabetes mellitus and hypothyroidism) that may contribute to hypertriglyceridemia.
- Rep: Advise females of reproductive potential to notify health care professional if pregnancy is planned or suspected, or if breastfeeding.
- Emphasize the importance of follow-up exams to determine effectiveness.

Evaluation/Desired Outcomes
- Lowering of serum triglyceride levels. Patients who do not have an adequate response after 2 mo of treatment should be withdrawn from therapy.

⚅ omeprazole (o-mep-ra-zole)
❋Losec, PriLOSEC, PriLOSEC OTC
Classification
Therapeutic: antiulcer agents
Pharmacologic: proton-pump inhibitors

Indications
GERD/maintenance of healing in erosive esophagitis. Duodenal ulcers (with or without anti-infectives for *Helicobacter pylori*). Short-term treatment of active benign gastric ulcer. Pathologic hypersecretory conditions, including Zollinger-Ellison syndrome. Reduction of risk of GI bleeding in critically ill patients. **OTC:** Heartburn occurring ≥twice/wk.

Action
Binds to an enzyme on gastric parietal cells in the presence of acidic gastric pH, preventing the final transport of hydrogen ions into the gastric lumen. **Therapeutic Effects:** Diminished accumulation of acid in the gastric lumen with lessened gastroesophageal reflux. Healing of duodenal ulcers.

Pharmacokinetics
Absorption: Rapidly absorbed following oral administration; immediate release formulation contains bicarbonate to prevent acid degradation.
Distribution: Good distribution into gastric parietal cells.
Protein Binding: 95%.
Metabolism and Excretion: Mostly metabolized by the liver via the CYP2C19 isoenzyme, and to a lesser extent by the CYP3A4 isoenzyme; ⚅ the CYP2C19 isoenzyme exhibits genetic polymorphism (15–20% of Asian patients and 3–5% of Caucasian and Black patients may be poor metabolizers and may have significantly ↑ omeprazole concentrations and an ↑ risk of adverse effects); inactive metabolites are excreted in urine (77%) and feces.
Half-life: 0.5–1 hr (↑ in liver disease to 3 hr).

TIME/ACTION PROFILE (antisecretory effects)

ROUTE	ONSET	PEAK	DURATION
PO-delayed release	within 1 hr	within 2 hr	72–96 hr

Contraindications/Precautions
Contraindicated in: Hypersensitivity to omeprazole or related drugs (benzimidazoles); Concurrent use of rilpivirine.
Use Cautiously in: Hepatic impairment (dose ↓ may be necessary); Patients using high-doses for >1 yr (↑ risk of hip, wrist, or spine fractures and fundic gland polyps); Patients using therapy for >3 yr (↑ risk of vitamin B$_{12}$ deficiency); Pre-existing risk of hypocalcemia; Lactation: Safety not established in breastfeeding; Pedi: Children <1 mo (safety and effectiveness not

established); Geri: Appears on Beers list. ↑ risk of *Clostridioides difficile* infection, pneumonia, GI malignancies, bone loss, and fractures in older adults. Avoid scheduled use for >8 wk in older adults unless for high-risk patients (e.g. oral corticosteroid or chronic NSAID use) or patients with erosive esophagitis, Barrett's esophagitis, pathological hypersecretory condition, or demonstrated need for maintenance therapy (e.g. failure of H_2 antagonist).

Adverse Reactions/Side Effects
CV: chest pain. **Derm:** ACUTE GENERALIZED EXANTHEMATOUS PUSTULOSIS, cutaneous lupus erythematosus, DRUG REACTION WITH EOSINOPHILIA AND SYSTEMIC SYMPTOMS (DRESS), itching, rash, STEVENS-JOHNSON SYNDROME, TOXIC EPIDERMAL NECROLYSIS. **F and E:** hypocalcemia (especially if treatment duration ≥3 mo), hypokalemia (especially if treatment duration ≥3 mo), hypomagnesemia (especially if treatment duration ≥3 mo). **GI:** <u>abdominal pain</u>, CLOSTRIDIOIDES DIFFICILE-ASSOCIATED DIARRHEA (CDAD), constipation, diarrhea, flatulence, fundic gland polyps, nausea, vomiting. **GU:** acute tubulointerstitial nephritis. **MS:** bone fracture. **Neuro:** dizziness, drowsiness, fatigue, headache, weakness. **Misc:** HYPERSENSITIVITY REACTIONS (including anaphylaxis, angioedema, or tubulointerstitial nephritis), systemic lupus erythematosus, vitamin B_{12} deficiency.

Interactions
Drug-Drug: May significantly ↓ levels and effectiveness of **rilpivirine**; concurrent use contraindicated. May ↑ levels and risk of toxicity of **antifungal agents**, **cilostazol**, **citalopram**, **diazepam**, **triazolam**, **cyclosporine**, **phenytoin**, **tacrolimus**, and **warfarin**; consider ↓ dose of cilostazol from 100 mg twice daily to 50 mg twice daily. May ↓ absorption of drugs requiring acid pH, including **ketoconazole**, **itraconazole**, **iron salts**, **dasatinib**, **erlotinib**, **nilotinib**, **atazanavir**, **nelfinavir**, and **mycophenolate mofetil**; avoid concurrent use with **atazanavir** and **nelfinavir**. May ↑ levels of **digoxin** and **methotrexate**. **Voriconazole** may ↑ levels. May ↓ the antiplatelet effects of **clopidogrel**; avoid concurrent use. **Rifampin** may ↓ levels and may ↓ response; avoid concurrent use. Hypomagnesemia and hypokalemia ↑ risk of **digoxin** toxicity.
Drug-Natural Products: St. John's wort may ↓ levels and may ↓ response; avoid concurrent use.

Route/Dosage
PO (Adults): *GERD/erosive esophagitis and maintenance of healing of erosive esophagitis:* 20 mg once daily. *Duodenal ulcers associated with H. pylori:* 40 mg once daily in the morning with clarithromycin for 2 wk, then 20 mg once daily for 2 wk *or* 20 mg twice daily with clarithromycin 500 mg twice daily and amoxicillin 1000 mg twice daily for 10 days (if ulcer is present at beginning of therapy, continue omeprazole 20 mg daily for 18 more days); has also been used with

clarithromycin and metronidazole. *Gastric ulcer:* 40 mg once daily for 4–6 wk. *Reduction of the risk of GI bleeding in critically ill patients:* 40 mg initially, then another 40 mg 6–8 hr later, followed by 40 mg once daily for up to 14 days. *Gastric hypersecretory conditions:* 60 mg once daily initially; may be increased up to 120 mg 3 times daily (doses >80 mg/day should be given in divided doses); *OTC:* 20 mg once daily for up to 14 days.
PO (Children 1–16 yr and ≥20 kg): *GERD/erosive esophagitis:* 20 mg once daily for 4–8 wk.
PO (Children 1–16 yr and 10–19 kg): *GERD/erosive esophagitis:* 10 mg once daily for 4–8 wk.
PO (Children 1–16 yr and 5–9 kg): *GERD/erosive esophagitis:* 5 mg once daily for 4–8 wk.
PO (Children 1 mo–<1 yr and ≥10 kg): *Erosive esophagitis:* 10 mg once daily for up to 6 wk.
PO (Children 1 mo–<1 yr and 5–9 kg): *Erosive esophagitis:* 5 mg once daily for up to 6 wk.
PO (Children 1 mo–<1 yr and 3–4 kg): *Erosive esophagitis:* 2.5 mg once daily for up to 6 wk.

Availability (generic available)
Delayed-release tablets: ✹ 10 mg, 20 mg^OTC. **Delayed-release capsules:** 10 mg, 20 mg, 40 mg. **Delayed-release powder for oral suspension (peach-mint flavor):** 2.5 mg/packet, 10 mg/packet. *In combination with:* metronidazole and clarithromycin in a compliance package (Losec 1-2-3 M); amoxicillin and clarithromycin in a compliance package (Losec 1-2-3-A) (both in Canada only); amoxicillin and rifabutin (Talicia); sodium bicarbonate (Konvomep, Zegerid [OTC]). See Appendix N.

NURSING IMPLICATIONS
Assessment
- Assess patient routinely for epigastric or abdominal pain and frank or occult blood in the stool, emesis, or gastric aspirate.
- Monitor bowel function. Report diarrhea, abdominal cramping, fever, and bloody stools to health care professional promptly as a sign of CDAD. May begin up to several wk following cessation of therapy.

Lab Test Considerations
- Monitor CBC with differential periodically during therapy.
- May cause ↑ AST, ALT, alkaline phosphatase, and bilirubin.
- May cause serum gastrin concentrations to ↑ during first 1–2 wk of therapy. Levels return to normal after discontinuation of omeprazole.
- Monitor INR and prothrombin time in patients taking warfarin.
- May cause hypomagnesemia. Monitor serum magnesium prior to and periodically during therapy.
- May cause false positive results in diagnostic investigations for neuroendocrine tumors due to ↑ serum

chromogranin A (CgA) levels secondary to drug-induced ↓ gastric acidity. Temporarily stop omeprazole at least 14 days before assessing CgA levels and consider repeating test if initial CgA levels are high.

Implementation

- Do not confuse Prilosec with Prozac or Pristiq. Do not confuse omeprazole with fomepizole.
- **PO:** Administer doses before meals, preferably in the morning. *DNC:* Swallow capsules and tablets whole; do not crush or chew. Capsules may be opened and sprinkled on cool applesauce, entire mixture should be ingested immediately and followed by a drink of water. Do not store for future use.
- *Powder for oral suspension:* Administer on empty stomach, at least 1 hr before a meal. Empty contents of 2.5-mg packet into 5 mL of water or contents of 10 mg packet into 15 mL of water. Stir. Leave 2–3 min to thicken. Stir and drink within 30 min. If material remains after drinking, add more water, stir and drink immediately. For patients with nasogastric or enteral feeding, suspend feeding for 3 hr before and 1 hr after administration. Empty packet contents into a small cup containing 5 mL of water for 2.5-mg dose or 15 mL water for 10-mg dose using a catheter tipped syringe. **Do not use other liquids or foods.** Immediately shake syringe and leave 2–3 min to thicken. Administer within 30 min. Refill the syringe with an equal amount of water. Shake and flush remaining contents from nasogastric or gastric tube into stomach.
- May be administered concurrently with antacids.

Patient/Family Teaching

- Instruct patient to take medication as directed for the full course of therapy, even if feeling better. Take missed doses as soon as remembered but not if almost time for next dose. Do not double doses.
- May cause occasional drowsiness or dizziness. Caution patient to avoid driving or other activities requiring alertness until response to medication is known.
- Instruct patient to notify healthcare professional of all Rx or OTC medications, vitamins, or herbal products being taken and consult health care professional before taking any new medications, especially St. John's wort.
- Advise patient to avoid alcohol, products containing aspirin or NSAIDs, and foods that may cause an increase in GI irritation.
- Advise patient to report onset of black, tarry stools; diarrhea; abdominal pain; or persistent headache to health care professional promptly.
- Instruct patient to notify health care professional of onset of black, tarry stools; diarrhea; abdominal pain; persistent headache; or if fever and diarrhea develop, especially if stool contains blood, pus, or mucus. Advise patient not to treat diarrhea without consulting health care professional.

- Rep: Advise females of reproductive potential to notify healthcare professional if pregnancy is planned or suspected, or if breastfeeding.

Evaluation/Desired Outcomes

- Decrease in abdominal pain or prevention of gastric irritation and bleeding. Healing of duodenal ulcers can be seen on x-ray examination or endoscopy.
- Decrease in symptoms of GERD and erosive esophagitis. Therapy is continued for 4–8 wk after initial episode.

---

ondansetron (on-dan-se-tron)
❦ Ondissolve ODF, ❦ Zofran,
❦ Zofran ODT, ~~Zuplenz~~
Classification
Therapeutic: antiemetics
Pharmacologic: 5-HT₃ antagonists

Indications
IV, PO: Prevention of nausea and vomiting associated with highly or moderately emetogenic chemotherapy. Prevention of postoperative nausea and vomiting. **PO:** Prevention of nausea and vomiting associated with radiation therapy.

Action
Blocks the effects of serotonin at 5-HT₃ receptor sites (selective antagonist) located in vagal nerve terminals and the chemoreceptor trigger zone in the CNS. **Therapeutic Effects:** Decreased incidence and severity of nausea and vomiting following chemotherapy, radiation, or surgery.

Pharmacokinetics
Absorption: IV administration results in complete bioavailability; 100% absorbed following oral administration.
Distribution: Unknown.
Metabolism and Excretion: Extensively metabolized by the liver (primarily by CYP3A4); 5% excreted unchanged by the kidneys.
Half-life: *Adults:* 3.5–5.5 hr; *Children 5 mo–12 yr:* 2.9 hr.

TIME/ACTION PROFILE (antiemetic effect)

ROUTE	ONSET	PEAK	DURATION
PO, IV	rapid	15–30 min	4–8 hr
IM	rapid	40 min	unknown

Contraindications/Precautions
Contraindicated in: Hypersensitivity; Orally disintegrating tablets contain aspartame and should not be used in patients with phenylketonuria; Congenital long QT syndrome; Concurrent use of apomorphine.
Use Cautiously in: Hepatic impairment; Abdominal surgery (may mask ileus); Phenylketonuria (orally disintegrating tablets contain phenylalanine); OB: Use during pregnancy only if potential maternal benefit justifies potential fetal risk; Lactation: Safety not established in

breastfeeding; Pedi: Safety and effectiveness not established in children ≤3 yr (PO) or <1 mo (parenteral).

Adverse Reactions/Side Effects

CV: myocardial ischemia, QT interval prolongation, TORSADES DE POINTES. **Derm:** STEVENS-JOHNSON SYNDROME, TOXIC EPIDERMAL NECROLYSIS. **GI:** constipation, diarrhea, ↑ liver enzymes, abdominal pain, dry mouth. **Neuro:** headache, dizziness, drowsiness, extrapyramidal reactions, fatigue, SEROTONIN SYNDROME, weakness.

Interactions

Drug-Drug: Use with **apomorphine** ↑ risk of severe hypotension and loss of consciousness; concurrent use contraindicated. **Carbamazepine**, **phenytoin**, and **rifampin** may ↓ levels. Drugs that affect serotonergic neurotransmitter systems, including **SSRIs, SNRIs, tricyclic antidepressants, MAOIs, fentanyl, lithium, buspirone, tramadol, methylene blue**, and **triptans**, ↑ risk of serotonin syndrome.

Route/Dosage

Prevention of Nausea/Vomiting Associated With Highly or Moderately Emetogenic Chemotherapy

PO (Adults): *Highly-emetogenic chemotherapy:* 24 mg 30 min prior to chemotherapy.

PO (Adults and Children >11 yr): *Moderately emetogenic chemotherapy:* 8 mg 30 min prior to chemotherapy and repeated 8 hr later; 8 mg every 12 hr may be given for 1–2 days following chemotherapy.

PO (Children 4–11 yr): *Moderately emetogenic chemotherapy:* 4 mg 30 min prior to chemotherapy and repeated 4 and 8 hr later; 4 mg every 8 hr may be given for 1–2 days following chemotherapy.

IV (Adults): 0.15 mg/kg (max dose = 16 mg) 30 min prior to chemotherapy, repeated 4 and 8 hr later.

IV (Children 6 mo–18 yr): 0.15 mg/kg (max dose = 16 mg) 30 min prior to chemotherapy, repeated 4 and 8 hr later.

Hepatic Impairment

PO, IM, IV (Adults): *Severe hepatic impairment:* Not to exceed 8 mg/day.

Prevention of Postoperative Nausea/Vomiting

PO (Adults): 16 mg 1 hr before induction of anesthesia.

IM, IV (Adults and Children >12 yr): 4 mg before induction of anesthesia or postoperatively.

IV (Children 1 mo–12 yr and >40 kg): 4 mg before induction of anesthesia or postoperatively.

IV (Children 1 mo–12 yr and ≤40 kg): 0.1 mg/kg before induction of anesthesia or postoperatively.

Hepatic Impairment

PO, IM, IV (Adults): *Severe hepatic impairment:* Not to exceed 8 mg/day.

Prevention of Nausea/Vomiting Associated With Radiation Therapy

PO (Adults): 8 mg 1–2 hr prior to radiation; may be repeated every 8 hr, depending on type, location, and extent of radiation.

Hepatic Impairment

PO, IM, IV (Adults): *Severe hepatic impairment:* Not to exceed 8 mg/day.

Availability (generic available)

Tablets: 4 mg, 8 mg, 24 mg. **Orally disintegrating tablets (contain aspartame) (strawberry flavor):** 4 mg, 8 mg. **Oral solution (strawberry flavor):** 4 mg/5 mL. **Solution for injection:** 2 mg/mL.

NURSING IMPLICATIONS

Assessment

- Assess patient for nausea, vomiting, abdominal distention, and bowel sounds prior to and following administration.
- Assess patient for extrapyramidal effects (involuntary movements, facial grimacing, rigidity, shuffling walk, trembling of hands) periodically during therapy.
- Monitor ECG in patients with hypokalemia, hypomagnesemia, HF, bradyarrhythmias, or patients taking concomitant medications that prolong the QT interval.
- Monitor for signs and symptoms of serotonin syndrome (mental status changes [agitation, hallucinations, delirium, coma], autonomic instability [tachycardia, labile BP, dizziness, diaphoresis, flushing, hyperthermia], neuromuscular symptoms [tremor, rigidity, myoclonus, hyperreflexia, incoordination], seizures, gastrointestinal symptoms [nausea, vomiting, diarrhea]). If symptoms occur, discontinue therapy.
- Assess for rash periodically during therapy. May cause Stevens-Johnson syndrome or toxic epidermal necrolysis. Discontinue therapy if severe or if accompanied with fever, general malaise, fatigue, muscle or joint aches, blisters, oral lesions, conjunctivitis, hepatitis, and/or eosinophilia.

Lab Test Considerations

- May cause transient ↑ in serum bilirubin, AST, and ALT levels.

Implementation

- First dose is administered prior to emetogenic event.
- **PO:** For orally disintegrating tablets, do not attempt to push through foil backing; with dry hands, peel back backing and remove tablet. Immediately place tablet on tongue; tablet will dissolve in seconds, then swallow with saliva. Administration of liquid is not necessary.

IV Administration

- **IV Push:** Administer undiluted (2 mg/mL) immediately before induction of anesthesia or postoperatively if nausea and vomiting occur shortly after surgery. *Rate:* Administer over at least 30 sec and preferably over 2–5 min.

- **Intermittent Infusion:** *Dilution:* Dilute doses for prevention of nausea and vomiting associated with chemotherapy in 50 mL of D5W, 0.9% NaCl, D5/0.9% NaCl, D5/0.45% NaCl. Solution is clear and colorless. Stable for 7 days at room temperature following dilution. *Concentration:* 1 mg/mL. *Rate:* Administer each dose over 15 min.

- **Y-Site Compatibility:** acetaminophen, aldesleukin, alemtuzumab, amifostine, amikacin, aminocaproic acid, amiodarone, anakinra, anidulafungin, argatroban, arsenic trioxide, ascorbic acid, atropine, azithromycin, aztreonam, benztropine, bivalirudin, bleomycin, bumetanide, buprenorphine, busulfan, butorphanol, calcium chloride, calcium gluconate, carboplatin, carmustine, caspofungin, cefazolin, cefotaxime, cefoxitin, ceftaroline, ceftazidime, ceftolozane/tazobactam, cefuroxime, chlorpromazine, ciprofloxacin, cisatracurium, cisplatin, cladribine, clindamycin, cyanocobalamin, cyclophosphamide, cyclosporine, cytarabine, dacarbazine, dactinomycin, daptomycin, daunorubicin hydrochloride, defibrotide, dexamethasone, dexmedetomidine, dexrazoxane, digoxin, diltiazem, diphenhydramine, dobutamine, docetaxel, dopamine, doxorubicin hydrochloride, doxorubicin liposomal, doxycycline, droperidol, enalaprilat, ephedrine, epinephrine, epirubicin, epoetin alfa, eptifibatide, erythromycin, esmolol, etoposide, etoposide phosphate, famotidine, fentanyl, filgrastim, floxuridine, fluconazole, fludarabine, folic acid, fosaprepitant, fosphenytoin, gemcitabine, gentamicin, glycopyrrolate, heparin, hetastarch, hydrocortisone, hydromorphone, idarubicin, ifosfamide, isavuconazonium, imipenem/cilastatin, irinotecan, isoproterenol, ketorolac, labetalol, LR, leucovorin calcium, levofloxacin, lidocaine, linezolid, magnesium sulfate, mannitol, melphalan, meperidine, mesna, methadone, methotrexate, metoclopramide, metoprolol, metronidazole, midazolam, mitomycin, mitoxantrone, morphine, moxifloxacin, multivitamins, mycophenolate, nafcillin, nalbuphine, naloxone, nicardipine, nitroglycerin, nitroprusside, norepinephrine, octreotide, oxacillin, oxaliplatin, oxytocin, paclitaxel, pamidronate, papaverine, penicillin G, pentamidine, pentostatin, phentolamine, phenylephrine, phytonadione, piperacillin/tazobactam, plazomicin, potassium acetate, potassium chloride, potassium phosphates, procainamide, prochlorperazine, promethazine, propranolol, protamine, pyridoxine, remifentanil, rocuronium, sodium acetate, sodium phosphates, succinylcholine, sufentanil, tacrolimus, tedizolid, telavancin, theophylline, thiotepa, tigecycline, tirofiban, tobramycin, topotecan, vancomycin, vasopressin, vecuronium, verapamil, vinblastine, vincristine, vinorelbine, voriconazole, zidovudine, zoledronic acid.

- **Y-Site Incompatibility:** acyclovir, allopurinol, aminophylline, amphotericin B deoxycholate, amphotericin B lipid complex, amphotericin B liposomal, ampicillin, ampicillin/sulbactam, azathioprine, blinatumomab, cefepime, chloramphenicol, dantrolene, ertapenem, foscarnet, furosemide, ganciclovir, gemtuzumab ozogamicin, indomethacin, lorazepam, meropenem/vaborbactam, methohexital, micafungin, milrinone, pantoprazole, pemetrexed, pentobarbital, phenobarbital, phenytoin, rituximab, sargramostim, sodium bicarbonate, thiopental, trastuzumab, trimethoprim/sulfamethoxazole.

Patient/Family Teaching

- Instruct patient to take ondansetron as directed.
- Advise patient to notify health care professional immediately if symptoms of irregular heartbeat, serotonin syndrome, or involuntary movement of eyes, face, or limbs occur.
- Rep: Advise females of reproductive potential to notify health care professional if pregnancy is planned or suspected or if breastfeeding.

Evaluation/Desired Outcomes

- Prevention of nausea and vomiting associated with emetogenic cancer chemotherapy.
- Prevention of postoperative nausea and vomiting.
- Prevention of nausea and vomiting due to radiation therapy.

---

oritavancin (oh-rit-a-**van**-sin)
Kimyrsa, Orbactiv
Classification
Therapeutic: anti-infectives
Pharmacologic: lipoglycopeptides

Indications

Acute bacterial skin and skin structure infections caused by or suspected to be caused by susceptible designated gram-positive bacteria.

Action

Binds to bacterial cell wall resulting in cell death. **Therapeutic Effects:** Bactericidal action against susceptible bacteria with resolution of infection. **Spectrum:** Active against *Staphylococcus aureus* (including methicillin-susceptible and resistant strains), *Streptococcus pyogenes*, *Streptococcus agalactiae*, *Streptococcus dysgalactiae*, *Streptococcus anginosus* (including *S. anginosus*, *S. intermidius*, and *S. constellatus*) and *Enterococcus faecalis* (vancomycin-susceptible strains only).

Pharmacokinetics

Absorption: IV administration results in complete bioavailability.
Distribution: Penetrates skin/skin structures.
Metabolism and Excretion: Slowly excreted unchanged in urine (5% in 2 wk) and feces (1% in 2 wk).
Half-life: 245 hr.

TIME/ACTION PROFILE (plasma concentrations)

ROUTE	ONSET	PEAK	DURATION
IV	rapid	end of infusion	at least 2 wk

Contraindications/Precautions

Contraindicated in: Hypersensitivity (cross-sensitivity with other glycopeptides may occur); Heparin use for 120 hr (5 days) following administration of oritavancin (causes false ↑ aPTT); Confirmed/suspected osteomyelitis (alternate treatment required).

Use Cautiously in: Severe renal impairment; Severe hepatic impairment; OB: Safety not established in pregnancy; Lactation: Safety not established in breastfeeding; Pedi: Safety and effectiveness not established in children; Geri: Older adults may have ↑ sensitivity to drug effects.

Adverse Reactions/Side Effects

CV: tachycardia. **GI:** ↑ liver enzymes, CLOSTRIDIOIDES DIFFICILE ASSOCIATED DIARRHEA (CDAD), nausea, vomiting. **Local:** infusion site reactions. **Neuro:** headache. **Misc:** HYPERSENSITIVITY REACTIONS (including anaphylaxis), infusion reactions (including infusion-related reaction resembling vancomycin flushing syndrome), limb/SUBQ abscess formation.

Interactions

Drug-Drug: ↑ risk of bleeding with **warfarin**; avoid concurrent use, if possible. Affects the activities of several CYP450 enzymes (careful monitoring of other **drugs metabolized by the CYP450 system** that have narrow therapeutic indices to assess for toxicity or ineffectiveness is recommended).

Route/Dosage

IV (Adults): 1200 mg single dose.

Availability

Lyophilized powder for injection (Orbactiv): 400 mg/vial. **Lyophilized powder for injection (Kimyrsa):** 1200 mg/vial.

NURSING IMPLICATIONS

Assessment

- Assess for infection (vital signs; appearance of wound, sputum, urine, and stool; WBC) at beginning of and during therapy.
- Obtain specimens for culture and sensitivity prior to therapy. First dose may be given before receiving results.
- Monitor bowel function. Diarrhea, abdominal cramping, fever, and bloody stools should be reported to health care professional promptly as a sign of CDAD. May begin up to 2 mo following cessation of therapy.
- Monitor for infusion-related reaction (resembling vancomycin flushing syndrome—flushing of upper

body, urticaria, pruritus, rash; chest pain, back pain, chills, tremor). May resolve with stopping or slowing infusion.

Lab Test Considerations

- Monitor hepatic function tests. May cause ↑ ALT, AST, and bilirubin.
- May cause hyperuricemia and hypoglycemia.
- Causes falsely ↑ aPTT for 120 hr after infusion. Avoid heparin administration during this time. Use a non-phospholipid dependent coagulation test such as Factor Xa assay if needed.
- Artificially prolongs PT and INR for up to 12 hr. May increase risk of bleeding with warfarin.

Implementation

- The two oritavancin products (*Orabactiv* and *Kimyrsa*) are different products. Directions for use are not interchangeable.

Orabactiv

- *Reconstitution:* Using three 400-mg vials, add 40 mL of sterile water for injection to each vial for a 10-mg/mL solution/vial. Swirl gently to avoid foaming and ensure powder is completely reconstituted. Solution is clear and colorless to pale yellow; do not administer solutions that are discolored or contain particulate matter. *Dilution:* Withdraw and discard 120 mL from 1000-mL bag of D5W. Withdraw 40 mL from each vial and add to D5W bag. Do not use 0.9% NaCl; may cause precipitation. *Concentration:* 1.2 mg/mL. Use within 6 hr at room temperature or 12 hr if refrigerated, including 3 hr infusion. *Rate:* Infuse over 3 hr.
- **Y-Site Incompatibility:** Do not mix with other solutions or medications. Flush line before and after infusion.

Kimyrsa

- *Reconstitution:* Add 40 mL sterile water for injection to 1200-mg vial. Swirl gently to avoid foaming. Solution is clear, colorless to pink; do not use solutions that are cloudy, discolored, or contain particulate matter. *Concentration:* 30 mg/mL. *Dilution:* Withdraw and discard 40 mL from a 250-mL IV bag of 0.9% NaCl or D5W. Withdraw 40 mL of the reconstituted vial and add to IV bag of 0.9% NaCl or D5W to bring volume to 250 mL. . *Concentration:* 4.8 mg/mL. Discard unused portion of reconstituted solution. Solution is stable for 4 hr at room temperature or 12 hr if refrigerated. Combined storage and infusion times should be within the stability times. *Rate:* Infuse over 1 hr.
- **Y-Site Compatibility:** 0.9% NaCl D5W.
- **Y-Site Incompatibility:** Drugs formulated at a basic or neutral pH., Do not use with other drugs. If same IV line must be used, flush line before and after infusion with 0.9% NaCl or D5W.

Patient/Family Teaching

- Explain purpose of oritavancin to patient.
- Instruct patient to notify health care professional if signs and symptoms of hypersensitivity reactions (rash, hives, dyspnea, facial swelling) occur.
- Instruct patient to notify health care professional immediately if diarrhea, abdominal cramping, fever, or bloody stools occur and not to treat with antidiarrheals without consulting health care professionals.
- Advise patient to notify health care professional of all Rx or OTC medications, vitamins, or herbal products being taken and to consult with health care professional before taking other medications.
- Rep: Advise females of reproductive potential to notify health care professional if pregnancy is planned or suspected or if breastfeeding.
- Instruct the patient to notify health care professional if symptoms do not improve.

Evaluation/Desired Outcomes

- Resolution of the signs and symptoms of infection. Length of time for complete resolution depends on the organism and site of infection.

---

oseltamivir (o-sel-tam-i-vir)
Tamiflu
Classification
Therapeutic: antivirals
Pharmacologic: neuraminidase inhibitors

Indications

Treatment of uncomplicated acute illness due to influenza infection in adults and children ≥2 wk who have had symptoms for ≤2 days. Prevention of influenza in patients ≥1 yr.

Action

Inhibits the enzyme neuraminidase, which may alter virus particle aggregation and release. **Therapeutic Effects:** Reduced duration or prevention of flu-related symptoms.

Pharmacokinetics

Absorption: Rapidly absorbed from the GI tract; 75% reaches systemic circulation as the active drug.
Distribution: Well distributed to tissues.
Metabolism and Excretion: Rapidly metabolized by the liver to oseltamivir carboxylate, the active drug. >99% excreted unchanged in urine.
Half-life: *Oseltamivir carboxylate:* 6–10 hr.

TIME/ACTION PROFILE (plasma concentrations)

ROUTE	ONSET	PEAK	DURATION
PO	unknown	unknown	12 hr

Contraindications/Precautions

Contraindicated in: Hypersensitivity; End-stage renal disease and not receiving dialysis.

Use Cautiously in: Renal impairment (↓ dose if CCr ≤60 mL/min); Hereditary fructose intolerance (75 mg of oral suspension contains 2 g of sorbitol); OB: Use during pregnancy only if potential maternal benefit justifies potential fetal risk; Lactation: Use during breastfeeding only if potential maternal benefit justifies potential risk to infant; Pedi: Children <2 wk (safety and effectiveness not established for treatment); children <1 yr (safety and effectiveness not established for prevention). Oral suspension contains sodium benzoate; avoid use in neonates.

Adverse Reactions/Side Effects

GI: nausea, vomiting. **Neuro:** abnormal behavior, agitation, confusion, delirium, hallucinations, insomnia, nightmares, SEIZURES, vertigo. **Resp:** bronchitis.

Interactions

Drug-Drug: May ↓ the therapeutic effect of **influenza virus vaccine**; avoid use 2 days prior to and 2 wk after vaccine administration.

Route/Dosage

Treatment of Influenza
PO (Adults and Children ≥13 yr): 75 mg twice daily for 5 days.
PO (Children 1–12 yr and >40 kg): 75 mg twice daily for 5 days.
PO (Children 1–12 yr and 23.1–40 kg): 60 mg twice daily for 5 days.
PO (Children 1–12 yr and 15.1–23 kg): 45 mg twice daily for 5 days.
PO (Children 1–12 yr and ≤15 kg): 30 mg twice daily for 5 days.
PO (Infants 2 wk–<1 yr): 3 mg/kg/dose twice daily for 5 days.

Renal Impairment
PO (Adults): *CCr 30–60 mL/min:* 30 mg twice daily for 5 days; *CCr 10–30 mL/min:* 30 mg once daily for 5 days; *CCr ≥10 mL/min and on hemodialysis:* 30 mg after each hemodialysis session (not to exceed 5 days); *CCr ≥10 mL/min and on peritoneal dialysis:* 30-mg single dose immediately after a dialysis exchange; *CCr <10 mL/min and not on dialysis:* Not recommended.

Influenza Prevention
PO (Adults and Children ≥13 yr): 75 mg once daily for ≥10 days.
PO (Children 1–12 yr and >40 kg): 75 mg once daily for 10 days.
PO (Children 1–12 yr and 23.1–40 kg): 60 mg once daily for 10 days.
PO (Children 1–12 yr and 15.1–23 kg): 45 mg once daily for 10 days.
PO (Children 1–12 yr and ≤15 kg): 30 mg once daily for 10 days.

Renal Impairment
PO (Adults): *CCr 30–60 mL/min:* 30 mg once daily for ≥10 days; *CCr 10–30 mL/min:* 30 mg every other day for ≥10 days; *CCr ≥10 mL/min and on hemodial-*

ysis: 30 mg after alternate hemodialysis sessions (treatment duration ≥10 days); *CCr ≥10 mL/min and on peritoneal dialysis:* 30 mg once weekly immediately after a dialysis exchange (treatment duration ≥10 days); *CCr <10 mL/min and not on dialysis:* Not recommended.

Availability (generic available)
Capsules: 30 mg, 45 mg, 75 mg. **Oral suspension (tutti-frutti flavor):** 6 mg/mL.

NURSING IMPLICATIONS
Assessment
- Monitor influenza symptoms (sudden onset of fever, cough, headache, fatigue, muscular weakness, sore throat). Additional supportive treatment may be indicated to treat symptoms.

Implementation
- Treatment with oseltamivir should be started as soon as possible from the first sign of flu symptoms within 2 days of exposure.
- Consider available information on influenza drug susceptibility patterns and treatment effects before using oseltamivir for prophylaxis.
- **PO:** May be administered with food or milk to minimize GI irritation.
- Use correct oral dosing device for measuring oral solution. Dosing errors have occurred due to oseltamivir dosing in mg and solution in mL. Make sure units of measure on prescription instructions match dosing device provided with the drug.
- If oral suspension is not available, capsules can be opened and mixed with flavored foods (regular or sugar-free chocolate syrup, corn syrup, caramel topping, light brown sugar dissolved in water). If correct dose and oral suspension are not available, pharmacist may compound emergency supply of oral suspension from 75 mg capsules.

Patient/Family Teaching
- Instruct patient to take oseltamivir as soon as influenza symptoms appear and to continue to take it as directed, for the full course of therapy, even if feeling better. Take missed doses as soon as remembered unless within 2 hr of next dose. Do not double doses.
- Caution patient that oseltamivir should not be shared with anyone, even if they have the same symptoms.
- Advise patient that oseltamivir is not a substitute for a flu shot. Patients should receive annual flu shot according to immunization guidelines.
- Advise patients to report behavioral changes (hallucinations, delirium, and abnormal behavior) to health care professional immediately.
- Advise patient to notify health care professional of all Rx or OTC medications, vitamins, or herbal products being taken and to consult with health care professional before taking other medications.

- Rep: Advise females of reproductive potential to notify health care professional if pregnancy is planned or suspected or if breastfeeding.

Evaluation/Desired Outcomes
- Reduced duration or prevention of flu-related symptoms.

☒ osimertinib (oh-si-mer-ti-nib)
Tagrisso
Classification
Therapeutic: antineoplastics
Pharmacologic: epidermal growth factor receptor (EGFR) inhibitors

Indications
☒ Metastatic epidermal growth factor receptor (EGFR) T790M mutation-positive non–small-cell lung cancer (NSCLC) in patients who have progressed on or after EGFR tyrosine kinase inhibitor therapy. ☒ First-line treatment of metastatic NSCLC in patients whose tumors have EGFR exon 19 deletions or exon 21 L858R mutations. ☒ Adjuvant therapy after tumor resection of NSCLC in patients whose tumors have EGFR exon 19 deletions or exon 21 L858R mutations.

Action
☒ Irreversibly binds to select mutant forms of EGFR (including T790M), resulting in inactivation of kinases that regulate proliferation and transformation; the T790M mutation is the most common mechanism of resistance to EGFR tyrosine kinase inhibitors. **Therapeutic Effects:** Decreased spread of NSCLC.

Pharmacokinetics
Absorption: Well absorbed following oral administration.
Distribution: Extensively distributed to tissues.
Protein Binding: 95%.
Metabolism and Excretion: Mostly metabolized by the liver via the CYP3A4 isoenzyme to two active metabolites; 68% excreted in feces (2% as unchanged drug); 14% excreted in urine (2% as unchanged drug).
Half-life: 48 hr.

TIME/ACTION PROFILE (plasma concentrations)

ROUTE	ONSET	PEAK	DURATION
Oral	unknown	6 hr	24 hr

Contraindications/Precautions
Contraindicated in: OB: Pregnancy; Lactation: Lactation.
Use Cautiously in: Congenital long QT syndrome, HF, electrolyte abnormalities, or taking QT interval prolonging medications; End stage renal disease (CCr <15 mL/min); Severe hepatic impairment; Rep: Women of

reproductive potential and men with female partners of reproductive potential; Pedi: Safety and effectiveness not established in children.

Adverse Reactions/Side Effects

CV: CARDIOMYOPATHY, cutaneous vasculitis, DEEP VEIN THROMBOSIS, QT interval prolongation. **Derm:** dry skin, nail disorders, pruritus, rash, ERYTHEMA MULTIFORME (EM), STEVENS-JOHNSON SYNDROME (SJS), urticaria. **EENT:** ↑ lacrimation, blepharitis, blurred vision, cataracts, dry eye, eye pain, keratitis. **F and E:** hypermagnesemia, hyponatremia. **GI:** constipation, diarrhea, nausea, stomatitis. **Hemat:** anemia, lymphopenia, NEUTROPENIA, THROMBOCYTOPENIA, APLASTIC ANEMIA. **Metab:** ↓ appetite. **MS:** back pain. **Neuro:** fatigue, headache, STROKE. **Resp:** cough, INTERSTITIAL LUNG DISEASE (ILD), PULMONARY EMBOLISM.

Interactions

Drug-Drug: Strong CYP3A4 inhibitors, including **itraconazole, nefazodone,** and **ritonavir,** may ↑ levels and the risk of toxicity; avoid concurrent use. **Strong CYP3A4 inducers,** including **carbamazepine, rifampin,** and **phenytoin,** may ↓ levels and its effectiveness; avoid concurrent use. May ↑ or ↓ **carbamazepine, cyclosporine, ergot derivatives, fentanyl, phenytoin,** or **quinidine**; avoid concurrent use. **QT interval prolonging drugs** may ↑ risk of torsades de pointes; avoid concurrent use. May ↑ levels of **P-glycoprotein substrates,** including **fexofenadine.** May ↑ levels of **breast cancer resistant protein substrates,** including **rosuvastatin.**
Drug-Natural Products: St. John's wort may ↓ levels and its effectiveness; avoid concurrent use.

Route/Dosage

PO (Adults): 80 mg once daily. In patients with metastatic disease, continue until disease progression or unacceptable toxicity. In adjuvant setting, continue until disease progression, unacceptable toxicity, or for up to 3 yr.

Availability

Tablets: 40 mg, 80 mg.

NURSING IMPLICATIONS

Assessment

- Assess for worsening respiratory symptoms (dyspnea, coughing, fever) during therapy; may indicate ILD or pneumonitis. If signs and symptoms occur, hold medication. If ILD confirmed, permanently discontinue osimertinib.
- Monitor cardiac status (ECG, electrolytes) periodically during therapy, especially in patients with congenital long QTc syndrome, HF, electrolyte abnormalities, or taking medications that prolong QTc interval. *If QTc interval >500 msec on at least 2 separate ECGs,* hold therapy until QTc interval is <481 msec or recovery to baseline if baseline is ≥481 msec, resume at 40-mg dose. *If QTc interval prolongation occurs with signs and symptoms of*

life-threatening arrhythmia, permanently discontinue therapy.
- Assess for signs and symptoms of cardiomyopathy (cardiac failure, pulmonary edema, ejection fraction decreased, stress cardiomyopathy) by echocardiogram, multigated acquisition (MUGA) scan prior to starting therapy and every 3 mo during therapy. *If asymptomatic and absolute decrease in left ventricular ejection fraction of 10% from baseline and below 50%,* withhold therapy for up to 4 wk. If improved to baseline, resume. If not improved to baseline, permanently discontinue. *If symptomatic HF develops,* permanently discontinue therapy.
- Monitor for symptoms of keratitis (eye inflammation, lacrimation, light sensitivity, blurred vision, eye pain, red eye) during therapy. If symptoms occur, refer to an ophthalmologist.
- Assess for skin rash during therapy. Hold osimertinib if SJS or EM are suspected. Discontinue osimertinib if SJS or EM are confirmed.

Lab Test Considerations

- Verify negative pregnancy test before starting therapy. ⧉ Patient selection is based on presence of EGFR exon mutations in tumor specimens. Information on FDA-approved tests for the detection of EGFR mutations is available at http://www.fda.gov/companiondiagnostics. Monitor CBC with differential before starting and periodically during therapy. May cause lymphopenia, thrombocytopenia, anemia, and neutropenia. *If ≥Grade 3 reaction occurs,* withhold osimertinib for up to 3 wk. *If improved to Grade 0–2,* resume at 80 mg or 40 mg daily. *If no improvement in 3 wk,* permanently discontinue osimertinib.
- May cause hyponatremia and hypermagnesemia.

Implementation

- **PO:** Administer once daily without regard to food.
- For patients with difficulty swallowing, disperse tablet in 60 mL (2 oz) of only non-carbonated water. Stir until tablet is completely dispersed and swallow immediately; do not crush, heat, or ultrasonicate during preparation. Rinse container with 4–8 oz of water and drink or administer through NG tube immediately. If administered via NG tube, disperse tablet in 15 mL of noncarbonated water, then use an additional 15 mL of water to transfer any residues in syringe. Administer 30 mL of solution via NG tube with 30 mL of water flushes.

Patient/Family Teaching

- Instruct patient to take osimertinib as directed. If dose missed, omit and take next dose as scheduled. Advise patient to read *Patient Information* prior to starting therapy and with each Rx dose refill in case of changes.
- Advise patient to notify health care professional if signs and symptoms of lung problems (worsening lung symptoms, trouble breathing, shortness of breath, cough, fever), heart problems (pounding or

racing heart, shortness of breath, swollen ankles or feet, lightheadedness, fainting), eye symptoms, rash (target lesions, severe blistering or peeling of skin), cutaneous vasculitis (multiple, non-blanching red papules on forearms, lower legs, or buttocks or large hives on trunk that do not go away within 24 hr and develop a bruised appearance), and aplastic anemia (new or persistent fevers, bruising, bleeding, pallor) occur.

- Instruct patient to notify health care professional of all Rx or OTC medications, vitamins, or herbal products being taken and consult health care professional before taking any new medications.
- Rep: May cause fetal harm. Caution females of reproductive potential to use effective contraception during and for 6 wk after final dose. Advise males with female partners of reproductive potential to use effective contraception during and for 4 mo after final dose. Advise females to avoid breastfeeding during and for 2 wk after final dose. May impair fertility in females and males.

Evaluation/Desired Outcomes
- Decreased spread of NSCLC.

---

ospemifene (os-**pem**-i-feen)
Osphena
Classification
Therapeutic: hormones
Pharmacologic: estrogen agonists/antagonists

Indications
Moderate to severe dyspareunia due to menopausal vulvar/vaginal atrophy. Moderate to severe vaginal dryness due to menopausal vulvar/vaginal atrophy.

Action
Has agonist (estrogen-like) effects on the endometrium of the uterus; effects are tissue-specific. **Therapeutic Effects:** Decreased dyspareunuia. Decreased vaginal dryness.

Pharmacokinetics
Absorption: Well absorbed following oral administration; food enhances absorption 2–3 fold.
Distribution: Extensively distributed to tissues.
Protein Binding: >99%.
Metabolism and Excretion: Mostly metabolized by the liver via the CYP3A4 and CYP2C9 isoenzymes; 75% excreted in feces, 7% in urine as metabolites; minimal amounts excreted unchanged in urine.
Half-life: 26 hr.

TIME/ACTION PROFILE (improvement in symptoms)

ROUTE	ONSET	PEAK	DURATION
PO	within 12 wk	unknown	unknown

Contraindications/Precautions
Contraindicated in: Hypersensitivity; Undiagnosed abnormal genital bleeding; History/suspicion of estrogen-dependent cancer; History of/current thromboembolic disorder, including deep vein thrombosis (DVT), pulmonary embolism (PE), MI, or stroke; Severe hepatic impairment; OB: Pregnancy; Lactation: Lactation.
Use Cautiously in: Patients with risk factors for cardiovascular disease, arterial vascular disease, or venous thromboembolism (including hypertension, obesity, family history, tobacco use, diabetes mellitus, history of DVT/PE, or systemic lupus erythematosus); Women with a uterus (estrogen use without a progestin ↑ risk of endometrial cancer); Known or suspected breast cancer.

Adverse Reactions/Side Effects
CV: DVT, MI. **Derm:** ↑ sweating, hot flush. **GU:** ENDOMETRIAL CANCER, genital/vaginal discharge. **MS:** muscle spasms. **Neuro:** STROKE. **Resp:** PE. **Misc:** HYPERSENSITIVITY REACTIONS (including angioedema).

Interactions
Drug-Drug: **Fluconazole** may ↑ levels and risk of toxicity; avoid concurrent use. **CYP3A4 or CYP2C9 inhibitors,** including **ketoconazole,** may ↑ levels and risk of toxicity. **Rifampin** may ↓ levels and effectiveness; avoid concurrent use. Avoid concurrent use of other **estrogens** or **estrogen agonist/antagonists** due to ↑ estrogen effects. May displace or be displaced by other **drugs that are highly protein bound.**

Route/Dosage
PO (Adults): 60 mg once daily.

Availability
Tablets: 60 mg.

NURSING IMPLICATIONS

Assessment
- Assess amount of pain during intercourse and vaginal dryness prior to and periodically during therapy.
- Determine methods previously used to treat dyspareunia.
- Assess BP before and periodically during therapy.
- Monitor for hypersensitivity reactions (angioedema, urticaria, rash, pruritus). If symptoms occur, discontinue ospemifene and treat symptomatically.

Implementation
- **PO:** Administer once daily with food.

Patient/Family Teaching
- Instruct patient to take ospemifene as directed. Advise patient to read *Patient Information* sheet before starting therapy and with each Rx refill in case of changes.
- Advise patient to report signs and symptoms of unusual vaginal bleeding, changes in vision or speech,

sudden new severe headaches, severe pains in chest or legs with or without shortness of breath, weakness, or fatigue promptly to health care professional immediately.

- Inform patient that ospemifene may cause hot flashes, vaginal discharge, muscle spasm, and increased sweating.
- Patients who still have a uterus should discuss addition of progestin with health care professional.
- Instruct patient to notify health care professional of all Rx or OTC medications, vitamins, or herbal products being taken and consult health care professional before taking any new medications.
- Advise patient to notify health care professional of medication regimen before treatment or surgery.
- Advise women to follow yearly exams (pelvic exam, breast exam, mammogram) to monitor for breast and uterine cancer.
- Caution patient that cigarette smoking, high BP, high cholesterol, diabetes, and being overweight during estrogen therapy may increase risk of heart disease.
- Ospemifene should not be taken during pregnancy or breastfeeding. Advise females of reproductive potential to notify health care professional if pregnancy is planned or suspected or if breastfeeding.
- Advise patient to discuss dose and need for ospemifene every 3–6 mo.

Evaluation/Desired Outcomes
- Decrease in pain during intercourse.
- Decreased vaginal dryness.

oxacillin, See PENICILLINS, PENICILLINASE RESISTANT.

oxaliplatin (ox-a-li-pla-tin)
~~Eloxatin~~
Classification
Therapeutic: antineoplastics
Pharmacologic: alkylating agents

Indications
Adjuvant treatment of stage III colon cancer in patients who have undergone complete resection of the primary tumor (in combination with 5-fluorouracil and leucovorin). Advanced colorectal cancer (in combination with 5-fluorouracil and leucovorin). **Unlabeled Use:** Ovarian cancer that has progressed despite treatment with other agents.

Action
Inhibits DNA replication and transcription by incorporating platinum into normal cross-linking (cell-cycle nonspecific). **Therapeutic Effects:** Death of rapidly replicating cells, particularly malignant ones.

Pharmacokinetics
Absorption: IV administration results in complete bioavailability.

Distribution: Extensive tissue distribution.
Protein Binding: >90% (platinum).
Metabolism and Excretion: Undergoes rapid and extensive nonenzymatic biotransformation; excreted mostly by the kidneys.
Half-life: 391 hrs.

TIME/ACTION PROFILE

ROUTE	ONSET	PEAK	DURATION
IV	unknown	unknown	unknown

Contraindications/Precautions
Contraindicated in: Hypersensitivity; Hypersensitivity to other platinum compounds; OB: Pregnancy; Lactation: Lactation.
Use Cautiously in: Renal impairment; HF, bradycardia, concomitant use of QT interval prolonging medications, hypokalemia, and hypomagnesemia; Rep: Women of reproductive potential and men with female partners of reproductive potential; Pedi: Safety and effectiveness not established in children; Geri: ↑ risk of adverse reactions in older adults.

Adverse Reactions/Side Effects
Adverse reactions are noted for the combination of oxaliplatin, 5-fluorouracil and leucovorin.
CV: chest pain, edema, QT interval prolongation, thromboembolism, TORSADES DE POINTES. **EENT:** visual abnormalities. **F and E:** dehydration, hypokalemia. **GI:** diarrhea, nausea, vomiting, abdominal pain, anorexia, gastroesophageal reflux, stomatitis. **Hemat:** anemia, NEUTROPENIA, THROMBOCYTOPENIA, leukopenia. **Local:** injection site reactions. **MS:** RHABDOMYOLYSIS, back pain. **Neuro:** fatigue, neurotoxicity, REVERSIBLE POSTERIOR LEUKOENCEPHALOPATHY SYNDROME. **Resp:** cough, dyspnea, PULMONARY FIBROSIS. **Misc:** ANAPHYLAXIS/ANAPHYLACTOID REACTIONS, fever.

Interactions
Drug-Drug: Concurrent use of **nephrotoxic agents** may ↑ toxicity. Concurrent use of QT interval prolonging medications, including **Class Ia antiarrhythmics** and **Class III antiarrhythmics** may ↑ risk of torsades de pointes.

Route/Dosage
IV (Adults): *Day 1:* 85 mg/m² with leucovorin 200 mg/m² at the same time over 2 hr, followed by 5-fluorouracil 400 mg/m² bolus over 2–4 min, then 5-fluorouracil 600 mg/m² as a 22-hr infusion. *Day 2:* leucovorin 200 mg/m² over 2 hr, followed by 5-fluorouracil 400 mg/m² bolus over 2–4 min, then 5-fluorouracil 600 mg/m² as a 22-hr infusion. Cycle is repeated every 2 wk. Dosage reduction/alteration may be required for neurotoxicity or other serious adverse effects.

Renal Impairment
IV (Adults): *CCr <30 mL/min:* ↓ dose on Day 1 to 65 mg/m².

Availability (generic available)

Lyophilized powder for injection: 50 mg/vial, 100 mg/vial. **Solution for injection:** 5 mg/mL.

NURSING IMPLICATIONS
Assessment

● Assess for peripheral sensory neuropathy. *Acute onset* occurs within hr to 1–2 days of dosing, resolves within 14 days, and frequently recurs with further dosing (transient paresthesia, dysesthesia, and hypoesthesia of hands, feet, perioral area, or throat). Symptoms may be precipitated or exacerbated by exposure to cold or cold objects; avoid ice during symptoms. May also cause jaw spasm, abnormal tongue sensation, dysarthria, eye pain, and a feeling of chest pressure. *Persistent* (>14 days) causes paresthesias, dysethesias, and hypoesthesias, but may also include deficits in proprioception that may interfere with daily activities (walking, writing, swallowing). Persistent neuropathy may occur without prior acute neuropathy and may improve upon discontinuation of oxaliplatin. **Adjuvant Therapy:** *For persistent Grade 2 neurosensory events that do not resolve,* reduce dose of oxaliplatin to 75 mg/m². *For patients with persistent Grade 3 neurosensory events,* consider discontinuing therapy. Do not alter infusional 5-fluorouracil/leucovorin regimen. *For Grade 4 neuropathy,* discontinue oxaliplatin. **Advanced Colorectal Cancer:** *For persistent Grade 2 neurosensory events that do not resolve, reduce dose to 65 mg/m². For patients with persistent Grade 3 neurosensory events,* consider discontinuing therapy. Do not alter infusional 5-fluorouracil/leucovorin regimen. *For Grade 4 neuropathy,* discontinue oxaliplatin.

● Assess for signs of pulmonary fibrosis (nonproductive cough, dyspnea, crackles, radiological; infiltrates). May be fatal. Discontinue oxaliplatin if pulmonary fibrosis occurs.

● Monitor for signs of anaphylaxis (rash, hives, swelling of lips or tongue, sudden cough). Epinephrine, corticosteroids, and antihistamines should be readily available.

● Monitor for signs and symptoms of reversible posterior leukoencephalopathy syndrome (headache, altered mental functioning, seizures, abnormal vision from blurriness to blindness, associated or not with hypertension).

● Monitor ECG in patients with HF, bradyarrhythmias, and electrolyte abnormalities and in patients taking drugs known to prolong the QT interval, including Class Ia and III antiarrhythmics.

● Monitor for signs and symptoms of GI adverse reactions (nausea, vomiting, diarrhea) during therapy. *If Grade 3 or 4 GI adverse reactions occur,* after recovery, reduce oxaliplatin dose to 75 mg/m² along with dose reduction of fluorouracil to 300 mg/m² as an IV bolus and 500 mg/m² as a 22-hr continuous infusion.

Lab Test Considerations

● Verify negative pregnancy test before starting therapy. Monitor WBC with differential, hemoglobin, platelet count, and blood chemistries (ALT, AST, bilirubin, and serum creatinine) at baseline and before each oxaliplatin cycle. **Adjuvant Therapy:** *For Grade 4 neutropenia or febrile neutropenia, or Grade 3 or 4 thrombocytopenia,* hold next dose until neutrophils ≥1.5 × 10⁹/L and platelets ≥75 × 10⁹/L. Reduce dose of oxaliplatin to 75 mg/m² and infusional 5-fluorouracil to 300 mg/m² bolus and 500 mg/m² 22-hr infusion. **Advanced Colorectal Cancer:** *After recovery from grade 3/4 gastrointestinal (despite prophylactic treatment), or grade 4 neutropenia, or febrile neutropenia, or grade 3/4 thrombocytopenia:* reduce dose of oxaliplatin to 65 mg/m² and 5-fluorouracil by 20% (300 mg/m² bolus and 500 mg/m² 22-hr infusion). Delay next dose until neutrophils ≥1.5 × 10⁹/L and platelets ≥75 × 10⁹/L. Monitor and correct electrolytes before starting therapy and periodically during therapy.

Implementation

● Monitor IV site frequently. Extravasation may result in local pain and inflammation that may be severe and lead to necrosis. If extravasation occurs, stop infusion immediately and disconnect (leave cannula/needle in place); gently aspirate extravasated solution (do not flush the line); remove needle/cannula; elevate extremity. Anti-inflammatory medication, such as high-dose oral dexamethasone, may reduce severity of the inflammatory reaction.

● Correct hypokalemia and hypermagnesemia before starting therapy.

● Premedicate patient with antiemetics with or without dexamethasone. Prehydration is not required.

IV Administration

● ***Reconstitution:*** Use only sterile water for injection or D5W to reconstitute powder. ***Concentration:*** To obtain final concentration of 5 mg/mL add 10 mL of diluent to 50-mg vial or 20 mL diluent to 100-mg vial. Gently swirl vial to dissolve powder. ***Dilution:*** Dilution with D5W (250 or 500 mL) is required prior to administration. Discard unused portion of vial. Solutions diluted in D5W are stable up to 6 hrs at room temperature or up to 24 hr under refrigeration. Solutions diluted for infusion do not require protection from light.

● **Intermittent Infusion:** Protect concentrated solution from light; do not freeze. ***Dilution:*** Must be further diluted with 250–500 mL of D5W. **Do not use 0.9% NaCl or any other chloride-containing solution for final solution.** Do not use aluminum needles or administration sets containing aluminum parts; aluminum may cause degradation of platinum compounds. May be stored in refrigerator for 24 hr or 6 hr at room temperature. Diluted solution is not light-sensitive. Do not administer solutions that are discolored or contain particulate matter. *Concentration:* 0.2–0.6 mg/mL. *Rate:* Administer oxaliplatin simultaneously with leucovorin in separate bags via Y-line over 120 min. Prolonging infusion time to 6 hr may decrease acute toxicities. Infusion times for fluorouracil and leucovorin do not need to change.

- **Y-Site Compatibility:** alemtuzumab, allopurinol, amifostine, amikacin, aminocaproic acid, aminophylline, amiodarone, amphotericin B deoxycholate, amphotericin B lipid complex, amphotericin B liposomal, ampicillin, ampicillin/sulbactam, anidulafungin, argatroban, atracurium, azithromycin, aztreonam, bivalirudin, bleomycin, bumetanide, buprenorphine, butorphanol, calcium gluconate, carboplatin, caspofungin, cefotetan, cefoxitin, ceftazidime, ceftriaxone, cefuroxime, chloramphenicol, ciprofloxacin, cisatracurium, cisplatin, clindamycin, cyclophosphamide, cyclosporine, cytarabine, dacarbazine, dactinomycin, daptomycin, daunorubicin hydrochloride, dexamethasone, dexmedetomidine, dexrazoxane, digoxin, diltiazem, diphenhydramine, dobutamine, docetaxel, dopamine, doxorubicin hydrochloride, doxorubicin liposomal, doxycycline, droperidol, enalaprilat, ephedrine, epinephrine, epirubicin, ertapenem, erythromycin, esmolol, etoposide, etoposide phosphate, famotidine, fentanyl, fluconazole, fludarabine, foscarnet, fosphenytoin, furosemide, gemcitabine, gemtuzumab ozogamicin, gentamicin, glycopyrrolate, granisetron, haloperidol, heparin, hetastarch, hydralazine, hydrocortisone, hydromorphone, idarubicin, ifosfamide, imipenem/cilastatin, insulin regular, irinotecan, isoproterenol, ketorolac, labetalol, leucovorin calcium, levofloxacin, levoleucovorin calcium, levorphanol, lidocaine, linezolid, lorazepam, magnesium sulfate, mannitol, meperidine, meropenem, mesna, methadone, methylprednisolone, metoclopramide, metoprolol, metronidazole, midazolam, milrinone, mitoxantrone, morphine, moxifloxacin, nafcillin, nalbuphine, naloxone, nicardipine, nitroglycerin, nitroprusside, norepinephrine, octreotide, ondansetron, paclitaxel, palonosetron, pemetrexed, pentamidine, phentolamine, phenylephrine, potassium acetate, potassium chloride, potassium phosphates, procainamide, prochlorperazine, promethazine, propranolol, rocuronium, sodium acetate, sodium bicarbonate, sodium phosphates, succinylcholine, sufentanil, tacrolimus, theophylline, thiotepa, tigecycline, tirofiban, tobramycin, topotecan, trimethoprim/sulfamethoxazole, vancomycin, vasopressin, vecuronium, verapamil, vinblastine, vincristine, vinorelbine, voriconazole, zidovudine, zoledronic acid.
- **Y-Site Incompatibility:** calcium chloride, cefepime, dantrolene, diazepam, sodium chloride-

Alkaline solutions, chloride-containing solutions. Infusion line should be flushed with D5W prior to administration of other solutions or medications.

Patient/Family Teaching

- Explain purpose of oxaliplatin to patient. Advise patient to read *Patient Information* before starting therapy and periodically during therapy in case of changes.
- Inform patients and caregivers of potential for peripheral neuropathy and potentiation by exposure to cold or cold objects. Advise patient to avoid cold drinks, use of ice in drinks or as ice packs, and to cover exposed skin prior to exposure to cold temperature or cold objects. Caution patients to cover themselves with a blanket during infusion, do not breathe deeply when exposed to cold air, wear warm clothing, and cover mouth and nose with a scarf or pull-down ski cap to warm the air that goes to their lungs, do not take things from the freezer or refrigerator without wearing gloves, drink fluids warm or at room temperature, always drink through a straw, do not use ice chips for nausea, be aware that most metals (car doors, mailbox) are cold; wear gloves to touch, do not run air conditioning at high levels in house or car, if hands get cold wash them with warm water. Advise health care professional of how you did since last treatment before next infusion.
- Instruct patient to notify health care professional immediately if signs of reversible posterior leukoencephalopathy syndrome, low blood cell counts (fever, persistent diarrhea, infection) or if persistent vomiting, signs of dehydration, cough or breathing difficulty, thirst, dry mouth, dizziness, decreased urination, signs of infection (fever, temperature of ≥100.5° F, cough that brings up mucus, chills or shivering, burning or pain on urination, pain on swallowing, sore throat, redness or swelling at intravenous site) or signs of allergic reactions occur.
- Rep: May cause fetal harm. Advise females of reproductive potential to use effective contraception during therapy and for at least 9 mo after final dose and to avoid breastfeeding during and for 3 mo after final dose. Advise males with female partners of reproductive potential to use effective contraception for 6 mo after final dose. May impair female and male fertility.

Evaluation/Desired Outcomes

- Decrease in size and spread of malignancies.

oxazepam (ox-az-e-pam)
~~Serax~~

Classification
Therapeutic: antianxiety agents, sedative/hypnotics
Pharmacologic: benzodiazepines

Schedule IV

Indications
Anxiety. Symptomatic treatment of alcohol withdrawal.

Action
Depresses the CNS, probably by potentiating GABA, an inhibitory neurotransmitter. **Therapeutic Effects:** Decreased anxiety. Diminished symptoms of alcohol withdrawal.

Pharmacokinetics
Absorption: Well absorbed following oral administration. Absorption is slower than with other benzodiazepines.

Distribution: Widely distributed. Crosses the blood-brain barrier. May cross the placenta and enter breast milk.

Metabolism and Excretion: Metabolized by the liver to inactive compounds.

Protein Binding: 97%.

Half-life: 5–15 hr.

TIME/ACTION PROFILE (sedation)

ROUTE	ONSET	PEAK	DURATION
PO	45–90 min	unknown	6–12 hr

Contraindications/Precautions
Contraindicated in: Hypersensitivity; Cross-sensitivity with other benzodiazepines may exist; Comatose patients or those with pre-existing CNS depression; Uncontrolled severe pain; Angle-closure glaucoma; Some products contain tartrazine and should be avoided in patients with known intolerance.

Use Cautiously in: Hepatic impairment (may be preferred over some benzodiazepines due to short half-life); History of suicide attempt or substance use disorder; Severe chronic obstructive pulmonary disease; Myasthenia gravis; OB: Use late in pregnancy can result in sedation (respiratory depression, lethargy, hypotonia) and/or withdrawal symptoms (hyperreflexia, irritability, restlessness, tremors, inconsolable crying, and feeding difficulties) in neonates; Lactation: Use while breast-feeding only if potential maternal benefit justifies potential risk to infant; Pedi: Children <6 yr (safety and effectiveness not established); Geri: Appears on Beers list. ↑ risk of cognitive impairment, delirium, falls, fractures, and motor vehicle accidents in older adults. If possible, avoid use in older adults.

Adverse Reactions/Side Effects
CV: tachycardia. **Derm:** rash. **EENT:** blurred vision. **GI:** constipation, diarrhea, drug-induced hepatitis, nausea, vomiting. **GU:** urinary problems. **Hemat:** leukopenia. **Neuro:** <u>dizziness</u>, <u>drowsiness</u>, confusion, depression, hangover, headache, impaired memory, paradoxical excitation, slurred speech. **Resp:** respiratory depression. **Misc:** physical dependence, psychological dependence, tolerance.

Interactions
Drug-Drug: Additive CNS depression with other **CNS depressants**, including **alcohol**, **antihistamines**, **antidepressants**, **opioid analgesics**, and other **sedative/hypnotics** (including other **benzodiazepines**). May ↓ the therapeutic effectiveness of **levodopa**. **Hormonal contraceptives** or **phenytoin** may ↓ effectiveness. **Theophylline** may ↓ sedative effects.

Drug-Natural Products: Concomitant use of **kava-kava**, **valerian**, **skullcap**, **chamomile**, or **hops** can ↑ CNS depression.

Route/Dosage
PO (Adults): *Antianxiety agent:* 10–30 mg 3–4 times daily. *Sedative/hypnotic/management of alcohol withdrawal:* 15–30 mg 3–4 times daily.

PO (Geriatric Patients): 5 mg 1–2 times daily initially or 10 mg 3 times daily; may be ↑ as needed.

Availability (generic available)
Capsules: 10 mg, 15 mg, 30 mg. **Tablets:** ❋ 10 mg, ❋ 15 mg, ❋ 30 mg.

NURSING IMPLICATIONS

Assessment
- Assess patient for anxiety and orientation, mood and behavior.
- Assess level of sedation (ataxia, dizziness, slurred speech) periodically during therapy.
- Assess regularly for continued need for treatment.
- Prolonged high-dose therapy may lead to psychological or physical dependence. Restrict the amount of drug available to patient.
- Assess risk for addiction, abuse, or misuse prior to administration and periodically during therapy.
- Geri: Assess CNS effects and risk of falls. Institute falls prevention strategies.

Lab Test Considerations
- Monitor CBC and liver function tests periodically during prolonged therapy.
- May cause decreased thyroidal uptake of ^{123}I and ^{131}I.

Implementation
- Medication should be tapered at the completion of therapy (taper by 0.5 mg every 3 days). Sudden cessation of medication may lead to withdrawal (insomnia, irritability, nervousness, tremors).
- **PO:** Administer with food if GI irritation becomes a problem.

Patient/Family Teaching
- Instruct patient to take oxazepam exactly as directed. Missed doses should be taken within 1 hr; if remembered later, omit and return to regular dosing schedule. Do not double or increase doses. If dose is less effective after a few wk, notify health care professional.

❋= Canadian drug name. ▓ = Genetic implication. ~~Strikethrough~~ = Discontinued. CAPITALS = life-threatening. <u>Underline</u> = most frequent.

- Inform patient that oxazepam is usually prescribed for short-term use; do not take more than prescribed or for a longer period than prescribed.
- Advise patient that oxazepam is a drug with known abuse potential. Protect it from theft, and never give to anyone other than the individual for whom it was prescribed. Store out of sight and reach of children, and in a location not accessible by others.
- Teach other methods to decrease anxiety, such as increased exercise, support group, relaxation techniques.
- May cause drowsiness or dizziness. Caution patient to avoid driving or other activities requiring alertness until response to medication is known.
- Advise patient to avoid the use of alcohol, other CNS depressants, including opioids, and to consult health care professional prior to the use of OTC preparations that contain antihistamines or alcohol. May cause overdose.
- Advise patient to notify health care professional of medication regimen prior to treatment or surgery.
- Rep: May cause fetal harm. Advise females of reproductive potential to use a nonhormonal method of contraception during use. Advise female patients to notify health care professional if pregnancy is planned or suspected or if breastfeeding. Monitor infants exposed to oxazepam during 2nd and 3rd trimester or immediately prior to or during childbirth for decreased fetal movement and/or fetal heart rate variability, "floppy infant syndrome," dependence, and symptoms of withdrawal (hypertonia, hyperreflexia, hypoventilation, irritability, tremors, diarrhea, vomiting); may occur shortly after delivery up to 3 wk after birth. Monitor breastfed infants for sedation and poor sucking. Encourage pregnant patients to enroll in the North American Antiepileptic Drug Pregnancy Registry by calling 1-888-233-2334; information is available at www.aedpregnancyregistry.org.
- Emphasize the importance of follow-up exams to monitor effectiveness of medication.
- Geri: Instruct patient and family how to reduce falls risk at home.

Evaluation/Desired Outcomes

- Decreased sense of anxiety.
- Increased ability to cope.
- Prevention or relief of acute agitation, tremor, and hallucinations during alcohol withdrawal.

BEERS

⚝ OXcarbazepine
(ox-kar-**baz**-e-peen)
Oxtellar XR, Trileptal
Classification
Therapeutic: anticonvulsants
Pharmacologic: carbamazepine analogues

Indications
Partial seizures (as monotherapy or adjunctive therapy). **Unlabeled Use:** Trigeminal neuralgia.

Action
Blocks sodium channels in neural membranes, stabilizing hyperexcitable states, inhibiting repetitive neuronal firing, and decreasing propagation of synaptic impulses. **Therapeutic Effects:** Decreased incidence of seizures.

Pharmacokinetics
Absorption: Rapidly absorbed after oral administration and rapidly converted to the active 10-hydroxy metabolite (MHD).
Distribution: Extensively distributed to tissues.
Metabolism and Excretion: Extensively converted to the active metabolite, MHD, which is then primarily excreted by the kidneys.
Half-life: *Oxcarbazepine:* 2 hr; *MHD:* 9 hr.

TIME/ACTION PROFILE (blood levels)

ROUTE	ONSET	PEAK	DURATION
PO	PO	rapid	4.5 hr†

†Steady-state levels of MHD are reached after 2–3 days during twice-daily dosing.

Contraindications/Precautions
Contraindicated in: Hypersensitivity to oxcarbazepine, carbamazepine, or eslicarbazepine.
Use Cautiously in: All patients (may ↑ risk of suicidal thoughts/behaviors); Renal impairment (dose ↓ recommended if CCr <30 mL/min); Severe hepatic impairment; Rep: Women of reproductive potential; OB: May be teratogenic (associated with oral clefts and cardiac abnormalities); levels of active metabolites may gradually ↓ during pregnancy which may ↑ seizure risk; use during pregnancy only if potential maternal benefit justifies potential fetal risk; Lactation: Use while breastfeeding only if potential maternal benefit justifies potential risk to infant; Pedi: Safety and effectiveness not established in children <2 yr (immediate-release) or <6 yr (extended-release); Geri: Appears on Beers list. May worsen or cause syndrome of inappropriate antidiuretic hormone (SIADH) secretion in older adults. Use with caution in older adults and closely monitor sodium concentrations when starting therapy or ↑ dose.
Exercise Extreme Caution in: ▓ Patients positive for HLA-B*1502 alleles (unless benefits clearly outweigh the risks) (↑ risk of serious skin reactions).

Adverse Reactions/Side Effects
Derm: acne, DRUG REACTION WITH EOSINOPHILIA AND SYSTEMIC SYMPTOMS (DRESS), rash, STEVENS-JOHNSON SYNDROME, TOXIC EPIDERMAL NECROLYSIS, urticaria. **EENT:** abnormal vision, diplopia, nystagmus. **Endo:** SIADH, hypothyroidism. **F and E:** ↑ thirst, hyponatremia. **GI:** abdominal pain, nausea, vomiting, dyspepsia. **Hemat:** lymphadenopathy. **Neuro:** ataxia, dizziness, drowsiness, gait disturbances, headache, tremor, ver-

tigo, cognitive symptoms, SEIZURES, SUICIDAL THOUGHTS. **Misc:** hypersensitivity reactions.

Interactions

Drug-Drug: May ↑ levels and risk of toxicity of **CYP2C19 substrates**, including **phenytoin** when used at doses greater than 1200 mg/day; may need to ↓ dose of phenytoin. May ↓ levels and effectiveness of **CYP3A4 substrates**, including **hormonal contraceptives**. **Carbamazepine**, **phenobarbital**, **phenytoin**, and **rifampin** may ↓ levels; monitor MHD levels during titration period; may need to adjust dose of oxcarbazepine.

Route/Dosage

(Immediate-release tablets and oral suspension can be interchanged at equal doses.).

PO (Adults): *Adjunctive therapy (immediate-release):* 300 mg twice daily, may ↑ by up to 600 mg/day at weekly intervals up to 1200 mg/day (up to 2400 mg/day may be needed); *Conversion to monotherapy (immediate-release):* 300 mg twice daily; may ↑ by 600 mg/day at weekly intervals, while other antiepileptic drugs are tapered over 3–6 wk; dose of oxcarbazepine should be ↑ up to 2400 mg/day over a period of 2–4 wk; *Initiation of monotherapy (immediate-release):* 300 mg twice daily, ↑ by 300 mg/day every 3rd day, up to 1200 mg/day. Maximum maintenance dose should be achieved over 2–4 wk; *Adjunctive therapy or monotherapy (extended-release):* 600 mg once daily for 1 wk; may ↑ by 600 mg/day at weekly intervals up to 1200–2400 mg once daily; *Concurrent use of strong CYP3A4 inducer (carbamazepine, phenobarbital, phenytoin, rifampin) (extended-release):* consider initiating therapy with 900 mg once daily.

PO (Children 2–16 yr): *Adjunctive therapy (immediate-release):* 4–5 mg/kg twice daily (up to 600 mg/day), ↑ over 2 wk to achieve 900 mg/day in patients 20–29 kg, 1200 mg/day in patients 29.1–39 kg and 1800 mg/day in patients >39 kg (range 6–51 mg/kg/day). In patients <20 kg, initial dose of 16–20 mg/kg/day may be used not to exceed 60 mg/kg/day. *Conversion to monotherapy (immediate-release):* 8–10 mg/kg given twice daily; may ↑ by 10 mg/kg/day at weekly intervals, whereas other antiepileptic drugs are tapered over 3–6 wk; dose of oxcarbazepine should be ↑ up to 600–900 mg/day in patients ≤20 kg, 900–1200 mg/day in patients 25–30 kg, 900–1500 mg/day in patients 35–40 kg. 1200–1500 mg/day in patients 45 kg, 1200–1800 mg/day in patients 50–55 kg, 1200–2100 mg/day in patients 60–65 kg, and 1500–2100 mg/day in patients 70 kg. Maximum maintenance dose should be achieved over 2–4 wk.

PO (Children 6–17 yr): *Adjunctive therapy or monotherapy (extended-release):* 8–10 mg/kg once daily (up to 600 mg/day) for 1 wk; may ↑ by 8–10 mg/kg/day at weekly intervals over 2–3 wk to achieve 900 mg/day in patients 20–29 kg, 1200 mg/day in patients

29.1–39 kg and 1800 mg/day in patients >39 kg; *Concurrent use of strong CYP3A4 inducer (carbamazepine, phenobarbital, phenytoin, rifampin) (extended-release):* consider initiating therapy with 12–15 mg/kg (max dose = 900 mg) once daily.

Renal Impairment

PO (Adults): *CCr<30 mL/min (immediate- and extended-release).* Initiate therapy at 300 mg/day and ↑ slowly to achieve desired response.

Availability (generic available)

Immediate-release tablets: 150 mg, 300 mg, 600 mg. **Extended-release tablets:** 150 mg, 300 mg, 600 mg. **Oral suspension (lemon-flavor):** 300 mg/5 mL.

NURSING IMPLICATIONS

Assessment

- Monitor closely for notable changes in behavior that could indicate the emergence or worsening of suicidal thoughts or behavior or depression.
- **Seizures:** Assess frequency, location, duration, and characteristics of seizure activity. Hyponatremia may increase frequency and severity of seizures.
- Monitor patient for CNS changes. May manifest as cognitive symptoms (psychomotor slowing, difficulty with concentration, speech or language problems), somnolence or fatigue, or coordination abnormalities (ataxia, gait disturbances).
- ⚭ Monitor for skin reactions (rash, erythema, urticaria, pruritus, fever, blistering). Patients with HLA-B*1502 alleles are at increased risk for Stevens-Johnson syndrome and toxic epidermal necrolysis. Discontinue oxcarbazepine if symptoms occur.
- Monitor for signs and symptoms of DRESS (fever, rash, lymphadenopathy, and/or facial swelling), associated with involvement of other organ systems (hepatitis, nephritis, hematologic abnormalities, myocarditis, myositis) during therapy. May resemble an acute viral infection. Eosinophilia is often present. Discontinue therapy if signs occur.

Lab Test Considerations

- Monitor ECG and serum electrolytes before and periodically during therapy. May cause hyponatremia. Usually occurs during the first 3 mo of therapy. May require dose reduction, fluid restriction, or discontinuation of therapy. Sodium levels return to normal within a few days of discontinuation.

Implementation

- Do not confuse oxcarbazepine with carbamazepine or oxaprozin.
- Implement seizure precautions as indicated.
- **PO:** Administer twice daily with or without food.
- Administer extended-release tablets on an empty stomach, at least 1 hr before or 2 hr after meals; giving with food increases risks of adverse effects.
  DNC: Swallow extended-release tablets whole, do not crush, break, or chew.

0

- Shake oral suspension well and prepare dose immediately after. Withdraw using oral dosing syringe supplied by manufacturer. May be mixed in a small glass of water just prior to administration or swallowed directly from syringe. Rinse syringe with warm water and allow to dry.

Patient/Family Teaching

- Instruct patient to take oxcarbazepine in equally spaced doses, as directed. Take missed doses as soon as possible but not just before next dose; do not double dose. Notify health care professional if more than 1 dose is missed. Medication should be gradually discontinued to prevent seizures. Instruct patient to read the *Medication Guide* before starting and with each Rx refill, changes may occur.
- May cause dizziness, drowsiness, or CNS changes. Advise patients to avoid driving or other activities requiring alertness until response to medication is known. Do not resume driving until physician gives clearance based on control of seizure disorder.
- Instruct patient to notify health care professional of all Rx or OTC medications, vitamins, or herbal products being taken and to consult with health care professional before taking other medications. Advise patient not to take alcohol or other CNS depressants, including opioids, concurrently with this medication.
- Advise patient and family to notify health care professional if thoughts about suicide or dying, attempts to commit suicide; new or worse depression; new or worse anxiety; feeling very agitated or restless; panic attacks; trouble sleeping; new or worse irritability; acting aggressive; being angry or violent; acting on dangerous impulses; an extreme increase in activity and talking, other unusual changes in behavior or mood occur.
- Instruct patient to notify health care professional of medication regimen before treatment or surgery. Rep: Advise females of reproductive potential to use an additional nonhormonal method of contraception during therapy and until next menstrual period. Instruct patient to notify health care professional if pregnancy is planned or suspected. Encourage patients who become pregnant to enroll in the North American Antiepileptic Drug Pregnancy Registry by calling 1-888-233-2334 or on the web at www.aedpregnancyregistry.org. Enrollment must be done by patients themselves.
- Advise patients to carry identification describing disease and medication regimen at all times.

Evaluation/Desired Outcomes

- Absence or reduction of seizure activity.

---

oxiconazole, See ANTIFUNGALS (TOPICAL).

OXYBUTYNIN (ox-i-byoo-ti-nin)
oxyBUTYnin (oral)
~~Ditropan~~, Ditropan XL
oxyBUTYnin (transdermal gel)
Gelnique
oxyBUTYnin (transdermal patch)
Oxytrol, Oxytrol for Women
Classification
Therapeutic: urinary tract antispasmodics
Pharmacologic: anticholinergics

Indications

Urinary symptoms that may be associated with neurogenic bladder including: Frequent urination, Urgency, Nocturia, Urge incontinence. Overactive bladder with symptoms of urge incontinence, urgency, and frequency.

Action

Inhibits the action of acetylcholine at postganglionic receptors. Has direct spasmolytic action on smooth muscle, including smooth muscle lining the GU tract, without affecting vascular smooth muscle. **Therapeutic Effects:** Increased bladder capacity. Delayed desire to void. Decreased urge incontinence, urinary urgency, and frequency and decreased number of urinary accidents associated with overactive bladder.

Pharmacokinetics

Absorption: Rapidly absorbed following oral administration, but undergoes extensive first-pass metabolism; extended-release tablets provide extended release. Transdermal absorption occurs by passive diffusion through intact skin and bypasses the first-pass effect.

Distribution: Highly bound (>99%) to plasma proteins. Widely distributed.

Metabolism and Excretion: Extensively metabolized by the liver via the CYP3A4 isoenzyme; one metabolite is pharmacologically active; metabolites are renally excreted with negligible (<0.1%) excretion of unchanged drug.

Half-life: 7–8 hr (oral and patch); 30–64 hr (gel).

TIME/ACTION PROFILE (urinary spasmolytic effect)

ROUTE	ONSET	PEAK	DURATION
PO	30–60 min	3–6 hr	6–10 hr (up to 24 hr with XL tablet)
TD-patch	within 24 hr	36 hr	3–4 days

Contraindications/Precautions

Contraindicated in: Hypersensitivity; Uncontrolled angle-closure glaucoma; Intestinal obstruction or atony; Urinary retention.

Use Cautiously in: Renal impairment; Hepatic impairment; Bladder outflow obstruction; Ulcerative colitis; Benign prostatic hyperplasia; Cardiovascular disease; Reflux esophagitis or gastrointestinal obstructive disorders; Patients with dementia receiving acetylcholinesterase inhibitors; Myasthenia gravis; Parkinson's disease (may worsen symptoms); Autonomic neuropathy (may worsen ↓ GI motility); OB: Safety not established in pregnancy; Lactation: Safety not established in breastfeeding; Pedi: Safety not established in children <18 yr (patch and gel) or <5 yr (oral); Geri: Poorly tolerated in older adults due to anticholinergic effects. Initiate treatment at lower doses.

Adverse Reactions/Side Effects

CV: chest pain, edema, tachycardia. **Derm:** ↓ sweating, *transdermal only:* application site reactions, hot flushes, pruritus. **EENT:** blurred vision, hoarseness. **GI:** <u>constipation</u>, <u>dry mouth</u>, nausea, abdominal pain, anorexia, diarrhea, dysphagia. **GU:** <u>urinary retention</u>, ↑ thirst. **Metab:** hyperthermia. **Neuro:** <u>dizziness</u>, <u>drowsiness</u>, agitation, confusion, hallucinations, headache. **Misc:** HYPERSENSITIVITY REACTIONS (including anaphylaxis and angioedema).

Interactions

Drug-Drug: ↑ anticholinergic effects with other **agents having anticholinergic properties**, including **amantadine**, **antidepressants**, **phenothiazines**, **disopyramide**, and **haloperidol**. Additive CNS depression with other **CNS depressants**, including **alcohol**, **antihistamines**, **antidepressants**, **opioids**, and **sedative/hypnotics**. **Ketoconazole**, **itraconazole**, **erythromycin**, and **clarithromycin** may ↑ effects. May ↓ the GI promotility effects of **metoclopramide**.

Route/Dosage

PO (Adults): *Immediate-release tablets:* 5 mg 2–3 times daily (not to exceed 5 mg 4 times daily) (may start with 2.5 mg 2–3 times daily in elderly). *Extended-release tablets:* 5–10 mg once daily; may ↑, as needed (in 5-mg increments) up to maximum dose of 30 mg/day.

PO (Children >5 yr): *Immediate-release tablets:* 5 mg 2–3 times daily (not to exceed 15 mg/day). *Extended-release tablets (children ≥6 yr):* 5 mg once daily; may ↑, as needed, (in 5-mg increments) up to maximum dose of 20 mg/day.

PO (Children 1–5 yr): 0.2 mg/kg/dose 2–3 times daily.

Transdermal (Adults): *Patch:* Apply one 3.9-mg system twice weekly (every 3–4 days); *Gel:* Apply contents of one sachet once daily.

Availability (generic available)

Immediate-release tablets: 2.5 mg, 5 mg. **Extended-release tablets:** 5 mg, 10 mg, 15 mg. **Syrup:** 5 mg/5 mL. **Transdermal gel:** 10%. **Transdermal patch:** 3.9 mg/24 hr^OTC.

NURSING IMPLICATIONS

Assessment

- Monitor voiding pattern and intake and output ratios, and assess abdomen for bladder distention prior to and periodically during therapy. Catheterization may be used to assess postvoid residual. Cystometry is usually performed to diagnose type of bladder dysfunction prior to prescription of oxybutynin.
- Geri: Assess geriatric patients for anticholinergic effects (sedation and weakness).

Implementation

- Do not confuse oxybutynin with oxycodone, Oxycontin, or oxymorphone.
- **PO:** Immediate-release tabs should be administered on an empty stomach; XL tablets may be given with or without food. *DNC:* Extended-release tablets should be swallowed whole; do not break, crush, or chew.
- **Transdermal patch:** Apply patch on same two days each wk (Sunday/Wednesday, Monday/Thursday) to hip, abdomen, or buttock in an area that is clean, dry, and without irritation. Patch should be worn continuously.
- **Transdermal gel:** Apply clear, colorless gel once daily to intact skin on abdomen (avoid area around navel), upper arms/shoulders, or thighs until dry. Rotate sites; do not use same site on consecutive days.

Patient/Family Teaching

- Instruct patient to take oxybutynin as directed. Take missed doses as soon as remembered unless almost time for next dose. Advise patient to read *Information for the Patient* prior to beginning therapy and with each Rx refill in case of new information.
- May cause drowsiness or blurred vision. Advise patient to avoid driving and other activities requiring alertness until response to medication is known.
- Advise patient to avoid concurrent use of alcohol and other CNS depressants while taking this medication.
- Instruct patient that frequent rinsing of mouth, good oral hygiene, and sugarless gum or candy may decrease dry mouth. Notify health care professional if mouth dryness persists >2 wk.
- Advise patient to stop taking oxybutynin and notify health care professional immediately if signs of angioedema and/or anaphylaxis (swelling of face, tongue, or throat; rash; dyspnea) occur.
- Inform patient that oxybutynin decreases the body's ability to perspire. Avoid strenuous activity in a warm environment because overheating may occur.
- Advise patient to notify health care professional if urinary retention occurs or if constipation persists. Discuss methods of preventing constipation, such as increasing dietary bulk, increasing fluid intake, and increasing mobility.
- Advise patient to notify health care professional of all Rx or OTC medications, vitamins, or herbal products

being taken and to consult with health care professional before taking other medications.

- Rep: Advise females of reproductive potential to notify health care professional if pregnancy is planned or suspected or if breastfeeding.
- Discuss need for continued medical follow-up. Periodic cystometry may be used to evaluate effectiveness. Ophthalmic exams should be performed periodically to detect glaucoma, especially in patients over 40 yr of age.
- **Transdermal patch:** Instruct patient on correct application and disposal of patch. Open pouch by tearing along arrows; apply immediately. Apply ½ patch to skin by removing ½ protective cover and applying firmly to skin. Apply 2nd half by bending in half and rolling patch onto skin while removing protective liner. Press patch firmly in place.
- Remove slowly; fold in half, sticky sides together, and discard. Wash site with mild soap and water or a small amount of baby oil.
- Advise patient referred for MRI to remove patch prior to test and give directions for replacing patch.
- **Transdermal gel:** Instruct patient on correct application of oxybutynin gel. Do not apply to recently shaved skin, skin with rashes, or areas treated with lotions, oils, or powders; may be used with sunscreen. Wash area with mild soap and water and dry completely before applying. Tear packet open just before use and squeeze entire contents into hand or directly onto application site of abdomen, arms/shoulders, or thighs. Amount of gel will be size of a nickel on the skin. Gently rub into skin until dry. Wash hands immediately following application. Avoid application near open fire or when smoking; medication is flammable. Do not shower, bathe, swim, exercise, or immerse the application site in water within 1 hr after application. Cover application site with clothing if close skin-to-skin contact at application site is anticipated.

Evaluation/Desired Outcomes

- Relief of bladder spasm and associated symptoms (frequency, urgency, nocturia, and incontinence) in patients with a neurogenic or overactive bladder.

REMS | HIGH ALERT

oxyCODONE (ox-i-koe-done)
Oxaydo, OxyCONTIN, ✦ Oxy IR, ✦ OxyNEO, Roxicodone, Roxybond, ✦ Supeudol, Xtampza ER
Classification
Therapeutic: opioid analgesics
Pharmacologic: opioid agonists, opioid agonists/nonopioid analgesic combinations

Schedule II

Indications
Moderate to severe pain. Pain severe enough to require daily, around-the-clock long-term opioid treatment and for which alternative treatment options are inadequate (extended-release) (children ≥11 yr should be tolerating a minimum opioid dose of ≥20 mg of oxycodone or equivalent for ≥5 days before initiating extended-release oxycodone therapy).

Action
Binds to opiate receptors in the CNS. Alters the perception of and response to painful stimuli, while producing generalized CNS depression. **Therapeutic Effects:** Decreased pain.

Pharmacokinetics
Absorption: Well absorbed from the GI tract.
Distribution: Widely distributed. Crosses the placenta; enters breast milk.
Protein Binding: 38–45%.
Metabolism and Excretion: Mostly metabolized by the liver by the CYP3A4 isoenzyme, and to a lesser extent by the CYP2D6 isoenzyme.
Half-life: 2–3 hr.

TIME/ACTION PROFILE (analgesic effects)

ROUTE	ONSET	PEAK	DURATION
PO	10–15 min	60–90 min	3–6 hr
PO-ER†	10–15 min	3 hr	12 hr

†Extended-release.

Contraindications/Precautions
Contraindicated in: Hypersensitivity; Some products contain alcohol or bisulfites and should be avoided in patients with known intolerance or hypersensitivity; Significant respiratory depression; Paralytic ileus; Acute or severe bronchial asthma; Acute, mild, intermittent, or postoperative pain (extended-release).
Use Cautiously in: Head trauma; ↑ intracranial pressure; Severe renal or hepatic disease; Hypothyroidism; Adrenal insufficiency; Alcoholism; Seizure disorders; Undiagnosed abdominal pain; Prostatic hyperplasia; Difficulty swallowing or GI disorders that may predispose patient to obstruction (↑ risk for GI obstruction); OB: Avoid chronic use; prolonged use of opioids during pregnancy can result in neonatal opioid withdrawal syndrome; Lactation: Use while breastfeeding only if potential maternal benefit justifies potential risk to infant; Pedi: Children <11 yr (safety and effectiveness of extended-release products not established); Geri: ↑ risk of respiratory depression in older adults; initial dose ↓ recommended.

Adverse Reactions/Side Effects
CV: orthostatic hypotension. **Derm:** flushing, sweating. **EENT:** blurred vision, diplopia, miosis. **Endo:** adrenal insufficiency. **GI:** constipation, choking, dry mouth, GI obstruction, nausea, vomiting. **GU:** urinary retention. **Neuro:** confusion, sedation, dizziness, dysphoria, euphoria, floating feeling, hallucinations, headache, un-

usual dreams. **Resp:** RESPIRATORY DEPRESSION (including central sleep apnea and sleep-related hypoxemia). **Misc:** physical dependence, psychological dependence, tolerance.

Interactions

Drug-Drug: Use with caution in patients receiving **MAO inhibitors** (may result in unpredictable reactions— ↓ initial dose of oxycodone to 25% of usual dose). Additive CNS depression with **alcohol, antihistamines,** and **sedative/hypnotics. Mixed agonist/ antagonist analgesics**, including **nalbuphine** or **butorphanol** and **partial agonist analgesics**, including **buprenorphine**, may ↓ oxycodone's analgesic effects and/or precipitate opioid withdrawal in physically dependent patients. Concurrent use of **CYP3A4 inhibitors** including **ritonavir, ketoconazole, itraconazole, fluconazole, clarithromycin, erythromycin, nefazodone, diltiazem, verapamil, nelfinavir,** and **fosamprenavir** ↑ levels and risk of opioid toxicity; careful monitoring during initiation, dose changes, or discontinuation of the inhibitor is recommended. Concurrent use with **CYP3A4 inducers** including **barbiturates, carbamazepine, efavirenz, corticosteroids, modafinil, nevirapine, oxcarbazepine, phenobarbital, phenytoin, rifabutin,** or **rifampin** may ↓ fentanyl levels and analgesia; if inducers are discontinued or dosage ↓, patients should be monitored for signs of opioid toxicity and necessary dose adjustments should be made. **CYP2D6 inhibitors** may ↑ levels. Use with **benzodiazepines** or other **CNS depressants** including other **opioids, non-benzodiazepine sedative/hypnotics, anxiolytics, general anesthetics, muscle relaxants, antipsychotics,** and **alcohol** may cause profound sedation, respiratory depression, coma, and death; reserve concurrent use for when alternative treatment options are inadequate. Drugs that affect serotonergic neurotransmitter systems, including **tricyclic antidepressants, SSRIs, SNRIs, MAO inhibitors, TCAs, tramadol, trazodone, mirtazapine, 5-HT₃ receptor antagonists, linezolid, methylene blue,** and **triptans,** ↑ risk of serotonin syndrome.

Route/Dosage

Larger doses may be required during chronic therapy. ER capsules are NOT bioequivalent to ER tablets.
PO (Adults ≥50 kg): *Opioid-naïve patients:* 5–10 mg every 3–4 hr initially, as needed. Once optimal analgesia is obtained, patients with chronic pain may be converted to an equivalent 24-hr dose given in 2 divided doses as extended-release tablets every 12 hr.
PO (Adults <50 kg): *Opioid-naïve patients:* 0.2 mg/kg every 3–4 hr initially, as needed. Once optimal analgesia is obtained, patients with chronic pain may be converted to an equivalent 24-hr dose given in 2 divided doses as extended-release tablets every 12 hr.

PO (Children ≥11 yr): 0.05–0.15 mg/kg every 4–6 hr as needed, as immediate-release product. Once optimal analgesia is obtained, patients with chronic pain may be converted to an equivalent 24-hr dose given in 2 divided doses as extended-release tablets every 12 hr.
Rect (Adults): 10–40 mg 3–4 times daily initially, as needed.

Hepatic Impairment
PO (Adults): ↓ initial dose by 50–66%.

Availability (generic available)

Immediate-release capsules: 5 mg. **Immediate-release tablets (Roxicodone):** 5 mg, 10 mg, 15 mg, 20 mg, 30 mg. **Immediate-release tablets (abuse-deterrent) (Oxaydo):** 5 mg, 7.5 mg. **Immediate-release tablets (abuse-deterrent) (Roxybond):** 5 mg, 15 mg, 30 mg. **Oral solution:** 5 mg/5 mL, 100 mg/5 mL (concentrated). **Extended-release capsules (abuse deterrent) (Xtampza ER):** 9 mg, 13.5 mg, 18 mg, 27 mg, 36 mg. **Extended-release tablets (abuse deterrent) (Oxycontin):** 10 mg, 15 mg, 20 mg, 30 mg, 40 mg, 60 mg, 80 mg. **Rectal suppositories:** ✹ 10 mg, ✹ 20 mg. *In combination with:* aspirin (Endodan, Percodan), acetaminophen (Endocet, Magnacet, Oxycet, Percocet, Xartemis XR); see Appendix N.

NURSING IMPLICATIONS
Assessment

● Assess type, location, and intensity of pain prior to and 1 hr (peak) after administration. When titrating opioid doses, increases of 25–50% should be administered until there is either a 50% reduction in the patient's pain rating on a numerical or visual analog scale or the patient reports satisfactory pain relief. A repeat dose can be safely administered at the time of the peak if previous dose is ineffective and side effects are minimal.
● Patients taking extended-release tablets may also be given supplemental short-acting opioid doses for breakthrough pain.
● An equianalgesic chart (see Appendix I) should be used when changing routes or when changing from one opioid to another.
● Assess BP, pulse, and respirations before and periodically during administration. If respiratory rate is <10/min, assess level of sedation. Physical stimulation may be sufficient to prevent significant hypoventilation. Dose may need to be decreased by 25–50%. Initial drowsiness will diminish with continued use. Monitor for respiratory depression, especially during initiation or following dose increase; serious, life-threatening, or fatal respiratory depression may occur. May cause sleep-related breathing disorders (central sleep apnea, sleep-related hypoxemia). Geri, Pedi: Assess geriatric and pediatric patients frequently; more sensitive to the effects of opioid anal-

gesics and may experience side effects and respiratory complications more frequently.

- Prolonged use may lead to physical and psychological dependence and tolerance. This should not prevent patient from receiving adequate analgesia. Patients who receive oxycodone for pain rarely develop psychological dependence. Progressively higher doses may be required to relieve pain with long-term therapy; may increase risk of overdose. Prolonged use of opioids should be reserved for patients whose pain remains severe enough to require them and alternative treatment options continue to be inadequate. Many acute pain conditions treated in the outpatient setting require no more than a few days of an opioid pain medicine.
- Assess bowel function routinely. Prevention of constipation should be instituted with increased intake of fluids and bulk, and laxatives to minimize constipating effects. Stimulant laxatives should be administered routinely if opioid use exceeds 2–3 days, unless contraindicated. Consider drugs for opioid induced constipation.
- Assess risk for opioid addiction, abuse, or misuse prior to administration. Abuse or misuse of extended-release preparations by crushing, chewing, snorting, or injecting dissolved product will result in uncontrolled delivery of oxycodone and can result in overdose and death. Abuse deterrent: *Oxaydo*, *Xtampza ER*, and *Oxycontin* are abuse deterrent formulations that are difficult to crush, and if crushed result in a gel.

Lab Test Considerations
- May ↑ plasma amylase and lipase levels.

Toxicity and Overdose
- If an opioid antagonist is required to reverse respiratory depression or coma, naloxone is the antidote. Dilute the 0.4-mg ampule of naloxone in 10 mL of 0.9% NaCl and administer 0.5 mL (0.02 mg) by IV push every 2 min. For children and patients weighing <40 kg, dilute 0.1 mg of naloxone in 10 mL of 0.9% NaCl for a concentration of 10 mcg/mL and administer 0.5 mcg/kg every 2 min. Titrate dose to avoid withdrawal, seizures, and severe pain.

Implementation
- *High Alert:* Accidental overdose of opioid analgesics has resulted in fatalities. Before administering, clarify all ambiguous orders. Pedi: Medication errors with opioid analgesics are common in pediatric patients; calculate doses carefully. Use appropriate measuring devices.
- Do not confuse short-acting oxycodone with long-acting Oxycontin. Do not confuse oxycodone with hydrocodone, oxybutynin, or oxymorphone. Do not confuse Oxycontin with MS Contin, oxybutynin, oxymorphone, or oxytocin.
- Explain therapeutic value of medication prior to administration to enhance the analgesic effect.

- Regularly administered doses may be more effective than prn administration. Analgesic is more effective if given before pain becomes severe.
- Coadministration with nonopioid analgesics may have additive analgesic effects and may permit lower doses.
- When converting from immediate-release to extended-release oxycodone administer total daily oral oxycodone dose once daily; dose of extended-release product can be titrated every 3–4 days (see Appendix I). To convert from another opioid to extended-release oxycodone, convert to total daily dose of oxycodone and then administer 50% of this dose as extended-release oxycodone once daily; can then titrate dose every 3–4 days. When converting from transdermal fentanyl, initiate extended-release oxycodone 18 hr after removing transdermal fentanyl patch; for each 25 mcg/hr fentanyl transdermal dose, the equianalgesic dose of extended-release hydromorphone is 12 mg once daily (should initiate at 50% of this calculated total daily dose given once daily).
- Oxycodone should be discontinued gradually after long-term use to prevent withdrawal symptoms. For patients on long-acting agents who are physically opioid-dependent, initiate the taper by a small enough increment (no greater than 10–25% of total daily dose) to avoid withdrawal symptoms, and proceed with dose-lowering at an interval of every 2–4 wk. Patients who have been taking opioids for briefer periods of time may tolerate a more rapid taper. Monitor frequently to manage pain and withdrawal symptoms (restlessness, lacrimation, rhinorrhea, yawning, perspiration, chills, myalgia, mydriasis, irritability, anxiety, backache, joint pain, weakness, abdominal cramps, insomnia, nausea, anorexia, vomiting, diarrhea, or increased blood pressure, respiratory rate, or heart rate). If withdrawal symptoms occur, pause the taper for a period of time or raise the dose of opioid analgesic to the previous dose, and then proceed with a slower taper. Also, monitor patients for changes in mood, emergence of suicidal thoughts, or use of other substances. A multimodal approach to pain management may optimize the treatment of chronic pain, as well as assist with the successful tapering of the opioid analgesic.
- **PO:** May be administered with food or milk to minimize GI irritation.
- Administer solution with properly calibrated measuring device.
- **Extended-Release:** *DNC:* Take 1 tablet at a time. Swallow extended-release tablet whole; do not crush, break, or chew. Taking broken, chewed, crushed, or dissolved extended-release tablets may lead to rapid release and absorption of a potentially fatal dose of oxycodone. Advise patients not to presoak, lick, or wet controlled-release tablets prior to placing in the mouth. Take each tablet with enough water to ensure complete swallowing immediately after placing in mouth. Dose of extended-release

preparations should be based on 24-hr opioid requirement determined with short-acting opioids then converted to extended-release form.

- Do not use *Oxaydo* for administration via nasogastric, gastric, or other feeding tubes as it may cause obstruction of feeding tubes.
- *REMS:* FDA strongly encourages health care professionals to complete a REMS-compliant education program that includes all the elements of the FDA Education *Blueprint for Health Care Providers Involved in the Management or Support of Patients with Pain,* available at www.fda.gov/OpioidAnalgesicREMSBlueprint. Information on programs can be found at 1-800-503-0784 or www.opioidanalgesicrems.com.
- Discuss availability of naloxone for emergency treatment of opioid overdose with the patient and caregiver and assess the potential need for access to naloxone, both when initiating and renewing therapy, especially if patient has household members (including children) or other close contacts at risk for accidental exposure or overdose. Consider prescribing naloxone, based on the patient's risk factors for overdose, such as concomitant use of CNS depressants, a history of opioid use disorder, or prior opioid overdose. However, the presence of risk factors for overdose should not prevent the proper management of pain in any patient.

Patient/Family Teaching

- *REMS:* Instruct patient on how and when to ask for and take pain medication. Do not stop taking without discussing with health care professional; may cause withdrawal symptoms if discontinued abruptly after prolonged use. Do not increase doses without discussing with health care professional, may lead to overdose. Discuss safe use, risks, and proper storage and disposal of opioid analgesics with patients and caregivers with each Rx. The Patient Counseling Guide is available at www.fda.gov/OpioidAnalgesic-REMSPCG.
- Advise patient that oxycodone is a drug with known abuse potential. Protect it from theft, and never give to anyone other than the individual for whom it was prescribed. Store out of sight and reach of children, and in a location not accessible by others.
- Educate patients and caregivers on how to recognize respiratory depression and emphasize the importance of calling 911 or getting emergency medical help right away in the event of a known or suspected overdose. Inform patients and caregivers about various ways to obtain naloxone as permitted by individual state naloxone dispensing and prescribing requirements or guidelines (by prescription, directly from a pharmacist, or as part of a community-based program).
- Advise patient to notify health care professional if pain control is not adequate or if severe or persistent side effects occur.

- Medication may cause drowsiness or dizziness. Advise patient to call for assistance when ambulating or smoking. Caution patient to avoid driving and other activities requiring alertness until response to medication is known.
- Advise patients taking *Oxycontin* tablets that empty matrix tablets may appear in stool.
- Advise patient to make position changes slowly to minimize orthostatic hypotension.
- Emphasize the importance of aggressive prevention of constipation with the use of oxycodone.
- Advise patient to avoid concurrent use of alcohol or other CNS depressants with this medication, may cause overdose.
- Instruct patient to notify health care professional of all Rx or OTC medications, vitamins, or herbal products being taken and consult health care professional before taking any new medications.
- Encourage patient to turn, cough, and breathe deeply every 2 hr to prevent atelectasis.
- Advise patient that good oral hygiene, frequent mouth rinses, and sugarless gum or candy may decrease dry mouth.
- Rep: Advise patient to notify health care professional if pregnancy is planned or suspected, or if breastfeeding. Inform patient of potential for neonatal opioid withdrawal syndrome with prolonged use during pregnancy. Monitor neonate for signs and symptoms of withdrawal symptoms (irritability, hyperactivity and abnormal sleep pattern, high pitched cry, tremor, vomiting, diarrhea, and/or failure to gain weight); usually occur the first days after birth. Monitor infants exposed to oxycodone through breast milk for excess sedation and respiratory depression. Chronic use may reduce fertility in females and males.
- Emphasize the importance of aggressive prevention of constipation with the use of oxycodone.

Evaluation/Desired Outcomes

- Decrease in severity of pain without a significant alteration in level of consciousness or respiratory status.

HIGH ALERT

oxytocin (ox-i-**toe**-sin)
Pitocin

Classification
Therapeutic: hormones
Pharmacologic: oxytocics

Indications

IV: Induction of labor at term. **IV:** Facilitation of threatened abortion. **IV, IM:** Postpartum control of bleeding after expulsion of the placenta.

Action

Stimulates uterine smooth muscle, producing uterine contractions similar to those in spontaneous labor. Has vasopressor and antidiuretic effects. **Therapeutic Effects:** Induction of labor. Control of postpartum bleeding.

Pharmacokinetics

Absorption: IV administration results in complete bioavailability.

Distribution: Widely distributed in extracellular fluid. Small amounts reach fetal circulation.

Metabolism and Excretion: Rapidly metabolized by liver and kidneys. Primarily excreted in urine as metabolites.

Half-life: 3–9 min.

TIME/ACTION PROFILE (reduction in uterine contractions)

ROUTE	ONSET	PEAK	DURATION
IV	immediate	unknown	1 hr
IM	3–5 min	unknown	30–60 min

Contraindications/Precautions

Contraindicated in: Hypersensitivity; Anticipated nonvaginal delivery.

Use Cautiously in: OB: 1st and 2nd stages of labor; slow infusion over 24 hr has caused water intoxication with seizure and coma or maternal death due to oxytocin's antidiuretic effect.

Adverse Reactions/Side Effects

Maternal adverse reactions are noted for IV use only. **CV:** *maternal:* hypotension; *fetal:* arrhythmias. **F and E:** *maternal:* hypochloremia, hyponatremia, water intoxication. **GU:** *maternal:* ↑ uterine motility, painful contractions, abruptio placentae, ↓ uterine blood flow. **Neuro:** *maternal:* COMA, SEIZURES; *fetal:* INTRACRANIAL HEMORRHAGE. **Resp:** *fetal:* ASPHYXIA, hypoxia. **Misc:** hypersensitivity reactions.

Interactions

Drug-Drug: Severe hypertension may occur if oxytocin follows administration of **vasopressors**.

Route/Dosage

Induction/Stimulation of Labor

IV (Adults): 0.5–1 milliunits/min; ↑ by 1–2 milliunits/min every 30–60 min until desired contraction pattern established; dose may be ↓ after desired frequency of contractions is reached and labor has progressed to 5–6 cm dilation.

Postpartum Hemorrhage

IV (Adults): 10 units infused at 20–40 milliunits/min. **IM (Adults):** 10 units after delivery of placenta.

Incomplete/Inevitable Abortion

IV (Adults): 10 units at a rate of 20–40 milliunits/min.

Availability (generic available)

Solution for injection: 10 units/mL.

NURSING IMPLICATIONS

Assessment

- Fetal maturity, presentation, and pelvic adequacy should be assessed prior to administration of oxytocin for induction of labor.
- Assess character, frequency, and duration of uterine contractions; resting uterine tone; and fetal heart rate frequently throughout administration. If contractions occur <2 min apart and are >50–65 mm Hg on monitor, if they last 60–90 sec or longer, or if a significant change in fetal heart rate develops, stop infusion and turn patient on her left side to prevent fetal anoxia. Notify health care professional immediately.
- Monitor maternal BP and pulse frequently and fetal heart rate continuously throughout administration.
- This drug occasionally causes water intoxication. Monitor patient for signs and symptoms (drowsiness, listlessness, confusion, headache, anuria) and notify physician or other health care professional if they occur.

Lab Test Considerations

- Monitor maternal electrolytes. Water retention may result in hypochloremia or hyponatremia.

Implementation

- Do not confuse oxytocin with Oxycontin.
- Do not administer oxytocin simultaneously by more than one route.
- **IM:** Ten units (1 mL) of oxytocin can be given after delivery of the placenta.

IV Administration

- **Continuous Infusion:** Rotate infusion container to ensure thorough mixing. Store solution in refrigerator, but do not freeze.
- Infuse via infusion pump for accurate dose. Oxytocin should be connected via Y-site injection to an IV of 0.9% NaCl for use during adverse reactions.
- Magnesium sulfate should be available if needed for relaxation of myometrium.
- Dose of oxytocin is determined by uterine response.
- **Induction of Labor:** *Dilution:* Dilute 1 mL (10 units) in 1 L of compatible infusion fluid (0.9% NaCl, D5W, or LR). *Concentration:* 10 milliunits/mL. *Rate:* Begin infusion at 0.5–2 milliunits/min (0.05–0.2 mL); increase in increments of 1–2 milliunits/min at 15–30-min intervals until contractions simulate normal labor. Gradually increase dose at 30–60 min intervals in increments of 1–2 milliunits/min until the desired contraction pattern has been established. Once desired frequency of contractions has been reached and labor has progressed to 5–6 cm dilation, dose may be reduced by similar increments.
- **Postpartum Bleeding:** *Dilution:* For control of postpartum bleeding, dilute 1–4 mL (10–40 units) in 1 L of compatible infusion fluid. *Concentration:* 10–40 milliunits/mL. *Rate:* Begin infusion at

a rate of 20–40 milliunits/min to control uterine atony. Adjust rate as indicated.

- **Incomplete or Inevitable Abortion:** *Dilution:* For incomplete or inevitable abortion, dilute 1 mL (10 units) in 500 mL of 0.9% NaCl or D5W. *Concentration:* 20 milliunits/mL. *Rate:* Infuse at a rate of 20–40 milliunits/min. Total dose should not exceed 30 units in a 12-hr period due to risk of water intoxication.

- **Y-Site Compatibility:** acetaminophen, acyclovir, allopurinol, amikacin, aminocaproic acid, aminophylline, amphotericin B liposomal, anidulafungin, argatroban, ascorbic acid, atropine, azathioprine, azithromycin, aztreonam, benztropine, bivalirudin, bumetanide, buprenorphine, butorphanol, calcium chloride, calcium gluconate, caspofungin, cefazolin, cefepime, cefotaxime, cefotetan, cefoxitin, ceftazidime, ceftriaxone, cefuroxime, chloramphenicol, ciprofloxacin, cisatracurium, clindamycin, cyclophosphamide, cyclosporine, daptomycin, dexamethasone, dexmedetomidine, digoxin, diphenhydramine, dobutamine, dopamine, doxycycline, droperidol, enalaprilat, ephedrine, epinephrine, epoetin alfa, eptifibatide, ertapenem, erythromycin, esmolol, famotidine, fentanyl, fluconazole, folic acid, foscarnet, fosphenytoin, furosemide, ganciclovir, gentamicin, glycopyrrolate, granisetron, heparin, hydrocortisone sodium succinate, hydromorphone, imipenem/cilastatin, isoproterenol, ketamine, ketorolac, labetalol, LR, leucovorin calcium, levofloxacin, lidocaine, linezolid, lorazepam, magnesium sulfate, mannitol, meperidine, meropenem, methadone, methylprednisolone, metoclopramide, metoprolol, metronidazole, midazolam, milrinone, morphine, moxifloxacin, multivitamins, mycophenolate, nafcillin, nalbuphine, naloxone, nicardipine, nitroglycerin, nitroprusside, norepinephrine, ondansetron, oxacillin, palonosetron, pamidronate, papaverine, penicillin G, pentamidine, pentobarbital, phenobarbital, phentolamine, phenylephrine, phytonadione, piperacillin/tazobactam, potassium acetate, potassium chloride, potassium phosphate, procainamide, prochlorperazine, promethazine, propranolol, protamine, pyridoxine, sodium acetate, sodium bicarbonate, sodium phosphate, succinylcholine, sufentanil, tacrolimus, theophylline, thiamine, tigecycline, tirofiban, tobramycin, vancomycin, vasopressin, verapamil, voriconazole, zidovudine, zoledronic acid.

- **Y-Site Incompatibility:** dantrolene, diazepam, dimenhydrinate, indomethacin, methohexital, phenytoin, trimethoprim/sulfamethoxazole.

- **Solution Compatibility:** dextrose/Ringer's or lactated Ringer's combinations, dextrose/saline combinations, Ringer's or lactated Ringer's injection, D5W, D10W, 0.45% NaCl, 0.9% NaCl.

Patient/Family Teaching

- Explain purpose of oxytocin to patient.
- Advise patient to expect contractions similar to menstrual cramps after administration has started.

Evaluation/Desired Outcomes

- Onset of effective contractions.
- Increase in uterine tone.
- Reduction in postpartum bleeding.

PACLitaxel (pak-li-tax-el)
~~Taxol~~

PACLitaxel protein-bound particles (albumin-bound)
Abraxane
Classification
Therapeutic: antineoplastics
Pharmacologic: taxoids

Indications
Paclitaxel: Advanced ovarian cancer (in combination with cisplatin). Non–small-cell lung cancer (NSCLC) when potentially curative surgery and/or radiation therapy is not an option. Metastatic breast cancer unresponsive to other therapy. Node-positive breast cancer when administered sequentially to standard combination chemotherapy that includes doxorubicin. Treatment of AIDS-related Kaposi's sarcoma. **Paclitaxel (albumin-bound):** Metastatic breast cancer after treatment failure or relapse where therapy included an anthracycline. Locally advanced or metastatic NSCLC when potentially curative surgery or radiation therapy is not an option (in combination with carboplatin). Metastatic pancreatic adenocarcinoma (in combination with gemcitabine).

Action
Interferes with the normal cellular microtubule function that is required for interphase and mitosis. **Therapeutic Effects:** Death of rapidly replicating cells, particularly malignant ones.

Pharmacokinetics
Absorption: IV administration results in complete bioavailability.
Distribution: Cross the placenta.
Protein Binding: 89–98%.
Metabolism and Excretion: Highly metabolized by the liver primarily by the CYP2C8 and CYP3A4 isoenzymes; <10% excreted unchanged in urine.
Half-life: *Paclitaxel:* 13–52 hr; *Paclitaxel protein-bound particles (albumin-bound):* 27 hr.

TIME/ACTION PROFILE (effect on WBCs)

ROUTE	ONSET	PEAK	DURATION
IV	unknown	11 days	3 wk

Contraindications/Precautions
Contraindicated in: Hypersensitivity to paclitaxel, other taxanes, or castor oil (paclitaxel); Severe hypersensitivity to paclitaxel protein-bound particles (paclitaxel protein-bound particles); AST >10× upper limit of normal (ULN) or total bilirubin >5× ULN (paclitaxel protein-bound particles); Moderate or severe hepatic impairment (pancreatic adenocarcinoma only for paclitaxel protein-bound particles); Known alcohol intolerance; Neutrophil count ≤1500/mm³ (for patients with ovarian, lung, breast, or pancreatic cancer) or

≤1000/mm³ (for patients with AIDS-related Kaposi's sarcoma); OB: Pregnancy; Lactation: Lactation.
Use Cautiously in: Moderate or severe hepatic impairment (↓ dose); Active infection; ↓ bone marrow reserve; Rep: Women of reproductive potential and men with female partners of reproductive potential; Pedi: Safety and effectiveness not established in children; Geri: Older adults may have ↑ risk of adverse reactions.

Adverse Reactions/Side Effects
CV: ECG changes, edema, hypotension, bradycardia. **Derm:** alopecia, STEVENS-JOHNSON SYNDROME, TOXIC EPIDERMAL NECROLYSIS. **GI:** ↑ liver enzymes, diarrhea, mucositis, nausea, vomiting, pancreatitis. **GU:** renal failure. **Hemat:** anemia, NEUTROPENIA, thrombocytopenia. **Local:** injection site reactions. **MS:** arthralgia, myalgia. **Neuro:** peripheral neuropathy, dizziness, headache, seizures. **Resp:** cough, dyspnea, interstitial pneumonia, PULMONARY EMBOLISM, PULMONARY FIBROSIS. **Misc:** HYPERSENSITIVITY REACTIONS (including anaphylaxis), SEPSIS.

Interactions
Drug-Drug: CYP3A4 inhibitors, including **atazanavir, clarithromycin, itraconazole, ketoconazole, nefazodone, nelfinavir,** and **ritonavir,** may ↑ levels and risk of toxicity; concurrent use should be undertaken with caution. **CYP3A4 inducers,** including **carbamazepine, rifampin,** and **phenytoin,** may ↓ levels and ↑ risk of treatment failure; concurrent use should be undertaken with caution. **Gemfibrozil** may ↑ levels and risk of toxicity; concurrent use should be undertaken with caution. ↑ risk of myelosuppression with other **antineoplastics** or **radiation therapy.** Myelosuppression ↑ when given after **cisplatin.** May ↑ levels and toxicity of **doxorubicin.** May ↓ antibody response to and ↑ risk of adverse reactions from **live-virus vaccines.**

Route/Dosage
Paclitaxel

Ovarian Cancer
IV (Adults): *Previously untreated patients:* 175 mg/m² over 3 hr every 3 wk or 135 mg/m² over 24 hr every 3 wk, followed by cisplatin; *Previously treated patients:* 135 mg/m² or 175 mg/m² over 3 hr every 3 wk.

Breast Cancer
IV (Adults): *Adjuvant treatment of node-positive breast cancer:* 175 mg/m² over 3 hr every 3 wk for 4 courses administered sequentially to doxorubicin-containing combination chemotherapy; *Failure of initial therapy for metastatic disease or relapse within 6 mo of adjuvant therapy:* 175 mg/m² over 3 hr every 3 wk.

NSCLC
IV (Adults): 135 mg/m² over 24 hr every 3 wk, followed by cisplatin.

AIDS-Related Kaposi's Sarcoma

IV (Adults): 135 mg/m² over 3 hr every 3 wk *or* 100 mg/m² over 3 hr every 2 wk (dose ↓/adjustment may be necessary in patients with advanced HIV infection).

Paclitaxel Protein-Bound Particles (albumin-bound)

Breast Cancer

IV (Adults): 260 mg/m² over 30 min every 3 wk.

Hepatic Impairment

IV (Adults): *Moderate hepatic impairment (AST levels <10 × ULN and bilirubin levels 1.51–3 × ULN):* 200 mg/m² over 30 min every 3 wk; dose may be ↑ to 260 mg/m² for the 3rd course based on individual tolerance; *Severe hepatic impairment (AST levels <10 × ULN and bilirubin levels 3.01–5 × ULN):* 200 mg/m² over 30 min every 3 wk; dose may be ↑ to 260 mg/m² for the 3rd course based on individual tolerance; *Severe hepatic impairment (AST levels >10 × ULN or bilirubin levels >5 × ULN):* Avoid use.

NSCLC

IV (Adults): 100 mg/m² over 30 min on Days 1, 8, and 15 of each 21-day cycle.

Hepatic Impairment

IV (Adults): *Moderate hepatic impairment (AST levels <10 × ULN and bilirubin levels 1.51–3 × ULN):* 80 mg/m² over 30 min on Days 1, 8, and 15 of each 21-day cycle; dose may be ↑ to 100 mg/m² for the 3rd course based on individual tolerance; *Severe hepatic impairment (AST levels <10 × ULN and bilirubin levels 3.01–5 × ULN):* 80 mg/m² over 30 min on Days 1, 8, and 15 of each 21-day cycle; dose may be ↑ to 100 mg/m² for the 3rd course based on individual tolerance; *Severe hepatic impairment (AST levels >10 × ULN or bilirubin levels >5 × ULN):* Avoid use.

Pancreatic Adenocarcinoma

IV (Adults): 125 mg/m² over 30–40 min on Days 1, 8, and 15 of each 28-day cycle.

Hepatic Impairment

IV (Adults): *Moderate or severe hepatic impairment:* Avoid use.

Availability

Paclitaxel (generic available)

Solution for injection: 6 mg/mL.

Paclitaxel Protein-Bound Particles (albumin-bound)

Lyophilized powder for injection: 100 mg/vial.

NURSING IMPLICATIONS

Assessment

- Monitor vital signs frequently, especially during first hr of the infusion.
- Monitor cardiovascular status especially during first 3 hr of infusion. Hypotension and bradycardia are

common but usually do not require treatment. Continuous ECG monitoring is recommended only for patients with serious underlying conduction abnormalities or those concurrently taking doxorubicin.

- Monitor for bone marrow depression. Assess for bleeding (bleeding gums, bruising, petechiae, guaiac stools, urine, and emesis) and avoid IM injections and taking rectal temperatures if platelet count is low. Apply pressure to venipuncture sites for 10 min. Assess for signs of infection during neutropenia. Anemia may occur. Monitor for dyspnea and orthostatic hypotension. Granulocyte-colony stimulating factor (G-CSF) may be used if necessary.

- Monitor intake and output, appetite, and nutritional intake. Paclitaxel causes nausea and vomiting in 50% of patients. Prophylactic antiemetics may be used. Adjust diet as tolerated to help maintain fluid and electrolyte balance and nutritional status.

- Assess patient for arthralgia and myalgia, which usually begin 2–3 days after therapy and resolve within 5 days. Pain is usually relieved by nonopioid analgesics but may be severe enough to require treatment with opioid analgesics.

- Assess for rash periodically during therapy. May cause Stevens-Johnson syndrome and toxic epidermal necrolysis. Discontinue therapy if severe or if accompanied with fever, general malaise, fatigue, muscle or joint aches, blisters, oral lesions, conjunctivitis, hepatitis, and/or eosinophilia.

- **Paclitaxel:** Monitor for hypersensitivity reactions continuously during the first 30 min and frequently thereafter. These occur frequently (19%), usually during the first 10 min of paclitaxel infusion, after the 1st or 2nd dose. Pretreatment is recommended for **all** patients and should include dexamethasone 20 mg PO (10 mg for patients with advanced HIV disease) 12 hr and 6 hr prior to paclitaxel, diphenhydramine 50 mg IV 30–60 min prior to paclitaxel. Most common manifestations are dyspnea, flushing, tachycardia, rash, hypotension, and chest pain. If these occur, stop infusion and notify health care professional. Treatment may include bronchodilators, epinephrine, antihistamines, and corticosteroids. Keep these agents and resuscitative equipment close by in the event of an anaphylactic reaction. Other manifestations of hypersensitivity reactions include flushing and rash.

- Assess for development of peripheral neuropathy. If severe symptoms occur, subsequent dose should be reduced by 20%.

- **Paclitaxel protein-bound (albumin-bound):** Consider premedication in patients who have had prior hypersensitivity reactions to paclitaxel protein-bound (albumin-bound). Do not re-challenge patients who experience a severe hypersensitivity reaction.

P

🍁 = Canadian drug name. ⬚⬚⬚ = Genetic implication. ~~Strikethrough~~ = Discontinued. CAPITALS = life-threatening. <u>Underline</u> = most frequent.

- Sensory neuropathy is dose- and schedule-dependent. *If ≥Grade 3 sensory neuropathy occurs*, withhold paclitaxel protein-bound (albumin-bound) until resolution to Grade 1 or 2 for metastatic breast cancer or until resolution to ≤Grade 1 for NSCLC and pancreatic cancer followed by a dose reduction for all subsequent courses of therapy.

Lab Test Considerations

- Verify negative pregnancy test before starting therapy.
- **Paclitaxel:** Monitor CBC and differential prior to and periodically during therapy. The nadir of leukopenia occurs in 11 days, with recovery by days 15– 21. *If neutrophil counts <500/mm³ for ≥1 wk*, reduce dose by 20% for subsequent courses.
- **Paclitaxel Protein-Bound Particles (albumin- bound):** Monitor CBC and differential frequently, including before starting therapy and prior to dosing on Day 1 (for breast cancer), 8, and 15 (for NSCLC and pancreatic cancer). For NSCLC: *If neutropenic fever (ANC <500/mm³ with fever >38°C) OR delay of next cycle by more than 7 days for ANC <1500/ mm³ OR ANC <500/mm³ for >7 days*, reduce dose on 1st occurrence to 75 mg/m² and on 2nd occurrence, reduce dose to 50 mg/m². For 3rd occurrence, discontinue therapy. Do not administer if neutrophil count is <1500/mm³. If severe neutropenia (neutrophils <500 cells/mm³ for seven days or more), reduce dose in subsequent courses. *If platelet count <50,000/mm³*, for 1st occurrence, reduce dose to 75 mg/m². Discontinue therapy at 2nd occurrence. For Pancreatic Cancer: *On Day 1, if ANC <1500 cells/mm³ OR platelet count <100,000 cells/mm³*, hold next dose until recovery. *On Day 8, if ANC 500 to <1000 cells/mm³ OR platelet count 50,000 to <75,000 cells/mm³*, reduce dose one level; *On Day 8, if ANC <500 cells/ mm³ OR <50,000 cells/mm³*, hold dose. *On Day 15, if Day 8 doses were reduced or given without modification, and ANC 500 to <1000 cells/mm³ OR platelet count 50,000 to <75,000 cells/mm³*, reduce dose 1 level from Day 8. *On Day 15, if Day 8 doses were reduced or given without modification, and ANC <500 cells/mm³ OR platelet count <50,000 cells/mm³*, hold doses. *On Day 15, if Day 8 doses were held and ANC ≥1000 cells/mm³ OR platelet count ≥75,000 cells/mm³*, reduce dose 1 level from Day 1. *On Day 15, if Day 8 doses were held and ANC 500 to <1000 cells/mm³ OR platelet count 50,000 to <75,000 cells/mm³*, reduce dose 2 levels from Day 1. On Day 15, if Day 8 doses were held and ANC <500 cells/mm³ OR platelet count <50,000 cells/mm³, hold doses. Monitor liver function studies (AST, ALT, LDH, bilirubin) prior to and periodically during therapy to detect hepatotoxicity.

Implementation

- Do not confuse paclitaxel with docetaxel or paclitaxel protein-bound particles.

Paclitaxel

IV Administration

- **Continuous Infusion:** Paclitaxel must be diluted prior to injection. *Dilution:* Dilute contents of 5- mL (30-mg) vials with the following diluents: 0.9% NaCl, D5W, D5/0.9% NaCl, or dextrose in Ringer's solution. *Concentration:* 0.3–1.2 mg/mL. Although haziness in solution is normal, inspect for particulate matter or discoloration before use. Use an in-line filter of not >0.22-micron pore size. Solutions are stable for 27 hr at room temperature and lighting. Do not use PVC containers or administration sets. *Rate:* Dose for *breast cancer, ovarian cancer, or AIDS-related Kaposi's sarcoma* is administered over 3 hr. Dose for *ovarian cancer* can also be administered as a 24-hr infusion.
- **Y-Site Compatibility:** acyclovir, alemtuzumab, allopurinol, amifostine, amikacin, aminophylline, amphotericin B lipid complex, ampicillin, ampicillin/ sulbactam, anidulafungin, argatroban, azithromycin, aztreonam, bivalirudin, bleomycin, bumetanide, buprenorphine, busulfan, butorphanol, calcium chloride, calcium gluconate, carboplatin, carmustine, caspofungin, cefazolin, cefepime, cefotaxime, cefotetan, cefoxitin, ceftazidime, ceftriaxone, cefuroxime, chloramphenicol, ciprofloxacin, cisatracurium, cisplatin, cladribine, clindamycin, cyclophosphamide, cyclosporine, cytarabine, dacarbazine, dactinomycin, dantrolene, daptomycin, daunorubicin hydrochloride, dexamethasone, dexmedetomidine, dexrazoxane, diltiazem, diphenhydramine, dobutamine, dopamine, doxorubicin hydrochloride, doxycycline, droperidol, enalaprilat, ephedrine, epinephrine, epirubicin, ertapenem, erythromycin, esmolol, etoposide, etoposide phosphate, famotidine, fentanyl, floxuridine, fluconazole, fludarabine, fluorouracil, foscarnet, fosphenytoin, furosemide, ganciclovir, gemcitabine, gentamicin, glycopyrrolate, granisetron, haloperidol, heparin, hetastarch, hydralazine, hydrocortisone, hydromorphone, ifosfamide, imipenem/cilastatin, insulin regular, irinotecan, isoproterenol, ketorolac, leucovorin calcium, levofloxacin, lidocaine, linezolid, lorazepam, magnesium sulfate, mannitol, meperidine, meropenem, mesna, methadone, methotrexate, metoclopramide, metoprolol, metronidazole, midazolam, milrinone, mitomycin, morphine, moxifloxacin, nafcillin, nalbuphine, naloxone, nicardipine, nitroglycerin, nitroprusside, norepinephrine, octreotide, ondansetron, oxaliplatin, palonosetron, pamidronate, pantoprazole, pemetrexed, pentamidine, pentobarbital, pentostatin, phenobarbital, phentolamine, phenylephrine, piperacillin/tazobactam, potassium acetate, potassium chloride, potassium phosphates, procainamide, prochlorperazine, promethazine, propofol, remifentanil, rituximab, sodium acetate, sodium bicarbonate, sodium phosphates, succinylcholine, sufentanil, tacrolimus, theophylline, thiopental, thiotepa, tigecycline, tirofiban, tobramycin, topotecan, trastu-

zumab, trimethoprim/sulfamethoxazole, vancomycin, vasopressin, vecuronium, verapamil, vinblastine, vincristine, vinorelbine, voriconazole, zidovudine, zoledronic acid.

- **Y-Site Incompatibility:** amiodarone, amphotericin B deoxycholate, amphotericin B liposomal, chlorpromazine, diazepam, digoxin, doxorubicin liposomal, gemtuzumab ozogamicin, hydroxyzine, idarubicin, indomethacin, labetalol, methylprednisolone, mitoxantrone, phenytoin, propranolol.

Paclitaxel Protein-Bound Particles (albumin-bound)

- **Dose Reduction for Pancreatic Cancer**: Full dose: 125 mm/m². 1st dose reduction: 100 mm/m². 2nd dose reduction: 75 mm/m². If additional dose reduction required: discontinue therapy.

IV Administration

- **Intermittent Infusion:** *Reconstitution:* Reconstitute by slowly adding 20 mL to each vial over at least 1 min for a concentration of 5 mg/mL. Direct solution to inside wall of vial to prevent foaming. Allow vial to sit for at least 5 min to ensure proper wetting of cake/powder. Gently swirl or invert vial for at least 2 min until powder is completely dissolved; avoid foaming. If foaming or clumping occurs, allow vial to stand for 15 min until foaming dissolves. Solution should be milky and homogenous without visible particles. If particles or settling are visible, gently invert vial to resuspend. Inject appropriate amount into sterile PVC IV bag. Do not use an in-line filter during administration. Do not administer solutions that are discolored or contain particulate matter. Reconstituted solution should be administered immediately but is stable for 8 hr if refrigerated. Discard unused portion. *Rate:* Administer over 30 min. Monitor infusion site closely for infiltration.
- **Y-Site Compatibility:** carboplatin, dexamethasone, gemcitabine, granisetron, palonosetron.

Patient/Family Teaching

- Explain purpose of paclitaxel to patient. Advise patient to read *Patient Information* before starting therapy and periodically during therapy in case of changes.
- Advise patient to notify health care professional immediately of rash, difficulty breathing, or symptoms of hypersensitivity reaction occurs.
- Instruct patient to notify health care professional promptly if fever; chills; cough; hoarseness; sore throat; signs of infection; lower back or side pain; painful or difficult urination; bleeding gums; bruising; petechiae; blood in stools, urine, or emesis; dyspnea; or orthostatic hypotension occurs. Caution patient to avoid crowds and persons with known infections. Instruct patient to use soft toothbrush and electric razor and to avoid falls. Caution patient not

to drink alcoholic beverages or to take medication containing aspirin or NSAIDs; may precipitate gastric bleeding.
- May cause dizziness. Caution patient to avoid driving or other activities requiring alertness until response to medication is known.
- Instruct patient to notify health care professional if abdominal pain, yellow skin, weakness, paresthesia, gait disturbances, or joint or muscle aches occur.
- Instruct patient to inspect oral mucosa for redness and ulceration. If mouth sores occur, advise patient to use sponge brush and rinse mouth with water after eating and drinking. Stomatitis usually resolves in 5–7 days.
- Discuss with patient the possibility of hair loss. Complete hair loss usually occurs between days 14 and 21 and is reversible after discontinuation of therapy. Explore coping strategies.
- Instruct patient not to receive any vaccinations without advice of health care professional.
- Rep: Advise females of reproductive potential to use a nonhormonal method of contraception during and for at least 6 mo after last dose of therapy and to avoid breastfeeding during and for 2 wk after last dose. Advise male patients with female partners of reproductive potential to use effective contraception during and for at least 3 mo after last dose. May impair fertility in females and males.
- Emphasize the need for periodic lab tests to monitor for side effects.

Evaluation/Desired Outcomes

- Decrease in size or spread of malignancy.

☒ **palbociclib** (pal-bo-si-klib)
Ibrance
Classification
Therapeutic: antineoplastics
Pharmacologic: kinase inhibitors

Indications

☒ Advanced or metastatic hormone receptor (HR)-positive, human epidermal growth factor 2 (HER2)-negative breast cancer as initial endocrine-based therapy (in combination with an aromatase inhibitor). ☒ Advanced or metastatic HR-positive, HER2-negative breast cancer in patients with disease progression following endocrine therapy (in combination with fulvestrant).

Action

Inhibits kinases (cyclin-dependent kinases 4 and 6) that are part of the signaling pathway for cell proliferation. **Therapeutic Effects:** Improved survival and decreased spread of breast cancer.

Pharmacokinetics

Absorption: 46% absorbed following oral administration.

Distribution: Unknown.

Metabolism and Excretion: Mostly metabolized (by CYP3A and sulfontransferase); 6.9% excreted unchanged in urine, 2.3% in feces.

Half-life: 29 hr.

TIME/ACTION PROFILE (improvement in progression-free survival)

ROUTE	ONSET	PEAK	DURATION
PO	within 4 mo	unknown	maintained throughout treatment

Contraindications/Precautions

Contraindicated in: OB: Pregnancy; Lactation: Lactation.

Use Cautiously in: Severe renal impairment; Severe hepatic impairment; Rep: Women of reproductive potential and men with female partners of reproductive potential; Pedi: Safety and effectiveness not established in children.

Adverse Reactions/Side Effects

Derm: alopecia. **EENT:** epistaxis. **GI:** stomatitis, vomiting, diarrhea, nausea. **GU:** ↓ fertility. **Hemat:** anemia, leukopenia, NEUTROPENIA, thrombocytopenia. **Metab:** ↓ appetite. **Neuro:** peripheral neuropathy, weakness. **Resp:** INTERSTITIAL LUNG DISEASE.

Interactions

Drug-Drug: Concurrent use with **CYP3A inhibitors** including **clarithromycin, itraconazole, ketoconazole, lopinavir/ritonavir, nefazodone, nelfinavir, posaconazole, ritonavir, verapamil,** and **voriconazole** ↑ levels and the risk of toxicity; avoid, if possible (if unavoidable, ↓ dose of palbociclib [resume original dose after 3–5 half-lives of offending drug have passed following discontinuation]). **Strong CYP3A inducers** including **carbamazepine, phenytoin, rifampin** can ↓ levels and effectiveness; concurrent use should be avoided. **Moderate CYP3A inducers** including **bosentan, efavirenz, etravirine, modafinil,** and **nafcillin** may also ↓ levels and effectiveness; avoid concurrent use. ↑ levels and effects/toxicity of **cyclosporine, dihydroergotamine, ergotamine, everolimus, fentanyl, midazolam, pimozide, quinidine, sirolimus,** and **tacrolimus;** if concurrent use is required dose ↓ may be necessary.

Drug-Natural Products: St. John's wort may ↓ levels and effectiveness; avoid concurrent use.

Drug-Food: Grapefruit/grapefruit juice ↑ levels and the risk of toxicity, avoid ingestion.

Route/Dosage

PO (Adults): 125 mg once daily for 21 days, followed by 7 days off; *Concurrent use of strong CYP3A4 inhibitor:* 75 mg once daily for 21 days, followed by 7 days off.

Hepatic Impairment

PO (Adults): *Severe hepatic impairment:* 75 mg once daily for 21 days, followed by 7 days off.

Availability (generic available)

Capsules: 75 mg, 100 mg, 125 mg.

NURSING IMPLICATIONS

Assessment

- Monitor for signs and symptoms of infection (fever, chills, dizziness, shortness of breath, weakness, increased bleeding or bruising) during therapy. Treat as medically appropriate. No dose adjustment is needed for Grade 1 or 2 non-hematologic toxicities. *For Grade ≥3 (if persisting despite medical treatment),* withhold palbociclib until symptoms resolve to Grade ≤1; Grade ≤2 (if not considered a safety risk for patient). Resume at next lower dose.

- Monitor for signs and symptoms of interstitial lung disease or pneumonitis (hypoxia, cough, dyspnea) during therapy. If symptoms are severe, permanently discontinue therapy.

Lab Test Considerations

- Verify negative pregnancy test before starting therapy.

- Monitor CBC prior to and at beginning of each cycle, on Day 15 of first 2 cycles, and as clinically indicated. May cause ↓ neutrophil counts; median time to first episode is 15 days and median duration of Grade ≥3 neutropenia was 7 days. May cause febrile neutropenia.

- No dose adjustment is needed for Grade 1 or 2 hematologic toxicities. *For Grade 3 Day 1 of cycle:* withhold palbociclib, repeat CBC monitoring within 1 wk. When recovered to Grade ≤2, start next cycle at same dose. *For Grade 3 Day 15 of first 2 cycles:* If Grade 3 on Day 15, continue palbociclib at current dose to complete cycle and repeat CBC on Day 22. *If Grade 4 on Day 22,* withhold palbociclib until recovery to Grade ≤2. Resume at next lower dose. Consider dose reduction in cases of prolonged (>1 wk) recovery from Grade 3 neutropenia or recurrent Grade 3 neutropenia on Day 1 of subsequent cycles. *For Grade 3 ANC (500– <1000/mm³) plus fever ≥38.5°C and/or infection,* withhold palbociclib until recovery to Grade ≤2. Resume at next lower dose. *For Grade 4,* withhold palbociclib until recovery to Grade ≤2. Resume at next lower dose.

- May cause ↓ WBC, lymphocytes, hemoglobin, and platelets.

Implementation

- **PO:** Administer once daily with food at the same time each day, for 21 consecutive days followed by 7 days off treatment, combination with letrozole once daily given throughout 28-day cycle. *DNC:* Swallow capsules whole; do not open, crush, or chew; do not swallow capsules that are broken, cracked, or not intact.

- If dose reduction needed for adverse reactions starting dose is 125 mg/day. 1st dose reduction is to 100 mg/day, 2nd dose reduction is to 75 mg/day; if further dose reduction needed, discontinue therapy.

Patient/Family Teaching
- Instruct patient to take palbociclib as directed. If a dose is vomited or missed, omit dose and take next dose at usual time; do not take an additional dose that day. Do not change dose or stop taking without consulting health care professional. Advise patient to read *Patient Information* before starting therapy and with each Rx refill in case of changes.
- Advise patient to avoid grapefruit or grapefruit products during therapy; may increase amount of palbociclib in blood.
- Advise patient to notify health care professional if signs and symptoms of infection occur.
- Instruct patient to notify health care professional of all Rx or OTC medications, vitamins, or herbal products being taken and to consult with health care professional before taking other medications, especially St. John's wort.
- Rep: Advise females of reproductive potential to use effective contraception and avoid breastfeeding during and for at least 3 wk after last dose. Advise patient to notify health care professional if pregnancy is planned or suspected. Advise males with female partners of reproductive potential to use effective contraception during and for at least 3 wk after last dose. Inform male patient that palbociclib may impair fertility.

Evaluation/Desired Outcomes
- Decrease in the spread of breast cancer.

---

palifermin (pa-liff-er-min)
Kepivance
Classification
Therapeutic: cytoprotective agents
Pharmacologic: keratinocyte growth factors

Indications
Severe oral mucositis (≥WHO grade 3) associated with myelotoxic therapy in patients requiring autologous hematopoietic stem cell support for hematologic malignancies.

Action
Enhances proliferation of epithelial cells. **Therapeutic Effects:** Decreased incidence/duration of mucositis.

Pharmacokinetics
Absorption: IV administration results in complete bioavailability.
Distribution: Unknown.
Metabolism and Excretion: Unknown.
Half-life: 4.5 hr.

TIME/ACTION PROFILE (plasma concentrations)

ROUTE	ONSET	PEAK	DURATION
IV	unknown	end of dose	unknown

Contraindications/Precautions
Contraindicated in: Hypersensitivity to palifermin or other *E. coli*–derived proteins; OB: Pregnancy; Lactation: Lactation.
Use Cautiously in: Allogeneic hematopoietic stem cell support (↑ risk of exacerbated mucositis); Pedi: Safety and effectiveness not established in children.

Adverse Reactions/Side Effects
Derm: erythema, pruritus, rash. **GI:** tongue thickening/discoloration. **GU:** ↓ fertility. **Metab:** ↑ amylase, ↑ lipase. **MS:** arthralgia. **Neuro:** dysesthesia, dysgeusia.

Interactions
Drug-Drug: Unfractionated heparin and **low-molecular weight heparin** ↑ levels (flush tubing with saline between use). Administration within 24 hr after **myelotoxic therapy (chemotherapy/radiation)** ↑ severity and duration of mucositis.

Route/Dosage
IV (Adults): 60 mcg/kg/day for 3 days before and 3 days after myelotoxic therapy.

Availability
Powder for injection: 6.25 mg/vial.

NURSING IMPLICATIONS
Assessment
- Assess level of oral mucositis prior to and periodically during therapy.

Lab Test Considerations
- May cause ↑ serum lipase and amylase; usually reversible.
- May cause proteinuria.

Implementation
- Do not administer palifermin within 24 hr before, during infusion, or 24 hr after infusion of myelotoxic chemotherapy.
- Administer doses for 3 consecutive days before (3rd dose 24–48 hr prior to chemotherapy) and 3 consecutive days after myelotoxic chemotherapy (4th dose on same day as hematopoietic stem cells infusion after infusion is completed and at least 4 days after most recent palifermin administration) for a total of 7 doses.

IV Administration
- **IV Push:** *Reconstitution:* Reconstitute palifermin powder by slowly injecting 1.2 mL of sterile water for injection aseptically. *Concentration:* 5 mg/mL. Swirl gently; do not shake or vigorously agitate. Solution should be clear and colorless; do not administer solution that is discolored or contains particulate matter. Dissolution usually takes less than 3 min. Administer immediately after reconstitution or refrigerate and administer within 24 hr. Do not freeze. Allow to reach room temperature for up to 1 hr. Protect

from light. Discard palifermin after expiration date or if left at room temperature for more than 1 hr. *Rate:* Administer via bolus injection. Do not use a filter.

- **Y-Site Incompatibility:** heparin. If heparin solution is used to maintain IV line, flush with 0.9% NaCl prior to and after use of palifermin.

Patient/Family Teaching

- Explain the purpose of palifermin to patient.
- Inform patient of evidence of tumor growth and stimulation in cell culture and animal models.
- Advise patient to notify health care professional if rash, erythema, edema, pruritus, oral/perioral dysesthesia (tongue discoloration, tongue thickening, alteration of taste) occur.
- Rep: May cause fetal harm. Advise females of reproductive potential to notify health care professional if pregnancy is planned or suspected and to avoid breastfeeding during therapy and for at least 2 wk after last dose. May impair female and male fertility.

Evaluation/Desired Outcomes

- Decrease in incidence and duration of oral mucositis in patients receiving myelotoxic therapy requiring hematopoietic stem cell support.

BEERS

paliperidone (pa-li-**per**-i-done)
Invega, Invega Hafyera, Invega Sustenna, Invega Trinza
Classification
Therapeutic: antipsychotics
Pharmacologic: benzisoxazoles

Indications

PO, IM: Acute and maintenance treatment of schizophrenia (Invega and Invega Sustenna). **IM:** Maintenance treatment of schizophrenia after patients have been adequately treated with Invega Sustenna for at least 4 mo (Invega Trinza). **IM:** Maintenance treatment of schizophrenia after patients have been adequately treated with either Invega Sustenna for at least 4 mo or Invega Trinza for at least one 3-mo cycle (Invega Hafyera). **PO, IM:** Acute treatment of schizoaffective disorder (as monotherapy or as adjunct to mood stabilizers and/or antidepressants) (Invega and Invega Sustenna).

Action

May act by antagonizing dopamine and serotonin in the CNS. Paliperidone is the active metabolite of risperidone. **Therapeutic Effects:** Decreased manifestations of schizophrenia. Decreased manifestations of schizoaffective disorder.

Pharmacokinetics

Absorption: 28% absorbed following oral administration, food ↑ absorption; slowly absorbed after IM administration (concentrations higher and more rapidly achieved with administration into deltoid muscle).

Distribution: Unknown.

Metabolism and Excretion: 59% excreted unchanged in urine; 32% excreted in urine as metabolites.

Half-life: *PO:* 23 hr; *IM (Sustenna):* 25–49 days; *IM (Trinza):* 84–139 days; *IM (Hafyera):* 148–159 days.

TIME/ACTION PROFILE (plasma concentrations)

ROUTE	ONSET	PEAK	DURATION
PO	unknown	24 hr	24 hr
IM —Sustenna	unknown	13 days	1 mo
IM —Trinza	unknown	30–33 days	3 mo
IM —Hafyera	unknown	29–32 days	6 mo

Contraindications/Precautions

Contraindicated in: Hypersensitivity to paliperidone or risperidone; Concurrent use of drugs known to cause QT interval prolongation (including quinidine, procainamide, sotalol, amiodarone, chlorpromazine, thioridazine, moxifloxacin); History of congenital QTc prolongation or other cardiac arrhythmias; Bradycardia, hypokalemia, hypomagnesemia (↑ risk of QTc prolongation); Pre-existing severe GI narrowing (due to nature of tablet formulation); CCr <50 mL/min (for IM).

Use Cautiously in: Patients with Parkinson's disease or dementia with Lewy Bodies (↑ sensitivity to effects of antipsychotics); History of suicide attempt; History of HF, MI, conduction abnormalities, stroke, TIA (↑ risk of orthostatic hypotension and syncope); Patients at risk for aspiration pneumonia or falls; History of seizures; Conditions which may ↑ body temperature (strenuous exercise, exposure to extreme heat, concurrent anticholinergics or risk of dehydration); ↓ GI transit time (may ↑ blood levels); May mask symptoms of some drug overdoses, intestinal obstruction, Reye's Syndrome, or brain tumor (due to antiemetic effect); Diabetes mellitus; Severe hepatic impairment; Renal impairment (dose ↓ recommended if CCr <80 mL/min); Low white blood cell count/absolute neutrophil count or history of drug-induced leukopenia/neutropenia (↑ risk of leukopenia/neutropenia); OB: Neonates at ↑ risk for extrapyramidal symptoms and withdrawal after delivery when exposed during the 3rd trimester; use only if maternal benefit outweighs fetal risk; Lactation: Use while breastfeeding only if potential maternal benefit justifies potential risk to infant; Pedi: Children <12 yr (safety and effectiveness not established); Geri: Appears on Beers list. ↑ risk of stroke, cognitive decline, and mortality in older adults with dementia. Avoid use in older adults, except for schizophrenia.

Adverse Reactions/Side Effects

CV: <u>palpitations, tachycardia (dose related)</u>, bradycardia, orthostatic hypotension, QT interval prolongation. **EENT:** blurred vision. **Endo:** galactorrhea, gynecomastia, hyperglycemia. **GI:** <u>abdominal pain</u>, dry mouth, dyspepsia, nausea, swollen tongue. **GU:** ↓ fertility (females), amenorrhea, impotence, priapism. **Hemat:** AGRANULOCYTOSIS, leukopenia, neutropenia. **Metab:** dyslipidemia, weight gain. **MS:** back pain, dystonia (dose related). **Neuro:** <u>drowsiness</u>, <u>extrapyramidal disorders</u> (dose related), <u>headache</u>, <u>insomnia</u>, akathisia, anxiety, confusion, dizziness, dysarthria, fatigue, NEUROLEPTIC MALIGNANT SYNDROME, SEIZURES, syncope, tardive dyskinesia, tremor (dose related), weakness. **Resp:** <u>dyspnea</u>, cough. **Misc:** fever, HYPERSENSITIVITY REACTIONS (including anaphylaxis and angioedema).

Interactions

Drug-Drug: ↑ risk of CNS depression with other **CNS depressants** including **alcohol**, **antihistamines**, **sedative/hypnotics**, or **opioid analgesics**. May antagonize the effects of **levodopa** or other **dopamine agonists**. ↑ risk of orthostatic hypotension with **antihypertensives**, **nitrates**, or other **agents that lower BP**. **Strong CYP3A4 inducers** or **strong P-glycoprotein inducers**, including **carbamazepine** or **rifampin** may ↓ levels/effects; avoid concurrent use with Invega Sustenna (if use of strong CYP3A4 or P-glycoprotein inducer necessary, consider using paliperidone ER tablets). **Valproic acid** may ↑ levels (may need to ↓ dose of paliperidone).

Drug-Natural Products: **St. John's wort** may ↓ levels/effects; avoid concurrent use with Invega Sustenna.

Route/Dosage

Schizophrenia

PO (Adults): 6 mg once daily; may titrate by 3 mg/day at intervals of at least 5 days (range 3–12 mg/day).
PO (Children 12–17 yr): 3 mg once daily; may titrate by 3 mg/day at intervals of at least 5 days (not to exceed 6 mg if <51 kg or 12 mg if ≥51 kg).
IM (Adults): *Invega Sustenna:* 234 mg initially, then 156 mg 1 wk later; continue with monthly maintenance dose of 117 mg (range of 39–234 mg based on efficacy and/or tolerability); *Invega Trinza:* Dose should be based on dose of previous 1-mo injection dose of Invega Sustenna. If last dose of Invega Sustenna was 78 mg: Administer 273 mg of Invega Trinza every 3 mo. If last dose of Invega Sustenna was 117 mg: Administer 410 mg of Invega Trinza every 3 mo. If last dose of Invega Sustenna was 156 mg: Administer 546 mg of Invega Trinza every 3 mo. If last dose of Invega Sustenna was 234 mg: Administer 819 mg of Invega Trinza every 3 mo. May adjust dose based on efficacy and/or tolerability (range: 273–819 mg). *Invega Hafyera:* Dose should be based on dose of previous 1-mo injection dose of Invega Sustenna or previous every 3-mo dose of Invega Trinza. If last dose of Invega Sustenna was 156 mg: Administer 1,092 mg of Invega Hafyera every 6 mo. If last dose of Invega Sustenna was 234 mg: Administer

1,560 mg of Invega Hafyera every 6 mo. If last dose of Invega Trinza was 546 mg: Administer 1,092 mg of Invega Hafyera every 6 mo. If last dose of Invega Trinza was 819 mg: Administer 1,560 mg of Invega Hafyera every 6 mo.

Renal Impairment

PO (Adults): *CCr 50–79 mL/min:* 3 mg/day initially; dose may be ↑ to maximum of 6 mg/day; *CCr 10–<50 mL/min:* 1.5 mg/day initially; dose may be ↑ to maximum of 3 mg/day.

Renal Impairment

IM (Adults): *CCr 50–79 mL/min:* Invega Sustenna: 156 mg initially, then 117 mg 1 wk later; continue with monthly maintenance dose of 78 mg; can adjust monthly maintenance dose to 39 mg, 78 mg, 117 mg, or 156 mg based on tolerability and response (max dose = 156 mg/month); Invega Trinza: once stabilized on Invega Sustenna, can then transition to appropriate dose of Invega Trinza (see above) *CCr <50 mL/min:* Contraindicated.

Schizoaffective Disorder

PO (Adults): 6 mg/day; may titrate by 3 mg/day at intervals of at least 4 days (range 3–12 mg/day).

Renal Impairment

PO (Adults): *CCr 50–79 mL/min:* 3 mg/day initially; dose may be ↑ to maximum of 6 mg/day; *CCr 10–<50 mL/min:* 1.5 mg/day initially; dose may be ↑ to maximum of 3 mg/day.

Availability (generic available)

Extended-release tablets (Invega): 1.5 mg, 3 mg, 6 mg, 9 mg. **Extended-release intramuscular injection (Invega Sustenna):** 39 mg/0.25 mL, ✹ 50 mg/0.5 mL, ✹ 75 mg/0.75 mL, 78 mg/0.5 mL, ✹ 100 mg/mL, 117 mg/0.75 mL, ✹ 150 mg/1.5 mL, 156 mg/mL, 234 mg/1.5 mL. **Extended-release intramuscular injection (Invega Trinza):** ✹ 175 mg/0.875 mL, ✹ 263 mg/1.315 mL, 273 mg/0.875 mL, ✹ 350 mg/1.75 mL, 410 mg/1.315 mL, ✹ 525 mg/2.625 mL, 546 mg/1.75 mL, 819 mg/2.625 mL. **Extended-release intramuscular injection (Invega Hafyera):** 1,092 mg/3.5 mL, 1,560 mg/5 mL.

NURSING IMPLICATIONS

Assessment

- Monitor patient's mental status (orientation, mood, behavior) before and periodically during therapy. Monitor closely for notable changes in behavior that could indicate the emergence or worsening of suicidal thoughts or behavior or depression, especially during early therapy. Restrict amount of drug available to patient.
- Assess weight and BMI initially and throughout therapy. Refer as appropriate for nutritional/weight and medical management.

- Monitor BP (sitting, standing, lying down) and pulse before and periodically during therapy. May cause prolonged QT interval, tachycardia, and orthostatic hypotension. Protect patient from falls.
- Observe patient when administering medication to ensure that medication is actually swallowed and not hoarded or cheeked.
- Monitor patient for onset of extrapyramidal side effects (*akathisia:* restlessness; *dystonia:* muscle spasms and twisting motions; or *pseudoparkinsonism:* mask-like face, rigidity, tremors, drooling, shuffling gait, dysphagia). Report these symptoms; reduction of dose or discontinuation of medication may be necessary.
- Monitor for tardive dyskinesia (involuntary rhythmic movement of mouth, face, and extremities). Report immediately; may be irreversible.
- Monitor for development of neuroleptic malignant syndrome (fever, muscle rigidity, delirium, respiratory distress, tachycardia, seizures, diaphoresis, hypertension or hypotension, cardiac arrhythmia, pallor, tiredness). Discontinue paliperidone and notify health care professional immediately if these symptoms occur.
- Monitor for symptoms related to hyperprolactinemia (menstrual abnormalities, galactorrhea, sexual dysfunction).
- Assess for falls risk. Drowsiness, orthostatic hypotension, and motor and sensory instability increase risk. Institute prevention if indicated.

Lab Test Considerations

- Monitor fasting blood glucose and cholesterol levels before and periodically during therapy.
- Monitor serum prolactin prior to and periodically during therapy. May cause ↑ serum prolactin levels.
- Monitor CBC frequently during initial mo of therapy in patients with pre-existing or history of low WBC. May cause leukopenia, neutropenia, or agranulocytosis. Discontinue therapy if this occurs.

Implementation

- *High Alert:* Do not confuse Invega Sustenna with Invega Trinza. Do no confuse Invega with Intuniv.
- **PO:** Administer once daily in the morning without regard to food. *DNC:* Tablets should be swallowed whole; do not crush, break, or chew.
- **IM:** *Invega Sustenna:* Administer initial and 2nd doses in deltoid using a 1½-inch, 22 gauge needle for patients ≥90 kg (≥200 lb) or 1-inch 23 gauge needle for patients <90 kg (<200 lb). Monthly maintenance doses can be administered in either deltoid or gluteal sites. For gluteal injection, use 1 ½-inch, 22 gauge needle regardless of patient weight. To avoid missed dose, may give 2nd dose 4 days before or after the 1-wk timepoint. Monthly doses may be given up to 7 days before or after the monthly timepoint. *After 1st mo, if missed dose is within 4 wk of scheduled dose,* administer 2nd dose of 156 mg as soon as possible. Give 3rd dose of

117 mg in either deltoid or gluteal muscle 5 wk after 1st injection (regardless of timing of 2nd injection). Then return to normal monthly injections in either deltoid or gluteal muscle. *If >4 wk and <7 wk since 1st injection,* resume by administering 156 mg dose in deltoid as soon as possible, a 2nd 156 mg dose in deltoid in 1 wk, followed by monthly doses in deltoid or gluteal sites. *If >7 mo since scheduled dose,* administer using initial dosing schedule. During regular monthly dose schedule, *if <6 wk since last injection,* administer previously stabilized dose as soon as possible, then monthly. *If >6 wk since last injection,* resume dose previously stabilized on, unless stabilized on 234 mg (then 1st two injections should be 156 mg). Administer 1 dose in deltoid as soon as possible, then another deltoid injection of same dose 1 wk later, then resume regular monthly schedule. *If >6 mo since last injection,* administer using initial dosing schedule.
- **IM:** *Invega Trinza:* Use only after at least 4 mo of monthly *Invega Sustenna* therapy. Prior to administration, shake the prefilled syringe vigorously for at least 15 sec within 5 min prior to administration to ensure a homogeneous suspension. *Deltoid injection:* For patients weighing <90 kg, use the 1-inch 22 gauge thin wall needle. For patients weighing ≥90 kg, use the 1½-inch 22 gauge thin wall needle. *Gluteal injection:* Regardless of patient weight, use 1½-inch 22 gauge thin wall needle. Initiate *Invega Trinza* when next 1-mo paliperidone dose is scheduled. *Avoid missed doses;* dose may be given 2 wk before or after 3 mo scheduled dose. *If more than 3½ mo (up to but <4 mo) since last dose,* administer previously administered dose as soon as possible, then continue with 3-mo injections. *If 4 mo up to and including 9 mo since last dose,* do NOT administer next dose. *If last dose was 273 mg,* administer 2 doses of 78 mg of *Invega Sustenna* one wk apart into deltoid muscle, then one dose of *Invega Trinza* 273 mg 1 mo after 2nd dose of *Invega Sustenna.* *If last dose was 410 mg,* administer 2 doses of 117 mg of *Invega Sustenna* 1 wk apart into deltoid muscle, then one dose of *Invega Trinza* 410 mg 1 mo after 2nd dose of *Invega Sustenna.* *If last dose was 819 mg,* administer 2 doses of 156 mg of *Invega Sustenna* 1 wk apart into deltoid muscle, then one dose of *Invega Trinza* 819 mg 1 mo after 2nd dose of *Invega Sustenna.* If >9 mo have elapsed since last injection of *Invega Trinza,* reinitiate treatment with *Invega Sustenna.* Then resume *Invega Trinza* after at least 4 mo of *Invega Sustenna.*
- **IM:** *Invega Hafyera* must be administered as a gluteal IM injection by a health care professional once every 6 mo. After shaking, solution is uniform, thick, and milky white; do not inject if discolored or contains particulate matter. Do not use needles from *Invega Sustenna* or *Invega Trinza;* may develop blockage. Begin *Invega Hafyera* only after therapy

has been established with either once-a-month *Invega Sustenna* for at least 4 mo OR every-3-mo *Invega Trinza* for at least 1 3-mo injection cycle. Begin within 1 wk before or after next scheduled dose for *Invega Sustenna* or 2 wk before or after *Invega Trinza* dose. May give *Invega Hafyera* injection up to 2 wk before or 3 wk after the scheduled 6-mo dose to avoid a missed dose. If >6 mo and 3 wk but <8 mo since last dose of *Invega Hafyera*, restart with *Invega Sustenna*. *If last dose of Invega Hafyera was 1092 mg,* administer *Invega Sustenna* 156 mg into deltoid muscle on Day 1. Then 1 mo after Day 1, administer *Invega Hafyera* 1092 mg into gluteal muscle. *If last dose of Invega Hafyera was 1560 mg,* administer *Invega Sustenna* 234 mg into deltoid muscle on Day 1. Then 1 mo after Day 1, administer *Invega Hafyera* 1560 mg into gluteal muscle. If 8 mo up to and including 11 mo since last dose of *Invega Hafyera*, restart with *Invega Sustenna*. *If last dose of Invega Hafyera was 1092 mg,* administer *Invega Sustenna* 156 mg into deltoid muscle on Day 1 and 156 mg on Day 8. Then 1 mo after Day 8, administer *Invega Hafyera* 1092 mg into gluteal muscle. *If last dose of Invega Hafyera was 1560 mg,* administer *Invega Sustenna* 156 mg into deltoid muscle on Day 1 and 156 mg on Day 8. Then 1 mo after Day 1, administer *Invega Hafyera* 1560 mg into gluteal muscle. If >11 mo since the last dose of *Invega Hafyera*, restart therapy with *Invega Sustenna*. *Invega Hafyera* can be resumed after therapy with *Invoga Sustenna* for at least 4 mo.

Patient/Family Teaching

- Instruct patient to take medication as directed. Advise patient that appearance of tablets in stool is normal and not of concern.
- Inform patient of the possibility of extrapyramidal symptoms, neuroleptic malignant syndrome, and tardive dyskinesia. Instruct patient to report these symptoms immediately to health care professional.
- Advise patient to change positions slowly to minimize orthostatic hypotension. Protect from falls.
- May cause drowsiness and dizziness. Caution patient to avoid driving or other activities requiring alertness until response to medication is known.
- Advise patient and family to notify health care professional if thoughts about suicide or dying, attempts to commit suicide; new or worse depression; new or worse anxiety; feeling very agitated or restless; panic attacks; trouble sleeping; new or worse irritability; acting aggressive; being angry or violent; acting on dangerous impulses; an extreme increase in activity and talking, other unusual changes in behavior or mood occur.
- Advise patient that extremes in temperature should also be avoided; this drug impairs body temperature regulation.

- Advise patient to notify health care professional of all Rx or OTC medications, vitamins, or herbal products being taken and to consult with health care professional before taking other medications, especially St. John's wort and alcohol.
- Advise patient to seek nutritional, weight, or medical management as needed for weight gain or cholesterol elevation.
- Instruct patient to notify health care professional promptly if sore throat, fever, unusual bleeding or bruising, rash, tremors, menstrual abnormalities, galactorrhea, or sexual dysfunction occur.
- Advise patient to notify health care professional of medication regimen before treatment or surgery.
- Rep: Advise females of reproductive potential to notify health care professional if pregnancy is planned or suspected, and to avoid breastfeeding. Encourage women who become pregnant while taking paliperidone to enroll in the National Pregnancy Registry for Atypical Antipsychotics at 1-866-961-2388 or visit http://womensmentalhealth.org/clinical-and-research-programs/pregnancyregistry/. Monitor neonates for extrapyramidal and/or withdrawal symptoms (agitation, hypertonia, hypotonia, tremor, somnolence, respiratory distress, feeding disorder) and manage symptoms appropriately. Monitor infants exposed to paliperidone through breast milk for excess sedation, failure to thrive, jitteriness, and extrapyramidal symptoms (tremors and abnormal muscle movements). May temporarily cause female infertility.
- Emphasize the importance of routine follow-up exams to monitor side effects and continued participation in psychotherapy to improve coping skills.

Evaluation/Desired Outcomes

- Decrease in excited, manic behavior.
- Decrease in positive symptoms (delusions, hallucinations) of schizophrenia.
- Decrease in negative symptoms (social withdrawal, flat, blunted affect) of schizophrenia.

palonosetron
(pa-lone-**o**-se-tron)
~~Aloxi~~
Classification
Therapeutic: antiemetics
Pharmacologic: 5-HT$_3$ antagonists

Indications

Prevention of acute and delayed nausea and vomiting caused by initial or repeat courses of moderately or highly emetogenic chemotherapy (moderately emetogenic chemotherapy for adults only). Prevention of postoperative nausea and vomiting for up to 24 hr after surgery.

Action

Blocks the effects of serotonin at receptor sites (selective antagonist) located in vagal nerve terminals and in the chemoreceptor trigger zones in the CNS. **Therapeutic Effects:** Decreased incidence and severity of nausea and vomiting following emetogenic chemotherapy or surgery.

Pharmacokinetics

Absorption: IV administration results in complete bioavailability.

Distribution: Well distributed to tissues.

Metabolism and Excretion: 50% metabolized by the liver via the CYP1A2, CYP2D6, and CYP3A4 isoenzymes to inactive metabolites; 40% excreted unchanged in urine.

Half-life: 40 hr.

TIME/ACTION PROFILE

ROUTE	ONSET	PEAK	DURATION
IV	within 30 min	unknown	7 days

Contraindications/Precautions

Contraindicated in: Hypersensitivity; cross sensitivity with other 5-HT$_3$ antagonists may occur.

Use Cautiously in: OB: Safety not established in pregnancy; Lactation: Use while breastfeeding only if potential maternal benefit justifies potential risk to infant; Pedi: Neonates <1 mo (safety and effectiveness not established).

Adverse Reactions/Side Effects

GI: constipation, diarrhea. **Neuro:** dizziness, headache.

Interactions

Drug-Drug: Drugs that affect serotonergic neurotransmitter systems, including **SSRIs**, **SNRIs**, **tricyclic antidepressants**, **MAO inhibitors**, **fentanyl**, **lithium**, **buspirone**, **tramadol**, **methylene blue**, and **triptans** ↑ risk of serotonin syndrome.

Route/Dosage

Prevention of Chemotherapy-Induced Nausea/Vomiting

IV (Adults): 0.25 mg given 30 min before start of chemotherapy.

IV (Children 1 mo–<17 yr): 20 mcg/kg (max dose = 1.5 mg) given 30 min before start of chemotherapy.

Prevention of Postoperative Nausea/Vomiting

IV (Adults): 0.075 mg given immediately before induction of anesthesia.

Availability (generic available)

Solution for injection: 0.05 mg/mL. *In combination with:* fosnetupitant (Akynzeo); netupitant (Akynzeo); see Appendix N.

NURSING IMPLICATIONS

Assessment

- Assess patient for nausea, vomiting, abdominal distention, and bowel sounds prior to and following administration.

Lab Test Considerations

- May cause transient ↑ in serum bilirubin, AST, and ALT levels.

Implementation

- 1st dose is administered prior to emetogenic event.
- Repeated dose within a 7-day period is not recommended.

IV Administration

- **IV Push:** Administer dose undiluted 30 min prior to chemotherapy or immediately prior to the induction of anesthesia. Flush line prior to and after administration with 0.9% NaCl. Do not administer solutions that are discolored or contain particulate matter.
- *Concentration:* 0.05 mg/mL. *Rate:* Administer over 30 sec in adults and 15 sec in children 30 min before starting chemotherapy and over 10 sec for postoperative nausea and vomiting.
- **Y-Site Compatibility:** alemtuzumab, amifostine, amikacin, aminocaproic acid, aminophylline, amiodarone, amphotericin B liposomal, ampicillin, ampicillin/sulbactam, anidulafungin, argatroban, atropine, azithromycin, aztreonam, bivalirudin, bleomycin, bumetanide, buprenorphine, busulfan, butorphanol, calcium acetate, calcium chloride, calcium gluconate, carboplatin, carmustine, caspofungin, cefazolin, cefepime, cefotaxime, cefotetan, cefoxitin, ceftazidime, ceftriaxone, cefuroxime, chloramphenicol, chlorpromazine, ciprofloxacin, cisatracurium, cisplatin, clindamycin, cyclophosphamide, cyclosporine, cytarabine, dacarbazine, dactinomycin, dantrolene, daptomycin, daunorubicin hydrochloride, dexamethasone, dexmedetomidine, dexrazoxane, digoxin, diltiazem, diphenhydramine, dobutamine, docetaxel, dopamine, doxorubicin hydrochloride, droperidol, enalaprilat, ephedrine, epinephrine, epirubicin, eptifibatide, erythromycin, esmolol, etoposide, etoposide phosphate, famotidine, fentanyl, fluconazole, fludarabine, fluorouracil, fosaprepitant, foscarnet, fosphenytoin, furosemide, gemcitabine, gentamicin, glycopyrrolate, haloperidol, heparin, hetastarch, hydralazine, hydrocortisone, hydromorphone, idarubicin, ifosfamide, insulin regular, irinotecan, isoproterenol, ketorolac, labetalol, LR, leucovorin calcium, levofloxacin, lidocaine, linezolid, lorazepam, magnesium sulfate, mannitol, melphalan, meperidine, meropenem, mesna, methadone, methotrexate, metoclopramide, metoprolol, metronidazole, midazolam, milrinone, mitomycin, mitoxantrone, morphine, moxifloxacin, nalbuphine, naloxone, neostigmine, nicardipine, nitroglycerin, nitroprusside, norepinephrine, octreotide, oxaliplatin, oxytocin, pacli-

taxel, paclitaxel protein bound, pamidronate, phenobarbital, phentolamine, phenylephrine, piperacillin/tazobactam, potassium acetate, potassium chloride, potassium phosphate, procainamide, prochlorperazine, promethazine, propofol, propranolol, remifentanil, rocuronium, sodium acetate, sodium bicarbonate, sodium phosphate, succinylcholine, sufentanil, tacrolimus, theophylline, thiotepa, tigecycline, tirofiban, tobramycin, topotecan, trimethoprim/sulfamethoxazole, vancomycin, vasopressin, vecuronium, verapamil, vinblastine, vincristine, vinorelbine, zidovudine.

- **Y-Site Incompatibility:** acyclovir, allopurinol, amphotericin B deoxycholate, diazepam, doxycycline, ganciclovir, gemtuzumab ozogamicin, imipenem/cilastatin, methylprednisolone, minocycline, nafcillin, pantoprazole, pentamidine, pentobarbital, phenytoin, thiopental.

Patient/Family Teaching
- Inform patient of purpose of medication.
- Advise patient to notify health care professional if nausea or vomiting occur.
- Rep: Advise females of reproductive potential to notify health care professional if pregnancy is planned or suspected or if breastfeeding.

Evaluation/Desired Outcomes
- Prevention of nausea and vomiting associated with initial and repeat courses of emetogenic cancer chemotherapy or surgery.

pamidronate (pa-mid-roe-nate)
Classification
Therapeutic: bone resorption inhibitors
Pharmacologic: bisphosphonates, hypocalcemics

Indications
Moderate to severe hypercalcemia associated with malignancy. Osteolytic bone lesions associated with multiple myeloma or breast cancer. Moderate to severe Paget's disease.

Action
Inhibits resorption of bone. **Therapeutic Effects:** Decreased serum calcium. Decreased skeletal destruction in multiple myeloma or breast cancer. Decreased skeletal complications in Paget's disease.

Pharmacokinetics
Absorption: IV administration results in complete bioavailability.
Distribution: Rapidly absorbed by bone. Reaches high concentrations in bone, liver, spleen, teeth, and tracheal cartilage. Approximately 50% of a dose is retained by bone and then slowly released.
Metabolism and Excretion: 50% is excreted unchanged in the urine.

Half-life: Elimination half-life from plasma is biphasic— 1st phase 1.6 hr, 2nd phase 27.2 hr. Elimination half-life from bone is 300 days.

TIME/ACTION PROFILE (effect on serum calcium)

ROUTE	ONSET	PEAK	DURATION
IV	24 hr	7 days	unknown

Contraindications/Precautions
Contraindicated in: Hypersensitivity to pamidronate, other bisphosphonates, or mannitol; OB: Pregnancy; Lactation: Lactation.
Use Cautiously in: Underlying cardiovascular disease, especially HF (initiate saline hydration cautiously); Invasive dental procedures, cancer, receiving chemotherapy or corticosteroids, poor oral hygiene, periodontal disease, dental disease, anemia, coagulopathy, infection, or poorly fitting dentures (may ↑ risk of jaw osteonecrosis); History of thyroid surgery (may be at ↑ risk for hypocalcemia); Renal impairment (dose ↓ recommended); Pedi: Safety and effectiveness not established in children.

Adverse Reactions/Side Effects
CV: arrhythmias, hypertension, syncope, tachycardia. **EENT:** blurred vision, conjunctivitis, eye pain/inflammation, rhinitis. **Endo:** hypothyroidism. **F and E:** hypocalcemia, hypokalemia, hypomagnesemia, hypophosphatemia, fluid overload. **GI:** nausea, abdominal pain, anorexia, constipation, vomiting. **GU:** nephrotoxicity. **Hemat:** leukopenia, anemia. **Local:** phlebitis at injection site. **MS:** muscle stiffness, pain, femur fractures, osteonecrosis (primarily of jaw). **Neuro:** fatigue. **Resp:** rales. **Misc:** fever.

Interactions
Drug-Drug: Hypokalemia and hypomagnesemia may ↑ risk of **digoxin** toxicity. **Calcium** and **vitamin D** will antagonize the beneficial effects of pamidronate. Concurrent use of **thalidomide** may ↑ risk of renal impairment.

Route/Dosage
Hypercalcemia of Malignancy
IV (Adults): *Moderate hypercalcemia:* 30–90 mg; may be repeated after 7 days.

Osteolytic Lesions from Multiple Myeloma
IV (Adults): 90 mg monthly.

Osteolytic Lesions from Metastatic Breast Cancer
IV (Adults): 90 mg every 3–4 wk.

Paget's Disease
IV (Adults): 90–180 mg/treatment; may be given as 30 mg daily for 3 days up to 30 mg/wk for 6 wk. Single doses of 60–90 mg may also be effective.

P

Availability (generic available)
Solution for injection: 3 mg/mL, 6 mg/mL, 9 mg/mL.

NURSING IMPLICATIONS
Assessment
- Monitor intake/output ratios and BP frequently during therapy. Assess for signs of fluid overload (edema, rales/crackles).
- Monitor symptoms of hypercalcemia (nausea, vomiting, anorexia, weakness, constipation, thirst, and cardiac arrhythmias).
- Observe for evidence of hypocalcemia (paresthesia, muscle twitching, laryngospasm, and Chvostek's or Trousseau's sign). Protect symptomatic patients by elevating and padding side rails; keep bed in low position.
- Monitor IV site for phlebitis (pain, redness, swelling). Symptomatic treatment should be used if this occurs.
- Assess for bone pain. Treatment with nonopioid or opioid analgesics may be necessary.

Lab Test Considerations
- Assess serum creatinine prior to each treatment. Withhold dose if renal function has deteriorated in patients treated for bone metastases.
- Monitor serum electrolytes (including calcium, phosphate, potassium, and magnesium), hemoglobin, and creatinine closely. Monitor CBC and platelet count during the first 2 wk of therapy. May cause hyperkalemia or hypokalemia, hypernatremia, and hematuria.
- Monitor renal function periodically during therapy.

Implementation
- Initiate a vigorous saline hydration, maintaining a urine output of 2000 mL/24 hr, concurrently with pamidronate therapy. Patients should be adequately hydrated, but avoid overhydration. Use caution in patients with underlying cardiovascular disease, especially HF. Do not use diuretics prior to treatment of hypovolemia.
- Patients with severe hypercalcemia should be started at the 90-mg dose.

IV Administration
- **Hypercalcemia:** *Dilution:* Dilute recommended dose in 1000 mL of 0.45% NaCl, 0.9% NaCl, or D5W. Solution is stable for 24 hr at room temperature. *Rate:* Administer 60-mg infusion over at least 4 hr and 90-mg infusion over 24 hr.
- **Multiple Myeloma:** *Dilution:* Dilute recommended dose in 500 mL of 0.45% NaCl, 0.9% NaCl, or D5W. *Rate:* Administer over 4 hr.
- **Paget's Disease:** Dilute recommended dose in 500 mL of 0.45% NaCl, 0.9% NaCl, or D5W.
- *Rate:* Administer over 4 hr.
- **Y-Site Compatibility:** acyclovir, alemtuzumab, allopurinol, amifostine, amikacin, aminophylline, amphotericin B lipid complex, amphotericin B liposomal, ampicillin, ampicillin/sulbactam, anidulafungin, argatroban, atracurium, azithromycin, aztreonam, bivalirudin, bleomycin, bumetanide, buprenorphine, butorphanol, carboplatin, carmustine, cefazolin, cefepime, cefotaxime, cefotetan, cefoxitin, ceftazidime, ceftriaxone, cefuroxime, chloramphenicol, chlorpromazine, ciprofloxacin, cisatracurium, cisplatin, clindamycin, cyclophosphamide, cyclosporine, cytarabine, dacarbazine, daptomycin, dexamethasone, dexmedetomidine, dexrazoxane, digoxin, diltiazem, diphenhydramine, dobutamine, docetaxel, dopamine, doxorubicin hydrochloride, doxorubicin liposomal, doxycycline, droperidol, enalaprilat, ephedrine, epinephrine, epirubicin, ertapenem, erythromycin, esmolol, etoposide, etoposide phosphate, famotidine, fentanyl, fluconazole, fludarabine, fluorouracil, foscarnet, fosphenytoin, furosemide, ganciclovir, gemcitabine, gentamicin, glycopyrrolate, granisetron, haloperidol, heparin, hydralazine, hydrocortisone, hydromorphone, ifosfamide, imipenem/cilastatin, insulin regular, isoproterenol, ketorolac, labetalol, levofloxacin, lidocaine, linezolid, lorazepam, magnesium sulfate, mannitol, melphalan, meperidine, meropenem, mesna, methotrexate, methylprednisolone, metoclopramide, metoprolol, metronidazole, midazolam, milrinone, mitoxantrone, morphine, moxifloxacin, mycophenolate, nafcillin, nalbuphine, naloxone, nicardipine, nitroglycerin, nitroprusside, norepinephrine, octreotide, ondansetron, oxytocin, paclitaxel, palonosetron, pemetrexed, pentamidine, pentobarbital, phenobarbital, phentolamine, phenylephrine, piperacillin/tazobactam, potassium acetate, potassium chloride, potassium phosphate, procainamide, prochlorperazine, promethazine, propranolol, remifentanil, rocuronium, sodium acetate, sodium bicarbonate, sodium phosphate, succinylcholine, sufentanil, tacrolimus, theophylline, thiopental, thiotepa, tigecycline, tirofiban, tobramycin, topotecan, trimethoprim/sulfamethoxazole, vancomycin, vasopressin, vecuronium, verapamil, vinblastine, vincristine, vinorelbine, voriconazole, zidovudine.
- **Y-Site Incompatibility:** amphotericin B deoxycholate, caspofungin, dantrolene, diazepam, leucovorin, phenytoin.
- **Additive Incompatibility:** Calcium-containing solutions, such as LR.

Patient/Family Teaching
- Advise patient to report signs of hypercalcemic relapse (bone pain, anorexia, nausea, vomiting, thirst, lethargy) or eye problems (pain, inflammation, blurred vision, conjunctivitis) to health care professional promptly.
- Advise patient to notify nurse of pain at the infusion site.
- Encourage patient to comply with dietary recommendations. Diet should contain adequate amounts of calcium and vitamin D.

- Advise patient to notify health care professional if bone pain is severe or persistent.
- Advise patient to maintain good oral hygiene and have regular dental examinations. Instruct patient to inform health care professional of pamidronate therapy prior to dental surgery.
- Emphasize the need for keeping follow-up exams to monitor progress, even after medication is discontinued, to detect relapse.
- Rep: May cause fetal harm. Advise females of reproductive potential to notify health care professional if pregnancy is planned or suspected and to avoid breastfeeding during therapy. May impair female and male fertility.

Evaluation/Desired Outcomes
- Lowered serum calcium levels.
- Decreased pain from lytic lesions.

---

pancrelipase (pan-kre-li-pase)
✦Cotazym, Creon, ✦Pancrease MT, Pancreaze, Pertzye, Viokace, Zenpep

Classification
Therapeutic: digestive agent
Pharmacologic: pancreatic enzymes

Indications
Pancreatic insufficiency associated with: Chronic pancreatitis, Pancreatectomy, Cystic fibrosis, GI bypass surgery, Ductal obstruction secondary to tumor.

Action
Contains lipolytic, amylolytic, and proteolytic activity. **Therapeutic Effects:** Increased digestion of fats, carbohydrates, and proteins in the GI tract.

Pharmacokinetics
Absorption: Unknown.
Distribution: Unknown.
Metabolism and Excretion: Unknown.
Half-life: Unknown.

TIME/ACTION PROFILE (digestant effects)

ROUTE	ONSET	PEAK	DURATION
PO	rapid	unknown	unknown

Contraindications/Precautions
Contraindicated in: Hypersensitivity to hog proteins.
Use Cautiously in: Gout, renal impairment, or hyperuricemia (may ↑ uric acid levels); OB: Systemic absorption during pregnancy expected to be minimal; significant fetal exposure not expected; Lactation: Systemic absorption expected to be minimal; significant exposure to breastfed infant not expected.

Adverse Reactions/Side Effects
Derm: hives, rash. **EENT:** nasal stuffiness. **GI:** abdominal pain (high doses only), diarrhea, nausea, stomach cramps, FIBROSING COLONOPATHY (high doses only), oral irritation. **GU:** hematuria. **Metab:** hyperuricemia. **Resp:** dyspnea, shortness of breath, wheezing. **Misc:** allergic reactions.

Interactions
Drug-Drug: Antacids (**calcium carbonate** or **magnesium hydroxide**) may ↓ effectiveness of pancrelipase. May ↓ the absorption of concurrently administered **iron supplements**.
Drug-Food: Alkaline foods destroy coating on enteric-coated products.

Route/Dosage
PO (Adults and Children ≥4 yr): Initiate with 500 lipase units/kg/meal; dose should be adjusted based on weight, clinical symptoms, and stool fat content; maximum dose = 2500 lipase units/kg/meal (or 10,000 lipase units/kg/day).
PO (Children >1 yr and <4 yr): Initiate with 1000 lipase units/kg/meal; dose should be adjusted based on weight, clinical symptoms, and stool fat content; maximum dose = 2500 lipase units/kg/meal (or 10,000 lipase units/kg/day).
PO (Children ≤1 yr): 2000–4000 lipase units per 120 mL of formula or breast milk.

Availability (generic available)
Tablets: 10,440 units lipase/39,150 units protease/39,150 units amylase, 20,880 units lipase/78,300 units protease/78,300 units amylase. **Delayed-release capsules:** 2600 units lipase/6200 units protease/10,850 units amylase, 3000 units lipase/9500 units protease/15,000 units amylase, 3000 units lipase/10,000 units protease/16,000 units amylase, 4000 units lipase/14,375 units protease/15,125 units amylase, 4200 units lipase/14,200 units protease/24,600 units amylase, 5000 units lipase/17,000 units protease/27,000 units amylase, 6000 units lipase/19,000 units protease/30,000 units amylase, 8000 units lipase/28,750 units protease/30,250 units amylase, ✦8000 units lipase/30,000 units protease/30,000 units amylase, 10,000 units lipase/34,000 units protease/55,000 units amylase, 10,500 units lipase/35,500 units protease/61,500 units amylase, 12,000 units lipase/38,000 units protease/60,000 units amylase, 13,800 units lipase/27,600 units protease/27,600 units amylase, 15,000 units lipase/51,000 units protease/82,000 units amylase, 16,000 units lipase/57,500 units protease/60,500 units amylase, 16,800 units lipase/56,800 units protease/98,400 units amylase, ✦20,000 units lipase/55,000 units protease/55,000 units amylase, 20,000 units lipase/68,000 units protease/109,000 units amylase, 20,700 units lipase/41,400 units protease/41,400 units amylase, 21,000 units lipase/54,700 units protease/83,900 units amylase, 23,000 units lipase/46,000 units protease/46,000 units amylase, 24,000 units lipase/76,000 units protease/120,000 units amylase, 25,000

units lipase/85,000 units protease/136,000 units amylase, 36,000 units lipase/114,000 units protease/180,000 units amylase, 40,000 units lipase/136,000 units protease/218,000 units amylase.

NURSING IMPLICATIONS
Assessment
* Assess patient's nutritional status (height, weight, skin-fold thickness, arm muscle circumference, and lab values) prior to and periodically throughout therapy.
* Monitor stools for high fat content (steatorrhea). Stools will be foul-smelling and frothy.
* Assess patient for allergy to pork; sensitivity to pancrelipase may exist.

Lab Test Considerations
* May cause ↑ serum and urine uric acid concentrations.

Implementation
* *Pancreaze* is not interchangeable with any other pancrelipase product.
* **PO:** Administer immediately before or with meals and snacks.
* *DNC:* Swallow tablets whole; do not crush, break, or chew.
* Swallow capsules whole. If unable to swallow, capsules may be opened and sprinkled on foods. Delayed-release capsules filled should not be chewed (sprinkle on soft, acidic foods that can be swallowed without chewing, such as applesauce or Jell-O) and followed immediately by water or juice to ensure complete ingestion. These medications should not be chewed or mixed with alkaline foods prior to ingestion or coating will be destroyed.
* Half of the prescribed *Pancreaze* and *Pertzye* dose for an individualized full meal should be given with each snack. The total daily dose should reflect approximately three meals plus two or three snacks per day.
* Do not mix contents of *Pancreaze*, *Pertzye*, or *Creon* capsules directly into breast milk or formula. Capsule contents may be sprinkled on small amounts of acidic soft food with a pH of 4.5 or less (applesauce) and given to the infant within 15 min. Contents of the capsule may also be administered directly to the mouth. Follow administration with breast milk or formula. Applesauce mixture of *Pertzye* can also be administered via a gastric tube.
* Do not mix *Zenpep* capsule contents directly into formula or breast milk prior to administration. Administer with applesauce, bananas, or pears (commercially prepared) and follow with breast milk or formula.

Patient/Family Teaching
* Encourage patients to comply with diet recommendations of health care professional (generally high-calorie, high-protein, low-fat). Dose should be adjusted for fat content of diet. Usually 300 mg of

pancrelipase is necessary to digest every 17 g of dietary fat. If a dose is missed, it should be omitted and next dose taken with next snack, as directed. Do not increase dose without consulting health care professional. Several days may be required to determine correct dose. Advise patient to read *Medication Guide* before starting therapy and with each Rx refill; information may be updated.
* Instruct patient not to chew tablets and to swallow them quickly with plenty of liquid to prevent mouth and throat irritation. Sit upright to enhance swallowing. Eating immediately after taking medication helps further ensure that the medication is swallowed and does not remain in contact with mouth and esophagus for a prolonged period. Patient should avoid sniffing powdered contents of capsules, as sensitization of nose and throat may occur (nasal stuffiness or respiratory distress).
* Advise patients and caregivers to notify health care professional if symptoms of fibrosing colonopathy (abdominal pain, distention, vomiting, constipation) occur. Symptoms occur more frequently with doses exceeding 6000 lipase units/kg of body weight per meal (10,000 lipase units/kg of body weight/day) and have been associated with colonic strictures in children below the age of 12 yr.
* Instruct patient to notify health care professional if joint pain, swelling of legs, gastric distress, or rash occurs.
* Rep: Advise female patients to notify health care professional if pregnancy is planned or suspected, or if breastfeeding.

Evaluation/Desired Outcomes
* Improved nutritional status in patients with pancreatic insufficiency.
* Normalization of stools in patients with steatorrhea.

⅜ panitumumab
(pan-i-**tu**-mu-mab)
   Vectibix
Classification
Therapeutic: antineoplastics
Pharmacologic: kinase inhibitors

Indications
⅜ Treatment of wild-type *RAS* (wild type in *KRAS* and *NRAS*) metastatic colorectal cancer that has failed fluoropyrimidine-, oxaliplatin-, and irinotecan-containing chemotherapy (to be used as monotherapy). ⅜ Treatment of wild-type *RAS* (wild type in *KRAS* and *NRAS*) metastatic colorectal cancer (as first-line therapy with FOLFOX).

Action
⅜ Binds to epidermal growth factor receptor resulting in inactivation of kinases that regulate proliferation and transformation. **Therapeutic Effects:** Decreased progression of colorectal cancer.

Pharmacokinetics

Absorption: IV administration results in complete bioavailability.
Distribution: Unknown.
Metabolism and Excretion: Unknown.
Half-life: 7.5 days.

TIME/ACTION PROFILE (plasma concentrations)

ROUTE	ONSET	PEAK	DURATION
IV	unknown	end of infusion	unknown

Contraindications/Precautions

Contraindicated in: Concurrent use of leucovorin; ⅹ *RAS:* mutant metastatic colorectal cancer or unknown *RAS* mutation status (↑ mortality and tumor progression); OB: Pregnancy; Lactation: Lactation.
Use Cautiously in: Rep: Women of reproductive potential; Pedi: Safety and effectiveness not established in children.

Adverse Reactions/Side Effects

CV: edema. **Derm:** acneiform dermatitis, dry skin, erythema, paronychia, pruritus, rash, skin exfoliation, skin fissures, abscesses, NECROTIZING FASCIITIS, photosensitivity. **EENT:** corneal perforation, eyelash growth, keratitis, ulcerative keratitis. **F and E:** hypocalcemia, hypomagnesemia. **GI:** abdominal pain, constipation, diarrhea, nausea, vomiting, stomatitis. **GU:** acute renal failure. **Neuro:** fatigue. **Resp:** cough, INTERSTITIAL LUNG DISEASE (ILD), PULMONARY FIBROSIS. **Misc:** INFUSION REACTIONS, SEPSIS.

Interactions

Drug-Drug: None reported.

Route/Dosage

IV (Adults): 6 mg/kg every 14 days.

Availability

Solution for injection: 20 mg/mL.

NURSING IMPLICATIONS

Assessment

● Assess for dermatologic toxicity (dermatitis acneiform, pruritus, erythema, rash, skin exfoliation, paronychia, dry skin, skin fissures). If severe, may lead to infection (sepsis, septic death, abscesses requiring incision and drainage). With severe reactions, hold panitumumab and monitor for inflammatory or infectious sequelae. *If severe dermatologic toxicities (Grade 3 or higher) or those considered intolerable occur,* hold panitumumab. *Upon 1st occurrence of a grade 3 dermatologic toxicity,* hold 1–2 doses; if skin improves to <Grade 3, reinitiate at original dose. *For 2nd occurrence of a grade 3 dermatologic toxicity,*

hold 1–2 doses; if skin improves to <Grade 3, reinitiate at 80% of original dose. *For 3rd occurrence of a grade 3 dermatologic toxicity,* hold 1–2 doses; if skin improves to <Grade 3, reinitiate at 60% of original dose. *For 4th occurrence of a grade 3 dermatologic toxicity,* permanently discontinue panitumumab.
● Monitor for severe infusion reactions (anaphylactic reaction, bronchospasm, fever, chills, hypotension). If severe reaction occurs, stop panitumumab; may require permanent discontinuation.
● Assess for pulmonary fibrosis (cough, wheezing, exertional dyspnea, ILD, pneumonitis, lung infiltrates). Permanently discontinue panitumumab if these signs occur.
● Monitor for diarrhea and dehydration during therapy.
● Monitor for evidence of keratitis, ulcerative keratitis, or corneal perforation. Interrupt or discontinue panitumumab for acute or worsening keratitis, ulcerative keratitis, or corneal perforation.

Lab Test Considerations

● ⅹ Patient selection is based on *RAS* status. Prior to administration, assess *RAS* mutational status in colorectal tumors and confirm the absence of a *RAS* mutation. Information on FDA-approved tests for the detection of *RAS* mutations in patients with metastatic colorectal cancer is available at: http://www.fda.gov/CompanionDiagnostics.
● Monitor electrolyte levels periodically during and for 8 wk after completion of therapy. May cause hypomagnesemia, hypocalcemia, and hypokalemia. Replace electrolytes as needed.

Implementation

● **Intermittent Infusion:** *Dilution:* Withdraw necessary amount of panitumumab. Dilute to a volume of 100 mL with 0.9% NaCl; dilute doses >1000 mg with 150 mL. *Concentration:* 10 mg/mL. Mix by inverting gently; do not shake. Administer via infusion pump using a low-protein binding 0.2 mcg or 0.22 mcg in-line filter. Solution is colorless and may contain a small amount of visible translucent to white, amorphous, proteinaceous particles. Do not administer solutions that are discolored or contain particulate matter. Store in refrigerator; do not freeze. Use diluted solution within 6 hr of preparation if stored at room temperature or within 24 hr if refrigerated. *Rate:* Administer over 60 min every 14 days. If 1st infusion is tolerated, subsequent infusions may be infused over 30–60 min. Administer doses >1000 mg over 90 min.
● *If mild to moderate infusion reaction (Grade 1 or 2) occurs,* decrease infusion rate by 50%. *If severe reaction (Grade 3 or 4) occurs,* immediately and permanently discontinue panitumumab.

P

- **Y-Site Incompatibility:** Flush line before and after administration with 0.9% NaCl. Do not mix with other medications or solutions.

Patient/Family Teaching

- Explain purpose of panitumumab to patient.
- May cause photosensitivity. Caution patient to wear sunscreen and hats and to limit sun exposure.
- Advise patient to notify health care professional if signs and symptoms of dermatologic toxicity, infusion reactions, pulmonary fibrosis, or ocular changes occur.
- Rep: May cause fetal harm. Advise females of reproductive potential to use effective contraception and to avoid breastfeeding during and for 2 months after last dose. May impair fertility in females.
- Emphasize the need for periodic blood tests to monitor electrolyte levels.

Evaluation/Desired Outcomes

- Decreased progression of colorectal cancer.

BEERS

☒ pantoprazole
(pan-**toe**-pra-zole)
✦Pantoloc, Protonix, ✦Tecta
Classification
Therapeutic: antiulcer agents
Pharmacologic: proton-pump inhibitors

Indications

Erosive esophagitis associated with GERD. Maintenance of healing of erosive esophagitis. Pathologic gastric hypersecretory conditions. **Unlabeled Use:** Adjunctive treatment of duodenal ulcers associated with *Helicobacter pylori*.

Action

Binds to an enzyme in the presence of acidic gastric pH, preventing the final transport of hydrogen ions into the gastric lumen. **Therapeutic Effects:** Diminished accumulation of acid in the gastric lumen, with lessened acid reflux. Healing of duodenal ulcers and esophagitis. Decreased acid secretion in hypersecretory conditions.

Pharmacokinetics

Absorption: Tablet is enteric-coated; absorption occurs only after tablet leaves the stomach.
Distribution: Unknown.
Protein Binding: 98%.
Metabolism and Excretion: Primarily metabolized by the CYP2C19 and CYP3A4 isoenzymes in the liver; ☒ the CYP2C19 isoenzyme exhibits genetic polymorphism (15–20% of Asian patients and 3–5% of Caucasian and Black patients may be poor metabolizers and may have significantly ↑ pantoprazole concentrations and an ↑ risk of adverse effects); inactive metabolites are excreted in urine (71%) and feces (18%).
Half-life: 1 hr.

TIME/ACTION PROFILE (effect on acid secretion)

ROUTE	ONSET†	PEAK	DURATION†
PO	2.5 hr	unknown	1 wk
IV	15–30 min	2 hr	unknown

†Onset = 51% inhibition; duration = return to normal following discontinuation.

Contraindications/Precautions

Contraindicated in: Hypersensitivity to pantoprazole or related drugs (benzimidazoles).
Use Cautiously in: Patients using high doses for >1 yr (↑ risk of hip, wrist, or spine fractures and fundic gland polyps); Patients using therapy for >3 yr (↑ risk of vitamin B_{12} deficiency); Pre-existing risk of hypocalcemia; OB: Use during pregnancy only if potential maternal benefit justifies potential fetal risk; Lactation: Use while breastfeeding only if potential maternal benefit justifies potential risk to infant; Pedi: Safety and effectiveness not established in children; Geri: Appears on Beers list. ↑ risk of *Clostridioides difficile* infection, pneumonia, GI malignancies, bone loss, and fractures in older adults. Avoid scheduled use for >8 wk in older adults unless for high-risk patients (e.g. oral corticosteroid or chronic NSAID use) or patients with erosive esophagitis, Barrett's esophagitis, pathological hypersecretory condition, or demonstrated need for maintenance therapy (e.g. failure of H_2 antagonist).

Adverse Reactions/Side Effects

Derm: ACUTE GENERALIZED EXANTHEMATOUS PUSTULOSIS, cutaneous lupus erythematosus, DRUG REACTION WITH EOSINOPHILIA AND SYSTEMIC SYMPTOMS (DRESS), STEVENS-JOHNSON SYNDROME, TOXIC EPIDERMAL NECROLYSIS. **Endo:** hyperglycemia. **F and E:** hypocalcemia (especially if treatment duration ≥3 mo), hypokalemia (especially if treatment duration ≥3 mo), hypomagnesemia (especially if treatment duration ≥3 mo). **GI:** abdominal pain, CLOSTRIDIOIDES DIFFICILE-ASSOCIATED DIARRHEA (CDAD), diarrhea, eructation, flatulence, fundic gland polyps. **GU:** acute tubulointerstitial nephritis. **Hemat:** vitamin B_{12} deficiency. **MS:** bone fracture. **Neuro:** headache. **Misc:** HYPERSENSITIVITY REACTIONS (including anaphylaxis, angioedema, or tubulointerstitial nephritis), systemic lupus erythematosis.

Interactions

Drug-Drug: May ↓ levels of **atazanavir** and **nelfinavir**; avoid concurrent use with either of these antiretrovirals. May ↓ absorption of drugs requiring acid pH, including **ketoconazole**, **itraconazole**, **ampicillin esters**, **iron salts**, **erlotinib**, and **mycophenolate mofetil**; concomitant use with **atazanavir** not recommended. May ↑ risk of bleeding with **warfarin** (monitor INR/PT). Hypomagnesemia and hypokalemia ↑ risk of **digoxin** toxicity. May ↑ **methotrexate** levels.

Route/Dosage

Gastroesophageal Reflux Disease

PO (Adults): *Short-term treatment of erosive esophagitis associated with GERD:* 40 mg once daily for up to 8 wk; *Maintenance of healing of erosive esophagitis:* 40 mg once daily.

PO (Children ≥5 yr): *15–39 kg:* 20 mg once daily for up to 8 wk; *≥40 kg:* 40 mg once daily for up to 8 wk.

IV (Adults): 40 mg once daily for 7–10 days.

Gastric Hypersecretory Conditions

PO (Adults): 40 mg twice daily, up to 120 mg twice daily.

IV (Adults): 80 mg every 12 hr (up to 240 mg/day).

Availability (generic available)

Delayed-release tablets: 20 mg, 40 mg. **Delayed-release oral suspension:** 40 mg/packet. **Powder for injection:** 40 mg/vial.

NURSING IMPLICATIONS

Assessment

● Assess patient routinely for epigastric or abdominal pain and for frank or occult blood in stool, emesis, or gastric aspirate.

Lab Test Considerations

● May cause abnormal liver function tests, including ↑ AST, ALT, alkaline phosphatase, and bilirubin.

● May cause hypomagnesemia. Monitor serum magnesium prior to and periodically during therapy.

Implementation

● Do not confuse Protonix with Lotronex or protamine.

● Patients receiving pantoprazole IV should be converted to PO dosing as soon as possible.

● Monitor bowel function. Diarrhea, abdominal cramping, fever, and bloody stools should be reported to health care professional promptly as a sign of CDAD. May begin up to several wk following cessation of therapy.

● **PO:** *DNC:* May be administered with or without food. Do not break, crush, or chew tablets.

● *Oral suspension:* Sprinkle granules on 1 tsp of applesauce or apple juice approximately 30 min prior to a meal. Do not crush or chew granules. Take sips of water to make sure granules are washed down into the stomach. Granules may also be emptied into a small cup or teaspoon containing one teaspoon of apple juice. Stir for 5 sec (granules will not dissolve) and swallow immediately. To make sure that entire dose is taken, rinse container once or twice with apple juice to remove any remaining granules. Swallow immediately. Do not use with anything other that applesauce or apple juice. For patients who have a *nasogastric tube* or gastrostomy tube in place, remove plunger from the barrel of a 60 mL catheter-tip syringe. Discard plunger. Connect catheter tip of syringe to a 16 French (or larger) tube. Hold syringe attached to tubing as high as possible while giving pantoprazole. Empty contents of packet into the bar-

rel of the syringe. Add 10 mL (2 tsp) of apple juice and gently tap and/or shake the barrel of the syringe to help rinse the syringe and tube. Repeat at least twice more using the same amount of apple juice (10 mL or 2 tsp) each time. No granules should remain in the syringe.

● Antacids may be used concurrently.

IV Administration

● **IV:** *Reconstitution:* Reconstitute each vial with 10 mL of 0.9% NaCl. Reconstituted solution is stable for 6 hr at room temperature.

● **IV Push:** *Dilution:* Administer undiluted. *Concentration:* 4 mg/mL. *Rate:* Administer over at least 2 min.

● **Intermittent Infusion:** *Dilution:* Dilute further with D5W, 0.9% NaCl, or LR. *Concentration:* 0.4–0.8 mg/mL. Diluted solution is stable for 24 hr at room temperature. *Rate:* Administer over 15 min at a rate of <3 mg/min.

● **Y-Site Compatibility:** acetazolamide, allopurinol, alprostadil, amifostine, aminocaproic acid, aminophylline, amphotericin B lipid complex, amphotericin B liposomal, ampicillin, ampicillin/sulbactam, anidulafungin, argatroban, arsenic trioxide, azithromycin, bleomycin, bumetanide, cangrelor, carboplatin, carmustine, ceftaroline, ceftolozane/tazobactam, ceftriaxone, cyclophosphamide, cytarabine, docetaxel, doxorubicin liposomal, doxycycline, eravacycline, ertapenem, fluorouracil, foscarnet, fosphenytoin, ganciclovir, granisetron, hetastarch, imipenem/cilastatin, irinotecan, isavuconazonium, meropenem/vaborbactam, mesna, methadone, methohexital, nafcillin, paclitaxel, penicillin G sodium, pentobarbital, phentolamine, phenylephrine, plazomicin, potassium chloride, procainamide, rifampin, succinylcholine, sufentanil, tedizolid, telavancin, theophylline, tigecycline, tirofiban, vasopressin, zidovudine, zoledronic acid.

● **Y-Site Incompatibility:** acetaminophen, alemtuzumab, atropine, aztreonam, blinatumomab, buprenorphine, butorphanol, calcium chloride, cefepime, cefotaxime, cefotetan, chloramphenicol, chlorpromazine, ciprofloxacin, cisatracurium, cisplatin, dacarbazine, dactinomycin, dantrolene, daptomycin, daunorubicin hydrochloride, dexamethasone, dexmedetomidine, dexrazoxane, diazepam, diltiazem, diphenhydramine, dobutamine, doxorubicin hydrochloride, droperidol, ephedrine, epirubicin, esmolol, estrogens,conjugated, etoposide, etoposide phosphate, famotidine, fentanyl, fluconazole, fludarabine, gemcitabine, gemtuzumab ozogamicin, glycopyrrolate, haloperidol, hydralazine, hydroxyzine, idarubicin, ifosfamide, indomethacin, ketorolac, labetalol, leucovorin calcium, levofloxacin, lidocaine, linezolid, lorazepam, melphalan, meperidine, methotrexate, methylprednisolone, metoprolol, metronidazole, milrinone, mitomycin, mitoxantrone, moxifloxacin, multivitamins, mycophenolate, nalbuphine, naloxone, nicardipine, ondansetron, palonosetron, pemetrexed, pentamidine, phenytoin, potassium acetate, potassium phosphates, prochlorperazine, promethazine, propranolol, remifentanil, rocuronium, sodium acetate, sodium phosphate, thiotepa, topotecan, vecuronium, verapamil, vinblastine, vincristine, vinorelbine, voriconazole, solutions containing zinc.

Patient/Family Teaching

- Instruct patient to take medication as directed for the full course of therapy, even if feeling better. Advise patient to read *Medication Guide* before starting therapy and with each Rx refill in case of changes.
- Advise patient to avoid alcohol, products containing aspirin or NSAIDs, and foods that may cause an increase in GI irritation.
- Advise patient to report onset of black, tarry stools; diarrhea; or abdominal pain to health care professional promptly. Instruct patient to notify health care professional immediately if rash, diarrhea, abdominal cramping, fever, or bloody stools occur and not to treat with antidiarrheals without consulting health care professional.
- Instruct patient to notify health care professional of all Rx or OTC medications, vitamins, or herbal products being taken and consult health care professional before taking any new medications.
- Rep: Advise females of reproductive potential to notify health care professional if pregnancy is planned or suspected, or if breastfeeding.

Evaluation/Desired Outcomes

- Decrease in abdominal pain, heartburn, gastric irritation, and bleeding in patients with GERD; may require up to 4 wk of therapy.
- Healing in patients with erosive esophagitis. Therapy is continued for up to 8 wk.

---

paricalcitol, See VITAMIN D COMPOUNDS.

BEERS

▨ PARoxetine
PARoxetine hydrochloride
(par-**ox**-e-teen)
  Paxil, Paxil CR
PARoxetine mesylate
  ~~Brisdelle~~, Pexeva
Classification
Therapeutic: antianxiety agents, antidepressants
Pharmacologic: selective serotonin reuptake inhibitors (SSRIs)

Indications
Paxil, Paxil CR, Pexeva: Treatment of the following disorders: Major depressive disorder, Panic disorder. **Paxil, Pexeva**: Treatment of the following disorders: Obsessive compulsive disorder (OCD), Generalized anxiety disorder. **Paxil, Paxil CR**: Social anxiety disorder. **Paxil**: Post-traumatic stress disorder (PTSD). **Paxil CR**: Premenstrual dysphoric disorder. **Paroxetine mesylate (7.5–mg capsule)**: Moderate to severe vasomotor symptoms associated with menopause.

Action
Inhibits neuronal reuptake of serotonin in the CNS, thus potentiating the activity of serotonin; has little effect on norepinephrine or dopamine; mechanism for benefit in treating vasomotor symptoms unknown. **Therapeutic Effects:** Antidepressant action. Decreased frequency of panic attacks, OCD, or anxiety. Improvement in manifestations of PTSD. Decreased dysphoria prior to menses. Decreased vasomotor symptoms in postmenopausal women.

Pharmacokinetics
Absorption: Completely absorbed following oral administration. Controlled-release tablets are enteric-coated and control medication release over 4–5 hr.
Distribution: Widely distributed throughout body fluids and tissues, including the CNS; cross the placenta and enter breast milk.
Protein Binding: 95%.
Metabolism and Excretion: Highly metabolized by the liver, primarily by the CYP2D6 isoenzyme; ⚕ the CYP2D6 isoenzyme exhibits genetic polymorphism; ~7% of population may be poor metabolizers and may have significantly ↑ paroxetine concentrations and an ↑ risk of adverse effects. 2% excreted unchanged in urine.
Half-life: 21 hr.

TIME/ACTION PROFILE (antidepressant action)

ROUTE	ONSET	PEAK	DURATION
PO	1–4 wk	unknown	unknown

Contraindications/Precautions
Contraindicated in: Hypersensitivity; Concurrent use of MAO inhibitors or MAO-inhibitor-like drugs (linezolid or methylene blue); Concurrent use of thioridazine or pimozide; Lactation: Lactation.
Use Cautiously in: Risk of suicide (may ↑ risk of suicide attempt/ideation especially during early treatment or dose adjustment); History of mania; History of seizures; History of bipolar disorder; Angle-closure glaucoma; Severe renal impairment; Severe hepatic impairment; OB: Use during the 1st trimester may be associated with an ↑ risk of cardiac malformations—consider fetal risk/maternal benefit; use during the 3rd trimester may result in neonatal serotonin syndrome requiring prolonged hospitalization, respiratory and nutritional support; Pedi: May ↑ risk of suicide attempt/

ideation especially during early treatment or dose adjustment; may be greater in children and adolescents (safety and effectiveness in children/adolescents not established); Geri: Appears on Beers list. May worsen or cause syndrome of inappropriate antidiuretic hormone (SIADH) secretion and/or hyponatremia in older adults. Use with caution in older adults and closely monitor sodium concentrations when starting therapy or ↑ dose.

Adverse Reactions/Side Effects

CV: chest pain, edema, hypertension, palpitations, postural hypotension, tachycardia, vasodilation. **Derm:** sweating, photosensitivity, pruritus, rash, STEVENS-JOHNSON SYNDROME (SJS). **EENT:** blurred vision, pharyngitis, rhinitis. **Endo:** SIADH. **F and E:** hyponatremia. **GI:** constipation, diarrhea, dry mouth, nausea, abdominal pain, dyspepsia, flatulence, taste disturbances, vomiting. **GU:** ↓ libido, delayed/absent orgasm, ejaculatory delay/failure, erectile dysfunction, genital disorders, infertility, urinary disorders, urinary frequency. **Hemat:** BLEEDING. **Metab:** ↓/↑ appetite, weight gain/loss. **MS:** back pain, bone fracture, myalgia, myopathy. **Neuro:** anxiety, dizziness, drowsiness, headache, insomnia, weakness, agitation, amnesia, confusion, depression, emotional lability, hangover, impaired concentration, malaise, NEUROLEPTIC MALIGNANT SYNDROME, paresthesia, SUICIDAL THOUGHTS, syncope, tremor. **Resp:** cough, yawning. **Misc:** chills, fever, SEROTONIN SYNDROME.

Interactions

Drug-Drug: Concurrent use with **MAO inhibitors** may result in serious, potentially fatal reactions (wait at least 2 wk after stopping MAO inhibitor before initiating paroxetine; wait at least 2 wk after stopping paroxetine before starting MAO inhibitors). Concurrent use with **MAO-inhibitor-like drugs**, such as **linezolid** or **methylene blue** may ↑ risk of serotonin syndrome; concurrent use contraindicated; do not start therapy in patients receiving **linezolid** or **methylene blue**; if **linezolid** or **methylene blue** need to be started in a patient receiving paroxetine, immediately discontinue paroxetine and monitor for signs/symptoms of serotonin syndrome for 2 wk or until 24 hr after last dose of linezolid or methylene blue, whichever comes first (may resume paroxetine therapy 24 hr after last dose of linezolid or methylene blue). Concurrent use with **pimozide** or **thioridazine** may ↑ risk of QT interval prolongation and torsades de pointes; concurrent use contraindicated. May ↓ metabolism and ↑ effects of certain **drugs that are metabolized by the liver**, including other **antidepressants, phenothiazines, class IC antiarrhythmics, risperidone, atomoxetine, theophylline,** and **quinidine.** Concurrent use should be undertaken with caution. **Cimetidine** ↑ blood levels. **Phenobarbital** and **phenytoin** may ↓ effectiveness. Concurrent use with **alcohol** is not recommended. May ↓ the effectiveness of **digoxin** and **ta-**

moxifen. ↑ risk of bleeding with **NSAIDs, aspirin, clopidogrel, prasugrel, ticagrelor, dabigatran, apixaban, edoxaban, rivaroxaban,** or **warfarin.** Drugs that affect serotonergic neurotransmitter systems, including **tricyclic antidepressants, SNRIs, fentanyl, lithium, buspirone, tramadol, meperidine, methadone, amphetamines,** and **triptans,** ↑ risk of serotonin syndrome.

Drug-Natural Products: ↑ risk of serotonergic side effects including serotonin syndrome with **St. John's wort, SAMe,** and **tryptophan.**

Route/Dosage

Depression
PO (Adults): 20 mg as a single dose in the morning; may ↑ by 10 mg/day at weekly intervals (not to exceed 50 mg/day). *Controlled-release tablets:* 25 mg once daily initially. May ↑ at weekly intervals by 12.5 mg (not to exceed 62.5 mg/day).

PO (Geriatric Patients or Debilitated Patients): 10 mg/day initially; may be slowly ↑ (not to exceed 40 mg/day). *Controlled-release tablets:* 12.5 mg once daily initially; may be slowly ↑ (not to exceed 50 mg/day).

Obsessive Compulsive Disorder
PO (Adults): 20 mg/day initially; ↑ by 10 mg/day at weekly intervals up to 40 mg (not to exceed 60 mg/day).

Panic Disorder
PO (Adults): 10 mg/day initially; ↑ by 10 mg/day at weekly intervals up to 40 mg (not to exceed 60 mg/day). *Controlled-release tablets:* 12.5 mg/day initially; ↑ by 12.5 mg/day at weekly intervals (not to exceed 75 mg/day).

Social Anxiety Disorder
PO (Adults): 20 mg/day. *Controlled-release tablets:* 12.5 mg/day initially; may ↑ by 12.5 mg/day weekly intervals (not to exceed 37.5 mg/day).

Generalized Anxiety Disorder
PO (Adults): 20 mg once daily initially; ↑ by 10 mg/day at weekly intervals (not to exceed 50 mg/day).

Post-Traumatic Stress Disorder
PO (Adults): 20 mg/day initially; may ↑ by 10 mg/day at weekly intervals (not to exceed 50 mg/day).

Premenstrual Dysphoric Disorder
PO (Adults): *Controlled-release tablets:* 12.5 mg once daily throughout menstrual cycle or during luteal phase of menstrual cycle only; may ↑ to 25 mg/day after 1 wk.

Menopausal Vasomotor Symptoms
PO (Adults): 7.5 mg once daily at bedtime.

Hepatic Impairment
PO (Adults): Paxil, Paxil CR, or **Pexeva:** *Severe hepatic impairment:* 10 mg/day initially; may slowly ↑

(not to exceed 40 mg/day). *Controlled-release tablets:* 12.5 mg once daily initially; may slowly ↑ (not to exceed 50 mg/day).

Renal Impairment
PO (Adults): Paxil, Paxil CR, or Pexeva: *Severe renal impairment:* 10 mg/day initially; may slowly ↑ (not to exceed 40 mg/day). *Controlled-release tablets:* 12.5 mg once daily initially; may slowly ↑ (not to exceed 50 mg/day).

Availability (generic available)
Paroxetine hydrochloride tablets: 10 mg, 20 mg, 30 mg, 40 mg. **Paroxetine hydrochloride controlled-release tablets:** 12.5 mg, 25 mg, 37.5 mg. **Paroxetine hydrochloride oral suspension (orange flavor):** 10 mg/5 mL. **Paroxetine mesylate capsules :** 7.5 mg. **Paroxetine mesylate tablets (Pexeva):** 10 mg, 20 mg, 30 mg.

NURSING IMPLICATIONS
Assessment
- Monitor appetite and nutritional intake. Weigh weekly. Notify health care professional of continued weight loss. Adjust diet as tolerated to support nutritional status.
- Assess for suicidal tendencies, especially during early therapy. Restrict amount of drug available to patient. Risk may be increased in children, adolescents, and adults ≤24 yr.
- Assess for serotonin syndrome (mental changes [agitation, hallucinations, coma], autonomic instability [tachycardia, labile BP, hyperthermia], neuromuscular aberrations [hyperreflexia, incoordination], and/or GI symptoms [nausea, vomiting, diarrhea]), especially in patients taking other serotonergic drugs (SSRIs, SNRIs, triptans).
- Monitor for development of neuroleptic malignant syndrome (fever, respiratory distress, tachycardia, seizures, diaphoresis, hypertension or hypotension, pallor, tiredness). Discontinue paroxetine and notify health care professional immediately if these symptoms occur.
- Assess for rash periodically during therapy. May cause SJS. Discontinue therapy if severe or if accompanied with fever, general malaise, fatigue, muscle or joint aches, blisters, oral lesions, conjunctivitis, hepatitis, and/or eosinophilia.
- Assess sexual function before starting paroxetine. Assess for changes in sexual function during treatment, including timing of onset; patient may not report.
- **Depression:** Monitor mental status (orientation, mood, behavior). Inform health care professional if patient demonstrates significant increase in anxiety, nervousness, or insomnia.
- **OCD:** Assess patient for frequency of obsessive-compulsive behaviors. Note degree to which these thoughts and behaviors interfere with daily functioning.
- **Panic Attacks:** Assess frequency and severity of panic attacks.
- **Social Anxiety Disorder:** Assess frequency and severity of episodes of anxiety.
- **PTSD:** Assess manifestations of post-traumatic stress disorder periodically during therapy.
- **Premenstrual Dysphoria:** Assess symptoms of premenstrual distress prior to and during therapy.

Lab Test Considerations
- Monitor CBC and differential periodically during therapy. Report leukopenia or anemia.

Implementation
- Do not confuse paroxetine with fluoxetine, duloxetine, or piroxicam. Do not confuse Paxil with Doxil, Plavix, or Trexall.
- Paroxetine mesylate (Pexeva) cannot be substituted with paroxetine (Paxil or Paxil CR) or generic paroxetine.
- Periodically reassess dose and continued need for therapy.
- **PO:** Administer as a single dose in the morning. May administer with food to minimize GI irritation.
- Swallow tablets whole. *DNC:* Do not crush, break, or chew. Shake suspension before administering.
- Taper to avoid potential withdrawal reactions.

Patient/Family Teaching
- Instruct patient to take paroxetine as directed. Take missed doses as soon as possible and return to regular dosing schedule. Do not double doses. Caution patient to consult health care professional before discontinuing paroxetine. Daily doses should be decreased slowly. Abrupt withdrawal may cause dizziness, sensory disturbances, agitation, anxiety, nausea, and sweating. Advise patient to read *Medication Guide* before starting and with each Rx refill in case of changes.
- May cause drowsiness or dizziness. Caution patient to avoid driving and other activities requiring alertness until response to the drug is known.
- Advise patient, family, and caregivers to look for suicidality, especially during early therapy or dose changes. Notify health care professional immediately if thoughts about suicide or dying, attempts to commit suicide, new or worse depression or anxiety, agitation or restlessness, panic attacks, insomnia, new or worse irritability, aggressiveness, acting on dangerous impulses, mania, or other changes in mood or behavior, or if symptoms of serotonin syndrome or neuroleptic malignant syndrome occur.
- Instruct patient to notify health care professional of all Rx or OTC medications, vitamins, or herbal products being taken and consult health care professional before taking any new medications and to

avoid alcohol or other CNS-depressant drugs, including opioids during therapy.
- Inform patient that frequent mouth rinses, good oral hygiene, and sugarless gum or candy may minimize dry mouth. Saliva substitute may be used. Consult dentist if dry mouth persists for more than 2 wk.
- Advise patient to notify health care professional if headache, weakness, nausea, anorexia, anxiety, or insomnia persists.
- Inform patient that paroxetine may cause symptoms of sexual dysfunction. In males, ejaculatory delay or failure, decreased libido, and erectile dysfunction may occur. In female patients, may result in decreased libido and delayed or absent orgasm. Advise patient to notify health care professional if symptoms occur.
- Rep: Advise females of reproductive potential to notify health care professional immediately if pregnancy is planned or suspected and to avoid breastfeeding during therapy. Use in the month before delivery has been associated with an increase in the risk of postpartum hemorrhage. Infants exposed to paroxetine during 1st trimester have increased risk of congenital malformations, particularly cardiovascular malformations. If used during pregnancy, should be tapered during 3rd trimester to avoid neonatal serotonin syndrome. Monitor infants exposed to paroxetine for excess sedation, restlessness, agitation, poor feeding, poor weight gain, respiratory distress; may ↑ risk of persistent pulmonary hypertension of the newborn. Inform patient of pregnancy exposure registry that monitors pregnancy outcomes in women exposed to antidepressants during pregnancy. Register patient by calling the National Pregnancy Registry for Antidepressants at 1-866-961-2388 or visiting online at https://womensmentalhealth.org/clinical-and-researchprograms/pregnancyregistry/antidepressants/.
- Emphasize the importance of follow-up exams to monitor progress. Encourage patient participation in psychotherapy to improve coping skills.

Evaluation/Desired Outcomes
- Increased sense of well-being.
- Renewed interest in surroundings. May require 1–4 wk of therapy to obtain antidepressant effects.
- Decrease in obsessive-compulsive behaviors.
- Decrease in frequency and severity of panic attacks.
- Decrease in frequency and severity of episodes of anxiety.
- Improvement in manifestations of PTSD.
- Decreased dysphoria prior to menses.

patiromer (pa-**tir**-oh-mer)
Veltassa
Classification
Therapeutic: antidotes, electrolyte modifiers
Pharmacologic: cationic exchange resins

Indications
Mild to moderate hyperkalemia (if severe, more immediate measures such as calcium IV or insulin/glucose IV should be instituted).

Action
Contains calcium-sorbitol counterion and ↑ fecal potassium excretion through binding of potassium in the lumen of the GI tract. **Therapeutic Effects:** Reduced serum potassium concentrations.

Pharmacokinetics
Absorption: Not systemically absorbed.
Distribution: Not distributed.
Metabolism and Excretion: Eliminated in the feces.
Half-life: Unknown.

TIME/ACTION PROFILE (↓ in serum potassium concentrations)

ROUTE	ONSET	PEAK	DURATION
PO	7–12 hr	unknown	24 hr

Contraindications/Precautions
Contraindicated in: Hypersensitivity; History of bowel impaction, bowel obstruction, or severe constipation (may be ineffective and worsen condition).
Use Cautiously in: Pedi: Safety and effectiveness not established in children.

Adverse Reactions/Side Effects
F and E: hypokalemia, hypomagnesemia. GI: constipation, diarrhea, flatulence, nausea.

Interactions
Drug-Drug: May ↓ absorption and effectiveness of **bisoprolol, carvedilol, ciprofloxacin, levothyroxine, metformin, mycophenolate mofetil, nebivolol, quinidine, telmisartan**, and **thiamine**; administer ≥3 hr before or after patiromer.

Route/Dosage
PO (Adults): 8.4 g once daily; titrate dose at ≥1 wk intervals by 8.4 g once daily as needed to achieve desired serum potassium concentration (max = 25.2 g once daily).

Availability
Powder for oral suspension: 8.4 g/pkt, 16.8 g/pkt, 25.2 g/pkt.

P

NURSING IMPLICATIONS
Assessment
* Monitor for bowel sounds and frequency and consistency of stools periodically during therapy. May cause constipation.

Lab Test Considerations
* Monitor serum potassium and magnesium periodically during therapy. May cause hypokalemia and hypomagnesemia. Consider magnesium supplements if hypomagnesemia occurs.

Implementation
* Due to delayed action, do not use patiromer as an emergency treatment of life-threatening hyperkalemia.
* PO: Administer immediately at least 3 hr before or 3 hr after other PO medications. Measure 1/3 cup of water. Pour half the water into a glass, then add patiromer and stir. Add the remaining half of the water and stir thoroughly. The powder will not dissolve and mixture will look cloudy. Add more water to the mixture as needed for desired consistency. Drink mixture immediately. If powder remains in the glass after drinking, add more water, stir and drink immediately. Repeat as needed to ensure the entire dose is administered. May use other beverages, or soft foods (apple sauce, yogurt, pudding) instead of water, to prepare mixture. Do not heat (microwave) or add to heated foods or liquids. Do not take in dry form. Stable for 3 mo at room temperature or until the package expiration date if refrigerated.

Patient/Family Teaching
* Instruct patient to take patiromer as directed and adhere to prescribed diet.
* Advise patient to take patiromer ≥3 hrs before or 3 hrs after other medications.
* Instruct patients to not heat (microwaved) or add to heated foods or liquids and should not be taken in its dry form.
* Rep: Advise females of reproductive potential to notify healthcare professional if pregnancy is planned or suspected or if breastfeeding. Patiromer is not absorbed systemically, so it is not expected to harm fetus.

Evaluation/Desired Outcomes
* Reduced serum potassium concentrations.

▓ PAZOPanib (pah-zoe-puh-nib)
Votrient
Classification
Therapeutic: antineoplastics
Pharmacologic: kinase inhibitors

Indications
Advanced renal cell carcinoma. Advanced soft tissue sarcoma in patients who have previously received chemotherapy.

Action
Acts as a tyrosine kinase inhibitor of several vascular endothelial growth factor receptors, platelet-derived growth factor receptor, fibroblast growth factor receptor, cytokine receptor, interleukin-2 receptor inducible T-cell kinase, leukocyte-specific protein tyrosine kinase, and transmembrane glycoprotein receptor tyrosine kinase. Overall effect is decreased angiogenesis in tumors. **Therapeutic Effects:** Decreased growth and spread of renal cell carcinoma. Improvement in progression-free survival.

Pharmacokinetics
Absorption: Well absorbed following oral administration; crushing tablet and ingesting food ↑ absorption.
Distribution: Unknown.
Protein Binding: >99%.
Metabolism and Excretion: Primarily metabolized by the liver via the CYP3A4 isoenzyme and to a lesser extent by the CYP1A2 and CYP2C8 isoenzymes; primarily eliminated in the feces, with <4% excreted by the kidneys.
Half-life: 30.9 hr.

TIME/ACTION PROFILE (plasma concentrations)

ROUTE	ONSET	PEAK	DURATION
PO	PO	2–4 hr	24 hr

Contraindications/Precautions
Contraindicated in: Severe hepatic impairment; History of hemoptysis, cerebral or GI bleeding in preceding 6 mo; Risk/history of arterial thrombotic events, including MI, angina or ischemic stroke within preceding 6 mo; OB: Pregnancy; Lactation: Lactation.
Use Cautiously in: Congenital prolonged QTc interval or concurrent medications/diseases that prolong the QTc interval (may ↑ risk of torsades de pointes); Electrolyte abnormalities (correct prior to use; may ↑ risk of potentially serious arrhythmia); Patients at risk for GI perforation/fistula; Surgery (interruption of therapy recommended); Hypertension (control before therapy is initiated); Hypothyroidism (may worsen condition); Moderate hepatic impairment (dose ↓ recommended); ▓ Patients of East Asian descent (↑ risk of neutropenia, thrombocytopenia, and palmar-plantar erythrodysesthesia); Rapidly growing tumors, high tumor burden, renal impairment, or dehydration (↑ risk of tumor lysis syndrome); ▓ Patients with genetically reduced UGT1A1 activity (presence of UGT1A1*28/*28 allele) (↑ risk of hyperbilirubinemia); ▓ Patients positive for HLA-B*5701 allele (↑ risk of hepatotoxicity); Rep: Women of reproductive potential and men with female partners of reproductive potential; Pedi: Safety and effectiveness not established in children; Geri: ↑ risk of hepatotoxicity in older adults.

Adverse Reactions/Side Effects

CV: bradycardia, hypertension, chest pain, DEEP VEIN THROMBOSIS (DVT), HF, MI, QT interval prolongation. **Derm:** hair color changes (depigmentation), alopecia, facial edema, impaired wound healing, palmar-plantar erythrodysesthesia (hand-foot syndrome), rash, skin depigmentation. **Endo:** hypothyroidism. **GI:** abdominal pain, anorexia, diarrhea, nausea, vomiting, ↓ weight, dyspepsia, GI PERFORATION/FISTULA, HEPATOTOXICITY, PANCREATITIS. **GU:** ↓ fertility, HEMOLYTIC UREMIC SYNDROME, proteinuria. **Hemat:** BLEEDING, neutropenia, thrombocytopenia, THROMBOTIC THROMBOCYTOPENIC PURPURA. **MS:** arthralgia, muscle spasms. **Neuro:** fatigue, weakness, dysgeusia, POSTERIOR REVERSIBLE ENCEPHALOPATHY SYNDROME (PRES), STROKE. **Resp:** INTERSTITIAL LUNG DISEASE (ILD), PULMONARY EMBOLISM (PE). **Misc:** TUMOR LYSIS SYNDROME.

Interactions

Drug-Drug: **Strong CYP3A4 inhibitors**, including **ketoconazole**, **ritonavir**, and **clarithromycin** may ↑ levels and risk of toxicity; avoid concurrent use; if concurrent use unavoidable, ↓ pazopanib dose. **Strong CYP3A4 inducers**, including **rifampin**, may ↓ levels and effectiveness; avoid concurrent use. May ↑ levels and risk of toxicity of **CYP3A4 substrates**, **CYP2D6 substrates**, or **CYP2C8 substrates** that have narrow therapeutic windows; concurrent use is not recommended. ↑ risk of hepatotoxicity with **simvastatin**. **Proton pump inhibitors** and **H₂ receptor antagonists** may ↓ levels; avoid concurrent use; use short-acting antacid instead. **Antacids** may ↓ levels; separate doses by several hrs. **QT interval prolonging drugs** may ↑ risk of QT interval prolongation; avoid concurrent use.
Drug-Food: **Grapefruit juice** may ↑ levels; avoid concurrent use.

Route/Dosage

PO (Adults): 800 mg once daily until disease progression or unacceptable toxicity; *Concurrent use of strong CYP3A4 inhibitors:* 400 mg once daily until disease progression or unacceptable toxicity.

Hepatic Impairment

PO (Adults): *Moderate hepatic impairment:* 200 mg once daily until disease progression or unacceptable toxicity.

Availability

Tablets: 200 mg.

NURSING IMPLICATIONS
Assessment

- Monitor BP during frequent therapy; may cause hypertension. BP should be well controlled prior to initiating therapy. If Grade 2 or 3 hypertension occurs, reduce dose and start or adjust antihypertensive

therapy. Permanently discontinue pazopanib if hypertension remains Grade 3 despite dose reduction(s) and adjustment of antihypertensive therapy. *If Grade 4 hypertension or hypertensive crisis occurs,* permanently discontinue pazopanib. Baseline and periodic evaluation of left ventricular ejection fraction is recommended in patients at risk of cardiac dysfunction. *If left ventricular systolic dysfunction is symptomatic or Grade 3,* hold pazopanib until improved to Grade <3. Resume therapy based on medical judgment. *If left ventricular systolic dysfunction is Grade 4,* permanently discontinue pazopanib.

- Obtain baseline ECG and monitor periodically during therapy. Maintain serum calcium, magnesium, and potassium within normal range during therapy. Monitor patients who are at risk of developing QTc interval prolongation (patients with a history of QT interval prolongation, patients taking antiarrhythmics or other medications that may prolong the QT interval, those with relevant preexisting cardiac disease). Monitor ECG and electrolytes (calcium, magnesium, potassium) at baseline and as indicated. Correct hypokalemia, hypomagnesemia, and hypocalcemia prior to starting and during therapy.

- Monitor for signs and symptoms of GI perforation and fistula (abdominal pain; swelling in stomach area; vomiting blood; black sticky stools; GI bleeding) during therapy. *If Grade 2 or 3 GI fistula occurs,* hold pazopanib and resume based on medical judgment. If Grade 4 fistula occurs, permanently discontinue pazopanib.

- Monitor for signs and symptoms of bleeding. *If Grade 2 symptoms occur,* hold pazopanib until improvement to Grade ≤1. Resume at reduced dose. *If Grade 2 symptoms recur after dose interruption and reduction or Grade 3 or 4 symptoms occur,* permanently discontinue pazopanib.

- Monitor for signs and symptoms of arterial thromboembolic events (MI, stroke). If symptoms occur, permanently discontinue pazopanib.

- Monitor for signs and symptoms of venous thromboembolic events (DVT, PE). *If Grade 3 symptoms occur,* hold pazopanib and resume at same dose if managed with appropriate therapy for at least 1 wk. *If Grade 4 symptoms occur,* permanently discontinue pazopanib.

- Monitor for pulmonary symptoms indicative of ILD/pneumonitis. Permanently discontinue pazopanib in patients who develop ILD or pneumonitis.

- Monitor for signs and symptoms of PRES (headache, seizure, lethargy, confusion, blindness, mild hypertension). Diagnosis is confirmed by MRI. Discontinue pazopanib permanently if PRES occurs.

P

Lab Test Considerations

- Verify negative pregnancy status prior to starting therapy.
- Monitor serum liver tests before initiation and wk 3, 5, 7, and 9, then at mo 3 and mo 4 if symptoms occur. Monitor periodically after mo 4. *If isolated ALT ↑ between 3 and 8 x the upper limit of normal (ULN)*, therapy may continue with weekly monitoring of liver function until ALT returns to Grade 1 or baseline. *If isolated ALT ↑ >8 x ULN,* stop therapy until ALT returns to Grade 1 or baseline. If benefit outweighs risk, may reintroduce at reduced dose of 400 mg/day with weekly serum liver tests for 8 wk. Following reintroduction, if ALT ↑ >3 x ULN recurs, permanently discontinue pazopanib. *If ALT ↑ occurs concurrently with ↑ serum bilirubin >2 x ULN,* discontinue pazopanib permanently. Monitor liver function tests until return to baseline. *Patients with only mild indirect hyperbilirubinemia (Gilbert's syndrome) and ↑ ALT >3 x ULN* should be managed as per recommendations for ↑ ALT.
- Monitor thyroid function periodically during therapy. May cause hypothyroidism.
- Obtain baseline urinalysis and monitor periodically with follow-up with 24-hr urine protein as indicated. *If 24-hr urine protein ≥ 3 g,* hold pazopanib until improvement to Grade ≤ 1. Resume at a reduced dose. Permanently discontinue if 24-hr urine protein ≥ 3 g does not improve or recurs despite dose reductions or if nephrotic syndrome is confirmed. May cause proteinuria. Discontinue therapy if Grade 4 proteinuria develops.
- May cause leukopenia, neutropenia, thrombocytopenia, and lymphocytopenia.
- May cause ↑ AST and ↓ serum phosphorous, sodium, and magnesium. May cause ↑ or ↓ serum glucose.

Implementation

- Do not confuse pazopanib with ponatinib.
- May impair wound healing. Hold pazopanib at least 1 wk prior to elective surgery. Do not administer for at least 2 wk following major surgery and until adequate wound healing.
- **Recommended Dose Reductions:** *For Renal Carcinoma,* 1st reduction: 400 mg once daily; 2nd reduction: 200 mg once daily. *For Soft Tissue Sarcoma,* 1st reduction: 600 mg once daily; 2nd reduction: 400 mg once daily.
- **PO:** Administer at least 1 hr before or 2 hr after a meal. *DNC:* Swallow tablets whole; do not crush tablets.

Patient/Family Teaching

- Instruct patient to take pazopanib on an empty stomach as directed. Take missed doses as soon as remembered; if less than 12 hr before next dose, omit dose. Advise patient to read the *Medication Guide* prior to taking pazopanib and with each Rx refill; new information may be available.
- Advise patient to avoid drinking grapefruit juice or eating grapefruit during therapy; may increase amounts of pazopanib absorbed.
- Advise patient to notify health care professional immediately if signs and symptoms of liver problems (yellowing of skin or whites of eyes, unusual darkening of urine, unusual tiredness, pain in the right upper stomach area), HF (shortness of breath), heart attack or stroke (chest pain or pressure; pain in arms, back, neck or jaw; shortness of breath; numbness or weakness on one side of body; trouble talking; headache; dizziness), blood clots (new chest pain, trouble breathing or shortness of breath that starts suddenly; leg pain; swelling of arms and hands, or legs and feet; cool or pale arm or leg), bleeding problems (unusual bleeding, bruising, wounds that do not heal), GI perforation or fistula, PRES (headaches, seizures, lack of energy, confusion, high BP, loss of speech, blindness or changes in vision, and problems thinking), severe increase in BP (severe chest pain, severe head ache, blurred vision, confusion, nausea and vomiting, severe anxiety, shortness of breath, seizures, unconsciousness), ILD (persistent cough, shortness of breath), tumor lysis syndrome (irregular heartbeat, seizures, confusion, muscle cramps or spasms, decrease in urine output) or severe infections (fever; cold symptoms such as runny nose or sore throat that do not go away; flu symptoms such as cough, tiredness, and body aches; pain when urinating; cuts, scrapes or wounds that are red, warm, swollen or painful) occur.
- Inform patient that diarrhea frequently occurs. Instruct patient on ways to manage diarrhea and to notify health care professional if moderate to severe diarrhea occurs.
- Inform patient that loss of color (depigmentation) of skin or hair may occur during therapy. Explore methods of coping.
- Instruct patient to notify health care professional of all Rx or OTC medications, vitamins, or herbal products being taken and consult health care professional before taking any new medications.
- Advise patient to notify health care professional of any impending surgery. Pazopanib must be stopped for at least 7 days prior to surgery due to the effects on healing and held for at least 2 wk after major surgery or until adequate healing.
- Rep: Advise females of reproductive potential and male patients with partners of reproductive potential to use effective contraception during therapy and for at least 2 wk after discontinuing therapy, and to notify health care professional immediately if pregnancy is suspected. Advise patient to avoid breastfeeding during therapy and for 2 wk after final dose. Inform patients that pazopanib may impair fertility for both men and women during therapy.

Evaluation/Desired Outcomes

- Decreased growth and spread of renal cell carcinoma.
- Improvement in spread of sarcoma.

---

pegfilgrastim (peg-fil-**gra**-stim)
Fulphila, Fylnetra, ✹ Lapelga, Neulasta, Neulasta Onpro, Nyvepria, Stimufend, Udenyca, Ziextenzo
Classification
Therapeutic: colony-stimulating factors

Indications

To decrease the incidence of infection (febrile neutropenia) in patients with nonmyeloid malignancies receiving myelosuppressive antineoplastics associated with a high risk of febrile neutropenia. **Neulasta and Udenyca:** To increase survival in patients acutely exposed to myelosuppressive doses of radiation.

Action

Filgrastim is a glycoprotein that binds to and stimulates neutrophils to divide and differentiate. Also activates mature neutrophils. Binding to a polyethylene glycol molecule prolongs its effects. **Therapeutic Effects:** Decreased incidence of infection in patients who are neutropenic from chemotherapy. Improved survival in patients acutely exposed to myelosuppressive doses of radiation.

Pharmacokinetics

Absorption: Well absorbed following SUBQ administration.
Distribution: Unknown.
Metabolism and Excretion: Unknown.
Half-life: 15–80 hr.

TIME/ACTION PROFILE

ROUTE	ONSET	PEAK	DURATION
SUBQ	unknown	unknown	unknown

Contraindications/Precautions

Contraindicated in: Hypersensitivity to filgrastim or *Escherichia coli*–derived proteins.
Use Cautiously in: Patients with breast or lung cancer receiving chemotherapy and/or radiotherapy (↑ risk of myelodysplastic syndrome or acute myeloid leukemia); Patients with sickle cell disease (↑ risk of sickle cell crisis); Malignancy with myeloid characteristics; OB: Use during pregnancy only if potential maternal benefit justifies potential fetal risk; Lactation: Use while breastfeeding only if potential maternal benefit justifies potential risk to infant.

Adverse Reactions/Side Effects

CV: aortitis. **GI:** SPLENIC RUPTURE. **GU:** glomerulonephritis. **Hemat:** ACUTE MYELOID LEUKEMIA, leukocytosis, MYELODYSPLASTIC SYNDROME, SICKLE CELL CRISIS, thrombocytopenia. **MS:** medullary bone pain. **Resp:** ADULT RESPIRATORY DISTRESS SYNDROME (ARDS). **Misc:** CAPILLARY LEAK SYNDROME, HYPERSENSITIVITY REACTIONS (including anaphylaxis).

Interactions

Drug-Drug: Simultaneous use with **antineoplastics** may have adverse effects on rapidly proliferating neutrophils; avoid use for 24 hr before and 24 hr following chemotherapy. **Lithium** may potentiate the release of neutrophils; concurrent use should be undertaken cautiously.

Route/Dosage

Patients with Cancer Receiving Myelosuppressive Chemotherapy

SUBQ (Adults and Children ≥45 kg): 6 mg per chemotherapy cycle.
SUBQ (Children 31–44 kg): 4 mg per chemotherapy cycle.
SUBQ (Children 21–30 kg): 2.5 mg per chemotherapy cycle.
SUBQ (Children 10–20 kg): 1.5 mg per chemotherapy cycle.
SUBQ (Children <10 kg): 0.1 mg/kg per chemotherapy cycle.

Patients Acutely Exposed to Myelosuppressive Doses of Radiation

SUBQ (Adults and Children ≥45 kg): 6 mg as soon as possible after suspected or confirmed exposure to radiation levels >2 gray (Gy), then 6 mg 1 wk later.
SUBQ (Children 31–44 kg): 4 mg as soon as possible after suspected or confirmed exposure to radiation levels >2 gray (Gy), then 4 mg 1 wk later.
SUBQ (Children 21–30 kg): 2.5 mg as soon as possible after suspected or confirmed exposure to radiation levels >2 gray (Gy), then 2.5 mg 1 wk later.
SUBQ (Children 10–20 kg): 1.5 mg as soon as possible after suspected or confirmed exposure to radiation levels >2 gray (Gy), then 1.5 mg 1 wk later.
SUBQ (Children <10 kg): 0.1 mg/kg as soon as possible after suspected or confirmed exposure to radiation levels >2 gray (Gy), then 0.1 mg/kg 1 wk later.

Availability

Solution for injection (prefilled syringes and autoinjectors): 6 mg/0.6 mL.

NURSING IMPLICATIONS

Assessment

- Assess patient for bone pain during therapy. Pain is usually mild to moderate and usually controllable with nonopioid analgesics, but may require opioid analgesics.
- Assess patient periodically for signs of ARDS (fever, lung infiltration, respiratory distress). If ARDS oc-

---

curs, treat condition and discontinue pegfilgrastim and/or withhold until symptoms resolve.
- Monitor for signs and symptoms of splenic rupture (left upper abdominal or shoulder pain) during therapy.
- Monitor for signs and symptoms of capillary leak syndrome (hypotension, hypoalbuminemia, edema, hemoconcentration). Treat symptomatically.
- Assess for signs and symptoms of aortitis (fever, abdominal pain, malaise, back pain, increased inflammatory markers [C-reactive protein, white blood cell count]). Discontinue pegfilgrastim if aortitis is suspected.
- May cause transient positive nuclear bone imaging changes.

Lab Test Considerations
- Obtain CBC and platelet count before chemotherapy. Monitor hematocrit, WBC, and platelet count regularly. May cause thrombocytopenia.
- May cause elevated LDH, alkaline phosphatase, and uric acid.

Implementation
- Do not confuse Neulasta with Lunesta or Nuedexta.
- Pegfilgrastim should not be administered between 14 days before and 24 hrs after administration of cytotoxic chemotherapy.
- Keep patients with sickle cell disease receiving pegfilgrastim well hydrated and monitor for sickle cell crisis. Discontinue therapy if sickle cell crisis occurs.
- **SUBQ:** Administer SUBQ once per chemotherapy cycle. Do not administer solutions that are discolored or contain particulate matter. Do not shake. Store refrigerated; allow to reach room temperature for at least 30 min and maximum of 48 hr, but protect from light.
- **On-body Injector:** Small, one-time use, lightweight, battery-powered, and waterproof up to 8 feet for 1 hr. Filled by health care professional with a prefilled syringe before application. The prefilled syringe with *Neulasta* and the *On-body Injector* are part of *Neulasta Onpro kit*. The *On-body Injector* is applied directly to skin using a self-adhesive backing. The *On-body Injector* uses sounds and lights to inform its status. The prefilled syringe gray needle cap contains dry natural rubber, derived from latex; do not use if allergic to latex. Apply to intact, non-irritated skin on abdomen or back of arm. Back of arm may only be used if there is a caregiver available to monitor the status of the *On-body Injector*. Approximately 27 hrs after the *On-body Injector* is applied, *Neulasta* will be delivered over approximately 45 min. Follow manufacturer's instructions for monitoring and removal. Instruct patients using the *On-body Injector* to notify health care professional immediately if they suspect the device may not have performed as intended in order to determine need for a replacement dose.

Patient/Family Teaching
- Instruct patient in technique for injection, care of medication, and disposal of equipment. Advise patient to read *Patient Information* before starting therapy and with each Rx refill in case of changes.
- Advise patient to notify health care professional immediately if signs of allergic reaction (shortness of breath, hives, rash, pruritus, laryngeal edema), ARDS (shortness of breath with or without a fever, trouble breathing, fast rate of breathing), kidney injury (swelling of face or ankles, blood in urine or dark-colored urine, urinate less than usual), capillary leak syndrome (swelling or puffiness and urinating less than usual, trouble breathing, swelling of abdomen and feeling of fullness, dizziness or feeling faint, general feeling of tiredness), myelodysplastic syndrome or acute myeloid leukemia (tiredness, fever, and easy bruising or bleeding), inflammation of the aorta (fever, abdominal pain, feeling tired, back pain), or signs of splenic rupture (left upper abdominal or shoulder tip pain) occur.
- Advise patients with sickle cell disease to maintain hydration and to notify health care professional promptly if symptoms of sickle cell crisis occur.
- Advise patient to notify health care professional of all Rx or OTC medications, vitamins, or herbal products being taken and to consult with health care professional before taking other medications.
- Rep: Advise females of reproductive potential to notify health care professional if pregnancy is planned or suspected, or if breastfeeding.
- Emphasize the importance of adherence with therapy and regular monitoring of blood counts.
- **Home Care Issues:** Instruct patient on correct disposal technique for home administration. Caution patient not to reuse needle, syringe, or drug product. Provide patient with a puncture-proof container for disposal of prefilled syringe.

Evaluation/Desired Outcomes
- Decreased incidence of infection in patients who are neutropenic from chemotherapy.
- Improved survival in patients acutely exposed to myelosuppressive doses of radiation.

peginterferon beta-1a
(peg-in-ter-**feer**-on **bay**-ta)
   Plegridy
Classification
Therapeutic: immune modifiers
Pharmacologic: interferons

Indications
Relapsing forms of multiple sclerosis (MS), including clinically isolated syndrome, relapsing-remitting disease, and active secondary progressive disease.

Action
Antiviral and immunoregulatory properties produced by interacting with specific receptor sites on cell sur-

faces may explain beneficial effects. Produced by recombinant DNA technology. Pegylation prolongs duration of action. **Therapeutic Effects:** Reduced incidence of relapse (neurologic dysfunction) and slowed physical disability.

Pharmacokinetics

Absorption: Extent of absorption following SUBQ or IM administration unknown.
Distribution: Widely distributed to tissues.
Metabolism and Excretion: Undergoes catabolism; excretion is mainly renal.
Half-life: 78 hr.

TIME/ACTION PROFILE (reduction in relapse rate)

ROUTE	ONSET	PEAK	DURATION
SUBQ	within one mo	24–36 wk	unknown
IM	unknown	unknown	unknown

Contraindications/Precautions

Contraindicated in: Hypersensitivity to natural or recombinant interferon beta or peginterferon.
Use Cautiously in: History of depression or suicidal ideation; Latex allergy; History of seizures; Renal impairment (risk of adverse reactions may be ↑); OB: Use during pregnancy only if potential maternal benefit justifies potential fetal risk; Lactation: Use while breastfeeding only if potential maternal benefit justifies potential risk to infant; Pedi: Safety and effectiveness not established in children; Geri: Safety and effectiveness not established in older adults.

Adverse Reactions/Side Effects

CV: HF. **Derm:** pruritus. **GI:** HEPATOTOXICITY, nausea, vomiting. **Hemat:** ↓ peripheral blood counts, HEMOLYTIC UREMIC SYNDROME, THROMBOTIC THROMBOCYTOPENIC PURPURA. **Local:** injection site reactions. **MS:** arthralgia, myalgia. **Neuro:** depression, headache, SEIZURES, SUICIDAL IDEATION, weakness. **Resp:** PULMONARY ARTERIAL HYPERTENSION (PAH). **Misc:** chills, fever, flu-like symptoms, AUTOIMMUNE DISORDERS, HYPERSENSITIVITY REACTIONS (including anaphylaxis).

Interactions

Drug-Drug: ↑ myelosuppression may occur with other **myelosuppressives** including **antineoplastics**. Concurrent use of **hepatotoxic agents** may ↑ the risk of hepatotoxicity (↑ liver enzymes).
Drug-Natural Products: Avoid concomitant use with **immunomodulating natural products** such as **astragalus**, **echinacea**, and **melatonin**.

Route/Dosage

IM, SUBQ (Adults): 63 mcg on Day 1, then 94 mcg on Day 15, then 125 mcg every 14 days.

Availability

Solution for injection (prefilled pens and prefilled syringes): 63 mcg/0.5 mL, 94 mcg/0.5 mL, 125 mcg/0.5 mL.

NURSING IMPLICATIONS

Assessment

- Assess frequency of exacerbations of symptoms of MS periodically during therapy.
- Monitor patient for signs of depression during therapy. If depression occurs, notify health care professional immediately.
- Monitor for injection site reactions (erythema, pain, pruritus, edema, bruising, drainage, necrosis). Avoid injecting near area of reaction.
- Monitor patient with significant cardiac disease for worsening symptoms during initiation and periodically during therapy.
- Assess patients who develop unexplained symptoms (dyspnea, new or increasing fatigue) for PAH. If other causes have been ruled out and a diagnosis of PAH is confirmed, discontinue therapy.

Lab Test Considerations

- Monitor serum AST, ALT, and bilirubin periodically during therapy.
- Monitor CBC with differential and platelet counts periodically during therapy. May cause anemia, ↓ lymphocyte, ↓ neutrophil, and ↓ platelet counts.

Implementation

- Administer prophylactic analgesics and/or antipyretics to prevent or minimize flu-like symptoms. Incidence of injection site reactions may be less with IM than with SUBQ dosing.
- Remove syringe from refrigerator and allow to warm to room temperature for 30 min before injection. Do not use warm water to warm. Solution is clear to slightly opalescent and colorless to slightly yellow. Do not administer solutions that are cloudy, discolored, or contain particulate matter.
- **SUBQ:** Inject SUBQ in abdomen, back of upper arm, or thigh every 14 days; rotate sites. Prefilled pens are for single dose; discard after use.
- For patients using SUBQ dosing for the first time, titrate using the *Plegridy Starter Pack* for use with the prefilled syringe. Kit is supplied separately and contains two titration devices (*Dose 1 for Day 1:* 63 mcg, orange clip; *Dose 2 for Day 15:* 94 mcg, blue clip; *Dose 3 for Day 29 and every 14 days after:* 125 mcg, gray clip) to be used only with prefilled syringes for SUBQ use.
- **IM:** Rotate injection sites between left and right thighs.
- Protective cover of prefilled syringe for IM use contains latex. Avoid handling by latex-sensitive individuals. Monitor for allergic reactions.

P

- For patients using IM dosing for the first time, titrate using the *Plegridy Titration Kit* for use with the pre-filled syringe. Kit is supplied separately and contains two titration devices (*Dose 1 for Day 1:* 63 mcg, yellow clip; *Dose 2 for Day 15:* 94 mcg, purple clip; *Dose 3 for Day 29 and every 14 days after:* 125 mcg, no clip) to be used only with prefilled syringes for IM use.

Patient/Family Teaching

- Instruct patient in correct technique for injection and care and disposal of equipment. Avoid injecting into areas of skin irritation, redness, bruising, infection, or scarring. Check injection site 2 hr after injection for redness, swelling, and tenderness. Notify health care professional if skin reaction does not clear in a few days. Caution patient not to reuse needles or syringes and provide patient with a puncture-resistant container for disposal.
- Instruct patient to take medication as directed; do not change dose or schedule without consulting health care professional. Advise patient to read *Medication Guide* prior to starting therapy and with each Rx refill in case of changes.
- Inform patient that flu-like symptoms (headache, fever, chills, myalgia, sweating, malaise, tiredness) may occur during therapy. Acetaminophen may be used for relief of fever and myalgias. Flu-like symptoms are not contagious.
- Advise patient to notify health care professional immediately if signs and symptoms of liver disease (yellowing of skin or whites of eyes, nausea, loss of appetite, tiredness, bleeding easily, confusion, sleepiness, dark-colored urine, pale stools), depression, suicidal thoughts, seizures, allergic reactions (itching; swelling of face, eyes, lips, tongue, throat; trouble breathing; feeling faint; anxiousness; rash; hives) or autoimmune diseases (easy bleeding or bruising, thyroid gland problems, autoimmune hepatitis) occur.
- Instruct patient to notify health care professional of all Rx or OTC medications, vitamins, or herbal products being taken and to consult with health care professional before taking other medications.
- Rep: Advise females of reproductive potential to notify health care professional if pregnancy is planned or suspected or if breastfeeding.

Evaluation/Desired Outcomes

- Decrease in the frequency of relapse (neurologic dysfunction) in patients with relapsing-remitting MS.

℥ **pegloticase** (peg-**loe**-ti-kase)
Krystexxa
Classification
Therapeutic: antigout agents
Pharmacologic: enzymes

Indications

Chronic gout in adults who have not responded to/cannot tolerate xanthine oxidase inhibitors, including allopurinol.

Action

Consists of recombinant uricase covalently bonded to monomethoxypoly(ethylene glycol); uricase catalyzes the oxidation of uric acid to allantoin, a water soluble by-product that is readily excreted in urine. **Therapeutic Effects:** ↓ serum uric acid levels with resultant ↓ in attacks of gout and its sequelae.

Pharmacokinetics

Absorption: IV administration results in complete bioavailability.
Distribution: Unknown.
Metabolism and Excretion: Unknown.
Half-life: Unknown.

TIME/ACTION PROFILE (effects on serum uric acid concentrations)

ROUTE	ONSET	PEAK	DURATION
IV	rapid	within 24 hr	>300 hr

Contraindications/Precautions

Contraindicated in: Serious hypersensitivity, including anaphylaxis; ℥ Glucose-6–phosphate dehydrogenase (G6PD) deficiency (↑ risk of hemolysis and methemoglobinemia).
Use Cautiously in: HF (may ↑ risk of exacerbation); Retreatment after a drug-free interval (↑ risk of allergic reactions, monitor carefully); OB: Use during pregnancy only if clearly needed; Lactation: Use while breastfeeding only if potential maternal benefit justifies potential risk to infant; Pedi: Safety and effectiveness not established in children; Geri: Older adults may be more sensitive to drug effects.

Adverse Reactions/Side Effects

CV: chest pain. **Derm:** contusion/ecchymoses. **EENT:** nasopharyngitis. **GI:** nausea, constipation, vomiting. **Hemat:** HEMOLYSIS, METHEMOGLOBINEMIA. **Metab:** gout flare. **Misc:** INFUSION REACTIONS, HYPERSENSITIVITY REACTIONS (including anaphylaxis).

Interactions

Drug-Drug: May interfere with the action of other **PEG-containing therapies**.

Route/Dosage

IV (Adults): 8 mg every 2 wk.

Availability

Solution for injection: 8 mg/mL.

NURSING IMPLICATIONS
Assessment

- Monitor for joint pain and swelling. Gout flares frequently occur upon initiation of therapy, but does not require discontinuation. Administer prophylactic doses of colchicine or an NSAID at least 1 wk before and concurrently during the first 6 mo of therapy.

● Monitor for signs and symptoms of anaphylaxis (wheezing, perioral or lingual edema, hemodynamic instability, rash, urticaria) during and following infusion. May occur with any infusion, including initial infusion; usually occurs with 2 hr of infusion. Delayed reactions have also been reported. Risk is higher in patients with uric acid level >6 mg/dL.

● Monitor for infusion reactions (rash, redness of skin, dyspnea, flushing, chest discomfort, chest pain) during and periodically after infusion. If infusion reaction occurs, slow or stop infusion; restart at slower rate. If severe reaction occurs, discontinue infusion and treat as needed. Risk is greater in patients who have lost therapeutic response. Monitor patient for at least 1 hr following infusion.

Lab Test Considerations

● ☷ Screen patients at risk for G6PD deficiency prior to starting therapy. Patients of African, Mediterranean (including Southern European and Middle Eastern), and Southern Asian ancestry are at increased risk for G6PD deficiency. Do not administer pegloticase to patients with G6PD deficiency.

● Monitor serum uric acid levels prior to infusion. Discontinue therapy if levels ↑ to >6 mg/dL, especially if 2 consecutive levels are >6 mg/dL.

Implementation

● Premedicate patient with antihistamines and corticosteroids prior to infusion to minimize risk of anaphylaxis and infusion reaction. Administer in a setting with professionals prepared to manage anaphylaxis and infusion reactions.

● May be administered with methotrexate.

● Discontinue all oral urate-lowering medications prior to and during therapy.

IV Administration

● **Intermittent Infusion:** Withdraw 1 mL of pegloticase from vial and inject into 250 mL bag of NaCl; discard unused portion. Invert bag several times to mix; do not shake. Solution is clear and colorless; do not administer solutions that are discolored or contain a precipitate. Solution is stable for 4 hr if refrigerated or at room temperature. Store in refrigerator and protect from light; do not freeze. Allow solution to reach room temperature before administering; do not use artificial heating. *Rate:* Infuse over 120 min. Do not administer via IV push or bolus.

● **Additive Incompatibility:** Do not mix with other medications.

Patient/Family Teaching

● Explain purpose of pegloticase to patient. Instruct patient to read *Medication Guide* before starting therapy before each infusion.

● Advise patient to notify health care professional immediately if signs of anaphylaxis or infusion reaction occur.

● ☷ Advise patient not to take pegloticase if they have G6PD deficiency.

● Inform patient that gout flares may initially ↑ during the first 3 mo of pegloticase. Advise patient to not to stop therapy but to take medication (colchicine, NSAID) to reduce flares regularly for the first few months of pegloticase therapy.

● Advise patient to notify health care professional of all Rx or OTC medications, vitamins, or herbal products being taken and to consult with health care professional before taking other medications.

● Instruct patient not to take oral urate-lowering medications before or during therapy.

● Rep: Advise females of reproductive potential to notify health care professional if pregnancy is planned or suspected and to avoid breastfeeding during therapy.

Evaluation/Desired Outcomes

● ↓ in uric acid levels with resultant improvement in gout symptoms in patients with chronic gout.

☷ pembrolizumab
(pem-broe-li-zoo-mab)
Keytruda
Classification
Therapeutic: antineoplastics
Pharmacologic: monoclonal antibodies, programmed death-1 inhibitors

Indications

Unresectable or metastatic melanoma. Adjuvant treatment of Stage IIB, IIC, or III melanoma following complete resection. ☷ First-line treatment of patients with stage III non–small-cell lung cancer (NSCLC), who are not candidates for surgical resection or definitive chemoradiation, or metastatic NSCLC and whose tumors express PD-L1 (tumor proportion score [TPS] ≥1%) and have no epidermal growth factor receptor (EGFR) or anaplastic lymphoma kinase (ALK) genomic tumor aberrations (as monotherapy). ☷ Metastatic NSCLC expressing PD-L1 (TPS ≥1%) that has progressed on or after platinum-containing chemotherapy (as monotherapy). Patients with EGFR or ALK genomic tumor aberrations should have disease progression on FDA-approved therapy for these aberrations prior to receiving pembrolizumab. Adjuvant treatment of Stage IB, II, or IIIA NSCLC following resection and platinum-based chemotherapy (as monotherapy). ☷ First-line treatment of metastatic non-squamous NSCLC with no EGFR or ALK genomic tumor aberrations (in combination with pemetrexed and platinum chemotherapy). First-line treatment of metastatic non-squamous NSCLC (in combination with carboplatin and either paclitaxel or nab-paclitaxel [albumin-bound]). Recurrent or metastatic head and neck squamous cell carcinoma (HNSCC) that has progressed on or after platinum-containing chemotherapy. First-line treatment of metastatic or unresectable, recurrent HNSCC (in combination with platinum and fluorouracil). ※ First-line treatment of metastatic or unresectable, recurrent HNSCC expressing PD-L1 (combined positive score [CPS] ≥1). Adults with relapsed or refractory classical Hodgkin lymphoma (cHL). Children with refractory cHL or cHL that has relapsed after ≥2 lines of therapy. Primary mediastinal large B-cell lymphoma that is refractory or that has relapsed after ≥2 prior lines of therapy (should not be used in patients who require urgent cytoreductive therapy). Locally advanced or metastatic urothelial carcinoma in patients who are not eligible for any platinum-containing chemotherapy. Locally advanced or metastatic urothelial carcinoma in patients who have disease progression during or following platinum-containing chemotherapy or within 12 mo of neoadjuvant or adjuvant treatment with platinum-containing chemotherapy. Locally advanced or metastatic urothelial carcinoma in patients who are not eligible for cisplatin-containing chemotherapy (in combination with enfortumab vedotin). Bacillus Calmette-Guerin (BCG)-unresponsive, high-risk, non-muscle invasive bladder cancer with carcinoma in situ with or without papillary tumors in patients who are not eligible for or have elected not to undergo cystectomy. ※ Unresectable or metastatic, microsatellite instability-high (MSI-H) or mismatch repair deficient (dMMR) solid tumors that have progressed following prior treatment and have no satisfactory alternative treatment options. ※ First-line treatment of unresectable or metastatic MSI-H or dMMR colorectal cancer. ※ First-line treatment of locally advanced unresectable or metastatic HER2-positive gastric or gastroesophageal junction adenocarcinoma (in combination with trastuzumab, fluoropyrimidine- and platinum-containing chemotherapy). ※ Locally advanced or metastatic esophageal or gastroesophageal junction (tumors with epicenter 1–5 cm above the gastroesophageal junction) carcinoma that is not amenable to surgical resection or definitive chemoradiation either as monotherapy after ≥1 prior line of systemic therapy for patients with tumors of squamous cell histology that express PD-L1 (CPS ≥10) or in combination with platinum- and fluoropyrimidine-based chemotherapy. ※ Recurrent or metastatic cervical cancer expressing PD-L1 (CPS ≥1) that has progressed on or after chemotherapy. ※ Persistent, recurrent, or metastatic cervical cancer expressing PD-L1 (CPS ≥1) (in combination with chemotherapy, with or without bevacizumab). Hepatocellular carcinoma in patients previously treated with sorafenib. Recurrent locally advanced or metastatic Merkel cell carcinoma. First-line treatment of advanced renal cell carcinoma (RCC) (in combination with axitinib or lenvatinib). Adjuvant treatment of RCC at intermediate-high or high risk of recurrence following nephrectomy, or following

nephrectomy and resection of metastatic lesions. ※ Advanced endometrial carcinoma that is mismatch repair proficient (pMMR) or not MSI-H in patients who have disease progression following prior systemic therapy in any setting and are not candidates for curative surgery or radiation (in combination with lenvatinib). ※ Advanced endometrial carcinoma that is MSI-H or dMMR in patients who have disease progression following prior systemic therapy in any setting and are not candidates for curative surgery or radiation. ※ Unresectable or metastatic tumor mutational burden-high (TMB-H) [≥10 mutations/megabase] solid tumors that have progressed following prior treatment and have no satisfactory alternative treatment options. Recurrent or metastatic cutaneous squamous cell carcinoma that is not curable by surgery or radiation. ※ Locally recurrent unresectable or metastatic triple-negative breast cancer (TNBC) in patients whose tumors express PD-L1 (CPS ≥10) (in combination with chemotherapy). High-risk early-stage TNBC (in combination with chemotherapy as neoadjuvant treatment, and then continued as a single agent as adjuvant treatment after surgery).

Action

Programmed death receptor-1 (PD-1) blocking antibody (an IgG4 kappa immunoglobulin) that binds to PD-1 and blocks its interaction with its ligands, PD-L1 and PD-L2, resulting in activation of the immune system and decreased tumor growth. **Therapeutic Effects:** Decreased spread of melanoma, NSCLC, HNSCC, cHL, urothelial carcinoma, MSI-H or dMMR solid tumors, MSI-H or dMMR colorectal cancer, gastric tumors, cervical cancer, endometrial cancer, esophageal cancer, primary mediastinal large B-cell lymphoma, hepatocellular carcinoma, Merkel cell carcinoma, RCC, TMB-H solid tumors, cutaneous squamous cell carcinoma, and TNBC.

Pharmacokinetics

Absorption: IV administration results in complete bioavailability.
Distribution: Unknown.
Metabolism and Excretion: Unknown.
Half-life: 26 days.

TIME/ACTION PROFILE (response)

ROUTE	ONSET	PEAK	DURATION
IV	within 3 mo	unknown	may persist for >8.8 mo

Contraindications/Precautions

Contraindicated in: OB: Pregnancy; Lactation: Lactation.

Use Cautiously in: Moderate or severe hepatic impairment; Solid organ transplant recipients (↑ risk of rejection); Allogeneic hematopoietic stem cell transplant recipients (↑ risk of transplantation complications); Rep: Women of reproductive potential; Pedi: Safety and effectiveness not established in children

<2 yr (cHL, MSI-H cancer, primary mediastinal large B-cell lymphoma, and Merkel cell carcinoma) <12 yr (melanoma), or children <18 yr (all other indications).

Adverse Reactions/Side Effects

CV: MYOCARDITIS, pericarditis, vasculitis. **Derm:** pruritus, rash, DRUG REACTION WITH EOSINOPHILIA AND SYSTEMIC SYMPTOMS (DRESS), STEVENS-JOHNSON SYNDROME (SJS), TOXIC EPIDERMAL NECROLYSIS (TEN). **EENT:** iritis, uveitis. **Endo:** hyperthyroidism, hypothyroidism, ADRENAL INSUFFICIENCY, hypoparathyroidism, hypophysitis, type 1 diabetes. **GI:** ↓ appetite, constipation, diarrhea, nausea, COLITIS, gastritis, HEPATITIS, pancreatitis. **GU:** nephritis. **Hemat:** anemia, hemolytic anemia. **MS:** arthralgia, back pain, extremity pain, myalgia, myositis, RHABDOMYOLYSIS. **Neuro:** dizziness, fatigue, headache, insomnia, autoimmune neuropathy, ENCEPHALITIS, Guillain-Barré syndrome, MENINGITIS, myasthenic syndrome, myelitis. **Resp:** PNEUMONITIS. **Misc:** INFUSION-RELATED REACTIONS, SEPSIS.

Interactions

Drug-Drug: None reported.

Route/Dosage

Melanoma

IV (Adults): 200 mg every 3 wk until disease progression or unacceptable toxicity *or* 400 mg every 6 wk until disease progression or unacceptable toxicity.

Adjuvant Treatment of Melanoma

IV (Adults): 200 mg every 3 wk until disease recurrence, unacceptable toxicity, or up to 12 mo *or* 400 mg every 6 wk until disease recurrence, unacceptable toxicity, or up to 12 mo.
IV (Children ≥12 yr): 2 mg/kg (max = 200 mg) every 3 wk until disease recurrence, unacceptable toxicity, or up to 12 mo.

Non-Small Cell Lung Cancer, Head and Neck Squamous Cell Carcinoma, Esophageal Cancer, or Locally Recurrent Unresectable or Metastatic Triple Negative Breast Cancer

IV (Adults): 200 mg every 3 wk until disease progression, unacceptable toxicity, or up to 24 mo *or* 400 mg every 6 wk until disease progression, unacceptable toxicity, or up to 24 mo. If being administered in combination with chemotherapy, should be administered prior to chemotherapy when given on the same day.

Adjuvant Treatment of Non-Small Cell Lung Cancer

IV (Adults): 200 mg every 3 wk until disease recurrence, unacceptable toxicity, or up to 12 mo *or* 400 mg every 6 wk until disease recurrence, unacceptable toxicity, or up to 12 mo.

Urothelial Carcinoma, Gastric Cancer, Cervical Cancer, Endometrial Carcinoma, Hepatocellular Cancer, Renal Cell Carcinoma, Cutaneous Squamous Cell Carcinoma, or Microsatellite Instability-High/Mismatch Repair Deficient Colorectal Cancer

IV (Adults): 200 mg every 3 wk until disease progression, unacceptable toxicity, or up to 24 mo *or* 400 mg every 6 wk until disease progression, unacceptable toxicity, or up to 24 mo. If being administered in combination with chemotherapy, bevacizumab, or trastuzumab, should be administered prior to these medications when given on the same day; if being administered in combination with enfortumab vedotin, should be administered after this medication when given on the same day.

Adjuvant Treatment of Renal Cell Carcinoma

IV (Adults): 200 mg every 3 wk until disease recurrence, unacceptable toxicity, or up to 12 mo *or* 400 mg every 6 wk until disease recurrence, unacceptable toxicity, or up to 12 mo.

Bacillus Calmette-Guerin-Unresponsive, High-Risk Non-Muscle Invasive Bladder Cancer

IV (Adults): 200 mg every 3 wk until persistent or recurrent high-risk non-muscle invasive bladder cancer, disease progression, unacceptable toxicity, or up to 24 mo *or* 400 mg every 6 wk until persistent or recurrent high-risk non-muscle invasive bladder cancer, disease progression, unacceptable toxicity, or up to 24 mo.

Classical Hodgkin Lymphoma, Microsatellite Instability-High/Mismatch Repair Deficient Cancer, Primary Mediastinal Large B-Cell Lymphoma, Merkel Cell Carcinoma, or Tumor Mutational Burden-High Cancer

IV (Adults): 200 mg every 3 wk until disease progression, unacceptable toxicity, or up to 24 mo *or* 400 mg every 6 wk until disease progression, unacceptable toxicity, or up to 24 mo.
IV (Children ≥2 yr): 2 mg/kg (max = 200 mg) every 3 wk until disease progression, unacceptable toxicity, or up to 24 mo.

High-Risk, Early-Stage Triple Negative Breast Cancer

IV (Adults): 200 mg every 3 wk for 24 wk (8 doses) (as neoadjuvant treatment in combination with chemotherapy) or until disease progression or unacceptable toxicity followed by 200 mg every 3 wk for up to 27 wk (9 doses) (as monotherapy as adjuvant treatment after surgery) *or* 400 mg every 6 wk for 24 wk (4 doses) (as neoadjuvant treatment in combination with chemotherapy) or until disease progression or unacceptable toxicity followed by 400 mg every 6 wk for up to 27 wk (5 doses) (as monotherapy as adjuvant treatment after surgery). If being administered in combination with chemotherapy, should be administered prior to chemotherapy when given on the same day.

Availability

Solution for injection: 25 mg/mL.

NURSING IMPLICATIONS

Assessment

- Monitor for signs and symptoms of immune-mediated pneumonitis (shortness of breath, chest pain, new or worse cough) periodically during therapy. Evaluate with x-ray. Treat with corticosteroids for ≥Grade 2 pneumonitis. *If Grade 2 immune-mediated pneumonitis occurs,* hold pembrolizumab. Resume therapy in patients with complete or partial resolution (Grades 0 to 1) after corticosteroid taper. *If Grades 3 or 4 or recurrent Grade 2 occur,* permanently discontinue therapy.

- Monitor for signs and symptoms of colitis (diarrhea, abdominal pain, mucus or blood in stool, with or without fever). *If Grades 2 or 3 immune-mediated colitis occur,* hold dose. Resume therapy in patients with complete or partial resolution (Grades 0 to 1) after corticosteroid taper. *If Grade 4 occurs,* permanently discontinue pembrolizumab.

- Assess for signs and symptoms of immune-mediated hepatitis (yellowing of skin or whites of eyes, unusual darkening of urine, unusual tiredness, pain in right upper stomach) before each dose.

- Monitor for signs and symptoms of infusion-related reactions (rigors, chills, wheezing, pruritus, flushing, rash, hypotension, hypoxemia, fever). *If Grades 1 or 2 infusion-related reactions occur,* hold or slow rate of infusion. *If Grades 3 or 4 reactions occur,* stop infusion and permanently discontinue therapy.

- Monitor for clinical signs and symptoms of hypophysitis (persistent or unusual headache, extreme weakness, dizziness or fainting, vision changes) during therapy. *If Grade 3 or 4 immune-mediated endocrinopathies occur,* hold dose until clinically stable.

- Assess for rash periodically during therapy. Topical emollients and/or topical corticosteroids may be adequate to treat mild to moderate non-exfoliative rashes. May cause SJS, TEN, and DRESS. *If rash, itching, blistering, or ulcers in mouth or other mucous membranes occur and SJS, TEN, or DRESS are suspected,* hold dose and refer for assessment and treatment. *If SJS, TEN, or DRESS are confirmed,* permanently discontinue therapy.

- Monitor for signs and symptoms of encephalitis (headache, fever, tiredness or weakness, confusion, memory problems, sleepiness, hallucinations, seizures, stiff neck) periodically during therapy. *If Grade 2 neurological toxicities occur,* hold therapy for patients with new-onset moderate to severe neurologic symptoms during diagnosis. *If Grade 3 or 4 neurological toxicities occur,* permanently

discontinue pembrolizumab and administer corticosteroids at dose of 1–2 mg/kg/day prednisone equivalents for immune-mediated encephalitis, followed by corticosteroid taper.

- Monitor for signs and symptoms of myocarditis (chest pain, dyspnea) during therapy. If Grade 2, 3 or 4 myocarditis occurs, permanently discontinue pembrolizumab.

Lab Test Considerations

- Verify negative pregnancy test prior to starting therapy. Patient selection is based on presence of positive PD-L1 expression in stage III NSCLC who are not candidates for surgical resection or definitive chemoradiation, metastatic NSCLC, first-line treatment of metastatic or unresectable, recurrent HNSCC, metastatic gastric cancer (if PD-L1 expression is not detected in an archival gastric cancer specimen, evaluate feasibility of obtaining a tumor biopsy for PD-L1 testing), previously treated recurrent locally advanced or metastatic esophageal cancer, and recurrent or metastatic cervical cancer. For MSI-H/dMMR indications, select patients for pembrolizumab as a single agent based on MSI-H/dMMR status in tumor specimens. For TMB-H, select patients for pembrolizumab as a single agent based on TMB-H status in tumor specimens. For combination therapy for non-MSI-H/dMMR advanced endometrial carcinoma, select patients for pembrolizumab in combination with lenvatinib based on MSI or MMR status in tumor specimens. For use of pembrolizumab in combination with chemotherapy, select patients based on the presence of positive PD-L1 expression in locally recurrent unresectable or metastatic TNBC. Information on FDA-approved tests used for patient selection is available at http://www.fda.gov/CompanionDiagnostics. An FDA-approved test for detection of MSI-H or dMMR is not currently available.

- Monitor for ↑ serum creatinine prior to and periodically during therapy. If Grade 2 or 3 increases in blood creatinine occur, hold pembrolizumab. Resume in patients with complete or partial resolution (Grade 0 to 1) after corticosteroid taper. Permanently discontinue if no complete or partial resolution within 12 wk of last dose or inability to reduce prednisone to ≤10 mg per day (or equivalent) within 12 wk of starting steroids. *If Grade 4 increases in blood creatinine occur,* permanently discontinue pembrolizumab.

- Monitor for abnormal liver tests prior to and periodically during therapy. For hepatitis with no tumor involvement: *If AST/ALT >3 and ≤8 times upper limit of normal (ULN) or total bilirubin >1.5 and ≤3 times ULN,* hold pembrolizumab. Resume with complete or partial resolution (Grade 0 to 1) after corticosteroid taper. Permanently discontinue if no complete or partial resolution within 12 wk of last dose or inability to reduce prednisone to ≤10 mg per day (or equivalent) within 12 wk of starting steroids. *If AST or ALT >8 times ULN or total bilirubin >3 times ULN,* permanently discontinue pembrolizumab. For hepatitis with tumor involvement of the liver: *If baseline AST/ALT is >1 and ≤3 times ULN and increases to >5 and ≤10 times ULN or baseline AST/ALT is >3 and ≤5 times ULN and increases to >8 and ≤10 times ULN,* hold pembrolizumab. *If AST/ALT >10 times ULN or total bilirubin >3 times ULN,* discontinue pembrolizumab permanently.

● Monitor for changes in thyroid function at start of and periodically during therapy, and as indicated based on clinical evaluation. Administer corticosteroids for ≥Grade 3 hyperthyroidism, withhold pembrolizumab for severe (Grade 3) hyperthyroidism and resume therapy when recovery to Grade 0 to 1. Permanently discontinue for life-threatening (Grade 4) hyperthyroidism. Manage hypothyroidism with thyroid replacement without interruption of therapy or corticosteroids.

● Monitor serum blood glucose. May cause hyperglycemia or other signs and symptoms of diabetes.

Implementation

IV Administration

● **Intermittent Infusion: *Dilution:*** Withdraw required volume of pembrolizumab and transfer to IV bag of 0.9% NaCl or D5W. Mix using gently inversion. Solution is clear to slightly opalescent, colorless to slightly yellow; do not administer solution if discolored or contains particulate matter other than translucent to white proteinaceous particles. Solution is stable at room temperature for up to 6 hr including infusion time and 96 hr if refrigerated. *Concentration:* 1 mg/mL to 10 mg/mL. *Rate:* Infuse through a sterile, non-pyrogenic, low-protein binding 0.2 micron to 5 micron in-line or add-on filter over 30 min.

● **Y-Site Incompatibility:** Do not administer other drugs through same infusion line.

Patient/Family Teaching

● Explain purpose of pembrolizumab to patient.
● Advise patient to notify health care professional immediately if signs and symptoms of pneumonitis, colitis, hepatitis, kidney problems (change in amount or color of urine), hormone gland problems (rapid heart beat, weight loss, increased sweating, weight gain, hair loss, feeling cold, constipation, deepening of voice, muscle aches, dizziness or fainting, persistent or unusual headache) occur.
● Instruct patient to notify health care professional of all Rx or OTC medications, vitamins, or herbal products being taken and to consult with health care professional before taking other medications.
● Rep: May cause fetal harm. Advise females of reproductive potential to use highly effective contraception and avoid breastfeeding during and for ≥4 mo after last dose.
● Emphasize importance of keeping scheduled appointments for blood work or other laboratory tests.

Evaluation/Desired Outcomes

● Decreased spread of melanoma, NSCLC, HNSCC, cHL, urothelial carcinoma, MSI-H or dMMR solid tumors, MSI-H or dMMR colorectal cancer, gastric tumors, cervical cancer, endometrial cancer, esophageal cancer, primary mediastinal large B-cell lymphoma, hepatocellular carcinoma, Merkel cell carcinoma, RCC, TMB-H solid tumors, cutaneous squamous cell carcinoma, and TNBC.

⚡ PEMEtrexed (pe-me-trex-ed)
Alimta, Pemfexy
Classification
Therapeutic: antineoplastics
Pharmacologic: antimetabolites, folate antagonists

Indications

Malignant pleural mesothelioma as initial therapy when tumor is unresectable or patient is not a candidate for surgery (in combination with cisplatin). ⚡ Metastatic non-squamous non–small-cell lung cancer (NSCLC) as initial therapy in patients without epidermal growth factor receptor or anaplastic lymphoma kinase genomic tumor aberrations (in combination with platinum-based therapy and pembrolizumab). Locally advanced or metastatic non-squamous NSCLC as initial therapy (in combination with cisplatin). Locally advanced or metastatic non-squamous NSCLC as maintenance treatment in patients whose disease has not progressed after 4 cycles of platinum-based first-line chemotherapy (as monotherapy). Recurrent, metastatic non-squamous NSCLC after previous chemotherapy (as monotherapy).

Action

Disrupts folate dependent metabolic processes involved in thymidine and purine synthesis. Converted intracellularly to polyglutamate form which increases duration of action. **Therapeutic Effects:** Decreases growth and spread of mesothelioma. Improved survival in patients with non-squamous NSCLC.

Pharmacokinetics

Absorption: IV administration results in complete bioavailability.
Distribution: Unknown.
Metabolism and Excretion: Minimal metabolism; 70–90% excreted unchanged in urine.
Half-life: 3.5 hr (normal renal function).

TIME/ACTION PROFILE (hematologic effects)

ROUTE	ONSET	PEAK	DURATION
IV	unknown	8–15 days	21 days

Contraindications/Precautions

Contraindicated in: Hypersensitivity; CCr <45 mL/min; OB: Pregnancy; Lactation: Lactation.

Use Cautiously in: Concurrent use of NSAIDs in patients with CCr 45–79 mL/min (avoid those with short half-lives); Third space fluid accumulation (ascites, pleural effusions); consider drainage prior to therapy; Hepatic impairment (dose alteration recommended); Rep: Women of reproductive potential and men with female partners of reproductive potential; Pedi: Safety and effectiveness not established in children.

Adverse Reactions/Side Effects

CV: chest pain. **Derm:** desquamation, rash, radiation recall, STEVENS-JOHNSON SYNDROME, TOXIC EPIDERMAL NECROLYSIS. **GI:** constipation, nausea, stomatitis, vomiting, anorexia, diarrhea, esophagitis, mouth pain. **GU:** ↓ fertility (men). **Hemat:** anemia, hemolytic anemia, leukopenia, thrombocytopenia. **Neuro:** neuropathy. **Resp:** pharyngitis, INTERSTITIAL PNEUMONITIS. **Misc:** fever, infection.

Interactions

Drug-Drug: NSAIDs, especially those with short half-lives, ↑ levels and risk of toxicity; avoid for 2 days before, day of, and 2 days after treatment. **Probenecid** ↑ levels. Concurrent use of **nephrotoxic agents** ↑ risk of nephrotoxicity.

Route/Dosage

Non-Squamous Non–Small-Cell Lung Cancer

IV (Adults): *Initial therapy (with cisplatin):* 500 mg/m² on Day 1 of each 21-day cycle for up to 6 cycles (administer before cisplatin); *Initial therapy (with platinum-based therapy and pembrolizumab):* 500 mg/m² on Day 1 of each 21-day cycle for 4 cycles (administer before carboplatin or cisplatin and after pembrolizumab). Following completion of platinum-based therapy, pemetrexed may be administered as monotherapy or with pembrolizumab as maintenance therapy until disease progression or unacceptable toxicity; *Maintenance treatment (as monotherapy) or disease recurrence (as monotherapy):* 500 mg/m² on Day 1 of each 21-day cycle until disease progression or unacceptable toxicity.

Mesothelioma

IV (Adults): 500 mg/m² on Day 1 of each 21-day cycle until disease progression or unacceptable toxicity.

Availability (generic available)

Lyophilized powder for injection: 100 mg/vial, 500 mg/vial, 1 g/vial. **Solution for injection:** 10 mg/mL, 25 mg/mL.

NURSING IMPLICATIONS

Assessment

- Monitor for rash during therapy. Pretreatment with dexamethasone 4 mg orally twice daily the day before, the day of, and the day after administration reduces incidence and severity or reaction.
- Monitor for hematologic and GI toxicities (mucositis, diarrhea). *If any Grade 3 or 4 toxicities, except mucositis or diarrhea, requiring hospitalization occur,* decrease doses of pemetrexed and cisplatin by 75%. *If Grade 3 or 4 mucositis occurs,* decrease pemetrexed dose by 50% and cisplatin by 100% of previous dose.
- Monitor for bone marrow depression. Assess for bleeding (bleeding gums, bruising, petechiae, guaiac stools, urine, and emesis) and avoid IM injections and taking rectal temperatures if platelet count is low. Apply pressure to venipuncture sites for 10 min. Assess for signs of infection during neutropenia. Anemia may occur; monitor for increased fatigue, dyspnea, and orthostatic hypotension.
- Assess for neurotoxicity during therapy. *If Grade 0–1 neurotoxicity occurs,* decrease pemetrexed and cisplatin doses by 100% of previous dose. *If Grade 2 neurotoxicity occurs,* decrease pemetrexed dose by 100% and cisplatin dose by 50% of previous dose. *If Grade 3 or 4 neurotoxicity occurs,* discontinue therapy.

Lab Test Considerations

- Verify negative pregnancy test before starting therapy. Monitor CBC and platelet counts for nadir and recovery and renal function, before each dose and on days 8 and 15 of each cycle and chemistry for renal and liver functions periodically. May cause neutropenia, thrombocytopenia, leukopenia, and anemia. A new cycle should not be started unless the ANC is ≥1500 cells/mm³, platelet count is ≥100,000 cells/mm³, and CCr is ≥45 mL/min. *If nadir of ANC is <500/mm³ and nadir of platelets are ≥50,000/mm³,* ↓ doses of pemetrexed and cisplatin by 75%. *If nadir of platelets is <50,000/mm³ regardless of ANC nadir,* ↓ pemetrexed and cisplatin doses by 50%.

Implementation

- Do not confuse pemetrexed with pralatrexate.
- Pemetrexed should be administered under supervision of a physician experienced in the use of chemotherapeutic agents.
- To reduce toxicity, 0.4–1 mg of folic acid must be taken daily for 7 days preceding 1st dose of pemetrexed and should continue during and for 21 days after last dose. Patients must also receive an injection of vitamin B₁₂ 1 mg IM during the wk preceding 1st dose of pemetrexed and every 3 cycles thereafter. Subsequent doses of vitamin B₁₂ may be given on same day as pemetrexed. Also administer dexamethasone 4 mg twice daily the day before,

the day of, and the day after pemetrexed administration.

IV Administration

- Prepare solution in a biologic cabinet. Wear gloves, gown, and mask while handling medication. Discard equipment in designated containers.
- **Intermittent Infusion:** *Reconstitution:* Calculate number of pemetrexed 500-mg vials needed; vials contain excess to facilitate delivery. Reconstitute 500 mg with 20 mL of preservative-free 0.9% NaCl. *Concentration:* 25 mg/mL. Swirl gently until powder is completely dissolved. Solution is clear and colorless to yellow or green-yellow. Do not administer if discolored or containing particulate matter. *Dilution:* Dilute further to 100 mL with preservative-free 0.9% NaCl. Solution is stable at room temperature or if refrigerated for up to 24 hr. *Rate:* Infuse over 10 min.
- **Y-Site Compatibility:** acyclovir, allopurinol, amifostine, amikacin, aminocaproic acid, aminophylline, amiodarone, amphotericin B lipid complex, amphotericin B liposomal, ampicillin, ampicillin/sulbactam, atracurium, azithromycin, aztreonam, bivalirudin, bleomycin, bumetanide, buprenorphine, butorphanol, carboplatin, carmustine, ceftriaxone, cefuroxime, cisatracurium, cisplatin, clindamycin, cyclophosphamide, cyclosporine, cytarabine, dactinomycin, daptomycin, dexamethasone, dexmedetomidine, dexrazoxane, digoxin, diltiazem, diphenhydramine, docetaxel, dopamine, doxorubicin liposomal, enalaprilat, ephedrine, epinephrine, eptifibatide, ertapenem, esmolol, etoposide, etoposide phosphate, famotidine, fentanyl, fluconazole, fludarabine, fluorouracil, foscarnet, fosphenytoin, furosemide, ganciclovir, glycopyrrolate, granisetron, haloperidol, heparin, hydrocortisone, hydromorphone, ifosfamide, imipenem/cilastatin, insulin regular, isoproterenol, ketorolac, labetalol, leucovorin calcium, levofloxacin, lidocaine, linezolid, lorazepam, magnesium sulfate, mannitol, meperidine, meropenem, mesna, methadone, methylprednisolone, metoclopramide, metoprolol, midazolam, milrinone, mitomycin, morphine, moxifloxacin, nafcillin, naloxone, nitroglycerin, norepinephrine, octreotide, oxaliplatin, paclitaxel, pamidronate, pentobarbital, phenobarbital, phentolamine, piperacillin/tazobactam, potassium acetate, potassium chloride, potassium phosphate, procainamide, promethazine, propranolol, remifentanil, rocuronium, sodium acetate, sodium bicarbonate, sodium phosphate, succinylcholine, sufentanil, tacrolimus, theophylline, thiopental, thiotepa, tigecycline, tirofiban, trimethoprim/sulfamethoxazole, vancomycin, vecuronium, verapamil, vinblastine, vincristine, vinorelbine, zidovudine, zoledronic acid.
- **Y-Site Incompatibility:** anidulafungin, calcium chloride, calcium gluconate, caspofungin, cefazolin, cefepime, cefotaxime, cefotetan, cefoxitin, ceftazidime, chloramphenicol, chlorpromazine, ciprofloxacin, D5W, dacarbazine, dantrolene, daunorubicin hydrochloride, diazepam, dobutamine, doxorubicin hydrochloride, doxycycline, droperidol, epirubicin, erythromycin, gemcitabine, gentamicin, hydralazine, idarubicin, irinotecan, metronidazole, minocycline, mitoxantrone, nalbuphine, nicardipine, nitroprusside, ondansetron, pantoprazole, pentamidine, phenytoin, prochlorperazine, tobramycin, topotecan, vasopressin.

Patient/Family Teaching

- Explain purpose of pemetrexed to patient.
- Emphasize the importance of taking prophylactic folic acid and vitamin B_{12} to reduce treatment-related hematologic and GI toxicity.
- Advise patient to notify health care professional immediately if signs and symptoms of infection (fever, sore throat), anemia, or neurotoxicity occur.
- Instruct patients to notify health care professional if persistent vomiting, diarrhea, or signs of dehydration appear.
- Instruct patient to notify health care professional of all Rx or OTC medications, vitamins, or herbal products being taken and consult health care professional before taking any new medications, especially NSAIDs, and to avoid alcohol during therapy.
- Rep: May cause fetal harm. Advise females of reproductive potential to use effective contraception during and for at least 6 mo after last dose of pemetrexed and to avoid breastfeeding during and for at least 1 wk after last dose. Advise males with female partners of reproductive potential to use effective contraception during and for at least 3 mo after last dose. If pregnancy is planned or suspected, notify health care professional promptly. May impair fertility in males.

Evaluation/Desired Outcomes

- Decreased growth and spread of mesothelioma or NSCLC.

PENICILLINS (pen-i-sill-ins)
penicillin G aqueous
　　Pfizerpen
penicillin G benzathine
　　Bicillin L-A
penicillin V
　　✿ Pen-VK
Classification
Therapeutic: anti-infectives
Pharmacologic: penicillins

Indications

Treatment of a wide variety of infections including: Pneumococcal pneumonia, Streptococcal pharyngitis,

Syphilis, Gonorrhea strains. Treatment of enterococcal infections (requires the addition of an aminoglycoside). Prevention of rheumatic fever. Should not be used as a single agent to treat anthrax. **Unlabeled Use:** Treatment of Lyme disease. Prevention of recurrent *Streptococcal pneumoniae* septicemia in children with sickle-cell disease.

Action

Bind to bacterial cell wall, resulting in cell death. **Therapeutic Effects:** Bactericidal action against susceptible bacteria. **Spectrum:** Active against: Most gram-positive organisms, including many streptococci (*Streptococcus pneumoniae*, group A beta-hemolytic streptococci), staphylococci (non–penicillinase-producing strains), and *Bacillus anthracis*; Some gram-negative organisms, such as *Neisseria meningitidis* and *Neisseria gonorrhoeae* (only penicillin susceptible strains); Some anaerobic bacteria and spirochetes including *Borellia burgdorferi*.

Pharmacokinetics

Absorption: Variably absorbed from the GI tract. *Penicillin V:* resists acid degradation in the GI tract. *Benzathine penicillin:* IM absorption is delayed and prolonged and results in sustained therapeutic blood levels.
Distribution: Widely distributed, although CNS penetration is poor in the presence of uninflamed meninges. Crosses the placenta and enters breast milk.
Metabolism and Excretion: Minimally metabolized by the liver, excreted mainly unchanged by the kidneys.
Half-life: 30–60 min.

TIME/ACTION PROFILE (plasma concentrations)

ROUTE	ONSET	PEAK	DURATION
Penicillin V PO	rapid	0.5–1 hr	4–6 hr
Penicillin G IM	rapid	0.25–0.5 hr	4–6 hr
Penicillin G IV	rapid	end of infusion	4–6 hr
Benzathine penicillin IM	delayed	12–24 hr	3 wk

Contraindications/Precautions

Contraindicated in: Previous hypersensitivity to penicillins (cross-sensitivity may exist with cephalosporins and other beta-lactams); Hypersensitivity to benzathine (benzathine preparation only); Some products may contain tartrazine and should be avoided in patients with known hypersensitivity.
Use Cautiously in: Severe renal impairment (dose ↓ recommended); OB: Although safety not established in pregnancy, has been used safely; Lactation: Safety not established in breastfeeding; Geri: Consider ↓ body mass, age-related ↓ in renal, hepatic, and cardiac function, comorbidities, and concurrent drug therapy when prescribing and dosing.

Adverse Reactions/Side Effects

Derm: rash, ACUTE GENERALIZED EXANTHEMATOUS PUSTULOSIS, DRUG REACTION WITH EOSINOPHILIA AND SYSTEMIC SYMPTOMS (DRESS), STEVENS-JOHNSON SYNDROME, TOXIC EPIDERMAL NECROLYSIS, urticaria. **GI:** diarrhea, epigastric distress, nausea, vomiting, CLOSTRIDIOIDES DIFFICILE-ASSOCIATED DIARRHEA (CDAD). **GU:** interstitial nephritis. **Hemat:** eosinophilia, hemolytic anemia, leukopenia. **Local:** pain at IM site, phlebitis at IV site. **Neuro:** SEIZURES. **Misc:** HYPERSENSITIVITY REACTIONS (including anaphylaxis and serum sickness), superinfection.

Interactions

Drug-Drug: May ↓ effectiveness of oral contraceptive agents. **Probenecid** ↓ renal excretion and ↑ blood levels of penicillin (therapy may be combined for this purpose). **Neomycin** may ↓ absorption of penicillin V. ↓ elimination of **methotrexate** and ↑ risk of serious toxicity.

Route/Dosage

Penicillin G

IM, IV (Adults): *Most infections:* 1–5 million units every 4–6 hr.
IM, IV (Children): 8333–16,667 units/kg every 4 hr; 12,550–25,000 units/kg every 6 hr; up to 250,000 units/kg/day in divided doses, some infections may require up to 300,000 units/kg/day.
IV (Infants >7 days): 25,000 units/kg every 8 hr; *Meningitis:* 50,000–75,000 units/kg every 6 hr.
IV (Infants <7 days): 25,000 units/kg every 12 hr; *Streptococcus B meningitis:* 100,000–150,000 units/kg/day in divided doses.

Penicillin G Benzathine

IM (Adults): *Streptococcal infections/erysipeloid:* 1.2 million units single dose. *Primary, secondary, and early latent syphilis:* 2.4 million units single dose. *Tertiary and late latent syphilis (not neurosyphilis):* 2.4 million units once weekly for 3 wk. *Prevention of rheumatic fever:* 1.2 million units every 3–4 wk.
IM (Children >27 kg): *Streptococcal infections/erysipeloid:* 900,000–1.2 million units (single dose). *Primary, secondary, and early latent syphilis:* up to 2.4 million units single dose. *Late latent or latent syphilis of undetermined duration:* 50,000 units/kg weekly for 3 wk. *Prevention of rheumatic fever:* 1.2 million units every 2–3 wk.
IM (Children <27 kg): *Streptococcal infections/erysipeloid:* 300,000–600,000 units single dose. *Primary, secondary, and early latent syphilis:* up to 2.4 million units single dose. *Late latent or latent syphilis of undetermined duration:* 50,000 units/kg weekly for 3 wk. *Prevention of rheumatic fever:* 1.2 million units every 2–3 wk.

Penicillin V Potassium

PO (Adults and Children ≥12 yr): *Most infections:* 125–500 mg every 6–8 hr. *Rheumatic fever prevention:* 125–250 mg every 12 hr.
PO (Children <12 yr): *Lyme disease:* 12.5 mg/kg every 6 hr (unlabeled); prevention of *Streptococcus*

pneumoniae sepsis in children with sickle cell disease—125 mg twice daily.

Availability

Penicillin G Potassium Aqueous (generic available)
Powder for injection : 5 million units/vial, 20 million units/vial. **Premixed solution for injection:** 1 million units/50 mL, 2 million units/50 mL, 3 million units/50 mL.

Penicillin G Sodium Aqueous (generic available)
Powder for injection: 5 million units/vial.

Penicillin G Benzathine
Suspension for IM injection: 600,000 units/mL.

Penicillin V Potassium (generic available)
Oral solution: 125 mg/5 mL, 250 mg/5 mL. **Tablets:** 250 mg, ✱ 300 mg, 500 mg.

NURSING IMPLICATIONS

Assessment
- Assess for infection (vital signs; appearance of wound, sputum, urine, and stool; WBC) at beginning of and during therapy.
- Obtain a history to determine previous use of and reactions to penicillins, cephalosporins, or other beta-lactam antibiotics. Persons with a negative history of penicillin sensitivity may still have an allergic response.
- Obtain specimens for culture and sensitivity before initiating therapy. 1st dose may be given before receiving results.
- Observe patient for signs and symptoms of anaphylaxis (rash, pruritus, laryngeal edema, wheezing). Discontinue drug and notify health care professional immediately if these symptoms occur. Keep epinephrine, an antihistamine, and resuscitation equipment close by in case of an anaphylactic reaction.
- Monitor bowel function. Diarrhea, abdominal cramping, fever, and bloody stools should be reported to health care professional promptly as a sign of CDAD. May begin up to several wk following cessation of therapy.

Lab Test Considerations
May cause positive direct Coombs' test results. Hyperkalemia may develop after large doses of penicillin G potassium. Monitor serum sodium concentrations in patient with hypertension or HF. Hypernatremia may develop after large doses of penicillin sodium. May cause ↑ AST, ALT, LDH, and serum alkaline phosphatase concentrations. May cause leukopenia and neutropenia, especially with prolonged therapy or hepatic impairment.

Implementation
- Do not confuse penicillin with penicillamine.
- **PO:** Administer around the clock. Penicillin V may be administered without regard for meals.
- Use calibrated measuring device for liquid preparations. Solution is stable for 14 days if refrigerated.
- **IM:** Reconstitute according to manufacturer's directions with sterile water for injection, D5W, or 0.9% NaCl.
- **IM:** Shake medication well before injection. Inject penicillin deep into a well-developed muscle mass at a slow, consistent rate to prevent blockage of the needle. Massage well. Accidental injury near or into a nerve can result in severe pain and dysfunction.
- Penicillin G potassium or sodium may be diluted with lidocaine (without epinephrine) 1% or 2% to minimize pain from IM injection.
- Never give penicillin G benzathine suspensions IV. May cause embolism or toxic reactions.

IV Administration
- **IV:** Change IV sites every 48 hr to prevent phlebitis.
- Administer slowly and observe patient closely for signs of hypersensitivity.
- **Intermittent Infusion:** *Dilution:* Doses of 3 million units or less should be diluted in at least 50 mL of D5W or 0.9% NaCl; doses of more than 3 million units should be diluted with 100 mL. *Concentration:* 100,000–500,000 units/mL (50,000 units/mL in neonates). *Rate:* Infuse over 1–2 hr in adults or 15–30 min in children.
- **Continuous Infusion:** Doses of 10 million units or more may be diluted in 1 or 2 L.
- *Rate:* Infuse over 24 hr.

Penicillin G Potassium
- **Y-Site Compatibility:** acyclovir, amiodarone, ascorbic acid, atropine, azathioprine, aztreonam, benztropine, bumetanide, buprenorphine, butorphanol, calcium chloride, calcium gluconate, cefazolin, cefotaxime, cefotetan, ceftazidime, ceftolozane/tazobactam, ceftriaxone, cefuroxime, chloramphenicol, chlorpromazine, clindamycin, cyanocobalamin, cyclophosphamide, cyclosporine, dexamethasone, digoxin, diltiazem, diphenhydramine, dopamine, enalaprilat, ephedrine, epinephrine, epoetin alfa, esmolol, famotidine, fentanyl, fluconazole, folic acid, foscarnet, furosemide, glycopyrrolate, heparin, hydrocortisone, hydromorphone, imipenem/cilastatin, indomethacin, insulin regular, isoproterenol, ketamine, ketorolac, LR, lidocaine, magnesium sulfate, mannitol, meperidine, meropenem/vaborbactam, methylprednisolone, metoclopramide, metoprolol, midazolam, morphine, multivitamins, nafcillin, nalbuphine, naloxone, nicardipine, nitroglycerin, nitroprusside, norepinephrine, ondansetron, oxacillin, oxytocin, penicillin G sodium, phenyleph-

P

rine, phytonadione, plazomicin, potassium chloride, procainamide, prochlorperazine, propranolol, pyridoxine, sodium bicarbonate, sufentanil, tacrolimus, theophylline, thiamine, tobramycin, vasopressin, verapamil.

- **Y-Site Incompatibility:** If aminoglycosides and penicillins must be administered concurrently, administer in separate sites at least 1 hr apart, dantrolene, diazepam, dobutamine, doxycycline, ganciclovir, haloperidol, minocycline, papaverine, pentamidine, pentobarbital, phenytoin, protamine, tranexamic acid, trimethoprim/sulfamethoxazole.

Penicillin G Sodium

- **Y-Site Compatibility:** ascorbic acid, atropine, azathioprine, aztreonam, benztropine, bumetanide, buprenorphine, butorphanol, calcium chloride, calcium gluconate, cefazolin, cefotaxime, cefotetan, cefoxitin, ceftazidime, ceftriaxone, cefuroxime, chloramphenicol, clindamycin, cyanocobalamin, cyclophosphamide, cyclosporine, dexamethasone, digoxin, diphenhydramine, dopamine, enalaprilat, ephedrine, epinephrine, epoetin alfa, esmolol, famotidine, fentanyl, fluconazole, folic acid, furosemide, glycopyrrolate, heparin, hydrocortisone, imipenem/cilastatin, indomethacin, insulin regular, isoproterenol, ketamine, ketorolac, LR, levofloxacin, lidocaine, magnesium sulfate, mannitol, meperidine, meropenem, methylprednisolone, metoclopramide, metoprolol, midazolam, morphine, multivitamins, nafcillin, nalbuphine, naloxone, nitroglycerin, nitroprusside, norepinephrine, ondansetron, oxacillin, oxytocin, pantoprazole, phenylephrine, phytonadione, potassium chloride, procainamide, prochlorperazine, propranolol, pyridoxine, sodium bicarbonate, sufentanil, theophylline, thiamine, vasopressin, verapamil.
- **Y-Site Incompatibility:** If aminoglycosides and penicillins must be administered concurrently, administer in separate sites at least 1 hr apart, dantrolene, diazepam, dobutamine, doxycycline, ganciclovir, haloperidol, labetalol, minocycline, morphine, papaverine, pentamidine, pentobarbital, phenytoin, protamine, tranexamic acid, trimethoprim/sulfamethoxazole.

Patient/Family Teaching

- Instruct patient to take medication around the clock and to finish drug completely as directed, even if feeling better. Advise patient that sharing this medication may be dangerous.
- Advise patient to report signs of superinfection (black, furry overgrowth on tongue; vaginal itching or discharge; loose or foul-smelling stools) and allergy.
- Instruct patient to notify health care professional if fever and diarrhea develop, especially if stool contains blood, pus, or mucus. Advise patient not to treat diarrhea without consulting health care professional.

- Instruct patient to notify health care professional if symptoms do not improve.
- Rep: Advise females of reproductive potential to notify health care professional if pregnancy is planned or suspected or if breastfeeding. Advise patient taking oral contraceptives to use an additional nonhormonal method of contraception during therapy with penicillin and until next menstrual period.
- Patient with an allergy to penicillin should be instructed to always carry an identification card with this information.

Evaluation/Desired Outcomes

- Resolution of signs and symptoms of infection. Length of time for complete resolution depends on the organism and site of infection.

PENICILLINS, PENICILLINASE RESISTANT
dicloxacillin (dye-klox-a-**sill**-in)
nafcillin (naf-**sill**-in)
oxacillin (ox-a-**sill**-in)
Classification
Therapeutic: anti-infectives
Pharmacologic: penicillinase resistant penicillins

Indications

Treatment of the following infections due to penicillinase-producing staphylococci: Respiratory tract infections, Sinusitis, Skin and skin structure infections. **Dicloxacillin:** Osteomyelitis. **Nafcillin, oxacillin:** Are also used to treat: Bone and joint infections, Urinary tract infections, Endocarditis, Septicemia, Meningitis.

Action

Bind to bacterial cell wall, leading to cell death. Not inactivated by penicillinase enzymes. **Therapeutic Effects:** Bactericidal action. **Spectrum:** Active against most gram-positive aerobic cocci but less so than penicillin. Spectrum is notable for activity against: Penicillinase-producing strains of *Staphylococcus aureus*, *Staphylococcus epidermidis*. Not active against methicillin-resistant staphylococci.

Pharmacokinetics

Absorption: *Dicloxacillin:* Rapidly but incompletely (35–76%) absorbed from the GI tract following oral administration. *Nafcillin and oxacillin:* IV administration results in complete bioavailability; well absorbed from IM sites.

Distribution: Widely distributed; penetration into CSF is minimal, but sufficient in the presence of inflamed meninges.

Metabolism and Excretion: *Dicloxacillin:* Some metabolism by the liver (6–10%) and some renal excretion of unchanged drug (60%); small amounts eliminated in the feces via the bile. *Nafcillin, oxacillin:* Partially metabolized by the liver (nafcillin

60%, oxacillin 49%), partially excreted unchanged by the kidneys.

Half-life: *Dicloxacillin:* 0.5–1.1 hr (↑ in severe hepatic and renal impairment); *Nafcillin:* Neonates: 1–5 hr; Children 1 mo–14 yr: 0.75–1.9 hr; Adults: 0.5–1.5 hr (↑ in renal impairment); *Oxacillin:* Neonates: 1.6 hr; Children up to 2 yr: 0.9–1.8 hr; Adults: 0.3–0.8 hr (↑ in severe hepatic impairment).

TIME/ACTION PROFILE (plasma concentrations)

ROUTE	ONSET	PEAK	DURATION
Dicloxacillin (PO)	30 min	30–120 min	6 hr
Nafcillin (IM)	30 min	60–120 min	4–6 hr
Nafcillin (IV)	rapid	end of infusion	4–6 hr
Oxacillin (IM)	rapid	30 min	4–6 hr
Oxacillin (IV)	rapid	end of infusion	4–6 hr

Contraindications/Precautions

Contraindicated in: Hypersensitivity to penicillins (cross-sensitivity with cephalosporins may exist).
Use Cautiously in: Severe renal impairment; Severe hepatic impairment; Lactation: Use while breastfeeding only if potential maternal benefit justifies potential risk to infant.

Adverse Reactions/Side Effects

Derm: <u>rash</u>, urticaria. **GI:** <u>diarrhea</u>, <u>nausea</u>, <u>vomiting</u>, ↑ liver enzymes, CLOSTRIDIOIDES DIFFICILE-ASSOCIATED DIARRHEA (CDAD). **GU:** acute kidney injury, hematuria, interstitial nephritis, proteinuria. **Hemat:** eosinophilia, leukopenia. **Local:** <u>pain at IM sites</u>, <u>phlebitis at IV sites</u>. **Neuro:** SEIZURES (high doses). **Misc:** HYPERSENSITIVITY REACTIONS (including anaphylaxis and serum sickness), superinfection.

Interactions

Drug-Drug: **Probenecid** ↓ renal excretion and ↑ levels (treatment may be combined for this purpose). May ↓ effectiveness of **oral contraceptive agents**. May ↓ elimination of **methotrexate** and ↑ risk of serious toxicity.

Route/Dosage

Dicloxacillin
PO (Adults and Children ≥40 kg): 125–250 mg every 6 hr (max dose = 2 g/day).
PO (Children <40 kg): 6.25–12.5 mg/kg every 6 hr; (up to 12.25 mg/kg every 6 hr has been used for osteomyelitis) (max dose = 2 g/day).

Nafcillin
IV (Adults): 500–2000 mg every 4–6 hr.
IM (Adults): 500 mg every 4–6 hr.

IM, IV (Children and Infants): 50–200 mg/kg/day divided every 4–6 hr (max dose = 12 g/day).
IM, IV (Neonates >2 kg): 25 mg/kg every 8 hr for the 1st 7 days of life, then 25 mg/kg every 6 hr.
IM, IV (Neonates 1.2–2 kg): 25 mg/kg every 12 hr for the 1st 7 days of life, then 25 mg/kg every 8 hr.
IM, IV (Neonates 0–4 wk, <1.2 kg): 25 mg/kg every 12 hr.

Oxacillin
IM, IV (Adults and Children ≥40 kg): 250–2000 mg every 4–6 hr (max dose = 12 g/day).
IM, IV (Children <40 kg): 100–200 mg/kg/day divided every 4–6 hr (max dose = 12 g/day).
IM, IV (Neonates ≥2 kg): 25 mg/kg every 8 hr for the 1st 7 days of life, then 25 mg/kg every 6 hr.
IM, IV (Neonates 1.2–2 kg): 25 mg/kg every 12 hr for the 1st 7 days of life, then 25 mg/kg every 8 hr.
IM, IV (Neonates <1.2 kg): 25 mg/kg every 12 hr.

Availability

Dicloxacillin (generic available)
Capsules: 250 mg, 500 mg.

Nafcillin (generic available)
Powder for injection: 1 g/vial, 2 g/vial, 10 g/vial.
Premixed infusion: 1 g/50 mL D5W, 2 g/100 mL D5W.

Oxacillin (generic available)
Powder for injection: 1 g/vial, 2 g/vial, 10 g/vial.
Premixed infusion: 1 g/50 mL D5W, 2 g/50 mL D5W.

NURSING IMPLICATIONS

Assessment

- Assess patient for infection (vital signs; appearance of wound, sputum, urine, and stool; WBC) at beginning of and throughout therapy.
- Obtain a history before initiating therapy to determine previous use of and reactions to penicillins, cephalosporins, or other beta-lactam antibiotics. Persons with a negative history of penicillin sensitivity may still have an allergic response.
- Obtain specimens for culture and sensitivity prior to initiating therapy. 1st dose may be given before receiving results.
- Observe patient for signs and symptoms of anaphylaxis (rash, pruritus, laryngeal edema, wheezing, abdominal pain). Discontinue the drug and notify health care professional immediately if these occur. Keep epinephrine, an antihistamine, and resuscitation equipment close by in the event of an anaphylactic reaction.
- Assess vein for signs of irritation and phlebitis. Change IV site every 48 hr to prevent phlebitis.
- Monitor bowel function. Diarrhea, abdominal cramping, fever, and bloody stools should be reported to health care professional promptly as a sign

of CDAD. May begin up to several wk following cessation of therapy.

Lab Test Considerations

- May cause leukopenia and neutropenia, especially with prolonged therapy or hepatic impairment.
- May cause positive direct Coombs' test result.
- May cause ↑ AST, ALT, LDH, and serum alkaline phosphatase concentrations.

Implementation

- **PO:** Administer around the clock on an empty stomach at least 1 hr before or 2 hr after meals. Take with a full glass of water; acidic juices may decrease absorption of penicillins.
- Use calibrated measuring device for liquid preparations. Shake well. Solution is stable for 14 days if refrigerated.

Nafcillin

IV Administration

- **IV, IM:** To reconstitute, add 3.4 mL to each 1-g vial or 6.8 mL to each 2-g vial, for a concentration of 250 mg/mL. Stable for 2−7 days if refrigerated.
- **IV Push:** *Dilution:* Dilute reconstituted solution with 15−30 mL of sterile water, 0.45% NaCl, or 0.9% NaCl for injection. *Concentration:* 100 mg/mL. *Rate:* Administer over 5−10 min.
- **Intermittent Infusion:** *Dilution:* Dilute with sterile water for injection, 0.9% NaCl, D5W, D10W, D5/0.25% NaCl, D5/0.45% NaCl, D5/0.9% NaCl, D5/LR, Ringer's or LR. Stable for 24 hr at room temperature, 96 hr if refrigerated. *Concentration:* 2−40 mg/mL. *Rate:* Infuse over at least 30−60 min to avoid vein irritation.
- **Y-Site Compatibility:** acyclovir, aminophylline, amphotericin B lipid complex, anidulafungin, argatroban, ascorbic acid, atracurium, atropine, aztreonam, benztropine, bivalirudin, bleomycin, bumetanide, buprenorphine, butorphanol, calcium chloride, calcium gluconate, carboplatin, carmustine, chlorpromazine, cisplatin, clindamycin, cyanocobalamin, cyclophosphamide, dactinomycin, daptomycin, dexamethasone, digoxin, dobutamine, docetaxel, dopamine, enalaprilat, ephedrine, epinephrine, epoetin alfa, erythromycin, etoposide, etoposide phosphate, famotidine, fentanyl, fludarabine, foscarnet, furosemide, ganciclovir, glycopyrrolate, granisetron, heparin, hetastarch, hydrocortisone, hydromorphone, imipenem/cilastatin, indomethacin, isoproterenol, ketorolac, lidocaine, linezolid, lorazepam, magnesium sulfate, mannitol, methylprednisolone, metoclopramide, metoprolol, metronidazole, milrinone, morphine, multivitamins, naloxone, nicardipine, nitroglycerin, nitroprusside, norepinephrine, octreotide, ondansetron, oxacillin, oxytocin, paclitaxel, pamidronate, pantoprazole, pemetrexed, penicillin G, pentobarbital, phenobarbital, phentolamine, phenylephrine, phytonadione, potassium acetate, potassium chloride, procainamide,

prochlorperazine, propofol, propranolol, sodium bicarbonate, sufentanil, tacrolimus, theophylline, thiamine, thiotepa, tigecycline, tirofiban, vasopressin, voriconazole, zidovudine, zoledronic acid.
- **Y-Site Incompatibility:** alemtuzumab, ampicillin, azathioprine, caspofungin, chloramphenicol, dantrolene, diazoxide, doxycycline, droperidol, epirubicin, folic acid, gemcitabine, haloperidol, hydralazine, hydroxyzine, idarubicin, irinotecan, meperidine, mitoxantrone, mycophenolate, palonosetron, pentamidine, phenytoin, promethazine, protamine, pyridoxine, succinylcholine, trimethoprim/sulfamethoxazole, vecuronium, vincristine, vinorelbine. If penicillins and aminoglycosides must be administered concurrently, administer at separate sites.

Oxacillin

IV Administration

- **IV, IM:** To reconstitute for IM or IV use, add 1.4 mL of sterile water for injection to each 250-mg vial, 2.7 mL to each 500-mg vial, 5.7 mL to each 1-g vial, 11.5 mL to each 2-g vial, and 23 mL to each 4-g vial, for a concentration of 250 mg/1.5 mL. Stable for 3 days at room temperature or 7 days if refrigerated.
- **IV Push:** *Dilution:* Further dilute each reconstituted 250-mg or 500-mg vial with 5 mL of sterile water or 0.9% NaCl for injection, 10 mL for each 1-g vial, 20 mL for each 2-g vial, and 40 mL for each 4-g vial. *Concentration:* 100 mg/mL. *Rate:* Administer slowly over 10 min.
- **Intermittent Infusion:** *Dilution:* Dilute with 0.9% NaCl, D5W, D5/0.9% NaCl, or LR. *Concentration:* 0.5−40 mg/mL. *Rate:* May be infused for up to 6 hr.
- **Y-Site Compatibility:** acyclovir, aminophylline, ascorbic acid, atracurium, atropine, aztreonam, benztropine, bumetanide, buprenorphine, butorphanol, chloramphenicol, chlorpromazine, clindamycin, cyanocobalamin, cyclophosphamide, cyclosporine, dexamethasone, digoxin, diltiazem, dopamine, enalaprilat, ephedrine, epinephrine, epoetin alfa, erythromycin, famotidine, fentanyl, fluconazole, folic acid, foscarnet, furosemide, glycopyrrolate, heparin, hydrocortisone, hydromorphone, imipenem/cilastatin, insulin regular, isoproterenol, ketorolac, labetalol, levofloxacin, lidocaine, mannitol, methotrexate, metoclopramide, metoprolol, midazolam, milrinone, morphine, multivitamins, nafcillin, naloxone, nitroglycerin, nitroprusside, norepinephrine, ondansetron, oxytocin, papaverine, penicillin G, pentobarbital, phenobarbital, phenylephrine, phytonadione, potassium chloride, procainamide, prochlorperazine, propranolol, sufentanil, tacrolimus, theophylline, thiamine, vancomycin, vasopressin, zidovudine.
- **Y-Site Incompatibility:** calcium chloride, calcium gluconate, dantrolene, diazepam, diazoxide, dobutamine, doxycycline, esmolol, haloperidol, hydrala-

zine, pentamidine, phenytoin, promethazine, pyridoxine, succinylcholine, trimethoprim/sulfamethoxazole. If penicillins and aminoglycosides must be administered concurrently, administer at separate sites.

Patient/Family Teaching

● Instruct patient to take medication around the clock and to finish the drug completely as directed, even if feeling better. Missed doses should be taken as soon as remembered. Advise patient that sharing of this medication may be dangerous.

● Advise patient to report signs of superinfection (black, furry overgrowth on the tongue; vaginal itching or discharge; loose or foul-smelling stools) and allergy.

● Instruct patient to notify health care professional if fever and diarrhea develop, especially if stool contains blood, pus, or mucus. Advise patient not to treat diarrhea without consulting health care professional.

● Instruct patient to notify health care professional if symptoms do not improve.

● Rep: Advise females of reproductive potential to notify health care professional if breastfeeding.

Evaluation/Desired Outcomes

● Resolution of the signs and symptoms of infection. Length of time for complete resolution depends on the organism and site of infection.

---

perindopril, See ANGIOTENSIN-CONVERTING ENZYME (ACE) INHIBITORS.

🅇 pertuzumab (per-**tue**-zue-mab)
Perjeta
Classification
Therapeutic: antineoplastics
Pharmacologic: HER2/neu receptor antagonists, monoclonal antibodies

Indications

🅇 HER2-positive metastatic breast cancer in patients who have not yet been treated with anti-HER2 agents or chemotherapy (in combination with docetaxel and trastuzumab [or trastuzumab hyaluronidase]). 🅇 Neoadjuvant treatment of HER2-positive locally advanced, inflammatory, or early stage breast cancer (either >2 cm in diameter or node-positive) (in combination with trastuzumab [or trastuzumab hyaluronidase] and chemotherapy). 🅇 Adjuvant treatment of HER2-positive early breast cancer at high risk of recurrence (in combination with trastuzumab [or trastuzumab hyaluronidase] and chemotherapy).

Action

A monoclonal antibody that attaches to and blocks the human epidermal growth factor receptor 2 protein (HER2), resulting in cell growth arrest and apoptosis. **Therapeutic Effects:** Decreased spread of breast cancer.

Pharmacokinetics

Absorption: IV administration results in complete bioavailability.
Distribution: Minimally distributed to tissues.
Metabolism and Excretion: Unknown.
Half-life: 18 days.

TIME/ACTION PROFILE

ROUTE	ONSET	PEAK	DURATION
IV	unknown	unknown	20 mo†

†Median duration of response.

Contraindications/Precautions

Contraindicated in: Hypersensitivity; OB: Pregnancy.
Use Cautiously in: 🅇 Asian patients (↑ incidence of febrile neutropenia); Lactation: Safety not established in breastfeeding; Rep: Women of reproductive potential; Pedi: Safety and effectiveness not established in children.

Adverse Reactions/Side Effects

May reflect combination treatment with docetaxel and trastuzumab.

CV: peripheral edema, HF. **Derm:** alopecia, rash, dry skin, nail disorder. **EENT:** ↑ lacrimation. **GI:** ↓ appetite, diarrhea, nausea, vomiting. **Hemat:** ANEMIA, LEUKOPENIA, NEUTROPENIA. **MS:** arthralgia, myalgia. **Neuro:** dizziness, dysgeusia, fatigue, headache, insomnia, peripheral neuropathy, weakness. **Resp:** dyspnea. **Misc:** chills, fever, HYPERSENSITIVITY REACTIONS (including anaphylaxis and angioedema), INFUSION REACTIONS.

Interactions

Drug-Drug: ↑ risk of bone marrow depression/immunosuppression with other **bone marrow depressants/immunosuppressants** or **radiation therapy**.

Route/Dosage

Metastatic Breast Cancer
IV (Adults): 840 mg initially, then 420 mg every 3 wk.

Neoadjuvant Treatment of Breast Cancer
IV (Adults): 840 mg initially, then 420 mg every 3 wk for 3–6 cycles given preoperatively. Following surgery, administer 420 mg every 3 wk to complete 1 yr of treatment (up to 18 cycles).

Adjuvant Treatment of Breast Cancer
IV (Adults): 840 mg initially, then 420 mg every 3 wk for 1 yr (up to 18 cycles) or until disease recurrence or unacceptable toxicity.

🍁 = Canadian drug name. 🅇 = Genetic implication. ~~Strikethrough~~ = Discontinued. CAPITALS = life-threatening. <u>Underline</u> = most frequent.

Availability

Solution for injection: 30 mg/mL.

NURSING IMPLICATIONS

Assessment

● Assess left ventricular ejection fraction (LVEF) before starting pertuzumab and at regular intervals during therapy. Metastatic Breast Cancer: *If pretreatment LVEF ≥50%, monitor prior to and about every 12 wk. If LVEF ↓ to <40% or 40–45% with a fall of ≥10% points below pretreatment value,* hold pertuzumab and trastuzumab (or trastuzumab hyaluronidase) for at least 3 wk. *If after 3 wk LVEF recovered to >45% or 40–45% with a fall of <10% points below pretreatment value,* resume pertuzumab and trastuzumab (or trastuzumab hyaluronidase). Early Breast Cancer: *If pretreatment LVEF ≥55%, monitor prior to and about every 12 wk or once neoadjuvant therapy. If LVEF ↓ to <50% with a fall of ≥10% points below pretreatment value,* hold pertuzumab and trastuzumab (or trastuzumab hyaluronidase) for at least 3 wk. *If after 3 wk LVEF recovered to >50% with a fall of <10% points below pretreatment value,* resume pertuzumab and trastuzumab (or trastuzumab hyaluronidase). For patients receiving anthracycline-based chemotherapy, a LVEF of ≥ 50% is required after completion of anthracyclines, before starting pertuzumab and trastuzumab.

● If trastuzumab is withheld or discontinued, withhold or discontinue pertuzumab. If docetaxel is discontinued, pertuzumab and trastuzumab therapy may continue. Dose reductions are not recommended for pertuzumab.

● Assess patient closely for 60 min after initial infusion and 30 min after subsequent infusions for signs and symptoms of infusion-associated reactions (pyrexia, chills, fatigue, headache, asthenia, hypersensitivity, vomiting). If a significant infusion-associated reaction occurs, slow or interrupt infusion and administer appropriate medical therapies. Monitor until complete resolution of signs and symptoms. If severe infusion reactions occur, consider discontinuation of pertuzumab.

● Monitor patient for signs and symptoms of hypersensitivity reactions (rash, hives, itching, dyspnea, swelling of throat, lips, tongue) occurs.

Lab Test Considerations

● Verify negative pregnancy status before starting therapy. Determine HER protein overexpression prior to therapy.

● Monitor CBC with differential periodically during therapy.

Implementation

IV Administration

● Administer pertuzumab, trastuzumab (or trastuzumab hyaluronidase) and docetaxel sequentially. Administer pertuzumab and trastuzumab or trastuzumab hyaluronidase in any order. Administer docetaxel after pertuzumab and trastuzumab or tras-

tuzumab hyaluronidase. Observe patient for 30 to 60 min after pertuzumab infusion and before any subsequent infusion of trastuzumab or docetaxel.

● **Intermittent Infusion:** *Dilution:* 0.9% NaCl; do not use D5W. Withdraw appropriate volume of pertuzumab and dilute in 250 mL using a PVC or non-PVC polyolefin infusion bag. Gently invert to mix; do not shake. If not administered immediately, may be refrigerated for 24 hr; do not freeze. *Rate:* Infuse initial 840 mg over 60 min, followed every 3 wk by 420 mg over 30–60 min.

● For delayed or missed doses, if time between 2 sequential infusions is <6 wk, administer 420 mg dose of pertuzumab; do not wait until next planned dose. If time between 2 sequential infusions ≥6 wk, readminister initial 840 mg dose over 60 min, followed every 3 wk by 420 mg dose over 30–60 min.

Patient/Family Teaching

● Explain purpose of medication to patient.

● Advise patient to report signs and symptoms of infusion-associated reactions immediately.

● Advise patient to notify health care professional immediately if signs and symptoms of left ventricular dysfunction (new onset or worsening shortness of breath, cough, swelling of the ankles/legs, swelling of the face, palpitations, weight gain of more than 5 pounds in 24 hr, dizziness or loss of consciousness) occur.

● Instruct patient to notify health care professional promptly if fever; chills; cough; hoarseness; sore throat; signs of infection; lower back or side pain; painful or difficult urination; bleeding gums; bruising; petechiae; blood in stools, urine, or emesis; increased fatigue; dyspnea. Caution patient to avoid crowds and persons with known infections. Instruct patient to use soft toothbrush and electric razor and to avoid falls. Caution patient not to drink alcoholic beverages or take medication containing aspirin or NSAIDs; may precipitate gastric bleeding.

● Instruct patient to notify health care professional of all Rx or OTC medications, vitamins, or herbal products being taken and consult health care professional before taking any new medications.

● Rep: May cause fetal harm. Advise females of reproductive potential to notify health care professional immediately if pregnancy is planned or suspected or if breastfeeding. Caution patient to use effective contraception during and for 7 mo following the last dose. Inform patients who become pregnant while receiving pertuzumab of pregnancy pharmacovigilance program to monitor infant outcomes. Encourage pregnant females who may be exposed to pertuzumab during pregnancy to report exposure to the Genentech Adverse Event Line at 1-888-835-2555. Monitor females who become pregnant for oligohydramnios.

Evaluation/Desired Outcomes

● Decreased spread of metastatic breast cancer.

pertuzumab/trastuzumab/ hyaluronidase
(per-**tue**-zue-mab/traz-**too**-zoo-mab/hye-al-yoor-**on**-i-dase)
Phesgo
Classification
Therapeutic: antineoplastics
Pharmacologic: HER2/neu receptor antagonists, monoclonal antibodies

Indications
Neoadjuvant treatment of human epidermal growth factor receptor 2 protein (HER2)-positive locally advanced, inflammatory, or early stage breast cancer (either >2 cm in diameter or node-positive) (in combination with chemotherapy). Adjuvant treatment of HER2-positive early breast cancer at high risk of recurrence (in combination with chemotherapy). HER2-positive metastatic breast cancer in patients who have not yet been treated with anti-HER2 agents or chemotherapy (in combination with docetaxel).

Action
Pertuzumab and trastuzumab: monoclonal antibody that binds to HER2 sites in breast cancer tissue and inhibits proliferation of cells that overexpress HER2; *Hyaluronidase:* Acts locally by depolymerizing hyaluronan, which increases permeability of the SUBQ tissue. **Therapeutic Effects:** Regression of breast cancer and metastases.

Pharmacokinetics
Pertuzumab
Absorption: 70% absorbed following SUBQ administration.
Distribution: Minimally distributed to tissues.
Metabolism and Excretion: Unknown.
Half-life: Unknown.
Trastuzumab
Absorption: 80% absorbed following SUBQ administration.
Distribution: Minimally distributed to tissues.
Metabolism and Excretion: Unknown.
Half-life: Unknown.

TIME/ACTION PROFILE (plasma concentrations)

ROUTE	ONSET	PEAK	DURATION
Pertuzumab (SUBQ)	unknown	4 days	unknown
Trastuzumab (SUBQ)	unknown	4 days	unknown

Contraindications/Precautions
Contraindicated in: Hypersensitivity; OB: Pregnancy.

Use Cautiously in: HF, uncontrolled hypertension, recent MI, arrhythmias, prior anthracycline exposure (equivalent to >360 mg/m² of doxorubicin); Pulmonary disease or extensive tumor involvement of lungs (↑ risk of pulmonary toxicity); Dyspnea at rest (↑ risk of hypersensitivity reaction); Lactation: Use while breastfeeding only if potential maternal benefit justifies potential risk to infant; Rep: Women of reproductive potential; Pedi: Safety and effectiveness not established in children.

Adverse Reactions/Side Effects
CV: arrhythmias, HF, hypertension, peripheral edema. **Derm:** alopecia, dry skin, rash, dermatitis, erythema, nail discoloration, palmar-plantar erythrodysesthesia syndrome. **EENT:** epistaxis, ↑ lacrimation, dry eyes, rhinorrhea. **Endo:** hypoglycemia. **F and E:** hyperkalemia, hyponatremia, hypernatremia, hypokalemia. **GI:** ↓ appetite, ↓ weight, ↑ liver enzymes, constipation, diarrhea, dyspepsia, hypoalbuminemia, nausea, stomatitis, vomiting, abdominal pain, hemorrhoids, hyperbilirubinemia. **GU:** ↑ serum creatinine, urinary tract infection. **Hemat:** anemia, leukopenia, lymphocytopenia, neutropenia, thrombocytopenia. **Local:** injection site pain, injection site reaction. **MS:** arthralgia, myalgia, muscle spasm, pain. **Neuro:** dizziness, dysgeusia, fatigue, headache, insomnia, paresthesia, peripheral neuropathy. **Resp:** cough, dyspnea, upper respiratory tract infection, ACUTE RESPIRATORY DISTRESS SYNDROME, INTERSTITIAL PNEUMONITIS, pleural effusion, PULMONARY EDEMA, PULMONARY FIBROSIS. **Misc:** fever, HYPERSENSITIVITY REACTIONS (including anaphylaxis and angioedema).

Interactions
Drug-Drug: Use of an **anthracycline (daunorubicin, doxorubicin, or idarubicin)** following therapy may ↑ risk of cardiotoxicity; if possible, avoid anthracycline-based therapy for up to 7 mo following completion of therapy.

Route/Dosage
Do not substitute Phesgo with or for pertuzumab, trastuzumab, ado-trastuzumab emtansine, or fam-trastuzumab deruxtecan.

Neoadjuvant Treatment of Breast Cancer
SUBQ (Adults): *Initial dose:* Pertuzumab 1,200 mg/trastuzumab 600 mg/hyaluronidase 10,000 units followed by maintenance dose in 3 wk; *Maintenance dose:* Pertuzumab 600 mg/trastuzumab 600 mg/hyaluronidase 20,000 units every 3 wk for 3–6 cycles as part of a treatment regimen for early breast cancer. Following surgery, continue pertuzumab/trastuzumab/hyaluronidase to complete 1 yr of treatment (up to 18 cycles) or until disease recurrence or unmanageable toxicity, whichever occurs first, as a part of a complete regimen for early breast cancer. In patients receiving an anthracycline-based regimen for early breast cancer,

administer pertuzumab/trastuzumab/hyaluronidase following completion of the anthracycline. In patients receiving docetaxel or paclitaxel, administer docetaxel or paclitaxel after pertuzumab/trastuzumab/hyaluronidase.

Adjuvant Treatment of Breast Cancer
SUBQ (Adults): *Initial dose:* Pertuzumab 1,200 mg/trastuzumab 600 mg/hyaluronidase 10,000 units followed by maintenance dose in 3 wk; *Maintenance dose:* Pertuzumab 600 mg/trastuzumab 600 mg/hyaluronidase 20,000 units every 3 wk for a total of 1 yr (up to 18 cycles) or until disease recurrence or unmanageable toxicity, whichever occurs first, as part of a complete regimen for early breast cancer. In patients receiving an anthracycline-based regimen for early breast cancer, administer pertuzumab/trastuzumab/hyaluronidase following completion of the anthracycline. In patients receiving docetaxel or paclitaxel, administer docetaxel or paclitaxel after pertuzumab/trastuzumab/hyaluronidase.

Metastatic Breast Cancer
SUBQ (Adults): *Initial dose:* Pertuzumab 1,200 mg/trastuzumab 600 mg/hyaluronidase 10,000 units followed by maintenance dose in 3 wk; *Maintenance dose:* Pertuzumab 600 mg/trastuzumab 600 mg/hyaluronidase 20,000 units every 3 wk until disease recurrence or unmanageable toxicity. Administer docetaxel after pertuzumab/trastuzumab/hyaluronidase.

Availability
Solution for injection: pertuzumab 60 mg, trastuzumab 60 mg, and hyaluronidase 2,000 units/mL, pertuzumab 80 mg, trastuzumab 40 mg, and hyaluronidase 2,000 units/mL.

NURSING IMPLICATIONS
Assessment
● Conduct a cardiac assessment, including history, physical examination, and determination of left ventricular ejection fraction (LVEF) by echocardiogram or MUGA scan before starting therapy. Assess LVEF at regular intervals. May cause hypertension, arrhythmias, left ventricular dysfunction, HF, cardiomyopathy and death. *For early breast cancer: with LVEF* ≥55%, monitor LVEF every 12 wk. Hold *Phesgo* for at least 3 wk for LVEF ↓ to <50% with a fall of ≥10% points below pretreatment value. Resume *Phesgo* after 3 wk if LVEF recovered to ≥50% or <10% points below pretreatment value. *For metastatic breast cancer with LVEF* ≥50%, monitor LVEF every 12 wk. Hold *Phesgo* for 3 wk for LVEF ↓ to either <40% or 40–45% with a fall of ≥10% points below pre-treatment value. Resume *Phesgo* after 3 wk if LVEF has recovered to either >45% or 40–45% with a fall of <10% points below pretreatment value. After repeat assessment within 3 wk, if LVEF has not improved, has declined further, and/or patient is symptomatic, permanently discontinue *Phesgo*. After completion of therapy, continue to monitor for cardiomyopathy

and assess LVEF measurements every 6 mo for at least 2 years.
● Monitor for at least 30 min after initial dose of *Phesgo* and 15 min after each maintenance dose for signs of hypersensitivity symptoms or administration-related reactions. If significant injection-related reaction occurs, slow or pause injection and administer symptomatic therapy. Have medications and emergency equipment available. For Grade 1 or 2 hypersensitivity reactions, premedicate with an analgesic, antipyretic, or antihistamine. Permanently discontinue *Phesgo* if anaphylaxis or severe injection-related reactions.
● Monitor for signs and symptoms of pulmonary toxicity (dyspnea, interstitial pneumonitis, pulmonary infiltrates, pleural effusions, non-cardiogenic pulmonary edema, pulmonary insufficiency and hypoxia, acute respiratory distress syndrome, pulmonary fibrosis) periodically during therapy.

Lab Test Considerations
● ✂ Patient selection is based on HER2 protein overexpression or HER2 gene amplification in tumor specimens using FDA-approved tests specific for breast cancer. Information on FDA-approved tests is available at http://www.fda.gov/CompanionDiagnostics.
● Obtain a negative pregnancy test before starting therapy.
● May exacerbate chemotherapy-induced neutropenia. May cause anemia, neutropenia, leukopenia, and febrile neutropenia.
● May cause ↑ serum creatinine, AST, ALT, bilirubin and ↓ albumin.
● May cause ↓ potassium and glucose and ↑ sodium and potassium.

Implementation
● *Phesgo* has different dose and administration instructions than pertuzumab IV, trastuzumab IV, and SUBQ trastuzumab when administered alone. Do not use other drugs in place of *Phesgo*. Must always be administered by health care professional.
● *In patients receiving anthracycline-based regimen for early breast cancer,* administer *Phesgo* following completion of the anthracycline. *In patients receiving Phesgo for early breast cancer with docetaxel or paclitaxel,* administer docetaxel or paclitaxel after *Phesgo*. *In patients receiving Phesgo for metastatic breast cancer with docetaxel,* administer docetaxel after *Phesgo*.
● **SUBQ:** Check label to make sure vial contains *Phesgo* and not IV pertuzumab, or IV trastuzumab, or SUBQ trastuzumab. Solution is clear to opalescent, and colorless to slightly brownish; do not administer solutions that are cloudy, discolored, or contain particulate matter. Do not dilute; do not shake. Attach 25–27 gauge 3/8–5/8 inch needle to syringe just before injection. Solution is stable for up to 4 hr at room temperature or 24 hr if refrigerated.

Inject into thighs only; alternate between right and left thigh with each dose. Inject initial dose of 15 mL over 8 min. Inject maintenance dose of 10 mL over 5 min. Inject at least 1 inch from previous site and avoid areas where skin is red, bruised, tender, or hard. Inject other SUBQ medications in different sites.

Patient/Family Teaching
- Explain purpose of *Phesgo* and regimen to patient.
- Advise patient to notify health care professional immediately if signs and symptoms of cardiomyopathy (new onset or worsening shortness of breath, cough, swelling of ankles or legs, swelling of face, palpitations, weight gain >5 pounds in 24 hr, dizziness, loss of consciousness) or hypersensitivity and administration-related reactions (dizziness, nausea, chills, fever, vomiting, diarrhea, urticaria, swelling of face or neck, breathing problems, chest pain) occur.
- Advise patient to notify health care professional of all Rx or OTC medications, vitamins, or herbal products being taken and to consult with health care professional before taking other medications.
- Rep: May cause fetal harm. Advise females of reproductive potential to use effective contraception and to avoid breastfeeding for 7 mo after last dose. If *Phesgo* is administered during pregnancy, or if a patient becomes pregnant while receiving *Phesgo* or within 7 mo following last dose of *Phesgo*, health care providers and patients should immediately report *Phesgo* exposure to pharmacovigilance program at Genentech at 1-888-835-2555.

Evaluation/Desired Outcomes
- Regression of breast cancer and metastases.

---

phenazopyridine
(fen-az-oh-**peer**-i-deen)
✶Phenazo, Pyridium

Classification
Therapeutic: nonopioid analgesics
Pharmacologic: urinary tract analgesics

Indications
Provides relief from the following urinary tract symptoms, which may occur in association with infection or following urologic procedures: Pain, Itching, Burning, Urgency, Frequency.

Action
Acts locally on the urinary tract mucosa to produce analgesic or local anesthetic effects. Has no antimicrobial activity. **Therapeutic Effects:** Diminished urinary tract discomfort.

Pharmacokinetics
Absorption: Well absorbed following oral administration.

Distribution: Unknown.
Metabolism and Excretion: Rapidly excreted unchanged in the urine.
Half-life: Unknown.

TIME/ACTION PROFILE (urinary analgesia)

ROUTE	ONSET	PEAK	DURATION
PO	unknown	5–6 hr	6–8 hr

Contraindications/Precautions
Contraindicated in: Hypersensitivity; Glomerulonephritis; Severe hepatitis, uremia, or renal failure; Renal impairment; Glucose-6-phosphate dehydrogenase deficiency.
Use Cautiously in: Hepatitis; OB: Safety not established in pregnancy; Lactation: Safety not established in breastfeeding.

Adverse Reactions/Side Effects
Derm: rash. **GI:** hepatotoxicity, nausea. **GU:** <u>bright-orange urine</u>, renal failure. **Hemat:** hemolytic anemia, methemoglobinemia. **Neuro:** headache, vertigo.

Interactions
Drug-Drug: None reported.

Route/Dosage
PO (Adults): 200 mg 3 times daily for 2 days.
PO (Children): 4 mg/kg 3 times daily for 2 days.

Availability (generic available)
Tablets: 95 mg^OTC, 100 mg, ✶100 mg^OTC, ✶200 mg^OTC, 200 mg.

NURSING IMPLICATIONS

Assessment
- Assess patient for urgency, frequency, and pain on urination prior to and during therapy.

Lab Test Considerations
- Renal function should be monitored periodically during course of therapy.
- Interferes with urine tests based on color reactions (glucose, ketones, bilirubin, steroids, protein).

Implementation
- *High Alert:* Do not confuse Pyridium with pyridoxine.
- Medication should be discontinued after pain or discomfort is relieved (usually 2 days for treatment of urinary tract infection). Concurrent antibiotic therapy should continue for full prescribed duration.
- PO: Administer medication with or following meals to decrease GI irritation. *DNC:* Do not crush, break, or chew tablet.

Patient/Family Teaching
- Instruct patient to take medication as directed. If a dose is missed, take as soon as remembered unless almost time for next dose.

P

- Advise patient that while phenazopyridine administration is stopped once pain or discomfort is relieved, concurrent antibiotic therapy must be continued for full duration of therapy. Do not save unused portion of phenazopyridine without consulting health care professional.
- Inform patient that drug causes reddish-orange discoloration of urine that may stain clothing or bedding. Sanitary napkin may be worn to avoid clothing stains. May also cause staining of soft contact lenses.
- Instruct patient to notify health care professional if rash, skin discoloration, or unusual tiredness occurs.
- Rep: Advise females of reproductive potential to notify health care professional if pregnancy is planned or suspected or if breastfeeding.

Evaluation/Desired Outcomes

- Decrease in pain and burning on urination.

BEERS

PHENobarbital
(fee-noe-**bar**-bi-tal)
~~Luminal~~, Sezaby
Classification
Therapeutic: anticonvulsants, sedative/hypnotics
Pharmacologic: barbiturates

Schedule IV

Indications

Tonic-clonic (grand mal), partial, and febrile seizures in children. Preoperative sedative and in other situations in which sedation may be required. Hypnotic (short-term).

Action

Produces all levels of CNS depression. Depresses the sensory cortex, decreases motor activity, and alters cerebellar function. Inhibits transmission in the nervous system and raises the seizure threshold. Capable of inducing (speeding up) enzymes in the liver that metabolize drugs, bilirubin, and other compounds. **Therapeutic Effects:** Anticonvulsant activity. Sedation.

Pharmacokinetics

Absorption: Absorption is slow but relatively complete (70–90%).
Distribution: Unknown.
Metabolism and Excretion: 75% metabolized by the liver, 25% excreted unchanged by the kidneys.
Half-life: *Neonates:* 1.8–8.3 days; *Infants:* 0.8–5.5 days; *Children:* 1.5–3 days; *Adults:* 2–6 days.

TIME/ACTION PROFILE (sedation†)

ROUTE	ONSET	PEAK	DURATION
PO	30–60 min	unknown	>6 hr
IM, SUBQ	10–30 min	unknown	4–6 hr
IV	5 min	30 min	4–6 hr

†Full anticonvulsant effects occur after 2–3 wk of chronic dosing unless a loading dose has been used.

Contraindications/Precautions

Contraindicated in: Hypersensitivity; Comatose patients or those with pre-existing CNS depression; Severe respiratory disease with dyspnea or obstruction; Uncontrolled severe pain; Known alcohol intolerance (elixir only); Lactation: Lactation.

Use Cautiously in: Hepatic impairment; Severe renal impairment; History of suicide attempt or drug abuse; OB: Chronic use during pregnancy results in drug dependency in the infant; may result in coagulation defects and fetal malformation; acute use at term may result in respiratory depression in the newborn; Geri: Appears on Beers list. Older adults have ↑ risk of physical dependence and risk of toxicity at lower doses. If possible, avoid use in older adults.

Adverse Reactions/Side Effects

CV: *IV:* hypotension. **Derm:** photosensitivity, rash, urticaria. **GI:** constipation, diarrhea, nausea, vomiting. **Local:** phlebitis at IV site. **MS:** arthralgia, myalgia. **Neuro:** hangover, delirium, depression, drowsiness, excitation, lethargy, neuralgia, vertigo. **Resp:** respiratory depression; *IV:* LARYNGOSPASM, bronchospasm. **Misc:** HYPERSENSITIVITY REACTIONS (including angioedema and serum sickness), physical dependence, psychological dependence.

Interactions

Drug-Drug: Additive CNS depression with other **CNS depressants**, including **alcohol**, **antihistamines**, **opioid analgesics**, and other **sedative/hypnotics**. May induce hepatic enzymes that metabolize other drugs, ↓ their effectiveness, including **hormonal contraceptives**, **warfarin**, **chloramphenicol**, **cyclosporine**, **dacarbazine**, **corticosteroids**, **tricyclic antidepressants**, **felodipine**, **clonazepam**, **carbamazepine**, **verapamil**, **theophylline**, **metronidazole**, and **quinidine**. May ↑ risk of hepatic toxicity of **acetaminophen**. **MAO inhibitors**, **valproic acid**, or **divalproex** may ↓ metabolism of phenobarbital, ↑ sedation. **Rifampin** may ↑ metabolism of and ↓ effects of phenobarbital. May ↑ risk of hematologic toxicity with **cyclophosphamide**.
Drug-Natural Products: Concomitant use of **kava-kava**, **valerian**, **chamomile**, or **hops** can ↑ CNS depression. **St. John's wort** may ↓ effects.

Route/Dosage

Status Epilepticus

IV (Adults and Children >1 mo): 15–18 mg/kg in a single or divided dose, maximum loading dose 20 mg/kg.
IV (Neonates): 15–20 mg/kg in a single dose. If clinically indicated, ≥15 minutes after completion of the initial loading dose, a 2nd loading dose may be administered over the subsequent 15 minutes as 20 mg/kg for term infants or 10–20 mg/kg for preterm infants.

Maintenance Anticonvulsant

IV, PO (Adults and Children >12 yr): 1–3 mg/kg/day as a single dose or 2 divided doses.

IV, PO (Children >5 yr): 2–3 mg/kg/day in 1–2 divided doses.
IV, PO (Children ≤5 yr): 3–5 mg/kg/day in 1–2 divided doses.

Sedation
PO, IM (Adults): 30–120 mg/day in 2–3 divided doses. *Preoperative sedation:* 100–200 mg IM 1–1.5 hr before the procedure.
PO (Children): 2 mg/kg 3 times daily. *Preoperative sedation:* 1–3 mg/kg PO/IM/IV 1–1.5 hr before the procedure.

Hypnotic
PO, SUBQ, IV, IM (Adults): 100–320 mg at bedtime.
IV, IM, SUBQ (Children): 3–5 mg/kg at bedtime.

Hyperbilirubinemia
PO (Adults): 90–180 mg/day in 2–3 divided doses.
PO (Children <12 yr): 3–8 mg/kg/day in 2–3 divided doses, doses up to 12 mg/kg/day have been used.

Availability (generic available)
Tablets: 15 mg, 16.2 mg, 30 mg, 32.4 mg, 60 mg, 64.8 mg, 97.2 mg, 100 mg. **Elixir:** 20 mg/5 mL. **Lyophilized powder for injection:** 100 mg/vial. **Solution for injection:** 65 mg/mL, 130 mg/mL.

NURSING IMPLICATIONS
Assessment
- Monitor respiratory status, pulse, and BP, and signs and symptoms of angioedema (swelling of lips, face, throat, dyspnea) frequently in patients receiving phenobarbital IV. Equipment for resuscitation and artificial ventilation should be readily available. Respiratory depression is dose-dependent.
- Prolonged therapy may lead to psychological or physical dependence. Restrict amount of drug available to patient, especially if depressed, suicidal, or with a history of addiction.
- Geri: Older adults may react to phenobarbital with marked excitement, depression, and confusion. Monitor for these adverse reactions.
- **Seizures:** Assess location, duration, and characteristics of seizure activity.
- **Sedation:** Assess level of consciousness and anxiety when used as a preoperative sedative.
- Assess postoperative patients for pain with a pain scale. Phenobarbital may increase sensitivity to painful stimuli.

Lab Test Considerations
- Patients on prolonged therapy should have hepatic and renal function and CBC evaluated periodically.
- Monitor serum folate concentrations periodically during therapy because of increased folate requirements of patients on long-term anticonvulsant therapy with phenobarbital.

- May cause ↓ serum bilirubin concentrations in neonates, in patients with congenital nonhemolytic unconjugated hyperbilirubinemia, and in epileptics.

Toxicity and Overdose
- Serum phenobarbital levels may be monitored when used as an anticonvulsant. Therapeutic blood levels are 10–40 mcg/mL. Symptoms of toxicity include confusion, drowsiness, dyspnea, slurred speech, and staggering.

Implementation
- Do not confuse phenobarbital with pentobarbital.
- Supervise ambulation and transfer of patients following administration. Two side rails should be raised and call bell within reach at all times. Keep bed in low position. Institute seizure and fall precautions.
- When changing from phenobarbital to another anticonvulsant, gradually decrease phenobarbital dose while concurrently increasing dose of replacement medication to maintain anticonvulsant effects.
- **PO:** Tablets may be crushed and mixed with food or fluids (do not administer dry) for patients with difficulty swallowing. Oral solution may be taken undiluted or mixed with water, milk, or fruit juice. Use calibrated measuring device for accurate measurement of liquid doses.
- **IM:** Injections should be given deep into the gluteal muscle to minimize tissue irritation. Do not inject >5 mL into any one site, because of tissue irritation.

IV Administration
- **IV:** Doses may require 15–30 min to reach peak concentrations in the brain. Administer minimal dose and wait for effectiveness before administering 2nd dose to prevent cumulative barbiturate-induced depression.
- **Intermittent Infusion:** *Reconstitution:* Reconstitute sterile powder for IV dose with 10 mL of 0.9% NaCl. *Dilution:* Do not use solution that is not absolutely clear within 5 min after reconstitution or that contains a precipitate. Discard powder or solution that has been exposed to air for longer than 30 min. If not administered immediately, place vial in original carton to protect from light. Stable for 8 hr at room temperature or 24 hr if refrigerated.
- Use a large peripheral vein to avoid local tissue toxicity. Solution is highly alkaline; avoid extravasation, which may cause tissue damage and necrosis. If extravasation occurs, injection of 5% procaine solution into affected area and application of moist heat may be ordered.
- *Concentration:* 130 mg/mL (undiluted). *Rate:* Do not inject IV faster than 60 mg/min. Infuse over 15–30 min. Infuse large loading doses over 60 min. Titrate slowly for desired response. Rapid administration may result in respiratory depression.
- **Y-Site Compatibility:** acyclovir, amikacin, aminocaproic acid, aminophylline, amphotericin B lipid

P

✸ = Canadian drug name. ▓ = Genetic implication. S̶t̶r̶i̶k̶e̶t̶h̶r̶o̶u̶g̶h̶ = Discontinued. CAPITALS = life-threatening. <u>Underline</u> = most frequent.

complex, amphotericin B liposomal, anidulafungin, argatroban, arsenic trioxide, ascorbic acid, atropine, azathioprine, aztreonam, benztropine, bivalirudin, bleomycin, bumetanide, butorphanol, calcium chloride, calcium gluconate, carboplatin, cefazolin, ceftazidime, ceftriaxone, chloramphenicol, cisplatin, clindamycin, cyanocobalamin, cyclophosphamide, cytarabine, dacarbazine, dactinomycin, daptomycin, dexamethasone, dexmedetomidine, dexrazoxane, digoxin, docetaxel, dopamine, doxorubicin liposomal, enalaprilat, epoetin alfa, eptifibatide, ertapenem, etoposide, etoposide phosphate, famotidine, fentanyl, fluconazole, fludarabine, fluorouracil, folic acid, fosphenytoin, furosemide, ganciclovir, gemcitabine, gentamicin, glycopyrrolate, granisetron, heparin, hetastarch, hydrocortisone, ibuprofen lysine, ifosfamide, indomethacin, insulin regular, irinotecan, ketorolac, labetalol, LR, leucovorin calcium, linezolid, lorazepam, magnesium sulfate, mannitol, meropenem, mesna, methadone, methotrexate, methylprednisolone, metoclopramide, metoprolol, metronidazole, milrinone, mitoxantrone, morphine, multivitamins, nafcillin, naloxone, nitroglycerin, nitroprusside, octreotide, oxacillin, oxytocin, paclitaxel, palonosetron, pamidronate, pemetrexed, pentobarbital, phenylephrine, phytonadione, piperacillin/tazobactam, potassium acetate, potassium chloride, procainamide, propofol, propranolol, rocuronium, sodium acetate, sodium bicarbonate, sufentanil, theophylline, thiotepa, tigecycline, tirofiban, tobramycin, vancomycin, vasopressin, vecuronium, vincristine, voriconazole, zoledronic acid.

- **Y-Site Incompatibility:** acetaminophen, alemtuzumab, amiodarone, amphotericin B deoxycholate, atracurium, buprenorphine, carmustine, caspofungin, cefotaxime, cefotetan, cefoxitin, cefuroxime, chlorpromazine, cyclophosphamide, dantrolene, diazepam, diltiazem, diphenhydramine, dobutamine, doxorubicin hydrochloride, doxycycline, epinephrine, epirubicin, esmolol, gemtuzumab ozogamicin, haloperidol, hydroxyzine, idarubicin, meperidine, midazolam, minocycline, mitomycin, mycophenolate, nalbuphine, nicardipine, norepinephrine, ondansetron, papaverine, pentamidine, phenytoin, prochlorperazine, promethazine, protamine, pyridoxine, succinylcholine, thiamine, topotecan, trimethoprim/sulfamethoxazole, verapamil, vinorelbine.

Patient/Family Teaching

- Advise patient to take medication as directed. Take missed doses as soon as remembered if not almost time for next dose; do not double doses.
- Advise patients on prolonged therapy not to discontinue medication without consulting health care professional. Abrupt withdrawal may precipitate seizures or status epilepticus.
- Medication may cause daytime drowsiness. Caution patient to avoid driving and other activities requiring alertness until response to medication is known. Do

not resume driving until physician gives clearance based on control of seizure disorder.
- Caution patient to avoid taking alcohol or other CNS depressants, including opioids, concurrently with this medication.
- Advise patient to notify health care professional if signs and symptoms of angioedema, fever, sore throat, mouth sores, unusual bleeding or bruising, nosebleeds, or petechiae occur.
- Teach sleep hygiene techniques (dark room, quiet, bedtime ritual, limit daytime napping, avoid nicotine and caffeine).
- Rep: Advise females of reproductive potential using oral contraceptives to use an additional nonhormonal contraceptive during therapy and until next menstrual period. Instruct patient to notify health care professional immediately if pregnancy is planned or suspected or if breastfeeding. Use during third trimester of pregnancy may cause withdrawal symptoms in the neonate, including seizures and hyperirritability; symptoms of withdrawal may be delayed in the neonate up to 14 days after birth. Monitor infant for respiratory depression if used during labor. A registry is available for women exposed to phenobarbital during pregnancy: Pregnant women may enroll themselves into the North American Antiepileptic Drug Pregnancy Registry (1-888-233-2334 or http://www.aedpregnancyregistry.org).
- Pedi: Advise parents or caregivers that child may experience irritability, hyperactivity, and/or sleep disturbances, which may diminish in a few days to a few wk or may persist until drug is stopped. An alternative medication can be considered. Instruct parents to monitor for skin rash occurring 7–20 days after treatment begins and to contact a health care provider if rash occurs. Teach family about symptoms of toxicity (staggering, drowsiness, slurred speech).

Evaluation/Desired Outcomes

- Decrease or cessation of seizure activity without excessive sedation. Several wk may be required to achieve maximum anticonvulsant effects.
- Preoperative sedation.
- Improvement in sleep patterns.
- Decrease in serum bilirubin levels.

REMS

phentermine/topiramate
(fen-ter-meen/toe-**pyre**-a-mate)
Qsymia
Classification
Therapeutic: weight control agents
Pharmacologic: appetite suppressants

Schedule IV

Indications

Weight management as part of a program including caloric restriction and increased exercise in adults with an initial body mass index (BMI) of ≥30 kg/m² *or a* BMI of ≥27 kg/m² with ≥1 other risk factor (hypertension, type 2 diabetes mellitus, or dyslipidemia). Weight management as part of a program including caloric restriction and increased exercise in children ≥12 years old with an initial BMI in the 95th percentile or greater standardized for age and sex.

Action
Phentermine: ↓ appetite and food consumption; *Topiramate:* ↓ appetite and enhances satiety. **Therapeutic Effects:** Weight loss.

Pharmacokinetics
Phentermine
Absorption: Extent of absorption following oral administration unknown.
Distribution: Unknown.
Metabolism and Excretion: Metabolized by the liver.
Half-life: 19–24 hr.
Topiramate
Absorption: 80% absorbed following oral administration.
Distribution: Unknown.
Metabolism and Excretion: Not extensively metabolized. 70% excreted unchanged in urine.
Half-life: 21 hr.

TIME/ACTION PROFILE (weight loss)

ROUTE	ONSET	PEAK	DURATION
PO	within 8 wk	16–32 wk	unknown

Contraindications/Precautions
Contraindicated in: Hypersensitivity/idiosyncrasy to sympathomimetics (contains tartrazine); Glaucoma; Hyperthyroidism; During/within 14 days of MAO inhibitors; End-stage renal disease on dialysis; Severe hepatic impairment; History of suicidal thought/active suicidal ideation; OB: Pregnancy; Lactation: Lactation.
Use Cautiously in: Diabetes (weight loss may ↑ risk of hypoglycemia); History of substance abuse; Ketogenic diet (↑ risk of kidney stones); Rep: Women of reproductive potential; Pedi: Children <12 yr (safety and effectiveness not established); may ↓ vertical growth; Geri: ↑ risk of adverse effects in older adults (consider age-related ↓ in cardiac, renal, and hepatic function, concurrent chronic disease states and medications).

Adverse Reactions/Side Effects
CV: tachycardia, hypotension, palpitations. **Derm:** alopecia, ERYTHEMA MULTIFORME, oligohydrosis (↓ sweating), STEVENS-JOHNSON SYNDROME, TOXIC EPIDERMAL NECROLYSIS. **EENT:** acute myopia, blurred vision, eye pain, secondary angle closure glaucoma, visual field defects. **Endo:** hypoglycemia. **F and E:** hypokalemia, metabolic acidosis. **GI:** altered taste, constipation, dry mouth, HEPATOTOXICITY. **GU:** ↑ serum creatinine, kidney stones. **Metab:** ↓ growth (children). **Neuro:** headache, insomnia, paresthesia, cognitive impairment, dizziness, mood disorders, SEIZURES (FOLLOWING ABRUPT DISCONTINUATION), SUICIDAL IDEATION. **Misc:** ALLERGIC REACTION, hyperthermia.

Interactions
Drug-Drug: ↑ risk of hypokalemia with **non-potassium sparing diuretics**. ↑ risk of CNS depression with **other CNS depressants** including **alcohol**, some **antihistamines**, **sedative/hypnotics**, **antipsychotics**, and **opioid analgesics**; avoid concurrent use of alcohol. Altered exposure to **oral contraceptives** may ↑ risk of irregular bleeding. **Carbamazepine** or **phenytoin** may ↓ levels. Concurrent use of topiramate with **valproic acid** may ↑ risk of hyperammonemia. Concurrent use of topiramate with **carbonic anhydrase inhibitors** may ↑ risk of metabolic acidosis and kidney stones. ↑ risk of hypotension with **antihypertensive** and **diuretics**. May ↓ **pioglitazone** levels.

Route/Dosage
PO (Adults): Phentermine 3.75 mg/topiramate 23 mg once daily for 14 days, then ↑ to phentermine 7.5 mg/topiramate 46 mg once daily for 12 wk, then assess weight loss. If patient has not lost at least 3% of baseline body weight, ↑ dose to phentermine 11.25 mg/topiramate 69 mg once daily for 14 days, then phentermine 15 mg/topiramate 92 mg once daily for 12 wk, then assess weight loss. If patient has not lost at least 5% of baseline body weight, discontinue therapy as success is unlikely. Discontinuation should proceed by taking the phentermine 15 mg/topiramate 92 mg capsule every other day for 1 wk and then discontinue therapy.
PO (Children ≥12 yr): Phentermine 3.75 mg/topiramate 23 mg once daily for 14 days, then ↑ to phentermine 7.5 mg/topiramate 46 mg once daily for 12 wk, then assess BMI. If patient has not experienced a reduction of at least 3% of baseline BMI, ↑ dose to phentermine 11.25 mg/topiramate 69 mg once daily for 14 days, then phentermine 15 mg/topiramate 92 mg once daily for 12 wk, then assess BMI. If patient has not experienced a reduction of at least 5% of baseline BMI, discontinue therapy as success is unlikely. Discontinuation should proceed by taking the phentermine 15 mg/topiramate 92 mg capsule every other day for 1 wk and then discontinue therapy. If weight loss exceeds 2 lb/wk, consider ↓ dose.

Renal Impairment
PO (Adults and Children ≥12 yr): *CCr <50 mL/min:* Not to exceed phentermine 7.5 mg/topiramate 46 mg once daily.

Hepatic Impairment
PO (Adults and Children): *Moderate hepatic impairment:* Not to exceed phentermine 7.5 mg/topiramate 46 mg once daily.

Availability

Capsules (contain tartrazine): phentermine 3.75 mg (immediate-release)/topiramate 23 mg (extended-release) (for titration only), phentermine 7.5 mg (immediate-release)/topiramate 46 mg (extended-release), phentermine 11.25 mg (immediate-release)/topiramate 69 mg (extended-release) (for titration only), phentermine 15 mg (immediate-release)/topiramate 92 mg (extended-release).

NURSING IMPLICATIONS

Assessment

● Monitor patients for weight loss and adjust concurrent medications (antihypertensives, antidiabetics, lipid-lowering agents) as needed. Evaluate weight loss after each 12 wk of therapy.

● Monitor closely for notable changes in behavior that could indicate the emergence or worsening of suicidal thoughts or behavior or depression. Discontinue phentermine/topiramate if these occur.

● Monitor BP and heart rate periodically during therapy; may cause increase in resting heart rate. May cause hypotension in patients treated with antihypertensives.

Lab Test Considerations

● Verify negative pregnancy test prior to starting therapy and monthly during therapy.

● Before starting and periodically during therapy with *Qsymia*, obtain a blood chemistry profile (serum bicarbonate, creatinine, and potassium) in all patients, and also blood glucose in patients with type 2 diabetes on antidiabetic medication.

● May cause hypoglycemia; monitor blood glucose closely in diabetic patients.

● May cause metabolic acidosis; monitor serum bicarbonate, prior to starting and periodically during therapy.

● May cause ↑ serum creatinine; peak increases observed after 4–8 wk of therapy. Monitor serum creatinine prior to and periodically during therapy; if persistent elevations occur, decrease dose or discontinue therapy.

● May cause hypokalemia; monitor serum potassium periodically during therapy.

Implementation

● *REMS: Qsymia* is only available through certified pharmacies that are enrolled in the Qsymia certified pharmacy network. Information can be obtained at www.QsymiaREMS.com or by calling 1-888-998-4887. **PO:** Administer once daily in the morning without regard to food. Avoid dosing in the evening; may cause insomnia.

Patient/Family Teaching

● Instruct patient to take phentermine/topiramate as directed. Do not stop taking without consulting health care professional. Discontinue gradually by taking 1 dose every other day for at least 1 wk

before stopping to prevent seizures. *REMS:* Explain *Qsymia* REMS requirements to patient.

● Advise patient to notify health care professional if sustained periods of heart pounding or racing while at rest; severe and persistent eye pain or significant changes in vision; changes in attention, concentration, memory, and/or difficulty finding words; factors that can increase risk of acidosis (prolonged diarrhea, surgery, high-protein/low-carbohydrate diet, and/or concomitant medications).

● Inform patients and families of risk of suicidal thoughts and behavior (behavioral changes, emerging or worsening signs and symptoms of depression, unusual changes in mood, or emergence of suicidal thoughts, behavior, or thoughts of self-harm). Advise that these should be reported to health care professional immediately.

● May cause changes in mental performance, motor performance, and/or vision. Caution patients to avoid driving and other activities requiring alertness until response to medication is known.

● Instruct patient to increase fluid intake to increase urinary output and decrease risk of kidney stones.

● Advise patient to monitor for decreased sweating and increased body temperature during physical activity, especially in hot weather.

● Instruct patient to notify health care professional of all Rx or OTC medications, vitamins, or herbal products being taken and consult health care professional before taking any new medications. Advise patient to avoid taking other CNS depressants, opioids, or alcohol.

● Rep: May cause fetal harm. Advise females of reproductive potential to use effective contraception and avoid breastfeeding during therapy. Advise female patients to notify health care professional if pregnancy is planned or suspected. For patients taking combined oral contraceptives, may cause irregular bleeding and spotting; advise patient to continue oral contraceptive and notify health care professional if spotting is concerning. *REMS:* Because of teratogenic risk, *Qsymia* is only available through a limited program under the REMS. Under the Qsymia REMS, only certified pharmacies may distribute *Qsymia*. Further information is available at www.QSYMIAREMS.com or by telephone at 1-888-998-4887.

Evaluation/Desired Outcomes

● Decrease in weight and BMI.

HIGH ALERT

phenylephrine (fen-il-eff-rin)

Biorphen, ✹Neo-Synephrine, Vazculep

Classification

Therapeutic: vasopressors

Pharmacologic: adrenergics, alpha adrenergic agonists, vasopressors

For ophthalmic use see Appendix B

Indications

Management of hypotension associated with shock that may persist after adequate fluid replacement. Management of hypotension associated with anesthesia. **Anesthesia adjunct.** Prolongation of the duration of spinal anesthesia. Localization of the effect of regional anesthesia.

Action

Constricts blood vessels by stimulating alpha-adrenergic receptors. **Therapeutic Effects:** Increased BP.

Pharmacokinetics

Absorption: Well absorbed from IM sites. IV administration results in complete bioavailability.
Distribution: Widely distributed to tissues.
Metabolism and Excretion: Metabolized by the liver into inactive metabolites.
Half-life: 2.5 hr.

TIME/ACTION PROFILE (vasopressor effects)

ROUTE	ONSET	PEAK	DURATION
IV	immediate	unknown	15–20 min
IM	10–15 min	unknown	0.5–2 hr
SUBQ	10–15 min	unknown	50–60 min

Contraindications/Precautions

Contraindicated in: Hypersensitivity to bisulfites.
Use Cautiously in: HF, coronary artery disease, or peripheral arterial disease; OB: Has been used safely during Caesarean section procedure; safety of use during first or second trimester of pregnancy not established; Lactation: Use while breastfeeding only if potential maternal benefit justifies potential risk to infant; Pedi: Safety and effectiveness not established in children.

Adverse Reactions/Side Effects

CV: ARRHYTHMIAS, bradycardia, chest pain, hypertension, ischemia, tachycardia. **Derm:** pruritus. **GI:** epigastric pain, nausea, vomiting. **Local:** phlebitis, sloughing at IV sites. **Neuro:** blurred vision, headache, insomnia, nervousness, tremor. **Resp:** dyspnea.

Interactions

Drug-Drug: Use with **general anesthetics** may result in myocardial irritability; use with extreme caution. Use with **MAO inhibitors**, **ergot alkaloids (methylergonovine)**, **oxytocics**, **tricyclic antidepressants**, **atropine**, **corticosteroids**, or **atomoxetine** results in severe hypertension. **Alpha-adrenergic blockers**, **PDE-5 inhibitors**, **calcium channel blockers**, **benzodiazepines**, **ACE inhibitors**, or **guanfacine** may antagonize vasopressor effects.

Route/Dosage

Hypotension

SUBQ, IM (Adults): 2–5 mg.
SUBQ, IM (Children): 0.1 mg/kg/dose every 1–2 hr as needed, maximum dose 5 mg.
IV (Adults): 0.2 mg (range 0.1–0.5 mg), may be repeated every 10–15 min *or* as an infusion at 100–180 mcg/min initially, 40–60 mcg/min maintenance.
IV (Children): 5–20 mcg/kg/dose every 10–15 min as needed or 0.1–0.5 mcg/kg/min infusion, titrate to effect.

Hypotension During Anesthesia

SUBQ, IM (Adults): 2–3 mg has been used 3–4 min before spinal anesthesia to prevent hypotension.
IM, SUBQ (Children): 0.5–1 mg/25 lb body weight.
IV (Adults): 40–100 mcg; may repeat every 1–2 min as needed (not to exceed total dose of 200 mcg); if BP remains low, initiate continuous infusion at 10–35 mcg/min (not to exceed 200 mcg/min).

Vasoconstrictor for Regional Anesthesia

Local (Adults): Add 1 mg to every 20 mL of local anesthetic (yields a 1:20,000 solution).

Prolongation of Spinal Anesthesia

Spinal (Adults): 2–5 mg added to anesthetic solution.

Availability (generic available)

Solution for injection: 0.1 mg/mL, 10 mg/mL. **Premixed infusion:** 20 mg/250 mL 0.9% NaCl, 25 mg/250 mL 0.9% NaCl, 40 mg/250 mL 0.9% NaCl, 50 mg/250 mL 0.9% NaCl.

NURSING IMPLICATIONS

Assessment

* Monitor BP every 2–3 min until stabilized and every 5 min thereafter during IV administration.
* Monitor ECG continuously for arrhythmias during IV administration.
* Assess IV site frequently throughout infusion. Antecubital or other large vein should be used to minimize risk of extravasation, which may cause tissue necrosis.

Implementation

* **High Alert:** Patient harm and fatalities have occurred from medication errors with phenylephrine. Prior to administration, have second practitioner independently check original order, dose calculations, concentration, route of administration, and infusion pump settings.

IV Administration

* **IV:** Blood volume depletion should be corrected, if possible, before initiation of IV phenylephrine.
* **IV Push:** *Dilution:* Dilute each 1 mg with 9 mL of sterile water for injection or D5W.

- For *Biorphen*, the **0.1 mg/mL** solution must NOT be diluted prior to administration.
- For *Biorphen* **10 mg/mL** solution, ***Dilution:*** dilute 1 mL (10 mg) with 99 mL of D5W or 0.9% NaCl before bolus or continuous infusion. ***Concentration:*** 100 mcg/mL. Solution is stable for 4 hr at room temperature or 24 hr if refrigerated. ***Rate:*** Administer each single dose over 1 min.
- **Continuous Infusion: *Dilution:*** Dilute 10 mg in 250 or 500 mL of D5W or 0.9% NaCl. For *Biorphen*, dilute 10 mg in 500 mL of D5W or 0.9% NaCl. ***Concentration:*** 20 or 40 mcg/mL. ***Rate:*** Titrate rate according to patient response. Infuse via infusion pump to ensure accurate dose rate.
- **Y-Site Compatibility:** alemtuzumab, amikacin, aminophylline, amiodarone, amphotericin B liposomal, anidulafungin, argatroban, arsenic trioxide, ascorbic acid, atracurium, atropine, azithromycin, aztreonam, benztropine, bivalirudin, bleomycin, bumetanide, buprenorphine, butorphanol, calcium chloride, calcium gluconate, cangrelor, carboplatin, carmustine, caspofungin, cefazolin, cefotaxime, cefotetan, cefoxitin, ceftazidime, ceftazidime/avibactam, ceftolozane/tazobactam, ceftriaxone, cefuroxime, chloramphenicol, cisatracurium, cisplatin, clindamycin, cyanocobalamin, cyclophosphamide, cyclosporine, cytarabine, dacarbazine, dactinomycin, daptomycin, daunorubicin hydrochloride, dexamethasone, dexmedetomidine, dexrazoxane, digoxin, diltiazem, diphenhydramine, dobutamine, docetaxel, dopamine, doxorubicin hydrochloride, doxycycline, enalaprilat, ephedrine, epinephrine, epirubicin, epoetin alfa, eptifibatide, eravacycline, ertapenem, erythromycin, esmolol, etomidate, etoposide, etoposide phosphate, famotidine, fentanyl, fluconazole, fludarabine, fluorouracil, folic acid, foscarnet, fosphenytoin, gentamicin, glycopyrrolate, granisetron, heparin, hetastarch, hydrocortisone, hydromorphone, idarubicin, ifosfamide, imipenem/cilastatin/relebactam, imipenem/cilastatin, irinotecan, isavuconazonium, isoproterenol, ketorolac, labetalol, LR, leucovorin calcium, levofloxacin, lidocaine, linezolid, lorazepam, magnesium sulfate, mannitol, meperidine, meropenem/vaborbactam, mesna, methadone, methotrexate, methylprednisolone, metoclopramide, metoprolol, metronidazole, micafungin, midazolam, milrinone, mitoxantrone, morphine, moxifloxacin, multivitamins, mycophenolate, nafcillin, nalbuphine, naloxone, nicardipine, nitroglycerin, nitroprusside, norepinephrine, octreotide, ondansetron, oritavancin, oxacillin, oxaliplatin, oxytocin, paclitaxel, palonosetron, pamidronate, pantoprazole, papaverine, penicillin G, pentobarbital, phenobarbital, phytonadione, piperacillin/tazobactam, plazomicin, potassium acetate, potassium chloride, procainamide, prochlorperazine, promethazine, propranolol, protamine, pyridoxine, remifentanil, rocuronium, sodium acetate, sodium bicarbonate, succinylcholine, sufentanil, tacrolimus, telavancin, theophylline, thiamine, thiotepa, tigecycline, tirofiban, tobramycin, topotecan, vancomycin, vasopressin, vecuronium, verapamil, vinblastine, vincristine, vinorelbine, voriconazole, zidovudine, zoledronic acid.
- **Y-Site Incompatibility:** acyclovir, amphotericin B deoxycholate, amphotericin B lipid complex, azathioprine, dantrolene, diazepam, ganciclovir, indomethacin, insulin regular, minocycline, mitomycin, pentamidine, phenytoin, thiopental, trimethoprim/sulfamethoxazole.
- **Anesthesia:** Phenylephrine 2–5 mg may be added to spinal anesthetic solution to prolong anesthesia.
- Phenylephrine 1 mg may be added to each 20 mL of local anesthetic to produce vasoconstriction.

Patient/Family Teaching
- Explain purpose of phenylephrine to patient.
- **IV:** Instruct patient to report headache, dizziness, dyspnea, or pain at IV infusion site promptly.
- Rep: Advise females of reproductive potential to notify health care professional if pregnancy is planned or suspected or if breastfeeding.

Evaluation/Desired Outcomes
- Increase in BP to normal range.
- Prolonged duration of spinal anesthesia.
- Localization of regional anesthesia.

ⅩⅩ phenytoin (fen-i-toyn)
Dilantin, Phenytek, ✤Tremytoine
Classification
Therapeutic: antiarrhythmics (group IB), anticonvulsants
Pharmacologic: hydantoins

Indications
Treatment/prevention of tonic-clonic (grand mal) seizures and complex partial seizures. **Unlabeled Use:** As an antiarrhythmic, particularly for ventricular arrhythmias associated with digoxin toxicity, prolonged QT interval, and surgical repair of congenital heart diseases in children. Management of neuropathic pain, including trigeminal neuralgia.

Action
Limits seizure propagation by altering ion transport. May also decrease synaptic transmission. Antiarrhythmic properties as a result of shortening the action potential and decreasing automaticity. **Therapeutic Effects:** Diminished seizure activity. Termination of ventricular arrhythmias.

Pharmacokinetics
Absorption: Absorbed slowly from the GI tract. Bioavailability differs among products; the Dilantin and Phenytek preparations are considered to be "extended" products. Other products are considered to be prompt release.
Distribution: Distributes into CSF and other body tissues and fluids. Enters breast milk; crosses the pla-

centa, achieving similar maternal/fetal levels. Preferentially distributes into fatty tissue.

Protein Binding: Adults 90–95%; ↓ protein binding in neonates (up to 20% free fraction available), infants (up to 15% free), and patients with hyperbilirubinemia, hypoalbuminemia, severe renal dysfunction or uremia.

Metabolism and Excretion: Mostly metabolized by the liver via the CYP2C9 isoenzyme, and to a lesser extent by the CYP2C19 isoenzyme; 爻 the CYP2C9 isoenzyme exhibits genetic polymorphism (intermediate or poor metabolizers may have significantly ↑ phenytoin concentrations and an ↑ risk of adverse reactions); minimal amounts excreted in the urine.

Half-life: 22 hr (range 7–42 hr).

TIME/ACTION PROFILE (anticonvulsant effect)

ROUTE	ONSET	PEAK	DURATION
PO	2–24 hr (1 wk)*	1.5–3 hr	6–12 hr
PO-ER	2–24 hr (1 wk)	4–12 hr	12–36 hr
IV	0.5–1 hr (1 wk)	rapid	12–24 hr

*() = time required for onset of action without a loading dose.

Contraindications/Precautions

Contraindicated in: Hypersensitivity; Hypersensitivity to propylene glycol (phenytoin injection only); History of hepatotoxicity related to phenytoin; Alcohol intolerance (phenytoin injection and liquid only); Sinus bradycardia, sinoatrial block, 2nd- or 3rd-degree heart block, or Stokes-Adams syndrome (phenytoin injection only); OB: Pregnancy (↑ risk of congenital anomalies; ↑ risk of hemorrhage in newborn if used at term).

Use Cautiously in: All patients (may ↑ risk of suicidal thoughts/behaviors); Hepatic or renal disease (↑ risk of adverse reactions; dose reduction recommended for hepatic impairment); Severe cardiac or respiratory disease (use of IV phenytoin may result in an ↑ risk of serious adverse reactions); Cardiac disease (↑ risk of cardiac arrest or bradycardia); 爻 CYP2C9 intermediate or poor metabolizers (↑ risk of phenytoin toxicity); Lactation: Use while breastfeeding only if potential maternal benefit justifies potential harm to infant; Pedi: Suspension contains sodium benzoate, a metabolite of benzyl alcohol that can cause potentially fatal gasping syndrome in neonates; Geri: Use of IV phenytoin may result in an ↑ risk of serious adverse reactions in older adults.

Exercise Extreme Caution in: 爻 Patients positive for human leukocyte antigen (HLA) allele, HLA-B*1502 allele or carriers of CYP2C9*3 variant (unless benefits clearly outweigh the risks) (↑ risk of serious skin reactions).

Adverse Reactions/Side Effects

CV: hypotension (↑ with IV phenytoin), bradycardia, CARDIAC ARREST, tachycardia. **Derm:** hypertrichosis, rash, ACUTE GENERALIZED EXANTHEMATOUS PUSTULOSIS, DRUG REACTION WITH EOSINOPHILIA AND SYSTEMIC SYMPTOMS (DRESS), exfoliative dermatitis, pruritus, purple glove syndrome, STEVENS-JOHNSON SYNDROME (SJS), TOXIC EPIDERMAL NECROLYSIS (TEN). **EENT:** diplopia, nystagmus. **GI:** gingival hyperplasia, nausea, constipation, drug-induced hepatitis, HEPATIC FAILURE, vomiting. **Hemat:** AGRANULOCYTOSIS, APLASTIC ANEMIA, leukopenia, lymphadenopathy, megaloblastic anemia, pure red cell aplasia, thrombocytopenia. **MS:** osteomalacia, osteoporosis. **Neuro:** ataxia, agitation, confusion, dizziness, drowsiness, dysarthria, dyskinesia, extrapyramidal syndrome, headache, insomnia, SUICIDAL THOUGHTS, vertigo, weakness.. **Misc:** ANGIOEDEMA, fever.

Interactions

Drug-Drug: Acute ingestion of **alcohol, amiodarone, benzodiazepines, capecitabine, chloramphenicol, chlordiazepoxide, cimetidine, disulfiram, estrogens, ethosuximide, felbamate, fluconazole, fluorouracil, fluoxetine, fluvastatin, fluvoxamine, halothane, isoniazid, itraconazole, ketoconazole, methylphenidate, miconazole, oxcarbazepine, omeprazole, phenothiazines, salicylates, sertraline, sulfonamides, trazodone, voriconazole,** and **warfarin** may ↑ levels. Chronic ingestion of **alcohol, barbiturates, carbamazepine, diazepam, diazoxide, fosamprenavir, nelfinavir, rifampin, ritonavir, sucralfate, theophylline,** and **vigabatrin** may ↓ levels. May ↓ the effects of **albendazole, amiodarone, apixaban, atorvastatin, benzodiazepines, carbamazepine, clozapine, cyclosporine, dabigatran, digoxin, edoxaban, efavirenz, estrogens, felbamate, fluvastatin, lacosamide, lamotrigine, lopinavir/ritonavir, methadone, mexiletine, nelfinavir, nifedipine, nimodipine, nisoldipine, oxcarbazepine, oral contraceptives, quetiapine, quinidine, rifampin, ritonavir, rivaroxaban, simvastatin, tacrolimus, theophylline, ticagrelor, topiramate, verapamil,** and **warfarin.** IV phenytoin and **dopamine** may cause additive hypotension. Additive CNS depression with other **CNS depressants,** including **alcohol, antihistamines, antidepressants, opioids,** and **sedative/hypnotics. Antacids** may ↓ absorption of orally administered phenytoin. ↑ systemic clearance of **methotrexate,** which has been associated with a worse event free survival; phenytoin use is not recommended in children undergoing chemotherapy for acute lymphocytic leukemia. May ↑ risk of hyperammonemia when used with **valproate.**

Drug-Natural Products: St. John's wort may ↓ levels.

Drug-Food: Phenytoin may ↓ absorption of **folic acid.** Concurrent administration of **enteral tube**

feedings may ↓ phenytoin absorption. **Folic acid** may ↓ levels.

Route/Dosage

IM administration is not recommended due to erratic absorption and pain on injection. Oral route should be used whenever possible.

Anticonvulsant

PO (Adults): Loading dose of 15–20 mg/kg as extended capsules in 3 divided doses given every 2–4 hr; maintenance dose 5–6 mg/kg/day given in 1–3 divided doses; usual dosing range = 200–1200 mg/day.
PO (Children 10–16 yr): 6–7 mg/kg/day in 2–3 divided doses.
PO (Children 7–9 yr): 7–8 mg/kg/day in 2–3 divided doses.
PO (Children 4–6 yr): 7.5–9 mg/kg/day in 2–3 divided doses.
PO (Children 0.5–3 yr): 8–10 mg/kg/day in 2–3 divided doses.
PO (Neonates up to 6 mo): 5–8 mg/kg/day in 2 divided doses, may require every 8 hr dosing.
IV (Adults): *Status epilepticus loading dose:* 15–20 mg/kg. Rate not to exceed 25–50 mg/min. *Maintenance dose:* same as PO dosing above.
IV (Children): *Status epilepticus loading dose:* 15–20 mg/kg at 1–3 mg/kg/min. *Maintenance dose:* same as PO dosing above.

Antiarrhythmic

IV (Adults): 50–100 mg every 10–15 min until arrhythmia is abolished, or a total of 15 mg/kg has been given, or toxicity occurs.
PO (Adults): Loading dose: 250 mg 4 times daily for 1 day, then 250 mg twice daily for 2 days, then maintenance at 300–400 mg/day in divided doses 1–4 times/day.
IV (Children): 1.25 mg/kg every 5 min, may repeat up to total loading dose of 15 mg/kg. *Maintenance dose:* 5–10 mg/kg/day in 2–3 divided doses IV or PO.

Availability (generic available)

Capsules: 30 mg, 100 mg, 200 mg, 300 mg. **Chewable tablets:** 50 mg. **Oral suspension:** ✹30 mg/5 mL, 100 mg/4 mL, 125 mg/5 mL. **Solution for injection:** 50 mg/mL.

NURSING IMPLICATIONS

Assessment

- Assess mental status (orientation, mood, behavior) before and periodically during therapy. Monitor closely for notable changes in behavior that could indicate the emergence or worsening of suicidal thoughts or behavior or depression.
- Assess oral hygiene. Vigorous cleaning beginning within 10 days of initiation of phenytoin therapy may help control gingival hyperplasia.
- Assess patient for phenytoin hypersensitivity syndrome (fever, skin rash, lymphadenopathy, angioedema). Rash usually occurs within the first 2 wk of

therapy. Hypersensitivity syndrome usually occurs at 3–8 wk but may occur up to 12 wk after initiation of therapy. May lead to renal failure, rhabdomyolysis, or hepatic necrosis; may be fatal.

- Observe patient for development of rash. Discontinue phenytoin at the first sign of skin reactions. Serious adverse reactions such as exfoliative, purpuric, or bullous rashes or the development of lupus erythematosus, SJS, or TEN preclude further use of phenytoin or fosphenytoin. ▓ SJS and TEN are significantly more common in patients with a particular HLA allele, HLA-B*1502 (occurs almost exclusively in patients with Asian ancestry, including Han Chinese, Filipinos, Malaysians, South Asian Indians, and Thais). Avoid using phenytoin or fosphenytoin as alternatives to carbamazepine for patients who test positive. If less serious skin eruptions (measles-like or scarlatiniform) occur, phenytoin may be resumed after complete clearing of the rash. If rash reappears, further use of fosphenytoin or phenytoin should be avoided.
- Monitor for signs and symptoms of DRESS (fever, rash, lymphadenopathy, and/or facial swelling), associated with involvement of other organ systems (hepatitis, nephritis, hematologic abnormalities, myocarditis, myositis) during therapy. May resemble an acute viral infection. Eosinophilia is often present. Discontinue therapy if signs occur.
- **Seizures:** Assess location, duration, frequency, and characteristics of seizure activity. EEG may be monitored periodically during therapy.
- Monitor BP, ECG, and respiratory function continuously during administration of IV phenytoin and throughout period when peak serum phenytoin levels occur (15–30 min after administration).
- **Arrhythmias:** Monitor ECG continuously during treatment of arrhythmias.

Lab Test Considerations

- Monitor CBC, serum calcium, albumin, and hepatic function tests prior to and monthly for the first several mo, then periodically during therapy.
- May cause ↑ serum alkaline phosphatase, GGT, and glucose levels.
- Monitor serum folate concentrations periodically during prolonged therapy.

Toxicity and Overdose

- Monitor serum phenytoin levels routinely. Therapeutic blood levels are 10–20 mcg/mL (8–15 mcg/mL in neonates) in patients with normal serum albumin and renal function. In patients with altered protein binding (neonates, patients with renal failure, hypoalbuminemia, acute trauma), free phenytoin serum concentrations should be monitored. Therapeutic serum free phenytoin levels are 1–2 mcg/mL.
- Progressive signs and symptoms of phenytoin toxicity include nystagmus, ataxia, confusion, nausea, slurred speech, and dizziness.

Implementation

- Implement seizure precautions.
- When transferring from phenytoin to another anti-convulsant, dose adjustments are made gradually over several wk.
- When substituting *fosphenytoin* for oral *phenytoin* therapy, the same total daily dose may be given as a single dose. Unlike parenteral phenytoin, fospheny-toin may be given safely by the IM route.
- **PO:** Administer with or immediately after meals to minimize GI irritation. Shake liquid preparations well before pouring. Use a calibrated measuring device for accurate dose. Chewable tablets must be crushed or chewed well before swallowing. Capsules may be opened and mixed with food or fluids for patients with difficulty swallowing. To prevent direct contact of alkaline drug with mucosa, have patient swallow a liquid first, follow with mixture of medication, then follow with a full glass of water or milk or with food.
- If patient is receiving enteral tube feedings, 2 hr should elapse between feeding and phenytoin administration. If phenytoin is administered via naso-gastric tube, flush tube with 2–4 oz water before and after administration.
- Do not interchange chewable phenytoin tablets with phenytoin sodium capsules; they are not bioequiva-lent.
- Capsules labeled "extended" may be used for once-a-day dose; those labeled "prompt" may result in toxic serum levels if used for once-a-day dose.

IV Administration

- **IV:** Slight yellow color will not alter solution potency. If refrigerated, may form precipitate, which dissolves after warming to room temperature. Discard solution that is not clear.
- To prevent precipitation and minimize local venous irritation, follow infusion with 0.9% NaCl through the same needle or catheter. Avoid extravasation; phenytoin is caustic to tissues; may lead to purple glove syndrome. Monitor infusion site closely.
- **IV Push:** Administer undiluted. *Rate:* Administer at a rate not to exceed 50 mg over 1 min in adults or 1–3 mg/kg/min in neonates. Rapid administration may result in severe hypotension, cardiovascular collapse, or CNS depression.
- **Intermittent Infusion:** *Dilution:* Administer by mixing with no more than 50 mL of 0.9% NaCl. *Concentration:* 1–10 mg/mL. Administer immediately following admixture. Use tubing with a 0.45- to 0.22-micron in-line filter. *Rate:* Complete infusion within 1 hr at a rate not to exceed 50 mg/min. In patients who may develop hypotension, patients with cardiovascular disease, or geriatric patients maximum rate of 25 mg/min [may be as low as 5–10 mg/min]. Maximum rate in neonates is 1–3 mg/kg/min. Monitor cardiac function and BP throughout infusion.

- **Y-Site Compatibility:** cisplatin.
- **Y-Site Incompatibility:** acetaminophen, acyclovir, alemtuzumab, amikacin, aminocaproic acid, aminophylline, amiodarone, amphotericin B deoxycholate, amphotericin B lipid complex, amphotericin B liposomal, ampicillin, ampicillin/sulbactam, anidulafungin, argatroban, arsenic trioxide, ascorbic acid, atropine, azathioprine, azithromycin, aztreonam, benztropine, bivalirudin, bleomycin, bumetanide, buprenorphine, butorphanol, calcium chloride, calcium gluconate, carboplatin, carmustine, caspofungin, cefazolin, cefepime, cefotaxime, cefotetan, cefoxitin, ceftazidime, ceftolozane/tazobactam, ceftriaxone, cefuroxime, chloramphenicol, chlorpromazine, ciprofloxacin, clindamycin, cyanocobalamin, cyclophosphamide, cyclosporine, cytarabine, dacarbazine, dactinomycin, dantrolene, daptomycin, daunorubicin hydrochloride, dexamethasone, dexmedetomidine, dexrazoxane, diazepam, digoxin, diltiazem, diphenhydramine, dobutamine, docetaxel, dopamine, doxorubicin hydrochloride, doxorubicin liposomal, doxycycline, enalaprilat, ephedrine, epinephrine, epirubicin, epoetin alfa, eptifibatide, ertapenem, erythromycin, etoposide, etoposide phosphate, fentanyl, fludarabine, fluorouracil, folic acid, fosphenytoin, furosemide, ganciclovir, gemcitabine, gemtuzumab ozogamicin, gentamicin, glycopyrrolate, granisetron, haloperidol, heparin, hetastarch, hydralazine, hydrocortisone, hydromorphone, hydroxyzine, idarubicin, ifosfamide, imipenem/cilastatin, indomethacin, insulin regular, irinotecan, isavuconazonium, isoproterenol, ketamine, ketorolac, labetalol, LR , leucovorin calcium, levofloxacin, lidocaine, linezolid, lorazepam, magnesium sulfate, mannitol, meperidine, meropenem, meropenem/vaborbactam, mesna, methadone, methotrexate, methylprednisolone, metoclopramide, metoprolol, metronidazole, micafungin, midazolam, milrinone, minocycline, mitoxantrone, morphine, moxifloxacin, multivitamins, mycophenolate, nafcillin, nalbuphine, naloxone, nicardipine, nitroglycerin, nitroprusside, norepinephrine, octreotide, ondansetron, oritavancin, oxacillin, oxytocin, paclitaxel, palonosetron, pamidronate, pantoprazole, papaverine, pemetrexed, penicillin G, pentamidine, pentobarbital, phenobarbital, phentolamine, phenylephrine, phytonadione, piperacillin/tazobactam, plazomicin, potassium acetate, potassium chloride, procainamide, prochlorperazine, promethazine, propofol, propranolol, protamine, pyridoxine, rocuronium, sodium acetate, sodium bicarbonate, succinylcholine, sufentanil, tacrolimus, tedizolid, theophylline, thiamine, thiotepa, tigecycline, tirofiban, tobramycin, topotecan, trimethoprim/sulfamethoxazole, vancomycin, vasopressin, vecuronium, verapamil, vinblastine, vincristine, vinorelbine, voriconazole, zoledronic acid.

P

- **Additive Incompatibility:** Do not admix with other solutions or medications, especially dextrose, because precipitation will occur.

Patient/Family Teaching

- Instruct patient to take phenytoin as directed, at the same time each day. If a dose is missed from a once-a-day schedule, take as soon as possible and return to regular dosing schedule. If taking several doses a day, take missed dose as soon as possible within 4 hr of next scheduled dose; do not double doses. Consult health care professional if doses are missed for 2 consecutive days. Abrupt withdrawal may lead to status epilepticus. Advise patient to read *Medication Guide* before starting therapy and with each Rx refill in case of changes.
- May cause drowsiness or dizziness. Caution patient to avoid driving or other activities requiring alertness until response to medication is known. Do not resume driving until health care professional gives clearance based on control of seizure disorder.
- Caution patient to avoid alcohol and CNS depressants. Advise patient to notify health care professional of all Rx or OTC medications, vitamins, or herbal products being taken and to consult with health care professional before taking other medications and alcohol.
- Instruct patient on importance of maintaining good dental hygiene and seeing dentist frequently for teeth cleaning to prevent tenderness, bleeding, and gingival hyperplasia. Starting oral hygiene program within 10 days of starting phenytoin therapy may minimize growth rate and severity of gingival enlargement. Patients under 23 yr of age and those taking doses >500 mg/day are at increased risk for gingival hyperplasia.
- Advise patient that brands of phenytoin may not be equivalent. Check with health care professional if brand or dose form is changed.
- Advise diabetic patients to monitor blood glucose carefully and to notify health care professional of significant changes.
- Instruct patient to notify health care professional of medication regimen prior to treatment or surgery.
- Advise patient not to take phenytoin within 2–3 hr of antacids.
- Advise patient to carry identification describing disease process and medication regimen at all times.
- Instruct patients that behavioral changes, skin rash, facial or perioral, swelling, shortness of breath, fever, sore throat, mouth ulcers, easy bruising, petechiae, unusual bleeding, abdominal pain, chills, pale stools, dark urine, jaundice, severe nausea or vomiting, drowsiness, slurred speech, unsteady gait, swollen glands, or persistent headache should be reported to health care professional immediately. Advise patient and family to notify health care professional if thoughts about suicide or dying, attempts to commit suicide; new or worse depression; new or worse anxiety; feeling very agitated or restless; panic attacks; trouble sleeping; new or worse irritability; acting aggressive; being angry or violent; acting on dangerous impulses; an extreme increase in activity and talking; other unusual changes in behavior or mood occur.
- Rep: May cause fetal harm. Advise female patients to use an additional nonhormonal method of contraception during therapy and until next menstrual period. Instruct patient to notify health care professional if pregnancy is planned or suspected. Encourage patients who become pregnant to enroll in the North American Antiepileptic Drug Pregnancy Registry that monitors pregnancy outcomes in women exposed to antiepileptic drugs, such as phenytoin, during pregnancy by calling 1-888-233-2334 or on the web at www.aedpregnancyregistry.org. Enrollment must be done by patients themselves. Monitor serum phenytoin concentrations periodically during pregnancy to determine need for dose adjustments. May cause depletion of vitamin K–dependent clotting factors in newborns. Administer vitamin K to mother before delivery and to neonate after birth to prevent bleeding related to decreased levels of vitamin K–dependent clotting factors which may occur in newborns exposed to phenytoin in utero.
- Emphasize the importance of routine exams to monitor progress. Patient should have routine physical exams, especially monitoring skin and lymph nodes, and EEG testing.

Evaluation/Desired Outcomes

- Decrease or cessation of seizures without excessive sedation.
- Suppression of arrhythmias.
- Relief of neuropathic pain.

phytonadione
(fye-toe-na-**dye**-one)
Classification
Therapeutic: antidotes, vitamins
Pharmacologic: fat-soluble vitamins

Indications

Prevention and treatment of hypoprothrombinemia, which may be associated with: Excessive doses of warfarin, Salicylates, Certain anti-infective agents, Nutritional deficiencies, Prolonged total parenteral nutrition. Prevention and treatment of vitamin K-deficiency bleeding in neonates.

Action

Acts as a vitamin K replacement. Required for hepatic synthesis of blood coagulation factors II (prothrombin), VII, IX, and X. **Therapeutic Effects:** Prevention of bleeding due to hypoprothrombinemia.

Pharmacokinetics

Absorption: Well absorbed following oral or SUBQ administration. Oral absorption requires presence of bile salts. Some vitamin K is produced by bacteria in the GI tract.

Distribution: Unknown.
Metabolism and Excretion: Rapidly metabolized by the liver.
Half-life: Unknown.

TIME/ACTION PROFILE

ROUTE	ONSET	PEAK†	DURATION‡
PO	6–12 hr	unknown	unknown
SUBQ	1–2 hr	3–6 hr	12–14 hr
IV	1–2 hr	3–6 hr	12 hr

†Control of hemorrhage.
‡Normal PT achieved.

Contraindications/Precautions

Contraindicated in: Hypersensitivity; Hypersensitivity or intolerance to benzyl alcohol (injection only).
Use Cautiously in: Hepatic impairment; Pedi: Use of injection formulations containing benzyl alcohol may lead to "gasping syndrome" in neonates and infants.
Exercise Extreme Caution in: Severe life-threatening reactions have occurred following IV administration, use other routes unless risk is justified.

Adverse Reactions/Side Effects

Derm: eczematous reactions, flushing, kernicterus, rash, scleroderma-like lesions, urticaria. **GI:** gastric upset, hyperbilirubinemia (large doses in very premature infants), unusual taste. **Hemat:** hemolytic anemia. **Local:** erythema, pain at injection site, swelling. **Misc:** HYPERSENSITIVITY REACTIONS.

Interactions

Drug-Drug: Large doses will counteract the effect of **warfarin**. Large doses of **salicylates** or broad-spectrum **anti-infectives** may ↑ vitamin K requirements. **Bile acid sequestrants**, **mineral oil**, and **sucralfate** may ↓ vitamin K absorption from the GI tract.

Route/Dosage

IV use of phytonadione should be reserved for patients with serious or life-threatening bleeding and elevated INR. Oral route is preferred in patients with elevated INRs and no serious or life-threatening bleeding. IM route should generally be avoided because of risk of hematoma formation.

Treatment of Hypoprothrombinemia due to Vitamin K Deficiency (from factors other than warfarin)

SUBQ, IV (Adults): 10 mg.
PO (Adults): 2.5–25 mg/day.
SUBQ, IV (Children >1 mo): 1–2 mg single dose.
PO (Children >1 mo): 2.5–5 mg/day.

Vitamin K Deficiency (Supratherapeutic INR) Secondary to Warfarin

PO (Adults): *INR ≥5 and <9 (no significant bleeding):* Hold warfarin and give 1–2.5 mg vitamin K; if more rapid reversal required, give ≤5 mg vitamin K;

INR >9 (no significant bleeding): Hold warfarin and give 2.5–5 mg vitamin K.
IV (Adults): *Elevated INR with serious or life-threatening bleeding:* 10 mg slow infusion.

Prevention of Hypoprothrombinemia during Total Parenteral Nutrition

IV (Adults): 5–10 mg once weekly.
IV (Children): 2–5 mg once weekly.

Prevention of Vitamin K-Deficiency Bleeding in Neonates

IM (Neonates): 0.5–1 mg, within 1 hr of birth, may repeat in 6–8 hr if needed. May be repeated in 2–3 wk if mother received previous anticonvulsant/anticoagulant/anti-infective/antitubercular therapy. 1–5 mg may be given IM to mother 12–24 hr before delivery.

Treatment of Vitamin K-Deficiency Bleeding in Neonates

IM, SUBQ (Neonates): 1–2 mg/day.

Availability (generic available)

Tablets: 5 mg. **Solution for injection:** 1 mg/0.5 mL, 10 mg/mL.

NURSING IMPLICATIONS

Assessment

- Monitor for frank and occult bleeding (guaiac stools, Hematest urine, and emesis). Monitor pulse and BP frequently; notify health care professional immediately if symptoms of internal bleeding or hypovolemic shock develop. Inform all personnel of patient's bleeding tendency to prevent further trauma. Apply pressure to all venipuncture sites for at least 5 min; avoid unnecessary IM injections.
- Pedi: Monitor for side effects and adverse reactions. Children may be especially sensitive to the effects and side effects of vitamin K. Neonates, especially premature neonates, may be more sensitive than older children.

Lab Test Considerations

- Monitor INR prior to and during vitamin K therapy to determine response to and need for further therapy.

Implementation

- The parenteral route is preferred for phytonadione therapy but, because of severe, potentially fatal hypersensitivity reactions, IV vitamin K is not recommended.
- Administration of whole blood or plasma may also be required in severe bleeding because of the delayed onset of this medication.
- Phytonadione is an antidote for warfarin overdose but does not counteract the anticoagulant activity of heparin.

IV Administration

- **Intermittent Infusion:** *Dilution:* Dilute in 0.9% NaCl, D5W, or D5/0.9% NaCl. *Rate:* Administer over 30–60 min. Rate should not exceed 1 mg/min.
- **Y-Site Compatibility:** amikacin, aminophylline, ascorbic acid, atracurium, atropine, azathioprine, aztreonam, benztropine, bumetanide, buprenorphine, butorphanol, calcium chloride, calcium gluconate, cefazolin, cefotaxime, cefotetan, cefoxitin, ceftazidime, ceftriaxone, cefuroxime, chloramphenicol, chlorpromazine, clindamycin, cyanocobalamin, cyclosporine, dexamethasone, digoxin, diphenhydramine, dopamine, doxycycline, enalaprilat, ephedrine, epinephrine, epoetin alfa, erythromycin, esmolol, famotidine, fentanyl, fluconazole, folic acid, furosemide, ganciclovir, gentamicin, glycopyrrolate, heparin, hydrocortisone, imipenem/cilastatin, indomethacin, insulin regular, isoproterenol, ketorolac, labetalol, LR, lidocaine, mannitol, meperidine, metoclopramide, metoprolol, metronidazole, midazolam, morphine, multivitamins, nafcillin, nalbuphine, naloxone, nitroglycerin, nitroprusside, norepinephrine, ondansetron, oxacillin, oxytocin, papaverine, penicillin G, pentamidine, pentobarbital, phenobarbital, phentolamine, phenylephrine, potassium chloride, procainamide, prochlorperazine, propranolol, pyridoxine, sodium bicarbonate, succinylcholine, sufentanil, theophylline, thiamine, tobramycin, vancomycin, vasopressin, verapamil.
- **Y-Site Incompatibility:** dantrolene, diazepam, magnesium sulfate, minocycline, phenytoin, trimethoprim/sulfamethoxazole.

Patient/Family Teaching

- Instruct patient to take phytonadione as directed. Take missed doses as soon as remembered unless almost time for next dose. Notify health care professional of missed doses.
- Cooking does not destroy substantial amounts of vitamin K. Patient should not drastically alter diet while taking vitamin K. See Appendix J for foods high in vitamin K.
- Caution patient to avoid IM injections and activities leading to injury. Use a soft toothbrush, do not floss, and shave with an electric razor until coagulation defect is corrected.
- Advise patient to report any symptoms of unusual bleeding or bruising (bleeding gums; nosebleed; black, tarry stools; hematuria; excessive menstrual flow).
- Advise patient to notify health care professional of all Rx or OTC medications, vitamins, or herbal products being taken and to consult with health care professional before taking other medications and alcohol.
- Advise patient to inform health care professional of medication regimen prior to treatment or surgery.
- Rep: Advise females of reproductive potential to notify health care professional if pregnancy is planned or suspected or if breastfeeding.

- Advise patient to carry identification at all times describing disease process.
- Emphasize the importance of frequent lab tests to monitor coagulation factors.

Evaluation/Desired Outcomes

- Prevention of spontaneous bleeding or cessation of bleeding in patients with hypoprothrombinemia secondary to impaired intestinal absorption or oral anticoagulant, salicylate, or anti-infective therapy.
- Prevention of hemorrhagic disease in the newborn.

BEERS

pimavanserin (pim-a-**van**-ser-in)
Nuplazid
Classification
Therapeutic: antipsychotics

Indications
Hallucinations and delusions associated with Parkinson's disease psychosis.

Action
Exact mechanism is unknown. May work by acting as an inverse agonist and antagonist primarily at 5-HT$_{2A}$ receptors and less at 5−HT$_{2C}$ receptors. **Therapeutic Effects:** Reduced frequency and/or severity of hallucinations and delusions in patients with Parkinson's disease psychosis.

Pharmacokinetics
Absorption: Unknown.
Distribution: Extensively distributed to tissues.
Protein Binding: 95%.
Metabolism and Excretion: Mostly metabolized by the liver (CYP3A4 and CYP3A5 isoenzymes) to an active metabolite. Primarily excreted in feces.
Half-life: 57 hr (pimavanserin); 200 hr (active metabolite).

TIME/ACTION PROFILE (plasma concentrations)

ROUTE	ONSET	PEAK	DURATION
PO	unknown	6 hr	unknown

Contraindications/Precautions
Contraindicated in: Hypersensitivity; QT interval prolongation; Concurrent use of agents that prolong the QT interval, including sotalol, quinidine, disopyramide, procainamide, amiodarone, thioridazine, chlorpromazine, moxifloxacin, and ziprasidone (↑ risk of serious arrhythmias); History of arrhythmias, including bradycardia; Hypokalemia or hypomagnesemia (↑ risk of serious arrhythmias); Congenital long QT syndrome (↑ risk of serious arrhythmias); Severe renal impairment (CCr <30 mL/min).
Use Cautiously in: OB: Safety not established in pregnancy; Lactation: Safety not established in breastfeeding; Pedi: Safety and effectiveness not established in

children; Geri: Appears on Beers list. ↑ risk of stroke, cognitive decline, and mortality in older adults with dementia. Avoid use in older adults, except for psychosis in Parkinson's disease.

Adverse Reactions/Side Effects
CV: peripheral edema, QT interval prolongation, TORSADES DE POINTES. **GI:** constipation, nausea. **Neuro:** confusion, gait disturbance, hallucinations. **Misc:** HYPERSENSITIVITY REACTIONS (including angioedema).

Interactions
Drug-Drug: Concurrent use of **amiodarone, sotalol, quinidine, disopyramide, procainamide, thioridazine, chlorpromazine, moxifloxacin,** and **ziprasidone** ↑ the risk of serious ventricular arrhythmias and should be avoided. **Strong CYP3A4 inhibitors,** including **clarithromycin, itraconazole,** and **ketoconazole,** may ↑ levels; ↓ dose of pimavanserin. **Strong CYP3A4 inducers,** including **carbamazepine, phenytoin,** and **rifampin** as well as **moderate CYP3A4 inducers,** including **efavirenz, modafinil, nafcillin,** and **thioridazine** may ↓ levels; avoid concurrent use.

Drug-Natural Products: St. John's wort may ↓ levels; avoid concurrent use.

Route/Dosage
PO (Adults): 34 mg once daily. *Concurrent use of strong CYP3A4 inhibitors:* 10 mg once daily.

Availability (generic available)
Capsules: 34 mg. **Tablets:** 10 mg.

NURSING IMPLICATIONS
Assessment
- Assess mental status (orientation, mood, behavior) before and periodically during therapy.

Implementation
- **PO:** Administer 2 tablets once daily without regard to food.
- Capsules can be taken whole, or opened and entire contents sprinkled over a tablespoon (15 mL) of applesauce, yogurt, pudding, or a liquid nutritional supplement. Consume immediately without chewing; do not store for future use.

Patient/Family Teaching
- Instruct patient to take pimavanserin as directed.
- Instruct patient to notify health care professional of all Rx or OTC medications, vitamins, or herbal products being taken and consult health care professional before taking any new medications, especially St. John's wort.
- Rep: Advise females of reproductive potential to notify health care professional if pregnancy is planned or suspected or if breastfeeding.

Evaluation/Desired Outcomes
- Reduced frequency and/or severity of hallucinations and delusions in patients with Parkinson's disease psychosis.

pimecrolimus
(pi-me-**cro**-li-mus)
Elidel
Classification
Therapeutic: immunosuppressants (topical)

Indications
Short-term and intermittent long-term management of mild to moderate atopic dermatitis unresponsive to or in patients intolerant of conventional treatment.

Action
Inhibits T-cell and mast cell activation by interfering with production of inflammatory cytokines. **Therapeutic Effects:** Decreased severity of atopic dermatitis.

Pharmacokinetics
Absorption: Minimally absorbed through intact skin.
Distribution: Local distribution after topical administration.
Metabolism and Excretion: Systemic metabolism and excretion are negligible with local application.
Half-life: Not applicable.

TIME/ACTION PROFILE (improvement in symptoms)

ROUTE	ONSET	PEAK	DURATION
topical	within 6 days	unknown	unknown

Contraindications/Precautions
Contraindicated in: Hypersensitivity; Should not be applied to areas of active cutaneous viral infections (↑ risk of dissemination); Concurrent use of occlusive dressings; Netherton's syndrome (↑ absorption of pimecrolimus); Lactation: Lactation.
Use Cautiously in: Clinical infection at treatment site (infection should be treated/cleared prior to use); Skin papillomas (warts); allow treatment/resolution prior to use; Natural/artificial sunlight (minimize exposure); OB: Use during pregnancy only if potential maternal benefit justifies potential fetal risk; Pedi: Children <2 yr (safety and effectiveness not established).

Adverse Reactions/Side Effects
Local: burning. **Misc:** ↑ risk of lymphoma/skin cancer.

Interactions
Drug-Drug: None reported.

Route/Dosage
Topical (Adults and Children ≥2 yr): Apply thin film twice daily; rub in gently and completely.

✦= Canadian drug name. 🔒 = Genetic implication. ~~Strikethrough~~ = Discontinued. CAPITALS = life-threatening. <u>Underline</u> = most frequent.

Availability (generic available)
Cream: 1%.

NURSING IMPLICATIONS

Assessment
● Assess skin lesions prior to and periodically during therapy. Discontinue therapy after signs and symptoms of atopic dermatitis have resolved. Resume treatment at the first signs and symptoms of recurrence.

Implementation
● **Topical:** Apply a thin layer to affected area twice daily and rub in gently and completely. May be used on all skin areas including head, neck, and intertriginous areas. Do not use with occlusive dressings.

Patient/Family Teaching
● Instruct patient on correct technique for application. Apply only as directed to external areas. Wash hands following application, unless hands are areas of application. Advise patient to read *Medication Guide* before starting and with each Rx refill in case of changes.
● Caution patient to avoid exposure to natural or artificial sunlight, including tanning beds, while using cream.
● Advise patient that pimecrolimus may cause skin burning. This occurs most commonly during 1st few days of application, is of mild to moderate severity, and improves within 5 days or as atopic dermatitis resolves.
● Rep: Advise females of reproductive potential to notify health care professional if pregnancy is planned or suspected or if breastfeeding.
● Advise patient to notify health care provider if no improvement is seen following 6 wk of treatment or at any time if condition worsens.

Evaluation/Desired Outcomes
● Resolution of signs and symptoms of atopic dermatitis.

---

piperacillin/tazobactam
(pi-**per**-a-sill-in/tay-zoe-**bak**-tam)
Zosyn
Classification
Therapeutic: anti-infectives
Pharmacologic: extended spectrum penicillins

Indications
Appendicitis and peritonitis. Skin and skin structure infections. Gynecologic infections. Community-acquired and nosocomial pneumonia.

Action
Piperacillin: Binds to bacterial cell wall membrane, causing cell death. Spectrum is extended compared with other penicillins. **Tazobactam:** Inhibits beta-lactamase, an enzyme that can destroy penicillins. **Therapeutic Effects:** Death of susceptible bacteria. **Spectrum:** Active against piperacillin-resistant, beta-lactamase–producing: *Bacteroides fragilis, E. coli, Acinetobacter baumanii, Klebsiella pneumoniae, Pseudomonas aeruginosa, Staphylococcus aureus, Haemophilus influenzae.*

Pharmacokinetics
Absorption: IV administration results in complete bioavailability.
Distribution: Widely distributed. Enters CSF well only when meninges are inflamed.
Metabolism and Excretion: Piperacillin (68%) and tazobactam (80%) are mostly excreted unchanged by the kidneys.
Half-life: *Adults:* 0.7–1.2 hr; *Children (6 mo–12 yr):* 0.7–0.9 hr; *Infants (2–5 mo):* 1.4 hr.

TIME/ACTION PROFILE (piperacillin plasma concentrations)

ROUTE	ONSET	PEAK	DURATION
IV	rapid	end of infusion	4–6 hr

Contraindications/Precautions
Contraindicated in: Hypersensitivity to penicillins, beta-lactams, cephalosporins, or tazobactam (cross-sensitivity may occur).
Use Cautiously in: Renal impairment (↑ risk of seizures) (dosage ↓ or increased interval recommended if CCr <40 mL/min); Seizure disorders; Sodium restriction; Critically ill patients (↑ risk of renal failure; use alternative antibiotic, if possible); OB: Safety not established in pregnancy; Lactation: Safety not established in breastfeeding; Pedi: Children <2 mo (safety and effectiveness not established).

Adverse Reactions/Side Effects
Derm: rash (↑ in patients with cystic fibrosis), ACUTE GENERALIZED EXANTHEMATOUS PUSTULOSIS, DRUG REACTION WITH EOSINOPHILIA AND SYSTEMIC SYMPTOMS (DRESS), STEVENS-JOHNSON SYNDROME, TOXIC EPIDERMAL NECROLYSIS, urticaria. **GI:** diarrhea, CLOSTRIDIOIDES DIFFICILE-ASSOCIATED DIARRHEA (CDAD), constipation, drug-induced hepatitis, nausea, vomiting. **GU:** interstitial nephritis, renal failure. **Hemat:** bleeding, leukopenia, neutropenia, thrombocytopenia. **Local:** pain, phlebitis at IV site. **Neuro:** confusion, dizziness, headache, insomnia, lethargy, SEIZURES (higher doses). **Misc:** fever (↑ in cystic fibrosis patients), hemophagocytic lymphohistiocytosis, HYPERSENSITIVITY REACTIONS (including anaphylaxis and serum sickness), superinfection.

Interactions
Drug-Drug: Probenecid ↓ renal excretion and ↑ blood levels. May alter excretion of **lithium. Potassium-losing diuretics, corticosteroids,** or **amphotericin B** may ↑ risk of hypokalemia. ↑ risk of hepatotoxicity with other **hepatotoxic agents.** May ↓ levels/

effects of **aminoglycosides** in patients with renal impairment. May ↑ levels and risk of toxicity from **methotrexate**. ↑ risk of acute kidney injury when concomitantly administered with **vancomycin**. May prolong the neuromuscular blockade associated with **vecuronium**.

Route/Dosage

Contains 2.84 mEq (65 mg) sodium/g of piperacillin; adult doses below expressed as combined piperacillin/tazobactam content.

Appendicitis/Peritonitis

IV (Adults and Children ≥2 mo and >40 kg): 3.375 g every 6 hr.
IV (Children ≥9 mo and ≤40 kg and normal renal function): 112.5 mg (100 mg piperacillin/12.5 mg tazobactam)/kg every 8 hr.
IV (Infants 2–9 mo and ≤40 kg and normal renal function): 90 mg (80 mg piperacillin/10 mg tazobactam)/kg every 8 hr.

Renal Impairment

IV (Adults): *CCr 20–40 mL/min:* 2.25 g every 6 hr; *CCr <20 mL/min:* 2.25 g every 8 hr; *Hemodialysis:* 2.25 g every 12 hr + 0.75 g following hemodialysis on hemodialysis days; *Continuous ambulatory peritoneal dialysis:* 2.25 g every 12 hr.

Nosocomial Pneumonia

IV (Adults and Children ≥2 mo and >40 kg): 4.5 g every 6 hr.
IV (Children ≥9 mo and ≤40 kg and normal renal function): 112.5 mg (100 mg piperacillin/12.5 mg tazobactam)/kg every 6 hr.
IV (Infants 2–9 mo and ≤40 kg and normal renal function): 90 mg (80 mg piperacillin/10 mg tazobactam)/kg every 6 hr.

Renal Impairment

IV (Adults): *CCr 20–40 mL/min:* 3.375 g every 6 hr; *CCr <20 mL/min:* 2.25 g every 6 hr; *Hemodialysis:* 2.25 g every 8 hr + 0.75 g following hemodialysis on hemodialysis days; *Continuous ambulatory peritoneal dialysis:* 2.25 g every 8 hr.

Skin and Skin Structure Infections, Gynecologic Infections, and Community-Acquired Pneumonia

IV (Adults): 3.375 g every 6 hr.

Renal Impairment

IV (Adults): *CCr 20–40 mL/min:* 2.25 g every 6 hr; *CCr <20 mL/min:* 2.25 g every 8 hr; *Hemodialysis:* 2.25 g every 12 hr + 0.75 g following hemodialysis on hemodialysis days; *Continuous ambulatory peritoneal dialysis:* 2.25 g every 12 hr.

Availability (generic available)

Powder for injection: 2.25 g (2 g piperacillin/0.25 g tazobactam)/vial, 3.375 g (3 g piperacillin/0.375 g tazobactam)/vial, 4.5 g (4 g piperacillin/0.5 g tazobac-

tam)/vial, 13.5 g (12 g piperacillin/1.5 g tazobactam)/vial, 40.5 g (36 g piperacillin/4.5 g tazobactam)/vial.
Premixed infusion: 2.25 g (2 g piperacillin/0.25 g tazobactam) in 50 mL, 3.375 g (3 g piperacillin/0.375 g tazobactam) in 50 mL, 4.5 g (4 g piperacillin/0.5 g tazobactam) in 100 mL.

NURSING IMPLICATIONS

Assessment

- Assess patient for infection (vital signs; appearance of wound, sputum, urine, and stool; WBC) at beginning of and during therapy.
- Obtain a history before initiating therapy to determine previous use of and reactions to penicillins or cephalosporins. Persons with a negative history of penicillin sensitivity may still have an allergic response.
- Obtain specimens for culture and sensitivity prior to initiating therapy. 1st dose may be given before receiving results.
- Observe patient for signs and symptoms of anaphylaxis (rash, pruritus, laryngeal edema, wheezing). Discontinue the drug and notify health care professional immediately if these occur. Keep epinephrine, an antihistamine, and resuscitation equipment close by in the event of an anaphylactic reaction.
- Monitor bowel function. Diarrhea, abdominal cramping, fever, and bloody stools should be reported to health care professional promptly as a sign of CDAD. May begin up to several wk following cessation of therapy.
- Assess for skin reactions (rash, fever, edema, mucosal erosions or ulcerations, red or inflamed eyes). Monitor patient with mild to moderate rash for progression. If rash becomes severe or systemic symptoms occur, discontinue piperacillin/tazobactam.
- Monitor for signs and symptoms of DRESS (fever, rash, lymphadenopathy, and/or facial swelling), associated with involvement of other organ systems (hepatitis, nephritis, hematologic abnormalities, myocarditis, myositis) during therapy. May resemble an acute viral infection. Eosinophilia is often present. Discontinue therapy if signs occur.
- Monitor for signs and symptoms of hemophagocytic lymphohistiocytosis (fever, rash, lymphadenopathy, hepatosplenomegaly, cytopenia); if these occur suspected, discontinue piperacillin/tazobactam immediately and treat as needed.

Lab Test Considerations

- Evaluate renal and hepatic function, CBC, serum potassium, and bleeding times prior to and routinely during therapy.
- May cause positive direct Coombs' test result.
- May cause ↑ BUN, serum creatinine, AST, ALT, serum bilirubin, alkaline phosphatase, and LDH.
- May cause leukopenia and neutropenia, especially with prolonged therapy or hepatic impairment.

P

- May cause prolonged prothrombin and partial thromboplastin time.
- May cause ↓ hemoglobin and hematocrit and thrombocytopenia, eosinophilia, leukopenia, and neutropenia. It also may cause proteinuria; hematuria; pyuria; hyperglycemia; ↓ total protein or albumin; and abnormalities in sodium, potassium, and calcium concentrations.

Implementation

IV Administration

- If a dose of piperacillin/tazobactam is required that does not equal 2.25 g, 3.375 g, or 4.5 g, premixed infusion should not be used.
- **Intermittent Infusion:** For patients weighing >40 kg: **Reconstitution:** Reconstitute 2.25 g, 3.375 g, and 4.5 g single-dose vials with 10 mL, 15 mL, and 20 mL, respectively of 0.9% NaCl, Sterile Water for Injection, or D5W. Swirl until dissolved. **Concentration:** 202.5 mg/mL (180 mg/mL of piperacillin and 22.5 mg/mL of tazobactam). **Dilution:** Dilute further in 50–150 mL of 0.9% NaCl, D5W, D6/0.9% NaCl, or LR. For patients weighing up to 40 kg: dilute to a concentration of 20 mg/mL to 80 mg/mL. Reconstituted vials stable for 24 hr at room temperature or 48 hr if refrigerated. Infusion stable for 24 hr at room temperature or 7 days if refrigerated. Premixed bags are stable for 24 hr at room temperature of 14 days if refrigerated. **Rate:** Infuse over 30 min.
- **Y-Site Compatibility:** acetaminophen, allopurinol, amifostine, aminocaproic acid, aminophylline, amphotericin B lipid complex, amphotericin B liposomal, anidulafungin, argatroban, arsenic trioxide, aztreonam, bivalirudin, bleomycin, bumetanide, buprenorphine, busulfan, butorphanol, calcium chloride, calcium gluconate, cangrelor, carboplatin, carmustine, cefepime, ceftolozane/tazobactam, chloramphenicol, clindamycin, cyclophosphamide, cyclosporine, cytarabine, dactinomycin, daptomycin, dexamethasone, dexmedetomidine, dexrazoxane, diazepam, digoxin, diphenhydramine, docetaxel, dopamine, enalaprilat, ephedrine, epinephrine, eptifibatide, eravacycline, erythromycin, esmolol, etoposide, etoposide phosphate, fentanyl, floxuridine, fluconazole, fludarabine, fluorouracil, foscarnet, fosphenytoin, furosemide, granisetron, heparin, hetastarch, hydrocortisone, hydromorphone, ifosfamide, isoproterenol, ketamine, ketorolac, leucovorin calcium, lidocaine, linezolid, lorazepam, magnesium sulfate, mannitol, melphalan, meperidine, meropenem/vaborbactam, mesna, methotrexate, methylprednisolone, metoclopramide, metoprolol, metronidazole, milrinone, morphine, naloxone, nitroglycerin, nitroprusside, norepinephrine, octreotide, ondansetron, oxytocin, paclitaxel, palonosetron, pemetrexed, pentobarbital, phenobarbital, phentolamine, phenylephrine, plazomicin, potassium acetate, potassium chloride, potassium phosphate, procainamide, remifentanil, rituximab, sar-

gramostim, sodium acetate, sodium bicarbonate, sodium phosphate, succinylcholine, sufentanil, tacrolimus, tedizolid, telavancin, theophylline, thiotepa, tigecycline, tirofiban, trimethoprim/sulfamethoxazole, vasopressin, vinblastine, vincristine, voriconazole, zidovudine, zoledronic acid.
- **Y-Site Incompatibility:** acyclovir, alemtuzumab, amiodarone, amphotericin B deoxycholate, caspofungin, chlorpromazine, ciprofloxacin, cisplatin, dacarbazine, dantrolene, daunorubicin hydrochloride, diltiazem, dobutamine, doxorubicin hydrochloride, doxorubicin liposomal, doxycycline, droperidol, epirubicin, famotidine, ganciclovir, gemcitabine, gemtuzumab ozogamicin, glycopyrrolate, haloperidol, hydralazine, hydroxyzine, idarubicin, insulin regular, irinotecan, labetalol, levofloxacin, methadone, midazolam, minocycline, mitomycin, mitoxantrone, mycophenolate, nalbuphine, nicardipine, pentamidine, phenytoin, prochlorperazine, promethazine, propranolol, rocuronium, thiopental, tobramycin, topotecan, tranexamic acid, trastuzumab, vecuronium, verapamil, vinorelbine.

Patient/Family Teaching

- Explain purpose of piperacillin/tazobactam to patient.
- Advise patient to report rash and signs of superinfection (black furry overgrowth on tongue, vaginal itching or discharge, loose or foul-smelling stools) and allergy.
- Caution patient to notify health care professional if fever and diarrhea occur, especially if stool contains blood, pus, or mucus. Advise patient not to treat diarrhea without consulting health care professional. May occur up to several wk after discontinuation of medication.
- Rep: Advise females of reproductive potential to notify health care professional if pregnancy is planned or suspected or if breastfeeding.

Evaluation/Desired Outcomes

- Resolution of the signs and symptoms of infection. Length of time for complete resolution depends on the organism and site of infection.

---

pitavastatin, See HMG-CoA REDUCTASE INHIBITORS (statins).

---

plecanatide (ple-kan-a-tide)
Trulance
Classification
Therapeutic: laxatives
Pharmacologic: guanylate cyclase-C agonists

Indications

Chronic idiopathic constipation. Irritable bowel syndrome with constipation.

Action
Locally ↑ cyclic guanosine monophosphate concentrations, which ↑ intestinal fluid and accelerates transit time. **Therapeutic Effects:** Increased frequency of complete spontaneous bowel movements.

Pharmacokinetics
Absorption: Minimally absorbed, action is primarily local.
Distribution: Stays within the GI tract with minimal distribution.
Metabolism and Excretion: Converted to its principal active metabolite within the GI tract. Plecanatide and active metabolite then degrade in intestinal lumen to smaller peptides and amino acids. Excretion information unknown.
Half-life: Unknown.

TIME/ACTION PROFILE (improvement in symptoms)

ROUTE	ONSET	PEAK	DURATION
PO	1 wk	2–12 wk	2 wk†

†Following discontinuation.

Contraindications/Precautions
Contraindicated in: Known/suspected mechanical GI obstruction; Pedi: Children <6 yr (↑ risk of dehydration).
Use Cautiously in: OB: Safety not established in pregnancy; fetal exposure to plecanatide or its active metabolite unlikely; Lactation: Use while breastfeeding only if potential maternal benefit justifies potential risk to infant; Pedi: Children 6–18 yr (safety and effectiveness not established).

Adverse Reactions/Side Effects
GI: ↑ liver enzymes, abdominal distention, diarrhea, flatulence.

Interactions
Drug-Drug: None reported.

Route/Dosage
PO (Adults): 3 mg once daily.

Availability
Tablets: 3 mg.

NURSING IMPLICATIONS
Assessment
● Monitor bowel function (frequency, consistency) periodically during therapy. If severe diarrhea occurs, withhold plecanatide and rehydrate patient.

Lab Test Considerations
● May cause ↑ ALT, and AST.

Implementation
● PO: Administer once daily without regard to food. Swallow tablet whole. Tablets can be crushed and mixed in applesauce or water and administered orally or with water in a nasogastric or gastric feeding tube. Do not mix with other foods or liquids.

Patient/Family Teaching
● Instruct patient to take plecanatide as directed. If a dose is missed, omit and take next dose at regular time; do not double doses.
● Instruct patient to notify health care professional of all Rx or OTC medications, vitamins, or herbal products being taken and consult health care professional before taking any new medications.
● Rep: Advise females of reproductive potential to notify health care professional if pregnancy is planned or suspected or if breastfeeding.

Evaluation/Desired Outcomes
● Increased frequency of complete spontaneous bowel movements.

---

polyethylene glycol 3350
(po-lee-**eth**-e-leen **glye**-kole)
✳ClearLax, ✳Comfilax, ✳Emolax, Gavilax, GlycoLax, ✳Hydralax, ✳Lax-a-Day, MiraLax, ✳PegaLax, ✳Relaxa, ✳RestoraLax
Classification
Therapeutic: laxatives
Pharmacologic: osmotics

Indications
Occasional constipation.

Action
Polyethylene glycol in solution acts as an osmotic agent, drawing water into the lumen of the GI tract. **Therapeutic Effects:** Evacuation of the GI tract without water or electrolyte imbalance.

Pharmacokinetics
Absorption: Nonabsorbable.
Distribution: Unknown.
Metabolism and Excretion: Excreted in fecal contents.
Half-life: Unknown.

TIME/ACTION PROFILE (bowel movement)

ROUTE	ONSET	PEAK	DURATION
PO	unknown	1–3 days	unknown

Contraindications/Precautions
Contraindicated in: GI obstruction; Gastric retention; Toxic colitis; Megacolon; Bowel perforation.
Use Cautiously in: Abdominal pain of uncertain cause, particularly if accompanied by fever; OB: Minimal systemic absorption; may be used during

✳= Canadian drug name. ℨ = Genetic implication. S̶t̶r̶i̶k̶e̶t̶h̶r̶o̶u̶g̶h̶ = Discontinued. CAPITALS = life-threatening. Underline = most frequent.

pregnancy when osmotic laxative needed; Lactation: Minimal systemic absorption; probably compatible with breastfeeding; Pedi: May be associated with metabolic acidosis and neuropsychiatric events in children.

Adverse Reactions/Side Effects

Derm: urticaria. **GI:** abdominal bloating, cramping, flatulence, nausea.

Interactions

Drug-Drug: None reported.

Route/Dosage

PO (Adults): 17 g (heaping tablespoon) in 8 oz of water once daily; may be used for up to 2 wk.
PO (Children >6 mo): 0.2–0.8 g/kg once daily, titrate to effect (max = 17 g/day).

Availability (generic available)

Oral powder: 17 g/dose (in 14-oz, 24-oz, and 26-oz containers).

NURSING IMPLICATIONS

Assessment

● Assess patient for abdominal distention, presence of bowel sounds, and usual pattern of bowel function.
● Assess color, consistency, and amount of stool produced.

Implementation

● Do not confuse polyethylene glycol with propylene glycol.
● PO: Dissolve powder in 8 oz of any beverage (hot or cold) prior to administration. Do not mix in starch-based thickeners used for patients with difficulty swallowing.

Patient/Family Teaching

● Inform patient that 2–4 days may be required to produce a bowel movement; best results require 1–2 wk of use. PEG should not be used for more than 2 wk. Prolonged, frequent, or excessive use may result in electrolyte imbalance and laxative dependence.
● Advise patient to notify health care professional if nausea, vomiting or abdominal pain, unusual cramps, bloating, diarrhea or a sudden change in bowel habits for >2 wk occurs. Advise patient to discontinue use and consult health care professional if severe diarrhea, rectal bleeding, abdominal pain, bloating, cramping, or nausea gets worse, or if they need to use for >1 wk.
● Rep: Advise females of reproductive potential to notify health care professional if pregnancy is planned or suspected or if breastfeeding.

Evaluation/Desired Outcomes

● A soft, formed bowel movement.

posaconazole (po-sa-**kon**-a-zole)

Noxafil, ✤Posanol

Classification
Therapeutic: antifungals
Pharmacologic: triazoles

Indications

PO, IV: Treatment of invasive aspergillosis (tablets and injection). **PO, IV:** Prevention of invasive *Aspergillus* and *Candida* infections in patients who are severely immunocompromised, such as hematopoietic stem cell transplant recipients with graft-versus-host disease or those with hematologic malignancies with prolonged neutropenia from chemotherapy (tablets, oral suspension, delayed-release oral suspension, and injection). **PO:** Treatment of oropharyngeal candidiasis (including candidiasis unresponsive to itraconazole or fluconazole) (oral suspension).

Action

Blocks ergosterol synthesis, a major component of fungal plasma membrane. **Therapeutic Effects:** Fungistatic/fungicidal action against susceptible fungi. **Spectrum:** *Aspergillus* spp. *Candida* spp.

Pharmacokinetics

Absorption: Well absorbed following oral administration; absorption is optimized by food; IV administration results in complete bioavailability.
Distribution: Extensive extravascular distribution and penetration into body tissues.
Protein Binding: >98%.
Metabolism and Excretion: Some metabolism via UDP glucuronidation; 66% eliminated unchanged in feces, 13% in urine (mostly as metabolites).
Half-life: 35 hr.

TIME/ACTION PROFILE (plasma concentrations)

ROUTE	ONSET	PEAK	DURATION
PO (suspension)	unknown	3–5 hr	8 hr
PO-ER	unknown	4–5 hr	24 hr
IV	unknown	2 hr	24 hr

Contraindications/Precautions

Contraindicated in: Hypersensitivity to posaconazole or other azole antifungals; Concurrent use of atorvastatin, ergot alkaloids, lovastatin, pimozide, quinidine, simvastatin, or sirolimus; Concurrent use of venetoclax at initiation and during the ramp-up phase; Hereditary fructose intolerance (for delayed-release oral suspension only).

Use Cautiously in: History of/predisposition to QTc prolongation including congenital QTc prolongation, concurrent medications that prolong QTc, or electrolyte abnormalities (hypokalemia, hypomagnesemia); correct pre-existing abnormalities prior to administration; Moderate-severe renal impairment (CCr <50 mL/min); use only if justified by risk/benefit assessment (IV form should be avoided, use oral form only); Severe diarrhea, vomiting, or renal impairment (monitor for breakthrough fungal infections); OB: Use during pregnancy only if potential maternal benefit justifies potential fetal risk; Lactation: Use while breastfeeding only if potential maternal benefit justifies potential risk to infant; Pedi: Children <18 yr (IV) or <13 yr (oral) (safety and effectiveness not established).

Adverse Reactions/Side Effects

CV: QT interval prolongation, TORSADES DE POINTES. **Endo:** adrenal insufficiency. **F and E:** hypokalemia, hypomagnesemia, hypocalcemia. **GI:** diarrhea, nausea, vomiting, HEPATOCELLULAR DAMAGE, PANCREATITIS. **Neuro:** headache. **Resp:** cough. **Misc:** fever, HYPERSENSITIVITY REACTIONS.

Interactions

Drug-Drug: May ↑ **cyclosporine**, **sirolimus**, and **tacrolimus** levels and risk of toxicity; use with sirolimus contraindicated; for cyclosporine and tacrolimus, ↓ dose initially and monitor levels frequently. May ↑ **quinidine** and **pimozide** levels and the risk for arrhythmias; concurrent use contraindicated. May ↑ levels and risk of toxicity from **ergot alkaloids**, including **ergotamine** and **dihydroergotamine**; concurrent use contraindicated. May ↑ levels of **simvastatin**, **atorvastatin**, or **lovastatin** and the risk for rhabdomyolysis; concurrent use contraindicated. May ↑ risk of tumor lysis syndrome, neutropenia, and serious infection during initiation or the ramp-up phase of **venetoclax** in patients with chronic lymphocytic leukemia or small lymphocytic leukemia; concurrent use contraindicated. **Rifabutin**, **phenytoin**, **cimetidine**, and **efavirenz** may ↓ levels and may ↓ effectiveness; avoid concurrent use. **Esomeprazole** and **metoclopramide** may ↓ levels and effectiveness. May ↑ **rifabutin** levels and risk of toxicity; avoid concurrent use. **QT interval prolonging drugs** may ↑ risk for QT interval prolongation and torsades de pointes; avoid concurrent use. May ↑ **digoxin** levels and risk of toxicity; monitor levels frequently. May ↑ **phenytoin**, **midazolam**, **ritonavir**, and **atazanavir** levels and risk of toxicity; monitor for excess clinical effect. May ↑ levels of and risk of neurotoxicity, syndrome of inappropriate antidiuretic hormone, and paralytic ileus with concurrent use of **vinca alkaloids**, including **vincristine** and **vinblastine**; consider using an alternative non-azole antifungal. May ↑ levels and risk of adverse cardiovascular reactions to **calcium channel blockers**; consider dosage reduction.

Route/Dosage

The oral suspension is NOT interchangeable with delayed-release tablets.

Treatment of Invasive Aspergillosis

May switch between use of IV and delayed-release tablets (another loading dose is not needed when switching between formulations).

PO (Adults and Children ≥13 yr): *Delayed-release tablets:* 300 mg twice daily on Day 1, then 300 mg once daily starting on Day 2 for a total of 6–12 wk.

IV (Adults and Children ≥13 yr): 300 mg twice daily on Day 1, then 300 mg once daily starting on Day 2 for a total of 6–12 wk.

Prophylaxis of Invasive *Aspergillus* and *Candida* Infections

PO (Adults and Children ≥13 yr): *Oral suspension:* 200 mg 3 times daily. Duration of therapy is based on recovery from neutropenia or immunosuppression.

PO (Adults and Children ≥2 yr and >40 kg): *Delayed-release tablets:* 300 mg twice daily on Day 1, then 300 mg once daily starting on Day 2. Duration of therapy is based on recovery from neutropenia or immunosuppression.

IV (Adults): 300 mg twice daily on Day 1, then 300 mg once daily starting on Day 2. Duration of therapy is based on recovery from neutropenia or immunosuppression.

IV (Children ≥2 yr): 6 mg/kg (max = 300 mg) twice daily on Day 1, then 6 mg/kg (max = 300 mg) once daily starting on Day 2. Duration of therapy is based on recovery from neutropenia or immunosuppression.

Treatment of Oropharyngeal Candidiasis

PO (Adults and Children ≥13 yr): *Oral suspension:* 100 mg twice daily on Day 1, then 100 mg once daily for the next 13 days. For refractory oropharyngeal candidiasis, give 400 mg twice daily; duration of therapy is based on the severity of the patient's underlying disease and clinical response.

Availability (generic available)

Delayed-release tablets: 100 mg. **Oral suspension (cherry-flavor):** 40 mg/mL. **Solution for injection:** 18 mg/mL.

NURSING IMPLICATIONS
Assessment

● Assess for signs and symptoms of fungal infection. If severe diarrhea or vomiting occurs, monitor closely for breakthrough fungal infection.

Lab Test Considerations
● Monitor liver function tests prior to and periodically during therapy. May cause ↑ ALT, ↑ AST, ↑ alkaline phosphatase, and ↑ total bilirubin levels; generally reversible on discontinuation. Discontinue posaconazole if clinical signs and symptoms of liver disease develop.

- Monitor electrolyte levels (potassium, magnesium, calcium) before starting and during therapy. Correct as necessary before and during therapy.
- If administered with tacrolimus or cyclosporine, monitor tacrolimus or cyclosporine whole blood trough concentrations frequently during and at discontinuation of posaconazole; adjust tacrolimus or cyclosporine dose accordingly.

Implementation

- Delayed-release tablet and oral suspension are not interchangeable. Tablets are the preferred oral formulation for prophylaxis because they achieve higher plasma concentrations of drug.
- **PO:** Administer delayed-release tablets with food. *DNC:* Swallow tablets whole; do not divide, crush, or chew.
- Shake suspension well before use. Use spoon provided to ensure accurate dose. Administer during or within 20 min of a full meal, liquid nutritional supplement, or an acidic carbonated beverage (ginger ale) to enhance absorption. Rinse spoon for administration with water after each use. Alternative therapy or close monitoring for breakthrough fungal infections should be considered for patients unable to eat a full meal or tolerate a nutritional supplement.

IV Administration
- **Intermittent Infusion:** Allow solution to reach room temperature before administering. *Dilution:* Dilute in D5W, D5/0.45% NaCl, D5/0.9% NaCl, D5/20 mEq potassium, 0.45% NaCl or 0.9% NaCl. *Concentration:* 1–2 mg/mL. Do not dilute with other solutions. Use immediately; stable for 24 hrs if refrigerated. Discard unused solution. Solution is clear, colorless to yellow; do not administer solutions that are discolored or contain particulate matter. Administer through a 0.22 micron polyethersulfone or polyvinylidene difluoride filter via central venous line, including a central venous catheter or peripherally inserted central catheter line. If no central catheter available, may be administered through a peripheral venous catheter by slow intravenous infusion over 30 min only as a single dose in advance of central venous line placement or to bridge the period during which a central venous line is replaced or is in use for other intravenous treatment. *Rate:* Infuse slowly over 90 min. Do not give as a bolus.
- **Y-Site Compatibility:** amikacin, caspofungin, ciprofloxacin, daptomycin, dobutamine, famotidine, filgrastim, gentamicin, hydromorphone, levofloxacin, lorazepam, meropenem, micafungin, morphine, norepinephrine, potassium chloride, vancomycin.

Patient/Family Teaching

- Instruct patient to take posaconazole during or immediately (within 20 min) following a full meal or liquid nutritional supplement in order to enhance absorption. Take missed doses as soon as remembered. Advise patient to read the *Patient Informa-*

tion before taking posaconazole and with each Rx refill in case of changes.
- Advise patient to notify health care professional if severe diarrhea or vomiting occurs; may decrease posaconazole blood levels and allow breakthrough fungal infections or if signs and symptoms of liver injury (itching, yellow eyes or skin, fatigue, flu-like symptoms) or change in heart rate or rhythm occur.
- Instruct patient to notify health care professional of all Rx or OTC medications, vitamins, or herbal products being taken and consult health care professional before taking any new medications.
- Rep: May cause fetal harm. Advise females of reproductive potential to notify health care professional if pregnancy is planned or suspected and to avoid breastfeeding during therapy.

Evaluation/Desired Outcomes

- Resolution of clinical and laboratory indications of fungal infections. Duration of therapy is based on recovery from infection or neutropenia or immunosuppression.

---

potassium and sodium phosphates
(po-**tas**-e-um/**soe**-dee-um **foss**-fates)

K-Phos Neutral, K-Phos No. 2

Classification
Therapeutic: antiurolithics, mineral and electrolyte replacements/supplements

Indications

Treatment and prevention of phosphate depletion in patients who are unable to ingest adequate dietary phosphate. Adjunct therapy of urinary tract infections with methenamine. Prevention of calcium urinary stones. Phosphate salts of potassium may be used in hypokalemic patients with metabolic acidosis or coexisting phosphorus deficiency.

Action

Phosphate is present in bone and is involved in energy transfer and carbohydrate metabolism. Serves as a buffer for the excretion of hydrogen ions by the kidneys. Dibasic potassium phosphate is converted in renal tubule to monobasic salt, resulting in urinary acidification, which is required for methenamine hippurate or mandelate to be active as urinary anti-infectives. Acidification of urine increases solubility of calcium, decreasing calcium stone formation. **Therapeutic Effects:** Replacement of phosphorus in deficiency states. Urinary acidification. Increased efficacy of methenamine. Decreased formation of calcium urinary tract stones.

Pharmacokinetics

Absorption: Well absorbed following oral administration. Vitamin D promotes GI absorption of phosphates.

Distribution: Phosphates enter extracellular fluids and are then actively transported to sites of action.
Metabolism and Excretion: Excreted mainly (>90%) by the kidneys.
Half-life: Unknown.

TIME/ACTION PROFILE (effects on serum phosphate levels)

ROUTE	ONSET	PEAK	DURATION
PO	unknown	unknown	unknown

Contraindications/Precautions

Contraindicated in: Hyperkalemia (potassium salts); Hyperphosphatemia; Hypocalcemia; Severe renal impairment; Untreated Addison's disease (potassium salts).
Use Cautiously in: Hyperparathyroidism; Cardiac disease; Hypernatremia (sodium phosphate only); Hypertension (sodium phosphate only); Mild or moderate renal impairment.

Adverse Reactions/Side Effects

Related to hyperphosphatemia, unless otherwise indicated.
CV: ARRHYTHMIAS, bradycardia, CARDIAC ARREST, ECG changes (absent P waves, widening of the QRS complex with biphasic curve, peaked T waves), edema. **GI:** <u>diarrhea</u>, abdominal pain, nausea, vomiting. **F and E:** hyperkalemia, hypernatremia, hyperphosphatemia, hypocalcemia, hypomagnesemia. **MS:** *hypocalcemia, hyperkalemia:* muscle cramps. **Neuro:** confusion, dizziness, flaccid paralysis, headache, heaviness of legs, paresthesias, tremor, weakness.

Interactions

Drug-Drug: Concurrent use of **potassium-sparing diuretics**, **ACE inhibitors**, or **angiotensin II receptor blockers** with potassium phosphate may result in hyperkalemia. Concurrent use of **corticosteroids** with sodium phosphate may result in hypernatremia. Concurrent administration of **calcium-, magnesium-,** or **aluminum-containing compounds** ↓ absorption of phosphates by formation of insoluble complexes. **Vitamin D** enhances the absorption of phosphates.
Drug-Food: **Oxalates** (in spinach and rhubarb) and **phytates** (in bran and whole grains) may ↓ absorption of phosphates by binding them in the GI tract.

Route/Dosage

Phosphorous Supplementation

PO (Adults and Children >4 yr): 250–500 mg (8–16 mmol) phosphorus (1–2 packets) 4 times daily.
PO (Children <4 yr): 250 mg (8 mmol) phosphorus (1 packet) 4 times daily.

Urinary Acidification

PO (Adults): 2 tablets 4 times/day.

Maintenance Phosphorus

PO (Adults): 50–150 mmol/day in divided doses.
PO (Children): 2–3 mmol/kg/day in divided doses.

Availability

Potassium and Sodium Phosphates

Tablets (K-Phos Neutral): elemental phosphorus 250 mg (8 mmol), sodium 298 mg (13 mEq), and potassium 45 mg (1.1 mEq). **Tablets (K-Phos No.2):** elemental phosphorus 250 mg (8 mmol), sodium 134 mg (5.8 mEq), and potassium 88 mg (2.3 mEq). **Powder for oral solution:** elemental phosphorus 250 mg (8 mmol), sodium 164 mg (7.1 mEq), and potassium 278 mg (7.1 mEq)/packet.

NURSING IMPLICATIONS

Assessment

- Assess patient for signs and symptoms of hypokalemia (weakness, fatigue, arrhythmias, presence of U waves on ECG, polyuria, polydipsia) and hypophosphatemia (anorexia, weakness, decreased reflexes, bone pain, confusion, blood dyscrasias) throughout therapy.
- Monitor intake and output ratios and daily weight. Report significant discrepancies.

Lab Test Considerations

- Monitor serum phosphate, potassium, sodium, and calcium levels prior to and periodically throughout therapy. Increased phosphate may cause hypocalcemia.
- Monitor renal function studies prior to and periodically throughout therapy.
- Monitor urinary pH in patients receiving potassium and sodium phosphate as a urinary acidifier.

Implementation

- **PO:** Tablets should be dissolved in a full glass of water. Allow mixture to stand for 2–5 min to ensure it is fully dissolved. Solutions prepared by pharmacy should not be further diluted.
- Medication should be administered after meals to minimize gastric irritation and laxative effect.
- Do not administer simultaneously with antacids containing aluminum, magnesium, or calcium.

Patient/Family Teaching

- Explain to the patient the purpose of the medication and the need to take as directed. Take missed doses as soon as remembered unless within 1 or 2 hr of the next dose. Explain that the tablets should not be swallowed whole. Tablets should be dissolved in water.
- Instruct patients in low-sodium diet (see Appendix J).
- Advise patient of the importance of maintaining a high fluid intake (drinking at least one 8-oz glass of water each hr) to prevent kidney stones.

P

✤ = Canadian drug name. ▨ = Genetic implication. ~~Strikethrough~~ = Discontinued. CAPITALS = life-threatening. <u>Underline</u> = most frequent.

- Instruct the patient to promptly report diarrhea, weakness, fatigue, muscle cramps, unexplained weight gain, swelling of lower extremities, shortness of breath, unusual thirst, or tremors.

Evaluation/Desired Outcomes

- Prevention and correction of serum phosphate and potassium deficiencies.
- Maintenance of acidic urine.
- Decreased urine calcium, which prevents formation of renal calculi.

potassium chloride

(poe-**tass**-ee-um **klor**-ide)

Klor-Con, Klor-Con M10, Klor-Con M15, Klor-Con M20, K̶-̶T̶a̶b̶, ✳ Micro-K, S̶l̶o̶w̶-̶K̶

Classification

Therapeutic: mineral and electrolyte replacements/supplements

Indications

Treatment/prevention of potassium depletion.

Action

Maintain acid-base balance, isotonicity, and electrophysiologic balance of the cell. Activator in many enzymatic reactions; essential to transmission of nerve impulses; contraction of cardiac, skeletal, and smooth muscle; gastric secretion; renal function; tissue synthesis; and carbohydrate metabolism. **Therapeutic Effects:** Replacement. Prevention of deficiency.

Pharmacokinetics

Absorption: Well absorbed following oral administration. IV administration results in complete availability.

Distribution: Enters extracellular fluid; then actively transported into cells.

Metabolism and Excretion: Excreted by the kidneys.

Half-life: Unknown.

TIME/ACTION PROFILE (↑ in serum potassium concentrations)

ROUTE	ONSET	PEAK	DURATION
PO	unknown	1–2 hr	unknown
IV	rapid	end of infusion	unknown

Contraindications/Precautions

Contraindicated in: Hyperkalemia; Severe renal impairment; Untreated Addison's disease; Some oral products may contain tartrazine (FDC yellow dye #5) or alcohol; avoid using in patients with known hypersensitivity or intolerance; Hyperkalemic familial periodic paralysis.

Use Cautiously in: Cardiac disease; Renal impairment; Diabetes mellitus (liquids may contain sugar);

Hypomagnesemia (may make correction of hypokalemia more difficult); GI hypomotility including dysphagia or esophageal compression from left atrial enlargement (tablets, capsules); Patients receiving potassium-sparing drugs.

Adverse Reactions/Side Effects

CV: ARRHYTHMIAS, ECG changes. **F and E:** hyperchloremia, hyperkalemia. **GI:** abdominal pain, diarrhea, flatulence, nausea, vomiting; *tablets, capsules only:* GI ulceration, stenotic lesions. **Local:** irritation at IV site. **Neuro:** confusion, paralysis, paresthesia, restlessness, weakness.

Interactions

Drug-Drug: Use with **potassium-sparing diuretics** or **ACE inhibitors** or **angiotensin II receptor antagonists** may lead to hyperkalemia. **Anticholinergics** may ↑ GI mucosal lesions in patients taking waxmatrix potassium chloride preparations.

Route/Dosage

Expressed as mEq of potassium.

Normal Daily Requirements

PO (Adults): 40–80 mEq/day.
PO (Children): 2–3 mEq/kg/day.
PO (Neonates): 2–6 mEq/kg/day.

Prevention of Hypokalemia During Diuretic Therapy

PO (Adults): 20–40 mEq/day in 1–2 divided doses; single dose should not exceed 20 mEq.
PO (Neonates , Infants and Children): 1–2 mEq/kg/day in 1–2 divided doses.

Treatment of Hypokalemia

PO (Adults): 40–100 mEq/day in divided doses.
PO (Neonates , Infants and Children): 2–5 mEq/kg/day in divided doses.
IV (Adults): 10–20 mEq/dose (maximum: 40 mEq/dose) to infuse over 2–3 hr (maximum infusion rate: 40 mEq/hr).
IV (Neonates, Infants and Children): 0.5–1 mEq/kg/dose (maximum 30 mEq/dose) as an infusion to infuse at 0.3–0.5 mEq/kg/hr (maximum infusion rate 1 mEq/kg/hr).

Availability

Extended-release capsules: 8 mEq, 10 mEq. **Extended-release tablets:** 8 mEq, 10 mEq, 15 mEq, 20 mEq. **Oral solution:** 20 mEq/15 mL, 40 mEq/15 mL. **Powder for oral solution:** 20 mEq/pkt. **Concentrate for injection:** 0.1 mEq/mL in 10-mEq ampules and vials, 0.2 mEq/mL in 10- and 20-mEq ampules and vials, 0.3 mEq/mL in 30-mEq ampules and vials, 0.4 mEq/mL in 20- and 40-mEq ampules and vials, 1.5 mEq/mL, 2 mEq/mL, 3 mEq/mL. **Solution for IV infusion:** 10 mEq/L in various dextrose and saline solutions in 250-, 500-, and 100-mL containers, 20 mEq/L in dextrose/saline/LRs in 250-, 500-, and 100-mL containers, 30 mEq/L in various dextrose and saline solutions in 250-, 500-, and 100-mL containers, 40 mEq/L in various dextrose and saline solutions in 250-, 500-, and 100-mL containers.

NURSING IMPLICATIONS

Assessment
- Assess for signs and symptoms of hypokalemia (weakness, fatigue, U wave on ECG, arrhythmias, polyuria, polydipsia) and hyperkalemia (see Toxicity and Overdose).
- Monitor pulse, BP, and ECG periodically during IV therapy.

Lab Test Considerations
- Monitor serum potassium before and periodically during therapy. Monitor renal function, serum bicarbonate, calcium, chloride, magnesium, phosphate, sodium), acid/base balance; and pH. Determine serum magnesium level if patient has refractory hypokalemia; hypomagnesemia should be corrected to facilitate effectiveness of potassium replacement. Monitor serum chloride because hypochloremia may occur if replacing potassium without concurrent chloride.

Toxicity and Overdose
- Symptoms of toxicity are those of hyperkalemia (slow, irregular heartbeat; fatigue; muscle weakness; paresthesia; confusion; dyspnea; peaked T waves; depressed ST segments; prolonged QT interval; widened QRS complexes; loss of P waves; and cardiac arrhythmias).
- Treatment includes discontinuation of potassium, administration of sodium bicarbonate to correct acidosis, dextrose and insulin to facilitate passage of potassium into cells, calcium salts to reverse ECG effects (in patients who are not receiving digoxin), sodium polystyrene used as an exchange resin, and/or dialysis for patient with impaired renal function.

Implementation
- **High Alert:** Medication errors involving too rapid infusion or bolus IV administration of potassium chloride have resulted in fatalities. See IV administration guidelines below.
- Renal tubular acidosis (hyperchloremic acidosis) may require other salts (potassium bicarbonate, potassium citrate, or potassium gluconate).
- If hypokalemia is secondary to diuretic therapy, consideration should be given to decreasing the dose of diuretic, unless there is a history of significant arrhythmias or concurrent digoxin therapy.
- **PO:** Administer with or after meals to decrease GI irritation.
- Use of tablets and capsules should be reserved for patients who cannot tolerate liquid preparations.
- Dissolve effervescent tablets in 3–8 oz of cold water. Ensure that effervescent tablet is fully dissolved. Powders and solutions should be diluted in 3–8 oz

of cold water or juice (do not use tomato juice if patient is on sodium restriction). Instruct patient to drink slowly over 5–10 min.
- Tablets and capsules should be taken with a meal and full glass of water. Do not chew or crush enteric-coated or extended-release tablets or capsules. Capsules can be opened and sprinkled on soft food (pudding, applesauce) and swallowed immediately with a glass of cool water or juice.
- **IV:** Potassium chloride is a vesicant/irritant (at concentrations >0.1 mEq/mL); ensure proper needle or catheter placement prior to and during IV infusion. Avoid extravasation. If extravasation occurs, stop infusion immediately; leave needle/cannula in place temporarily but do NOT flush the line; gently aspirate extravasated solution, then remove needle/cannula; elevate extremity; apply dry warm compresses; initiate hyaluronidase antidote. *Hyaluronidase* For adults, inject a total of 1 mL (15 units/mL) intradermally or SUBQ as 5 separate 0.2 mL injections (using a tuberculin syringe) around the site of extravasation; if IV catheter remains in place, administer IV through the infiltrated catheter; may repeat in 30 to 60 min if no resolution. *High Alert:* Never administer potassium IV push or bolus.
- **Continuous Infusion: *High Alert:*** Do not administer concentrations of ≥1.5 mEq/mL undiluted; may cause cardiac arrest. Concentrated products have black caps on vials or black stripes above constriction on ampules and are labeled with a warning about dilution requirement. Each single dose must be diluted and thoroughly mixed in 100–1000 mL of IV solution. Usually limited to 80 mEq/L via peripheral line (200 mEq/L via central line).
- Concentrations of 0.1 and 0.4 mEq/mL are intended for administration via calibrated infusion device and do not require dilution.
- ***Rate: High Alert:*** Infuse slowly, at a rate up to 10 mEq/hr in adults or 0.5 mEq/kg/hr in children in general care areas. Check hospital policy for maximum infusion rates (maximum rate in monitored setting 40 mEq/hr in adults or 1 mEq/kg/hr in children in a peripheral line. May use higher concentrations via central line). Use an infusion pump.
- **Solution Compatibility:** May be diluted in D5W, D10W, D5LR, D5/0.9% NaCl, D5/0.45% NaCl, 0.9% NaCl, 0.45% 0.9% NaCl, and LR. Commercially available premixed with many of the above IV solutions.
- **Y-Site Compatibility:** acetaminophen, acyclovir, alemtuzumab, allopurinol, alprostadil, amifostine, amikacin, aminocaproic acid, aminophylline, amphotericin B liposomal, anidulafungin, argatroban, arsenic trioxide, ascorbic acid, atropine, azathioprine, aztreonam, benztropine, bivalirudin, bleomycin, bumetanide, buprenorphine, butorphanol, calcium gluconate, cangrelor, carboplatin, carmustine, caspofungin, cefazolin, cefotaxime, cefotetan, cefoxi-

P

tin, ceftaroline, ceftazidime, ceftazidime/avibactam, ceftolozane/tazobactam, ceftriaxone, cefuroxime, chloramphenicol, chlorpromazine, ciprofloxacin, cisatracurium, cisplatin, cladribine, clindamycin, cyclophosphamide, cyclosporine, cytarabine, dacarbazine, dactinomycin, daptomycin, daunorubicin hydrochloride, dexamethasone, dexmedetomidine, dexrazoxane, digoxin, diltiazem, diphenhydramine, dobutamine, docetaxel, dopamine, doxorubicin hydrochloride, doxorubicin liposomal, doxycycline, enalaprilat, ephedrine, epinephrine, epirubicin, epoetin alfa, eptifibatide, ertapenem, erythromycin, esmolol, etoposide, etoposide phosphate, famotidine, fentanyl, filgrastim, fluconazole, fludarabine, folic acid, foscarnet, fosphenytoin, furosemide, gemcitabine, gemtuzumab ozogamicin, gentamicin, granisetron, heparin, hetastarch, hydrocortisone, hydromorphone, ibuprofen lysine, idarubicin, ifosfamide, imipenem/cilastatin, indomethacin, insulin aspart, insulin regular, irinotecan, isavuconazonium, isoproterenol, ketamine, ketorolac, labetalol, leucovorin calcium, levofloxacin, lidocaine, linezolid, lorazepam, magnesium sulfate, mannitol, melphalan, meperidine, meropenem, meropenem/vaborbactam, mesna, methadone, methotrexate, methylprednisolone, metoclopramide, metoprolol, metronidazole, micafungin, midazolam, milrinone, mitomycin, mitoxantrone, morphine, moxifloxacin, multivitamin, mycophenolate, nafcillin, nalbuphine, naloxone, nicardipine, nitroglycerin, nitroprusside, norepinephrine, octreotide, ondansetron, oritavancin, oxacillin, oxaliplatin, oxytocin, paclitaxel, palonosetron, pamidronate, pantoprazole, papaverine, penicillin G, pentobarbital, phenobarbital, phentolamine, phenylephrine, phytonadione, piperacillin/tazobactam, plazomicin, posaconazole, potassium acetate, procainamide, prochlorperazine , promethazine, propofol, propranolol, protamine, pyridoxine, remifentanil, rituximab, rocuronium, sargramostim, sodium acetate, sodium bicarbonate, succinylcholine, sufentanil, tacrolimus, tedizolid, telavancin, theophylline, thiotepa, tigecycline, tirofiban, tobramycin, topotecan, trastuzumab, vancomycin, vasopressin, vecuronium, verapamil, vinblastine, vincristine, vinorelbine, voriconazole, zidovudine, zoledronic acid.

- **Y-Site Incompatibility:** amphotericin B deoxycholate, blinatumomab, dantrolene, diazepam, haloperidol, pentamidine, phenytoin, trimethoprim/sulfamethoxazole.

Patient/Family Teaching

- Explain to patient purpose of the medication and the need to take as directed, especially when concurrent digoxin or diuretics are taken. A missed dose should be taken as soon as remembered within 2 hr; if not, return to regular dose schedule. Do not double dose.
- Emphasize correct method of administration. GI irritation or ulceration may result from chewing en-

teric-coated tablets or insufficient dilution of liquid or powder forms.

- Instruct patient to avoid salt substitutes or low-salt milk or food unless approved by health care professional. Patient should be advised to read all labels to prevent excess potassium intake.
- Advise patient regarding sources of dietary potassium (see Appendix J). Encourage compliance with recommended diet.
- Instruct patient to report dark, tarry, or bloody stools; weakness; unusual fatigue; or tingling of extremities. Notify health care professional if nausea, vomiting, diarrhea, or stomach discomfort persists. Dose may require adjustment.
- Emphasize the importance of regular follow-up exams to monitor serum levels and progress.

Evaluation/Desired Outcomes

- Prevention and correction of serum potassium depletion.

pramipexole (pra-mi-**pex**-ole)

❋ Mirapex, Mirapex ER

Classification
Therapeutic: antiparkinson agents
Pharmacologic: dopamine agonists

Indications
Parkinson's disease. Restless leg syndrome (immediate-release only).

Action
Stimulates dopamine receptors in the striatum of the brain. **Therapeutic Effects:** Decreased tremor and rigidity in Parkinson's disease. Decreased leg restlessness.

Pharmacokinetics
Absorption: >90% absorbed following oral administration.

Distribution: Widely distributed.

Metabolism and Excretion: 90% excreted unchanged in urine.

Half-life: 8 hr ($\uparrow$ in geriatric patients and patients with renal impairment).

TIME/ACTION PROFILE (plasma concentrations)

ROUTE	ONSET	PEAK	DURATION
PO	unknown	2 hr	8 hr
PO-ER	unknown	6 hr	24 hr

Contraindications/Precautions
Contraindicated in: Hypersensitivity; Major psychotic disorder; Impulsive control/compulsive behaviors.

Use Cautiously in: Renal impairment ($\uparrow$ dosing interval recommended if CCr <60 mL/min [immediate-release] or CCr <50 mL/min [extended-release]); OB: Safety not established in pregnancy; Lactation: Use while breastfeeding only if potential maternal benefit justifies potential risk to infant; may inhibit lactation; Pedi: Safety and effectiveness not established in children.

Adverse Reactions/Side Effects

CV: orthostatic hypotension. **Derm:** pruritus. **Endo:** syndrome of inappropriate antidiuretic hormone. **GI:** constipation, dry mouth, dyspepsia, nausea. **GU:** urinary frequency. **MS:** leg cramps, muscle pain, postural deformities, RHABDOMYOLYSIS. **Neuro:** amnesia, dizziness, drowsiness, hallucinations, weakness, abnormal dreams, aggression, agitation, confusion, delirium, delusions, disorientation, dyskinesia, extrapyramidal syndrome, headache, hypertonia, impulse control disorders (gambling, sexual, uncontrolled spending, binge/compulsive eating), insomnia, paranoid ideation, psychosis, SLEEP ATTACKS, unsteadiness/falling. **Misc:** tooth disease.

Interactions

Drug-Drug: Concurrent **levodopa** ↑ risk of hallucinations and dyskinesia. **Cimetidine**, **diltiazem**, **triamterene**, **verapamil**, **quinidine**, **quinine**, and **cisplatin** may ↑ levels. Effectiveness may be ↓ by **dopamine antagonists**, including **butyrophenones**, **metoclopramide**, **phenothiazines**, or **thioxanthenes**.

Route/Dosage

When switching from immediate-release to extended-release product, the same total daily dose can be used.

Parkinson's Disease

PO (Adults): *Immediate-release:* 0.125 mg 3 times daily initially; may be ↑ every 5–7 days (range 1.5–4.5 mg/day in 3 divided doses); *Extended-release:* 0.375 mg once daily; may be ↑ to 0.75 mg once daily in 5–7 days, and then ↑ every 5–7 days by 0.75 mg/day (max dose = 4.5 mg/day).

Renal Impairment

PO (Adults Immediate-release): *CCr 35–59 mL/min:* 0.125 mg twice daily initially, may be ↑ every 5–7 days up to 1.5 mg twice daily; *CCr 15–34 mL/min:* 0.125 mg daily initially, may be ↑ every 5–7 days up to 1.5 mg daily.

Renal Impairment

PO (Adults Extended-release): *CCr 30–50 mL/min:* 0.375 mg every other day; may consider ↑ dose to 0.375 mg once daily after 1 wk based on response and tolerability; may ↑ in 0.375 mg increments after 1 wk (max dose = 2.25 mg/day).

Restless Leg Syndrome

PO (Adults): 0.125 mg daily 1–3 hr before bedtime. May be ↑ at 4–7 day intervals to 0.25 mg daily, then up to 0.5 mg daily.

Renal Impairment

PO (Adults Immediate-release): *CCr 20–60 mL/min:* 0.125 mg daily 1–3 hr before bedtime. May be ↑ at 14-day intervals to 0.25 mg daily, then up to 0.5 mg daily.

Availability (generic available)

Immediate-release tablets: 0.125 mg, 0.25 mg, 0.5 mg, 0.75 mg, 1 mg, 1.5 mg. **Extended-release tablets:** 0.375 mg, 0.75 mg, 1.5 mg, 2.25 mg, 3 mg, 3.75 mg, 4.5 mg.

NURSING IMPLICATIONS

Assessment

- Assess patient for signs and symptoms of psychotic-like behavior (confusion, paranoid ideation, delusions, hallucinations, psychotic-like behavior, disorientation, aggressive behavior, agitation, delirium, hallucinations). Risk of symptoms increases with age. Notify health care professional if these occur.
- Monitor ECG and BP frequently during dose adjustment and periodically during therapy.
- Assess patient for drowsiness and sleep attacks. Drowsiness is a common side effect of pramipexole, but sleep attacks or episodes of falling asleep during activities that require active participation may occur without warning. Assess patient for concomitant medications that have sedating effects or may increase serum pramipexole levels (see Interactions). May require discontinuation of therapy.
- **Parkinson's Disease:** Assess patient for signs and symptoms of Parkinson's disease (tremor, muscle weakness and rigidity, ataxia) before and throughout therapy.
- **Restless Leg Syndrome:** Assess sleep patterns and frequency of restless leg disturbances.

Implementation

- An attempt to reduce the dose of levodopa/carbidopa may be made cautiously during pramipexole therapy.
- Taper or discontinuation may cause withdrawal symptoms (apathy, anxiety, depression, fatigue, insomnia, sweating, pain); symptoms do not respond to levodopa. Trial readministration of pramipexole at lowest dose may be considered.
- **PO:** Administer with meals to minimize nausea; usually resolves with continued therapy. *DNC:* Swallow extended-release tablets whole; do not crush, break, or chew.

Patient/Family Teaching

- Instruct patient to take medication as directed. Take missed doses or immediate-release product as soon as remembered if it is not almost time for next dose. If extended release tablets are missed, skip dose and take next regular dose. Do not double doses. Consult health care professional before reducing dose or discontinuing medication; may cause withdrawal symptoms, fever, confusion, or severe muscle stiffness. Advise patient to read the *Patient Information* sheet before taking and with each Rx refill, as changes may occur.

- May cause drowsiness and unexpected episodes of falling asleep. Caution patient to avoid driving or other activities requiring alertness until response to medication is known. Advise patient to notify health care professional if episodes of falling asleep occur.
- Advise patient to change position slowly to minimize orthostatic hypotension. May occur more frequently during initial therapy.
- Instruct patient to notify health care professional of all Rx or OTC medications, vitamins, or herbal products being taken and consult health care professional before taking any new medications.
- Advise patient to have periodic skin exams to check for lesions that may be melanoma.
- Advise patient to notify health care professional if new or increased gambling, sexual, or other intense urges or psychotic-like behaviors occur.
- Rep: Advise females of reproductive potential to notify health care professional if pregnancy is planned or suspected or if breastfeeding. Pramipexole may inhibit lactation.

Evaluation/Desired Outcomes
- Decreased tremor and rigidity in Parkinson's disease.
- Decrease in restless legs and improved sleep.

---

prasterone (pras-ter-one)
Intrarosa
Classification
Therapeutic: none assigned
Pharmacologic: steroids

Indications
Moderate to severe dyspareunia.

Action
Inactive steroid that is converted into active androgens and/or estrogens. Exact mechanism in treatment of vulvar and vaginal atrophy in menopausal women not fully established. **Therapeutic Effects:** Reduced severity of dyspareunia.

Pharmacokinetics
Absorption: Unknown.
Distribution: Unknown.
Metabolism and Excretion: Metabolized via dehydrogenase, reductase, and aromatase to estradiol and testosterone.
Half-life: Unknown.

TIME/ACTION PROFILE (reduction in severity of dyspareunia)

ROUTE	ONSET	PEAK	DURATION
Vag	unknown	12 wk	unknown

Contraindications/Precautions
Contraindicated in: Undiagnosed abnormal genital bleeding; Current or history of breast cancer.
Use Cautiously in: None reported.

Adverse Reactions/Side Effects
GU: vaginal discharge.

Interactions
Drug-Drug: None reported.

Route/Dosage
Vag (Adults): Insert one vaginal insert at bedtime.

Availability
Vaginal insert: 6.5 mg.

NURSING IMPLICATIONS
Assessment
- Assess for pain during intercourse periodically during therapy.

Implementation
- **Vag:** Insert vaginal insert at bedtime using applicator provided. Vaginal inserts can be stored at room temperature or refrigerated.

Patient/Family Teaching
- Explain purpose of prasterone to patient. Instruct patient to read *Instructions for Use* before inserting prasterone.
- Inform patient that vaginal discharge and abnormal PAP smear findings may occur with prasterone.
- Advise patient to notify health care professional of all Rx or OTC medications, vitamins, or herbal products being taken and to consult with health care professional before taking other medications during therapy.

Evaluation/Desired Outcomes
- Decreased pain during intercourse.

BEERS

prasugrel (pra-soo-grel)
Effient
Classification
Therapeutic: antiplatelet agents
Pharmacologic: thienopyridines

Indications
Reduction of thrombotic cardiovascular events (including stent thrombosis) in patients with acute coronary syndrome who will be managed with percutaneous coronary intervention (PCI) including patients with unstable angina (UA) or non-ST-elevation myocardial infarction (NSTEMI). Reduction of thrombotic cardiovascular events (including stent thrombosis) in patients with ST-elevation myocardial infarction (STEMI) when managed with either primary/delayed PCI.

Action

Acts by irreversibly binding its active metabolite to the $P2Y_{12}$ class of ADP receptors on platelets; inhibiting platelet activation and aggregation. **Therapeutic Effects:** Decreased thrombotic events including cardiovascular death, nonfatal MI, and nonfatal stroke.

Pharmacokinetics

Absorption: Well absorbed following oral administration (79%), then rapidly converted to an active metabolite.

Distribution: Unknown.

Protein Binding: *Active metabolite:* 98%.

Metabolism and Excretion: Active metabolite is metabolized to two inactive compounds; 68% excreted in the urine and 27% in feces as inactive metabolites.

Half-life: *Active metabolite:* 7 hr (range 2–15 hr).

TIME/ACTION PROFILE (effect on platelet function)

ROUTE	ONSET	PEAK	DURATION
PO	within 1 hr	2 hr	5–9 days†

†Following discontinuation.

Contraindications/Precautions

Contraindicated in: Hypersensitivity; Active pathological bleeding; History of transient ischemic attack or stroke.

Use Cautiously in: Patients about to undergo coronary artery bypass grafting (CABG) (↑ risk of bleeding; discontinue at least 7 days prior to surgery); Premature discontinuation (↑ risk of stent thrombosis, MI, and death); Body weight <60 kg, propensity to bleed, severe hepatic impairment, concurrent use of medications that ↑ the risk of bleeding (↑ risk of bleeding); Hypotension in the setting of recent coronary angiography, PCI, CABG, or other surgical procedure (suspect bleeding but do not discontinue prasugrel); OB: Use during pregnancy only if potential maternal benefit justifies potential fetal risk; Lactation: Use while breastfeeding only if potential maternal benefit justifies potential risk to infant; Pedi: Safety and effectiveness not established in children; Geri: Appears on Beers list. ↑ risk of major bleeding compared to clopidogrel, especially in patients ≥75 yrs old. Use with caution in older adults, especially in patients ≥75 yrs old. If used in patients ≥75 yrs old, consider using a lower dose (5 mg once daily).

Adverse Reactions/Side Effects

CV: atrial fibrillation, bradycardia, hypertension, hypotension, peripheral edema. **Derm:** rash. **GI:** diarrhea, nausea. **Hemat:** BLEEDING, leukopenia, THROMBOTIC THROMBOCYTOPENIC PURPURA. **Metab:** hyperlipidemia. **MS:** back pain, extremity pain, non-cardiac chest pain. **Neuro:** dizziness, fatigue, headache. **Resp:** cough, dyspnea. **Misc:** fever, HYPERSENSITIVITY REACTIONS (including angioedema).

Interactions

Drug-Drug: ↑ risk of bleeding with **warfarin** and **NSAIDs**. **Opioids** may ↓ absorption of active metabolite and ↓ antiplatelet effects; consider using parenteral antiplatelet in patients with acute coronary syndrome if concurrent use of opioids needed.

Route/Dosage

Aspirin 75–325 mg/daily should be taken concurrently.

PO (Adults ≥60 kg): 60 mg initially as a loading dose, then 10 mg once daily.

PO (Adults <60 kg): 60 mg initially as a loading dose, then consider maintenance dose of 5 mg once daily.

Availability (generic available)

Tablets: 5 mg, 10 mg.

NURSING IMPLICATIONS

Assessment

- Assess patient for symptoms of stroke, peripheral vascular disease, or MI periodically during therapy.
- Monitor patient for signs of thrombotic thrombocytopenic purpura (thrombocytopenia, microangiopathic hemolytic anemia, neurologic findings, renal dysfunction, fever). May rarely occur, even after short exposure (<2 wk). Requires prompt treatment.

Lab Test Considerations
- Monitor bleeding time during therapy. Prolonged bleeding time, which is time- and dose-dependent, is expected.
- Monitor CBC with differential and platelet count periodically during therapy. Thrombocytopenia and anemia may rarely occur.

Implementation

- Discontinue prasugrel 7 days before planned surgical procedures.
- Patients should take aspirin 75–325 mg daily with prasugrel.
- *In patients with UA or NSTEMI*, dose is usually administered at time of diagnosis or at time of PCI.
- *In patients with STEMI* presenting within 12 hrs of symptom onset, loading dose is usually administered at time of diagnosis or at time of PCI.
- **PO:** Administer once daily without regard to food. *DNC:* Swallow tablets whole; do not break.

Patient/Family Teaching

- Instruct patient to take medication as directed. Take missed doses as soon as possible unless almost time for next dose; do not double doses. Do not discontinue without consulting health care professional. Advise patient to read *Medication Guide* before taking and with each Rx refill; in case of changes. Instruct patient to keep prasugrel in original container

P

with dessicant, and keep tightly capped to protect from moisture.

- Inform patient that they will bleed and bruise more easily and will take longer to stop bleeding. Notify health care professional immediately if you have unexpected bleeding or bleeding that lasts a long time, bleeding that is severe or you cannot control, pink or brown urine, red or black stool (looks like tar), bruises that happen without a known cause or get larger, cough up blood or blood clots, vomit blood or your vomit looks like "coffee grounds."
- Advise patient to notify health care professional promptly if fever, weakness, skin paleness, purple skin patches, yellowing of skin or eyes, chills, sore throat, neurological changes, or unusual bleeding or bruising, swelling of lips, difficulty breathing, rash, or hives occur.
- Advise patient to notify health care professional and dentists of medication regimen prior to treatment or surgery.
- Instruct patient to notify health care professional of all Rx or OTC medications, vitamins, or herbal products being taken and consult health care professional before taking any new medications, especially NSAIDs.
- Rep: Advise female patient to notify health care professional if pregnancy is planned or suspected and to avoid breastfeeding during therapy.

Evaluation/Desired Outcomes
- Prevention of stroke, MI, and vascular death in patients at risk.

---

pravastatin, See HMG-CoA REDUCTASE INHIBITORS (statins).

BEERS

prazosin (pra-zoe-sin)
~~Minipress~~
Classification
Therapeutic: antihypertensives
Pharmacologic: peripherally acting antiadrenergics

Indications
Mild to moderate hypertension. **Unlabeled Use:** Urinary outflow obstruction in patients with benign prostatic hyperplasia.

Action
Dilates both arteries and veins by blocking postsynaptic alpha$_1$-adrenergic receptors. Decreases contractions in smooth muscle of prostatic capsule. **Therapeutic Effects:** Lowering of BP. Decreased symptoms of prostatic hyperplasia (urinary urgency, urinary hesitancy, nocturia).

Pharmacokinetics
Absorption: 60% absorbed following oral administration.
Distribution: Widely distributed.
Protein Binding: 97%.
Metabolism and Excretion: Extensively metabolized by the liver. Minimal (5–10%) renal excretion of unchanged drug.
Half-life: 2–3 hr.

TIME/ACTION PROFILE (antihypertensive effects)

ROUTE	ONSET	PEAK	DURATION
PO	2 hr	2–4 hr†	10 hr

†Following single dose; maximal antihypertensive effects occur after 3–4 wk of chronic dosing.

Contraindications/Precautions
Contraindicated in: Hypersensitivity.
Use Cautiously in: Renal impairment (↑ sensitivity to effects; dose ↓ may be required); Angina pectoris; Patients undergoing cataract surgery (↑ risk of intraoperative floppy iris syndrome); OB: Use during pregnancy only if potential maternal benefit justifies potential fetal risk; other antihypertensives preferred in pregnancy; Lactation: Use while breastfeeding only if potential maternal benefit justifies potential risk to infant; Pedi: Safety and effectiveness not established in children; Geri: Appears on Beers list. ↑ risk of orthostatic hypotension in older adults. Avoid use for treatment of hypertension in older adults.

Adverse Reactions/Side Effects
CV: first-dose orthostatic hypotension, palpitations, angina, edema, syncope. **EENT:** blurred vision, intraoperative floppy iris syndrome. **GI:** abdominal cramps, diarrhea, dry mouth, nausea, vomiting. **GU:** erectile dysfunction, priapism. **Neuro:** dizziness, headache, weakness, depression, drowsiness.

Interactions
Drug-Drug: Additive hypotension with acute ingestion of **alcohol**, other **antihypertensives**, or **nitrates**. Antihypertensive effects may be ↓ by **NSAIDs**.

Route/Dosage
Hypertension
PO (Adults): 1 mg 2–3 times daily (give 1st dose at bedtime) for initial 3 days of therapy, then ↑ gradually to maintenance dose of 6–15 mg/day in 2–3 divided doses (not to exceed 20–40 mg/day).

Benign Prostatic Hyperplasia
PO (Adults): 1–5 mg twice daily.

Availability (generic available)
Capsules: 1 mg, 2 mg, 5 mg. **Tablets:** ❋ 1 mg, ❋ 2 mg, ❋ 5 mg.

NURSING IMPLICATIONS

Assessment
- Assess for first-dose orthostatic reaction (dizziness, weakness) and syncope. May occur 30 min – 2 hr after initial dose and occasionally thereafter. Incidence may be dose related. Volume-depleted or sodium-restricted patients may be more sensitive. Observe patient closely during this period; take precautions to prevent injury. 1st dose may be given at bedtime to minimize this reaction.
- Monitor intake and output ratios and daily weight; assess for edema daily, especially at beginning of therapy.
- **Hypertension:** Monitor BP and pulse frequently during initial dose adjustment and periodically during therapy. Report significant changes.
- Monitor frequency of prescription refills to determine adherence.
- **Benign Prostatic Hyperplasia:** Assess patient for symptoms of prostatic hyperplasia (urinary hesitancy, feeling of incomplete bladder emptying, interruption of urinary stream, impairment of size and force of urinary stream, terminal urinary dribbling, straining to start flow, dysuria, urgency) before and periodically during therapy.
- Rule out prostatic carcinoma before therapy; symptoms are similar.

Implementation
- May be used in combination with diuretics or beta blockers to minimize sodium and water retention. If these are added to prazosin therapy, reduce dose of prazosin initially and titrate to effect.
- **PO:** Administer daily dose at bedtime, without regards to meals, at the same time each day. If necessary, dose may be increased to twice daily.

Patient/Family Teaching
- Instruct patient to take medication at the same time each day. Take missed doses as soon as remembered. If not remembered until next day, omit; do not double doses.
- Advise patient to weigh self twice weekly and assess feet and ankles for fluid retention.
- May cause dizziness or drowsiness. Advise patient to avoid driving or other activities requiring alertness until response to the medication is known.
- Caution patient to avoid sudden changes in position to decrease orthostatic hypotension. Alcohol, CNS depressants, standing for long periods, hot showers, and exercising in hot weather should be avoided because of enhanced orthostatic effects.
- Advise patient to notify health care professional of all Rx or OTC medications, vitamins, or herbal products being taken and to consult with health care professional before taking other medications, especially NSAIDs and cough, cold, or allergy remedies.

- Instruct patient to notify health care professional of medication regimen before any surgery.
- Advise patient to notify health care professional immediately if erection lasts for 4 hr or longer or if frequent dizziness, fainting, or swelling of feet or lower legs occurs.
- Rep: Advise females of reproductive potential to notify health care professional if pregnancy is planned or suspected or if breastfeeding.
- Emphasize the importance of follow-up exams to evaluate effectiveness of medication.
- **Hypertension:** Emphasize the importance of continuing to take this medication as directed, even if feeling well. Medication controls but does not cure hypertension.
- Encourage patient to comply with additional interventions for hypertension (weight reduction, low-sodium diet, smoking cessation, moderation of alcohol consumption, regular exercise, and stress management).
- Instruct patient and family on proper technique for BP monitoring. Advise them to check BP at least weekly and to report significant changes.

Evaluation/Desired Outcomes
- Decrease in BP without appearance of side effects.
- Decrease in symptoms of prostatic hyperplasia.

---

prednisoLONE, See CORTICOSTEROIDS (SYSTEMIC).

---

predniSONE, See CORTICOSTEROIDS (SYSTEMIC).

---

pregabalin (pre-gab-a-lin)
Lyrica, Lyrica CR
Classification
Therapeutic: analgesics, anticonvulsants
Pharmacologic: gamma aminobutyric acid (GABA) analogues, nonopioid analgesics

Schedule V

Indications
Immediate-release and extended-release: Treatment of the following conditions: Neuropathic pain associated with diabetic peripheral neuropathy, Postherpetic neuralgia. **Immediate-release:** Treatment of the following conditions: Fibromyalgia, Neuropathic pain associated with spinal cord injury, Partial-onset seizures (adjunctive therapy).

Action
Binds to calcium channels in CNS tissues which regulate neurotransmitter release. Does not bind to opioid

receptors. **Therapeutic Effects:** Decreased neuropathic or postherpetic pain. Decreased partial-onset seizures.

Pharmacokinetics

Absorption: Well absorbed (>90%) following oral administration.

Distribution: Well distributed to tissues; probably crosses the blood-brain barrier.

Metabolism and Excretion: Minimally metabolized; 90% excreted unchanged in urine.

Half-life: 6 hr.

TIME/ACTION PROFILE (↓ post-herpetic pain)

ROUTE	ONSET	PEAK	DURATION
PO	unknown	2–4 wk	unknown

Contraindications/Precautions

Contraindicated in: Hypersensitivity; Known/suspected myopathy; Severe renal impairment (CCr <30 mL/min) (extended-release only); Lactation: Lactation.

Use Cautiously in: All patients (may ↑ risk of suicidal thoughts/behaviors); Renal impairment (dose alteration recommended for CCr <60 mL/min); HF; History of drug dependence/drug-seeking behavior; Respiratory impairment (↑ risk of respiratory depression); OB: Safety not established in pregnancy; Pedi: Children <1 mo (safety and effectiveness not established); Geri: Consider age-related ↓ in renal function when determining dose in older adults.

Adverse Reactions/Side Effects

CV: peripheral edema, PR interval prolongation. **Derm:** bullous pemphigoid, STEVENS-JOHNSON SYNDROME. **EENT:** blurred vision, double vision, vertigo. **GI:** dry mouth, abdominal pain, constipation, diarrhea, nausea, vomiting. **Hemat:** thrombocytopenia. **Metab:** ↑ appetite, weight gain. **MS:** ↑ creatine kinase. **Neuro:** dizziness, drowsiness, headache, impaired attention/concentration/thinking, SUICIDAL THOUGHTS/BEHAVIORS. **Resp:** RESPIRATORY DEPRESSION. **Misc:** fever, HYPERSENSITIVITY REACTIONS (including angioedema).

Interactions

Drug-Drug: Concurrent use with **pioglitazone** may ↑ risk of fluid retention. ↑ risk of CNS and respiratory depression with other **CNS depressants** including **opioids, alcohol, benzodiazepines**, or other **sedatives/hypnotics.**

Route/Dosage

Diabetic Neuropathic Pain

PO (Adults): *Immediate-release:* 50 mg 3 times daily, ↑ over 7 days up to 100 mg 3 times daily. *Extended-release:* 165 mg once daily after an evening meal; ↑ to 330 mg once daily after an evening meal within 1 wk.

Renal Impairment

PO (Adults): *CCr 30–60 mL/min:* Immediate-release: 75–300 mg/day in 2–3 divided doses; Extended-release: 82.5–330 mg once daily after an evening meal; *CCr 15–30 mL/min:* Immediate-release: 25–150 mg/day in 1–2 divided doses; *CCr <15 mL/min:* Immediate-release: 25–75 mg/day as a single daily dose.

Postherpetic Neuralgia

PO (Adults): *Immediate-release:* 75 mg twice daily or 50 mg 3 times daily initially, may ↑ over 7 days to 300 mg/day in 2–3 divided doses; after 2–4 wk may ↑ to 600 mg/day in 2–3 divided doses. *Extended-release:* 165 mg once daily after an evening meal; ↑ to 330 mg once daily after an evening meal within 1 wk; if pain is persistent after 2–4 wk, may then ↑ dose of up to 660 mg once daily after an evening meal.

Renal Impairment

PO (Adults): *CCr 30–60 mL/min:* Immediate-release: 75–300 mg/day in 2–3 divided doses; Extended-release: 82.5–330 mg once daily after an evening meal; *CCr 15–30 mL/min:* Immediate-release: 25–150 mg/day in 1–2 divided doses; *CCr <15 mL/min:* Immediate-release: 25–75 mg/day as a single daily dose.

Fibromyalgia

PO (Adults): *Immediate-release:* 75 mg twice daily initially, may ↑ to 150 mg twice daily within 1 wk based on efficacy and tolerability. May ↑ to 225 twice daily.

Renal Impairment

PO (Adults): *CCr 30–60 mL/min:* Immediate-release: 75–300 mg/day in 2–3 divided doses *CCr 15–30 mL/min:* Immediate-release: 25–150 mg/day in 1–2 divided doses; *CCr <15 mL/min:* Immediate-release: 25–75 mg/day as a single daily dose.

Spinal Cord Injury Neuropathic Pain

PO (Adults): *Immediate-release:* 75 mg twice daily initially, may be ↑ to 150 mg twice daily within 1 wk based on efficacy and tolerability; if insufficient pain relief after 2–3 wk, may ↑ to 300 twice daily.

Renal Impairment

PO (Adults): *CCr 30–60 mL/min:* Immediate-release: 75–300 mg/day in 2–3 divided doses; *CCr 15–30 mL/min:* Immediate-release: 25–150 mg/day in 1–2 divided doses; *CCr <15 mL/min:* Immediate-release: 25–75 mg/day as a single daily dose.

Partial Onset Seizures

PO (Adults): *Immediate-release:* 75 mg twice daily or 50 mg 3 times daily initially; may gradually ↑ on a weekly basis up to a max dose of 600 mg/day (in 2–3 divided doses).

PO (Children ≥1 mo and ≥30 kg): *Immediate-release:* 2.5 mg/kg/day in 2–3 divided doses; may gradually ↑ on a weekly basis up to a max dose of 10 mg/kg/day in 2–3 divided doses (max = 600 mg/day).

PO (Children ≥1 mo and <30 kg): *Immediate-release:* 3.5 mg/kg/day in 2–3 divided doses for patients ≥4 yr old or in 3 divided doses for patients 1 mo-<4 yr old; may gradually ↑ on a weekly basis up to a max dose of 14 mg/kg/day in 2–3 divided doses for patients ≥4 yr old or in 3 divided doses for patients 1 mo–<4 yr old.

Renal Impairment
PO (Adults): *CCr 30–60 mL/min:* Immediate-release: 75–300 mg/day in 2–3 divided doses; *CCr 15–30 mL/min:* Immediate-release: 25–150 mg/day in 1–2 divided doses; *CCr <15 mL/min:* Immediate-release: 25–75 mg/day as a single daily dose.

Availability (generic available)
Immediate-release capsules: 25 mg, 50 mg, 75 mg, 100 mg, 150 mg, 200 mg, 225 mg, 300 mg. **Extended-release tablets:** 82.5 mg, 165 mg, 330 mg. **Oral solution:** 20 mg/mL.

NURSING IMPLICATIONS
Assessment
* Monitor closely for notable changes in behavior that could indicate the emergence or worsening of suicidal thoughts or behavior, or depression.
* **Diabetic Peripheral Neuropathy, Postherpetic Neuralgia, Fibromyalgia, and Spinal Cord Injury Pain:** Assess location, characteristics, and intensity of pain periodically during therapy.
* **Seizures:** Assess location, duration, and characteristics of seizure activity.

Lab Test Considerations
* May cause ↑ creatine kinase levels.
* May cause ↓ platelet count.

Implementation
* Do not confuse Lyrica with Lopressor or Hydrea.
* Pregabalin should be discontinued gradually over at least 1 wk. Abrupt discontinuation may cause insomnia, nausea, headache, anxiety, sweating, and diarrhea when used for pain and may cause increase in seizure frequency when treating seizures.
* **PO:** May be administered without regard to meals. Oral solution may be stored at room temperature.

Patient/Family Teaching
* Instruct patient to take medication as directed. Take missed doses as soon as remembered unless almost time for next dose; do not double doses. Do not discontinue abruptly. Advise patient to read the *Patient Information Leaflet* prior to taking pregabalin and with each Rx refill in case of changes.
* May cause dizziness, drowsiness, and blurred vision. Caution patient to avoid driving or activities requiring alertness until response to medication is known. Advise patient to notify health care professional if changes in vision occur. Patients with seizures should not resume driving until health care professional gives clearance based on control of seizure disorder.
* Instruct patient to promptly report unexplained muscle pain, tenderness, or weakness, especially if

accompanied by malaise or fever. Discontinue therapy if myopathy is diagnosed or suspected or if markedly elevated creatine kinase levels occur.
* Advise patient and family to notify health care professional if thoughts about suicide or dying, attempts to commit suicide; new or worse depression; new or worse anxiety; feeling very agitated or restless; panic attacks; trouble sleeping; new or worse irritability; acting aggressive; being angry or violent; acting on dangerous impulses; an extreme increase in activity and talking, other unusual changes in behavior or mood occur.
* Inform patient that pregabalin may cause edema and weight gain.
* Advise patient to notify health care professional of all Rx or OTC medications, vitamins, or herbal products being taken and to consult with health care professional before taking other medications.
* Caution patient to avoid alcohol or other CNS depressants, including opioids, with pregabalin, may cause respiratory depression and overdose.
* Instruct patient to notify health care professional of medication regimen before treatment or surgery.
* Rep: Advise females of reproductive potential to notify health care professional if pregnancy is planned or suspected and to avoid breastfeeding during therapy. May impair male fertility. Encourage patients who become pregnant to enroll in the NAAED Pregnancy Registry by calling 1-800-233-2334. Information can be found at http://www.aedpregnancyregistry.org/.
* Advise patient to carry identification describing disease process and medication regimen at all times.

Evaluation/Desired Outcomes
* Decrease in intensity of chronic pain.
* Decrease in the frequency or cessation of seizures.

prochlorperazine
(proe-klor-**pair**-a-zeen)
~~Compazine~~, Compro,
✢ Prochlorazine
Classification
Therapeutic: antiemetics, antipsychotics
Pharmacologic: phenothiazines

Indications
Nausea and vomiting.

Action
Alters the effects of dopamine in the CNS. Possesses significant anticholinergic and alpha-adrenergic blocking activity. Depresses the chemoreceptor trigger zone in the CNS. **Therapeutic Effects:** Diminished nausea and vomiting.

Pharmacokinetics

Absorption: Absorption from tablet is variable; may be better with oral liquid formulations. Well absorbed after IM administration.

Distribution: Widely distributed, high concentrations in the CNS.

Protein Binding: ≥90%.

Metabolism and Excretion: Highly metabolized by the liver and GI mucosa.

Half-life: Unknown.

TIME/ACTION PROFILE (antiemetic effect)

ROUTE	ONSET	PEAK	DURATION
PO	30–40 min	unknown	3–4 hr
Rect	60 min	unknown	3–4 hr
IM	10–20 min	10–30 min	3–4 hr
IV	rapid (min)	10–30 min	3–4 hr

Contraindications/Precautions

Contraindicated in: Hypersensitivity; Cross-sensitivity with other phenothiazines may exist; Angle-closure glaucoma; Bone marrow depression; Severe liver or cardiovascular disease; Hypersensitivity to bisulfites or benzyl alcohol (some parenteral products); Pedi: Children <2 yr or <9.1 kg.

Use Cautiously in: Diabetes mellitus; Respiratory disease; Prostatic hypertrophy; CNS tumors; Seizure disorder; Intestinal obstruction; At risk for falls; OB: Safety not established in pregnancy; Lactation: Safety not established in breastfeeding; Geri: Dose ↓ recommended; ↑ risk of mortality in older adults treated for dementia-related psychosis.

Adverse Reactions/Side Effects

CV: ECG changes, hypotension, tachycardia. **Derm:** photosensitivity, pigment changes, rash. **EENT:** blurred vision, dry eyes, lens opacities. **Endo:** galactorrhea. **GI:** constipation, dry mouth, anorexia, hepatitis, ileus. **GU:** pink or reddish-brown discoloration of urine, urinary retention. **Hemat:** AGRANULOCYTOSIS, leukopenia. **Metab:** hyperthermia. **Neuro:** extrapyramidal reactions, NEUROLEPTIC MALIGNANT SYNDROME, sedation, tardive dyskinesia. **Misc:** allergic reactions.

Interactions

Drug-Drug: Additive hypotension with **antihypertensives**, **nitrates**, or acute ingestion of **alcohol**. Additive CNS depression with other **CNS depressants**, including **alcohol**, **antidepressants**, **antihistamines**, **opioid analgesics**, **sedative/hypnotics**, or **general anesthetics**. Additive anticholinergic effects with other **drugs possessing anticholinergic properties**, including **antihistamines**, some **antidepressants**, **atropine**, **haloperidol**, and other **phenothiazines**. **Lithium** ↑ risk of extrapyramidal reactions. May mask early signs of **lithium** toxicity. ↑ risk of agranulocytosis with **antithyroid agents**. ↓ beneficial effects of **levodopa**. **Antacids** may ↓ absorption.

Drug-Natural Products: Concomitant use of **kava-kava**, **valerian**, **chamomile**, or **hops** can ↑

CNS depression. ↑ anticholinergic effects with **angel's trumpet**, **jimson weed**, and **scopolia**.

Route/Dosage

Pediatric dose should not exceed 10 mg on the 1st day and then should not exceed 20 mg/day in children 2–5 yr or 25 mg/day in children 6–12 yr.

PO (Adults and Children ≥12 yr): 5–10 mg 3–4 times daily (not to exceed 40 mg/day).

PO (Children 18–39 kg): 2.5 mg 3 times daily *or* 5 mg twice daily (not to exceed 15 mg/day).

PO (Children 14–17 kg): 2.5 mg 2–3 times daily (not to exceed 10 mg/day).

PO (Children 9–13 kg): 2.5 mg 1–2 times daily (not to exceed 7.5 mg/day).

IM (Adults and Children ≥12 yr): 5–10 mg every 3–4 hr as needed. *Nausea/vomiting associated with surgery:* 5–10 mg; may be repeated once.

IM (Children 2–12 yr): 132 mcg (0.132 mg)/kg; usually only 1 dose is required.

IV (Adults and Children ≥12 yr): 2.5–10 mg (not to exceed 40 mg/day). *Nausea/vomiting associated with surgery:* 5–10 mg; may be repeated once.

Rect (Adults): 25 mg twice daily.

Rect (Children 18–39 kg): 2.5 mg 3 times daily or 5 mg twice daily (not to exceed 15 mg/day).

Rect (Children 14–17 kg): 2.5 mg 2–3 times daily (not to exceed 10 mg/day).

Rect (Children 9–13 kg): 2.5 mg 1–2 times daily (not to exceed 7.5 mg/day).

Availability (generic available)

Tablets: 5 mg, 10 mg. **Solution for injection:** 5 mg/mL (edisylate). **Suppositories:** ✱ 10 mg, 25 mg.

NURSING IMPLICATIONS

Assessment

- Monitor BP (sitting, standing, lying down), ECG, pulse, and respiratory rate before and frequently during the period of dosage adjustment. May cause Q-wave and T-wave changes in ECG.

- Assess patient for level of sedation after administration.

- Monitor patient for onset of akathisia (restlessness or desire to keep moving) and extrapyramidal side effects (*parkinsonian:* difficulty speaking or swallowing, loss of balance control, pill rolling, mask-like face, shuffling gait, rigidity, tremors; and *dystonic:* muscle spasms, twisting motions, twitching, inability to move eyes, weakness of arms or legs) every 2 mo during therapy and 8–12 wk after therapy has been discontinued. Report these symptoms; reduction in dose or discontinuation may be necessary. Trihexyphenidyl or diphenhydramine may be used to control these symptoms.

- Monitor for tardive dyskinesia (uncontrolled rhythmic movement of mouth, face, and extremities; lip smacking or puckering; puffing of cheeks; uncontrolled chewing; rapid or worm-like movements of tongue). Report immediately; may be irreversible.

- Monitor for development of neuroleptic malignant syndrome (fever, respiratory distress, tachycardia, seizures, diaphoresis, hypertension or hypotension, pallor, tiredness, severe muscle stiffness, loss of bladder control). Notify health care professional immediately if these symptoms occur.
- Assess for falls risk. Drowsiness, orthostatic hypotension, and motor and sensory instability increase risk. Institute prevention if indicated.
- **Antiemetic:** Assess patient for nausea and vomiting before and 30–60 min after administration.

Lab Test Considerations
- CBC and liver function tests should be evaluated periodically during therapy. May cause blood dyscrasias, especially between wk 4 and 10 of therapy. Hepatotoxicity is more likely to occur between wk 2 and 4 of therapy. May recur if medication is restarted. Liver function abnormalities may require discontinuation of therapy.
- May cause false-positive or false-negative pregnancy test results and false-positive urine bilirubin test results.
- May cause ↑ serum prolactin levels.

Implementation

- To prevent contact dermatitis, avoid getting solution on hands.
- Phenothiazines should be discontinued 48 hr before and not resumed for 24 hr after myelography; they lower seizure threshold.
- **PO:** Administer with food, milk, or a full glass of water to minimize gastric irritation.
- **IM:** Do not inject SUBQ. Inject slowly, deep into well-developed muscle. Keep patient recumbent for at least 30 min after injection to minimize hypotensive effects. Slight yellow color will not alter potency. Do not administer solution that is markedly discolored or that contains a precipitate.

IV Administration
- **IV Push:** *Concentration:* Dilute to a concentration of 1 mg/mL. *Rate:* Administer at a rate of 1 mg/min; not to exceed 5 mg/min.
- **Intermittent Infusion:** *Dilution:* Dilute 20 mg in up to 1 L dextrose, saline, Ringer's or LR, dextrose/saline, dextrose/Ringer's, or lactated Ringer's combinations.
- **Continuous Infusion:** Has been used as infusion with 20 mg/L of compatible solution.
- **Y-Site Compatibility:** acetaminophen, alemtuzumab, amikacin, amiodarone, anidulafungin, argatroban, arsenic trioxide, ascorbic acid, atracurium, atropine, azithromycin, benztropine, bleomycin, bumetanide, buprenorphine, butorphanol, carboplatin, carmustine, caspofungin, chlorpromazine, cisatracurium, cisplatin, cladribine, cyanocobalamin, cyclophosphamide, cyclosporine, cytarabine, dacarbazine, dactinomycin, daptomycin, daunorubi-

cin hydrochloride, dexmedetomidine, dexrazoxane, digoxin, diltiazem, diphenhydramine, dobutamine, docetaxel, dopamine, doxorubicin hydrochloride, doxorubicin liposomal, doxycycline, enalaprilat, ephedrine, epinephrine, epirubicin, eptifibatide, erythromycin, esmolol, etoposide, famotidine, fentanyl, fluconazole, gentamicin, glycopyrrolate, granisetron, hetastarch, hydrocortisone, hydromorphone, idarubicin, ifosfamide, irinotecan, isoproterenol, labetalol, LR, leucovorin calcium, lidocaine, linezolid, magnesium sulfate, mannitol, melphalan, meperidine, methotrexate, methylprednisolone, metoclopramide, metoprolol, metronidazole, milrinone, mitoxantrone, morphine, moxifloxacin, multivitamins, mycophenolate, nafcillin, nalbuphine, naloxone, nicardipine, nitroglycerin, norepinephrine, octreotide, ondansetron, oxacillin, oxaliplatin, oxytocin, paclitaxel, palonosetron, pamidronate, papaverine, penicillin G, phentolamine, phenylephrine, phytonadione, potassium acetate, potassium chloride, procainamide, promethazine, propofol, propranolol, protamine, pyridoxine, remifentanil, rituximab, rocuronium, sargramostim, sodium acetate, succinylcholine, sufentanil, tacrolimus, theophylline, thiamine, thiotepa, tigecycline, tirofiban, tobramycin, topotecan, trastuzumab, vancomycin, vasopressin, vecuronium, verapamil, vinblastine, vincristine, vinorelbine, zoledronic acid.
- **Y-Site Incompatibility:** acyclovir, aldesleukin, allopurinol, amifostine, aminophylline, amphotericin B deoxycholate, amphotericin B lipid complex, amphotericin B liposomal, ampicillin, ampicillin/sulbactam, azathioprine, aztreonam, bivalirudin, calcium chloride, cefazolin, cefepime, cefotaxime, cefotetan, cefoxitin, ceftazidime, ceftriaxone, cefuroxime, chloramphenicol, clindamycin, dantrolene, dexamethasone, epoetin alfa, ertapenem, etoposide phosphate, filgrastim, fludarabine, fluorouracil, folic acid, foscarnet, fosphenytoin, furosemide, ganciclovir, gemcitabine, gemtuzumab ozogamicin, heparin, imipenem/cilastatin, indomethacin, insulin regular, ketorolac, levofloxacin, midazolam, minocycline, mitomycin, nitroprusside, pantoprazole, pemetrexed, pentamidine, pentobarbital, phenobarbital, phenytoin, piperacillin/tazobactam, sodium bicarbonate, trimethoprim/sulfamethoxazole.

Patient/Family Teaching

- Instruct patient to take medication as directed, not to skip doses or double up on missed doses. Take missed doses as soon as remembered unless almost time for next dose. If more than 2 doses are scheduled each day, missed dose should be taken within about 1 hr of the ordered time. Abrupt withdrawal may lead to gastritis, nausea, vomiting, dizziness, headache, tachycardia, and insomnia.
- Inform patient of possibility of extrapyramidal symptoms and tardive dyskinesia. Instruct patient to re-

port these symptoms immediately to health care professional.

- Advise patient to change positions slowly to minimize orthostatic hypotension. Protect from falls.
- May cause drowsiness. Caution patient to avoid driving or other activities requiring alertness until response to medication is known.
- Caution patient to avoid alcohol and CNS depressants. Advise patient to notify health care professional of all Rx or OTC medications, vitamins, or herbal products being taken and to consult with health care professional before taking other medications and alcohol.
- Advise patient to use sunscreen and protective clothing when exposed to the sun to prevent photosensitivity reactions. Extremes in temperature should also be avoided, because this drug impairs body temperature regulation.
- Instruct patient to use frequent mouth rinses, good oral hygiene, and sugarless gum or candy to minimize dry mouth. Consult health care professional if dry mouth continues for >2 wk.
- Advise patient not to take prochlorperazine within 2 hr of antacids or antidiarrheal medication.
- Advise patient that increasing bulk and fluids in the diet and exercise may help minimize the constipating effects of this medication.
- Inform patient that this medication may turn urine pink to reddish-brown.
- Advise patient to notify health care professional of medication regimen before treatment or surgery.
- Instruct patient to notify health care professional promptly if sore throat, fever, unusual bleeding or bruising, skin rashes, weakness, tremors, visual disturbances, dark-colored urine, or clay-colored stools are noted.
- Rep: Advise female patients to notify health care professional if pregnancy is planned or suspected or if breastfeeding. Maternal use of phenothiazines may cause jaundice or hyper- or hyporeflexia in newborn infants. Use during 3rd trimester may ↑ risk for abnormal muscle movements (extrapyramidal symptoms) and withdrawal symptoms in newborns following delivery; may include agitation, feeding disorder, hypertonia, hypotonia, respiratory distress, somnolence, and tremor; may be self-limiting or require hospitalization. Monitor infants breastfed by a mother taking prochlorperazine for drowsiness, skin reactions, and hypotension.
- Emphasize the importance of routine follow-up exams to monitor response to medication and detect side effects. Periodic ocular exams are indicated. Encourage continued participation in psychotherapy as ordered by health care professional.

Evaluation/Desired Outcomes

- Relief of nausea and vomiting.

progesterone
(proe-**jess**-te-rone)
Crinone, Endometrin, Prometrium
Classification
Therapeutic: hormones
Pharmacologic: progestins

Indications

Crinone, Prometrium, and Oil for Injection: Secondary amenorrhea. **Oil for injection:** Abnormal uterine bleeding. **Prometrium:** Prevention of endometrial hyperplasia in postmenopausal women who have not had a hysterectomy (with estrogen). **Crinone and Endometrin:** Part of assisted reproductive technology in the management of infertility.

Action

Produces: Secretory changes in the endometrium, Increase in basal body temperature, Histologic changes in vaginal epithelium, Relaxation of uterine smooth muscle, Mammary alveolar tissue growth, Pituitary inhibition, Withdrawal bleeding in the presence of estrogen. **Therapeutic Effects:** Restoration of hormonal balance with control of uterine bleeding. Successful outcome in assisted reproduction.

Pharmacokinetics

Absorption: Micronization increases oral and vaginal absorption.
Distribution: Unknown.
Protein Binding: ≥90%.
Metabolism and Excretion: Metabolized by the liver; 50–60% eliminated by kidneys; 10% eliminated in feces.
Half-life: Several min.

TIME/ACTION PROFILE (plasma concentrations)

ROUTE	ONSET	PEAK	DURATION
PO	unknown	2–4 hr	unknown
Vaginal	unknown	34.8–55 hr	unknown
IM	unknown	19.6–28 hr	unknown

Contraindications/Precautions

Contraindicated in: Hypersensitivity; Hypersensitivity to parabens or sesame oil/seeds (IM suspension only); Hypersensitivity to peanuts (Prometrium only); Undiagnosed vaginal bleeding; Thromboembolic disease; Cerebrovascular disease; Severe hepatic impairment; Breast or genital cancer; Missed abortion; OB: Pregnancy.
Use Cautiously in: History of hepatic impairment; Cardiovascular disease; Depression; Lactation: Use while breastfeeding only if potential maternal benefit justifies potential risk to infant.

Adverse Reactions/Side Effects

CV: DEEP VEIN THROMBOSIS, edema, MI, thrombophlebitis. **Derm:** chloasma, melasma, rash. **EENT:** retinal thrombosis. **Endo:** amenorrhea, breakthrough bleeding, breast tenderness, changes in menstrual flow, galactorrhea, spotting. **GI:** ↓ weight, constipation, hepatitis, nausea. **GU:** cervical erosions, pelvic pain, vaginal discharge. **Local:** irritation or pain at IM injection site. **Metab:** ↑ weight. **Neuro:** depression, headache, STROKE. **Resp:** PULMONARY EMBOLISM. **Misc:** gingival bleeding, HYPERSENSITIVITY REACTIONS (including anaphylaxis and angioedema).

Interactions
Drug-Drug: May ↓ effectiveness of **bromocriptine** when used concurrently for galactorrhea and amenorrhea.

Route/Dosage
Secondary Amenorrhea
PO (Adults): 400 mg once daily in the evening for 10 days.
Vag (Adults): 45 mg (1 applicatorful of 4% gel) once every other day for up to 6 doses; may be ↑ to 90 mg (1 applicatorful of 8% gel) once every other day for up to 6 doses.
IM (Adults): 100–150 mg (single dose) or 5–10 mg once daily for 6–8 days given 8–10 days before expected menstrual period.

Abnormal Uterine Bleeding
IM (Adults): 5–10 mg once daily for 6 days.

Prevention of Endometrial Hyperplasia
PO (Adults): 200 mg once daily at bedtime for 12 days sequentially per 28-day cycle.

Assisted Reproductive Technology
Vag (Adults): *Patients who require progesterone supplementation:* 90 mg (1 applicatorful of 8% gel) once daily; if pregnancy occurs, may continue for up to 10–12 wk *or* 100 mg insert 2 or 3 times daily starting the day after oocyte retrieval and continuing for up to 10 wk total duration; *Patients with partial or complete ovarian failure who require progesterone replacement (intravaginal gel):* 90 mg (1 applicatorful of 8% gel) twice daily; if pregnancy occurs, may continue for up to 10–12 wk.

Availability (generic available)
Capsules (Prometrium): 100 mg, 200 mg. **Oil for injection:** 50 mg/mL. **Vaginal gel (Crinone):** 4%, 8%. **Vaginal insert (Endometrin):** 100 mg. *In combination with:* estradiol (Bijuva). See Appendix N.

NURSING IMPLICATIONS
Assessment
- Monitor BP periodically during therapy.
- Monitor intake and output ratios and weekly weight. Report significant discrepancies or steady weight gain.
- **Amenorrhea:** Assess patient's usual menstrual history. Administration of drug usually begins 8–10

days before anticipated menstruation. Withdrawal bleeding usually occurs 48–72 hr after course of therapy. Therapy should be discontinued if menses occur during injection series.
- **Dysfunctional Bleeding:** Monitor pattern and amount of vaginal bleeding (pad count). Bleeding should end by 6th day of therapy. Therapy should be discontinued if menses occur during injection series.

Lab Test Considerations
- Monitor hepatic function before and periodically during therapy.
- May cause ↑ alkaline phosphatase levels.
- May ↓ pregnanediol excretion concentrations.
- May cause ↑ serum concentrations of low-density lipoprotein cholesterol and ↓ concentrations of high-density lipoprotein cholesterol.
- May alter thyroid function test results.

Implementation
- **PO:** Administer at bedtime. For patients who experience difficulty swallowing the capsules, take with a full glass of water while in the standing position.
- **IM:** Shake vial before preparing IM dose. Administer deep IM. Rotate sites.
- **Vag:** Vaginal gel and insert are administered with disposable applicator provided by manufacturer.
- If dose increase is required from 4% gel to 8% gel, doubling the volume of the 4% gel will not accomplish dose increase; changing to 8% gel is required.

Patient/Family Teaching
- Explain purpose of progesterone to patient.
- Advise patient to report signs and symptoms of fluid retention (swelling of ankles and feet, weight gain), thromboembolic disorders (pain, swelling, tenderness in extremities, headache, chest pain, blurred vision), mental depression, or hepatic impairment (yellowed skin or eyes, pruritus, dark urine, light-colored stools) to health care professional.
- Instruct patient to notify health care professional if change in vaginal bleeding pattern or spotting occurs.
- Caution patient to use sunscreen and protective clothing to prevent photosensitivity reactions.
- Advise patient to notify health care professional of medication regimen before treatment or surgery.
- Rep: Advise females of reproductive potential to notify health care professional immediately if pregnancy is planned or suspected, or if breastfeeding.
- Emphasize the importance of routine follow-up physical exams, including BP; breast, abdomen, and pelvic examinations; and Pap smears.
- **Vag:** Instruct patient not to use vaginal gel concurrently with other vaginal agents. If these agents must be used concurrently, administer at least 6 hr before or after vaginal gel. Small, white globules may ap-

pear as a vaginal discharge possibly due to gel accumulation, even several days after use.

Evaluation/Desired Outcomes

• Reduction of uterine bleeding.
• Successful outcome in assisted reproduction.

propofol (proe-poe-fol)
Diprivan
Classification
Therapeutic: general anesthetics

Indications

Induction of general anesthesia in children >3 yr and adults. Maintenance of balanced anesthesia when used with other agents in children >2 mo and adults. Initiation and maintenance of monitored anesthesia care. Sedation of intubated, mechanically ventilated patients in intensive care units (ICUs).

Action

Short-acting hypnotic. Mechanism of action is unknown. Produces amnesia. Has no analgesic properties. **Therapeutic Effects:** Induction and maintenance of anesthesia.

Pharmacokinetics

Absorption: IV administration results in complete bioavailability.
Distribution: Rapidly and widely distributed. Crosses the blood-brain barrier well; rapidly redistributed to other tissues.
Protein Binding: 95–99%.
Metabolism and Excretion: Rapidly metabolized by the liver. Primarily excreted in urine as metabolites.
Half-life: 3–12 hr (blood-brain equilibration half-life 2.9 min).

TIME/ACTION PROFILE (loss of consciousness)

ROUTE	ONSET	PEAK	DURATION†
IV	40 sec	unknown	3–5 min

†Time to recovery is 8 min (up to 19 min if opioid analgesics have been used).

Contraindications/Precautions

Contraindicated in: Hypersensitivity to propofol, soybean oil, egg lecithin, or glycerol; OB: Crosses placenta; may cause neonatal depression; may affect child's brain development when used during 3rd trimester.
Use Cautiously in: Cardiovascular disease; Lipid disorders (emulsion may have detrimental effect); ↑ intracranial pressure; Cerebrovascular disorders; Hypovolemic patients (lower induction and maintenance dosage ↓ recommended); Lactation: Safety not established in breastfeeding; Pedi: Not recommended for induction of anesthesia in children <3 yr, or for mainte-

nance of anesthesia in infants <2 mo; not for ICU or pre-procedure sedation; may affect brain development in children <3 yr; Geri: Lower induction and maintenance dose ↓ recommended in older adults.

Adverse Reactions/Side Effects

CV: bradycardia, hypotension, hypertension. **Derm:** flushing. **GI:** abdominal cramping, hiccups, nausea, vomiting. **GU:** discoloration of urine (green). **Local:** burning, pain, stinging, coldness, numbness, tingling at IV site. **MS:** involuntary muscle movements, perioperative myoclonia. **Neuro:** dizziness, headache. **Resp:** APNEA, cough. **Misc:** fever, PROPOFOL INFUSION SYNDROME.

Interactions

Drug-Drug: Additive CNS and respiratory depression with **alcohol**, **antihistamines**, **opioid analgesics**, and **sedative/hypnotics** (dose ↓ may be required). **Theophylline** may antagonize the CNS effects of propofol. Cardiorespiratory instability can occur when used with **acetazolamide**. Serious bradycardia can occur with concurrent use of **fentanyl** in children. ↑ risk of hypertriglyceridemia with **intravenous fat emulsion**.

Route/Dosage

General Anesthesia

IV (Adults <55 yr): *Induction:* 40 mg every 10 sec until induction achieved (2–2.5 mg/kg total). *Maintenance:* 100–200 mcg/kg/min. Rates of 150–200 mcg/kg/min are usually required during first 10–15 min after induction, then ↓ by 30–50% during first 30 min of maintenance. Rates of 50–100 mcg/kg/min are associated with optimal recovery time. May also be given intermittently in increments of 25–50 mg.
IV (Geriatric Patients, Cardiac Patients, Debilitated Patients, or Hypovolemic Patients): *Induction:* 20 mg every 10 sec until induction achieved (1–1.5 mg/kg total). *Maintenance:* 50–100 mcg/kg/min (dose in cardiac anesthesia ranges from 50–150 mcg/kg/min depending on concurrent use of opioid).
IV (Adults Undergoing Neurosurgical Procedures): *Induction:* 20 mg every 10 sec until induction achieved (1–2 mg/kg total). *Maintenance:* 100–200 mcg/kg/min.
IV (Children ≥3 yr–16 yr): *Induction:* 2.5–3.5 mg/kg, use lower dose for children ASA III or IV.
IV (Children 2 mo–16 yr): *Maintenance:* 125–300 mcg/kg/min (following first 30 min of maintenance, rate should be ↓ if possible), younger children may require larger infusion rates compared to older children.

Monitored Anesthesia Care Sedation

IV (Adults <55 yr): *Initiation:* 100–150 mcg/kg/min infusion or 0.5 mg/kg as slow injection. *Maintenance:* 25–75 mcg/kg/min infusion or incremental boluses of 10–20 mg.
IV (Geriatric Patients, Debilitated Patients, or ASA III/IV Patients): *Initiation:* Use slower infusion or injection rates. *Maintenance:* 20% less than the

usual adult infusion dose; rapid/repeated bolus dosing should be avoided.

ICU Sedation
IV (Adults): 5 mcg/kg/min for a minimum of 5 min. Additional increments of 5–10 mcg/kg/min over 5–10 min may be given until desired response is obtained. (Range 5–50 mcg/kg/min.) Dose should be reassessed every 24 hr.

Availability (generic available)
Lipid emulsion for injection: 10 mg/mL.

NURSING IMPLICATIONS
Assessment
- Assess respiratory status, pulse, and BP continuously throughout propofol therapy. Frequently causes apnea lasting ≥60 sec. Maintain patent airway and adequate ventilation. Propofol should be used only by individuals experienced in endotracheal intubation, and equipment for this procedure should be readily available.
- Assess level of sedation and level of consciousness throughout and following administration.
- When using for ICU sedation, wake-up and assessment of CNS function should be done daily during maintenance to determine minimum dose required for sedation. Maintain a light level of sedation during these assessments; do not discontinue. Abrupt discontinuation may cause rapid awakening with anxiety, agitation, and resistance to mechanical ventilation.
- Assess injection site for pain; may be minimized if larger veins of the forearm or antecubital fossa are used, especially in pediatric patients. Pain may be reduced by a prior injection of intravenous lidocaine (1 mL of a 1% solution). Monitor for extravasation.
- Monitor for propofol infusion syndrome (severe metabolic acidosis, hyperkalemia, lipemia, rhabdomyolysis, hepatomegaly, cardiac and renal failure). Most frequent with prolonged, high-dose infusions (>5 mg/kg/hr for >48 hr) but has also been reported following large-dose, short-term infusions during surgical anesthesia. If prolonged sedation or increasing dose is required, or metabolic acidosis occurs, consider alternative means of sedation.

Toxicity and Overdose
- If overdose occurs, monitor pulse, respiration, and BP continuously. Maintain patent airway and assist ventilation as needed. If hypotension occurs, treatment includes IV fluids, repositioning, and vasopressors.

Implementation
- Do not confuse Diprivan with Diflucan.
- Dose is titrated to patient response.
- Propofol has no effect on the pain threshold. Adequate analgesia should *always* be used when propofol is used as an adjunct to surgical procedures.

IV Administration
- **IV Push:** *Dilution:* Usually administered undiluted. If dilution is necessary, use only D5W. Shake well before use. Solution is opaque, making detection of contaminants difficult. Do not use if separation of the emulsion is evident. Contains no preservatives; maintain sterile technique and administer immediately after preparation. *Concentration:* Undiluted: 10 mg/mL. If dilution is necessary, dilute to concentration ≥2 mg/mL.
- Discard unused portions and IV lines at the end of anesthetic procedure or within 6 hr. For ICU sedation, discard after 12 hr if administered directly from vial or after 6 hr if transferred to a syringe or other container. Do not administer via filter <5–micron pore size.
- Aseptic technique is essential. Solution is capable of rapid growth of bacterial contaminants. Infections and subsequent deaths have been reported. *Rate:* Administer over 3–5 min. Titrate to desired level of sedation. Frequently causes pain, burning, and stinging at injection site; use larger veins of the forearm, antecubital fossa, or a dedicated IV catheter. Lidocaine 10–20 mg IV may be administered prior to injection to minimize pain. Pedi: Induction doses may be administered over 20–30 sec.
- **Intermittent/Continuous Infusion:** *Dilution:* Administer undiluted. Allow 3 to 5 min between dose adjustments to allow for and assess the clinical effects. *Concentration:* 10 mg/mL. *Rate:* Based on patient's weight (see Route/Dosage section).
- **Solution Compatibility:** D5W, LR, D5/LR, D5/0.45% NaCl, D5/0.2% NaCl.
- **Y-Site Compatibility:** acyclovir, aminophylline, ampicillin, aztreonam, bumetanide, buprenorphine, butorphanol, calcium gluconate, carboplatin, cefazolin, cefepime, cefotaxime, cefotetan, cefoxitin, ceftaroline, cefuroxime, chlorpromazine, cisplatin, clindamycin, cyclophosphamide, cyclosporine, cytarabine, dexamethasone, dexmedetomidine, diphenhydramine, droperidol, enalaprilat, epinephrine, esmolol, famotidine, fentanyl, fluconazole, fluorouracil, furosemide, glycopyrrolate, granisetron, haloperidol, heparin, hydrocortisone, hydromorphone, ifosfamide, imipenem/cilastatin, insulin regular, isoproterenol, ketamine, labetalol, lorazepam, mannitol, meperidine, milrinone, nafcillin, nalbuphine, naloxone, nitroprusside, norepinephrine, paclitaxel, palonosetron, pentobarbital, phenobarbital, potassium chloride, prochlorperazine, propranolol, sodium bicarbonate, sufentanil, tigecycline.
- **Y-Site Incompatibility:** acetaminophen, amikacin, calcium chloride, ciprofloxacin, cisatracurium, diazepam, digoxin, doxorubicin hydrochloride, eravacycline, gentamicin, isavuconazonium, LR, levofloxacin, methotrexate, methylprednisolone,

P

---

metoclopramide, metronidazole, mitoxantrone, phenytoin, plazomicin, tobramycin, verapamil.

Patient/Family Teaching

- Inform patient that this medication will decrease mental recall of the procedure.
- May cause drowsiness or dizziness. Advise patient to request assistance prior to ambulation and transfer and to avoid driving or other activities requiring alertness for 24 hr following administration.
- Advise patient to avoid alcohol or other CNS depressants, including opioids, without the advice of a health care professional for 24 hr following administration.
- Rep: Advise females of reproductive potential to notify health care professional if pregnancy is planned or suspected or if breastfeeding. Monitor neonates for hypotension and sedation following maternal exposure to propofol.

Evaluation/Desired Outcomes

- Induction and maintenance of anesthesia.
- Sedation in mechanically ventilated patients in an intensive care setting.

HIGH ALERT

ⵊ propranolol
(proe-**pran**-oh-lole)
Hemangeol, ~~Inderal~~, Inderal LA, Inderal XL, InnoPran XL

Classification
Therapeutic: antianginals, antiarrhythmics (Class II), antihypertensives, vascular headache suppressants
Pharmacologic: beta blockers

Indications

Hypertension, angina, arrhythmias, hypertrophic cardiomyopathy, thyrotoxicosis, essential tremors, pheochromocytoma (all but Hemangeol). Prevention and management of MI, and the prevention of vascular headaches (all but Hemangeol). Proliferating infantile hemangioma requiring systemic therapy (Hemangeol only). **Unlabeled Use:** Also used to manage alcohol withdrawal, aggressive behavior, antipsychotic-associated akathisia, situational anxiety, and esophageal varices. Post-traumatic stress disorder (PTSD).

Action

Blocks stimulation of beta₁ (myocardial) and beta₂ (pulmonary, vascular, and uterine)-adrenergic receptor sites; its mechanism for the treatment of infantile hemangiomas is unknown. **Therapeutic Effects:** Decreased heart rate and BP. Suppression of arrhythmias. Prevention of MI. Prevention of vascular headaches. Hemangioma resolution.

Pharmacokinetics

Absorption: Well absorbed but undergoes extensive first-pass hepatic metabolism.

Distribution: Moderate CNS penetration. Crosses the placenta; enters breast milk.
Protein Binding: 93%.
Metabolism and Excretion: Almost completely metabolized by the liver (primarily for CYP2D6 isoenzyme) ⵊ (the CYP2D6 enzyme system exhibits genetic polymorphism; ~7% of population may be poor metabolizers and may have significantly ↑ propranolol concentrations and an ↑ risk of adverse effects).
Half-life: 3.4–6 hr.

TIME/ACTION PROFILE (cardiovascular effects)

ROUTE	ONSET	PEAK	DURATION
PO	30 min	60–90 min†	6–12 hr
PO–ER	unknown	6 hr	24 hr
IV	immediate	1 min	4–6 hr

†Following single dose, full effect not seen until several wk of therapy.

Contraindications/Precautions

Contraindicated in: Hypersensitivity; Uncompensated HF; Pulmonary edema; Cardiogenic shock; Bradycardia, sick sinus syndrome, or heart block (unless pacemaker present); Premature infants with corrected age <5 wk (Hemangeol only); Asthma or history of bronchospasm (Hemangeol only); BP <50/30 mmHg (Hemangeol only); Pheochromocytoma (Hemangeol only); Pedi: Infants <2 kg (Hemangeol only).
Use Cautiously in: Renal or hepatic impairment; Pulmonary disease (including asthma); Diabetes mellitus (may mask signs of hypoglycemia); Thyrotoxicosis (may mask symptoms); History of severe allergic reactions (may ↑ intensity of response); Skeletal muscle disease (may exacerbate myopathy); OB: Crosses the placenta and may cause fetal/neonatal bradycardia, hypotension, hypoglycemia, or respiratory depression. May also ↓ blood supply to the placenta, ↑ the risk for premature birth or fetal death, and cause intrauterine growth retardation. May ↑ risk of cardiac and pulmonary complications in the infant during the neonatal time frame. Lactation: Safety not established in breastfeeding; Pedi: ↑ risk of hypoglycemia in children, especially during periods of fasting such as before surgery, during prolonged exertion, or with coexisting renal insufficiency; Geri: Older adults may have ↑ sensitivity to beta blockers; initial dose reduction and careful titration recommended.

Adverse Reactions/Side Effects

CV: ARRHYTHMIAS, BRADYCARDIA, HF, orthostatic hypotension, peripheral vasoconstriction, PULMONARY EDEMA. **Derm:** ERYTHEMA MULTIFORME, EXFOLIATIVE DERMATITIS, itching, rash, STEVENS-JOHNSON SYNDROME (SJS), TOXIC EPIDERMAL NECROLYSIS. **EENT:** blurred vision, dry eyes, nasal stuffiness. **Endo:** hyperglycemia, hypoglycemia (↑ in children). **GI:** constipation, diarrhea, nausea. **GU:** erectile dysfunction, ↓ libido. **MS:** arthralgia, back pain, muscle cramps, myopathy.
Neuro: fatigue, weakness, anxiety, depression, dizzi-

ness, drowsiness, insomnia, memory loss, mental status changes, nervousness, nightmares, paresthesia. **Resp:** bronchospasm, wheezing. **Misc:** drug-induced lupus syndrome, HYPERSENSITIVITY REACTIONS (including anaphylaxis).

Interactions

Drug-Drug: General anesthesia, **IV phenytoin**, and **verapamil** may cause additive myocardial depression. Additive bradycardia may occur with **digoxin**. Additive hypotension may occur with other **antihypertensives**, acute ingestion of **alcohol**, or **nitrates**. Levels may be ↓ with chronic **alcohol** use. Concurrent use with **amphetamines**, **cocaine**, **ephedrine**, **epinephrine**, **norepinephrine**, **phenylephrine**, or **pseudoephedrine** may result in unopposed alpha-adrenergic stimulation (excessive hypertension, bradycardia). Concurrent **thyroid** administration may ↓ effectiveness. May alter the effectiveness of **insulin** or **oral hypoglycemics** (dose adjustments may be necessary). May ↓ effectiveness of **beta-adrenergic bronchodilators** and **theophylline**. May ↓ beneficial beta cardiovascular effects of **dopamine** or **dobutamine**. Use cautiously within 14 days of **MAO inhibitor** therapy (may result in hypertension). **Cimetidine** may ↑ blood levels and toxicity. Concurrent **NSAIDs** may ↓ antihypertensive action. **Smoking** ↑ metabolism and ↓ effects; smoking cessation may ↑ effects. May ↑ levels of **lidocaine** and **bupivacaine**.

Route/Dosage

PO (Adults): *Antianginal:* 80–320 mg/day in 2–4 divided doses or once daily as extended/sustained-release capsules. *Antihypertensive:* 40 mg twice daily initially; may be ↑ as needed (usual range 120–240 mg/day; doses up to 1 g/day have been used); *or* 80 mg once daily as extended/sustained-release capsules, ↑ as needed up to 120 mg. *InnoPran XL* dosing form is designed to be given once daily at bedtime. *Antiarrhythmic:* 10–30 mg 3–4 times daily. *Prevention of MI:* 180–240 mg/day in divided doses. *Hypertrophic cardiomyopathy:* 20–40 mg 3–4 times daily. *Adjunct therapy of pheochromocytoma:* 20 mg 3 times daily to 40 mg 3–4 times daily concurrently with alpha-blocking therapy, started 3 days before surgery is planned. *Vascular headache prevention:* 20 mg 4 times daily *or* 80 mg/day as extended/sustained-release capsules; may be ↑ as needed up to 240 mg/day. *Management of tremor:* 40 mg twice daily; may be ↑ up to 120 mg/day (up to 320 mg have been used).

PO (Children): *Antihypertensive/antiarrhythmic:* 0.5–1 mg/kg/day in 2–4 divided doses; may be ↑ as needed (usual range for maintenance dose is 2–4 mg/kg/day in 2 divided doses).

PO (Children 5 wk–5 mo): *Infantile hemangioma:* 0.6 mg/kg twice daily (at least 9 hr apart); after 1 wk, ↑ to 1.1 mg/kg twice daily; after another wk, ↑ to 1.7 mg/kg twice daily and maintain for 6 mo.

IV (Adults): *Antiarrhythmic:* 1–3 mg; may be repeated after 2 min and again in 4 hr if needed.
IV (Children): *Antiarrhythmic:* 10–100 mcg (0.01–0.1 mg)/kg (up to 1 mg/dose); may be repeated every 6–8 hr if needed.

Availability (generic available)

Immediate-release tablets: 10 mg, 20 mg, 40 mg, 60 mg, 80 mg. **Extended-release capsules:** 60 mg, 80 mg, 120 mg, 160 mg. **Oral solution:** 20 mg/5 mL, 40 mg/5 mL. **Oral solution (Hemangeol):** 4.28 mg/mL. **Solution for injection:** 1 mg/mL. *In combination with:* hydrochlorothiazide (generic only).

NURSING IMPLICATIONS

Assessment

- Monitor BP and pulse frequently during dose adjustment period and periodically during therapy.
- Abrupt withdrawal of propranolol may precipitate life-threatening arrhythmias, hypertension, or myocardial ischemia. Drug should be tapered over a 2-wk period before discontinuation. Assess patient carefully during tapering and after medication is discontinued. Consider that patients taking propranolol for non-cardiac indications may have undiagnosed cardiac disease. Abrupt discontinuation or withdrawal over too-short a period of time (less than 9 days) should be avoided.
- Pedi: Assess pediatric patients for signs and symptoms of hypoglycemia, particularly when oral foods and fluids are restricted.
- Patients receiving **propranolol IV** must have continuous ECG monitoring and may have pulmonary capillary wedge pressure (PCWP) or central venous pressure (CVP) monitoring during and for several hrs after administration.
- Assess for orthostatic hypotension when assisting patient up from supine position.
- Monitor intake and output ratios and daily weight. Assess patient routinely for evidence of fluid overload (peripheral edema, dyspnea, rales/crackles, fatigue, weight gain, jugular venous distention).
- Assess for rash periodically during therapy. May cause SJS. Discontinue therapy if severe or if accompanied with fever, general malaise, fatigue, muscle or joint aches, blisters, oral lesions, conjunctivitis, hepatitis and/or eosinophilia.
- **Angina:** Assess frequency and characteristics of anginal attacks periodically during therapy.
- **Vascular Headache Prophylaxis:** Assess frequency, severity, characteristics, and location of vascular headaches periodically during therapy.
- **PTSD:** Assess frequency of symptoms (flashbacks, nightmares, efforts to avoid thoughts or activities that may trigger memories of the trauma, and hypervigilance) periodically during therapy.
- **Infantile Hemangioma:** Monitor heart rate and BP for 2 hr after propranolol initiation or dose in-

P

---

creases. May worsen bradycardia or hypotension. Discontinue if symptomatic bradycardia (<80 beats per min) or hypotension (systolic BP <50 mmHg) occurs.

Lab Test Considerations

● May cause ↑ BUN, serum lipoprotein, potassium, triglyceride, and uric acid levels.

● May cause ↑ ANA titers.

● May cause ↓ or ↑ in blood glucose levels. In labile diabetic patients, hypoglycemia may be accompanied by precipitous ↑ of BP.

Toxicity and Overdose

● Monitor patients receiving beta blockers for signs of overdose (bradycardia, severe dizziness or fainting, severe drowsiness, dyspnea, bluish fingernails or palms, seizures). Notify health care professional immediately if these signs occur.

● Hypotension may be treated with modified Trendelenburg position and IV fluids unless contraindicated. Vasopressors (epinephrine, norepinephrine, dopamine, dobutamine) may also be used. Hypotension does not respond to beta agonists.

● Glucagon has been used to treat bradycardia and hypotension.

Implementation

● *High Alert:* IV vasoactive medications are inherently dangerous. Before administering intravenously, have second practitioner independently check the original order, dose calculations, and infusion pump settings. Also, patient harm or fatalities have occurred when switching from oral to IV propranolol; oral and parenteral doses are not interchangeable. IV dose is 1/10 of the oral dose. Change to oral therapy as soon as possible.

● *High Alert:* Do not confuse Inderal with Adderall .

● **PO:** Take apical pulse prior to administering. If <50 bpm or if arrhythmia occurs, hold medication and notify health care professional.

● Administer with meals or directly after eating to enhance absorption.

● *DNC:* Swallow extended release tablets whole; do not crush, break, or chew.Propranolol tablets may be crushed and mixed with food.

● Administer *Innopran XL* tablets at bedtime and take consistently either on an empty stomach for with food. Avoid discontinuing abruptly, especially in patients with ischemic heart disease. Gradually decrease dose over 1 – 2 wk. If angina markedly worsens or acute coronary insufficiency develops, promptly resume therapy, at least temporarily and take other measures for management of unstable angina.

● Mix propranolol oral solution with liquid or semisolid food (water, juices, applesauce, puddings). To ensure entire dose is taken, rinse glass with more liquid or have patient consume all of the applesauce or pudding. Do not store after mixing.

● Administer *Hemangeol* during or right after a feeding to prevent hypoglycemia. Skip dose if child is not eating or is vomiting. Administer using oral syringe provided; if necessary may be diluted in small amount of milk or fruit juice and given in baby's bottle.

IV Administration

● **IV Push:** *Dilution:* Administer undiluted or dilute each 1 mg in 10 mL of D5W for injection. *Concentration:* Undiluted: 1 mg/mL. Diluted in 10 mL of D5W: 0.1 mg/mL. *Rate:* Administer at 0.5 mg/min for adults to avoid hypotension and cardiac arrest; do not exceed 1 mg/min. Pedi: Administer over 10 min.

● **Intermittent Infusion:** *Dilution:* May be diluted in 50 mL of 0.9% NaCl, D5W, D5/0.45% NaCl, D5/0.9% NaCl, or LR. *Concentration:* Depends on dose. *Rate:* Infuse over 10 – 15 min.

● **Y-Site Compatibility:** acyclovir, alemtuzumab, alteplase, amikacin, aminocaproic acid, aminophylline, amiodarone, anidulafungin, argatroban, arsenic trioxide, ascorbic acid, atropine, azathioprine, aztreonam, benztropine, bivalirudin, bleomycin, bumetanide, buprenorphine, butorphanol, calcium chloride, calcium gluconate, carboplatin, carmustine, caspofungin, cefazolin, cefotaxime, cefotetan, cefoxitin, ceftazidime, ceftriaxone, cefuroxime, chloramphenicol, chlorpromazine, cisplatin, clindamycin, cyanocobalamin, cyclophosphamide, cyclosporine, cytarabine, dacarbazine, dactinomycin, daptomycin, daunorubicin hydrochloride, dexamethasone, dexmedetomidine, dexrazoxane, digoxin, diltiazem, diphenhydramine, dobutamine, docetaxel, dopamine, doxorubicin hydrochloride, doxorubicin liposomal, doxycycline, enalaprilat, ephedrine, epinephrine, epirubicin, epoetin alfa, eptifibatide, ertapenem, erythromycin, esmolol, etoposide, etoposide phosphate, famotidine, fentanyl, fluconazole, fludarabine, fluorouracil, folic acid, foscarnet, fosphenytoin, furosemide, ganciclovir, gemcitabine, gemtuzumab ozogamicin, gentamicin, glycopyrrolate, granisetron, heparin, hetastarch, hydrocortisone, hydromorphone, idarubicin, ifosfamide, imipenem/cilastatin, irinotecan, isoproterenol, ketorolac, labetalol, LR, leucovorin calcium, levofloxacin, lidocaine, linezolid, lorazepam, magnesium sulfate, mannitol, meperidine, meropenem, mesna, methadone, methohexital, methotrexate, methylprednisolone, metoclopramide, metoprolol, metronidazole, midazolam, milrinone, mitoxantrone, morphine, moxifloxacin, multivitamins, mycophenolate, nafcillin, nalbuphine, naloxone, nicardipine, nitroglycerin, nitroprusside, norepinephrine, octreotide, ondansetron, oxacillin, oxaliplatin, oxytocin, palonosetron, pamidronate, papaverine, pemetrexed, penicillin G, pentamidine, pentobarbital, phenobarbital, phentolamine, phenylephrine, phytonadione, potassium acetate, potassium chloride, procainamide, prochlorperazine, promethazine, propofol, protamine, pyridoxine, rocuronium, sodium acetate, sodium bicarbonate, succinylcholine, sufentanil, tacrolimus, theophylline, thiamine, thiotepa, tigecycline, tirofiban, tobramycin, topotecan, vancomycin, vasopressin, vecuronium, verapamil, vinblastine, vincristine, vinorelbine, voriconazole, zoledronic acid.

- **Y-Site Incompatibility:** amphotericin B deoxycholate, amphotericin B lipid complex, amphotericin B liposomal, dantrolene, diazepam, indomethacin, insulin regular, mitomycin, paclitaxel, pantoprazole, phenytoin, piperacillin/tazobactam, trimethoprim/sulfamethoxazole.

Patient/Family Teaching

- Instruct patient to take medication as directed, at the same time each day, even if feeling well; do not skip or double up on missed doses. Take missed doses as soon as possible up to 4 hr before next dose (8 hr with extended-release propranolol). Inform patient that abrupt withdrawal can cause life-threatening arrhythmias, hypertension, or myocardial ischemia. Advise parent to read medication guide prior to starting and with each Rx refill in case of changes in *Hemangeol.*
- Advise patient to make sure enough medication is available for weekends, holidays, and vacations. A written prescription may be kept in wallet in case of emergency.
- Teach patient and family how to check pulse daily and BP biweekly. Advise patient to hold dose and contact health care professional if pulse is <50 bpm or BP changes significantly.
- May cause drowsiness or dizziness. Caution patients to avoid driving or other activities that require alertness until response to the drug is known.
- Advise patients to change positions slowly to minimize orthostatic hypotension, especially during initiation of therapy or when dose is increased.
- Caution patient that this medication may increase sensitivity to cold.
- Instruct patient to notify health care professional of all Rx or OTC medications, vitamins, or herbal products being taken and to consult health care professional before taking other Rx, OTC, or herbal products, especially NSAIDs and cold preparations, concurrently with this medication.
- Advise diabetic patients to closely monitor blood sugar, especially if weakness, malaise, irritability, or fatigue occurs. Medication may mask some signs of hypoglycemia, but dizziness and sweating may still occur. Acute hypertension may occur following insulin-induced hypoglycemia in patients receiving propranolol. Instruct parents/caregivers of children receiving *Hemangeol* how to recognize signs of hypoglycemia, and to notify health care professional and take child to nearest emergency department if hypoglycemia is suspected.
- Advise patient to notify health care professional if slow pulse, difficulty breathing, wheezing, cold hands and feet, dizziness, light-headedness, confusion, depression, rash, fever, sore throat, unusual bleeding, or bruising occurs.
- Instruct patient to inform health care professional of medication regimen prior to treatment or surgery.
- Rep: Advise females of reproductive potential to notify health care professional if pregnancy is planned or suspected or if breastfeeding. Monitor neonates exposed to propranolol during pregnancy for bradycardia, hypotension, hypoglycemia, and respiratory depression. May also ↓ blood supply to placenta, ↑ risk for premature birth or fetal death, and cause intrauterine growth retardation. May ↑ risk of cardiac and pulmonary complications in the infant during the neonatal time frame.
- Advise patient to carry identification describing disease process and medication regimen at all times.
- **Hypertension:** Reinforce the need to continue additional therapies for hypertension (weight loss, sodium restriction, stress reduction, regular exercise, moderation of alcohol consumption, and smoking cessation). Medication controls but does not cure hypertension.
- **Angina:** Caution patient to avoid overexertion with decrease in chest pain.
- **Vascular Headache Prophylaxis:** Caution patient that sharing this medication may be dangerous.
- **PTSD:** Advise patient that medication may relieve distressing symptoms but that psychotherapy is the primary treatment for the disorder. Refer patient and family to a PTSD support group.

Evaluation/Desired Outcomes

- Decrease in BP.
- Control of arrhythmias without appearance of detrimental side effects.
- Reduction in frequency of anginal attacks.
- Increase in activity tolerance.
- Prevention of MI.
- Prevention of vascular headaches.
- Management of thyrotoxicosis.
- Management of pheochromocytoma.
- Decrease in tremors.
- Management of hypertrophic cardiomyopathy.
- Decrease in symptoms associated with PTSD.
- Resolution of infantile hemangioma (Hemangeol only).

protamine (proe-ta-meen)

Classification
Therapeutic: antidotes
Pharmacologic: antiheparins

Indications

Acute management of severe heparin overdosage. Used to neutralize heparin received during dialysis, cardiopulmonary bypass, and other procedures. **Unlabeled**

Use: Management of overdose of heparin-like compounds.

Action

A strong base that forms a complex with heparin (an acid). **Therapeutic Effects:** Inactivation of heparin.

Pharmacokinetics

Absorption: IV administration results in complete bioavailability.
Distribution: Unknown.
Metabolism and Excretion: Metabolic fate not known. Protamine-heparin complex eventually degrades.
Half-life: 7 min.

TIME/ACTION PROFILE (reversal of heparin effect)

ROUTE	ONSET	PEAK	DURATION
IV	30 sec–1 min	unknown	2 hr†

†Depends on body temperature.

Contraindications/Precautions

Contraindicated in: Hypersensitivity to protamine or fish.
Use Cautiously in: Patients who have received previous protamine-containing insulin or vasectomized men (↑ risk of hypersensitivity reactions); OB: Safety not established in pregnancy; use during pregnancy only if clearly needed; Lactation: Safety not established in breastfeeding; use while breastfeeding only if clearly needed.

Adverse Reactions/Side Effects

CV: bradycardia, hypertension, hypotension. **Derm:** flushing. **GI:** nausea, vomiting. **Hemat:** bleeding. **MS:** back pain. **Resp:** dyspnea, pulmonary hypertension. **Misc:** HYPERSENSITIVITY REACTIONS (including anaphylaxis and angioedema).

Interactions

Drug-Drug: None reported.

Route/Dosage

IV (Adults and Children): *Heparin overdose:* 1 mg/ 100 units of heparin. If given >30 min after heparin, give 0.5 mg/100 units of heparin (not to exceed 100 mg/2 hr). Further doses should be determined by coagulation tests. If heparin was administered subcutaneously, use 1–1.5 mg protamine per 100 units of heparin, give 25–50 mg of the protamine dose slowly followed by a continuous infusion over 8–16 hr. *Enoxaparin overdose (unlabeled use)* 1 mg/each mg of enoxaparin to be neutralized. *Dalteparin overdose (unlabeled use):* 1 mg/100 anti-Xa units of dalteparin. If required, a 2nd dose of 0.5 mg/100 anti-Xa units of dalteparin may be given 2–4 hr later if laboratory assessment indicates need.

Availability (generic available)

Solution for injection: 10 mg/mL.

NURSING IMPLICATIONS

Assessment

- Assess for bleeding and hemorrhage during therapy. Hemorrhage may recur 8–9 hr after therapy because of rebound effects of heparin. Rebound may occur as late as 18 hr after therapy in patients heparinized for cardiopulmonary bypass.
- Assess for allergy to fish (salmon), previous reaction to or use of protamine insulin or protamine sulfate. Vasectomized and infertile men also have higher risk of hypersensitivity reaction.
- Observe patient for signs and symptoms of hypersensitivity reaction (hives, edema, coughing, wheezing). Keep epinephrine, an antihistamine, and resuscitative equipment close by in the event of anaphylaxis.
- Assess for hypovolemia before initiation of therapy. Failure to correct hypovolemia may result in cardiovascular collapse from peripheral vasodilating effects of protamine sulfate.

Lab Test Considerations

- Monitor clotting factors, activated clotting time (ACT), activated partial thromboplastin time (aPTT), and thrombin time (TT) 5–15 min after therapy and again as necessary.

Implementation

- Do not confuse protamine with Protonix.
- Discontinue heparin infusion. In milder cases, overdose may be treated by heparin withdrawal alone.
- In severe cases, fresh frozen plasma or whole blood may also be required to control bleeding.
- Dose varies with type of heparin, route of heparin therapy, and amount of time elapsed since discontinuation of heparin.
- Do not administer >100 mg in 2 hr without rechecking clotting studies, as protamine sulfate has its own anticoagulant properties.

IV Administration

- **IV Push:** *Dilution:* May be administered undiluted. If further dilution is desired, D5W or 0.9% NaCl may be used. *Concentration:* 10 mg/mL. *Rate:* Administer by slow IV push over 1–3 min. Rapid infusion rate may result in hypotension, bradycardia, flushing, or feeling of warmth. If these symptoms occur, stop infusion and notify health care professional. No more than 50 mg should be administered within a 10-min period.
- **Y-Site Compatibility:** acetaminophen, amikacin, aminophylline, ascorbic acid, atropine, azathioprine, aztreonam, benztropine, bumetanide, buprenorphine, butorphanol, calcium chloride, calcium gluconate, chlorpromazine, clindamycin, cyclosporine, digoxin, diphenhydramine, dobutamine, dopamine, doxycycline, enalaprilat, ephedrine, epinephrine, epoetin alfa, erythromycin, esmolol, famotidine, fentanyl, fluconazole, ganciclovir, gentamicin, glycopyrrolate, imipenem/cilastatin, isoproterenol, labetalol, LR, lidocaine, magnesium sul-

fate, mannitol, meperidine, metoclopramide, metoprolol, midazolam, morphine, multivitamins, nalbuphine, naloxone, nitroglycerin, nitroprusside, norepinephrine, ondansetron, oxytocin, papaverine, phentolamine, phenylephrine, phytonadione, potassium chloride, procainamide, prochlorperazine, promethazine, propranolol, pyridoxine, sodium bicarbonate, succinylcholine, sufentanil, theophylline, thiamine, tobramycin, vancomycin, vasopressin, verapamil.

- **Y-Site Incompatibility:** ampicillin, ampicillin/sulbactam, cefazolin, cefotaxime, cefotetan, cefoxitin, ceftazidime, ceftriaxone, cefuroxime, chloramphenicol, dantrolene, dexamethasone, diazepam, folic acid, furosemide, heparin, hydrocortisone, indomethacin, insulin regular, ketorolac, methylprednisolone, nafcillin, oxacillin, penicillin G, pentamidine, pentobarbital, phenobarbital, phenytoin, trimethoprim/sulfamethoxazole.

Patient/Family Teaching
- Explain purpose of the medication to patient. Instruct patient to report recurrent bleeding immediately.
- Advise patient to avoid activities that may result in bleeding (shaving, brushing teeth, receiving injections or rectal temperatures, or ambulating) until risk of hemorrhage has passed.
- Rep: Advise females of reproductive potential to notify health care professional if pregnancy is planned or suspected or if breastfeeding.

Evaluation/Desired Outcomes
- Control of bleeding.
- Normalization of clotting factors in heparinized patients.

prucalopride (proo-kal-oh-pride)
Motegrity, ✲Resotran
Classification
Therapeutic: prokinetic agents
Pharmacologic: 5-HT$_4$ agonists

Indications
Treatment of chronic idiopathic constipation.

Action
Acts as a selective serotonin type 4 (5-HT$_4$) receptor agonist, which stimulates colonic peristalsis and leads to increased bowel motility. **Therapeutic Effects:** Increased frequency of complete spontaneous bowel movements.

Pharmacokinetics
Absorption: >90% absorbed following oral administration.
Distribution: Extensively distributed to tissues.

Metabolism and Excretion: Primarily excreted by the kidneys, with 60–65% being excreted unchanged in the urine, and 5% in feces.
Half-life: 24 hr.

TIME/ACTION PROFILE (plasma concentrations)

ROUTE	ONSET	PEAK	DURATION
PO	unknown	2–3 hr	24 hr

Contraindications/Precautions
Contraindicated in: Hypersensitivity; Intestinal perforation or obstruction, obstructive ileus, Crohn's disease, ulcerative colitis, or toxic megacolon/megarectum; End-stage renal disease requiring dialysis.
Use Cautiously in: Depression; Severe renal impairment (CCr <30 mL/min) (↓ dose); OB: Use during pregnancy only if potential maternal benefit justifies potential fetal risk; Lactation: Use while breastfeeding only if potential maternal benefit justifies potential risk to infant; Pedi: Safety and effectiveness not established in children; Geri: May need to ↓ dose in older adults due to age-related ↓ in renal function.

Adverse Reactions/Side Effects
GI: <u>abdominal pain</u>, <u>diarrhea</u>, nausea, abdominal distension, flatulence, vomiting. **Neuro:** <u>headache</u>, depression, dizziness, fatigue, SUICIDAL THOUGHTS/BEHAVIOR.

Interactions
Drug-Drug: None reported.

Route/Dosage
PO (Adults): 2 mg once daily.
Renal Impairment
PO (Adults): *CCr <30 mL/min:* 1 mg once daily.

Availability
Tablets: 1 mg, 2 mg.

NURSING IMPLICATIONS
Assessment
- Assess bowel sounds and frequency, quantity, and consistency of stools periodically during therapy.
- Monitor for signs and symptoms of persistent worsening of depression or the emergence of suicidal thoughts and behaviors.

Implementation
- **PO:** Administer once daily without regard to food.

Patient/Family Teaching
- Instruct patient to take prucalopride as directed. Advise patient to read *Patient Information* before starting therapy and with each Rx refill in case of changes.
- Advise patient and family members to discontinue prucalopride and notify health care professional im-

mediately if suicidal ideation and behavior (unusual changes in mood or behavior, persistent worsening of depression, feeling sad or hopeless, thoughts or attempts at self harm, emergence of suicidal thoughts or behavior) occur.
- Instruct patient to notify health care professional of all Rx or OTC medications, vitamins, or herbal products being taken and consult health care professional before taking any new medications.
- Rep: Advise females of reproductive potential to notify health care professional if pregnancy is planned or suspected, or if breastfeeding. Inform patient of pregnancy exposure registry that monitors pregnancy outcomes in women exposed to prucalopride during pregnancy. Register patients by contacting MotherToBaby Pregnancy Studies conducted by the Organization of Teratology Information Specialists at 1-877-311-8972 or visiting https://mothertobaby .org/pregnancy-studies/.

Evaluation/Desired Outcomes
- Increased frequency of complete spontaneous bowel movements.

pseudoephedrine
(soo-doe-e-**fed**-rin)
Silfedrine Children's, ~~Sudafed 12 Hour~~, Sudafed 24 Hour, Sudafed Children's, SudoGest, SudoGest 12 Hour
Classification
Therapeutic: allergy, cold, and cough remedies, nasal drying agents/decongestants
Pharmacologic: adrenergics, alpha adrenergic agonists

Indications
Symptomatic management of nasal congestion associated with acute viral upper respiratory tract infections. Used in combination with antihistamines in the management of allergic conditions. Used to open obstructed eustachian tubes in chronic otic inflammation or infection.

Action
Stimulates alpha- and beta-adrenergic receptors. Produces vasoconstriction in the respiratory tract mucosa (alpha-adrenergic stimulation) and possibly bronchodilation (beta$_2$-adrenergic stimulation). **Therapeutic Effects:** Reduction of nasal congestion, hyperemia, and swelling in nasal passages.

Pharmacokinetics
Absorption: Well absorbed after oral administration.
Distribution: Appears to enter the CSF.
Metabolism and Excretion: Partially metabolized by the liver. 55–75% excreted unchanged by the kidneys (depends on urine pH).

Half-life: Children: 3.1 hr; Adults: 9–16 hr (depends on urine pH).

TIME/ACTION PROFILE (decongestant effects)

ROUTE	ONSET	PEAK	DURATION
PO	15–30 min	unknown	4–6 hr
PO-ER	60 min	unknown	12 hr

Contraindications/Precautions
Contraindicated in: Hypersensitivity to sympathomimetic amines; Hypertension, severe coronary artery disease; Concurrent MAO inhibitor therapy; Known alcohol intolerance (some liquid products).
Use Cautiously in: Hyperthyroidism; Diabetes mellitus; Prostatic hyperplasia; Ischemic heart disease; Glaucoma; OB, Lactation: Safety not established; Pedi: Avoid OTC cough and cold products containing this medication in children <4 yr.

Adverse Reactions/Side Effects
CV: palpitations, CARDIOVASCULAR COLLAPSE, hypertension, tachycardia. **Derm:** diaphoresis. **GI:** anorexia, dry mouth. **GU:** dysuria. **Neuro:** anxiety, nervousness, dizziness, drowsiness, excitability, fear, hallucinations, headache, insomnia, restlessness, SEIZURES, weakness. **Resp:** respiratory difficulty.

Interactions
Drug-Drug: Concurrent use with **MAO inhibitors** may cause hypertensive crisis. Additive adrenergic effects with other **adrenergics**. Concurrent use with **beta blockers** may result in hypertension or bradycardia. **Drugs that acidify the urine** may ↓ effectiveness. **Phenothiazines** and **tricyclic antidepressants** potentiate pressor effects. **Drugs that alkalinize the urine (sodium bicarbonate, high-dose antacid therapy)** may intensify effectiveness.
Drug-Food: Foods that acidify the urine may ↓ effectiveness. **Foods that alkalinize the urine** may intensify effectiveness (see lists in Appendix J).

Route/Dosage
PO (Adults and Children >12 yr): 60 mg every 6 hr as needed (not to exceed 240 mg/day) *or* 120 mg extended-release preparation every 12 hr *or* 240 mg extended-release preparation every 24 hr.
PO (Children 6–12 yr): 30 mg every 6 hr as needed (not to exceed 120 mg/day).
PO (Children 4–5 yr): 15 mg every 6 hr (not to exceed 60 mg/day).

Availability (generic available)
Tablets: 30 mg^{OTC}, 60 mg^{OTC}. **Extended-release tablets:** 120 mg^{OTC}, 240 mg^{OTC}. **Capsules:** ❀ 60 mg^{OTC}. **Extended-release capsules:** ❀ 240 mg^{OTC}. **Liquid (grape and others):** 15 mg/5 mL^{OTC}, 30 mg/5 mL^{OTC}. *In combination with:* antihistamines, acetaminophen, cough suppressants, and expectorants^{OTC}. See Appendix N.

NURSING IMPLICATIONS

Assessment

- Assess congestion (nasal, sinus, eustachian tube) before and periodically during therapy.
- Monitor pulse and BP before beginning therapy and periodically during therapy.
- Assess lung sounds and character of bronchial secretions. Maintain fluid intake of 1500–2000 mL/day to decrease viscosity of secretions.

Implementation

- Do not confuse Sudafed with sotalol or Sudafed PE.
- Administer pseudoephedrine at least 2 hr before bedtime to minimize insomnia.
- **PO:** *DNC:* Extended-release tablets and capsules should be swallowed whole; do not crush, break, or chew.Contents of the capsule can be mixed with jam or jelly and swallowed without chewing for patients with difficulty swallowing.

Patient/Family Teaching

- Instruct patient to take medication as directed and not to take more than recommended. Take missed doses within 1 hr; if remembered later, omit. Do not double doses. Caution parents to avoid OTC cough and cold products in children <4 yr.
- Instruct patient to notify health care professional if nervousness, slow or fast heart rate, breathing difficulties, hallucinations, or seizures occur, because these symptoms may indicate overdose.
- Instruct patient to contact health care professional if symptoms do not improve within 7 days or if fever is present.
- Rep: Avoid use during 1st trimester of pregnancy because of potential fetal harm. Prolonged use later in pregnancy should also be avoided. Avoid use during breastfeeding.

Evaluation/Desired Outcomes

- Decreased nasal, sinus, or eustachian tube congestion.

---

pyrazinamide
(peer-a-**zin**-a-mide)
✳ Tebrazid
Classification
Therapeutic: antituberculars

Indications

Active tuberculosis (TB) (in combination with other agents).

Action

Converted to pyrazinoic acid in susceptible strains of Mycobacterium, which lowers the pH of the environment. **Therapeutic Effects:** Bacteriostatic action against susceptible mycobacteria. **Spectrum:** Active against mycobacteria only.

Pharmacokinetics

Absorption: Well absorbed after oral administration.
Distribution: Widely distributed. Reaches high concentrations in the CNS (same as plasma).
Metabolism and Excretion: Mostly metabolized by the liver. Metabolite (pyrazinoic acid) has antimycobacterial activity; 3–4% excreted unchanged by the kidneys.
Half-life: *Pyrazinamide:* 9.5 hr. *Pyrazinoic acid:* 12 hr. Both are ↑ in renal impairment.

TIME/ACTION PROFILE (plasma concentrations)

ROUTE	ONSET	PEAK	DURATION
PO	unknown	1–2 hr (4–5 hr†)	24 hr

†For pyrazinoic acid.

Contraindications/Precautions

Contraindicated in: Hypersensitivity; Cross-sensitivity with ethionamide, isoniazid, niacin, or nicotinic acid may exist; Severe hepatic impairment.
Use Cautiously in: Gout; Renal failure; Diabetes mellitus; Acute intermittent porphyria; OB: Use during pregnancy only if clearly needed; Lactation: Use while breastfeeding only if potential maternal benefit justifies potential risk to infant.

Adverse Reactions/Side Effects

Derm: acne, photosensitivity, rash. **GI:** anorexia, diarrhea, HEPATOTOXICITY, nausea, vomiting. **GU:** dysuria. **Hemat:** anemia, thrombocytopenia. **Metab:** hyperuricemia. **MS:** arthralgia, gouty arthritis.

Interactions

Drug-Drug: Concurrent use with **rifampin** may result in life-threatening hepatotoxicity; avoid concurrent use. May ↓ levels and effectiveness of **cyclosporine**. May ↓ effectiveness of **antigout agents**.

Route/Dosage

PO (Adults and Children): 15–30 mg/kg/day as a single dose. Up to 60 mg/kg/day has been used in isoniazid-resistant TB (not to exceed 2 g/day as a single dose or 3 g/day in divided doses). May also be given as 50–70 mg/kg 2–3 times weekly (not to exceed 2 g/dose on daily regimen, 3 g/dose for 3-times-weekly regimen, or 4 g/dose for twice-weekly regimen). *Patients with HIV:* 20–40 mg/kg/day for first 2 mo of therapy (maximum: 2 g/day); further dosing depends on regimen employed.

Availability (generic available)

Tablets: 500 mg.

NURSING IMPLICATIONS

Assessment

- Perform mycobacterial studies and susceptibility tests before and periodically during therapy to detect possible resistance.

Lab Test Considerations

- Evaluate hepatic function before and every 2–4 wk during therapy. Increased AST and ALT may not be predictive of clinical hepatitis and may return to normal levels during treatment. Patients with impaired liver function should receive pyrazinamide therapy only if crucial to treatment.
- Monitor serum uric acid concentrations during therapy. May cause ↑ resulting in precipitation of acute gout.
- May interfere with urine ketone determinations.

Implementation

- **PO:** May be given concurrently with isoniazid.

Patient/Family Teaching

- Advise patient to take medication as directed and not to skip doses or double up on missed doses. Take

missed doses as soon as remembered unless almost time for next dose. Emphasize the importance of continuing therapy even after symptoms have subsided. Length of therapy depends on regimen being used and underlying disease states.

- Inform patients with diabetes that pyrazinamide may interfere with urine ketone measurements.
- Advise patients to notify health care professional if no improvement is noticed after 2–3 wk of therapy or if fever, anorexia, malaise, nausea, vomiting, darkened urine, yellowish discoloration of the skin and eyes, pain, or swelling of the joints occurs.
- Advise patients to use sunscreen and protective clothing to prevent photosensitivity reactions.
- Rep: Advise females of reproductive potential to notify health care professional if pregnancy is planned or suspected or if breastfeeding. Monitor infants exposed to pyrazinamide via breast milk for jaundice.
- Emphasize the importance of regular follow-up exams to monitor progress and check for side effects.

Evaluation/Desired Outcomes

- Resolution of signs and symptoms of TB.
- Negative sputum cultures.

BEERS

QUEtiapine (kwet-**eye**-a-peen)
SEROquel, SEROquel XR
Classification
Therapeutic: antipsychotics, mood stabilizers

Indications
Schizophrenia. Depressive episodes with bipolar disorder. Acute manic episodes associated with bipolar I disorder (as monotherapy [for adults or adolescents] or with lithium or divalproex [adults only]). Maintenance treatment of bipolar I disorder (with lithium or divalproex). Adjunctive treatment of depression.

Action
Probably acts by serving as an antagonist of dopamine and serotonin. Also antagonizes histamine H_1 receptors and alpha$_1$-adrenergic receptors. **Therapeutic Effects:** Decreased manifestations of psychoses, depression, or acute mania.

Pharmacokinetics
Absorption: Well absorbed after oral administration.
Distribution: Widely distributed.
Metabolism and Excretion: Extensively metabolized by the liver via the CYP3A4 isoenzyme to norquetiapine (active metabolite with anticholinergic properties); <1% excreted unchanged in the urine.
Half-life: 6 hr.

TIME/ACTION PROFILE (antipsychotic effects)

ROUTE	ONSET	PEAK	DURATION
PO	unknown	unknown	8–12 hr
PO-XR	unknown	unknown	unknown

Contraindications/Precautions
Contraindicated in: Hypersensitivity; Concurrent use of agents that prolong the QT interval, including dofetilide, sotalol, quinidine, disopyramide, amiodarone, dronedarone, thioridazine, chlorpromazine, droperidol, moxifloxacin, mefloquine, pentamidine, arsenic trioxide, tacrolimus, ziprasidone, erythromycin, citalopram, escitalopram, and clarithromycin (↑ risk of serious arrhythmias); History of arrhythmias, including bradycardia; Hypokalemia or hypomagnesemia (↑ risk of serious arrhythmias); Congenital long QT syndrome (↑ risk of serious arrhythmias).
Use Cautiously in: Cardiovascular disease, cerebrovascular disease, dehydration, or hypovolemia (↑ risk of hypotension); History of seizures or Alzheimer's dementia; Diabetes (may ↑ risk of hyperglycemia); Patients at risk for aspiration pneumonia or falls; Hepatic impairment (dose ↓ may be necessary); Hypothyroidism (may be exacerbated); History of suicide attempt; Low white blood cell count or history of drug-induced leukopenia/neutropenia (↑ risk of leukopenia/neutro-

penia); Urinary retention, prostatic hypertrophy, constipation, or ↑ intraocular pressure; OB: Neonates at ↑ risk for extrapyramidal symptoms and withdrawal after delivery when exposed during the 3rd trimester; use only if potential maternal benefit justifies potential fetal risk; Lactation: Use while breastfeeding only if potential maternal benefit justifies potential risk to infant; Pedi: May ↑ risk of suicide attempt/ideation especially during early treatment or dose adjustment; risk may be greater in children or adolescents; Geri: Appears on Beers list. ↑ risk of stroke, cognitive decline, and mortality in older adults with dementia. Avoid use in older adults, except for schizophrenia, bipolar disorder, adjunctive treatment of major depressive disorder, or psychosis in Parkinson's disease.

Adverse Reactions/Side Effects
CV: ↑ BP (children), palpitations, peripheral edema, postural hypotension. **Derm:** ACUTE GENERALIZED EXANTHEMATOUS PUSTULOSIS, DRUG REACTION WITH EOSINOPHILIA AND SYSTEMIC SYMPTOMS (DRESS), STEVENS-JOHNSON SYNDROME (SJS), sweating. **EENT:** ear pain, pharyngitis, rhinitis. **Endo:** hyperglycemia, hyperprolactinemia, hypothyroidism. **GI:** anorexia, constipation, dry mouth, dyspepsia, GI OBSTRUCTION, PANCREATITIS. **GU:** ↓ fertility (females). **Hemat:** ↓ hemoglobin, AGRANULOCYTOSIS, leukopenia, neutropenia. **Metab:** weight gain, hyperlipidemia, hypertriglyceridemia. **MS:** rhabdomyolysis. **Neuro:** dizziness, cognitive impairment, extrapyramidal symptoms, NEUROLEPTIC MALIGNANT SYNDROME, sedation, SEIZURES, tardive dyskinesia. **Resp:** cough, dyspnea. **Misc:** flu-like syndrome.

Interactions
Drug-Drug: QT interval prolonging medications, including **macrolide antibiotics** (**erythromycin, clarithromycin**), **dofetilide, sotalol, quinidine, disopyramide, procainamide, thioridazine, chlorpromazine, droperidol, moxifloxacin, mefloquine, pentamidine, arsenic trioxide, citalopram, escitalopram, tacrolimus,** and **ziprasidone** may ↑ the risk of serious ventricular arrhythmias and should be avoided. ↑ CNS depression may occur with **alcohol, antihistamines, opioid analgesics,** and **sedative/hypnotics.** ↑ risk of hypotension with acute ingestion of **alcohol** or **antihypertensives. CYP3A inducers,** including **phenytoin, carbamazepine, barbiturates, rifampin,** or **corticosteroids** may ↓ levels and effects. **CYP3A inhibitors,** including **ketoconazole, itraconazole, fluconazole, protease inhibitors,** or **erythromycin** may ↑ levels and risk of toxicity. Concurrent use of **anticholinergic medications** may ↑ risk of anticholinergic adverse reactions.

Route/Dosage
Schizophrenia
PO (Adults): *Immediate release:* 25 mg twice daily on Day 1, ↑ by 25–50 mg 2–3 times daily on Days 2 and

Q

3, up to 300–400 mg/day in 2–3 divided doses by Day 4 (not to exceed 800 mg/day); *Extended release:* 300 mg once daily, ↑ by 300 mg/day (not to exceed 800 mg/day); elderly patients or patients with hepatic impairment should be started on immediate-release product and converted to extended-release product once effective dose is reached.

PO (Children 13–17 yr): *Immediate release:* 25 mg twice daily on Day 1, ↑ to 50 mg twice daily on Day 2, then ↑ to 100 mg twice daily on Day 3, then ↑ to 150 mg twice daily on Day 4, then ↑ to 200 mg twice daily on Day 5; may then ↑ by no more than 100 mg/day (not to exceed 800 mg/day).

Acute Manic Episodes Associated With Bipolar I Disorder

PO (Adults): *Immediate release:* 50 mg twice daily on Day 1, then ↑ to 100 mg twice daily on Day 2, then ↑ to 150 mg twice daily on Day 3, then ↑ to 200 mg twice daily on Day 4; may then ↑ by no more than 200 mg/day up to 400 mg twice daily on Day 6 if needed; *Extended release:* 300 mg once daily on Day 1, then 600 mg once daily on Day 2, then 400–800 mg once daily starting on Day 3.

PO (Children 10–17 yr): *Immediate release:* 25 mg twice daily on Day 1, then ↑ to 50 mg twice daily on Day 2, then ↑ to 100 mg twice daily on Day 3, then ↑ to 150 mg twice daily on Day 4, then ↑ to 200 mg twice daily on Day 5; may then ↑ by no more than 100 mg/day (not to exceed 600 mg/day).

Acute Depressive Episodes Associated With Bipolar Disorder

PO (Adults): *Immediate release or extended release:* 50 mg once daily at bedtime on Day 1, then ↑ to 100 mg daily at bedtime on Day 2, then ↑ to 200 mg daily at bedtime on Day 3, then ↑ to 300 mg daily at bedtime thereafter.

Maintenance Treatment of Bipolar I Disorder

PO (Adults): Continue at the dose required to maintain symptom remission (usual dosage: 400–800 mg/day given as once daily dose [extended release] or in two divided doses [immediate release]).

PO (Children 10–17 yr): Continue at the lowest dose required to maintain symptom remission.

Depression

PO (Adults): *Extended release:* 50 mg once daily on Days 1 and 2, then ↑ to 150 mg once daily starting on Day 3 (not to exceed 300 mg/day).

Availability (generic available)

Immediate-release tablets: 25 mg, 50 mg, 100 mg, 200 mg, 300 mg, 400 mg. **Extended-release tablets:** 50 mg, 150 mg, 200 mg, 300 mg, 400 mg.

NURSING IMPLICATIONS

Assessment

- Monitor mental status (mood, orientation, behavior) before and periodically during therapy.

- Assess for suicidal tendencies, especially during early therapy. Restrict amount of drug available to patient. Risk may be increased in children, adolescents, and adults ≤24 yr.
- Assess weight and BMI initially and during therapy.
- Monitor BP (sitting, standing, lying) and pulse before and frequently during initial dose titration. If hypotension occurs during dose titration, return to the previous dose.
- Observe patient carefully to ensure medication is swallowed and not hoarded or cheeked.
- Monitor for onset of extrapyramidal side effects (*akathisia:* restlessness; *dystonia:* muscle spasms and twisting motions; or *pseudoparkinsonism:* mask-like faces, rigidity, tremors, drooling, shuffling gait, dysphagia). Report these symptoms; reduction of dose or discontinuation may be necessary. Trihexyphenidyl or benztropine may be used to control these symptoms.
- Monitor for tardive dyskinesia (involuntary rhythmic movement of mouth, face, and extremities). Report immediately; may be irreversible.
- Monitor for development of neuroleptic malignant syndrome (fever, respiratory distress, tachycardia, seizures, diaphoresis, hypertension or hypotension, pallor, tiredness). Notify health care professional immediately if these symptoms occur.
- Assess for rash periodically during therapy. May cause SJS. Discontinue therapy if severe or if accompanied with fever, general malaise, fatigue, muscle or joint aches, blisters, oral lesions, conjunctivitis, hepatitis, and/or eosinophilia.
- Monitor for signs of pancreatitis (nausea, vomiting, anorexia, persistent severe abdominal pain, sometimes radiating to the back) during therapy.
- Monitor for symptoms related to hyperprolactinemia (menstrual abnormalities, galactorrhea, sexual dysfunction).
- Assess for falls risk. Drowsiness, orthostatic hypotension, and motor and sensory instability increase risk. Institute prevention if indicated.
- Monitor for signs and symptoms of DRESS (fever, rash, lymphadenopathy, and/or facial swelling), associated with involvement of other organ systems (hepatitis, nephritis, hematologic abnormalities, myocarditis, myositis) during therapy. May resemble an acute viral infection. Eosinophilia is often present. Discontinue therapy if signs occur.

Lab Test Considerations

- May cause asymptomatic ↑ in AST and ALT.
- May also cause anemia, thrombocytopenia, leukocytosis, and leukopenia.
- May cause ↑ total cholesterol and triglycerides.
- Obtain fasting blood glucose and cholesterol levels initially and during therapy.
- Monitor serum prolactin prior to and periodically during therapy. May cause ↑ serum prolactin levels.

Implementation

- Do not confuse quetiapine with olanzapine. Do not confuse Seroquel with Seroquel XR.
- If therapy is reinstituted after an interval of ≥1 wk off, follow initial titration schedule.
- **PO:** May be administered without regard to food. *DNC:* Extended-release tablets should be swallowed whole, do not break, crush, or chew.

Patient/Family Teaching

- Instruct patient to take medication as directed. Take missed doses as soon as remembered unless almost time for next dose; do not double doses. Consult health care professional prior to stopping quetiapine; should be discontinued gradually. Stopping abruptly may cause insomnia, nausea, and vomiting.
- Advise patient and caregiver that quetiapine should not be given to elderly patients with dementia-related psychosis; may ↑ risk of death.
- Inform patient of the possibility of extrapyramidal symptoms. Instruct patient to report symptoms immediately to health care professional.
- Advise patient to change positions slowly to minimize orthostatic hypotension. Protect from falls.
- May cause drowsiness. Caution patient to avoid driving or other activities requiring alertness until response to medication is known.
- Advise patient to avoid extremes in temperature; this drug impairs body temperature regulation.
- Advise patient to notify health care professional of all Rx or OTC medications, vitamins, or herbal products being taken and to consult with health care professional before taking other medications and alcohol, especially other CNS depressants, including opioids.
- Advise patient and family to notify health care professional if thoughts about suicide or dying, attempts to commit suicide; new or worse depression; new or worse anxiety; feeling very agitated or restless; panic attacks; trouble sleeping; new or worse irritability; acting aggressive; being angry or violent; acting on dangerous impulses; an extreme increase in activity and talking; other unusual changes in behavior or mood occur.
- Refer patient for nutritional, weight, or medical management of dyslipidemia as indicated.
- Advise patient to notify health care professional of medication regimen before treatment or surgery.
- Instruct patient to notify health care professional promptly of sore throat, fever, unusual bleeding or bruising, constipation, or rash.
- Rep: Advise females of reproductive potential to notify health care professional if pregnancy is planned or suspected, and to avoid breastfeeding during therapy. Encourage women who become pregnant while taking quetiapine to enroll in the National Pregnancy Registry for Atypical Antipsychotics at 1-866-961-2388 or visit https://womensmentalhealth.org/research/pregnancyregistry/. Monitor neonates for extrapyramidal and/or withdrawal symptoms and manage symptoms appropriately. May lead to temporary, reversible infertility in females.
- Emphasize importance of routine follow-up exams to monitor side effects and continued participation in psychotherapy as indicated to improve coping skills. Ophthalmologic exams should be performed before and every 6 mo during therapy.

Evaluation/Desired Outcomes

- Decrease in excited, manic, behavior.
- Decrease in signs of depression in patients with bipolar disorder.
- Decrease in manic episodes in patients with bipolar I disorder.
- Decrease in positive symptoms (delusions, hallucinations) of schizophrenia.
- Decrease in negative symptoms (social withdrawal, flat, blunt affect) of schizophrenia.

quinapril, See ANGIOTENSIN-CONVERTING ENZYME (ACE) INHIBITORS.

RABEprazole (ra-bep-ra-zole)
Aciphex, ~~Aciphex Sprinkle~~, ✿Pariet
Classification
Therapeutic: antiulcer agents
Pharmacologic: proton-pump inhibitors

Indications
Gastroesophageal reflux disease (GERD). Duodenal ulcers (including combination therapy with clarithromycin and amoxicillin to eradicate *Helicobacter pylori* and prevent recurrence). Pathological hypersecretory conditions, including Zollinger-Ellison syndrome.

Action
Binds to an enzyme in the presence of acidic gastric pH, preventing the final transport of hydrogen ions into the gastric lumen. **Therapeutic Effects:** Diminished accumulation of acid in the gastric lumen, with lessened acid reflux. Healing of duodenal ulcers and esophagitis. Decreased acid secretion in hypersecretory conditions.

Pharmacokinetics
Absorption: Delayed-release tablet is designed to allow rabeprazole, which is not stable in gastric acid, to pass through the stomach intact. Subsequently 52% is absorbed after oral administration.
Distribution: Unknown.
Protein Binding: 96.3%.
Metabolism and Excretion: Mostly metabolized by the CYP3A4 and CYP2C19 isoenzymes in the liver; ▓ (the CYP2C19 enzyme system exhibits genetic polymorphism; 15–20% of Asian patients and 3–5% of Caucasian and Black patients may be poor metabolizers and may have significantly ↑ rabeprazole concentrations and an ↑ risk of adverse effects); 10% excreted in feces; remainder excreted in urine as inactive metabolites.
Half-life: 1–2 hr.

TIME/ACTION PROFILE (acid suppression)

ROUTE	ONSET	PEAK	DURATION
PO	within 1 hr	unknown	24 hr†

†Suppression continues to increase over the first wk of therapy.

Contraindications/Precautions
Contraindicated in: Hypersensitivity to rabeprazole or related drugs (benzimidazoles); Concurrent use of rilpivirine.
Use Cautiously in: Severe hepatic impairment (dose reduction may be necessary); Patients using high doses for >1 yr (↑ risk of hip, wrist, or spine fractures and fundic gland polyps); Patients using therapy for >3 yr (↑ risk of vitamin B$_{12}$ deficiency); Pre-existing risk of hypocalcemia; OB: Safety not established in pregnancy; Lactation: Use while breastfeeding only if potential maternal benefit justifies potential risk to infant; Pedi: Children <12 yr (safety and effectiveness not established); Geri: Appears on Beers list. ↑ risk of *Clostridioides*

difficile infection, pneumonia, GI malignancies, bone loss, and fractures in older adults. Avoid scheduled use for >8 wk in older adults unless for high-risk patients (e.g., oral corticosteroid or chronic NSAID use) or patients with erosive esophagitis, Barrett's esophagitis, pathological hypersecretory condition, or demonstrated need for maintenance therapy (e.g., failure of H$_2$ antagonist).

Adverse Reactions/Side Effects
Derm: ACUTE GENERALIZED EXANTHEMATOUS PUSTULOSIS (AGEP), cutaneous lupus erythematosus, DRUG REACTION WITH EOSINOPHILIA AND SYSTEMIC SYMPTOMS (DRESS), photosensitivity, rash, STEVENS-JOHNSON SYNDROME (SJS), TOXIC EPIDERMAL NECROLYSIS (TEN). **F and E:** hypocalcemia (especially if treatment duration ≥3 mo), hypokalemia (especially if treatment duration ≥3 mo), hypomagnesemia (especially if treatment duration ≥3 mo). **GI:** abdominal pain, CLOSTRIDIOIDES DIFFICILE-ASSOCIATED DIARRHEA (CDAD), constipation, diarrhea, fundic gland polyps, nausea. **GU:** acute tubulointerstitial nephritis. **MS:** bone fracture, neck pain. **Neuro:** dizziness, headache, malaise. **Misc:** chills, fever, HYPERSENSITIVITY REACTIONS (including anaphylaxis, angioedema, or tubulointerstitial nephritis), systemic lupus erythematosus, vitamin B$_{12}$ deficiency.

Interactions
Drug-Drug: May ↓ absorption of drugs requiring acid pH, including **ketoconazole**, **itraconazole**, **atazanavir**, **iron salts**, **erlotinib**, **dasatinib**, **nelfinavir**, **nilotinib**, **rilpivirine**, and **mycophenolate mofetil**; concurrent use with **rilpivirine** contraindicated; avoid concurrent use with **nelfinavir**. May ↑ levels of **digoxin**, **methotrexate**, and **tacrolimus**. Hypomagnesemia and hypokalemia ↑ risk of **digoxin** toxicity. May ↑ the risk of bleeding with **warfarin** (monitor INR).

Route/Dosage

Gastroesophageal Reflux Disease
PO (Adults): *Healing of erosive or ulcerative GERD:* 20 mg once daily for 4–8 wk; *Maintenance of healing of erosive or ulcerative GERD:* 20 mg once daily; *Symptomatic GERD:* 20 mg once daily for 4 wk (additional 4 wk may be considered for nonresponders).
PO (Children ≥12 yr): *Short-term treatment of symptomatic GERD:* 20 mg once daily for up to 8 wk.
PO (Children 1–11 yr): *≥15 kg:* 10 mg once daily for up to 12 wk (given as sprinkle); *<15 kg:* 5 mg once daily for up to 12 wk (given as sprinkle); may ↑ up to 10 mg once daily if inadequate response.

Duodenal Ulcers
PO (Adults): *Healing of duodenal ulcers:* 20 mg once daily for up to 4 wk.

H. pylori Eradication to Reduce the Risk of Duodenal Ulcer Recurrence (Triple Therapy)
PO (Adults): 20 mg twice daily for 7 days, with amoxicillin 1000 mg twice daily for 7 days and clarithromycin 500 mg twice daily for 7 days.

Pathological Hypersecretory Conditions Including Zollinger-Ellison Syndrome

PO (Adults): 60 mg once daily initially; may be adjusted as needed and continued as necessary; doses up to 100 mg daily or 60 mg twice daily have been used.

Availability (generic available)
Delayed-release capsules (sprinkle): 10 mg.
Delayed-release tablets: ✤ 10 mg, 20 mg.

NURSING IMPLICATIONS
Assessment
- Assess routinely for epigastric or abdominal pain and frank or occult blood in the stool, emesis, or gastric aspirate.
- Monitor bowel function. Report diarrhea, abdominal cramping, fever, and bloody stools to health care professional promptly as a sign of CDAD. May begin up to several wk following cessation of therapy.
- Monitor for rash or other cutaneous reactions. May cause SJS, TEN, DRESS, and AGEP. Discontinue rabeprazole at the first sign of severe cutaneous adverse reactions.

Lab Test Considerations
- Monitor CBC with differential periodically during therapy.
- May cause hypomagnesemia. Monitor serum magnesium prior to and periodically during therapy.

Implementation
- **_High Alert:_** Do not confuse rabeprazole with aripiprazole. Do not confuse Aciphex with Accupril or Aricept.
- **PO:** Administer without regard to food, preferably in the morning. _DNC:_ Tablets should be swallowed whole; do not break, crush, or chew.
- For treatment of duodenal ulcers, take after a meal.
- For _Helicobacter pylori_ eradication, take tablets with food.
- Capsules may be opened and sprinkled on a small amount of soft food (apple sauce, fruit, or vegetable-based baby food, yogurt) or empty contents into small amount of liquid (infant formula, apple juice, pediatric electrolyte solution). Food or liquid should be at or below room temperature. Whole dose should be taken within 15 min of being sprinkled. Granules should not be chewed or crushed. Dose should be taken 30 min before a meal. Do not store mixture for future use.

Patient/Family Teaching
- Instruct patient to take medication as directed for the full course of therapy, even if feeling better. Take missed doses as soon as remembered but not if almost time for next dose. Do not double doses.
- May cause occasional drowsiness or dizziness. Caution patient to avoid driving or other activities requiring alertness until response to medication is known.
- Advise patient to avoid alcohol, products containing aspirin or NSAIDs, and foods that may cause an increase in GI irritation.
- Caution patients to wear sunscreen and protective clothing to prevent photosensitivity reactions.
- Advise patient to report onset of black, tarry stools; diarrhea; abdominal pain; or persistent headache to health care professional promptly.
- Instruct patient to notify health care professional of all Rx or OTC medications, vitamins, or herbal products being taken and consult health care professional before taking any new medications.
- Instruct patient to notify health care professional of onset of black, tarry stools; diarrhea; abdominal pain; or persistent headache or if fever and diarrhea develop, especially if stool contains blood, pus, or mucus. Advise patient not to treat diarrhea without consulting health care professional.
- Rep: Advise females of reproductive potential to notify health care professional if pregnancy is planned or suspected or if breastfeeding.

Evaluation/Desired Outcomes
- Decrease in abdominal pain or prevention of gastric irritation and bleeding.
- Decrease in symptoms of GERD.
- Decreased acid secretion in hypersecretory conditions.

raloxifene (ra-lox-i-feen)
Evista
Classification
Therapeutic: bone resorption inhibitors
Pharmacologic: selective estrogen receptor modulators

Indications
Treatment and prevention of osteoporosis in postmenopausal women. Reduction of the risk of breast cancer in postmenopausal women with osteoporosis and those at high risk for invasive breast cancer.

Action
Binds to estrogen receptors, producing estrogen-like effects on bone, resulting in reduced resorption of bone and decreased bone turnover. **Therapeutic Effects:** Prevention of osteoporosis in patients at risk. Decreased risk of breast cancer.

Pharmacokinetics
Absorption: Although well absorbed (>60%), after oral administration, extensive first-pass metabolism results in 2% bioavailability.
Distribution: Extensively distributed to tissues.
Protein Binding: 95%.

✤= Canadian drug name. ▨ = Genetic implication. ~~Strikethrough~~ = Discontinued. CAPITALS = life-threatening. <u>Underline</u> = most frequent.

Metabolism and Excretion: Extensively metabolized by the liver; undergoes enterohepatic cycling; excreted primarily in feces.

Half-life: 27.7 hr.

TIME/ACTION PROFILE (effects on bone turnover)

ROUTE	ONSET	PEAK	DURATION
PO	unknown	3 mo	unknown

Contraindications/Precautions

Contraindicated in: Hypersensitivity; History of thromboembolic events.

Use Cautiously in: Potential immobilization (↑ risk of thromboembolic events); History of stroke or transient ischemic attack; Atrial fibrillation; Hypertension; Cigarette smoking.

Adverse Reactions/Side Effects

CV: DEEP VEIN THROMBOSIS, MI. **Derm:** hot flush. **EENT:** retinal vein thrombosis. **MS:** leg cramps. **Neuro:** STROKE. **Resp:** PULMONARY EMBOLISM.

Interactions

Drug-Drug: Cholestyramine ↓ absorption; avoid concurrent use. May alter effects of **warfarin** and other **highly protein-bound drugs**. Concurrent systemic **estrogen** therapy is not recommended.

Route/Dosage

PO (Adults): 60 mg once daily.

Availability (generic available)

Tablets: 60 mg.

NURSING IMPLICATIONS

Assessment

- Assess patient for bone mineral density with x-ray, serum, and urine bone turnover markers (bone-specific alkaline phosphatase, osteocalcin, and collagen breakdown products) before and periodically during therapy.

Lab Test Considerations

- May cause ↑ reduced serum total cholesterol, low-density lipoprotein cholesterol, fibrinogen, and apolipoprotein B.
- May cause ↑ hormone-binding globulin (sex steroid-binding globulin, thyroxine-binding globulin, corticosteroid-binding globulin) with ↑ total hormone concentrations.
- May cause small ↓ in serum total calcium, inorganic phosphate, total protein, and albumin.
- May also cause slight decrease in platelet count.

Implementation

- **PO:** May be administered without regard to meals.
- Calcium supplementation should be added to diet if daily intake is inadequate.

Patient/Family Teaching

- Instruct patient to take raloxifene as directed. Discuss the importance of adequate calcium and vita-

min D intake or supplementation. Instruct patient to read the *Medication Guide* when initiating therapy and again with each prescription refill in case of changes.

- Advise patient to discontinue smoking and alcohol consumption.
- Emphasize the importance of regular weight-bearing exercise. Advise patient that raloxifene should be discontinued at least 72 hr before and during prolonged immobilization (recovery from surgery, prolonged bedrest). Instruct patient to avoid prolonged restrictions of movement during travel because of the increased risk of venous thrombosis.
- Advise patient that raloxifene will not reduce hot flashes or flushes associated with estrogen deficiency and may cause hot flashes.
- Instruct patient to notify health care professional immediately if leg pain or a feeling of warmth in the lower leg (calf); swelling of the legs, hands, or feet; sudden chest pain; shortness of breath or coughing up blood; or sudden change in vision, such as loss of vision or blurred vision occur. Being still for a long time (sitting still during a long car or airplane trip, being in bed after surgery) can increase risk of blood clots.

Evaluation/Desired Outcomes

- Prevention of osteoporosis in postmenopausal women.
- Reduced risk of breast cancer in postmenopausal women with osteoporosis and those at high risk for invasive breast cancer.

raltegravir (ral-**teg**-ra-veer)
Isentress, Isentress HD

Classification
Therapeutic: antiretrovirals
Pharmacologic: integrase strand transfer inhibitors (INSTIs)

Indications

HIV-1 infection (in combination with other antiretrovirals).

Action

Inhibits HIV-1 integrase, which is required for viral replication. **Therapeutic Effects:** Evidence of decreased viral replication and reduced viral load with slowed progression of HIV and its sequelae.

Pharmacokinetics

Absorption: Well absorbed following oral administration.

Distribution: Unknown.

Metabolism and Excretion: Mostly metabolized by the uridine diphosphate glucuronosyltransferase (UGT) A1A enzyme system; 23% excreted in urine as parent drug and metabolite.

Half-life: 9 hr.

TIME/ACTION PROFILE (plasma concentrations)

ROUTE	ONSET	PEAK	DURATION
PO	unknown	3 hr	12 hr

Contraindications/Precautions

Contraindicated in: Lactation: Breastfeeding not recommended in women with HIV.

Use Cautiously in: Phenylketonuria (chewable tablets contain phenylalanine); OB: Considered a preferred integrase strand transfer inhibitor for pregnant patients living with HIV who are antiretroviral-naive, who have had antiretroviral therapy in the past but are restarting, or who require a new antiretroviral therapy regimen; Pedi: Preterm neonates (safety and effectiveness not established); Geri: Choose dose carefully in older adults, considering concurrent disease states, drug therapy, and age-related ↓ in hepatic and renal function.

Adverse Reactions/Side Effects

CV: MI. **Derm:** rash, STEVENS-JOHNSON SYNDROME (SJS), TOXIC EPIDERMAL NECROLYSIS. **GI:** diarrhea, abdominal pain, gastritis, hepatitis, nausea, vomiting. **GU:** renal failure/impairment. **Hemat:** anemia, neutropenia. **Metab:** lipodystrophy. **MS:** ↑ creatine kinase, myopathy, RHABDOMYOLYSIS. **Neuro:** headache, depression, dizziness, fatigue, insomnia, SUICIDAL THOUGHTS, weakness. **Misc:** fever, immune reconstitution syndrome.

Interactions

Drug-Drug: Concurrent use with **strong inducers of the UGT A1A enzyme system**, including **rifampin**, may ↓ levels and effectiveness. Concurrent use with **strong inhibitors of the UGT A1A enzyme system**, including **atazanavir**, may ↑ levels and the risk of toxicity. ↑ risk of rhabdomyolysis/myopathy with **HMG-CoA reductase inhibitors**. **Proton pump inhibitors** may ↑ levels and the risk of toxicity. **Efavirenz**, **etravirine**, and **tipranavir/ritonavir** may ↓ levels and effectiveness. Administration with **antacids**, containing **magnesium** or **aluminum** ↓ absorption of raltegravir; separate administration of raltegravir and magnesium- or aluminum-containing antacids by ≥6 hr.

Route/Dosage

Do not substitute the chewable tablets or oral suspension for the film-coated tablets.

PO (Adults): *Treatment-naive patients or patients who are virologically suppressed on an initial regimen of raltegravir 400 mg twice daily:* Two 600-mg tablets (1200 mg) once daily or 400 mg twice daily; *Treatment-experienced patients:* 400 mg twice daily; *Concurrent use of rifampin (either treatment-naive or treatment-experienced patients):* 800 mg twice daily.

PO (Children ≥40 kg and either treatment-naive or virologically suppressed on an initial regimen of raltegravir 400 mg twice daily): *Tablet:* Two 600-mg tablets (1200 mg) once daily or 400 mg twice daily; *Chewable tablets:* 300 mg twice daily.

PO (Children 28–39 kg): *Tablet:* 400 mg twice daily; *Chewable tablets (if unable to swallow tablet):* 200 mg twice daily.

PO (Children 25–27 kg): *Tablet:* 400 mg twice daily; *Chewable tablets (if unable to swallow tablet):* 150 mg twice daily.

PO (Children ≥4 wk and 20–<25 kg): *Chewable tablets:* 150 mg twice daily.

PO (Children ≥4 wk and 14–19 kg): *Oral suspension:* 100 mg twice daily; *Chewable tablets:* 100 mg twice daily.

PO (Children ≥4 wk and 10–13 kg): *Oral suspension:* 80 mg twice daily; *Chewable tablets:* 75 mg twice daily.

PO (Children ≥4 wk and 8–9 kg): *Oral suspension:* 60 mg twice daily; *Chewable tablets:* 50 mg twice daily.

PO (Children ≥4 wk and 6–7 kg): *Oral suspension:* 40 mg twice daily; *Chewable tablets:* 50 mg twice daily.

PO (Children ≥4 wk and 4–5 kg): *Oral suspension:* 30 mg twice daily; *Chewable tablets:* 25 mg twice daily.

PO (Children ≥4 wk and 3–<4 kg): *Oral suspension:* 25 mg twice daily; *Chewable tablets:* 25 mg twice daily.

PO (Neonates 1–4 wk and 4–<5 kg): *Oral suspension:* 15 mg twice daily.

PO (Neonates 1–4 wk and 3–<4 kg): *Oral suspension:* 10 mg twice daily.

PO (Neonates 1–4 wk and 2–<3 kg): *Oral suspension:* 8 mg twice daily.

PO (Neonates 0–1 wk and 4–<5 kg): *Oral suspension:* 7 mg once daily.

PO (Neonates 0–1 wk and 3–<4 kg): *Oral suspension:* 5 mg once daily.

PO (Neonates 0–1 wk and 2–<3 kg): *Oral suspension:* 4 mg once daily.

Availability

Tablets: 400 mg, 600 mg. **Chewable tablets (orange-banana):** 25 mg, 100 mg. **Packet for oral suspension (banana flavor):** 100 mg/pkt.

NURSING IMPLICATIONS

Assessment

- Assess patient for change in severity of HIV symptoms and for symptoms of opportunistic infections during therapy.
- Monitor for anxiety, depression (especially in patients with a history of psychiatric illness), suicidal ideation, and paranoia during therapy.

R

- Assess for rash periodically during therapy. May cause SJS. Discontinue therapy if severe or if accompanied with fever, general malaise, fatigue, muscle or joint aches, blisters, oral lesions, conjunctivitis, hepatitis, and/or eosinophilia.

Lab Test Considerations
- Monitor viral load and CD4 counts regularly during therapy.
- May cause ↓ absolute neutrophil count, hemoglobin, and platelet counts.
- May cause ↑ serum glucose, AST, ALT, GGT, total bilirubin, alkaline phosphatase, pancreatic amylase, serum lipase, and CK concentrations.

Implementation
- Tablets are not interchangeable with chewable tablets or packets for oral suspension.
- **PO:** May be administered without regard to meals.
- *DNC:* Swallow tablets whole; do not break, crush, or chew.
- Chewable tablets may be chewed or swallowed. For children with difficulty chewing the 25 mg chewable tablet, tablet may be crushed. Place the tablet(s) in a small, clean cup. For each tablet, add a teaspoonful (5 mL) of liquid (water, juice, breast milk). Within 2 min, tablet(s) will absorb liquid and fall apart. Using a spoon, crush any remaining pieces of the tablet(s). Immediately administer the entire dose orally. If any portion of dose is left in the cup, add another teaspoonful (5 mL) of liquid, swirl and administer immediately.
- *Oral suspension:* Pour packet for oral solution into 10 mL of water and mix in provided mixing cup. Gently swirl for 45 sec until mix is uniform; do not shake. Once mixed, administer with syringe orally within 30 min of mixing. Discard unused solution.

Patient/Family Teaching
- Emphasize the importance of taking raltegravir as directed, at evenly spaced times throughout day. Do not take more than prescribed amount and do not stop taking without consulting health care professional. Take missed doses as soon as remembered unless almost time for next dose. Do not double doses. Advise patient to read *Patient Information* sheet before starting therapy and with each Rx renewal in case of changes.
- Instruct patient that raltegravir should not be shared with others.
- Instruct patient to notify health care professional of all Rx or OTC medications, vitamins, or herbal products being taken and consult health care professional before taking any new medications.
- Inform patient that raltegravir does not cure AIDS or prevent associated or opportunistic infections. Raltegravir does not reduce the risk of transmission of HIV to others through sexual contact or blood contamination. Caution patient to use a condom during sexual contact and to avoid sharing needles or donating blood to prevent spreading the AIDS virus to others. Advise patient that the long-term effects of raltegravir are unknown at this time.
- Advise patient to notify health care professional if they develop any unusual symptoms, if any known symptom persists or worsen, or if signs and symptoms of rhabdomyolysis (unexplained muscle pain, tenderness, weakness), rash, or depression or suicidal thoughts occur.
- Immune reconstitution syndrome may trigger opportunistic infections or autoimmune disorders. Notify health care professional if symptoms occur.
- Rep: Advise females of reproductive potential to notify health care professional if pregnancy is planned or suspected. Inform pregnant women about the pregnancy exposure registry to monitor pregnancy outcomes. Enroll patient in the Antiretroviral Pregnancy Registry by calling 1-800-258-4263. Advise female patient to avoid breastfeeding during therapy.
- Emphasize the importance of regular follow-up exams and blood counts to determine progress and monitor for side effects.

Evaluation/Desired Outcomes
- Delayed progression of AIDS and decreased opportunistic infections in patients with HIV.
- Decrease in viral load and improvement in CD4 cell counts.

---

ramipril, See ANGIOTENSIN-CONVERTING ENZYME (ACE) INHIBITORS.

⚡ ramucirumab
(ra-mue-**sir**-ue-mab)
Cyramza
Classification
Therapeutic: antineoplastics
Pharmacologic: vascular endothelial growth factor antagonists

Indications
Advanced gastric cancer or gastroesophageal junction adenocarcinoma following unsuccessful combination treatment that included a fluoropyrimidine or platinum compound (as monotherapy or in combination with paclitaxel). ⚡ First-line treatment of metastatic non–small cell lung cancer (NSCLC) in patients whose tumors have epidermal growth factor receptor (EGFR) exon 19 deletions or exon 21 (L858R) substitution mutations (in combination with erlotinib). Metastatic NSCLC with disease progression on or after platinum-based chemotherapy (in combination with docetaxel). Metastatic colorectal cancer with disease progression on or after treatment with bevacizumab, oxaliplatin, and a fluoropyrimidine (in combination with irinotecan, folinic acid, and 5–fluorouracil [FOLFIRI]). Hepatocellular carcinoma in patients with an alpha fetopro-

tein of ≥400 ng/mL who have been previously treated with sorafenib.

Action

A monoclonal antibody that binds to vascular endothelial growth factor receptor 2, antagonizing its effects, resulting in decreased angiogenesis. **Therapeutic Effects:** Decreased growth and spread of gastric cancer, gastroesophageal junction adenocarcinoma, NSCLC, colorectal cancer, and hepatocellular carcinoma.

Pharmacokinetics

Absorption: IV administration results in complete bioavailability.
Distribution: Minimally distributed to tissues.
Metabolism and Excretion: Unknown.
Half-life: Unknown.

TIME/ACTION PROFILE (improved survival)

ROUTE	ONSET	PEAK	DURATION
IV	within 1 mo	7–8 mo	24 mo

Contraindications/Precautions

Contraindicated in: OB: Pregnancy; Lactation: Lactation.
Use Cautiously in: Child-Pugh Class B or C cirrhosis (use only if benefits outweigh risk of further deterioration); Surgery (discontinue prior to surgery, reinstate when healing is complete); Serious or non-healing wounds; Hypertension (must be controlled prior to treatment); Rep: Women of reproductive potential; Pedi: Safety and effectiveness not established in children.

Adverse Reactions/Side Effects

CV: hypertension, CARDIAC ARREST, MI. **Derm:** impaired wound healing. **Endo:** hypothyroidism. **F and E:** hyponatremia. **GI:** diarrhea, GI OBSTRUCTION/PERFORATION, worsened cirrhosis/hepatorenal syndrome. **GU:** ↓ fertility (females), nephrotic syndrome, proteinuria. **Hemat:** BLEEDING, neutropenia. **Neuro:** encephalopathy, headache, POSTERIOR REVERSIBLE ENCEPHALOPATHY SYNDROME (PRES), STROKE. **Misc:** INFUSION-RELATED REACTIONS.

Interactions

Drug-Drug: ↑ risk of bleeding with **anticoagulants**, **antiplatelet agents** and **NSAIDs**.

Route/Dosage

Gastric Cancer or Hepatocellular Carcinoma

IV (Adults): 8 mg/kg every 2 wk until disease progression or unacceptable toxicity.

Non−Small Cell Lung Cancer

IV (Adults): *First-line treatment in tumors with EGFR exon 19 deletions or exon 21 (L858R) substitution mutations:* 10 mg/kg every 2 wk until disease

progression or unacceptable toxicity; *Disease progression on or after platinum-based therapy:* 10 mg/kg on Day 1 of a 21-day cycle prior to docetaxel; continued until disease progression or unacceptable toxicity.

Colorectal Cancer

IV (Adults): 8 mg/kg every 2 wk prior to FOLFIRI administration; continued until disease progression or unacceptable toxicity.

Availability

Solution for injection: 10 mg/mL.

NURSING IMPLICATIONS

Assessment

- Monitor for infusion-related reactions (rigors/tremors, back pain/spasms, chest pain and/or tightness, chills, flushing, dyspnea, wheezing, hypoxia, paresthesia, bronchospasm, supraventricular tachycardia, hypotension) during infusion. Reduce infusion rate by 50% for Grade 1 or 2 reactions, and immediately and permanently discontinue ramucirumab if Grade 3 or 4 reactions occur.
- Monitor BP prior to and at least every 2 wk during therapy. Hold therapy for severe hypertension until BP is under control. Permanently discontinue if unable to control hypertension.
- Avoid administration for at least 28 days prior to and 28 days after surgery or until wound is healed.
- If arterial thromboembolic events (MI, cardiac arrest, stroke, cerebral ischemia) occur, permanently discontinue.
- Monitor for signs and symptoms of bleeding (bleeding, lightheadedness) during therapy. *If Grade 3 or 4 bleeding occurs,* permanently discontinue medication.
- Monitor for signs and symptoms of GI perforation (severe diarrhea, vomiting, severe abdominal pain) during therapy. Discontinue medication permanently if perforation occurs.

Lab Test Considerations

- Verify negative pregnancy test before starting therapy. Monitor urinary protein periodically during therapy. Hold ramucirumab for urine protein ≥2 g/24 hr. Reinitiate therapy at reduced dose (reduce 8 mg dose to 6 mg/kg and 10 mg to 8 mg) every 2 wk once urinary protein levels <2 g/24 hr. If protein level returns to ≥2 g/24 hr hold therapy until urine protein <2 g per 24 hr and reduce dose (reduce 6 mg to 5 mg/kg and 8 mg to 6 mg) every 2 wk once urinary protein levels return to <2 g/24 hr. Discontinue therapy permanently if urine protein level >3 g/24 hr or if nephrotic syndrome occurs.

Implementation

- Hold ramucirumab therapy for at least 4 wk before elective surgery and for at least 2 wk after major surgery until adequate wound healing occurs.

- Prior to each dose, premedicate all patients with IV histamine H$_1$ antagonist (diphenhydramine). Premedicate patients who have experienced a Grade 1 or 2 infusion reaction with dexamethasone and acetaminophen prior to each infusion.

IV Administration

- **Intermittent Infusion:** Withdraw required volume from vial. *Dilution:* Dilute with 0.9% NaCl for a final volume of 250 mL. Do not use dextrose-containing solutions. Gently invert to ensure adequate mixing. Solution is clear to slightly opalescent and colorless to slightly yellow; do not administer solutions that are discolored or contain particulate material. Solution is stable for 24 hr if refrigerated or 4 hr at room temperature. Discard unused solution. *Rate:* Infuse over 60 min via infusion pump through a separate infusion line using a 0.22 micron filter; do not administer as IV push or bolus. Flush line with 0.9% NaCl at end of infusion. If 1st infusion is tolerated, administer all subsequent infusions over 30 min.
- **Y-Site Incompatibility:** Do not dilute with other solutions or infuse with other electrolyte solutions or medications.

Patient/Family Teaching

- Explain purpose of ramucirumab to patient.
- Advise patient to notify health care professional if bleeding or lightheadedness occur.
- Instruct patient in self BP monitoring and advise patient to notify health care professional if signs and symptoms of hypertension (elevated BP, severe headache, lightheadedness, neurologic symptoms) or if severe diarrhea, vomiting, or severe abdominal pain occur.
- Advise patient to notify health care professional of medication regimen prior to surgery; must be stopped for at least 4 wk before elective surgery and for at least 2 wk after major surgery until adequate wound healing occurs; may impair wound healing.
- Rep: May cause fetal harm. Advise females of reproductive potential to use effective contraception during and for at least 3 mo after last dose and avoid breastfeeding for 2 mo after last dose. Notify health care professional if pregnancy is suspected. Advise patient that ramucirumab may impair fertility in females.

Evaluation/Desired Outcomes

- Decreased growth and spread of cancer.

---

ranolazine (ra-nole-a-zeen)

Aspruzyo Sprinkle, ✤ Corzyna, Ra-nexa

Classification
Therapeutic: antianginals

Indications

Chronic angina pectoris.

Action

Does not ↓ BP or heart rate; remainder of mechanism is not known. **Therapeutic Effects:** Decreased frequency of angina.

Pharmacokinetics

Absorption: Highly variable.
Distribution: Unknown.
Metabolism and Excretion: Metabolized by the liver primarily by the CYP3A isoenzyme and to a lesser extent by the CYP2D6 isoenzyme; <5% excreted unchanged in urine and feces.
Half-life: 7 hr.

TIME/ACTION PROFILE (plasma concentrations)

ROUTE	ONSET	PEAK	DURATION
PO	unknown	2–5 hr	12 hr

Contraindications/Precautions

Contraindicated in: Hypersensitivity; Concurrent use of potent CYP3A inhibitors; Concurrent use of CYP3A inducers; Hepatic impairment; Lactation: Lactation.

Use Cautiously in: Renal impairment; OB: Use during pregnancy only if potential maternal benefit justifies potential fetal risk; Pedi: Safety and effectiveness not established in children; Geri: ↑ risk of adverse reactions in patients >75 yr.

Adverse Reactions/Side Effects

CV: palpitations, QT interval prolongation, TORSADES DE POINTES. EENT: tinnitus. GI: abdominal pain, constipation, dry mouth, nausea, vomiting. GU: acute renal failure. **Neuro:** dizziness, headache.

Interactions

Drug-Drug: Ketoconazole, itraconazole, clarithromycin, nefazodone, nelfinavir, and ritonavir significantly ↑ levels; concurrent use contraindicated. Rifampin, rifabutin, rifapentin, phenobarbital, phenytoin, and carbamazepine significantly ↓ levels; concurrent use contraindicated. Verapamil, diltiazem, aprepitant, erythromycin, and fluconazole ↑ levels (do not exceed ranolazine dose of 500 mg twice daily). Cyclosporine may ↑ levels. Paroxetine may ↑ levels. May ↑ levels of simvastatin. May ↓ metabolism and ↑ effects of metoprolol, tricyclic antidepressants, and antipsychotics; dosage adjustments may be necessary. May ↑ digoxin levels; dose adjustment may be required.
Drug-Natural Products: St. John's wort significantly ↓ levels (contraindicated).
Drug-Food: Grapefruit juice↑ levels (do not exceed ranolazine dose of 500 mg twice daily).

Route/Dosage

PO (Adults): 500 mg twice daily initially, may be ↑ to 1000 mg twice daily.

Availability (generic available)
Extended-release tablets: 500 mg, 1000 mg. **Extended-release granules:** 500 mg/pkt, 1000 mg/pkt.

NURSING IMPLICATIONS
Assessment
- Assess location, duration, intensity, and precipitating factors of anginal pain.
- Monitor ECG at baseline and periodically during therapy to evaluate effects on QT interval.

Lab Test Considerations
- Monitor renal function after starting and periodically during therapy in patients with moderate to severe renal impairment (CCr <60 mL/min) for ↑ serum creatinine accompanied by ↑ BUN. Usually has a rapid onset, but does not progress during therapy and is reversible with discontinuation of ranolazine. If acute renal failure develops, discontinue ranolazine.
- May cause transient eosinophilia.
- May cause small mean ↓ in hematocrit.

Implementation
- Ranolazine should be used in combination with calcium channel blockers, beta blockers, or nitrates.
- Do not administer with grapefruit juice or grapefruit products.
- **PO:** May be administered without regard to food. *DNC:* Tablets should be swallowed whole; do not break, crush, or chew.
- Sprinkle granules on one tablespoonful of soft food (applesauce or yogurt) and consume immediately. Do not crush or chew granules.
- *Nasogastric (NG) tube:* Add content of a sachet to a plastic catheter tip syringe and add 50 mL of water. Gently shake syringe for approximately 15 seconds. Promptly deliver through a 12 French or larger NG tube. Ensure no granules are left in the syringe. Rinse with additional water (about 15 mL) if needed.
- *Gastrostomy/Gastric (G) tube:* Add content of a sachet to a plastic catheter tip syringe and add 30 mL of water. Gently shake syringe for approximately 15 seconds. Promptly deliver through a 12 French or larger G-tube. Rinse with 20 mL of water in the syringe. Ensure no granules are left in the syringe. Rinse with additional water (about 15 mL) if needed.

Patient/Family Teaching
- Instruct patient to take ranolazine as directed. If a dose is missed, take the usual dose at the next scheduled time; do not double doses. Explain to patient that ranolazine is used for chronic therapy and will not help an acute angina episode.
- Advise patient to avoid grapefruit juice and grapefruit products when taking ranolazine.
- May cause dizziness and light-headedness. Caution patient to avoid driving and other activities requiring alertness until response to medication is known.

- Advise patient to notify health care professional if fainting occurs.
- Inform patient that ranolazine may cause changes in the ECG. Patient should inform health care professional if they have a personal or family history of QTc prolongation, congenital long QT syndrome, or proarrhythmic conditions such as hypokalemia.
- Instruct patient to notify health care professional of all Rx or OTC medications, vitamins, or herbal products being taken and consult health care professional before taking any new medications.
- Rep: Advise females of reproductive potential to notify health care professional if pregnancy is planned or suspected, or if breastfeeding.

Evaluation/Desired Outcomes
- Decrease in frequency of angina attacks.

---

rasagiline (ra-sa-ji-leen)
Azilect
Classification
Therapeutic: antiparkinson agents
Pharmacologic: monoamine oxidase type B inhibitors

Indications
Parkinson's disease.

Action
Irreversibly inactivates monoamine oxidase (MAO) by binding to it at type B (brain sites); inactivation of MAO leads to increased amounts of dopamine available in the CNS. Differs from selegiline by its nonamphetamine characteristics. **Therapeutic Effects:** Improvement in symptoms of Parkinson's disease, allowing increase in function.

Pharmacokinetics
Absorption: 36% absorbed following oral administration.
Distribution: Extensively distributed to tissues; readily crosses the blood-brain barrier.
Metabolism and Excretion: Extensively metabolized by the liver primarily by the CYP1A2 isoenzyme to an inactive metabolite; <1% excreted in urine.
Half-life: 1.3 hr; does not correlate with duration of MAO-B inhibition.

TIME/ACTION PROFILE

ROUTE	ONSET	PEAK	DURATION
PO	rapid	1 hr	40 days*

*Recovery of MAO-B function.

Contraindications/Precautions
Contraindicated in: Hypersensitivity; Concurrent use of meperidine, tramadol, methadone, or another MAO inhibitor; Moderate to severe hepatic impairment;

R

Elective surgery requiring general anesthesia; Pheo-chromocytoma; Psychotic disorder.

Use Cautiously in: Mild hepatic impairment; OB: Safety not established in pregnancy; Lactation: Safety not established in breastfeeding; Pedi: Safety and effectiveness not established in children.

Adverse Reactions/Side Effects

CV: <u>orthostatic hypotension (may ↑ levodopa-induced hypotension)</u>, ↑ BP, chest pain, syncope. **Derm:** ↑ melanoma risk, alopecia, ecchymosis, rash. **EENT:** conjunctivitis, rhinitis. **GI:** ↓ weight, anorexia, dizziness, dyspepsia, gastroenteritis, vomiting. **GU:** ↓ libido, albuminuria. **Hemat:** leukopenia. **MS:** arthralgia, arthritis, neck pain. **Neuro:** depression, dizziness, drowsiness, dyskinesia (may ↑ levodopa-induced dyskinesia), hallucinations, impulse control disorders (gambling, sexual), malaise, paresthesia, sleep driving, vertigo. **Resp:** asthma. **Misc:** fever, flu-like syndrome.

Interactions

Drug-Drug: Concurrent use of **meperidine**, **tramadol**, **methadone**, or other **MAO inhibitors** may ↑ risk of serotonin syndrome; concurrent use contraindicated. **CYP1A2 inhibitors**, including **ciprofloxacin**, may ↑ levels and risk of toxicity; dose adjustment is recommended. **Dextromethorphan** may ↑ risk of psychosis/bizarre behavior; avoid concurrent use. ↑ risk of adverse reactions with **mirtazapine** and **cyclobenzaprine**; avoid concurrent use. Hypertensive crisis may occur with **sympathomimetic amines**, including **amphetamines**, **pseudoephedrine**, **phenylephrine**, or **ephedrine**; avoid concurrent use. ↑ risk of serotonin syndrome with **tricyclic antidepressants**, **SSRIs**, and **SNRIs**; rasagiline should be discontinued ≥14 days prior to initiation of antidepressants (**fluoxetine** should be discontinued ≥5 wk prior to rasagiline therapy). **Drug-Natural Products:** St. John's wort may ↑ risk of serotonin syndrome; avoid concurrent use. **Drug-Food:** Ingestion of foods containing high amounts of **tyramine** (>150 mg) (e.g., cheese) may result in life-threatening hypertensive crisis.

Route/Dosage

PO (Adults): *Monotherapy or as adjunct therapy in patients not taking levodopa:* 1 mg once daily; *Concurrent levodopa therapy:* 0.5 mg once daily, may ↑ to 1 mg once daily; *Concurrent use of ciprofloxacin or other CYP1A2 inhibitors:* 0.5 mg once daily.

Hepatic Impairment

PO (Adults): *Mild hepatic impairment:* 0.5 mg once daily.

Availability (generic available)

Tablets: 0.5 mg, 1 mg.

NURSING IMPLICATIONS

Assessment

- Assess signs and symptoms of Parkinson's disease (tremor, muscle weakness and rigidity, ataxic gait) prior to and periodically during therapy.

- Monitor BP periodically during therapy.
- Assess skin for melanomas periodically during therapy.
- Assess for serotonin syndrome (mental changes [agitation, hallucinations, coma], autonomic instability [tachycardia, labile BP, hyperthermia], neuromuscular aberrations [hyperreflexia, incoordination], and/or GI symptoms [nausea, vomiting, diarrhea]), especially in patients taking other serotonergic drugs (SSRIs, SNRIs, triptans).
- Monitor for drowsiness or sleepiness. May cause patients to fall asleep while engaged in activities of daily living, including the operation of motor vehicles.

Lab Test Considerations

- May cause albuminuria, leukopenia, and abnormal liver function tests.

Toxicity and Overdose

- Concurrent ingestion of tyramine-rich foods and many medications may result in a life-threatening hypertensive crisis. Signs and symptoms of hypertensive crisis include chest pain, tachycardia or bradycardia, severe headache, neck stiffness or soreness, nausea and vomiting, sweating, photosensitivity, and enlarged pupils.

Implementation

- Do not confuse Azilect with Aricept. Do not confuse rasagiline with repaglinide.
- If used in combination with levodopa, a reduction in levodopa dose may be considered based on individual results.
- **PO:** Administer once daily.

Patient/Family Teaching

- Instruct patient to take rasagiline as directed. Missed doses should be omitted and next dose taken at usual time the following day. Do not double doses. Do not discontinue abruptly; may cause elevated temperature, muscular rigidity, altered consciousness, and autonomic instability.
- Caution patient to avoid alcohol, CNS depressants, and foods or beverages containing tyramine (see Appendix J) during and for at least 2 wk after therapy has been discontinued; they may precipitate a hypertensive crisis. Contact health care professional immediately if symptoms of hypertensive crisis or serotonin syndrome develop.
- Instruct patient to notify health care professional of all Rx or OTC medications, vitamins, or herbal products being taken and consult health care professional before taking any new medications. Caution patient to avoid use of St. John's wort and analgesics meperidine, tramadol, or methadone during therapy.
- Caution patient to avoid elective surgery requiring general anesthesia, cocaine, or local anesthesia containing sympathomimetic vasoconstrictors within 14 days of discontinuing rasagiline. If surgery is necessary sooner, benzodiazepines, rocuronium, fentanyl, morphine, and codeine may be used cautiously.

- May cause dizziness or drowsiness. Caution patient to avoid driving and other activities requiring alertness until response to medication is known.
- Caution patient to change positions slowly to minimize orthostatic hypotension. Geriatric patients are at increased risk for this side effect.
- Advise patient to monitor for melanomas frequently and on a regular basis.
- Caution patient to notify health care professional if new skin lesions, agitation, aggression, delirium, hallucinations, sleep driving, or new or increased gambling, sexual, or other intense urges occur.
- Inform patient that rasagiline may cause falling asleep while engaged in activities of daily living, including the operation of motor vehicles, conversations, and eating. Notify health care professional if periods of daytime sleepiness occur.
- Advise patient to notify health care professional immediately if severe headache, neck stiffness, heart racing, or palpitations occur.
- Rep: Advise female patients to notify health care professionals if pregnancy is planned or suspected, or if breastfeeding.

Evaluation/Desired Outcomes
- Improvement in symptoms of Parkinson's disease, allowing increase in function.

☒ rasburicase (ras-**byoor**-i-case)
Elitek, ✦ Fasturtec
Classification
Therapeutic: antigout agents, antihyperuricemics
Pharmacologic: enzymes

Indications
Initial management of increased uric acid levels in patients with leukemia, lymphoma, or other malignancies who are being treated with antineoplastics, which are expected to produce hyperuricemia.

Action
An enzyme that promotes the conversion of uric acid to allantoin, an inactive, water-soluble compound. Produced by recombinant DNA technology. **Therapeutic Effects:** Decreased sequelae of hyperuricemia (nephropathy, arthropathy).

Pharmacokinetics
Absorption: IV administration results in complete bioavailability.
Distribution: Well distributed to tissues.
Metabolism and Excretion: Unknown.
Half-life: 18 hr.

TIME/ACTION PROFILE (↓ in uric acid)

ROUTE	ONSET	PEAK	DURATION
IV	rapid	unknown	4–24 hr

Contraindications/Precautions
Contraindicated in: ☒ Glucose-6–phosphate dehydrogenase (G6PD) deficiency (↑ risk of severe hemolysis); Previous allergic reaction, hemolysis, or methemoglobinemia from rasburicase; OB: Pregnancy; Lactation: Lactation.
Use Cautiously in: None reported.

Adverse Reactions/Side Effects
Derm: rash. **GI:** abdominal pain, constipation, diarrhea, mucositis, nausea, vomiting. **Hemat:** HEMOLYSIS, METHEMOGLOBINEMIA, neutropenia. **Neuro:** headache. **Resp:** respiratory distress. **Misc:** fever, HYPERSENSITIVITY REACTIONS (including anaphylaxis), sepsis.

Interactions
Drug-Drug: None reported.

Route/Dosage
IV (Adults and Children): 0.2 mg/kg daily as a single dose for 5 days.

Availability
Lyophilized powder for injection: 1.5 mg/vial, 7.5 mg/vial.

NURSING IMPLICATIONS
Assessment
- Monitor patients for signs of allergic reactions and anaphylaxis (chest pain, dyspnea, hypotension, urticaria). If these signs occur, rasburicase should be immediately and permanently discontinued.

Lab Test Considerations
- Monitor patients for hemolysis. ☒ Screen patients at higher risk for G6PD deficiency (patients of African American or Mediterranean ancestry) prior to therapy. If hemolysis occurs, discontinue and do not restart rasburicase.
- Monitor patients for methemoglobinemia. Discontinue rasburicase and do not restart in patients who develop methemoglobinemia.
- May cause spuriously low uric acid levels in blood samples left at room temperature. Collect blood for uric acid levels in pre-chilled tubes containing heparin and immediately immerse and maintain in an ice water bath. Uric acid must be analyzed in plasma. Plasma samples must be assayed within 4 hr of collection.

Implementation
- Chemotherapy is initiated 4–24 hr after 1st dose of rasburicase.

IV Administration
- **Intermittent Infusion:** Determine number of vials of rasburicase needed based on patient's weight and dose/kg. *Reconstitution:* Reconstitute in diluent provided. Add 1 mL of diluent provided to each vial and mix by swirling very gently. Do not shake or vor-

R

✦ = Canadian drug name. ☒ = Genetic implication. ~~Strikethrough~~ = Discontinued. CAPITALS = life-threatening. <u>Underline</u> = most frequent.

tex. Reconstitute 7.5 mg vial with 5 mL of diluent. Solution should be clear and colorless. Do not use solutions that are discolored or contain particulate matter. *Dilution:* Remove dose from reconstituted vials and inject into infusion bag of 0.9% NaCl for a final total volume of 50 mL. Administer within 24 hr of reconstitution. Store reconstituted or diluted solution in refrigerator for up to 24 hr. *Rate:* Administer over 30 min. Do not administer as a bolus.

• **Y-Site Incompatibility:** Infuse through a separate line. Do not use a filter with infusion. If separate line is not possible, flush line with at least 15 mL of 0.9% NaCl prior to rasburicase infusion.

Patient/Family Teaching

• Inform patient and family of purpose of rasburicase infusion.

• Rep: May cause fetal harm. Advise females of reproductive potential to notify health care professional if pregnancy is planned or suspected and to avoid breastfeeding during and for 2 wk after last dose.

Evaluation/Desired Outcomes

• Decrease in plasma uric acid levels in pediatric patients receiving antineoplastics expected to result in tumor lysis and subsequent elevation of plasma uric acid levels. More than 1 course of therapy or administration beyond 5 days is not recommended.

---

regorafenib (re-goe-raf-e-nib)
Stivarga
Classification
Therapeutic: antineoplastics
Pharmacologic: kinase inhibitors

Indications

Metastatic colorectal cancer that has failed previous treatment that included a fluoropyrimidine, oxaliplatin, irinotecan, an anti-VEGF therapy, and additional anti-EGFR therapy if tumor is of the *RAS* wild type. Locally advanced, unresectable, or metastatic gastrointestinal stromal tumor in patients who have previously been treated with imatinib and sunitinib. Hepatocellular carcinoma in patients who have previously been treated with sorafenib.

Action

Inhibits kinases, which are responsible for many phases of cell function and proliferation. **Therapeutic Effects:** Decreased progression of hepatocellular carcinoma and metastatic colorectal cancer with improved survival. Decreased progression of gastrointestinal stromal tumor.

Pharmacokinetics

Absorption: Well absorbed following oral administration (69–83%).
Distribution: Unknown.
Protein Binding: *Regorafenib:* >99.5%, *M-2 metabolite:* 99.8%, *M-5 metabolite:* 99.95%.

Metabolism and Excretion: Primarily metabolized by the liver via the CYP3A4 isoenzyme and UGT1A9; 2 metabolites (M-2 and M-5) have antineoplastic activity. Undergoes enterohepatic circulation. 47% excreted in feces as parent compound, 24% as metabolites; 19% excreted in urine (mostly as inactive metabolites).
Half-life: *Regorafenib:* 28 hr, *M-2 metabolite:* 25 hr, *M-5 metabolite:* 51 hr.

TIME/ACTION PROFILE (improved survival)

ROUTE	ONSET	PEAK	DURATION
PO	3 mo	3 mo	up to 10 mo

Contraindications/Precautions

Contraindicated in: Severe hepatic impairment; OB: Pregnancy; Lactation: Lactation.
Use Cautiously in: History of hypertension or cardiovascular disease (BP should be controlled prior to treatment); Elective surgical procedures (discontinue 2 wk prior to surgery); Asian patients (↑ risk of palmar-plantar erythrodysesthesia); Rep: Women of reproductive potential and men with female partners of reproductive potential; Pedi: Safety and effectiveness not established in children.

Adverse Reactions/Side Effects

CV: HYPERTENSION, MYOCARDIAL ISCHEMIA/INFARCTION. **Derm:** alopecia, ERYTHEMA MULTIFORME, impaired wound healing, PALMAR-PLANTAR ERYTHRODYSESTHESIA, rash, STEVENS-JOHNSON SYNDROME (SJS), TOXIC EPIDERMAL NECROLYSIS (TEN). **EENT:** dysphonia. **Endo:** hypothyroidism. **F and E:** hypocalcemia, hypokalemia, hypophosphatemia, hyponatremia. **GI:** ↓ appetite, ↓ weight, ↑ lipase, diarrhea, mucositis, ↑ amylase, ↑ liver enzymes, dry mouth, GI FISTULA/PERFORATION, HEPATOTOXICITY, reflux. **GU:** proteinuria, ↓ fertility. **Hemat:** anemia, BLEEDING, lymphopenia, THROMBOCYTOPENIA. **MS:** pain, musculoskeletal stiffness. **Neuro:** fatigue, dysgeusia, headache, POSTERIOR REVERSIBLE ENCEPHALOPATHY SYNDROME (PRES), tremor. **Misc:** fever, INFECTION.

Interactions

Drug-Drug: **Strong CYP3A4 inhibitors,** including **clarithromycin, itraconazole, ketoconazole, posaconazole,** and **voriconazole,** ↑ levels and the risk of toxicity, avoid concurrent use. **Strong CYP3A4 inducers,** including **carbamazepine, phenobarbital, phenytoin,** and **rifampin,** ↓ levels and effectiveness, avoid concurrent use. May ↑ risk of bleeding with **warfarin.** May ↑ levels and risk of toxicity of **breast cancer resistance protein (BCRP) substrates,** including **methotrexate, fluvastatin,** or **atorvastatin.**
Drug-Natural Products: St. John's wort ↓ levels and effectiveness; avoid concurrent use.
Drug-Food: Grapefruit juice ↑ levels and the risk of toxicity; avoid concurrent use.

Route/Dosage

PO (Adults): 160 mg daily on days 1–21 of a 28-day cycle. Continue until disease progression or unacceptable toxicity.

Availability

Tablets: 40 mg.

NURSING IMPLICATIONS

Assessment

- Monitor BP prior to and weekly during the first 6 wk, then every cycle of therapy. Do not initiate regorafenib until BP is well controlled.
- Assess for myocardial ischemia or infarction during therapy.
- Assess for bleeding during therapy. Interrupt therapy if severe hemorrhage occurs.
- Assess for rash periodically during therapy. May cause SJS or TEN. Discontinue therapy if severe or if accompanied with fever, general malaise, fatigue, muscle or joint aches, blisters, oral lesions, conjunctivitis, hepatitis, and/or eosinophilia.
- Monitor for signs and symptoms of PRES (seizures, headache, visual disturbances, confusion, altered mental function) during therapy. Diagnosis via MRI. Discontinue regorafenib in patients who develop PRES.

Lab Test Considerations

- Obtain liver function test (ALT, AST, bilirubin) before starting, at least every 2 wk during first 2 mo of therapy, and monthly thereafter. Monitor liver function tests weekly in patients with ↑ liver function tests until improvement to <3× the upper limit of normal (ULN) or baseline.
- May cause anemia, thrombocytopenia, neutropenia, and lymphopenia.
- May cause hypocalcemia, hypokalemia, hyponatremia, and hypophosphatemia.
- May cause proteinuria, ↑ serum lipase, and ↑ serum amylase.
- May cause ↑ INR. Monitor INR levels more frequently in patients receiving warfarin.

Implementation

- **High Alert:** Fatalities have occurred with incorrect administration of chemotherapeutic agents. Before administering, clarify all ambiguous orders; double-check single, daily, and course-of-therapy dose limits. Therapy should be initiated by physician experienced in the treatment of patients with colorectal cancer.
- May impair wound healing. Hold therapy for at least 2 wk before elective surgery and for at least 2 wk after major surgery until adequate wound healing occurs.
- **PO:** Administer four 40 mg tablets once daily at same time of day with a whole glass of water for the

first 21 days of each 28-day cycle. *DNC:* Swallow tablets whole with a low-fat meal that contains <30% fat and <600 calories.

- **Dose modifications:** *Interrupt therapy for* Grade 2 hand-foot skin reaction (HFSR) that is recurrent or does not improve in 7 days despite dose reduction; interrupt therapy for a minimum of 7 days for Grade 3 (HFSR), symptomatic Grade 2 hypertension, any Grade 3 or 4 adverse reactions.
- *Reduce dose to 120 mg daily for* 1st occurrence of Grade 2 HFSR of any duration, after 1st recovery of any Grade 3 or 4 adverse reaction, for Grade 3 ↑ AST or ALT; only resume if potential benefit outweighs risk of hepatotoxicity.
- *Reduce dose to 80 mg daily for* reoccurrence of Grade 2 HFSR at 120 mg dose, after recovery of any Grade 3 or 4 adverse reaction at 120 mg dose (except hepatotoxicity).
- *Discontinue regorafenib permanently for* failure to tolerate 80 mg dose, any occurrence of ↑ AST or ALT >20 × ULN, any occurrence of ↑ AST or ALT >3 × ULN with concurrent bilirubin >2 × ULN, reoccurrence of ↑ AST or ALT >5 × ULN despite reduction to 120 mg dose, any Grade 4 adverse reaction; only resume if the potential benefits outweigh the risks.

Patient/Family Teaching

- Instruct patient to take tablets at the same time each day with a low-fat meal. Take missed doses on the same day as soon as remembered; do not take 2 doses on the same day to make up for a missed dose. Store medicine in original container; do not place in daily or weekly pill boxes. Discard remaining tablets 28 days after opening bottle. Tightly close bottle after each opening and keep desiccant in bottle. Advise patient to read *Patient Information* before starting therapy and with each Rx refill in case of changes.
- Advise patient to avoid drinking grapefruit juice or eating grapefruit during regorafenib therapy.
- Advise patient to notify health care professional immediately if signs and symptoms of liver problems (yellowing of skin or white part of eyes, nausea, vomiting, dark tea-colored urine, change in sleep pattern), bleeding, skin changes (redness, pain, blisters, bleeding, swelling), hypertension (severe headache, lightheadedness, neurologic symptoms), myocardial ischemia or infarction (chest pain, shortness of breath, dizziness, fainting), or GI perforation or fistula (severe abdominal pain, persistent swelling of abdomen, high fever, chills, nausea, vomiting, severe diarrhea, dehydration) occur.
- Advise patient to notify health care provider of therapy prior to surgery or if had recent surgery.
- Advise patient to maintain adequate hydration to minimize risk and to notify health care professional

R

promptly if signs and symptoms of PRES (headache, seizures, weakness, confusion, high BP, blindness or change in vision, problems thinking) occur.

● Instruct patient to notify health care professional of all Rx or OTC medications, vitamins, or herbal products being taken and consult health care professional before taking any new medications, especially St. John's wort.

● Rep: May cause fetal harm. Advise women of reproductive potential and men of the need for effective contraception during and for at least 2 mo after completion of therapy. Notify health care provider immediately if pregnancy is planned or suspected and to avoid breastfeeding during therapy.

● Emphasize importance of monitoring lab values to monitor for adverse reactions.

Evaluation/Desired Outcomes

● Decreased progression of hepatocellular carcinoma and metastatic colorectal cancer.

● Decreased progression of gastrointestinal stromal tumor.

relugolix/estradiol/ norethindrone

(rel-ue-**goe**-lix/es-tra-**dye**-ole/nor-**eth**-in-drone)

Myfembree

Classification

Therapeutic: hormones

Pharmacologic: GnRH antagonist, estrogens, progestins

Indications

Heavy menstrual bleeding associated with uterine fibroids in premenopausal women. Moderate to severe pain associated with endometriosis in premenopausal women.

Action

Relugolix: reversibly binds to gonadotropin-releasing hormone (GnRH) receptors in the pituitary gland, causing a decrease in the release of luteinizing hormone and follicle-stimulating hormone, which subsequently leads to decreased serum concentrations of estradiol and progesterone; *Estradiol:* an estrogen that reduces the ↑ in bone resorption and resultant bone loss that can occur due to a ↓ in circulating estrogen concentrations from relugolix; *Norethindrone:* a progestin that protects the uterus from estrogen-induced endometrial hyperplasia. **Therapeutic Effects:** Reduction in menstrual blood loss in premenopausal women with uterine fibroids. Reduction in pain in premenopausal women with endometriosis.

Pharmacokinetics

Relugolix

Absorption: 12% absorbed following oral administration.

Distribution: Unknown.

Metabolism and Excretion: Primarily metabolized in the liver via the CYP3A4 isoenzyme (and to a lesser extent by CYP2C8). Primarily excreted in feces (81%; 4.2% as unchanged drug), with 4.1% excreted in urine (2.2% as unchanged drug).

Half-life: 61 hr.

Estradiol

Absorption: Well absorbed following oral administration.

Distribution: Widely distributed to tissues.

Metabolism and Excretion: Mostly metabolized by the liver and other tissues. Enterohepatic recirculation occurs, and more absorption may occur from the GI tract.

Half-life: 16.6 hr.

Norethindrone

Absorption: Rapidly absorbed following oral administration.

Distribution: Widely distributed to tissues.

Metabolism and Excretion: Mostly metabolized by the liver. Metabolites primarily excreted in the urine (>50%), with 20–40% being excreted in feces.

Half-life: 8–9 hr.

TIME/ACTION PROFILE (plasma concentrations)

ROUTE	ONSET	PEAK	DURATION
PO (relugolix)	unknown	2 hr	unknown
PO (estradiol)	unknown	7 hr	unknown
PO (norethindrone)	unknown	1 hr	unknown

Contraindications/Precautions

Contraindicated in: Hypersensitivity; Women >35 years old who smoke; Current or history of deep vein thrombosis or pulmonary embolism; Cerebrovascular disease, cardiovascular disease, or peripheral vascular disease; Subacute bacterial endocarditis with valvular disease or atrial fibrillation; Inherited or acquired hypercoagulopathies; Uncontrolled hypertension; Headaches with focal neurological symptoms or migraine headaches with aura if >35 years old; Osteoporosis; Current or history of breast cancer or other hormone-sensitive malignancy; Increased risk for hormone-sensitive malignancy; Hepatic impairment; Undiagnosed abnormal uterine bleeding; OB: Pregnancy.

Use Cautiously in: Underlying cardiovascular disease; Obesity; History of low trauma fracture or risk factors for osteoporosis or bone loss, including taking medications that may ↓ bone mineral density; History of suicidal ideation, depression, or anxiety; Submucosal uterine fibroids (↑ risk of prolapse or expulsion); Prediabetes or diabetes; Hypertriglyceridemia; Hypothyroidism or hypoadrenalism (may need to ↑ doses of thyroid hormone or cortisol replacement therapy; Lactation: Use while breastfeeding only if potential maternal benefit justifies potential risk to infant; Rep: Women of reproductive potential; Pedi: Safety and effectiveness not established in children.

Adverse Reactions/Side Effects

CV: DEEP VEIN THROMBOSIS, edema, hypertension, MI. **Derm:** hot flush, hyperhidrosis, night sweats, alopecia. **Endo:** hyperglycemia. **GI:** ↑ liver enzymes, cholecystitis, diarrhea, dyspepsia, nausea. **GU:** ↓ libido, amenorrhea, uterine bleeding, uterine fibroid expulsion/prolapse, vulvovaginal dryness. **Metab:** hypercholesterolemia, hypertriglyceridemia. **MS:** ↓ bone mineral density, arthralgia. **Neuro:** headache, anxiety, depression, dizziness, fatigue, irritability, STROKE, SUICIDAL THOUGHTS/BEHAVIORS. **Resp:** PULMONARY EMBOLISM. **Misc:** BREAST CANCER, HYPERSENSITIVITY REACTIONS (including anaphylaxis and angioedema).

Interactions

Drug-Drug: Corticosteroids, anticonvulsants, or **proton pump inhibitors** may ↑ risk of bone mineral density reduction and osteoporosis. **Hormonal contraceptives** may ↓ effectiveness of relugolix/estradiol/norethindrone and ↑ risk of thromboembolic events; avoid concurrent use. **P-glycoprotein (P-gp) inhibitors** may ↑ relugolix levels and risk of toxicity; avoid concurrent use. If concurrent use unavoidable, administer relugolix/estradiol/norethindrone first and then administer P-gp inhibitor ≥6 hr later. **Combined P-gp and strong CYP3A4 inducers** may ↓ relugolix/estradiol/norethindrone levels and effectiveness; avoid concurrent use.

Route/Dosage

PO (Adults): One tablet once daily. Start as early as possible after the onset of menses but no later than 7 days after menses has started. Duration of therapy not to exceed 24 mo.

Availability

Tablets: relugolix 40 mg/estradiol 1 mg/norethindrone 0.5 mg.

NURSING IMPLICATIONS

Assessment

● Monitor for signs and symptoms of thrombotic events (sudden unexplained partial or complete loss of vision, proptosis, diplopia, papilledema, retinal vascular lesions). Discontinue therapy immediately if an arterial or venous thrombotic, cardiovascular, or cerebrovascular event occurs or is suspected. Assess for retinal vein thrombosis. Risk is greatest among women over 35 yr of age who smoke and women with uncontrolled hypertension, dyslipidemia, vascular disease, or obesity. Discontinue *Myfembree* at least 4 to 6 wk before surgery of the type associated with an increased risk of thromboembolism, or during periods of prolonged immobilization, if feasible.

● May cause bone loss. Assess bone mineral density (BMD) by dual-energy x-ray absorptiometry (DXA)

at baseline and periodically in women with heavy menstrual bleeding associated with uterine fibroids. In women with moderate to severe pain associated with endometriosis, annual DXA is recommended while taking *Myfembree*. Consider discontinuing *Myfembree* if risk associated with bone loss exceeds the potential benefit of therapy. May add calcium and vitamin D supplement to increase BMD.

● Assess patients with a history of suicidal ideation, depression, and mood disorders prior to starting therapy for mood changes and depressive symptoms including shortly after initiating treatment, to determine whether the risks of continuing therapy outweigh the benefits. Patients with new or worsening depression, anxiety, or other mood changes should be referred to a mental health professional. Advise patients to seek immediate medical attention for suicidal ideation and behavior. Re-evaluate the benefits and risks of continuing *Myfembree* if such events occur.

● Monitor for signs and symptoms of hypersensitivity reactions (anaphylaxis, urticaria, angioedema). Immediately discontinue therapy if a hypersensitivity reaction occurs.

Lab Test Considerations

● Validate negative pregnancy test before starting therapy.

● Monitor blood sugar frequently. May decrease glucose tolerance and increase blood glucose.

● Monitor lipid levels and consider discontinuing therapy if hypercholesterolemia or hypertriglyceridemia worsens.

Implementation

● Begin therapy as soon as possible after the onset of menses but no later than 7 days after menses has started. If *Myfembree* is started later in the menstrual cycle, irregular and/or heavy bleeding may initially occur.

● Total duration of *Myfembree* therapy is 24 mo.

● **PO:** Administer one tablet orally once daily at the same time, without regard to food.

Patient/Family Teaching

● Instruct patient to take medication as directed at the same time each day. Take missed doses as soon as possible the same day and then resume regular dosing the next day at the usual time. Advise patient to read *Patient Information* before starting therapy and with each Rx refill in case of changes.

● Inform patient of the potential for bone loss, including the scans and possible supplementation with calcium and vitamin D.

● May cause hair thinning or loss. Discuss with patient the possibility of hair loss. Explore methods of coping. May consider discontinuing therapy.

● Instruct patient to notify health care professional of all Rx or OTC medications, vitamins, or herbal prod-

R

ucts being taken and consult health care professional before taking any new medications.

- Advise patient to notify health care professional immediately if signs and symptoms of thromboembolism (leg pain or swelling that will not go away; sudden shortness of breath; double vision; bulging of the eyes; sudden blindness, partial or complete; pain or pressure in your chest, arm, or jaw; sudden, severe headache unlike your usual headaches; weakness or numbness in an arm or leg; trouble speaking); suicidal thoughts (thoughts about suicide or dying, attempts to commit suicide, new or worse depression, new or worse anxiety, other unusual changes in behavior or mood) or liver problems (jaundice, dark, amber-colored urine, feeling tired, nausea and vomiting, generalized swelling, right upper abdomen pain, bruising easily) occur.
- Rep: May cause early pregnancy loss if administered to pregnant women. Advise females of reproductive potential to use effective non-hormonal contraception during therapy and for one wk after final dose. Women who take *Myfembree* may experience amenorrhea or a reduction in amount, intensity, or duration of menstrual bleeding; may delay ability to recognize pregnancy. Avoid concomitant use of hormonal contraceptives with *Myfembree*. The use of estrogen-containing hormonal contraceptives can increase estrogen levels which may increase risk of estrogen-associated adverse events and decrease the efficacy of *Myfembree*. Inform patient of pregnancy exposure registry that monitors pregnancy outcomes in women exposed to *Myfembree*. during pregnancy. Pregnant females exposed to *Myfembree*. and health care providers are encouraged to call the Myfembree Pregnancy Exposure Registry at 1-855-428-0707.

Evaluation/Desired Outcomes
- Reduction in menstrual blood loss in premenopausal women with uterine fibroids.
- Moderate to severe pain associated with endometriosis in premenopausal women.

remdesivir (rem-de-si-vir)
Veklury
Classification
Therapeutic: antivirals
Pharmacologic: nucleoside analogues

Indications
Coronavirus 2019 (COVID-19) infection in patients who are hospitalized. COVID-19 infection in patients who are not hospitalized, have mild to moderate COVID-19, and are at high risk for progression to severe COVID-19, including hospitalization or death.

Action
As an adenosine nucleotide prodrug, remdesivir is metabolized to an active nucleoside triphosphate metabolite, after being distributed into cells. Remdesivir triphosphate acts as an adenosine triphosphate (ATP) analog and competes with ATP for incorporation into RNA chains by the SARS-CoV-2 RNA-dependent RNA polymerase, which results in delayed chain termination during viral RNA replication. **Therapeutic Effects:** Reduced time to recovery in hospitalized patients (hospital discharge, hospitalized but not requiring supplemental oxygen and no longer requiring ongoing care) from COVID-19 infection. Reduction in risk of hospitalization or all-cause mortality in nonhospitalized patients.

Pharmacokinetics
Absorption: IV administration results in complete bioavailability.
Distribution: Unknown.
Metabolism and Excretion: Remdesivir is a prodrug that is metabolized intracellularly to the active metabolite, remdesivir triphosphate. Primarily excreted in urine (74%, 10% as unchanged drug), with 18% of drug being excreted in feces.
Half-life: *Nucleoside triphosphate metabolite:* 20 hr.

TIME/ACTION PROFILE (median time to recovery)

ROUTE	ONSET	PEAK	DURATION
IV	unknown	11 days	unknown

Contraindications/Precautions
Contraindicated in: Hypersensitivity.
Use Cautiously in: OB: Safety not established in pregnancy; Lactation: Safety not established in breastfeeding; Pedi: Children <28 days or weighing <3 kg (safety and effectiveness not established).

Adverse Reactions/Side Effects
Endo: hyperglycemia. **GI:** nausea, ↑ liver enzymes, constipation. **GU:** acute kidney injury. **Hemat:** anemia. **Resp:** RESPIRATORY FAILURE. **Misc:** fever, HYPERSENSITIVITY REACTIONS (including anaphylaxis and angioedema), infusion reactions.

Interactions
Drug-Drug: Chloroquine or hydroxychloroquine may ↓ antiviral effects; avoid concurrent use.

Route/Dosage
IV (Adults and Children ≥40 kg): *Hospitalized patients:* 200 mg on Day 1, then 100 mg once daily starting on Day 2. Treatment duration = 10 days (patients requiring invasive mechanical ventilation and/or extracorporeal membrane oxygenation [ECMO]); 5 days (patients not requiring invasive mechanical ventilation and/or ECMO) (if these patients are not improving after 5 days, treatment may be continued for another 5 days). *Nonhospitalized patients:* 200 mg on Day 1, then 100 mg once daily on Days 2 and 3.
IV (Children ≥28 days and 3–<40 kg): *Hospitalized patients:* 5 mg/kg on Day 1, then 2.5 mg/kg once daily starting on Day 2. Treatment duration = 10 days

(patients requiring invasive mechanical ventilation and/or ECMO); 5 days (patients not requiring invasive mechanical ventilation and/or ECMO) (if these patients are not improving after 5 days, treatment may be continued for another 5 days). *Nonhospitalized patients:* 5 mg/kg on Day 1, then 2.5 mg/kg once daily on Days 2 and 3.

Availability

Lyophilized powder for injection: 100 mg/vial. **Solution for injection:** 5 mg/mL.

NURSING IMPLICATIONS

Assessment

● Monitor for signs and symptoms of COVID-19 infection (fever, cough, shortness of breath) before and periodically during therapy.

● Monitor for signs and symptoms of hypersensitivity reactions (hypotension, tachycardia, bradycardia, dyspnea, wheezing, angioedema, rash, nausea, vomiting, diaphoresis, shivering) during therapy and for at least 1 hr after infusion is complete. Slowing infusion rate to maximum time of 120 min may prevent reactions. If clinically significant symptoms occur, immediately discontinue infusion and begin symptomatic treatment.

Lab Test Considerations
Monitor hepatic function before starting and during therapy as clinically appropriate. *If ALT ≥5 × upper limit of normal (ULN),* do not start remdesivir therapy. *If ALT ≥5 × ULN during therapy or ALT elevation accompanied by signs or symptoms of liver inflammation or increasing conjugated bilirubin, alkaline phosphatase, or INR,* hold dose. Resume when ALT <5 × ULN. Monitor prothrombin time before starting and during therapy as clinically appropriate.

Implementation

● Do not administer with chloroquine or hydroxychloroquine; may decrease antiviral activity.

● Administer remdesivir only in settings in which health care professionals have immediate access to medications to treat a severe infusion or hypersensitivity reaction, such as anaphylaxis, and the ability to activate the emergency medical system.

IV Administration

● **Intermittent Infusion: Remdesivir powder for Injection, 100 mg:** *Reconstitution:* Reconstitute lyophilized powder with 19 mL of Sterile Water for Injection. Discard vial if vacuum does not pull Sterile Water for Injection into vial. Shake vial for 30 sec. Allow contents to settle for 2–3 min for a clear solution. If contents not completely dissolved, shake for 30 sec and allow to settle for 2–3 min. Repeat until solution is clear. *Concentration:* 5 mg/mL. Reconstituted solution is stable for 4 hr at room temperature or 24 hr if refrigerated. *Dilution:* Dilute

with 100 mL or 250 mL of 0.9% NaCl. *For 200 mg dose,* withdraw and discard 40 mL from the 250 mL or 100 mL 0.9% NaCl infusion bag. Withdraw 40 mL of reconstituted solution and inject into infusion bag. *For 100 mg dose,* withdraw and discard 20 mL from the 250 mL or 100 mL 0.9% NaCl infusion bag. Withdraw 20 mL of reconstituted solution and inject into infusion bag. Gently invert bag 20 times to mix; do not shake. Solution is stable for 24 hr at room temperature or 48 hr if refrigerated. **Remdesivir solution for Injection, 100 mg/20 mL (5 mg/mL):** Allow vials to reach room temperature; stable for 12 hr at room temperature before dilution. Solution is clear and colorless to yellow; do not use solutions that are cloudy, discolored, or contain particulate matter. *Dilution: For 200 mg dose,* withdraw and discard 40 ml from 250 mL infusion bag of 0.9% NaCl. Inject 5 mL air into vial and withdraw 40 mL remdesivir solution; last 5 mL may require force to withdraw. Inject remdesivir solution into infusion bag. *For 100 mg dose,* withdraw and discard 20 ml from 250 mL infusion bag of 0.9% NaCl. Inject 10 mL air into vial and withdraw 20 mL remdesivir solution; last 5 mL may require force to withdraw. Inject remdesivir solution into infusion bag. Gently invert bag 20 times to mix; do not shake. Solution is stable for 24 hr at room temperature or 48 hr if refrigerated. *Rate: Infuse 250 mL* over 30 min for rate of 8.33 mL/min, over 60 min for rate of 4.17 mL/min, or over 120 min for rate of 2.08 mL/min. *Infuse 100 mL* over 30 min for rate of 3.33 mL/min, over 60 min for rate of 1.67 mL/min, or over 120 min for rate of 0.83 mL/min.

Patient/Family Teaching

● Explain purpose of remdesivir to patient.

● Advise patient to notify health care professional immediately if signs and symptoms of hypersensitivity reactions (low blood pressure, changes in heartbeat, shortness of breath, wheezing, swelling of lips, face, or throat, rash, nausea, vomiting, sweating, shivering) occur.

● Instruct patient to notify health care professional of all Rx or OTC medications, vitamins, or herbal products being taken and to consult health care professional before taking other Rx, OTC, or herbal products, especially chloroquine or hydroxychloroquine.

● Rep: Advise females of reproductive potential to notify health care professional if pregnancy is planned or suspected or if breastfeeding during therapy.

Evaluation/Desired Outcomes

● Reduced time to recovery (hospital discharge, hospitalized but not requiring supplemental oxygen and no longer requiring ongoing care) from COVID-19 infection.

R

reteplase, See THROMBOLYTIC AGENTS.

---

revefenacin (rev-e-fen-a-sin)
    Yupelri
    Classification
    Therapeutic: bronchodilators
    Pharmacologic: anticholinergics

Indications
Maintenance treatment of COPD (not for acute [rescue] use).

Action
Acts as an anticholinergic by inhibiting the M_3 receptor in bronchial smooth muscle, which leads to bronchodilation. **Therapeutic Effects:** Bronchodilation with lessened symptoms of COPD.

Pharmacokinetics
Absorption: 3% systemically absorbed following oral inhalation.
Distribution: Extensively distributed to tissues.
Metabolism and Excretion: Rapidly hydrolyzed to an active metabolite. Primarily eliminated in feces (88%) with less than 5% excreted in urine.
Half-life: 22–70 hr.

TIME/ACTION PROFILE (plasma concentrations)

ROUTE	ONSET	PEAK	DURATION
Nebulization	rapid	14–41 min	24 hr

Contraindications/Precautions
Contraindicated in: Hypersensitivity; Hepatic impairment.
Use Cautiously in: Narrow-angle glaucoma; Prostatic hyperplasia or bladder neck obstruction; OB: Safety not established in pregnancy; Lactation: Use while breastfeeding only if potential maternal benefit justifies potential risk to infant; Pedi: Safety and effectiveness not established in children.

Adverse Reactions/Side Effects
Neuro: headache. **Resp:** cough, paradoxical bronchospasm. **Misc:** HYPERSENSITIVITY REACTIONS (including anaphylaxis and angioedema).

Interactions
Drug-Drug: May ↑ risk of anticholinergic effects with other **anticholinergics. Rifampin** or **cyclosporine** may ↑ levels of active metabolite; concurrent use not recommended.

Route/Dosage
Inhaln (Adults): 175 mcg via nebulization once daily.

Availability
Solution for inhalation: 175 mcg/3 mL.

NURSING IMPLICATIONS

Assessment
- Assess lung sounds, pulse, and BP before administration and during peak of medication. Note amount, color, and character of sputum produced. Closely monitor patients on higher dose for adverse effects.
- Monitor pulmonary function tests before initiating and periodically during therapy to determine effectiveness.
- Observe for paradoxical bronchospasm (wheezing, dyspnea, tightness in chest) during therapy. If condition occurs, hold medication and notify health care professional immediately.
- Monitor patient for signs of hypersensitivity reactions (rash, hives, severe itching, swelling of face, mouth, and tongue, difficulty breathing or swallowing) during therapy. Discontinue therapy and consider alternative if reaction occurs.

Implementation
- **Inhaln:** Administer once daily by oral inhalation via a standard jet nebulizer connected to an air compressor.

Patient/Family Teaching
- Instruct patient to use medication as directed. Do not discontinue therapy without discussing with health care professional, even if feeling better. Use a rapid-acting bronchodilator if symptoms occur before next dose is due. Caution patient not to use more than once a day; may cause adverse effects, paradoxical bronchospasm, or loss of effectiveness of medication. Instruct patient to review *Patient Information* before starting therapy and with each Rx refill in case of changes.
- Caution patient not to use medication to treat acute symptoms. Use a rapid-acting inhaled beta-adrenergic bronchodilator for relief of acute asthma attacks. Notify health care professional immediately if symptoms get worse or more inhalations than usual are needed from rescue inhaler.
- Instruct patient to contact health care professional immediately if shortness of breath is not relieved by medication or nausea, vomiting, shakiness, headache, fast or irregular heartbeat, sleeplessness, or signs and symptoms of narrow angle glaucoma (eye pain or discomfort, blurred vision, visual halos or colored images, red eyes) or urinary retention (difficulty passing urine, painful urination) occur.
- Advise patient to consult health care professional before taking any Rx, OTC, or herbal products or alcohol concurrently with this therapy. Caution patient also to avoid smoking and other respiratory irritants.
- Rep: Advise females of reproductive potential to notify health care professional if pregnancy is planned or suspected or if breastfeeding.

Evaluation/Desired Outcomes
- Bronchodilation with decreased airflow obstruction.

Rh$_o$(D) IMMUNE GLOBULIN
(arr aych oh dee im-**yoon glob** -yoo-lin)

Rh$_o$(D) immune globulin standard dose IM
HyperRHO S/D Full Dose, RhoGAM

Rh$_o$(D) immune globulin micro-dose IM
HyperRHO S/D Mini-Dose, MICRhoGAM

Rh$_o$(D) immune globulin IV
WinRho SDF

Rh$_o$(D) immune globulin micro-dose IM, IV
Rhophylac

Classification
Therapeutic: vaccines/immunizing agents
Pharmacologic: immune globulins

Indications
IM, IV: Administered to Rh$_o$(D)-negative patients who have been exposed to Rh$_o$(D)-positive blood by: Pregnancy or delivery of a Rh$_o$(D)-positive infant, Abortion of a Rh$_o$(D)-positive fetus, Fetal-maternal hemorrhage due to amniocentesis, other obstetrical manipulative procedure, or intra-abdominal trauma while carrying a Rh$_o$(D)-positive fetus, Transfusion of Rh$_o$(D)-positive blood or blood products to a Rh$_o$(D)-negative patient.
IV: Management of immune thrombocytopenic purpura (ITP).

Action
Prevent production of anti-Rh$_o$(D) antibodies in Rh$_o$(D)-negative patients who were exposed to Rh$_o$(D)-positive blood. Increase platelet counts in patients with ITP. **Therapeutic Effects:** Prevention of antibody response and hemolytic disease of the newborn (erythroblastosis fetalis) in future pregnancies of women who have conceived a Rh$_o$(D)-positive fetus. Prevention of Rh$_o$(D) sensitization following transfusion accident. Decreased bleeding in patients with ITP.

Pharmacokinetics
Absorption: IV administration results in complete bioavailability. Well absorbed from IM sites.
Distribution: Unknown.
Metabolism and Excretion: Unknown.
Half-life: 25–30 days.

TIME/ACTION PROFILE (plasma concentrations)

ROUTE	ONSET	PEAK	DURATION
IM	rapid	5–10 days	unknown
IV†	unknown	2 hr	unknown

†When given for ITP, platelet counts start to rise in 1–2 days, peak after 5–7 days, and last for 30 days.

Contraindications/Precautions
Contraindicated in: Prior hypersensitivity reaction to human immune globulin; Rh$_o$(D)- or Du-positive patients.
Use Cautiously in: ITP patients with pre-existing anemia (decrease dose if Hgb <10 g/dL). May also cause disseminated intravascular coagulation in ITP patients.

Adverse Reactions/Side Effects
CV: hypertension, hypotension. **Derm:** rash. **GI:** diarrhea, nausea, vomiting. **GU:** acute renal failure. **Hemat:** anemia; *ITP:* DISSEMINATED INTRAVASCULAR COAGULATION, INTRAVASCULAR HEMOLYSIS. **Local:** pain at injection site. **MS:** arthralgia, myalgia. **Neuro:** dizziness, headache. **Misc:** fever.

Interactions
Drug-Drug: May ↓ antibody response to some live-virus vaccines (**measles**, **mumps**, **rubella**).

Route/Dosage
Rh$_o$(D) Immune Globulin (for IM use only)
Following Delivery
IM (Adults): *HyperRHO S/D Full Dose, RhoGAM:* 1 vial standard dose (300 mcg) within 72 hr of delivery.

Before Delivery
IM (Adults): *HyperRHO S/D Full Dose, RhoGAM:* 1 vial standard dose (300 mcg) at 26–28 wk.

Termination of Pregnancy (<13 wk Gestation)
IM (Adults): *HyperRHO S/D Mini-Dose, MICRhoGAM:* 1 vial of microdose (50 mcg) within 72 hr.

Termination of Pregnancy (>13 wk Gestation)
IM (Adults): *RhoGAM:* 1 vial standard dose (300 mcg) within 72 hr.

Large Fetal-Maternal Hemorrhage (>15 mL)
IM (Adults): *RhoGAM:* 20 mcg/mL of Rh$_o$(D)-positive fetal RBCs.

Transfusion Accident
IM (Adults): *HyperRHO S/D Full Dose, RhoGAM:* (Volume of Rh-positive blood administered × Hct of donor blood)/15 = number of vials of standard dose (300 mcg) preparation (round to next whole number of vials).

Rh$_o$(D) Immune Globulin IV (for IM or IV Use)
Following Delivery
IM, IV (Adults): *WinRho SDF:* 120 mcg within 72 hr of delivery. *Rhophylac:* 300 mcg within 72 hr of delivery.

Prior to Delivery
IM, IV (Adults): *WinRho SDF, Rhophylac:* 300 mcg at 28 wk; if initiated earlier in pregnancy, repeat every 12 wk.

R

Following Amniocentesis or Chorionic Villus Sampling

IM, IV (Adults): *WinRho SDF (before 34 wk gestation):* 300 mcg immediately; repeat every 12 wk during pregnancy. *Rhophylac:* 300 mcg within 72 hr of procedure.

Termination of Pregnancy, Amniocentesis, or Any Other Manipulation

IM, IV (Adults): *WinRho SDF:* 120 mcg within 72 hr after event.

Large Fetal-Maternal Hemorrhage/Transfusion Accident

IM (Adults): *WinRho SDF:* 1200 mcg every 12 hr until total dose is given (total dose determined by amount of blood loss/hemorrhage).
IV (Adults): *WinRho SDF:* 600 mcg every 8 hr until total dose is given (total dose determined by amount of blood loss/hemorrhage).

Immune Thrombocytopenic Purpura

IV (Adults and Children): *WinRho SDF, Rhophylac:* 50 mcg/kg initially (if Hgb <10 g/dL, ↓ dose to 25–40 mcg/kg); further dosing/frequency determined by clinical response (range 25–60 mcg/kg). Each dose may be given as a single dose or in 2 divided doses on separate days.

Availability

Rh₀(D) Immune Globulin (for IM Use)

Solution for injection (prefilled syringes): 50 mcg (microdose—MICRhoGAM, HyperRHO S/D Mini-Dose), 300 mcg (standard dose—RhoGAM, HyperRHO S/D Full Dose).

Rh₀(D) Immune Globulin Intravenous (for IM or IV Use)

Injection: 300 mcg/vial, 500 mcg/vial, 3000 mcg/vial.
Prefilled syringes: 300 mcg/2 mL.

NURSING IMPLICATIONS

Assessment

- **IV:** Assess vital signs periodically during therapy in patients receiving IV Rh₀(D) immune globulin.
- **ITP:** Monitor patient for signs and symptoms of intravascular hemolysis (back pain, shaking chills, fever, hemoglobinuria), anemia, and renal insufficiency. If transfusions are required, use Rh₀(D)-negative packed red blood cells to prevent exacerbation of intravascular hemolysis.

Lab Test Considerations

- *Pregnancy:* Type and crossmatch of mother and newborn's cord blood must be performed to determine need for medication. Mother must be Rh₀(D)-negative and Du-negative. Infant must be Rh₀(D)-positive. If there is doubt regarding infant's blood type or if father is Rh₀(D)-positive, medication should be given.
- An infant born to a woman treated with Rh₀(D) immune globulin antepartum may have a weakly posi-

tive direct Coombs' test result on cord or infant blood.

- *ITP:* Monitor platelet counts, RBC counts, hemoglobin, and reticulocyte levels to determine effectiveness of therapy.

Implementation

- Do not give to infant, to Rh₀(D)-positive individual, or to Rh₀(D)-negative individual previously sensitized to the Rh₀(D) antigen. However, there is no more risk than when given to a woman who is not sensitized. When in doubt, administer Rh₀(D) immune globulin.
- Do not confuse IM and IV formulations. Rh immune globulin for IV administration is labeled "Rh Immune Globulin Intravenous." Rh Immune Globulin Intravenous may be given IM; however, Rh Immune Globulin (microdose and standard dose) is for IM use only and cannot be given IV.
- When using prefilled syringes, allow solution to reach room temperature before administration.
- **IM:** Reconstitute Rh₀(D) immune globulin IV for IM use immediately before use with 1.25 mL of 0.9% NaCl. Inject diluent onto inside wall of vial and wet pellet by gently swirling until dissolved. Do not shake.
- Administer into the deltoid muscle. Dose should be given within 3 hr but may be given up to 72 hr after delivery, miscarriage, abortion, or transfusion.

IV Administration

- **IV Push:** Reconstitute Rh₀(D) immune globulin IV for IV administration immediately before use with 2.5 mL of 0.9% NaCl. Inject diluent onto inside wall of vial and wet pellet by gently swirling until dissolved. Do not shake. *Rate:* Administer over 3–5 min.

Patient/Family Teaching

- **Pregnancy:** Explain to patient that the purpose of this medication is to protect future Rh₀(D)-positive infants.
- **ITP:** Explain purpose of medication to patient.

Evaluation/Desired Outcomes

- Prevention of erythroblastosis fetalis in future Rh₀(D)-positive infants.
- Prevention of Rh₀(D) sensitization following incompatible transfusion.
- Decreased bleeding episodes in patients with ITP.

⚙ **ribociclib** (rye-boe-**sye**-klib)
Kisqali
Classification
Therapeutic: antineoplastics
Pharmacologic: kinase inhibitors

Indications

⚙ Advanced or metastatic hormone receptor (HR)-positive, human epidermal growth factor 2 (HER2)-negative breast cancer (as initial endocrine-based therapy) (in combination with an aromatase inhibitor). ⚇ Advanced or metastatic HR-positive, HER2-negative breast cancer (as initial endocrine-based therapy or following disease progression on endocrine therapy in postmenopausal women or in men) (in combination with fulvestrant).

Action
Inhibits kinases (cyclin-dependent kinases 4 and 6) that are part of the signaling pathway for cell proliferation. **Therapeutic Effects:** Improved survival and decreased spread of breast cancer.

Pharmacokinetics
Absorption: 66% absorbed following oral administration.
Distribution: Extensively distributed to the tissues.
Metabolism and Excretion: Mostly metabolized in the liver by the CYP3A4 isoenzyme; 17% excreted unchanged in feces, 12% in urine.
Half-life: 32 hr.

TIME/ACTION PROFILE (plasma concentrations)

ROUTE	ONSET	PEAK	DURATION
PO	unknown	1–4 hr	unknown

Contraindications/Precautions
Contraindicated in: QT interval prolongation (QT interval ≥450 msec); Uncorrected hypokalemia or hypomagnesemia; Recent MI, HF, unstable angina, or bradycardia; OB: Pregnancy; Lactation: Lactation.
Use Cautiously in: Severe renal impairment (↓ dose); Moderate or severe hepatic impairment (↓ dose); Rep: Women of reproductive potential; Pedi: Safety and effectiveness not established in children.

Adverse Reactions/Side Effects
CV: peripheral edema, QT interval prolongation, syncope. **Derm:** alopecia, pruritus, rash, DRUG REACTION WITH EOSINOPHILIA AND SYSTEMIC SYMPTOMS (DRESS), STEVENS-JOHNSON SYNDROME (SJS), TOXIC EPIDERMAL NECROLYSIS (TEN). **F and E:** hypokalemia, hypophosphatemia. **GI:** ↑ liver enzymes, abdominal pain, constipation, diarrhea, nausea, stomatitis, vomiting, hyperbilirubinemia. **GU:** ↑ serum creatinine, ↓ fertility (males). **Hemat:** anemia, NEUTROPENIA, THROMBOCYTOPENIA. **Metab:** ↓ appetite. **MS:** back pain. **Neuro:** fatigue, headache, insomnia. **Resp:** dyspnea, INTERSTITIAL LUNG DISEASE (ILD). **Misc:** fever.

Interactions
Drug-Drug: Strong CYP3A4 inhibitors, including **clarithromycin, conivaptan, itraconazole, ketoconazole, lopinavir/ritonavir, nefazodone, nelfinavir, posaconazole, ritonavir,** or **voriconazole** may ↑ levels and the risk of toxicity; avoid concurrent use, if possible (if unavoidable, ↓ dose of ribociclib).

Strong CYP3A4 inducers, including **carbamazepine, phenytoin,** or **rifampin** can ↓ levels and effectiveness; avoid concurrent use. May ↑ levels and effects/toxicity of **cyclosporine, dihydroergotamine, ergotamine, everolimus, fentanyl, midazolam, pimozide, quinidine, sirolimus** and **tacrolimus;** if concurrent use is required, dose ↓ may be necessary. **QT-interval-prolonging medications,** including **amiodarone, chloroquine, clarithromycin, disopyramide, haloperidol, methadone, moxifloxacin, ondansetron, pimozide, procainamide, quinidine, sotalol,** and **tamoxifen** may ↑ risk of QT interval prolongation; avoid concurrent use.
Drug-Natural Products: St. John's wort may ↓ levels and effectiveness; avoid concurrent use.
Drug-Food: Grapefruit/grapefruit juice or pomegranate/pomegranate juice may ↑ levels and the risk of toxicity; avoid ingestion.

Route/Dosage
PO (Adults): 600 mg once daily for 21 days, followed by 7 days off to complete a 28-day treatment cycle; continue treatment cycles until disease progression or unacceptable toxicity. *Concurrent use of strong CYP3A4 inhibitor:* 400 mg once daily for 21 days, followed by 7 days off to complete a 28-day treatment cycle; continue treatment cycles until disease progression or unacceptable toxicity.

Renal Impairment
PO (Adults): *Severe renal impairment:* 200 mg once daily for 21 days, followed by 7 days off to complete a 28-day treatment cycle; continue treatment cycles until disease progression or unacceptable toxicity.

Hepatic Impairment
PO (Adults): *Moderate or severe hepatic impairment:* 400 mg once daily for 21 days, followed by 7 days off to complete a 28-day treatment cycle; continue treatment cycles until disease progression or unacceptable toxicity.

Availability
Tablets: 200 mg.

NURSING IMPLICATIONS
Assessment
● Monitor ECG prior to starting therapy. Avoid administering ribociclib to patient with QT interval >450 msec. Repeat ECG on Day 14 of first cycle, beginning of 2nd cycle, and as indicated. *If QT interval >480 msec,* suspend therapy. *If QT interval prolongation resolves to <481 msec,* resume therapy at same dose level. *If QT ≥481 msec recurs,* interrupt dose until QT interval resolves to <481 msec; then resume ribociclib at next lower dose level. *If QT interval >500 msec,* withhold therapy if >500 msec on at least 2 separate ECGs (within same visit). *If QT interval prolongation resolves to <481 msec,* re-

sume therapy at next lower dose. *If QT interval prolongation is either >500 msec or >60 msec change from baseline AND associated with any of the following: Torsades de Pointes, polymorphic ventricular tachycardia, unexplained syncope, or signs and symptoms of serious arrhythmia,* permanently discontinue ribociclib.

- Monitor for signs and symptoms of ILD/pneumonitis (hypoxia, cough, dyspnea) during therapy. *If Grade 1 symptoms (asymptomatic) occur,* continue dose and treat symptoms. *If Grade 2 symptoms (symptomatic) occur,* hold therapy until ≤Grade 1. Resume at next lower dose. *If Grade 2 recurs,* discontinue ribociclib permanently. *If Grade 3 (severe symptomatic) or Grade 4 symptoms (life-threatening) occur,* permanently discontinue therapy.
- Monitor for signs and symptoms of cutaneous reactions (rash, erythema, purpura) during therapy. *If reactions are Grade 1 (< 10% body surface area [BSA] with active skin toxicity, no signs of systemic involvement) or Grade 2 (10–30% BSA with active skin toxicity, no signs of systemic involvement),* continue at same dose and initiate medical therapy and monitor as clinically indicated. *If Grade 3 reaction (severe rash not responsive to medical management; >30% BSA with active skin toxicity, signs of systemic involvement present; SJS) occurs,* hold ribociclib until the cause of the reaction has been determined. If the cause is SJS, TEN, or DRESS, permanently discontinue therapy. If cause is not SJS, TEN, DRESS, hold dose until recovery to Grade ≤ 1, then resume ribociclib at same dose level. If the cutaneous adverse reaction still recurs at Grade 3, resume ribociclib at the next lower dose level. *If Grade 4 reaction (any % BSA associated with extensive superinfection, with IV antibiotics indicated; life-threatening consequences; TEN) occurs,* permanently discontinue ribociclib.

Lab Test Considerations
- Verify negative pregnancy test prior to starting therapy.
- Monitor serum electrolytes (potassium, calcium, phosphorous, magnesium) prior to starting therapy, at beginning of first 6 cycles, and as indicated. Correct abnormalities before starting therapy.
- Monitor liver function before starting therapy, every 2 wk for first 2 cycles, at beginning of each subsequent 4 cycles, and as indicated. **For AST and/or ALT ↑ from baseline, WITHOUT ↑ total bilirubin >2 × upper limit of normal (ULN):** *Grade 1 (>ULN to 3 × ULN),* No dose adjustment. *Grade 2 (>3 to 5 × ULN),* Baseline at <Grade 2: Hold dose until recovery to ≤baseline grade, then resume at same dose. *If Grade 2 recurs,* resume ribociclib at next lower dose. Do not interrupt dose for Grade 2 at baseline. *Grade 3 (>5 to 20 × ULN),* withhold dose until recovery to ≤baseline grade, then resume at next lower dose. *If Grade 3 recurs,* discontinue ribociclib. *Grade 4 (>20 × ULN),* discontinue ribo-

ciclib. **Combined ↑ in AST and/or ALT WITH total bilirubin ↑, in absence of cholestasis:** *If ALT and/or AST >3 × ULN along with total bilirubin >2 × ULN irrespective of baseline grade,* discontinue ribociclib.
- Monitor CBC before starting therapy, every 2 wk for first 2 cycles, at beginning of each subsequent 4 cycles, and as indicated. *If Grade 1 or 2 (ANC 1000/mm³ to <lower limit of normal) occurs,* no dose adjustment required. *If Grade 3 (ANC 500–1000/mm³) occurs,* interrupt dose until recovery to Grade ≤2. Resume therapy at same dose. *If toxicity recurs at Grade 3,* hold dose until recovery, then resume ribociclib at next lower dose. *If Grade 3 febrile neutropenia occurs,* suspend therapy until recovery of neutropenia to Grade ≤2. Resume therapy at next lower dose. *If Grade 4 (ANC <500/mm³) occurs,* withhold therapy until recovery to Grade ≤2. Resume ribociclib at next lower dose.

Implementation
- **Dose Reduction Schedule:** Starting dose: 600 mg/day. First dose reduction: 400 mg/day. Second dose reduction: 200 mg/day.
- **PO:** Administer once daily, at the same time each day, preferably in the morning, without regard to food. *DNC:* Swallow tablets whole; do not crush, break, or chew. Do not administer tablets that are broken, cracked, or not intact.
- Pre/perimenopausal women or men taking ribociclib and an aromatase inhibitor should also be treated with a luteinizing hormone-releasing hormone (LHRH) agonist. Men taking ribociclib plus fulvestrant should be treated with an LHRH agonist.

Patient/Family Teaching
- Instruct patient to take ribociclib as directed. If patient vomits after taking dose or misses dose, do not take more that day. Take next dose next day at usual time. Advise patient to read *Patient Information* prior to starting and with each Rx refill in case of changes.
- Advise patient to avoid eating pomegranate or grapefruit and to avoid drinking pomegranate or grapefruit juice during therapy.
- Advise patient to notify health care professional if signs and symptoms of heart rhythm problems (change in heartbeat [fast or irregular], dizziness, feeling faint), low white blood cell counts (fever and chills), or liver problems (yellowing of skin or whites of eyes, jaundice, dark or brown, tea-colored urine, feeling very tired, loss of appetite, pain on upper right side of abdomen, unusual bleeding or bruising) or skin reactions occur.
- Instruct patient to notify health care professional of all Rx or OTC medications, vitamins, or herbal products being taken and to consult with health care professional before taking other medications.
- Rep: May cause fetal harm. Advise females of reproductive potential to use effective contraception and

to avoid breastfeeding during and for at least 3 wk after last dose of therapy. Inform male patients that ribociclib may impair fertility.

Evaluation/Desired Outcomes

● Improved survival and decreased spread of breast cancer.

---

rifabutin (riff-a-**byoo**-tin)
Mycobutin
Classification
Therapeutic: agents for atypical mycobacterium

Indications

Prevention of disseminated *Mycobacterium avium* complex (MAC) disease in patients with advanced HIV infection.

Action

Appears to inhibit DNA-dependent RNA polymerase in susceptible organisms. **Therapeutic Effects:** Antimycobacterial action against susceptible organisms. **Spectrum:** Active against *M. avium* and most strains of *M. tuberculosis*.

Pharmacokinetics

Absorption: Well absorbed following oral administration (50–85%). Absorption ↓ in patients with HIV (20%).
Distribution: Widely distributed to body tissues and fluids.
Metabolism and Excretion: Mostly metabolized by the liver; <5% excreted unchanged by the kidneys.
Half-life: 45 hr.

TIME/ACTION PROFILE (plasma concentrations)

ROUTE	ONSET	PEAK	DURATION
PO	rapid	2–4 hr	24 hr

Contraindications/Precautions

Contraindicated in: Hypersensitivity. Cross-sensitivity with other rifamycins (rifampin) may occur; Active tuberculosis; Concurrent use of ritonavir; Lactation: Lactation.
Use Cautiously in: OB: Use during pregnancy only if potential maternal benefit justifies potential fetal risk; Pedi: Safety and effectiveness not established in children.

Adverse Reactions/Side Effects

CV: chest pain, chest pressure. **Derm:** ACUTE GENERALIZED EXANTHEMATOUS PUSTULOSIS, DRUG REACTION WITH EOSINOPHILIA AND SYSTEMIC SYMPTOMS (DRESS), rash, skin discoloration, STEVENS-JOHNSON SYNDROME (SJS), TOXIC EPIDERMAL NECROLYSIS (TEN). **EENT:** ocular disturbances. **GI:** altered taste, CLOSTRIDIOIDES DIFFICILE-

ASSOCIATED DIARRHEA (CDAD), drug-induced hepatitis. **Hemat:** hemolysis, neutropenia, thrombocytopenia. **MS:** arthralgia, myositis. **Resp:** dyspnea. **Misc:** brownorange discoloration of body fluids (urine, tears, saliva), flu-like syndrome.

Interactions

Drug-Drug: Ritonavir may significantly ↑ levels; concurrent use contraindicated. May ↓ levels and effectiveness of **efavirenz**, **nelfinavir**, **nevirapine**, **corticosteroids**, **disopyramide**, **quinidine**, **opioid analgesics**, **oral hypoglycemic agents**, **warfarin**, **estrogens**, **estrogen-containing contraceptives**, **phenytoin**, **verapamil**, **fluconazole**, **theophylline**, **zidovudine**, and **chloramphenicol**. May ↓ levels and effectiveness of **bictegravir** and **tenofovir alafenamide**; concurrent use with **bictegravir/emtricitabine/tenofovir alafenamide** is not recommended. May ↓ levels and effectiveness of **doravirine**; ↑ doravirine dose. May ↓ levels and effectiveness of **rilpivirine** and **tenofovir alafenamide**; concurrent use with **rilpivirine/tenofovir alafenamide/emtricitabine** is not recommended. **Efavirenz** and **nevirapine** may ↑ levels.

Route/Dosage

PO (Adults): 300 mg once daily. If GI upset occurs, may give as 150 mg twice daily with food.

Availability (generic available)

Capsules: 150 mg. *In combination with:* amoxicillin and omeprazole (Talicia). See Appendix N.

NURSING IMPLICATIONS

Assessment

● Monitor patient for signs of active tuberculosis (purified protein derivative [PPD], chest x-ray, sputum culture, blood culture, urine culture, biopsy of suspicious lymph nodes) prior to and during therapy. Rifabutin must not be administered to patients with active tuberculosis.

● Monitor bowel function. Diarrhea, abdominal cramping, fever, and bloody stools should be reported to health care professional promptly as a sign of CDAD. May begin up to several wk following cessation of therapy.

● Assess patient for skin rash frequently during therapy. Discontinue rifabutin at first sign of rash; may be life-threatening. SJS, TEN, or DRESS may develop. Treat symptomatically; may recur once treatment is stopped.

● Monitor for signs and symptoms of hypersensitivity reactions (hypotension, urticaria, angioedema, acute bronchospasm, conjunctivitis, thrombocytopenia, neutropenia), or flu-like syndrome (weakness, fatigue, muscle pain, nausea, vomiting, headache, fever, chills, aches, rash, itching, sweats, dizziness, shortness of breath, chest pain, cough, syncope, palpitations). If symptoms occur, discontinue rifabutin.

🍁 = Canadian drug name. ▓ = Genetic implication. ~~Strikethrough~~ = Discontinued. CAPITALS = life-threatening. <u>Underline</u> = most frequent.

Lab Test Considerations
● Monitor CBC periodically during therapy. May cause neutropenia and thrombocytopenia.

Implementation
● Do not confuse rifabutin with rifapentine.
● **PO:** May be administered without regard to meals. High-fat meals slow rate but not extent of absorption. May be mixed with foods such as applesauce. If GI upset occurs, administer with food.

Patient/Family Teaching
● Advise patient to take medication as directed. Do not skip doses or double up on missed doses. Emphasize the importance of continuing therapy even if asymptomatic.
● Advise patient to notify health care professional promptly if signs and symptoms of neutropenia (sore throat, fever, signs of infection), thrombocytopenia (unusual bleeding or bruising), or hepatitis (yellow eyes and skin, nausea, vomiting, anorexia, unusual tiredness, weakness) occur.
● Caution patient to avoid the use of alcohol during this therapy, because this may increase the risk of hepatotoxicity.
● Instruct patient to notify health care professional immediately if diarrhea, abdominal cramping, fever, or bloody stools occur and not to treat with antidiarrheals without consulting health care professionals.
● Instruct patient to report symptoms of myositis (myalgia, arthralgia), uveitis (intraocular inflammation), or hypersensitivity reactions to health care professional promptly.
● Inform patient that skin, saliva, sputum, sweat, tears, urine, and feces may become brown-orange and that soft contact lenses may become permanently discolored.
● Rep: Advise females of reproductive potential to notify health care professional if pregnancy is planned or suspected and to avoid breastfeeding during therapy.
● Emphasize the importance of regular follow-up exams to monitor progress and to check for side effects.

Evaluation/Desired Outcomes
● Prevention of disseminated MAC in patients with advanced HIV infection.

---

rifAMPin (rif-am-pin)
Rifadin, ~~Rimactane~~, ✳Rofact
Classification
Therapeutic: antituberculars
Pharmacologic: rifamycins

Indications
Active tuberculosis (with other agents). Elimination of meningococcal carriers. **Unlabeled Use:** Prevention of disease caused by *Haemophilus influenzae* type B in close contacts. Synergy with other antimicrobial agents for *S. aureus* infections.

Action
Inhibits RNA synthesis by blocking RNA transcription in susceptible organisms. **Therapeutic Effects:** Bactericidal action against susceptible organisms. **Spectrum:** Broad spectrum notable for activity against: *Mycobacterium* spp., *Staphylococcus aureus, H. influenzae, Legionella pneumophila, Neisseria meningitidis.*

Pharmacokinetics
Absorption: Well absorbed following oral administration.
Distribution: Widely distributed; enters CSF.
Protein Binding: 80%.
Metabolism and Excretion: Mostly metabolized by the liver; 60% eliminated in feces via biliary elimination.
Half-life: 3 hr.

TIME/ACTION PROFILE (plasma concentrations)

ROUTE	ONSET	PEAK	DURATION
PO	rapid	2–4 hr	12–24 hr
IV	rapid	end of infusion	12–24 hr

Contraindications/Precautions
Contraindicated in: Hypersensitivity; Concurrent use of atazanavir, darunavir, fosamprenavir, lurasidone, praziquantel, or tipranavir.
Use Cautiously in: History of liver disease (↑ risk of hepatotoxicity); Chronic liver disease, poor nutritional status, or prolonged use of antibacterial drugs or anticoagulants (↑ risk of vitamin K deficiency and subsequent coagulation disorders); Diabetes; Concurrent use of other hepatotoxic agents; OB: Safety not established in pregnancy; Lactation: Safety not established in breastfeeding.

Adverse Reactions/Side Effects
Derm: ACUTE GENERALIZED EXANTHEMATOUS PUSTULOSIS, DRUG REACTION WITH EOSINOPHILIA AND SYSTEMIC SYMPTOMS (DRESS), pruritus, rash, STEVENS-JOHNSON SYNDROME, TOXIC EPIDERMAL NECROLYSIS. **EENT:** red discoloration of tears. **GI:** abdominal pain, diarrhea, flatulence, heartburn, nausea, vomiting, HEPATOTOXICITY, red discoloration of saliva and teeth. **GU:** red discoloration of urine. **Hemat:** bleeding, hemolytic anemia, thrombocytopenia, THROMBOTIC MICROANGIOPATHY (including thrombotic thrombocytopenic purpura and hemolytic uremia syndrome). **MS:** arthralgia, muscle weakness, myalgia. **Neuro:** ataxia, confusion, drowsiness, fatigue, headache, weakness. **Resp:** INTERSTITIAL LUNG DISEASE. **Misc:** flu-like syndrome, HYPERSENSITIVITY REACTIONS (including angioedema).

Interactions
Drug-Drug: Significantly ↓ levels and effectiveness of atazanavir, darunavir, fosamprenavir, lurasidone, praziquantel, and tipranavir; concurrent use contraindicated. Significantly ↓ levels and effectiveness of efavirenz, quinine, sofosbuvir, ticagrelor, and

zidovudine; avoid concomitant use. Significantly ↓ levels and effectiveness of **hormonal contraceptives**; use nonhormonal birth control during rifampin therapy. May ↓ levels and effectiveness of numerous drugs, including **chloramphenicol, clarithromycin, cyclosporine, diazepam, diltiazem, disopyramide, doxycycline, fluconazole, glipizide, glyburide, haloperidol, ketoconazole, levothyroxine, losartan, lovastatin, metoprolol, mexiletine, morphine, moxifloxacin, nifedipine, nortriptyline, ondansetron, oxycodone, phenytoin, prednisolone, propafenone, propranolol, quinidine, simvastatin, tamoxifen, theophylline, toremifene, verapamil,** and **zolpidem**. May ↑ levels of active metabolite of **clopidogrel**, which may ↑ risk of bleeding; avoid concomitant use. May ↓ levels and effectiveness of **warfarin**; monitor INR regularly during concurrent therapy. May significantly ↓ levels and effectiveness of **itraconazole**; avoid use 2 wk before and during itraconazole therapy. May significantly ↓ levels and effectiveness of **irinotecan**; avoid use 2 wk before and during irinotecan therapy. May ↓ levels and effectiveness of **digoxin**; closely monitor serum digoxin concentrations and ↑ digoxin dose by 20–40%, if needed. May significantly ↓ levels and effectiveness of **tacrolimus**; monitor tacrolimus whole blood concentrations regularly and ↑ tacrolimus dose as necessary. May ↓ levels and effectiveness of **methadone**, which may ↑ risk of withdrawal symptoms. Absorption may be ↓ by **antacids**; administer rifampin ≥1 hr prior to antacids. **Probenecid** and **trimethoprim/sulfamethoxazole** may ↑ levels and risk of toxicity. Concurrent use with **atovaquone** may ↓ atovaquone levels and effectiveness and ↑ levels and risk of toxicity of rifampin; avoid concomitant use. May ↓ levels and effectiveness of **dapsone**; may also ↑ levels and toxicity of the active metabolite of **dapsone**, which could ↑ the risk of methemoglobinemia.

Route/Dosage
Tuberculosis
PO, IV (Adults): 600 mg/day or 10 mg/kg/day (up to 600 mg/day) single dose; may also be given twice weekly.
PO, IV (Children and Infants): 10–20 mg/kg/day single dose or divided every 12 hr (not to exceed 600 mg/day); may also be given twice weekly.

Asymptomatic Carriers of MenIngococcus
PO, IV (Adults): 600 mg every 12 hr for 2 days.
PO, IV (Children ≥1 mo): 10 mg/kg every 12 hr for 2 days (max: 600 mg/dose).
PO (Infants <1 mo): 5 mg/kg every 12 hr for 2 days.

H. influenzae Prophylaxis
PO (Adults): 600 mg/day for 4 days.
PO (Children): 20 mg/kg/day for 4 days (max: 600 mg/dose).
PO (Neonates): 10 mg/kg/day for 4 days.

Synergy for *S. aureus* Infections
PO (Adults): 300–600 mg twice daily.
PO (Children and Neonates): 5–20 mg/kg/day divided every 12 hr (max: 600 mg/dose).

Availability (generic available)
Capsules: 150 mg, 300 mg. **Powder for injection:** 600 mg/vial.

NURSING IMPLICATIONS
Assessment
- Perform mycobacterial studies and susceptibility tests prior to and periodically during therapy to detect possible resistance.
- Assess lung sounds and character and amount of sputum periodically during therapy.
- Monitor for signs and symptoms of DRESS (fever, rash, lymphadenopathy, and/or facial swelling), associated with involvement of other organ systems (hepatitis, nephritis, hematologic abnormalities, myocarditis, myositis) during therapy. May resemble an acute viral infection. Eosinophilia is often present. Discontinue therapy if signs occur.
- Monitor for signs and symptoms of hypersensitivity reactions (fever, rash, urticaria, angioedema, hypotension, acute bronchospasm, conjunctivitis, thrombocytopenia, neutropenia, elevated liver transaminases), or flu-like syndrome (weakness, fatigue, muscle pain, nausea, vomiting, headache, chills, aches, itching, sweats, dizziness, shortness of breath, chest pain, cough, syncope, palpitations). Discontine rifampin if symptoms occur.

Lab Test Considerations
- Evaluate renal function, CBC, and urinalysis periodically and during therapy.
- Monitor hepatic function at least monthly during therapy. May cause ↑ BUN, AST, ALT, and serum alkaline phosphatase, bilirubin, and uric acid concentrations.
- May cause false-positive direct Coombs' test results. May interfere with folic acid and vitamin B assays.
- May interfere with dexamethasone suppression test results; discontinue rifampin 15 days prior to test.
- May interfere with methods for determining serum folate and vitamin B levels and with urine tests based on color reaction.
- Monitor coagulation tests (PT, INR, aPTT) during therapy in patients at risk for vitamin K deficiency.

Implementation
- Do not confuse rifampin with rifaximin or Rifamate.
- May use vitamin K supplementation in patients at risk for vitamin K deficiency.
- **PO:** Administer medication on an empty stomach at least 1 hr before or 2 hr after meals with a full glass (240 mL) of water. If GI irritation becomes a problem, may be administered with food. Antacids may

also be taken 1 hr prior to administration. Capsules may be opened and contents mixed with applesauce or jelly for patients with difficulty swallowing.

● Pharmacist can compound a syrup for patients unable to swallow solids.

IV Administration

● Avoid extravasation; may cause local irritation and inflammation due to extravascular infiltration of the infusion. If these occur, discontinue infusion and restart at another site.

● IV doses are the same doses as oral.

● **Intermittent Infusion:** *Reconstitution:* Reconstitute each 600-mg vial with 10 mL of sterile water for injection for a concentration of 60 mg/mL. Swirl gently to dissolve. *Dilution:* Dilute further in 100 mL or 500 mL of D5W or 0.9% NaCl. Reconstituted vials are stable for 24 hr at room temperature. Infusion is stable at room temperature for 4 hr (in D5W) or 24 hr (in 0.9% NaCl). *Concentration:* Not to exceed 60 mg/mL. *Rate:* Administer solutions diluted in 100 mL over 30 min and solutions diluted in 500 mL over 3 hr.

● **Y-Site Compatibility:** amiodarone, bumetanide, ciprofloxacin, daptomycin, midazolam, pantoprazole, tigecycline, vancomycin.

● **Y-Site Incompatibility:** diltiazem.

Patient/Family Teaching

● Advise patient to take medication once daily (unless biweekly regimens are used), as directed, and not to skip doses or double up on missed doses. Emphasize the importance of continuing therapy even after symptoms have subsided. Length of therapy for tuberculosis depends on regimen being used and underlying disease states. Patients on short-term prophylactic therapy should also be advised of the importance of compliance with therapy.

● Advise patient to notify health care professional promptly if signs and symptoms of hepatitis (yellow eyes and skin, nausea, vomiting, anorexia, unusual tiredness, weakness) or of thrombocytopenia (unusual bleeding or bruising) occur.

● Caution patient to avoid the use of alcohol during this therapy, because this may increase the risk of hepatotoxicity.

● Instruct patient to report the occurrence of flu-like symptoms (fever, chills, myalgia, headache) promptly.

● Rifampin may occasionally cause drowsiness. Caution patient to avoid driving or other activities requiring alertness until response to medication is known.

● Inform patient that saliva, sputum, teeth, sweat, tears, urine, and feces may become red-orange to red-brown and that soft contact lenses may become permanently discolored.

● Rep: Advise females of reproductive potential to notify health care professional if pregnancy is planned or suspected and to avoid breastfeeding during therapy.

● Emphasize the importance of regular follow-up exams to monitor progress and to check for side effects.

Evaluation/Desired Outcomes

● Decreased fever and night sweats.
● Diminished cough and sputum production.
● Negative sputum cultures.
● Increased appetite.
● Weight gain.
● Reduced fatigue.
● Sense of well-being in patients with tuberculosis.
● Prevention of meningococcal meningitis.
● Prevention of *H. influenzae* type B infection. Prophylactic course is usually short term.

---

rifAXIMin (ri-fax-i-min)

Xifaxan, ✶Zaxine

Classification
Therapeutic: anti-infectives
Pharmacologic: rifamycins

Indications

Travelers' diarrhea due to noninvasive strains of *Escherichia coli*. Reduction in risk of overt hepatic encephalopathy recurrence. Treatment of irritable bowel syndrome with diarrhea.

Action

Inhibits bacterial RNA synthesis by binding to bacterial DNA-dependent RNA polymerase. **Therapeutic Effects:** Decreased severity of travelers' diarrhea. Decreased episodes of overt hepatic encephalopathy. Decreased signs/symptoms of irritable bowel syndrome with diarrhea. **Spectrum:** *Escherichia coli* (enterotoxigenic and enteroaggregative strains).

Pharmacokinetics

Absorption: Poorly absorbed (<0.4%); action is primarily in GI tract.
Distribution: 80–90% concentrated in gut.
Metabolism and Excretion: Almost exclusively excreted unchanged in feces.
Half-life: 6 hr.

TIME/ACTION PROFILE

ROUTE	ONSET	PEAK	DURATION
PO	unknown	unknown	unknown

Contraindications/Precautions

Contraindicated in: Hypersensitivity to rifaximin or other rifamycins; Diarrhea with fever or bloody stools; Diarrhea caused by other infectious agents; Lactation: Lactation.

Use Cautiously in: OB: Use during pregnancy only if potential maternal benefit justifies potential fetal risk; Pedi: Safety not established in children <18 yr (hepatic encephalopathy or irritable bowel syndrome with diarrhea) or <12 yr (travelers' diarrhea).

Adverse Reactions/Side Effects

CV: <u>peripheral edema</u>. **GI:** CLOSTRIDIOIDES DIFFICILE-AS-SOCIATED DIARRHEA (CDAD). **Neuro:** <u>dizziness</u>.

Interactions

Drug-Drug: **P-glycoprotein inhibitors,** including **cyclosporine,** may ↑ levels and risk of toxicity. May cause fluctuations in INR when used with **warfarin**; closely monitor INR.

Route/Dosage

Travelers' Diarrhea

PO (Adults and Children ≥ 12 yr): 200 mg 3 times daily for 3 days.

Hepatic Encephalopathy

PO (Adults): 550 mg twice daily.

Irritable Bowel Syndrome With Diarrhea

PO (Adults): 550 mg 3 times daily for 14 days; if recurrence of symptoms, may treat up to an additional 2 times.

Availability

Tablets: 200 mg, 550 mg.

NURSING IMPLICATIONS

Assessment

- **Traveler's Diarrhea:** Assess frequency and consistency of stools and bowel sounds prior to and during therapy.
- Assess fluid and electrolyte balance and skin turgor for dehydration.
- **Hepatic Encephalopathy:** Assess mental status periodically during therapy.
- **Irritable Bowel Syndrome With Diarrhea:** Assess frequency and consistency of stools and other irritable bowel syndrome symptoms (bloating, cramping) daily.
- Monitor bowel function. Diarrhea, abdominal cramping, fever, and bloody stools should be reported to health care professional promptly as a sign of CDAD. May begin up to several wk following cessation of therapy.

Lab Test Considerations

- May cause lymphocytosis, monocytosis, and neutropenia.

Implementation

- Do not confuse rifaximin with rifampin.
- **PO:** Administer with or without food.

Patient/Family Teaching

- Instruct patient to take rifaximin as directed and to complete therapy, even if feeling better. Caution patient to stop taking rifaximin if diarrhea symptoms get worse, persist more than 24–48 hr, or are accompanied by fever or blood in the stool. Consult health care professional if these occur. Advise pa-

tient not to treat diarrhea without consulting health care professional. May occur up to several wk after discontinuation of medication.
- May cause dizziness. Caution patient to avoid driving and other activities requiring alertness until response to medication is known.
- Rep: Advise females of reproductive potential to notify health care professional if pregnancy is planned or suspected or if breastfeeding.

Evaluation/Desired Outcomes

- Decreased severity of travelers' diarrhea.
- Reduction in risk of overt hepatic encephalopathy recurrence.
- Reduction in symptoms of irritable bowel syndrome with diarrhea.

---

rilpivirine (ril-pi-vir-een)

Edurant

Classification

Therapeutic: antiretrovirals
Pharmacologic: non-nucleoside reverse transcriptase inhibitors

---

Indications

Treatment-naïve patients with HIV infection with HIV-1 RNA ≤ 100,000 copies/mL at start of therapy. Short-term treatment of HIV infection in patients with an HIV-1 RNA < 50 copies/mL who are on a stable antiretroviral regimen with no history of treatment failure and with no known or suspected resistance to either cabotegravir or rilpivirine (in combination with cabotegravir) (to be used as either oral lead-in to assess the tolerability of rilpivirine prior to administration of cabotegravir/rilpivirine extended-release injection or oral therapy for patients who will miss planned injection dosing with cabotegravir/rilpivirine extended-release injection).

Action

Inhibits HIV-replication by non-competitively inhibiting HIV reverse transcriptase. **Therapeutic Effects:** Slowed progression of HIV infection and decreased occurrence of sequelae. Increases CD4 cell counts and decreases viral load.

Pharmacokinetics

Absorption: Well absorbed following oral administration.
Distribution: Unknown.
Protein Binding: 99.7%.
Metabolism and Excretion: Mostly metabolized by the liver by the CYP3A isoenzyme; 25% excreted in feces unchanged, <1% excreted unchanged in urine.
Half-life: 50 hr.

R

TIME/ACTION PROFILE (plasma concentrations)

ROUTE	ONSET	PEAK	DURATION
PO	unknown	4–5 hr	24 hr

Contraindications/Precautions

Contraindicated in: Concurrent use of CYP3A inducers or proton pump inhibitors; Lactation: Breastfeeding not recommended in patients with HIV.

Use Cautiously in: Concurrent use of drugs that ↑ risk of torsades de pointes (may ↑ risk of arrhythmias); History of depression or suicide attempt; Hepatitis B or C; Pedi: Children <12 yr (safety and effectiveness not established).

Adverse Reactions/Side Effects

Derm: DRUG REACTION WITH EOSINOPHILIA AND SYSTEMIC SYMPTOMS (DRESS), rash. **Endo:** Grave's disease. **GI:** autoimmune hepatitis, hepatotoxicity. **MS:** polymyositis. **Neuro:** depression (↑ in children), dizziness, Guillain-Barré syndrome, headache, insomnia. **Misc:** immune reconstitution syndrome.

Interactions

Drug-Drug: CYP3A inducers, including **carbamazepine**, **dexamethasone** (more than a single dose), **oxcarbazepine**, **phenobarbital**, **phenytoin**, **rifampin**, or **rifapentine**, ↓ levels and effectiveness and promote virologic resistance; concurrent use contraindicated. **Proton pump inhibitors**, including **esomeprazole, lansoprazole, omeprazole, pantoprazole**, and **rabeprazole**, ↓ levels and effectiveness and may ↑ resistance; concurrent use contraindicated. Concurrent use with **antacids** may ↓ levels and effectiveness; use with caution, administer at least 2 hr before or 4 hr after rilpivirine. Concurrent use with **H₂ antagonists** may ↓ levels and effectiveness; use with caution, administer at least 12 hr before or 4 hr after rilpivirine. **Rifabutin** may ↓ levels; ↑ rilpivirine dose to 50 mg once daily during concurrent use. **Efavirenz, etravirine**, and **nevirapine** may ↓ levels; avoid concurrent use. **Darunavir/ritonavir, lopinavir/ritonavir, atazanavir/ritonavir, fosamprenavir/ritonavir, tipranavir/ritonavir, atazanavir, fosamprenavir**, and **nelfinavir** may ↑ levels. **Clarithromyin** or **erythromycin** may ↑ levels; consider using azithromycin. **Fluconazole, itraconazole, ketoconazole, posaconazole**, and **voriconazole** may ↑ levels; rilpivirine may ↓ **ketoconazole** levels. Concurrent use with **QT interval-prolonging drugs** may ↑ risk of serious arrhythmias. May ↓ levels of **methadone**; monitor clinical effects.

Drug-Natural Products: Concurrent use of St. John's wort ↓ blood levels and effectiveness and promote virologic resistance; concurrent use contraindicated.

Route/Dosage

Treatment-Naïve Patients With HIV Infection

PO (Adults and Children ≥12 yr and ≥35 kg): 25 mg once daily; *Pregnant patients on stable rilpivirine regimen prior to pregnancy and virologically suppressed (HIV RNA <50 copies/mL):* 25 mg once daily; *Concurrent rifabutin therapy:* 50 mg once daily (↓ dose to 25 mg once daily when rifabutin discontinued).

Combination Therapy With Cabotegravir for HIV Infection

PO (Adults and Children ≥12 yr and ≥35 kg): *Oral lead-in therapy to assess tolerability of rilpivirine:* 25 mg once daily (with oral cabotegravir 30 mg once daily) for ≥28 days, then switch to cabotegravir/rilpivirine extended-release injection. *To replace planned missed cabotegravir/rilpivirine extended-release injections for patients on monthly dosing schedule (if patient plans to miss scheduled monthly injection by >7 days):* 25 mg once daily (with oral cabotegravir 30 mg once daily) initiated at the same time as missed injection of cabotegravir/rilpivirine and then continued until day the cabotegravir/rilpivirine extended-release injection is restarted (oral replacement therapy can be continued for up to 2 mo). *To replace planned missed cabotegravir/rilpivirine extended-release injections for patients on every 2-mo dosing schedule (if patient plans to miss scheduled every 2-mo injection by >7 days):* 25 mg once daily (with oral cabotegravir 30 mg once daily) initiated the same time as missed injection of cabotegravir/rilpivirine and then continued until day the cabotegravir/rilpivirine extended-release injection is restarted (oral replacement therapy can be continued for up to 2 mo).

Availability

Tablets: 25 mg. *In combination with:* cabotegravir (Cabenuva); dolutegravir (Juluca); emtricitabine and tenofovir alafenamide (Odefsey); emtricitabine and tenofovir disoproxil fumarate (Complera). See Appendix N.

NURSING IMPLICATIONS

Assessment

- Assess for change in severity of HIV symptoms and for symptoms of opportunistic infections during therapy.
- Monitor closely for notable changes in behavior that could indicate the emergence or worsening of suicidal thoughts or behavior or depression.
- Assess for rash periodically during therapy. May cause DRESS. Discontinue therapy if severe or if accompanied with fever, general malaise, fatigue, muscle or joint aches, blisters, oral lesions, conjunctivitis, hepatitis, and/or eosinophilia.

Lab Test Considerations

- Monitor viral load and CD4 cell count regularly during therapy.
- Monitor liver function tests before and periodically during therapy in patients with underlying liver dis-

ease, hepatitis B or C, or marked ↑ transaminase. May cause ↑ serum creatinine, AST, ALT, total bilirubin, total cholesterol, LDL, and triglycerides.

Implementation

- **PO:** Administer once daily with a meal.
- When administered with cabotegravir, administer rilpivirine with cabotegravir once daily at same time with a meal. Take last PO dose on same day as cabotegravir injection is started. If patient plans to miss a scheduled cabotegravir injection by >7 days, take daily PO therapy to replace up to 2 consecutive monthly injection visits. Take 1st PO dose 1 mo after last injection.

Patient/Family Teaching

- Emphasize the importance of taking rilpivirine as directed, at the same time each day. It must always be used in combination with other antiretroviral drugs. Do not take more than prescribed amount and do not stop taking without consulting health care professional. Take missed doses with a meal if remembered <12 hr of the time it is usually taken, then return to regular schedule. If more than 12 hr from time dose is usually taken, omit dose and resume dosing schedule; do not double doses. Advise patient to read *Patient Information* prior to starting therapy and with each Rx refill in case of changes.
- Advise patient to take antacids 2 hr before or 4 hr after and H₂ antagonists 12 hr before or 4 hr after rilpivirine.
- Instruct patient that rilpivirine should not be shared with others.
- Inform patient that rilpivirine does not cure AIDS or prevent associated or opportunistic infections. Rilpivirine may reduce the risk of transmission of HIV to others through sexual contact or blood contamination. Caution patient to use a condom and to avoid sharing needles or donating blood to prevent spreading the AIDS virus to others. Advise patient that the long-term effects of rilpivirine are unknown at this time.
- Inform patients and families of risk of suicidal thoughts and behavior and advise that behavioral changes, emergency or worsening signs and symptoms of depression, unusual changes in mood, or emergence of suicidal thoughts, behavior, or thoughts of self-harm should be reported to health care professional immediately.
- Immune reconstitution syndrome may trigger opportunistic infections or autoimmune disorders. Notify health care professional if symptoms or rash occur.
- May cause dizziness. Caution patient to avoid driving or other activities requiring alertness until response to medication is known.
- Advise patient to notify health care professional of all Rx or OTC medications, vitamins, or herbal products being taken and to consult with health care professional before taking other medications, especially St. John's wort.
- Rep: Advise patient taking oral contraceptives to use a nonhormonal method of birth control during rilpivirine therapy. If pregnancy is suspected notify health care professional promptly. Encourage health care professionals to enroll pregnant women in the Antiretroviral Pregnancy Registry by calling 1-800-258-4263. Advise female patient to avoid breastfeeding.
- Emphasize the importance of regular follow-up exams and blood counts to determine progress and monitor for side effects.

Evaluation/Desired Outcomes

- Delayed progression of AIDS and decreased opportunistic infections in patients with HIV.
- Decrease in viral load and increase in CD4 cell counts.

rimegepant (ri-meg-je-pant)
Nurtec
Classification
Therapeutic: vascular headache suppressants
Pharmacologic: calcitonin gene-related peptide receptor antagonists

Indications
Acute treatment of migraine with or without aura. Preventive treatment of episodic migraines.

Action
Binds to and inhibits the calcitonin gene-related peptide (CGRP) receptor, which reduces the neuroinflammatory and vasodilatory effects of CGRP. **Therapeutic Effects:** Reduction in pain and other bothersome symptoms associated with migraine. Reduction in number of monthly migraine days.

Pharmacokinetics
Absorption: 64% absorbed following oral administration. High-fat foods may delay and reduce extent of absorption.
Distribution: Extensively distributed to tissues.
Protein Binding: 96%.
Metabolism and Excretion: Primarily metabolized in liver via the CYP3A4 isoenzyme, and to a lesser extent by the CYP2C9 isoenzyme. Primarily excreted as unchanged drug in feces (42%) and urine (51%).
Half-life: 11 hr.

TIME/ACTION PROFILE (relief of migraine pain)

ROUTE	ONSET	PEAK	DURATION
PO	0.5 hr	2 hr	up to 48 hr

✦ = Canadian drug name. ▩ = Genetic implication. ~~Strikethrough~~ = Discontinued. CAPITALS = life-threatening. Underline = most frequent.

Contraindications/Precautions

Contraindicated in: Hypersensitivity; Severe hepatic impairment; End-stage renal disease (CCr <15 mL/min).

Use Cautiously in: OB: Safety not established in pregnancy; Lactation: Safety not established in breastfeeding; Pedi: Safety and effectiveness not established in children.

Adverse Reactions/Side Effects

GI: nausea. **Misc:** hypersensitivity reactions.

Interactions

Drug-Drug: Strong CYP3A4 inhibitors, including **itraconazole** may significantly ↑ levels and risk of toxicity; avoid concurrent use. **Moderate CYP3A4 inhibitors** may ↑ levels and risk of toxicity; avoid another dose of rimegepant within 48 hr during concurrent use. **Strong CYP3A4 inducers**, including **rifampin** or **moderate CYP3A4 inducers**, may ↓ levels and effectiveness; avoid concurrent use. **P-glycoprotein inhibitors**, including **cyclosporine** or **quinidine**, may ↑ levels and risk of toxicity; avoid another dose of rimegepant within 48 hr during concurrent use.

Route/Dosage

Acute Migraine Treatment

PO (Adults): 75 mg as single dose (max dose = 75 mg/24 hr). Should not be used to treat >18 migraines in 30-day period.

Preventive Treatment of Episodic Migraines

PO (Adults): 75 mg every other day.

Availability

Orally disintegrating tablets (ODTs) (menthol flavor): 75 mg.

NURSING IMPLICATIONS

Assessment

- Assess pain location, character, intensity, duration, and associated symptoms (photophobia, phonophobia, nausea, vomiting) during migraine attack.
- Monitor frequency of migraine headaches in patients using rimegepant for prophylaxis.

Implementation

- Use dry hands when opening blister pack. Peel back foil covering of one blister and gently remove the ODT. Do not push ODT through foil. As soon as blister is opened, remove ODT and place on tongue; ODT may also be placed under tongue. ODT will disintegrate in saliva so that it can be swallowed without additional liquid. Take ODT immediately after opening blister pack. Do not store ODT outside the blister pack for future use.
- **PO: Treatment**: Administer ODT once daily as needed for migraine attacks. Limit dose to one ODT/day and no more than 18 doses in a 30-day period.
- **Prophylaxis**: Administer one ODT every other day for prevention of migraine headaches.

Patient/Family Teaching

- Instruct patient to take rimegepant as soon as symptoms of a migraine attack appear, but it may be administered any time during an attack. Do not use more than 75 mg in any 24-hr period.
- Instruct patient using rimegepant for prevention to take as directed.
- Advise patient to avoid alcohol, which aggravates headaches, during rimegepant use.
- Advise patient that lying down in a darkened room following rimegepant administration may further help relieve headache.
- Inform patients of potential for hypersensitivity reaction and that these reactions can occur days after administration of rimegepant. Advise patients to notify health care professional immediately if signs or symptoms of hypersensitivity reactions (shortness of breath, rash) occur. Rimegepant should be discontinued if hypersensitivity reaction occurs.
- Advise patient to notify health care professional of all Rx or OTC medications, vitamins, or herbal products being taken and to consult with health care professional before taking other medications.
- Advise females of reproductive potential to notify health care professional if pregnancy is planned or suspected or if breastfeeding. Inform patient of the pregnancy exposure registry that monitors pregnancy outcomes in women exposed to *Nurtec* during pregnancy. For more information, health care professionals or patients are encouraged to contact: 1-877-366-0324, email nurtecpregnancyregistry@ppd.com, or visit nurtecpregnancyregistry.com.

Evaluation/Desired Outcomes

- Relief of migraine attack.
- Reduction in frequency of migraine headaches.

risankizumab
(ris-an-kiz-ue-mab)
Skyrizi
Classification
Therapeutic: antipsoriatics
Pharmacologic: interleukin antagonists, monoclonal antibodies

Indications

Moderate to severe plaque psoriasis in patients who are candidates for phototherapy or systemic therapy. Active psoriatic arthritis (as monotherapy or in combination with non-biologic disease-modifying antirheumatic drugs [DMARDs]). Moderately to severely active Crohn's disease.

Action

Binds to the p19 protein subunit of the interleukin (IL)-23 cytokine to prevent its interaction with the IL-23 receptor. This cytokine is normally involved in inflammatory and immune responses. Binding to interleukins antagonizes their effects, inhibiting the release of proinflammatory cytokines and chemokines. **Therapeutic Effects:** Decrease in area and severity of psoriatic lesions. Improvement in clinical and symptomatic parameters of psoriatic arthritis. Improvement in clinical and endoscopic remission rates in Crohn's disease.

Pharmacokinetics

Absorption: 89% absorbed following SUBQ administration. IV administration results in complete bioavailability.

Distribution: Well distributed to tissues.

Metabolism and Excretion: Broken down by catabolic processes into peptides and amino acids.

Half-life: *Plaque psoriasis:* 28 days; *Crohn's disease:* 21 days.

TIME/ACTION PROFILE (plasma concentrations)

ROUTE	ONSET	PEAK	DURATION
SUBQ	unknown	3–14 days	12 wk
IV	unknown	unknown	unknown

Contraindications/Precautions

Contraindicated in: Hypersensitivity; Active, untreated infection.

Use Cautiously in: History of tuberculosis (possibility of reactivation); Cirrhosis (for Crohn's disease only); OB: Use during pregnancy only if potential maternal benefit justifies potential fetal risk; Lactation: Safety not established in breastfeeding; Pedi: Safety and effectiveness not established in children.

Exercise Extreme Caution in: Chronic infection or history of recurrent infection.

Adverse Reactions/Side Effects

GI: hepatotoxicity (in Crohn's disease). **Local:** injection site reactions. **Neuro:** fatigue, headache. **Misc:** infection, HYPERSENSITIVITY REACTIONS (including anaphylaxis).

Interactions

Drug-Drug: May ↓ antibody response to and ↑ risk of adverse reactions from **live vaccines**; avoid use during therapy.

Route/Dosage

Plaque Psoriasis and Psoriatic Arthritis

SUBQ (Adults): 150 mg initially and 4 wk later, then 150 mg every 12 wk.

Crohn's Disease

IV (Adults): *Induction:* 600 mg initially and then at Week 4 and Week 8. At Week 12, begin Maintenance therapy (SUBQ) (see below).

SUBQ (Adults): *Maintenance:* 180 mg or 360 mg at Week 12, and then every 8 wk.

Availability

Solution for SUBQ injection (prefilled pens): 150 mg/mL. Solution for SUBQ injection (prefilled syringes): 75 mg/0.83 mL, 150 mg/mL. **Solution for SUBQ injection (prefilled cartridge with on-body injector):** 360 mg/2.4 mL. **Solution for IV injection:** 60 mg/mL.

NURSING IMPLICATIONS

Assessment

- Assess patient for tuberculosis (TB) before starting, during, and after therapy. Do not administer risankizumab to patient with active TB. Consider anti-TB therapy before starting therapy in patients with a past history of latent or active TB in whom an adequate course of treatment cannot be confirmed.
- Assess skin lesions before and periodically during therapy.
- Monitor for signs and symptoms of infection (fever, chills, cough, dyspnea, skin infections) periodically during therapy.
- Monitor for signs and symptoms of hypersensitivity reactions (fainting; dizziness; feeling lightheaded; chest tightness; swelling of face, eyelids, lips, mouth, tongue, or throat; skin rash; hives; trouble breathing or throat tightness; itching) during therapy.

Lab Test Considerations

- *For Crohn's disease:* assess liver enzymes and bilirubin levels prior to starting therapy and periodically for at least 12 wk.

Implementation

- Complete all age-appropriate vaccinations as recommended by current immunization guidelines before starting therapy.
- Before injecting, remove carton from refrigerator and without removing prefilled pen or prefilled syringe(s) from the carton, allow risankizumab to reach room temperature out of direct sunlight: 30–90 min for prefilled pen and 15–30 min for the prefilled syringe(s). Solution is colorless to slightly yellow and clear to slightly opalescent; may contain a few translucent to white particles. Do not use if solution is cloudy, discolored, or contains large particles. Do not freeze or shake.
- May use pen, prefilled syringe, or prefilled cartridge with supplied on-body injector for SUBQ injections. Follow manufacturer's *Instructions for Use* for each method.
- **SUBQ:** Inject into abdomen or thigh; may inject in upper, outer arm if administered by health care professional or caregiver. Do not inject into areas where skin is tender, bruised, erythematous, indurated or affected by psoriasis. If using 75 mg/0.83 mL syringes, 150 mg dose requires two syringes. Inject in different locations.

IV Administration

- **Induction:** Administered by a health care professional. *Dilution:* Withdraw 10 mL of risankizumab from vial and inject into IV bag or glass bottle containing D5W (600 mg/10 mL in 100 mL, or 250 mL, or 500 mL). *Concentration:* Approximately 1.2 mg/mL to 6 mg/mL. Discard any remaining solution in the vial. Do not shake vial or diluted solution. Allow diluted solution to warm to room temperature (if stored refrigerated) prior to administration. Complete infusion within 8 hr of dilution. Solution is stable for 8 hr at room temperature and up to 20 hr if refrigerated and protected from light. *Rate:* Infuse over at least 1 hr.

- At Week 12, begin SUBQ maintenance therapy.
- **Y-Site Incompatibility:** Do not administer with other medications or solutions.

Patient/Family Teaching

- Instruct patient caregiver in correct injection technique and disposal of equipment. Administer at Week 0, Week 4, and every 12 wk thereafter. If a dose is missed, administer as soon as possible, then resume dosing at the regular scheduled time.
- Advise patient to notify health care professional if signs and symptoms of infection (fever, sweats, chills, cough, shortness of breath, blood in mucus [phlegm], muscle aches, warm, red, or painful skin or sores different from psoriasis, weight loss, diarrhea or stomach pain, burning on urination, urinating more often than usual) occur.
- Advise patient to avoid live vaccines during therapy.
- Instruct patient to notify health care professional of all Rx or OTC medications, vitamins, or herbal products being taken and to consult health care professional before taking other Rx, OTC, or herbal products.
- Rep: Advise females of reproductive potential to notify health care professional if pregnancy is planned or suspected or if breastfeeding. Delay live virus immunizations in infants exposed in utero for a minimum of 5 mo after birth. Inform patient of pregnancy exposure registry that monitors outcomes in women who become pregnant while treated with risankizumab. Encourage patient to enroll by calling 1-877-302-2161.

Evaluation/Desired Outcomes

- Decrease in area and severity of psoriatic lesions.
- Improvement in clinical and symptomatic parameters of psoriatic arthritis.
- Improvement in clinical and endoscopic remission rates in Crohn's disease.

risedronate (ris-ed-roe-nate)

Actonel, ✤Actonel DR, Atelvia

Classification
Therapeutic: bone resorption inhibitors
Pharmacologic: bisphosphonates

Indications

Prevention and treatment of postmenopausal and corticosteroid-induced osteoporosis. Treatment of Paget's disease in men and women. Treatment of osteoporosis in men.

Action

Inhibits bone resorption by binding to bone hydroxyapatite, which inhibits osteoclast activity. **Therapeutic Effects:** Reversal of the progression of osteoporosis with decreased fractures and other sequelae. Reduced bone turnover and resorption; normalization of serum alkaline phosphatase with reduced complications of Paget's disease.

Pharmacokinetics

Absorption: Rapidly but poorly absorbed following oral administration (0.63% bioavailability).
Distribution: 60% of absorbed dose distributes to bone.
Metabolism and Excretion: 40% of absorbed dose is excreted unchanged by kidneys; unabsorbed drug is excreted in feces.
Half-life: *Initial:* 1.5 hr; *terminal:* 220 hr (reflects dissociation from bone).

TIME/ACTION PROFILE (effects on serum alkaline phosphatase)

ROUTE	ONSET	PEAK	DURATION
PO	within days	30 days	up to 16 mo

Contraindications/Precautions

Contraindicated in: Hypersensitivity; Severe renal impairment (CCr <30 mL/min); Hypocalcemia; Abnormalities of the esophagus, which delay esophageal emptying (i.e., strictures, achalasia); Inability to stand/sit upright for at least 30 min; OB: Pregnancy.
Use Cautiously in: History of upper GI disorders; Other disturbances of bone or mineral metabolism (correct abnormalities before initiating therapy); Dietary deficiencies (supplemental vitamin D and calcium may be required); Invasive dental procedures, cancer, receiving chemotherapy, corticosteroids, angiogenesis inhibitors, poor oral hygiene, periodontal disease, dental disease, anemia, coagulopathy, infection, or poorly fitting dentures (may ↑ risk of jaw osteonecrosis); Lactation: Use while breastfeeding only if potential maternal benefit justifies potential risk to infant.

Adverse Reactions/Side Effects

CV: chest pain, edema. **Derm:** rash, STEVENS-JOHNSON SYNDROME, TOXIC EPIDERMAL NECROLYSIS. **EENT:** amblyopia, conjunctivitis, dry eyes, eye pain/inflammation, tinnitus. **GI:** abdominal pain, diarrhea, belching, colitis, constipation, dysphagia, esophageal cancer, esophageal ulcer, esophagitis, gastric ulcer, nausea. **MS:** arthralgia, musculoskeletal pain, femur fractures, osteonecrosis (primarily of jaw). **Neuro:** weakness. **Resp:** asthma exacerbation. **Misc:** flu-like syndrome.

Interactions

Drug-Drug: Concurrent use with **NSAIDs** or **aspirin** ↑ risk of GI irritation. Absorption is ↓ by **calcium**

supplements or antacids. **Proton pump inhibitors and H₂ antagonists** may cause a faster release of drug from the delayed-release product that can ↑ levels; concurrent use not recommended.

Drug-Food: Food ↓ absorption (administer at least 30 min before breakfast).

Route/Dosage

Prevention and Treatment of Postmenopausal Osteoporosis

PO (Adults): 5 mg once daily (immediate-release tablets) *or* 35 mg once weekly (immediate- or delayed-release tablets) *or* 75 mg taken on 2 consecutive days for a total of 2 tablets each mo (immediate-release tablets) *or* 150 mg once monthly (immediate-release tablets).

Prevention and Treatment of Glucocorticoid-Induced Osteoporosis

PO (Adults): 5 mg once daily (immediate-release tablets).

Treatment of Osteoporosis in Men

PO (Adults): 35 mg once weekly (immediate-release tablets).

Treatment of Paget's Disease

PO (Adults): 30 mg once daily for 2 mo (immediate-release tablets); retreatment may be considered after 2 mo off therapy.

Availability (generic available)

Immediate-release tablets: 5 mg, 30 mg, 35 mg, 150 mg. **Delayed-release tablets (Atelvia):** 35 mg.

NURSING IMPLICATIONS

Assessment

- Perform a routine oral exam prior to initiation of therapy. Dental exam with appropriate preventative dentistry should be considered prior to therapy. Patients with history of tooth extraction, poor oral hygiene, gingival infections, diabetes, or use of a dental appliance or those taking immunosuppressive therapy, angiogenesis inhibitors, or systemic corticosteroids are at greater risk for osteonecrosis of the jaw.
- **Osteoporosis:** Assess patients via bone density study for low bone mass before and periodically during therapy.
- **Paget's disease:** Assess for symptoms of Paget's disease (bone pain, headache, decreased visual and auditory acuity, increased skull size).

Lab Test Considerations

- *Osteoporosis:* Assess serum calcium before and periodically during therapy. Hypocalcemia and vitamin D deficiency should be treated before initiating alendronate therapy. May cause mild, transient ↑ of calcium and phosphate.

- *Paget's disease:* Monitor alkaline phosphatase prior to and periodically during therapy to monitor effectiveness of therapy.

Implementation

- Do not confuse Actonel with Actos.
- **PO:** Administer *Actonel* first thing in the morning with 6–8 oz of water, 30 min prior to other medications, beverages, or food. Waiting longer than 30 min will improve absorption. Administer *Atelvia* right after breakfast with at least 4 oz of water. *DNC:* Swallow tablet whole; do not crush, break, or chew.
- Calcium-, magnesium-, or aluminum-containing agents may interfere with absorption of risedronate and should be taken at a different time of day with food.
- Avoid administering delayed-release product with proton pump inhibitors or H₂ antagonists; may allow a faster release and increased drug level.

Patient/Family Teaching

- Instruct patient on the importance of taking as directed. Risedronate should be taken with 6–8 oz of water (mineral water, orange juice, coffee, and other beverages decrease absorption). *If a dose of Actonel 35 is missed,* take 1 tablet the morning remembered, then return to the 1 tablet/wk on the originally scheduled day; do not take 2 pills at once. *If 1 or both tablets of Actonel 75 are missed and the next month's scheduled doses are more than 7 days away:* if both Actonel 75 doses are missed, take 1 the morning remembered and 1 the next morning. If only 1 Actonel 75 tablet is missed: take the missed tablet on the morning of the day after you remember, then return to original schedule. Do not take more than two 75 mg tablets within 7 days. *If 1 or both tablets of Actonel 75 are missed and the next month's scheduled doses are within 7 days,* omit and return to schedule next mo. *If 1 or both tablets of Actonel 150 are missed and the next month's scheduled doses are more than 7 days away,* take the missed tablet on the morning of the day after you remember, then return to original schedule. Do not take more than two 150-mg tablets within 7 days. *If 1 or both tablets of Actonel 75 are missed and the next month's scheduled doses are within 7 days,* omit and return to schedule next mo. Encourage patient to read the *Medication Guide* before starting therapy and with each Rx refill in case of changes.
- Caution patients to remain upright for 30 min following dose to facilitate passage to stomach and minimize risk of esophageal irritation.
- Advise patient to eat a balanced diet and consult health care professional about the need for supplemental calcium and vitamin D (see Appendix J).

R

- Inform patient that severe musculoskeletal pain may occur within days, mo, or yr after starting risedronate. Symptoms my resolve completely after discontinuation or slow or incomplete resolution may occur. Notify health care professional if severe pain occurs.
- Advise patient to notify health care professional of all Rx or OTC medications, vitamins, or herbal products being taken and to consult with health care professional before taking other medications.
- Encourage patient to participate in regular exercise and to modify behaviors that increase the risk of osteoporosis (stop smoking, reduce alcohol consumption).
- Advise patient to practice good mouth care during therapy and to notify health care professional if signs and symptoms of osteonecrosis of the jaw (jaw pain, toothache, sores on gums) occur.
- Advise patient to inform health care professional of risedronate therapy prior to dental surgery.
- Rep: May cause fetal harm. Advise females of reproductive potential to notify health care professional if pregnancy is planned or suspected and to avoid breastfeeding during therapy. May impair female and male fertility.

Evaluation/Desired Outcomes
- Reversal of the progression of osteoporosis with decreased fractures and other sequelae. For patients at low risk of fracture, discontinue after 3 to 5 yr of use.
- Decrease in serum alkaline phosphatase and the progression of Paget's disease.

BEERS

risperiDONE (riss-per-i-done)
Perseris, RisperDAL, RisperDAL Consta, RisperDAL M-TAB, Rykindo, Uzedy
Classification
Therapeutic: antipsychotics, mood stabilizers
Pharmacologic: benzisoxazoles

Indications
PO, IM, SUBQ: Schizophrenia. **PO:** Acute manic or mixed episodes associated with bipolar I disorder (as monotherapy or in combination with lithium or valproate). **IM:** Maintenance treatment of bipolar I disorder (as monotherapy or in combination with lithium or valproate). **PO:** Irritability associated with autistic disorder.

Action
May act by antagonizing dopamine and serotonin in the CNS. **Therapeutic Effects:** Decreased symptoms of psychoses, bipolar mania, or autism.

Pharmacokinetics
Absorption: 70% after administration of tablets, solution, or orally disintegrating tablets. Following IM administration, small initial release of drug, followed by 3-wk lag; the rest of release starts at 3 wk and lasts 4–6 wk. Following SUBQ administration, initial release of drug occurs at 4–6 hr, with the rest of release occurring at 10–14 days after administration.

Distribution: Unknown.

Metabolism and Excretion: Primarily metabolized by the liver by the CYP2D6 isoenzyme to 9-hydroxyrisperidone (has similar pharmacological properties as risperidone). Risperidone and its active metabolite are renally eliminated.

Half-life: *Extensive metabolizers:* 3 hr for risperidone, 21 hr for 9-hydroxyrisperidone. *Poor metabolizers:* 20 hr for risperidone and 30 hr for 9-hydroxyrisperidone; *SUBQ:* 9–11 days.

TIME/ACTION PROFILE (clinical effects)

ROUTE	ONSET	PEAK	DURATION
PO	1–2 wk	unknown	up to 6 wk†
IM	3 wk	4–6 wk	up to 6 wk†
SUBQ	2 wk	6–8 wk	unknown

†After discontinuation.

Contraindications/Precautions
Contraindicated in: Hypersensitivity to risperidone or paliperidone; Lactation: Lactation.

Use Cautiously in: Renal or hepatic impairment (initial dose ↓ recommended); Underlying cardiovascular disease (↑ risk of arrhythmias and hypotension); History of seizures; History of drug abuse; Diabetes or risk factors for diabetes (may worsen glucose control); Patients at risk for aspiration or falls; Renal impairment; Hepatic impairment; OB: Neonates at ↑ risk for extrapyramidal symptoms and withdrawal after delivery when exposed during the 3rd trimester; use during pregnancy only if potential maternal benefit justifies potential fetal risk; Pedi: Safety and effectiveness not established in children <13 yr (schizophrenia), <10 yr (bipolar disorder), or <5 yr (autism) ; Geri: Appears on Beers list. ↑ risk of stroke, cognitive decline, and mortality in older adults with dementia. Avoid use in older adults, except for schizophrenia or bipolar disorder.

Adverse Reactions/Side Effects
CV: arrhythmias, orthostatic hypotension, syncope, tachycardia. **Derm:** itching/skin rash, ↑ pigmentation, dry skin, photosensitivity, seborrhea, STEVENS-JOHNSON SYNDROME, sweating, TOXIC EPIDERMAL NECROLYSIS. **EENT:** pharyngitis, rhinitis, visual disturbances. **Endo:** galactorrhea, hyperglycemia. **F and E:** polydipsia. **GI:** constipation, diarrhea, dry mouth, nausea, ↑ salivation, abdominal pain, anorexia, dyspepsia, dysphagia, vomiting. **GU:** ↓ libido, dysmenorrhea/menorrhagia, ↓ fertility (females), amenorrhea, difficulty urinating, gynecomastia, impotence, polyuria, priapism. **Hemat:** AGRANULOCYTOSIS, leukopenia, neutropenia. **Metab:** weight gain, dyslipidemia, weight loss. **MS:** arthralgia, back pain. **Neuro:** ↑ dreams, ↑ sleep duration, aggressive behavior, dizziness, extrapyramidal reactions, headache, insomnia, sedation, fatigue, impaired tem-

perature regulation, nervousness, NEUROLEPTIC MALIG-
NANT SYNDROME, SEIZURES, tardive dyskinesia. **Resp:**
cough, dyspnea. **Misc:** HYPERSENSITIVITY REACTIONS (including anaphylaxis and angioedema).

Interactions

Drug-Drug: May ↓ the antiparkinsonian effects of **levodopa** or other **dopamine agonists**. **Strong
CYP3A4 inducers,** including **carbamazepine, phenytoin, rifampin,** and **phenobarbital** may ↑ metabolism and may ↓ effectiveness; dose adjustments may be
necessary. **Fluoxetine** and **paroxetine** ↑ blood levels
and may ↑ effects; dose adjustments may be necessary.
Clozapine ↓ metabolism and may ↑ effects of risperidone. ↑ CNS depression may occur with other **CNS depressants,** including **alcohol, antihistamines, sed-
ative/hypnotics,** or **opioid analgesics**. Concurrent
use with **methylphenidate** may ↑ risk of extrapyramidal symptoms.

Drug-Natural Products: Kava, valerian, or chamomile can ↑ CNS depression.

Route/Dosage

Schizophrenia

PO (Adults): 1 mg twice daily, ↑ by 1–2 mg/day no
more frequently than every 24 hr to 4–8 mg daily.
PO (Children 13–17 yr): 0.5 mg once daily, ↑ by
0.5–1.0 mg no more frequently than every 24 hr to 3
mg daily. May administer half the daily dose twice daily
if drowsiness persists.
IM (Adults): 25 mg every 2 wk; some patients may
benefit from a higher dose of 37.5 or 50 mg every 2 wk.
IM (Geriatric Patients): 25 mg every 2 wk.
SUBQ (Adults): *Currently taking (switching from) 2
mg/day of oral risperidone:* Uzedy: 50 mg once
monthly or 100 mg every 2 mo; *Currently taking
(switching from) 3 mg/day of oral risperidone:* Perseris: 90 mg once monthly; Uzedy: 75 mg once monthly
or 150 mg every 2 mo; *Currently taking (switching
from) 4 mg/day of oral risperidone:* Perseris: 120 mg
once monthly; Uzedy: 100 mg once monthly or 200 mg
every 2 mo; *Currently taking (switching from) 5 mg/
day of oral risperidone:* Uzedy: 125 mg once monthly
or 250 mg every 2 mo; *Concurrent use of strong
CYP2D6 inhibitor (e.g., fluoxetine or paroxetine):*
Perseris: Initiate 90 mg once monthly 2–4 wk before
starting strong CYP2D6 inhibitor therapy; Uzedy: When
initiation of strong CYP2D6 inhibitor is expected, place
patients on a lower dose of risperidone prior to the
planned start of the strong CYP2D6 inhibitor. When a
strong CYP2D6 inhibitor is initiated in patients already
receiving the lowest risperidone dose (50 mg once
monthly or 100 mg every 2 mo), continue treatment
with these doses unless clinical judgment requires interruption of treatment. *Concurrent use of strong
CYP3A4 inducer:* Perseris: If receiving 90 mg once
monthly regimen, ↑ dose to 120 mg once monthly (and

consider using additional oral risperidone); if receiving
120 mg once monthly regimen, consider using additional oral risperidone; Uzedy: Upon initiation of therapy with a strong CYP3A4 inducer, closely monitor patients during the first 4–8 wk since the dose of Uzedy
may need to be adjusted. A dose ↑ of Uzedy or additional oral risperidone may be considered.

Hepatic/Renal Impairment

PO (Adults): *Severe renal impairment (CCr <30
mL/min) or severe hepatic impairment:* Start with 0.5
mg twice daily; ↑ by 0.5 mg twice daily, up to 1.5 mg
twice daily; then ↑ at weekly intervals if necessary.

Hepatic/Renal Impairment

IM (Adults): Start with 0.5 mg PO twice daily for 1st
wk, then ↑ to 1 mg PO twice daily or 2 mg PO once
daily during 2nd wk. If 2 mg/day PO dose is well tolerated, can initiate 12.5 mg or 25 mg IM every 2 wk.

Hepatic/Renal Impairment

SUBQ (Adults): *Perseris:* Titrate patients up to at least
3 mg/day of oral risperidone before initiating Perseris.
If patient tolerates this dose of oral risperidone, consider SUBQ dose of 90 mg once monthly. *Uzedy:* Titrate
patients up to at least 2 mg/day of oral risperidone before initiating Uzedy. If patient tolerates this dose of oral
risperidone, consider SUBQ dose of 50 mg once
monthly.

Acute Manic or Mixed Episodes Associated With Bipolar I Disorder

PO (Adults): 2–3 mg/day as a single daily dose, dose
may be ↑ at 24-hr intervals by 1 mg (range 1–5 mg/
day).
PO (Children 13–17 yr): 0.5 mg once daily, ↑ by
0.5–1 mg no more frequently than every 24 hr to 2.5
mg daily. May administer half the daily dose twice daily
if drowsiness persists.
PO (Geriatric Patients): Start with 0.5 mg twice daily;
↑ by 0.5 mg twice daily, up to 1.5 mg twice daily; then
↑ at weekly intervals if necessary. May also be given as a
single daily dose after initial titration.

Hepatic/Renal Impairment

PO (Adults): *Severe renal impairment (CCr <30
mL/min) or severe hepatic impairment:* Start with 0.5
mg twice daily; ↑ by 0.5 mg twice daily, up to 1.5 mg
twice daily; then ↑ at weekly intervals if necessary.

Maintenance Treatment of Bipolar I Disorder

IM (Adults): 25 mg every 2 wk; some patients may
benefit from a higher dose of 37.5 or 50 mg every 2 wk.
IM (Geriatric Patients): 25 mg every 2 wk.

Hepatic/Renal Impairment

IM (Adults): Start with 0.5 mg PO twice daily for 1st
wk, then ↑ to 1 mg PO twice daily or 2 mg PO once
daily during 2nd wk. If 2 mg/day PO dose is well tolerated, can initiate 12.5 mg or 25 mg IM every 2 wk.

R

Irritability Associated With Autistic Disorder

PO (Children 5–16 yr weighing <20 kg): 0.25 mg/day initially. After at least 4 days of therapy, may ↑ to 0.5 mg/day. Dose ↑ in increments of 0.25 mg/day may be considered at 2 wk or longer intervals. May be given as a single or divided dose.

PO (Children 5–16 yr weighing >20 kg): 0.5 mg/day initially. After at least 4 days of therapy, may ↑ to 1 mg/day. Dose ↑ in increments of 0.5 mg/day may be considered at 2 wk or longer intervals. May be given as a single or divided dose.

Hepatic/Renal Impairment

PO (Adults): *Severe renal impairment (CCr <30 mL/min) or severe hepatic impairment:* Start with 0.5 mg twice daily; ↑ by 0.5 mg twice daily, up to 1.5 mg twice daily; then ↑ at weekly intervals if necessary.

Availability (generic available)

Immediate-release tablets: 0.25 mg, 0.5 mg, 1 mg, 2 mg, 3 mg, 4 mg. **Orally disintegrating tablets (Risperdal M-Tabs):** 0.25 mg, 0.5 mg, 1 mg, 2 mg, 3 mg, 4 mg. **Oral solution:** 1 mg/mL. **Extended-release suspension for IM injection (Risperdal Consta, Rykindo):** 12.5 mg/vial kit, 25 mg/vial kit, 37.5 mg/vial kit, 50 mg/vial kit. **Extended-release suspension for SUBQ injection (Perseris):** 90 mg/vial kit, 120 mg/vial kit. **Extended-release suspension for SUBQ injection (Uzedy):** 50 mg/0.14 mL, 75 mg/0.14 mL, 100 mg/0.28 mL, 125 mg/0.35 mL, 150 mg/0.42 mL, 200 mg/0.56 mL, 250 mg/0.7 mL.

NURSING IMPLICATIONS

Assessment

- Monitor patient's mental status (orientation, mood, behavior) and mood before and periodically during therapy. Monitor closely for notable changes in behavior that could indicate the emergence or worsening of suicidal thoughts or behavior or depression, especially during early therapy. Restrict amount of drug available to patient.
- Assess weight and BMI initially and throughout therapy. Monitor for symptoms of hyperglycemia (polydipsia, polyuria, polyphagia, weakness) periodically during therapy.
- Monitor BP (sitting, standing, lying down) and pulse before and frequently during initial dose titration. May cause prolonged QT interval, tachycardia, and orthostatic hypotension. If hypotension occurs, dose may need to be decreased.
- Observe patient when administering medication to ensure medication is swallowed and not hoarded or cheeked.
- Monitor patient for onset of extrapyramidal side effects (*akathisia:* restlessness; *dystonia:* muscle spasms and twisting motions; or *pseudoparkinsonism:* mask-like face, rigidity, tremors, drooling, shuffling gait, dysphagia). Report these symptoms; reduction of dose or discontinuation may be necessary. Trihexyphenidyl or benztropine may be used to control symptoms.
- Monitor for tardive dyskinesia (involuntary rhythmic movement of mouth, face, and extremities). Report immediately; may be irreversible.
- Monitor for development of neuroleptic malignant syndrome (fever, respiratory distress, tachycardia, seizures, diaphoresis, hypertension or hypotension, pallor, tiredness). Notify health care professional immediately if these symptoms occur.
- Monitor for symptoms related to hyperprolactinemia (menstrual abnormalities, galactorrhea, sexual dysfunction).
- Assess for falls risk. Drowsiness, orthostatic hypotension, and motor and sensory instability increase risk. Institute prevention if indicated.
- Monitor weight during therapy. May cause weight gain in children and adolescents.
- Monitor for skin rash during therapy. May require discontinuation of therapy.

Lab Test Considerations

- May cause ↑ serum prolactin levels.
- May cause ↑ AST and ALT.
- May also cause anemia, thrombocytopenia, leukocytosis, and leukopenia.
- Obtain fasting blood glucose and cholesterol levels initially and periodically during therapy.
- Monitor CBC frequently during initial mo of therapy in patients with pre-existing or history of low WBC. May cause leukopenia, neutropenia, or agranulocytosis. Discontinue therapy if this occurs.
- Monitor serum prolactin prior to and periodically during therapy. May cause ↑ serum prolactin levels.

Implementation

- Do not confuse risperidone with ropinirole. Do not confuse Risperdal with Restoril or ropinirole.
- When switching from other antipsychotics, discontinue previous agents when starting risperidone and minimize the period of overlapping antipsychotic agents.
- If therapy is reinstituted after an interval off risperidone, follow initial titration schedule.
- For IM use, establish tolerance with oral dosing before IM use and continue oral dosing for 3 wk following initial IM injection. *Risperdal Consta:* Take oral doses for 3 wk, starting with the 1st dose of risperidone. Then discontinue PO doses. *Rykindo:* Take oral doses for 7 days, starting with day of 1st dose of risperidone. After 7 days, discontinue PO doses. Do not increase dose more frequently than every 4 wk.
- **PO:** Daily doses can be taken in the morning or evening.
- For orally disintegrating tablets, open blister pack by pealing back foil to expose tablet; do not try to push tablet through foil. Use dry hands to remove tablet from blister and immediately place entire tablet on tongue. Tablets disintegrate in mouth within sec and can be swallowed with or without liquid. Do not attempt to split or chew tablet. Do not try to store tablets once removed from blister.

- Oral solution can be administered directly from calibrated oral dosing syringe or mixed with water, coffee, orange juice, or low-fat milk; do not mix with cola or tea.
- **SUBQ:** Mix *Perseris* according to manufacturer's instructions. May be injected into abdomen or back of upper arm; avoid areas with nodules, lesions, excessive pigment, irritation, redness, bruising, infection, or scarring. Hold syringe upright for several sec to allow air bubbles to rise; depress the plunger to expel excess air. Pinch skin to avoid IM injection. Do not rub site after injection. Advise patient that they may have a lump for several wk; will decrease in size over time. Instruct patient not to rub or massage injection site and avoid constriction by belts or clothing waistbands.
- **IM:** Reconstitute with 2 mL of diluent provided by manufacturer. Administer via deep deltoid (1-in. needle) or gluteal (2-in. needle) injection using enclosed safety needle; alternate arms or buttocks with each injection. Allow solution to warm to room temperature prior to injection. Administer immediately after mixed with diluent; shake well to mix suspension. Must be administered within 6 hr of reconstitution. Store dose pack in refrigerator.
- Do not combine dose strengths in a single injection.

Patient/Family Teaching

- Instruct patient to take medication as directed.
- Inform patient of the possibility of extrapyramidal symptoms. Instruct patient to report these symptoms immediately to health care professional.
- Advise patient to change positions slowly to minimize orthostatic hypotension. Protect from falls.
- May cause drowsiness. Caution patient to avoid driving or other activities requiring alertness until response to medication is known.
- Advise patient and family to notify health care professional if thoughts about suicide or dying, attempts to commit suicide; new or worse depression; new or worse anxiety; feeling very agitated or restless; panic attacks; trouble sleeping; new or worse irritability; acting aggressive; being angry or violent; acting on dangerous impulses; an extreme increase in activity and talking; other unusual changes in behavior or mood occur.
- Advise patient to use sunscreen and protective clothing when exposed to the sun to prevent photosensitivity reactions. Extremes in temperature should also be avoided; this drug impairs body temperature regulation.
- Instruct patient to notify health care professional of all Rx or OTC medications, vitamins, or herbal products being taken and consult health care professional before taking any new medications. Caution patient to avoid concurrent use of alcohol and other CNS depressants.

- Advise patient to notify health care professional of medication regimen before treatment or surgery.
- Instruct patient to notify health care professional promptly if sore throat, fever, unusual bleeding or bruising, rash, tremors, or symptoms of hyperglycemia occur.
- Rep: May cause fetal harm. Advise females or reproductive potential to notify health care professional if pregnancy is planned or suspected, and to avoid breastfeeding. Encourage women who become pregnant while taking risperidone to enroll in the National Pregnancy Registry for Atypical Antipsychotics at 1-866-961-2388 or visit http://womensmentalhealth.org/research/pregnancyregistry/. Monitor neonates for extrapyramidal and/or withdrawal symptoms. Monitor infants exposed to risperidone through breast milk for excess sedation, failure to thrive, jitteriness, and extrapyramidal symptoms (tremors and abnormal muscle movements). May impair fertility in females; usually reversible.
- Emphasize the importance of routine follow-up exams to monitor side effects and continued participation in psychotherapy to improve coping skills.

Evaluation/Desired Outcomes

- Decrease in excited, manic behavior.
- Decrease in positive symptoms (delusions, hallucinations) of schizophrenia.
- Decreased aggression toward others, deliberate self-injury, temper tantrums, and mood changes in children with autism.
- Decrease in negative symptoms (social withdrawal, flat, blunted affects) of schizophrenia.
- Decrease in autism symptoms.

ritlecitinib (rit-le-sye-ti-nib)
Litfulo
Classification
Therapeutic: none assigned
Pharmacologic: kinase inhibitors

Indications
Severe alopecia areata.

Action
Irreversibly inhibits Janus kinase 3 and the tyrosine kinase expressed in the hepatocellular carcinoma (TEC) kinase family by blocking the adenosine triphosphate binding site, both of which may inhibit T cell activation. **Therapeutic Effects:** Reduction in scalp hair loss.

Pharmacokinetics
Absorption: 64% absorbed following oral administration.
Distribution: Unknown.
Metabolism and Excretion: Metabolized by multiple pathways, including glutathione S-transferase and

several CYP450 enzymes (CYP3A, CYP2C8, CYP1A2, and CYP2C9). Primarily excreted as metabolites in the urine (66%), with 20% excreted in the feces.
Half-life: 1.3–2.3 hr.

TIME/ACTION PROFILE (reduction in scalp hair loss)

ROUTE	ONSET	PEAK	DURATION
PO	6–8 wk	unknown	≥24 wk

Contraindications/Precautions

Contraindicated in: Hypersensitivity; Active, serious infection; Severe hepatic impairment; Lactation: Lactation.

Use Cautiously in: Chronic, recurrent infection; Previous exposure to tuberculosis (TB); History of serious or opportunistic infection; Lived or traveled in areas of endemic TB or mycoses; Predisposed to infection; >50 yr old with ≥1 cardiovascular risk factor (may ↑ risk of all-cause mortality, cardiovascular death, MI, stroke, and thrombosis); Current or past history of smoking (↑ risk of malignancy, cardiovascular death, MI, or stroke); Known malignancy (other than a successfully treated non-melanoma skin cancer or cervical cancer); OB: Safety not established in pregnancy; Pedi: Children <12 yr (safety and effectiveness not established); Geri: Infection risk may be ↑ in older adults.

Adverse Reactions/Side Effects

CV: ARTERIAL THROMBOSIS, CARDIOVASCULAR DEATH, DEEP VEIN THROMBOSIS, MI. **Derm:** acne, atopic dermatitis, folliculitis, rash, urticaria. **GI:** diarrhea, ↑ liver enzymes, stomatitis. **Hemat:** anemia, lymphopenia, thrombocytopenia. **MS:** ↑ creatine kinase. **Neuro:** headache, dizziness, STROKE. **Resp:** PULMONARY EMBOLISM. **Misc:** fever, HYPERSENSITIVITY REACTIONS (including anaphylaxis), INFECTION (including TB, bacterial, invasive fungal, viral, and other infections due to opportunistic pathogens), MALIGNANCY.

Interactions

Drug-Drug: May ↑ risk of adverse reactions and ↓ antibody response to **live vaccines**; avoid concurrent use. May ↑ levels and risk of toxicity of **CYP3A substrates**. May ↑ levels and risk of toxicity of **CYP1A2 substrates**. **Strong CYP3A inducers,** including **rifampin,** may ↓ levels and effectiveness; concurrent use not recommended.

Route/Dosage

PO (Adults): 50 mg once daily.

Availability

Capsules: 50 mg.

NURSING IMPLICATIONS

Assessment

• Assess scalp for hair regrowth periodically during therapy.

• Monitor for signs and symptoms of infection during and after therapy. If a patient develops a serious or opportunistic infection, interrupt ritlecitinib, promptly complete diagnostic testing appropriate for an immunocompromised patient, and start antimicrobial therapy. May resume ritlecitinib once the infection is controlled.

• Screen patient for TB before starting therapy. Do not administer ritlecitinib to patients with active TB. Start anti-TB therapy before starting ritlecitinib in patients with a new diagnosis of latent TB or previously untreated latent TB.

• May cause viral reactivation (herpes virus reactivation). If a patient develops herpes zoster, consider holding therapy until episode resolves.

• Screen for viral hepatitis before starting ritlecitinib.

• Monitor for signs and symptoms of a hypersensitivity reaction (dyspnea, feeling faint or dizzy, swelling of lips, tongue, or throat; urticaria, hives, rash) during therapy. Discontinue ritlecitinib if reaction occurs.

Lab Test Considerations

• Monitor absolute lymphocyte counts (ALC) and platelet counts before starting therapy, at 4 wk after start of therapy, then according to routine patient management. If ALC is <500/mm³, hold doses; may be restarted once ALC returns to above this value. If platelet count is <50,000/mm³, discontinue therapy.

• Monitor liver enzymes before starting and periodically during therapy. If increases in ALT or AST are observed and drug-induced liver injury is suspected, hold ritlecitinib until diagnosis is determined.

• May cause ↑ CK.

Implementation

• Verify that all vaccinations, including prophylactic herpes zoster, are current before starting therapy.

• **PO:** Administer once daily without regard to food. *DNC:* Swallow capsules whole; do not crush, split, or chew.

Patient/Family Teaching

• Instruct patient to take ritlecitinib as directed. If a dose is missed, administer dose as soon as possible, unless it is <8 hr before next dose; then skip missed dose and resume dosing at the regular scheduled time. If therapy is held, a temporary interruption for <6 wk is not expected to result in significant loss of regrown scalp hair. Advise patient to read *Medication Information* before starting ritlecitinib and with each Rx refill in case of changes.

• Advise patient to notify health care professional if signs and symptoms of infections (fever; sweating; chills; muscle aches; cough or shortness of breath; blood in phlegm; weight loss; warm, red, or painful skin or sores on the body; diarrhea or stomach pain; burning on urination or urinating more often than usual; feeling very tired), heart attack or stroke (chest discomfort lasting more than a few minutes, or that goes away and comes back; severe tightness, pain, pressure, or heaviness in chest, throat, neck, or jaw; pain or discomfort in arms, back, neck, jaw, or stomach; shortness of breath with or without chest discomfort; breaking out in a cold sweat; nausea or vomiting; light-headedness; weakness in one part or on one side of body; slurred speech), blood clots (swelling, pain or tenderness in one or both legs; sudden, unexplained chest or upper back pain; shortness of breath or difficulty breathing; changes in vision, especially in one eye only), or hypersensitivity reactions occur.

- Inform patient that ritlecitinib may increase risk of cancer (lymphoma, lung cancer). Advise patient to have periodic skin examinations and to tell health care professional if they have ever had any type of cancer.
- Instruct patient to notify health care professional of all Rx or OTC medications, vitamins, or herbal products being taken and consult health care professional before taking any new medications.
- Advise patient to avoid live attenuated vaccines during or shortly before starting therapy.
- Rep: Advise females of reproductive potential to notify health care professional if pregnancy is planned or suspected and to avoid breastfeeding during therapy and for 14 hr after last dose. If patient becomes pregnant while receiving ritlecitinib, health care professional should report pregnancy exposure the Pregnancy Exposure Registry by calling 1-877-390-2940.

Evaluation/Desired Outcomes
- Decrease in scalp hair loss.

ritonavir (ri-toe-na-veer)
Norvir
Classification
Therapeutic: antiretrovirals
Pharmacologic: protease inhibitors

Indications
HIV infection (in combination with other antiretrovirals).

Action
Inhibits the action of HIV protease and prevents the cleavage of viral polyproteins. **Therapeutic Effects:** Increased CD4 cell counts and decreased viral load with subsequent slowed progression of HIV infection and its sequelae.

Pharmacokinetics
Absorption: Appears to be well absorbed after oral administration.
Distribution: Poor CNS penetration.
Protein Binding: 98–99%.
Metabolism and Excretion: Primarily metabolized in the liver by the CYP3A4 and CYP2D6 isoen-

zymes; one metabolite has antiretroviral activity; 3.5% excreted unchanged in urine.
Half-life: 3–5 hr.

TIME/ACTION PROFILE (plasma concentrations)

ROUTE	ONSET	PEAK	DURATION
PO	rapid	4 hr*	12 hr

*Nonfasting.

Contraindications/Precautions
Contraindicated in: Hypersensitivity; Concurrent use of alfuzosin, amiodarone, apalutamide, colchicine, dihydroergotamine, dronedarone, ergotamine, flecainide, fluticasone, lomitapide, lovastatin, lurasidone, meperidine, methylergonovine, midazolam (PO), pimozide, propafenone, quinidine, ranolazine, simvastatin, sildenafil (Revatio), St. John's wort, triazolam, or voriconazole; Lactation: Breastfeeding not recommended in patients with HIV.
Use Cautiously in: Hepatic impairment or a history of hepatitis; Diabetes mellitus; Hemophilia (↑ risk of bleeding); Structural heart disease, conduction abnormalities, ischemic heart disease, or HF (↑ risk of heart block); Pedi: Children <1 mo (safety and effectiveness not established).

Adverse Reactions/Side Effects
CV: heart block, orthostatic hypotension, PR interval prolongation, syncope. **Derm:** rash, skin eruptions, STEVENS-JOHNSON SYNDROME (SJS), sweating, TOXIC EPIDERMAL NECROLYSIS (TEN), urticaria. **EENT:** pharyngitis, throat irritation. **Endo:** hyperglycemia. **F and E:** dehydration. **GI:** abdominal pain, altered taste, anorexia, diarrhea, nausea, vomiting, constipation, dyspepsia, flatulence. **GU:** renal impairment. **Metab:** fat redistribution, hyperlipidemia. **MS:** ↑ creatine kinase, myalgia. **Neuro:** abnormal thinking, weakness, dizziness, headache, malaise, paresthesia, SEIZURES, somnolence. **Resp:** bronchospasm. **Misc:** fever, HYPERSENSITIVITY REACTIONS (including anaphylaxis and angioedema), immune reconstitution syndrome.

Interactions
Drug-Drug: ↑ levels and risk of toxicity from some antiarrhythmics (**amiodarone, dronedarone, flecainide, pimozide, propafenone, quinidine**), ergot derivatives (**dihydroergotamine, ergotamine, methylergonovine**), **fluticasone (inhalation), lomitapide, lurasidone, meperidine, ranolazine, sildenafil (Revatio), alfuzosin, lovastatin, simvastatin, voriconazole, midazolam (oral)**, and **triazolam**; concurrent use contraindicated. May ↑ **colchicine** levels; concurrent use in patients with renal or hepatic impairment contraindicated; ↓ dose of colchicine in patients without renal or hepatic impairment. **Apalutamide** may ↓ levels and promote resistance; concurrent use contraindicated. ↑ levels of **maraviroc;**

↓ maraviroc dose to 150 mg twice daily. ↑ levels of **clarithromycin**; ↓ clarithromycin dose if CCr <60 mL/min. ↑ levels of **rifabutin**; ↓ rifabutin dose to 150 mg every other day or 3 times weekly. May also ↑ levels and effects of some **opioid analgesics (fentanyl, hydrocodone, oxycodone, tramadol)**; some **NSAIDs (diclofenac, ibuprofen, indomethacin)**; some **antiarrhythmics (disopyramide, lidocaine, mexiletine)**; many **antidepressants (amitriptyline, clomipramine, desipramine, imipramine, nortriptyline, nefazodone, sertraline, trazodone, fluoxetine, paroxetine, venlafaxine)**; some **antiemetics (dronabinol, ondansetron)**; some **beta blockers (metoprolol, pindolol, propranolol, timolol)**; many **calcium channel blockers (amlodipine, diltiazem, felodipine, isradipine, nicardipine, nifedipine, nimodipine, nisoldipine, verapamil)**; some **immunosuppressants (cyclosporine, tacrolimus)**; some **antipsychotics (chlorpromazine, haloperidol, perphenazine, risperidone, thioridazine)**; and also **atazanavir, darunavir, fosamprenavir, quinidine, tipranavir, bedaquiline, methamphetamine**, and **warfarin**; dosage ↓ may be necessary. May ↑ **vincristine** and **vinblastine** levels; consider holding or switching to another antiretroviral regimen that does not contain a CYP3A or P-glycoprotein inhibitor. May ↑ **dasatinib** and **nilotinib** levels; may need to ↓ doses of dasatinib and nilotinib. May ↑ **venetoclax** and **ibrutinib** levels and ↑ risk of tumor lysis syndrome; avoid concurrent use. May ↑ **abemaciclib** and **neratinib** levels and risk of toxicity; avoid concurrent use. May ↑ levels and risk of toxicity of **glecaprevir/pibrentasvir** and **sofosbuvir/velpatasvir/voxilaprevir, ombitasvir**, and **paritaprevir**; avoid concurrent use. May ↑ levels of systemic, inhaled, nasal, or ophthalmic **corticosteroids (betamethasone, budesonide, ciclesonide, dexamethasone, fluticasone, methylprednisolone, mometasone, prednisone**, or **triamcinolone**; consider alternative corticosteroid such as beclomethasone or prednisolone. ↓ levels and effects of **hormonal contraceptives, zidovudine, bupropion**, and **theophylline**; dose alteration or alternative therapy may be necessary. Levels may be ↑ by **clarithromycin** or **fluoxetine**. ↑ risk of heart block with **beta blockers, verapamil, diltiazem, digoxin**, or **atazanavir**. May ↑ concentrations of phosphodiesterase type 5 inhibitors, causing hypotension, visual changes, priapism; ↓ starting doses not to exceed 25 mg within 48 hr for **sildenafil** (Viagra), 2.5 mg every 72 hr for **vardenafil** and 10 mg every 72 hr for **tadalafil**. May ↑ risk of adverse effects with **salmeterol**; concurrent use not recommended. ↑ risk of myopathy with **atorvastatin** or **rosuvastatin**; use lowest possible dose of statin. May ↑ **bosentan** levels; initiate bosentan at 62.5 mg once daily or every other day; if patient already receiving bosentan, discontinue bosentan at least 36 hr before initiation of ritonavir and then restart bosentan at least 10 days later at 62.5 mg once daily or every other day. May ↑ **tadalafil (Adcirca)**

levels; initiate tadalafil (Adcirca) at 20 mg once daily; if patient already receiving tadalafil (Adcirca), discontinue tadalafil (Adcirca) at least 24 hr before initiation of ritonavir and then restart tadalafil (Adcirca) at least 7 days later at 20 mg once daily. May ↑ **colchicine** levels; ↓ dose of colchicine; do not administer colchicine if patients have renal or hepatic impairment. May ↑ **quetiapine** levels; ↓ quetiapine dose to ⅙ of current dose. **Dexamethasone** may ↓ levels/effects; consider use of alternative corticosteroid, such as beclomethasone or prednisolone. **Encorafenib** and **ivosidenib** may ↑ risk of QT interval prolongation; avoid concurrent use, if possible. If concurrent use necessary, ↓ dose of encorafenib and ivosidenib. Concurrent use with **elagolix** may ↑ elagolix levels and ↓ ritonavir levels; do use with elagolix 200 mg twice daily for longer than 1 mo; do not use with elagolix 150 mg once daily for longer than 6 mo. May ↑ levels of active metabolite of **fostamatinib**, which can ↑ risk of hepatotoxicity and neutropenia; may need to ↓ dose of fostamatinib.
Drug-Natural Products: St. John's wort may ↓ levels and promote resistance; concurrent use contraindicated.

Drug-Food: Food ↑ absorption.

Route/Dosage

PO (Adults): 300 mg twice daily for 2–3 days, then 400 mg twice daily for 2–3 days, then 500 mg twice daily for 2–3 days, then 600 mg twice daily as maintenance.

PO (Children >1 mo): 250 mg/m² twice daily initially; ↑ by 50 mg/m² twice daily every 2–3 days up to 400 mg/m² twice daily (if unable to get up to 400 mg/m² twice daily, consider alternative antiretroviral therapy).

Availability (generic available)

Tablets: 100 mg. **Oral powder:** 100 mg/pkt.

NURSING IMPLICATIONS

Assessment

- Assess patient for change in severity of HIV symptoms and for symptoms of opportunistic infections during therapy.
- Assess patient for rash (mild to moderate rash usually occurs in the 2nd wk of therapy and resolves within 1–2 wk of continued therapy). If rash is severe (extensive erythematous or maculopapular rash with moist desquamation or angioedema) or accompanied by systemic symptoms (serum sickness-like reaction, SJS, TEN), therapy must be discontinued immediately.

Lab Test Considerations
- Monitor viral load and CD4 counts regularly during therapy.
- Monitor for hyperglycemia, new onset diabetes mellitus, or an exacerbation of diabetes mellitus. May cause hyperglycemia.
- Monitor serum triglycerides and total cholesterol prior to and periodically during therapy. May cause

↑ serum AST, ALT, GGT, total bilirubin, CK, triglycerides, and uric acid concentrations.

Implementation

- Do not confuse ritonavir with Retrovir.
- **PO:** Administer with a meal or light snack. *DNC:* Swallow tablets whole; do not crush, break, or chew. Store tablets at room temperature.
- Oral powder may be mixed with applesauce, vanilla pudding, water, chocolate milk, or infant formula to reduce the bitter flavor. Administer within 2 hr of preparation or discard.
- May be administered via feeding tubes compatible with ethanol and propylene glycol, such as silicone and polyvinyl chloride; do not use with polyurethane feeding tubes due to potential incompatibility.
- If nausea occurs on dose of 600 mg twice daily, may titrate by 300 mg twice daily for 1 day, then 400 mg twice daily for 2 days, then 500 mg twice daily for 1 day, then 600 mg twice daily thereafter.
- Patients initiating concurrent therapy with nucleoside analogues may have less GI intolerance by initiating ritonavir for 2 wk and then adding the nucleoside analogue.

Patient/Family Teaching

- Emphasize the importance of taking ritonavir as directed, at evenly spaced times during day. Do not take more than prescribed amount, and do not stop taking without consulting health care professional. Take missed doses as soon as remembered; do not double doses.
- Instruct patient that ritonavir should not be shared with others.
- Advise patient to notify health care professional of all Rx or OTC medications, vitamins, or herbal products being taken and consult health care professional before taking any new medications, especially St. John's wort.
- Inform patient that ritonavir does not cure HIV or prevent associated or opportunistic infections. Ritonavir may reduce the risk of transmission of HIV to others through sexual contact or blood contamination. Caution patient to use a condom during sexual contact and to avoid sharing needles or donating blood to prevent spreading HIV to others. Advise patient that the long-term effects of ritonavir are unknown at this time.
- Inform patient that ritonavir may cause hyperglycemia. Advise patient to notify health care professional if increased thirst or hunger; unexplained weight loss; increased urination; fatigue; or dry, itchy skin occurs.
- Instruct patient to notify health care professional immediately if rash occurs.
- Inform patient that redistribution and accumulation of body fat may occur, causing central obesity, dorsocervical fat enlargement (buffalo hump), peripheral wasting, breast enlargement, and cushingoid appearance. The cause and long-term effects are not known.
- Rep: Advise patient taking oral contraceptives to use a nonhormonal method of birth control during ritonavir therapy. If pregnancy is suspected notify health care professional promptly. Encourage pregnant women to enroll in the Antiretroviral Pregnancy Registry by calling 1-800-258-4263. Advise female patient to avoid breastfeeding during therapy.
- Emphasize the importance of regular follow-up exams and blood counts to determine progress and monitor for side effects.

Evaluation/Desired Outcomes

- Delayed progression of AIDS and decreased opportunistic infections in patients with HIV.
- Decrease in viral load and improvement in CD4 cell counts.

ⅩⅩ **riTUXimab** (ri-tux-i-mab)
Riabni, Rituxan, ✹ Riximyo, Ruxience, Truxima
Classification
Therapeutic: antineoplastics
Pharmacologic: monoclonal antibodies

R

Indications

Riabni, Rituxan, Ruxience, and Truxima: Treatment of the following conditions: ⅩⅩ Relapsed or refractory, low-grade or follicular, CD20-positive, B-cell non-Hodgkin's lymphoma (NHL) (as monotherapy). ⅩⅩ Previously untreated follicular, CD20-positive, B-cell NHL in combination with first-line chemotherapy and, in patients achieving a complete or partial response to rituximab in combination with chemotherapy, as single-agent maintenance therapy. ⅩⅩ Non-progressing, low-grade, CD20-positive, B-cell NHL following treatment with cyclophosphamide, vincristine, and prednisone (as monotherapy). ⅩⅩ Previously untreated diffuse large B-cell, CD20-positive, NHL (in combination with CHOP or another anthracycline-based chemotherapy regimen). ⅩⅩ CD-20 positive chronic lymphocytic leukemia (CLL) (in combination with fludarabine and cyclophosphamide). Moderately to severely active rheumatoid arthritis in patients who have had an inadequate response to ≥1 TNF antagonist therapies (with methotrexate). Granulomatosis with polyangiitis (Wegener's granulomatosis) and microscopic polyangiitis (in combination with glucocorticoids). **Rituxan only:** Treatment of the following condition: Moderate to severe pemphigus vulgaris. ⅩⅩ Previously untreated, advanced stage, CD20-positive diffuse large B-cell lymphoma, Burkitt lymphoma, Burkitt-like lymphoma, or mature B-cell acute leukemia (in combination with chemotherapy).

Action
Binds to the CD20 antigen on the surface of lymphoma cells, preventing the activation process for cell cycle initiation and differentiation. **Therapeutic Effects:** Death of lymphoma cells. Prolonged progression-free survival in CLL. Reduced signs and symptoms of rheumatoid arthritis. Achievement of complete remission in granulomatosis with polyangiitis, microscopic polyangiitis, and pemphigus vulgaris.

Pharmacokinetics
Absorption: IV administration results in complete bioavailability.
Distribution: Binds specifically to CD20 binding sites on lymphoma cells.
Metabolism and Excretion: Unknown.
Half-life: 59.8–174 hr (depending on tumor burden).

TIME/ACTION PROFILE (B-cell depletion)

ROUTE	ONSET	PEAK	DURATION
IV	within 14 days	3–4 wk	6–9 mo†

†Duration of depletion after 4 wk of treatment.

Contraindications/Precautions
Contraindicated in: Hypersensitivity to murine (mouse) proteins; OB: Can pass placental barrier potentially causing fetal B-cell depletion. Use during pregnancy only if clearly needed; Lactation: Lactation.
Use Cautiously in: Pre-existing bone marrow depression; Hepatitis B virus (HBV) infection (may reactivate infection during and for several mo after treatment); Systemic lupus erythematosus (may cause fatal progressive multifocal leukoencephalopathy [PML]); HIV infection (may ↑ risk of HIV-associated lymphoma); Rep: Women of reproductive potential; Pedi: Safety and effectiveness not established for children <6 mo (mature B-cell lymphomas and B-cell acute leukemia), <2 yr (granulomatosis with polyangiitis and microscopic polyangiitis), and <18 yr (all other indications).

Adverse Reactions/Side Effects
CV: hypotension, ARRHYTHMIAS, peripheral edema. **Derm:** flushing, STEVENS-JOHNSON SYNDROME (SJS), TOXIC EPIDERMAL NECROLYSIS (TEN), urticaria. **Endo:** hyperglycemia. **F and E:** hypocalcemia. **GI:** abdominal pain, altered taste, dyspepsia, HBV REACTIVATION. **GU:** renal failure. **Hemat:** ANEMIA, NEUTROPENIA, THROMBOCYTOPENIA. **MS:** arthralgia, back pain. **Neuro:** headache, PML. **Resp:** bronchospasm, cough, dyspnea. **Misc:** HYPERSENSITIVITY REACTIONS (including anaphylaxis and angioedema), infection, INFUSION REACTIONS, TUMOR LYSIS SYNDROME.

Interactions
Drug-Drug: May ↓ antibody response to or ↑ risk of adverse reactions to **live vaccines**; avoid use during treatment; inactive vaccines should be administered ≥4 wk prior to start of therapy.

Route/Dosage

Relapsed or Refractory, Low-Grade or Follicular, CD20-Positive, B-Cell Non-Hodgkin's Lymphoma
IV (Adults): 375 mg/m² once weekly for 4 or 8 doses; may retreat with 375 mg/m² once weekly for 4 doses.

Previously Untreated Follicular, CD20–Positive, B-Cell Non-Hodgkin's Lymphoma
IV (Adults): 375 mg/m² given on Day 1 of each cycle of chemotherapy with cyclophosphamide, vincristine, and prednisone for up to 8 doses; if patients experience complete or partial response, give 375 mg/m² (as monotherapy) every 8 wk for 12 doses (initiate this maintenance therapy 8 wk after completion of rituximab + cyclophosphamide/vincristine/prednisone regimen).

Non-Progressing Low-Grade, CD20–Positive, B-Cell Non-Hodgkin's Lymphoma
IV (Adults): For patients who have not progressed following 6–8 cycles of chemotherapy with cyclophosphamide, vincristine, and prednisone, 375 mg/m² given once weekly for 4 doses given every 6 mo for up to 16 doses.

Diffuse Large B-Cell Non-Hodgkin's Lymphoma
IV (Adults): 375 mg/m² given on Day 1 of each cycle of chemotherapy for up to 8 infusions.

Previously Untreated Mature B-Cell Lymphomas and B-Cell Acute Leukemia
IV (Children ≥6 mo): 375 mg/m²/dose in combination with systemic Lymphome Malin B chemotherapy regimen; administer 2 doses during each of the two induction courses (Day –2 and Day 1), and one dose during each of the two consolidation cycles (Day 1) (6 doses total).

Chronic Lymphocytic Leukemia
IV (Adults): 375 mg/m² given on the day before initiating chemotherapy with fludarabine and cyclophosphamide, then 500 mg/m² on Day 1 of cycles 2–6 (every 28 days).

Rheumatoid Arthritis
IV (Adults): 1000 mg every 2 wk for 2 doses; subsequent courses should be administered every 24 wk (not sooner than every 16 wk).

Granulomatosis With Polyangiitis and Microscopic Polyangiitis
IV (Adults): *Induction treatment:* 375 mg/m² once weekly for 4 wk; *Follow-up treatment in patients who have achieved disease control with induction treatment:* 500 mg every 2 wk for 2 doses (should be started 16–24 wk after last rituximab induction dose; if achieved disease control with another agent, start follow-up treatment within 4 wk after last induction dose of that agent), then 500 mg every 6 mo thereafter.
IV (Children ≥2 yr): *Induction treatment:* 375 mg/m² once weekly for 4 wk; *Follow-up treatment in pa-*

tients who have achieved disease control with induction treatment: 250 mg/m² every 2 wk for 2 doses (should be started 16–24 wk after last rituximab induction dose; if achieved disease control with another agent, start follow-up treatment within 4 wk after last induction dose of that agent), then 250 mg/m² every 6 mo thereafter.

Pemphigus Vulgaris
IV (Adults): 1000 mg every 2 wk for 2 doses, then maintenance dose of 500 mg infusion at month 12 and then every 6 mo thereafter. Upon relapse, administer 1000 mg.

Availability
Solution for injection: 10 mg/mL.

NURSING IMPLICATIONS
Assessment
- Monitor patient for fever, chills/rigors, nausea, urticaria, fatigue, headache, pruritus, bronchospasm, dyspnea, sensation of tongue or throat swelling, rhinitis, vomiting, hypotension, flushing, and pain at disease sites. Infusion-related events occur frequently within 30 min–2 hr of beginning 1st infusion and may resolve with slowing or discontinuing infusion and treatment with IV saline, diphenhydramine, and acetaminophen. Patients with increased risk (females, patients with pulmonary infiltrates, chronic lymphocytic leukemia, or mantle cell leukemia) may have more severe reactions, which may be fatal. Signs of severe reactions include hypotension, angioedema, hypoxia, or bronchospasm and may require interruption of infusion. May result in pulmonary infiltrates, adult respiratory distress syndrome, MI, ventricular fibrillation, and cardiogenic shock. Monitor closely. Incidence decreases with subsequent infusions.
- Monitor patient for tumor lysis syndrome due to rapid reduction in tumor volume (acute renal failure, hyperkalemia, hypocalcemia, hyperuricemia, or hypophosphatemia) usually occurring 12–24 hr after 1st infusion. Risks are higher in patients with greater tumor burden; may be fatal. Correct electrolyte abnormalities, monitor renal function and fluid balance, and administer supportive care, including dialysis, as indicated.
- Assess for signs and symptoms of hypersensitivity reactions (hypotension, bronchospasm, angioedema) during administration. May respond to decrease in infusion rate. Premedication with diphenhydramine and acetaminophen is recommended. Treatment includes diphenhydramine, acetaminophen, bronchodilators, or IV saline as indicated. Epinephrine, antihistamines, and corticosteroids should be readily available in the event of a severe reaction. If severe reactions occur, discontinue infusion; may be resumed at 50% of the rate when symptoms have resolved completely.

- Monitor ECG during and immediately after infusion in patients with pre-existing cardiac conditions (arrhythmias, angina) or patients who have developed arrhythmias during previous infusions of rituximab. Life-threatening arrhythmias may occur.
- Assess for signs of PML (hemiparesis, apathy, confusion, cognitive deficiencies, and ataxia) periodically during therapy.
- Assess for infection during and for 1 yr after therapy. Bacterial, fungal, and new or reactivated viral infections may occur. Screen patient for HBV infection prior to therapy. Discontinue rituximab and any concomitant chemotherapy in patients who develop viral hepatitis or other serious infections, and institute appropriate treatment.
- Assess for mucocutaneous reactions periodically during therapy. May cause SJS and TEN. Discontinue therapy if severe or if accompanied with fever, general malaise, fatigue, muscle or joint aches, blisters, oral lesions, conjunctivitis, hepatitis, and/or eosinophilia.

Lab Test Considerations
- Verify negative pregnancy status before starting therapy. Monitor CBC and platelet count before starting and regularly during therapy and frequently in patients with blood dyscrasias. May cause anemia, thrombocytopenia, or neutropenia.
- Frequently causes B-cell depletion with an associated ↓ in serum immunoglobulins in a minority of patients; does not appear to cause an increased incidence of infection.
- Obtain HBsAg and anti-HBc to screen patient for HBV infection before initiating therapy. May cause reactivation of HBV up to 24 mo after therapy.

Implementation
- Do not confuse rituximab with infliximab. Do not confuse Rituxan with Rituxan Hycela.
- Transient hypotension may occur during infusion; antihypertensive medications may be held for 12 hr before infusion.
- **Rheumatoid Arthritis:** Administer 100 mg methylprednisolone IV or equivalent 30 min prior to each infusion to minimize infusion reactions.
- **Granulomatosis With Polyangiitis and Microscopic Polyangiitis:** Administer methylprednisolone 1000 mg IV per day for 1 to 3 days followed by oral prednisone 1 mg/kg/day (not to exceed 80 mg/day and tapered per clinical need) to treat severe vasculitis symptoms. Begin regimen within 14 days prior to or with the initiation of rituximab and may continue during and after the 4-wk course of rituximab treatment.
- Prophylaxis against *Pneumocystis jiroveci* pneumonia and herpes virus recommended during treatment and for up to 12 mo following treatment as appropriate for patients with CLL, and during and for at least 6 mo following last rituximab infusion for pa-

tients with granulomatosis with polyangiitis and microscopic polyangiitis.

IV Administration
- **Intermittent Infusion:** *Dilution:* Dilute with 0.9% NaCl or D5W. *Concentration:* 1–4 mg/mL. Gently invert bag to mix. Solution is clear to slightly opalescent and colorless to slightly yellow; do not administer solutions that are cloudy, discolored, or contain particulate matter. Discard unused portion remaining in vial. Solution is stable for 12 hr at room temperature and for 24 hr if refrigerated. *Rate:* Do not administer as an IV push or bolus.
- *First infusion:* Administer at an initial rate of 50 mg/hr. If hypersensitivity or infusion-related events do not occur, rate may be escalated in 50-mg/hr increments every 30 min to a maximum of 400 mg/hr.
- *Subsequent infusions:* May be administered at an initial rate of 100 mg/hr and increased by 100-mg/hr increments at 30-min intervals to a maximum of 400 mg/hr.
- For previously untreated NHL and B-cell NHL, if no Grade 3 or 4 infusion-related reactions occurred in Cycle 1, may administer via 90-min infusion using glucocorticoids. Begin at rate of 20% of dose over 30 min, with remaining 80% dose over 60 min. If tolerated, then can be used for remainder of therapy.
- **Y-Site Compatibility:** acyclovir, amifostine, amikacin, aminophylline, ampicillin, ampicillin/sulbactam, aztreonam, bleomycin, bumetanide, buprenorphine, busulfan, butorphanol, calcium gluconate, carboplatin, carmustine, cefazolin, cefotaxime, cefotetan, cefoxitin, ceftazidime, ceftriaxone, cefuroxime, chlorpromazine, cisplatin, clindamycin, cyclophosphamide, cytarabine, dactinomycin, daunorubicin hydrochloride, dexamethasone, dexrazoxane, digoxin, diphenhydramine, dobutamine, docetaxel, dopamine, doxorubicin liposomal, doxycycline, droperidol, enalaprilat, etoposide phosphate, famotidine, fentanyl, filgrastim, floxuridine, fluconazole, fludarabine, fluorouracil, ganciclovir, gemcitabine, gentamicin, granisetron, haloperidol, heparin, hydrocortisone, hydromorphone, idarubicin, ifosfamide, imipenem/cilastatin, irinotecan, leucovorin calcium, lorazepam, magnesium sulfate, mannitol, meperidine, mesna, methotrexate, methylprednisolone, metoclopramide, metronidazole, mitomycin, mitoxantrone, morphine, nalbuphine, paclitaxel, pentamidine, piperacillin/tazobactam, potassium chloride, prochlorperazine, promethazine, sargramostim, theophylline, thiotepa, tobramycin, trimethoprim/sulfamethoxazole, vinblastine, vincristine, vinorelbine, zidovudine.
- **Y-Site Incompatibility:** aldesleukin, ciprofloxacin, cyclosporine, doxorubicin hydrochloride, furosemide, levofloxacin, minocycline, ondansetron, sodium bicarbonate, topotecan, vancomycin.

Patient/Family Teaching
- Inform patient of the purpose of the medication. Advise patient to read the *Medication Guide* prior to

starting therapy and before each infusion in case of changes.
- Advise patient to report infusion-related events or symptoms of hypersensitivity reactions immediately.
- Instruct patient to notify health care professional promptly if fever; chills; cough; hoarseness; sore throat; signs of infection; lower back or side pain; painful or difficult urination; bleeding gums; bruising; petechiae; blood in stools, urine, or emesis; increased fatigue; dyspnea; orthostatic hypotension; or painful ulcers or sores on your skin, lips, or in mouth, blisters, peeling skin, rash, pustule occurs. Caution patient to avoid crowds and persons with known infections. Instruct patient to use soft toothbrush and electric razor and to avoid falls. Caution patient not to drink alcoholic beverages or take medication containing aspirin or NSAIDs; may precipitate gastric bleeding.
- Advise patient to consult health care professional prior to receiving any vaccinations.
- Rep: May cause fetal harm. Advise females of reproductive potential to use effective contraception during and for 12 mo following therapy, and to avoid breastfeeding during and for at least 6 mo after last dose. Observe newborns and infants of women taking rituximab during pregnancy for signs of infection.

Evaluation/Desired Outcomes
- Decrease in spread of malignancy.
- Reduced signs and symptoms of rheumatoid arthritis.
- Achievement of complete remission in granulomatosis with polyangiitis and microscopic polyangiitis.

rivaroxaban (ri-va-**rox**-a-ban)
Xarelto
Classification
Therapeutic: anticoagulants
Pharmacologic: antithrombotics, factor Xa inhibitors

Indications
Prevention of deep vein thrombosis (DVT) that may lead to pulmonary embolism (PE) following knee or hip replacement surgery. Prevention of venous thromboembolism (VTE) and VTE-related death during hospitalization and following hospital discharge in patients admitted for an acute medical illness who are at risk for thromboembolic complications and not at high risk of bleeding. Treatment of DVT or PE. Reduction in risk of recurrence of DVT and/or PE in patients at continued risk for recurrent DVT or PE after completion of initial treatment for at least 6 mo. Reduction in risk of stroke/systemic embolism in patients with nonvalvular atrial fibrillation (AF). Reduction in risk of major cardiovascular events (cardiovascular death, MI, and stroke) in patients with chronic coronary artery disease (in combination with aspirin). Reduction in risk of major

thrombotic vascular events (MI, ischemic stroke, acute limb ischemia, and major amputation of a vascular etiology) in patients with peripheral artery disease (PAD), including patients who have recently undergone a lower extremity revascularization procedure due to symptomatic PAD (in combination with aspirin). Treatment of VTE and the reduction in the risk of recurrent VTE in pediatric patients from birth to <18 years after ≥5 days of initial parenteral anticoagulant treatment. Thromboprophylaxis in pediatric patients ≥2 years old with congenital heart disease who have undergone the Fontan procedure.

Action

Acts as selective factor X inhibitor that blocks the active site of factor Xa, inactivating the cascade of coagulation. **Therapeutic Effects:** Treatment and prevention of thromboembolic events and major cardiovascular events.

Pharmacokinetics

Absorption: Well absorbed (80%) following oral administration; absorption occurs in the stomach and ↓ as it enters the small intestine.
Distribution: Unknown.
Metabolism and Excretion: 51% metabolized by the liver; 36% excreted unchanged in urine. Metabolites do not have anticoagulant activity.
Half-life: 5–9 hr.

TIME/ACTION PROFILE (anticoagulant effect)

ROUTE	ONSET	PEAK	DURATION
PO	unknown	2–4 hr†	24 hr

†Plasma concentrations.

Contraindications/Precautions

Contraindicated in: Hypersensitivity; Active major bleeding; Severe renal impairment (adults) (CCr <15 mL/min [DVT/PE treatment or prevention]); Prosthetic heart valves; Transcatheter aortic valve replacement (↑ risk of death and bleeding); Moderate to severe hepatic impairment or any liver pathology resulting in altered coagulation (adults); PE with hemodynamic instability or requiring thrombolysis or pulmonary embolectomy; Concurrent use of drugs that are combined P-glycoprotein (P-gp) inducers/strong CYP3A4 inducers or combined P-gp inhibitors/strong CYP3A4 inhibitors; Triple positive antiphospholipid syndrome (↑ risk of thrombosis); Lactation: Lactation; Pedi: Moderate or severe renal impairment (eGFR: <50 mL/min/1.73 m²) (children ≥1 yr); serum creatinine above 97.5th percentile (children <1 yr); Pedi: Hepatic impairment in children; Pedi: Children <6 mo and any of the following (<37 wk of gestation at birth; <10 days of oral feeding; or <2.6 kg).
Use Cautiously in: Neuroaxial spinal anesthesia or spinal puncture, especially if concurrent with an in-

dwelling epidural catheter, drugs affecting hemostasis, history of traumatic/repeated spinal puncture or spinal deformity (↑ risk of spinal hematoma); CCr ≤50 mL/min (AF) (↓ dose); Use of feeding tube (proper placement of tube must be documented to ensure absorption); OB: Use during pregnancy only if potential maternal benefit justifies potential fetal risk; Rep: Women of reproductive potential with abnormal uterine bleeding (↑ risk of uterine bleeding); Geri: Appears on Beers list. ↑ risk of bleeding in older adults. Avoid use for long-treatment of AF or VTE in favor of safer anticoagulant options.

Adverse Reactions/Side Effects

CV: syncope. **Derm:** blister, pruritus. **Hemat:** BLEEDING. **Local:** wound secretion. **MS:** extremity pain, muscle spasm.

Interactions

Drug-Drug: Concurrent use of drugs that are combined P-gp inhibitors/strong CYP3A4 inhibitors, including **ketoconazole**, **itraconazole**, **lopinavir/ritonavir**, **ritonavir**, and **conivaptan** may ↑ levels; avoid concomitant use. Concurrent use of drugs that are combined P-gp inducers/strong CYP3A4 inducers, including **carbamazepine**, **phenytoin**, or **rifampin** may ↓ levels; avoid concomitant use. Concurrent use of drugs that are combined P-gp inhibitors/moderate CYP3A4 inhibitors, including **erythromycin**, in patients with renal impairment (CCr 15–79 mL/min) may ↑ levels; avoid concomitant use. ↑ risk of bleeding with other **anticoagulants**, **aspirin**, **clopidogrel**, **ticagrelor**, **prasugrel**, **fibrinolytics**, **NSAIDs**, **SNRIs**, or **SSRIs**.
Drug-Natural Products: St. John's wort may ↓ levels; avoid concomitant use.

Route/Dosage

Prevention of Deep Vein Thrombosis Following Knee or Hip Replacement Surgery

PO (Adults): 10 mg once daily, initiated 6–10 hr postoperatively (when hemostasis is achieved) continued for 35 days after hip replacement or 12 days after knee replacement.

Prevention of Venous Thromboembolism in Acutely Ill Medical Patients at Risk for Thromboembolic Complications Not at High Risk of Bleeding

PO (Adults): 10 mg once daily while in the hospital and after hospital discharge for a total of 31–39 days.

Treatment of Deep Vein Thrombosis or Pulmonary Embolism

PO (Adults): 15 mg twice daily with food for 21 days, then 20 mg once daily with food for remainder of treatment period.

Reduction in Risk of Recurrent Deep Vein Thrombosis and/or Pulmonary Embolism in Patients at Continued Risk for Recurrent Deep Vein Thrombosis and/or Pulmonary Embolism

PO (Adults): 10 mg once daily to be initiated after ≥6 mo of standard anticoagulant treatment.

Reduction in Risk of Stroke/Systemic Embolism in Nonvalvular Atrial Fibrillation

PO (Adults): 20 mg once daily with evening meal.

Renal Impairment

PO (Adults): *CCr ≤50 mL/min:* 15 mg once daily with evening meal.

Reduction in Risk of Major Cardiovascular Events in Patients With Chronic Coronary Artery Disease or Reduction in Risk of Major Thrombotic Vascular Events in Peripheral Arterial Disease, Including Patients After Lower Extremity Revascularization Due to Symptomatic Peripheral Arterial Disease

PO (Adults): 2.5 mg twice daily.

Treatment of Venous Thromboembolism and Reduction in Risk of Recurrent Venous Thromboembolism in Pediatric Patients

PO (Children Birth–<18 yr and ≥50 kg): *Oral suspension or tablets:* 20 mg once daily with food to be initiated after ≥5 days of initial parenteral anticoagulation therapy. Continue therapy for ≥3 mo (unless <2 yr with catheter-related thrombosis).

PO (Children Birth–<18 yr and 30–49.9 kg): *Oral suspension or tablets:* 15 mg once daily with food to be initiated after ≥5 days of initial parenteral anticoagulation therapy. Continue therapy for ≥3 mo (unless <2 yr with catheter-related thrombosis).

PO (Children Birth–<18 yr and 12–29.9 kg): *Oral suspension:* 5 mg twice daily with feeding or food to be initiated after ≥5 days of initial parenteral anticoagulation therapy. Continue therapy for ≥3 mo (unless <2 yr with catheter-related thrombosis).

PO (Children Birth–<18 yr and 10–11.9 kg): *Oral suspension:* 3 mg three times daily with feeding or food to be initiated after ≥5 days of initial parenteral anticoagulation therapy. Continue therapy for ≥3 mo (unless <2 yr with catheter-related thrombosis).

PO (Children Birth–<18 yr and 9–9.9 kg): *Oral suspension:* 2.8 mg three times daily with feeding or food to be initiated after ≥5 days of initial parenteral anticoagulation therapy. Continue therapy for ≥3 mo (unless <2 yr with catheter-related thrombosis).

PO (Children Birth–<18 yr and 8–8.9 kg): *Oral suspension:* 2.4 mg three times daily with feeding or food to be initiated after ≥5 days of initial parenteral anticoagulation therapy. Continue

therapy for ≥3 mo (up to 12 mo) unless <2 yr with catheter-related VTE in which duration should be 1 mo (up to 3 mo).

PO (Children Birth–<18 yr and 7–7.9 kg): *Oral suspension:* 1.8 mg three times daily with feeding or food to be initiated after ≥5 days of initial parenteral anticoagulation therapy. Continue therapy for ≥3 mo (up to 12 mo) unless <2 yr with catheter-related VTE in which duration should be 1 mo (up to 3 mo).

PO (Children Birth–<18 yr and 5–6.9 kg): *Oral suspension:* 1.6 mg three times daily with feeding or food to be initiated after ≥5 days of initial parenteral anticoagulation therapy. Continue therapy for ≥3 mo (up to 12 mo) unless <2 yr with catheter-related VTE in which duration should be 1 mo (up to 3 mo).

PO (Children Birth–<18 yr and 4–4.9 kg): *Oral suspension:* 1.4 mg three times daily with feeding or food to be initiated after ≥5 days of initial parenteral anticoagulation therapy. Continue therapy for ≥3 mo (up to 12 mo) unless <2 yr with catheter-related VTE in which duration should be 1 mo (up to 3 mo).

PO (Children Birth–<18 yr and 3–3.9 kg): *Oral suspension:* 0.9 mg three times daily with feeding or food to be initiated after ≥5 days of initial parenteral anticoagulation therapy. Continue therapy for ≥3 mo (up to 12 mo) unless <2 yr with catheter-related VTE in which duration should be 1 mo (up to 3 mo).

PO (Children Birth–<18 yr and 2.6–2.9 kg): *Oral suspension:* 0.8 mg three times daily with feeding or food to be initiated after ≥5 days of initial parenteral anticoagulation therapy. Continue therapy for ≥3 mo (up to 12 mo) unless <2 yr with catheter-related VTE in which duration should be 1 mo (up to 3 mo).

Thromboprophylaxis in Pediatric Patients With Congenital Heart Disease After Fontan Procedure

PO (Children ≥2 yr and ≥50 kg): *Oral suspension or tablets:* 10 mg once daily.

PO (Children ≥2 yr and 30–49.9 kg): *Oral suspension:* 7.5 mg once daily.

PO (Children ≥2 yr and 20–29.9 kg): *Oral suspension:* 2.5 mg twice daily.

PO (Children ≥2 yr and 12–19.9 kg): *Oral suspension:* 2 mg twice daily.

PO (Children ≥2 yr and 10–11.9 kg): *Oral suspension:* 1.7 mg twice daily.

PO (Children ≥2 yr and 8–9.9 kg): *Oral suspension:* 1.6 mg twice daily.

PO (Children ≥2 yr and 7–7.9 kg): *Oral suspension:* 1.1 mg twice daily.

Availability

Tablets: 2.5 mg, 10 mg, 15 mg, 20 mg. **Oral suspension:** 1 mg/mL.

NURSING IMPLICATIONS
Assessment
- Assess for signs of bleeding and hemorrhage (bleeding gums; nosebleed; unusual bruising; black, tarry stools; hematuria; fall in hematocrit or BP; guaiac-positive stools); bleeding from surgical site. Notify health care professional if these occur. May use prothrombin concentrate complex, activated prothrombin complex concentrate or recombinant factor VIIa attempt to reverse life-threatening bleeding; efficacy and safety studies have not been done.
- Monitor patients with epidural catheters frequently for signs and symptoms of neurologic impairment (midline back pain, sensory and motor deficits [numbness, tingling, weakness in lower limbs], bowel and/or bladder dysfunction). Epidural catheter should not be removed earlier than 18 hr in young patients aged 20–45 yr and 26 hr in elderly patients aged 60–76 yr after last administration of rivaroxaban; next dose should be at least 6 hr after catheter removal.

Lab Test Considerations
- May cause ↑ serum AST, ALT, total bilirubin, and GGT levels.
- Monitor renal function periodically during therapy.

Toxicity and Overdose
- Antidote is andexanet alfa; effects persist for at least 24 hr after last dose. Other agents and hemodialysis do not have a significant effect. Consider using prothrombin complex concentrate or Factor VIIa.

Implementation
- *When switching from warfarin to rivaroxaban,* discontinue warfarin and start rivaroxaban as soon as INR <3.0 in adults and <2.5 in pediatric patients to avoid periods of inadequate anticoagulation. *When switching from anticoagulants other than warfarin to rivaroxaban,* for adult or pediatric patients, start rivaroxaban 0–2 hr prior to next scheduled evening dose and omit dose of other anticoagulant. For continuous heparin, discontinue heparin and administer rivaroxaban at same time. *When switching from rivaroxaban to warfarin or other anticoagulants,* for adult and pediatric patients currently taking rivaroxaban and transitioning to an anticoagulant with rapid onset, discontinue rivaroxaban and give 1st dose of the other anticoagulant (oral or parenteral) at the time that the next rivaroxaban dose was due. May discontinue rivaroxaban and begin both parenteral anticoagulant and warfarin at time of next rivaroxaban dose. Once rivaroxaban is discontinued, INR testing may be done reliably 24 hr after last dose.
- Discontinue at least 24 hr prior to surgery and other interventions. Restart as soon as hemostasis has been re-established.
- If rivaroxaban must be discontinued for other than bleeding, consider replacing with another anticoagulant; discontinuation increases risk of thrombotic events.
- To ensure a therapeutic dose is maintained, monitor child's weight and review dose regularly, especially for children below 12 kg.
- **PO:** *Prophylaxis of DVT following surgery:* Administer 1st dose 6–10 hr after surgery, once hemostasis has been established. To increase absorption, all doses should be taken with feeding or food. Do not break or split tablets.
- If unable to swallow tablet, 15 mg and 20 mg tablets may be crushed, mixed with applesauce, and administered immediately after mixing. Follow dose immediately with food.
- If administering crushed tablet via nasogastric (NG) or gastric feeding tube, check placement of tube. Rivaroxaban is absorbed from the GI tract, not the small intestine. Suspend crushed tablet in 50 mL water and administer. Follow administration of 15-mg or 20-mg tablet immediately with food.
- Crushed tablets are stable in water or applesauce for up to 4 hr.
- Oral suspension may be given through NG or gastric feeding tube. After administration, flush feeding tube with water.
- *Reduction in Risk of Stroke in Nonvalvular AF:* Administer with evening meal.
- *Treatment of DVT and/or PE:* Administer with food, at the same time each day.
- *Reduction in the Risk of Recurrence of DVT and/or PE in Patients at Continued Risk for DVT and/or PE, Prophylaxis of VTE in Acutely Ill Medical Patients at Risk for Thromboembolic Complications Not at High Risk of Bleeding, or Reduction of Risk of Major Cardiovascular Events (Cardiovascular Death, MI, and Stroke) in Chronic Coronary Artery Disease or PAD:* Administer without regard for food.

Patient/Family Teaching
- Instruct patient to take medication as directed. *Adults:* Take missed doses as soon as remembered that day. If taking 2.5 mg twice daily, take a single 2.5 mg dose at next scheduled dose. If taking 15 mg twice daily, may take two 15-mg tablets to achieve 30 mg daily dose, then return to regular schedule. If taking 10 mg, 15 mg, or 20 mg once daily, take missed dose immediately; do not double dose. *Pediatric Patients:* If taken once a day, take missed dose as soon as possible once noticed, but only on the same day. If not possible, skip dose and continue with next dose as prescribed; do not take two doses to make up for a missed dose. If rivaroxaban is taken two times a day, take missed morning dose as soon as possible once it is noticed; a missed morn-

ing dose may be taken together with the evening dose. A missed evening dose can only be taken in the same evening. If rivaroxaban is taken three times a day, if a dose is missed, patient should skip missed dose and go back to the regular dosing schedule at the usual time without compensating for missed dose. If patient vomits or spits up dose within 30 min after receiving dose, give a new dose; if >30 min after dose is taken, do not readminister dose; take next dose as scheduled. If patient vomits or spits up dose repeatedly, contact child's doctor right away. Inform health care professional of missed doses at time of checkup or lab tests. Inform patients that anticoagulant effect may persist for 2–5 days following discontinuation. Advise patient to read the *Medication Guide* before starting therapy and with each Rx refill in case of changes. Caution patients not to discontinue medication early without consulting health care professional.
* Advise patient to report any symptoms of unusual bleeding or bruising (bleeding gums; nosebleed; black, tarry stools; hematuria; excessive menstrual flow) and symptoms of spinal or epidural hematoma (tingling; numbness, especially in lower extremities; muscular weakness) to health care professional immediately.
* Instruct patient not to drink alcohol or take other Rx, OTC, or herbal products, especially those containing aspirin, NSAIDs, or St. John's wort, or to start or stop any new medications during rivaroxaban therapy without advice of health care professional.
* Rep: Advise females of reproductive potential to notify health care professional if pregnancy is planned or suspected, or if breastfeeding. Monitor for bleeding in fetus and/or neonate of women taking rivaroxaban during pregnancy. In pregnant women, rivaroxaban should be used only if potential benefit justifies the potential risk to the mother and fetus.

Evaluation/Desired Outcomes
* Prevention of blood clots and subsequent PE following knee/hip replacement surgery. Duration of treatment is 35 days for patients with hip replacement and 12 days for patients with knee replacement surgery.
* Treatment and prevention of thromboembolic events and major cardiovascular events.

---

rivastigmine (rye-va-**stig**-meen)
Exelon
Classification
Therapeutic: anti-Alzheimer's agents
Pharmacologic: cholinergics (cholinesterase inhibitors)

Indications
PO: Mild to moderate dementia associated with Alzheimer's disease. **Transdermal:** Mild, moderate, or severe dementia associated with Alzheimer's disease. Mild

to moderate dementia associated with Parkinson's disease.

Action
Enhances cholinergic function by reversible inhibition of cholinesterase. **Therapeutic Effects:** Decreased dementia (temporary) associated with Alzheimer's disease and Parkinson's disease. Enhanced cognitive ability.

Pharmacokinetics
Absorption: Well absorbed following oral administration. Transdermal patch is slowly absorbed over 8 hr.
Distribution: Widely distributed to tissues.
Metabolism and Excretion: Rapidly and extensively metabolized by the liver; metabolites are excreted by the kidneys.
Half-life: *PO:* 1.5 hr; *Transdermal:* 24 hr.

TIME/ACTION PROFILE (improvement in dementia)

ROUTE	ONSET	PEAK	DURATION
PO	within 2 wk	up to 12 wk	unknown
Transdermal	unknown	unknown	unknown

Contraindications/Precautions
Contraindicated in: Hypersensitivity to rivastigmine or other carbamates; History of application site reactions with transdermal product suggestive of allergic contact dermatitis.
Use Cautiously in: History of asthma or obstructive pulmonary disease; History of GI bleeding; Sick sinus syndrome or other supraventricular cardiac conduction abnormalities; Moderate or severe renal impairment (dose ↓ may be needed); Mild or moderate hepatic impairment (dose ↓ may be needed); Patients weighing <50 kg (dose ↓ may be needed); OB: Safety not established in pregnancy; Lactation: Use during breastfeeding only if potential maternal benefit justifies potential risk to infant; Pedi: Safety and effectiveness not established in children.

Adverse Reactions/Side Effects
CV: edema, HF, hypotension. **Derm:** allergic dermatitis. **GI:** anorexia, diarrhea, nausea, vomiting, ↓ weight, abdominal pain, dyspepsia, flatulence. **Local:** application reactions (for transdermal patch only). **Neuro:** weakness, dizziness, drowsiness, headache, tremor. **Misc:** fever.

Interactions
Drug-Drug: Nicotine may ↓ levels and effectiveness.

Route/Dosage
PO (Adults): 1.5 mg twice daily initially; after at least 2 wk, dose may be ↑ to 3 mg twice daily. Further increments may be made at 2-wk intervals up to 6 mg twice daily.
Transdermal (Adults): *Initial Dose:* 4.6 mg/24-hr transdermal patch initially; ↑ to 9.5 mg/24-hr transder-

mal patch after at least 4 wk; may ↑ to 13.3 mg/24-hr transdermal patch if needed (is recommended effective dose for patients with severe Alzheimer's disease).

Hepatic Impairment
Transdermal (Adults): *Mild to moderate hepatic impairment:* Do not exceed dose of 4.6 mg/24 hr.

Availability (generic available)
Capsules: 1.5 mg, 3 mg, 4.5 mg, 6 mg. **Transdermal patch:** 4.6 mg/24 hr, 9.5 mg/24 hr, 13.3 mg/24 hr.

NURSING IMPLICATIONS
Assessment
- Assess cognitive function (memory, attention, reasoning, language, ability to perform simple tasks) periodically throughout therapy.
- Monitor patient for nausea, vomiting, anorexia, and weight loss. Notify health care professional if these side effects occur.
- Monitor for hypersensitivity skin reactions; may occur after oral or transdermal administration. If allergic contact dermatitis is suspected after transdermal use, may switch to oral rivastigmine after negative allergy testing. If disseminated hypersensitivity reaction of the skin occurs, discontinue therapy.

Implementation
- Patients switching from oral doses of <6 mg to transdermal doses should use 4.6 mg/24 hr patch. Patients taking oral doses of 6–12 mg may be converted directly to 9.5 mg/24 hr patch. Apply patch on the day following the last oral dose.
- **PO:** Administer in the morning and evening with food.
- **Transdermal:** Apply patch to clean, dry, hairless area that will not be rubbed by tight clothing. Upper or lower back is recommended, may also use upper arm or chest. Do not apply to red, irritated, or cut skin. Rotate sites to prevent irritation, do not use same site within 14 days. Remove adhesive liner and apply by pressing patch firmly until edges stick well. May be worn during bathing and hot weather. Each 24 hr, remove old patch and discard by folding in half and apply new patch to a new area.

Patient/Family Teaching
- **PO:** Emphasize the importance of taking rivastigmine at regular intervals as directed.
- Caution patient and caregiver that rivastigmine may cause dizziness. Caution patient to avoid driving or other activities requiring alertness until response to medication is known.
- Advise patient and caregiver to notify health care professional if nausea, vomiting, anorexia, or weight loss occur. If adverse effects become intolerable during treatment with *transdermal patch*, instruct patient to discontinue patches for several

days and then restart at same or next lower dose level. If treatment is interrupted for more than several days, lowest dose level should be used when restarting and titrate according to Route and Dosage section.
- Advise patient and caregiver to notify health care professional of medication regimen prior to treatment or surgery.
- Inform patient and caregiver that improvement in cognitive functioning may take wk to mo and that the degenerative process is not reversed.
- Rep: Advise females of reproductive potential to notify health care professional if pregnancy is planned or suspected or if breastfeeding.
- **Transdermal:** Instruct patient and caregiver on the correct application, rotation, and discarding of patch. Patch should be folded in half and discarded out of reach of children and pets; medication remains in discarded patch. Replace missed doses immediately and apply next patch at usual time. Advise patient and caregiver to avoid contact with eyes and to wash hands after applying patch. Avoid exposure to heat sources (excessive sunlight, saunas, heating pads) for long periods.
- Advise patient and caregiver to notify health care professional if skin reactions occur.
- Advise patient referred for MRI test to discuss patch with referring health care professional and MRI facility to determine if removal of patch is necessary prior to test and for directions for replacing patch.

Evaluation/Desired Outcomes
- Temporary improvement in cognitive function (memory, attention, reasoning, language, ability to perform simple tasks) in patients with Alzheimer's disease.
- Improvement in cognitive function and overall functioning in patients with Parkinson's disease.

---

rizatriptan (riz-a-**trip**-tan)
Maxalt, Maxalt-MLT, RizaFilm
Classification
Therapeutic: vascular headache suppressants
Pharmacologic: 5-HT₁ agonists

Indications
Acute treatment of migraine with or without aura.

Action
Acts as an agonist at specific 5-HT₁ receptor sites in intracranial blood vessels and sensory trigeminal nerves. **Therapeutic Effects:** Cranial vessel vasoconstriction with associated decrease in release of neuropeptides and resultant decrease in migraine headache.

R

Pharmacokinetics

Absorption: Completely absorbed after oral administration, but first-pass metabolism results in 45% bioavailability.

Distribution: Unknown.

Metabolism and Excretion: Primarily metabolized by monoamine oxidase-A (MAO-A); minor conversion to an active compound; 14% excreted unchanged in urine.

Half-life: 2–3 hr.

TIME/ACTION PROFILE (plasma concentrations)

ROUTE	ONSET	PEAK	DURATION
PO	30 min	1–1.5 hr	unknown

Contraindications/Precautions

Contraindicated in: Hypersensitivity; Ischemic or vasospastic cardiovascular, cerebrovascular, or peripheral vascular syndromes; History of significant cardiovascular disease; Uncontrolled hypertension; Should not be used within 24 hr of other 5-HT$_1$ agonists or ergot-type compounds (dihydroergotamine); Basilar or hemiplegic migraine; Concurrent MAO-A inhibitor therapy or within 2 wk of discontinuing MAO-A inhibitor therapy; Phenylketonuria (orally disintegrating tablet [ODT] contains aspartame).

Use Cautiously in: Severe renal impairment, especially in patients on dialysis; Moderate hepatic impairment; OB: Safety not established in pregnancy; Lactation: Safety not established in breastfeeding; Pedi: Safety and effectiveness not established in children <12 yr (oral films) or <6 yr (tablets and ODTs).

Exercise Extreme Caution in: Cardiovascular risk factors (hypertension, hypercholesterolemia, cigarette smoking, obesity, diabetes, strong family history, menopausal women or men >40 yr); use only if cardiovascular status has been evaluated and determined to be safe and 1st dose is administered under supervision.

Adverse Reactions/Side Effects

CV: chest pain, CORONARY ARTERY VASOSPASM, MI, myocardial ischemia, VENTRICULAR ARRHYTHMIAS. **Derm:** TOXIC EPIDERMAL NECROLYSIS. **GI:** dry mouth, nausea. **Neuro:** dizziness, drowsiness, weakness. **Misc:** HYPERSENSITIVITY REACTIONS (including angioedema).

Interactions

Drug-Drug: Concurrent use with **MAO-A inhibitors** ↑ levels and adverse reactions (concurrent use or use within 2 wk of MAO inhibitor is contraindicated). Concurrent use with other **5-HT agonists** or **ergot-type compounds (dihydroergotamine)** may result in ↑ vasoactive properties (avoid use within 24 hr of each other). **Propranolol** ↑ levels and risk of adverse reactions (↓ dose of rizatriptan; rizatriptan not recommended in children <40 kg). ↑ risk of serotonin syndrome when used with **SSRIs** or **SNRIs**.

Drug-Natural Products: ↑ risk of serotonergic side effects including serotonin syndrome with **St. John's wort** and **SAMe**.

Route/Dosage

PO (Adults): *Tablet or ODT:* 5–10 mg (use 5-mg dose in patients receiving propranolol); may be repeated in 2 hr; not to exceed 3 doses/24 hr. *Oral film:* 10 mg administered on the tongue; may be repeated in 2 hr; not to exceed 3 doses/24 hr.

PO (Children 6–17 yr and ≥40 kg): *Tablet or ODT:* 10 mg single dose (use 5-mg dose in patients receiving propranolol).

PO (Children 6–17 yr and <40 kg): *Tablet or ODT:* 5 mg single dose (do NOT use in patients receiving propranolol).

PO (Children 12–17 yr and ≥40 kg): *Oral film:* 10 mg administered on the tongue as single dose.

Availability (generic available)

Tablets: 5 mg, 10 mg. **ODTs (Maxalt-MLT) (peppermint flavor):** 5 mg, 10 mg. **Oral films:** 10 mg.

NURSING IMPLICATIONS

Assessment

- Assess pain location, character, intensity, and duration and associated symptoms (photophobia, phonophobia, nausea, vomiting) during migraine attack.
- Assess for serotonin syndrome (mental changes [agitation, hallucinations, coma], autonomic instability [tachycardia, labile BP, hyperthermia], neuromuscular aberrations [hyper reflexia, incoordination], and/or GI symptoms [nausea, vomiting, diarrhea]), especially in patients taking other serotonergic drugs (SSRIs, SNRIs).
- Assess cardiovascular status in triptan-naive patients with multiple cardiovascular risk factors (increased age, diabetes, hypertension, smoking, obesity, strong family history of coronary artery disease) before receiving rizatriptan. For patients with multiple cardiovascular risk factors who have a negative cardiovascular evaluation, consider administering the 1st dose of rizatriptan in a medically supervised setting and performing an ECG immediately following administration. Periodic cardiovascular evaluation in intermittent long-term users of rizatriptan may be used.

Implementation

- If migraine headache returns, a second dose may be administered 2 hr after first dose. Maximum daily dose should not exceed 30 mg in any 24-hr period.
- PO: *DNC:* Tablets should be swallowed whole with liquid.
- ODTs should be left in the package until use. Remove from the blister pouch. Do not push tablet through the blister; peel open the blister pack with dry hands and place tablet on tongue. Tablet will dissolve rapidly and be swallowed with saliva. No liquid is needed to take the ODT.

- Place the oral film on tongue, where it will disintegrate within approximately 2 min and can be swallowed with saliva. No liquid is needed.

Patient/Family Teaching

- Inform patient that rizatriptan should be used only during a migraine attack. It is meant to be used for relief of migraine attacks but not to prevent or reduce the number of attacks.
- Instruct patient to administer rizatriptan as soon as symptoms of a migraine attack appear, but it may be administered at any time during an attack. If migraine symptoms return, a 2nd dose may be used. Allow at least 2 hr between doses, and do not use more than 30 mg in any 24-hr period.
- If patient has no response to first dose of rizatriptan, reconsider diagnosis of migraine before rizatriptan is administered to treat any subsequent attacks.
- Caution patient not to take rizatriptan within 24 hr of other vascular headache suppressants.
- Advise patient that lying down in a darkened room after rizatriptan administration may further help relieve headache.
- Advise patient that overuse (use more than 10 days/mo) may lead to exacerbation of headache (migraine-like daily headaches, or as a marked increase in frequency of migraine attacks). May require gradual withdrawal of rizatriptan and treatment of symptoms (transient worsening of headache).
- Advise patient to notify health care professional before next dose of rizatriptan if pain or tightness in the chest occurs during use. If pain is severe or does not subside, notify health care professional immediately. If feelings of tingling, heat, flushing, heaviness, pressure, drowsiness, dizziness, tiredness, or sickness develop, discuss with health care professional at next visit.
- May cause dizziness or drowsiness. Caution patient to avoid driving or other activities requiring alertness until response to medication is known.
- Caution patient to avoid alcohol, which aggravates headaches, during rizatriptan use.
- Advise patient to notify health care professional of all Rx or OTC medications, vitamins, or herbal products being taken and to consult with health care professional before taking other medications.
- Advise patient to notify health care professional immediately if signs or symptoms of serotonin syndrome occur.
- Rep: Advise females of reproductive potential to notify health care professional if pregnancy is planned or suspected or if breastfeeding.

Evaluation/Desired Outcomes

- Relief of migraine attack.

rolapitant (rol-ap-i-tant)
Varubi
Classification
Therapeutic: antiemetics
Pharmacologic: neurokinin antagonists

Indications
To prevent delayed nausea and vomiting associated with initial/repeat courses of emetogenic cancer chemotherapy (in combination with dexamethasone and a 5-HT$_3$ antagonist).

Action
Acts as a selective antagonist at substance P/neurokinin 1 (NK$_1$) receptors in the brain. **Therapeutic Effects:** Decreased nausea and vomiting associated with chemotherapy. Augments the antiemetic effects of dexamethasone and 5-HT$_3$ antagonists.

Pharmacokinetics
Absorption: Well absorbed following oral administration.
Distribution: Extensively distributed to tissues.
Protein Binding: 99.8%.
Metabolism and Excretion: Mostly metabolized, primarily by the CYP3A4 isoenzyme; one metabolite, C4−pyrrolidine-hydroxylated rolapitant (M19), has antiemetic activity. Excretion is mainly via hepatic/biliary elimination. 14% excreted in urine (8% as metabolites), 73% in feces (38% as unchanged drug).
Half-life: *Rolapitant:* 7 days; *M19:* 7 days.

TIME/ACTION PROFILE (plasma concentrations)

ROUTE	ONSET	PEAK	DURATION
PO	within 30 min	4 hr	unknown

Contraindications/Precautions
Contraindicated in: Concurrent use of CYP2D6 substrates with a narrow therapeutic index.
Use Cautiously in: Concurrent use of other CYP2D6 substrates; Severe hepatic impairment (avoid if possible; if unavoidable, monitor carefully); OB: Safety not established in pregnancy; Lactation: Safety not established in breastfeeding; Pedi: Safety and effectiveness not established in children; Geri: Older adults may be more sensitive to drug effects.

Adverse Reactions/Side Effects
CV: dizziness. **GI:** ↓ appetite, abdominal pain, dyspepsia, hiccups, stomatitis. **GU:** ↓ fertility (females). **Hemat:** anemia, neutropenia. **Misc:** infusion reactions.

Interactions
Drug-Drug: ↑ levels and risk of serious cardiac toxicity with **CYP2D6 substrates** with a narrow therapeutic index, including **thioridazine** and **pimozide**; concur-

rent use contraindicated. May ↑ levels and risk of toxicity of other **CYP2D6 substrates** for an extended period of time (≥28 days). May ↑ levels and risk of toxicity of **breast cancer resistance protein (BCRP) substrates**, including **irinotecan, methotrexate, rosuvastatin**, and **topotecan**; dose reduction may be necessary. May ↑ levels and risk of toxicity of **P-glycoprotein (P-gp) substrates**, including **digoxin**; avoid concurrent use with P-gp substrates with a narrow therapeutic index. **Strong CYP3A4 inducers**, including **rifampin**, may ↓ levels and effectiveness; avoid concurrent use.

Route/Dosage
PO (Adults): 180 mg administered within 2 hr prior to start of chemotherapy.

Availability
Tablets: 90 mg.

NURSING IMPLICATIONS
Assessment
- Assess nausea, vomiting, appetite, bowel sounds, and abdominal pain prior to and following administration.

Lab Test Considerations
- May cause ↓ WBC.

Implementation
- **PO:** Administer 2 hr before starting chemotherapy without regard to food. Due to long action, administer no more frequently than once every 14 days. Given with dexamethasone and a 5-HT₃ antagonist.

Patient/Family Teaching
- Instruct patient to take rolapitant as directed. Direct patient to read the *Patient Package Insert* before starting therapy and each time Rx renewed in case of changes.
- Instruct patient to notify health care professional of all Rx or OTC medications, vitamins, or herbal products being taken and consult health care professional before taking any new medications.
- Advise patient and family to use general measures to decrease nausea (begin with sips of liquids and small, nongreasy meals; provide oral hygiene; remove noxious stimuli from environment).
- Rep: Advise females of reproductive potential to notify health care professional if pregnancy is planned or suspected, or if breastfeeding. May impair fertility in females; impairment is reversible.

Evaluation/Desired Outcomes
- Decreased delayed nausea and vomiting associated with emetogenic chemotherapy.

romosozumab
(roe-moe-**soz**-ue-mab)
Evenity
Classification
Therapeutic: bone resorption inhibitors
Pharmacologic: sclerostin inhibitors

Indications
Treatment of osteoporosis in postmenopausal women who are at high risk for a fracture or have failed or are intolerant to other medications used to treat osteoporosis.

Action
Inhibits sclerostin, which leads to increased bone formation and decreased bone resorption. **Therapeutic Effects:** Reduction in vertebral and non-vertebral fractures and improvement in bone mineral density.

Pharmacokinetics
Absorption: Unknown.
Distribution: Minimally distributed to tissues.
Metabolism and Excretion: Degraded into small peptides and amino acids; elimination pathway unknown.
Half-life: 12.8 days.

TIME/ACTION PROFILE (plasma concentrations)

ROUTE	ONSET	PEAK	DURATION
SUBQ	unknown	5 days	4 wk

Contraindications/Precautions
Contraindicated in: Hypersensitivity; Hypocalcemia (correct before administration); MI or stroke in past year (↑ risk of cardiovascular death, MI, or stroke).
Use Cautiously in: Patients with risk factors for cardiovascular disease; Severe renal impairment (CCr 15–29 mL/min), or receiving dialysis (monitor serum calcium concentrations and calcium and vitamin D intake); Invasive dental procedures, cancer, receiving chemotherapy, corticosteroids, or angiogenesis inhibitors, poor oral hygiene, diabetes, gingival infections, periodontal disease, dental disease, anemia, coagulopathy, infection, or poorly fitting dentures (↑ risk of jaw osteonecrosis); Geri: Older adults may be more sensitive to drug effects.

Adverse Reactions/Side Effects
CV: CARDIOVASCULAR DEATH, MI, peripheral edema. **F and E:** hypocalcemia. **Local:** injection site reactions. **MS:** arthralgia, atypical femoral fracture, muscle spasm, osteonecrosis of the jaw. **Neuro:** headache, insomnia, paresthesia, STROKE. **Misc:** HYPERSENSITIVITY REACTIONS (including anaphylaxis and angioedema).

Interactions
Drug-Drug: None reported.

Route/Dosage
SUBQ (Adults): 210 mg once monthly for 12 mo.

Availability
Solution for injection (prefilled syringes): 105 mg/1.17 mL.

NURSING IMPLICATIONS
Assessment
- Assess patients for low bone mass before and periodically during therapy.
- Assess cardiac history. Avoid administration in patients who have had an MI or stroke within the preceding year. Discontinue romosozumab if MI or stroke occurs.
- Monitor for signs and symptoms of hypocalcemia (spasms, twitches, or cramps in muscles; numbness or tingling in fingers, toes, or around mouth) periodically during therapy.
- Perform a routine oral exam prior to initiation of therapy. Dental exam with appropriate preventative dentistry should be considered prior to therapy. Patients with history of tooth extraction, poor oral hygiene, gingival infections, diabetes, cancer, receiving radiation, anemia, coagulopathy, or use of a dental appliance or those taking immunosuppressive therapy, angiogenesis inhibitors, or systemic corticosteroids are at greater risk for osteonecrosis of the jaw.

Implementation
- Duration of therapy is limited to 1 yr due to ↓ effectiveness. If continued therapy is needed, continue therapy with an anti-resorptive agent.
- Supplement patient with calcium and vitamin D during therapy.
- If a dose is missed, administer as soon as possible and reschedule monthly from date of last dose.
- **SUBQ:** Administer by a health care professional. Allow romosozumab to warm to room temperature for at least 30 min; do not warm in any other way. Solution is clear to opalescent, colorless to light yellow; do not administer solutions that are cloudy, discolored, or contain particulate matter. Do not shake. Dose requires 2 injections in separate sites; thigh, abdomen, outer area of upper arm. Do not inject into areas where the skin is tender, bruised, red, or hard. Avoid injecting into areas with scars or stretch marks. Refrigerate solution in original carton to protect from light; do not freeze. Stable for 30 days at room temperature.

Patient/Family Teaching
- Explain purpose of romosozumab to patient.
- Advise patient to notify health care professional immediately if signs and symptoms of MI or hypersensitivity occur.
- Advise patient to eat a balanced diet and consult health care professional about the need for supplemental calcium and vitamin D.
- Encourage patient to participate in regular exercise and to modify behaviors that increase the risk of osteoporosis (stop smoking, reduce alcohol consumption).

- Advise patient to notify health care professional if signs and symptoms if osteonecrosis of the jaw (pain, numbness, swelling of or drainage from the jaw, mouth, or teeth) or hypocalcemia (spasms, twitches, or cramps in muscles; numbness or tingling in fingers, toes, or around mouth) or thigh, hip, or groin pain occur.
- Advise parents to notify health care professional of all Rx or OTC medications, vitamins, or herbal products being taken and to consult with health care professional before taking other medications.

Evaluation/Desired Outcomes
- Reduction in vertebral and non-vertebral fractures and improvement in bone mineral density.

---

rOPINIRole (roe-pin-i-role)
~~Requip, Requip XL~~
Classification
Therapeutic: antiparkinson agents
Pharmacologic: dopamine agonists

Indications
Parkinson's disease. Restless leg syndrome (immediate-release only).

Action
Stimulates dopamine receptors in the brain. **Therapeutic Effects:** Decreased tremor and rigidity in Parkinson's disease. Decreased leg restlessness.

Pharmacokinetics
Absorption: 55% absorbed following oral administration.
Distribution: Widely distributed to tissues.
Metabolism and Excretion: Extensively metabolized by the liver primarily by the CYP1A2 isoenzyme; <10% excreted unchanged in urine.
Half-life: 6 hr.

TIME/ACTION PROFILE

ROUTE	ONSET	PEAK	DURATION
PO	unknown	unknown	8 hr

Contraindications/Precautions
Contraindicated in: Hypersensitivity; Major psychotic disorder; Impulsive control/compulsive behaviors.
Use Cautiously in: Hepatic impairment (slower titration may be required); Severe cardiovascular disease; OB: Safety not established in pregnancy; Lactation: Use while breastfeeding only if potential maternal benefit justifies potential risk to infant; may inhibit lactation; Pedi: Safety and effectiveness not established in children; Geri: ↑ risk of hallucinations in older adults.

R

Adverse Reactions/Side Effects

CV: <u>orthostatic hypotension</u>, hypertension, peripheral edema, syncope. **Derm:** sweating. **EENT:** abnormal vision. **GI:** constipation, dry mouth, dyspepsia, nausea, vomiting. **Neuro:** <u>dizziness</u>, <u>syncope</u>, aggression, agitation, confusion, delirium, delusions, disorientation, drowsiness, dyskinesia, fatigue, hallucinations, headache, impulse control disorders (gambling, sexual, uncontrolled spending, binge/compulsive eating), insomnia, paranoid ideation, psychosis, SLEEP ATTACKS, somnolence, weakness.

Interactions

Drug-Drug: **CYP1A2 inhibitors**, including **ciprofloxacin** may ↑ levels and risk of toxicity. **CYP1A2 inducers**, including **cigarette smoke** may ↓ levels and effectiveness. **Estrogens** may ↑ levels and risk of toxicity. **Phenothiazines, butyrophenones, thioxanthenes**, or **metoclopramide** may ↓ effectiveness. May ↑ effects of **levodopa**; consider ↓ dose of levodopa.

Route/Dosage

Parkinson's Disease

PO (Adults): *Immediate-release:* 0.25 mg 3 times daily for 1 wk, then 0.5 mg 3 times daily for 1 wk, then 0.75 mg 3 times daily for 1 wk, then 1 mg 3 times daily for 1 wk; then may ↑ by 1.5 mg/day every wk up to 9 mg/day; then may ↑ by up to 3 mg/day every wk up to 24 mg/day; *Extended-release:* 2 mg once daily for 1–2 wk; may ↑ by 2 mg/day; do not exceed 8 mg/day in patients with advanced Parkinson's disease or 12 mg/day in patients with early Parkinson's disease.

Renal Impairment

PO (Adults): *Hemodialysis:* Immediate release: 0.25 mg 3 times daily; may ↑ dose as needed based on response and tolerability (not to exceed 18 mg/day).

Restless Leg Syndrome

PO (Adults): *Immediate-release:* 0.25 mg once daily initially, 1–3 hr before bedtime. After 2 days, ↑ to 0.5 mg once daily and to 1 mg once daily by the end of first wk of dosing, then ↑ by 0.5 mg weekly, up to 4 mg/day as needed/tolerated.

Renal Impairment

PO (Adults): *Hemodialysis:* Immediate release 0.25 mg once daily; may ↑ dose as needed based on response and tolerability (not to exceed 3 mg/day).

Availability (generic available)

Immediate-release tablets: 0.25 mg, 0.5 mg, 1 mg, 2 mg, 3 mg, 4 mg, 5 mg. **Extended-release tablets:** 2 mg, 4 mg, 6 mg, 8 mg, 12 mg.

NURSING IMPLICATIONS

Assessment

- Assess BP periodically during therapy.
- Assess patient for drowsiness and sleep attacks. Drowsiness is a common side effect of ropinirole, but sleep attacks or episodes of falling asleep during activities that require active participation may occur without warning. Assess patient for concomitant medications that have sedating effects or may increase serum ropinirole levels (see Interactions). May require discontinuation of therapy.
- Assess patient for signs and symptoms of psychotic-like behavior (confusion, paranoid ideation, delusions, hallucinations, psychotic-like behavior, disorientation, aggressive behavior, agitation, delirium, hallucinations). Risk of symptoms increases with age. Notify health care professional if these occur.
- **Parkinson's Disease:** Assess patient for signs and symptoms of Parkinson's disease (tremor, muscle weakness and rigidity, ataxic gait) prior to and during therapy.
- **Restless Leg Syndrome:** Assess sleep patterns and frequency of restless leg disturbances.
- Monitor for *augmentation* (earlier onset of symptoms in the evening or afternoon), increase in symptoms, and spread of symptoms to involve other extremities and *rebound* (new onset of symptoms in the early morning hr). If symptoms occur, consider dose adjustment or discontinuation of therapy.

Lab Test Considerations

- May cause ↑ BUN.

Implementation

- Do not confuse ropinirole with Risperdal or risperidone.
- **PO:** May be administered with or without food. Administration with food may decrease nausea. *DNC:* Swallow extended-release tablets whole; do not break, crush, or chew.
- Taper or discontinuation may cause withdrawal symptoms (apathy, anxiety, depression, fatigue, insomnia, sweating, pain); symptoms do not respond to levodopa. Trial readministration of ropinirole at lowest dose may be considered.

Patient/Family Teaching

- Instruct patient to take medication exactly as directed. Missed doses should be taken as soon as possible, but not if almost time for next dose. Do not double doses. Do not stop abruptly; may cause hyperpyrexia and confusion. Taper doses gradually over 7 days.
- Caution patient to change positions slowly to minimize orthostatic hypotension.
- May cause drowsiness and unexpected episodes of falling asleep. Caution patient to avoid driving or other activities requiring alertness until response to medication is known. Advise patient to notify health care professional if episodes of falling asleep occur.
- Advise patient to avoid alcohol and other CNS depressants concurrently with ropinirole.
- Advise patient that increasing fluids, sugarless gum or candy, ice, or saliva substitutes may help minimize dry mouth. Consult health care professional if dry mouth continues for >2 wk.
- Advise patient to have periodic skin exams to check for lesions that may be melanoma.

- Advise patient to notify health care professional if new or increased gambling, sexual, or other impulse control disorders or psychotic-like behaviors occur.
- Rep: Advise females of reproductive potential to notify health care professional if pregnancy is planned or suspected, or if breastfeeding. Advise patients that ropinirole could inhibit lactation because ropinirole inhibits prolactin secretion.

Evaluation/Desired Outcomes
- Decreased tremor and rigidity in Parkinson's disease.
- Decrease in restless legs and improved sleep.

---

rosuvastatin, See HMG-CoA REDUCTASE INHIBITORS (statins).

░ rucaparib (roo-kap-a-rib)
Rubraca
Classification
Therapeutic: antineoplastics
Pharmacologic: enzyme inhibitors

Indications
Maintenance treatment of recurrent epithelial ovarian, fallopian tube, or primary peritoneal cancer in patients who have experienced a complete or partial response to platinum-based chemotherapy. ░ Deleterious *BRCA* mutation-associated metastatic, castration-resistant prostate cancer in patients who have been treated with androgen-receptor directed therapy and a taxane-based chemotherapy regimen.

Action
Acts as a poly (ADP-ribose) polymerase (PARP) inhibitor, thereby disrupting DNA transcription, cell cycle regulation and DNA repair. **Therapeutic Effects:** Decreased growth and spread of epithelial ovarian, fallopian tube, primary peritoneal, or prostate cancer.

Pharmacokinetics
Absorption: 30–45% absorbed following oral administration; bioavailability increased but delayed with high-fat meal.
Distribution: Extensively distributed to tissues.
Metabolism and Excretion: Extensively metabolized primarily by the CYP2D6 isoenzyme and to a lesser extent by the CYP1A2 and CYP3A4 isoenzymes; information regarding mode of elimination unknown.
Half-life: 17–19 hr.

TIME/ACTION PROFILE (plasma concentrations)

ROUTE	ONSET	PEAK	DURATION
PO	unknown	2 hr	unknown

Contraindications/Precautions
Contraindicated in: OB: Pregnancy; Lactation: Lactation.
Use Cautiously in: Severe hepatic impairment; Severe renal impairment or dialysis; Rep: Women of reproductive potential and men with female partners of reproductive potential; Pedi: Safety and effectiveness not established in children.

Adverse Reactions/Side Effects
Derm: <u>photosensitivity</u>, <u>rash</u>, palmar-plantar erythrodysaesthesia syndrome, pruritus. **Endo:** hypercholesterolemia. **GI:** ↓ appetite, ↑ liver function tests, <u>abdominal pain</u>, constipation, <u>diarrhea</u>, <u>nausea</u>, <u>vomiting</u>. **GU:** ↑ serum creatinine. **Hemat:** anemia, lymphocytopenia, neutropenia, thrombocytopenia, MYELODYSPLASTIC SYNDROME/ACUTE MYELOID LEUKEMIA. **Neuro:** <u>dizziness</u>, dysgeusia, <u>fatigue</u>. **Resp:** dyspnea. **Misc:** <u>fever</u>.

Interactions
Drug-Drug: May ↑ levels and toxicity of **CYP1A2 substrates**, **CYP2C9 substrates**, **CYP2C19 substrates**, and **CYP3A substrates**; if concurrent administration unavoidable, consider ↓ dose of CYP1A2, CYP2C9, CYP2C19, or CYP3A substrate; if concurrent administration with warfarin unavoidable, monitor INR more frequently.

Route/Dosage
PO (Adults): 600 mg twice daily until disease progression or unacceptable toxicity.

Availability
Tablets: 200 mg, 250 mg, 300 mg.

NURSING IMPLICATIONS
Assessment
- Monitor for signs and symptoms of myelodysplastic syndrome/acute myeloid leukemia during therapy. May require discontinuation of therapy.

Lab Test Considerations
- Select patients for maintenance treatment of recurrent ovarian cancer or for maintenance treatment of recurrent ovarian cancer based on the presence of a deleterious *BRCA* mutation (germline and/or somatic). For patient selection for *BRCA*-mutated ovarian cancer, information on the FDA-approved test for the detection of a tumor *BRCA* mutation in patients with ovarian cancer is available at: http://www.fda.gov/CompanionDiagnostics.Verify negative pregnancy test prior to starting therapy.Monitor CBC prior to and monthly during therapy. Do not start rucaparib until hematologic toxicity from previous chemotherapy has recovered to ≤Grade 1. For prolonged hematologic toxicities, interrupt rucaparib and monitor CBC weekly until recovery. If levels have not recovered to ≤Grade 1 after 4 wk, refer patient to hematologist for further investigations, including

bone marrow analysis and blood sample for cytogenetics. If myelodysplastic syndrome/acute myeloid leukemia is confirmed, discontinue rucaparib.
- May cause anemia, thrombocytopenia, lymphocytopenia, and neutropenia.
- May cause ↑ serum creatinine, ALT, AST, and cholesterol.

Implementation
- Patients receiving rucaparib for metastatic, castration-resistant prostate cancer should also receive a gonadotropin-releasing hormone analog concurrently or should have had bilateral orchiectomy.
- **Recommended Dose Modifications for Adverse Reactions:** *Starting dose:* 600 mg twice daily. *1st dose reduction:* 500 mg twice daily. *2nd dose reduction:* 400 mg twice daily. *3rd dose reduction:* 300 mg twice daily.
- **PO:** Administer 2 tablets twice daily approximately 12 hr apart, without regard to food.

Patient/Family Teaching
- Instruct patient to take rucaparib as directed. If a dose is missed, omit and take next dose at scheduled time. Do not replace vomited doses.
- Advise patient to notify health care professional if signs and symptoms of myelodysplastic syndrome/ acute myeloid leukemia (weakness, feeling tired, fever, weight loss, frequent infections, bruising, bleeding easily, breathlessness, blood in urine or stool) occur.
- Advise patient to wear protective clothing and sunscreen to prevent photosensitivity reactions.
- Instruct patient to notify health care professional of all Rx or OTC medications, vitamins, or herbal products being taken and consult health care professional before taking any new medications.
- Rep: May cause fetal harm. Advise females of reproductive potential to use effective contraception during and for 6 mo following last dose of rucaparib and to avoid breastfeeding during and for 2 wk after last dose. Advise males with female partners of reproductive potential to use effective contraception during and for 3 mo after last dose. Advise males to avoid donating sperm during therapy and for 3 mo after last dose.

Evaluation/Desired Outcomes
- Decrease in growth and spread of ovarian, fallopian tube, primary peritoneal, or prostate cancer.

ruxolitinib (topical)
(**rux**-oh-**li**-ti-nib)
Opzelura
Classification
Therapeutic: none assigned
Pharmacologic: kinase inhibitors

Indications
Short-term and non-continuous chronic treatment of mild to moderate atopic dermatitis in non-immuno-compromised patients whose disease is not adequately controlled with topical prescription therapies or when those therapies are not advisable. Nonsegmental vitiligo.

Action
Inhibits Janus kinase 1 and 2 which are normally involved in the signaling of hematopoiesis and immune processes. **Therapeutic Effects:** Decreased severity of atopic dermatitis. Reduction in depigmented areas in nonsegmental vitiligo.

Pharmacokinetics
Absorption: Systemic absorption occurs following topical administration and is dependent on dose and surface area of application.
Distribution: Unknown.
Protein Binding: 97%.
Metabolism and Excretion: Primarily metabolized in the liver via the CYP3A4 isoenzyme, with minor contribution from CYP2C9. Primarily excreted in the urine (74%), with 22% excreted in the feces. Less than 1% excreted as unchanged drug.
Half-life: 116 hr.

TIME/ACTION PROFILE (plasma concentrations)

ROUTE	ONSET	PEAK	DURATION
Topical	unknown	unknown	unknown

Contraindications/Precautions
Contraindicated in: Active, serious infection; Risk factor for thrombosis; Lactation: Lactation.
Use Cautiously in: Chronic or recurrent infection; History of a serious infection or opportunistic infection; Exposure to tuberculosis; Resided or traveled in areas of endemic tuberculosis or endemic mycoses; Immunocompromised; OB: Other agents preferred for the topical treatment of atopic dermatitis and vitiligo in pregnancy; Pedi: Children <12 yr (safety and effectiveness not established).

Adverse Reactions/Side Effects
CV: ARTERIAL THROMBOSIS, DEEP VEIN THROMBOSIS. **Derm:** acne, erythema, folliculitis, NON-MELANOMA SKIN CANCER, pruritus, urticaria. **EENT:** nasopharyngitis, rhinorrhea, tonsillitis. **GI:** diarrhea. **Hemat:** anemia, eosinophilia, neutropenia, thrombocytopenia. **Metab:** hyperlipidemia. **Neuro:** headache. **Resp:** PULMONARY EMBOLISM. **Misc:** fever, INFECTION (including reactivation tuberculosis and other opportunistic infections due to bacterial, fungal, viral, and mycobacterial pathogens).

Interactions
Drug-Drug: Strong CYP3A4 inhibitors, including **ketoconazole**, may ↑ levels and risk of toxicity; avoid concurrent use.

Route/Dosage

Atopic Dermatitis

Topical (Adults and Children ≥12 yr): Apply a thin layer twice daily to affected area(s) of up to 20% body surface area. Discontinue once signs/symptoms resolve. Reassess therapy if signs/symptoms have not resolved within 8 wk. Do not use more than one 60-g tube per wk or one 100-g tube per 2 wk.

Nonsegmental Vitiligo

Topical (Adults and Children ≥12 yr): Apply a thin layer twice daily to affected area(s) of up to 10% body surface area. Reassess need for continued therapy if no meaningful improvement with repigmentation by 24 wk. Do not use more than one 60-g tube per wk or one 100-g tube per 2 wk.

Availability

Cream: 1.5%.

NURSING IMPLICATIONS

Assessment

- Assess area of skin affected before applying and periodically during therapy.
- Monitor signs and symptoms of infection during and after therapy. Interrupt ruxolitinib if serious infection, an opportunistic infection, or sepsis occurs. Do not resume ruxolitinib until the infection is controlled.
- Evaluate patients for latent and active TB infection before administration. Monitor for signs and symptoms of TB during therapy.
- Monitor for signs and symptoms of viral reactivation during therapy. If herpes zoster occurs during therapy, consider holding therapy until episode resolves.
- Assess for hepatitis B and C before starting therapy. Avoid therapy in patients with active hepatitis B or hepatitis C.

Lab Test Considerations

- Monitor CBC periodically during therapy. May cause thrombocytopenia, anemia, and neutropenia. If severe levels occur, discontinue therapy.
- May cause increases in total cholesterol, low-density lipoprotein cholesterol, and triglycerides.

Implementation

- **Topical: Atopic dermatitis:** Apply a thin layer of ruxolitinib twice daily to affected areas of up to 20% body surface area. Stop using when signs and symptoms of atopic dermatitis (itch, rash, and redness) resolve. If signs and symptoms do not improve within 8 wk, re-examine affected area.

- **Nonsegmental Vitiligo:** Apply a thin layer of ruxolitinib twice daily to affected areas of up to 10% body surface area; may require >24 wk. If repigmentation meaningful by 24 wk, re-evaluate affected area.

Patient/Family Teaching

- Instruct patient to apply cream as directed. Wash hands after applying, unless hands are being treated. Ruxolitinib is only for use on the skin only; do not use in eyes, mouth, or vagina. Advise patient to read Medication Guide before starting therapy and with each Rx refill in case of changes.
- Advise patient to notify health care professional promptly if signs and symptoms of infection (fever, sweating, chills, muscle aches, cough or shortness of breath, blood in phlegm, weight loss, warm, red, or painful skin or sores on body, diarrhea or stomach pain, burning during urination or urinating more often than usual, feeling very tired), heart attack or stroke (discomfort in center of chest that lasts > a few minutes, or that goes away and comes back, severe tightness, pain, pressure, or heaviness in chest, throat, neck, or jaw, pain or discomfort in arms, back, neck, jaw, or stomach, shortness of breath with or without chest discomfort, breaking out in a cold sweat, nausea or vomiting, feeling lightheaded, weakness in one part or on one side of body, slurred speech), blood clots (swelling, pain, or tenderness in one or both legs, sudden, unexplained chest or upper back pain, shortness of breath or difficulty breathing) or low blood counts (unusual bleeding, shortness of breath, bruising, fever, tiredness) occur.
- Advise patient to wear protective clothing and sunscreen and to exposure to sunlight and UV light to decrease risk of developing skin cancer.
- Instruct patient to notify health care professional of all Rx or OTC medications, vitamins, or herbal products being taken and consult health care professional before taking any new medications during therapy.
- Rep: Advise females of reproductive potential to notify health care professional if pregnancy is planned or suspected and to avoid breastfeeding during and for 4 wk after last dose. There is a pregnancy registry that monitors pregnancy outcomes in pregnant persons exposed to ruxolitinib during pregnancy. Pregnant persons exposed to ruxolitinib and health care providers should report ruxolitinib exposure by calling 1-855-463-3463.

Evaluation/Desired Outcomes

- Decreased severity of atopic dermatitis.
- Reduction in depigmented areas in nonsegmental vitiligo.

ⅩⅩⅩ sacubitril/valsartan
(sa-**ku**-bi-tril/val-**sar**-tan)
Entresto
Classification
Therapeutic: vasodilators, heart failure agents
Pharmacologic: angiotensin II receptor antagonists, neprilysin inhibitors

Indications
Chronic HF in adults. Symptomatic HF in children ≥1 yr with systemic left ventricular systolic dysfunction.

Action
Sacubitril: a pro-drug converted to LBQ657, its active moiety. LBQ657 inhibits the enzyme neprilysin. Neprilysin degrades vasoactive peptides, including natriuretic peptides, bradykinin, and adrenomedullin resulting in ↑ levels of these peptides, causing vasodilation and ↓ extracellular fluid volume via sodium excretion. *Valsartan:* Blocks vasoconstrictor and aldosterone-producing effects of angiotensin II at receptor sites, including vascular smooth muscle and the adrenal glands. **Therapeutic Effects:** Reduction in cardiovascular death and hospitalizations due to HF in adults. Reduction in NT-proBNP concentrations in children.

Pharmacokinetics
Sacubitril
Absorption: ≥60% absorbed following oral administration.
Distribution: Widely distributed to tissues.
Protein Binding: 94–97%.
Metabolism and Excretion: Rapidly converted to LBQ657, its active form. LBQ657 is not significantly metabolized; 52–68% excreted in urine, primarily as LBQ657; 37–48% excreted in feces, primarily as LBQ657.
Half-life: *Sacubitril:* 1.4 hr. *LBQ657:* 11.5 hr.
Valsartan
Absorption: Absorption in combinations with sacubitril is greater than 10–35% absorbed following oral administration of single-entity formulation.
Distribution: Widely distributed to tissues.
Protein Binding: 94–97%.
Metabolism and Excretion: Minimally metabolized by the liver; 13% excreted in urine, 86% in feces.
Half-life: 9.9 hr.

TIME/ACTION PROFILE (plasma concentrations)

ROUTE	ONSET	PEAK	DURATION
Sacubitril (PO)	unknown	0.5 hr	12 hr
LBQ657	unknown	2 hr	12 hr
Valsartan (PO)	unknown	1.5 hr	12 hr

Contraindications/Precautions
Contraindicated in: Hypersensitivity, hereditary angioedema, or history of angioedema from previous ACE inhibitors or ARBs; Concurrent use of ACE inhibitors during or for 36 hr before or after; Concurrent use with aliskiren in patients with diabetes or moderate to severe renal impairment (CCr <60 mL/min); Severe hepatic impairment; OB: Pregnancy; Lactation: Lactation.
Use Cautiously in: Volume- or salt-depleted patients or patients receiving high doses of diuretics (correct deficits before initiating therapy or initiate at lower doses); ⅩⅩ Black patients (may not be effective); Renal impairment due to primary renal disease or HF (may worsen renal function); Rep: Women of reproductive potential; Pedi: Children <1 yr (safety and effectiveness not established).

Adverse Reactions/Side Effects
CV: hypotension. **F and E:** hyperkalemia. **Neuro:** dizziness. **Resp:** cough. **Misc:** ANGIOEDEMA.

Interactions
Drug-Drug: NSAIDs and selective COX-2 inhibitors may ↑ the risk of renal impairment. ↑ risk of hypotension with other antihypertensives and diuretics. Concurrent use of potassium-sparing diuretics, potassium-containing salt substitutes, or potassium supplements may ↑ risk of hyperkalemia. ↑ risk of hyperkalemia, renal dysfunction, hypotension, and syncope with concurrent use of ACE inhibitors or aliskiren; avoid concurrent use with aliskiren in patients with diabetes or CCr <60 mL/min; avoid concurrent use with ACE inhibitors. May ↑ lithium levels and risk of toxicity.

Route/Dosage
PO (Adults): Sacubitril 49 mg/valsartan 51 mg twice daily initially; double dose in 2–4 wk to target dose of sacubitril 97 mg/valsartan 103 mg as tolerated. *Patients not currently receiving ARBs inhibitors or angiotensin II receptor blockers or receiving low doses of these agents:* Sacubitril 24 mg/valsartan 26 mg twice daily initially; double dose every 2–4 wk to target dose of sacubitril 97 mg/valsartan 103 mg as tolerated.
PO (Children ≥1 yr and ≥50 kg): Sacubitril 49 mg/valsartan 51 mg twice daily initially; ↑ dose in 2 wk to sacubitril 72 mg/valsartan 78 mg twice daily as tolerated, then ↑ dose again in 2 wk to target dose of sacubitril 97 mg/valsartan 103 mg twice daily as tolerated. *Patients not currently receiving ACE inhibitors or angiotensin II receptor blockers or receiving low doses of these agents:* Sacubitril 24 mg/valsartan 26 mg twice daily initially; ↑ dose in 2 wk to sacubitril 49 mg/valsartan 51 mg twice daily as tolerated, then ↑ dose again in 2 wk to sacubitril 72 mg/valsartan 78 mg twice daily as tolerated, then ↑ dose again in 2 wk to target dose of sacubitril 97 mg/valsartan 103 mg twice daily as tolerated.
PO (Children ≥1 yr and 40–<50 kg): Sacubitril 24 mg/valsartan 26 mg twice daily initially; ↑ dose in 2 wk

to sacubitril 49 mg/valsartan 51 mg twice daily as tolerated, then ↑ dose again in 2 wk to target dose of sacubitril 72 mg/valsartan 78 mg twice daily as tolerated. *Patients not currently receiving ACE inhibitors or angiotensin II receptor blockers or receiving low doses of these agents:* 0.8 mg/kg (represents combined mg dose of sacubitril and valsartan) of oral suspension twice daily initially; ↑ dose in 2 wk to 1.6 mg/kg (represents combined mg dose of sacubitril and valsartan) of oral suspension twice daily as tolerated, then ↑ dose in 2 wk to 2.3 mg/kg (represents combined mg dose of sacubitril and valsartan) of oral suspension twice daily as tolerated, then ↑ dose again in 2 wk to target dose of 3.1 mg/kg (represents combined mg dose of sacubitril and valsartan) of oral suspension twice daily as tolerated.

PO (Children ≥1 yr and <40 kg): 1.6 mg/kg (represents combined mg dose of sacubitril and valsartan) of oral suspension twice daily initially, then ↑ dose in 2 wk to 2.3 mg/kg (represents combined mg dose of sacubitril and valsartan) of oral suspension twice daily as tolerated, then ↑ dose again in 2 wk to target dose of 3.1 mg/kg (represents combined mg dose of sacubitril and valsartan) of oral suspension twice daily as tolerated. *Patients not currently receiving ACE inhibitors or angiotensin II receptor blockers or receiving low doses of these agents:* 0.8 mg/kg (represents combined mg dose of sacubitril and valsartan) of oral suspension twice daily initially; ↑ dose in 2 wk to 1.6 mg/kg (represents combined mg dose of sacubitril and valsartan) of oral suspension twice daily as tolerated, then ↑ dose in 2 wk to 2.3 mg/kg (represents combined mg dose of sacubitril and valsartan) of oral suspension twice daily as tolerated, then ↑ dose again in 2 wk to target dose of 3.1 mg/kg (represents combined mg dose of sacubitril and valsartan) of oral suspension twice daily as tolerated.

Hepatic/Renal Impairment
PO (Adults): *Severe renal impairment (CCr <30 mL/min/1.73 m²) or moderate hepatic impairment:* Sacubitril 24 mg/valsartan 26 mg twice daily initially; double dose every 2–4 wk to target dose of sacubitril 97 mg/valsartan 103 mg as tolerated.

Hepatic/Renal Impairment
PO (Children ≥1 yr and ≥50 kg): *Severe renal impairment (CCr <30 mL/min/1.73 m²) or moderate hepatic impairment :* Sacubitril 24 mg/valsartan 26 mg twice daily initially; ↑ dose in 2 wk to sacubitril 49 mg/valsartan 51 mg twice daily as tolerated, then ↑ dose again in 2 wk to sacubitril 72 mg/valsartan 78 mg twice daily as tolerated, then ↑ dose again in 2 wk to target dose of sacubitril 97 mg/valsartan 103 mg twice daily as tolerated.

Hepatic/Renal Impairment
PO (Children ≥1 yr and 40–<50 kg): *Severe renal impairment (CCr <30 mL/min/1.73 m²) or moderate hepatic impairment:* 0.8 mg/kg (represents combined mg dose of sacubitril and valsartan) of oral suspension twice daily initially; ↑ dose in 2 wk to 1.6 mg/kg (represents combined mg dose of sacubitril and valsartan) of oral suspension twice daily as tolerated, then ↑ dose in 2 wk to 2.3 mg/kg (represents combined mg dose of sacubitril and valsartan) of oral suspension twice daily as tolerated, then ↑ dose again in 2 wk to target dose of 3.1 mg/kg (represents combined mg dose of sacubitril and valsartan) of oral suspension twice daily as tolerated.

Hepatic/Renal Impairment
PO (Children ≥1 yr and <40 kg): *Severe renal impairment (CCr <30 mL/min/1.73 m²) or moderate hepatic impairment:* 0.8 mg/kg (represents combined mg dose of sacubitril and valsartan) of oral suspension twice daily initially; ↑ dose in 2 wk to 1.6 mg/kg (represents combined mg dose of sacubitril and valsartan) of oral suspension twice daily as tolerated, then ↑ dose in 2 wk to 2.3 mg/kg (represents combined mg dose of sacubitril and valsartan) of oral suspension twice daily as tolerated, then ↑ dose again in 2 wk to target dose of 3.1 mg/kg (represents combined mg dose of sacubitril and valsartan) of oral suspension twice daily as tolerated.

Availability
Tablets: sacubitril 24 mg/valsartan 26 mg, sacubitril 49 mg/valsartan 51 mg, sacubitril 97 mg/valsartan 103 mg.

NURSING IMPLICATIONS
Assessment
* Assess BP (lying, sitting, standing) and pulse frequently during initial dose adjustment and periodically throughout therapy. Correct volume or salt depletion prior to administration of therapy. If hypotension occurs, consider reducing dose of diuretics, concomitant antihypertensive agents, and treatment of other causes of hypotension (hypovolemia). If hypotension persists, reduce the dose or temporarily discontinue therapy. Permanent discontinuation of therapy is usually not required.
* Monitor daily weight and assess patient routinely for resolution of fluid overload (peripheral edema, rales/crackles, dyspnea, weight gain, jugular venous distention).
* Monitor frequency of prescription refills to determine compliance.
* Assess patients for signs of angioedema (dyspnea, orofacial swelling); may occur more frequently in Black patients. If signs occur, discontinue therapy, provide supportive therapy, and monitor for airway compromise.

Lab Test Considerations
* Monitor renal function. May cause ↑ in BUN and serum creatinine. May require ↓ dose.

S

- May cause hyperkalemia. May require ↓ dose.
- May cause ↓ in hemoglobin and hematocrit.

Implementation
- **PO:** Administer twice daily.
- If switching from an ACE inhibitor to *Entresto*, allow 36 hr between last ACE inhibitor dose and starting *Entresto*. For patients unable to swallow pills, a suspension can be made by a pharmacist.

Patient/Family Teaching
- Instruct patient to take *Entresto* as directed, at the same time each day, even if feeling well. Take missed doses as soon as remembered if not almost time for next dose; do not double doses. Warn patient not to discontinue therapy unless directed by health care professional. Advise patient to read *Patient Information* before starting therapy and with each Rx refill in case of changes.
- Caution patient to avoid salt substitutes containing potassium or foods containing high levels of potassium or sodium unless directed by health care professional. See Appendix J.
- Instruct patient to notify health care professional if swelling of face, eyes, lips, or tongue or if difficulty swallowing or breathing occur.
- May cause dizziness. Caution patient to avoid driving or other activities requiring alertness until response to medication is known.
- Instruct patient to notify health care professional of all Rx or OTC medications, vitamins, or herbal products being taken and to avoid concurrent use of Rx, OTC, and herbal products, especially NSAIDs, potassium supplements or salt substitute, ACE inhibitors, ARBs, lithium, or aliskiren, without consulting health care professional.
- Instruct patient to notify health care professional of medication regimen before treatment or surgery.
- Rep: May cause fetal harm. Advise females of reproductive potential to use contraception and avoid breastfeeding during therapy. Notify health care professional if pregnancy is planned or suspected. *Entresto* should be discontinued as soon as possible when pregnancy is detected.
- Emphasize the importance of follow-up exams to evaluate effectiveness of medication.

Evaluation/Desired Outcomes
- Decreased HF-related hospitalizations in adults with HF.
- Decreased NT-proBNP concentrations in children with HF.

---

safinamide (sa-fin-a-mide)
✤ Onstryv, Xadago
Classification
Therapeutic: antiparkinson agents
Pharmacologic: monoamine oxidase type B inhibitors

Indications
Adjunctive treatment to levodopa/carbidopa in patients with Parkinson's disease who are experiencing "off" episodes.

Action
Irreversibly inhibits monoamine oxidase (MAO) B, which leads to ↑ dopamine levels in the CNS. **Therapeutic Effects:** Increased amount of "on" time without dyskinesia or with non-troublesome dyskinesia.

Pharmacokinetics
Absorption: 95% absorbed following oral administration.
Distribution: Extensively distributed to the tissues; readily crosses the blood-brain barrier.
Metabolism and Excretion: Extensively metabolized by hydrolytic oxidation or oxidative cleavage to inactive metabolites; 76% excreted in urine (primarily as inactive metabolites).
Half-life: 20–26 hr.

TIME/ACTION PROFILE (plasma concentrations)

ROUTE	ONSET	PEAK	DURATION
PO	unknown	2–3 hr	24 hr

Contraindications/Precautions
Contraindicated in: Hypersensitivity; Concurrent use of other MAO inhibitors; Concurrent use of opioids, SNRIs, TCAs, cyclobenzaprine, methylphenidate, amphetamine, or St. John's wort; Concurrent use of dextromethorphan; Severe hepatic impairment; Psychotic disorder; Lactation: Lactation.
Use Cautiously in: Retinal disease; Moderate hepatic impairment (do not exceed maximum recommended dose); OB: Use during pregnancy only if potential maternal benefit justifies potential fetal risk; Pedi: Safety and effectiveness not established in children.

Adverse Reactions/Side Effects
CV: hypertension, orthostatic hypotension. **EENT:** visual changes. **GI:** ↑ liver enzymes, nausea. **Neuro:** dyskinesia, ↑ fall risk, anxiety, drowsiness, hallucinations, impulse control disorders (gambling, sexual, binge eating), insomnia, paresthesia, psychosis, sleep attacks, sleep driving. **Resp:** cough. **Misc:** hypersensitivity reactions.

Interactions
Drug-Drug: Concurrent use of other **MAO inhibitors**, including **linezolid** and **isoniazid**, may ↑ risk of hypertensive crises and is contraindicated; separate administration by ≥14 days. Concurrent use of **meperidine**, **methadone**, **tramadol**, **SSRIs**, **SNRIs**, **TCAs**, **cyclobenzaprine**, **methylphenidate**, or **amphetamine** may ↑ risk of serotonin syndrome and is contraindicated; separate administration by ≥14 days; SSRIs may be used at the lowest dose possible. Concurrent use with **dextromethorphan** may result in psychosis/

bizarre behavior and is contraindicated. Hypertensive crisis may occur with cough and cold products containing **sympathomimetic amines** including **pseudoephedrine** and **phenylephrine**; monitor patient's BP closely. May ↑ levels/toxicity of **imatinib, irinotecan, lapatinib, methotrexate, mitoxantrone, rosuvastatin, sulfasalazine,** and **topotecan**; monitor closely for adverse effects. **Dopamine antagonists,** including **antipsychotics** and **metoclopramide** may ↓ effectiveness of safinamide.

Drug-Natural Products: Concurrent use with **St. John's wort** may ↑ risk of serotonin syndrome; concurrent use contraindicated.

Drug-Food: Ingestion of foods containing high amounts of **tyramine** (>150 mg) (e.g., cheese) may result in hypertensive crisis.

Route/Dosage
PO (Adults): 50 mg once daily; after 2 wk, may ↑ dose to 100 mg once daily.

Hepatic Impairment
PO (Adults): *Moderate hepatic impairment:* Do not exceed 50 mg/day; *Severe hepatic impairment:* Contraindicated.

Availability (generic available)
Tablets: 50 mg, 100 mg.

NURSING IMPLICATIONS

Assessment
● Assess signs and symptoms of Parkinson's disease (tremor, muscle weakness and rigidity, ataxic gait) prior to and during therapy.
● Monitor for new-onset hypertension or hypertension not adequately controlled after starting safinamide. Sustained BP elevation may require dose reduction.
● Assess for serotonin syndrome (mental changes [agitation, hallucinations, coma], autonomic instability [tachycardia, labile BP, hyperthermia], neuromuscular aberrations [hyperreflexia, incoordination], and/or GI symptoms [nausea, vomiting, diarrhea]), especially in patients taking other serotonergic drugs (SSRIs, SNRIs, triptans).

Toxicity and Overdose
● Concurrent ingestion of tyramine-rich foods and many medications may result in a life-threatening hypertensive crisis. Signs and symptoms of hypertensive crisis include chest pain, tachycardia or bradycardia, severe headache, neck stiffness or soreness, nausea and vomiting, sweating, photosensitivity, and enlarged pupils.

Implementation
● **PO:** Administer once daily, at the same time each day, without regard to food.

Patient/Family Teaching
● Instruct patient to take safinamide as directed. Missed doses should be omitted and next dose taken at usual time the following day. Do not double doses. Do not discontinue abruptly; may cause elevated temperature, muscular rigidity, altered consciousness, and autonomic instability. Advise patient to read *Patient Information* before starting therapy and with each Rx refill in case of changes.
● Caution patient to avoid alcohol, CNS depressants, and foods or beverages containing tyramine (see Appendix J) during and for at least 2 wk after therapy has been discontinued; they may precipitate a hypertensive crisis. Contact health care professional immediately if symptoms of hypertensive crisis or serotonin syndrome develop.
● Instruct patient to notify health care professional of all Rx or OTC medications, vitamins, or herbal products being taken and consult health care professional before taking any new medications. Caution patient to avoid use of St. John's wort, cough or cold products containing dextromethorphan, and analgesics meperidine, tramadol, or methadone during therapy.
● May cause drowsiness and unexpected episodes of falling asleep. Caution patient to avoid driving or other activities requiring alertness until response to medication is known. Advise patient to notify health care professional if episodes of falling asleep occur.
● Advise patient to notify health care professional if new or increased gambling, sexual, or other impulse control disorders or psychotic-like behaviors occur.
● Rep: Advise female patients to notify health care professionals if pregnancy is planned or suspected or if breastfeeding.

Evaluation/Desired Outcomes
● Improvement in symptoms of Parkinson's disease, allowing increase in function.

---

salmeterol (sal-me-te-role)
Serevent Diskus
Classification
Therapeutic: bronchodilators
Pharmacologic: adrenergics

Indications
As concomitant therapy for the treatment of asthma and the prevention of bronchospasm in patients who are currently taking but are inadequately controlled on an inhaled corticosteroid. Prevention of exercise-induced bronchospasm. Maintenance treatment to prevent bronchospasm in COPD.

Action
Produces accumulation of cyclic adenosine monophosphate at beta$_2$-adrenergic receptors. Relatively specific

for beta$_2$ (pulmonary) receptors. **Therapeutic Effects:** Bronchodilation.

Pharmacokinetics
Absorption: Minimal systemic absorption follows inhalation.
Distribution: Action is primarily local.
Metabolism and Excretion: Metabolized in the liver via the CYP3A4 isoenzyme; 60% excreted in feces, 25% excreted in urine.
Half-life: 3–4 hr.

TIME/ACTION PROFILE (bronchodilation)

ROUTE	ONSET	PEAK	DURATION
Inhaln	10–25 min	3–4 hr	12 hr†

†9 hr in adolescents.

Contraindications/Precautions
Contraindicated in: Hypersensitivity to salmeterol or milk proteins; Acute attack of asthma (onset of action is delayed); Patients not receiving a inhaled corticosteroid (↑ risk of asthma-related death); Patients whose asthma is currently controlled on low- or medium-dose inhaled corticosteroid therapy.
Use Cautiously in: Cardiovascular disease (including angina and hypertension); Seizure disorders; Diabetes; Glaucoma; Hyperthyroidism; Pheochromocytoma; Excessive use (may lead to tolerance and paradoxical bronchospasm); OB: Use during pregnancy only if potential maternal benefit justifies potential fetal risk; may inhibit contractions during labor; Lactation: Use while breastfeeding only if potential maternal benefit justifies potential risk to infant; Pedi: Children <4 yr (safety and effectiveness not established).

Adverse Reactions/Side Effects
CV: palpitations, tachycardia. **GI:** abdominal pain, diarrhea, nausea. **MS:** muscle cramps/soreness. **Neuro:** headache, nervousness, tremor. **Resp:** cough, paradoxical bronchospasm.

Interactions
Drug-Drug: Beta blockers may ↓ therapeutic effects. **MAO inhibitors** and **tricyclic antidepressants** may potentiate cardiovascular effects. **Strong CYP3A4 inhibitors**, including **ketoconazole, itraconazole, ritonavir, atazanavir, clarithromycin, nefazodone**, or **nelfinavir**, may ↑ levels and the risk of toxicity; concurrent use not recommended.
Drug-Natural Products: Use with caffeine-containing herbs (**cola nut, guarana, mate, tea, coffee**) ↑ stimulant effect.

Route/Dosage
Asthma
Inhaln (Adults and Children ≥4 yr): 50 mcg (1 inhalation) twice daily (approximately 12 hr apart).

Prevention of Exercise-Induced Bronchospasm
Inhaln (Adults and Children ≥4 yr): 50 mcg (1 inhalation) ≥30 min before exercise; additional doses should not be used for ≥12 hr.

COPD
Inhaln (Adults): 50 mcg (1 inhalation) twice daily (approximately 12 hr apart).

Availability
Powder for oral inhalation: 50 mcg/blister. *In combination with:* fluticasone (Advair Diskus, Advair HFA, AirDuo Digihaler, AirDuo RespiClick, Wixela Inhub). See Appendix N.

NURSING IMPLICATIONS
Assessment
- Assess lung sounds, pulse, and BP before administration and periodically during therapy.
- Monitor pulmonary function tests before initiating therapy and periodically during therapy.
- Observe for paradoxical bronchospasm (wheezing, dyspnea, tightness in chest) and hypersensitivity reaction (rash; urticaria; swelling of the face, lips, or eyelids). Frequently occurs with first use of new canister or vial. If condition occurs, withhold medication and notify physician or other health care professional immediately.

Lab Test Considerations
- May cause ↑ serum glucose concentrations; occurs rarely with recommended doses and is more pronounced with frequent use of high doses.
- May cause ↓ serum potassium concentrations, which are usually transient and dose related; rarely occurs at recommended doses and is more pronounced with frequent use of high doses.

Toxicity and Overdose
- Symptoms of overdose include persistent agitation, chest pain or discomfort, decreased BP, dizziness, hyperglycemia, hypokalemia, seizures, tachyarrhythmias, persistent trembling, and vomiting.
- Treatment includes discontinuing salmeterol and other beta-adrenergic agonists and providing symptomatic, supportive therapy. Cardioselective beta blockers are used cautiously because they may induce bronchospasm.

Implementation
- Salmeterol should be used along with an inhaled corticosteroid, not as monotherapy. Patients taking salmeterol twice daily should not use additional doses for exercise-induced bronchospasm.
- **Inhaln:** Once removed from foil overwrap, discard diskus when every blister has been used or 6 wk have passed, whichever comes first.

Patient/Family Teaching
- Advise patient to take salmeterol as directed. Do not use more than the prescribed dose. If a regularly

scheduled dose is missed, use as soon as possible and resume regular schedule. Do not double doses. If symptoms occur before next dose is due, use a rapid-acting inhaled bronchodilator.

● Instruct patient using *powder for inhalation* never to exhale into diskus device and always to hold device in a level horizontal position. Mouthpiece should be kept dry; never wash.

● Caution patient not to use salmeterol to treat acute symptoms. A rapid-acting inhaled beta-adrenergic bronchodilator should be used for relief of acute asthma attacks.

● Advise patients on chronic therapy not to use additional salmeterol to prevent exercise-induced bronchospasm. Patients using salmeterol for prevention of exercise-induced bronchospasm should not use additional doses of salmeterol for 12 hr after prophylactic administration.

● Advise patient to notify health care professional immediately if difficulty in breathing persists after use of salmeterol, if condition worsens, if more inhalations of rapid-acting bronchodilator than usual are needed to relieve an acute attack, or if using 4 or more inhalations of a rapid-acting bronchodilator for 2 or more consecutive days or more than 1 canister in an 8-wk period.

● Salmeterol should be used with inhaled corticosteroids and is not a substitute for corticosteroids or adrenergic bronchodilators. Advise patients using inhalation or systemic corticosteroids to consult health care professional before stopping or reducing therapy.

● Rep: Advise females of reproductive potential to notify health care professional if pregnancy is planned or suspected or if breastfeeding.

● Emphasize the importance of regular follow-up exams to determine progress during therapy.

Evaluation/Desired Outcomes

● Prevention of bronchospasm or reduction of frequency of acute asthma attacks in patients with chronic asthma. Improvement in asthma control can occur within 15 min of starting therapy, but full benefit may take 1 wk or longer. Time to onset and degree of symptom relief will vary with individual.

● Prevention of exercise-induced asthma.

● Prevention of bronchospasm in COPD.

---

sarilumab (sar-il-ue-mab)
Kevzara
Classification
Therapeutic: antirheumatics, immunosuppressants
Pharmacologic: interleukin antagonists

Indications
Moderately to severely active rheumatoid arthritis in patients who have not responded to ≥1 disease-modifying antirheumatic drugs (DMARD) (as monotherapy or in combination with methotrexate or other non-biologic DMARDs). Polymyalgia rheumatica in patients who had an inadequate response to corticosteroids or cannot tolerate a corticosteroid taper.

Action
Acts as an inhibitor of interleukin-6 (IL-6) receptors by binding to them. IL-6 is a mediator of various inflammatory processes. **Therapeutic Effects:** Slowed progression of rheumatoid arthritis. Sustained remission in polymyalgia rheumatica.

Pharmacokinetics
Absorption: Well absorbed via SUBQ injection.
Distribution: Well distributed to tissues.
Metabolism and Excretion: Metabolic pathway has not been defined. Elimination is predominantly through the linear, non-saturable proteolytic pathway at high concentrations; at lower concentrations, elimination is predominately through non-linear saturable target-mediated pathway.
Half-life: *200 mg every 2 wk dose:* up to 10 days; *150 mg every 2 wk dose:* up to 8 days.

TIME/ACTION PROFILE (plasma concentrations)

ROUTE	ONSET	PEAK	DURATION
SUBQ	unknown	2–4 days	28–43 days

Contraindications/Precautions
Contraindicated in: Hypersensitivity; Active infection; Active hepatic disease/impairment; Absolute neutrophil count (ANC) <2000/mm³ (<500/mm³ while on therapy) or platelet count <150,000/mm³ (<50,000/mm³ while on therapy); Concurrent use with biological DMARDs.

Use Cautiously in: Chronic or recurrent infection; History of serious or opportunistic infection; Exposure to tuberculosis; Lived in or traveled to areas of endemic tuberculosis or endemic mycoses; Diverticulitis or concomitant use of NSAIDs or corticosteroids (↑ risk for GI perforation); Severe renal impairment; Geri: ↑ risk of infections; OB: Use during pregnancy only if potential maternal benefit justifies potential fetal risk; Lactation: Use while breastfeeding only if potential maternal benefit justifies potential risk to infant; Pedi: Safety and effectiveness not established in children.

Adverse Reactions/Side Effects
GI: ↑ liver enzymes, GI PERFORATION. **Hemat:** NEUTROPENIA, THROMBOCYTOPENIA. **Local:** injection site reactions. **Metab:** dyslipidemia. **Misc:** INFECTION (including tuberculosis [TB], disseminated fungal infections, and infections with opportunistic pathogens), hypersensitivity reactions, MALIGNANCY.

Interactions

Drug-Drug: May alter the activity of CYP450 enzymes; the effects of the following drugs should be monitored: **cyclosporine**, **theophylline**, **warfarin**, **hormonal contraceptives**, **atorvastatin**, and **lovastatin**. May ↓ antibody response to and ↑ risk of adverse reactions to **live virus vaccines**; avoid concurrent use.

Route/Dosage

Rheumatoid Arthritis

SUBQ (Adults): 200 mg every 2 wk.

Polymyalgia Rheumatica

SUBQ (Adults): 200 mg every 2 wk (in combination with a corticosteroid taper). May be used as monotherapy once corticosteroid taper is completed.

Availability

Solution for SUBQ injection (prefilled syringes and prefilled pens): 150 mg/1.14 mL, 200 mg/1.14 mL.

NURSING IMPLICATIONS

Assessment

- Assess for signs of infection (fever, dyspnea, flu-like symptoms, frequent or painful urination, redness or swelling at the site of a wound), including TB, prior to injection. Sarilumab is contraindicated in patients with active infection. Monitor new infections closely; most common are upper respiratory tract infections, bronchitis, and urinary tract infections. Signs and symptoms of inflammation may be lessened due to suppression from sarilumab. Infections may be fatal, especially in patients taking immunosuppressive therapy. If patient develops a serious infection, discontinue sarilumab until infection is controlled.
- Monitor for signs and symptoms of viral reactivation: herpes zoster (rash, blisters), hepatitis B (jaundice, dark urine, light-colored stools, fatigue, weakness, loss of appetite, nausea, vomiting, stomach pain) during therapy.

Lab Test Considerations

- Assess lipid parameters approximately 4 to 8 wk after starting therapy, then at approximately 6-mo intervals. May cause increases in LDL cholesterol, HDL cholesterol, and/or triglycerides.
- **Rheumatoid Arthritis:** Monitor neutrophil count prior to, and 4 and 8 wk after starting, and every 3 mo during therapy. Base dose modifications on measures from end of dosing interval. *If ANC >1000 cells/mm³*, maintain current dose of sarilumab. *If ANC 500–1000 cells/mm³*, withhold therapy until ANC >1000. Resume at 150 mg every 2 wk and ↑ to 200 mg every 2 wk as appropriate. If ANC <500 cells/mm³, discontinue sarilumab.
- Monitor platelet count prior to, and 4 and 8 wk after starting, and every 3 mo during therapy. *If platelet count 50,000–100,000 cells/mm³*, suspend therapy until platelets >100,000. Resume at 150 mg

every 2 wk and ↑ to 200 mg every 2 wk as appropriate.
- Monitor serum AST and ALT prior to, and 4 and 8 wk after starting, and every 3 mo during therapy. *If ALT > upper limits of normal (ULN) to 3 × ULN or less,* consider modifying dose of concomitant DMARDs as clinically appropriate. *If ALT >3 × ULN to 5 × ULN or less,* hold therapy until ALT <3 × ULN. Resume at 150 mg every 2 wk and ↑ to 200 mg every 2 wk as appropriate. *If ALT >5 × ULN,* discontinue sarilumab.
- Monitor serum lipid levels 4–8 wk following start of therapy, then at 6-mo intervals. Manage with clinical guidelines for hyperlipidemia. **Polymyalgia Rheumatica:** Discontinue sarilumab if neutropenia (ANC <1,000 per mm³ at the end of the dosing interval), thrombocytopenia (platelet count <100,000 per mm³) or AST or ALT elevations >3 x ULN occur.

Implementation

- Administer a tuberculin skin test prior to administration of sarilumab. Patients with latent TB should be treated for TB prior to therapy.
- Other DMARDs should be continued during sarilumab therapy.
- **SUBQ:** Refrigerate in original carton to protect from light. If using a prefilled pen, allow to sit at room temperature for 60 min before injecting; do not use other methods of warming. If using a prefilled syringe, allow to sit at room temperature for 30 min before injecting; do not use other methods of warming. Do not freeze or shake. May be stored for up to 14 days in original carton at room temperature. Inject full amount in syringe. Rotate injection sites; avoid areas where skin is tender, damaged, or has bruises or scars. Solution is clear and colorless to pale yellow; do not administer solutions that are discolored or contain particulate matter.

Patient/Family Teaching

- Instruct patient on the purpose for sarilumab. If a dose is missed, contact health care professional to schedule next infusion. Instruct patient and caregiver in correct technique for SUBQ injections and care and disposal of equipment. Advise patient to read the *Medication Guide* before starting and with each Rx refill in case of changes.
- Caution patient to notify health care professional immediately if signs of infection (fever, sweating, chills, muscle aches, cough, shortness of breath, blood in phlegm, weight loss, warm, red or painful skin or sores, diarrhea or stomach pain, burning on urination, urinary frequency, feeling tired), fever and stomach-area pain that does not go away, change in bowel habits, severe rash, swollen face, or difficulty breathing occur. If signs and symptoms of anaphylaxis occur, discontinue injections and notify health care professional immediately.
- Advise patient to avoid receiving live vaccines during therapy.

- Instruct patient to notify health care professional of all Rx or OTC medications, vitamins, or herbal products being taken and consult health care professional before taking any new medications.
- Instruct patient to notify health care professional of medication regimen prior to treatment or surgery.
- Rep: Advise females of reproductive potential to notify health care professional if pregnancy is planned or suspected, or if breastfeeding, Encourage women who become pregnant while taking sarilumab to participate in the pregnancy registry by calling 1-877-311-8972.

Evaluation/Desired Outcomes
- Slowed progression of rheumatoid arthritis.
- Sustained remission in polymyalgia rheumatica.

BEERS

scopolamine (scoe-**pol**-a-meen)
Transderm-Scop
Classification
Therapeutic: antiemetics
Pharmacologic: anticholinergics

Indications
Prevention of motion sickness. Prevention of postoperative nausea and vomiting.

Action
Inhibits the muscarinic activity of acetylcholine. Corrects the imbalance of acetylcholine and norepinephrine in the CNS, which may be responsible for motion sickness. **Therapeutic Effects:** Reduction of postoperative nausea and vomiting. Reduction of spasms.

Pharmacokinetics
Absorption: Well absorbed following transdermal administration.
Distribution: Crosses the blood-brain barrier.
Metabolism and Excretion: Mostly metabolized by the liver.
Half-life: 8 hr.

TIME/ACTION PROFILE (antiemetic, sedative properties)

ROUTE	ONSET	PEAK	DURATION
Transdermal	4 hr	unknown	72 hr

Contraindications/Precautions
Contraindicated in: Hypersensitivity; Angle-closure glaucoma; Acute hemorrhage; Tachycardia secondary to cardiac insufficiency or thyrotoxicosis; OB: Pregnant women with severe pre-eclampsia (may ↑ risk of seizures).
Use Cautiously in: Possible intestinal obstruction; Prostatic hyperplasia; Chronic renal, hepatic, pulmonary, or cardiac disease; OB: Use during pregnancy

only if potential maternal benefit justifies potential fetal risk; Lactation: Use while breastfeeding only if potential maternal benefit justifies potential risk to infant; Pedi: ↑ risk of adverse reactions in children; Geri: Appears on Beers list. ↑ risk of adverse reactions in older adults due to anticholinergic effects. Avoid use in older adults.

Adverse Reactions/Side Effects
CV: <u>tachycardia</u>, palpitations. **Derm:** ↓ sweating. **EENT:** <u>blurred vision</u>, mydriasis, photophobia. **GI:** <u>dry mouth</u>, constipation. **GU:** <u>urinary hesitancy</u>, urinary retention. **Neuro:** <u>drowsiness</u>, confusion.

Interactions
Drug-Drug: ↑ anticholinergic effects with **antihistamines**, **antidepressants**, **quinidine**, or **disopyramide**. ↑ CNS depression with **alcohol**, **antidepressants**, **antihistamines**, **opioid analgesics**, or **sedative/hypnotics**. May alter the absorption of other **orally administered drugs** by slowing motility of the GI tract. May ↑ GI mucosal lesions in patients taking oral **wax-matrix potassium chloride preparations**.
Drug-Natural Products: ↑ anticholinergic effects with **jimson weed** and **scopolia**.

Route/Dosage
Transdermal (Adults): *Motion sickness:* Apply 1 patch 4 hr prior to travel and then every 3 days (as needed); *Preoperative:* Apply 1 patch the evening before surgery (remove 24 hr after surgery).

Availability (generic available)
Transdermal system: 1.5 mg scopolamine/patch releases 0.5 mg scopolamine over 3 days.

NURSING IMPLICATIONS
Assessment
- Monitor for nausea and vomiting before and during therapy.
- Assess patient for signs of urinary retention periodically during therapy.

Implementation
- **Transdermal:** Apply at least 4 hr (US product) before exposure to travel to prevent motion sickness.

Patient/Family Teaching
- **Transdermal:** Instruct patient on application of transdermal patches. Apply at least 4 hr (US product) before exposure to travel to prevent motion sickness. Wash hands and dry thoroughly before and after application. Apply to hairless, clean, dry area behind ear; avoid areas with cuts or irritation. Apply pressure over system to ensure contact with skin. System is effective for 3 days. If system becomes dislodged, replace with a new system on another site behind the ear. System is waterproof and not affected by bathing or showering.

S

- Instruct patient to remove patch and notify health care professional immediately if symptoms of acute angle-closure glaucoma (pain or reddening of the eyes with pupil dilation) occur.
- Caution patients engaging in underwater sports of potentially distorting effects of scopolamine.
- Advise patient referred for MRI test to discuss patch with referring health care professional and MRI facility to determine if removal of patch is necessary prior to test and for directions for replacing patch.
- Instruct patient to take medication as directed. Take missed doses as soon as remembered. Do not double doses.
- May cause drowsiness or blurred vision. Caution patient to avoid driving or other activities requiring alertness until response to medication is known.
- Advise patient to use caution when exercising and in hot weather; overheating may result in heatstroke.
- Advise patient to avoid concurrent use of alcohol and other CNS depressants, including opioids, with this medication.
- Inform patient that frequent mouth rinses, good oral hygiene, and sugarless gum or candy may minimize dry mouth.
- Rep: Advise patient to notify health care professional if pregnancy is planned or suspected, or if breastfeeding. When the transdermal patch is used to prevent nausea and vomiting associated with surgery, dose adjustments are required prior to cesarean delivery. Avoid use of transdermal patches in pregnant patients with severe preeclampsia; may cause eclamptic seizures. Monitor for dry mouth, drowsiness, blurred vision, and dilation of the pupils in infant of a mother using transdermal scopolamine. May decrease milk production.

Evaluation/Desired Outcomes

- Prevention of motion sickness.
- Prevention of postoperative nausea and vomiting.

---

secnidazole (sek-nid-a-zole)
Solosec
Classification
Therapeutic: anti-infectives
Pharmacologic: imidazoles

Indications
Bacterial vaginosis. Trichomoniasis.

Action
Disrupts DNA synthesis in susceptible organisms. **Therapeutic Effects:** Resolution of bacterial vaginosis. Resolution of trichomoniasis. **Spectrum:** Active against *Bacteroides spp.*, *Gardnerella vaginalis*, *Prevotella spp.*, *Mobiluncus spp.*, and *Trichomonas vaginalis*.

Pharmacokinetics
Absorption: Rapidly and completely absorbed following oral administration.

Distribution: Extensively distributed to tissues.
Metabolism and Excretion: Primarily metabolized by CYP450 system in liver; 15% excreted unchanged in urine.
Half-life: 17 hr.

TIME/ACTION PROFILE (plasma concentrations)

ROUTE	ONSET	PEAK	DURATION
PO	rapid	4 hr	unknown

Contraindications/Precautions
Contraindicated in: Hypersensitivity; cross-sensitivity with other imidazoles may occur; Cockayne syndrome (↑ risk of hepatotoxicity and death); Lactation: Lactation.

Use Cautiously in: OB: Safety not established in pregnancy; Pedi: Children <12 yr (safety and effectiveness not established).

Adverse Reactions/Side Effects
GI: abdominal pain, diarrhea, metallic taste, nausea, vomiting. **GU:** vulvovaginal candidiasis, vulvovaginal pruritus. **Neuro:** headache.

Interactions
Drug-Drug: **Alcohol** or preparations containing **ethanol** or **propylene glycol** may lead to nausea, vomiting, diarrhea, abdominal pain, dizziness, and headache. Avoid use during secnidazole therapy and for ≥2 days after completing therapy.

Route/Dosage

Bacterial Vaginosis
PO (Adults and Children ≥12 yr): 2-g single dose.

Trichomoniasis
PO (Adults and Children ≥12 yr): 2-g single dose. Any sexual partners should also be treated with a 2-g single dose.

Availability
Oral granules: 2 g/pkt.

NURSING IMPLICATIONS

Assessment

- Assess for symptoms of bacterial vaginosis (thin white or gray vaginal discharge; pain, itching, or burning in the vagina; strong fish-like odor, especially after sex; burning on urination; and itching around the outside of the vagina) before and periodically following secnidazole.
- Assess for symptoms of trichomoniasis (foul-smelling vaginal discharge, genital itching, painful urination) before and periodically following secnidazole.

Lab Test Considerations

- Obtain specimen for culture and sensitivity before starting therapy.

Implementation

- **PO:** Administer packet once without regard to meals. Open packet and sprinkle entire contents onto applesauce, yogurt, or pudding. Granules will not dissolve. Consume all of the mixture within 30 min without chewing or crunching granules. May be followed with a glass of water to aid in swallowing. Granules are not intended to be dissolved in any liquid.

Patient/Family Teaching

• Instruct patient in correct technique for taking secnidazole. Advise patient to read *Patient Information* before taking secnidazole.

• Advise patient to notify health care professional if signs and symptoms of vulvovaginal candidiasis (vaginal itching, white or yellowish discharge [discharge may be lumpy or look like cottage cheese]) occur. May require treatment with antifungal agents.

• Advise patient to avoid alcohol during and for 2 days after last dose of secnidazole. May cause nausea, vomiting, diarrhea, abdominal pain, dizziness, and headache when taken with alcohol.

• Advise patient to notify health care professional of all Rx or OTC medications, vitamins, or herbal products being taken and to consult with health care professional before taking other medications during therapy.

• Rep: Advise females of reproductive potential to notify health care professional if pregnancy is planned or suspected. Advise female patient to avoid breastfeeding for at least 96 hr (4 days) following secnidazole dose.

Evaluation/Desired Outcomes

• Resolution of bacterial vaginosis.
• Resolution of trichomoniasis.

---

selegiline (se-le-ji-leen)
~~Eldepryl~~, Emsam, Zelapar

Classification
Therapeutic: antiparkinson agents, antidepressants
Pharmacologic: monoamine oxidase type B inhibitors

Indications

PO: Parkinson's disease (with levodopa or levodopa/carbidopa) in patients who fail to respond to levodopa/carbidopa alone (in combination with levodopa or levodopa/carbidopa). **Transdermal:** Major depressive disorder.

Action

Following conversion by MAO to its active form, selegiline inactivates MAO by irreversibly binding to it at type B (brain) sites; results in higher levels of monoamine neurotransmitters in the brain (dopamine, serotonin, norepinephrine). **Therapeutic Effects:** Increased response to levodopa/dopamine therapy in Parkinson's disease. Decreased symptoms of depression.

Pharmacokinetics

Absorption: Well absorbed following oral administration. 25–30% of patch content is absorbed; levels are higher than those following oral administration because there is less first-pass hepatic metabolism.

Distribution: Widely distributed to tissues; crosses the blood-brain barrier.

Metabolism and Excretion: Mostly metabolized by the liver, primarily by the CYP2A6, CYP2C9, and CYP3A4/5 isoenzymes to N-desmethylselegiline, amphetamine, and methamphetamine as well as inactive metabolites. Primarily excreted in urine as metabolites.

Half-life: *Oral:* 10 hr; *Transdermal:* 20 hr.

TIME/ACTION PROFILE (beneficial effects in Parkinson's disease)

ROUTE	ONSET	PEAK	DURATION
PO	2–3 days†	40–90 min†	unknown
Orally disintegrating	5 min†	10–15 min†	unknown
Transdermal	unknown	≥2 wk‡	unknown

† Beneficial effects in Parkinson's disease; ‡ Antidepressant effects

Contraindications/Precautions

Contraindicated in: Hypersensitivity; Pheochromocytoma; Major psychotic disorder; Concurrent use of opioids, other MAO inhibitors, St. John's wort, cyclobenzaprine, or dextromethorphan; Lactation: Lactation.

Use Cautiously in: History of peptic ulcer disease; Phenylketonuria (orally disintegrating tablets only); Elective surgery; May ↑ risk of suicide attempt/ideation, especially during early treatment or dose adjustment (transdermal only); History of mania (transdermal only); OB: Safety not established in pregnancy; Pedi: Safety and effectiveness not established in children; Geri: ↑ risk of orthostatic hypotension in older adults.

Adverse Reactions/Side Effects

CV: orthostatic hypotension. **Derm:** *Transdermal:* application site reactions, acne, ecchymoses, pruritus, sweating. **GI:** nausea, abdominal pain, diarrhea, dry mouth. **Neuro:** aggression, agitation, confusion, delirium, delusions, disorientation, dizziness, fainting, hallucinations, headache, insomnia, paranoia, psychosis, sedation, SEROTONIN SYNDROME, urges (gambling, sexual), vivid dreams.

Interactions

Drug-Drug: Use with **opioid analgesic** (e.g. **meperidine**) or **cyclobenzaprine** may ↑ risk of serotonin syndrome; concurrent use contraindicated. Selegiline should be discontinued for ≥2 wk before initiating any of these medications. Use with other **MAO inhibitors**, including **linezolid**, may ↑ risk of hypertensive crises; concurrent use contraindicated. Selegiline should be discontinued for ≥2 wk before initiating any other medication with MAO inhibitor properties.

S

Use with products containing **dextromethorphan** may lead to episodes of psychosis or bizarre behavior; concurrent use contraindicated. Drugs that affect serotonergic neurotransmitter systems, including **tricyclic antidepressants**, **SSRIs**, **SNRIs**, **fentanyl**, **buspirone**, **amphetamines**, and **triptans** may ↑ risk of serotonin syndrome; avoid concurrent use with any antidepressant. Selegiline should be discontinued for ≥14 days before initiating any antidepressant. Fluoxetine should be discontinued for ≥5 wk before initiating selegiline. May initially ↑ risk of side effects (primarily dyskinesia) of **levodopa/carbidopa** (dose of levodopa/carbidopa may need to be ↓ by 10–30%). **Antipsychotics** and **metoclopramide** may ↓ effectiveness. **Drug-Natural Products:** Use with **St. John's wort** may ↑ risk of serotonin syndrome; concurrent use contraindicated.
Drug-Food: Doses >10 mg/day (tablets/capsules), >2.5 mg/day (orally disintegrating tablets), or >6 mg/24 hr (transdermal) may produce hypertensive reactions with **tyramine-containing foods** (see Appendix J).

Route/Dosage

Parkinson's Disease
PO (Adults): *Capsules or tablets:* 5 mg twice daily with breakfast and lunch (some patients may require further dividing of doses—2.5 mg 4 times daily).
Orally disintegrating tablets: 1.25 mg once daily for ≥6 wk. After 6 wk, may ↑ to 2.5 mg once daily if effect not achieved and patient is tolerating medication.

Depression
Transdermal (Adults): Apply 6 mg/24-hr patch once daily initially; if necessary, may be ↑ at 2-wk intervals in increments of 3 mg/24-hr patch (max dose = 12 mg/24 hr).

Availability (generic available)
Capsules: 5 mg. **Tablets:** 5 mg. **Orally disintegrating tablets (contain phenylalanine) (Zelapar) (grapefruit-flavor):** 1.25 mg. **Transdermal patch (Emsam):** 6 mg/24 hr, 9 mg/24 hr, 12 mg/24 hr.

NURSING IMPLICATIONS

Assessment
- **Parkinson's Disease:** Assess patient for signs and symptoms of Parkinson's disease (tremor, muscle weakness and rigidity, ataxic gait) prior to and during therapy.
- Assess BP periodically during therapy.
- **Depression:** Assess mental status, mood changes, and anxiety level frequently. Assess for suicidal tendencies, agitation, irritability, and unusual changes in behavior especially during early therapy. Assess for any personal or family history of bipolar disorder, mania, or hypomania before starting therapy. Monitor pediatric patients face-to-face weekly during first 4 wk, every other wk for 4 wk, at 12 wk, and as clinically indicated during therapy. Restrict amount of drug available to patient.

- Monitor BP and pulse rate before and frequently during therapy for depression. Report significant changes promptly.

Toxicity and Overdose
- Concurrent ingestion of tyramine-rich foods and many medications may result in a life-threatening hypertensive crisis. Signs and symptoms of hypertensive crisis include chest pain, tachycardia or bradycardia, severe headache, neck stiffness or soreness, nausea and vomiting, sweating, photosensitivity, and enlarged pupils. If hypertensive crisis occurs, discontinue selegiline and administer labetalol 20 mg slowly IV to control hypertension. Manage fever with external cooling. Monitor patient closely until symptoms have stabilized.

Implementation
- Do not confuse selegiline with Salagen. Do not confuse Zelapar with Zyprexa or Zydis.
- An attempt to reduce the dose of levodopa/carbidopa by 10–30% may be made after 2–3 days of selegiline therapy.
- **PO:** Administer 5-mg tablet with breakfast and lunch.
- Administer *orally disintegrating tablets* in the morning, before breakfast and without liquid. Remove tablet gently from blister pack with clean, dry hands immediately before administering. Do not attempt to push tablet through backing. Tablet will disintegrate within sec when placed on tongue. Avoid food or liquid within 5 min of administering orally disintegrating tablets.
- **Transdermal:** Apply system to dry, intact skin on the upper torso such as chest, back, upper thigh, or outer surface of the upper arm once every 24 hr at the same time each day. Avoid areas that are hairy, oily, irritated, broken, scarred, or calloused. Wash area gently with soap and warm water; rinse thoroughly. Allow skin to dry completely before application. Apply immediately after removing from package. Do not alter the system (i.e., cut) in any way before application. Remove liner from adhesive layer and press firmly in place with palm of hand for 30 sec, especially around the edges, to make sure contact is complete. Remove used system and fold so that adhesive edges are together. Only 1 selegiline patch should be worn at a time. Dispose away from children and pets. Apply new system to a different site. Wash hands thoroughly with soap and water to remove any medicine that may have gotten on them.

Patient/Family Teaching
- Instruct patient to take medication as directed. Take missed doses as soon as possible, but not if late afternoon or evening or almost time for next dose. Do not double doses. Caution patient that taking more than the prescribed dose may increase side effects and place patient at risk for hypertensive crisis if foods containing tyramine are consumed (see Appendix J).

- Advise patients taking selegiline ≥20 mg/day to avoid large amounts of tyramine-containing foods (see Appendix J), alcoholic beverages, large quantities of caffeine-containing beverages, or OTC or herbal cough or cold medications.
- Caution patient and caregiver that selegiline may cause drowsiness and dizziness. Monitor and assist with ambulation and caution patient to avoid driving and other activities requiring alertness until response to medication is known.
- Inform patient and family of the signs and symptoms of MAO inhibitor–induced hypertensive crisis (severe headache, chest pain, nausea, vomiting, photosensitivity, enlarged pupils). Advise patient to notify health care professional immediately if severe headache or any other unusual symptoms occur. At least 14 days should elapse between discontinuation of selegiline and start of MAO inhibitor therapy.
- Caution patient to change positions slowly to minimize orthostatic hypotension.
- Advise patient to notify health care professional of signs and symptoms of serotonin syndrome (mental status changes [agitation, hallucinations, delirium, and coma], autonomic instability [tachycardia, labile BP, dizziness, diaphoresis, flushing, hyperthermia], neuromuscular changes [tremor, rigidity, myoclonus, hyperreflexia, incoordination], seizures, and/or GI symptoms [nausea, vomiting, diarrhea]).
- Instruct patient to notify health care professional of all Rx or OTC medications, vitamins, or herbal products being taken and to consult with health care professional before taking other medications. Caution patient to avoid use of St. John's wort and the analgesics meperidine, tramadol, or methadone during therapy.
- Advise patient to notify health care professional if agitation, aggression, delirium, hallucinations, new or increased gambling, sexual, or other intense urges occur.
- Advise patient that increasing fluids, sugarless gum or candy, ice, or saliva substitutes may help minimize dry mouth. Consult health care professional if dry mouth continues for >2 wk.
- Rep: Advise females of reproductive potential to notify health care professional if pregnancy is planned or suspected. Advise patient to avoid breastfeeding during and for 7 days after final dose.
- **Transdermal:** Instruct patient to apply patch as directed. Advise patients and caregivers to read the *Medication Guide about Using Antidepressants in Children and Teenagers*. Inform patient that improvement may be noticed after 1 to several wk of therapy. Advise patient not to discontinue therapy without consulting health care professional.
- Caution patient to avoid alcohol and CNS depressants during and for at least 2 wk after therapy has been discontinued; they may precipitate a hypertensive crisis. Contact health care professional immediately if symptoms of hypertensive crisis develop. Patients taking 9 mg/24 hr or 12 mg/24 hr must avoid foods or beverages containing tyramine (see Appendix J) from the 1st day of the increased dose through 2 wk after discontinuation of selegiline transdermal therapy.
- Advise patient to avoid exposing application site to external sources of direct heat such as heating pads, electric blankets, heat lamps, saunas, hot tubs, heated water beds, and prolonged direct sunlight.
- Caution patient to change positions slowly to minimize orthostatic hypotension. Geriatric patients are at increased risk for this side effect.
- Advise patient referred for MRI test to discuss patch with referring health care professional and MRI facility to determine if removal of patch is necessary prior to test and for directions for replacing patch.
- Advise patients and caregivers to notify health care professional if severe headache, neck stiffness, heart racing or palpitations, anxiety, agitation, panic attacks, insomnia, irritability, hostility, aggressiveness, impulsivity, akathisia, hypomania, mania, change in behavior, worsening of depression, or suicidal ideation occur, especially during initial therapy or during changes in dose.
- Advise patient to notify health care professional of medication regimen before treatment or surgery. If possible, therapy should be discontinued at least 2 wk before surgery.

Evaluation/Desired Outcomes

- Improved response to levodopa/carbidopa in patients with Parkinson's disease.
- Improved mood in depressed patients.
- Decreased anxiety.
- Increased appetite.
- Improved energy level.
- Improved sleep. Evaluate effectiveness of therapy periodically.

---

semaglutide (sem-a-**gloo**-tide)
Ozempic, Rybelsus, Wegovy

Classification
Therapeutic: antidiabetics, weight control agents
Pharmacologic: glucagon-like peptide-1 (GLP-1) receptor agonists

Indications

Ozempic and Rybelsus: Type 2 diabetes mellitus (as adjunct to diet and exercise). **Ozempic:** To reduce the risk of major adverse cardiovascular events in patients with type 2 diabetes mellitus and established cardiovascular disease (injection only). **Wegovy:** Chronic weight management in: Adults who are obese (body mass index [BMI] ≥30 kg/m²) *OR* are overweight (BMI ≥27 kg/m²) with ≥1 weight-related comorbid condition (e.g., hypertension, dyslipidemia, type 2 diabetes) (as adjunct to reduced-calorie diet and increased physical activity). Pediatric patients ≥12 yr old who are obese (initial BMI ≥95th percentile standardized for age and sex) (as adjunct to reduced-calorie diet and increased physical activity).

Action

Acts as an acylated human glucagon-like peptide-1 (GLP-1, an incretin) receptor agonist; increases intracellular cyclic AMP (cAMP) leading to insulin release when glucose is elevated, which then subsides as blood glucose decreases toward euglycemia. Also decreases glucagon secretion and delays gastric emptying. Also helps to suppress appetite, leading to decreased caloric intake. **Therapeutic Effects:** Improved glycemic control. Reduction in risk of cardiovascular death, non-fatal MI, or non-fatal stroke. Reduction in body weight.

Pharmacokinetics

Absorption: 89% absorbed following SUBQ injection; 0.4–1% absorbed following oral administration. **Distribution:** Minimally distributed to tissues. **Protein Binding:** >99%. **Metabolism and Excretion:** Endogenously metabolized; eliminated in the urine (3% as unchanged drug) and feces. **Half-life:** 1 wk.

TIME/ACTION PROFILE (plasma concentrations)

ROUTE	ONSET	PEAK	DURATION
SUBQ	unknown	1–3 days	unknown
PO	unknown	1 hr	unknown

Contraindications/Precautions

Contraindicated in: Hypersensitivity; Personal or family history of medullary thyroid carcinoma; Multiple endocrine neoplasia syndrome type 2; Type 1 diabetes; Diabetic ketoacidosis.

Use Cautiously in: History of pancreatitis; Diabetic retinopathy (↑ risk of complications); History of angioedema or anaphylaxis to another GLP-1 receptor agonist; History of suicidal attempt or active suicidal ideations; OB: Use during pregnancy only if potential maternal benefit justifies potential fetal risk; insulin recommended for glucose management in pregnancy; Lactation: Use while breastfeeding only if potential maternal benefit justifies potential risk to infant; Rep: Women of reproductive potential; Pedi: Safety and effectiveness not established in children <12 yr (Wegovy) or <18 yr (Ozempic or Rybelsus).

Adverse Reactions/Side Effects

CV: ↑ heart rate. **Derm:** hair loss. **EENT:** retinopathy complications. **Endo:** hypoglycemia, MEDULLARY THYROID CARCINOMA. **GI:** abdominal pain, constipation, diarrhea, nausea, vomiting, ↓ appetite, ↑ amylase, ↑ lipase, abdominal distention, cholecystitis, cholelithiasis,

dyspepsia, flatulence, PANCREATITIS, vomiting. **GU:** acute kidney injury. **Local:** injection site reactions. **Neuro:** fatigue, headache, dizziness, SUICIDAL BEHAVIOR/IDEATION (Wegovy only). **Misc:** HYPERSENSITIVITY REACTIONS (including anaphylaxis and angioedema).

Interactions

Drug-Drug: Concurrent use with **agents that increase insulin secretion**, including **sulfonylureas** or **insulin**, may ↑ the risk of serious hypoglycemia; use cautiously and consider dose ↓ of agent increasing insulin secretion. May alter absorption of concomitantly administered **oral medications** due to delayed gastric emptying.

Route/Dosage

Type 2 Diabetes

PO (Adults): 3 mg once daily for 30 days, then 7 mg once daily; after 30 days, may ↑ to 14 mg once daily if additional glycemic control needed.

SUBQ (Adults): *Ozempic:* 0.25 mg once weekly initially for 4 wk, then 0.5 mg once weekly for 1 wk; may then ↑ dose after ≥4 wk, if needed, to 1 mg once weekly; may then ↑ dose after ≥4 wk, if needed, to 2 mg once weekly.

Reduction in Risk of Major Adverse Cardiovascular Events in Patients With Type 2 Diabetes Mellitus and Established Cardiovascular Disease

SUBQ (Adults): *Ozempic:* 0.25 mg once weekly initially for 4 wk, then 0.5 mg once weekly for 1 wk; may then ↑ dose after 4 wk, if needed, up to 1 mg once weekly.

Chronic Weight Management

SUBQ (Adults and Children ≥12 yr): *Wegovy:* 0.25 mg once weekly initially for 4 wk, then 0.5 mg once weekly for 4 wk, then 1 mg once weekly for 4 wk, then 1.7 mg once weekly for 4 wk, then 2.4 mg once weekly thereafter.

Availability

Tablets (Rybelsus): 3 mg, 7 mg, 14 mg. **Solution for injection (Ozempic) (prefilled pens):** 2 mg/3 mL (delivers doses of 0.25 mg or 0.5 mg), 4 mg/3 mL (delivers dose of 1 mg), 8 mg/3 mL (delivers dose of 2 mg). **Solution for injection (Wegovy) (prefilled pens):** 0.25 mg/0.5 mL, 0.5 mg/0.5 mL, 1 mg/0.5 mL, 1.7 mg/0.75 mL, 2.4 mg/0.75 mL.

NURSING IMPLICATIONS

Assessment

- Observe patient taking concurrent insulin for signs and symptoms of hypoglycemic reactions (sweating, hunger, weakness, dizziness, tremor, tachycardia, anxiety, headache, blurred vision, slurred speech, irritability).
- Monitor for pancreatitis (persistent severe abdominal pain, sometimes radiating to the back, with or without vomiting). If pancreatitis is suspected, dis-

continue semaglutide; if confirmed, do not restart semaglutide.

- Monitor weight before and periodically during therapy.
- Monitor for signs and symptoms of hypersensitivity reactions (swelling of face, lips, tongue or throat; problems breathing or swallowing; severe rash or itching; fainting or feeling dizzy; very rapid heartbeat) during therapy.
- Monitor heart rate regularly during therapy. If a sudden sustained increase in resting heart rate occurs, discontinue semaglutide.

Lab Test Considerations
- Monitor serum HbA$_{1c}$ periodically during therapy to evaluate effectiveness.
- *Wegovy:* In patients with type 2 diabetes, monitor blood glucose prior to starting and during therapy.
- May ↑ lipase and pancreatic amylase.

Implementation

- Patients stabilized on a diabetic regimen who are exposed to stress, fever, trauma, infection, or surgery may require administration of insulin.
- Patients treated with PO *Rybelsus* 14 mg daily can be transitioned to *Ozempic* SUBQ 0.5 mg once-weekly. Patients can start *Ozempic* the day after their last dose of *Rybelsus*. Patients treated with once weekly *Ozempic* 0.5 mg SUBQ can be transitioned to PO *Rybelsus* 7 mg or 14 mg. Patients can start *Rybelsus* up to 7 days after last injection of *Ozempic*. There is no equivalent dose of *Rybelsus* for *Ozempic* 1 mg.
- **PO:** Administer at least 30 min before first food, beverage, or other oral medications of the day with no >4 oz of plain water only. Waiting <30 min, or taking *Rybelsus* with food, beverages (other than plain water), or other PO medications decreases absorption and will lessen effects. Waiting >30 min to eat may increase absorption. *DNC:* Swallow tablets whole; do not split, crush, or chew.
- *Wegovy:* If dose escalation is not tolerated, may delay dose escalation for 4 wk. If patients do not tolerate maintenance dose of 2.4 mg once-weekly, dose can be temporarily decreased to 1.7 mg once-weekly, for a maximum of 4 wk. After 4 wk, increase to maintenance dose of 2.4 mg once-weekly. Discontinue *Wegovy:* if patient cannot tolerate 2.4 mg dose.
- **SUBQ:** Administer once weekly on same day each wk, any time of day without regard to meals. May change day of injection as long as time between doses is >48 hr. Inject into abdomen, thigh, or upper arm, rotating sites each wk. Solution is clear and colorless; do not administer solutions that are cloudy, discolored, or contain particulate matter. Store pens in refrigerator in original box until administration to protect from light; do not freeze. *Wegovy:* single-use pens are stable for up to 28 days.

Ozempic multi-dose pens are stable if refrigerated without the needle for 56 days after 1st use. Use a new needle for each injection.

Patient/Family Teaching

- Instruct patient to take semaglutide as directed. If a PO dose is missed, omit dose and take next dose the following day. Instruct patient in correct technique for injection and disposal of materials. Follow manufacturer's instructions for pen use. Pen should never be shared between patients, even if needle is changed. Administer missed *Ozempic* doses as soon as remembered within 5 days of missed dose; if >5 days, skip dose and administer next dose on regular scheduled day. Administer missed *Wegovy* doses as soon as remembered. If 1 dose is missed and next scheduled dose is >2 days away (48 hr), administer *Wegovy* as soon as possible. If one dose is missed and the next scheduled dose is <2 days away (48 hr), omit dose and resume dosing on regularly scheduled day of wk. If >2 consecutive doses are missed, resume dosing as scheduled or restart *Wegovy* and follow dose escalation schedule; may reduce occurrence of GI symptoms. Advise patient to read the *Medication Guide* before starting therapy and with each Rx refill in case of changes.
- Advise patient taking insulin and semaglutide to never mix insulin and semaglutide together. Give as 2 separate injections. Both injections may be given in the same body area, but should not be given right next to each other.
- Explain to patient that this medication controls hyperglycemia but does not cure diabetes. Therapy is long-term.
- Review signs of hypoglycemia and hyperglycemia with patient. If hypoglycemia occurs, advise patient to take a glass of orange juice or 2–3 tsp of sugar, honey, or corn syrup dissolved in water and notify health care professional.
- Encourage patient to follow prescribed diet, medication, and exercise regimen to prevent hypoglycemic or hyperglycemic episodes.
- Instruct patient in proper testing of serum glucose and ketones. These tests should be closely monitored during periods of stress or illness, and health care professional should be notified if significant changes occur.
- Advise patient to notify health care professional of all Rx or OTC medications, vitamins, or herbal products being taken and consult health care professional before taking any new medications.
- Advise patient to notify health care professional and discontinue semaglutide immediately if signs of pancreatitis (nausea, vomiting, abdominal pain radiating to back), palpitations while at rest, or hypersensitivity (swelling of face, lips, tongue or throat; problems breathing or swallowing, severe rash or

S

itching, fainting or feeling dizzy, very rapid heartbeat) occur.
- Inform patient of risk of benign and malignant thyroid C-cell tumors. Advise patient to notify health care professional if symptoms of thyroid tumors (lump in neck, hoarseness, trouble swallowing, shortness of breath) occur.
- Advise patient to inform health care professional of medication regimen before treatment or surgery.
- Advise patient to carry a form of sugar (sugar packets, candy) and identification describing disease process and medication regimen at all times.
- Rep: Insulin is the preferred method of controlling blood glucose during pregnancy. Advise females of reproductive potential and males with female partners of reproductive potential to discontinue semaglutide in women at least 2 mo before a planned pregnancy to allow for long washout period of semaglutide. Counsel female patients to notify health care professional if pregnancy is planned or suspected or if breastfeeding. Inform patient of pregnancy exposure registry that monitors pregnancy outcomes in women exposed to semaglutide during pregnancy. Pregnant women exposed to semaglutide and health care professionals are encouraged to contact Novo Nordisk at 1-877-390-2760 or www.wegovypregnancyregistry.com.
- Emphasize the importance of routine follow-up exams.

Evaluation/Desired Outcomes
- Improved glycemic control.
- Reduction in risk of cardiovascular death, non-fatal MI, or non-fatal stroke.
- Reduction in body weight.

---

senna (sen-na)
Ex-Lax, Senokot
Classification
Therapeutic: laxatives
Pharmacologic: stimulant laxatives

Indications
Treatment of constipation, particularly when associated with: Slow transit time, Constipating drugs, Irritable or spastic bowel syndrome, Neurologic constipation.

Action
Active components of senna (sennosides) alter water and electrolyte transport in the large intestine, resulting in accumulation of water and increased peristalsis.
Therapeutic Effects: Laxative action.

Pharmacokinetics
Absorption: Minimally absorbed following oral administration.
Distribution: Unknown.
Metabolism and Excretion: Unknown.
Half-life: Unknown.

TIME/ACTION PROFILE (laxative effect)

ROUTE	ONSET	PEAK	DURATION
PO	6–12 hr†	unknown	3–4 days

†May take as long as 24 hr.

Contraindications/Precautions
Contraindicated in: Hypersensitivity; Abdominal pain of unknown cause, especially if associated with fever; Rectal fissures; Ulcerated hemorrhoids; Known alcohol intolerance (some liquid products).
Use Cautiously in: Chronic use (may lead to laxative dependence); Possible intestinal obstruction; OB: Other agents recommended for treatment of constipation in pregnancy (↑ risk of electrolyte abnormalities).

Adverse Reactions/Side Effects
F and E: electrolyte abnormalities (chronic use or dependence). **GI:** <u>cramping</u>, <u>diarrhea</u>, nausea. **GU:** pink-red or brown-black discoloration of urine. **Misc:** laxative dependence.

Interactions
Drug-Drug: May ↓ absorption of other **orally administered drugs** because of ↓ transit time.

Route/Dosage
Larger doses have been used to treat/prevent opioid-induced constipation. Consult labeling of individual OTC products for more specific dosing information.
PO (Adults): 17.2–50 mg 1–2 times daily.
PO (Children 12–17 yr): 17.6–26.4 mg 1–2 times daily.
PO (Children 6–11 yr): 8.8–13.2 mg 1–2 times daily.
PO (Children 2–6 yr): 4.4–6.6 mg 1–2 times daily.

Availability (generic available)
Tablets: 8.6 mg^OTC, 15 mg ^OTC, 17.2 mg^OTC, 25 mg^OTC.
Syrup: 8.8 mg/5 mL^OTC.

NURSING IMPLICATIONS
Assessment
- Assess patient for abdominal distention, presence of bowel sounds, and usual pattern of bowel function.
- Assess color, consistency, and amount of stool produced.

Implementation
- **PO:** Take with a full glass of water. Administer at bedtime for evacuation 6–12 hr later. Administer on an empty stomach for more rapid results.
- Shake oral solution well before administering.

Patient/Family Teaching
- Advise patient that laxatives should be used only for short-term therapy. Long-term therapy may cause electrolyte imbalance and dependence.
- Encourage patient to use other forms of bowel regulation, such as increasing bulk in the diet, increasing fluid intake, and increasing mobility. Normal bowel

habits are individualized and may vary from 3 times/day to 3 times/wk.
- Inform patient that this medication may cause a change in urine color to pink, red, violet, yellow, or brown.
- Instruct patients with cardiac disease to avoid straining during bowel movements (Valsalva maneuver).
- Advise patient not to use laxatives when abdominal pain, nausea, vomiting, or fever is present.
- Rep: Advise females of reproductive potential to notify health care professional if pregnancy is planned or suspected.

Evaluation/Desired Outcomes
- A soft, formed bowel movement.

---

sertaconazole, See ANTIFUNGALS (TOPICAL).

BEERS

sertraline (ser-tra-leen)
Zoloft
Classification
Therapeutic: antidepressants
Pharmacologic: selective serotonin reuptake inhibitors (SSRIs)

Indications
Major depressive disorder. Panic disorder. Obsessive-compulsive disorder (OCD). Post-traumatic stress disorder (PTSD). Social anxiety disorder (social phobia). Premenstrual dysphoric disorder. **Unlabeled Use:** Generalized anxiety disorder.

Action
Inhibits neuronal uptake of serotonin in the CNS, thus potentiating the activity of serotonin. Has little effect on norepinephrine or dopamine. **Therapeutic Effects:** Antidepressant action. Decreased incidence of panic attacks. Decreased obsessive and compulsive behavior. Decreased feelings of intense fear, helplessness, or horror. Decreased social anxiety. Decrease in premenstrual dysphoria.

Pharmacokinetics
Absorption: Appears to be well absorbed after oral administration.
Distribution: Extensively distributed throughout body tissues.
Protein Binding: 98%.
Metabolism and Excretion: Extensively metabolized by the liver; one metabolite has some antidepressant activity; 14% excreted unchanged in feces.
Half-life: 24 hr.

TIME/ACTION PROFILE (antidepressant effect)

ROUTE	ONSET	PEAK	DURATION
PO	within 2–4 wk	unknown	unknown

Contraindications/Precautions
Contraindicated in: Hypersensitivity; Concurrent use of MAO inhibitors or MAO inhibitor-like drugs (linezolid or methylene blue); Concurrent use of pimozide; Oral concentrate contains alcohol; avoid in patients with known intolerance.
Use Cautiously in: Severe renal impairment; Severe hepatic impairment; History of mania; History of suicide attempt; Angle-closure glaucoma; OB: Use during 3rd trimester may result in neonatal serotonin syndrome requiring prolonged hospitalization, respiratory and nutritional support. Use during pregnancy only if potential maternal benefit justifies potential fetal risk; Pedi: May ↑ risk of suicide attempt/ideation, especially during early treatment or dose adjustment; risk may be greater in children or adolescents; Geri: Appears on Beers list. May worsen or cause syndrome of inappropriate antidiuretic hormone (SIADH) secretion and/or hyponatremia in older adults. Use with caution in older adults and closely monitor sodium concentrations when starting therapy or ↑ dose.

Adverse Reactions/Side Effects
CV: chest pain, palpitations, QT interval prolongation, TORSADES DE POINTES. **Derm:** ↑ sweating, hot flashes, rash. **EENT:** pharyngitis, rhinitis, tinnitus, visual abnormalities. **Endo:** diabetes, SIADH. **F and E:** ↑ thirst, hyponatremia. **GI:** diarrhea, dry mouth, nausea, abdominal pain, altered taste, anorexia, constipation, dyspepsia, flatulence, vomiting. **GU:** ↓ libido, delayed/absent orgasm, ejaculatory delay/failure, erectile dysfunction, menstrual disorders, urinary disorders, urinary frequency. **Hemat:** BLEEDING. **Metab:** ↑ appetite. **MS:** back pain, myalgia. **Neuro:** dizziness, drowsiness, fatigue, headache, insomnia, tremor, agitation, anxiety, confusion, emotional lability, hypertonia, hypoesthesia, impaired concentration, manic reaction, nervousness, paresthesia, SUICIDAL THOUGHTS, twitching, weakness, yawning. **Misc:** fever.

Interactions
Drug-Drug: Serious, potentially fatal reactions (hyperthermia, rigidity, myoclonus, autonomic instability, with fluctuating vital signs and extreme agitation, which may proceed to delirium and coma) may occur with concurrent **MAO inhibitors**. MAO inhibitors should be stopped at least 14 days before sertraline therapy. Sertraline should be stopped at least 14 days before MAO inhibitor therapy. Concurrent use with **MAO-inhibitor–like drugs**, such as **linezolid** or **methylene blue**, may ↑ risk of serotonin syndrome; concurrent use contraindicated; do not start therapy in

S

✢= Canadian drug name. ⅜ = Genetic implication. S̶t̶r̶i̶k̶e̶t̶h̶r̶o̶u̶g̶h̶ = Discontinued. CAPITALS = life-threatening. <u>Underline</u> = most frequent.

patients receiving **linezolid** or **methylene blue**; if **linezolid** or **methylene blue** need to be started in a patient receiving sertraline, immediately discontinue sertraline and monitor for signs/symptoms of serotonin syndrome for 2 wk or until 24 hr after last dose of linezolid or methylene blue, whichever comes first (may resume sertraline therapy 24 hr after last dose of linezolid or methylene blue). May ↑ **pimozide** levels and the risk of QT interval prolongation and ventricular arrhythmias; concurrent use contraindicated. Drugs that affect serotonergic neurotransmitter systems, including **tricyclic antidepressants, SNRIs, fentanyl, lithium, buspirone, tramadol, meperidine, methadone, amphetamines**, and **triptans**, ↑ risk of serotonin syndrome. May ↑ sensitivity to **adrenergics** and ↑ the risk of serotonin syndrome. Concurrent use with **alcohol** is not recommended. May ↑ levels/effects of **warfarin, phenytoin, tricyclic antidepressants**, some **benzodiazepines (alprazolam)**, or **clozapine**. ↑ risk of bleeding with **NSAIDs, aspirin, clopidogrel, prasugrel, ticagrelor, dabigatran, apixaban, edoxaban, rivaroxaban**, or **warfarin**. **Cimetidine** ↑ blood levels and effects. Concurrent use of **QT interval prolonging medications** may ↑ risk of QT interval prolongation and torsades de pointes; avoid concurrent use.

Drug-Natural Products: ↑ risk of serotonergic side effects including serotonin syndrome with **St. John's wort** and **SAMe**.

Route/Dosage

Depression

PO (Adults): 50 mg once daily in the morning or evening initially; after several wk may be ↑ at weekly intervals up to 200 mg/day, depending on response.

Obsessive Compulsive Disorder

PO (Adults): 50 mg once daily in the morning or evening initially; after several wk, may be ↑ at weekly intervals up to 200 mg/day, depending on response.
PO (Children 13–17 yr): 50 mg once daily.
PO (Children 6–12 yr): 25 mg once daily.

Panic Disorder

PO (Adults): 25 mg once daily initially, may ↑ after 1 wk to 50 mg once daily.

Post-Traumatic Stress Disorder

PO (Adults): 25 mg once daily for 7 days, then ↑ to 50 mg once daily; may then be ↑ if needed at intervals of at least 7 days (range 50–200 mg once daily).

Social Anxiety Disorder

PO (Adults): 25 mg once daily initially, then 50 mg once daily; may be ↑ at weekly intervals up to 200 mg/day.

Premenstrual Dysphoric Disorder

PO (Adults): 50 mg/day initially either daily or daily during luteal phase of cycle. Daily dosing may be titrated upward in 50-mg increments at the beginning of a cycle. In luteal phase–only dosing a 50 mg/day titra-

tion step for 3 days at the beginning of each luteal phase dosing period should be used (range 50–150 mg/day).

Availability (generic available)

Tablets: 25 mg, 50 mg, 100 mg. **Capsules:** ✿ 25 mg, ✿ 50 mg, ✿ 100 mg, 150 mg, 200 mg. **Oral solution (concentrated) (contains 12% alcohol):** 20 mg/mL.

NURSING IMPLICATIONS

Assessment

- Assess for suicidal tendencies, especially during early therapy. Restrict amount of drug available to patient. Risk may be increased in children, adolescents, and adults ≤24 yr. After starting therapy, children, adolescents, and young adults should be seen by health care professional at least weekly for 4 wk, every 3 wk for next 4 wk, and on advice of health care professional thereafter.
- Monitor appetite and nutritional intake. Weigh weekly. Notify health care professional of continued weight loss. Adjust diet as tolerated to support nutritional status.
- Assess for serotonin syndrome (mental changes [agitation, hallucinations, coma], autonomic instability [tachycardia, labile BP, hyperthermia], neuromuscular aberrations [hyper-reflexia, incoordination], and/or GI symptoms [nausea, vomiting, diarrhea]), especially in patients taking other serotonergic drugs (SSRIs, SNRIs, triptans). If symptoms occur, discontinue sertraline.
- Assess sexual function before starting sertraline. Assess for changes in sexual function during treatment, including timing of onset; patient may not report.
- **Depression:** Monitor mood changes. Inform health care professional if patient demonstrates significant increase in anxiety, nervousness, or insomnia.
- Assess for suicidal tendencies, especially during early therapy. Restrict amount of drug available to patient.
- **OCD:** Assess patient for frequency of obsessive-compulsive behaviors. Note degree to which these thoughts and behaviors interfere with daily functioning.
- **Panic Attacks:** Assess frequency and severity of panic attacks.
- **PTSD:** Assess patient for feelings of fear, helplessness, and horror. Determine effect on social and occupational functioning.
- **Social Anxiety Disorder:** Assess patient for symptoms of social anxiety disorder (blushing, sweating, trembling, tachycardia during interactions with new people, people in authority, or groups) periodically during therapy.
- **Premenstrual Dysphoric Disorder:** Assess patient for symptoms of premenstrual dysphoric disorder (feeling angry, tense, or tired; crying easily, feeling sad or hopeless; arguing with family or friends for no reason; difficulty sleeping or paying attention;

feeling out of control or unable to cope; having cramping, bloating, food craving, or breast tenderness) periodically during therapy.

Lab Test Considerations
● May cause false-positive urine screening tests for benzodiazepines.
● May cause hyperglycemia and diabetes mellitus; monitor serum glucose if clinical symptoms occur.

Implementation
● Do not confuse sertraline with cetirizine or Soriatane.
● Periodically reassess dose and continued need for therapy.
● **PO:** Administer as a single dose in the morning or evening.
● For oral concentrate, use dropper provided to remove oral concentrate and mix with 4 oz (1/2 cup) of water, ginger ale, lemon/lime soda, lemonade, or orange juice ONLY. Do not mix with other liquids. Take immediately after mixing. Do not mix in advance. Slight haze may appear after mixing; this is normal. Dropper dispenser contains dry natural rubber; advise patient with latex allergy.

Patient/Family Teaching
● Instruct patient to take sertraline as directed. Take missed doses as soon as possible and return to regular dosing schedule. Do not double doses. Do not stop abruptly; may cause dysphoric mood, irritability, agitation, dizziness, sensory disturbances (paresthesias such as electric shock sensations), anxiety, confusion, headache, lethargy, emotional lability, insomnia, and hypomania.
● May cause drowsiness or dizziness. Caution patient to avoid driving and other activities requiring alertness until response to the drug is known.
● Advise patient, family, and caregivers to look for suicidality, especially during early therapy or dose changes. Notify health care professional immediately if thoughts about suicide or dying, attempts to commit suicide; new or worse depression or anxiety; agitation or restlessness; panic attacks; insomnia; new or worse irritability, aggressiveness, acting on dangerous impulses, mania, or other changes in mood or behavior or if symptoms of serotonin syndrome occur.
● Advise patient to avoid alcohol or other CNS depressant drugs during therapy and to consult with health care professional before taking other medications and to avoid alcohol or other CNS depressant drugs, including opioids, during therapy.
● Instruct patient to notify health care professional of all Rx or OTC medications, vitamins, or herbal products being taken and consult health care professional before taking any new medications, especially St. John's wort or SAMe.

● Inform patient that frequent mouth rinses, good oral hygiene, and sugarless gum or candy may minimize dry mouth. If dry mouth persists for more than 2 wk, consult health care professional regarding use of saliva substitute.
● Advise patient to wear sunscreen and protective clothing to prevent photosensitivity reactions.
● Advise patient to notify health care professional if headache, weakness, nausea, anorexia, anxiety, or insomnia persists, or if bleeding (bruising, hematoma, epistaxis, petechiae) occurs.
● Inform patient that sertraline may cause symptoms of sexual dysfunction. In males, ejaculatory delay or failure, decreased libido, and erectile dysfunction may occur. In female patients, may result in decreased libido and delayed or absent orgasm. Advise patient to notify health care professional if symptoms occur.
● Rep: Advise females of reproductive potential to notify health care professional immediately if pregnancy is planned or suspected or if breastfeeding. If used during pregnancy, should be tapered during 3rd trimester to avoid neonatal serotonin syndrome. Use in the month before delivery may increase risk of postpartum hemorrhage. Monitor infants exposed to sertraline for excess sedation, restlessness, agitation, poor feeding, poor weight gain, respiratory distress; may ↑ risk of persistent pulmonary hypertension of the newborn. Inform patient of pregnancy exposure registry that monitors pregnancy outcomes in women exposed to antidepressants during pregnancy. Register patients by calling the National Pregnancy Registry for Antidepressants at 1-866-961-2388 or visiting online at https://womensmentalhealth.org/research/pregnancyregistry/antidepressants.
● Emphasize the importance of follow-up exams to monitor progress. Encourage patient participation in psychotherapy to improve coping skills.

Evaluation/Desired Outcomes
● Increased sense of well-being.
● Renewed interest in surroundings. May require 1–4 wk of therapy to obtain antidepressant effects.
● Decrease in obsessive-compulsive behaviors.
● Decrease in frequency and severity of panic attacks.
● Decrease in symptoms of PTSD.
● Decrease in social anxiety disorder.
● Decrease in symptoms of premenstrual dysphoric disorder.

sevelamer (se-**vel**-a-mer)
Renagel, Renvela
Classification
Therapeutic: electrolyte modifiers
Pharmacologic: phosphate binders

S

Indications
Hyperphosphatemia associated with end-stage renal disease.

Action
A polymer that binds phosphate in the GI tract, preventing its absorption. **Therapeutic Effects:** Decreased serum phosphate levels and reduction in the consequences of hyperphosphatemia (ectopic calcification, secondary hyperparathyroidism with osteitis fibrosa).

Pharmacokinetics
Absorption: Not absorbed; action is local (in GI tract).
Distribution: Unknown.
Metabolism and Excretion: Eliminated in feces.
Half-life: Unknown.

TIME/ACTION PROFILE (↓ in serum phosphate concentrations)

ROUTE	ONSET	PEAK	DURATION
PO	5 days	2 wk	unknown

Contraindications/Precautions
Contraindicated in: Hypersensitivity; Hypophosphatemia; Bowel obstruction.
Use Cautiously in: Dysphagia, swallowing disorders, severe GI motility disorders, or major GI tract surgery (avoid use of tablets); OB: Not systemically absorbed; no fetal exposure expected. May ↓ levels of folate and fat-soluble minerals; consider supplementation during pregnancy; Lactation: Not systemically absorbed; no expected presence in breast milk. May ↓ levels of folate and fat-soluble minerals; consider supplementation while breastfeeding; Pedi: Safety and effectiveness not established in children <18 yr (Renagel) and children <6 yr (Renvela).

Adverse Reactions/Side Effects
GI: diarrhea, dyspepsia, vomiting, BLEEDING GI ULCER, BOWEL OBSTRUCTION/NECROSIS/PERFORATION, choking (tablet), colitis, constipation, dysphagia (tablet), ESOPHAGEAL OBSTRUCTION (tablet), flatulence, nausea, ulceration.

Interactions
Drug-Drug: May ↓ absorption of other drugs and ↓ effectiveness, especially **drugs whose efficacy is dependent on tightly controlled blood levels**. ↓ absorption of **ciprofloxacin.**

Route/Dosage
PO (Adults): 800–1600 mg 3 times daily with meals; may titrate by 800 mg every 2 wk to achieve target serum phosphorus levels.
PO (Children ≥6 yr and BSA ≥1.2 m²): *Renvela:* 1600 mg 3 times daily with meals; may titrate by 800 mg every 2 wk to achieve target serum phosphorus levels.
PO (Children ≥6 yr and BSA 0.75–<1.2 m²): *Renvela:* 800 mg 3 times daily with meals; may titrate by

400 mg every 2 wk to achieve target serum phosphorus levels.

Availability (generic available)
Powder for oral suspension: 800 mg/pkt, 2400 mg/pkt. **Tablets:** 400 mg, 800 mg.

NURSING IMPLICATIONS
Assessment
● Assess patient for GI side effects periodically during therapy.

Lab Test Considerations
● Monitor serum phosphorous, calcium, bicarbonate, and chloride levels periodically during therapy.

Implementation
● Do not confuse Renagel with Renvela.
● Doses of concurrent medications, especially antiarrhythmics, should be spaced at least 1 hr before or 3 hr after sevelamer.
● **PO:** Administer with meals. *DNC:* Do not break, chew, or crush tablets; contents expand in water.
● Use suspension for patients with swallowing disorders. Place contents of powder packet in a cup and mix thoroughly with at least 1 oz of water for the 800-mg dose or 2 oz of water for the 2400-mg dose packet. Stir mixture vigorously (it does not dissolve) and drink entire preparation within 30 min or resuspend the preparation right before drinking.

Patient/Family Teaching
● Instruct patient to take sevelamer with meals as directed and to adhere to prescribed diet.
● Caution patient to space concurrent medications at least 1 hr before or 3 hr after sevelamer.
● Advise patient to notify health care professional if GI effects (worsening of existing constipation, bloody stools) occur.
● Rep: Advise patient to notify health care professional if pregnancy is planned or suspected, or if breastfeeding. Sevelamer is not systemically absorbed, but may decrease serum levels of fat-soluble vitamins and folic acid in pregnant women. May consider supplementation.

Evaluation/Desired Outcomes
● Decrease in serum phosphorous concentration to ≤6 mg/dL. Dose adjustment is based on serum phosphorous concentrations.

---

sildenafil (sil-den-a-fil)
Liqrev, Revatio, Viagra
Classification
Therapeutic: erectile dysfunction agents, vasodilators
Pharmacologic: phosphodiesterase type 5 inhibitors

Indications

Viagra: Erectile dysfunction (ED). **Revatio and Liqrev:** Pulmonary arterial hypertension (PAH) (WHO Group I).

Action

Viagra: Enhances effects of nitric oxide released during sexual stimulation. Nitric oxide activates guanylate cyclase, which produces increased levels of cyclic guanosine monophosphate (cGMP). cGMP produces smooth muscle relaxation of the corpus cavernosum, which promotes increased blood flow and subsequent erection. cGMP also leads to vasodilation of the pulmonary vasculature. Sildenafil inhibits the enzyme phosphodiesterase type 5 (PDE5), PDE5 inactivates cGMP. *Revatio and Liqrev:* Produces vasodilation of the pulmonary vascular bed. **Therapeutic Effects:** *Viagra:* Enhanced blood flow to the corpus cavernosum and erection sufficient to allow sexual intercourse. Requires sexual stimulation. *Revatio and Liqrev:* Improved exercise tolerance (or pulmonary hemodynamics) and delayed worsening of disease.

Pharmacokinetics

Absorption: Rapidly absorbed (41%) after oral administration; IV administration results in complete bioavailability.

Distribution: Widely distributed to tissues; negligible amount in semen.

Protein Binding: 96%.

Metabolism and Excretion: Primarily metabolized by the liver via the CYP3A4 isoenzyme; one metabolite is active and accounts for 20% or more of drug effect. Metabolites excreted mostly (80%) in feces; 13% excreted in urine.

Half-life: 4 hr (for sildenafil and active metabolite).

TIME/ACTION PROFILE (vasodilation, ability to produce erection)

ROUTE	ONSET	PEAK	DURATION
PO	within 1 hr	30–120 min	up to 4 hr

Contraindications/Precautions

Contraindicated in: Hypersensitivity; Concurrent use of nitrates or riociguat; Pulmonary veno-occlusive disease.

Use Cautiously in: Serious underlying cardiovascular disease (including history of MI, stroke, or serious arrhythmia within 6 mo); cardiac failure, or coronary artery disease with unstable angina; History of HF, coronary artery disease, uncontrolled hypertension (BP >170/110 mm Hg) or hypotension (BP <90/50 mm Hg), dehydration, autonomic dysfunction, or severe left ventricular outflow obstruction; Pulmonary hypertension secondary to sickle cell anemia (may ↑ risk of vaso-occlusive crises); Concurrent treatment with antihypertensives or glipizide; Renal impairment (CCr <30

mL/min, hepatic impairment; all result in ↑ blood levels; ↓ dose required with Viagra); Anatomic penile deformity (angulation, cavernosal fibrosis, Peyronie disease); Conditions associated with priapism (sickle cell anemia, multiple myeloma, leukemia); Bleeding disorders or active peptic ulceration; History of sudden severe vision loss or at risk for non-arteritic ischemic optic neuropathy (low cup-to-disc ratio in eye, age >50 yr, diabetes, hypertension, coronary artery disease, hyperlipidemia, and smoking); may ↑ risk of recurrence; Retinitis pigmentosa; Alpha adrenergic blockers (patients should be on stable dose of alpha blockers before starting sildenafil); OB: *Revatio and Liqrev:* Use during pregnancy only if potential maternal benefit justifies potential fetal risk; Lactation: *Revatio and Liqrev:* Safety not established; Pedi: *Revatio and Liqrev:* Safety and effectiveness not established in children <18 yr (Liqrev) or <1 yr (Revatio); Geri: Older adults may have ↑ levels and may require lower doses.

Adverse Reactions/Side Effects

CV: hypotension, MI, SUDDEN DEATH, vaso-occlusive crises. **Derm:** flushing, rash. **EENT:** epistaxis, hearing loss, nasal congestion, vision loss. **GI:** dyspepsia, diarrhea. **GU:** priapism, urinary tract infection. **MS:** myalgia. **Neuro:** headache, dizziness, insomnia, paresthesia. **Misc:** HYPERSENSITIVITY REACTIONS (including anaphylaxis).

Interactions

Drug-Drug: Concurrent use of **nitrates** may cause serious, life-threatening hypotension and is contraindicated. Concurrent use of **riociguat** may result in severe hypotension; concurrent use contraindicated. **CYP3A4 inhibitors**, including **cimetidine**, **erythromycin**, **tacrolimus**, **ketoconazole**, **itraconazole**, and **protease inhibitor antiretrovirals**, including **nelfinavir** and **ritonavir**, may ↑ levels and the risk of toxicity, including hypotension (initial dose of sildenafil for ED should be ↓ to 25 mg) (concurrent use of strong CYP3A inhibitors not recommended with oral Revatio). ↑ risk of hypotension with **alpha adrenergic blockers** and acute ingestion of **alcohol**. CYP3A4 inducers, including **rifampin**, **bosentan**, **barbiturates**, **carbamazepine**, **phenytoin**, **efavirenz**, **nevirapine**, **rifampin**, or **rifabutin**, may ↓ levels and effectiveness; dose adjustments may be necessary in the treatment of PAH. May ↑ levels and the risk of toxicity of **bosentan**. Use cautiously with **glipizide**. May ↑ the risk of bleeding with **warfarin**.

Route/Dosage

Erectile Dysfunction

PO (Adults): *Viagra:* 50 mg taken 1 hr before sexual activity (range 25–100 mg taken 30 min–4 hr before sexual activity); not more than once daily; *Concurrent use of Viagra with alpha-blocker antihypertensives:*

do not use 50–100 mg dose within 4 hr of alpha blocker, 25-mg dose may be taken anytime.

PO (Geriatric Patients ≥65 yr or with concurrent enzyme inhibitors): *Viagra:* 25 mg taken 1 hr before sexual activity (range 25–100 mg taken 30 min–4 hr before sexual activity); not more than once daily.

Hepatic/Renal Impairment
PO (Adults): *Viagra:* 25 mg taken 1 hr before sexual activity (range 25–100 mg taken 30 min–4 hr before sexual activity); not more than once daily.

Pulmonary Arterial Hypertension

IV therapy is indicated for patients unable to take PO therapy
PO (Adults): *Revatio or Liqrev:* 20 mg 3 times daily; may ↑ in 20-mg increments to 80 mg 3 times daily based on clinical response and tolerability.

PO (Children ≥1 yr and >45 kg): *Revatio:* 20 mg 3 times daily; may ↑ to 40 mg 3 times daily based on clinical response and tolerability.

PO (Children ≥1 yr and 21–45 kg): *Revatio:* 20 mg 3 times daily.

PO (Children ≥1 yr and ≤20 kg): *Revatio:* 10 mg 3 times daily.

IV (Adults): *Revatio:* 10 mg 3 times daily.

Availability (generic available)
Tablets (Revatio): 20 mg. **Tablets (Viagra):** 25 mg, 50 mg, 100 mg. **Oral suspension (Revatio) (grape flavor):** 10 mg/mL. **Oral suspension (Liqrev) (strawberry flavor):** 10 mg/mL. **Solution for injection (Revatio):** 0.8 mg/mL.

NURSING IMPLICATIONS
Assessment
- **Viagra:** Determine the presence of ED before administration. Sildenafil has no effect in the absence of sexual stimulation.
- **Revatio:** Monitor hemodynamic parameters and exercise tolerance prior to and periodically during therapy.

Implementation
- Do not confuse Viagra with Allegra.
- **PO:** Dose for *ED* is usually administered 1 hr before sexual activity. May be administered 30 min–4 hr before sexual activity.
- Dose for *PAH* is administered 3 times daily without regard to food. Doses should be spaced 4–6 hr apart.
- Use syringe provided for accurate dosing of oral suspension. Shake well before using. *Revatio* oral suspension is stable for 60 days from date of reconstitution; *Liqrev* oral suspension is stable for 90 days after opening the bottle.

IV Administration
- **IV Push:** Administer undiluted. Solution is clear and colorless; do not administer solutions that are cloudy, discolored, or contain a precipitate. *Rate:* Administer as a bolus three times daily.

Patient/Family Teaching
- Instruct patient to take sildenafil as directed. For *ED,* take approximately 1 hr before sexual activity and not more than once per day. If taking sildenafil for *PAH,* take missed doses as soon as remembered unless almost time for next dose; do not double doses.
- Advise patient that *Viagra* is not indicated for use in women.
- Caution patient not to take sildenafil concurrently with alpha-adrenergic blockers (unless on a stable dose of nitrates). If chest pain occurs after taking sildenafil, instruct patient to seek immediate medical attention. Advise patient taking sildenafil for *PAH* to notify health care professional of all Rx or OTC medications, vitamins, or herbal products being taken and to consult with health care professional before taking other medications.
- Instruct patient to notify health care professional promptly if erection lasts longer than 4 hr or if experiencing sudden or decreased vision loss in 1 or both eyes or loss or decrease in hearing, ringing in the ears, or dizziness.
- Inform patient that sildenafil offers no protection against sexually transmitted diseases. Counsel patient that protection against sexually transmitted diseases and HIV infection should be considered.
- Rep: Advise females of reproductive potential to notify health care professional if pregnancy is planned or suspected or if breastfeeding.

Evaluation/Desired Outcomes
- Male erection sufficient to allow intercourse.
- Increased exercise tolerance.

silodosin (si-lo-do-sin)
Rapaflo
Classification
Therapeutic: benign prostatic hyperplasia (BPH) agents
Pharmacologic: alpha-adrenergic blockers

Indications
Benign prostatic hyperplasia (BPH).

Action
Blocks postsynaptic $alpha_1$-adrenergic receptors. Decreases contractions in the smooth muscle of the prostatic capsule. **Therapeutic Effects:** Decreased signs and symptoms of BPH (urinary urgency, hesitancy, nocturia).

Pharmacokinetics
Absorption: 32% absorbed following oral administration.
Distribution: Well distributed to tissues.
Protein Binding: 97%.
Metabolism and Excretion: Extensively metabolized by the liver by the CYP3A4 isoenzyme, UGT2B7, and other metabolic pathways; 33.5% excreted in urine and 54.9% in feces.

Half-life: 13.3 hr.

TIME/ACTION PROFILE (effect on BPH symptoms)

ROUTE	ONSET	PEAK	DURATION
PO	rapid	24 hr	24 hr*

*Following discontinuation.

Contraindications/Precautions

Contraindicated in: Hypersensitivity; Severe renal impairment (CrCl <30 mL/min); Severe hepatic impairment; Concurrent use of strong CYP3A4 inhibitors. **Use Cautiously in:** Cataract surgery (may cause intraoperative floppy iris syndrome); Moderate renal impairment (lower dose recommended); Geri: ↑ risk of orthostatic hypotension in older adults; Pedi: Safety and effectiveness not established in children.

Adverse Reactions/Side Effects

CV: orthostatic hypotension. **Derm:** pruritus, rash, urticaria. **GI:** diarrhea. **GU:** retrograde ejaculation. **Neuro:** dizziness, headache. **Misc:** allergic reactions.

Interactions

Drug-Drug: Strong CYP3A4 inhibitors, including **ketoconazole**, **clarithromycin**, **itraconazole**, and **ritonavir**, significantly ↑ levels and risk of toxicity; concurrent use contraindicated. **Moderate CYP3A4 inhibitors**, including **diltiazem**, **erythromycin**, and **verapamil**, may ↑ levels and risk of toxicity; use cautiously. Concurrent use with **antihypertensives** (including **calcium channel blockers** and **thiazide diuretics**), other **alpha blockers**, and **PDE-5 inhibitors** (including **sildenafil**, **tadalafil**, and **vardenafil**) ↑ the risk of dizziness and orthostatic hypotension. **P-glycoprotein inhibitors**, including **cyclosporine**, may ↑ levels and the risk of toxicity; concurrent use not recommended.

Route/Dosage

PO (Adults): 8 mg once daily.

Renal Impairment
PO (Adults): *CCr 30–50 mL/min:* 4 mg once daily.

Availability (generic available)

Capsules: 4 mg, 8 mg.

NURSING IMPLICATIONS

Assessment

- Assess patient for symptoms of BPH (urinary hesitancy, feeling of incomplete bladder emptying, interruption of urinary stream, impairment of size and force of urinary stream, terminal urinary dribbling, straining to start flow, frequency, dysuria, nocturia, urgency) before and periodically during therapy.
- Assess patient for orthostatic reaction and syncope. Monitor BP (lying and standing) and during initial therapy and periodically thereafter.

- Rule out prostate cancer before initiating therapy; symptoms are similar.

Implementation

- **High Alert:** Do not confuse Rapaflo with Rapamune. Do not confuse silodosin with sirolimus.
- **PO:** Administer with food at the same meal each day.
- If unable to swallow capsule, may open capsule and sprinkle powder inside on a tablespoonful of applesauce. Swallow immediately, within 5 min, without chewing; follow with 8 oz of cool water to ensure complete dose is swallowed. Use cool applesauce, soft enough to be swallowed without chewing. Do not store for future use or subdivide capsule contents.

Patient/Family Teaching

- Instruct patient to take medication as directed with the same meal each day.
- May cause dizziness. Caution patient to avoid driving or other activities requiring alertness until response to the medication is known.
- Caution patient to avoid sudden changes in position to decrease orthostatic hypotension, especially patients with low BP or concurrently taking antihypertensives. Geri: Assess risk for falls; instruct patient and family in preventing falls at home.
- Instruct patient to notify health care professional of all Rx or OTC medications, vitamins, or herbal products being taken and consult health care professional before taking any new medications, especially cough, cold, or allergy remedies.
- Instruct patient to notify health care professional of medication regimen before any surgery. Patients planning cataract surgery should notify ophthalmologist of silodosin therapy prior to surgery.
- Inform patient that silodosin may cause retrograde ejaculation (orgasm with reduced or no semen). This does not pose a safety concern and is reversible with discontinuation.
- Emphasize the importance of follow-up exams to evaluate effectiveness of medication.

Evaluation/Desired Outcomes

- Decreased symptoms of BPH.

---

simvastatin, See HMG-CoA REDUCTASE INHIBITORS (statins).

---

sirolimus (systemic)
(sir-**oh**-li-mus)
   Rapamune
Classification
Therapeutic: immunosuppressants

Indications

Prevention of organ rejection in kidney transplantation (in combination with corticosteroids and cyclosporine). Lymphangioleiomyomatosis.

Action

Inhibits T-lymphocyte activation/proliferation, which occurs as a response to antigenic and cytokine stimulation; antibody production is also inhibited. **Therapeutic Effects:** Decreased incidence and severity of organ rejection. Improvement in pulmonary function in lymphangioleiomyomatosis.

Pharmacokinetics

Absorption: 14% absorbed following oral administration.

Distribution: Concentrates in erythrocytes; distributes to heart, intestines, kidneys, liver, lungs, muscle, spleen, and testes in high concentrations.

Protein Binding: 92%.

Metabolism and Excretion: Extensively metabolized in the liver via the CYP3A4 isoenzyme; 91% excreted in feces.

Half-life: 62 hr.

TIME/ACTION PROFILE (plasma concentrations)

ROUTE	ONSET	PEAK	DURATION
PO	rapid	1–2 hr	24 hr

Contraindications/Precautions

Contraindicated in: Hypersensitivity; Alcohol intolerance/sensitivity (solution contains ethanol); Severe hepatic impairment; OB: Pregnancy.

Use Cautiously in: Mild or moderate hepatic impairment; Lactation: Use while breastfeeding only if the potential maternal benefit justifies the potential risk to the infant; Rep: Women of reproductive potential; Pedi: Children <13 yr (safety and effectiveness not established).

Adverse Reactions/Side Effects

Reflects combined therapy with corticosteroids and cyclosporine.

CV: edema, hypotension, pericardial effusion. **Derm:** acne, rash, ↓ wound healing, thrombocytopenic purpura. **Endo:** hyperglycemia. **F and E:** hypokalemia. **GI:** ascites, hepatotoxicity. **GU:** amenorrhea, infertility (males), menorrhagia, ovarian cysts, renal impairment. **Hemat:** leukopenia, thrombocytopenia, anemia. **Metab:** hypercholesterolemia, hypertriglyceridemia. **MS:** arthralgia. **Neuro:** insomnia, tremor, PROGRESSIVE MULTIFOCAL LEUKOENCEPHALOPATHY (PML). **Resp:** INTERSTITIAL LUNG DISEASE, PULMONARY HYPERTENSION. **Misc:** ANGIOEDEMA, INFECTION (including activation of latent viral infections such as BK virus-associated nephropathy and *Clostridioides difficile*-associated diarrhea), lymphocele, LYMPHOMA.

Interactions

Drug-Drug: Cyclosporine (modified) significantly ↑ levels and the risk of toxicity; administer sirolimus 4 hr after cyclosporine. **Strong CYP3A4 inhibitors,** including **ketoconazole, voriconazole, itraconazole, clarithromycin,** and **erythromycin,** may ↑ levels and the risk of toxicity; avoid concurrent use. **Diltiazem, verapamil, nicardipine, clotrimazole, fluconazole, metoclopramide, cimetidine, danazol, letermovir,** and **protease inhibitors** may ↑ levels and the risk of toxicity; monitor sirolimus levels and adjust dose as necessary. **Strong CYP3A4 inducers,** including **rifampin** and **rifabutin,** may ↓ levels and effectiveness; avoid concurrent use. **Carbamazepine, phenobarbital, phenytoin,** and **rifapentine** may ↓ levels and effectiveness. Risk of renal impairment may be ↑ by concurrent use of other **nephrotoxic agents.** Concurrent use with **tacrolimus** and **corticosteroids** in lung transplantation may ↑ risk of anastomotic dehiscence; fatalities have been reported (not approved for this use). Concurrent use with **tacrolimus** and **corticosteroids** in liver transplantation may ↑ risk of hepatic artery thrombosis; fatalities have been reported (not approved for this use). Concurrent use with **ACE inhibitors** may ↑ risk of angioedema. May ↓ antibody response to and ↑ risk of adverse reactions to **live-virus vaccines;** avoid vaccination. May ↑ **verapamil** levels and the risk of toxicity. **Cannabidiol** may ↑ levels and the risk of toxicity; monitor sirolimus levels and adjust dose as necessary.

Drug-Natural Products: Concomitant use with **echinacea** and **melatonin** may interfere with immunosuppression. **St. John's wort** may ↓ levels and effectiveness.

Drug-Food: Grapefruit juice may ↑ levels and the risk of toxicity; avoid concurrent ingestion.

Route/Dosage

Kidney Transplantation

PO (Adults and Children ≥13 yr): 6 mg loading dose, followed by 2 mg/day maintenance dose. *Dosing following cyclosporine withdrawal:* Patients at low to moderate risk for rejection after transplantation may be withdrawn from cyclosporine over 4–8 wk beginning 2–4 mo after transplant. Thereafter, sirolimus dose should be titrated upward to maintain a whole blood trough level of 12–14 ng/mL. Clinical assessment should also be used to gauge dose. Dose changes can be made at 7–14 day intervals. The following formula may also be used: sirolimus maintenance dose = current dose × (target concentration/current concentration). If a large ↑ is needed, a loading dose may be given and blood levels reassessed 3–4 days later. Loading dose may be calculated by the following formula: sirolimus loading dose = 3 × (new maintenance dose-current maintenance dose). Loading doses >40 mg should be spread over 2 days.

PO (Adults and Children ≥13 yr and <40 kg): 3 mg/m² loading dose, followed by 1 mg/m²/day maintenance dose. *See adjustments above for doses following cyclosporine withdrawal.*

Hepatic Impairment

PO (Adults and Children): *Mild or moderate hepatic impairment:* ↓ maintenance dose by 33%; loading dose is unchanged; *Severe hepatic impairment:* ↓ maintenance dose by 50%; loading dose is unchanged.

Lymphangioleiomyomatosis

PO (Adults): 2 mg once daily. Monitor whole blood trough level in 10–20 days and titrate dose to maintain level of 5–15 ng/mL. The following formula may also be used to adjust dose: sirolimus maintenance dose = current dose × (target concentration/current concentration). Further dose changes can be made at 7–14 day intervals. Once stable dose achieved, should monitor whole blood trough levels at least every 3 mo.

Hepatic Impairment

(Adults): *Mild or moderate hepatic impairment:* ↓ dose by 33%; *Severe hepatic impairment:* ↓ dose by 50%.

Availability (generic available)

Oral solution (contains alcohol): 1 mg/mL. **Tablet:** 0.5 mg, 1 mg, 2 mg.

NURSING IMPLICATIONS

Assessment

- Monitor BP closely during therapy. Hypertension is a common complication of sirolimus therapy and should be treated.
- Assess for any new signs or symptoms that may be suggestive of PML, an opportunistic infection of the brain that leads to death or severe disability; withhold dose and notify health care professional promptly. Symptoms of PML may include hemiparesis, apathy, confusion, cognitive deficiencies, and ataxia. Consider decreasing the amount of immunosuppression in these patients.
- **Lymphangioleiomyomatosis:** Monitor for signs and symptoms of lymphangioleiomyomatosis (wheezing; cough, which may be bloody; shortness of breath; chest pain; pneumothorax) periodically during therapy.

Lab Test Considerations

- Monitor sirolimus blood levels when dose forms are changed and in patients likely to have altered drug metabolism, patients ≥13 yr who weigh <40 kg, patients with hepatic impairment, and during concurrent administration of drugs that may interact with sirolimus. Trough concentrations of ≥15 ng/mL are associated with an ↑ in adverse effects.
- Monitor patients for hyperlipidemia. May require additional interventions to treat hyperlipidemia.
- May cause anemia, leukopenia, thrombocytopenia, and hypokalemia.

- May cause ↑ AST, ↑ ALT, hypophosphatemia, and hyperglycemia.

Implementation

- Therapy with sirolimus should be started as soon as possible post-transplant. Concurrent therapy with cyclosporine and corticosteroids is recommended. Sirolimus should be taken 4 hr after cyclosporine (Modified, Neoral).
- Sirolimus should be ordered only by health care professionals skilled in immunosuppressive therapy, with the staff and facilities to manage renal transplant patients.
- **PO:** Administer consistently with or without food. *DNC:* Swallow tablet whole; do not crush, break, or chew. Do not administer with or mix with grapefruit juice.
- To dilute from bottle, use amber oral dose syringe to withdraw prescribed amount. Empty sirolimus from syringe into a glass or plastic container holding at least 2 oz (60 mL) of water or orange juice; do not use other liquids. Stir vigorously and drink at once. Refill container with at least 4 oz of additional liquid, stir vigorously, and drink at once.
- Store bottles in refrigerator. Protect from light. Solution may develop a slight haze when refrigerated; allow to stand at room temperature and shake gently until haze disappears. Sirolimus may remain in syringe at room temperature or refrigerated for up to 24 hr. Discard syringe after 1 use. Oral solution must be used within 1 mo of opening bottle.

Patient/Family Teaching

- Instruct patient to take sirolimus at the same time each day, as directed. Advise patient to avoid taking with or diluting with grapefruit juice. Do not skip or double up on missed doses. Do not discontinue medication without advice of health care professional.
- Advise patient to avoid grapefruit and grapefruit juice during therapy.
- Reinforce the need for lifelong therapy to prevent transplant rejection. Review symptoms of rejection for transplanted organ and stress need to notify health care professional immediately if they occur.
- Advise patient to notify health care professional if swelling of your face, eyes, or mouth; trouble breathing or wheezing; throat tightness; chest pain or tightness; feeling dizzy or faint; rash or peeling of skin; swelling of hands or feet; or symptoms of PML occur.
- Advise patient to wear sunscreen and protective clothing and limit time in sunlight and UV light due to increased risk of skin cancer.
- Caution patient to notify health care professional if signs of infection occur.

- Advise patient to avoid vaccinations with a live virus during therapy; sirolimus may decrease vaccine effectiveness.
- Rep: May cause fetal harm. Advise females of reproductive potential of the risk of taking sirolimus during pregnancy. Caution women of reproductive potential to use effective contraception prior to, during, and for 12 wk following therapy. May cause male and female infertility.
- Emphasize the importance of repeated lab tests during sirolimus therapy.

Evaluation/Desired Outcomes

- Prevention of transplanted kidney rejection.
- Reduction in symptoms of lymphangioleiomyomatosis.

SITagliptin (sit-a-glip-tin)
Januvia
Classification
Therapeutic: antidiabetics
Pharmacologic: enzyme inhibitors

Indications
Type 2 diabetes mellitus (as an adjunct to diet and exercise).

Action
Inhibits the enzyme dipeptidyl peptidase-4 (DPP-4), which slows the inactivation of incretin hormones, resulting in increased levels of active incretin hormones. These hormones are released by the intestine throughout the day and are involved in regulation of glucose homeostasis. Increased/prolonged incretin levels result in an increase in insulin release and decrease in glucagon levels. **Therapeutic Effects:** Improved control of blood glucose.

Pharmacokinetics
Absorption: 87% absorbed following oral administration.
Distribution: Extensively distributed to tissues.
Metabolism and Excretion: Undergoes minor metabolism by the liver via the CYP3A4 and CYP2C8 isoenzymes to inactive metabolites; 87% excreted in the urine (79% as unchanged drug), with 13% excreted in the feces.
Half-life: 12.4 hr.

TIME/ACTION PROFILE (plasma concentrations)

ROUTE	ONSET	PEAK	DURATION
PO	rapid	1–4 hr	24 hr

Contraindications/Precautions
Contraindicated in: Hypersensitivity; Type 1 diabetes mellitus.
Use Cautiously in: Renal impairment (↓ dose for CCr <45 mL/min); History of pancreatitis; History of

angioedema to another DPP-4 inhibitor; History of HF or renal impairment (↑ risk of HF); OB: Safety not established in pregnancy; Lactation: Safety not established in breastfeeding; Pedi: Safety and effectiveness not established in children; Geri: Consider age-related ↓ in renal function when determining dose in older adults.

Adverse Reactions/Side Effects
CV: HF. **Derm:** bullous pemphigoid, rash, STEVENS-JOHNSON SYNDROME (SJS), urticaria. **EENT:** nasopharyngitis. **GI:** diarrhea, nausea, PANCREATITIS. **GU:** acute renal failure. **MS:** arthralgia, back pain, myalgia, RHABDOMYOLYSIS. **Neuro:** headache. **Resp:** upper respiratory tract infection. **Misc:** HYPERSENSITIVITY REACTIONS (including anaphylaxis and angioedema).

Interactions
Drug-Drug: May slightly ↑ levels of **digoxin**; monitoring recommended. ↑ risk of hypoglycemia when used with **insulin**, **glyburide**, **glipizide**, or **glimepiride**; may need to ↓ dose of insulin or sulfonylurea.

Route/Dosage
PO (Adults): 100 mg once daily.
Renal Impairment
PO (Adults): *CCr 30– <45 mL/min:* 50 mg once daily; *CCr <30 mL/min, hemodialysis, or peritoneal dialysis:* 25 mg once daily.

Availability
Tablets: 25 mg, 50 mg, 100 mg. *In combination with:* ertugliflozin (Steglujan); metformin (Janumet); metformin XR (Janumet XR). See Appendix N.

NURSING IMPLICATIONS
Assessment

- Observe patient for signs and symptoms of hypoglycemic reactions (abdominal pain, sweating, hunger, weakness, dizziness, headache, tremor, tachycardia, anxiety).
- Monitor for signs of pancreatitis (nausea, vomiting, anorexia, persistent severe abdominal pain, sometimes radiating to the back) during therapy. If pancreatitis occurs, discontinue sitagliptin and monitor serum and urine amylase, amylase/CCr ratio, electrolytes, serum calcium, glucose, and lipase.
- Assess for rash periodically during therapy. May cause SJS. Discontinue therapy if severe or if accompanied with fever, general malaise, fatigue, muscle or joint aches, blisters, oral lesions, conjunctivitis, hepatitis, and/or eosinophilia.

Lab Test Considerations
- Monitor hemoglobin A1C prior to and periodically during therapy.
- Monitor renal function prior to and periodically during therapy.

Implementation
- Do not confuse sitagliptin with saxagliptin or sumatriptan. Do not confuse Januvia with Jantoven or Janumet.

- Patients stabilized on a diabetic regimen who are exposed to stress, fever, trauma, infection, or surgery may require administration of insulin.
- **PO:** May be administered once daily without regard to food.

Patient/Family Teaching

- Instruct patient to take sitagliptin as directed. Take missed doses as soon as remembered, unless it is almost time for next dose; do not double doses. Advise patient to read the *Medication Guide* before starting and with each Rx refill in case of changes.
- Explain to patient that sitagliptin helps control hyperglycemia but does not cure diabetes. Therapy is usually long term.
- Instruct patient not to share this medication with others, even if they have the same symptoms; it may harm them.
- Encourage patient to follow prescribed diet, medication, and exercise regimen to prevent hyperglycemic or hypoglycemic episodes.
- Review signs of hypoglycemia and hyperglycemia with patient. If hypoglycemia occurs, advise patient to take a glass of orange juice or 2–3 tsp of sugar, honey, or corn syrup dissolved in water, and notify health care professional.
- Instruct patient in proper testing of blood glucose and urine ketones. These tests should be monitored closely during periods of stress or illness and health care professional notified if significant changes occur.
- Advise patient to stop taking sitagliptin and notify health care professional promptly if symptoms of hypersensitivity reactions (rash; hives; swelling of face, lips, tongue, and throat; difficulty in breathing or swallowing) or pancreatitis occur.
- Advise patient to notify health care professional of all Rx or OTC medications, vitamins, or herbal products being taken and to consult with health care professional before taking other medications.
- Rep: Advise females with reproductive potential to notify health care professional if pregnancy is planned or suspected, or if breastfeeding.

Evaluation/Desired Outcomes

- Improved hemoglobin A1C, fasting plasma glucose and 2-hr postprandial glucose levels.

---

sodium bicarbonate
(**soe**-dee-um bye-**kar**-boe-nate)
Classification
Therapeutic: antiulcer agents
Pharmacologic: alkalinizing agents

Indications

PO, IV: Management of metabolic acidosis. **PO, IV:** Used to alkalinize urine and promote excretion of cer-

tain drugs in overdosage situations (phenobarbital, aspirin). **PO:** Antacid. **Unlabeled Use:** Stabilization of acid-base status in cardiac arrest and treatment of life-threatening hyperkalemia.

Action

Acts as an alkalinizing agent by releasing bicarbonate ions. Following oral administration, releases bicarbonate, which is capable of neutralizing gastric acid. **Therapeutic Effects:** Alkalinization. Neutralization of gastric acid.

Pharmacokinetics

Absorption: Following oral administration, excess bicarbonate is absorbed and results in metabolic alkalosis and alkaline urine. IV administration results in complete bioavailability.

Distribution: Widely distributed into extracellular fluid.

Metabolism and Excretion: Sodium and bicarbonate are excreted by the kidneys.

Half-life: Unknown.

TIME/ACTION PROFILE (PO = antacid effect; IV = alkalinization)

ROUTE	ONSET	PEAK	DURATION
PO	immediate	30 min	1–3 hr
IV	immediate	rapid	unknown

Contraindications/Precautions

Contraindicated in: Metabolic or respiratory alkalosis; Hypocalcemia; Hypernatremia; Excessive chloride loss; As an antidote following ingestion of strong mineral acids; Patients on sodium-restricted diets (oral use as an antacid only); Renal failure (oral use as an antacid only); Severe abdominal pain of unknown cause, especially if associated with fever (oral use as an antacid only).

Use Cautiously in: HF; Renal impairment; Concurrent corticosteroid therapy; Chronic use as an antacid (may cause metabolic alkalosis and possible sodium overload); Pedi: May ↑ risk of cerebral edema in children with diabetic ketoacidosis.

Adverse Reactions/Side Effects

CV: edema. **F and E:** metabolic alkalosis, hypernatremia, hypocalcemia, hypokalemia. **GI:** *PO:* flatulence, gastric distention. **Local:** irritation at IV site. **Neuro:** cerebral hemorrhage (with rapid injection in infants), tetany.

Interactions

Drug-Drug: Following oral administration, may ↓ absorption of **ketoconazole**. Concurrent use with **calcium-containing antacids** may lead to milk-alkali syndrome. Urinary alkalinization may result in ↓ **salicylate** or **barbiturate** blood levels; ↑ blood levels of **quinidine, mexiletine, flecainide,** or **ampheta-**

S

mines; ↑ risk of crystalluria from **fluoroquinolones**; ↓ effectiveness of **methenamine**. May negate the protective effects of **enteric-coated products** (do not administer within 1–2 hr of each other).

Route/Dosage
Contains 12 mEq of sodium/g.

Alkalinization of Urine
PO (Adults): 48 mEq (4 g) initially, then 12–24 mEq (1–2 g) every 4 hr (up to 48 mEq every 4 hr) or 1 tsp of powder every 4 hr as needed.
PO (Children): 1–10 mEq/kg/day (84–840 mg/kg/day) in divided doses.
IV (Adults and Children): 2–5 mEq/kg as a 4–8-hr infusion.

Antacid
PO (Adults): *Tablets/powder:* 325 mg–2 g 1–4 times daily or ½ tsp every 2 hr as needed. *Effervescent powder:* 3.9–10 g in water after meals; patients >60 yr should receive 1.9–3.9 g after meals.

Systemic Alkalinization/Cardiac Arrest
IV (Adults and Children and Infants): *Cardiac arrest/urgent situations:* 1 mEq/kg; may repeat 0.5 mEq/kg every 10 min. *Less urgent situations:* 2–5 mEq/kg as a 4–8-hr infusion.

Renal Tubular Acidosis
PO (Adults): 0.5–2 mEq/kg/day in 4–5 divided doses.
PO (Children): 2–3 mEq/kg/day in 3–4 divided doses.

Availability (generic available)
Oral powder: (20.9 mEq Na/½ tsp) in 120-, 240-, 480-, and 2400-g containers^OTC. **Tablets:** 325 mg (3.9 mEq Na/tablet)^OTC, ❖ 500 mg (6.0 mEq Na/tablet^OTC, 650 mg (7.7 mEq Na/tablet)^OTC. **Solution for injection:** 4.2% (0.5 mEq/mL), 8.4% (1 mEq/mL).

NURSING IMPLICATIONS

Assessment
- **IV:** Assess fluid balance (intake and output, daily weight, edema, lung sounds) throughout therapy. Report symptoms of fluid overload (hypertension, edema, dyspnea, rales/crackles, frothy sputum) if they occur.
- Assess patient for signs of acidosis (disorientation, headache, weakness, dyspnea, hyperventilation), alkalosis (confusion, irritability, paresthesia, tetany, altered breathing pattern), hypernatremia (edema, weight gain, hypertension, tachycardia, fever, flushed skin, mental irritability), or hypokalemia (weakness, fatigue, U wave on ECG, arrhythmias, polyuria, polydipsia) throughout therapy.
- Observe IV site closely. Avoid extravasation, as tissue irritation or cellulitis may occur. If infiltration occurs, confer with physician or other health care professional regarding warm compresses and infiltration of site with lidocaine or hyaluronidase.

- **Antacid:** Assess patient for epigastric or abdominal pain and frank or occult blood in the stool, emesis, or gastric aspirate.

Lab Test Considerations
- Monitor serum sodium, potassium, calcium, bicarbonate concentrations, serum osmolarity, acid-base balance, and renal function prior to and periodically throughout therapy.
- Obtain arterial blood gases frequently in emergency situations and during parenteral therapy.
- Monitor urine pH frequently when used for urinary alkalinization.
- Antagonizes effects of pentagastrin and histamine during gastric acid secretion test. Avoid administration during the 24 hr preceding the test.

Implementation
- This medication may cause premature dissolution of enteric-coated tablets in the stomach.
- **PO:** Tablets must be taken with a full glass of water.
- When used in treatment of peptic ulcers, may be administered 1 and 3 hr after meals and at bedtime.

IV Administration
- **IV Push:** Used in cardiac arrest or urgent situations. *Dilution:* Use premeasured ampules or prefilled syringes to ensure accurate dose. *Rate:* Administer by rapid bolus. Flush IV line before and after administration to prevent incompatible medications used in arrest management from precipitating.
- **Continuous Infusion:** *Dilution:* May be diluted in dextrose, saline, and dextrose/saline combinations. Premixed infusions are already diluted and ready to use. *Rate:* May be administered over 4–8 hr.
- **Y-Site Compatibility:** acyclovir, amifostine, amikacin, aminophylline, asparaginase, atropine, aztreonam, bivalirudin, bumetanide, cefazolin, cefepime, ceftazidime, ceftriaxone, chloramphenicol, cimetidine, cladribine, clindamycin, cyclophosphamide, cyclosporine, cytarabine, daptomycin, daunorubicin hydrochloride, dexamethasone, dexmedetomidine, digoxin, docetaxel, doxorubicin hydrochloride, enalaprilat, ertapenem, erythromycin, esmolol, etoposide, etoposide phosphate, famotidine, fentanyl, filgrastim, fluconazole, fludarabine, furosemide, gemcitabine, gentamicin, granisetron, heparin, hydrocortisone, ifosfamide, indomethacin, insulin regular, ketorolac, labetalol, levofloxacin, lidocaine, linezolid, lorazepam, magnesium sulfate, melphalan, mesna, methylprednisolone, metoclopramide, metoprolol, metronidazole, milrinone, morphine, nafcillin, nitroglycerin, nitroprusside, paclitaxel, palonosetron, pantoprazole, pemetrexed, penicillin G potassium, phenylephrine, phytonadione, piperacillin/tazobactam, potassium chloride, procainamide, propranolol, propofol, protamine, remifentanil, tacrolimus, thiotepa, tirofiban, tobramycin, vasopressin, voriconazole.

- **Y-Site Incompatibility:** allopurinol, amiodarone, amphotericin B, ampicillin, anidulafungin, calcium chloride, calcium gluconate, caspofungin, cefotaxime, cefoxitin, cefuroxime, diazepam, diphenhydramine, dobutamine, doxorubicin liposomal, doxycycline, epinephrine, ganciclovir, haloperidol, hydroxyzine, idarubicin, imipenem/cilastatin, isoproterenol, lansoprazole, leucovorin, meperidine, midazolam, nalbuphine, norepinephrine, ondansetron, phenytoin, prochlorperazine, promethazine, sargramostim, trimethoprim/sulfamethoxazole, verapamil, vincristine, vinorelbine.
- **Solution Incompatibility:** Do not add to LR or Ionosol products, as compatibility varies with concentration.

Patient/Family Teaching

- Instruct patient to take medication as directed. Take missed doses as soon as remembered unless almost time for next dose.
- Review symptoms of electrolyte imbalance with patients on chronic therapy; instruct patient to notify health care professional if these symptoms occur.
- Advise patient not to take milk products concurrently with this medication. Renal calculi or hypercalcemia (milk-alkali syndrome) may result.
- Emphasize the importance of regular follow-up examinations to monitor serum electrolyte levels and acid-base balance and to monitor progress.
- **Antacid:** Advise patient to avoid routine use of sodium bicarbonate for indigestion. Dyspepsia that persists >2 wk should be evaluated by a health care professional.
- Advise patient on sodium-restricted diet to avoid use of baking soda as a home remedy for indigestion.
- Instruct patient to notify health care professional if indigestion is accompanied by chest pain, difficulty breathing, or diaphoresis or if stools become dark and tarry.

Evaluation/Desired Outcomes

- Increase in urinary pH.
- Clinical improvement of acidosis.
- Enhanced excretion of selected overdoses and poisonings.
- Decreased gastric discomfort.

---

sodium phenylbutyrate/ taurursodiol

(**sow**-dee-um fen-il-**byoo**-ti-rate/ taur-**ur**-so-**dye**-ol)
   Relyvrio
   Classification
Therapeutic: agents for amyotrophic lateral sclerosis, none assigned
Pharmacologic: histone deacetylase inhibitors, bile acid replacements

---

Indications
Amyotrophic lateral sclerosis (ALS).

Action
Sodium phenylbutyrate: Acts as a histone deacetylase inhibitor. Its mechanism of benefit in ALS is unknown. *Taurursodiol:* A bile acid. Its mechanism of benefit in ALS is unknown. **Therapeutic Effects:** Slowed decline in motor, bulbar, and respiratory function.

Pharmacokinetics
Absorption: Extent of absorption following oral administration unknown. High-fat meal decreases absorption of sodium phenylbutyrate.
Distribution: Unknown.
Protein Binding: *Sodium phenylbutyrate:* 82%; *Taurursodiol:* 98%.
Metabolism and Excretion: Sodium phenylbutyrate is metabolized in the liver and kidney. Taurursodiol undergoes enterohepatic recirculation. Sodium phenylbutyrate primarily (80–100%) excreted in urine as a metabolite. Excretion pathway of taurursodiol unknown.
Half-life: *Sodium phenylbutyrate:* 0.46 hr; *Taurursodiol:* 4.3 hr.

TIME/ACTION PROFILE (plasma concentrations)

ROUTE	ONSET	PEAK	DURATION
Sodium phenylbutyrate (PO)	unknown	30 min	unknown
Taurursodiol (PO)	unknown	4.5 hr	unknown

Contraindications/Precautions
Contraindicated in: Moderate or severe renal impairment; Moderate or severe hepatic impairment.
Use Cautiously in: Biliary disorders (↑ risk of diarrhea); Pancreatic disorders, intestinal malabsorption, or intestinal disorders (may cause ↓ absorption); HF, renal disease, or hypertension (↑ sodium content); OB: Safety not established in pregnancy; Lactation: Safety not established in breastfeeding; Pedi: Safety and effectiveness not established in children.

Adverse Reactions/Side Effects
GI: ↑ salivation, abdominal pain, diarrhea, nausea. **Neuro:** dizziness, fatigue. **Resp:** upper respiratory tract infection.

Interactions
Drug-Drug: Absorption may be ↓ by **bile acid sequestrants**, including **cholestyramine, colesevelam,** and **colestipol,** as well as **aluminum-based antacids**; avoid concurrent use. **Bile salt export pump inhibitors,** including **cyclosporine** may ↑

S

levels and risk of toxicity; avoid concurrent use. **Probenecid** may ↑ levels of active metabolite and risk of toxicity; avoid concurrent use. **Histone deacetylase inhibitors**, including **belinostat**, **romidepsin**, and **vorinostat** may ↑ risk of toxicity; avoid concurrent use. **OATP1B3 inhibitors** may ↑ risk of toxicity; avoid concurrent use.

Route/Dosage
PO (Adults): 1 packet once daily for 3 wks, then 1 packet twice daily thereafter.

Availability
Powder for oral suspension: sodium phenylbutyrate 3 g and taurursodiol 1 g/packet.

NURSING IMPLICATIONS

Assessment
● Assess symptoms of ALS before starting and periodically during therapy.

Implementation
● **PO:** Administer *Relyvrio* before a snack or meal. Empty contents of packet in a cup containing 8 oz of room temperature water and stir vigorously. Take orally or administer via feeding tube within 1 hr of preparation. Reconstituted suspension may be stored for up to 1 hr at room temperature. Discard any unused suspension after 1 hr.

Patient/Family Teaching
● Instruct patient and caregiver to take *Relyvrio* as directed. Advise patient to read *Patient Information* before starting therapy and with each Rx refill in case of changes.
● Advise patient to notify their health care professional if they have new or worsening diarrhea.
● Inform patient that 2 packets of *Relyvrio* contain 928 mg sodium. Advise patient to limit sodium intake if they are sensitive to sodium (HF, severe renal insufficiency, or other conditions associated with sodium retention) should limit their sodium intake.
● Inform patient to avoid aluminum-based antacids during therapy; may interfere with the absorption of *Relyvrio*.
● Advise patient to monitor for diarrhea; notify health care professional if diarrhea becomes severe.
● Instruct patient to notify health care professional of all Rx or OTC medications, vitamins, or herbal products being taken and to consult health care professional before taking any other Rx, OTC, or herbal products.
● Rep: Advise females of reproductive potential to notify health care professional if pregnancy is planned or suspected or if breastfeeding.

Evaluation/Desired Outcomes
● Slowed decline in motor, bulbar, and respiratory function.

sodium polystyrene sulfonate
(soe-dee-um po-lee-stye-reen sul-fon-ate)
❋ Kayexalate, SPS
Classification
Therapeutic: hypokalemic, electrolyte modifiers
Pharmacologic: cationic exchange resins

Indications
Mild to moderate hyperkalemia (if severe, more immediate measures such as sodium bicarbonate IV, calcium, or glucose/insulin infusion should be instituted).

Action
Exchanges sodium ions for potassium ions in the intestine (each 1 g is exchanged for 1 mEq potassium). **Therapeutic Effects:** Reduction of serum potassium concentrations.

Pharmacokinetics
Absorption: Distributed throughout the intestine but is nonabsorbable.
Distribution: Not distributed.
Metabolism and Excretion: Eliminated in the feces.
Half-life: Unknown.

TIME/ACTION PROFILE (decrease in serum potassium concentrations)

ROUTE	ONSET	PEAK	DURATION
PO	2–12 hr	unknown	6–24 hr
Rectal	2–12 hr	unknown	4–6 hr

Contraindications/Precautions
Contraindicated in: Life-threatening hyperkalemia (other, more immediate measures should be instituted); Hypersensitivity to saccharin or parabens (some products); Ileus; Abnormal bowel function (↑ risk for intestinal necrosis); Postoperative patients with no bowel movement (↑ risk for intestinal necrosis); History of impaction, chronic constipation, inflammatory bowel disease, ischemic colitis, vascular intestinal atherosclerosis, previous bowel resection, or bowel obstruction (↑ risk for intestinal necrosis); Known alcohol intolerance (suspension only).
Use Cautiously in: HF; Hypertension; Edema; Sodium restriction; Constipation.

Adverse Reactions/Side Effects
CV: edema. **F and E:** hypocalcemia, hypokalemia, hypomagnesemia. **GI:** constipation, fecal impaction, anorexia, gastric irritation, INTESTINAL NECROSIS, ischemic colitis, nausea, vomiting.

Interactions
Drug-Drug: May ↓ absorption of any other orally administered medication; administer sodium polystyrene sulfonate ≥3 hr before or after other oral medications (≥6 hr for patients with gastroparesis). Administration

with **calcium** or **magnesium-containing antacids** may ↓ resin-exchanging ability and ↑ risk of systemic alkalosis. Hypokalemia may enhance **digoxin** toxicity. Use with **sorbitol** may ↑ risk of colonic necrosis; concurrent use not recommended.

Route/Dosage
4 level tsp = 15 g (4.1 mEq sodium/g).
PO (Adults): 15 g 1–4 times daily in water (up to 40 g 4 times daily).
Rect (Adults): 30–50 g as a retention enema; repeat as needed every 6 hr.
PO, Rect (Children): 1 g/kg/dose every 6 hr.

Availability (generic available)
Oral suspension: 15 g sodium polystyrene sulfonate with 20 g sorbitol/60 mL, 15 g sodium polystyrene sulfonate with 14.1 g sorbitol/60 mL. **Powder for suspension:** 15 g/bottle, 454 g/bottle.

NURSING IMPLICATIONS
Assessment
● Monitor response of symptoms of hyperkalemia (fatigue, muscle weakness, paresthesia, confusion, dyspnea, peaked T waves, depressed ST segments, prolonged QT segments, widened QRS complexes, loss of P waves, and cardiac arrhythmias). Assess for development of hypokalemia (weakness, fatigue, arrhythmias, flat or inverted T waves, prominent U waves).
● Monitor intake and output ratios and daily weight. Assess for symptoms of fluid overload (dyspnea, rales/crackles, jugular venous distention, peripheral edema). Concurrent low-sodium diet may be ordered for patients with HF (see Appendix J).
● In patients receiving concurrent digoxin, assess for symptoms of digoxin toxicity (anorexia, nausea, vomiting, visual disturbances, arrhythmias).
● Assess abdomen and note character and frequency of stools. Discontinue sodium polystyrene sulfonate if patient becomes constipated. Concurrent sorbitol or laxatives may be ordered to prevent constipation or impaction. Some products contain sorbitol to prevent constipation. Patient should ideally have 1–2 watery stools each day during therapy. Monitor for intestinal necrosis if sorbitol is added.

Lab Test Considerations
● Monitor serum potassium daily during therapy. Notify health care professional when potassium ↓ to 4–5 mEq/L.
● Monitor renal function and electrolytes (especially sodium, calcium, bicarbonate, and magnesium) prior to and periodically throughout therapy.

Implementation
● Consult health care professional regarding discontinuation of medications that may increase serum

potassium (angiotensin-converting enzyme inhibitors, potassium-sparing diuretics, potassium supplements, salt substitutes).
● Administer PO doses at least 3 hr before or 3 hr after other medications (patients with gastroparesis may require a 6-hr separation).
● An osmotic laxative (sorbitol) is usually administered concurrently to prevent constipation.
● **PO:** For oral or nasogastric tube administration, shake commercially available suspension well before use. Solution is stable for 24 hr when refrigerated. When using powder, add prescribed amount to 3–4 mL water/g of powder. Shake well. Do not mix in orange juice or in any fruit juice known to contain potassium. Do not heat solution to enhance dissolution of powder; heating impairs exchange resin properties. Chilling and adding syrup may improve palatability. May also be added to food. Resin cookie or candy recipes are available; discuss with pharmacist or dietitian.
● **Retention Enema:** Precede retention enema with cleansing enema. Administer solution via rectal tube or 28-French Foley catheter with 30-mL balloon. Insert tube at least 20 cm and tape in place.
● For retention enema, add powder to 100 mL of prescribed solution (usually sorbitol or 20% dextrose in water). Shake well to dissolve powder thoroughly; should be of liquid consistency. Position patient on left side and elevate hips on pillow if solution begins to leak. Follow administration of medication with additional 50–100 mL of diluent to ensure administration of complete dose. Encourage patient to retain enema as long as possible, at least 30–60 min.
● After retention period, irrigate colon with 1–2 L of non-sodium-containing solution. Y-connector with tubing may be attached to Foley or rectal tube; cleansing solution is administered through 1 port of the Y and allowed to drain by gravity through the other port.

Patient/Family Teaching
● Explain purpose and method of administration of medication to patient.
● Advise patient to avoid taking antacids or laxatives during therapy, unless approved by health care professional; may cause systemic alkalosis.
● Advise females of reproductive potential to notify health care professional if pregnancy is planned or suspected or if breastfeeding.
● Inform patient of need for frequent lab tests to monitor effectiveness.

Evaluation/Desired Outcomes
● Normalization of serum potassium levels.

S

☒ sofosbuvir/velpatasvir
(soe-**fos**-bue-vir/vel-**pat**-as-vir)
Epclusa
Classification
Therapeutic: antivirals
Pharmacologic: NS5B inhibitors, NS5A inhibitors

Indications
☒ Chronic hepatitis C virus (HCV) genotype 1, 2, 3, 4, 5, or 6 infection in patients without cirrhosis or with compensated cirrhosis. ☒ Chronic HCV genotype 1, 2, 3, 4, 5, or 6 infection in patients with decompensated cirrhosis (in combination with ribavirin).

Action
Sofosbuvir: inhibits the HCV NS5B RNA-dependent RNA polymerase, resulting in inhibition of viral replication. *Velpatasvir:* inhibits the HCV NS5A protein, resulting in inhibition of viral replication. **Therapeutic Effects:** Decreased levels of HCV with sustained virologic response and lessened sequelae of chronic HCV infection.

Pharmacokinetics
Sofosbuvir
Absorption: Rapidly metabolized following absorption (extensive first-pass effect).
Distribution: Unknown.
Metabolism and Excretion: Extensively metabolized primarily to GS-461203, an active antiviral moiety, then converted to GS-331007, which does not have antiviral activity. 80% excreted in urine mostly as GS-331007 (3.5% as unchanged drug), 14% excreted in feces, 2.5% excreted in expired air.
Half-life: *Sofosbuvir:* 0.4 hr; *GS-331007:* 25 hr.
Velpatasvir
Absorption: Well absorbed following oral administration.
Distribution: Unknown.
Protein Binding: >99.5%.
Metabolism and Excretion: Primarily metabolized in the liver via the CYP2B6, CYP2C8, and CYP3A4 isoenzymes. Primarily undergoes biliary excretion, with 94% excreted in feces and 0.4% eliminated in urine.
Half-life: 47 hr.

TIME/ACTION PROFILE (plasma concentrations)

ROUTE	ONSET	PEAK	DURATION
sofosbuvir (PO)	unknown	0.5–1 hr	24 hr
velpatasvir (PO)	unknown	3 hr	24 hr

Contraindications/Precautions
Contraindicated in: Situations when ribavirin is contraindicated (when ribavirin required); Concurrent use with other drugs/regimens containing sofosbuvir; Receiving immunosuppressant or chemotherapy medications (↑ risk of hepatitis B virus [HBV] reactivation); OB: Pregnant women or men whose partners are pregnant (when ribavirin is required; ribavirin may cause fetal harm); Lactation: Lactation (when ribavirin required).
Use Cautiously in: OB: Safety not established in pregnancy (when ribavirin not required); Lactation: Safety not established in breastfeeding (when ribavirin not required); Pedi: Children <3 yo (safety and effectiveness not established); Geri: Older adults may be more sensitive to drug's effects.

Adverse Reactions/Side Effects
Without Ribavirin
Derm: rash **GI:** ↑ lipase, HBV reactivation, nausea. **Neuro:** <u>fatigue</u>, <u>headache</u>, insomnia, irritability.

With Ribavirin
Derm: rash. **GI:** <u>diarrhea</u>, nausea, HBV reactivation, ↑ lipase. **Hemat:** <u>anemia</u>. **Neuro:** <u>fatigue</u>, <u>headache</u>, <u>insomnia</u>.

Interactions
Drug-Drug: Concurrent use of **P-glycoprotein inducers** may ↓ levels and effectiveness of sofosbuvir and velpatasvir; concurrent use not recommended. Concurrent use of **moderate to strong CYP2B6, CYP2C8, or CYP3A4 inducers** may ↓ levels and effectiveness of velpatasvir; concurrent use not recommended. **Amiodarone** may ↑ risk of symptomatic bradycardia when used with sofosbuvir-containing regimens; concurrent use not recommended; if amiodarone necessary, monitor patients in inpatient setting for first 48 hr of concomitant use and then monitor heart rate on outpatient basis for at least the first 2 wk of treatment; follow same monitoring procedure if discontinuing amiodarone immediately before initiation of sofosbuvir/velpatasvir. **Acid-reducing agents** may ↓ levels and effectiveness of velpatasvir; separate administration from **antacids**, including **magnesium hydroxide** and **aluminum hydroxide** by 4 hr; administer **H₂-receptor antagonists** simultaneously or 12 hr apart from sofosbuvir/velpatasvir (dose of H₂ antagonist should not exceed famotidine 40 mg twice daily or equivalent); concurrent use with **proton-pump inhibitors** not recommended (if proton pump inhibitor necessary, administer sofosbuvir/velpatasvir with food and take 4 hr before **omeprazole** 20 mg; use with other proton pump inhibitors not studied). May ↑ levels and risk of toxicity of **digoxin**; therapeutic monitoring of serum digoxin concentrations recommended. May ↑ levels and risk of toxicity of **topotecan**; concurrent use not recommended. **Carbamazepine, phenytoin, phenobarbital, oxcarbazepine, rifabutin,** and **rifampin** may ↓ levels and effectiveness of sofosbuvir and velpatasvir; concurrent use not recommended. **Efavirenz** may ↓ levels and effectiveness of velpatasvir; concurrent use not recommended. May ↑ levels/toxicity of **tenofovir disoproxil fumarate**; monitor closely. **Tipranavir/ritonavir** may ↓ levels and effectiveness of sofos-

buvir and velpatasvir; concurrent use not recommended. May ↑ levels and risk of toxicity of **rosuvastatin** and **atorvastatin**; rosuvastatin dose should not exceed 10 mg/day; monitor closely for atorvastatin-induced myopathy or rhabdomyolysis. May cause fluctuations in INR when used with **warfarin**; closely monitor INR. May ↑ risk of hypoglycemia when used with certain **antidiabetic agents**.

Drug-Natural Products: St. John's wort may ↓ levels and effectiveness of sofosbuvir and velpatasvir; concurrent use not recommended.

Route/Dosage

Dosing recommendations below may also be followed for patients coinfected with HIV.

PO (Adults): *Patients without cirrhosis or with compensated cirrhosis (including liver transplant recipients):* One 400-mg/100-mg tablet once daily for 12 wk; *Patients with decompensated cirrhosis:* One 400-mg/100-mg tablet once daily for 12 wk in combination with ribavirin.

PO (Children ≥3 yr or ≥30 kg): *Patients without cirrhosis or with compensated cirrhosis (including liver transplant recipients):* One 400-mg/100-mg tablet once daily for 12 wk *or* two 200-mg/50-mg tablets once daily for 12 wk *or* two 200-mg/50-mg pellet packets once daily for 12 wk; *Patients with decompensated cirrhosis:* One 400-mg/100-mg tablet once daily for 12 wk in combination with ribavirin *or* two 200-mg/50-mg tablets once daily for 12 wk in combination with ribavirin *or* two 200-mg/50-mg pellet packets once daily for 12 wk in combination with ribavirin.

PO (Children ≥3 yr or 17–<30 kg): *Patients without cirrhosis or with compensated cirrhosis (including liver transplant recipients):* one 200-mg/50-mg tablet once daily for 12 wk *or* one 200-mg/50-mg pellet packet once daily for 12 wk; *Patients with decompensated cirrhosis:* one 200-mg/50-mg tablet once daily for 12 wk in combination with ribavirin *or* one 200-mg/50-mg pellet packet once daily for 12 wk in combination with ribavirin.

PO (Children ≥3 yr or <17 kg): *Patients without cirrhosis or with compensated cirrhosis (including liver transplant recipients):* one 150-mg/37.5-mg pellet packet once daily for 12 wk; *Patients with decompensated cirrhosis:* one 150-mg/37.5-mg pellet packet once daily for 12 wk in combination with ribavirin.

Availability

Tablets: sofosbuvir 200 mg/velpatasvir 50 mg, sofosbuvir 400 mg/velpatasvir 100 mg. **Oral pellets:** sofosbuvir 150 mg/velpatasvir 37.5 mg per pkt, sofosbuvir 200 mg/velpatasvir 50 mg per pkt.

NURSING IMPLICATIONS

Assessment

● Monitor for signs and symptoms of HBV reactivation (jaundice, dark urine, light-colored stools, fatigue, weakness, loss of appetite, nausea, vomiting, stomach pain) during therapy.

Lab Test Considerations

● Measure hepatitis B surface antigen (HBsAg) and hepatitis core antibody (anti-HBc) in all patients before starting HCV therapy. May cause HBV reactivation. Monitor for clinical and laboratory signs of hepatitis flare (↑ AST, ALT, bilirubin, liver failure, death) or HBV reactivation (rapid ↑ in serum HBV DNA level) during HCV treatment and post-treatment follow-up.

● May cause ↑ serum lipase and amylase levels.

● May cause ↑ CK and indirect bilirubin levels.

Implementation

● **PO:** Administer one tablet daily without regard to food for 12 wk.

● Do not chew oral pellets; causes a bitter aftertaste. May be administered directly into mouth and swallowed whole or taken with food. In pediatric patients <6 years of age, administer oral pellets with food to increase tolerability and palatability. Sprinkle oral pellets on one or more spoonfuls of non-acidic soft food (pudding, chocolate syrup, ice cream) at or below room temperature. Take oral pellets within 15 min of gently mixing with food and swallow entire contents without chewing.

● Administer antacids 4 hr apart from sofosbuvir/velpatasvir. May administer simultaneously or 12 hr apart with H₂-receptor antagonists at doses not to exceed famotidine 40 mg twice daily. Avoid administration with proton pump inhibitors; if medically necessary, administer sofosbuvir/velpatasvir with food and 4 hr before omeprazole 20 mg.

Patient/Family Teaching

● Instruct patient to take *Epclusa* as directed. Do not skip or miss doses or stop medication without consulting health care professional. Advise patient to read *Patient Information* before starting and with each Rx refill in case of changes.

● Advise patient to notify health care professional if they have a history of HBV. May cause reactivation.

● Instruct patient to notify health care professional of all Rx or OTC medications, vitamins, or herbal products being taken and consult health care professional before taking any new medications, especially St. John's wort.

● Rep: Advise patients to notify health care professional if pregnancy is planned or suspected, or if breastfeeding. Advise females of reproductive potential who take *Epclusa* with ribavirin to use effective contraception during and for 6 mo after therapy is completed. Notify health care professional immediately if pregnancy is suspected.

Evaluation/Desired Outcomes

● Decreased levels of HCV with sustained virologic response and lessened sequelae of chronic HCV infection.

solifenacin (so-li-**fen**-a-sin)
VESIcare, VESIcare LS
Classification
Therapeutic: urinary tract antispasmodics
Pharmacologic: anticholinergics

Indications
Overactive bladder with symptoms (urge incontinence, urgency, frequency) (tablets only). Neurogenic detrusor overactivity (suspension only).

Action
Acts as a muscarinic (cholinergic) receptor antagonist; antagonizes bladder smooth muscle contraction. **Therapeutic Effects:** Decreased symptoms of overactive bladder. Improved maximum cystometric capacity in neurogenic detrusor overactivity.

Pharmacokinetics
Absorption: 90% absorbed following oral administration.
Distribution: Extensively distributed to tissues.
Protein Binding: 98%.
Metabolism and Excretion: Extensively metabolized by liver via the CYP3A4 isoenzyme. 69% excreted in urine as metabolites, 22% in feces.
Half-life: *Tablets:* 45–68 hr; *Suspension:* 26 hr.

TIME/ACTION PROFILE (plasma concentrations)

ROUTE	ONSET	PEAK	DURATION
Oral	unknown	3–8 hr	24 hr

Contraindications/Precautions
Contraindicated in: Hypersensitivity; Urinary retention; Gastric retention; Uncontrolled angle-closure glaucoma; Severe hepatic impairment; History of QT interval prolongation or concurrent use of QT interval prolonging medications.
Use Cautiously in: Moderate hepatic impairment (lower dose recommended); Renal impairment; Bladder outflow obstruction; GI obstructive disorders, severe constipation, or ulcerative colitis; Myasthenia gravis; Angle-closure glaucoma; OB: Safety not established in pregnancy; Lactation: Safety not established in breastfeeding; Pedi: Children <2 yr (safety and effectiveness not established).

Adverse Reactions/Side Effects
CV: palpitations, QT interval prolongation, tachycardia. **EENT:** blurred vision. **GI:** constipation, dry mouth, abdominal pain, dyspepsia, nausea. **GU:** urinary tract infection. **MS:** muscle weakness. **Neuro:** confusion, drowsiness, hallucinations, headache. **Misc:** HYPERSENSITIVITY REACTIONS (including anaphylaxis and angioedema).

Interactions
Drug-Drug: **Strong CYP3A4 inhibitors,** including **ketoconazole,** may significantly ↑ levels and risk of toxicity. **QT interval prolonging medications** may ↑ risk of QT interval prolongation; avoid concurrent use.

Route/Dosage
Overactive Bladder
PO (Adults): *Tablets:* 5 mg once daily, may ↑ to 10 mg once daily; *Concurrent use of strong CYP3A4 inhibitors:* Tablets: Not to exceed 5 mg once daily.

Renal Impairment
PO (Adults): *CCr <30 mL/min:* Tablets: Not to exceed 5 mg once daily.

Hepatic Impairment
PO (Adults): *Moderate hepatic impairment:* Tablets: Not to exceed 5 mg once daily.

Neurogenic Detrusor Overactivity
PO (Children ≥2 yr and >60 kg): *Suspension:* 5 mg once daily, may ↑ to 10 mg once daily; *Concurrent use of strong CYP3A4 inhibitors:* Suspension: Not to exceed 5 mg once daily.
PO (Children ≥2 yr and 46–60 kg): *Suspension:* 4 mg once daily, may ↑ to 8 mg once daily; *Concurrent use of strong CYP3A4 inhibitors:* Suspension: Not to exceed 4 mg once daily.
PO (Children ≥2 yr and 31–45 kg): *Suspension:* 3 mg once daily, may ↑ to 6 mg once daily; *Concurrent use of strong CYP3A4 inhibitors:* Suspension: Not to exceed 3 mg once daily.
PO (Children ≥2 yr and 16–30 kg): *Suspension:* 3 mg once daily, may ↑ to 5 mg once daily; *Concurrent use of strong CYP3A4 inhibitors:* Suspension: Not to exceed 3 mg once daily.
PO (Children ≥2 yr and 9–15 kg): *Suspension:* 2 mg once daily, may ↑ to 4 mg once daily; *Concurrent use of strong CYP3A4 inhibitors:* Suspension: Not to exceed 2 mg once daily.

Renal Impairment
PO (Children ≥2 yr): *CCr <30 mL/min:* >60 kg: Not to exceed 5 mg once daily (suspension); 46–60 kg: Not to exceed 4 mg once daily (suspension); 16–45 kg: Not to exceed 3 mg once daily (suspension); 9–15 kg: Not to exceed 2 mg once daily (suspension).

Hepatic Impairment
PO (Children ≥2 yr): *Moderate hepatic impairment:* >60 kg: Not to exceed 5 mg once daily (suspension); 46–60 kg: Not to exceed 4 mg once daily (suspension); 16–45 kg: Not to exceed 3 mg once daily (suspension); 9–15 kg: Not to exceed 2 mg once daily (suspension).

Availability (generic available)
Tablets (Vesicare): 5 mg, 10 mg. **Oral suspension (orange flavor) (Vesicare LS):** 1 mg/mL.

NURSING IMPLICATIONS
Assessment
- **Overactive Bladder:** Monitor voiding pattern and assess symptoms of overactive bladder (urinary ur-

gency, urinary incontinence, urinary frequency) to
and periodically during therapy.
● **Neurogenic Detrusor Overactivity:** Measure
bladder capacity as directed.

Implementation
● **PO:** Administer once daily without regard to food.
Tablets must be swallowed whole; do not break,
crush, or chew.
● Administer suspension once daily followed by water
or milk. Shake before use. Use calibrated measuring
device to ensure accurate dose.

Patient/Family Teaching
● Instruct patient to take solifenacin as directed. Advise patient to read the *Patient Information* before
starting therapy and with each prescription refill.
Overactive bladder: if a dose is missed, skip dose
and take next day; do not take 2 doses in same day.
Neurogenic Detrusor Overactivity: take missed
doses as soon as remembered if within 12 hr; if >12
hr since missed dose, omit dose and take next dose
at usual time.
● Do not share solifenacin with others; may be dangerous.
● May cause dizziness and blurred vision. Caution patient to avoid driving and other activities that require
alertness until response to medication is known.
● Advise patient to notify health care professional immediately if hives; rash; swelling or lips, face,
tongue, or throat; or trouble breathing occurs.
● Inform patient of potential anticholinergic side effects (constipation, urinary retention, blurred vision,
heat prostration in a hot environment).
● Instruct patient to notify health care professional of
all Rx or OTC medications, vitamins, or herbal products being taken and consult health care professional before taking any new medications.
● Rep: Advise females of reproductive potential to notify health care professional if pregnancy is planned
or suspected or if breastfeeding.

Evaluation/Desired Outcomes
● Decrease in symptoms of overactive bladder (urge
urinary incontinence, urgency, frequency).
● Improved bladder capacity in neurogenic detrusor
overactivity.

---

solriamfetol (sol-ri-am-fe-tol)
Sunosi
Classification
Therapeutic: central nervous system stimu-
lants
Pharmacologic: dopamine norepinephrine
reuptake inhibitors

Schedule IV

Indications
Excessive daytime sleepiness due to narcolepsy or obstructive sleep apnea.

Action
Selective dopamine and norepinephrine reuptake inhibitor. **Therapeutic Effects:** Improved wakefulness.

Pharmacokinetics
Absorption: 95% absorbed following oral adminis-
tration; high-fat food delays absorption.
Distribution: Extensively distributed to tissues.
Metabolism and Excretion: Undergoes minimal
metabolism; primarily excreted in urine as unchanged
drug (95%).
Half-life: 7 hr.

TIME/ACTION PROFILE (plasma concentrations)

ROUTE	ONSET	PEAK	DURATION
PO	unknown	1.25–3 hr	unknown

Contraindications/Precautions
Contraindicated in: Concurrent use or use within
14 days of discontinuation of MAO inhibitors; End-stage
renal disease.
Use Cautiously in: Cardiovascular disease, cerebrovascular disease, or hypertension; Moderate or severe renal impairment (↓ dose recommended); Psychoses or bipolar disorder; History of drug
(especially stimulants) or alcohol abuse; OB: Use
during pregnancy only if potential maternal benefit
justifies potential fetal risk; Lactation: Use while
breastfeeding only if potential maternal benefit justifies potential risk to infant; Pedi: Safety and effectiveness not established in children; Geri: Because of reduced renal function, older adults may be at ↑ risk of
adverse reactions.

Adverse Reactions/Side Effects
CV: ↑ BP, ↑ HR, palpitations. **Derm:** ↑ sweating. **GI:** ↓
appetite, abdominal pain, constipation, diarrhea, dry
mouth, nausea. **Neuro:** <u>headache</u>, anxiety, dizziness,
insomnia, irritability.

Interactions
Drug-Drug: Concurrent use with or within 14 days
of discontinuation of **MAO inhibitors** may ↑ risk of
hypertensive crises; concurrent use contraindicated.
Use cautiously with other **drugs that increase BP or
HR. Dopaminergic drugs** may have synergistic effects.

Route/Dosage
PO (Adults): *Narcolepsy:* 75 mg once daily; may ↑
dose to 150 mg once daily, if needed, after ≥3 days.
Obstructive sleep apnea: 37.5 mg once daily; may
double dose at intervals of at least every 3 days, if
needed (max dose = 150 mg/day).

✦= Canadian drug name. ⁙ = Genetic implication. ~~Strikethrough~~ = Discontinued. CAPITALS = life-threatening. <u>Underline</u> = most frequent.

Renal Impairment
PO (Adults): *Moderate renal impairment (eGFR 30–59 mL/min/1.73 m²) (for either narcolepsy or obstructive sleep apnea):* 37.5 mg once daily; may ↑ dose to 75 mg once daily after ≥7 days, if needed. *Severe renal impairment (eGFR 15–29 mL/min/1.73 m²) (for either narcolepsy or obstructive sleep apnea):* 37.5 mg once daily.

Availability
Tablets: 75 mg, 150 mg.

NURSING IMPLICATIONS

Assessment
* Observe and document frequency of narcoleptic episodes.
* Assess BP and control hypertension before starting therapy. Monitor BP during therapy and treat new-onset hypertension and exacerbations of pre-existing hypertension.

Implementation
* **PO:** Administer once daily upon awakening without regard to food.

Patient/Family Teaching
* Instruct patient to take solriamfetol as directed. Avoid taking medication within 9 hr of planned bedtime; may impair ability to fall asleep.
* Advise patient that sharing this medication with others, even those with same symptoms, is dangerous and illegal. Advise patient that solriamfetol is a drug with known abuse potential. Protect it from theft; store out of sight and reach of children, and in a location not accessible by others.
* Advise patient to notify health care professional if anxiety, insomnia, irritability, agitation, or signs of psychosis or bipolar disorders occur.
* Advise patient to notify health care professional of all Rx or OTC medications, vitamins, or herbal products being taken and to consult with health care professional before taking other medications. If alcohol is used during therapy, intake should be limited to moderate amounts.
* Rep: Advise females of reproductive potential to notify health care professional if pregnancy is planned or suspected or if breastfeeding. Monitor breastfed infants for agitation, insomnia, anorexia, and reduced weight gain. Encourage women who become pregnant to enroll in the pregnancy exposure registry to monitor outcomes for women exposed to solriamfetol during pregnancy by calling 1-877-283-6220 or contacting www.SunosiPregnancyRegistry.com.

Evaluation/Desired Outcomes
* Improved ability to stay awake.

---

spironolactone, See DIURETICS (POTASSIUM-SPARING).

---

streptomycin, See AMINOGLYCOSIDES.

---

sucralfate (soo-kral-fate)
Carafate, ✤ Cytogard, ✤ Sulcrate, ✤ Sulcrate Plus
Classification
Therapeutic: antiulcer agents
Pharmacologic: GI protectants

Indications
Short-term management of duodenal ulcers. Maintenance (preventive) therapy of duodenal ulcers. **Unlabeled Use:** Management of gastric ulcer or gastroesophageal reflux. Prevention of gastric mucosal injury caused by high-dose aspirin or other NSAIDs in patients with rheumatoid arthritis or in high-stress situations (e.g., intensive care unit). **Suspension:** Mucositis/stomatitis/rectal or oral ulcerations from various etiologies.

Action
Aluminum salt of sulfated sucrose reacts with gastric acid to form a thick paste, which selectively adheres to the ulcer surface. **Therapeutic Effects:** Protection of ulcers, with subsequent healing.

Pharmacokinetics
Absorption: Systemic absorption is minimal (<5%).
Distribution: Unknown.
Metabolism and Excretion: >90% is eliminated in the feces.
Half-life: 6–20 hr.

TIME/ACTION PROFILE (mucosal protectant effect)

ROUTE	ONSET	PEAK	DURATION
PO	1–2 hr	unknown	6 hr

Contraindications/Precautions
Contraindicated in: Hypersensitivity.
Use Cautiously in: Renal failure (accumulation of aluminum can occur); Diabetes (↑ risk of hyperglycemia with suspension); Impaired swallowing (↑ risk of tablet aspiration).

Adverse Reactions/Side Effects
Derm: pruritus, rash. **Endo:** hyperglycemia (with suspension). **GI:** constipation, diarrhea, dry mouth, gastric discomfort, indigestion, nausea. **Neuro:** dizziness, drowsiness. **Misc:** HYPERSENSITIVITY REACTIONS (including anaphylaxis and angioedema).

Interactions
Drug-Drug: May ↓ absorption of **phenytoin, fat-soluble vitamins,** or **tetracycline.** ↓ effectiveness when used with **antacids** or **cimetidine.** ↓ absorption of **fluoroquinolones** (separate administration by 2 hr).

Route/Dosage

Treatment of Ulcers
PO (Adults): 1 g 4 times daily, given 1 hr before meals and at bedtime; or 2 g twice daily, on waking and at bedtime.

PO (Adults): 1 g twice daily, given 1 hr before a meal.

Gastroesophageal Reflux
PO (Adults): 1 g 4 times daily, given 1 hr before meals and at bedtime.

PO (Children): 40–80 mg/kg/day divided every 6 hr, given 1 hr before meals and at bedtime.

Stomatitis
PO (Adults and Children): 5–10 mL of suspension, swish and spit or swish and swallow 4 times daily.

Proctitis
Rect (Adults): 2 g of suspension given as an enema once or twice daily.

Availability (generic available)
Oral suspension (cherry flavor): 1 g/10 mL, ✲ 200 mg/mL. **Tablets:** 1 g.

NURSING IMPLICATIONS

Assessment
- Assess patient routinely for abdominal pain and frank or occult blood in the stool.

Implementation
- **PO:** Administer on an empty stomach, 1 hr before meals and at bedtime. Tablet may be broken or dissolved in water before ingestion. Shake suspension well before administration.
- Oral suspension is only for oral use; do not administer IV. Shake well before use. Store at room temperature, do not freeze.
- If antacids are also required for pain, administer 30 min before or after sucralfate dose.

Patient/Family Teaching
- Advise patient to continue with course of therapy for 4–8 wk, even if feeling better, to ensure ulcer healing. If a dose is missed, take as soon as remembered unless almost time for next dose; do not double doses.
- Advise patient that increase in fluid intake, dietary bulk, and exercise may prevent drug-induced constipation.
- Emphasize the importance of routine examinations to monitor progress.

Evaluation/Desired Outcomes
- Decrease in abdominal pain.
- Prevention and healing of duodenal ulcers, seen by x-ray examination and endoscopy.

---

sulbactam/durlobactam
(sul-**bak**-tam/der-low-**bak**-tam)
Xacduro
Classification
Therapeutic: anti-infectives
Pharmacologic: beta-lactamase inhibitors

Indications
Hospital-acquired bacterial pneumonia and ventilator-associated bacterial pneumonia caused by susceptible isolates of *Acinetobacter baumannii-calcoaceticus* complex.

Action
Sulbactam is a beta-lactam antibiotic and a beta-lactamase inhibitor that inhibits *Acinetobacter baumannii-calcoaceticus* complex penicillin-binding proteins. Durlobactam is a beta-lactamase inhibitor that protects sulbactam from being degraded by certain serine-beta-lactamases. **Therapeutic Effects:** Bactericidal action against susceptible bacteria. **Spectrum:** Active against the following gram-negative pathogen: *Acinetobacter baumannii-calcoaceticus* complex.

Pharmacokinetics
Absorption: IV administration results in complete bioavailability.

Distribution: Well distributed to tissues.

Metabolism and Excretion: Undergoes minimal metabolism. Primarily excreted by the kidneys, with 75–85% of sulbactam and 78% of durlobactam being excreted as unchanged drug.

Half-life: *Sulbactam:* 2–3 hr; *Durlobactam:* 2–3 hr.

TIME/ACTION PROFILE (plasma concentrations)

ROUTE	ONSET	PEAK	DURATION
IV	rapid	end of infusion	6 hr

Contraindications/Precautions
Contraindicated in: Hypersensitivity to sulbactam, durlobactam, or any beta-lactam antibiotic.

Use Cautiously in: Renal impairment (↓ dose if CCr <45 mL/min); CCr ≥130 mL/min; OB: Safety not established in pregnancy; Lactation: Safety not established in breastfeeding; Pedi: Safety and effectiveness not established in children; Geri: Consider age-related ↓ in renal function in determining dose in older adults.

Adverse Reactions/Side Effects
CV: arrhythmia. **F and E:** hypokalemia. **GI:** ↑ liver enzymes, diarrhea, CLOSTRIDIOIDES DIFFICILE-ASSOCIATED DIARRHEA (CDAD), constipation. **GU:** acute kidney injury. **Hemat:** anemia, thrombocytopenia. **Misc:** HYPERSENSITIVITY REACTIONS (including anaphylaxis).

S

✲ = Canadian drug name. ▓ = Genetic implication. S̶t̶r̶i̶k̶e̶t̶h̶r̶o̶u̶g̶h̶ = Discontinued. CAPITALS = life-threatening. Underline = most frequent.

Interactions

Drug-Drug: Probenecid may ↓ renal excretion and ↑ levels of sulbactam; concurrent use not recommended.

Route/Dosage

IV (Adults): *CCr 45–129 mL/min:* Sulbactam 1 g/durlobactam 1 g every 6 hr for 7–14 days. *CCr ≥130 mL/min:* Sulbactam 1 g/durlobactam 1 g every 4 hr for 7–14 days.

Renal Impairment

IV (Adults): *CCr 30–44 mL/min:* Sulbactam 1 g/durlobactam 1 g every 8 hr for 7–14 days. *CCr 15–29 mL/min:* Sulbactam 1 g/durlobactam 1 g every 12 hr for 7–14 days. *CCr <15 mL/min (at baseline before initiating therapy):* Sulbactam 1 g/durlobactam 1 g every 12 hr for first 3 doses, then sulbactam 1 g/durlobactam 1 g every 24 hr to complete a total treatment course of 7–14 days. *CCr <15 mL/min (after initiating therapy):* Sulbactam 1 g/durlobactam 1 g every 24 hr for 7–14 days.

Availability

Lyophilized powder for injection: sulbactam 1 g/vial + durlobactam 0.5 g/vial (2 vials supplied).

NURSING IMPLICATIONS

Assessment

- Assess patient for infection (vital signs, wound appearance, sputum, urine, stool, and WBCs) at beginning and throughout therapy.
- Obtain a history before initiating therapy to determine previous use of, and reactions to, penicillins or cephalosporins. Persons with a negative history of penicillin sensitivity may still have an allergic response.
- Obtain specimens for culture and sensitivity before therapy. First dose may be given before receiving results.
- Monitor for signs and symptoms of hypersensitivity (rash, pruritus, laryngeal edema, wheezing). Discontinue drug and notify health care professional immediately if these occur. Keep epinephrine, an antihistamine, and resuscitation equipment close by in the event of an anaphylactic reaction.
- Monitor bowel function. Report diarrhea, abdominal cramping, fever, and bloody stools to health care professional promptly as a sign of CDAD. May begin up to several mo following cessation of therapy.
- Monitor for rash; may lead to severe skin reactions.

Implementation

IV Administration

- **Intermittent Infusion:** *Xacduro* kit includes one clear single-dose vial of sulbactam 1 g and two amber single-dose vials of durlobactam 0.5 g as sterile powders. *Reconstitution:* Reconstitute *sulbactam* 1 g 5 mL of sterile water for injection and gently shake to dissolve. Solution is clear, colorless to

slightly yellow; do not use solutions that are cloudy, discolored, or contain particulate matter. Dilution must occur within 1 hr of reconstitution. Reconstitute *durlobactam* 0.5 g single-dose vial with 2.5 mL of sterile water for injection and gently shake to dissolve. Solution is clear, light yellow to orange; do not use solutions that are cloudy, discolored, or contain particulate matter. Dilution must occur within 1 hour of reconstitution. To prepare *Xacduro* dose, withdraw 5 mL of reconstituted sulbactam and 5 mL (2.5 mL from each vial) of reconstituted durlobactam. Add withdrawn volume of both sulbactam and durlobactam to a 100 mL bag of 0.9% NaCl. Discard unused portion. Store solution in refrigerator. Allow solutions to reach room temperature over 15–30 min before administering. Solutions are stable for 24 hr if refrigerated. *Rate:* Infuse over 3 hr.
- **Y-Site Incompatibility:** Do not mix with other drugs or solutions.

Patient/Family Teaching

- Explain purpose of *Xacduro* to patient.
- Advise patient to report rash, signs of superinfection (furry overgrowth on the tongue, vaginal itching or discharge, loose or foul-smelling stools), and allergy.
- Caution patient to notify health care professional if fever and diarrhea occur, especially if stool contains blood, pus, or mucus. Advise patient not to treat diarrhea without consulting health care professional. May occur up to several wk after discontinuation of medication.
- Rep: Advise females of reproductive potential to notify health care professional if pregnancy is planned or suspected or if breastfeeding.
- Instruct the patient to notify health care professional if symptoms do not improve.

Evaluation/Desired Outcomes

- Resolution of signs and symptoms of infection. Length of time for complete resolution depends on the organism and site of infection.

---

sulconazole, See ANTIFUNGALS (TOPICAL).

※ sulfaSALAzine

(sul-fa-**sal**-a-zeen)

Azulfidine, Azulfidine EN-tabs, ✦ Salazopyrin

Classification

Therapeutic: antirheumatics (DMARD), gastrointestinal anti-inflammatories

Indications

Mild to moderate ulcerative colitis or as adjunctive therapy in severe ulcerative colitis. Rheumatoid arthritis unresponsive or intolerant to salicylates and/or NSAIDs.

Action
Locally acting anti-inflammatory action in the colon, where activity is probably a result of inhibition of prostaglandin synthesis. **Therapeutic Effects:** Reduction in the symptoms of ulcerative colitis or rheumatoid arthritis.

Pharmacokinetics
Absorption: 10–15% absorbed after oral administration.
Distribution: Widely distributed; crosses the placenta and enters breast milk.
Protein Binding: 99%.
Metabolism and Excretion: Split by intestinal bacteria into sulfapyridine and 5-aminosalicylic acid. Some absorbed sulfasalazine is excreted by bile back into intestines; 15% excreted unchanged by the kidneys. Sulfapyridine also excreted mostly by the kidneys.
Half-life: 6 hr.

TIME/ACTION PROFILE (plasma concentrations)

ROUTE	ONSET	PEAK	DURATION
PO	1 hr	1.5–6 hr	6–12 hr

Contraindications/Precautions
Contraindicated in: Hypersensitivity reactions to sulfonamides, salicylates, or sulfasalazine; Cross-sensitivity with furosemide, sulfonylurea hypoglycemic agents, or carbonic anhydrase inhibitors may exist; ⚎ Glucose-6–phosphate dehydrogenase deficiency (↑ risk of hemolysis); Hypersensitivity to bisulfites (mesalamine enema only); Urinary tract or intestinal obstruction; Porphyria.
Use Cautiously in: Severe hepatic impairment; Severe renal impairment; History of porphyria; Blood dyscrasias; OB: Neural tube defects have been reported; use during pregnancy only if potential maternal benefit justifies potential fetal risk; Lactation: May compete with bilirubin for binding sites on plasma proteins in the newborn and cause kernicterus; bloody stools or diarrhea reported in breastfed infants; Pedi: Children <2 yr (safety and effectiveness not established).

Adverse Reactions/Side Effects
Derm: rash, ACUTE GENERALIZED EXANTHEMATOUS PUSTULOSIS, DRUG REACTION WITH EOSINOPHILIA AND SYSTEMIC SYMPTOMS (DRESS), EXFOLIATIVE DERMATITIS, photosensitivity, STEVENS-JOHNSON SYNDROME (SJS), TOXIC EPIDERMAL NECROLYSIS (TEN), yellow discoloration. **GI:** anorexia, diarrhea, nausea, vomiting, drug-induced hepatitis. **GU:** crystalluria, infertility, oligospermia, orange-yellow discoloration of urine, renal impairment. **Hemat:** AGRANULOCYTOSIS, APLASTIC ANEMIA, blood dyscrasias, eosinophilia, hemolytic anemia, megaloblastic anemia, thrombocytopenia. **Neuro:** headache, peripheral neuropathy. **Resp:** pneumonitis. **Misc:** fever, HY-PERSENSITIVITY REACTIONS (including anaphylaxis and angioedema).

Interactions
Drug-Drug: May ↑ action/risk of toxicity from **oral hypoglycemic agents**, **phenytoin**, **methotrexate**, **zidovudine**, or **warfarin**. ↑ risk of drug-induced hepatitis with other **hepatotoxic agents**. ↑ risk of crystalluria with **methenamine**. May ↓ metabolism and ↑ effects/toxicity of **mercaptopurine** or **thioguanine**.
Drug-Food: May ↓ **iron** and **folic acid** absorption.

Route/Dosage
Ulcerative Colitis
PO (Adults): 1 g every 6–8 hr (may start with 500 mg every 6–12 hr), followed by maintenance dose of 500 mg every 6 hr.
PO (Children >2 yr): *Initial:* 6.7–10 mg/kg every 4 hr *or* 10–15 mg/kg every 6 hr *or* 13.3–20 mg/kg every 8 hr. *Maintenance:* 7.5 mg/kg every 6 hr (not to exceed 2 g/day).

Rheumatoid Arthritis
PO (Adults): 500 mg–1 g/day (as delayed-release tablets) for 1 wk, then ↑ by 500 mg/day every wk up to 2 g/day in 2 divided doses; if no benefit seen after 12 wk, ↑ to 3 g/day in 2 divided doses.
PO (Children ≥6 yr): 30–50 mg/kg/day in 2 divided doses (as delayed-release tablets); initiate therapy at 25% of planned maintenance dose and ↑ every 7 days until maintenance dose is reached (not to exceed 2 g/day).

Availability (generic available)
Tablets: 500 mg. **Delayed-release (enteric-coated) tablets (Azulfidine EN-tabs):** 500 mg.

NURSING IMPLICATIONS
Assessment
- Assess patient for allergy to sulfonamides and salicylates. Discontinue therapy if rash, difficulty breathing, swelling of face or lips, or fever occur.
- Monitor intake and output ratios. Fluid intake should be sufficient to maintain a urine output of at least 1200–1500 mL daily to prevent crystalluria and stone formation.
- Assess for rash periodically during therapy. May cause SJS, TEN, and DRESS. Discontinue therapy if severe or if accompanied by fever, general malaise, fatigue, muscle or joint aches, blisters, oral lesions, conjunctivitis, hepatitis, and/or eosinophilia.
- **Ulcerative Colitis:** Assess abdominal pain and frequency, quantity, and consistency of stools at the beginning of and during therapy.
- **Rheumatoid Arthritis:** Assess range of motion and degree of swelling and pain in affected joints before and periodically during therapy.

S

Lab Test Considerations

• Monitor urinalysis, BUN, and serum creatinine before and periodically during therapy. May cause crystalluria and urinary cell calculi formation. Discontinue sulfasalazine if renal function declines.

• Monitor CBC with differential and liver function tests before and every 2nd wk during first 3 mo of therapy, monthly during the 2nd 3 mo, and every 3 mo thereafter or as clinically indicated. Discontinue sulfasalazine if blood dyscrasias occur.

• Serum sulfapyridine levels may be monitored; concentrations >50 μg/mL may be associated with increased incidence of adverse reactions.

• Higher than recommended doses can interfere with a variety of lab assays that use nicotinamide adenine dinucleotide or nicotinamide adenine dinucleotide phosphate (CK, AST/ALT, ammonia, thyroxine, glucose).

Implementation

• Do not confuse sulfasalazine with cefuroxime or sulfadiazine.

• Varying dosing regimens of sulfasalazine may be used to minimize GI side effects.

• **PO:** Administer after meals or with food to minimize GI irritation, with a full glass of water. *DNC:* Swallow enteric-coated tablets whole; do not crush or chew.

Patient/Family Teaching

• Instruct patient on the correct method of administration. Advise patient to take medication as directed, even if feeling better. Take missed doses as soon as remembered unless almost time for next dose.

• May cause dizziness. Caution patient to avoid driving or other activities that require alertness until response to medication is known.

• Advise patient to notify health care professional if skin rash, sore throat, fever, mouth sores, unusual bleeding or bruising, wheezing, fever, or hives occur.

• Caution patient to use sunscreen and protective clothing to prevent photosensitivity reactions.

• Inform patient that this medication may cause orange-yellow discoloration of urine and skin, which is not significant. May permanently stain contact lenses yellow.

• Instruct patient to notify health care professional if symptoms worsen or do not improve. If symptoms of acute intolerance (cramping, acute abdominal pain, bloody diarrhea, fever, headache, rash) occur, discontinue therapy and notify health care professional immediately.

• Rep: May cause fetal harm. Advise females of reproductive potential to notify health care professional if pregnancy is planned or suspected, and to avoid breastfeeding during therapy. Neural tube defects have been reported in infants of women taking sulfasalazine during pregnancy. Monitor newborns for kernicterus if mother taking sulfasalazine; monitor breastfed infants for bloody stool or diarrhea. Inform male patient that sulfasalazine may cause infertility; usually reversible.

• Instruct patient to notify health care professional if symptoms do not improve after 1–2 mo of therapy.

Evaluation/Desired Outcomes

• Decrease in diarrhea and abdominal pain.

• Return to normal bowel pattern in patients with ulcerative colitis. Effects may be seen within 3–21 days. The usual course of therapy is 3–6 wk.

• Maintenance of remission in patients with ulcerative colitis.

• Decrease in pain and inflammation and increase in mobility in patients with rheumatoid arthritis.

SUMAtriptan (soo-ma-**trip**-tan)
Imitrex, ✦ Imitrex DF, Imitrex STATdose, Onzetra Xsail, Tosymra, Zembrace SymTouch

Classification
Therapeutic: vascular headache suppressants
Pharmacologic: 5-HT$_1$ agonists

Indications
SUBQ, PO, Intranasal: Acute treatment of migraine attacks. **SUBQ:** Acute treatment of cluster headache episodes.

Action
Acts as a selective agonist of 5-HT$_1$ at specific vascular serotonin receptor sites, causing vasoconstriction in large intracranial arteries. **Therapeutic Effects:** Relief of acute attacks of migraine.

Pharmacokinetics
Absorption: Well absorbed (97%) after SUBQ administration. Absorption after oral administration is incomplete and significant amounts undergo substantial hepatic metabolism, resulting in poor bioavailability (14%). Well absorbed after intranasal administration.
Distribution: Well distributed to tissues.
Metabolism and Excretion: Mostly metabolized (80%) by the liver.
Half-life: 2 hr.

TIME/ACTION PROFILE (relief of migraine)

ROUTE	ONSET	PEAK	DURATION
PO	within 30 min	2–4 hr	up to 24 hr
SUBQ	30 min	up to 2 hr	up to 24 hr
Nasal	within 60 min	2 hr	unknown

Contraindications/Precautions
Contraindicated in: Hypersensitivity to sumatriptan or latex (needle shield of prefilled syringe contains rubber [latex derivative]); Ischemic heart disease or signs and symptoms of ischemic heart disease, Prinzmetal's angina, or uncontrolled hypertension; Stroke or transient ischemic attack; Peripheral vascular disease (including, but not limited to, ischemic bowel disease);

Concurrent MAO inhibitor therapy; Hemiplegic or basilar migraine; Concurrent use of (within 24 hr) ergotamine-containing or ergot-type drugs or other 5HT$_1$ agonists; Severe hepatic impairment.

Use Cautiously in: OB: Use during pregnancy only if potential maternal benefit justifies potential fetal risk; Lactation: Use while breastfeeding only if potential maternal benefit justifies potential risk to infant; Rep: Women of reproductive potential; Pedi: Safety and effectiveness not established in children; Geri: ↑ risk of cardiovascular complications in older adults.

Exercise Extreme Caution in: Cardiovascular risk factors (hypertension, hypercholesterolemia, smoking, obesity, diabetes, family history, menopausal women or men >40 yr); use only if cardiovascular status has been evaluated and determined to be safe and 1st dose is administered under supervision.

Adverse Reactions/Side Effects

CV: angina, chest pressure, chest tightness, coronary vasospasm, ECG changes, MI, transient hypertension. **Derm:** tingling, warm sensation, burning sensation, cool sensation, flushing. **EENT:** alterations in vision, nasal sinus discomfort, throat discomfort. **GI:** abdominal discomfort, dysphagia. **Local:** injection site reaction. **MS:** jaw discomfort, muscle cramps, myalgia, neck pain, neck stiffness. **Neuro:** dizziness, vertigo, anxiety, drowsiness, fatigue, feeling of heaviness, feeling of tightness, headache, malaise, numbness, tight feeling in head, weakness. **Misc:** HYPERSENSITIVITY REACTIONS (including anaphylaxis and angioedema).

Interactions

Drug-Drug: The risk of vasospastic reactions may be ↑ by concurrent use of **ergotamine** or **dihydroergotamine** (avoid within 24 hr of each other). Avoid concurrent use with other **5HT$_1$ agonists**. **MAO inhibitors** may ↑ levels; do not use within 2 wk of discontinuing MAO inhibitor. ↑ risk of serotonin syndrome with **SSRIs, SNRIs, TCAs, meperidine, bupropion,** or **buspirone**; avoid concurrent use.

Drug-Natural Products: ↑ risk of serotonergic side effects including serotonin syndrome with **St. John's wort** and **SAMe**.

Route/Dosage

PO (Adults): 25 mg initially; if response is inadequate at 2 hr, up to 100 mg may be given (initial doses of 25–50 mg may be more effective than 25 mg). If headache recurs, doses may be repeated every 2 hr (not to exceed 300 mg/day). If PO therapy is to follow SUBQ injection, additional PO sumatriptan may be taken every 2 hr (not to exceed 200 mg/day).

SUBQ (Adults): 6 mg; may repeat after 1 hr (not to exceed 12 mg in 24 hr); *Zembrace SymTouch:* 3 mg; may repeat after 1 hr (not to exceed 12 mg/24 hr).

Intranasal (Adults): *Nasal spray (Imitrex):* Single dose of 5, 10, or 20 mg in 1 nostril; may be repeated in 2 hr (not to exceed 40 mg/24 hr or treatment of >5 episodes/mo); *Nasal spray (Tosymra):* Single dose of 10 mg in 1 nostril; may be repeated in 1 hr (not to exceed 30 mg/24 hr); *Nasal powder:* 11 mg in each nostril; may be repeated in 2 hr (not to exceed 44 mg/24 hr or treatment of >4 episodes/mo).

Hepatic Impairment

PO (Adults): 25 mg initially; if response is inadequate at 2 hr, up to 50 mg may be given (initial doses of 25–50 mg may be more effective than 25 mg). If headache recurs, doses may be repeated every 2 hr (not to exceed 300 mg/day). If PO therapy is to follow SUBQ injection, additional PO sumatriptan may be taken every 2 hr (not to exceed 200 mg/day); no single oral dose should exceed 50 mg.

Availability (generic available)

Nasal powder capsules (Onzetra Xsail): 11 mg. **Nasal spray (Imitrex, Tosymra):** 5 mg/spray, 10 mg/spray, 20 mg/spray. **Solution for injection (autoinjectors):** 3 mg/0.5 mL, 4 mg/0.5 mL, 6 mg/0.5 mL. **Tablets:** 25 mg, 50 mg, 100 mg. *In combination with:* naproxen (Treximet); see Appendix N.

NURSING IMPLICATIONS

Assessment

- Assess pain location, intensity, duration, and associated symptoms (photophobia, phonophobia, nausea, vomiting) during migraine attack.
- Give initial SUBQ dose under observation to patients with potential for coronary artery disease including postmenopausal women, men >40 yr, patients with risk factors for coronary artery disease such as hypertension, hypercholesterolemia, obesity, diabetes, smoking, or family history. Monitor BP before and for 1 hr after initial injection. If angina occurs, monitor ECG for ischemic changes.
- Monitor for serotonin syndrome in patients taking SSRIs or SNRIs concurrently with sumatriptan.

Implementation

- Do not confuse sumatriptan with sitagliptin or zolmitriptan.
- **PO:** Tablets should be swallowed whole; *DNC:* do not crush, break, or chew. Tablets are film-coated to prevent contact with tablet contents, which have an unpleasant taste and may cause nausea and vomiting.
- **SUBQ:** Administer as a single injection. Solution is clear and colorless or pale yellow; do not use if dark-colored or cloudy or if beyond expiration date.
- **Intranasal:** 10-mg dose may be administered as 2 sprays of 5 mg in 1 nostril or 1 spray in each nostril.
- **Nasal Powder:** Remove clear device cap from the reusable delivery device, then remove a disposable nosepiece from foil pouch and click nosepiece into device body. Press fully and promptly release white

S

piercing button on device body to pierce capsule inside nosepiece. White piercing button should only be pressed once and released prior to administration to each nostril. Insert nosepiece into nostril making a tight seal. Rotate device to place mouthpiece into the mouth. Patient blows forcefully through mouthpiece to deliver the sumatriptan powder into nasal cavity. Vibration (e.g., a rattling noise) may occur, and indicates that patient is blowing forcefully, as directed. Once medication in the first nosepiece has been administered, remove and discard nosepiece.

Patient/Family Teaching

- Inform patient that sumatriptan should be used only *during* a migraine attack. It is meant to be used for relief of migraine attacks but not to prevent or reduce the number of attacks.
- Instruct patient to administer sumatriptan as soon as symptoms of a migraine attack appear, but it may be administered at any time during an attack. If migraine symptoms return, a 2nd injection may be used. Allow at least 1 hr between doses, and do not use more than 2 injections in any 24-hr period. Additional sumatriptan doses are not likely to be effective, and alternative medications may be used. If no relief from 1st dose, unlikely 2nd dose will provide relief. Advise patient to read *Patient Information* prior to using and with each Rx refill; new information may be available.
- Advise patient that lying down in a darkened room after sumatriptan administration may further help relieve headache.
- Advise patient that overuse (use more than 10 days/mo) may lead to exacerbation of headache (migraine-like daily headaches, or as a marked increase in frequency of migraine attacks). May require gradual withdrawal of sumatriptan and treatment of symptoms (transient worsening of headache).
- Advise patient to notify health care professional before next dose of sumatriptan if pain or tightness in chest occurs during use. If pain is severe or does not subside, notify health care professional immediately. If wheezing; heart throbbing; swelling of eyelids, face, or lips; skin rash; skin lumps; or hives occur, notify health care professional immediately, and do not take more sumatriptan without approval of health care professional. If usual dose fails to relieve 3 consecutive headaches, or if frequency and/or severity increases, notify health care professional. If feelings of tingling, heat, flushing, heaviness, pressure, drowsiness, dizziness, tiredness, or sickness develop, discuss with health care professional at next visit.
- Sumatriptan may cause dizziness or drowsiness. Caution patient to avoid driving or other activities requiring alertness until response to medication is known.
- Advise patient to avoid alcohol, which aggravates headaches, during sumatriptan use.

- Instruct patient to notify health care professional of all Rx or OTC medications, vitamins, or herbal products being taken and consult health care professional before taking any new medications. Patients concurrently taking SSRI or SNRI antidepressants should notify health care professional promptly if signs of serotonin syndrome (mental status changes: agitation, hallucinations, coma; autonomic instability: tachycardia, labile BP, hyperthermia; neuromuscular aberrations: hyper-reflexia, incoordination; and/or gastrointestinal symptoms: nausea, vomiting, diarrhea) occur.
- Rep: Caution patient not to use sumatriptan if pregnancy is planned or suspected or if breastfeeding. Adequate contraception should be used during therapy.
- SUBQ: Instruct patient on the proper technique for loading, administering, and discarding the *Imitrex STATdose pen* autoinjector. Patient information pamphlet is provided. Instructional video is available from the manufacturer.
- Inform patient that pain or redness at the injection site usually lasts less than 1 hr.
- **Intranasal:** Instruct patient in proper technique for intranasal administration. Usual dose is a single spray in 1 nostril. If headache returns, a 2nd dose may be administered in ≥2 hr. Do not administer 2nd dose if no relief was provided by 1st dose without consulting health care professional.

Evaluation/Desired Outcomes

- Relief of migraine attack.

SUNItinib (su-ni-ti-nib)
Sutent
Classification
Therapeutic: antineoplastics
Pharmacologic: kinase inhibitors

Indications

Gastrointestinal stromal tumor that has progressed on or has intolerance to imatinib. Advanced renal cell carcinoma. Adjuvant treatment of patients at high risk of recurrent renal cell carcinoma following nephrectomy. Advanced pancreatic neuroendocrine tumors.

Action

Inhibits multiple receptor tyrosine kinases, which are enzymes implicated in tumor growth, abnormal vascular growth, and tumor metastases. **Therapeutic Effects:** Decreased tumor spread.

Pharmacokinetics

Absorption: Well absorbed following oral administration.

Distribution: Extensively distributed to tissues.

Protein Binding: *Sunitinib:* 95%; *primary active metabolite:* 90%.

Metabolism and Excretion: Metabolized by the liver via the CYP3A4 isoenzyme to its primary active metabolite. This metabolite is further metabolized by CYP3A4. Excretion is primarily fecal.

Half-life: *Sunitinib:* 40–60 hr; *primary active metabolite:* 80–110 hr.

TIME/ACTION PROFILE (plasma concentrations)

ROUTE	ONSET	PEAK	DURATION
PO	unknown	6–12 hr	24 hr

Contraindications/Precautions

Contraindicated in: Hypersensitivity; New York Heart Association class II-IV HF; OB: Pregnancy; Lactation: Lactation.

Use Cautiously in: Renal impairment; Hepatic impairment; Concurrent use of bisphosphonates or a history of dental disease (may ↑ risk of osteonecrosis of the jaw [ONJ]); History of myocardial ischemia or MI; Left ventricular ejection fraction <50% and >20% below baseline with no signs/symptoms of HF (need to interrupt therapy or ↓ dose); Diabetes (↑ risk of hypoglycemia); History of QT interval prolongation, use of antiarrhythmics, cardiac disease, bradycardia, or electrolyte disturbances; Rep: Women of reproductive potential and men with female partners of reproductive potential; Pedi: Safety and effectiveness not established in children.

Adverse Reactions/Side Effects

CV: hypertension, DEEP VEIN THROMBOSIS, HF, MI, peripheral edema, QT interval prolongation, TORSADES DE POINTES. **Derm:** alopecia, ERYTHEMA MULTIFORME, hair color change, hand-foot syndrome, impaired wound healing, NECROTIZING FASCIITIS, rash, skin discoloration, STEVENS-JOHNSON SYNDROME, TOXIC EPIDERMAL NECROLYSIS. **EENT:** epistaxis. **Endo:** hypoglycemia, hypothyroidism, adrenal insufficiency, hyperthyroidism. **F and E:** dehydration, hypophosphatemia. **GI:** diarrhea, dyspepsia, HEPATOTOXICITY, nausea, stomatitis, vomiting, ↑ lipase/amylase, ↑ liver enzymes, anorexia, cholecystitis, constipation, esophagitis, GI PERFORATION, oral pain. **GU:** HEMOLYTIC UREMIC SYNDROME, ↓ fertility, nephrotic syndrome, proteinuria, renal failure. **Hemat:** anemia, HEMORRHAGE, lymphopenia, neutropenia, thrombocytopenia, THROMBOTIC THROMBOCYTOPENIC PURPURA. **Metab:** hyperuricemia. **MS:** arthralgia, back pain, limb pain, myalgia, osteonecrosis (primarily ONJ). **Neuro:** fatigue, dizziness, dysgeusia, headache, POSTERIOR REVERSIBLE ENCEPHALOPATHY SYNDROME (PRES). **Resp:** PULMONARY EMBOLISM. **Misc:** fever, TUMOR LYSIS SYNDROME.

Interactions

Drug-Drug: **Strong CYP3A4 inhibitors**, including **ketoconazole**, may ↑ levels and the risk of toxicity; avoid concurrent use, if possible. If concurrent use necessary, ↓ sunitinib dose. **Strong CYP3A4 inducers**, including **rifampin**, may ↓ levels and effective-

ness; avoid concurrent use, if possible. If concurrent use necessary, ↑ sunitinib dose. Concurrent use with **alendronate, ibandronate, pamidronate, risedronate**, or **zoledronic acid** may ↑ risk of jaw osteonecrosis. ↑ risk of microangiopathic hemolytic anemia when used with **bevacizumab**; concurrent use not recommended. Concurrent use of other **QT-interval prolonging medications** may ↑ risk of torsades de pointes.

Drug-Natural Products: **St. John's wort** may ↓ levels and effectiveness; avoid concurrent use.

Drug-Food: **Grapefruit juice** may ↑ levels and the risk of toxicity; avoid concurrent use.

Route/Dosage

Gastrointestinal Stromal Tumor and Renal Cell Carcinoma

PO (Adults): 50 mg once daily for 4 wk, followed by 2 wk off; continue until disease progression or unacceptable toxicity. *Concurrent use of strong CYP3A4 inhibitors:* 37.5 mg once daily for 4 wk, followed by 2 wk off; continue until disease progression or unacceptable toxicity. *Concurrent use of strong CYP3A4 inducers:* 87.5 mg once daily for 4 wk, followed by 2 wk off; continue until disease progression or unacceptable toxicity.

Renal Impairment

PO (Adults): *End-stage renal disease (on hemodialysis):* No initial adjustment required; subsequent dosage ↑ (up to 2-fold) may be required due to reduced exposure.

Adjuvant Treatment of Renal Cell Carcinoma

PO (Adults): 50 mg once daily for 4 wk, followed by 2 wk off for a total of nine 6-wk cycles. *Concurrent use of strong CYP3A4 inhibitors:* 37.5 mg once daily for 4 wk, followed by 2 wk off for a total of nine 6-wk cycles. *Concurrent use of strong CYP3A4 inducers:* 87.5 mg once daily for 4 wk, followed by 2 wk off for a total of nine 6-wk cycles.

Renal Impairment

PO (Adults): *End-stage renal disease (on hemodialysis):* No initial adjustment required; subsequent dosage ↑ (up to 2-fold) may be required due to reduced exposure.

Pancreatic Neuroendocrine Tumor

PO (Adults): 37.5 mg once daily until disease progression or unacceptable toxicity. *Concurrent use of strong CYP3A4 inhibitors:* 25 mg once daily until disease progression or unacceptable toxicity. *Concurrent use of strong CYP3A4 inducers:* 62.5 mg once daily until disease progression or unacceptable toxicity.

Renal Impairment

PO (Adults): *End-stage renal disease (on hemodialysis):* No initial adjustment required; subsequent dosage ↑ (up to 2-fold) may be required due to reduced exposure.

S

Availability (generic available)
Capsules: 12.5 mg, 25 mg, 37.5 mg, 50 mg.

NURSING IMPLICATIONS
Assessment
- Monitor for signs of HF (dyspnea, edema, jugular venous distention) during therapy. Assess LVEF at baseline and periodically during therapy in patients with cardiac events in the previous 12 mo and a baseline ejection fraction in patients without cardiovascular risk factors. *If asymptomatic cardiomyopathy (LVEF >20% but <50% below baseline or below lower limit of normal if baseline was not obtained)* occurs, hold sunitinib until resolution to Grade 0 or 1 or baseline. Resume at a reduced dose. *If clinically manifested HF occurs,* discontinue sunitinib permanently.
- Monitor for hypertension and treat with standard antihypertensive therapy. *If Grade 3 hypertension occurs,* hold sunitinib until resolution to Grade 0 or 1 or baseline. Resume at a reduced dose. *If Grade 4 hypertension occurs,* permanently discontinue therapy.
- Monitor for signs and symptoms of bleeding (epistaxis, GI bleeding) during therapy. If Grade 3 or 4 hemorrhage occurs, hold sunitinib until resolution to Grade 0 to 1 or baseline. Either resume at reduced dose or discontinue depending on the severity and persistence of adverse reaction.
- Perform an oral examination before starting and periodically during therapy. Monitor for signs and symptoms of ONJ (tooth or jaw pain, swelling of the jaw) during therapy. Patients taking bisphosphonates, who have dental disease, or undergo invasive dental procedures, are at increased risk. Hold sunitinib for at least 3 wk before scheduled dental surgery or invasive dental procedures, if possible. Hold therapy for development of ONJ until complete resolution occurs.
- Monitor ECG and electrolytes periodically during therapy; may cause QT interval prolongation and torsades de pointes.
- Monitor for rash. If progressive skin rash with blisters or mucosal lesions or necrotizing fasciitis occurs, discontinue and do not restart sunitinib.
- Monitor for signs and symptoms of PRES (hypertension, headache, decreased alertness, altered mental functioning, visual loss, including cortical blindness) during therapy. An MRI is necessary to confirm diagnosis. Discontinue sunitinib in patients developing PRES.

Lab Test Considerations
- Monitor CBC with platelet count and serum chemistries including phosphate at the beginning of each treatment cycle. May cause neutropenia, lymphopenia, anemia, and thrombocytopenia. May cause ↑ serum creatinine, hypokalemia, and hyperuricemia.
- Monitor ALT, AST, and bilirubin before starting therapy, during each cycle of treatment, and as clinically

indicated. *If Grade 3 hepatotoxicity occurs,* hold sunitinib until resolution to Grade 0 or 1 or baseline. Resume therapy at reduced dose. If Grade 3 hepatotoxicity recurs or Grade 4 hepatotoxicity occurs, permanently discontinue sunitinib. May cause ↑ AST, ALT, alkaline phosphatase, total and indirect bilirubin, amylase, and lipase.
- Monitor thyroid function at baseline and in patients with symptoms of hypothyroidism or hyperthyroidism. May be treated with standard medical practice.
- Monitor urinalysis for urine protein at baseline and periodically during therapy. Follow up with 24-hr urine protein as clinically indicated. *If ≥3 grams proteinuria in 24 hr in the absence of nephrotic syndrome occurs,* hold sunitinib until resolution to Grade 0 or 1 or baseline. Resume therapy at reduced dose. *If nephrotic syndrome or recurrent proteinuria of ≥3 grams per 24 hr despite dose reductions occurs,* permanently discontinue sunitinib.
- Monitor blood glucose levels periodically during and after therapy. Assess if antidiabetic drug dose needs to be adjusted to minimize the risk of hypoglycemia.

Implementation
- Do not confuse sunitinib with sorafenib.
- **Recommended Dose Modifications:** For patients with gastrointestinal stromal tumor and advanced renal cell carcinoma: *First dose reduction,* 37.5 once daily. *Second dose reduction,* 25 mg once daily. For patients with adjuvant renal cell carcinoma: *First dose reduction,* 37.5 mg once daily. For patients with pancreatic neuroendocrine tumor: *First dose reduction,* 25 mg once daily.
- **PO:** Administer once daily with or without food.

Patient/Family Teaching
- Instruct patient to take sunitinib as directed. Take missed doses as soon as remembered if within 12 hr of missed dose. If >12 hr since missed dose, omit dose and take next dose at regular time. Do not take more than 1 dose at a time. Tell your health care professional about the missed dose.
- Advise patient to avoid grapefruit juice and grapefruit products during therapy.
- Instruct patient to notify health care professional promptly if signs and symptoms of liver failure (itching, yellow eyes or skin, dark urine, pain or discomfort in the right upper stomach area), rash, bleeding (painful, swollen abdomen, black, sticky stools, bloody urine, vomiting blood, headache, coughing up blood, change in your mental status), ONJ (tooth or jaw pain, jaw swelling) or tumor lysis syndrome (nausea, shortness of breath, irregular heartbeat, clouding of urine, tiredness) occur.
- Advise patient that GI disorders (diarrhea, nausea, stomatitis, dyspepsia, vomiting) are common and may require antiemetic and antidiarrheal medications.

- Inform patient that sunitinib may cause discoloration (yellow) of skin and depigmentation of hair or skin.
- Instruct patient to notify health care professional of all Rx or OTC medications, vitamins, or herbal products being taken and consult health care professional before taking any new medications, especially St. John's wort.
- Advise patient to notify health care professionals of therapy. Therapy must be stopped for at least 3 wk before scheduled dental surgery, invasive dental procedures, or elective surgeries and then held for at least 2 wk after major surgery until adequate wound healing.
- Advise patient to notify health care professional if bleeding or swelling occur.
- Rep: May cause fetal harm. Advise females of reproductive potential to use effective contraception during and after therapy and to avoid breastfeeding during and for 4 wk after last dose. Advise males with female partners of reproductive potential to use effective contraception during and for 7 wk after last dose. May impair male and female fertility.

Evaluation/Desired Outcomes

- Decrease in tumor spread.

---

suvorexant (soo-voe-**rex**-ant)
Belsomra
Classification
Therapeutic: sedative/hypnotics
Pharmacologic: orexin receptor antagonists

Schedule IV

Indications

Insomnia associated with difficulty in sleep onset and/or maintenance.

Action

Antagonizes the effects of orexins A and B, naturally occurring neuropeptides that promote wakefulness, by binding to their receptors. **Therapeutic Effects:** Improved sleep.

Pharmacokinetics

Absorption: 82% absorbed following oral administration; a high-fat meal will delay absorption and sleep onset. ↑ absorption in obese females.
Distribution: Well distributed to tissues.
Protein Binding: >99%.
Metabolism and Excretion: Extensively metabolized by the liver via the CYP3A isoenzyme and to a lesser extent by the CYP2C19 isoenzyme to inactive metabolites. 66% excreted in feces, 23% in urine, mostly as metabolites.
Half-life: 12 hr (↑ in hepatic impairment).

TIME/ACTION PROFILE (sleep)

ROUTE	ONSET	PEAK	DURATION
PO	30 min (delayed by food)	unknown	7 hr†

†Excess sedation may persist for several days after discontinuation.

Contraindications/Precautions

Contraindicated in: Narcolepsy; Severe hepatic impairment.
Use Cautiously in: History of substance abuse or drug dependence; Obese patients (↑ levels, especially in women, dose ↓ may be warranted); History of or concurrent psychiatric diagnoses; Underlying pulmonary disease; OB: Use during pregnancy only if potential maternal benefit justifies potential fetal risk; Lactation: Use while breastfeeding only if potential maternal benefit justifies potential risk to infant; Pedi: Safety and effectiveness not established in children; Geri: ↑ risk of falls in older adults.

Adverse Reactions/Side Effects

Adverse reactions, especially related to CNS depression are dose-related, especially at the 20-mg dose.
Neuro: drowsiness, cataplexy, complex sleep behaviors (including sleep driving, sleep walking, or engaging in other activities while sleeping), daytime drowsiness, hallucinations (during sleep), sleep paralysis, worsening of depression/suicidal ideation.

Interactions

Drug-Drug: Strong CYP3A inhibitors, including **clarithromycin, conivaptan, itraconazole, ketoconazole, nefazodone, nelfinavir, posaconazole,** and **ritonavir,** ↑ risk of excessive sedation; avoid concurrent use. **Moderate CYP3A inhibitors,** including **aprepitant, atazanavir, ciprofloxacin, diltiazem, erythromycin, fluconazole, fosamprenavir, imatinib,** and **verapamil,** may result in ↑ sedation; ↓ suvorexant dose. Risk of CNS depression, next-day impairment, "sleep-driving," and other complex behaviors while not fully awake ↑ with other **CNS depressants,** including **alcohol,** some **antihistamines, opioids,** other **sedative/hypnotics** (including **benzodiazepines**), and **tricyclic antidepressants;** dose adjustments may be necessary. **CYP3A inducers,** including **carbamazepine, phenytoin,** and **rifampin,** may ↓ levels and effectiveness. May alter **digoxin** levels; closely monitor serum digoxin concentrations.
Drug-Food: Grapefruit juice may ↑ levels and excess sedation; ↓ suvorexant dose.

Route/Dosage

PO (Adults): 10 mg within 30 min of going to bed; if well tolerated but not optimally effective, dose may be ↑ the following night, not to exceed 20 mg (dose may not be repeated on a single night and should be when

≥7 hr of sleep time is anticipated before planned awakening). *Concurrent use of moderate CYP3A inhibitors:* 5 mg initially, dose may be ↑ to 10 mg if lower dose is tolerated but not optimally effective. Lowest effective dose should be used.

Availability

Tablets: 5 mg, 10 mg, 15 mg, 20 mg.

NURSING IMPLICATIONS

Assessment

- Assess mental status, sleep patterns, and potential for abuse prior to administration. Prolonged use of >7–10 days may lead to physical and psychological dependence. Limit amount of drug available to the patient.
- Assess alertness at time of peak effect. Notify health care professional if desired sedation does not occur.

Implementation

- Before administering, reduce external stimuli and provide comfort measures to increase effectiveness of medication.
- Protect patient from injury. Raise bed side rails. Assist with ambulation. Remove patient's cigarettes.
- Use lowest effective dose.
- PO: Administer no more than once/night and within 30 min of going to bed. Take only if at least 7 hr remaining before awaking. *DNC:* Swallow tablets whole with full glass of water. For faster onset of sleep, do not administer with or immediately after a meal.

Patient/Family Teaching

- Instruct patient to take suvorexant as directed. Advise patient not to take suvorexant unless able to stay in bed a full night (7 hr) before being active again. Do not take more than the amount prescribed because of the habit-forming potential. Not recommended for use longer than 7–10 days. Instruct patient to read the *Medication Guide* for correct product before taking and with each Rx refill, changes may occur.
- Because of rapid onset, advise patient to go to bed immediately after taking suvorexant.
- May cause daytime drowsiness or dizziness. Advise patient to avoid driving or other activities requiring alertness for at least 8 hr after dosing until response to this medication is known.
- Caution patient that complex sleep-related behaviors (sleep-driving) may occur while asleep. Inform families and advise to notify health care professional if these behaviors occur.
- Instruct patient to notify health care professional of all Rx or OTC medications, vitamins, or herbal products being taken and to avoid concurrent use of Rx, OTC, and herbal products without consulting health care professional.
- Caution patient to avoid concurrent use of alcohol or other CNS depressants, including opioids.
- Advise patient to notify health care professional if depression worsens or suicidal thoughts occur.
- Advise patient to notify health care professional immediately if signs of anaphylaxis (swelling of the tongue or throat, trouble breathing, and nausea and vomiting) occur.
- Rep: Advise females of reproductive potential to notify health care professional if pregnancy is planned or suspected or if breastfeeding.

Evaluation/Desired Outcomes

- Relief of insomnia.

⚠ TACROLIMUS
tacrolimus (oral, IV)
(ta-**kroe**-li-mus)
♣Advagraf, Astagraf XL,
♣Envarsus PA, Envarsus XR, Prograf
tacrolimus (topical)
Protopic
Classification
Therapeutic: immunosuppressants

Indications
PO, IV: Prevention of organ rejection in patients who have undergone allogeneic liver, kidney, heart, or lung transplantation (in combination with other immunosuppressants) (extended-release only indicated for kidney transplant). **Topical:** Moderate to severe atopic dermatitis in patients who do not respond to or cannot tolerate alternative, conventional therapies.

Action
Inhibit T-lymphocyte activation. **Therapeutic Effects:** Prevention of transplanted organ rejection. Improvement in signs/symptoms of atopic dermatitis.

Pharmacokinetics
Absorption: Absorption following oral administration is erratic and incomplete (bioavailability ranges 5–67%); minimal amounts absorbed following topical use.
Distribution: Crosses the placenta and enters breast milk.
Protein Binding: 99%.
Metabolism and Excretion: 99% metabolized by the liver; <1% excreted unchanged in the urine.
Half-life: *Liver transplant patients:* 11.7 hr; *healthy volunteers:* 21.2 hr.

TIME/ACTION PROFILE
(immunosuppression)

ROUTE	ONSET	PEAK	DURATION
PO	rapid	1.3–3.2 hr*	12 hr
PO-ER	unknown	unknown	24 hr
IV	rapid	unknown	8–12 hr
Topical†	unknown	1–2 wk	unknown

*Blood level.
†Improvement in atopic dermatitis.

Contraindications/Precautions
Contraindicated in: Hypersensitivity to tacrolimus or to castor oil (a component in the injection); Concurrent use with cyclosporine (↑ risk of nephrotoxicity); Concurrent use of sirolimus (↑ risk of mortality and adverse reactions); Congenital long QT syndrome; Weakened/compromised immune system; Malignant or premalignant skin condition; Lactation: Lactation.
Use Cautiously in: Heart failure, bradycardia, or electrolyte disorders (hypokalemia, hypomagnesemia,

hypocalcemia); Concurrent use of other drugs known to prolong the QT interval; Severe infection, graft-versus-host disease, or human leukocyte antigen mismatch (↑ risk of thrombotic microangiopathy); Renal or hepatic impairment (dose ↓ may be required; if oliguria occurs, wait 48 hr before initiating tacrolimus); Exposure to sunlight/UV light (may ↑ risk of malignant skin changes); Superficial skin infections; Rep: Women and men of reproductive potential; OB: Hyperkalemia and renal impairment may occur in the newborn; use during pregnancy only if potential maternal benefit justifies potential fetal risk; Pedi: Higher end of dosing range is required to maintain adequate blood levels in children.

Adverse Reactions/Side Effects
Noted primarily for PO and IV use.
CV: hypertension, peripheral edema, QT interval prolongation. **Derm:** pruritus, rash, alopecia, herpes simplex, hirsutism, impaired wound healing, photosensitivity, sweating. **EENT:** abnormal vision, amblyopia, sinusitis, tinnitus. **Endo:** hyperglycemia, hyperlipidemia. **F and E:** hyperkalemia, hypomagnesemia, hyperphosphatemia, hypocalcemia, hyponatremia, hypophosphatemia, metabolic acidosis, metabolic alkalosis. **GI:** ↑ liver enzymes, abdominal pain, anorexia, ascites, constipation, diarrhea, dyspepsia, nausea, vomiting, ↑ appetite, cholangitis, cholestatic jaundice, dysphagia, flatulence, GI BLEEDING, GI PERFORATION, oral thrush, peritonitis. **GU:** nephrotoxicity, urinary tract infection, ↓ fertility. **Hemat:** anemia, leukocytosis, leukopenia, thrombocytopenia, coagulation defects, pure red cell aplasia, thrombotic microangiopathy (including hemolytic uremic syndrome and thrombotic thrombocytopenia purpura). **Local:** *topical:* burning, stinging. **MS:** arthralgia, hypertonia, leg cramps, muscle spasm, myalgia, myasthenia, osteoporosis. **Neuro:** dizziness, headache, insomnia, paresthesia, tremor, abnormal dreams, agitation, anxiety, confusion, depression, emotional lability, hallucinations, neuropathy, POSTERIOR REVERSIBLE ENCEPHALOPATHY SYNDROME (PRES), psychoses, SEIZURES, somnolence. **Resp:** cough, pleural effusion, asthma, bronchitis, pharyngitis, pneumonia, pulmonary edema. **Misc:** generalized pain, chills, fever, HYPERSENSITIVITY REACTIONS (including anaphylaxis), INFECTION (including activation of latent viral infections such as BK virus-associated nephropathy), MALIGNANCY (including lymphoma and skin cancer).

Interactions
Noted primarily for PO and IV use, but should be considered for topical use.

Drug-Drug: Risk of nephrotoxicity is ↑ by concurrent use of **aminoglycosides**, **amphotericin B**, **cisplatin**, **nucleotide reverse transcriptase inhibitors**, **protease inhibitors**, or **cyclosporine** (allow 24 hr to pass after stopping cyclosporine before starting tacrolimus). Concurrent use of **potassium-spar-**

T

ing diuretics, **ACE inhibitors**, or **angiotensin II receptor blockers** ↑ risk of hyperkalemia. **Strong CYP3A4 inhibitors**, including **chloramphenicol, clarithromycin, cobicistat, itraconazole, ketoconazole, nefazodone, posaconazole, protease inhibitors,** and **voriconazole**, may significantly ↑ levels; ↓ tacrolimus dose by 2/3 when used with voriconazole or posaconazole; closely monitor tacrolimus whole blood trough concentrations. **Mild CYP3A4 inhibitors** and **moderate CYP3A4 inhibitors,** including **amiodarone, calcium channel blockers, cimetidine, clotrimazole, danazol, erythromycin, ethinyl estradiol, fluconazole, imatinib, isavuconazonium, lansoprazole, letermovir, nilotinib,** and **omeprazole,** may ↑ levels and risk of toxicity; closely monitor tacrolimus whole blood trough concentrations and adjust tacrolimus dose, if needed. **Magnesium/aluminum hydroxide** and **metoclopramide** may ↑ levels and risk of toxicity; closely monitor tacrolimus whole blood trough concentrations and adjust tacrolimus dose, if needed. **Strong CYP3A4 inducers,** including **carbamazepine, phenobarbital, phenytoin, rifabutin,** and **rifampin,** may ↓ levels; ↑ tacrolimus dose and closely monitor tacrolimus whole blood trough concentrations. **Mild CYP3A4 inducers** and **moderate CYP3A4 inducers,** including **methylprednisolone** or **prednisone,** may ↓ levels; closely monitor tacrolimus whole blood trough concentrations and adjust tacrolimus dose, if needed. **Vaccinations** may be less effective if given concurrently with tacrolimus (avoid use of live-virus vaccines). May ↑ levels of **mycophenolate mofetil** or **mycophenolic acid. Caspofungin** may ↓ levels; closely monitor tacrolimus whole blood trough concentrations and adjust tacrolimus dose, if needed. **Cannabidiol** may ↑ levels and the risk of toxicity; monitor tacrolimus levels and adjust dose as necessary. **Drug-Natural Products:** Concomitant use with **astragalus, echinacea,** and **melatonin** may interfere with immunosuppression. **St. John's wort** may ↓ levels; ↑ tacrolimus dose and closely monitor tacrolimus whole blood trough concentrations. **Schisandra sphenanthera** may significantly ↑ levels; closely monitor tacrolimus whole blood trough concentrations. **Drug-Food:** Food ↓ the rate and extent of GI absorption. **Grapefruit juice** may ↑ levels and risk of toxicity; avoid concurrent use.

Route/Dosage

Because of the potential risk for anaphylaxis, the IV route of administration should be reserved for those patients unable to take the drug orally. Extended-release capsules are not interchangeable with immediate-release capsules/granules or other extended-release products. When converting between immediate-release capsules and granules, the total daily dose should remain the same. Black patients may require a higher dose to achieve desired tacrolimus trough concentrations. Patients with cystic fibrosis may also require a

higher dose for lung transplantation due to a reduced bioavailability.

Kidney Transplantation

PO (Adults): *Immediate-release capsules (in combination with azathioprine):* 0.2 mg/kg/day in 2 divided doses initially; titrate to achieve recommended whole blood trough concentration; *Immediate-release capsules (in combination with mycophenolate mofetil and IL-2 antagonist):* 0.1 mg/kg/day in 2 divided doses initially; titrate to achieve recommended whole blood trough concentration; *Extended-release capsules (AstagrafXL) (in combination with basiliximab induction):* 0.15 mg/kg once daily (to be started either before or within 48 hr of completion of transplant); *Extended-release capsules (AstagrafXL) (without basiliximab induction):* 0.1 mg/kg given as single dose preoperatively within 12 hr prior to reperfusion, followed by 0.2 mg/kg once daily started postoperatively at least 4 hr after preoperative dose and within 12 hr after reperfusion; *Conversion from immediate-release capsules to extended-release capsules (Envarsus XR):* Initiate extended-release treatment with a once-daily dose that is 80% of the total daily dose of the immediate-release product (also appropriate for Black patients).

PO (Children): *Immediate-release capsules or suspension:* 0.3 mg/kg/day in 2 divided doses initially; titrate to achieve recommended whole blood trough concentration.

IV (Adults): 0.03–0.05 mg/kg/day as a continuous infusion initially; titrate to achieve recommended blood concentration.

Liver Transplantation

PO (Adults): *Immediate-release capsules:* 0.1–0.15 mg/kg/day in 2 divided doses initially; titrate to achieve recommended blood concentration.

PO (Children): *Immediate-release capsules:* 0.15–0.2 mg/kg/day in 2 divided doses initially; titrate to achieve recommended blood concentration. *Suspension:* 0.2 mg/kg/day in 2 divided doses initially; titrate to achieve recommended blood concentration.

IV (Adults): 0.03–0.05 mg/kg/day as a continuous infusion initially; titrate to achieve recommended blood concentration.

IV (Children): 0.03–0.05 mg/kg/day.

Heart Transplantation

PO (Adults): *Immediate-release capsules:* 0.075 mg/kg/day in 2 divided doses initially; titrate to achieve recommended blood concentration.

PO (Children): *Immediate-release capsules or suspension (without antibody induction treatment):* 0.3 mg/kg/day in 2 divided doses initially; titrate to achieve recommended whole blood trough concentration. *Immediate-release capsules or suspension (with antibody induction treatment):* 0.1 mg/kg/day in 2 divided doses initially; titrate to achieve recommended whole blood trough concentration.

IV (Adults): 0.01 mg/kg/day as a continuous infusion initially; titrate to achieve recommended blood concentration.

Lung Transplantation

PO (Adults): *Immediate-release capsules:* 0.075 mg/kg/day in 2 divided doses initially; titrate to achieve recommended blood concentration.

PO (Children): *Immediate-release capsules or suspension (without antibody induction treatment):* 0.3 mg/kg/day in 2 divided doses initially; titrate to achieve recommended whole blood trough concentration. *Immediate-release capsules or suspension (with antibody induction treatment):* 0.1 mg/kg/day in 2 divided doses initially; titrate to achieve recommended whole blood trough concentration.

IV (Adults): 0.01–0.03 mg/kg/day as a continuous infusion initially; titrate to achieve recommended blood concentration.

Atopic Dermatitis

Topical (Adults): Apply 0.03% or 0.1% ointment twice daily. Discontinue when signs/symptoms of atopic dermatitis resolve.

Topical (Children ≥2–15 yr): Apply 0.03% ointment twice daily. Discontinue when signs/symptoms of atopic dermatitis resolve.

Availability (generic available)

Capsules: 0.5 mg, 1 mg, 5 mg. **Extended-release capsules (Astragraf XL):** 0.5 mg, 1 mg, ✸ 3 mg, 5 mg. **Extended-release tablets (Envarsus XR):** 0.75 mg, 1 mg, 4 mg. **Granules for oral suspension:** 0.2 mg/pkt, 1 mg/pkt. **Solution for injection:** 5 mg/mL. **Topical ointment:** 0.03%, 0.1%.

NURSING IMPLICATIONS

Assessment

- Assess for symptoms of PRES (headache, altered mental status, seizures, visual disturbances, hypertension) periodically during therapy. Confirm diagnosis by radiologic procedure. If PRES is suspected or diagnosed, maintain BP control and immediately reduce immunosuppression. Symptoms are usually reversed on reduction or discontinuation of immunosuppression.
- **Prevention of Organ Rejection:** Monitor BP closely during therapy. Hypertension is a common complication of tacrolimus therapy and should be treated.
- Observe patients receiving IV tacrolimus for the development of anaphylaxis (rash, pruritus, laryngeal edema, wheezing) for at least 30 min and frequently thereafter. If signs develop, stop infusion and initiate treatment.
- **Atopic Dermatitis:** Assess skin lesions prior to and periodically during therapy.

- Use only for short time, not continuously, and in the minimum dose possible to decrease risk of developing skin cancer.

Lab Test Considerations
- Tacrolimus blood level monitoring may be helpful in the evaluation of rejection and toxicity, dose adjustments, and assessment of compliance. *For kidney transplantation*, during the first 3 mo, most patients maintained tacrolimus whole blood concentrations between 7–20 ng/mL and then between 5–15 ng/mL through 1 yr. *For de novo kidney transplantation*, during the first mo, most patients maintained tacrolimus whole blood concentrations between 6–11 ng/mL and then between 4–11 ng/mL through month 1. *For heart transplantation*, from wk 1 to 3 mo, most patients maintained tacrolimus trough whole blood concentrations between 8–20 ng/mL and then between 6–18 ng/mL from 3–18 mo post-transplant.
- Monitor serum creatinine, potassium, and glucose closely. ↑ serum creatinine and ↓ urine output may indicate nephrotoxicity. May also cause insulin-dependent post-transplant diabetes mellitus (▒ incidence is higher in Black and Hispanic patients).
- May also cause hyperuricemia, hypokalemia, hyperkalemia, hypomagnesemia, metabolic acidosis, metabolic alkalosis, hyperlipidemia, hyperphosphatemia, hypophosphatemia, hypocalcemia, and hyponatremia.
- Monitor CBC. May cause anemia, leukocytosis, and thrombocytopenia.

Implementation

- Do not confuse Prograf with Prozac. Do not confuse tacrolimus with tamsulosin.
- Do not confuse immediate-release tacrolimus with extended-release tacrolimus.
- Should only be prescribed by health care professionals experienced with immunosuppressive therapy and organ transplant patients.
- Begin therapy with tacrolimus no sooner than 6 hr post-transplantation. Concurrent therapy with corticosteroids is recommended in the early postoperative period.
- Tacrolimus should not be used concomitantly with cyclosporine. Tacrolimus or cyclosporine should be discontinued at least 24 hr before starting the other.
- Oral therapy is preferred because of the risk of anaphylactic reactions with IV tacrolimus. IV therapy should be replaced with oral therapy as soon as possible.
- Adults should be started at the lower end of the dose range; children require higher doses to maintain blood trough concentrations similar to adults.
- Immediate and extended-release capsules are not interchangeable.
- **PO:** Oral doses can be initiated 8–12 hr after discontinuation of IV doses. May be taken without re-

gard to food, but should be consistent, with or without food and at same time each day.

- Take extended-release capsules at the same time each day, preferably in the morning, on an empty stomach at least 1 hr before or 2 hr after breakfast. *DNC:* Swallow capsules whole; do not chew, divide, or crush.
- **Topical:** Do not use continuously for a long time.
- **Topical:** Wash hands before applying. Apply a thin layer of ointment twice daily to affected skin. Use smallest amount of ointment needed to control signs and symptoms of eczema. Do not cover treated area with bandages, dressings, or wraps. If not treating areas on hands, wash hands with soap and water after applying to remove any ointment on hands.

IV Administration
- **Continuous Infusion:** *Dilution:* Dilute in 0.9% NaCl or D5W. *Concentration:* 0.004–0.02 mg/mL. May be stored in polyethylene or glass containers for 24 hr following dilution. Do not store in PVC containers. Do not administer solutions that are discolored or contain particulate matter. *Rate:* Administer daily dose as a continuous infusion over 24 hr.
- **Y-Site Compatibility:** alemtuzumab, amifostine, amikacin, aminocaproic acid, aminophylline, amiodarone, amphotericin B lipid complex, amphotericin B liposomal, anidulafungin, argatroban, arsenic trioxide, azithromycin, aztreonam, benztropine, bivalirudin, bleomycin, bumetanide, buprenorphine, busulfan, butorphanol, calcium acetate, calcium chloride, calcium gluconate, carboplatin, carmustine, caspofungin, cefazolin, cefotaxime, cefotetan, cefoxitin, ceftazidime, ceftolozane/tazobactam, ceftriaxone, cefuroxime, chloramphenicol, chlorpromazine, ciprofloxacin, cisatracurium, cisplatin, clindamycin, cyclophosphamide, cyclosporine, cytarabine, dacarbazine, dactinomycin, daptomycin, daunorubicin hydrochloride, dexamethasone, dexmedetomidine, dexrazoxane, digoxin, diltiazem, diphenhydramine, dobutamine, docetaxel, dopamine, doxorubicin hydrochloride, doxorubicin liposomal, doxycycline, droperidol, enalaprilat, ephedrine, epinephrine, epirubicin, ertapenem, erythromycin, esmolol, etoposide, etoposide phosphate, famotidine, fentanyl, fluconazole, fludarabine, foscarnet, fosphenytoin, gemcitabine, gentamicin, glycopyrrolate, granisetron, haloperidol, heparin, hetastarch, hydralazine, hydrocortisone, hydromorphone, idarubicin, ifosfamide, imipenem/cilastatin, insulin regular, irinotecan, isavuconazonium, isoproterenol, ketorolac, labetalol, leucovorin calcium, levofloxacin, lidocaine, linezolid, lorazepam, magnesium sulfate, mannitol, meperidine, meropenem, mesna, methadone, methotrexate, methylprednisolone, metoclopramide, metoprolol, metronidazole, micafungin, midazolam, milrinone, mitomycin, mitoxantrone, morphine, moxifloxacin, multivitamins, mycophenolate, nafcillin, nalbuphine, naloxone, nicardipine, nitroglycerin, nitroprusside, norepinephrine, octreotide, ondansetron, oxacillin, oxaliplatin, oxytocin, paclitaxel, palonosetron, pamidronate, pemetrexed, penicillin G potassium, pentamidine, phentolamine, phenylephrine, piperacillin, piperacillin/tazobactam, potassium acetate, potassium chloride, potassium phosphate, procainamide, prochlorperazine, promethazine, propranolol, remifentanil, rocuronium, sodium acetate, sodium bicarbonate, sodium phosphate, succinylcholine, sufentanil, tedizolid, theophylline, thiotepa, tigecycline, tirofiban, tobramycin, topotecan, vancomycin, vasopressin, vecuronium, verapamil, vinblastine, vincristine, vinorelbine, voriconazole, zidovudine, zoledronic acid.
- **Y-Site Incompatibility:** acyclovir, allopurinol, azathioprine, cefepime, dantrolene, diazepam, esomeprazole, folic acid, ganciclovir, gemtuzumab ozogamicin, iron sucrose, levothyroxine, phenytoin, thiopental.

Patient/Family Teaching

- Instruct patient to take tacrolimus at the same time each day, with or without food, as directed. Do not skip or double up on missed doses. Do not discontinue medication without advice of health care professional. Take missed doses of extended-release capsule as soon as remembered unless more than 14 hr after scheduled dose; do not double doses. Advise patient to read the *Patient Information* before starting tacrolimus and with each Rx refill in case of changes. Instruct patient to inspect capsules with each new Rx, before taking. Contact health care professional if appearance of capsules or dose has changed.
- Advise patient to avoid grapefruit and grapefruit juice and alcohol during therapy.
- Reinforce the need for lifelong therapy to prevent transplant rejection. Review symptoms of rejection for transplanted organ and stress need to notify health care professional immediately if they occur.
- Advise patient to avoid eating raw oysters or other shellfish; make sure they are fully cooked before eating.
- Instruct patient to notify health care professional if signs of diabetes mellitus (frequent urination, increased thirst or hunger), infection (fever; sweats; chills; cough or flu-like symptoms; muscle aches; warm, red, painful areas on skin), neurotoxicity (vision changes, deliriums, or tremors), or PRES occur.
- Advise patient to wear protective clothing and sunscreen to avoid photosensitivity reactions.
- Instruct patient to avoid exposure to chicken pox, measles, mumps, and rubella. If exposed, see health care professional for prophylactic therapy.
- Instruct patient to notify health care professional of all Rx or OTC medications, vitamins, or herbal products being taken and consult health care professional before taking any new medications.

- Inform patient of the risk of lymphoma or skin cancer with tacrolimus therapy.
- Rep: May cause fetal harm. Advise females of reproductive potential to notify health care professional if pregnancy is planned or suspected or if breastfeeding. Encourage females who become pregnant and males who have fathered a pregnancy during treatment with tacrolimus to enroll in the pregnancy registry to collect information about birth outcomes by calling 1-877-955-6877 or https://www.transplantpregnancyregistry.org/.
- Emphasize the importance of repeated lab tests during tacrolimus therapy.
- **Topical:** Instruct patient to apply ointment as directed. Advise patient to read the *Medication Guide* prior to starting and with each Rx renewal; new information may be available.
- Advise patient not to bathe, shower, or swim right after applying; may wash off ointment. May use moisturizers with ointment. Instruct patient to check with health care professional first about products to use. If moisturizers are used, apply them after application of ointment.
- Advise patients to contact health care professional if their symptoms do not improve after 6 wk of therapy, if their symptoms worsen, or they develop a skin infection.
- Instruct patient to use ointment only on areas of skin with atopic dermatitis.
- Advise patient to stop using the ointment when the signs/symptoms of atopic dermatitis go away.
- Advise patient to limit sun exposure during treatment.
- Advise patient of the risk of using topical tacrolimus during pregnancy.
- Inform patient of the risk of lymphoma or skin cancer with topical tacrolimus therapy.

Evaluation/Desired Outcomes
- Prevention of transplanted organ rejection.
- Management of atopic dermatitis.

tadalafil (ta-da-la-fil)
Adcirca, Alyq, Cialis, Tadliq
Classification
Therapeutic: erectile dysfunction agents, vasodilators
Pharmacologic: phosphodiesterase type 5 inhibitors

Indications
Cialis: Treatment of: Erectile dysfunction (ED), Benign prostatic hyperplasia (BPH). *Adcirca, Alyq, and Tadliq:* Pulmonary arterial hypertension (PAH).

Action
Increases cyclic guanosine monophosphate (cGMP) levels by inhibiting phosphodiesterase type 5 an enzyme

responsible for the breakdown of cGMP. cGMP produces smooth muscle relaxation of the corpus cavernosum, which in turn promotes increased blood flow and subsequent erection. cGMP also leads to vasodilation of the pulmonary vasculature. **Therapeutic Effects:** *Cialis:* Enhanced blood flow to the corpus cavernosum and erection sufficient to allow sexual intercourse. Improved signs and symptoms of BPH. *Adcirca, Alyq, and Tadliq:* Improved exercise tolerance in PAH.

Pharmacokinetics
Absorption: Well absorbed following oral administration.
Distribution: Extensive tissue distribution; penetrates semen.
Protein Binding: 94%.
Metabolism and Excretion: Mostly metabolized by the liver via the CYP3A4 isoenzyme system; metabolites are excreted in feces (61%) and urine (36%).
Half-life: 17.5 hr.

TIME/ACTION PROFILE (vasodilation, improved erectile function)

ROUTE	ONSET	PEAK	DURATION
PO	rapid	0.5–6 hr	36

Contraindications/Precautions
Contraindicated in: Hypersensitivity; Concurrent use of nitrates or riociguat; Unstable angina, recent history of stroke, life-threatening heart failure within 6 mo, uncontrolled hypertension, arrhythmias, stroke within 6 mo or MI within 90 days; Any other cardiovascular pathology precluding sexual activity; Known hereditary degenerative retinal disorders; Severe hepatic impairment; Severe renal impairment (Adcirca, Alyq, and Tadliq); Severe renal impairment (CCr <30 mL/min) (Cialis once-daily dosing); Pedi: Children or newborns.
Use Cautiously in: Left ventricular outflow obstruction; Penile deformity; Renal impairment; Underlying conditions predisposing to priapism including sickle cell anemia, multiple myeloma, or leukemia; Bleeding disorders or active peptic ulcer disease; History of sudden severe vision loss or nonarteritic ischemic optic neuropathy; may ↑ risk of recurrence; Low cup-to-disk ratio, age >50 yr, diabetes, hypertension, coronary artery disease, hyperlipidemia, or smoking (↑ risk of nonarteritic ischemic optic neuropathy); Geri: ↑ risk of diarrhea in older adults.

Adverse Reactions/Side Effects
CV: hypotension, peripheral edema. **Derm:** flushing. **EENT:** hearing loss, nasal congestion, vision loss. **GI:** diarrhea, dyspepsia. **GU:** ↓ fertility, priapism. **MS:** back pain, limb pain, myalgia. **Neuro:** headache.

Interactions
Drug-Drug: Concurrent use of **nitrates** may cause serious, life-threatening hypotension and is contraindi-

cated. Concurrent use of **riociguat** may result in severe hypotension; concurrent use contraindicated. ↑ risk of hypotension with **alpha-adrenergic blockers** and acute ingestion of **alcohol**; discontinue alpha-adrenergic blocker therapy ≥1 day before starting Cialis for BPH. **Strong CYP3A4 inhibitors**, including **ritonavir**, **ketoconazole**, and**itraconazole**, may ↑ levels and the risk of toxicity (dose adjustments recommended with Cialis; avoid concurrent use with Adcirca, Alyq, and Tadliq). **CYP3A4 inducers** may ↓ levels and its effectiveness; avoid concurrent use with Adcirca, Alyq, or Tadliq.

Route/Dosage

Cialis (for ED)
PO (Adults): 10 mg prior to sexual activity (range 5–20 mg; not to exceed one dose/24 hr) *or* 2.5 mg once daily (max: 5 mg/day); *Concurrent use of strong CYP3A4 inhibitors:* single dose should not exceed 10 mg in any 72-hr period; for once-daily dose regimen, should not exceed 2.5 mg/day.

Renal Impairment
PO (Adults): *CCr 30–50 mL/min (as-needed dosing):* Initial dose should not exceed 5 mg/day; maximum dose should not exceed 10 mg in 48 hr; *CCr <30 mL/min (as-needed dosing):* Maximum dose should not exceed 5 mg in 72 hr; *CCr <30 mL/min (once-daily dosing):* Not recommended for use.

Hepatic Impairment
PO (Adults): *Mild or moderate hepatic impairment:* Daily dose should not exceed 10 mg (once-daily dose regimen not recommended) *Severe hepatic impairment:* Not recommended for use.

Cialis (for BPH or ED/BPH)
PO (Adults): 5 mg once daily; *Concurrent use of strong CYP3A4 inhibitors:* Should not exceed 2.5 mg once daily.

Renal Impairment
PO (Adults): *CCr 30–50 mL/min:* Initial dose should not exceed 2.5 mg/day; maximum dose should not exceed 5 mg/day; *CCr <30 mL/min:* Not recommended for use.

Hepatic Impairment
PO (Adults): Not recommended for use.

Adcirca, Alyq, and Tadliq (for PAH)
PO (Adults): 40 mg once daily; *If receiving ritonavir for ≥1 wk:* start 20 mg once daily; may then ↑ to 40 mg once daily based on tolerability; *If initiating ritonavir while on Adcirca, Alyq, or Tadliq:* stop Adcirca, Alyq, or Tadliq ≥24 hr before starting ritonavir; may reinitiate Adcirca, Alyq, or Tadliq at 20 mg once daily after ≥1 wk of therapy with ritonavir; may then ↑ to 40 mg once daily based on tolerability.

Renal Impairment
(Adults): *CCr 31–80 mL/min:* Start 20 mg once daily; may then ↑ to 40 mg once daily based on tolerability.

Hepatic Impairment
PO (Adults): *Mild or moderate hepatic impairment:* Start with 20 mg once daily.

Availability (generic available)
Tablets (Cialis): 2.5 mg, 5 mg, 10 mg, 20 mg. **Tablets (Adcirca or Alyq):** 20 mg. **Oral suspension (Tadliq) (peppermint flavor):** 20 mg/5 mL. *In combination with:* finasteride (Entadfi). See Appendix N.

NURSING IMPLICATIONS

Assessment
- *Cialis for ED*: Determine ED before administration. Tadalafil has no effect in the absence of sexual stimulation.
- *Cialis for BPH*: Assess for symptoms of BPH (urinary hesitancy, feeling of incomplete bladder emptying, interruption of urinary stream, impairment of size and force of urinary stream, terminal urinary dribbling, straining to start flow, dysuria, urgency) before and periodically during therapy.
- Digital rectal examinations should be performed before and periodically during therapy for BPH.
- *Adcirca, Alyq, Tadliq*: Monitor hemodynamic parameters and exercise tolerance prior to and periodically during therapy.

Implementation
- **PO:** Administer dose *as needed for ED* at least 30 min prior to sexual activity; effectiveness may continue for 36 hr.
- Administer dose for *PAH, BPH, ED/BPH, or daily for ED* once daily at the same time each day.
- May be administered without regard to food. *DNC:* Swallow tablets whole; do not crush, break, or chew.
- Shake suspension well for 30 sec before measuring dose.

Patient/Family Teaching
- Instruct patient to take tadalafil as needed for ED at least 30 min before sexual activity and not more than once per day. Inform patient that sexual stimulation is required for an erection to occur after taking tadalafil. Instruct patient to take tadalafil for PAH as directed. Advise patient to read *Patient Information* before starting therapy and with each Rx refill in case of changes.
- Advise patient that tadalafil is not indicated for use in women.
- Caution patient not to take tadalafil concurrently with alpha adrenergic blockers (unless on a stable dose) or nitrates. If chest pain occurs after taking tadalafil, instruct patient to seek immediate medical attention.
- Advise patient to avoid excess alcohol intake (≥5 units) in combination with tadalafil; may increase risk of orthostatic hypotension, increased heart rate, decreased standing BP, dizziness, headache.
- Instruct patient to notify health care professional promptly if erection lasts longer than 4 hr, if they are

not satisfied with their sexual performance or develop unwanted side effects, or if they experience sudden or decreased vision loss in one or both eyes or loss or decrease in hearing, ringing in the ears, or dizziness.

- Advise patient to notify health care professional of all Rx or OTC medications, vitamins, or herbal products being taken and to consult with health care professional before taking other medications.
- Inform patient that tadalafil offers no protection against sexually transmitted diseases. Counsel patient that protection against sexually transmitted diseases and HIV infection should be considered.
- Rep: Advise females of reproductive potential to notify health care professional if pregnancy is planned or suspected or if breastfeeding.

Evaluation/Desired Outcomes

- Male erection sufficient to allow intercourse.
- Decrease in urinary symptoms of BPH.
- Increased exercise tolerance in PAH.

※ tamoxifen (ta-mox-i-fen)
Soltamox
Classification
Therapeutic: antineoplastics
Pharmacologic: antiestrogens

Indications
※ Estrogen-receptor positive metastatic breast cancer. ※ Adjuvant treatment of early-stage estrogen-receptor positive breast cancer. To reduce the occurrence of contralateral breast cancer when used as adjuvant therapy for breast cancer. Prevention of breast cancer in high-risk patients. To reduce risk of invasive breast cancer in women with ductal carcinoma *in situ* following breast surgery and radiation.

Action
Competes with estrogen for binding sites in breast and other tissues. Reduces DNA synthesis and estrogen response. **Therapeutic Effects:** Suppression of tumor growth. Reduced incidence of breast cancer in high-risk patients.

Pharmacokinetics
Absorption: Well absorbed after oral administration.
Distribution: Widely distributed to tissues.
Metabolism and Excretion: Primarily metabolized by the liver via the CYP3A isoenzyme into N-desmethyltamoxifen and via the CYP2D6 isoenzyme into 4-hydroxytamoxifen. Both of these metabolites are further metabolized into endoxifen (N-desmethyltamoxifen via CYP2D6 and 4-hydroxytamoxifen via CYP3A). Both endoxifen and 4-hydroxytamoxifen are 30- to 100-fold more potent than tamoxifen in suppressing estrogen-dependent cell proliferation. ※ The CYP2D6 enzyme

system exhibits genetic polymorphism (~7% of population may be poor metabolizers and may have significantly ↓ endoxifen concentrations and ↓ effectiveness of tamoxifen). Slowly eliminated in the feces. Minimal amounts excreted in the urine.
Half-life: 7 days.

TIME/ACTION PROFILE (tumor response)

ROUTE	ONSET	PEAK	DURATION
PO	4–10 wk	several mo	several wk

Contraindications/Precautions
Contraindicated in: Hypersensitivity; Concurrent warfarin therapy with history of deep vein thrombosis (DVT) or pulmonary embolism (PE) (patients with ductal carcinoma *in situ* or at high risk for breast cancer only); OB: Pregnancy; Lactation: Lactation.
Use Cautiously in: ↓ bone marrow reserve; History of thromboembolic events; Rep: Women of reproductive potential;.

Adverse Reactions/Side Effects
CV: DVT, edema. **Derm:** hot flashes. **EENT:** blurred vision. **F and E:** hypercalcemia. **GI:** nausea, vomiting. **GU:** UTERINE MALIGNANCIES, vaginal bleeding. **Hemat:** leukopenia, thrombocytopenia. **MS:** bone pain. **Neuro:** confusion, depression, headache, STROKE, weakness.. **Resp:** PE. **Misc:** tumor flare.

Interactions
Drug-Drug: **Estrogens** may ↓ effectiveness of concurrently administered tamoxifen. **Bromocriptine** may ↑ levels and risk of toxicity. May ↑ the anticoagulant effect of **warfarin.** Risk of thromboembolic events is ↑ by concurrent use of other **antineoplastics.**

Route/Dosage
Metastatic Breast Cancer
PO (Adults): 20 mg once daily *or* 20 mg twice daily.

Adjuvant Treatment of Breast Cancer
PO (Adults): 20 mg once daily for 5–10 yr.

Prevention of Breast Cancer in High-Risk Women or Ductal Carcinoma *in Situ*
PO (Adults): 20 mg once daily for 5 yr.

Availability (generic available)
Oral solution (licorice aniseed flavor): 10 mg/5 mL. **Tablets:** 10 mg, 20 mg.

NURSING IMPLICATIONS
Assessment
- Assess for an increase in bone or tumor pain. Confer with health care professional regarding analgesics. This transient pain usually resolves despite continued therapy.

Lab Test Considerations
- Verify negative pregnancy test before starting therapy. Monitor CBC, platelets, and calcium levels be-

T

fore and during therapy. May cause transient hypercalcemia in patients with metastases to the bone. An estrogen receptor assay should be assessed before initiation of therapy.

- Monitor serum cholesterol and triglyceride concentrations in patients with pre-existing hyperlipidemia. May cause ↑ concentrations.
- Monitor hepatic function tests and thyroxine (T₄) periodically during therapy. May cause ↑ serum hepatic enzyme and thyroxine concentrations.
- Gynecologic examinations should be performed regularly; may cause variations in Papanicolaou and vaginal smears.

Implementation

- **PO:** Administer with food or fluids if GI irritation becomes a problem. Consult health care professional if patient vomits shortly after administration of medication to determine need for repeat dose.

Patient/Family Teaching

- Instruct patient to take medication as directed. If a dose is missed, it should be omitted. Advise patient to read *Medication Guide* before starting therapy and with each Rx refill in case of changes.
- If skin lesions are present, inform patient that lesions may temporarily increase in size and number and may have increased erythema.
- Advise patient to report bone pain to health care professional promptly. This pain may be severe. Analgesics should be ordered to control pain. Inform patient that this may be an indication of the drug's effectiveness and will resolve over time.
- Instruct patient to monitor weight weekly. Weight gain or peripheral edema should be reported to health care professional.
- Advise patient that medication may cause hot flashes. Notify health care professional if these become bothersome.
- Instruct patient to notify health care professional promptly if pain or swelling of legs, shortness of breath, weakness, sleepiness, confusion, nausea, vomiting, weight gain, dizziness, headache, loss of appetite, or blurred vision occurs. Patient should also report menstrual irregularities, vaginal bleeding, pelvic pain or pressure.
- Rep: May cause fetal harm. Advise females of reproductive potential to use a nonhormonal method of contraception during and for 2 mo after last dose of tamoxifen and to avoid breastfeeding for 3 mo after last dose. May cause female infertility.

Evaluation/Desired Outcomes

- Decrease in the size or spread of breast cancer. Observable effects of therapy may not be seen for 4–10 wk after initiation.
- Reduced incidence of breast cancer in high-risk patients.

⚠ **tamsulosin** (tam-**soo**-loe-sin)
Flomax, ✿ Flomax CR

Classification
Therapeutic: benign prostatic hyperplasia (BPH) agents
Pharmacologic: alpha-adrenergic blockers

Indications
Benign prostatic hyperplasia (BPH).

Action
Decreases contractions in smooth muscle of the prostatic capsule by preferentially binding to alpha₁-adrenergic receptors. **Therapeutic Effects:** Decreased symptoms of BPH (urinary urgency, hesitancy, nocturia).

Pharmacokinetics
Absorption: >90% absorbed after oral administration.
Distribution: Widely distributed to tissues.
Protein Binding: 94–99%.
Metabolism and Excretion: Primarily metabolized by the liver via the CYP3A4 and CYP2D6 isoenzymes; ⚠ the CYP2D6 enzyme system exhibits genetic polymorphism (~7% of population may be poor metabolizers and may have significantly ↑ tamsulosin concentrations and an ↑ risk of adverse effects). <10% excreted unchanged in urine.
Half-life: 14 hr.

TIME/ACTION PROFILE (↑ in urine flow)

ROUTE	ONSET	PEAK	DURATION
PO	unknown	2 wk	unknown

Contraindications/Precautions
Contraindicated in: Hypersensitivity.
Use Cautiously in: Patients at risk for prostate cancer (symptoms may be similar); Patients undergoing cataract surgery (↑ risk of intraoperative floppy iris syndrome); Sulfa allergy; ⚠ CYP2D6 poor metabolizers (especially when using higher dose of 0.8 mg/day).

Adverse Reactions/Side Effects
CV: orthostatic hypotension. **EENT:** intraoperative floppy iris syndrome, rhinitis. **GU:** priapism, retrograde/diminished ejaculation. **Neuro:** dizziness, headache.

Interactions
Drug-Drug: Cimetidine may ↑ levels and the risk of toxicity. ↑ risk of hypotension with **doxazosin, prazosin,** and**terazosin**; concurrent use should be avoided. ↑ risk of hypotension with **sildenafil, tadalafil,** and **vardenafil**. Strong **CYP3A4 inhibitors** and **CYP2D6 inhibitors** may ↑ levels and the risk of toxicity; concurrent use should be avoided.

Route/Dosage
PO (Adults): 0.4 mg once daily after a meal; may ↑ after 2–4 wk to 0.8 mg/day.

Availability (generic available)

Capsules: 0.4 mg. *In combination with:* dutasteride (Jalyn); see Appendix N.

NURSING IMPLICATIONS

Assessment

- Assess patient for symptoms of BPH (urinary hesitancy, feeling of incomplete bladder emptying, interruption of urinary stream, impairment of size and force of urinary stream, terminal urinary dribbling, straining to start flow, dysuria, urgency) before and periodically during therapy.
- Assess patient for first-dose orthostatic hypotension and syncope. Incidence may be dose related. Observe patient closely during this period and take precautions to prevent injury.
- Monitor intake and output ratios and daily weight, and assess for edema daily, especially at beginning of therapy. Report weight gain or edema.
- Rectal exams prior to and periodically throughout therapy to assess prostate size are recommended.

Implementation

- Do not confuse tamsulosin with tacrolimus.
- **PO:** Administer daily dose 30 min after the same meal each day. *DNC:* Swallow capsules whole; do not open, crush, or chew.
- If dose is interrupted for several days at either the 0.4-mg or 0.8-mg dose, restart therapy with the 0.4-mg/day dose.

Patient/Family Teaching

- Instruct patient to take tamsulosin as directed. Emphasize the importance of continuing to take this medication, even if feeling well. Instruct patient to take medication at the same time each day. If a dose is missed, take as soon as remembered unless almost time for next dose. Do not double doses. Advise patient to read *Patient Information* before starting tamsulosin and with each Rx refill in case of changes.
- May cause dizziness. Advise patient to avoid driving or other activities requiring alertness until response to medication is known.
- Caution patient to change positions slowly to minimize orthostatic hypotension.
- Instruct patient to notify health care professional of all Rx or OTC medications, vitamins, or herbal products being taken and consult health care professional before taking any new medications, especially cough, cold, or allergy remedies.
- Inform patient that tamsulosin may cause abnormal ejaculation including ejaculation failure, ejaculation disorder, retrograde ejaculation, and ejaculation decrease, which may impair fertility. Symptoms are reversible when medication is discontinued.
- Emphasize the importance of follow-up visits to determine effectiveness of therapy.

Evaluation/Desired Outcomes

- Decrease in urinary symptoms of BPH (urinary urgency, hesitancy, nocturia).

REMS

tapentadol (ta-pen-ta-dol)
Nucynta, Nucynta ER, ✸Nucynta IR
Classification
Therapeutic: analgesics (centrally acting), opioid analgesics
Pharmacologic: opioid agonists

Schedule II

Indications

Acute pain that is severe enough to require an opioid analgesic and for which alternative treatments are inadequate. Moderate to severe chronic pain in opioid-tolerant patients requiring use of daily, around-the-clock long-term opioid treatment and for which alternative treatment options are inadequate (extended-release only). Diabetic pain associated with diabetic peripheral neuropathy in patients requiring around-the-clock opioid analgesia for an extended time (extended-release only).

Action

Acts as a mu-opioid receptor agonist. Also inhibits the reuptake of norepinephrine. **Therapeutic Effects:** Decrease in pain severity.

Pharmacokinetics

Absorption: 32% absorbed following oral administration.
Distribution: Widely distributed.
Metabolism and Excretion: Undergoes extensive first-pass hepatic metabolism (97%); metabolites have no analgesic activity; metabolized drug is 99% renally excreted.
Half-life: 4 hr.

TIME/ACTION PROFILE (analgesic effect)

ROUTE	ONSET	PEAK	DURATION
PO	unknown	1 hr	4–6 hr

Contraindications/Precautions

Contraindicated in: Hypersensitivity; Significant respiratory depression in unmonitored settings or where resuscitative equipment is not readily available; Paralytic ileus; Severe renal impairment; Severe hepatic impairment; Concurrent use of MAO inhibitors or use of MAO inhibitors in the preceding 2 wk; Acute or severe bronchial asthma; Acute, mild, intermittent, or postoperative pain (extended-release only); OB: Not recommended for use during labor and delivery; Pedi: Children ≥6 yr and ≥40 kg with renal or hepatic impairment.

T

✸= Canadian drug name. ⬚ = Genetic implication. S̶t̶r̶i̶k̶e̶t̶h̶r̶o̶u̶g̶h̶ = Discontinued. CAPITALS = life-threatening. <u>Underline</u> = most frequent.

Use Cautiously in: Conditions associated with hypoxia, hypercapnea, or ↓ respiratory reserve, including asthma, chronic obstructive pulmonary disease, cor pulmonale, extreme obesity, sleep apnea syndrome, myxedema, kyphoscoliosis, CNS depression, use of other CNS depressants, or coma (↑ risk of further respiratory depression); use smallest effective dose; History of substance abuse or addiction disorder; Seizure disorders; Moderate hepatic impairment; OB: Prolonged use of opioids during pregnancy can result in neonatal opioid withdrawal syndrome; Lactation: Use while breastfeeding only if potential maternal benefit justifies potential risk to infant; Pedi: Safety and effectiveness not established in children <18 yr (extended release) or <6 yr and <(immediate release); Geri: ↑ risk of respiratory depression in older adults (dose ↓ suggested).

Adverse Reactions/Side Effects
CV: hypotension. **Endo:** adrenal insufficiency. **GI:** diarrhea, nausea, vomiting. **GU:** ↓ fertility. **Neuro:** allodynia, dizziness, headache, hyperalgesia, SEIZURES, somnolence. **Resp:** RESPIRATORY DEPRESSION (including central sleep apnea and sleep-related hypoxemia). **Misc:** HYPERSENSITIVITY REACTIONS (including anaphylaxis and angioedema).

Interactions
Drug-Drug: Concurrent use of **MAO inhibitors** or use of MAO inhibitors in the preceding 2 wk can result in potentially life-threatening adverse cardiovascular reactions due to additive effects on norepinephrine levels; concurrent use or use of MAO inhibitors in preceding 2 wk contraindicated. Use with **benzodiazepines** or other **CNS depressants**, including other **opioids**, **nonbenzodiazepine sedative/hypnotics**, **anxiolytics**, **general anesthetics**, **muscle relaxants**, **antipsychotics**, and **alcohol**, may cause profound sedation, respiratory depression, coma, and death; reserve concurrent use for when alternative treatment options are inadequate. **Alcohol** may ↑ levels and ↑ the risk of toxicity. **Mixed agonist/antagonist analgesics**, including **nalbuphine** and **butorphanol**, and **partial agonist analgesics**, including **buprenorphine**, may ↓ tapentadol's analgesic effects and/or precipitate opioid withdrawal in physically dependent patients. Drugs that affect serotonergic neurotransmitter systems, including **tricyclic antidepressants**, **SSRIs**, **SNRIs**, **MAO inhibitors**, **TCAs**, **tramadol**, **trazodone**, **mirtazapine**, **5-HT₃ receptor antagonists**, **linezolid**, **methylene blue**, and **triptans**, ↑ risk of serotonin syndrome.

Route/Dosage
When switching from immediate-release to extended-release product, the same total daily dose can be used.

PO (Adults): *Immediate release:* 50 mg, 75 mg, or 100 mg initially, then every 4–6 hr as needed and tolerated. If adequate analgesia is not achieved within first hr of first dose, additional dose may be given. Doses

should not exceed 700 mg on the first day or 600 mg/day thereafter; *Extended release:* 50 mg twice daily; titrate dose up to 100–250 mg twice daily (not to exceed dose of 500 mg/day).
PO (Children ≥6 yr and ≥80 kg): *Immediate release:* 50 mg every 4 hr; may ↑ to 75 mg every 4 hr as needed and tolerated. If adequate analgesia still not achieved, may ↑ to 100 mg every 4 hr to maintain analgesia without intolerable side effects (not to exceed 7.5 mg/kg/day). Duration of treatment should not exceed 3 days.
PO (Children ≥6 yr and 60–79 kg): *Immediate release:* 50 mg every 4 hr; may ↑ to 75 mg every 4 hr as needed and tolerated (not to exceed 7.5 mg/kg/day). Duration of treatment should not exceed 3 days.
PO (Children ≥6 yr and 40–59 kg): *Immediate release:* 50 mg every 4 hr (not to exceed 7.5 mg/kg/day). Duration of treatment should not exceed 3 days.

Hepatic Impairment
PO (Adults): *Moderate hepatic impairment:* Immediate release: 50 mg every 8 hr initially, then titrate to maintain analgesia without intolerable side effects; Extended-release: 50 mg once daily; may titrate up to maximum dose of 100 mg once daily, if needed.

Availability
Immediate-release tablets: 50 mg, 75 mg, 100 mg.
Extended-release tablets: 50 mg, 100 mg, 150 mg, 200 mg, 250 mg.

NURSING IMPLICATIONS
Assessment
- Assess type, location, and intensity of pain before and 1 hr (peak) after administration.
- **High Alert:** Assess level of consciousness, BP, pulse, and respirations before and periodically during administration. If respiratory rate is <10/min, assess level of sedation. Physical stimulation may be sufficient to prevent significant hypoventilation. Subsequent doses may need to be decreased by 25–50%. Initial drowsiness will diminish with continued use. Monitor for respiratory depression, especially during initiation or following dose increase; serious, life-threatening, or fatal respiratory depression may occur. May cause sleep-related breathing disorders (central sleep apnea, sleep-related hypoxemia). Geri, Pedi: Assess geriatric and pediatric patients frequently; more sensitive to the effects of opioid analgesics and may experience side effects and respiratory complications more frequently
- Patients taking extended-release tapentadol may require additional short-acting or rapid-onset opioid doses for breakthrough pain. Doses of short-acting opioids should be equivalent to 10–20% of 24 hr total and given every 2 hr as needed.
- Assess bowel function routinely. Prevention of constipation should be instituted with increased intake of fluids and bulk and with laxatives to minimize constipating effects. Administer stimulant laxatives routinely if opioid use exceeds 2–3 days, unless

contraindicated. Consider drugs for opioid-induced constipation.

• Prolonged use may lead to physical and psychological dependence and tolerance, although these may be milder than with opioids. This should not prevent patient from receiving adequate analgesia. Patients who receive tapentadol for pain rarely develop psychological dependence.

• Monitor patient for seizures. May occur within recommended dose range. Risk is increased in patients with a history of seizures and in patients taking antidepressants (SSRIs, SNRIs, TCAs) or other drugs that decrease the seizure threshold.

• Monitor for serotonin syndrome (mental-status changes [agitation, hallucinations, coma]), autonomic instability [tachycardia, labile BP, hyperthermia], neuromuscular aberrations [hyperreflexia, incoordination], and/or gastrointestinal symptoms [nausea, vomiting, diarrhea] in patients taking SSRIs, SNRIs, triptans, TCAs, or MAO inhibitors concurrently with tapentadol.

• Assess risk for opioid addiction, abuse, or misuse prior to administration. Abuse or misuse of extended-release preparations by crushing, chewing, snorting, or injecting dissolved product will result in uncontrolled delivery of tapentadol and can result in overdose and death.

• Monitor for symptoms of opioid-induced hyperalgesia (increased pain upon opioid dose increase, decreased pain upon opioid dose decrease, or pain from ordinarily nonpainful stimuli (allodynia). If a patient is suspected to be experiencing opioid-induced hyperalgesia, consider appropriately decreasing the dose of the current opioid analgesic, or using opioid rotation (safely switching patient to a different opioid moiety).

Toxicity and Overdose

• Overdose may cause respiratory depression. Naloxone may reverse some, but not all, of the symptoms of overdose. Treatment should be symptomatic and supportive. Maintain adequate respiratory exchange.

Implementation

• Explain therapeutic value of medication prior to administration to enhance the analgesic effect.

• Initial immediate-release dose of 50 mg, 75 mg, or 100 mg is individualized based on pain severity, previous experience with similar drugs, and ability to monitor patient. 2nd dose may be administered as soon as 1 hr after first dose if adequate pain relief is not obtained with first dose.

• Medication should be discontinued gradually after long-term use to prevent withdrawal symptoms. For patients on long-acting agents who are physically opioid-dependent, initiate the taper by a small enough increment (e.g., no greater than 10% to 25% of total daily dose) to avoid withdrawal symp-

toms, and proceed with dose-lowering at an interval of every 2 to 4 wk. Patients who have been taking opioids for briefer periods of time may tolerate a more rapid taper. Monitor frequently to manage pain and withdrawal symptoms (restlessness, lacrimation, rhinorrhea, yawning, perspiration, chills, myalgia, mydriasis, irritability, anxiety, backache, joint pain, weakness, abdominal cramps, insomnia, nausea, anorexia, vomiting, diarrhea, or increased blood pressure, respiratory rate, or heart rate). If withdrawal symptoms occur, pause the taper for a period of time or raise the dose of opioid analgesic to the previous dose, and then proceed with a slower taper. Also, monitor patients for changes in mood, emergence of suicidal thoughts, or use of other substances. A multimodal approach to pain management may optimize the treatment of chronic pain, as well as assist with the successful tapering of the opioid analgesic.

• **PO:** Tapentadol may be administered without regard to meals.

• *DNC:* Swallow extended-release tablets whole; do not crush, break, or chew.

• Use calibrated syringe to administer correct dose of oral solution.

• *REMS:* FDA strongly encourages health care professionals to complete a REMS-compliant education program that includes all the elements of the FDA Education *Blueprint for Health Care Providers Involved in the Management or Support of Patients with Pain,* available at www.fda.gov/OpioidAnalgesicREMSBlueprint. Information on programs can be found at 1-800-503-0784 or www.opioidanalgesicrems.com.

• Discuss availability of naloxone for emergency treatment of opioid overdose with the patient and caregiver and assess the potential need for access to naloxone, both when initiating and renewing therapy, especially if patient has household members (including children) or other close contacts at risk for accidental exposure or overdose. Consider prescribing naloxone, based on the patient's risk factors for overdose, such as concomitant use of CNS depressants, a history of opioid use disorder, or prior opioid overdose. However, the presence of risk factors for overdose should not prevent the proper management of pain in any patient.

Patient/Family Teaching

• *REMS:* Instruct patient on how and when to ask for and take pain medication and to take tapentadol as directed; do not adjust dose without consulting health care professional. Report breakthrough pain and adverse reactions to health care professional. Do not take tapentadol if pain is mild or can be controlled with other pain medications such as NSAIDs or acetaminophen. Do not stop abruptly; may cause withdrawal symptoms (anxiety, sweating, insomnia,

T

rigors, pain, nausea, tremors, diarrhea, upper respiratory symptoms, hallucinations). Decrease dose gradually. Advise patient to read the *Medication Guide* prior to taking tapentadol and with each Rx refill, in case of changes. Discuss safe use, risks, and proper storage and disposal of opioid analgesics with patients and caregivers with each Rx. The Patient Counseling Guide (PCG) is available at www.fda.gov/OpioidAnalgesicREMSPCG.

● Advise patient that tapentadol is a drug with known abuse potential. Protect it from theft, and never give to anyone other than the individual for whom it was prescribed; may be dangerous. Store out of sight and reach of children, and in a location not accessible by others.

● May cause dizziness and drowsiness. Caution patient to avoid driving or other activities requiring alertness until response to medication is known.

● Inform patient that tapentadol may cause seizures. Stop taking tapentadol and notify health care professional immediately if seizures occur.

● Advise patient to change positions slowly to minimize orthostatic hypotension.

● Caution patient to avoid concurrent use of alcohol or other CNS depressants, including other opioids, with this medication.

● Educate patients and caregivers on how to recognize respiratory depression and emphasize the importance of calling 911 or getting emergency medical help right away in the event of a known or suspected overdose. Inform patients and caregivers about various ways to obtain naloxone as permitted by individual state naloxone dispensing and prescribing requirements or guidelines (by prescription, directly from a pharmacist, or as part of a community-based program).

● Instruct patient to notify health care professional of all Rx or OTC medications, vitamins, or herbal products being taken and consult health care professional before taking any new medications.

● Advise patient to notify health care professional if signs of serotonin syndrome occur.

● Encourage patient to turn, cough, and breathe deeply every 2 hr to prevent atelectasis.

● Rep: Advise patient to notify health care professional if pregnancy is planned or suspected, or if breastfeeding. Inform patient of potential for neonatal opioid withdrawal syndrome with prolonged use during pregnancy. Monitor neonate for signs and symptoms of withdrawal symptoms (irritability, hyperactivity and abnormal sleep pattern, high pitched cry, tremor, vomiting, diarrhea, and/or failure to gain weight); usually occur the first days after birth. Monitor infants exposed to tapentadol through breast milk for excess sedation and respiratory depression. Chronic use may reduce fertility in females and males.

Evaluation/Desired Outcomes

● Decrease in severity of pain without a significant alteration in level of consciousness or respiratory status.

tavaborole, See ANTIFUNGALS (TOPICAL).

tedizolid (ted-eye-zoe-lid)
Sivextro
Classification
Therapeutic: anti-infectives
Pharmacologic: oxazolidinones

Indications
Treatment of acute bacterial skin and skin structure infections.

Action
Inhibits bacterial protein synthesis at the level of the 23S ribosome of the 50S subunit. **Therapeutic Effects:** Bacteriostatic action against enterococci, staphylococci and streptococci, resulting in resolution of infection. **Spectrum:** Active against *Staphylococcus aureus* including methicillin-resistant strains (MRSA), *Streptococcus pyogenes*, *Streptococcus agalactiae*, *Streptococcus anginosus* group (including *Streptococcus anginosus*, *Streptococcus intermedius*, *Streptococcus constellatus*), and *Enterococcus faecalis*.

Pharmacokinetics
Absorption: IV administration results in complete bioavailability; well absorbed (91%) following oral administration.
Distribution: Well distributed to tissues.
Metabolism and Excretion: Rapidly converted by phosphatases to its active form; primarily excreted in feces (82%) and urine (18%) (<3% excreted unchanged in urine or feces).
Half-life: 12 hr.

TIME/ACTION PROFILE (plasma concentrations)

ROUTE	ONSET	PEAK	DURATION
PO	unknown	2.5 hr	24 hr
IV	rapid	end of infusion	24 hr

Contraindications/Precautions
Contraindicated in: Uncontrolled hypertension, pheochromocytoma, thyrotoxicosis, or concurrent use of sympathomimetic agents, vasopressors, or dopaminergic agents (↑ risk of hypertensive response); Carcinoid syndrome (↑ risk of serotonin syndrome); OB: Pregnancy.
Use Cautiously in: Neutropenia (safety and efficacy not established if WBC <1000 cells/mm³); Lactation: Use while breastfeeding only if potential maternal benefit justifies potential risk to infant; Pedi: Children <12 yr (safety and effectiveness not established).

Adverse Reactions/Side Effects
GI: CLOSTRIDIOIDES DIFFICILE-ASSOCIATED DIARRHEA (CDAD), diarrhea, nausea, vomiting. **Neuro:** dizziness, headache. **Misc:** infusion reactions.

Interactions
Drug-Drug: ↑ risk of hypertensive response with **MAO inhibitors, sympathomimetics** (e.g., **pseudoephedrine**), **vasopressors** (e.g., **epinephrine, norepinephrine**), and **dopaminergic agents** (e.g., **dopamine, dobutamine**); concurrent or recent use should be avoided. ↑ risk of serotonin syndrome with **SSRIs, TCAs, triptans, meperidine, bupropion,** or **buspirone**; avoid concurrent use. May ↑ levels of **methotrexate, topotecan,** or **rosuvastatin**; discontinue these medications temporarily during tedizolid treatment.

Route/Dosage
PO, IV (Adults and Children ≥12 yr): 200 mg once daily for 6 days.

Availability
Tablets: 200 mg. **Lyophilized powder for injection:** 200 mg/vial.

NURSING IMPLICATIONS
Assessment
- Assess for infection (vital signs; appearance of wound, sputum, urine, and stool; WBC) at beginning of and during therapy.
- Obtain specimens for culture and sensitivity prior to initiating therapy. First dose may be given before receiving results.
- Monitor bowel function. Diarrhea, abdominal cramping, fever, and bloody stools should be reported to health care professional promptly as a sign of CDAD. May begin up to several mo following cessation of therapy.

Lab Test Considerations
- Consider alternate therapies in patients with neutrophil counts <1000 cells/mm³.
- May cause anemia.

Implementation
- Dose adjustment is not necessary when switching from IV to oral formulation.
- **PO:** May be administered with or without food.

IV Administration
- **Intermittent Infusion:** *Reconstitution:* Reconstitute each vial with 4 mL of sterile water for injection. Gently swirl and let vial stand until completely dissolved; avoid shaking. *Dilution:* Dilute further with 250 mL of 0.9% NaCl by slowly injecting reconstituted solution into 250 mL bag. Gently invert bag to mix; avoid shaking to minimize foaming. Solution is clear and colorless to pale yellow; do not administer solutions that are discolored or contain particu-

late material. Must be used within 24 hr of reconstitution at room temperature or under refrigeration. *Rate:* Infuse over 1 hr.
- **Y-Site Compatibility:** amikacin, amiodarone, ampicillin/sulbactam, anidulafungin, azithromycin, aztreonam, bumetanide, cefazolin, cefepime, ceftazidime, ceftazidime/avibactam, ceftolozane/tazobactam, ceftriaxone, cefuroxime, ciprofloxacin, cisatracurium, daptomycin, dexamethasone, dexmedetomidine, digoxin, diltiazem, dopamine, epinephrine, eptifibatide, ertapenem, esomeprazole, famotidine, fentanyl, fosphenytoin, furosemide, heparin, hydrocortisone, hydromorphone, imipenem/cilastatin, insulin regular, labetalol, levofloxacin, lidocaine, lorazepam, mannitol, meperidine, meropenem, meropenem/vaborbactam, mesna, methylprednisolone, metoclopramide, metronidazole, micafungin, midazolam, milrinone, morphine, naloxone, nitroglycerin, norepinephrine, ondansetron, pantoprazole, penicillin G potassium, phenylephrine, piperacillin/tazobactam, plazomicin, potassium chloride, potassium phosphate, rocuronium, sodium bicarbonate, sodium phosphate, tacrolimus, tigecycline, vancomycin, vasopressin, vecuronium.
- **Y-Site Incompatibility:** albumin (human), calcium chloride, calcium gluconate, caspofungin, ceftaroline, cyclosporine, diphenhydramine, dobutamine, doxycycline, esmolol, gentamicin, Hartmann's solution, isavuconazonium, LR, magnesium sulfate, nicardipine, phenytoin, tobramycin.

Patient/Family Teaching
- Advise patients taking oral tedizolid to take as directed, for full course of therapy, even if feeling better. Take missed doses as soon as remembered up to 8 hr before next dose; if less than 8 hr before next dose, wait until next scheduled dose. Do not double dose.
- Advise patient to notify health care professional of all Rx or OTC medications, vitamins, or herbal products being taken and to consult with health care professional before taking other medications.
- Instruct patient to notify health care professional if changes in vision occur or immediately if diarrhea, abdominal cramping, fever, or bloody stools occur and not to treat with antidiarrheals without consulting health care professionals.
- Rep: May cause fetal harm. Advise females of reproductive potential to notify health care professional if pregnancy is planned or suspected, or if breastfeeding.
- Advise patient to notify health care professional if no improvement is seen in a few days.

Evaluation/Desired Outcomes
- Resolution of signs and symptoms of infection. Length of time for complete resolution depends on organism and site of infection.

✦ = Canadian drug name. ▓ = Genetic implication. ~~Strikethrough~~ = Discontinued. CAPITALS = life-threatening. <u>Underline</u> = most frequent.

telavancin (tel-a-van-sin)
Vibativ
Classification
Therapeutic: anti-infectives
Pharmacologic: lipoglycopeptides

Indications
Complicated skin/skin structure infections caused by susceptible bacteria. Hospital-acquired and ventilator-associated bacterial pneumonia caused by *Staphylococcus aureus*.

Action
Inhibits bacterial cell wall synthesis by interfering with the polymerization and cross-linking of peptidoglycan. **Therapeutic Effects:** Bactericidal action against susceptible organisms. **Spectrum:** Active against *Staphylococcus aureus* (including methicillin-susceptible and -resistant strains), *Streptococcus pyogenes*, *Streptococcus agalactiae*, *Streptococcus anginosus* (including *S. anginosus*, *S. intermedius*, and *S. constellatus*), and *Enterococcus faecalis* (vancomycin-susceptible strains only).

Pharmacokinetics
Absorption: IV administration results in complete bioavailability.
Distribution: Minimal distribution to tissues.
Metabolism and Excretion: Metabolism is not known; 76% excreted unchanged in urine <1% in feces.
Half-life: 8 hr.

TIME/ACTION PROFILE (plasma concentrations)

ROUTE	ONSET	PEAK	DURATION
IV	unknown	end of infusion	24 hr

Contraindications/Precautions
Contraindicated in: Hypersensitivity; Congenital long QT syndrome, known prolongation of the QT interval, uncompensated HF, or severe left ventricular hypertrophy (↑ risk of fatal arrhythmias); Concurrent use of unfractionated heparin (aPTT may be falsely ↑ for up to 18 hr after telavancin therapy); OB: Pregnancy.
Use Cautiously in: Renal impairment (dose ↓ recommended for CCr ≤50 mL/min) (efficacy may be ↓ in patients with complicated skin/skin structure infections and CCr ≤50 mL/min) (↑ risk of mortality in patients with hospital-acquired or ventilator-associated pneumonia and CCr ≤50 mL/min; use only if benefit outweighs risk); Diabetes, HF, hypertension (↑ risk of renal impairment); Lactation: Use while breastfeeding only if potential maternal benefit justifies potential risk to infant; Pedi: Safety and effectiveness not established in children (may be associated with poor outcomes in children <1 yr who have immature renal function);

Geri: Consider age-related ↓ in renal function in older adults.

Adverse Reactions/Side Effects
CV: QT interval prolongation. **GI:** nausea, taste disturbance, vomiting, abdominal pain, CLOSTRIDIOIDES DIFFICILE-ASSOCIATED DIARRHEA (CDAD). **GU:** foamy urine, nephrotoxicity. **Neuro:** dizziness. **Misc:** ANAPHYLAXIS, infusion reactions.

Interactions
Drug-Drug: Concurrent use of **QT interval prolonging medications** may ↑ risk of arrhythmias. Concurrent use of **NSAIDs, ACE inhibitors**, and **loop diuretics** may ↑ risk of nephrotoxicity.

Route/Dosage
Complicated Skin/Skin Structure Infections
IV (Adults): 10 mg/kg ever 24 hr for 7–14 days.
Renal Impairment
IV (Adults): *CCr 30–50 mL/min:* 7.5 mg/kg every 24 hr; *CCr 10–≤30 mL/min:* 10 mg/kg every 48 hr.

Hospital-Acquired/Ventilator-Associated Bacterial Pneumonia
IV (Adults): 10 mg/kg ever 24 hr for 7–21 days.
Renal Impairment
IV (Adults): *CCr 30–50 mL/min:* 7.5 mg/kg every 24 hr; *CCr 10–≤30 mL/min:* 10 mg/kg every 48 hr.

Availability
Lyophilized powder for injection: 750 mg/vial.

NURSING IMPLICATIONS
Assessment
- Assess for infection (vital signs; appearance of wound, sputum, urine, and stool; WBC) at beginning of and throughout therapy.
- Obtain specimens for culture and sensitivity prior to therapy. First dose may be given before receiving results.
- Monitor bowel function. Diarrhea, abdominal cramping, fever, and bloody stools should be reported to health care professional promptly as a sign of CDAD. May begin up to several wk following cessation of therapy.
- Monitor for infusion-related reactions (resembling vancomycin flushing syndrome—flushing of upper body, urticaria, pruritus, rash). May resolve with stopping or slowing infusion.
- Observe patient for signs and symptoms of anaphylaxis (rash, pruritus, laryngeal edema, wheezing). Discontinue drug and notify health care professional immediately if symptoms occur. Keep epinephrine, an antihistamine, and resuscitation equipment close by in case of anaphylactic reaction.

Lab Test Considerations
- Verify negative pregnancy test before starting therapy. Monitor renal function (serum creatinine, CCr)

prior to, every 48–72 hr during, and at the end of therapy. May cause nephrotoxicity. If renal function decreases, reassess need for telavancin.
- May interfere with prothrombin time, INR, aPTT, activated clotting time, and coagulation-based factor Xa tests. Collect blood samples for these tests as close to next dose of telavancin as possible.
- Interferes with urine qualitative dipstick protein assays and quantitative dye methods; may use microalbumin assays.

Implementation

IV Administration
- **Intermittent Infusion:** *Reconstitution:* Reconstitute the 750-mg vial with 45 mL of D5W, sterile water for injection, or 0.9% NaCl for concentrations of 15 mg/mL. Reconstitution time is usually under 2 min but may require up to 20 min. Mix thoroughly with contents dissolved completely. Do not administer solution that is discolored or contains particulate matter. Discard vial if vacuum did not pull diluent into vial. Time in vial plus time in bag should not exceed 4 hr at room temperature or 72 hr if refrigerated. *Dilution:* For doses of 150–800 mg, dilute further with 100–250 mL of D5W, 0.9% NaCl, or LR. *Concentration:* For doses <150 mg or >800 mg, dilute for a final concentration of 0.6–8 mg/mL. *Rate:* Administer over at least 60 min to minimize infusion reactions. Flush line with D5W, 0.9% NaCl, or LR before and after administration.
- **Y-Site Compatibility:** amphotericin B lipid complex, ampicillin/sulbactam, azithromycin, calcium gluconate, caspofungin, cefepime, ceftazidime, ceftriaxone, ciprofloxacin, dexamethasone, diltiazem, dobutamine, dopamine, doxycycline, ertapenem, famotidine, fluconazole, gentamicin, hydrocortisone, labetalol, magnesium sulfate, mannitol, meropenem, metoclopramide, milrinone, norepinephrine, ondansetron, pantoprazole, phenylephrine, piperacillin/tazobactam, potassium chloride, potassium phosphate, sodium bicarbonate, sodium phosphate, tigecycline, tobramycin, vasopressin.
- **Y-Site Incompatibility:** amphotericin B deoxycholate, amphotericin B liposomal, digoxin, esomeprazole, furosemide, levofloxacin, micafungin.

Patient/Family Teaching
- Instruct patient to notify health care professional immediately if diarrhea, abdominal cramping, fever, or bloody stools occur and not to treat with antidiarrheals without consulting health care professionals.
- Inform patient that common side effects include taste disturbance, nausea, vomiting, headache, and foamy urine. Notify health care professional if signs of infusion reaction occur.
- Instruct patient to notify health care professional of all Rx or OTC medications, vitamins, or herbal prod-

ucts being taken and consult health care professional before taking any new medications.
- Rep: May cause fetal harm. Advise females of reproductive potential to use effective contraception during and for 2 days after last dose and to notify health care professional if pregnancy is suspected. Inform patient of pregnancy exposure registry that monitors pregnancy outcomes in women exposed to telavancin during pregnancy. Encourage pregnant patients to enroll in the VIBATIV pregnancy registry by calling 1-877-484-2700. May impair fertility in males.
- Instruct the patient to notify health care professional if symptoms do not improve.

Evaluation/Desired Outcomes
- Resolution of the signs and symptoms of infection. Length of time for complete resolution depends on the organism and site of infection.

telmisartan, See ANGIOTENSIN II RECEPTOR ANTAGONISTS.

tenecteplase, See THROMBOLYTIC AGENTS.

tenofovir alafenamide
(te-**noe**-fo-veer al-a-**fen**-a-mide)
Vemlidy
Classification
Therapeutic: antiretrovirals
Pharmacologic: nucleoside reverse transcriptase inhibitors

Indications
Chronic hepatitis B virus (HBV) infection in patients with compensated liver disease.

Action
Converted by hydrolysis to tenofovir and subsequently phosphorylated to the active metabolite, tenofovir diphosphate, which inhibits replication of HBV through incorporation into viral DNA by the HBV reverse transcriptase resulting in disruption of DNA synthesis. **Therapeutic Effects:** Decreased progression/sequelae of chronic HBV infection.

Pharmacokinetics
Absorption: Tenofovir alafenamide is a prodrug, which is hydrolyzed into tenofovir; absorption enhanced by high-fat meals.
Distribution: Unknown.
Metabolism and Excretion: Tenofovir is phosphorylated to tenofovir diphosphate (active metabolite); 32% excreted in feces, <1% in urine.

Half-life: 0.51 hr.

TIME/ACTION PROFILE (plasma concentrations)

ROUTE	ONSET	PEAK	DURATION
PO	unknown	0.5 hr	24 hr

Contraindications/Precautions

Contraindicated in: End-stage renal disease (CCr <15 mL/min) (not receiving hemodialysis); Decompensated hepatic impairment.

Use Cautiously in: Coinfection with HIV and chronic HBV; Renal impairment or receiving nephrotoxic medications (↑ risk of renal impairment); OB: Use during pregnancy only if potential maternal benefit justifies potential fetal risk; Lactation: Use while breastfeeding only if potential maternal benefit justifies potential risk to infant; Pedi: Children <12 yr (safety and effectiveness not established).

Adverse Reactions/Side Effects

GI: ↑ amylase, ↑ liver enzymes, abdominal pain, LACTIC ACIDOSIS/HEPATOMEGALY WITH STEATOSIS, nausea. **GU:** ACUTE RENAL FAILURE/FANCONI SYNDROME, glycosuria. **Metab:** hyperlipidemia. **MS:** ↑ creatine kinase, back pain. **Neuro:** fatigue, headache. **Resp:** cough.

Interactions

Drug-Drug: Nephrotoxic agents, including **NSAIDs,** ↑ risk of nephrotoxicity; avoid concurrent use. Medications that compete for active tubular secretion, including **acyclovir, cidofovir, ganciclovir, valacyclovir, valganciclovir,** or **aminoglycosides,** may ↑ levels and the risk of toxicity; avoid concurrent use. **Carbamazepine, oxcarbazepine, phenobarbital, phenytoin, rifabutin, rifampin,** or **rifapentine** may ↓ levels and its effectiveness; concurrent use with oxcarbazepine, phenobarbital, phenytoin, rifabutin, rifampin, or rifapentine not recommended; ↑ tenofovir alafenamide dose to 50 mg once daily when used with carbamazepine.

Drug-Natural Products: St. John's wort may ↓ levels and its effectiveness; concurrent use not recommended.

Route/Dosage

PO (Adults and Children ≥12 yr): 25 mg once daily.

Renal Impairment
PO (Adults and Children ≥12 yr): *Hemodialysis:* Administer dose after dialysis session.

Availability

Tablets: 25 mg. *In combination with:* bictegravir and emtricitabine (Biktarvy); darunavir, cobicistat, and emtricitabine (Symtuza); elvitegravir, cobicistat, and emtricitabine (Genvoya); emtricitabine (Descovy); emtricitabine and rilpivirine (Odefsey). See Appendix N.

NURSING IMPLICATIONS

Assessment

- Monitor signs of hepatitis (jaundice, fatigue, anorexia, pruritus) during therapy. Upon discontinuation of therapy, monitor for exacerbations of HBV for at least several mo after stopping therapy.

Lab Test Considerations

- Test patient for HIV-1 infection before starting therapy; *Vemlidy* should not be used alone in patient with HIV-1 infection.
- Monitor liver function tests and HBV levels during and following therapy. If therapy is discontinued, may cause severe exacerbation of HBV. Lactic acidosis may occur with hepatic toxicity causing hepatic steatosis; may be fatal, especially in women.
- May cause renal impairment. Monitor serum creatinine, estimated CCr, urine glucose, and urine protein before starting and periodically during therapy. Also assess serum phosphorous in patients with chronic kidney disease. Discontinue medication in patients who develop clinically significant ↓ in renal function or evidence of Fanconi syndrome.
- May cause ↑ ALT, AST, serum CK, serum amylase, LDL cholesterol, and glycosuria.

Implementation

- **PO:** Administer once daily with food.

Patient/Family Teaching

- Instruct patient to take medication as directed. Avoid missing doses. Advise patient to read *Patient Information* before starting and with each Rx refill in case of changes.
- Advise patient to notify health care professional immediately if symptoms of lactic acidosis (feel very weak or tired, have unusual [not normal] muscle pain, have trouble breathing, have stomach pain with nausea or vomiting, feel cold, especially in your arms and legs, feel dizzy or lightheaded, have a fast or irregular heartbeat) or severe liver problems (yellow skin or whites eyes, dark "tea-colored" urine, light-colored bowel stools, loss of appetite, nausea, pain, aching, or tenderness in right side of abdomen) occur.
- Instruct patient to notify health care professional of all Rx or OTC medications, vitamins, or herbal products being taken and consult health care professional before taking any new medications.
- Rep: Advise females of reproductive potential to notify health care professional if pregnancy is planned or suspected or if breastfeeding. Advise patient taking oral contraceptives to use a nonhormonal method of birth control during therapy. Inform patient of pregnancy exposure registry that monitors pregnancy outcomes in women exposed to *Vemlidy* during pregnancy. Register patient in the Antiretroviral Pregnancy Registry by calling 1-800-258-4263.

Evaluation/Desired Outcomes
- Decreased progression/sequelae of chronic HBV infection.

BEERS

terazosin (ter-ay-zoe-sin)
~~Hytrin~~
Classification
Therapeutic: antihypertensives
Pharmacologic: peripherally acting antiadrenergics

Indications
Mild to moderate hypertension (as monotherapy or in combination with other antihypertensives). Benign prostatic hyperplasia (BPH).

Action
Dilates both arteries and veins by blocking postsynaptic alpha₁-adrenergic receptors. Decreases contractions in smooth muscle of the prostatic capsule. **Therapeutic Effects:** Lowering of BP. Decreased symptoms of BPH (urinary urgency, hesitancy, nocturia).

Pharmacokinetics
Absorption: Well absorbed after oral administration.
Distribution: Unknown.
Metabolism and Excretion: 50% metabolized by the liver. 10% excreted unchanged by the kidneys. 20% excreted unchanged in feces. 40% eliminated in bile.
Half-life: 12 hr.

TIME/ACTION PROFILE

ROUTE	ONSET†	PEAK‡	DURATION†
PO-hypertension	15 min	6–8 wk	24 hr
PO-BPH	2–6 wk	unknown	unknown

†After single dose.
‡After multiple oral dosing.

Contraindications/Precautions
Contraindicated in: Hypersensitivity.
Use Cautiously in: Deyhdration, volume or sodium depletion (↑ risk of hypotension); Patients undergoing cataract surgery (↑ risk of intraoperative floppy iris syndrome); OB: Other antihypertensive agents preferred during pregnancy; Lactation: Safety not established in breastfeeding; Pedi: Safety and effectiveness not established in children; Geri: Appears on Beers list. ↑ risk of orthostatic hypotension in older adults. Avoid use for treatment of hypertension in older adults.

Adverse Reactions/Side Effects
CV: first-dose orthostatic hypotension, arrhythmias, chest pain, palpitations, peripheral edema, tachycardia. **Derm:** pruritus. **EENT:** nasal congestion, blurred vision, conjunctivitis, intraoperative floppy iris syndrome, sinusitis. **GI:** nausea, abdominal pain, diarrhea, dry

mouth, vomiting. **GU:** erectile dysfunction, urinary frequency. **Metab:** weight gain. **MS:** arthralgia, back pain, extremity pain. **Neuro:** dizziness, headache, weakness, drowsiness, nervousness, paresthesia. **Resp:** dyspnea. **Misc:** fever.

Interactions
Drug-Drug: ↑ risk of hypotension with **sildenafil**, **tadalafil**, **vardenafil**, other **antihypertensives**, **nitrates**, or acute ingestion of **alcohol**. **NSAIDs**, **sympathomimetics**, or **estrogens** may ↓ effects of antihypertensive therapy.

Route/Dosage
Hypertension
PO (Adults): 1 mg initially, then slowly ↑ up to 5 mg/day (usual range 1–5 mg/day); may be given as single dose or in 2 divided doses (not to exceed 20 mg/day).

Benign Prostatic Hyperplasia
PO (Adults): 1 mg at bedtime; gradually may be ↑ up to 5–10 mg/day.

Availability (generic available)
Capsules: 1 mg, 2 mg, 5 mg, 10 mg. **Tablets:** ✸ 1 mg, ✸ 2 mg, ✸ 5 mg, ✸ 10 mg.

NURSING IMPLICATIONS
Assessment
- Assess for first-dose orthostatic reaction (dizziness, weakness) and syncope. May occur 30 min–2 hr after initial dose and occasionally thereafter. Incidence may be dose related. Volume-depleted or sodium-restricted patients may be more sensitive. Observe patient closely during this period; take precautions to prevent injury. First dose may be given at bedtime to minimize this reaction.
- Monitor intake and output ratios and daily weight; assess for edema daily, especially at beginning of therapy.
- **Hypertension:** Monitor BP and pulse frequently during initial dose adjustment and periodically during therapy. Report significant changes.
- Monitor frequency of prescription refills to determine adherence.
- **BPH:** Assess patient for symptoms of BPH (urinary hesitancy, feeling of incomplete bladder emptying, interruption of urinary stream, impairment of size and force of urinary stream, terminal urinary dribbling, straining to start flow, dysuria, urgency) before and periodically during therapy.
- Rule out prostatic carcinoma before therapy; symptoms are similar.

Implementation
- May be used in combination with diuretics or beta blockers to minimize sodium and water retention. If these are added to terazosin therapy, reduce dose of terazosin initially and titrate to effect.

✸ = Canadian drug name. ▓ = Genetic implication. ~~Strikethrough~~ = Discontinued. CAPITALS = life-threatening. <u>Underline</u> = most frequent.

- **PO:** Administer daily dose at bedtime. If necessary, dose may be increased to twice daily.

Patient/Family Teaching

- Instruct patient to take medication at the same time each day. Take missed doses as soon as remembered. If not remembered until next day, omit; do not double doses.
- Advise patient to weigh self twice weekly and assess feet and ankles for fluid retention.
- May cause dizziness or drowsiness. Advise patient to avoid driving or other activities requiring alertness until response to the medication is known.
- Caution patient to avoid sudden changes in position to decrease orthostatic hypotension. Alcohol, CNS depressants, including opioids, standing for long periods, hot showers, and exercising in hot weather should be avoided because of enhanced orthostatic effects.
- Advise patient to notify health care professional of all Rx or OTC medications, vitamins, or herbal products being taken and to consult with health care professional before taking other medications, especially NSAIDs, cough, cold, or allergy remedies.
- Instruct patient to notify health care professional of medication regimen before any surgery.
- Advise patient to notify health care professional if frequent dizziness, fainting, or swelling of feet or lower legs occurs.
- Rep: Advise females of reproductive potential to notify health care professional if pregnancy is planned or suspected or if breastfeeding. Terazosin is not a preferred antihypertensive for use during pregnancy; consider transitioning to a preferred agent in patients planning to become pregnant.
- Emphasize the importance of follow-up exams to evaluate effectiveness of medication.
- **Hypertension:** Emphasize the importance of continuing to take this medication as directed, even if feeling well. Medication controls but does not cure hypertension.
- Encourage patient to comply with additional interventions for hypertension (weight reduction, low-sodium diet, smoking cessation, moderation of alcohol consumption, regular exercise, and stress management).
- Instruct patient and family on proper technique for BP monitoring. Advise them to check BP at least weekly and to report significant changes.

Evaluation/Desired Outcomes

- Decrease in BP without appearance of side effects.
- Decreased symptoms of BPH. May require 2–6 wk of therapy before effects are noticeable.

---

terbinafine, See ANTIFUNGALS (TOPICAL).

---

terbutaline (ter-byoo-ta-leen)
✹Bricanyl Turbuhaler
Classification
Therapeutic: bronchodilators
Pharmacologic: adrenergics

Indications
Management of reversible airway disease due to asthma (SUBQ used for short-term control and oral agent as long-term control). **Unlabeled Use:** Management of preterm labor (tocolytic) (terbutaline injection may only be used for the short-term [≤72 hr]) management of preterm labor to prolong pregnancy and allow for the administration of antenatal steroids).

Action
Results in the accumulation of cyclic adenosine monophosphate (cAMP) at beta-adrenergic receptors. Produces bronchodilation. Inhibits the release of mediators of immediate hypersensitivity reactions from mast cells. Relatively selective for beta$_2$ (pulmonary)-adrenergic receptor sites, with less effect on beta$_1$ (cardiac)-adrenergic receptors. **Therapeutic Effects:** Bronchodilation.

Pharmacokinetics
Absorption: 35–50% absorbed following oral administration but rapidly undergoes first-pass metabolism. Well absorbed following SUBQ administration.
Distribution: Unknown.
Metabolism and Excretion: Partially metabolized by the liver; 60% excreted unchanged by the kidneys.
Half-life: 5.7 hr.

TIME/ACTION PROFILE (bronchodilation)

ROUTE	ONSET	PEAK	DURATION
PO	within 60–120 min	within 2–3 hr	4–8 hr
SUBQ	within 15 min	within 0.5–1 hr	1.5–4 hr

Contraindications/Precautions
Contraindicated in: Hypersensitivity to adrenergic amines.
Use Cautiously in: Cardiac disease; Hypertension; Hyperthyroidism; Diabetes; Glaucoma; OB: Use for bronchodilation in pregnancy only if potential maternal benefit justifies potential fetal risk; Geri: Older adults are more susceptible to adverse reactions (may require dose ↓).

Adverse Reactions/Side Effects
CV: angina, arrhythmias, hypertension, myocardial ischemia, tachycardia. **Endo:** hyperglycemia. **F and E:** hypokalemia. **GI:** nausea, vomiting. **Neuro:** nervousness, restlessness, tremor, headache, insomnia. **Resp:** pulmonary edema.

Interactions
Drug-Drug: Concurrent use with other **adrenergics** (sympathomimetic) will have additive adrenergic side

effects. Use with **MAO inhibitors** may lead to hypertensive crisis. **Beta blockers** may negate its therapeutic effect.

Drug-Natural Products: Use with caffeine-containing herbs (**cola nut, guarana, mate, tea, coffee**) ↑ stimulant effect.

Route/Dosage
Asthma
PO (Adults and Children >15 yr): 2.5–5 mg 3 times daily, given every 6 hr (not to exceed 15 mg/24 hr).
PO (Children 12–15 yr): 2.5 mg 3 times daily (given every 6 hr) (not to exceed 7.5 mg/24 hr).
PO (Children <12 yr): 0.05 mg/kg 3 times daily; may ↑ gradually (not to exceed 0.15 mg/kg 3–4 times daily or 5 mg/24 hr).
SUBQ (Adults and Children ≥12 yr): 250 mcg; may repeat in 15–30 min (not to exceed 500 mcg/4 hr).
SUBQ (Children <12 yr): 0.005–0.01 mg/kg; may repeat in 15–20 min.

Tocolysis (off-label)
IV (Adults): 2.5–10 mcg/min infusion; ↑ by 5 mcg/min every 10 min until contractions stop (not to exceed 30 mcg/min). After contractions have stopped for 30 min, ↓ infusion rate to lowest effective amount and maintain for 4–8 hr.

Availability (generic available)
Tablets: 2.5 mg, 5 mg. **Solution for injection:** 1 mg/mL.

NURSING IMPLICATIONS
Assessment
- **Bronchodilator:** Assess lung sounds, respiratory pattern, pulse, and BP before administration and during peak of medication. Note amount, color, and character of sputum produced, and notify health care professional of abnormal findings.
- Monitor pulmonary function tests before initiating therapy and periodically throughout therapy to determine effectiveness of medication.
- **Preterm Labor:** Monitor maternal pulse and BP, frequency and duration of contractions, and fetal heart rate. Notify health care professional if contractions persist or increase in frequency or duration or if symptoms of maternal or fetal distress occur. Maternal side effects include tachycardia, palpitations, tremor, anxiety, and headache.
- Assess maternal respiratory status for symptoms of pulmonary edema (increased rate, dyspnea, rales/crackles, frothy sputum).
- Monitor mother and neonate for symptoms of hypoglycemia (anxiety; chills; cold sweats; confusion; cool, pale skin; difficulty in concentration; drowsiness; excessive hunger; headache; irritability; nausea; nervousness; rapid pulse; shakiness; unusual

tiredness; or weakness) and mother for hypokalemia (weakness, fatigue, U wave on ECG, arrhythmias).

Lab Test Considerations
- May cause transient ↓ in serum potassium concentrations with higher than recommended doses.
- Monitor maternal serum glucose and electrolytes. May cause hypokalemia and hypoglycemia. Monitor neonate's serum glucose, because hypoglycemia may also occur in neonates.

Toxicity and Overdose
- Symptoms of overdose include persistent agitation, chest pain or discomfort, decreased BP, dizziness, hyperglycemia, hypokalemia, seizures, tachyarrhythmias, persistent trembling, and vomiting.
- Treatment includes discontinuing beta-adrenergic agonists and symptomatic, supportive therapy. Cardioselective beta blockers are used cautiously because they may induce bronchospasm.

Implementation
- **PO:** Administer with meals to minimize gastric irritation.
- Tablet may be crushed and mixed with food or fluids for patients with difficulty swallowing.
- **SUBQ:** Administer SUBQ injections in lateral deltoid area. Do not use solution if discolored.

IV Administration
- **Continuous Infusion:** *Dilution:* May be diluted in D5W, 0.9% NaCl, or 0.45% NaCl. *Concentration:* 1 mg/mL (undiluted). *Rate:* Use infusion pump to ensure accurate dose. Begin infusion at 10 mcg/min. Increase dosage by 5 mcg every 10 min until contractions cease. Maximum dose is 80 mcg/min. Begin to taper dose in 5-mcg decrements after a 30–60 min contraction-free period is attained. Switch to oral dose form after patient is contraction-free 4–8 hr on the lowest effective dose.
- **Y-Site Compatibility:** insulin regular.

Patient/Family Teaching
- Instruct patient to take medication as directed. If on a scheduled dosing regimen, take a missed dose as soon as possible; space remaining doses at regular intervals. Do not double doses. Caution patient not to exceed recommended dose; may cause adverse effects, paradoxical bronchospasm, or loss of effectiveness of medication.
- Instruct patient to contact health care professional immediately if shortness of breath is not relieved by medication or is accompanied by diaphoresis, dizziness, palpitations, or chest pain.
- Advise patient to consult health care professional before taking any OTC medications or alcoholic beverages concurrently with this therapy. Caution patient also to avoid smoking and other respiratory irritants.

- **Preterm Labor:** Notify health care professional immediately if labor resumes or if significant side effects occur.

Evaluation/Desired Outcomes

- Prevention or relief of bronchospasm.
- Increase in ease of breathing.
- Control of preterm labor in a fetus of 20–36 wk gestational age.

terconazole, See ANTIFUNGALS (VAGINAL).

teriflunomide
(ter-i-**floo**-noe-mide)
Aubagio
Classification
Therapeutic: anti-multiple sclerosis agents
Pharmacologic: immune response modifiers, pyrimidine synthesis inhibitors

Indications

Relapsing forms of multiple sclerosis (MS), including clinically isolated syndrome, relapsing-remitting disease, and active secondary progressive disease.

Action

Inhibits an enzyme required for pyrimidine synthesis; has antiproliferative and anti-inflammatory effects. **Therapeutic Effects:** ↓ incidence and severity of relapses in MS, with a decrease in disability progression.

Pharmacokinetics

Absorption: Well absorbed following oral administration.
Distribution: Well distributed to tissues.
Protein Binding: >99%.
Metabolism and Excretion: Metabolized via hydrolysis to inactive metabolites. 38% excreted in feces, and 23% excreted in urine.
Half-life: 18–19 days.

TIME/ACTION PROFILE (decrease in disability progression)

ROUTE	ONSET	PEAK	DURATION
PO	3–6 mo	unknown	unknown

Contraindications/Precautions

Contraindicated in: Hypersensitivity to teriflunomide or leflunomide; Severe hepatic impairment; Concurrent use of leflunomide; Live virus vaccinations; Active acute or chronic infection; Rep: Women of reproductive potential not using effective contraception; OB: Pregnancy; Lactation: Lactation.
Use Cautiously in: Mild or moderate hepatic impairment; Severe immunodeficiency, bone marrow disease or severe uncontrolled infection; Concurrent use of neurotoxic medications or diabetes mellitus (↑ risk

of peripheral neuropathy); Hypertension (control before therapy is initiated); Rep: Women of reproductive potential and men with female partners of reproductive potential; Pedi: Safety and effectiveness not established in children; Geri: ↑ risk of peripheral neuropathy in older adults.

Adverse Reactions/Side Effects

CV: hypertension. **Derm:** alopecia, DRUG REACTION WITH EOSINOPHILIA AND SYSTEMIC SYMPTOMS (DRESS), STEVENS-JOHNSON SYNDROME (SJS), TOXIC EPIDERMAL NECROLYSIS (TEN). **F and E:** hyperkalemia, hypophosphatemia. **GI:** ↑ liver enzymes, diarrhea, nausea, HEPATOTOXICITY. **GU:** acute renal failure (urate nephropathy). **Hemat:** leukopenia, neutropenia, thrombocytopenia. **Neuro:** paresthesia, peripheral neuropathy. **Misc:** HYPERSENSITIVITY REACTIONS (including anaphylaxis, angioedema, and urticaria), INFECTION (including latent tuberculosis [TB] and viral infections).

Interactions

Drug-Drug: May ↑ levels and the risk of toxicity of **CYP2C8 substrates**, including **paclitaxel, pioglitazone**, and **repaglinide**. May ↓ levels and effectiveness of **CYP1A2 substrates**, including **alosetron, duloxetine, theophylline**, and **tizanidine**. May ↓ response to and ↑ risk of adverse reactions from **live vaccines**; avoid live vaccinations and consider long half-life of teriflunomide before administering. May ↑ levels and the risk of toxicity of **ethinyl estradiol** and **levonorgestrel**. May ↑ risk the of bleeding with **warfarin**. ↑ risk of additive immunosuppression with other **immunosuppressants or antineoplastics**; consider long half-life of teriflunomide. **Breast cancer resistant protein inhibitors**, including **cyclosporine, eltrombopag**, and **gefitinib**, may ↑ levels and the risk of toxicity.

Route/Dosage

PO (Adults): 7 mg once daily *or* 14 mg once daily.

Availability (generic available)

Film-coated tablets: 7 mg, 14 mg.

NURSING IMPLICATIONS

Assessment

- Assess BP before starting and periodically during therapy. Treat hypertension as needed.
- Assess for rash periodically during therapy. May cause SJS or TEN. Discontinue therapy if severe or if accompanied with fever, general malaise, fatigue, muscle or joint aches, blisters, oral lesions, conjunctivitis, hepatitis and/or eosinophilia.
- Monitor for signs and symptoms of DRESS (fever, rash, lymphadenopathy and/or facial swelling, eosinophilia, in association with other organ system involvement, such as hepatitis, nephritis, hematologic abnormalities, myocarditis, or myositis, sometimes resembling an acute viral infection). Discontinue teriflunomide if DRESS is confirmed.

Lab Test Considerations

- Verify negative pregnancy test before starting therapy. Monitor liver function tests (transaminases, bilirubin) within 6 mo of starting therapy and monthly after teriflunomide therapy begins. Do not administer if ALT >2 × upper limit of normal (ULN). Consider discontinuing therapy if serum transaminase ↑ >3 × ULN is confirmed. Monitor serum transaminase and bilirubin in patients with symptoms of liver dysfunction. If liver injury is suspected, discontinue teriflunomide, begin accelerated elimination procedure, and monitor liver function tests weekly until normal.
- Monitor CBC with platelet count within 6 mo prior to starting and periodically during therapy based on signs and symptoms of infection. Mean decrease in WBC occurs during first 6 wk and remains low during therapy.
- Monitor INR closely in patients taking warfarin.

Implementation

- Administer a tuberculin skin test prior to administration of teriflunomide. Patients with active latent TB should be treated for TB prior to therapy.
- **PO:** Administer once daily without regard to food.
- **Drug Elimination Procedure:** Females of reproductive potential who wish to become pregnant, females who become pregnant during therapy, and males who want to father a child must continue teriflunomide and go through one of the drug elimination procedures. Either of the following procedures is recommended to achieve nondetectable plasma levels <0.02 mg/L after stopping treatment with teriflunomide; 1) Administer cholestyramine 8 g 3 times daily (every 8 hr) for 11 days. If cholestyramine 8 g is not well tolerated, cholestyramine 4 g 3 times/day can be used; *or* 2) Administration of 50 g oral activated charcoal powder every 12 hr for 11 days. (Days do not need to be consecutive unless rapid lowering of levels is desired.) Verify plasma levels <0.02 mg/L by 2 separate tests at least 14 days apart. Plasma levels may take up to 2 yr to reach nondetectable levels without drug elimination procedure.

Patient/Family Teaching

- Instruct patient to take teriflunomide as directed. Advise patient to read *Medication Guide* before starting therapy and with each Rx refill in case of changes.
- Advise patient to notify health care professional promptly if symptoms of liver problems (nausea, vomiting, stomach pain, loss of appetite, tiredness, skin or whites of eyes yellowing, dark urine), serious skin problems (redness or peeling), infection (fever, tiredness, body aches, chills, nausea, vomiting), or interstitial lung disease (cough, dyspnea, with or without fever) occur.

- Instruct patient to notify health care professional if symptoms of peripheral neuropathy (numbness and tingling in hands and feet different from symptoms of MS), kidney problems (flank pain), high potassium level (nausea or racing heartbeat), or high BP occur.
- Instruct patient to notify health care professional of all Rx or OTC medications, vitamins, or herbal products being taken and consult health care professional before taking any new medications.
- Instruct patient to avoid vaccinations with live vaccines during and following therapy without consulting health care professional.
- Discuss the possibility of hair loss with patient. Explore methods of coping.
- Rep: May cause fetal harm. Effective birth control should be used during therapy and until blood levels of teriflunomide are low enough. If pregnancy is planned or suspected, or if breastfeeding, notify health care professional immediately; an accelerated elimination procedure may be used to decrease blood levels more rapidly. Male patients with female partners of reproductive potential who plan to become pregnant may also use this method. If female partner does not plan to become pregnant, use effective birth control until blood levels are low enough; may require 2 yr. Females of reproductive potential are recommended to undergo accelerated elimination procedure upon discontinuation of teriflunomide. Inform patient of pregnancy exposure registry that monitors pregnancy outcomes in women exposed to teriflunomide during pregnancy. Patients who become pregnant should be encouraged to enroll in the Aubagio Pregnancy Registry at 1-800-745-4447 to collect information about mother and baby's health. Advise patient to avoid breastfeeding during therapy.

Evaluation/Desired Outcomes

- Decrease in the number of MS flares (relapses) and slowing of physical problems caused by MS.

BEERS REMS

TESTOSTERONE
(tess-**toss**-te-rone)
testosterone cypionate
Depo-Testosterone
testosterone enanthate
✤Delatestryl , Xyosted
testosterone nasal gel
Natesto
testosterone pellets
Testopel
testosterone transdermal gel
Androgel, Testim, Vogelxo

T

testosterone transdermal solution
~~Axiron~~

testosterone undecanoate
Aveed, Jatenzo, Kyzatrex, Tlando
Classification
Therapeutic: hormones
Pharmacologic: androgens

Schedule III

Indications
Hypogonadism in men with low testosterone serum concentrations. Delayed puberty in men (enanthate and pellets). Androgen-responsive breast cancer in postmenopausal women (palliative) (enanthate). **Unlabeled Use:** Part of masculinizing hormone therapy in Female to Male (FtM) transgender patients.

Action
Responsible for the normal growth and development of male sex organs. Maintenance of male secondary sex characteristics: Growth and maturation of the prostate, seminal vesicles, penis, scrotum, Development of male hair distribution, Vocal cord thickening, Alterations in body musculature and fat distribution. **Therapeutic Effects:** Correction of hormone deficiency in male hypogonadism: Initiation of male puberty. Suppression of tumor growth in some forms of breast cancer. Increased male characteristics in FtM transgender patients.

Pharmacokinetics
Absorption: Well absorbed from IM or SUBQ sites, through skin, or through nasal mucosa. Cypionate, enanthate, and undecanoate salts are absorbed slowly. Skin serves as reservoir for sustained release of testosterone into systemic circulation; 10% absorbed into systemic circulation during 24-hr period.
Distribution: Crosses the placenta.
Protein Binding: 98%.
Metabolism and Excretion: Metabolized by the liver. 90% eliminated in urine as metabolites.
Half-life: *Enanthate (IM), nasal gel, pellets, topical gel, topical solution, undecanoate:* 10–100 min; *cypionate:* 8 days; *enanthate (SUBQ):* Unknown.

TIME/ACTION PROFILE (androgenic effects†)

ROUTE	ONSET	PEAK	DURATION
IM—cypionate, enanthate	unknown	unknown	2–4 wk
IM—undecanoate	unknown	unknown	10 wk
SUBQ —enanthate	unknown	unknown	unknown
Nasal gel	unknown	unknown	3 mo
Oral	unknown	unknown	unknown
Pellets	unknown	unknown	3–6 mo
Transdermal (solution)	unknown	14 days	7–10 days
Transdermal (gel)	30 min	unknown	24 hr

†Response is highly variable among individuals; may take mo.

Contraindications/Precautions
Contraindicated in: Hypersensitivity; Men with breast or prostate cancer; Age-related hypogonadism (undecanoate [PO]); Some products contain benzyl alcohol and should be avoided in patients with known hypersensitivity; Women (pellets, nasal gel, tablets, topical gel, topical solution); OB: Pregnancy; Lactation: Lactation.

Use Cautiously in: Diabetes mellitus; Established cardiovascular disease or risk factors for cardiovascular disease; Hypertension; Renal or hepatic impairment; Benign prostatic hyperplasia; Hypercalcemia; Obesity or chronic lung disease (↑ risk of sleep apnea); Polycythemia; Nasal disorders, nasal/sinus surgery, nasal fracture in previous 6 mo, nasal fracture that caused deviated anterior nasal septum, mucosal inflammatory disorders (e.g., Sjogren's syndrome), or sinus disorders (nasal gel); Pedi: Prepubertal males exposed to testosterone may experience premature development of secondary sexual characteristics, aggression, and other side effects; Geri: Appears on Beers list. ↑ risk of prostatic hyperplasia/carcinoma in older adults. Avoid use in older adults, except for confirmed hypogonadism with clinical symptoms.

Adverse Reactions/Side Effects
CV: edema, DEEP VEIN THROMBOSIS, ↑ blood pressure, MI. **Derm:** male pattern baldness. **EENT:** deepening of voice; *nasal gel:* epistaxis, nasal scabbing, nasopharyngitis, rhinorrhea. **Endo:** *women:* change in libido, clitoral enlargement, ↓ breast size; *men:* acne, facial hair, gynecomastia, erectile dysfunction, oligospermia, priapism. **F and E:** hypercalcemia, hyperkalemia, hyperphosphatemia. **GI:** abdominal cramps, changes in appetite, HEPATOTOXICITY, nausea, vomiting; *buccal:* bitter taste, gingivitis, gum edema, gum tenderness. **GU:** ↓ fertility, ↓ sperm count, menstrual irregularities, nocturia, priapism, prostatic enlargement, urinary hesitancy, urinary incontinence. **Hemat:** ↑ hematocrit. **Local:** chronic skin irritation (transdermal), pain at injection/implantation site, pulmonary oil microembolism reactions (IM). **Metab:** hyperlipidemia. **Neuro:** anxiety, confusion, depression, fatigue, headache, STROKE, SUICIDAL THOUGHTS/BEHAVIOR, vertigo. **Resp:** PULMONARY EMBOLISM, sleep apnea. **Misc:** HYPERSENSITIVITY REACTIONS (including anaphylaxis).

Interactions
Drug-Drug: May ↑ action of **warfarin**, **oral hypoglycemic agents**, and **insulin**. Concurrent use with **corticosteroids** may ↑ risk of edema formation.

Route/Dosage
Replacement Therapy
IM (Adults): 50–400 mg every 2–4 wk (enanthate or cypionate); 750 mg initially, then at wk 4, then every 10 wk (undecanoate).
SUBQ (Adults): 75 mg once weekly (enanthate).
Intranasal (Adults): 1 actuation (5.5 mg) in each nostril 3 times daily.

PO (Adults): *Jatenzo:* 158 mg twice daily; may titrate up to 396 mg twice daily based on serum testosterone concentrations. *Kyzatrex:* 200 mg twice daily; may titrate up to 400 mg twice daily based on serum testosterone concentrations. *Tlando:* 225 mg twice daily.

Transdermal (Adults): *Androgel 1% or Testim:* 5 g (contains 50 mg of testosterone; 5 mg systemically absorbed) applied once daily (morning preferable); if needed, may be ↑ to maximum of 10 g (contains 100 mg of testosterone; 10 mg systemically absorbed); *Androgel 1.62%:* 40.5 mg of testosterone (2 pump actuations) applied once daily (morning preferable); dose may be adjusted down to a minimum of 20.25 mg or up to a maximum of 81 mg of testosterone, if needed (dose based on serum testosterone levels) *Vogelxo:* 50 mg of testosterone (1 tube, 1 packet, or 4 pump actuations) applied once daily; dose may be adjusted up to a maximum of 100 mg of testosterone, if needed (dose based on serum testosterone levels).

SUBQ (for SUBQ implantation) (pellets) (Adults): 150–450 mg every 3–6 mo.

Topical (Adults): 60 mg (2 pump actuations) applied once daily; may be ↑ up to 120 mg (4 pump actuations) based on serum testosterone concentrations.

Delayed Male Puberty

IM (Children): 50–200 mg every 2–4 wk for up to 6 mo (enanthate).

SUBQ (for SUBQ implantation) (pellets) (Children): 150–450 mg every 3–6 mo.

Palliative Management of Breast Cancer

IM (Adults): 200–400 mg every 2–4 wk (enanthate).

Availability (generic available)

Capsules (Jatenzo): 158 mg, 198 mg, 237 mg. **Capsules (Kyzatrex):** 100 mg, 150 mg, 200 mg. **Capsules (Tlando):** 112.5 mg. **Nasal gel:** 5.5 mg/pump actuation. **Pellets:** 75 mg. **Solution for intramuscular injection (cypionate) (in oil):** 100 mg/mL, 200 mg/mL. **Solution for intramuscular injection (enanthate) (in oil):** 200 mg/mL. **Solution for intramuscular injection (undecanoate) (in oil) (Aveed):** 250 mg/mL. **Solution for SUBQ injection (enanthate) (autoinjector) (Xyosted):** 50 mg/0.5 mL, 75 mg/0.5 mL, 100 mg/0.5 mL. **Transdermal gel (Androgel):** 20.25 mg/packet (1.62%), 25 mg/packet (1%), 40.5 mg/packet (1.62%), 50 mg/packet (1%), 75-g metered dose pump (each pump dispenses 60 metered 12.5-mg doses [1%]), 88-g metered dose pump (each pump dispenses 60 metered 20.25-mg doses [1.62%]). **Transdermal gel (Testim):** 50 mg/unit–dose tube (1%). **Transdermal gel (Vogelxo):** 50 mg/packet or unit–dose tube (1%), 75-g metered dose pump (each pump dispenses 60 metered 12.5-mg doses [1%]). **Transdermal solution:** 30 mg/pump actuation.

NURSING IMPLICATIONS
Assessment

● Monitor intake and output ratios, weigh patient twice weekly, and assess patient for edema. Report significant changes indicative of fluid retention.

● Assess for abuse using higher doses than prescribed and usually in conjunction with other anabolic androgenic steroids. May result in heart attack, heart failure, stroke, depression, hostility, aggression, liver toxicity, and infertility. Measure serum testosterone if abuse is suspected.

● **Men:** Monitor for precocious puberty in boys (acne, darkening of skin, development of male secondary sex characteristics—increase in penis size, frequent erections, growth of body hair). Bone age determinations should be measured every 6 mo to determine rate of bone maturation and effects on epiphyseal closure.

● Monitor for breast enlargement, persistent erections, and increased urge to urinate in men. Monitor for difficulty urinating in elderly men, because prostate enlargement may occur.

● **Women:** Assess for virilism (deepening of voice, unusual hair growth or loss, clitoral enlargement, acne, menstrual irregularity).

● In women with metastatic breast cancer, monitor for symptoms of hypercalcemia (nausea, vomiting, constipation, lethargy, loss of muscle tone, thirst, polyuria).

Lab Test Considerations

● Prior to therapy, measure serum testosterone in the morning on at least two separate days. Normal range (300–1050 ng/dL). Monitor serum testosterone concentrations 4–12 wk after starting therapy. Discontinue therapy is concentrations are consistently outside of normal range.

● Monitor hemoglobin and hematocrit periodically during therapy; may cause polycythemia.

● Monitor hepatic function tests, prostate specific antigen and serum cholesterol levels periodically during therapy. May cause ↑ serum AST, ALT, and bilirubin, ↑ cholesterol levels, and suppress clotting factors II, V, VII, and X.

● Monitor serum and urine calcium levels and serum alkaline phosphatase concentrations in women with metastatic breast cancer.

● Monitor serum sodium, chloride, potassium, and phosphate concentrations (may be ↑).

● Monitor blood glucose closely in patients with diabetes who are receiving oral hypoglycemic agents or insulin.

● *Transdermal Solution:* Measure serum testosterone concentrations after initiation of therapy to ensure desired concentrations (300–1050 ng/dL) are achieved. Adjust dose based on serum testosterone concentration from a single blood draw 2–8 hr af-

T

ter applying and at least 14 days after starting treatment or following dose adjustment. If concentration is below 300 ng/dL, daily dose may be increased from 60 mg (2 pump actuations) to 90 mg (3 pump actuations) or from 90 mg to 120 mg (4 pump actuations). If concentration exceeds 1050 ng/dL, the daily testosterone dose should be decreased from 60 mg (2 pump actuations) to 30 mg (1 pump actuation) as instructed by health care professional. If concentration consistently exceeds 1050 ng/dL at lowest daily dose of 30 mg (1 pump actuation), discontinue therapy.

- *Nasal gel:* Monitor serum testosterone concentrations after 1 mo and periodically during therapy. If total testosterone concentrations consistently exceed 1050 ng/dL, discontinue therapy. If total testosterone concentrations are consistently below 300 ng/dL, consider alternative therapy.

Implementation

- Range-of-motion exercises should be done with all bedridden patients to prevent mobilization of calcium from the bone.
- **PO:** Administer twice daily, in the morning and evening, with food.
- **IM:** Administer IM deep into gluteal muscle. Crystals may form when vials are stored at low temperatures; warming and shaking vial will redissolve crystals. Use of a wet syringe or needle may cause solution to become cloudy but will not affect its potency.
- **SUBQ:** Pellets are to be implanted SUBQ by a health care professional.
- **Transdermal: Solution:** Apply to axilla using applicator at the same time each morning, to clean, dry, intact skin. Do not apply to other parts of the body including to the scrotum, penis, abdomen, shoulders, or upper arms. Prime pump when using for first time by depressing pump 3 times, discard any product dispensed directly into a basin, sink, or toilet, and then wash liquid away thoroughly. Prime only prior to first use of each pump. After priming, completely depress pump once with nozzle over applicator cup to dispense 30 mg of testosterone. Apply in 30 mg (1 pump actuation) increments. Place actuator into the axilla and wipe steadily down and up into the axilla. If solution drips or runs, wipe back up with applicator cup. Do not rub into skin with fingers or hand. Repeat process for each 30-mg dose needed. When repeat application to same axilla, allow axilla to dry completely before more is applied. Rinse applicator under room temperature, running water and pat dry with a tissue. Allow axilla to dry completely prior to dressing. Solution has an alcohol base and is flammable until dry. Apply deodorant prior to application of testosterone solution. Avoid swimming or washing for 2 hr after application. Wash hands immediately with soap and water after application.
- **Transdermal: Gel:** Apply gel once daily, preferably in the morning, to clean dry intact skin of shoulders

and upper arms (*Androgel, Testim,* and *Vogelxo*) or abdomen (Androgel only) or front or inner thighs (Fortesta). Gel should not be applied to scrotum (5–30 times more permeable than other sites). Refer to the chart on the pump label to determine how many full pump depressions are required for the daily prescribed dose.

- The dose of Fortesta should be titrated based on the serum testosterone concentration from a single blood draw 2 hr after applying Fortesta and at approximately 14 days and 35 days after starting treatment or following dose adjustment.
- **Intranasal:** Prime pump by inverting, depressing pump 10 times, and discarding any amount dispensed directly into a sink and washing gel away thoroughly with warm water. Wipe tip with a clean, dry tissue. If gel gets on hands, wash hands with warm water and soap. Priming should be done only prior to first use of each dispenser. Blow nose. Place right index finger on pump of actuator and while in front of a mirror, slowly advance tip of actuator into left nostril upwards until finger on the pump reaches the base of the nose. Tilt the actuator so that the opening on the tip of the actuator is in contact with the lateral wall of the nostril to ensure that the gel is applied to the nasal wall. Slowly depress the pump until it stops. Remove the actuator from the nose while wiping the tip along the inside of the lateral nostril wall to fully transfer the gel. Repeat with right nostril. Press on the nostrils at a point just below bridge of the nose and lightly massage. Refrain from blowing nose or sniffing for 1 hr after administration.

Patient/Family Teaching

- Advise patient to report the following signs and symptoms promptly: *in male patients,* priapism (sustained and often painful erections), difficulty urinating, or gynecomastia; *in female patients,* virilism (which may be reversible if medication is stopped as soon as changes are noticed) or hypercalcemia (nausea, vomiting, constipation, and weakness); *in male or female patients,* edema (unexpected weight gain, swelling of feet), hepatitis (yellowing of skin or eyes and abdominal pain), or unusual bleeding or bruising.
- Instruct patient to use testosterone as directed. Do not use higher than prescribed doses. Explain rationale for prohibiting use of testosterone for increasing athletic performance. Testosterone is neither safe nor effective for this use and has a potential risk of serious side effects.
- Advise diabetic patients to monitor blood closely for alterations in blood glucose concentrations.
- Emphasize the importance of regular follow-up physical exams, lab tests, and x-ray exams to monitor progress.
- Radiologic bone age determinations should be evaluated every 6 mo in prepubertal children to deter-

mine rate of bone maturation and effects on epiphyseal centers.

- Rep: May cause fetal harm. Advise females of reproductive potential to notify health care professional immediately if pregnancy is planned or suspected or if breastfeeding. May impair fertility.
- **Transdermal: Gel or Solution:** Explain application to patient.
- Advise patient that women and children should avoid contact with unclothed or unwashed application site. Patients should cover the application site(s) with clothing (T-shirt) after solution has dried. For direct skin-to-skin contact, patient should wash application site thoroughly with soap and water to remove any testosterone residue. If unwashed or unclothed skin with testosterone solution comes in direct contact with skin of another person, wash area of contact with soap and water as soon as possible.
- **Intranasal:** Advise patient to notify health care professional if nasal signs or symptoms (nasopharyngitis, rhinorrhea, epistaxis, nasal discomfort, nasal scabbing) occur.

Evaluation/Desired Outcomes
- Resolution of the signs of androgen deficiency without side effects. Therapy is usually limited to 3–6 mo followed by bone growth or maturation determinations.
- Decrease in the size and spread of breast malignancy in postmenopausal women. In antineoplastic therapy, response may require 3 mo of therapy; if signs of disease progression appear, therapy should be discontinued.
- Increased male characteristics in FtM transgender patients.

TETRACYCLINES
doxycycline (dox-i-**sye**-kleen)
Acticlate, ✿Apprilon, Doryx, Doxy, ✿Doxycin, ✿Doxytab, Oracea, ✿Periostat, Vibramycin
minocycline (min-oh-**sye**-kleen)
Amzeeq, Minocin, Minolira, Solodyn, Ximino, Zilxi
tetracycline (te-tra-**sye**-kleen)
~~Sumycin~~

Classification
Therapeutic: anti-infectives
Pharmacologic: tetracyclines

Indications
Treatment of various infections caused by unusual organisms, including: *Mycoplasma, Chlamydia, Rickettsia, Borellia burgdorferi.* Gonorrhea and syphilis in penicillin-allergic patients. Prevention of exacerbations of chronic bronchitis. Treatment of inhalational anthrax

(postexposure) and cutaneous anthrax (doxycycline only). Treatment of acne. Malaria prophylaxis (doxycycline only). Inflammatory lesions of non-nodular acne vulgaris (Solodyn and Ximino). Rosacea (Zilxi).

Action
Inhibits bacterial protein synthesis at the level of the 30S bacterial ribosome. **Therapeutic Effects:** Bacteriostatic action against susceptible bacteria. **Spectrum:** Includes activity against some gram-positive pathogens: *Bacillus anthracis, Clostridioides perfringens, Clostridioides tetani, Listeria monocytogenes, Nocardia, Propionibacterium acnes, Actinomyces israelii.* Active against some gram-negative pathogens: *Haemophilus influenzae, Legionella pneumophila, Yersinia enterocolitica, Yersinia pestis, Neisseria gonorrboeae, Neisseria meningitidis.* Also active against several other pathogens, including: *Mycoplasma, Treponema pallidum, Chlamydia, Rickettsia, B. burgdorferi.*

Pharmacokinetics
Absorption: *Tetracycline:* 60–80% absorbed following oral administration. *Doxycycline:* Well absorbed from the GI tract. *Minocycline:* Well absorbed from the GI tract; minimal absorption following topical administration.

Distribution: Widely distributed, some penetration into CSF.

Metabolism and Excretion: *Doxycycline:* 20–40% excreted unchanged by the urine; some inactivation in the intestine and some enterohepatic circulation with excretion in bile and feces. *Minocycline:* 5–20% excreted unchanged by the urine; some metabolism by the liver with enterohepatic circulation and excretion in bile and feces. *Tetracycline:* Excreted mostly unchanged by the kidneys.

Half-life: *Doxycycline:* 14–17 hr (↑ in severe renal impairment). *Minocycline:* 11–26 hr. *Tetracycline:* 6–12 hr.

TIME/ACTION PROFILE (plasma concentrations)

ROUTE	ONSET	PEAK	DURATION
Doxycycline-PO	1–2 hr	1.5–4 hr	12 hr
Doxycycline-IV	rapid	end of infusion	12 hr
Minocycline-PO	rapid	2–3 hr	6–12 hr
Minocycline-PO—ER	unknown	3.5–4 hr	24 hr
Tetracycline-PO	1–2 hr	2–4 hr	6–12 hr

Contraindications/Precautions
Contraindicated in: Hypersensitivity to any of the tetracyclines; Some products contain alcohol or bisulfites; avoid in patients with known hypersensitivity or in-

---

✿ = Canadian drug name. ▓ = Genetic implication. ~~Strikethrough~~ = Discontinued. CAPITALS = life-threatening. <u>Underline</u> = most frequent.

tolerance; OB: Risk of permanent staining of teeth in infant if used during last half of pregnancy (doxycycline may be used to treat anthrax in pregnant women due to the seriousness of the disease); Lactation: Lactation; Pedi: Children <8 yr (permanent staining of teeth) (unless used for anthrax; doxycycline may be used to treat anthrax in children due to the seriousness of the disease).

Use Cautiously in: Renal impairment; Hepatic impairment (minocycline); Nephrogenic diabetes insipidus; Rep: Women of reproductive potential (↑ risk of intracranial hypertension if overweight or have a previous history of intracranial hypertension); Pedi: Children <9 yr (safety and effectiveness of topical formulation not established).

Adverse Reactions/Side Effects

Derm: erythema (topical minocycline only), photosensitivity, DRUG RASH WITH EOSINOPHILIA AND SYSTEMIC SYMPTOMS (DRESS), dry skin (topical minocycline only), ERYTHEMA MULTIFORME, EXFOLIATIVE DERMATITIS, hyperpigmentation of skin and mucous membranes (minocycline only), itching (topical minocycline only), rash, skin peeling (topical minocycline only), STEVENS-JOHNSON SYNDROME (SJS), TOXIC EPIDERMAL NECROLYSIS (TEN). **EENT:** vestibular reactions (minocycline only). **Endo:** *minocycline:* thyroid disorders. **GI:** diarrhea, nausea, PANCREATITIS, vomiting, CLOSTRIDIOIDES DIFFI-CILE-ASSOCIATED DIARRHEA (CDAD), dysphagia, esophagitis, glossitis, HEPATOTOXICITY. **Hemat:** blood dyscrasias. **MS:** *minocycline:* lupus-like syndrome. **Local:** *doxycycline, minocycline:* phlebitis at IV site. **Neuro:** intracranial hypertension; *minocycline:* dizziness.. **Misc:** HYPERSENSITIVITY REACTIONS (including anaphylaxis and angioedema), superinfection.

Interactions

Drug-Drug: May ↑ effect of **warfarin**. May ↓ effectiveness of **estrogen-containing hormonal contraceptives**. **Antacids**, **calcium**, **iron**, **zinc**, **aluminum**, and **magnesium** form insoluble compounds (chelates) and ↓ absorption of tetracyclines. **Sucralfate** may bind to tetracycline and ↓ its absorption from the GI tract. **Cholestyramine** or **colestipol** ↓ oral absorption of tetracyclines. **Adsorbent antidiarrheals** may ↓ absorption of tetracyclines. **Barbiturates**, **carbamazepine**, or **phenytoin** may ↓ activity of doxycycline. **Isotretinoin** may ↑ risk of intracranial hypertension with doxycycline; avoid concomitant use.

Drug-Food: **Calcium** in foods or **dairy products** ↓ absorption by forming insoluble compounds (chelates).

Route/Dosage

Doxycycline

PO (Adults and Children >8 yr and >45 kg): *Most infections:* 100 mg every 12 hr on the 1st day, then 100–200 mg once daily or 50–100 mg every 12 hr; *Gonorrhea:* 100 mg every 12 hr for 7 days or 200 mg once daily for 7 days (delayed-release tablets) or 300

mg followed 1 hr later by another 300-mg dose; *Uncomplicated urethral, endocervical, or rectal infection caused by Chlamydia trachomatis:* 100 mg every 12 hr for 7 days; *Syphilis (early):* 100 mg every 12 hr for 14 days; *Syphilis (>1 yr duration):* 100 mg every 12 hr for 4 wk; *Malaria prophylaxis:* 100 mg once daily; *Lyme disease:* 100 mg twice daily; *Periodontitis:* 20 mg twice daily; *Rosacea:* 40 mg once daily in morning.

PO (Children >8 yr and ≤45 kg): *Most infections:* 2.2 mg/kg every 12 hr on the 1st day, then 2.2–4.4 mg/kg once daily or 1.1–2.2 mg/kg every 12 hr; *Malaria prophylaxis:* 2 mg/kg once daily.

PO, IV (Adults and Children >45 kg): *Inhalational anthrax (postexposure):* 100 mg IV every 12 hr; change to 100 mg PO every 12 hr when clinically appropriate for a total of 60 days; one or two other anti-infectives may be added initially, depending on clinical situation; *Cutaneous anthrax:* 100 mg PO every 12 hr for 60 days; some patients may require IV therapy initially depending on clinical situation.

PO, IV (Children ≤45 kg): *Inhalational anthrax (postexposure):* 2.2 mg/kg IV every 12 hr; change to 2.2 mg/kg PO every 12 hr when clinically appropriate for a total of 60 days; one or two other anti-infectives may be added initially, depending on clinical situation; *Cutaneous anthrax:* 2.2 mg/kg every 12 hr for 60 days; some patients may require IV therapy initially depending on clinical situation.

Minocycline

PO (Adults): 100–200 mg initially, then 100 mg every 12 hr or 50 mg every 6 hr.

PO, IV (Children ≥8 yr): 4 mg/kg initially, then 2 mg/kg every 12 hr.

PO (Adults and Children ≥12 yr [Solodyn and Ximino]): *126–136 kg*—135 mg once daily for 12 wk; *111–125 kg:* 115 mg once daily for 12 wk; *97–110 kg:* 105 mg once daily for 12 wk; *85–96 kg:* 90 mg once daily for 12 wk; *72–84 kg:* 80 mg once daily for 12 wk; *60–71 kg:* 65 mg once daily for 12 wk; *50–59 kg:* 55 mg once daily for 12 wk; *45–49 kg:* 45 mg once daily for 12 wk.

IV (Adults): 200 mg initially, then 100 mg every 12 hr (max dose = 400 mg/day).

Topical (Adults): *Zilxi:* Apply to affected area(s) once daily ≥1 hr before bedtime.

Topical (Adults and Children ≥9 yr): *Amzeeq:* Apply to affected area(s) once daily ≥1 hr before bedtime.

Tetracycline

PO (Adults): 250–500 mg every 6 hr or 500 mg–1 g every 12 hr. *Chronic treatment of acne:* 500 mg–2 g/day for 3 wk, then ↓ to 125 mg–1 g/day.

PO (Children ≥8 yr): 6.25–12.5 mg/kg every 6 hr or 12.5–25 mg/kg every 12 hr.

Availability

Doxycycline (generic available)

Immediate-release tablets: 20 mg, 50 mg, 75 mg, 100 mg, 150 mg. **Immediate-release capsules:** 50

mg, 75 mg, 100 mg, 150 mg. **Delayed-release tablets:** 50 mg, 60 mg, 75 mg, 80 mg, 100 mg, 120 mg, 150 mg, 200 mg. **Delayed-release capsules:** 40 mg. **Oral suspension (raspberry flavor):** 25 mg/5 mL. **Syrup (apple-raspberry flavor):** 50 mg/5 mL. **Powder for injection:** 100 mg/vial, 200 mg/vial.

Minocycline (generic available)
Immediate-release tablets: 50 mg, 75 mg, 100 mg. **Immediate-release capsules:** 50 mg, 75 mg, 100 mg. **Extended-release tablets:** 45 mg, 55 mg, 65 mg, 80 mg, 90 mg, 105 mg, 115 mg, 135 mg. **Extended-release capsules:** 45 mg, 90 mg, 135 mg. **Lyophilized powder for injection:** 100 mg/vial. **Topical foam (Amneeq):** 4%. **Topical foam (Zilxi):** 1.5%.

Tetracycline (generic available)
Capsules: 250 mg, 500 mg.

NURSING IMPLICATIONS

Assessment
- Assess for infection (vital signs; appearance of wound, sputum, urine, and stool; WBC) at beginning of and throughout therapy.
- Obtain specimens for culture and sensitivity before initiating therapy. First dose may be given before receiving results.
- Monitor bowel function. Diarrhea, abdominal cramping, fever, and bloody stools should be reported to health care professional promptly as a sign of CDAD. May begin up to several wk following cessation of therapy.
- Assess for rash periodically during therapy. May cause SJS or TEN. Discontinue therapy if severe or if accompanied by fever, general malaise, fatigue, muscle or joint aches, blisters, oral lesions, conjunctivitis, hepatitis, and/or eosinophilia.
- Monitor for signs and symptoms of DRESS (fever, rash, lymphadenopathy, and/or facial swelling), associated with involvement of other organ systems (hepatitis, nephritis, hematologic abnormalities, myocarditis, myositis) during therapy. May resemble an acute viral infection. Eosinophilia is often present. Discontinue therapy if signs occur.
- **IV:** Assess IV site frequently; may cause thrombophlebitis.

Lab Test Considerations
- Monitor renal and hepatic function and CBC periodically during long-term therapy.
- May cause ↑ AST, ALT, serum alkaline phosphatase, bilirubin, and amylase concentrations. Tetracyclines, except doxycycline, may cause ↑ serum BUN.

Implementation
- Do not confuse Oracea with Orencia.
- **PO:** Administer around the clock. Administer at least 1 hr before or 2 hr after meals. *Doxycycline and minocycline* may be taken with food or milk if GI ir-

ritation occurs. Administer with a full glass of liquid and at least 1 hr before going to bed to avoid esophageal ulceration. Use calibrated measuring device for liquid preparations. Shake liquid preparations well. Do not administer within 1–3 hr of other medications.
- *DNC:* Do not open, break, crush or chew extended release capsules and tablets.
- Avoid administration of calcium, zinc, antacids, magnesium- or aluminum-containing medications, sodium bicarbonate, or iron supplements within 1–3 hr of oral tetracyclines.

Doxycycline
- The *Oracea* product is only indicated for rosacea, not for infections.
- **PO: Public Health Emergency—Exposure to Anthrax:** To prepare doses for infants and children exposed to anthrax, place one 100-mg tablet in a small bowl and crush to a fine powder with a metal spoon, leaving no large pieces. Add 4 level teaspoons of low-fat milk, low-fat chocolate milk, regular chocolate milk, chocolate pudding, or apple juice. Mix food or drink and doxycycline powder until powder dissolves. Mixture is stable in a covered container for 24 hr if refrigerated (if made with milk or pudding) or at room temperature (if made with juice). Number of teaspoons to administer/dose is based on child's weight (0–12.5 lb—1/2 tsp; 12.5–25 lb—1 tsp; 25–37.5 lb—1 1/2 tsp; 37.5–50 lb—2 tsp; 50–62.5 lb—2 1/2 tsp; 62.5–75 lb—3 tsp; 75–87.5 lb—3 1/2 tsp; 87.5–100 lb—4 tsp).
- Capsules may be administered by carefully opening and sprinkling capsule contents on a spoonful of applesauce. Swallow applesauce immediately without chewing and followed with a cool 8-oz glass of water to ensure complete swallowing of capsule contents. Applesauce should not be hot and should be soft enough to be swallowed without chewing. If mixture cannot be taken immediately, discard; do not store for later use.

IV Administration
- **Intermittent Infusion:** *Reconstitution:* Reconstitute each 100 mg with 10 mL of sterile water or 0.9% NaCl for injection. *Dilution:* Dilute further in 100–1000 mL of 0.9% NaCl, D5W, D5/LR, Ringer's, or lactated Ringer's solution. Solution is stable for 12 hr at room temperature and 72 hr if refrigerated. If diluted with D5/LR or lactated Ringer's solution, administer within 6 hr. Protect solution from direct sunlight. *Concentration:* Concentrations of <1 mcg/mL or >1 mg/mL are not recommended. *Rate:* Administer over a minimum of 1–4 hr. Avoid rapid administration. Avoid extravasation.
- **Y-Site Compatibility:** acyclovir, alemtuzumab, amifostine, amikacin, aminophylline, amiodarone,

T

---

anidulafungin, argatroban, arsenic trioxide, ascorbic acid, atropine, azithromycin, aztreonam, benztropine, bivalirudin, bleomycin, bumetanide, buprenorphine, butorphanol, calcium chloride, calcium gluconate, cangrelor, carboplatin, carmustine, caspofungin, cefotaxime, ceftolozane/tazobactam, ceftriaxone, chlorpromazine, cisatracurium, cisplatin, clindamycin, cyanocobalamin, cyclophosphamide, cyclosporine, cytarabine, dacarbazine, dactinomycin, daptomycin, daunorubicin hydrochloride, dexmedetomidine, dexrazoxane, digoxin, diltiazem, diphenhydramine, dobutamine, docetaxel, dopamine, doxorubicin hydrochloride, enalaprilat, ephedrine, epinephrine, epirubicin, epoetin alfa, eptifibatide, ertapenem, esmolol, etoposide, etoposide phosphate, famotidine, fentanyl, filgrastim, fluconazole, fludarabine, fosphenytoin, gemcitabine, gentamicin, glycopyrrolate, granisetron, hetastarch, hydromorphone, idarubicin, ifosfamide, imipenem/cilastatin, insulin regular, irinotecan, isavuconazonium, isoproterenol, labetalol, LR, leucovorin calcium, levofloxacin, lidocaine, linezolid, lorazepam, magnesium sulfate, mannitol, melphalan, meperidine, meropenem/vaborbactam, mesna, methadone, metoclopramide, metoprolol, metronidazole, midazolam, milrinone, mitoxantrone, morphine, multivitamins, mycophenolate, nalbuphine, naloxone, nicardipine, nitroglycerin, nitroprusside, norepinephrine, octreotide, ondansetron, oxaliplatin, oxytocin, paclitaxel, pamidronate, pantoprazole, papaverine, pentamidine, phentolamine, phenylephrine, phytonadione, plazomicin, potassium chloride, procainamide, prochlorperazine, promethazine, propofol, propranolol, protamine, pyridoxine, remifentanil, rituximab, rocuronium, sargramostim, sodium acetate, succinylcholine, sufentanil, tacrolimus, telavancin, theophylline, thiamine, thiotepa, tirofiban, tobramycin, topotecan, trastuzumab, vancomycin, vasopressin, vecuronium, verapamil, vinblastine, vincristine, vinorelbine, voriconazole, zoledronic acid.

- **Y-Site Incompatibility:** allopurinol, aminocaproic acid, amphotericin B lipid complex, amphotericin B liposomal, ampicillin, ampicillin/sulbactam, azathioprine, cefazolin, cefotetan, cefoxitin, ceftazidime, cefuroxime, chloramphenicol, dantrolene, dexamethasone, diazepam, erythromycin, fluorouracil, folic acid, furosemide, ganciclovir, gemtuzumab ozogamicin, heparin, hydrocortisone, indomethacin, ketorolac, methotrexate, methylprednisolone, nafcillin, oxacillin, palonosetron, pemetrexed, penicillin G, pentobarbital, phenobarbital, phenytoin, piperacillin/tazobactam, potassium acetate, sodium bicarbonate, tedizolid, trimethoprim/sulfamethoxazole.

Minocycline

IV Administration

- IV doses are indicated only when oral therapy is not adequate or tolerated. Resume oral doses as soon as possible.

- **Intermittent Infusion:** Reconstitute vial with 5 mL of sterile water for injection. *Dilution:* 100 mL– 1,000 mL 0.9% NaCl, D5W, or D5/0.9% NaCl, or in 250 mL– 1000 mL LR, but not with other solutions containing calcium; precipitate may form, especially in neutral and alkaline solutions. Solutions are stable for 4 hr at room temperature or 24 hr if refrigerated. *Rate:* Infuse over 60 min. Do not infuse rapidly.

- **Y-Site Incompatibility:** Do not administer with other medications or solutions. Flush line between doses.

Patient/Family Teaching

- Instruct patient to take medication around the clock and to finish the drug completely as directed, even if feeling better. Take missed doses as soon as possible unless it is almost time for next dose; do not double doses. Advise patient that sharing of this medication may be dangerous.

- Advise patient to avoid taking milk or other dairy products concurrently with oral tetracyclines. Also avoid taking antacids, zinc, calcium, magnesium- or aluminum-containing medications, sodium bicarbonate, and iron supplements within 1–3 hr of oral tetracyclines.

- Instruct patient to notify health care professional immediately if rash, diarrhea, abdominal cramping, fever, or bloody stools occur and not to treat with antidiarrheals without consulting health care professionals.

- *Minocycline* commonly causes dizziness or unsteadiness. Caution patient to avoid driving or other activities requiring alertness until response to medication is known. Notify health care professional if these symptoms occur.

- Caution patient to use sunscreen and protective clothing to prevent photosensitivity reactions.

- Advise patient to report the signs of superinfection (black, furry overgrowth on the tongue; vaginal itching or discharge; loose or foul-smelling stools) or intracranial hypertension (headache, blurred vision, diplopia, vision loss). Women who are overweight, of reproductive potential, or have a history of intracranial hypertension are at greater risk for developing tetracycline-associated intracranial hypertension. Skin rash, pruritus, and urticaria should also be reported.

- Advise patient to notify health care professional of all Rx or OTC medications, vitamins, or herbal products being taken and to consult with health care professional before taking other medications.

- Instruct patient to notify health care professional of medication regimen before treatment or surgery.

- Rep: Advise females of reproductive potential to use a nonhormonal method of contraception while taking tetracyclines and until next menstrual period. Men attempting to father a child should not take minocycline. May cause yellow-brown discoloration and softening of teeth and bones if administered prenatally. Not recommended during pregnancy or lactation unless used for the treatment of anthrax.

- Instruct patient to notify health care professional if symptoms do not improve within a few days for systemic preparations.
- Caution patient to discard outdated or decomposed tetracyclines; they may be toxic.
- **Malaria Prophylaxis:** Advise patient to avoid being bitten by mosquitoes by using protective measures, especially from dusk to dawn (e.g., staying in well-screened areas, using mosquito nets, covering the body with clothing, and using an effective insect repellant). Doxycycline prophylaxis should begin 1–2 days before travel to the malarious area, continued daily while in the malarious area, and after leaving the malarious area, should be continued for 4 more wk to avoid development of malaria. Do not exceed 4 mo.

Evaluation/Desired Outcomes

- Resolution of the signs and symptoms of infection. Length of time for complete resolution depends on the organism and site of infection.
- Decrease in acne lesions.
- Treatment of inhalation anthrax (postexposure) or treatment of cutaneous anthrax (doxycycline).
- Prevention of malaria.
- Reduction in inflammatory lesions associated with rosacea.

REMS

thalidomide (tha-lid-oh-mide)
Thalomid
Classification
Therapeutic: immunosuppressants

Indications

Cutaneous manifestations of moderate to severe erythema nodosum leprosum. Prevention (maintenance) and suppression of recurrent erythema nodosum leprosum. Newly diagnosed multiple myeloma (in combination with dexamethasone). **Unlabeled Use:** Bechet's syndrome. HIV-associated wasting syndrome. Aphthous stomatitis (including HIV associated). Crohn's disease.

Action

May suppress excess levels of tumor necrosis factor-alpha and alter leukocyte migration by altering characteristics of cell surfaces. **Therapeutic Effects:** Decreased skin lesions in erythema nodosum leprosum and prevention of recurrence. Slowed progression of multiple myeloma.

Pharmacokinetics

Absorption: 67–93% absorbed following oral administration.
Distribution: Well distributed to tissues.

Metabolism and Excretion: Hydrolyzed in plasma to multiple metabolites. Primarily excreted in the urine (92%; <4% as unchanged drug).
Half-life: 5–7 hr.

TIME/ACTION PROFILE (plasma concentrations)

ROUTE	ONSET	PEAK	DURATION
PO	unknown	2–5 hr	unknown

Contraindications/Precautions

Contraindicated in: Hypersensitivity; Seizure disorders; Concurrent use of pembrolizumab in patients with multiple myeloma (↑ risk of mortality); OB: Pregnancy; Lactation: Lactation.
Use Cautiously in: Rep: Women of reproductive potential and men with female sexual partners of reproductive potential; Pedi: Children <12 yr (safety and effectiveness not established).

Adverse Reactions/Side Effects

CV: bradycardia, edema, orthostatic hypotension, thromboembolic events (↑ risk with dexamethasone in multiple myeloma). **Derm:** DRUG REACTION WITH EOSINOPHILIA AND SYSTEMIC SYMPTOMS (DRESS), rash, STEVENS-JOHNSON SYNDROME, TOXIC EPIDERMAL NECROLYSIS, photosensitivity. **GI:** constipation. **Hemat:** neutropenia, thrombocytopenia. **Neuro:** dizziness, drowsiness, peripheral neuropathy, SEIZURES. **Misc:** HYPERSENSITIVITY REACTIONS (including anaphylaxis and angioedema), TUMOR LYSIS SYNDROME.

Interactions

Drug-Drug: ↑ CNS depression with concurrent use of **barbiturates**, **sedative/hypnotics**, **alcohol**, **chlorpromazine**, or other **CNS depressants**. Concurrent use of **agents that may cause peripheral neuropathy** ↑ risk of peripheral neuropathy.
Drug-Natural Products: Concurrent use with **echinacea** and **melatonin** may interfere with immunosuppression.

Route/Dosage

Erythema Nodosum Leprosum

PO (Adults ≥50 kg): 100–300 mg once daily initially; up to 400 mg/day has been used, depending on previous response. Every 3–6 mo, attempts should be made to taper and discontinue in decrements of 50 mg every 2–4 wk.
PO (Adults <50 kg): 100 mg once daily initially; up to 400 mg/day has been used, depending on previous response. Every 3–6 mo, attempts should be made to taper and discontinue in decrements of 50 mg every 2–4 wk.

Multiple Myeloma

PO (Adults): 200 mg once daily in 28-day treatment cycles.

✱ = Canadian drug name. � = Genetic implication. S̶t̶r̶i̶k̶e̶t̶h̶r̶o̶u̶g̶h̶ = Discontinued. CAPITALS = life-threatening. Underline = most frequent.

Availability

Capsules: 50 mg, 100 mg, 150 mg, 200 mg.

NURSING IMPLICATIONS

Assessment

- Assess monthly for initial 3 mo and periodically during therapy to detect early signs of peripheral neuropathy (numbness, tingling, or pain in hands and feet). Commonly occurs with prolonged therapy, but has occurred following short-term use or following completion of therapy. May be severe and irreversible. Electrophysiologic testing may be done at baseline and every 6 mo to detect asymptomatic peripheral neuropathy. If symptoms occur, discontinue thalidomide immediately to limit further damage. Reinstate therapy only if neuropathy returns to baseline.
- Monitor for signs of hypersensitivity reaction (erythematous macular rash, fever, tachycardia, hypotension). May require discontinuation of therapy if severe. If reaction recurs when dosing is resumed, discontinue thalidomide.
- Monitor for signs and symptoms of bleeding (petechiae, epistaxis, gastrointestinal bleeding) during therapy. May require dose interruption, reduction, or discontinuation.
- Monitor for side effects (constipation, oversedation, peripheral neuropathy); may require discontinuation or dose reduction until side effects resolve.
- **Multiple Myeloma:** Assess for venous thromboembolism (dyspnea, chest pain, arm or leg swelling) periodically during therapy, especially in patients concurrently taking dexamethasone. Consider prophylaxis depending on patient risk factors.

Lab Test Considerations

- Assess pregnancy status prior to starting therapy. Pregnancy tests with a sensitivity of at least 50 mIU/mL must be done within 10–14 days and within 24 hr of starting therapy. Once treatment has started, pregnancy tests should occur weekly during first 4 wk of use, then every 4 wk in females with a regular menstrual cycle and every 2 wk in females with an irregular cycle. Monitor WBC with differential and platelet count during therapy. May cause ↓ WBC. Do not initiate therapy with an absolute neutrophil count (ANC) ≤750/mm³. If ANC ↓ to ≤750/mm³ during therapy, re-evaluate medication regimen; if neutropenia persists, consider discontinuing therapy. May cause thrombocytopenia.
- May cause ↑ viral load levels in patients with HIV.

Implementation

- Do not confuse Thalomid with thiamine.
- ***REMS:*** Due to teratogenic effects, thalidomide may be prescribed only by prescribers registered in the *Thalomid REMS* program. Required components of the *Thalomid REMS* program include prescribers must be certified with the *Thalomid REMS* program by enrolling and complying with the REMS require-

ments; patients must sign a Patient-Physician Agreement Form and comply with the REMS requirements. Female patients of reproductive potential who are not pregnant must comply with the pregnancy testing and contraception requirements, and males must comply with contraception requirements. Pharmacies must be certified with the *Thalomid REMS* program, must only dispense to patients who are authorized to receive *Thalomid*, and must comply with REMS requirements. Information about *Thalomid* and the *Thalomid REMS* program is available at www.thalomidrems.com or by calling the REMS Call Center at 1-888-423-5436. Thalidomide is started within 24 hr of a negative pregnancy test with a sensitivity of at least 50 mIU/mL. Pregnancy testing must occur weekly during first month of therapy, then monthly thereafter in women with a regular menstrual cycle. For women with irregular menses, pregnancy testing should occur every 2 wk. If pregnancy occurs, thalidomide should be discontinued immediately. Any suspected fetal exposure must be reported to the FDA and the manufacturer, and patient should be referred to an obstetrician/gynecologist experienced in reproductive toxicity. Even a single dose (1 capsule [regardless of strength]) taken by a pregnant woman during her pregnancy can cause severe birth defects.

- If health care professionals or other caregivers are exposed to body fluids from patients receiving thalidomide, use appropriate precautions, such as wearing gloves to prevent the potential cutaneous exposure to thalidomide or washing the exposed area with soap and water.
- Corticosteroids may be used concurrently with thalidomide for patients with moderate to severe neuritis associated with a severe erythema nodosum leprosum reaction. Use of corticosteroids can be tapered and discontinued when neuritis resolves.
- **PO:** Administer once daily with water, preferably at bedtime and at least 1 hr after the evening meal. If divided doses are used, administer at least 1 hr after meals.

Patient/Family Teaching

- Instruct patient to take thalidomide as directed. Do not discontinue without notifying health care professional; dose should be tapered gradually. Explain *Thalomid REMS* program to patient.
- Advise patient that thalidomide should not be shared with others.
- Frequently causes drowsiness or dizziness. Caution patient to avoid driving or other activities requiring alertness until response to medication is known.
- Advise patient to change positions slowly to minimize orthostatic hypotension.
- Caution patient to use sunscreen and protective clothing to prevent photosensitivity reactions.
- Advise patient to notify health care professional immediately if pain, numbness, tingling, or burning in

hands or feet or shortness of breath, chest pain, swelling of arms or legs occur.

- Instruct patient not to donate blood and male patients not to donate sperm while taking thalidomide and for 1 mo following discontinuation.
- Rep: May cause fetal harm. Inform females of reproductive potential that they must use one highly effective method (IUD, hormonal contraceptive, tubal ligation, partner's vasectomy) and one additional method (latex condom, diaphragm, cervical cap) AT THE SAME TIME for at least 4 wk before, during therapy and interruptions of therapy, and for 4 wk following discontinuation of therapy, even with a history of infertility, unless due to a hysterectomy or patient has been postmenopausal naturally for 24 consecutive mo. Advise female patients to avoid breastfeeding during therapy. Males receiving thalidomide with female partners of reproductive potential must always use a latex condom during and for up to 4 wk following discontinuation, even if they have undergone a successful vasectomy. Thalidomide must be discontinued if pregnancy is suspected or confirmed. Suspected fetal exposure must be reported to FDA via MedWatch at 1-800-FDA-1088 and to manufacturer at 1-888-668-2528. Inform females there is a Pregnancy Exposure Registry that monitors pregnancy outcomes in females exposed to thalidomide during pregnancy and that they can contact the Pregnancy Exposure Registry by calling 1-888-423-5436. May impair male fertility.
- Advise patient to notify health care professional of all Rx or OTC medications, vitamins, or herbal products being taken and to consult with health care professional before taking other medications. Concomitant use of HIV-protease inhibitors, modafinil, penicillins, rifampin, rifabutin, phenytoin, carbamazepine, or certain herbal supplements such as St. John's wort with hormonal contraceptive agents may reduce the effectiveness of contraception during and for up to one mo after discontinuation of these concomitant therapies. Women requiring treatment with one or more of these drugs must use two other effective or highly effective methods of contraception or abstain from heterosexual sexual contact while taking thalidomide.

Evaluation/Desired Outcomes

- Resolution of the signs and symptoms of active erythema nodosum leprosum reaction. Usually requires at least 2 wk of therapy; then taper medication in 50-mg decrements every 2–4 wk.
- Prevention of recurrent erythema nodosum leprosum. Tapering off medication should be attempted every 3–6 mo in decrements of 50 mg every 2–4 wk.
- Decrease in serum and urine paraprotein measurements in patients with multiple myeloma.

thiamine (thye-a-min)
vitamin B1
Classification
Therapeutic: vitamins
Pharmacologic: water-soluble vitamins

Indications
Treatment of thiamine deficiencies (beriberi). Prevention of Wernicke's encephalopathy. Dietary supplement in patients with GI disease, alcoholism, or cirrhosis.

Action
Required for carbohydrate metabolism. **Therapeutic Effects:** Replacement in deficiency states.

Pharmacokinetics
Absorption: Well absorbed from the GI tract by an active process. Excessive amounts are not absorbed completely. Also well absorbed from IM sites.
Distribution: Widely distributed to tissues.
Metabolism and Excretion: Metabolized by the liver. Excess amounts are excreted unchanged by the kidneys.
Half-life: Unknown.

TIME/ACTION PROFILE (time for symptoms of deficiency—edema and heart failure—to resolve†)

ROUTE	ONSET	PEAK	DURATION
PO, IM, IV	hr	days	days–wk

†Confusion and psychosis take longer to respond.

Contraindications/Precautions
Contraindicated in: Hypersensitivity; Known alcohol intolerance or bisulfite hypersensitivity (elixir only).
Use Cautiously in: Wernicke's encephalopathy (condition may be worsened unless thiamine is administered before glucose).

Adverse Reactions/Side Effects
Adverse reactions and side effects are extremely rare and are usually associated with IV administration or extremely large doses.
CV: hypotension, VASCULAR COLLAPSE. **Derm:** cyanosis, pruritus, sweating, tingling, urticaria, warmth. **EENT:** tightness of the throat. **GI:** nausea. **Neuro:** restlessness, weakness. **Resp:** pulmonary edema, respiratory distress. **Misc:** ANGIOEDEMA.

Interactions
Drug-Drug: None reported.

Route/Dosage
Thiamine Deficiency (Beriberi)
PO (Adults): 5–10 mg 3 times daily.
PO (Children): 10–50 mg/day in divided doses.

T

✳ = Canadian drug name. ⚇ = Genetic implication. ~~Strikethrough~~ = Discontinued. CAPITALS = life-threatening. <u>Underline</u> = most frequent.

IM, IV (Adults): 5–100 mg 3 times daily.
IM, IV (Children): 10–25 mg/day.

Dietary Supplement
PO (Adults): 1–1.6 mg/day.
PO (Children 4–10 yr): 0.9–1 mg/day.
PO (Children birth–3 yr): 0.3–0.7 mg/day.

Availability (generic available)
Tablets: 5 mg^OTC, 10 mg^OTC, 25 mg^OTC, 50 mg^OTC, 100 mg^OTC, 250 mg^OTC, 500 mg^OTC. **Injection:** 100 mg/mL.

NURSING IMPLICATIONS
Assessment
● Assess for signs and symptoms of thiamine deficiency (anorexia, GI distress, irritability, palpitations, tachycardia, edema, paresthesia, muscle weakness and pain, depression, memory loss, confusion, psychosis, visual disturbances, elevated serum pyruvic acid levels).
● Assess patient's nutritional status (diet, weight) prior to and during therapy.
● Monitor patients receiving IV thiamine for anaphylaxis (wheezing, urticaria, edema).

Lab Test Considerations
● May interfere with certain methods of testing serum theophylline, uric acid, and urobilinogen concentrations.

Implementation
● Do not confuse thiamine with Thalomid.
● Because of infrequency of single B-vitamin deficiencies, combinations are commonly administered.
● **IM, IV:** Parenteral administration is reserved for patients in whom oral administration is not feasible.
● **IM:** Administration may cause tenderness and induration at injection site. Cool compresses may decrease discomfort.

IV Administration
● **IV:** Sensitivity reactions and death have occurred from IV administration. An intradermal test dose is recommended in patients with suspected sensitivity. Monitor site for erythema and induration.
● **IV Push:** *Concentration:* Administer undiluted at 100 mg/mL. *Rate:* Administer at a rate of 100 mg over 5 min.
● **Continuous Infusion:** *Dilution:* May be diluted in dextrose/Ringer's or LR combinations, dextrose/saline combinations, D5W, D10W, Ringer's and LR injection, 0.9% NaCl, or 0.45% NaCl. Usually administered with other vitamins.
● **Y-Site Compatibility:** amikacin, ascorbic acid, atracurium, atropine, aztreonam, benztropine, bumetanide, buprenorphine, butorphanol, calcium chloride, calcium gluconate, cefazolin, cefotaxime, cefotetan, cefoxitin, ceftriaxone, cefuroxime, chlorpromazine, clindamycin, cyanocobalamin, cyclosporine, dexamethasone, digoxin, diphenhydramine, dobutamine, dopamine, doxycycline, enalaprilat, ephedrine, epinephrine, erythromycin, esmolol, famotidine, fentanyl, gentamicin, glycopyrrolate, heparin, insulin regular, isoproterenol, labetalol, lidocaine, magnesium sulfate, mannitol, meperidine, metoclopramide, metoprolol, morphine, multivitamins, nafcillin, nalbuphine, naloxone, nitroglycerin, nitroprusside, norepinephrine, oxacillin, oxytocin, papaverine, penicillin G, pentamidine, phentolamine, phenylephrine, phytonadione, potassium chloride, procainamide, prochlorperazine, promethazine, propranolol, protamine, pyridoxine, succinylcholine, sufentanil, theophylline, tobramycin, vancomycin, vasopressin, verapamil.
● **Y-Site Incompatibility:** aminophylline, azathioprine, ceftazidime, chloramphenicol, dantrolene, diazepam, folic acid, furosemide, ganciclovir, hydrocortisone, imipenem/cilastatin, indomethacin, methylprednisolone, pentobarbital, phenobarbital, phenytoin, sodium bicarbonate, trimethoprim/sulfamethoxazole.

Patient/Family Teaching
● Encourage patient to comply with dietary recommendations of health care professional. Explain that the best source of vitamins is a well-balanced diet with foods from the four basic food groups.
● Teach patient that foods high in thiamine include cereals (whole grain and enriched), meats (especially pork), and fresh vegetables; loss is variable during cooking.
● Caution patients self-medicating with vitamin supplements not to exceed RDA. The effectiveness of megadoses of vitamins for treatment of various medical conditions is unproven and may cause side effects.
● Rep: Thiamine requirements are increased in during pregnancy, especially in women with prolonged nausea and vomiting. RDA for thiamine during lactation is 1.4 mg.

Evaluation/Desired Outcomes
● Prevention of or decrease in the signs and symptoms of vitamin B deficiency.
● Decrease in the symptoms of neuritis, ocular signs, ataxia, edema, and heart failure may be seen within hrs of administration and may disappear within a few days.
● Confusion and psychosis may take longer to respond and may persist if nerve damage has occurred.

HIGH ALERT

THROMBOLYTIC AGENTS
alteplase (**al**-te-plase)
Activase, ✦Activase rt-PA, Cathflo Activase
reteplase (**re**-te-plase)
Retavase
tenecteplase (te-**nek**-te-plase)
TNKase
Classification
Therapeutic: thrombolytics
Pharmacologic: plasminogen activators

Indications
Alteplase, reteplase, tenecteplase: Acute MI. **Alteplase:** Acute ischemic stroke. Acute massive pulmonary emboli (PE). **Alteplase:** Occluded central venous access devices.

Action
Directly activate plasminogen, converting it to plasmin, which is then able to degrade fibrin present in clots. **Therapeutic Effects:** Lysis of thrombi in coronary arteries, with preservation of ventricular function or improvement of ventricular function (and ↓ risk of HF or death). Lysis of PE. Lysis of thrombi causing ischemic stroke, reducing risk of neurologic sequelae. Restoration of cannula or catheter patency and function.

Pharmacokinetics
Absorption: IV administration results in complete bioavailability. Intracoronary administration or administration into occluded catheters or cannulae has a more localized effect.
Distribution: Minimally distributed to tissues.
Metabolism and Excretion: *Alteplase, tenecteplase:* Rapidly metabolized by the liver. *Reteplase:* Cleared primarily by the liver and kidneys.
Half-life: *Alteplase:* 35 min; *reteplase:* 13–16 min; *tenecteplase:* 20–24 min (initial phase), 90–130 min (terminal phase).

TIME/ACTION PROFILE (fibrinolysis)

ROUTE	ONSET	PEAK	DURATION
Alteplase IV	30 min	60 min	unknown
Reteplase IV	30 min	30–90 min	48 hr
Tenecteplase IV	rapid	unknown	unknown

Contraindications/Precautions
Contraindicated in: Active internal bleeding; History of cerebrovascular accident; Recent (within 2 mo) intracranial or intraspinal injury or trauma; Intracranial neoplasm, AV malformation, or aneurysm; Severe uncontrolled hypertension; Known bleeding tendencies; Hypersensitivity; cross-sensitivity with other thrombolytics may occur.
Use Cautiously in: Recent (within 10 days) major surgery, trauma, GI, or GU bleeding; Left heart thrombus; Severe renal impairment; Severe hepatic impairment; Hemorrhagic ophthalmic conditions; Septic phlebitis; Previous puncture of a noncompressible vessel; Subacute bacterial endocarditis or acute pericarditis; OB, Lactation, Pedi: Safety not established; Geri: ↑ risk of intracranial bleeding in patients >75 yr.
Exercise Extreme Caution in: Patients receiving concurrent anticoagulant therapy (↑ risk of intracranial bleeding).

Adverse Reactions/Side Effects
CV: hypotension, reperfusion arrhythmias. **Derm:** ecchymoses, flushing, urticaria. **EENT:** epistaxis, gingival bleeding. **GI:** nausea, vomiting. **Hemat:** BLEEDING. **Local:** hemorrhage at injection sites, phlebitis at IV site. **MS:** musculoskeletal pain. **Neuro:** INTRACRANIAL HEMORRHAGE. **Resp:** bronchospasm, hemoptysis. **Misc:** fever, HYPERSENSITIVITY REACTIONS (including anaphylaxis).

Interactions
Drug-Drug: Concurrent use of **aspirin**, other **NSAIDs**, **warfarin**, **heparin**, **low-molecular-weight heparins**, **direct thrombin inhibitors**, **eptifibatide**, **tirofiban**, **clopidogrel**, **ticagrelor**, **prasugrel**, **dipyridamole** may ↑ risk of bleeding, although these agents are frequently used together or in sequence. Effects may be ↓ by **antifibrinolytic agents**, including **aminocaproic acid** or **tranexamic acid**.
Drug-Natural Products: ↑ anticoagulant effect and bleeding risk with **anise**, **arnica**, **chamomile**, **clove**, **dong quai**, **fenugreek**, **feverfew**, **garlic**, **ginger**, **ginkgo**, **Panax ginseng**, **licorice**, and others.

Route/Dosage

Alteplase

Myocardial Infarction (Accelerated or Front-Loading Infusion)
IV (Adults): 15 mg bolus, then 0.75 mg/kg (up to 50 mg) over 30 min, then 0.5 mg/kg (up to 35 mg) over next 60 min; usually accompanied by heparin therapy.

Myocardial Infarction (3-Hr Infusion)
IV (Adults >65 kg): 60 mg over 1st hr (6–10 mg given as a bolus over first 1–2 min), 20 mg over the 2nd hr, and 20 mg over the 3rd hr for a total dose of 100 mg.
IV (Adults <65 kg): 0.75 mg/kg over 1st hr (0.075–0.125 mg/kg given as a bolus over first 1–2 min), 0.25 mg/kg over the 2nd hr, and 0.25 mg/kg over the 3rd hr for a total dose of 1.25 mg/kg (not to exceed 100 mg total).

Pulmonary Embolism
IV (Adults): 100 mg over 2 hr; follow with heparin.

Acute Ischemic Stroke
IV (Adults): 0.9 mg/kg (not to exceed 90 mg), given as an infusion over 1 hr, with 10% of the dose given as a bolus over the 1st min.

Occluded Venous Access Devices
IV (Adults and Children >30 kg): 2 mg/2 mL instilled into occluded catheter; if unsuccessful, may repeat once after 2 hr.
IV (Adults and Children <30 kg): 110% of the lumen volume (not to exceed 2 mg in 2 mL) instilled into occluded catheter; if unsuccessful, may repeat once after 2 hr.

Reteplase
IV (Adults): 10 units, followed 30 min later by an additional 10 units.

T

Tenecteplase

IV (Adults <60 kg): 30 mg as a single dose.
IV (Adults ≥60 kg and <70 kg): 35 mg as a single dose.
IV (Adults ≥70 kg and <80 kg): 40 mg as a single dose.
IV (Adults ≥80 kg and <90 kg): 45 mg as a single dose.
IV (Adults ≥90 kg): 50 mg as a single dose.

Availability

Alteplase

Powder for injection: 2 mg/vial, 50 mg/vial, 100 mg/vial.

Reteplase

Powder for injection: 10 units/vial.

Tenecteplase

Powder for injection: 50 mg/vial.

NURSING IMPLICATIONS

Assessment

- Begin therapy as soon as possible after the onset of symptoms.
- Monitor vital signs, including temperature, continuously for coronary thrombosis and at least every 4 hr during therapy for other indications. Do not use lower extremities to monitor BP. Notify health care professional if systolic BP >180 mm Hg or diastolic BP >110 mm Hg. Should not be given if hypertension is uncontrolled. Inform health care professional if hypotension occurs. Hypotension may result from the drug, hemorrhage, or cardiogenic shock.
- Assess patient carefully for bleeding every 15 min during the 1st hr of therapy, every 15–30 min during the next 8 hr, and at least every 4 hr for the duration of therapy. Frank bleeding may occur from sites of invasive procedures or from body orifices. Internal bleeding may also occur (decreased neurologic status; abdominal pain with coffee-grounds emesis or black, tarry stools; hematuria; joint pain). If uncontrolled bleeding occurs, stop medication and notify health care professional immediately.
- Assess neurologic status during therapy. Altered sensorium or neurologic changes may be indicative of intracranial bleeding.
- **MI:** Monitor ECG continuously. Notify health care professional if significant arrhythmias occur. Monitor cardiac enzymes. Radionuclide myocardial scanning and/or coronary angiography may be ordered 7–10 days after therapy to monitor effectiveness of therapy.
- Assess intensity, character, location, and radiation of chest pain. Note presence of associated symptoms (nausea, vomiting, diaphoresis). Notify health care professional if chest pain is unrelieved or recurs.
- Monitor heart sounds and breath sounds frequently. Inform health care professional if signs of HF occur (rales/crackles, dyspnea, S_3 heart sound, jugular venous distention).

- **Acute Ischemic Stroke:** Assess neurologic status. Determine time of onset of stroke symptoms. Alteplase must be administered within 3–4.5 hr of onset (within 3 hr in patients older than 80 yr, those taking oral anticoagulants, those with a baseline National Institutes of Health Stroke Scale score 25, or those with both a history of stroke and diabetes).
- **PE:** Monitor pulse, BP, hemodynamics, and respiratory status (rate, degree of dyspnea, arterial blood gases).
- **Cannula/Catheter Occlusion:** Monitor ability to aspirate blood as indicator of patency. Ensure that patient exhales and holds breath when connecting and disconnecting IV syringe to prevent air embolism.

Lab Test Considerations

- Hematocrit, hemoglobin, platelet count, fibrin/fibrin degradation product titer, fibrinogen concentration, PT, thrombin time, and aPTT may be evaluated before and frequently during therapy. Bleeding time may be assessed before therapy if patient has received platelet inhibitors.
- Obtain type and crossmatch and have blood available at all times in case of hemorrhage.
- Stools should be tested for occult blood loss and urine for hematuria periodically during therapy.

Toxicity and Overdose

- **High Alert:** If local bleeding occurs, apply pressure to site. If severe or internal bleeding occurs, discontinue infusion. Clotting factors and/or blood volume may be restored through infusions of whole blood, packed RBCs, fresh frozen plasma, or cryoprecipitate. Do not administer dextran; it has antiplatelet activity. Aminocaproic acid may be used as an antidote.

Implementation

- **High Alert:** Overdose and underdose of thrombolytic medications have resulted in patient harm or death. Have second practitioner independently check original order, dose calculations, and infusion pump settings.
- Do not confuse Activase with Cathflo Activase or TNKase. Do not confuse TNKase with t-PA.
- Thrombolytic agents should be used only in settings in which hematologic function and clinical response can be adequately monitored.
- Starting two IV lines before therapy is recommended: one for the thrombolytic agent, the other for any additional infusions.
- Avoid invasive procedures, such as IM injections or arterial punctures, with this therapy. If such procedures must be performed, apply pressure to all arterial and venous puncture sites for at least 30 min. Avoid venipunctures at noncompressible sites (jugular vein, subclavian site).
- Acetaminophen may be ordered to control fever.

Alteplase

IV Administration

- **Intermittent Infusion:** Vials are packaged with sterile water for injection (without preservatives) to be used as diluent. Do not use bacteriostatic water for injection. *Reconstitution:* Reconstitute 20-mg vials with 20-mL and 50-mg vials with 50 mL using an 18-gauge needle. Avoid excess agitation during dilution; swirl or invert gently to mix. Solution may foam upon reconstitution. Bubbles will resolve upon standing a few min. Solution will be clear to pale yellow. Stable for 8 hr at room temperature. *Concentration:* May be administered as reconstituted (1 mg/mL). *Dilution:* May be further diluted immediately before use in an equal amount of 0.9% NaCl or D5W. *Rate:* Flush line with 20–30 mL of saline at completion of infusion to ensure entire dose is received. See Route and Dosage section for specific rates.
- **Y-Site Compatibility:** eptifibatide, lidocaine, propranolol, tobramycin, vancomycin.
- **Y-Site Incompatibility:** bivalirudin, cangrelor, dobutamine, dopamine, heparin, nitroglycerin.
- **Cathflo Activase:** Reconstitute by withdrawing 2.2 mL of sterile water (provided) and injecting into *Cathflo Activase* vial, directing diluent into powder for a concentration of 1 mg/mL. Allow slight foaming to dissipate by letting vial stand undisturbed. Do not use bacteriostatic water. Mix by gently swirling to dissolve; complete dissolution should occur within 3 min. Do not shake. Solution should be colorless to pale yellow. Use solution within 8 hr.
- Withdraw 2.0 mL of reconstituted solution and instill into occluded catheter. After 30 min dwell time, attempt to aspirate blood. If catheter remains occluded, allow 120 min dwell time. If catheter function is not restored after one dose, 2nd dose may be instilled. If catheter function is restored, aspirate 4–5 mL of blood to remove *Cathflo Activase* and residual clot. Gently irrigate catheter with 0.9% NaCl.

Reteplase

IV Administration

- **IV Push:** *Reconstitution:* Reconstitute using diluent, needle, syringe, and dispensing pin provided. Reconstitute only with sterile water for injection without preservatives. Solution is colorless. Do not administer solutions that are discolored or contain a precipitate. Slight foaming may occur; allow vial to stand undisturbed for several min to dissipate bubbles. Reconstitute immediately before use. Stable for 4 hr at room temperature. *Concentration:* Administer undiluted. *Rate:* Administer each bolus over 2 min into an IV line containing D5W; flush line before and after bolus.
- **Y-Site Incompatibility:** bivalirudin, cangrelor, heparin; No other medication should be infused or injected into line used for reteplase.

Tenecteplase

IV Administration

- **IV Push:** Vials are packaged with sterile water for injection (without preservatives) to be used as diluent. Do not use bacteriostatic water for injection. Do not discard shield assembly. *Reconstitution:* To reconstitute aseptically withdraw 10 mL of diluent and inject into the tenecteplase vial, directing the stream into the powder. Slight foaming may occur; large bubbles will dissipate if left standing undisturbed for several min. Swirl gently until contents are completely dissolved; do not shake. *Concentration:* Solution containing 5 mg/mL is clear and colorless to pale yellow. Withdraw dose from reconstituted vial with the syringe and discard unused portion. Once dose is in syringe, stand the shield vertically on a flat surface (with green side down) and passively recap the red hub cannula. Remove the entire shield assembly, including the red hub cannula, by twisting counterclockwise. Shield assembly also contains the clear-ended blunt plastic cannula; retain for split septum IV access. Reconstitute immediately before use. May be refrigerated and administered within 8 hr. *Rate:* Administer as a single IV bolus over 5 sec.
- **Y-Site Incompatibility:** Precipitate forms in line when administered with dextrose-containing solutions. Flush line with saline-containing solution prior to and following administration of tenecteplase.

Patient/Family Teaching

- Explain purpose of medication and the need for close monitoring to patient and family. Instruct patient to report hypersensitivity reactions (rash, dyspnea) and bleeding or bruising.
- Explain need for bedrest and minimal handling during therapy to avoid injury. Avoid all unnecessary procedures such as shaving and vigorous tooth brushing.
- Rep: Advise females of reproductive potential to notify health care professional if pregnancy is planned or suspected or if breastfeeding.

Evaluation/Desired Outcomes

- Lysis of thrombi and restoration of blood flow.
- Prevention of neurologic sequelae in acute ischemic stroke.
- Cannula or catheter patency.

BEERS

ticagrelor (tye-ka-grel-or)
Brilinta
Classification
Therapeutic: antiplatelet agents
Pharmacologic: platelet aggregation inhibitors

Indications

To reduce the risk of cardiovascular death, MI, and stroke in patients with acute coronary syndrome (ACS) or a history of MI. Also reduces the risk of stent thrombosis in patients who have received an intracoronary stent for ACS (in combination with aspirin). To reduce the risk of first MI or stroke in patients with coronary artery disease who are at high risk for such events (in combination with aspirin). To reduce the risk of stroke in patients with acute ischemic stroke (NIH Stroke Scale score ≤5) or high-risk transient ischemic attack (TIA) (in combination with aspirin).

Action

Both parent drug and its active metabolite inhibit platelet aggregation by reversibly interacting with platelet $P2Y_{12}$ADP-receptors, preventing signal transduction and platelet activation. **Therapeutic Effects:** Reduction in risk of cardiovascular death, MI, and stroke associated with ACS. Reduction in stent thrombosis. Reduction in risk of first MI or stroke in high-risk patients with coronary artery disease. Reduction in risk of stroke in patients with acute ischemic stroke or TIA.

Pharmacokinetics

Absorption: 36% absorbed following oral administration.
Distribution: Well distributed to tissues.
Protein Binding: 99%.
Metabolism and Excretion: Mostly metabolized in the liver by the CYP3A4 isoenzyme, with some metabolism by the CYP3A5 isoenzyme) with conversion to an active metabolite (AR-C124910XX); excretion primarily via biliary secretion; <1% excreted unchanged or as active metabolite in urine.
Half-life: *Ticagrelor:* 7 hr; *Active metabolite:* 9 hr.

TIME/ACTION PROFILE (inhibition of platelet aggregation)

ROUTE	ONSET	PEAK	DURATION
PO	within 30 min	4 hr	5 days†

† Following discontinuation.

Contraindications/Precautions

Contraindicated in: Hypersensitivity; Active bleeding; History of intracranial bleeding; Severe hepatic impairment (↑ risk of bleeding); Impending coronary artery bypass graft surgery or other surgery (discontinue 5 days prior); Use of thrombolytics for treatment of acute ischemic stroke; Lactation: Lactation.
Use Cautiously in: Moderate hepatic impairment; History of sick sinus syndrome, 2nd- or 3rd-degree heart block, or bradycardia-related syncope in the absence of a pacemaker; Hypotension following recent coronary artery bypass graft surgery or percutaneous coronary intervention in patients receiving ticagrelor (consider bleeding as a cause); OB: Use during pregnancy only if potential maternal benefit justifies potential fetal risk; Pedi: Safety and effectiveness not established in children; Geri: Appears on Beers list. ↑ risk of

major bleeding compared to clopidogrel, especially in patients ≥75 yr old. Use with caution in older adults, especially in patients ≥75 yr old.

Adverse Reactions/Side Effects

CV: bradycardia, heart block. **Endo:** gynecomastia. **Hemat:** BLEEDING. **Resp:** dyspnea, central sleep apnea, Cheyne-Stokes respiration. **Misc:** HYPERSENSITIVITY REACTIONS (including angioedema).

Interactions

Drug-Drug: Strong CYP3A4/5 inhibitors, including **atazanavir, clarithromycin, itraconazole, ketoconazole, nefazodone, nelfinavir, ritonavir**, and **voriconazole**, ↑ levels and the risk of bleeding; avoid concurrent use. **Strong CYP3A inducers**, including **carbamazepine, dexamethasone, phenobarbital, phenytoin**, and **rifampin**, may ↓ levels and effectiveness; avoid concurrent use. **P-glycoprotein inhibitors**, including **cyclosporine**, may ↑ levels and the risk of bleeding. Concurrent use of **lovastatin** or **simvastatin** in doses >40 mg/day ↑ risk of statin-related adverse reactions. Effectiveness is ↓ by **aspirin** >100 mg/day (maintain aspirin at 75–100 mg/day). May alter **digoxin** levels (monitoring recommended). Risk of bleeding ↑ by **anticoagulants, fibrinolytics**, and chronic **NSAIDs**. **Opioids** may ↓ absorption of ticagrelor and its active metabolite and ↓ antiplatelet effects; consider using parenteral antiplatelet in patients with acute coronary syndrome if concurrent use of opioids needed.

Route/Dosage

Acute Coronary Syndrome or History of Myocardial Infarction

PO (Adults): *Loading dose:* 180 mg; followed by *maintenance dose:* 90 mg twice daily for 1 yr, then 60 mg twice daily.

Coronary Artery Disease Without a History of Myocardial Infarction or Stroke

PO (Adults): 60 mg twice daily.

Acute Ischemic Stroke or Transient Ischemic Attack

PO (Adults): *Loading dose:* 180 mg; followed by *maintenance dose:* 90 mg twice daily for up to 30 days.

Availability (generic available)

Tablets: 60 mg, 90 mg.

NURSING IMPLICATIONS

Assessment

- Assess patient for symptoms of stroke, peripheral vascular disease, or MI periodically during therapy.
- Observe patient for signs and symptoms of hypersensitivity reactions (rash, facial swelling, pruritus, laryngeal edema, wheezing). Discontinue drug and notify health care professional immediately if symptoms occur. Keep epinephrine, an antihistamine,

and resuscitation equipment close by in case of ana-phylactic reaction.

Lab Test Considerations
- May cause ↑ serum uric acid and ↑ serum creatinine.
- May cause false negative results in heparin-induced platelet aggregation assay for patients with heparin-induced thrombocytopenia.

Implementation
- **PO:** Administer without regard to food.
- For patients unable to swallow, tablets can be crushed and mixed with water. Mixture can also be administered via a nasogastric tube.
- Patients who have received a loading dose of clopidogrel may be started on ticagrelor.
- For acute ischemic stroke or TIA, administer a loading dose of aspirin (300–325 mg) and a daily maintenance dose of aspirin (75–100 mg) with ticagrelor.
- Discontinue ticagrelor 5 days before planned surgical procedures with a major risk of bleeding. If ticagrelor must be temporarily discontinued, restart as soon as possible. Premature discontinuation of therapy may increase risk of MI, stent thrombosis, and death.

Patient/Family Teaching
- Instruct patient to take ticagrelor exactly as directed. Take missed doses as soon as possible unless almost time for next dose; do not double doses. Do not discontinue ticagrelor without consulting health care professional; may increase risk of cardiovascular events. Advise patient to read the *Medication Guide* before starting therapy and with each Rx refill in case of changes.
- Advise patient that daily aspirin should not exceed 100 mg and to avoid taking other medications that contain aspirin.
- Inform patient that they will bleed and bruise more easily and it will take longer to stop bleeding. Advise patient to notify health care professional promptly if unusual, prolonged, or excessive bleeding or blood in stool or urine occurs.
- Inform patient that ticagrelor may cause shortness of breath, which usually resolves during therapy. Advise patient to notify health care professional if unexpected or severe shortness of breath or symptoms of hypersensitivity reactions occur.
- Advise patient to notify health care professional of medication regimen prior to treatment or surgery or dental procedure. Prescriber should be consulted before stopping ticagrelor.
- Instruct patient to notify health care professional of all Rx or OTC medications, vitamins, or herbal products being taken and consult health care professional before taking any new medications, especially aspirin or NSAIDs.
- Rep: Advise females of reproductive potential to notify health care professional if pregnancy is planned or suspected and to avoid breastfeeding during therapy.

Evaluation/Desired Outcomes
- Decreased thrombotic cardiovascular events in patients with ACS.
- Reduction in risk of first MI or stroke in high-risk patients with coronary artery disease.
- Reduction in risk of stroke in patients with acute ischemic stroke or TIA.

---

tigecycline (tye-gi-**sye**-kleen)
Tygacil
Classification
Therapeutic: anti-infectives
Pharmacologic: glycylcyclines

Indications
Complicated skin/skin structure infections, complicated intra-abdominal infections, or community-acquired bacterial pneumonia caused by susceptible bacteria (should only be used when alternative treatments are not suitable; should NOT be used for diabetic foot infections).

Action
Inhibits bacterial protein synthesis by binding to the 30S ribosomal subunit. **Therapeutic Effects:** Resolution of infection. **Spectrum:** Active against the following gram-positive bacteria: *Enterococcus faecalis* (vancomycin-susceptible strains only), *Staphylococcus aureus* (methicillin-sensitive and methicillin-resistant strains), *Streptococcus agalactiae*, *Streptococcus anginosus*, *Streptococcus pneumoniae* (penicillin-susceptible isolates), and *Streptococcus pyogenes*. Also active against these gram-negative organisms: *Citrobacter freundii*, *Enterobacter cloacae*, *Escherichia coli*, *Haemophilus influenzae*, *Legionella pneumophila*, *Klebsiella oxytoca*, and *Klebsiella pneumoniae*. Additionally active against the following anaerobes: *Bacteroides fragilis*, *Bacteroides thetaiotaomicron*, *Bacteroides uniformis*, *Bacteroides vulgatus*, *Clostridium perfringens*, and *Peptostreptococcus micros*.

Pharmacokinetics
Absorption: IV administration results in complete bioavailability.
Distribution: Widely distributed with good penetration into gall bladder, lung, and colon.
Metabolism and Excretion: Minimal metabolism; primary route of elimination is biliary/fecal excretion of unchanged drug and metabolites (59%), 33% renal (22% unchanged).

T

Half-life: 27.1 hr (after 1 dose); 42.4 hr after multiple doses.

TIME/ACTION PROFILE (plasma concentrations)

ROUTE	ONSET	PEAK	DURATION
IV	rapid	end of infusion	12 hr

Contraindications/Precautions

Contraindicated in: Hypersensitivity; Diabetic foot infections; Hospital-acquired or ventilator-associated pneumonia; Pedi: Children.

Use Cautiously in: Complicated intra-abdominal infections due to perforation; Severe hepatic impairment (↓ maintenance dose recommended); OB: Use during pregnancy only if potential maternal benefit outweighs potential fetal risk; may cause permanent teeth discoloration and suppress bone growth in fetus, especially when used during 2nd or 3rd trimester; Lactation: Use while breastfeeding only if potential maternal benefit justifies potential risk to infant; Geri: Older adults may be more sensitive to adverse effects.

Adverse Reactions/Side Effects

Derm: STEVENS-JOHNSON SYNDROME (SJS). **Endo:** hyperglycemia, hypoglycemia. **F and E:** hypocalcemia, hyponatremia. **GI:** nausea, vomiting, ↑ liver enzymes, anorexia, CLOSTRIDIOIDES DIFFICILE-ASSOCIATED DIARRHEA (CDAD), dry mouth, jaundice, PANCREATITIS. **GU:** ↑ serum creatinine. **Hemat:** hypofibrinogenemia. **Local:** injection site reactions. **Neuro:** dysgeusia, somnolence. **Resp:** pneumonia. **Misc:** DEATH, HYPERSENSITIVITY REACTIONS (including anaphylaxis).

Interactions

Drug-Drug: May ↓ the effectiveness of **hormonal contraceptives**. Effects on **warfarin** are unknown; monitoring recommended. May ↑ trough levels and risk of toxicity of **calcineurin inhibitors**, including **cyclosporine** and **tacrolimus**.

Route/Dosage

IV (Adults): 100 mg initially, then 50 mg every 12 hr for 5–14 days (skin/skin structure infections and intra-abdominal infections) or 7–14 days (pneumonia).

Hepatic Impairment

IV (Adults): *Severe hepatic impairment:* 100 mg initially, then 25 mg every 12 hr.

Availability (generic available)

Lyophilized powder for injection: 50 mg/vial.

NURSING IMPLICATIONS

Assessment

- Assess for infection (vital signs; appearance of wound, sputum, urine, and stool; WBC) at beginning of and throughout therapy.
- Obtain specimens for culture and sensitivity before initiating therapy. 1st dose may be given before receiving results.

- Before initiating therapy, obtain a history of tetracycline hypersensitivity; may also have an allergic response to tigecycline.
- Monitor bowel function. Diarrhea, abdominal cramping, fever, and bloody stools should be reported to health care professional promptly as a sign of CDAD. May begin up to several wk following cessation of therapy.
- Assess patient for signs of pancreatitis (nausea, vomiting, abdominal pain, increased serum lipase or amylase) periodically during therapy. May require discontinuation of therapy.
- Assess for rash periodically during therapy. May cause SJS. Discontinue therapy if severe or if accompanied with fever, general malaise, fatigue, muscle or joint aches, blisters, oral lesions, conjunctivitis, hepatitis and/or eosinophilia.

Lab Test Considerations

- Monitor baseline blood coagulation parameters, including fibrinogen, before starting therapy and regularly during therapy. May cause anemia, leukocytosis, and thrombocythemia.
- May cause ↑ serum alkaline phosphatase, amylase, bilirubin, LDH, AST, and ALT.
- May cause hyperglycemia, hypokalemia, hypoproteinemia, hypocalcemia, hyponatremia, and ↑ BUN.

Implementation

- May cause yellow-brown discoloration and softening of teeth and bones if administered prenatally or during early childhood. Not recommended for children under 8 yr of age or during pregnancy or lactation unless used for the treatment of anthrax.

IV Administration

- **Intermittent Infusion:** Reconstitute each vial with 5.3 mL of 0.9% NaCl or D5W to achieve a concentration of 10 mg/mL. *Dilution:* Dilute further in 100 mL of D5W, LR, or 0.9% NaCl. Reconstituted solution should be yellow to orange in color. Do not administer solutions that are discolored or contain particulate matter. Infusion is stable for up to 24 hr at room temperature or for up to 48 hr if refrigerated. *Concentration:* Final concentration of infusion should be ≤1 mg/mL. *Rate:* Infuse over 30–60 min. Flush line before and after infusion with 0.9% NaCl or D5W.
- **Y-Site Compatibility:** acetylcysteine, acyclovir, allopurinol, amifostine, amikacin, aminocaproic acid, aminophylline, amphotericin B liposomal, ampicillin, ampicillin/sulbactam, argatroban, arsenic trioxide, azithromycin, aztreonam, bivalirudin, bumetanide, buprenorphine, busulfan, butorphanol, calcium chloride, calcium gluconate, cangrelor, carboplatin, carmustine, caspofungin, cefazolin, cefepime, cefotaxime, cefotetan, cefoxitin, ceftazidime, ceftolozane/tazobactam, ceftriaxone, cefuroxime, ciprofloxacin, cisatracurium, cisplatin, clindamycin, cyclophosphamide, cyclosporine, cytarabine, dacarbazine, dactinomycin, daptomycin, daunorubicin hy-

drochloride, dexamethasone, dexmedetomidine, dexrazoxane, digoxin, diltiazem, diphenhydramine, dobutamine, docetaxel, dopamine, doxorubicin hydrochloride, doxorubicin liposomal, droperidol, enalaprilat, epinephrine, eptifibatide, ertapenem, erythromycin, esmolol, etoposide, etoposide phosphate, famotidine, fentanyl, fluconazole, fludarabine, fluorouracil, foscarnet, fosphenytoin, furosemide, ganciclovir, gemcitabine, gentamicin, glycopyrrolate, granisetron, haloperidol, heparin, hydrocortisone, hydromorphone, ifosfamide, imipenem/cilastatin, insulin regular, irinotecan, isavuconazonium, isoproterenol, ketorolac, labetalol, LR, leucovorin calcium, levofloxacin, lidocaine, linezolid, lorazepam, magnesium sulfate, mannitol, melphalan, meperidine, meropenem, meropenem/vaborbactam, mesna, methohexital, methotrexate, metoclopramide, metoprolol, metronidazole, midazolam, milrinone, mitomycin, mitoxantrone, morphine, moxifloxacin, mycophenolate, nafcillin, nalbuphine, naloxone, nitroglycerin, nitroprusside, norepinephrine, octreotide, ondansetron, oxaliplatin, oxytocin, paclitaxel, palonosetron, pamidronate, pantoprazole, pemetrexed, pentamidine, pentobarbital, phenobarbital, phenylephrine, piperacillin/tazobactam, plazomicin, potassium acetate, potassium chloride, potassium phosphate, procainamide, prochlorperazine, promethazine, propofol, propranolol, remifentanil, rocuronium, sodium acetate, sodium bicarbonate, sodium phosphate, succinylcholine, sufentanil, tacrolimus, tedizolid, telavancin, theophylline, thiopental, thiotepa, tirofiban, tobramycin, topotecan, trimethoprim/sulfamethoxazole, vancomycin, vasopressin, vecuronium, vinblastine, vincristine, vinorelbine, zidovudine, zoledronic acid.

- **Y-Site Incompatibility:** amiodarone, amphotericin B deoxycholate, bleomycin, chloramphenicol, chlorpromazine, dantrolene, diazepam, epirubicin, esomeprazole, hydralazine, idarubicin, nicardipine, phenytoin, verapamil.

Patient/Family Teaching
- Advise patient that full course of therapy should be completed, even if feeling better. Skipping doses or not completing full course of therapy may result in decreased effectiveness and increased risk of bacterial resistance.
- Instruct patient to notify health care professional if fever and diarrhea develop, especially if stool contains blood, pus, or mucus. Advise patient not to treat diarrhea without consulting health care professional.
- Advise patient to report the signs of superinfection (black, furry overgrowth on the tongue, vaginal itching or discharge, loose or foul-smelling stools). Skin rash, pruritus, and urticaria should also be reported.

- Rep: Advise females of reproductive potential to use a nonhormonal method of contraception while taking tigecycline and until next menstrual period. Use during the second and third trimesters may cause permanent yellow-gray-brown discoloration of the teeth and reversible inhibition of bone growth. Advise patient to avoid breastfeeding during and for 9 days after last dose of tigecycline. Advise patient to notify health care professional if pregnancy is planned or suspected.

Evaluation/Desired Outcomes
- Resolution of signs and symptoms of infection.

tildrakizumab
(til-dra-**kiz**-ue-mab)
Ilumya
Classification
Therapeutic: antipsoriatics
Pharmacologic: interleukin antagonists, monoclonal antibodies

Indications
Moderate to severe plaque psoriasis in patients who are candidates for phototherapy or systemic therapy.

Action
Binds to the p19 protein subunit of the interleukin (IL)-23 cytokine to prevent its interaction with the IL-23 receptor. This cytokine is normally involved in inflammatory and immune responses. Binding to interleukins antagonizes their effects, inhibiting the release of proinflammatory cytokines and chemokines. **Therapeutic Effects:** Decrease in area and severity of psoriatic lesions.

Pharmacokinetics
Absorption: 73–80% absorbed following SUBQ administration.
Distribution: Well distributed to tissues.
Metabolism and Excretion: Broken down by catabolic processes into peptides and amino acids.
Half-life: 23 days.

TIME/ACTION PROFILE (plasma concentrations)

ROUTE	ONSET	PEAK	DURATION
SUBQ	unknown	6 days	12 wk

Contraindications/Precautions
Contraindicated in: Hypersensitivity; Active, untreated infection.
Use Cautiously in: History of tuberculosis (TB) (possibility of reactivation); OB: Use during pregnancy only if potential maternal benefit justifies potential fetal risk; Lactation: Use while breastfeeding only if potential maternal benefit justifies potential risk to infant; Pedi: Safety and effectiveness not established in children.

Exercise Extreme Caution in: Chronic infection or history of recurrent infection.

Adverse Reactions/Side Effects
GI: diarrhea. **Local:** injection site reactions. **Misc:** infection, HYPERSENSITIVITY REACTIONS (including angioedema and urticaria).

Interactions
Drug-Drug: May ↓ antibody response to and ↑ risk of adverse reactions from **live vaccines**; avoid use during therapy.

Route/Dosage
SUBQ (Adults): 100 mg initially and 4 wk later, then 100 mg every 12 wk.

Availability
Solution for injection (prefilled syringes): 100 mg/mL.

NURSING IMPLICATIONS
Assessment
- Assess affected area(s) prior to and periodically during therapy.
- Assess patient for latent TB with a tuberculin skin test prior to initiation of therapy. Treatment of latent TB should be started before therapy with tildrakizumab. Monitor patients for signs and symptoms of active TB during and after therapy.
- Assess for signs of infection (fever, dyspnea, flu-like symptoms, frequent or painful urination, redness or swelling at the site of a wound), including tuberculosis, prior to injection. Monitor new infections closely; most common are upper respiratory tract infections, bronchitis, and urinary tract infections.

Implementation
- Do not confuse Ilumya with Ilaris.
- Injection should be administered by a health care professional.
- Update immunizations to current prior to initiating therapy.
- **SUBQ:** Allow prefilled syringe to sit in carton at room temperature for 30 min prior to injection. Solution is clear to slightly opalescent, colorless to slightly yellow; do not administer solutions that are cloudy, discolored, or contain particulate matter. Air bubbles in solution do not need removal; do not shake. Inject into abdomen, thigh, or upper arm. Do not inject within 2 inches of umbilicus, or into skin that is tender, bruised, erythematous, indurated, affected by psoriasis or into scars, stretch marks, or blood vessels. Follow manufacturer's directions for retractable needle syringe. Store in refrigerator in original carton until time of use; do not freeze. May be stored at room temperature in original carton for up to 30 days.

Patient/Family Teaching
- Explain purpose of tildrakizumab to patient. If a dose is missed, administer as soon as possible. Resume dosing at regularly scheduled interval. Advise patient and caregiver to read the *Medication Guide* before starting therapy and with each Rx refill in case of changes.
- Advise patient to notify health care professional if signs and symptoms of hypersensitivity reaction (feel faint, swelling of face, eyelids, lips, mouth, tongue or throat, skin rash, trouble breathing or throat tightness, chest tightness and infection (fever; sweats; chills; sore throat; cough; shortness of breath); blood in phlegm (mucus); muscle aches; warm, red, or painful skin or sores different from psoriasis; weight loss; diarrhea or stomach pain; burning during urination or urinating more often than normal) occur.
- Instruct patient to avoid receiving live vaccines during therapy.
- Instruct patient to notify health care professional of all Rx or OTC medications, vitamins, or herbal products being taken and consult health care professional before taking any new medications.
- Rep: Advise females of reproductive potential to notify health care professional if pregnancy is planned or suspected or if breastfeeding.

Evaluation/Desired Outcomes
- Decrease in extent and severity of psoriatic lesions.

tioconazole, See ANTIFUNGALS (VAGINAL).

tiotropium (tye-o-**trope**-ee-yum)
♣ Spiriva, Spiriva Handihaler, Spiriva Respimat
Classification
Therapeutic: bronchodilators
Pharmacologic: anticholinergics

Indications
Long-term maintenance treatment of bronchospasm due to COPD. Reduction of exacerbations in patients with COPD. Long-term maintenance treatment of asthma.

Action
Acts as anticholinergic by selectively and reversibly inhibiting M_3 receptors in smooth muscle of airways. **Therapeutic Effects:** Decreased incidence and severity of bronchospasm in COPD and asthma.

Pharmacokinetics
Absorption: *Handihaler:* 19% absorbed following inhalation; *Respimat:* 33% absorbed following inhalation.
Distribution: Extensive tissue distribution; due to route of administration ↑ concentrations occur in lung.

Metabolism and Excretion: 74% excreted unchanged in urine; 25% of absorbed drug is metabolized.

Half-life: 5–6 days.

TIME/ACTION PROFILE (bronchodilation)

ROUTE	ONSET	PEAK	DURATION
Inhaln	rapid	5 min	24 hr

Contraindications/Precautions

Contraindicated in: Hypersensitivity to tiotropium or ipratropium.

Use Cautiously in: Hypersensitivity to atropine or milk proteins; Narrow-angle glaucoma, prostatic hyperplasia, bladder neck obstruction (may worsen condition); CCr ≤60 mL/min (monitor closely); OB: Safety not established in pregnancy; Lactation: Safety not established in breastfeeding; Pedi: Children <6 yr (safety and effectiveness not established).

Adverse Reactions/Side Effects

CV: tachycardia. **Derm:** rash. **EENT:** glaucoma. **GI:** <u>dry mouth</u>, constipation. **GU:** urinary difficulty, urinary retention. **Resp:** paradoxical bronchospasm. **Misc:** HYPERSENSITIVITY REACTIONS (including angioedema).

Interactions

Drug-Drug: Should not be used concurrently with **ipratropium** due to risk of additive anticholinergic effects.

Route/Dosage

Inhaln (Adults): *Handihaler:* 18 mcg once daily; *Respimat:* 2 inhalations of 2.5 mcg once daily.

Inhaln (Adults and Children ≥6 yr): *Respimat:* 2 inhalations of 1.25 mcg once daily.

Availability (generic available)

Dry powder capsules for inhalation (Handihaler): 18 mcg. **Inhalation solution (Respimat):** 1.25 mcg/inhalation in cartridge (delivers 28 or 60 metered inhalations), 2.5 mcg/inhalation in cartridge (delivers 28 or 60 metered inhalations).

NURSING IMPLICATIONS

Assessment

- **Inhaln:** Assess respiratory status (rate, breath sounds, degree of dyspnea, pulse) before administration and at peak of medication effect. Consult health care professional about alternative medication if severe bronchospasm is present; onset of action is too slow for patients in acute distress. If paradoxical bronchospasm (wheezing) occurs, hold medication and notify health care professional immediately.

Implementation

- Do not confuse Spiriva with Apidra or Inspra.
- **Inhaln:** See Appendix C for administration of inhalation medications.

Patient/Family Teaching

- Instruct patient to take medication as directed. Capsules are for inhalation only and must not be swallowed. Take missed doses as soon as remembered unless almost time for the next dose; space remaining doses evenly during day. Do not double doses.
- Advise patient that tiotropium is not to be used for acute bronchospasm attacks, but may be continued during an acute exacerbation.
- Advise patient to notify health care professional immediately if signs and symptoms of angioedema (swelling of the lips, tongue, or throat, itching, rash) or signs of glaucoma (eye pain or discomfort, blurred vision, visual halos or colored images in association with red eyes from conjunctival congestion and corneal edema) occur.
- Caution patient to avoid spraying medication in eyes; may cause blurring of vision and pupil dilation.
- Advise patient that rinsing mouth after using inhaler, good oral hygiene, and sugarless gum or candy may minimize dry mouth; usually resolves with continued treatment.
- Instruct patient to notify health care professional of all Rx or OTC medications, vitamins, or herbal products being taken and consult health care professional before taking any new medications, including eye drops.
- Rep: Advise females of reproductive potential to inform health care professional if pregnancy is planned or suspected or if breastfeeding.
- **Handihaler:** Instruct patient in proper use and cleaning of the Handihaler inhaler. Review the *Patient's Instructions for Use* guide with patient. Capsules should be stored in sealed blisters; remove immediately before use or effectiveness of capsules is reduced. Tear blister strip carefully to expose only one capsule at a time. Discard capsules that are inadvertently exposed to air. *Spiriva* should be administered only via the Handihaler and the Handihaler should not be used with other medications. When disposing of capsule, tiny amount of powder left in capsule is normal.
- **Respimat:** Advise patient to prime inhaler by actuating inhaler toward the ground until an aerosol cloud is visible, then repeat process 3 more times. If not used for >3 days, actuate inhaler once to prepare inhaler for use. If not used for >21 days, actuate inhaler until an aerosol cloud is visible, then repeat 3 more times to prepare inhaler for use. Discard 3 mo from 1st use.

Evaluation/Desired Outcomes

- Decreased dyspnea.
- Improved breath sounds.
- Fewer exacerbations in patients with COPD and asthma.

T

tirzepatide (tir-**zep**-a-tide)
Mounjaro
Classification
Therapeutic: antidiabetics
Pharmacologic: glucagon-like peptide-1 (GLP-1) receptor agonistsglucose-dependent insulinotropic polypeptide (GIP) receptor agonists

Indications
Type 2 diabetes mellitus (as adjunct to diet and exercise).

Action
Acts as a glucose-dependent insulinotropic polypeptide (GIP) receptor and glucagon-like peptide-1 (GLP-1) receptor agonist; increases insulin secretion and reduces glucagon secretion, both in a glucose-dependent manner. Also slows gastric emptying. **Therapeutic Effects:** Improved glycemic control.

Pharmacokinetics
Absorption: 80% absorbed following subcutaneous administration.
Distribution: Minimally distributed to tissues.
Protein Binding: 99%.
Metabolism and Excretion: Metabolized by proteolytic cleavage, beta-oxidation, and amide hydrolysis. Excreted in the urine and feces, with very little being eliminated as unchanged drug.
Half-life: 5 days.

TIME/ACTION PROFILE (plasma concentrations)

ROUTE	ONSET	PEAK	DURATION
SUBQ	unknown	8–72 hr	unknown

Contraindications/Precautions
Contraindicated in: Hypersensitivity; Personal or family history of medullary thyroid carcinoma; Multiple endocrine neoplasia syndrome type 2; Type 1 diabetes; Severe gastroparesis.
Use Cautiously in: History of pancreatitis; Diabetic retinopathy (↑ risk of complications); History of angioedema or anaphylaxis to another GLP-1 receptor agonist; OB: Use during pregnancy only if potential maternal benefit justifies potential fetal risk; insulin recommended for glucose management in pregnancy; Lactation: Use while breastfeeding only if potential maternal benefit justifies potential risk to infant; Pedi: Safety and effectiveness not established in children.

Adverse Reactions/Side Effects
CV: ↑ heart rate. **EENT:** retinopathy complications. **Endo:** hypoglycemia, MEDULLARY THYROID CARCINOMA. **GI:** diarrhea, nausea, ↑ amylase, ↑ lipase, abdominal distension, abdominal pain, cholecystitis, cholelithiasis, constipation, dyspepsia, flatulence, gastroesophageal reflux disease, PANCREATITIS, vomiting. **GU:** acute kidney injury. **Local:** injection site reactions. **Metab:** ↓ appetite. **Misc:** HYPERSENSITIVITY REACTIONS (including anaphylaxis and angioedema).

Interactions
Drug-Drug: Concurrent use with **agents that increase insulin secretion**, including **sulfonylureas** or **insulin**, may ↑ the risk of serious hypoglycemia; use cautiously and consider dose ↓ of agent increasing insulin secretion. May alter absorption of concomitantly administered **oral medications**, including **oral hormonal contraceptives**, due to delayed gastric emptying; advise patients taking oral hormonal contraceptive to switch to a non-oral contraceptive method or add a barrier contraceptive method for 4 wk after initiating therapy and for 4 wk after each dose escalation of tirzepatide.

Route/Dosage
SUBQ (Adults): 2.5 mg once weekly initially for 4 wk, then ↑ to 5 mg once weekly; may then ↑ dose in 2.5 mg/wk increments every 4 wks, if needed, to achieve glycemic goals (max weekly dose = 15 mg/wk).

Availability
Solution for injection (prefilled pens): 2.5 mg/0.5 mL, 5 mg/0.5 mL, 7.5 mg/0.5 mL, 10 mg/0.5 mL, 12.5 mg/0.5 mL, 15 mg/0.5 mL.

NURSING IMPLICATIONS
Assessment
- Observe patient taking concurrent insulin for signs and symptoms of hypoglycemic reactions (sweating, hunger, weakness, dizziness, tremor, tachycardia, anxiety, headache, blurred vision, slurred speech, irritability).
- If thyroid nodules or elevated serum calcitonin are noted, patient should be referred to an endocrinologist.
- Monitor for pancreatitis (persistent severe abdominal pain, sometimes radiating to the back, with or without vomiting). If pancreatitis is suspected, discontinue tirzepatide; if confirmed, do not restart tirzepatide.
- Monitor for signs and symptoms of hypersensitivity reactions (anaphylaxis, angioedema) during therapy.

Lab Test Considerations
- Monitor serum A_{1c} periodically during therapy to evaluate effectiveness.
- May ↑ lipase and pancreatic amylase.

Implementation
- Patients stabilized on a diabetic regimen who are exposed to stress, fever, trauma, infection, or surgery may require administration of insulin.
- **SUBQ:** Administer once weekly at any time of the day, without regard to food. Day of wk may be changed as long as at least 72 hr before next dose. Inject into abdomen, thigh, or upper arm. Rotate in-

jection sites with each dose. Solution is clear and colorless to slightly yellow; do not administer solutions that are cloudy, discolored or contain particulate matter. Store pens at room temperature for up to 21 days; do not freeze. Store in the original carton to protect from light.

- When using with insulin, administer as separate injections; never mix. If injecting tirzepatide and insulin in same body region, injections should not be close to each other.

Patient/Family Teaching

- Instruct patient on use of pen and to take tirzepatide as directed. Follow manufacturer's instructions for pen use. Pen should never be shared between patients, even if needle is changed. Store pen in refrigerator; do not freeze. After initial use, pen may be stored at room temperature up to 14 days. Advise patient to read the *Medication Guide* before starting tirzepatide and with each Rx refill in case of changes.
- Take missed dose as soon as remembered as long as 3 days (72 hr) until next scheduled dose. If less than 3 days until next scheduled dose, skip and take next scheduled dose.
- Advise patient taking insulin and tirzepatide to never mix insulin and tirzepatide together. Give as 2 separate injections. Both injections may be given in the same body area, but should not be given right next to each other.
- Explain to patient that this medication controls hyperglycemia but does not cure diabetes. Therapy is long-term.
- Review signs of hypoglycemia and hyperglycemia with patient. If hypoglycemia occurs, advise patient to take a glass of orange juice or 2–3 tsp of sugar, honey, or corn syrup dissolved in water and notify health care professional.
- Encourage patient to follow prescribed diet, medication, and exercise regimen to prevent hypoglycemic or hyperglycemic episodes.
- Instruct patient in proper testing of serum glucose and ketones. These tests should be closely monitored during periods of stress or illness, and health care professional should be notified if significant changes occur.
- Advise patient to notify health care professional if changes in vision occur during therapy.
- Advise patient to notify health care professional of all Rx or OTC medications, vitamins, or herbal products being taken and consult health care professional before taking any new medications.
- Advise patient to notify health care professional immediately if signs of pancreatitis (nausea, vomiting, abdominal pain) or hypersensitivity (swelling of face, lips, tongue or throat, problems breathing or swallowing, severe rash or itching, fainting or feeling dizzy, very rapid heartbeat) occur.

- Inform patient of risk of benign and malignant thyroid C-cell tumors. Advise patient to notify health care professional if symptoms of thyroid tumors (lump in neck, hoarseness, trouble swallowing, shortness of breath) occur.
- Advise patient to inform health care professional of medication regimen before treatment or surgery.
- Advise patient to carry a form of sugar (sugar packets, candy) and identification describing disease process and medication regimen at all times.
- Rep: Insulin is the preferred method of controlling blood glucose during pregnancy. Counsel females of reproductive potential to notify health care professional if pregnancy is planned or suspected or if breastfeeding. Advise patients using oral hormonal contraceptives to switch to a non-oral contraceptive method, or add a barrier method of contraception for 4 wk after initiation and for 4 wk after each dose escalation.
- Emphasize the importance of routine follow-up exams.

Evaluation/Desired Outcomes

- Improved glycemic control.

tisotumab vedotin
(tye-**sot**-ue-mab ve-**doe**-tin)
  Tivdak
Classification
Therapeutic: antineoplastics
Pharmacologic: antimicrotubulars, tissue factor-directed antibody drug conjugates

Indications

Recurrent or metastatic cervical cancer with disease progression during or after chemotherapy.

Action

Acts as an antibody-drug conjugate (ADC) composed of a human IgG1 monoclonal antibody that is directed against tissue factor (located on the cell surface of cancer cells). Monomethyl auristatin E (MMAE) (an agent that disrupts microtubules and subsequently causes apoptosis) is attached to the antibody via a cleavable linker. The ADC binds to tissue factor on the cancer cells; the complex is then internalized, and then the MMAE is cleaved and released inside the cancer cells. **Therapeutic Effects:** Reduced progression of recurrent or metastatic cervical cancer.

Pharmacokinetics

Absorption: IV administration results in complete bioavailability.
Distribution: Minimally distributed to tissues.
Metabolism and Excretion: Monoclonal antibody component is degraded into smaller peptides via catabolism. MMAE is primarily metabolized in the liver

via the CYP3A4 isoenzyme. 17% of MMAE excreted in feces, and 6% excreted in urine, primarily as unchanged drug.

Half-life: *ADC:* 4 days; *MMAE:* 2.5 days.

TIME/ACTION PROFILE (plasma concentrations)

ROUTE	ONSET	PEAK	DURATION
IV	unknown	ADC: end of infusion; MMAE: 2–3 days	unknown

Contraindications/Precautions

Contraindicated in: Moderate or severe hepatic impairment; OB: Pregnancy; Lactation: Lactation.

Use Cautiously in: Rep: Women of reproductive potential and men with female partners of reproductive potential; Pedi: Safety and effectiveness not established in children.

Adverse Reactions/Side Effects

CV: DEEP VEIN THROMBOSIS. **Derm:** alopecia, pruritus, rash, STEVENS-JOHNSON SYNDROME (SJS). **EENT:** blepharitis, conjunctival abrasion/erosion, conjunctival hemorrhage, conjunctival hyperemia, conjunctival scar, conjunctivitis, corneal bleeding, corneal erosion, corneal scar, dry eye, epistaxis, keratitis, ocular hyperemia, blepharitis. **Endo:** hypoglycemia. **F and E:** hypomagnesemia, hyponatremia. **GI:** ↓ appetite, ↓ weight, ↑ liver enzymes, abdominal pain, constipation, diarrhea, hypoalbuminemia, nausea, vomiting, ileus. **GU:** ↑ serum creatinine, urinary tract infection, ↓ fertility (males). **Hemat:** ↑ activated partial thromboplastin time, ↑ prothrombin time, anemia, HEMORRHAGE, leukopenia, lymphocytopenia, neutropenia. **Metab:** hyperuricemia. **MS:** ↑creatine kinase, arthralgia, myalgia, muscle weakness. **Neuro:** fatigue, peripheral neuropathy. **Resp:** pneumonia, PNEUMONITIS, PULMONARY EMBOLISM. **Misc:** fever.

Interactions

Drug-Drug: Strong CYP3A4 inhibitors, including **ketoconazole,** may ↑ levels and risk of toxicity of MMAE; monitor closely.

Route/Dosage

IV (Adults ≥100 kg): 200 mg every 3 wk; continue until disease progression or unacceptable toxicity.
IV (Adults <100 kg): 2 mg/kg every 3 wk; continue until disease progression or unacceptable toxicity.

Availability

Lyophilized powder for injection: 40 mg/vial.

NURSING IMPLICATIONS

Assessment

- May cause changes in the corneal epithelium and conjunctiva resulting in changes in vision, including severe vision loss, and corneal ulceration; usually begin within first 1–2 mo of therapy. Refer patients to an eye care provider for an ophthalmic exam including visual acuity and slit lamp exam at baseline, prior to each dose, and as clinically indicated. Adhere to premedication and required eye care to reduce the risk of ocular adverse reactions. Promptly refer patients to an eye care provider for any new or worsening ocular signs and symptoms. *If superficial punctate* **keratitis** *occurs,* monitor patient. *For first occurrence of* confluent superficial keratitis, hold tisotumab dose until superficial punctate keratitis or normal, then resume therapy at next lower dose. *For second occurrence of confluent superficial keratitis,* permanently discontinue tisotumab. *For first occurrence of* **conjunctival ulceration,** hold dose until complete conjunctival re-epithelialization, then resume therapy at next lower dose. *For second occurrence of conjunctival ulceration,* permanently discontinue tisotumab. *If* **conjunctival or corneal scarring or symblepharon** *occur,* permanently discontinue tisotumab. *If Grade 1* **conjunctivitis and other ocular adverse reactions** *occur,* monitor patient. *For first occurrence of Grade 2 conjunctivitis and other ocular adverse reactions,* hold dose until Grade ≤1, then resume therapy at same dose. For second occurrence, hold dose until Grade ≤1, then resume therapy at next lower dose level. If no resolution to Grade ≤1, permanently discontinue. *For third occurrence of Grade 3 or 4 conjunctivitis,* permanently discontinue tisotumab.

- Monitor for signs and symptoms of neuropathy, (paresthesia, tingling or a burning sensation, neuropathic pain, muscle weakness, dysesthesia) during therapy; usually occurs within first 2–3 mo of therapy. *If Grade 2 peripheral neuropathy occurs,* hold dose until Grade ≤1, then resume therapy at next lower dose. If Grade 3 or 4 peripheral neuropathy occurs, permanently discontinue tisotumab.

- Monitor for signs and symptoms of hemorrhage. *If pulmonary or CNS hemorrhage occurs,* permanently discontinue tisotumab. *For Grade 2 hemorrhage in any other location,* hold tisotumab until bleeding has resolved then resume at same dose. *For first occurrence of Grade 3 hemorrhage in any other location,* hold tisotumab until bleeding has resolved then resume at same dose. *For second occurrence of Grade 3 or Grade 4 hemorrhage,* permanently discontinue tisotumab.

- Monitor for signs and symptoms of pneumonitis (hypoxia, cough, dyspnea or interstitial infiltrates on radiologic exams) during therapy. *If Grade 2 pneumonitis occurs,* hold dose until Grade ≤1 for persistent or recurrent pneumonitis, consider resuming therapy at next lower dose. If Grade 3 or 4 pneumonitis occurs, discontinue tisotumab permanently.

- Monitor for signs or symptoms of severe cutaneous adverse reactions (target lesions, worsening skin reactions, blistering or peeling of the skin, painful sores in mouth, nose, throat, or genital area, fever or flu-like symptoms, swollen lymph nodes). If signs or symptoms occur, hold *Tivdak* until cause has been determined. Permanently discontinue *Tivdak* for confirmed Grade 3 or 4 severe cutaneous adverse reactions, including SJS.

Lab Test Considerations
- Verify negative pregnancy test before starting therapy.
- May cause ↓ hemoglobin, ↓ lymphocytes, ↓ leukocytes, and ↓ neutrophils.
- May cause ↑ serum creatinine, AST, ALT, LDH, urate, alkaline phosphatase, and CK levels.
- May cause ↓ blood glucose, sodium, magnesium, and albumin.
- May cause ↑ PT, INR, and aPTT.

Implementation
- After examination with a slit lamp, administer first drop of topical corticosteroid eye drops in each eye prior to each infusion. Instruct patient to continue to administer eye drops in each eye for 72 hr after each infusion.
- Administer topical ocular vasoconstrictor drops in each eye immediately prior to each infusion. Change cold packs as needed during infusion to ensure eye area remains cold.
- Use cooling eye pads during the infusion.
- **Recommended Dose Reductions:** *Starting dose:* 2 mg/kg. *First dose reduction:* 1.3 mg/kg. *Second dose reduction:* 0.9 mg/kg.

IV Administration
- **IV:** Solution should be prepared in a biologic cabinet. Wear gloves, gown, and mask while handling medication. If powder or solution comes in contact with skin or mucosa, wash thoroughly with soap and water. Discard equipment in specially designated containers.
- **Intermittent Infusion:** *Reconstitution:* Reconstitute each 40 mg vial with 4 mL of sterile water for injection. Slowly swirl each vial until contents are completely dissolved; do not shake. Allow reconstituted vial(s) to settle. Do not expose to direct sunlight. Reconstituted solution is clear to slightly opalescent, colorless to brownish-yellow; do not administer solutions that are cloudy, discolored, or contain particulate matter. Add to diluent immediately. Reconstituted solution is stable for 8 hr at room temperature or 24 hr if refrigerated; do not freeze. *Concentration:* 10 mg/mL. *Dilution:* Dilute further with D5W, 0.9% NaCl, or LR. Mix by gentle inversion. *Concentration:* 0.7 mg/mL to 2.4 mg/mL. Diluted solution is clear to slightly opalescent, colorless to brownish-yellow; do not administer solutions that are cloudy, discolored, or contain particulate matter. *If diluted with 0.9% NaCl,* solution is stable up to 18 hr if refrigerated. *If diluted with D5W,* solution is stable up to 24 hr if refrigerated. *If diluted with LR,* solution is stable up to 12 hr if refrigerated. Do not freeze. Once removed from refrigerator, complete infusion within 4 hr. *Rate:* Infuse over 30 min through an IV line containing a 0.2 micron in-line filter. Do not administer as IV push or bolus.
- **Y-Site Incompatibility:** Do not mix with or administer with other medications.

Patient/Family Teaching
- Explain purpose of tisotumab to patient. Advise patient to read *Medication Guide* before starting and periodically during therapy in case of changes.
- Inform patient of potential eye problems and eye drop regimen. Instruct patient to use steroid eye drops before each infusion and as prescribed for 72 hr after each infusion. Instruct patient to use vasoconstrictor eye drops right before each infusion. Instruct patient to administer topical lubricating eye drops for duration of therapy and for 30 days after last dose of tisotumab. Advise patient to notify health care professional if new or worsening vision changes or eye problems develop during therapy.
- Advise patients to avoid wearing contact lenses unless advised by their eye care provider for the entire duration of therapy.
- Advise patient to notify health care professional immediately if signs and symptoms of bleeding (blood in stools or black stools, blood in urine, cough up or vomit blood, unusual vaginal bleeding, any unusual or heavy bleeding), lung problems (trouble breathing, shortness of breath, cough), severe skin reactions (skin reactions that look like rings [target lesions] rash or itching that continues to get worse; blistering or peeling of skin; painful sores or ulcers in mouth, nose, throat, or genital area; fever or flu-like symptoms; swollen lymph nodes) or peripheral neuropathy (numbness in hands or feet, muscle weakness) occur.
- Discuss with patient the possibility of hair loss. Explore methods of coping. May also cause darkening of skin and fingernails.
- Instruct patient to notify health care professional of all Rx or OTC medications, vitamins, or herbal products being taken and consult health care professional before taking any new medications.
- Rep: May cause fetal harm. Advise females of reproductive potential to use effective contraception during and for 2 mo after last dose and to avoid breastfeeding during and for 3 wk after last dose. Advise males with female partners of reproductive potential to use effective contraception during and for 4 mo after last dose. May impair male fertility.

Evaluation/Desired Outcomes
- Reduced progression of recurrent or metastatic cervical cancer.

✦ = Canadian drug name. ▓ = Genetic implication. S̶t̶r̶i̶k̶e̶t̶h̶r̶o̶u̶g̶h̶ = Discontinued. CAPITALS = life-threatening. U̲n̲d̲e̲r̲l̲i̲n̲e̲ = most frequent.

tobramycin, See AMINOGLYCOSIDES.

tocilizumab (toe-si-liz-oo-mab)
Actemra, Actemra ACTPen
Classification
Therapeutic: antirheumatics, immunosuppressants
Pharmacologic: interleukin antagonists

Indications
Moderately to severely active rheumatoid arthritis in patients who have not responded to ≥1 disease-modifying antirheumatic drug [DMARD] (as monotherapy or in combination with methotrexate or other non-biologic DMARDs). Active systemic juvenile idiopathic arthritis (as monotherapy or in combination with methotrexate). Active polyarticular juvenile idiopathic arthritis (as monotherapy or in combination with methotrexate). Giant cell arteritis. Chimeric antigen receptor T cell-induced severe or life-threatening cytokine release syndrome. Systemic sclerosis-associated interstitial lung disease (ILD). Coronavirus disease 2019 (COVID-19) in hospitalized patients who are receiving systemic corticosteroids and require supplemental oxygen, non-invasive or invasive mechanical ventilation, or extracorporeal membrane oxygenation.

Action
Acts as an inhibitor of interleukin-6 (IL-6) receptors by binding to them. IL-6 is a mediator of various inflammatory processes. **Therapeutic Effects:** Slowed progression of rheumatoid arthritis, systemic/polyarticular juvenile idiopathic arthritis, giant cell arteritis. Resolution of cytokine release syndrome. Slowing in rate of decline in pulmonary function in systemic sclerosis-associated ILD. Reduced mortality and prolonged time to mechanical ventilation in COVID-19.

Pharmacokinetics
Absorption: IV administration results in complete bioavailability; 80% absorbed following SUBQ administration.
Distribution: Minimally distributed to tissues.
Metabolism and Excretion: Unknown.
Half-life: *4 mg/kg dose:* up to 11 days; *8 mg/kg:* up to 13 days.

TIME/ACTION PROFILE (improvement)

ROUTE	ONSET	PEAK	DURATION
IV	within 1 mo	4 mo	unknown
SUBQ	unknown	unknown	unknown

Contraindications/Precautions
Contraindicated in: Hypersensitivity; Active infection (for all indications other than COVID-19); Active hepatic disease/impairment; Absolute neutrophil count (ANC) <2000/mm³ (<500/mm³ while on therapy) or platelet count below 100,000/mm³ (<50,000/mm³ while on therapy) (for rheumatoid arthritis, giant cell arteritis, systemic sclerosis-associated ILD, polyarticular juvenile idiopathic arthritis, and systemic juvenile idiopathic arthritis); ANC <1000/mm³ or platelet count below 50,000/mm³ (for COVID-19); Lactation: Lactation.

Use Cautiously in: Patients at risk for GI perforation, including patients with diverticulitis; Renal impairment; Hepatic impairment; Patients with risk factors for tuberculosis (TB); OB: Use during pregnancy only if potential maternal benefit justifies potential fetal risk; Pedi: Children <2 yr (safety and effectiveness not established); Geri: ↑ risk of adverse reactions in older adults.

Adverse Reactions/Side Effects
CV: hypertension. **Derm:** rash, STEVENS-JOHNSON SYNDROME. **EENT:** nasopharyngitis. **GI:** ↑ liver enzymes, GI PERFORATION, HEPATOTOXICITY. **Hemat:** NEUTROPENIA, THROMBOCYTOPENIA. **Metab:** hyperlipidemia. **Neuro:** headache, dizziness. **Misc:** INFECTION (including tuberculosis, disseminated fungal infections and infections with opportunistic pathogens), HYPERSENSITIVITY REACTIONS (including anaphylaxis), infusion reactions.

Interactions
Drug-Drug: May alter the activity of CYP450 enzymes; the effects of the following drugs should be monitored: **cyclosporine**, **theophylline**, **warfarin**, **hormonal contraceptives**, **atorvastatin**, and **lovastatin**. Concurrent use of other hepatotoxic medications, including **methotrexate**, may ↑ risk of hepatotoxicity. May ↓ antibody response to and ↑ risk of adverse reactions to **live virus vaccines**; do not administer concurrently.

Route/Dosage

Rheumatoid Arthritis
IV (Adults): 4 mg/kg every 4 wk; may ↑ to 8 mg/kg every 4 wk based on clinical response.
SUBQ (Adults ≥100 kg): 162 mg once weekly.
SUBQ (Adults <100 kg): 162 mg every 2 wk, may ↑ to every wk based on clinical response.

Systemic Juvenile Idiopathic Arthritis
IV (Children ≥2 yr and ≥30 kg): 8 mg/kg every 2 wk.
IV (Children ≥2 yr and <30 kg): 12 mg/kg every 2 wk.
SUBQ (Children ≥2 yr and ≥30 kg): 162 mg once weekly.
SUBQ (Children ≥2 yr and <30 kg): 162 mg every 2 wk.

Polyarticular Juvenile Idiopathic Arthritis
IV (Children ≥2 yr and ≥30 kg): 8 mg/kg every 4 wk.
IV (Children ≥2 yr and <30 kg): 10 mg/kg every 4 wk.
SUBQ (Children ≥2 yr and ≥30 kg): 162 mg every 2 wk.

SUBQ (Children ≥2 yr and <30 kg): 162 mg every 3 wk.

Giant Cell Arteritis
IV (Adults): 6 mg/kg (max = 600 mg/dose) every 4 wk (with a tapering course of corticosteroids).
SUBQ (Adults): 162 mg once weekly (with a tapering course of corticosteroids); may also consider giving 162 mg every 2 wk (with a tapering course of corticosteroids) based on clinical response.

Cytokine Release Syndrome
IV (Adults and Children ≥2 yr and ≥30 kg): 8 mg/kg (max = 800 mg/dose) initially; if patient does not clinically improve after initial dose, up to 3 additional doses may be administered every 8 hr.
IV (Adults and Children ≥2 yr and <30 kg): 12 mg/kg initially; if patient does not clinically improve after initial dose, up to 3 additional doses may be administered every 8 hr.

Systemic Sclerosis-Associated Interstitial Lung Disease
SUBQ (Adults): 162 mg once weekly.

COVID-19
IV (Adults): 8 mg/kg (max = 800 mg) as single dose; if clinical signs/symptoms worsen or do not improve, may administer another 8 mg/kg (max = 800 mg) dose ≥8 hr after initial dose.

Availability
Solution for intravenous injection: 20 mg/mL. **Solution for SUBQ injection (autoinjectors or prefilled syringes):** 162 mg/0.9 mL.

NURSING IMPLICATIONS
Assessment
● Assess pain and range of motion before and periodically during therapy.
● Assess for signs of infection (fever, dyspnea, flu-like symptoms, frequent or painful urination, redness or swelling at the site of a wound), including tuberculosis, prior to injection. Tocilizumab is contraindicated in patients with active infection. Monitor new infections closely; most common are upper respiratory tract infections, bronchitis, and urinary tract infections. Signs and symptoms of inflammation may be lessened due to suppression from tocilizumab. Infections may be fatal, especially in patients taking immunosuppressive therapy. If patient develops a serious infection, discontinue tocilizumab until infection is controlled.
● Monitor for injection site reactions (redness and/or itching, rash, hemorrhage, bruising, pain, or swelling). Rash will usually disappear within a few days. Application of a towel soaked in cold water may relieve pain or swelling.
● Monitor patient for signs of anaphylaxis (urticaria, dyspnea, facial edema) following injection. Medica-

tions (antihistamines, corticosteroids, epinephrine) and equipment should be readily available in the event of a severe reaction. Discontinue tocilizumab immediately if anaphylaxis or other severe allergic reaction occurs.
● In patients with COVID-19, monitor for signs and symptoms of new infections during and after therapy. Evaluate patients for risk factors for TB. In patients with COVID-19, it is not necessary to test for latent infection before starting therapy. For all other indications, assess patient for latent TB with a tuberculin skin test prior to initiation of therapy. Treatment of latent TB should be started before therapy with tocilizumab.
● Assess for signs and symptoms of systemic fungal infections (fever, malaise, weight loss, sweats, cough, dyspnea, pulmonary infiltrates, serious systemic illness with or without concomitant shock). Ascertain if patient lives in or has traveled to areas of endemic mycoses. Consider empiric antifungal treatment for patients at risk of histoplasmosis and other invasive fungal infections until the pathogens are identified. Consult with an infectious diseases specialist. Consider stopping tocilizumab until the infection has been diagnosed and adequately treated.

Lab Test Considerations
● Assess CBC with platelet count prior to initiating therapy and after 4–8 wk, then every 3 mo during therapy. Do not administer tocilizumab to patients with an ANC <2000/mm³, platelet count <100,000/mm³, or ALT or AST above 1.5 x the upper limit of normal (ULN).
● If ANC >1000/mm³, maintain dose. If ANC 500–1000/mm³, interrupt IV tocilizumab until ANC >1000/mm³, then resume at 4 mg/kg and ↑ to 8 mg/kg as clinically appropriate or reduce SUBQ tocilizumab to every other wk and increase frequency to every wk as clinically appropriate. If ANC <500/mm³, discontinue tocilizumab.
● If platelet count 50,000–100,000/mm³, interrupt dosing until platelet count >100,000/mm³, then resume IV dosing at 4 mg/kg and ↑ to 8 mg/kg as clinically appropriate or reduce SUBQ tocilizumab to every other wk and increase frequency to every wk as clinically appropriate. If platelet count <50,000/mm³, discontinue tocilizumab.
● Do not start tocilizumab for patients with COVID-19 who have ANC <1000 per mm³, platelet count <50,000 mm³, or ALT or AST >10 times ULN.
● **For rheumatoid arthritis, giant cell arteritis and ILD,** obtain liver test panel (ALT, AST, alkaline phosphatase, and total bilirubin before starting therapy, every 4–8 wk after start of therapy for first 6 mo and every 3 mo thereafter. If liver enzymes persistently ↑ >1–3 × ULN, reduce IV tocilizumab dose to 4 mg/kg and reduce SUBQ injection to every other wk or interrupt until AST/ALT have normal-

T

ized. *If >3–5 × ULN* (confirmed by repeat testing), interrupt tocilizumab until <3 × ULN and follow recommendations for ↑ >1–3 × ULN. *If persistent ↑ >1–3 × ULN or >5 × ULN*, discontinue tocilizumab. **For Systemic Juvenile Idiopathic Arthritis and Polyarticular Juvenile Idiopathic Arthritis,** monitor liver test panel at the time of the 2nd administration and thereafter every 4–8 wk for polyarticular juvenile idiopathic arthritis and every 2–4 wk for systemic juvenile idiopathic arthritis.

- Monitor lipid levels after 4–8 wk of therapy, then follow clinical guidelines for management of hyperlipidemia. May cause ↑ total cholesterol, triglycerides, LDL cholesterol, and/or HDL cholesterol.

Implementation

- Administer a tuberculin skin test prior to administration of tocilizumab (for all indications other than COVID-19). Patients with latent TB should be treated for TB prior to therapy.
- Immunizations should be current prior to initiating therapy. Patients on tocilizumab may receive concurrent vaccinations, except for live vaccines.
- Do not administer solutions that are discolored or contain particulate matter. Discard unused solution.
- Other DMARDs should be continued during tocilizumab therapy.
- When transitioning from IV therapy to SUBQ administration, administer first SUBQ dose instead of next scheduled IV dose.
- **Children:** Do not change dose based on single visit weight; weight fluctuates.
- To switch from IV to SUBQ, administer next dose SUBQ instead of IV.
- **SUBQ:** Solution is clear and colorless to pale yellow; do not administer solutions that are discolored or contain particulate matter. Rotate injection sites; avoid sites with moles, scars, areas where skin is tender, bruised, red, hard, or not intact.

IV Administration

- **Intermittent Infusion:** *Dilution:* Withdraw volume of 0.9% NaCl or 0.45% NaCl from a 100-mL bag (50 mL bag for children <30 kg) equal to volume of solution required for patient's dose. Slowly add tocilizumab from each vial to infusion bag. Invert slowly to mix; avoid foaming. Do not infuse solutions that are discolored or contain particulate matter. Diluted solution is stable for 24 hr if refrigerated or at room temperature; protect from light. Allow solution to reach room temperature before infusing. *Rate:* Infuse over 60 min. Do not administer via IV push or bolus.
- **Y-Site Incompatibility:** Do not infuse concomitantly in the same line with other drugs.

Patient/Family Teaching

- Instruct patient on the purpose for tocilizumab. If a dose is missed, contact health care professional to schedule next infusion. Instruct patient and caregiver in correct technique for SUBQ injections and

care and disposal of equipment. Advise patient and caregiver to read *Medication Guide* before starting therapy and with each Rx refill in case of changes.
- Caution patient to notify health care professional immediately if signs of infection (fever, sweating, chills, muscle aches, cough, shortness of breath, blood in phlegm, weight loss, warm, red or painful skin or sores, diarrhea or stomach pain, burning on urination, urinary frequency, feeling tired), fever and stomach-area pain that does not go away, change in bowel habits, severe rash, swollen face, or difficulty breathing occurs while taking. If signs and symptoms of anaphylaxis occur, discontinue injections and notify health care professional immediately.
- Instruct patient to notify health care professional of all Rx or OTC medications, vitamins, or herbal products being taken and consult health care professional before taking any new medications.
- Instruct patient to notify health care professional of medication regimen prior to treatment or surgery.
- Rep: Advise females of reproductive potential to notify health care professional if pregnancy is planned or suspected, or if breastfeeding. Inform patient of pregnancy exposure registry that monitors pregnancy outcomes in women exposed to tocilizumab during pregnancy. Register patient by calling 1-877-311-8972; health care professional or patient can call to register.

Evaluation/Desired Outcomes

- Decreased pain and swelling with decreased rate of joint destruction in patients with rheumatoid arthritis, systemic idiopathic juvenile arthritis, polyarticular juvenile idiopathic arthritis, or giant cell arteritis.
- Slowing in rate of decline in pulmonary function in systemic sclerosis-associated ILD.
- Reduced mortality and prolonged time to mechanical ventilation in COVID-19.

⚹ **tofacitinib** (toe-fa-**sye**-ti-nib)
Xeljanz, Xeljanz XR
Classification
Therapeutic: antirheumatics
Pharmacologic: kinase inhibitors

Indications

Moderately to severely active rheumatoid arthritis in patients who have had an inadequate response/intolerance to ≥1 tumor necrosis factor (TNF) blocker (as monotherapy or in combination with nonbiologic disease-modifying antirheumatic drugs [DMARDs]) (not to be used with biologic DMARDs or potent immunosuppressants including azathioprine and cyclosporine) (immediate-release and extended-release tablets only). Active psoriatic arthritis in patients who have had an inadequate response/intolerance to ≥1 TNF blocker (in combination with other nonbiologic DMARDs) (not to be used with biologic DMARDs or potent immunosuppressants including azathioprine and cyclosporine) (immediate-release and extended-release tablets only). Active ankylosing spondylitis in patients who have had an inadequate response/intolerance to ≥1 TNF blocker (not to be used with biologic DMARDs or potent immunosuppressants including azathioprine and cyclosporine) (immediate-release and extended-release tablets only). Moderately to severely active ulcerative colitis in patients who have had an inadequate response/intolerance to ≥1 TNF blocker (not to be used with biologic therapies or potent immunosuppressants including azathioprine and cyclosporine) (immediate-release and extended-release tablets only). Active polyarticular course juvenile idiopathic arthritis in patients who have had an inadequate response/intolerance to ≥1 TNF blocker (not to be used with biologic DMARDs or potent immunosuppressants including azathioprine and cyclosporine) (immediate-release tablets and oral solution only).

Action
Acts as a Janus kinase inhibitor. Some results of inhibition include decreased hematopoiesis and immune cell function. Decreases circulating killer cells, increases B cell count, and decreases serum C-reactive protein. **Therapeutic Effects:** Improvement in clinical and symptomatic parameters of rheumatoid arthritis, psoriatic arthritis, ankylosing spondylitis, ulcerative colitis, and polyarticular course juvenile idiopathic arthritis.

Pharmacokinetics
Absorption: 74% absorbed following oral administration.
Distribution: Well distributed to tissues.
Metabolism and Excretion: Primarily metabolized by the liver via the CYP3A4 isoenzyme, with some contribution from the CYP2C19 isoenzyme. 30% renal excretion of the parent drug.
Half-life: 3 hr.

TIME/ACTION PROFILE (clinical improvement)

ROUTE	ONSET	PEAK	DURATION
PO	within 2 wk	3 mo	unknown
PO-ER	unknown	unknown	unknown

Contraindications/Precautions
Contraindicated in: Active infection; Administration of live vaccines; Severe hepatic impairment; Increased risk for thrombosis; History of MI or stroke; Lymphocyte count <500 cells/mm³, absolute neutrophil count (ANC) <1000 cells/mm³, or Hgb <9 g/dL; Lactation: Lactation.
Use Cautiously in: Patients with rheumatoid arthritis who are >50 yr old and have ≥1 cardiovascular risk factor (↑ risk of all-cause mortality, cardiovascular death, MI, stroke, and thrombosis); Current or past history of smoking (↑ risk of malignancy, cardiovascular death, MI, or stroke); Known malignancy; Risk of GI perforation; Chronic lung disease (↑ risk of infection); ⚅ Japanese patients (↑ risk of herpes zoster); OB: Use during pregnancy only if potential maternal benefit justifies potential fetal risk; Pedi: Safety and effectiveness not established in children <18 yr (rheumatoid arthritis, psoriatic arthritis, and ulcerative colitis) or <2 yr (active polyarticular course juvenile idiopathic arthritis); Geri: Infection risk may be ↑ in older adults.

Adverse Reactions/Side Effects
CV: ARTERIAL THROMBOSIS, CARDIOVASCULAR DEATH, DEEP VEIN THROMBOSIS, MI, peripheral edema. **Derm:** erythema, pruritus, rash. **F and E:** dehydration. **GI:** ↑ liver enzymes, abdominal pain, diarrhea, dyspepsia, gastritis, GI PERFORATION, vomiting. **GU:** ↑ serum creatinine. **Hemat:** anemia, neutropenia. **Metab:** hyperlipidemia. **MS:** arthralgia, joint swelling, musculoskeletal pain, tendonitis. **Neuro:** fatigue, headache, insomnia, paresthesia, STROKE. **Resp:** PULMONARY EMBOLISM. **Misc:** DEATH, fever, HYPERSENSITIVITY REACTIONS (including angioedema and urticaria), INFECTION (including tuberculosis [TB], bacterial, invasive fungal infections, viral, and other infections due to opportunistic pathogens), MALIGNANCY.

Interactions
Drug-Drug: May ↑ risk of adverse reactions and ↓ antibody response to **live vaccines**; avoid concurrent use. **Strong CYP3A4 inhibitors**, including **ketoconazole**, or **moderate CYP3A4 inhibitors/strong CYP2C19 inhibitors**, including **fluconazole**, may ↑ levels and the risk of toxicity; dose ↓ recommended. **Strong CYP3A4 inducers**, including **rifampin**, may ↓ levels and effectiveness; avoid concurrent use. ↑ risk of immunosuppression when used concurrently with other potent **immunosuppressants**, including **azathioprine, cyclosporine, tacrolimus, antineoplastics**, or **radiation therapy**.

Route/Dosage
Rheumatoid Arthritis, Psoriatic Arthritis, and Ankylosing Spondylitis
PO (Adults): *Immediate-release tablets:* 5 mg twice daily; *Extended-release tablets:* 11 mg once daily; *Concurrent use of strong CYP3A4 inhibitors or concurrent use of moderate CYP3A4 inhibitor with a strong CYP2C19 inhibitor:* 5 mg once daily (immediate-release tablets); if taking 11 mg once daily (extended-release tablets), then switch to 5 mg once daily (immediate-release tablets).

Renal Impairment
PO (Adults): *Moderate or severe renal impairment:* 5 mg once daily (immediate-release); if taking 11 mg once daily (extended-release tablets), then switch to 5 mg once daily (immediate-release tablets). For patients undergoing hemodialysis, administer dose after dialysis session.

Hepatic Impairment

PO (Adults): *Moderate hepatic impairment:* 5 mg once daily (immediate-release tablets); if taking 11 mg once daily (extended-release tablets), then switch to 5 mg once daily (immediate-release tablets).

Ulcerative Colitis

PO (Adults): *Immediate-release tablets:* Induction: 10 mg twice daily for ≥8 wk; based on therapeutic response, may transition to maintenance dose or continue 10 mg twice daily for an additional 8 wk. Discontinue therapy if inadequate response achieved after 16 wk using 10 mg twice daily. Maintenance: 5 mg twice daily; if patient experiences loss of response on 5 mg twice daily, then use 10 mg twice daily after assessing the benefits and risks and use for the shortest duration; use lowest effective dose to maintain response; *Extended-release tablets:* Induction: 22 mg once daily for ≥8 wk; based on therapeutic response, may transition to maintenance dose or continue 22 mg once daily for an additional 8 wk. Discontinue therapy if inadequate response achieved after 16 wk using 22 mg once daily. Maintenance: 11 mg once daily; if patient experiences loss of response on 11 mg once daily, then use 22 mg once daily after assessing the benefits and risks and use for the shortest duration; use lowest effective dose to maintain response; *Concurrent use of strong CYP3A4 inhibitors or concurrent use of moderate CYP3A4 inhibitor with a strong CYP2C19 inhibitor:* if taking 10 mg twice daily (immediate-release tablets), ↓ to 5 mg twice daily (immediate-release tablets); if taking 5 mg twice daily (immediate-release tablets), ↓ to 5 mg once daily (immediate-release tablets). If taking 22 mg once daily (extended-release tablets), then ↓ to 11 mg once daily (extended-release tablets); if taking 11 mg once daily (extended-release tablets), then switch to 5 mg once daily (immediate-release tablets).

Renal Impairment

PO (Adults): *Moderate or severe renal impairment:* if taking 10 mg twice daily (immediate-release tablets), ↓ to 5 mg twice daily (immediate-release tablets); if taking 5 mg twice daily (immediate-release tablets), ↓ to 5 mg once daily (immediate-release tablets). If taking 22 mg once daily (extended-release tablets), then ↓ to 11 mg once daily (extended-release tablets); if taking 11 mg once daily (extended-release tablets), then switch to 5 mg once daily (immediate-release tablets). For patients undergoing hemodialysis, administer dose after dialysis session.

Hepatic Impairment

PO (Adults): *Moderate hepatic impairment:* if taking 10 mg twice daily (immediate-release tablets), ↓ to 5 mg twice daily (immediate-release tablets); if taking 5 mg twice daily (immediate-release tablets), ↓ to 5 mg once daily (immediate-release tablets). If taking 22 mg once daily (extended-release tablets), then ↓ to 11 mg once daily (extended-release tablets); if taking 11 mg once daily (extended-release tablets), then switch to 5 mg once daily (immediate-release).

Active Polyarticular Course Juvenile Idiopathic Arthritis

PO (Children ≥ 2 yr and ≥40 kg): *Immediate-release tablets or oral solution:* 5 mg twice daily. *Concurrent use of strong CYP3A4 inhibitors or concurrent use of moderate CYP3A4 inhibitor with a strong CYP2C19 inhibitor:* 5 mg once daily (immediate-release tablets or oral solution).

PO (Children ≥ 2 yr and 20–<40 kg): *Oral solution:* 4 mg twice daily. *Concurrent use of strong CYP3A4 inhibitors or concurrent use of moderate CYP3A4 inhibitor with a strong CYP2C19 inhibitor:* 4 mg once daily (oral solution).

PO (Children ≥ 2 yr and 10–<20 kg): *Oral solution:* 3.2 mg twice daily. *Concurrent use of strong CYP3A4 inhibitors or concurrent use of moderate CYP3A4 inhibitor with a strong CYP2C19 inhibitor:* 3.2 mg once daily (oral solution).

Renal Impairment

PO (Children ≥ 2 yr): *Moderate or severe renal impairment:* ≥40 kg: 5 mg once daily (immediate-release tablets or oral solution); 20–<40 kg: 4 mg once daily (oral solution). 10–<20 kg: 3.2 mg once daily (oral solution). For patients undergoing hemodialysis, administer dose after dialysis session.

Hepatic Impairment

PO (Children ≥2 yr): *Moderate hepatic impairment:* ≥40 kg: 5 mg once daily (immediate-release tablets or oral solution); 20–<40 kg: 4 mg once daily (oral solution). 10–<20 kg: 3.2 mg once daily (oral solution).

Availability (generic available)

Immediate-release tablets: 5 mg, 10 mg. **Extended-release tablets:** 11 mg, 22 mg. **Oral solution (grape flavor):** 1 mg/mL.

NURSING IMPLICATIONS

Assessment

- Assess pain and range of motion before and periodically during therapy.
- Assess for signs of infection (fever, dyspnea, flu-like symptoms, frequent or painful urination, redness or swelling at the site of a wound), including tuberculosis, prior to and periodically during therapy. Interrupt therapy if patient develops an active infection. Monitor new infections closely; most common are pneumonia, cellulitis, herpes zoster, urinary tract infection, diverticulitis, and appendicitis. Infections may be fatal, especially in patients taking immunosuppressive therapy.
- Assess for signs and symptoms of systemic fungal infections (fever, malaise, weight loss, sweats, cough, dyspnea, pulmonary infiltrates, serious systemic illness with or without concomitant shock). Ascertain if patient lives in or has traveled to areas of endemic mycoses. Consider empiric antifungal treatment for patients at risk of histoplasmosis and other invasive fungal infections until the pathogens are identified.

Consult with an infectious diseases specialist. Consider stopping tofacitinib until the infection has been diagnosed and adequately treated.

- Assess patient for latent TB with a tuberculin skin test prior to initiation of therapy. Treatment of latent TB should be started before therapy with tofacitinib.

Lab Test Considerations

- Monitor CBC prior to and periodically during therapy. Do not initiate tofacitinib in patients with lymphocyte count <500 cells/mm³, an ANC <1000 cells/mm³, or who have Hgb <9 g/dL.
- Monitor lymphocyte count at baseline and every 3 mo thereafter. *If lymphocyte count ≥500 cells/mm³* maintain dose. *If lymphocyte count <500 cells/mm³ and confirmed by repeat testing,* discontinue tofacitinib.
- Monitor neutrophil count at baseline, after 4–8 wk of therapy, and every 3 mo thereafter. *If ANC >1000 cells/mm³,* maintain dose. *If ANC 500–1000 cells/mm³,* for persistent decreases in this range, interrupt dosing until ANC >1000 cells/mm³. *If ANC <500 cells/mm³ and confirmed by repeat testing,* discontinue tofacitinib.
- Monitor Hgb at baseline, after 4–8 wk of therapy, and every 3 mo thereafter. *If ↓ in Hgb ≤2 g/dL and Hgb ≥9.0 g/dL and confirmed by repeat testing,* maintain dose. *If ↓ in Hgb >2 dL and Hgb <8.0 g/dL,* interrupt administration of tofacitinib until hemoglobin values have normalized.
- Monitor liver enzymes prior to and periodically during therapy.
- Monitor total cholesterol, LDL cholesterol, and HDL cholesterol 4–8 wk following initiation of therapy.

Implementation

- Administer a tuberculin skin test prior to administration of tofacitinib. Patients with active latent TB should be treated for TB prior to therapy.
- Immunizations should be current prior to initiating therapy. Patients on tofacitinib should not receive live vaccines.
- Screen patient for viral hepatitis before starting therapy.
- Extended-release tablets are not interchangeable with oral solution.
- *To switch from immediate release to extended release,* patients treated with *Xeljanz* 5 mg twice daily may be switched to *Xeljanz XR* 11 mg once daily the day following the last dose of *Xeljanz* 5 mg.
- PO: Administer twice daily without regard to food. *DNC:* Swallow extended release tablets whole; do not crush, break, or chew.
- Oral solution is clear and colorless. Administer oral solution using the included press-in bottle adapter and oral dosing syringe.

Patient/Family Teaching

- Instruct patient to take tofacitinib as directed. Advise patient to read *Medication Guide* before starting and with each Rx refill in case of changes.
- Caution patient to notify health care professional immediately if signs of infection (fever, sweating, chills, muscle aches, cough, shortness of breath, blood in phlegm, weight loss, warm, red, or painful skin or sores, diarrhea or stomach pain, burning on urination or urinating more often than normal, feeling very tired) or stomach or intestinal perforation (fever, stomach-area pain that does not go away, change in bowel habits) occur.
- Advise patient to notify health care professional of all Rx or OTC medications, vitamins, or herbal products being taken and to consult with health care professional before taking other medications.
- Instruct patient to notify health care professional of medication regimen prior to treatment or surgery.
- Inform patient of increased risk of lymphoma and other cancers. Advise patient to have periodic skin exams for new lesions of skin cancer.
- Rep: Advise females of reproductive potential to notify health care professional if pregnancy is planned or suspected and to avoid breastfeeding during therapy and for at least 18 hr after the last dose of oral solution or 36 hr after the last dose of extended release tablets. Inform patient of pregnancy exposure registry that monitors pregnancy outcomes in women exposed to tofacitinib during pregnancy. Encourage patients who become pregnant during therapy to enroll in the pregnancy registry by calling 1-877-311-8972. May impair female fertility.
- Emphasize the importance of follow-up lab tests to monitor for adverse reactions.

Evaluation/Desired Outcomes

- Decreased pain and swelling with improved physical functioning and decreased rate of joint destruction in patients with rheumatoid arthritis, psoriatic arthritis, ankylosing spondylitis, and polyarticular course juvenile idiopathic arthritis.
- Decrease in diarrhea and abdominal pain in patients with ulcerative colitis.

tolnaftate, See ANTIFUNGALS (TOPICAL).

tolterodine (tol-ter-oh-deen)
Detrol, Detrol LA
Classification
Therapeutic: urinary tract antispasmodics
Pharmacologic: anticholinergics

Indications
Overactive bladder with symptoms of urinary frequency, urgency, or urge incontinence.

Action
Acts as a competitive muscarinic receptor antagonist resulting in inhibition of cholinergically mediated bladder contraction. **Therapeutic Effects:** Decreased urinary frequency, urgency, and urge incontinence.

Pharmacokinetics
Absorption: Well absorbed (77%) following oral administration.
Distribution: Extensively distributed to tissues.
Protein Binding: 96.3%.
Metabolism and Excretion: Extensively metabolized by the liver, via the CYP2D6 isoenzyme; ‡‡ (the CYP2D6 enzyme system exhibits genetic polymorphism; ~7% of population may be poor metabolizers and may have significantly ↑ tolterodine concentrations and an ↑ risk of adverse effects); one metabolite (5-hydroxymethyltolterodine) is active; other metabolites are excreted in urine.
Half-life: *Tolterodine:* 1.9–3.7 hr; *5-hydroxymethyltolterodine:* 2.9–3.1 hr.

TIME/ACTION PROFILE (effects on bladder function)

ROUTE	ONSET	PEAK	DURATION
PO	unknown	unknown	12 hr

Contraindications/Precautions
Contraindicated in: Hypersensitivity to tolterodine or fesoterodine; Urinary retention; Gastric retention; Severe hepatic impairment; End-stage renal disease (CCr <10 mL/min); Uncontrolled angle-closure glaucoma; Lactation: Lactation.
Use Cautiously in: GI obstructive disorders, including pyloric stenosis (↑ risk of gastric retention); Significant bladder outflow obstruction (↑ risk of urinary retention); Controlled angle-closure glaucoma; Myasthenia gravis; Mild to moderate hepatic impairment (↓ dose); Severe renal impairment (CCr 10–30 mL/min) (↓ dose); OB: Use during pregnancy only if potential maternal benefit justifies potential fetal risk; Pedi: Safety and effectiveness not established in children.

Adverse Reactions/Side Effects
EENT: blurred vision, dry eyes. **GI:** dry mouth, constipation, dyspepsia. **Neuro:** dizziness, headache, sedation. **Misc:** HYPERSENSITIVITY REACTIONS (including anaphylaxis and angioedema).

Interactions
Drug-Drug: **Strong CYP3A4 inhibitors,** including **erythromycin, clarithromycin, cyclosporine, itraconazole, ketoconazole,** and **vinblastine,** may ↑ levels and the risk of toxicity.

Route/Dosage
Immediate-Release Tablets
PO (Adults): 2 mg twice daily; may be lowered depending on response; *Concurrent use of strong CYP3A4 inhibitors:* 1 mg twice daily.
Hepatic/Renal Impairment
PO (Adults): *Mild to moderate hepatic impairment or severe renal impairment (CCr 10–30 mL/min):* 1 mg twice daily.
Extended-Release Capsules
PO (Adults): 4 mg once daily; may be lowered depending on response; *Concurrent use of strong CYP3A4 inhibitors:* 2 mg once daily.
Hepatic/Renal Impairment
PO (Adults): *Mild to moderate hepatic impairment or severe renal impairment (CCr 10–30 mL/min):* 2 mg once daily.

Availability (generic available)
Extended-release capsules: 2 mg, 4 mg. **Tablets:** 1 mg, 2 mg.

NURSING IMPLICATIONS
Assessment
- Assess patient for urinary urgency, frequency, and urge incontinence periodically during therapy.
- Monitor for signs and symptoms of anaphylaxis and angioedema (difficulty breathing, upper airway obstruction, fall in BP, rash, swelling of face or neck). Have emergency equipment readily available.

Implementation
- **PO:** Administer without regard to food.
- *DNC:* Extended-release capsules should be swallowed whole; do not open, crush, dissolve, or chew.

Patient/Family Teaching
- Instruct patient to take tolterodine as directed.
- May cause dizziness and blurred vision. Caution patient to avoid driving or other activities requiring alertness until response to medication is known.
- Instruct patient to notify health care professional immediately if rash or signs and symptoms of anaphylaxis or angioedema occur.
- Rep: Advise females of reproductive potential to notify health care professional if pregnancy is planned or suspected or if breastfeeding.

Evaluation/Desired Outcomes
- Decreased urinary frequency, urgency, and urge incontinence.

REMS

tolvaptan (tol-**vap**-tan)
✦Jinarc, Jynarque, Samsca
Classification
Therapeutic: electrolyte modifiers
Pharmacologic: vasopressin antagonists

Indications

Samsca: Significant hypervolemic and euvolemic hyponatremia (serum sodium <125 mEq/L or less marked symptomatic hyponatremia that has resisted correction by fluid restriction), including patients with HF and syndrome of inappropriate antidiuretic hormone. **Jynarque:** Patients at risk of rapidly progressing autosomal dominant polycystic kidney disease.

Action

Acts as a selective vasopressin V2-receptor antagonist, resulting in increased renal water excretion and increased serum sodium. **Therapeutic Effects:** Correction of hyponatremia (Samsca). Slowed deterioration of renal function (Jynarque).

Pharmacokinetics

Absorption: 40% absorbed following oral administration.

Distribution: Well distributed to tissues.

Protein Binding: >99%.

Metabolism and Excretion: Extensively metabolized in the liver via the CYP3A4 isoenzyme; 59% excreted in the feces (19% as unchanged drug), with 40% excreted in the urine (<1% as unchanged drug).

Half-life: 12 hr.

TIME/ACTION PROFILE

ROUTE	ONSET	PEAK	DURATION
PO	within 8 hr	2–4 hr†	7 days

† Plasma concentrations.

Contraindications/Precautions

Contraindicated in: Hypersensitivity; Hepatic impairment; Urgent need to acutely raise serum sodium (Samsca); Patients who cannot appropriately sense/respond to thirst; Hypovolemia; Uncorrected abnormal serum sodium concentrations (Jynarque); Anuria; Uncorrected urinary outflow obstruction; Lactation: Lactation.

Use Cautiously in: Severe malnutrition, alcoholism or advanced liver disease (↑ risk of osmotic demyelination; correct electrolyte abnormalities at a slower rates); Cirrhosis (↑ risk of GI bleeding, use only when the need to treat outweighs risk); OB: Use during pregnancy only if potential maternal benefit justifies potential fetal risk; Pedi: Safety and effectiveness not established in children; Geri: Older adults may have ↑ sensitivity to effects.

Adverse Reactions/Side Effects

CV: palpitations. **Derm:** dry skin, rash. **Endo:** <u>hyperglycemia</u>. **F and E:** <u>thirst</u>, hypernatremia, hypovolemia. **GI:** <u>constipation</u>, <u>diarrhea</u>, <u>dry mouth</u>, ↓ appetite, dyspepsia, HEPATOTOXICITY. **GU:** <u>polyuria</u>. **Metab:** hyperuricemia. **Neuro:** <u>dizziness</u>, <u>weakness</u>, osmotic demyelination. **Misc:** HYPERSENSITIVITY REACTIONS (including anaphylaxis).

Interactions

Drug-Drug: Strong CYP3A inhibitors, including **ketoconazole, clarithromycin, itraconazole, nelfinavir, ritonavir,** and **nefazodone,** as well as **moderate CYP3A inhibitors,** including **erythromycin, fluconazole, aprepitant, diltiazem,** and **verapamil,** may ↑ levels and risk of toxicity; avoid concurrent use. **CYP3A inducers,** including **rifampin,** may ↓ levels and effectiveness; avoid concurrent use with Jynarque; dosage adjustments may be necessary with Samsca. **P-glycoprotein inhibitors,** including **cyclosporine,** may ↑ levels and risk of toxicity; dosage adjustments may be necessary. May ↑ risk of hyperkalemia with **angiotensin II receptor blockers, ACE inhibitors,** and **potassium-sparing diuretics. Diuretics** may ↑ risk of too rapidly correcting serum sodium concentrations. May inhibit effects of **desmopressin;** avoid concurrent use.

Drug-Food: Grapefruit juice may ↑ levels and the risk of toxicity; avoid concurrent use.

Route/Dosage

Samsca and Jynarque should not be used interchangeably.

Hyponatremia (Samsca)

PO (Adults): 15 mg once daily initially; may ↑ at intervals of ≥1 day to 30 mg once daily, up to a maximum of 60 mg once daily. Do not use for longer than 30 days.

Autosomal Dominant Polycystic Kidney Disease (Jynarque and Jinarc)

PO (Adults): 60 mg/day initially (taken as 45 mg upon wakening and then 15 mg 8 hr later); may be ↑ after at least 1 wk to 90 mg/day (taken as 60 mg upon wakening and then 30 mg 8 hr later); may then be ↑ after at least 1 wk to 120 mg/day (taken as 90 mg upon wakening and then 30 mg 8 hr later); *Concurrent use of moderate CYP3A inhibitors:* 30 mg/day initially (taken as 15 mg upon wakening and then 15 mg 8 hr later); may be ↑ after at least 1 wk to 45 mg/day (taken as 30 mg upon wakening and then 15 mg 8 hr later); may then be ↑ after at least 1 wk to 60 mg/day (taken as 45 mg upon wakening and then 15 mg 8 hr later).

Availability (generic available)

Tablets (Jynarque): 15 mg, 30 mg, 45 mg, 60 mg, 90 mg. **Tablets (Samsca):** 15 mg, 30 mg.

NURSING IMPLICATIONS

Assessment

- Monitor neurologic status and assess for signs and symptoms of osmotic demyelination syndrome (trouble speaking, dysphagia, drowsiness, confusion, mood changes, involuntary movements, weakness, seizures), especially during initiation and after titration. If a rapid ↑ in sodium or symptoms occur, discontinue tolvaptan and consider administration of hypotonic fluid.

T

- Monitor fluid balance. If hypovolemia occurs interrupt or discontinue tolvaptan and provide supportive care (monitor vital signs, balance fluid and electrolytes).
- Monitor for signs and symptoms of liver injury (fatigue, anorexia, right upper abdominal discomfort, dark urine, jaundice) periodically during therapy. If symptoms occur, discontinue therapy.

Lab Test Considerations
- Monitor serum sodium levels frequently during initiation and dose titration and periodically during therapy. Too rapid correction of hyponatremia (>12 mEq/L/24 hr) can cause osmotic demyelination syndrome.
- Monitor serum potassium in patients with serum potassium >5 mEq/L or taking medication known to ↑ potassium.
- Monitor ALT, AST, and bilirubin 2 wk and 4 wk after starting therapy, then monthly for first 18 mo and every 3 mo thereafter. If ALT, AST, or bilirubin increase to >2 × upper limit of normal (ULN), immediately discontinue *Jynarque;* repeat tests as soon as possible (within 48–72 hr). If levels stabilize or resolve, *Jynarque* may be reinitiated with increased frequency of monitoring as long as ALT and AST remain below 3 times ULN. Do not restart in patients with signs or symptoms of hepatic injury or whose ALT or AST ever exceeds 3 x ULN during therapy with tolvaptan, unless another explanation for liver injury exists and the injury has resolved. In patients with a stable, low baseline AST or ALT, an increase >2 x baseline, even if <2 x ULN, may indicate early liver injury. Suspend and promptly (48–72 hr) reevaluate liver enzymes before reinitiating therapy with more frequent monitoring.

Implementation
- Initiate and reinitiate therapy in a hospital.
- *REMS:* REMS requirements are for *Jynarque* product. Avoid fluid restriction during first 24 hr of therapy.
- PO: Administer once daily without regard to meals.

Patient/Family Teaching
- Instruct patient to take tolvaptan as directed. Avoid drinking grapefruit juice during therapy; may cause ↑ levels. Take missed doses as soon as remembered, but not if just before next dose; do not double doses. Do not stop and restart therapy. Restarting therapy may require hospitalization.
- *REMS:* Explain requirements of Jynarque REMS program (patient must enroll, comply with ongoing monitoring requirements, must get Jynarque from pharmacies participating in REMS program).
- Inform patients they can continue fluid ingestion in response to thirst during therapy and should have water available to drink at all times during therapy. Following discontinuation of therapy, resume fluid restriction.

- Advise patient to notify health care professional immediately if signs and symptoms of hepatotoxicity (feeling tired, fever, loss of appetite, rash, nausea, itching, right upper abdomen pain or tenderness, yellowing of skin and white part of eye, vomiting, dark urine) occur.
- Advise patient to notify health care professional of all Rx or OTC medications, vitamins, or herbal products being taken and to consult with health care professional before taking other medications.
- Advise patient to notify health care professional if signs of dehydration (vomiting, diarrhea, inability to drink normally, dizziness, feeling faint) or bleeding (vomiting bright red blood, dark blood clots, or coffee-ground-like material; black, tarry stools; bloody stools).
- Rep: Advise females of reproductive potential to notify health care professional if pregnancy is planned or suspected, and to avoid breastfeeding.

Evaluation/Desired Outcomes
- Normalization of serum sodium levels. Therapy should be limited to 30 days (Samsca).
- Slowed deterioration of renal function (Jynarque).

---

topiramate (toe-**peer**-a-mate)
Eprontia, Qudexy XR, Topamax, Topamax Sprinkle, Trokendi XR
Classification
Therapeutic: anticonvulsants, mood stabilizers

Indications
Partial-onset seizures (as monotherapy or adjunctive therapy). Primary generalized tonic-clonic seizures (as monotherapy or adjunctive therapy). Seizures due to Lennox-Gastaut syndrome (as adjunctive therapy). Prevention of migraine headache. **Unlabeled Use:** Adjunct in treatment of bipolar disorder. Infantile spasms.

Action
Action may be due to: Blockade of sodium channels in neurons, Enhancement of gamma-aminobutyrate, an inhibitory neurotransmitter, Prevention of activation of excitatory receptors. **Therapeutic Effects:** Decreased incidence of seizures. Decreased incidence/severity of migraine headache.

Pharmacokinetics
Absorption: 80% absorbed following oral administration.
Distribution: Minimally distributed to tissues.
Metabolism and Excretion: Not extensively metabolized. 70% excreted unchanged in urine.
Half-life: *Immediate release:* 21 hr; *Extended release:* 31 hr.

TIME/ACTION PROFILE (plasma concentrations†)

ROUTE	ONSET	PEAK	DURATION
PO	unknown	2 hr	12 hr
PO-ER	unknown	24 hr	unknown

†After single dose.

Contraindications/Precautions

Contraindicated in: Hypersensitivity; Recent alcohol use (within 6 hr before and after use of extended-release product); Metabolic acidosis (on metformin) (with extended-release product only).

Use Cautiously in: All patients (may ↑ risk of suicidal thoughts/behaviors); Renal impairment (dose ↓ recommended if CCr <70 mL/min/1.73 m²); Hepatic impairment; Dehydration; Patients predisposed to metabolic acidosis; Sulfa allergy; Rep: Women of reproductive potential; OB: Use during pregnancy only if potential maternal benefit justifies potential fetal risk; Lactation: Use while breastfeeding only if potential maternal benefit justifies potential risk to infant; Pedi: Safety and effectiveness not established in children <2 yr (immediate-release) and <6 yr (extended-release); children are more prone to oligohydrosis, hyperthermia, metabolic acidosis, ↓ bone mineral density, and ↓ growth; Geri: Consider age-related ↓ in renal/hepatic impairment, concurrent disease states and drug therapy in older adults.

Adverse Reactions/Side Effects

Derm: oligohydrosis (↑ in children), STEVENS-JOHNSON SYNDROME, TOXIC EPIDERMAL NECROLYSIS. **EENT:** abnormal vision, diplopia, nystagmus, ↑ intraocular pressure, acute myopia/secondary angle closure glaucoma, mydriasis, ocular pain, ocular redness, retinal detachment, visual field defects. **Endo:** ↓ growth (children). **F and E:** hyperchloremic metabolic acidosis. **GI:** nausea, abdominal pain, anorexia, constipation, dry mouth, hyperammonemia. **GU:** kidney stones. **Hemat:** BLEEDING, leukopenia. **Metab:** weight loss, hyperthermia (↑ in children). **MS:** ↓ bone mineral density (↑ in children). **Neuro:** ataxia, cognitive disorders, dizziness, drowsiness, fatigue, impaired concentration/memory, nervousness, paresthesia, psychomotor slowing, sedation, speech problems, aggressive reaction, agitation, anxiety, confusion, depression, encephalopathy, malaise, mood problems, SEIZURES, SUICIDAL THOUGHTS, tremor. **Misc:** fever.

Interactions

Drug-Drug: Alcohol use within 6 hr before or after use of Trokendi XR may significantly alter topiramate levels; use during this time frame contraindicated. **Phenytoin**, **carbamazepine**, or **valproic acid** may ↓ levels and effectiveness. May ↑ levels and the risk of toxicity of **phenytoin**, **amitriptyline**, or **lithium**. May ↓ levels and effectiveness of **hormonal contraceptives**,

risperidone, or **valproic acid**. ↑ risk of CNS depression with **alcohol** or other **CNS depressants**. **Carbonic anhydrase inhibitors** (e.g. **acetazolamide** or **zonisamide**) may ↑ risk of metabolic acidosis and kidney stones. Concurrent use with **valproic acid** may ↑ risk of hyperammonemia, encephalopathy, and hypothermia. ↑ risk of bleeding with **aspirin**, **clopidogrel**, **ticagrelor**, **prasugrel**, **warfarin**, **dabigatran**, **rivaroxaban**, **apixaban**, **edoxaban**, **NSAIDs**, or **SSRIs**.

Route/Dosage

Epilepsy (monotherapy)

PO (Adults and Children ≥10 yr): *Immediate-release:* 25 mg twice daily initially, gradually ↑ at weekly intervals to 200 mg twice daily over a 6-wk period; *Extended-release (Qudexy XR or Trokendi XR):* 50 mg once daily initially, gradually ↑ at weekly intervals to 400 mg once daily over a 6-wk period.

PO (Children 2–<10 yr [6–<10 yr for Trokendi XR] and >38 kg): *Immediate-release:* 25 mg once daily in the evening initially, gradually ↑ at weekly intervals to 125 mg twice daily over a 5–7-wk period; if needed may continue to titrate dose on a weekly basis up to 200 mg twice daily; *Extended-release (Qudexy XR or Trokendi XR):* 25 mg once daily for 1 wk, then ↑ to 50 mg once daily for 1 wk, then ↑ by 25–50 mg/day at weekly intervals over a 5–7-wk period to target dose of 250–400 mg once daily.

PO (Children 2–<10 yr [6–<10 yr for Trokendi XR] and 32–38 kg): *Immediate-release:* 25 mg once daily in the evening initially, gradually ↑ at weekly intervals to 125 mg twice daily over a 5–7-wk period; if needed, may continue to titrate dose on a weekly basis up to 175 mg twice daily; *Extended-release (Qudexy XR or Trokendi XR):* 25 mg once daily for 1 wk, then ↑ to 50 mg once daily for 1 wk, then ↑ by 25–50 mg/day at weekly intervals over a 5–7-wk period to target dose of 250–350 mg once daily.

PO (Children 2–<10 yr [6–<10 yr for Trokendi XR] and 23–31 kg): *Immediate-release:* 25 mg once daily in the evening initially, gradually ↑ at weekly intervals to 100 mg twice daily over a 5–7-wk period; if needed; may continue to titrate dose on a weekly basis up to 175 mg twice daily; *Extended-release (Qudexy XR or Trokendi XR):* 25 mg once daily for 1 wk, then ↑ to 50 mg once daily for 1 wk, then ↑ by 25–50 mg/day at weekly intervals over a 5–7-wk period to target dose of 200–350 mg once daily.

PO (Children 2–<10 yr [6–<10 yr for Trokendi XR] and 12–22 kg): *Immediate-release:* 25 mg once daily in the evening initially, gradually ↑ at weekly intervals to 100 mg twice daily over a 5–7-wk period; if needed, may continue to titrate dose on a weekly basis up to 150 mg twice daily; *Extended-release (Qudexy XR or Trokendi XR):* 25 mg once daily for 1 wk, then ↑ to 50 mg once daily for 1 wk, then ↑ by 25–50 mg/

T

day at weekly intervals over a 5–7-wk period to target dose of 200–300 mg once daily.

PO (Children 2–<10 yr [6–<10 yr for Trokendi XR] and ≤11 kg): *Immediate-release:* 25 mg once daily in the evening initially, gradually ↑ at weekly intervals to 75 mg twice daily over a 5–7-wk period; if needed, may continue to titrate dose on a weekly basis up to 125 mg twice daily; *Extended-release (Qudexy XR or Trokendi XR):* 25 mg once daily for 1 wk, then ↑ to 50 mg once daily for 1 wk, then ↑ by 25–50 mg/day at weekly intervals over a 5–7-wk period to target dose of 150–250 mg once daily.

Renal Impairment
PO (Adults): *CCr <10 mL/min:* ↓ dose by 50%.

Epilepsy (adjunctive therapy)
PO (Adults and Children ≥17 yr): *Immediate-release:* 25–50 mg/day initially, ↑ by 25–50 mg/day at weekly intervals up to 200–400 mg/day in 2 divided doses (200–400 mg/day in 2 divided doses for partial seizures or Lennox-Gastaut syndrome and 400 mg/day in 2 divided doses for primary generalized tonic-clonic seizures); *Extended-release (Qudexy XR or Trokendi XR):* 25–50 mg once daily initially, ↑ by 25–50 mg/day at weekly intervals up to 200–400 mg once daily (for partial seizures or Lennox-Gastaut syndrome) and 400 mg once daily (for primary generalized tonic-clonic seizures).

PO (Children 2–16 yr): *Immediate-release and extended-release (Qudexy XR):* 25 mg once daily at night initially for first wk, ↑ at 1–2 wk intervals by 1–3 mg/kg/day up to 5–9 mg/kg/day in 2 divided doses.

PO (Children 6–16 yr): *Extended-release (Trokendi XR):* 25 mg once daily at night initially for first wk, ↑ at 1–2 wk intervals by 1–3 mg/kg/day up to 5–9 mg/kg/day given once daily at night.

Renal Impairment
PO (Adults): *CCr <70 mL/min:* ↓ dose by 50%.

Migraine Prevention
PO (Adults and Children ≥12 yr): *Immediate-release:* 25 mg at night initially, ↑ by 25 mg/day at weekly intervals up to target dose of 100 mg/day in 2 divided doses; *Extended-release (Qudexy XR):* 25 mg once daily initially, ↑ by 25 mg/day at weekly intervals up to target dose of 100 mg once daily.

Renal Impairment
PO (Adults): *CCr <70 mL/min:* ↓ dose by 50%.

Availability (generic available)
Immediate-release tablets: 25 mg, 50 mg, 100 mg, 200 mg. **Extended-release capsules (Qudexy XR):** 25 mg, 50 mg, 100 mg, 150 mg, 200 mg. **Extended-release capsules (Trokendi XR):** 25 mg, 50 mg, 100 mg, 200 mg. **Oral solution (mixed berry flavor):** 25 mg/mL. **Sprinkle capsules:** 15 mg, 25 mg. *In combination with:* phentermine (Qsymia). See Appendix N.

NURSING IMPLICATIONS
Assessment
- Monitor closely for notable changes in behavior that could indicate the emergence or worsening of suicidal thoughts or behavior or depression.
- Pedi: Monitor growth rate (height and weight) in pediatric patients; may have negative effects on height and weight.
- **Seizures:** Assess location, duration, and characteristics of seizure activity.
- **Migraines:** Assess pain location, intensity, duration, and associated symptoms (photophobia, phonophobia, nausea, vomiting) during migraine attack. Monitor frequency and intensity of pain on pain scale.
- **Bipolar Disorder:** Assess mental status (mood, orientation, behavior) and cognitive abilities before and periodically during therapy.

Lab Test Considerations
- Monitor CBC with differential and platelet count before therapy to determine baseline levels and periodically during therapy. Frequently causes anemia.
- Monitor hepatic function periodically during therapy. May cause ↑ AST and ALT levels.
- Evaluate serum bicarbonate prior to and periodically during therapy. Monitor for signs and symptoms of metabolic acidosis (hyperventilation, fatigue, anorexia, cardiac arrhythmias, stupor). If metabolic acidosis occurs, dosing taper or discontinuation may be necessary.

Implementation
- Implement seizure precautions.
- Do not confuse Topamax with Toprol XL.
- **PO:** May be administered without regard to meals.
- *DNC:* Do not break/crush tablets because of bitter taste.
- Contents of the sprinkle capsules can be sprinkled on a small amount (teaspoon) of soft food, such as applesauce, custard, ice cream, oatmeal, pudding, or yogurt. To open, hold the capsule upright so that you can read the word "TOP." Carefully twist off the clear portion of the capsule. It may be best to do this over the small portion of the food onto which you will be pouring the sprinkles. Sprinkle the entire contents of the capsule onto the food. Be sure the patient swallows the entire spoonful of the sprinkle/food mixture immediately without chewing. Follow with fluids immediately to make sure all of the mixture is swallowed. Never store a sprinkle/food mixture for use at another time.
- A 6 mg/mL oral suspension may be compounded by pharmacy for pediatric patients.
- *DNC:* Swallow extended-release capsules *(Trokendi XR)* whole; do not sprinkle on food, break, crush, dissolve, or chew.
- *DNC:* Swallow extended-release capsules *(Qudexy XR)* whole; may be opened and sprinkled on soft food; do not crush or chew. Swallow immediately; do not save for later.

Patient/Family Teaching

- Instruct patient to take topiramate exactly as directed. Take missed doses as soon as possible but not just before next dose; do not double doses. Notify health care professional if more than 1 dose is missed. Medication should be gradually discontinued to prevent seizures and status epilepticus. Instruct patient to read the *Medication Guide* before starting and with each Rx refill in case of changes.
- May cause decreased sweating and increased body temperature. Advise patients, especially parents of pediatric patients, to provide adequate hydration and monitoring, especially during hot weather.
- May cause dizziness, drowsiness, confusion, and difficulty concentrating. Caution patients to avoid driving or other activities requiring alertness until response to medication is known.
- Advise patient to maintain a fluid intake of 2000–3000 mL of fluid/day to prevent the formation of kidney stones.
- Instruct patient to notify health care professional immediately if periorbital pain or blurred vision occur. Medication should be discontinued if ocular symptoms occur. May lead to permanent loss of vision.
- Advise patient and family to notify health care professional if thoughts about suicide or dying, attempts to commit suicide; new or worse depression; new or worse anxiety; feeling very agitated or restless; panic attacks; trouble sleeping; new or worse irritability; acting aggressive; being angry or violent; acting on dangerous impulses; an extreme increase in activity and talking; other unusual changes in behavior or mood; or rash occur.
- Inform patients that topiramate may cause encephalopathy. If signs and symptoms (unexplained lethargy, vomiting, changes in mental status) occur, notify health care professional.
- Caution patient to make position changes slowly to minimize orthostatic hypotension.
- Instruct patient to notify health care professional of all Rx or OTC medications, vitamins, or herbal products being taken and consult health care professional before taking any new medications.
- Advise patient not to take alcohol or other CNS depressants concurrently with this medication. Avoid alcohol 6 hr before and 6 hr after taking *Trokendi XR*.
- Instruct patient to notify health care professional of medication regimen before treatment or surgery.
- Advise patient to use sunscreen and wear protective clothing to prevent photosensitivity reactions.
- Rep: May cause fetal harm. Infants exposed to topiramate during pregnancy are at increased risk for cleft lip and/or cleft palate and for being small for gestational age. Advise patient to use a nonhormonal form of contraception while taking topiramate; may make hormonal contraceptives less effective. Notify

health care professional if pregnancy is planned or suspected or if breastfeeding. If pregnancy occurs, encourage patient to enroll in the North American Drug Pregnancy Registry by calling 1-888-233-2334 or online at http://www.aedpregnancyregistry.org/.
- Advise patient to carry identification describing disease and medication regimen at all times.

Evaluation/Desired Outcomes

- Absence or reduction of seizure activity.
- Decrease in incidence and severity of migraine headaches.
- Remission of manic symptoms.

HIGH ALERT

topotecan (toe-poe-**tee**-kan)
Hycamtin
Classification
Therapeutic: antineoplastics
Pharmacologic: enzyme inhibitors

Indications

IV: Metastatic ovarian cancer that has not responded to previous chemotherapy. Small cell lung cancer unresponsive to first line therapy. Stage IV-B persistent or recurrent cervical cancer not amenable to treatment with surgery or radiation (with cisplatin). **PO:** Relapsed small cell lung cancer in patients with a complete or partial prior response and who are at least 45 days from the end of first-line chemotherapy.

Action

Interferes with DNA synthesis by inhibiting the enzyme topoisomerase. **Therapeutic Effects:** Death of rapidly replicating cells, particularly malignant ones.

Pharmacokinetics

Absorption: IV administration results in complete bioavailability. 40% absorbed following oral administration.

Distribution: Well distributed to tissues.

Metabolism and Excretion: Small amounts metabolized by the liver. 18–33% excreted in feces and 20–50% excreted in urine (primarily as metabolites).

Half-life: *PO:* 3–6 hr; *IV:* 2–3 hr.

TIME/ACTION PROFILE (effects on WBCs)

ROUTE	ONSET	PEAK	DURATION
PO	unknown	1–2 hr	24 hr
IV	within days	11 days	7 days

Contraindications/Precautions

Contraindicated in: Hypersensitivity; OB: Pregnancy; Lactation: Lactation.

Use Cautiously in: Renal impairment ($\downarrow$ dose if CCr <40 mL/min); Platelet count <25,000 cells/mm^3 ($\downarrow$ dose); History of interstitial lung disease (ILD), pul-

T

monary fibrosis, lung cancer, thoracic radiation, or use of pneumotoxic drugs or colony stimulating factors; Rep: Women of reproductive potential; Geri: Older adults may require dose ↓ due to age-related ↓ in renal function.

Adverse Reactions/Side Effects

Derm: alopecia. **GI:** abdominal pain, diarrhea, nausea, vomiting, ↑ liver enzymes, anorexia, constipation, stomatitis. **Hemat:** anemia, leukopenia, thrombocytopenia. **MS:** arthralgia. **Neuro:** headache, fatigue, weakness. **Resp:** dyspnea, ILD.

Interactions

Drug-Drug: **P-glycoprotein inhibitors**, including **amiodarone**, **azithromycin**, **captopril**, **carvedilol**, **clarithromycin**, **conivaptan**, **cyclosporine**, **diltiazem**, **dronedarone**, **erythromycin**, **felodipine**, **itraconazole**, **ketoconazole**, **lopinavir**, **ritonavir**, **quinidine**, **ranolazine**, **ticagrelor**, or **verapamil** may ↑ levels and the risk of toxicity; avoid concurrent use. Neutropenia is prolonged by concurrent use of **filgrastim** (do not use filgrastim until day 6; 24 hr following completion of topotecan). ↑ myelosuppression with other **antineoplastics** (especially **cisplatin**) or **radiation therapy**. May ↓ antibody response to and ↑ risk of adverse reactions from **live virus vaccines**.

Route/Dosage

PO (Adults): 2.3 mg/m²/day for 5 days starting on day 1 of a 21-day course (round calculated oral dose to nearest 0.25 mg and prescribe the minimum number of 1 mg and 0.25 mg capsules with the same number of capsules prescribed for each of the 5 days).

IV (Adults): *Ovarian and Small Cell Lung Cancer:* 1.5 mg/m²/day for 5 days starting on day 1 of a 21-day course; *Cervical Cancer:* 75 mg/m² on Days 1, 2, and 3 followed by cisplatin on Day 1 and repeated every 21 days.

Renal Impairment

PO (Adults): *CCr 30–49 mL/min:* 1.5 mg/m²/day for 5 days starting on day 1 of a 21-day course; dose may be ↑ after first course by 0.4 mg/m²/day if no severe hematologic or GI toxicities occur; *CCr <30 mL/min:* 0.6 mg/m²/day for 5 days starting on day 1 of a 21-day course; dose may be ↑ after first course by 0.4 mg/m²/day if no severe hematologic or GI toxicities occur.

Renal Impairment

IV (Adults): *CCr 20–39 mL/min:* 0.75 mg/m²/day for 5 days starting on day 1 of a 21-day course. *Cervical Cancer:* Administer at standard doses only if serum creatinine ≤1.5 mg/dL. Do not administer if serum creatinine >1.5 mg/dL.

Availability (generic available)

Capsules: 0.25 mg, 1 mg. **Powder for injection:** 4 mg/vial. **Solution for injection:** 1 mg/mL.

NURSING IMPLICATIONS

Assessment

- Monitor vital signs frequently during administration.
- Monitor for bone marrow depression. Assess for bleeding (bleeding gums, bruising, petechiae; guaiac stools, urine, and emesis) and avoid IM injections and taking rectal temperatures if platelet count is low. Apply pressure to venipuncture sites for 10 min. Assess for signs of infection during neutropenia. Anemia may occur. Monitor for increased fatigue, dyspnea, and orthostatic hypotension.
- Nausea and vomiting are common. Pretreatment with antiemetics should be considered.
- Assess IV site frequently for extravasation, which causes mild local erythema and bruising.
- Monitor for signs and symptoms of ILD (cough, fever, dyspnea, hypoxia). Discontinue topotecan if ILD is confirmed.

Lab Test Considerations

- Verify negative pregnancy test before starting therapy. Monitor CBC with differential and platelet count prior to administration and frequently during therapy. Baseline neutrophil count of ≥1500 cells/mm³ and platelet count of ≥100,000 cells/mm³ are required before first dose. The nadir of neutropenia occurs in 11 days, with a duration of 7 days. The nadir of thrombocytopenia occurs in 15 days, with a duration of 5 days. The nadir of anemia occurs in 15 days. Subsequent doses should not be administered until neutrophils recover to >1000 cells/mm³, platelets recover to >100,000 cells/mm³, and hemoglobin levels recover to 9 g/dL. **When topotecan used as a single agent,** ↓ dose to 1.25 mg/m² if *neutrophil <500 cells/mm³*, or administer granulocyte-colony stimulating factor (G-CSF) starting no sooner than 24 hr following the last dose or *platelet counts <25,000 cells/mm³* during previous cycle. **When topotecan used with cisplatin,** ↓ dose to 0.6 mg/m² (and to 0.45 mg/m² if necessary) for febrile neutropenia (*neutrophil counts <1,000 cells/mm³ with temperature of ≥38°C (100.4°F)*, or administer G-CSF starting no sooner than 24 hr following the last dose or *platelet counts <25,000 cells/mm³* during previous cycle.
- Monitor liver function. May cause transient ↑ in AST, ALT, and bilirubin concentrations.

Implementation

- ***High Alert:*** Check dose carefully before administration.
- **PO:** May be taken without regard to food. *DNC:* Capsules must be swallowed whole; do not open, crush, or chew. If patient vomits after taking dose, do not replace dose.
- Do not administer capsules to patients with Grade 3 or 4 diarrhea. When recovered to ≤Grade 1, resume with dose ↓ by 0.4 mg/m²/day for subsequent courses.

IV Administration

- Solution should be prepared in a biologic cabinet. Wear gloves, gown, and mask while handling IV medication. Discard IV equipment in specially designated containers.
- **Intermittent Infusion:** *Reconstitution:* Reconstitute each vial with 4 mL of sterile water for injection. *Dilution:* Dilute further in D5W or 0.9% NaCl. Infusion is stable for 24 hr at room temperature or up to 7 days if refrigerated. Solution is yellow to yellow-green. *Concentration:* 10–50 mcg/mL. *Rate:* Infuse over 30 min.
- **Y-Site Compatibility:** alemtuzumab, amikacin, amiodarone, anidulafungin, argatroban, aztreonam, bivalirudin, buprenorphine, butorphanol, calcium chloride, carboplatin, caspofungin, cefazolin, cefotaxime, cefotetan, cefoxitin, ceftriaxone, cefuroxime, chloramphenicol, chlorpromazine, ciprofloxacin, cisatracurium, cisplatin, cyclophosphamide, cyclosporine, dacarbazine, dactinomycin, daptomycin, daunorubicin hydrochloride, dexmedetomidine, dexrazoxane, diltiazem, diphenhydramine, dobutamine, docetaxel, dopamine, doxorubicin hydrochloride, doxorubicin liposomal, doxycycline, droperidol, enalaprilat, ephedrine, epinephrine, erythromycin, esmolol, etoposide, etoposide phosphate, famotidine, fentanyl, fluconazole, fludarabine, furosemide, gemcitabine, gemtuzumab ozogamicin, gentamicin, glycopyrrolate, granisetron, haloperidol, heparin, hetastarch, hydralazine, hydrocortisone, hydromorphone, idarubicin, ifosfamide, insulin regular, isoproterenol, labetalol, leucovorin, levofloxacin, lidocaine, linezolid, lorazepam, magnesium sulfate, mannitol, meperidine, methylprednisolone, metoclopramide, metoprolol, metronidazole, midazolam, milrinone, mitoxantrone, morphine, moxifloxacin, nalbuphine, naloxone, nitroglycerin, nitroprusside, norepinephrine, octreotide, ondansetron, oxaliplatin, paclitaxel, palonosetron, pamidronate, pentamidine, phenylephrine, potassium chloride, procainamide, prochlorperazine, promethazine, propranolol, remifentanil, succinylcholine, sufentanil, tacrolimus, theophylline, thiotepa, tigecycline, tirofiban, tobramycin, vancomycin, vasopressin, vecuronium, verapamil, vinblastine, vincristine, vinorelbine, voriconazole, zidovudine, zoledronic acid.
- **Y-Site Incompatibility:** acyclovir, allopurinol, amifostine, aminophylline, amphotericin B deoxycholate, amphotericin B lipid complex, ampicillin, ampicillin/sulbactam, bumetanide, calcium gluconate, cefepime, ceftazidime, clindamycin, dantrolene, dexamethasone, diazepam, digoxin, ertapenem, fluorouracil, foscarnet, fosphenytoin, ganciclovir, hydrocortisone, imipenem/cilastatin, ketorolac, meropenem, methohexital, mitomycin, nafcillin, pantoprazole, pemetrexed, pentobarbital, phenobarbital, phenytoin, piperacillin/tazobactam, potassium acetate, potassium phosphate, rituximab, sodium bicarbonate, sodium phosphate, thiopental, trastuzumab, trimethoprim/sulfamethoxazole.

Patient/Family Teaching

- Instruct patient to take as directed. If patient vomits after taking, do not replace dose; notify health care professional. Do not take missed doses; take next scheduled dose and notify health care professional. If any capsules are broken or leaking, do not touch with bare hands; dispose of capsules and wash hands with soap and water. Patient should be instructed to read the *Patient Information* guide prior to first dose and with each Rx refill in case of changes.
- May cause drowsiness or sleepiness during and for several days after therapy. Caution patient to avoid driving and other activities requiring alertness until response to medication is known.
- Instruct patient to notify health care professional if fever; chills; sore throat; signs of infection; bleeding gums; bruising; petechiae; blood in urine, stool; emesis; or signs and symptoms of interstitial lung disease occur. Caution patient to avoid crowds and persons with known infections. Instruct patient to use soft toothbrush and electric razor. Patient should be cautioned not to drink alcoholic beverages or take products containing aspirin or NSAIDs.
- May cause diarrhea. Advise patient to notify health care professional if diarrhea with fever or stomach pain or cramps or diarrhea that occurs more than 3 times/day.
- Advise patient to notify health care professional of all Rx or OTC medications, vitamins, or herbal products being taken and to consult with health care professional before taking other medications.
- Discuss with patient the possibility of hair loss. Explore methods of coping.
- Instruct patient not to receive any vaccinations without advice of health care professional.
- Rep: May cause fetal harm. Advise females of reproductive potential to use effective contraception during and for 6 months after last dose of topotecan and to avoid breastfeeding during and for 1 wk after last dose. Advise males with female partners of reproductive potential to use effective contraception during and for 3 months after last dose. May impair fertility in females and males.
- Emphasize the need for periodic lab tests to monitor for side effects.

Evaluation/Desired Outcomes

- Decrease in size and spread of malignancy.

---

torsemide (tore-se-mide)

~~Demadex~~, Soaanz

Classification
Therapeutic: antihypertensives
Pharmacologic: loop diuretics

Indications

Edema due to: HF, Hepatic or renal disease. Hypertension.

Action

Inhibits the reabsorption of sodium and chloride from the loop of Henle and distal renal tubule. Increases renal excretion of water, sodium, chloride, magnesium, hydrogen, and calcium. Effectiveness persists in impaired renal function. **Therapeutic Effects:** Diuresis and subsequent mobilization of excess fluid (edema, pleural effusions). Decreased BP.

Pharmacokinetics

Absorption: 80% absorbed after oral administration.
Distribution: Widely distributed to tissues.
Protein Binding: ≥99%.
Metabolism and Excretion: Primarily metabolized by the liver via the CYP2C9 isoenzyme, with minor metabolism via the CYP2C8 and CYP2C18 isoenzymes. 80% metabolized by liver, 20% excreted in urine.
Half-life: 3.5 hr.

TIME/ACTION PROFILE (diuretic effect)

ROUTE	ONSET	PEAK	DURATION
PO	within 60 min	60–120 min	6–8 hr

Contraindications/Precautions

Contraindicated in: Hypersensitivity; Cross-sensitivity with thiazide diuretics and sulfonamides may occur; Hepatic coma; Anuria.
Use Cautiously in: Severe hepatic impairment (may precipitate hepatic coma; concurrent use with potassium-sparing diuretics may be necessary); Electrolyte depletion; Severe renal impairment and hypoproteinemia (↑ risk of ototoxicity); Diabetes mellitus; Increasing azotemia; OB: Safety not established in pregnancy; Lactation: Safety not established in breastfeeding; Pedi: Safety and effectiveness not established in children; Geri: Older adults may have ↑ risk of side effects, especially hypotension and electrolyte imbalance, at usual doses.

Adverse Reactions/Side Effects

CV: hypotension. **Derm:** photosensitivity, rash, STEVENS-JOHNSON SYNDROME (SJS), TOXIC EPIDERMAL NECROLYSIS (TEN). **EENT:** hearing loss, tinnitus. **Endo:** hyperglycemia. **F and E:** dehydration, hypochloremia, hypokalemia, hypomagnesemia, hyponatremia, hypovolemia, metabolic alkalosis, hypocalcemia. **GI:** constipation, diarrhea, dry mouth, dyspepsia, nausea, vomiting. **GU:** acute renal failure, excessive urination, renal impairment. **Metab:** hyperuricemia. **MS:** arthralgia, muscle cramps, myalgia. **Neuro:** dizziness, headache, nervousness.

Interactions

Drug-Drug: ↑ hypotension with **antihypertensives**, **nitrates**, or acute ingestion of **alcohol**. ↑ risk of hypokalemia with other **diuretics**, **amphotericin B**, **stimulant laxatives**, and **corticosteroids**. Hypokalemia may ↑ risk of **digoxin** toxicity and ↑ risk of arrhythmia in patients taking drugs that prolong the QT interval. **CYP2C9 inhibitors**, including **amiodarone**, **fluconazole**, and **miconazole**, may ↑ levels and the risk of toxicity. **CYP2C9 inducers**, including **rifampin**, may ↓ levels and effectiveness. May ↑ levels and the risk of toxicity of **CYP2C9 substrates**, including **celecoxib**, **phenytoin**, or **warfarin**. ↑ risk of nephrotoxicity with other **nephrotoxic drugs**, including **aminoglycosides**, **cisplatin**, **NSAIDs**, **ACE inhibitors**, **angiotensin II receptor blockers**, and **radiocontrast agents**. May ↑ the risk of **lithium** toxicity. ↑ risk of ototoxicity with **aminoglycosides**. **NSAIDs** may ↓ effectiveness. May ↑ the risk of **salicylate** toxicity (with use of high-dose **salicylate** therapy). **Cholestyramine** may ↓ absorption.

Route/Dosage

Heart Failure

PO (Adults): *Generic or Soaanz:* 20 mg once daily; dose may be doubled until desired effect is obtained (max = 200 mg/day).

Chronic Renal Failure

PO (Adults): *Generic or Soaanz:* 20 mg once daily; dose may be doubled until desired effect is obtained (max = 200 mg/day).

Hepatic Cirrhosis

PO (Adults): *Generic only:* 5–10 mg once daily (with aldosterone antagonist or potassium-sparing diuretic); dose may be doubled until desired effect is obtained (max = 40 mg/day).

Hypertension

PO (Adults): *Generic only:* 2.5–5 mg once daily, may be ↑ to 10 mg once daily after 4–6 wk (if still not effective, add another agent).

Availability (generic available)

Tablets: 5 mg, 10 mg, 20 mg, 40 mg, 60 mg, 100 mg.

NURSING IMPLICATIONS

Assessment

- Assess fluid status during therapy. Monitor daily weight, intake and output ratios, amount and location of edema, lung sounds, skin turgor, and mucous membranes. Notify health care professional if thirst, dry mouth, lethargy, weakness, hypotension, or oliguria occurs.

- Monitor BP and pulse before and during administration. Monitor frequency of prescription refills to determine adherence in patients treated for hypertension.

- Assess patients receiving digoxin for anorexia, nausea, vomiting, muscle cramps, paresthesia, and confusion. Patients taking digoxin are at increased risk of digoxin toxicity due to potassium-depleting effect of the diuretic. Potassium supplements or potassium-sparing diuretics may be used concurrently to prevent hypokalemia.
- Assess patient for tinnitus and hearing loss. Audiometry is recommended for patients receiving prolonged high-dose IV therapy. Hearing loss is most common following rapid or high-dose IV administration in patients with decreased renal function or those taking other ototoxic drugs.
- Assess for allergy to sulfonamides.
- Assess patient for skin rash frequently during therapy. Discontinue torsemide at first sign of rash; may be life-threatening. SJS or TEN may develop. Treat symptomatically; may recur once treatment is stopped.
- Geri: Diuretic use is associated with increased risk for falls in older adults. Assess falls risk and implement fall prevention strategies.

Lab Test Considerations
- Monitor electrolytes, renal and hepatic function, serum glucose, and uric acid levels before and periodically during therapy. May cause ↓ serum sodium, potassium, calcium, and magnesium concentrations. May also cause ↑ BUN, serum glucose, serum creatinine, and uric acid levels.

Implementation
- Administer medication in the morning to prevent disruption of sleep cycle.
- **PO:** May be taken with food or milk to minimize gastric irritation.

Patient/Family Teaching
- Instruct patient to take torsemide as directed. Take missed doses as soon as possible; do not double doses.
- Caution patient to change positions slowly to minimize orthostatic hypotension. Caution patient that the use of alcohol, exercise during hot weather, or standing for long periods during therapy may enhance orthostatic hypotension.
- Instruct patient to consult health care professional regarding a diet high in potassium (see Appendix J).
- Advise patient to contact health care professional if they gain more than 2–3 lb/day.
- Instruct patient to notify health care professional of all Rx or OTC medications, vitamins, or herbal products being taken and to consult health care professional before taking any OTC medications concurrently with this therapy.
- Instruct patient to notify health care professional of medication regimen prior to treatment or surgery.

- Caution patient to use sunscreen and protective clothing to prevent photosensitivity reactions.
- Advise patient to contact health care professional immediately if rash muscle weakness, cramps, nausea, dizziness, numbness, or tingling of extremities occurs.
- Advise diabetic patients to monitor blood glucose closely; may cause increased blood glucose levels.
- Rep: Advise females of reproductive potential to notify health care professional if pregnancy is planned or suspected or if breastfeeding.
- Emphasize the importance of routine follow-up examinations.
- **Hypertension:** Advise patients on antihypertensive regimen to continue taking medication even if feeling better. Torsemide controls but does not cure hypertension.
- Reinforce the need to continue additional therapies for hypertension (weight loss, exercise, restricted sodium intake, stress reduction, regular exercise, moderation of alcohol consumption, cessation of smoking).

Evaluation/Desired Outcomes
- Decrease in edema.
- Decrease in abdominal girth and weight.
- Increase in urinary output.
- Decrease in BP.

REMS

☷traMADol (tra-ma-dol)
ConZip, ✹Durela, Qdolo, ✹Ralivia, ✹Tridural, U̶l̶t̶r̶a̶m̶, U̶l̶t̶r̶a̶m̶ ̶E̶R̶, ✹Zytram XL

Classification
Therapeutic: analgesics (centrally acting), opioid analgesics
Pharmacologic: opioid agonists

Schedule IV

Indications
Moderate to moderately severe pain (extended-release formulations indicated for patients who require around-the-clock pain management).

Action
Acts as a μ-opioid receptor agonist. Inhibits reuptake of serotonin and norepinephrine in the CNS. **Therapeutic Effects:** Decreased pain.

Pharmacokinetics
Absorption: *Immediate-release:* 75% absorbed after oral administration; *Extended-release:* 85–90% (compared with immediate-release).
Distribution: Crosses the placenta; enters breast milk.

Metabolism and Excretion: ⧸ Mostly metabolized by the liver (primarily by the CYP2D6 and CYP3A4 isoenzymes); primarily metabolized by the CYP2D6 isoenzyme to active metabolite with analgesic activity (M1); CYP2D6 enzyme system exhibits genetic polymorphism; ~7% of population may be poor metabolizers and may have significantly ↑ concentrations of tramadol and ↓ concentrations of M1 metabolite. 1–10% of Whites, 3–4% of Blacks, and 1–2% of East Asians may be CYP2D6 ultra-rapid metabolizers and have significantly ↑ concentrations of M1 metabolite. 30% eliminated unchanged in the urine.

Half-life: *Tramadol (immediate release):* 6–8 hr, *Extended release:* 7.9 hr; *Active metabolite:* 7–9 hr; both are ↑ in renal or hepatic impairment.

TIME/ACTION PROFILE (analgesia)

ROUTE	ONSET	PEAK	DURATION
PO-immediate release	1 hr	2–3 hr	4–6 hr
PO-extended release	unknown	12 hr	24 hr

Contraindications/Precautions

Contraindicated in: Hypersensitivity; Cross-sensitivity with opioids may occur; Significant respiratory depression; Acute or severe bronchial asthma (in unmonitored setting or in absence of resuscitative equipment); Known or suspected GI obstruction (including paralytic ileus); Concurrent use of monoamine oxidase (MAO) inhibitors (or use within the past 14 days); Patients who are acutely intoxicated with alcohol, sedatives/hypnotics, centrally acting analgesics, opioid analgesics, or psychotropic agents; Patients who are physically dependent on opioid analgesics (may precipitate withdrawal); ⧸ Ultra-rapid metabolizers of CYP2D6 (↑ risk of respiratory depression and death); CCr <30 mL/min or hepatic impairment (extended release); Lactation: Lactation; Pedi: Children <12 yr, children <18 yr following tonsillectomy and/or adenoidectomy, and children 12–18 yr who are postoperative; have obstructive sleep apnea, obesity, severe pulmonary disease, or neuromuscular disease; or are taking other medications that cause respiratory depression (↑ risk of respiratory depression and death).

Use Cautiously in: History of epilepsy or risk factors for seizures; Diabetes mellitus (↑ risk of hypoglycemia); Renal impairment (↑ dosing interval recommended if CCr <30 mL/min); Hepatic impairment (↑ dosing interval recommended in patients with cirrhosis); Suicidal or prone to addiction (↑ risk of suicide); Excessive use of alcohol (↑ risk of suicide); ↑ intracranial pressure or head trauma; History of opioid dependence or recent use of large doses of opioids; OB: Use during pregnancy only if potential maternal benefit justifies potential fetal risk; Geri: *Immediate release:* Not to exceed 300 mg/day in patients >75 yr; *Extended release:* Use with extreme caution in patients >75 yr. ↑ risk of hyponatremia in females >65 yr.

Adverse Reactions/Side Effects

Derm: pruritus, sweating. **EENT:** visual disturbances. **Endo:** hypoglycemia. **F and E:** hyponatremia. **GI:** constipation, nausea, abdominal pain, anorexia, diarrhea, dry mouth, dyspepsia, flatulence, vomiting. **GU:** ↓ fertility, menopausal symptoms, urinary retention/frequency. **Neuro:** dizziness, headache, somnolence, anxiety, confusion, coordination disturbance, euphoria, hypertonia, malaise, nervousness, SEIZURES, sleep disorder, stimulation, weakness. **Resp:** RESPIRATORY DEPRESSION (including central sleep apnea and sleep-related hypoxemia). **Misc:** physical dependence, psychological dependence, tolerance.

Interactions

Drug-Drug: MAO inhibitors ↑ risk of adverse reactions; concurrent use or use within previous 14 days contraindicated. ↑ risk of CNS depression when used concurrently with other **CNS depressants**, including **alcohol, antihistamines, sedative/hypnotics, opioid analgesics, anesthetics,** or **psychotropic agents.** Mixed agonist/antagonist analgesics, including **nalbuphine** or **butorphanol,** and **partial agonist analgesics,** including **buprenorphine,** may ↓ tramadol's analgesic effects and/or precipitate opioid withdrawal in physically dependent patients. ↑ risk of seizures with high doses of **penicillins, cephalosporins, phenothiazines, opioid analgesics,** or **antidepressants.** Carbamazepine ↑ metabolism and ↓ effectiveness of tramadol (increased doses may be required). CYP2D6 inhibitors, including **quinidine, fluoxetine, paroxetine,** and **bupropion,** may ↓ levels of active metabolite (M1) and lead to ↓ analgesic effects. CYP3A4 inhibitors, including **erythromycin, clarithromycin, ketoconazole, itraconazole,** and **protease inhibitors,** may allow for a greater degree of metabolism via CYP2D6 and ↑ levels of the active metabolite (M1) leading to respiratory depression. CYP3A4 inducers may ↓ levels and effectiveness. Drugs that affect serotonergic neurotransmitter systems, including **SSRIs, SNRIs, MAO inhibitors, TCAs, trazodone, mirtazapine, 5-HT$_3$ receptor antagonists, linezolid, methylene blue,** and **triptans,** ↑ risk of serotonin syndrome.

Drug-Natural Products: Concomitant use of **kava-kava, valerian,** or **chamomile** can ↑ CNS depression. ↑ risk of serotonin syndrome when used with **St. John's wort.**

Route/Dosage

Immediate Release

PO (Adults ≥18 yr): *Rapid titration:* 50–100 mg every 4–6 hr (not to exceed 400 mg/day [300 mg in patients >75 yr]). *Gradual titration:* 25 mg/day initially, ↑ by 25 mg/day every 3 days to reach dose of 25 mg 4 times daily, then ↑ by 50 mg/day every 3 days to reach dose of 50 mg 4 times daily; may then use 50–100 mg every 4–6 hr (maximum dose = 400 mg/day).

Renal Impairment
PO (Adults): *CCr <30 mL/min:* ↑ dosing interval to every 12 hr (not to exceed 200 mg/day).

Hepatic Impairment
PO (Adults): *Severe hepatic impairment:* 50 mg every 12 hr.

Extended Release
PO (Adults): *Not currently receiving immediate-release:* 100 mg once daily initially, may then titrate every 5 days up to 300 mg/day; *Currently receiving immediate-release:* calculate 24-hr total dose of immediate-release product and give same dose (rounded down to next lowest 100-mg increment) of ER once daily (maximum dose = 300 mg/day).

Availability (generic available)
Immediate-release tablets: 50 mg, 100 mg. **Extended-release capsules (Conzip):** 100 mg, 200 mg, 300 mg. **Extended-release tablets:** ✿ 75 mg, 100 mg, ✿ 150 mg, 200 mg, 300 mg, ✿ 400 mg. **Oral solution (grape flavor):** 5 mg/mL. *In combination with:* acetaminophen; celecoxib (Seglentis). See Appendix N.

NURSING IMPLICATIONS
Assessment
- Assess type, location, and intensity of pain before and 2–3 hr (peak) after administration.
- Assess BP and respiratory rate before and periodically during administration. Respiratory depression has not occurred with recommended doses.
- Assess bowel function routinely. Prevention of constipation should be instituted with increased intake of fluids and bulk and with laxatives to minimize constipating effects. Administer stimulant laxatives routinely if opioid use exceeds 2–3 days, unless contraindicated. Consider drugs for opioid-induced constipation.
- Prolonged use may lead to physical and psychological dependence and tolerance, although these may be milder than with other opioids. This should not prevent patient from receiving adequate analgesia. Patients who receive tramadol for pain rarely develop psychological dependence. If tolerance develops, changing to an opioid agonist may be required to relieve pain. Prolonged use of opioids should be reserved for patients whose pain remains severe enough to require them and alternative treatment options continue to be inadequate. Many acute pain conditions treated in the outpatient setting require no more than a few days of an opioid pain medicine.
- Monitor for signs and symptoms of hyponatremia (confusion, disorientation) during therapy, especially during early therapy. If signs and symptoms of hyponatremia occur, begin treatment (fluid restriction) and discontinue tramadol.

- Monitor patient for seizures. May occur within recommended dose range. Risk is increased with higher doses and in patients taking antidepressants (SSRIs, SNRIs, TCAs, or MAO inhibitors), opioid analgesics, or other drugs that decrease the seizure threshold. Also monitor for serotonin syndrome (mental-status changes [e.g., agitation, hallucinations, coma], autonomic instability [e.g., tachycardia, labile BP, hyperthermia], neuromuscular aberrations [e.g., hyperreflexia, incoordination] and/or GI symptoms [e.g., nausea, vomiting, diarrhea] in patients taking these drugs concurrently).
- Assess risk for opioid addiction, abuse, or misuse prior to administration. Abuse or misuse of extended-release preparations by crushing, chewing, snorting, or injecting dissolved product will result in uncontrolled delivery of tramadol and can result in overdose and death.

Lab Test Considerations
- May cause ↑ serum creatinine, ↑ liver enzymes, ↓ hemoglobin, and proteinuria.
- May cause hyponatremia and hypoglycemia. Monitor blood glucose levels in patients with predisposing risk factors, including diabetes, renal insufficiency, or in elderly patients.

Toxicity and Overdose
- Overdose may cause respiratory depression and seizures. Naloxone may reverse some, but not all, of the symptoms of overdose. Treatment should be symptomatic and supportive. Maintain adequate respiratory exchange. Hemodialysis is not helpful because it removes only a small portion of administered dose. Seizures may be managed with barbiturates or benzodiazepines; naloxone increases risk of seizures.

Implementation
- **High Alert:** Do not confuse tramadol with trazodone.
- Tramadol is considered to provide more analgesia than codeine 60 mg but less than combined aspirin 650 mg/codeine 60 mg for acute postoperative pain.
- For chronic pain, daily doses of 250 mg of tramadol provide pain relief similar to that of 5 doses/day of acetaminophen 300 mg/codeine 30 mg, 5 doses/day of aspirin 325 mg/codeine 30 mg, or 2–3 doses/day of acetaminophen 500 mg/oxycodone 5 mg.
- Explain therapeutic value of medication before administration to enhance the analgesic effect.
- Regularly administered doses may be more effective than as-needed administration. Analgesic is more effective if given before pain becomes severe.
- Tramadol should be discontinued gradually after long-term use to prevent withdrawal symptoms. For patients on long-acting agents who are physically opioid-dependent, initiate the taper by a small enough increment (no greater than 10%–25% of

T

total daily dose) to avoid withdrawal symptoms, and proceed with dose-lowering at an interval of every 2–4 wk. Patients who have been taking opioids for briefer periods of time may tolerate a more rapid taper. Monitor frequently to manage pain and withdrawal symptoms (restlessness, lacrimation, rhinorrhea, yawning, perspiration, chills, myalgia, mydriasis, irritability, anxiety, backache, joint pain, weakness, abdominal cramps, insomnia, nausea, anorexia, vomiting, diarrhea, or increased blood pressure, respiratory rate, or heart rate). If withdrawal symptoms occur, pause the taper for a period of time or raise the dose of opioid analgesic to the previous dose, and then proceed with a slower taper. Also, monitor patients for changes in mood, emergence of suicidal thoughts, or use of other substances. A multimodal approach to pain management may optimize the treatment of chronic pain, as well as assist with the successful tapering of the opioid analgesic.

- **PO:** Tramadol may be administered without regard to meals. **DNC:** Swallow extended-release tablets and capsules whole; do not crush, break, dissolve, or chew.
- **REMS:** FDA strongly encourages health care professionals to complete a REMS-compliant education program that includes all the elements of the FDA Education *Blueprint for Health Care Providers Involved in the Management or Support of Patients with Pain,* available at www.fda.gov/OpioidAnalgesicREMSBlueprint. Information on programs can be found at 1-800-503-0784 or www.opioidanalgesicrems.com.
- Discuss availability of naloxone for emergency treatment of opioid overdose with the patient and caregiver and assess the potential need for access to naloxone, both when initiating and renewing therapy, especially if patient has household members (including children) or other close contacts at risk for accidental exposure or overdose. Consider prescribing naloxone, based on the patient's risk factors for overdose, such as concomitant use of CNS depressants, a history of opioid use disorder, or prior opioid overdose. However, the presence of risk factors for overdose should not prevent the proper management of pain in any patient.

Patient/Family Teaching

- **REMS:** Instruct patient on how and when to ask for pain medication. Do not stop taking without discussing with health care professional; may cause withdrawal symptoms if discontinued abruptly after prolonged use. Do not increase doses without discussing with health care professional; may lead to overdose. Discuss safe use, risks, and proper storage and disposal of opioid analgesics with patients and caregivers with each Rx. The Patient Counseling Guide is available at https://opioidanalgesicrems.com/patientCounselingGuide.html.

- May cause dizziness and drowsiness. Caution patient to avoid driving or other activities requiring alertness until response to medication is known.
- Advise patient that tramadol is a drug with known abuse potential. Protect it from theft, and never give to anyone other than the individual for whom it was prescribed. Store out of sight and reach of children, and in a location not accessible by others.
- Educate patients and caregivers on how to recognize respiratory depression and emphasize the importance of calling 911 or getting emergency medical help right away in the event of a known or suspected overdose. Inform patients and caregivers about ways to obtain naloxone as permitted by individual state naloxone dispensing and prescribing requirements or guidelines (by prescription, directly from a pharmacist, or as part of a community-based program).
- Advise patient to change positions slowly to minimize orthostatic hypotension.
- Caution patient to avoid concurrent use of alcohol or other CNS depressants, including other opioids, with this medication. Advise patient to notify health care professional before taking other RX, OTC, or herbal products concurrently.
- Advise patient to notify health care professional if seizures or if symptoms of serotonin syndrome occur.
- Encourage patient to turn, cough, and breathe deeply every 2 hr to prevent atelectasis.
- Rep: Advise patient to notify health care professional if pregnancy is planned or suspected and to avoid breastfeeding during therapy. Inform patient of potential for neonatal opioid withdrawal syndrome with prolonged use during pregnancy. Monitor neonate for signs and symptoms of withdrawal symptoms (irritability, hyperactivity and abnormal sleep pattern, high pitched cry, tremor, vomiting, diarrhea, and/or failure to gain weight); usually occur the first days after birth. Monitor infants exposed to tramadol through breast milk for excess sedation and respiratory depression. Neonatal seizures, fetal death, and still birth have been reported with tramadol immediate-release products. Chronic use may reduce fertility in females and males.
- Emphasize the importance of aggressive prevention of constipation with the use of tramadol.

Evaluation/Desired Outcomes

- Decrease in severity of pain without a significant alteration in level of consciousness or respiratory status.

---

trandolapril, See ANGIOTENSIN-CONVERTING ENZYME (ACE) INHIBITORS.

HIGH ALERT

⌘ trastuzumab
(traz-**too**-zoo-mab)
Herceptin, Herzuma, Kanjinti, Ogivri, Ontruzant, Trazimera
Classification
Therapeutic: antineoplastics
Pharmacologic: monoclonal antibodies

Indications
⌘ HER2-overexpressing metastatic gastric or gastroesophageal adenocarcinoma in patients who have not received prior treatment for metastatic disease (in combination with cisplatin and capecitabine or 5-fluorouracil). ⌘ HER2-overexpressing node-positive or node-negative breast cancer (as part of one of the following regimens: doxorubicin, cyclophosphamide, and either paclitaxel or docetaxel; or docetaxel and carboplatin) (as adjuvant therapy). ⌘ HER2-overexpressing node-positive or node-negative breast cancer (to be used alone after multi-modality anthracycline-based therapy) (as adjuvant therapy). ⌘ HER2-overexpressing metastatic breast cancer (as first-line therapy) (in combination with paclitaxel). ⌘ HER2-overexpressing metastatic breast cancer in patients who have already received ≥1 other chemotherapy regimens for metastatic disease (as monotherapy).

Action
⌘ A monoclonal antibody that binds to HER2 sites in breast cancer tissue and inhibits proliferation of cells that overexpress HER2 protein. **Therapeutic Effects:** Regression of breast, gastric, or gastroesophageal cancer and metastases.

Pharmacokinetics
Absorption: IV administration results in complete bioavailability.
Distribution: Unknown.
Metabolism and Excretion: Unknown.
Half-life: Unknown.

TIME/ACTION PROFILE (plasma concentrations)

ROUTE	ONSET	PEAK	DURATION
IV	unknown	unknown	unknown

Contraindications/Precautions
Contraindicated in: OB: Pregnancy; Lactation: Lactation.
Use Cautiously in: Pre-existing pulmonary conditions; Hypersensitivity to trastuzumab, Chinese hamster ovary cell proteins, or other components of the product; Hypersensitivity to benzyl alcohol (use sterile water for injection instead of bacteriostatic water, which accompanies the vial); Rep: Women of reproductive po-

tential; Pedi: Safety not established in children; Geri: Older adults may have ↑ risk of cardiotoxicity.
Exercise Extreme Caution in: Patients with pre-existing cardiac dysfunction.

Adverse Reactions/Side Effects
CV: ARRHYTHMIAS, HF, hypertension, tachycardia. **Derm:** rash, acne, herpes simplex. **EENT:** pharyngitis, rhinitis, sinusitis. **F and E:** edema. **GI:** abdominal pain, anorexia, diarrhea, nausea, vomiting. **Hemat:** anemia, leukopenia. **MS:** pain, arthralgia, bone pain. **Neuro:** depression, dizziness, headache, insomnia, neuropathy, paresthesia, peripheral neuritis, weakness. **Resp:** cough, dyspnea, INTERSTITIAL PNEUMONITIS, PULMONARY EDEMA, PULMONARY FIBROSIS. **Misc:** chills, fever, INFECTION, flu-like syndrome, HYPERSENSITIVITY REACTIONS (including anaphylaxis and angioedema).

Interactions
Drug-Drug: Concurrent use of **anthracyclines**, including **daunorubicin**, **doxorubicin**, or **idarubicin**, may ↑ risk of cardiotoxicity. **Paclitaxel** may ↑ levels and risk of toxicity.

Route/Dosage

Adjuvant Treatment of Breast Cancer
IV (Adults): *During and following paclitaxel, docetaxel, or docetaxel/carboplatin:* 4 mg/kg initially, then 2 mg/kg once weekly during chemotherapy for the first 12 wk (paclitaxel or docetaxel) or 18 wk (docetaxel/carboplatin); 1 wk after the last weekly dose, give 6 mg/kg every 3 wk. Do not exceed treatment duration of 1 yr; *As single agent within 3 wk following completion of multi-modality, anthracycline-based chemotherapy regimens:* 8 mg/kg initially, then 6 mg/kg every 3 wk. Do not exceed treatment duration of 1 yr.

Metastatic Breast Cancer
IV (Adults): 4 mg/kg initially, then 2 mg/kg once weekly until disease progression.

Metastatic Gastric Cancer
IV (Adults): 8 mg/kg initially, then 6 mg/kg every 3 wk until disease progression.

Availability
Lyophilized powder for injection: 150 mg/vial, 420 mg/vial.

NURSING IMPLICATIONS
Assessment
● Assess for infusion-related symptoms (chills, fever, nausea, vomiting, pain [in some cases at tumor sites], headache, dizziness, dyspnea, hypotension, rash, and asthenia) following initial infusion. Severe reactions (bronchospasm, anaphylaxis, angioedema, hypoxia, severe hypotension) may occur during or immediately following the initial infusion. May be treated with epinephrine, corticosteroids, diphenhydramine, bron-

T

chodilators, and oxygen. Discontinue if dyspnea or severe hypotension occurs and discontinue permanently if severe reaction occurs.

● Assess for signs and symptoms of HF (dyspnea, increased cough, paroxysmal nocturnal dyspnea, peripheral edema, S_3 gallop, reduced ejection fraction) prior to and frequently during therapy. Baseline cardiac assessment of history, physical exam, and left ventricular ejection fraction (LVEF) with ECG or multiple gated acquisition scan. Monitor LVEF every 3 mo and at completion of therapy, every 6 mo for 2 yr. Withhold trastuzumab for ≥16% absolute decrease in LVEF from pretreatment values or an LVEF value below institutional limits of normal and ≥10% absolute decrease in LVEF from pretreatment values. Repeat LVEF measures every 4 wk if dose is withheld. HF associated with trastuzumab may be severe, resulting in cardiac failure, death, and stroke. Trastuzumab should be discontinued upon the development of significant HF.

● Monitor patient for signs of pulmonary hypersensitivity reactions (dyspnea, pulmonary infiltrates, pleural effusion, noncardiogenic pulmonary edema, pulmonary insufficiency, hypoxia, acute respiratory distress syndrome). Patients with symptomatic pulmonary disease or extensive lung tumor involvement are at increased risk. Infusion should be discontinued if severe symptoms occur.

Lab Test Considerations

● Verify negative pregnancy test before starting therapy. 🏶 *HER2* protein overexpression is used to determine whether treatment with trastuzumab is indicated. *HER2* protein overexpression is detected by Hercep-Test (IHC assay) and PathVysion (FISH assay).

● May cause anemia and leukopenia.

Implementation

● *High Alert:* Do not confuse trastuzumab with ado-trastuzumab.

● *High Alert:* Fatalities have occurred with chemotherapeutic agents. Before administering, clarify all ambiguous orders; double check single, daily, and course-of-therapy dose limits; have second practitioner independently double check original order, dose calculations and infusion pump settings.

● May be administered in the outpatient setting.

● *If a dose is missed by ≤1 wk,* administer usual maintenance dose as soon as possible. Do not wait until next planned cycle. Administer subsequent maintenance doses 7 days or 21 days later according to the weekly or three-weekly schedules, respectively. *If a dose is missed by >1 wk,* administer a reloading dose as soon as possible. Administer subsequent maintenance doses 7 days or 21 days later according to weekly or three-weekly schedules, respectively.

IV Administration

● **Intermittent Infusion:** *Reconstitution:* Reconstitute each vial with 20 mL of bacteriostatic water for injection, directing the stream of diluent into lyophilized cake of trastuzumab. *Concentration:* 21 mg/mL. Swirl the vial gently; do not shake. May foam slightly; allow the vial to stand undisturbed for 5 min. Solution should be clear to slightly opalescent and colorless to pale yellow, without particulate matter. Label vial immediately in the area marked "Do not use after" with the date 28 days from the date of reconstitution. Stable for 24 hr at room temperature or 28 days if refrigerated. If patient is allergic to benzyl alcohol, use sterile water for injection for reconstitution. Use immediately and discard any unused portion. *Dilution:* Calculate to volume required for the desired dose, withdraw, and add it to an infusion containing 250 mL of 0.9% NaCl. Invert bag gently to mix. *Rate:* Infuse the 4 mg/kg loading dose over 90 min and the weekly 2 mg/kg dose over 30 min or 6 mg/kg dose over 30–90 min every 3 wk, or 8 mg/kg dose over 90 min if the loading dose was well tolerated. Do not administer as an IV push or bolus.

● **Y-Site Compatibility:** acyclovir, amifostine, aminophylline, ampicillin, ampicillin/sulbactam, bleomycin, bumetanide, buprenorphine, busulfan, butorphanol, calcium gluconate, carboplatin, carmustine, cefazolin, ceftazidime, ceftriaxone, cefuroxime, ciprofloxacin, cisplatin, cyclophosphamide, cytarabine, dactinomycin, daunorubicin hydrochloride, dexamethasone, digoxin, diphenhydramine, dobutamine, docetaxel, dopamine, doxorubicin hydrochloride, doxorubicin liposomal, doxycycline, droperidol, enalaprilat, etoposide phosphate, famotidine, fentanyl, filgrastim, fluconazole, fluorouracil, ganciclovir, gemcitabine, gentamicin, granisetron, haloperidol, heparin, hydrocortisone, hydromorphone, ifosfamide, imipenem/cilastatin, leucovorin calcium, lorazepam, magnesium sulfate, mannitol, meperidine, mesna, methotrexate, methylprednisolone, metoclopramide, metronidazole, mitomycin, mitoxantrone, paclitaxel, pentamidine, potassium chloride, prochlorperazine, promethazine, remifentanil, sargramostim, sodium bicarbonate, theophylline, thiotepa, tobramycin, trimethoprim/sulfamethoxazole, vancomycin, vinblastine, vincristine, vinorelbine, zidovudine.

● **Y-Site Incompatibility:** aldesleukin, amikacin, aztreonam, cefotaxime, cefotetan, cefoxitin, chlorpromazine, clindamycin, cyclosporine, fludarabine, furosemide, idarubicin, irinotecan, levofloxacin, morphine, nalbuphine, ondansetron, piperacillin/tazobactam, topotecan.

● **Additive Incompatibility:** Do not dilute trastuzumab with or add to solutions containing dextrose. Do not mix or dilute with other drugs.

Patient/Family Teaching

● Explain purpose of trastuzumab to patient.

● Instruct patient to notify health care professional promptly if new onset or worsening shortness of breath, cough, swelling of the ankles/legs, swelling of the face, palpitations, weight gain of more than 5 pounds in 24 hr, dizziness or loss of consciousness occur. Caution patient to avoid crowds and persons with known infections.

● Advise patient not to receive any vaccinations without advice of health care professional.

● Rep: May cause fetal harm. Advise females of reproductive potential to notify health care professional immediately if pregnancy is planned or suspected or if breastfeeding. Caution patient to use effective contraception during and for 7 mo following last dose. Monitor infants exposed to trastuzumab for oligohydramnios, pulmonary hypoplasia, skeletal abnormalities, and neonatal death. Advise women who are breastfeeding to discontinue nursing or discontinue trastuzumab. Encourage women who may be exposed during pregnancy to report exposure to the Genentech Adverse Event Line at 1-888-835-2555.

Evaluation/Desired Outcomes

● Regression of breast, gastric, or gastroesophageal cancer and metastases.

⸚ trastuzumab/hyaluronidase
(traz-**too**-zoo-mab/hye-al-yoor-**on**-i-dase)

Herceptin Hylecta, ✽Herceptin SC

Classification
Therapeutic: antineoplastics
Pharmacologic: monoclonal antibodies

Indications

⸚ Human epidermal growth factor receptor 2 (HER2)-overexpressing node-positive or node-negative breast cancer (as part of one of the following regimens: doxorubicin, cyclophosphamide, and either paclitaxel or docetaxel; or docetaxel and carboplatin) (as adjuvant therapy). ⸚ HER2-overexpressing node-positive or node-negative breast cancer (to be used alone after multimodality anthracycline-based therapy) (as adjuvant therapy). ⸚ HER2-overexpressing metastatic breast cancer (as first-line therapy) (in combination with paclitaxel). ⸚ HER2-overexpressing metastatic breast cancer in patients who have already received ≥1 other chemotherapy regimens for metastatic disease (as monotherapy).

Action

Trastuzumab: ⸚A monoclonal antibody that binds to *HER2* sites in breast cancer tissue and inhibits proliferation of cells that overexpress *HER2* protein; *Hyaluronidase:* Acts locally by depolymerizing hyaluronan, which increases permeability of the SUBQ tissue. **Therapeutic Effects:** Regression of breast cancer and metastases.

Pharmacokinetics

Absorption: 77% absorbed following SUBQ administration.

Distribution: Minimally distributed to tissues.
Metabolism and Excretion: Unknown.
Half-life: Unknown.

TIME/ACTION PROFILE (plasma concentrations)

ROUTE	ONSET	PEAK	DURATION
SUBQ	Unknown	1–4 days	Unknown

Contraindications/Precautions

Contraindicated in: OB: Pregnancy.

Use Cautiously in: Pulmonary disease or extensive tumor involvement of lungs (↑ risk of pulmonary toxicity); Dyspnea at rest (↑ risk of hypersensitivity reaction); Lactation: Use while breastfeeding only if potential maternal benefit justifies potential risk to infant; Rep: Women of reproductive potential; Pedi: Safety and effectiveness in children not established; Geri: Older adults may have ↑ risk of cardiac dysfunction.

Exercise Extreme Caution in: Pre-existing cardiac dysfunction.

Adverse Reactions/Side Effects

CV: <u>edema</u>, ARRHYTHMIAS, HF, hypertension, SUDDEN CARDIAC DEATH. **Derm:** <u>alopecia</u>, <u>flushing</u>, <u>rash</u>, erythema, pruritus, skin discoloration. **EENT:** epistaxis. **GI:** ↓ <u>appetite</u>, <u>abdominal pain</u>, <u>constipation</u>, <u>diarrhea</u>, dyspepsia, <u>nausea</u>, stomatitis, <u>vomiting</u>, ↑ liver enzymes. **GU:** menstrual abnormalities, urinary tract infection. **Hemat:** <u>anemia</u>, <u>leukopenia</u>, NEUTROPENIA. **Local:** injection site pain. **MS:** arthralgia, <u>myalgia</u>. **Neuro:** dizziness, dysgeusia, <u>headache</u>, <u>peripheral neuropathy</u>, insomnia. **Resp:** <u>cough</u>, <u>upper respiratory tract infection</u>, ACUTE RESPIRATORY DISTRESS SYNDROME, dyspnea, INTERSTITIAL PNEUMONITIS, pleural effusion, PULMONARY EDEMA, PULMONARY FIBROSIS. **Misc:** <u>fatigue</u>, <u>fever</u>, HYPERSENSITIVITY REACTIONS (including anaphylaxis and angioedema).

Interactions

Drug-Drug: Concurrent administration of myelosuppressive **chemotherapy drugs** may worsen degree of neutropenia. Concurrent **anthracycline** (**daunorubicin, doxorubicin,** or **idarubicin**) therapy may ↑ risk of cardiotoxicity; if possible, avoid anthracycline-based therapy for up to 7 mo after stopping trastuzumab hyaluronidase.

Route/Dosage

Do not substitute with or for ado-trastuzumab emtansine. Dosage and route of administration is different from trastuzumab.

SUBQ (Adults): Trastuzumab 600 mg/hyaluronidase 10,000 units every 3 wk for 52 wk or disease recurrence, whichever occurs first (for adjuvant therapy) or until disease progression (for metastatic disease).

T

Availability

Solution for injection: trastuzumab 120 mg and hyaluronidase 2,000 units/mL.

NURSING IMPLICATIONS

Assessment

● Conduct thorough cardiac assessment, including history, physical examination, and determination of left ventricular ejection fraction (LVEF) by echocardiogram or MUGA scan immediately before starting therapy. Determine LVEF measurements every 3 mo during and upon completion of therapy. Repeat LVEF measures at 4 wk intervals if trastuzumab hyaluronidase is held for LVEF dysfunction. Conduct LVEF measurements every 6 mo for at least 2 years following completion of therapy. *If ≥16% absolute ↓ in LVEF from pretreatment values or LVEF is below institutional limits of normal and ≥10% absolute ↓ in LVEF from pretreatment values,* hold trastuzumab hyaluronidase for at least 4 wk. Therapy may be resumed if, within 4–8 wk, LVEF returns to normal limits and absolute ↓ from baseline is ≤15%. *If persistent (>8 wk) LVEF decline or suspension of trastuzumab hyaluronidase for >3 occasions for cardiomyopathy,* permanently discontinue trastuzumab hyaluronidase.
● Monitor patient for signs and symptoms of pulmonary toxicity (dyspnea, pulmonary infiltrates, pleural effusion, noncardiogenic pulmonary edema, pulmonary insufficiency, hypoxia, acute respiratory distress syndrome). Patients with symptomatic pulmonary disease or extensive lung tumor involvement are at increased risk. Infusion should be discontinued if severe symptoms occur.
● Monitor for signs and symptoms of hypersensitivity reactions especially during first administration. Permanently discontinue trastuzumab hyaluronidase in patients with anaphylaxis or severe hypersensitivity reactions.

Lab Test Considerations

● Verify negative pregnancy status before starting therapy. ▣ Patient selection is based on *HER2* protein overexpression or *HER2* gene amplification in tumor specimens. Assessment of *HER2* protein overexpression and *HER2* gene amplification should be performed using FDA-approved tests specific for breast cancer by laboratories with demonstrated proficiency. Information on FDA-approved tests for the detection of *HER2* protein overexpression and *HER2* gene amplification is available at: http://www.fda.gov/CompanionDiagnostics.

Implementation

● *High Alert:* Do not confuse trastuzumab hyaluronidase (Herceptin Hylecta) with trastuzumab (Herceptin) or with ado-trastuzumab (Kadcyla).
● Extending therapy beyond 1 yr is not recommended.
● Before administration, check the vial to ensure that drug being administered is trastuzumab hyaluronidase and not IV trastuzumab or ado-trastuzumab.

● **SUBQ:** Injection should be administered by a health care professional. Solution does to not need to be diluted. Solution is colorless to yellowish and clear to opalescent; do not administer solutions that are cloudy, discolored, or contain particulate matter. Syringes are for single use only. Attach the hypodermic injection needle to the syringe immediately prior to administration to avoid clogging the needle, then adjust volume to 5 mL. Solution is compatible with polypropylene and polycarbonate syringe material and stainless steel transfer and injection needles. Solution is stable for 24 hr if refrigerated or 4 hr at room temperature; protect from light. Do not freeze or shake. Alternate injection between right and left thigh. Give new injection at least 2.5 cm from previous injection site. Avoid areas where skin is red, bruised, tender, or hard, or areas where there are moles or scars. Administer dose over 2–5 min.

Patient/Family Teaching

● Explain purpose of trastuzumab hyaluronidase to patient.
● Advise patients to contact a health care professional immediately if signs and symptoms of HF (new onset or worsening shortness of breath, cough, swelling of the ankles/legs, swelling of face, palpitations, weight gain >5 pounds in 24 hr, dizziness, loss of consciousness) or hypersensitivity reactions (dizziness, nausea, chills, fever, vomiting, diarrhea, urticaria, angioedema, breathing problems, chest pain) occur.
● Rep: May cause fetal harm (oligohydramnios, pulmonary hypoplasia, skeletal abnormalities, neonatal death). Advise females of reproductive potential to use effective contraception during and for 7 mo after last dose. Monitor women who received trastuzumab hyaluronidase during pregnancy or within 7 mo prior to conception for oligohydramnios. If oligohydramnios occurs, perform fetal testing. Advise patients to notify health care professional if pregnancy is suspected or if breastfeeding. Inform patient of *Pregnancy Pharmacovigilance Program.* Patients who become pregnant during or with 7 mo of therapy should call immediately to report exposure to Genentech at 1-888-835-2555.

Evaluation/Desired Outcomes

● Regression of breast cancer and metastases.

---

traZODone (traz-oh-done)
~~Desyrel~~
Classification
Therapeutic: antidepressants

Indications

Major depression. **Unlabeled Use:** Insomnia.

Action

Alters the effects of serotonin in the CNS. **Therapeutic Effects:** Antidepressant action, which may develop only over several wk.

Pharmacokinetics

Absorption: Well absorbed after oral administration.
Distribution: Widely distributed to tissues.
Protein Binding: 89–95%.
Metabolism and Excretion: Extensively metabolized by the liver via the CYP3A4 isoenzyme; minimal excretion of unchanged drug by the kidneys.
Half-life: 5–9 hr.

TIME/ACTION PROFILE (antidepressant effect)

ROUTE	ONSET	PEAK	DURATION
PO	1–2 wk	2–4 wk	wk

Contraindications/Precautions

Contraindicated in: Hypersensitivity; Recovery period after MI; Concurrent electroconvulsive therapy; Concurrent use of MAO inhibitors or MAO inhibitor-like drugs (linezolid or methylene blue); Angle-closure glaucoma; Lactation: Lactation.
Use Cautiously in: Cardiovascular disease; Suicidal behavior; Severe renal impairment (dose ↓ recommended); Severe hepatic impairment (dose ↓ recommended); OB: Other agents preferred for treatment of depression or insomnia in pregnancy; Pedi: Safety and effectiveness not established in children; suicide risk may be greater in children and adolescents; Geri: Initial dose ↓ recommended in older adults.

Adverse Reactions/Side Effects

CV: hypotension, arrhythmias, chest pain, hypertension, palpitations, QT interval prolongation, tachycardia. **Derm:** rash. **EENT:** blurred vision, tinnitus. **GI:** dry mouth, constipation, diarrhea, excess salivation, flatulence, nausea, vomiting. **GU:** erectile dysfunction, hematuria, priapism, urinary frequency. **Hemat:** anemia, leukopenia. **MS:** myalgia. **Neuro:** drowsiness, confusion, dizziness, dysgeusia, fatigue, hallucinations, headache, insomnia, nightmares, slurred speech, SUICIDAL THOUGHTS, syncope, tremor, weakness.

Interactions

Drug-Drug: Serious, potentially fatal reactions (hyperthermia, rigidity, myoclonus, autonomic instability, with fluctuating vital signs and extreme agitation, which may proceed to delirium and coma) may occur with concurrent **MAO inhibitors**. MAO inhibitors should be stopped at least 14 days before trazodone therapy. Trazodone should be stopped at least 14 days before MAO inhibitor therapy. Concurrent use with **MAO-inhibitor like drugs**, such as **linezolid** or **methylene blue**, may ↑ risk of serotonin syndrome; concurrent use contraindicated; do not start therapy in patients receiving **linezolid** or **methylene blue**; if **linezolid** or **methylene blue** need to be started in a patient receiving trazodone, immediately discontinue trazodone and monitor for signs/symptoms of serotonin syndrome for

2 wk or until 24 hr after last dose of linezolid or methylene blue, whichever comes first (may resume trazodone therapy 24 hr after last dose of linezolid or methylene blue). May ↑ **digoxin** or **phenytoin** levels and the risk of toxicity. ↑ CNS depression with other **CNS depressants**, including **alcohol**, **opioid analgesics**, and **sedative/hypnotics**. ↑ risk of hypotension with **antihypertensives**, acute ingestion of **alcohol**, or **nitrates**. **Fluoxetine** may ↑ levels and the risk of toxicity. **CYP3A4 inhibitors**, including **ritonavir** and **ketoconazole**, may ↑ levels and the risk of toxicity. **CYP3A4 inducers**, including **carbamazepine**, may ↓ levels and its effectiveness. Drugs that affect serotonergic neurotransmitter systems, including **tricyclic antidepressants**, **fentanyl**, **buspirone**, **tramadol** and **triptans**, may ↑ the risk of serotonin syndrome. ↑ risk of bleeding with **NSAIDs**, **aspirin**, **clopidogrel**, **prasugrel**, **ticagrelor**, or **warfarin**.
Drug-Natural Products: Concomitant use of **kava-kava**, **valerian**, or **chamomile** can ↑ CNS depression. ↑ risk of serotonergic side effects including serotonin syndrome with **St. John's wort** and **SAMe**.

Route/Dosage

Depression
PO (Adults): 150 mg/day in 3 divided doses; ↑ by 50 mg/day every 3–4 days until desired response (not to exceed 400 mg/day in outpatients or 600 mg/day in hospitalized patients).
PO (Geriatric Patients): 75 mg/day in divided doses initially; may be ↑ every 3–4 days.

Insomnia
PO (Adults): 25–100 mg at bedtime.

Availability (generic available)
Tablets: 50 mg, 100 mg, 150 mg, 300 mg.

NURSING IMPLICATIONS

Assessment

- Monitor BP and pulse rate before and during initial therapy. Monitor ECGs in patients with pre-existing cardiac disease before and periodically during therapy to detect arrhythmias.
- Assess for possible sexual dysfunction.
- Assess for serotonin syndrome (mental changes [agitation, hallucinations, coma], autonomic instability [tachycardia, labile BP, hyperthermia], neuromuscular aberrations [hyper-reflexia, incoordination], and/or GI symptoms [nausea, vomiting, diarrhea]), especially in patients taking other serotonergic drugs (SSRIs, SNRIs, triptans).
- **Depression:** Assess mental status (orientation, mood, and behavior) frequently.
- Assess for suicidal tendencies, especially during early therapy. Restrict amount of drug available to patient. Risk may be increased in children, adolescents, and adults ≤24 yr. After starting therapy, chil-

T

dren, adolescents, and young adults should be seen by health care professional at least weekly for 4 wk, every 3 wk for next 4 wk, and on advice of health care professional thereafter.

Lab Test Considerations
● Assess CBC and renal and hepatic function before and periodically during therapy. Slight, clinically insignificant ↓ in leukocyte and neutrophil counts may occur.

Implementation
● Do not confuse trazodone with tramadol.
● **PO:** Administer with or immediately after meals to minimize side effects (nausea, dizziness) and allow maximum absorption of trazodone. A larger portion of the total daily dose may be given at bedtime to decrease daytime drowsiness and dizziness.

Patient/Family Teaching
● Instruct patient to take medication as directed. If a dose is missed, take as soon as remembered. Do not take if within 4 hr of next scheduled dose; do not double doses. Consult health care professional before discontinuing medication; gradual dose reduction is necessary to prevent aggravation of condition. Advise patient to read *Medication Guide* prior starting therapy and with each Rx refill in case of changes.
● May cause drowsiness and blurred vision. Caution patient to avoid driving and other activities requiring alertness until response to drug is known.
● Caution patient to change positions slowly to minimize orthostatic hypotension.
● Advise patient to avoid concurrent use of alcohol or other CNS depressant drugs.
● Advise patient, family, and caregivers to look for suicidality, especially during early therapy or dose changes. Notify health care professional immediately if thoughts about suicide or dying, attempts to commit suicide, new or worse depression or anxiety, agitation or restlessness, panic attacks, insomnia, new or worse irritability, aggressiveness, acting on dangerous impulses, mania, or other changes in mood or behavior or if symptoms of serotonin syndrome occur.
● Advise patient to notify health care professional of all Rx or OTC medications, vitamins, or herbal products being taken and to consult with health care professional before taking other medications, especially aspirin and NSAIDs.
● Inform patient that frequent rinses, good oral hygiene, and sugarless candy or gum may diminish dry mouth. Health care professional should be notified if this persists >2 wk. An increase in fluid intake, fiber, and exercise may prevent constipation.
● Advise patient to notify health care professional of medication regimen before treatment or surgery.
● Instruct patient to notify health care professional if priapism, irregular heartbeat, fainting, confusion, skin rash, or tremors occur or if dry mouth, nausea

and vomiting, dizziness, headache, muscle aches, constipation, or diarrhea becomes pronounced.
● Instruct patient to notify health care professional if signs of serotonin syndrome (mental status changes: agitation, hallucinations, coma; autonomic instability: tachycardia, labile BP, hyperthermia; neuromuscular aberrations: hyperreflexia, incoordination; and/or gastrointestinal symptoms: nausea, vomiting, diarrhea) occur.
● Rep: Advise females of reproductive potential to notify health care professional if pregnancy is planned and to not breastfeeding during therapy.
● Emphasize the importance of follow-up exams to evaluate progress.

Evaluation/Desired Outcomes
● Resolution of depression.
● Increased sense of well-being.
● Renewed interest in surroundings.
● Increased appetite.
● Improved energy level.
● Improved sleep.

triamcinolone, See CORTICOSTEROIDS (NASAL).

triamcinolone, See CORTICOSTEROIDS (SYSTEMIC).

triamcinolone, See CORTICOSTEROIDS (TOPICAL/LOCAL).

triamterene, See DIURETICS (POTASSIUM-SPARING).

BEERS

☒ trimethoprim/ sulfamethoxazole
(trye-**meth**-oh-prim/sul-fa-meth-**ox**-a-zole)
Bactrim, Bactrim DS, ✦Septra, ✦Sulfatrim, ✦Sulfatrim DS, Sulfatrim Pediatric
Classification
Therapeutic: anti-infectives, antiprotozoals
Pharmacologic: folate antagonists, sulfonamides

Indications
Treatment of: Bronchitis, *Shigella* enteritis, Otitis media, *Pneumocystis jirovecii* pneumonia (PJP), Urinary tract infections, Traveler's diarrhea. Prevention of PJP in patients with HIV. **Unlabeled Use:** Biliary tract infections, osteomyelitis, burn and wound infections,

chlamydial infections, endocarditis, gonorrhea, intra-abdominal infections, nocardiosis, rheumatic fever prophylaxis, sinusitis, eradication of meningococcal carriers, prophylaxis of urinary tract infections, and an alternative agent in the treatment of chancroid. Prevention of bacterial infections in immunosuppressed patients.

Action
Combination inhibits the metabolism of folic acid in bacteria at two different points. **Therapeutic Effects:** Bactericidal action against susceptible bacteria. **Spectrum:** Active against many strains of gram-positive aerobic pathogens including: *Streptococcus pneumoniae, Staphylococcus aureus.* Has activity against many aerobic gram-negative pathogens, such as: *Enterobacter, Klebsiella, Morganella morganii, Escherichia coli, Proteus mirabilis, Proteus vulgaris, Shigella, Haemophilus influenzae. Pneumocystis jirovecii.* Not active against *Pseudomonas aeruginosa.*

Pharmacokinetics
Absorption: Well absorbed from the GI tract.
Distribution: Widely distributed to tissues. Crosses the blood-brain barrier.
Metabolism and Excretion: Some metabolism by the liver (20%); remainder excreted unchanged by the kidneys.
Half-life: *Trimethoprim (TMP):* 6–11 hr; *sulfamethoxazole (SMX):* 9–12 hr, both prolonged in renal failure.

TIME/ACTION PROFILE (plasma concentrations)

ROUTE	ONSET	PEAK	DURATION
PO	rapid	2–4 hr	6–12 hr
IV	rapid	end of infusion	6–12 hr

Contraindications/Precautions
Contraindicated in: Hypersensitivity to sulfonamides or trimethoprim; History of drug-induced immune thrombocytopenia due to sulfonamides or trimethoprim; Megaloblastic anemia secondary to folate deficiency; Severe renal impairment; Severe hepatic impairment; Concurrent use with dofetilide; Lactation: Avoid breastfeeding in infants who have glucose-6–phosphate dehydrogenase (G6PD) deficiency or hyperbilirubinemia; Pedi: Children <2 mo (can cause kernicterus).
Use Cautiously in: Mild or moderate renal impairment (dose ↓ required if CCr <30 mL/min); Mild or moderate hepatic impairment; ⚡ G6PD deficiency (↑ risk hemolysis); HIV (↑ incidence of adverse reactions); Concurrent use with other products containing propylene glycol (IV only) (↑ risk of lactic acidosis); OB: ↑ risk of neural tube defects, cardiovascular malformations, urinary tract defects, oral clefts, and club

foot in fetus when used during pregnancy; use during pregnancy only if potential maternal benefit justifies potential fetal risk; Lactation: Use while breastfeeding only if potential maternal benefit justifies potential risk to infant; Geri: Appears on Beers list. Use with caution in older adults taking an angiotensin-converting enzyme inhibitor, angiotensin II receptor blocker, or angiotensin receptor/neprilysin inhibitor, and in those with a reduced CCr because of ↑ risk of hyperkalemia.

Adverse Reactions/Side Effects
CV: hypotension. **Derm:** rash, ACUTE FEBRILE NEUTROPHILIC DERMATOSIS, ACUTE GENERALIZED EXANTHEMATOUS PUSTULOSIS, DRUG REACTION WITH EOSINOPHILIA AND SYSTEMIC SYMPTOMS (DRESS), ERYTHEMA MULTIFORME, FEBRILE NEUTROPHILIC DERMATOSIS, photosensitivity, STEVENS-JOHNSON SYNDROME (SJS), TOXIC EPIDERMAL NECROLYSIS. **Endo:** hypoglycemia. **F and E:** hyperkalemia, hyponatremia. **GI:** nausea, vomiting, cholestatic jaundice, CLOSTRIDIOIDES DIFFICILE-ASSOCIATED DIARRHEA (CDAD), diarrhea, HEPATIC NECROSIS, hepatitis, pancreatitis, stomatitis. **GU:** crystalluria. **Hemat:** AGRANULOCYTOSIS, APLASTIC ANEMIA, hemolytic anemia, leukopenia, megaloblastic anemia, thrombocytopenia. **Local:** phlebitis at IV site. **Neuro:** fatigue, hallucinations, headache, insomnia, kernicterus (neonates), mental depression. **Misc:** fever, HYPERSENSITIVITY REACTIONS (including anaphylaxis and respiratory failure).

Interactions
Drug-Drug: May ↑ **dofetilide** levels and the risk of QT interval prolongation with arrhythmias; concurrent use contraindicated. May ↑ levels and the risk of toxicity of **phenytoin**; closely monitor phenytoin levels. May ↑ levels of and the risk of bleeding from **warfarin**; closely monitor INR. May ↑ hypoglycemic effects of **sulfonylureas, pioglitazone, repaglinide,** and **metformin.** May ↑ toxicity of **methotrexate**; avoid concurrent use. ↑ risk of thrombocytopenia from **thiazide diuretics**, especially in older adults. May ↑ risk of nephrotoxicity associated with **cyclosporine**; avoid concurrent use. May ↑ levels and the risk of toxicity of **digoxin**, especially in older adults; closely monitor digoxin levels. **Indomethacin** may ↑ levels and the risk of toxicity; avoid concurrent use. **ACE inhibitors** may ↑ risk of hyperkalemia; avoid concurrent use. May ↓ the effects of **tricyclic antidepressants.** May ↑ risk of myelosuppression with **zidovudine.** May ↑ **procainamide** levels and the risk of QT interval prolongation with arrhythmias; closely monitor procainamide levels.

Route/Dosage
Dosing based on TMP content.

Bacterial Infections
PO, IV (Adults and Children >2 mo): *Mild to moderate infections:* 6–12 mg TMP/kg/day divided every 12 hr; *Serious infection/PJP:* 15–20 mg TMP/kg/day divided every 6–8 hr.

PO (Adults): *Urinary tract infection/chronic bronchitis:* 1 double-strength tablet (160 mg TMP/800 mg SMX) every 12 hr for 10–14 days.

Urinary Tract Infection Prophylaxis

PO, IV (Adults and Children >2 mo): 2 mg TMP/kg/dose once daily or 5 mg TMP/kg/dose twice weekly.

P. jirovecii Pneumonia Prevention

PO (Adults): 1 double-strength tablet (160 mg TMP/800 mg SMX) once daily (may also be given 3 times weekly).

PO (Children >1 mo): 150 mg TMP/m²/day divided every 12 hr or given as a single dose on 3 consecutive days/wk (not to exceed 320 mg TMP/1600 mg SMX per day).

Availability (generic available)

Tablets: ✿ 20 mg TMP/100 mg SMX, 80 mg TMP/400 mg SMX, 160 mg TMP/800 mg SMX (double-strength). **Oral suspension (cherry, grape flavors):** 40 mg TMP/200 mg SMX per 5 mL. **Solution for injection:** 16 mg TMP/80 mg SMX per mL (contains 40% propylene glycol).

NURSING IMPLICATIONS

Assessment

- Assess for infection (vital signs; appearance of wound, sputum, urine, and stool; WBC) at beginning of and during therapy.
- Obtain specimens for culture and sensitivity before initiating therapy. First dose may be given before receiving results.
- Inspect IV site frequently. Phlebitis is common.
- Assess patient for allergy to sulfonamides.
- Monitor intake and output ratios. Fluid intake should be sufficient to maintain a urine output of at least 1200–1500 mL daily to prevent crystalluria and stone formation.
- Monitor bowel function. Diarrhea, abdominal cramping, fever, and bloody stools should be reported to health care professional promptly as a sign of CDAD. May begin up to several wk following cessation of therapy.
- Assess for rash periodically during therapy. May cause SJS. Discontinue therapy if severe or if accompanied with fever, general malaise, fatigue, muscle or joint aches, blisters, oral lesions, conjunctivitis, hepatitis, and/or eosinophilia.

Lab Test Considerations

- Monitor CBC and urinalysis periodically during therapy.
- May produce ↑ serum bilirubin, serum potassium, serum creatinine, and alkaline phosphatase.
- May cause hypoglycemia.

Implementation

- Do not confuse DS (double-strength) formulations with single-strength formulations.
- Do not administer medication IM.

- **PO:** Administer around the clock with a full glass of water. Use calibrated measuring device for liquid preparations.

IV Administration

- **Intermittent Infusion:** *Dilution:* Dilute each 5 mL of trimethoprim/sulfamethoxazole with 125 mL of D5W (stable for 24 hr at room temperature). May also dilute each 5 mL of drug with 75 mL of D5W if fluid restriction is required (stable for 6 hr at room temperature). Do not refrigerate. *Concentration:* Should not exceed 1.06 mg/mL. *Rate:* Infuse over 60–90 min.

- **Y-Site Compatibility:** acyclovir, aldesleukin, alemtuzumab, allopurinol, amifostine, aminocaproic acid, amphotericin B deoxycholate, amphotericin B liposomal, anidulafungin, argatroban, arsenic trioxide, azithromycin, bivalirudin, bleomycin, cangrelor, carboplatin, carmustine, cefepime, ceftaroline, cisplatin, cyclophosphamide, cytarabine, dactinomycin, daptomycin, defibrotide, dexmedetomidine, diltiazem, docetaxel, doxorubicin liposomal, eptifibatide, ertapenem, etoposide, etoposide phosphate, filgrastim, fludarabine, fluorouracil, fosphenytoin, gemcitabine, gemtuzumab ozogamicin, granisetron, hetastarch, hydromorphone, ifosfamide, irinotecan, leucovorin calcium, levofloxacin, linezolid, lorazepam, melphalan, meropenem, mesna, methotrexate, metronidazole, milrinone, mitomycin, mitoxantrone, octreotide, oxaliplatin, paclitaxel, palonosetron, pamidronate, pemetrexed, perphenazine, piperacillin/tazobactam, potassium acetate, remifentanil, rituximab, sargramostim, sodium acetate, thiotepa, tigecycline, tirofiban, trastuzumab, vecuronium, vinblastine, vincristine, voriconazole, zidovudine, zoledronic acid.

- **Y-Site Incompatibility:** amikacin, aminophylline, amphotericin B lipid complex, ampicillin, ampicillin/sulbactam, ascorbic acid, atropine, azathioprine, benztropine, blinatumomab, bumetanide, buprenorphine, butorphanol, calcium chloride, calcium gluconate, caspofungin, cefazolin, cefotaxime, cefoxitin, ceftazidime, ceftriaxone, cefuroxime, chloramphenicol, chlorpromazine, clindamycin, cyanocobalamin, cyclosporine, dacarbazine, dantrolene, daunorubicin hydrochloride, dexamethasone, dexrazoxane, diazepam, digoxin, diphenhydramine, dobutamine, dopamine, doxorubicin hydrochloride, doxycycline, ephedrine, epinephrine, epirubicin, epoetin alfa, erythromycin, famotidine, fentanyl, fluconazole, folic acid, furosemide, ganciclovir, gentamicin, glycopyrrolate, haloperidol, hydralazine, hydrocortisone, hydroxyzine, idarubicin, imipenem/cilastatin, indomethacin, insulin regular, isoproterenol, ketamine, ketorolac, LR, lidocaine, mannitol, methadone, methylprednisolone, metoclopramide, metoprolol, midazolam, minocycline, multivitamins, mycophenolate, nafcillin, nalbuphine, naloxone, nitroglycerin, nitroprusside, norepinephrine, ondansetron, oritavancin, oxacillin, oxytocin, papaverine, penicillin G, pentamidine, pentobarbital, phenobarbital, phentol-amine, phenylephrine, phenytoin, phytonadione, po-tassium chloride, procainamide, prochlorperazine, promethazine, propranolol, protamine, pyridoxine, sodium bicarbonate, succinylcholine, sufentanil, theophylline, thiamine, tobramycin, topotecan, van-comycin, verapamil, vinorelbine.

Patient/Family Teaching

- Instruct patient to take medication around the clock and to finish drug completely as directed, even if feeling well. Take missed doses as soon as remem-bered unless almost time for next dose. Advise pa-tient that sharing of this medication may be danger-ous.

- Instruct patient to notify health care professional if rash or fever and diarrhea develop, especially if di-arrhea contains blood, mucus, or pus. Advise patient not to treat diarrhea without consulting health care professional.

- Caution patient to use sunscreen and protective clothing to prevent photosensitivity reactions.

- Advise patient to notify health care professional if skin rash, sore throat, fever, mouth sores, or un-usual bleeding or bruising occurs.

- Advise patient to notify health care professional of all Rx or OTC medications, vitamins, or herbal products being taken and to consult with health care profes-sional before taking other medications.

- Instruct patient to notify health care professional if symptoms do not improve within a few days.

- Rep: May cause fetal harm. Advise females of repro-ductive potential to notify health care professional if pregnancy is planned or suspected, or if breastfeed-ing. Fetal exposure during pregnancy may lead to in-creased risk of congenital malformations, neural tube defects, cardiovascular malformations, urinary tract defects, oral clefts, and club foot.

- Emphasize importance of regular follow-up exams to monitor blood counts in patients on prolonged therapy.

- **Home Care Issues:** Instruct family or caregiver on dilution, rate, and administration of drug and proper care of IV equipment.

Evaluation/Desired Outcomes

- Resolution of the signs and symptoms of infection. Length of time for complete resolution depends on organism and site of infection.

- Resolution of symptoms of traveler's diarrhea.

- Prevention of PJP pneumonia in patients with HIV.

ubrogepant (ue-**broe**-je-pant)
Ubrelvy

Classification
Therapeutic: vascular headache suppressants
Pharmacologic: calcitonin gene-related peptide receptor antagonists

Indications
Acute treatment of migraine with or without aura.

Action
Binds to and antagonizes the calcitonin gene-related peptide (CGRP) receptor, which reduces the neuroinflammatory and vasodilatory effects of CGRP. **Therapeutic Effects:** Relief of pain associated with acute migraine attacks.

Pharmacokinetics
Absorption: Rapidly absorbed. Absorption delayed by high-fat food.
Distribution: Widely distributed to tissues.
Metabolism and Excretion: Primarily metabolized by the liver via the CYP3A4 isoenzyme to inactive metabolites. Eliminated in bile/feces (42% as unchanged drugs) and urine (6% as unchanged drug).
Half-life: 5–7 hr.

TIME/ACTION PROFILE (pain relief)

ROUTE	ONSET	PEAK	DURATION
PO	30–60 min	2 hr	24 hr

Contraindications/Precautions
Contraindicated in: Hypersensitivity; Concurrent use of strong CYP3A4 inhibitors; End-stage renal disease (CCr <15 mL/min).
Use Cautiously in: Severe renal impairment (CCr 15–29 mL/min); Severe hepatic impairment (↓ dose); OB: Safety not established in pregnancy; Lactation: Safety not established in breastfeeding; Pedi: Safety and effectiveness not established in children.

Adverse Reactions/Side Effects
GI: dry mouth, nausea. **Neuro:** drowsiness. **Misc:** HYPERSENSITIVITY REACTIONS (including anaphylaxis and facial/throat edema).

Interactions
Drug-Drug: Strong CYP3A4 inhibitors, including **clarithromycin, itraconazole**, or **ketoconazole** may significantly ↑ levels and the risk of toxicity; concurrent use contraindicated. **Moderate CYP3A4 inhibitors** as well as **weak CYP3A4 inhibitors**, including **ciprofloxacin, cyclosporine, fluconazole, fluvoxamine**, or **verapamil**, may ↑ levels and the risk of toxicity; ↓ ubrogepant dose. **Strong CYP3A4 inducers**, including **phenobarbital, phenytoin**, or **rifampin**, may significantly ↓ levels and effectiveness; avoid concurrent use. **Moderate CYP3A4 inducers** or **weak CYP3A4 inducers** may ↓ levels and effectiveness; ↑ ubrogepant dose. **P-glycoprotein (P-gp) in-**hibitors as well as **breast cancer resistant protein (BCRP) inhibitors**, including **carvedilol, eltrombopag**, or **quinidine**, may ↑ levels and the risk of toxicity; ↓ ubrogepant dose.
Drug-Natural Products: St. John's wort may ↓ levels and effectiveness; avoid concurrent use.
Drug-Food: Grapefruit juice may ↑ levels and the risk of toxicity; ↓ ubrogepant dose.

Route/Dosage
PO (Adults): 50 mg or 100 mg initially; if response is inadequate at 2 hr, may repeat dose (not to exceed 200 mg/24 hr). *Concurrent use of moderate CYP3A4 inhibitors:* 50 mg initially (not to exceed 50 mg/24 hr). *Concurrent use of weak CYP3A4 inhibitors:* 50 mg initially; if response is inadequate at 2 hr, may repeat dose (not to exceed 100 mg/24 hr). *Concurrent use of weak or moderate CYP3A4 inducers:* 100 mg initially; if response is inadequate at 2 hr, may repeat dose (not to exceed 200 mg/24 hr). *Concurrent use of P-gp or BCRP inhibitors:* 50 mg initially; if response is inadequate at 2 hr, may repeat dose (not to exceed 100 mg/24 hr).

Renal Impairment
PO (Adults): *CCr 15–29 mL/min:* 50 mg initially; if response is inadequate at 2 hr, may repeat dose (not to exceed 100 mg/24 hr).

Hepatic Impairment
PO (Adults): *Severe hepatic impairment:* 50 mg initially; if response is inadequate at 2 hr, may repeat dose (not to exceed 100 mg/24 hr).

Availability
Tablets: 50 mg, 100 mg.

NURSING IMPLICATIONS
Assessment
- Assess pain location, character, intensity, and duration and associated symptoms (photophobia, phonophobia, nausea, vomiting) during migraine attack.

Implementation
- **PO:** Administer without regard to food. If needed, a second dose may be taken at least 2 hr after initial dose.

Patient/Family Teaching
- Instruct patient to take ubrogepant as soon as symptoms of a migraine attack appear, but it may be administered any time during an attack. If migraine symptoms return, a second dose may be used. Allow at least 2 hr between doses, and do not use more than 100 mg in any 24-hr period. Advise patient to read *Patient Information* before starting therapy and with each Rx refill in case of changes.
- Inform patient that ubrogepant should only be used during a migraine attack. It is meant to be used for relief of migraine attacks but not to prevent or reduce the number of attacks.
- Advise patient to avoid grapefruit and grapefruit juice during therapy. Instruct patient not take a sec-

ond tablet within 24 hr if grapefruit or grapefruit juice was consumed.
- May cause dizziness or drowsiness. Caution patient to avoid driving or other activities requiring alertness until response to medication is known.
- Advise patient to avoid alcohol, which aggravates headaches, during ubrogepant use.
- Advise patient that lying down in a darkened room following ubrogepant administration may further help relieve headache.
- Advise patient to notify health care professional of all Rx or OTC medications, vitamins, or herbal products being taken and to consult with health care professional before taking other medications, especially St. John's wort.
- Advise patient to notify health care professional immediately if signs and symptoms of hypersensitivity reactions (anaphylaxis, dyspnea, facial or throat swelling, rash, hives, itching) occur.
- Rep: Advise females of reproductive potential to notify health care professional if pregnancy is planned or suspected or if breastfeeding. Inform patient of pregnancy exposure registry that monitors outcomes in women who become pregnant while taking ubrogepant. Encourage patients to enroll by calling 1-833-277-0206 or visiting http://empresspregnancyregistry.com.

Evaluation/Desired Outcomes
- Relief of migraine attack.

ulipristal, See CONTRACEPTIVES, HORMONAL.

umeclidinium
(ue-mek-li-**din**-ee-um)
Incruse Ellipta
Classification
Therapeutic: bronchodilators
Pharmacologic: anticholinergics

Indications
Maintenance treatment of COPD.

Action
Acts as an anticholinergic by inhibiting M3 muscarinic receptors in bronchial smooth muscle resulting in bronchodilation. **Therapeutic Effects:** Bronchodilation with decreased airflow obstruction.

Pharmacokinetics
Absorption: Minimal oral absorption; remainder of absorption occurs in lungs.
Distribution: Unknown.
Metabolism and Excretion: Primarily metabolized by the liver via the CYP2D6 isoenzyme; metabolites do not contribute to bronchodilation.

Half-life: 11 hr.

TIME/ACTION PROFILE (bronchodilation)
ROUTE	ONSET	PEAK	DURATION
inhaln	1 hr	2–12 hr	24 hr

Contraindications/Precautions
Contraindicated in: Severe/acute symptoms of airflow obstruction; Severe hypersensitivity to milk proteins or other ingredients; Concurrent use with other anticholinergics.
Use Cautiously in: Narrow-angle glaucoma (may cause acute angle closure); Urinary retention, prostatic hyperplasia, bladder-neck obstruction; Severe hepatic impairment; OB: Safety not established in pregnancy; Lactation: Use while breastfeeding only if potential maternal benefit outweighs potential risk to infant; Pedi: Safety and effectiveness not established in children; Geri: Older adults may be more sensitive to drug effects.

Adverse Reactions/Side Effects
CV: chest pain. EENT: acute narrow-angle glaucoma, cough, nasopharyngitis. GU: urinary retention. MS: arthralgia. Resp: PARADOXICAL BRONCHOSPASM. Misc: HYPERSENSITIVITY REACTIONS (including anaphylaxis and angioedema).

Interactions
Drug-Drug: ↑ risk of anticholinergic adverse reactions when used concurrently with other **anticholinergics**; avoid concurrent use.

Route/Dosage
Inhaln (Adults): One inhalation (62.5 mcg) once daily.

Availability
Powder for inhalation in blister strips (contains lactose): 62.5 mcg/blister. *In combination with:* vilanterol (Anoro Ellipta), fluticasone and vilanterol (Trelegy Ellipta). See Appendix N.

NURSING IMPLICATIONS
Assessment
- Assess respiratory status (rate, breath sounds, degree of dyspnea, pulse) before administration and at peak of medication. Consult health care professional about alternative medication if severe bronchospasm is present; onset of action is too slow for patients in acute distress. If paradoxical bronchospasm (wheezing) occurs, withhold medication and notify health care professional immediately.

Implementation
- **Inhaln:** Follow manufacturer's instructions for use of inhaler. Breathe out; do not blow into mouthpiece. Close lips around mouthpiece. Breathe in a long, steady deep breath. Continue to hold breath as long as possible while removing inhaler from mouth. Slide cover over mouthpiece.

*= Canadian drug name. §§ = Genetic implication. ~~Strikethrough~~ = Discontinued. CAPITALS = life-threatening. <u>Underline</u> = most frequent.

Patient/Family Teaching

- Instruct patient in the correct use of inhaler. Advise patient not to discontinue without consulting health care professional; symptoms may recur.
- Inform patient that umeclidinium should not be used for treating sudden breathing problems.
- Advise patient to notify health care professional if worsening symptoms; decreasing effectiveness of inhaled, short-acting beta$_2$-agonists; need for more inhalations than usual of inhaled, short-acting beta$_2$-agonists; or significant decrease in lung function occur.
- Instruct patient to notify health care professional of all Rx or OTC medications, vitamins, or herbal products being taken and to avoid concurrent use of Rx, OTC, and herbal products without consulting health care professional.
- Advise patient to notify health care professional if signs and symptoms of worsening narrow-angle glaucoma (eye pain or discomfort, blurred vision, visual halos, colored images associated with red dyes from conjunctival congestion, corneal edema) or worsening urinary retention (difficulty passing urine, painful urination) occur.
- Rep: Advise females of reproductive potential to notify health care professional if pregnancy is planned or suspected or if breastfeeding.

Evaluation/Desired Outcomes

- Decrease in the number of flare-ups or the worsening of COPD symptoms (exacerbations).

upadacitinib
(ue-**pad**-a-sye-ti-nib)
Rinvoq
Classification
Therapeutic: antirheumatics
Pharmacologic: kinase inhibitors

Indications

Moderately to severely active rheumatoid arthritis in patients who have had an inadequate response/intolerance to ≥1 tumor necrosis factor (TNF) blocker (not to be used with other Janus kinase [JAK] inhibitors, biologic disease modifying antirheumatic drugs [DMARDs] or potent immunosuppressants [including azathioprine or cyclosporine]). Active psoriatic arthritis in patients who have had an inadequate response/intolerance to ≥1 TNF blocker (not to be used with other JAK inhibitors, biologic DMARDs or potent immunosuppressants [including azathioprine or cyclosporine]). Refractory, moderate to severe atopic dermatitis in patients whose disease is not adequately controlled with other systemic drug products, including biologics, or when use of those therapies are not recommended (not to be used with other JAK inhibitors, biologic immunomodulators, or other immunosuppressants). Moderately to severely active ulcerative colitis in patients who have had an inadequate response/intolerance to ≥1

TNF blocker (not to be used with other JAK inhibitors, biological therapies, or potent immunosuppressants [including azathioprine or cyclosporine]). Moderately to severely active Crohn's disease in patients who have had an inadequate response/intolerance to ≥1 TNF blocker (not to be used with other JAK inhibitors, biological therapies, or potent immunosuppressants [including azathioprine or cyclosporine]). Active ankylosing spondylitis in patients who have had an inadequate response/intolerance to ≥1 TNF blocker (not to be used with other JAK inhibitors, biologic DMARDs, or potent immunosuppressants [including azathioprine or cyclosporine]). Active non-radiographic axial spondyloarthritis in patients with objective signs of inflammation who have had an inadequate response or intolerance to TNF blocker therapy (not to be used with other JAK inhibitors, biologic DMARDs, or potent immunosuppressants [including azathioprine or cyclosporine]).

Action

Inhibits JAK enzymes, which prevents the activation of signal transducers, and activators of transcription, which ultimately results in decreased hematopoiesis and immune cell function. **Therapeutic Effects:** Improvement in clinical and symptomatic parameters of rheumatoid arthritis, psoriatic arthritis, atopic dermatitis, ulcerative colitis, Crohn's disease, ankylosing spondylitis, and non-radiographic axial spondyloarthritis.

Pharmacokinetics

Absorption: Well absorbed following oral administration.

Distribution: Unknown.

Metabolism and Excretion: Primarily metabolized by the liver via the CYP3A4 isoenzyme and to a lesser extent by the CYP2D6 isoenzyme; 38% excreted in feces and 24% excreted in urine as unchanged drug.

Half-life: 8–14 hr.

TIME/ACTION PROFILE (clinical improvement)

ROUTE	ONSET	PEAK	DURATION
PO	within 2 wk	3 mo	unknown

Contraindications/Precautions

Contraindicated in: Hypersensitivity; Active infection; Lymphocyte count <500 cells/mm^3, absolute neutrophil count (ANC) <1000 cells/mm^3, or Hgb <8 g/dL; Increased risk for thrombosis; History of MI or stroke; Severe hepatic impairment; End-stage renal disease (CCr <15 mL/min) (atopic dermatitis and ulcerative colitis only); OB: Pregnancy; Lactation: Lactation.

Use Cautiously in: Patients who are >50 yr old and have ≥1 cardiovascular risk factor (↑ risk of all-cause mortality, cardiovascular death, MI, stroke, and thrombosis); Current or past history of smoking (↑ risk of malignancy, cardiovascular death, MI, or stroke); Known malignancy; Previously exposed to tuberculosis (TB); History of serious or opportunistic infection; Re-

---

sided or traveled in areas of endemic TB or endemic mycoses; Underlying conditions that predispose to infection; History of diverticulitis or use of NSAIDs (↑ risk of GI perforation); End-stage renal disease; Rep: Women of reproductive potential; Pedi: Safety and effectiveness not established in children <18 yr (rheumatoid arthritis, psoriatic arthritis, and ulcerative colitis) or <12 yr (atopic dermatitis).

Adverse Reactions/Side Effects
CV: ARTERIAL THROMBOSIS, CARDIOVASCULAR DEATH, DEEP VEIN THROMBOSIS, MI. GI: ↑ liver enzymes, GI PERFORATION, nausea. Hemat: anemia, lymphopenia, NEUTROPENIA. Metab: dyslipidemia. MS: ↑ creatine kinase. Neuro: STROKE. Resp: cough, PULMONARY EMBOLISM. Misc: DEATH, fever, HYPERSENSITIVITY REACTIONS (including anaphylaxis and angioedema), INFECTION (including TB, bacterial, invasive fungal, viral, or opportunistic infections), MALIGNANCY.

Interactions
Drug-Drug: May ↑ risk of adverse reactions and ↓ antibody response to live vaccines; avoid concurrent use. Strong CYP3A4 inhibitors, including ketoconazole or clarithromycin, may ↑ levels and the risk of toxicity; avoid concurrent use. Strong CYP3A4 inducers, including rifampin, may ↓ levels and effectiveness; concurrent use not recommended. NSAIDs may ↑ risk of GI perforation; concurrent use requires careful monitoring. ↑ risk of immunosuppression when used concurrently with other potent immunosuppressants including azathioprine, cyclosporine, tacrolimus, antineoplastics, or radiation therapy.
Drug-Food: Grapefruit or grapefruit juice may ↑ levels and the risk of toxicity; avoid concurrent use.

Route/Dosage
Rheumatoid Arthritis, Psoriatic Arthritis, Ankylosing Spondylitis, or Non-Radiographic Axial Spondyloarthritis
PO (Adults): 15 mg once daily.

Atopic Dermatitis
PO (Geriatric Patients ≥65 yr): 15 mg once daily.
PO (Adults and Children 12–64 and ≥40 kg): 15 mg once daily. If adequate response not achieved, may ↑ to 30 mg once daily. If adequate response not achieved with 30 mg once daily, discontinue therapy. Concurrent use of strong CYP3A4 inhibitors: 15 mg once daily.

Renal Impairment
(Adults and Children ≥12 yr and ≥40 kg): CCr 15–<30 mL/min: 15 mg once daily. CCr <15 mL/min: Not recommended.

Ulcerative Colitis
PO (Adults): Induction therapy: 45 mg once daily for 8 wk. Maintenance therapy: 15 mg once daily; may ↑ to 30 mg once daily if patients have refractory, severe, or extensive disease. If adequate response not achieved with 30 mg once daily, discontinue therapy. Concurrent use of strong CYP3A4 inhibitors: ↓ induction therapy dose to 30 mg once daily for 8 wk. For maintenance therapy, do not exceed 15 mg once daily.

Renal Impairment
PO (Adults): CCr 15–<30 mL/min: Induction therapy: 30 mg once daily for 8 wk. Maintenance therapy: 15 mg once daily. CCr <15 mL/min: Not recommended.

Crohn's Disease
PO (Adults): Induction therapy: 45 mg once daily for 12 wk. Maintenance therapy: 15 mg once daily; may ↑ to 30 mg once daily if patients have refractory, severe, or extensive disease. If adequate response not achieved with 30 mg once daily, discontinue therapy. Concurrent use of strong CYP3A4 inhibitors: ↓ induction therapy dose to 30 mg once daily for 12 wk. For maintenance therapy, do not exceed 15 mg once daily.

Renal Impairment
PO (Adults): CCr 15–<30 mL/min: Induction therapy: 30 mg once daily for 12 wk. Maintenance therapy: 15 mg once daily. CCr <15 mL/min: Not recommended.

Availability
Extended-release tablets: 15 mg, 30 mg, 45 mg.

NURSING IMPLICATIONS
Assessment
- Assess pain and range of motion before and periodically during therapy.
- Assess for signs of infection (fever, dyspnea, flu-like symptoms, frequent or painful urination, redness or swelling at the site of a wound), including TB and hepatitis B virus, prior to and periodically during therapy. Upadacitinib is contraindicated in patients with active infection. Monitor new infections closely; most common are upper respiratory tract infections, bronchitis, and urinary tract infections. Infections may be fatal, especially in patients taking immunosuppressive therapy. If patient develops a serious infection, including serious opportunistic infection, interrupt therapy until infection is controlled.
- Assess patient for latent TB with a tuberculin skin test prior to initiation of therapy. Treatment of latent TB should be started before therapy with upadacitinib.
- Assess skin for new lesions periodically during therapy; risk of skin cancer is increased.
- Monitor for signs and symptoms of thrombosis (swelling, pain or tenderness in the leg, sudden unexplained chest pain, shortness of breath) during therapy.
- Monitor patients at risk for GI perforation (patients with a history of diverticulitis and those taking con-

upadacitinib **1239**

comitant medications, including NSAIDs or cortico-steroids). Evaluate promptly patients presenting with new-onset abdominal pain for early identification of GI perforation.

Lab Test Considerations
- Verify negative pregnancy test before starting therapy.
- Monitor neutrophil count at baseline and periodically during therapy. Do not start therapy and interrupt therapy if ANC <1000 cells/mm^3 and restart therapy once ANC returns above this value.
- Monitor lymphocyte count at baseline and periodically during therapy. Do not start therapy and interrupt therapy if absolute lymphocyte count (ALC) <500 cells/mm^3 and restart therapy once ALC returns above this value.
- May cause anemia. Monitor Hgb at baseline and periodically during therapy. Do not start therapy and interrupt therapy if Hgb <8 g/dL.
- May cause ↑ in total cholesterol, LDL cholesterol, and HDL cholesterol. Monitor levels 12 wk after starting therapy and periodically thereafter for hyperlipidemia.
- Monitor liver enzymes at baseline and periodically thereafter. If AST or ALT are ↑ and drug-induced liver injury is suspected, hold upadacitinib.

Implementation
- Immunizations, including prophylactic zoster vaccinations, should be current before starting therapy. Patients on upadacitinib may receive concurrent vaccinations, except for live vaccines.
- Administer a tuberculin skin test prior to administration of upadacitinib. Patients with active latent TB should be treated for TB prior to therapy.
- Screen patient for viral hepatitis before starting therapy.
- **PO:** Administer once daily without regard to food. *DNC:* Swallow tablets whole; do not split, crush, or chew.

Patient/Family Teaching
- Instruct patient to take upadacitinib as directed. Advise patient to read *Patient Information* before starting therapy and with each Rx refill in case of changes.
- Caution patient to avoid grapefruit or grapefruit juice during therapy.
- Advise patient to avoid live vaccines during therapy.
- Caution patient to notify health care professional immediately if signs of infection (fever, sweating, chills, muscle aches, cough, shortness of breath, blood in phlegm, weight loss, warm, red, or painful skin or sores, diarrhea or stomach pain, burning on urination or urinating more often than normal, feeling very tired), blood clots, or stomach or intestinal perforation (fever, stomach-area pain that does not go away, change in bowel habits) occur.
- Advise patient to notify health care professional of all Rx or OTC medications, vitamins, or herbal products

being taken and to consult with health care professional before taking other medications.
- Instruct patient to notify health care professional of medication regimen prior to treatment or surgery.
- Inform patient of increased risk of lymphoma and other cancers. Advise patient to have periodic skin exams for new lesions of skin cancer.
- Instruct patients to contact their health care professional if medication residue is observed repeatedly in stool or ostomy output.
- Rep: May cause fetal harm. Advise females of reproductive potential to use effective contraception during and for 4 wk after final dose and to avoid breastfeeding during and for 6 days after last dose. Advise patient to notify health care professional immediately if pregnancy is planned or suspected. If pregnancy occurs during therapy report to the AbbVie Inc.'s Adverse Event reporting line at 1-800-633-9110, or FDA at 1-800-FDA-1088 or www.fda.gov/medwatch.
- Emphasize the importance of regular lab tests to monitor for adverse drug reactions.

Evaluation/Desired Outcomes
- Improved physical function and decreased fatigue in patients with of rheumatoid arthritis, psoriatic arthritis, atopic dermatitis, ulcerative colitis, Crohn's disease, ankylosing spondylitis, and non-radiographic axial spondyloarthritis.

✗ ustekinumab
(uss-te-**kin**-oo-mab)
   Stelara
Classification
Therapeutic: antipsoriatics
Pharmacologic: interleukin antagonists, monoclonal antibodies

Indications
Moderate to severe plaque psoriasis in patients who are candidates for phototherapy or systemic therapy. Active psoriatic arthritis (as monotherapy or with methotrexate). Moderately to severely active Crohn's disease. Moderately to severely active ulcerative colitis.

Action
Binds to the p40 protein subunit used by both the interleukin (IL) 12 and IL-23 cytokines. These cytokines that are involved in inflammatory and immune responses, including natural killer cell activation and CD4+ T-cell differentiation and activation. Binding to interleukins antagonizes their effects, disrupting IL-12 and IL-23 mediated signaling and cytokine cascades. **Therapeutic Effects:** Decrease in area and severity of psoriatic lesions. Decreased progression of psoriatic arthritis. Reduced signs and symptoms and maintenance of clinical remission of Crohn's disease and ulcerative colitis.

Pharmacokinetics

Absorption: Well absorbed following SUBQ administration. IV administration results in complete bioavailability.

Distribution: Minimally distributed to tissues.

Metabolism and Excretion: Broken down by catabolic processes into peptides and amino acids.

Half-life: *Psoriasis:* 15–46 days; *Crohn's disease:* 19 days.

TIME/ACTION PROFILE (plasma concentrations)

ROUTE	ONSET	PEAK	DURATION
45 mg SUBQ	unknown	13.5 days	12 wk
90 mg SUBQ	unknown	7 days	12 wk
IV	unknown	unknown	unknown

Contraindications/Precautions

Contraindicated in: Hypersensitivity; Active untreated infection.

Use Cautiously in: History of known malignancy or tuberculosis (TB) (possibility of reactivation); >60 yr, history of prolonged immunosuppressant therapy, or history of PUVA treatment (↑ risk of skin cancer); OB: Use during pregnancy only if potential maternal benefit justifies potential fetal risk; Lactation: Use while breastfeeding only if potential maternal benefit justifies potential risk to infant; Pedi: Safety and effectiveness not established in children <18 yr (Crohn's disease) or <6 yr (psoriasis or psoriatic arthritis).

Exercise Extreme Caution in: Chronic infection or history of recurrent infection.

Adverse Reactions/Side Effects

Local: erythema. **Neuro:** fatigue, headache, POSTERIOR REVERSIBLE ENCEPHALOPATHY SYNDROME. **Resp:** eosinophilic pneumonia, interstitial pneumonia, RESPIRATORY FAILURE. **Misc:** HYPERSENSITIVITY REACTIONS (including anaphylaxis and angioedema), INFECTION, MALIGNANCY.

Interactions

Drug-Drug: May ↓ antibody response to and ↑ risk of adverse reactions from **live vaccines**. May ↓ desired antibody response to **non-live vaccines**. May affect the activity of CYP450 drug-metabolizing enzymes; when treatment is started during concurrent **CYP450 substrates**, especially those with a narrow therapeutic indices, including **warfarin** and **cyclosporine**; appropriate monitoring and dose adjustment should be carried out.

Route/Dosage

Plaque Psoriasis

SUBQ (Adults and Children ≥6 yr and >100 kg): 90 mg initially and 4 wk later, then 90 mg every 12 wk.

SUBQ (Adults ≤100 kg): 45 mg initially and 4 wk later, then 45 mg every 12 wk.

SUBQ (Children ≥6 yr and 60–100 kg): 45 mg initially and 4 wk later, then 45 mg every 12 wk.

SUBQ (Children ≥6 yr and <60 kg): 0.75 mg/kg initially and 4 wk later, then 0.75 mg/kg every 12 wk.

Psoriatic Arthritis

SUBQ (Adults): 45 mg initially and 4 wk later, then 45 mg every 12 wk.

SUBQ (Adults and Children ≥6 yr and >100 kg and with coexistent moderate to severe plaque psoriasis): 90 mg initially and 4 wk later, then 90 mg every 12 wk.

SUBQ (Children ≥6 yr and ≥60 kg): 45 mg initially and 4 wk later, then 45 mg every 12 wk.

SUBQ (Children ≥6 yr and <60 kg): 0.75 mg/kg initially and 4 wk later, then 0.75 mg/kg every 12 wk.

Crohn's Disease and Ulcerative Colitis

IV, SUBQ (Adults >85 kg): 520 mg IV infusion, then 90 mg SUBQ 8 wk later and then 90 mg every 8 wk.

IV, SUBQ (Adults 56–85 kg): 390 mg IV infusion, then 90 mg SUBQ 8 wk later and then 90 mg every 8 wk.

IV, SUBQ (Adults ≤55 kg): 260 mg IV infusion, then 90 mg SUBQ 8 wk later and then 90 mg every 8 wk.

Availability

Solution for intravenous injection: 5 mg/mL. **Solution for SUBQ injection:** 45 mg/0.45 mL (vials and prefilled syringes), 90 mg/1 mL (prefilled syringes).

NURSING IMPLICATIONS

Assessment

- Assess affected area(s) prior to and periodically during therapy.
- Assess for signs of infection (fever, dyspnea, flu-like symptoms, frequent or painful urination, redness or swelling at the site of a wound), including tuberculosis, prior to injection. Ustekinumab is contraindicated in patients with active infection. New infections should be monitored closely; most common are upper respiratory tract infections, bronchitis, and urinary tract infections. Infections may be fatal, especially in patients taking immunosuppressive therapy. ⚇ Patients genetically deficient in IL-12/IL-23 are particularly vulnerable to disseminated infections; diagnostic testing should be considered.
- Assess patient for latent TB with a tuberculin skin test prior to initiation of therapy. Treatment of latent TB should be started before therapy with ustekinumab.
- Monitor for signs and symptoms of hypersensitivity reaction and anaphylaxis (rash, chest tightness, feeling faint, difficulty breathing, throat tightness, swelling of face, eyelids, tongue, or throat) during therapy.

U

Implementation

- Administer a tuberculin skin test prior to administration of ustekinumab. Patients with active latent TB should be treated for TB prior to therapy.
- Immunizations should be current prior to initiating therapy. Patients on ustekinumab may receive concurrent vaccinations, except for live vaccines.
- **SUBQ:** Should be administered by health care professional unless patient or caregiver has been trained to administer injection. Administer using a 27 gauge, 1/2 inch needle in upper arm, gluteal region, thigh, or abdomen; rotate site. Do not administer in areas that are tender, bruised, erythematous, or indurated. Solution is colorless to light yellow and may contain a few small translucent or white particles; do not administer solutions that are discolored, cloudy, or contain other particulate matter. Do not shake. Store solution in refrigerator; do not freeze.
- Inform patients with a latex allergy that needle cover on the prefilled syringe contains latex.

IV Administration

- **Intermittent Infusion:** Withdraw equal amount as dose from 250 mL bag of 0.9% NaCl or 0.45% NaCl. Withdraw 26 mL from each vial of ustekinumab and add to 250 mL bag; mix gently. Solution is clear and colorless to light yellow; do not administer solutions that are discolored or contain particulate matter. Solution is stable for 7 hr at room temperature. Discard remaining solution. *Rate:* Infuse over at least 1 hr through a 0.2 micrometer in-line, sterile, non-pyrogenic, low protein-binding filter.
- **Y-Site Incompatibility:** Do not infuse in same IV line with other agents.

Patient/Family Teaching

- Instruct patient on correct technique for self-injection, care and disposal of equipment. Review *Medication Guide* with patient before starting therapy and with each injection.
- Inform patient that ustekinumab may lower ability to fight and increase risk for infections. Advise patient to notify health care professional immediately if signs of anaphylaxis or infection (fever, sweats, chills, muscle aches, cough, shortness of breath, blood in phlegm, weight loss, warm, red, or painful sores, diarrhea or stomach pain, burning or urination or urinary frequency, tiredness) occur.
- Inform patient that ustekinumab may increase for cancer. Advise patient to obtain preventative screening.
- Advise patient to notify health care professional if signs of reversible posterior encephalopathy syndrome (headache, seizures, confusion, visual problems) occur.
- Instruct patient to notify health care professional of all Rx or OTC medications, vitamins, or herbal products being taken and consult health care professional before taking any new medications.
- Instruct patient to notify health care professional of medication regimen prior to treatment or surgery.
- Rep: Advise females of reproductive potential to notify health care professional if pregnancy is planned or suspected or if breastfeeding.

Evaluation/Desired Outcomes

- Decrease in extent and severity of psoriatic lesions.
- Decreased progression of psoriatic arthritis.
- Reduced signs and symptoms and maintenance of clinical remission of Crohn's disease or ulcerative colitis.

valACYclovir

(val-ay-**sye**-kloe-veer)

Valtrex

Classification

Therapeutic: antivirals

Indications

Treatment of herpes zoster (shingles). Treatment/suppression of genital herpes. Reduction of transmission of genital herpes. Treatment of chickenpox. Treatment of herpes labialis (cold sores).

Action

Rapidly converted to acyclovir. Acyclovir interferes with viral DNA synthesis. **Therapeutic Effects:** Inhibited viral replication, decreased viral shedding, reduced time to healing of lesions. Reduced transmission of genital herpes.

Pharmacokinetics

Absorption: 54% bioavailable as acyclovir after oral administration of valacyclovir.

Distribution: CSF concentrations of acyclovir are 50% of plasma concentrations.

Metabolism and Excretion: Rapidly converted to acyclovir via intestinal/hepatic metabolism. Primarily excreted in the urine as acyclovir.

Half-life: 2.5–3.3 hr; up to 14 hr in renal impairment (acyclovir).

TIME/ACTION PROFILE (plasma concentrations†)

ROUTE	ONSET	PEAK	DURATION
PO	unknown	1.5–2.5 hr	8–24 hr

†Acyclovir.

Contraindications/Precautions

Contraindicated in: Hypersensitivity to valacyclovir or acyclovir.

Use Cautiously in: Renal impairment (↓ dose/↑ dosing interval recommended if CCr <50 mL/min); Pedi: Safety and effectiveness not established in children <18 yr (herpes zoster or genital herpes), <12 yr (herpes labialis), or <2 yr (chickenpox); Geri: Dose ↓ may be necessary in older adults due to ↑ risk of acute renal failure and CNS side effects.

Adverse Reactions/Side Effects

GI: <u>nausea</u>, abdominal pain, anorexia, constipation, diarrhea. **GU:** crystalluria, RENAL FAILURE. **Hemat:** THROMBOTIC THROMBOCYTOPENIC PURPURA/HEMOLYTIC UREMIC SYNDROME (very high doses in immunosuppressed patients). **Neuro:** <u>headache</u>, agitation, confusion, delirium, dizziness, encephalopathy, hallucinations, SEIZURES, weakness.

Interactions

Drug-Drug: **Probenecid** and **cimetidine** may ↑ levels and the risk of toxicity, especially in patients with renal impairment. Concurrent use of other **nephrotoxic drugs** ↑ risk of adverse renal effects.

Route/Dosage

Herpes Zoster

PO (Adults): 1 g 3 times daily for 7 days.

Renal Impairment

PO (Adults): *CCr 30–49 mL/min:* 1 g every 12 hr. *CCr 10–29 mL/min:* 1 g every 24 hr. *CCr <10 mL/ min:* 500 mg every 24 hr.

Genital Herpes

PO (Adults): *Initial treatment:* 1 g twice daily for 10 days. *Recurrence:* 500 mg twice daily for 3 days. *Suppression of recurrence:* 1 g once daily or 500 mg once daily in patients experiencing <10 recurrences/yr. *Suppression of recurrence in HIV-infected patients:* 500 mg every 12 hr. *Reduction of transmission:* 500 mg once daily for source partner.

Renal Impairment

PO (Adults): *CCr 10–29 mL/min:* 1 g every 24 hr for initial treatment of genital herpes, 500 mg every 24 hr for treatment of recurrent episodes of genital herpes, 500 mg every 48 hr for suppression of genital herpes in patients with 9 or fewer recurrences/yr, 500 mg every 24 hr for suppression of genital herpes in patients with ≥10 recurrences/yr or HIV-infected patients. *CCr <10 mL/min:* 500 mg every 24 hr for initial treatment of genital herpes, 500 mg every 24 hr for treatment of recurrent episodes of genital herpes, 500 mg every 48 hr for suppression of genital herpes in patients with 9 or fewer recurrences/yr, 500 mg every 24 hr for suppression of genital herpes in patients with ≥10 recurrences/yr or HIV-infected patients.

Herpes Labialis

PO (Adults and Children ≥12 yr): 2 g initially, then 2 g 12 hr later.

Renal Impairment

PO (Adults): *CCr 30–49 mL/min:* 1 g initially, then 1 g 12 hr later. *CCr 10–29 mL/min:* 500 mg initially, then 500 mg 12 hr later. *CCr <10 mL/min:* 500 mg as a single dose.

Chickenpox

PO (Children ≥2 yr): 20 mg/kg 3 times daily for 5 days (not to exceed 1 g 3 times daily).

Availability (generic available)

Tablets: 500 mg, 1 g.

V

NURSING IMPLICATIONS

Assessment

- Assess lesions before and daily during therapy.
- Monitor patient for signs of thrombotic thrombocytopenic purpura/hemolytic uremic syndrome (thrombocytopenia, microangiopathic hemolytic anemia, neurologic findings, renal dysfunction, fever). Requires prompt treatment; may be fatal.

Implementation

- **High Alert:** Do not confuse valacyclovir with valganciclovir. Do not confuse Valtrex with Valcyte.
- **PO:** May be administered without regard to meals.
- **Herpes Zoster:** Implement valacyclovir therapy as soon as possible after the onset of signs or symptoms of herpes zoster; most effective if started within 48 hr of the onset of zoster rash. Efficacy of treatment started >72 hr after rash onset is unknown.
- **Genital Herpes and Herpes Labialis:** Implement treatment for genital herpes as soon as possible after onset of symptoms (tingling, itching, burning).
- **Chicken Pox:** Initiate therapy at the earliest sign or symptom; preferably within 24 hr of onset of rash.

Patient/Family Teaching

- Instruct patient to take valacyclovir exactly as directed for the full course of therapy. Take missed doses as soon as remembered if not just before next dose; do not double doses. Advise patient to read the *Patient Information* before starting therapy.
- Advise patient to maintain adequate hydration during therapy.
- Advise patient to notify health care professional promptly if nervous system symptoms (aggressive behavior, unsteady movement, shaky movements, confusion, speech problems, hallucinations, seizures, coma) occur.
- Instruct patient to notify health care professional of all Rx or OTC medications, vitamins, or herbal products being taken and consult health care professional before taking any new medications.
- Rep: Instruct females of reproductive potential to notify health care professional if pregnancy is planned or suspected, or if breastfeeding.
- **Herpes Zoster:** Inform patient that valacyclovir does not prevent the spread of infection to others. Precautions should be taken around others who have not had chickenpox or varicella vaccine, or are immunosuppressed, until all lesions have crusted.
- **Genital Herpes and Herpes Labialis:** Inform patient that valacyclovir does not prevent the spread of herpes labialis to others. Advise patient to avoid contact with others while lesions or symptoms are present. Valacyclovir reduces transmission of genital herpes to others. Advise patient to practice safe sex (avoid sexual intercourse when lesions are present and wear a condom made of latex or polyurethane during sexual contact).

Evaluation/Desired Outcomes

- Decrease in time to full crusting, loss of vesicles, loss of ulcers, and development of crusts in patients with acute herpes zoster (shingles).
- Decrease in time to full crusting, loss of vesicles, loss of ulcers, and development of crusts in patients with genital herpes.
- Decrease in frequency of outbreaks in patients with genital herpes.
- Decrease in time to full crusting, loss of vesicles, loss of ulcers, and development of crusts in patients with herpes labialis. Decrease in transmission of genital herpes.
- Treatment of chickenpox.

✄ **valbenazine** (val-ben-a-zeen)
Ingrezza
Classification
Therapeutic: none assigned
Pharmacologic: reversible monoamine depleters

Indications

Tardive dyskinesia. Chorea associated with Huntington's disease.

Action

Acts as a reversible inhibitor of the vesicular monoamine transporter 2, which inhibits the reuptake of serotonin, norepinephrine, and dopamine into vesicles in presynaptic neurons. **Therapeutic Effects:** Reduced severity of tardive dyskinesia. Reduction in chorea.

Pharmacokinetics

Absorption: 49% absorbed following oral administration.
Distribution: Well distributed to tissues.
Protein Binding: >99%.
Metabolism and Excretion: ✄ Rapidly and extensively metabolized by the liver via hydrolysis to the active metabolite, α-dihydrotetrabenazine (α-HTBZ); also metabolized via the CYP3A4 isoenzyme to form other minor metabolites. α-HTBZ is further metabolized, in part, via the CYP2D6 isoenzyme. The CYP2D6 isoenzyme exhibits genetic polymorphism; 7% of population may be poor metabolizers and may have significantly ↑ concentrations and an ↑ risk of adverse effects. 60% eliminated in urine (<2% as unchanged drug) and 30% eliminated in feces (<2% as unchanged drug).
Half-life: 15–22 hr (valbenazine and α-HTBZ).

TIME/ACTION PROFILE (plasma concentrations)

ROUTE	ONSET	PEAK	DURATION
PO	unknown	0.5–1 hr	unknown

Contraindications/Precautions

Contraindicated in: Hypersensitivity; Congenital long QT syndrome or history of torsades de pointes; Lactation: Lactation.

Use Cautiously in: Patients with Huntington's disease with history of depression or suicidal thoughts/attempts; ▓ Poor CYP2D6 metabolizers or taking strong CYP2D6 inhibitor (may need to ↓ valbenazine dose); Moderate or severe hepatic impairment (↓ dose); OB: Safety not established in pregnancy; Pedi: Safety and effectiveness not established in children.

Adverse Reactions/Side Effects

EENT: blurred vision. **GI:** constipation, nausea, vomiting, xerostomia. **GU:** urinary retention. **MS:** arthralgia, bradykinesia. **Neuro:** fatigue, sedation/somnolence, akathisia, balance difficulty, depression, dizziness, gait disturbances, headache, NEUROLEPTIC MALIGNANT SYNDROME (NMS), parkinsonism, restlessness, SUICIDAL THOUGHTS/BEHAVIORS, tremor, unsteady gait. **Misc:** HYPERSENSITIVITY REACTIONS (including angioedema).

Interactions

Drug-Drug: **MAO inhibitors** may ↑ risk of serotonin syndrome and/or ↓ the effect of valbenazine; avoid concurrent use. **Strong CYP3A4 inhibitors**, including **itraconazole**, **ketoconazole**, or **clarithromycin** may ↑ levels of valbenazine and its active metabolite (α-HTBZ) and the risk of toxicity; ↓ valbenazine dose. **Strong CYP2D6 inhibitors**, including **fluoxetine**, **paroxetine**, or **quinidine** may ↑ levels of the active metabolite (α-HTBZ) and the risk of toxicity; may need to ↓ valbenazine dose. **Strong CYP3A4 inducers**, including **rifampin**, **carbamazepine**, or **phenytoin** may ↓ levels and effectiveness; concurrent use not recommended. May ↑ levels and the risk of toxicity of **digoxin**.

Drug-Natural Products: **St. John's wort** may ↓ levels and effectiveness; concurrent use not recommended.

Route/Dosage

Tardive Dyskinesia

PO (Adults): 40 mg once daily; after 1 wk, ↑ to 80 mg once daily. *Known CYP2D6 poor metabolizer:* 40 mg once daily (with no additional titration). *Concurrent use of strong CYP3A4 inhibitors or strong CYP2D6 inhibitors:* 40 mg once daily (with no additional titration).

Hepatic Impairment

PO (Adults): *Moderate or severe hepatic impairment:* 40 mg once daily (with no additional titration).

Chorea Associated with Huntington's Disease

PO (Adults): 40 mg once daily; ↑ by 20 mg/day every 2 wk until achieve recommended dose of 80 mg once daily. *Known CYP2D6 poor metabolizer:* 40 mg once

daily (with no additional titration). *Concurrent use of strong CYP3A4 inhibitors or strong CYP2D6 inhibitors:* 40 mg once daily (with no additional titration).

Hepatic Impairment

PO (Adults): *Moderate or severe hepatic impairment:* 40 mg once daily (with no additional titration).

Availability

Capsules: 40 mg, 60 mg, 80 mg.

NURSING IMPLICATIONS

Assessment

- Monitor for changes in signs and symptoms of tardive dyskinesia (uncontrolled rhythmic movement of mouth, face, and extremities; lip smacking or puckering; puffing of cheeks; uncontrolled chewing; rapid or worm-like movements of tongue, excessive eye blinking) periodically during therapy.
- Monitor patients with Huntington's disease for new or worsening depression, and suicidal ideation or behaviors. If these reactions occur and do not resolve, consider discontinuing therapy.
- Monitor for signs and symptoms of hypersensitivity (angioedema involving the larynx, glottis, lips, and eyelids). If signs and symptoms of hypersensitivity occur discontinue valbenazine.
- Monitor for signs and symptoms of NMS (hyperpyrexia, muscle rigidity, altered mental status, evidence of autonomic instability [irregular pulse or blood pressure, tachycardia, diaphoresis, cardiac arrhythmia]). Immediately discontinue valbenazine if symptoms occur. Recurrence of NMS has been reported with resumption of therapy. If therapy with valbenazine is needed after recovery from NMS, patients should be monitored for signs of recurrence.

Implementation

- **PO:** Administer once daily without regard to food.

Patient/Family Teaching

- Instruct patient to take valbenazine as directed. Do not stop taking valbenazine without consulting health care professional. Advise patient to read *Patient Information* before starting and with each Rx refill in case of changes.
- May cause drowsiness. Caution patient to avoid driving and other activities requiring alertness until response to medication is known.
- Advise patient to notify health care professional if symptoms of NMS, heart rhythm problems (fast, slow, or irregular heartbeat, shortness of breath, dizziness, fainting) or if a fast or irregular heartbeat occurs.
- Instruct patient to notify health care professional of all Rx or OTC medications, vitamins, or herbal products being taken and consult health care professional before taking any new medications.

V

- Rep: May cause fetal harm. Advise females of reproductive potential to notify health care professional if pregnancy is planned or suspected and to avoid breastfeeding during and for 5 days after last dose of therapy.

Evaluation/Desired Outcomes

- Decrease in severity of uncontrolled movements.
- Reduction in chorea.

valGANciclovir
(val-gan-**sye**-kloe-veer)
Valcyte
Classification
Therapeutic: antivirals

Indications

Treatment of cytomegalovirus (CMV) retinitis in patients with AIDS. Prevention of CMV disease in kidney, kidney/pancreas and heart transplant patients at risk.

Action

Valganciclovir is a prodrug, which is rapidly converted to ganciclovir by intestinal and hepatic enzymes. CMV virus converts ganciclovir to its active form (ganciclovir phosphate) inside host cell, where it inhibits viral DNA polymerase. **Therapeutic Effects:** Antiviral effect directed preferentially against CMV-infected cells.

Pharmacokinetics

Absorption: 59.4% absorbed following oral administration, rapidly converted to ganciclovir.
Distribution: Widely distributed to tissues, including CSF.
Metabolism and Excretion: Rapidly converted to ganciclovir; ganciclovir is mostly excreted by the kidneys.
Half-life: 4.1 hr (intracellular half-life of ganciclovir phosphate is 18 hr).

TIME/ACTION PROFILE (ganciclovir plasma concentrations)

ROUTE	ONSET	PEAK	DURATION
PO	rapid	2 hr	12–24 hr

Contraindications/Precautions

Contraindicated in: Hypersensitivity to valganciclovir or ganciclovir; Hemodialysis; Undergoing liver transplantation; Lactation: Lactation.
Use Cautiously in: Renal impairment (dosage ↓ recommended if CCr <60 mL/min); Pre-existing bone marrow depression; Previous or concurrent myelosuppressive drug therapy or radiation therapy; Rep: Women of reproductive potential and men with female partners of reproductive potential; OB: Use during pregnancy only if potential maternal benefit justifies potential fetal risk; Pedi: Children <4 mo (safety and effectiveness not established); Geri: Age-related ↓ in renal function requires dosage ↓ in older adults.

Adverse Reactions/Side Effects

GI: abdominal pain, diarrhea, nausea, vomiting. **GU:** ↓ fertility, renal impairment. **Hemat:** anemia, aplastic anemia, bone marrow depression, NEUTROPENIA, pancytopenia, THROMBOCYTOPENIA. **Neuro:** headache, insomnia, agitation, ataxia, confusion, dizziness, hallucinations, paresthesia, peripheral neuropathy, psychosis, sedation, SEIZURES. **Misc:** fever, HYPERSENSITIVITY REACTIONS (including anaphylaxis), INFECTION.

Interactions

Drug-Drug: ↑ risk of hematologic toxicity with **zidovudine. Probenecid** may ↑ levels and risk of toxicity. Patients with renal impairment may experience accumulation of metabolites of **mycophenolate** and valganciclovir.
Drug-Food: Food ↑ absorption.

Route/Dosage

Treatment of CMV Disease

PO (Adults): *Induction:* 900 mg twice daily for 21 days; *Maintenance treatment or patients with inactive CMV retinitis:* 900 mg once daily.

Renal Impairment

CCr 40–59 mL/min (Adults): *Induction:* 450 mg twice daily for 21 days; *Maintenance treatment or patients with inactive CMV retinitis:* 450 mg once daily.

Renal Impairment

CCr 25–39 mL/min (Adults): *Induction:* 450 mg once daily for 21 days; *Maintenance treatment or patients with inactive CMV retinitis:* 450 mg every 2 days.

Renal Impairment

CCr 10–24 mL/min (Adults): *Induction:* 450 mg every 2 days for 21 days; *Maintenance treatment or patients with inactive CMV retinitis:* 450 mg twice weekly.

Prevention of CMV Disease in Transplant Patients

PO (Adults): *Kidney/pancreas or heart transplant:* 900 mg once daily, starting 10 days prior to transplant and continued for 100 days after; *Kidney transplant:* 900 mg once daily, starting 10 days prior to transplant and continued for 200 days after.
PO (Children 4 mo–16 yr): *Kidney transplant:* Dose is based on body surface area (BSA) and CCr. Dose = 7 × BSA × CCr (see prescribing information for equations used for BSA and CCr); all calculated doses should be rounded to nearest 25 mg (max = 900 mg) and administered as oral solution; should be started 10 days prior to transplant and continued for 200 days after.
PO (Children 4 mo–16 yr): *Heart transplant:* Dose is based on BSA and CCr. Dose = 7 × BSA × CCr (see

prescribing information for equations used for BSA and CCr); all calculated doses should be rounded to nearest 25 mg (max = 900 mg) and administered as oral solution; should be started 10 days prior to transplant and continued for 100 days after.

Renal Impairment
PO (Adults): *CCr 40–59 mL/min:* 450 mg once daily; *CCr 25–39 mL/min:* 450 mg every 2 days; *CCr 12–24 mL/min:* 450 mg twice weekly.

Availability (generic available)
Tablets: 450 mg. **Oral solution (tutti-frutti flavor):** 50 mg/mL.

NURSING IMPLICATIONS

Assessment
- Diagnosis of CMV retinitis should be determined by ophthalmoscopy prior to treatment with valganciclovir.
- Culture for CMV (urine, blood, throat) may be taken prior to administration. However, a negative CMV culture does not rule out CMV retinitis. If symptoms do not respond after several wk, resistance to valganciclovir may have occurred. Ophthalmologic exams should be performed weekly during induction and every 2 wk during maintenance or more frequently if the macula or optic nerve is threatened. Progression of CMV retinitis may occur during or following ganciclovir treatment.
- Assess for signs of infection (fever, chills, cough, hoarseness, lower back or side pain, sore throat, difficult or painful urination). Notify health care professional if these symptoms occur.
- Assess for bleeding (bleeding gums, bruising, petechiae, or guaiac stools, urine, and emesis). Avoid IM injections and taking rectal temperatures. Apply pressure to venipuncture sites for 10 min.

Lab Test Considerations
- Verify negative pregnancy test before starting therapy.
- May cause granulocytopenia, anemia, and thrombocytopenia. Monitor neutrophil and platelet count closely during therapy. Do not administer if absolute neutrophil count <500/mm³, platelet count <25,000/mm³, or Hgb <8 g/dL. Recovery begins within 3–7 days of discontinuation of therapy.
- Monitor BUN and serum creatinine at least once every 2 wk during therapy. May cause ↑ in serum creatinine.

Implementation
- Do not confuse valganciclovir with valacyclovir. Do not confuse Valcyte with Valtrex.
- **PO:** Administer tablets and oral solution with food. Adults should take tablets, not oral solution. Handle valganciclovir tablets carefully. *DNC:* Do not break or crush. Avoid direct contact with broken

or crushed tablets. If contact with the skin or mucous membranes occurs, wash thoroughly with soap and water and rinse eyes thoroughly with plain water.
- Oral solution (50 mg/mL) must be prepared by the pharmacist prior to dispensing to the patient. Shake well prior to use. Use oral dispenser provided for accurate dose. Store oral solution in refrigerator for no longer than 49 days.

Patient/Family Teaching
- Instruct patient to take valganciclovir with food, as directed. Take missed doses as soon as remembered, unless almost time for next dose; do not double doses. Advise patient to read *Patient Information* before starting therapy and with each Rx refill in case of changes.
- Inform patient that valganciclovir is not a cure for CMV retinitis. Progression of retinitis may continue in immunocompromised patients during and following therapy. Advise patients to have regular ophthalmic exams at least every 4–6 wk. Duration of therapy for CMV prevention is based on the duration and degree of immunosuppression.
- May cause seizures, sedation, dizziness, ataxia, and/or confusion. Caution patient not to drive or do other activities requiring alertness until response to medication is known.
- Advise patient to notify health care professional if fever; chills; sore throat; other signs of infection; bleeding gums; bruising; petechiae; or blood in urine, stool, or emesis occurs. Caution patient to avoid crowds and persons with known infections. Instruct patient to use soft toothbrush and electric razor. Patient should be cautioned not to drink alcoholic beverages or take products containing aspirin or NSAIDs.
- Caution patient to use sunscreen and protective clothing to prevent photosensitivity reactions.
- Rep: May cause fetal harm. Advise females of reproductive potential to use effective contraception during and for at least 30 days following therapy and to avoid breastfeeding. Advise males with female partners of reproductive potential to use a barrier method of contraception during and for at least 90 days following therapy. Advise patient to notify health care professional immediately if pregnancy is suspected. May cause temporary or permanent infertility.
- Emphasize the importance of frequent follow-up exams to monitor blood counts.

Evaluation/Desired Outcomes
- Management of the symptoms of CMV retinitis in patients with AIDS.
- Prevention of CMV disease in kidney, kidney/pancreas and heart transplant patients at risk.

⚡VALPROATES
divalproex sodium
(dye-val-**proe**-ex **soe**-dee-um)
Depakote, Depakote ER, Depakote
Sprinkle, ✤Epival
valproate sodium
(val-**proe**-ate **soe**-dee-um)
~~Depacon~~
valproic acid (val-**proe**-ik **as**-id)
~~Depakene~~
Classification
Therapeutic: anticonvulsants, vascular headache suppressants

Indications
Monotherapy and adjunctive therapy for simple and
complex absence seizures. Monotherapy and adjunctive
therapy for complex partial seizures. Adjunctive therapy
for patients with multiple seizure types, including absence seizures. **Divalproex sodium only.** Manic episodes associated with bipolar disorder. Prevention of
migraine headache.

Action
Increase levels of GABA, an inhibitory neurotransmitter
in the CNS. **Therapeutic Effects:** Suppression of seizure activity. Decreased manic episodes. Decreased frequency of migraine headaches.

Pharmacokinetics
Absorption: Well absorbed following oral administration; divalproex is enteric-coated, and absorption is
delayed. Extended-release form produces lower blood
levels. IV administration results in complete bioavailability.
Distribution: Rapidly distributed into plasma and
extracellular water. Cross blood-brain barrier.
Protein Binding: 80–90% (↓ in neonates, elderly,
renal impairment, or chronic hepatic impairment).
Metabolism and Excretion: Mostly metabolized
by the liver; minimal amounts excreted unchanged in
urine.
Half-life: Adults: 9–16 hr.

TIME/ACTION PROFILE (onset = anticonvulsant effect; peak = blood levels)

ROUTE	ONSET	PEAK	DURATION
PO—liquid	2–4 days	15–120 min	6–24 hr
PO—capsules	2–4 days	1–4 hr	6–24 hr
PO—delayed-release products	2–4 days	3–5 hr	12–24 hr
PO—extended-release products	2–4 days	7–14 hr	24 hr
IV	2–4 days	end of infusion	6–24 hr

Contraindications/Precautions
Contraindicated in: Hypersensitivity; Hepatic impairment; ⚡ Known/suspected urea cycle disorders
(may result in fatal hyperammonemic encephalopathy);
⚡ Mitochondrial disorders caused by mutations in mitochondrial DNA polymerase gamma (↑ risk for potentially fatal hepatotoxicity); Rep: Women of reproductive
potential not using effective contraception (for migraine prophylaxis only); OB: Pregnancy (for migraine
prophylaxis only); Lactation: Lactation; Pedi: Children
<2 yr with suspected mitochondrial disorder caused by
mutations in mitochondrial DNA polymerase gamma
(↑ risk for potentially fatal hepatotoxicity).
Use Cautiously in: All patients (may ↑ risk of suicidal thoughts/behaviors); Bleeding disorders; Renal
impairment; Hepatic impairment; Organic brain disease; Bone marrow depression; Rep: Women of reproductive potential (use for seizure disorders or bipolar
disorders only if other medications are ineffective,
poorly tolerated, or inappropriate); OB: Pregnancy
(may cause fetal harm including ↓ IQ, neurodevelopmental disorders [including autism spectrum disorders
and attention deficit/hyperactivity disorder], neural
tube defects, hearing impairment/loss, and other major
congenital malformations); use for seizure disorders or
bipolar disorders only if other medications are ineffective, poorly tolerated, or inappropriate; Geri: ↑ risk of
adverse effects in older adults.

Adverse Reactions/Side Effects
CV: peripheral edema. **Derm:** alopecia, DRUG REACTION
WITH EOSINOPHILIA AND SYSTEMIC SYMPTOMS (DRESS),
rash. **EENT:** visual disturbances. **GI:** abdominal pain,
anorexia, diarrhea, indigestion, nausea, vomiting, constipation, HEPATOTOXICITY, PANCREATITIS. **Hemat:**
thrombocytopenia, leukopenia. **Metab:** ↑ appetite, HY-
PERAMMONEMIA, weight gain. **Neuro:** agitation, dizziness, headache, insomnia, sedation, tremor, ataxia,
confusion, depression, HYPOTHERMIA, SUICIDAL
THOUGHTS.

Interactions
Drug-Drug: ↑ risk of bleeding with **warfarin. Aspirin, carbamazepine, chlorpromazine, cimetidine,
erythromycin,** or **felbamate** may ↑ levels and the risk
of toxicity. ↑ risk of CNS depression with other **CNS depressants,** including **alcohol, antihistamines, antidepressants, opioid analgesics, MAO inhibitors,**
and **sedative/hypnotics. MAO inhibitors** and other
antidepressants may ↓ seizure threshold and ↓ effectiveness of valproate. **Carbamazepine, ertapenem,
imipenem, meropenem, methotrexate, phenobarbital, phenytoin, estrogen-containing contraceptives,** or **rifampin** may ↓ levels and effectiveness. May
↑ levels and the risk of toxicity of **carbamazepine, diazepam, amitriptyline, nortriptyline, ethosuximide, lamotrigine, phenobarbital, phenytoin, rufi-
namide, topiramate,** or **zidovudine;** dosage
adjustments of these medications may be necessary.
May ↑ levels and the risk of toxicity of **propofol;** ↓

dose of propofol. Concurrent use with **topiramate** may ↑ the risk of hypothermia and hyperammonemia with or without encephalopathy. **Cholestyramine** may ↓ levels and effectiveness; separate administration by 3 hr. Concurrent use with **cannabidiol** may ↑ risk of liver enzyme elevation; monitor liver enzymes closely during concomitant therapy.

Route/Dosage

Regular-release and delayed-release formulations usually given in 2–4 divided doses daily; extended-release formulation (Depakote ER) usually given once daily.

Seizure Disorders

PO (Adults and Children >10 yr): *Single-agent therapy (complex partial seizures):* Initial dose of 10–15 mg/kg/day in 1–4 divided doses; ↑ by 5–10 mg/kg/day weekly until therapeutic response achieved (not to exceed 60 mg/kg/day); when daily dose exceeds 250 mg, give in divided doses. *Polytherapy (complex partial seizures):* Initial dose of 10–15 mg/kg/day; ↑ by 5–10 mg/kg/day weekly until therapeutic response achieved (not to exceed 60 mg/kg/day); when daily dosage exceeds 250 mg, give in divided doses.

PO (Adults and Children >2 yr [>10 yr for Depakote ER]): *Simple and complex absence seizures:* Initial dose of 15 mg/kg/day in 1–4 divided doses; ↑ by 5–10 mg/kg/day weekly until therapeutic response achieved (not to exceed 60 mg/kg/day); when daily dose exceeds 250 mg, give in divided doses.

IV (Adults and Children): Give same daily dose and at same frequency as was given orally; switch to oral formulation as soon as possible.

Rect (Adults and Children): Dilute syrup 1:1 with water for use as a retention enema. Give 17–20 mg/kg load, maintenance 10–15 mg/kg/dose every 8 hr.

Bipolar Disorder

PO (Adults): *Depakote:* Initial dose of 750 mg/day in divided doses initially, titrated rapidly to desired clinical effect or trough plasma levels of 50–125 mcg/mL (not to exceed 60 mg/kg/day). *Depakote ER:* Initial dose of 25 mg/kg once daily; titrated rapidly to desired clinical effect of trough plasma levels of 85–125 mcg/mL (not to exceed 60 mg/kg/day).

Migraine Prevention

PO (Adults and Children ≥16 yr): *Depakote:* 250 mg twice daily (up to 1000 mg/day). *Depakote ER:* 500 mg once daily for 1 wk, then ↑ to 1000 mg once daily.

Availability

Valproic Acid (generic available)
Capsules: 250 mg. **Oral solution:** 250 mg/5 mL.

Valproate Sodium (generic available)
Solution for injection: 100 mg/mL.

Divalproex Sodium (generic available)
Delayed-release tablets (Depakote): 125 mg, 250 mg, 500 mg. **Extended-release tablets (Depakote ER):** 250 mg, 500 mg. **Sprinkle capsules:** 125 mg.

NURSING IMPLICATIONS

Assessment

- **Seizures:** Assess location, duration, frequency, and characteristics of seizure activity. Institute seizure precautions.
- **Bipolar Disorder:** Assess mood, ideation, and behavior frequently.
- **Migraine Prophylaxis:** Monitor frequency and intensity of migraine headaches.
- Geri: Assess older adults for excessive somnolence.
- Assess for suicidal tendencies, especially during early therapy. Restrict amount of drug available to patient. Risk may be increased in children, adolescents, and adults ≤24 yr.
- Monitor for signs and symptoms of pancreatitis (abdominal pain, nausea, vomiting, anorexia). If pancreatitis occurs, valproates should be discontinued and alternate therapy initiated.
- Monitor for signs and symptoms of DRESS (fever, rash, lymphadenopathy, hepatitis, nephritis, hematological abnormalities, myocarditis, myositis, eosinophilia). If symptoms occur and DRESS is confirmed, discontinue valproate and do not restart.

Lab Test Considerations
- Monitor CBC, platelet count, and bleeding time prior to and periodically during therapy. May cause leukopenia and thrombocytopenia.
- Monitor hepatic function (LDH, AST, ALT, and bilirubin) and serum ammonia concentrations prior to and periodically during therapy. May cause hepatotoxicity; monitor closely, especially during initial 6 mo of therapy; fatalities have occurred. Therapy should be discontinued if hyperammonemia occurs.
- May interfere with accuracy of thyroid function tests.
- May cause false-positive results in urine ketone tests.

Toxicity and Overdose
- Therapeutic serum levels range from 50–100 mcg/mL (50–125 mcg/mL for mania). Doses are gradually ↑ until a predose serum concentration of at least 50 mcg/mL is reached. However, a good correlation among daily dose, serum level, and therapeutic effects has not been established. Monitor patients receiving near the maximum recommended 60 mg/kg/day for toxicity.

Implementation
- Do not confuse *Depakote ER* and regular dose forms. *Depakote ER* produces lower blood levels than *Depakote* dosing forms. If switching from *Depakote* to *Depakote ER*, increase dose by 8–20%.

V

- Single daily doses are usually administered at bedtime because of sedation.
- **PO:** Administer with or immediately after meals to minimize GI irritation. *DNC:* Swallow extended-release and delayed-release tablets and capsules whole; do not open, break, or chew; will cause mouth or throat irritation and destroy extended release mechanism. Do not administer tablets with milk or carbonated beverages (may cause premature dissolution). Delayed-release divalproex sodium may cause less GI irritation than valproic acid capsules.
- Geri: Reduce starting dose in older adults. Increase doses more slowly and with regular monitoring for fluid and nutritional intake, dehydration, somnolence, and other adverse reactions.
- Shake liquid preparations well before pouring. Use calibrated measuring device to ensure accurate dose. Oral solution may be mixed with food or other liquids to improve taste.
- Sprinkle capsules may be swallowed whole or opened and entire capsule contents sprinkled on a teaspoonful of soft, cool food (applesauce, pudding). Do not chew mixture. Administer immediately; do not store for future use.
- To convert from valproic acid to divalproex sodium, initiate divalproex sodium at same total daily dose and dosing schedule as valproic acid. Once patient is stabilized on divalproex sodium, attempt administration 2–3 times daily.
- **Rect:** Dilute syrup 1:1 with water for use as a retention enema.

IV Administration
- **Intermittent Infusion:** *Dilution:* May be diluted in at least 50 mL of D5W, 0.9% NaCl, or LR. Solution is stable for 24 hr at room temperature. *Concentration:* 2 mg/mL. *Rate:* Infuse over 60 min (≤20 mg/min). Rapid infusion may cause increased side effects. Has been given as an infusion of ≤15 mg/kg over 5–10 min (1.5–3 mg/kg/min). Rapid loading doses of 20 to 40 mg/kg have been administered over 1 to 5 min. In pediatric patients, an infusion rate of 1.5 to 3 mg/kg/minute has been recommended.
- **Y-Site Compatibility:** cefepime, ceftazidime, dexamethasone, dobutamine, dopamine, fosphenytoin, insulin aspart, lorazepam, magnesium sulfate, mannitol, meropenem, methylprednisolone, naloxone, pentobarbital, thiopental.
- **Y-Site Incompatibility:** diazepam, midazolam, phenytoin, vancomycin.

Patient/Family Teaching
- Instruct patient to take medication as directed. If a dose is missed on a once-a-day schedule, take as soon as remembered that day. If on a multiple-dose schedule, take it within 6 hr of the scheduled time, then space remaining doses throughout the remainder of the day. Abrupt withdrawal may lead to status epilepticus. Advise patient to read the *Medication Guide* before starting therapy and with each Rx refill in case of changes.
- May cause drowsiness or dizziness. Caution patient to avoid driving or other activities requiring alertness until effects of medication are known. Tell patient not to resume driving until physician gives clearance based on control of seizure disorder.
- Instruct patient to notify health care professional of all Rx or OTC medications, vitamins, or herbal products being taken and consult health care professional before taking any new medications, especially CNS depressants or opioids. Caution patient to avoid alcohol during therapy.
- Advise patient and family to notify health care professional if thoughts about suicide or dying, attempts to commit suicide; new or worse depression; new or worse anxiety; feeling very agitated or restless; panic attacks; trouble sleeping; new or worse irritability; acting aggressive; being angry or violent; acting on dangerous impulses; an extreme increase in activity and talking, other unusual changes in behavior or mood occur.
- Instruct patient to notify health care professional of medication regimen prior to treatment or surgery.
- Advise patient to notify health care professional if anorexia, abdominal pain, severe nausea and vomiting, yellow skin or eyes, fever, sore throat, malaise, weakness, facial edema, lethargy, unusual bleeding or bruising, pregnancy, or loss of seizure control occurs. Children <2 yr of age are especially at risk for fatal hepatotoxicity.
- Rep: May cause fetal harm. Advise females of reproductive potential to use effective contraception during therapy and to notify health care professional immediately if pregnancy is planned or suspected, or if breastfeeding. Dietary folic acid supplementation prior to conception and during first trimester of pregnancy decreases the risk for congenital neural tube defects in the general population. May cause abnormal clotting and hepatic failure in pregnant woman and neonate. May cause adverse effects on neurodevelopment, including increases in autism spectrum disorders and attention deficit/hyperactivity disorder, decreased IQ, neural tube defects, and hearing impairment/loss. Advise pregnant patients taking valproates to enroll in the North American Anti Epileptic Drug Pregnancy Registry to monitor pregnancy outcomes by calling 1-888-233-2334; call must be made by patient. Registry website is www.aedpregnancyregistry.org. May cause male infertility. Monitor breastfed infant for signs of liver damage including jaundice and unusual bruising or bleeding.
- Advise patient to carry identification at all times describing medication regimen.
- Emphasize the importance of routine exams to monitor progress.

Evaluation/Desired Outcomes
- Decreased seizure activity.
- Decreased incidence of manic episodes in patients with bipolar disorders.
- Decreased frequency of migraine headaches.

valproate sodium, See VALPROATES.

valproic acid, See VALPROATES.

valsartan, See ANGIOTENSIN II RECEPTOR ANTAGONISTS.

vancomycin (van-koe-mye-sin)
Firvanq, Vancocin
Classification
Therapeutic: anti-infectives

Indications
IV: Potentially life-threatening infections when less toxic anti-infectives are contraindicated. Particularly useful in staphylococcal infections, including: endocarditis, meningitis, osteomyelitis, pneumonia, septicemia, soft-tissue infections in patients who have allergies to penicillin or its derivatives or when sensitivity testing demonstrates resistance to methicillin. **PO:** Staphylococcal enterocolitis or diarrhea due to *Clostridioides difficile*. **IV:** Part of endocarditis prophylaxis in high-risk patients who are allergic to penicillin.

Action
Binds to bacterial cell wall, resulting in cell death. **Therapeutic Effects:** Bactericidal action against susceptible organisms. **Spectrum:** Active against gram-positive pathogens, including: Staphylococci (including methicillin-resistant strains of *Staphylococcus aureus*), Group A beta-hemolytic streptococci, *Streptococcus pneumoniae*, *Corynebacterium*, *Clostridioides difficile*, *Enterococcus faecalis*, *Enterococcus faecium*.

Pharmacokinetics
Absorption: Poorly absorbed from the GI tract.
Distribution: Widely distributed to tissues. Some penetration (20–30%) of CSF.
Metabolism and Excretion: Oral doses excreted primarily in the feces; IV vancomycin eliminated almost entirely by the kidneys.
Half-life: *Neonates:* 6–10 hr; *Children 3 mo–3 yr:* 4 hr; *Children >3 yr:* 2–2.3 hr; *Adults:* 5–8 hr (↑ in renal impairment).

TIME/ACTION PROFILE (plasma concentrations)

ROUTE	ONSET	PEAK	DURATION
IV	rapid	end of infusion	12–24 hr

Contraindications/Precautions
Contraindicated in: Hypersensitivity.
Use Cautiously in: Renal impairment (dose ↓ required if CCr ≤80 mL/min); Hearing impairment; Intestinal obstruction or inflammation (↑ systemic absorption when given orally); OB: Pharmacokinetics of IV vancomycin may be altered in pregnancy (volume of distribution may be ↑); systemic absorption of PO vancomycin expected to be minimal; Lactation: Use while breastfeeding only if potential maternal benefit justifies potential risk to infant.

Adverse Reactions/Side Effects
CV: hypotension. **Derm:** ACUTE GENERALIZED EXANTHEMATOUS PUSTULOSIS, DRUG REACTION WITH EOSINOPHILIA AND SYSTEMIC SYMPTOMS, LINEAR IGA BULLOUS DERMATOSIS, rash, STEVENS-JOHNSON SYNDROME, TOXIC EPIDERMAL NECROLYSIS. **EENT:** ototoxicity. **GI:** nausea, vomiting. **GU:** nephrotoxicity. **Hemat:** eosinophilia, leukopenia. **Local:** phlebitis. **MS:** back and neck pain. **Misc:** chills, fever, HYPERSENSITIVITY REACTIONS (including anaphylaxis), vancomycin flushing syndrome (with rapid infusion).

Interactions
Drug-Drug: May cause additive ototoxicity and nephrotoxicity with other **ototoxic** and **nephrotoxic drugs**, including **aspirin, aminoglycosides, cyclosporine, cisplatin**, and **loop diuretics**. May enhance neuromuscular blockade from **nondepolarizing neuromuscular blocking agents**. ↑ risk of histamine flush when used with **general anesthetics** in children.

Route/Dosage
Serious Systemic Infections
IV (Adults): 500 mg every 6 hr *or* 1 g every 12 hr (up to 4 g/day).
IV (Children >1 mo): 40 mg/kg/day divided every 6–8 hr. *Staphylococcal CNS infection:* 60 mg/kg/day divided every 6 hr, maximum dose: 1 g/dose.
IV (Neonates 1 wk–1 mo and >2000 g): 15–20 mg/kg every 8 hr.
IV (Neonates 1 wk–1 mo and 1200–2000 g): 10–15 mg/kg every 8–12 hr.
IV (Neonates 1 wk–1 mo and <1200 g): 15 mg/kg every 24 hr.
IV (Neonates <1 wk and >2000 g): 10–15 mg/kg every 8–12 hr.
IV (Neonates <1 wk and 1200–2000 g): 10–15 mg/kg every 12–18 hr.

IV (Neonates <1 wk and <1200 g): 15 mg/kg every 24 hr.
IT (Adults): 20 mg/day.
IT (Children): 5–20 mg/day.
IT (Neonates): 5–10 mg/day.

Renal Impairment
IV (Adults): An initial loading dose of 750 mg–1 g (not less than 15 mg/kg); serum level monitoring is optimal for choosing maintenance dose in patients with renal impairment; these guidelines may be helpful. *CCr 50–80 mL/min:* 1 g every 1–3 days; *CCr 10–50 mL/min:* 1 g every 3–7 days; *CCr <10 mL/min:* 1 g every 7–14 days.

Endocarditis Prophylaxis in Penicillin-Allergic Patients
IV (Adults and Adolescents): 1 g single dose 1 hr preprocedure.
IV (Children): 20 mg/kg single dose 1 hr preprocedure.

Diarrhea Due to *C. difficile*
PO (Adults): 125 mg every 6 hr for 10 days.
PO (Children): 40 mg/kg/day divided into 3 or 4 doses for 7–10 days (not to exceed 2 g/day).

Staphylococcal Enterocolitis
PO (Adults): 500–2000 mg/day in 3–4 divided doses for 7–10 days.
PO (Children): 40 mg/kg/day in 3–4 divided doses for 7–10 days (not to exceed 2 g/day).

Availability (generic available)
Capsules: 125 mg, 250 mg. **Powder for oral solution (grape flavor):** 3.75 g/bottle, 7.5 g/bottle, 15 g/bottle. **Premixed infusion:** 500 mg/100 mL D5W, 750 mg/150 mL D5W, 1000 mg/200 mL D5W or 0.9% NaCl, 1250 mg/200 mL D5W, 1500 mg/300 mL D5W, 1750 mg/350 mL D5W, 2000 mg/400 mL D5W. **Solution for injection:** 250 mg/vial, 500 mg/vial, 750 mg/vial, 1 g/vial, 1.5 g/vial, 5 g/vial, 10 g/vial, 100 g/vial.

NURSING IMPLICATIONS
Assessment
- Assess patient for infection (vital signs; appearance of wound, sputum, urine, and stool; WBC) at beginning of and throughout therapy.
- Obtain specimens for culture and sensitivity prior to initiating therapy. First dose may be given before receiving results.
- Monitor IV site closely. Vancomycin is irritating to tissues and causes necrosis and severe pain with extravasation. Rotate infusion site.
- Monitor BP during IV infusion.
- Evaluate eighth cranial nerve function by audiometry and serum vancomycin levels prior to and throughout therapy in patients with borderline renal function or those >60 yr of age. Prompt recognition and intervention are essential in preventing permanent damage.
- Monitor intake and output ratios and daily weight. Cloudy or pink urine may be a sign of nephrotoxicity.

- Assess patient for signs of superinfection (black, furry overgrowth on tongue; vaginal itching or discharge; loose or foul-smelling stools). Report occurrence.
- Observe patient for signs and symptoms of anaphylaxis (rash, pruritus, laryngeal edema, wheezing). Discontinue drug and notify health care professional immediately if these problems occur. Keep epinephrine, an antihistamine, and resuscitation equipment close by in case of an anaphylactic reaction.
- *C. difficile*-**Associated Diarrhea:** Assess bowel status (bowel sounds, frequency and consistency of stools, presence of blood in stools) throughout therapy.

Lab Test Considerations
- Monitor for casts, albumin, or cells in the urine or decreased specific gravity, CBC, and renal function periodically during therapy.
- May cause ↑ BUN levels.

Toxicity and Overdose
- Trough concentrations should not exceed 10 mcg/mL (mild to moderate infections) or 15–20 mcg/mL (for severe infections).

Implementation
- Vancomycin must be given orally for treatment of staphylococcal enterocolitis and *C. difficile*-associated diarrhea. Orally administered vancomycin is not effective for other types of infections.
- **PO:** Use calibrated measuring device for liquid preparations. Shake well before use. Oral solution is stable for 14 days if refrigerated.

IV Administration
- **Intermittent Infusion:** *Dilution:* To reconstitute, add 10 mL of sterile water for injection to 500-mg vial or 20 mL of sterile water for injection to 1-g vial for a concentration of 50 mg/mL. Dilute further with at least 100 mL of 0.9% NaCl, D5W, D5/0.9% NaCl, or LR for every 500 mg of vancomycin being administered. Reconstituted vials stable for 14 days if refrigerated. Infusion is stable for 96 hr if refrigerated. *Concentration:* ≤5 mg/mL. *Rate:* Infuse over at least 60 min (90 min for doses >1 g). Do not administer rapidly or as a bolus, to minimize risk of thrombophlebitis, hypotension, and vancomycin flushing syndrome (sudden, severe hypotension; flushing and/or maculopapular rash of face, neck, chest, and upper extremities). May need to slow infusion further to 1.5–2 hr if vancomycin flushing syndrome occurs.
- **IT:** *Dilution:* Dilute with preservative-free NS. *Concentration:* 1–5 mg/mL. *Rate:* Directly instill into ventricular cerebrospinal fluid.
- **Y-Site Compatibility:** acetaminophen, acetylcysteine, acyclovir, aldesleukin, alemtuzumab, allopurinol, alprostadil, amifostine, amikacin, aminocaproic acid, amiodarone, anidulafungin, argatroban, arsenic trioxide, ascorbic acid, atracurium, atropine, azithromycin, benztropine, bleomycin, bumetanide,

buprenorphine, butorphanol, calcium chloride, calcium gluconate, carboplatin, carmustine, caspofungin, ceftolozane/tazobactam, chlorpromazine, ciprofloxacin, cisatracurium, cisplatin, clindamycin, cyanocobalamin, cyclophosphamide, cyclosporine, cytarabine, dactinomycin, daunorubicin hydrochloride, dexamethasone, dexmedetomidine, dexrazoxane, digoxin, diltiazem, diphenhydramine, dobutamine, docetaxel, dopamine, doxorubicin hydrochloride, doxorubicin liposomal, doxycycline, enalaprilat, ephedrine, epinephrine, epirubicin, eptifibatide, eravacycline, ertapenem, erythromycin, esmolol, etoposide, etoposide phosphate, famotidine, fentanyl, filgrastim, fluconazole, fludarabine, folic acid, fosphenytoin, gemcitabine, gentamicin, glycopyrrolate, granisetron, hetastarch, hydromorphone, ifosfamide, insulin regular, irinotecan, isavuconazonium, isoproterenol, ketamine, labetalol, levofloxacin, lidocaine, linezolid, lorazepam, magnesium sulfate, mannitol, melphalan, meperidine, meropenem/vaborbactam, mesna, methadone, metoclopramide, metoprolol, metronidazole, midazolam, milrinone, mitoxantrone, morphine, multivitamins, mycophenolate, nalbuphine, naloxone, nicardipine, nitroglycerin, nitroprusside, norepinephrine, octreotide, ondansetron, oxaliplatin, oxytocin, paclitaxel, palonosetron, pamidronate, papaverine, pemetrexed, pentamidine, pentobarbital, phenobarbital, phentolamine, phenylephrine, phytonadione, plazomicin, potassium acetate, potassium chloride, procainamide, prochlorperazine, promethazine, propranolol, protamine, pyridoxine, remifentanil, rifampin, sodium acetate, sodium bicarbonate, sodium citrate, succinylcholine, sufentanil, tacrolimus, tedizolid, thiamine, thiotepa, tigecycline, tirofiban, tobramycin, trastuzumab, vasopressin, vecuronium, verapamil, vinblastine, vincristine, vinorelbine, voriconazole, zidovudine, zoledronic acid.

- **Y-Site Incompatibility:** albumin, human, aminophylline, amphotericin B deoxycholate, amphotericin lipid complex, amphotericin B liposomal, azathioprine, bivalirudin, chloramphenicol, dantrolene, daptomycin, diazepam, epoetin alfa, fluorouracil, furosemide, ganciclovir, gemtuzumab ozogamicin, ibuprofen lysine, idarubicin, indomethacin, ketorolac, leucovorin calcium, methylprednisolone, mitomycin, moxifloxacin, phenytoin, rituximab, trimethoprim/sulfamethoxazole, valproate sodium.

Patient/Family Teaching

- Advise patients on oral vancomycin to take as directed. Take missed doses as soon as remembered unless almost time for next dose; do not double dose.
- Instruct patient to report signs of hypersensitivity, tinnitus, vertigo, or hearing loss.
- Advise patient to notify health care professional if no improvement is seen in a few days.
- Patients with a history of rheumatic heart disease or valve replacement need to be taught importance of using antimicrobial prophylaxis prior to invasive dental or medical procedures.
- Rep: Advise females of reproductive potential to notify health care professional if pregnancy is planned or suspected or if breastfeeding.

Evaluation/Desired Outcomes

- Resolution of signs and symptoms of infection. Length of time for complete resolution depends on organism and site of infection.
- Endocarditis prophylaxis.

REMS

vandetanib (van-det-a-nib)
Caprelsa
Classification
Therapeutic: antineoplastics
Pharmacologic: kinase inhibitors

Indications
Symptomatic/progressive medullary thyroid cancer in patients with unresectable, locally advanced, or metastatic disease.

Action
Inhibits tyrosine kinase; results in inhibited action of epidermal growth factor (EGFR), vascular endothelial cell growth factor and other kinase-based actions. Inhibits endothelial cell migration/proliferation/survival and new blood vessel formation. Also inhibits EGFR-dependent cell survival. **Therapeutic Effects:** Decreased spread of thyroid cancer.

Pharmacokinetics
Absorption: Well absorbed following oral administration.
Distribution: Extensively distributed to tissues.
Metabolism and Excretion: Mostly metabolized by the liver; 44% excreted in feces, 25% in urine.
Half-life: 19 days.

TIME/ACTION PROFILE (plasma concentrations)

ROUTE	ONSET	PEAK	DURATION
PO	unknown	4–10 hr	24 hr

Contraindications/Precautions
Contraindicated in: Congenital long QT syndrome or QTcF interval >450 msec; Hypocalcemia (serum calcium should be within normal range), hypokalemia (serum potassium should be >4.0 mEq/L and within normal range), or hypomagnesemia (serum magnesium should be within normal range); Severe renal im-

pairment (CCr <30 mL/min); OB: Pregnancy; Lactation: Lactation.

Use Cautiously in: Diarrhea (↑ risk of electrolyte abnormalities and risk of arrhythmias); Renal impairment (dose ↓ recommended for CCr 30–<50 mL/min with close monitoring of QT interval); Moderate or severe hepatic impairment; Rep: Women of reproductive potential; Pedi: Safety and effectiveness not established in children.

Exercise Extreme Caution in: Concurrent use of other drugs know to prolong QT interval (avoid if possible; if medically necessary, monitoring is required).

Adverse Reactions/Side Effects

CV: hypertension, HF, QT interval prolongation, TORSADES DE POINTES. **Derm:** acne, photosensitivity reaction, rash, impaired wound healing, pruritus, STEVENS-JOHNSON SYNDROME, TOXIC EPIDERMAL NECROLYSIS. **Endo:** hypothyroidism. **F and E:** hypocalcemia. **GI:** ↓ appetite, abdominal pain, diarrhea, nausea, dyspepsia, GI PERFORATION, vomiting. **GU:** proteinuria, renal failure. **Hemat:** BLEEDING. **Neuro:** fatigue, headache, depression, insomnia, REVERSIBLE POSTERIOR LEUKOENCEPHALOPATHY SYNDROME (RPLS), STROKE. **Resp:** INTERSTITIAL LUNG DISEASE (ILD), upper respiratory tract infection.

Interactions

Drug-Drug: **Strong CYP3A4 inducers**, including **carbamazepine, dexamethasone, phenobarbital, phenytoin, rifabutin, rifampin, rifapentine**, and **phenobarbital**, may ↓ levels and effectiveness; avoid concurrent use. Concurrent use with **QT interval prolonging drugs**, including some **antiarrhythmics** (**amiodarone, disopyramide, procainamide, sotalol, dofetilide**) **chloroquine, clarithromycin, granisetron, haloperidol, methadone, moxifloxacin**, and **pimozide** may ↑ risk of QT interval prolongation and torsades de pointes; avoid concurrent use. May ↑ levels and the risk of toxicity of **metformin** and **digoxin**.

Drug-Natural Products: St. John's wort may ↓ levels and effectiveness; avoid concurrent use.

Route/Dosage

PO (Adults): 300 mg once daily.

Renal Impairment

PO (Adults): *CCr 30–<50 mL/min:* 200 mg once daily. *CCr <30 mL/min:* Not recommended.

Availability

Tablets: 100 mg, 300 mg.

NURSING IMPLICATIONS

Assessment

- May prolong the QT interval. Obtain ECG at baseline, at 2–4 wk, at 8–12 wk after starting therapy and every 3 mo thereafter. Use these parameters to assess QT interval following dose reduction for QT interval prolongation or dose interruption >2 wk. May

require more frequent monitoring if diarrhea occurs.

- Assess patient for rash periodically during therapy. Mild to moderate skin reactions may include rash, acne, dry skin, dermatitis, and pruritus and may be treated with topical or systemic corticosteroids, oral antihistamines, and topical and systemic antibiotics. Treatment of severe rash (Grade 3 or greater) may include systemic corticosteroids and discontinuation of treatment until improved. Upon improvement, may be restarted at a reduced dose.
- Assess for signs and symptoms of ILD (hypoxia, pleural effusion, cough, dyspnea). If radiological changes occur with few or no symptoms, therapy may continue. If symptoms are moderate, consider interrupting therapy until symptoms improve. If symptoms are severe, discontinue therapy; permanent discontinuation should be considered. Treat with antibiotics and corticosteroids.
- Assess for signs and symptoms of HF (intake and output rations, daily weight, peripheral edema, rales and crackles upon lung auscultation, dyspnea) periodically during therapy.
- Monitor BP during therapy. Control hypertension during therapy.
- Monitor for diarrhea. If severe diarrhea develops, hold therapy until resolved.
- Monitor for signs and symptoms of RPLS (seizures, headache, visual disturbances, confusion, altered mental status); discontinue therapy if symptoms occur.

Lab Test Considerations

- Verify negative pregnancy test before starting therapy.
- Monitor serum calcium, potassium, and magnesium periodically during therapy. Maintain serum potassium at ≥4 mEq/L. Maintain serum calcium and magnesium within normal limits. May require more frequent monitoring if diarrhea occurs.
- Monitor TSH at baseline, at 2–4 wk, at 8–12 wk, and every 3 mo thereafter in patients with thyroidectomy. If symptoms of hypothyroidism occur, check TSH levels and adjust thyroid replacement.
- May cause ↓ serum glucose, WBC, hemoglobin, neutrophils, and platelets.
- May cause ↑ serum ALT, serum creatinine, serum bilirubin, and serum glucose.

Implementation

- *REMS:* Due to the cardiac risks, only prescribers and pharmacies certified with the Caprelsa REMS program are able to prescribe and dispense vandetanib. To learn about the specific REMS requirements and to enroll in the CAPRELSA REMS Program, call 1-800-817-2722 or visit www.caprelsarems.com.
- Correct hypocalcemia, hypokalemia, and hypomagnesemia prior to therapy.

- **PO:** May be administered daily without regard to food. **DNC:** Swallow tablets whole; do not crush, break, or chew. If unable to swallow tablet, tablet may be dispersed in a glass containing 2 oz of non-carbonated water and stirred for approximately 10 min until tablet is dispersed (will not completely dissolve). No other liquids should be used. Swallow dispersion immediately, then mix any residue with 4 oz of non-carbonated water and swallow. Dispersion may also be administered through nasogastric or gastrostomy tubes. Avoid direct contact with crushed tablets with skin or mucous membranes. Wash thoroughly to avoid exposure.

Patient/Family Teaching

- Instruct patient to take vandetanib as directed. Take missed doses as soon as remembered unless within 12 hr of next dose. Instruct patient to read *Medication Guide* prior to starting therapy and with each Rx refill in case of changes.
- Advise patients to notify health care professional if rash or signs and symptoms of interstitial lung disease or reversible posterior leukoencephalopathy syndrome. If diarrhea occurs, instruct patient to treat with antidiarrheal medications and notify health care professional if diarrhea becomes severe or persistent.
- May cause tiredness, weakness, or blurred vision. Caution patients to avoid driving or other activities requiring alertness until response to medication is known.
- Caution patient to wear sunscreen and protective clothing during and for 4 mo after therapy is discontinued to prevent photosensitivity reactions.
- Advise patient to notify health care professional of all Rx or OTC medications, vitamins, or herbal products being taken and to consult with health care professional before taking other medications, especially St. John's wort.
- May impair wound healing. Advise patient to notify health care professionals of therapy. Therapy must be stopped for at least 1 month before elective dental surgery, invasive dental procedures, or elective surgeries and then held for at least 2 wk after major surgery until adequate wound healing.
- Rep: May cause fetal harm. Advise females of reproductive potential to use effective contraception during and for 4 mo after therapy and to avoid breastfeeding during therapy and for 4 month after final dose. May impair female and male fertility.
- Emphasize the importance of regular follow-up exams, ECGs, and blood counts to determine progress and monitor for side effects.

Evaluation/Desired Outcomes

- Decreased spread of thyroid cancer.

vardenafil (var-**den**-a-fil)
✢ Levitra, ✢ Staxyn

Classification
Therapeutic: erectile dysfunction agents
Pharmacologic: phosphodiesterase type 5 inhibitors

Indications
Erectile dysfunction (ED).

Action
Increases cyclic guanosine monophosphate (cGMP) levels by inhibiting phosphodiesterase type 5, an enzyme responsible for the breakdown of cGMP. cGMP produces smooth muscle relaxation of the corpus cavernosum, which in turn promotes increased blood flow and subsequent erection. **Therapeutic Effects:** Enhanced blood flow to the corpus cavernosum and erection sufficient to allow sexual intercourse. Requires sexual stimulation.

Pharmacokinetics
Absorption: 15% absorbed following oral administration; absorption is rapid.
Distribution: Extensive tissue distribution; penetrates semen.
Protein Binding: 95%.
Metabolism and Excretion: Mostly metabolized by the liver via the CYP3A4 isoenzyme and to a lesser extent the CYP2C isoenzyme. M1 metabolite has antierectile dysfunction activity. Parent drug and metabolites are mostly excreted in feces. 2–6% renally eliminated.
Half-life: 4–6 hr.

TIME/ACTION PROFILE

ROUTE	ONSET	PEAK	DURATION
PO	rapid	0.5–2 hr	4 hr

Contraindications/Precautions
Contraindicated in: Hypersensitivity; Concurrent use of nitrates or riociguat; Unstable angina, recent history of stroke, life-threatening arrhythmias, HF or MI within 6 mo; End-stage renal disease requiring dialysis; Known hereditary degenerative retinal disorders; Moderate hepatic impairment (orally disintegrating tablets only); Severe hepatic impairment; Congenital or acquired QT prolongation or concurrent use of Class IA or III antiarrhythmics.
Use Cautiously in: Other serious underlying cardiovascular disease or left ventricular outflow obstruction; Penile deformity; Underlying conditions predisposing to priapism, including sickle cell anemia, multiple myeloma, or leukemia; Bleeding disorders or active peptic ulcer diseases; History of sudden severe vision loss or non-arteritic ischemic optic neuropathy (NAION); may ↑ risk of recurrence; Low cup-to-disk

V

✢ = Canadian drug name. ⚌ = Genetic implication. ~~Strikethrough~~ = Discontinued. CAPITALS = life-threatening. Underline = most frequent.

ratio, age >50 yr, diabetes, hypertension, coronary artery disease, hyperlipidemia, or smoking (↑ risk of NAION); Geri: Older adults may have ↑ levels; ↓ dose required.

Adverse Reactions/Side Effects

Derm: flushing. **EENT:** HEARING LOSS, rhinitis, sinusitis, VISION LOSS. **GI:** dyspepsia, nausea. **GU:** priapism. **Neuro:** headache, amnesia, dizziness. **Misc:** flu syndrome.

Interactions

Drug-Drug: Concurrent use of **nitrates** may cause serious, life-threatening hypotension and is contraindicated. Concurrent use of **riociguat** may result in severe hypotension; concurrent use contraindicated. Concurrent use of Class IA antiarrhythmics (such as **quinidine** or **procainamide**) or **Class III antiarrhythmics** (such as **amiodarone** or **sotalol**) ↑ risk of serious arrhythmias and should be avoided. Concurrent use of alpha-adrenergic blockers may cause serious hypotension; lowest doses of each should be used initially. **Strong CYP3A4 inhibitors,** including **atazanavir, clarithromycin, cobicistat, itraconazole, ketoconazole,** and **ritonavir,** may ↑ levels and the risk of toxicity; concurrent use of **moderate CYP3A4 inhibitors,** including **erythromycin,** may also ↑ levels and the risk of toxicity; avoid concurrent use with Staxyn; dose of Levitra must be ↓. ↑ risk of hypotension with **alpha-adrenergic blockers** and acute ingestion of **alcohol**; patients should be on stable dose of alpha blockers before starting vardenafil (should start therapy with tablets [orally disintegrating tablets should not be used]).

Route/Dosage

The tablets and orally disintegrating tablets are not interchangeable; the orally disintegrating tablets provide a higher level of systemic exposure compared to the tablets.

Tablets

PO (Adults): 10 mg taken 1 hr prior to sexual activity (range 5–20 mg; not to exceed one dose/24 hr); *Concurrent use of cobicistat or ritonavir:* single dose should not exceed 2.5 mg in any 72-hr period; *Concurrent use of atazanavir, clarithromycin, ketoconazole 400 mg daily, or itraconazole 400 mg daily:* single dose should not exceed 2.5 mg/24 hr; *Concurrent use of ketoconazole 200 mg daily, itraconazole 200 mg daily, or erythromycin:* single dose should not exceed 5 mg/24 hr; *Concurrent use of stable alpha-blocker therapy (not on potent CYP3A4 inhibitor):* 5 mg initial dose; titrate as tolerated; *Concurrent use of stable alpha-blocker and potent CYP3A4 inhibitor therapy:* 2.5 mg initial dose; titrate as tolerated. **PO (Geriatric Patients ≥65 yr):** 5 mg initial dose; titrate as tolerated.

Hepatic Impairment

PO (Adults): *Moderate hepatic impairment:* May start with 5 mg dose (not to exceed 10 mg).

Orally Disintegrating Tablets

PO (Adults): 10 mg taken 1 hr prior to sexual activity (not to exceed one dose/24 hr).

Availability (generic available)

Tablets: 2.5 mg, 5 mg, 10 mg, 20 mg. **Orally disintegrating tablets (peppermint flavor):** 10 mg.

NURSING IMPLICATIONS

Assessment

* Assess for the presence of ED before administration. Vardenafil has no effect in the absence of sexual stimulation.

Implementation

* *Tablets* and *orally disintegrating tablets* are not interchangeable.
* **PO:** *Tablets* are usually administered 1 hr before sexual activity. May be administered 30 min to 4 hr before sexual activity.
* Administer *orally disintegrating tablets* 1 hr before sexual activity. These tablets should be left in the package until use. Remove from the blister pouch. Do not push tablet through the blister; peel open the blister pack with dry hands and place tablet on tongue. Tablet will dissolve rapidly and be swallowed with saliva. No liquid is needed to take the orally disintegrating tablet.
* May be administered without regard to food.

Patient/Family Teaching

* Instruct patient to take vardenafil approximately 30 min–1 hr before sexual activity and not more than once per day. Inform patient that sexual stimulation is required for an erection to occur after taking vardenafil.
* Advise patient that vardenafil is not indicated for use in women.
* Caution patient not to take vardenafil concurrently with alpha adrenergic blockers (unless on a stable dose) or nitrates. If chest pain occurs after taking vardenafil, instruct patient to seek immediate medical attention.
* Instruct patient to notify health care professional promptly if erection lasts longer than 4 hr or if sudden or decreased vision loss in one or both eyes, or loss or decrease in hearing, ringing in the ears, or dizziness occurs.
* Instruct patient to notify health care professional of all Rx or OTC medications, vitamins, or herbal products being taken and consult health care professional before taking any new medications.
* Inform patient that vardenafil offers no protection against sexually transmitted diseases. Counsel patient that protection against sexually transmitted diseases and HIV infection should be considered.

Evaluation/Desired Outcomes

* Male erection sufficient to allow intercourse.

varenicline (systemic)
(var-**en**-i-kleen)
✤ Champix, ~~Chantix~~

Classification
Therapeutic: smoking deterrents
Pharmacologic: nicotine agonists

Indications
Smoking cessation (in combination with nonpharmacologic support).

Action
Selectively binds to alpha$_4$, beta$_2$ nicotinic acetylcholine receptors, acting as a nicotine agonist; prevents the binding of nicotine to receptors. **Therapeutic Effects:** Decreased desire to smoke.

Pharmacokinetics
Absorption: 100% absorbed following oral administration.
Distribution: Unknown.
Metabolism and Excretion: Minimally metabolized; 92% excreted in urine unchanged.
Half-life: 24 hr.

TIME/ACTION PROFILE

ROUTE	ONSET	PEAK	DURATION
PO	unknown	3–4 hr	24 hr

Contraindications/Precautions
Contraindicated in: Hypersensitivity; Lactation: Lactation.
Use Cautiously in: Severe renal impairment (↓ dose recommended if CCr <30 mL/min); Stable cardiovascular disease (may ↑ risk of cardiovascular events); Psychiatric illness; Seizure disorders; OB: Use during pregnancy only if potential maternal benefit outweighs potential fetal risk; Pedi: Safety not established in children; Geri: Consider age-related ↓ in renal function in older adults.

Adverse Reactions/Side Effects
CV: MI, syncope. **Derm:** flushing, hyperhidrosis, acne, dermatitis, dry skin, STEVENS-JOHNSON SYNDROME (SJS). **EENT:** blurred vision, visual disturbances. **GI:** diarrhea, gingivitis, nausea, ↑ appetite, ↑ liver enzymes, constipation, dyspepsia, dysphagia, enterocolitis, eructation, flatulence, gallbladder disorder, GI bleeding, vomiting. **Hemat:** anemia. **MS:** arthralgia, back pain, musculoskeletal pain, muscle cramps, myalgia, restless legs. **Neuro:** ↓ attention span, depression, dizziness, insomnia, irritability, restlessness, abnormal dreams, aggression, agitation, amnesia, anxiety, delusions, disorientation, dissociation, hallucinations, HOMICIDAL THOUGHTS/BEHAVIOR, hostility, mania, migraine, mood changes, panic, paranoia, psychosis, SEIZURES,

sleepwalking, STROKE, SUICIDAL THOUGHTS/BEHAVIOR. **Misc:** accidental injury, chills, fever, HYPERSENSITIVITY REACTIONS (including angioedema), mild physical dependence.

Interactions
Drug-Drug: Smoking cessation may ↓ metabolism of **theophylline**, **warfarin**, and **insulin** resulting in ↑ effects; careful monitoring is recommended. Risk of adverse reactions (nausea, vomiting, dizziness, fatigue, headache) may be ↑ with **nicotine** replacement therapy (nicotine transdermal patches). Concomitant use with **alcohol** may ↑ risk of worsening neuropsychiatric events.

Route/Dosage
PO (Adults): Treatment is started one wk prior to planned smoking cessation (may also begin dosing and then quit smoking between days 8 and 35 of treatment); 0.5 mg once daily on the first three days, then 0.5 mg twice daily for the next 4 days, then 1 mg twice daily.

Renal Impairment
PO (Adults): *CCr <30 mL/min:* 0.5 mg daily, may ↑ to 0.5 mg twice daily.

Availability (generic available)
Tablets: 0.5 mg, 1 mg.

NURSING IMPLICATIONS

Assessment
- Assess for desire to stop smoking.
- Monitor for nausea. Usually dose-dependent. May require dose reduction.
- Assess mental status and mood changes, especially during initial few mo of therapy and during dose changes. Risk may be increased in children, adolescents, and adults ≤24 yr. Inform health care professional if patient demonstrates significant increase in signs of depression (depressed mood, loss of interest in usual activities, significant change in weight and/or appetite, insomnia or hypersomnia, psychomotor agitation or retardation, increased fatigue, feelings of guilt or worthlessness, slowed thinking or impaired concentration, suicide attempt or suicidal or homicidal ideation). Restrict amount of drug available to patient.
- Assess for rash periodically during therapy. May cause SJS. Discontinue therapy if severe or if accompanied with fever, general malaise, fatigue, muscle or joint aches, blisters, oral lesions, conjunctivitis, hepatitis and/or eosinophilia.

Lab Test Considerations
- May cause anemia.

Implementation
- **PO:** Administer after eating with a full glass of water.

V

✤ = Canadian drug name. ▧ = Genetic implication. ~~Strikethrough~~ = Discontinued. CAPITALS = life-threatening. <u>Underline</u> = most frequent.

Patient/Family Teaching

● Instruct patient to take varenicline as directed. Set a date to stop smoking. Start taking varenicline 1 wk before quit date. Patient may also begin varenicline and then quit smoking between days 8 and 35 of therapy. Begin with 0.5 mg/day for the first 3 days, then for the next 4 days take one 0.5 mg tablet in the morning and in the evening. After first 7 days, increase to 1 mg tablet in the morning and evening. Advise patient to read *Medication Guide* before starting therapy and with each Rx refill in case of changes.

● Encourage patient to attempt to quit, even if they had early lapses after quit day.

● Advise patient to stop taking varenicline and contact health care professional promptly if agitation, depressed mood, any changes in behavior that are not typical of nicotine withdrawal, or if suicidal thoughts or behavior; rash with mucosal lesions or skin reaction, or chest pain, pressure, or dyspnea occur. Encourage patient to reduce amount of alcohol consumed until effects of medication are known.

● Provide patient with educational materials and counseling to support attempts to quit smoking.

● Caution patient not to share varenicline with others. May be harmful.

● May cause blurred vision, dizziness, and disturbance in attention. Caution patient to avoid driving and other activities requiring alertness until response to medication is known.

● Inform patient that nausea, insomnia, and vivid, unusual, or strange dreams may occur and are usually transient. Advise patient to notify health care professional if these symptoms are persistent and bothersome; dose reduction may be considered.

● Instruct patient to notify health care professional of all Rx or OTC medications, vitamins, or herbal products being taken and consult health care professional before taking any new medications. Inform patient that some medications may require dose adjustments after quitting smoking.

● Rep: Advise females of reproductive potential to notify health care professional if pregnancy is planned or suspected or if breastfeeding. Monitor breastfed infants for seizures and excessive vomiting.

Evaluation/Desired Outcomes

● Smoking cessation. Patients who have successfully stopped smoking at the end of 12 wk should take an additional 12-wk course to increase the likelihood of long-term abstinence. Patients who do not succeed in stopping smoking during 12 wk of initial therapy or who relapse after treatment should be encouraged to make another attempt once factors contributing to the failed attempt have been identified and addressed.

vasopressin (vay-soe-press-in)
~~Pitressin~~, Vasostrict

Classification
Therapeutic: hormones
Pharmacologic: antidiuretic hormones, vasopressors

Indications

Central diabetes insipidus due to deficient antidiuretic hormone. Vasodilatory shock. **Unlabeled Use:** Gastrointestinal hemorrhage.

Action

Alters the permeability of the renal collecting ducts, allowing reabsorption of water. Directly stimulates musculature of GI tract. In high doses acts as a nonadrenergic peripheral vasoconstrictor. **Therapeutic Effects:** Decreased urine output and increased urine osmolality in diabetes insipidus. Increased BP.

Pharmacokinetics

Absorption: IM absorption may be unpredictable. IV administration results in complete bioavailability.
Distribution: Well distributed to tissues.
Metabolism and Excretion: Rapidly degraded by the liver and kidneys; <5% excreted unchanged by the kidneys.
Half-life: <10 min.

TIME/ACTION PROFILE (antidiuretic effect)

ROUTE	ONSET	PEAK	DURATION
IM, SUBQ	unknown	unknown	2–8 hr
IV	unknown	unknown	30–60 min

Contraindications/Precautions

Contraindicated in: Hypersensitivity to 8-L arginine vasopressin or chlorobutanol (only in multidose vial); Chronic renal failure.

Use Cautiously in: Perioperative polyuria (↑ sensitivity to vasopressin effects); Comatose patients; Seizures; Migraine headaches; Asthma; HF; Cardiovascular disease; Renal impairment; OB: Higher doses (0.07 units/min) for vasodilatory shock may be needed in 2nd and 3rd trimesters; Lactation: Safety not established in breastfeeding; Geri: Older adults may have ↑ sensitivity to effects.

Adverse Reactions/Side Effects

CV: angina, chest pain, MI. **Derm:** paleness, perioral blanching, sweating. **Endo:** diabetes insipidus. **F and E:** water intoxication (higher doses). **GI:** abdominal cramps, belching, diarrhea, flatulence, heartburn, nausea, vomiting. **Neuro:** "pounding" sensation in head, dizziness, trembling. **Misc:** allergic reactions, fever.

Interactions

Drug-Drug: Antidiuretic effect may be ↓ by concurrent administration of **clozapine**, **lithium**, **demeclocycline**, **foscarnet**. Antidiuretic effect may be ↑ by concurrent administration of **cyclophosphamide**, **enalapril**, **felbamate**, **haloperidol**, **ifosfamide**, **pentamidine**, **tricyclic antidepressants**, **SSRIs**, or **vincristine**. Vasopressor effect may be ↑ by concurrent administration of **ganglionic blocking agents**, **indomethacin**, or **catecholamines**. **Furosemide** ↑ urine flow.

Route/Dosage
Diabetes Insipidus
IM, SUBQ (Adults): 5–10 units 2–4 times daily.
IM, SUBQ (Children): 2.5–10 units 2–4 times daily.
IV (Adults and Children): 0.0005 units/kg/hr, double dose every 30 min as needed to a maximum of 0.01 units/kg/hr.

Vasodilatory Shock
IV (Adults): 0.01 units/min, titrate by 0.005 units/min every 10–15 min until target BP achieved (max dose = 0.07 units/min).
IV (Infants and Children): 0.0003–0.002 units/kg/min, titrate to effect.

GI Hemorrhage
IV (Adults): 0.2–0.4 units/min then titrate to maximum dose of 0.9 units/min; if bleeding stops, continue same dose for 12 hr, then taper off over 24–48 hr.
IV (Children): 0.002–0.005 units/kg/min then titrate to maximum dose of 0.01 units/kg/min; if bleeding stops, continue same dose for 12 hr, then taper off over 24–48 hr.

Availability (generic available)
Premixed infusion: 20 units/100 mL D5W, 40 units/100 mL D5W, 60 units/100 mL D5W. **Solution for injection:** 20 units/mL.

NURSING IMPLICATIONS
Assessment
- Monitor BP, HR, and ECG periodically throughout therapy and continuously throughout cardiopulmonary resuscitation.
- **Diabetes Insipidus:** Monitor urine osmolality and urine volume frequently to determine effects of medication. Assess patient for symptoms of dehydration (excessive thirst, dry skin and mucous membranes, tachycardia, poor skin turgor). Weigh patient daily, monitor intake and output, and assess for edema.

Lab Test Considerations
- Monitor urine specific gravity during therapy.
- Monitor serum electrolyte concentrations periodically during therapy.

Toxicity and Overdose
- Signs and symptoms of water intoxication include confusion, drowsiness, headache, weight gain, difficulty urinating, seizures, and coma.
- Treatment of overdose includes water restriction and temporary discontinuation of vasopressin until polyuria occurs. If symptoms are severe, administra-

tion of mannitol, hypertonic dextrose, urea, and/or furosemide may be used.

Implementation
- Aqueous vasopressin injection may be administered SUBQ or IM for diabetes insipidus.
- Administer 1–2 glasses of water at the time of administration to minimize side effects (blanching of skin, abdominal cramps, nausea).

IV Administration
- **Continuous Infusion:** *Dilution:* Dilute 2.5 mg (no fluid restriction) or 5 mg (fluid restriction) of vasopressin in 500 mL or 100 mL respectively of 0.9% NaCl or D5W. Solution is clear and colorless; do not administer solutions that are cloudy, discolored, or contain particulate matter. *Concentration:* 0.1 units/mL or 1 unit/mL. Solution is stable for 18 hr at room temperature or 24 hr if refrigerated. *Rate:* See Route/Dosage section.
- **Y-Site Compatibility:** acyclovir, alemtuzumab, allopurinol, amifostine, amikacin, aminocaproic acid, aminophylline, amiodarone, amphotericin B liposomal, anidulafungin, argatroban, arsenic trioxide, ascorbic acid, atracurium, atropine, azathioprine, azithromycin, aztreonam, benztropine, bivalirudin, bleomycin, bumetanide, buprenorphine, busulfan, butorphanol, calcium chloride, calcium gluconate, carboplatin, carmustine, caspofungin, cefazolin, cefepime, cefotaxime, cefotetan, cefoxitin, ceftaroline, ceftazidime, ceftazidime/avibactam, ceftolozane/tazobactam, ceftriaxone, cefuroxime, chloramphenicol, chlorpromazine, ciprofloxacin, cisatracurium, cisplatin, clindamycin, cyanocobalamin, cyclophosphamide, cyclosporine, cytarabine, dacarbazine, dactinomycin, daptomycin, dexamethasone, dexmedetomidine, dexrazoxane, digoxin, diltiazem, diphenhydramine, dobutamine, docetaxel, dopamine, doxorubicin hydrochloride, doxorubicin liposomal, doxycycline, droperidol, enalaprilat, ephedrine, epinephrine, epirubicin, epoetin alfa, eravacycline, ertapenem, erythromycin, esmolol, etoposide, etoposide phosphate, famotidine, fentanyl, fluconazole, fludarabine, fluorouracil, folic acid, foscarnet, fosphenytoin, ganciclovir, gemcitabine, gentamicin, glycopyrrolate, granisetron, heparin, hetastarch, hydrocortisone, hydromorphone, idarubicin, ifosfamide, imipenem/cilastatin, irinotecan, isavuconazonium, isoproterenol, ketorolac, labetalol, LR, leucovorin calcium, levofloxacin, lidocaine, linezolid, lorazepam, magnesium sulfate, mannitol, melphalan, meperidine, meropenem, meropenem/vaborbactam, mesna, methadone, methohexital, methotrexate, methylprednisolone, metoclopramide, metoprolol, metronidazole, micafungin, midazolam, milrinone, mitomycin, mitoxantrone, morphine, moxifloxacin, multivitamins, mycophenolate, nafcillin, nalbuphine, naloxone, nicardipine, nitroglyc-

V

erin, nitroprusside, norepinephrine, octreotide, ondansetron, oxacillin, oxaliplatin, oxytocin, paclitaxel, palonosetron, pamidronate, pantoprazole, papaverine, penicillin G, pentamidine, pentobarbital, phenobarbital, phentolamine, phenylephrine, phytonadione, piperacillin/tazobactam, plazomicin, potassium acetate, potassium chloride, potassium phosphate, procainamide, prochlorperazine, promethazine, propranolol, protamine, pyridoxine, remifentanil, rocuronium, sodium acetate, sodium bicarbonate, sodium phosphate, succinylcholine, sufentanil, tacrolimus, tedizolid, telavancin, theophylline, thiamine, thiopental, thiotepa, tigecycline, tirofiban, tobramycin, topotecan, vancomycin, vecuronium, verapamil, vinblastine, vincristine, vinorelbine, voriconazole, zidovudine, zoledronic acid.

- **Y-Site Incompatibility:** amphotericin B lipid complex, dantrolene, diazepam, gemtuzumab ozogamicin, indomethacin, pemetrexed, phenytoin.

Patient/Family Teaching

- Explain purpose of vasopressin to patient.
- Advise patient to drink 1–2 glasses of water at time of administration to minimize side effects (blanching of skin, abdominal cramps, nausea). Inform patient that these side effects are not serious and usually disappear in a few min.
- Caution patient to avoid concurrent use of alcohol while taking vasopressin.
- Rep: Advise females of reproductive potential to notify health care professional if pregnancy is planned or suspected or if breastfeeding. Due to increased clearance of vasopressin in the second and third trimester, the dose of vasopressin may need to be increased. May produce tonic uterine contractions that could threaten the continuation of pregnancy.
- Patients with diabetes insipidus should carry identification at all times describing disease process and medication regimen.

Evaluation/Desired Outcomes

- Decrease in urine volume.
- Relief of polydipsia.
- Increased urine osmolality in patients with central diabetes insipidus.
- Increase in BP.

vedolizumab
(ve-doe-**liz**-yoo-mab)
  Entyvio
Classification
Therapeutic: gastrointestinal anti-inflammatories
Pharmacologic: monoclonal antibodies, integrin receptor antagonists

Indications
Moderately to severely active ulcerative colitis or Crohn's disease that has not responded adequately to/

lost response to/become intolerant to tumor necrosis factor (TNF) blockers or immunomodulators; or has become intolerant to/dependant on corticosteroids and failed to induce/maintain beneficial response/remission, improved endoscopic appearance (ulcerative colitis) or achieved corticosteroid-free remission.

Action
A monoclonal antibody that binds to certain integrins, blocking their interaction with substances involved in mucosal cell adhesion, also inhibits migration of memory T-lymphocytes across endothelium into inflamed GI tissue. **Therapeutic Effects:** Decreased chronic GI inflammation and symptomatology associated with ulcerative colitis and Crohn's disease.

Pharmacokinetics
Absorption: IV administration results in complete bioavailability.
Distribution: Minimally distributed to tissues.
Metabolism and Excretion: Unknown.
Half-life: 25 days.

TIME/ACTION PROFILE (clinical improvement)

ROUTE	ONSET	PEAK	DURATION
IV	within 6 wk	unknown	up to 8 wk

Contraindications/Precautions
Contraindicated in: Hypersensitivity; Active severe infection; Live-virus vaccinations; Concurrent use of natalizumab; Concurrent use of TNF blockers.
Use Cautiously in: OB: Use during pregnancy only if potential maternal benefits justify potential fetal risk; Lactation: Use while breastfeeding only if potential maternal benefit justifies potential risk to infant; Pedi: Safety and effectiveness not established in children.

Adverse Reactions/Side Effects
Derm: pruritus, rash. **GI:** ↑ liver enzymes, oropharyngeal pain. **MS:** arthralgia, back pain, extremity pain. **Neuro:** headache, fatigue, PROGRESSIVE MULTIFOCAL LEUKOENCEPHALOPATHY (PML). **Resp:** cough. **Misc:** fever, HYPERSENSITIVITY REACTIONS (including anaphylaxis), INFECTION, INFUSION REACTIONS.

Interactions
Drug-Drug: May ↓ antibody response to and ↑ risk of adverse reactions from **live-virus vaccines** (complete immunizations prior to treatment). Concurrent use with **natalizumab** may ↑ risk of infections and PML and should be avoided. Concurrent use with **TNF blockers** may ↑ risk of infections and should be avoided.

Route/Dosage
Ulcerative Colitis
IV (Adults): 300 mg initially, then 2 and 6 wk later, then every 8 wk; treatment may be continued if beneficial response is obtained by wk 14.

SUBQ (Adults): 108 mg every 2 wk (may switch to SUBQ dosing at Week 6 after receiving the first two IV doses [at Week 0 and Week 2] if demonstrated clinical response or remission); treatment may be continued if beneficial response is obtained by Week 14.

Crohn's Disease
IV (Adults): 300 mg initially, then 2 and 6 wk later, then every 8 wk; treatment may be continued if beneficial response is obtained by Week 14.

Availability
Lyophilized powder for intravenous injection: 300 mg/vial. **Solution for SUBQ injection (prefilled syringes or pens):** 108 mg/0.68 mL.

NURSING IMPLICATIONS
Assessment
- Assess abdominal pain and frequency, quantity, and consistency of stools at beginning and during therapy.
- Assess for signs of hypersensitivity or infusion-related reactions (dyspnea, bronchospasm, urticaria, flushing, rash, swelling of lips, tongue, throat, or face, wheezing, hypertension, tachycardia). If anaphylaxis or serious allergic reactions occur, discontinue vedolizumab and treat symptoms.
- Assess for new signs or symptoms suggestive of PML, an opportunistic infection of the brain caused by the JC virus, leading to death or severe disability; hold dose and notify health care professional promptly. Monitor during therapy and for at least 6 mo following discontinuation. PML symptoms may begin gradually but usually over days to wk and leads to death or severe disability over wk to mo. Symptoms include progressive weakness on one side of body or clumsiness of limbs, disturbance of vision, changes in thinking, memory and orientation leading to confusion and personality changes. Diagnosis is usually made via gadolinium-enhanced MRI and CSF analysis. Withhold vedolizumab at first sign of PML.

Lab Test Considerations
- May cause ↑ AST, ALT, and serum bilirubin. Discontinue in patients with jaundice or other evidence of liver injury.

Implementation
- Perform test for latent tuberculosis (TB). If positive, begin treatment for TB prior to starting vedolizumab therapy. Monitor for TB throughout therapy, even if latent TB test is negative.
- Ensure patient is up to date according to current immunization guidelines before starting therapy.
- Following the first two IV doses administered at Week 0 and Week 2, may be switched to SUBQ injection at Week 6. *Week 6 and thereafter:* Administer 108 mg SUBQ once every 2 wk. Discontinue therapy in patients who show no evidence of therapeutic

benefit by Week 14. May be switched from IV infusion to SUBQ injection, for patients in clinical response or remission beyond Week 6. To switch patients to SUBQ injection, administer first SUBQ dose in place of the next scheduled IV infusion and every 2 wk thereafter. Inspect the solution visually for particulate matter and discoloration prior to administration. Solution in *Entyvio* in prefilled syringe or *Entyvio Pen* is clear to moderately opalescent, colorless to slightly yellow solution; do not use with visible particulate matter or discoloration.
- **SUBQ:** Administer each SUBQ injection at a different anatomic location (such as thighs, any quadrant of abdomen, or upper arms) than the previous injection. Do not inject into moles, scars, bruises, or areas where the skin is tender, erythematous, or indurated.

IV Administration
- **Intermittent Infusion:** *Reconstitution:* Reconstitute with 4.8 mL sterile water for injection, 0.9% NaCl, or LR using 21- to 25-gauge needle. Direct stream to wall of vial to prevent excessive foaming. Gently swirl vial for at least 15 sec to dissolve; do not invert or shake vigorously. Allow to sit for up to 20 min at room temperature for reconstitution and settling of foam. If not fully dissolved after 20 min, allow another 10 min. Do not use vial if not dissolved within 30 min. Solution is clear or opalescent, colorless to light brownish-yellow; do not administer solutions that are cloudy, discolored or contain particulate matter. Swirl gently and invert vial 3 times prior to withdrawing. Use immediately after reconstitution. Reconstituted solution is stable for 8 hr if refrigerated. Withdraw 5 mL (300 mg) using 21- to 25-gauge needle. Discard unused portion. *Dilution:* 250 mL 0.9% NaCl or LR. Gently mix bag. Use as soon as possible. Use solutions diluted with LR immediately or store in refrigerator up to 6 hr. Solutions diluted with 0.9% NaCl are stable up to 12 hr at room temperature or 24 hr if refrigerated; do not freeze. *Rate:* Infuse over 30 min; do not administer as IV push or bolus. Flush line with 30 mL of 0.9% NaCl or LR after infusion.
- **Y-Site Incompatibility:** Do not administer with other solutions or medications.

Patient/Family Teaching
- Explain purpose of vedolizumab to patient. Advise patient to read *Medication Guide* prior to therapy.
- Instruct patient and/or caregiver in proper technique to administer SUBQ injection. If SUBQ injection is interrupted or if a scheduled dose(s) of SUBQ *Entyvio* is missed, inject next SUBQ dose as soon as possible and then every 2 wk thereafter. In the event of incomplete dose administration (patient attempts administration of dose with *Entyvio Pen* but is uncertain if a full dose was administered), instruct the patient to call their pharmacy or health care professional.

V

- Instruct patient to report symptoms of PML (progressive weakness on one side of the body or clumsiness of limbs; disturbance of vision; changes in thinking, memory, and orientation leading to confusion and personality changes), hypersensitivity reactions, hepatotoxicity (yellowing of the skin and eyes, unusual darkening of the urine, anorexia, nausea, feeling tired or weak, vomiting, right upper abdominal pain), or worsening of symptoms (new or sudden change in your thinking, eyesight, balance, or strength or other problems) that persist over several days to health care professional immediately.
- Inform patient of risk of infection. Advise patient to notify health care professional if symptoms of infection (fever, chills, muscle aches, shortness of breath, runny nose, cough, sore throat, red or painful skin or open cuts or sores, tiredness, pain during urination) occur.
- Advise patient to avoid live and oral vaccines during therapy.
- Advise patient to notify health care professional of all Rx or OTC medications, vitamins, or herbal products being taken and to consult with health care professional before taking other medications.
- Rep: Advise females of reproductive potential to notify health care professional if pregnancy is planned or suspected, or if breastfeeding. Encourage pregnant women to join Entyvio Pregnancy Registry by calling 1-877-825-3327. Registry monitors pregnancy outcomes in women exposed to vedolizumab during pregnancy.

Evaluation/Desired Outcomes

- Decreased chronic GI inflammation and symptomatology associated with ulcerative colitis and Crohn's disease. Discontinue therapy if no improvement by Week 14.

⚠ vemurafenib (vem-u-raf-e-nib)
Zelboraf

Classification
Therapeutic: antineoplastics
Pharmacologic: kinase inhibitors

Indications

⚠ Unresectable or metastatic melanoma with BRAF V600E mutation. ⚠ Erdheim-Chester disease ECD with BRAFV600E mutation.

Action

Inhibits mutated forms of the enzyme kinase. Inhibits proliferation that occurs in conjunction with activated BRAF proteins. **Therapeutic Effects:** Decreased spread of melanoma and Erdheim-Chester disease.

Pharmacokinetics

Absorption: Some absorption follows oral administration; bioavailability is not known.
Distribution: Widely distributed to tissues.
Protein Binding: >99%.

Metabolism and Excretion: Mostly metabolized by the liver via the CYP3A4 isoenzyme system; primarily excreted in the feces, with 1% eliminated in urine.
Half-life: 57 hr.

TIME/ACTION PROFILE (plasma concentrations)

ROUTE	ONSET	PEAK	DURATION
PO	unknown	3 hr	12 hr

Contraindications/Precautions

Contraindicated in: Underlying electrolyte abnormalities (↑ risk of serious arrhythmias; correct prior to administration); Congenital or acquired prolonged QT syndromes; Baseline QTc interval >500 msec; Concurrent use of QT-interval prolonging drugs; OB: Pregnancy; Lactation: Lactation.

Use Cautiously in: Severe renal impairment; Severe hepatic impairment; Receiving radiation therapy prior to, during, or after therapy (↑ risk of radiation sensitization/recall); Rep: Women of reproductive potential; Pedi: Safety and effectiveness not established in children; Geri: ↑ risk of cutaneous squamous cell carcinoma, nausea, ↓ appetite, peripheral edema, keratoacanthoma, and atrial fibrillation in older adults.

Adverse Reactions/Side Effects

CV: peripheral edema, QT interval prolongation, TORSADES DE POINTES. **Derm:** alopecia, dry skin, photosensitivity (↑ in females), pruritus, rash (↑ in females), SKIN CANCER, skin papilloma, DRUG REACTION WITH EOSINOPHILIA AND SYSTEMIC SYMPTOMS (DRESS), keratoacanthoma (↑ in males), STEVENS-JOHNSON SYNDROME (SJS), TOXIC EPIDERMAL NECROLYSIS (TEN). **EENT:** iritis, retinal vein occlusion, uveitis. **GI:** ↓ appetite, HEPATOTOXICITY, nausea. **GU:** ↑ serum creatinine (↑ in females), acute interstitial nephritis, acute tubular necrosis. **MS:** arthralgia (↑ in females), myalgia, Dupuytren's contracture, back pain, pain, plantar fascial fibromatosis. **Neuro:** fatigue, weakness, dysgeusia, headache. **Resp:** cough. **Misc:** fever, HYPERSENSITIVITY REACTIONS (including anaphylaxis), radiation sensitization/recall.

Interactions

Drug-Drug: **QT interval prolonging drugs** may ↑ the risk of QT interval prolongation with arrhythmias; concurrent use contraindicated. Concurrent use with **CYP1A2 substrates with narrow therapeutic indices** not recommended. Consider dose ↓ of substrates. **Strong CYP3A inhibitors**, including **atazanavir, clarithromycin, itraconazole, ketoconazole, nefazodone, nelfinavir, ritonavir,** and **voriconazole,** may ↑ levels and the risk of toxicity; avoid concurrent use; if concurrent use is necessary, consider ↓ vemurafenib dose. **Strong CYP3A inducers,** including **carbamazepine, phenobarbital, phenytoin, rifabutin, rifampin,** and **rifapentine,** may ↓ levels and effectiveness; avoid concurrent use; if concurrent use necessary, ↑ vemurafenib dose. May ↑ risk of bleeding with **warfarin**. Concurrent use with

ipilimumab may ↑ risk of hepatotoxicity. May ↑ **digoxin** levels and the risk of toxicity.

Route/Dosage
PO (Adults): 960 mg (4 tablets) twice daily until disease progression or unacceptable toxicity; *Concurrent use of strong CYP3A4 inducers:* 1200 mg (5 tablets) twice daily until disease progression or unacceptable toxicity.

Availability
Tablets: 240 mg.

NURSING IMPLICATIONS
Assessment
* Perform dermatologic evaluation prior to initiation and every 2 mo during therapy. Excise any suspicious lesions, send for dermapathologic evaluation, and treat with standard care. Continue monitoring for 6 mo following discontinuation of therapy.
* Monitor ECG 15 days after initiation of therapy, monthly during first 3 mo, every 3 mo thereafter, and more often if clinically indicated.
* Monitor for hypersensitivity reactions (rash, erythema, hypotension). Permanently discontinue therapy if severe reaction occurs.
* Monitor for signs and symptoms of uveitis periodically during therapy. May require treatment with steroid and mydriatic ophthalmic drops.
* Assess patient for rash (mild to moderate rash usually occurs in the 2nd wk of therapy and resolves within 1–2 wk of continued therapy). If rash is severe (extensive erythematous or maculopapular rash with moist desquamation or angioedema) or accompanied by systemic symptoms (serum sickness-like reaction, SJS, TEN), therapy must be discontinued immediately.

Lab Test Considerations
* ⚄ Information on FDA-approved tests for the detection of BRAF V600 mutations in melanoma is available at www.fda.gov/CompanionDiagnostics.
* Monitor serum potassium, magnesium, and calcium before starting therapy and after dose modification.
* Monitor AST, ALT, alkaline phosphatase, and bilirubin before starting therapy, monthly during therapy, and as clinically indicated. May require dose reduction, treatment interruption, or discontinuation.
* Monitor serum creatinine before starting and periodically during therapy.

Implementation
* **PO:** Administer (four 240-mg tablets) twice daily, without regard to food. Take first dose in the morning with 2nd dose about 12 hr later. *DNC:* Swallow tablets whole; do not crush or chew.
* Adverse reactions or QTc prolongation may occur requiring dose modification. *If Grade 1 or 2 (tolerable) occur,* maintain dose at 960 mg twice daily. *If*

Grade 2 (Intolerable) or Grade 3, 1st appearance occurs, interrupt therapy until Grade 0–1. Resume dosing at 720 mg twice daily. *If 2nd appearance,* interrupt therapy until Grade 0–1. Resume dosing at 480 mg twice daily. *If 3rd appearance,* discontinue permanently. *If Grade 4, 1st appearance occurs,* discontinue permanently or interrupt therapy until Grade 0–1. Resume dosing at 480 twice daily. *If 2nd appearance,* discontinue permanently. Doses below 480 mg twice daily are not recommended.

Patient/Family Teaching
* Instruct patient to take vemurafenib as directed. If vomiting occurs, do not take an additional dose; take next dose as scheduled. Take missed doses as soon as remembered up to 4 hr before next dose; do not double dose.
* ⚄ Inform patient that assessment of BRAF mutation is required for selection of patients.
* Instruct patient to stop taking vemurafenib and notify health care professional immediately if signs and symptoms of allergic reaction (rash or redness all over body; feeling faint; difficulty breathing or swallowing; throat tightness or hoarseness; fast heartbeat; swelling of face, lips, or tongue) or severe skin reactions (blisters on skin; blisters or sores in mouth; peeling of skin, fever, redness or swelling of face, hands, or soles of feet) occur.
* Advise patient to wear broad spectrum UVA/UVB sunscreen, lip balm (SPF ≥30), and protective clothing, and to avoid sun exposure to prevent photosensitivity reactions. Severe photosensitivity reactions may require dose modifications.
* Advise patient to notify health care professional if signs and symptoms of liver dysfunction (yellow skin or whites of eyes; feeling tired; urine turns dark or brown; nausea or vomiting; loss of appetite; pain on right side of stomach) or eye problems (eye pain, swelling, or redness; blurred vision; vision changes) occur.
* Instruct patient to notify health care professional of all Rx or OTC medications, vitamins, or herbal products being taken and consult health care professional before taking any new medications.
* Inform patient that regular assessments of skin and assessments for signs and symptoms of other malignancies must be done during and for up to 6 mo after therapy. Advise patient to notify health care professional immediately if any changes in skin occur.
* Rep: Advise women of reproductive potential to use effective contraception during and for at least 2 wk after last dose of vemurafenib, and to avoid breastfeeding during and for 2 wk after last dose.

Evaluation/Desired Outcomes
* Decreased spread of melanoma.

✳ = Canadian drug name. ⚄ = Genetic implication. ~~Strikethrough~~ = Discontinued. CAPITALS = life-threatening. <u>Underline</u> = most frequent.

venlafaxine (ven-la-**fax**-een)
~~Effexor~~, Effexor XR

Classification
Therapeutic: antidepressants, antianxiety agents
Pharmacologic: selective serotonin/norepinephrine reuptake inhibitors

Indications
Major depressive disorder. Generalized anxiety disorder (Effexor XR only). Social anxiety disorder (extended release only). Panic disorder (extended release only). **Unlabeled Use:** Premenstrual dysphoric disorder.

Action
Inhibits serotonin and norepinephrine reuptake in the CNS. **Therapeutic Effects:** Decrease in depressive symptomatology, with fewer relapses/recurrences. Decreased anxiety. Decrease in panic attacks.

Pharmacokinetics
Absorption: 92–100% absorbed after oral administration.
Distribution: Extensive distribution into body tissues.
Metabolism and Excretion: Extensively metabolized on first pass through the liver (primarily through the CYP2D6 isoenzyme); ‡ the CYP2D6 isoenzyme exhibits genetic polymorphism (~7% of population may be poor metabolizers and may have significantly ↑ venlafaxine concentrations and an ↑ risk of adverse effects). One metabolite, O-desmethylvenlafaxine (ODV), has antidepressant activity. 5% of venlafaxine is excreted unchanged in urine; 30% of the active metabolite is excreted in urine.
Half-life: *Venlafaxine:* 3–5 hr; *ODV:* 9–11 hr (both are ↑ in hepatic/renal impairment).

TIME/ACTION PROFILE (antidepressant action)

ROUTE	ONSET	PEAK	DURATION
PO	within 2 wk	2–4 wk	unknown

Contraindications/Precautions
Contraindicated in: Hypersensitivity; Concurrent use of MAO inhibitors or MAO inhibitor-like drugs (linezolid or methylene blue); Lactation: Lactation.
Use Cautiously in: Cardiovascular disease, including hypertension; Hepatic or renal impairment (↓ dose recommended); History of seizures or neurologic impairment; History of mania; History of drug abuse; Angle-closure glaucoma; OB: Use during pregnancy only if potential maternal benefit justifies potential fetal risk (potential for discontinuation syndrome or toxicity in the neonate when venlafaxine is taken during the 3rd trimester); Pedi: Safety and effectiveness not established in children; ↑ risk of suicidal thinking and behavior (suicidality) in children and adolescents with major depressive disorder and other psychiatric disorders.

Adverse Reactions/Side Effects
CV: chest pain, hypertension, palpitations, tachycardia. **Derm:** ecchymoses, itching, photosensitivity, skin rash. **EENT:** rhinitis, visual disturbances, epistaxis, tinnitus. **GI:** abdominal pain, altered taste, anorexia, constipation, diarrhea, dry mouth, dyspepsia, nausea, vomiting, weight loss. **GU:** ↓ libido, delayed/absent orgasm, ejaculatory delay/failure, erectile dysfunction, urinary frequency, urinary retention. **Hemat:** BLEEDING. **Neuro:** abnormal dreams, anxiety, dizziness, headache, insomnia, nervousness, paresthesia, weakness, abnormal thinking, agitation, confusion, depersonalization, drowsiness, emotional lability, NEUROLEPTIC MALIGNANT SYNDROME, SEIZURES, SUICIDAL THOUGHTS, twitching, worsening depression. **Misc:** chills, discontinuation syndrome, SEROTONIN SYNDROME, yawning.

Interactions
Drug-Drug: Concurrent use with **MAO inhibitors** may result in serious, potentially fatal reactions (wait at least 2 wk after stopping MAO inhibitor before initiating venlafaxine; wait at least 1 wk after stopping venlafaxine before starting MAO inhibitors). Concurrent use with **MAO-inhibitor like drugs**, such as **linezolid** or **methylene blue**, may ↑ risk of serotonin syndrome; concurrent use contraindicated; do not start therapy in patients receiving **linezolid** or **methylene blue**; if linezolid or methylene blue need to be started in a patient receiving venlafaxine, immediately discontinue venlafaxine and monitor for signs/symptoms of serotonin syndrome for 2 wk or until 24 hr after last dose of linezolid or methylene blue, whichever comes first (may resume venlafaxine therapy 24 hr after last dose of linezolid or methylene blue). Concurrent use with **alcohol** or other **CNS depressants**, including **sedatives/hypnotics**, **antihistamines**, and **opioid analgesics**, in depressed patients is not recommended. Drugs that affect serotonergic neurotransmitter systems, including **tricyclic antidepressants**, **SNRIs**, **fentanyl**, **lithium**, **buspirone**, **tramadol**, **meperidine**, **methadone**, **amphetamines**, and **triptans**, ↑ risk of serotonin syndrome. **Lithium** may have ↑ serotonergic effects with venlafaxine; use cautiously in patients receiving venlafaxine. May ↑ levels and the risk of toxicity of **desipramine** and **haloperidol**. **Cimetidine** may ↑ the effects of venlafaxine (may be more pronounced in geriatric patients, those with hepatic or renal impairment, or those with pre-existing hypertension). **Ketoconazole** may ↑ the effects of venlafaxine. ↑ risk of bleeding with **NSAIDs**, **aspirin**, **clopidogrel**, **prasugrel**, **ticagrelor**, **dabigatran**, **apixaban**, **edoxaban**, **rivaroxaban**, or **warfarin**.
Drug-Natural Products: Concomitant use of **kava-kava**, **valerian**, **chamomile**, or **hops** can ↑ CNS depression. ↑ risk of serotonergic side effects including serotonin syndrome with **St. John's wort** and **SAMe**.

Route/Dosage

Major Depressive Disorder

PO (Adults): *Tablets:* 75 mg/day in 2–3 divided doses; may ↑ by up to 75 mg/day every 4 days, up to 225 mg/day (not to exceed 375 mg/day in 3 divided doses); *Extended-release capsules:* 75 mg once daily (some patients may be started at 37.5 mg once daily) for 4–7 days; may ↑ by up to 75 mg/day at intervals of not less than 4 days (not to exceed 225 mg/day).

Renal Impairment

PO (Adults): *CCr 10–70 mL/min:* ↓ daily dose by 25% (immediate release); *CCr 30–89 mL/min:* ↓ daily dose by 25–50% (extended release); *CCr <30 mL/ min:* ↓ daily dose by ≥50% (extended release); *Hemodialysis:* ↓ daily dose by ≥50%.

Hepatic Impairment

PO (Adults): *Mild, moderate, or severe hepatic impairment:* ↓ daily dose by 50%.

General Anxiety Disorder

PO (Adults): *Extended-release capsules:* 75 mg once daily (some patients may be started at 37.5 mg once daily) for 4–7 days; may ↑ by up to 75 mg/day at intervals of not less than 4 days (not to exceed 225 mg/day).

Renal Impairment

PO (Adults): *CCr 10–70 mL/min:* ↓ daily dose by 25% (immediate release); *CCr 30–89 mL/min:* ↓ daily dose by 25–50% (extended release); *CCr <30 mL/ min:* ↓ daily dose by ≥50% (extended release); *Hemodialysis:* ↓ daily dose by ≥50%.

Hepatic Impairment

PO (Adults): *Mild, moderate, or severe hepatic impairment:* ↓ daily dose by 50%.

Social Anxiety Disorder

PO (Adults): *Extended-release capsules:* 75 mg once daily.

Renal Impairment

PO (Adults): *CCr 10–70 mL/min:* ↓ daily dose by 25% (immediate release); *CCr 30–89 mL/min:* ↓ daily dose by 25–50% (extended release); *CCr <30 mL/ min:* ↓ daily dose by ≥50% (extended release); *Hemodialysis:* ↓ daily dose by ≥50%.

Hepatic Impairment

PO (Adults): *Mild, moderate, or severe hepatic impairment:* ↓ daily dose by 50%.

Panic Disorder

PO (Adults): *Extended-release capsules:* 37.5 mg once daily for 7 days; may then ↑ to 75 mg once daily; may then ↑ by 75 mg/day every 7 days (not to exceed 225 mg/day).

Hepatic Impairment

PO (Adults): *Mild, moderate, or severe hepatic impairment:* ↓ daily dose by 50%.

Renal Impairment

PO (Adults): *CCr 10–70 mL/min:* ↓ daily dose by 25% (immediate release); *CCr 30–89 mL/min:* ↓ daily dose by 25–50% (extended release); *CCr <30 mL/ min:* ↓ daily dose by ≥50% (extended release); *Hemodialysis:* ↓ daily dose by ≥50%.

Availability (generic available)

Immediate-release tablets: 25 mg, 37.5 mg, 50 mg, 75 mg, 100 mg. **Extended-release capsules:** 37.5 mg, 75 mg, 150 mg. **Extended-release tablets:** 37.5 mg, 75 mg, 150 mg, 225 mg.

NURSING IMPLICATIONS

Assessment

- Screen patients for a personal or family history of bipolar disorder, mania, or hypomania before starting therapy.
- Assess mental status and mood changes. Inform health care professional if patient demonstrates significant increase in anxiety, nervousness, or insomnia.
- Assess suicidal tendencies, especially in early therapy. Restrict amount of drug available to patient. Risk may be increased in children, adolescents, and adults ≤24 yr.
- Monitor BP before and periodically during therapy. Sustained hypertension may be dose-related; decrease dose or discontinue therapy if this occurs.
- Monitor appetite and nutritional intake. Weigh weekly. Report continued weight loss. Adjust diet as tolerated to support nutritional status.
- Assess for serotonin syndrome (mental changes [agitation, hallucinations, coma], autonomic instability [tachycardia, labile BP, hyperthermia], neuromuscular aberrations [hyper-reflexia, incoordination], and/or GI symptoms [nausea, vomiting, diarrhea]), especially in patients taking other serotonergic drugs (SSRIs, SNRIs, triptans).
- Assess sexual function before starting venlafaxine. Assess for changes in sexual function during treatment, including timing of onset; patient may not report.

Lab Test Considerations

- Monitor CBC with differential and platelet count periodically during therapy. May cause anemia, leukocytosis, leukopenia, thrombocytopenia, basophilia, and eosinophilia.
- May cause an ↑ in serum alkaline phosphatase, bilirubin, AST, ALT, BUN, and creatinine.
- May also cause ↑ serum cholesterol.
- May cause electrolyte abnormalities (hyperglycemia or hypoglycemia, hyperkalemia or hypokalemia, hyperuricemia, hyperphosphatemia or hypophosphatemia, and hyponatremia).

V

✿ = Canadian drug name. ▓ = Genetic implication. S̶t̶r̶i̶k̶e̶t̶h̶r̶o̶u̶g̶h̶ = Discontinued. CAPITALS = life-threatening. U̲n̲d̲e̲r̲l̲i̲n̲e̲ = most frequent.

- May cause false-positive immunoassay screening tests for phencyclidine and amphetamine.

Implementation

- Do not confuse Effexor XR (venlafaxine) with Enablex (darifenacin).
- **PO:** Administer venlafaxine with food.
- *DNC:* Swallow extended-release capsules and tablets whole; do not crush, break, or chew.
- Extended-release capsules may be opened and contents sprinkled on a spoonful of applesauce. Take immediately and follow with a glass of water. Do not store mixture for later use.

Patient/Family Teaching

- Instruct patient to take venlafaxine as directed at the same time each day. Take missed doses as soon as possible unless almost time for next dose. Do not double doses or discontinue abruptly. Patients taking venlafaxine for >6 wk should have dose gradually decreased before discontinuation to prevent dizziness, nausea, headache, irritability, insomnia, diarrhea, anxiety, fatigue, abnormal dreams, and hyperhidrosis; discontinuation may take several mo.
- Advise patient, family, and caregivers to look for suicidality, especially during early therapy or dose changes. Notify health care professional immediately if thoughts about suicide or dying, attempts to commit suicide; new or worse depression or anxiety; agitation or restlessness; panic attacks; insomnia; new or worse irritability; aggressiveness; acting on dangerous impulses, mania, or other changes in mood or behavior or if symptoms of serotonin syndrome occur.
- May cause drowsiness or dizziness. Caution patient to avoid driving or other activities requiring alertness until response to the drug is known.
- Instruct patient to notify health care professional of all Rx or OTC medications, vitamins, or herbal products being taken and consult health care professional before taking any new medications. Caution patient to avoid taking alcohol or other CNS-depressant drugs, including opioids, during therapy.
- Instruct patient to notify health care professional if signs of allergy (rash, hives) occur.
- Inform patient that venlafaxine may cause symptoms of sexual dysfunction. In males, ejaculatory delay or failure, decreased libido, and erectile dysfunction may occur. In female patients, may result in decreased libido and delayed or absent orgasm. Advise patient to notify health care professional if symptoms occur.
- Rep: Advise females of reproductive potential to notify health care professional immediately if pregnancy is planned or suspected or if breastfeeding. Use during last month of pregnancy increases risk of postpartum hemorrhage. If used during pregnancy, should be tapered during 3rd trimester to avoid neonatal serotonin syndrome. Monitor infants exposed to venlafaxine for excess sedation, restlessness, agitation, poor feeding, poor weight gain, respiratory distress; may ↑ risk of persistent pulmonary hypertension of the newborn. Inform patient of pregnancy exposure registry that monitors pregnancy outcomes in women exposed to antidepressants during pregnancy. Register patients by calling the National Pregnancy Registry for Antidepressants at 1-844-405-6185 or visiting online at https://womensmentalhealth.org/research/pregnancyregistry/antidepressants/.
- Emphasize the importance of follow-up exams to monitor progress.

Evaluation/Desired Outcomes

- Increased sense of well-being.
- Renewed interest in surroundings. Need for therapy should be periodically reassessed. Therapy is usually continued for several mo.
- Decreased anxiety.

verapamil (ver-ap-a-mil)

~~Calan~~, Calan SR, ✤ Isoptin SR, Verelan, Verelan PM

Classification

Therapeutic: antianginals, antiarrhythmics (class IV), antihypertensives, vascular headache suppressants
Pharmacologic: calcium channel blockers

Indications

Hypertension. Chronic stable angina. Vasospastic (Prinzmetal's) angina. Atrial fibrillation or atrial flutter. Supraventricular tachycardia. **Unlabeled Use:** Prevention of migraine headache.

Action

Inhibits the transport of calcium into myocardial and vascular smooth muscle cells, resulting in inhibition of excitation-contraction coupling and subsequent contraction. Decreases sinoatrial and atrioventricular nodal conduction and prolongs atrioventricular node refractory period in conduction tissue. **Therapeutic Effects:** Reduction in BP. Reduction in frequency and severity of angina episodes. Reduction of ventricular rate during atrial fibrillation or atrial flutter. Prevention and/or termination of supraventricular tachycardia.

Pharmacokinetics

Absorption: 90% absorbed after oral administration, but much is rapidly metabolized, resulting in bioavailability of 20–25%.
Distribution: Well distributed to tissues.
Protein Binding: 90%.
Metabolism and Excretion: Primarily metabolized by the liver via the CYP3A4 isoenzyme. Primarily excreted in urine (4% as unchanged drug).
Half-life: 4.5–12 hr.

TIME/ACTION PROFILE (cardiovascular effects)

ROUTE	ONSET	PEAK	DURATION
PO	1–2 hr	30–90 min†	3–7 hr
PO-extended release	unknown	5–7 hr	24 hr
IV	1–5 min‡	3–5 min	2 hr‡

†Single dose; effects from multiple doses may not be evident for 24–48 hr.

‡Antiarrhythmic effects; hemodynamic effects begin 3–5 min after injection and persist for 10–20 min.

Contraindications/Precautions

Contraindicated in: Hypersensitivity; Sick sinus syndrome; 2nd- or 3rd-degree heart block (unless an artificial pacemaker is in place); Systolic BP <90 mm Hg; HF, severe left ventricular dysfunction, or cardiogenic shock, unless associated with supraventricular tachyarrhythmias; Concurrent IV beta blocker therapy; Lactation: Lactation.

Use Cautiously in: Severe hepatic impairment (dose ↓ recommended); History of serious ventricular arrhythmias; OB: Safety not established in pregnancy; Geri: Dose ↓/slower IV infusion rates recommended in older adults (↑ risk of hypotension).

Adverse Reactions/Side Effects

CV: ARRHYTHMIAS, bradycardia, chest pain, HF, hypotension, palpitations, peripheral edema, syncope, tachycardia. **Derm:** dermatitis, erythema multiforme, flushing, photosensitivity, pruritus/urticaria, rash, STEVENS-JOHNSON SYNDROME (SJS), sweating. **EENT:** blurred vision, disturbed equilibrium, epistaxis, tinnitus. **Endo:** gynecomastia, hyperglycemia. **GI:** ↑ liver enzymes, anorexia, constipation, diarrhea, dry mouth, dyspepsia, nausea, vomiting. **GU:** dysuria, nocturia, polyuria, sexual dysfunction, urinary frequency. **Hemat:** anemia, leukopenia, thrombocytopenia. **Metab:** weight gain. **MS:** joint stiffness, muscle cramps. **Neuro:** abnormal dreams, anxiety, confusion, dizziness/lightheadedness, drowsiness, dysgeusia, extrapyramidal reactions, headache, jitteriness, nervousness, paresthesia, psychiatric disturbances, tremor, weakness. **Resp:** cough, dyspnea. **Misc:** gingival hyperplasia.

Interactions

Drug-Drug: Additive hypotension may occur when used concurrently with **fentanyl**, other **antihypertensives**, **nitrates**, acute ingestion of **alcohol**, or **quinidine**. Antihypertensive effects may be ↓ by concurrent use of **NSAIDs**. May ↑ levels and the risk of toxicity of **digoxin**. Concurrent use with **beta blockers**, **digoxin**, **clonidine**, or **ivabradine** may result in bradycardia or conduction defects; avoid concurrent use with ivabradine. ↑ risk of hypotension and bradycardia with **erythromycin**, **clarithromycin**, or **ritonavir**. May ↑ levels and the risk of toxicity of **cyclosporine**, **quinidine**, **theophylline**, or

carbamazepine. **Rifampin** and **phenobarbital** may ↓ levels and effectiveness. ↑ the muscle-paralyzing effects of **nondepolarizing neuromuscular-blocking agents**. May alter **lithium** levels. May ↑ risk of bleeding with **aspirin**. May ↑ levels and the risk of toxicity of **sirolimus**, **temsirolimus**, or **everolimus**; consider ↓ dose of sirolimus, temsirolimus, everolimus, and verapamil. ↑ risk of myopathy with **simvastatin** and **lovastatin**; do not exceed 10 mg/day of simvastatin and 20 mg/day of lovastatin.

Drug-Natural Products: ↑ **caffeine** levels with caffeine-containing herbs (**cola nut**, **guarana**, **mate**, **tea**, **coffee**).

Drug-Food: Grapefruit juice ↑ levels and the risk of toxicity.

Route/Dosage

PO (Adults): 80–120 mg 3 times daily, ↑ as needed. *Patients with hepatic impairment or geriatric patients:* 40 mg 3 times daily initially. *Extended-release preparations:* 120–240 mg/day as a single dose; may be ↑ as needed (range 240–480 mg/day).

PO (Children ≤15 yr): 4–8 mg/kg/day in divided doses.

IV (Adults): 5–10 mg (75–150 mcg/kg); may repeat with 10 mg (150 mcg/kg) after 15–30 min.

IV (Children 1–15 yr): 2–5 mg (100–300 mcg/kg); may repeat after 30 min (initial dose not to exceed 5 mg; repeat dose not to exceed 10 mg).

IV (Children <1 yr): 0.75–2 mg (100–200 mcg/kg); may repeat after 30 min.

Availability (generic available)

Immediate-release tablets: 40 mg, 80 mg, 120 mg. **Extended-release capsules (Verelan):** 120 mg, 180 mg, 240 mg, 360 mg. **Extended-release capsules (Verelan PM):** 100 mg, 200 mg, 300 mg. **Extended-release tablets:** 120 mg, 180 mg, 240 mg. **Solution for injection:** 2.5 mg/mL. *In combination with:* trandolapril.

NURSING IMPLICATIONS

Assessment

● Monitor BP and pulse before therapy, during dosage titration, and periodically throughout therapy. Monitor ECG periodically during prolonged therapy. Verapamil may cause prolonged PR interval.

● Monitor intake and output ratios and daily weight. Assess for signs of HF (peripheral edema, rales/crackles, dyspnea, weight gain, jugular venous distention).

● Patients receiving digoxin concurrently with calcium channel blockers should have routine serum digoxin levels and be monitored for signs and symptoms of digoxin toxicity.

● Assess for rash periodically during therapy. May cause SJS. Discontinue therapy if severe or if accompanied with fever, general malaise, fatigue, muscle

V

or joint aches, blisters, oral lesions, conjunctivitis, hepatitis, and/or eosinophilia.

- **Angina:** Assess location, duration, intensity, and precipitating factors of patient's anginal pain.
- **Arrhythmias:** Monitor ECG continuously during administration. Notify health care professional promptly if bradycardia or prolonged hypotension occurs. Emergency equipment and medication should be available. Monitor BP and pulse before and frequently during administration.

Lab Test Considerations
- Total serum calcium concentrations are not affected by calcium channel blockers.
- Monitor serum potassium periodically. Hypokalemia ↑ risk of arrhythmias and should be corrected.
- Monitor renal and hepatic functions periodically during long-term therapy. May cause ↑ hepatic enzymes after several days of therapy, which return to normal on discontinuation of therapy.

Implementation
- **PO:** Administer verapamil with meals or milk to minimize gastric irritation.
- **DNC:** Swallow extended-release tablets and capsules whole; do not open, crush, break, or chew. Empty tablets that appear in stool are not significant.

IV Administration
- **IV:** Patients should remain recumbent for at least 1 hr after IV administration to minimize hypotensive effects.
- **IV Push:** *Dilution:* Administer undiluted. *Concentration:* 2.5 mg/mL. *Rate:* Administer over 2 min. Geri: Administer over 3 min.
- **Y-Site Compatibility:** alemtuzumab, amikacin, aminocaproic acid, amphotericin B lipid complex, anidulafungin, argatroban, arsenic trioxide, ascorbic acid, atracurium, atropine, azithromycin, aztreonam, benztropine, bivalirudin, bleomycin, bumetanide, buprenorphine, butorphanol, calcium chloride, calcium gluconate, cangrelor, carboplatin, carmustine, caspofungin, cefazolin, cefotaxime, cefotetan, cefoxitin, ceftriaxone, cefuroxime, chlorpromazine, ciprofloxacin, cisplatin, clindamycin, cyanocobalamin, cyclophosphamide, cyclosporine, cytarabine, dacarbazine, dactinomycin, daptomycin, daunorubicin hydrochloride, dexamethasone, dexmedetomidine, dexrazoxane, digoxin, diltiazem, diphenhydramine, dobutamine, docetaxel, dopamine, doxorubicin hydrochloride, doxorubicin liposomal, doxycycline, enalaprilat, ephedrine, epinephrine, epirubicin, epoetin alfa, eptifibatide, erythromycin, esmolol, etoposide, etoposide phosphate, famotidine, fentanyl, fluconazole, fludarabine, gemcitabine, gemtuzumab ozogamicin, gentamicin, glycopyrrolate, granisetron, heparin, hetastarch, hydrocortisone, hydromorphone, idarubicin, ifosfamide, imipenem/cilastatin, insulin regular, insulin aspart, irinotecan, isoproterenol, ketorolac, labetalol, LR, leucovorin calcium, levofloxacin, lidocaine, linezolid, lorazepam, magnesium sulfate, mannitol, meperidine, mesna, methadone, methotrexate, methylprednisolone, metoclopramide, metoprolol, metronidazole, midazolam, milrinone, mitomycin, mitoxantrone, morphine, moxifloxacin, multivitamins, mycophenolate, nalbuphine, naloxone, nitroglycerin, nitroprusside, norepinephrine, octreotide, ondansetron, oxaliplatin, oxytocin, paclitaxel, palonosetron, pamidronate, papaverine, pemetrexed, penicillin G, pentamidine, phentolamine, phenylephrine, phytonadione, potassium acetate, potassium chloride, procainamide, prochlorperazine, promethazine, propranolol, protamine, pyridoxine, rocuronium, sodium acetate, succinylcholine, sufentanil, tacrolimus, theophylline, thiamine, tirofiban, tobramycin, topotecan, vancomycin, vasopressin, vecuronium, vinblastine, vincristine, vinorelbine, voriconazole, zoledronic acid.
- **Y-Site Incompatibility:** acyclovir, albumin, human, aminophylline, amiodarone, amphotericin B deoxycholate, amphotericin B liposomal, ampicillin, ampicillin/sulbactam, azathioprine, ceftazidime, chloramphenicol, dantrolene, diazepam, ertapenem, fluorouracil, folic acid, foscarnet, fosphenytoin, furosemide, ganciclovir, indomethacin, pantoprazole, pentobarbital, phenobarbital, phenytoin, piperacillin/tazobactam, propofol, sodium bicarbonate, thiotepa, tigecycline, trimethoprim/sulfamethoxazole.

Patient/Family Teaching
- Advise patient to take medication as directed, even if feeling well. Take missed doses as soon as possible unless almost time for next dose; do not double doses. May need to be discontinued gradually.
- Advise patient to avoid large amounts (6–8 glasses of grapefruit juice/day) during therapy.
- Instruct patient on correct technique for monitoring pulse. Instruct patient to contact health care professional if heart rate is <50 bpm.
- Caution patient to change positions slowly to minimize orthostatic hypotension.
- May cause drowsiness or dizziness. Advise patient to avoid driving or other activities requiring alertness until response to the medication is known.
- Instruct patient on importance of maintaining good dental hygiene and seeing dentist frequently for teeth cleaning to prevent tenderness, bleeding, and gingival hyperplasia (gum enlargement).
- Instruct patient to notify health care professional of all Rx or OTC medications, vitamins, or herbal products being taken and consult health care professional before taking any new medications, especially cold preparations.
- Advise patient to notify health care professional if irregular heartbeats, rash, dyspnea, swelling of hands and feet, pronounced dizziness, nausea, constipation, or hypotension occurs or if headache is severe or persistent.
- Caution patient to wear protective clothing and use sunscreen to prevent photosensitivity reactions.

- Rep: Advise females of reproductive potential to notify health care professional if pregnancy is planned or suspected and avoid breastfeeding during therapy.
- **Angina:** Instruct patient on concurrent nitrate or beta blocker therapy to continue taking both medications as directed and use SL nitroglycerin as needed for anginal attacks.
- Advise patient to contact health care professional if chest pain does not improve, worsens after therapy, or occurs with diaphoresis; if shortness of breath occurs; or if severe, persistent headache occurs.
- Caution patient to discuss exercise restrictions with health care professional before exertion.
- **Hypertension:** Encourage patient to comply with other interventions for hypertension (weight reduction, low-sodium diet, smoking cessation, moderation of alcohol consumption, regular exercise, and stress management). Medication controls but does not cure hypertension.
- Instruct patient and family in proper technique for monitoring BP. Advise patient to take BP weekly and to report significant changes to health care professional.

Evaluation/Desired Outcomes

- Decrease in BP.
- Decrease in frequency and severity of anginal attacks.
- Decrease in need for nitrate therapy.
- Increase in activity tolerance and sense of well-being.
- Suppression and prevention of atrial tachyarrhythmias.
- Prevention and/or termination of supraventricular tachycardia.

BEERS

vilazodone (vil-az-oh-done)
Viibryd
Classification
Therapeutic: antidepressants
Pharmacologic: selective serotonin reuptake inhibitors (SSRIs), benzofurans

Indications
Major depressive disorder.

Action
Increases serotonin activity in the CNS by inhibiting serotonin reuptake. Also binds selectively with high affinity to 5-HT$_{1A}$ receptors and is a 5-HT$_{1A}$ receptor partial agonist. **Therapeutic Effects:** Improvement in symptoms of depression.

Pharmacokinetics
Absorption: 72% absorbed following oral administration with food.

Distribution: Unknown.
Protein Binding: 96–99%.
Metabolism and Excretion: Mostly metabolized by the liver, primarily by the CYP3A4 isoenzyme; 1% excreted unchanged in urine.
Half-life: 25 hr.

TIME/ACTION PROFILE (plasma concentrations)

ROUTE	ONSET	PEAK	DURATION
PO	unknown	4–5 hr	unknown

Contraindications/Precautions
Contraindicated in: Concurrent use of MAO inhibitors or MAO inhibitor-like drugs (linezolid or methylene blue).
Use Cautiously in: History of seizure disorder; History of suicide attempt/suicidal ideation; Bipolar disorder (may ↑ risk of mania/hypomania); Angle-closure glaucoma; OB: Use during pregnancy only if potential maternal benefit justifies potential fetal risk; Lactation: Use while breastfeeding only if potential maternal benefit justifies potential risk to infant; Pedi: Safety and effectiveness not established in children; ↑ risk of suicidal thinking/behavior in children, adolescents, and young adults; Geri: Appears on Beers list. May worsen or cause syndrome of inappropriate antidiuretic hormone (SIADH) secretion and/or hyponatremia in older adults. Use with caution in older adults and closely monitor sodium concentrations when starting therapy or ↑ dose.

Adverse Reactions/Side Effects
Endo: SIADH. **F and E:** hyponatremia. **GI:** diarrhea, nausea, dry mouth, PANCREATITIS, vomiting. **GU:** ↓ libido, delayed/absent orgasm, ejaculatory delay/failure, erectile dysfunction. **Hemat:** BLEEDING. **Neuro:** insomnia, abnormal dreams, dizziness, NEUROLEPTIC MALIGNANT-LIKE SYNDROME, restlessness, SEIZURES, sleep paralysis, SUICIDAL THOUGHTS. **Misc:** SEROTONIN SYNDROME.

Interactions
Drug-Drug: Concurrent use with, or use within 14 days of starting or stopping, **MAO inhibitors** may ↑ risk of neuroleptic malignant syndrome or serotonin syndrome and should be avoided. Concurrent use with **MAO-inhibitor like drugs**, such as **linezolid** or **methylene blue**, may ↑ risk of serotonin syndrome; concurrent use contraindicated; do not start therapy in patients receiving **linezolid** or **methylene blue**; if **linezolid** or **methylene blue** need to be started in a patient receiving vilazodone, immediately discontinue vilazodone and monitor for signs/symptoms of serotonin syndrome for 2 wk or until 24 hr after last dose of linezolid or methylene blue, whichever comes first (may resume vilazodone therapy 24 hr after last dose of

V

linezolid or methylene blue). Drugs that affect serotonergic neurotransmitter systems, including **tricyclic antidepressants**, **SNRIs**, **fentanyl**, **lithium**, **buspirone**, **tramadol**, **meperidine**, **methadone**, **amphetamines**, and **triptans**, ↑ risk of serotonin syndrome. ↑ risk of bleeding with **NSAIDs**, **aspirin**, **clopidogrel**, **prasugrel**, **ticagrelor**, **dabigatran**, **apixaban**, **edoxaban**, **rivaroxaban**, or **warfarin**. **Strong CYP3A4 inhibitors**, including **ketoconazole**, may ↑ levels and the risk of toxicity. **Moderate CYP3A4 inhibitors**, including **erythromycin**, may ↑ levels and the risk of toxicity; ↓ dose to 20 mg daily if toxicity occurs. **Strong CYP3A4 inducers**, including **carbamazepine**, may ↓ levels and effectiveness. **Drug-Natural Products:** ↑ risk of serotonin syndrome with **St. John's wort**.

Route/Dosage

PO (Adults): 10 mg once daily for one wk, then 20 mg once daily for one wk; dose may be ↑ to 40 mg once daily (recommended dose = 20–40 mg/day). *Concurrent use of strong CYP3A4 inhibitors:* not to exceed 20 mg/day; *Concurrent use of strong CYP3A4 inducers (if used for >14 days):* may need to ↑ dose up to 2-fold (daily dose should not exceed 80 mg).

Availability (generic available)

Tablets: 10 mg, 20 mg, 40 mg.

NURSING IMPLICATIONS

Assessment

- Assess mental status and mood changes. Inform health care professional if patient demonstrates significant ↑ in anxiety, nervousness, or insomnia.
- Prior to starting therapy, screen patient for bipolar disorder (detailed psychiatric history, including family/personal history of suicide, bipolar disorder, depression). Use cautiously in patients with a positive history.
- Assess suicidal tendencies, especially in early therapy. Restrict amount of drug available to patient. Risk may be ↑ in children, adolescents, and adults ≤24 yr.
- Assess for signs and symptoms of hyponatremia (headache, difficulty concentrating, memory impairment, confusion, weakness, unsteadiness). May require discontinuation of therapy.
- Assess for serotonin syndrome (mental changes [agitation, hallucinations, coma], autonomic instability [tachycardia, labile BP, hyperthermia], neuromuscular aberrations [hyper-reflexia, incoordination], and/or GI symptoms [nausea, vomiting, diarrhea]), especially in patients taking other serotonergic drugs (SSRIs, SNRIs, triptans).
- Monitor for development of neuroleptic malignant syndrome (fever, muscle rigidity, altered mental status, respiratory distress, tachycardia, seizures, diaphoresis, hypertension or hypotension, pallor, tiredness, loss of bladder control). Discontinue vila-

zodone and notify health care professional immediately if these symptoms occur.
- Assess sexual function before starting vilazodone. Assess for changes in sexual function during treatment, including timing of onset; patient may not report.

Lab Test Considerations

- Monitor serum sodium concentrations periodically during therapy. May cause hyponatremia potentially as a result of SIADH.
- May cause altered anticoagulant effects. Monitor patients receiving warfarin, NSAIDs, or aspirin concurrently.

Implementation

- **PO:** Administer vilazodone with food; administration without food can result in inadequate drug concentrations and may ↓ effectiveness.
- When discontinuing therapy, decrease dose gradually; 40 mg once daily to 20 mg once daily for 4 days, followed by 10 mg once daily for 3 days. Taper patients taking 20 mg once daily dose to 10 mg once daily for 7 days. Stopping abruptly may cause flu-like symptoms (headache, sweating, and nausea), anxiety, high or low mood, irritability, feeling restless or sleepy, dizziness, electric shock-like sensations, tremor, and confusion.

Patient/Family Teaching

- Instruct patient to take vilazodone as directed at the same time each day. Take missed doses as soon as possible unless almost time for next dose. Do not double doses or discontinue abruptly. Gradually ↓ dose before discontinuation. Advise patient to read *Medication Guide* before starting therapy and with each Rx refill; new information may be available.
- Advise patient, family, and caregivers to look for activation of mania/hypomania and suicidality, especially during early therapy or dose changes. Notify health care professional immediately if thoughts about suicide or dying, attempts to commit suicide; new or worse depression or anxiety; agitation or restlessness; panic attacks; insomnia; new or worse irritability; aggressiveness; acting on dangerous impulses, mania, or other changes in mood or behavior or if symptoms of serotonin syndrome occur.
- Caution patient of the risk of serotonin syndrome and neuroleptic malignant syndrome, especially when taking triptans, tramadol, tryptophan supplements, and other serotonergic or antipsychotic agents.
- May cause dizziness. Caution patient to avoid driving or other activities requiring alertness until response to the drug is known.
- Instruct patient to notify health care professional of all Rx or OTC medications, vitamins, or herbal products being taken and to avoid concurrent use of Rx, OTC, and herbal products, especially NSAIDs, aspirin, and warfarin, without consulting health care professional.

- Caution patient to avoid taking alcohol or other CNS-depressant drugs, including opioids, during therapy.
- Inform patient that vilazodone may cause symptoms of sexual dysfunction. In males, ejaculatory delay or failure, decreased libido, and erectile dysfunction may occur. In female patients, may result in decreased libido and delayed or absent orgasm. Advise patient to notify health care professional if symptoms occur.
- Rep: Advise females of reproductive potential to notify health care professional immediately if pregnancy is planned or suspected or if breastfeeding. Use during last month of pregnancy increases risk of postpartum hemorrhage. If used during pregnancy, should be tapered during 3rd trimester to avoid neonatal serotonin syndrome. Monitor infants exposed to vilazodone for excess sedation, restlessness, agitation, poor feeding, poor weight gain, respiratory distress; may ↑ risk of persistent pulmonary hypertension of the newborn. Inform patient of pregnancy exposure registry that monitors pregnancy outcomes in women exposed to antidepressants during pregnancy. Register patients by calling the National Pregnancy Registry for Antidepressants at 1-844-405-6185 or visiting online at https://womensmentalhealth.org/research/pregnancyregistry/antidepressants/.
- Emphasize the importance of follow-up exams to monitor progress. Encourage patient participation in psychotherapy.

Evaluation/Desired Outcomes

- ↑ sense of well-being.
- Renewed interest in surroundings. Need for therapy should be periodically reassessed. Therapy is usually continued for several mo.
- ↓ anxiety.

HIGH ALERT

vinBLAStine (vin-**blass**-teen)
Classification
Therapeutic: antineoplastics
Pharmacologic: vinca alkaloids

Indications
Palliative treatment of the following: Hodgkin's lymphoma, Lymphocytic lymphoma, Histiocytic lymphoma, Advanced mycosis fungoides, Testicular carcinoma, Kaposi's sarcoma, Breast cancer.

Action
Binds to proteins of mitotic spindle, causing metaphase arrest. Cell replication is stopped as a result (cell cycle–specific for M phase). **Therapeutic Effects:** Death of rapidly replicating cells, particularly malignant ones.

Pharmacokinetics
Absorption: IV administration results in complete bioavailability.

Distribution: Does not cross the blood-brain barrier well.
Metabolism and Excretion: Converted by the liver to an active antineoplastic compound; excreted in the feces via biliary excretion, with some renal elimination.
Half-life: 24 hr.

TIME/ACTION PROFILE (effects on WBC counts)

ROUTE	ONSET	PEAK	DURATION
IV	5–7 days	10 days	7–14 days

Contraindications/Precautions
Contraindicated in: Hypersensitivity; OB: Pregnancy; Lactation: Lactation.
Use Cautiously in: Infection; ↓ bone marrow reserve; Hepatic impairment (↓ dose by 50% if serum bilirubin >3 mg/dL); Rep: Women of reproductive potential;.

Adverse Reactions/Side Effects
Derm: alopecia, dermatitis, vesiculation. **Endo:** syndrome of inappropriate antidiuretic hormone (SIADH). **GI:** nausea, vomiting, anorexia, constipation, diarrhea, stomatitis. **GU:** gonadal suppression. **Hemat:** anemia, leukopenia, thrombocytopenia. **Local:** phlebitis at IV site. **Metab:** hyperuricemia. **Neuro:** depression, neuritis, paresthesia, peripheral neuropathy, SEIZURES, weakness. **Resp:** BRONCHOSPASM.

Interactions
Drug-Drug: Additive bone marrow depression with other **antineoplastics** or **radiation therapy**. Bronchospasm may occur in patients who have been previously treated with **mitomycin**. May ↓ antibody response to **live-virus vaccines** and ↑ risk of adverse reactions. May ↓ **phenytoin** levels.

Route/Dosage
IV (Adults): *Initial:* 3.7 mg/m² (100 mcg/kg), single dose; ↑ weekly as tolerated by 1.8 mg/m² (50 mcg/kg) to maximum of 18.5 mg/m² (usual dose is 5.5–7.4 mg/m²). *Maintenance:* 10 mg 1–2 times/mo or one increment less than last dose every 7–14 days.
IV (Children): *Initial:* 2.5 mg/m², single dose; ↑ weekly as tolerated by 1.25 mg/m² to maximum of 7.5 mg/m². *Maintenance:* one increment less than last dose every 7 days.

Availability (generic available)
Solution for injection: 1 mg/mL.

NURSING IMPLICATIONS
Assessment
- Monitor BP, pulse, and respiratory rate during therapy. Bronchospasm can be life-threatening and may occur at time of infusion or several hr to wk later.

✳ = Canadian drug name. ⚅ = Genetic implication. S̶t̶r̶i̶k̶e̶t̶h̶r̶o̶u̶g̶h̶ = Discontinued. CAPITALS = life-threatening. Underline = most frequent.

- Monitor for bone marrow depression. Assess for bleeding (bleeding gums, bruising, petechiae, guaiac stools, urine, and emesis) and avoid IM injections and taking rectal temperatures if platelet count is low. Apply pressure to venipuncture sites for 10 min. Assess for signs of infection during neutropenia. Anemia may occur. Monitor for increased fatigue, dyspnea, and orthostatic hypotension.
- May cause nausea and vomiting. Monitor intake and output, appetite, and nutritional intake. Prophylactic antiemetics may be used. Adjust diet as tolerated.
- Vinblastine is a vesicant. Assess injection site frequently for redness, irritation, or inflammation. If extravasation occurs, infusion must be stopped and restarted elsewhere to avoid damage to SUBQ tissue. Standard treatment includes infiltration with hyaluronidase and application of heat.
- Monitor for symptoms of gout (increased uric acid, joint pain, edema). Encourage patient to drink at least 2 L of fluid per day. Allopurinol or alkalinization of urine may be used to decrease uric acid levels.

Lab Test Considerations
- Monitor CBC prior to and routinely throughout therapy. If WBC <2000, subsequent doses are usually withheld until WBC is ≥4000. The nadir of leukopenia occurs in 5–10 days and recovery usually occurs 7–14 days later. Thrombocytopenia may also occur in patients who have received radiation or other chemotherapy agents.
- Monitor liver function studies (AST, ALT, LDH, bilirubin) and renal function studies (BUN, serum creatinine) prior to and periodically throughout therapy.
- May cause ↑ uric acid. Monitor periodically during therapy.

Implementation
- **High Alert:** Fatalities have occurred with chemotherapeutic agents. Before administering, clarify all ambiguous orders; double check single, daily, and course-of-therapy dose limits; have second practitioner independently double check original order, dose calculations, and infusion pump settings. Do not administer SUBQ, IM, or intrathecally (IT). IT administration is fatal. Vinblastine must be dispensed in an overwrap stating, "For IV use only." Overwrap should remain in place until immediately before administration.
- **High Alert:** Do not confuse vinblastine with vincristine.
- Solution should be prepared in a biologic cabinet. Wear gloves, gown, and mask while handling medication. Discard IV equipment in specially designated containers. Prepare in a minibag, not a syringe.
- Do not inject into extremities with impaired circulation; may cause thrombophlebitis.

IV Administration
- **IV Push: *Dilution:*** Dilute each 10 mg with 10 mL of 0.9% NaCl for injection with phenol or benzyl alcohol. Solution is clear. Reconstituted medication is stable for 28 days if refrigerated. *Concentration:* 1 mg/mL. *Rate:* Administer each single dose over 1 min through Y-site injection of a free-flowing infusion of 0.9% NaCl or D5W.
- **Intermittent Infusion: *Dilution:*** Dilute in 25 to 50 mL of 0.9% NaCl, D5W, or LR. Dilution in large volumes (100–250 mL) or prolonged infusion (≥30 min) increases chance of vein irritation and extravasation.
- **Y-Site Compatibility:** acyclovir, alemtuzumab, allopurinol, amifostine, amikacin, aminophylline, amiodarone, amphotericin B deoxycholate, amphotericin B lipid complex, ampicillin, ampicillin/sulbactam, anidulafungin, argatroban, arsenic trioxide, aztreonam, bivalirudin, bleomycin, bumetanide, buprenorphine, busulfan, butorphanol, calcium chloride, calcium gluconate, carboplatin, carmustine, caspofungin, cefazolin, cefotaxime, cefotetan, cefoxitin, ceftazidime, ceftriaxone, cefuroxime, chloramphenicol, chlorpromazine, ciprofloxacin, cisatracurium, cisplatin, clindamycin, cyclophosphamide, cyclosporine, dacarbazine, dactinomycin, daptomycin, daunorubicin hydrochloride, dexamethasone, dexmedetomidine, dexrazoxane, digoxin, diltiazem, diphenhydramine, dobutamine, docetaxel, dopamine, doxorubicin hydrochloride, doxorubicin liposomal, doxycycline, droperidol, enalaprilat, ephedrine, epinephrine, epirubicin, ertapenem, erythromycin, esmolol, etoposide, etoposide phosphate, famotidine, fentanyl, filgrastim, fluconazole, fludarabine, fluorouracil, foscarnet, fosphenytoin, ganciclovir, gemcitabine, gentamicin, glycopyrrolate, granisetron, haloperidol, heparin, hetastarch, hydralazine, hydrocortisone, hydromorphone, idarubicin, ifosfamide, imipenem/cilastatin, insulin regular, irinotecan, isoproterenol, ketorolac, labetalol, leucovorin calcium, levofloxacin, lidocaine, linezolid, lorazepam, magnesium sulfate, mannitol, melphalan, meperidine, meropenem, mesna, methadone, methotrexate, metoclopramide, metoprolol, metronidazole, midazolam, milrinone, mitomycin, mitoxantrone, morphine, moxifloxacin, nafcillin, nalbuphine, naloxone, nitroglycerin, nitroprusside, norepinephrine, octreotide, ondansetron, oxaliplatin, paclitaxel, palonosetron, pamidronate, pemetrexed, pentamidine, pentobarbital, phenobarbital, phentolamine, phenylephrine, piperacillin/tazobactam, potassium acetate, potassium chloride, potassium phosphate, procainamide, prochlorperazine, promethazine, propranolol, remifentanil, rituximab, sargramostim, sodium acetate, sodium bicarbonate, sodium phosphate, succinylcholine, sufentanil, tacrolimus, theophylline, thiopental, thiotepa, tigecycline, tirofiban, tobramycin, topotecan, trastuzumab, trimethoprim/sulfamethoxazole, vancomycin, vasopressin, vecuronium, verapamil, vincristine, vinorelbine, voriconazole, zidovudine, zoledronic acid.

- **Y-Site Incompatibility:** amphotericin B liposomal, cefepime, dantrolene, diazepam, furosemide, gemtuzumab ozogamicin, pantoprazole, phenytoin.

Patient/Family Teaching

- Advise patient to notify health care professional if fever; chills; sore throat; signs of infection; bleeding gums; bruising; petechiae; or blood in urine, stool, or emesis occurs. Caution patient to avoid crowds and persons with known infections. Instruct patient to use soft toothbrush and electric razor. Caution patient not to drink alcoholic beverages or take products containing aspirin or NSAIDs.
- Instruct patient to inspect oral mucosa for redness and ulceration. Advise patient that, if ulceration occurs, to avoid spicy foods, use sponge brush, and rinse mouth with water after eating and drinking. Topical agents may be used if mouth pain interferes with eating. Stomatitis pain may require treatment with opioid analgesics.
- Instruct patient to report symptoms of neurotoxicity (paresthesia, pain, difficulty walking, persistent constipation).
- Advise patient that jaw pain, pain in organs containing tumor tissue, nausea, and vomiting may occur. Avoid constipation and report other adverse reactions.
- Discuss with patient the possibility of hair loss. Explore coping strategies.
- Instruct patient not to receive any vaccinations without advice of health care professional.
- Advise patient to notify health care professional of all Rx or OTC medications, vitamins, or herbal products being taken and to consult with health care professional before taking other medications.
- Rep: May cause fetal harm. Advise females of reproductive potential to notify health care professional if pregnancy is planned or suspected and to avoid breastfeeding during therapy. Contraception should be used during and for at least 2 mo after therapy is concluded. If chemotherapy is indicated, avoid during the first trimester, leave a 3-wk time period between the last chemotherapy dose and anticipated delivery, and do not administer chemotherapy beyond week 33 of gestation. If treatment cannot be deferred until after delivery in patients with early stage Hodgkin's lymphoma, may be administered safely and effectively in the latter phase of pregnancy. Advise patient to enroll in the pregnancy registry for all cancers diagnosed during pregnancy at Cooper Health (877-635-4499).
- Emphasize need for periodic lab tests to monitor for side effects.

Evaluation/Desired Outcomes

- Regression of malignancy without the appearance of detrimental side effects.

HIGH ALERT

vinCRIStine (vin-kriss-teen)

~~Vincasar PFS~~

Classification
Therapeutic: antineoplastics
Pharmacologic: vinca alkaloids

Indications

Used alone and in combination with other treatment modalities (antineoplastics, surgery, or radiation therapy) in treatment of: Hodgkin's disease, Leukemias, Neuroblastoma, Malignant lymphomas, Rhabdomyosarcoma, Wilms' tumor, Other tumors.

Action

Binds to proteins of mitotic spindle, causing metaphase arrest. Cell replication is stopped as a result (cell cycle–specific for M phase). Has little or no effect on bone marrow. **Therapeutic Effects:** Death of rapidly replicating cells, particularly malignant ones.

Pharmacokinetics

Absorption: IV administration results in complete bioavailability.

Distribution: Rapidly and widely distributed; extensively bound to tissues.

Metabolism and Excretion: Metabolized by the liver and eliminated in the feces via biliary excretion.

Half-life: 10.5–37.5 hr.

TIME/ACTION PROFILE (effects on blood counts†)

ROUTE	ONSET	PEAK	DURATION
IV	unknown	4 days	7 days

†Usually mild.

Contraindications/Precautions

Contraindicated in: Hypersensitivity; OB: Pregnancy; Lactation: Lactation.

Use Cautiously in: Infection; ↓ bone marrow reserve; Hepatic impairment (50% dose ↓ recommended if serum bilirubin >3 mg/dL); Rep: Women of reproductive potential;.

Adverse Reactions/Side Effects

Derm: alopecia. **EENT:** cortical blindness, diplopia. **Endo:** syndrome of inappropriate antidiuretic hormone (SIADH). **GI:** nausea, vomiting, abdominal cramps, anorexia, constipation, ileus, stomatitis. **GU:** gonadal suppression, nocturia, oliguria, urinary retention. **Hemat:** anemia, leukopenia, thrombocytopenia (mild and brief). **Local:** phlebitis at IV site, tissue necrosis (from extravasation). **Metab:** hyperuricemia. **Neuro:** ascending peripheral neuropathy, agitation, insomnia, mental depression, mental status changes. **Resp:** bronchospasm.

V

✳ = Canadian drug name. ⚇ = Genetic implication. ~~Strikethrough~~ = Discontinued. CAPITALS = life-threatening. <u>Underline</u> = most frequent.

Interactions

Drug-Drug: Bronchospasm may occur in patients who have been previously treated with **mitomycin**. **L-asparaginase** may ↓ hepatic metabolism of vincristine (give vincristine 12–24 hr prior to asparaginase). May ↓ antibody response to **live-virus vaccines** and ↑ risk of adverse reactions.

Route/Dosage

IV (Adults): 10–30 mcg/kg (0.4–1.4 mg/m²); may repeat weekly (not to exceed 2 mg/dose).
IV (Children >10 kg): 1.5–2 mg/m² single dose; may repeat weekly.
IV (Children <10 kg): 50 mcg/kg single dose; may repeat weekly.

Availability (generic available)

Solution for injection: 1 mg/mL.

NURSING IMPLICATIONS

Assessment

- Monitor BP, pulse, and respiratory rate during therapy. Report significant changes.
- Monitor neurologic status. Assess for paresthesia (numbness, tingling, pain), loss of deep tendon reflexes (Achilles reflex is usually first involved), weakness (wrist drop or footdrop, gait disturbances), cranial nerve palsies (jaw pain, hoarseness, ptosis, visual changes), autonomic dysfunction (ileus, difficulty voiding, orthostatic hypotension, impaired sweating), and CNS dysfunction (decreased level of consciousness, agitation, hallucinations). Notify physician if these symptoms develop, as they may persist for mo.
- Monitor intake and output ratios and daily weight; report significant discrepancies. Decreased urine output with concurrent hyponatremia may indicate SIADH, which usually responds to fluid restriction.
- Assess infusion site frequently for redness, irritation, or inflammation. If extravasation occurs, infusion must be stopped and restarted elsewhere to avoid damage to SUBQ tissue. Cellulitis and discomfort may be minimized by infiltration with hyaluronidase and application of moderate heat or by application of cold compresses.
- Assess nutritional status. An antiemetic may be used to minimize nausea and vomiting.
- Monitor for symptoms of gout (increased uric acid, joint pain, edema). Encourage patient to drink at least 2 liters of fluid per day. Allopurinol or alkalinization of urine may be used to decrease uric acid levels.

Lab Test Considerations

- Monitor CBC prior to and periodically throughout therapy. May cause slight leukopenia 4 days after therapy, which resolves within 7 days. Platelet count may ↑ or ↓.

- Monitor liver function studies (AST, ALT, LDH, bilirubin) and renal function studies (BUN, creatinine) prior to and periodically throughout therapy.
- May cause ↑ uric acid. Monitor periodically during therapy.

Implementation

- **High Alert:** Fatalities have occurred with chemotherapeutic agents. Before administering, clarify all ambiguous orders; double check single, daily, and course-of-therapy dose limits; have second practitioner independently double check original order, dose calculations, and infusion pump settings. Do not administer SUBQ, IM, or intrathecally (IT). IT administration is fatal. Vincristine must be dispensed in an overwrap stating "For IV use only." Overwrap should remain in place until immediately before administration.
- **High Alert:** Do not confuse vincristine with vinblastine.
- Solution should be prepared in a biologic cabinet. Wear gloves, gown, and mask while handling medication. Discard IV equipment in specially designated containers.

IV Administration

- **IV Push: Dilution:** Does not need to be reconstituted. **Concentration:** Administer undiluted at 1 mg/mL. **Rate:** Administer each dose IV push over 1 min through Y-site injection of a free-flowing infusion of 0.9% NaCl or D5W.
- **Y-Site Compatibility:** acyclovir, alemtuzumab, allopurinol, amifostine, amikacin, aminophylline, amiodarone, amphotericin B lipid complex, amphotericin B liposomal, ampicillin, ampicillin/sulbactam, anidulafungin, argatroban, azithromycin, aztreonam, bivalirudin, bleomycin, bumetanide, buprenorphine, butorphanol, calcium chloride, calcium gluconate, carboplatin, carmustine, caspofungin, cefazolin, cefotetan, cefoxitin, ceftazidime, ceftriaxone, cefuroxime, chlorpromazine, ciprofloxacin, cisatracurium, cladribine, cisplatin, cladribine, clindamycin, cyclophosphamide, cyclosporine, cytarabine, dactinomycin, daptomycin, daunorubicin hydrochloride, dexamethasone, dexmedetomidine, dexrazoxane, digoxin, diltiazem, diphenhydramine, dobutamine, docetaxel, dopamine, doxorubicin hydrochloride, doxorubicin liposomal, doxycycline, droperidol, enalaprilat, ephedrine, epinephrine, epirubicin, ertapenem, erythromycin, esmolol, etoposide, etoposide phosphate, famotidine, fentanyl, filgrastim, fluconazole, fludarabine, fluorouracil, foscarnet, fosphenytoin, fosphenytoin, ganciclovir, gemcitabine, gentamicin, granisetron, haloperidol, heparin, hetastarch, hydrocortisone, hydromorphone, ifosfamide, imipenem/cilastatin, insulin regular, isoproterenol, ketorolac, labetalol, leucovorin calcium, levofloxacin, lidocaine, linezolid, lorazepam, magnesium sulfate, mannitol, melphalan, meperidine, merope-

nem, mesna, methotrexate, methoprednisolone, metoclopramide, metoprolol, metronidazole, midazolam, milrinone, mitomycin, mitoxantrone, morphine, moxifloxacin, nalbuphine, naloxone, nicardipine, nitroglycerin, nitroprusside, norepinephrine, octreotide, ondansetron, oxaliplatin, paclitaxel, palonosetron, pemetrexed, pentamidine, pentobarbital, phenobarbital, phenylephrine, piperacillin/tazobactam, potassium acetate, potassium chloride, potassium phosphate, procainamide, prochlorperazine, promethazine, propranolol, remifentanil, rituximab, rocuronium, sargramostim, sodium acetate, sodium phosphate, succinylcholine, sufentanil, tacrolimus, theophylline, thiopental, thiotepa, tigecycline, tirofiban, tobramycin, topotecan, trastuzumab, trimethoprim/sulfamethoxazole, vancomycin, vasopressin, vecuronium, verapamil, vinblastine, vinorelbine, voriconazole, zidovudine, zoledronic acid.

- **Y-Site Incompatibility:** amphotericin B deoxycholate, cefepime, diazepam, idarubicin, nafcillin, pantoprazole, phenytoin.

Patient/Family Teaching

- Instruct patient to notify health care professional immediately if redness, swelling, or pain at injection site occurs.
- Instruct patient to report symptoms of neurotoxicity (paresthesia, pain, difficulty walking, persistent constipation). Inform patient that increased fluid intake, dietary fiber, and exercise may minimize constipation. Stool softeners or laxatives may be used. Patient should inform health care professional if severe constipation or abdominal discomfort occurs, as this may be a sign of neuropathy.
- Advise patient to notify health care professional if fever; chills; sore throat; signs of infection; bleeding gums; bruising; petechiae; blood in urine, stool, or emesis; or mouth sores occur. Caution patient to avoid crowds and persons with known infections.
- Discuss with patient the possibility of hair loss. Explore coping strategies.
- Instruct patient not to receive any vaccinations without advice of health care professional.
- Rep: May cause fetal harm. Advise females of reproductive potential to notify health care professional if pregnancy is planned or suspected and to avoid breastfeeding during therapy. Contraception should be used during and for at least 2 mo after therapy is concluded.
- Emphasize need for periodic lab tests to monitor for side effects.

Evaluation/Desired Outcomes

- Regression of malignancy without the appearance of detrimental side effects.

---

vinorelbine (vine-oh-**rel**-been)
~~Navelbine~~

Classification
Therapeutic: antineoplastics
Pharmacologic: vinca alkaloids

Indications
Inoperable non-small-cell lung cancer (as monotherapy or in combination with cisplatin).

Action
Binds to a protein (tubulin) of cellular microtubules, where it interferes with microtubule assembly. Cell replication is stopped as a result (cell cycle–specific for M phase). **Therapeutic Effects:** Death of rapidly replicating cells, particularly malignant ones.

Pharmacokinetics
Absorption: IV administration results in complete bioavailability.
Distribution: Highly bound to platelets and lymphocytes.
Metabolism and Excretion: Mostly metabolized by the liver. At least one metabolite is active. Large amounts eliminated in feces; 11% excreted unchanged by the kidneys.
Half-life: 28–44 hr.

TIME/ACTION PROFILE (effect on WBCs)

ROUTE	ONSET	PEAK	DURATION
IV	unknown	7–10 days	7–15 days

Contraindications/Precautions
Contraindicated in: Hypersensitivity; Active infection; ↓ bone marrow reserve; OB: Pregnancy; Lactation: Lactation.
Use Cautiously in: Hepatic impairment (dose ↓ recommended if total bilirubin >2 m g/dL); Debilitated patients (↑ risk of hyponatremia); Granulocytopenia (temporarily discontinue or reduce dose); Rep: Women of reproductive potential; Pedi: Safety and effectiveness not established in children.

Adverse Reactions/Side Effects
CV: chest pain. **Derm:** alopecia, rash. **F and E:** hyponatremia. **GI:** constipation, nausea, ↑ in liver enzymes, abdominal pain, anorexia, diarrhea, vomiting. **Hemat:** anemia, neutropenia, thrombocytopenia. **Local:** <u>irritation at IV site</u>, phlebitis. **MS:** arthralgia, back pain, jaw pain, myalgia. **Neuro:** <u>fatigue</u>, neurotoxicity. **Resp:** shortness of breath.

Interactions
Drug-Drug: ↑ bone marrow depression with other **antineoplastics** or **radiation therapy.** Concurrent use with **cisplatin** ↑ risk and severity of bone marrow

V

---

depression. Concurrent use with **mitomycin** or **chest radiation** ↑ risk of pulmonary reactions.

Route/Dosage
IV (Adults): 30 mg/m² once weekly.

Hepatic Impairment
IV (Adults): *Total bilirubin 2.1–3 mg/dL:* 15 mg/m² once weekly; *total bilirubin ≥3 mg/dL:* 7.5 mg/m² once weekly.

Availability (generic available)
Solution for injection: 10 mg/mL.

NURSING IMPLICATIONS
Assessment
- Monitor BP, pulse, and respiratory rate during therapy. Note significant changes. Acute shortness of breath and severe bronchospasm may occur infrequently shortly after administration. Treatment with corticosteroids, bronchodilators, and supplemental oxygen may be required, especially in patients with a history of pulmonary disease.
- Assess frequently for signs of infection (sore throat, temperature, cough, mental status changes), especially when nadir of granulocytopenia is expected.
- Monitor neurologic status. Assess for paresthesia (numbness, tingling, pain), loss of deep tendon reflexes (Achilles reflex is usually first involved), weakness (wrist drop or footdrop, gait disturbances), cranial nerve palsies (jaw pain, hoarseness, ptosis, visual changes), autonomic dysfunction (constipation, difficulty voiding, orthostatic hypotension, impaired sweating), and CNS dysfunction (decreased level of consciousness, agitation, hallucinations). These symptoms may persist for mo. The incidence of neurotoxicity associated with vinorelbine is less than that of other vinca alkaloids.
- Monitor intake and output and daily weight for significant discrepancies.
- Assess nutritional status. Mild to moderate nausea is common. An antiemetic may be used to minimize nausea and vomiting.
- Monitor for symptoms of gout (increased uric acid, joint pain, edema). Encourage patient to drink at least 2 L of fluid/day. Allopurinol and alkalinization of urine may decrease uric acid levels.

Lab Test Considerations
- Monitor CBC prior to each dose and routinely during therapy. The nadir of granulocytopenia usually occurs 7–10 days after vinorelbine administration and recovery usually follows within 7–15 days. If granulocyte count is <1500/mm³, dose reduction or temporary interruption of vinorelbine may be warranted. If repeated episodes of fever and/or sepsis occur during granulocytopenia, future dose of vinorelbine should be modified. May also cause mild to moderate anemia. Thrombocytopenia rarely occurs.
- Monitor liver function studies (AST, ALT, LDH, bilirubin) and renal function studies (BUN, creatinine)

prior to and periodically during therapy. May cause ↑ uric acid; monitor periodically during therapy.

Implementation
- **High Alert:** Fatalities have occurred with chemotherapeutic agents. Before administering, clarify all ambiguous orders; double check single, daily, and course-of-therapy dose limits; have second practitioner independently double check original order, dose calculations, and infusion pump settings.
- Solution should be prepared in a biologic cabinet. Wear gloves, gown, and mask while handling medication. Discard IV equipment in specially designated containers.
- Assess infusion site frequently for redness, irritation, or inflammation. Vinorelbine is a vesicant. If extravasation occurs, infusion must be stopped and restarted elsewhere to avoid damage to SUBQ tissue. Treatment of extravasation includes application of warm compresses applied over the area immediately for 30–60 min, then alternating on/off every 15 min for 1 day to increase systemic absorption of the drug. Hyaluronidase 150 units diluted in 1–2 mL of 0.9% NaCl, 1 mL for each mL extravasated, should be injected through existing IV cannula or SUBQ if the needle has been removed to enhance absorption and dispersion of the extravasated drug.

IV Administration
- **IV Push:** *Dilution:* Dilute vinorelbine with 0.9% NaCl or D5W. *Concentration:* 1.5–3 mg/mL. *Rate:* Infuse over 6–10 min into Y-site closest to bag of a free-flowing IV or into a central line.
- Flush vein with at least 75–125 mL of 0.9% NaCl or D5W administered over 10 min or more following administration of vinorelbine.
- **Intermittent Infusion:** *Dilution:* Dilute vinorelbine with 0.9% NaCl, D5W, 0.45% NaCl, D5/0.45% NaCl, Ringer's or lactated Ringer's injection. Solution should be colorless to pale yellow. Do not administer solutions that are discolored or contain particulate matter. Diluted solution is stable for 24 hr at room temperature. *Concentration:* 0.5–2 mg/mL. *Rate:* Infuse over 6–10 min (up to 30 min) into Y-site closest to bag of a free-flowing IV or into a central line.
- Flush vein with at least 75–125 mL of 0.9% NaCl or D5W administered over 10 min or more following administration of vinorelbine.
- **Y-Site Compatibility:** amikacin, aztreonam, bleomycin, bumetanide, buprenorphine, butorphanol, calcium gluconate, carboplatin, carmustine, cefotaxime, ceftazidime, chlorpromazine, cisplatin, clindamycin, cyclophosphamide, cytarabine, dacarbazine, dactinomycin, daunorubicin hydrochloride, dexamethasone, diphenhydramine, doxorubicin hydrochloride, doxorubicin liposomal, doxycycline, droperidol, enalaprilat, etoposide, famotidine, filgrastim, floxuridine, fluconazole, fludarabine, gemcitabine, gentamicin, granisetron, haloperidol, hydrocortisone, hydromorphone, idarubicin, ifosfamide, imipenem/cilastatin,

lorazepam, mannitol, melphalan, meperidine, mesna, methotrexate, metoclopramide, metronidazole, mitoxantrone, morphine, nalbuphine, ondansetron, oxaliplatin, potassium chloride, prochlorperazine, promethazine, tobramycin, vancomycin, vinblastine, vincristine, zidovudine.

- **Y-Site Incompatibility:** acyclovir, allopurinol, aminophylline, amphotericin B deoxycholate, ampicillin, cefazolin, ceftriaxone, cefuroxime, fluorouracil, furosemide, ganciclovir, lansoprazole, methylprednisolone, mitomycin, sodium bicarbonate, thiotepa, trimethoprim/sulfamethoxazole.

Patient/Family Teaching

- Instruct patient to report symptoms of neurotoxicity (paresthesia, pain, difficulty walking, persistent constipation).
- Inform patient that increased fluid intake, dietary fiber, and exercise may minimize constipation. Stool softeners or laxatives may be necessary. Patient should be advised to report severe constipation or abdominal discomfort, as this may be a sign of ileus, which may occur as a consequence of neuropathy.
- Advise patient to notify health care professional if fever; chills; sore throat; signs of infection; bleeding gums; bruising; petechiae; blood in urine, stool, or emesis; or mouth sores occur.
- Caution patient to avoid crowds and persons with known infections.
- Rep: May cause fetal harm. Advise females of reproductive potential to use effective contraception during and for at least 2 mo after last dose of vinorelbine and to avoid breastfeeding during and for 9 days after last dose.
- Discuss with patient the possibility of hair loss and explore coping strategies.
- Instruct patient not to receive any vaccinations without advice of health care professional.
- Emphasize the need for periodic lab tests to monitor for side effects.

Evaluation/Desired Outcomes

- Decrease in the size or spread of malignancy without detrimental side effects.

VITAMIN B₁₂ PREPARATIONS

cyanocobalamin
(sye-an-oh-koe-**bal**-a-min)
  Nascobal

hydroxocobalamin
(hye-drox-oh-koe-**bal**-a-min)
  Cyanokit
Classification
Therapeutic: antianemics, vitamins
Pharmacologic: water-soluble vitamins

Indications

Vitamin B₁₂ deficiency (parenteral product or nasal spray should be used when deficiency is due to malabsorption). Pernicious anemia (only parenteral products should be used for initial therapy; nasal or oral products are not indicated until patients have achieved hematologic remission following parenteral therapy and have no signs of CNS involvement). Part of the Schilling test (vitamin B₁₂ absorption test) (diagnostic). Cyanide poisoning (Cyanokit only).

Action

Necessary coenzyme for metabolic processes, including fat and carbohydrate metabolism and protein synthesis. Required for cell production and hematopoiesis. **Therapeutic Effects:** Corrects manifestations of pernicious anemia (megaloblastic indices, GI lesions, and neurologic damage). Corrects vitamin B₁₂ deficiency. Reverses symptoms of cyanide toxicity (Cyanokit only).

Pharmacokinetics

Absorption: Oral absorption in GI tract requires intrinsic factor and calcium; well absorbed after IM, SUBQ, and nasal administration. IV administration results in complete bioavailability.

Distribution: Stored in the liver and bone marrow.

Metabolism and Excretion: Primarily excreted unchanged in urine.

Half-life: *Cyanocobalamin:* 6 days (400 days in liver); *Hydroxocobalamin:* 26–31 hr.

TIME/ACTION PROFILE (reticulocytosis)

ROUTE	ONSET	PEAK	DURATION
Cyanocobalamin IM, SUBQ, nasal	unknown	3–10 days	unknown
Hydroxocobalamin IM	unknown	unknown	unknown

Contraindications/Precautions

Contraindicated in: Hypersensitivity; Lactation: *Cyanokit:* Lactation; Pedi: Avoid using preparations containing benzyl alcohol in premature infants (associated with fatal "gasping syndrome").

Use Cautiously in: Hereditary optic nerve atrophy (accelerates nerve damage); Uremia, folic acid deficiency, concurrent infection, iron deficiency (response to B₁₂ will be impaired); Renal impairment (when using aluminum-containing products); OB: *Cyanokit:* Use during pregnancy only if potential maternal benefit justifies potential fetal risk; Pedi: *Cyanokit:* Safety and effectiveness not established in children.

Adverse Reactions/Side Effects

CV: HF; *Cyanokit:* hypertension, chest pain, tachycardia. **Derm:** itching; *Cyanokit:* erythema, rash. **EENT:** *Cyanokit:* dry throat, eye redness, eye swelling. **GI:** diarrhea; *Cyanokit:* abdominal discomfort, dyspepsia, dysphagia, hematochezia, nausea, vomiting. **F and E:** hypokalemia. **GU:** *Cyanokit:* red urine, acute renal

V

failure. **Hemat:** thrombocytosis. **Local:** pain at IM site. **Neuro:** headache; *Cyanokit:* dizziness, memory impairment, restlessness. **Resp:** pulmonary edema; *Cyanokit:* dyspnea. **Misc:** HYPERSENSITIVITY REACTIONS (including anaphylaxis).

Interactions
Drug-Drug: Chloramphenicol and **antineoplastics** may ↓ hematologic response to vitamin B$_{12}$. **Colchicine, aminosalicylic acid, cimetidine,** and excess intake of **alcohol** or **vitamin C** may ↓ oral absorption/effectiveness of vitamin B$_{12}$.

Route/Dosage
Cyanocobalamin (oral products are usually not recommended due to poor absorption and should be used only if patient refuses the IM, deep SUBQ, or intranasal route of administration)
PO (Adults and Children): *Vitamin B$_{12}$ deficiency:* amount depends on deficiency (up to 1000 mcg/day have been used).
PO (Adults): *Pernicious anemia (for hematologic remission only):* 1000–2000 mcg once daily.
IM, SUBQ (Adults): *Vitamin B$_{12}$ deficiency:* 30 mcg once daily for 5–10 days, then 100–200 mcg once monthly. *Pernicious anemia:* 100 mcg once daily for 6–7 days; if improvement, give same dose every other day for 7 doses, then every 3–4 days for 2–3 wk; once hematologic values return to normal (remission), can give maintenance dose of 100 mcg once monthly (doses up to 1000 mcg have been used for maintenance) (could alternatively use oral or intranasal formulations below for maintenance at specified doses).
Schilling test: Flushing dose is 1000 mcg.
IM, SUBQ (Children): *Vitamin B$_{12}$ deficiency:* 0.2 mcg/kg once daily for 2 days, then 1000 mcg once daily for 2–7 days, then 100 mcg once weekly for 1 mo. *Pernicious anemia:* 30–50 mcg once daily for ≥2 wk (to a total dose of 1000–5000 mcg), then give maintenance dose of 100 mcg once monthly (doses up to 1000 mcg have been used for maintenance).
Intranasal (Adults): *Vitamin B$_{12}$ deficiency:* 500 mcg (one spray) in one nostril once weekly. *Pernicious anemia (for hematologic remission only):* 500 mcg (one spray) in one nostril once weekly.

Hydroxocobalamin
IM (Adults): *Vitamin B$_{12}$ deficiency:* 30 mcg once daily for 5–10 days, then 100–200 mcg once monthly. *Pernicious anemia:* 100 mcg once daily for 6–7 days; if improvement, give same dose every other day for 7 doses, then every 3–4 days for 2–3 wk; once hematologic values return to normal (remission), give maintenance dose of 100 mcg once monthly. *Schilling test:* Flushing dose is 1000 mcg.
IM (Children): *Vitamin B$_{12}$ deficiency:* 100 mcg once daily for ≥2 wk (to achieve total dose of 1000–5000 mcg), then 30–50 mcg once monthly. *Pernicious anemia:* 30–50 mcg once daily for ≥2 wk (to

achieve total dose of 1000–5000 mcg), then 100 mcg once monthly.
IV (Adults): *Cyanide poisoning (Cyanokit only):* 5 g over 15 min; another 5 g dose may be infused over 15–120 min depending upon severity of poisoning (maximum cumulative dose = 10 g).

Availability
Cyanocobalamin (generic available)
Tablets: 100 mcg^{OTC}, 250 mcg^{OTC}, 500 mcg^{OTC}, 1000 mcg^{OTC}. **Extended-release tablets:** 1000 mcg^{OTC}. **Sublingual tablets:** 2500 mcg^{OTC}. **Lozenges:** 50 mcg^{OTC}, 100 mcg^{OTC}, 250 mcg^{OTC}, 500 mcg^{OTC}. **Nasal spray:** 500 mcg/0.1 mL actuation (8 sprays/bottle). **Solution for injection:** 1000 mcg/mL.

Hydroxocobalamin (generic available)
Solution for intramuscular injection: 1000 mcg/mL. **Powder for intravenous injection (Cyanokit):** 5 g/vial.

NURSING IMPLICATIONS
Assessment
- Assess patient for signs of vitamin B$_{12}$ deficiency (pallor; neuropathy; psychosis; red, inflamed tongue) before and periodically during therapy.

Lab Test Considerations
- Monitor plasma folic acid, vitamin B$_{12}$, and iron levels, hemoglobin, hemtaocrit, and reticulocyte count before treatment, 1 mo after the start of therapy, and then every 3–6 mo. Evaluate serum potassium level in patients receiving vitamin B$_{12}$ for pernicious anemia for hypokalemia during the first 48 hr of treatment. Serum potassium and platelet counts should be monitored routinely during the course of therapy.
- **Cyanokit:** Management of cyanide poisoning should also include establishment of airway, ensuring adequate oxygenation and hydration, cardiovascular support, and seizure management. Monitor BP and heart rate continuously during and after infusion and immediately report significant changes. The maximal ↑ in BP usually occurs toward the end of the infusion. BP usually returns to baseline within 4 hr of drug administration.

Implementation
- Usually administered in combination with other vitamins; solitary vitamin B$_{12}$ deficiencies are rare.
- Administration of vitamin B$_{12}$ by the oral route is useful only for nutritional deficiencies. Patients with small-bowel disease, malabsorption syndrome, or gastric or ileal resections require parenteral administration.
- **PO:** Administer with meals to increase absorption.
- May be mixed with fruit juices. Administer immediately after mixing; ascorbic acid alters stability.
- **Intranasal:** Dose should not be administered within 1 hr of hot food or liquids (these substances may result in the formation of nasal secretions, which may result in ↓ effectiveness of nasal spray).
- **IM, SUBQ:** Vials should be protected from light.

- If SUBQ route used, deep SUBQ administration is preferred.

IV Administration
- **IV:** IV route should only be used with Cyanokit.
- **Intermittent Infusion:** *Dilution:* Dilute each Cyanokit vial with 200 mL of 0.9% NaCl, D5W, or LR. Gently invert the vial for at least 60 sec prior to infusion. Reconstituted vial can be hung for infusion and is stable for 6 hr at room temperature. Discard any unused solution after 6 hr. *Rate:* Administer initial 5 g dose over 15 min. Administer additional 5 g dose over 15–120 min.
- **Y-Site Incompatibility:** ascorbic acid, blood products, diazepam, dobutamine, dopamine, fentanyl, nitroglycerin, pentobarbital, propofol, sodium thiosulfate, thiopental.

Patient/Family Teaching
- Encourage patient to comply with diet recommendations of health care professional. Explain that the best source of vitamins is a well-balanced diet with foods from the four basic food groups.
- Foods high in vitamin B_{12} include meats, seafood, egg yolk, and fermented cheeses; few vitamins are lost with ordinary cooking.
- Patients self-medicating with vitamin supplements should be cautioned not to exceed RDA. Effectiveness of megadoses for treatment of various medical conditions is unproved and may cause side effects.
- Inform patients with pernicious anemia of the lifelong need for vitamin B_{12} replacement.
- Emphasize the importance of follow-up exams to evaluate progress.
- Rep: Advise females of reproductive potential to notify health care professional if pregnancy is planned or suspected or if breastfeeding.
- **Intranasal:** Instruct patient in proper administration technique. Review *Patient Information Sheet* and demonstrate use of actuator. Unit must be primed with 3 strokes upon using for the first time. Unit must be primed with 1 stroke before each of the remaining doses. Advise patient to clear nose, then place tip approximately 1 inch into nostril and press pump once, firmly and quickly. After dose, remove unit from nose and massage dosed nostril gently for a few sec. Vial delivers 8 doses. Unit should be stored at room temperature and protected from light.
- **Intermittent Infusion:** Advise patient that skin redness may last up to 2 wk and that their urine may remain red for up to 5 wk after drug administration. Instruct patient to avoid sun exposure while their skin is red. Advise patient to contact health care professional if skin or urine redness persist after these time periods. Advise patient that a rash may develop from 7–28 days after drug administration. It will usually resolve without treatment within a few wk. Advise patient to contact health care professional if rash persists after this time period.

Evaluation/Desired Outcomes
- Resolution of the symptoms of vitamin B_{12} deficiency.
- Increase in reticulocyte count.
- Improvement in manifestations of pernicious anemia.
- Resolution of symptoms of cyanide poisoning.

VITAMIN D COMPOUNDS
calcifediol (kal-si-fe-**dye**-ol)
  Rayaldee
calcitriol (kal-si-**trye**-ole)
  Rocaltrol
cholecalciferol (kol-e-kal-**sif**-e-role)
  Delta-D3, ✤ Euro D
doxercalciferol
(**dox**-er-kal-**sif**-e-role)
  Hectorol
ergocalciferol
(**er**-goe-kal-**sif**-e-role)
  Drisdol
paricalcitol (par-i-**kal**-si-tole)
  Zemplar
Classification
Therapeutic: vitamins
Pharmacologic: fat-soluble vitamins

Indications
Cholecalciferol: Secondary hyperparathyroidism in patients with stage 3 or 4 chronic kidney disease and serum total 25-hydroxyvitamin D levels <30 ng/mL.
Calcitriol: Treatment of the following conditions: Hypocalcemia in chronic renal dialysis; Hypocalcemia in patients with hypoparathyroidism or pseudohypoparathyroidism; Secondary hyperparathyroidism and resulting metabolic bone disease in predialysis patients with moderate to severe renal insufficiency. **Cholecalciferol:** Treatment or prevention of vitamin D deficiency. **Doxercalciferol:** Treatment of the following conditions: Secondary hyperparathyroidism in patients undergoing chronic renal dialysis (IV and PO); Secondary hyperparathyroidism in patients with Stage 3 or 4 chronic kidney disease (PO only). **Ergocalciferol:** Treatment of the following conditions: Familial hypophosphatemia; Hypoparathyroidism; Vitamin D–resistant rickets. **Paricalcitol:** Prevention and treatment of secondary hyperparathyroidism in patients with Stage 3 or 4 (PO) or Stage 5 (PO and IV) chronic kidney disease.

Action
Calcifediol is a prohormone of the active form of vitamin D_3, calcitriol. Cholecalciferol requires activation in the liver and kidneys to create the active form of vitamin D_3 (calcitriol). Doxercalciferol and ergocalciferol require activation in the liver to create the active form of vitamin D_2. Paricalcitol is a synthetic analogue of calcitriol. Vitamin D promotes the absorption of calcium

V

and ↓ parathyroid hormone concentration. **Therapeutic Effects:** Treatment and prevention of deficiency states, particularly bone manifestations. Improved calcium and phosphorous homeostasis in patients with chronic kidney disease.

Pharmacokinetics

Absorption: *Calcifediol, calcitriol, doxercalciferol, ergocalciferol, paricalcitol:* Well absorbed following oral administration. *Doxercalciferol, paricalcitol:* IV administration results in complete bioavailability.
Distribution: Calcitriol and paricalcitol cross the placenta; calcitriol also enters breast milk.
Protein Binding: *Calcifediol:* >98%; *Calcitriol and paricalcitol:* 99.9%.
Metabolism and Excretion: *Calcifediol:* Converted to calcitriol by the 1-alpha-hydroxylase enzyme, CYP27B1, in kidney; also metabolized by CYP24A1 to inactive metabolites; primarily excreted in feces. *Calcitriol:* Undergoes enterohepatic recycling and is excreted mostly in bile. *Cholecalciferol:* Converted by the liver and kidneys to calcitriol (active form of vitamin D_3). *Ergocalciferol:* Converted to active form of vitamin D_2 by sunlight, the liver, and the kidneys. *Doxercalciferol:* Converted by the liver to the active form of vitamin D_2. *Paricalcitol:* mostly metabolized by the liver and excreted via hepatobiliary elimination.
Half-life: *Calcifediol:* 25 days. *Calcitriol:* 5–8 hr. *Cholecalciferol:* 14 hr. *Doxercalciferol:* 32–37 hr (up to 96 hr). *Paricalcitol:* 14–20 hr.

TIME/ACTION PROFILE (effects on serum calcium)

ROUTE	ONSET	PEAK	DURATION
Calcifediol-PO	2 wk	20 wk	unknown
Calcitriol-PO	2–6 hr	2–6 hr	3–5 days
Cholecalciferol-PO	unknown	unknown	unknown
Doxercalciferol PO	unknown	8 wk	1 wk
Doxercalciferol-IV	unknown	8 wk	1 wk
Ergocalciferol-PO	12–24 hr	unknown	up to 6 mo
Paricalcitol-PO	unknown	2–4 wk	unknown
Paricalcitol IV	unknown	up to 2 wk	unknown

Contraindications/Precautions

Contraindicated in: Hypersensitivity; Hypercalcemia; Vitamin D toxicity; Concurrent use of magnesium-containing antacids or other vitamin D supplements; **Ergocalciferol**: Known intolerance to tartrazine; **Cholecalciferol and ergocalciferol**: Malabsorption problems.
Use Cautiously in: Calcitriol, doxercalciferol, paricalcitol: Patients receiving digoxin; OB: Safety not established in pregnancy; Lactation: Use while breastfeeding only if potential maternal benefit outweighs potential risk to infant; Pedi: Safety and effectiveness of calcifediol and doxercalciferol not established in children.

Adverse Reactions/Side Effects

Seen primarily as manifestations of toxicity (hypercalcemia).

CV: *calcifediol:* arrhythmias, edema, HF, hypertension; *doxercalciferol:* bradycardia; *paricalcitol:* palpitations. **Derm:** pruritus. **EENT:** conjunctivitis, photophobia, rhinorrhea. **F and E:** HYPERCALCEMIA; *calcifediol:* hyperkalemia, hyperphosphatemia, polydipsia. **GI:** abdominal pain, anorexia, constipation, ↓ appetite, ↓ weight, dry mouth, ↑ liver enzymes, nausea, PANCREATITIS, polydipsia, vomiting. **GU:** albuminuria, azotemia, ↓ libido, nocturia, polyuria. **Hemat:** *calcifediol:* anemia. **Local:** pain at injection site. **Metab:** hyperthermia. **MS:** bone pain, muscle pain; *doxercalciferol:* arthralgia; *paricalcitol:* metastatic calcification. **Neuro:** *calcifediol:* dysgeusia, headache, SEIZURES, somnolence, weakness; *calcifediol:* confusion; *doxercalciferol:* dizziness, malaise. **Resp:** *doxercalciferol and ergocalciferol:* dyspnea. **Misc:** *calcitriol:* allergic reactions, chills, fever; *doxercalciferol:* HYPERSENSITIVITY REACTIONS (including anaphylaxis, angioedema, hypotension, dyspnea, and cardiac arrest).

Interactions

Drug-Drug: Cholestyramine, colestipol, or **mineral oil** ↓ absorption of vitamin D analogues. **Calcium-containing drugs, thiazide diuretics**, and other **vitamin D analogs** may ↑ risk of hypercalcemia. **Corticosteroids** ↓ effectiveness of vitamin D analogues. Using calcifediol, calcitriol, doxercalciferol, or paricalcitol with **digoxin** may ↑ risk of arrhythmias. Vitamin D requirements ↓ by **phenytoin, fosphenytoin, sucralfate, barbiturates**, and **primidone**. Concurrent use with **magnesium-containing drugs** may lead to hypermagnesemia. Concurrent use of **calcium-containing drugs** may ↑ risk of hypercalcemia. **Agents that induce liver enzymes (phenobarbital, rifampin)** and **agents that inhibit liver enzymes (atazanavir, clarithromycin, erythromycin, itraconazole, ketoconazole, nefazodone, nelfinavir, ritonavir, verapamil, voriconazole)** may alter requirements for calcifediol, doxercalciferol, and paricalcitol (monitoring of calcium and phosphorus recommended).
Drug-Food: Ingestion of **foods high in calcium content** (see Appendix J) may lead to hypercalcemia.

Route/Dosage

Calcifediol

PO (Adults): 30 mcg once daily at bedtime; if desired intact PTH level (iPTH) remains elevated after 3 mo, ↑ to 60 mcg once daily at bedtime. Maintenance dose should target total 25-hydroxyvitamin D levels of 30–100 ng/mL, iPTH levels within desired therapeutic range, serum calcium <9.8 mg/dL, and serum phosphorus ≤5.5 mg/dL.

Calcitriol

PO (Adults): *Hypocalcemia during dialysis:* 0.25 mcg once daily or every other day; if needed, may ↑ by 0.25 mcg/day at 4–8-wk intervals (typical dosage = 0.5–1 mcg/day). *Hypoparathyroidism:* 0.25 mcg once daily initially; if needed, may ↑ dose by 0.25 mcg/day at 2–4-wk intervals (typical dosage = 0.5–2 mcg/day).

Predialysis patients: 0.25 mcg once daily (up to 0.5 mcg/day).

PO (Children): *Hypocalcemia during dialysis:* 0.25–2 mcg once daily. *Hypoparathyroidism (children ≥6 yr):* 0.25 mcg once daily initially; if needed, may ↑ dose by 0.25 mcg/day at 2–4-wk intervals (typical dosage = 0.5–2 mcg/day). *Hypoparathyroidism (children 1–5 yr):* 0.25–0.75 mcg once daily. *Hypoparathyroidism (children <1 yr):* 0.04–0.08 mcg/kg/day. *Predialysis patients (children ≥3 yr):* 0.25 mcg once daily (up to 0.5 mcg/day). *Predialysis patients (children <3 yr):* 10–15 ng/kg/day.

IV (Adults): *Hypocalcemia during dialysis:* 0.5 mcg (0.01 mcg/kg) 3 times weekly. May be ↑ by 0.25–0.5 mcg/dose at 2–4-wk intervals (typical maintenance dose = 0.5–3.0 mcg 3 times weekly [0.01–0.05 mcg/kg 3 times weekly]).

IV (Children): *Hypocalcemia during dialysis:* 0.01–0.05 mcg/kg 3 times weekly.

Cholecalciferol

PO (Adults): 400–1000 units once daily.

PO (Infants): *Exclusively or partially breastfed:* 400 units once daily.

Doxercalciferol

PO (Adults): *Dialysis patients:* 10 mcg 3 times weekly (at dialysis); dose may be adjusted by 2.5 mcg at 8-wk intervals based on iPTH concentrations (maximum dose = 20 mcg 3 times weekly). *Non-dialysis patients:* 1 mcg once daily; dose may be adjusted by 0.5 mcg at 2-wk intervals based on iPTH concentrations (maximum dose = 3.5 mcg/day).

IV (Adults): 4 mcg 3 times weekly at the end of dialysis; dose may be adjusted by 1–2 mcg at 8-wk intervals based on iPTH concentrations (maximum dose = 6 mcg 3 times weekly).

Ergocalciferol

PO (Adults): *Vitamin D–resistant rickets:* 12,000–500,000 units/day (to be used with phosphate supplement). *Familial hypophosphatemia:* 10,000–80,000 units/day (with phosphorus 1–2 g/day). *Hypoparathyroidism:* 50,000–200,000 units/day (to be used with calcium supplement).

PO (Children): *Vitamin D–resistant rickets:* 40,000–80,000 units/day (to be used with phosphate supplement). *Familial hypophosphatemia:* 10,000–80,000 units/day (with phosphorus 1–2 g/day). *Hypoparathyroidism:* 50,000–200,000 units/day (to be used with calcium supplement).

PO (Infants): *Exclusively or partially breastfed:* 400 units once daily.

Paricalcitol

Stage 3 or 4 Chronic Kidney Disease

PO (Adults): *Baseline iPTH concentration ≤500 pg/mL:* Initiate with 1 mcg once daily or 2 mcg 3 times weekly; dose can be adjusted at 2–4-wk intervals based on iPTH, calcium, and phosphate concentrations. *Baseline iPTH concentration >500 pg/mL:* Initiate with 2 mcg once daily or 4 mcg 3 times weekly; dose can be adjusted at 2–4-wk intervals based on iPTH, calcium, and phosphate concentrations.

Stage 5 Chronic Kidney Disease

PO (Adults): Initial dose (in mcg) is based on following equation: baseline iPTH concentration (pg/mL)/80; dose should be given 3 times weekly; dose can be adjusted at 2–4-wk intervals based on iPTH, calcium, and phosphate concentrations.

IV (Adults and Children ≥5 yr): 0.04–0.1 mcg/kg 3 times weekly during dialysis; dose can be adjusted by 2–4 mcg at 2–4-wk intervals based on iPTH, calcium, and phosphate concentrations (doses up to 0.24 mcg/kg have been used).

Availability

Calcifediol

Extended-release capsules: 30 mcg.

Calcitriol (generic available)

Capsules: 0.25 mcg, 0.5 mcg. **Oral solution:** 1 mcg/mL.

Cholecalciferol (generic available)

Capsules: 1,000 units^OTC, 2,000 units^OTC, 5,000 units^OTC, 10,000 units^OTC, 25,000 units^OTC, 50,000 units^OTC. **Chewable tablets:** 400 units^OTC. **Oral solution:** 400 units/mL^OTC, 5,000 units/mL^OTC. **Tablets:** 400 units^OTC, 1,000 units^OTC, 2,000 units^OTC, 3,000 units^OTC, 5,000 units^OTC, 50,000 units^OTC. *In combination with:* alendronate (Fosamax Plus D), see Appendix N.

Doxercalciferol (generic available)

Capsules: 0.5 mcg, 1 mcg, 2.5 mcg. **Solution for injection:** 2 mcg/mL.

Ergocalciferol (generic available)

Capsules: 50,000 units. **Oral solution:** 8000 units/mL^Rx, OTC. **Tablets:** 400 units, 2,000 units.

Paricalcitol (generic available)

Capsules: 1 mcg, 2 mcg, 4 mcg. **Solution for injection:** 2 mcg/mL, 5 mcg/mL.

NURSING IMPLICATIONS

Assessment

- Assess for symptoms of vitamin deficiency prior to and periodically during therapy.
- Monitor for signs and symptoms of hypercalcemia (feeling tired, difficulty thinking clearly, loss of appetite, nausea, vomiting, constipation, increased thirst, increased urination, weight loss) during therapy. May increase risk of cardiac arrhythmias and seizures. May require frequent monitoring and change in dose.
- Assess patient for bone pain and weakness prior to and during therapy.
- Observe patient carefully for evidence of hypocalcemia (paresthesia, muscle twitching, laryngospasm,

colic, cardiac arrhythmias, and Chvostek's or Trousseau's sign). Protect symptomatic patient by raising and padding side rails; keep bed in low position.
- Monitor serum and signs and symptoms of digoxin toxicity (abdominal pain, anorexia, nausea, vomiting, visual disturbances, bradycardia, other arrhythmias) during therapy in patients taking concomitant digoxin. Hypercalcemia may increase risk of digoxin toxicity in patients taking digoxin.
- **Calcifediol:** Monitor for signs and symptoms of adynamic bone disease (fractures) during therapy. May develop if intact PTH levels are abnormally low due to suppression.
- Pedi: Monitor height and weight; growth arrest may occur in prolonged high-dose therapy.
- **Rickets/Osteomalacia:** Assess patient for bone pain and weakness prior to and during therapy.

Lab Test Considerations
- Ensure serum calcium is <9.8 mg/dL before starting *calcifediol* therapy. During *calcifediol* therapy, monitor serum calcium, phosphorus, total 25-hydroxyvitamin D, and iPTH levels at least every 3 mo after starting therapy or dose adjustment, and then at least every 6–12 mo. During *calcitriol* therapy, serum calcium and phosphate concentrations should be drawn twice weekly initially. Serum calcium, magnesium, alkaline phosphatase, and iPTH should then be monitored at least monthly. During *cholecalciferol* therapy, serum calcium, phosphate, and alkaline phosphatase concentrations should be monitored periodically. During *doxercalciferol* therapy, serum ionized calcium, phosphate, and iPTH concentrations should be monitored prior to initiation of therapy, and then weekly during the first 12 wk of therapy, then periodically. Alkaline phosphatase should be monitored periodically. During *ergocalciferol* therapy, serum calcium and phosphate concentrations should be monitored every 2 wk. During oral *paricalcitol* therapy, serum calcium, phosphate, and iPTH concentrations should be monitored at least every 2 wk for the first 3 mo of therapy or after any dosage adjustment, then monthly for 3 mo, then every 3 mo. During IV *paricalcitol* therapy, serum calcium and phosphate concentrations should be monitored twice weekly initially until dosage stabilized, and then at least monthly. Serum iPTH concentrations should be monitored every 3 mo.
- The serum calcium × phosphate product (Ca × P) should not exceed 70 mg²/dL² (55 mg²/dL² for doxercalciferol) (patients may be at ↑ risk of calcification).
- Calcitriol may cause false ↑ cholesterol levels.

Toxicity and Overdose
- Toxicity is manifested as hypercalcemia, hypercalciuria, and hyperphosphatemia. Assess patient for appearance of nausea, vomiting, anorexia, weakness, constipation, headache, bone pain, and metallic taste. Later symptoms include polyuria, polydipsia, photophobia, rhinorrhea, pruritus, and cardiac arrhythmias. Notify health care professional immediately if these signs of hypervitaminosis D occur.

Treatment usually consists of discontinuation of calcitriol, a low-calcium diet, use of low-calcium dialysate in peritoneal dialysis patients, and administration of a laxative. IV hydration and loop diuretics may be ordered to increase urinary excretion of calcium. Hemodialysis may also be used.

Implementation
- **PO:** May be administered without regard to meals. Measure solution accurately with calibrated dropper provided by manufacturer. May be mixed with juice, cereal, or food, or dropped directly into mouth. Calcitriol capsules or solution should be protected from light.
- **Calcifediol:** *DNC:* Administer at bedtime; swallow capsules whole, do not open, crush, or chew.

IV Administration
- **IV Push:** Administer *doxercalciferol* and *paricalcitol* undiluted by rapid injection through the catheter at the end of a hemodialysis period.

Patient/Family Teaching
- Advise patient to take medication as directed. Take missed doses as soon as remembered that day, unless almost time for next dose; do not double up on doses. If a *calcifediol* dose is missed, omit and take next dose at the next regularly scheduled time; do not double doses.
- Review diet modifications with patient. See Appendix J for foods high in calcium and vitamin D. Renal patients must still consider renal failure diet in food selection. Health care professional may order concurrent calcium supplement.
- Encourage patient to comply with dietary recommendations of health care professional. Explain that the best source of vitamins is a well-balanced diet with foods from the 4 basic food groups and the importance of sunlight exposure. See Appendix J for foods high in vitamin D.
- Patients self-medicating with vitamin supplements should be cautioned not to exceed RDA. The effectiveness of megadoses for treatment of various medical conditions is unproved and may cause side effects.
- Instruct patient to notify health care professional of all Rx or OTC medications, vitamins, or herbal products being taken and to consult health care professional before taking other Rx, OTC, or herbal products.
- Advise patient to avoid concurrent use of antacids containing magnesium.
- Review symptoms of overdose and instruct patient to report these promptly to health care professional.
- Emphasize the importance of follow-up exams to evaluate progress.
- **Calcifediol:** Advise patient to notify health care professional if signs and symptoms of hypercalcemia occur.
- Emphasize importance of routine lab tests.
- Rep: Advise patient to notify health care professional if pregnancy is planned or suspected or if breastfeeding. Monitor infants exposed to calcifediol through breast milk for signs and symptoms of hypercalcemia, including seizures, vomiting, constipa-

tion and weight loss. Consider monitoring of serum calcium in the infant.

Evaluation/Desired Outcomes

- Normalization of serum calcium and parathyroid hormone levels.
- Resolution or prevention of vitamin D deficiency.
- Improvement in symptoms of vitamin D–resistant rickets.
- **Calcifediol:** Serum total hydroxyvitamin D levels between 30 and 100 ng/mL, iPTH levels within therapeutic range, serum calcium (corrected for low albumin) within normal range and serum phosphorus <5.5 mg/dL.

📑 voriconazole (vor-i-kon-a-zole)
Vfend
Classification
Therapeutic: antifungals
Pharmacologic: azoles

Indications

Invasive aspergillosis. Candidemia (in patients without neutropenia) and serious *Candida* infections in skin, bladder, abdomen, kidney, and wounds. Esophageal candidiasis. Scedosporiosis and fusariosis in patients intolerant of or refractory to other therapies.

Action

Inhibits fungal ergosterol synthesis leading to production of abnormal fungal plasma membrane. **Therapeutic Effects:** Antifungal activity. **Spectrum:** Spectrum is notable for activity against: *Aspergillus* spp., *Candida* spp., *Scedosporium apiospermum, Fusarium* spp.

Pharmacokinetics

Absorption: 96% absorbed following oral administration; IV administration results in complete bioavailability.

Distribution: Widely distributed to tissues.

Metabolism and Excretion: Primarily metabolized by liver via the CYP2C19, CYP2C9, and CYP3A4 isoenzymes; <2% excreted unchanged in urine. 📑 The CYP2C19 isoenzyme exhibits genetic polymorphism; 15–20% of Asian patients and 3–5% of Caucasian and Black patients may be poor metabolizers and may have significantly ↑ voriconazole concentrations and an ↑ risk of adverse effects.

Half-life: Dose-dependent (adults: 6–9 hr); ↑ in hepatic impairment.

TIME/ACTION PROFILE (plasma concentrations)

ROUTE	ONSET	PEAK	DURATION
PO	rapid	1–2 hr	12 hr
IV	rapid	end of infusion	12 hr

Contraindications/Precautions

Contraindicated in: Concurrent use of dihydroergotamine, carbamazepine, efavirenz (≥400 mg/day), ergotamine, ivabradine, lurasidone, naloxegol, phenobarbital, pimozide, rifabutin, rifampin, ritonavir (400 mg every 12 hr), quinidine, sirolimus, St. John's wort, tolvaptan, and venetoclax; Tablets contain lactose and should be avoided in patients with galactose intolerance, Lapp lactase deficiency, or glucose-galactose malabsorption; Severe hepatic impairment; OB: Pregnancy.

Use Cautiously in: Mild to moderate hepatic impairment (↓ IV and PO maintenance doses); Renal impairment (CCr <50 mL/min) (Vehicle in IV formulation can accumulate resulting in toxicity; avoid use of IV unless potential benefit greatly outweighs potential risk, use oral form only); Congenital/acquired QT interval prolongation, HF, sinus bradycardia, hypokalemia, hypomagnesemia, or symptomatic arrhythmias; Hematologic malignancy (↑ risk of hepatotoxicity); Rep: Women of reproductive potential; Lactation: Use while breastfeeding only if potential maternal benefit justifies potential risk to infant; Pedi: Children <2 yr (safety and effectiveness not established); suspension contains benzyl alcohol, which may cause potentially fatal "gasping syndrome" in neonates; ↑ risk of photosensitivity reactions in children.

Adverse Reactions/Side Effects

CV: changes in BP, peripheral edema, QT interval prolongation, tachycardia. **Derm:** DRUG REACTION WITH EOSINOPHILIA AND SYSTEMIC SYMPTOMS (DRESS), MELANOMA, photosensitivity, rash, SQUAMOUS CELL CARCINOMA, STEVENS-JOHNSON SYNDROME (SJS), TOXIC EPIDERMAL NECROLYSIS. **EENT:** visual disturbances, eye hemorrhage. **Endo:** ADRENAL INSUFFICIENCY. **F and E:** hyperglycemia, hypokalemia, hypomagnesemia. **GI:** abdominal pain, diarrhea, HEPATOTOXICITY, nausea, pancreatitis, vomiting. **MS:** fluorosis, periostitis. **Neuro:** dizziness, hallucinations, headache. **Misc:** chills, fever, infusion reactions.

Interactions

Drug-Drug: **Carbamazepine, phenobarbital,** and **rifampin** may significantly ↓ levels and effectiveness; concurrent use contraindicated. May significantly ↑ levels of **ivabradine, pimozide,** and **quinidine,** which can ↑ the risk of QT interval prolongation and torsades de pointes; concurrent use contraindicated. May significantly ↑ levels and risk of toxicity of **dihydroergotamine, ergotamine, lurasidone, sirolimus,** and **tolvaptan;** concurrent use contraindicated. May ↑ levels of **naloxegol,** which could precipitate symptoms of opioid withdrawal; concurrent use contraindicated. Concurrent use with **efavirenz** at doses of ≥400 mg every 24 hr is contraindicated, since it may significantly ↑ efavirenz levels and significantly ↓ voriconazole levels; if used together, ↑ oral maintenance dose of vori-

V

---

conazole to 400 mg every 12 hr and ↓ dose of efavirenz to 300 mg daily. Concurrent use with **ritonavir** at dose of 400 mg every 12 hr is contraindicated, since ritonavir may significantly ↓ voriconazole levels; use with ritonavir at dose of 100 mg every 12 hr; should also be avoided, if possible. Concurrent use with **rifabutin** may significantly ↑ rifabutin levels and significantly ↓ voriconazole levels; if used together, ↑ oral maintenance dose of voriconazole to 400 mg every 12 hr and ↓ dose of efavirenz to 300 mg daily. Concurrent use with **venetoclax** at initiation and during ramp-up phase in patients with chronic lymphocytic leukemia or small lymphocytic leukemia is contraindicated because may ↑ risk of tumor lysis syndrome. **Fluconazole** may ↑ levels and the risk of toxicity; avoid concurrent use. May ↑ levels and the risk of toxicity of **cyclosporine**; ↓ cyclosporine dose by 50%. May ↑ levels and the risk of toxicity of **tacrolimus**; ↓ tacrolimus dose to ⅓ of the starting dose. May ↑ levels and the risk of toxicity of **glasdegib**; avoid concurrent use. May ↑ levels and the risk of toxicity of tyrosine kinase inhibitors, including **axitinib**, **bosutinib**, **cabozantinib**, **ceritinib**, **cobimetinib**, **dabrafenib**, **dasatinib**, **ibrutinib**, **nilotinib**, **ribociclib**, and **sunitinib**; if concurrent use cannot be avoided, ↓ dose of tyrosine kinase inhibitor. May ↑ levels and the risk of toxicity of **eszopiclone**; ↓ dose of eszopiclone. May ↑ levels and the risk of toxicity of **tretinoin**; closely monitor patient for signs/symptoms of pseudotumor cerebri or hypercalcemia. May ↑ levels and the risk of toxicity of **HMG-CoA reductase inhibitors**, some **benzodiazepines** (**alprazolam**, **midazolam**, **triazolam**), **fentanyl**, **oxycodone**, **NSAIDs** (**ibuprofen**, **diclofenac**), some **calcium channel blockers**, **sulfonylureas** (**glipizide**, **glyburide**), **phenytoin**, **warfarin**, and **vinca alkaloids** (**vincristine**, **vinblastine**); dose ↓ may be needed and careful monitoring required during concurrent use. May ↑ **methadone** levels and ↑ risk of QT interval prolongation. May ↑ levels of **corticosteroids** and ↑ risk of adrenal suppression. May ↑ levels and the risk of toxicity of **ivacaftor**; ↓ ivacaftor dose. Concurrent use with **hormonal contraceptives** containing **ethinyl estradiol** and **norethindrone** may ↑ voriconazole, ethinyl estradiol, and norethindrone levels. May ↑ levels and the risk of toxicity of **everolimus**; concurrent use not recommended. May ↑ levels and the risk of toxicity of **omeprazole**; if patient receiving ≥40 mg/day of omeprazole, ↓ omeprazole dose by 50%. Similar effects may occur with other **proton-pump inhibitors**. May ↑ levels and the risk of toxicity of **protease-inhibitors** and **non-nucleoside reverse transcriptase inhibitors**; frequent monitoring recommended. **Non-nucleoside reverse transcriptase inhibitors** may induce or inhibit the metabolism of voriconazole; frequent monitoring recommended. **Letermovir** may ↓ levels and effectiveness; avoid concurrent use. Use with **methotrexate** may ↑ risk of photosensitivity reactions.

Drug-Natural Products: St. John's wort may significantly ↓ levels and effectiveness; concurrent use contraindicated.

Route/Dosage

Invasive Aspergillosis, Scedosporiosis, or Fusariosis

IV, PO (Adults ≥40 kg): *Loading dose (IV):* 6 mg/kg IV every 12 hr for 2 doses, followed by *maintenance dose (IV)* of 4 mg/kg IV every 12 hr (use 5 mg/kg IV every 12 hr if concurrently using with phenytoin). Continue IV therapy for ≥7 days, then switch to oral maintenance dose once patient has clinically improved and can tolerate oral medications. *Maintenance dose (PO):* 200 mg PO every 12 hr (use 400 mg PO every 12 hr if concurrently using with phenytoin or efavirenz); if response inadequate, may ↑ to 300 mg every 12 hr. Total duration of therapy: ≥6–12 wk.

IV, PO (Adults <40 kg): *Loading dose (IV):* 6 mg/kg IV every 12 hr for 2 doses, followed by *maintenance dose (IV)* of 4 mg/kg IV every 12 hr (use 5 mg/kg IV every 12 hr if concurrently using with phenytoin). Continue IV therapy for ≥7 days, then switch to oral maintenance dose once patient has clinically improved and can tolerate oral medications. *Maintenance dose (PO):* 100 mg PO every 12 hr (use 200 mg PO every 12 hr if concurrently using with phenytoin; use 400 mg PO every 12 hr if concurrently using with efavirenz); if response inadequate, may ↑ to 150 mg every 12 hr. Total duration of therapy: ≥6–12 wk.

IV, PO (Children ≥15 yr): *Loading dose (IV):* 6 mg/kg IV every 12 hr for 2 doses, followed by *maintenance dose (IV)* of 4 mg/kg IV every 12 hr. Continue IV therapy for ≥7 days, then switch to oral maintenance dose once patient has clinically improved and can tolerate oral medications. *Maintenance dose (PO):* 200 mg every 12 hr; if response inadequate, may ↑ to 300 mg every 12 hr. Total duration of therapy: ≥6–12 wk.

IV, PO (Children 12–14 yr and ≥50 kg): *Loading dose (IV):* 6 mg/kg IV every 12 hr for 2 doses, followed by *maintenance dose (IV)* of 4 mg/kg IV every 12 hr. Continue IV therapy for ≥7 days, then switch to oral maintenance dose once patient has clinically improved and can tolerate oral medications. *Maintenance dose (PO):* 200 mg every 12 hr; if response inadequate, may ↑ to 300 mg every 12 hr. Total duration of therapy: ≥6–12 wk.

IV, PO (Children 12–14 yr and <50 kg): *Loading dose (IV):* 9 mg/kg IV every 12 hr for 2 doses, followed by *maintenance dose (IV)* of 8 mg/kg IV every 12 hr; if response inadequate, may ↑ maintenance dose by 1 mg/kg. Continue IV therapy for ≥7 days, then switch to oral maintenance dose once patient has clinically improved and can tolerate oral medications. *Maintenance dose (PO):* 9 mg/kg every 12 hr (not to exceed 350 mg every 12 hr); if response inadequate, may ↑ by 1 mg/kg or 50 mg (not to exceed 350 mg every 12 hr). Total duration of therapy: ≥6–12 wk.

IV, PO (Children 2–11 yr): *Loading dose (IV):* 9 mg/kg IV every 12 hr for 2 doses, followed by *mainte-*

nance dose (IV) of 8 mg/kg IV every 12 hr; if response inadequate, may ↑ maintenance dose by 1 mg/kg. Continue IV therapy for ≥7 days, then switch to oral maintenance dose once patient has clinically improved and can tolerate oral medications. *Maintenance dose (PO):* 9 mg/kg every 12 hr (not to exceed 350 mg every 12 hr); if response inadequate, may ↑ by 1 mg/kg or 50 mg (not to exceed 350 mg every 12 hr). Total duration of therapy: ≥6–12 wk.

Hepatic Impairment
IV, PO (Adults): *Mild or moderate hepatic impairment:* Use standard IV loading dose, ↓ maintenance doses (IV or PO) by 50%; *Severe hepatic impairment:* Not recommended.

Candidemia in Non-Neutropenic Patients or Other Deep Tissue *Candida* Infections
IV, PO (Adults ≥40 kg): *Loading dose (IV):* 6 mg/kg IV every 12 hr for 2 doses, followed by *maintenance dose (IV)* of 3–4 mg/kg IV every 12 hr (use 5 mg/kg IV every 12 hr if concurrently using with phenytoin). Switch to oral dosing once patient has clinically improved and can tolerate oral medications. *Maintenance dose (PO):* 200 mg PO every 12 hr (use 400 mg PO every 12 hr if concurrently using with phenytoin or efavirenz); if response inadequate, may ↑ to 300 mg every 12 hr. Total duration of therapy: ≥14 days following resolution of symptoms or following last positive culture, whichever is longer.

IV, PO (Adults <40 kg): *Loading dose (IV):* 6 mg/kg IV every 12 hr for 2 doses, followed by *maintenance dose (IV)* of 3–4 mg/kg IV every 12 hr (use 5 mg/kg IV every 12 hr if concurrently using with phenytoin). Switch to oral dosing once patient has clinically improved and can tolerate oral medications. *Maintenance dose (PO):* 100 mg PO every 12 hr (use 200 mg PO every 12 hr if concurrently using with phenytoin; use 400 mg PO every 12 hr if using concurrently with efavirenz); if response inadequate, may ↑ to 150 mg every 12 hr. Total duration of therapy: ≥14 days following resolution of symptoms or following last positive culture, whichever is longer.

IV, PO (Children ≥15 yr): *Loading dose (IV):* 6 mg/kg IV every 12 hr for 2 doses, followed by *maintenance dose (IV)* of 3–4 mg/kg IV every 12 hr. Switch to oral dosing once patient has clinically improved and can tolerate oral medications. *Maintenance dose (PO):* 200 mg every 12 hr; if response inadequate, may ↑ to 300 mg every 12 hr. Total duration of therapy: ≥14 days following resolution of symptoms or following last positive culture, whichever is longer.

IV, PO (Children 12–14 yr and ≥50 kg): *Loading dose (IV):* 6 mg/kg IV every 12 hr for 2 doses, followed by *maintenance dose (IV)* of 3–4 mg/kg IV every 12 hr. Switch to oral dosing once patient has clinically improved and can tolerate oral medications. *Maintenance dose (PO):* 200 mg every 12 hr; if response in-

adequate, may ↑ to 300 mg every 12 hr. Total duration of therapy: ≥14 days following resolution of symptoms or following last positive culture, whichever is longer.

IV, PO (Children 12–14 yr and <50 kg): *Loading dose (IV):* 9 mg/kg IV every 12 hr for 2 doses, followed by *maintenance dose (IV)* of 8 mg/kg IV every 12 hr; if response inadequate, may ↑ maintenance dose by 1 mg/kg. Switch to oral dosing once patient has clinically improved and can tolerate oral medications. *Maintenance dose (PO):* 9 mg/kg every 12 hr (not to exceed 350 mg every 12 hr); if response inadequate, may ↑ by 1 mg/kg or 50 mg (not to exceed 350 mg every 12 hr). Total duration of therapy: ≥14 days following resolution of symptoms or following last positive culture, whichever is longer.

IV, PO (Children 2–11 yr): *Loading dose (IV):* 9 mg/kg IV every 12 hr for 2 doses, followed by *maintenance dose (IV)* of 8 mg/kg IV every 12 hr; if response inadequate, may ↑ maintenance dose by 1 mg/kg. Switch to oral dosing once patient has clinically improved and can tolerate oral medications. *Maintenance dose (PO):* 9 mg/kg every 12 hr (not to exceed 350 mg every 12 hr); if response inadequate, may ↑ by 1 mg/kg or 50 mg (not to exceed 350 mg every 12 hr). Total duration of therapy: ≥14 days following resolution of symptoms or following last positive culture, whichever is longer.

Hepatic Impairment
IV, PO (Adults): *Mild or moderate hepatic impairment:* Use standard IV loading dose, ↓ maintenance doses (IV or PO) by 50%; *Severe hepatic impairment:* Not recommended.

Esophageal Candidiasis
PO (Adults ≥40 kg): 200 mg every 12 hr (use 400 mg every 12 hr if concurrently using with phenytoin or efavirenz); if response inadequate, may ↑ to 300 mg every 12 hr. Duration of therapy: ≥14 days and for ≥7 days following resolution of symptoms.

PO (Adults <40 kg): 100 mg every 12 hr (use 200 mg every 12 hr if concurrently using with phenytoin; use 400 mg every 12 hr if using concurrently with efavirenz); if response inadequate, may ↑ to 150 mg every 12 hr. Duration of therapy: ≥14 days and for ≥7 days following resolution of symptoms.

PO (Children ≥15 yr): 200 mg every 12 hr; if response inadequate, may ↑ to 300 mg every 12 hr. Duration of therapy: ≥14 days and for ≥7 days following resolution of symptoms.

PO (Children 12–14 yr and ≥50 kg): 200 mg every 12 hr; if response inadequate, may ↑ to 300 mg every 12 hr. Duration of therapy: ≥14 days and for ≥7 days following resolution of symptoms.

IV, PO (Children 12–14 yr and <50 kg): Initiate therapy with *maintenance dose (IV)* of 4 mg/kg IV every 12 hr; if response inadequate, may ↑ maintenance dose by 1 mg/kg. Switch to oral dosing once pa-

V

tient has clinically improved and can tolerate oral medications. *Maintenance dose (PO):* 9 mg/kg every 12 hr (not to exceed 350 mg every 12 hr); if response inadequate, may ↑ by 1 mg/kg or 50 mg (not to exceed 350 mg every 12 hr). Total duration of therapy: ≥14 days and for ≥7 days following resolution of symptoms.
IV, PO (Children 2–11 yr): Initiate therapy with *maintenance dose (IV)* of 4 mg/kg IV every 12 hr; if response inadequate, may ↑ maintenance dose by 1 mg/kg. Switch to oral dosing once patient has clinically improved and can tolerate oral medications. *Maintenance dose (PO):* 9 mg/kg every 12 hr (not to exceed 350 mg every 12 hr); if response inadequate, may ↑ by 1 mg/kg or 50 mg (not to exceed 350 mg every 12 hr). Total duration of therapy: ≥14 days and for ≥7 days following resolution of symptoms.

Hepatic Impairment
IV, PO (Adults): *Mild or moderate hepatic impairment:* Use standard IV loading dose, ↓ maintenance doses (IV or PO) by 50%; *Severe hepatic impairment:* Not recommended.

Availability (generic available)
Tablets: 50 mg, 200 mg. **Oral suspension (orange flavor):** 40 mg/mL. **Powder for injection:** 200 mg/vial.

NURSING IMPLICATIONS
Assessment
- Monitor for signs and symptoms of fungal infections prior to and during therapy.
- Obtain specimens for culture and histopathology prior to therapy to isolate and identify organism. Therapy may be started before results are received.
- Monitor visual function including visual acuity, visual field, and color perception in patients receiving more than 28 days of therapy. Vision usually returns to normal within 14 days after discontinuation of therapy.
- Monitor for allergic reactions during infusion of voriconazole (flushing, fever, sweating, tachycardia, chest tightness, dyspnea, faintness, nausea, pruritus, rash). Symptoms occur immediately upon start of infusion. May require discontinuation.
- Monitor patients with risk factors for acute pancreatitis (recent chemotherapy, hematopoietic stem cell transplantation) for the signs of pancreatitis (abdominal pain, ↑ serum amylase and lipase).
- Assess for rash periodically during therapy. May cause SJS. Discontinue therapy if severe or if accompanied with fever, general malaise, fatigue, muscle or joint aches, blisters, oral lesions, conjunctivitis, hepatitis and/or eosinophilia.

Lab Test Considerations
- Monitor liver function tests (AST, ALT, and bilirubin) prior to, weekly during first mo and monthly during therapy. If abnormal liver function tests occur, monitor for development of severe hepatic injury. Discontinue therapy if markedly ↑ or clinical signs and symptoms of liver disease develop.
- Monitor renal function (serum creatinine) during therapy.

Implementation
- Once patient can tolerate oral medication, PO voriconazole may be used.
- Correct electrolyte disturbances (hypokalemia, hypomagnesemia, hypocalcemia) prior to initiation and during therapy.
- **PO:** Administer at least 1 hr before or 1 hr after a meal.
- Shake suspension well (approximately 10 sec) before measuring suspension. Use oral dispenser provided to ensure accurate dose. Do not mix suspension with other medicine, flavored liquid, or syrup. Store suspension at room temperature up to 14 days, then discard.

IV Administration
- Do not administer voriconazole with blood products or concentrated electrolytes, even in separate lines. Non-concentrated electrolytes can be infused at same time, but separate lines must be used. TPN can be administered simultaneously but must be via separate line or via a different port in a multi-lumen catheter.
- **Intermittent Infusion:** *Reconstitution:* Reconstitute each 200-mg vial with 19 mL of sterile water for injection to achieve concentration of 10 mg/mL. Calculate volume of 10 mg/mL solution required for patient dose. *Dilution:* Withdraw and discard equal volume of diluent from infusion bag or bottle to be used. Withdraw required volume of voriconazole solution from vial(s) and add to appropriate volume of 0.9% NaCl, LR, D5/LR, D5/0.45% NaCl, D5W, 0.45% NaCl, or D5/0.9% NaCl. Reconstituted solution stable for 24 hr if refrigerated. Discard partially used vials. *Concentration:* Final concentration of infusion should be 0.5–5 mg/mL. *Rate:* Infuse over 1–3 hr at a rate not to exceed 3 mg/kg/hr.
- **Y-Site Compatibility:** acyclovir, alemtuzumab, allopurinol, amifostine, amikacin, aminocaproic acid, aminophylline, amiodarone, amphotericin B liposomal, ampicillin, ampicillin/sulbactam, anidulafungin, argatroban, arsenic trioxide, azithromycin, aztreonam, bivalirudin, bleomycin, buprenorphine, butorphanol, bumetanide, calcium acetate, calcium chloride, calcium gluconate, cangrelor, carboplatin, carmustine, caspofungin, cefazolin, cefotaxime, cefotetan, cefoxitin, ceftaroline, ceftazidime, ceftriaxone, chloramphenicol, chlorpromazine, ciprofloxacin, cisatracurium, cisplatin, clindamycin, cyclophosphamide, cytarabine, dacarbazine, dactinomycin, daptomycin, daunorubicin hydrochloride, dexamethasone, dexmedetomidine, dexrazoxane, digoxin, diltiazem, diphenhydramine, dobutamine, docetaxel, dopamine, doxycycline, droperidol, enalaprilat, ephedrine, epinephrine, epirubicin,

ertapenem, erythromycin, esmolol, etoposide, etoposide phosphate, famotidine, fentanyl, fluconazole,
fludarabine, fluorouracil, foscarnet, fosphenytoin,
furosemide, ganciclovir, gemcitabine, gentamicin,
glycopyrrolate, granisetron, haloperidol, heparin,
hydralazine, hydrocortisone, ifosfamide, imipenem/
cilastatin, insulin regular, irinotecan, isoproterenol,
ketorolac, labetalol, leucovorin calcium, levofloxacin, lidocaine, linezolid, lorazepam, magnesium sulfate, mannitol, melphalan, meperidine, meropenem,
mesna, methadone, methohexital, methotrexate,
methylprednisolone, metoclopramide, metoprolol,
metronidazole, midazolam, milrinone, mitomycin,
morphine, mycophenolate, nafcillin, nalbuphine,
naloxone, nicardipine, nitroglycerin, norepinephrine, octreotide, ondansetron, oxaliplatin, oxytocin,
paclitaxel, pamidronate, pentamidine, pentobarbital,
phenobarbital, phenylephrine, piperacillin/tazobac-
tam, potassium acetate, potassium chloride, potassium phosphate, procainamide, promethazine, propranolol, remifentanil, rocuronium, sodium acetate,
sodium bicarbonate, sodium phosphate, succinylcholine, sufentanil, tacrolimus, theophylline, thiotepa, tirofiban, tobramycin, topotecan, trimetho-
prim/sulfamethoxazole, vancomycin, vasopressin,
vecuronium, verapamil, vinblastine, vincristine, vinorelbine, zidovudine, zoledronic acid.
- **Y-Site Incompatibility:** amphotericin B deoxycholate, amphotericin B lipid complex, busulfan, cefepime, cyclosporine, dantrolene, diazepam, doxorubicin hydrochloride, gemtuzumab ozogamicin,
idarubicin, mitoxantrone, moxifloxacin, nitroprusside, pantoprazole, phenytoin, thiopental.

Patient/Family Teaching
- Advise patient to take voriconazole as directed, on
an empty stomach. Advise patient to read *Patient Information* before starting voriconazole and with
each Rx refill in case of changes.
- May cause blurred vision, photophobia, and dizziness. Caution patient to avoid driving and other activities requiring alertness until response to medication is known. Also advise patient to avoid driving at
night during voriconazole therapy.
- Advise patient to avoid direct sunlight, sunlamps and
tanning beds during voriconazole therapy. Use sunscreen and protective clothing to prevent severe sunburn. Advise patient to have dermatologic evaluation
on a regular basis to allow early detection and management of premalignant lesions; squamous cell carcinoma of the skin and melanoma have been reported during long-term therapy.
- Instruct patient to notify health care professional of
all Rx or OTC medications, vitamins, or herbal products being taken and consult health care professional before taking any new medications.

- Advise patient to notify health care professional if
rash or signs and symptoms of allergic reaction occur.
- Rep: May cause fetal harm. Advise females of reproductive potential to use effective contraception and
notify health care professional if pregnancy is
planned or suspected, or if breastfeeding. Monitor
for adverse reactions if voriconazole is administered
concurrently with oral contraceptives. If pregnancy
is detected, discontinue medication as soon as possible.

Evaluation/Desired Outcomes
- Resolution of fungal infections.

voxelotor (vox-el-oh-tor)
Oxbryta
Classification
Therapeutic: none assigned
Pharmacologic: hemoglobin S polymerization
inhibitors

Indications
Sickle cell disease.

Action
Binds to hemoglobin S (HgbS) (sickle hemoglobin)
and improves affinity of HgbS for oxygen. Through this
increased affinity, it inhibits polymerization of HgbS,
which inhibits sickling of red blood cells, improves de-
formability of red blood cells, and reduces viscosity of
whole blood. **Therapeutic Effects:** Increase in Hgb of
more than 1 g/dL compared to baseline.

Pharmacokinetics
Absorption: Absorption increased with high-fat,
high-calorie meal.
Distribution: Primarily distributed into red blood
cells.
Protein Binding: 99.8%.
Metabolism and Excretion: Primarily metabolized in liver via the CYP3A4 isoenzyme, with minor metabolism by the CYP2C19, CYP2B6, and CYP2C9 isoenzymes; also undergoes glucuronidation. Primarily
excreted in feces (33% as unchanged drug), with 35%
excreted in urine (mostly as metabolites).
Half-life: 35.5 hr.

TIME/ACTION PROFILE (whole blood concentrations)

ROUTE	ONSET	PEAK	DURATION
PO	unknown	6–18 hr	unknown

Contraindications/Precautions
Contraindicated in: Serious hypersensitivity; Lactation: Lactation.

�= Canadian drug name. ⚇ = Genetic implication. ~~Strikethrough~~ = Discontinued. CAPITALS = life-threatening. <u>Underline</u> = most frequent.

Use Cautiously in: Severe hepatic impairment (↓ dose); OB: Use during pregnancy only if potential maternal benefit justifies potential fetal risk; Pedi: Children <4 yr (safety and effectiveness not established).

Adverse Reactions/Side Effects

Derm: rash, DRUG REACTION WITH EOSINOPHILIA AND SYSTEMIC SYMPTOMS (DRESS). **GI:** abdominal pain, diarrhea, nausea. **Neuro:** fatigue, headache. **Misc:** fever, hypersensitivity reactions.

Interactions

Drug-Drug: **Strong CYP3A4 inducers**, including **rifampin**, or **moderate CYP3A4 inducers**, including **efavirenz**, may ↓ levels and effectiveness; avoid concurrent use. If concurrent use unavoidable, ↑ voxelotor dosage. May ↑ levels and the risk of toxicity of **CYP3A4 substrates** with narrow therapeutic index, including **midazolam**; avoid concurrent use. If concurrent use unavoidable, ↓ CYP3A4 substrate.

Route/Dosage

PO (Adults and Children ≥12 yr): 1500 mg once daily. *Concurrent use of strong CYP3A4 inducers:* 2500 mg once daily. *Concurrent use of moderate CYP3A4 inducers:* 2000 mg once daily.
PO (Children 4–<12 yr and ≥40 kg): 1500 mg once daily. *Concurrent use of strong CYP3A4 inducers:* 2500 mg (five 500-mg tablets) once daily *or* 2400 mg (eight 300-mg oral tablets for suspension) once daily. *Concurrent use of moderate CYP3A4 inducers:* 2000 mg (four 500-mg tablets) once daily *or* 2100 mg (seven 300-mg oral tablets for suspension) once daily.
PO (Children 4–<12 yr and 20–<40 kg): 900 mg once daily. *Concurrent use of strong CYP3A4 inducers:* 1500 mg once daily. *Concurrent use of moderate CYP3A4 inducers:* 1200 mg once daily.
PO (Children 4–<12 yr and 10–<20 kg): 600 mg once daily. *Concurrent use of strong or moderate CYP3A4 inducers:* 900 mg once daily.

Hepatic Impairment
PO (Adults and Children ≥12 yr): *Severe hepatic impairment:* 1000 mg once daily.

Hepatic Impairment
PO (Children 4–<12 yr and ≥40 kg): *Severe hepatic impairment:* 1000 mg (two 500-mg tablets) once daily *or* 900 mg (three 300-mg oral tablets for suspension) once daily.

Hepatic Impairment
PO (Children 4–<12 yr and 20–<40 kg): *Severe hepatic impairment:* 600 mg once daily.

Hepatic Impairment
PO (Children 4–<12 yr and 10–<20 kg): *Severe hepatic impairment:* 300 mg once daily.

Availability

Tablets: 300 mg, 500 mg. **Tablets for oral suspension (grape flavor):** 300 mg.

NURSING IMPLICATIONS

Assessment

- Monitor for signs and symptoms of hypersensitivity reaction (rash, urticaria, mild shortness of breath, mild facial swelling, eosinophilia) during therapy. If symptoms occur, treat symptoms and discontinue therapy; do not restart therapy.
- Monitor for DRESS (a combination of skin rash, fever, peripheral eosinophilia, and internal systemic organ involvement [hepatic, renal, pulmonary]). If signs occur, discontinue voxelotor and do not reinitiate.

Lab Test Considerations
- May interfere with measurement of Hgb subtypes (HgbA, HgbS, and HgbF) by high-performance liquid chromatography. If precise quantitation of Hgb species is required, perform chromatography when the patient is not receiving voxelotor therapy.

Implementation

- **PO:** Administer once daily without regard to food. *DNC:* Swallow tablets whole; do not cut, crush, or chew.
- Disperse tablets for oral suspension immediately before administration in a cup and in room-temperature clear liquid (drinking water, clear soda, apple juice, clear electrolyte drinks, clear flavored drinks, clear sports drinks) before swallowing. *DNC:* Do not swallow whole, cut, crush, or chew the tablets for oral suspension. After tablets start to disintegrate, swirl contents of cup until tablets are dispersed, wait 1 to 5 min, swirl contents of cup again, and then orally administer contents of cup. Tablet(s) will not completely dissolve; small tablet clumps remain in the mixture. Resuspend any residue left in cup in more clear drink and administer. Repeat until no tablet residue is left in the cup. May be substituted for tablets in adults and pediatric patients >12 yr with difficulty swallowing tablets.

Patient/Family Teaching

- Instruct patient to take as directed. If a dose is missed, omit and continue with dosing on the next day. Advise patient to read *Patient Information* before starting therapy and with each Rx refill in case of changes.
- Advise patient to notify health care professional if signs and symptoms of hypersensitivity reactions (rash, hives, shortness of breath, swelling of face) occur.
- Advise patient to notify health care professional of all Rx or OTC medications, vitamins, or herbal products being taken and to consult with health care professional before taking other medications.
- Rep: Advise females of reproductive potential to notify health care professional if pregnancy is planned or suspected and to avoid breastfeeding during and for at least 2 wk after last dose.

Evaluation/Desired Outcomes

- Increase in Hgb of more than 1 g/dL compared to baseline.

BEERS HIGH ALERT

⊠ **warfarin** (war-fa-rin)
~~Coumadin~~, Jantoven
Classification
Therapeutic: anticoagulants
Pharmacologic: coumarins

Indications

Prophylaxis and treatment of: Venous thrombosis, Pulmonary embolism, Atrial fibrillation with embolization. Management of MI. Prevention of thrombus formation and embolization after prosthetic valve placement.

Action

Interferes with hepatic synthesis of vitamin K–dependent clotting factors (II, VII, IX, and X). **Therapeutic Effects:** Prevention of thromboembolic events.

Pharmacokinetics

Absorption: Well absorbed from the GI tract after oral administration.
Distribution: Minimally distributed to tissues.
Protein Binding: 99%.
Metabolism and Excretion: Primarily metabolized by the liver via the CYP2C9 isoenzyme, with some metabolism via the CYP3A4 isoenzyme; ⊠ the CYP2C9 isoenzyme exhibits genetic polymorphism (intermediate or poor metabolizers may have significantly ↑ (S)-warfarin concentrations and an ↑ risk of adverse reactions).
Half-life: 42 hr.

TIME/ACTION PROFILE (effects on coagulation tests)

ROUTE	ONSET	PEAK	DURATION
PO	36–72 hr	5–7 days†	2–5 days‡

†At a constant dose
‡After discontinuation

Contraindications/Precautions

Contraindicated in: Uncontrolled bleeding; Open wounds; Active ulcer disease; Recent brain, eye, or spinal cord injury or surgery; Severe hepatic impairment; Uncontrolled hypertension; OB: Pregnancy.
Use Cautiously in: Malignancy; History of ulcer, liver disease, or acute kidney injury; History of poor compliance; ⊠ Asian patients or those who carry the CYP2C9*2 allele and/or the CYP2C9*3 allele, or with the VKORC1 AA genotype (↑ risk of bleeding with standard dosing; lower initial doses should be considered); Rep: Women of reproductive potential; Pedi: Has been used safely in children, but may require more frequent PT/INR assessments; Geri: Appears on Beers list. ↑ risk of major bleeding when compared to direct acting oral anticoagulants (DOACs) in older adults. Avoid starting as initial therapy for treatment of nonvalvular atrial fibrillation or venous thromboembolism unless alternative

options (DOACs) are contraindicated or there are significant barriers to their use. If already using warfarin, it may be reasonable to continue treatment, especially if INR is well controlled (i.e., >70% time in therapeutic range) and no adverse effects.

Adverse Reactions/Side Effects

Derm: dermal necrosis. **GI:** cramps, nausea. **GU:** CALCIPHYLAXIS. **Hemat:** BLEEDING. **Misc:** fever.

Interactions

Drug-Drug: Androgens, **capecitabine, cefotetan, chloramphenicol, clopidogrel, disulfiram, fluconazole, fluoroquinolones, itraconazole, metronidazole** (including vaginal use), **thrombolytics, eptifibatide, tirofiban, sulfonamides, quinidine, quinine, NSAIDs, valproates,** and **aspirin** may ↑ the response to warfarin and ↑ the risk of bleeding. Chronic use of **acetaminophen** may ↑ the risk of bleeding. Chronic **alcohol** ingestion may ↓ action of warfarin; if chronic **alcohol** abuse results in significant liver damage, action of warfarin may be ↑ due to ↓ production of clotting factor. Acute **alcohol** ingestion may ↑ action of warfarin. **Barbiturates, carbamazepine, rifampin,** and **hormonal contraceptives containing estrogen** may ↓ the anticoagulant response to warfarin. **Many other drugs** may affect the activity of warfarin.
Drug-Natural Products: St. John's wort ↓ effect. ↑ bleeding risk with **anise, arnica, chamomile, clove, dong quai, fenugreek, feverfew, garlic, ginger, ginkgo, Panax ginseng, licorice,** and others.
Drug-Food: Ingestion of large quantities of **foods high in vitamin K content** (see list in Appendix J) may antagonize the anticoagulant effect of warfarin.

Route/Dosage

⊠ **PO (Adults):** 2–5 mg/day for 2–4 days; then adjust daily dose by results of INR. Initiate therapy with lower doses in older adults or in Asian patients or those with CYP2C9*2 and/or CYP2C9*3 alleles or VKORC1 AA genotype.
PO (Children >1 mo): *Initial loading dose:* 0.2 mg/kg (maximum dose: 10 mg) for 2–4 days then adjust daily dose by results of INR, use 0.1 mg/kg if hepatic impairment is present. *Maintenance dose range:* 0.05–0.34 mg/kg/day.

Availability (generic available)

Tablets: 1 mg, 2 mg, 2.5 mg, 3 mg, 4 mg, 5 mg, 6 mg, 7.5 mg, 10 mg.

NURSING IMPLICATIONS

Assessment

● Assess for signs of bleeding and hemorrhage (bleeding gums; nosebleed; unusual bruising; tarry, black stools; hematuria; fall in hematocrit or BP; guaiac-positive stools, urine, or nasogastric aspirate).

W

- Assess for evidence of additional or increased thrombosis. Symptoms depend on area of involvement.

Lab Test Considerations
- Monitor PT, INR, and other clotting factors frequently during therapy; monitor more frequently in patients with renal impairment. Therapeutic PT ranges 1.3–1.5 times greater than control; however, the INR, a standardized system that provides a common basis for communicating and interpreting PT results, is usually referenced. Normal INR (not on anticoagulants) is 0.8–1.2. An INR of 2.5–3.5 is recommended for patients at very high risk of embolization (for example, patients with mitral valve replacement and ventricular hypertrophy). Lower levels are acceptable when risk is lower. Heparin may affect the PT/INR; draw blood for PT/INR in patients receiving both heparin and warfarin at least 5 hr after the IV bolus dose, 4 hr after cessation of IV infusion, or 24 hr after SUBQ heparin injection. ✖ Asian patients and those who carry the CYP2C9*2 allele and/or the CYP2C9*3 allele, or those with VKORC1 AA genotype may require more frequent monitoring and lower doses.
- Geri: Patients over 60 yr exhibit greater than expected PT/INR response. Monitor for side effects at lower therapeutic ranges.
- Pedi: Achieving and maintaining therapeutic PT/INR ranges may be more difficult in pediatric patients. Assess PT/INR levels more frequently.
- Monitor hepatic function and CBC before and periodically throughout therapy.
- Monitor stool and urine for occult blood before and periodically during therapy.

Toxicity and Overdose
- Withholding 1 or more doses of warfarin is usually sufficient if INR is excessively elevated or if minor bleeding occurs. If overdose occurs or anticoagulation needs to be immediately reversed, the antidote is vitamin K (phytonadione). Administration of whole blood or plasma also may be required in severe bleeding because of the delayed onset of vitamin K.

Implementation
- **High Alert:** Do not confuse Jantoven with Janumet or Januvia .
- Because of the large number of medications capable of significantly altering warfarin's effects, careful monitoring is recommended when new agents are started or other agents are discontinued. Interactive potential should be evaluated for all new medications (Rx, OTC, and herbal products).
- **PO:** Administer medication at same time each day. Medication requires 3–5 days to reach effective levels; usually begun while patient is still on heparin.

- Do not interchange brands; potencies may not be equivalent.

Patient/Family Teaching
- Instruct patient to take medication as directed. Take missed doses as soon as remembered that day; do not double doses. Inform health care professional of missed doses at time of checkup or lab tests. Inform patients that anticoagulant effect may persist for 2–5 days following discontinuation. Advise patient to read *Medication Guide* before starting therapy and with each Rx refill in case of changes.
- Review foods high in vitamin K (see Appendix J). Patient should have consistent limited intake of these foods, as vitamin K is the antidote for warfarin, and alternating intake of these foods will cause PT levels to fluctuate. Advise patient to avoid cranberry juice or products during therapy.
- Caution patient to avoid IM injections and activities leading to injury. Instruct patient to use a soft toothbrush, not to floss, and to shave with an electric razor during warfarin therapy. Advise patient that venipunctures and injection sites require application of pressure to prevent bleeding or hematoma formation.
- Advise patient to report any symptoms of unusual bleeding or bruising (bleeding gums; nosebleed; black, tarry stools; hematuria; excessive menstrual flow) and pain, color, or temperature change to any area of your body to health care professional immediately. ✖ Patients with a deficiency in protein C and/or S mediated anticoagulant response may be at greater risk for tissue necrosis.
- Instruct patient not to drink alcohol or take other Rx, OTC, or herbal products, especially those containing aspirin or NSAIDs, or to start or stop any new medications during warfarin therapy without advice of health care professional.
- Rep: May cause fetal harm. Advise females of reproductive potential to use effective contraception during and for 1 month after last dose. Advise patient to notify health care professional if pregnancy is planned or suspected or if breastfeeding.
- Instruct patient to carry identification describing medication regimen at all times and to inform all health care personnel caring for patient on anticoagulant therapy before lab tests, treatment, or surgery.
- Emphasize the importance of frequent lab tests to monitor coagulation factors.

Evaluation/Desired Outcomes
- Prolonged PT (1.3–2.0 times the control; may vary with indication) or INR of 2–4.5 without signs of hemorrhage.

zaleplon (za-lep-lon)
~~Sonata~~
Classification
Therapeutic: sedative/hypnotics

Schedule IV

Indications
Short-term management of insomnia in patients unable to get ≥4 hr of sleep; especially useful in sleep initiation disorders.

Action
Produces CNS depression by binding to GABA receptors in the CNS. Has no analgesic properties. **Therapeutic Effects:** Induction of sleep.

Pharmacokinetics
Absorption: Rapidly absorbed following oral administration.
Distribution: Well distributed to tissues.
Metabolism and Excretion: Extensively metabolized in the liver (mostly by aldehyde oxidase and some by the CYP3A4 isoenzyme).
Half-life: 1 hr.

TIME/ACTION PROFILE

ROUTE	ONSET	PEAK	DURATION
PO	within min	unknown	3–4 hr

Contraindications/Precautions
Contraindicated in: Hypersensitivity; History of experiencing complex sleep behaviors with zaleplon; Severe hepatic impairment; OB: Pregnancy; Lactation: Lactation.

Use Cautiously in: Mild or moderate hepatic impairment or weight ≤50 kg (initiate therapy at lowest dose); Impaired respiratory function; History of suicide attempt; Pedi: Safety and effectiveness not established in children; Geri: Appears on Beers list. ↑ risk of cognitive impairment, delirium, falls, fractures, and motor vehicle accidents in older adults. Avoid use in older adults.

Adverse Reactions/Side Effects
CV: peripheral edema. **Derm:** photosensitivity. **EENT:** abnormal vision, altered sense of smell, ear pain, epistaxis, hearing sensitivity, ocular pain. **GI:** abdominal pain, anorexia, colitis, dyspepsia, nausea. **GU:** dysmenorrhea. **Neuro:** abnormal thinking, amnesia, anxiety, behavior changes, COMPLEX SLEEP BEHAVIORS (including sleep driving, sleep walking, or engaging in other activities while sleeping), depersonalization, dizziness, drowsiness, hallucinations, headache, hyperesthesia, impaired memory (briefly following dose), impaired psychomotor function (briefly following dose), malaise, nightmares, paresthesia, tremor, vertigo, weakness. **Misc:** fever.

Interactions
Drug-Drug: **Cimetidine** may ↑ levels and the risk of toxicity; initiate therapy at a lower dose. Additive CNS depression with other **CNS depressants**, including **alcohol, antihistamines, opioid analgesics**, other **sedative/hypnotics, phenothiazines**, and **tricyclic antidepressants**. CYP3A4 inducers, including **rifampin, phenytoin, carbamazepine**, and **phenobarbital**, may ↓ levels and effectiveness.
Drug-Natural Products: Concomitant use of **kava-kava, valerian, chamomile**, or **hops** can ↑ CNS depression.
Drug-Food: Concurrent ingestion of a **high-fat meal** slows the rate of absorption.

Route/Dosage
PO (Adults <65 yr): 10 mg (range 5–20 mg) at bedtime.

Hepatic Impairment
PO (Adults): Initiate therapy at 5 mg at bedtime (not to exceed 10 mg at bedtime).

Availability (generic available)
Capsules: 5 mg, 10 mg.

NURSING IMPLICATIONS
Assessment
● Assess mental status, sleep patterns, and potential for abuse prior to administering this medication. Zaleplon is used to treat short-term difficulty in falling asleep; decreases time to sleep onset. May not increase total sleep time or decrease number of wakenings after falling asleep. Prolonged use of >7–10 days may lead to physical and psychological dependence. Limit amount of drug available to the patient.
● Assess alertness at time of peak effect. Notify health care professional if desired sedation does not occur.
● Assess patient for pain. Medicate as needed. Untreated pain decreases sedative effects.

Implementation
● Do not confuse Sonata with Soriatane.
● Before administering, reduce external stimuli and provide comfort measures to increase effectiveness of medication.
● Protect patient from injury. Supervise ambulation and transfer of patients after administration. Remove cigarettes. Side rails should be raised and call bell within reach at all times.
● PO: *DNC:* Tablets should be swallowed whole with full glass of water immediately before bedtime or after going to bed and experiencing difficulty falling asleep. Do not administer with or immediately after a high-fat or heavy meal.

Patient/Family Teaching
● Instruct patient to take zaleplon as directed. Do not take more than the amount prescribed because of

Z

the habit-forming potential. Not recommended for use longer than 7–10 days. Rebound insomnia (1–2 nights) may occur when stopped. If used for 2 wk or longer, abrupt withdrawal may result in dysphoria, insomnia, abdominal or muscle cramps, vomiting, sweating, tremors, and seizures.

- Because of rapid onset, advise patient to go to bed immediately after taking zaleplon.
- May cause daytime drowsiness or dizziness. Advise patient to avoid driving or other activities requiring alertness until response to this medication is known.
- Inform patient that amnesia may occur, but can be avoided if zaleplon is only taken when patient is able to get >4 hr sleep.
- Caution patient that complex sleep-related behaviors (sleep-driving, making phone calls, preparing and eating food, having sex, sleep walking) may occur while asleep. Inform patient to notify health care professional if sleep-related behaviors (may include sleep-driving—driving while not fully awake after ingestion of a sedative-hypnotic product, with no memory of the event) occur.
- Caution patient to avoid concurrent use of alcohol or other CNS depressants, including opioids.
- Rep: May cause fetal harm. Use is not recommended during pregnancy or breastfeeding. Advise females of reproductive potential to notify health care professional if pregnancy is planned or suspected, or if breastfeeding.

Evaluation/Desired Outcomes
- Improved ability to fall asleep; decreased time to sleep onset.

---

zavegepant (za-ve-je-pant)
Zavzpret
Classification
Therapeutic: vascular headache suppressants
Pharmacologic: calcitonin gene-related peptide receptor antagonists

Indications
Acute treatment of migraine with or without aura.

Action
Binds to and inhibits the calcitonin gene-related peptide (CGRP) receptor, which reduces the neuroinflammatory and vasodilatory effects of CGRP. **Therapeutic Effects:** Reduction in pain and other bothersome symptoms associated with migraine.

Pharmacokinetics
Absorption: 5% absorbed following intranasal administration.
Distribution: Extensively distributed to tissues.
Protein Binding: 90%.
Metabolism and Excretion: Primarily metabolized in liver via the CYP3A4 isoenzyme, and to a lesser extent by the CYP2D6 isoenzyme. Primarily excreted as unchanged drug in feces (80%) and urine (11%).

Half-life: 6.55 hr.

TIME/ACTION PROFILE (relief of migraine pain)

ROUTE	ONSET	PEAK	DURATION
IN	0.5 hr	2 hr	up to 48 hr

Contraindications/Precautions
Contraindicated in: Hypersensitivity; Severe hepatic impairment; Severe renal impairment (CCr <30 mL/min).
Use Cautiously in: OB: Safety not established in pregnancy; Lactation: Safety not established in breastfeeding; Pedi: Safety and effectiveness not established in children.

Adverse Reactions/Side Effects
EENT: nasal discomfort. **GI:** taste disorders, nausea, vomiting. **Misc:** hypersensitivity reactions.

Interactions
Drug-Drug: **Organic anion transporting polypeptide 1B3 (OATP1B3) inhibitors** or **sodium taurocholate co-transporting polypeptide (NTCP) transporter inhibitors,** including **rifampin** may ↑ levels and risk of toxicity; avoid concurrent use. **Organic anion transporting polypeptide 1B3 (OATP1B3) inducers** or **sodium taurocholate co-transporting polypeptide (NTCP) transporter inducers** may ↓ levels and effectiveness; avoid concurrent use. **Intranasal decongestants** may ↓ absorption of zavegepant; avoid concurrent use. If concurrent use unavoidable, administer intranasal decongestant ≥1 hr after zavegepant.

Route/Dosage
Intranasal (Adults): Single dose of 10 mg in one nostril.

Availability
Nasal spray: 10 mg/spray.

NURSING IMPLICATIONS
Assessment
- Assess pain location, character, intensity, duration, and associated symptoms (photophobia, phonophobia, nausea, vomiting) of migraine pain.
- Monitor frequency of migraine headaches.
- Monitor for signs and symptoms of hypersensitivity reactions (anaphylaxis, dyspnea, rash, pruritus, urticaria, facial edema). If a hypersensitivity reaction occurs, discontinue zavegepant and begin therapy as needed.

Implementation
- **Intranasal:** Administer a single 10 mg spray in one nostril, as needed. Do not administer more than one spray in each 24 hr period.

Patient/Family Teaching
- Instruct patient to administer zavegepant as directed. Do not test or prime the nasal spray before use. Ad-

vise patient to read the *Patient Information* before starting therapy and with each Rx refill in case of changes.
- Advise patient to avoid using intranasal decongestants with zavegepant; may decrease the absorption of zavegepant. If concurrent use is unavoidable, administer intranasal decongestants at least 1 hr after zavegepant administration.
- Advise patient to notify health care professional immediately if signs or symptoms of hypersensitivity reactions (shortness of breath, rash, swelling of the face, mouth, tongue, or throat) occur.
- Advise patient to notify health care professional of all Rx or OTC medications, vitamins, or herbal products being taken and to consult with health care professional before taking other medications.
- Rep: Advise females of reproductive potential to notify health care professional if pregnancy is planned or suspected or if breastfeeding.

Evaluation/Desired Outcomes
- Decrease in pain and symptoms associated with migraine headaches.

zidovudine (zye-**doe**-vue-deen)
Retrovir
Classification
Therapeutic: antiretrovirals
Pharmacologic: nucleoside reverse transcriptase inhibitors

Indications
HIV infection (in combination with other antiretrovirals). Reduction of maternal/fetal transmission of HIV. **Unlabeled Use:** Chemoprophylaxis after occupational exposure to HIV.

Action
Following intracellular conversion to its active form, inhibits viral RNA synthesis by inhibiting the enzyme DNA polymerase (reverse transcriptase). Prevents viral replication. **Therapeutic Effects:** Virustatic action against selected retroviruses. Slowed progression and decreased sequelae of HIV infection. Decreased viral load and improved CD4 cell counts. Decreased transmission of HIV to infants born to HIV-infected mothers.

Pharmacokinetics
Absorption: Well absorbed following oral administration.
Distribution: Widely distributed; enters the CNS.
Metabolism and Excretion: Mostly (75%) metabolized by the liver; 15–20% excreted unchanged by the kidneys.
Half-life: 1 hr.

TIME/ACTION PROFILE (plasma concentrations)

ROUTE	ONSET	PEAK	DURATION
PO	unknown	0.5–1.5 hr	4 hr
IV	rapid	end of infusion	4 hr

Contraindications/Precautions
Contraindicated in: Hypersensitivity; Lactation: Breastfeeding not recommended in mothers with HIV. **Use Cautiously in:** ↓ bone marrow reserve (dose ↓ required for anemia or granulocytopenia); Women and obese patients (↑ risk of lactic acidosis and severe hepatomegaly); Severe renal impairment; Severe hepatic impairment; Latex allergy (IV only); Geri: Select dose carefully due to potential for age-related ↓ in hepatic, renal, or cardiac function in older adults.

Adverse Reactions/Side Effects
Derm: nail pigmentation. **Endo:** gynecomastia. **F and E:** LACTIC ACIDOSIS. **GI:** abdominal pain, diarrhea, nausea, anorexia, dyspepsia, HEPATOMEGALY (with steatosis), oral mucosa pigmentation, PANCREATITIS, vomiting. **Hemat:** anemia, granulocytopenia, pure red-cell aplasia, thrombocytosis. **Metab:** lipoatrophy. **MS:** back pain, myopathy. **Neuro:** headache, weakness, ↓ mental acuity, anxiety, confusion, depression, dizziness, insomnia, restlessness, SEIZURES, syncope, tremor. **Misc:** immune reconstitution syndrome.

Interactions
Drug-Drug: ↑ bone marrow depression with other **agents having bone marrow–depressing properties, antineoplastics, radiation therapy,** or **ganciclovir.** ↑ neurotoxicity may occur with **acyclovir.** Toxicity may be ↑ by concurrent administration of **probenecid** or **fluconazole.** Levels are ↓ by **clarithromycin.**

Route/Dosage
HIV Infection
PO (Adults): 100 mg every 4 hr while awake or 200 mg 3 times daily or 300 mg twice daily (depends on combination and clinical situation).
PO (Children 4 wk–<18 yr): *4–8.9 kg:* 12 mg/kg twice daily or 8 mg/kg 3 times daily; *9–29.9 kg:* 9 mg/kg twice daily or 6 mg/kg 3 times daily; ≥*30 kg:* 300 mg twice daily or 200 mg 3 times daily.
IV (Adults and Children >12 yr): 1 mg/kg every 4 hr. Change to oral therapy as soon as possible.
IV (Children): 120 mg/m² every 6 hr (not to exceed 160 mg/dose) or 20 mg/m²/hr as a continuous infusion.

Prevention of Maternal/Fetal Transmission of HIV Infection
PO (Adults >14 wk Pregnant): 100 mg 5 times daily until onset of labor.

Z

IV (Adults during Labor and Delivery): 2 mg/kg over 1 hr, then continuous infusion of 1 mg/kg/hr until umbilical cord is clamped.

PO (Neonates): 2 mg/kg every 6 hr until 6 wk of age.

IV (Neonates): 1.5 mg/kg every 6 hr until 6 wk of age.

Availability (generic available)

Tablets: 300 mg. **Capsules:** 100 mg. **Oral solution:** 50 mg/5 mL. **Solution for injection:** 10 mg/mL. *In combination with:* lamivudine (Combivir); abacavir and lamivudine; see Appendix N.

NURSING IMPLICATIONS

Assessment

- Assess patient for change in severity of symptoms of HIV and for symptoms of opportunistic infections during therapy.

Lab Test Considerations

- Monitor viral load and CD4 counts prior to and periodically during therapy.
- Monitor CBC every 2 wk during the first 8 wk of therapy in patients with advanced HIV disease, and decrease to every 4 wk after the first 2 mo if zidovudine is well tolerated or monthly during the first 3 mo and every 3 mo thereafter unless indicated in patients who are asymptomatic or have early symptoms. Commonly causes granulocytopenia and anemia. Anemia may occur 2–4 wk after initiation of therapy. Anemia may respond to epoetin administration (see epoetin monograph). Granulocytopenia usually occurs after 6–8 wk of therapy. Consider dose reduction, discontinuation of therapy, or blood transfusions if hemoglobin <7.5 g/dL or reduction of >25% from baseline and/or granulocyte count <750/mm³ or reduction of >50% from baseline. Therapy may be gradually resumed when bone marrow recovery is evident.
- May cause ↑ serum AST, ALT, and alkaline phosphatase levels. Lactic acidosis may occur with hepatic toxicity, causing hepatic steatosis; may be fatal, especially in women.
- Monitor serum amylase, lipase, and triglycerides periodically during therapy. Elevated serum levels may indicate pancreatitis and require discontinuation.

Implementation

- Do not confuse Retrovir (zidovudine) with ritonavir.
- **PO:** Administer doses around the clock.
- For neonates, use a syringe with 0.1-mL graduations to ensure accurate dosing of the oral solution.
- **IV:** Patient should receive the IV infusion only until oral therapy can be administered.

IV Administration

- **Intermittent Infusion:** *Retrovir* vial stoppers contain latex; may cause allergic reactions in latex-sensitive individuals. *Dilution:* Remove calculated dose from the vial and dilute with D5W or 0.9% NaCl. Do not use solutions that are discolored. Stable for 24 hr at room temperature or 48 hr if refrigerated. *Concentration:* Not to exceed 4 mg/mL. *Rate:* Infuse at a constant rate over 1 hr in adults or over 30 min in neonates. Avoid rapid infusion or bolus injection.

- **Continuous Infusion:** Has also been administered via continuous infusion.

- **Y-Site Compatibility:** acyclovir, alemtuzumab, allopurinol, amifostine, amikacin, aminocaproic acid, amiodarone, amphotericin B deoxycholate, amphotericin B lipid complex, amphotericin B liposomal, anidulafungin, argatroban, arsenic trioxide, azithromycin, aztreonam, bivalirudin, bleomycin, carboplatin, carmustine, caspofungin, cefepime, ceftazidime, ceftriaxone, cisatracurium, cisplatin, clindamycin, cyclophosphamide, cytarabine, dacarbazine, dactinomycin, daptomycin, daunorubicin hydrochloride, dexamethasone, dexmedetomidine, diltiazem, dobutamine, docetaxel, dopamine, doxorubicin hydrochloride, doxorubicin liposomal, epirubicin, eptifibatide, ertapenem, erythromycin, etoposide, etoposide phosphate, filgrastim, fluconazole, fludarabine, fluorouracil, foscarnet, fosphenytoin, gemcitabine, gentamicin, granisetron, heparin, hetastarch, hydromorphone, idarubicin, ifosfamide, imipenem/cilastatin, irinotecan, leucovorin calcium, levofloxacin, linezolid, lorazepam, melphalan, meperidine, meropenem, mesna, methadone, methotrexate, metoclopramide, metronidazole, milrinone, mitomycin, mitoxantrone, morphine, mycophenolate, nafcillin, nicardipine, octreotide, ondansetron, oxacillin, oxaliplatin, oxytocin, paclitaxel, palonosetron, pamidronate, pantoprazole, pemetrexed, pentamidine, phenylephrine, piperacillin/tazobactam, potassium acetate, potassium chloride, remifentanil, rituximab, rocuronium, sargramostim, sodium acetate, tacrolimus, thiotepa, tigecycline, tirofiban, tobramycin, topotecan, trastuzumab, trimethoprim/sulfamethoxazole, vancomycin, vasopressin, vecuronium, vinblastine, vincristine, vinorelbine, voriconazole, zoledronic acid.

- **Y-Site Incompatibility:** dexrazoxane, gemtuzumab ozogamicin.

Patient/Family Teaching

- Instruct patient to take zidovudine as directed, around the clock, even if sleep is interrupted. Emphasize the importance of compliance with therapy, not taking more than prescribed amount, and not discontinuing without consulting health care professional. Take missed doses as soon as remembered unless almost time for next dose; do not double doses. Inform patient that long-term effects of zidovudine are unknown at this time.
- Instruct patient that zidovudine should not be shared with others.
- Zidovudine may cause dizziness or fainting. Caution patient to avoid driving or other activities requiring alertness until response to medication is known.
- Inform patient that zidovudine does not cure HIV and may reduce the risk of transmission of HIV to

others through sexual contact or blood contamination. Caution patient to use a condom during sexual contact and avoid sharing needles or donating blood to prevent spreading the AIDS virus to others.

- Instruct patient to notify health care professional promptly if signs of pancreatitis (nausea, vomiting, abdominal pain), lactic acidosis (feel very weak or tired; feel cold, especially in arms and legs; unusual muscle pain; feel dizzy or lightheaded; trouble breathing; fast or irregular heartbeat; stomach pain with nausea and vomiting), liver problems (yellowing of skin or white part of eyes; loss of appetite; nausea; dark or "tea-colored" urine; pain, aching, or tenderness on right side of abdomen; light-colored stools) or immune reconstitution syndrome (signs and symptoms of an infection, *Mycobacterium avium* infection, cytomegalovirus, *Pneumocystis jirovecii* pneumonia, tuberculosis) occur.
- Instruct patient to notify health care professional promptly if fever, sore throat, signs of infection, muscle weakness, or shortness of breath occurs. Caution patient to avoid crowds and persons with known infections. Instruct patient to use soft toothbrush, to use caution when using toothpicks or dental floss, and to have dental work done prior to therapy or deferred until blood counts return to normal.
- Advise patient to notify health care professional of all Rx or OTC medications, vitamins, or herbal products being taken and to consult with health care professional before taking other medications.
- Inform patient that redistribution and accumulation of body fat may occur, causing central obesity, dorsocervical fat enlargement (buffalo hump), peripheral wasting, breast enlargement, and cushingoid appearance. The cause and long-term effects are not known.
- Rep: Advise females of reproductive potential to notify health care professional if pregnancy is planned or suspected and avoid breastfeeding. Advise patient taking oral contraceptives to use a nonhormonal method of birth control during therapy. Inform patient of pregnancy exposure registry that monitors pregnancy outcomes in women exposed to zidovudine during pregnancy. Enroll patients in the Antiretroviral Pregnancy Registry by calling 1-800-258-4263.
- Emphasize the importance of regular follow-up exams and blood counts to determine progress and monitor for side effects.

Evaluation/Desired Outcomes

- Decrease in viral load and increase in CD4 counts in patients with HIV.
- Delayed progression of AIDS and decreased opportunistic infections in patients with HIV.
- Reduction of maternal/fetal transmission of HIV.

ziprasidone (zi-pra-si-done)
Geodon, ✷Zeldox

Classification
Therapeutic: antipsychotics, mood stabilizers
Pharmacologic: piperazine derivatives

Indications
Schizophrenia; IM form is reserved for control of acutely agitated patients. Acute manic or mixed episodes associated with bipolar I disorder (oral only). Maintenance treatment of bipolar I disorder (as adjunct to lithium or valproate) (oral only).

Action
Effects probably mediated by antagonism of dopamine type 2 (D2) and serotonin type 2 (5-HT$_2$). Also antagonizes α_2 adrenergic receptors. **Therapeutic Effects:** Diminished schizophrenic behavior. Reduced symptoms of mania.

Pharmacokinetics
Absorption: 60% absorbed following oral administration; 100% absorbed from IM sites.
Distribution: Well distributed to tissues.
Protein Binding: 99%.
Metabolism and Excretion: 99% metabolized by the liver; <1% excreted unchanged in urine.
Half-life: *PO:* 7 hr; *IM:* 2–5 hr.

TIME/ACTION PROFILE (plasma concentrations)

ROUTE	ONSET	PEAK	DURATION
PO	within hrs	1–3 days†	unknown
IM	rapid	60 min	unknown

†Steady state achieved following continuous use.

Contraindications/Precautions
Contraindicated in: Hypersensitivity; History of QT interval prolongation (persistent QTc interval >500 msec); arrhythmias, recent MI or uncompensated HF; Concurrent use of other drugs known to prolong the QT interval including quinidine, dofetilide, sotalol, other class Ia and III antiarrhythmics, pimozide, sotalol, thioridazine, chlorpromazine, pentamidine, arsenic trioxide, mefloquine, tacrolimus, droperidol, and moxifloxacin; Hypokalemia or hypomagnesemia.
Use Cautiously in: Concurrent diuretic therapy or diarrhea (may ↑ the risk of hypotension, hypokalemia, or hypomagnesemia); Hepatic impairment; History of cardiovascular or cerebrovascular disease; Hypotension, concurrent antihypertensive therapy, dehydration, or hypovolemia (may ↑ risk of orthostatic hypotension); At risk for aspiration pneumonia or falls; History of suicide attempt; OB: Neonates at ↑ risk for extrapyramidal symptoms and withdrawal after delivery when exposed during the 3rd trimester; use during preg-

Z

nancy only if potential maternal benefit justifies potential fetal risk; Lactation: Use while breastfeeding only if potential maternal benefit justifies potential risk to infant; Pedi: Safety and effectiveness not established in children; Geri: Appears on Beers list. ↑ risk of stroke, cognitive decline, and mortality in older adults with dementia. Avoid use in older adults, except for schizophrenia or bipolar disorder.

Adverse Reactions/Side Effects

CV: orthostatic hypotension, QT interval prolongation. **Derm:** DRUG REACTION WITH EOSINOPHILIA AND SYSTEMIC SYMPTOMS (DRESS), rash, STEVENS-JOHNSON SYNDROME (SJS), urticaria. **EENT:** rhinorrhea. **Endo:** galactorrhea, hyperglycemia. **GI:** constipation, diarrhea, nausea, dysphagia. **GU:** amenorrhea, impotence. **Hemat:** AGRANULOCYTOSIS, leukopenia, neutropenia. **Metab:** hyperlipidemia, weight gain. **Neuro:** dizziness, drowsiness, restlessness, extrapyramidal reactions, NEUROLEPTIC MALIGNANT SYNDROME, seizures, syncope, tardive dyskinesia. **Resp:** cough.

Interactions

Drug-Drug: Concurrent use of **quinidine, dofetilide, other class Ia and III antiarrhythmics, pimozide, sotalol, thioridazine, chlorpromazine, pentamidine, arsenic trioxide, mefloquine, tacrolimus, droperidol, moxifloxacin**, or other agents that prolong the QT interval may result in potentially life-threatening adverse drug reactions; concurrent use contraindicated. Additive CNS depression may occur with **alcohol, antidepressants, antihistamines, opioid analgesics**, or **sedative/hypnotics**. Levels and effectiveness may be ↓ by **carbamazepine**. Levels and effects may be ↑ by **ketoconazole**.

Route/Dosage

Schizophrenia

PO (Adults): 20 mg twice daily initially; dose increments may be made at 2-day intervals up to 80 mg twice daily.
IM (Adults): 10–20 mg as needed up to 40 mg/day; may be given as 10 mg every 2 hr or 20 mg every 4 hr.

Acute Manic or Mixed Episodes Associated with Bipolar I Disorder

PO (Adults): 40 mg twice on first day, then 60 or 80 mg twice daily on 2nd day, then 40–80 mg twice daily.

Maintenance Treatment of Bipolar I Disorder (as adjunct to lithium or valproate)

PO (Adults): Continue same dose on which patient was initially stabilized (range: 40–80 mg twice daily).

Availability (generic available)

Capsules: 20 mg, 40 mg, 60 mg, 80 mg. **Lyophilized powder for injection:** 20 mg/vial.

NURSING IMPLICATIONS

Assessment

- Monitor patient's mental status (orientation, mood, behavior) prior to and periodically during therapy.

- Assess weight and BMI initially and periodically during therapy.
- Monitor BP (sitting, standing, lying) and pulse rate prior to and frequently during initial dose titration. Patients found to have persistent QTc interval measurements of >500 msec should have ziprasidone discontinued. Patients who experience dizziness, palpitations, or syncope may require further evaluation (i.e., Holter monitoring).
- Assess for rash during therapy. May be treated with antihistamines or corticosteroids. Usually resolves upon discontinuation of ziprasidone. Medication should be discontinued if no alternative etiology for rash is found. May cause SJS or DRESS. Discontinue therapy if severe or if accompanied with fever, general malaise, fatigue, muscle or joint aches, blisters, oral lesions, conjunctivitis, hepatitis, and/or eosinophilia.
- Observe carefully when administering medication to ensure medication is actually taken and not hoarded or cheeked.
- Monitor for onset of akathisia (restlessness or desire to keep moving) and extrapyramidal side effects (*parkinsonian*: difficulty speaking or swallowing, loss of balance control, pill rolling of hands, mask-like face, shuffling gait, rigidity, tremors and dystonic muscle spasms, twisting motions, twitching, inability to move eyes, weakness of arms or legs) every 2 mo during therapy and 8–12 wk after therapy has been discontinued. Notify health care professional if these symptoms occur, as reduction in dose or discontinuation of medication may be necessary. Trihexyphenidyl or benztropine may be used to control these symptoms.
- Although not yet reported for ziprasidone, monitor for possible tardive dyskinesia (uncontrolled rhythmic movement of mouth, face, and extremities, lip smacking or puckering, puffing of cheeks, uncontrolled chewing, rapid or worm-like movements of tongue). Report these symptoms immediately; may be irreversible.
- Monitor frequency and consistency of bowel movements. Increasing bulk and fluids in the diet may help to minimize constipation.
- Ziprasidone lowers the seizure threshold. Institute seizure precautions for patients with history of seizure disorder.
- Monitor for development of neuroleptic malignant syndrome (fever, respiratory distress, tachycardia, seizures, diaphoresis, hypertension or hypotension, pallor, tiredness). Notify health care professional immediately if these symptoms occur.
- Monitor for symptoms related to hyperprolactinemia (menstrual abnormalities, galactorrhea, sexual dysfunction).
- Assess for falls risk. Drowsiness, orthostatic hypotension, and motor and sensory instability increase risk. Institute prevention if indicated.

Lab Test Considerations
● Monitor serum potassium and magnesium prior to and periodically during therapy. Patients with low potassium or magnesium should have levels treated and checked prior to resuming therapy. Obtain fasting blood glucose and cholesterol levels initially and periodically during therapy.
● Monitor CBC frequently during initial mo of therapy in patients with pre-existing or history of low WBC. May cause leukopenia, neutropenia, or agranulocytosis. Discontinue therapy if this occurs.
● Monitor serum prolactin prior to and periodically during therapy. May cause ↑ serum prolactin levels.

Implementation
● Dose adjustments should be made at intervals of no less than 2 days. Usually patients should be observed for several wk before dose titration.
● Patients on parenteral therapy should be converted to oral doses as soon as possible.
● **PO:** Administer capsules with food or milk to decrease gastric irritation. *DNC:* Swallow capsules whole; do not open, crush, or chew.
● **IM:** *Reconstitution:* Add 1.2 mL of sterile water for injection to the vial; shake vigorously until all drug is dissolved for a concentration of 20 mg/mL. Discard unused portion. Do not mix with other products or solutions. Do not administer solutions that are discolored or contain particulate matter.

Patient/Family Teaching
● Instruct patient to take medication as directed, at the same time each day. Do not discontinue medication without discussing with health care professional, even if feeling well. Patients on long-term therapy may need to discontinue gradually.
● Inform patient of possibility of extrapyramidal symptoms. Instruct patient to report these symptoms immediately.
● Advise patient to change positions slowly to minimize orthostatic hypotension. Protect from falls.
● May cause seizures and drowsiness. Caution patient to avoid driving or other activities requiring alertness until response to medication is known.
● Advise patient to notify health care professional of all Rx or OTC medications, vitamins, or herbal products being taken and to consult with health care professional before taking other medications. Caution patient to avoid concurrent use of alcohol and other CNS depressants, including opioids.
● Advise patient to notify health care professional of medication regimen prior to treatment or surgery.
● Instruct patient to notify health care professional promptly if dizziness, loss of consciousness, palpitations, menstrual abnormalities, galactorrhea, or sexual dysfunction occur.
● Rep: Advise females of reproductive potential to notify health care professional if pregnancy is planned or suspected, and to avoid breastfeeding during therapy. Monitor neonates exposed to ziprasidone during third trimester for extrapyramidal and/or withdrawal symptoms. Some neonates recovered within hrs or days without specific treatment; others required prolonged hospitalization. Monitor infants exposed through breast milk for excess sedation, irritability, poor feeding, and extrapyramidal symptoms (tremors and abnormal muscle movements). May impair fertility in females. Inform patient of pregnancy exposure registry that monitors pregnancy outcomes in women exposed to atypical antipsychotics. Register patients by contacting the National Pregnancy Registry for Atypical Antipsychotics at 1-866-961-2388 or online at http://womensmentalhealth.org/research/pregnancyregistry/.
● Advise patient of need for continued medical follow-up for psychotherapy, eye exams, and laboratory tests.

Evaluation/Desired Outcomes
● Decrease in acute excited, manic behavior.
● Decrease in positive (delusions, hallucinations) and negative symptoms (social withdrawal, flat, blunted affect) of schizophrenia.
● Management of signs and symptoms of Bipolar I Disorder.

---

zoledronic acid
(zoe-led-**dron**-ic **as**-id)
✤Aclasta, Reclast, ✤Zometa
Classification
Therapeutic: bone resorption inhibitors, electrolyte modifiers, hypocalcemics
Pharmacologic: bisphosphonates

Indications
Hypercalcemia of malignancy. Multiple myeloma and metastatic bone lesions from solid tumors. Paget's disease. Treatment of osteoporosis in men. Treatment and prevention of osteoporosis in postmenopausal women. Treatment and prevention of glucocorticoid-induced osteoporosis in patients expected to be on glucocorticoids for ≥12 mo.

Action
Inhibits bone resorption. Inhibits increased osteoclast activity and skeletal calcium release induced by tumors. **Therapeutic Effects:** Decreased serum calcium. Decreased serum alkaline phosphatase. Decreased fractures, radiation/surgery to bone, or spinal cord compression in patients with multiple myeloma or metastatic bone lesions. Decreased hip, vertebral, or non-vertebral osteoporosis-related fractures in postmenopausal women. Increased bone mass in men, postmenopausal women, and patients on prolonged corticosteroid therapy.

Pharmacokinetics

Absorption: IV administration results in complete bioavailability.

Distribution: Concentrated in and binds to bone.

Metabolism and Excretion: Mostly excreted unchanged by the kidneys.

Half-life: 167 hr.

TIME/ACTION PROFILE (effect on serum calcium)

ROUTE	ONSET	PEAK	DURATION
IV	within 4 days	4–7 days	30 days

Contraindications/Precautions

Contraindicated in: Hypersensitivity to zoledronic acid or other bisphosphonates; Severe renal impairment (CCr <35 mL/min) or acute renal failure; Hypocalcemia (correct before administering); adequate supplemental calcium and vitamin D required; OB: Pregnancy.

Use Cautiously in: History of aspirin-induced asthma; Chronic renal impairment; Chronic renal impairment, concurrent use of diuretics or nephrotoxic drugs, or dehydration (↑ risk of renal impairment; correct deficits prior to use); Concurrent use of nephrotoxic drugs; Invasive dental procedures, cancer, receiving chemotherapy, corticosteroids, or angiogenesis inhibitors, undergoing radiation, poor oral hygiene, periodontal disease, dental disease, anemia, coagulopathy, infection, or poorly fitting dentures (may ↑ risk of osteonecrosis of the jaw [ONJ]); Lactation: Use while breastfeeding only if potential maternal benefit justifies potential risk to infant; Pedi: Potential for long-term retention in bone in children; use in children only if potential benefit outweighs potential risk; Geri: ↑ risk of renal impairment in older adults.

Adverse Reactions/Side Effects

CV: hypotension, chest pain, leg edema. **Derm:** pruritus, rash, STEVENS-JOHNSON SYNDROME, TOXIC EPIDERMAL NECROLYSIS. **EENT:** conjunctivitis. **F and E:** hypophosphatemia, hypocalcemia, hypokalemia, hypomagnesemia. **GI:** abdominal pain, constipation, diarrhea, nausea, vomiting, dysphagia. **GU:** ↓ fertility (females), renal impairment/failure. **Hemat:** anemia. **MS:** musculoskeletal pain, femur fractures, osteonecrosis (primarily ONJ). **Neuro:** agitation, anxiety, confusion, insomnia. **Resp:** asthma exacerbation. **Misc:** fever, flu-like syndrome.

Interactions

Drug-Drug: Concurrent use of **loop diuretics**, **calcitonin**, or **aminoglycosides** ↑ risk of hypocalcemia. Concurrent use of **NSAIDs** may ↑ risk of nephrotoxicity.

Route/Dosage

Paget's Disease

IV (Adults): 5 mg as a single dose (information regarding retreatment unknown).

Treatment of Osteoporosis in Men or Postmenopausal Women or Treatment/Prevention of Glucocorticoid-Induced Osteoporosis

IV (Adults): 5 mg once yearly.

Prevention of Osteoporosis in Postmenopausal Women

IV (Adults): 5 mg every 2 yr.

Hypercalcemia of Malignancy

IV (Adults): 4 mg; may be repeated after 7 days.

Multiple Myeloma or Bone Metastases from Solid Tumors

IV (Adults): 4 mg every 3–4 wk (has been used for up to 15 mo).

Availability (generic available)

Premixed infusion: 4 mg/100 mL, 5 mg/100 mL. **Solution for injection:** 0.8 mg/mL.

NURSING IMPLICATIONS

Assessment

- Monitor intake and output ratios. Initiate a vigorous saline hydration promptly and maintain a urine output of 2 L/day during therapy. Patients should be adequately hydrated, but avoid overhydration. Do not use diuretics prior to treatment of hypovolemia.
- Assess for acute-phase reaction (fever, myalgia, flu-like symptoms, headache, arthralgia). Usually occur within 3 days of dose and resolve within 3 days of onset, but may take 7–14 days to resolve; incidence decreases with repeat dosing.
- Perform a routine oral exam prior to initiation of therapy. Dental exam with appropriate preventative dentistry should be considered prior to therapy. Patients with history of tooth extraction, poor oral hygiene, gingival infections, diabetes, cancer, receiving radiation, anemia, coagulopathy, or use of a dental appliance or those taking immunosuppressive therapy, angiogenesis inhibitors, or systemic corticosteroids are at greater risk for ONJ.
- **Hypercalcemia:** Monitor symptoms of hypercalcemia (nausea, vomiting, anorexia, weakness, constipation, thirst, cardiac arrhythmias).
- Observe for evidence of hypocalcemia (paresthesia, muscle twitching, laryngospasm, Chvostek's or Trousseau's sign).
- **Paget's Disease:** Assess for symptoms of Paget's disease (bone pain, headache, decreased visual and auditory acuity, increased skull size) periodically during therapy.
- **Osteoporosis:** Assess patients via bone density study for low bone mass before and periodically during therapy.

Lab Test Considerations

- Verify negative pregnancy test before starting therapy.
- Monitor CCr, calculated based on actual body weight using the Cockcroft-Gault formula, prior to each treatment. Patients with a normal serum creatinine

prior to treatment, who develop an increase of 0.5 mg/dL within 2 wk of next dose should have next dose withheld until serum creatinine is within 10% of baseline value. Patients with an abnormal serum creatinine prior to treatment who have an increase of 1.0 mg/dL within 2 wk of next dose should have next dose withheld until serum creatinine is within 10% of baseline value.

- Assess serum calcium, phosphate, and magnesium before and periodically during therapy. If hypocalcemia, hypophosphatemia, or hypomagnesemia occur, temporary supplementation may be required. Hypocalcemia and vitamin D deficiency should be treated before initiating zoledronic acid therapy.
- Monitor CBC with differential and hemoglobin and hematocrit closely during therapy.
- *Paget's Disease:* Monitor serum alkaline phosphatase prior to and periodically during therapy to monitor effectiveness.

Implementation

- Vigorous saline hydration alone may be sufficient to treat mild, asymptomatic hypercalcemia. Adequate rehydration is required prior to administration.
- Patients on long-term therapy should have 1200 mg of oral calcium and 800–1000 units of vitamin D each day.
- Patients treated for *Paget's disease* should receive 1500 mg elemental calcium and 800 units of vitamin D daily, particularly during the 2 wk after dosing. Patients with osteoporosis should take 1200 mg of calcium and 800–1000 units of vitamin D daily. Patients with multiple myeloma and bone metastasis of solid tumors take an oral calcium supplement of 500 mg and a multiple vitamin containing 400 international units of vitamin D daily.
- Administration of acetaminophen or ibuprofen following administration may reduce the incidence of acute-phase reaction symptoms.

IV Administration

- **Intermittent Infusion: *Dilution:*** Dilute 4-mg dose further with 100 mL of 0.9% NaCl or D5W. If not used immediately, may be refrigerated for up to 24 hr. *Reclast* comes ready to use 5 mg in 100-mL solution. If refrigerated, allow solution to reach room temperature prior to administration. Do not administer solution that is discolored or contains particulate matter. *Rate:* Administer as a single infusion over at least 15 min. Rapid infusions increase risk of renal deterioration and renal failure.
- **Y-Site Compatibility:** acyclovir, allopurinol, amifostine, amikacin, aminocaproic acid, aminophylline, amiodarone, amphotericin B lipid complex, amphotericin B liposomal, ampicillin, ampicillin/sulbactam, anidulafungin, argatroban, arsenic trioxide, azithromycin, aztreonam, bivalirudin, bleomycin, bumetanide, buprenorphine, busulfan, butor-

phanol, carboplatin, carmustine, caspofungin, cefazolin, cefepime, cefotaxime, cefotetan, cefoxitin, ceftazidime, ceftriaxone, cefuroxime, chloramphenicol, chlorpromazine, ciprofloxacin, cisatracurium, cisplatin, clindamycin, cyclophosphamide, cyclosporine, cytarabine, dacarbazine, dactinomycin, daptomycin, daunorubicin hydrochloride, dexamethasone, dexmedetomidine, dexrazoxane, digoxin, diltiazem, diphenhydramine, dobutamine, docetaxel, dopamine, doxorubicin hydrochloride, doxorubicin liposomal, doxycycline, droperidol, enalaprilat, ephedrine, epinephrine, epirubicin, eptifibatide, ertapenem, erythromycin, esmolol, etoposide, etoposide phosphate, famotidine, fentanyl, fluconazole, fludarabine, fluorouracil, foscarnet, fosphenytoin, furosemide, ganciclovir, gemcitabine, gentamicin, glycopyrrolate, granisetron, haloperidol, heparin, hydralazine, hydrocortisone, hydromorphone, idarubicin, ifosfamide, imipenem/cilastatin, insulin regular, irinotecan, isoproterenol, ketorolac, labetalol, levofloxacin, lidocaine, linezolid, lorazepam, magnesium sulfate, mannitol, melphalan, meperidine, meropenem, mesna, methadone, methotrexate, methylprednisolone, metoclopramide, metoprolol, metronidazole, midazolam, milrinone, mitomycin, mitoxantrone, morphine, moxifloxacin, mycophenolate, nafcillin, nalbuphine, naloxone, nicardipine, nitroglycerin, nitroprusside, norepinephrine, octreotide, ondansetron, oxaliplatin, oxytocin, paclitaxel, pantoprazole, pemetrexed, pentamidine, pentobarbital, phenobarbital, phenylephrine, piperacillin/tazobactam, potassium acetate, potassium chloride, potassium phosphate, procainamide, prochlorperazine, promethazine, propranolol, remifentanil, rocuronium, sodium acetate, sodium bicarbonate, sodium phosphate, succinylcholine, sufentanil, tacrolimus, theophylline, thiopental, thiotepa, tigecycline, tirofiban, tobramycin, topotecan, trimethoprim/sulfamethoxazole, vancomycin, vecuronium, verapamil, vinblastine, vincristine, vinorelbine, voriconazole, zidovudine.
- **Y-Site Incompatibility:** alemtuzumab, calcium-containing solutions, dantrolene, diazepam, gemtuzumab ozogamicin, phenytoin. Manufacturer recommends administration as a single infusion in a line separate from all other drugs.
- **Additive Incompatibility:** Do not mix with solutions containing calcium, such as Lactated Ringer's solution.

Patient/Family Teaching

- Explain the purpose of zoledronic acid to patient. Advise patient to read *Medication Guide* prior to each administration in case of changes.
- Advise patients of the importance of adequate hydration. Patient should be instructed to drink at least two glasses of water prior to receiving dose.

Z

- Advise patient to notify health care professional of all Rx or OTC medications, vitamins, or herbal products being taken and to consult with health care professional before taking other medications.
- Advise patient to eat a balanced diet and consult health care professional about the need for supplemental calcium and vitamin D.
- Inform patient that severe musculoskeletal pain may occur within days, mo, or yr after starting zoledronic acid. Symptoms may resolve completely after discontinuation or slow or incomplete resolution may occur. Notify health care professional if severe pain occurs.
- Encourage patient to participate in regular exercise and to modify behaviors that increase the risk of osteoporosis (stop smoking, reduce alcohol consumption).
- Advise patient to notify health care professional if signs and symptoms of ONJ (pain, numbness, swelling of or drainage from the jaw, mouth, or teeth) or hypocalcemia (spasms, twitches, or cramps in muscles; numbness or tingling in fingers, toes, or around mouth) or thigh, hip, or groin pain occur.
- Advise patient to inform health care professional of zoledronic acid therapy prior to dental surgery.
- Rep: May cause fetal harm. Advise females of reproductive potential to use effective contraception and avoid breastfeeding during and after therapy. May impair fertility in females.
- Emphasize the importance of lab tests to monitor progress.

Evaluation/Desired Outcomes

- Decrease in serum calcium.
- Decrease in serum alkaline phosphatase and the progression of Paget's disease.
- Reversal of the progression of osteoporosis with decreased fractures and other sequelae. Discontinuation after 3–5 yr should be considered for postmenopausal women with low risk for fractures.

ZOLMitriptan (zole-mi-**trip**-tan)
Zomig, ✿ Zomig Rapimelt, ~~Zomig ZMT~~

Classification
Therapeutic: vascular headache suppressants
Pharmacologic: 5-HT₁ agonists

Indications
Acute treatment of migraine headache.

Action
Acts as an agonist at specific 5-HT₁ receptor sites in intracranial blood vessels and sensory trigeminal nerves. **Therapeutic Effects:** Relief of acute attacks of migraine.

Pharmacokinetics
Absorption: Well absorbed (40%) following oral and intranasal administration.

Distribution: Unknown.

Metabolism and Excretion: Mostly metabolized by the liver; some conversion to metabolites that are more active than zolmitriptan. 8% excreted unchanged in urine.

Half-life: 3 hr (for zolmitriptan and active metabolite).

TIME/ACTION PROFILE (relief of headache)

ROUTE	ONSET	PEAK	DURATION
PO	unknown	1.5 hr*	unknown
Intranasal	unknown	3 hr	unknown

*3 hr for orally disintegrating tablets.

Contraindications/Precautions
Contraindicated in: Hypersensitivity; Significant underlying heart disease (including ischemic heart disease, history of MI, coronary artery vasospasm, uncontrolled hypertension); Stroke or transient ischemic attack; Peripheral vascular disease (including, but not limited to ischemic bowel disease); Concurrent (or within 24 hr) use of other 5-HT agonists, ergotamine, or ergot-type medications; Concurrent (or within 2 wk) use of MAO inhibitors; Hemiplegic or basilar migraine; Symptomatic Wolff-Parkinson-White syndrome or other arrhythmias; Moderate to severe hepatic impairment (nasal spray only).

Use Cautiously in: Cardiovascular risk factors (hypertension, hypercholesterolemia, cigarette smoking, obesity, diabetes, strong family history, menopausal females or males >40 yr [use only if cardiovascular status has been evaluated and determined to be safe and 1st dose is administered under supervision]); Hepatic impairment (use lower doses of oral); OB: Safety not established in pregnancy; Lactation: Use while breastfeeding only if potential maternal benefit justifies potential risk to infant; Pedi: Safety and effectiveness not established in children <18 yr (oral); children <12 yr (intranasal).

Adverse Reactions/Side Effects
CV: angina, chest pain/pressure/tightness/heaviness, hypertension, MI, palpitations. **Derm:** sweating, warm/cold sensation. **EENT:** throat pain/tightness/pressure. **GI:** dry mouth, dyspepsia, dysphagia, nausea. **MS:** myalgia, myasthenia. **Neuro:** dizziness, drowsiness, hypesthesia, paresthesia, vertigo, weakness.

Interactions
Drug-Drug: Because of ↑ risk of cerebral vasospasm, avoid concurrent use of other **5-HT agonists** (**naratriptan, sumatriptan, rizatriptan**) and/or **ergot-type preparations** (**dihydroergotamine**). Concurrent use of **MAO inhibitors** ↑ blood levels and risk of toxicity (avoid use within 2 wk of MAO inhibitors). Blood levels may be ↑ by **hormonal contraceptives**. **Cimetidine** ↑ half-life of zolmitriptan and its active metabolite. ↑ risk of serotonin syndrome with **SSRIs**,

SNRIs, TCAs, **triptans, meperidine, bupropion**, or **buspirone**; avoid concurrent use.
Drug-Natural Products: ↑ risk of serotonergic side effects including serotonin syndrome with **St. John's wort** and **SAMe**.

Route/Dosage
PO (Adults): 1.25 – 2.5 mg initially; if headache returns, dose may be repeated after 2 hr (not to exceed 10 mg/24 hr); *Concurrent use of cimetidine:* Single dose not to exceed 2.5 mg (not to exceed 5 mg/24 hr).

Hepatic Impairment
PO (Adults): *Moderate to severe hepatic impairment (oral tablets only):* 1.25 mg initially; if headache returns, dose may be repeated after 2 hr (not to exceed 5 mg/24 hr).
Intranasal (Adults and Children ≥12 yr): Single 2.5 mg initially (maximum single dose = 5 mg); may be repeated after 2 hr (not to exceed 10 mg/24 hr); *Concurrent use of cimetidine:* Single dose not to exceed 2.5 mg (not to exceed 5 mg/24 hr).

Availability (generic available)
Tablets: 2.5 mg, 5 mg. **Orally disintegrating tablets:** 2.5 mg, 5 mg. **Nasal spray:** 2.5 mg/100 mcL unit-dose spray device (package of 6), 5 mg/100 mcL unit-dose spray device (package of 6).

NURSING IMPLICATIONS
Assessment
- Assess pain location, intensity, duration, and associated symptoms (photophobia, phonophobia, nausea, vomiting) during migraine attack.
- Monitor for serotonin syndrome in patients taking SSRIs or SNRIs concurrently with zolmitriptan.

Implementation
- Do not confuse zolmitriptan with sumatriptan.
- **PO:** Initial dose is 2.5 mg. Lower doses can be achieved by breaking 2.5-mg tablet.
- Orally disintegrating tablets should be left in the package until use. Remove from the blister pouch. Do not push tablet through the blister; peel open the blister pack with dry hands and place tablet on tongue. Do not break orally disintegrating tablet. Tablet will dissolve rapidly and be swallowed with saliva. No liquid is needed to take the orally disintegrating tablet.
- **Intranasal:** Remove cap from nasal spray. Hold upright and block one nostril. Tilt head slightly back, insert device into opposite nostril, and depress plunger. May repeat in 2 hr.

Patient/Family Teaching
- Inform patient that zolmitriptan should be used only during a migraine attack. It is meant to be used to relieve migraine attack, not to prevent or reduce the number of attacks.
- Instruct patient to administer zolmitriptan as soon as symptoms appear, but it may be administered any time during an attack. If migraine symptoms return, a 2nd dose may be used. Allow at least 2 hr between doses, and do not use more than 10 mg in any 24-hr period.
- If dose does not relieve headache, additional zolmitriptan doses are not likely to be effective; notify health care professional.
- Advise patient that lying down in a darkened room following zolmitriptan administration may further help relieve headache.
- May cause dizziness or drowsiness. Caution patient to avoid driving or other activities requiring alertness until response to medication is known.
- Advise patient to notify health care professional prior to next dose of zolmitriptan if pain or tightness in the chest occurs during use. If pain is severe or does not subside, notify health care professional immediately. If wheezing; heart throbbing; swelling of eyelids, face, or lips; skin rash; skin lumps; or hives occur, notify health care professional immediately and do not take more zolmitriptan without approval of health care professional. If feelings of tingling, heat, flushing, heaviness, pressure, drowsiness, dizziness, tiredness, or sickness develop, discuss with health care professional at next visit.
- Advise patient to avoid alcohol, which aggravates headaches, during zolmitriptan use.
- Advise patient that overuse (use more than 10 days/mo) may lead to exacerbation of headache (migraine-like daily headaches, or as a marked increase in frequency of migraine attacks). May require gradual withdrawal of zolmitriptan and treatment of symptoms (transient worsening of headache).
- Advise patient to notify health care professional of all Rx or OTC medications, vitamins, or herbal products being taken and to consult with health care professional before taking other medications. Patients concurrently taking SSRI or SNRI antidepressants should notify health care professional promptly if signs of serotonin syndrome (mental status changes: agitation, hallucinations, coma; autonomic instability: tachycardia, labile BP, hyperthermia; neuromuscular aberrations: hyper-reflexia, incoordination; and/or gastrointestinal symptoms: nausea, vomiting, diarrhea) occur.
- Rep: Advise females of reproductive potential to notify health care professional if pregnancy is planned or suspected, or if breastfeeding. Holding breastfeeding for 24 hr after the maternal dose will minimize infant exposure via breast milk.

Evaluation/Desired Outcomes
- Relief of migraine attack.

Z

✱ = Canadian drug name. ▨ = Genetic implication. ~~Strikethrough~~ = Discontinued. CAPITALS = life-threatening. <u>Underline</u> = most frequent.

zolpidem (zole-pi-dem)
Ambien, Ambien CR, Edluar,
✦Sublinox
Classification
Therapeutic: sedative/hypnotics

Schedule IV

Indications
Insomnia with difficulties in sleep initiation (generic sublingual tablets are indicated for insomnia when a middle-of-the-night awakening is followed by difficulty returning to sleep).

Action
Produces CNS depression by binding to GABA receptors. Has no analgesic properties. **Therapeutic Effects:** Sedation and induction of sleep.

Pharmacokinetics
Absorption: Rapidly absorbed following oral administration. Controlled-release formulation releases 10 mg immediately, then another 2.5 mg later.
Distribution: Unknown.
Metabolism and Excretion: Converted to inactive metabolites, which are excreted by the kidneys; clearance of sublingual tablet lower in women than in men.
Half-life: 2.5–3 hr (↑ in older adults and patients with hepatic impairment).

TIME/ACTION PROFILE (sedation)

ROUTE	ONSET	PEAK*	DURATION
PO	rapid	30 min–2 hr	6–8 hr
PO-ER	rapid	2–4 hr	6–8 hr
SL	rapid	unknown	unknown

*Food delays peak levels and effects.

Contraindications/Precautions
Contraindicated in: Hypersensitivity; History of experiencing complex sleep behaviors with zolpidem; Severe hepatic impairment (↑ risk of hepatic encephalopathy).
Use Cautiously in: History of previous psychiatric illness, suicide attempt, drug or alcohol abuse; Mild or moderate hepatic impairment (↑ risk of hepatic encephalopathy; initial dose ↓ recommended); Pulmonary disease; Sleep apnea; Myasthenia gravis; OB: May ↑ risk of respiratory depression in neonates after birth; Lactation: May cause excess sedation in breastfed infants; use while breastfeeding only if potential maternal benefit justifies potential risk in infants; Pedi: Safety and effectiveness not established in children; Geri: Appears on Beers list. ↑ risk of cognitive impairment, delirium, falls, fractures, and motor vehicle accidents in older adults. Avoid use in older adults.

Adverse Reactions/Side Effects
EENT: blurred vision, double vision. **GI:** diarrhea, nausea, vomiting. **Neuro:** daytime drowsiness, dizziness,

abnormal thinking, agitation, amnesia, behavior changes, COMPLEX SLEEP BEHAVIORS (including sleep driving, sleep walking, or engaging in other activities while sleeping), delirium, hallucinations, prolonged reaction time. **Resp:** respiratory depression. **Misc:** HYPERSENSITIVITY REACTIONS (including anaphylaxis), physical dependence, psychological dependence, tolerance.

Interactions
Drug-Drug: CNS and respiratory depression may ↑ with **sedatives/hypnotics**, **alcohol**, **phenothiazines**, **tricyclic antidepressants**, **opioids**, or **antihistamines**. **CYP3A4 inducers**, including **rifampin**, may ↓ levels and effectiveness. **CYP3A4 inhibitors**, including **ketoconazole**, may ↑ levels and the risk of toxicity; consider ↓ zolpidem dose.
Drug-Natural Products: Concomitant use of **kava-kava**, **valerian**, or **chamomile** can ↑ CNS depression. **St. John's wort** may ↓ levels; avoid concurrent use.
Drug-Food: Food ↓ and delays absorption.

Route/Dosage
PO, SL (Adults): *Tablets or SL tablets (Edluar):* 5 mg (for women) and 5–10 mg (for men) at bedtime; may ↑ to 10 mg at bedtime if 5-mg dose not effective; *SL tablets (generic):* 1.75 mg (for women) or 3.5 mg (for men) once upon awakening in the middle of the night; *Extended-release tablets:* 6.25 mg (for women) and 6.25–12.5 mg (for men) at bedtime; may ↑ to 12.5 mg at bedtime if 6.25-mg dose not effective.
PO, SL (Geriatric Patients, Debilitated Patients, or Patients with Mild/Moderate Hepatic Impairment): *Tablets or SL tablets (Edluar):* Do not exceed dose of 5 mg at bedtime; *Extended-release tablets:* Do not exceed dose of 6.25 mg at bedtime.
SL (Geriatric Patients, Patients Taking Concomitant CNS Depressants, or Patients with Mild/Moderate Hepatic Impairment): *SL tablets (generic):* Do not exceed dose of 1.75 mg at bedtime (in either men or women).

Availability (generic available)
Immediate-release tablets: 5 mg, 10 mg. **Immediate-release capsules:** 7.5 mg. **Extended-release tablets:** 6.25 mg, 12.5 mg. **Sublingual tablets (Edluar):** 5 mg, 10 mg. **Sublingual tablets:** 1.75 mg, 3.5 mg.

NURSING IMPLICATIONS
Assessment
- Assess mental status, sleep patterns, and potential for abuse prior to administration. Prolonged use of >7–10 days may lead to physical and psychological dependence. Limit amount of drug available to the patient.
- Assess alertness at time of peak effect. Notify health care professional if desired sedation does not occur.
- Assess patient for pain. Medicate as needed. Untreated pain decreases sedative effects.

- Monitor respiratory drive; increased risk of respiratory depression should be considered before prescribing zolpidem in patients with respiratory impairment, including sleep apnea and myasthenia gravis, or with concomitant opioid use.

Implementation

- **High Alert:** Do not confuse zolpidem with Zyloprim.
- Before administering, reduce external stimuli and provide comfort measures to increase effectiveness of medication.
- Protect patient from injury. Raise bed side rails. Assist with ambulation. Remove patient's cigarettes.
- Use lowest effective dose.
- **PO:** Swallow tablets whole with full glass of water. For faster onset of sleep, do not administer with or immediately after a meal.
- **DNC:** Swallow extended-release tablets whole; do not crush, break, or chew.
- **SL:** To open the blister pack, separate the individual blisters at the perforations. Peel off top layer of paper and push tablet through foil. Place the tablet under the tongue, allow to disintegrate; do not swallow or take with water.
- Only take if at least 4 hr left prior to time to awakening.

Patient/Family Teaching

- Instruct patient to take zolpidem as directed. Take as a single dose and do not readminister during the same night. Advise patient not to take zolpidem unless able to stay in bed a full night (7–8 hr) before being active again. Do not take more than the amount prescribed because of the habit-forming potential. Not recommended for use longer than 7–10 days. If used for 2 wk or longer, abrupt withdrawal may result in fatigue, nausea, flushing, light-headedness, uncontrolled crying, vomiting, GI upset, panic attack, or nervousness. Instruct patient to read *Patient Information* for correct product before taking and with each Rx refill in case of changes.
- Because of rapid onset, advise patient to go to bed immediately after taking zolpidem.
- May cause daytime drowsiness or dizziness. Advise patient to avoid driving or other activities requiring alertness until response to this medication is known.
- Caution patient that complex sleep-related behaviors (sleep-driving) may occur while asleep.
- Advise patient to notify health care professional immediately if signs of anaphylaxis (swelling of the tongue or throat, trouble breathing, and nausea and vomiting) occur.
- Caution patient to avoid concurrent use of alcohol or other CNS depressants, including opioids.
- Rep: Advise females of reproductive potential to notify health care professional if pregnancy is planned or suspected or if breastfeeding. Monitor neonates

exposed to zolpidem during pregnancy and breastfeeding for signs of excess sedation, hypotonia, and respiratory depression.

Evaluation/Desired Outcomes

- Relief of insomnia.
- Re-evaluate insomnia after 7–10 days of therapy.

---

zuranolone (zoo-**ran**-oh-lone)
Zurzuvae
Classification
Therapeutic: antidepressants
Pharmacologic: corticosteroids, gamma aminobutyric acid (GABA) enhancers

Indications
Postpartum depression.

Action
Although not fully understood, thought to be related to positive allosteric modulation of GABA-A receptors. **Therapeutic Effects:** Reduction in depressive symptoms.

Pharmacokinetics
Absorption: Extent of absorption following oral administration unknown. Absorption increased with fat-containing foods.
Distribution: Extensively distributed to tissues.
Metabolism and Excretion: Extensively metabolized in the liver via the CYP3A4 isoenzyme to inactive metabolites. 45% excreted in urine and 41% excreted in feces primarily as metabolites.
Half-life: 19.7–24.6 hr.

TIME/ACTION PROFILE (reduction in depressive symptoms)

ROUTE	ONSET	PEAK	DURATION
PO	3 days	unknown	at least 45 days

Contraindications/Precautions
Contraindicated in: OB: Pregnancy.
Use Cautiously in: Moderate or severe renal impairment; Severe hepatic impairment; Rep: Women of reproductive potential; Lactation: Enters breast milk; use while breastfeeding only if potential maternal benefit justifies potential risk to infant; Pedi: Safety and effectiveness not established in children.

Adverse Reactions/Side Effects
Derm: rash. **EENT:** nasopharyngitis, sinus congestion. **GI:** abdominal pain, diarrhea, dry mouth. **GU:** urinary tract infection. **MS:** muscle twitching, myalgia. **Neuro:** dizziness, sedation, anxiety, confusion, fatigue, gait disturbances, memory impairment, SUICIDAL THOUGHTS/BEHAVIORS, tremor. **Misc:** physical dependence.

Interactions

Drug-Drug: Use with **benzodiazepines** or other **CNS depressants**, including **opioids, non-benzodiazepine sedative/hypnotics, anxiolytics, muscle relaxants**, and **alcohol** may cause profound sedation, loss of consciousness, and/or respiratory depression; avoid concurrent use, if possible; if concurrent use unavoidable, ↓ zuranolone dose. **Strong CYP3A4 inhibitors**, including **itraconazole**, may ↑ levels and risk of toxicity; ↓ zuranolone dose. **Strong CYP3A4 inducers**, including **rifampin**, may ↓ levels and effectiveness; avoid concurrent use.

Route/Dosage

PO (Adults): 50 mg once daily in the evening for 14 days. If patients experience CNS adverse effects within the 14-day period, consider ↓ dose to 40 mg once daily in the evening within the 14-day period. *Concurrent use of strong CYP3A4 inhibitors:* 30 mg once daily in the evening for 14 days.

Renal Impairment

PO (Adults): *eGFR <60 mL/min/1.73 m²:* 30 mg once daily in the evening for 14 days.

Hepatic Impairment

PO (Adults): *Severe hepatic impairment:* 30 mg once daily in the evening for 14 days.

Availability

Capsules: 20 mg, 25 mg, 30 mg.

NURSING IMPLICATIONS

Assessment

● Monitor mood changes. Inform health care professional if patient demonstrates significant increase in anxiety, nervousness, or insomnia.
● Assess for suicidal tendencies, especially in patients ≤24 yr.

Implementation

● Administer once daily in the evening for 14 days with fat-containing food (400 to 1,000 calories, 25% to 50% fat).

Patient/Family Teaching

● Instruct patient to take medication as directed. If an evening dose is missed, take next dose at the regular time the following evening. Do not take extra capsules on the same day to make up for the missed dose. Continue taking zuranolone once daily until remainder of 14-day treatment course is completed.

Advise patient to read Medication Guide before starting zuranolone.
● Inform patients that zuranolone causes driving impairment due to CNS depressant effects. Caution patient to avoid driving and other activities requiring alertness until at least 12 hr after zuranolone administration for the duration of the 14-day treatment course. Inform patients that they may not be able to assess their own driving competence or the degree of driving impairment caused by zuranolone.
● Instruct patient to notify health care professional of all Rx or OTC medications, vitamins, or herbal products being taken and consult health care professional before taking any new medications. Advise patient to avoid taking other CNS depressants, including alcohol, benzodiazepines, opioids, and tricyclic antidepressants; may cause falls, somnolence, cognitive impairment, and the risk of respiratory depression.
● Advise patient, family, and caregivers to look for suicidality, especially during early therapy or dose changes. Notify health care professional immediately if thoughts about suicide or dying, attempts to commit suicide, new or worsening depression or anxiety, agitation or restlessness, panic attacks, insomnia, new or worsening irritability, aggressiveness, acting on dangerous impulses, mania, or other changes in mood or behavior occur.
● Rep: May cause fetal harm. Advise females of reproductive potential to use effective contraception during treatment with zuranolone and for one wk after the final dose. Advise a pregnant woman of the potential risk to an infant exposed to zuranolone in utero. Advise females with reproductive potential to notify health care professional if pregnancy is planned or suspected or if breastfeeding. There is a pregnancy exposure registry that monitors pregnancy outcomes in women exposed to antidepressants, including zuranolone, during pregnancy. Health care professionals are encouraged to register patients by calling the National Pregnancy Registry for Antidepressants at 1-866-961-2388 or visiting online at https://womensmentalhealth.org/research/pregnancyregistry/antidepressants/.

Evaluation/Desired Outcomes

● Increased sense of well-being.
● Renewed interest in surroundings.

Drugs Approved in Canada

These monographs describe medications approved for use in Canada by the Therapeutic Products Directorate, a division of Health Canada's Health Products and Food Branch. The medications are not approved by the United States Food and Drug Administration; however, similar formulations carrying different generic or brand names might be available in the U.S.

alfacalcidol (al-fa-kal-si-dol)

✤One-Alpha

Classification
Therapeutic: vitamins
Pharmacologic: vitamin D analogues

Indications

Management of hypocalcemia, secondary hyperparathyroidism and osteodystrophy associated with chronic renal failure.

Action

Stimulates intestinal absorption of calcium and phosphorus, reabsorption of calcium from bone and renal reabsorption of calcium. Does not require renal activation. **Therapeutic Effects:** Improved calcium and phosphorus homeostasis in patients with chronic kidney disease.

Pharmacokinetics

Absorption: Completely absorbed following oral administration.
Distribution: Unknown.
Protein Binding: Extensively protein bound.
Metabolism and Excretion: Following absorption, 50% is rapidly converted by liver to active metabolite $(1.25-(OH)_2D$; 13% renally excreted.
Half-life: 3 hr.

TIME/ACTION PROFILE (levels of active metabolite)

ROUTE	ONSET†	PEAK	DURATION‡
PO	6 hr	12 hr	few days–1 wk
IV	unknown	4 hr	few days–1 wk

†Effect on intestinal calcium absorption, bone pain and muscle weakness improve within 2 wk–3 mo.
‡Effect on serum calcium levels following discontinuation.

Contraindications/Precautions

Contraindicated in: Concurrent use of other vitamin D analogs or magnesium-containing antacids; Lactation: Avoid breastfeeding.
Use Cautiously in: OB: Potential benefits should be weighed against hazards to fetus and mother; Pedi: Safety and effectiveness not established.

Adverse Reactions/Side Effects

CNS: headache, drowsiness, weakness. **CV:** ARRHYTHMIAS, hypertension. **EENT:** conjunctivitis, photophobia.
GI: constipation, nausea, anorexia, dry mouth, metallic taste, pancreatitis, polydipsia, vomiting. **Derm:** pruritus, rash. **F and E:** HYPERCALCEMIA, hyperphosphatemia, hyperthermia, ↑ thirst. **GU:** albuminuria, hypercalcuria, ↓ libido, nocturia, polyuria. **Metab:** ectopic calcification, hypercholesterolemia, hyperthermia. **MS:** bone pain, muscle pain.

Interactions

Drug-Drug: Hypercalcemia ↑ risk of toxicity from **digoxin**. ↑ risk of toxicity and adverse reactions with concurrent use of other **vitamin D analogs**. Concurrent use of **bile acid sequestrants**, including **cholestyramine**, or **mineral oil** ↓ absorption and effectiveness. Concurrent use of **barbiturates** and other **anticonvulsants** may ↓ effectiveness; larger doses of alfacalcidol may be required.

Route/Dosage

PO (Adults): *Pre-dialysis patients:* 0.25 mcg/day for 2 mo initially; if necessary, dose increments of 0.25 mg/day may be made at 2 mo intervals (usual range 0.5–1.0 mcg/day); *dialysis patients:* 1 mcg/day, if necessary dose increments of 0.5 mcg/day may be made at 2–4 wk intervals (usual range 1–2 mcg/day, up to 3 mcg/day). When normalization occurs, dose should be ↓ to minimum amount required to maintain normal serum calcium levels.
IV (Adults): *Dialysis patients:* 1 mcg during each dialysis session (2–3 times weekly); if necessary, dose may be ↑ weekly by 1 mcg per dialysis session up to 12 mcg/wk (range 1.5–12 mcg/wk). When normalization occurs, dose should be ↓ to minimum amount required to maintain normal serum calcium levels.

Availability

Soft gel capsules: 0.25 mcg, 1 mcg; **Oral drops:** 2 mcg/mL; **Solution for injection (contains ethanol and propylene glycol):** 2 mcg/mL.

NURSING IMPLICATIONS

Assessment

- Assess for signs of vitamin D deficiency prior to and during treatment.
- Assess for bone pain and weakness during therapy; usually decreases within 2 wk to 3 mo.

Lab Test Considerations
- *For pre-dialysis patients:* Monitor serum calcium and phosphate levels monthly and electrolytes peri-

odically during treatment. *For dialysis patients:* Monitor serum calcium at least twice weekly during dose titration. If hypercalcemia occurs decrease dose of alfacalcidol by 50% and stop all calcium supplements until calcium levels return to normal. May cause ↑ plasma phosphorous levels. Maintain serum phosphate levels <2.0 mmol/L. Monitor inorganic phosphorus, magnesium, alkaline phosphatase, creatinine, BUN, 24-hr urinary calcium and protein as needed.

Toxicity and Overdose
- Toxicity is manifested as hypercalcemia, hypercalciuria, and hyperphosphatemia. Assess for appearance of nausea, vomiting, anorexia, weakness, constipation, headache, bone pain, and metallic taste. Later symptoms include polyuria, polydipsia, photophobia, rhinorrhea, pruritus, and cardiac arrhythmias. Notify health care professional immediately if these signs of hypervitaminosis D occur. Treatment usually consists of discontinuation of alfacalcidol, a low-calcium diet, stopping calcium supplements. Persistent or markedly elevated serum calcium levels in hemodialysis patients may be corrected by dialysis against a calcium-free dialysate.

Implementation
- **PO:** Administer with food. Use calibrated dropper with oral for accurate dose. Oral solution may be mixed with water or milk.
- **IV:** Administer IV during hemodialysis. Shake well before use. Keep refrigerated. Single use vials; discard unused portion.

Patient/Family Teaching
- Advise patient to take medication as directed. Do not stop taking without consulting with health care professional.
- Advise patient and family to notify health care professional if signs and symptoms of hypercalcemia occur.
- Review diet modifications with patient. See Appendix J for foods high in calcium and vitamin D. Renal patients must still consider renal failure diet in food selection. Health care professional may order concurrent calcium supplement.
- Encourage patient to comply with dietary recommendations. Explain that best source of vitamins is a well-balanced diet with foods from all 4 basic food groups, and sunlight exposure for vitamin D.
- Advise patient to avoid concurrent use of antacids containing magnesium during therapy.
- Instruct patient to notify health care professional of all Rx or OTC medications, vitamins, or herbal products being taken and to consult health care professional before taking any other Rx, OTC, or herbal products.
- Rep: Advise females of reproductive potential to notify health care professional if pregnancy is planned or suspected or if breastfeeding.

- Emphasize the importance of follow-up exams to evaluate progress.

Evaluation
- Improved levels of calcium and phosphorous in patients with kidney disease.

bezafibrate (bezz-uh-**fibe**-rate)
❦Bezalip SR
Classification
Therapeutic: lipid-lowering agents
Pharmacologic: fibric acid derivatives

Indications
Use in conjunction with diet and other modalities in the treatment of hypercholesterolemia (Type IIa and IIb mixed hyperlipidemia, to decrease serum TG, LDL cholesterol and apolipoprotein B and increase HDL cholesterol, and apolipoprotein A). Treatment of adults with hypertriglyceridemia (Type IV and V hyperlipidemias) at risk of pancreatitis and other sequelae.

Action
Inhibits triglyceride synthesis. **Therapeutic Effects:** Lowered cholesterol and triglycerides, increased HDL, with decreased risk of pancreatitis and other sequelae.

Pharmacokinetics
Absorption: Well absorbed (100%) following oral administration.
Distribution: Unknown.
Metabolism and Excretion: 50% metabolized, 50% excreted unchanged in urine, remainder as metabolites. 3% excreted in feces.
Half-life: 1–2 hr.

TIME/ACTION PROFILE (blood levels)

ROUTE	ONSET	PEAK	DURATION
PO	unknown	3–4 hr	24 hr

Contraindications/Precautions
Contraindicated in: Hypersensitivity/photosensitivity to bezafibrate or other fibric acid or fibrate derivatives; Severe hepatic or renal impairment (CCr <60 mL/min), primary biliary cirrhosis, gallstone or gallbladder disease or hypoalbuminemia; OB: Avoid use during pregnancy (discontinue several mo prior to conception); Lactation: Discontinue breastfeeding.
Use Cautiously in: History of liver disease; Doses >400 mg/day in conjunction with HMG CoA reductase inhibitors (statins) with any risk factors (renal impairment, infection, trauma, surgery, hormonal or electrolyte imbalance) ↑ risk for rhabdomyolysis; Geri: Consider age-related ↓ in renal function; avoid in patients >70 yr; Pedi: Limited experience in children at a dose of 10–20 mg/kg/day.

Adverse Reactions/Side Effects
CNS: dizziness, headache. **GI:** dyspepsia, flatulence, gastritis, ↓ appetite, abdominal distension, abdominal

pain, cholestasis, constipation, diarrhea, nausea. **GU:** erectile dysfunction, renal failure. **Derm:** alopecia, photosensitivity reaction, pruritus, rash, urticaria. **MS:** muscle cramps, muscular weakness, myalgia, RHABDOMYOLYSIS. **Misc:** hypersensitivity reactions including ANAPHYLAXIS.

Interactions

Drug-Drug: ↑ risk of bleeding with **oral anticoagulants;** ↓ dose of anticoagulant by 50% with frequent monitoring. **Cyclosporine** ↑ risk of severe myositis/ rhabdomyolysis; combination therapy should be undertaken with caution. Concurrent use of **immunosuppressants** may ↑ risk of reversible renal impairment. ↑ risk of myopathy with **HMG CoA reductase inhibitors (statins);** combination therapy should be undertaken with extreme caution and must be discontinued at the first signs of myopathy and should not be undertaken in the presence of predisposing factors including impaired renal function, severe infection, trauma, surgery, hormonal /electrolyte imbalance or ↑ alcohol intake. ↑ risk of serious hypoglycemia with **insulin** or **sulfonylureas**. Concurrent use with **MAO inhibitors** may ↑ risk of hepatotoxicity. **Cholestyramine** and other **bile-acid sequestrants** may ↓ absorption; separate administration by ≥2 hr. Effectiveness may be ↓ by concurrent **estrogen**.

Route/Dosage
PO (Adults): 400 mg once daily.

Availability
Sustained-release tablet: 400 mg.

NURSING IMPLICATIONS
Assessment
● Obtain a diet history with regard to fat consumption. Before starting benzafibrate, every attempt should be made to obtain a normal triglyceride level with diet, exercise and weight loss.
● Assess for cholelithiasis. If gallbladder studies are indicated, and gallstones are found, discontinue therapy.

Lab Test Considerations
● Monitor serum lipids prior to and periodically during therapy.
● Monitor AST and ALT serums periodically during therapy to assess for ↑ levels. Discontinue therapy if levels rise >3 times normal value.
● If patient develops muscle tenderness during therapy, monitor CPK levels. If CPK levels are markedly ↑ or myopathy occurs, discontinue therapy.

Implementation
● **PO:** Administer without regard to meals. *DNC:* Swallow sustained-release tablets whole; do not crush, break, or chew.

Patient/Family Teaching
● Instruct the patient to take the medication as directed, and to not share medication. Missed doses should be taken as soon as remembered; do not double dose. Medication helps control but does not cure elevated serum triglyceride levels.
● Advise patient that medication should be taken in conjunction with diet restrictions of fat, cholesterol, carbohydrates, and alcohol, as well as an exercise regimen, and cessation of smoking.
● Instruct patient to notify health care professional of unexplained muscle pain or weakness, tiredness, fever, nausea, vomiting, abdominal pain.
● Instruct patient to notify health care professional of all Rx or OTC medications, vitamins, or herbal products being taken and to consult health care professional before taking any other Rx, OTC, or herbal products.
● Rep: Advise females of reproductive potential to immediately notify health care professional if pregnancy is planned or suspected.
● Emphasize importance of follow-up appointments, and lab tests to evaluate effectiveness.

Evaluation
● A decrease in serum triglyceride and LDL cholesterol levels.
● An increase in HDL levels.

buserelin (bue-se-**rel**-in)
❋Suprefact
Classification
Therapeutic: antineoplastics, hormones
Pharmacologic: luteinizing hormone-releasing hormone (LHRH) analogues

Indications
Subcutaneous injection: Initial and maintenance palliative treatment of advanced hormone-dependent prostate cancer (usually given with an anti-androgen). *Nasal solution:* Maintenance palliative treatment of advanced hormone-dependent prostate cancer (usually given with an anti-androgen). *Nasal solution:* Nonsurgical treatment of endometriosis (course of treatment 6–9 mo).

Action
Acts as a synthetic analog of endogenous gonadotropin-releasing hormone (GnRH/LHRH). Chronic use results in inhibited secretion of gonadotropin release and gonadal steroid production. The overall effect is due to down-regulation of pituitary LHRH receptors. In males, testosterone synthesis and release is decreased. In females, secretion of estrogen is decreased. **Therapeutic Effects:** Decreased spread of advanced prostate cancer. Decreased sequelae of endometriosis (pain, dysmenorrhea).

Pharmacokinetics

Absorption: *SUBQ:* 70%; *intranasal:* 1–3%; *implant:* drug is slowly absorbed over 2–3 mo.
Distribution: Accumulates in liver, kidneys and anterior pituitary lobe; enters breast milk in small amounts.
Metabolism and Excretion: Metabolized in liver, kidneys and by enzymes on membranes in the pituitary gland.
Half-life: *SUBQ:* 80 min; *intranasal:* 1–2 hr; *implant:* 20–30 days.

TIME/ACTION PROFILE

ROUTE	ONSET	PEAK	DURATION
prostate cancer †	7 days	4 mo	until discontinuation
endometriosis ‡ (intranasal)	unknown	unknown	duration of treatment

† ↓ in testosterone levels.
‡ Symptom improvement.

Contraindications/Precautions

Contraindicated in: Hypersensitivity; Nonhormonal-dependent prostate cancer or previous orchiectomy; Females with undiagnosed vaginal bleeding; OB: Pregnancy (avoid use); Lactation: Avoid breastfeeding (small amounts enter breast milk; injection contains benzyl alcohol).
Use Cautiously in: Prostate cancer with urinary tract obstruction or spinal lesions; Pedi: Safety and effectiveness not established (injection contains benzyl alcohol).

Adverse Reactions/Side Effects

CNS: depression, dizziness. **CV:** hypertension. **Endo:** glucose intolerance. **Hemat:** anemia. **Local:** injection site reactions. **MS:** osteoporosis (long-term use). **Misc:** transient exacerbation of metastatic prostate cancer or endometriosis.

Prostate cancer

CNS: headache (nasal solution). **EENT:** nasal irritation (nasal spray). **GU:** ↓ libido, impotence. **Derm:** hot flushes. **Endo:** gynecomastia, testosterone flare. **MS:** bone pain.

Endometriosis

CNS: headache, weakness, insomnia. **CV:** edema. **GI:** constipation, gastrointestinal disorders, nausea. **GU:** ↓ libido, vaginal dryness, menorrhagia. **Derm:** hot flushes, acne. **Endo:** suppression of ovulation. **MS:** back pain.

Interactions

Drug-Drug: Risk of serious arrhythmias may be ↑ by concurrent **amiodarone, disopyramide, dofetilide, flecainide ibitilide, propafenone quinidine, sotalol, antipsychotics** (including **chlorpromazine**) **antidepressants** (including **amitriptyline** and **nor-** triptyline), **opioids** (including **methadone**), **macrolide anti-infectives** (including **azithromycin, erythromycin** and **clarithromycin**), **fluoroquinolones** (including **moxifloxacin**), **azole antifungals, 5-HT3 antagonists** (including **ondansetron**), **beta-2 receptor agonists** (including **salbutamol**), **pentamidine,** and **quinine**.

Route/Dosage

Prostate cancer

SUBQ (Adults): *Initial treatment:* 500 mcg every 8 hr for 7 days, *Maintenance treatment:* 200 mcg daily.
Intranasal (Adults): *Maintenance treatment:* 400 mcg (200 mcg in each nostril) 3 times daily.

Endometriosis

Intranasal (Adults): 400 mcg (200 mcg in each nostril) 3 times daily. Treatment is usually continued for 6 mo; not to exceed 9 mo.

Availability

Solution for subcutaneous injection (contains benzyl alcohol): 1000 mcg/mL; **Intranasal Solution:** 1000 mcg/mL (delivers 100 mcg per actuation).

NURSING IMPLICATIONS

Assessment

- **Cancer:** Monitor patients with vertebral metastases for increased back pain and decreased sensory/motor function.
- Monitor intake and output ratios and assess for bladder distention in patients with urinary tract obstruction during initiation of therapy.
- **Endometriosis:** Assess for signs and symptoms of endometriosis before and periodically during therapy. Amenorrhea usually occurs within 8 wk of initial administration and menses usually resume 8 wk after completion.

Lab Test Considerations

- Monitor serum testosterone levels every 3 mo during treatment with male patients. When treatment begins, testosterone levels can temporarily markedly ↑ and patients may need another medication to ↓ levels.
- Monitor blood glucose in patients with diabetes frequently; may affect blood glucose levels.
- Verify negative pregnancy test before starting therapy for women.

Implementation

Prostate Cancer

- **SUBQ:** Only use syringes that come with kit for accurate dose. Inject into fatty tissue of abdomen, arm, or leg 3 times/day for 7 days; then daily during maintenance.
- **Intranasal:** When used as maintenance, begin nasal spray in each nostril 3 times daily. If patient also receives decongestant nasal spray, wait 30 min to give buserelin spray before or after the decongestant.

Endometriosis

- **Intranasal:** One spray in each nostril 3 times daily for 6–9 mo.

Patient/Family Teaching

- Inform male patients that they may experience breast swelling and tenderness, decreased libido, hot flashes and sweats, impotence and weight gain. Notify health care professional if these symptoms occur.
- Inform female patients that they may experience decreased libido, constipation, painful sexual intercourse, menopausal symptoms, changes in hair growth. Notify health care professional if these symptoms occur.
- Rep: Caution both male and female patients to use contraception while taking this drug. Advise females of reproductive potential to inform health care professional if pregnancy is suspected. Buserelin may cause fetal harm.
- **SUBQ:** Instruct patient in proper technique for self-injection, care and disposal of equipment. Use only syringes included in kit. Instruct patients that syringes may only be used once, and then discarded.
- **Intranasal:** Instruct patient on proper nasal spray technique. Prime pump before use.
- Advise patients that the nasal spray can cause nose bleeds, and may change smell and taste senses.

Evaluation

- Decrease in the spread of prostate cancer.
- Decrease in lesions and pain in endometriosis.

---

cannabidiol (ka-**na**-bi-dye-ole)

delta-9–tetrahydrocannabinol (THC)
(**del**-ta nine tet-re-hye-dro-ka-**na**-bi-nole)
♣Sativex
Classification
Therapeutic: analgesic adjuncts, therapeutic antispasticity agents
Pharmacologic: cannabinoids

Indications

Adjunct treatment of spasticity in adults with multiple sclerosis (MS) who have not responded to other therapies. Analgesic adjunct in the management of neuropathic pain in patients with MS or advanced cancer who have not responded to opioids or other analgesics for severe pain.

Action

Acts on cannabinoid receptors located in pain pathways in the brain, spinal cord, and peripheral nerve terminals. Has analgesic and muscle relaxant properties.
Therapeutic Effects: Decreased pain and spasticity.

Pharmacokinetics

Absorption: Buccal absorption is slower than inhalation.
Distribution: Highly lipid soluble, distributes and accumulates in fatty tissues. Cannabinoids enter breast milk in considerable amounts.
Metabolism and Excretion: Some first-pass hepatic metabolism occurs; highly metabolized by the CYP450 enzyme system. Metabolites can be stored in fatty tissues and rereleased over time (up to weeks); one metabolite of THC is pharmacologically active (11-hydroxy-THC). Further metabolism occurs in renal and biliary systems.
Half-life: Bi-exponential half-lives with short initial phases of *Cannabidiol:* 1.4–1.8 hr; *THC:* 1.3–1.7 hr *11–hydroxy-THC:* 1.9–2.1 hr; terminal elimination half-life of *cannabinoids:* 24–26 hr or more.

TIME/ACTION PROFILE (analgesic and antispasticity effects)

ROUTE	ONSET	PEAK†	DURATION
cannabidiol	unknown	1.6–2.8 hr	up to 12 hr
THC	unknown	1.6–2.4 hr	up to 12 hr

†Blood levels peak more quickly when administered under the tongue.

Contraindications/Precautions

Contraindicated in: Allergy/hypersensitivity to cannabinoids, propylene glycol or peppermint oil; Serious cardiovascular disease, including ischemic heart disease, arrhythmias, poorly controlled hypertension or severe heart failure; History of schizophrenia/psychoses; Patients of reproductive potential who are not using reliable contraception; Sore/inflamed mucosa (may alter absorption); OB: Pregnancy (avoid use); Lactation: Avoid breastfeeding (cannabinoids enter breast milk in considerable amounts); Pedi: Safety and effectiveness not established.
Use Cautiously in: Epilepsy/recurrent seizures; Substance use; Perioperative state (consider possible changes in cardiovascular status); History of depression/suicide attempt or ideation; Significant hepatic/renal impairment; Rep: Women of reproductive potential (reliable contraception must be ensured); Cancer patients with urinary tract pathology (↑ risk of urinary tract adverse reactions); Geri: Use cautiously.

Adverse Reactions/Side Effects

CNS: dizziness, fatigue, confusion, depression, disorientation, drowsiness, euphoria, hallucinations, psychotic reactions, suicidal ideation, weakness. **CV:** hypertension, palpitations, tachycardia, postural hypotension. **GI:** appetite change, constipation, dry mouth, dysgeusia, mucosal/teeth discoloration, nausea

---

♣= Canadian drug name. ⚭ = Genetic implication. ~~Strikethrough~~ = Discontinued. CAPITALS = life-threatening. <u>Underline</u> = most frequent.

(↑ in cancer patients), stomatitis. **GU:** urinary retention (↑ in cancer patients). **Local:** application site irritation. **Misc:** physical dependence, psychological dependence.

Interactions
Drug-Drug: ↑ risk of CNS depression with other **CNS depressants** including **alcohol**, some **antidepressants**, some **antihistamines**, **benzodiazepines**, **GABA inhibitors**, **sedative/hypnotics**, **opioids**, and **psychotropics/antipsychotics**. Cannabidiol inhibits the CYP450 enzyme system; may ↑ effects of **amitriptyline**, **alfentanil**, **fentanyl** and **sufentanil**.
Drug-Natural Products: ↑ risk of intoxication with other forms of **cannabis**.

Route/Dosage
Buccal (Adults): *Day 1:* One spray in the morning and one in the evening; may ↑ by 1 spray/day on subsequent days. If unacceptable effects occur, temporarily discontinue and restart at a lower # of sprays/day or use longer intervals between sprays. Titrate to optimal maintenance dose (usual range 4–8 sprays/day, usually not more than 12 sprays/day; higher doses have been used/tolerated). Adjust dose to changes in patient condition.

Availability
Buccal spray contains ethanol (50% v/v), propylene glycol and peppermint oil: Each ml contains *Cannabidiol:* 25 mg and *THC:* 27 mg/ml. Delivers 100 microliters/spray, each spray provides cannabidiol 2.5 mg and THC 2.7 mg.

NURSING IMPLICATIONS
Assessment
- Assess patient's pain level before and after cannabidiol.

Implementation
- Prime pump before first use. Shake vial gently and remove protective cap. Hold vial in an upright position and press firmly and quickly on the actuator 2 or 3 times, until a fine spray appears. Point spray into a tissue, away from patient.
- Administer one spray 2 times/day, in morning and in evening, on first day. Administer under tongue or in buccal area. Rotate sites in mouth to avoid irritation. Effects should be noticed in about 30 min. Do not spray the back of throat or into nose. After first day, increase dose by 1 spray every 24 hr, spacing doses evenly. No more than 12 doses should be used over a 24-hr period. Space each spray by at least 15 min.

Patient/Family Teaching
- Caution patient to use medication as directed.
- Instruct patient on correct spray technique. Instruct patient to rotate sites in the mouth between the tongue and buccal locations.
- Instruct patient to store unopened bottles in refrigerator. Do not freeze. Keep away from sources of heat such as direct sunlight or flames (product is flammable). Opened bottles may be stored at room temperature. Keep out of reach of children.
- Inform patient that any unused contents should be discarded after 28 days. Do not dispose of medications in wastewater (e.g., down the sink or in the toilet) or in household garbage. Consult pharmacist how to dispose of expired or unneeded medication.
- Caution patient to avoid alcohol while taking cannabidiol.
- Rep: Advise females of reproductive potential to notify health care professional if pregnancy is planned or suspected or if breastfeeding.

Evaluation
- Decrease in pain.
- Decrease in muscle spasticity.

---

cilazapril (sye-lay-za-pril)
✦Inhibace
Classification
Therapeutic: antihypertensives
Pharmacologic: ACE inhibitors

Indications
Alone or with other agents in the management of hypertension. HF.

Action
ACE inhibitors block the conversion of angiotensin I to the vasoconstrictor angiotensin II. ACE inhibitors also prevent the degradation of bradykinin and other vasodilatory prostaglandins. ACE inhibitors also ↑ plasma renin levels and ↓ aldosterone levels. Net result is systemic vasodilation. **Therapeutic Effects:** Lowering of BP in hypertensive patients. Improved symptoms in patients with HF.

Pharmacokinetics
Absorption: Well absorbed following oral administration, rapidly converted to active metabolite, cilazaprilat (57% bioavailability for cilazaprilat).
Distribution: Enters breast milk.
Metabolism and Excretion: Cilazaprilat is eliminated unchanged by the kidneys (91%).
Half-life: *Early elimination phase:* 0.9 hr; *terminal elimination phase (enzyme-bound cilazaprilat):* 36–49 hr.

TIME/ACTION PROFILE (effects on hemodynamics)

ROUTE	ONSET	PEAK	DURATION
PO (hypertension)	within 1 hr	3–7 hr	12–24 hr
PO (heart failure)	1–2 hr	2–4 hr	24 hr

Contraindications/Precautions
Contraindicated in: Hypersensitivity; History of angioedema with previous use of ACE inhibitors; Concur-

rent use with aliskiren in patients with diabetes or moderate to severe renal impairment (CCr <60 mL/min); OB: Can cause injury or death of fetus: if pregnancy occurs, discontinue immediately; Lactation: Discontinue drug or use formula.

Use Cautiously in: Renal impairment, hepatic impairment, hypovolemia, hyponatremia, concurrent diuretic therapy; ☒ Black patients with hypertension (monotherapy less effective, may require additional therapy; ↑ risk of angioedema); Rep: Women of reproductive potential; Surgery/anesthesia (hypotension may be exaggerated); Geri: Initial dose ↓ recommended for most agents due to age-related ↓ in renal function; Pedi: Safety and effectiveness not established.

Exercise Extreme Caution in: Family history of angioedema.

Adverse Reactions/Side Effects

CNS: dizziness, drowsiness, fatigue, headache, insomnia, vertigo, weakness. **Resp:** <u>cough</u>, dyspnea. **CV:** <u>hypotension</u>, chest pain, edema, tachycardia. **Endo:** hyperuricemia. **GI:** <u>taste disturbances</u>, abdominal pain, anorexia, constipation, diarrhea, nausea, vomiting. **GU:** erectile dysfunction, proteinuria, renal dysfunction, renal failure. **Derm:** flushing, pruritis, rashes. **F and E:** hyperkalemia. **Hemat:** AGRANULOCYTOSIS. **MS:** back pain, muscle cramps, myalgia. **Misc:** ANGIOEDEMA, fever.

Interactions

Drug-Drug: Excessive hypotension may occur with concurrent use of **diuretics** or other **antihypertensives** or **alcohol**. ↑ risk of hyperkalemia with concurrent use of **potassium supplements**, **potassium-sparing diuretics**, or **potassium-containing salt substitutes**. ↑ risk of hyperkalemia, renal impairment, hypotension, and syncope with concurrent use of **angiotensin II receptor antagonists** or **aliskiren**; avoid concurrent use with aliskiren in patients with diabetes or CCr <60 mL/min. **NSAIDs** and selective **COX-2 inhibitors** may blunt the antihypertensive effect and ↑ the risk of renal dysfunction. ↑ levels and may ↑ risk of **lithium** toxicity.

Route/Dosage

Hypertension

PO (Adults ≤65 yr): *As monotherapy:* 2.5 mg once daily initially, may be increased every 2 wk by 2.5 mg/day; usual dose 2.5–5 mg once daily, not to exceed 10 mg/day. Twice daily administration may be necessary in some patients; *With diuretics:* 0.5 mg once daily initially, titrate carefully.
PO (Adults >65 yr): *As monotherapy:* 1.25 mg once daily initially, titrate carefully.

Renal Impairment

PO (Adults): *CCr >40 mL/min:* 1 mg once daily initially, titrate carefully, not to exceed 5 mg once daily; *CCr 10–40 mL/min:* 0.5 mg once daily initially, titrate carefully, not to exceed 2.5 mg once daily; *CCr <10 mL/min:* not recommended.

Hepatic Impairment

PO (Adults): 0.5 mg once daily or less.

Heart Failure

PO (Adults): After considering concurrent diuretic therapy/salt/volume depletion, *Initial dose:* 0.5 mg/day with careful monitoring, after 5 days dose may be ↑ to 1 mg/day, dose may then be carefully titrated as needed/tolerated up to 2.5 mg/day; rarely patients may require 5 mg/day.

Renal Impairment

PO (Adults): *CCr 10–40 mL/min:* 0.25–0.5 mg once daily; *CCr <10 mL/min:* not recommended.

Availability

Tablets: 1 mg, 2.5 mg, 5 mg. *In combination with:* hydrochlorothiazide 12.5 mg (Inhibace Plus).

NURSING IMPLICATIONS

Assessment

- Assess patient for signs of angioedema; dyspnea and facial swelling.
- **Hypertension:** Monitor BP and pulse frequently during initial dose adjustment and periodically during therapy. Notify health care professional of significant changes.
- **Heart Failure:** Monitor daily weight and assess frequently for fluid overload (dyspnea, rales/crackles, weight gain, jugular venous distention).

Lab Test Considerations

- Monitor BUN, creatinine, and serum electrolyte levels periodically during therapy.
- Monitor CBC periodically. May cause agranulocytosis.
- May cause ↑ AST, ALT, alkaline phosphatase, serum bilirubin, uric acid, and glucose.

Implementation

- **PO:** Tablets may be taken before or after meals.

Patient/Family Teaching

- Instruct patient to take cilazapril as directed. Take missed dose as soon as remembered. If not until the following day, skip missed dose. Do not double doses.
- Caution patient to change positions slowly to minimize hypotension. Use of alcohol, standing for long periods, exercising, and hot weather may ↑ orthostatic hypotension.
- May cause dizziness. Caution patient to avoid driving and other activities requiring alertness until response to medication is known.

✿ = Canadian drug name. ☒ = Genetic implication. ~~Strikethrough~~ = Discontinued. CAPITALS = life-threatening. <u>Underline</u> = most frequent.

- Instruct patient on proper technique for monitoring blood pressure. Advise patient to check BP and weight weekly and record and report results to health care professional.
- Provide patient with additional interventions for hypertension control (weight reduction, low sodium diet, cessation of smoking, exercise regimen, stress management, and moderation of alcohol consumption). Medication controls but does not cure hypertension.
- Instruct patient to notify health care professional of all Rx or OTC medications, vitamins, or herbal products being taken and consult health care professional before taking any new medications, especially cough, cold, or allergy remedies.
- Rep: Advise females of reproductive potential to use contraception and to notify health care professional if planning or suspecting pregnancy. Discontinue medication immediately if pregnancy is confirmed.

Evaluation

- Decrease in blood pressure.
- Decrease in signs and symptoms of heart failure.

cloxacillin (klox-a-**sill**-in)
Classification
Therapeutic: anti-infectives
Pharmacologic: penicillinase resistant penicillins

Indications
Treatment of the following infections due to penicillinase-producing staphylococci: respiratory tract infections, sinusitis, septicemia, endocarditis, osteomyelitis, skin and skin structure infections.

Action
Bind to bacterial cell wall, leading to cell death. Not inactivated by penicillinase enzymes. **Therapeutic Effects:** Bactericidal action. **Spectrum:** Active against most gram-positive aerobic cocci. Spectrum is notable for activity against: Penicillinase-producing strains of *Staphylococcus aureus* and *Staphylococcus epidermidis*. Not active against methicillin-resistant bacteria (MRSA).

Pharmacokinetics
Absorption: IV administration results in complete bioavailability. Moderately absorbed (50%) following oral administration.
Distribution: Widely distributed; penetration into CSF is minimal but sufficient in the presence of inflamed meninges; crosses the placenta and enters breast milk.
Metabolism and Excretion: Some metabolism by the liver (9–22%) and some renal excretion of unchanged drug (20%).
Half-life: 0.5–1.1 hr (↑ in severe hepatic impairment, renal impairment, and in neonates).

TIME/ACTION PROFILE

ROUTE	ONSET	PEAK	DURATION
PO	30 min	30–120 min	6 hr
IM	unknown	unknown	6 hr
IV	rapid	end of injection/infusion	6 hr

Contraindications/Precautions
Contraindicated in: Previous hypersensitivity to penicillin (cross-sensitivity exists with cephalosporins and other beta-lactam antibiotics).
Use Cautiously in: Severe renal or hepatic impairment; OB: Safety not established; Pedi: Safety in premature and newborn infants not established.

Adverse Reactions/Side Effects
CNS: SEIZURES. **GI:** diarrhea, epigastric distress, nausea, vomiting, CLOSTRIDIOIDES DIFFICILE-ASSOCIATED DIARRHEA (CDAD). **GU:** interstitial nephritis. **Derm:** rash, urticaria. **Hemat:** eosinophilia, leukopenia. **Misc:** allergic reactions including ANAPHYLAXIS and SERUM SICKNESS, superinfection.

Interactions
Drug-Drug: May ↓ effectiveness of **oral contraceptive agents**. **Probenecid** ↓ renal excretion and ↑ levels (therapy may be combined for this purpose). Concurrent use with **methotrexate** ↓ methotrexate elimination and ↑ risk of serious toxicity.
Drug-Food: Food ↓ oral absorption by 50%.

Route/Dosage
PO (Adults): 250–500 mg every 6 hr.
PO (Children >1 mo): 50–100 mg/kg/day divided every 6 hr up to a maximum of 4 g/day.
IM, IV (Adults): 250–500 mg every 6 hr, maximum dose 6 g/day.
IM, IV (Children up to 20 kg): 25–50 mg/kg/day in 4 equally divided doses every 6 hr.

Availability
Capsules: ✹ 250 mg, ✹ 500 mg; **Oral solution:** ✹ 125 mg/5 mL; **Powder for injection (requires reconstitution/dilution:** ✹ 250 mg/vial, ✹ 500 mg/vial, ✹ 1 g/vial, ✹ 2 g/vial.

NURSING IMPLICATIONS
Assessment

- Assess for infection (vital signs; appearance of wound, sputum, urine, and stool; WBC) at beginning of and throughout therapy.
- Obtain a history before initiating therapy to determine previous use of and reactions to cephalosporins or other beta-lactam antibiotics. Persons with no history of penicillin sensitivity may still have an allergic response.
- Obtain specimens for culture and sensitivity prior to initiating therapy. First dose may be given before receiving results.

- Observe patient for signs and symptoms of anaphylaxis (rash, pruritus, laryngeal edema, wheezing, abdominal pain). Discontinue drug and notify health care professional immediately if these occur. Keep epinephrine, an antihistamine, and resuscitation equipment close by in event of an anaphylactic reaction.
- Monitor bowel function. Diarrhea, abdominal cramping, fever, and bloody stools should be reported to health care professional promptly as a sign of Clostridioides difficile-associated diarrhea (CDAD). May begin up to several wk following cessation of therapy.

Lab Test Considerations

- May cause leukopenia and neutropenia, especially with prolonged therapy or hepatic impairment.
- May cause positive direct Coombs' test result.
- May cause ↑ AST, ALT, LDH, and serum alkaline phosphatase concentrations.

Implementation

- **PO:** Administer around the clock on an empty stomach at least 1 hr before or 2 hr after meals. Take with a full glass of water; acidic juices may decrease absorption of penicillins. Swallow capsules whole; do not crush, chew, or open capsules.
- Use calibrated measuring device for liquid preparations. Shake well. Solution is stable for 14 days if refrigerated.
- **IM:** Reconstitute by adding 1.9 mL and 1.7 mL sterile water to 250 mg and 500 mg respectively, for concentrations of 125 mg/mL and 250 mg/mL. Shake well to dissolve. Stable for 24 hr at room temperature or 48 hr if refrigerated.
- **IV:** For IV use, reconstitute 250 mg vial with 4.9 mL, 500 mg vial with 4.8 mL, and 1000 mg vial with 9.6 mL sterile water for concentrations of 50 mg/mL, 100 mg/mL, and 100 mg/mL respectively. Shake well. Use reconstituted solution immediately. Infuse over 2−4 min.
- **IV:** Reconstitute for infusion with sterile water for injection using 3.4 mL for 1000 mg, 6.8 mL for 2000 mg, and 34 mL for 10,000 mg, resulting in 250 mg/mL. Add to an appropriate infusion fluid in amount calculated to give desired dose. Shake well to dissolve. Use solution immediately. Infuse over 30−40 min.
- **Y-Site Compatibility:** epinephrine ketamine.
- **Y-Site Incompatibility:** pantoprazole, rocuronium.

Patient/Family Teaching

- Instruct patient to take medication around the clock and to finish the drug completely as directed, even if feeling better. Missed doses should be taken as soon as remembered. Advise patient that sharing of this medication may be dangerous.

- Advise patient to report signs of superinfection (black, furry overgrowth on the tongue; vaginal itching or discharge; loose or foul-smelling stools) and allergy.
- Instruct patient to notify health care professional if fever and diarrhea develop, especially if stool contains blood, pus, or mucus. Advise patient not to treat diarrhea without consulting health care professional.
- Rep: Advise females of reproductive potential to notify health care professional if pregnancy is planned or suspected or if breastfeeding. Advise patient taking oral contraceptives to use an additional nonhormonal method of contraception during therapy with penicillin and until next menstrual period.
- Instruct patient to notify health care professional if symptoms do not improve.

Evaluation

- Resolution of the signs and symptoms of infection. Length of time for complete resolution depends on the organism and site of infection.

cyproterone (sy-proe-te-rone)
🍁Androcur
Classification
Therapeutic: antineoplastics, hormones
Pharmacologic: antiandrogens

Indications
Palliative treatment of advanced prostate cancer.

Action
Has antiandrogenic and progestogenic/antigonadotropic properties, resulting in blocked binding of the active metabolite of testosterone on the surface of prostatic cancer cells and decreased production of testicular testosterone. **Therapeutic Effects:** Decreased spread of prostate cancer.

Pharmacokinetics
Absorption: Completely absorbed following oral administration. Absorption after IM depot injection is delayed and prolonged.
Distribution: Unknown.
Metabolism and Excretion: Metabolized by the CYP3A enzyme system; excreted in feces (60%) and urine (33%), as unchanged drug and metabolites.
Half-life: *PO:* 38 hr; *IM:* 4 days.

TIME/ACTION PROFILE (blood levels)

ROUTE	ONSET	PEAK	DURATION
PO	unknown	3–4 hr	8–12 hr
IM (depot)	unknown	3–4 days	1–2 wk

Contraindications/Precautions
Contraindicated in: Hypersensitivity; Liver disease/hepatic impairment/liver tumors (not due to prostate

cancer); Dubin Johnson syndrome; Rotor syndrome; History of meningioma; Wasting diseases (not related to prostate cancer); Severe depression; Thromboembolism; OB: Not indicated for use in women; Pedi: Not recommended for use in children <18 yr.

Use Cautiously in: History of cardiovascular disease; Renal impairment.

Adverse Reactions/Side Effects

CNS: fatigue, weakness, depression, MENINGIOMAS. **Resp:** cough, dyspnea, pulmonary microembolism. **CV:** edema, heart failure, hypotension, myocardial infarction, syncope, tachycardia, THROMBOEMBOLISM, vasovagal reactions. **GI:** anorexia, constipation, diarrhea, HEPATOTOXICITY, LIVER TUMORS, nausea, vomiting. **Derm:** ↑ sweating, dry skin, hot flashes, patchy hair loss. **Endo:** adrenal suppression, antiandrogen withdrawal syndrome, gynecomastia. **F and E:** hypercalcemia. **GU:** impotence, infertility. **Hemat:** anemia, thrombocytopenia. **Metab:** glucose intolerance, hyperlipidemia. **MS:** osteoporosis (long term use). **Misc:** allergic reactions.

Interactions

Drug-Drug: Antiandrogenic effect may be ↓ by **alcohol**. Effectiveness/long-term survival may be ↓ by concurrent **GnRH agonist** treatment. ↑ risk of myopathy with **HMG CoA reductase inhibitors (statins)**. Blood levels and effects may be ↑ by **strong inhibitors of CYP3A4** including **clotrimazole**, **itraconazole**, **ketoconazole** and **ritonavir**. Blood levels and effectiveness may be ↓ by **inducers of CYP3A4** including **phenytoin**, and **rifampicin**. Use cautiously with other **drugs that are substrates of the P450 enzymes**.

Drug-Natural Products: Blood levels and effectiveness may be ↓ by **St. John's wort.**

Route/Dosage

PO (Adults): 200–300 mg/day in 2–3 divided doses, not to exceed 300 mg/day; *After orchiectomy:* 100–200 mg/day.

IM (Adults): 300 mg once weekly; *After orchiectomy:* 300 mg every 2 wk.

Availability

Tablets: 50 mg. *In combination with:* Ethinyl estradiol (Diane-35, Cyestra-35, Cleo-35).

NURSING IMPLICATIONS

Assessment

- Assess for signs and symptoms of thromboembolism (chest pain, dyspnea, vital signs, level of consciousness). Discontinue therapy if symptoms occur.
- Monitor mood changes, especially during first 6–8 wk. Note degree to which these thoughts and behaviors interfere with daily functioning. Inform health care professional if patient demonstrates significant increase in anxiety, nervousness, or insomnia.

Lab Test Considerations

- Monitor PSA during therapy. May cause increase in PSA. If PSA increase occurs discontinue therapy and monitor for 6–8 wk for withdrawal response prior to any decision to proceed with other prostate cancer therapy.
- May impair carbohydrate metabolism. Monitor fasting blood glucose and glucose tolerance tests periodically during therapy, especially in patients with diabetes. May require dose changes in insulin or oral antidiabetic agents.
- Monitor CBC and platelet count periodically during therapy.
- Monitor liver function tests prior to and periodically during therapy and if symptoms of hepatotoxicity occur. May develop several wk to mo after therapy starts. Discontinue therapy if hepatotoxicity occurs.
- Monitor adrenocortical function tests by serum cortisol assay periodically during therapy.

Implementation

- **PO:** Take by mouth two or three times a day with or just after meals as directed. Dose is usually lower after orchiectomy.

Patient/Family Teaching

- Instruct patient to take cyproterone as directed. Take missed doses as soon as remembered, unless almost time for next dose, then skip missed dose and resume usual dosing schedule. Do not double dose.
- Inform patient that benign breast lumps may occur; they generally subside 1–3 mo after discontinuation of therapy and/or after dose reduction. Dose reduction should be weighed against the risk of inadequate tumor control.
- Advise patient to avoid alcohol during therapy.
- May cause fatigue and lassitude during first few wk of therapy; then diminishes. Caution patient to avoid driving and other activities requiring alertness until response to medication is known.
- Inform patient that sperm count and volume of ejaculate decrease with therapy. Infertility is common but is reversible when therapy is discontinued.
- Discuss with patient potential for patchy hair loss. Explore methods of coping.
- Instruct patient to notify health care professional of all Rx or OTC medications, vitamins, or herbal products being taken and consult health care professional before taking any new medications, especially St. John's wort.
- Rep: Advise patient to notify health care professional if pregnancy is planned or suspected or if breastfeeding.
- Emphasize the importance of follow-up appointments and blood tests to monitor progression of treatment.

Evaluation

- Decreased spread of prostate cancer.

danaparoid sodium

(da-**nap**-a-roid)

✦Orgaran

Classification

Therapeutic: anticoagulants

Pharmacologic: heparins (low molecular weight)

Indications

Prevention of thromboembolic phenomena including deep vein thrombosis and pulmonary emboli after surgical procedures known to increase the risk of such complications (knee/hip replacement, abdominal surgery). Management of non-hemorrhagic stroke. Treatment/prevention of thromboembolic phenomena in patients with a history of heparin-induced thrombocytopenia (HIT).

Action

Potentiates the inhibitory effect of antithrombin on factor Xa and thrombin. Danaparoid sodium is a heparinoid. **Therapeutic Effects:** Prevention of thrombus formation.

Pharmacokinetics

Absorption: 100% absorbed after SUBQ administration; IV administration results in complete bioavailability.

Distribution: Unknown.

Metabolism and Excretion: Excreted mostly by the kidneys.

Half-life: 25 hr.

TIME/ACTION PROFILE (anticoagulant effect)

ROUTE	ONSET	PEAK	DURATION
SUBQ	unknown	2–5 hr	12 hr

Contraindications/Precautions

Contraindicated in: Hypersensitivity to danaparoid sodium, pork products, or sulfites; Uncontrolled bleeding; Imminent/threatened abortion; Lactation: Avoid breastfeeding.

Use Cautiously in: Severe hepatic or renal impairment (dosage ↓ may be necessary in severe renal impairment); Retinopathy (hypertensive or diabetic); Untreated hypertension; Recent history of ulcer disease; Spinal/epidural anesthesia; History of congenital or acquired bleeding disorder; Malignancy; History of thrombocytopenia related to heparin (HIT), has been used successfully; OB: Safe use in pregnancy has not been established; Geri: Dosage ↓ may be necessary in severe renal impairment; Pedi: Safety not established.

Exercise Extreme Caution in: Severe uncontrolled hypertension; Bacterial endocarditis, bleeding disorders; GI bleeding/ulceration/pathology; Hemor-

rhagic stroke; Recent CNS or ophthalmologic surgery; Active GI bleeding/ulceration.

Adverse Reactions/Side Effects

CNS: dizziness, headache, insomnia. **CV:** edema. **GI:** constipation, nausea, reversible increase in liver enzymes, vomiting. **GU:** urinary retention. **Derm:** ecchymoses, pruritus, rash, urticaria. **Hemat:** BLEEDING, anemia, thrombocytopenia. **Local:** erythema at injection site, hematoma, irritation, pain. **Misc:** fever.

Interactions

Drug-Drug: Risk of bleeding may be ↑ by concurrent use of other **anticoagulants** including **warfarin** or **drugs that affect platelet function**, including **aspirin**, **NSAIDs**, **dipyridamole**, some **penicillins**, **clopidogrel**, **ticlopidine**, and **dextran**.

Route/Dosage

Prophylaxis of DVT (non HIT patients)

SUBQ (Adults): 750 anti-factor Xa IU every 12 hr starting 1–4 hr preop and at least 2 hr postop for 7–10 days or until ambulatory (up to 14 days). *Prophylaxis of DVT following Orthopedic, Major Abdominal Surgery, and Thoracic Surgery:* 750 anti-factor Xa units, twice daily up to 14 days, initiate 1–4 hr preop. **IV, SUBQ (Adults):** *Prophylaxis of Deep Vein Thrombosis in Non-hemorrhagic Stroke Patients:* up to 1000 anti-Xa units IV, followed by 750 anti-Xa units subcutaneously, twice daily for 7–14 days.

HIT

IV, SUBQ (Adults): *DVT prophylaxis, current HIT, ≤90 kg:* 750 anti-Xa units SC two or three times daily for 7–10 days (initial bolus of 1250 anti-Xa units IV may be used); *DVT prophylaxis, current HIT, >90 kg:* 1250 anti-Xa units SC two or three times daily for 7–10 days (initial bolus of 1250 anti-Xa units IV may be used); *DVT prophylaxis, past (>3 mo) HIT, ≤90 kg:* 750 anti-Xa units SC two or three times daily for 7–10 days; *DVT prophylaxis, past (>3 mo) HIT, >90 kg:* 750 anti-Xa units SC three times daily or 1250 anti-Xa units SC twice daily for 7–10 days; *Established pulmonary embolism or DVT, thrombus <5 days, >90 kg:* 3750 anti-Xa units IV bolus, then 400 anti-Xa units/hr for 4 hr, then 300 anti-Xa units/hr for 4 hr, then 150–200 anti-Xa units/hr for 5–7 days or 1750 anti-Xa units SC twice daily for 4–7 days; *Established pulmonary embolism or DVT, thrombus <5 days, 55–90 kg:* 2250–2500 anti-Xa units IV bolus, then 400 anti-Xa units/hr for 4 hr, then 300 anti-Xa units/hr for 4 hr, then 150–200 anti-Xa units/hr for 5–7 days or 2000 anti-Xa units SC twice daily for 4–7 days; *Established pulmonary embolism or DVT, thrombus <5 days, <55 kg:* 1250–1500 anti-Xa units IV bolus, then 400 anti-Xa units/hr for 4 hr, then 300 anti-Xa units/hr for 4 hr, then 150–200 anti-Xa units/hr for 5–7 days or 1500 anti-Xa units SC twice daily for 4–7 days; *Estab-*

lished pulmonary embolism or DVT, thrombus ≥5 days, >90 kg: 1250 anti-Xa units IV bolus, then 750 anti-Xa units SC three times daily or 1250 anti-Xa units twice daily; *Established pulmonary embolism or DVT, thrombus ≥5 days, ≤90 kg:* 1250 anti-Xa units IV bolus, then 750 anti-Xa units SC 2–3 times daily; *Surgical prophylaxis, nonvascular surgery, >90 kg:* 750 anti-Xa units SC 1–4 hr before procedure, repeat ≥6 hr after procedure, then 1250 anti-Xa units SC twice daily for 7–10 days; *Surgical prophylaxis, nonvascular surgery, ≤90 kg:* 750 anti-Xa units SC 1–4 hr before procedure, repeat ≥6 hr after procedure, then 750 anti-Xa units SC twice daily for 7–10 days; *Surgical prophylaxis, embolectomy, >90 kg:* 2250–2500 anti-Xa units IV bolus before procedure, then 150–200 anti-Xa units/hr IV starting ≥6 hr after procedure for 5–7 days or 750 anti-Xa units 2–3 times daily or change to oral anticoagulants after several days; *Surgical prophylaxis, embolectomy, 55–90 kg:* 2250–2500 anti-Xa units IV bolus before procedure, then 1250 anti-Xa units SC twice daily starting ≥6 hr after procedure, then 750 anti-Xa units 2–3 times daily or change to oral anticoagulants after several days; *Cardiac catheterization >90 kg:* 3750 anti-Xa units IV bolus prior to procedure; *Cardiac catheterization <90 kg:* 2500 anti-Xa units IV bolus prior to procedure; *Percutaneous transluminal coronary angioplasty:* 2500 anti-Xa units IV prior to procedure, then 150–200 anti-Xa units/hr IV for 1–2 days after procedure, may be followed by 750 anti-Xa units SC for several days; *Intra-aortic balloon pump catherization, >90 kg:* 3750 anti-Xa units IV bolus before procedure, then 150–200 anti-Xa units/hr IV or a 2nd bolus of 1250 anti-Xa units IV or 750 anti-Xa units SC two or three times daily or 1250 anti-Xa units SC twice daily; *Intra-aortic balloon pump catherization, <90 kg:* 2500 anti-Xa units IV bolus before procedure, then 150–200 anti-Xa units/hr IV or a 2nd bolus of 1250 anti-Xa units IV or 750 anti-Xa units SC two or three times daily or 1250 anti-Xa units SC twice daily; *Peripheral vascular bypass:* 2250–2500 anti-Xa units IV bolus before procedure, then 150–200 anti-Xa units/hr IV started ≥6 hr after procedure for 5–7 days or 750 anti-Xa units SC two or three times daily or change to oral anticoagulants; *Hemodialysis, every other day or less frequently:* 3750 anti-Xa units IV bolus before first 2 hemodialysis, then 3000 anti-Xa units IV bolus (if plasma antifactory Xa level <300 U/L) or 2500 anti-Xa units IV (if plasma antifactory Xa levels 350–400); *Hemodialysis, every other day or less frequently, <55kg:* 2500 anti-Xa units IV bolus before first 2 hemodialysis, then 2000 anti-Xa units IV bolus (if plasma antifactory Xa level <300 U/L), or 1500 anti-Xa units IV (if plasma antifactory Xa levels 350–400); *Hemodialysis, daily:* 3750 anti-Xa units IV before first dialysis, then 2500 before second dialysis; *Hemodialysis, daily, <55kg:* 2500 anti-Xa units IV before first dialysis, then 2000 before second dialysis; *Hemofiltration, 55–90kg:* 2500 anti-Xa units IV bolus, then 600/h for 4h, then 400/h for 4/

h, then 200–600/h to maintain plasma antifactory Xa levels of 500–1000 U/L; *Hemofiltration, <55kg:* 2000 anti-Xa units IV bolus, then 400/h for 4h, then 150–400/h to maintain plasma antifactory Xa levels of 500–1000 U/L.

Availability
Solution for injection (contains sulfites): 750 antifactor Xa units/0.6 mL ampule.

NURSING IMPLICATIONS
Assessment
- Assess for signs of bleeding and hemorrhage (bleeding gums; nosebleed; unusual bruising; black, tarry stools; hematuria; fall in hematocrit or BP; guaiac-positive stools); bleeding from surgical site. Notify health care professional if these occur.
- Assess for evidence of additional or increased thrombosis. Symptoms will depend on area of involvement. Monitor neurological status frequently for signs of neurological impairment. May require urgent treatment.
- Monitor patient for hypersensitivity reactions (chills, fever, urticaria).
- Monitor patients with epidural catheters frequently for signs and symptoms of neurologic impairment.
- **SUBQ:** Observe injection sites for hematomas, ecchymosis, or inflammation.

Lab Test Considerations
- Monitor CBC, and stools for occult blood periodically during therapy. Monitor platelet count every other day for first wk, twice weekly for next 2 wk, and weekly thereafter. If thrombocytopenia occurs, monitor closely. If hematocrit decreases unexpectedly, assess patient for potential bleeding sites.
- Special monitoring of clotting times (aPTT) is not necessary.
- May cause ↑ in AST, ALT, and alkaline phosphatase levels.

Toxicity and Overdose
- Danaparoid sodium is not reversed with protamine sulfate. If overdose occurs, discontinue danaparoid sodium. Transfusion with fresh frozen plasma and plasmapheresis has been used if bleeding is uncontrollable.

Implementation
- Cannot be used interchangeably (unit for unit) with unfractionated heparin or other low-molecular-weight heparins.
- Conversion to oral anticoagulant therapy (unless it is contraindicated) should not be started until adequate antithrombotic control with parenteral danaparoid sodium has been achieved; conversion may take up to 5 days.
- **SUBQ:** Administer deep into SUBQ tissue. Alternate injection sites daily between the left and right anterolateral and left and right posterolateral abdominal

wall. Inject entire length of needle at a 45° or 90° angle into a skin fold held between thumb and forefinger; hold skin fold throughout injection. Do not aspirate or massage. Rotate sites frequently. Do not administer IM because of danger of hematoma formation. Solution should be clear; do not inject solution containing particulate matter.

- If excessive bruising occurs, ice cube massage of site before injection may lessen bruising.

IV Administration
- **IV Push:** SUBQ is preferred route. *Dilution:* If administered IV, give as a bolus. May dilute with 0.9% NaCl, D5/0.9% NaCl, Ringer's, LR, and mannitol. Stable for up to 48 hr at room temperature.
- **Y-Site Incompatibility:** Administer separately; do not mix with other drugs.

Patient/Family Teaching
- Instruct patient in correct technique for self-injection, care and disposal of equipment.
- Advise patient to report any symptoms of unusual bleeding or bruising, dizziness, itching, rash, fever, swelling, or difficulty breathing to health care professional immediately.
- Instruct patient not to take aspirin, naproxen, or ibuprofen without consulting health care professional while on danaparoid sodium therapy.
- Rep: Advise females of reproductive potential to notify health care professional if pregnancy is planned or suspected or if breastfeeding.

Evaluation
- Prevention of deep vein thrombosis and pulmonary emboli.

---

domperidone (dom-**per**-i-done)
Classification
Therapeutic: gastric stimulant
Pharmacologic: butyrophenones, dopamine antagonists

Indications
Management of symptoms associated with GI motility disorders including subacute/chronic gastritis and diabetic gastroparesis. Treatment of nausea/vomiting associated with dopamine agonist antiparkinson therapy. **Unlabeled Use:** To stimulate lactation.

Action
Acts as a peripheral dopamine receptor blocker. Increases GI motility, peristalsis, and lower esophageal sphincter pressure. Facilitates gastric emptying and decreases small bowel transit time. Also increases prolactin levels. **Therapeutic Effects:** Improved GI motility. Decreased nausea/vomiting associated with dopamine agonist antiparkinson therapy.

Pharmacokinetics
Absorption: Well absorbed following oral administration.
Distribution: Does not cross the blood-brain barrier; enters breast milk in low concentrations.
Metabolism and Excretion: Undergoes extensive first-pass hepatic metabolism; much via the CYP3A4 enzyme system. 31% excreted in urine, 66% in feces.
Half-life: 7 hr.

TIME/ACTION PROFILE

ROUTE	ONSET	PEAK	DURATION
PO	unknown	30 min (blood levels)	6–8 hr

Contraindications/Precautions
Contraindicated in: Known hypersensitivity/intolerance; Concurrent use of ketoconazole; Prolactinoma; Conditions where GI stimulation is dangerous including GI hemorrhage/mechanical obstruction/perforation; Lactation: Breastfeeding is not recommended unless potential benefits outweigh potential risks.
Use Cautiously in: History of breast cancer; Hepatic impairment; Severe renal impairment (dose adjustment may be necessary during chronic therapy); OB: Use only if expected benefit outweighs potential hazard; Pedi: Safety and effectiveness not established.

Adverse Reactions/Side Effects
CNS: headache, insomnia. **GI:** dry mouth. **GU:** amenorrhea, impotence. **Derm:** hot flashes, rash. **Endo:** galactorrhea, gynecomastia, hyperprolactinemia.

Interactions
Drug-Drug: Ketoconazole ↑ levels and the risk of cardiovascular toxicity; concurrent use contraindicated; other **azole antifungals, macrolide anti-infectives,** and **protease inhibitors** may have similar effects. Risk of adverse cardiovascular reactions may be ↑ by concurrent use of **drugs known to ↑ QT interval** including **antiarrhythmics,** some **fluoroquinolones, antipsychotics, beta-2 adrenergic agonists, antimalarials, SSRIs, tri/tetracyclic antidepressants,** and **nefazodone** and should be undertaken cautiously, especially if other risk factors for *torsade de pointes* exists. Effectiveness may be ↓ by concurrent use of **anticholinergics.** Due to effects on gastric motility, absorption of drugs from the small intestine may be accelerated, while absorption of drugs from the stomach may be slowed, especially **sustained-release** or **enteric-coated** formulations. Concurrent use with **MAOIs** should be undertaken with caution.
Drug-Food: Grapefruit juice may ↑ levels.

Route/Dosage
PO (Adults): *Upper GI motility disorders:* 10 mg 3 times daily; *Nausea/vomiting due to dopamine ago-*

nist antiparkinson agents: 10 mg 3 times daily; higher doses may be required during dose titration.

Renal Impairment
PO (Adults): Depending on degree of impairment, dosing during chronic therapy should be reduced to once or twice daily.

Availability
Tablets: 10 mg.

NURSING IMPLICATIONS
Assessment
● Assess for nausea, vomiting, abdominal distention, and bowel sounds before and after administration.
● Monitor BP (sitting, standing, lying down) and pulse before and periodically during therapy. May cause prolonged QT interval, tachycardia, and orthostatic hypotension, especially in patients older than 60 yr or taking >30 mg/day.
● Monitor for symptoms related to hyperprolactinemia (menstrual abnormalities, galactorrhea, sexual dysfunction).

Lab Test Considerations
● May cause ↑ serum ALT, AST, and cholesterol.
● Monitor serum prolactin prior to and periodically during therapy. May cause ↑ serum prolactin levels.

Implementation
● Use lowest effective dose.
● Administer 3 times daily, 15–30 min before meals and at bedtime.

Patient/Family Teaching
● Instruct patient to take as directed. Advise patient to avoid grapefruit juice during therapy.
● Advise patient to notify health care professional if galactorrhea (excessive or spontaneous flow of breast milk), gynecomastia (excessive development of male mammary gland), menstrual irregularities (spotting or delayed periods), palpitations, irregular heartbeat (arrhythmia), dizziness, or fainting occur.
● Rep: Advise females of reproductive potential to notify health care professional if pregnancy is planned or suspected or if breastfeeding.

Evaluation
● Prevention or relief of nausea and vomiting.
● Decreased symptoms of gastric stasis.

---

flupentixol (floo-**pen**-tiks-ol)
✦Fluanxol
Classification
Therapeutic: antipsychotics
Pharmacologic: thioxanthenes

Indications
Maintenance treatment of schizophrenia in patients whose symptomatology does not include excitement,

agitation, or hyperactivity. Not indicated for the treatment of dementia in the elderly.

Action
Alters the effects of dopamine in the CNS. Has some anticholinergic and alpha-adrenergic blocking activity. **Therapeutic Effects:** Diminished signs and symptoms of schizophrenia.

Pharmacokinetics
Absorption: *Flupentixol dihydrochloride:* 40% absorbed following oral administration; *Flupentixol decanoate:* slowly released from IM injection sites.
Distribution: Distributes to lungs, liver, and spleen; enter CNS; extensive tissue distribution.
Protein Binding: 99%.
Metabolism and Excretion: Mostly metabolized, metabolites do not have antipsychotic activity. Most metabolites are excreted in feces, some renal elimination.
Half-life: *Flupentixol dihydrochloride:* 35 hr; *Flupentixol decanoate:* 3 wk.

TIME/ACTION PROFILE (antipsychotic effect)

ROUTE	ONSET	PEAK	DURATION
PO	within 2–3 days	3–8 hr (blood level)	8 hr
IM (depot)	24–72 hr	4–7 days (blood level)	2–4 wk

Contraindications/Precautions
Contraindicated in: Hypersensitivity to flupentixol or other thioxanthines (cross-sensitivity with phenothiazines may occur); CNS depression due to any cause, including comatose states, cortical brain damage (known or suspected), or circulatory collapse; Opiate, alcohol, or barbiturate intoxication; Hepatic impairment, cerebrovascular insufficiency, or severe cardiovascular pathology; Concurrent use of other drugs known to prolong QT interval; Pedi: Safety and effectiveness not established; not recommended.
Use Cautiously in: Brain tumors or intestinal obstruction (may mask symptoms); Patients exposed to extreme heat or organophosphorous insecticides; Risk factors for/history of stroke; Any risk factors for QT prolongation including hypokalmia, hypomagnesemia, genetic predisposition, cardiovascular disease history (including bradycardia), recent MI, HF, or arrhythmias; Known/suspected glaucoma; History of seizures (may ↓ seizure threshold); Parkinson's disease (may worsen symptoms); Geri: Consider age-related ↓ in renal, cardiac, and hepatic function; OB: Use only if expected benefit outweighs potential risks to infant; Lactation: Safe use not established; low levels in breast milk are not expected to affect infant if therapeutic doses are used.

Adverse Reactions/Side Effects

CNS: dizziness, NEUROLEPTIC MALIGNANT SYNDROME. **EENT:** blurred vision. **CV:** extrapyramidal symptoms, tachycardia, hypotension, QT INTERVAL PROLONGATION, sedation, tardive dyskinesia, THROMBOEMBOLISM. **GI:** constipation, dry mouth, excess salivation, hepatotoxicity. **GU:** ↓ libido, urinary retention. **Derm:** photosensitivity reactions, rash, sweating. **Endo:** glucose intolerance, hyperprolactinemia, menstrual irregularity. **Hemat:** agranulocytosis, granulocytopenia, neutropenia. **Metab:** weight change. **MS:** osteoporosis (long term use).

Interactions

Drug-Drug: ↑ CNS depression with other **CNS depressants** including **alcohol**, some **antidepressants**, some **antihistamines**, **anxiolytics**, **benzodiazepines**, and **sedative/hypnotics**. ↑ risk of QT prolongation and serious arrhythmias with **Class Ia and III antiarrhythmics** (including **quinidine**, **amiodarone**, and **sotalol**), some **antipsychotics** (including **thioridazine**), some **macrolides** (including **erythromycin**), and some **fluoroquinolones** (including **moxifloxacin**); concurrent use should be avoided. Concurrent use of **diuretics** and other **drugs affecting electrolytes** may ↑ risk of QT interval prolongation and serious arrhythmias. ↑ risk of anticholinergic adverse reactions, including paralytic ileus when used concurrently with other **anticholinergics** or **drugs with anticholinergic side effects**. May ↓ metabolism and ↑ effects of **tricyclic antidepressants**. ↑ risk of extrapyramidal symptoms with **metoclopramide**. May ↓ effectiveness of **levodopa** and **dopamine agonists**.

Route/Dosage

PO (Adults): 1 mg 3 times daily initially; ↑ by 1 mg every 2–3 days until desired response, usual effective dose is 3–6 mg/day in divided doses (up to 12 mg/day has been used); if insomnia occurs, evening dose may be ↓.

IM (Adults): Initiate with a 5–20 mg test dose (use 5 mg dose in elderly/frail/cachectic patients) as the 2% injection. Patients previously treated with long-acting neuroleptic injections may tolerate initial doses of 20 mg. A 2nd 20 mg dose may be given 4–10 days later and then 20–40 mg every 2–3 wk depending on response. Oral flupentixol should be continued, but gradually decreased in the first wk following depot injection. Guidelines for conversion from PO to depot IM injection: daily oral dose (mg) × 4 = dose of depot injection (mg) given every 2 wk *or* daily oral dose (mg) × 8 = depot injection (mg) given every 4 wk.

Availability

Tablets (flupentixol dihydrochloride): 0.5 mg, 3 mg, 5 mg; **Depot injection (flupentixol decanoate: contains medium-chain triglycerides [coconut oil]):** 20 mg/mL (2%), 100 mg/mL (10%).

NURSING IMPLICATIONS

Assessment

- Assess mental status (orientation, mood, behavior) before and periodically during therapy.
- Monitor BP (sitting, standing, lying), ECG, pulse, and respiratory rate before and frequently during the period of dose adjustment. May cause QT prolongation.
- Observe carefully when administering oral medication to ensure that medication is actually taken and not hoarded.
- Assess weight and BMI initially and during therapy.
- Assess fluid intake and bowel function. Increased bulk and fluids in the diet help minimize constipation.
- Monitor for onset of akathisia (restlessness or desire to keep moving) and extrapyramidal side effects (*parkinsonian:* difficulty speaking or swallowing, loss of balance control, pill rolling, mask-like face, shuffling gait, rigidity, tremors; *dystonic:* muscle spasms, twisting motions, twitching, inability to move eyes, weakness of arms or legs) every 2 mo during therapy and 8–12 wk after therapy has been discontinued. Reduction in dose or discontinuation of medication may be necessary. Benztropine or diphenhydramine may be used to control these symptoms.
- Monitor for tardive dyskinesia (uncontrolled rhythmic movement of mouth, face, and extremities; lip smacking or puckering; puffing of cheeks; uncontrolled chewing; rapid or worm-like movements of tongue). Report immediately; may be irreversible.
- Monitor for development of neuroleptic malignant syndrome (fever, respiratory distress, tachycardia, seizures, diaphoresis, arrhythmias, hypertension or hypotension, pallor, tiredness, severe muscle stiffness, loss of bladder control). Report immediately.
- Monitor for symptoms related to hyperprolactinemia (menstrual abnormalities, galactorrhea, sexual dysfunction).

Lab Test Considerations

- Monitor CBC and liver function tests periodically during treatment. May cause ↑ AST, ALT, and alkaline phosphatase.
- Monitor blood glucose prior to and periodically during therapy. May cause hyperglycemia.
- Monitor serum prolactin prior to and periodically during therapy. May cause ↑ serum prolactin levels.
- May cause false-positive pregnancy tests.

Implementation

- **PO:** Initially, take tablets 3 times daily, without regard to food. Dose will increase for first few days until desired results. Maintenance dose is usually taken in morning.
- When converting to IM doses, PO dose is usually continued in decreasing doses for first wk.

- **IM:** Inject deep IM preferably into gluteus maximus. Solution is a yellow viscous oil, aspirate prior to injection to ensure dose is not injected IV. Do not administer solutions that are discolored, hazy, or contain particulate matter.
- For large doses or pain with large volume, flupentizol decanoate BP 10% (100 mg/mL) may be used instead of flupentixol decanoate BP 2% (20 mg/mL).

Patient/Family Teaching

- Instruct patient to take as directed. If a dose is missed, omit and take next dose as scheduled. Discontinuation should be gradual; abrupt discontinuation may cause withdrawal symptoms (nausea, vomiting, anorexia, diarrhea, rhinorrhea, sweating, myalgias, paraesthesias, insomnia, restlessness, anxiety, agitation, vertigo, feelings of warmth and coldness, tremor). Symptoms begin within 1 to 4 days of withdrawal and abate within 7 to 14 days. Advise patient to read *Patient Information* leaflet prior to starting therapy and with each Rx refill in case of changes.
- Inform patient of possibility of extrapyramidal symptoms and tardive dyskinesia. Caution patient to report these symptoms immediately to health care professional.
- Advise patient to change positions slowly to minimize orthostatic hypotension.
- Medication may cause drowsiness. Caution patient to avoid driving or other activities requiring alertness until response to medication is known.
- Advise patient to notify health care professional of all Rx or OTC medications, vitamins, or herbal products being taken and to consult with health care professional before taking other medications.
- Caution patient to avoid concurrent use of alcohol and other CNS depressants.
- Instruct patient to notify health care professional promptly if sore throat, fever, unusual bleeding or bruising, rash, weakness, tremors, visual disturbances, dark-colored urine, or clay-colored stools occur.
- Instruct patient to avoid sun exposure and to wear protective clothing and sunscreen when outdoors.
- Advise patient to notify health care professional of medication regimen before treatment or surgery.
- Rep: Advise females of reproductive potential to notify health care professional if pregnancy is planned or suspected or if breastfeeding.

Evaluation

- Decreased symptoms of schizophrenia (delusions, hallucinations, social withdrawal, flat, blunt affect).

---

fusidic acid (fyoo-**sid**-ik as-id)
✤Fucidin, ✤ Fucithalmic
Classification
Therapeutic: anti-infectives

Indications
Topical: Local treatment of primary and secondary bacterial skin infections including impetigo contagiosa, erythrasma and secondary skin infections such as infected wounds/burns. **Ophth:** Treatment of superficial eye infections.

Action
Inhibits bacterial protein synthesis. **Therapeutic Effects:** Resolution of localized bacterial infections. Not active against Gram-negative organisms; active against Staphylococci, Streptococci, and Corynebacterium.

Pharmacokinetics
Absorption: Unknown.
Distribution: Systemically absorbed drug crosses the placenta and enters breast milk.
Metabolism and Excretion: Absorbed drug is extensively metabolized.
Half-life: 5–6 hr.

TIME/ACTION PROFILE

ROUTE	ONSET	PEAK	DURATION
Top	unknown	unknown	6–8 hr
Ophth	unknown	unknown	12 hr

Contraindications/Precautions
Contraindicated in: Hypersensitivity to fusidic acid or other components of the formulation (topical ointment contains lanolin).
Use Cautiously in: OB: Potential benefits should be weighed against the possible hazards to the fetus (crosses the placenta); Lactation: Safe use during breastfeeding has not been established (enters breast milk).

Adverse Reactions/Side Effects
Derm: mild local irritation.

Interactions
Drug-Drug: None noted.

Route/Dosage
Topical (Adults and Children): Apply to affected area 3–4 times daily.
Ophth (Adults and Children): One drop into conjunctival sac of both eyes every 12 hr for 7 days.

Availability
Topical cream: 2% (20 mg/g); **Topical ointment (contains lanolin):** 2% (20 mg/g); **Ophthalmic viscous drops (microcrystalline suspension):** 1%. *In combination with:* hydrocortisone (Fucidin H).

NURSING IMPLICATIONS
Assessment
- Inspect involved areas of skin and mucous membranes before and frequently during therapy. Increased skin irritation may indicate need to discontinue medication.

Implementation
- Do not confuse topical product with ophthalmic product.
- **Topical:** Consult health care professional for proper cleansing technique before applying medication. Apply small amount to cover affected area completely. Avoid the use of occlusive wrappings or dressings unless directed by health care professional.
- **Ophth:** Administer 1 drop into conjunctival sac of both eyes every 12 hr for 7 days. See Appendix C for instructions.

Patient/Family Teaching
- Instruct patient to apply medication as directed for full course of therapy, even if feeling better. Emphasize the importance of avoiding the eyes.
- Advise patient to report increased skin irritation or lack of response to therapy to health care professional.

Evaluation
- Resolution of skin or eye infection.

---

gliclazide (glik-la-zide)
✦Diamicron MR
Classification
Therapeutic: antidiabetics
Pharmacologic: sulfonylureas

Indications
Control of blood sugar in type 2 diabetes mellitus when control of diet and exercise fails or when insulin is not an option. Requires some pancreatic function.

Action
Lowers blood glucose by stimulating the release of insulin from the pancreas and increasing sensitivity to insulin at receptor sites. **Therapeutic Effects:** Lowering of blood glucose in diabetic patients.

Pharmacokinetics
Absorption: Well absorbed following oral administration (97%).
Distribution: Unknown.
Protein Binding: 95%.
Metabolism and Excretion: Extensively metabolized, metabolites are mostly eliminated (60–70%) in urine, 10–20% in feces; <1% excreted unchanged in urine.
Half-life: *Tablets:* 10.4 hr; *modified-release tablets:* 16 hr.

TIME/ACTION PROFILE (effect on blood sugar)

ROUTE	ONSET	PEAK	DURATION
PO	unknown	4–6 hr (blood levels)	12–24 hr

Contraindications/Precautions
Contraindicated in: Hypersensitivity; cross-sensitivity with other sulfonylureas may occur; Unstable diabetes, type 1 diabetes mellitus, diabetic ketoacidosis, diabetic coma or pre-coma; Severe hepatic or renal impairment; Concurrent use of oral/oromucosal miconazole, alcohol or alcohol-containing medications, or systemic phenylbutazone; OB: Should not be used during pregnancy; insulin is preferred; Lactation: Should not be used during lactation; insulin is preferred.
Use Cautiously in: Glucose 6-phosphate dehydrogenase deficiency (↑ risk of hemolytic anemia); Infection, stress, or changes in diet may alter requirements for control of blood sugar or require use of insulin; Impaired thyroid, pituitary, or adrenal function; Malnutrition, high fever, prolonged nausea, or vomiting; Pedi: Safety and effectiveness not established.

Adverse Reactions/Side Effects
Endo: hypoglycemia. **GI:** ↑ liver enzymes, abdominal pain, diarrhea, dyspepsia, nausea, vomiting. **Derm:** photosensitivity, rash.

Interactions
Drug-Drug: Concurrent use of **alcohol, angiotensin converting-enzyme inhibitors, antituberculars, azole antifungals, beta-blockers, clarithromycin, clofibrate, disopyramide, H2–receptor antagonists, MAO inhibitors, NSAIDs, phenylbutazone, salicylates,** long-acting **sulfonamides, warfarin,** may ↑ risk of hypoglycemia. ↑ risk of hypoglycemia with other **antidiabetic agents** including **alpha glucosidase inhibitors, biguanides,** and **insulin**. Concurrent use of **chlorpromazine, corticosteroids, danazol, diuretics** (including **thiazides,** and **furosemide), hormonal contraceptives (estrogen** and **progestogen), nicotinic acid** (pharmacologic doses), **ritodrine, salbutamol, terbutaline,** or **tetracosactrin** may ↑ risk of hyperglycemia and lead to loss of diabetic control. May ↑ risk of bleeding with **warfarin**. Concurrent use with **alcohol** may result in a disulfiram-like reaction and should be avoided. **Beta-blockers** may ↓ some symptoms of hyperglycemia.

Route/Dosage
PO (Adults): *Tablets:* 80–320 mg/day, doses >160 mg/day should be divided and given twice daily; *modified-release tablets:* 30 mg daily, may be ↑ in 30-mg increments every 2 wk until blood sugar is controlled up to 120 mg/day.

Availability
Tablets (contain lactose): 80 mg; **Modified-release tablets:** 30 mg, 60 mg.

✦= Canadian drug name. ⋦ = Genetic implication. S̶t̶r̶i̶k̶e̶t̶h̶r̶o̶u̶g̶h̶ = Discontinued. CAPITALS = life-threatening. <u>Underline</u> = most frequent.

NURSING IMPLICATIONS
Assessment
- Observe for signs and symptoms of hypoglycemia (hunger, weakness, sweating, dizziness, tachycardia, anxiety).
- Assess patient for allergy to sulfonylureas.

Lab Test Considerations
- Monitor serum glucose and glycosylated hemoglobin periodically during therapy to evaluate effectiveness of treatment.
- Monitor liver function periodically in patients with mild to moderate liver dysfunction. May cause ↑ AST, ALT, alkaline phosphatase, and LDH.
- Monitor renal function periodically in patients with mild to moderate renal dysfunction. May cause ↑ creatinine and hyponatremia.

Toxicity and Overdose
- Overdose is manifested by symptoms of hypoglycemia. Mild hypoglycemia may be treated with administration of oral glucose. Treat severe hypoglycemia with IV D50W followed by continuous IV infusion of more dilute dextrose solution at a rate sufficient to keep serum glucose at approximately 100 mg/dL.

Implementation
- Patients on a diabetic regimen exposed to stress, fever, infection, trauma, or surgery may require administration of insulin.
- **PO:** Administer with meals at the same time every day.

Patient/Family Teaching
- Instruct patient to take gliclazides as directed at the same time every day.
- Explain to patient that this medication does not cure diabetes and must be used in conjunction with a prescribed diet, exercise regimen, to prevent hypoglycemic and hyperglycemic events.
- Instruct patient on proper technique for home glucose monitoring. Monitor closely during periods of stress or illness and notify health care professional if significant changes occur.
- Review signs of hypoglycemia and hyperglycemia with patient. If hypoglycemia occurs, advise patient to drink a glass of orange juice or ingest 2–3 tsp of sugar, honey, or corn syrup dissolved in water or an appropriate number of glucose tablets and notify health care professional.
- Encourage patient to follow prescribed diet, medication, and exercise regimen to prevent hypoglycemic or hyperglycemic episodes.
- Concurrent use of alcohol may cause a disulfiram-like reaction (abdominal cramps, nausea, flushing, headaches, and hypoglycemia).
- Instruct patient to avoid sun exposure and to wear protective clothing and sunscreen when outdoors.
- Caution patient to avoid other medications, especially aspirin and alcohol, while on this therapy without consulting health care professional.

- Advise patient to notify health care professional promptly if unusual weight gain, swelling of ankles, drowsiness, shortness of breath, muscle cramps, weakness, sore throat, rash, or unusual bleeding or bruising occurs.
- Advise patient to inform health care professional of medication regimen prior to treatment or surgery.
- Advise patient to carry sugar packets or candy, and identification describing diabetes diagnosis and medication regimen.
- Rep: Insulin is the recommended method of controlling blood sugar during pregnancy. Counsel female patients to use a form of contraception other than oral contraceptives and to notify health care professional promptly if pregnancy is planned or suspected.
- Emphasize the importance of routine follow-up exams.

Evaluation
- Control of blood glucose levels to avoid episodes of hypoglycemia and hyperglycemia.

methotrimeprazine
(meth-oh-try-**mep**-ra-zeen)
❖Methoprazine, ❖ Nozinan
Classification
Therapeutic: antipsychotics, nonopioid analgesics
Pharmacologic: phenothiazines

Indications
Management of psychotic disturbances. Management of conditions associated with anxiety/tension. As an analgesic and adjunct in pain due to cancer, zona, trigeminal neuralgia, intercostal neuralgia, phantom limb pain, and muscular discomforts. Used as a preoperative sedative. As an antiemetic. As a sedative in the treatment of insomnia.

Action
Sedation. **Therapeutic Effects:** Reduction in severity of pain.

Pharmacokinetics
Absorption: Well absorbed after PO/IM administration. IV administration results in complete bioavailability.
Distribution: Enters CSF and crosses the placenta. Minimal amounts enter breast milk.
Metabolism and Excretion: Mostly metabolized by the liver. Some metabolites are active; 1% excreted unchanged by the kidneys.
Half-life: 15–30 hr.

TIME/ACTION PROFILE

ROUTE	ONSET	PEAK	DURATION
PO (blood levels)	unknown	2.7–2.9 hr	8–12 hr
IM (analgesia)	unknown	20–40 min	8 hr (up to 24 hr in children)

Contraindications/Precautions

Contraindicated in: Blood dyscrasias; Hepatic impairment; Hypersensitivity to methotrimeprazine, phenothiazines or sulfites; Comatose patients or those who have overdosed on CNS depressants including alcohol, analgesics, opioids, or sedative/hypnotics; OB: Third-trimester use may result in agitation, hypotonia, tremor, somnolence, respiratory distress, and feeding disturbances in newborn and should be avoided.

Use Cautiously in: History of seizures; History of glaucoma or prostatic hypertrophy (↑ risk of anticholinergic adverse reactions); Bradycardia, electrolyte abnormalities, congenital/acquired prolonged QT interval or concurrent use of drugs that may prolong QT interval (↑ risk of serious arrhythmias); Underlying cardiovascular disease including stroke, arteriosclerosis, or thromboembolism (↑ risk of adverse cardiovascular effects); Geri: Initial dosage ↓ recommended, ↑ risk of death in elderly patients with dementia; Lactation: Safety not established; Pedi: Safety not established.

Adverse Reactions/Side Effects

CNS: amnesia, drowsiness, excess sedation, disorientation, euphoria, extrapyramidal reactions, headache, NEUROLEPTIC MALIGNANT SYNDROME, SEIZURES, slurred speech, tardive dyskinesia, weakness. **EENT:** nasal congestion. **CV:** orthostatic hypotension, bradycardia, palpitations, tachycardia. **GI:** constipation, abdominal discomfort, dry mouth, nausea, vomiting. **GU:** difficulty in urination. **Endo:** hyperglycemia, hyperprolactinemia. **Hemat:** blood dyscrasias. **Local:** pain at injection site. **Misc:** chills.

Interactions

Drug-Drug: ↑ CNS depression with other **CNS depressants**, including **alcohol**, **antihistamines**, **antidepressants**, **opioids**, or **sedative/hypnotics**; ↓ dose of these agents by 50% initially. ↑ anticholinergic effects with **antihistamines**, **antidepressants**, **phenothiazines**, **quinidine**, **disopyramide**, **atropine**, or **scopolamine**; ↓ doses of concurrent atropine or scopolamine. Reverses vasopressor effects of **epinephrine**; avoid concurrent use—if vasopressor required, use phenylephrine or norepinephrine. ↑ risk of hypotension with acute ingestion of **alcohol**, **nitrates**, **MAO inhibitors**, or **antihypertensives**. Concurrent use with **succinylcholine** may result in tachycardia, hypotension, CNS stimulation, delirium, and ↑ extrapyramidal symptoms.

Drug-Natural Products: Concomitant use of **kava**, **valerian**, **skullcap**, **chamomile**, or **hops** ↑ risk of CNS depression.

Route/Dosage

PO (Adults): *Minor conditions:* 6–25 mg/day in 3 divided doses (if sedation occurs, use smaller daytime doses and a larger dose at bedtime); *Night time sedative:* 10–25 mg as a single bedtime dose; *Psychoses/intense pain:* 50–75 mg/day in 2–3 divided doses, dose

may be titrated upward to desired effect (doses of 1 g/day have been used, if daily dose exceeds 100–200 mg, administer in divided doses and keep patient at bedrest).

PO (Children): 0.25 mg/kg/day in 2–3 divided doses (not to exceed 40 mg/day in children <12 yr).

IM (Adults): *Postoperative analgesic adjunct:* 10–25 mg every 8 hr; if given with opioids, ↓ opioid dose by 50%.

IM (Children): *Analgesia:* 62.5–125 mcg (0.0625–0.125 mg)/kg/day single dose or divided doses, change to oral medication as soon as possible.

IV (Children): *Palliative care setting:* 62.5 mcg (0.0625 mg)/kg/day in 250 mL of 5% dextrose solution as a slow infusion (20–40 drops/min).

Availability

Tablets: 2 mg, 5 mg, 25 mg, 50 mg; **Solution for injection:** 25 mg/mL.

NURSING IMPLICATIONS
Assessment

- Assess type, location, and intensity of pain before and 30 min after administration.
- Monitor BP frequently after injection. Orthostatic hypotension, fainting, syncope, and weakness frequently occur from 10 min to 12 hr after administration. Patient should remain supine for 6–12 hr after injection.
- Assess weight and BMI initially and throughout therapy.
- Observe patient carefully for extrapyramidal side effects (*parkinsonian:* difficulty speaking or swallowing, loss of balance control, pill rolling, mask-like face, shuffling gait, rigidity, tremors; *dystonic:* muscle spasms, twisting motions, twitching, inability to move eyes, weakness of arms or legs). Usually occur only after prolonged or high-dose therapy. Usually resolve with dose decrease or administration of antiparkinsonian agent.
- Monitor for tardive dyskinesia (involuntary rhythmic movement of mouth, face, and extremities). Report immediately and discontinue therapy; may be irreversible.
- Monitor for development of neuroleptic malignant syndrome (fever, respiratory distress, tachycardia, seizures, diaphoresis, hypertension or hypotension, pallor, tiredness). Discontinue methotrimeprazine and notify health care professional immediately if these symptoms occur.
- Methotrimeprazine potentiates the action of other CNS depressants but can be given in conjunction with modified doses of opioid analgesics for management of severe pain. This medication does not significantly depress respiratory status and can be useful where pulmonary reserve is low.
- Monitor for symptoms related to hyperprolactinemia (menstrual abnormalities, galactorrhea, sexual dysfunction).

✿= Canadian drug name. ※ = Genetic implication. S̶t̶r̶i̶k̶e̶t̶h̶r̶o̶u̶g̶h̶ = Discontinued. CAPITALS = life-threatening. <u>Underline</u> = most frequent.

D R U G S

A P P R O V E D

I N

C A N A D A

Lab Test Considerations

- Monitor CBC prior to and periodically during therapy and liver function tests should be evaluated periodically throughout long-term (>30 days) therapy.
- Monitor blood glucose prior to and periodically during therapy. May cause hyperglycemia.
- Monitor serum prolactin prior to and periodically during therapy. May cause ↑ serum prolactin levels.

Implementation

- **PO:** May be administered during day or only at night depending on indication.
- **IM:** Do not inject SUBQ. Inject slowly into deep, well-developed muscle. Rotate injection sites.
- **Intermittent Infusion:** For patients in palliative care, may be infused as 0.0625 mg/kg/day in 250 mL of D5W. *Rate:* Infuse slowly 20–40 drops per min.
- **Y-Site Compatibility:** fentanyl hydromorphone, methadone, morphine, sufentanil.
- **Y-Site Incompatibility:** heparin.

Patient/Family Teaching

- Instruct patient on how and when to ask for pain medication.
- Instruct patient to take medication as directed. Take missed doses as soon as remembered unless almost time for next dose; do not double dose. Advise patient to read *Patient Information* leaflet prior to starting therapy and with each Rx refill in case of changes.
- Advise patients to make position changes slowly and to remain recumbent for 6–12 hr after administration to minimize orthostatic hypotension.
- May cause drowsiness. Caution patient to request assistance with ambulation and transfer and to avoid driving or other activities requiring alertness until response to the medication is known.
- Advise patient to notify health care professional of all Rx or OTC medications, vitamins, or herbal products being taken and to consult with health care professional before taking other medications.
- Caution patient to avoid taking alcohol or other CNS depressants concurrently with this medication.
- Advise patient to use sunscreen and protective clothing when exposed to the sun. Extremes of temperature should also be avoided because this drug impairs body temperature regulation.
- Instruct patient to use frequent mouth rinses, good oral hygiene, and sugarless gum or candy to minimize dry mouth.
- Instruct patient to notify health care professional promptly if sore throat, fever, unusual bleeding or bruising, rash, weakness, tremors, dark-colored urine, or clay-colored stools or signs of blood clots (swelling, pain, and redness in an arm or leg that can be warm to touch, sudden chest pain, difficulty breathing, heart palpitations) occur.

Evaluation

- Decrease in severity of pain.
- Sedation.

moclobemide
(moe-**kloe**-be-mide)
✤Manerix

Classification
Therapeutic: antidepressants
Pharmacologic: monamine oxidase (MAO) inhibitors, benzamides

Indications
Treatment of depression.

Action
Short-acting, reversible inhibitor of monoamine oxidase type A. Increases concentrations of serotonin, norepinephrine, and dopamine. **Therapeutic Effects:** Decreased symptoms of depression, with improved mood and quality of life.

Pharmacokinetics
Absorption: 98% absorbed following oral administration, but undergoes first-pass hepatic metabolism resulting in 90% bioavailability.
Distribution: Unknown.
Metabolism and Excretion: Extensively metabolized (partially by CYP2C19 and CYP2D6), very small amounts are pharmacologically active, less than 1% excreted unchanged in urine.
Half-life: 1.5 hr (↑ with dose).

TIME/ACTION PROFILE

ROUTE	ONSET	PEAK	DURATION
PO	days–several wk (antidepressant effect)	0.5–3.5 hr (blood levels)	24 hr (MAO-A inhibition)

Contraindications/Precautions
Contraindicated in: Known hypersensitivity; Acute confusional states; Concurrent use of tricyclic antidepressants; Concurrent use of SSRIs or other MAO inhibitors; Concurrent use of dextromethorphan, meperidine, selegiline, or thioridazine; Pedi: Safety not established, use is not recommended.
Use Cautiously in: History of suicide attempt or ideation; History of thyrotoxicosis or pheochromocytoma (possible risk of hypertensive reaction); Severe hepatic impairment (↓ dose required); Renal impairment; OB: Should not be used unless anticipated benefits justify potential harm to fetus; Lactation: Not recommended unless anticipated benefits justify potential harm to infant.

Adverse Reactions/Side Effects
CNS: agitation, insomnia, restlessness, SUICIDAL IDEATION, tremor. **CV:** hypotension.

Interactions
Drug-Drug: ↑ levels and risk of QT prolongation with **thioridazine**, avoid concurrent use. Concurrent use with **selegiline** greatly ↑ sensitivity to tyramine and is

contraindicated. Concurrent use with **tricyclic antidepressants** may result in severe adverse reactions and is contraindicated. Should not be used with **SSRIs** or other **MAO inhibitors**; when making a switch allow 4–5 half-lives of previous drug; for **fluoxetine** wait at least 5 wk. Excessive **alcohol** should be avoided. **Cimetidine** ↓ metabolism and ↑ blood levels, ↓ moclobemide dose by 50%. Because of the potential for interactions with **anesthetics**, especially local anesthetics containing **epinephrine**, moclobemide should be discontinued at least 2 days prior to procedures. Concurrent use with **opioids** should be avoided; dosage adjustments may be necessary. Concurrent use of **sympathomimetics** including **ephedrine** and **amphetamines** may ↑ blood pressure and should be avoided. Concurrent use with **dextromethorphan** may result in vertigo, tremor, nausea and vomiting and should be avoided. Concurrent use with **antihypertensives** should be carefully monitored. **Drug-Food:** Ingestion of large amounts of **tyramine-containing foods**, including some cheeses and **Marmite yeast extract** may result in hypertension and arrhythmias and should be undertaken with caution.

Route/Dosage
PO (Adults): 150 mg twice daily initially; may be ↑ gradually after one wk as needed/tolerated up to 600 mg/day.

Hepatic Impairment
PO (Adults): *Severe hepatic impairment or concurrent enzyme inhibitor (cimetidine):* ↓ daily dose to ⅓ to ½ of standard dose.

Availability
Tablets: 100 mg, 150 mg, 300 mg.

NURSING IMPLICATIONS
Assessment
- Assess mental status for orientation, mood, behavior, and anxiety. Assess for suicidal tendencies. Restrict amount of drug available to patient.
- Monitor BP and pulse before and frequently during therapy. Report significant changes promptly.
- Monitor mood changes. Assess for suicidal tendencies, especially during early therapy. Restrict amount of drug available to patient.
- Monitor intake and output ratios and daily weight. Assess patient for peripheral edema and urinary retention.

Lab Test Considerations
- Monitor liver and kidney function periodically during treatment.
- Monitor serum glucose closely in diabetic patients; hypoglycemia may occur.

Toxicity and Overdose
- Concurrent ingestion of tyramine-rich foods and many medications may result in a life-threatening hypten-

sive crisis. Signs and symptoms of hypertensive crisis include chest pain, tachycardia, severe headache, nausea and vomiting, photosensitivity, and enlarged pupils. Treatment includes IV phentolamine.
- Symptoms of overdose include anxiety, irritability, tachycardia, hypertension or hypotension, respiratory distress, dizziness, drowsiness, hallucinations, confusion, seizures, fever, and diaphoresis. Treatment includes induction of vomiting or gastric lavage and supportive therapy as symptoms arise.

Implementation
- Administer after meals. Swallow tablet whole; do not crush, break, or chew. Dose may be adjusted gradually during the first wk of therapy.

Patient/Family Teaching
- Instruct patient to take medication as directed. Take missed doses if remembered unless almost time for next dose; do not double doses. Do not discontinue abruptly; withdrawal symptoms (nausea, vomiting, malaise, nightmares, agitation, psychosis, seizures) may occur. Advise patient to read *Patient Information* leaflet prior to starting and with each Rx refill in case of changes.
- Caution patient to avoid alcohol, CNS depressants, OTC drugs, and foods or beverages containing tyramine (see Appendix J) during and for at least 2 wk after therapy has been discontinued; they may precipitate a hypertensive crisis. Contact health care professional immediately if symptoms of hypertensive crisis develop.
- Caution patient to notify health care professional if neck stiffness, changes in vision, diarrhea, constipation, rapid/pounding heartbeat, sudden and severe headache, stiff neck, confusion, disorientation, slurred speech, behavioral changes, seizures.
- Advise patient and family to notify health care professional if thoughts about suicide or dying, attempts to commit suicide; new or worse depression; new or worse anxiety; feeling very agitated or restless; panic attacks; trouble sleeping; new or worse irritability; acting aggressive; being angry or violent; acting on dangerous impulses; an extreme increase in activity and talking; other unusual changes in behavior or mood occur.
- Instruct patient to carry identification describing medication regimen.
- Rep: Advise females of reproductive potential to notify health care professional if pregnancy is planned or suspected or if breastfeeding.
- Encourage patient to participate in psychotherapy in conjunction with taking medication.

Evaluation
- Improved mood in depressed patients.
- Decreased anxiety.

🍁 = Canadian drug name. ⚏ = Genetic implication. ~~Strikethrough~~ = Discontinued. CAPITALS = life-threatening. <u>Underline</u> = most frequent.

D
R
U
G
S

A
P
P
R
O
V
E
D

I
N

C
A
N
A
D
A

pinaverium (pin-ah-**veer**-ee-um)
✦Dicetel
Classification
Therapeutic: anti-irritable bowel syndrome agents
Pharmacologic: calcium channel blockers

Indications
Management of symptoms of irritable bowel syndrome, (IBS) including abdominal pain, bowel disturbances and discomfort. Treatment of symptoms related to biliary tract disorders.

Action
Acts as a calcium channel blocker with specific selectivity for intestinal smooth muscle. Relaxes gastrointestinal (mainly colon) and biliary tracts, inhibits colonic motor response to food/pharmacologic stimulation. **Therapeutic Effects:** Decreased symptoms of IBS.

Pharmacokinetics
Absorption: Poorly absorbed (1–10%).
Distribution: Distributes selectively to digestive tract.
Protein Binding: 97%.
Metabolism and Excretion: Minimal enterohepatic cycling, eliminated almost entirely in feces. Some metabolism.
Half-life: 1.5 hr.

TIME/ACTION PROFILE (blood levels)

ROUTE	ONSET	PEAK	DURATION
PO	unknown	1 hr	unknown

Contraindications/Precautions
Contraindicated in: Known hypersensitivity; Galactose intolerance/Lapp lactase deficiency/glucose-galactose malabsorption (tablets contain lactose); Lactation: Avoid use if breastfeeding; Pedi: Safety and effectiveness not established, use is not recommended.
Use Cautiously in: Pre-existing esophageal lesions/hiatal hernia (glass of water and snack should be taken with each dose); OB: Should be used only if essential to welfare of patient.

Adverse Reactions/Side Effects
All less than 1%. **CNS:** drowsiness, headache, vertigo. **GI:** constipation, diarrhea, distention, dry mouth, epigastric pain/fullness, esophageal irritation, nausea. **Derm:** rash.

Interactions
Drug-Drug: Concurrent use of **anticholinergics** may ↑ spasmolytic effects.

Route/Dosage
PO (Adults): 50 mg 3 times daily; may be ↑ as needed/tolerated up to 100 mg 3 times daily.

Availability
Tablets (contain lactose): 50 mg, 100 mg.

NURSING IMPLICATIONS
Assessment
● Assess for symptoms of IBS (abdominal pain or discomfort, bloating, constipation).
● Assess for lactose intolerance; product contains lactose.

Implementation
● **PO:** Administer tablet with a glass of water and food. Swallow tablet whole, do not crush, chew, or suck. If >3 tablets/day prescribed, take additional tablets with glass of water and a snack. May be irritating to esophagus. Do not take the tablet while lying down or just before bedtime.

Patient/Family Teaching
● Instruct patient to take pinaverium as directed. Take missed doses as soon as remembered unless almost time for next dose; do not double doses.
● Caution patient to inform health care professional if the following side effects persist or worsen: stomach pain or fullness, nausea, constipation or diarrhea, heartburn, headache, dry mouth, dizziness, skin rash.
● Instruct patient to avoid alcohol intake while taking this medication.
● Rep: Advise females of reproductive potential to inform health care professional if pregnancy is planned or suspected or if breastfeeding.

Evaluation
● A decrease in symptoms of irritable bowel syndrome. The length of treatment depends on the condition being treated.

prucalopride succinate
(proo-**kal**-o-pride)
✦Resotran
Classification
Therapeutic: prokinetic agents
Pharmacologic: dihydrobenzofurancarboxamides

Indications
Treatment of chronic idiopathic constipation in adult females who do not respond to laxatives.

Action
Acts as a serotonin (5–HT$_4$) receptor agonist with prokinetic properties. Enhances peristalsis and gastrointestinal propulsion. **Therapeutic Effects:** Laxative effect.

Pharmacokinetics
Absorption: Rapidly absorbed (90%) following oral administration.

Distribution: Rapidly and extensively distributed, enters breast milk.

Metabolism and Excretion: 60% excreted unchanged in urine, 3–8% unchanged in feces, minor amounts are extensively metabolized.

Half-life: 24 hr.

TIME/ACTION PROFILE (normalization of bowel movements)

ROUTE	ONSET	PEAK	DURATION
PO	3–4 days	1–4 wk	unknown

Contraindications/Precautions

Contraindicated in: Hypersensitivity; Renal impairment requiring dialysis; Intestinal obstruction/perforation (structural or functional), obstructive ileus, severe gastrointestinal inflammatory disease, including Crohn's disease, ulcerative colitis, toxic megacolon/megarectum; Galactose intolerance, Lapp lactase deficiency or glucose/galactose malabsorption (tablets contain lactose); OB: Not recommended for use during pregnancy; Lactation: Not recommended for use while breastfeeding; Pedi: Safety and effectiveness not established; not recommended for use.

Use Cautiously in: Severe/clinically stable concurrent chronic diseases including liver, cardiovascular or lung disease, neurological or psychiatric disorders, cancer, AIDS or other disorders or insulin-dependent diabetes mellitus; History of arrhythmias or cardiovascular disease, ischemic heart disease, pre-excitation syndromes (including Wolff Parkinson-White syndrome, Lown-Ganong-Levine syndrome, or AV nodal disorders (↑ risk of arrhythmias); Severe renal impairment (↓ dose recommended); Geri: Due to age-related ↓ in renal function, ↓ dose is recommended.

Adverse Reactions/Side Effects

CNS: <u>headache</u>, dizziness, fatigue. **CV:** ↓ PR interval, palpitations, tachycardia. **GI:** <u>abdominal pain</u>, diarrhea, <u>nausea</u>, vomiting.

Interactions

Drug-Drug: Severe diarrhea may ↓ effectiveness of **oral hormonal contraceptives**; additional method of contraception recommended. Blood levels and effects are ↑ by concurrent CYP3A4 and P-gp inhibitors including **ketoconazole**, **verapamil**, **cyclosporine**, and **quinidine**. Beneficial effects may be ↓ by concurrent use of **anticholinergics**.

Route/Dosage

PO (Adults): 2 mg once daily. If no bowel movement occurs in 3–4 days, add-on laxatives should be considered. If benefit is not obtained after 4 wk, prucalopride succinate should be discontinued.

PO (Adults >65 yr): 1 mg once daily.

Renal Impairment

PO (Adults): *GFR <30 mL/min/1.73m²:* 1 mg once daily.

Availability

Tablets (contain lactose): 1 mg, 2 mg.

NURSING IMPLICATIONS
Assessment
- Assess for symptoms of chronic constipation (abdominal pain or discomfort, bloating, constipation).

Implementation
- **PO:** Medication should be taken with food or on an empty stomach at the same time each day.

Patient/Family Teaching
- Instruct patient to take prucalopride succinate as directed.
- Caution the patient to discontinue the medication and notify health care professional with occurrence of severe diarrhea, signs of heart attack, black tarry stools, vomiting of blood or material that looks like coffee grounds.
- Advise patient on a nutritional regimen and hydration, and exercise to decrease constipation.
- Inform patient that if no bowel movement within 3 days of treatment, a "rescue" laxative may be added occasionally while taking prucalopride succinate.
- Rep: Advise females of reproductive potential who are taking prucalopride succinate to use an effective method of birth control during treatment. If pregnancy occurs while taking this medication, contact health care professional immediately.

Evaluation
- A soft, formed bowel movement.

---

trimebutine (try-meh-boo-teen)
✤Modulon
Classification
Therapeutic: lower gastrointestinal tract motility regulators, spasmolytics

Indications
Symptomatic treatment of irritable bowel syndrome (IBS). Treatment of postoperative paralytic ileus.

Action
Acts as a spasmolytic. **Therapeutic Effects:** ↓ symptoms of IBS. Resumption of intestinal transit following abdominal surgical procedures.

Pharmacokinetics
Absorption: Rapidly absorbed following oral administration.

Distribution: Unknown.

✤ = Canadian drug name. ⅀ = Genetic implication. S̶t̶r̶i̶k̶e̶t̶h̶r̶o̶u̶g̶h̶ = Discontinued. CAPITALS = life-threatening. <u>Underline</u> = most frequent.

Metabolism and Excretion: Extensively metabolized, <2.4% excreted unchanged in urine.
Half-life: 2.7–3.1 hr.

TIME/ACTION PROFILE (symptom relief)

ROUTE	ONSET	PEAK	DURATION
PO	within 3 days–2 wk	1 hr (blood level)	>1 wk (following discontinuation)

Contraindications/Precautions
Contraindicated in: Hypersensitivity.
Use Cautiously in: OB: Not recommended for use; Pedi: Children <12 yr (safety and effectiveness not established).

Adverse Reactions/Side Effects
CNS: dizziness, drowsiness, fatigue, headache. **GI:** diarrhea, dry mouth, dysgeusia, dyspepsia, epigastric pain, nausea. **Derm:** hot/cold sensation, rash.

Interactions
Drug-Drug: None known.

Route/Dosage
PO (Adults): 200 mg 3 times daily.

Availability
Tablets: 100 mg, 200 mg.

NURSING IMPLICATIONS
Assessment
- Assess for symptoms of irritable bowel syndrome (cramping, constipation and diarrhea, mucus in stools).
- Assess for abdominal distention and assess bowel sounds.
- Monitor intake and output and record.

Implementation
- PO: Administer three times daily before meals.

Patient/Family Teaching
- Instruct patient to take trimebutine as directed.
- Rep: Advise females of reproductive potential to inform health care professional if pregnancy is planned or suspected or if breastfeeding.

Evaluation
- Decrease signs and symptoms of irritable bowel disease.

zopiclone (zoe-pi-clone)
✦Imovane
Classification
Therapeutic: sedative/hypnotics
Pharmacologic: cyclopyrrolones

Indications
Short-term treatment of insomnia characterized by difficulty falling asleep and frequent/early awakenings.

Action
Interacts with GABA-receptor complexes; not a benzodiazepine. **Therapeutic Effects:** Improved sleep with decreased latency and increased maintenance of sleep.

Pharmacokinetics
Absorption: Rapidly absorbed (75%) following oral administration.
Distribution: Rapidly distributed from extravascular compartment. Enters breast milk in concentrations that are 50% of plasma levels.
Metabolism and Excretion: Extensively metabolized (mostly by the CYP3A4 enzyme system), metabolites have minimal sedative/hypnotic activity; 4–5% excreted unchanged in urine.
Half-life: 5 hr.

TIME/ACTION PROFILE

ROUTE	ONSET	PEAK	DURATION
PO	rapid	2 hr	6 hr

Contraindications/Precautions
Contraindicated in: Hypersensitivity; Myasthenia gravis; Severe hepatic impairment; Severe respiratory impairment (including sleep apnea); Galactose intolerance (5 mg tablet contains lactose); OB: May cause fetal harm, neonatal CNS depression or withdrawal; Lactation: Breastfeeding not recommended.
Use Cautiously in: Renal, hepatic, or pulmonary impairment (dosage ↓ may be recommended); Past history of paradoxical reactions to sedative/hypnotics or alcohol or violent behavior; History of depression or suicidal ideation; Geri: ↑ sensitivity may ↑ the risk of falls, confusion, or anterograde amnesia (use lowest effective dose); Pedi: Safety and effectiveness not established.
Exercise Extreme Caution in: History of substance/alcohol abuse.

Adverse Reactions/Side Effects
CV: abnormal thinking, behavioral changes, sleep-driving. **GI:** bitter taste, anorexia, constipation, dry mouth, dyspepsia. **Misc:** allergic reactions including ANAPHYLAXIS, ANAPHYLACTOID REACTIONS, and ANGIOEDEMA.

Interactions
Drug-Drug: ↑ risk of CNS depression with other **CNS depressants** including **antihistamines**, **antidepressants**, **opioids**, **sedative/hypnotics**, and **antipsychotics**. ↑ levels and risk of CNS depression with **drugs that inhibit the CYP3A4 enzyme system**, including **erythromycin ketoconazole**, **itraconazole**, **clarithromycin**, **nefazodone**, **ritonavir**, and **nelfinavir**; ↓ dose may be necessary. Levels and effectiveness may be ↓ by **drugs that induce the CYP3A4 enzyme system**, including **carbamazepine**, **phenobarbital**, **phenytoin**, **rifampicin**, and **rifampin**; dose ↑ may be necessary.

Route/Dosage
PO (Adults): 5–7.5 mg taken immediately before bedtime; not to exceed 7.5 mg or 7–10 days use. Geri: 3.75 mg initially taken immediately before bedtime; may be ↑ up to 7.5 mg if needed.

Hepatic/Renal Impairment
PO (Adults): 3.75 mg initially taken immediately before bedtime; may be ↑ up to 7.5 mg if needed.

Availability
Tablets: 5 mg, 7.5 mg.

NURSING IMPLICATIONS
Assessment
- Assess mental status, sleep patterns, and previous use of sedative/hypnotics. Prolonged use of >7–10 days may lead to physical and psychological dependence.
- Assess alertness at time of peak of drug. Notify health care professional if desired sedation does not occur.
- Assess patient for pain. Medicate as needed. Untreated pain decreases sedative effects.

Implementation
- Before administering, reduce external stimuli and provide comfort measures to increase effectiveness of medication.
- Protect patient from injury. Raise bed side rails. Assist with ambulation. Remove cigarettes from patients.
- Use lowest effective dose.
- **PO:** Tablets should be swallowed with full glass of water. For faster onset of sleep, do not administer with or immediately after a meal.

Patient/Family Teaching
- Instruct patient to take zopiclone as directed. Advise patient not to take zopiclone unless able to stay in bed a full night (7–8 hr) before being active again. Do not take more than the amount prescribed because of the habit-forming potential. Not recommended for use longer than 7–10 days. If used for 2 wk or longer, abrupt withdrawal may result in fatigue, nausea, flushing, light-headedness, uncontrolled crying, vomiting, GI upset, panic attack, or nervousness. Instruct patient to read *Patient Information* for correct product before taking and with each Rx refill, changes may occur.
- Because of rapid onset, advise patient to go to bed immediately after taking zopiclone.
- May cause daytime drowsiness or dizziness. Advise patient to avoid driving or other activities requiring alertness until response to this medication is known.
- Caution patient that complex sleep-related behaviors (sleep-driving) may occur while asleep.
- Advise patient to notify health care professional immediately if signs of anaphylaxis (swelling of the

tongue or throat, trouble breathing, and nausea and vomiting) occur.
- Caution patient to avoid concurrent use of alcohol or other CNS depressants.

Evaluation
- Relief of insomnia by improved falling asleep and decreased frequency of nocturnal and early morning awakenings.

zuclopenthixol
(zoo-kloe-pen-**thix**-ole)
✹Clopixol, ✹ Clopixol-Acuphase, ✹ Clopixol Depot
Classification
Therapeutic: antipsychotics
Pharmacologic: thioxanthenes

Indications
Management of schizophrenia; *oral:* initial and maintenance management; *IM (acuphase):* initial treatment of acute psychotic episodes or exacerbation of psychosis due to schizophrenia; *IM (depot):* maintenance management of schizophrenia.

Action
Has high affinity for dopamine D_1 and D_2 receptors, α_1–adrenergic and 5–HT_2 receptors. Dopaminergic blockade produces neuroleptic activity. **Therapeutic Effects:** Decreases psychoses due to schizophrenia.

Pharmacokinetics
Absorption: *PO:* well absorbed following oral administration; *IM (depot and acuphase):* slowly absorbed from IM sites.
Distribution: Enters breast milk.
Metabolism and Excretion: Mostly metabolized (partially by the CYP2D6 enzyme system), metabolites do not have antipsychotic activity; minimal amounts excreted unchanged in urine.
Half-life: *PO:* 20 hr.

TIME/ACTION PROFILE (antipsychotic effect)

ROUTE	ONSET	PEAK	DURATION
PO	within hrs	4 hr (blood level)	8–24 hr
IM (acetate [Acuphase])	2–4 hr	8 hr (sedation)	2–3 days
IM (decanoate [Depot])	within 3 days	3–7 days (blood level)	2–4 wk

Contraindications/Precautions
Contraindicated in: Treatment of dementia; Narrow angle glaucoma; Pedi: Safety and effectiveness not established, use not recommended.

✹ = Canadian drug name. ✗ = Genetic implication. ~~Strikethrough~~ = Discontinued. CAPITALS = life-threatening. <u>Underline</u> = most frequent.

Use Cautiously in: Hepatic or renal impairment; Electrolyte abnormalities, including hypokalemia, hypomagnesemia, concurrent diuretic therapy or drugs affecting QT interval or cardiovascular disease/history (↑ risk of serious arrhythmias); Intestinal pathology or brain lesions (antiemetic effect may mask symptoms); History of seizures (may ↓ threshold); Parkinson's disease (may cause deterioration); Risk factors/history of stroke; Abrupt discontinuation (should be tapered); **Geri:** Consider age-related ↓ in renal, hepatic, and cardiovascular function, concurrent disease states and drug therapies; **OB:** Infants exposed in the third trimester may exhibit extrapyramidal and withdrawal reactions including agitation, hypertonia, hypotonia, tremor, somnolence, respiratory distress, and feeding disorders; do not use in pregnancy unless expected benefit to the mother outweighs potential fetal risks; **Lactation:** Enters breast milk; safety not established.

Adverse Reactions/Side Effects

CNS: dizziness, extrapyramidal symptoms, fatigue, sedation, NEUROLEPTIC MALIGNANT SYNDROME, tardive dyskinesia, syncope, weakness. **EENT:** abnormal vision accommodation. **CV:** arrhythmias, hypotension, tachycardia, THROMBOEMBOLISM. **GI:** constipation, dry mouth, diarrhea, thirst, vomiting. **Derm:** ↑ sweating, photosensitivity reactions. **Endo:** hyperprolactinemia, hyperglycemia. **GU:** ↓ libido, abnormal urination. **Hemat:** anemia, granulocytopenia. **Metab:** weight change. **MS:** myalgia.

Interactions

Drug-Drug: ↑ risk of CNS depression with other **CNS depressants** including **alcohol**, some **antihistamines**, some **antidepressants**, **anxiolytics**, **barbiturates**, **benzodiazepines**, and **sedative/hypnotics**. ↑ levels and risk of toxicity with **CYP2D6 inhibitors**. Concurrent use of **diuretics**, **lithium**, **Class Ia and III antiarrhythmics** including **amiodarone**, **sotalol**, and **quinidine**; some **antipsychotics** including **thioridazine**, some **macrolides** including **erythromycin**; and some **fluoroquinolones** including **moxifloxacin** ↑ risk of QT interval prolongation and serious arrhythmias; concurrent use should be avoided. ↑ risk of anticholinergic adverse reactions with other **anticholinergic drugs**. ↑ risk of hypotension with **antihypertensives** and **diuretics**. Concurrent use with **tricyclic antidepressants** may result in altered metabolism and effects of both. ↑ risk of extrapyramidal symptoms with **metoclopramide**. May ↓ beneficial effects of **levodopa** and **dopamine agonists**.

Route/Dosage

PO (Adults): *Acute psychoses:* 10–50 mg/day in 2–3 divided doses initially; may be ↑ by 10–20 mg/day every 2–3 days, titrate according to response. Usual dose range is 20–60 mg/day; doses >100 mg/day are not recommended. Dose should be ↓ to lowest dose needed to control symptoms (usual range 20–40 mg/

day). Once maintenance dose is established, may be given as a single daily dose.

IM (Adults): *Zuclopenthixol acetate [Acuphase]:* 50–150 mg, may be repeated every 2–3 days if necessary, some patients may need an additional dose 1–2 days after first injection only; care must be taken to avoid overmedicating due to delay in absorption and antipsychotic effects. Maximum cumulative dose should not exceed 400 mg or four injections. *Zuclopenthixol acetate (Acuphase)* dose form is not meant for long-term use, duration should not exceed 2 wk. If injection volume exceeds 2 mL, dose should be divided and given in two sites. If oral maintenance is to be used, treatment with tablets should be initiated 2–3 days following the last dose of the *Zuclopenthixol acetate (Acuphase)* dose form; if *Zuclopenthixol decanoate (Depot)* dose form is to be used for maintenance, may be given concurrently with the last injection of *Zuclopenthixol acetate (Acuphase)* dose form. *Suggested transfer regimen to oral dosing:* If *Zuclopenthixol acetate (Acuphase)* dose was 50 mg, daily oral dose could be 20 mg; if *Zuclopenthixol acetate (Acuphase)* dose was 100 mg, then daily oral dose could be 40 mg; if *Zuclopenthixol acetate (Acuphase)* dose was 150 mg, then daily oral dose could be 60 mg. *Suggested transfer regimen to Zuclopenthixol decanoate (Depot) dosing:* If *Zuclopenthixol acetate (Acuphase)* dose was 50 mg, then IM dose of *Zuclopenthixol decanoate (Depot)* could be 100 mg every 2 wk; if *Zuclopenthixol acetate (Acuphase)* dose was 100 mg, then IM dose of *Zuclopenthixol decanoate (Depot)* could be 200 mg every 2 wk; if *Zuclopenthixol acetate (Acuphase)* dose was 150 mg, then IM dose of *Zuclopenthixol decanoate (Depot)* could be 300 mg every 2 wk.

IM (Adults): *Zuclopenthixol decanoate [depot]:* Usual maintenance dose is 150–300 mg every 2–4 wk, regimens should be individualized according to response, care must be taken not to overmedicate due to delayed/prolonged absorption and effects. If injection volume exceeds 2 mL, dose should be divided and given in two sites.

Availability

Zuclopenthixol hydrochloride tablets—contain castor oil: 10 mg, 25 mg; **Zuclopenthixol acetate injection (Acuphase)—contains medium-chain triglycerides:** 50 mg/mL; **Zuclopenthixol decanoate injection (Depot)—contains medium-chain triglycerides:** 200 mg/mL.

NURSING IMPLICATIONS
Assessment

- Assess mental status (orientation, mood, behavior) before and periodically during therapy.
- Observe carefully when administering oral medication to ensure that medication is actually taken and not hoarded.
- Assess weight and BMI initially and during therapy.

- Assess fluid intake and bowel function. Increased bulk and fluids in the diet help minimize constipation.
- Monitor for onset of akathisia (restlessness or desire to keep moving) and extrapyramidal side effects (*parkinsonian:* difficulty speaking or swallowing, loss of balance control, pill rolling, mask-like face, shuffling gait, rigidity, tremors; *dystonic:* muscle spasms, twisting motions, twitching, inability to move eyes, weakness of arms or legs) every 2 mo during therapy and 8–12 wk after therapy has been discontinued. Reduction in dose or discontinuation of medication may be necessary. Benztropine or diphenhydramine may be used to control these symptoms.
- Monitor for tardive dyskinesia (uncontrolled rhythmic movement of mouth, face, and extremities; lip smacking or puckering; puffing of cheeks; uncontrolled chewing; rapid or worm-like movements of tongue). Report immediately; may be irreversible.
- Monitor for development of neuroleptic malignant syndrome (fever, respiratory distress, tachycardia, seizures, diaphoresis, arrhythmias, hypertension or hypotension, pallor, tiredness, severe muscle stiffness, loss of bladder control). Report immediately.
- Monitor for symptoms related to hyperprolactinemia (menstrual abnormalities, galactorrhea, sexual dysfunction).

Lab Test Considerations

- Monitor CBC and liver function tests every 6 mo and periodically as needed during treatment. May cause ↑ AST, ALT, and alkaline phosphatase.
- Monitor blood glucose prior to and periodically during therapy. May cause hyperglycemia.
- Monitor serum prolactin prior to and periodically during therapy. May cause ↑ serum prolactin levels.

Implementation

- **PO:** Administer tablets before or after meals.
- **IM:** Administer deep in large muscle. A test dose may be ordered for first administration.

Patient/Family Teaching

- Instruct patient to take as directed. If a dose is missed, omit and take next dose as scheduled. Discontinuation should be gradual.
- Inform patient of possibility of extrapyramidal symptoms and tardive dyskinesia. Caution patient to report these symptoms immediately to health care professional.
- Advise patient to change positions slowly to minimize orthostatic hypotension.
- Medication may cause drowsiness. Caution patient to avoid driving or other activities requiring alertness until response to medication is known.
- Advise patient to notify health care professional of all Rx or OTC medications, vitamins, or herbal products being taken and to consult with health care professional before taking other medications.
- Instruct patient to notify health care professional promptly if sore throat, fever, unusual bleeding or bruising, rash, weakness, tremors, visual disturbances, dark-colored urine, or clay-colored stools occur.
- Instruct patient to avoid sun exposure and to wear protective clothing and sunscreen when outdoors.
- Advise patient to notify health care professional of medication regimen before treatment or surgery.
- Rep: Advise females of reproductive potential to notify health care professional if pregnancy is planned or suspected or if breastfeeding or planning to breastfeed.

Evaluation

- Decreased symptoms of schizophrenia (delusions, hallucinations, social withdrawal, flat, blunt affect).

Natural/Herbal Products

The following monographs introduce some commonly used natural products. Because the amounts of active ingredients in these agents are not standardized or currently subject to FDA guidelines for medicines, *Davis's Drug Guide for Nurses*, although respectful of patients' right to choose from a variety of therapeutic options, does not endorse their routine use unless supervised by a knowledgeable health care professional. Users should take into account the possibility of adverse reactions and interactions and consider the relative lack of data supporting widespread use of these products. Doses are poorly standardized, and individuals are advised to read package labels carefully to ensure safe and efficacious use.

aloe (al-oh)
Other Name(s):
Aloe vera, Cape aloe, Aloe latex, Burn plant, Curacao aloe
Classification
Therapeutic: laxatives, wound/ulcer/decubiti healing agent

Common Uses
PO: Cathartic laxative. **Topical:** Use on burns/sunburns, wounds, irritated skin, psoriasis; topical anti-infective.

Action
PO: Exerts a laxative effect by causing increased mucous secretion and peristalsis. The cathartic effects occur within 10 hr. Water and electrolyte reabsorption are inhibited. **Topical:** May help accelerate wound healing through inhibition of thromboxane A2 and increased microcirculation preventing ischemia in wounds, although the evidence is inconsistent. May have some activity against gram-positive, gram-negative bacteria and yeast. **Therapeutic Effects:** Relief of constipation. Improved wound healing.

Pharmacokinetics
Absorption: Unknown.
Distribution: Unknown.
Metabolism and Excretion: Unknown.
Half-life: Unknown.

TIME/ACTION PROFILE

ROUTE	ONSET	PEAK	DURATION
PO, Topical	unknown	unknown	unknown

Contraindications/Precautions
Contraindicated in: Intestinal obstruction; Inflammatory intestinal diseases (including Crohn's disease); Appendicitis and abdominal pain of unknown origin; OB: Safety not established; Pedi: Oral aloe not appropriate for children <12 yr. Topically applied aloe gel-containing formulations have been safely used in clinical trials.

Use Cautiously in: Renal disease; Fluid or electrolyte abnormalities; Diabetes; Alcohol-containing products should be used cautiously in patients with known intolerance or liver disease; Pedi: Cautious use in children >12 yr.

Adverse Reactions/Side Effects
Derm: Contact dermatitis, skin irritation. **Endo:** hypoglycemia. **F and E:** dehydration, HYPOKALEMIA. **GI:** Cramping, diarrhea, laxative dependence (chronic use). **GU:** hematuria.

Interactions
Natural Product-Drug: Combining oral aloe with potassium-wasting drugs (e.g., **diuretics**, other **laxatives**, **corticosteroids**, **cisplatin**, **amphotericin B**) may worsen hypokalemia. Hypokalemia may ↑ risk of toxicity from **digoxin** and some **antiarrhythmics**. May have additive effects with **antidiabetic** agents. May ↑ bleeding risk with **warfarin**. Alcohol-containing preparations may interact with **disulfiram** and **metronidazole**.
Natural-Natural: ↑ hypokalemia risk with **licorice** and **horsetail**. Additive effects with stimulant laxative herbs and herbs with hypoglycemic potential. ↑ bleeding risk with antiplatelet herbs.

Route/Commonly Used Doses
PO (Adults): *Constipation:* 100–200 mg aloe or 50 mg of aloe extract taken in the evening. Do not use for >1–2 wk without medical advice; *Juice:* 1 teaspoonful tid after meals.
Topical (Adults): Aloe gel can be applied liberally to affected areas 2–3 times daily.

Availability
Alone or in combination with other herbal medicinals^OTC; Capsules^OTC; Juice^OTC; Tincture (1:10 in 50% alcohol)^OTC; Topical or gel or applied directly from cut plant.

NURSING IMPLICATIONS
Assessment
- **Constipation:** Assess for abdominal distention, presence of bowel sounds, and usual pattern of elimination.
- Assess color, consistency, and amount of stool produced.

- **Topical:** Perform baseline skin assessment prior to applying aloe to minor wounds, burns, and abrasions. Observe the size, character, and location of the affected area prior to the application of aloe.
- Note topical response assessing for increased inflammation, drainage, pain, warmth, and/or pruritus.

Lab Test Considerations
- Monitor serum potassium in patients with chronic use and CBC in patients who self-medicate and experience bloody diarrhea or have ulcerative colitis or Crohn's disease.

Implementation
- **PO:** Administer laxative at bedtime to induce a bowel movement in the morning.
- **Topical:** Wash hands and then apply liberally to affected area of skin. Cover broken areas of skin with a light non-adhering dressing (e.g., band-aid dressing with *Telfa* lining) to facilitate keeping area clean. Do not apply an occlusive dressing over site of application.

Patient/Family Teaching
- **Constipation:** Instruct patients with pre-existing intestinal disorders (e.g., ulcerative colitis, Crohn's disease, irritable bowel syndrome) not to take aloe juice without the advice of a health care professional.
- Counsel patients that the oral juice should not be taken if they are experiencing abdominal pain, nausea, vomiting, or fever.
- Inform patients that occasional constipation may not be an issue but persistent constipation may represent a more serious health problem and to consult their health care professional.
- Advise patients to expect laxative response to the oral juice in 8–12 hr.
- Caution patients that the laxative effects may be dramatic and that accompanying dehydration and electrolyte imbalances may occur. If severe diarrhea occurs or persists, seek out treatment from their health care professional.
- Advise patients other than those with spinal cord injury that laxatives should only be used for short-term therapy. Although this is considered by some to be a natural way of correcting constipation it still carries the risk of electrolyte imbalance and dependency with chronic use.
- Encourage patients to use other forms of bowel regulation: increasing bulk in the diet, increasing fluid intake, and increasing mobility, as appropriate. Normal bowel habits are individualized and may vary from 3 times/day to 3 times/wk.
- Advise patients to consume 1500–2000 mL/day of fluids during therapy to prevent dehydration.
- Caution patients with a known cardiac history not to take this herbal supplement without the advice of their health care professional because of the risk of hypokalemia worsening arrhythmias.

- Caution patients with cardiac history to avoid straining during bowel movements (Valsalva maneuver).
- **Topical:** Advise patients that topical applications should only be used for minor burns, abrasions, or wounds. Wounds of larger size or more serious burns should be treated by a health care professional.
- Instruct patients using topical application on a non-intact skin surface about signs and symptoms of infection (milky or discolored drainage, redness, warmth, swelling, pain) and to promptly seek out treatment of a health care professional if this occurs.
- Counsel patients that if improvement in the wound is not occurring or it worsens, stop treatment with aloe vera and seek the advice of a health care professional.
- Warn patients with risk factors for delayed wound healing (e.g., diabetic patients, vascular disease) not to self-medicate with aloe vera without the approval of their health care professional.

Evaluation
- A soft, formed bowel movement.
- Evacuation of the colon.
- Relief of sunburn pain.
- Wound healing in small localized burns or abrasions.

arnica (ar-ni-cuh)
Other Name(s):
Arnica montana, leopard's bane, mountain tobacco, mountain snuff, wolf's bane
Classification
Therapeutic: anti-inflammatories, immune stimulants

Common Uses
Topical treatment of insect bites, bruises, acne, boils, sprains, muscle, and joint pain.

Action
Polysaccharides in arnica may produce a slight anti-inflammatory and analgesic effect. Some antibacterial effects are seen, in addition to a counterirritant effect, which may aid in wound healing. **Therapeutic Effects:** Decreased inflammation. Pain relief.

Pharmacokinetics
Absorption: Systemic absorption may occur following topical application to broken skin.
Distribution: Unknown.
Metabolism and Excretion: Unknown.
Half-life: Unknown.

TIME/ACTION PROFILE

ROUTE	ONSET	PEAK	DURATION
Topical	unknown	unknown	unknown

Contraindications/Precautions

Contraindicated in: Not for oral use (except in highly diluted homeopathic preparations); Arnica allergy; Avoid use on broken skin; Infectious or inflammatory GI conditions; OB: Pregnancy and lactation.
Use Cautiously in: Infectious or inflammatory GI conditions; Surgery (discontinue use 2 wk prior to procedure due to antiplatelet effects).

Adverse Reactions/Side Effects

GI: abdominal pain, diarrhea (if taken orally), vomiting. **Derm:** edematous dermatitis with pustules (chronic treatment of damaged skin), eczema (prolonged use). **Misc:** local allergic reactions.

Interactions

Natural Product-Drug: Alcohol-containing preparations may interact with **disulfiram** and **metronidazole.** May potentiate the effects of **anticoagulants** and **antiplatelet agents,** increasing the risk of bleeding.
Natural-Natural: May increase risk of bleeding with **clove, garlic, ginger, ginkgo,** and **ginseng.**

Route/Commonly Used Doses

Topical (Adults): *Topical:* rub or massage arnica tincture, cream, or gel onto injured area 2–3 times a day. Do not apply to broken skin; *Compress:* dilute 1 tablespoon of arnica tincture in ½ L water. Wet a gauze pad with solution and apply to affected area for 15 min. For use in poultices, dilute tincture 3–10 times with water.

Availability

Cream, tincture, salve, ointment, gel, and oil^{OTC} is rendered as **oil**^OTC; **Topical (preparations should contain not more than 20–25% arnica tincture or 15% arnica oil)**^OTC**; Homeopathic preparations**^OTC**.**

NURSING IMPLICATIONS

Assessment

- Inspect skin for breaks prior to application to ensure arnica is applied only to an intact surface. Note the size, character, and location of affected area prior to application of arnica.
- After application, monitor affected area for signs of allergic response.

Toxicity and Overdose

- Systemic absorption may result in nausea, vomiting, organ damage, hypertension, cardiotoxicity, arrhythmias, muscular weakness, collapse, vertigo, renal dysfunction, coma, and death. If ingested orally, induce emesis and gastric lavage to remove undigested contents. Supportive care may be necessary. Do not take orally or apply to non-intact skin to avoid systemic absorption.

Implementation

- Clean skin with a non-alcohol containing cleanser prior to applying arnica. Apply topically to affected area, or site of injury, ensuring skin is intact.
- Do not take orally or apply to an open wound because of potential for systemic absorption with toxicity.

Patient/Family Teaching

- Teach patients to inspect the affected area for breaks in the skin and not to apply arnica to any areas where the skin is broken.
- Warn patients that use on non-intact skin and oral ingestion may cause life-threatening toxicity.
- Advise patients that arnica should only be used for short periods of time in the treatment of minor aches and pains associated with local muscle, joint, or skin pain. Prolonged use may cause allergic/hypersensitivity reactions to develop.
- Instruct patients taking antihypertensive agents to avoid concurrent use of arnica.
- Rep: Advise females of reproductive potential to notify health care professional if pregnancy is planned or suspected. Arnica should be avoided during pregnancy.

Evaluation

- Relief of, or improvement in, minor aches and pains associated with muscle or joint overuse, or sprains and/or local skin irritation from insect bites, bruises, boils, or acne.

bilberry (bill-beh-ree)

Other Name(s):
Vaccinium myrtillus, Tegens
Classification
Therapeutic: ocular agents, vascular agents

Common Uses

Visual acuity improvement, atherosclerosis, venous insufficiency, varicose veins, diabetes mellitus, diarrhea, hemorrhoids, peptic ulcer disease, osteoarthritis, and chronic fatigue syndrome.

Action

Anthocyanidins in bilberry have a variety of effects including increased glycosaminoglycans synthesis, decreased vascular permeability, reduced membrane thickness, redistribution of microvascular blood flow, and formation of interstitial fluid. **Therapeutic Effects:** Decreased inflammation. Decreased edema. Decreased blood glucose. Improved circulation.

Pharmacokinetics

Absorption: Unknown.
Distribution: Unknown.
Metabolism and Excretion: Eliminated by the kidneys.

Half-life: Unknown.

TIME/ACTION PROFILE

ROUTE	ONSET	PEAK	DURATION
PO	unknown	unknown	unknown

Contraindications/Precautions

Contraindicated in: Hypersensitivity or allergy to bilberry; Leaves are potentially toxic with chronic use of 1.5 g/kg/day.

Use Cautiously in: Diabetic patients; Patients at risk for bleeding; OB: Avoid use in pregnancy due to lack of safety data.

Adverse Reactions/Side Effects

Endo: low blood sugar. **GI:** diarrhea, upset stomach. **Hemat:** bleeding, bruising.

Interactions

Natural Product-Drug: May ↑ effects of **anticoagulants and antiplatelet drugs** and ↓ platelet activity. May ↑ effects of **antidiabetic agents** and cause hypoglycemia.

Natural-Natural: Avoid use with chromium-containing herbs and supplements (bilberry contains chromium). Avoid use with herbs with hypoglycemic properties.

Route/Commonly Used Doses

PO (Adults): *General use:* 80–160 mg of aqueous extract three times daily. *Retinopathy:* 160 mg of bilberry extract (Tegens®) has been taken twice daily for one mo. *Chronic venous insufficiency:* A bilberry extract equivalent to 173 mg of anthocyanins has been taken daily for 30 days.

Availability

Liquid extract; **Tablets**; **Softgel capsules** 160 mg.

NURSING IMPLICATIONS

Assessment

● Monitor BP periodically during therapy, coagulation panel, blood glucose.

Lab Test Considerations

● Monitor coagulation studies in patients on anticoagulants and antiplatelet agents.
● Monitor blood glucose periodically during therapy. May cause hypoglycemia.

Implementation

● Administer without regard to food.

Patient/Family Teaching

● Instruct patient to take bilberry as directed.

Evaluation

● Improvement in vascular insufficiency.
● Decrease in diarrhea.

black cohosh (blak coe-hosh)
Remifemin
Other Name(s):
baneberry black snakeroot, bugbane, phytoestrogen, rattle root, rattle-weed, rattle top, squaw root
Classification
Therapeutic: menopausal agents

Do not confuse black cohosh with blue or white cohosh

Common Uses

Management of menopausal symptoms. Premenstrual discomfort. Dysmenorrhea. Mild sedative. Rheumatism.

Action

Therapeutic effects are produced by glycosides isolated from the fresh or dried rhizome with attached roots. Mechanism of action is unclear. **Therapeutic Effects:** May decrease symptoms of menopause, including hot flashes, sweating, sleep disturbance, and anxiety. Has no effect on vaginal epithelium.

Pharmacokinetics

Absorption: Unknown.
Distribution: Unknown.
Metabolism and Excretion: Unknown.
Half-life: Unknown.

TIME/ACTION PROFILE

ROUTE	ONSET	PEAK	DURATION
PO	unknown	unknown	unknown

Contraindications/Precautions

Contraindicated in: OB: Pregnancy and lactation.

Use Cautiously in: Breast cancer (may increase risk of metastasis); Hormone-sensitive cancers; Protein S deficiency (increased risk for thrombosis); Liver disease.

Adverse Reactions/Side Effects

Neuro: dizziness, headache, SEIZURES (in combination with evening primrose and chasteberry). **GI:** GI upset, hepatotoxicity. **Derm:** rash. **Misc:** breast tenderness, cramping, vaginal spotting/bleeding, weight gain.

Interactions

Natural Product-Drug: Unknown effects when combined with hormone replacement therapy and **antiestrogens** (e.g., **tamoxifen**). Concurrent use with **hepatotoxic drugs** may ↑ risk of liver damage. **Alcohol-containing preparations** may interact with **disulfiram** and **metronidazole**. May ↓ cytotoxic effects of **cisplatin**. May precipitate hypotension when used in combination with **antihypertensives**.

Natural-Natural: May ↑ risk of hepatotoxicity when used with **chaparral**, **comfrey**, **kava-kava**, and **niacin**.

Route/Commonly Used Doses

PO (Adults): *Tablets (Remifemin):* 20 mg twice daily. *Liquid extract:* 0.3–2 mL 2–3 times daily. *Tincture:* 2–4 mL 2–3 times daily. *Dried rhizome:* 0.3–2 g 3 times daily. Do not use for more than 6 mo.

Availability

Alone or in combination with other herbal medicinals^{OTC}; **Tablets (Remifemin 20 mg [best studied black cohosh product])**^{OTC}; **Liquid extract (1:1 in 90% alcohol)**^{OTC}; **Tincture (1:10 in 60% alcohol)**^{OTC}; **Dried rhizome.**

NURSING IMPLICATIONS
Assessment

● Assess frequency and severity of menopausal symptoms.
● Monitor BP for patients on antihypertensive drugs; may increase effects and cause hypotension.
● Assess for history of seizures or liver disease.

Implementation

● Administration with food may help to minimize nausea.

Patient/Family Teaching

● Advise patients with seizures, liver dysfunction, excessive alcohol intake, cancer, or other medical problems to consult their health care professional prior to initiating self-therapy with this herb.
● Advise patient to consult health care professional before taking with other estrogen replacements.
● Advise patient to notify health care professional if pregnancy is planned or suspected. Avoid use during pregnancy; may induce a miscarriage.

Evaluation

● Resolution of menopausal vasomotor symptoms.

---

chondroitin (konn-**droy**-tinn)

Other Name(s):
chondroitin polysulfate, CPS, CDS
Classification
Therapeutic: nonopioid analgesics

Common Uses

Osteoarthritis. Ischemic heart disease. Hyperlipidemia. Osteoporosis. **Ophth:** In combination with sodium hyaluronate, for use as a surgical aid in cataract extraction or lens implantation, and as a lubricant.

Action

May serve as a building block of articular cartilage. May protect cartilage against degradation. May have antiatherogenic properties. **Therapeutic Effects:** Improvement in osteoarthritis symptoms.

Pharmacokinetics

Absorption: 8–18% is absorbed orally.
Distribution: Unknown.
Metabolism and Excretion: Unknown.
Half-life: Unknown.

TIME/ACTION PROFILE

ROUTE	ONSET	PEAK	DURATION
PO	unknown	unknown	unknown

Contraindications/Precautions

Contraindicated in: OB: Pregnancy and lactation.
Use Cautiously in: Asthma (may exacerbate symptoms); Clotting disorders (may ↑ risk of bleeding); Prostate cancer (may ↑ risk of metastasis or recurrence).

Adverse Reactions/Side Effects

GI: diarrhea, heartburn, nausea. **Hemat:** bleeding (antiplatelet effect). **Misc:** allergic reactions, edema, hair loss.

Interactions

Natural Product-Drug: Use of chondroitin with **anticoagulant** and **antiplatelet** drugs, **thrombolytics**, **NSAIDs**, some **cephalosporins**, and **valproates** may ↑ risk of bleeding.
Natural-Natural: Herbs with anticoagulant or antiplatelet properties may ↑ bleeding risk when combined with chondroitin, including: **anise**, **arnica**, **chamomile**, **clove**, **dong quai**, **fenugreek**, **feverfew**, **ginger**, **ginkgo**, **Panax ginseng**, **licorice**, and others.

Route/Commonly Used Doses

PO (Adults): *Osteoarthritis:* 800–2000 mg daily, as a single dose or in 2–3 divided doses. *Prevention of recurrent myocardial infarction:* 10 g daily in 3 divided doses for 3 mo followed by 1.5 g daily in 3 divided doses as maintenance therapy.
IM (Adults): *Osteoarthritis:* 50 mg twice weekly for 8 wk every 4 mo.

Availability

Tablets^{OTC}; Capsules^{OTC}; Injection (not available in US); Ophthalmic Drops Rx in combination with sodium hyaluronate (Viscoat).

NURSING IMPLICATIONS
Assessment

● Evaluate drug profile before starting therapy with this herbal supplement. If the patient is taking anticoagulants or antiplatelet drugs, avoid use of this herb.
● Monitor pain (type, location, and intensity) and range of motion on an ongoing basis as an indicator of drug efficacy.
● Assess for gastric discomfort and instruct patient to seek out the advice of a health care professional if persistent gastric discomfort occurs.

CAPITALS = life-threatening; <u>Underline</u> = most frequent.

- Assess for signs of bleeding and discontinue herbal supplement promptly and seek out health care professional for follow-up.

Implementation
- **PO:** Administer with food.

Patient/Family Teaching
- Advise patients that this herbal supplement is usually taken with glucosamine.
- Caution patients who take aspirin or NSAIDs or other non-prescription medications not to take this herbal supplement without conferring with their health care professional.
- Instruct patients that this medication works by building up cartilage and that this requires that the medication be taken consistently over a period of time. It is not recommended as a supplemental pain medication.
- Advise female patients to notify health care professional if pregnancy is planned or suspected or if breast feeding; avoid use.

Evaluation
- Improvement in pain and range of motion.
- Reduced need for supplemental or breakthrough pain medication.

echinacea *Echinacea purpurea* (ek-i-nay-sha)
Other Name(s):
American coneflower, black sampson, black susan, *brauneria angustifolia*, kansas snakeroot, purple coneflower, red sunflower, *rudbeckia*, sampson root, scurvy root
Classification
Therapeutic: immune stimulants

Common Uses
Bacterial and viral infections. Prevention and treatment of colds, coughs, flu, and bronchitis. Fevers. Wounds and burns. Inflammation of the mouth and pharynx. Urinary tract infections. Vaginal candidiasis.

Action
Medicinal parts derived from the roots, leaves, or whole plant of perennial herb (Echinacea). *Echinacea purpurea herba* has been reported to promote wound healing, which may be due to an increase in white blood cells, spleen cells, and increased activity of granulocytes, as well as an increase in helper T cells and cytokines. *E. purpurea radix* has been shown to have antibacterial, antiviral, anti-inflammatory, and immune-modulating effects. **Therapeutic Effects:** Resolution of respiratory and urinary tract infections. Decreased duration and intensity of common cold. Improved wound healing. Stimulates phagocytosis; inhibits action of hyaluronidase (secreted by bacteria),

which helps bacteria gain access to healthy cells. Externally, has antifungal and bacteriostatic properties.

Pharmacokinetics
Absorption: Unknown.
Distribution: Unknown.
Metabolism and Excretion: Unknown.
Half-life: Unknown.

TIME/ACTION PROFILE

ROUTE	ONSET	PEAK	DURATION
PO	unknown	unknown	unknown

Contraindications/Precautions
Contraindicated in: Multiple sclerosis, leukosis, collagenoses, AIDS, tuberculosis, autoimmune diseases; Hypersensitivity and cross-sensitivity in patients allergic to plants in *Asteraceae/Compositae* plant family (daisies, chrysanthemums, marigolds, etc.); OB: Pregnancy and lactation.
Use Cautiously in: Diabetes; Pedi: May increase risk of rash in children; Tinctures should be used cautiously in alcoholics or patients with liver disease; Do not take longer than 8 wk: may suppress immune function.

Adverse Reactions/Side Effects
CNS: dizziness, fatigue, headache, somnolence. **EENT:** sore throat, tingling sensation on tongue. **GI:** abdominal pain, constipation, diarrhea, heartburn, nausea, vomiting. **Derm:** allergic reaction, rash (more common in children). **Misc:** fever.

Interactions
Natural Product-Drug: May possibly interfere with **immunosuppressants** because of its immuno-stimulant activity. May ↑ risk for hepaotoxicity from **anabolic steroids**, **methotrexate**, or **ketoconazole** when taken with echinacea. May ↑ **midazolam** availability.
Natural-Natural: May ↑ risk for hepatotoxicity when taken with **kava**.

Route/Commonly Used Doses
PO (Adults): *Tablets:* 6.78 mg tablets, take 2 tabs 3 times daily. *Capsules:* 500–1000 mg 3 times a day for 5–7 days. *Fluid extract:* 1–2 mL tid; solid form (6.5:1): 150–300 mg tid. Should not be used for more than 8 wk at a time. *Tea:* ½ tsp comminuted drug, steeped and strained after 10 min, 1 cup 5–6 times daily on the first day, titrating down to 1 cup daily over the next 5 days. *Echinacea purpuren herb juice:* 6–9 mL/day. *Liquid:* 20 drops every 2 hr for the first day of symptoms, then 3 times daily for up to 10 days.
Topical (Adults): *Ointment, lotion, tincture used externally:* 1.5–7.5 mL tincture, 2–5 g dried root.

Availability
Capsules^OTC; Tablets ^OTC; Dried Root^OTC; **The dried root can be steeped and strained in boiling water**

and taken as a tea^OTC; Liquid extract^OTC; 1:1 in 45% alcohol^OTC; Tincture^OTC; 1:5 in 45% alcohol^OTC; Blended teas^OTC; *Echinacea purpuren* herb juice^OTC.

NURSING IMPLICATIONS

Assessment
- Assess wound for size, appearance, and drainage prior to the start of and periodically during therapy.
- Assess frequency of common mild illnesses (such as a cold) in response to use.

Implementation
- Tinctures may contain significant concentrations of alcohol and may not be suitable for children, alcoholics, patients with liver disease, or those taking disulfiram, metronidazole, some cephalosporins, or sulfonylurea oral antidiabetic agents.
- Prolonged use of this agent may cause overstimulation of the immune system, and use beyond 8 wk is not recommended. Therapy of 10–14 days is usually considered sufficient.
- May be taken without regard to food.

Patient/Family Teaching
- Herb is more effective for treatment than prevention of colds. Take at first sign of symptoms.
- Advise patient to seek immediate treatment for an illness that does not improve after taking this herb.
- Instruct patient that the usual course of therapy is 10–14 days and 8 wk is the maximum.
- Inform patient that use of this herb is not recommended in severe illnesses (e.g., AIDS, tuberculosis) or autoimmune diseases (e.g., multiple sclerosis, collagen diseases, etc.).
- Caution patient that prolonged use of this herb may result in overstimulation of the immune system, possibly with subsequent immunosuppression.
- Instruct patient to consult health care professional before taking any prescription or OTC medications concurrently with echinacea.
- Keep tincture in a dark bottle away from sunlight. Should be taken several times a day.
- Store herb in airtight container away from sunlight.
- Rep: Advise females of reproductive potential to avoid pregnancy or breast feeding during use.

Evaluation
- Improved wound healing.
- Infrequent common illnesses.
- Illnesses of shorter duration and less severity.

feverfew (fee-vurr-fyoo)
Other Name(s):
Altamisa, Bachelor's Buttons, *Chrysanthemum parethenium*, Featerfoiul, Featherfew, Featherfoil, Flirtwort Mid-summer Daisy, *Pyrethrum parthenium*, Santa Maria, *Tanaceti parthenii*, Wild chamomile, Wild quinine

Classification
Therapeutic: vascular headache suppressants

Common Uses
PO: Migraine headache prophylaxis. **Topical:** Toothaches and as an antiseptic.

Action
The sesquiterpene lactone, parthenolide, may provide feverfew's migraine prophylaxis effects. Feverfew may also have antiplatelet and vasodilatory effects and block prostaglandin synthesis. **Therapeutic Effects:** May reduce the symptoms and frequency of migraine headaches.

Pharmacokinetics
Absorption: Unknown.
Distribution: Unknown.
Metabolism and Excretion: Unknown.
Half-life: Unknown.

TIME/ACTION PROFILE

ROUTE	ONSET	PEAK	DURATION
PO	2–4 mo	unknown	unknown

Contraindications/Precautions
Contraindicated in: OB: Pregnancy and lactation; Feverfew hypersensitivity or allergy to *Asteraceae/Compositae* family plants, including ragweed, chrysanthemums, daisies, and marigolds.
Use Cautiously in: Use >4 mo (safety and efficacy not established).

Adverse Reactions/Side Effects
CNS: "Post-Feverfew Syndrome" (anxiety, headache, insomnia, muscle and joint aches). **CV:** *with long-term use:* tachycardia. GI: diarrhea, heartburn, mouth ulceration and soreness (from chewing fresh leaves), nausea, vomiting. **Derm:** contact dermatitis (when used topically).

Interactions
Natural Product-Drug: Use of feverfew with **anticoagulant** and **antiplatelet** drugs, **thrombolytics**, **NSAIDs**, some **cephalosporins**, and **valproates** may increase risk of bleeding. Concomitant use with NSAIDs may also reduce feverfew effectiveness.
Natural-Natural: Use with **anise**, **arnica**, **chamomile**, **clove**, **dong quai**, **fenugreek**, **garlic**, **ginger**, **gingko**, **licorice**, and *Panax ginseng* may increase anticoagulant potential of feverfew.

Route/Commonly Used Doses
PO (Adults): 50–100 mg feverfew extract daily (standardized to 0.2–0.35% parthenolide) or 50–125 mg freeze-dried leaf daily with or after food.

Availability

Feverfew extract standardized to 0.2-0.35% parthenolide^OTC^; **Fresh leaf**^OTC^; **Freeze-dried leaf**^OTC^.

NURSING IMPLICATIONS

Assessment

- Monitor frequency, intensity, and duration of migraine headaches prior to and during ongoing therapy.
- Assess for mouth ulcers or skin ulcerations during therapy.

Implementation

- Take with food or on a full stomach.

Patient/Family Teaching

- Instruct patients to take this medication on a consistent basis to prevent migraine headaches. This herbal supplement is not for treatment of migraines.
- Warn patients about mouth ulcers and sores and that if this occurs to seek the advice of a health care professional. Encourage proper oral hygiene.
- Advise patients not to abruptly stop this product because of the possibility of post-feverfew syndrome. Inform patients that anxiety, headache, insomnia, and muscle aches may indicate withdrawal. Feverfew should be gradually tapered.
- Review dietary and medication profile of patient to identify potential interactions. Instruct patient about other herbs that may interact with feverfew.
- Counsel patients on anticoagulants not to take feverfew except as directed by their health care provider.
- Advise patients to avoid using NSAIDs as this may reduce the effectiveness of feverfew.
- Instruct patients to look for signs of bleeding such as unusual bruising or inability to clot after a cut and to seek the advice of a health care professional if this occurs.
- Inform patients that feverfew should reduce the number of migraines and severity of symptoms but that duration of the migraine may not be affected.

Evaluation

- Reduction in the frequency and severity of migraine headaches.

garlic (gar-lik)

Other Name(s):
Alli sativa bulbus, *Allium sativum*
Classification
Therapeutic: lipid-lowering agents

Common Uses

PO: Hypertension, hyperlipidemia, cardiovascular disease prevention, colorectal and gastric cancer prevention. **Topical:** Dermal fungal infections including tinea corporis, cruris, and pedis.

Action

May have HMG-CoA inhibitor properties in lowering cholesterol, but less effectively than statin drugs; vaso-

dilatory and antiplatelet properties. **Therapeutic Effects:** Decreased cholesterol levels. Decreased platelet aggregation.

Pharmacokinetics

Absorption: Garlic oil is well absorbed.
Distribution: Unknown.
Metabolism and Excretion: Kidney and lungs.
Half-life: Unknown.

TIME/ACTION PROFILE

ROUTE	ONSET	PEAK	DURATION
PO	4–25 wk	unknown	unknown

Contraindications/Precautions

Contraindicated in: Bleeding disorders. Discontinue use 1–2 wk prior to surgery.
Use Cautiously in: Diabetes, gastrointestinal infection or inflammation.

Adverse Reactions/Side Effects

CNS: dizziness. **GI:** bad breath, diarrhea, flatulence, Irritation of the mouth, esophagus, and stomach, nausea, vomiting. **Derm:** Contact dermatitis and other allergic reactions (asthma, rash, anaphylaxis [rare]), Diaphoresis. **Hemat:** Chronic use or excessive dose may lead to ↓ hemoglobin production and lysis of RBCs, platelet dysfunction, prolonged bleeding time. **Misc:** body odor.

Interactions

Natural Product-Drug: Use of garlic with **anticoagulants**, **antiplatelet agents**, and **thrombolytics** may ↑ risk of bleeding. May ↓ the effectiveness of **contraceptive drugs** and **cyclosporine**. May ↓ plasma concentrations of **saquinavir**, **nevirapine**, **delavirdine**, and **efavirenz**. May ↓ **isoniazid** levels by 65%.
Natural-Natural: Herbs with anticoagulant or antiplatelet properties may increase bleeding risk when combined with garlic, including: **angelica, anise, asafoetida, bogbean, boldo, capsicum, celery, chamomile, clove, danshen, dong quai, fenugreek, feverfew, ginger, ginkgo,** *Panax ginseng,* **horse chestnut, horseradish, licorice, meadowsweet, papain, passionflower, poplar, prickly ash, onion, quassia, red clover, turmeric, wild carrot, wild lettuce, willow,** and others.

Route/Commonly Used Doses

PO (Adults): 200–400 mg tid of standardized garlic powder extract with 1.3% allin. *Fresh garlic:* 1–7 cloves per day. One clove contains approximately 4 g of garlic.
Topical (Adults): *Tinea infections:* 0.4% cream, 0.6% gel, or 1% gel applied bid x 7 days.

Availability

Capsules^OTC^; **Tablets**^OTC^; **Topical cream**; **Topical gel**; **Fresh garlic**^OTC^.

NURSING IMPLICATIONS
Assessment
- Obtain usual dietary intake from patient, especially in regard to fat consumption.
- Assess patient's reason for using this herbal remedy and knowledge about hyperlipidemia.
- Ascertain the amount of garlic the patient consumes on a regular basis.

Implementation
- Take orally as fresh clove, capsule, or tablet.
- Do not exceed recommended dose.

Patient/Family Teaching
- Instruct patients about the need to follow a healthy diet (low in fat and high in vegetables and fruits) in conjunction with garlic. Other lipid-reducing strategies, such as exercise and smoking cessation, should also be employed.
- Inform patients that there are other more effective agents for lipid reduction available.
- Caution patients about the potential for bleeding and not to take this herbal remedy without notifying their health care provider if they are taking other medications. Instruct patients undergoing elective surgery to stop using garlic 2 wk prior to surgery and to notify the surgeon that they are taking garlic in the event of emergent surgery.
- Notify patients that allergies may occur and to discontinue use if symptoms develop.
- Emphasize the need for follow-up exams with a health care professional to assess effectiveness of the regimen.

Evaluation
- Normalization of lipid profile.
- Prevention of cardiac disease.

---

ginger *Zingiber officinale*
(jin-jer)
Other Name(s):
Calicut, cochin, gengibre, ginger root, imber, ingwerwurzel, ingwer, Jamaica ginger, jenjibre, kankyo, jiang, zingiber
Classification
Therapeutic: antianemics

Common Uses
Prevention and treatment of nausea and vomiting associated with motion sickness, loss of appetite, pregnancy, surgery, and chemotherapy. Prevention of postoperative nausea and vomiting. May be used for dyspepsia, flatulence, relief of joint pain in rheumatoid arthritis, cramping, and diarrhea. Migraine headache. Tonic (toning/strengthening agent) in gout, gas, respi-

ratory infections, anti-inflammatory, stimulant (tones the gut, increases saliva and gastric juices, acts as anticoagulant, decreases blood cholesterol).

Action
Antiemetic effect due to increasing GI motility and transport; may act on serotonin receptors. Shown to be hypoglycemic, hypotensive, or hypertensive, and positive inotropic agent. Inhibits prostaglandins and platelets, lowers cholesterol, and improves appetite and digestion. **Therapeutic Effects:** ↓ nausea and vomiting due to motion sickness, surgery, and chemotherapy. ↓ joint pain and improvement of joint motion in rheumatoid arthritis. Antioxidant.

Pharmacokinetics
Absorption: Unknown.
Distribution: Unknown.
Metabolism and Excretion: Unknown.
Half-life: Unknown.

TIME/ACTION PROFILE

ROUTE	ONSET	PEAK	DURATION
PO	unknown	unknown	unknown

Contraindications/Precautions
Contraindicated in: Lactation (if using large amounts); Gallstones.
Use Cautiously in: Pregnancy (preliminary evidence that ginger might affect fetal sex hormones); Patients with ↑ risk of bleeding; Diabetes; Anticoagulant therapy; Cardiovascular disease.

Adverse Reactions/Side Effects
GI: minor heartburn. **Derm:** dermatitis (when used topically).

Interactions
Natural Product-Drug: May ↑ risk of bleeding when used with **anticoagulants**, **antiplatelet agents**, and **thrombolytics**. May have additive effects with **antidiabetic agents** (causing hypoglycemia) and **calcium channel blockers** (causing hypotension).
Natural-Natural: May theoretically ↑ risk of bleeding when used with other **herbs** that have anticoagulant or antiplatelet activities.

Route/Commonly Used Doses
PO (Adults): *Motion sickness:* 1000 mg dried ginger root taken 30 min–4 hr before travel or 250 mg qid. *Postoperative nausea prevention:* 1000 mg ginger taken 1 hr before induction or anesthesia. *Chemotherapy-induced nausea:* 2–4 g/day. Up to 2 g freshly powdered drug has been used as an antiemetic (not to exceed 4 g/day). *Migraine headache:* 500 mg at onset then 500 mg every 4 hr up to 1.5–2 g/day for 3–4 days. *Osteoarthritis:* 170 mg tid or 255 mg bid of ginger extract. *Whole root rhizome:* 0.25–1 g for other

illnesses. *Tea:* pour 150 mL boiling water over 0.5–1 g of ginger and strain after 5 min. *Tincture:* 0.25–3 mL.

Availability

Alone or in combination with other herbal medicinalsᴼᵀᶜ; **Dried powdered root**ᴼᵀᶜ; **Syrup**ᴼᵀᶜ; **Tincture**ᴼᵀᶜ; **Tablets**ᴼᵀᶜ; **Capsules (≥550 mg)**ᴼᵀᶜ; **Spice**ᴼᵀᶜ; **Tea**ᴼᵀᶜ.

NURSING IMPLICATIONS

Assessment

- Assess patient for nausea, vomiting, abdominal distention, and pain prior to and after administration of the herb when used as an antiemetic agent.
- Assess pain location, duration, intensity, and associated symptoms (photophobia, phonophobia, nausea, vomiting) during migraine attack.
- Assess pain, swelling, and range of motion in affected joints prior to and after administration when used in the treatment of arthritis.
- Assess patient for epigastric pain prior to and after administration when used as a gastroprotective agent.
- Monitor BP and heart rate in patients with cardiovascular disease including hypertension.

Lab Test Considerations

- Monitor blood glucose and coagulation panels periodically during therapy.

Implementation

- Administer ginger prior to situations where nausea or vomiting is anticipated (e.g., motion sickness).
- Dose form and strengths vary with each disease state. Ensure that proper formulation and dose are administered for the indicated use.

Patient/Family Teaching

- Instruct patients receiving anticoagulants not to take this herb without the advice of health care professional (increased risk of bleeding).
- Advise patient to stop the herb immediately if palpitations occur and notify health care professional.
- Advise patient to observe for easy bruising or other signs of bleeding. If they occur, stop the herb immediately and notify health care professional.
- Counsel patients with a history of gallbladder disease to use this herb only under the supervision of health care professional.
- Instruct patient to consult health care professional before taking any Rx, OTC, or other herbal products concurrently with ginger.
- Herb is meant to be used as a tonic, not for long-term use.

Evaluation

- Prevention of nausea and vomiting.
- Relief of epigastric pain.
- Improved joint mobility and relief of pain.
- Relief of migraine headache.

ginkgo (ging-ko)

Other Name(s):
Bai guo ye, fossil tree, ginkgo folium, Japanese silver apricot, kew tree, maidenhair-tree, *salisburia adiantifolia*, yinhsing

Classification
Therapeutic: antiplatelet agents, central nervous system stimulants

Common Uses

Symptomatic relief of organic brain dysfunction (dementia syndromes, short-term memory deficits, inability to concentrate, depression). Intermittent claudication. Vertigo and tinnitus of vascular origin. Improvement of peripheral circulation. Premenstrual syndrome.

Action

Improves tolerance to hypoxemia, especially in cerebral tissue. Inhibits development of cerebral edema and accelerates its regression. Improves memory, blood flow (microcirculation), compensation of disequilibrium, and rheological properties of blood. Inactivates toxic oxygen radicals. Antagonizes platelet-activating factor. Interferes with bronchoconstriction and phagocyte chemotaxis. **Therapeutic Effects:** Symptomatic relief of dementia syndromes. Inhibits arterial spasm, decreases capillary fragility and blood viscosity. Improves venous tone, relaxes vascular smooth muscle.

Pharmacokinetics

Absorption: 70–100% absorption.
Distribution: Unknown.
Metabolism and Excretion: Unknown.
Half-life: Unknown.

TIME/ACTION PROFILE

ROUTE	ONSET	PEAK	DURATION
PO	unknown	unknown	unknown

Contraindications/Precautions

Contraindicated in: Hypersensitivity; Pregnancy and lactation.
Use Cautiously in: Bleeding disorders; Children (fresh seeds have caused seizures and death); Diabetes; Epilepsy; Surgery (discontinue use 2 wk prior).

Adverse Reactions/Side Effects

CNS: CEREBRAL BLEEDING, dizziness, headache, seizure, vertigo. **CV:** palpitations. **GI:** flatulence, stomach upset. **Derm:** allergic skin reaction. **Hemat:** bleeding. **Misc:** hypersensitivity reactions.

Interactions

Natural Product-Drug: Theoretically may potentiate effects of **anticoagulants**, **thrombolytics**, **anti-**

platelet agents, and **MAO inhibitors**. May also ↑ risk of bleeding with some **cephalosporins**, **valproic acid**, and **NSAIDs**. May ↓ effectiveness of **anticonvulsants**. May alter **insulin** metabolism requiring dose adjustments of antidiabetic drugs.

Natural-Natural: May ↑ risk of bleeding when used with other **herbs** with antiplatelet effects (including **angelica**, **arnica**, **chamomile**, **feverfew**, **garlic**, **ginger**, and **licorice**).

Route/Commonly Used Doses

Organic Brain Syndromes

PO (Adults): 120–240 mg ginkgo leaf extract daily in 2 or 3 doses.

Intermittent Claudication

PO (Adults): 120–240 mg ginkgo leaf extract daily in 2 or 3 doses.

Vertigo and Tinnitus

PO (Adults): 120–160 mg ginkgo leaf extract daily in 2 or 3 doses.

Cognitive Function Improvement

PO (Adults): 120–600 mg per day.

Premenstrual Syndrome

PO (Adults): 80 mg BID starting on the 16th day of the menstrual cycle until the 5th day of the next cycle.

Availability

Ginkgo leaf extract (acetone/water) 22–27% flavonoid glycosides, 5–7% terpene lactones, 2.6–3.2% bilobalide, <5 ppm of ginkgolic acids.

NURSING IMPLICATIONS

Assessment

- Assess cognitive function (memory, attention, reasoning, language, ability to perform simple tasks) prior to and periodically during therapy. Exclude other treatable causes of dementia prior to instituting treatment with ginkgo.
- Assess frequency, duration, and severity of muscle cramps (claudication) experienced by the patient prior to and periodically throughout therapy.
- Assess for headache and neurologic changes (thromboembolism).

Implementation

- **PO:** Start dose at 120 mg per day and increase as needed to minimize side effects.
- May be administered without regard to food. Administer at same time each day.
- Use of dried leaf preparations in the form of a tea is not recommended because of insufficient quantity of active ingredients.
- Advise patients to avoid crude ginkgo plant parts, which can cause severe allergic reactions.

Patient/Family Teaching

- Advise patient to observe for easy bruising and other signs of bleeding and report to health care professional if they occur.
- Caution patient to keep this herb out of the reach of children; may cause seizures.
- Caution patient to avoid handling the pulp or seed coats because of the risk of contact dermatitis. Wash skin under free-flowing water promptly if contact does occur.
- Instruct patient not to exceed recommended doses; large doses may result in toxicity (restlessness, diarrhea, nausea and vomiting, headache).
- Notify patients receiving anticoagulant or antiplatelet therapy not to take this medication without approval of health care professional and frequent monitoring.
- Instruct patient to consult health care professional before taking any prescription or OTC medications concurrently with ginkgo.

Evaluation

- Improvement in walking distances pain-free.
- Improvement in tinnitus and vertigo.
- Improvement in short-term memory, attention span, and ability to perform simple tasks.
- Improvement in sexual function.
- Decreased symptoms of premenstrual syndrome.
- Administration for a minimum of 6–8 wk of 80 mg (tid) (not <6 wk) is required to determine response.

ginseng *Panax ginseng* (jin-seng)

Other Name(s):
Asian ginseng, Chinese ginseng, hong shen, Japanese ginseng, Korean ginseng, red ginseng, renshen, white ginseng

Classification
Therapeutic: none assigned

Common Uses

Improving physical and mental stamina. General tonic to energize during times of fatigue and inability to concentrate. Sedative, sleep aid, antidepressant. Diabetes. Enhanced sexual performance/aphrodisiac. Increased longevity. Adjunctive treatment of cancer. Increased immune response. Increased appetite.

Action

Main active ingredient is ginsenoside from the dried root. Serves as CNS stimulant and depressant. Enhances immune function. Interferes with platelet aggregation and coagulation. Has analgesic, anti-inflammatory, and estrogen-like effects. **Therapeutic Effects:** Improves mental and physical ability. May improve appetite,

CAPITALS = life-threatening; Underline = most frequent.

memory, sleep pattern. May reduce fasting blood glucose level in diabetic patients.

Pharmacokinetics
Absorption: Unknown.
Distribution: Unknown.
Metabolism and Excretion: Unknown.
Half-life: Unknown.

TIME/ACTION PROFILE

ROUTE	ONSET	PEAK	DURATION
PO	unknown	unknown	unknown

Contraindications/Precautions
Contraindicated in: Pregnancy (androgenization of fetus); Lactation; Children; Manic-depressive disorders and psychosis; Hypertension; Asthma; Infection; Organ transplant recipients (can interfere with immunosuppressive therapy); Hormone-sensitive cancers.
Use Cautiously in: Autoimmune diseases; Cardiovascular disease; Diabetes (may have hypoglycemic effects); Patients receiving anticoagulants; Bleeding disorders; Schizophrenia (may cause agitation).

Adverse Reactions/Side Effects
CNS: insomnia, agitation, depression, dizziness, euphoria, headaches, nervousness. **CV:** hypertension, tachycardia. **GI:** diarrhea. **GU:** amenorrhea, vaginal bleeding. **Derm:** skin eruptions. **Endo:** estrogen-like effects. **Misc:** fever, mastalgia, STEVENS-JOHNSON SYNDROME.

Interactions
Natural Product-Drug: May ↓ anticoagulant activity of **warfarin**. May interfere with **MAO inhibitors** treatment and cause headache, tremulousness, and manic episodes. May enhance blood glucose lowering effects of **oral hypoglycemics** and **insulin**. May interfere with **immunosuppressant** therapy. Use with caution when taking **estrogens**.
Natural-Natural: May ↑ risk of bleeding when used with **herbs** that have antiplatelet or anticoagulant activities. May prolong the QT interval when used with **bitter orange**, **country mallow**, and **ephedra** and ↑ risk of life-threatening arrhythmias. May ↑ risk of hypoglycemia when used with herbs with hypoglycemic potential.
Natural-Food: May potentiate effects of **caffeine** in **coffee** or **tea** and CNS stimulant effects of **mate**.

Route/Commonly Used Doses
PO (Adults): *Capsule:* 200–600 mg/day; *extract:* 100–300 mg 3 times daily; *crude root:* 1–2 g/day; *infusion: tea:* 1–2 g root daily (½ tbsp/cup water) up to 3 times daily (*P. ginseng* tea bag usually contains 1500 mg of ginseng root). Do not use for longer than 3 mo. *Cold/flu prevention:* 100 mg daily 4 wk prior to influenza vaccination and continued for 8 wk; *Chronic bronchitis:* 100 mg BID for 9 days combined with antibiotic therapy; *Erectile dysfunction:* 900 mg TID; *Type 2 diabetes:* 200 mg daily.

Availability (generic available)
Root powder^OTC; Extract in alcohol^OTC; Capsules^OTC; Tea bags^OTC.

NURSING IMPLICATIONS
Assessment
- Assess level of energy, attention span, and fatigue person is experiencing prior to initiating and periodically during therapy.
- Assess appetite; sleep duration; and perceived quality, emotional lability, and work efficiency prior to and during therapy.
- Patients with chronic medical problems should not use this herb without the advice of health care professional.
- Assess for ginseng toxicity (nervousness, insomnia, palpitations, and diarrhea).
- Monitor patients with diabetes more frequently for hypoglycemia until response to the agent is ascertained.
- Assess for the development of ginseng abuse syndrome (occurs when large doses of the herb are taken concomitantly with other psychomotor stimulants such as coffee and tea. May present as diarrhea, hypertension, restlessness, insomnia, skin eruptions, depression, appetite suppression, euphoria, and edema).

Implementation
- May be taken without regard to food.
- Take at the same time daily and do not increase dose above the recommended amount because of potential toxic effects.

Patient/Family Teaching
- Caution patients with cardiovascular disease, hypertension or hypotension, or on steroid therapy to avoid the use of this herb.
- Instruct patient in the symptoms of ginseng toxicity and to reduce dose or stop use of the herb if they occur.
- Advise patient to limit the amount of caffeine consumed.
- Advise patients with diabetes to monitor blood sugar levels until response to this agent is known.
- Teach patient about the signs and symptoms of hepatitis (yellow skin or whites of eyes, dark urine, light-colored stools, lack of appetite for several days or longer, nausea, abdominal pain) and to stop use of the herb and promptly contact health care professional if they occur. (This herb is hepatoprotectant at low doses, but hepatodestructive at high doses.).
- Caution patient not to exceed recommended doses because of potential side effects and toxicity.
- Instruct patient to discontinue ginseng if diarrhea develops.
- Instruct patient to consult health care professional before taking any Rx or OTC medications concurrently with ginseng.

- Rep: Advise females of reproductive potential to avoid use of ginseng if pregnancy is planned or suspected or if breast feeding.

Evaluation

- Improved energy level and sense of well-being.
- Improved quality of sleep.
- Improved concentration and work efficiency.
- Improved appetite.
- May need to take for several wk before seeing results.
- Recommended course of therapy is 3 wk. A repeated course is feasible. Do not use for longer than 3 mo.

---

glucosamine
(glew-**kos**-ah-meen)
Other Name(s):
2-amino-2-deoxyglucose sulfate, chitosamine
Classification
Therapeutic: antirheumatics

Common Uses
Osteoarthritis. Temporomandibular joint (TMJ) arthritis. Glaucoma.

Action
May stop or slow osteoarthritis progression by stimulating cartilage and synovial tissue metabolism. **Therapeutic Effects:** Decreased pain and improved joint function.

Pharmacokinetics
Absorption: 0.9% absorbed.
Distribution: Unknown.
Metabolism and Excretion: 74% eliminated via first-pass metabolism.
Half-life: Unknown.

TIME/ACTION PROFILE

ROUTE	ONSET	PEAK	DURATION
PO	unknown	unknown	unknown

Contraindications/Precautions
Contraindicated in: Shellfish allergy (glucosamine is often derived from marine exoskeletons); Pregnancy and lactation.
Use Cautiously in: Diabetes (may worsen glycemic control); Asthma (may exacerbate symptoms); Surgery (may affect blood glucose levels, discontinue glucosamine 2 wk before elective procedures).

Adverse Reactions/Side Effects
GI: constipation, diarrhea, heartburn, nausea. **CNS:** drowsiness, headache. **Derm:** skin reactions. **Endo:** hyperglycemia.

Interactions
Natural Product-Drug: May antagonize the effects of **antidiabetics**. May induce resistance to some chemotherapy drugs such as **etoposide**, **teniposide**, and **doxorubicin**. May increase anticoagulant effects of **warfarin**.
Natural-Natural: None known.

Route/Commonly Used Doses
PO (Adults): 500 mg three times daily.
Topical (Adults): use cream as needed for up to 8 wk.

Availability
Tablets 500 mg^OTC; **Capsules** 500 mg^OTC; **Topical cream** 30 mg/g in combination with other ingredients^OTC.

NURSING IMPLICATIONS
Assessment

- Assess for shellfish allergy prior to initiating therapy.
- Monitor pain (type, location, and intensity) and range of motion periodically during therapy.
- Assess bowel function periodically during therapy. Constipation may be reduced by increased fluid intake and bulk in diet; bulk laxatives may be added if necessary.

Lab Test Considerations

- Monitor serum glucose levels periodically during therapy for patients with diabetes.

Implementation

- Administer prior to meals.

Patient/Family Teaching

- Instruct patients that effects of this drug come from stimulating cartilage and synovial tissue metabolism and that the supplement must be taken on a regular basis to achieve benefit. Do not use as an intermittent pain medication.
- Caution patients with a shellfish allergy that this herbal supplement should not be used.
- Advise patient to notify health care professional if gastric discomfort develops and persists.
- Advise diabetic patients to monitor glucose values closely during initial therapy.

Evaluation

- Improvement in pain and range of motion.

---

green tea (green tee)
Other Name(s):
Camellia sinensis
Classification
Therapeutic: central nervous system stimulants

Common Uses

Bladder, esophageal, ovarian, and pancreatic cancer risk reduction, mental alertness, hypotension, cervical dysplasia associated with human papillomavirus infection, hyperlipidemia, weight loss, protection of the skin from sun damage, genital warts, dental caries, Parkinson's disease.

Action

Caffeine in green tea stimulates the CNS and cardiovascular system through adenosine receptor blockade and phosphodiesterase inhibition. **Therapeutic Effects:** Improved cognitive performance and mental alertness.

Pharmacokinetics

Absorption: Unknown.
Distribution: Unknown.
Metabolism and Excretion: Unknown.
Half-life: Unknown.

TIME/ACTION PROFILE

ROUTE	ONSET	PEAK	DURATION
PO	unknown	unknown	unknown

Contraindications/Precautions

Contraindicated in: Allergy/hypersensitivity; Pregnancy and lactation (doses >200 mg/day due to caffeine content).

Use Cautiously in: Patients with caffeine sensitivity. Long-term use of doses >250 mg/day may produce tolerance, psychological dependence, tachyarrhythmias, and sleep disturbances; Iron deficiency anemia (may worsen); Diabetes (may impair glucose control); Cardiac conditions (may induce arrhythmias in sensitive individuals); Bleeding disorders.

Adverse Reactions/Side Effects

CV: arrhythmia, tachycardia. **CNS:** agitation, dizziness, excitement, insomnia, tremors. **GI:** abdominal pain, diarrhea, hepatotoxicity, nausea, vomiting. **F and E:** hypokalemia. **Endo:** hyperglycemia. **Hemat:** prolonged bleeding time.

Interactions

Natural Product-Drug: Green tea may ↓ effects of **adenosine**. ↑ risk of bleeding with **anticoagulants** or **antiplatelet** agents. ↑ effects of **CNS stimulants**. May impair glucose control from **antidiabetic** agents. Abrupt withdrawal can ↑ **lithium** levels. May ↓ **dipyridamole** — induced vasodilation. **Verapamil** can ↑ caffeine concentrations by 25%. Additive effects with **methylxanthines**.
Natural-Natural: ↑ risk of adverse cardiovascular effects with **bitter orange**. ↑ risk of hepatotoxicity with hepatotoxic herbs or supplements. ↑ risk of seizures, hypertension, or stroke with **ephedra** and **creatine**.

Route/Commonly Used Doses

PO (Adults): Range: 1–10 cups/day. One cup provides approximately 60 mg of caffeine.

Availability

Tea leaves.

NURSING IMPLICATIONS

Assessment

- Monitor BP and heart rate periodically during therapy.

Lab Test Considerations

- Monitor serum glucose, homocysteine, and uric acid levels periodically during therapy.
- Monitor liver and kidney function periodically during therapy.

Implementation

- May be taken as tea or as an extract in capsules.

Patient/Family Teaching

- Rep: Advise females of reproductive potential to limit green tea due to the caffeine content.

Evaluation

- Improvement in memory.

---

lutein (loo-tee-in)

Other Name(s):
carotenoid epsilon-carotene-3, e-lutein, luteina, xanthophyll, zeaxanthin
Classification
Therapeutic: ocular agents

Common Uses

Prevention of vision loss or eye disease.

Action

Lutein is a pigment called carotenoid, and is one of two major carotenoids found in the human eye. It functions as a light filter, protecting the tissue from sun damage. **Therapeutic Effects:** Decreased risk of development of AMD and cataracts.

Pharmacokinetics

Absorption: Unknown.
Distribution: Unknown.
Metabolism and Excretion: Unknown.
Half-life: Unknown.

TIME/ACTION PROFILE

ROUTE	ONSET	PEAK	DURATION
PO	Unknown	Unknown	Unknown

Contraindications/Precautions

Contraindicated in: Hypersensitivity.
Use Cautiously in: Cystic fibrosis; Pregnancy and lactation.

Adverse Reactions/Side Effects

Derm: carotendermia.

Interactions

Natural Product-Drug: There are no known natural-drug interactions. Advise patients to speak to medical practitioners before starting any new supplement if they are on medication.

Natural-Natural: Taking with **beta-carotene** or **Vitamin E** may reduce the absorptions of these vitamins.

Route/Commonly Used Doses
PO (Adults): 10–20 mg/day.

Availability
Capules^OTC; Tablets^OTC.

NURSING IMPLICATIONS
Assessment
● Instruct patients to have yearly ophthalmic examinations.

Implementation
● PO: Orally as a capsule or tablets as a single daily dose.

Patient/Family Teaching
● Advise patient to take as directed.

Evaluation
● Decreased risk of macular degeneration or cataracts.

---

melatonin (mel-uh-**toh**-nin)
Other Name(s):
pineal hormone, N-acetyl-5–methoxtryptamine
Classification
Therapeutic: sedative/hypnotics

Common Uses
Sleep disorders (including insomnia, jet lag and circadian rhythm disorders).

Action
Melatonin is a hormone secreted from the pineal gland in a 24-hour circadian rhythm, regulating the normal sleep/wake cycle. As a supplement, melatonin has both phase-shifting and sleep-promoting properties. In addition to promoting sleep, physiologic roles of melatonin include regulation of the secretion of growth hormone and gonadotropic hormones. It also possesses antioxidant activity. **Therapeutic Effects:** Improved sleep pattern.

Pharmacokinetics
Absorption: Unknown.
Distribution: Unknown.
Metabolism and Excretion: Unknown.
Half-life: Unknown.

TIME/ACTION PROFILE

	ONSET	PEAK	DURATION
PO	unknown	unknown	unknown

Contraindications/Precautions
Contraindicated in: Hypersensitivity; Pregnancy and lactation.
Use Cautiously in: Seizure disorders; Diabetes; Hypertension.

Adverse Reactions/Side Effects
CV: hypotension. **GI:** abdominal cramps, nausea, vomiting. **Neuro:** dizziness, drowsiness, headache.

Interactions
Natural Product-Drug: Additive sedation with **CNS depressants**. May ↑ bleeding risk with **antiplatelet agents** and **anticoagulants**. May interfere with the glucose-lowering effects of **hypoglycemic agents**. May decrease effectiveness of **nifedipine**.
Natural-Natural: May have additive sedative effects with herbs that have sedative properties including **5–HTP, kava, St.John's wort, valerian** and others. May increase risk of bleeding with herbs that have antiplatelet/anticoagulant properties such as **clove, garlic, ginger, gingko, ginseng** and others.

Route/Commonly Used Doses
PO (Adults): 0.3–10 mg daily at bedtime.

Availability
Capsules^OTC; Tablets^OTC; Sublingual Tablets^OTC; Gummies^OTC.

NURSING IMPLICATIONS
Assessment
● Assess sleep patterns before and periodically throughout therapy.

Lab Test Considerations
● Monitor blood glucose, coagulation panel, hormone panel, and lipid panel periodically during therapy.

Implementation
● PO: Administer before bedtime.

Patient/Family Teaching
● Instruct patient to take at bedtime as directed.
● Causes drowsiness. Caution patient to avoid driving and other activities requiring alertness until response to medication is known.
● Caution patient to avoid concurrent use of alcohol or other CNS depressants.
● Advise female patient to notify health care professional if pregnancy is planned or suspected or if breast feeding.

Evaluation
● Relief of insomnia.

CAPITALS = life-threatening; Underline = most frequent.

milk thistle (milk this-ul)

Other Name(s):
Holy thistle, Lady's thistle, Mary Thistle, Silybin, Silymarin
Classification
Therapeutic: antidotes

Common Uses
Cirrhosis, chronic hepatitis, gallstones, psoriasis, liver cleansing and detoxification, treatment of liver toxicity due to Amanita mushroom poisoning (European IV formulation), and chemicals. Dyspepsia (in combination with other herbs). Diabetes.

Action
The active component, silymarin, has antioxidant and hepatoprotectant actions. Silymarin helps prevent toxin penetration and stimulates hepatocyte regeneration. **Therapeutic Effects:** Liver detoxification. Improved dyspepsia symptoms. Decreased fasting blood glucose.

Pharmacokinetics
Absorption: 23–47% absorbed after oral administration.
Distribution: Unknown.
Metabolism and Excretion: Hepatic metabolism by cytochrome P450 3A4.
Half-life: 6 hr.

TIME/ACTION PROFILE

ROUTE	ONSET	PEAK	DURATION
PO	5–30 days or more	unknown	unknown

Contraindications/Precautions
Contraindicated in: Pregnancy and lactation (insufficient information available); Allergy to chamomile, ragweed, asters, chrysanthemums, and other members of the family *Asteraceae/Compositae*.
Use Cautiously in: Hormone-sensitive cancers/conditions (milk thistle plant parts may have estrogenic effects).

Adverse Reactions/Side Effects
GI: anorexia, bloating, Laxative effect, nausea. **Misc:** Allergic reactions.

Interactions
Natural Product-Drug: In vitro, milk thistle extract inhibited the drug-metabolizing enzyme **cytochrome P450 3A4**. Interactions have not been reported in humans, but milk thistle should be used cautiously with other drugs metabolized by 3A4, such as **cyclosporine**, **carbamazepine**, **HMG-CoA inhibitors**, **ketoconazole**, and **alprazolam**.
Natural-Natural: Herbs with hypoglycemic potential may have additive hypoglycemic effects.

Route/Commonly Used Doses
PO (Adults): *Hepatic cirrhosis:* 420 mg/day of extract containing 70–80% silymarin; *Chronic active hepatitis:* 140 mg tid of silymarin; 240 mg bid of silibinin; *Diabetes:* 200 mg tid of silymarin; *Tea:* 3–4 times daily 30 min before meals. Tea is not recommended as silymarin is not sufficiently water soluble.
IV (Adults): 20–50 mg/kg over 24 hr, 48 hr post–mushroom ingestion (IV formulation not available in US).

Availability
Capsules^OTC; Tablets^OTC; Crude drug^OTC; Tea^OTC; Extract^OTC.

NURSING IMPLICATIONS
Assessment
- Assess patients for signs of liver failure (jaundice, mental status changes, abdominal distention, ascites, generalized edema).
- Evaluate consistency and frequency of bowel movements.

Lab Test Considerations
- Monitor liver function, lipid profile, and blood glucose periodically during therapy.

Implementation
- **PO:** Orally as an extract, capsule, tablets, or as a dried fruit as a single daily dose or divided into three doses.
- Tea is not recommended as milk thistle is not water-soluble.

Patient/Family Teaching
- Inform patient of symptoms of liver failure; advise patient to report worsening symptomatology promptly to health care professional.
- Advise patients to avoid alcohol and follow diet for liver or gall bladder disease being treated.
- Emphasize the need for blood tests to monitor liver function tests.

Evaluation
- Normalization of liver function tests.
- Reduction in jaundice, abdominal distention, fatigue, and other symptoms associated with liver disease.

saw palmetto
(saw pal-**met**-toe)
Other Name(s):
American Dwarf Palm Tree, Cabbage Palm, Ju-Zhong, Palmier Nain, Sabal, Sabal Fructus, Saw Palmetto Berry, *Serenoa repens*
Classification
Therapeutic: benign prostatic hyperplasia (BPH) agents

Common Uses

Benign prostatic hyperplasia.

Action

Exerts antiandrogenic, anti-inflammatory, and antiproliferative properties in prostate tissue resulting in improvement in BPH symptoms such as frequent urination, hesitancy, urgency, and nocturia. Comparable in efficacy to finasteride but may be less effective than prazosin. **Therapeutic Effects:** Decreased urinary symptoms of BPH.

Pharmacokinetics

Absorption: Unknown.
Distribution: Unknown.
Metabolism and Excretion: Unknown.
Half-life: Unknown.

TIME/ACTION PROFILE

ROUTE	ONSET	PEAK	DURATION
PO	1–2 mo	unknown	48 wk (longest studied treatment duration)

Contraindications/Precautions

Contraindicated in: Pregnancy and lactation.
Use Cautiously in: Prior to surgery (discontinue 2 wk before to prevent bleeding).

Adverse Reactions/Side Effects

CNS: dizziness, headache. **GI:** constipation, diarrhea, nausea, vomiting.

Interactions

Natural Product-Drug: Hormonal action may interfere with other hormonal therapies (**testosterone**, **hormonal contraceptives**). Avoid use with **antiplatelet** or **anticoagulant drugs** (may ↑ bleeding risk).
Natural-Natural: Concomitant use with herbs that affect platelet aggregation such as **ginger**, **garlic**, **gingko**, and **ginseng** may ↑ bleeding risk.

Route/Commonly Used Doses

PO (Adults): *Lipophilic extract (80–90% fatty acids):* 160 mg twice daily or 320 mg once daily. *Whole berries:* 1–2 g daily. *Liquid extract from berry pulp:* 1–2 mL three times daily. *Tea (efficacy is questionable due to lipophilicity of active constituents):* 1 cup three times daily. Tea is prepared by steeping 0.5–1 g dried berry in 150 mL boiling water for 5–10 min.

Availability

Lipophilic extract (80-90% fatty acids)[OTC];
Whole berries[OTC]; **Liquid extract**[OTC].

NURSING IMPLICATIONS

Assessment

- Assess patient for symptoms of benign prostatic hypertrophy (BPH) (urinary hesitancy, feeling of incomplete bladder emptying, interruption in urinary stream, impairment in size and force of urinary stream, terminal urinary dribbling, straining to start flow, dysuria, urgency) before and periodically during therapy.
- Perform rectal exams prior to and periodically during therapy to assess prostate size are recommended.

Implementation

- Take on a full stomach to minimize GI effects.

Patient/Family Teaching

- Advise patients to start therapy with saw palmetto only after evaluation by a health care professional who will provide continued follow-up care.
- Inform patients that saw palmetto does not alter the size of the prostate but still should relieve the symptoms associated with BPH.
- Advise patient that taking saw palmetto with food may reduce GI effects and improve tolerability.

Evaluation

- Decrease in urinary symptoms of BPH.

St. John's wort (*Hypericum perforatum*)

(saynt **jonz** wort)
Other Name(s):
Amber, Demon chaser, Goatweed, Hardhay, Klamath weed, Rosin rose, Tipton weed
Classification
Therapeutic: antidepressants

Common Uses

PO: Management of mild to moderate depression and obsessive compulsive disorder (OCD). (Not effective for major depression.) **Topical:** Inflammation of the skin, blunt injury, wounds, and burns. Other uses are for capillary strengthening, decreasing uterine bleeding, and reducing tumor size.

Action

Derived from *Hypericum perforatum*; the active component is *hypericin*. **PO:** Antidepressant action may be due to ability to inhibit reuptake of serotonin and other neurotransmitters. **Topical:** Anti-inflammatory, antifungal, antiviral, and antibacterial properties. **Therapeutic Effects: PO:** Decreased signs and symptoms of depression. **Topical:** Decreased inflammation of burns or other wounds.

CAPITALS = life-threatening; Underline = most frequent.

Pharmacokinetics

Absorption: Unknown.
Distribution: Unknown.
Metabolism and Excretion: Unknown.
Half-life: *Hypericum constituents:* 24.8–26.5 hr.

TIME/ACTION PROFILE

ROUTE	ONSET	PEAK	DURATION
PO	10–14 days	within 4–6 wk	unknown

Contraindications/Precautions

Contraindicated in: Pregnancy and lactation.
Use Cautiously in: Children 6–17 years: use orally no longer than 8 wk; History of phototoxicity; Surgery (discontinue 2 wk prior to surgical procedures); Alzheimer's disease (may induce psychosis); Patients undergoing general anesthesia (may cause cardiovascular collapse); History of suicide attempt, severe depression, schizophrenia, or bipolar disorder (can induce hypomania or psychosis).

Adverse Reactions/Side Effects

CNS: dizziness, restlessness, sleep disturbances. **CV:** hypertension. **GI:** abdominal pain, bloating, diarrhea, dry mouth, feeling of fullness, flatulence, nausea, vomiting. **Neuro:** neuropathy. **Derm:** allergic skin reactions (hives, itching, skin rash), phototoxicity. **Misc:** serotonin syndrome.

Interactions

Natural Product-Drug: Concurrent use with **alcohol** or other **antidepressants** (including **SSRIs** and **MAO inhibitors**) may ↑ risk of adverse CNS reactions. May ↓ the effectiveness and serum concentrations of **digoxin**, **alprazolam**, **amitriptyline**, **imatinib**, **irinotecan**, **warfarin**, and **protease inhibitors**. Use with **MAO Inhibitors**, **tramadol**, **pentazocine**, and **selective serotonin agonists** could result in serotonin syndrome. May ↓ effectiveness of **oral contraceptives**. May ↓ plasma **cyclosporine** and **tacrolimus** levels by 30–70% and cause acute transplant rejection. May ↑ metabolism of **phenytoin** and **phenobarbital** and cause loss of seizure control. Avoid use of St. John's wort and **MAO Inhibitors** within 2 wk of each other.
Natural-Natural: May ↑ risk of serotonin syndrome when taken with **tryptophan** and **SAM-e**.

Route/Commonly Used Doses

PO (Adults): *Mild Depression:* 300 mg of St. John's wort (standardized to 0.3% hypericin) 3 times daily or 250 mg twice daily of 0.2% hypericin extract. *OCD:* 450 mg twice daily of extended release preparation.
Topical (Adults): 0.2–1 mg total hypericin daily.

Availability

Preparations for Oral Use

Dried herb^(OTC); Dried (hydroalcoholic) extract^(OTC); Oil^(OTC); Tincture^(OTC).

Preparations for Topical Application

Liquid^(OTC); Semisolid^(OTC).

NURSING IMPLICATIONS

Assessment

- **Depression:** Assess for depression periodically during therapy.
- **Inflammation:** Assess skin or skin lesions periodically during therapy.

Implementation

- **PO:** Tea can be prepared by mixing 2–4 dried herbs in 150 mL of boiling water and steeping for 10 min.

Patient/Family Teaching

- Instruct patient to take St. John's wort as directed.
- Patients with depression should be evaluated by health care professional. Standard therapy may be of greater benefit for moderate to severe depression.
- Instruct patient to consult health care professional before taking other Rx, OTC, or herbal products concurrently with St. John's wort. May reduce the therapeutic effectiveness of other drugs. May potentiate effect of sedatives and side effects of other antidepressants. Do not take within 2 wk of MAO inhibitor therapy.
- Caution patients to avoid sun exposure and use protective sunscreen to reduce the risk of photosensitivity reactions.
- Inform patient to purchase herbs from a reputable source and that products and their contents vary among different manufacturers.
- Caution patient not to use alcohol while taking St. John's wort.
- Advise patient to notify health care professional of medication regimen prior to treatment or surgery.
- Inform patient that St. John's wort is usually taken for a period of 4–6 wk. If no improvement is seen, another therapy should be considered.

Evaluation

- Decrease in signs and symptoms of depression or anxiety.
- Improvement in skin inflammation.

---

turmeric (tur-mur-rik)

Other Name(s):

curcuma, curcumin, curcuminoid, turmeric root

Classification
Therapeutic: anti-inflammatories

Common Uses
Osteoarthritis. Dyspepsia. Pruritus.

Action
Turmeric is a spice that contains a chemical called curcumin, which may reduce swelling. As a supplement, turmeric may have both pain relief and anti-inflammatory properties. **Therapeutic Effects:** Decreased inflammation.

Pharmacokinetics
Absorption: Unknown.
Distribution: Unknown.
Metabolism and Excretion: Unknown.
Half-life: Unknown.

TIME/ACTION PROFILE

	ONSET	PEAK	DURATION
PO	unknown	unknown	unknown

Contraindications/Precautions
Contraindicated in: Hypersensitivity; Pregnancy and lactation.
Use Cautiously in: Diabetes; Coagulation disorders; Liver disorders.

Adverse Reactions/Side Effects
GI: diarrhea, nausea, vomiting. **Neuro:** dizziness.

Interactions
Natural Product-Drug: May increase bleeding risk with **antiplatelet agents** and **anticoagulants**. Turmeric is an antioxidant, there are concerns it may decrease the effects of some cancer medications (**alkylating agents** or **Topoisomerase I inhibitors**). May interfere with the glucose lowering effects of **hypoglycemic agents** and cause blood sugar to drop. May affect absorption of **talinolol**, ↓ the effects. May affect absorption of **amlodipine**, ↑ the effects. May affect absorption of **tamoxifex**, ↓ the effects. Turmeric should be used cautiously with other drugs metabolized by the liver (**Cytochrome P450**). Large amounts of turmeric may decrease effects of **estrogen**.
Natural-Natural: May have affect absorption of iron. May increase risk of bleeding with herbs that have antiplatelet/anticoagulant properties such as **clove**, **garlic**, **ginger**, **gingko**, **ginseng** and others. Avoid using with other with herbs that affect blood glucose such as **chromium**, **fenugreek**, **garlic**, **ginseng** and others.

Route/Commonly Used Doses
PO (Adults): 1–2 g per day.

Availability
Capsules^OTC; Tablets^OTC.

NURSING IMPLICATIONS
Assessment

Lab Test Considerations
- Monitor blood glucose, coagulation panel, hormone panel, and lipid panel periodically during therapy.

Implementation
- **PO:** Orally as a capsule or tablets as a single daily dose or divided into three doses.
- It is sometimes prepared as a topical cream or gel.

Patient/Family Teaching
- Advise patient to report worsening symptomatology promptly to health care professional.
- Rep: Advise females of reproductive potential to notify health care professional if pregnancy is planned or suspected or if breast feeding.

Evaluation
- Relief of pain and inflammation.

valerian (vuh-lare-ee-en)
Other Name(s):
Amantilla, All-Heal, Baldrian, Baldrianwurzel, Belgium Valerian, Common Valerian, Fragrant Valerian, Garden Heliotrope, Garden Valerian, Indian Valerian, Mexican Valerian, Pacific Valerian, Tagara, Valeriana, *Valeriana officinalis*, *Valerianae radix*, Valeriana rhizome, Valeriane
Classification
Therapeutic: antianxiety agents, sedative/hypnotics

Common Uses
Insomnia. Anxiety.

Action
May increase concentrations of the inhibitory CNS transmitter GABA. **Therapeutic Effects:** Improvement in sleep quality.

Pharmacokinetics
Absorption: Unknown.
Distribution: Unknown.
Metabolism and Excretion: Unknown.
Half-life: Unknown.

TIME/ACTION PROFILE

ROUTE	ONSET	PEAK	DURATION
PO	30–60 min	2 hr	unknown

Contraindications/Precautions
Contraindicated in: Pregnancy and lactation.
Use Cautiously in: Alcohol use (may have additive sedative effects); Surgery (discontinue use 2 wk prior to elective procedures); Children (do not use longer than 8 wk).

Adverse Reactions/Side Effects

CNS: drowsiness, headache. **GI:** dry mouth. **Misc:** Benzodiazepine-like withdrawal symptoms with discontinuation after long-term use.

Interactions

Natural Product-Drug: Additive CNS depression with **alcohol, antihistamines, anesthetic agents, sedative hypnotics,** and other **CNS depressants.** Alcohol-containing preparations may interact with **disulfiram** and **metronidazole.**

Natural-Natural: Additive sedative effects can occur when used with herbal supplements with sedative properties such as **kava, l-tryptophan, melatonin, SAMe,** and **St. John's wort.**

Route/Commonly Used Doses

PO (Adults): *Tea:* 1 cup tea 1–5 times daily. Tea is made by steeping 2–3 g root in 150 mL boiling water for 5–10 min then straining. *Tincture:* 1–3 mL 1–5 times daily. *Extract:* 400–900 mg up to 2 hr before bedtime or 300–450 mg divided tid.

Availability

Capsules^OTC^; Extract^OTC^; Tea^OTC^; Tincture^OTC^.

NURSING IMPLICATIONS

Assessment

- Assess degree of anxiety and level of sedation prior to and periodically throughout therapy.
- Assess sleep patterns.

- Assess response in the elderly population where drowsiness and loss of balance may pose a significant risk for injury.

Implementation

- Take 1–2 hr before bedtime if used for nighttime hypnotic.
- Administer orally three to five times daily to control anxiety.

Patient/Family Teaching

- Encourage patients to avoid stimulants such as caffeine and to provide an environment that promotes restful sleep.
- May cause drowsiness. Caution patient to avoid driving or other activities requiring alertness until response to drug is known.
- Caution patient to avoid use of alcohol and other medications or herbals that have a sedative effect; may increase drowsiness.
- Advise patients to discontinue 2 wk prior to elective surgical procedures.
- Inform patients that dependence with withdrawal symptoms may develop with prolonged use.
- Rep: Advise females of reproductive potential to avoid valerian if pregnancy is planned or suspected or breast feeding.

Evaluation

- Decreased anxiety level.
- Improvement in sleep with a feeling of restfulness without drowsiness upon awakening.

BEERS CRITERIA

The Beers criteria for potentially inappropriate medication use in adults 65 and older in the United States is a compilation of drugs and drug classes found to increase the risk of adverse events in older adults. Frequently, older adults are more sensitive to the medications or their side effects. These adverse events have significant economic and quality of life costs for society and individuals and can result in more frequent hospitalizations, permanent injury, or death. Often, the potential for adverse events can be minimized by prescribing safer alternatives or prescribing at the lowest effective dose.

ALPRAZolam (avoid use) (Xanax, Xanax XR)

amiodarone (avoid use as first-line therapy for atrial fibrillation unless heart failure or significant left ventricular hypertrophy present) (Nexterone, Pacerone)

amitriptyline (avoid use) (Elavil)

amoxapine (avoid use)

ARIPiprazole (avoid use, except in schizophrenia, bipolar disorder, or adjunctive treatment of major depressive disorder) (Abilify, Abilify Asimtufii, Abilify Maintena, Abilify MyCite, Aristada, Aristada Initio)

asenapine (avoid use, except in schizophrenia or bipolar disorder) (Saphris, Secuado)

aspirin (avoid use for primary prevention of cardiovascular disease; avoid chronic use for pain (at doses >325 mg/day) unless other alternatives are not effective and the patient can take a gastroprotective agent; avoid short-term use for pain (at doses >325 mg/day) in combination with oral or parenteral corticosteroids, anticoagulants, or antiplatelet agents unless other alternatives are not effective and the patient can take a gastroprotective agent)

atropine (avoid use of all formulations except for ophthalmic formulations) (Atropen)

benztropine (avoid use of oral formulation)

brexpiprazole (avoid use, except in schizophrenia, adjunctive treatment of major depressive disorder, or agitation associated with dementia due to Alzheimer's disease) (Rexulti)

bumetanide (use with caution) (Burinex)

butalbital (avoid use)

canagliflozin (use with caution) (Invokana)

carBAMazepine (use with caution) (Carbatrol, Epitol, Equetro, TEGretol, TEGretol CR, TEGretol XR)

cariprazine (avoid use, except in schizophrenia, bipolar disorder. or adjunctive treatment of major depressive disorder) (Vraylar)

carisoprodol (avoid use) (Soma)

chlordiazePOXIDE (avoid use)

chlordiazePOXIDE-amitriptyline (avoid use)

chlorothiazide (use with caution) (Diuril)

chlorpheniramine (avoid use) (Chlor-Trimeton, Chlor-Trimeton Allergy, Ed Chlorphed Jr)

chlorproMAZINE (avoid use, except in schizophrenia, bipolar disorder, or for short-term use as an antiemetic)

chlorthalidone (use with caution) (Thalitone)

chlorzoxazone (avoid use) (Lorzone)

citalopram (use with caution) (CeleXA)

clidinium-chlordiazepoxide (avoid use) (Librax)

cloBAZam (avoid use) (Onfi, Sympazan)

clomiPRAMINE (avoid use) (Anafranil)

clonazePAM (avoid use) (KlonoPIN, Rivotril)

cloNIDine (avoid use for first-line treatment of hypertension) (Catapres-TTS, Duraclon, Kapvay, Nexiclon XR)

clorazepate (avoid use)

cloZAPine (avoid use, except in schizophrenia, bipolar disorder, or psychosis in Parkinson disease) (Clozaril, Versacloz)

---

cyclobenzaprine (avoid use) (Amrix, Fexmid)

cyproheptadine (avoid use)

dabigatran (use caution in selecting over apixaban for long-term treatment of nonvalvular atrial fibrillation or venous thromboembolism) (Pradaxa)

dapagliflozin (use with caution) (Farxiga, Forxiga)

desipramine (avoid use) (Norpramin)

desmopressin (avoid use for treatment of nocturia or nocturnal polyuria) (Bipazen, DDAVP, DDAVP Melt, Nocdurna, Octostim)

dessicated thyroid (avoid use) (Adthyza, Armour Thyroid)

desvenlafaxine (use with caution) (Pristiq)

dexlansoprazole (avoid scheduled use for >8 wk unless for high-risk patients [e.g., oral corticosteroid or chronic NSAID use] or patients with erosive esophagitis, Barrett's esophagitis, pathological hypersecretory condition, or demonstrated need for maintenance treatment [e.g., failure of H_2 antagonist]) (Dexilant)

dextromethorphan-quinidine (use with caution) (Nuedexta)

diazePAM (avoid use) (Diastat, Valium, Valtoco)

diclofenac (avoid chronic use unless other alternatives are not effective and the patient can take a gastroprotective agent; avoid short-term use in combination with oral or parenteral corticosteroids, anticoagulants, or antiplatelet agents unless other alternatives are not effective and the patient can take a gastroprotective agent) (Cambia, Flector, Lofena, Pennsaid, Voltaren, Zipsor, Zorvolex)

dicyclomine (avoid use) (Bentyl)

diflunisal (avoid chronic use unless other alternatives are not effective and the patient can take a gastroprotective agent; avoid short-term use in combination with oral or parenteral corticosteroids, anticoagulants, or antiplatelet agents unless other alternatives are not effective and the patient can take a gastroprotective agent)

digoxin (avoid use for first-line treatment of atrial fibrillation or heart failure; if used, avoid using dose >0.125 mg/day) (Lanoxin)

dimenhyDRINATE (avoid use) (Dramamine, Driminate, Gravol)

diphenhydrAMINE (avoid use of oral formulations) (Benadryl)

dipyridamole (avoid use of short-acting formulation) (Persantine)

doxazosin (avoid use for treatment of hypertension) (Cardura, Cardura XL)

doxepin (avoid use of dose >6 mg/day) (Silenor, Sinequan)

doxylamine (avoid use)

dronedarone (avoid use in patients with permanent atrial fibrillation or HF) (Multaq)

DULoxetine (use with caution) (Cymbalta)

empagliflozin (use with caution) (Jardiance)

ergoloid mesylates (avoid use)

ertugliflozin (use with caution) (Steglatro)

escitalopram (use with caution) (Cipralex, Lexapro)

BEERS CRITERIA continued

esomeprazole (avoid scheduled use for >8 wk unless for high-risk patients [e.g., oral corticosteroid or chronic NSAID use], or patients with erosive esophagitis, Barrett's esophagitis, pathological hypersecretory condition, or demonstrated need for maintenance treatment [e.g., failure of H_2 antagonist]) (NexIUM, NexIUM 24HR)

estazolam (avoid use)

estrogens (with or without progestins) (avoid use of systemic estrogens; intravaginal formulations acceptable to use for treatment of dyspareunia, recurrent lower urinary tract infections, and other vaginal symptoms)

eszopiclone (avoid use) (Lunesta)

etodolac (avoid chronic use unless other alternatives are not effective and the patient can take a gastroprotective agent; avoid short-term use in combination with oral or parenteral corticosteroids, anticoagulants, or antiplatelet agents unless other alternatives are not effective and the patient can take a gastroprotective agent)

FLUoxetine (use with caution) (PROzac)

fluPHENAZine (avoid use, except in schizophrenia)

flurbiprofen (avoid chronic use unless other alternatives are not effective and the patient can take a gastroprotective agent; avoid short-term use in combination with oral or parenteral corticosteroids, anticoagulants, or antiplatelet agents unless other alternatives are not effective and the patient can take a gastroprotective agent)

fluvoxaMINE (use with caution) (Luvox)

furosemide (use with caution) (Furoscix, Lasix)

glimepiride (avoid use as first- or second-line monotherapy or as add-on treatment unless there are significant barriers to the use of safer and more effective agents; if a sulfonylurea is used, glipizide is preferred) (Amaryl)

glipiZIDE (avoid use as first- or second-line monotherapy or as add-on treatment unless there are significant barriers to the use of safer and more effective agents; if a sulfonylurea is used, this is the preferred agent) (Glucotrol XL)

glyBURIDE (avoid use as first- or second-line monotherapy or as add-on treatment unless there are significant barriers to the use of safer and more effective agents; if a sulfonylurea is used, glipizide is preferred) (Glynase)

growth hormone (avoid use, except for confirmed growth hormone deficiency due to an established etiology)

guanFACINE (avoid use for treatment of hypertension) (Intuniv, Intuniv XR)

haloperidol (avoid use, except in schizophrenia, bipolar disorder, or for short-term use as antiemetic) (Haldol Decanoate)

hydroCHLOROthiazide (use with caution)

hydrOXYzine (avoid use) (Atarax, Vistaril)

hyoscyamine (avoid use) (Anaspaz, Levbid, Levsin, Nulev, Oscimin, Symax)

ibuprofen (avoid chronic use unless other alternatives are not effective and the patient can take a gastroprotective agent; avoid short-term use in combination with oral or parenteral corticosteroids, anticoagulants, or antiplatelet agents unless other alternatives are not effective and the patient can take a gastroprotective agent) (Advil, Motrin)

iloperidone (avoid use, except in schizophrenia) (Fanapt)

imipramine (avoid use)

indomethacin (avoid chronic use unless other alternatives are not effective and the patient can take a gastroprotective agent; avoid short-term use in combination with oral or parenteral corticosteroids, anticoagulants, or antiplatelet agents unless other alternatives are not effective and the patient can take a gastroprotective agent) (Indocin)

insulin (avoid use of regimens containing only short- or rapid-acting insulin without concurrent use of basal or long-acting insulin)

ketorolac (avoid chronic use unless other alternatives are not effective and the patient can take a gastroprotective agent; avoid short-term use in combination with oral or parenteral corticosteroids, anticoagulants, or antiplatelet agents unless other alternatives are not effective and the patient can take a gastroprotective agent) (Sprix, Toradol)

lansoprazole (avoid scheduled use for >8 wk unless for high-risk patients [e.g., oral corticosteroid or chronic NSAID use], or patients with erosive esophagitis, Barrett's esophagitis, pathological hypersecretory condition, or demonstrated need for maintenance treatment [e.g., failure of H_2 antagonist]) (Prevacid, Prevacid 24HR, Prevacid SoluTab)

levomilnacipran (use with caution) (Fetzima)

LORazepam (avoid use) (Ativan, Loreev XR)

lumateperone (avoid use, except in schizophrenia or bipolar disorder) (Caplyta)

lurasidone (avoid use, except in schizophrenia or bipolar disorder) (Latuda)

meclizine (avoid use) (Antivert, Bonine)

megestrol (avoid use)

meloxicam (avoid chronic use unless other alternatives are not effective and the patient can take a gastroprotective agent; avoid short-term use in combination with oral or parenteral corticosteroids, anticoagulants, or antiplatelet agents unless other alternatives are not effective and the patient can take a gastroprotective agent)

meperidine (avoid use) (Demerol)

meprobamate (avoid use)

metaxalone (avoid use)

methocarbamol (avoid use) (Robaxin)

methylTESTOSTERone (avoid use, except for confirmed hypogonadism with clinical symptoms) (Methitest)

metoclopramide (avoid use, except in gastroparesis [use should generally not exceed 12 wk]) (Gimoti, Metonia, Reglan)

midazolam (avoid use) (Nayzilam, Seizalam)

milnacipran (use with caution) (Savella)

mineral oil (avoid oral use) (Fleet Oil)

mirtazapine (use with caution) (Remeron, Remeron RD, Remeron SolTab)

nabumetone (avoid chronic use unless other alternatives are not effective and the patient can take a gastroprotective agent; avoid short-term use in combination with oral or parenteral corticosteroids, anticoagulants, or antiplatelet agents unless other alternatives are not effective and the patient can take a gastroprotective agent) (Relafen DS)

naproxen (avoid chronic use unless other alternatives are not effective and the patient can take a gastroprotective agent; avoid short-term use in combination with oral or parenteral corticosteroids, anticoagulants, or antiplatelet agents unless other alternatives are not effective and the patient can take a gastroprotective agent) (Aleve, Anaprox, Anaprox DS, Maxidol, Naprelan, Naprosyn)

NIFEdipine (avoid use of immediate-release formulation) (Adalat XL, Procardia XL)

nitrofurantoin (avoid use if CCr <30 mL/min or for long-term suppression of urinary tract infections) (Furadantin, Macrobid, Microdantin)

nortriptyline (avoid use) (Aventyl, Pamelor)

OLANZapine (avoid use, except in schizophrenia, bipolar disorder, or for short-term use as antiemetic) (ZyPREXA, ZyPREXA Relprevv, ZyPREXA Zydis)

olanzapine-fluoxetine (avoid use, except in bipolar disorder or treatment-resistant depression) (Symbyax)

olanzapine-samidorphan (avoid use, except in schizophrenia or bipolar disorder) (Lybalvi)

omeprazole (avoid scheduled use for >8 wk unless for high-risk patients [e.g., oral corticosteroid or chronic NSAID use], or patients with erosive esophagitis, pathological hypersecretory condition, or demonstrated need for maintenance treatment [e.g., failure of H_2 antagonist]) (Losec, PriLOSEC, PriLOSEC OTC)

orphenadrine (avoid use)

oxaprozin (avoid chronic use unless other alternatives are not effective and the patient can take a gastroprotective agent; avoid short-term use in combination with oral or parenteral corticosteroids, anticoagulants, or antiplatelet agents unless other alternatives are not effective and the patient can take a gastroprotective agent) (Daypro)

oxazepam (avoid use)

OXcarbazepine (use with caution) (Oxtellar XR, Trileptal)

paliperidone (avoid use, except in schizophrenia) (Invega, Invega Hafyera, Invega Sustenna, Invega Trinza)

pantoprazole (avoid scheduled use for >8 wk unless for high-risk patients [e.g., oral corticosteroid or chronic NSAID use], or patients with erosive esophagitis, Barrett's esophagitis, pathological hypersecretory condition, or demonstrated need for maintenance treatment [e.g., failure of H_2 antagonist]) (Pantoloc, Protonix, Tecta)

PARoxetine (avoid use) (Paxil, Paxil CR, Pexeva)

perphenazine (avoid use, except in schizophrenia or for short-term use as antiemetic)

perphenazine-amitriptyline (avoid use, except in schizophrenia or major depressive disorder with anxiety/agitation)

PHENobarbital (avoid use) (Sezaby)

pimavanserin (avoid use, except in psychosis in Parkinson disease) (Nuplazid)

piroxicam (avoid chronic use unless other alternatives are not effective and the patient can take a gastroprotective agent; avoid short-term use in combination with oral or parenteral corticosteroids, anticoagulants, or antiplatelet agents unless other alternatives are not effective and the patient can take a gastroprotective agent) (Feldene)

prasugrel (use with caution, especially in patients 75 years old; if used in patients 75 years old, consider using a lower dose [5 mg]) (Effient)

prazosin (avoid use for treatment of hypertension) (Minipress)

primidone (avoid use) (Mysoline)

promethazine (avoid use) (Histanil, Phenergan, Promethegan)

QUEtiapine (avoid use, except in schizophrenia, bipolar disorder, adjunctive treatment of major depressive disorder, or psychosis in Parkinson disease) (SEROquel, SEROquel XR)

RABEprazole (avoid scheduled use for >8 wk unless for high-risk patients [e.g., oral corticosteroid or chronic NSAID use], or patients with erosive esophagitis, Barrett esophagitis, or pathological hypersecretory condition, or demonstrated need for maintenance treatment [e.g., failure of H_2 antagonist]) (Aciphex, Pariet)

risperiDONE (avoid use, except in schizophrenia or bipolar disorder) (Perseris, RisperDAL, RisperDAL Consta, RisperDAL M-TAB, Rykindo, Uzedy)

rivaroxaban (avoid use for long-term treatment of atrial fibrillation or venous thromboembolism in favor of safer anticoagulant options) (Xarelto)

scopolamine (avoid use) (Transderm-Scop)

sertraline (use with caution) (Zoloft)

sulindac (avoid chronic use unless other alternatives are not effective and the patient can take a gastroprotective agent; avoid short-term use in combination with oral or parenteral corticosteroids, anticoagulants, or antiplatelet agents unless other alternatives are not effective and the patient can take a gastroprotective agent)

temazepam (avoid use) (Restoril)

terazosin (avoid use for treatment of hypertension)

testosterone (avoid use, except for confirmed hypogonadism with clinical symptoms) (Androgel, Aveed, Delatestryl, Depo-Testosterone, Fortesta, Jatenzo, Kyzatrex, Natesto, Testim, Testopel, Tlando, Vogelxo, Xyosted)

thioridazine (avoid use, except in schizophrenia)

thiothixene (avoid use, except in schizophrenia)

ticagrelor (use with caution, especially in patients 75 years old) (Brilinta)

torsemide (use with caution) (Soaanz)

traMADol (use with caution) (ConZip, Durela, Qdolo, Ralivia, Tridural, Zytram XL)

triazolam (avoid use) (Halcion)

trihexyphenidyl (avoid use)

trimethoprim-sulfamethoxazole (use with caution in patients taking an angiotensin-converting enzyme inhibitor, angiotensin receptor blocker, or angiotensin receptor/neprilysin inhibitor, and in those with a reduced CCr) (Bactrim, Bactrim DS, Septra, Sulfatrim, Sulfatrim DS, Sulfatrim Pediatric)

venlafaxine (use with caution) (Effexor XR)

vilazodone (use with caution) (Viibryd)

vortioxetine (use with caution) (Trintellix)

warfarin (avoid starting as initial therapy for treatment of nonvalvular atrial fibrillation or venous thromboembolism unless alternative options [direct oral anticoagulants] are contraindicated or there are significant barriers to their use; if already using, may be reasonable to continue treatment, especially if INR is well-controlled [i.e., >70% time in therapeutic range] and no adverse effects) (Jantoven)

zaleplon (avoid use)

ziprasidone (avoid use, except in schizophrenia or bipolar disorder) (Geodon, Zeldox)

zolpidem (avoid use) (Ambien, Ambien CR, Edluar, Sublinox)

The 2023 American Geriatrics Society Beers Criteria Update Expert Panel. American Geriatrics Society 2023 updated AGS Beers Criteria for potentially inappropriate medication use in older adults. *J Am Geriatr Soc.* 2023;71(7):2052–2081.

DRUGS ASSOCIATED WITH INCREASED RISK OF FALLS IN THE ELDERLY

Many factors are associated with falls in the elderly, including frailty, disease, vision, polypharmacy, and certain medications. Below is a list of drugs associated with falls. Assess geriatric patients on these medications for fall risk and implement fall reduction strategies.

ACE Inhibitors
benazepril (Lotensin)
captopril
enalapril (Vasotec)
fosinopril
lisinopril (Prinivil, Zestril)
moexipril
perindopril
quinapril (Accupril)
ramipril (Altace)
trandolapril

Angiotensin II Receptor Antagonists
azilsartan (Edarbi)
candesartan (Atacand)
eprosartan
irbesartan (Avapro)
losartan (Cozaar)
olmesartan (Benicar)
telmisartan (Micardis)
valsartan (Diovan)

Antiarrhythmics
digoxin (Lanoxin)
disopyramide (Norpace)

Anticonvulsants
carbamazepine (Carbatrol, Epitol, Equetro, Tegretol)
ethosuximide (Zarontin)
felbamate (Felbatol)
gabapentin (Gralise, Neurontin)
lamotrigine (Lamictal)
levetiracetam (Keppra, Spritam)
methsuximide (Celontin)
phenobarbital
phenytoin (Dilantin, Phenytek)
pregabalin (Lyrica)
primidone (Mysoline)
tiagabine (Gabitril)
topiramate (Qudexy XR, Topamax, Trokendi XR)
valproate (Depakote)
zonisamide (Zonegran)

Antidepressants
amitriptyline
amoxapine
bupropion (Aplenzin, Forfivo XL, Wellbutrin XL)
citalopram (Celexa)
clomipramine (Anafranil)
desipramine (Norpramin)
doxepin (Silenor)
duloxetine (Cymbalta, Drizalma Sprinkle)
escitalopram (Lexapro)
fluoxetine (Prozac)
fluvoxamine
imipramine (Tofranil)
isocarboxazid (Marplan)
maprotiline
mirtazapine (Remeron)
nefazodone
paroxetine (Paxil, Pexeva)
phenelzine (Nardil)
protriptyline (Vivactil)
sertraline (Zoloft)
tranylcypromine (Parnate)

trazodone
trimipramine
venlafaxine (Effexor XR)

Antihistamines/Antinauseants
dimenhydrinate (Dramamine)
diphenhydramine (Benadryl)
hydroxyzine (Vistaril)
meclizine (Bonine)
metoclopramide (Reglan)
prochlorperazine (Compro)
promethazine
scopolamine patch (Transderm Scop)

Antiparkinsonian Agents
amantadine (Gocovri, Osmolex ER)
bromocriptine (Parlodel)
entacapone (Comtan)
levodopa/carbidopa (Duopa, Rytary, Sinemet, Sinemet CR)
pramipexole (Mirapex, Mirapex ER)
selegiline (Zelapar)

Antipsychotics (Atypical)
aripiprazole (Abilify, Abilify Maintena, Aristada, Aristada Initio)
clozapine (Clozaril, Versacloz)
olanzapine (Zyprexa, Zyprexa Relprevv, Zyprexa Zydis)
paliperidone (Invega, Invega Sustenna, Invega Trinza)
quetiapine (Seroquel, Seroquel XR)
risperidone (Perseris, Risperdal, Risperdal Consta)
ziprasidone (Geodon)

Antipsychotics (Typical)
chlorpromazine
fluphenazine
haloperidol (Haldol)
loxapine (Adasuve)
perphenazine
pimozide
thioridazine
thiothixene
trifluoperazine

Anxiolytics
buspirone
meprobamate

Benzodiazepines (Long-Acting)
chlordiazepoxide (Librium)
clonazepam (Klonopin)
clorazepate (Tranxene)
diazepam (Valium)
flurazepam

Benzodiazepines (Intermediate-Acting)
alprazolam (Xanax, Xanax XR)
estazolam
lorazepam (Ativan)
oxazepam
temazepam (Restoril)

Benzodiazepines (Short-Acting)
triazolam (Halcion)

Beta Blockers
acebutolol
atenolol (Tenormin)
bisoprolol
carvedilol (Coreg, Coreg CR)
labetalol (Trandate)
metoprolol (Kasprago Sprinkle, Lopressor, Toprol XL)
propranolol (Inderal LA, InnoPran XL)
timolol

Calcium Channel Blockers
amlodipine (Katerzia, Norvasc)
diltiazem (Cardizem, Cardizem CD, Cardizem LA, Cartia XT, Taztia XT, Tiazac)
felodipine
isradipine
nicardipine (Cardene)
nifedipine (Adalat CC, Procardia XL)
nisoldipine (Sular)
verapamil (Calan SR, Verelan, Verelan PM)

Diuretics
amiloride/hydrochlorothiazide
bumetanide (Bumex)
furosemide (Lasix)
hydrochlorothiazide (Microzide)
triamterene/hydrochlorothiazide (Dyazide, Maxzide)

Opioid Analgesics
codeine
fentanyl (Abstral, Actiq, Duragesic, Fentora, Ionsys, Lazanda, Sublimaze, Subsys)
hydrocodone (Hysingla ER, Zohydro ER)
hydromorphone (Dilaudid)
levorphanol
meperidine (Demerol)
methadone (Dolophine, Methadose)
morphine (Duramorph, Infumorph, Kadian, Mitigo, Morphabond ER, MS Contin)
oxycodone (Oxaydo, OxyContin, Roxicodone, Xtampza ER)
oxymorphone (Opana)

Skeletal Muscle Relaxants
baclofen (Gablofen, Lioresal, Ozobax)

Vasodilators
doxazosin (Cardura, Cardura XL)
hydralazine
isosorbide dinitrate/mononitrate (Dilatrate SR, Isordil, Monoket)
nitroglycerin (GoNitro, Minitran, Nitro-Dur, Nitrolingual, Nitromist, Nitrostat)
prazosin (Minipress)
terazosin

American Geriatrics Society, British Geriatrics Society, and American Academy of Orthopedic Surgeons Panel on Falls Prevention. Guideline for the prevention of falls in older persons. J Am Geriatr Soc. 49:664–672, 2001.
Hoel RW, Giddings Connolly RM, Takahashi PY. Polypharmacy management in older patients. Mayo Clin Proc 96:242–256, 2021.

DO NOT CRUSH!

Do not crush any oral medication that is labeled as:

Antineoplastic **(AN)**
Buccal **(BU)**
Delayed Release **(DR)**
Enteric Coated **(EC)**
Extended Release **(ER)**
Effervescent Tablet **(EVT)**
Film coated **(FC)**
Mucous Membrane Irritant **(MMI)**
Orally Disintegrating Tablets **(ODT)**
Sublingual **(SL)**

Do not crush any oral medication that ends in the following letters:

CD CR ER LA SR XL XR XT

MEDICATIONS THAT SHOULD NOT BE CRUSHED:

Abilify MyCite
Absorica Capsule **(MMI)**
Acamprosate Tablet **(DR)**
Aciphex Tablet **(DR)**
Actiq Lozenge **(chewing or swallowing may ↓ bioavailability)**
Actonel Tablet **(FC, MMI)**
Adderall XR Capsule **(ER)**—see code "C"
Adzenys XR-ODT Tablet **(ER, ODT)**—see codes "A," "E"
Aemcolo Tablet **(DR)**
Afinitor Tablet **(AN, MMI)**—see code "H"
Akeega Tablet **(AN)**
Alecensa Capsule **(AN)**
Alkindi Sprinkle—see code "C"
Allegra-D Allergy & Congestion 12-Hour or 24-Hour Tablet **(ER)**
Altoprev Tablet **(ER)**
Alunbrig Tablet **(AN, FC)**
Ambien CR Tablet **(ER, FC)**
Amitiza Capsule **(gelatin coated)**
Amnesteem Capsule **(MMI)**
Amoxicillin/Clavulanate ER Tablet **(ER)**—see codes "A," "B"
Ampyra Capsule **(ER, FC)**
Amrix Capsule **(ER)**—see code "C"
Antara Capsule
Antivert Tablet
Aplenzin Tablet **(ER)**
Apriso Capsule **(ER)**
Aptensio XR Capsule **(ER)**—see codes "A," "C"
Aptivus Capsule **(oil emulsion within spheres)**
Aricept 23-mg Tablet **(crushing may ↑ rate of absorption)**
Arthrotec Tablet—see code "F"
Aspirin/Dipyridamole ER Capsule **(ER)**
Aspruzyo Sprinkle **(FC)**
Astagraf XL Capsule **(ER)**—see code "A"
Atelvia Tablet **(DR, MMI)**
Austedo XR Tablet **(ER, FC)**
Avodart Capsule **(liquid filled, MMI)**—see codes "F," "H"
Azulfidine EN Tablet **(DR)**
Bafiertam Capsule **(DR)**
Balversa Tablet **(AN, FC)**
Bayer Low-Dose Aspirin Tablet **(EC)**
Belbuca Buccal Film **(BU) (chewing or swallowing may ↓ bioavailability)**—see code "E"
Belsomra Tablet **(ER)**
Benzonatate Capsule **(chewing or crushing may cause local anesthesia of mucous membranes, which could lead to choking)**

Biltricide Tablet **(crushing, breaking, or chewing can leave bitter taste)**—see code "B"
Binosto Tablet **(EVT)**—see codes "A," "G"
Bonjesta Tablet **(ER)**
Bosulif Tablet **(AN, FC)**
Briviact Tablet **(FC)**—see code "A"
Brukinsa Capsule **(AN)**
Budesonide DR Capsule **(DR)**—see code "C"
Cabometyx Tablet **(AN)**
Calquence Capsule/Tablet **(AN)**
Caprelsa Tablet **(AN, FC, MMI) (may be dissolved in water)**
Carbaglu Tablet **(dissolve in water)**
Carbatrol Capsule **(ER)**—see codes "A," "C"
Carbidopa/Levodopa ER Tablet **(ER)**—see code "B"
Cardizem CD/LA Capsule **(ER)**
Cardizem Tablet **(FC)**
Cardura XL Tablet **(ER)**
Cartia XT Capsule **(ER)**
Cefaclor ER Tablet **(ER, FC)**—see code "A"
Cefuroxime Tablet **(crushing, breaking, or chewing can leave bitter taste)**
Cellcept Capsule/Tablet **(FC)**—see codes "A," "H"
Cerdelga Capsule
Chlor-Trimeton Allergy 12-Hour Tablet **(ER)**
Cholbam Capsule—see code "C"
Cibinqo Tablet **(FC)**
Claravis Capsule **(liquid filled, MMI)**
Clarinex-D 12-Hour/24-Hour Tablet **(ER)**
Clarithromycin ER Tablet **(ER, FC)**
Claritin-D Allergy & Congestion 12-Hour/24-Hour Tablet **(ER)**
Colazal Capsule—see code "C"
Colestid Tablet—see code "A"
Cometriq Capsule **(AN)**
Concerta Tablet **(ER)**—see code "A"
Contrave Tablet **(ER)**
Conzip Capsule **(ER) (crushing, chewing, or dissolving can leave bitter taste)**—see code "A"
Copiktra Capsule **(AN)**
Coreg CR Capsule **(ER)**—see code "C"
Cotellic Tablet **(AN, FC)**
Cotempla XR-ODT Tablet **(ER, ODT)**—see codes "A," "E"
Creon Capsule **(DR, MMI)**—see code "C"
Cresemba Capsule **(opening the capsule may ↓ absorption)**
Cyclophosphamide Capsule/Tablet **(AN)**—see code "H"
Cymbalta Capsule **(DR)**
Darifenacin ER Tablet **(ER)**
Daurismo Tablet **(AN, FC)**
Delzicol Capsule **(DR)**—see code "C"
Depakote Tablet **(DR)**—see code "A"
Depakote ER Tablet **(ER)**—see code "A"
Depakote Sprinkle Capsule—see code "C"
Detrol LA Capsule **(ER)**
Dexedrine Capsule **(ER)**—see code "A"
Dexilant Capsule **(DR)**—see code "C"
Diacomit Capsule—see code "A"
Diclegis Tablet **(DR)**
Diclofenac ER Tablet **(ER)**

Diflunisal Tablet **(FC, MMI)**
Doryx Tablet **(DR)**—see code "A"
Doryx MPC Tablet **(DR)**—see code "A"
Drisdol Capsule **(liquid filled)**—see code "A"
Droxia Capsule—see code "H"
Duavee Tablet **(FC)**—see code "H"
Duexis Tablet **(FC, MMI)**
Dulcolax Tablet **(EC)**—see code "D"
EC-Naprosyn Tablet **(DR, EC)**—see code "D"
Ecotrin Tablet **(EC, MMI)**
Edluar SL Tablet **(SL)**—see code "E"
Effer-K Tablet **(EVT)**—see code "G"
Effexor XR Capsule **(ER)**—see code "C"
Elepsia XR Tablet **(ER)**—see code "A"
Emend Capsule—see code "A"
Envarsus XR Tablet **(ER)**—see code "A"
Equetro Capsule **(ER)**—see codes "A," "C"
Ergomar SL Tablet **(SL)**—see code "E"
Erivedge Capsule **(AN)**—see code "F"
Erleada Tablet **(AN, FC)**
Ery-Tab Tablet **(DR)**—see code "A"
Erythromycin DR Capsule **(DR)**—see codes "A," "C"
Evekeo ODT—see codes "A," "E"
Exjade Tablet **(dissolve in water, orange juice, or apple juice)**
Ezallor Sprinkle—see code "C"
Feldene Capsule **(MMI)**
Felodipine Tablet **(ER)**
Fenoglide Tablet
Fentora Buccal Tablet **(BU) (crushing could ↓ effectiveness)**
Ferrous Gluconate Tablet **(MMI)**
Fetzima Capsule **(ER)**
Flomax Capsule
Fluoxetine DR Capsule **(DR)**—see code "A"
Fluvoxamine ER Capsule **(ER)**
Focalin XR Capsule **(ER)**—see code "C"
Forfivo XL Tablet **(FC)**
Fosamax Tablet **(MMI)**
Fosamax Plus D Tablet **(MMI)**
Fotivda Capsule **(AN)**
Galafold Capsule
Galantamine ER Capsule **(ER)**—see code "A"
Geodon Capsule
Gleevec Tablet **(MMI) (may dissolve in water or apple juice)**—see code "H"
Gleostine Capsule **(AN, gelatin coated)**—see code "H"
Glucotrol XL Tablet **(ER)**
Glumetza Tablet **(ER)**—see code "A"
Gocovri Capsule **(ER)**—see codes "A," "C"
Gralise Tablet **(ER, FC)**—see code "A"
Hetlioz Capsule—see code "A"
Horizant Tablet **(ER)**—see code "A"
Hycamtin Capsule **(AN)**
Hydrea Capsule **(AN)**—see code "H"
Hydromorphone ER Tablet **(ER) (crushing, chewing or dissolving may ↑ risk of fatal overdose)**—see code "A"

DO NOT CRUSH! continued

MEDICATIONS THAT SHOULD NOT BE CRUSHED:

Hysingla ER Tablet **(ER) (crushing, chewing or dissolving may ↑ risk of fatal overdose)**
Ibandronate Tablet **(MMI)**
Ibrance Capsule/Tablet **(AN, FC)**
Iclusig Tablet **(AN, FC)**
Idhifa Tablet **(AN, FC)**
Imbruvica Capsule/Tablet **(AN, FC)**—see code "A"
Inderal LA Capsule **(ER)**—see code "A"
Indomethacin ER Capsule **(ER)**—see codes "A," "C"
Inlyta Tablet **(AN, FC)**
Innopran XL Capsule **(ER)**—see code "A"
Inqovi Tablet **(AN, FC)**
Intelence Tablet **(may dissolve in water)**
Intuniv Tablet **(ER)**
Invega Tablet **(ER)**
Invokamet XR Tablet **(ER, FC)**
Iressa Tablet **(AN, FC) (may dissolve in water)**
Isentress Tablet **(FC)**—see code "A"
Isentress HD Tablet **(FC)**—see code "A"
Isosorbide Mononitrate ER Tablet **(ER)**—see code "B"
Jalyn Capsule **(MMI)**—see codes "F," "H"
Janumet XR Tablet **(ER, FC)**
Jaypirca Tablet **(AN, FC)**
Jentadueto XR Tablet **(ER, FC)**
Jornay PM Capsule **(ER)**—see codes "A," "C"
Juxtapid Capsule
K-Tab Tablet **(ER, FC)**—see code "A"
Kaletra Tablet **(FC)**—see code "A"
Kalydeco Tablet **(FC)**—see code "A"
Kapvay Tablet **(ER)**
Kaspargo Capsule **(ER)**
Kazano Tablet **(FC)**
Keppra Tablet **(FC) (crushing, breaking, or chewing can leave bitter taste)**—see code "A"
Keppra XR Tablet **(ER, FC)**—see code "A"
Ketoprofen ER Capsule **(ER, MMI)**
Kisqali Tablet **(AN, FC)**
Klor-Con Tablet **(ER, FC)**—see code "B"
Klor-Con M Tablet **(ER)**—see codes "A," "B"
Kombiglyze XR Tablet **(ER, FC)**
Korlym Tablet
Koselugo Capsule **(AN)**
Krazati Tablet **(AN, FC)**
Lamictal XR Tablet **(ER)**
Lenvima Capsule **(AN) (may dissolve in water or apple juice)**
Lescol XL Tablet **(ER)**
Letairis Tablet **(FC)**—see code "F"
Levbid Tablet **(ER)**—see codes "A," "B"
Lialda Tablet **(DR)**
Linzess Capsule **(gelatin coated)**—see code "C"
Lipofen Capsule
Litfulo Capsule
Lithobid Tablet **(ER, FC)**—see code "A"
Lorbrena Tablet **(AN, FC)**—see code "H"
Loreev XR Capsule—see codes "A," "C"
Lovaza Capsule **(liquid filled)**

Lumakras Tablet **(AN, FC) (may dissolve in water)**
Lunesta Tablet **(FC) (crushing, breaking, or chewing can leave bitter taste)**
Lupkynis Capsule
Lybalvi Tablet **(FC)**
Lynparza Tablet **(AN, FC)**
Lyrica CR Tablet **(ER, FC)**—see code "A"
Lytgobi Tablet **(AN)**
Mavenclad Tablet **(AN)**—see code "H"
Mavyret Pellets **(mix with food, not liquid)**
Mayzent Tablet **(FC)**
Mekinist Tablet **(AN, FC)**—see code "A"
Mestinon Tablet **(ER)**—see code "A"
Minolira Tablet **(ER)**—see code "B"
Mirapex ER Tablet **(ER)**
Motpoly XR Capsule **(ER)**—see code "A"
Motrin Tablet **(crushing, breaking, or chewing can leave bitter taste)**—see code "A"
MS Contin Tablet **(ER) (crushing, chewing, or dissolving may ↑ risk of fatal overdose)**—see code "A"
Mucinex Tablet **(ER)**—see code "A"
Mucinex D Tablet **(ER)**—see codes "A," "B"
Mucinex DM Tablet **(ER)**—see code "A"
Mycapssa Capsule **(DR)**
Mydayis Capsule **(ER)**—see code "C"
Myfortic Tablet **(DR)**—see codes "A," "H"
Myrbetriq Tablet **(ER, FC)**—see code "A"
Mytesi Tablet **(DR, FC)**
Namenda XR Capsule **(ER)**—see codes "A," "C"
Namzaric Capsule **(ER)**—see code "C"
Naprelan Tablet **(ER, FC)**—see code "A"
Nerlynx Tablet **(AN)**
Neurontin Capsule/Tablet **(FC)**—see codes "A," "B," "C"
Nexiclon XR Tablet **(ER)**—see code "B"
Nexium Capsule **(DR)**—see code "C"
Nexium 24HR Capsule/Tablet **(DR)**—see codes "A," "C"
Niacin ER Tablet **(ER)**
Nicorette Lozenge—see code "E"
Ninlaro Capsule **(AN)**
Nitrostat SL Tablet **(SL)**—see code "E"
Norpace CR Capsule **(ER)**
Northera Capsule
Norvir Tablet **(FC)**—see code "A"
Noxafil Tablet **(DR, FC)**—see code "A"
Nubeqa Tablet **(AN, FC)**
Nucynta ER Tablet **(ER, FC) (crushing, chewing or dissolving may ↑ risk of fatal overdose)**
Ofev Capsule **(crushing or chewing can leave bitter taste)**
Ojjaara Tablet **(AN)**
Onureg Tablet **(AN, FC)**
Opfolda Capsule—see code "C"
Opsumit Tablet **(FC)**

Oravig Buccal Tablet **(BU)**
Orenitram Tablet **(ER)**
Orphenadrine Citrate ER Tablet **(ER)**
Oseni Tablet **(FC)**
Oserdu Tablet **(AN, FC)**
Osmolex ER Tablet **(ER)**—see code "A"
Otezla Tablet **(FC)**
Oxaydo Tablet **(may obstruct feeding tubes if crushed)**—see code "A"
Oxbryta Tablet **(FC)**—see code "A"
Oxtellar XR Tablet **(ER)**—see code "A"
Oxybutynin ER Tablet **(ER)**—see code "A"
OxyContin Tablet **(ER, FC) (crushing, chewing or dissolving may ↑ risk of fatal overdose)**
Oxymorphone ER Tablet **(ER, FC) (crushing, chewing or dissolving may ↑ risk of fatal overdose)**
Pancreaze Capsule **(DR, MMI)**—see code "C"
Paxil Tablet **(FC)**—see codes "A," "B"
Paxil CR Tablet **(ER, FC)**—see code "A"
Paxlovid Tablet
Pemazyre Tablet **(AN)**
Pentasa Tablet **(ER)**—see code "C"
Pentoxifylline ER Tablet **(ER)**
Pertzye Capsule **(DR, MMI)**—see code "C"
Piqray Tablet
Pomalyst Capsule **(AN)**
Pradaxa Capsule **(breaking, chewing, or emptying may ↑ bioavailability)**
Prevacid 24HR Capsule **(DR)**
Prevacid Capsule **(DR)**—see code "C"
Prevacid SoluTab Tablet **(ODT) (may dissolve in water to administer via nasogastric tube)**
Prevymis Tablet **(FC)**
Prilosec OTC Tablet **(DR)**
Pristiq Tablet **(ER)**
Procardia XL Tablet **(ER, FC)**
Procysbi Capsule **(DR)**—see code "C"
Promacta Tablet **(FC)**—see code "A"
Protonix Tablet **(DR)**—see code "A"
Pylera Capsule **(MMI)**
Qinlock Tablet **(AN)**
Qtern Tablet **(FC)**
Quedexy XR Capsule **(ER)**—see codes "A," "C"
Ranexa Tablet **(ER, FC)**
Rapamune Tablet **(FC)**—see code "A"
Rayaldee Capsule **(ER)**
Rayos Tablet **(DR)**—see code "A"
Relexxi Tablet **(ER)**
Renagel Tablet **(FC) (expands in liquid when crushed or broken)**—see code "A"
Renvela Tablet **(FC) (expands in liquid when crushed or broken)**—see code "A"
Retevmo Capsule **(AN)**
Revlimid Capsule—see code "F"
Reyataz Capsule **(gelatin coated)**
Rezlidhia Capsule **(AN)**
Rinvoq Tablet **(ER)**

MEDICATIONS THAT SHOULD NOT BE CRUSHED:

Ritalin LA Capsule **(ER)**—see codes "A," "C"
Ropinirole ER Tablet **(ER, FC)**
Roweepra Tablet **(crushing or chewing can leave bitter taste)**—see code "A"
Rozlytrek Capsule **(AN)**
Rukobia Tablet **(ER, FC)**
Rybelsus Tablet
Rydapt Capsule **(AN, liquid filled)**
Rytary Capsule **(ER)**—see code "C"
Rythmol SR Capsule **(ER)**
Saphris SL Tablet **(SL)**—see code "E"
Scemblix Tablet **(AN, FC)**—see code "B"
Sensipar Tablet **(FC) (cutting tablets may cause variable dosing accuracy)**
Seroquel XR Tablet **(ER)**
Sikos Tablet **(FC) (may dissolve in water)**—see code "H"
Solodyn Tablet **(ER, FC)**
Sotyktu Tablet **(FC)**
Sporanox Capsule—see code "A"
Spritam ODT **(ODT)**—see code "E"
Sprycel Tablet **(AN)**
Stalevo Tablet **(FC)**
Stivarga Tablet **(AN, FC)**
Strattera Capsule **(contents can cause ocular irritation)**
Suboxone SL Film **(SL)**—see code "E"
Sudafed 12-Hour/24-Hour Tablet **(ER)**—see code "A"
Sular Tablet **(ER, FC)**
Symdeko Tablet
Synjardy XR Tablet **(SR)**
Tabrecta Tablet **(AN, FC)**
Tafinlar Capsule **(AN)**
Tafinlar Tablet for Suspension **(AN) (dissolve in water)**
Tagrisso Tablet **(AN, FC) (may dissolve in water)**
Talzenna Capsule **(AN)**
Tasigna Capsule **(AN)**—see code "C"
Taztia XT Capsule **(ER)**—see code "C"
Tazverik Tablet **(AN, FC)**
Tecfidera Capsule **(DR)**

Tegretol XR Tablet **(ER)**—see code "A"
Temodar Capsule **(AN, MMI)**—see code "H"
Tepmetko Tablet **(AN) (may dissolve in water)**
Theo-24 Capsule **(ER)**—see codes "A," "C"
Tiazac Capsule **(ER)**—see code "C"
Tibsovo Tablet **(AN, FC)**
Tivicay PD Tablet **(may dissolve in water)**
Tolsura Capsule **(gelatin coated)**—see code "A"
Topamax Capsule, Tablet **(FC) (crushing, breaking, or chewing can leave bitter taste)**—see codes "A," "C"
Toprol XL Tablet **(ER)**—see code "B"
Toviaz Tablet **(ER, FC)**
Trazodone Tablet **(crushing or chewing can leave bitter taste)**—see code "B"
Treximet Tablet **(FC) (crushing, chewing, or breaking may cause rapid absorption)**
Trikafta Tablet
Trilipix Capsule **(DR)**
Triumeq PD Tablet **(dissolve in water)**
Trokendi XR Capsule **(ER)**—see code "A"
Tukysa Tablet **(AN)**
Turalio Capsule **(AN)**
Tylenol 8-Hour Arthritis Pain Tablet **(ER)**
Uceris Tablet **(ER)**
Uptravi Tablet **(FC)**
Urocit-K Tablet **(ER)**
Uroxatral Tablet **(ER)**
Valcyte Tablet **(FC)**—see codes "A," "F," "H"
Valproic Acid Capsule **(MMI)**—see code "A"
Vanflyta Tablet **(AN, FC)**
Vascepa Capsule
Venclexta Tablet **(AN, FC)**
Veozah Tablet **(FC)**
Verapamil ER Tablet **(ER)**
Verelan Capsule **(DR)**—see code "C"
Verelan PM Capsule **(ER)**—see code "C"

Verzenio Tablet **(AN)**
Vesicare Tablet **(FC) (crushing, breaking, or chewing can leave bitter taste)**—see code "A"
Vijoice Tablet **(AN) (may dissolve in water)**
Vimovo Tablet **(DR)**
Vimpat Tablet **(FC)**—see code "A"
Viokace Tablet **(MMI)**
Vitrakvi Capsule **(AN)**—see code "A"
Vonjo Capsule **(AN)**
Votrient Tablet **(AN, FC) (crushing may ↑ bioavailability)**
Vumenty Capsule **(DR)**
Vyndamax Capsule **(liquid filled)**
Vyndaqel Capsule **(liquid filled)**
Welireg Tablet **(AN, FC)**
Wellbutrin SR/XL Tablet **(ER, FC)**
Xalcori Capsule **(AN)**
Xanax XR Tablet **(ER)**—see code "A"
Xeljanz XR Tablet **(ER)**—see code "A"
Xeloda Tablet **(AN, FC)**
Xenleta Tablet **(FC)**
Xigduo XR Tablet **(ER, FC)**
Ximino Capsule **(ER)**
Xospata Tablet **(AN)**
Xpovio Tablet **(AN)**
Xtampza ER Capsule **(ER)**—see code "C"
Xtandi Capsule, Tablet **(AN)**
Yargesa Capsule—see code "C"
Yonsa Tablet **(AN)**
Yosprala Tablet **(DR, FC)**
Zavesca Capsule—see code "C"
Zegerid Capsule—see code "A"
Zejula Capsule/Tablet **(AN, FC)**
Zelboraf Tablet **(AN, FC)**
Zenatane Capsule **(gelatin coated, MMI)**
Zenpep Capsule **(DR, MMI)**—see code "C"
Zopoaia Capsule
Zileuton ER Tablet **(ER)**
Zolinza Capsule **(AN, MMI)**
Zortress Tablet **(AN, MMI)**—see code "H"
Zubsolv SL Tablet **(SL)**—see code "E"
Zydelig Tablet **(AN, FC)**
Zytiga Tablet **(AN, FC)**

CODES:

A: Liquid forms are available
B: Tablets that are scored may be broken in half
C: Capsule can be opened—contents may be used/ sprinkled on certain foods or liquids as recommended by the manufacturer

D: Do not take with antacids or milk products
E: Disintegrates on or under the tongue—do not chew
F: Women of reproductive potential should not handle crushed or broken tablets or the contents of opened capsules

G: Effervescent tablets must be dissolved in the volume of diluent recommended by the manufacturer
H: Avoid direct contact with skin as may enhance tumor development

LIST OF CONFUSED DRUG NAMES

Drug Name	Confused Drug Name
Abelcet	amphotericin B
Accupril	Aciphex
acetaminophen	acetaZOLAMIDE
acetaZOLAMIDE	acetaminophen
acetic acid for irrigation	glacial acetic acid
Aciphex	Accupril
Aciphex	Aricept
Activase	Cathflo Activase
Activase	TNKase
Actonel	Actos
Actos	Actonel
Adacel (Tdap)	Daptacel (DTaP)
Adderall	Adderall XR
Adderall XR	Adderall
ado-trastuzumab emtansine	trastuzumab
Afrin (oxymetazoline)	Afrin (saline)
Afrin (saline)	Afrin (oxymetazoline)
Aggrastat	argatroban
Allegra (fexofenadine)	Allegra Anti-Itch Cream (diphenhydramine/ allantoin)
Allegra	Viagra
Allegra Anti-Itch Cream (diphenhydramine/ allantoin)	Allegra (fexofenadine)
ALPRAZolam	clonazePAM
ALPRAZolam	LORazepam
amantadine	amiodarone
Ambien	ambrisentan
Ambisome	amphotericin B
ambrisentan	Ambien
aMILoride	amLODIPine
amiodarone	amantadine
amLODIPine	aMILoride
amphotericin B	Abelcet
amphotericin B	Ambisome
amphotericin B	amphotericin B liposomal
amphotericin B liposomal	amphotericin B
antacid	Atacand
anticoagulant citrate dextrose solution formula A	anticoagulant sodium citrate solution
anticoagulant sodium citrate solution	anticoagulant citrate dextrose solution formula A
Apidra	Spiriva
apixaban	axitinib
argatroban	Aggrastat
Aricept	Aciphex
Aricept	Azilect
ARIPiprazole	proton pump inhibitors
ARIPiprazole	RABEprazole
Arista AH (absorbable hemostatic agent)	Arixtra
Arixtra	Arista AH (absorbable hemostatic agent)
Atacand	antacid
atomoxetine	atorvastatin

Drug Name	Confused Drug Name
atorvastatin	atomoxetine
azaCITIDine	azaTHIOprine
axitinib	apixaban
azaTHIOprine	azaCITIDine
Azilect	Aricept
B & O (belladonna and opium)	Beano
BabyBIG	HBIG (hepatitis B immune globulin)
Beano	B & O (belladonna and opium)
Benadryl	benazepril
benazepril	Benadryl
Betadine (with povidone-iodine)	Betadine (without povidone-iodine)
Betadine (without povidone-iodine)	Betadine (with povidone-iodine)
betaine (anhydrous form)	betaine HCl
betaine HCl	betaine (anhydrous form)
Bicillin C-R	Bicillin L-A
Bicillin L-A	Bicillin C-R
Brevibloc	Brevital
Brevital	Brevibloc
Brilinta	Briviact
Briviact	Brilinta
BUPivacaine	ROPivacaine
buprenorphine	HYDROmorphone
buPROPion	busPIRone
busPIRone	buPROPion
captopril	carvedilol
carBAMazepine	OXcarbazepine
CARBOplatin	CISplatin
Cardene	Cardizem
Cardizem	Cardene
carvedilol	captopril
Cathflo Activase	Activase
ceFAZolin	cefoTEtan
ceFAZolin	cefOXitin
ceFAZolin	cefTAZidime
ceFAZolin	cefTRIAXone
cefoTEtan	ceFAZolin
cefoTEtan	cefOXitin
cefoTEtan	cefTAZidime
cefoTEtan	cefTRIAXone
cefOXitin	ceFAZolin
cefOXitin	cefoTEtan
cefOXitin	cefTAZidime
cefOXitin	cefTRIAXone
cefTAZidime	ceFAZolin
cefTAZidime	cefoTEtan
cefTAZidime	cefOXitin
cefTAZidime	cefTRIAXone
cefTRIAXone	ceFAZolin
cefTRIAXone	cefoTEtan
cefTRIAXone	cefOXitin
cefTRIAXone	cefTAZidime
cefuroxime	sulfaSALAzine
CeleBREX	CeleXA

Brand names always start with an upper case letter. Some brand names incorporate tall man letters in initial characters and may not be readily recognized as brand names. Brand name products appear in black; generic/other products appear in red.

Drug Name	Confused Drug Name	Drug Name	Confused Drug Name
CeleBREX	Cerebyx	desmopressin	vasopressin
CeleXA	CeleBREX	dexAMETHasone	dexmedeTOMIDine
CeleXA	Cerebyx	Dexilant	DULoxetine
CeleXA	ZyPREXA	dexmedeTOMIDine	dexAMETHasone
Cerebyx	CeleBREX	dexmethylphenidate	methadone
Cerebyx	CeleXA	diazePAM	dilTIAZem
cetirizine	sertraline	Diflucan	Diprivan
cetirizine	stavudine	dilTIAZem	diazePAM
chlordiazePOXIDE	chlorproMAZINE	dimenhyDRINATE	diphenhydrAMINE
chlorproMAZINE	chlordiazePOXIDE	diphenhydrAMINE	dimenhyDRINATE
CISplatin	CARBOplatin	Diprivan	Diflucan
citalopram	escitalopram	disopyramide	desipramine
Claritin-D	Claritin-D 24	DOBUTamine	DOPamine
Claritin-D 24	Claritin-D	DOCEtaxel	PACLitaxel
cloBAZam	clonazePAM	DOPamine	DOBUTamine
clomiPHENE	clomiPRAMINE	Doxil	Paxil
clomiPRAMINE	clomiPHENE	DOXOrubicin	DAUNOrubicin
clonazePAM	ALPRAZolam	DOXOrubicin	DOXOrubicin liposomal
clonazePAM	cloBAZam	DOXOrubicin	IDArubicin
clonazePAM	cloNIDine	DOXOrubicin liposomal	DOXOrubicin
clonazePAM	cloZAPine	Dramamine (dimenhyDRINATE)	Dramamine (ginger root)
clonazePAM	LORazepam	Dramamine (dimenhyDRINATE)	Dramamine (meclizine)
cloNIDine	clonazePAM	Dramamine (ginger root)	Dramamine (dimenhyDRINATE)
cloNIDine	cloZAPine	Dramamine (ginger root)	Dramamine (meclizine)
cloNIDine	KlonoPIN	Dramamine (meclizine)	Dramamine (dimenhyDRINATE)
cloZAPine	clonazePAM	Dramamine (meclizine)	Dramamine (ginger root)
cloZAPine	cloNIDine	droNABinol	droPERidol
Clozaril	Colazal	droPERidol	droNABinol
coagulation factor IX (recombinant)	factor IX complex, vapor heated	Dulcolax (bisacodyl)	Dulcolax (docusate sodium)
coenzyme Q10	Cometriq	Dulcolax (docusate sodium)	Dulcolax (bisacodyl)
Colace	Cozaar	DULoxetine	Dexilant
Colazal	Clozaril	DULoxetine	FLUoxetine
colchicine	Cortrosyn	DULoxetine	PARoxetine
Cometriq	coenzyme Q10	elvitegravir, cobicistat, emtricitabine, and tenofovir alafenamide	elvitegravir, cobicistat, emtricitabine, and tenofovir disoproxil fumarate
Cortrosyn	colchicine	elvitegravir, cobicistat, emtricitabine, and tenofovir disoproxil fumarate	elvitegravir, cobicistat, emtricitabine, and tenofovir alafenamide
Cozaar	Colace	Enbrel	Levbid
Cozaar	Zocor	Engerix-B adult	Engerix-B pediatric/adolescent
cycloPHOSphamide	cycloSERINE	Engerix-B pediatric/adolescent	Engerix-B adult
cycloPHOSphamide	cycloSPORINE	ePHEDrine	EPINEPHrine
cycloSERINE	cycloPHOSphamide	EPINEPHrine	ePHEDrine
cycloSERINE	cycloSPORINE	epiRUBicin	eriBULin
cycloSPORINE	cycloPHOSphamide	eriBULin	epiRUBicin
cycloSPORINE	cycloSERINE	escitalopram	citalopram
Cymbalta	Symbyax	factor IX complex, vapor heated	coagulation factor IX (recombinant)
dabigatran	vigabatrin		
DACTINomycin	DAPTOmycin		
Daptacel (DTaP)	Adacel (Tdap)		
DAPTOmycin	DACTINomycin		
DAUNOrubicin	DOXOrubicin		
DAUNOrubicin	IDArubicin		
Depakote	Depakote ER		
Depakote ER	Depakote		
DEPO-Medrol	SOLU-Medrol		
Depo-Provera	Depo-subQ provera 104		
Depo-subQ provera 104	Depo-Provera		
desipramine	disopyramide		

Brand names always start with an upper case letter. Some brand names incorporate tall man letters in initial characters and may not be readily recognized as brand names. Brand name products appear in black; generic/other products appear in red.

LIST OF CONFUSED DRUG NAMES continued

MEDICATION SAFETY TOOLS | List of Confused Drug Names

Drug Name	Confused Drug Name
Fanapt	Xanax
Farxiga	Fetzima
fentaNYL	SUFentanil
Fetzima	Farxiga
flavoxATE	fluvoxaMINE
Flonase	Flovent
Flovent	Flonase
flumazenil	influenza virus vaccine
FLUoxetine	DULoxetine
FLUoxetine	PARoxetine
fluPHENAZine	fluvoxaMINE
fluvoxaMINE	flavoxATE
fluvoxaMINE	fluPHENAZine
Fluzone High-Dose Quadrivalent	Fluzone Quadrivalent
Fluzone Quadrivalent	Fluzone High-Dose Quadrivalent
fomepizole	omeprazole
gabapentin	gemfibrozil
gemfibrozil	gabapentin
gentamicin	gentian violet
gentian violet	gentamicin
glacial acetic acid	acetic acid for irrigation
glipiZIDE	glyBURIDE
glyBURIDE	glipiZIDE
guaiFENesin	guanFACINE
guanFACINE	guaiFENesin
HBIG (hepatitis B immune globulin)	BabyBIG
heparin	Hespan
Hespan	heparin
HMG-CoA reductase inhibitors ("statins")	nystatin
HumaLOG	HumuLIN
HumaLOG	NovoLOG
HumaLOG Mix 75/25	HumuLIN 70/30
HumuLIN	HumaLOG
HumuLIN	NovoLIN
HumuLIN 70/30	HumaLOG Mix 75/25
HumuLIN R U-100	HumuLIN R U-500
HumuLIN R U-500	HumuLIN R U-100
hydrALAZINE	hydroCHLOROthiazide
hydrALAZINE	HYDROmorphone
hydrALAZINE	hydrOXYzine
Hydrea	Lyrica
hydroCHLOROthiazide	hydrALAZINE
hydroCHLOROthiazide	hydrOXYzine
hydroCHLOROthiazide	hydroxychloroquine
HYDROcodone	oxyCODONE
HYDROmorphone	buprenorphine
HYDROmorphone	hydrALAZINE
HYDROmorphone	hydrOXYzine
HYDROmorphone	morphine
HYDROmorphone	oxyMORphone
hydroxychloroquine	hydroCHLOROthiazide
hydroxychloroquine	hydroxyurea
hydroxyurea	hydroxychloroquine

Drug Name	Confused Drug Name
hydroxyurea	hydrOXYzine
hydroxyurea	Ure-Na (palatable form of oral urea)
hydrOXYzine	hydrALAZINE
hydrOXYzine	hydroCHLOROthiazide
hydrOXYzine	HYDROmorphone
hydrOXYzine	hydroxyurea
IDArubicin	DAUNOrubicin
IDArubicin	DOXOrubicin
IDArubicin	idaruCIZUmab
idaruCIZUmab	IDArubicin
Ilaris	Ilumya
Ilumya	Ilaris
inFLIXimab	riTUXimab
influenza virus vaccine	flumazenil
influenza virus vaccine	perflutren lipid microspheres
influenza virus vaccine	tuberculin purified protein derivative (PPD)
Inspra	Spiriva
Intuniv	Invega
Invega	Intuniv
ISOtretinoin	tretinoin
Jantoven	Janumet
Jantoven	Januvia
Janumet	Jantoven
Janumet	Januvia
Janumet	Sinemet
Januvia	Jantoven
Januvia	Janumet
Kaletra	Keppra
Keppra	Kaletra
Ketalar	ketorolac
ketamine	ketorolac
ketorolac	Ketalar
ketorolac	ketamine
ketorolac	methadone
KlonoPIN	cloNIDine
labetalol	LaMICtal
labetalol	lamoTRIgine
LaMICtal	labetalol
lamiVUDine	lamoTRIgine
lamoTRIgine	labetalol
lamoTRIgine	lamiVUDine
lamoTRIgine	levETIRAcetam
lamoTRIgine	levothyroxine
Lanoxin	levothyroxine
Lanoxin	naloxone
lanthanum carbonate	lithium carbonate
Lantus	Latuda
Lasix	Wakix
Latuda	Lantus
leucovorin calcium	Leukeran
leucovorin calcium	LEVOleucovorin
Leukeran	leucovorin calcium
Leukeran	Myleran
Levbid	Enbrel

Brand names always start with an upper case letter. Some brand names incorporate tall man letters in initial characters and may not be readily recognized as brand names. Brand name products appear in black; generic/other products appear in red.

1362

Drug Name	Confused Drug Name	Drug Name	Confused Drug Name
Levemir	Lovenox	metyraPONE	metyroSINE
levETIRAcetam	lamoTRIgine	metyroSINE	metyraPONE
levETIRAcetam	levOCARNitine	miFEPRIStone	miSOPROStol
levETIRAcetam	levOFLOXacin	migALAstat	migLUstat
levOCARNitine	levETIRAcetam	migLUstat	migALAstat
levOFLOXacin	levETIRAcetam	miSOPROStol	miFEPRIStone
LEVOleucovorin	leucovorin calcium	mitoMYcin	mitoXANTRONE
levothyroxine	lamoTRIgine	mitoXANTRONE	mitoMYcin
levothyroxine	Lanoxin	mitoXANTRONE	MTX Patch (lidocaine and menthol)
levothyroxine	liothyronine	morphine	HYDROmorphone
linaCLOtide	linaGLIPtin	morphine - non-concentrated oral liquid	morphine - oral liquid concentrate
linaGLIPtin	linaCLOtide		
liothyronine	levothyroxine	morphine - oral liquid concentrate	morphine - non-concentrated oral liquid
Lipitor	ZyrTEC		
lithium carbonate	lanthanum carbonate	Motrin	Neurontin
Lopressor	Lyrica	MS Contin	OxyCONTIN
LORazepam	ALPRAZolam	MTX Patch (lidocaine and menthol)	methotrexate
LORazepam	clonazePAM		
LORazepam	Lovaza	MTX Patch (lidocaine and menthol)	mitoXANTRONE
Lotronex	Protonix		
Lovaza	LORazepam	Mucinex D	Mucinex DM
Lovenox	Levemir	Mucinex DM	Mucinex D
Lunesta	Neulasta	Myleran	Leukeran
Lupron Depot-3 Month	Lupron Depot-Ped	nalbuphine	naloxone
Lupron Depot-Ped	Lupron Depot-3 Month	naloxone	Lanoxin
Lyrica	Hydrea	naloxone	nalbuphine
Lyrica	Lopressor	neratinib	nilotinib
Malarone	mefloquine	neratinib	niraparib
medroxyPROGESTERone	methylPREDNISolone	Neulasta	Lunesta
medroxyPROGESTERone	methylTESTOSTERone	Neulasta	Nuedexta
mefloquine	Malarone	Neurontin	Motrin
memantine	methadone	NexAVAR	NexIUM
metFORMIN	metroNIDAZOLE	NexIUM	NexAVAR
methadone	dexmethylphenidate	niCARdipine	NIFEdipine
methadone	ketorolac	niCARdipine	niMODipine
methadone	memantine	NIFEdipine	niCARdipine
methadone	methylphenidate	NIFEdipine	niMODipine
methadone	metOLazone	nilotinib	neratinib
methazolAMIDE	methIMAzole	nilotinib	niraparib
methazolAMIDE	metOLazone	niMODipine	niCARdipine
methIMAzole	methazolAMIDE	niMODipine	NIFEdipine
methIMAzole	metOLazone	niraparib	neratinib
methotrexate	metOLazone	niraparib	nilotinib
methotrexate	MTX Patch (lidocaine and menthol)	nizatidine	tiZANidine
		NovoLIN	HumuLIN
methylphenidate	methadone	NovoLIN	NovoLOG
methylPREDNISolone	medroxyPROGESTERone	NovoLIN 70/30	NovoLOG Mix 70/30
methylPREDNISolone	methylTESTOSTERone	NovoLOG	HumaLOG
methylTESTOSTERone	medroxyPROGESTERone	NovoLOG	NovoLIN
methylTESTOSTERone	methylPREDNISolone	NovoLOG Flexpen	NovoLOG Mix 70/30 Flexpen
metOLazone	methadone		
metOLazone	methazolAMIDE	NovoLOG Mix 70/30	NovoLIN 70/30
metOLazone	methIMAzole	NovoLOG Mix 70/30 Flexpen	NovoLOG Flexpen
metOLazone	methotrexate		
metoprolol succinate	metoprolol tartrate	Nuedexta	Neulasta
metoprolol tartrate	metoprolol succinate	nystatin	HMG-CoA reductase inhibitors ("statins")
metroNIDAZOLE	metFORMIN		

Brand names always start with an upper case letter. Some brand names incorporate tall man letters in initial characters and may not be readily recognized as brand names. Brand name products appear in black; generic/other products appear in red.

LIST OF CONFUSED DRUG NAMES continued

Drug Name	Confused Drug Name	Drug Name	Confused Drug Name
OLANZapine	QUEtiapine	Pristiq	PriLOSEC
omeprazole	fomepizole	Prograf	Proscar
Oracea	Orencia	Prograf	PROzac
Orencia	Oracea	propylene glycol	polyethylene glycol
Os-Cal	Asacol	Proscar	Prograf
oxaprozin	OXcarbazepine	Proscar	Provera
OXcarbazepine	carBAMazepine	protamine	Protonix
OXcarebazepine	oxaprozin	proton pump inhibitors	ARIPiprazole
oxyBUTYnin	oxyCODONE	Protonix	Lotronex
oxyBUTYnin	OxyCONTIN	Protonix	protamine
oxyBUTYnin	oxyMORphone	Provera	Proscar
oxyCODONE	HYDROcodone	Provera	PROzac
oxyCODONE	oxyBUTYnin	PROzac	PriLOSEC
oxyCODONE	OxyCONTIN	PROzac	Prograf
oxyCODONE	oxyMORphone	PROzac	Provera
OxyCONTIN	MS Contin	Pyridium	pyridoxine
OxyCONTIN	oxyBUTYnin	pyRIDostigmine	pyridoxine
OxyCONTIN	oxyCODONE	pyridoxine	pralodixime
OxyCONTIN	oxyMORphone	pyridoxine	Pyridium
OxyCONTIN	oxytocin	pyridoxine	pyRIDostigmine
oxyMORphone	HYDROmorphone	QUEtiapine	OLANZapine
oxyMORphone	oxyBUTYnin	quiNIDine	quiNINE
oxyMORphone	oxyCODONE	quiNINE	quiNIDine
oxyMORphone	OxyCONTIN	RABEprazole	ARIPiprazole
oxytocin	OxyCONTIN	Rapaflo	Rapamune
PACLitaxel	DOCEtaxel	Rapamune	Rapaflo
PACLitaxel	PACLitaxel protein-bound particles	rasagiline	repaglinide
		Remeron	Rozerem
PACLitaxel protein-bound particles	PACLitaxel	Renagel	Renvela
		Renvela	Renagel
PARoxetine	DULoxetine	repaglinide	rasagiline
PARoxetine	FLUoxetine	Restoril	RisperDAL
PARoxetine	piroxicam	Retrovir	ritonavir
Paxil	Doxil	ribavirin	riboflavin
Paxil	Plavix	riboflavin	ribavirin
Paxil	Trexall	rifabutin	rifapentine
PAZOPanib	PONATinib	rifAMPin	rifAXIMin
PEMEtrexed	PRALAtrexate	rifapentine	rifabutin
penicillAMINE	penicillin	rifAXIMin	rifAMPin
penicillin	penicillAMINE	RisperDAL	Restoril
PENTobarbital	PHENobarbital	RisperDAL	rOPINIRole
perflutren lipid microspheres	influenza virus vaccine	risperiDONE	rOPINIRole
		ritonavir	Retrovir
PHENobarbital	PENTobarbital	Rituxan	Rituxan Hycela
piroxicam	PARoxetine	Rituxan Hycela	Rituxan
Plavix	Paxil	riTUXimab	inFLIXimab
Plavix	Pradaxa	romiDEPsin	romiPLOStim
polyethylene glycol	propylene glycol	romiPLOStim	romiDEPsin
PONATinib	PAZOPanib	rOPINIRole	RisperDAL
potassium acetate	sodium acetate	rOPINIRole	risperiDONE
Pradaxa	Plavix	ROPivacaine	BUPivacaine
PRALAtrexate	PEMEtrexed	Rozerem	Razadyne
pralidoxime	pyridoxine	Rozerem	Remeron
prednisoLONE	predniSONE	Salagen	selegiline
predniSONE	prednisoLONE	SandIMMUNE	SandoSTATIN
PriLOSEC	Pristiq	SandoSTATIN	SandIMMUNE
PriLOSEC	PROzac	selegiline	Salagen

Brand names always start with an upper case letter. Some brand names incorporate tall man letters in initial characters and may not be readily recognized as brand names. Brand name products appear in black; generic/other products appear in red.

Drug Name	Confused Drug Name	Drug Name	Confused Drug Name
SEROquel	SEROquel XR	Toprol-XL	Topamax
SEROquel XR	SEROquel	Toujeo	Tradjenta
sertraline	cetirizine	Toujeo	Tresiba
silodosin	sirolimus	Toujeo	Trulicity
Sinemet	Janumet	t-PA	TNKase
sirolimus	silodosin	Tracleer	Tricor
SITagliptin	SUMAtriptan	Tradjenta	Toujeo
Slynd	Syeda	Tradjenta	Tresiba
sodium acetate	potassium acetate	Tradjenta	Trulicity
Solu-CORTEF	SOLU-Medrol	traMADol	traZODone
SOLU-Medrol	DEPO-Medrol	trastuzumab	ado-trastuzumab emtansine
SOLU-Medrol	Solu-CORTEF	traZODone	traMADol
SORAfenib	SUNItinib	Tresiba	Tarceva
sotalol	Sudafed	Tresiba	Toujeo
Spiriva	Apidra	Tresiba	Tradjenta
Spiriva	Inspra	Tresiba	Trulicity
Spravato	Steglatro	tretinoin	ISOtretinoin
stavudine	cetirizine	Trexall	Paxil
Steglatro	Spravato	Tricor	Tracleer
Sudafed	sotalol	tromethamine	Trophamine
Sudafed	Sudafed PE	Trophamine	tromethamine
Sudafed 12 Hour	Sudafed 12 Hour Pressure + Pain	Trulicity	Toujeo
Sudafed 12 Hour Pressure + Pain	Sudafed 12 Hour	Trulicity	Tradjenta
Sudafed PE	Sudafed	Trulicity	Tresiba
SUFentanil	fentaNYL	tuberculin purified protein derivative (PPD)	influenza virus vaccine
sulfADIAZINE	sulfaSALAzine	tuberculin purified protein derivative (PPD)	tetanus diphtheria toxoid (Td)
sulfaSALAzine	cefuroxime	Tylenol	Tylenol PM
sulfaSALAzine	sulfADIAZINE	Tylenol PM	Tylenol
SUMAtriptan	SITagliptin	Ure-Na (palatable form of oral urea)	hydroxyurea
SUMAtriptan	ZOLMitriptan	valACYclovir	valGANciclovir
SUNItinib	SORAfenib	Valcyte	Valtrex
Syeda	Slynd	valGANciclovir	valACYclovir
Symbyax	Cymbalta	Valtrex	Valcyte
tacrolimus	tamsulosin	vasopressin	desmopressin
tamsulosin	tacrolimus	Venofer	Vfend
Tarceva	Tresiba	Venofer	Vimpat
TEGretol	TEGretol XR	Vfend	Venofer
TEGretol XR	TEGretol	Vfend	Vimpat
tetanus diphtheria toxoid (Td)	tuberculin purified protein derivative (PPD)	Viagra	Allegra
Thalomid	thiamine	vigabatrin	dabigatran
thiamine	Thalomid	Vimpat	Venofer
Thrombate III	thrombin topical (recombinant)	Vimpat	Vfend
thrombin topical (recombinant)	Thrombate III	vinBLAStine	vinCRIStine
tiaGABine	tiZANidine	vinCRIStine	vinBLAStine
Tiazac	Ziac	Viracept	Viramune
tiZANidine	tiaGABine	Viramune	Viracept
tiZANidine	nizatidine	Wakix	Lasix
TNKase	Activase	Wellbutrin SR	Wellbutrin XL
TNKase	t-PA	Wellbutrin XL	Wellbutrin SR
Tobradex	Tobrex	Xanax	Fanapt
Tobrex	Tobradex	Xeloda	Xenical
Topamax	Toprol-XL	Xenical	Xeloda
		Yasmin	Yaz

Brand names always start with an upper case letter. Some brand names incorporate tall man letters in initial characters and may not be readily recognized as brand names. Brand name products appear in black; generic/other products appear in red.

LIST OF CONFUSED DRUG NAMES continued

Drug Name	Confused Drug Name	Drug Name	Confused Drug Name
Yaz	Yasmin	Zovirax	Zyvox
Zegerid	Zestril	Zyloprim	zolpidem
Zelapar	ZyPREXAZydis	ZyPREXA	CeleXA
Zestril	Zegerid	ZyPREXA	Zestril
Zestril	Zetia	ZyPREXA	ZyrTEC
Zestril	ZyPREXA	ZyPREXA Zydis	Zelapar
Zetia	Zestril	ZyrTEC	Lipitor
Ziac	Tiazac	ZyrTEC	Zocor
Zocor	Cozaar	ZyrTEC	ZyPREXA
Zocor	ZyrTEC	ZyrTEC	ZyrTEC-D
ZOLMitriptan	SUMAtriptan	ZyrTEC-D	ZyrTEC
zolpidem	Zyloprim	Zyvox	Zovirax

Brand names always start with an upper case letter. Some brand names incorporate tall man letters in initial characters and may not be readily recognized as brand names. Brand name products appear in black; generic/other products appear in red.

FDA-APPROVED LIST OF GENERIC DRUG NAMES WITH TALL MAN (MIXED CASE) LETTERS

Drug Name with Tall Man (Mixed Case) Letters	Confused with
buPROPion	busPIRone
busPIRone	buPROPion
clomiPHENE	clomiPRAMINE
clomiPRAMINE	clomiPHENE
cycloSERINE	cycloSPORINE
cycloSPORINE	cycloSERINE
DAUNOrubicin	DOXOrubicin
dimenhyDRINATE	diphenhydrAMINE
diphenhydrAMINE	dimenhyDRINATE
DOBUTamine	DOPamine
DOPamine	DOBUTamine
DOXOrubicin	DAUNOrubicin
glipiZIDE	glyBURIDE
glyBURIDE	glipiZIDE
hydrALAZINE	hydrOXYzine—HYDROmorphone
HYDROmorphone	hydrOXYzine—hydrALAZINE
hydrOXYzine	hydrALAZINE—HYDROmorphone
medroxyPROGESTERone	methylPREDNISolone—methylTESTOSTERone
methylPREDNISolone	medroxyPROGESTERone—methylTESTOSTERone
methylTESTOSTERone	medroxyPROGESTERone—methylPREDNISolone
mitoXANTRONE	Not specified
niCARdipine	NIFEdipine
NIFEdipine	niCARdipine
prednisoLONE	predniSONE
predniSONE	prednisoLONE
risperiDONE	rOPINIRole
rOPINIRole	risperiDONE
vinBLAStine	vinCRIStine
vinCRIStine	vinBLAStine

ISMP LIST OF ADDITIONAL DRUG NAMES WITH TALL MAN (MIXED CASE) LETTERS

Drug Name with Tall Man (Mixed Case) Letters	Confused with
ALPRAZolam	LORazepam—clonazePAM
aMILoride	amLODIPine
amLODIPine	aMILoride
ARIPiprazole	RABEprazole
azaCITIDine	azaTHIOprine
azaTHIOprine	azaCITIDine
BUPivacaine	ROPivacaine
carBAMazepine	OXcarbazepine
CARBOplatin	CISplatin
ceFAZolin	cefoTEtan—cefOXitin—cefTAZidime—cefTRIAXone
cefoTEtan	ceFAZolin—cefOXitin—cefTAZidime—cefTRIAXone
cefOXitin	ceFAZolin—cefoTEtan—cefTAZidime—cefTRIAXone
cefTAZidime	ceFAZolin—cefoTEtan—cefOXitin—cefTRIAXone
cefTRIAXone	ceFAZolin—cefoTEtan—cefOXitin—cefTAZidime
CeleBREX*	CeleXA*
CeleXA*	CeleBREX*
chlordiazePOXIDE	chlorproMAZINE
chlorproMAZINE	chlordiazePOXIDE
CISplatin	CARBOplatin
cloBAZam	clonazePAM
clonazePAM	ALPRAZolam—cloBAZam—cloNIDine—cloZAPine—LORazepam
cloNIDine	clonazePAM—cloZAPine—KlonoPIN*
cloZAPine	clonazePAM—cloNIDine
cycloPHOSphamide	cycloSERINE—cycloSPORINE
cycloSERINE	cycloPHOSphamide—cycloSPORINE
cycloSPORINE	cycloPHOSphamide—cycloSERINE
DACTINomycin	DAPTOmycin
DAPTOmycin	DACTINomycin
DEPO-Medrol*	SOLU-Medrol*
dexAMETHasone	dexmedeTOMIDine
dexmedeTOMIDine	dexAMETHasone
diazePAM	dilTIAZem
dilTIAZem	diazePAM
DOCEtaxel	PACLitaxel
DOXOrubicin	IDArubicin
droNABinol	droPERidol
droPERidol	droNABinol
DULoxetine	FLUoxetine—PARoxetine
ePHEDrine	EPINEPHrine
EPINEPHrine	ePHEDrine
epiRUBicin	eriBULin
eriBULin	epiRUBicin
fentaNYL	SUFentanil
flavoxATE	fluvoxaMINE
FLUoxetine	DULoxetine—PARoxetine

*Brand names always start with an upper case letter. Some brand names incorporate tall man letters in initial characters and may not be readily recognized as brand names. An asterisk follows all brand names in IMSP List of Additional Drug Names with Tall Man Letters.

© US Food and Drug Administration (FDA) and Institute for Safe Medication Practices (ISMP). FDA and ISMP Lists of Look-Alike Drug Names with Recommended Tall Man Letters. ISMP; 2023.

ISMP LIST OF ADDITIONAL DRUG NAMES WITH TALL MAN (MIXED CASE) LETTERS continued

Drug Name with Tall Man (Mixed Case) Letters	Confused with
fluPHENAZine	fluvoxaMINE
fluvoxaMINE	flavoxATE—fluPHENAZine
guaiFENesin	guanFACINE
guanFACINE	guaiFENesin
HumaLOG*	HumuLIN*
HumuLIN*	HumaLOG*
hydrALAZINE	hydroCHLOROthiazide—hydrOXYzine
hydroCHLOROthiazide	hydrALAZINE—hydrOXYzine
HYDROcodone	oxyCODONE
HYDROmorphone	morphine—oxyMORphone
hydrOXYzine	hydrALAZINE—hydroCHLOROthiazide
IDArubicin	DOXOrubicin—idaruCIZUmab
idaruCIZUmab	IDArubicin
inFLIXimab	riTUXimab
ISOtretinoin	tretinoin
KlonoPIN*	cloNIDine
LaMICtal*	LamISIL*
LamISIL*	LaMICtal*
lamiVUDine	lamoTRIgine
lamoTRIgine	lamiVUDine
levETIRAcetam	levOCARNitine—levOFLOXacin
levOCARNitine	levETIRAcetam
levOFLOXacin	levETIRAcetam
LEVOleucovorin	leucovorin
LORazepam	ALPRAZolam—clonazePAM
metFORMIN	metroNIDAZOLE
methazolAMIDE	methiMAZOLE—metOLazone
methiMAZOLE	methazolAMIDE—metOLazone
metOLazone	methazolAMIDE—methiMAZOLE
metroNIDAZOLE	metFORMIN
metyraPONE	metyroSINE
metyroSINE	metyraPONE
miFEPRIStone	miSOPROStol
migALAstat	migLUstat
migLUstat	migALAstat
miSOPROStol	miFEPRIStone
mitoMYcin	mitoXANTRONE
mitoXANTRONE	mitoMYcin
NexAVAR*	NexIUM*
NexIUM*	NexAVAR*
niCARdipine	NIFEdipine—niMODipine
NIFEdipine	niCARdipine—niMODipine
niMODipine	niCARdipine—NIFEdipine
NovoLIN*	NovoLOG*
NovoLOG*	NovoLIN*
OLANZapine	QUEtiapine
OXcarbazepine	carBAMazepine
oxyBUTYnin	oxyCODONE—OxyCONTIN*—oxyMORphone
oxyCODONE	HYDROcodone—oxyBUTYnin—OxyCONTIN*—oxyMORphone
OxyCONTIN*	oxyBUTYnin—oxyCODONE—oxyMORphone
oxyMORphone	HYDROmorphone—oxyBUTYnin—oxyCODONE—OxyCONTIN*
PACLitaxel	DOCEtaxel
PARoxetine	DULoxetine—FLUoxetine
PAZOPanib	PONATinib
PEMEtrexed	PRALAtrexate
penicillAMINE	penicillin
PENTobarbital	PHENobarbital
PHENobarbital	PENTobarbital
PONATinib	PAZOPanib
PRALAtrexate	PEMEtrexed
PriLOSEC*	PROzac*
PROzac*	PriLOSEC*
QUEtiapine	OLANZapine
quiNIDine	quiNINE
quiNINE	quiNIDine
RABEprazole	ARIPiprazole
rifAMPin	rifAXIMin
rifAXIMin	rifAMPin
RisperDAL*	rOPINIRole
risperiDONE	rOPINIRole
riTUXimab	inFLIXimab
romiDEPsin	romiPLOStim
romiPLOStim	romiDEPsin
rOPINIRole	RisperDAL*—risperiDONE
SandIMMUNE*	SandoSTATIN*
SandoSTATIN*	SandIMMUNE*
SAXagliptin	SITagliptin
SINEquan*	SEROquel*
SITagliptin	SAXagliptin—SUMAtriptan
Solu—CORTEF*	SOLU—Medrol*
SOLU—Medrol*	Solu—CORTEF*—DEPO-Medrol*
SORAfenib	SUNItinib
SUFentanil	fentaNYL
sulfADIAZINE	sulfaSALAzine
sulfaSALAzine	sulfADIAZINE
SUMAtriptan	SITagliptin—ZOLMitriptan
SUNItinib	SORAfenib
tiaGABine	tiZANidine
tiZANidine	tiaGABine
traMADol	traZODone
traZODone	traMADol
valACYclovir	valGANciclovir
valGANciclovir	valACYclovir
ZOLMitriptan	SUMAtriptan
ZyPREXA*	ZyrTEC*
ZyrTEC*	ZyPREXA*

*Brand names always start with an upper case letter. Some brand names incorporate tall man letters in initial characters and may not be readily recognized as brand names. An asterisk follows all brand names in IMSP List of Additional Drug Names with Tall Man Letters.

© US Food and Drug Administration (FDA) and Institute for Safe Medication Practices (ISMP). FDA and ISMP Lists of Look-Alike Drug Names with Recommended Tall Man Letters. ISMP; 2023.

PEDIATRIC INTRAVENOUS MEDICATION QUICK REFERENCE CHART

Risk of fluid overload in infants and children is always a consideration when administering IV medications. The following table provides maximum concentrations—the smallest amount of fluid necessary for diluting specific medications—and the maximum rate at which the medications be given.

Drug	Maximum Concentration	Maximum Rate
acetaminophen	10 mg/mL	Infuse over 15 min
acetazolamide	100 mg/mL	500 mg/min
acyclovir	10 mg/mL	Infuse over 1 hr
adenosine	3 mg/mL	Give over 1–2 sec
allopurinol	6 mg/mL	Infuse over 30 min
amikacin	10 mg/mL	Infuse over 30–60 min
aminocaproic acid	20 mg/mL	Infuse over 10–60 min
aminophylline	25 mg/mL (IV push) 1 mg/mL (intermittent infusion)	Infuse over 15–30 min
amphotericin B deoxycholate	0.1 mg/mL (peripherally) 0.25 mg/mL (centrally)	Infuse over 2–6 hr (peripherally or centrally)
amphotericin B lipid complex	2 mg/mL	2.5 mg/kg/hr
amphotericin B liposomal	2 mg/mL	Infuse over 2 hr
ampicillin	100 mg/mL	IV push: Dose ≤500 mg: Give over 3–5 min; Dose >500 mg: Give over 10–15 min Intermittent infusion: Infuse over 20 min (neonates) or 10–15 min (infants, children, and adolescents)
ampicillin/sulbactam	30 mg/mL (ampicillin)	IV push: Give over 10–15 min Intermittent infusion: Infuse over 15–30 min
anidulafungin	0.77 mg/mL	≤1.1 mg/min
atropine	1 mg/mL	Give over 1 min
azathioprine	10 mg/mL (IV push) <10 mg/mL (intermittent infusion)	IV push: Give over 5 min Intermittent infusion: Infuse over 30–60 min
azithromycin	2 mg/mL	Infuse over 1 hr
aztreonam	20 mg/mL	IV push: Give over 3–5 min Intermittent infusion: Infuse over 20–60 min
belimumab	4 mg/mL	Infuse over 1 hr
bezlotoxumab	10 mg/mL	Infuse over 1 hr
brivaracetam	10 mg/mL	Give over 2–15 min
bumetanide	0.25 mg/mL (IV push) 0.04 mg/mL (intermittent infusion)	Give over 1–2 min
caffeine citrate	20 mg/mL	Infuse over 10–20 min
calcium chloride	20 mg/mL	100 mg/min
calcium gluconate	50 mg/mL	100 mg/min
caspofungin	0.5 mg/mL	Infuse over 1 hr
cefazolin	138 mg/mL (IV push) 20 mg/mL (intermittent infusion)	IV push: Give over 3–5 min Intermittent infusion: Infuse over 10–60 min
cefepime	160 mg/mL	Intermittent infusion: Infuse over 30 min Extended infusion: Infuse over 3–4 hr
cefotaxime	200 mg/mL (IV push) 60 mg/mL (intermittent infusion)	IV push: Give over 3–5 min Intermittent infusion: Infuse over 15–30 min
cefoxitin	180 mg/mL (IV push) 125 mg/mL (intermittent infusion)	IV push: Give over 3–5 min Intermittent infusion: Infuse over 15–60 min
ceftaroline	12 mg/mL	Neonates and infants <2 mo: Infuse over 30–60 min; Infants 2 mo, children, and adolescents: Infuse over 5–60 min
ceftazidime	180 mg/mL (IV push) 40 mg/mL (intermittent infusion) 30 mg/mL (continuous infusion)	IV push: Give over 3–5 min Intermittent infusion: Infuse over 15–30 min
ceftazidime/avibactam	Ceftazidime 40 mg/mL and avibactam 10 mg/mL	Infuse over 2 hr
ceftolozane/tazobactam	Ceftolozane 16.3 mg/mL and tazobactam 8.1 mg/mL	Ceftolozane dose <2 g: Infuse over 1 hr; Ceftolozane dose of 2 g: Infuse over 3 hr
ceftriaxone	40 mg/mL	IV push: Give over 2–5 min Intermittent infusion: Infuse over 1 hr (neonates) or 30 min (infants, children, and adolescents)
cefuroxime	100 mg/mL (IV push) 137 mg/mL (intermittent infusion)	IV push: Give over 3–5 min Intermittent infusion: Infuse over 15–30 min
cetirizine	10 mg/mL	Give over 1–2 min
chlorothiazide	28 mg/mL	IV push: Give over 3–5 min Intermittent infusion: Infuse over 30 min
chlorpromazine	1 mg/mL	0.5 mg/min
ciprofloxacin	2 mg/mL	Infuse over 60 min

PEDIATRIC INTRAVENOUS MEDICATION QUICK REFERENCE CHART
continued

Drug	Maximum Concentration	Maximum Rate
clindamycin	18 mg/mL	30 mg/min
cyclosporine	2.5 mg/mL	Infuse over 2–6 hr
dalbavancin	5 mg/mL	Infuse over 30 min
dexamethasone	10 mg/mL	Dose ≤10 mg: Give over 1–4 min Dose >10 mg: Infuse over 15–30 min
dexmedetomidine	4 mcg/mL	Infuse loading dose over 10–20 min
diazepam	5 mg/mL	1–2 mg/min
digoxin	100 mcg/mL	Infuse over 5–10 min
diphenhydramine	50 mg/mL	IV push: ≤25 mg/min Intermittent infusion: Infuse over 10–15 min
enalaprilat	1.25 mg/mL	Give over 5 min
ertapenem	20 mg/mL	Infuse over 30 min
erythromycin	5 mg/mL	Infuse over 20–120 min
esomeprazole	0.8 mg/mL	Infuse over 10–30 min
ethacrynic acid	2 mg/mL	Infuse over 5–30 min
famotidine	4 mg/mL (IV push) 0.2 mg/mL (intermittent infusion)	IV push: Give over 2 min Intermittent infusion: Infuse over 15–30 min
fentanyl	50 mcg/mL	Give over 3–5 min; infuse larger doses (>5 mcg/kg) over 5–10 min
fluconazole	2 mg/mL	Infuse over 1–2 hr
flumazenil	0.1 mg/mL	0.2 mg/min
fosaprepitant	1 mg/mL	Infants 6 mo and children <12 yr: Infuse over 60 min; Children 12–17 yr: Infuse over 30 min
foscarnet	12 mg/mL (peripherally) 24 mg/mL (centrally)	60 mg/kg/hr
fosphenytoin	25 mg/mL	2 mg/kg/min
furosemide	10 mg/mL	0.5 mg/kg/min
ganciclovir	10 mg/mL	Infuse over 1 hr
gentamicin	10 mg/mL	Infuse over 30–120 min
glycopyrrolate	0.2 mg/mL	Give over 1–2 min
granisetron	1 mg/mL (IV push) 50 mcg/mL (intermittent infusion)	IV push: Give over 30 sec Intermittent infusion: Infuse over 30–60 min
hydralazine	20 mg/mL	Give over 1–2 min
hydrocortisone	50 mg/mL (IV push) 5 mg/mL (intermittent infusion)	IV push: Give over 30 sec Intermittent infusion: Infuse over 20–30 min
hydromorphone	4 mg/mL	Give over 2–3 min
ibuprofen	4 mg/mL	Infuse over 10 min
ibuprofen lysine	5 mg/mL	Infuse over 15 min
imipenem/cilastatin	5 mg/mL	Dose ≤500 mg: Infuse over 20–30 min; Dose >500 mg: Infuse over 40–60 min
indomethacin	1 mg/mL	Infuse over 20–30 min
infliximab	4 mg/mL	Infuse over 2 hr
ketamine	50 mg/mL (IV push) 2 mg/mL (continuous infusion)	IV push: 0.5 mg/kg/min
ketorolac	30 mg/mL	Give over 1–5 min
labetalol	5 mg/mL (IV push) 1 mg/mL (continuous infusion)	IV push: 10 mg/min
lacosamide	10 mg/mL	Infuse over 30–60 min
levetiracetam	20 mg/mL (neonates) 50 mg/mL (infants, children, and adolescents)	Neonates: Concentration ≤15 mg/mL: Infuse over 10–15 min; Concentration of 20 mg/mL: 1 mg/kg/min Infants, children, and adolescents: Concentration ≤15 mg/mL: Infuse over 15 min; Concentration of 50 mg/mL: Infuse over 5–10 min
levocarnitine	8 mg/mL	Give over 2–3 min
levothyroxine	100 mcg/mL	Give over 2–3 min
linezolid	2 mg/mL	Infuse over 30–120 min
lorazepam	2 mg/mL	2 mg/min or 0.05 mg/kg over 2–5 min
magnesium sulfate	200 mg/mL	Infuse over 10–20 min
meperidine	10 mg/mL	Give over 5 min
meropenem	50 mg/mL (IV push) 20 mg/mL (intermittent or extended infusion)	IV push: Give over 3–5 min Intermittent infusion: Infuse over 15–30 min Extended infusion: Infuse over 3–4 hr
methylprednisolone	125 mg/mL (IV push) 2.5 mg/mL (intermittent infusion)	IV push: Give over 1–5 min Intermittent infusion: Infuse over 15–60 min
metoclopramide	5 mg/mL (IV push) 0.4 mg/mL (intermittent infusion)	IV push: Dose ≤10 mg: Give over 1–2 min Intermittent infusion: Dose >10 mg: Infuse over 15 min
metronidazole	5 mg/mL	Infuse over 30–60 min
micafungin	1.5 mg/mL	Infuse over 1 hr

Drug	Maximum Concentration	Maximum Rate
midazolam	5 mg/mL	Give over 20–30 sec (5 min in neonates)
milrinone	200 mcg/mL	Loading dose: Give over 10 min
morphine	5 mg/mL (IV push or intermittent infusion) 1 mg/mL (continuous infusion)	IV push: Give over 4–5 min Intermittent infusion: Infuse over 15–30 min
mycophenolate	6 mg/mL	Infuse over 2 hr
nafcillin	125 mg/mL	IV push: Give over 5–10 min Intermittent infusion: Infuse over 30–60 min
naloxone	0.04 mg/mL (IV push) 400 mcg/mL (continuous infusion)	Give over 30 sec
ondansetron	2 mg/mL (IV push) 1 mg/mL (intermittent infusion)	IV push: Give over 2–5 min Intermittent infusion: Infuse over 15–30 min
oxacillin	100 mg/mL (IV push) 40 mg/mL (intermittent infusion)	IV push: Give over 10 min Intermittent infusion: Infuse over 15–30 min
palonosetron	30 mcg/mL	Prevention of chemotherapy-induced nausea/vomiting: Infuse over 15 min Prevention of postoperative nausea/vomiting: Give over 10 sec
pantoprazole	4 mg/mL (IV push) 0.8 mg/mL (intermittent infusion)	IV push: Give over 2 min Intermittent infusion: Infuse over 15 min
penicillin G	150,000 units/mL	Infuse over 15–30 min
pentamidine	6 mg/mL	Infuse over 1–2 hr
pentobarbital	50 mg/mL	50 mg/min
phenobarbital	65 mg/mL	30 mg/min
phenytoin	10 mg/mL	Neonates: 1 mg/kg/min; Infants, children, and adolescents: 3 mg/kg/min
phytonadione	10 mg/mL	1 mg/min
piperacillin/tazobactam	Piperacillin 80 mg/mL and tazobactam 10 mg/mL	Intermittent infusion: Infuse over 30 min Extended infusion: Neonates: Infuse over 3 hr; Infants, children, and adolescents: Infuse over 4 hr
posaconazole	2 mg/mL	Infuse over 90 min
potassium chloride	80 mEq/L (peripherally) 300 mEq/L (centrally)	≤0.5 mEq/kg/hr
propranolol	1 mg/mL	Infuse over 10 min
protamine	10 mg/mL	5 mg/min
remdesivir	1.25 mg/mL	Infuse over 30–120 min
rifampin	6 mg/mL	Infuse over 30–270 min
rocuronium	10 mg/mL	Give over 10 sec
tacrolimus	0.02 mg/mL	Infuse over 2–24 hr
tedizolid	0.8 mg/mL	Infuse over 1 hr
tobramycin	10 mg/mL	Infuse over 20–60 min
trimethoprim/sulfamethoxazole	1 mL drug per 15 mL diluent	Infuse over 60–90 min
valproate sodium	50 mg/mL	3 mg/kg/min
vancomycin	10 mg/mL	Infuse over 60 min
verapamil	2.5 mg/mL	Give over 2–3 min
voriconazole	5 mg/mL	3 mg/kg/hr
zidovudine	4 mg/mL	Infuse over 30–60 min

Lexicomp Online. Waltham, MA: UpToDate, Inc.; July 30, 2021. https://online.lexi.com. Accessed October 21, 2023.

MEDICATION SAFETY TOOLS | Pediatric Intravenous Medication Quick Reference Chart

Appendices

APPENDIX A

Recent Drug Approvals

To view full-text monographs of drugs that have been recently released from the FDA or to learn about changes to dosage forms, please visit www.DrugGuide.com.

✄ capivasertib
(kap-**eye**-va-**ser**-tib)
Truqap
Classification
Therapeutic: antineoplastics
Pharmacologic: kinase inhibitors

Indications
✄ Hormone receptor-positive, human epidermal growth factor receptor 2 (HER2)-negative, locally advanced or metastatic breast cancer with ≥1 *PIK3CA/AKT1/PTEN*-alteration following progression on ≥1 endocrine-based regimen in the metastatic setting or recurrence on or within 12 months of completing adjuvant therapy (in combination with fulvestrant).

Contraindications/Precautions
Contraindicated in: Hypersensitivity; Severe renal impairment; Severe hepatic impairment; OB: Pregnancy; Lactation: Lactation.
Use Cautiously in: Insulin-dependent diabetes; Diabetes, obesity, elevated fasting glucose (>160 mg/dL), elevated A1c, concurrent use of corticosteroids, or infection; Moderate hepatic impairment; Rep: Women of reproductive potential and men with female partners of reproductive potential; Pedi: Safety and effectiveness not established in children.

Adverse Reactions/Side Effects
Derm: dermatitis, dry skin, eczema, pruritus, rash, skin discoloration, urticaria, DRUG REACTION WITH EOSINOPHILIA AND SYSTEMIC SYMPTOMS (DRESS), ERYTHEMA MULTIFORME, palmar-plantar erythrodysesthesia.
Endo: HYPERGLYCEMIA. **F and E:** hypocalcemia, hypokalemia, dehydration, ketoacidosis. **GI:** ↑ liver enzymes, DIARRHEA, nausea, stomatitis, vomiting. **GU:** ↑ serum creatinine, urinary tract infection. **Hemat:** anemia, leukopenia, lymphopenia, neutropenia, thrombocytopenia. **Metab:** ↓ appetite, hypertriglyceridemia. **Neuro:** fatigue, headache.

Route/Dosage
PO (Adults): 400 mg twice daily for 4 days, followed by 3 days off; continue until disease progression or unacceptable toxicity. *Concurrent use with strong or moderate CYP3A4 inhibitor:* 320 mg twice daily for 4 days, followed by 3 days off; continue until disease progression or unacceptable toxicity.

etrasimod (e-tras-i-mod)
Velsipity
Classification
Therapeutic: gastrointestinal anti-inflammatories
Pharmacologic: receptor modulators

Indications
Moderately to severely active ulcerative colitis.

Contraindications/Precautions
Contraindicated in: MI, unstable angina, stroke, transient ischemic attack, decompensated HF requiring hospitalization, or Class III or IV HF within the past 6 mo; History or presence of Mobitz type II 2nd- or 3rd-degree heart block, sick sinus syndrome, or sinoatrial block, unless the patient has a functioning pacemaker; Active infection; ✄ Concurrent use of moderate or strong CYP2C8 or CYP3A4 inhibitors in poor CYP2C9 metabolizers; Severe hepatic impairment; OB: Pregnancy.
Use Cautiously in: QT interval prolongation (>450 msec in males, >470 msec females) or concurrent use of QT interval prolonging medications; Heart rate <50 bpm; Cardiac arrhythmias requiring use of class Ia or III antiarrhythmics; Ischemic heart disease, class I or II HF, cardiac arrest, cerebrovascular disease, or uncontrolled hypertension; Symptomatic bradycardia, recurrent cardiogenic syncope, or severe untreated sleep apnea; Mobitz type I 2nd-degree AV block, unless the patient has a functioning pacemaker; Immunocompromised or taking other immunosuppressant medications (↑ risk of progressive multifocal leukoencephalopathy [PML]); Lactation: Use while breast feeding only if potential maternal benefit justifies potential risk to infant; Rep: Women of reproductive potential; Pedi: Safety and effectiveness not established in children.

Adverse Reactions/Side Effects
CV: bradycardia, heart block, hypertension. **EENT:** macular edema, vision abnormalities. **GI:** ↑ liver enzymes, nausea. **GU:** urinary tract infection. **Hemat:** lymphopenia. **Metab:** hypercholesterolemia. **MS:** arthralgia. **Neuro:** POSTERIOR REVERSIBLE ENCEPHALOPATHY SYNDROME (PRES), dizziness, headache, PML.
Resp: ↓ pulmonary function. **Misc:** INFECTION (including bacterial and viral), immune reconstitution inflammatory syndrome, MALIGNANCY.

Route/Dosage
PO (Adults): 2 mg once daily.

---

fruquintinib (frew-kwin-ti-nib)
Fruzaqla
Classification
Therapeutic: antineoplastics
Pharmacologic: vascular endothelial growth-factor antagonists, kinase inhibitors

Indications
Metastatic colorectal cancer in patients who have been previously treated with fluoropyrimidine-, oxaliplatin-, and irinotecan-based chemotherapy; an antivascular endothelial growth factor (VEGF) therapy; and, if *RAS* wild-type and medically appropriate, an anti-epidermal growth factor receptor therapy.

Contraindications/Precautions
Contraindicated in: Severe hepatic impairment; OB: Pregnancy; Lactation: Lactation.

Use Cautiously in: Uncontrolled hypertension; Cardiovascular disease; History of thromboembolism; Aspirin hypersensitivity (contains tartrazine); Moderate hepatic impairment; Rep: Women of reproductive potential and men with female partners of reproductive potential; Pedi: Safety and effectiveness not established in children.

Adverse Reactions/Side Effects
CV: hypertension. **Derm:** palmar plantar erythrodysesthesia, impaired wound healing, rash. **EENT:** dysphonia, throat pain. **Endo:** hyperglycemia, hypothyroidism. **F and E:** hypocalcemia, hypokalemia, hypomagenesemia, hyponatremia. **GI:** ↑ liver enzymes, abdominal pain, anorexia, diarrhea, HEPATOTOXICITY, hyperbilirubinemia, hypoalbuminemia, stomatitis, GI PERFORATION. **GU:** ↑ serum creatinine, proteinuria. **Hemat:** ↑ activated partial thromboplastin time, anemia, BLEEDING, lymphopenia, thrombocytopenia, ARTERIAL THROMBOEMBOLIC EVENTS. **Metab:** hypercholesterolemia, hypertriglyceridemia, hyperuricemia. **MS:** arthralgia, pain. **Neuro:** POSTERIOR REVERSIBLE ENCEPHALOPATHY SYNDROME (PRES). **Misc:** fatigue, INFECTION, HYPERSENSITIVITY REACTIONS, proctalgia.

Route/Dosage
PO (Adults): 5 mg once daily for 21 days of each 28-day cycle; continue until disease progression or unacceptable toxicity.

---

gepirone (ge-pi-rone)
Exxua
Classification
Therapeutic: antidepressants
Pharmacologic: 5-HT$_1$ agonists

Indications
Major depressive disorder.

Contraindications/Precautions
Contraindicated in: Hypersensitivity; QTc interval >450 msec at baseline; Congenital long QT syndrome; Concurrent use of strong CYP3A4 inhibitors; Severe hepatic impairment; Concurrent use (or within 14 days) of MAO inhibitors or MAO inhibitor–like drugs (linezolid or methylene blue).

Use Cautiously in: History of suicide attempt; Uncontrolled or significant cardiac disease, recent MI, HF, unstable angina, bradyarrhythmias, uncontrolled hypertension, 2nd- or 3rd-degree heart block, severe aortic stenosis, or uncontrolled hypothyroidism (↑ risk of torsades de pointes); Electrolyte abnormalities (correct before initiating therapy); Bipolar disorder; Family history of bipolar disorder, depression, or suicide; Moderate or severe renal impairment; Moderate hepatic impairment; OB: Use during 3rd trimester may result in neonatal serotonin syndrome requiring prolonged hospitalization, respiratory and nutritional support. Use during pregnancy only if potential maternal benefit justifies potential fetal risk; Lactation: Safety not established in breast feeding; Pedi: Safety and effectiveness not established in children. May ↑ risk of suicide attempt/ideation, especially during early treatment or dose adjustment; risk may be greater in children or adolescents; Geri: Maximum dose of 36.3 mg/day in older adults.

Adverse Reactions/Side Effects
CV: palpitations, peripheral edema, QT interval prolongation, tachycardia. **Derm:** ↑ sweating. **EENT:** nasal congestion, nasopharyngitis. **GI:** diarrhea, nausea, abdominal pain, constipation, dry mouth, dyspepsia, vomiting. **GU:** breast tenderness. **Metab:** ↑ appetite, ↑ weight. **Neuro:** dizziness, headache, insomnia, sedation, agitation, confusion, fatigue, jitteriness, paresthesia. **Resp:** dyspnea, upper respiratory tract infection. **Misc:** hypersensitivity reactions.

Route/Dosage
PO (Adults): 18.2 mg once daily; may ↑ to 36.3 mg once daily on Day 4 based on clinical response and tolerability. May then further ↑ to 54.5 mg once daily after Day 7, and then to 72.6 mg once daily after Day 14. *Concurrent use of moderate CYP3A4 inhibitor:* ↓ gepirone dose by 50%.

PO (Geriatric Patients): 18.2 mg once daily; may ↑ to 36.3 mg once daily after Day 7 based on clinical response and tolerability (max dose = 36.3 mg/day). *Concurrent use of moderate CYP3A4 inhibitor:* ↓ gepirone dose by 50%.

Renal Impairment
PO (Adults): *CCr <50 mL/min:* 18.2 mg once daily; may ↑ to 36.3 mg once daily after Day 7 based on clinical response and tolerability (max dose = 36.3 mg/day). *Concurrent use of moderate CYP3A4 inhibitor:* ↓ gepirone dose by 50%.

Hepatic Impairment

PO (Adults): *Moderate hepatic impairment:* 18.2 mg once daily; may ↑ to 36.3 mg once daily after Day 7 based on clinical response and tolerability (max dose = 36.3 mg/day). *Concurrent use of moderate CYP3A4 inhibitor:* ↓ gepirone dose by 50%.

---

nalmefene (nal-me-feen)
Opvee
Classification
Therapeutic: antidotes
Pharmacologic: opioid antagonists

Indications
Emergency treatment of known or suspected overdose caused by natural or synthetic opioids and characterized by respiratory and/or CNS depression.

Contraindications/Precautions
Contraindicated in: Known hypersensitivity.
Use Cautiously in: Overdosage of buprenorphine (may not completely reverse respiratory depression; may required repeated doses); Pedi: Children <12 yr (safety and effectiveness not established).
Exercise Extreme Caution in: Patients known to be physically dependent on opioid agents or who have undergone surgery with large doses of opioid analgesics (especially those with severe cardiovascular disease or who have received cardiovascular medications) (↑ risk of withdrawal and cardiovascular complications).

Adverse Reactions/Side Effects
CV: hypertension, hypotension, tachycardia. **Derm:** ↑ sweating, erythema, hot flush. **EENT:** nasal discomfort, nasal congestion, oropharyngeal pain, rhinitis, throat irritation. **GI:** nausea, abdominal pain, dry mouth, vomiting. **Metab:** ↓ appetite. **Neuro:** headache, agitation, anxiety, claustrophobia, dizziness, dysgeusia, fatigue, insomnia, paresthesia, recurrent CNS depression. **Resp:** dyspnea, recurrent respiratory depression. **Misc:** chills, fever, postoperative pain.

Route/Dosage
Intranasal (Adults and Children ≥12 yr): One spray (2.7 mg) in one nostril; if desired response not achieved, may repeat dose every 2–5 min.

---

nirsevimab (nir-sev-i-mab)
Beyfortus
Classification
Therapeutic: vaccines/immunizing agents
Pharmacologic: immune globulins, monoclonal antibodies

Indications
Prevention of respiratory syncytial virus (RSV) lower respiratory tract disease in the following individuals: Neonates and infants born during or entering their first RSV season; Children up to 24 months of age who remain vulnerable to severe RSV disease through their second RSV season.

Contraindications/Precautions
Contraindicated in: Serious hypersensitivity reactions; Pedi: Children >24 mo (safety and effectiveness not established).
Use Cautiously in: Thrombocytopenia any coagulation disorder or receiving anticoagulation therapy.

Adverse Reactions/Side Effects
Derm: rash. **Local:** injection site reaction. **Misc:** HYPERSENSITIVITY REACTIONS (including anaphylaxis).

Route/Dosage

Neonates and Infants Born During or Entering Their First RSV Season

IM (Neonates and Infants <8 mo and ≥5 kg): 100 mg as single dose; *Undergoing cardiac surgery with cardiopulmonary bypass (>90 days since initial dose):* Administer additional 50 mg single dose; *Undergoing cardiac surgery with cardiopulmonary bypass (≤90 days since initial dose):* Administer additional 100 mg single dose.
IM (Neonates and Infants <8 mo and <5 kg): 50 mg as single dose. *Undergoing cardiac surgery with cardiopulmonary bypass (regardless of time since initial dose):* Administer additional 50 mg single dose.

Children Who Remain at Increased Risk for Severe RSV Disease in Their Second RSV Season

IM (Infants and Children 8–19 mo): 200 mg as a single dose. *Undergoing cardiac surgery with cardiopulmonary bypass (>90 days since initial dose):* Administer additional 100 mg single dose; *Undergoing cardiac surgery with cardiopulmonary bypass (≤90 days since initial dose):* Administer additional 200 mg single dose.

---

rezafungin (re-za-fun-jin)
Rezzayo
Classification
Therapeutic: antifungals
Pharmacologic: echinocandins

Indications
Candidemia and invasive candidiasis in patients who have limited or no alternative treatment options.

Contraindications/Precautions
Contraindicated in: Hypersensitivity to rezafungin or other echinocandins.
Use Cautiously in: OB: Safety during pregnancy not established; Lactation: Safety during breast feeding not established; Pedi: Safety and effectiveness not established in children.

Adverse Reactions/Side Effects
CV: edema. **Derm:** erythema, photosensitivity. **F and E:** hypokalemia, hypomagnesemia, hypophosphatemia. **GI:** diarrhea, ↑ liver enzymes, abdominal pain, constipation, dysphagia, GI BLEEDING, nausea, vomiting. **GU:** acute kidney injury. **Hemat:** anemia, disseminated intravascular coagulation. **Neuro:** dizziness, headache, insomnia, peripheral neuropathy, tremor. **Misc:** fever, infusion-related reactions.

Route/Dosage
IV (Adults): 400 mg initially on Day 1, then 200 mg once weekly beginning on Day 8 for up to four doses (including the dose on Day 1).

---

roflumilast (topical)
(row-**floo**-mi-last)
Zoryve
Classification
Therapeutic: antipsoriatics
Pharmacologic: phosphodiesterase inhibitors

Indications
Plaque psoriasis (including intertriginous areas).

Contraindications/Precautions
Contraindicated in: Moderate to severe hepatic impairment.
Use Cautiously in: OB: Safety not established in pregnancy; Lactation: Use while breast feeding only if potential maternal benefits justify potential risk to infant; Pedi: Children <12 yr (safety and effectiveness not established).

Adverse Reactions/Side Effects
GI: diarrhea, nausea. **Local:** pain, urticaria. **Neuro:** headache, insomnia.

Route/Dosage
Topical (Adults and Children ≥12 yr): Apply to affected area(s) once daily.

---

sotagliflozin (soe-ta-gli-**floe**-zin)
Inpefa
Classification
Therapeutic: none assigned
Pharmacologic: sodium-glucose co-transporter 1 (SGLT1) inhibitors, sodium-glucose co-transporter 2 (SGLT2) inhibitors

Indications
To reduce the risk of cardiovascular death, hospitalization for HF and urgent HF visits in patients with HF. To reduce the risk of cardiovascular death, hospitalization for HF and urgent HF visits in patients with type 2 diabetes mellitus, chronic kidney disease, and other cardiovascular risk factors.

Contraindications/Precautions
Contraindicated in: Hypersensitivity; Type 1 diabetes; Moderate or severe hepatic impairment; eGFR <15 mL/min/1.73 m² or hemodialysis; Rep: SGLT2 inhibitors are not recommended for the treatment of HF in women of reproductive potential; OB: 2nd and 3rd trimesters of pregnancy. SGLT2 inhibitors are not recommended for the treatment of HF during pregnancy; Lactation: Lactation.
Use Cautiously in: History of type 1 or 2 diabetes, pancreatitis, pancreatic surgery, acute febrile illness, reduced caloric intake due to illness or surgery, surgical procedures, volume depletion, or alcohol abuse (↑ risk of ketoacidosis); Hypovolemia, chronic kidney disease (eGFR <60 mL/min/1.73 m²), or concurrent use of loop diuretics (↑ risk of volume depletion or hypotension); History of genital mycotic infections; OB: Safety not established during 1st trimester of pregnancy; Pedi: Safety and effectiveness not established in children; Geri: Older adults may have ↑ risk of hypovolemia and hypotension.

Adverse Reactions/Side Effects
CV: hypotension. **Endo:** hypoglycemia (↑ with other medications). **F and E:** dehydration, KETOACIDOSIS. **GI:** diarrhea. **GU:** urinary tract infection (including pyelonephritis), acute kidney injury, genital mycotic infection, NECROTIZING FASCIITIS OF PERINEUM (FOURNIER'S GANGRENE). **Neuro:** dizziness.

Route/Dosage
PO (Adults): 200 mg once daily, then after 2 wk, ↑ to 400 mg once daily.

---

tapinarof (ta-**pin**-ar-of)
Vtama
Classification
Therapeutic: antipsoriatics
Pharmacologic: aryl hydrocarbon receptor agonists

Indications
Plaque psoriasis.

Contraindications/Precautions
Contraindicated in: None.
Use Cautiously in: OB: Safety not established in pregnancy; Lactation: Use while breast feeding only if potential maternal benefit justifies potential risk to infant; Pedi: Safety and effectiveness not established in children.

Adverse Reactions/Side Effects
Derm: contact dermatitis, folliculitis, pruritus, urticaria. **Neuro:** headache.

Route/Dosage
Topical (Adults): Apply to affected area(s) once daily.

taurolidine/heparin
(ta-**roe**-li-dyne/**hep**-a-rin)
Defencath
Classification
Therapeutic: anti-infectives, anticoagulants
Pharmacologic: antithrombotics

Indications
To reduce the incidence of catheter-related bloodstream infections in patients with kidney failure receiving chronic hemodialysis (HD) through a central venous catheter.

Contraindications/Precautions
Contraindicated in: Known heparin-induced thrombocytopenia; Known hypersensitivity to taurolidine, heparin, the citrate excipient, or pork products. **Use Cautiously in:** Pedi: Safety and effectiveness not established in children.

Adverse Reactions/Side Effects
GI: nausea, vomiting. **Hemat:** BLEEDING, HEPARIN-INDUCED THROMBOCYTOPENIA. **MS:** musculoskeletal chest pain. **Neuro:** dizziness. **Misc:** hemodialysis catheter malfunction, loss of catheter patency, hypersensitivity reactions.

Route/Dosage
Not intended for systemic administration or for use as a catheter lock flush.

Intracatheter (Adults): Instill a sufficient volume of catheter lock solution (containing heparin 1000 units/mL and taurolidine 13.5 mg/mL) into each HD catheter lumen at the conclusion of each HD session; prior to initiation of the next HD session, aspirate and discard solution from the catheter.

teplizumab (tep-**liz**-ue-mab)
Tzield
Classification
Therapeutic: antidiabetics
Pharmacologic: monoclonal antibodies

Indications
To delay the onset of Stage 3 type 1 diabetes in patients with Stage 2 type 1 diabetes.

Contraindications/Precautions
Contraindicated in: Active or chronic infection (excluding localized skin infection); Laboratory or clinical evidence of acute infection with Epstein-Barr virus or cytomegalovirus; Lymphocyte count <1000 cells/mcL; Hemoglobin <10 g/dL; Platelet count <150,000 cells/mcL; Absolute neutrophil count <1500 cells/mcL; Elevated ALT or AST >2 times upper limit of normal (ULN) or bilirubin >1.5 times ULN; OB: Pregnancy.
Use Cautiously in: Lactation: Safety not established during breast feeding; Rep: Women of reproductive potential; Pedi: Children <8 yr (safety and effectiveness not established).

Adverse Reactions/Side Effects
Derm: rash. **F and E:** ↓ bicarbonate, hypocalcemia. **GI:** ↑ liver enzymes, diarrhea, nausea. **Hemat:** anemia, leukopenia, lymphopenia, thrombocytopenia, neutropenia. **Neuro:** headache. **Misc:** cytokine release syndrome, HYPERSENSITIVITY REACTIONS (including angioedema), infection.

Route/Dosage
IV (Adults and Children >8 yr): *Day 1:* 65 mcg/m^2 as single dose; *Day 2:* 125 mcg/m^2 as single dose; *Day 3:* 250 mcg/m^2 as single dose; *Day 4:* 500 mcg/m^2 as single dose; *Day 5–14:* 1,030 mcg/m^2 once daily.

terlipressin (ter-li-**pres**-sin)
Terlivaz
Classification
Therapeutic: hormones
Pharmacologic: antidiuretic hormones

Indications
Hepatorenal syndrome in patients with a rapid reduction in kidney function.

Contraindications/Precautions
Contraindicated in: Hypoxia or worsening respiratory symptoms; Acute-on-chronic liver failure Grade 3; Coronary, peripheral, or mesenteric ischemia; Severe cardiovascular conditions or cerebrovascular disease, and ischemic disease; OB: Pregnancy.
Use Cautiously in: High prioritization for liver transplantation (adverse effects may ↑ risk of ineligibility); Lactation: Safety not established in breast feeding; Pedi: Safety and effectiveness not established in children.

Adverse Reactions/Side Effects
CV: bradycardia, edema, MYOCARDIAL ISCHEMIA, PERIPHERAL ISCHEMIA. **Derm:** cyanosis. **GI:** abdominal pain, diarrhea, nausea, GI ISCHEMIA/OBSTRUCTION. **Neuro:** CEREBROVASCULAR ISCHEMIA. **Resp:** dyspnea, RESPIRATORY FAILURE, pleural effusion. **Misc:** SEPSIS.

Route/Dosage

IV (Adults): 0.85 mg every 6 hr on Days 1–3, then adjust dose as follows based on SCr starting on Day 4: ↓ *SCr by ≥30% from baseline: Continue 0.85 mg every 6 hr until 24 hr after patient achieves second consecutive SCr ≤1.5 mg/dL ≥2 hr apart or* for maximum of 14 days; ↓ *SCr by <30% from baseline:* ↑ *dose to 1.7 mg every 6 hr and continue until 24 hr after patient achieves second consecutive SCr ≤1.5 mg/dL ≥2 hr apart or* for maximum of 14 days; *SCr at or above baseline:* Discontinue therapy.

---

vonoprazan (von-oh-pra-zan)
Voquezna
Classification
Therapeutic: antiulcer agents
Pharmacologic: potassium-competitive acid blockers

Indications

Treatment of erosive esophagitis and relief of heartburn associated with erosive esophagitis. Maintenance of healed erosive esophagitis and relief of heartburn associated with erosive esophagitis. Treatment of *Helicobacter pylori* infection (in combination with amoxicillin or with amoxicillin and clarithromycin).

Contraindications/Precautions

Contraindicated in: Hypersensitivity; Concurrent use of rilpivirine-containing products; Severe renal impairment (for treatment of *Helicobacter pylori* infection); Moderate or severe hepatic impairment (for treatment of *Helicobacter pylori* infection); Lactation: Lactation.

Use Cautiously in: Patients using high doses for >1 yr (↑ risk of hip, wrist, or spine fractures and fundic gland polyps); Severe renal impairment (↓ dose recommended for treatment of erosive esophagitis); Moderate or severe hepatic impairment (↓ dose recommended for treatment of erosive esophagitis); OB: Safety not established in pregnancy; Pedi: Safety and effectiveness not established in children.

Adverse Reactions/Side Effects

CV: hypertension. **Derm:** STEVENS-JOHNSON SYNDROME, TOXIC EPIDERMAL NECROLYSIS. **F and E:** hypocalcemia (especially if treatment duration ≥3 mo), hypokalemia (especially if treatment duration ≥3 mo), hypomagnesemia (especially if treatment duration ≥3 mo). **GI:** abdominal distension, abdominal pain, CLOSTRIDIOIDES DIFFICILE-ASSOCIATED DIARRHEA, diarrhea, dyspepsia, fundic gland polyps, gastritis, nausea. **GU:** acute tubulointerstitial nephritis, urinary tract infection. **Hemat:** vitamin B$_{12}$ deficiency. **MS:** bone fracture. **Misc:** HYPERSENSITIVITY REACTIONS (including anaphylaxis).

Route/Dosage
Treatment of Erosive Esophagitis and Relief of Heartburn Associated with Erosive Esophagitis

PO (Adults): 20 mg once daily for 8 wk.

Renal Impairment
PO (Adults): *CCr <30 mL/min:* 10 mg once daily for 8 wk.

Hepatic Impairment
PO (Adults): *Moderate or severe hepatic impairment:* 10 mg once daily for 8 wk.

Maintenance of Healed Erosive Esophagitis and Relief of Heartburn Associated with Erosive Esophagitis

PO (Adults): 10 mg once daily for up to 6 mo.

Treatment of *Helicobacter pylori* Infection

PO (Adults): *In combination with amoxicillin (dual therapy) or amoxicillin and clarithromycin (triple therapy):* 20 mg twice daily for 14 days.

Renal Impairment
PO (Adults): *CCr <30 mL/min:* Not recommended.

Hepatic Impairment
PO (Adults): *Moderate or severe hepatic impairment:* Not recommended.

REMS

zilucoplan (zil-ue-koe-plan)
Zilbrysq
Classification
Therapeutic: anti-myasthenics
Pharmacologic: complement inhibitors

Indications
Generalized myasthenia gravis in patients who are anti-acetylcholine receptor antibody positive.

Contraindications/Precautions
Contraindicated in: Unresolved *Neisseria meningitidis* infection.

Use Cautiously in: OB: Safety not established in pregnancy; Lactation: Safety not established in breast feeding; Pedi: Safety and effectiveness not established in children.

Adverse Reactions/Side Effects
GI: diarrhea, nausea, pancreatic cysts, PANCREATITIS, vomiting. **Hemat:** eosinophilia. **Local:** injection site reactions. **Misc:** INFECTION (including *Neisseria meningitidis*, *Streptococcus pneumoniae*, and *Haemophilus influenzae*).

Route/Dosage
SUBQ (Adults ≥77 kg): 32.4 mg once daily.
SUBQ (Adults 56–<77 kg): 23 mg once daily.
SUBQ (Adults <56 kg): 16.6 mg once daily.

DISCONTINUED DRUGS

Generic Name (Brand Name)	Reason for Discontinuation
alfentanil (Alfenta)	Discontinued by manufacturer
aliskiren/amlodipine (Tekamlo)	Discontinued by manufacturer
amlodipine/celecoxib (Consensi)	Discontinued by manufacturer
attapulgite (🍁 Children's Kaopectate)	Discontinued by manufacturer
brompheniramine (🍁 Dimetane)	Discontinued by manufacturer
carteolol (Cartrol)	Discontinued by manufacturer
choline and magnesium salicylates (Trilisate)	Discontinued by manufacturer
copanlisib (Aliqopa)	Discontinued by manufacturer
cortisone (🍁 Cortone)	Discontinued by manufacturer
didanosine (Videx)	Discontinued by manufacturer
dimercaprol	Discontinued by manufacturer
dolasetron (Anzemet)	Discontinued by manufacturer
edetate calcium disodium	Discontinued by manufacturer
eflornithine (topical) (Vaniqa)	Discontinued by manufacturer
estramustine (Emcyt)	Discontinued by manufacturer
etidronate (Didronel)	Discontinued by manufacturer
fenoldopam (Corlopam)	Discontinued by manufacturer
ferric pyrophosphate citrate (Triferic)	Discontinued by manufacturer
flunisolide (Aerospan)	Discontinued by manufacturer
flurazepam (Dalmane)	Discontinued by manufacturer
gemifloxacin (Factive)	Discontinued by manufacturer
glycopyrrolate (inhalation) (Lonhala Magnair)	Discontinued by manufacturer
HYDROXYprogesterone caproate (Makena)	Discontinued by manufacturer
indacaterol (Arcapta Neohaler)	Discontinued by manufacturer
indinavir (Crixivan)	Discontinued by manufacturer
ingenol (Picato)	Discontinued by manufacturer
insulin detemir (Levemir)	Discontinued by manufacturer
lactitol (Pizensy)	Discontinued by manufacturer
lamivudine/raltegravir (Dutrebis)	Discontinued by manufacturer
levamlodipine (Conjupri)	Discontinued by manufacturer
lindane	Discontinued by manufacturer
lixisenatide (Adlyxin)	Discontinued by manufacturer
lucinactant (Surfaxin)	Discontinued by manufacturer
macimorelin (Macrilen)	Discontinued by manufacturer
mechlorethamine (Mustargen)	Discontinued by manufacturer
metaproterenol (Alupent)	Discontinued by manufacturer
methyldopa (Aldomet)	Discontinued by manufacturer

🍁= Canadian drug name. ☒ = Genetic implication. ~~Strikethrough~~ = Discontinued. CAPITALS = life-threatening. <u>Underline</u> = most frequent.

DISCONTINUED DRUGS (continued)

Generic Name (Brand Name)	Reason for Discontinuation
moxetumumab pasudotox (Lumoxiti)	Discontinued by manufacturer
muromonab-CD3 (Orthoclone OKT3)	Discontinued by manufacturer
nabilone (Cesamet)	Discontinued by manufacturer
netilmicin (Netromycin)	Discontinued by manufacturer
omacetaxine (Synribo)	Discontinued by manufacturer
ombitasvir/paritaprevir/ritonavir/ dasabuvir (✽ Holkira Pak)	Discontinued by manufacturer
pancuronium (Pavulon)	Discontinued by manufacturer
panobinostat (Farydak)	Discontinued by manufacturer
physostigmine (Antilirium)	Discontinued by manufacturer
propantheline (Pro-Banthine)	Discontinued by manufacturer
quinupristin/dalfopristin (Synercid)	Discontinued by manufacturer
rosiglitazone (Avandia)	Discontinued by manufacturer
saquinavir (Invirase)	Discontinued by manufacturer
stavudine (Zerit)	Discontinued by manufacturer
streptozocin (Zanosar)	Discontinued by manufacturer
tacrine (Cognex)	Discontinued by manufacturer
tenapanor (Ibsrela)	Discontinued by manufacturer
testosterone transdermal system (Androderm)	Discontinued by manufacturer
tiludronate (Skelid)	Discontinued by manufacturer
TOLBUTamide (Orinase)	Discontinued by manufacturer
tolmetin (Tolectin)	Discontinued by manufacturer
vincristine liposome (Marqibo)	Discontinued by manufacturer

Ophthalmic Medications

General Info: See Appendix C for administration techniques for ophthalmic agents.

Consult health care professional regarding:

- Concurrent use of contact lenses (medication or additives may be absorbed by the lens).
- Concurrent administration of other ophthalmic agents (order and spacing may be important).

ADRs = adverse reactions.

DRUG NAME	DOSE	NOTES
Anesthetics		
Uses: Provide brief local anesthesia to allow measurement of intraocular pressure, removal of foreign bodies, or other superficial procedures.		
CAUTIONS: Repeated use may result in ↑ risk of CNS and cardiovascular toxicity; cross-sensitivity with some local anesthetics may occur.		
chlorprocaine (Iheezo)	**Adults:** 3 drops of 3% gel (single dose).	● ADRs: conjunctival hyperemia, mydriasis, irritation
lidocaine (Akten)	**Adults and children:** 2 drops of 3.5% gel (single dose).	● Does not interact with ophthalmic cholinesterase inhibitors ● ADRs: ophthalmic: irritation; systemic: irregular heartbeat, CNS depression
proparacaine (Alcaine)	**Adults and children:** 1–2 drops of 0.5% solution (single dose).	● Does not interact with ophthalmic cholinesterase inhibitors ● ADRs: ophthalmic: irritation; systemic: irregular heartbeat, CNS depression
tetracaine (Altacaine)	**Adults:** 1–2 drops of 0.5% solution (single dose).	● May interact with ophthalmic cholinesterase inhibitors, resulting in ↑ duration of action and risk of toxicity ● ADRs: ophthalmic: irritation; systemic: irregular heartbeat, CNS depression
Antihistamines		
Uses: Various forms of allergic conjunctivitis.		
alcaftadine (Lastacaft [OTC])	**Adults and children ≥2 yr:** 1 drop of 0.25% solution once daily.	● ADRs: transient burning/stinging, headache
azelastine	**Adults and children ≥3 yr:** 1 drop of 0.05% solution twice daily.	● ADRs: transient burning/stinging, headache, bitter taste
bepotastine (Bepreve)	**Adults and children ≥2 yr:** 1 drop of 1.5% solution twice daily.	● ADRs: taste disturbance, headache, local irritation
cetirizine (Zerviate)	**Adults and children ≥2 yr:** 1 drop of 0.24% solution twice daily (given 8 hr apart).	● ADRs: transient burning/stinging, ↓ visual acuity
epinastine	**Adults and children ≥2 yr:** 1 drop of 0.05% solution twice daily.	● ADRs: headache, local irritation
ketotifen (Acuvue Theravision, Alaway [OTC], Zaditor)	**Adults and children ≥3 yr:** 1 drop of 0.025% solution twice daily (given 8–12 hr apart). **Adults and children ≥11 yr:** Drug-eluting contact lens: 1 lens in each eye once daily.	● ADRs: local irritation, eye pain (contact lens)
olopatadine (Pataday [OTC])	**Adults and children ≥2 yr:** *0.1% solution:* 1 drop twice daily (given 6–8 hr apart); *0.2% solution:* 1 drop once daily; *0.7% solution:* 1 drop once daily.	● ADRs: headache, conjunctival irritation

DRUG NAME	DOSE	NOTES

Antibacterials

Uses: Localized superficial ophthalmic infections (e.g., bacterial conjunctivitis).
CAUTIONS: Small amounts may be absorbed and result in hypersensitivity reactions.

DRUG NAME	DOSE	NOTES
azithromycin (AzaSite)	**Adults and children ≥1 yr:** 1 drop of 1% solution twice daily (given 8–12 hr apart) for 2 days, then once daily for 5 more days.	• When used to treat ocular chlamydial infections, concurrent systemic therapy is required • ADRs: eye irritation
bacitracin	**Adults and children:** ¼–½-in. ointment strip every 3–4 hr for acute infections or 2–3 times daily for mild to moderate infections.	• ADRs: eye irritation
besifloxacin (Besivance)	**Adults and children ≥1 yr:** 1 drop of 0.6% suspension 3 times daily (given 4–12 hr apart) for 7 days.	• ADRs: headache, eye irritation
ciprofloxacin (Ciloxan)	**Adults and children of all ages (solution) or ≥2 yr (ointment):** *Bacterial conjunctivitis:* Solution: 1–2 drops of 0.3% solution every 2 hr while awake for 2 days, then every 4 hr while awake for 5 more days; Ointment: ½-in. strip 3 times daily for 2 days, then twice daily for 5 more days; *Corneal ulcers:* Solution: 2 drops of 0.3% solution every 15 min for 6 hr, then every 30 min while awake for rest of day, then every hr while awake for next 24 hr, then every 4 hr while awake for next 12 days or longer if re-epithelialization does not occur.	• May cause harmless white crystalline precipitate that resolves over time • ADRs: altered taste, systemic allergic reactions, photophobia, discomfort
erythromycin	**Adults and children:** *Treatment of infections:* ½-in. ointment strip 2–6 times daily. **Infants:** *Prophylaxis of ophthalmia neonatorum:* ½-in. ointment strip in each eye as a single dose.	• ADRs: irritation
gatifloxacin (Zymaxid)	**Adults and children ≥1 yr:** 1 drop of 0.5% solution every 2 hr while awake (up to 8 times/day) for 1 day, then 2–4 times daily while awake for 6 more days.	• ADRs: irritation, headache, ↓ visual acuity, taste disturbance
gentamicin	**Adults and children:** *Solution:* 1–2 drops of 0.3% solution every 2–4 hr.	• ADRs: irritation, burning, stinging, blurred vision (ointment)
levofloxacin	**Adults and children ≥6 yr:** 1–2 drops of 0.5% solution every 2 hr while awake for 2 days (up to 8 times/day); then every 4 hr while awake for 5 more days (up to 4 times/day).	• ADRs: altered taste, systemic allergic reactions, photophobia
moxifloxacin (Vigamox)	**Adults and children:** 1 drop of 0.5% solution 3 times daily for 7 days.	• ADRs: irritation, ↓ visual acuity
ofloxacin (Ocuflox)	**Adults and children ≥1 yr:** *Bacterial conjunctivitis:* 1–2 drops of 0.3% solution every 2–4 hr while awake for 2 days, then 4 times daily for 5 more days; *Corneal ulcer:* 1–2 drops of 0.3% solution every 30 min while awake and every 4–6 hr while sleeping for 2 days, then every hr while awake for 4–6 more days, then 4 times daily until cured.	• ADRs: altered taste, systemic allergic reactions, photophobia
sulfacetamide	**Adults and children ≥2 mo:** *Solution:* 1–2 drops of 10% solution every 2–3 hr while awake (less frequently at night) for 7–10 days; *Ointment:* ½-in. strip every 3–4 hr and at bedtime for 7–10 days.	• Cross-sensitivity with other sulfonamides (including thiazides) may occur • ADRs: local irritation

DRUG NAME	DOSE	NOTES
tobramycin (Tobrex)	**Adults and children ≥2 mo:** *Solution:* 1–2 drops of 0.3% solution every 2–4 hr depending on severity of infection; *Ointment:* ½-in. strip every 8–12 hr.	• Ointment may retard corneal wound healing • ADRs: irritation, burning, stinging, blurred vision (ointment)

Antifungal

Uses: Fungal blepharitis, conjunctivitis, and keratitis.
CAUTIONS: Small amounts may be absorbed and result in hypersensitivity reactions.

natamycin (Natacyn)	**Adults:** *Fungal keratitis:* 1 drop of 5% suspension every 1–2 hr for 3–4 days, then 6–8 times/day for 2–3 wk; *Fungal blepharitis or conjunctivitis:* 1 drop of 5% suspension every 4–6 hr for 2–3 wk.	• ADRs: irritation, swelling

Antiparasitic

Uses: Demodex blepharitis.

lotilaner (Xdemvy)	**Adults:** 1 drop of 0.25% solution every 12 hr for 6 wk.	• ADRs: burning, stinging

Antivirals

Uses: Herpetic conjunctivitis and keratitis.
CAUTIONS: Small amounts may be absorbed and result in hypersensitivity reactions.

ganciclovir (Zirgan)	**Adults and children ≥2 yr:** 1 drop of 0.15% gel 5 times daily (every 3 hr while awake) until corneal ulcer heals, then 3 times daily for 7 days.	• ADRs: blurred vision, irritation, keratopathy
trifluridine	**Adults and children ≥6 yr:** 1 drop of 1% solution every 2 hr while awake (up to 9 drops/day) until re-epithelialization occurs, then every 4 hr while awake for 7 more days (not to exceed 21 days).	• ADRs: burning, stinging, keratopathy

Artificial Tears/Ocular Lubricants (sterile buffered isotonic solutions/ointments)

Uses: Artificial tears: keep the eyes moist with isotonic solutions and wetting agents in the management of dry eyes due to lack of tears; also provide lubrication for artificial eyes. Ocular lubricants: provide lubrication and protection in a variety of conditions including exposure keratitis, ↓ corneal sensitivity, corneal erosions, keratitis sicca, during/following ocular surgery or removal of a foreign body.

Artificial tears (Bion Tears, Genteal Tears, HypoTears, LiquiTears, Murine Tears, Nature's Tears, Soothe, Systane, ✿ Teardrops,, Tears Naturale, Viva-Drops)	**Adults and children:** *Artificial tears:* Solution: 1–2 drops 3–4 times daily; Insert: 1 insert 1–2 times daily; *Ocular lubricants:* small amount instilled into conjunctiva several times daily.	• May alter effects of other concurrently administered ophthalmic medications • ADRs: photophobia, lid edema stinging (insert only), transient blurred vision, eye discomfort

Beta Blockers

Uses: Treatment of open-angle glaucoma and other forms of ocular hypertension (↓ formation of aqueous humor).
CAUTIONS: Systemic absorption is minimal but may occur. Systemic absorption may result in additive adverse cardiovascular effects (bradycardia, hypotension), especially when used with other cardiovascular agents (antihypertensives, antiarrhythmics). Other systemic adverse reactions may occur, including bronchospasm or delirium (geriatric patients). Concurrent use with ophthalmic epinephrine may ↓ effectiveness.

betaxolol (Betoptic S)	**Adults and children:** 1 drop of 0.25% suspension or solution twice daily.	• ADRs: conjunctivitis, ↓ visual acuity, ocular burning, rash (may be less likely than others to cause bronchospasm if systemically absorbed)
carteolol	**Adults:** 1 drop of 1% solution twice daily.	• ADRs: ocular burning, ↓ visual acuity
levobunolol	**Adults:** 1–2 drops of 0.5% solution once daily.	• ADRs: conjunctivitis, ↓ visual acuity, ocular burning, rash

DRUG NAME	DOSE	NOTES
timolol (Betimol, Istalol, Timoptic, Timoptic Ocudose, Timoptic-XE)	**Adults:** *Solution:* 1 drop of 0.25–0.5% solution 1–2 times daily; *Gel-forming solution:* 1 drop of 0.25–0.5% solution once daily. **Children:** *Solution:* 1 drop of 0.25–0.5% solution twice daily; *Gel-forming solution:* 1 drop of 0.25–0.5% solution once daily.	● ADRs: conjunctivitis, ↓ visual acuity, ocular burning, rash

Carbonic Anhydrase Inhibitors

Uses: Treatment of open-angle glaucoma and other forms of ocular hypertension (↓ formation of aqueous humor).
CAUTIONS: May exacerbate kidney stones; should not be used in patients with CCr <30 mL/min; may have cross-sensitivity with sulfonamides.

brinzolamide (Azopt)	**Adults:** 1 drop of 1% suspension 3 times daily.	● ADRs: burning, stinging, unusual taste
dorzolamide	**Adults and children:** 1 drop of 2% solution 3 times daily.	● ADRs: bitter taste, ocular irritation, or allergy

Cholinergics (direct-acting)

Uses: Treatment of open-angle glaucoma (facilitates the outflow of aqueous humor); also used to facilitate miosis after ophthalmic surgery or before examination (to counteract mydriatics). Pilocarpine (Vuity™) used in treatment of presbyopia.
CAUTIONS: Conditions in which pupillary constriction occurs should be avoided. If significant systemic absorption occurs, bronchospasm, sweating, and ↑ urination and salivation may occur.

acetylcholine (Miochol-E)	**Adults:** 0.5–2 mL instilled into anterior chamber before or after securing one or more sutures.	● ADRs: corneal edema, corneal clouding
carbachol (Miostat)	**Adults:** 0.5 mL instilled into anterior chamber before or after securing sutures.	● ADRs: blurred vision, altered vision, stinging, eye pain
pilocarpine (Qlosi, Vuity)	**Adults:** *Presbyopia:* Vuity: 1 drop of 1.25% solution once daily. An additional drop (in each eye) may be administered 3–6 hr after 1st dose; Qlosi: 1 drop of 0.4% solution once daily, or as needed, up to twice daily. An additional drop (in each eye) may be administered 2–3 hr after 1st dose. **Adults and children ≥2 yr:** *Glaucoma:* 1 drop of 1–4% solution up to 4 times daily; *Counteracting mydriatic sympathomimetics:* 1 drop of 1–4% solution (may be repeated prior to surgery). **Children <2 yr:** *Glaucoma:* 1 drop of 1% solution 3 times daily.	● ADRs: blurred vision, altered vision, stinging, eye pain, headache

Cholinergics (cholinesterase inhibitors)

Uses: Treatment of open-angle glaucoma not controlled with short-acting miotics or other agents; also used in varying doses for accommodative esotropia (diagnosis and treatment).
CAUTIONS: Enhances neuromuscular blockade from succinylcholine; intensifies the actions of cocaine and some other local anesthetics; additive toxicity with antimyasthenics, anticholinergics, and cholinesterase inhibitors (including some pesticides). Use cautiously in patients with history or risk of retinal detachment.

echothiophate (Phospholine Iodide)	**Adults:** 1 drop of 0.125% solution 1–2 times daily.	● Irreversible cholinesterase inhibitor ● May cause hyperactivity in patients with Down syndrome ● ADRs: blurred vision, change in vision, brow ache, miosis, eyelid twitching, watering eyes

Corticosteroids

Uses: Management of inflammatory eye conditions including allergic conjunctivitis, nonspecific superficial keratitis, anterior endogenous uveitis; management of infectious conjunctivitis (with anti-infectives); management of corneal injury; suppression of graft rejection following keratoplasty; management of postoperative inflammation; management of dry eye disease; management of macular edema.
CAUTIONS: Use cautiously in patients with infectious ocular processes (avoid in herpes simplex keratitis), especially fungal and viral ocular infections (may mask symptoms); diabetes, glaucoma, or epithelial compromise.

DRUG NAME	DOSE	NOTES
dexamethasone (Dextenza, Dexycu, Maxidex, Ozurdex)	**Adults and children:** *Solution:* 1–2 drops of 0.1% solution every hr during the day and every 2 hr during the night, gradually ↓ the dose to 1 drop every 4 hr, then to 3–4 times daily; *Suspension:* 1–2 drops of 0.1% suspension up to 4–6 times daily; *Implant*— one 0.7-mg implant injected into affected eye; *Insert:* one 0.4-mg insert (releases 0.4 mg dose for up to 30 days); *Suspension for injection:* 0.005 mL of 9% suspension injected into posterior chamber at end of ocular surgery.	● As condition improves, ↓ frequency of administration of ophthalmic solution/suspension ● ADRs: corneal thinning, ↑ intraocular pressure, irritation
difluprednate (Durezol)	**Adults and children:** *Postoperative inflammation:* 1 drop of 0.05% emulsion 4 times daily beginning 24 hr after surgery and continued for 2 wk, then 2 times daily for 1 wk, then taper; *Uveitis:* 1 drop of 0.05% emulsion 4 times daily for 14 days, then taper.	● As condition improves, ↓ frequency of administration ● ADRs: blepharitis, photophobia, ↓ visual acuity
fluorometholone (Flarex, FML, FML Forte)	**Adults and children ≥2 yr:** *Suspension 1–2 drops of 0.1% suspension 4 times daily (up to 2 drops every 2 hr during initial 24–48 hr) or 1 drop of 0.25% suspension 2–4 times daily (up to 1 drop every 4 hr during initial 24–48 hr).*	● As condition improves, ↓ frequency of administration ● ADRs: corneal thinning, ↑ intraocular pressure, irritation
loteprednol (Alrex, Eysuvis, Inveltys, Lotemax, Lotemax SM)	**Adults:** *Allergic conjunctivitis:* Alrex: 1 drop of 0.2% suspension 4 times daily; *Dry eye disease:* Eysuvis: 1–2 drops of 0.25% suspension 4 times daily for up to 2 wk; *Inflammatory conditions:* Lotemax: 1–2 drops of 0.5% suspension 4 times daily (up to 1 drop every hr may be used in first wk); *Postoperative inflammation/pain:* Lotemax gel/suspension: 1–2 drops of 0.5% gel/suspension 4 times daily beginning 24 hr after surgery and continued for 2 wk or 1 drop of 0.38% gel 3 times daily beginning 24 hr after surgery and continued for 2 wk; Lotemax ointment: ½-in. strip 4 times daily beginning 24 hr after surgery and continued for 2 wk; Inveltys suspension: 1–2 drops of 1% suspension 2 times daily beginning 24 hr after surgery and continued for 2 wk. **Children:** *Postoperative inflammation/pain:* Lotemax gel: 1–2 drops of 0.5% gel 4 times daily beginning 24 hr after surgery and continued for 2 wk.	● ADRs: corneal thinning, ↑ intraocular pressure, irritation
prednisolone (Pred Forte, Pred Mild)	**Adults and children:** 1–2 drops of 0.12–1% solution/suspension 2–4 times daily.	● As condition improves, ↓ frequency of administration ● ADRs: corneal thinning, ↑ intraocular pressure, irritation

Cycloplegic Mydriatics

Uses: Preparation for cycloplegic refraction; induction of mydriasis; management of uveitis (not tropicamide).
CAUTIONS: Use cautiously in patients with a history of glaucoma; systemic absorption may cause anticholinergic effects such as confusion, unusual behavior, flushing, hallucinations, slurred speech, drowsiness, swollen stomach (infants), tachycardia, or dry mouth.

atropine (Isopto Atropine)	**Adults and children ≥3 mo:** *Cycloplegia/mydriasis:* Solution: 1–2 drops of 1% solution 40 min before procedure; Ointment: 0.3–0.5 cm strip 1–2 times daily.	● Effects on accommodation may last 6 days; mydriasis may last 12 days ● ADRs: irritation, blurred vision, photophobia

DRUG NAME	DOSE	NOTES
cyclopentolate (Cyclogyl)	**Adults:** 1–2 drops of 0.5–2% solution; may repeat in 5–10 min. **Children:** 1 drop of 0.5–2% solution; may be followed 5–10 min later by 1 drop of 0.5–1% solution.	• Peak of cycloplegia is within 25–75 min and lasts 6–24 hr • Peak of mydriasis is within 30–60 min and may last several days • 2% solution used for heavily pigmented iris • ADRs: irritation, blurred vision, photophobia
homatropine	**Adults:** *Cycloplegic refraction:* 1–2 drops of 2–5% solution, may repeat in 5–10 min for 2 more doses; *Uveitis:* 1–2 drops of 2–5% solution 2–3 times daily (up to every 4 hr). **Children ≥3 mo:** *Cycloplegic refraction:* 1–2 drops of 2% solution, may repeat in 10–15 min if needed; *Uveitis:* 1–2 drops of 2% solution 2–3 times daily (up to every 4 hr).	• Cycloplegia and mydriasis may last for 24–72 hr • ADRs: irritation, blurred vision, photophobia
tropicamide (Mydriacyl)	**Adults and children:** 1–2 drops of 0.5–1% solution.	• Stronger solution/repeated dosing may be required in patients with dark irises • Peak effect occurs in 20–40 min • Cycloplegia lasts 2–6 hr; mydriasis lasts up to 7 hr • ADRs: irritation, blurred vision, photophobia

Immunomodulators

Uses: Management of keratoconjunctivitis sicca and vernal keratoconjunctivitis.
CAUTIONS: Tear production is not ↑ during concurrent use of ophthalmic NSAIDs or punctal plugs.

cyclosporine (Cequa, Restasis, Verkazia, Vevye)	**Adults and children ≥16 yr:** *Keratoconjunctivitis sicca:* Restasis: 1 drop of 0.05% emulsion every 12 hr. **Adults:** *Keratoconjunctivitis sicca:* Cequa: 1 drop of 0.09% solution every 12 hr; Vevye: 1 drop of 0.1% solution every 12 hr. **Adults and children ≥4 yr:** *Vernal keratoconjunctivitis:* Verkazia: 1 drop of 0.1% emulsion 4 times daily until signs/symptoms resolve.	• Emulsion should be inverted to obtain uniform opaque appearance prior to use. • ADRs: irritation, blurred vision, conjunctival hyperemia
lifitegrast (Xiidra)	**Adults:** 1 drop of 5% solution every 12 hr.	• Emulsion should be inverted to obtain uniform opaque appearance prior to use. • ADRs: headache, irritation, blurred vision, metallic taste

Mast Cell Stabilizers

Uses: Management of vernal keratoconjunctivitis and allergic conjunctivitis.
CAUTIONS: Require several days of treatment before effects are seen.

cromolyn	**Adults and children ≥4 yr:** 1–2 drops of 4% solution 4–6 times daily.	• ADRs: irritation
lodoxamide (Alomide)	**Adults and children ≥2 yr:** 1–2 drops of 0.1% solution 4 times daily for up to 3 mo.	• ADRs: blurred vision, foreign body sensation, irritation
nedocromil (Alocril)	**Adults and children ≥3 yr:** 1–2 drops of 2% solution twice daily throughout period of exposure to allergen.	• ADRs: headache, ocular burning, unpleasant taste, nasal congestion

Nonsteroidal Anti-inflammatory Drugs

Uses: Management of pain/inflammation following surgery (bromfenac, diclofenac, ketorolac, nepafenac), allergic conjunctivitis (ketorolac), inhibition of perioperative miosis (flurbiprofen).
CAUTIONS: Cross-sensitivity with systemic NSAIDs may occur; concurrent use of anticoagulants, other NSAIDs, thrombolytics, some cephalosporins, and valproates may ↑ the risk of bleeding. May slow/delay healing. Avoid contact lens use.

DRUG NAME	DOSE	NOTES
bromfenac (Bromsite, Prolensa)	**Adults:** *Generic:* 1 drop of 0.09% solution once daily starting 1 day before surgery and continued on day of surgery and for 2 wk after surgery; *Bromsite* 1 drop of 0.075% solution twice daily starting 1 day before surgery and continued on day of surgery and for 2 wk after surgery; *Prolensa:* 1 drop of 0.07% solution once daily starting 1 day before surgery and continued on day of surgery and for 2 wk after surgery.	• Contains sulfites • ADRs: irritation, headache
diclofenac	**Adults:** *Cataract surgery:* 1 drop of 0.1% solution 4 times daily starting 24 hr after surgery and for 2 wk after surgery; *Corneal refractive surgery:* 1–2 drops of 0.1% solution within hour before surgery, within 15 min after surgery, then continue 4 times daily for up to 3 days.	• ADRs: irritation, allergic reactions
flurbiprofen	**Adults:** 1 drop of 0.03% solution every 30 min, beginning 2 hr prior to surgery (4 drops total in each eye).	• ADRs: irritation, allergic reactions
ketorolac (Acular, Acular LS, Acuvail)	**Adults and children ≥2 yr:** *Allergic conjunctivitis:* Acular: 1 drop of 0.5% solution 4 times daily; *Postoperative pain/inflammation:* Acular: 1 drop of 0.5% solution 4 times daily starting 24 hr after cataract surgery and for 2 wk after surgery; Acular LS: 1 drop of 0.4% solution 4 times daily for up to 4 days after corneal refractive surgery; Acuvail: 1 drop of 0.45% solution twice daily starting 1 day before cataract surgery and continued for 2 wk after surgery.	• ADRs: irritation, allergic reactions
nepafenac (Ilevro, Nevanac)	**Adults and children ≥10 yr:** *Ilevro:* 1 drop of 0.3% suspension once daily starting one day before cataract surgery and continued for 2 wk after surgery; instill 1 additional drop 30–120 min before surgery; *Nevanac:* 1 drop of 0.1% suspension 3 times daily starting one day before cataract surgery and continued for 2 wk after surgery.	• ADRs: irritation, photophobia, headache, hypertension, nausea/vomiting

Ocular Decongestants/Vasoconstrictors

Uses: ↓ ocular congestion due to irritation by vasoconstricting conjunctival blood vessels; stronger solutions have mydriatic effects. Treatment of acquired blepharoptosis (Upneeq™).

CAUTIONS: Systemic absorption may result in adverse cardiovascular effects; excessive/prolonged use may produce rebound hyperemia; use caution in patients at risk for acute angle-closure glaucoma; cardiovascular effects may be exaggerated by MAO inhibitors and dose adjustment may be required within 21 days of MAO inhibitors; ↑ risk of arrhythmias with inhalation anesthetics.

naphazoline	**Adults:** 1–2 drops of 0.012% solution up to 4 times daily (for up to 3 days) or 1–2 drops of 0.1% solution every 3–4 hr as needed.	• ADRs: ophthalmic-rebound hyperemia; systemic-dizziness, headache, nausea, sweating, weakness
oxymetazoline (Upneeq)	**Adults:** 1 drop of 0.1% solution once daily.	• ADRs: ophthalmic-rebound hyperemia; systemic-headache, insomnia, nervousness, tachycardia
phenylephrine	**Adults and children:** *Mydriasis:* 1 drop of 2.5–10% solution, may repeat in 3–5 min as needed (max = 3 drops/eye).	• ADRs: ophthalmic-blurred vision, irritation; systemic-dizziness, tachycardia, hypertension, paleness, sweating, trembling
tetrahydrozoline (Visine [OTC])	**Adults:** 1–2 drops of 0.05% solution 2–4 times daily.	• ADRs: ophthalmic–irritation; systemic–tachycardia, hypertension

DRUG NAME	DOSE	NOTES

Prostaglandin Agonists

Uses: Treatment of open-angle glaucoma (↑ outflow of aqueous humor).
CAUTIONS: May change eye color to brown; will form precipitate with thimerosal-containing products; can be used with other agents to ↓ intraocular pressure.

DRUG NAME	DOSE	NOTES
bimatoprost (Durysta, Lumigan)	**Adults and children ≥16 yr:** 1 drop of 0.01– 0.03% solution once daily in the evening. **Adults:** One implant in anterior chamber of affected eye.	• ADRs: local irritation, foreign body sensation, ↑ eyelash growth, ↑ brown pigmentation in iris
latanoprost (Iyuzeh, Xalatan, Xelpros)	**Adults:** 1 drop of 0.005% solution/emulsion once daily in the evening.	• ADRs: local irritation, foreign body sensation, ↑ eyelash growth, ↑ brown pigmentation in iris
latanoprostene (Vyzulta)	**Adults and children >16 yr:** 1 drop of 0.024% solution once daily in the evening.	• ADRs: conjunctival hyperemia, local irritation, eye pain, ↑ eyelash growth, ↑ brown pigmentation in iris
omidenepag isopropyl (Omlonti)	**Adults:** 1 drop of 0.002% solution once daily in the evening.	• ADRs: conjunctival hyperemia, photophobia, blurred vision, dry eye, eye pain, headache, ↑ eyelash growth, ↑ brown pigmentation in iris
tafluprost (Zioptan)	**Adults:** 1 drop of 0.0015% solution once daily in the evening.	• ADRs: local irritation, foreign body sensation, ↑ eyelash growth, ↑ brown pigmentation in iris
travoprost (Travatan Z)	**Adults and children ≥16 yr:** 1 drop of 0.004% solution once daily in the evening.	• ADRs: local irritation, foreign body sensation, ↑ eyelash growth, ↑ brown pigmentation in iris

Rho Kinase Inhibitor

Uses: Treatment of open-angle glaucoma or ocular hypertension (↑ outflow of aqueous humor).
CAUTIONS: Can be used with other agents to ↓ intraocular pressure.

DRUG NAME	DOSE	NOTES
netarsudil (Rhopressa)	**Adults:** 1 drop of 0.02% solution once daily in the evening.	• ADRs: conjunctival hyperemia, corneal verticillata, conjunctival hemorrhage eye pain

Semifluorinated Alkan

Uses: Dry eye disease.

DRUG NAME	DOSE	NOTES
perfluorohexyloctane (Miebo)	**Adults:** 1 drop of 100% solution 4 times daily.	• ADRs: blurred vision

Sympathomimetics

Uses: Treatment of open-angle glaucoma and other forms of intraocular hypertension (↓ formation of aqueous humor); brimonidine also available as over-the-counter product to ↓ ocular redness.
CAUTIONS: Systemic absorption may result in adverse cardiovascular and CNS reactions (especially in patients with cardiovascular disease); avoid use in patients predisposed to acute angle-closure glaucoma.

DRUG NAME	DOSE	NOTES
apraclonidine (Iopidine)	**Adults:** *Open-angle glaucoma:* 1–2 drops of 0.5% solution 3 times daily; *Postoperative reduction of intraocular pressure:* 1 drop of 1% solution 1 hr before surgery and upon completion of surgery.	• A selective alpha-adrenergic agonist • Monitor pulse and blood pressure • Avoid concurrent use with MAO inhibitors • ADRs: ophthalmic-irritation, mydriasis; systemic-allergic reactions, arrhythmias, bradycardia, drowsiness, dry nose, fainting, headache, nervousness, weakness
brimonidine (Alphagan P, Lumify [OTC])	**Adults and children ≥2 yr:** *Glaucoma:* 1 drop of 0.1–0.2% solution 3 times daily (8 hr apart). **Adults and children ≥5 yr:** *Ocular redness (Lumify™):* 1 drop of 0.025% solution every 6–8 hr as needed (up to 4 times daily).	• A selective alpha-adrenergic agonist • Avoid concurrent use with MAO inhibitors • Tricyclic antidepressants may ↓ effectiveness; additive CNS depression may occur with other CNS depressants, additive adverse cardiovascular effects with other cardiovascular agents • ADRs: ophthalmic-irritation; systemic-drowsiness, dizziness, dry mouth, headache, weakness, muscular pain

Medication Administration Techniques

Subcutaneous Injection Sites

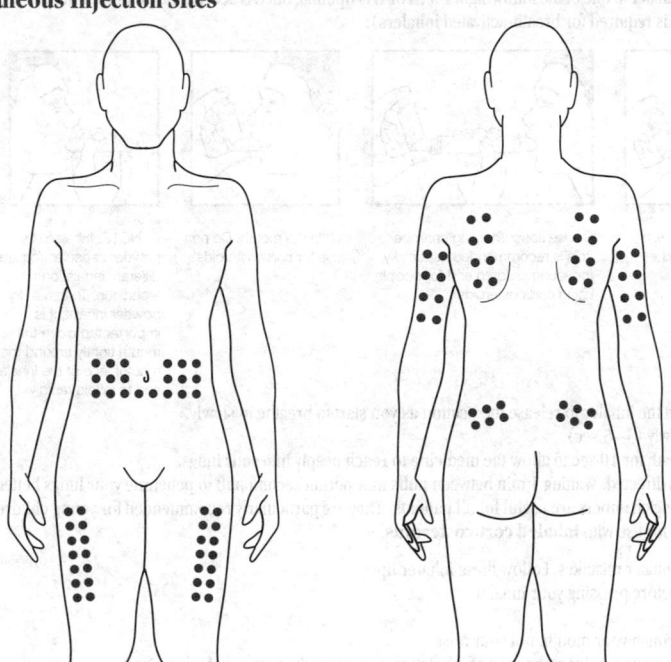

Administration of Ophthalmic Medications

For instillation of ophthalmic solutions, instruct patient to lie down or tilt head back and look at ceiling. Pull down on lower lid, creating a small pocket, and instill solution into pocket. With systemically acting drugs, apply pressure to the inner canthus for 1–2 min to minimize systemic absorption. Instruct patient to gently close eye. Wait 5 min before instilling second drop or any other ophthalmic solutions.

For instillation of ophthalmic ointment, instruct patient to hold tube in hand for several minutes to warm. Squeeze a small amount of ointment (¼–½ in.) inside lower lid. Instruct patient to close eye gently and roll eyeball around in all directions with eye closed. Wait 10 min before instilling any other ophthalmic ointments.

Do not touch cap or tip of container to eye, fingers, or any surface.

Administration of Medications with Metered-Dose Inhalers

Instruct patient on the proper use of the metered-dose inhaler. There are 3 methods of using a metered-dose inhaler. Shake inhaler well. (1) Take a drink of water to moisten the throat; place the inhaler mouthpiece 2 finger-widths away from mouth; tilt head back slightly. While activating the inhaler, take a slow, deep breath for 3–5 sec; hold the breath for 10 sec; and breathe out slowly. (2) Exhale and close lips firmly around mouthpiece. Administer during second half of inhalation, and hold breath for as long as possible to ensure deep instillation of medication. (3) Use of spacer. Consult health care professional to determine method desired prior to instruction. Allow 1–2 min between inhalations. Rinse mouth with water or mouthwash after each use to minimize dry mouth and hoarseness. breath for 10 sec; and breathe out slowly. (2) Exhale and close lips firmly around mouthpiece. Administer during second half of inhalation, and hold breath for as long as possible to ensure deep instillation of medication. (3) Use of spacer. Consult health care professional to determine method desired prior to instruction. Allow 1–2 min between inhalations. Rinse mouth with water or mouthwash after each use to minimize dry mouth and hoarseness. Wash inhalation assembly at least daily in warm running water.

For use of dry powder inhalers, turn head away from inhaler and exhale (do not blow into inhaler). Do not shake. Close mouth tightly around the mouthpiece of the inhaler and inhale rapidly.

Steps for Using Your Inhaler*

1. Remove the cap and hold inhaler upright.
2. Shake the inhaler.
3. Tilt your head back slightly and breathe out slowly.
4. Position the inhaler in one of the following ways (A or B is optimal, but C is acceptable for those who have difficulty with A or B. C is required for breath-activated inhalers):

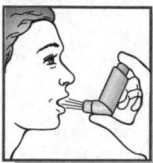 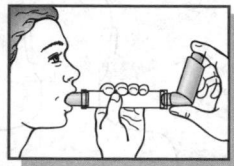 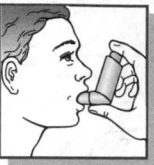 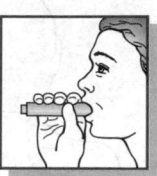

A. Open mouth with inhaler 1 to 2 inches away.

B. Use space/holding chamber (this is recommended especially for young children and for people using corticosteroids).

C. In the mouth. Do not use for corticosteroids.

D. NOTE: Inhaled dry powder capsules require a different inhalation technique. To use a dry powder inhaler, it is important to close the mouth tightly around the mouthpiece of the inhaler and to inhale rapidly.

5. Press down on the inhaler to release medication as you start to breathe in slowly.
6. Breathe in slowly (3–5 sec).
7. Hold your breath for 10 sec to allow the medicine to reach deeply into your lungs.
8. Repeat puff as directed. Waiting 1 min between puffs may permit second puff to penetrate your lungs better.
9. Spacers/holding chambers are useful for all patients. They are particularly recommended for young children and older adults and for use with **inhaled corticosteroids**.

Avoid common inhaler mistakes. Follow these inhaler tips:
● Breathe out before pressing your inhaler.
● Inhale slowly.
● Breathe in through your mouth, not your nose.
● Press down on your inhaler at the start of inhalation (or within the first sec of inhalation).
● Keep inhaling as you press down on your inhaler.
● Press your inhaler only once while you are inhaling (one breath for each puff).
● Make sure you breathe in evenly and deeply.
● If you are using a short-acting bronchodilator inhaler and a corticosteroid inhaler, use the bronchodilator first, and allow 5 min to elapse before using the corticosteroid.

Other inhalers have become available in addition to the one illustrated here. Different types of inhalers may require different techniques.

Administration of Medications by Nebulizer

Administer in a location where patient can sit comfortably for 10–15 min. Plug in compressor. Mix medication as directed, or empty unit-dose vials into nebulizer. Do not mix different types of medications without checking with health care professional. Assemble mask or mouthpiece and connect tubing to port on compressor. Have patient sit in a comfortable upright position. Make sure that mask fits properly over nose and mouth and that mist does not flow into eyes, or put mouthpiece into mouth. Turn on compressor. Instruct patient to take slow deep breaths. If possible, patient should hold breath for 10 sec before slowly exhaling. Continue this process until medication chamber is empty. Wash mask in hot soapy water; rinse well and allow to air dry before next use.

Administration of Nasal Sprays

Clear nasal passages of secretions prior to use. If nasal passages are blocked, use a decongestant immediately prior to use to ensure adequate penetration of the spray. Keep head upright. Breathe in through nose during administration. Sniff hard for a few minutes after administration.

---

*Source: Expert Panel Report 3: Guidelines for the Diagnosis and Management of Asthma. National Asthma Education and Prevention Program, National Heart, Lung, and Blood Institute, 2007.

Intramuscular Injection Sites

Deltoid site

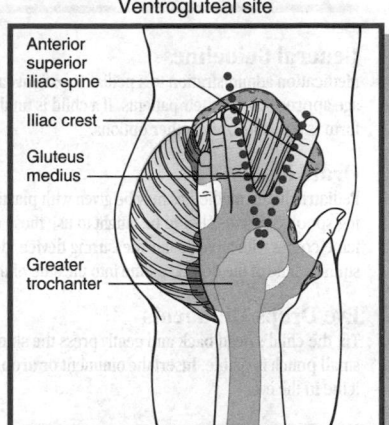

- Acromial process
- Deltoid muscle
- Scapula
- Humerus
- Deep brachial artery
- Radial nerve

Ventrogluteal site

- Anterior superior iliac spine
- Iliac crest
- Gluteus medius
- Greater trochanter

Vastus lateralis site

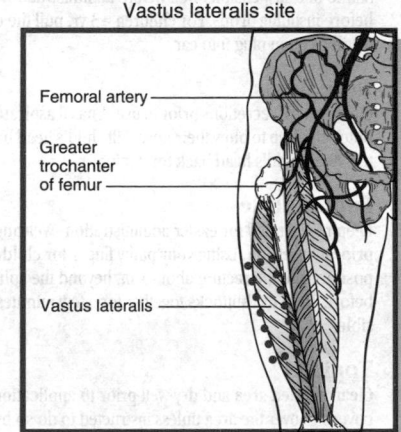

- Femoral artery
- Greater trochanter of femur
- Vastus lateralis

The deltoid and ventrogluteal sites are the preferred sites for adults; the vastus lateralis site is preferred in children under 2 yr of age.

Administering Medications to Children

General Guidelines
Medication administration to a pediatric patient can be challenging. Prescribers should order dosage forms that are age appropriate for their patients. If a child is unable to take a particular dosage form, ask the pharmacist if another form is available or for other options.

Oral Liquids
Pediatric liquid medicines may be given with plastic medicine cups, oral syringes, oral droppers, or cylindrical dosing spoons. Parents should be taught to use these calibrated devices rather than using household utensils. If a medicine comes with a particular measuring device, do not use it with another product. For young children, it is best to squirt a little of the dose at a time into the side of the cheek away from the bitter taste buds at the back of the tongue.

Eye Drops/Ointments
Tilt the child's head back and gently press the skin under the lower eyelid and pull the lower lid away slightly until a small pouch is visible. Insert the ointment or drop (1 at a time) and close the eye for a few minutes to keep the medicine in the eye.

Ear Drops
Shake otic suspensions well before administration. For children <3 yr, pull the outer ear outward and downward before instilling drops. For children ≥3 yr, pull the outer ear outward and upward. Keep child on side for 2 min and instill a cotton plug into ear.

Nose Drops
Clear nose of secretions prior to use. A nasal aspirator (bulb syringe) may be used in infants and young children. Ask older children to blow their nose. Tilt child's head back over a pillow and squeeze dropper without touching the nostril. Keep child's head back for 2 min.

Suppositories
Keep refrigerated for easier administration. Wearing gloves, moisten the rounded end with water or petroleum jelly prior to insertion. Using your pinky finger for children <3 yr and your index finger for those ≥3 yr, insert the suppository into the rectum about 1 in. beyond the sphincter. If the suppository slides out, insert it a little farther than before. Hold the buttocks together for a few minutes and have the child hold their position for about 20 min, if possible.

Topicals
Clean affected area and dry well prior to application. Apply a thin layer to the skin and rub in gently. Do not apply coverings over the area unless instructed to do so by the prescriber.

Metered-Dose Inhalers
Generally the same principles apply in children as in adults, except the use of spacers is recommended for young children (see Appendix C).

Formulas Helpful for Calculating Doses

Ratio and Proportion

A ratio is the same as a fraction and can be expressed as a fraction (½) or in the algebraic form (1:2). This relationship is stated as *one is to two*.

A proportion is an equation of equal fractions or ratios.

$$\frac{1}{2} = \frac{4}{8}$$

To calculate doses, begin each proportion with the two known values, for example 15 grains = 1 gram (known equivalent) or 10 milligrams = 2 milliliters (dose available) on one side of the equation. Next, make certain that the units of measure on the opposite side of the equation are the same as the units of the known values and are placed on the same level of the equation.

Problem A:
$$\frac{15 \text{ gr}}{1 \text{ g}} = \frac{10 \text{ gr}}{x \text{ g}}$$

Problem B:
$$\frac{10 \text{ mg}}{2 \text{ mL}} = \frac{5 \text{ mg}}{x \text{ mL}}$$

Once the proportion is set up correctly, cross-multiply the opposing values of the proportion.

Problem A:
$$\frac{15 \text{ gr}}{1 \text{ g}} \diagup\!\!\!\!\diagdown \frac{10 \text{ gr}}{x \text{ g}}$$

$$15x = 10$$

Problem B:
$$\frac{10 \text{ mg}}{2 \text{ mL}} \diagup\!\!\!\!\diagdown \frac{5 \text{ mg}}{x \text{ mL}}$$

$$10x = 10$$

Next, divide each side of the equation by the number with the x to determine the answer. Then, add the unit of measure corresponding to x in the original equation.

Problem A:
$$\frac{15x}{15} = \frac{10}{15}$$

$$x = \frac{2}{3} \text{ or } 0.6 \text{ g}$$

Problem B:
$$\frac{10x}{10} = \frac{10}{10}$$

$$x = 1 \text{ mL}$$

Calculation of IV Drip Rate

To calculate the drip rate for an intravenous infusion, 3 values are needed:

I. The amount of solution and corresponding time for infusion. May be ordered as:

$$1000 \text{ mL over 8 hr}$$

or

$$125 \text{ mL/hr}$$

II. The equivalent in time to convert hr to min.

$$1 \text{ hr} = 60 \text{ min}$$

III. The drop factor or number of drops that equal 1 mL of fluid. (This information can be found on the IV tubing box.)

$$10 \text{ gtt} = 1 \text{ mL}$$

Set up the problem by placing each of the 3 values in a proportion.

$$\frac{125 \text{ mL}}{1 \text{ hr}} \times \frac{1 \text{ hr}}{60 \text{ min}} \times \frac{10 \text{ gtt}}{1 \text{ mL}}$$

Units of measure can be canceled out from the upper and lower levels of the equation. The units cancel, leaving:

$$\frac{125}{1} \times \frac{1}{60 \text{ min}} \times \frac{10 \text{ gtt}}{1}$$

Next, multiply each level across and divide the numerator by the denominator for the answer.

$$\frac{125}{1} \times \frac{1}{6 \text{ min}} \times \frac{1 \text{ gtt}}{1}$$

$$125/6 = 20.8 \text{ or } 21 \text{ gtt/min}$$

Calculation of Creatinine Clearance (CCr) in Adults from Serum Creatinine

$$\text{Men: } CCr = \frac{\text{ideal body weight (kg)} \times (140 - \text{age})}{72 \times \text{serum creatinine (mg/dL)}}$$

$$\text{Women: } CCr = 0.85 \times \text{calculation for men}$$

Calculation of Body Surface Area (BSA) in Adults and Children

Dubois method:

$$\text{SA (cm}^2) = \text{wt (kg)}^{0.425} \times 71.84$$

$$\text{SA (m}^2) \text{ K} \times \sqrt[3]{\text{wt}^2 \text{ (kg)}} \text{ (common K value 0.1 for toddlers, 0.103 for neonates)}$$

Simplified method:

$$\text{BSA (m}^2) = \sqrt{\frac{\text{ht (cm)} \times \text{wt (kg)}}{3600}}$$

Body Mass Index

$$\text{BMI} = \text{wt (kg)/ht (m}^2)$$

Pediatric Dosage Calculations

Most drugs in children are dosed according to body weight (mg/kg) or body surface area (BSA) (mg/m^2). Care must be taken to properly convert body weight from pounds to kilograms (1 kg = 2.2 lb) before calculating doses based on body weight. Doses are often expressed as mg/kg/day or mg/kg/dose; therefore, orders written "mg/kg/d," which is confusing, *require further clarification from the prescriber.*

Chemotherapeutic drugs are commonly dosed according to body surface area, which requires an extra verification step (BSA calculation) prior to dosing. Medications are available in multiple concentrations, therefore *orders written in "mL" rather than "mg" are not acceptable and require further clarification.*

Dosing also varies by indication; therefore, diagnostic information is helpful when calculating doses. The following examples are typically encountered when dosing medication in children.

Example 1.
Amoxicillin oral suspension will be given to a 1-yr-old child weighing 22 lb for otitis media at a dose of 40 mg/kg/day in 2 divided doses. The suspension is available at a concentration of 400 mg/5 mL. How many milliliters should be administered to the child for each dose?

Step 1. Convert pounds to kg:	22 lb × 1 kg/2.2 lb = 10 kg
Step 2. Calculate the dose in mg:	10 kg × 40 mg/kg/day = 400 mg/day
Step 3. Divide the dose by the frequency:	400 mg/day ÷ 2 = 200 mg/day
Step 4. Convert the mg dose to mL:	200 mg/dose ÷ 400 mg/5 mL = **2.5 mL**

Example 2.
Ceftriaxone is being prescribed for a 5-yr-old child weighing 18 kg for meningitis at a dose of 100 mg/kg IV once daily. After reconstitution, the concentration of ceftriaxone solution in the vial is 40 mg/mL. How many milliliters of the solution should be administered to this child for each dose?

Step 1. Calculate the dose in mg:	18 kg × 100 mg/kg/day = 1800 mg/day
Step 2. Divide the dose by the frequency:	1800 mg/day ÷ 1 (daily) = 1800 mg/dose
Step 3. Convert the mg dose to mL:	1800 mg/dose ÷ 40 mg/mL = **45 mL**

Example 3.
Vincristine is being administered to a 4-yr-old child (height 97 cm; weight 37 lb) with leukemia at a dose of 2 mg/m^2. Vincristine is available in a vial at a concentration of 1 mg/mL. How many milliliters should be administered to this child for each dose?

Step 1. Convert pounds to kg:	37 lb × 1 kg/2.2 lb = 16.8 kg
Step 2. Calculate BSA:	$\sqrt{16.8 \text{ kg} \times 97 \text{ cm}/3600}$ = 0.67 m^2
Step 3. Calculate the dose in mg:	2 mg/m^2 × 0.67 m^2 = 1.34 mg
Step 4. Calculate the dose in mL:	1.34 mg ÷ 1 mg/mL = **1.34 mL**

APPENDIX G

Normal Values of Common Laboratory Tests

SERUM TESTS

HEMATOLOGIC	MEN	WOMEN
Hemoglobin	14–17.3 g/dL	11.7–15.5 g/dL
Hematocrit	42–52%	36–48%
Red blood cells (RBC)	4.51–6.01 million/mm³	4.01–5.51 million/mm³
Mean corpuscular volume (MCV)	77–97 (micrometer)³	78–102 (micrometer)³
Mean corpuscular hemoglobin (MCH)	27–35 picogram	27–35 picogram
Mean corpuscular hemoglobin concentration (MCHC)	32–36 g/dL	32–36 g/dL
Erythrocyte sedimentation rate (ESR)	≤20 mm/hr	≤30 mm/hr
Leukocytes (WBC)	4500–11,100/mm³	4500–11,100/mm³
Neutrophils	40–75% (2700–6500/mm³)	40–75% (2700–6500/mm³)
Bands	3–8% (150–700/mm³)	3–8% (150–700/mm³)
Eosinophils	0–5.5% (50–400/mm³)	0–5.5% (50–500/mm³)
Basophils	0–1% (0–100/mm³)	0–1% (0–100/mm³)
Monocytes	4–9% (200–400/mm³)	4–9% (200–400/mm³)
Lymphocytes	14–44% (1500–3700/mm³)	14–44% (1500–3700/mm³)
T lymphocytes	60–80% of lymphocytes	60–80% of lymphocytes
B lymphocytes	10–20% of lymphocytes	10–20% of lymphocytes
Platelets	150,000–450,000/mm³	150,000–450,000/mm³
Prothrombin time (PT)	10–13 sec	10–13 sec
Partial thromboplastin time (PTT)	30–45 sec	30–45 sec
Bleeding time (duke)	1–3 min	1–3 min
(ivy)	2–7 min	2–7 min
(template)	2.5–10 min	2.5–10 min

CHEMISTRY	MEN	WOMEN
Sodium	135–145 mEq/L	135–145 mEq/L
Potassium	3.5–5.3 mEq/L	3.5–5.3 mEq/L
Chloride	97–107 mEq/L	97–107 mEq/L
Bicarbonate (HCO₃)	19–25 mEq/L	19–25 mEq/L
Total calcium	8.4–10.2 mg/dL or 4.5–5.5 mEq/L	8.4–10.2 mg/dL or 4.5–5.5 mEq/L
Ionized calcium	4.64–5.52 mg/dL or 2.1–2.6 mEq/L	4.64–5.52 mg/dL or 2.1–2.6 mEq/L
Phosphorus/phosphate	2.5–4.5 mg/dL	2.5–4.5 mg/dL
Magnesium	1.6–2.2 mg/dL or 1.5–2.5 mEq/L	1.6–2.2 mg/dL or 1.5–2.5 mEq/L
Glucose	65–99 mg/dL	65–99 mg/dL
Osmolality	275–295 mOsm/kg	275–295 mOsm/kg
Ammonia (NH₃)	10–80 mcg/dL	10–80 mcg/dL
Amylase	100–300 U/L	100–300 U/L
Creatine phosphokinase total (CK, CPK)	50–204 U/L	36–160 U/L
Creatine kinase isoenzymes, MB fraction	0–4% in MI	0–4% in MI
Lactic dehydrogenase (LDH)	90–156 U/L	90–156 U/L
Protein, total	6–8 g/d	6–8 g/d
Albumin	3.7–5.1 g/dL	3.7–5.1 g/dL

HEPATIC	MEN	WOMEN
AST	20–40 U/L	15–30 U/L
ALT	19–36 IU/mL	24–36 IU/mL
Total bilirubin	0.3–1.2 mg/dL	0.3–1.2 mg/dL
Conjugated bilirubin	0.0–0.3 mg/dL	0.0–0.3 mg/dL
Unconjugated (indirect) bilirubin	0.2–1.1 mg/dL	0.2–1.1 mg/dL
Alkaline phosphatase	35–142 U/L	25–125 U/L

RENAL	MEN	WOMEN
BUN	8–21 mg/dL	8–21 mg/dL
Creatinine	0.61–1.21 mg/dL	0.51–1.11 mg/dL
Uric acid	4.0–8.2 mg/dL	2.5–7.3 mg/dL

ARTERIAL BLOOD GASES	MEN	WOMEN
pH	7.35–7.45	7.35–7.45
Po₂	80–95 mm Hg	80–95 mm Hg
Pco₂	35–45 mm Hg	35–45 mm Hg
O₂ saturation	95–99%	95–99%
Base excess	+3–(−2)	+3–(−2)
Bicarbonate (HCO₃⁻)	22–26 mEq/L	22–26 mEq/L

URINE TESTS

URINE	MEN	WOMEN
pH	4.5–8.0	4.5–8.0
Specific gravity	1.005–1.03	1.005–1.03

Controlled Substances Schedules

General

A controlled substance is any type of drug that the federal government has categorized as having significant potential for abuse or addiction. While controlled substances are regulated in both the United States (U.S.) and Canada, differences exist between the two countries with respect to scheduling and enforcement.

IN THE UNITED STATES:

The Drug Enforcement Agency (DEA), an arm of the United States Justice Department, classifies controlled substances according to five schedules, based on whether they have a currently accepted medical use in treatment in the United States, the potential for abuse and dependence liability (physical and psychological) of the medication, and likelihood of causing dependence when abused. Some states may have stricter prescription regulations. Physicians, dentists, podiatrists, and veterinarians may prescribe controlled substances. Nurse practitioners and physician assistants may also prescribe controlled substances with limitations that vary from state to state.

Schedule I (C-I)

Potential for abuse is so high as to be unacceptable. Have no currently accepted medical use in the United States. May be used for research with appropriate limitations. Examples are marijuana, LSD, and heroin.

Schedule II (C-II)

High potential for abuse which may lead to severe physical and psychological dependence (amphetamines, opioid analgesics, certain barbiturates). Outpatient prescriptions must be in writing. In emergencies, telephone orders may be acceptable if a written prescription is provided within 72 hr. No refills are allowed.

Schedule III (C-III)

Substances in this schedule have a potential for abuse less than substances in Schedules I or II, and abuse may lead to moderate or low physical dependence or high psychological dependence (certain nonbarbiturate sedatives, certain nonamphetamine CNS stimulants, and certain opioid analgesics). Outpatient prescriptions can be refilled 5 times within 6 mo from date of issue if authorized by prescriber. Telephone orders are acceptable.

Schedule IV (C-IV)

Less abuse potential than Schedule III with minimal liability for physical or psychological dependence (certain sedatives/hypnotics, certain antianxiety agents, certain nonamphetamine CNS stimulants, some barbiturates, and benzodiazepines). Outpatient prescriptions can be refilled 6 times within 6 mo from date of issue if authorized by prescriber. Telephone orders are acceptable.

Schedule V (C-V)

Minimal abuse potential. Number of outpatient refills determined by prescriber. Some products (cough suppressants with small amounts of codeine, antidiarrheals containing paregoric, pregabalin) may be available without prescription to patients >18 yr of age.

IN CANADA:

The federal *Controlled Drugs and Substances Act (CDSA)* along with the *Narcotic Control Regulations*, Part G of the *Food and Drug Regulations*, and the *Benzodiazepines and Other Targeted Substances Regulations* regulate narcotics, controlled drugs, and targeted substances.

The CDSA classifies controlled substances according to eight schedules and three classes of precursors. While a few examples are listed below, a complete list of drugs scheduled in Canada's Controlled Drugs and Substances act can be accessed at: http://laws-lois.justice.gc.ca/eng/acts/C%2D38.8/

Schedule I

— opioids and derivatives and related drugs (e.g., morphine, oxycodone, heroin)

Schedule II

— cannabis (marijuana) and derivatives

Schedule III

— amphetamines and related drugs and substances (e.g., methylphenidate, LSD)

Schedule IV
— barbiturates and derivatives, anabolic steroids and related drugs, and benzodiazepines (e.g., diazepam)

Schedule VI
— precursors Class A (e.g., pseudoephedrine and salts)
— precursors Class B (e.g., acetone, toluene)
— precursors Class C (mixtures of the above)

Schedules VII & VIII
— cannabis and its resins in varying amounts
(Note: In Canada marijuana may be used for medical purposes. It is regulated by the Access to Cannabis for Medical Purposes Regulations, which can be accessed at: http://www.laws-lois.justice.gc.ca/eng/regulations/SOR-2016-230/page-1.html)

The CDSA federally regulates conditions of sale, distribution, and accountability relating to controlled substances. Provincial legislation compliments how patients access controlled substances from regulated health professionals. As such, it is imperative for an individual to become familiar with legislation pertaining to the specific province he/she is working in. Some federal regulations are as follows:

Narcotic drug — Two subcategories of prescription narcotics — "Straight" Narcotics and Verbal Prescription Narcotics
(e.g., codeine, morphine, fentanyl, oxycodone)

Straight Narcotics
- All single active ingredient products containing a narcotic, along with all narcotics for parenteral use and narcotic compounds containing more than one narcotic entity or less than two non-narcotic ingredients.
- Prescription can be written, faxed, or generated electronically in an authorized provincial electronic health record and must be signed and dated by prescriber.
- Refills are not permitted, but a prescription may be dispensed in divided portions. Prescription transfers from one pharmacist to another are not permitted.

Verbal Prescription Narcotic
(e.g., Tylenol No. 2 and Tylenol No. 3)
- Refers to oral combination products containing only one narcotic and two or more non-narcotic ingredients in a therapeutic dose. (Excluding diacetylmorphine, oxycodone, hydrocodone, methadone, or pentazocine. This means that an oral combination product that contains these drugs cannot be classified as a Verbal Prescription Narcotic.)
- Similar rules as above but prescriptions may also be verbal.

Exempted Codeine Preparations
(e.g., Tylenol No. 1)
- Under federal regulations, products containing codeine (meaning codeine phosphate or its equivalent) may be purchased over the counter, without a prescription, provided they have two other medicinal ingredients and a **maximum** of 8 mg of codeine per solid oral dose unit or 20 mg per 30 mL of liquid.
- The product may not be supplied if there are reasonable grounds to suspect the product will be used for other than recognized medical or dental purposes.

Controlled Drugs — Part 1
(e.g., Dexedrine, Ritalin, pentobarbital, secobarbital)
- Refers to drugs listed in Part I of the Schedule to Part G of the Food and Drug Regulations.
- Prescription may be written or verbal; no refills allowed if prescription is verbal.
- Refills are permitted if the number of repeats and the frequency or interval between refills is specified. Prescription transfers are not permitted.

Controlled Drugs — Parts 2 and 3
(e.g., other barbiturates and anabolic steroids)
- Refers to drugs listed in Parts II and III of the Schedule to Part G of the Food and Drug Regulations.
- Prescription may be written or verbal.

- Refills are permitted if prescribed in writing or verbally and the number of repeats and frequency or interval between refills is specified. Prescription transfers are not permitted.

Benzodiazepines and Other Targeted Substances
(e.g., lorazepam, diazepam)
- Refers to all benzodiazepines except flunitrazepam, which is listed in Schedule III of the Act as an illicit substance.
- Prescriptions may be written or verbal. Refills are permitted if the prescription is less than 1 yr old and the prescriber specifies the number of times it can be refilled. If the prescriber indicated the interval between refills, the pharmacist cannot refill the prescription if that interval has expired. Prescription transfers are permitted, but only once.

References:

1. Minister of Justice (2023). Controlled Drugs and Substances Act. Available at http://laws-lois.justice.gc.ca/PDF/C-38.8.pdf
2. National Association of Pharmacy Regulatory Authorities (www.napra.org)
3. U.S. Department of Justice, Drug Enforcement Administration (2023). Controlled Substance Schedules. https://www.deadiversion.usdog.gov/schedules/

APPENDIX I

Equianalgesic Dosing Guidelines

OPIOID ANALGESICS STARTING ORAL DOSE COMMONLY USED FOR SEVERE PAIN

NAME	EQUIANALGESIC DOSE		STARTING ORAL DOSE		COMMENTS	PRECAUTIONS AND CONTRAINDICATIONS
	ORAL*	PARENTERAL†	ADULTS	CHILDREN		
Morphine-like agonists (mu agonists)						
morphine	30 mg	10 mg	15–30 mg	0.3 mg/kg	Standard of comparison for opioid analgesics. Sustained release preparations (MS Contin) release over 8–12 hr. Other formulations (MS Contin) last 12–24 hr. Generic sustained release morphine preparations are now available.	For all opioids, caution in patients with impaired ventilation, bronchial asthma, ↑ intracranial pressure, liver failure.
hydromorphone (Dilaudid)	7.5 mg	1.5 mg	Opioid naïve: 4–8 mg	0.06 mg/kg	Slightly shorter duration than morphine. Sustained release preparations release over 24 hr.	
fentanyl	—	0.1 mg	—			
oxycodone	20 mg	—	10–20 mg	0.2 mg/kg		
methadone	10 mg	5 mg	5–10 mg	0.2 mg/kg	Good oral potency, long plasma half-life (24–36 hr).	Accumulates with repeated dosing, requiring decreases in dose size and frequency, especially on days 2–5. Use with caution in older adults.
levorphanol	2 mg (acute), 1 mg (chronic)	—	2–4 mg	0.04 mg/kg	Long plasma half-life (12–16 hr, but may be as long as 90–120 hr after one wk of dosing).	Accumulates on days 2 and 3. Use with caution in older adults.
oxymorphone (Opana)	10 mg	—	—	—	—	
meperidine (Demerol)	300 mg	100 mg	Not Recommended	—	Slightly shorter acting than morphine; accumulates with repetitive dosing causing CNS excitation; avoid in children with impaired renal function or who are receiving monoamine oxidase inhibitors.‡	Use with caution. Normeperidine (toxic metabolite) accumulates with repetitive dosing causing CNS excitation and a high risk of seizure. Avoid in children, renal impairment, and patients on monoamine oxidase inhibitors.‡

	EQUIANALGESIC DOSE		STARTING ORAL DOSE		
NAME	**ORAL***	**PARENTERAL†**	**ADULTS**	**CHILDREN**	**PRECAUTIONS AND CONTRAINDICATIONS**
Centrally acting mu agonists tramadol (UltramConZip)	120 mg	—	50–100 mg every 4–6 hr	—	Prodrug; significant serotonin reuptake inhibition. Maximum dose: IR 400 mg/day; ER 300 mg/day.	Caution with pre-existing seizure disorder, concurrent use of medications that ↓ seizure threshold, or medications that ↑ risk of serotonin syndrome.
tapentadol (Nucynta)	100 mg	—	50–100 mg every 4–6 hr	—	Sustained release preparation (Nucynta ER) releases over 12 hr. Blocks reuptake of norepinephrine > serotonin.)	Caution with pre-existing seizure disorder or concurrent use of medications that ↓ seizure threshold.
Mixed agonists–antagonists (kappa agonists) nalbuphine	—	10 mg	10 mg every 3–6 hr	0.1–0.2 mg/kg every 3–4 hr	Not available orally; not scheduled under Controlled Substances Act. Kappa agonist, partial mu antagonist.	Incidence of psychotomimetic effects lower than with pentazocine; may precipitate withdrawal in opioid-dependent patients.
butorphanol	—	2 mg	1–4 mg every 3–4 hr (IM); 0.5–2 mg every 3–4 hr (IV)	—	Kappa agonist, partial mu antagonist. Also available in nasal spray.	Likenalbuphine.
Partial agonist buprenorphine (Buprenex)	—	0.4 mg	0.3 mg every 6–8 hr (IM/IV)	2–12 yr: 0.2–0.6 mg every 4–6 hr (IM/IV)	Sublingual tablets now available both plain and with naloxone for opioid-dependent patient management for specially certified physicians. These tablets are not approved as analgesics. Also available as a long-acting transdermal patch (Butrans), and buccal film (Belbuca).	May precipitate withdrawal in opioid-dependent patients; not readily reversed by naloxone; avoid in labor.

*Starting dose should be lower for older adults.
†These are standard parenteral doses for acute pain in adults and can also be used to convert doses for IV infusions and repeated small IV boluses. For single IV boluses, use half the IM dose. IV doses for children >6 mo. = parenteral equianalgesic dose times weight (kg)/100.
‡Irritating to tissues with repeated IM injections.
Kishner, S. (2022). Opioid equivalents and conversions. Medscape. https://emedicine.medscape.com/article/2138678-overview?form=fpf

GUIDELINES FOR PATIENT-CONTROLLED INTRAVENOUS OPIOID ADMINISTRATION FOR ADULTS WITH ACUTE PAIN

DRUG*	USUAL STARTING DOSE AFTER LOADING	USUAL DOSE RANGE	USUAL LOCKOUT (MIN)	USUAL LOCKOUT RANGE (MIN)
Morphine (1 mg/mL)	1 mg	0.5–2.5 mg	8	5–10
Hydromorphone (0.2 mg/mL)	0.2 mg	0.05–0.4 mg	8	5–10
Fentanyl (50 mcg/mL)	20 mcg	10–50 mcg	6	5–8

*Standard concentrations for most PCA machines are listed in parentheses.
Modified from *American Pain Society, Principles of Analgesic Use in the Treatment of Acute Pain and Cancer Pain*, ed.7. American Pain Society, 2016.

FENTANYL TRANSDERMAL DOSE BASED ON DAILY MORPHINE DOSE*

ORAL 24-HR MORPHINE (mg/day)	TRANSDERMAL FENTANYL (mg/day)	FENTANYL TRANSDERMAL (mcg/hr)
30–90	0.6	25
91–150	1.2	50
151–210	1.8	75
211–270	2.4	100
271–330	3.0	125
331–390	3.6	150
391–450	4.2	175
451–510	4.8	200
511–570	5.4	225
571–630	6.0	250
631–690	6.6	275
691–750	7.2	300
For each additional 60 mg/day	+0.6	+25

*A 10-mg IM or 60-mg oral dose of morphine every 4 hr for 24 hr (total of 60 mg/day IM or 360 mg/day oral) was considered approximately equivalent to fentanyl transdermal 100 mcg/hr.

Food Sources for Specific Nutrients

Potassium-Rich Foods

artichoke
avocado
bananas
beet greens
bok choy
breadfruit
cantaloupe
cassava
coconut water
dried fruits
durian
grapefruit
honey dew
jack fruit

kiwi
kohlrabi
lima beans
mango
meats
milk
dried peas and beans
nuts
oranges/orange juice
papaya
peach
pear
plantains
pomegranate fruit and juice

potatoes (white and sweet)
prunes/prune juice
pummelo
pumpkin
rutabaga
salt substitute
spinach
sunflower seeds
Swiss chard
tomatoes/tomato juice
vegetable juice
winter squash (acorn, butternut, hubbard)

Sodium-Rich Foods

baking mixes (pancakes, muffins)
barbecue sauce
buttermilk
salted butter/margarine
canned chili
canned seafood
canned soups

canned spaghetti sauce
cured meats
dry onion soup mix
"fast" foods
frozen dinners
macaroni and cheese
microwave dinners
Parmesan cheese

pickles
salad dressings (prepared)
salt
salted pretzels, potato chips
sauerkraut
tomato ketchup

Calcium-Rich Foods

almond (milk/nuts)
calcium fortified foods
canned salmon/sardines
cheese
cream soups (with milk)

greens: collard/mustard/turnip
kale
milk
soy (beans/milk)
spinach

tofu
yogurt

Vitamin K-Rich Foods

asparagus
beet greens
broccoli
brussel sprouts
cabbage

collard greens
dandelion leaves
garden cress
green tea leaves
kale

mustard greens
parsley
spinach
Swiss chard
turnip greens

Low-Sodium Foods

canned pumpkin
egg yolk
fresh vegetables
fruit
grits (not instant)

honey
jams and jellies
low-calorie mayonnaise
macaroons
puffed wheat and rice

dried peas and beans
sherbet
unsalted nuts
whiskey

Foods that Acidify Urine

cheeses
corn
cranberries
eggs
fish

grains (breads and cereals)
lentils
meats
nuts (Brazil, filberts, walnuts)
pasta

plums
poultry
prunes
rice

Foods that Alkalinize Urine

all fruits except cranberries,
prunes, plums

all vegetables (except corn)
milk

nuts (almonds, chesnuts)

Foods Containing Tyramine

aged cheeses (blue, Boursault,
brick, Brie, Camembert,
cheddar, Emmenthaler,
Gruyère, mozzarella, Parmesan,
Romano, Roquefort, Stilton,
Swiss)
American processed cheese
avocados (especially over-ripe)
bananas
bean curd
beer and ale

caffeine-containing beverages
(coffee, tea, colas)
caviar
chocolate
distilled spirits
fermented sausage (bologna,
salami, pepperoni, summer
sausage)
liver
meats prepared with tenderizer
miso soup
over-ripe fruit

peanuts
raisins
raspberries
red wine (especially Chianti)
sauerkraut
sherry
shrimp paste
smoked or pickled fish
soy sauce
vermouth
yeasts
yogurt

Iron-Rich Foods

cereals
clams
dried beans and peas

dried fruit
leafy green vegetables
lean red meats

molasses (blackstrap)
organ meats

Vitamin D-Rich Foods

canned salmon, sardines, tuna
cereals

fish
fish liver oils

fortified milk
nonfat dry milk

Foods that Interact With/Inhibit the CYP3A4 Isoenzyme

grapefruit
grapefruit juice

Seville oranges
tangelos

Insulins and Insulin Therapy

The goal of insulin therapy for patients with diabetes is to provide coverage that most closely resembles endogenous insulin production and results in the best glycemic control without hypoglycemia. Although daytime control of hyperglycemia may be accomplished with bolus doses of rapid-acting insulin analogs, elevations in fasting glucose may remain a problem. If fasting blood glucose levels remain elevated, the basal insulin dose (intermediate or long-acting) may have to be adjusted.

Most insulins used today are recombinant DNA human insulins. Produced through genetic engineering, synthetic human insulin is "manufactured" by yeast or nonpathogenic *E. coli*. In recent years, pharmaceutical companies have developed several new types and formulations of insulin.

Different insulins are distinguished by how quickly they are absorbed, the time and length of peak activity, and overall duration of action. Onset, peak, and duration of action times are approximate and vary according to individual factors such as injection site, blood supply, concurrent illnesses, lifestyle, and exercise level. These factors can vary from patient to patient and can vary in any patient from day to day.

There are 5 kinds of insulins: rapid-acting, short-acting, intermediate-acting, long-acting, and combination insulins.

Rapid-Acting Insulins
Rapid-acting insulins are analogs of regular insulin. An analog is a chemical structure very similar to another but differing in one component. Admelog/Humalog/Lyumjev (lispro), Apidra (glulisine), and Fiasp/Novolog (aspart) are rapid-acting insulin analogs. The amino acid sequences of these analogs are nearly identical to human insulin. They differ in the positioning of certain proteins, which allows them to enter the bloodstream rapidly—within 15 min of subcutaneous injection. This closely mimics the body's own insulin response and allows greater flexibility in eating schedules for diabetic patients. Also, because these insulins leave the bloodstream quickly, the risk of hypoglycemic episodes several hours after the meal is lessened. The peak time for rapid-acting insulins is 1–2 hr and the duration is 3–4 hr. Rapid-acting insulin solutions are clear. Insulin aspart, insulin glulisine, and insulin lispro (100 units/mL only) can be given intravenously in selected situations under medical supervision.

Short-Acting Insulins
Regular insulin is a short-acting insulin and is available commercially as Humulin R or Novolin R. The onset of regular insulin is 0.5–1 hr; its peak activity occurs 2–4 hr after subcutaneous injection and its duration of action is 5–7 hr. This time/action profile makes rigid meal scheduling necessary, as the patient must estimate that a meal will occur within 45 min of injection. Short-acting insulin solutions are clear. Regular insulin (100 units/mL only) can be given intravenously.

Intermediate-Acting Insulins
Intermediate-acting insulin contains protamine, which delays onset, peak, and duration of action to provide basal insulin coverage. Basal insulins are given to control blood glucose levels throughout the day when not eating. Commercially, intermediate-acting insulins are available as Humulin N or Novolin N. (The "N" stands for NPH.) Action starts between 2 and 4 hr after injecting. Peak activity occurs between 4 and 10 hr. Duration of action lasts 10–16 hr. The addition of protamine causes the cloudy appearance of intermediate-acting insulins and results in the formulation being a suspension rather than a solution. This is why these insulins must be gently mixed before administering. Intermediate-acting insulins can be mixed with short- or rapid-acting insulins to provide both basal and bolus coverage. Intermediate-acting insulins should not be administered intravenously.

Long-Acting Insulins
Long-acting insulins have the most delayed onset and the longest duration of all insulins. Products include Basaglar/Lantus/Semglee/Toujeo (glargine), Levemir (detemir), and Tresiba (degludec). Peaks are not as prominent in long-acting insulins. In fact, insulin glargine has no real peak action because it forms slowly dissolving crystals in the subcutaneous tissue. The onset of action of insulin glargine and insulin detemir is 3–4 hr and for insulin degludec is within 2 hr after subcutaneous injection. Full activity occurs within 4 to 5 hr and remains constant for 24 hr. Even though these insulins are clear solutions, they cannot be diluted or mixed with any other insulin or solution. Mixing these insulins with other insulin products can alter the onset of action and time to peak effect. If bolus insulin is to be given at the same time as insulin glargine, insulin detemir, or insulin degludec, two separate syringes and injection sites must be used. Long-acting insulins should not be administered intravenously.

Combination Insulins

Various combinations of premixed insulins are available, containing fixed proportions of two different insulins, usually a short- and an intermediate-acting insulin. Typically the intermediate-acting insulin makes up 70–75% of the mixture, with rapid- or short-acting insulin making up the remainder. Onset, peak, and duration vary according to each specific product. Brand names of these products include Humulin 70/30 (70% NPH, 30% regular), Humalog Mix 75/25 (75% insulin lispro protamine suspension and 25% insulin lispro), Humalog Mix 50/50 (50% insulin lispro protamine suspension and 50% insulin lispro), and Novolin 70/30 (70% NPH, 30% regular), or Novolog Mix 70/30 (70% insulin aspart protamine suspension and 30% insulin aspart).

BRAND NAME	GENERIC NAME	TYPE OF INSULIN	ONSET/PEAK/DURATION
Humalog Mix 75/25	insulin lispro protamine	Combination	15–30 min/2.8 hr/24 hr
Humalog Mix 50/50	suspension & insulin lispro injection mixtures	Combination	
Novolog Mix 70/30	insulin aspart protamine suspension & insulin aspart injection mixtures	Combination	15 min/1–4 hr/18–24 hr
Humulin 70/30	NPH/regular insulin mixture	Combination	30 min/2–12 hr/24 hr
Novolin 70/30	NPH/regular insulin mixture	Combination	30 min/2–12 hr/24 hr
Apidra	insulin glulisine	Rapid-Acting	Within 15 min/1–2 hr/3–4 hr
Admelog, Humalog, or Lyumjev	insulin lispro	Rapid-Acting	Within 15 min/1–2 hr/3–4 hr
Fiasp or Novolog	insulin aspart	Rapid-Acting	Within 15 min/1–2 hr/3–4 hr
Humulin R	regular insulin (SUBQ)	Short-Acting	½–1 hr/2–4 hr/5–7 hr
Novolin R	regular insulin (SUBQ)	Short-Acting	½–1 hr/2–4 hr/5–7 hr
Humulin R	regular insulin (IV)	Short-Acting	10–30 min/15–30 min/30–60 min
Novolin R	regular insulin (IV)	Short-Acting	10–30 min/15–30 min/30–60 min
Humulin N	NPH	Intermediate-Acting	2–4 hr/4–10 hr/10–16 hr
Novolin N	NPH	Intermediate-Acting	2–4 hr/4–10 hr/10–16 hr
Levemir	insulin detemir	Long-Acting	3–4 hr/3–14 hr/6–24 hr
Basaglar, Lantus, Semglee, or Toujeo	insulin glargine	Long-Acting	3–4 hr/No Peak/24 hr
Tresiba	insulin degludec	Long-Acting	Within 2 hr/12 hr/up to 42 hr

Differences in U.S. and Canadian Pharmaceutical Practices

In the United States (U.S.) and Canada, most drugs are prescribed and used similarly. However, certain processes and actions of the U.S. and Canadian pharmaceutical industries differ in significant ways, affecting both consumers and health care providers. Safety, marketing, and availability are three of these issues.

Safety

Controversy related to the importation of medications from Canada by U.S. consumers has sometimes raised concerns about the safety of these drugs. These fears are unfounded; in fact, the Canadian approval and manufacturing processes are very similar to U.S. processes. Both countries have pharmaceutical-related standards, laws, and policies to ensure that chemical entities marketed for human diseases and conditions are safe and effective. The process of taking a new drug from the laboratory to the pharmacy shelves includes:

Scientific development. The process begins with research. Scientists develop a new molecular entity targeted at a specific disease, symptom, or condition.

Patenting. A manufacturer applies for a patent, which prevents other drug companies from manufacturing a chemically identical drug. Patent protection lasts 17 years in the U.S. and 20 years in Canada. After a patent expires, any manufacturer can make generic versions of the chemical; generic drugs typically cost much less than the brand-name drugs.

Preclinical testing. Before a drug is taken by human subjects, preclinical testing of the chemical is performed first on animals. Testing helps identify drug action, toxicity effects, side effects, adverse reactions, dose amounts and routes, and administration procedures. This phase can last anywhere from 3 to 5 years.

Permission to begin clinical testing. Once a drug is found to have demonstrable positive health effects and is safe for animal consumption, a manufacturer seeks permission to begin clinical studies with human subjects. In the U.S., this process is called New Drug Application (NDA) and is administered by the Food and Drug Administration (FDA). In Canada, the process is referred to as a Clinical Trial Application (CTA) and is administered by Health Canada.

Clinical trials. Clinical trials are initiated to establish the potential benefits and risks for humans. Several subphases are required in the clinical trials phase whereby increasingly larger sample sizes are necessary.

Phase 0: A new designation for first-in-human trials, which are designed to assess whether the drug affects humans in a manner that is expected.

Phase 1: Between 20 and 80 healthy volunteers are recruited to assess safety, tolerance, dose ranges, pharmacokinetics, and pharmacodynamics.

Phase 2: Up to 300 patient volunteers with the drug-targeted disease are enrolled to assess efficacy and toxicity. Variables from Phase I trials may also be assessed.

Phase 3: Between 1000 and 3000 patient volunteers are entered into a randomized, double-blinded study designed to confirm drug effectiveness, comparability with existing treatments, and further exploration of potential and real side effects.

Ongoing surveillance of a drug for rare or long-term effects, or Phase 4 in Canada, continues after approval is received and marketing begun.

Approval. The results of the clinical studies are reviewed by Health Canada in Canada and by the FDA in the U.S. These regulatory bodies assess all aspects of a drug, including the labeling. The approval process is often deemed excessively long by physicians and patients who are anxious to try new remedies for refractory or terminal diseases. Efforts are ongoing to shorten the process in both countries. For example, Health Canada is collaborating with the FDA to develop a harmonized system for new drug submissions. A jointly planned Common Electronic Submissions Gateway (CESG) has been developed to allow submissions to be sent to both Canada and the U.S. in a common platform, while the review of these submissions continues to be a separate process.[1]

Marketing. Once a drug has been approved, it can be prescribed to consumers or, if it does not require a prescription, purchased by them.

Postmarketing surveillance. More clinical data become available when a drug is marketed and used by many people for longer periods of time. Pharmacovigilance is the term used to refer to the process of ongoing assessment of a drug's safety and effectiveness during this phase. In Canada, this includes Adverse Drug Reaction reporting by consumers and health professionals as described in "Detecting and Managing Adverse Drug Reactions."

Differences Between Canadian and U.S. Drug Pricing and Marketing
One major difference between Canadian and U.S drug regulatory processes is pricing. In Canada, the Patented Medicine Prices Review Board (PMPRB) regulates the prices that manufacturers can charge for prescription and nonprescription medicines. This is to ensure that prices are not excessive. No such control exists in the U.S., with postrebate prices for medications in the U.S. being approximately 10–15% higher than in Canada.[2]
Another difference is in advertising. In the U.S., manufacturers can market drugs directly, and forcefully, to consumers, a controversial privilege that has resulted in consumers requesting specific medications despite not necessarily understanding all of the risks and benefits. In Canada, such advertising is limited and subject to the approval of the Advertising Standards Canada (ASC) agency and the Pharmaceutical Advertising Advisory Board (PAAB). To address this issue in the U.S., the Institute of Medicine (IOM) has recommended that the FDA ban direct-to-consumer advertising during the first 2 years after a drug is marketed. Such a delay may help to prevent large numbers of people experiencing side effects not observed in the clinical trials, such as occurred with sildenafil (Viagra) when several patients died or developed vision problems in the first months after marketing began.

Natural Health Products
In Canada, Natural Health Products (NHPs) are regulated by Health Canada under the Natural Health Products Regulations. All NHPs must have a product license, and the Canadian sites that manufacture, package, label, and import these products must have a site license. A Natural Product Number (NPN) or Homeopathic Medicine Number (DIN-HM) is issued for the product only after it has been reviewed by Health Canada for its safety and efficacy. The term "Natural Product" refers to vitamins and mineral supplements, herbal remedies, traditional and homeopathic medicines, probiotics and other products such as amino acids, enzymes, essential fatty acids, protein supplements, or personal care items for consumption that contain natural ingredients.

In the U.S., the FDA classifies natural products as food products under the Dietary Supplements Health Education Act, so claims about the ability of a supplement to diagnose, prevent, treat, or cure a disease is prohibited. It is not necessary, however, for natural products to undergo review or approval or for testing to be done for identity and purity of active ingredients.

Drug Schedule, Availability, and Pregnancy Category Differences
In Canada, drug schedules are used to classify medication according to accessibility. The Canadian drug schedules as defined by NAPRA (the National Pharmacy Regulatory Authorities) are:

- **Schedule I**: Available only by prescription and provided by a pharmacist.
- **Schedule II**: Available only from a pharmacist; does not require a prescription; must be kept in an area with no public access (i.e., behind-the-counter).
- **Schedule III**: Available via open access in a pharmacy only (i.e., over-the-counter) to guarantee access to a pharmacist; does not require a prescription.
- **Unscheduled**: Can be sold in any store without professional supervision.

Each province and territory in Canada decides where to schedule each individual drug (except opioids and controlled substances), frequently changing schedules as new evidence is obtained. (Note: The province of Québec has not adopted this national model.)

The U.S., in contrast, categorizes medications according to two general classes:

- **Prescription Only**: Available only by prescription and provided by a pharmacist.
- **Over-the-Counter (OTC)**: Available via open access in the pharmacy.

As a result of these differences in accessibility some potentially dangerous drugs (such as insulin and codeine-containing cough medicines) are available only with a prescription in the U.S. and available without a prescription but in consultation with a pharmacist in Canada. Similarly, some Canadian drugs are available in combinations not found in the U.S. (see Appendix N for new Canadian combination drugs). There can also be significant variation within Canada due to each province and territory independently scheduling drugs, with the exception of narcotics and controlled substances. Other differences also exist with respect to drug availability between the two countries.

SOURCES CITED
1. Rawson, Nigel, S.B. "New Drug Approval Times and Safety Warnings in the United States and Canada, 1992–2011." J Popul Ther Clin Pharmacol Vol 20(2):e67–e81; April 22, 2013.

1412 APPENDIX L

2. Kanavos P, Ferrario A, Vandoros S, Anderson GF. "Higher US branded drug prices and spending compared to other countries may stem partly from quick uptake of new drugs." Health Affairs (Millwood). 2013; 32(4):753–761. doi:10.1377/hlthaff.2012.0920

ADDITIONAL REFERENCES

Common Electronic Submissions Gateway. https://www.canada.ca/en/health-canada/services/drugs-health-products/drug-products/applications-submissions/guidance-documents/common-electronic-submissions-gateway.html (accessed 10 October 2023).

Health Canada. https://www.canada.ca/en/health-canada.html (accessed 10 October 2023).

Natural and Non-Prescription Health Products. https://www.canada.ca/en/health-canada/services/drugs-health-products/natural-non-prescription/regulation.html (accessed 10 October 2023).

U.S. Food and Drug Administration. http://www.fda.gov (accessed 10 October 2023).

APPENDIX M

Routine Pediatric and Adult Immunizations

Immunization recommendations change frequently. For the latest recommendations see http://www.cdc.gov/vaccines/schedules/hcp/index.html. For Canadian recommendations see the Canadian Immunization Guide (Public Health Agency of Canada) https://www.canada.ca/en/public-health/services/publications/healthy-living/canadian-immunization-guide-part-1-key-immunization-information/page-13-recommended-immunization-schedules.html

ROUTINE PEDIATRIC IMMUNIZATIONS (0–18 yr)

GENERIC NAME (BRAND NAMES)	ROUTE/DOSAGE	CONTRAINDICATIONS/PRECAUTIONS	ADVERSE REACTIONS/SIDE EFFECTS	NOTES
COVID-19 (mRNA) vaccine (Moderna, Novavax, Pfizer BioNTech)	Age 6 mo–<5 yr: *Moderna:* 0.25 mL (25 mcg) IM initially, then at 4–8 wk after 1st dose; *Pfizer BioNTech:* 0.3 mL (3 mcg) IM initially, then at 3–8 wk after 1st dose, and at ≥8 wk after 2nd dose Age 5–<12 yr: *Moderna:* 0.25 mL (25 mcg) IM × 1 dose; *Pfizer BioNTech:* 0.3 mL (10 mcg) IM × 1 dose Age ≥12 yr: *Moderna:* 0.5 mL (50 mcg) IM x 1 dose; *Novavax:* 0.5 mL (5 mcg rS protein and 50 mcg Matrix-M adjuvant) IM initially, then 3–8 wk after 1st dose; *Pfizer BioNTech:* 0.3 mL (30 mcg) IM × 1 dose	Contraindications: Severe allergic reaction (e.g., anaphylaxis) after a previous dose or to a component of the vaccine. Precautions: History of diagnosed nonsevere allergy to a component of the vaccine; history of immediate nonsevere allergic reaction (regardless of severity and occurring within 4 hr) to a previous dose; moderate or severe acute illness with or without fever; history of multisystem inflammatory syndrome or history of myocarditis or pericarditis within 3 wk after a dose of any COVID-19 vaccine.	Local reactions: pain; tenderness; swelling; erythema of injection site. Systemic reactions: fever; fatigue/malaise; headache; chills; myalgia; arthralgia; in children <3 yr, irritability/crying sleepiness, and anorexia; localized axillary lymphadenopathy on the side of injection; myocarditis/pericarditis (especially in males age 12–39 yr).	Please see the latest guidance from the CDC for patients who are moderately or severely immunocompromised.¹ Observe for ≥15 min after vaccine dose and for 30 min if history of nonsevere, immediate allergic reaction to previous dose of COVID-19 vaccine.
Diphtheria toxoid, tetanus toxoid, and acellular pertussis vaccine—DTaP (Daptacel, Infanrix)	5-dose series: 0.5 mL IM at age 2 mo, 4 mo, 6 mo, 15–18 mo, and 4–6 yr (1st dose may be given as early as age 6 wk; 4th dose may be given as early as age 12 mo).	Contraindications: Severe allergic reaction (e.g., anaphylaxis) after a previous dose or to vaccine component; encephalopathy within 7 days of administration of previous dose of Tdap, DTP, or DTaP vaccines. Precautions: Guillain-Barré syndrome within 6 wk after previous dose of tetanus-toxoid-containing vaccine; history of Arthus-type hypersensitivity reaction to vaccine components; progressive neurologic disorder; moderate or severe acute illness with or without fever; allergy to latex; syncope.	Injection site reactions (pain, redness, swelling; fever; drowsiness; irritability/fussiness; crying; lethargy; anorexia.	Individual components may be given as separate injections if unusual reactions occur. The same product should be used for all doses when possible. Do not give to children ≥7 yr.

GENERIC NAME (BRAND NAMES)	ROUTE/DOSAGE	CONTRAINDICATIONS	ADVERSE REACTIONS/ SIDE EFFECTS	NOTES
Haemophilus influenzae type b vaccination — Hib(ActHIB), Hiberix, PedvaxHIB)	*ActHIB or Hiberix*: 4-dose series (0.5 mL/dose IM) (3-dose primary series at age 2 mo, 4 mo, and 6 mo, followed by a booster dose* at 12–15 mo). *PedvaxHIB*: 3-dose series (0.5 mL/dose IM) (2-dose primary series at age 2 mo and 4 mo, followed by a booster dose at 12–15 mo).	Contraindications: Severe allergic reaction (e.g., anaphylaxis) after a previous dose or to vaccine component; history of severe allergic reaction to dry natural latex. Precautions: Moderate or severe acute illness with or without fever.	Sleepiness; fever; injection site reactions (pain, redness, swelling); crying; diarrhea, vomiting.	Please see the latest guidance from the CDC for children undergoing chemotherapy, hematopoietic stem cell transplant, anatomic or functional asplenia, splenectomy, HIV, immunoglobulin deficiency, and early component deficiency.
Hepatitis A vaccine — HepA(Havrix, Vaqta)	2-dose series: 0.5 mL IM at 12–23 mo, then 0.5 mL IM of either Vaqta 6–18 mo after the 1st dose OR Havrix 6–12 mo after the 1st dose.	Contraindications: Severe allergic reaction (e.g., anaphylaxis) to a previous dose or to vaccine component (including neomycin). Precautions: Moderate or severe acute illness with or without fever; latex allergy; syncope.	Injection site soreness; headache; anorexia; fever; malaise.	Also recommended in children ≥1 yr who live in areas with high rates of hepatitis A or are in other high-risk groups (e.g., chronic liver disease, HIV, illicit drug users, experiencing homelessness, adolescent males who have sex with other males, close personal contact within first 60 days of arrival of international adoptee from country where hepatitis A is endemic).
Hepatitis B vaccine — HepB (Engerix-B, Recombivax HB)	*Infants born to HBsAg-negative mothers* (3-dose series): Birth weight >2000 g: 0.5 mL IM within 24 hr of birth, at age 1–2 mo, and at age 6–18 mo; Birth weight <2,000 g: 0.5 mL at chronological age of 1 mo or at hospital discharge, at age 1–2 mo, and then at age 6–18 mo. *Infants born to HBsAg-positive mothers*: Birth weight >2000 g (3-dose series): 0.5 mL IM within 12 hr of birth, at age 1–2 mo, and then at age 6 mo. Birth weight <2000 g (4-dose series): 0.5 mL IM within 12 hr of birth, at age 1 mo, at age 2–3 mo, and then at age 6 mo.	Contraindications: Severe allergic reaction (e.g., anaphylaxis) after a previous dose or to vaccine component (including yeast). Precautions: Moderate or severe acute illness with or without fever.	Injection site reactions; fatigue; dizziness; headache; fever.	Determine mother's HBsAg status to guide vaccine administration.
Human papillomavirus vaccine, 9-valent — HPV9 (Gardasil 9)	0.5 mL IM at age 11–12 yr; if initiated before age 15 yr, give 2 doses (1st dose may be given as early as age 9 yr), with 2nd dose being given 6–12 mo after 1st dose. Minimum interval is 5 mo. If initiated at ≥age 15 yr, give 3-dose series (minimum intervals: dose 1 to dose 2: 4 wk; dose 2 to dose 3: 12 wk; dose 1 to dose 3: 5 mo).	Contraindications: Serious allergic reaction (e.g., anaphylaxis) after a previous dose or to vaccine component (including yeast). Precautions: Moderate or severe acute illness with or without fever.	Injection site reactions; dizziness; fever; headache; syncope.	Immunocompromised patients: 3-dose series is indicated even with initiation of vaccination at age 9–14 yr. If history of sexual abuse or assault, then start at age 9 yr.
Influenza vaccine (Afluria Quadrivalent, Fluad Quadrivalent, Fluarix Quadrivalent, Flublok Quadrivalent, Flucelvax Quadrivalent, FluLaval Quadrivalent, Fluzone High-Dose Quadrivalent, Fluzone Quadrivalent)	For the 2023–2024 influenza season: Age 6 mo–8 yr and have received fewer than 2 influenza vaccine doses before July 1, 2023, or if vaccination history is unknown: 2 doses separated by at ≥4 wk; age 6 mo–8 yr and have received ≥2 influenza doses before July 1, 2023: 1 dose; age ≥9 yr: 1 dose	Contraindications: Severe allergic reaction (e.g., anaphylaxis) after a previous dose or to a vaccine component. Precautions: Guillain-Barré syndrome within 6 wk after a previous dose of any type of influenza vaccine; moderate or severe acute illness with or without fever.	Injection site reactions; headache; fatigue; fever; myalgia; possible neurologic toxicity.	Minimum age for inactivated vaccine is 6 mo, live/attenuated vaccine is 2 yr, and recombinant influenza vaccine is 18 yr. There are multiple contraindications and precautions for the various influenza vaccines; refer to the CDC or manufacturer information.

GENERIC NAME (BRAND NAMES)	ROUTE/DOSAGE	CONTRAINDICATIONS	ADVERSE REACTIONS/ SIDE EFFECTS	NOTES
Measles, mumps, and rubella vaccine—MMR (M-M-R II, Priorix)	2-dose series: 0.5 mL SUBQ at age 12–15 mo and at age 4–6 yr (2nd dose may be given earlier if ≥4 wk have elapsed since the 1st dose).	Contraindications: Severe allergic reaction (e.g., anaphylaxis) after a previous dose or to vaccine component; severe immunodeficiency; pregnancy. Precautions: Recent receipt of antibody-containing blood product; history of thrombocytopenia or thrombocytopenic purpura; moderate or severe acute illness with or without fever.	Injection site reactions; irritability; fever; rash; diarrhea, vomiting.	If unusual reactions occur, individual components may be given as separate injections. Immunosuppression may ↓ antibody response to injection and ↑ the risk of viral transmission. Do not administer IM or IV.
Meningococcal conjugate vaccine *Serogroups A, C, W, and Y conjugate vaccines:* MenQuadfi [MenACWY-TT], Menveo [MenACWY-CRM]) *Serogroup B vaccines:* Bexsero [MenB-4C], Trumenba [MenB-FHbp]	*MenQuadfi or Menveo:* 0.5 mL IM single dose at age 11–12 yr with a booster dose at age 16 yr; if received 1st dose at age 13–15 yr, should receive booster dose at age 16–18 yr [with an interval of ≥8 wk between doses] if received 1st dose at age ≥16 yr, no booster dose needed. Single dose of MenQuadfi or Menveo should be given to previously unvaccinated college freshmen (≤21 yr) living in dormitories. *Bexsero or Trumenba:* Young adults age 16–23 yr who are not at ↑ risk for meningococcal disease may be given 2 doses of either Bexsero (≥1 mo apart) or Trumenba (6 mo apart) (based on shared decision-making).	Contraindications: Severe allergic reaction (e.g., anaphylaxis) after a previous dose or to vaccine component. Precautions: Pregnancy; latex sensitivity (MenB-4C only); moderate or severe illness with or without fever; Guillain-Barré syndrome (if there is a previous history).	Injection site reactions; anorexia; arthralgia; diarrhea; fatigue; fever; headache; myalgia; nausea; irritability; drowsiness; vomiting	Special situations for use of serogroups A, C, W, and Y conjugate vaccines outside the recommended age range include anatomic or functional asplenia (including sickle cell disease); HIV; persistent complement component deficiency; complement inhibitor (e.g., eculizumab, ravulizumab) use; travel to countries with hyperendemic or epidemic meningococcal disease; 1st-yr college students who live in residential housing (if not previously vaccinated at age ≥16 yr); military recruits; and adolescent vaccination of children who received MenACWY prior to age 10 yr. Special situations for use of serogroups B vaccine include anatomic or functional asplenia (including sickle cell disease); persistent complement component deficiency; and complement inhibitor (e.g., eculizumab, ravulizumab) use. Bexsero and Trumenba are not interchangeable.
Pneumococcal conjugate vaccine, 15-valent or 20-valent—PCV15 or PCV20 (PCV15, Vaxneuvance) (PCV20, Prevnar 20)	4-dose series: 0.5 mL IM at age 2 mo, 4 mo, 6 mo, and 12–15 mo.	Contraindications: Severe allergic reaction (e.g., anaphylaxis) after a previous dose or to vaccine component (including diphtheria toxoid). Precautions: Moderate or severe acute illness with or without fever.	Injection site reactions; arthralgia; chills; anorexia; fatigue; fever; headache; insomnia; irritability; myalgia.	One dose may also be given to previously unvaccinated healthy children age 24–59 mo; two doses (given ≥8 wk apart) may also be given to previously unvaccinated children age 24–59 mo with conditions that ↑ the risk of pneumococcal disease.
Pneumococcal polysaccharide vaccine—PPSV23 (Pneumovax 23)	0.5 mL IM or SUBQ ≥8 wk after final dose of PCV in high-risk children age ≥2 yr.	Contraindications: Severe allergic reaction (e.g., anaphylaxis) after a previous dose or to vaccine component; age <2 yr. Precautions: Moderate or severe acute illness with or without fever.	Injection site reactions; headache; fatigue; myalgia; fever.	

GENERIC NAME (BRAND NAMES)	ROUTE/DOSAGE	CONTRAINDICATIONS	ADVERSE REACTIONS/ SIDE EFFECTS	NOTES
Polio vaccine, inactivated—IPV (IPOL)	*4-dose series:* 0.5 mL IM or SUBQ at age 2 mo, 4 mo, 6–18 mo, and 4–6 yr. Administer the final dose on or after age 4 yr and ≥6 mo after the previous dose.	Contraindications: Severe allergic reaction (e.g., anaphylaxis) after a previous dose or to vaccine component (including neomycin, 2-phenoxyethanol, formaldehyde, streptomycin, or polymyxin B); moderate or severe illness with fever. Precautions: Illness with or without fever.	Injection site reactions; anorexia; fatigue; fever; irritability; vomiting.	Oral polio vaccine (OPV) is no longer recommended for use in the United States.
Rotavirus vaccine (Rotarix, RotaTeq)	*Rotarix:* 2-dose series of 1 mL PO at age 6 wk and then ≥4 wk later. Complete series by age 24 wk. *RotaTeq:* 3-dose series of 2 mL PO at age 2 mo, 4 mo, and 6 mo. Complete series by age 32 wk.	Contraindications: Severe allergic reaction (e.g., anaphylaxis) after a previous dose or to vaccine component; latex allergy (Rotarix only); history of uncorrected congenital malformation of GI tract (Rotarix only); history of intussusception; severe combined immunodeficiency disease. Precautions: Chronic GI disease; spina bifida (Rotarix only); moderate or severe acute illness with or without fever.	Diarrhea; fever; anorexia; vomiting; cough; runny nose; irritability.	First dose of either product may be given as early as age 6 wk. Series should not be started when age ≥15 wk. Series should be completed with same product, when possible. If RotaTeq used in any of the doses, a total of 3 doses should be given. Delay vaccine if infants are suffering from acute diarrhea or vomiting. Rotavirus shedding occurs in stool after vaccination, which should be considered if close contacts are immunocompromised.
Tetanus toxoid, **reduced** diphtheria toxoid, and acellular pertussis vaccine absorbed (Tdap, Adacel, Boostrix)	0.5 mL IM at age 11–12 yr if previously completed DTaP series, then followed by booster doses of either Td or Tdap every 10 yr; one-time dose may be given if age ≥7 yr if did not previously complete DTaP series.	Contraindications: Severe allergic reaction (e.g., anaphylaxis) after a previous dose or to vaccine component; encephalopathy within 7 days of administration of previous dose of Tdap, DTP, or DtaP vaccines. Precautions: Guillain-Barré syndrome within 6 wk after previous dose of tetanus-toxoid–containing vaccine; history of Arthus-type hypersensitivity; progressive or unstable neurological disorder; uncontrolled seizures, or progressive encephalopathy; moderate or severe acute illness with or without fever.	Injection site reactions; abdominal pain; fever; rash; arthralgia; chills; diarrhea; fatigue; headache; myalgia; nausea; vomiting.	Should also be given to pregnant adolescents during each pregnancy (preferably during 27–36 wk gestation) regardless of interval since prior Td or Tdap.

GENERIC NAME (BRAND NAMES)	ROUTE/DOSAGE	CONTRAINDICATIONS	ADVERSE REACTIONS/ SIDE EFFECTS	NOTES
Varicella vaccine (Var, Varivax)	*2-dose series:* 0.5 mL IM or SUBQ at age 12–15 mo and at 4–6 yr (2nd dose may be given earlier if ≥3 mo have elapsed since 1st dose); if age 7–18 yr with no evidence of immunity, 2 doses should be given (≥3 mo apart if age 7–12 yr or ≥4–8 wk apart if age ≥13 yr).	Contraindications: Severe allergic reaction (e.g., anaphylaxis) after a previous dose or to vaccine component (including gelatin or neomycin); severe immunosuppression; pregnancy or planning to become pregnant in next 3 mo. Precautions: Recent receipt of antibody-containing blood product; receipt of specific antiviral drugs 24 hr before vaccination (avoid use for 14 days after vaccination); use of salicylates (avoid use for 6 wk after vaccination); moderate or severe acute illness with or without fever.	Injection site reactions; anorexia; chills; diarrhea; fatigue; fever; rash; headache; irritability; nausea; vomiting.	Immunosuppression may ↓ antibody response to injection and ↑ the risk of viral transmission.

Nursing Implications:

Assessment
Assess previous immunization history and history of hypersensitivity.
Assess for history of latex allergy. Some prefilled syringes may use latex components and should be avoided in those with hypersensitivity.
Assess for immunocompromising conditions, pregnancy, allergy to vaccine components, history of acute or moderate illness, previous adverse reactions.
Review for any changes in vaccines.
Assess for special situations that may lead to a change in usual vaccine administration. Regularly evaluate any changes on the CDC website.

Implementation
Administer each immunization by appropriate route:
PO: Rotavirus.
SUBQ: measles, mumps, rubella, polio, varicella, pneumococcal polysaccharide.
IM: COVID-19, diphtheria, tetanus toxoid, pertussis, polio, Haemophilus b, hepatitis B, meningococcal conjugate, hepatitis A, pneumococcal conjugate, pneumococcal polysaccharide, influenza injection, human papillomavirus, varicella.

Patient/Family Teaching
Provide patient or patient's legal representative a copy of the CDC Vaccine Information Statement and review the information related to the vaccine from the CDC prior to administering the vaccine.
Inform parent(s) or legal guardian of potential and reportable side effects of immunization.
Notify the health care professional if patient develops fever higher than $39.4°$ C ($103°$ F); difficulty breathing; hives; itching; swelling of eyes, face, or inside of nose; sudden, severe tiredness or weakness; or convulsions.
Review next scheduled immunization with parent.

Evaluation
Prevention of diseases through active immunity.

ROUTINE ADULT IMMUNIZATIONS

GENERIC NAME (BRAND NAMES)	INDICATIONS	DOSAGE/ROUTE	CONTRAINDICATIONS	ADVERSE REACTIONS/SIDE EFFECTS
COVID-19 (mRNA) vaccine (Moderna, Novavax, Pfizer BioNTech)	All adults	Age ≥12 yr: Moderna: 0.5 mL (50 mcg) IM × 1 dose; Novavax: 0.5 mL (5 mcg rS protein and 50 mcg Matrix-M adjuvant) IM initially, then 3–8 wk after 1st dose; Pfizer-BioNTech: 0.3 mL (30 mcg) IM × 1 dose.	Contraindications: Severe allergic reaction (e.g., anaphylaxis) after a previous dose or to a component of the vaccine. Precautions: History of diagnosed non-severe allergy to a component of the vaccine; history of immediate nonsevere allergic reaction (regardless of severity and occurring within 4 hr) to a previous dose; moderate or severe acute illness with or without fever; history of multisystem inflammatory syndrome or history of myocarditis or pericarditis within 3 wk after a dose of any COVID-19 vaccine.	Local reactions: pain; tenderness; swelling; erythema of injection site. Systemic reactions: fever; fatigue/malaise; headache; chills; myalgia; arthralgia; localized axillary lymphadenopathy on the side of injection; myocarditis/pericarditis (especially in males age 12–39 yrs).
Hepatitis A vaccine—HepA (Havrix, Vaqta)	Chronic liver disease; HIV; experiencing homelessness; users of injection/noninjection illicit drugs; men who have sex with men; working with hepatitis A virus in a research laboratory setting; health care facilities providing services to injection or noninjection drug users or group homes and nonresidential day care facilities for developmentally disabled persons; pregnancy (if at risk for infection or severe outcome from infection during pregnancy); travel to endemic areas; unvaccinated individuals who anticipate close personal contact with an international adoptee during the initial 60 days after their arrival in the U.S. from a country with intermediate or high endemicity.	2-dose series: 1 mL IM initially, then 1 mL IM 6–12 mo (Havrix) or 6–18 mo (Vaqta) after initial dose.	Contraindications: Severe allergic reaction (e.g., anaphylaxis) after a previous dose or to a component of the vaccine (including neomycin). Precautions: Moderate or severe acute illness with or without fever; syncope.	Injection site reactions; anorexia; nausea; fatigue; ↓ appetite, fever; irritability; headache.

GENERIC NAME (BRAND NAMES)	INDICATIONS	DOSAGE/ROUTE	CONTRAINDICATIONS	ADVERSE REACTIONS/ SIDE EFFECTS
Hepatitis B vaccine — HepB (Engerix-B, Heplisav-B, PreHevbrio, Recombivax HB)	Chronic liver disease; sex partners of persons with chronic hepatitis B virus infection; sexually active persons not in mutually monogamous relationships; persons seeking evaluation or treatment for a sexually transmitted infection; men who have sex with men; experiencing homelessness; receive clotting factor concentrates; users of injection/ noninjection illicit drugs; household contacts of persons with chronic hepatitis B infection; residents and staff of facilities for developmentally disabled persons; health care and public safety personnel with reasonably anticipated risk for exposure to blood or blood-contaminated body fluids; hemodialysis, peritoneal dialysis, home dialysis, and predialysis patients; diabetes mellitus (19–59 yr; ≥60 yr through shared decision making); incarcerated persons; pregnancy (if at risk for infection or severe outcome from infection during pregnancy); travel to endemic areas.	*Recombivax HB, and Engerix-B, and PreHevbrio (3-dose series)*: 1 mL IM initially, then 1 mL IM at 1 mo and 6 mo after initial dose. *Heplisav-B (2-dose series)*: 0.5 mL IM initially, then 0.5 mL IM ≥4 wk later.	Contraindications: Severe allergic reaction (e.g., anaphylaxis) after a previous dose or to a component of the vaccine (including yeast); pregnancy (Heplisav-B and PreHevbrio not recommended). Precautions: Moderate or severe acute illness with or without fever.	Injection site reactions; fatigue; dizziness; headache; fever.
Human papillomavirus vaccine, 9-valent — HPV9 (Gardasil 9)	All previously unvaccinated or partially vaccinated adults ≤45 years of age.	If age ≥15 yr at initial vaccination, give 3-dose series: 0.5 mL IM initially, then 0.5 mL IM at 1–2 mo and 6 mo after initial dose.	Contraindications: Severe allergic reaction (e.g., anaphylaxis) after a previous dose or to a component of the vaccine (including yeast); pregnancy.	Injection site reactions; dizziness; fever; headache; syncope.
Influenza vaccine (Afluria Quadrivalent, Fluad Quadrivalent, Fluarix Quadrivalent, Flublok Quadrivalent, Flucelvax Quadrivalent, Flu-Laval Quadrivalent, Fluzone High-Dose Quadrivalent, Fluzone Quadrivalent)	All adults.	All ages (all vaccines except for Fluzone High-Dose Quadrivalent): 0.5 mL IM annually. ≥65 yr: Any one of quadrivalent high-dose inactivated influenza vaccine, quadrivalent recombinant influenza vaccine, or quadrivalent adjuvanted inactivated influenza vaccine is preferred.	Contraindications: Severe allergic reaction (e.g., anaphylaxis) after a previous dose or to a component of the vaccine. Precautions: Guillain-Barré syndrome within 6 wk of influenza vaccine; moderate or severe acute illness with or without fever. If patient experiences anaphylactic reaction to eggs or egg-containing foods, any vaccine other than Flublok Quadrivalent or Flucelvax Quadrivalent should be administered and supervised by health care professional with experience in recognition and management of severe allergic conditions.	Fever; headache; injection site reactions; malaise; drowsiness; myalgia.

GENERIC NAME (BRAND NAMES)	INDICATIONS	DOSAGE/ROUTE	CONTRAINDICATIONS	ADVERSE REACTIONS/ SIDE EFFECTS
Measles, mumps, and rubella vaccine—MMR (M-M-R II, Priorix)	Adults born in or after 1957 with unreliable documentation of previous vaccination (unless have laboratory evidence of immunity to all 3 diseases); health care workers born before 1957 who do not have laboratory evidence of immunity to measles, mumps, or rubella.	Adults born in or after 1957 with unreliable documentation of previous vaccination: 1 or 2 doses of 0.5 mL SUBQ (with ≥28 days between doses); high-risk groups should receive a total of 2 doses (with ≥28 days between doses).	Contraindications: Severe allergic reaction (e.g., anaphylaxis) after a previous dose or to a component of the vaccine (including gelatin and neomycin); severe immunodeficiency; active untreated tuberculosis; pregnancy. Precautions: Recent receipt or antibody-containing blood product; history of thrombocytopenia or thrombocytopenic purpura; moderate or severe acute illness with or without fever.	Injection site reactions; arthralgia; fever; rash; encephalitis. Immunosuppression may ↓ antibody response to injection and ↑ the risk of viral transmission (live vaccine).
Meningococcal conjugate vaccine Serogroups A, C, W, and Y conjugate vaccines: MenQuadfi [MenACWY-TT]), Menveo [MenACWY-CRM] Serogroup B vaccines: Bexsero [MenB-4C], Trumenba [MenB-FHbp]	Serogroups A, C, W, and Y conjugate vaccines: 1st-year college students living in residential housing if they have not previously received a dose on or after their 16th birthday; military recruits; anatomic or functional asplenia (including sickle cell disease); persistent complement component deficiency; HIV; persistent complement component deficiency; complement inhibitor use; travel in areas in which meningococcal disease is hyperendemic or epidemic; microbiologists routinely exposed to Neisseria meningitidis; persons at risk during a community outbreak. Serogroup B vaccines: Anatomic or functional asplenia (including sickle cell disease); persistent complement component deficiency; complement inhibitor use. May also administer to young adults aged 16–23 yr who are not at ↑ risk for meningococcal disease (based on shared decision making).	Serogroups A, C, W, and Y conjugate vaccines: Adults not previously vaccinated with functional or anatomic asplenia, HIV, persistent complement deficiency, or complement inhibitor use: 0.5 mL IM initially, then 0.5 mL IM ≥8 wk later. Repeat dose every 5 yr if person remains at ↑ risk. Adults not previously vaccinated who are traveling to areas where meningococcal disease is endemic/hyperendemic, or microbiologists routinely exposed to Neisseria meningitidis: 0.5 mL IM × 1 dose. Repeat dose every 5 yr if person remains at ↑ risk. Military recruits: 0.5 mL IM × 1 dose. Adults not previously vaccinated who are 1st-year college students living in residential housing: 0.5 mL IM × 1 dose. Serogroup B vaccines: Patients at ↑ risk for serogroup B meningococcal disease: Bexsero: 0.5 mL IM initially, then 0.5 mL IM ≥1 mo after initial dose; Trumenba: 0.5 mL IM initially, then 0.5 mL IM 1–2 mo, and 6 mo after initial dose. Patients age 16–23 yr who are not at risk for serogroup B meningococcal disease: Bexsero: 0.5 mL IM initially, then 0.5 mL IM ≥1 mo after initial dose; Trumenba: 0.5 mL IM initially, then 0.5 mL IM 6 mo after initial dose.	Serogroups A, C, W, and Y conjugate vaccines: Contraindications: Severe allergic reaction (e.g., anaphylaxis) after a previous dose or to a component of the vaccine (including diphtheria toxoid or CRM197-containing vaccine [MenACWY-CRM only] or tetanus toxoid [MenACWY-TT only]). Precautions: Moderate or severe acute illness with or without fever. Serogroup B vaccines: Contraindications: Severe allergic reaction (e.g., anaphylaxis) after a previous dose or to a component of the vaccine. Precautions: Pregnancy; latex sensitivity (MenB-4C only); moderate or severe illness with or without fever.	Injection site reactions; anorexia; arthralgia; diarrhea; fatigue; fever; headache; myalgia; nausea; irritability; malaise.

GENERIC NAME (BRAND NAMES)	INDICATIONS	DOSAGE/ROUTE	CONTRAINDICATIONS	ADVERSE REACTIONS/ SIDE EFFECTS
Pneumococcal conjugate vaccine, 15-valent or 20-valent — PCV15 or PCV20 (PCV15, Vaxneuvance, PCV20, Prevnar 20)	All adults ≥65 yr: who have not previously received a dose of PCV13, PCV15, or PCV20; whose previous vaccination history is unknown; who have previously received only PCV7, PCV13, or PPSV23; or who have previously received both PCV13 and PPSV23 was received at age ≥65 yr. Adults 19–64 yr with alcoholism, chronic heart/liver/lung disease, chronic renal failure, cigarette smoking, cochlear implant, congenital or acquired asplenia, cerebrospinal fluid leak, diabetes, malignancy, HIV, immunodeficiency, solid organ transplants, or sickle cell disease.	0.5 mL IM x 1 dose. Patients who have not previously received a dose of PCV13, PCV15, or PCV20 or whose previous vaccination history is unknown: 1 dose of PCV15 OR 1 dose of PCV20. If PCV15 is used, this should be followed by a dose of PPSV23 given ≥1 yr after the PCV15 dose.	Contraindications: Severe allergic reaction (e.g., anaphylaxis) after a previous dose or to a component of the vaccine (including neomycin). Precautions: Moderate or severe acute illness with or without fever; syncope.	Arthralgia; injection site reactions; chills; anorexia; fatigue; fever; headache; insomnia; irritability; myalgia; rash.
Pneumococcal polysaccharide vaccine — PPSV23 (Pneumovax 23)	All adults ≥65 yr: who have not previously received a dose of PCV13, PCV15, or PCV20; whose previous vaccination history is unknown; who have previously received only PCV7, PCV13, or PPSV23; or who have previously received both PCV13 and PPSV23 was received at age ≥65 yr. Adults 19–64 yr with alcoholism, chronic heart/liver/lung disease, chronic renal failure, cigarette smoking, cochlear implant, congenital or acquired asplenia, cerebrospinal fluid leak, diabetes, malignancy, HIV, immunodeficiency, solid organ transplants, or sickle cell disease.	0.5 mL IM or SUBQ x 1 dose. Patients who have not previously received a dose of PCV13, PCV15, PCV20 or whose previous vaccination history is unknown: 1 dose of PCV15 OR 1 dose of PCV20. If PCV15 is used, this should be followed by a dose of PPSV23 given ≥1 yr after the PCV15 dose. A minimum interval of 8 wk between PCV15 and PPSV23 can be considered for adults with an immunocompromising condition, cochlear implant, or cerebrospinal fluid leak.	Contraindications: Severe allergic reaction (e.g., anaphylaxis) after a previous dose or to a component of the vaccine. Precautions: Moderate or severe acute illness with or without fever.	Chills; fever; injection site reactions; fatigue; myalgia.
Respiratory syncytial virus vaccine — RSV (Abrysvo, Arexvy)	Age ≥60 yr (based on shared decision-making); pregnancy (during wk 32–36) (Abrysvo only).	0.5 mL IM x 1 dose.	Contraindications: Severe allergic reaction (e.g., anaphylaxis) after a previous dose or to a component of the vaccine. Precautions: Immunocompromising conditions; syncope.	Injection site pain; fatigue; myalgia; headache; arthralgia.

GENERIC NAME (BRAND NAMES)	INDICATIONS	DOSAGE/ROUTE	CONTRAINDICATIONS	ADVERSE REACTIONS/ SIDE EFFECTS
Smallpox and monkeypox vaccine—Mpox (Jynneos)	Age ≥18 yr and the following risk factors for Mpox infection: 1) persons who are gay, bisexual, and other men who have sex with men, transgender, or nonbinary people who in the past 6 mo have had: a) a new diagnosis of ≥1 sexually transmitted infection; b) >1 sex partner; c) sex at a commercial sex venue; d) sex in association with a large public event in a geographic area where Mpox transmission is occurring; 2) Persons who are sexual partners of the persons described above; 3) Persons who anticipate experiencing any of the situations described above.	0.1 mL intradermally initially, then 0.1 mL intradermally 4 wk later.	Contraindications: Severe allergic reaction (e.g., anaphylaxis) after a previous dose or to a component of the vaccine. Precautions: Moderate or severe acute illness, with or without fever.	Change in appetite; nausea; injection site reactions; chills; fatigue; headache; arthralgia, myalgia
Tetanus toxoid, **reduced** diphtheria toxoid and acellular pertussis vaccine absorbed—Tdap (Adacel, Boostrix)	Single dose should be given to replace one of the every 10-yr Td boosters in all adults who did not previously receive a dose of Tdap or if their vaccine status is unknown. Single dose should also be given as soon as feasible to all pregnant women (preferred during 27–36 wks gestation), close contacts of infants <12 mo, and health care workers with direct patient contact.	Previously did not receive Tdap at or after age 11 years: 1 dose of Tdap (0.5 mL IM), then Td or Tdap every 10 yr.	Contraindications: Severe allergic reaction (e.g., anaphylaxis) after a previous dose or to a component of the vaccine; encephalopathy within 7 days of administration of previous dose of DTP, DTaP, or Tdap. Precautions: Guillain-Barré syndrome within 6 wk after a previous dose; history of Arthus-type sensitivity; moderate or severe acute illness with or without fever; progressive or unstable neurological disorder; uncontrolled seizures; progressive encephalopathy.	Abdominal pain; arthralgia; chills, diarrhea; fatigue, headache; myalgia, nausea; pain at injection site; vomiting.
Tetanus-diphtheria—Td (Tenivac, TDVax)	All adults who lack written documentation of a primary series consisting of ≥3 doses of tetanus—and diphtheria—toxoid-containing vaccine; booster dose should be given to all adults every 10 yr. (see info above regarding use of Tdap to replace one dose of Td in booster series).	Previously did not receive Tdap at or after age 11 yr: 1 dose of Tdap, then Td (0.5 mL IM) or Tdap every 10 yr. If adult did not receive the primary vaccination for tetanus, diphtheria, or pertussis: 1 dose of Tdap followed by 1 dose of Td or Tdap ≥4 wk later, and then 1 dose of Td or Tdap 6–12 mo later, then Td or Tdap every 10 yr thereafter.	Contraindications: Severe allergic reaction (e.g., anaphylaxis) after a previous dose or to a component of the vaccine. Precautions: Guillain-Barré syndrome within 6 wk after a previous dose; history of Arthus-type sensitivity; moderate or severe acute illness with or without fever.	Injection site reactions; arthralgia; chills; diarrhea; fatigue; headache; myalgia; nausea.

GENERIC NAME (BRAND NAMES)	INDICATIONS	DOSAGE/ROUTE	CONTRAINDICATIONS	ADVERSE REACTIONS/ SIDE EFFECTS
Varicella vaccine—Var (Varivax)	Any adult with no evidence of immunity to varicella.	*2-dose series:* 0.5 mL SUBQ initially, then 0.5 mL SUBQ 4–8 wk after initial dose.	Contraindications: Severe allergic reaction (e.g., anaphylaxis) after a previous dose or to a component of the vaccine (including gelatin or neomycin); pregnancy or planning to become pregnant in next 3 mo; severe immunodeficiency; active febrile illness; active, untreated tuberculosis. Precautions: Recent receipt of antibody-containing blood product; use of antiviral drugs 24 hr before vaccination (avoid for 14 days after vaccination), use of aspirin-containing products; moderate or severe acute illness with or without fever.	Fever; rash; injection site reactions. Immunosuppression may ↓ antibody response to injection and ↑ the risk of viral transmission (live vaccine).
Zoster vaccine (Shingrix)	All adults ≥50 yr (regardless of previous history of herpes zoster or vaccination with Zostavax or varicella vaccine).	*2-dose series:* 0.5 mL SUBQ initially, then 0.5 mL SUBQ 2–6 mo after initial dose.	Contraindications: Severe allergic reaction (e.g., anaphylaxis) after a previous dose or to a component of the vaccine (including gelatin or neomycin); severe immunosuppression (in the absence of severe immunosuppression, HIV is not a contraindication); pregnancy (also avoid becoming pregnant for 4 wk after immunization). Precautions: Moderate to severe illness in persons with acute herpes zoster (vaccination should be delayed until the acute stage has resolved and symptoms abate).	Injection-site reactions; myalgia; fatigue. Immunosuppression may ↓ antibody response to injection and ↑ the risk of viral transmission (live vaccine).

It is recommended that the health care provider regularly review vaccine information on the Centers for Disease Control and Prevention website, as recommendations and guidelines can change. This information is not all-encompassing, and each vaccine has additional information. Regularly review for special conditions, catch-up immunization schedule, and guidelines for immunocompromising conditions.
Source: Adapted from the recommendations of the Department of Health and Human Services, Centers for Disease Control and Prevention: http://www.cdc.gov/vaccines/schedules/hcp/index.html.

Bibliography

American Geriatrics Society, British Geriatrics Society, and American Academy of Orthopedic Surgeons Panel on Falls Prevention. Guideline for the prevention of falls in older persons. J Am Geriatr Soc. 2001;49:664–672.

Blumenthal M, et al. The Complete German Commission E Monographs: Therapeutic Guide to Herbal Medicines. Integrative Medical Communications; 1998.

Clinical Resource. Meds That Should Not Be Crushed. Pharmacist's Letter/Pharmacy Technician's Letter/Prescriber's Letter. February 2023.

Facts and Comparisons. Wolters Kluwer Clinical Drug Information, Inc., Hudson, OH.

Fetrow CW, Avila JR. Professional's Handbook of Complementary & Alternative Medicines. 3rd ed. Lippincott Williams & Wilkins; 2004.

Kuhn MA, Winston D. Herbal Therapy and Supplements: A Scientific and Traditional Approach. 2nd ed. Lippincott Williams & Wilkins; 2007.

Lexi-Comp, Inc: (Lexi-Drugs [Comp + Specialties]). Lexi-Comp, Inc., Hudson, OH.

MICROMEDEX® 2023 (Healthcare Series).

National Institutes of Health Office of Dietary Supplements. Vitamin and Mineral Fact Sheets, Bethesda, MD. https://ods.od.nih.gov/factsheets/list-VitaminsMinerals.

National Kidney Foundation: A–Z Guide for High Potassium Foods, National Kidney Foundation. https://www.kidney.org/atoz/content/potassium.

PDR for Herbal Medicines. 4th ed. Thomson Healthcare; 2011.

Pennington JAT, Spungen J. Bowes and Church's Food Values of Portions Commonly Used. 19th ed. Lippincott Williams & Wilkins; 2010.

Pflipsen MC, Vega Colon KM. Anaphylaxis: Recognition and management. Am Fam Physician 2020;102:355–362.

The 2023 American Geriatrics Society Beers Criteria Update Expert Panel. American Geriatrics Society 2023 updated AGS Beers Criteria for potentially inappropriate medication use in older adults. J Am Geriatr Soc 2023; 71:(7)2052–2081.

Van Leeuwen AM, Bladh, ML. Davis's Comprehensive Manual of Laboratory and Diagnostic Tests with Nursing Implications. 10th ed. FA Davis Company; 2023.

https://www.fda.gov/drugs.

https://www.ismp.org/.

Comprehensive Index*

*Entries for **generic** names appear in **boldface type**. Trade names appear in regular type, with Canadian names preceded by a maple leaf icon (🍁). **CLASSIFICATIONS** appear in **BOLDFACE SMALL CAPS**. *Combination Drugs* appear in *italics* and can be accessed in Appendix N online at fadavis.com, herbal products are preceded by a yin-yang icon (☯), and drugs with genetic implications are preceded by a double-helix icon (〰️).

*Entries for **generic** names appear in **boldface** type. Trade names appear in regular type, with Canadian names preceded by a maple leaf icon (✳). **CLASSIFICATIONS** appear in **BOLDFACE SMALL CAPS**. *Combination Drugs* appear in *italics* and can be accessed in Appendix N online at fadavis.com, herbal products are preceded by a yin-yang icon (◐), and drugs with genetic implications are preceded by a double-helix icon (⧖).

*Entries for **generic** names appear in **boldface type**. Trade names appear in regular type, with Canadian names preceded by a maple leaf icon (✤). CLASSIFICATIONS appear in **BOLDFACE SMALL CAPS**. *Combination Drugs* appear in *italics* and can be accessed in Appendix N online at fadavis.com, herbal products are preceded by a yin-yang icon (☯), and drugs with genetic implications are preceded by a double-helix icon (⚇).

*Entries for **generic** names appear in **boldface type**. Trade names appear in regular type, with Canadian names preceded by a maple leaf icon (🍁). **CLASSIFICATIONS** appear in **BOLDFACE SMALL CAPS**. *Combination Drugs* appear in *italics* and can be accessed in Appendix N online at fadavis.com, herbal products are preceded by a yin-yang icon (☯), and drugs with genetic implications are preceded by a double-helix icon (⚕).

---

*Entries for **generic** names appear in **boldface type**. Trade names appear in regular type, with Canadian names preceded by a maple leaf icon (✹). CLASSIFICATIONS appear in **BOLDFACE SMALL CAPS**. *Combination Drugs* appear in *italics* and can be accessed in Appendix N online at fadavis.com, herbal products are preceded by a yin-yang icon (◐), and drugs with genetic implications are preceded by a double-helix icon (⚮).

C O M P R E H E N S I V E   I N D E X

*Entries for **generic** names appear in **boldface type**. Trade names appear in regular type, with Canadian names preceded by a maple leaf icon (🍁). CLASSIFICATIONS appear in **BOLDFACE SMALL CAPS**. *Combination Drugs* appear in *italics* and can be accessed in Appendix N online at fadavis.com, herbal products are preceded by a yin-yang icon (◐), and drugs with genetic implications are preceded by a double-helix icon (⚇).

*Entries for **generic** names appear in **boldface type**. Trade names appear in regular type, with Canadian names preceded by a maple leaf icon (❋). **CLASSIFICATIONS** appear in **BOLDFACE SMALL CAPS**. *Combination Drugs* appear in *italics* and can be accessed in Appendix N online at fadavis.com, herbal products are preceded by a yin-yang icon (◐), and drugs with genetic implications are preceded by a double-helix icon (⚏).

---

*Entries for **generic** names appear in **boldface type**. Trade names appear in regular type, with Canadian names preceded by a maple leaf icon (✽). **CLASSIFICATIONS** appear in **BOLDFACE SMALL CAPS**. *Combination Drugs* appear in *italics* and can be accessed in Appendix N online at fadavis.com, herbal products are preceded by a yin-yang icon (◑), and drugs with genetic implications are preceded by a double-helix icon (⚕).

*Entries for **generic** names appear in **boldface type**. Trade names appear in regular type, with Canadian names preceded by a maple leaf icon (✽). **CLASSIFICATIONS** appear in **BOLDFACE SMALL CAPS**. *Combination Drugs* appear in *italics* and can be accessed in Appendix N online at fadavis.com, herbal products are preceded by a yin-yang icon (☯), and drugs with genetic implications are preceded by a double-helix icon (§§§).

C O M P R E H E N S I V E   I N D E X

*Entries for **generic** names appear in **boldface type**. Trade names appear in regular type, with Canadian names preceded by a maple leaf icon (🍁). CLASSIFICATIONS appear in **BOLDFACE SMALL CAPS**. *Combination Drugs* appear in *italics* and can be accessed in Appendix N online at fadavis.com, herbal products are preceded by a yin-yang icon (🌀), and drugs with genetic implications are preceded by a double-helix icon (⚌).

Ketalar, 1362
ketamine, 1362, 1370
ketoconazole, 160
Ketodan, 160
🍁Ketoderm, 160
Ketoprofen ER Capsule, 1358
ketorolac, 735, 1354, 1362–1363, 1370, 1389
ketotifen, 1383
Kevzara, 1123
☯kew tree, 1342
Keytruda, 995
Khedezla, 424
Kimyrsa, 946
KINASE INHIBITORS
 ⚕**abemaciclib, 83**
 ⚕**abrocitinib, 87**
 ⚕**afatinib, 106**
 ⚕**alectinib, 109**
 ⚕**alpelisib, 119**
 baricitinib, 203
 ⚕**binimetinib, 221**
 ⚕**brigatinib, 239**
 ⚕**capivasertib, 1375**
 ⚕**ceritinib, 318**
 ⚕**cobimetinib, 344**
 ⚕**dabrafenib, 391**
 deucravacitinib, 426
 ⚕**encorafenib, 507**
 ⚕**everolimus, 544**
 fruquintinib, 1376
 ⚕**lapatinib, 753**
 ⚕**lenvatinib, 763**
 ⚕**neratinib, 897**
 ⚕**nilotinib, 905**
 ⚕**palbociclib, 969**
 ⚕**panitumumab, 980**
 ⚕**PAZOPanib, 988**
 ⚕**regorafenib, 1072**
 ⚕**ribociclib, 1080**
 ritlecitinib, 1097
 ruxolitinib (topical), 1116
 SUNITinib, 1158
 ⚕**tofacitinib, 1210**
 upadacitinib, 1238
 vandetanib, 1253
 ⚕**vemurafenib, 1262**
Kisqali, 1080
Kisqali Tablet, 1358
Kitabis Pak, 127
☯Klamath weed, 1349
KlonoPIN, 334, 1353, 1361–1362, 1367–1368
Klonopin, 1356
Klor-Con, 1034
Klor-Con M15, 1034
Klor-Con M10, 1034

Klor-Con M20, 1034
Klor-Con M Tablet, 1358
Klor-Con Tablet, 1358
Kloxxado, 891
🍁Koffex DM, 433
Kombiglyze XR Tablet, 1358
Konvomep Oral Suspension, App N
☯Korean ginseng, 1343
Korlym, 859
Korlym Tablet, 1358
Koselugo Capsule, 1358
K-Phos Neutral, 1032
K-Phos No. 2, 1032
Krazati Tablet, 1358
Kristalose, 744
Krystexxa, 994
K-Tab, 1034
K-Tab Tablet, 1358
Kurvelo, 353, App N
Kyleena, 354
Kytril, 640
Kyzatrex, 1184, 1355

L

labetalol, 738, 1356, 1362, 1370
lacosamide, 740, 1370
lactic acid/citric acid/ potassium bitartrate, 743
Lactinex, App N
lactitol, 1381
lactulose, 744
☯Lady's thistle, 1348
Lagevrio, 873
LaMICtal, 747, 1362, 1368
Lamictal, 1356
LaMICtal ODT, 747
LaMICtal XR, 747
Lamictal XR Tablet, 1358
🍁Lamisil, 160
Lam**ISIL**, 1368
Lamisil AT, 160
lami**VUD**ine, 745, 1362, 1368
lamivudine/raltegravir, 1381
lamo**TRIG**ine, 747, 1362–1363, 1368
lamotrigine, 1356
🍁Lancora, 729
Lanoxin, 442, 1353, 1356, 1362–1363
lansoprazole, 750, 1354
lanthanum, 752
lanthanum carbonate, 1362–1363
Lantus, 706, 1362
Lantus SoloStar, 706

⚕**lapatinib, 753**
🍁Lapelga, 991
Larin 1/20, 353, App N
Larin 1.5/30, 353, App N
Larin 24 Fe, 353
Larin Fe 1/20, 353
Larin Fe 1.5/30, 353
Larin Fe 1/20 Phase I, App N
Larin Fe 1.5/30 Phase I, App N
Larin Fe 1/20 Phase II, App N
Larin Fe 1.5/30 Phase II, App N
Larin 24 Fe Phase I, App N
Larin 24 Fe Phase II, App N
Lasix, 612, 1354, 1356, 1362, 1365
Lastacaft [OTC], 1383
latanoprost, 1390
latanoprostene, 1390
Latuda, 800, 1354, 1362
🍁Lax-a-Day, 1029
LAXATIVES, 69
☯**aloe, 1333**
 bisacodyl, 223
 DOCUSATE, 462
 docusate calcium, 462
 docusate sodium, 462
 lactulose, 744
 magnesium chloride (12% Mg; 9.8 mEq Mg/g), 804
 magnesium citrate (16.2% Mg; 4.4 mEq Mg/g), 804
 magnesium gluconate (5.4% Mg; 4.4 mEq/g), 804
 magnesium hydroxide (41.7% Mg; 34.3 mEq Mg/ g), 804
 magnesium oxide (60.3% Mg; 49.6 mEq Mg/g), 804
 MAGNESIUM SALTS (ORAL), 804
 methylnaltrexone, 838
 naldemedine, 889
 ⚕**naloxegol, 890**
 plecanatide, 1028
 polyethylene glycol 3350, 1029
 senna, 1132
Layolis Fe, 353
Layolis Fe Phase I, App N
Layolis Fe Phase II, App N
Lazanda, 1356
lecanemab, 755
Leena, 354
Leena Phase I, App N
Leena Phase II, App N
Leena Phase III, App N
lefamulin, 756

*Entries for **generic** names appear in **boldface type**. Trade names appear in regular type, with Canadian names preceded by a maple leaf icon (🍁). **CLASSIFICATIONS** appear in **BOLDFACE SMALL CAPS**. *Combination Drugs* appear in *italics* and can be accessed in Appendix N online at fadavis.com, herbal products are preceded by a yin-yang icon (☯), and drugs with genetic implications are preceded by a double-helix icon (⚕).

---

*Entries for **generic** names appear in **boldface type.** Trade names appear in regular type, with Canadian names preceded by a maple leaf icon (❀). **CLASSIFICATIONS** appear in **BOLDFACE SMALL CAPS.** *Combination Drugs* appear in *italics* and can be accessed in Appendix N online at fadavis.com, herbal products are preceded by a yin-yang icon (❂), and drugs with genetic implications are preceded by a double-helix icon (☒).

*Entries for **generic** names appear in **boldface type**. Trade names appear in regular type, with Canadian names preceded by a maple leaf icon (✿). **CLASSIFICATIONS** appear in **BOLDFACE SMALL CAPS**. *Combination Drugs* appear in *italics* and can be accessed in Appendix N online at fadavis.com, herbal products are preceded by a yin-yang icon (◐), and drugs with genetic implications are preceded by a double-helix icon (⬚).

---

*Entries for **generic** names appear in **boldface type**. Trade names appear in regular type, with Canadian names preceded by a maple leaf icon (✳). **CLASSIFICATIONS** appear in **BOLDFACE SMALL CAPS**. *Combination Drugs* appear in *italics* and can be accessed in Appendix N online at fadavis.com, herbal products are preceded by a yin-yang icon (☯), and drugs with genetic implications are preceded by a double-helix icon (⚛).

*Entries for **generic** names appear in **boldface type**. Trade names appear in regular type, with Canadian names preceded by a maple leaf icon (✽). **CLASSIFICATIONS** appear in **BOLDFACE SMALL CAPS**. *Combination Drugs* appear in *italics* and can be accessed in Appendix N online at fadavis.com, herbal products are preceded by a yin-yang icon (◉), and drugs with genetic implications are preceded by a double-helix icon (፠).

*Entries for **generic** names appear in **boldface type**. Trade names appear in regular type, with Canadian names preceded by a maple leaf icon (🍁). **CLASSIFICATIONS** appear in **BOLDFACE SMALL CAPS**. *Combination Drugs* appear in *italics* and can be accessed in Appendix N online at fadavis.com, herbal products are preceded by a yin-yang icon (☯), and drugs with genetic implications are preceded by a double-helix icon (⚮).

COMPREHENSIVE INDEX